ICD-10-PCS Code Book

2022

Anne B. Casto, RHIA, CCS
Consulting Editor

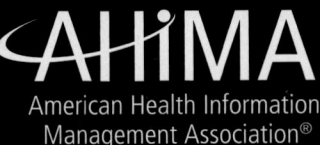

AHIMA
American Health Information
Management Association®

ISBN: 978-1-58426-846-8
AHIMA Product No.: AC222021

AHIMA Staff:
Rachel Schratz, MA, Assistant Editor
Christine Scheid, Content Development Manager
Megan Grennan, Director, Content Production and AHIMA Press
James Pinnick, Vice President, Content and Product Development

Cover image: © knikola, Shutterstock

Limit of Liability/Disclaimer of Warranty: This book is sold, as is, without warranty of any kind, either express or implied. While every precaution has been taken in the preparation of this book, the publisher and author assume no responsibility for errors or omissions. Neither is any liability assumed for damages resulting from the use of the information or instructions contained herein. It is further stated that the publisher and author are not responsible for any damage or loss to your data or your equipment that results directly or indirectly from your use of this book.

The Centers for Medicare and Medicaid Services (CMS) and the National Center for Health Statistics (NCHS), two departments within the US Federal Government's Department of Health and Human Services (HHS) provide the *International Classification of Diseases, Tenth Revision, Clinical Modification* (ICD-10-CM) for coding and reporting. ICD-10-CM is the US modification to the World Health Organization's (WHO) International Classification of Diseases, Tenth Revision (ICD-10).

Coding Clinic for ICD-10-CM and ICD-10-PCS is a publication of the American Hospital Association (AHA).

Unless otherwise noted, art pieces were created by Jason Isley and Cognition Studio, Inc, and are all copyright of the American Health Information Management Association.

The websites listed in this book were current and valid as of the date of publication. However, webpage addresses and the information on them may change at any time. The user is encouraged to perform his or her own general web searches to locate any site addresses listed here that are no longer valid.

All copyrights and trademarks mentioned in this book are the possession of their respective owners. AHIMA makes no claim of ownership by mentioning products that contain such marks.

For more information about AHIMA Press publications, including updates, https://www.ahima.org/education-events/ education-by-product/books/.

American Health Information Management Association
233 North Michigan Avenue, 21st Floor
Chicago, Illinois 60601-5809
ahima.org

Contents

About the Consulting Editor

Anne B. Casto, RHIA, CCS, is the president of Casto Consulting, LLC. Casto Consulting, LLC is a consulting firm that provides services to hospitals and other healthcare stakeholders primarily in the areas of reimbursement and coding. Casto Consulting, LLC specializes in linking coding and billing practices to positive revenue cycle outcomes. Additionally, the firm provides guidance to consulting firms, healthcare organizations and healthcare insurers regarding reimbursement methodologies and Medicare regulations.

Additionally, Ms. Casto is a lecturer in the HIMS department at The Ohio State University, School of Health and Rehabilitation Sciences. Over the past 20 years, Ms. Casto has taught numerous courses in the areas of healthcare reimbursement, coding, and revenue cycle management.

Prior to her current roles, Ms. Casto was the vice president of clinical information for Cleverley & Associates where she worked very closely with APC regulations and guidelines, preparing hospitals for the implementation of the Medicare OPPS. Ms. Casto was also the clinical information product manager for CHIPS/Ingenix. She joined CHIPS/Ingenix in 1998 and spent the majority of her time developing coding compliance products for the inpatient and outpatient settings.

Ms. Casto has been responsible for inpatient and outpatient coding activities in several large hospitals including Mt. Sinai Medical Center (NYC), Beth Israel Medical Center (NYC), and The Ohio State University. She worked extensively with CMI, quality measures, physician documentation, and coding accuracy efforts at these facilities.

Ms. Casto received her degree in Health Information Management at The Ohio State University in 1995. She received her Certified Coding Specialist credential in 1998 from the American Health Information Management Association. In 2009 Ms. Casto received her ICD-10-CM/PCS Trainer certificate from AHIMA. Ms. Casto is the author of an AHIMA-published textbook entitled *Principles of Healthcare Reimbursement*. Additionally, Ms. Casto was a contributing author to the published AHIMA books: *Severity DRGs and Reimbursement; A MS-DRG Primer* and *Effective Management of Coding Services.*

Ms. Casto received the AHIMA Legacy Award, part of the FORE Triumph Awards, in 2007 which honors a significant contribution to the knowledge base of the HIM field through an insightful publication. Additionally, Ms. Casto was honored with the Ohio Health Information Management Association's Distinguished Member Award in 2008 and the Ohio Health Information Management Association's Professional Achievement Award in 2011.

Acknowledgments

Many thanks to my family for their support during this project. Thanks to Dr. Susan White, The Ohio State University; your data manipulation skills are second to none. I thank the reviewers for their thoughtful comments and suggestions. Many thanks to Linda Hyde, RHIA, and Rachael D'Andrea, MS, RHIA, CDIP, CHTS-TR, CPHQ, for their very thorough technical review of the book.

ICD-10-PCS Overview

The International Classification of Diseases, Tenth Revision, Procedure Coding System (ICD-10-PCS) was created to accompany the World Health Organization's (WHO) ICD-10 diagnosis classification. This coding system was developed to replace ICD-9-CM procedure codes for reporting inpatient procedures. ICD-10-PCS was designed to enable each code to have a standard structure and be very descriptive, and yet flexible enough to accommodate future needs.

History of ICD-10-PCS

The WHO has maintained the International Classification of Diseases (ICD) for recording cause of death since 1893. It has updated the ICD periodically to reflect new discoveries in epidemiology and changes in medical understanding of disease. The International Classification of Diseases Tenth Revision (ICD-10), published in 1992, is the latest revision of the ICD. The WHO authorized the National Center for Health Statistics (NCHS) to develop a clinical modification of ICD-10 for use in the United States. This version of ICD-10 is called ICD-10-CM, and is intended to replace the previous US clinical modification, ICD-9-CM, that had been in use since 1979. ICD-9-CM contains a procedure classification; ICD-10-CM does not.

The Centers for Medicare and Medicaid Services (CMS), the agency responsible for maintaining the inpatient procedure code set in the United States, contracted with 3M Health Information Systems in 1993 to design and then develop a procedure classification system to replace Volume 3 of ICD-9-CM. ICD-10-PCS is the result. ICD-10-PCS was initially released in 1998. It has been updated annually since that time.

ICD-10-PCS Design

ICD-10-PCS is fundamentally different from previous procedure classification systems in its structure, organization, and capabilities. It was designed and developed to adhere to recommendations made by the National Committee on Vital and Health Statistics (NCVHS). It also incorporates input from a wide range of organizations, individual physicians, healthcare professionals, and researchers. Several structural attributes were recommended for a new procedure coding system. These attributes include a multiaxial structure, completeness, and expandability.

Multiaxial Structure

The key attribute that provides the framework for all other structural attributes is multiaxial code structure. *Multiaxial code structure* makes it possible for the ICD-10-PCS to be complete, expandable, and provide a high degree of flexibility and functionality.

ICD-10-PCS codes are composed of seven characters. Each character represents a category of information that can be specified about the procedure performed. A character defines both the category of information and its physical position in the code. A character's position can be understood as a semi-independent axis of classification that allows different specific values to be inserted into that space, and whose physical position remains stable. Within a defined code range, a character retains the general meaning that it confers on any value in that position.

Completeness

Completeness is considered a key structural attribute for a new procedure coding system. The specific recommendation for completeness included that a unique code be available for each significant procedure, that each code retain its unique definition, and that codes that have been deleted are not reused.

In ICD-10-PCS, a unique code is constructed for every significantly different procedure. Within each section, a character defines a consistent component of a code, and contains all applicable values for that character. The values define individual expressions (Open, Percutaneous) of the character's general meaning (approach) that are then used to construct unique procedure codes. Because all approaches by which a procedure is performed are assigned a separate approach value, every procedure which uses a different approach will have its own unique code. This is true of the other characters as well. The same procedure performed on a different body part has its own unique code; the same procedure performed using a different device has its own unique code, and so on.

Because ICD-10-PCS codes are constructed of individual values rather than lists of fixed codes and text descriptions, the unique, stable definition of a code in the system is retained. New values may be added to the system to represent a specific new approach or device or qualifier, but whole codes by design cannot be given new meanings and reused.

Expandability

Expandability was also recommended as a key structural attribute. The specific recommendation for expandability included that the system be capable of accommodating new procedures and technology and that these new codes could be added to the system without disrupting the existing structure.

ICD-10-PCS is designed to be easily updated as new codes are required for new procedures and new techniques. Changes to ICD-10-PCS can all be made within the existing structure because whole codes are not added. Instead, a new value for a character can be added to the system as needed. Likewise, an existing value for a character can be added to a table(s) in the system.

ICD-10-PCS Additional Characteristics

ICD-10-PCS possesses several additional characteristics in response to government and industry recommendations. These characteristics are

- Standardized terminology within the coding system
- Standardized level of specificity
- No diagnostic information
- No explicit "not otherwise specified" (NOS) code options
- Limited use of "not elsewhere classified" (NEC) code options

Standardized Terminology

Words commonly used in clinical vocabularies may have multiple meanings. This can cause confusion and result in inaccurate data. ICD-10-PCS is standardized and self-contained. Characters and values used in the system are defined in the system. For example, the word *excision* is used to describe a wide variety of surgical procedures. In ICD-10-PCS, the word *excision* describes a single, precise surgical objective, defined as "cutting out or off, without replacement, a portion of a body part."

No Eponyms or Common Procedure Names

The terminology used in ICD-10-PCS is standardized to provide precise and stable definitions of all procedures performed. This standardized terminology is used in all ICD-10-PCS code descriptions. As a result, ICD-10-PCS code descriptions do not include eponyms or common procedure names.

In ICD-10-PCS, physicians' names are not included in a code description, nor are procedures identified by common terms or acronyms such as appendectomy or CABG. Instead, such procedures are coded to the root operation that accurately identifies the objective of the procedure.

ICD-10-PCS assigns procedure codes according to the root operation that matches the objective of the procedure. By relying on the universal objectives defined in root operations rather than eponyms or specific procedure titles that change or become obsolete, ICD-10-PCS preserves the capacity to define past, present, and future procedures accurately using stable terminology in the form of characters and values.

No Combination Codes

With rare exceptions, ICD-10-PCS does not define multiple procedures with one code. This is to preserve standardized terminology and consistency across the system. A procedure that meets the reporting criteria for a separate procedure is coded separately in ICD-10-PCS. This allows the system to respond to changes in technology and medical practice with the maximum degree of stability and flexibility.

Standardized Level of Specificity

ICD-10-PCS provides a standardized level of specificity for each code, so each code represents a single procedure variation. In general, ICD-10-PCS code descriptions are much more specific than previous procedure classification systems but sometimes an ICD-10-PCS code description is actually less specific. ICD-10-PCS provides a standardized level of specificity that can be predicted across the system.

Diagnosis Information Excluded

Another key feature of ICD-10-PCS is that information pertaining to a diagnosis is excluded from the code descriptions. Adding diagnosis information limits the flexibility and functionality of a procedure coding system. It has the effect of placing a code "off limits" because the diagnosis in the medical record does not match the diagnosis in the procedure code description. The code cannot be used even though the procedural part of the code description precisely matches the procedure performed. Diagnosis information is not contained in any ICD-10-PCS code. The diagnosis codes, not the procedure codes, will specify the reason the procedure is performed.

Not Otherwise Specified (NOS) Code Options Restricted

The standardized level of specificity designed into ICD-10-PCS restricts the use of broadly applicable NOS or unspecified code options in the system. A minimal level of specificity is required to construct a valid code.

Limited Not Elsewhere Classified (NEC) Code Options

NEC options are provided in ICD-10-PCS, but only for specific, limited use. In the Medical and Surgical section, two significant NEC options are the root operation value Q, Repair, and the device value Y, Other Device. The root operation Repair is a true NEC value. It is used only when the procedure performed is not one of the other root operations in the Medical and Surgical section. Other Device, on the other hand, is intended to be used to temporarily define new devices that do not have a specific value assigned, until one can be added to the system. No categories of medical or surgical devices are permanently classified to Other Device.

ICD-10-PCS Code Structure

Undergirding ICD-10-PCS is a logical, consistent structure that informs the system as a whole, down to the level of a single code. This means the process of constructing codes in ICD-10-PCS is also logical and consistent: the spaces of the code, called *characters* are filled with individual letters and numbers, called *values*.

Characters

All codes in ICD-10-PCS are seven characters long. Each character in the seven-character code represents an aspect of the procedure. The following are two examples of the code structure: one from the Medical and Surgical section and one from the Ancillary section.

Medical and Surgical Code Structure

Character 1	Character 2	Character 3	Character 4	Character 5	Character 6	Character 7
Section	Body System	Operation	Body Part	Approach	Device	Qualifier

Imaging Section Code Structure

Character 1	Character 2	Character 3	Character 4	Character 5	Character 6	Character 7
Section	Body System	Type	Body Part	Contrast	Qualifier	Qualifier

An ICD-10-PCS code is best understood as the result of a process rather than as an isolated, fixed quantity. The process consists of assigning values from among the valid choices for that part of the system, according to the rules governing the construction of codes.

Values

One of 34 possible values can be assigned to each character in a code: the numbers 0 through 9 and the alphabet (except the letters I and O, because they are easily confused with the numbers 1 and 0). A finished code looks like this: 02103D4.

This code is derived by choosing a specific value for each of the seven characters. Based on details about the procedure performed, values for each character specifying the section, body system, root operation, body part, approach, device, and qualifier are assigned. Because the definition of each character is a function of its physical position in the code, the same value placed in a different position in the code means something different. The value 0 in the first character means something different than 0 in the second character, or 0 in the third character, and so on.

Code Structure Example

The following example defines each character using the code 0LB50ZZ, Excision of right lower arm and wrist tendon, Open approach. This example comes from the Medical and Surgical section of ICD-10-PCS.

Character 1: Section

The first character in the code determines the broad procedure category, or section, where the code is found. In this example, the section is Medical and Surgical. 0 is the value that represents Medical and Surgical in the first character.

Character 1	Character 2	Character 3	Character 4	Character 5	Character 6	Character 7
Section	Body System	Root Operation	Body Part	Approach	Device	Qualifier
0						

Character 2: Body System

The second character defines the body system—the general physiological system or anatomical region involved. Examples of body systems include Lower Arteries, Central Nervous System, and Respiratory System. In this example, the body system is Tendons, represented by the value L.

Character 1	Character 2	Character 3	Character 4	Character 5	Character 6	Character 7
Section	Body System	Root Operation	Body Part	Approach	Device	Qualifier
0	L					

Character 3: Root Operation

The third character defines the root operation, or the objective of the procedure. Some examples of root operations are Bypass, Drainage, and Reattachment. In this example code, the root operation is Excision. When used in the third character of the code, the value B represents Excision.

Character 1	Character 2	Character 3	Character 4	Character 5	Character 6	Character 7
Section	Body System	Root Operation	Body Part	Approach	Device	Qualifier
0	L	B				

Character 4: Body Part

The fourth character defines the body part or specific anatomical site where the procedure was performed. The body system (second character) provides only a general indication of the procedure site. The body part and body system values together provide a precise description of the procedure site. Examples of body parts are Kidney, Tonsils, and Thymus. In this example, the body part value is 5, Lower Arm and Wrist, Right. When the second character is L, the value 5 when used in the fourth character of the code represents the right lower arm and wrist tendon.

Character 1	Character 2	Character 3	Character 4	Character 5	Character 6	Character 7
Section	Body System	Root Operation	Body Part	Approach	Device	Qualifier
0	L	B	5			

Character 5: Approach

The fifth character defines the approach, or the technique used to reach the procedure site. Seven different approach values are used in the Medical and Surgical section to define the approach. Examples of approaches include Open and Percutaneous Endoscopic. In this example code, the approach is Open and is represented by the value 0.

Character 1	Character 2	Character 3	Character 4	Character 5	Character 6	Character 7
Section	Body System	Root Operation	Body Part	Approach	Device	Qualifier
0	L	B	5	0		

Character 6: Device

Depending on the procedure performed, there may be a device left in place at the end of the procedure. The sixth character defines the device. Device values fall into four basic categories:

- Grafts and Prostheses
- Implants
- Simple or Mechanical Appliances
- Electronic Appliances

In this example, there is no device used in the procedure. The value Z is used to represent No Device, as shown here:

Character 1	Character 2	Character 3	Character 4	Character 5	Character 6	Character 7
Section	Body System	Operation	Body Part	Approach	Device	Qualifier
0	L	B	5	0	Z	

Character 7: Qualifier

The seventh character defines a qualifier for the code. A qualifier specifies an additional attribute of the procedure, if applicable. Examples of qualifiers include Diagnostic and Stereotactic. Qualifier choices vary depending on the previous values selected. In this example, there is no specific qualifier applicable to this procedure, so the value is No Qualifier, represented by the letter Z.

Character 1	Character 2	Character 3	Character 4	Character 5	Character 6	Character 7
Section	Body System	Operation	Body Part	Approach	Device	Qualifier
0	L	B	5	0	Z	Z

0LB50ZZ is the complete specification of the procedure "Excision of right lower arm and wrist tendon, open approach."

ICD-10-PCS Organization and Official Conventions

The *ICD-10-PCS Code Book*, 2022 Edition is based on the official International Classification of Diseases, Tenth Revision, Procedure Classification System, issued by the US Department of Health and Human Services (HHS) and CMS. This book is consistent with the content of the government's version of ICD-10-PCS and follows the official conventions.

Index

The Alphabetic Index is provided to assist the user with locating the appropriate table to construct procedure codes. Each table contains all the information required to construct valid procedure codes. Coders should not code from the PCS Index alone; the PCS code tables should always be consulted before assigning a PCS procedure code.

Main Terms

Main terms in the Alphabetic Index reflect the root operations, third character, of procedures. The Index includes not only root operation terms, but also other common procedural terms, anatomical sites, and device terms. The main terms are listed alphabetically. After the coder has located the correct main term and subterm in the Alphabetic Index, he or she is provided with the first three to four digits of the procedure code. The coder should then move to the Tables section of the code book and locate the appropriate table to complete the code construction. Even if the entire seven-digit code is provided in the Index, the coder should still reference the Tables to ensure the correct PCS code has been constructed.

See Reference

Common procedure terms are often listed with the *see* reference. The coder is instructed to follow the reference provided in order to locate the appropriate table to construct the code. For example, the *see* reference is present for the main term Colectomy. The Index excerpt is as follows:

Colectomy

see Excision, Gastrointestinal System 0DB

see Resection, Gastrointestinal System 0DT

In this example, the coder should review the definition of the root operations Excision and Resection to determine which is consistent with the medical record documentation. The coder should then proceed to the corresponding table as suggested by the *see* reference.

Use Reference

Anatomical site terms and device terms are often listed with the *use* reference. The coder is instructed to follow the reference provided in order to locate the appropriate main term for the procedure in question. For example, the *use* reference is present for the main term Inferior rectus muscle. The Index excerpt is as follows:

> **Inferior rectus muscle**
>
> > *use* Muscle, Extraocular, Left
> >
> > *use* Muscle, Extraocular, Right

In this example, the coder should identify the root operation for the procedure, and then look for the subterm that identifies the body part indicated in the *use* reference. For example, the procedure is excision of the inferior rectus muscle. The coder would locate the main term Excision. The Index excerpt is as follows:

> **Excision**
>
> Muscle
>
> > Extraocular
> >
> > > Left 08BM
> > >
> > > Right 08BL

In this example, the coder knows that the Code Table 08B is the correct table because the previous review of the *use* reference identified that the inferior rectus muscle is an extraocular muscle. The coder can now proceed to the 08B Table to finish constructing the PCS code.

In addition to the *use* reference, the coder may also consult appendix D for Body Part Table or appendix E for the Device Table.

Code Tables

ICD-10-PCS contains 17 sections of Code Tables, represented by the numbers 0 through 9 and the letters B through D, F through H and X. The Tables are organized by general type of procedure. The three main sections of tables include:

1. **Medical and Surgical section**
   - Medical and Surgical (first character 0)
2. **Medical and Surgical Related sections**
   - Obstetrics (first character 1)
   - Placement (first character 2)
   - Administration (first character 3)
   - Measurement and Monitoring (first character 4)
   - Extracorporeal or Systemic Assistance and Performance (first character 5)
   - Extracorporeal or Systemic Therapies (first character 6)
   - Osteopathic (first character 7)
   - Other Procedures (first character 8)
   - Chiropractic (first character 9)
3. **Ancillary sections**
   - Imaging (first character B)
   - Nuclear Medicine (first character C)
   - Radiation Therapy (first character D)
   - Physical Rehabilitation and Diagnostic Audiology (first character F)
   - Mental Health (first character G)
   - Substance Abuse (first character H)
   - New Technology (first character X)

Each code table is defined by the first three characters of the PCS code. Each of these characters is displayed above the table. The table consists of all the options for characters 4 through 7. The root operation or root

type, character 3, is present along with its official definition. Table 097 is provided here as an example of the table structure.

0 **Medical and Surgical**

9 **Ear, Nose, Sinus**

7 **Dilation: Expanding an orifice or the lumen of a tubular body part**

Body Part Character 4	Approach Character 5	Device Character 6	Qualifier Character 7
F Eustachian Tube, Right **G** Eustachian Tube, Left	**0** Open **7** Via Natural or Artificial Opening **8** Via Natural or Artificial Opening Endoscopic	**D** Intraluminal Device **Z** No Device	**Z** No Qualifier
F Eustachian Tube, Right **G** Eustachian Tube, Left	**3** Percutaneous **4** Percutaneous Endoscopic	**Z** No Device	**Z** No Qualifier

There can be multiple rows within the table for the first three characters, so the coder must carefully review all the applicable rows. Additionally, a table may cover multiple pages. Therefore, the coder must continue to review the code table options until the end of the table is reached to ensure the correct PCS code has been constructed.

Code Listing

Code Listings for the Medical and Surgical and Obstetrics sections are included in this manual to assist coders with ensuring that the intended code has been selected for reporting. The Code Listings are presented in alphanumeric order. Within the Code Listing, several additional conventions are included to assist coders with navigating the Medicare Code Editor (MCE) edits, official coding guidelines, and other reporting requirements such as the Inpatient Prospective Payment System (IPPS) Hospital-Acquired Conditions (HACs) related codes. The Code Listings are combined with the Tables section of the code book. In the Medical and Surgical section, the Code Listing appears after each body system. For the Obstetrics section, the Code Listing appears at the end of the section.

ICD-10-PCS Additional Conventions

The use of symbols has been added to this code book to alert the user to Medicare reimbursement logic and edits that are impacted by procedure coding. Some codes may be included in multiple reimbursement issues and, therefore, may have more than one symbol. For a quick reference review the legend at the bottom of each page of the Code Listing (Medical/Surgical section and Obstetrics section) as well as the inside cover of the code book. The symbols are described in detail here.

Medicare Code Edits

Hospital inpatient Medicare claims paid under the IPPS are processed through the Medicare Code Editor (MCE) prior to payment by the Medicare administrative contractor (MAC). The code edits are intended to ensure that all claims processed by the MAC are accurate and complete. The information in this manual is based on the MCE v39.

Several of the MCE edits pertain to procedures. We have included identification of the codes included in these edits in this manual to assist users with preparing accurate and complete claims. The MCE edits included in this manual:

- Sex conflict
- Medicare non-covered procedures
- Medicare limited coverage procedures

Note: It is important to remember these edits are Medicare edits and may not apply to other third-party payers claim processing.

Sex Conflict Edit

The sex conflict edit is activated when the sex of the patient and the type of procedure performed does not match. The following symbols are used to identify female-only and male-only procedures.

♀ **Female-only** procedure: This symbol appears to the left of the applicable code in the code listing.

♂ **Male-only** procedure: This symbol appears to the left of the applicable code in the code listing.

Medicare Non-covered Procedure

Medicare does not reimburse for all ICD-10-PCS procedures. There are some procedures that are never reimbursed, and there are some procedures that are only reimbursed when certain specified diagnosis codes are also included on the claim. Non-covered procedures are designated by a red triangle symbol ▲ located next to the code description for the applicable code. If there is conditional logic for the non-coverage, it is provided to the right of the red triangle.

Medicare Limited Coverage Procedures

For certain procedures whose medical complexity and serious nature incur extraordinary associated costs, Medicare limits coverage to a portion of the cost. The limited coverage edit indicates this type of limited coverage. Limited coverage procedures are designated by a lime green triangle symbol ▲ located next to the code description for the applicable code. If there is conditional logic for the limited coverage, it is provided to the right of the lime green triangle.

MS-DRG Procedure Designations

The MS-DRG system is utilized within the IPPS to determine the unadjusted reimbursement amount for Medicare hospital inpatient claims. The MS-DRG Definitions Manual includes the logic for MS-DRG refinement and selection as well as logic based on the IPPS final rules released each August. The information in this manual is based on the MS-DRG v39. *Note:* It is important to remember that these edits are Medicare edits and may not apply to other third-party payers claim processing.

Non-Operating Room Procedures

Within the MS-DRG logic, CMS designates the PCS codes that impact MS-DRG assignment. In the MS-DRG system, operating room (OR) procedures impact MS-DRG assignment resulting in the admission being assigned to a surgical MS-DRG. Typically, non-OR procedures do not impact the MS-DRG assignment; in the basic sense they do not convert medical MS-DRGs to surgical MS-DRGs. However, there are some exceptions. Throughout the Medical and Surgical and Obstetrics sections, non-OR procedures that impact MS-DRG assignment and result in a surgical admission are indicated with a purple dot ●. The purple dot symbol is located to the left of the applicable code in the code listing.

Hospital-Acquired Conditions Related Procedures

As part of the Medicare Value-Based Purchasing program, CMS has implemented a Paying for Value program entitled Hospital-Acquired Conditions (HACs) Present on Admission Indicator Program. This program is designed to reduce reimbursements to facilities where the value of the medical or surgical services have been comprised due to preventable conditions. Reimbursement for admissions that meet the HAC Present on Admission Indicator Program criteria will be reduced. In this manual, the HAC-associated procedures are identified with an orange rectangle HAC with HAC. The orange rectangle is located below the code description in the code listing. If there is conditional logic for the procedure code, it is included to the right of the orange rectangle.

Cluster Codes Required

Within the MS-DRG logic CMS has designated codes that must be reported with specified other codes in order to fully report a complete procedure. For these procedures, such as simultaneous pancreas and kidney transplants, if the correct cluster of codes is not reported, the desired MS-DRG will not be calculated for the encounter. Cluster codes are identified with a green box with a plus sign in the middle ⊞. The green box with a code-specific note is located below the code description for applicable code in the code listing.

IPPS New Services and Technology Add-On Payment

Sections 1886(d)(5)(K) and (L) of the Social Security Act established a process to identify new medical services and technologies utilized in the hospital inpatient setting. The New Services and Technology Add-on Payment policy ensures that adequate payment for new medical services and technologies is provided for under IPPS reimbursement. Each year in the IPPS Final Rule, CMS designates which new services and technologies qualify for add-on payment. Additionally, the corresponding PCS codes that should be used to report the new services and technologies are identified. The fiscal year 2022 IPPS new services and technologies are provided in Appendix H. Appendix H is an on-line appendix.

AHA Coding Clinic for ICD-10-CM and ICD-10-PCS

The American Hospital Association began publishing coding guidance for ICD-10-CM and ICD-10-PCS in the fourth quarter of 2012. In this code book we identify procedure codes that are discussed in the *Coding Clinic* guidance fourth quarter 2012 through second quarter 2021. Within the Code Listing the following sky blue note alerts the coder to

review the AHA *Coding Clinic* prior to assignment of the code to ensure appropriate and accurate reporting. The quarter of publication, year and page number(s) are provided in the note.

AHA CC: 4Q; 2012; pg#-pg#

For sections of the PCS Code Book that do not have Code Listings, the AHA *Coding Clinic* references are listed in the Introduction of the section.

AHA Coding Clinic Crosswalk for Deleted Codes

Deleted Code	Coding Clinic Reference	Replacement Code
047K3Z6	4Q, 2016, 88-89	047K3ZZ
04CK3Z6	4Q, 2016, 88-89	04CK3ZZ
04V03E6	4Q, 2016, 91-92	04V03EZ
04V03F6	4Q, 2016, 92-94	04V03FZ
0B5S0ZZ	2Q, 2016, 17-18	See 0B5T0ZZ
0BQR0ZZ	2Q, 2016, 22-23	See 0BQT0ZZ
0BQR4ZZ	3Q, 2014, 28	See 0BQT4ZZ
0BQS0ZZ	2Q, 2016, 22-23	See 0BQT0ZZ
0BQS4ZZ	3Q, 2014, 28	See 0BQT4ZZ
0NQS0ZZ	3Q, 2016, 29-30	See 0NQR0ZZ
0NSS04Z	3Q, 2014, 23-24	See 0NSR04Z
0NSS0ZZ	1Q, 2017, 20-21	See 0NSR0ZZ
0NR80JZ	3Q, 2017, 17	See 0NR70JZ

ICD-10-PCS Coding Guidelines

The ICD-10-PCS Coding Guidelines are presented here in the introduction and throughout this manual. Within the manual, the Medical and Surgical Section Guidelines are presented after the Introduction of the Medical and Surgical section. The Obstetric Section Guidelines are presented after the Introduction of the Obstetrics section. Lastly, the New Technology Guidelines are presented after the Introduction of the New Technology section.

Throughout the Code Listings, applicable guidelines are identified via an instruction note in order to remind users to reference the coding guidelines prior to code reporting. The instruction note *Review Coding Guideline...* followed by the guideline reference number is included after the section header for applicable sections or after the code description for applicable codes. It is imperative to review the ICD-10-PCS coding guidelines to ensure the procedure code being reported is accurate and complete.

ICD-10-PCS Official Guidelines for Coding and Reporting, 2022

The Centers for Medicare and Medicaid Services (CMS) and the National Center for Health Statistics (NCHS), two departments within the US federal government's Department of Health and Human Services (DHHS) provide the following guidelines for coding and reporting using the International Classification of Diseases, 10th Revision, Procedure Coding System (ICD-10-PCS). These guidelines should be used as a companion document to the official version of the ICD-10-PCS as published on the CMS website. The ICD-10-PCS is a procedure classification published by the United States for classifying procedures performed in hospital inpatient health care settings.

These guidelines have been approved by the four organizations that make up the Cooperating Parties for the ICD-10-PCS: the American Hospital Association (AHA), the American Health Information Management Association (AHIMA), CMS, and NCHS.

These guidelines are a set of rules that have been developed to accompany and complement the official conventions and instructions provided within the ICD-10-PCS itself. They are intended to provide direction that is applicable in most circumstances. However, there may be unique circumstances where exceptions are applied. The instructions and conventions of the classification take precedence over guidelines. These guidelines are based on the coding and sequencing instructions in the Tables, Index, and Definitions of ICD-10-PCS, but provide additional instruction. Adherence to these guidelines when assigning ICD-10-PCS procedure codes is required under the Health Insurance Portability and Accountability Act (HIPAA). The procedure codes have been adopted under HIPAA for hospital inpatient healthcare settings. A joint effort between the healthcare provider and the coder is essential to achieve complete and accurate documentation, code assignment, and reporting of diagnoses and procedures. These guidelines have been developed to assist both the healthcare provider and the coder in identifying those procedures that are to be reported. The importance of consistent, complete documentation in the medical record cannot be overemphasized. Without such documentation, accurate coding cannot be achieved.

Conventions

A1. ICD-10-PCS codes are composed of seven characters. Each character is an axis of classification that specifies information about the procedure performed. Within a defined code range, a character specifies the same type of information in that axis of classification.

Example: The fifth axis of classification specifies the approach in sections 0 through 4 and 7 through 9 of the system.

A2. One of 34 possible values can be assigned to each axis of classification in the seven-character code: they are the numbers 0 through 9 and the alphabet (except the letters I and O because they are easily confused with the numbers 1 and 0). The number of unique values used in an axis of classification differs as needed.

Example: Where the fifth axis of classification specifies the approach, seven different approach values are currently used to specify the approach.

A3. The valid values for an axis of classification can be added to as needed.

Example: If a significantly distinct type of device is used in a new procedure, a new device value can be added to the system.

A4. As with words in their context, the meaning of any single value is a combination of its axis of classification and any preceding values on which it may be dependent.

Example: The meaning of a body part value in the Medical and Surgical section is always dependent on the body system value. The body part value 0 in the Central Nervous body system specifies Brain and the body part value 0 in the Peripheral Nervous body system specifies Cervical Plexus.

A5. As the system is expanded to become increasingly detailed, over time more values will depend on preceding values for their meaning.

Example: In the Lower Joints body system, the device value 3 in the root operation Insertion specifies Infusion Device and the device value 3 in the root operation Replacement specifies Ceramic Synthetic Substitute.

A6. The purpose of the Alphabetic Index is to locate the appropriate table that contains all information necessary to construct a procedure code. The PCS Tables should always be consulted to find the most appropriate valid code.

A7. It is not required to consult the Index first before proceeding to the Tables to complete the code. A valid code may be chosen directly from the Tables.

A8. All seven characters must be specified to be a valid code. If the documentation is incomplete for coding purposes, the physician should be queried for the necessary information.

A9. Within a PCS Table, valid codes include all combinations of choices in characters 4 through 7 contained in the same row of the table. In the example below, 0JHT3VZ is a valid code, and 0JHW3VZ is *not* a valid code.

Section:	0	Medical and Surgical
Body System:	J	Subcutaneous Tissue and Fascia
Operation:	H	Insertion: Putting in a nonbiological appliance that monitors, assists, performs, or prevents a physiological function but does not physically take the place of a body part

Body Part (4th)	Approach (5th)	Device (6th)	Qualifier (7th)
S Subcutaneous Tissue and Fascia, Head and Neck **V** Subcutaneous Tissue and Fascia, Upper Extremity **W** Subcutaneous Tissue and Fascia, Lower Extremity	**0** Open **3** Percutaneous	**1** Radioactive Element **3** Infusion Device **Y** Other Device	**Z** No Qualifier
T Subcutaneous Tissue and Fascia, Trunk	**0** Open **3** Percutaneous	**1** Radioactive Element **3** Infusion Device **V** Infusion Pump **Y** Other Device	**Z** No Qualifier

A10. "And," when used in a code description, means "and/or," except when used to describe a combination of multiple body parts for which separate values exist for each body part (e.g., Skin and Subcutaneous Tissue used as a qualifier, where there are separate body part values for "Skin" and "Subcutaneous Tissue").

Example: Lower Arm and Wrist Muscle means lower arm and/or wrist muscle.

A11. Many of the terms used to construct PCS codes are defined within the system. It is the coder's responsibility to determine what the documentation in the medical record equates to in the PCS definitions. The physician is not expected to use the terms used in PCS code descriptions, nor is the coder required to query the physician when the correlation between the documentation and the defined PCS terms is clear.

Example: When the physician documents "partial resection" the coder can independently correlate "partial resection" to the root operation Excision without querying the physician for clarification.

Medical and Surgical Section Guidelines (section 0)

B2. Body System
General guidelines
B2.1a

The procedure codes in Anatomical Regions, General, Anatomical Regions, Upper Extremities and Anatomical Regions, Lower Extremities can be used when the procedure is performed on an anatomical region rather than a specific body part, or on the rare occasion when no information is available to support assignment of a code to a specific body part.

Examples: Chest tube drainage of the pleural cavity is coded to the root operation Drainage found in the body system Anatomical Regions, General. Suture repair of the abdominal wall is coded to the root operation Repair in the body system Anatomical Regions, General. Amputation of the foot is coded to the root operation Detachment in the body system Anatomical Regions, Lower Extremities.

B2.1b

Where the general body part values "upper" and "lower" are provided as an option in the Upper Arteries, Lower Arteries, Upper Veins, Lower Veins, Muscles and Tendons body systems, "upper" or "lower "specifies body parts located above or below the diaphragm respectively.

Example: Vein body parts above the diaphragm are found in the Upper Veins body system; vein body parts below the diaphragm are found in the Lower Veins body system.

B3. Root Operation
General guidelines
B3.1a

In order to determine the appropriate root operation, the full definition of the root operation as contained in the PCS Tables must be applied.

B3.1b

Components of a procedure specified in the root operation definition or explanation as integral to that root operation are not coded separately. Procedural steps necessary to reach the operative site and close the operative site, including anastomosis of a tubular body part, are also not coded separately.

Example: Resection of a joint as part of a joint replacement procedure is included in the root operation definition of Replacement and is not coded separately. Laparotomy performed to reach the site of an open liver biopsy is not coded separately. In a resection of sigmoid colon with anastomosis of descending colon to rectum, the anastomosis is not coded separately.

Multiple procedures
B3.2

During the same operative episode, multiple procedures are coded if:

    a. The same root operation is performed on different body parts as defined by distinct values of the body part character.

        Examples: Diagnostic excision of liver and pancreas are coded separately. Excision of lesion in the ascending colon and excision of lesion in the transverse colon are coded separately.

    b. The same root operation is repeated in multiple body parts, and those body parts are separate and distinct body parts classified to a single ICD-10-PCS body part value.

        Examples: Excision of the sartorius muscle and excision of the gracilis muscle are both included in the upper leg muscle body part value, and multiple procedures are coded. Extraction of multiple toenails are coded separately.

c. Multiple root operations with distinct objectives are performed on the same body part.

Example: Destruction of sigmoid lesion and bypass of sigmoid colon are coded separately.

d. The intended root operation is attempted using one approach but is converted to a different approach.

Example: Laparoscopic cholecystectomy converted to an open cholecystectomy is coded as percutaneous endoscopic Inspection and open Resection.

Discontinued or incomplete procedures
B3.3

If the intended procedure is discontinued or otherwise not completed, code the procedure to the root operation performed. If a procedure is discontinued before any other root operation is performed, code the root operation Inspection of the body part or anatomical region inspected.

Example: A planned aortic valve replacement procedure is discontinued after the initial thoracotomy and before any incision is made in the heart muscle, when the patient becomes hemodynamically unstable. This procedure is coded as an open Inspection of the mediastinum.

Biopsy procedures
B3.4a

Biopsy procedures are coded using the root operations Excision, Extraction, or Drainage and the qualifier Diagnostic. *Examples:* Fine needle aspiration biopsy of fluid in the lung is coded to the root operation Drainage with the qualifier Diagnostic. Biopsy of bone marrow is coded to the root operation Extraction with the qualifier Diagnostic. Lymph node sampling for biopsy is coded to the root operation Excision with the qualifier Diagnostic.

Biopsy followed by more definitive treatment
B3.4b

If a diagnostic Excision, Extraction, or Drainage procedure (biopsy) is followed by a more definitive procedure, such as Destruction, Excision or Resection at the same procedure site, both the biopsy and the more definitive treatment are coded.

Example: Biopsy of breast followed by partial mastectomy at the same procedure site, both the biopsy and the partial mastectomy procedure are coded.

Overlapping body layers
B3.5

If root operations Excision, Extraction, Repair or Inspection are performed on overlapping layers of the musculoskeletal system, the body part specifying the deepest layer is coded.

Example: Excisional debridement that includes skin and subcutaneous tissue and muscle is coded to the muscle body part.

Bypass procedures
B3.6a

Bypass procedures are coded by identifying the body part bypassed "from" and the body part bypassed "to." The fourth character body part specifies the body part bypassed from, and the qualifier specifies the body part bypassed to.

Example: Bypass from stomach to jejunum, stomach is the body part and jejunum is the qualifier.

B3.6b

Coronary artery bypass procedures are coded differently than other bypass procedures as described in the previous guideline. Rather than identifying the body part bypassed from, the body part identifies the number of coronary artery sites bypassed to, and the qualifier specifies the vessel bypassed from.

Example: Aortocoronary artery bypass of the left anterior descending coronary artery and the obtuse marginal coronary artery is classified in the body part axis of classification as two coronary arteries and the qualifier specifies the aorta as the body part bypassed from.

B3.6c

If multiple coronary arteries are bypassed, a separate procedure is coded for each coronary artery that uses a different device and/or qualifier.

Example: Aortocoronary artery bypass and internal mammary coronary artery bypass are coded separately.

Control vs. more definitive root operations

B3.7

The root operation Control is defined as, "Stopping, or attempting to stop, postprocedural or other acute bleeding." Control is the root operation coded when the procedure performed to achieve hemostasis, beyond what would be considered integral to a procedure, utilizes techniques (e.g. cautery, application of substances or pressure, suturing or ligation or clipping of bleeding points at the site) that are not described by a more specific root operation definition, such as Bypass, Detachment, Excision, Extraction, Reposition, Replacement, or Resection. If a more specific root operation definition applies to the procedure performed, then the more specific root operation is coded instead of Control.

Examples: Silver nitrate cautery to treat acute nasal bleeding is coded to the root operation Control. Liquid embolization of the right internal iliac artery to treat acute hematoma by stopping blood flow is coded to the root operation Occlusion. Suctioning of residual blood to achieve hemostasis during a transbronchial cryobiopsy is considered integral to the cryobiopsy procedure and is not coded separately.

Excision vs. Resection

B3.8

PCS contains specific body parts for anatomical subdivisions of a body part, such as lobes of the lungs or liver and regions of the intestine. Resection of the specific body part is coded whenever all of the body part is cut out or off, rather than coding Excision of a less specific body part.

Example: Left upper lung lobectomy is coded to Resection of Upper Lung Lobe, Left rather than Excision of Lung, Left.

Excision for graft

B3.9

If an autograft is obtained from a different procedure site in order to complete the objective of the procedure, a separate procedure is coded, except when the seventh character qualifier value in the ICD-10-PCS table fully specifies the site from which the autograft was obtained.

Examples: Coronary bypass with excision of saphenous vein graft, excision of saphenous vein is coded separately. Replacement of breast with autologous deep inferior epigastric artery perforator (DIEP) flap, excision of the DIEP flap is not coded separately. The seventh character qualifier value Deep Inferior Epigastric Artery Perforator Flap in the Replacement table fully specifies the site of the autograft harvest.

Fusion procedures of the spine

B3.10a

The body part coded for a spinal vertebral joint(s) rendered immobile by a spinal fusion procedure is classified by the level of the spine (e.g. thoracic). There are distinct body part values for a single vertebral joint and for multiple vertebral joints at each spinal level.

Example: Body part values specify Lumbar Vertebral Joint, Lumbar Vertebral Joints, 2 or More and Lumbosacral Vertebral Joint.

B3.10b

If multiple vertebral joints are fused, a separate procedure is coded for each vertebral joint that uses a different device and/or qualifier.

Example: Fusion of lumbar vertebral joint, posterior approach, anterior column and fusion of lumbar vertebral joint, posterior approach, posterior column are coded separately.

B3.10c

Combinations of devices and materials are often used on a vertebral joint to render the joint immobile. When combinations of devices are used on the same vertebral joint, the device value coded for the procedure is as follows:

- If an interbody fusion device is used to render the joint immobile (containing bone graft or bone graft substitute), the procedure is coded with the device value Interbody Fusion Device
- If bone graft is the *only* device used to render the joint immobile, the procedure is coded with the device value Nonautologous Tissue Substitute or Autologous Tissue Substitute
- If a mixture of autologous and nonautologous bone graft (with or without biological or synthetic extenders or binders) is used to render the joint immobile, code the procedure with the device value Autologous Tissue Substitute

Examples: Fusion of a vertebral joint using a cage style interbody fusion device containing morsellized bone graft is coded to the device Interbody Fusion Device. Fusion of a vertebral joint using a bone dowel interbody fusion device

made of cadaver bone and packed with a mixture of local morsellized bone and demineralized bone matrix is coded to the device Interbody Fusion Device. Fusion of a vertebral joint using both autologous bone graft and bone bank bone graft is coded to the device Autologous Tissue Substitute.

Inspection procedures
B3.11a

Inspection of a body part(s) performed in order to achieve the objective of a procedure is not coded separately.

Example: Fiberoptic bronchoscopy performed for irrigation of bronchus, only the irrigation procedure is coded.

B3.11b

If multiple tubular body parts are inspected, the most distal body part (the body part furthest from the starting point of the inspection) is coded. If multiple non-tubular body parts in a region are inspected, the body part that specifies the entire area inspected is coded.

Examples: Cystoureteroscopy with inspection of bladder and ureters is coded to the ureter body part value. Exploratory laparotomy with general inspection of abdominal contents is coded to the peritoneal cavity body part value.

B3.11c

When both an Inspection procedure and another procedure are performed on the same body part during the same episode, if the Inspection procedure is performed using a different approach than the other procedure, the Inspection procedure is coded separately.

Example: Endoscopic Inspection of the duodenum is coded separately when open Excision of the duodenum is performed during the same procedural episode.

Occlusion vs. Restriction for vessel embolization procedures
B3.12

If the objective of an embolization procedure is to completely close a vessel, the root operation Occlusion is coded. If the objective of an embolization procedure is to narrow the lumen of a vessel, the root operation Restriction is coded.

Examples: Tumor embolization is coded to the root operation Occlusion, because the objective of the procedure is to cut off the blood supply to the vessel. Embolization of a cerebral aneurysm is coded to the root operation Restriction, because the objective of the procedure is not to close off the vessel entirely, but to narrow the lumen of the vessel at the site of the aneurysm where it is abnormally wide.

Release procedures
B3.13

In the root operation Release, the body part value coded is the body part being freed and not the tissue being manipulated or cut to free the body part.

Example: Lysis of intestinal adhesions is coded to the specific intestine body part value.

Release vs. Division
B3.14

If the sole objective of the procedure is freeing a body part without cutting the body part, the root operation is Release. If the sole objective of the procedure is separating or transecting a body part, the root operation is Division.

Examples: Freeing a nerve root from surrounding scar tissue to relieve pain is coded to the root operation Release. Severing a nerve root to relieve pain is coded to the root operation Division.

Reposition for fracture treatment
B3.15

Reduction of a displaced fracture is coded to the root operation Reposition and the application of a cast or splint in conjunction with the Reposition procedure is not coded separately. Treatment of a nondisplaced fracture is coded to the procedure performed.

Examples: Casting of a nondisplaced fracture is coded to the root operation Immobilization in the Placement section.

Putting a pin in a nondisplaced fracture is coded to the root operation Insertion.

Transplantation vs. Administration
B3.16

Putting in a mature and functioning living body part taken from another individual or animal is coded to the root operation Transplantation. Putting in autologous or nonautologous cells is coded to the Administration section.

Example: Putting in autologous or nonautologous bone marrow, pancreatic islet cells or stem cells is coded to the Administration section.

Transfer procedures using multiple tissue layers
B3.17

The root operation Transfer contains qualifiers that can be used to specify when a transfer flap is composed of more than one tissue layer, such as a musculocutaneous flap. For procedures involving transfer of multiple tissue layers including skin, subcutaneous tissue, fascia or muscle, the procedure is coded to the body part value that describes the deepest tissue layer in the flap, and the qualifier can be used to describe the other tissue layer(s) in the transfer flap.

Example: A musculocutaneous flap transfer is coded to the appropriate body part value in the body system Muscles, and the qualifier is used to describe the additional tissue layer(s) in the transfer flap.

Excision/Resection followed by replacement
B3.18

If an Excision or Resection of a body part is followed by a Replacement procedure, code both procedures to identify each distinct objective, except when the Excision or Resection is considered integral and preparatory for the Replacement procedure.

Examples: Mastectomy followed by reconstruction, both Resection and Replacement of the breast are coded to fully capture the distinct objectives of the procedures performed. Maxillectomy with obturator reconstruction, both Excision and Replacement of the maxilla are coded to fully capture the distinct objectives of the procedures performed. Excisional debridement of tendon with skin graft, both the Excision of the tendon and the Replacement of the skin with a graft are coded to fully capture the distinct objectives of the procedures performed. Esophagectomy followed by reconstruction with colonic interposition, both the Resection and the Transfer of the large intestine to function as the esophagus are coded to fully capture the distinct objectives of the procedures performed.

Examples: Resection of a joint as part of a joint replacement procedure is considered integral and preparatory for the Replacement of the joint and the Resection is not coded separately. Resection of a valve as part of a valve replacement procedure is considered integral and preparatory for the valve Replacement and the Resection is not coded separately.

B4. Body Part
General guidelines
B4.1a

If a procedure is performed on a portion of a body part that does not have a separate body part value, code the body part value corresponding to the whole body part.

Example: A procedure performed on the alveolar process of the mandible is coded to the mandible body part.

B4.1b

If the prefix "peri" is combined with a body part to identify the site of the procedure, and the site of the procedure is not further specified, then the procedure is coded to the body part named. This guideline applies only when a more specific body part value is not available.

Examples: A procedure site identified as perirenal is coded to the kidney body part when the site of the procedure is not further specified. A procedure site described in the documentation as peri-urethral, and the documentation also indicates that it is the vulvar tissue and not the urethral tissue that is the site of the procedure, then the procedure is coded to the vulva body part. A procedure site documented as involving the periosteum is coded to the corresponding bone body part.

B4.1c

If a procedure is performed on a continuous section of a tubular body part, code the body part value corresponding to the anatomically most proximal (closest to the heart) portion of the tubular body part.

Examples: A procedure performed on a continuous section of artery from the femoral artery to the external iliac artery with the point of entry at the femoral artery is coded to the external iliac body part. A procedure performed on a continuous

section of artery from the femoral artery to the external iliac artery with the point of entry at the external iliac artery is also coded to the external iliac artery body part.

Branches of body parts
B4.2

Where a specific branch of a body part does not have its own body part value in PCS, the body part is typically coded to the closest proximal branch that has a specific body part value. In the cardiovascular body systems, if a general body part is available in the correct root operation table, and coding to a proximal branch would require assigning a code in a different body system, the procedure is coded using the general body part value.

Examples: A procedure performed on the mandibular branch of the trigeminal nerve is coded to the trigeminal nerve body part value. Occlusion of the bronchial artery is coded to the body part value Upper Artery in the body system Upper Arteries, and not to the body part value Thoracic Aorta, Descending in the body system Heart and Great Vessels.

Bilateral body part values
B4.3

Bilateral body part values are available for a limited number of body parts. If the identical procedure is performed on contralateral body parts, and a bilateral body part value exists for that body part, a single procedure is coded using the bilateral body part value. If no bilateral body part value exists, each procedure is coded separately using the appropriate body part value.

Example: The identical procedure performed on both fallopian tubes is coded once using the body part value Fallopian Tube, Bilateral. The identical procedure performed on both knee joints is coded twice using the body part values Knee Joint, Right and Knee Joint, Left.

Coronary arteries
B4.4

The coronary arteries are classified as a single body part that is further specified by number of arteries treated. One procedure code specifying multiple arteries is used when the same procedure is performed, including the same device and qualifier values.

Examples: Angioplasty of two distinct coronary arteries with placement of two stents is coded as Dilation of Coronary Artery, Two Arteries, with Two Intraluminal Devices. Angioplasty of two distinct coronary arteries, one with stent placed and one without, is coded separately as Dilation of Coronary Artery, One Artery with Intraluminal Device, and Dilation of Coronary Artery, One Artery with no device.

Tendons, ligaments, bursae and fascia near a joint
B4.5

Procedures performed on tendons, ligaments, bursae and fascia supporting a joint are coded to the body part in the respective body system that is the focus of the procedure. Procedures performed on joint structures themselves are coded to the body part in the joint body systems.

Example: Repair of the anterior cruciate ligament of the knee is coded to the knee bursa and ligament body part in the Bursae and Ligaments body system. Knee arthroscopy with shaving of articular cartilage is coded to the knee joint body part in the Lower Joints body system.

Skin, subcutaneous tissue and fascia overlying a joint
B4.6

If a procedure is performed on the skin, subcutaneous tissue or fascia overlying a joint, the procedure is coded to the following body part:

- Shoulder is coded to Upper Arm
- Elbow is coded to Lower Arm
- Wrist is coded to Lower Arm
- Hip is coded to Upper Leg
- Knee is coded to Lower Leg
- Ankle is coded to Foot

Fingers and toes
B4.7

If a body system does not contain a separate body part value for fingers, procedures performed on the fingers are coded to the body part value for the hand. If a body system does not contain a separate body part value for toes, procedures performed on the toes are coded to the body part value for the foot.

Example: Excision of finger muscle is coded to one of the hand muscle body part values in the Muscles body system.

Upper and lower intestinal tract
B4.8

In the Gastrointestinal body system, the general body part values Upper Intestinal Tract and Lower Intestinal Tract are provided as an option for the root operations such as Change, Insertion, Inspection, Removal and Revision. Upper Intestinal Tract includes the portion of the gastrointestinal tract from the esophagus down to and including the duodenum, and Lower Intestinal Tract includes the portion of the gastrointestinal tract from the jejunum down to and including the rectum and anus.

Example: In the root operation Change table, change of a device in the jejunum is coded using the body part Lower Intestinal Tract.

B5. Approach
Open approach with percutaneous endoscopic assistance
B5.2a

Procedures performed using the open approach with percutaneous endoscopic assistance are coded to the approach Open.

Example: Laparoscopic-assisted sigmoidectomy is coded to the approach Open.

Percutaneous endoscopic approach with extension of incision
B5.2b

Procedures performed using the percutaneous endoscopic approach, with incision or extension of an incision to assist in the removal of all or a portion of a body part or to anastomose a tubular body part to complete the procedure, are coded to the approach value Percutaneous Endoscopic.

Examples: Laparoscopic sigmoid colectomy with extension of stapling port for removal of specimen and direct anastomosis is coded to the approach value Percutaneous Endoscopic. Laparoscopic nephrectomy with midline incision for removing the resected kidney is coded to the approach value Percutaneous Endoscopic. Robotic-assisted laparoscopic prostatectomy with extension of incision for removal of the resected prostate is coded to the approach value Percutaneous Endoscopic.

External approach
B5.3a

Procedures performed within an orifice on structures that are visible without the aid of any instrumentation are coded to the approach External.

Example: Resection of tonsils is coded to the approach External.

B5.3b

Procedures performed indirectly by the application of external force through the intervening body layers are coded to the approach External.

Example: Closed reduction of fracture is coded to the approach External.

Percutaneous procedure via device
B5.4

Procedures performed percutaneously via a device placed for the procedure are coded to the approach Percutaneous.

Example: Fragmentation of kidney stone performed via percutaneous nephrostomy is coded to the approach Percutaneous.

B6. Device
General guidelines
B6.1a

A device is coded only if a device remains after the procedure is completed. If no device remains, the device value No Device is coded. In limited root operations, the classification provides the qualifier values Temporary and Intraoperative,

for specific procedures involving clinically significant devices, where the purpose of the device is to be utilized for a brief duration during the procedure or current inpatient stay. If a device that is intended to remain after the procedure is completed requires removal before the end of the operative episode in which it was inserted (for example, the device size is inadequate or a complication occurs), both the insertion and removal of the device should be coded.

B6.1b

Materials such as sutures, ligatures, radiological markers and temporary post-operative wound drains are considered integral to the performance of a procedure and are not coded as devices.

B6.1c

Procedures performed on a device only and not on a body part are specified in the root operations Change, Irrigation, Removal and Revision, and are coded to the procedure performed.

Example: Irrigation of percutaneous nephrostomy tube is coded to the root operation Irrigation of indwelling device in the Administration section.

Drainage device
B6.2

A separate procedure to put in a drainage device is coded to the root operation Drainage with the device value Drainage Device.

Obstetric Section Guidelines (section 1)

C. Obstetrics Section
Products of conception
C1

Procedures performed on the products of conception are coded to the Obstetrics section. Procedures performed on the pregnant female other than the products of conception are coded to the appropriate root operation in the Medical and Surgical section.

Example: Amniocentesis is coded to the products of conception body part in the Obstetrics section. Repair of obstetric urethral laceration is coded to the urethra body part in the Medical and Surgical section.

Procedures following delivery or abortion
C2

Procedures performed following a delivery or abortion for curettage of the endometrium or evacuation of retained products of conception are all coded in the Obstetrics section, to the root operation Extraction and the body part Products of Conception, Retained. Diagnostic or therapeutic dilation and curettage performed during times other than the postpartum or post-abortion period are all coded in the Medical and Surgical section, to the root operation Extraction and the body part Endometrium.

Radiation Therapy Section Guidelines (section D)

D. Radiation Therapy Section
Brachytherapy
D1.a

Brachytherapy is coded to the modality Brachytherapy in the Radiation Therapy section. When a radioactive brachytherapy source is left in the body at the end of the procedure, it is coded separately to the root operation Insertion with the device value Radioactive Element.

Example: Brachytherapy with implantation of a low dose rate brachytherapy source left in the body at the end of the procedure is coded to the applicable treatment site in section D, Radiation Therapy, with the modality Brachytherapy, the modality qualifier value, Low Dose Rate, and the applicable isotope value and qualifier value. The implantation of the brachytherapy source is coded separately to the device value Radioactive Element in the appropriate Insertion table of the Medical and Surgical section. The Radiation Therapy section code identifies the specific modality and isotope of the brachytherapy, and the root operation Insertion code identifies the implantation of the brachytherapy source that remain in the body at the end of the procedure.

Exception: Implantation of Cesium-131 brachytherapy seeds embedded in a collagen matrix to the treatment site after resection of brain tumor is coded to the root operation Insertion with the device value Radioactive Element, Cesium-131 Collagen Implant. The procedure is coded to the root operation Insertion only, because the device value

identifies both the implantation of the radioactive element and a specific brachytherapy isotope that is not included in the Radiation Therapy section tables.

D1.b

A separate procedure to place a temporary applicator for delivering the brachytherapy is coded to the root operation Insertion and the device value Other Device.

Examples: Intrauterine brachytherapy applicator placed as a separate procedure from the brachytherapy procedure is coded to Insertion of Other Device, and the brachytherapy is coded separately using the modality Brachytherapy in the Radiation Therapy section. Intrauterine brachytherapy applicator placed concomitantly with delivery of the brachytherapy dose is coded with a single code using the modality Brachytherapy in the Radiation Therapy section.

New Technology Section Guidelines (section X)

E. New Technology Section

General guidelines

E1.a

Section X codes fully represent the specific procedure described in the code title, and do not require any additional codes from other sections of ICD-10-PCS. When section X contains a code title which describes a specific new technology procedure, and it is the only procedure performed, only the section X code is reported for the procedure. There is no need to report an additional code in another section of ICD-10-PCS.

Example: XW043A6 Introduction of Cefiderocol Anti-infective into Central Vein, Percutaneous Approach, New Technology Group 6, can be coded to indicate that Cefiderocol Anti-infective was administered via a central vein. A separate code from table 3E0 in the Administration section of ICD-10-PCS is not coded in addition to this code.

E1.b

When multiple procedures are performed, New Technology section X codes are coded following the multiple procedures guideline.

Examples: Dual filter cerebral embolic filtration used during transcatheter aortic valve replacement (TAVR), X2A5312 Cerebral Embolic Filtration, Dual Filter in Innominate Artery and Left Common Carotid Artery, Percutaneous Approach, New Technology Group 2, is coded for the cerebral embolic filtration, along with an ICD-10-PCS code for the TAVR procedure. An extracorporeal flow reversal circuit for embolic neuroprotection placed during a transcarotid arterial revascularization procedure, a code from table X2A, Assistance of the Cardiovascular System is coded for the use of the extracoporeal flow reversal circuit, along with an ICD-10-PCS code for the transcarotid arterial revascularization procedure.

F. Selection of Principal Procedure

The following instructions should be applied in the selection of principal procedure and clarification on the importance of the relation to the principal diagnosis when more than one procedure is performed:

1. Procedure performed for definitive treatment of both principal diagnosis and secondary diagnosis

   a. Sequence procedure performed for definitive treatment most related to principal diagnosis as principal procedure.

2. Procedure performed for definitive treatment and diagnostic procedures performed for both principal diagnosis and secondary diagnosis

   a. Sequence procedure performed for definitive treatment most related to principal diagnosis as principal procedure

3. A diagnostic procedure was performed for the principal diagnosis and a procedure is performed for definitive treatment of a secondary diagnosis.

   a. Sequence diagnostic procedure as principal procedure, since the procedure most related to the principal diagnosis takes precedence.

4. No procedures performed that are related to principal diagnosis; procedures performed for definitive treatment and diagnostic procedures were performed for secondary diagnosis

   a. Sequence procedure performed for definitive treatment of secondary diagnosis as principal procedure, since there are no procedures (definitive or nondefinitive treatment) related to principal diagnosis.

Amniocentesis
see Drainage, Products of
Conception 1090

Amnioinfusion
see Introduction of substance in or
on, Products of Conception 3E0E

Amnioscopy 10J08ZZ

Amniotomy
see Drainage, Products of
Conception 1090

**AMPLATZER® Muscular VSD
Occluder**
use Synthetic Substitute

Amputation
see Detachment

AMS 800® Urinary Control System
use Artificial Sphincter in Urinary
System

Anal orifice
use Anus

Analog radiography
see Plain Radiography

Anastomosis
see Bypass

Anatomical snuffbox
use Muscle, Lower Arm and Wrist,
Left
use Muscle, Lower Arm and Wrist,
Right

**Andexanet Alfa, Factor Xa Inhibitor
Reversal Agent**
use Coagulation Factor Xa,
Inactivated

Andexxa
use Coagulation Factor Xa,
Inactivated

AneuRx® AAA Advantage®
use Intraluminal Device

Angiectomy
see Excision, Heart and Great
Vessels 02B
see Excision, Upper Arteries 03B
see Excision, Lower Arteries 04B
see Excision, Upper Veins 05B
see Excision, Lower Veins 06B

Angiocardiography
Combined right and left heart
see Fluoroscopy, Heart, Right and
Left B216
Left Heart
see Fluoroscopy, Heart, Left B215
Right Heart
see Fluoroscopy, Heart, Right B214
SPY system intravascular
fluorescence
see Monitoring, Physiological
Systems 4A1

Angiography
see Computerized Tomography (CT
Scan), Artery
see Fluoroscopy, Artery
see Magnetic Resonance Imaging
(MRI), Artery
see Plain Radiography, Artery

Angioplasty
see Dilation, Heart and Great
Vessels 027
see Repair, Heart and Great Vessels
02Q
see Replacement, Heart and Great
Vessels 02R
see Dilation, Upper Arteries 037
see Repair, Upper Arteries 03Q
see Replacement, Upper Arteries
03R
see Dilation, Lower Arteries 047
see Repair, Lower Arteries 04Q
see Replacement, Lower Arteries
04R
see Supplement, Heart and Great
Vessels 02U

Angioplasty *(continued)*
see Supplement, Upper Arteries 03U
see Supplement, Lower Arteries 04U

Angiorrhaphy
see Repair, Heart and Great Vessels
02Q
see Repair, Upper Arteries 03Q
see Repair, Lower Arteries 04Q

Angioscopy
02JY4ZZ
03JY4ZZ
04JY4ZZ

Angiotensin II
use Synthetic Human Angiotensin II

Angiotripsy
see Occlusion, Upper Arteries 03L
see Occlusion, Lower Arteries 04L

Angular artery
use Artery, Face

Angular vein
use Vein, Face, Left
use Vein, Face, Right

Annular ligament
use Bursa and Ligament, Elbow, Left
use Bursa and Ligament, Elbow,
Right

Annuloplasty
see Repair, Heart and Great Vessels
02Q
see Supplement, Heart and Great
Vessels 02U

Annuloplasty ring
use Synthetic Substitute

Anoplasty
see Repair, Anus 0DQQ
see Supplement, Anus 0DUQ

Anorectal junction
use Rectum

Anoscopy 0DJD8ZZ

Ansa cervicalis
use Nerve, Cervical Plexus

Antabuse therapy HZ93ZZZ

Antebrachial fascia
use Subcutaneous Tissue and Fascia,
Lower Arm, Left
use Subcutaneous Tissue and Fascia,
Lower Arm, Right

Anterior (pectoral) lymph node
use Lymphatic, Axillary, Left
use Lymphatic, Axillary, Right

Anterior cerebral artery
use Artery, Intracranial

Anterior cerebral vein
use Vein, Intracranial

Anterior choroidal artery
use Artery, Intracranial

Anterior circumflex humeral artery
use Artery, Axillary, Left
use Artery, Axillary, Right

Anterior communicating artery
use Artery, Intracranial

Anterior cruciate ligament (ACL)
use Bursa and Ligament, Knee, Left
use Bursa and Ligament, Knee,
Right

Anterior crural nerve
use Nerve, Femoral

Anterior facial vein
use Vein, Face, Left
use Vein, Face, Right

Anterior intercostal artery
use Artery, Internal Mammary, Left
use Artery, Internal Mammary,
Right

Anterior interosseous nerve
use Nerve, Median

Anterior lateral malleolar artery
use Artery, Anterior Tibial, Left
use Artery, Anterior Tibial, Right

Anterior lingual gland
use Gland, Minor Salivary

Anterior medial malleolar artery
use Artery, Anterior Tibial, Left
use Artery, Anterior Tibial, Right

Anterior spinal artery
use Artery, Vertebral, Left
use Artery, Vertebral, Right

Anterior tibial recurrent artery
use Artery, Anterior Tibial, Left
use Artery, Anterior Tibial, Right

Anterior ulnar recurrent artery
use Artery, Ulnar, Left
use Artery, Ulnar, Right

Anterior vagal trunk
use Nerve, Vagus

Anterior vertebral muscle
use Muscle, Neck, Left
use Muscle, Neck, Right

**Anti-SARS-CoV-2 hyperimmune
globulin**
use Hyperimmune Globulin

**Antibacterial Envelope (TYRX)
(AIGISRx)**
use Anti-Infective Envelope

Antibiotic-eluting Bone Void Filler
XW0V0P7

Antigen-free air conditioning
see Atmospheric Control,
Physiological Systems 6A0

Antihelix
use Ear, External, Bilateral
use Ear, External, Left
use Ear, External, Right

Antimicrobial envelope
use Anti-Infective Envelope

Antitragus
use Ear, External, Bilateral
use Ear, External, Left
use Ear, External, Right

Antrostomy
see Drainage, Ear, Nose, Sinus 099

Antrotomy
see Drainage, Ear, Nose, Sinus 099

Antrum of Highmore
use Sinus, Maxillary, Left
use Sinus, Maxillary, Right

Aortic annulus
use Valve, Aortic

Aortic arch
use Thoracic Aorta, Ascending/Arch

Aortic intercostal artery
use Upper Artery

Aortography
see Plain Radiography, Upper
Arteries B30
see Fluoroscopy, Upper Arteries B31
see Plain Radiography, Lower
Arteries B40
see Fluoroscopy, Lower Arteries B41

Aortoplasty
see Repair, Aorta, Thoracic,
Descending 02QW
see Repair, Aorta, Thoracic,
Ascending/Arch 02QX
see Replacement, Aorta, Thoracic,
Descending 02RW
see Replacement, Aorta, Thoracic,
Ascending/Arch 02RX
see Supplement, Aorta, Thoracic,
Descending 02UW
see Supplement, Aorta, Thoracic,
Ascending/Arch 02UX
see Repair, Aorta, Abdominal 04Q0
see Replacement, Aorta,
Abdominal 04R0
see Supplement, Aorta, Abdominal
04U0

Apalutamide Antineoplastic
XW0DXJ5

Apical (subclavicular) lymph node
use Lymphatic, Axillary, Left
use Lymphatic, Axillary, Right

**ApiFix® Minimally Invasive
Deformity Correction (MID-C)
System**
use Posterior (Dynamic)
Distraction Device in New
Technology

Apneustic center *use* Pons

Appendectomy
see Excision, Appendix 0DBJ
see Resection, Appendix 0DTJ

Appendicolysis
see Release, Appendix 0DNJ

Appendicotomy
see Drainage, Appendix 0D9J

Application
see Introduction of substance in
or on

aprevo™
use Interbody Fusion Device,
Customizable in New Technology

Aquablation therapy, prostate
XV508A4

Aquapheresis 6A550Z3

Aqueduct of Sylvius
use Cerebral Ventricle

Aqueous humour
use Anterior Chamber, Left
use Anterior Chamber, Right

Arachnoid mater, intracranial
use Cerebral Meninges

Arachnoid mater, spinal
use Spinal Meninges

Arcuate artery
use Artery, Foot, Left
use Artery, Foot, Right

Areola
use Nipple, Left
use Nipple, Right

**AROM (artificial rupture of
membranes)** 10907ZC

Arterial canal (duct)
use Artery, Pulmonary, Left

Arterial pulse tracing
see Measurement, Arterial 4A03

Arteriectomy
see Excision, Heart and Great
Vessels 02B
see Excision, Upper Arteries 03B
see Excision, Lower Arteries 04B

Arteriography
see Plain Radiography, Heart B20
see Fluoroscopy, Heart B21
see Plain Radiography, Upper
Arteries B30
see Fluoroscopy, Upper Arteries
B31
see Plain Radiography, Lower
Arteries B40
see Fluoroscopy, Lower Arteries B41

Arterioplasty
see Repair, Heart and Great Vessels
02Q
see Replacement, Heart and Great
Vessels 02R
see Repair, Upper Arteries 03Q
see Replacement, Upper Arteries
03R
see Repair, Lower Arteries 04Q
see Replacement, Lower Arteries
04R
see Supplement, Upper Arteries
03U
see Supplement, Lower Arteries
04U
see Supplement, Heart and Great
Vessels 02U

Arteriorrhaphy
see Repair, Heart and Great Vessels
02Q
see Repair, Upper Arteries 03Q
see Repair, Lower Arteries 04Q

Arterioscopy
   see Inspection, Artery, Lower 04JY
   see Inspection, Artery, Upper 03JY
   see Inspection, Great Vessel 02JY
Arthrectomy
   see Excision, Upper Joints 0RB
   see Resection, Upper Joints 0RT
   see Excision, Lower Joints 0SB
   see Resection, Lower Joints 0ST
Arthrocentesis
   see Drainage, Upper Joints 0R9
   see Drainage, Lower Joints 0S9
Arthrodesis
   see Fusion, Upper Joints 0RG
   see Fusion, Lower Joints 0SG
Arthrography
   see Plain Radiography, Skull and
     Facial Bones BN0
   see Plain Radiography, Non-Axial
     Upper Bones BP0
   see Plain Radiography, Non-Axial
     Lower Bones BQ0
Arthrolysis
   see Release, Upper Joints 0RN
   see Release, Lower Joints 0SN
Arthropexy
   see Repair, Upper Joints 0RQ
   see Reposition, Upper Joints 0RS
   see Repair, Lower Joints 0SQ
   see Reposition, Lower Joints 0SS
Arthroplasty
   see Repair, Upper Joints 0RQ
   see Replacement, Upper Joints 0RR
   see Repair, Lower Joints 0SQ
   see Replacement, Lower Joints 0SR
   see Supplement, Lower Joints 0SU
   see Supplement, Upper Joints 0RU
Arthroplasty, radial head
   see Replacement, Radius, Left 0PRJ
   see Replacement, Radius, Right
     0PRH
Arthroscopy
   see Inspection, Upper Joints 0RJ
   see Inspection, Lower Joints 0SJ
Arthrotomy
   see Drainage, Upper Joints 0R9
   see Drainage, Lower Joints 0S9
Articulating Spacer (Antibiotic)
   use Articulating Spacer in Lower
     Joints
Artificial anal sphincter (AAS)
   use Artificial Sphincter in
     Gastrointestinal System
Artificial bowel sphincter
   (neosphincter)
   use Artificial Sphincter in
     Gastrointestinal System
Artificial Sphincter
   Insertion of device in
     Anus 0DHQ
     Bladder 0THB
     Bladder Neck 0THC
     Urethra 0THD
   Removal of device from
     Anus 0DPQ
     Bladder 0TPB
     Urethra 0TPD
   Revision of device in
     Anus 0DWQ
     Bladder 0TWB
     Urethra 0TWD
Artificial urinary sphincter (AUS)
   use Artificial Sphincter in Urinary
     System
Aryepiglottic fold
   use Larynx
Arytenoid cartilage
   use Larynx
Arytenoid muscle
   use Muscle, Neck, Left
   use Muscle, Neck, Right

Arytenoidectomy
   see Excision, Larynx 0CBS
Arytenoidopexy
   see Repair, Larynx 0CQS
Ascenda Intrathecal Catheter
   use Infusion Device
Ascending aorta
   use Thoracic Aorta, Ascending/
     Arch
Ascending palatine artery
   use Artery, Face
Ascending pharyngeal artery
   use Artery, External Carotid, Left
   use Artery, External Carotid, Right
aScope™ Duodeno
   see New Technology, Hepatobiliary
     System and Pancreas XFJ
Aspiration, fine needle
   Fluid or gas
     see Drainage
   Tissue biopsy
     see Excision
     see Extraction
Assessment
   Activities of daily living
     see Activities of Daily Living
       Assessment, Rehabilitation
       F02
   Hearing
     see Hearing Assessment,
       Diagnostic Audiology F13
   Hearing aid
     see Hearing Aid Assessment,
       Diagnostic Audiology F14
   Intravascular perfusion, using
     indocyanine green (ICG) dye
     see Monitoring, Physiological
       Systems 4A1
   Motor function
     see Motor Function Assessment,
       Rehabilitation F01
   Nerve function
     see Motor Function Assessment,
       Rehabilitation F01
   Speech
     see Speech Assessment,
       Rehabilitation F00
   Vestibular
     see Vestibular Assessment,
       Diagnostic Audiology F15
   Vocational
     see Activities of Daily Living
       Treatment, Rehabilitation
       F08
Assistance
   Cardiac
     Continuous
       Balloon Pump 5A02210
       Impeller Pump 5A0221D
       Other Pump 5A02216
       Pulsatile Compression
         5A02215
     Intermittent
       Balloon Pump 5A02110
       Impeller Pump 5A0211D
       Other Pump 5A02116
       Pulsatile Compression
         5A02115
   Circulatory
     Continuous
       Hyperbaric 5A05221
       Supersaturated 5A0522C
     Intermittent
       Hyperbaric 5A05121
       Supersaturated 5A0512C
   Respiratory
     24-96 Consecutive Hours
       Continuous Negative Airway
         Pressure 5A09459
       Continuous Positive Airway
         Pressure 5A09457

Assistance *(continued)*
   Respiratory *(continued)*
     24-96 Consecutive Hours
       (continued)
       High Nasal Flow/Velocity
         5A0945A
       Intermittent Negative Airway
         Pressure 5A0945B
       Intermittent Positive Airway
         Pressure 5A09458
       No Qualifier 5A0945Z
     Continuous, Filtration 5A0920Z
     Greater than 96 Consecutive
       Hours
       Continuous Negative Airway
         Pressure 5A09559
       Continuous Positive Airway
         Pressure 5A09557
       High Nasal Flow/Velocity
         5A0955A
       Intermittent Negative Airway
         Pressure 5A0955B
       Intermittent Positive Airway
         Pressure 5A09558
       No Qualifier 5A0955Z
     Less than 24 Consecutive Hours
       Continuous Negative Airway
         Pressure 5A09359
       Continuous Positive Airway
         Pressure 5A09357
       High Nasal Flow/Velocity
         5A0935A
       Intermittent Negative Airway
         Pressure 5A0935B
       Intermittent Positive Airway
         Pressure 5A09358
       No Qualifier 5A0935Z
Associating liver partition and
   portal vein ligation (ALPPS)
   see Division, Hepatobiliary System
     and Pancreas 0F8
   see Resection, Hepatobiliary
     System and Pancreas 0FT
Assurant (Cobalt) stent
   use Intraluminal Device
Atezolizumab Antineoplastic XW0
Atherectomy
   see Extirpation, Heart and Great
     Vessels 02C
   see Extirpation, Upper Arteries
     03C
   see Extirpation, Lower Arteries
     04C
Atlantoaxial joint
   use Joint, Cervical Vertebral
Atmospheric Control 6A0Z
AtriClip LAA Exclusion System
   use Extraluminal Device
Atrioseptoplasty
   see Repair, Heart and Great Vessels
     02Q
   see Replacement, Heart and Great
     Vessels 02R
   see Supplement, Heart and Great
     Vessels 02U
Atrioventricular node
   use Conduction Mechanism
Atrium dextrum cordis
   use Atrium, Right
Atrium pulmonale
   use Atrium, Left
Attain Ability® lead
   use Cardiac Lead, Pacemaker in
     02H
   use Cardiac Lead, Defibrillator in
     02H
Attain StarFix® (OTW) lead
   use Cardiac Lead, Defibrillator in
     02H
   use Cardiac Lead, Pacemaker in
     02H

Audiology, diagnostic
   see Hearing Assessment, Diagnostic
     Audiology F13
   see Hearing Aid Assessment,
     Diagnostic Audiology F14
   see Vestibular Assessment,
     Diagnostic Audiology F15
Audiometry
   see Hearing Assessment, Diagnostic
     Audiology F13
Auditory tube
   use Eustachian Tube, Left
   use Eustachian Tube, Right
Auerbach's (myenteric) plexus
   use Nerve, Abdominal Sympathetic
Auricle
   use Ear, External, Bilateral
   use Ear, External, Left
   use Ear, External, Right
Auricularis muscle
   use Muscle, Head
Autograft
   use Autologous Tissue Substitute
Autologous artery graft
   use Autologous Arterial Tissue in
     Heart and Great Vessels
   use Autologous Arterial Tissue in
     Lower Arteries
   use Autologous Arterial Tissue in
     Lower Veins
   use Autologous Arterial Tissue in
     Upper Arteries
   use Autologous Arterial Tissue in
     Upper Veins
Autologous vein graft
   use Autologous Venous Tissue in
     Heart and Great Vessels
   use Autologous Venous Tissue in
     Lower Arteries
   use Autologous Venous Tissue in
     Lower Veins
   use Autologous Venous Tissue in
     Upper Arteries
   use Autologous Venous Tissue in
     Upper Veins
Automated Chest Compression
   (ACC) 5A1221J
AutoPulse® Resuscitation System
   5A1221J
Autotransfusion
   see Transfusion
Autotransplant
   Adrenal tissue
     see Reposition, Endocrine
       System 0GS
   Kidney
     see Reposition, Urinary System
       0TS
   Pancreatic tissue
     see Reposition, Pancreas
       0FSG
   Parathyroid tissue
     see Reposition, Endocrine
       System 0GS
   Thyroid tissue
     see Reposition, Endocrine
       System 0GS
   Tooth
     see Reattachment, Mouth and
       Throat 0CM
Avulsion
   see Extraction
AVYCAZ® (ceftazidime-avibactam)
   use Other Anti-infective
Axial Lumbar Interbody Fusion
   System
   use Interbody Fusion Device in
     Lower Joints
AxiaLIF® System
   use Interbody Fusion Device in
     Lower Joints

Axicabtagene Ciloeucel
use Axicabtagene Ciloleucel
Immunotherapy
Axicabtagene Ciloleucel
Immunotherapy XW0
Axillary fascia
use Subcutaneous Tissue and Fascia,
Upper Arm, Left
use Subcutaneous Tissue and Fascia,
Upper Arm, Right
Axillary nerve
use Nerve, Brachial Plexus
AZEDRA®
use Iobenguane I-131 Antineoplastic

B

BAK/C® Interbody Cervical Fusion
System
use Interbody Fusion Device in
Upper Joints
BAL (bronchial alveolar lavage),
diagnostic
see Drainage, Respiratory System
0B9
Balanoplasty
see Repair, Penis 0VQS
see Supplement, Penis 0VUS
Balloon atrial septostomy (BAS)
02163Z7
Balloon Pump
Continuous, Output 5A02210
Intermittent, Output 5A02110
Bandage, Elastic
see Compression
Banding
see Occlusion
see Restriction
Banding, esophageal varices
see Occlusion, Vein, Esophageal
06L3
Banding, laparoscopic (adjustable)
gastric
Initial procedure 0DV64CZ
Surgical correction
see Revision of device in,
Stomach 0DW6
Bard® Composix® (E/X)(LP) mesh
use Synthetic Substitute
Bard® Composix® Kugel® patch
use Synthetic Substitute
Bard® Dulex™ mesh
use Synthetic Substitute
Bard® Ventralex™ hernia patch
use Synthetic Substitute
Barium swallow
see Fluoroscopy, Gastrointestinal
System BD1
Baroreflex Activation Therapy®
(BAT®)
Stimulator Generator in
Subcutaneous Tissue and Fascia
use Stimulator Lead in Upper
Arteries
Barricaid® Annular Closure Device
(ACD)
use Synthetic Substitute
Bartholin's (greater vestibular)
gland
use Gland, Vestibular
Basal (internal) cerebral vein
use Vein, Intracranial
Basal metabolic rate (BMR)
see Measurement, Physiological
Systems 4A0Z
Basal nuclei
use Basal Ganglia
Base of Tongue
use Pharynx
Basilar artery
use Artery, Intracranial

Basis pontis
use Pons
Beam Radiation
Abdomen DW03
Intraoperative DW033Z0
Adrenal Gland DG02
Intraoperative DG023Z0
Bile Ducts DF02
Intraoperative DF023Z0
Bladder DT02
Intraoperative DT023Z0
Bone
Intraoperative DP0C3Z0
Other DP0C
Bone Marrow D700
Intraoperative D7003Z0
Brain D000
Intraoperative D0003Z0
Brain Stem D001
Intraoperative D0013Z0
Breast
Left DM00
Intraoperative DM003Z0
Right DM01
Intraoperative DM013Z0
Bronchus DB01
Intraoperative DB013Z0
Cervix DU01
Intraoperative DU013Z0
Chest DW02
Intraoperative DW023Z0
Chest Wall DB07
Intraoperative DB073Z0
Colon DD05
Intraoperative DD053Z0
Diaphragm DB08
Intraoperative DB083Z0
Duodenum DD02
Intraoperative DD023Z0
Ear D900
Intraoperative D9003Z0
Esophagus DD00
Intraoperative DD003Z0
Eye D800
Intraoperative D8003Z0
Femur DP09
Intraoperative DP093Z0
Fibula DP0B
Intraoperative DP0B3Z0
Gallbladder DF01
Intraoperative DF013Z0
Gland
Adrenal DG02
Intraoperative DG023Z0
Parathyroid DG04
Intraoperative DG043Z0
Pituitary DG00
Intraoperative DG003Z0
Thyroid DG05
Intraoperative DG053Z0
Glands
Intraoperative D9063Z0
Salivary D906
Head and Neck DW01
Intraoperative DW013Z0
Hemibody DW04
Intraoperative DW043Z0
Humerus DP06
Intraoperative DP063Z0
Hypopharynx D903
Intraoperative D9033Z0
Ileum DD04
Intraoperative DD043Z0
Jejunum DD03
Intraoperative DD033Z0
Kidney DT00
Intraoperative DT003Z0
Larynx D90B
Intraoperative D90B3Z0
Liver DF00
Intraoperative DF003Z0

Beam Radiation (continued)
Lung DB02
Intraoperative DB023Z0
Lymphatics
Abdomen D706
Intraoperative D7063Z0
Axillary D704
Intraoperative D7043Z0
Inguinal D708
Intraoperative D7083Z0
Neck D703
Intraoperative D7033Z0
Pelvis D707
Intraoperative D7073Z0
Thorax D705
Intraoperative D7053Z0
Mandible DP03
Intraoperative DP033Z0
Maxilla DP02
Intraoperative DP023Z0
Mediastinum DB06
Intraoperative DB063Z0
Mouth D904
Intraoperative D9043Z0
Nasopharynx D90D
Intraoperative D90D3Z0
Neck and Head DW01
Intraoperative DW013Z0
Nerve
Intraoperative D0073Z0
Peripheral D007
Nose D901
Intraoperative D9013Z0
Oropharynx D90F
Intraoperative D90F3Z0
Ovary DU00
Intraoperative DU003Z0
Palate
Hard D908
Intraoperative D9083Z0
Soft D909
Intraoperative
D9093Z0
Pancreas DF03
Intraoperative DF033Z0
Parathyroid Gland DG04
Intraoperative DG043Z0
Pelvic Bones DP08
Intraoperative DP083Z0
Pelvic Region DW06
Intraoperative DW063Z0
Pineal Body DG01
Intraoperative DG013Z0
Pituitary Gland DG00
Intraoperative DG003Z0
Pleura DB05
Intraoperative DB053Z0
Prostate DV00
Intraoperative DV003Z0
Radius DP07
Intraoperative DP073Z0
Rectum DD07
Intraoperative DD073Z0
Rib DP05
Intraoperative DP053Z0
Sinuses D907
Intraoperative D9073Z0
Skin
Abdomen DH08
Intraoperative DH083Z0
Arm DH04
Intraoperative DH043Z0
Back DH07
Intraoperative DH073Z0
Buttock DH09
Intraoperative DH093Z0
Chest DH06
Intraoperative DH063Z0
Face DH02
Intraoperative DH023Z0
Leg DH0B
Intraoperative DH0B3Z0

Beam Radiation (continued)
Skin (continued)
Neck DH03
Intraoperative DH033Z0
Skull DP00
Intraoperative DP003Z0
Spinal Cord D006
Intraoperative D0063Z0
Spleen D702
Intraoperative D7023Z0
Sternum DP04
Intraoperative DP043Z0
Stomach DD01
Intraoperative DD013Z0
Testis DV01
Intraoperative DV013Z0
Thymus D701
Intraoperative D7013Z0
Thyroid Gland DG05
Intraoperative DG053Z0
Tibia DP0B
Intraoperative DP0B3Z0
Tongue D905
Intraoperative D9053Z0
Trachea DB00
Intraoperative DB003Z0
Ulna DP07
Intraoperative DP073Z0
Ureter DT01
Intraoperative DT013Z0
Urethra DT03
Intraoperative DT033Z0
Uterus DU02
Intraoperative DU023Z0
Whole Body DW05
Intraoperative DW053Z0
Bedside swallow F00ZJWZ
Berlin Heart Ventricular Assist
Device
use Implantable Heart Assist System
in Heart and Great Vessels
Bezlotoxumab Monoclonal Antibody
XW0
Biceps brachii muscle
use Muscle, Upper Arm, Left
use Muscle, Upper Arm, Right
Biceps femoris muscle
use Muscle, Upper Leg, Left
use Muscle, Upper Leg, Right
Bicipital aponeurosis
use Subcutaneous Tissue and Fascia,
Lower Arm, Left
use Subcutaneous Tissue and Fascia,
Lower Arm, Right
Bicuspid valve
use Valve, Mitral
Bili light therapy
see Phototherapy, Skin 6A60
Bioactive embolization coil(s)
use Intraluminal Device, Bioactive
in Upper Arteries
Bioengineered Allogeneic Construct,
Skin XHRPXF7
Biofeedback GZC9ZZZ
BioFire® FilmArray® Pneumonia
Panel XXEBXQ6
Biopsy
see Drainage with qualifier
Diagnostic
see Excision with qualifier Diagnostic
see Extraction with qualifier
Diagnostic
BiPAP
see Assistance, Respiratory v5A09
Bisection
see Division
Biventricular external heart assist
system
use Short-term External Heart
Assist System in Heart and Great
Vessels

Blepharectomy
see Excision, Eye 08B
see Resection, Eye 08T
Blepharoplasty
see Repair, Eye 08Q
see Replacement, Eye 08R
see Reposition, Eye 08S
see Supplement, Eye 08U
Blepharorrhaphy
see Repair, Eye 08Q
Blepharotomy
see Drainage, Eye 089
Blinatumomab
use Other Antineoplastic
BLINCYTO® (blinatumomab)
use Other Antineoplastic
Block, Nerve, anesthetic injection
3E0T3BZ
Blood glucose monitoring system
use Monitoring Device
Blood pressure
see Measurement, Arterial 4A03
BMR (basal metabolic rate)
see Measurement, Physiological
Systems 4A0Z
Body of femur
use Femoral Shaft, Left
use Femoral Shaft, Right
Body of fibula
use Fibula, Left
use Fibula, Right
Bone anchored hearing device
use Hearing Device, Bone
Conduction in 09H
use Hearing Device in Head and Facial
Bones
Bone bank bone graft
use Nonautologous Tissue
Substitute
Bone Growth Stimulator
Insertion of device in
Bone
Facial 0NHW
Lower 0QHY
Nasal 0NHB
Upper 0PHY
Skull 0NH0
Removal of device from
Bone
Facial 0NPW
Lower 0QPY
Nasal 0NPB
Upper 0PPY
Skull 0NP0
Revision of device in
Bone
Facial 0NWW
Lower 0QWY
Nasal 0NWB
Upper 0PWY
Skull 0NW0
Bone marrow transplant
see Transfusion, Circulatory 302
**Bone morphogenetic protein 2
(BMP 2)**
use Recombinant Bone
Morphogenetic Protein
**Bone screw (interlocking)(lag)
(pedicle)(recessed)**
use Internal Fixation Device in
Head and Facial Bones
use Internal Fixation Device in
Lower Bones
use Internal Fixation Device in Upper
Bones
Bony labyrinth
use Ear, Inner, Left
use Ear, Inner, Right
Bony orbit
use Orbit, Left
use Orbit, Right

Bony vestibule
use Ear, Inner, Left
use Ear, Inner, Right
Botallo's duct
use Artery, Pulmonary, Left
Bovine pericardial valve
use Zooplastic Tissue in Heart and
Great Vessels
Bovine pericardium graft
use Zooplastic Tissue in Heart and
Great Vessels
BP (blood pressure)
see Measurement, Arterial 4A03
Brachial (lateral) lymph node
use Lymphatic, Axillary, Left
use Lymphatic, Axillary, Right
Brachialis muscle
use Muscle, Upper Arm, Left
use Muscle, Upper Arm, Right
Brachiocephalic artery
use Artery, Innominate
Brachiocephalic trunk
use Artery, Innominate
Brachiocephalic vein
use Vein, Innominate, Left
use Vein, Innominate, Right
Brachioradialis muscle
use Muscle, Lower Arm and Wrist,
Left
use Muscle, Lower Arm and Wrist,
Right
Brachytherapy
Abdomen DW13
Adrenal Gland DG12
Back
Lower DW1L
Upper DW1K
Bile Ducts DF12
Bladder DT12
Bone Marrow D710
Brain D010
Brain Stem D011
Breast
Left DM10
Right DM11
Bronchus DB11
Cervix DU11
Chest DW12
Chest Wall DB17
Colon DD15
Cranial Cavity DW10
Diaphragm DB18
Duodenum DD12
Ear D910
Esophagus DD10
Extremity
Lower DW1Y
Upper DW1X
Eye D810
Gastrointestinal Tract DW1P
Gallbladder DF11
Genitourinary Tract
DW1R
Gland
Adrenal DG12
Parathyroid DG14
Pituitary DG10
Thyroid DG15
Glands, Salivary D916
Head and Neck DW11
Hypopharynx D913
Ileum DD14
Jejunum DD13
Kidney DT10
Larynx D91B
Liver DF10
Lung DB12
Lymphatics
Abdomen D716
Axillary D714
Inguinal D718

Brachytherapy (*continued*)
Lymphatics (*continued*)
Neck D713
Pelvis D717
Thorax D715
Mediastinum DB16
Mouth D914
Nasopharynx D91D
Neck and Head DW11
Nerve, Peripheral D017
Nose D911
Oropharynx D91F
Ovary DU10
Palate
Hard D918
Soft D919
Pancreas DF13
Parathyroid Gland DG14
Pelvic Region DW16
Pineal Body DG11
Pituitary Gland DG10
Pleura DB15
Prostate DV10
Rectum DD17
Respiratory Tract DW1Q
Sinuses D917
Spinal Cord D016
Spleen D712
Stomach DD11
Testis DV11
Thymus D711
Thyroid Gland DG15
Tongue D915
Trachea DB10
Ureter DT11
Urethra DT13
Uterus DU12
Brachytherapy, CivaSheet®
see Brachytherapy with qualifier
Unidirectional Source
see Insertion with device
Radioactive Element
Brachytherapy seeds
use Radioactive Element
Breast procedures, skin only
use Skin, Chest
Brexanolone XW0
Brexucabtagene Autoleucel
use Brexucabtagene Autoleucel
Immunotherapy
**Brexucabtagene Autoleucel
Immunotherapy** XW0
Broad ligament
use Uterine Supporting Structure
**Bromelain-enriched Proteolytic
Enzyme** XW0
Bronchial artery
use Upper Artery
Bronchography
see Fluoroscopy, Respiratory
System BB1
see Plain Radiography, Respiratory
System BB0
Bronchoplasty
see Repair, Respiratory System 0BQ
see Supplement, Respiratory System
0BU
Bronchorrhaphy
see Repair, Respiratory System 0BQ
Bronchoscopy 0BJ08ZZ
Bronchotomy
see Drainage, Respiratory System
0B9
Bronchus Intermedius
use Main Bronchus, Right
BRYAN® Cervical Disc System
use Synthetic Substitute
Buccal gland
use Buccal Mucosa
Buccinator lymph node
use Lymphatic, Head

Buccinator muscle
use Muscle, Facial
Buckling, scleral with implant
see Supplement, Eye 08U
Bulbospongiosus muscle
use Muscle, Perineum
Bulbourethral (Cowper's) gland
use Urethra
Bundle of His
use Conduction Mechanism
Bundle of Kent
use Conduction Mechanism
Bunionectomy
see Excision, Lower Bones 0QB
Bursectomy
see Excision, Bursae and
Ligaments 0MB
see Resection, Bursae and
Ligaments 0MT
Bursocentesis
see Drainage, Bursae and Ligaments
0M9
Bursography
see Plain Radiography, Non-Axial
Upper Bones BP0
see Plain Radiography, Non-Axial
Lower Bones BQ0
Bursotomy
see Division, Bursae and Ligaments
0M8
see Drainage, Bursae and Ligaments
0M9
BVS 5000 Ventricular Assist Device
use Short-term External Heart
Assist System in Heart and Great
Vessels
Bypass
Anterior Chamber
Left 08133
Right 08123
Aorta
Abdominal 0410
Thoracic
Ascending/Arch 021X
Descending 021W
Artery
Anterior Tibial
Left 041Q
Right 041P
Axillary
Left 03160
Right 03150
Brachial
Left 0318
Right 0317
Common Carotid
Left 031J0
Right 031H0
Common Iliac
Left 041D
Right 041C
Coronary
Four or More Arteries
0213
One Artery 0210
Three Arteries 0212
Two Arteries 0211
External Carotid
Left 031N0
Right 031M0
External Iliac
Left 041J
Right 041H
Femoral
Left 041L
Right 041K
Foot
Left 041W
Right 041V
Hepatic 0413
Innominate 03120

Bypass *(continued)*
  Artery *(continued)*
    Internal Carotid
      Left 031L0
      Right 031K0
    Internal Iliac
      Left 041F
      Right 041E
    Intracranial 031G0
    Peroneal
      Left 041U
      Right 041T
    Popliteal
      Left 041N
      Right 041M
    Posterior Tibial
      Left 041S
      Right 041R
    Pulmonary
      Left 021R
      Right 021Q
    Pulmonary Trunk 021P
    Radial
      Left 031C
      Right 031B
    Splenic 0414
    Subclavian
      Left 03140
      Right 03130
    Temporal
      Left 031T0
      Right 031S0
    Ulnar
      Left 031A
      Right 0319
  Atrium
    Left 0217
    Right 0216
  Bladder 0T1B
  Cavity, Cranial 0W110J
  Cecum 0D1H
  Cerebral Ventricle 0016
  Colon
    Ascending 0D1K
    Descending 0D1M
    Sigmoid 0D1N
    Transverse 0D1L
  Duct
    Common Bile 0F19
    Cystic 0F18
    Hepatic
      Common 0F17
      Left 0F16
      Right 0F15
    Lacrimal
      Left 081Y
      Right 081X
    Pancreatic 0F1D
      Accessory 0F1F
  Duodenum 0D19
  Ear
    Left 091E0
    Right 091D0
  Esophagus 0D15
    Lower 0D13
    Middle 0D12
    Upper 0D11
  Fallopian Tube
    Left 0U16
    Right 0U15
  Gallbladder 0F14
  Ileum 0D1B
  Intestine
    Large 0D1E
    Small 0D18
  Jejunum 0D1A
  Kidney Pelvis
    Left 0T14
    Right 0T13
  Pancreas 0F1G

Bypass *(continued)*
  Pelvic Cavity 0W1J
  Peritoneal Cavity 0W1G
  Pleural Cavity
    Left 0W1B
    Right 0W19
  Spinal Canal 001U
  Stomach 0D16
  Trachea 0B11
  Ureter
    Left 0T17
    Right 0T16
  Ureters, Bilateral 0T18
  Vas Deferens
    Bilateral 0V1Q
    Left 0V1P
    Right 0V1N
  Vein
    Axillary
      Left 0518
      Right 0517
    Azygos 0510
    Basilic
      Left 051C
      Right 051B
    Brachial
      Left 051A
      Right 0519
    Cephalic
      Left 051F
      Right 051D
    Colic 0617
    Common Iliac
      Left 061D
      Right 061C
    Esophageal 0613
    External Iliac
      Left 061G
      Right 061F
    External Jugular
      Left 051Q
      Right 051P
    Face
      Left 051V
      Right 051T
    Femoral
      Left 061N
      Right 061M
    Foot
      Left 061V
      Right 061T
    Gastric 0612
    Hand
      Left 051H
      Right 051G
    Hemiazygos 0511
    Hepatic 0614
    Hypogastric
      Left 061J
      Right 061H
    Inferior Mesenteric 0616
    Innominate
      Left 0514
      Right 0513
    Internal Jugular
      Left 051N
      Right 051M
    Intracranial 051L
    Portal 0618
    Renal
      Left 061B
      Right 0619
    Saphenous
      Left 061Q
      Right 061P
    Splenic 0611
    Subclavian
      Left 0516
      Right 0515
    Superior Mesenteric 0615

Bypass *(continued)*
  Vein *(continued)*
    Vertebral
      Left 051S
      Right 051R
    Vena Cava
      Inferior 0610
      Superior 021V
    Ventricle
      Left 021L
      Right 021K
Bypass, cardiopulmonary 5A1221Z

C

Caesarean section
  see Extraction, Products of Conception 10D0
Calcaneocuboid joint
  use Joint, Tarsal, Left
  use Joint, Tarsal, Right
Calcaneocuboid ligament
  use Bursa and Ligament, Foot, Left
  use Bursa and Ligament, Foot, Right
Calcaneofibular ligament
  use Bursa and Ligament, Ankle, Left
  use Bursa and Ligament, Ankle, Right
Calcaneus
  use Tarsal, Left
  use Tarsal, Right
Cannulation
  see Bypass
  see Dilation
  see Drainage
  see Irrigation
Canthorrhaphy
  see Repair, Eye 08Q
Canthotomy
  see Release, Eye 08N
Capitate bone
  use Carpal, Left
  use Carpal, Right
Caplacizumab XW0
Capsulectomy, lens
  see Excision, Eye 08B
Capsulorrhaphy, joint
  see Repair, Lower Joints 0SQ
  see Repair, Upper Joints 0RQ
Caption Guidance system X2JAX47
Cardia
  use Esophagogastric Junction
Cardiac contractility modulation lead
  use Cardiac Lead in Heart and Great Vessels
Cardiac event recorder
  use Monitoring Device
Cardiac Lead
  Defibrillator
    Atrium
      Left 02H7
      Right 02H6
    Pericardium 02HN
    Vein, Coronary 02H4
    Ventricle
      Left 02HL
      Right 02HK
  Insertion of device in
    Atrium
      Left 02H7Z
      Right 02H6
    Pericardium 02HN
    Vein, Coronary 02H4
    Ventricle
      Left 02HL
      Right 02HK

Cardiac Lead *(continued)*
  Pacemaker
    Atrium
      Left 02H7
      Right 02H6
    Pericardium 02HN
    Vein, Coronary 02H4
    Ventricle
      Left 02HL
      Right 02HK
  Removal of device from, Heart 02PA
  Revision of device in, Heart 02WA
Cardiac plexus
  use Nerve, Thoracic Sympathetic
Cardiac Resynchronization Defibrillator Pulse Generator
  Abdomen 0JH8
  Chest 0JH6
Cardiac Resynchronization Pacemaker Pulse Generator
  Abdomen 0JH8
  Chest 0JH6
Cardiac resynchronization therapy (CRT) lead
  use Cardiac Lead, Defibrillator in 02H
  use Cardiac Lead, Pacemaker in 02H
Cardiac Rhythm Related Device
  Insertion of device in
    Abdomen 0JH8
    Chest 0JH6
  Removal of device from, Subcutaneous Tissue and Fascia, Trunk 0JPT
  Revision of device in, Subcutaneous Tissue and Fascia, Trunk 0JWT
Cardiocentesis
  see Drainage, Pericardial Cavity 0W9D
Cardioesophageal junction
  use Esophagogastric Junction
Cardiolysis
  see Release, Heart and Great Vessels 02N
CardioMEMS® pressure sensor
  use Monitoring Device, Pressure Sensor in 02H
Cardiomyotomy
  see Division, Esophagogastric Junction 0D84
Cardioplegia
  see Introduction of substance in or on, Heart 3E08
Cardiorrhaphy
  see Repair, Heart and Great Vessels 02Q
Cardioversion 5A2204Z
Caregiver training F0FZ
Carmat total artificial heart (TAH)
  use Biologic with Synthetic Substitute, Autoregulated Electrohydraulic in 02R
Caroticotympanic artery
  use Artery, Internal Carotid, Left
  use Artery, Internal Carotid, Right
Carotid (artery) sinus (baroreceptor) lead
  use Stimulator Lead in Upper Arteries
Carotid glomus
  use Carotid Bodies, Bilateral
  use Carotid Body, Left
  use Carotid Body, Right
Carotid sinus
  use Artery, Internal Carotid, Left
  use Artery, Internal Carotid, Right

Carotid sinus nerve
 use Nerve, Glossopharyngeal
Carotid WALLSTENT® Monorail® Endoprosthesis
 use Intraluminal Device
Carpectomy
 see Excision, Upper Bones 0PB
 see Resection, Upper Bones 0PT
Carpometacarpal ligament
 use Bursa and Ligament, Hand, Left
 use Bursa and Ligament, Hand, Right
Casirivimab (REGN10933) and Imdevimab (REGN10987)
 use REGN-COV2 Monoclonal Antibody
Casting
 see Immobilization
CAT scan
 see Computerized Tomography (CT Scan)
Catheterization
 see Dilation
 see Drainage
 Heart
  see Measurement, Cardiac 4A02
 see Irrigation
 see Insertion of device in
 Umbilical vein, for infusion 06H033T
Cauda equina
 use Spinal Cord, Lumbar
Cauterization
 see Destruction
 see Repair
Cavernous plexus
 use Nerve, Head and Neck Sympathetic
CBMA (Concentrated Bone Marrow Aspirate)
 use Concentrated Bone Marrow Aspirate
CBMA (Concentrated Bone Marrow Aspirate) injection, intramuscular XK02303
Cecectomy
 see Excision, Cecum 0DBH
 see Resection, Cecum 0DTH
Cecocolostomy
 see Bypass, Gastrointestinal System 0D1
 see Drainage, Gastrointestinal System 0D9
Cecopexy
 see Repair, Cecum 0DQH
 see Reposition, Cecum 0DSH
Cecoplication
 see Restriction, Cecum 0DVH
Cecorrhaphy
 see Repair, Cecum 0DQH
Cecostomy
 see Bypass, Cecum 0D1H
 see Drainage, Cecum 0D9H
Cecotomy
 see Drainage, Cecum 0D9H
Cefiderocol Anti-Infective XW0
Ceftazidime-avibactam
 use Other Anti-infective
Ceftolozane/Tazobactam Anti-Infective XW0
Celiac (solar) plexus
 use Nerve, Abdominal Sympathetic
Celiac ganglion
 use Nerve, Abdominal Sympathetic
Celiac lymph node
 use Lymphatic, Aortic
Celiac trunk
 use Artery, Celiac
Central axillary lymph node
 use Lymphatic, Axillary, Left
 use Lymphatic, Axillary, Right

Central venous pressure
 see Measurement, Venous 4A04
Centrimag® Blood Pump
 use Short-term External Heart Assist System in Heart and Great Vessels
Cephalogram BN00ZZZ
CERAMENT® G
 use Antibiotic-eluting Bone Void Filler
Ceramic on ceramic bearing surface
 use Synthetic Substitute, Ceramic in 0SR
Cerclage
 see Restriction
Cerebral aqueduct (Sylvius)
 use Cerebral Ventricle
Cerebral Embolic Filtration
 Dual Filter X2A5312
 Extracorporeal Flow Reversal Circuit X2A
 Single Deflection Filter X2A6325
Cerebrum
 use Brain
Cervical esophagus
 use Esophagus, Upper
Cervical facet joint
 use Joint, Cervical Vertebral
 use Joint, Cervical Vertebral, 2 or more
Cervical ganglion
 use Nerve, Head and Neck Sympathetic
Cervical interspinous ligament
 use Bursa and Ligament, Head and Neck
Cervical intertransverse ligament
 use Bursa and Ligament, Head and Neck
Cervical ligamentum flavum
 use Bursa and Ligament, Head and Neck
Cervical lymph node
 use Lymphatic, Neck, Left
 use Lymphatic, Neck, Right
Cervicectomy
 see Excision, Cervix 0UBC
 see Resection, Cervix 0UTC
Cervicothoracic facet joint
 use Joint, Cervicothoracic Vertebral
Cesarean section
 see Extraction, Products of Conception 10D0
Cesium-131 Collagen Implant
 use Radioactive Element, Cesium-131 Collagen Implant in 00H
Change device in
 Abdominal Wall 0W2FX
 Back
  Lower 0W2LX
  Upper 0W2KX
 Bladder 0T2BX
 Bone
  Facial 0N2WX
  Lower 0Q2YX
  Nasal 0N2BX
  Upper 0P2YX
 Bone Marrow 072TX
 Brain 0020X
 Breast
  Left 0H2UX
  Right 0H2TX
 Bursa and Ligament
  Lower 0M2YX
  Upper 0M2XX
 Cavity, Cranial 0W21X
 Chest Wall 0W28X
 Cisterna Chyli 072LX
 Diaphragm 0B2TX
 Duct
  Hepatobiliary 0F2BX
  Pancreatic 0F2DX

Change device in *(continued)*
 Ear
  Left 092JX
  Right 092HX
 Epididymis and Spermatic Cord 0V2MX
 Extremity
  Lower
   Left 0Y2BX
   Right 0Y29X
  Upper
   Left 0X27X
   Right 0X26X
 Eye
  Left 0821X
  Right 0820X
 Face 0W22X
 Fallopian Tube 0U28X
 Gallbladder 0F24X
 Gland
  Adrenal 0G25X
  Endocrine 0G2SX
  Pituitary 0G20X
  Salivary 0C2AX
 Head 0W20X
 Intestinal Tract
  Lower 0D2DXUZ
  Upper 0D20XUZ
 Jaw
  Lower 0W25X
  Upper 0W24X
 Joint
  Lower 0S2YX
  Upper 0R2YX
 Kidney 0T25X
 Larynx 0C2SX
 Liver 0F20X
 Lung
  Left 0B2LX
  Right 0B2KX
 Lymphatic 072NX
  Thoracic Duct 072KX
 Mediastinum 0W2CX
 Mesentery 0D2VX
 Mouth and Throat 0C2YX
 Muscle
  Lower 0K2YX
  Upper 0K2XX
 Nasal Mucosa and Soft Tissue 092KX
 Neck 0W26X
 Nerve
  Cranial 002EX
  Peripheral 012YX
 Omentum 0D2UX
 Ovary 0U23X
 Pancreas 0F2GX
 Parathyroid Gland 0G2RX
 Pelvic Cavity 0W2JX
 Penis 0V2SX
 Pericardial Cavity 0W2DX
 Perineum
  Female 0W2NX
  Male 0W2MX
 Peritoneal Cavity 0W2GX
 Peritoneum 0D2WX
 Pineal Body 0G21X
 Pleura 0B2QX
 Pleural Cavity
  Left 0W2BX
  Right 0W29X
 Products of Conception 10207
 Prostate and Seminal Vesicles 0V24X
 Retroperitoneum 0W2HX
 Scrotum and Tunica Vaginalis 0V28X
 Sinus 092QX
 Skin 0H2PX
 Skull 0N20X
 Spinal Canal 002UX
 Spleen 072PX

Change device in *(continued)*
 Subcutaneous Tissue and Fascia
  Head and Neck 0J2SX
  Lower Extremity 0J2WX
  Trunk 0J2TX
  Upper Extremity 0J2VX
 Tendon
  Lower 0L2YX
  Upper 0L2XX
 Testis 0V2DX
 Thymus 072MX
 Thyroid Gland 0G2KX
 Trachea 0B21
 Tracheobronchial Tree 0B20X
 Ureter 0T29X
 Urethra 0T2DX
 Uterus and Cervix 0U2DXHZ
 Vagina and Cul-de-sac 0U2HXGZ
 Vas Deferens 0V2RX
 Vulva 0U2MX
Change device in or on
 Abdominal Wall 2W03X
 Anorectal 2Y03X5Z
 Arm
  Lower
   Left 2W0DX
   Right 2W0CX
  Upper
   Left 2W0BX
   Right 2W0AX
 Back 2W05X
 Chest Wall 2W04X
 Ear 2Y02X5Z
 Extremity
  Lower
   Left 2W0MX
   Right 2W0LX
  Upper
   Left 2W09X
   Right 2W08X
 Face 2W01X
 Finger
  Left 2W0KX
  Right 2W0JX
 Foot
  Left 2W0TX
  Right 2W0SX
 Genital Tract, Female 2Y04X5Z
 Hand
  Left 2W0FX
  Right 2W0EX
 Head 2W00X
 Inguinal Region
  Left 2W07X
  Right 2W06X
 Leg
  Lower
   Left 2W0RX
   Right 2W0QX
  Upper
   Left 2W0PX
   Right 2W0NX
 Mouth and Pharynx 2Y00X5Z
 Nasal 2Y01X5Z
 Neck 2W02X
 Thumb
  Left 2W0HX
  Right 2W0GX
 Toe
  Left 2W0VX
  Right 2W0UX
 Urethra 2Y05X5Z
Chemoembolization
 see Introduction of substance in or on
Chemosurgery, Skin 3E00XTZ
Chemothalamectomy
 see Destruction, Thalamus 0059
Chemotherapy, Infusion for cancer
 see Introduction of substance in or on

Chest compression (CPR), external
 Manual 5A12012
 Mechanical 5A1221J
Chest x-ray
 see Plain Radiography, Chest BW03
Chiropractic Manipulation
 Abdomen 9WB9X
 Cervical 9WB1X
 Extremities
  Lower 9WB6X
  Upper 9WB7X
 Head 9WB0X
 Lumbar 9WB3X
 Pelvis 9WB5X
 Rib Cage 9WB8X
 Sacrum 9WB4X
 Thoracic 9WB2X
Choana
 use Nasopharynx
Cholangiogram
 see Plain Radiography, Hepatobiliary System and Pancreas BF0
 see Fluoroscopy, Hepatobiliary System and Pancreas BF1
Cholecystectomy
 see Excision, Gallbladder 0FB4
 see Resection, Gallbladder 0FT4
Cholecystojejunostomy
 see Bypass, Hepatobiliary System and Pancreas 0F1
 see Drainage, Hepatobiliary System and Pancreas 0F9
Cholecystopexy
 see Repair, Gallbladder 0FQ4
 see Reposition, Gallbladder 0FS4
Cholecystoscopy 0FJ44ZZ
Cholecystostomy
 see Drainage, Gallbladder 0F94
 see Bypass, Gallbladder 0F14
Cholecystotomy
 see Drainage, Gallbladder 0F94
Choledochectomy
 see Excision, Hepatobiliary System and Pancreas 0FB
 see Resection, Hepatobiliary System and Pancreas 0FT
Choledocholithotomy
 see Extirpation, Duct, Common Bile 0FC9
Choledochoplasty
 see Repair, Hepatobiliary System and Pancreas 0FQ
 see Replacement, Hepatobiliary System and Pancreas 0FR
 see Supplement, Hepatobiliary System and Pancreas 0FU
Choledochoscopy 0FJB8ZZ
Choledochotomy
 see Drainage, Hepatobiliary System and Pancreas 0F9
Cholelithotomy
 see Extirpation, Hepatobiliary System and Pancreas 0FC
Chondrectomy
 see Excision, Lower Joints 0SB
 see Excision, Upper Joints 0RB
 Knee
  see Excision, Lower Joints 0SB
 Semilunar cartilage
  see Excision, Lower Joints 0SB
Chondroglossus muscle
 use Muscle, Tongue, Palate, Pharynx
Chorda tympani
 use Nerve, Facial
Chordotomy
 see Division, Central Nervous System and Cranial Nerves 008

Choroid plexus
 use Cerebral Ventricle
Choroidectomy
 see Excision, Eye 08B
 see Resection, Eye 08T
Ciliary body
 use Eye, Left
 use Eye, Right
Ciliary ganglion
 use Nerve, Head and Neck Sympathetic
cilta-cel *use* Ciltacabtagene Autoleucel
Ciltacabtagene Autoleucel XW0
Circle of Willis
 use Artery, Intracranial
Circumcision 0VTTXZZ
Circumflex iliac artery
 use Artery, Femoral, Left
 use Artery, Femoral, Right
CivaSheet®
 use Radioactive Element
CivaSheet® Brachytherapy
 see Brachytherapy with qualifier Unidirectional Source
 see Insertion with device Radioactive Element
Clamp and rod internal fixation system (CRIF)
 use Internal Fixation Device in Lower Bones
 use Internal Fixation Device in Upper Bones
Clamping
 see Occlusion
Claustrum
 use Basal Ganglia
Claviculectomy
 see Excision, Upper Bones 0PB
 see Resection, Upper Bones 0PT
Claviculotomy
 see Division, Upper Bones 0P8
 see Drainage, Upper Bones 0P9
Clipping, aneurysm
 see Occlusion using Extraluminal Device
 see Restriction using Extraluminal Device
Clitorectomy, clitoridectomy
 see Excision, Clitoris 0UBJ
 see Resection, Clitoris 0UTJ
Clolar
 use Clofarabine
Closure
 see Occlusion
 see Repair
Clysis
 see Introduction of substance in or on
Coagulation
 see Destruction
Coagulation Factor Xa, Inactivated XW0
Coagulation Factor Xa, (Recombinant) Inactivated
 use Coagulation Factor Xa, Inactivated
COALESCE® radiolucent interbody fusion device
 use Interbody Fusion Device, Radiolucent Porous in New Technology
CoAxia NeuroFlo catheter
 use Intraluminal Device
Cobalt/chromium head and polyethylene socket
 use Synthetic Substitute, Metal on Polyethylene in 0SR
Cobalt/chromium head and socket
 use Synthetic Substitute, Metal in 0SR

Coccygeal body
 use Coccygeal Glomus
Coccygeus muscle
 use Muscle, Trunk, Left
 use Muscle, Trunk, Right
Cochlea
 use Ear, Inner, Left
 use Ear, Inner, Right
Cochlear implant (CI), multiple channel (electrode)
 use Hearing Device, Multiple Channel Cochlear Prosthesis in 09H
Cochlear implant (CI), single channel (electrode)
 use Hearing Device, Single Channel Cochlear Prosthesis in 09H
Cochlear Implant Treatment F0BZ0
Cochlear nerve
 use Nerve, Acoustic
COGNIS® CRT-D
 use Cardiac Resynchronization Defibrillator Pulse Generator in 0JH
COHERE® radiolucent interbody fusion device
 use Interbody Fusion Device, Radiolucent Porous in New Technology
Colectomy
 see Excision, Gastrointestinal System 0DB
 see Resection, Gastrointestinal System 0DT
Collapse
 see Occlusion
Collection from
 Breast, Breast Milk 8E0HX62
 Indwelling Device
  Circulatory System
   Blood 8C02X6K
   Other Fluid 8C02X6L
  Nervous System
   Cerebrospinal Fluid 8C01X6J
   Other Fluid 8C01X6L
 Integumentary System, Breast Milk 8E0HX62
 Reproductive System, Male, Sperm 8E0VX63
Colocentesis
 see Drainage, Gastrointestinal System 0D9
Colofixation
 see Repair, Gastrointestinal System 0DQ
 see Reposition, Gastrointestinal System 0DS
Cololysis
 see Release, Gastrointestinal System 0DN
Colonic Z-Stent®
 use Intraluminal Device
Colonoscopy 0DJD8ZZ
Colopexy
 see Repair, Gastrointestinal System 0DQ
 see Reposition, Gastrointestinal System 0DS
Coloplication
 see Restriction, Gastrointestinal System 0DV
Coloproctectomy
 see Excision, Gastrointestinal System 0DB
 see Resection, Gastrointestinal System 0DT
Coloproctostomy
 see Bypass, Gastrointestinal System 0D1
 see Drainage, Gastrointestinal System 0D9

Colopuncture
 see Drainage, Gastrointestinal System 0D9
Colorrhaphy
 see Repair, Gastrointestinal System 0DQ
Colostomy
 see Bypass, Gastrointestinal System 0D1
 see Drainage, Gastrointestinal System 0D9
Colpectomy
 see Excision, Vagina 0UBG
 see Resection, Vagina 0UTG
Colpocentesis
 see Drainage, Vagina 0U9G
Colpopexy
 see Repair, Vagina 0UQG
 see Reposition, Vagina 0USG
Colpoplasty
 see Repair, Vagina 0UQG
 see Supplement, Vagina 0UUG
Colporrhaphy
 see Repair, Vagina 0UQG
Colposcopy 0UJH8ZZ
Columella
 use Nasal Mucosa and Soft Tissue
Common digital vein
 use Vein, Foot, Left
 use Vein, Foot, Right
Common facial vein
 use Vein, Face, Left
 use Vein, Face, Right
Common fibular nerve
 use Nerve, Peroneal
Common hepatic artery
 use Artery, Hepatic
Common iliac (subaortic) lymph node
 use Lymphatic, Pelvis
Common interosseous artery
 use Artery, Ulnar, Left
 use Artery, Ulnar, Right
Common peroneal nerve
 use Nerve, Peroneal
Complete (SE) stent
 use Intraluminal Device
Compression
 see Restriction
 Abdominal Wall 2W13X
 Arm
  Lower
   Left 2W1DX
   Right 2W1CX
  Upper
   Left 2W1BX
   Right 2W1AX
 Back 2W15X
 Chest Wall 2W14X
 Extremity
  Lower
   Left 2W1MX
   Right 2W1LX
  Upper
   Left 2W19X
   Right 2W18X
 Face 2W11X
 Finger
  Left 2W1KX
  Right 2W1JX
 Foot
  Left 2W1TX
  Right 2W1SX
 Hand
  Left 2W1FX
  Right 2W1EX
 Head 2W10X
 Inguinal Region
  Left 2W17X
  Right 2W16X

Compression *(continued)*
  Leg
    Lower
      Left 2W1RX
      Right 2W1QX
    Upper
      Left 2W1PX
      Right 2W1NX
  Neck 2W12X
  Thumb
    Left 2W1HX
    Right 2W1GX
  Toe
    Left 2W1VX
    Right 2W1UX
Computer-aided Assessment, Intracranial Vascular Activity XXE0X07
Computer-aided Guidance, Transthoracic Echocardiography X2JAX47
Computer-aided Mechanical Aspiration X2C
Computer-aided Triage and Notification, Pulmonary Artery Flow XXE3X27
Computer-assisted Intermittent Aspiration
  see New Technology, Cardiovascular System X2C
Computer Assisted Procedure
  Extremity
    Lower
      No Qualifier 8E0YXBZ
      With Computerized Tomography 8E0YXBG
      With Fluoroscopy 8E0YXBF
      With Magnetic Resonance Imaging 8E0YXBH
    Upper
      No Qualifier 8E0XXBZ
      With Computerized Tomography 8E0XXBG
      With Fluoroscopy 8E0XXBF
      With Magnetic Resonance Imaging 8E0XXBH
  Head and Neck Region
    No Qualifier 8E09XBZ
    With Computerized Tomography 8E09XBG
    With Fluoroscopy 8E09XBF
    With Magnetic Resonance Imaging 8E09XBH
  Trunk Region
    No Qualifier 8E0WXBZ
    With Computerized Tomography 8E0WXBG
    With Fluoroscopy 8E0WXBF
    With Magnetic Resonance Imaging 8E0WXBH
Computerized Tomography (CT Scan)
  Abdomen BW20
    Chest and Pelvis BW25
  Abdomen and Chest BW24
  Abdomen and Pelvis BW21
  Airway, Trachea BB2F
  Ankle
    Left BQ2H
    Right BQ2G
  Aorta
    Abdominal B420
      Intravascular Optical Coherence B420Z2Z
    Thoracic B320
      Intravascular Optical Coherence B320Z2Z
  Arm
    Left BP2F
    Right BP2E

Computerized Tomography (CT Scan) *(continued)*
  Artery
    Celiac B421
      Intravascular Optical Coherence B421Z2Z
    Common Carotid
      Bilateral B325
      Intravascular Optical Coherence B325Z2Z
    Coronary
      Bypass Graft
        Multiple B223
          Intravascular Optical Coherence B223Z2Z
        Multiple B221
          Intravascular Optical Coherence B221Z2Z
      Internal Carotid
        Bilateral B328
          Intravascular Optical Coherence B328Z2Z
      Intracranial B32R
        Intravascular Optical Coherence B32RZ2Z
      Lower Extremity
        Bilateral B42H
          Intravascular Optical Coherence B42HZ2Z
        Left B42G
          Intravascular Optical Coherence B42GZ2Z
        Right B42F
          Intravascular Optical Coherence B42FZ2Z
      Pelvic B42C
        Intravascular Optical Coherence B42CZ2Z
      Pulmonary
        Left B32T
          Intravascular Optical Coherence B32TZ2Z
        Right B32S
          Intravascular Optical Coherence B32SZ2Z
      Renal
        Bilateral B428
          Intravascular Optical Coherence B428Z2Z
        Transplant B42M
          Intravascular Optical Coherence B42MZ2Z
      Superior Mesenteric B424
        Intravascular Optical Coherence B424Z2Z
      Vertebral
        Bilateral B32G
          Intravascular Optical Coherence B32GZ2Z
  Bladder BT20
  Bone
    Facial BN25
    Temporal BN2F
  Brain B020
  Calcaneus
    Left BQ2K
    Right BQ2J
  Cerebral Ventricle B028
  Chest, Abdomen and Pelvis BW25
  Chest and Abdomen BW24
  Cisterna B027
  Clavicle
    Left BP25
    Right BP24
  Coccyx BR2F
  Colon BD24
  Ear B920
  Elbow
    Left BP2H
    Right BP2G

Computerized Tomography (CT Scan) *(continued)*
  Extremity
    Lower
      Left BQ2S
      Right BQ2R
    Upper
      Bilateral BP2V
      Left BP2U
      Right BP2T
  Eye
    Bilateral B827
    Left B826
    Right B825
  Femur
    Left BQ24
    Right BQ23
  Fibula
    Left BQ2C
    Right BQ2B
  Finger
    Left BP2S
    Right BP2R
  Foot
    Left BQ2M
    Right BQ2L
  Forearm
    Left BP2K
    Right BP2J
  Gland
    Adrenal, Bilateral BG22
    Parathyroid BG23
    Parotid, Bilateral B926
    Salivary, Bilateral B92D
    Submandibular, Bilateral B929
    Thyroid BG24
  Hand
    Left BP2P
    Right BP2N
  Hands and Wrists, Bilateral BP2Q
  Head BW28
  Head and Neck BW29
  Heart
    Intravascular Optical Coherence B226Z2Z
    Right and Left B226
  Hepatobiliary System, All BF2C
  Hip
    Left BQ21
    Right BQ20
  Humerus
    Left BP2B
    Right BP2A
  Intracranial Sinus B522
    Intravascular Optical Coherence B522Z2Z
  Joint
    Acromioclavicular, Bilateral BP23
    Finger
      Left BP2DZZZ
      Right BP2CZZZ
    Foot
      Left BQ2Y
      Right BQ2X
    Hand
      Left BP2DZZZ
      Right BP2CZZZ
    Sacroiliac BR2D
    Sternoclavicular
      Bilateral BP22
      Left BP21
      Right BP20
    Temporomandibular, Bilateral BN29
    Toe
      Left BQ2Y
      Right BQ2X
  Kidney
    Bilateral BT23
    Left BT22

Computerized Tomography (CT Scan) *(continued)*
  Kidney *(continued)*
    Right BT21
    Transplant BT29
  Knee
    Left BQ28
    Right BQ27
  Larynx B92J
  Leg
    Left BQ2F
    Right BQ2D
  Liver BF25
  Liver and Spleen BF26
  Lung, Bilateral BB24
  Mandible BN26
  Nasopharynx B92F
  Neck BW2F
  Neck and Head BW29
  Orbit, Bilateral BN23
  Oropharynx B92F
  Pancreas BF27
  Patella
    Left BQ2W
    Right BQ2V
  Pelvic Region BW2G
  Pelvis BR2C
    Chest and Abdomen BW25
  Pelvis and Abdomen BW21
  Pituitary Gland B029
  Prostate BV23
  Ribs
    Left BP2Y
    Right BP2X
  Sacrum BR2F
  Scapula
    Left BP27
    Right BP26
  Sella Turcica B029
  Shoulder
    Left BP29
    Right BP28
  Sinus
    Intracranial B522
      Intravascular Optical Coherence B522Z2Z
    Paranasal B922
  Skull BN20
  Spinal Cord B02B
  Spine
    Cervical BR20
    Lumbar BR29
    Thoracic BR27
  Spleen and Liver BF26
  Thorax BP2W
  Tibia
    Left BQ2C
    Right BQ2B
  Toe
    Left BQ2Q
    Right BQ2P
  Trachea BB2F
  Tracheobronchial Tree
    Bilateral BB29
    Left BB28
    Right BB27
  Vein
    Pelvic (Iliac)
      Left B52G
        Intravascular Optical Coherence B52GZ2Z
      Right B52F
        Intravascular Optical Coherence B52FZ2Z
    Pelvic (Iliac) Bilateral B52H
      Intravascular Optical Coherence B52HZ2Z
    Portal B52T
      Intravascular Optical Coherence B52TZ2Z

Computerized Tomography (CT Scan) *(continued)*
  Vein *(continued)*
    Pulmonary
      Bilateral B52S
        Intravascular Optical Coherence B52SZ2Z
      Left B52R
        Intravascular Optical Coherence B52RZ2Z
      Right B52Q
        Intravascular Optical Coherence B52QZ2Z
    Renal
      Bilateral B52L
        Intravascular Optical Coherence B52LZ2Z
      Left B52K
        Intravascular Optical Coherence B52KZ2Z
      Right B52J
        Intravascular Optical Coherence B52JZ2Z
    Spanchnic B52T
      Intravascular Optical Coherence B52TZ2Z
    Vena Cava
      Inferior B529
        Intravascular Optical Coherence B529Z2Z
      Superior B528
        Intravascular Optical Coherence B528Z2Z
    Ventricle, Cerebral B028
    Wrist
      Left BP2M
      Right BP2L

Concentrated Bone Marrow Aspirate (CBMA) injection, intramuscular XK02303

Concerto II CRT-D
  use Cardiac Resynchronization Defibrillator Pulse Generator in 0JH

Condylectomy
  see Excision, Head and Facial Bones 0NB
  see Excision, Lower Bones 0QB
  see Excision, Upper Bones 0PB

Condyloid process
  use Mandible, Left
  use Mandible, Right

Condylotomy
  see Division, Head and Facial Bones 0N8
  see Division, Lower Bones 0Q8
  see Division, Upper Bones 0P8
  see Drainage, Head and Facial Bones 0N9
  see Drainage, Lower Bones 0Q9
  see Drainage, Upper Bones 0P9

Condylysis
  see Release, Head and Facial Bones 0NN
  see Release, Lower Bones 0QN
  see Release, Upper Bones 0PN

Conization, cervix
  see Excision, Cervix 0UBC

Conjunctivoplasty
  see Repair, Eye 08Q
  see Replacement, Eye 08R

CONSERVE® PLUS Total Resurfacing Hip System
  use Resurfacing Device in Lower Joints

Construction
  Auricle, ear
    see Bypass, Urinary System 0T1
  Ileal conduit
    see Replacement, Ear, Nose, Sinus 09R

Consulta CRT-D
  use Cardiac Resynchronization Defibrillator Pulse Generator in 0JH

Consulta CRT-P
  use Cardiac Resynchronization Pacemaker Pulse Generator in 0JH

Contact Radiation
  Abdomen DWY37ZZ
  Adrenal Gland DGY27ZZ
  Bile Ducts DFY27ZZ
  Bladder DTY27ZZ
  Bone, Other DPYC7ZZ
  Brain D0Y07ZZ
  Brain Stem D0Y17ZZ
  Breast
    Left DMY07ZZ
    Right DMY17ZZ
  Bronchus DBY17ZZ
  Cervix DUY17ZZ
  Chest DWY27ZZ
  Chest Wall DBY77ZZ
  Colon DDY57ZZ
  Diaphragm DBY87ZZ
  Duodenum DDY27ZZ
  Ear D9Y07ZZ
  Esophagus DDY07ZZ
  Eye D8Y07ZZ
  Femur DPY97ZZ
  Fibula DPYB7ZZ
  Gallbladder DFY17ZZ
  Gland
    Adrenal DGY27ZZ
    Parathyroid DGY47ZZ
    Pituitary DGY07ZZ
    Thyroid DGY57ZZ
  Glands, Salivary D9Y67ZZ
  Head and Neck DWY17ZZ
  Hemibody DWY47ZZ
  Humerus DPY67ZZ
  Hypopharynx D9Y37ZZ
  Ileum DDY47ZZ
  Jejunum DDY37ZZ
  Kidney DTY07ZZ
  Larynx D9YB7ZZ
  Liver DFY07ZZ
  Lung DBY27ZZ
  Mandible DPY37ZZ
  Maxilla DPY27ZZ
  Mediastinum DBY67ZZ
  Mouth D9Y47ZZ
  Nasopharynx D9YD7ZZ
  Neck and Head DWY17ZZ
  Nerve, Peripheral D0Y77ZZ
  Nose D9Y17ZZ
  Oropharynx D9YF7ZZ
  Ovary DUY07ZZ
  Palate
    Hard D9Y87ZZ
    Soft D9Y97ZZ
  Pancreas DFY37ZZ
  Parathyroid Gland DGY47ZZ
  Pelvic Bones DPY87ZZ
  Pelvic Region DWY67ZZ
  Pineal Body DGY17ZZ
  Pituitary Gland DGY07ZZ
  Pleura DBY57ZZ
  Prostate DVY07ZZ
  Radius DPY77ZZ
  Rectum DDY77ZZ
  Rib DPY57ZZ
  Sinuses D9Y77ZZ
  Skin
    Abdomen DHY87ZZ
    Arm DHY47ZZ
    Back DHY77ZZ
    Buttock DHY97ZZ
    Chest DHY67ZZ
    Face DHY27ZZ

Contact Radiation *(continued)*
  Skin *(continued)*
    Leg DHYB7ZZ
    Neck DHY37ZZ
  Skull DPY07ZZ
  Spinal Cord D0Y67ZZ
  Sternum DPY47ZZ
  Stomach DDY17ZZ
  Testis DVY17ZZ
  Thyroid Gland DGY57ZZ
  Tibia DPYB7ZZ
  Tongue D9Y57ZZ
  Trachea DBY07ZZ
  Ulna DPY77ZZ
  Ureter DTY17ZZ
  Urethra DTY37ZZ
  Uterus DUY27ZZ
  Whole Body DWY57ZZ

ContaCT software *(Measurement of intracranial arterial flow)* 4A03X5D

CONTAK RENEWAL® 3 RF (HE) CRT-D
  use Cardiac Resynchronization Defibrillator Pulse Generator in 0JH

Contegra Pulmonary Valved Conduit
  use Zooplastic Tissue in Heart and Great Vessels

CONTEPO™
  use Fosfomycin Anti-infective

Continuous Glucose Monitoring (CGM) device
  use Monitoring Device

Continuous Negative Airway Pressure
  24-96 Consecutive Hours, Ventilation 5A09459
  Greater than 96 Consecutive Hours, Ventilation 5A09559
  Less than 24 Consecutive Hours, Ventilation 5A09359

Continuous Positive Airway Pressure
  24-96 Consecutive Hours, Ventilation 5A09457
  Greater than 96 Consecutive Hours, Ventilation 5A09557
  Less than 24 Consecutive Hours, Ventilation 5A09357

Continuous renal replacement therapy (CRRT) 5A1D90Z

Contraceptive Device
  Change device in, Uterus and Cervix 0U2DXHZ
  Insertion of device in
    Cervix 0UHC
    Subcutaneous Tissue and Fascia
      Abdomen 0JH8
      Chest 0JH6
      Lower Arm
        Left 0JHH
        Right 0JHG
      Lower Leg
        Left 0JHP
        Right 0JHN
      Upper Arm
        Left 0JHF
        Right 0JHD
      Upper Leg
        Left 0JHM
        Right 0JHL
    Uterus 0UH9
  Removal of device from
    Subcutaneous Tissue and Fascia
      Lower Extremity 0JPW
      Trunk 0JPT
      Upper Extremity 0JPV
    Uterus and Cervix 0UPD

Contraceptive Device *(continued)*
  Revision of device in
    Subcutaneous Tissue and Fascia
      Lower Extremity 0JWW
      Trunk 0JWT
      Upper Extremity 0JWV
    Uterus and Cervix 0UWD

Contractility Modulation Device
  Abdomen 0JH8
  Chest 0JH6

Control, Epistaxis
  see Control bleeding in, Nasal Mucosa and Soft Tissue 093K

Control bleeding in
  Abdominal Wall 0W3F
  Ankle Region
    Left 0Y3L
    Right 0Y3K
  Arm
    Lower
      Left 0X3F
      Right 0X3D
    Upper
      Left 0X39
      Right 0X38
  Axilla
    Left 0X35
    Right 0X34
  Back
    Lower 0W3L
    Upper 0W3K
  Buttock
    Left 0Y31
    Right 0Y30
  Cavity, Cranial 0W31
  Chest Wall 0W38
  Elbow Region
    Left 0X3C
    Right 0X3B
  Extremity
    Lower
      Left 0Y3B
      Right 0Y39
    Upper
      Left 0X37
      Right 0X36
  Face 0W32
  Femoral Region
    Left 0Y38
    Right 0Y37
  Foot
    Left 0Y3N
    Right 0Y3M
  Gastrointestinal Tract 0W3P
  Genitourinary Tract 0W3R
  Hand
    Left 0X3K
    Right 0X3J
  Head 0W30
  Inguinal Region
    Left 0Y36
    Right 0Y35
  Jaw
    Lower 0W35
    Upper 0W34
  Knee Region
    Left 0Y3G
    Right 0Y3F
  Leg
    Lower
      Left 0Y3J
      Right 0Y3H
    Upper
      Left 0Y3D
      Right 0Y3C
  Mediastinum 0W3C
  Nasal Mucosa and Soft Tissue 093K
  Neck 0W36
  Oral Cavity and Throat 0W33
  Pelvic Cavity 0W3J

Control bleeding in (continued)
  Pericardial Cavity 0W3D
  Perineum
    Female 0W3N
    Male 0W3M
  Peritoneal Cavity 0W3G
  Pleural Cavity
    Left 0W3B
    Right 0W39
  Respiratory Tract 0W3Q
  Retroperitoneum 0W3H
  Shoulder Region
    Left 0X33
    Right 0X32
  Wrist Region
    Left 0X3H
    Right 0X3G
Control bleeding using Tourniquet, External *see* Compression, Anatomical Regions 2W1
Conus arteriosus
  use Ventricle, Right
Conus medullaris
  use Spinal Cord, Lumbar
Convalescent Plasma (Nonautologous) *see* New Technology, Anatomical Regions XW1
Conversion
  Cardiac rhythm 5A2204Z
  Gastrostomy to jejunostomy feeding device
    see Insertion of device in, Jejunum 0DHA
Cook Biodesign® Fistula Plug(s)
  use Nonautologous Tissue Substitute
Cook Biodesign® Hernia Graft(s)
  use Nonautologous Tissue Substitute
Cook Biodesign® Layered Graft(s)
  use Nonautologous Tissue Substitute
Cook Zenapro™ Layered Graft(s)
  use Nonautologous Tissue Substitute
Cook Zenith AAA Endovascular Graft
  use Intraluminal Device
Cook Zenith® Fenestrated AAA Endovascular Graft
  use Intraluminal Device, Branched or Fenestrated, One or Two Arteries in 04V
  use Intraluminal Device, Branched or Fenestrated, Three or More Arteries in 04V
Coracoacromial ligament
  use Bursa and Ligament, Shoulder, Left
  use Bursa and Ligament, Shoulder, Right
Coracobrachialis muscle
  use Muscle, Upper Arm, Left
  use Muscle, Upper Arm, Right
Coracoclavicular ligament
  use Bursa and Ligament, Shoulder, Left
  use Bursa and Ligament, Shoulder, Right
Coracohumeral ligament
  use Bursa and Ligament, Shoulder, Left
  use Bursa and Ligament, Shoulder, Right
Coracoid process
  use Scapula, Left
  use Scapula, Right
Cordotomy
  see Division, Central Nervous System and Cranial Nerves 008

Core needle biopsy
  see Excision with qualifier Diagnostic
CoreValve transcatheter aortic valve
  use Zooplastic Tissue in Heart and Great Vessels
Cormet Hip Resurfacing System
  use Resurfacing Device in Lower Joints
Corniculate cartilage
  use Larynx
CoRoent® XL
  use Interbody Fusion Device in Lower Joints
Coronary arteriography
  see Fluoroscopy, Heart B21
  see Plain Radiography, Heart B20
Corox (OTW) Bipolar Lead
  use Cardiac Lead, Defibrillator in 02H
  use Cardiac Lead, Pacemaker in 02H
Corpus callosum
  use Brain
Corpus cavernosum
  use Penis
Corpus spongiosum
  use Penis
Corpus striatum
  use Basal Ganglia
Corrugator supercilii muscle
  use Muscle, Facial
Cortical strip neurostimulator lead
  use Neurostimulator Lead in Central Nervous System and Cranial Nerves
Corvia IASD®
  use Synthetic Substitute
COSELA™ *use* Trilaciclib
Costatectomy
  see Excision, Upper Bones 0PB
  see Resection, Upper Bones 0PT
Costectomy
  see Excision, Upper Bones 0PB
  see Resection, Upper Bones 0PT
Costocervical trunk
  use Artery, Subclavian, Left
  use Artery, Subclavian, Right
Costochondrectomy
  see Excision, Upper Bones 0PB
  see Resection, Upper Bones 0PT
Costoclavicular ligament
  use Bursa and Ligament, Shoulder, Left
  use Bursa and Ligament, Shoulder, Right
Costosternoplasty
  see Repair, Upper Bones 0PQ
  see Replacement, Upper Bones 0PR
  see Supplement, Upper Bones 0PU
Costotomy
  see Division, Upper Bones 0P8
  see Drainage, Upper Bones 0P9
Costotransverse joint
  use Joint, Thoracic Vertebral
Costotransverse ligament
  use Rib(s) Bursa and Ligament
Costovertebral joint
  use Joint, Thoracic Vertebral
Costoxiphoid ligament
  use Sternum Bursa and Ligament
Counseling
  Family, for substance abuse, Other Family Counseling HZ63ZZZ
  Group
    12-Step HZ43ZZZ
    Behavioral HZ41ZZZ
    Cognitive HZ40ZZZ
    Cognitive-Behavioral HZ42ZZZ
    Confrontational HZ48ZZZ
    Continuing Care HZ49ZZZ
    Infectious Disease

Counseling (continued)
  Group (continued)
    Post-Test HZ4CZZZ
    Pre-Test HZ4CZZZ
    Interpersonal HZ44ZZZ
    Motivational Enhancement HZ47ZZZ
    Psychoeducation HZ46ZZZ
    Spiritual HZ4BZZZ
    Vocational HZ45ZZZ
  Individual
    12-Step HZ33ZZZ
    Behavioral HZ31ZZZ
    Cognitive HZ30ZZZ
    Cognitive-Behavioral HZ32ZZZ
    Confrontational HZ38ZZZ
    Continuing Care HZ39ZZZ
    Infectious Disease
      Post-Test HZ3CZZZ
      Pre-Test HZ3CZZZ
    Interpersonal HZ34ZZZ
    Motivational Enhancement HZ37ZZZ
    Psychoeducation HZ36ZZZ
    Spiritual HZ3BZZZ
    Vocational HZ35ZZZ
  Mental Health Services
    Educational GZ60ZZZ
    Other Counseling GZ63ZZZ
    Vocational GZ61ZZZ
Countershock, cardiac 5A2204Z
Cowper's (bulbourethral) gland
  use Urethra
CPAP (continuous positive airway pressure)
  see Assistance, Respiratory 5A09
Craniectomy
  see Excision, Head and Facial Bones 0NB
  see Resection, Head and Facial Bones 0NT
Cranioplasty
  see Repair, Head and Facial Bones 0NQ
  see Replacement, Head and Facial Bones 0NR
  see Supplement, Head and Facial Bones 0NU
Craniotomy
  see Drainage, Central Nervous System and Cranial Nerves 009
  see Division, Head and Facial Bones 0N8
  see Drainage, Head and Facial Bones 0N9
Creation
  Perineum
    Female 0W4N0
    Male 0W4M0
  Valve
    Aortic 024F0
    Mitral 024G0
    Tricuspid 024J0
Cremaster muscle
  use Muscle, Perineum
CRESEMBA® (isavuconazonium sulfate)
  use Other Anti-infective
Cribriform plate
  use Bone, Ethmoid, Left
  use Bone, Ethmoid, Right
Cricoid cartilage
  use Trachea
Cricoidectomy
  see Excision, Larynx 0CBS
Cricothyroid artery
  use Artery, Thyroid, Left
  use Artery, Thyroid, Right
Cricothyroid muscle
  use Muscle, Neck, Left
  use Muscle, Neck, Right

Crisis Intervention GZ2ZZZZ
CRRT (Continuous renal replacement therapy) 5A1D90Z
Crural fascia
  use Subcutaneous Tissue and Fascia, Upper Leg, Left
  use Subcutaneous Tissue and Fascia, Upper Leg, Right
Crushing, nerve
  Cranial
    see Destruction, Central Nervous System and Cranial Nerves 005
  Peripheral
    see Destruction, Peripheral Nervous System 015
Cryoablation
  see Destruction
Cryotherapy
  see Destruction
Cryptorchidectomy
  see Excision, Male Reproductive System 0VB
  see Resection, Male Reproductive System 0VT
Cryptorchiectomy
  see Excision, Male Reproductive System 0VB
  see Resection, Male Reproductive System 0VT
Cryptotomy
  see Division, Gastrointestinal System 0D8
  see Drainage, Gastrointestinal System 0D9
CT scan
  see Computerized Tomography (CT Scan)
CT sialogram
  see Computerized Tomography (CT Scan), Ear, Nose, Mouth and Throat B92
Cubital lymph node
  use Lymphatic, Upper Extremity, Left
  use Lymphatic, Upper Extremity, Right
Cubital nerve
  use Nerve, Ulnar
Cuboid bone
  use Tarsal, Left
  use Tarsal, Right
Cuboideonavicular joint
  use Joint, Tarsal, Left
  use Joint, Tarsal, Right
Culdocentesis
  see Drainage, Cul-de-sac 0U9F
Culdoplasty
  see Repair, Cul-de-sac 0UQF
  see Supplement, Cul-de-sac 0UUF
Culdoscopy 0UJH8ZZ
Culdotomy
  see Drainage, Cul-de-sac 0U9F
Culmen
  use Cerebellum
Cultured epidermal cell autograft
  use Autologous Tissue Substitute
Cuneiform cartilage
  use Larynx
Cuneonavicular joint
  use Joint, Tarsal, Left
  use Joint, Tarsal, Right
Cuneonavicular ligament
  use Bursa and Ligament, Foot, Left
  use Bursa and Ligament, Foot, Right
Curettage
  see Excision
  see Extraction
Cutaneous (transverse) cervical nerve
  use Nerve, Cervical Plexus

CVP (central venous pressure)
   see Measurement, Venous 4A04
Cyclodiathermy
   see Destruction, Eye 085
Cyclophotocoagulation
   see Destruction, Eye 085
CYPHER® Stent
   use Intraluminal Device, Drug-
      eluting in Heart and Great Vessels
Cystectomy
   see Excision, Bladder 0TBB
   see Resection, Bladder 0TTB
Cystocele repair
   see Repair, Subcutaneous Tissue
      and Fascia, Pelvic Region 0JQC
Cystography
   see Fluoroscopy, Urinary System
      BT1
   see Plain Radiography, Urinary
      System BT0
Cystolithotomy
   see Extirpation, Bladder 0TCB
Cystopexy
   see Repair, Bladder 0TQB
   see Reposition, Bladder 0TSB
Cystoplasty
   see Repair, Bladder 0TQB
   see Replacement, Bladder 0TRB
   see Supplement, Bladder 0TUB
Cystorrhaphy
   see Repair, Bladder 0TQB
Cystoscopy 0TJB8ZZ
Cystostomy
   see Bypass, Bladder 0T1B
Cystostomy tube
   use Drainage Device
Cystotomy
   see Drainage, Bladder 0T9B
Cystourethrography
   see Fluoroscopy, Urinary System
      BT1
   see Plain Radiography, Urinary
      System BT0
Cystourethroplasty
   see Repair, Urinary System 0TQ
   see Replacement, Urinary System
      0TR
   see Supplement, Urinary System 0TU
**Cytarabine and Daunorubicin
   Liposome Antineoplastic** XW0

D

DBS lead
   use Neurostimulator Lead in Central
      Nervous System and Cranial
      Nerves
**DeBakey Left Ventricular Assist
   Device**
   use Implantable Heart Assist System
      in Heart and Great Vessels
Debridement
   Excisional
      see Excision
   Non-excisional
      see Extraction
Decompression, Circulatory 6A15
Decortication, lung
   see Extirpation, Respiratory
      System 0BC
   see Release, Respiratory System
      0BN
Deep brain neurostimulator lead
   use Neurostimulator Lead in Central
      Nervous System and Cranial
      Nerves
Deep cervical fascia
   use Subcutaneous Tissue and Fascia,
      Neck, Left
   use Subcutaneous Tissue and Fascia,
      Neck, Right

Deep cervical vein
   use Vein, Vertebral, Left
   use Vein, Vertebral, Right
Deep circumflex iliac artery
   use Artery, External Iliac, Left
   use Artery, External Iliac, Right
Deep facial vein
   use Vein, Face, Left
   use Vein, Face, Right
**Deep femoral (profunda femoris)
   vein**
   use Vein, Femoral, Left
   use Vein, Femoral, Right
Deep femoral artery
   use Artery, Femoral, Left
   use Artery, Femoral, Right
**Deep Inferior Epigastric Artery
   Perforator Flap**
   Replacement
      Bilateral 0HRV077
      Left 0HRU077
      Right 0HRT077
   Transfer
      Left 0KXG
      Right 0KXF
Deep palmar arch
   use Artery, Hand, Left
   use Artery, Hand, Right
Deep transverse perineal muscle
   use Muscle, Perineum
Deferential artery
   use Artery, Internal Iliac, Left
   use Artery, Internal Iliac, Right
Defibrillator Generator
   Abdomen 0JH8
   Chest 0JH6
Defibrotide Sodium Anticoagulant
   XW0
**Defibtech Automated Chest
   Compression** (ACC) device
   5A1221J
Defitelio
   use Defibrotide Sodium
      Anticoagulant
Delivery
   Cesarean
      see Extraction, Products of
         Conception 10D0
   Forceps
      see Extraction, Products of
         Conception 10D0
   Manually assisted 10E0XZZ
   Products of Conception
      10E0XZZ
   Vacuum assisted
      see Extraction, Products of
         Conception 10D0
Delta frame external fixator
   use External Fixation Device, Hybrid
      in 0PH
   use External Fixation Device, Hybrid
      in 0PS
   use External Fixation Device,
      Hybrid in 0QH
   use External Fixation Device,
      Hybrid in 0QS
**Delta III Reverse shoulder
   prosthesis**
   use Synthetic Substitute,
      Reverse Ball and Socket in
      0RR
Deltoid fascia
   use Subcutaneous Tissue and Fascia,
      Upper Arm, Left
   use Subcutaneous Tissue and Fascia,
      Upper Arm, Right
Deltoid ligament
   use Bursa and Ligament, Ankle,
      Left
   use Bursa and Ligament, Ankle,
      Right

Deltoid muscle
   use Muscle, Shoulder, Left
   use Muscle, Shoulder, Right
**Deltopectoral (infraclavicular)
   lymph node**
   use Lymphatic, Upper Extremity,
      Left
   use Lymphatic, Upper Extremity,
      Right
Denervation
   Cranial nerve
      see Destruction, Central Nervous
         System and Cranial
         Nerves 005
   Peripheral nerve
      see Destruction, Peripheral
         Nervous System 015
Dens
   use Cervical Vertebra
Densitometry
   Plain Radiography
      Femur
         Left BQ04ZZ1
         Right BQ03ZZ1
      Hip
         Left BQ01ZZ1
         Right BQ00ZZ1
      Spine
         Cervical BR00ZZ1
         Lumbar BR09ZZ1
         Thoracic BR07ZZ1
         Whole BR0GZZ1
   Ultrasonography
      Elbow
         Left BP4HZZ1
         Right BP4GZZ1
      Hand
         Left BP4PZZ1
         Right BP4NZZ1
      Shoulder
         Left BP49ZZ1
         Right BP48ZZ1
      Wrist
         Left BP4MZZ1
         Right BP4LZZ1
Denticulate (dentate) ligament
   use Spinal Meninges
Depressor anguli oris muscle
   use Muscle, Facial
Depressor labii inferioris muscle
   use Muscle, Facial
Depressor septi nasi muscle
   use Muscle, Facial
Depressor supercilii muscle
   use Muscle, Facial
Dermabrasion
   see Extraction, Skin and Breast
      0HD
Dermis
   use Skin
Descending genicular artery
   use Artery, Femoral, Left
   use Artery, Femoral, Right
Destruction
   Acetabulum
      Left 0Q55
      Right 0Q54
   Adenoids 0C5Q
   Ampulla of Vater 0F5C
   Anal Sphincter 0D5R
   Anterior Chamber
      Left 08533ZZ
      Right 08523ZZ
   Anus 0D5Q
   Aorta
      Abdominal 0450
      Thoracic
         Ascending/Arch 025X
         Descending 025W
   Aortic Body 0G5D
   Appendix 0D5J

Destruction (continued)
   Artery
      Anterior Tibial
         Left 045Q
         Right 045P
      Axillary
         Left 0356
         Right 0355
      Brachial
         Left 0358
         Right 0357
      Celiac 0451
      Colic
         Left 0457
         Middle 0458
         Right 0456
      Common Carotid
         Left 035J
         Right 035H
      Common Iliac
         Left 045D
         Right 045C
      External Carotid
         Left 035N
         Right 035M
      External Iliac
         Left 045J
         Right 045H
      Face 035R
      Femoral
         Left 045L
         Right 045K
      Foot
         Left 045W
         Right 045V
      Gastric 0452
      Hand
         Left 035F
         Right 035D
      Hepatic 0453
      Inferior Mesenteric
         045B
      Innominate 0352
      Internal Carotid
         Left 035L
         Right 035K
      Internal Iliac
         Left 045F
         Right 045E
      Internal Mammary
         Left 0351
         Right 0350
      Intracranial 035G
      Lower 045Y
      Peroneal
         Left 045U
         Right 045T
      Popliteal
         Left 045N
         Right 045M
      Posterior Tibial
         Left 045S
         Right 045R
      Pulmonary
         Left 025R
         Right 025Q
      Pulmonary Trunk 025P
      Radial
         Left 035C
         Right 035B
      Renal
         Left 045A
         Right 0459
      Splenic 0454
      Subclavian
         Left 0354
         Right 0353
      Superior Mesenteric 0455
      Temporal
         Left 035T
         Right 035S

12

Destruction *(continued)*
Subcutaneous Tissue and
Fascia *(continued)*
Hand
Left 0J5K
Right 0J5J
Lower Arm
Left 0J5H
Right 0J5G
Lower Leg
Left 0J5P
Right 0J5N
Neck
Left 0J55
Right 0J54
Pelvic Region 0J5C
Perineum 0J5B
Scalp 0J50
Upper Arm
Left 0J5F
Right 0J5D
Upper Leg
Left 0J5M
Right 0J5L
Tarsal
Left 0Q5M
Right 0Q5L
Tendon
Abdomen
Left 0L5G
Right 0L5F
Ankle
Left 0L5T
Right 0L5S
Foot
Left 0L5W
Right 0L5V
Hand
Left 0L58
Right 0L57
Head and Neck 0L50
Hip
Left 0L5K
Right 0L5J
Knee
Left 0L5R
Right 0L5Q
Lower Arm and Wrist
Left 0L56
Right 0L55
Lower Leg
Left 0L5P
Right 0L5N
Perineum 0L5H
Shoulder
Left 0L52
Right 0L51
Thorax
Left 0L5D
Right 0L5C
Trunk
Left 0L5B
Right 0L59
Upper Arm
Left 0L54
Right 0L53
Upper Leg
Left 0L5M
Right 0L5L
Testis
Bilateral 0V5C
Left 0V5B
Right 0V59
Thalamus 0059
Thymus 075M
Thyroid Gland 0G5K
Left Lobe 0G5G
Right Lobe 0G5H
Tibia
Left 0Q5H
Right 0Q5G

Destruction *(continued)*
Toe Nail 0H5RXZZ
Tongue 0C57
Tonsils 0C5P
Tooth
Lower 0C5X
Upper 0C5W
Trachea 0B51
Tunica Vaginalis
Left 0V57
Right 0V56
Turbinate, Nasal 095L
Tympanic Membrane
Left 0958
Right 0957
Ulna
Left 0P5L
Right 0P5K
Ureter
Left 0T57
Right 0T56
Urethra 0T5D
Uterine Supporting Structure
0U54
Uterus 0U59
Uvula 0C5N
Vagina 0U5G
Valve
Aortic 025F
Mitral 025G
Pulmonary 025H
Tricuspid 025J
Vas Deferens
Bilateral 0V5Q
Left 0V5P
Right 0V5N
Vein
Axillary
Left 0558
Right 0557
Azygos 0550
Basilic
Left 055C
Right 055B
Brachial
Left 055A
Right 0559
Cephalic
Left 055F
Right 055D
Colic 0657
Common Iliac
Left 065D
Right 065C
Coronary 0254
Esophageal 0653
External Iliac
Left 065G
Right 065F
External Jugular
Left 055Q
Right 055P
Face
Left 055V
Right 055T
Femoral
Left 065N
Right 065M
Foot
Left 065V
Right 065T
Gastric 0652
Hand
Left 055H
Right 055G
Hemiazygos 0551
Hepatic 0654
Hypogastric
Left 065J
Right 065H
Inferior Mesenteric 0656

Destruction *(continued)*
Vein *(continued)*
Innominate
Left 0554
Right 0553
Internal Jugular
Left 055N
Right 055M
Intracranial 055L
Lower 065Y
Portal 0658
Pulmonary
Left 025T
Right 025S
Renal
Left 065B
Right 0659
Saphenous
Left 065Q
Right 065P
Splenic 0651
Subclavian
Left 0556
Right 0555
Superior Mesenteric
0655
Upper 055Y
Vertebral
Left 055S
Right 055R
Vena Cava
Inferior 0650
Superior 025V
Ventricle
Left 025L
Right 025K
Vertebra
Cervical 0P53
Lumbar 0Q50
Thoracic 0P54
Vesicle
Bilateral 0V53
Left 0V52
Right 0V51
Vitreous
Left 08553ZZ
Right 08543ZZ
Vocal Cord
Left 0C5V
Right 0C5T
Vulva 0U5M
Detachment
Arm
Lower
Left 0X6F0Z
Right 0X6D0Z
Upper
Left 0X690Z
Right 0X680Z
Elbow Region
Left 0X6C0ZZ
Right 0X6B0ZZ
Femoral Region
Left 0Y680ZZ
Right 0Y670ZZ
Finger
Index
Left 0X6P0Z
Right 0X6N0Z
Little
Left 0X6W0Z
Right 0X6V0Z
Middle
Left 0X6R0Z
Right 0X6Q0Z
Ring
Left 0X6T0Z
Right 0X6S0Z
Foot
Left 0Y6N0Z
Right 0Y6M0Z

Detachment *(continued)*
Forequarter
Left 0X610ZZ
Right 0X600ZZ
Hand
Left 0X6K0Z
Right 0X6J0Z
Hindquarter
Bilateral 0Y640ZZ
Left 0Y630ZZ
Right 0Y620ZZ
Knee Region
Left 0Y6G0ZZ
Right 0Y6F0ZZ
Leg
Lower
Left 0Y6J0Z
Right 0Y6H0Z
Upper
Left 0Y6D0Z
Right 0Y6C0Z
Shoulder Region
Left 0X630ZZ
Right 0X620ZZ
Thumb
Left 0X6M0Z
Right 0X6L0Z
Toe
1st
Left 0Y6Q0Z
Right 0Y6P0Z
2nd
Left 0Y6S0Z
Right 0Y6R0Z
3rd
Left 0Y6U0Z
Right 0Y6T0Z
4th
Left 0Y6W0Z
Right 0Y6V0Z
5th
Left 0Y6Y0Z
Right 0Y6X0Z
Determination, Mental status
GZ14ZZZ
Detorsion
see Release
see Reposition
**Detoxification Services, for
substance abuse** HZ2ZZZZ
Device Fitting F0DZ
Diagnostic Audiology
see Audiology, Diagnostic
Diagnostic imaging
see Imaging, Diagnostic
Diagnostic radiology
see Imaging, Diagnostic
Dialysis
Hemodialysis *see* Performance,
Urinary 5A1D
Peritoneal 3E1M39Z
Diaphragma sellae
use Dura Mater
**Diaphragmatic pacemaker
generator**
use Stimulator Generator in
Subcutaneous Tissue and
Fascia
**Diaphragmatic Pacemaker
Lead**
Insertion of device in, Diaphragm
0BHT
Removal of device from, Diaphragm
0BPT
Revision of device in, Diaphragm
0BWT
Digital radiography, plain
see Plain Radiography
Dilation
Ampulla of Vater 0F7C
Anus 0D7Q

15

Dilation (continued)

Aorta
  Abdominal 0470
  Thoracic
    Ascending/Arch 027X
    Descending 027W
Artery
  Anterior Tibial
    Left 047Q
      Sustained Release Drug-
        eluting Intraluminal
        Device X27Q385
        Four or More X27Q3C5
        Three X27Q3B5
        Two X27Q395
    Right 047P
      Sustained Release Drug-
        eluting Intraluminal
        Device X27P385
        Four or More X27P3C5
        Three X27P3B5
        Two X27P395
  Axillary
    Left 0376
    Right 0375
  Brachial
    Left 0378
    Right 0377
  Celiac 0471
  Colic
    Left 0477
    Middle 0478
    Right 0476
  Common Carotid
    Left 037J
    Right 037H
  Common Iliac
    Left 047D
    Right 047C
  Coronary
    Four or More Arteries 0273
    One Artery 0270
    Three Arteries 0272
    Two Arteries 0271
  External Carotid
    Left 037N
    Right 037M
  External Iliac
    Left 047J
    Right 047H
  Face 037R
  Femoral
    Left 047L
      Sustained Release Drug-
        eluting Intraluminal
        Device X27J385
        Four or More X27J3C5
        Three X27J3B5
        Two X27J395
    Right 047K
      Sustained Release Drug-
        eluting Intraluminal
        Device X27H385
        Four or More X27H3C5
        Three X27H3B5
        Two X27H395
  Foot
    Left 047W
    Right 047V
  Gastric 0472
  Hand
    Left 037F
    Right 037D
  Hepatic 0473
  Inferior Mesenteric 047B
  Innominate 0372
  Internal Carotid
    Left 037L
    Right 037K
  Internal Iliac
    Left 047F

Dilation (continued)

Artery (continued)
  Internal Iliac (continued)
    Right 047E
  Internal Mammary
    Left 0371
    Right 0370
  Intracranial 037G
  Lower 047Y
  Peroneal
    Left 047U
      Sustained Release Drug-
        eluting Intraluminal
        Device X27U385
        Four or More X27U3C5
        Three X27U3B5
        Two X27U395
    Right 047T
      Sustained Release Drug-
        eluting Intraluminal
        Device X27T385
        Four or More X27T3C5
        Three X27T3B5
        Two X27T395
  Popliteal
    Left 047N
    Left Distal
      Sustained Release Drug-
        eluting Intraluminal
        Device X27N385
        Four or More X27N3C5
        Three X27N3B5
        Two X27N395
    Left Proximal
      Sustained Release Drug-
        eluting Intraluminal
        Device X27L385
        Four or More X27L3C5
        Three X27L3B5
        Two X27L395
    Right 047M
    Right Distal
      Sustained Release Drug-
        eluting Intraluminal
        Device X27M385
        Four or More X27M3C5
        Three X27M3B5
        Two X27M395
    Right Proximal
      Sustained Release Drug-
        eluting Intraluminal
        Device X27K385
        Four or More X27K3C5
        Three X27K3B5
        Two X27K395
  Posterior Tibial
    Left 047S
      Sustained Release Drug-
        eluting Intraluminal
        Device X27S385
        Four or More X27S3C5
        Three X27S3B5
        Two X27S395
    Right 047R
      Sustained Release Drug-
        eluting Intraluminal
        Device X27R385
        Four or More X27R3C5
        Three X27R3B5
        Two X27R395
  Pulmonary
    Left 027R
    Right 027Q
  Pulmonary Trunk 027P
  Radial
    Left 037C
    Right 037B
  Renal
    Left 047A
    Right 0479
  Splenic 0474

Dilation (continued)

Artery (continued)
  Subclavian
    Left 0374
    Right 0373
  Superior Mesenteric 0475
  Temporal
    Left 037T
    Right 037S
  Thyroid
    Left 037V
    Right 037U
  Ulnar
    Left 037A
    Right 0379
  Upper 037Y
  Vertebral
    Left 037Q
    Right 037P
Bladder 0T7B
Bladder Neck 0T7C
Bronchus
  Lingula 0B79
  Lower Lobe
    Left 0B7B
    Right 0B76
  Main
    Left 0B77
    Right 0B73
  Middle Lobe, Right 0B75
  Upper Lobe
    Left 0B78
    Right 0B74
Carina 0B72
Cerebral Ventricle 0076
Cecum 0D7H
Cervix 0U7C
Colon
  Ascending 0D7K
  Descending 0D7M
  Sigmoid 0D7N
  Transverse 0D7L
Duct
  Common Bile 0F79
  Cystic 0F78
  Hepatic
    Common 0F77
    Left 0F76
    Right 0F75
  Lacrimal
    Left 087Y
    Right 087X
  Pancreatic 0F7D
    Accessory 0F7F
  Parotid
    Left 0C7C
    Right 0C7B
Duodenum 0D79
Esophagogastric Junction 0D74
Esophagus 0D75
  Lower 0D73
  Middle 0D72
  Upper 0D71
Eustachian Tube
  Left 097G
  Right 097F
Fallopian Tube
  Left 0U76
  Right 0U75
Fallopian Tubes, Bilateral 0U77
Hymen 0U7K
Ileocecal Valve 0D7C
Ileum 0D7B
Intestine
  Large 0D7E
    Left 0D7G
    Right 0D7F
  Small 0D78
Jejunum 0D7A
Kidney Pelvis
  Left 0T74

Dilation (continued)

Kidney Pelvis (continued)
  Right 0T73
Larynx 0C7S
Pharynx 0C7M
Rectum 0D7P
Stomach 0D76
  Pylorus 0D77
Trachea 0B71
Ureter
  Left 0T77
  Right 0T76
Ureters, Bilateral 0T78
Urethra 0T7D
Uterus 0U79
Vagina 0U7G
Valve
  Aortic 027F
  Mitral 027G
  Pulmonary 027H
  Tricuspid 027J
Vas Deferens
  Bilateral 0V7Q
  Left 0V7P
  Right 0V7N
Vein
  Axillary
    Left 0578
    Right 0577
  Azygos 0570
  Basilic
    Left 057C
    Right 057B
  Brachial
    Left 057A
    Right 0579
  Cephalic
    Left 057F
    Right 057D
  Colic 0677
  Common Iliac
    Left 067D
    Right 067C
  Esophageal 0673
  External Iliac
    Left 067G
    Right 067F
  External Jugular
    Left 057Q
    Right 057P
  Face
    Left 057V
    Right 057T
  Femoral
    Left 067N
    Right 067M
  Foot
    Left 067V
    Right 067T
  Gastric 0672
  Hand
    Left 057H
    Right 057G
  Hemiazygos 0571
  Hepatic 0674
  Hypogastric
    Left 067J
    Right 067H
  Inferior Mesenteric 0676
  Innominate
    Left 0574
    Right 0573
  Internal Jugular
    Left 057N
    Right 057M
  Intracranial 057L
  Lower 067Y
  Portal 0678
  Pulmonary
    Left 027T
    Right 027S

Dilation (continued)
  Vein (continued)
    Renal
      Left 067B
      Right 0679
    Saphenous
      Left 067Q
      Right 067P
    Splenic 0671
    Subclavian
      Left 0576
      Right 0575
    Superior Mesenteric 0675
    Upper 057Y
    Vertebral
      Left 057S
      Right 057R
    Vena Cava
      Inferior 0670
      Superior 027V
    Ventricle
      Left 027L
      Right 027K
Direct Lateral Interbody Fusion (DLIF) device
  use Interbody Fusion Device in Lower Joints
Disarticulation
  see Detachment
Discectomy, diskectomy
  see Excision, Lower Joints 0SB
  see Excision, Upper Joints 0RB
  see Resection, Lower Joints 0ST
  see Resection, Upper Joints 0RT
Discography
  see Fluoroscopy, Axial Skeleton, Except Skull and Facial Bones BR1
  see Plain Radiography, Axial Skeleton, Except Skull and Facial Bones BR0
Dismembered pyeloplasty
  see Repair, Kidney Pelvis
Distal humerus
  use Humeral Shaft, Left
  use Humeral Shaft, Right
Distal humerus, involving joint
  use Joint, Elbow, Left
  use Joint, Elbow, Right
Distal radioulnar joint
  use Joint, Wrist, Left
  use Joint, Wrist, Right
Diversion
  see Bypass
Diverticulectomy
  see Excision, Gastrointestinal System 0DB
Division
  Acetabulum
    Left 0Q85
    Right 0Q84
  Anal Sphincter 0D8R
  Basal Ganglia 0088
  Bladder Neck 0T8C
  Bone
    Ethmoid
      Left 0N8G
      Right 0N8F
    Frontal 0N81
    Hyoid 0N8X
    Lacrimal
      Left 0N8J
      Right 0N8H
    Nasal 0N8B
    Occipital 0N87
    Palatine
      Left 0N8L
      Right 0N8K
    Parietal
      Left 0N84
      Right 0N83

Division (continued)
  Bone (continued)
    Pelvic
      Left 0Q83
      Right 0Q82
    Sphenoid 0N8C
    Temporal
      Left 0N86
      Right 0N85
    Zygomatic
      Left 0N8N
      Right 0N8M
  Brain 0080
  Bursa and Ligament
    Abdomen
      Left 0M8J
      Right 0M8H
    Ankle
      Left 0M8R
      Right 0M8Q
    Elbow
      Left 0M84
      Right 0M83
    Foot
      Left 0M8T
      Right 0M8S
    Hand
      Left 0M88
      Right 0M87
    Head and Neck 0M80
    Hip
      Left 0M8M
      Right 0M8L
    Knee
      Left 0M8P
      Right 0M8N
    Lower Extremity
      Left 0M8W
      Right 0M8V
    Perineum 0M8K
    Rib(s) 0M8G
    Shoulder
      Left 0M82
      Right 0M81
    Spine
      Lower 0M8D
      Upper 0M8C
    Sternum 0M8F
    Upper Extremity
      Left 0M8B
      Right 0M89
    Wrist
      Left 0M86
      Right 0M85
  Carpal
    Left 0P8N
    Right 0P8M
  Cerebral Hemisphere 0087
  Chordae Tendineae 0289
  Clavicle
    Left 0P8B
    Right 0P89
  Coccyx 0Q8S
  Conduction Mechanism 0288
  Esophagogastric Junction 0D84
  Femoral Shaft
    Left 0Q89
    Right 0Q88
  Femur
    Lower
      Left 0Q8C
      Right 0Q8B
    Upper
      Left 0Q87
      Right 0Q86
  Fibula
    Left 0Q8K
    Right 0Q8J
  Gland, Pituitary 0G80
  Glenoid Cavity
    Left 0P88

Division (continued)
  Glenoid Cavity (continued)
    Right 0P87
  Humeral Head
    Left 0P8D
    Right 0P8C
  Humeral Shaft
    Left 0P8G
    Right 0P8F
  Hymen 0U8K
  Kidneys, Bilateral 0T82
  Liver 0F80
    Left Lobe 0F82
    Right Lobe 0F81
  Mandible
    Left 0N8V
    Right 0N8T
  Maxilla 0N8R
  Metacarpal
    Left 0P8Q
    Right 0P8P
  Metatarsal
    Left 0Q8P
    Right 0Q8N
  Muscle
    Abdomen
      Left 0K8L
      Right 0K8K
    Facial 0K81
    Foot
      Left 0K8W
      Right 0K8V
    Hand
      Left 0K8D
      Right 0K8C
    Head 0K80
    Hip
      Left 0K8P
      Right 0K8N
    Lower Arm and Wrist
      Left 0K8B
      Right 0K89
    Lower Leg
      Left 0K8T
      Right 0K8S
    Neck
      Left 0K83
      Right 0K82
    Papillary 028D
    Perineum 0K8M
    Shoulder
      Left 0K86
      Right 0K85
    Thorax
      Left 0K8J
      Right 0K8H
    Tongue, Palate, Pharynx 0K84
    Trunk
      Left 0K8G
      Right 0K8F
    Upper Arm
      Left 0K88
      Right 0K87
    Upper Leg
      Left 0K8R
      Right 0K8Q
  Nerve
    Abdominal Sympathetic 018M
    Abducens 008L
    Accessory 008R
    Acoustic 008N
    Brachial Plexus 0183
    Cervical 0181
    Cervical Plexus 0180
    Facial 008M
    Femoral 018D
    Glossopharyngeal 008P
    Head and Neck Sympathetic 018K
    Hypoglossal 008S
    Lumbar 018B
    Lumbar Plexus 0189

Division (continued)
  Nerve (continued)
    Lumbar Sympathetic 018N
    Lumbosacral Plexus 018A
    Median 0185
    Oculomotor 008H
    Olfactory 008F
    Optic 008G
    Peroneal 018H
    Phrenic 0182
    Pudendal 018C
    Radial 0186
    Sacral 018R
    Sacral Plexus 018Q
    Sacral Sympathetic 018P
    Sciatic 018F
    Thoracic 0188
    Thoracic Sympathetic 018L
    Tibial 018G
    Trigeminal 008K
    Trochlear 008J
    Ulnar 0184
    Vagus 008Q
  Orbit
    Left 0N8Q
    Right 0N8P
  Ovary
    Bilateral 0U82
    Left 0U81
    Right 0U80
  Pancreas 0F8G
  Patella
    Left 0Q8F
    Right 0Q8D
  Perineum, Female 0W8NXZZ
  Phalanx
    Finger
      Left 0P8V
      Right 0P8T
    Thumb
      Left 0P8S
      Right 0P8R
    Toe
      Left 0Q8R
      Right 0Q8Q
  Radius
    Left 0P8J
    Right 0P8H
  Ribs
    1 to 2 0P81
    3 or More 0P82
  Sacrum 0Q81
  Scapula
    Left 0P86
    Right 0P85
  Skin
    Abdomen 0H87XZZ
    Back 0H86XZZ
    Buttock 0H88XZZ
    Chest 0H85XZZ
    Ear
      Left 0H83XZZ
      Right 0H82XZZ
    Face 0H81XZZ
    Foot
      Left 0H8NXZZ
      Right 0H8MXZZ
    Hand
      Left 0H8GXZZ
      Right 0H8FXZZ
    Inguinal 0H8AXZZ
    Lower Arm
      Left 0H8EXZZ
      Right 0H8DXZZ
    Lower Leg
      Left 0H8LXZZ
      Right 0H8KXZZ
    Neck 0H84XZZ
    Perineum 0H89XZZ
    Scalp 0H80XZZ

Division (continued)

Skin (continued)
 Upper Arm
  Left 0H8CXZZ
  Right 0H8BXZZ
 Upper Leg
  Left 0H8JXZZ
  Right 0H8HXZZ
Skull 0N80
Spinal Cord
 Cervical 008W
 Lumbar 008Y
 Thoracic 008X
Sternum 0P80
Stomach, Pylorus 0D87
Subcutaneous Tissue and Fascia
 Abdomen 0J88
 Back 0J87
 Buttock 0J89
 Chest 0J86
 Face 0J81
 Foot
  Left 0J8R
  Right 0J8Q
 Hand
  Left 0J8K
  Right 0J8J
 Head and Neck 0J8S
 Lower Arm
  Left 0J8H
  Right 0J8G
 Lower Extremity 0J8W
 Lower Leg
  Left 0J8P
  Right 0J8N
 Neck
  Left 0J85
  Right 0J84
 Pelvic Region 0J8C
 Perineum 0J8B
 Scalp 0J80
 Trunk 0J8T
 Upper Arm
  Left 0J8F
  Right 0J8D
 Upper Extremity 0J8V
 Upper Leg
  Left 0J8M
  Right 0J8L
Tarsal
 Left 0Q8M
 Right 0Q8L
Tendon
 Abdomen
  Left 0L8G
  Right 0L8F
 Ankle
  Left 0L8T
  Right 0L8S
 Foot
  Left 0L8W
  Right 0L8V
 Hand
  Left 0L88
  Right 0L87
 Head and Neck 0L80
 Hip
  Left 0L8K
  Right 0L8J
 Knee
  Left 0L8R
  Right 0L8Q
 Lower Arm and Wrist
  Left 0L86
  Right 0L85
 Lower Leg
  Left 0L8P
  Right 0L8N
 Perineum 0L8H
 Shoulder
  Left 0L82

Division (continued)

Tendon (continued)
 Shoulder (continued)
  Right 0L81
 Thorax
  Left 0L8D
  Right 0L8C
 Trunk
  Left 0L8B
  Right 0L89
 Upper Arm
  Left 0L84
  Right 0L83
 Upper Leg
  Left 0L8M
  Right 0L8L
Thyroid Gland Isthmus 0G8J
Tibia
 Left 0Q8H
 Right 0Q8G
Turbinate, Nasal 098L
Ulna
 Left 0P8L
 Right 0P8K
Uterine Supporting Structure 0U84
Vertebra
 Cervical 0P83
 Lumbar 0Q80
 Thoracic 0P84

Doppler study
 see Ultrasonography
Dorsal digital nerve
 use Nerve, Radial
Dorsal metacarpal vein
 use Vein, Hand, Left
 use Vein, Hand, Right
Dorsal metatarsal artery
 use Artery, Foot, Left
 use Artery, Foot, Right
Dorsal metatarsal vein
 use Vein, Foot, Left
 use Vein, Foot, Right
Dorsal root ganglion
 use Cervical Spinal Cord
 use Lumbar Spinal Cord
 use Spinal Cord
 use Thoracic Spinal Cord
Dorsal scapular artery
 use Artery, Subclavian, Left
 use Artery, Subclavian, Right
Dorsal scapular nerve
 use Nerve, Brachial Plexus
Dorsal venous arch
 use Vein, Foot, Left
 use Vein, Foot, Right
Dorsalis pedis artery
 use Artery, Anterior Tibial, Left
 use Artery, Anterior Tibial, Right
DownStream® System
 5A0512C
 5A0522C

Drainage
 Abdominal Wall 0W9F
 Acetabulum
  Left 0Q95
  Right 0Q94
 Adenoids 0C9Q
 Ampulla of Vater 0F9C
 Anal Sphincter 0D9R
 Ankle Region
  Left 0Y9L
  Right 0Y9K
 Anterior Chamber
  Left 0893
  Right 0892
 Anus 0D9Q
 Aorta, Abdominal 0490
 Aortic Body 0G9D
 Appendix 0D9J

Drainage (continued)

Arm
 Lower
  Left 0X9F
  Right 0X9D
 Upper
  Left 0X99
  Right 0X98
Artery
 Anterior Tibial
  Left 049Q
  Right 049P
 Axillary
  Left 0396
  Right 0395
 Brachial
  Left 0398
  Right 0397
 Celiac 0491
 Colic
  Left 0497
  Middle 0498
  Right 0496
 Common Carotid
  Left 039J
  Right 039H
 Common Iliac
  Left 049D
  Right 049C
 External Carotid
  Left 039N
  Right 039M
 External Iliac
  Left 049J
  Right 049H
 Face 039R
 Femoral
  Left 049L
  Right 049K
 Foot
  Left 049W
  Right 049V
 Gastric 0492
 Hand
  Left 039F
  Right 039D
 Hepatic 0493
 Inferior Mesenteric 049B
 Innominate 0392
 Internal Carotid
  Left 039L
  Right 039K
 Internal Iliac
  Left 049F
  Right 049E
 Internal Mammary
  Left 0391
  Right 0390
 Intracranial 039G
 Lower 049Y
 Peroneal
  Left 049U
  Right 049T
 Popliteal
  Left 049N
  Right 049M
 Posterior Tibial
  Left 049S
  Right 049R
 Radial
  Left 039C
  Right 039B
 Renal
  Left 049A
  Right 0499
 Splenic 0494
 Subclavian
  Left 0394
  Right 0393
 Superior Mesenteric 0495

Drainage (continued)

Artery (continued)
 Temporal
  Left 039T
  Right 039S
 Thyroid
  Left 039V
  Right 039U
 Ulnar
  Left 039A
  Right 0399
 Upper 039Y
 Vertebral
  Left 039Q
  Right 039P
Auditory Ossicle
 Left 099A
 Right 0999
Axilla
 Left 0X95
 Right 0X94
Back
 Lower 0W9L
 Upper 0W9K
Basal Ganglia 0098
Bladder 0T9B
Bladder Neck 0T9C
Bone
 Ethmoid
  Left 0N9G
  Right 0N9F
 Frontal 0N91
 Hyoid 0N9X
 Lacrimal
  Left 0N9J
  Right 0N9H
 Nasal 0N9B
 Occipital 0N97
 Palatine
  Left 0N9L
  Right 0N9K
 Parietal
  Left 0N94
  Right 0N93
 Pelvic
  Left 0Q93
  Right 0Q92
 Sphenoid 0N9C
 Temporal
  Left 0N96
  Right 0N95
 Zygomatic
  Left 0N9N
  Right 0N9M
Bone Marrow 079T
Brain 0090
Breast
 Bilateral 0H9V
 Left 0H9U
 Right 0H9T
Bronchus
 Lingula 0B99
 Lower Lobe
  Left 0B9B
  Right 0B96
 Main
  Left 0B97
  Right 0B93
 Middle Lobe, Right 0B95
 Upper Lobe
  Left 0B98
  Right 0B94
Buccal Mucosa 0C94
Bursa and Ligament
 Abdomen
  Left 0M9J
  Right 0M9H
 Ankle
  Left 0M9R
  Right 0M9Q

Drainage *(continued)*

Bursa and Ligament *(continued)*
Elbow
Left 0M94
Right 0M93
Foot
Left 0M9T
Right 0M9S
Hand
Left 0M98
Right 0M97
Head and Neck 200M90
Hip
Left 0M9M
Right 0M9L
Knee
Left 0M9P
Right 0M9N
Lower Extremity
Left 0M9W
Right 0M9V
Perineum 0M9K
Rib(s) 0M9G
Shoulder
Left 0M92
Right 0M91
Spine
Lower 0M9D
Upper 0M9C
Sternum 0M9F
Upper Extremity
Left 0M9B
Right 0M99
Wrist
Left 0M96
Right 0M95
Buttock
Left 0Y91
Right 0Y90
Carina 0B92
Carotid Bodies, Bilateral 0G98
Carotid Body
Left 0G96
Right 0G97
Carpal
Left 0P9N
Right 0P9M
Cavity, Cranial 0W91
Cecum 0D9H
Cerebellum 009C
Cerebral Hemisphere 0097
Cerebral Meninges 0091
Cerebral Ventricle 0096
Cervix 0U9C
Chest Wall 0W98
Choroid
Left 089B
Right 089A
Cisterna Chyli 079L
Clavicle
Left 0P9B
Right 0P99
Clitoris 0U9J
Coccygeal Glomus 0G9B
Coccyx 0Q9S
Colon
Ascending 0D9K
Descending 0D9M
Sigmoid 0D9N
Transverse 0D9L
Conjunctiva
Left 089T
Right 089S
Cord
Bilateral 0V9H
Left 0V9G
Right 0V9F
Cornea
Left 0899
Right 0898
Cul-de-sac 0U9F

Drainage *(continued)*

Diaphragm 0B9T
Disc
Cervical Vertebral 0R93
Cervicothoracic Vertebral 0R95
Lumbar Vertebral 0S92
Lumbosacral 0S94
Thoracic Vertebral 0R99
Thoracolumbar Vertebral 0R9B
Duct
Common Bile 0F99
Cystic 0F98
Hepatic
Common 0F97
Left 0F96
Right 0F95
Lacrimal
Left 089Y
Right 089X
Pancreatic 0F9D
Accessory 0F9F
Parotid
Left 0C9C
Right 0C9B
Duodenum 0D99
Dura Mater 0092
Ear
External
Left 0991
Right 0990
External Auditory Canal
Left 0994
Right 0993
Inner
Left 099E
Right 099D
Middle
Left 0996
Right 0995
Elbow Region
Left 0X9C
Right 0X9B
Epididymis
Bilateral 0V9L
Left 0V9K
Right 0V9J
Epidural Space, Intracranial 0093
Epiglottis 0C9R
Esophagogastric Junction 0D94
Esophagus 0D95
Lower 0D93
Middle 0D92
Upper 0D91
Eustachian Tube
Left 099G
Right 099F
Extremity
Lower
Left 0Y9B
Right 0Y99
Upper
Left 0X97
Right 0X96
Eye
Left 0891
Right 0890
Eyelid
Lower
Left 089R
Right 089Q
Upper
Left 089P
Right 089N
Face 0W92
Fallopian Tube
Left 0U96
Right 0U95
Fallopian Tubes, Bilateral 0U97
Femoral Region
Left 0Y98
Right 0Y97

Drainage *(continued)*

Femoral Shaft
Left 0Q99
Right 0Q98
Femur
Lower
Left 0Q9C
Right 0Q9B
Upper
Left 0Q97
Right 0Q96
Fibula
Left 0Q9K
Right 0Q9J
Finger Nail 0H9Q
Foot
Left 0Y9N
Right 0Y9M
Gallbladder 0F94
Gingiva
Lower 0C96
Upper 0C95
Gland
Adrenal
Bilateral 0G94
Left 0G92
Right 0G93
Lacrimal
Left 089W
Right 089V
Minor Salivary 0C9J
Parotid
Left 0C99
Right 0C98
Pituitary 0G90
Sublingual
Left 0C9F
Right 0C9D
Submaxillary
Left 0C9H
Right 0C9G
Vestibular 0U9L
Glenoid Cavity
Left 0P98
Right 0P97
Glomus Jugulare 0G9C
Hand
Left 0X9K
Right 0X9J
Head 0W90
Humeral Head
Left 0P9D
Right 0P9C
Humeral Shaft
Left 0P9G
Right 0P9F
Hymen 0U9K
Hypothalamus 009A
Ileocecal Valve 0D9C
Ileum 0D9B
Inguinal Region
Left 0Y96
Right 0Y95
Intestine
Large 0D9E
Left 0D9G
Right 0D9F
Small 0D98
Iris
Left 089D
Right 089C
Jaw
Lower 0W95
Upper 0W94
Jejunum 0D9A
Joint
Acromioclavicular
Left 0R9H
Right 0R9G

Drainage *(continued)*

Joint *(continued)*
Ankle
Left 0S9G
Right 0S9F
Carpal
Left 0R9R
Right 0R9Q
Carpometacarpal
Left 0R9T
Right 0R9S
Cervical Vertebral 0R91
Cervicothoracic Vertebral 0R94
Coccygeal 0S96
Elbow
Left 0R9M
Right 0R9L
Finger Phalangeal
Left 0R9X
Right 0R9W
Hip
Left 0S9B
Right 0S99
Knee
Left 0S9D
Right 0S9C
Lumbar Vertebral 0S90
Lumbosacral 0S93
Metacarpophalangeal
Left 0R9V
Right 0R9U
Metatarsal-Phalangeal
Left 0S9N
Right 0S9M
Occipital-cervical 0R90
Sacrococcygeal 0S95
Sacroiliac
Left 0S98
Right 0S97
Shoulder
Left 0R9K
Right 0R9J
Sternoclavicular
Left 0R9F
Right 0R9E
Tarsal
Left 0S9J
Right 0S9H
Tarsometatarsal
Left 0S9L
Right 0S9K
Temporomandibular
Left 0R9D
Right 0R9C
Thoracic Vertebral 0R96
Thoracolumbar Vertebral 0R9A
Toe Phalangeal
Left 0S9Q
Right 0S9P
Wrist
Left 0R9P
Right 0R9N
Kidney
Left 0T91
Right 0T90
Kidney Pelvis
Left 0T94
Right 0T93
Knee Region
Left 0Y9G
Right 0Y9F
Larynx 0C9S
Leg
Lower
Left 0Y9J
Right 0Y9H
Upper
Left 0Y9D
Right 0Y9C

Drainage (continued)

Subcutaneous Tissue and
Fascia (continued)
Neck (continued)
Right 0J94
Pelvic Region 0J9C
Perineum 0J9B
Scalp 0J90
Upper Arm
Left 0J9F
Right 0J9D
Upper Leg
Left 0J9M
Right 0J9L
Subdural Space, Intracranial 0094
Tarsal
Left 0Q9M
Right 0Q9L
Tendon
Abdomen
Left 0L9G
Right 0L9F
Ankle
Left 0L9T
Right 0L9S
Foot
Left 0L9W
Right 0L9V
Hand
Left 0L98
Right 0L97
Head and Neck 0L90
Hip
Left 0L9K
Right 0L9J
Knee
Left 0L9R
Right 0L9Q
Lower Arm and Wrist
Left 0L96
Right 0L95
Lower Leg
Left 0L9P
Right 0L9N
Perineum 0L9H
Shoulder
Left 0L92
Right 0L91
Thorax
Left 0L9D
Right 0L9C
Electrocautery
Right 0L99
Upper Arm
Left 0L94
Right 0L93
Upper Leg
Left 0L9M
Right 0L9L
Testis
Bilateral 0V9C
Left 0V9B
Right 0V99
Thalamus 0099
Thymus 079M
Thyroid Gland 0G9K
Left Lobe 0G9G
Right Lobe 0G9H
Tibia
Left 0Q9H
Right 0Q9G
Toe Nail 0H9R
Tongue 0C97
Tonsils 0C9P
Tooth
Lower 0C9X
Upper 0C9W
Trachea 0B91
Tunica Vaginalis
Left 0V97
Right 0V96

Drainage (continued)

Turbinate, Nasal 099L
Tympanic Membrane
Left 0998
Right 0997
Ulna
Left 0P9L
Right 0P9K
Ureter
Left 0T97
Right 0T96
Ureters, Bilateral 0T98
Urethra 0T9D
Uterine Supporting Structure 0U94
Uterus 0U99
Uvula 0C9N
Vagina 0U9G
Vas Deferens
Bilateral 0V9Q
Left 0V9P
Right 0V9N
Vein
Axillary
Left 0598
Right 0597
Azygos 0590
Basilic
Left 059C
Right 059B
Brachial
Left 059A
Right 0599
Cephalic
Left 059F
Right 059D
Colic 0697
Common Iliac
Left 069D
Right 069C
Esophageal 0693
External Iliac
Left 069G
Right 069F
External Jugular
Left 059Q
Right 059P
Face
Left 059V
Right 059T
Femoral
Left 069N
Right 069M
Foot
Left 069V
Right 069T
Gastric 0692
Hand
Left 059H
Right 059G
Hemiazygos 0591
Hepatic 0694
Hypogastric
Left 069J
Right 069H
Inferior Mesenteric 0696
Innominate
Left 0594
Right 0593
Internal Jugular
Left 059N
Right 059M
Intracranial 059L
Lower 069Y
Portal 0698
Renal
Left 069B
Right 0699
Saphenous
Left 069Q
Right 069P
Splenic 0691

Drainage (continued)

Vein (continued)
Subclavian
Left 0596
Right 0595
Superior Mesenteric 0695
Upper 059Y
Vertebral
Left 059S
Right 059R
Vena Cava, Inferior 0690
Vertebra
Cervical 0P93
Lumbar 0Q90
Thoracic 0P94
Vesicle
Bilateral 0V93
Left 0V92
Right 0V91
Vitreous
Left 0895
Right 0894
Vocal Cord
Left 0C9V
Right 0C9T
Vulva 0U9M
Wrist Region
Left 0X9H
Right 0X9G

Dressing

Abdominal Wall 2W23X4Z
Arm
Lower
Left 2W2DX4Z
Right 2W2CX4Z
Upper
Left 2W2BX4Z
Right 2W2AX4Z
Back 2W25X4Z
Chest Wall 2W24X4Z
Extremity
Lower
Left 2W2MX4Z
Right 2W2LX4Z
Upper
Left 2W29X4Z
Right 2W28X4Z
Face 2W21X4Z
Finger
Left 2W2KX4Z
Right 2W2JX4Z
Foot
Left 2W2TX4Z
Right 2W2SX4Z
Hand
Left 2W2FX4Z
Right 2W2EX4Z
Head 2W20X4Z
Inguinal Region
Left 2W27X4Z
Right 2W26X4Z
Leg
Lower
Left 2W2RX4Z
Right 2W2QX4Z
Upper
Left 2W2PX4Z
Right 2W2NX4Z
Neck 2W22X4Z
Thumb
Left 2W2HX4Z
Right 2W2GX4Z
Toe
Left 2W2VX4Z
Right 2W2UX4Z

Driver stent (RX) (OTW)
use Intraluminal Device

Drotrecogin alfa, infusion
see Introduction of Recombinant
Human-activated
Protein C

Duct of Santorini
use Duct, Pancreatic, Accessory

Duct of Wirsung
use Duct, Pancreatic

Ductogram, mammary
see Plain Radiography, Skin,
Subcutaneous Tissue and Breast
BH0

Ductography, mammary
see Plain Radiography, Skin,
Subcutaneous Tissue and Breast
BH0

Ductus deferens
use Vas Deferens
use Vas Deferens, Bilateral
use Vas Deferens, Left
use Vas Deferens, Right

Duodenal ampulla
use Ampulla of Vater

Duodenectomy
see Excision, Duodenum 0DB9
see Resection, Duodenum 0DT9

Duodenocholedochotomy
see Drainage, Gallbladder 0F94

Duodenocystostomy
see Bypass, Gallbladder 0F14
see Drainage, Gallbladder 0F94

Duodenoenterostomy
see Bypass, Gastrointestinal System
0D1
see Drainage, Gastrointestinal
System 0D9

Duodenojejunal flexure
use Jejunum

Duodenolysis
see Release, Duodenum 0DN9

Duodenorrhaphy
see Repair, Duodenum 0DQ9

Duodenoscopy, single-use (aScope™
Duodeno) (EXALT™ Model D)
see New Technology,
Hepatobiliary System and
Pancreas XFJ

Duodenostomy
see Bypass, Duodenum 0D19
see Drainage, Duodenum 0D99

Duodenotomy
see Drainage, Duodenum 0D99

**DuraGraft® Endothelial Damage
Inhibitor**
use Endothelial Damage Inhibitor

**DuraHeart Left Ventricular Assist
System**
use Implantable Heart Assist System
in Heart and Great Vessels

Dural venous sinus
use Vein, Intracranial

Dura mater, intracranial
use Dura Mater

Dura mater, spinal
use Spinal Meninges

Durata® Defibrillation Lead
use Cardiac Lead, Defibrillator in
02H

Durvalumab Antineoplastic XW0

DynaNail®
use Internal Fixation Device,
Sustained Compression in 0RG
use Internal Fixation Device,
Sustained Compression in 0SG

DynaNail Mini®
use Internal Fixation Device,
Sustained Compression in 0RG
use Internal Fixation Device,
Sustained Compression in 0SG

**Dynesys® Dynamic Stabilization
System**
use Spinal Stabilization Device,
Pedicle-Based in 0RH
use Spinal Stabilization Device,
Pedicle-Based in 0SH

E

E-Luminexx™ (Biliary)(Vascular) Stent
use Intraluminal Device

Earlobe
use Ear, External, Bilateral
use Ear, External, Left
use Ear, External, Right

ECCO2R (Extracorporeal Carbon Dioxide Removal) 5A0920Z

Echocardiogram
see Ultrasonography, Heart B24

Echography
see Ultrasonography

EchoTip® Insight™ Portosystemic Pressure Gradient Measurement System 4A044B2

ECMO
see Performance, Circulatory 5A15

ECMO, intraoperative
see Performance, Circulatory 5A15A

Eculizumab XW0

EDWARDS INTUITY Elite valve system
use Zooplastic Tissue, Rapid Deployment in New Technology

EEG (electroencephalogram)
see Measurement, Central Nervous 4A00

EGD (esophagogastroduodenoscopy) 0DJ08ZZ

Eighth cranial nerve
use Nerve, Acoustic

Ejaculatory duct
use Vas Deferens
use Vas Deferens, Bilateral
use Vas Deferens, Left
use Vas Deferens, Right

EKG (electrocardiogram)
see Measurement, Cardiac 4A02

EKOS™ EkoSonic® Endovascular System
see Fragmentation, Artery

Eladocagene exuparvovec XW0Q316

Electrical bone growth stimulator (EBGS)
use Bone Growth Stimulator in Head and Facial Bones
use Bone Growth Stimulator in Lower Bones
use Bone Growth Stimulator in Upper Bones

Electrical muscle stimulation (EMS) lead
use Stimulator Lead in Muscles

Electrocautery
Destruction
see Destruction
Repair
see Repair

Electroconvulsive Therapy
Bilateral-Multiple Seizure GZB3ZZZ
Bilateral-Single Seizure GZB2ZZZ
Electroconvulsive Therapy, Other GZB4ZZZ
Unilateral-Multiple Seizure GZB1ZZZ
Unilateral-Single Seizure GZB0ZZZ

Electroencephalogram (EEG)
see Measurement, Central Nervous 4A00

Electromagnetic Therapy
Central Nervous 6A22
Urinary 6A21

Electronic muscle stimulator lead
use Stimulator Lead in Muscles

Electrophysiologic stimulation (EPS)
see Measurement, Cardiac 4A02

Electroshock therapy
see Electroconvulsive Therapy

Elevation, bone fragments, skull
see Reposition, Head and Facial Bones 0NS

Eleventh cranial nerve
use Nerve, Accessory

Ellipsys® vascular access system
see New Technology, Cardiovascular System X2K

Eluvia™ Drug-Eluting Vascular Stent System
use Intraluminal Device, Sustained Release Drug-eluting in New Technology
use Intraluminal Device, Sustained Release Drug-eluting, Two in New Technology
use Intraluminal Device, Sustained Release Drug-eluting, Three in New Technology
use Intraluminal Device, Sustained Release Drug-eluting, Four or More in New Technology

ELZONRIS™
use Tagraxofusp-erzs Antineoplastic

Embolectomy
see Extirpation

Embolization
see Occlusion
see Restriction

Embolization coil(s)
use Intraluminal Device

EMG (electromyogram)
see Measurement, Musculoskeletal 4A0F

Encephalon
use Brain

Endarterectomy
see Extirpation, Lower Arteries 04C
see Extirpation, Upper Arteries 03C

Endeavor® (III)(IV) (Sprint) Zotarolimus-eluting Coronary Stent System
use Intraluminal Device, Drug-eluting in Heart and Great Vessels

EndoAVF procedure, using magnetic-guided radiofrequency
see Bypass, Upper Arteries 031

EndoAVF procedure, using thermal resistance energy
see New Technology, Cardiovascular System X2K

Endologix AFX® Endovascular AAA System
use Intraluminal Device

EndoSure® sensor
use Monitoring Device, Pressure Sensor in 02H

ENDOTAK RELIANCE® (G) Defibrillation Lead
use Cardiac Lead, Defibrillator in 02H

Endothelial damage inhibitor, applied to vein graft XY0VX83

Endotracheal tube (cuffed)(double-lumen)
use Intraluminal Device, Endotracheal Airway in Respiratory System

Endovascular fistula creation, using magnetic-guided radiofrequency
see Bypass, Upper Arteries 031

Endovascular fistula creation, using thermal resistance energy
see New Technology, Cardiovascular System X2K

Endurant® II AAA stent graft system
use Intraluminal Device

Endurant® Endovascular Stent Graft
use Intraluminal Device

Engineered Chimeric Antigen Receptor T-cell Immunotherapy
Allogeneic XW0
Autologous XW0

Enlargement
see Dilation
see Repair

EnRhythm
use Pacemaker, Dual Chamber in 0JH

ENROUTE® Transcarotid Neuroprotection System
see New Technology, Cardiovascular System X2A

ENSPRYNG™
use Satralizumab-mwge

Enterorrhaphy
see Repair, Gastrointestinal System 0DQ

Enterra gastric neurostimulator
use Stimulator Generator, Multiple Array in 0JH

Enucleation
Eyeball
see Resection, Eye 08T
Eyeball with prosthetic implant
see Replacement, Eye 08R

Ependyma
use Cerebral Ventricle

Epicel® cultured epidermal autograft
use Autologous Tissue Substitute

Epic™ Stented Tissue Valve (aortic)
use Zooplastic Tissue in Heart and Great Vessels

Epidermis
use Skin

Epididymectomy
see Excision, Male Reproductive System 0VB
see Resection, Male Reproductive System 0VT

Epididymoplasty
see Repair, Male Reproductive System 0VQ
see Supplement, Male Reproductive System 0VU

Epididymorrhaphy
see Repair, Male Reproductive System 0VQ

Epididymotomy
see Drainage, Male Reproductive System 0V9

Epidural space, spinal
use Spinal Canal

Epiphysiodesis
see Insertion of device in Lower Bones 0QH
see Insertion of device in Upper Bones 0PH
see Repair, Lower Bones 0QQ
see Repair, Upper Bones 0PQ

Epiploic foramen
use Peritoneum

Epiretinal Visual Prosthesis
Left 08H105Z
Right 08H005Z

Episiorrhaphy
see Repair, Perineum, Female 0WQN

Episiotomy
see Division, Perineum, Female 0W8N

Epithalamus
use Thalamus

Epitrochlear lymph node
use Lymphatic, Upper Extremity, Left
use Lymphatic, Upper Extremity, Right

EPS (electrophysiologic stimulation)
see Measurement, Cardiac 4A02

Eptifibatide, infusion
see Introduction of Platelet Inhibitor

ERCP (endoscopic retrograde cholangiopancreatography)
see Fluoroscopy, Hepatobiliary System and Pancreas BF1

Erdafitinib Antineoplastic XW0DXL5

Erector spinae muscle
use Muscle, Trunk, Left
use Muscle, Trunk, Right

ERLEADA®
use Apalutamide Antineoplastic

Esketamine Hydrochloride XW097M5

Esophageal artery
use Upper Artery

Esophageal obturator airway (EOA)
use Intraluminal Device, Airway in Gastrointestinal System

Esophageal plexus
use Nerve, Thoracic Sympathetic

Esophagectomy
see Excision, Gastrointestinal System 0DB
see Resection, Gastrointestinal System 0DT

Esophagocoloplasty
see Repair, Gastrointestinal System 0DQ
see Supplement, Gastrointestinal System 0DU

Esophagoenterostomy
see Bypass, Gastrointestinal System 0D1
see Drainage, Gastrointestinal System 0D9

Esophagoesophagostomy
see Bypass, Gastrointestinal System 0D1
see Drainage, Gastrointestinal System 0D9

Esophagogastrectomy
see Excision, Gastrointestinal System 0DB
see Resection, Gastrointestinal System 0DT

Esophagogastroduodenoscopy (EGD) 0DJ08ZZ

Esophagogastroplasty
see Repair, Gastrointestinal System 0DQ
see Supplement, Gastrointestinal System 0DU

Esophagogastroscopy 0DJ68ZZ

Esophagogastrostomy
see Bypass, Gastrointestinal System 0D1
see Drainage, Gastrointestinal System 0D9

Esophagojejunoplasty
see Supplement, Gastrointestinal System 0DU

Esophagojejunostomy
see Bypass, Gastrointestinal System 0D1
see Drainage, Gastrointestinal System 0D9

Esophagomyotomy
see Division, Esophagogastric Junction 0D84

Esophagoplasty
  see Repair, Gastrointestinal System 0DQ
  see Replacement, Esophagus 0DR5
  see Supplement, Gastrointestinal System 0DU

Esophagoplication
  see Restriction, Gastrointestinal System 0DV

Esophagorrhaphy
  see Repair, Gastrointestinal System 0DQ

Esophagoscopy 0DJ08ZZ

Esophagotomy
  see Drainage, Gastrointestinal System 0D9

Esteem® implantable hearing system
  use Hearing Device in Ear, Nose, Sinus

ESWL (extracorporeal shock wave lithotripsy)
  see Fragmentation

Ethmoidal air cell
  use Sinus, Ethmoid, Left
  use Sinus, Ethmoid, Right

Ethmoidectomy
  see Excision, Ear, Nose, Sinus 09B
  see Excision, Head and Facial Bones 0NB
  see Resection, Ear, Nose, Sinus 09T
  see Resection, Head and Facial Bones 0NT

Ethmoidotomy
  see Drainage, Ear, Nose, Sinus 099

Evacuation
  Hematoma
    see Extirpation
  Other Fluid
    see Drainage

Evera (XT)(S)(DR/VR)
  use Defibrillator Generator in 0JH

Everolimus-eluting coronary stent
  use Intraluminal Device, Drug-eluting in Heart and Great Vessels

Evisceration
  Eyeball
    see Resection, Eye 08T
  Eyeball with prosthetic implant
    see Replacement, Eye 08R

Ex-PRESS™ mini glaucoma shunt
  use Synthetic Substitute

EXALT™ Model D Single-Use Duodenoscope
  see New Technology, Hepatobiliary System and Pancreas XFJ

Examination
  see Inspection

Exchange
  see Change device in

Excision
  Abdominal Wall 0WBF
  Acetabulum
    Left 0QB5
    Right 0QB4
  Adenoids 0CBQ
  Ampulla of Vater 0FBC
  Anal Sphincter 0DBR
  Ankle Region
    Left 0YBL
    Right 0YBK
  Anus 0DBQ
  Aorta
    Abdominal 04B0
    Thoracic
      Ascending/Arch 02BX
      Descending 02BW
  Aortic Body 0GBD
  Appendix 0DBJ

Excision *(continued)*
  Arm
    Lower
      Left 0XBF
      Right 0XBD
    Upper
      Left 0XB9
      Right 0XB8
  Artery
    Anterior Tibial
      Left 04BQ
      Right 04BP
    Axillary
      Left 03B6
      Right 03B5
    Brachial
      Left 03B8
      Right 03B7
    Celiac 04B1
    Colic
      Left 04B7
      Middle 04B8
      Right 04B6
    Common Carotid
      Left 03BJ
      Right 03BH
    Common Iliac
      Left 04BD
      Right 04BC
    External Carotid
      Left 03BN
      Right 03BM
    External Iliac
      Left 04BJ
      Right 04BH
    Face 03BR
    Femoral
      Left 04BL
      Right 04BK
    Foot
      Left 04BW
      Right 04BV
    Gastric 04B2
    Hand
      Left 03BF
      Right 03BD
    Hepatic 04B3
    Inferior Mesenteric 04BB
    Innominate 03B2
    Internal Carotid
      Left 03BL
      Right 03BK
    Internal Iliac
      Left 04BF
      Right 04BE
    Internal Mammary
      Left 03B1
      Right 03B0
    Intracranial 03BG
    Lower 04BY
    Peroneal
      Left 04BU
      Right 04BT
    Popliteal
      Left 04BN
      Right 04BM
    Posterior Tibial
      Left 04BS
      Right 04BR
    Pulmonary
      Left 02BR
      Right 02BQ
    Pulmonary Trunk 02BP
    Radial
      Left 03BC
      Right 03BB
    Renal
      Left 04BA
      Right 04B9
    Splenic 04B4

Excision *(continued)*
  Artery *(continued)*
    Subclavian
      Left 03B4
      Right 03B3
    Superior Mesenteric 04B5
    Temporal
      Left 03BT
      Right 03BS
    Thyroid
      Left 03BV
      Right 03BU
    Ulnar
      Left 03BA
      Right 03B9
    Upper 03BY
    Vertebral
      Left 03BQ
      Right 03BP
  Atrium
    Left 02B7
    Right 02B6
  Auditory Ossicle
    Left 09BA
    Right 09B9
  Axilla
    Left 0XB5
    Right 0XB4
  Back
    Lower 0WBL
    Upper 0WBK
  Basal Ganglia 00B8
  Bladder 0TBB
  Bladder Neck 0TBC
  Bone
    Ethmoid
      Left 0NBG
      Right 0NBF
    Frontal 0NB1
    Hyoid 0NBX
    Lacrimal
      Left 0NBJ
      Right 0NBH
    Nasal 0NBB
    Occipital 0NB7
    Palatine
      Left 0NBL
      Right 0NBK
    Parietal
      Left 0NB4
      Right 0NB3
    Pelvic
      Left 0QB3
      Right 0QB2
    Sphenoid 0NBC
    Temporal
      Left 0NB6
      Right 0NB5
    Zygomatic
      Left 0NBN
      Right 0NBM
  Brain 00B0
  Breast
    Bilateral 0HBV
    Left 0HBU
    Right 0HBT
    Supernumerary 0HBY
  Bronchus
    Lingula 0BB9
    Lower Lobe
      Left 0BBB
      Right 0BB6
    Main
      Left 0BB7
      Right 0BB3
    Middle Lobe, Right 0BB5
    Upper Lobe
      Left 0BB8
      Right 0BB4
  Buccal Mucosa 0CB4

Excision *(continued)*
  Bursa and Ligament
    Abdomen
      Left 0MBJ
      Right 0MBH
    Ankle
      Left 0MBR
      Right 0MBQ
    Elbow
      Left 0MB4
      Right 0MB3
    Foot
      Left 0MBT
      Right 0MBS
    Hand
      Left 0MB8
      Right 0MB7
    Head and Neck 0MB0
    Hip
      Left 0MBM
      Right 0MBL
    Knee
      Left 0MBP
      Right 0MBN
    Lower Extremity
      Left 0MBW
      Right 0MBV
    Rib(s) 0MBG
    Perineum 0MBK
    Shoulder
      Left 0MB2
      Right 0MB1
    Spine
      Lower 0MBD
      Upper 0MBC
    Sternum 0MBF
    Upper Extremity
      Left 0MBB
      Right 0MB9
    Wrist
      Left 0MB6
      Right 0MB5
  Buttock
    Left 0YB1
    Right 0YB0
  Carina 0BB2
  Carotid Bodies, Bilateral 0GB8
  Carotid Body
    Left 0GB6
    Right 0GB7
  Carpal
    Left 0PBN
    Right 0PBM
  Cecum 0DBH
  Cerebellum 00BC
  Cerebral Hemisphere 00B7
  Cerebral Meninges 00B1
  Cerebral Ventricle 00B6
  Cervix 0UBC
  Chest Wall 0WB8
  Chordae Tendineae 02B9
  Choroid
    Left 08BB
    Right 08BA
  Cisterna Chyli 07BL
  Clavicle
    Left 0PBB
    Right 0PB9
  Clitoris 0UBJ
  Coccygeal Glomus 0GBB
  Coccyx 0QBS
  Colon
    Ascending 0DBK
    Descending 0DBM
    Sigmoid 0DBN
    Transverse 0DBL
  Conduction Mechanism 02B8
  Conjunctiva
    Left 08BTXZ
    Right 08BSXZ

24

Excision *(continued)*

Head 0KB0
Hip
  Left 0KBP
  Right 0KBN
Lower Arm and Wrist
  Left 0KBB
  Right 0KB9
Lower Leg
  Left 0KBT
  Right 0KBS
Neck
  Left 0KB3
  Right 0KB2
Papillary 02BD
Perineum 0KBM
Shoulder
  Left 0KB6
  Right 0KB5
Thorax
  Left 0KBJ
  Right 0KBH
Tongue, Palate, Pharynx 0KB4
Trunk
  Left 0KBG
  Right 0KBF
Upper Arm
  Left 0KB8
  Right 0KB7
Upper Leg
  Left 0KBR
  Right 0KBQ
Nasal Mucosa and Soft Tissue
  09BK
Nasopharynx 09BN
Neck 0WB6
Nerve
  Abdominal Sympathetic 01BM
  Abducens 00BL
  Accessory 00BR
  Acoustic 00BN
  Brachial Plexus 01B3
  Cervical 01B1
  Cervical Plexus 01B0
  Facial 00BM
  Femoral 01BD
  Glossopharyngeal 00BP
  Head and Neck Sympathetic
    01BK
  Hypoglossal 00BS
  Lumbar 01BB
  Lumbar Plexus 01B9
  Lumbar Sympathetic 01BN
  Lumbosacral Plexus 01BA
  Median 01B5
  Oculomotor 00BH
  Olfactory 00BF
  Optic 00BG
  Peroneal 01BH
  Phrenic 01B2
  Pudendal 01BC
  Radial 01B6
  Sacral 01BR
  Sacral Plexus 01BQ
  Sacral Sympathetic 01BP
  Sciatic 01BF
  Thoracic 01B8
  Thoracic Sympathetic 01BL
  Tibial 01BG
  Trigeminal 00BK
  Trochlear 00BJ
  Ulnar 01B4
  Vagus 00BQ
Nipple
  Left 0HBX
  Right 0HBW
Omentum 0DBU
Oral Cavity and Throat 0WB3
Orbit
  Left 0NBQ
  Right 0NBP

Excision *(continued)*

Ovary
  Bilateral 0UB2
  Left 0UB1
  Right 0UB0
Palate
  Hard 0CB2
  Soft 0CB3
Pancreas 0FBG
Para-aortic Body 0GB9
Paraganglion Extremity 0GBF
Parathyroid Gland 0GBR
  Inferior
    Left 0GBP
    Right 0GBN
  Multiple 0GBQ
  Superior
    Left 0GBM
    Right 0GBL
Patella
  Left 0QBF
  Right 0QBD
Penis 0VBS
Pericardium 02BN
Perineum
  Female 0WBN
  Male 0WBM
Peritoneum 0DBW
Phalanx
  Finger
    Left 0PBV
    Right 0PBT
  Thumb
    Left 0PBS
    Right 0PBR
  Toe
    Left 0QBR
    Right 0QBQ
Pharynx 0CBM
Pineal Body 0GB1
Pleura
  Left 0BBP
  Right 0BBN
Pons 00BB
Prepuce 0VBT
Prostate 0VB0
Radius
  Left 0PBJ
  Right 0PBH
Rectum 0DBP
Retina
  Left 08BF3Z
  Right 08BE3Z
Retroperitoneum
  0WBH
Ribs
  1 to 2 0PB1
  3 or More 0PB2
Sacrum 0QB1
Scapula
  Left 0PB6
  Right 0PB5
Sclera
  Left 08B7XZ
  Right 08B6XZ
Scrotum 0VB5
Septum
  Atrial 02B5
  Nasal 09BM
  Ventricular 02BM
Shoulder Region
  Left 0XB3
  Right 0XB2
Sinus
  Accessory 09BP
  Ethmoid
    Left 09BV
    Right 09BU
  Frontal
    Left 09BT
    Right 09BS

Excision *(continued)*

Sinus *(continued)*
  Mastoid
    Left 09BC
    Right 09BB
  Maxillary
    Left 09BR
    Right 09BQ
  Sphenoid
    Left 09BX
    Right 09BW
Skin
  Abdomen 0HB7XZ
  Back 0HB6XZ
  Buttock 0HB8XZ
  Chest 0HB5XZ
  Ear
    Left 0HB3XZ
    Right 0HB2XZ
  Face 0HB1XZ
  Foot
    Left 0HBNXZ
    Right 0HBMXZ
  Hand
    Left 0HBGXZ
    Right 0HBFXZ
  Inguinal 0HBAXZ
  Lower Arm
    Left 0HBEXZ
    Right 0HBDXZ
  Lower Leg
    Left 0HBLXZ
    Right 0HBKXZ
  Neck 0HB4XZ
  Perineum 0HB9XZ
  Scalp 0HB0XZ
  Upper Arm
    Left 0HBCXZ
    Right 0HBBXZ
  Upper Leg
    Left 0HBJXZ
    Right 0HBHXZ
Skull 0NB0
Spinal Cord
  Cervical 00BW
  Lumbar 00BY
  Thoracic 00BX
Spinal Meninges 00BT
Spleen 07BP
Sternum 0PB0
Stomach 0DB6
  Pylorus 0DB7
Subcutaneous Tissue and Fascia
  Abdomen 0JB8
  Back 0JB7
  Buttock 0JB9
  Chest 0JB6
  Face 0JB1
  Foot
    Left 0JBR
    Right 0JBQ
  Hand
    Left 0JBK
    Right 0JBJ
  Lower Arm
    Left 0JBH
    Right 0JBG
  Lower Leg
    Left 0JBP
    Right 0JBN
  Neck
    Left 0JB5
    Right 0JB4
  Pelvic Region 0JBC
  Perineum 0JBB
  Scalp 0JB0
  Upper Arm
    Left 0JBF
    Right 0JBD
  Upper Leg
    Left 0JBM

Excision *(continued)*

Subcutaneous Tissue and
Fascia *(continued)*
  Upper Leg *(continued)*
    Right 0JBL
Tarsal
  Left 0QBM
  Right 0QBL
Tendon
  Abdomen
    Left 0LBG
    Right 0LBF
  Ankle
    Left 0LBT
    Right 0LBS
  Foot
    Left 0LBW
    Right 0LBV
  Hand
    Left 0LB8
    Right 0LB7
  Head and Neck
    0LB0
  Hip
    Left 0LBK
    Right 0LBJ
  Knee
    Left 0LBR
    Right 0LBQ
  Lower Arm and Wrist
    Left 0LB6
    Right 0LB5
  Lower Leg
    Left 0LBP
    Right 0LBN
  Perineum 0LBH
  Shoulder
    Left 0LB2
    Right 0LB1
  Thorax
    Left 0LBD
    Right 0LBC
  Trunk
    Left 0LBB
    Right 0LB9
  Upper Arm
    Left 0LB4
    Right 0LB3
  Upper Leg
    Left 0LBM
    Right 0LBL
Testis
  Bilateral 0VBC
  Left 0VBB
  Right 0VB9
Thalamus 00B9
Thymus 07BM
Thyroid Gland
  Left Lobe 0GBG
  Right Lobe 0GBH
Thyroid Gland Isthmus 0GBJ
Tibia
  Left 0QBH
  Right 0QBG
Toe Nail 0HBRXZ
Tongue 0CB7
Tonsils 0CBP
Tooth
  Lower 0CBX
  Upper 0CBW
Trachea 0BB1
Tunica Vaginalis
  Left 0VB7
  Right 0VB6
Turbinate, Nasal 09BL
Tympanic Membrane
  Left 09B8
  Right 09B7
Ulna
  Left 0PBL
  Right 0PBK

Excision *(continued)*
Ureter
Left 0TB7
Right 0TB6
Urethra 0TBD
Uterine Supporting Structure 0UB4
Uterus 0UB9
Uvula 0CBN
Vagina 0UBG
Valve
Aortic 02BF
Mitral 02BG
Pulmonary 02BH
Tricuspid 02BJ
Vas Deferens
Bilateral 0VBQ
Left 0VBP
Right 0VBN
Vein
Axillary
Left 05B8
Right 05B7
Azygos 05B0
Basilic
Left 05BC
Right 05BB
Brachial
Left 05BA
Right 05B9
Cephalic
Left 05BF
Right 05BD
Colic 06B7
Common Iliac
Left 06BD
Right 06BC
Coronary 02B4
Esophageal 06B3
External Iliac
Left 06BG
Right 06BF
External Jugular
Left 05BQ
Right 05BP
Face
Left 05BV
Right 05BT
Femoral
Left 06BN
Right 06BM
Foot
Left 06BV
Right 06BT
Gastric 06B2
Hand
Left 05BH
Right 05BG
Hemiazygos 05B1
Hepatic 06B4
Hypogastric
Left 06BJ
Right 06BH
Inferior Mesenteric 06B6
Innominate
Left 05B4
Right 05B3
Internal Jugular
Left 05BN
Right 05BM
Intracranial 05BL
Lower 06BY
Portal 06B8
Pulmonary
Left 02BT
Right 02BS
Renal
Left 06BB
Right 06B9

Excision *(continued)*
Vein *(continued)*
Saphenous
Left 06BQ
Right 06BP
Splenic 06B1
Subclavian
Left 05B6
Right 05B5
Superior Mesenteric 06B5
Upper 05BY
Vertebral
Left 05BS
Right 05BR
Vena Cava
Inferior 06B0
Superior 02BV
Ventricle
Left 02BL
Right 02BK
Vertebra
Cervical 0PB3
Lumbar 0QB0
Thoracic 0PB4
Vesicle
Bilateral 0VB3
Left 0VB2
Right 0VB1
Vitreous
Left 08B53Z
Right 08B43Z
Vocal Cord
Left 0CBV
Right 0CBT
Vulva 0UBM
Wrist Region
Left 0XBH
Right 0XBG
EXCLUDER® AAA Endoprosthesis
use Intraluminal Device
use Intraluminal Device, Branched or Fenestrated, One or Two Arteries in 04V
use Intraluminal Device, Branched or Fenestrated, Three or More Arteries in 04V
EXCLUDER® IBE Endoprosthesis
use Intraluminal Device, Branched or Fenestrated, One or Two Arteries in 04V
Exclusion, Left atrial appendage (LAA)
see Occlusion, Atrium, Left 02L7
Exercise, rehabilitation
see Motor Treatment, Rehabilitation F07
Exploration
see Inspection
Express® (LD) Premounted Stent System
use Intraluminal Device
Express® Biliary SD Monorail® Premounted Stent System
use Intraluminal Device
Express® SD Renal Monorail® Premounted Stent System
use Intraluminal Device
Extensor carpi radialis muscle
use Muscle, Lower Arm and Wrist, Left
Extensor carpi radialis muscle
use Muscle, Lower Arm and Wrist, Right
Extensor carpi ulnaris muscle
use Muscle, Lower Arm and Wrist, Left
use Muscle, Lower Arm and Wrist, Right
Extensor digitorum brevis muscle
use Muscle, Foot, Left
use Muscle, Foot, Right

Extensor digitorum longus muscle
use Muscle, Lower Leg, Left
use Muscle, Lower Leg, Right
Extensor hallucis brevis muscle
use Muscle, Foot, Left
use Muscle, Foot, Right
Extensor hallucis longus muscle
use Muscle, Lower Leg, Left
use Muscle, Lower Leg, Right
External anal sphincter
use Anal Sphincter
External auditory meatus
use Ear, External Auditory Canal, Left
use Ear, External Auditory Canal, Right
External fixator
use External Fixation Device in Head and Facial Bones
use External Fixation Device in Lower Bones
use External Fixation Device in Lower Joints
use External Fixation Device in Upper Bones
use External Fixation Device in Upper Joints
External maxillary artery
use Artery, Face
External naris
use Nasal Mucosa and Soft Tissue
External oblique aponeurosis
use Subcutaneous Tissue and Fascia, Trunk
External oblique muscle
use Muscle, Abdomen, Left
use Muscle, Abdomen, Right
External popliteal nerve
use Nerve, Peroneal
External pudendal artery
use Artery, Femoral, Left
use Artery, Femoral, Right
External pudendal vein
use Vein, Saphenous, Left
use Vein, Saphenous, Right
External urethral sphincter
use Urethra
Extirpation
Acetabulum
Left 0QC5
Right 0QC4
Adenoids 0CCQ
Ampulla of Vater 0FCC
Anal Sphincter 0DCR
Anterior Chamber
Left 08C3
Right 08C2
Anus 0DCQ
Aorta
Abdominal 04C0
Thoracic
Ascending/Arch 02CX
Descending 02CW
Aortic Body 0GCD
Appendix 0DCJ
Artery
Anterior Tibial
Left 04CQ
Right 04CP
Axillary
Left 03C6
Right 03C5
Brachial
Left 03C8
Right 03C7
Celiac 04C1
Colic
Left 04C7
Middle 04C8
Right 04C6

Extirpation *(continued)*
Artery *(continued)*
Common Carotid
Left 03CJ
Right 03CH
Common Iliac
Left 04CD
Right 04CC
Coronary
Four or More Arteries 02C3
One Artery 02C0
Three Arteries 02C2
Two Arteries 02C1
External Carotid
Left 03CN
Right 03CM
External Iliac
Left 04CJ
Right 04CH
Face 03CR
Femoral
Left 04CL
Right 04CK
Foot
Left 04CW
Right 04CV
Gastric 04C2
Hand
Left 03CF
Right 03CD
Hepatic 04C3
Inferior Mesenteric 04CB
Innominate 03C2
Internal Carotid
Left 03CL
Right 03CK
Internal Iliac
Left 04CF
Right 04CE
Internal Mammary
Left 03C1
Right 03C0
Intracranial 03CG
Lower 04CY
Peroneal
Left 04CU
Right 04CT
Popliteal
Left 04CN
Right 04CM
Posterior Tibial
Left 04CS
Right 04CR
Pulmonary
Left 02CR
Right 02CQ
Pulmonary Trunk 02CP
Radial
Left 03CC
Right 03CB
Renal
Left 04CA
Right 04C9
Splenic 04C4
Subclavian
Left 03C4
Right 03C3
Superior Mesenteric 04C5
Temporal
Left 03CT
Right 03CS
Thyroid
Left 03CV
Right 03CU
Ulnar
Left 03CA
Right 03C9
Upper 03CY
Vertebral
Left 03CQ
Right 03CP

Extirpation *(continued)*
  Atrium
    Left 02C7
    Right 02C6
  Auditory Ossicle
    Left 09CA
    Right 09C9
  Basal Ganglia 00C8
  Bladder 0TCB
  Bladder Neck
    0TCC
  Bone
    Ethmoid
      Left 0NCG
      Right 0NCF
    Frontal 0NC1
    Hyoid 0NCX
    Lacrimal
      Left 0NCJ
      Right 0NCH
    Nasal 0NCB
    Occipital 0NC7
    Palatine
      Left 0NCL
      Right 0NCK
    Parietal
      Left 0NC4
      Right 0NC3
    Pelvic
      Left 0QC3
      Right 0QC2
    Sphenoid 0NCC
    Temporal
      Left 0NC6
      Right 0NC5
    Zygomatic
      Left 0NCN
      Right 0NCM
  Brain 00C0
  Breast
    Bilateral 0HCV
    Left 0HCU
    Right 0HCT
  Bronchus
    Lingula 0BC9
    Lower Lobe
      Left 0BCB
      Right 0BC6
    Main
      Left 0BC7
      Right 0BC3
    Middle Lobe, Right
      0BC5
    Upper Lobe
      Left 0BC8
      Right 0BC4
  Buccal Mucosa 0CC4
  Bursa and Ligament
    Abdomen
      Left 0MCJ
      Right 0MCH
    Ankle
      Left 0MCR
      Right 0MCQ
    Elbow
      Left 0MC4
      Right 0MC3
    Foot
      Left 0MCT
      Right 0MCS
    Hand
      Left 0MC8
      Right 0MC7
    Head and Neck
      0MC0
    Hip
      Left 0MCM
      Right 0MCL
    Knee
      Left 0MCP
      Right 0MCN

Extirpation *(continued)*
  Bursa and Ligament *(continued)*
    Lower Extremity
      Left 0MCW
      Right 0MCV
    Perineum 0MCK
    Rib(s) 0MCG
    Shoulder
      Left 0MC2
      Right 0MC1
    Spine
      Lower 0MCD
      Upper 0MCC
    Sternum 0MCF
    Upper Extremity
      Left 0MCB
      Right 0MC9
    Wrist
      Left 0MC6
      Right 0MC5
  Carina 0BC2
  Carotid Bodies, Bilateral
    0GC8
  Carotid Body
    Left 0GC6
    Right 0GC7
  Carpal
    Left 0PCN
    Right 0PCM
  Cavity, Cranial 0WC1
  Cecum 0DCH
  Cerebellum 00CC
  Cerebral Hemisphere 00C7
  Cerebral Meninges 00C1
  Cerebral Ventricle 00C6
  Cervix 0UCC
  Chordae Tendineae 02C9
  Choroid
    Left 08CB
    Right 08CA
  Cisterna Chyli 07CL
  Clavicle
    Left 0PCB
    Right 0PC9
  Clitoris 0UCJ
  Coccygeal Glomus 0GCB
  Coccyx 0QCS
  Colon
    Ascending 0DCK
    Descending 0DCM
    Sigmoid 0DCN
    Transverse 0DCL
  Computer-aided Mechanical
    Aspiration X2C
  Conduction Mechanism 02C8
  Conjunctiva
    Left 08CTXZZ
    Right 08CSXZZ
  Cord
    Bilateral 0VCH
    Left 0VCG
    Right 0VCF
  Cornea
    Left 08C9XZZ
    Right 08C8XZZ
  Cul-de-sac 0UCF
  Diaphragm 0BCT
  Disc
    Cervical Vertebral 0RC3
    Cervicothoracic Vertebral 0RC5
    Lumbar Vertebral 0SC2
    Lumbosacral 0SC4
    Thoracic Vertebral 0RC9
    Thoracolumbar Vertebral 0RCB
  Duct
    Common Bile 0FC9
    Cystic 0FC8
    Hepatic
      Common 0FC7
      Left 0FC6
      Right 0FC5

Extirpation *(continued)*
  Duct *(continued)*
    Lacrimal
      Left 08CY
      Right 08CX
    Pancreatic 0FCD
      Accessory 0FCF
    Parotid
      Left 0CCC
      Right 0CCB
  Duodenum 0DC9
  Dura Mater 00C2
  Ear
    External
      Left 09C1
      Right 09C0
    External Auditory Canal
      Left 09C4
      Right 09C3
    Inner
      Left 09CE
      Right 09CD
    Middle
      Left 09C6
      Right 09C5
  Endometrium 0UCB
  Epididymis
    Bilateral 0VCL
    Left 0VCK
    Right 0VCJ
  Epidural Space, Intracranial 00C3
  Epiglottis 0CCR
  Esophagogastric Junction 0DC4
  Esophagus 0DC5
    Lower 0DC3
    Middle 0DC2
    Upper 0DC1
  Eustachian Tube
    Left 09CG
    Right 09CF
  Eye
    Left 08C1XZZ
    Right 08C0XZZ
  Eyelid
    Lower
      Left 08CR
      Right 08CQ
    Upper
      Left 08CP
      Right 08CN
  Fallopian Tube
    Left 0UC6
    Right 0UC5
  Fallopian Tubes, Bilateral 0UC7
  Femoral Shaft
    Left 0QC9
    Right 0QC8
  Femur
    Lower
      Left 0QCC
      Right 0QCB
    Upper
      Left 0QC7
      Right 0QC6
  Fibula
    Left 0QCK
    Right 0QCJ
  Finger Nail 0HCQXZZ
  Gallbladder 0FC4
  Gastrointestinal Tract
    0WCP
  Genitourinary Tract
    0WCR
  Gingiva
    Lower 0CC6
    Upper 0CC5
  Gland
    Adrenal
      Bilateral 0GC4
      Left 0GC2
      Right 0GC3

Extirpation *(continued)*
  Gland *(continued)*
    Lacrimal
      Left 08CW
      Right 08CV
    Minor Salivary 0CCJ
    Parotid
      Left 0CC9
      Right 0CC8
    Pituitary 0GC0
    Sublingual
      Left 0CCF
      Right 0CCD
    Submaxillary
      Left 0CCH
      Right 0CCG
    Vestibular 0UCL
  Glenoid Cavity
    Left 0PC8
    Right 0PC7
  Glomus Jugulare 0GCC
  Humeral Head
    Left 0PCD
    Right 0PCC
  Humeral Shaft
    Left 0PCG
    Right 0PCF
  Hymen 0UCK
  Hypothalamus 00CA
  Ileocecal Valve 0DCC
  Ileum 0DCB
  Intestine
    Large 0DCE
      Left 0DCG
      Right 0DCF
    Small 0DC8
  Iris
    Left 08CD
    Right 08CC
  Jaw
    Lower 0WC5
    Upper 0WC4
  Jejunum 0DCA
  Joint
    Acromioclavicular
      Left 0RCH
      Right 0RCG
    Ankle
      Left 0SCG
      Right 0SCF
    Carpal
      Left 0RCR
      Right 0RCQ
    Carpometacarpal
      Left 0RCT
      Right 0RCS
    Cervical Vertebral 0RC1
    Cervicothoracic Vertebral 0RC4
    Coccygeal 0SC6
    Elbow
      Left 0RCM
      Right 0RCL
    Finger Phalangeal
      Left 0RCX
      Right 0RCW
    Hip
      Left 0SCB
      Right 0SC9
    Knee
      Left 0SCD
      Right 0SCC
    Lumbar Vertebral 0SC0
    Lumbosacral 0SC3
    Metacarpophalangeal
      Left 0RCV
      Right 0RCU
    Metatarsal-Phalangeal
      Left 0SCN
      Right 0SCM
    Occipital-cervical 0RC0
    Sacrococcygeal 0SC5

Extirpation (continued)
Spinal Meninges 00CT
Spleen 07CP
Sternum 0PC0
Stomach 0DC6
  Pylorus 0DC7
Subarachnoid Space, Intracranial 00C5
Subcutaneous Tissue and Fascia
  Abdomen 0JC8
  Back 0JC7
  Buttock 0JC9
  Chest 0JC6
  Face 0JC1
  Foot
    Left 0JCR
    Right 0JCQ
  Hand
    Left 0JCK
    Right 0JCJ
  Lower Arm
    Left 0JCH
    Right 0JCG
  Lower Leg
    Left 0JCP
    Right 0JCN
  Neck
    Left 0JC5
    Right 0JC4
  Pelvic Region 0JCC
  Perineum 0JCB
  Scalp 0JC0
  Upper Arm
    Left 0JCF
    Right 0JCD
  Upper Leg
    Left 0JCM
    Right 0JCL
Subdural Space, Intracranial 00C4
Tarsal
  Left 0QCM
  Right 0QCL
Tendon
  Abdomen
    Left 0LCG
    Right 0LCF
  Ankle
    Left 0LCT
    Right 0LCS
  Foot
    Left 0LCW
    Right 0LCV
  Hand
    Left 0LC8
    Right 0LC7
  Head and Neck 0LC0
  Hip
    Left 0LCK
    Right 0LCJ
  Knee
    Left 0LCR
    Right 0LCQ
  Lower Arm and Wrist
    Left 0LC6
    Right 0LC5
  Lower Leg
    Left 0LCP
    Right 0LCN
  Perineum 0LCH
  Shoulder
    Left 0LC2
    Right 0LC1
  Thorax
    Left 0LCD
    Right 0LCC
  Trunk
    Left 0LCB
    Right 0LC9
  Upper Arm
    Left 0LC4
    Right 0LC3

Extirpation (continued)
Tendon (continued)
  Upper Leg
    Left 0LCM
    Right 0LCL
Testis
  Bilateral 0VCC
  Left 0VCB
  Right 0VC9
Thalamus 00C9
Thymus 07CM
Thyroid Gland 0GCK
  Left Lobe 0GCG
  Right Lobe 0GCH
Tibia
  Left 0QCH
  Right 0QCG
Toe Nail 0HCRXZZ
Tongue 0CC7
Tonsils 0CCP
Tooth
  Lower 0CCX
  Upper 0CCW
Trachea 0BC1
Tunica Vaginalis
  Left 0VC7
  Right 0VC6
Turbinate, Nasal 09CL
Tympanic Membrane
  Left 09C8
  Right 09C7
Ulna
  Left 0PCL
  Right 0PCK
Ureter
  Left 0TC7
  Right 0TC6
Urethra 0TCD
Uterine Supporting Structure 0UC4
Uterus 0UC9
Uvula 0CCN
Vagina 0UCG
Valve
  Aortic 02CF
  Mitral 02CG
  Pulmonary 02CH
  Tricuspid 02CJ
Vas Deferens
  Bilateral 0VCQ
  Left 0VCP
  Right 0VCN
Vein
  Axillary
    Left 05C8
    Right 05C7
  Azygos 05C0
  Basilic
    Left 05CC
    Right 05CB
  Brachial
    Left 05CA
    Right 05C9
  Cephalic
    Left 05CF
    Right 05CD
  Colic 06C7
  Common Iliac
    Left 06CD
    Right 06CC
  Coronary 02C4
  Esophageal 06C3
  External Iliac
    Left 06CG
    Right 06CF
  External Jugular
    Left 05CQ
    Right 05CP
  Face
    Left 05CV
    Right 05CT

Extirpation (continued)
Vein (continued)
  Femoral
    Left 06CN
    Right 06CM
  Foot
    Left 06CV
    Right 06CT
  Gastric 06C2
  Hand
    Left 05CH
    Right 05CG
  Hemiazygos 05C1
  Hepatic 06C4
  Hypogastric
    Left 06CJ
    Right 06CH
  Inferior Mesenteric 06C6
  Innominate
    Left 05C4
    Right 05C3
  Internal Jugular
    Left 05CN
    Right 05CM
  Intracranial 05CL
  Lower 06CY
  Portal 06C8
  Pulmonary
    Left 02CT
    Right 02CS
  Renal
    Left 06CB
    Right 06C9
  Saphenous
    Left 06CQ
    Right 06CP
  Splenic 06C1
  Subclavian
    Left 05C6
    Right 05C5
  Superior Mesenteric 06C5
  Upper 05CY
  Vertebral
    Left 05CS
    Right 05CR
Vena Cava
  Inferior 06C0
  Superior 02CV
Ventricle
  Left 02CL
  Right 02CK
Vertebra
  Cervical 0PC3
  Lumbar 0QC0
  Thoracic 0PC4
Vesicle
  Bilateral 0VC3
  Left 0VC2
  Right 0VC1
Vitreous
  Left 08C5
  Right 08C4
Vocal Cord
  Left 0CCV
  Right 0CCT
Vulva 0UCM
Extracorporeal shock wave lithotripsy
see Fragmentation
Extracranial-intracranial bypass (EC-IC)
see Bypass, Upper Arteries 031
Extracorporeal Carbon Dioxide Removal (ECCO2R) 5A0920Z
Extraction
Acetabulum
  Left 0QD50ZZ
  Right 0QD40ZZ
Ampulla of Vater 0FDC

Extraction (continued)
Anus 0DDQ
Appendix 0DDJ
Auditory Ossicle
  Left 09DA0ZZ
  Right 09D90ZZ
Bone
  Ethmoid
    Left 0NDG0ZZ
    Right 0NDF0ZZ
  Frontal 0ND10ZZ
  Hyoid 0NDX0ZZ
  Lacrimal
    Left 0NDJ0ZZ
    Right 0NDH0ZZ
  Nasal 0NDB0ZZ
  Occipital 0ND70ZZ
  Palatine
    Left 0NDL0ZZ
    Right 0NDK0ZZ
  Parietal
    Left 0ND40ZZ
    Right 0ND30ZZ
  Pelvic
    Left 0QD30ZZ
    Right 0QD20ZZ
  Sphenoid 0NDC0ZZ
  Temporal
    Left 0ND60ZZ
    Right 0ND50ZZ
  Zygomatic
    Left 0NDN0ZZ
    Right 0NDM0ZZ
Bone Marrow 07DT
  Iliac 07DR
  Sternum 07DQ
  Vertebral 07DS
Brain 00D0
Breast
  Bilateral 0HDV
  Left 0HDU
  Right 0HDT
  Supernumerary 0HDY
Bronchus
  Lingula 0BD9
  Lower Lobe
    Left 0BDB
    Right 0BD6
  Main
    Left 0BD7
    Right 0BD3
  Middle Lobe, Right 0BD5
  Upper Lobe
    Left 0BD8
    Right 0BD4
Bursa and Ligament
  Abdomen
    Left 0MDJ
    Right 0MDH
  Ankle
    Left 0MDR
    Right 0MDQ
  Elbow
    Left 0MD4
    Right 0MD3
  Foot
    Left 0MDT
    Right 0MDS
  Hand
    Left 0MD8
    Right 0MD7
  Head and Neck 0MD0
  Hip
    Left 0MDM
    Right 0MDL
  Knee
    Left 0MDP
    Right 0MDN
  Lower Extremity
    Left 0MDW
    Right 0MDV

Extraction (continued)

Bursa and Ligament (continued)
  Perineum 0MDK
  Rib(s) 0MDG
  Shoulder
    Left 0MD2
    Right 0MD1
  Spine
    Lower 0MDD
    Upper 0MDC
  Sternum 0MDF
  Upper Extremity
    Left 0MDB
    Right 0MD9
  Wrist
    Left 0MD6
    Right 0MD5
Carina 0BD2
Carpal
  Left 0PDN0ZZ
  Right 0PDM0ZZ
Cecum 0DDH
Cerebral Hemisphere 00D7
Cerebral Meninges 00D1
Cisterna Chyli 07DL
Clavicle
  Left 0PDB0ZZ
  Right 0PD90ZZ
Coccyx 0QDS0ZZ
Colon
  Ascending 0DDK
  Descending 0DDM
  Sigmoid 0DDN
  Transverse 0DDL
Cornea
  Left 08D9XZZ
  Right 08D8XZ
Duct
  Common Bile 0FD9
  Cystic 0FD8
  Hepatic
    Common 0FD7
    Left 0FD6
    Right 0FD5
  Pancreatic 0FDD
    Accessory 0FDF
Duodenum 0DD9
Dura Mater 00D2
Endometrium 0UDB
Esophagogastric Junction 0DD4
Esophagus 0DD5
  Lower 0DD3
  Middle 0DD2
  Upper 0DD1
Femoral Shaft
  Left 0QD90ZZ
  Right 0QD80ZZ
Femur
  Lower
    Left 0QDC0ZZ
    Right 0QDB0ZZ
  Upper
    Left 0QD70ZZ
    Right 0QD60ZZ
Fibula
  Left 0QDK0ZZ
  Right 0QDJ0ZZ
Finger Nail 0HDQXZZ
Gallbladder 0FD4
Glenoid Cavity
  Left 0PD80ZZ
  Right 0PD70ZZ
Hair 0HDSXZZ
Humeral Head
  Left 0PDD0ZZ
  Right 0PDC0ZZ
Humeral Shaft
  Left 0PDG0ZZ
  Right 0PDF0ZZ
Ileocecal Valve 0DDC
Ileum 0DDB

Intestine
  Large 0DDE
    Left 0DDG
    Right 0DDF
  Small 0DD8
Jejunum 0DDA
Kidney
  Left 0TD1
  Right 0TD0
Lens
  Left 08DK3ZZ
  Right 08DJ3ZZ
Liver 0FD0
  Left Lobe 0FD2
  Right Lobe 0FD1
Lung
  Bilateral 0BDM
  Left 0BDL
  Lower Lobe
    Left 0BDJ
    Right 0BDF
  Middle Lobe, Right 0BDD
  Right 0BDK
  Upper Lobe
    Left 0BDG
    Right 0BDC
Lung Lingula 0BDH
Lymphatic
  Aortic 07DD
  Axillary
    Left 07D6
    Right 07D5
  Head 07D0
  Inguinal
    Left 07DJ
    Right 07DH
  Internal Mammary
    Left 07D9
    Right 07D8
  Lower Extremity
    Left 07DG
    Right 07DF
  Mesenteric 07DB
  Neck
    Left 07D2
    Right 07D1
  Pelvis 07DC
  Thoracic Duct 07DK
  Thorax 07D7
  Upper Extermity
    Left 07D4
    Right 07D3
Mandible
  Left 0NDV0ZZ
  Right 0NDT0ZZ
Maxilla 0NDR0ZZ
Metacarpal
  Left 0PDQ0ZZ
  Right 0PDP0ZZ
Metatarsal
  Left 0QDP0ZZ
  Right 0QDN0ZZ
Muscle
  Abdomen
    Left 0KDL0ZZ
    Right 0KDK0ZZ
  Facial 0KD10ZZ
  Foot
    Left 0KDW0ZZ
    Right 0KDV0ZZ
  Hand
    Left 0KDD0ZZ
    Right 0KDC0ZZ
  Head 0KD00ZZ
  Hip
    Left 0KDP0ZZ
    Right 0KD90ZZ
  Lower Arm and Wrist
    Left 0KDB0ZZ
    Right 0KD90ZZ

Muscle (continued)
  Lower Leg
    Left 0KDT0ZZ
    Right 0KDS0ZZ
  Neck
    Left 0KD30ZZ
    Right 0KD20ZZ
  Perineum 0KDM0ZZ
  Shoulder
    Left 0KD60ZZ
    Right 0KD50ZZ
  Thorax
    Left 0KDJ0ZZ
    Right 0KDH0ZZ
  Tongue, Palate, Pharynx
    0KD40ZZ
  Trunk
    Left 0KDG0ZZ
    Right 0KDF0ZZ
  Upper Arm
    Left 0KD80ZZ
    Right 0KD70ZZ
  Upper Leg
    Left 0KDR0ZZ
    Right 0KDQ0ZZ
Nerve
  Abdominal Sympathetic 01DM
  Abducens 00DL
  Accessory 00DR
  Acoustic 00DN
  Brachial Plexus 01D3
  Cervical 01D1
  Cervical Plexus 01D0
  Facial 00DM
  Femoral 01DD
  Glossopharyngeal 00DP
  Head and Neck Sympathetic
    01DK
  Hypoglossal 00DS
  Lumbar 01DB
  Lumbar Plexus 01D9
  Lumbar Sympathetic 01DN
  Lumbosacral Plexus 01DA
  Median 01D5
  Oculomotor 00DH
  Olfactory 00DF
  Optic 00DG
  Peroneal 01DH
  Phrenic 01D2
  Pudendal 01DC
  Radial 01D6
  Sacral 01DR
  Sacral Plexus 01DQ
  Sacral Sympathetic 01DP
  Sciatic 01DF
  Thoracic 01D8
  Thoracic Sympathetic 01DL
  Tibial 01DG
  Trigeminal 00DK
  Trochlear 00DJ
  Ulnar 01D4
  Vagus 00DQ
Orbit
  Left 0NDQ0ZZ
  Right 0NDP0ZZ
Ova 0UDN
Pancreas 0FDG
Patella
  Left 0QDF0ZZ
  Right 0QDD0ZZ
Phalanx
  Finger
    Left 0PDV0ZZ
    Right 0PDT0ZZ
  Thumb
    Left 0PDS0ZZ
    Right 0PDR0ZZ
  Toe
    Left 0QDR0ZZ
    Right 0QDQ0ZZ

Pleura
  Left 0BDP
  Right 0BDN
Products of Conception
  Ectopic 10D2
  Extraperitoneal 10D00Z2
  High 10D00Z0
  High Forceps 10D07Z5
  Internal Version 10D07Z7
  Low 10D00Z1
  Low Forceps
    10D07Z3
  Mid Forceps 10D07Z4
  Other 10D07Z8
  Retained 10D1
  Vacuum 10D07Z6
Radius
  Left 0PDJ0ZZ
  Right 0PDH0ZZ
Rectum 0DDP
Ribs
  1 to 2 0PD10ZZ
  3 or More 0PD20ZZ
Sacrum 0QD10ZZ
Scapula
  Left 0PD60ZZ
  Right 0PD50ZZ
Septum, Nasal 09DM
Sinus
  Accessory 09DP
  Ethmoid
    Left 09DV
    Right 09DU
  Frontal
    Left 09DT
    Right 09DS
  Mastoid
    Left 09DC
    Right 09DB
  Maxillary
    Left 09DR
    Right 09DQ
  Sphenoid
    Left 09DX
    Right 09DW
Skin
  Abdomen 0HD7XZZ
  Back 0HD6XZZ
  Buttock 0HD8XZZ
  Chest 0HD5XZZ
  Ear
    Left 0HD3XZZ
    Right 0HD2XZZ
  Face 0HD1XZZ
  Foot
    Left 0HDNXZZ
    Right 0HDMXZZ
  Hand
    Left 0HDGXZZ
    Right 0HDFXZZ
  Inguinal 0HDAXZZ
  Lower Arm
    Left 0HDEXZZ
    Right 0HDDXZZ
  Lower Leg
    Left 0HDLXZZ
    Right 0HDKXZZ
  Neck 0HD4XZZ
  Perineum 0HD9XZZ
  Scalp 0HD0XZZ
  Upper Arm
    Left 0HDCXZZ
    Right 0HDBXZZ
  Upper Leg
    Left 0HDJXZZ
    Right 0HDHXZZ
Skull 0ND00ZZ
Spinal Meninges 00DT
Spleen 07DP
Sternum 0PD00ZZ

Extraction *(continued)*
  Stomach 0DD6
    Pylorus 0DD7
  Subcutaneous Tissue and Fascia
    Abdomen 0JD8
    Back 0JD7
    Buttock 0JD9
    Chest 0JD6
    Face 0JD1
    Foot
      Left 0JDR
      Right 0JDQ
    Hand
      Left 0JDK
      Right 0JDJ
    Lower Arm
      Left 0JDH
      Right 0JDG
    Lower Leg
      Left 0JDP
      Right 0JDN
    Neck
      Left 0JD5
      Right 0JD4
    Pelvic Region 0JDC
    Perineum 0JDB
    Scalp 0JD0
    Upper Arm
      Left 0JDF
      Right 0JDD
    Upper Leg
      Left 0JDM
      Right 0JDL
  Tarsal
    Left 0QDM0ZZ
    Right 0QDL0ZZ
  Tendon
    Abdomen
      Left 0LDG0ZZ
      Right 0LDF0ZZ
    Ankle
      Left 0LDT0ZZ
      Right 0LDS0ZZ
    Foot
      Left 0LDW0ZZ
      Right 0LDV0ZZ
    Hand
      Left 0LD80ZZ
      Right 0LD70ZZ
    Head and Neck
      0LD00ZZ
    Hip
      Left 0LDK0ZZ
      Right 0LDJ0ZZ
    Knee
      Left 0LDR0ZZ
      Right 0LDQ0ZZ
    Lower Arm and Wrist
      Left 0LD60ZZ
      Right 0LD50ZZ
    Lower Leg
      Left 0LDP0ZZ
      Right 0LDN0ZZ
    Perineum 0LDH0ZZ
    Shoulder
      Left 0LD20ZZ
      Right 0LD10ZZ
    Thorax
      Left 0LDD0ZZ
      Right 0LDC0ZZ
    Trunk
      Left 0LDB0ZZ
      Right 0LD90ZZ
    Upper Arm
      Left 0LD40ZZ
      Right 0LD30ZZ
    Upper Leg
      Left 0LDM0ZZ
      Right 0LDL0ZZ
  Thymus 07DM

Extraction *(continued)*
  Tibia
    Left 0QDH0ZZ
    Right 0QDG0ZZ
  Toe Nail 0HDRXZZ
  Tooth
    Lower 0CDXXZ
    Upper 0CDWXZ
  Trachea 0BD1
  Turbinate, Nasal 09DL
  Tympanic Membrane
    Left 09D8
    Right 09D7
  Ulna
    Left 0PDL0ZZ
    Right 0PDK0ZZ
  Vein
    Basilic
      Left 05DC
      Right 05DB
    Brachial
      Left 05DA
      Right 05D9
    Cephalic
      Left 05DF
      Right 05DD
    Femoral
      Left 06DN
      Right 06DM
    Foot
      Left 06DV
      Right 06DT
    Hand
      Left 05DH
      Right 05DG
    Lower 06DY
    Saphenous
      Left 06DQ
      Right 06DP
    Upper 05DY
  Vertebra
    Cervical 0PD30ZZ
    Lumbar 0QD00ZZ
    Thoracic 0PD40ZZ
  Vocal Cord
    Left 0CDV
    Right 0CDT
Extradural space, intracranial
  use Epidural Space, Intracranial
Extradural space, spinal
  use Spinal Canal
EXtreme Lateral Interbody Fusion (XLIF) device
  use Interbody Fusion Device in Lower Joints

F

Face lift
  see Alteration, Face 0W02
Facet replacement spinal stabilization device
  use Spinal Stabilization Device, Facet Replacement in 0RH
  use Spinal Stabilization Device, Facet Replacement in 0SH
Facial artery
  use Artery, Face
Factor Xa Inhibitor Reversal Agent, Andexanet Alfa
  use Coagulation Factor Xa, Inactivated
False vocal cord
  use Larynx
Falx cerebri
  use Dura Mater
Fascia lata
  use Subcutaneous Tissue and Fascia, Upper Leg, Left

Fascia lata *(continued)*
  use Subcutaneous Tissue and Fascia, Upper Leg, Right
Fasciaplasty, fascioplasty
  see Repair, Subcutaneous Tissue and Fascia 0JQ
  see Replacement, Subcutaneous Tissue and Fascia 0JR
Fasciectomy
  see Excision, Subcutaneous Tissue and Fascia 0JB
  see Release
Fasciorrhaphy
  see Repair, Subcutaneous Tissue and Fascia 0JQ
Fasciotomy
  see Division, Subcutaneous Tissue and Fascia 0J8
  see Drainage, Subcutaneous Tissue and Fascia 0J9
  see Release
Feeding Device
  Change device in
    Lower 0D2DXUZ
    Upper 0D20XUZ
  Insertion of device in
    Duodenum 0DH9
    Esophagus 0DH5
    Ileum 0DHB
    Intestine, Small 0DH8
    Jejunum 0DHA
    Stomach 0DH6
  Removal of device from
    Esophagus 0DP5
    Intestinal Tract
      Lower 0DPD
      Upper 0DP0
    Stomach 0DP6
  Revision of device in
    Intestinal Tract
      Lower 0DWD
      Upper 0DW0
    Stomach 0DW6
Femoral head
  use Femur, Upper, Left
  use Femur, Upper, Right
Femoral lymph node
  use Lymphatic, Lower Extremity, Left
  use Lymphatic, Lower Extremity, Right
Femoropatellar joint
  use Joint, Knee, Left
  use Joint, Knee, Left, Femoral Surface
  use Joint, Knee, Right
  use Joint, Knee, Right, Femoral Surface
Femorotibial joint
  use Joint, Knee, Left
  use Joint, Knee, Left, Tibial Surface
  use Joint, Knee, Right
  use Joint, Knee, Right, Tibial Surface
FETROJA®
  use Cefiderocol Anti-infective
FGS (fluorescence-guided surgery)
  see Fluorescence Guided Procedure
Fibular artery
  use Artery, Peroneal, Left
  use Artery, Peroneal, Right
Fibular sesamoid
  use Metatarsal, Left
  use Metatarsal, Right
Fibularis brevis muscle
  use Muscle, Lower Leg, Left
  use Muscle, Lower Leg, Right
Fibularis longus muscle
  use Muscle, Lower Leg, Left
  use Muscle, Lower Leg, Right

Fifth cranial nerve
  use Nerve, Trigeminal
Filum terminale
  use Spinal Meninges
Fimbriectomy
  see Excision, Female Reproductive System 0UB
  see Resection, Female Reproductive System 0UT
Fine needle aspiration
  Fluid or gas
    see Drainage
  Tissue biopsy
    see Excision
    see Extraction
First cranial nerve
  use Nerve, Olfactory
First intercostal nerve
  use Nerve, Brachial Plexus
Fistulization
  see Bypass
  see Drainage
  see Repair
Fitting
  Arch bars, for fracture reduction
    see Reposition, Mouth and Throat 0CS
  Arch bars, for immobilization
    see Immobilization, Face 2W31
  Artificial limb
    see Device Fitting, Rehabilitation F0D
  Hearing aid
    see Device Fitting, Rehabilitation F0D
  Ocular prosthesis F0DZ8UZ
  Prosthesis, limb
    see Device Fitting, Rehabilitation F0D
  Prosthesis, ocular F0DZ8UZ
Fixation, bone
  External, with fracture reduction
    see Reposition
  External, without fracture reduction
    see Insertion
  Internal, with fracture reduction
    see Reposition
  Internal, without fracture reduction
    see Insertion
FLAIR® Endovascular Stent Graft
  use Intraluminal Device
Flexible Composite Mesh
  use Synthetic Substitute
Flexor carpi radialis muscle
  use Muscle, Lower Arm and Wrist, Left
  use Muscle, Lower Arm and Wrist, Right
Flexor carpi ulnaris muscle
  use Muscle, Lower Arm and Wrist, Left
  use Muscle, Lower Arm and Wrist, Right
Flexor digitorum brevis muscle
  use Muscle, Foot, Left
  use Muscle, Foot, Right
Flexor digitorum longus muscle
  use Muscle, Lower Leg, Left
  use Muscle, Lower Leg, Right
Flexor hallucis brevis muscle
  use Muscle, Foot, Left
  use Muscle, Foot, Right
Flexor hallucis longus muscle
  use Muscle, Lower Leg, Left
  use Muscle, Lower Leg, Right
Flexor pollicis longus muscle
  use Muscle, Lower Arm and Wrist, Left
  use Muscle, Lower Arm and Wrist, Right

Flow Diverter embolization device
use Intraluminal Device, Flow
Diverter in 03V
FlowSense Noninvasive Thermal Sensor
see Measurement, Central Nervous
Cerebrospinal Fluid Shunt
Fluorescence Guided Procedure
Extremity
Lower 8E0Y
Upper 8E0X
Head and Neck Region 8E09
Aminolevulinic Acid 8E09
No Qualifier 8E09
Trunk Region 8E0W
Fluorescent Pyrazine, Kidney
XT25XE5
Fluoroscopy
Abdomen and Pelvis BW11
Airway, Upper BB1DZZZ
Ankle
Left BQ1
Right BQ1G
Aorta
Abdominal B410
Laser, Intraoperative B410
Thoracic B310
Laser, Intraoperative B310
Thoraco-Abdominal B31P
Laser, Intraoperative B31P
Aorta and Bilateral Lower
Extremity Arteries B41D
Laser, Intraoperative B41D
Arm
Left BP1FZZZ
Right BP1EZZZ
Artery
Brachiocephalic-Subclavian
Right B311
Laser, Intraoperative B311
Bronchial B31L
Laser, Intraoperative B31L
Bypass Graft, Other B21F
Cervico-Cerebral Arch B31Q
Laser, Intraoperative B31Q
Common Carotid
Bilateral B315
Laser, Intraoperative B315
Left B314
Laser, Intraoperative B314
Right B313
Laser, Intraoperative B313
Coronary
Bypass Graft
Multiple B213
Laser, Intraoperative B213
Single B212
Laser, Intraoperative
B212
Multiple B211
Laser, Intraoperative B211
Single B210
Laser, Intraoperative B210
External Carotid
Bilateral B31C
Laser, Intraoperative B31C
Left B31B
Laser, Intraoperative B31B
Right B319
Laser, Intraoperative B319
Hepatic B412
Laser, Intraoperative B412
Inferior Mesenteric B415
Laser, Intraoperative B415
Intercostal B31L
Laser, Intraoperative B31L
Internal Carotid
Bilateral B318
Laser, Intraoperative B318
Left B317
Laser, Intraoperative B317

Fluoroscopy (continued)
Artery (continued)
Internal Carotid (continued)
Right B316
Laser, Intraoperative B316
Internal Mammary Bypass Graft
Left B218
Right B217
Intra-Abdominal
Laser, Intraoperative B41B
Other B41B
Intracranial B31R
Laser, Intraoperative B31R
Lower
Laser, Intraoperative B41J
Other B41J
Lower Extremity
Bilateral and Aorta B41D
Laser, Intraoperative B41D
Left B41G
Laser, Intraoperative B41G
Right B41F
Laser, Intraoperative B41F
Lumbar B419
Laser, Intraoperative B419
Pelvic B41C
Laser, Intraoperative B41C
Pulmonary
Left B31T
Laser, Intraoperative B31T
Right B31S
Laser, Intraoperative
B31S
Pulmonary Trunk B31U
Laser, Intraoperative B31U
Renal
Bilateral B418
Laser, Intraoperative B418
Left B417
Laser, Intraoperative B417
Right B416
Laser, Intraoperative B416
Spinal B31M
Laser, Intraoperative B31M
Splenic B413
Laser, Intraoperative B413
Subclavian
Laser, Intraoperative B312
Left B312
Superior Mesenteric
B414
Laser, Intraoperative B414
Upper
Laser, Intraoperative B31N
Other B31N
Upper Extremity
Bilateral B31K
Laser, Intraoperative B31K
Left B31J
Laser, Intraoperative B31J
Right B31H
Laser, Intraoperative B31H
Vertebral
Bilateral B31G
Laser, Intraoperative B31G
Left B31F
Laser, Intraoperative B31F
Right B31D
Laser, Intraoperative
B31D
Bile Duct BF10
Pancreatic Duct and Gallbladder
BF14
Bile Duct and Gallbladder BF13
Biliary Duct BF11
Bladder BT10
Kidney and Ureter BT14
Left BT1F
Right BT1D
Bladder and Urethra BT1B
Bowel, Small BD1

Fluoroscopy (continued)
Calcaneus
Left BQ1KZZZ
Right BQ1JZZZ
Clavicle
Left BP15ZZZ
Right BP14ZZZ
Coccyx BR1F
Colon BD14
Corpora Cavernosa BV10
Dialysis Fistula B51W
Dialysis Shunt B51W
Diaphragm BB16ZZZ
Disc
Cervical BR11
Lumbar BR13
Thoracic BR12
Duodenum BD19
Elbow
Left BP1H
Right BP1G
Epiglottis B91G
Esophagus BD11
Extremity
Lower BW1C
Upper BW1J
Facet Joint
Cervical BR14
Lumbar BR16
Thoracic BR15
Fallopian Tube
Bilateral BU12
Left BU11
Right BU10
Fallopian Tube and Uterus
BU18
Femur
Left BQ14ZZZ
Right BQ13ZZZ
Finger
Left BP1SZZZ
Right BP1RZZZ
Foot
Left BQ1MZZZ
Right BQ1LZZZ
Forearm
Left BP1KZZZ
Right BP1JZZZ
Gallbladder BF12
Bile Duct and Pancreatic Duct
BF14
Gallbladder and Bile Duct
BF13
Gastrointestinal, Upper BD1
Hand
Left BP1PZZZ
Right BP1NZZZ
Head and Neck BW19
Heart
Left B215
Right B214
Right and Left B216
Hip
Left BQ11
Right BQ10
Humerus
Left BP1BZZZ
Right BP1AZZZ
Ileal Diversion Loop BT1C
Ileal Loop, Ureters and Kidney
BT1G
Intracranial Sinus B512
Joint
Acromioclavicular, Bilateral
BP13ZZZ
Finger
Left BP1D
Right BP1C
Foot
Left BQ1Y
Right BQ1X

Fluoroscopy (continued)
Joint (continued)
Hand
Left BP1D
Right BP1C
Lumbosacral BR1B
Sacroiliac BR1D
Sternoclavicular
Bilateral BP12ZZZ
Left BP11ZZZ
Right BP10ZZZ
Temporomandibular
Bilateral BN19
Left BN18
Right BN17
Thoracolumbar BR18
Toe
Left BQ1Y
Right BQ1X
Kidney
Bilateral BT13
Ileal Loop and Ureter BT1G
Left BT12
Right BT11
Ureter and Bladder BT14
Left BT1F
Right BT1D
Knee
Left BQ18
Right BQ17
Larynx B91J
Leg
Left BQ1FZZZ
Right BQ1DZZZ
Liver BF15
Lung
Bilateral BB14ZZZ
Left BB13ZZZ
Right BB12ZZZ
Mediastinum BB1CZZZ
Mouth BD1B
Neck and Head BW19
Oropharynx BD1B
Pancreatic Duct BF1
Gallbladder and Bile Buct
BF14
Patella
Left BQ1WZZZ
Right BQ1VZZZ
Pelvis BR1C
Pelvis and Abdomen BW11
Pharynix B91G
Ribs
Left BP1YZZZ
Right BP1XZZZ
Sacrum BR1F
Scapula
Left BP17ZZZ
Right BP16ZZZ
Shoulder
Left BP19
Right BP18
Sinus, Intracranial B512
Spinal Cord B01B
Spine
Cervical BR10
Lumbar BR19
Thoracic BR17
Whole BR1G
Sternum BR1H
Stomach BD12
Toe
Left BQ1QZZZ
Right BQ1PZZZ
Tracheobronchial Tree
Bilateral BB19YZZ
Left BB18YZZ
Right BB17YZZ
Ureter
Ileal Loop and Kidney
BT1G

Fluoroscopy *(continued)*
  Ureter *(continued)*
    Kidney and Bladder BT14
      Left BT1F
      Right BT1D
    Left BT17
    Right BT16
  Urethra BT15
  Urethra and Bladder BT1B
  Uterus BU16
  Uterus and Fallopian Tube BU18
  Vagina BU19
  Vasa Vasorum BV18
  Vein
    Cerebellar B511
    Cerebral B511
    Epidural B510
    Jugular
      Bilateral B515
      Left B514
      Right B513
    Lower Extremity
      Bilateral B51D
      Left B51C
      Right B51B
    Other B51V
    Pelvic (Iliac)
      Left B51G
      Right B51F
    Pelvic (Iliac) Bilateral B51H
    Portal B51T
    Pulmonary
      Bilateral B51S
      Left B51R
      Right B51Q
    Renal
      Bilateral B51L
      Left B51K
      Right B51J
    Spanchnic B51T
    Subclavian
      Left B517
      Right B516
    Upper Extremity
      Bilateral B51P
      Left B51N
      Right B51M
  Vena Cava
    Inferior B519
    Superior B518
  Wrist
    Left BP1M
    Right BP1L
Fluoroscopy, laser intraoperative
  Fluoroscopy, Heart B21
  Fluoroscopy, Lower Arteries B41
  Fluoroscopy, Upper Arteries B31
Flushing
  see Irrigation
Foley catheter
  use Drainage Device
Fontan completion procedure Stage II
  see Bypass, Vena Cava, Inferior 0610
Foramen magnum
  use Occipital Bone
Foramen of Monro (intraventricular)
  use Cerebral Ventricle
Foreskin
  use Prepuce
Formula™ Balloon-Expandable Renal Stent System
  use Intraluminal Device
Fosfomycin Anti-infective XW0
Fosfomycin injection
  use Fosfomycin Anti-infective
Fossa of Rosenmuller
  use Nasopharynx

Fourth cranial nerve
  use Nerve, Trochlear
Fourth ventricle
  use Cerebral Ventricle
Fovea
  use Retina, Left
  use Retina, Right
Fragmentation
  Ampulla of Vater 0FFC
  Anus 0DFQ
  Appendix 0DFJ
  Artery
    Anterior Tibial
      Left 04FQ3Z
      Right 04FP3Z
    Axillary
      Left 03F63Z
      Right 03F53Z
    Brachial
      Left 03F83Z
      Right 03F73Z
    Common Iliac
      Left 04FD3Z
      Right 04FC3Z
    Coronary
      Four or More Arteries 02F33ZZ
      One Artery 02F03ZZ
      Three Arteries 02F23ZZ
      Two Arteries 02F13ZZ
    External Iliac
      Left 04FJ3Z
      Right 04FH3Z
    Femoral
      Left 04FL3Z
      Right 04FK3Z
    Innominate 03F23Z
    Internal Iliac
      Left 04FF3Z
      Right 04FE3Z
    Intracranial 03FG3Z
    Lower 04FY3Z
    Peroneal
      Left 04FU3Z
      Right 04FT3Z
    Popliteal
      Left 04FN3Z
      Right 04FM3Z
    Posterior Tibial
      Left 04FS3Z
      Right 04FR3Z
    Pulmonary
      Left 02FR3Z
      Right 02FQ3Z
    Pulmonary Trunk 02FP3Z
    Radial
      Left 03FC3Z
      Right 03FB3Z
    Subclavian
      Left 03F43Z
      Right 03F33Z
    Ulnar
      Left 03FA3Z
      Right 03F93Z
    Upper 03FY3Z
  Bladder 0TFB
  Bladder Neck 0TFC
  Bronchus
    Lingula 0BF9
    Lower Lobe
      Left 0BFB
      Right 0BF6
    Main
      Left 0BF7
      Right 0BF3
    Middle Lobe, Right 0BF5
    Upper Lobe
      Left 0BF8
      Right 0BF4
  Carina 0BF2
  Cavity, Cranial 0WF1

Fragmentation *(continued)*
  Cecum 0DFH
  Cerebral Ventricle 00F6
  Colon
    Ascending 0DFK
    Descending 0DFM
    Sigmoid 0DFN
    Transverse 0DFL
  Duct
    Common Bile 0FF9
    Cystic 0FF8
    Hepatic
      Common 0FF7
      Left 0FF6
      Right 0FF5
    Pancreatic 0FFD
      Accessory 0FFF
    Parotid
      Left 0CFC
      Right 0CFB
  Duodenum 0DF9
  Epidural Space, Intracranial 00F3
  Esophagus 0DF5
  Fallopian Tube
    Left 0UF6
    Right 0UF5
  Fallopian Tubes, Bilateral 0UF7
  Gallbladder 0FF4
  Gastrointestinal Tract 0WFP
  Genitourinary Tract 0WFR
  Ileum 0DFB
  Intestine
    Large 0DFE
      Left 0DFG
      Right 0DFF
    Small 0DF8
  Jejunum 0DFA
  Kidney Pelvis
    Left 0TF4
    Right 0TF3
  Mediastinum 0WFC
  Oral Cavity and Throat 0WF3
  Pelvic Cavity 0WFJ
  Pericardial Cavity 0WFD
  Pericardium 02FN
  Peritoneal Cavity 0WFG
  Pleural Cavity
    Left 0WFB
    Right 0WF9
  Rectum 0DFP
  Respiratory Tract 0WFQ
  Spinal Canal 00FU
  Stomach 0DF6
  Subarachnoid Space, Intracranial 00F5
  Subdural Space, Intracranial 00F4
  Trachea 0BF1
  Ureter
    Left 0TF7
    Right 0TF6
  Urethra 0TFD
  Uterus 0UF9
  Vein
    Axillary
      Left 05F83Z
      Right 05F73Z
    Basilic
      Left 05FC3Z
      Right 05FB3Z
    Brachial
      Left 05FA3Z
      Right 05F93Z
    Cephalic
      Left 05FF3Z
      Right 05FD3Z
    Common Iliac
      Left 06FD3Z
      Right 06FC3Z
    External Iliac
      Left 06FG3Z
      Right 06FF3Z

Fragmentation *(continued)*
  Vein *(continued)*
    Femoral
      Left 06FN3Z
      Right 06FM3Z
    Hypogastric
      Left 06FJ3Z
      Right 06FH3Z
    Innominate
      Left 05F43Z
      Right 05F33Z
    Lower 06FY3Z
    Pulmonary
      Left 02FT3Z
      Right 02FS3Z
    Saphenous
      Left 06FQ3Z
      Right 06FP3Z
    Subclavian
      Left 05F63Z
      Right 05F53Z
    Upper 05FY3Z
  Vitreous
    Left 08F5
    Right 08F4
Fragmentation, Ultrasonic
  see Fragmentation, Artery
Freestyle (Stentless) Aortic Root Bioprosthesis
  use Zooplastic Tissue in Heart and Great Vessels
Frenectomy
  see Excision, Mouth and Throat 0CB
  see Resection, Mouth and Throat 0CT
Frenoplasty, frenuloplasty
  see Repair, Mouth and Throat 0CQ
  see Replacement, Mouth and Throat 0CR
  see Supplement, Mouth and Throat 0CU
Frenotomy
  see Drainage, Mouth and Throat 0C9
  see Release, Mouth and Throat 0CN
Frenulotomy
  see Drainage, Mouth and Throat 0C9
  see Release, Mouth and Throat 0CN
Frenulum labii inferioris
  use Lip, Lower
Frenulum labii superioris
  use Lip, Upper
Frenulum linguae
  use Tongue
Frenulumectomy
  see Excision, Mouth and Throat 0CB
  see Resection, Mouth and Throat 0CT
Frontal lobe
  use Cerebral Hemisphere
Frontal vein
  use Vein, Face, Left
  use Vein, Face, Right
Frozen elephant trunk (FET) technique, aortic arch replacement
  see New Technology, Cardiovascular System X2R
  see Replacement, Heart and Great Vessels 02R
Frozen elephant trunk (FET) technique, thoracic aorta restriction
  see New Technology, Cardiovascular System X2V
  see Restriction, Heart and Great Vessels 02V

FUJIFILM EP-7000X System for Oxygen Saturation Endoscopic Imaging (OXEI)
see New Technology, Gastrointestinal System XD2

Fulguration
see Destruction

Fundoplication, gastroesophageal
see Restriction, Esophagogastric Junction 0DV4

Fundus uteri
use Uterus

Fusion
Acromioclavicular
 Left 0RGH
 Right 0RGG
Ankle
 Left 0SGG
 Right 0SGF
Carpal
 Left 0RGR
 Right 0RGQ
Carpometacarpal
 Left 0RGT
 Right 0RGS
Cervical Vertebral 0RG1
 2 or more 0RG2
  Interbody Fusion Device
   Nanotextured Surface XRG2092
   Radiolucent Porous XRG20F3
  Interbody Fusion Device, Nanotextured Surface XRG1092
   Radiolucent Porous XRG10F3
Cervicothoracic Vertebral 0RG4
 Interbody Fusion Device
  Nanotextured Surface XRG4092
  Radiolucent Porous XRG40F3
Coccygeal 0SG6
Elbow
 Left 0RGM
 Right 0RGL
Finger Phalangeal
 Left 0RGX
 Right 0RGW
Hip
 Left 0SGB
 Right 0SG9
Knee
 Left 0SGD
 Right 0SGC
Lumbar Vertebral 0SG0
 2 or more 0SG1
  Interbody Fusion Device
   Customizable XRGC
   Nanotextured Surface XRGC092
   Radiolucent Porous XRGC0F3
  Interbody Fusion Device
   Customizable XRGB
   Nanotextured Surface XRGB092
   Radiolucent Porous XRGB0F3
Lumbosacral 0SG3
 Interbody Fusion Device
  Customizable XRGD
  Nanotextured Surface XRGD092
  Radiolucent Porous XRGD0F3
Metacarpophalangeal
 Left 0RGV
 Right 0RGU
Metatarsal-Phalangeal
 Left 0SGN
 Right 0SGM

Fusion *(continued)*
Occipital-cervical 0RG0
 Interbody Fusion Device
  Nanotextured Surface XRG0092
  Radiolucent Porous XRG00F3
Sacrococcygeal 0SG5
Sacroiliac
 Left 0SG8
 Right 0SG7
Shoulder
 Left 0RGK
 Right 0RGJ
Sternoclavicular
 Left 0RGF
 Right 0RGE
Tarsal
 Left 0SGJ
 Right 0SGH
Tarsometatarsal
 Left 0SGL
 Right 0SGK
Temporomandibular
 Left 0RGD
 Right 0RGC
Thoracic Vertebral 0RG6
 2 to 7 0RG7
  Interbody Fusion Device Nanotextured Surface XRG7092
   Radiolucent Porous XRG70F3
 8 or more 0RG8
  Interbody Fusion Device
   Nanotextured Surface XRG8092
   Radiolucent Porous XRG80F3
  Interbody Fusion Device
   Nanotextured Surface XRG6092
   Radiolucent Porous XRG60F3
Thoracolumbar Vertebral 0RGA
 Interbody Fusion Device
  Customizable XRGA
  Nanotextured Surface XRGA092
  Radiolucent Porous XRGA0F3
Toe Phalangeal
 Left 0SGQ
 Right 0SGP
Wrist
 Left 0RGP
 Right 0RGN

Fusion screw (compression)(lag) (locking)
use Internal Fixation Device in Lower Joints
use Internal Fixation Device in Upper Joints

G

Gait training
see Motor Treatment, Rehabilitation F07

Galea aponeurotica
use Subcutaneous Tissue and Fascia, Scalp

Gammaglobulin
use Globulin

GammaTile™
use Radioactive Element, Cesium-131 Collagen Implant in 00H

GAMUNEX-C, for COVID-19 treatment
use High-Dose Intravenous Immune Globulin

Ganglion impar (ganglion of Walther)
use Nerve, Sacral Sympathetic

Ganglionectomy
Destruction of lesion
 see Destruction
Excision of lesion
 see Excision

Gasserian ganglion
use Nerve, Trigeminal

Gastrectomy
Partial
 see Excision, Stomach 0DB6
Total
 see Resection, Stomach 0DT6
Vertical (sleeve)
 see Excision, Stomach 0DB6

Gastric electrical stimulation (GES) lead
use Stimulator Lead in Gastrointestinal System

Gastric lymph node
use Lymphatic, Aortic

Gastric pacemaker lead
use Stimulator Lead in Gastrointestinal System

Gastric plexus
use Nerve, Abdominal Sympathetic

Gastrocnemius muscle
use Muscle, Lower Leg, Left
use Muscle, Lower Leg, Right

Gastrocolic ligament
use Omentum

Gastrocolic omentum
use Omentum

Gastrocolostomy
see Bypass, Gastrointestinal System 0D1
see Drainage, Gastrointestinal System 0D9

Gastroduodenal artery
use Artery, Hepatic

Gastroduodenectomy
see Excision, Gastrointestinal System 0DB
see Resection, Gastrointestinal System 0DT

Gastroduodenoscopy 0DJ08ZZ

Gastroenteroplasty
see Repair, Gastrointestinal System 0DQ
see Supplement, Gastrointestinal System 0DU

Gastroenterostomy
see Bypass, Gastrointestinal System 0D1
see Drainage, Gastrointestinal System 0D9

Gastroesophageal (GE) junction
use Esophagogastric Junction

Gastrogastrostomy
see Bypass, Stomach 0D16
see Drainage, Stomach 0D96

Gastrohepatic omentum
use Omentum

Gastrojejunostomy
see Bypass, Stomach 0D16
see Drainage, Stomach 0D96

Gastrolysis
see Release, Stomach 0DN6

Gastropexy
see Repair, Stomach 0DQ6
see Reposition, Stomach 0DS6

Gastrophrenic ligament
use Omentum

Gastroplasty
see Repair, Stomach 0DQ6
see Supplement, Stomach 0DU6

Gastroplication
see Restriction, Stomach 0DV6

Gastropylorectomy
see Excision, Gastrointestinal System 0DB

Gastrorrhaphy
see Repair, Stomach 0DQ6

Gastroscopy 0DJ68ZZ

Gastrosplenic ligament
use Omentum

Gastrostomy
see Bypass, Stomach 0D16
see Drainage, Stomach 0D96

Gastrotomy
see Drainage, Stomach 0D96

Gemellus muscle
use Muscle, Hip, Left
use Muscle, Hip, Right

Geniculate ganglion
use Nerve, Facial

Geniculate nucleus
use Thalamus

Genioglossus muscle
use Muscle, Tongue, Palate, Pharynx

Genioplasty
see Alteration, Jaw, Lower 0W05

Genitofemoral nerve
use Nerve, Lumbar Plexus

GIAPREZA™
use Synthetic Human Angiotensin II

Gilteritinib Antineoplastic XW0DXV5

Gingivectomy
see Excision, Mouth and Throat 0CB

Gingivoplasty
see Repair, Mouth and Throat 0CQ
see Replacement, Mouth and Throat 0CR
see Supplement, Mouth and Throat 0CU

Glans penis
use Prepuce

Glenohumeral joint
use Joint, Shoulder, Left
use Joint, Shoulder, Right

Glenohumeral ligament
use Bursa and Ligament, Shoulder, Left
use Bursa and Ligament, Shoulder, Right

Glenoid fossa (of scapula)
use Glenoid Cavity, Left
use Glenoid Cavity, Right

Glenoid ligament (labrum)
use Shoulder Joint, Left
use Shoulder Joint, Right

Globus pallidus
use Basal Ganglia

Glomectomy
see Excision, Endocrine System 0GB
see Resection, Endocrine System 0GT

Glossectomy
see Excision, Tongue 0CB7
see Resection, Tongue 0CT7

Glossoepiglottic fold
use Epiglottis

Glossopexy
see Repair, Tongue 0CQ7
see Reposition, Tongue 0CS7

Glossoplasty
see Repair, Tongue 0CQ7
see Replacement, Tongue 0CR7
see Supplement, Tongue 0CU7

Glossorrhaphy
see Repair, Tongue 0CQ7

Glossotomy
see Drainage, Tongue 0C97

Glottis
use Larynx

Gluteal Artery Perforator Flap
Replacement
Bilateral 0HRV079
Left 0HRU079
Right 0HRT079
Transfer
Left 0KXG
Right 0KXF
Gluteal lymph node
use Lymphatic, Pelvis
Gluteal vein
use Vein, Hypogastric, Left
use Vein, Hypogastric, Right
Gluteus maximus muscle
use Muscle, Hip, Left
use Muscle, Hip, Right
Gluteus medius muscle
use Muscle, Hip, Left
use Muscle, Hip, Right
Gluteus minimus muscle
use Muscle, Hip, Left
use Muscle, Hip, Right
GORE® DUALMESH®
use Synthetic Substitute
GORE EXCLUDER® AAA Endoprosthesis
use Intraluminal Device
use Intraluminal Device, Branched or Fenestrated, One or Two Arteries in 04V
use Intraluminal Device, Branched or Fenestrated, Three or More Arteries in 04V
GORE EXCLUDER® IBE Endoprosthesis
use Intraluminal Device, Branched or Fenestrated, One or Two Arteries in 04V
GORE TAG® Thoracic Endoprosthesis
use Intraluminal Device
Gracilis muscle
use Muscle, Upper Leg, Left
use Muscle, Upper Leg, Right
Graft
see Replacement
see Supplement
Great auricular nerve
use Nerve, Cervical Plexus
Great cerebral vein
use Vein, Intracranial
Great(er) saphenous vein
use Vein, Saphenous, Left
use Vein, Saphenous, Right
Greater alar cartilage
use Nasal Mucosa and Soft Tissue
Greater occipital nerve
use Nerve, Cervical
Greater Omentum
use Omentum
Greater splanchnic nerve
use Nerve, Thoracic Sympathetic
Greater superficial petrosal nerve
use Nerve, Facial
Greater trochanter
use Femur, Upper, Left
use Femur, Upper, Right
Greater tuberosity
use Humeral Head, Left
use Humeral Head, Right
Greater vestibular (Bartholin's) gland
use Gland, Vestibular
Greater wing
use Bone, Sphenoid
GS-5734 *use* Remdesivir Anti-infective
Guedel airway
use Intraluminal Device, Airway in Mouth and Throat

Guidance, catheter placement
EKG
see Measurement, Physiological Systems 4A0
Fluoroscopy
see Fluoroscopy, Veins B51
Ultrasound
see Ultrasonography, Veins B54

H

Hallux
use Toe, 1st, Left
use Toe, 1st, Right
Hamate bone
use Carpal, Left
use Carpal, Right
Hancock Bioprosthesis (aortic) (mitral) valve
use Zooplastic Tissue in Heart and Great Vessels
Hancock Bioprosthetic Valved Conduit
use Zooplastic Tissue in Heart and Great Vessels
Harmony™ transcatheter pulmonary valve (TPV) placement 02RH38M
Harvesting, stem cells
see Pheresis, Circulatory 6A55
hdIVIG (high-dose intravenous immunogloblin), for COVID-19 treatment
use High-Dose Intravenous Immune Globulin
Head of fibula
use Fibula, Left
use Fibula, Right
Hearing Aid Assessment F14Z
Hearing Assessment F13Z
Hearing Device
Bone Conduction
Left 09HE
Right 09HD
Insertion of device in
Left 0NH6
Right 0NH5
Multiple Channel Cochlear Prosthesis
Left 09HE
Right 09HD
Removal of device from, Skull 0NP0
Revision of device in, Skull 0NW0
Single Channel Cochlear Prosthesis
Left 09HE
Right 09HD
Hearing Treatment F09Z
Heart Assist System
Implantable
Insertion of device in, Heart 02HA
Removal of device from, Heart 02PA
Revision of device in, Heart 02WA
Short-term External
Insertion of device in, Heart 02HA
Removal of device from, Heart 02PA
Revision of device in, Heart 02WA
HeartMate II® Left Ventricular Assist Device (LVAD)
use Implantable Heart Assist System in Heart and Great Vessels
HeartMate 3™ LVAS
use Implantable Heart Assist System in Heart and Great Vessels
HeartMate XVE® Left Ventricular Assist Device (LVAD)
use Implantable Heart Assist System in Heart and Great Vessels

HeartMate® implantable heart assist system
see Insertion of device in, Heart 02HA
Helix
use Ear, External, Bilateral
use Ear, External, Left
use Ear, External, Right
Hematopoietic cell transplant (HCT)
see Transfusion, Circulatory 302
Hemicolectomy
see Resection, Gastrointestinal System 0DT
Hemicystectomy
see Excision, Urinary System 0TB
Hemigastrectomy
see Excision, Gastrointestinal System 0DB
Hemiglossectomy
see Excision, Mouth and Throat 0CB
Hemilaminectomy
see Excision, Lower Bones 0QB
see Excision, Upper Bones 0PB
Hemilaminotomy
see Drainage, Lower Bones 0Q9
see Drainage, Upper Bones 0P9
see Excision, Lower Bones 0QB
see Excision, Upper Bones 0PB
see Release, Central Nervous System and Cranial Nerves 00N
see Release, Lower Bones 0QN
see Release, Peripheral Nervous System 01N
see Release, Upper Bones 0PN
Hemilaryngectomy
see Excision, Larynx 0CBS
Hemimandibulectomy
see Excision, Head and Facial Bones 0NB
Hemimaxillectomy
see Excision, Head and Facial Bones 0NB
Hemipylorectomy
see Excision, Gastrointestinal System 0DB
Hemispherectomy
see Excision, Central Nervous System and Cranial Nerves 00B
see Resection, Central Nervous System and Cranial Nerves 00T
Hemithyroidectomy
see Resection, Endocrine System 0GT
see Excision, Endocrine System 0GB
Hemodialysis
see Performance, Urinary 5A1D
Hemolung® Respiratory Assist System (RAS) 5A0920Z
Hemospray® Endoscopic Hemostat
use Mineral-based Topical Hemostatic Agent
Hepatectomy
see Excision, Hepatobiliary System and Pancreas 0FB
see Resection, Hepatobiliary System and Pancreas 0FT
Hepatic artery proper
use Artery, Hepatic
Hepatic flexure
use Colon, Transverse
Hepatic lymph node
use Lymphatic, Aortic
Hepatic plexus
use Nerve, Abdominal Sympathetic
Hepatic portal vein
use Vein, Portal
Hepaticoduodenostomy
see Bypass, Hepatobiliary System and Pancreas 0F1
see Drainage, Hepatobiliary System and Pancreas 0F9

Hepaticotomy
see Drainage, Hepatobiliary System and Pancreas 0F9
Hepatocholedochostomy
see Drainage, Duct, Common Bile 0F99
Hepatogastric ligament
use Omentum
Hepatopancreatic ampulla
use Ampulla of Vater
Hepatopexy
see Repair, Hepatobiliary System and Pancreas 0FQ
see Reposition, Hepatobiliary System and Pancreas 0FS
Hepatorrhaphy
see Repair, Hepatobiliary System and Pancreas 0FQ
Hepatotomy
see Drainage, Hepatobiliary System and Pancreas 0F9
Herculink (RX) Elite Renal Stent System
use Intraluminal Device
Herniorrhaphy
see Repair, Anatomical Regions, General 0WQ
see Repair, Anatomical Regions, Lower Extremities 0YQ
With synthetic substitute
see Supplement, Anatomical Regions, General 0WU
see Supplement, Anatomical Regions, Lower Extremities 0YU
HIG (hyperimmune globulin), for COVID-19 treatment
use Hyperimmune Globulin
High-Dose intravenous Immune Globulin, for COVID-19 treatment XW1
High-dose intravenous immunoglobulin (hdIVIG), for COVID-19 treatment
use High-Dose Intravenous Immune Globulin
Hip (joint) liner
use Liner in Lower Joints
HIPEC (hyperthermic intraperitoneal chemotherapy) 3E0M30Y
hIVIG (hyperimmune intravenous immunoglobulin), for COVID-19 treatment,
use Hyperimmune Globulin
Holter monitoring 4A12X45
Holter valve ventricular shunt
use Synthetic Substitute
Human angiotensin II, synthetic
use Synthetic Human Angiotensin II
Humeroradial joint
use Joint, Elbow, Left
use Joint, Elbow, Right
Humeroulnar joint
use Joint, Elbow, Left
use Joint, Elbow, Right
Humerus, distal
use Humeral Shaft, Left
use Humeral Shaft, Right
Hydrocelectomy
see Excision, Male Reproductive System 0VB
Hydrotherapy
Assisted exercise in pool
see Motor Treatment, Rehabilitation F07
Whirlpool
see Activities of Daily Living Treatment, Rehabilitation F08
Hymenectomy
see Excision, Hymen 0UBK
see Resection, Hymen 0UTK

Hymenoplasty
see Repair, Hymen 0UQK
see Supplement, Hymen 0UUK
Hymenorrhaphy
see Repair, Hymen 0UQK
Hymenotomy
see Division, Hymen 0U8K
see Drainage, Hymen 0U9K
Hyoglossus muscle
use Muscle, Tongue, Palate,
Pharynx
Hyoid artery
use Artery, Thyroid, Left
use Artery, Thyroid, Right
Hyperalimentation
see Introduction of substance in or on
Hyperbaric oxygenation
Decompression sickness
treatment
see Decompression, Circulatory
6A15
Wound treatment
see Assistance, Circulatory 5A05
Hyperimmune globulin
use Globulin
**Hyperimmune globulin, for
COVID-19 treatment** XW1
**Hyperimmune intravenous
immunoglobulin (hIVIG), for
COVID-19 treatment**
use Hyperimmune Globulin
Hyperthermia
Radiation Therapy
Abdomen DWY38ZZ
Adrenal Gland DGY28ZZ
Bile Ducts DFY28ZZ
Bladder DTY28ZZ
Bone, Other DPYC8ZZ
Bone Marrow D7Y08ZZ
Brain D0Y08ZZ
Brain Stem D0Y18ZZ
Breast
Left DMY08ZZ
Right DMY18ZZ
Bronchus DBY18ZZ
Cervix DUY18ZZ
Chest DWY28ZZ
Chest Wall DBY78ZZ
Colon DDY58ZZ
Diaphragm DBY88ZZ
Duodenum DDY28ZZ
Ear D9Y08ZZ
Esophagus DDY08ZZ
Eye D8Y08ZZ
Femur DPY98ZZ
Fibula DPYB8ZZ
Gallbladder DFY18ZZ
Gland
Adrenal DGY28ZZ
Parathyroid DGY48ZZ
Pituitary DGY08ZZ
Thyroid DGY58ZZ
Glands, Salivary D9Y68ZZ
Head and Neck DWY18ZZ
Hemibody DWY48ZZ
Humerus DPY68ZZ
Hypopharynx D9Y38ZZ
Ileum DDY48ZZ
Jejunum DDY38ZZ
Kidney DTY08ZZ
Larynx D9YB8ZZ
Liver DFY08ZZ
Lung DBY28ZZ
Lymphatics
Abdomen D7Y68ZZ
Axillary D7Y48ZZ
Inguinal D7Y88ZZ
Neck D7Y38ZZ
Pelvis D7Y78ZZ
Thorax D7Y58ZZ
Mandible DPY38ZZ

Hyperthermia *(continued)*
Radiation Therapy *(continued)*
Maxilla DPY28ZZ
Mediastinum DBY68ZZ
Mouth D9Y48ZZ
Nasopharynx D9YD8ZZ
Neck and Head DWY18ZZ
Nerve, Peripheral D0Y78ZZ
Nose D9Y18ZZ
Oropharynx D9YF8ZZ
Ovary DUY08ZZ
Palate
Hard D9Y88ZZ
Soft D9Y98ZZ
Pancreas DFY38ZZ
Parathyroid Gland DGY48ZZ
Pelvic Bones DPY88ZZ
Pelvic Region DWY68ZZ
Pineal Body DGY18ZZ
Pituitary Gland DGY08ZZ
Pleura DBY58ZZ
Prostate DVY08ZZ
Radius DPY78ZZ
Rectum DDY78ZZ
Rib DPY58ZZ
Sinuses D9Y78ZZ
Skin
Abdomen DHY88ZZ
Arm DHY48ZZ
Back DHY78ZZ
Buttock DHY98ZZ
Chest DHY68ZZ
Face DHY28ZZ
Leg DHYB8ZZ
Neck DHY38ZZ
Skull DPY08ZZ
Spinal Cord D0Y68ZZ
Spleen D7Y28ZZ
Sternum DPY48ZZ
Stomach DDY18ZZ
Testis DVY18ZZ
Thymus D7Y18ZZ
Thyroid Gland DGY58ZZ
Tibia DPYB8ZZ
Tongue D9Y58ZZ
Trachea DBY08ZZ
Ulna DPY78ZZ
Ureter DTY18ZZ
Urethra DTY38ZZ
Uterus DUY28ZZ
Whole Body DWY58ZZ
Whole Body 6A3Z
**Hyperthermic intraperitoneal
chemotherapy (HIPEC)**
3E0M30Y
Hypnosis GZFZZZZ
Hypogastric artery
use Artery, Internal Iliac, Left
use Artery, Internal Iliac, Right
Hypopharynx
use Pharynx
Hypophysectomy
see Excision, Gland, Pituitary
0GB0
see Resection, Gland, Pituitary
0GT0
Hypophysis
use Gland, Pituitary
Hypothalamotomy
see Destruction, Thalamus 0059
Hypothenar muscle
use Muscle, Hand, Left
use Muscle, Hand, Right
Hypothermia, Whole Body 6A4Z
Hysterectomy
Supracervical
see Resection, Uterus 0UT9
Total
see Resection, Uterus 0UT9
Hysterolysis
see Release, Uterus 0UN9

Hysteropexy
see Repair, Uterus 0UQ9
see Reposition, Uterus 0US9
Hysteroplasty
see Repair, Uterus 0UQ9
Hysterorrhaphy
see Repair, Uterus 0UQ9
Hysteroscopy 0UJD8ZZ
Hysterotomy
see Drainage, Uterus 0U99
Hysterotrachelectomy
see Resection, Cervix 0UTC
see Resection, Uterus 0UT9
Hysterotracheloplasty
see Repair, Uterus 0UQ9
Hysterotrachelorrhaphy
see Repair, Uterus 0UQ9

I

IABP (Intra-aortic balloon pump)
see Assistance, Cardiac 5A02
**IAEMT (Intraoperative anesthetic
effect monitoring and titration)**
see Monitoring, Central Nervous 4A10
**IASD® (InterAtrial Shunt Device),
Corvia**
use Synthetic Substitute
**Idarucizumab, Pradaxa®
(dabigatran) reversal agent**
use Other Therapeutic Substance
Ide-cel
use Idecabtagene Vicleucel
Immunotherapy
Idecabtagene Vicleucel
use Idecabtagene Vicleucel
Immunotherapy
**Idecabtagene Vicleucel
Immunotherapy** XW0
IGIV-C, for COVID-19 treatment
use Hyperimmune Globulin
IHD (Intermittent hemodialysis)
5A1D70Z
Ileal artery
use Artery, Superior Mesenteric
Ileectomy
see Excision, Ileum 0DBB
see Resection, Ileum 0DTB
Ileocolic artery
use Artery, Superior Mesenteric
Ileocolic vein
use Vein, Colic
Ileopexy
see Repair, Ileum 0DQB
see Reposition, Ileum 0DSB
Ileorrhaphy
see Repair, Ileum 0DQB
Ileoscopy 0DJD8ZZ
Ileostomy
see Bypass, Ileum 0D1B
see Drainage, Ileum 0D9B
Ileotomy
see Drainage, Ileum 0D9B
Ileoureterostomy
see Bypass, Urinary System 0T1
Iliac crest
use Bone, Pelvic, Left
use Bone, Pelvic, Right
Iliac fascia
use Subcutaneous Tissue and Fascia,
Upper Leg, Left
use Subcutaneous Tissue and Fascia,
Upper Leg, Right
Iliac lymph node
use Lymphatic, Pelvis
Iliacus muscle
use Muscle, Hip, Left
use Muscle, Hip, Right
Iliofemoral ligament
use Bursa and Ligament, Hip, Left
use Bursa and Ligament, Hip, Right

Iliohypogastric nerve
use Nerve, Lumbar Plexus
Ilioinguinal nerve
use Nerve, Lumbar Plexus
Iliolumbar artery
use Artery, Internal Iliac, Left
use Artery, Internal Iliac, Right
Iliolumbar ligament
use Bursa and Ligament, Lower
Spine
Iliotibial tract (band)
use Subcutaneous Tissue and Fascia,
Upper Leg, Left
use Subcutaneous Tissue and Fascia,
Upper Leg, Right
Ilium
use Bone, Pelvic, Left
use Bone, Pelvic, Right
Ilizarov external fixator
use External Fixation Device, Ring
in 0PH
use External Fixation Device, Ring
in 0PS
use External Fixation Device, Ring
in 0QH
use External Fixation Device, Ring
in 0QS
Ilizarov-Vecklich device
use External Fixation Device,
Limb Lengthening in
0QH
use External Fixation Device, Limb
Lengthening in 0PH
Imaging, diagnostic
see Computerized Tomography
(CT Scan)
see Fluoroscopy
see Magnetic Resonance Imaging
(MRI)
see Plain Radiography
see Ultrasonography
**Imdevimab (REGN10987) and
Casirivimab (REGN10933)**
use REGN-COV2 Monoclonal
Antibody
IMFINZI®
use Durvalumab Antineoplastic
IMI/REL
use Imipenem-cilastatin-relebactam
Anti-infective
**Imipenem-cilastatin-relebactam
Anti-infective** XW0
Immobilization
Abdominal Wall 2W33X
Arm
Lower
Left 2W3DX
Right 2W3CX
Upper
Left 2W3BX
Right 2W3AX
Back 2W35X
Chest Wall 2W34X
Extremity
Lower
Left 2W3MX
Right 2W3LX
Upper
Left 2W39X
Right 2W38X
Face 2W31X
Finger
Left 2W3KX
Right 2W3JX
Foot
Left 2W3TX
Right 2W3SX
Hand
Left 2W3FX
Right 2W3EX
Head 2W30X

Immobilization (*continued*)
  Inguinal Region
    Left 2W37X
    Right 2W36X
  Leg
    Lower
      Left 2W3RX
      Right 2W3QX
    Upper
      Left 2W3PX
      Right 2W3NX
  Neck 2W32X
  Thumb
    Left 2W3H
    Right 2W3GX
  Toe
    Left 2W3VX
    Right 2W3UX
Immunization
  see Introduction of Serum, Toxoid, and Vaccine
Immunoglobulin
  use Globulin
Immunotherapy
  see Introduction of Immunotherapeutic Substance
Immunotherapy, antineoplastic
  Interferon
    see Introduction of Low-dose Interleukin-2
  Interleukin-2, high-dose
    see Introduction of High-dose Interleukin-2
  Interleukin-2, low-dose
    see Introduction of Low-dose Interleukin-2
  Monoclonal antibody
    see Introduction of Monoclonal Antibody
  Proleukin, high-dose
    see Introduction of High-dose Interleukin-2
  Proleukin, low-dose
    see Introduction of Low-dose Interleukin-2
Impella® heart pump
  use Short-term External Heart Assist System in Heart and Great Vessels
Impeller Pump
  Continuous, Output 5A0221D
  Intermittent, Output 5A0211D
Implantable cardioverter-defibrillator (ICD)
  use Defibrillator Generator in 0JH
Implantable drug infusion pump (anti-spasmodic) (chemotherapy)(pain)
  use Infusion Device, Pump in Subcutaneous Tissue and Fascia
Implantable glucose monitoring device
  use Monitoring Device
Implantable hemodynamic monitor (IHM)
  use Monitoring Device, Hemodynamic in 0JH
Implantable hemodynamic monitoring system (IHMS)
  use Monitoring Device, Hemodynamic in 0JH
Implantable Miniature Telescope™ (IMT)
  use Synthetic Substitute, Intraocular Telescope in 08R
Implantation
  see Insertion
  see Replacement
Implanted (venous)(access) port
  use Vascular Access Device, Totally Implantable in Subcutaneous Tissue and Fascia

IMV (intermittent mandatory ventilation)
  see Assistance, Respiratory 5A09
In Vitro Fertilization 8E0ZXY1
Incision, abscess
  see Drainage
Incudectomy
  see Excision, Ear, Nose, Sinus 09B
  see Resection, Ear, Nose, Sinus 09T
Incudopexy
  see Reposition, Ear, Nose, Sinus 09S
  see Repair, Ear, Nose, Sinus 09Q
Incus
  use Auditory Ossicle, Left
  use Auditory Ossicle, Right
Induction of labor
  Artificial rupture of membranes
    see Drainage, Pregnancy 109
  Oxytocin
    see Introduction of Hormone
InDura, intrathecal catheter (1P) (spinal)
  use Infusion Device
Inferior cardiac nerve
  use Nerve, Thoracic Sympathetic
Inferior cerebellar vein
  use Vein, Intracranial
Inferior cerebral vein
  use Vein, Intracranial
Inferior epigastric artery
  use Artery, External Iliac, Left
  use Artery, External Iliac, Right
Inferior epigastric lymph node
  use Lymphatic, Pelvis
Inferior genicular artery
  use Artery, Popliteal, Left
  use Artery, Popliteal, Right
Inferior gluteal artery
  use Artery, Internal Iliac, Left
  use Artery, Internal Iliac, Right
Inferior gluteal nerve
  use Nerve, Sacral Plexus
Inferior hypogastric plexus
  use Nerve, Abdominal Sympathetic
Inferior labial artery
  use Artery, Face
Inferior longitudinal muscle
  use Muscle, Tongue, Palate, Pharynx
Inferior mesenteric ganglion
  use Nerve, Abdominal Sympathetic
Inferior mesenteric lymph node
  use Lymphatic, Mesenteric
Inferior mesenteric plexus
  use Nerve, Abdominal Sympathetic
Inferior oblique muscle
  use Muscle, Extraocular, Left
  use Muscle, Extraocular, Right
Inferior pancreaticoduodenal artery
  use Artery, Superior Mesenteric
Inferior phrenic artery
  use Aorta, Abdominal
Inferior rectus muscle
  use Muscle, Extraocular, Left
  use Muscle, Extraocular, Right
Inferior suprarenal artery
  use Artery, Renal, Left
  use Artery, Renal, Right
Inferior tarsal plate
  use Eyelid, Lower, Left
  use Eyelid, Lower, Right
Inferior thyroid vein
  use Vein, Innominate, Left
  use Vein, Innominate, Right
Inferior tibiofibular joint
  use Joint, Ankle, Left
  use Joint, Ankle, Right
Inferior turbinate
  use Turbinate, Nasal

Inferior ulnar collateral artery
  use Artery, Brachial, Left
  use Artery, Brachial, Right
Inferior vesical artery
  use Artery, Internal Iliac, Left
  use Artery, Internal Iliac, Right
Infraauricular lymph node
  use Lymphatic, Head
Infraclavicular (deltopectoral) lymph node
  use Lymphatic, Upper Extremity, Left
  use Lymphatic, Upper Extremity, Right
Infrahyoid muscle
  use Muscle, Neck, Left
  use Muscle, Neck, Right
Infraparotid lymph node
  use Lymphatic, Head
Infraspinatus fascia
  use Subcutaneous Tissue and Fascia, Upper Arm, Left
  use Subcutaneous Tissue and Fascia, Upper Arm, Right
Infraspinatus muscle
  use Muscle, Shoulder, Left
  use Muscle, Shoulder, Right
Infundibulopelvic ligament
  use Uterine Supporting Structure
Infusion
  see Introduction of substance in or on
Infusion Device, Pump
  Insertion of device in
    Abdomen 0JH8
    Back 0JH7
    Chest 0JH6
    Lower Arm
      Left 0JHH
      Right 0JHG
    Lower Leg
      Left 0JHP
      Right 0JHN
    Trunk 0JHT
    Upper Arm
      Left 0JHF
      Right 0JHD
    Upper Leg
      Left 0JHM
      Right 0JHL
  Removal of device from
    Lower Extremity 0JPW
    Trunk 0JPT
    Upper Extremity 0JPV
  Revision of device in
    Lower Extremity 0JWW
    Trunk 0JWT
    Upper Extremity 0JWV
Infusion, glucarpidase
  Central vein 3E043GQ
  Peripheral vein 3E033GQ
Inguinal canal
  use Inguinal Region, Bilateral
  use Inguinal Region, Left
  use Inguinal Region, Right
Inguinal triangle
  use Inguinal Region, Bilateral
  use Inguinal Region, Left
  use Inguinal Region, Right
Injection
  see Introduction of substance in or on
Injection, Concentrated Bone Marrow Aspirate (CBMA), intramuscular XK02303
Injection reservoir, port
  use Vascular Access Device, Totally Implantable in Subcutaneous Tissue and Fascia
Injection reservoir, pump
  use Infusion Device, Pump in Subcutaneous Tissue and Fascia

Insemination, artificial 3E0P7LZ
Insertion
  Antimicrobial envelope
    see Introduction of Anti-infective
  Aqueous drainage shunt
    see Bypass, Eye 081
    see Drainage, Eye 089
  Products of Conception 10H0
  Spinal Stabilization Device
    see Insertion of device in, Upper Joints 0RH
    see Insertion of device in, Lower Joints 0SH
Insertion of device in
  Abdominal Wall 0WHF
  Acetabulum
    Left 0QH5
    Right 0QH4
  Anal Sphincter 0DHR
  Ankle Region
    Left 0YHL
    Right 0YHK
  Anus 0DHQ
  Aorta
    Abdominal 04H0
    Thoracic
      Ascending/Arch 02HX
      Descending 02HW
  Arm
    Lower
      Left 0XHF
      Right 0XHD
    Upper
      Left 0XH9
      Right 0XH8
  Artery
    Anterior Tibial
      Left 04HQ
      Right 04HP
    Axillary
      Left 03H6
      Right 03H5
    Brachial
      Left 03H8
      Right 03H7
    Celiac 04H1
    Colic
      Left 04H7
      Middle 04H8
      Right 04H6
    Common Carotid
      Left 03HJ
      Right 03HH
    Common Iliac
      Left 04HD
      Right 04HC
    Coronary
      Four or More Arteries 02H3
      One Artery 02H0
      Three Arteries 02H2
      Two Arteries 02H1
    External Carotid
      Left 03HN
      Right 03HM
    External Iliac
      Left 04HJ
      Right 04HH
    Face 03HR
    Femoral
      Left 04HL
      Right 04HK
    Foot
      Left 04HW
      Right 04HV
    Gastric 04H2
    Hand
      Left 03HF
      Right 03HD
    Hepatic 04H3

Internal thoracic artery
  use Artery, Internal Mammary, Left
  use Artery, Internal Mammary, Right
  use Artery, Subclavian, Left
  use Artery, Subclavian, Right
Internal urethral sphincter
  use Urethra
Interphalangeal (IP) joint
  use Joint, Finger Phalangeal, Left
  use Joint, Finger Phalangeal, Right
  use Joint, Toe Phalangeal, Left
  use Joint, Toe Phalangeal, Right
Interphalangeal ligament
  use Bursa and Ligament, Foot, Left
  use Bursa and Ligament, Foot, Right
  use Bursa and Ligament, Hand, Left
  use Bursa and Ligament, Hand, Right
Interrogation, cardiac rhythm related device
  Interrogation only
    see Measurement, Cardiac 4B02
  With cardiac function testing
    see Measurement, Cardiac 4A02
Interruption
  see Occlusion
Interspinalis muscle
  use Muscle, Trunk, Left
  use Muscle, Trunk, Right
Interspinous ligament, cervical
  use Head and Neck Bursa and Ligament
Interspinous ligament, lumbar
  use Lower Spine Bursa and Ligament
Interspinous ligament, thoracic
  use Upper Spine Bursa and Ligament
Interspinous process spinal stabilization device
  use Spinal Stabilization Device, Interspinous Process in 0RH
  use Spinal Stabilization Device, Interspinous Process in 0SH
InterStim® Therapy lead
  use Neurostimulator Lead in Peripheral Nervous System
InterStim® II Therapy neurostimulator
  use Stimulator Generator, Single Array in 0JH
InterStim™ Micro Therapy neurostimulator
  use Stimulator Generator, Single Array Rechargeable in 0JH
Intertransversarius muscle
  use Muscle, Trunk, Left
  use Muscle, Trunk, Right
Intertransverse ligament, cervical
  use Head and Neck Bursa and Ligament
Intertransverse ligament, lumbar
  use Lower Spine Bursa and Ligament
Intertransverse ligament, thoracic
  use Upper Spine Bursa and Ligament
Interventricular foramen (Monro)
  use Cerebral Ventricle
Interventricular septum
  use Septum, Ventricular
Intestinal lymphatic trunk
  use Cisterna Chyli
Intracranial Arterial Flow, Whole Blood mRNA XXE5XT7
Intraluminal Device
  Airway
    Esophagus 0DH5
    Mouth and Throat 0CHY

Intraluminal Device *(continued)*
  Airway *(continued)*
    Nasopharynx 09HN
  Bioactive
    Occlusion
      Common Carotid
        Left 03LJ
        Right 03LH
      External Carotid
        Left 03LN
        Right 03LM
      Internal Carotid
        Left 03LL
        Right 03LK
      Intracranial 03LG
      Vertebral
        Left 03LQ
        Right 03LP
    Restriction
      Common Carotid
        Left 03VJ
        Right 03VH
      External Carotid
        Left 03VN
        Right 03VM
      Internal Carotid
        Left 03VL
        Right 03VK
      Intracranial 03VG
      Vertebral
        Left 03VQ
        Right 03VP
  Endobronchial Valve
    Lingula 0BH9
    Lower Lobe
      Left 0BHB
      Right 0BH6
    Main
      Left 0BH7
      Right 0BH3
    Middle Lobe, Right 0BH5
    Upper Lobe
      Left 0BH8
      Right 0BH4
  Endotracheal Airway
    Change device in, Trachea 0B21XEZ
    Insertion of device in, Trachea 0BH1
  Pessary
    Change device in, Vagina and Cul-de-sac 0U2HXGZ
    Insertion of device in Cul-de-sac 0UHF
    Vagina 0UHG
Intramedullary (IM) rod (nail)
  use Internal Fixation Device, Intramedullary in Lower Bones
  use Internal Fixation Device, Intramedullary in Upper Bones
Intramedullary skeletal kinetic distractor (ISKD)
  use Internal Fixation Device, Intramedullary in Lower Bones
  use Internal Fixation Device, Intramedullary in Upper Bones
Intraocular Telescope
  Left 08RK30Z
  Right 08RJ30Z
Intra.OX 8E02XDZ
Intraoperative Radiation Therapy (IORT)
  Anus DDY8CZZ
  Bile Ducts DFY2CZZ
  Bladder DTY2CZZ
  Brain D0Y0CZZ
  Brain Stem D0Y1CZZ
  Cervix DUY1CZZ
  Colon DDY5CZZ
  Duodenum DDY2CZZ

Intraoperative Radiation Therapy (IORT) *(continued)*
  Gallbladder DFY1CZZ
  Ileum DDY4CZZ
  Jejunum DDY3CZZ
  Kidney DTY0CZZ
  Larynx D9YBCZZ
  Liver DFY0CZZ
  Mouth D9Y4CZZ
  Nasopharynx D9YDCZZ
  Nerve, Peripheral D0Y7CZZ
  Ovary DUY0CZZ
  Pancreas DFY3CZZ
  Pharynx D9YCCZZ
  Prostate DVY0CZZ
  Rectum DDY7CZZ
  Spinal Cord D0Y6CZZ
  Stomach DDY1CZZ
  Ureter DTY1CZZ
  Urethra DTY3CZZ
  Uterus DUY2CZZ
Intrauterine device (IUD)
  use Contraceptive Device in Female Reproductive System
Intravascular fluorescence angiography (IFA)
  see Monitoring, Physiological Systems 4A1
Intravascular Lithotripsy (IVL)
  see Fragmentation
Intravascular ultrasound assisted thrombolysis
  see Fragmentation, Artery
Introduction of substance in or on
  Artery
    Central 3E06
      Analgesics 3E06
      Anesthetic, Intracirculatory 3E06
      Anti-infective 3E06
      Anti-inflammatory 3E06
      Antiarrhythmic 3E06
      Antineoplastic 3E06
      Destructive Agent 3E06
      Diagnostic Substance, Other 3E06
      Electrolytic Substance 3E06
      Hormone 3E06
      Hypnotics 3E06
      Immunotherapeutic 3E06
      Nutritional Substance 3E06
      Platelet Inhibitor 3E06
      Radioactive Substance 3E06
      Sedatives 3E06
      Serum 3E06
      Thrombolytic 3E06
      Toxoid 3E06
      Vaccine 3E06
      Vasopressor 3E06
      Water Balance Substance 3E06
    Coronary 3E07
      Diagnostic Substance, Other 3E07
      Platelet Inhibitor 3E07
      Thrombolytic 3E07
    Peripheral 3E05
      Analgesics 3E05
      Anesthetic, Intracirculatory 3E05
      Anti-infective 3E052
      Anti-inflammatory 3E05
      Antiarrhythmic 3E05
      Antineoplastic 3E05
      Destructive Agent 3E05
      Diagnostic Substance, Other 3E05

Introduction of substance in or on *(continued)*
  Artery *(continued)*
    Peripheral 3E05 *(continued)*
      Electrolytic Substance 3E05
      Hormone 3E05
      Hypnotics 3E05
      Immunotherapeutic 3E05
      Nutritional Substance 3E05
      Platelet Inhibitor 3E05
      Radioactive Substance 3E05
      Sedatives 3E05
      Serum 3E05
      Thrombolytic 3E05
      Toxoid 3E05
      Vaccine 3E05
      Vasopressor 3E05
      Water Balance Substance 3E05
  Biliary Tract 3E0J
    Analgesics 3E0J
    Anesthetic, Agent 3E0J
    Anti-infective 3E0J
    Anti-inflammatory 3E0J
    Antineoplastic 3E0J
    Destructive Agent 3E0J
    Diagnostic Substance, Other 3E0J
    Electrolytic Substance 3E0J
    Gas 3E0J
    Hypnotics 3E0J
    Islet Cells, Pancreatic 3E0J
    Nutritional Substance 3E0J
    Radioactive Substance 3E0J
    Sedatives 3E0J
    Water Balance Substance 3E0J
  Bone 3E0V
    Analgesics 3E0V3NZ
    Anesthetic, Agent 3E0V3BZ
    Anti-infective 3E0V32
    Anti-inflammatory 3E0V33Z
    Antineoplastic 3E0V30
    Destructive Agent 3E0V3TZ
    Diagnostic Substance, Other 3E0V3KZ
    Electrolytic Substance 3E0V37Z
    Hypnotics 3E0V3NZ
    Nutritional Substance 3E0V36Z
    Radioactive Substance 3E0V3HZ
    Sedatives 3E0V3NZ
    Water Balance Substance 3E0V37Z
  Bone Marrow 3E0A3GC
    Antineoplastic 3E0A30
  Brain 3E0Q
    Analgesics 3E0Q
    Anesthetic, Agent 3E0Q
    Anti-infective 3E0Q
    Anti-inflammatory 3E0Q
    Antineoplastic 3E0Q
    Destructive Agent 3E0Q
    Diagnostic Substance, Other 3E0Q
    Electrolytic Substance 3E0Q
    Gas 3E0Q
    Hypnotics 3E0Q
    Nutritional Substance 3E0Q
    Radioactive Substance 3E0Q
    Sedatives 3E0Q
    Stem Cells
      Embryonic 3E0Q
      Somatic 3E0Q
    Water Balance Substance 3E0Q
  Cranial Cavity 3E0Q
    Analgesics 3E0Q
    Anesthetic Agent 3E0Q
    Anti-infective 3E0Q

Cranial Cavity 3E0Q (continued)
Anti-inflammatory 3E0Q
Antineoplastic 3E0Q
Destructive Agent 3E0Q
Diagnostic Substance, Other
3E0Q
Electrolytic Substance 3E0Q
Gas 3E0Q
Hypnotics 3E0Q
Nutritional Substance
3E0Q
Radioactive Substance 3E0Q
Sedatives 3E0Q
Stem Cells
Embryonic 3E0Q
Somatic 3E0Q
Water Balance Substance 3E0Q
Ear 3E0B
Analgesics 3E0B
Anesthetic Agentl 3E0B
Anti-infective 3E0B
Anti-inflammatory 3E0B
Antineoplastic 3E0B
Destructive Agent 3E0B
Diagnostic Substance, Other
3E0B
Hypnotics 3E0B
Radioactive Substance 3E0B
Sedatives 3E0B
Epidural Space 3E0S3GC
Analgesics 3E0S3NZ
Anesthetic Agent 3E0S3BZ
Anti-infective 3E0S32
Anti-inflammatory 3E0S33Z
Antineoplastic 3E0S30
Destructive Agent 3E0S3TZ
Diagnostic Substance, Other
3E0S3KZ
Electrolytic Substance 3E0S37Z
Gas 3E0S
Hypnotics 3E0S3NZ
Nutritional Substance 3E0S36Z
Radioactive Substance 3E0S3HZ
Sedatives 3E0S3NZ
Water Balance Substance
3E0S37Z
Eye 3E0C
Analgesics 3E0C
Anesthetic Agent 3E0C
Anti-infective 3E0C
Anti-inflammatory 3E0C
Antineoplastic 3E0C
Destructive Agent 3E0C
Diagnostic Substance, Other
3E0C
Gas 3E0C
Hypnotics 3E0C
Pigment 3E0C
Radioactive Substance
3E0C
Sedatives 3E0C
Gastrointestinal Tract
Lower 3E0H
Analgesics 3E0H
Anesthetic Agent 3E0H
Anti-infective 3E0H
Anti-inflammatory 3E0H
Antineoplastic 3E0H
Destructive Agent 3E0H
Diagnostic Substance, Other
3E0H
Electrolytic Substance 3E0H
Gas 3E0H
Hypnotics 3E0H
Nutritional Substance 3E0H
Radioactive Substance 3E0H
Sedatives 3E0H
Water Balance Substance
3E0H

Gastrointestinal Tract (continued)
Upper 3E0G
Analgesics 3E0G
Anesthetic Agent 3E0G
Anti-infective 3E0G
Anti-inflammatory 3E0G
Antineoplastic 3E0G
Destructive Agent 3E0G
Diagnostic Substance, Other
3E0G
Electrolytic Substance 3E0G
Gas 3E0G
Hypnotics 3E0G
Nutritional Substance 3E0G
Radioactive Substance 3E0G
Sedatives 3E0G
Water Balance Substance
3E0G
Genitourinary Tract 3E0K
Analgesics 3E0K
Anesthetic Agent 3E0K
Anti-infective 3E0K
Anti-inflammatory 3E0K
Antineoplastic 3E0K
Destructive Agent 3E0K
Diagnostic Substance, Other
3E0K
Electrolytic Substance 3E0K
Gas 3E0K
Hypnotics 3E0K
Nutritional Substance 3E0K
Radioactive Substance 3E0K
Sedatives 3E0K
Water Balance Substance 3E0K
Heart 3E08
Diagnostic Substance. Other
3E08
Platelet Inhibitor 3E08
Thrombolytic 3E08
Joint 3E0U
Analgesics 3E0U3NZ
Anesthetic Agent 3E0U3BZ
Anti-infective 3E0U
Anti-inflammatory 3E0U33Z
Antineoplastic 3E0U30
Destructive Agent 3E0U3TZ
Diagnostic Substance, Other
3E0U3KZ
Electrolytic Substance 3E0U37Z
Gas 3E0U3SF
Hypnotics 3E0U3NZ
Nutritional Substance 3E0U36Z
Radioactive Substance 3E0U3HZ
Sedatives 3E0U3NZ
Water Balance Substance
3E0U37Z
Lymphatic 3E0W3GC
Analgesics 3E0W3NZ
Anesthetic Agent 3E0W3BZ
Anti-infective 3E0W32
Anti-inflammatory 3E0W33Z
Antineoplastic 3E0W30
Destructive Agent 3E0W3TZ
Diagnostic Substance, Other
3E0W3KZ
Electrolytic Substance 3E0W37Z
Hypnotics 3E0W3NZ
Nutritional Substance 3E0W36Z
Radioactive Substance
3E0W3HZ
Sedatives 3E0W3NZ
Water Balance Substance
3E0W37Z
Mouth 3E0D
Analgesics 3E0D
Anesthetic Agent 3E0D
Anti-infective 3E0D
Anti-inflammatory 3E0D
Antiarrhythmic 3E0D

Mouth 3E0D (continued)
Antineoplastic 3E0D
Destructive Agent 3E0D
Diagnostic Substance, Other
3E0D
Electrolytic Substance 3E0D
Hypnotics 3E0D
Nutritional Substance 3E0D
Radioactive Substance 3E0D
Sedatives 3E0D
Serum 3E0D
Toxoid 3E0D
Vaccine 3E0D
Water Balance Substance 3E0D
Mucous Membrane 3E00XGC
Analgesics 3E00XNZ
Anesthetic Agent 3E00XBZ
Anti-infective 3E00X2
Anti-inflammatory 3E00X3Z
Antineoplastic 3E00X0
Destructive Agent 3E00XTZ
Diagnostic Substance, Other
3E00XKZ
Hypnotics 3E00XNZ
Pigment 3E00XMZ
Sedatives 3E00XNZ
Serum 3E00X4Z
Toxoid 3E00X4Z
Vaccine 3E00X4Z
Muscle 3E023GC
Analgesics 3E023NZ
Anesthetic Agent 3E023BZ
Anti-infective 3E0232
Anti-inflammatory 3E0233Z
Antineoplastic 3E0230
Destructive Agent 3E023TZ
Diagnostic Substance, Other
3E023KZ
Electrolytic Substance 3E0237Z
Hypnotics 3E023NZ
Nutritional Substance 3E0236Z
Radioactive Substance 3E023HZ
Sedatives 3E023NZ
Serum 3E0234Z
Toxoid 3E0234Z
Vaccine 3E0234Z
Water Balance Substance
3E0237Z
Nerve
Cranial 3E0X3GC
Anesthetic Agent 3E0X3BZ
Anti-inflammatory 3E0X33Z
Destructive Agent 3E0X3TZ
Peripheral 3E0T3GC
Anesthetic Agent 3E0T3BZ
Anti-inflammatory 3E0T33Z
Destructive Agent 3E0T3TZ
Plexus 3E0T3GC Agent
3E0T3BZ
Anti-inflammatory 3E0T33Z
Destructive Agent 3E0T3TZ
Nose 3E09
Analgesics 3E09
Anesthetic Agent 3E09
Anti-infective 3E09
Anti-inflammatory 3E09
Antineoplastic 3E09
Destructive Agent 3E09
Diagnostic Substance, Other
3E09
Hypnotics 3E09
Radioactive Substance 3E09
Sedatives 3E09
Serum 3E09
Toxoid 3E09
Vaccine 3E09
Pancreatic Tract 3E0J
Analgesics 3E0J
Anesthetic Agent 3E0J

Pancreatic Tract 3E0J (continued)
Anti-infective 3E0J
Anti-inflammatory 3E0J
Antineoplastic 3E0J0
Destructive Agent 3E0J
Diagnostic Substance, Other
3E0J
Electrolytic Substance 3E0J
Gas 3E0J
Hypnotics 3E0J
Islet Cells, Pancreatic 3E0JU
Nutritional Substance 3E0J
Radioactive Substance 3E0J
Sedatives 3E0J
Water Balance Substance 3E0J
Pericardial Cavity 3E0Y
Analgesics 3E0Y3NZ
Anesthetic Agent 3E0Y3BZ
Anti-infective 3E0Y32
Anti-inflammatory 3E0Y33Z
Antineoplastic 3E0Y
Destructive Agent 3E0Y3TZ
Diagnostic Substance, Other
3E0Y3KZ
Electrolytic Substance 3E0Y37Z
Gas 3E0Y
Hypnotics 3E0Y3NZ
Nutritional Substance 3E0Y36Z
Radioactive Substance 3E0Y3HZ
Sedatives 3E0Y3NZ
Water Balance Substance
3E0Y37Z
Peritoneal Cavity 3E0M
Adhesion Barrier 3E0M
Analgesics 3E0M3NZ
Anesthetic Agent 3E0M3BZ
Anti-infective 3E0M32
Anti-inflammatory 3E0M33Z
Antineoplastic 3E0M
Destructive Agent 3E0M3TZ
Diagnostic Substance, Other
3E0M3KZ
Electrolytic Substance 3E0M37Z
Gas 3E0M
Hypnotics 3E0M3NZ
Nutritional Substance 3E0M36Z
Radioactive Substance 3E0M3HZ
Sedatives 3E0M3NZ
Water Balance Substance
3E0M37Z
Pharynx 3E0D
Analgesics 3E0D
Anesthetic Agent 3E0D
Anti-infective 3E0D
Anti-inflammatory 3E0D
Antiarrhythmic 3E0D
Antineoplastic 3E0D
Destructive Agent 3E0D
Diagnostic Substance, Other
3E0D
Electrolytic Substance 3E0D
Hypnotics 3E0D
Nutritional Substance 3E0D
Radioactive Substance 3E0D
Sedatives 3E0D
Serum 3E0D
Toxoid 3E0D
Vaccine 3E0D
Water Balance Substance 3E0D
Pleural Cavity 3E0L
Adhesion Barrier 3E0L
Analgesics 3E0L3NZ
Anesthetic Agent 3E0L3BZ
Anti-infective 3E0L32
Anti-inflammatory 3E0L33Z
Antineoplastic 3E0L
Destructive Agent 3E0L3TZ
Diagnostic Substance, Other
3E0L3KZ

Introduction of substance in or on (continued)

Pleural Cavity 3E0L (continued)
- Electrolytic Substance 3E0L37Z
- Gas 3E0L
- Hypnotics 3E0L3NZ
- Nutritional Substance 3E0L36Z
- Radioactive Substance 3E0L3HZ
- Sedatives 3E0L3NZ
- Water Balance Substance 3E0L37Z

Products of Conception 3E0E
- Analgesics 3E0E
- Anesthetic Agent 3E0E
- Anti-infective 3E0E2
- Anti-inflammatory 3E0E
- Antineoplastic 3E0E0
- Destructive Agent 3E0E
- Diagnostic Substance, Other 3E0E
- Electrolytic Substance 3E0E
- Gas 3E0E
- Hypnotics 3E0E
- Nutritional Substance 3E0E
- Radioactive Substance 3E0E
- Sedatives 3E0E
- Water Balance Substance 3E0E

Reproductive
- Female 3E0P
  - Adhesion Barrier 3E0P0
  - Analgesics 3E0P
  - Anesthetic Agent 3E0P
  - Anti-infective 3E0P
  - Anti-inflammatory 3E0P
  - Antineoplastic 3E0P
  - Destructive Agent 3E0P
  - Diagnostic Substance, Other 3E0P
  - Electrolytic Substance 3E0P
  - Gas 3E0P
  - Hormone 3E0P
  - Hypnotics 3E0P
  - Nutritional Substance 3E0P
  - Ovum, Fertilized 3E0P
  - Radioactive Substance 3E0P
  - Sedatives 3E0P
  - Sperm 3E0P
  - Water Balance Substance 3E0P
- Male 3E0N
  - Analgesics 3E0N
  - Anesthetic Agent 3E0N
  - Anti-infective 3E0N
  - Anti-inflammatory 3E0N
  - Antineoplastic 3E0N0
  - Destructive Agent 3E0N
  - Diagnostic Substance, Other 3E0N
  - Electrolytic Substance 3E0N
  - Gas 3E0N
  - Hypnotics 3E0N
  - Nutritional Substance 3E0N
  - Radioactive Substance 3E0N
  - Sedatives 3E0N
  - Water Balance Substance 3E0N

Respiratory Tract 3E0F
- Analgesics 3E0F
- Anesthetic Agent 3E0F
- Anti-infective 3E0F
- Anti-inflammatory 3E0F
- Antineoplastic 3E0F
- Destructive Agent 3E0F
- Diagnostic Substance, Other 3E0F
- Electrolytic Substance 3E0F
- Gas 3E0F
- Hypnotics 3E0F
- Nutritional Substance 3E0F
- Radioactive Substance 3E0F
- Sedatives 3E0F
- Water Balance Substance 3E0F

Introduction of substance in or on (continued)

Skin 3E00XGC
- Analgesics 3E00XNZ
- Anesthetic Agent 3E00XBZ
- Anti-infective 3E00X2
- Anti-inflammatory 3E00X3Z
- Antineoplastic 3E00X0
- Destructive Agent 3E00XTZ
- Diagnostic Substance, Other 3E00XKZ
- Hypnotics 3E00XNZ
- Pigment 3E00XMZ
- Sedatives 3E00XNZ
- Serum 3E00X4Z
- Toxoid 3E00X4Z
- Vaccine 3E00X4Z

Spinal Canal 3E0R3GC
- Analgesics 3E0R3NZ
- Anesthetic Agent 3E0R3BZ
- Anti-infective 3E0R32
- Anti-inflammatory 3E0R33Z
- Antineoplastic 3E0R30
- Destructive Agent 3E0R3TZ
- Diagnostic Substance, Other 3E0R3KZ
- Electrolytic Substance 3E0R37Z
- Gas 3E0R
- Hypnotics 3E0R3NZ
- Nutritional Substance 3E0R36Z
- Radioactive Substance 3E0R3HZ
- Sedatives 3E0R3NZ
- Stem Cells
  - Embryonic 3E0R
  - Somatic 3E0R
- Water Balance Substance 3E0R37Z

Subcutaneous Tissue 3E013GC
- Analgesics 3E013NZ
- Anesthetic Agent 3E013BZ
- Anti-infective 3E01
- Anti-inflammatory 3E0133Z
- Antineoplastic 3E0130
- Destructive Agent 3E013TZ
- Diagnostic Substance, Other 3E013KZ
- Electrolytic Substance 3E0137Z
- Hormone 3E013V
- Hypnotics 3E013NZ
- Nutritional Substance 3E0136Z
- Radioactive Substance 3E013HZ
- Sedatives 3E013NZ
- Serum 3E0134Z
- Toxoid 3E0134Z
- Vaccine 3E0134Z
- Water Balance Substance 3E0137Z

Vein
- Central 3E04
  - Analgesics 3E04
  - Anesthetic, Intracirculatory 3E04
  - Anti-infective 3E04
  - Anti-inflammatory 3E04
  - Antiarrhythmic 3E04
  - Antineoplastic 3E04
  - Destructive Agent 3E04
  - Diagnostic Substance, Other 3E04
  - Electrolytic Substance 3E04
  - Hormone 3E04
  - Hypnotics 3E04
  - Immunotherapeutic 3E04
  - Nutritional Substance 3E04
  - Platelet Inhibitor 3E04
  - Radioactive Substance 3E04
  - Sedatives 3E04
  - Serum 3E04
  - Thrombolytic 3E04
  - Toxoid 3E04
  - Vaccine 3E04

Introduction of substance in or on (continued)

Vein (continued)
- Central 3E04 (continued)
  - Vasopressor 3E04
  - Water Balance Substance 3E04
- Peripheral 3E03
  - Analgesics 3E03
  - Anesthetic, Intracirculatory 3E03
  - Anti-infective 3E03
  - Anti-inflammatory 3E03
  - Antiarrhythmic 3E03
  - Antineoplastic 3E03
  - Destructive Agent 3E03
  - Diagnostic Substance, Other 3E03
  - Electrolytic Substance 3E03
  - Hormone 3E03
  - Hypnotics 3E03
  - Immunotherapeutic 3E03
  - Islet Cells, Pancreatic 3E03
  - Nutritional Substance 3E03
  - Platelet Inhibitor 3E03
  - Radioactive Substance 3E03
  - Sedatives 3E03
  - Serum 3E03
  - Thrombolytic 3E03
  - Toxoid 3E03
  - Vaccine 3E03
  - Vasopressor 3E03
  - Water Balance Substance 3E03

Intubation
- Airway
  - *see* Insertion of device in, Esophagus 0DH5
  - *see* Insertion of device in, Mouth and Throat 0CHY
  - *see* Insertion of device in, Trachea 0BH1
- Drainage device
  - *see* Drainage
- Feeding Device
  - *see* Insertion of device in, Gastrointestinal System 0DH

INTUITY Elite valve system, EDWARDS
- *use* Zooplastic Tissue, Rapid Deployment Technique in New Technology

Iobenguane I-131 Antineoplastic XW0

Iobenguane I-131, High Specific Activity (HSA)
- *use* Iobenguane I-131 Antineoplastic

IPPB (intermittent positive pressure breathing)
- *see* Assistance, Respiratory 5A09

IRE (Irreversible Electroporation)
- *see* Destruction, Hepatobiliary System and Pancreas 0F5

Iridectomy
- *see* Excision, Eye 08B
- *see* Resection, Eye 08T

Iridoplasty
- *see* Repair, Eye 08Q
- *see* Replacement, Eye 08R
- *see* Supplement, Eye 08U

Iridotomy
- *see* Drainage, Eye 089

Irreversible Electroporation (IRE)
- *see* Destruction, Hepatobiliary System and Pancreas 0F5

Irrigation
- Biliary Tract, Irrigating Substance 3E1J
- Brain, Irrigating Substance 3E1Q38Z

Irrigation (continued)
- Cranial Cavity, Irrigating Substance 3E1Q38Z
- Ear, Irrigating Substance 3E1B
- Epidural Space, Irrigating Substance 3E1S38Z
- Eye, Irrigating Substance 3E1C
- Gastrointestinal Tract
  - Lower, Irrigating Substance 3E1H
  - Upper, Irrigating Substance 3E1G
- Genitourinary Tract, Irrigating Substance 3E1K
- Irrigating Substance 3C1ZX8Z
- Joint, Irrigating Substance 3E1U
- Mucous Membrane, Irrigating Substance 3E10
- Nose, Irrigating Substance 3E19
- Pancreatic Tract, Irrigating Substance 3E1J
- Pericardial Cavity, Irrigating Substance 3E1Y38Z
- Peritoneal Cavity
  - Dialysate 3E1M39Z
  - Irrigating Substance 3E1M
- Pleural Cavity, Irrigating Substance 3E1L38Z
- Reproductive
  - Female, Irrigating Substance 3E1P
  - Male, Irrigating Substance 3E1N
- Respiratory Tract, Irrigating Substance 3E1F
- Skin, Irrigating Substance 3E10
- Spinal Canal, Irrigating Substance 3E1R38Z

Isavuconazole (isavuconazonium sulfate)
- *use* Other Anti-Infective

ISC-REST kit
- ISCDx XXE5XT7
- QIAGEN Access Anti-SARS-CoV-2 Total Test XXE5XV7
- QIAstat-Dx Respiratory SARS-CoV-2 Panel XXE97U7

Ischiatic nerve
- *use* Nerve, Sciatic

Ischiocavernosus muscle
- *use* Muscle, Perineum

Ischiofemoral ligament
- *use* Bursa and Ligament, Hip, Left
- *use* Bursa and Ligament, Hip, Right

Ischium
- *use* Bone, Pelvic, Left
- *use* Bone, Pelvic, Right

Isolation 8E0ZXY6

Isotope Administration, Other Radiation, Whole Body DWY5G

Itrel (3)(4) neurostimulator
- *use* Stimulator Generator, Single Array in 0JH

J

Jakafi®
- *use* Ruxolitinib

Jejunal artery
- *use* Artery, Superior Mesenteric

Jejunectomy
- *see* Excision, Jejunum 0DBA
- *see* Resection, Jejunum 0DTA

Jejunocolostomy
- *see* Bypass, Gastrointestinal System 0D1
- *see* Drainage, Gastrointestinal System 0D9

Jejunopexy
- *see* Repair, Jejunum 0DQA
- *see* Reposition, Jejunum 0DSA

Jejunostomy
see Bypass, Jejunum 0D1A
see Drainage, Jejunum 0D9A
Jejunotomy
see Drainage, Jejunum 0D9A
Joint fixation plate
use Internal Fixation Device in
Lower Joints
use Internal Fixation Device in
Upper Joints
Joint liner (insert)
use Liner in Lower Joints
Joint spacer (antibiotic)
use Spacer in Lower Joints
use Spacer in Upper Joints
Jugular body
use Glomus Jugulare
Jugular lymph node
use Lymphatic, Neck, Left
use Lymphatic, Neck, Right

K

Kappa
use Pacemaker, Dual Chamber in
0JH
Kcentra
use 4-Factor Prothrombin Complex
Concentrate
Keratectomy, kerectomy
see Excision, Eye 08B
see Resection, Eye 08T
Keratocentesis
see Drainage, Eye 089
Keratoplasty
see Repair, Eye 08Q
see Replacement, Eye 08R
see Supplement, Eye 08U
Keratotomy
see Drainage, Eye 089
see Repair, Eye 08Q
KEVZARA® use Sarilumab
**Keystone Heart TriGuard 3™
CEPD (cerebral embolic
protection device)** X2A6325
Kirschner wire (K-wire)
use Internal Fixation Device in
Head and Facial Bones
use Internal Fixation Device in
Lower Bones
use Internal Fixation Device in
Lower Joints
use Internal Fixation Device in
Upper Bones
use Internal Fixation Device in
Upper Joints
Knee (implant) insert
use Liner in Lower Joints
KUB x-ray
see Plain Radiography, Kidney,
Ureter and Bladder BT04
Kuntscher nail
use Internal Fixation Device,
Intramedullary in Lower
Bones
use Internal Fixation Device,
Intramedullary in Upper
Bones
KYMRIAH®
use Tisagenlecleucel
Immunotherapy

L

Labia majora
use Vulva
Labia minora
use Vulva
Labial gland
use Lip, Lower
use Lip, Upper

Labiectomy
see Excision, Female Reproductive
System 0UB
see Resection, Female Reproductive
System 0UT
see Release, Central Nervous
System 00N
see Release, Peripheral Nervous
System 01N
Lacrimal canaliculus
use Duct, Lacrimal, Left
use Duct, Lacrimal, Right
Lacrimal punctum
use Duct, Lacrimal, Left
use Duct, Lacrimal, Right
Lacrimal sac
use Duct, Lacrimal, Left
use Duct, Lacrimal, Right
**LAGB (laparoscopic adjustable
gastric banding)**
Initial procedure 0DV64CZ
Surgical correction
see Revision of device in,
Stomach 0DW6
Laminectomy
see Excision, Lower Bones 0QB
see Excision, Upper Bones 0PB
see Release, Central Nervous
System and Cranial Nerves 00N
see Release, Peripheral Nervous
System 01N
Laminotomy
see Drainage, Lower Bones 0Q9
see Drainage, Upper Bones 0P9
see Excision, Lower Bones 0QB
see Excision, Upper Bones 0PB
see Release, Central Nervous
System and Cranial Nerves
00N
see Release, Lower Bones 0QN
see Release, Peripheral Nervous
System 01N
see Release, Upper Bones 0PN
**LAP-BAND® adjustable gastric
banding system**
use Extraluminal Device
**Laparoscopic-assisted transanal
pull-through**
see Excision, Gastrointestinal
System 0DB
see Resection, Gastrointestinal
System 0DT
Laparoscopy
see Inspection
Laparotomy
Drainage
see Drainage, Peritoneal Cavity
0W9G
Exploratory
see Inspection, Peritoneal Cavity
0WJG
Laryngectomy
see Excision, Larynx 0CBS
see Resection, Larynx 0CTS
Laryngocentesis
see Drainage, Larynx 0C9S
Laryngogram
see Fluoroscopy, Larynx B91J
Laryngopexy
see Repair, Larynx 0CQS
Laryngopharynx
use Pharynx
Laryngoplasty
see Repair, Larynx 0CQS
see Replacement, Larynx 0CRS
see Supplement, Larynx 0CUS
Laryngorrhaphy
see Repair, Larynx 0CQS
Laryngoscopy 0CJS8ZZ
Laryngotomy
see Drainage, Larynx 0C9S

Laser Interstitial Thermal Therapy
Adrenal Gland DGY2KZZ
Anus DDY8KZZ
Bile Ducts DFY2KZZ
Brain D0Y0KZZ
Brain Stem D0Y1KZZ
Breast
Left DMY0KZZ
Right DMY1KZZ
Bronchus DBY1KZZ
Chest Wall DBY7KZZ
Colon DDY5KZZ
Diaphragm DBY8KZZ
Duodenum DDY2KZZ
Esophagus DDY0KZZ
Gallbladder DFY1KZZ
Gland
Adrenal DGY2KZZ
Parathyroid DGY4KZZ
Pituitary DGY0KZZ
Thyroid DGY5KZZ
Ileum DDY4KZZ
Jejunum DDY3KZZ
Liver DFY0KZZ
Lung DBY2KZZ
Mediastinum DBY6KZZ
Nerve, Peripheral D0Y7KZZ
Pancreas DFY3KZZ
Parathyroid Gland DGY4KZZ
Pineal Body DGY1KZZ
Pituitary Gland DGY0KZZ
Pleura DBY5KZZ
Prostate DVY0KZZ
Rectum DDY7KZZ
Spinal Cord D0Y6KZZ
Stomach DDY1KZZ
Thyroid Gland DGY5KZZ
Trachea DBY0KZZ
Lateral (brachial) lymph node
use Lymphatic, Axillary, Left
use Lymphatic, Axillary, Right
Lateral canthus
use Eyelid, Upper, Left
use Eyelid, Upper, Right
Lateral collateral ligament (LCL)
use Bursa and Ligament, Knee, Left
use Bursa and Ligament, Knee,
Right
Lateral condyle of femur
use Femur, Lower, Left
use Femur, Lower, Right
Lateral condyle of tibia
use Tibia, Left
use Tibia, Right
Lateral cuneiform bone
use Tarsal, Left
use Tarsal, Right
Lateral epicondyle of femur
use Femur, Lower, Left
use Femur, Lower, Right
Lateral epicondyle of humerus
use Humeral Shaft, Left
use Humeral Shaft, Right
Lateral femoral cutaneous nerve
use Nerve, Lumbar Plexus
Lateral malleolus
use Fibula, Left
use Fibula, Right
Lateral meniscus
use Joint, Knee, Left
use Joint, Knee, Right
Lateral nasal cartilage
use Nasal Mucosa and Soft Tissue
Lateral plantar artery
use Artery, Foot, Left
use Artery, Foot, Right
Lateral plantar nerve
use Nerve, Tibial
Lateral rectus muscle
use Muscle, Extraocular, Left
use Muscle, Extraocular, Right

Lateral sacral artery
use Artery, Internal Iliac, Left
use Artery, Internal Iliac, Right
Lateral sacral vein
use Vein, Hypogastric, Left
use Vein, Hypogastric, Right
Lateral sural cutaneous nerve
use Nerve, Peroneal
Lateral tarsal artery
use Artery, Foot, Left
use Artery, Foot, Right
Lateral temporomandibular ligament
use Bursa and Ligament, Head and
Neck
Lateral thoracic artery
use Artery, Axillary, Left
use Artery, Axillary, Right
Latissimus dorsi muscle
use Muscle, Trunk, Left
use Muscle, Trunk, Right
**Latissimus Dorsi Myocutaneous
Flap**
Replacement
Bilateral 0HRV075
Left 0HRU075
Right 0HRT075
Transfer
Left 0KXG
Right 0KXF
Lavage
see Irrigation
Bronchial alveolar, diagnostic
see Drainage, Respiratory
System 0B9
Least splanchnic nerve
use Nerve, Thoracic Sympathetic
Lefamulin Anti-infective XW0
Left ascending lumbar vein
use Vein, Hemiazygos
Left atrioventricular valve
use Valve, Mitral
Left auricular appendix
use Atrium, Left
Left colic vein
use Vein, Colic
Left coronary sulcus
use Heart, Left
Left gastric artery
use Artery, Gastric
Left gastroepiploic artery
use Artery, Splenic
Left gastroepiploic vein
use Vein, Splenic
Left inferior phrenic vein
use Vein, Renal, Left
Left inferior pulmonary vein
use Vein, Pulmonary, Left
Left jugular trunk
use Lymphatic, Thoracic Duct
Left lateral ventricle
use Cerebral Ventricle
Left ovarian vein
use Vein, Renal, Left
Left second lumbar vein
use Vein, Renal, Left
Left subclavian trunk
use Lymphatic, Thoracic Duct
Left subcostal vein
use Vein, Hemiazygos
Left superior pulmonary vein
use Vein, Pulmonary, Left
Left suprarenal vein
use Vein, Renal, Left
Left testicular vein
use Vein, Renal, Left
Lengthening
Bone, with device
see Insertion of Limb
Lengthening Device
Muscle, by incision
see Division, Muscles 0K8

Lengthening (continued)
Tendon, by incision
  see Division, Tendons 0L8
Leptomeninges, intracranial
  use Cerebral Meninges
Leptomeninges, spinal
  use Spinal Meninges
Lesser alar cartilage
  use Nasal Mucosa and Soft Tissue
Lesser occipital nerve
  use Nerve, Cervical Plexus
Lesser Omentum
  use Omentum
Lesser saphenous vein
  use Saphenous Vein, Left
  use Saphenous Vein, Right
Lesser splanchnic nerve
  use Nerve, Thoracic
    Sympathetic
Lesser trochanter
  use Femur, Upper, Left
  use Femur, Upper, Right
Lesser tuberosity
  use Humeral Head, Left
  use Humeral Head, Right
Lesser wing
  use Bone, Sphenoid
Leukopheresis, therapeutic
  see Pheresis, Circulatory 6A55
Levator anguli oris muscle
  use Muscle, Facial
Levator ani muscle
  use Perineum Muscle
Levator labii superioris alaeque nasi muscle
  use Muscle, Facial
Levator labii superioris muscle
  use Muscle, Facial
Levator palpebrae superioris muscle
  use Eyelid, Upper, Left
  use Eyelid, Upper, Right
Levator scapulae muscle
  use Muscle, Neck, Left
  use Muscle, Neck, Right
Levator veli palatini muscle
  use Muscle, Tongue, Palate,
    Pharynx
Levatores costarum muscle
  use Muscle, Thorax, Left
  use Muscle, Thorax, Right
Lifeline ARM Automated Chest Compression (ACC) device 5A1221J
LifeStent® (Flexstar)(XL) Vascular Stent System
  use Intraluminal Device
Lifileucel use Lifileucel
  Immunotherapy
Lifileucel Immunotherapy XW0
Ligament of head of fibula
  use Bursa and Ligament, Knee, Left
  use Bursa and Ligament, Knee,
    Right
Ligament of the lateral malleolus
  use Bursa and Ligament, Ankle,
    Left
  use Bursa and Ligament, Ankle,
    Right
Ligamentum flavum, cervical
  use Head and Neck Bursa and
    Ligament
Ligamentum flavum, lumbar
  use Lower Spine Bursa and Ligament
Ligamentum flavum, thoracic
  use Upper Spine Bursa and Ligament
Ligation
  see Occlusion
Ligation, hemorrhoid
  see Occlusion, Lower Veins,
    Hemorrhoidal Plexus
Light Therapy GZJZZZZ

Liner
Removal of device from
  Hip
    Left 0SPB09Z
    Right 0SP909Z
  Knee
    Left 0SPD09Z
    Right 0SPC09Z
Revision of device in
  Hip
    Left 0SWB09Z
    Right 0SW909Z
  Knee
    Left 0SWD09Z
    Right 0SWC09Z
Supplement
  Hip
    Left 0SUB09Z
      Acetabular Surface
        0SUE09Z
      Femoral Surface 0SUS09Z
    Right 0SU909Z
      Acetabular Surface
        0SUA09Z
      Femoral Surface 0SUR09Z
  Knee
    Left 0SUD09
      Femoral Surface 0SUU09Z
      Tibial Surface 0SUW09Z
    Right 0SUC09
      Femoral Surface 0SUT09Z
      Tibial Surface 0SUV09Z
Lingual artery
  use Artery, External Carotid, Left
  use Artery, External Carotid, Right
Lingual tonsil
  use Pharynx
Lingulectomy, lung
  see Excision, Lung Lingula 0BBH
  see Resection, Lung Lingula 0BTH
Lisocabtagene Maraleucel
  use Lisocabtagene Maraleucel
    Immunotherapy
Lisocabtagene Maraleucel Immunotherapy XW0
Lithoplasty
  see Fragmentation
Lithotripsy
  see Fragmentation
With removal of fragments
  see Extirpation
LITT (laser interstitial thermal therapy)
  see Laser Interstitial Thermal
    Therapy
LIVIAN™ CRT-D
  use Cardiac Resynchronization
    Defibrillator Pulse Generator in
    0JH
Lobectomy
  see Excision, Central Nervous
    System and Cranial Nerves 00B
  see Excision, Endocrine System 0GB
  see Excision, Hepatobiliary System
    and Pancreas 0FB
  see Excision, Respiratory System
    0BB
  see Resection, Endocrine System 0GT
  see Resection, Hepatobiliary System
    and Pancreas 0FT
  see Resection, Respiratory System
    0BT
Lobotomy
  see Division, Brain 0080
Localization
  see Map
  see Imaging
Locus ceruleus
  use Pons
Long thoracic nerve
  use Nerve, Brachial Plexus

Loop ileostomy
  see Bypass, Ileum 0D1B
Loop recorder, implantable
  use Monitoring Device
Lower GI series
  see Fluoroscopy, Colon
    BD14
Lower Respiratory Fluid Nucleic Acid-base Microbial Detection XXEBXQ6
LTX Regional Anticoagulant
  use Nafamostat Anticoagulant
LUCAS® Chest Compression System 5A1221J
Lumbar artery
  use Aorta, Abdominal
Lumbar facet joint
  use Joint, Lumbar Vertebral
Lumbar ganglion
  use Nerve, Lumbar Sympathetic
Lumbar lymph node
  use Lymphatic, Aortic
Lumbar lymphatic trunk
  use Cisterna Chyli
Lumbar splanchnic nerve
  use Nerve, Lumbar Sympathetic
Lumbosacral facet joint
  use Joint, Lumbosacral
Lumbosacral trunk
  use Nerve, Lumbar
Lumpectomy
  see Excision
Lunate bone
  use Carpal, Left
  use Carpal, Right
Lunotriquetral ligament
  use Bursa and Ligament, Hand,
    Left
  use Bursa and Ligament, Hand,
    Right
Lurbinectedin XW0
Lymphadenectomy
  see Excision, Lymphatic and Hemic
    Systems 07B
  see Resection, Lymphatic and
    Hemic Systems 07T
Lymphadenotomy
  see Drainage, Lymphatic and Hemic
    Systems 079
Lymphangiectomy
  see Excision, Lymphatic and Hemic
    Systems 07B
  see Resection, Lymphatic and
    Hemic Systems 07T
Lymphangiogram
  see Plain Radiography, Lymphatic
    System B70
Lymphangioplasty
  see Repair, Lymphatic and Hemic
    Systems 07Q
  see Supplement, Lymphatic and
    Hemic Systems 07U
Lymphangiorrhaphy
  see Repair, Lymphatic and Hemic
    Systems 07Q
Lymphangiotomy
  see Drainage, Lymphatic and Hemic
    Systems 079
Lysis
  see Release

M

Macula
  use Retina, Left
  use Retina, Right
MAGEC® Spinal Bracing and Distraction System
  use Magnetically Controlled
    Growth Rod(s) in New
    Technology

Magnet extraction, ocular foreign body
  see Extirpation, Eye 08C
Magnetic-guided radiofrequency endovascular fistula
Radial Artery, Left 031C
Radial Artery, Right 031B
Ulnar Artery, Left 031A
Ulnar Artery, Right 0319
Magnetic Resonance Imaging (MRI)
Abdomen BW30
Ankle
  Left BQ3H
  Right BQ3G
Aorta
  Abdominal B430
  Thoracic B330
Arm
  Left BP3F
  Right BP3E
Artery
  Celiac B431
  Cervico-Cerebral Arch B33Q
  Common Carotid, Bilateral B335
  Coronary
    Bypass Graft, Multiple
      B233
    Multiple B231
  Internal Carotid, Bilateral B338
  Intracranial B33R
  Lower Extremity
    Bilateral B43H
    Left B43G
    Right B43F
  Pelvic B43C
  Renal, Bilateral B438
  Spinal B33M
  Superior Mesenteric B434
  Upper Extremity
    Bilateral B33K
    Left B33J
    Right B33H
  Vertebral, Bilateral B33G
Bladder BT30
Brachial Plexus BW3P
Brain B030
Breast
  Bilateral BH32
  Left BH31
  Right BH30
Calcaneus
  Left BQ3K
  Right BQ3J
Chest BW33Y
Coccyx BR3F
Connective Tissue
  Lower Extremity BL31
  Upper Extremity BL30
Corpora Cavernosa BV30
Disc
  Cervical BR31
  Lumbar BR33
  Thoracic BR32
Ear B930
Elbow
  Left BP3H
  Right BP3G
Eye
  Bilateral B837
  Left B836
  Right B835
Femur
  Left BQ34
  Right BQ33
Fetal Abdomen BY33
Fetal Extremity BY35
Fetal Head BY30
Fetal Heart BY31
Fetal Spine BY34
Fetal Thorax BY32
Fetus, Whole BY36

Measurement *(continued)*
 Peripheral Nervous *(continued)*
  Electrical Activity 4A01
  Stimulator 4B01XVZ
 Positive Blood Culture Fluorescence
  Hybridization for Organism
  Identification, Concentration and
  Susceptibility XXE5XN6
 Products of Conception
  Cardiac
   Electrical Activity 4A0H
    Rate 4A0H
    Rhythm 4A0H
    Sound 4A0HH
  Nervous
   Conductivity 4A0J
   Electrical Activity 4A0J
   Pressure 4A0J
 Respiratory
  Capacity 4A09
  Flow 4A09
  Pacemaker 4B09X
  Rate 4A09
  Resistance 4A09
  Total Activity 4A09
  Volume 4A09
 Sleep 4A0ZXQZ
 Temperature 4A0Z
 Urinary
  Contractility 4A0D
  Flow 4A0D
  Pressure 4A0D
  Resistance 4A0D
  Volume 4A0D
 Venous
  Flow
   Central 4A04
   Peripheral 4A04
   Portal 4A04
   Pulmonary 4A04
  Pressure
   Central 4A04
   Peripheral 4A04
   Portal 4A04
   Pulmonary 4A04
  Pulse
   Central 4A04
   Peripheral 4A04
   Portal 4A04
   Pulmonary 4A04
  Saturation, Peripheral 4A04
 Visual
  Acuity 4A07X0Z
  Mobility 4A07X7Z
  Pressure 4A07XBZ
 Whole Blood Nucleic Acid-base
  Microbial Detection XXE5XM5
Meatoplasty, urethra
 see Repair, Urethra 0TQD
Meatotomy
 see Drainage, Urinary System 0T9
Mechanical chest compression
 (mCPR) 5A1221J
Mechanical Initial Specimen
 Diversion Technique Using
 Active Negative Pressure (blood
 collection) XXE5XR7
Mechanical ventilation
 see Performance, Respiratory 5A19
Medial canthus
 use Eyelid, Lower, Left
 use Eyelid, Lower, Right
Medial collateral ligament (MCL)
 use Bursa and Ligament, Knee, Left
 use Bursa and Ligament, Knee, Right
Medial condyle of femur
 use Femur, Lower, Left
 use Femur, Lower, Right
Medial condyle of tibia
 use Tibia, Left
 use Tibia, Right

Medial cuneiform bone
 use Tarsal, Left
 use Tarsal, Right
Medial epicondyle of femur
 use Femur, Lower, Left
 use Femur, Lower, Right
Medial epicondyle of humerus
 use Humeral Shaft, Left
 use Humeral Shaft, Right
Medial malleolus
 use Tibia, Left
 use Tibia, Right
Medial meniscus
 use Joint, Knee, Left
 use Joint, Knee, Right
Medial plantar artery
 use Artery, Foot, Left
 use Artery, Foot, Right
Medial plantar nerve
 use Nerve, Tibial
Medial popliteal nerve
 use Nerve, Tibial
Medial rectus muscle
 use Muscle, Extraocular, Left
 use Muscle, Extraocular, Right
Medial sural cutaneous nerve
 use Nerve, Tibial
Median antebrachial vein
 use Vein, Basilic, Left
 use Vein, Basilic, Right
Median cubital vein
 use Vein, Basilic, Left
 use Vein, Basilic, Right
Median sacral artery
 use Aorta, Abdominal
Mediastinal cavity
 use Mediastinum
Mediastinal lymph node
 use Lymphatic, Thorax
Mediastinal space
 use Mediastinum
Mediastinoscopy 0WJC4ZZ
Medication Management
 GZ3ZZZZ
 for substance abuse
  Antabuse HZ83ZZZ
  Bupropion HZ87ZZZ
  Clonidine HZ86ZZZ
  Levo-alpha-acetyl-methadol
   (LAAM) HZ82ZZZ
  Methadone Maintenance
   HZ81ZZZ
  Naloxone HZ85ZZZ
  Naltrexone HZ84ZZZ
  Nicotine Replacement HZ80ZZZ
  Other Replacement Medication
   HZ89ZZZ
  Psychiatric Medication
   HZ88ZZZ
Meditation 8E0ZXY5
Medtronic Endurant® II AAA stent
 graft system
 use Intraluminal Device
Meissner's (submucous) plexus
 use Nerve, Abdominal Sympathetic
Melody® transcatheter pulmonary
 valve
 use Zooplastic Tissue in Heart and
  Great Vessels
Membranous urethra
 use Urethra
Meningeorrhaphy
 see Repair, Cerebral Meninges
  00Q1
 see Repair, Spinal Meninges
  00QT
Meniscectomy, knee
 see Excision, Joint, Knee, Left
  0SBD
 see Excision, Joint, Knee, Right
  0SBC

Mental foramen
 use Mandible, Left
 use Mandible, Right
Mentalis muscle
 use Muscle, Facial
Mentoplasty
 see Alteration, Jaw, Lower 0W05
Meropenem-vaborbactam Anti-
 infective XW0
Mesenterectomy
 see Excision, Mesentery 0DBV
Mesenteriorrhaphy,
 mesenterorrhaphy
 see Repair, Mesentery 0DQV
Mesenteriplication
 see Repair, Mesentery 0DQV
Mesoappendix
 use Mesentery
Mesocolon
 use Mesentery
Metacarpal ligament
 use Bursa and Ligament, Hand,
  Left
 use Bursa and Ligament, Hand,
  Right
Metacarpophalangeal ligament
 use Bursa and Ligament, Hand, Left
 use Bursa and Ligament, Hand,
  Right
Metal on metal bearing surface
 use Synthetic Substitute, Metal in
  0SR
Metatarsal ligament
 use Bursa and Ligament, Foot, Left
 use Bursa and Ligament, Foot,
  Right
Metatarsectomy
 see Excision, Lower Bones 0QB
 see Resection, Lower Bones 0QT
Metatarsophalangeal (MTP) joint
 use Joint, Metatarsal-Phalangeal,
  Left
 use Joint, Metatarsal-Phalangeal,
  Right
Metatarsophalangeal ligament
 use Bursa and Ligament, Foot, Left
 use Bursa and Ligament, Foot,
  Right
Metathalamus
 use Thalamus
Micro-Driver stent (RX) (OTW)
 use Intraluminal Device
MicroMed HeartAssist
 use Implantable Heart Assist
  System in Heart and Great
  Vessels
Micrus CERECYTE microcoil
 use Intraluminal Device, Bioactive
  in Upper Arteries
Midcarpal joint
 use Joint, Carpal, Left
 use Joint, Carpal, Right
Middle cardiac nerve
 use Nerve, Thoracic Sympathetic
Middle cerebral artery
 use Artery, Intracranial
Middle cerebral vein
 use Vein, Intracranial
Middle colic vein
 use Vein, Colic
Middle genicular artery
 use Artery, Popliteal, Left
 use Artery, Popliteal, Right
Middle hemorrhoidal vein
 use Vein, Hypogastric, Left
 use Vein, Hypogastric, Right
Middle rectal artery
 use Artery, Internal Iliac, Left
 use Artery, Internal Iliac, Right
Middle suprarenal artery
 use Aorta, Abdominal

Middle temporal artery
 use Artery, Temporal, Left
 use Artery, Temporal, Right
Middle turbinate
 use Turbinate, Nasal
Mineral-based Topical Hemostatic
 Agent XW0
MIRODERM™ Biologic Wound
 Matrix
 use Skin Substitute, Porcine Liver
  Derived in New Technology
MitraClip valve repair system
 use Synthetic Substitute
Mitral annulus
 use Valve, Mitral
Mitroflow® Aortic Pericardial Heart
 Valve
 use Zooplastic Tissue in Heart and
  Great Vessels
Mobilization, adhesions
 see Release
Molar gland
 use Buccal Mucosa
MolecuLight i:X® wound imaging
 see Other Imaging, Anatomical
  Regions BW5
Monitoring
 Arterial
  Flow
   Coronary 4A13
   Peripheral 4A13
   Pulmonary 4A13
  Pressure
   Coronary 4A13
   Peripheral 4A13
   Pulmonary 4A13
  Pulse
   Coronary 4A13
   Peripheral 4A13
   Pulmonary 4A13
  Saturation, Peripheral 4A13
  Sound, Peripheral 4A13
 Cardiac
  Electrical Activity 4A12
   Ambulatory 4A12X45
   No Qualifier 4A12X4Z
  Output 4A12
  Rate 4A12
  Rhythm 4A12
  Sound 4A12
  Total Activity, Stress
   4A12XM4
  Vascular Perfusion, Indocyanine
   Green Dye 4A12XSH
 Central Nervous
  Conductivity 4A10
  Electrical Activity
   Intraoperative 4A10
   No Qualifier 4A10
  Pressure 4A100BZ
   Intracranial 4A10
  Saturation, Intracranial 4A10
  Temperature, Intracranial
   4A10
 Gastrointestinal
  Motility 4A1B
  Pressure 4A1B
  Secretion 4A1B
  Vascular Perfusion,
   Indocyanine Green Dye
   4A1BXSH
 Kidney, Fluorescent Pyrazine
  XT25XE5
 Lymphatic
  Flow
   Indocyanine Green Dye
    4A16
   No Qualifier A416
  Pressure 4A16
 Oxygen Saturation Endoscopic
  Imaging (OXEI) XD2

Monitoring (continued)
Peripheral Nervous
Conductivity
Motor 4A11
Sensory 4A11
Electrical Activity
Intraoperative 4A11
No Qualifier 4A11
Products of Conception
Cardiac
Electrical Activity 4A1H
Rate 4A1H
Rhythm 4A1H
Sound 4A1H
Nervous
Conductivity 4A1J
Electrical Activity 4A1J
Pressure 4A1J
Respiratory
Capacity 4A19
Flow 4A19
Rate 4A19
Resistance 4A19
Volume 4A19
Skin and Breast
Vascular Perfusion,
Indocyanine Green Dye
4A1GXSH
Sleep 4A1ZXQZ
Temperature 4A1Z
Urinary
Contractility 4A1D
Flow 4A1D
Pressure 4A1D
Resistance 4A1D
Volume 4A1D
Venous
Flow
Central 4A14
Peripheral 4A14
Portal 4A14
Pulmonary 4A14
Pressure
Central 4A14
Peripheral 4A14
Portal 4A14
Pulmonary 4A14
Pulse
Central 4A14
Peripheral 4A14
Portal 4A14
Pulmonary 4A14
Saturation
Central 4A14
Portal 4A14
Pulmonary 4A14
Monitoring Device, Hemodynamic
Abdomen 0JH8
Chest 0JH6
**Mosaic Bioprosthesis (aortic)
(mitral) valve**
use Zooplastic Tissue in Heart and
Great Vessels
Motor Function Assessment F01
Motor Treatment F07
MR Angiography
see Magnetic Resonance Imaging
(MRI), Heart B23
see Magnetic Resonance
Imaging (MRI), Lower
Arteries B43
see Magnetic Resonance Imaging
(MRI), Upper Arteries B33
**MULTI-LINK (VISION)(MINI-
VISION)(ULTRA) Coronary
Stent System**
use Intraluminal Device
Multiple sleep latency test
4A0ZXQZ
Musculocutaneous nerve
use Nerve, Brachial Plexus

Musculopexy
see Repair, Muscles 0KQ
see Reposition, Muscles 0KS
Musculophrenic artery
use Artery, Internal Mammary, Left
use Artery, Internal Mammary,
Right
Musculoplasty
see Repair, Muscles 0KQ
see Supplement, Muscles 0KU
Musculorrhaphy
see Repair, Muscles 0KQ
Musculospiral nerve
use Nerve, Radial
Myectomy
see Excision, Muscles 0KB
see Resection, Muscles 0KT
Myelencephalon
use Medulla Oblongata
Myelogram
CT
see Computerized Tomography
(CT Scan), Central Nervous
System B02
MRI
see Magnetic Resonance Imaging
(MRI), Central Nervous
System B03
Myenteric (Auerbach's) plexus
use Nerve, Abdominal Sympathetic
Myocardial Bridge Release
see Release, Artery, Coronary
Myomectomy
see Excision, Female Reproductive
System 0UB
Myometrium
use Uterus
Myopexy
see Repair, Muscles 0KQ
see Reposition, Muscles 0KS
Myoplasty
see Repair, Muscles 0KQ
see Supplement, Muscles 0KU
Myorrhaphy
see Repair, Muscles 0KQ
Myoscopy
see Inspection, Muscles 0KJ
Myotomy
see Division, Muscles 0K8
see Drainage, Muscles 0K9
Myringectomy
see Excision, Ear, Nose, Sinus 09B
see Resection, Ear, Nose, Sinus 09T
Myringoplasty
see Repair, Ear, Nose, Sinus 09Q
see Replacement, Ear, Nose, Sinus
09R
see Supplement, Ear, Nose, Sinus
09U
Myringostomy
see Drainage, Ear, Nose, Sinus 099
Myringotomy
see Drainage, Ear, Nose, Sinus 099

N

NA-1 (Nerinitide)
use Nerinitide
Nafamostat Anticoagulant
XY0YX37
Nail bed
use Finger Nail
use Toe Nail
Nail plate
use Finger Nail
use Toe Nail
**nanoLOCK™ interbody fusion
device**
use Interbody Fusion Device,
Nanotextured Surface in New
Technology

Narcosynthesis GZGZZZZ
Narsoplimab Monoclonal Antibody
XW0
Nasal cavity
use Nasal Mucosa and Soft Tissue
Nasal concha
use Turbinate, Nasal
Nasalis muscle
use Muscle, Facial
Nasolacrimal duct
use Duct, Lacrimal, Left
use Duct, Lacrimal, Right
Nasopharyngeal airway (NPA)
use Intraluminal Device, Airway in
Ear, Nose, Sinus
Navicular bone
use Tarsal, Left
use Tarsal, Right
**Near Infrared Spectroscopy,
Circulatory System** 8E02
Neck of femur
use Femur, Upper, Left
use Femur, Upper, Right
**Neck of humerus (anatomical)
(surgical)**
use Humeral Head, Left
use Humeral Head, Right
Neovasc Reducer™
use Reduction Device in New
Technology
Nephrectomy
see Excision, Urinary System
0TB
see Resection, Urinary System 0TT
Nephrolithotomy
see Extirpation, Urinary System
0TC
Nephrolysis
see Release, Urinary System 0TN
Nephropexy
see Repair, Urinary System 0TQ
see Reposition, Urinary System
0TS
Nephroplasty
see Repair, Urinary System 0TQ
see Supplement, Urinary System
0TU
Nephropyeloureterostomy
see Bypass, Urinary System 0T1
see Drainage, Urinary System
0T9
Nephrorrhaphy
see Repair, Urinary System 0TQ
Nephroscopy, transurethral
0TJ58ZZ
Nephrostomy
see Bypass, Urinary System 0T1
see Drainage, Urinary System
0T9
Nephrotomography
see Fluoroscopy, Urinary System
BT1
see Plain Radiography, Urinary
System BT0
Nephrotomy
see Division, Urinary System
0T8
see Drainage, Urinary System
0T9
Nerinitide XW0
Nerve conduction study
see Measurement, Central Nervous
4A00
see Measurement, Peripheral
Nervous 4A01
Nerve Function Assessment F01
Nerve to the stapedius
use Nerve, Facial
Nesiritide
use Human B-type Natriuretic
Peptide

Neurectomy
see Excision, Central Nervous
System and Cranial Nerves
00B
see Excision, Peripheral Nervous
System 01B
Neurexeresis
see Extraction, Central Nervous
System and Cranial Nerves
00D
see Extraction, Peripheral Nervous
System 01D
Neurohypophysis
use Gland, Pituitary
Neurolysis
see Release, Central Nervous
System and Cranial Nerves
00N
see Release, Peripheral Nervous
System 01N
**Neuromuscular electrical
stimulation (NEMS) lead**
use Stimulator Lead in Muscles
Neurophysiologic monitoring
see Monitoring, Central Nervous
4A10
Neuroplasty
see Repair, Central Nervous System
and Cranial Nerves 00Q
see Repair, Peripheral Nervous
System 01Q
see Supplement, Central Nervous
System and Cranial Nerves 00U
see Supplement, Peripheral Nervous
System 01U
Neurorrhaphy
see Repair, Central Nervous System
and Cranial Nerves 00Q
see Repair, Peripheral Nervous
System 01Q
Neurostimulator Generator
Insertion of device in, Skull
0NH00NZ
Removal of device from, Skull
0NP00NZ
Revision of device in, Skull
0NW00NZ
**Neurostimulator generator, multiple
channel**
use Stimulator Generator, Multiple
Array in 0JH
**Neurostimulator generator, multiple
channel rechargeable**
use Stimulator Generator,
Multiple Array Rechargeable
in 0JH
**Neurostimulator generator, single
channel**
use Stimulator Generator, Single
Array in 0JH
**Neurostimulator generator, single
channel rechargeable**
use Stimulator Generator, Single
Array Rechargeable in 0JH
Neurostimulator Lead
Insertion of device in
Brain 00H0
Cerebral Ventricle 00H6
Nerve
Cranial 00HE
Peripheral 01HY
Spinal Canal 00HU
Spinal Cord 00HV
Vein
Azygos 05H0
Innominate
Left 05H4
Right 05H3
Removal of device from
Brain 00P0
Cerebral Ventricle 00P6

Neurostimulator Lead (*continued*)
  Removal of device from (*continued*)
    Nerve
      Cranial 00PE
      Peripheral 01PY
    Spinal Canal 00PU
    Spinal Cord 00PV
    Vein
      Azygos 05P0
      Innominate
        Left 05P4
        Right 05HP3
  Revision of device in
    Brain 00W0
    Cerebral Ventricle 00W6
    Nerve
      Cranial 00WE
      Peripheral 01WY
    Spinal Canal 00WU
    Spinal Cord 00WV
    Vein
      Azygos 05W0
      Innominate
        Left 05W4
        Right 05HW3
Neurostimulator Lead in Oropharynx XWHD7Q7
Neurotomy
  see Division, Central Nervous System and Cranial Nerves 008
  see Division, Peripheral Nervous System and Cranial Nerves 018
Neurotripsy
  see Destruction, Central Nervous System and Cranial Nerves 005
  see Destruction, Peripheral Nervous System 015
Neutralization plate
  use Internal Fixation Device in Head and Facial Bones
  use Internal Fixation Device in Lower Bones
  use Internal Fixation Device in Upper Bones
New Technology
  Amivantamab Monoclonal Antibody XW0
  Antibiotic-eluting Bone Void Filler XW0V0P7
  Aorta
    Thoracic Arch using Branched Synthetic Substitute with Intraluminal Device X2RX0N7
    Thoracic Descending using Branched Synthetic Substitute with Intraluminal Device X2VW0N7
  Apalutamide Antineoplstic XW0DJX5
  Atezolizumab Antineoplastic XW0
  Axicabtagene Ciloleucel Immunotherapy XW0
  Bezlotoxumab Monoclonal Antibody XW0
  Bioengineered Allogeneic Construct, Skin XHRPXF7
  Brexanolone XW0
  Brexucabtagene Autoleucel Immunotherapy XW0
  Bromelain-enriched Proteolytic Enzyme XW0
  Caplacizumab XW0
  Cefiderocol Anti-infective XW0
  Ceftolozane/Tazobactam Anti-infective XW0
  Cerebral Embolic Filtration
    Dual Filter X2A5312
    Extracorporeal Flow Reversal Circuit X2A
    Single Deflection Filter X2A6325

New Technology (*continued*)
  Ciltacabtagene Autoleucel XW0
  Coagulation Factor Xa, Inactivated XW0
  Computer-aided Assessment, Intracranial Vascular Activity XXE0X07
  Computer-aided Guidance, Transthoracic Echocardiography X2JAX47
  Computer-aided Mechanical Aspiration X2C
  Computer-aided Triage and Notification, Pulmonary Artery Flow XXE3X27
  Concentrated Bone Marrow Aspirate XK02303
  Coronary Sinus, Reduction Device X2V73Q7
  Cytarabine and Daunorubicin Liposome Antineoplastic XW0
  Defibrotide Sodium Anticoagulant XW0
  Destruction, Prostate, Robotic Waterjet Ablation XV508A4
  Dilation
    Anterior Tibial
      Left
        Sustained Release Drug-eluting Intraluminal Device X27Q385
        Four or More X27Q3C5
        Three X27Q3B5
        Two X27Q395
      Right
        Sustained Release Drug-eluting Intraluminal Device X27P385
        Four or More X27P3C5
        Three X27P3B5
        Two X27P395
    Femoral
      Left
        Sustained Release Drug-eluting Intraluminal Device X27J385
        Four or More X27J3C5
        Three X27J3B5
        Two X27J395
      Right
        Sustained Release Drug-eluting Intraluminal Device X27H385
        Four or More X27H3C5
        Three X27H3B5
        Two X27H395
    Peroneal
      Left
        Sustained Release Drug-eluting Intraluminal Device X27U385
        Four or More X27U3C5
        Three X27U3B5
        Two X27U395
      Right
        Sustained Release Drug-eluting Intraluminal Device X27T385
        Four or More X27T3C5
        Three X27T3B5
        Two X27T395
    Popliteal
      Left Distal
        Sustained Release Drug-eluting Intraluminal Device X27N385
        Four or More X27N3C5
        Three X27N3B5
        Two X27N395

New Technology (*continued*)
  Dilation (*continued*)
    Popliteal (*continued*)
      Left Proximal
        Sustained Release Drug-eluting Intraluminal Device X27L385
        Four or More X27L3C5
        Three X27L3B5
        Two X27L395
      Right Distal
        Sustained Release Drug-eluting Intraluminal Device X27M385
        Four or More X27M3C5
        Three X27M3B5
        Two X27M395
      Right Proximal
        Sustained Release Drug-eluting Intraluminal Device X27K385
        Four or More X27K3C5
        Three X27QK3B5
        Two X27K395
    Posterior Tibial
      Left
        Sustained Release Drug-eluting Intraluminal Device X27S385
        Four or More X27S3C5
        Three X27S3B5
        Two X27S395
      Right
        Sustained Release Drug-eluting Intraluminal Device X27R385
        Four or More X27R3C5
        Three X27R3B5
        Two X27R395
  Durvalumab Antineoplastic XW0
  Eculizumab XW0
  Eladocagene exuparvovec XW0Q316
  Endothelial Damage Inhibitor XY0VX83
  Engineered Chimeric Antigen Receptor T-cell Immunotherapy
    Allogeneic XW0
    Autologous XW0
  Erdafitinib Antineoplastic XW0DXL5
  Esketamine Hydrochloride XW097M5
  Fosfomycin Anti-infective XW0
  Fusion
    Cervical Vertebral
      2 or more
        Nanotextured Surface XRG2092
        Radiolucent Porous XRG20F3
        Interbody Fusion Device
          Nanotextured Surface XRG1092
          Radiolucent Porous XRG10F3
    Cervicothoracic Vertebral
      Nanotextured Surface XRG4092
      Radiolucent Porous XRG40F3
    Lumbar Vertebral
      2 or more
        Customizable XRGC
        Nanotextured Surface XRGC092
        Radiolucent Porous XRGC0F3
        Interbody Fusion Device
          Customizable XRGB
          Nanotextured Surface XRGB092
          Radiolucent Porous XRGB0F3

New Technology (*continued*)
  Fusion (*continued*)
    Lumbosacral
      Customizable XRGD
      Nanotextured Surface XRGD092
      Radiolucent Porous XRGD0F3
    Occipital-cervical
      Nanotextured Surface XRG0092
      Radiolucent Porous XRG00F3
    Thoracic Vertebral
      2 to 7
        Nanotextured Surface XRG7092
        Radiolucent Porous XRG70F3
      8 or more
        Nanotextured Surface XRG8092
        Radiolucent Porous XRG80F3
      Interbody Fusion Device
        Nanotextured Surface XRG6092
        Radiolucent Porous XRG60F3
    Thoracolumbar Vertebral
      Customizable XRGA
      Nanotextured Surface XRGA092
      Radiolucent Porous XRGA0F3
  Gilteritinib Antineoplastic XW0DXV5
  High-Dose Intravenous Immune Globulin, for COVID-19 treatment XW1
  Hyperimmune Globulin, for COVID-19 treatment XW1
  Idecabtagene Vicleucel Immunotherapy XW0
  Imipenem-cilastatin-relebactam Anti-infective XW0
  Intracranial Arterial Flow, Whole Blood mRNA XXE5XT7
  Iobenguane I-131 Antineoplastic XW0
  Kidney, Fluorescent Pyrazine XT25XE5
  Lefamulin Anti-infective XW0
  Lifileucel Immunotherapy XW0
  Lisocabtagene Maraleucel Immunotherapy XW0
  Lower Respiratory Fluid Nucleic Acid-base Microbial Detection XXEBXQ6
  Lurbinectedin XW0
  Mechanical Initial Specimen Diversion Technique Using Active Negative Pressure (blood collection) XXE5XR7
  Meropenem-vaborbactam Anti-infective XW0
  Mineral-based Topical Hemostatic Agent XW0
  Nafamostat Anticoagulant XY0YX37
  Narsoplimab Monoclonal Antibody XW0
  Nerinitide XW0
  Neurostimulator Lead in Oropharynx XWHD7Q7
  Omadacycline Anti-infective XW0
  Other New Technology Therapeutic Substance XW0
  Oxygen Saturation Endoscopic Imaging (OXEI) XD2
  Plasma, Convalescent (Nonautologous) XW1
  Plazomicin Anti-infective XW0

Occlusion (*continued*)

Duct (*continued*)

Hepatic

Common 0FL7

Left 0FL6

Right 0FL5

Lacrimal

Left 08LY

Right 08LX

Pancreatic 0FLD

Accessory 0FLF

Parotid

Left 0CLC

Right 0CLB

Duodenum 0DL9

Esophagogastric Junction 0DL4

Esophagus 0DL5

Lower 0DL3

Middle 0DL2

Upper 0DL1

Fallopian Tube

Left 0UL6

Right 0UL5

Fallopian Tubes, Bilateral 0UL7

Ileocecal Valve 0DLC

Ileum 0DLB

Intestine

Large 0DLE

Left 0DLG

Right 0DLF

Small 0DL8

Jejunum 0DLA

Kidney Pelvis

Left 0TL4

Right 0TL3

Left atrial appendage (LAA)

see Occlusion, Atrium, Left 02L7

Lymphatic

Aortic 07LD

Axillary

Left 07L6

Right 07L5

Head 07L0

Inguinal

Left 07LJ

Right 07LH

Internal Mammary

Left 07L9

Right 07L8

Lower Extremity

Left 07LG

Right 07LF

Mesenteric 07LB

Neck

Left 07L2

Right 07L1

Pelvis 07LC

Thoracic Duct 07LK

Thorax 07L7

Upper Extremity

Left 07L4

Right 07L3

Rectum 0DLP

Stomach 0DL6

Pylorus 0DL7

Trachea 0BL1

Ureter

Left 0TL7

Right 0TL6

Urethra 0TLD

Vagina 0ULG

Valve, Pulmonary 02LH

Vas Deferens

Bilateral 0VLQ

Left 0VLP

Right 0VLN

Vein

Axillary

Left 05L8

Right 05L7

Occlusion (*continued*)

Vein (*continued*)

Azygos 05L0

Basilic

Left 05LC

Right 05LB

Brachial

Left 05LA

Right 05L9

Cephalic

Left 05LF

Right 05LD

Colic 06L7

Common Iliac

Left 06LD

Right 06LC

Esophageal 06L3

External Iliac

Left 06LG

Right 06LF

External Jugular

Left 05LQ

Right 05LP

Face

Left 05LV

Right 05LT

Femoral

Left 06LN

Right 06LM

Foot

Left 06LV

Right 06LT

Gastric 06L2

Hand

Left 05LH

Right 05LG

Hemiazygos 05L1

Hepatic 06L4

Hypogastric

Left 06LJ

Right 06LH

Inferior Mesenteric 06L6

Innominate

Left 05L4

Right 05L3

Internal Jugular

Left 05LN

Right 05LM

Intracranial 05LL

Lower 06LY

Portal 06L8

Pulmonary

Left 02LT

Right 02LS

Renal

Left 06LB

Right 06L9

Saphenous

Left 06LQ

Right 06LP

Splenic 06L1

Subclavian

Left 05L6

Right 05L5

Superior Mesenteric 06L5

Upper 05LY

Vertebral

Left 05LS

Right 05LR

Vena Cava

Inferior 06L0

Superior 02LV

Occlusion, REBOA (resuscitative endovascular balloon occlusion of the aorta)

02LW3DJ

04L03DJ

Occupational therapy

see Activities of Daily Living Treatment, Rehabilitation F08

Octagam 10%, for COVID-19 treatment

use High-Dose Intravenous Immune Globulin

Odentectomy

see Excision, Mouth and Throat 0CB

see Resection, Mouth and Throat 0CT

Odontoid process

use Cervical Vertebra

Olecranon bursa

use Bursa and Ligament, Elbow, Left

use Bursa and Ligament, Elbow, Right

Olecranon process

use Ulna, Left

use Ulna, Right

Olfactory bulb

use Nerve, Olfactory

Omadacycline Anti-infective XW0

Omentectomy, omentumectomy

see Excision, Gastrointestinal System 0DB

see Resection, Gastrointestinal System 0DT

Omentofixation

see Repair, Gastrointestinal System 0DQ

Omentoplasty

see Repair, Gastrointestinal System 0DQ

see Replacement, Gastrointestinal System 0DR

see Supplement, Gastrointestinal System 0DU

Omentorrhaphy

see Repair, Gastrointestinal System 0DQ

Omentotomy

see Drainage, Gastrointestinal System 0D9

Omnilink Elite Vascular Balloon Expandable Stent System

use Intraluminal Device

Onychectomy

see Excision, Skin and Breast 0HB

see Resection, Skin and Breast 0HT

Onychoplasty

see Repair, Skin and Breast 0HQ

see Replacement, Skin and Breast 0HR

Onychotomy

see Drainage, Skin and Breast 0H9

Oophorectomy

see Excision, Female Reproductive System 0UB

see Resection, Female Reproductive System 0UT

Oophoropexy

see Repair, Female Reproductive System 0UQ

see Reposition, Female Reproductive System 0US

Oophoroplasty

see Repair, Female Reproductive System 0UQ

see Supplement, Female Reproductive System 0UU

Oophororrhaphy

see Repair, Female Reproductive System 0UQ

Oophorostomy

see Drainage, Female Reproductive System 0U9

Oophorotomy

see Drainage, Female Reproductive System 0U9

see Division, Female Reproductive System 0U8

Oophorrhaphy

see Repair, Female Reproductive System 0UQ

Open Pivot (mechanical) valve

use Synthetic Substitute

Open Pivot Aortic Valve Graft (AVG)

use Synthetic Substitute

Ophthalmic artery

use Intracranial Artery

Ophthalmic nerve

use Nerve, Trigeminal

Ophthalmic vein

use Vein, Intracranial

Opponensplasty

Tendon replacement

see Replacement, Tendons 0LR

Tendon transfer

see Transfer, Tendons 0LX

Optic chiasma

use Nerve, Optic

Optic disc

use Retina, Left

use Retina, Right

Optic foramen

use Bone, Sphenoid

Optical coherence tomography, intravascular

see Computerized Tomography (CT Scan)

Optimizer™ III implantable pulse generator

use Contractility Modulation Device in 0JH

Orbicularis oculi muscle

use Eyelid, Upper, Left

use Eyelid, Upper, Right

Orbicularis oris muscle

use Muscle, Facial

Orbital Atherectomy

see Extirpation, Heart and Great Vessels 02C

Orbital fascia

use Subcutaneous Tissue and Fascia, Face

Orbital portion of ethmoid bone

use Orbit, Left

use Orbit, Right

Orbital portion of frontal bone

use Orbit, Left

use Orbit, Right

Orbital portion of lacrimal bone

use Orbit, Left

use Orbit, Right

Orbital portion of maxilla

use Orbit, Left

use Orbit, Right

Orbital portion of palatine bone

use Orbit, Left

use Orbit, Right

Orbital portion of sphenoid bone

use Orbit, Left

use Orbit, Right

Orbital portion of zygomatic bone

use Orbit, Left

use Orbit, Right

Orchectomy, orchidectomy, orchiectomy

see Excision, Male Reproductive System 0VB

see Resection, Male Reproductive System 0VT

Orchidoplasty, orchioplasty

see Repair, Male Reproductive System 0VQ

see Replacement, Male Reproductive System 0VR

see Supplement, Male Reproductive System 0VU

Orchidorrhaphy, orchiorrhaphy

see Repair, Male Reproductive System 0VQ

Orchidotomy, orchiotomy, orchotomy
see Drainage, Male Reproductive System 0V9
Orchiopexy
see Repair, Male Reproductive System 0VQ
see Reposition, Male Reproductive System 0VS
Oropharyngeal airway (OPA)
use Intraluminal Device, Airway in Mouth and Throat
Oropharynx
use Pharynx
Ossiculectomy
see Excision, Ear, Nose, Sinus 09B
see Resection, Ear, Nose, Sinus 09T
Ossiculotomy
see Drainage, Ear, Nose, Sinus 099
Ostectomy
see Excision, Head and Facial Bones 0NB
see Excision, Lower Bones 0QB
see Excision, Upper Bones 0PB
see Resection, Head and Facial Bones 0NT
see Resection, Lower Bones 0QT
see Resection, Upper Bones 0PT
Osteoclasis
see Division, Head and Facial Bones 0N8
see Division, Lower Bones 0Q8
see Division, Upper Bones 0P8
Osteolysis
see Release, Head and Facial Bones 0NN
see Release, Lower Bones 0QN
see Release, Upper Bones 0PN
Osteopathic Treatment
Abdomen 7W09X
Cervical 7W01X
Extremity
Lower 7W06X
Upper 7W07X
Head 7W00X
Lumbar 7W03X
Pelvis 7W05X
Rib Cage 7W08X
Sacrum 7W04X
Thoracic 7W02X
Osteopexy
see Repair, Head and Facial Bones 0NQ
see Repair, Lower Bones 0QQ
see Repair, Upper Bones 0PQ
see Reposition, Head and Facial Bones 0NS
see Reposition, Lower Bones 0QS
see Reposition, Upper Bones 0PS
Osteoplasty
see Repair, Head and Facial Bones 0NQ
see Repair, Lower Bones 0QQ
see Repair, Upper Bones 0PQ
see Replacement, Head and Facial Bones 0NR
see Replacement, Lower Bones 0QR
see Replacement, Upper Bones 0PR
see Supplement, Head and Facial Bones 0NU
see Supplement, Lower Bones 0QU
see Supplement, Upper Bones 0PU
Osteorrhaphy
see Repair, Head and Facial Bones 0NQ
see Repair, Lower Bones 0QQ
see Repair, Upper Bones 0PQ

Osteotomy, ostotomy
see Division, Head and Facial Bones 0N8
see Division, Lower Bones 0Q8
see Division, Upper Bones 0P8
see Drainage, Head and Facial Bones 0N9
see Drainage, Lower Bones 0Q9
see Drainage, Upper Bones 0P9
Other Imaging
Bile Duct, Indocyanine Green Dye, Intraoperative BF50200
Bile Duct and Gallbladder, Indocyanine Green Dye, Intraoperative BF53200
Extremity
Lower BW5CZ1Z
Upper BW5JZ1Z
Gallbladder, Indocyanine Green Dye, Intraoperative BF52200
Gallbladder and Bile Duct, Indocyanine Green Dye, Intraoperative BF53200
Head and Neck BW59Z1Z
Hepatobiliary System, All, Indocyanine Green Dye, Intraoperative BF5C200
Liver, Indocyanine Green Dye, Intraoperative BF55200
Liver and Spleen, Indocyanine Green Dye, Intraoperative BF56200
Neck and Head BW59Z1Z
Pancreas, Indocyanine Green Dye, Intraoperative BF57200
Spleen and Liver, Indocyanine Green Dye, Intraoperative BF56200
Trunk BW52Z1Z
Other New Technology Therapeutic Substance XW0
Otic ganglion
use Nerve, Head and Neck Sympathetic
OTL-101
use Hematopoietic Stem/Progenitor Cells, Genetically Modified
OTL-103
use Hematopoietic Stem/Progenitor Cells, Genetically Modified
OTL-200
use Hematopoietic Stem/Progenitor Cells, Genetically Modified
Otoplasty
see Repair, Ear, Nose, Sinus 09Q
see Replacement, Ear, Nose, Sinus 09R
see Supplement, Ear, Nose, Sinus 09U
Otoscopy
see Inspection, Ear, Nose, Sinus 09J
Oval window
use Ear, Middle, Left
use Ear, Middle, Right
Ovarian artery
use Aorta, Abdominal
Ovarian ligament
use Uterine Supporting Structure
Ovariectomy
see Excision, Female Reproductive System 0UB
see Resection, Female Reproductive System 0UT
Ovariocentesis
see Drainage, Female Reproductive System 0U9
Ovariopexy
see Repair, Female Reproductive System 0UQ
see Reposition, Female Reproductive System 0US

Ovariotomy
see Division, Female Reproductive System 0U8
see Drainage, Female Reproductive System 0U9
Ovatio™ CRT-D
use Cardiac Resynchronization Defibrillator Pulse Generator in 0JH
Oversewing
Gastrointestinal ulcer
see Repair, Gastrointestinal System 0DQ
Pleural bleb
see Repair, Respiratory System 0BQ
Oviduct
use Fallopian Tube, Left
use Fallopian Tube, Right
Oximetry, Fetal pulse 10H073Z
OXINIUM
use Synthetic Substitute, Oxidized Zirconium on Polyethylene in 0SR
Oxygen Saturation Endoscopic Imaging (OXEI) XD2
Oxygenation
Extracorporeal membrane (ECMO)
see Performance, Circulatory 5A15
Hyperbaric
see Assistance, Circulatory 5A05
Supersaturated
see Assistance, Circulatory 5A05

P

Pacemaker
Dual Chamber
Abdomen 0JH8
Chest 0JH6
Intracardiac
Insertion of device in
Atrium
Left 02H7
Right 02H6
Vein, Coronary 02H4
Ventricle
Left 02HL
Right 02HK
Removal of device from Heart 02PA
Revision of device in Heart 02WA
Single Chamber
Abdomen 0JH8
Chest 0JH6
Single Chamber Rate Responsive
Abdomen 0JH8
Chest 0JH6
Packing
Abdominal Wall 2W43X5Z
Anorectal 2Y43X5Z
Arm
Lower
Left 2W4DX5Z
Right 2W4CX5Z
Upper
Left 2W4BX5Z
Right 2W4AX5Z
Back 2W45X5Z
Chest Wall 2W44X5Z
Ear 2Y42X5Z
Extremity
Lower
Left 2W4MX5Z
Right 2W4LX5Z
Upper
Left 2W49X5Z
Right 2W48X5Z
Face 2W41X5Z

Packing (*continued*)
Finger
Left 2W4KX5Z
Right 2W4JX5Z
Foot
Left 2W4TX5Z
Right 2W4SX5Z
Genital Tract, Female 2Y44X5Z
Hand
Left 2W4FX5Z
Right 2W4EX5Z
Head 2W40X5Z
Inguinal Region
Left 2W47X5Z
Right 2W46X5Z
Leg
Lower
Left 2W4RX5Z
Right 2W4QX5Z
Upper
Left 2W4PX5Z
Right 2W4NX5Z
Mouth and Pharynx 2Y40X5Z
Nasal 2Y41X5Z
Neck 2W42X5Z
Thumb
Left 2W4HX5Z
Right 2W4GX5Z
Toe
Left 2W4VX5Z
Right 2W4UX5Z
Urethra 2Y45X5Z
Paclitaxel-eluting coronary stent
use Intraluminal Device, Drug-eluting in Heart and Great Vessels
Paclitaxel-eluting peripheral stent
use Intraluminal Device, Drug-eluting in Lower Arteries
use Intraluminal Device, Drug-eluting in Upper Arteries
Palatine gland
use Buccal Mucosa
Palatine tonsil
use Tonsils
Palatine uvula
use Uvula
Palatoglossal muscle
use Muscle, Tongue, Palate, Pharynx
Palatopharyngeal muscle
use Muscle, Tongue, Palate, Pharynx
Palatoplasty
see Repair, Mouth and Throat 0CQ
see Replacement, Mouth and Throat 0CR
see Supplement, Mouth and Throat 0CU
Palatorrhaphy
see Repair, Mouth and Throat 0CQ
Palmar (volar) digital vein
use Vein, Hand, Left
use Vein, Hand, Right
Palmar (volar) metacarpal vein
use Vein, Hand, Left
use Vein, Hand, Right
Palmar cutaneous nerve
use Nerve, Median
use Nerve, Radial
Palmar fascia (aponeurosis)
use Subcutaneous Tissue and Fascia, Hand, Left
use Subcutaneous Tissue and Fascia, Hand, Right
Palmar interosseous muscle
use Muscle, Hand, Left
use Muscle, Hand, Right

Palmar ulnocarpal ligament
   use Bursa and Ligament, Wrist, Left
   use Bursa and Ligament, Wrist, Right
Palmaris longus muscle
   use Muscle, Lower Arm and Wrist, Left
   use Muscle, Lower Arm and Wrist, Right
Pancreatectomy
   see Excision, Pancreas 0FBG
   see Resection, Pancreas 0FTG
Pancreatic artery
   use Artery, Splenic
Pancreatic plexus
   use Nerve, Abdominal Sympathetic
Pancreatic vein
   use Vein, Splenic
Pancreaticoduodenostomy
   see Bypass, Hepatobiliary System and Pancreas 0F1
Pancreaticosplenic lymph node
   use Lymphatic, Aortic
Pancreatogram, endoscopic retrograde
   see Fluoroscopy, Pancreatic Duct BF18
Pancreatolithotomy
   see Extirpation, Pancreas 0FCG
Pancreatotomy
   see Division, Pancreas 0F8G
   see Drainage, Pancreas 0F9G
Panniculectomy
   see Excision, Skin, Abdomen 0HB7
   see Excision, Subcutaneous Tissue and Fascia, Abdomen 0JB8
Paraaortic lymph node
   use Lymphatic, Aortic
Paracentesis
   Eye
      see Drainage, Eye 089
   Peritoneal Cavity
      see Drainage, Peritoneal Cavity 0W9G
   Tympanum
      see Drainage, Ear, Nose, Sinus 099
Parapharyngeal space
   use Neck
Pararectal lymph node
   use Lymphatic, Mesenteric
Parasternal lymph node
   use Lymphatic, Thorax
Parathyroidectomy
   see Excision, Endocrine System 0GB
   see Resection, Endocrine System 0GT
Paratracheal lymph node
   use Lymphatic, Thorax
Paraurethral (Skene's) gland
   use Gland, Vestibular
Parenteral nutrition, total
   see Introduction of Nutritional Substance
Parietal lobe
   use Cerebral Hemisphere
Parotid lymph node
   use Lymphatic, Head
Parotid plexus
   use Nerve, Facial
Parotidectomy
   see Excision, Mouth and Throat 0CB
   see Resection, Mouth and Throat 0CT
Pars flaccida
   use Tympanic Membrane, Left
   use Tympanic Membrane, Right

Partial joint replacement
   Hip
      see Replacement, Lower Joints 0SR
   Knee
      see Replacement, Lower Joints 0SR
   Shoulder
      see Replacement, Upper Joints 0RR
Partially absorbable mesh
   use Synthetic Substitute
Patch, blood, spinal 3E0R3GC
Patellapexy
   see Repair, Lower Bones 0QQ
   see Reposition, Lower Bones 0QS
Patellaplasty
   see Repair, Lower Bones 0QQ
   see Replacement, Lower Bones 0QR
   see Supplement, Lower Bones 0QU
Patellar ligament
   use Bursa and Ligament, Knee, Left
   use Bursa and Ligament, Knee, Right
Patellar tendon
   use Tendon, Knee, Left
   use Tendon, Knee, Right
Patellectomy
   see Excision, Lower Bones 0QB
   see Resection, Lower Bones 0QT
Patellofemoral joint
   use Joint, Knee, Left
   use Joint, Knee, Left, Femoral Surface
   use Joint, Knee, Right
   use Joint, Knee, Right, Femoral Surface
pAVF (percutaneous arteriovenous fistula), using magnetic-guided radiofrequency
   see Bypass, Upper Arteries 031
pAVF (percutaneous arteriovenous fistula), using thermal resistance energy
   see New Technology, Cardiovascular System X2K
Pectineus muscle
   use Muscle, Upper Leg, Left
   use Muscle, Upper Leg, Right
Pectoral (anterior) lymph node
   use Lymphatic, Axillary, Left
   use Lymphatic, Axillary, Right
Pectoral fascia
   use Subcutaneous Tissue and Fascia, Chest
Pectoralis major muscle
   use Muscle, Thorax, Left
   use Muscle, Thorax, Right
Pectoralis minor muscle
   use Muscle, Thorax, Left
   use Muscle, Thorax, Right
Pedicle-based dynamic stabilization device
   use Spinal Stabilization Device, Pedicle-Based in 0RH
   use Spinal Stabilization Device, Pedicle-Based in 0SH
PEEP (positive end expiratory pressure)
   see Assistance, Respiratory 5A09
PEG (percutaneous endoscopic gastrostomy) 0DH63UZ
PEJ (percutaneous endoscopic jejunostomy) 0DHA3UZ
Pelvic splanchnic nerve
   use Nerve, Abdominal Sympathetic
   use Nerve, Sacral Sympathetic

Penectomy
   see Excision, Male Reproductive System 0VB
   see Resection, Male Reproductive System 0VT
Penile urethra
   use Urethra
Penumbra Indigo® Aspiration System
   see New Technology, Cardiovascular System X2C
PERCEPT™ neurostimulator
   use Stimulator Generator, Multiple Array in 0JH
Perceval sutureless valve
   use Zooplastic Tissue, Rapid Deployment Technique in New Technology
Percutaneous endoscopic gastrojejunostomy (PEG/J) tube
   use Feeding Device in Gastrointestinal System
Percutaneous endoscopic gastrostomy (PEG) tube
   use Feeding Device in Gastrointestinal System
Percutaneous nephrostomy catheter
   use Drainage Device
Percutaneous transluminal coronary angioplasty (PTCA)
   see Dilation, Heart and Great Vessels 027
Performance
   Biliary
      Multiple, Filtration 5A1C60Z
      Single, Filtration 5A1C00Z
   Cardiac
      Continuous
         Output 5A1221Z
         Pacing 5A1223Z
      Intermittent, Pacing 5A1213Z
      Single, Output, Manual 5A12012
   Circulatory
      Continuous
         Central Membrane 5A1522F
         Peripheral Veno-arterial Membrane 5A1522G
         Peripheral Veno-venous Membrane 5A1522H
      Intraoperative
         Central Membrane 5A15A2F
         Peripheral Veno-arterial Membrane 5A15A2G
         Peripheral Veno-venous Membrane 5A15A2H
   Respiratory
      24-96 Consecutive Hours, Ventilation 5A1945Z
      Greater than 96 Consecutive Hours, Ventilation 5A1955Z
      Less than 24 Consecutive Hours, Ventilation 5A1935Z
      Single, Ventilation, Nonmechanical 5A19054
   Urinary
      Continuous, Greater than 18 hours per day, Filtration 5A1D90Z
      Intermittent, Less than 6 hours per day, Filtration 5A1D70Z
      Prolonged Intermittent, 6-18 hours per day, Filtration 5A1D80Z
Perfusion
   see Introduction of substance in or on
Perfusion, donor organ
   Heart 6AB50BZ
   Kidney(s) 6ABT0BZ
   Liver 6ABF0BZ
   Lung(s) 6ABB0BZ

Pericardiectomy
   see Excision, Pericardium 02BN
   see Resection, Pericardium 02TN
Pericardiocentesis
   see Drainage, Pericardial Cavity 0W9D
Pericardiolysis
   see Release, Pericardium 02NN
Pericardiophrenic artery
   use Artery, Internal Mammary, Left
   use Artery, Internal Mammary, Right
Pericardioplasty
   see Repair, Pericardium 02QN
   see Replacement, Pericardium 02RN
   see Supplement, Pericardium 02UN
Pericardiorrhaphy
   see Repair, Pericardium 02QN
Pericardiostomy
   see Drainage, Pericardial Cavity 0W9D
Pericardiotomy
   see Drainage, Pericardial Cavity 0W9D
Perimetrium
   use Uterus
Peripheral Intravascular Lithotripsy (Peripheral IVL)
   see Fragmentation
Peripheral parenteral nutrition
   see Introduction of Nutritional Substance
Peripherally inserted central catheter (PICC)
   use Infusion Device
Peritoneal dialysis 3E1M39Z
Peritoneocentesis
   see Drainage, Peritoneal Cavity 0W9G
   see Drainage, Peritoneum 0D9W
Peritoneoplasty
   see Repair, Peritoneum 0DQW
   see Replacement, Peritoneum 0DRW
   see Supplement, Peritoneum 0DUW
Peritoneoscopy 0DJW4ZZ
Peritoneotomy
   see Drainage, Peritoneum 0D9W
Peritoneumectomy
   see Excision, Peritoneum 0DBW
Peroneus brevis muscle
   use Muscle, Lower Leg, Left
   use Muscle, Lower Leg, Right
Peroneus longus muscle
   use Muscle, Lower Leg, Left
   use Muscle, Lower Leg, Right
Pessary ring
   use Intraluminal Device, Pessary in Female Reproductive System
PET scan
   see Positron Emission Tomographic (PET) Imaging
Petrous part of temporal bone
   use Bone, Temporal, Left
   use Bone, Temporal, Right
Phacoemulsification, lens
   With IOL implant
      see Replacement, Eye 08R
   Without IOL implant
      see Extraction, Eye 08D
Phagenyx® System XWHD7Q7
Phalangectomy
   see Excision, Lower Bones 0QB
   see Excision, Upper Bones 0PB
   see Resection, Lower Bones 0QT
   see Resection, Upper Bones 0PT

Phallectomy
  see Excision, Penis 0VBS
  see Resection, Penis 0VTS
Phalloplasty
  see Repair, Penis 0VQS
  see Supplement, Penis 0VUS
Phallotomy
  see Drainage, Penis 0V9S
Pharmacotherapy, for substance abuse
  Antabuse HZ93ZZZ
  Bupropion HZ97ZZZ
  Clonidine HZ96ZZZ
  Levo-alpha-acetyl-methadol (LAAM) HZ92ZZZ
  Methadone Maintenance HZ91ZZZ
  Naloxone HZ95ZZZ
  Naltrexone HZ94ZZZ
  Nicotine Replacement HZ90ZZZ
  Psychiatric Medication HZ98ZZZ
  Replacement Medication, Other HZ99ZZZ
Pharyngeal constrictor muscle
  use Muscle, Tongue, Palate, Pharynx
Pharyngeal plexus
  use Nerve, Vagus
Pharyngeal recess
  use Nasopharynx
Pharyngeal tonsil
  use Adenoids
Pharyngogram
  see Fluoroscopy, Pharynix B91G
Pharyngoplasty
  see Repair, Mouth and Throat 0CQ
  see Replacement, Mouth and Throat 0CR
  see Supplement, Mouth and Throat 0CU
Pharyngorrhaphy
  see Repair, Mouth and Throat 0CQ
Pharyngotomy
  see Drainage, Mouth and Throat 0C9
Pharyngotympanic tube
  use Eustachian Tube, Left
  use Eustachian Tube, Right
Pheresis
  Erythrocytes 6A55
  Leukocytes 6A55
  Plasma 6A55
  Platelets 6A55
  Stem Cells
    Cord Blood 6A55
    Hematopoietic 6A55
Phlebectomy
  see Excision, Lower Veins 06B
  see Excision, Upper Veins 05B
  see Extraction, Lower Veins 06D
  see Extraction, Upper Veins 05D
Phlebography
  see Plain Radiography, Veins B50
  Impedance 4A04X51
Phleborrhaphy
  see Repair, Lower Veins 06Q
  see Repair, Upper Veins 05Q
Phlebotomy
  see Drainage, Lower Veins 069
  see Drainage, Upper Veins 059
Photocoagulation
  For Destruction
    see Destruction
  For Repair
    see Repair
Photopheresis, therapeutic
  see Phototherapy, Circulatory 6A65
Phototherapy
  Circulatory 6A65
  Skin 6A60

Phototherapy *(continued)*
  Ultraviolet light
    see Ultraviolet Light Therapy, Physiological Systems 6A8
Phrenectomy, phrenoneurectomy
  see Excision, Nerve, Phrenic 01B2
Phrenemphraxis
  see Destruction, Nerve, Phrenic 0152
Phrenic nerve stimulator generator
  use Stimulator Generator in Subcutaneous Tissue and Fascia
Phrenic nerve stimulator lead
  use Diaphragmatic Pacemaker Lead in Respiratory System
Phreniclasis
  see Destruction, Nerve, Phrenic 0152
Phrenicoexeresis
  see Extraction, Nerve, Phrenic 01D2
Phrenicotomy
  see Division, Nerve, Phrenic 0182
Phrenicotripsy
  see Destruction, Nerve, Phrenic 0152
Phrenoplasty
  see Repair, Respiratory System 0BQ
  see Supplement, Respiratory System 0BU
Phrenotomy
  see Drainage, Respiratory System 0B9
Physiatry
  see Motor Treatment, Rehabilitation F07
Physical medicine
  see Motor Treatment, Rehabilitation F07
Physical therapy
  see Motor Treatment, Rehabilitation F07
PHYSIOMESH™ Flexible Composite Mesh
  use Synthetic Substitute
Pia mater, intracranial
  use Cerebral Meninges
Pia mater, spinal
  use Spinal Meninges
Pinealectomy
  see Excision, Pineal Body 0GB1
  see Resection, Pineal Body 0GT1
Pinealoscopy 0GJ14ZZ
Pinealotomy
  see Drainage, Pineal Body 0G91
Pinna
  use Ear, External, Bilateral
  use Ear, External, Left
  use Ear, External, Right
Pipeline™ (Flex) embolization device
  use Intraluminal Device, Flow Diverter in 03V
Piriform recess (sinus)
  use Pharynx
Piriformis muscle
  use Muscle, Hip, Right
  use Muscle, Hip, Left
PIRRT (Prolonged intermittent renal replacement therapy) 5A1D80Z
Pisiform bone
  use Carpal, Left
  use Carpal, Right
Pisohamate ligament
  use Bursa and Ligament, Hand, Left
  use Bursa and Ligament, Hand, Right

Pisometacarpal ligament
  use Bursa and Ligament, Hand, Left
  use Bursa and Ligament, Hand, Right
Pituitectomy
  see Excision, Gland, Pituitary 0GB0
  see Resection, Gland, Pituitary 0GT0
Plain film radiology
  see Plain Radiography
Plain Radiography
  Abdomen BW00ZZZ
  Abdomen and Pelvis BW01ZZZ
  Abdominal Lymphatic
    Bilateral B701
    Unilateral B700
  Airway, Upper BB0DZZZ
  Ankle
    Left BQ0H
    Right BQ0G
  Aorta
    Abdominal B400
    Thoracic B300
    Thoraco-Abdominal B30P
  Aorta and Bilateral Lower Extremity Arteries B40D
  Arch
    Bilateral BN0DZZZ
    Left BN0CZZZ
    Right BN0BZZZ
  Arm
    Left BP0FZZZ
    Right BP0EZZZ
  Artery
    Brachiocephalic-Subclavian, Right B301
    Bronchial B30L
    Bypass Graft, Other B20F
    Cervico-Cerebral Arch B30Q
    Common Carotid
      Bilateral B305
      Left B304
      Right B303
    Coronary
      Bypass Graft
        Multiple B203
        Single B202
      Multiple B201
      Single B200
    External Carotid
      Bilateral B30C
      Left B30B
      Right B309
    Hepatic B402
    Inferior Mesenteric B405
    Intercostal B30L
    Internal Carotid
      Bilateral B308
      Left B307
      Right B306
    Internal Mammary Bypass Graft
      Left B208
      Right B207
    Intra-Abdominal, Other B40B
    Intracranial B30R
    Lower, Other B40J
    Lower Extremity
      Bilateral and Aorta B40D
      Left B40G
      Right B40F
    Lumbar B409
    Pelvic B40C
    Pulmonary
      Left B30T
      Right B30S
    Renal
      Bilateral B408
      Left B407
      Right B406
      Transplant B40M

Plain Radiography *(continued)*
  Artery *(continued)*
    Spinal B30M
    Splenic B403
    Subclavian, Left B302
    Superior Mesenteric B404
    Upper, Other B30N
    Upper Extremity
      Bilateral B30K
      Left B30J
      Right B30H
    Vertebral
      Bilateral B30G
      Left B30F
      Right B30D
  Bile Duct BF00
  Bile Duct and Gallbladder BF03
  Bladder BT00
    Kidney and Ureter BT04
  Bladder and Urethra BT0B
  Bone
    Facial BN05ZZZ
    Nasal BN04ZZZ
  Bones, Long, All BW0BZZZ
  Breast
    Bilateral BH02ZZZ
    Left BH01ZZZ
    Right BH00ZZZ
  Calcaneus
    Left BQ0KZZZ
    Right BQ0JZZZ
  Chest BW03ZZZ
  Clavicle
    Left BP05ZZZ
    Right BP04ZZZ
  Coccyx BR0FZZZ
  Corpora Cavernosa BV00
  Dialysis Fistula B50W
  Dialysis Shunt B50W
  Disc
    Cervical BR01
    Lumbar BR03
    Thoracic BR02
  Duct
    Lacrimal
      Bilateral B802
      Left B801
      Right B800
    Mammary
      Multiple
        Left BH06
        Right BH05
      Single
        Left BH04
        Right BH03
  Elbow
    Left BP0H
    Right BP0G
  Epididymis
    Left BV02
    Right BV01
  Extremity
    Lower BW0CZZZ
    Upper BW0JZZZ
  Eye
    Bilateral B807ZZZ
    Left B806ZZZ
    Right B805ZZZ
  Facet Joint
    Cervical BR04
    Lumbar BR06
    Thoracic BR05
  Fallopian Tube
    Bilateral BU02
    Left BU01
    Right BU00
  Fallopian Tube and Uterus BU08
  Femur
    Left, Densitometry BQ04ZZ1
    Right, Densitometry BQ03ZZ1

Plain Radiography (continued)

Finger
- Left BP0SZZZ
- Right BP0RZZZ

Foot
- Left BQ0MZZZ
- Right BQ0LZZZ

Forearm
- Left BP0KZZZ
- Right BP0JZZZ

Gallbladder and Bile Duct
- BF03

Gland

Parotid
- Bilateral B906
- Left B905
- Right B904

Salivary
- Bilateral B90D
- Left B90C
- Right B90B

Submandibular
- Bilateral B909
- Left B908
- Right B907

Hand
- Left BP0PZZZ
- Right BP0NZZZ

Heart
- Left B205
- Right B204
- Right and Left B206

Hepatobiliary System, All
- BF0C

Hip
- Left BQ01
  - Densitometry BQ01ZZ1
- Right BQ00
  - Densitometry BQ00ZZ1

Humerus
- Left BP0BZZZ
- Right BP0AZZZ

Ileal Diversion Loop BT0C

Intracranial Sinus B502

Joint

Acromioclavicular, Bilateral
- BP03ZZZ

Finger
- Left BP0D
- Right BP0C

Foot
- Left BQ0Y
- Right BQ0X

Hand
- Left BP0D
- Right BP0C

Lumbosacral BR0BZZZ

Sacroiliac BR0D

Sternoclavicular
- Bilateral BP02ZZZ
- Left BP01ZZZ
- Right BP00ZZZ

Temporomandibular
- Bilateral BN09
- Left BN08
- Right BN07

Thoracolumbar BR08ZZZ

Toe
- Left BQ0Y
- Right BQ0X

Kidney
- Bilateral BT03
- Left BT02
- Right BT01
- Ureter and Bladder BT04

Knee
- Left BQ08
- Right BQ07

Leg
- Left BQ0FZZZ
- Right BQ0DZZZ

Plain Radiography (continued)

Lymphatic

Head B704

Lower Extremity
- Bilateral B70B
- Left B709
- Right B708

Neck B704

Pelvic B70C

Upper Extremity
- Bilateral B707
- Left B706
- Right B705

Mandible BN06ZZZ

Mastoid B90HZZZ

Nasopharynx B90FZZZ

Optic Foramina
- Left B804ZZZ
- Right B803ZZZ

Orbit
- Bilateral BN03ZZZ
- Left BN02ZZZ
- Right BN01ZZZ

Oropharynx B90FZZZ

Patella
- Left BQ0WZZZ
- Right BQ0VZZZ

Pelvis BR0CZZZ

Pelvis and Abdomen BW01ZZZ

Prostate BV03

Retroperitoneal Lymphatic
- Bilateral B701
- Unilateral B700

Ribs
- Left BP0YZZZ
- Right BP0XZZZ

Sacrum BR0FZZZ

Scapula
- Left BP07ZZZ
- Right BP06ZZZ

Shoulder
- Left BP09
- Right BP08

Sinus
- Intracranial B502
- Paranasal B902ZZZ

Skull BN00ZZZ

Spinal Cord B00B

Spine
- Cervical, Densitometry BR00ZZ1
- Lumbar, Densitometry BR09ZZ1
- Thoracic, Densitometry BR07ZZ1
- Whole, Densitometry BR0GZZ1

Sternum BR0HZZZ

Teeth
- All BN0JZZZ
- Multiple BN0HZZZ

Testicle
- Left BV06
- Right BV05

Toe
- Left BQ0QZZZ
- Right BQ0PZZZ

Tooth, Single BN0GZZZ

Tracheobronchial Tree
- Bilateral BB09YZZ
- Left BB08Y
- Right BB07Y

Ureter
- Bilateral BT08
- Kidney and Bladder BT04
- Left BT07
- Right BT06

Urethra BT05

Urethra and Bladder BT0B

Uterus BU06

Uterus and Fallopian Tube BU08

Vagina BU09

Vasa Vasorum BV08

Plain Radiography (continued)

Vein

Cerebellar B501

Cerebral B501

Epidural B500

Jugular
- Bilateral B505
- Left B504
- Right B503

Lower Extremity
- Bilateral B50D
- Left B50C
- Right B50B
- Other B50V

Pelvic (Iliac)
- Left B50G
- Right B50F

Pelvic (Iliac) Bilateral B50H

Portal B50T

Pulmonary
- Bilateral B50S
- Left B50R
- Right B50Q

Renal
- Bilateral B50L
- Left B50K
- Right B50J

Spanchnic B50T

Subclavian
- Left B507
- Right B506

Upper Extremity
- Bilateral B50P
- Left B50N
- Right B50M

Vena Cava
- Inferior B509
- Superior B508

Whole Body BW0KZZZ

Infant BW0MZZZ

Whole Skeleton BW0LZZZ

Wrist
- Left BP0M
- Right BP0L

Planar Nuclear Medicine Imaging

Abdomen CW10

Abdomen and Chest CW14

Abdomen and Pelvis CW11

Anatomical Regions, Multiple CW1YYZZ

Anatomical Region, Other CW1ZZZZ

Bladder, Kidneys and Ureters CT13

Bladder and Ureters CT1H

Blood C713

Bone Marrow C710

Brain C010

Breast CH1YYZZ
- Bilateral CH12
- Left CH11
- Right CH10

Bronchi and Lungs CB12

Central Nervous System C01YYZZ

Cerebrospinal Fluid C015

Chest CW13

Chest and Abdomen CW14

Chest and Neck CW16

Digestive System CD1YYZZ

Ducts, Lacrimal, Bilateral C819

Ear, Nose, Mouth and Throat C91YYZZ

Endocrine System CG1YYZZ

Extremity

Lower CW1D
- Bilateral CP1F
- Left CP1D
- Right CP1C

Upper CW1M
- Bilateral CP1B
- Left CP19
- Right CP18

Planar Nuclear Medicine Imaging (continued)

Eye C81YYZZ

Gallbladder CF14

Gastrointestinal Tract CD17
- Upper CD15

Gland
- Adrenal, Bilateral CG14
- Parathyroid CG11
- Thyroid CG12

Glands, Salivary, Bilateral C91B

Head and Neck CW1B

Heart C21YYZZ
- Right and Left C216

Hepatobiliary System, All CF1C

Hepatobiliary System and Pancreas CF1YYZZ

Kidneys, Ureters and Bladder CT13

Liver CF15

Liver and Spleen CF16

Lungs and Bronchi CB12

Lymphatics
- Head C71J
- Head and Neck C715
- Lower Extremity C71P
- Neck C71K
- Pelvic C71D
- Trunk C71M
- Upper Chest C71L
- Upper Extremity C71N

Lymphatics and Hematologic System C71YYZZ

Musculoskeletal System
- All CP1Z
- Other CP1YYZZ

Myocardium C21G

Neck and Chest CW16

Neck and Head CW1B

Pancreas and Hepatobiliary System CF1YYZZ

Pelvic Region CW1J

Pelvis CP16

Pelvis and Abdomen CW11

Pelvis and Spine CP17

Reproductive System, Male CV1YYZZ

Respiratory System CB1YYZZ

Skin CH1YYZZ

Skull CP11

Spine CP15

Spine and Pelvis CP17

Spleen C712

Spleen and Liver CF16

Subcutaneous Tissue CH1YYZZ

Testicles, Bilateral CV19

Thorax CP14

Ureters, Kidneys and Bladder CT13

Ureters and Bladder CT1H

Urinary System CT1YYZZ

Veins C51YYZZ
- Central C51R
- Lower Extremity
  - Bilateral C51D
  - Left C51C
  - Right C51B
- Upper Extremity
  - Bilateral C51Q
  - Left C51P
  - Right C51N

Whole Body CW1N

Plantar digital vein
- use Vein, Foot, Left
- use Vein, Foot, Right

Plantar fascia (aponeurosis)
- use Subcutaneous Tissue and Fascia, Foot, Left
- use Subcutaneous Tissue and Fascia, Foot, Right

Plantar metatarsal vein
use Vein, Foot, Left
use Vein, Foot, Right
Plantar venous arch
use Vein, Foot, Left
use Vein, Foot, Right
Plaque Radiation
Abdomen DWY3FZZ
Adrenal Gland DGY2FZZ
Anus DDY8FZZ
Bile Ducts DFY2FZZ
Bladder DTY2FZZ
Bone, Other DPYCFZZ
Bone Marrow D7Y0FZZ
Brain D0Y0FZZ
Brain Stem D0Y1FZZ
Breast
    Left DMY0FZZ
    Right DMY1FZZ
Bronchus DBY1FZZ
Cervix DUY1FZZ
Chest DWY2FZZ
Chest Wall DBY7FZZ
Colon DDY5FZZ
Diaphragm DBY8FZZ
Duodenum DDY2FZZ
Ear D9Y0FZZ
Esophagus DDY0FZZ
Eye D8Y0FZZ
Femur DPY9FZZ
Fibula DPYBFZZ
Gallbladder DFY1FZZ
Gland
    Adrenal DGY2FZZ
    Parathyroid DGY4FZZ
    Pituitary DGY0FZZ
    Thyroid DGY5FZZ
Glands, Salivary D9Y6FZZ
Head and Neck DWY1FZZ
Hemibody DWY4FZZ
Humerus DPY6FZZ
Ileum DDY4FZZ
Jejunum DDY3FZZ
Kidney DTY0FZZ
Larynx D9YBFZZ
Liver DFY0FZZ
Lung DBY2FZZ
Lymphatics
    Abdomen D7Y6FZZ
    Axillary D7Y4FZZ
    Inguinal D7Y8FZZ
    Neck D7Y3FZZ
    Pelvis D7Y7FZZ
    Thorax D7Y5FZZ
Mandible DPY3FZZ
Maxilla DPY2FZZ
Mediastinum DBY6FZZ
Mouth D9Y4FZZ
Nasopharynx D9YDFZZ
Neck and Head DWY1FZZ
Nerve, Peripheral D0Y7FZZ
Nose D9Y1FZZ
Ovary DUY0FZZ
Palate
    Hard D9Y8FZZ
    Soft D9Y9FZZ
Pancreas DFY3FZZ
Parathyroid Gland DGY4FZZ
Pelvic Bones DPY8FZZ
Pelvic Region DWY6FZZ
Pharynx D9YCFZZ
Pineal Body DGY1FZZ
Pituitary Gland DGY0FZZ
Pleura DBY5FZZ
Prostate DVY0FZZ
Radius DPY7FZZ
Rectum DDY7FZZ
Rib DPY5FZZ
Sinuses D9Y7FZZ
Skin
    Abdomen DHY8FZZ

Plaque Radiation *(continued)*
Skin *(continued)*
    Arm DHY4FZZ
    Back DHY7FZZ
    Buttock DHY9FZZ
    Chest DHY6FZZ
    Face DHY2FZZ
    Foot DHYCFZZ
    Hand DHY5FZZ
    Leg DHYBFZZ
    Neck DHY3FZZ
Skull DPY0FZZ
Spinal Cord D0Y6FZZ
Spleen D7Y2FZZ
Sternum DPY4FZZ
Stomach DDY1FZZ
Testis DVY1FZZ
Thymus D7Y1FZZ
Thyroid Gland DGY5FZZ
Tibia DPYBFZZ
Tongue D9Y5FZZ
Trachea DBY0FZZ
Ulna DPY7FZZ
Ureter DTY1FZZ
Urethra DTY3FZZ
Uterus DUY2FZZ
Whole Body DWY5FZZ
Plasma, Convalescent
    (Nonautologous) XW1
Plasmapheresis, therapeutic
see Pheresis, Physiological Systems
    6A5
Plateletpheresis, therapeutic
see Pheresis, Physiological Systems
    6A5
Platysma muscle
use Muscle, Neck, Left
use Muscle, Neck, Right
Plazomicin Anti-infective XW0
Pleurectomy
see Excision, Respiratory System
    0BB
see Resection, Respiratory System
    0BT
Pleurocentesis
see Drainage, Anatomical Regions,
    General 0W9
Pleurodesis, pleurosclerosis
Chemical injection
    see Introduction of substance in
        or on, Pleural Cavity 3E0L
Surgical
    see Destruction, Respiratory
        System 0B5
Pleurolysis
see Release, Respiratory System
    0BN
Pleuroscopy 0BJQ4ZZ
Pleurotomy
see Drainage, Respiratory System
    0B9
Plica semilunaris
use Conjunctiva, Left
use Conjunctiva, Right
Plication
see Restriction
Pneumectomy
see Excision, Respiratory System
    0BB
see Resection, Respiratory System
    0BT
Pneumocentesis
see Drainage, Respiratory System
    0B9
Pneumogastric nerve
use Nerve, Vagus
Pneumolysis
see Release, Respiratory System 0BN
Pneumonectomy
see Resection, Respiratory System
    0BT

Pneumonolysis
see Release, Respiratory System
    0BN
Pneumonopexy
see Repair, Respiratory System 0BQ
see Reposition, Respiratory System
    0BS
Pneumonorrhaphy
see Repair, Respiratory System
    0BQ
Pneumonotomy
see Drainage, Respiratory System
    0B9
Pneumotaxic center
use Pons
Pneumotomy
see Drainage, Respiratory System
    0B9
Pollicization
see Transfer, Anatomical Regions,
    Upper Extremities 0XX
Polyclonal hyperimmune globulin
use Globulin
Polyethylene socket
use Synthetic Substitute,
    Polyethylene in 0SR
Polymethylmethacrylate
    (PMMA)
use Synthetic Substitute
Polypectomy, gastrointestinal
see Excision, Gastrointestinal
    System 0DB
Polypropylene mesh
use Synthetic Substitute
Polysomnogram 4A1ZXQZ
Pontine tegmentum
use Pons
Popliteal ligament
use Bursa and Ligament, Knee, Left
use Bursa and Ligament, Knee,
    Right
Popliteal lymph node
use Lymphatic, Lower Extremity,
    Left
use Lymphatic, Lower Extremity,
    Right
Popliteal vein
use Vein, Femoral, Left
use Vein, Femoral, Right
Popliteus muscle
use Muscle, Lower Leg, Left
use Muscle, Lower Leg, Right
Porcine (bioprosthetic) valve
use Zooplastic Tissue in Heart and
    Great Vessels
Positive Blood Culture Fluorescence
    Hybridization for Organism
    Identification, Concentration
    and Susceptibility XXE5XN6
Positive end expiratory pressure
see Performance, Respiratory
    5A19
Positron Emission Tomographic
    (PET) Imaging
Brain C030
Bronchi and Lungs CB32
Central Nervous System C03YYZZ
Heart C23YYZZ
Lungs and Bronchi CB32
Myocardium C23G
Respiratory System CB3YYZZ
Whole Body CW3NYZZ
Positron emission tomography
see Positron Emission Tomographic
    (PET) Imaging
Postauricular (mastoid) lymph
    node
use Lymphatic, Neck, Left
use Lymphatic, Neck, Right
Postcava
use Vena Cava, Inferior

Posterior (subscapular) lymph node
use Lymphatic, Axillary, Left
use Lymphatic, Axillary, Right
Posterior auricular artery
use Artery, External Carotid, Left
use Artery, External Carotid, Right
Posterior auricular nerve
use Nerve, Facial
Posterior auricular vein
use Vein, External Jugular, Left
use Vein, External Jugular, Right
Posterior cerebral artery
use Artery, Intracranial
Posterior chamber
use Eye, Left
use Eye, Right
Posterior circumflex humeral
    artery
use Artery, Axillary, Left
use Artery, Axillary, Right
Posterior communicating artery
use Artery, Intracranial
Posterior cruciate ligament (PCL)
use Bursa and Ligament, Knee, Left
use Bursa and Ligament, Knee,
    Right
Posterior (Dynamic) Distraction
    Device
Lumbar XNS0
Thoracic XNS4
Posterior facial (retromandibular)
    vein
use Vein, Face, Left
use Vein, Face, Right
Posterior femoral cutaneous nerve
use Nerve, Sacral Plexus
Posterior inferior cerebellar artery
    (PICA)
use Artery, Intracranial
Posterior interosseous nerve
use Nerve, Radial
Posterior labial nerve
use Nerve, Pudendal
Posterior scrotal nerve
use Nerve, Pudendal
Posterior spinal artery
use Artery, Vertebral, Left
use Artery, Vertebral, Right
Posterior tibial recurrent artery
use Artery, Anterior Tibial, Left
use Artery, Anterior Tibial,
    Right
Posterior ulnar recurrent artery
use Artery, Ulnar, Left
use Artery, Ulnar, Right
Posterior vagal trunk
use Nerve, Vagus
PPN (peripheral parenteral
    nutrition)
see Introduction of Nutritional
    Substance
Praxbind® (idarucizumab),
    Pradaxa® (dabigatran) reversal
    agent
use Other Therapeutic Substance
Preauricular lymph node
use Lymphatic, Head
Precava
use Vena Cava, Superior
PRECICE intramedullary limb
    lengthening system
use Internal Fixation Device,
    Intramedullary Limb
    Lengthening in 0PH
use Internal Fixation Device,
    Intramedullary Limb
    Lengthening in 0QH
Prepatellar bursa
use Bursa and Ligament, Knee, Left
use Bursa and Ligament, Knee,
    Right

Preputiotomy
see Drainage, Male Reproductive System 0V9

Pressure support ventilation
see Performance, Respiratory 5A19

PRESTIGE® Cervical Disc
use Synthetic Substitute

Pretracheal fascia
use Subcutaneous Tissue and Fascia, Neck, Left
use Subcutaneous Tissue and Fascia, Neck, Right

Prevertebral fascia
use Subcutaneous Tissue and Fascia, Neck, Left
use Subcutaneous Tissue and Fascia, Neck, Right

PrimeAdvanced neurostimulator (SureScan)(MRI Safe)
use Stimulator Generator, Multiple Array in 0JH

Princeps pollicis artery
use Artery, Hand, Left
use Artery, Hand, Right

Probing, duct
Diagnostic
see Inspection
Dilation
see Dilation

PROCEED™ Ventral Patch
use Synthetic Substitute

Procerus muscle
use Muscle, Facial

Proctectomy
see Excision, Rectum 0DBP
see Resection, Rectum 0DTP

Proctoclysis
see Introduction of substance in or on, Gastrointestinal Tract, Lower 3E0H

Proctocolectomy
see Excision, Gastrointestinal System 0DB
see Resection, Gastrointestinal System 0DT

Proctocolpoplasty
see Repair, Gastrointestinal System 0DQ
see Supplement, Gastrointestinal System 0DU

Proctoperineoplasty
see Repair, Gastrointestinal System 0DQ
see Supplement, Gastrointestinal System 0DU

Proctoperineorrhaphy
see Repair, Gastrointestinal System 0DQ

Proctopexy
see Repair, Rectum 0DQP
see Reposition, Rectum 0DSP

Proctoplasty
see Repair, Rectum 0DQP
see Supplement, Rectum 0DUP

Proctorrhaphy
see Repair, Rectum 0DQP

Proctoscopy 0DJD8ZZ

Proctosigmoidectomy
see Excision, Gastrointestinal System 0DB
see Resection, Gastrointestinal System 0DT

Proctosigmoidoscopy 0DJD8ZZ

Proctostomy
see Drainage, Rectum 0D9P

Proctotomy
see Drainage, Rectum 0D9P

Prodisc-C
use Synthetic Substitute

Prodisc-L
use Synthetic Substitute

Production, atrial septal defect
see Excision, Septum, Atrial 02B5

Profunda brachii
use Artery, Brachial, Left
use Artery, Brachial, Right

Profunda femoris (deep femoral) vein
use Vein, Femoral, Left
use Vein, Femoral, Right

PROLENE Polypropylene Hernia System (PHS)
use Synthetic Substitute

Prolonged intermittent renal replacement therapy (PIRRT) 5A1D80Z

Pronator quadratus muscle
use Muscle, Lower Arm and Wrist, Left
use Muscle, Lower Arm and Wrist, Right

Pronator teres muscle
use Muscle, Lower Arm and Wrist, Left
use Muscle, Lower Arm and Wrist, Right

Prostatectomy
see Excision, Prostate 0VB0
see Resection, Prostate 0VT0

Prostatic urethra
use Urethra

Prostatomy, prostatotomy
see Drainage, Prostate 0V90

Protecta XT CRT-D
use Cardiac Resynchronization Defibrillator Pulse Generator in 0JH

Protecta XT DR (XT VR)
use Defibrillator Generator in 0JH

Protégé® RX Carotid Stent System
use Intraluminal Device

Proximal radioulnar joint
use Joint, Elbow, Left
use Joint, Elbow, Right

Psoas muscle
use Muscle, Hip, Left
use Muscle, Hip, Right

PSV (pressure support ventilation)
see Performance, Respiratory 5A19

Psychoanalysis GZ54ZZZ

Psychological Tests
Cognitive Status GZ14ZZZ
Developmental GZ10ZZZ
Intellectual and Psychoeducational GZ12ZZZ
Neurobehavioral Status GZ14ZZZ
Neuropsychological GZ13ZZZ
Personality and Behavioral GZ11ZZZ

Psychotherapy
Family, Mental Health Services GZ72ZZZ
Group
GZHZZZZ
Mental Health Services GZHZZZZ
Individual
see Psychotherapy, Individual, Mental Health Services
for substance abuse
12-Step HZ53ZZZ
Behavioral HZ51ZZZ
Cognitive HZ50ZZZ
Cognitive-Behavioral HZ52ZZZ
Confrontational HZ58ZZZ
Interactive HZ55ZZZ

Psychotherapy (continued)
Individual (continued)
see Psychotherapy, Individual, Mental Health Services (continued)
Interpersonal HZ54ZZZ
Motivational Enhancement HZ57ZZZ
Psychoanalysis HZ5BZZZ
Psychodynamic HZ5CZZZ
Psychoeducation HZ56ZZZ
Psychophysiological HZ5DZZZ
Supportive HZ59ZZZ
Mental Health Services
Behavioral GZ51ZZZ
Cognitive GZ52ZZZ
Cognitive-Behavioral GZ58ZZZ
Interactive GZ50ZZZ
Interpersonal GZ53ZZZ
Psychoanalysis GZ54ZZZ
Psychodynamic GZ55ZZZ
Psychophysiological GZ59ZZZ
Supportive GZ56ZZZ

PTCA (percutaneous transluminal coronary angioplasty)
see Dilation, Heart and Great Vessels 027

Pterygoid muscle
use Muscle, Head

Pterygoid process
use Bone, Sphenoid

Pterygopalatine (sphenopalatine) ganglion
use Nerve, Head and Neck Sympathetic

Pubis
use Bone, Pelvic, Left
use Bone, Pelvic, Right

Pubofemoral ligament
use Bursa and Ligament, Hip, Left
use Bursa and Ligament, Hip, Right

Pudendal nerve
use Nerve, Sacral Plexus

Pull-through, laparoscopic-assisted transanal
see Excision, Gastrointestinal System 0DB
see Resection, Gastrointestinal System 0DT

Pull-through, rectal
see Resection, Rectum 0DTP

Pulmoaortic canal
use Artery, Pulmonary, Left

Pulmonary annulus
use Valve, Pulmonary

Pulmonary artery wedge monitoring
see Monitoring, Arterial 4A13

Pulmonary plexus
use Nerve, Thoracic Sympathetic
use Nerve, Vagus

Pulmonic valve
use Valve, Pulmonary

Pulpectomy
see Excision, Mouth and Throat 0CB

Pulverization
see Fragmentation

Pulvinar
use Thalamus

Pump reservoir
use Infusion Device, Pump in Subcutaneous Tissue and Fascia

Punch biopsy
see Excision with qualifier Diagnostic

Puncture
see Drainage

Puncture, lumbar
see Drainage, Spinal Canal 009U

Pure-Vu® System XDPH8K7

Pyelography
see Fluoroscopy, Urinary System BT1
see Plain Radiography, Urinary System BT0

Pyeloileostomy, urinary diversion
see Bypass, Urinary System 0T1

Pyeloplasty
see Repair, Urinary System 0TQ
see Replacement, Urinary System 0TR
see Supplement, Urinary System 0TU

Pyeloplasty, dismembered
see Repair, Kidney Pelvis

Pyelorrhaphy
see Repair, Urinary System 0TQ

Pyeloscopy 0TJ58ZZ

Pyelostomy
see Drainage, Urinary System 0T9
see Bypass, Urinary System 0T1

Pyelotomy
see Drainage, Urinary System 0T9

Pylorectomy
see Excision, Stomach, Pylorus 0DB7
see Resection, Stomach, Pylorus 0DT7

Pyloric antrum
use Stomach, Pylorus

Pyloric canal
use Stomach, Pylorus

Pyloric sphincter
use Stomach, Pylorus

Pylorodiosis
see Dilation, Stomach, Pylorus 0D77

Pylorogastrectomy
see Excision, Gastrointestinal System 0DB
see Resection, Gastrointestinal System 0DT

Pyloroplasty
see Repair, Stomach, Pylorus 0DQ7
see Supplement, Stomach, Pylorus 0DU7

Pyloroscopy 0DJ68ZZ

Pylorotomy
see Drainage, Stomach, Pylorus 0D97

Pyramidalis muscle
use Muscle, Abdomen, Left
use Muscle, Abdomen, Right

Q

Quadrangular cartilage
use Septum, Nasal

Quadrant resection of breast
see Excision, Skin and Breast 0HB

Quadrate lobe
use Liver

Quadratus femoris muscle
use Muscle, Hip, Left
use Muscle, Hip, Right

Quadratus lumborum muscle
use Muscle, Trunk, Left
use Muscle, Trunk, Right

Quadratus plantae muscle
use Muscle, Foot, Left
use Muscle, Foot, Right

Quadriceps (femoris)
  use Muscle, Upper Leg, Left
  use Muscle, Upper Leg, Right
Quarantine 8E0ZXY6

R

Radial artery arteriovenous fistula, using Thermal Resistance Energy X2K
Radial collateral carpal ligament
  use Bursa and Ligament, Wrist, Left
  use Bursa and Ligament, Wrist, Right
Radial collateral ligament
  use Bursa and Ligament, Elbow, Left
  use Bursa and Ligament, Elbow, Right
Radial notch
  use Ulna, Left
  use Ulna, Right
Radial recurrent artery
  use Artery, Radial, Left
  use Artery, Radial, Right
Radial vein
  use Vein, Brachial, Left
  use Vein, Brachial, Right
Radialis indicis
  use Artery, Hand, Left
  use Artery, Hand, Right
Radiation Therapy
  see Beam Radiation
  see Brachytherapy
  see Other Radiation
  see Stereotactic Radiosurgery
Radiation treatment
  see Radiation Therapy
Radiocarpal joint
  use Joint, Wrist, Left
  use Joint, Wrist, Right
Radiocarpal ligament
  use Bursa and Ligament, Wrist, Left
  use Bursa and Ligament, Wrist, Right
Radiography
  see Plain Radiography
Radiology, analog
  see Plain Radiography
Radiology, diagnostic
  see Imaging, Diagnostic
Radioulnar ligament
  use Bursa and Ligament, Wrist, Left
  use Bursa and Ligament, Wrist, Right
Range of motion testing
  see Motor Function Assessment, Rehabilitation F01
Rapid ASPECTS XXE0X07
REALIZE® Adjustable Gastric Band
  use Extraluminal Device
Reattachment
  Abdominal Wall 0WMF0ZZ
  Ampulla of Vater 0FMC
  Ankle Region
    Left 0YML0ZZ
    Right 0YMK0ZZ
  Arm
    Lower
      Left 0XMF0ZZ
      Right 0XMD0ZZ
    Upper
      Left 0XM90ZZ
      Right 0XM80ZZ
  Axilla
    Left 0XM50ZZ
    Right 0XM40ZZ
  Back
    Lower 0WML0ZZ
    Upper 0WMK0ZZ

Reattachment (*continued*)
  Bladder 0TMB
  Bladder Neck 0TMC
  Breast
    Bilateral 0HMVXZZ
    Left 0HMUXZZ
    Right 0HMTXZZ
  Bronchus
    Lingula 0BM90ZZ
    Lower Lobe
      Left 0BMB0ZZ
      Right 0BM60ZZ
    Main
      Left 0BM70ZZ
      Right 0BM30ZZ
    Middle Lobe, Right 0BM50ZZ
    Upper Lobe
      Left 0BM80ZZ
      Right 0BM40ZZ
  Bursa and Ligament
    Abdomen
      Left 0MMJ
      Right 0MMH
    Ankle
      Left 0MMR
      Right 0MMQ
    Elbow
      Left 0MM4
      Right 0MM3
    Foot
      Left 0MMT
      Right 0MMS
    Hand
      Left 0MM8
      Right 0MM7
    Head and Neck 0MM0
    Hip
      Left 0MMM
      Right 0MML
    Knee
      Left 0MMP
      Right 0MMN
    Lower Extremity
      Left 0MMW
      Right 0MMV
    Perineum 0MMK
    Rib(s) 0MMG
    Shoulder
      Left 0MM2
      Right 0MM1
    Spine
      Lower 0MMD
      Upper 0MMC
    Sternum 0MMF
    Upper Extremity
      Left 0MMB
      Right 0MM9
    Wrist
      Left 0MM6
      Right 0MM5
  Buttock
    Left 0YM10ZZ
    Right 0YM00ZZ
  Carina 0BM20ZZ
  Cecum 0DMH
  Cervix 0UMC
  Chest Wall 0WM80ZZ
  Clitoris 0UMJXZZ
  Colon
    Ascending 0DMK
    Descending 0DMM
    Sigmoid 0DMN
    Transverse 0DML
  Cord
    Bilateral 0VMH
    Left 0VMG
    Right 0VMF
  Cul-de-sac 0UMF
  Diaphragm 0BMT0ZZ

Reattachment (*continued*)
  Duct
    Common Bile 0FM9
    Cystic 0FM8
    Hepatic
      Common 0FM7
      Left 0FM6
      Right 0FM5
    Pancreatic 0FMD
      Accessory 0FMF
  Duodenum 0DM9
  Ear
    Left 09M1XZZ
    Right 09M0XZZ
  Elbow Region
    Left 0XMC0ZZ
    Right 0XMB0ZZ
  Esophagus 0DM5
  Extremity
    Lower
      Left 0YMB0ZZ
      Right 0YM90ZZ
    Upper
      Left 0XM70ZZ
      Right 0XM60ZZ
  Eyelid
    Lower
      Left 08MRXZZ
      Right 08MQXZZ
    Upper
      Left 08MPXZZ
      Right 08MNXZZ
  Face 0WM20ZZ
  Fallopian Tube
    Left 0UM6
    Right 0UM5
  Fallopian Tubes, Bilateral 0UM7
  Femoral Region
    Left 0YM80ZZ
    Right 0YM70ZZ
  Finger
    Index
      Left 0XMP0ZZ
      Right 0XMN0ZZ
    Little
      Left 0XMW0ZZ
      Right 0XMV0ZZ
    Middle
      Left 0XMR0ZZ
      Right 0XMQ0ZZ
    Ring
      Left 0XMT0ZZ
      Right 0XMS0ZZ
  Foot
    Left 0YMN0ZZ
    Right 0YMM0ZZ
  Forequarter
    Left 0XM10ZZ
    Right 0XM00ZZ
  Gallbladder 0FM4
  Gland
    Left 0GM2
    Right 0GM3
  Hand
    Left 0XMK0ZZ
    Right 0XMJ0ZZ
  Hindquarter
    Bilateral 0YM40ZZ
    Left 0YM30ZZ
    Right 0YM20ZZ
  Hymen 0UMK
  Ileum 0DMB
  Inguinal Region
    Left 0YM60ZZ
    Right 0YM50ZZ
  Intestine
    Large 0DME
      Left 0DMG
      Right 0DMF
    Small 0DM8

Reattachment (*continued*)
  Jaw
    Lower 0WM50ZZ
    Upper 0WM40ZZ
  Jejunum 0DMA
  Kidney
    Left 0TM1
    Right 0TM0
  Kidney Pelvis
    Left 0TM4
    Right 0TM3
  Kidneys, Bilateral 0TM2
  Knee Region
    Left 0YMG0ZZ
    Right 0YMF0ZZ
  Leg
    Lower
      Left 0YMJ0ZZ
      Right 0YMH0ZZ
    Upper
      Left 0YMD0ZZ
      Right 0YMC0ZZ
  Lip
    Lower 0CM10ZZ
    Upper 0CM00ZZ
  Liver 0FM0
    Left Lobe 0FM2
    Right Lobe 0FM1
  Lung
    Left 0BML0ZZ
    Lower Lobe
      Left 0BMJ0ZZ
      Right 0BMF0ZZ
    Middle Lobe, Right 0BMD0ZZ
    Right 0BMK0ZZ
    Upper Lobe
      Left 0BMG0ZZ
      Right 0BMC0ZZ
  Lung Lingula 0BMH0ZZ
  Muscle
    Abdomen
      Left 0KML
      Right 0KMK
    Facial 0KM1
    Foot
      Left 0KMW
      Right 0KMV
    Hand
      Left 0KMD
      Right 0KMC
    Head 0KM0
    Hip
      Left 0KMP
      Right 0KMN
    Lower Arm and Wrist
      Left 0KMB
      Right 0KM9
    Lower Leg
      Left 0KMT
      Right 0KMS
    Neck
      Left 0KM3
      Right 0KM2
    Perineum 0KMM
    Shoulder
      Left 0KM6
      Right 0KM5
    Thorax
      Left 0KMJ
      Right 0KMH
    Tongue, Palate, Pharynx 0KM4
    Trunk
      Left 0KMG
      Right 0KMF
    Upper Arm
      Left 0KM8
      Right 0KM7
    Upper Leg
      Left 0KMR
      Right 0KMQ

Reattachment (*continued*)
  Nasal Mucosa and Soft Tissue
    09MKXZZ
  Neck 0WM60ZZ
  Nipple
    Left 0HMXXZZ
    Right 0HMWXZZ
  Ovary
    Bilateral 0UM2
    Left 0UM1
    Right 0UM0
  Palate, Soft 0CM30ZZ
  Pancreas 0FMG
  Parathyroid Gland
    0GMR
    Inferior
      Left 0GMP
      Right 0GMN
    Multiple 0GMQ
    Superior
      Left 0GMM
      Right 0GML
  Penis 0VMSXZZ
  Perineum
    Female 0WMN0ZZ
    Male 0WMM0ZZ
  Rectum 0DMP
  Scrotum 0VM5XZZ
  Shoulder Region
    Left 0XM30ZZ
    Right 0XM20ZZ
  Skin
    Abdomen 0HM7XZZ
    Back 0HM6XZZ
    Buttock 0HM8XZZ
    Chest 0HM5XZZ
    Ear
      Left 0HM3XZZ
      Right 0HM2XZZ
    Face 0HM1XZZ
    Foot
      Left 0HMNXZZ
      Right 0HMMXZZ
    Hand
      Left 0HMGXZZ
      Right 0HMFXZZ
    Inguinal 0HMAXZZ
    Lower Arm
      Left 0HMEXZZ
      Right 0HMDXZZ
    Lower Leg
      Left 0HMLXZZ
      Right 0HMKXZZ
    Neck 0HM4XZZ
    Perineum 0HM9XZZ
    Scalp 0HM0XZZ
    Upper Arm
      Left 0HMCXZZ
      Right 0HMBXZZ
    Upper Leg
      Left 0HMJXZZ
      Right 0HMHXZZ
  Stomach 0DM6
  Tendon
    Abdomen
      Left 0LMG
      Right 0LMF
    Ankle
      Left 0LMT
      Right 0LMS
    Foot
      Left 0LMW
      Right 0LMV
    Hand
      Left 0LM8
      Right 0LM7
    Head and Neck
      0LM0
    Hip
      Left 0LMK
      Right 0LMJ

Reattachment (*continued*)
  Tendon (*continued*)
    Knee
      Left 0LMR
      Right 0LMQ
    Lower Arm and
      Wrist
      Left 0LM6
      Right 0LM5
    Lower Leg
      Left 0LMP
      Right 0LMN
    Perineum 0LMH
    Shoulder
      Left 0LM2
      Right 0LM1
    Thorax
      Left 0LMD
      Right 0LMC
    Trunk
      Left 0LMB
      Right 0LM9
    Upper Arm
      Left 0LM4
      Right 0LM3
    Upper Leg
      Left 0LMM
      Right 0LML
  Testis
    Bilateral 0VMC
    Left 0VMB
    Right 0VM9
  Thumb
    Left 0XMM0ZZ
    Right 0XML0ZZ
  Thyroid Gland
    Left Lobe 0GMG
    Right Lobe 0GMH
  Toe
    1st
      Left 0YMQ0ZZ
      Right 0YMP0ZZ
    2nd
      Left 0YMS0ZZ
      Right 0YMR0ZZ
    3rd
      Left 0YMU0ZZ
      Right 0YMT0ZZ
    4th
      Left 0YMW0ZZ
      Right 0YMV0ZZ
    5th
      Left 0YMY0ZZ
      Right 0YMX0ZZ
  Tongue 0CM70ZZ
  Tooth
    Lower 0CMX
    Upper 0CMW
  Trachea 0BM10ZZ
  Tunica Vaginalis
    Left 0VM7
    Right 0VM6
  Ureter
    Left 0TM7
    Right 0TM6
  Ureters, Bilateral 0TM8
  Urethra 0TMD
  Uterine Supporting Structure
    0UM4
  Uterus 0UM9
  Uvula 0CMN0ZZ
  Vagina 0UMG
  Vulva 0UMMXZZ
  Wrist Region
    Left 0XMH0ZZ
    Right 0XMG0ZZ
REBOA (resuscitative
  endovascular balloon occlusion
  of the aorta)
  02LW3DJ
  04L03DJ

Rebound HRD® (Hernia Repair
  Device)
  use Synthetic Substitute
RECELL® cell suspension
  autograft
  see Replacement, Skin and Breast
    0HR
Recession
  see Repair
  see Reposition
Reclosure, disrupted abdominal wall
  0WQFXZZ
Reconstruction
  see Repair
  see Replacement
  see Supplement
Rectectomy
  see Excision, Rectum 0DBP
  see Resection, Rectum 0DTP
Rectocele repair
  see Repair, Subcutaneous Tissue
    and Fascia, Pelvic Region
    0JQC
Rectopexy
  see Repair, Gastrointestinal System
    0DQ
  see Reposition, Gastrointestinal
    System 0DS
Rectoplasty
  see Repair, Gastrointestinal System
    0DQ
  see Supplement, Gastrointestinal
    System 0DU
Rectorrhaphy
  see Repair, Gastrointestinal System
    0DQ
Rectoscopy 0DJD8ZZ
Rectosigmoid junction
  use Colon, Sigmoid
Rectosigmoidectomy
  see Excision, Gastrointestinal
    System 0DB
  see Resection, Gastrointestinal
    System 0DT
Rectostomy
  see Drainage, Rectum 0D9P
Rectotomy
  see Drainage, Rectum 0D9P
Rectus abdominis muscle
  use Muscle, Abdomen, Left
  use Muscle, Abdomen, Right
Rectus femoris muscle
  use Muscle, Upper Leg,
    Left
  use Muscle, Upper Leg, Right
Recurrent laryngeal nerve
  use Nerve, Vagus
Reducer® System
  use Reduction Device in New
    Technology
Reduction
  Dislocation
    see Reposition
  Fracture
    see Reposition
  Intussusception, intestinal
    see Reposition, Gastrointestinal
    System 0DS
  Mammoplasty
    see Excision, Skin and Breast 0HB
  Prolapse
    see Reposition
  Torsion
    see Reposition
  Volvulus, gastrointestinal
    see Reposition, Gastrointestinal
    System 0DS
Reduction Device, Coronary Sinus
  X2V73Q7
Refusion
  see Fusion

Rehabilitation
  see Activities of Daily Living
    Assessment, Rehabilitation
    F02
  see Activities of Daily Living
    Treatment, Rehabilitation
    F08
  see Caregiver Training,
    Rehabilitation F0F
  see Cochlear Implant Treatment,
    Rehabilitation F0B
  see Device Fitting, Rehabilitation
    F0D
  see Hearing Treatment,
    Rehabilitation F09
  see Motor Function Assessment,
    Rehabilitation F01
  see Motor Treatment, Rehabilitation
    F07
  see Speech Assessment,
    Rehabilitation F00
  see Speech Treatment,
    Rehabilitation F06
  see Vestibular Treatment,
    Rehabilitation F0C
Reimplantation
  see Reattachment
  see Reposition
  see Transfer
Reinforcement
  see Repair
  see Supplement
Relaxation, scar tissue
  see Release
Release
  Acetabulum
    Left 0QN5
    Right 0QN4
  Adenoids 0CNQ
  Ampulla of Vater 0FNC
  Anal Sphincter 0DNR
  Anterior Chamber
    Left 08N33ZZ
    Right 08N23ZZ
  Anus 0DNQ
  Aorta
    Abdominal 04N0
    Thoracic
      Ascending/Arch 02NX
      Descending 02NW
  Aortic Body 0GND
  Appendix 0DNJ
  Artery
    Anterior Tibial
      Left 04NQ
      Right 04NP
    Axillary
      Left 03N6
      Right 03N5
    Brachial
      Left 03N8
      Right 03N7
    Celiac 04N1
    Colic
      Left 04N7
      Middle 04N8
      Right 04N6
    Common Carotid
      Left 03NJ
      Right 03NH
    Common Iliac
      Left 04ND
      Right 04NC
    Coronary
      Four or More Arteries 02N3
      One Artery 02N0
      Three Arteries 02N2
      Two Arteries 02N1
    External Carotid
      Left 03NN
      Right 03NM

Release (continued)

Artery (continued)

External Iliac
  Left 04NJ
  Right 04NH
Face 03NR
Femoral
  Left 04NL
  Right 04NK
Foot
  Left 04NW
  Right 04NV
Gastric 04N2
Hand
  Left 03NF
  Right 03ND
Hepatic 04N3
Inferior Mesenteric
  04NB
Innominate 03N2
Internal Carotid
  Left 03NL
  Right 03NK
Internal Iliac
  Left 04NF
  Right 04NE
Internal Mammary
  Left 03N1
  Right 03N0
Intracranial 03NG
Lower 04NY
Peroneal
  Left 04NU
  Right 04NT
Popliteal
  Left 04NN
  Right 04NM
Posterior Tibial
  Left 04NS
  Right 04NR
Pulmonary
  Left 02NR
  Right 02NQ
Pulmonary Trunk
  02NP
Radial
  Left 03NC
  Right 03NB
Renal
  Left 04NA
  Right 04N9
Splenic 04N4
Subclavian
  Left 03N4
  Right 03N3
Superior Mesenteric 04N5
Temporal
  Left 03NT
  Right 03NS
Thyroid
  Left 03NV
  Right 03NU
Ulnar
  Left 03NA
  Right 03N9
Upper 03NY
Vertebral
  Left 03NQ
  Right 03NP
Atrium
  Left 02N7
  Right 02N6
Auditory Ossicle
  Left 09NA
  Right 09N9
Basal Ganglia 00N8
Bladder 0TNB
Bladder Neck 0TNC
Bone
  Ethmoid
    Left 0NNG

Release (continued)

Bone (continued)

Ethmoid (continued)
  Right 0NNF
Frontal 0NN1
Hyoid 0NNX
Lacrimal
  Left 0NNJ
  Right 0NNH
Nasal 0NNB
Occipital 0NN7
Palatine
  Left 0NNL
  Right 0NNK
Parietal
  Left 0NN4
  Right 0NN3
Pelvic
  Left 0QN3
  Right 0QN2
Sphenoid 0NNC
Temporal
  Left 0NN6
  Right 0NN5
Zygomatic
  Left 0NNN
  Right 0NNM
Brain 00N0
Breast
  Bilateral 0HNV
  Left 0HNU
  Right 0HNT
Bronchus
  Lingula 0BN9
  Lower Lobe
    Left 0BNB
    Right 0BN6
  Main
    Left 0BN7
    Right 0BN3
  Middle Lobe, Right
    0BN5
  Upper Lobe
    Left 0BN8
    Right 0BN4
Buccal Mucosa 0CN4
Bursa and Ligament
  Abdomen
    Left 0MNJ
    Right 0MNH
  Ankle
    Left 0MNR
    Right 0MNQ
  Elbow
    Left 0MN4
    Right 0MN3
  Foot
    Left 0MNT
    Right 0MNS
  Hand
    Left 0MN8
    Right 0MN7
  Head and Neck 0MN0
  Hip
    Left 0MNM
    Right 0MNL
  Knee
    Left 0MNP
    Right 0MNN
  Lower Extremity
    Left 0MNW
    Right 0MNV
  Perineum 0MNK
  Rib(s) 0MNG
  Shoulder
    Left 0MN2
    Right 0MN1
  Spine
    Lower 0MND
    Upper 0MNC
  Sternum 0MNF

Release (continued)

Bursa and Ligament (continued)

Upper Extremity
  Left 0MNB
  Right 0MN9
Wrist
  Left 0MN6
  Right 0MN5
Carina 0BN2
Carotid Bodies, Bilateral 0GN8
Carotid Body
  Left 0GN6
  Right 0GN7
Carpal
  Left 0PNN
  Right 0PNM
Cecum 0DNH
Cerebellum 00NC
Cerebral Hemisphere 00N7
Cerebral Meninges 00N1
Cerebral Ventricle 00N6
Cervix 0UNC
Chordae Tendineae 02N9
Choroid
  Left 08NB
  Right 08NA
Cisterna Chyli 07NL
Clavicle
  Left 0PNB
  Right 0PN9
Clitoris 0UNJ
Coccygeal Glomus 0GNB
Coccyx 0QNS
Colon
  Ascending 0DNK
  Descending 0DNM
  Sigmoid 0DNN
  Transverse 0DNL
Conduction Mechanism 02N8
Conjunctiva
  Left 08NTXZZ
  Right 08NSXZZ
Cord
  Bilateral 0VNH
  Left 0VNG
  Right 0VNF
Cornea
  Left 08N9XZZ
  Right 08N8XZZ
Cul-de-sac 0UNF
Diaphragm 0BNT
Disc
  Cervical Vertebral 0RN3
  Cervicothoracic Vertebral
    0RN5
  Lumbar Vertebral 0SN2
  Lumbosacral 0SN4
  Thoracic Vertebral 0RN9
  Thoracolumbar Vertebral
    0RNB
Duct
  Common Bile 0FN9
  Cystic 0FN8
  Hepatic
    Common 0FN7
    Left 0FN6
    Right 0FN5
  Lacrimal
    Left 08NY
    Right 08NX
  Pancreatic 0FND
    Accessory 0FNF
  Parotid
    Left 0CNC
    Right 0CNB
Duodenum 0DN9
Dura Mater 00N2
Ear
  External
    Left 09N1
    Right 09N0

Release (continued)

Ear (continued)

External Auditory Canal
  Left 09N4
  Right 09N3
Inner
  Left 09NE
  Right 09ND
Middle
  Left 09N6
  Right 09N5
Epididymis
  Bilateral 0VNL
  Left 0VNK
  Right 0VNJ
Epiglottis 0CNR
Esophagogastric Junction
  0DN4
Esophagus 0DN5
  Lower 0DN3
  Middle 0DN2
  Upper 0DN1
Eustachian Tube
  Left 09NG
  Right 09NF
Eye
  Left 08N1XZZ
  Right 08N0XZZ
Eyelid
  Lower
    Left 08NR
    Right 08NQ
  Upper
    Left 08NP
    Right 08NN
Fallopian Tube
  Left 0UN6
  Right 0UN5
Fallopian Tubes, Bilateral
  0UN7
Femoral Shaft
  Left 0QN9
  Right 0QN8
Femur
  Lower
    Left 0QNC
    Right 0QNB
  Upper
    Left 0QN7
    Right 0QN6
Fibula
  Left 0QNK
  Right 0QNJ
Finger Nail 0HNQXZZ
Gallbladder 0FN4
Gingiva
  Lower 0CN6
  Upper 0CN5
Gland
  Adrenal
    Bilateral 0GN4
    Left 0GN2
    Right 0GN3
  Lacrimal
    Left 08NW
    Right 08NV
  Minor Salivary 0CNJ
  Parotid
    Left 0CN9
    Right 0CN8
  Pituitary 0GN0
  Sublingual
    Left 0CNF
    Right 0CND
  Submaxillary
    Left 0CNH
    Right 0CNG
  Vestibular 0UNL
Glenoid Cavity
  Left 0PN8
  Right 0PN7

Release *(continued)*
Septum
  Atrial 02N5
  Nasal 09NM
  Ventricular 02NM
Sinus
  Accessory 09NP
  Ethmoid
    Left 09NV
    Right 09NU
  Frontal
    Left 09NT
    Right 09NS
  Mastoid
    Left 09NC
    Right 09NB
  Maxillary
    Left 09NR
    Right 09NQ
  Sphenoid
    Left 09NX
    Right 09NW
Skin
  Abdomen 0HN7XZZ
  Back 0HN6XZZ
  Buttock 0HN8XZZ
  Chest 0HN5XZZ
  Ear
    Left 0HN3XZZ
    Right 0HN2XZZ
  Face 0HN1XZZ
  Foot
    Left 0HNNXZZ
    Right 0HNMXZZ
  Hand
    Left 0HNGXZZ
    Right 0HNFXZZ
  Inguinal 0HNAXZZ
  Lower Arm
    Left 0HNEXZZ
    Right 0HNDXZZ
  Lower Leg
    Left 0HNLXZZ
    Right 0HNKXZZ
  Neck 0HN4XZZ
  Perineum 0HN9XZZ
  Scalp 0HN0XZZ
  Upper Arm
    Left 0HNCXZZ
    Right 0HNBXZZ
  Upper Leg
    Left 0HNJXZZ
    Right 0HNHXZZ
Spinal Cord
  Cervical 00NW
  Lumbar 00NY
  Thoracic 00NX
Spinal Meninges 00NT
Spleen 07NP
Sternum 0PN0
Stomach 0DN6
  Pylorus 0DN7
Subcutaneous Tissue and
  Fascia
  Abdomen 0JN8
  Back 0JN7
  Buttock 0JN9
  Chest 0JN6
  Face 0JN1
  Foot
    Left 0JNR
    Right 0JNQ
  Hand
    Left 0JNK
    Right 0JNJ
  Lower Arm
    Left 0JNH
    Right 0JNG
  Lower Leg
    Left 0JNP
    Right 0JNN

Release *(continued)*
Subcutaneous Tissue and Fascia
(continued)
  Neck
    Left 0JN5
    Right 0JN4
  Pelvic Region
    0JNC
  Perineum 0JNB
  Scalp 0JN0
  Upper Arm
    Left 0JNF
    Right 0JND
  Upper Leg
    Left 0JNM
    Right 0JNL
Tarsal
  Left 0QNM
  Right 0QNL
Tendon
  Abdomen
    Left 0LNG
    Right 0LNF
  Ankle
    Left 0LNT
    Right 0LNS
  Foot
    Left 0LNW
    Right 0LNV
  Hand
    Left 0LN8
    Right 0LN7
  Head and Neck 0LN0
  Hip
    Left 0LNK
    Right 0LNJ
  Knee
    Left 0LNR
    Right 0LNQ
  Lower Arm and Wrist
    Left 0LN6
    Right 0LN5
  Lower Leg
    Left 0LNP
    Right 0LNN
  Perineum 0LNH
  Shoulder
    Left 0LN2
    Right 0LN1
  Thorax
    Left 0LND
    Right 0LNC
  Trunk
    Left 0LNB
    Right 0LN9
  Upper Arm
    Left 0LN4
    Right 0LN3
  Upper Leg
    Left 0LNM
    Right 0LNL
Testis
  Bilateral 0VNC
  Left 0VNB
  Right 0VN9
Thalamus 00N9
Thymus 07NM
Thyroid Gland
  0GNK
  Left Lobe 0GNG
  Right Lobe
    0GNH
Tibia
  Left 0QNH
  Right 0QNG
Toe Nail 0HNRXZZ
Tongue 0CN7
Tonsils 0CNP
Tooth
  Lower 0CNX
  Upper 0CNW

Release *(continued)*
Trachea 0BN1
Tunica Vaginalis
  Left 0VN7
  Right 0VN6
Turbinate, Nasal 09NL
Tympanic Membrane
  Left 09N8
  Right 09N7
Ulna
  Left 0PNL
  Right 0PNK
Ureter
  Left 0TN7
  Right 0TN6
Urethra 0TND
Uterine Supporting Structure 0UN4
Uterus 0UN9
Uvula 0CNN
Vagina 0UNG
Valve
  Aortic 02NF
  Mitral 02NG
  Pulmonary 02NH
  Tricuspid 02NJ
Vas Deferens
  Bilateral 0VNQ
  Left 0VNP
  Right 0VNN
Vein
  Axillary
    Left 05N8
    Right 05N7
  Azygos 05N0
  Basilic
    Left 05NC
    Right 05NB
  Brachial
    Left 05NA
    Right 05N9
  Cephalic
    Left 05NF
    Right 05ND
  Colic 06N7
  Common Iliac
    Left 06ND
    Right 06NC
  Coronary 02N4
  Esophageal 06N3
  External Iliac
    Left 06NG
    Right 06NF
  External Jugular
    Left 05NQ
    Right 05NP
  Face
    Left 05NV
    Right 05NT
  Femoral
    Left 06NN
    Right 06NM
  Foot
    Left 06NV
    Right 06NT
  Gastric 06N2
  Hand
    Left 05NH
    Right 05NG
  Hemiazygos 05N1
  Hepatic 06N4
  Hypogastric
    Left 06NJ
    Right 06NH
  Inferior Mesenteric 06N6
  Innominate
    Left 05N4
    Right 05N3
  Internal Jugular
    Left 05NN
    Right 05NM
  Intracranial 05NL

Release *(continued)*
Vein *(continued)*
  Lower 06NY
  Portal 06N8
  Pulmonary
    Left 02NT
    Right 02NS
  Renal
    Left 06NB
    Right 06N9
  Saphenous
    Left 06NQ
    Right 06NP
  Splenic 06N1
  Subclavian
    Left 05N6
    Right 05N5
  Superior Mesenteric 06N5
  Upper 05NY
  Vertebral
    Left 05NS
    Right 05NR
Vena Cava
  Inferior 06N0
  Superior 02NV
Ventricle
  Left 02NL
  Right 02NK
Vertebra
  Cervical 0PN3
  Lumbar 0QN0
  Thoracic 0PN4
Vesicle
  Bilateral 0VN3
  Left 0VN2
  Right 0VN1
Vitreous
  Left 08N53ZZ
  Right 08N43ZZ
Vocal Cord
  Left 0CNV
  Right 0CNT
Vulva 0UNM
Relocation
see Reposition
Remdesivir Anti-infective XW0
Removal
Abdominal Wall 2W53X
Anorectal 2Y53X5
Arm
  Lower
    Left 2W5DX
    Right 2W5CX
  Upper
    Left 2W5BX
    Right 2W5AX
Back 2W55X
Chest Wall 2W54X
Ear 2Y52X5Z
Extremity
  Lower
    Left 2W5MX
    Right 2W5LX
  Upper
    Left 2W59X
    Right 2W58X
Face 2W51X
Finger
  Left 2W5KX
  Right 2W5JX
Foot
  Left 2W5TX
  Right 2W5SX
Genital Tract, Female
  2Y54X5Z
Hand
  Left 2W5FX
  Right 2W5EX
Head 2W50X
Inguinal Region
  Left 2W57X

Removal *(continued)*

Inguinal Region *(continued)*
Right 2W56X
Leg
Lower
Left 2W5RX
Right 2W5QX
Upper
Left 2W5PX
Right 2W5NX
Mouth and Pharynx 2Y50X5Z
Nasal 2Y51X5Z
Neck 2W52X
Thumb
Left 2W5HX
Right 2W5GX
Toe
Left 2W5VX
Right 2W5UX
Urethra 2Y55X5Z

Removal of device from
Abdominal Wall 0WPF
Acetabulum
Left 0QP5
Right 0QP4
Anal Sphincter 0DPR
Anus 0DPQ
Artery
Lower 04PY
Upper 03PY
Back
Lower 0WPL
Upper 0WPK
Bladder 0TPB
Bone
Facial 0NPW
Lower 0QPY
Nasal 0NPB
Pelvic
Left 0QP3
Right 0QP2
Upper 0PPY
Bone Marrow 07PT
Brain 00P0
Breast
Left 0HPU
Right 0HPT
Bursa and Ligament
Lower 0MPY
Upper 0MPX
Carpal
Left 0PPN
Right 0PPM
Cavity, Cranial 0WP1
Cerebral Ventricle 00P6
Chest Wall 0WP8
Cisterna Chyli 07PL
Clavicle
Left 0PPB
Right 0PP9
Coccyx 0QPS
Diaphragm 0BPT
Disc
Cervical Vertebral 0RP3
Cervicothoracic Vertebral 0RP5
Lumbar Vertebral 0SP2
Lumbosacral 0SP4
Thoracic Vertebral 0RP9
Thoracolumbar Vertebral 0RPB
Duct
Hepatobiliary 0FPB
Pancreatic 0FPD
Ear
Inner
Left 09PE
Right 09PD
Left 09PJ
Right 09PH
Epididymis and Spermatic Cord 0VPM

Esophagus 0DP5
Extremity
Lower
Left 0YPB
Right 0YP9
Upper
Left 0XP7
Right 0XP6
Eye
Left 08P1
Right 08P0
Face 0WP2
Fallopian Tube 0UP8
Femoral Shaft
Left 0QP9
Right 0QP8
Femur
Lower
Left 0QPC
Right 0QPB
Upper
Left 0QP7
Right 0QP6
Fibula
Left 0QPK
Right 0QPJ
Finger Nail 0HPQX
Gallbladder 0FP4
Gastrointestinal Tract 0WPP
Genitourinary Tract 0WPR
Gland
Adrenal 0GP5
Endocrine 0GPS
Pituitary 0GP0
Salivary 0CPA
Glenoid Cavity
Left 0PP8
Right 0PP7
Great Vessel 02PY
Hair 0HPSX
Head 0WP0
Heart 02PA
Humeral Head
Left 0PPD
Right 0PPC
Humeral Shaft
Left 0PPG
Right 0PPF
Intestinal Tract
Lower 0DPD
Upper 0DP0
Jaw
Lower 0WP5
Upper 0WP4
Joint
Acromioclavicular
Left 0RPH
Right 0RPG
Ankle
Left 0SPG
Right 0SPF
Carpal
Left 0RPR
Right 0RPQ
Carpometacarpal
Left 0RPT
Right 0RPS
Cervical Vertebral 0RP1
Cervicothoracic Vertebral 0RP4
Coccygeal 0SP6
Elbow
Left 0RPM
Right 0RPL
Finger Phalangeal
Left 0RPX
Right 0RPW
Hip
Left 0SPB
Acetabular Surface 0SPE
Femoral Surface 0SPS

Joint *(continued)*
Hip *(continued)*
Right 0SP9
Acetabular Surface 0SPA
Femoral Surface 0SPR
Knee
Left 0SPD
Femoral Surface 0SPU
Tibial Surface 0SPW
Right 0SPC
Femoral Surface 0SPT
Tibial Surface 0SPV
Lumbar Vertebral 0SP0
Lumbosacral 0SP3
Metacarpophalangeal
Left 0RPV
Right 0RPU
Metatarsal-Phalangeal
Left 0SPN
Right 0SPM
Occipital-cervical 0RP0
Sacrococcygeal 0SP5
Sacroiliac
Left 0SP8
Right 0SP7
Shoulder
Left 0RPK
Right 0RPJ
Sternoclavicular
Left 0RPF
Right 0RPE
Tarsal
Left 0SPJ
Right 0SPH
Tarsometatarsal
Left 0SPL
Right 0SPK
Temporomandibular
Left 0RPD
Right 0RPC
Thoracic Vertebral 0RP6
Thoracolumbar Vertebral 0RPA
Toe Phalangeal
Left 0SPQ
Right 0SPP
Wrist
Left 0RPP
Right 0RPN
Kidney 0TP5
Larynx 0CPS
Lens
Left 08PK3
Right 08PJ3
Liver 0FP0
Lung
Left 0BPL
Right 0BPK
Lymphatic 07PN
Thoracic Duct 07PK
Mediastinum 0WPC
Mesentery 0DPV
Metacarpal
Left 0PPQ
Right 0PPP
Metatarsal
Left 0QPP
Right 0QPN
Mouth and Throat 0CPY
Muscle
Extraocular
Left 08PM
Right 08PL
Lower 0KPY
Upper 0KPX
Nasal Mucosa and Soft Tissue 09PK
Neck 0WP6
Nerve
Cranial 00PE
Peripheral 01PY

Omentum 0DPU
Ovary 0UP3
Pancreas 0FPGZ
Parathyroid Gland 0GPR0
Patella
Left 0QPF
Right 0QPD
Pelvic Cavity 0WPJ
Penis 0VPS
Pericardial Cavity 0WPD
Perineum
Female 0WPN
Male 0WPM
Peritoneal Cavity 0WPG
Peritoneum 0DPW
Phalanx
Finger
Left 0PPV
Right 0PPT
Thumb
Left 0PPS
Right 0PPR
Toe
Left 0QPR
Right 0QPQ
Pineal Body 0GP10
Pleura 0BPQ
Pleural Cavity
Left 0WPB
Right 0WP9
Products of Conception 10P0
Prostate and Seminal Vesicles 0VP4
Radius
Left 0PPJ
Right 0PPH
Rectum 0DPP1
Respiratory Tract 0WPQZ
Retroperitoneum 0WPH
Ribs
1 to 2 0PP1
3 or More 0PP2
Sacrum 0QP1
Scapula
Left 0PP6
Right 0PP5
Scrotum and Tunica Vaginalis 0VP8
Sinus 09PY0
Skin 0HPPX
Skull 0NP0
Spinal Canal 00PU
Spinal Cord 00PV
Spleen 07PP
Sternum 0PP0
Stomach 0DP6
Subcutaneous Tissue and Fascia
Head and Neck 0JPS
Lower Extremity 0JPW
Trunk 0JPT
Upper Extremity 0JPV
Tarsal
Left 0QPM
Right 0QPL
Tendon
Lower 0LPY
Upper 0LPX
Testis 0VPD
Thymus 07PM
Thyroid Gland 0GPK0
Tibia
Left 0QPH
Right 0QPG
Toe Nail 0HPRXZ
Trachea 0BP1
Tracheobronchial Tree 0BP0
Tympanic Membrane
Left 09P80
Right 09P70

63

Removal of device from *(continued)*

Ulna
  Left 0PPL
  Right 0PPK
Ureter 0TP9
Urethra 0TPD
Uterus and Cervix
  0UPD
Vagina and Cul-de-sac
  0UPH
Vas Deferens 0VPR
Vein
  Azygos 05P0
  Innominate
    Left 05P4
    Right 05P3
  Lower 06PY
  Upper 05PY
Vertebra
  Cervical 0PP3
  Lumbar 0QP0
  Thoracic 0PP4
Vulva 0UPM

Renal calyx
use Kidney
use Kidneys, Bilateral
use Kidney, Left
use Kidney, Right
Renal capsule
use Kidney
use Kidneys, Bilateral
use Kidney, Left
use Kidney, Right
Renal cortex
use Kidney
use Kidneys, Bilateral
use Kidney, Left
use Kidney, Right
Renal dialysis
see Performance, Urinary 5A1D
Renal nerve
use Abdominal Sympathetic
  Nerve
Renal plexus
use Nerve, Abdominal
  Sympathetic
Renal segment
use Kidney
use Kidneys, Bilateral
use Kidney, Left
use Kidney, Right
Renal segmental artery
use Artery, Renal, Left
use Artery, Renal, Right
Reopening, operative site
Control of bleeding
  see Control bleeding in
Inspection only
  see Inspection
Repair
Abdominal Wall 0WQF
Acetabulum
  Left 0QQ5
  Right 0QQ4
Adenoids 0CQQ
Ampulla of Vater 0FQC
Anal Sphincter 0DQR
Ankle Region
  Left 0YQL
  Right 0YQK
Anterior Chamber
  Left 08Q33
  Right 08Q23
Anus 0DQQ
Aorta
  Abdominal 04Q0
  Thoracic
    Ascending/Arch 02QX
    Descending 02QW
Aortic Body 0GQD
Appendix 0DQJ

Repair *(continued)*

Arm
  Lower
    Left 0XQF
    Right 0XQD
  Upper
    Left 0XQ9
    Right 0XQ8
Artery
  Anterior Tibial
    Left 04QQ
    Right 04QP
  Axillary
    Left 03Q6
    Right 03Q5
  Brachial
    Left 03Q8
    Right 03Q7
  Celiac 04Q1
  Colic
    Left 04Q7
    Middle 04Q8
    Right 04Q6
  Common Carotid
    Left 03QJ
    Right 03QH
  Common Iliac
    Left 04QD
    Right 04QC
  Coronary
    Four or More Arteries
      02Q3
    One Artery 02Q0
    Three Arteries
      02Q2
    Two Arteries 02Q1
  External Carotid
    Left 03QN
    Right 03QM
  External Iliac
    Left 04QJ
    Right 04QH
  Face 03QR
  Femoral
    Left 04QL
    Right 04QK
  Foot
    Left 04QW
    Right 04QV
  Gastric 04Q2
  Hand
    Left 03QF
    Right 03QD
  Hepatic 04Q3
  Inferior Mesenteric 04QB
  Innominate 03Q2
  Internal Carotid
    Left 03QL
    Right 03QK
  Internal Iliac
    Left 04QF
    Right 04QE
  Internal Mammary
    Left 03Q1
    Right 03Q0
  Intracranial 03QG
  Lower 04QY
  Peroneal
    Left 04QU
    Right 04QT
  Popliteal
    Left 04QN
    Right 04QM
  Posterior Tibial
    Left 04QS
    Right 04QR
  Pulmonary
    Left 02QR
    Right 02QQ
  Pulmonary Trunk
    02QP

Repair *(continued)*

Artery *(continued)*
  Radial
    Left 03QC
    Right 03QB
  Renal
    Left 04QA
    Right 04Q9
  Splenic 04Q4
  Subclavian
    Left 03Q4
    Right 03Q3
  Superior Mesenteric
    04Q5
  Temporal
    Left 03QT
    Right 03QS
  Thyroid
    Left 03QV
    Right 03QU
  Ulnar
    Left 03QA
    Right 03Q9
  Upper 03QY
  Vertebral
    Left 03QQ
    Right 03QP
Atrium
  Left 02Q7
  Right 02Q6
Auditory Ossicle
  Left 09QA
  Right 09Q9
Axilla
  Left 0XQ5
  Right 0XQ4
Back
  Lower 0WQL
  Upper 0WQK
Basal Ganglia 00Q8
Bladder 0TQB
Bladder Neck
  0TQC
Bone
  Ethmoid
    Left 0NQG
    Right 0NQF
  Frontal 0NQ1
  Hyoid 0NQX
  Lacrimal
    Left 0NQJ
    Right 0NQH
  Nasal 0NQB
  Occipital 0NQ7
  Palatine
    Left 0NQL
    Right 0NQK
  Parietal
    Left 0NQ4
    Right 0NQ3
  Pelvic
    Left 0QQ3
    Right 0QQ2
  Sphenoid 0NQC
  Temporal
    Left 0NQ6
    Right 0NQ
  Zygomatic
    Left 0NQN
    Right 0NQM
Brain 00Q0
Breast
  Bilateral 0HQV
  Left 0HQU
  Right 0HQT
  Supernumerary
    0HQY
Bronchus
  Lingula 0BQ9
  Lower Lobe
    Left 0BQB

Repair *(continued)*

Bronchus *(continued)*
  Lower Lobe *(continued)*
    Right 0BQ6
  Main
    Left 0BQ7
    Right 0BQ3
  Middle Lobe, Right
    0BQ5
  Upper Lobe
    Left 0BQ8
    Right 0BQ4
Buccal Mucosa 0CQ4
Bursa and Ligament
  Abdomen
    Left 0MQJ
    Right 0MQH
  Ankle
    Left 0MQR
    Right 0MQQ
  Elbow
    Left 0MQ4
    Right 0MQ3
  Foot
    Left 0MQT
    Right 0MQS
  Hand
    Left 0MQ8
    Right 0MQ7
  Head and Neck 0MQ0
  Hip
    Left 0MQM
    Right 0MQL
  Knee
    Left 0MQP
    Right 0MQN
  Lower Extremity
    Left 0MQW
    Right 0MQV
  Perineum 0MQK
  Rib(s) 0MQG
  Shoulder
    Left 0MQ2
    Right 0MQ1
  Spine
    Lower 0MQD
    Upper 0MQC
  Sternum 0MQF
  Upper Extremity
    Left 0MQB
    Right 0MQ9
  Wrist
    Left 0MQ6
    Right 0MQ5
Buttock
  Left 0YQ1
  Right 0YQ0
Carina 0BQ2
Carotid Bodies, Bilateral 0GQ8
Carotid Body
  Left 0GQ6
  Right 0GQ7
Carpal
  Left 0PQN
  Right 0PQM
Cecum 0DQH
Cerebellum 00QC
Cerebral Hemisphere
  00Q7
Cerebral Meninges 00Q1
Cerebral Ventricle 00Q6
Cervix 0UQC
Chest Wall 0WQ8
Chordae Tendineae 02Q9
Choroid
  Left 08QB
  Right 08QA
Cisterna Chyli 07QL
Clavicle
  Left 0PQB
  Right 0PQ9

Replantation, scalp
see Reattachment, Skin, Scalp
0HM0
Reposition
Acetabulum
Left 0QS5
Right 0QS4
Ampulla of Vater 0FSC
Anus 0DSQ
Aorta
Abdominal 04S0
Thoracic
Ascending/Arch 02SX0ZZ
Descending 02SW0ZZ
Artery
Anterior Tibial
Left 04SQ
Right 04SP
Axillary
Left 03S6
Right 03S5
Brachial
Left 03S8
Right 03S7
Celiac 04S1
Colic
Left 04S7
Middle 04S8
Right 04S6
Common Carotid
Left 03SJ
Right 03SH
Common Iliac
Left 04SD
Right 04SC
Coronary
One Artery 02S00ZZ
Two Arteries 02S10ZZ
External Carotid
Left 03SN
Right 03SM
External Iliac
Left 04SJ
Right 04SH
Face 03SR
Femoral
Left 04SL
Right 04SK
Foot
Left 04SW
Right 04SV
Gastric 04S2
Hand
Left 03SF
Right 03SD
Hepatic 04S3
Inferior Mesenteric
04SB
Innominate 03S2
Internal Carotid
Left 03SL
Right 03SK
Internal Iliac
Left 04SF
Right 04SE
Internal Mammary
Left 03S1
Right 03S0
Intracranial 03SG
Lower 04SY
Peroneal
Left 04SU
Right 04ST
Popliteal
Left 04SN
Right 04SM
Posterior Tibial
Left 04SS
Right 04SR
Pulmonary
Left 02SR0ZZ

Reposition *(continued)*
Artery *(continued)*
Pulmonary *(continued)*
Right 02SQ0ZZ
Pulmonary Trunk
02SP0ZZ
Radial
Left 03SC
Right 03SB
Renal
Left 04SA
Right 04S9
Splenic 04S4
Subclavian
Left 03S4
Right 03S3
Superior Mesenteric
04S5
Temporal
Left 03ST
Right 03SS
Thyroid
Left 03SV
Right 03SU
Ulnar
Left 03SA
Right 03S9
Upper 03SY
Vertebral
Left 03SQ
Right 03SP
Auditory Ossicle
Left 09SA
Right 09S9
Bladder 0TSB
Bladder Neck
0TSC
Bone
Ethmoid
Left 0NSG
Right 0NSF
Frontal 0NS1
Hyoid 0NSX
Lacrimal
Left 0NSJ
Right 0NSH
Nasal 0NSB
Occipital 0NS7
Palatine
Left 0NSL
Right 0NSK
Parietal
Left 0NS4
Right 0NS3
Pelvic
Left 0QS3
Right 0QS2
Sphenoid 0NSC
Temporal
Left 0NS6
Right 0NS5
Zygomatic
Left 0NSN
Right 0NSM
Breast
Bilateral 0HSV0ZZ
Left 0HSU0ZZ
Right 0HST0ZZ
Bronchus
Lingula 0BS90ZZ
Lower Lobe
Left 0BSB0ZZ
Right 0BS60ZZ
Main
Left 0BS70ZZ
Right 0BS30ZZ
Middle Lobe, Right
0BS50ZZ
Upper Lobe
Left 0BS80ZZ
Right 0BS40ZZ

Reposition *(continued)*
Bursa and Ligament
Abdomen
Left 0MSJ
Right 0MSH
Ankle
Left 0MSR
Right 0MSQ
Elbow
Left 0MS4
Right 0MS3
Foot
Left 0MST
Right 0MSS
Hand
Left 0MS8
Right 0MS7
Head and Neck
0MS0
Hip
Left 0MSM
Right 0MSL
Knee
Left 0MSP
Right 0MSN
Lower Extremity
Left 0MSW
Right 0MSV
Perineum 0MSK
Rib(s) 0MSG
Shoulder
Left 0MS2
Right 0MS1
Spine
Lower 0MSD
Upper 0MSC
Sternum 0MSF
Upper Extremity
Left 0MSB
Right 0MS9
Wrist
Left 0MS6
Right 0MS5
Carina 0BS20ZZ
Carpal
Left 0PSN
Right 0PSM
Cecum 0DSH
Cervix 0USC
Clavicle
Left 0PSB
Right 0PS9
Coccyx 0QSS
Colon
Ascending 0DSK
Descending 0DSM
Sigmoid 0DSN
Transverse 0DSL
Cord
Bilateral 0VSH
Left 0VSG
Right 0VSF
Cul-de-sac 0USF
Diaphragm 0BST0ZZ
Duct
Common Bile
0FS9
Cystic 0FS8
Hepatic
Common 0FS7
Left 0FS6
Right 0FS5
Lacrimal
Left 08SY
Right 08SX
Pancreatic 0FSD
Accessory 0FSF
Parotid
Left 0CSC
Right 0CSB
Duodenum 0DS9ZZ

Reposition *(continued)*
Ear
Bilateral 09S2ZZ
Left 09S1ZZ
Right 09S0ZZ
Epiglottis 0CSR
Esophagus 0DS5ZZ
Eustachian Tube
Left 09SG
Right 09SF
Eyelid
Lower
Left 08SR
Right 08SQ
Upper
Left 08SP
Right 08SN
Fallopian Tube
Left 0US6
Right 0US5
Fallopian Tubes, Bilateral
0US7
Femoral Shaft
Left 0QS9
Right 0QS8
Femur
Lower
Left 0QSC
Right 0QSB
Upper
Left 0QS7
Right 0QS6
Fibula
Left 0QSK
Right 0QSJ
Gallbladder 0FS4
Gland
Adrenal
Left 0GS2
Right 0GS3
Lacrimal
Left 08SW
Right 08SV
Glenoid Cavity
Left 0PS8
Right 0PS7
Hair 0HSSXZZ
Humeral Head
Left 0PSD
Right 0PSC
Humeral Shaft
Left 0PSG
Right 0PSF
Ileum 0DSB
Intestine
Large 0DSE
Small 0DS8
Iris
Left 08SD3ZZ
Right 08SC3ZZ
Jejunum 0DSAZZ
Joint
Acromioclavicular
Left 0RSHZ
Right 0RSGZ
Ankle
Left 0SSG
Right 0SSF
Carpal
Left 0RSR
Right 0RSQ
Carpometacarpal
Left 0RST
Right 0RSS
Cervical Vertebral 0RS1
Cervicothoracic Vertebral
0RS4
Coccygeal 0SS6
Elbow
Left 0RSM
Right 0RSL

Humeral Shaft
  Left 0PTG0ZZ
  Right 0PTF0ZZ
Hymen 0UTK
Ileocecal Valve
  0DTC
Ileum 0DTB
Intestine
  Large 0DTE
    Left 0DTG
    Right 0DTF
  Small 0DT8
Iris
  Left 08TD3ZZ
  Right 08TC3ZZ
Jejunum 0DTA
Joint
  Acromioclavicular
    Left 0RTH0ZZ
    Right 0RTG0ZZ
  Ankle
    Left 0STG0ZZ
    Right 0STF0ZZ
  Carpal
    Left 0RTR0ZZ
    Right 0RTQ0ZZ
  Carpometacarpal
    Left 0RTT0ZZ
    Right 0RTS0ZZ
  Cervicothoracic Vertebral
    0RT40ZZ
  Coccygeal
    0ST60ZZ
  Elbow
    Left 0RTM0ZZ
    Right 0RTL0ZZ
  Finger Phalangeal
    Left 0RTX0ZZ
    Right 0RTW0ZZ
  Hip
    Left 0STB0ZZ
    Right 0ST90ZZ
  Knee
    Left 0STD0ZZ
    Right 0STC0ZZ
  Metacarpophalangeal
    Left 0RTV0ZZ
    Right 0RTU0ZZ
  Metatarsal-Phalangeal
    Left 0STN0ZZ
    Right 0STM0ZZ
  Sacrococcygeal
    0ST50ZZ
  Sacroiliac
    Left 0ST80ZZ
    Right 0ST70ZZ
  Shoulder
    Left 0RTK0ZZ
    Right 0RTJ0ZZ
  Sternoclavicular
    Left 0RTF0ZZ
    Right 0RTE0ZZ
  Tarsal
    Left 0STJ0ZZ
    Right 0STH0ZZ
  Tarsometatarsal
    Left 0STL0ZZ
    Right 0STK0ZZ
  Temporomandibular
    Left 0RTD0ZZ
    Right 0RTC0ZZ
  Toe Phalangeal
    Left 0STQ0ZZ
    Right 0STP0ZZ
  Wrist
    Left 0RTP0ZZ
    Right 0RTN0ZZ
Kidney
  Left 0TT1
  Right 0TT0

Kidney Pelvis
  Left 0TT4
  Right 0TT3
Kidneys, Bilateral
  0TT2
Larynx 0CTS
Lens
  Left 08TK3ZZ
  Right 08TJ3ZZ
Lip
  Lower 0CT1
  Upper 0CT0
Liver 0FT0
  Left Lobe 0FT2
  Right Lobe 0FT1
Lung
  Bilateral 0BTM
  Left 0BTL
  Lower Lobe
    Left 0BTJ
    Right 0BTF
  Middle Lobe, Right 0BTD
  Right 0BTK
  Upper Lobe
    Left 0BTG
    Right 0BTC
Lung Lingula 0BTH
Lymphatic
  Aortic 07TD
  Axillary
    Left 07T6
    Right 07T5
  Head 07T0
  Inguinal
    Left 07TJ
    Right 07TH
  Internal Mammary
    Left 07T9
    Right 07T8
  Lower Extremity
    Left 07TG
    Right 07TF
  Mesenteric 07TB
  Neck
    Left 07T2
    Right 07T1
  Pelvis 07TC
  Thoracic Duct 07TK
  Thorax 07T7
  Upper Extremity
    Left 07T4
    Right 07T3
Mandible
  Left 0NTV0ZZ
  Right 0NTT0ZZ
Maxilla 0NTR0ZZ
Metacarpal
  Left 0PTQ0ZZ
  Right 0PTP0ZZ
Metatarsal
  Left 0QTP0ZZ
  Right 0QTN0ZZ
Muscle
  Abdomen
    Left 0KTL
    Right 0KTK
  Extraocular
    Left 08TM
    Right 08TL
  Facial 0KT1
  Foot
    Left 0KTW
    Right 0KTV
  Hand
    Left 0KTD
    Right 0KTC
  Head 0KT0
  Hip
    Left 0KTP
    Right 0KTN

Muscle *(continued)*
  Lower Arm and Wrist
    Left 0KTB
    Right 0KT9
  Lower Leg
    Left 0KTT
    Right 0KTS
  Neck
    Left 0KT3
    Right 0KT2
  Papillary 02TD
  Perineum 0KTM
  Shoulder
    Left 0KT6
    Right 0KT5
  Thorax
    Left 0KTJ
    Right 0KTH
  Tongue, Palate, Pharynx
    0KT4
  Trunk
    Left 0KTG
    Right 0KTF
  Upper Arm
    Left 0KT8
    Right 0KT7
  Upper Leg
    Left 0KTR
    Right 0KTQ
Nasal Mucosa and Soft Tissue
  09TK
Nasopharynx 09TN
Nipple
  Left 0HTXXZZ
  Right 0HTWXZZ
Omentum 0DTU
Orbit
  Left 0NTQ0ZZ
  Right 0NTP0ZZ
Ovary
  Bilateral 0UT2
  Left 0UT1
  Right 0UT0
Palate
  Hard 0CT2
  Soft 0CT3
Pancreas 0FTG
Para-aortic Body 0GT9
Paraganglion Extremity 0GTF
Parathyroid Gland 0GTR
  Inferior
    Left 0GTP
    Right 0GTN
  Multiple 0GTQ
  Superior
    Left 0GTM
    Right 0GTL
Patella
  Left 0QTF0ZZ
  Right 0QTD0ZZ
Penis 0VTS
Pericardium 02TN
Phalanx
  Finger
    Left 0PTV0ZZ
    Right 0PTT0ZZ
  Thumb
    Left 0PTS0ZZ
    Right 0PTR0ZZ
  Toe
    Left 0QTR0ZZ
    Right 0QTQ0ZZ
Pharynx 0CTM
Pineal Body 0GT1
Prepuce 0VTT
Products of Conception, Ectopic 10T2
Prostate 0VT0
Radius
  Left 0PTJ0ZZ
  Right 0PTH0ZZ

Rectum 0DTP
Ribs
  1 to 2 0PT10ZZ
  3 or More 0PT20ZZ
Scapula
  Left 0PT60ZZ
  Right 0PT50ZZ
Scrotum 0VT5
Septum
  Atrial 02T5
  Nasal 09TM
  Ventricular 02TM
Sinus
  Accessory 09TP
  Ethmoid
    Left 09TV
    Right 09TU
  Frontal
    Left 09TT
    Right 09TS
  Mastoid
    Left 09TC
    Right 09TB
  Maxillary
    Left 09TR
    Right 09TQ
  Sphenoid
    Left 09TX
    Right 09TW
Spleen 07TP
Sternum 0PT00ZZ
Stomach 0DT6
  Pylorus 0DT7
Tarsal
  Left 0QTM0ZZ
  Right 0QTL0ZZ
Tendon
  Abdomen
    Left 0LTG
    Right 0LTF
  Ankle
    Left 0LTT
    Right 0LTS
  Foot
    Left 0LTW
    Right 0LTV
  Hand
    Left 0LT8
    Right 0LT7
  Head and Neck
    0LT0
  Hip
    Left 0LTK
    Right 0LTJ
  Knee
    Left 0LTR
    Right 0LTQ
  Lower Arm and
    Wrist
    Left 0LT6
    Right 0LT5
  Lower Leg
    Left 0LTP
    Right 0LTN
  Perineum 0LTH
  Shoulder
    Left 0LT2
    Right 0LT1
  Thorax
    Left 0LTD
    Right 0LTC
  Trunk
    Left 0LTB
    Right 0LT9
  Upper Arm
    Left 0LT4
    Right 0LT3
  Upper Leg
    Left 0LTM
    Right 0LTL

Resection *(continued)*

Testis
Bilateral 0VTC
Left 0VTB
Right 0VT9
Thymus 07TM
Thyroid Gland 0GTK
Left Lobe 0GTG
Right Lobe 0GTH
Thyroid Gland Isthmus 0GTJ
Tibia
Left 0QTH0ZZ
Right 0QTG0ZZ
Toe Nail 0HTRXZZ
Tongue 0CT7
Tonsils 0CTP
Tooth
Lower 0CTX0Z
Upper 0CTW0Z
Trachea 0BT1
Tunica Vaginalis
Left 0VT7
Right 0VT6
Turbinate, Nasal 09TL
Tympanic Membrane
Left 09T8
Right 09T7
Ulna
Left 0PTL0ZZ
Right 0PTK0ZZ
Ureter
Left 0TT7
Right 0TT6
Urethra 0TTD
Uterine Supporting Structure
0UT4
Uterus 0UT9
Uvula 0CTN
Vagina 0UTG
Valve, Pulmonary 02TH
Vas Deferens
Bilateral 0VTQ
Left 0VTP
Right 0VTN
Vesicle
Bilateral 0VT3
Left 0VT2
Right 0VT1
Vitreous
Left 08T53ZZ
Right 08T43ZZ
Vocal Cord
Left 0CTV
Right 0CTT
Vulva 0UTM

Resection, Left ventricular outflow tract obstruction (LVOT)
see Dilation, Ventricle, Left 027L

Resection, Subaortic membrane (Left ventricular outflow tract obstruction)
see Dilation, Ventricle, Left 027L

Restoration, Cardiac, Single, Rhythm 5A2204Z

RestoreAdvanced neurostimulator (SureScan)(MRI Safe)
use Stimulator Generator, Multiple Array Rechargeable in 0JH

RestoreSensor neurostimulator (SureScan)(MRI Safe)
use Stimulator Generator, Multiple Array Rechargeable in 0JH

RestoreUltra neurostimulator (SureScan)(MRI Safe)
use Stimulator Generator, Multiple Array Rechargeable in 0JH

Restriction
Ampulla of Vater 0FVC
Anus 0DVQ

Restriction *(continued)*

Aorta
Abdominal 04V0
Intraluminal Device, Branched or Fenestrated 04V0
Thoracic
Ascending/Arch, Intraluminal Device, Branched or Fenestrated 02VX
Descending, Intraluminal Device, Branched or Fenestrated 02VW
Artery
Anterior Tibial
Left 04VQ
Right 04VP
Axillary
Left 03V6
Right 03V5
Brachial
Left 03V8
Right 03V7
Celiac 04V1
Colic
Left 04V7
Middle 04V8
Right 04V6
Common Carotid
Left 03VJ
Right 03VH
Common Iliac
Left 04VD
Right 04VC
External Carotid
Left 03VN
Right 03VM
External Iliac
Left 04VJ
Right, 04VHZ
Face 03VR
Femoral
Left 04VL
Right 04VK
Foot
Left 04VW
Right 04VV
Gastric 04V2
Hand
Left 03VF
Right 03VD
Hepatic 04V3
Inferior Mesenteric 04VB
Innominate 03V2
Internal Carotid
Left 03VL
Right 03VK
Internal Iliac
Left 04VF
Right 04VE
Internal Mammary
Left 03V1
Right 03V0
Intracranial 03VG
Lower 04VY
Peroneal
Left 04VU
Right 04VT
Popliteal
Left 04VN
Right 04VM
Posterior Tibial
Left 04VS
Right 04VR
Pulmonary
Left 02VR
Right 02VQ
Pulmonary Trunk 02VP
Radial
Left 03VC
Right 03VB

Restriction *(continued)*

Artery *(continued)*
Renal
Left 04VA
Right 04V9
Splenic 04V4
Subclavian
Left 03V4
Right 03V3
Superior Mesenteric 04V5
Temporal
Left 03VT
Right 03VS
Thyroid
Left 03VV
Right 03VU
Ulnar
Left 03VA
Right 03V9
Upper 03VY
Vertebral
Left 03VQ
Right 03VP
Bladder 0TVB
Bladder Neck 0TVC
Bronchus
Lingula 0BV9
Lower Lobe
Left 0BVB
Right 0BV6
Main
Left 0BV7
Right 0BV3
Middle Lobe, Right 0BV5
Upper Lobe
Left 0BV8
Right 0BV4
Carina 0BV2
Cecum 0DVH
Cervix 0UVC
Cisterna Chyli 07VL
Colon
Ascending 0DVK
Descending 0DVM
Sigmoid 0DVN
Transverse 0DVL
Duct
Common Bile 0FV9
Cystic 0FV8
Hepatic
Common 0FV7
Left 0FV6
Right 0FV5
Lacrimal
Left 08VY
Right 08VX
Pancreatic 0FVD
Accessory 0FVF
Parotid
Left 0CVC
Right 0CVB
Duodenum 0DV9
Esophagogastric Junction 0DV4
Esophagus 0DV5
Lower 0DV3
Middle 0DV2
Upper 0DV1
Heart 02VA
Ileocecal Valve 0DVC
Ileum 0DVB
Intestine
Large 0DVE
Left 0DVG
Right 0DVF
Small 0DV8
Jejunum 0DVA
Kidney Pelvis
Left 0TV4

Restriction *(continued)*

Kidney Pelvis *(continued)*
Right 0TV3
Lymphatic
Aortic 07VD
Axillary
Left 07V6
Right 07V5
Head 07V0
Inguinal
Left 07VJ
Right 07VH
Internal Mammary
Left 07V9
Right 07V8
Lower Extremity
Left 07VG
Right 07VF
Mesenteric 07VB
Neck
Left 07V2
Right 07V1
Pelvis 07VC
Thoracic Duct 07VK
Thorax 07V7
Upper Extremity
Left 07V4
Right 07V3
Rectum 0DVP
Stomach 0DV6
Pylorus 0DV7
Trachea 0BV1
Ureter
Left 0TV7
Right 0TV6
Urethra 0TVD
Valve, Mitral 02VG
Vein
Axillary
Left 05V8
Right 05V7
Azygos 05V0
Basilic
Left 05VC
Right 05VB
Brachial
Left 05VA
Right 05V9
Cephalic
Left 05VF
Right 05VD
Colic 06V7Z
Common Iliac
Left 06VD
Right 06VC
Esophageal 06V3
External Iliac
Left 06VG
Right 06VF
External Jugular
Left 05VQ
Right 05VP
Face
Left 05VV
Right 05VT
Femoral
Left 06VN
Right 06VM
Foot
Left 06VV
Right 06VT
Gastric 06V2
Hand
Left 05VH
Right 05VG
Hemiazygos 05V1
Hepatic 06V4
Hypogastric
Left 06VJ
Right 06VH

Resuscitation (continued)
  Vein (continued)
    Inferior Mesenteric 06V6
    Innominate
      Left 05V4
      Right 05V3
    Internal Jugular
      Left 05VN
      Right 05VM
    Intracranial 05VL
    Lower 06VY
    Portal 06V8
    Pulmonary
      Left 02VT
      Right 02VS
    Renal
      Left 06VB
      Right 06V9
    Saphenous
      Left 06VQ
      Right 06VP
    Splenic 06V1
    Subclavian
      Left 05V6
      Right 05V5
    Superior Mesenteric 06V5
    Upper 05VY
    Vertebral
      Left 05VS
      Right 05VR
    Vena Cava
      Inferior 06V0
      Superior 02VV
    Ventricle, Left 02VL
Resurfacing Device
  Removal of device from
    Left 0SPB0BZ
    Right 0SP90BZ
  Revision of device in
    Left 0SWB0BZ
    Right 0SW90BZ
  Supplement
    Left 0SUB0BZ
      Acetabular Surface 0SUE0BZ
      Femoral Surface
        0SUS0BZ
    Right 0SU90BZ
      Acetabular Surface 0SUA0BZ
      Femoral Surface
        0SUR0BZ
Resuscitation
  Cardiopulmonary
    see Assistance, Cardiac 5A02
  Cardioversion 5A2204Z
  Defibrillation 5A2204Z
  Endotracheal intubation
    see Insertion of device in,
      Trachea 0BH1
  External chest compression, manual
    5A12012
  External chest compression,
    mechanical 5A1221J
  Pulmonary 5A19054
Resuscitative endovascular balloon
  occlusion of the aorta (REBOA)
  02LW3DJ
  04L03DJ
Resuture, Heart valve prosthesis
  see Revision of device in, Heart and
    Great Vessels 02W
Retained placenta, manual
  removal
  see Extraction, Products of
    Conception, Retained 10D1
Retraining
  Cardiac
    see Motor Treatment,
      Rehabilitation F07
  Vocational
    see Activities of Daily Living
      Treatment, Rehabilitation F08

Retrogasserian rhizotomy
  see Division, Nerve, Trigeminal
    008K
Retroperitoneal cavity
  use Retroperitoneum
Retroperitoneal lymph node
  use Lymphatic, Aortic
Retroperitoneal space
  use Retroperitoneum
Retropharyngeal lymph node
  use Lymphatic, Neck, Left
  use Lymphatic, Neck, Right
Retropharyngeal space *use* Neck
Retropubic space
  use Pelvic Cavity
Reveal (LINQ) (DX)(XT)
  use Monitoring Device
Reverse® Shoulder Prosthesis
  use Synthetic Substitute, Reverse
    Ball and Socket in 0RR
Reverse total shoulder replacement
  see Replacement, Upper Joints
    0RR
Revision
  Correcting a portion of existing
    device
    see Revision of device in
  Removal of device without
    replacement
    see Removal of device from
  Replacement of existing device
    see Removal of device from
    see Root operation to place
      new device, e.g., Insertion,
      Replacement, Supplement
Revision of device in
  Abdominal Wall 0WWF
  Acetabulum
    Left 0QW5
    Right 0QW4
  Anal Sphincter 0DWR
  Anus 0DWQ
  Artery
    Lower 04WY
    Upper 03WYM
  Auditory Ossicle
    Left 09WA
    Right 09W9
  Back
    Lower 0WWL
    Upper 0WWK
  Bladder 0TWB
  Bone
    Facial 0NWW
    Lower 0QWY
    Nasal 0NWB
    Pelvic
      Left 0QW3
      Right 0QW2
    Upper 0PWY
  Bone Marrow 07WT
  Brain 00W0
  Breast
    Left 0HWU
    Right 0HWT
  Bursa and Ligament
    Lower 0MWY
    Upper 0MWX
  Carpal
    Left 0PWN
    Right 0PWM
  Cavity, Cranial 0WW1
  Cerebral Ventricle
    00W6
  Chest Wall 0WW8
  Cisterna Chyli 07WL
  Clavicle
    Left 0PWB
    Right 0PW9
  Coccyx 0QWS
  Diaphragm 0BWTM

Revision of device in (continued)
  Disc
    Cervical Vertebral 0RW3
    Cervicothoracic Vertebral
      0RW5
    Lumbar Vertebral
      0SW2
    Lumbosacral 0SW4
    Thoracic Vertebral
      0RW9
    Thoracolumbar Vertebral
      0RWB
  Duct
    Hepatobiliary 0FWB
    Pancreatic 0FWD
  Ear
    Inner
      Left 09WE
      Right 09WD
    Left 09WJ
    Right 09WH
  Epididymis and Spermatic Cord
    0VWM
  Esophagus 0DW5D
  Extremity
    Lower
      Left 0YWB
      Right 0YW9
    Upper
      Left 0XW7
      Right 0XW6
  Eye
    Left 08W1
    Right 08W0
  Face 0WW2
  Fallopian Tube 0UW8
  Femoral Shaft
    Left 0QW9
    Right 0QW8
  Femur
    Lower
      Left 0QWC
      Right 0QWB
    Upper
      Left 0QW7
      Right 0QW6
  Fibula
    Left 0QWK
    Right 0QWJ
  Finger Nail 0HWQX
  Gallbladder 0FW4
  Gastrointestinal Tract
    0WWP
  Genitourinary Tract 0WWR
  Gland
    Adrenal 0GW50
    Endocrine 0GWS
    Pituitary 0GW00
    Salivary 0CWA
  Glenoid Cavity
    Left 0PW8
    Right 0PW7
  Great Vessel 02WY
  Hair 0HWSX
  Head 0WW0
  Heart 02WA
  Humeral Head
    Left 0PWD
    Right 0PWC
  Humeral Shaft
    Left 0PWG
    Right 0PWF
  Intestinal Tract
    Lower 0DWD
    Upper 0DW0
  Intestine
    Large 0DWE
    Small 0DW8
  Jaw
    Lower 0WW5
    Upper 0WW4

Revision of device in (continued)
  Joint
    Acromioclavicular
      Left 0RWH
      Right 0RWG
    Ankle
      Left 0SWG
      Right 0SWF
    Carpal
      Left 0RWR
      Right 0RWQ
    Carpometacarpal
      Left 0RWT
      Right 0RWS
    Cervical Vertebral 0RW1
    Cervicothoracic Vertebral
      0RW4
    Coccygeal 0SW6
    Elbow
      Left 0RWM
      Right 0RWL
    Finger Phalangeal
      Left 0RWX
      Right 0RWW
    Hip
      Left 0SWB
        Acetabluar Surface 0SWE
        Femoral Surface 0SWS
      Right 0SW9
        Acetabluar Surface 0SWA
        Femoral Surface 0SWR
    Knee
      Left 0SWD
        Femoral Surface 0SWU
        Tibial Surface 0SWW
      Right 0SWC
        Femoral Surface 0SWT
        Tibial Surface 0SWV
    Lumbar Vertebral 0SW0
    Lumbosacral 0SW3
    Metacarpophalangeal
      Left 0RWV
      Right 0RWU
    Metatarsal-Phalangeal
      Left 0SWN
      Right 0SWM
    Occipital-cervical 0RW0
    Sacrococcygeal 0SW5
    Sacroiliac
      Left 0SW8
      Right 0SW7
    Shoulder
      Left 0RWK
      Right 0RWJ
    Sternoclavicular
      Left 0RWF
      Right 0RWE
    Tarsal
      Left 0SWJ
      Right 0SWH
    Tarsometatarsal
      Left 0SWL
      Right 0SWK
    Temporomandibular
      Left 0RWD
      Right 0RWC
    Thoracic Vertebral 0RW6
    Thoracolumbar Vertebral
      0RWA
    Toe Phalangeal
      Left 0SWQ
      Right 0SWP
    Wrist
      Left 0RWP
      Right 0RWN
  Kidney 0TW5
  Larynx 0CWS
  Lens
    Left 08WKJ
    Right 08WJ
  Liver 0FW0

Salpingotomy
 see Drainage, Female Reproductive System 0U9
Salpinx
 use Fallopian Tube, Left
 use Fallopian Tube, Right
Saphenous nerve
 use Nerve, Femoral
SAPIEN transcatheter aortic valve
 use Zooplastic Tissue in Heart and Great Vessels
Sarilumab XW0
SARS-CoV-2 Antibody Detection, Serum/Plasma Nanoparticle Fluorescence XXE5XV7
SARS-CoV-2 Polymerase Chain Reaction, Nasopharyngeal Fluid XXE97U7
Sartorius muscle
 use Muscle, Upper Leg, Left
 use Muscle, Upper Leg, Right
Satralizumab-mwge XW01397
SAVAL below-the-knee (BTK) drug-eluting stent system
 use Intraluminal Device, Sustained Release Drug-eluting in New Technology
 use Intraluminal Device, Sustained Release Drug-eluting, Four or More in New Technology
 use Intraluminal Device, Sustained Release Drug-eluting, Three in New Technology
 use Intraluminal Device, Sustained Release Drug-eluting, Two in New Technology
Scalene muscle
 use Muscle, Neck, Left
 use Muscle, Neck, Right
Scan
 Computerized Tomography (CT)
 see Computerized Tomography (CT Scan)
 Radioisotope
 see Planar Nuclear Medicine Imaging
Scaphoid bone
 use Carpal, Left
 use Carpal, Right
Scapholunate ligament
 use Bursa and Ligament, Wrist, Left
 use Bursa and Ligament, Wrist, Right
Scaphotrapezium ligament
 use Bursa and Ligament, Hand, Left
 use Bursa and Ligament, Hand, Right
Scapulectomy
 see Excision, Upper Bones 0PB
 see Resection, Upper Bones 0PT
Scapulopexy
 see Repair, Upper Bones 0PQ
 see Reposition, Upper Bones 0PS
Scarpa's (vestibular) ganglion
 use Nerve, Acoustic
Sclerectomy
 see Excision, Eye 08B
Sclerotherapy, mechanical
 see Destruction
Sclerotherapy, via injection of sclerosing agent
 see Introduction, Destructive Agent
Sclerotomy
 see Drainage, Eye 089
Scrotectomy
 see Excision, Male Reproductive System 0VB
 see Resection, Male Reproductive System 0VT

Scrotoplasty
 see Repair, Male Reproductive System 0VQ
 see Supplement, Male Reproductive System 0VU
Scrotorrhaphy
 see Repair, Male Reproductive System 0VQ
Scrototomy
 see Drainage, Male Reproductive System 0V9
Sebaceous gland
 use Skin
Second cranial nerve
 use Nerve, Optic
Section, cesarean
 see Extraction, Pregnancy 10D
Secura (DR) (VR)
 use Defibrillator Generator in 0JH
Sella Turcica
 use Bone, Sphenoid
Semicircular canal
 use Ear, Inner, Left
 use Ear, Inner, Right
Semimembranosus muscle
 use Muscle, Upper Leg, Left
 use Muscle, Upper Leg, Right
Semitendinosus muscle
 use Muscle, Upper Leg, Left
 use Muscle, Upper Leg, Right
Sentinel™ Cerebral Protection System (CPS) X2A5312
Seprafilm
 use Adhesion Barrier
Septal cartilage
 use Septum, Nasal
Septectomy
 see Excision, Ear, Nose, Sinus 09B
 see Excision, Heart and Great Vessels 02B
 see Resection, Ear, Nose, Sinus 09T
 see Resection, Heart and Great Vessels 02T
Septoplasty
 see Repair, Ear, Nose, Sinus 09Q
 see Repair, Heart and Great Vessels 02Q
 see Replacement, Ear, Nose, Sinus 09R
 see Replacement, Heart and Great Vessels 02R
 see Reposition, Ear, Nose, Sinus 09S
 see Supplement, Ear, Nose, Sinus 09U
 see Supplement, Heart and Great Vessels 02U
Septostomy, balloon atrial 02163Z7
Septotomy
 see Drainage, Ear, Nose, Sinus 099
Sequestrectomy, bone
 see Extirpation
Serratus anterior muscle
 use Muscle, Thorax, Left
 use Muscle, Thorax, Right
Serratus posterior muscle
 use Muscle, Trunk, Left
 use Muscle, Trunk, Right
Seventh cranial nerve
 use Nerve, Facial
Sheffield hybrid external fixator
 use External Fixation Device, Hybrid in 0PH
 use External Fixation Device, Hybrid in 0PS
 use External Fixation Device, Hybrid in 0QH
 use External Fixation Device, Hybrid in 0QS

Sheffield ring external fixator
 use External Fixation Device, Ring in 0PH
 use External Fixation Device, Ring in 0PS
 use External Fixation Device, Ring in 0QH
 use External Fixation Device, Ring in 0QS
Shirodkar cervical cerclage 0UVC7ZZ
Shockwave Intravascular Lithotripsy (Shockwave IVL)
 see Fragmentation
Shock Wave Therapy, Musculoskeletal 6A93
Short gastric artery
 use Artery, Splenic
Shortening
 see Excision
 see Repair
 see Reposition
Shunt creation
 see Bypass
Sialoadenectomy
 Complete
 see Resection, Mouth and Throat 0CT
 Partial
 see Excision, Mouth and Throat 0CB
Sialodochoplasty
 see Repair, Mouth and Throat 0CQ
 see Replacement, Mouth and Throat 0CR
 see Supplement, Mouth and Throat 0CU
Sialoectomy
 see Excision, Mouth and Throat 0CB
 see Resection, Mouth and Throat 0CT
Sialography
 see Plain Radiography, Ear, Nose, Mouth and Throat B90
Sialolithotomy
 see Extirpation, Mouth and Throat 0CC
Sigmoid artery
 use Artery, Inferior Mesenteric
Sigmoid flexure
 use Colon, Sigmoid
Sigmoid vein
 use Vein, Inferior Mesenteric
Sigmoidectomy
 see Excision, Gastrointestinal System 0DB
 see Resection, Gastrointestinal System 0DT
Sigmoidorrhaphy
 see Repair, Gastrointestinal System 0DQ
Sigmoidoscopy 0DJD8ZZ
Sigmoidotomy
 see Drainage, Gastrointestinal System 0D9
Single lead pacemaker (atrium) (ventricle)
 use Pacemaker, Single Chamber in 0JH
Single lead rate responsive pacemaker (atrium)(ventricle)
 use Pacemaker, Single Chamber Rate Responsive in 0JH
Single-use Duodenoscope XFJ
Single-use Oversleeve with Intraoperative Colonic Irrigation XDPH8K7
Sinoatrial node
 use Conduction Mechanism

Sinogram
 Abdominal Wall
 see Fluoroscopy, Abdomen and Pelvis BW11
 Chest Wall
 see Plain Radiography, Chest BW03
 Retroperitoneum
 see Fluoroscopy, Abdomen and Pelvis BW11
Sinusectomy
 see Excision, Ear, Nose, Sinus 09B
 see Resection, Ear, Nose, Sinus 09T
Sinusoscopy 09JY4ZZ
Sinusotomy
 see Drainage, Ear, Nose, Sinus 099
Sinus venosus
 use Atrium, Right
Sirolimus-eluting coronary stent
 use Intraluminal Device, Drug-eluting in Heart and Great Vessels
Sixth cranial nerve
 use Nerve, Abducens
Size reduction, breast
 see Excision, Skin and Breast 0HB
SJM Biocor® Stented Valve System
 use Zooplastic Tissue in Heart and Great Vessels
Skene's (paraurethral) gland
 use Gland, Vestibular
Skin Substitute, Porcine Liver Derived, Replacement XHRPXL2
Sling
 Fascial, orbicularis muscle (mouth)
 see Supplement, Muscle, Facial 0KU1
 Levator muscle, for urethral suspension
 see Reposition, Bladder Neck 0TSC
 Pubococcygeal, for urethral suspension
 see Reposition, Bladder Neck 0TSC
 Rectum
 see Reposition, Rectum 0DSP
Small bowel series
 see Fluoroscopy, Bowel, Small BD13
Small saphenous vein
 use Vein, Saphenous, Left
 use Vein, Saphenous, Right
Snapshot_NIR 8E02XDZ
Snaring, polyp, colon
 see Excision, Gastrointestinal System 0DB
Solar (celiac) plexus
 use Nerve, Abdominal Sympathetic
Soleus muscle
 use Muscle, Lower Leg, Left
 use Muscle, Lower Leg, Right
Soliris®
 see Eculizumab
Spacer
 Insertion of device in
 Disc
 Lumbar Vertebral 0SH2
 Lumbosacral 0SH4
 Joint
 Acromioclavicular
 Left 0RHH
 Right 0RHG
 Ankle
 Left 0SHG
 Right 0SHF

Spacer *(continued)*
Insertion of device in *(continued)*
Joint *(continued)*
Carpal
Left 0RHR
Right 0RHQ
Carpometacarpal
Left 0RHT
Right 0RHS
Cervical Vertebral 0RH1
Cervicothoracic Vertebral
0RH4
Coccygeal 0SH6
Elbow
Left 0RHM
Right 0RHL
Finger Phalangeal
Left 0RHX
Right 0RHW
Hip
Left 0SHB
Right 0SH9
Knee
Left 0SHD
Right 0SHC
Lumbar Vertebral 0SH0
Lumbosacral 0SH3
Metacarpophalangeal
Left 0RHV
Right 0RHU
Metatarsal-Phalangeal
Left 0SHN
Right 0SHM
Occipital-cervical 0RH0
Sacrococcygeal 0SH5
Sacroiliac
Left 0SH8
Right 0SH7
Shoulder
Left 0RHK
Right 0RHJ
Sternoclavicular
Left 0RHF
Right 0RHE
Tarsal
Left 0SHJ
Right 0SHH
Tarsometatarsal
Left 0SHL
Right 0SHK
Temporomandibular
Left 0RHD
Right 0RHC
Thoracic Vertebral 0RH6
Thoracolumbar Vertebral
0RHA
Toe Phalangeal
Left 0SHQ
Right 0SHP
Wrist
Left 0RHP
Right 0RHN
Removal of device from
Acromioclavicular
Left 0RPH
Right 0RPG
Ankle
Left 0SPG
Right 0SPF
Carpal
Left 0RPR
Right 0RPQ
Carpometacarpal
Left 0RPT
Right 0RPS
Cervical Vertebral 0RP1
Cervicothoracic Vertebral
0RP4
Coccygeal 0SP6
Elbow
Left 0RPM

Spacer *(continued)*
Removal of device from *(continued)*
Elbow *(continued)*
Right 0RPL
Finger Phalangeal
Left 0RPX
Right 0RPW
Hip
Left 0SPB
Right 0SP9
Knee
Left 0SPD
Right 0SPC
Lumbar Vertebral 0SP0
Lumbosacral 0SP3
Metacarpophalangeal
Left 0RPV
Right 0RPU
Metatarsal-Phalangeal
Left 0SPN
Right 0SPM
Occipital-cervical 0RP0
Sacrococcygeal 0SP5
Sacroiliac
Left 0SP8
Right 0SP7
Shoulder
Left 0RPK
Right 0RPJ
Sternoclavicular
Left 0RPF
Right 0RPE
Tarsal
Left 0SPJ
Right 0SPH
Tarsometatarsal
Left 0SPL
Right 0SPK
Temporomandibular
Left 0RPD
Right 0RPC
Thoracic Vertebral 0RP6
Thoracolumbar Vertebral
0RPA
Toe Phalangeal
Left 0SPQ
Right 0SPP
Wrist
Left 0RPP
Right 0RPN
Revision of device in
Acromioclavicular
Left 0RWH
Right 0RWG
Ankle
Left 0SWG
Right 0SWF
Carpal
Left 0RWR
Right 0RWQ
Carpometacarpal
Left 0RWT
Right 0RWS
Cervical Vertebral 0RW1
Cervicothoracic Vertebral
0RW4
Coccygeal 0SW6
Elbow
Left 0RWM
Right 0RWL
Finger Phalangeal
Left 0RWX
Right 0RWW
Hip
Left 0SWB
Right 0SW9
Knee
Left 0SWD
Right 0SWC
Lumbar Vertebral 0SW0
Lumbosacral 0SW3

Spacer *(continued)*
Revision of device in *(continued)*
Metacarpophalangeal
Left 0RWV
Right 0RWU
Metatarsal-Phalangeal
Left 0SWN
Right 0SWM
Occipital-cervical 0RW0
Sacrococcygeal 0SW5
Sacroiliac
Left 0SW8
Right 0SW7
Shoulder
Left 0RWK
Right 0RWJ
Sternoclavicular
Left 0RWF
Right 0RWE
Tarsal
Left 0SWJ
Right 0SWH
Tarsometatarsal
Left 0SWL
Right 0SWK
Temporomandibular
Left 0RWD
Right 0RWC
Thoracic Vertebral 0RW6
Thoracolumbar Vertebral 0RWA
Toe Phalangeal
Left 0SWQ
Right 0SWP
Wrist
Left 0RWP
Right 0RWN
Spacer, Articulating (Antibiotic)
use Articulating Spacer in Lower
Joints
Spacer, Static (Antibiotic)
use Spacer in Lower Joints
Spectroscopy
Intravascular Near Infrared 8E023DZ
Near Infrared
see Physiological Systems and
Anatomical Regions 8E0
Speech Assessment F00
Speech therapy
see Speech Treatment,
Rehabilitation F06
Speech Treatment F06
Sphenoidectomy
see Excision, Ear, Nose, Sinus 09B
see Excision, Head and Facial
Bones 0NB
see Resection, Ear, Nose, Sinus 09T
see Resection, Head and Facial
Bones 0NT
Sphenoidotomy
see Drainage, Ear, Nose, Sinus 099
Sphenomandibular ligament
use Bursa and Ligament, Head and
Neck
**Sphenopalatine (pterygopalatine)
ganglion**
use Nerve, Head and Neck
Sympathetic
Sphincterorrhaphy, anal
see Repair, Anal Sphincter 0DQR
Sphincterotomy, anal
see Division, Anal Sphincter 0D8R
see Drainage, Anal Sphincter
0D9R
Spinal cord neurostimulator lead
use Neurostimulator Lead in Central
Nervous System and Cranial
Nerves
**Spinal growth rod(s), magnetically
controlled**
use Magnetically Controlled Growth
Rod(s) in New Technology

Spinal nerve, cervical
use Nerve, Cervical
Spinal nerve, lumbar
use Nerve, Lumbar
Spinal nerve, sacral
use Nerve, Sacral
Spinal nerve, thoracic
use Nerve, Thoracic
Spinal Stabilization Device
Facet Replacement
Cervical Vertebral 0RH1
Cervicothoracic Vertebral 0RH4
Lumbar Vertebral 0SH0
Lumbosacral 0SH3
Occipital-cervical 0RH0
Thoracic Vertebral 0RH6
Thoracolumbar Vertebral 0RHA
Interspinous Process
Cervical Vertebral 0RH1
Cervicothoracic Vertebral
0RH4
Lumbar Vertebral 0SH0
Lumbosacral 0SH3
Occipital-cervical 0RH0
Thoracic Vertebral 0RH6
Thoracolumbar Vertebral 0RHA
Pedicle-Based
Cervical Vertebral 0RH1
Cervicothoracic Vertebral
0RH4
Lumbar Vertebral 0SH0
Lumbosacral 0SH3
Occipital-cervical 0RH0
Thoracic Vertebral 0RH6
Thoracolumbar Vertebral
0RHA
SpineJack® system
use Synthetic Substitute,
Mechanically Expandable
(Paired) in New Technology
Spinous process
use Vertebra, Cervical
use Vertebra, Lumbar
use Vertebra, Thoracic
Spiral ganglion
use Nerve, Acoustic
Spiration IBV™ Valve System
use Intraluminal Device,
Endobronchial Valve in
Respiratory System
Splenectomy
see Excision, Lymphatic and Hemic
Systems 07B
see Resection, Lymphatic and
Hemic Systems 07T
Splenic flexure
use Colon, Transverse
Splenic plexus
use Nerve, Abdominal Sympathetic
Splenius capitis muscle
use Muscle, Head
Splenius cervicis muscle
use Muscle, Neck, Left
use Muscle, Neck, Right
Splenolysis
see Release, Lymphatic and Hemic
Systems 07N
Splenopexy
see Repair, Lymphatic and Hemic
Systems 07Q
see Reposition, Lymphatic and
Hemic Systems 07S
Splenoplasty
see Repair, Lymphatic and Hemic
Systems 07Q
Splenorrhaphy
see Repair, Lymphatic and Hemic
Systems 07Q
Splenotomy
see Drainage, Lymphatic and Hemic
Systems 079

Splinting, musculoskeletal
  see Immobilization, Anatomical
    Regions 2W3
SPRAVATO™
  use Esketamine Hydrochloride
SPY system intravascular
  fluorescence angiography
  see Monitoring, Physiological
    Systems 4A1
SPY PINPOINT fluorescence
  imaging system
  see Monitoring, Physiological
    Systems 4A1
  see Other Imaging, Hepatobiliary
    System and Pancreas BF5
SPY system intraoperative
  fluorescence cholangiography
  see Other Imaging, Hepatobiliary
    System and Pancreas BF5
Staged hepatectomy
  see Division, Hepatobiliary System
    and Pancreas 0F8
  see Resection, Hepatobiliary
    System and Pancreas 0FT
Stapedectomy
  see Excision, Ear, Nose, Sinus 09B
  see Resection, Ear, Nose, Sinus 09T
Stapediolysis
  see Release, Ear, Nose, Sinus 09N
Stapedioplasty
  see Repair, Ear, Nose, Sinus 09Q
  see Replacement, Ear, Nose, Sinus
    09R
  see Supplement, Ear, Nose, Sinus 09U
Stapedotomy
  see Drainage, Ear, Nose, Sinus 099
Stapes
  use Auditory Ossicle, Left
  use Auditory Ossicle, Right
Static Spacer (Antibiotic)
  use Spacer in Lower Joints
STELARA®
  use Other New Technology
    Therapeutic Substance
Stellate ganglion
  use Nerve, Head and Neck
    Sympathetic
Stem cell transplant
  see Transfusion, Circulatory 302
Stensen's duct
  use Duct, Parotid, Left
  use Duct, Parotid, Right
Stent retriever thrombectomy
  see Extirpation, Upper Arteries 03C
Stent, intraluminal (cardiovascular)
    (gastrointestinal)(hepatobiliary)
    (urinary)
  use Intraluminal Device
Stented tissue valve
  use Zooplastic Tissue in Heart and
    Great Vessels
Stereotactic Radiosurgery
  Abdomen DW23
  Adrenal Gland DG22
  Bile Ducts DF22
  Bladder DT22
  Bone Marrow D720
  Brain D020
  Brain Stem D021
  Breast
    Left DM20
    Right DM21
  Bronchus DB21
  Cervix DU21
  Chest DW22
  Chest Wall DB27
  Colon DD25
  Diaphragm DB28
  Duodenum DD22
  Ear D920
  Esophagus DD20

Stereotactic
  Radiosurgery (*continued*)
  Eye D820
  Gallbladder DF21
  Gamma Beam
    Abdomen DW23JZZ
    Adrenal Gland DG22JZZ
    Bile Ducts DF22JZZ
    Bladder DT22JZZ
    Bone Marrow D720JZZ
    Brain D020JZZ
    Brain Stem D021JZZ
    Breast
      Left DM20JZZ
      Right DM21JZZ
    Bronchus DB21JZZ
    Cervix DU21JZZ
    Chest DW22JZZ
    Chest Wall DB27JZZ
    Colon DD25JZZ
    Diaphragm DB28JZZ
    Duodenum DD22JZZ
    Ear D920JZZ
    Esophagus DD20JZZ
    Eye D820JZZ
    Gallbladder DF21JZZ
    Gland
      Adrenal DG22JZZ
      Parathyroid DG24JZZ
      Pituitary DG20JZZ
      Thyroid DG25JZZ
    Glands, Salivary D926JZZ
    Head and Neck DW21JZZ
    Ileum DD24JZZ
    Jejunum DD23JZZ
    Kidney DT20JZZ
    Larynx D92BJZZ
    Liver DF20JZZ
    Lung DB22JZZ
    Lymphatics
      Abdomen D726JZZ
      Axillary D724JZZ
      Inguinal D728JZZ
      Neck D723JZZ
      Pelvis D727JZZ
      Thorax D725JZZ
    Mediastinum DB26JZZ
    Mouth D924JZZ
    Nasopharynx D92DJZZ
    Neck and Head DW21JZZ
    Nerve, Peripheral D027JZZ
    Nose D921JZZ
    Ovary DU20JZZ
    Palate
      Hard D928JZZ
      Soft D929JZZ
    Pancreas DF23JZZ
    Parathyroid Gland DG24JZZ
    Pelvic Region DW26JZZ
    Pharynx D92CJZZ
    Pineal Body DG21JZZ
    Pituitary Gland DG20JZZ
    Pleura DB25JZZ
    Prostate DV20JZZ
    Rectum DD27JZZ
    Sinuses D927JZZ
    Spinal Cord D026JZZ
    Spleen D722JZZ
    Stomach DD21JZZ
    Testis DV21JZZ
    Thymus D721JZZ
    Thyroid Gland DG25JZZ
    Tongue D925JZZ
    Trachea DB20JZZ
    Ureter DT21JZZ
    Urethra DT23JZZ
    Uterus DU22JZZ
  Gland
    Adrenal DG22
    Parathyroid DG24
    Pituitary DG20

Stereotactic
  Radiosurgery (*continued*)
  Gland (*continued*)
    Thyroid DG25
  Glands, Salivary D926
  Head and Neck DW21
  Ileum DD24
  Jejunum DD23
  Kidney DT20
  Larynx D92B
  Liver DF20
  Lung DB22
  Lymphatics
    Abdomen D726
    Axillary D724
    Inguinal D728
    Neck D723
    Pelvis D727
    Thorax D725
  Mediastinum DB26
  Mouth D924
  Nasopharynx D92D
  Neck and Head DW21
  Nerve, Peripheral D027
  Nose D921
  Other Photon
    Abdomen DW23DZZ
    Adrenal Gland DG22DZZ
    Bile Ducts DF22DZZ
    Bladder DT22DZZ
    Bone Marrow D720DZZ
    Brain D020DZZ
    Brain Stem D021DZZ
    Breast
      Left DM20DZZ
      Right DM21DZZ
    Bronchus DB21DZZ
    Cervix DU21DZZ
    Chest DW22DZZ
    Chest Wall DB27DZZ
    Colon DD25DZZ
    Diaphragm DB28DZZ
    Duodenum DD22DZZ
    Ear D920DZZ
    Esophagus DD20DZZ
    Eye D820DZZ
    Gallbladder DF21DZZ
    Gland
      Adrenal DG22DZZ
      Parathyroid DG24DZZ
      Pituitary DG20DZZ
      Thyroid DG25DZZ
    Glands, Salivary D926DZZ
    Head and Neck DW21DZZ
    Ileum DD24DZZ
    Jejunum DD23DZZ
    Kidney DT20DZZ
    Larynx D92BDZZ
    Liver DF20DZZ
    Lung DB22DZZ
    Lymphatics
      Abdomen D726DZZ
      Axillary D724DZZ
      Inguinal D728DZZ
      Neck D723DZZ
      Pelvis D727DZZ
      Thorax D725DZZ
    Mediastinum DB26DZZ
    Mouth D924DZZ
    Nasopharynx D92DDZZ
    Neck and Head DW21DZZ
    Nerve, Peripheral D027DZZ
    Nose D921DZZ
    Ovary DU20DZZ
    Palate
      Hard D928DZZ
      Soft D929DZZ
    Pancreas DF23DZZ
    Parathyroid Gland DG24DZZ
    Pelvic Region DW26DZZ
    Pharynx D92CDZZ

Stereotactic
  Radiosurgery (*continued*)
  Other Photon (*continued*)
    Pineal Body DG21DZZ
    Pituitary Gland DG20DZZ
    Pleura DB25DZZ
    Prostate DV20DZZ
    Rectum DD27DZZ
    Sinuses D927DZZ
    Spinal Cord D026DZZ
    Spleen D722DZZ
    Stomach DD21DZZ
    Testis DV21DZZ
    Thymus D721DZZ
    Thyroid Gland DG25DZZ
    Tongue D925DZZ
    Trachea DB20DZZ
    Ureter DT21DZZ
    Urethra DT23DZZ
    Uterus DU22DZZ
  Ovary DU20
  Palate
    Hard D928
    Soft D929
  Pancreas DF23
  Parathyroid Gland DG24
  Particulate
    Abdomen DW23HZZ
    Adrenal Gland DG22HZZ
    Bile Ducts DF22HZZ
    Bladder DT22HZZ
    Bone Marrow D720HZZ
    Brain D020HZZ
    Brain Stem D021HZZ
    Breast
      Left DM20HZZ
      Right DM21HZZ
    Bronchus DB21HZZ
    Cervix DU21HZZ
    Chest DW22HZZ
    Chest Wall DB27HZZ
    Colon DD25HZZ
    Diaphragm DB28HZZ
    Duodenum DD22HZZ
    Ear D920HZZ
    Esophagus DD20HZZ
    Eye D820HZZ
    Gallbladder DF21HZZ
    Gland
      Adrenal DG22HZZ
      Parathyroid DG24HZZ
      Pituitary DG20HZZ
      Thyroid DG25HZZ
    Glands, Salivary D926HZZ
    Head and Neck DW21HZZ
    Ileum DD24HZZ
    Jejunum DD23HZZ
    Kidney DT20HZZ
    Larynx D92BHZZ
    Liver DF20HZZ
    Lung DB22HZZ
    Lymphatics
      Abdomen D726HZZ
      Axillary D724HZZ
      Inguinal D728HZZ
      Neck D723HZZ
      Pelvis D727HZZ
      Thorax D725HZZ
    Mediastinum DB26HZZ
    Mouth D924HZZ
    Nasopharynx D92DHZZ
    Neck and Head DW21HZZ
    Nerve, Peripheral D027HZZ
    Nose D921HZZ
    Ovary DU20HZZ
    Palate
      Hard D928HZZ
      Soft D929HZZ
    Pancreas DF23HZZ
    Parathyroid Gland DG24HZZ
    Pelvic Region DW26HZZ

Stereotactic
  Radiosurgery *(continued)*
    Particulate *(continued)*
      Pharynx D92CHZZ
      Pineal Body DG21HZZ
      Pituitary Gland DG20HZZ
      Pleura DB25HZZ
      Prostate DV20HZZ
      Rectum DD27HZZ
      Sinuses D927HZZ
      Spinal Cord D026HZZ
      Spleen D722HZZ
      Stomach DD21HZZ
      Testis DV21HZZ
      Thymus D721HZZ
      Thyroid Gland DG25HZZ
      Tongue D925HZZ
      Trachea DB20HZZ
      Ureter DT21HZZ
      Urethra DT23HZZ
      Uterus DU22HZZ
    Pelvic Region DW26
    Pharynx D92C
    Pineal Body DG21
    Pituitary Gland DG20
    Pleura DB25
    Prostate DV20
    Rectum DD27
    Sinuses D927
    Spinal Cord D026
    Spleen D722
    Stomach DD21
    Testis DV21
    Thymus D721
    Thyroid Gland DG25
    Tongue D925
    Trachea SB20
    Ureter DT21
    Urethra DT23
    Uterus DU22

Steripath® Micro™ Blood Collection System XXE5XR7
Sternoclavicular ligament
  use Bursa and Ligament, Shoulder, Left
  use Bursa and Ligament, Shoulder, Right
Sternocleidomastoid artery
  use Artery, Thyroid, Left
  use Artery, Thyroid, Right
Sternocleidomastoid muscle
  use Muscle, Neck, Left
  use Muscle, Neck, Right
Sternocostal ligament
  use Sternum Bursa and Ligament
Sternotomy
  see Division, Sternum 0P80
  see Drainage, Sternum 0P90
Stimulation, cardiac
  Cardioversion 5A2204Z
  Electrophysiologic testing
    see Measurement, Cardiac 4A02
Stimulator Generator
  Insertion of device in
    Abdomen 0JH8
    Back 0JH7
    Chest 0JH6
    Multiple Array
      Abdomen 0JH8
      Back 0JH7
      Chest 0JH6
    Multiple Array Rechargeable
      Abdomen 0JH8
      Back 0JH7
      Chest 0JH6
  Removal of device from,
    Subcutaneous Tissue and Fascia, Trunk 0JPT
  Revision of device in, Subcutaneous Tissue and Fascia, Trunk 0JWT

Stimulator Generator *(continued)*
  Single Array
    Abdomen 0JH8
    Back 0JH7
    Chest 0JH6
  Single Array Rechargeable
    Abdomen 0JH8
    Back 0JH7
    Chest 0JH6
Stimulator Lead
  Insertion of device in
    Anal Sphincter 0DHR
    Artery
      Left 03HL
      Right 03HK
    Bladder 0THB
    Muscle
      Lower 0KHY
      Upper 0KHX
    Stomach 0DH6
    Ureter 0TH9
  Removal of device from
    Anal Sphincter 0DPR
    Artery, Upper 03PY
    Bladder 0TPB
    Muscle
      Lower 0KPY
      Upper 0KPX
    Stomach 0DP6
    Ureter 0TP9
  Revision of device in
    Anal Sphincter 0DWR
    Artery, Upper 03WY
    Bladder 0TWB
    Muscle
      Lower 0KWY
      Upper 0KWX
    Stomach 0DW6
    Ureter 0TW9
Stoma
  Excision
    Abdominal Wall 0WBFXZ2
    Neck 0WB6XZ2
  Repair
    Abdominal Wall 0WQFXZ2
    Neck 0WQ6XZ2
Stomatoplasty
  see Repair, Mouth and Throat 0CQ
  see Replacement, Mouth and Throat 0CR
  see Supplement, Mouth and Throat 0CU
Stomatorrhaphy
  see Repair, Mouth and Throat 0CQ
StrataGraft®
  use Bioengineered Allogeneic Construct
Stratos LV
  use Cardiac Resynchronization Pacemaker Pulse Generator in 0JH
Stress test
  4A02XM4
  4A12XM4
Stripping
  see Extraction
Study
  Electrophysiologic stimulation, cardiac
    see Measurement, Cardiac 4A02
  Ocular motility 4A07X7Z
  Pulmonary airway flow measurement
    see Measurement, Respiratory 4A09
  Visual acuity 4A07X0Z
Styloglossus muscle
  use Muscle, Tongue, Palate, Pharynx
Stylomandibular ligament
  use Bursa and Ligament, Head and Neck

Stylopharyngeus muscle
  use Muscle, Tongue, Palate, Pharynx
Subacromial bursa
  use Bursa and Ligament, Shoulder, Left
  use Bursa and Ligament, Shoulder, Right
Subaortic (common iliac) lymph node
  use Lymphatic, Pelvis
Subarachnoid space, spinal
  use Spinal Canal
Subclavicular (apical) lymph node
  use Lymphatic, Axillary, Left
  use Lymphatic, Axillary, Right
Subclavius muscle
  use Muscle, Thorax, Left
  use Muscle, Thorax, Right
Subclavius nerve
  use Nerve, Brachial Plexus
Subcostal artery
  use Upper Artery
Subcostal muscle
  use Muscle, Thorax, Left
  use Muscle, Thorax, Right
Subcostal nerve
  use Nerve, Thoracic
Subcutaneous injection reservoir, port
  use Vascular Access Device, Totally Implantable in Subcutaneous Tissue and Fascia
Subcutaneous Defibrillator Lead
  Insertion of device in, Subcutaneous Tissue and Fascia, Chest 0JH6
  Removal of device from, Subcutaneous Tissue and Fascia, Trunk 0JPT
  Revision of device in, Subcutaneous Tissue and Fascia, Trunk 0JWT
Subcutaneous injection reservoir, pump
  use Infusion Device, Pump in Subcutaneous Tissue and Fascia
Subdermal progesterone implant
  use Contraceptive Device in Subcutaneous Tissue and Fascia
Subdural space, spinal
  use Spinal Canal
Submandibular ganglion
  use Nerve, Facial
  use Nerve, Head and Neck Sympathetic
Submandibular gland
  use Gland, Submaxillary, Left
  use Gland, Submaxillary, Right
Submandibular lymph node
  use Lymphatic, Head
Submandibular space
  use Subcutaneous Tissue and Fascia, Face
Submaxillary ganglion
  use Nerve, Head and Neck Sympathetic
Submaxillary lymph node
  use Lymphatic, Head
Submental artery
  use Artery, Face
Submental lymph node
  use Lymphatic, Head
Submucous (Meissner's) plexus
  use Nerve, Abdominal Sympathetic
Suboccipital nerve
  use Nerve, Cervical
Suboccipital venous plexus
  use Vein, Vertebral, Left
  use Vein, Vertebral, Right

Subparotid lymph node
  use Lymphatic, Head
Subscapular (posterior) lymph node
  use Lymphatic, Axillary, Left
  use Lymphatic, Axillary, Right
Subscapular aponeurosis
  use Subcutaneous Tissue and Fascia, Upper Arm, Left
  use Subcutaneous Tissue and Fascia, Upper Arm, Right
Subscapular artery
  use Artery, Axillary, Left
  use Artery, Axillary, Right
Subscapularis muscle
  use Muscle, Shoulder, Left
  use Muscle, Shoulder, Right
Substance Abuse Treatment
  Counseling
    Family, for substance abuse, Other Family Counseling HZ63ZZZ
    Group
      12-Step HZ43ZZZ
      Behavioral HZ41ZZZ
      Cognitive HZ40ZZZ
      Cognitive-Behavioral HZ42ZZZ
      Confrontational HZ48ZZZ
      Continuing Care HZ49ZZZ
      Infectious Disease
        Post-Test HZ4CZZZ
        Pre-Test HZ4CZZZ
      Interpersonal HZ44ZZZ
      Motivational Enhancement HZ47ZZZ
      Psychoeducation HZ46ZZZ
      Spiritual HZ4BZZZ
      Vocational HZ45ZZZ
    Individual
      12-Step HZ33ZZZ
      Behavioral HZ31ZZZ
      Cognitive HZ30ZZZ
      Cognitive-Behavioral HZ32ZZZ
      Confrontational HZ38ZZZ
      Continuing Care HZ39ZZZ
      Infectious Disease
        Post-Test HZ3CZZZ
        Pre-Test HZ3CZZZ
      Interpersonal HZ34ZZZ
      Motivational Enhancement HZ37ZZZ
      Psychoeducation HZ36ZZZ
      Spiritual HZ3BZZZ
      Vocational HZ35ZZZ
  Detoxification Services, for substance abuse HZ2ZZZZ
  Medication Management
    Antabuse HZ83ZZZ
    Bupropion HZ87ZZZ
    Clonidine HZ86ZZZ
    Levo-alpha-acetyl-methadol (LAAM) HZ82ZZZ
    Methadone Maintenance HZ81ZZZ
    Naloxone HZ85ZZZ
    Naltrexone HZ84ZZZ
    Nicotine Replacement HZ80ZZZ
    Other Replacement Medication HZ89ZZZ
    Psychiatric Medication HZ88ZZZ
  Pharmacotherapy
    Antabuse HZ93ZZZ
    Bupropion HZ97ZZZ
    Clonidine HZ96ZZZ
    Levo-alpha-acetyl-methadol (LAAM) HZ92ZZZ
    Methadone Maintenance HZ91ZZZ
    Naloxone HZ95ZZZ
    Naltrexone HZ94ZZZ
    Nicotine Replacement HZ90ZZZ

Substance Abuse
    Treatment (continued)
    Pharmacotherapy (continued)
      Psychiatric Medication HZ98ZZZ
      Replacement Medication, Other
        HZ99ZZZ
    Psychotherapy
      12-Step HZ53ZZZ
      Behavioral HZ51ZZZ
      Cognitive HZ50ZZZ
      Cognitive-Behavioral HZ52ZZZ
      Confrontational HZ58ZZZ
      Interactive HZ55ZZZ
      Interpersonal HZ54ZZZ
      Motivational Enhancement
        HZ57ZZZ
      Psychoanalysis HZ5BZZZ
      Psychodynamic HZ5CZZZ
      Psychoeducation HZ56ZZZ
      Psychophysiological HZ5DZZZ
      Supportive HZ59ZZZ
Substantia nigra
  use Basal Ganglia
Subtalar (talocalcaneal) joint
  use Joint, Tarsal, Left
  use Joint, Tarsal, Right
Subtalar ligament
  use Bursa and Ligament, Foot, Left
  use Bursa and Ligament, Foot,
    Right
Subthalamic nucleus
  use Basal Ganglia
Suction curettage (D&C),
    nonobstetric
  see Extraction, Endometrium 0UDB
Suction curettage, obstetric post-
    delivery
  see Extraction, Products of
    Conception, Retained 10D1
Superficial circumflex iliac vein
  use Vein, Saphenous, Left
  use Vein, Saphenous, Right
Superficial epigastric artery
  use Artery, Femoral, Left
  use Artery, Femoral, Right
Superficial epigastric vein
  use Vein, Saphenous, Left
  use Vein, Saphenous, Right
Superficial Inferior Epigastric
    Artery Flap
  Replacement
    Bilateral 0HRV078
    Left 0HRU078
    Right 0HRT078
  Transfer
    Left 0KXG
    Right 0KXF
Superficial palmar arch
  use Artery, Hand, Left
  use Artery, Hand, Right
Superficial palmar venous arch
  use Vein, Hand, Left
  use Vein, Hand, Right
Superficial temporal artery
  use Artery, Temporal, Left
  use Artery, Temporal, Right
Superficial transverse perineal
    muscle
  use Muscle, Perineum
Superior cardiac nerve
  use Nerve, Thoracic Sympathetic
Superior cerebellar vein
  use Vein, Intracranial
Superior cerebral vein
  use Vein, Intracranial
Superior clunic (cluneal) nerve
  use Nerve, Lumbar
Superior epigastric artery
  use Artery, Internal Mammary, Left
  use Artery, Internal Mammary,
    Right

Superior genicular artery
  use Artery, Popliteal, Left
  use Artery, Popliteal, Right
Superior gluteal artery
  use Artery, Internal Iliac, Left
  use Artery, Internal Iliac, Right
Superior gluteal nerve
  use Nerve, Lumbar Plexus
Superior hypogastric plexus
  use Nerve, Abdominal Sympathetic
Superior labial artery
  use Artery, Face
Superior laryngeal artery
  use Artery, Thyroid, Left
  use Artery, Thyroid, Right
Superior laryngeal nerve
  use Nerve, Vagus
Superior longitudinal muscle
  use Muscle, Tongue, Palate,
    Pharynx
Superior mesenteric ganglion
  use Nerve, Abdominal Sympathetic
Superior mesenteric lymph node
  use Lymphatic, Mesenteric
Superior mesenteric plexus
  use Nerve, Abdominal Sympathetic
Superior oblique muscle
  use Muscle, Extraocular, Left
  use Muscle, Extraocular, Right
Superior olivary nucleus
  use Pons
Superior rectal artery
  use Artery, Inferior Mesenteric
Superior rectal vein
  use Vein, Inferior Mesenteric
Superior rectus muscle
  use Muscle, Extraocular, Left
  use Muscle, Extraocular, Right
Superior tarsal plate
  use Eyelid, Upper, Left
  use Eyelid, Upper, Right
Superior thoracic artery
  use Artery, Axillary, Left
  use Artery, Axillary, Right
Superior thyroid artery
  use External Carotid Artery, Left
  use External Carotid Artery,
    Right
  use Thyroid, Left
  use Thyroid, Right
Superior turbinate
  use Turbinate, Nasal
Superior ulnar collateral artery
  use Artery, Brachial, Left
  use Artery, Brachial, Right
Supersaturated Oxygen therapy
  5A0512C
  5A0522C
Supplement
  Abdominal Wall 0WUF
  Acetabulum
    Left 0QU5
    Right 0QU4
  Ampulla of Vater 0FUC
  Anal Sphincter 0DUR
  Ankle Region
    Left 0YUL
    Right 0YUK
  Anus 0DUQ
  Aorta
    Abdominal 04U0
    Thoracic
      Ascending/Arch 02UX
      Descending 02UW
  Arm
    Lower
      Left 0XUF
      Right 0XUD
    Upper
      Left 0XU9
      Right 0XU8

Supplement (continued)
  Artery
    Anterior Tibial
      Left 04UQ
      Right 04UP
    Axillary
      Left 03U6
      Right 03U5
    Brachial
      Left 03U8
      Right 03U7
    Celiac 04U1
    Colic
      Left 04U7
      Middle 04U8
      Right 04U6
    Common Carotid
      Left 03UJ
      Right 03UH
    Common Iliac
      Left 04UD
      Right 04UC
    Coronary
      Four or More Arteries 02U3
      One Artery 02U0
      Three Arteries 02U2
      Two Arteries 02U1
    External Carotid
      Left 03UN
      Right 03UM
    External Iliac
      Left 04UJ
      Right 04UH
    Face 03UR
    Femoral
      Left 04UL
      Right 04UK
    Foot
      Left 04UW
      Right 04UV
    Gastric 04U2
    Hand
      Left 03UF
      Right 03UD
    Hepatic 04U3
    Inferior Mesenteric 04UB
    Innominate 03U2
    Internal Carotid
      Left 03UL
      Right 03UK
    Internal Iliac
      Left 04UF
      Right 04UE
    Internal Mammary
      Left 03U1
      Right 03U0
    Intracranial 03UG
    Lower 04UY
    Peroneal
      Left 04UU
      Right 04UT
    Popliteal
      Left 04UN
      Right 04UM
    Posterior Tibial
      Left 04US
      Right 04UR
    Pulmonary
      Left 02UR
      Right 02UQ
    Pulmonary Trunk 02UP
    Radial
      Left 03UC
      Right 03UB
    Renal
      Left 04UA
      Right 04U9
    Splenic 04U4
    Subclavian
      Left 03U4
      Right 03U3

Supplement (continued)
  Artery (continued)
    Superior Mesenteric
      04U5
    Temporal
      Left 03UT
      Right 03US
    Thyroid
      Left 03UV
      Right 03UU
    Ulnar
      Left 03UA
      Right 03U9
    Upper 03UY
    Vertebral
      Left 03UQ
      Right 03UP
  Atrium
    Left 02U7
    Right 02U6
  Auditory Ossicle
    Left 09UA
    Right 09U9
  Axilla
    Left 0XU5
    Right 0XU4
  Back
    Lower 0WUL
    Upper 0WUK
  Bladder 0TUB
  Bladder Neck 0TUC
  Bone
    Ethmoid
      Left 0NUG
      Right 0NUF
    Frontal 0NU1
    Hyoid 0NUX
    Lacrimal
      Left 0NUJ
      Right 0NUH
    Nasal 0NUB
    Occipital 0NU7
    Palatine
      Left 0NUL
      Right 0NUK
    Parietal
      Left 0NU4
      Right 0NU3
    Pelvic
      Left 0QU3
      Right 0QU2
    Sphenoid 0NUC
    Temporal
      Left 0NU6
      Right 0NU5
    Zygomatic
      Left 0NUN
      Right 0NUM
  Breast
    Bilateral 0HUV
    Left 0HUU
    Right 0HUT
  Bronchus
    Lingula 0BU9
    Lower Lobe
      Left 0BUB
      Right 0BU6
    Main
      Left 0BU7
      Right 0BU3
    Middle Lobe, Right
      0BU5
    Upper Lobe
      Left 0BU8
      Right 0BU4
  Buccal Mucosa
    0CU4
  Bursa and Ligament
    Abdomen
      Left 0MUJ
      Right 0MUH

Supplement (continued)
Vein (continued)
Basilic
Left 05UC
Right 05UB
Brachial
Left 05UA
Right 05U9
Cephalic
Left 05UF
Right 05UD
Colic 06U7
Common Iliac
Left 06UD
Right 06UC
Esophageal 06U3
External Iliac
Left 06UG
Right 06UF
External Jugular
Left 05UQ
Right 05UP
Face
Left 05UV
Right 05UT
Femoral
Left 06UN
Right 06UM
Foot
Left 06UV
Right 06UT
Gastric 06U2
Hand
Left 05UH
Right 05UG
Hemiazygos 05U1
Hepatic 06U4
Hypogastric
Left 06UJ
Right 06UH
Inferior Mesenteric 06U6
Innominate
Left 05U4
Right 05U3
Internal Jugular
Left 05UN
Right 05UM
Intracranial 05UL
Lower 06UY
Portal 06U8
Pulmonary
Left 02UT
Right 02US
Renal
Left 06UB
Right 06U9
Saphenous
Left 06UQ
Right 06UP
Splenic 06U1
Subclavian
Left 05U6
Right 05U5
Superior Mesenteric
06U5
Upper 05UY
Vertebral
Left 05US
Right 05UR
Vena Cava
Inferior 06U0
Superior 02UV
Ventricle
Left 02UL
Right 02UK
Vertebra
Cervical 0PU3
Lumbar 0QU0
Mechanically Expandable
(Paired) Synthetic
Substitute XNU0356

Supplement (continued)
Vertebra (continued)
Thoracic 0PU4
Mechanically Expandable
(Paired) Synthetic
Substitute XNU4356
Vesicle
Bilateral 0VU3
Left 0VU2
Right 0VU1
Vocal Cord
Left 0CUV
Right 0CUT
Vulva 0UUM
Wrist Region
Left 0XUH
Right 0XUG
Supraclavicular (Virchow's) lymph node
use Lymphatic, Neck, Left
use Lymphatic, Neck, Right
Supraclavicular nerve
use Nerve, Cervical Plexus
Suprahyoid lymph node
use Lymphatic, Head
Suprahyoid muscle
use Muscle, Neck, Left
use Muscle, Neck, Right
Suprainguinal lymph node
use Lymphatic, Pelvis
Supraorbital vein
use Vein, Face, Left
use Vein, Face, Right
Suprarenal gland
use Gland, Adrenal
use Gland, Adrenal, Bilateral
use Gland, Adrenal, Left
use Gland, Adrenal, Right
Suprarenal plexus
use Nerve, Abdominal Sympathetic
Suprascapular nerve
use Nerve, Brachial Plexus
Supraspinatus fascia
use Subcutaneous Tissue and Fascia, Upper Arm, Left
use Subcutaneous Tissue and Fascia, Upper Arm, Right
Supraspinatus muscle
use Muscle, Shoulder, Left
use Muscle, Shoulder, Right
Supraspinous ligament
use Bursa and Ligament, Lower Spine
use Bursa and Ligament, Upper Spine
Suprasternal notch
use Sternum
Supratrochlear lymph node
use Lymphatic, Upper Extremity, Left
use Lymphatic, Upper Extremity, Right
Sural artery
use Artery, Popliteal, Left
use Artery, Popliteal, Right
Surpass Streamline™ Flow Diverter
use Intraluminal Device, Flow Diverter in 03V
Suspension
Bladder Neck
see Reposition, Bladder Neck 0TSC
Kidney
see Reposition, Urinary System 0TS
Urethra
see Reposition, Urinary System 0TS
Urethrovesical
see Reposition, Bladder Neck 0TSC
Uterus
see Reposition, Uterus 0US9

Suspension (continued)
Uterus (continued)
Vagina
see Reposition, Vagina 0USG
Sustained Release Drug-eluting Intraluminal Device
Dilation
Anterior Tibial
Left X27Q385
Right X27P385
Femoral
Left X27J385
Right X27H385
Peroneal
Left X27U385
Right X27T385
Popliteal
Left Distal X27N385
Left Proximal X27L385
Right Distal X27M385
Right Proximal X27K385
Posterior Tibial
Left X27S385
Right X27R385
Four or More
Anterior Tibial
Left X27Q3C5
Right X27P3C5
Femoral
Left X27J3C5
Right X27H3C5
Peroneal
Left X27U3C5
Right X27T3C5
Popliteal
Left Distal X27N3C5
Left Proximal X27L3C5
Right Distal X27M3C5
Right Proximal X27K3C5
Posterior Tibial
Left X27S3C5
Right X27R3C5
Three
Anterior Tibial
Left X27Q3B5
Right X27P3B5
Femoral
Left X27J3B5
Right X27H3B5
Peroneal
Left X27U3B5
Right X27T3B5
Popliteal
Left Distal X27N3B5
Left Proximal X27L3B5
Right Distal X27M3B5
Right Proximal X27K3B5
Posterior Tibial
Left X27S3B5
Right X27R3B5
Two
Anterior Tibial
Left X27Q395
Right X27P395
Femoral
Left X27J395
Right X27H395
Peroneal
Left X27U395
Right X27T395
Popliteal
Left Distal X27N395
Left Proximal X27L395
Right Distal X27M395
Right Proximal X27K395
Posterior Tibial
Left X27S395
Right X27R395
Suture
Laceration repair
see Repair

Suture (continued)
Ligation
see Occlusion
Suture Removal
Extremity
Lower 8E0YXY8
Upper 8E0XXY8
Head and Neck Region 8E09XY8
Trunk Region 8E0WXY8
Sutureless valve, Perceval
use Zooplastic Tissue, Rapid Deployment Technique in New Technology
Sweat gland
use Skin
Sympathectomy
see Excision, Peripheral Nervous System 01B
SynCardia Total Artificial Heart
use Synthetic Substitute
SynCardia (temporary) total artificial heart (TAH) use Synthetic Substitute, Pneumatic in 02R
Synchra CRT-P
use Cardiac Resynchronization Pacemaker Pulse Generator in 0JH
SynchroMed pump
use Infusion Device, Pump in Subcutaneous Tissue and Fascia
Synechiotomy, iris
see Release, Eye 08N
Synovectomy
Lower joint
see Excision, Lower Joints 0SB
Upper joint
see Excision, Upper Joints 0RB
Systemic Nuclear Medicine Therapy
Abdomen CW70
Anatomical Regions, Multiple CW7YYZZ
Chest CW73
Thyroid CW7G
Whole Body CW7N
Synthetic Human Angiotensin II
XW0

T

Tagraxofusp-erzs Antineoplastic
XW0
Takedown
Arteriovenous shunt
see Removal of device from, Upper Arteries 03P
Arteriovenous shunt, with creation of new shunt
see Bypass, Upper Arteries 031
Stoma
see Excision
see Reposition
Talent® Converter
use Intraluminal Device
Talent® Occluder
use Intraluminal Device
Talent® Stent Graft (abdominal) (thoracic)
use Intraluminal Device
Talocalcaneal (subtalar) joint
use Joint, Tarsal, Left
use Joint, Tarsal, Right
Talocalcaneal ligament
use Bursa and Ligament, Foot, Left
use Bursa and Ligament, Foot, Right
Talocalcaneonavicular joint
use Joint, Tarsal, Left
use Joint, Tarsal, Right
Talocalcaneonavicular ligament
use Bursa and Ligament, Foot, Left

Talocalcaneonavicular ligament *(continued)*
use Bursa and Ligament, Foot, Right

Talocrural joint
use Joint, Ankle, Left
use Joint, Ankle, Right

Talofibular ligament
use Bursa and Ligament, Ankle, Left
use Bursa and Ligament, Ankle, Right

Talus bone
use Tarsal, Left
use Tarsal, Right

TandemHeart® System
use Short-term External Heart Assist System in Heart and Great Vessels

Tarsectomy
see Excision, Lower Bones 0QB
see Resection, Lower Bones 0QT

Tarsometatarsal ligament
use Bursa and Ligament, Foot, Left
use Bursa and Ligament, Foot, Right

Tarsorrhaphy
see Repair, Eye 08Q

Tattooing
Cornea 3E0CXMZ
Skin
see Introduction of substance in or on, Skin 3E00

TAXUS® Liberté® Paclitaxel-eluting Coronary Stent System
use Intraluminal Device, Drug-eluting in Heart and Great Vessels

TBNA (transbronchial needle aspiration)
Fluid or gas
see Drainage, Respiratory System 0B9
Tissue biopsy
see Extraction, Respiratory System 0BD

Tecartus™
use Brexucabtagene Autoleucel Immunotherapy

TECENTRIQ®
use Atezolizumab Antineoplastic

Telemetry 4A12X4Z
Ambulatory 4A12X45

Temperature gradient study 4A0ZXKZ

Temporal lobe
use Cerebral Hemisphere

Temporalis muscle
use Muscle, Head

Temporoparietalis muscle
use Muscle, Head

Tendolysis
see Release, Tendons 0LN

Tendonectomy
see Excision, Tendons 0LB
see Resection, Tendons 0LT

Tendonoplasty, tenoplasty
see Repair, Tendons 0LQ
see Replacement, Tendons 0LR
see Supplement, Tendons 0LU

Tendorrhaphy
see Repair, Tendons 0LQ

Tendototomy
see Division, Tendons 0L8
see Drainage, Tendons 0L9

Tenectomy, tenonectomy
see Excision, Tendons 0LB
see Resection, Tendons 0LT

Tenolysis
see Release, Tendons 0LN

Tenontorrhaphy
see Repair, Tendons 0LQ

Tenontotomy
see Division, Tendons 0L8
see Drainage, Tendons 0L9

Tenorrhaphy
see Repair, Tendons 0LQ

Tenosynovectomy
see Excision, Tendons 0LB
see Resection, Tendons 0LT

Tenotomy
see Division, Tendons 0L8
see Drainage, Tendons 0L9

Tensor fasciae latae muscle
use Muscle, Hip, Left
use Muscle, Hip, Right

Tensor veli palatini muscle
use Muscle, Tongue, Palate, Pharynx

Tenth cranial nerve
use Nerve, Vagus

Tentorium cerebelli
use Dura Mater

Teres major muscle
use Muscle, Shoulder, Left
use Muscle, Shoulder, Right

Teres minor muscle
use Muscle, Shoulder, Left
use Muscle, Shoulder, Right

Terlipressin XW0

TERLIVAZ®
use Terlipressin

Termination of pregnancy
Aspiration curettage 10A07ZZ
Dilation and curettage 10A07ZZ
Hysterotomy 10A00ZZ
Intra-amniotic injection 10A03ZZ
Laminaria 10A07ZW
Vacuum 10A07Z6

Testectomy
see Excision, Male Reproductive System 0VB
see Resection, Male Reproductive System 0VT

Testicular artery
use Aorta, Abdominal

Testing
Glaucoma 4A07XBZ
Hearing
see Hearing Assessment, Diagnostic Audiology F13
Mental health
see Psychological Tests
Muscle function, electromyography (EMG)
see Measurement, Musculoskeletal 4A0F
Muscle function, manual
see Motor Function Assessment, Rehabilitation F01
Neurophysiologic monitoring, intra-operative
see Monitoring, Physiological Systems 4A1
Range of motion
see Motor Function Assessment, Rehabilitation F01
Vestibular function
see Vestibular Assessment, Diagnostic Audiology F15

Thalamectomy
see Excision, Thalamus 00B9

Thalamotomy
see Drainage, Thalamus 0099

Thenar muscle
use Muscle, Hand, Left
use Muscle, Hand, Right

Therapeutic Massage
Musculoskeletal System 8E0KX1Z
Reproductive System
Prostate 8E0VX1C
Rectum 8E0VX1D

Therapeutic occlusion coil(s)
use Intraluminal Device

Thermography 4A0ZXKZ

Thermotherapy, prostate
see Destruction, Prostate 0V50

Third cranial nerve
use Nerve, Oculomotor

Third occipital nerve
use Nerve, Cervical

Third ventricle
use Cerebral Ventricle

Thoracectomy
see Excision, Anatomical Regions, General 0WB

Thoracentesis
see Drainage, Anatomical Regions, General 0W9

Thoracic aortic plexus
use Nerve, Thoracic Sympathetic

Thoracic esophagus
use Esophagus, Middle

Thoracic facet joint
use Joint, Thoracic Vertebral

Thoracic ganglion
use Nerve, Thoracic Sympathetic

Thoracoacromial artery
use Artery, Axillary, Left
use Artery, Axillary, Right

Thoracocentesis
see Drainage, Anatomical Regions, General 0W9

Thoracolumbar facet joint
use Joint, Thoracolumbar Vertebral

Thoracoplasty
see Repair, Anatomical Regions, General 0WQ
see Supplement, Anatomical Regions, General 0WU

Thoracostomy tube
use Drainage Device

Thoracostomy, for lung collapse
see Drainage, Respiratory System 0B9

Thoracotomy
see Drainage, Anatomical Regions, General 0W9

Thoraflex™ Hybrid device *use* Branched Synthetic Substitute with Intraluminal Device in New Technology

Thoratec IVAD (Implantable Ventricular Assist Device)
use Implantable Heart Assist System in Heart and Great Vessels

Thoratec Paracorporeal Ventricular Assist Device
use Short-term External Heart Assist System in Heart and Great Vessels

Thrombectomy
see Extirpation

Thrombolysis, Ultrasound assisted
see Fragmentation, Artery

Thymectomy
see Excision, Lymphatic and Hemic Systems 07B
see Resection, Lymphatic and Hemic Systems 07T

Thymopexy
see Repair, Lymphatic and Hemic Systems 07Q
see Reposition, Lymphatic and Hemic Systems 07S

Thymus gland
use Thymus

Thyroarytenoid muscle
use Muscle, Neck, Left
use Muscle, Neck, Right

Thyrocervical trunk
use Artery, Thyroid, Left
use Artery, Thyroid, Right

Thyroid cartilage
use Larynx

Thyroidectomy
see Excision, Endocrine System 0GB
see Resection, Endocrine System 0GT

Thyroidorrhaphy
see Repair, Endocrine System 0GQ

Thyroidoscopy 0GJK4ZZ

Thyroidotomy
see Drainage, Endocrine System 0G9

Tibial insert
use Liner in Lower Joints

Tibial sesamoid
use Metatarsal, Left
use Metatarsal, Right

Tibialis anterior muscle
use Muscle, Lower Leg, Left
use Muscle, Lower Leg, Right

Tibialis posterior muscle
use Muscle, Lower Leg, Left
use Muscle, Lower Leg, Right

Tibiofemoral joint
use Joint, Knee, Left
use Joint, Knee, Left, Tibial Surface
use Joint, Knee, Right
use Joint, Knee, Right, Tibial Surface

Tibioperoneal trunk
use Popliteal Artery, Left
use Popliteal Artery, Right

Tisagenlecleucel
use Tisagenlecleucel Immunotherapy

Tisagenlecleucel Immunotherapy XW0

Tissue bank graft
use Nonautologous Tissue Substitute

Tissue Expander
Insertion of device in
Breast
Bilateral 0HHV
Left 0HHU
Right 0HHT
Nipple
Left 0HHX
Right 0HHW
Subcutaneous Tissue and Fascia
Abdomen 0JH8
Back 0JH7
Buttock 0JH9
Chest 0JH6
Face 0JH1
Foot
Left 0JHR
Right 0JHQ
Hand
Left 0JHK
Right 0JHJ
Lower Arm
Left 0JHH
Right 0JHG
Lower Leg
Left 0JHP
Right 0JHN
Neck
Left 0JH5
Right 0JH4
Pelvic Region 0JHC
Perineum 0JHB
Scalp 0JH0
Upper Arm
Left 0JHF
Right 0JHD
Upper Leg
Left 0JHM
Right 0JHL

Tissue Expander (*continued*)
Removal of device from
Breast
Left 0HPU
Right 0HPT
Subcutaneous Tissue and Fascia
Head and Neck 0JPS
Lower Extremity 0JPW
Trunk 0JPT
Upper Extremity 0JPV
Revision of device in
Breast
Left 0HWU
Right 0HWT
Subcutaneous Tissue and Fascia
Head and Neck 0JWS
Lower Extremity 0JWW
Trunk 0JWT
Upper Extremity 0JWV
Tissue expander (inflatable) (injectable)
use Tissue Expander in Skin and Breast
use Tissue Expander in Subcutaneous Tissue and Fascia
Tissue Plasminogen Activator (tPA) (r-tPA)
use Thrombolytic Other
Titanium Sternal Fixation System (TSFS)
use Internal Fixation Device, Rigid Plate in 0PS
use Internal Fixation Device, Rigid Plate in 0PH
Tocilizumab XW0
Tomographic (Tomo) Nuclear Medicine Imaging
Abdomen CW20
Abdomen and Chest CW24
Abdomen and Pelvis CW21
Anatomical Regions, Multiple CW2YYZZ
Bladder, Kidneys and Ureters CT23
Brain C020
Breast CH2YYZZ
Bilateral CH22
Left CH21
Right CH20
Bronchi and Lungs CB22
Central Nervous System C02YYZZ
Cerebrospinal Fluid C025
Chest CW23
Chest and Abdomen CW24
Chest and Neck CW26
Digestive System CD2YYZZ
Endocrine System CG2YYZZ
Extremity
Lower CW2D
Bilateral CP2F
Left CP2D
Right CP2C
Upper CW2M
Bilateral CP2B
Left CP29
Right CP28
Gallbladder CF24
Gastrointestinal Tract CD27
Gland, Parathyroid CG21
Head and Neck CW2B
Heart C22YYZZ
Right and Left C226
Hepatobiliary System and Pancreas CF2YYZZ
Kidneys, Ureters and Bladder CT23
Liver CF25
Liver and Spleen CF26
Lungs and Bronchi CB22
Lymphatics and Hematologic System C72YYZZ
Musculoskeletal System, Other CP2YYZZ

Tomographic (Tomo) Nuclear Medicine Imaging (*continued*)
Myocardium C22G
Neck and Chest CW26
Neck and Head CW2B
Pancreas and Hepatobiliary System CF2YYZZ
Pelvic Region CW2J
Pelvis CP26
Pelvis and Abdomen CW21
Pelvis and Spine CP27
Respiratory System CB2YYZZ
Skin CH2YYZZ
Skull CP21
Skull and Cervical Spine CP23
Spine
Cervical CP22
Cervical and Skull CP23
Lumbar CP2H
Thoracic CP2G
Thoracolumbar CP2J
Spine and Pelvis CP27
Spleen C722
Spleen and Liver CF26
Subcutaneous Tissue CH2YYZZ
Thorax CP24
Ureters, Kidneys and Bladder CT23
Urinary System CT2YYZZ
Tomography, computerized
see Computerized Tomography (CT Scan)
Tongue, base of
use Pharynx
Tonometry 4A07XBZ
Tonsillectomy
see Excision, Mouth and Throat 0CB
see Resection, Mouth and Throat 0CT
Tonsillotomy
see Drainage, Mouth and Throat 0C9
Total Anomalous Pulmonary Venous Return (TAPVR) repair
see Bypass, Atrium, Left 0217
see Bypass, Vena Cava, Superior 021V
Total artificial (replacement) heart
use Synthetic Substitute
Total parenteral nutrition (TPN)
see Introduction of Nutritional Substance
Tourniquet, External
see Compression, Anatomical Regions 2W1
Trachectomy
see Excision, Trachea 0BB1
see Resection, Trachea 0BT1
Trachelectomy
see Excision, Cervix 0UBC
see Resection, Cervix 0UTC
Trachelopexy
see Repair, Cervix 0UQC
see Reposition, Cervix 0USC
Tracheloplasty
see Repair, Cervix 0UQC
Trachelorrhaphy
see Repair, Cervix 0UQC
Trachelotomy
see Drainage, Cervix 0U9C
Tracheobronchial lymph node
use Lymphatic, Thorax
Tracheoesophageal fistulization 0B110D6
Tracheolysis
see Release, Respiratory System 0BN
Tracheoplasty
see Repair, Respiratory System 0BQ
see Supplement, Respiratory System 0BU
Tracheorrhaphy
see Repair, Respiratory System 0BQ

Tracheoscopy 0BJ18ZZ
Tracheostomy
see Bypass, Respiratory System 0B1
Tracheostomy Device
Bypass, Trachea 0B11
Change device in, Trachea 0B21XFZ
Removal of device from, Trachea 0BP1
Revision of device in, Trachea 0BW1
Tracheostomy tube
use Tracheostomy Device in Respiratory System
Tracheotomy
see Drainage, Respiratory System 0B9
Traction
Abdominal Wall 2W63X
Arm
Lower
Left 2W6DX
Right 2W6CX
Upper
Left 2W6BX
Right 2W6AX
Back 2W65X
Chest Wall 2W64X
Extremity
Lower
Left 2W6MX
Right 2W6LX
Upper
Left 2W69X
Right 2W68X
Face 2W61X
Finger
Left 2W6KX
Right 2W6JX
Foot
Left 2W6TX
Right 2W6SX
Hand
Left 2W6FXZ
Right 2W6EXZ
Head 2W60X
Inguinal Region
Left 2W67X
Right 2W66X
Leg
Lower
Left 2W6RX
Right 2W6QX
Upper
Left 2W6PX
Right 2W6NX
Neck 2W62X
Thumb
Left 2W6HX
Right 2W6GX
Toe
Left 2W6VX
Right 2W6UX
Tractotomy
see Division, Central Nervous System and Cranial Nerves 008
Tragus
use Ear, External, Bilateral
use Ear, External, Left
use Ear, External, Right
Training, caregiver
see Caregiver Training
TRAM (transverse rectus abdominis myocutaneous) flap reconstruction
Free
see Replacement, Skin and Breast 0HR
Pedicled
see Transfer, Muscles 0KX

Transcatheter Pulmonary Valve (TPV) placement
In conduit 02RH38L
Native site 02RH38M
Transdermal Glomerular Filtration Rate (GFR) Measurement System XT25XE5
Transection
see Division
Transfer
Buccal Mucosa 0CX4
Bursa and Ligament
Abdomen
Left 0MXJ
Right 0MXH
Ankle
Left 0MXR
Right 0MXQ
Elbow
Left 0MX4
Right 0MX3
Foot
Left 0MXT
Right 0MXS
Hand
Left 0MX8
Right 0MX7
Head and Neck 0MX0
Hip
Left 0MXM
Right 0MXL
Knee
Left 0MXP
Right 0MXN
Lower Extremity
Left 0MXW
Right 0MXV
Perineum 0MXK
Rib(s) 0MXG
Shoulder
Left 0MX2
Right 0MX1
Spine
Lower 0MXD
Upper 0MXC
Sternum 0MXF
Upper Extremity
Left 0MXB
Right 0MX9
Wrist
Left 0MX6
Right 0MX5
Finger
Left 0XXP0ZM
Right 0XXN0ZL
Gingiva
Lower 0CX6
Upper 0CX5
Immunotherapy
see New Technology, Anatomical Regions XW2
Intestine
Large 0DXE
Small 0DX8
Lip
Lower 0CX1
Upper 0CX0
Muscle
Abdomen
Left 0KXL
Right 0KXK
Extraocular
Left 08XM
Right 08XL
Facial 0KX1
Foot
Left 0KXW
Right 0KXV
Hand
Left 0KXD

Transfer (continued)
 Muscle (continued)
  Hand (continued)
   Right 0KXC
  Head 0KX0
  Hip
   Left 0KXP
   Right 0KXN
  Lower Arm and Wrist
   Left 0KXB
   Right 0KX9
  Lower Leg
   Left 0KXT
   Right 0KXS
  Neck
   Left 0KX3
   Right 0KX2
  Perineum 0KXM
  Shoulder
   Left 0KX6
   Right 0KX5
  Thorax
   Left 0KXJ
   Right 0KXH
  Tongue, Palate, Pharynx
   0KX4
  Trunk
   Left 0KXG
   Right 0KXF
  Upper Arm
   Left 0KX8
   Right 0KX7
  Upper Leg
   Left 0KXR
   Right 0KXQ
 Nerve
  Abducens 00XL
  Accessory 00XR
  Acoustic 00XN
  Cervical 01X1
  Facial 00XM
  Femoral 01XD
  Glossopharyngeal 00XP
  Hypoglossal 00XS
  Lumbar 01XB
  Median 01X5
  Oculomotor 00XH
  Olfactory 00XF
  Optic 00XG
  Peroneal 01XH
  Phrenic 01X2
  Pudendal 01XC
  Radial 01X6
  Sciatic 01XF
  Thoracic 01X8
  Tibial 01XG
  Trigeminal 00XK
  Trochlear 00XJ
  Ulnar 01X4
  Vagus 00XQ
 Palate, Soft 0CX3
 Prepuce 0VXT
 Skin
  Abdomen 0HX7XZZ
  Back 0HX6XZZ
  Buttock 0HX8XZZ
  Chest 0HX5XZZ
  Ear
   Left 0HX3XZZ
   Right 0HX2XZZ
  Face 0HX1XZZ
  Foot
   Left 0HXNXZZ
   Right 0HXMXZZ
  Hand
   Left 0HXGXZZ
   Right 0HXFXZZ
  Inguinal 0HXAXZZ
  Lower Arm
   Left 0HXEXZZ
   Right 0HXDXZZ

Transfer (continued)
 Skin (continued)
  Lower Leg
   Left 0HXLXZZ
   Right 0HXKXZZ
  Neck 0HX4XZZ
  Perineum 0HX9XZZ
  Scalp 0HX0XZZ
  Upper Arm
   Left 0HXCXZZ
   Right 0HXBXZZ
  Upper Leg
   Left 0HXJXZZ
   Right 0HXHXZZ
 Stomach 0DX6
 Subcutaneous Tissue and Fascia
  Abdomen 0JX8
  Back 0JX7
  Buttock 0JX9
  Chest 0JX6
  Face 0JX1
  Foot
   Left 0JXR
   Right 0JXQ
  Hand
   Left 0JXK
   Right 0JXJ
  Lower Arm
   Left 0JXH
   Right 0JXG
  Lower Leg
   Left 0JXP
   Right 0JXN
  Neck
   Left 0JX5
   Right 0JX4
  Pelvic Region 0JXC
  Perineum 0JXB
  Scalp 0JX0
  Upper Arm
   Left 0JXF
   Right 0JXD
  Upper Leg
   Left 0JXM
   Right 0JXL
 Tendon
  Abdomen
   Left 0LXG
   Right 0LXF
  Ankle
   Left 0LXT
   Right 0LXS
  Foot
   Left 0LXW
   Right 0LXV
  Hand
   Left 0LX8
   Right 0LX7
  Head and Neck 0LX0
  Hip
   Left 0LXK
   Right 0LXJ
  Knee
   Left 0LXR
   Right 0LXQ
  Lower Arm and Wrist
   Left 0LX6
   Right 0LX5
  Lower Leg
   Left 0LXP
   Right 0LXN
  Perineum 0LXH
  Shoulder
   Left 0LX2
   Right 0LX1
  Thorax
   Left 0LXD
   Right 0LXC
  Trunk
   Left 0LXB
   Right 0LX9

Transfer (continued)
 Tendon (continued)
  Upper Arm
   Left 0LX4
   Right 0LX3
  Upper Leg
   Left 0LXM
   Right 0LXL
 Tongue 0CX7
Transfusion
 Immunotherapy see New
  Technology, Anatomical Regions
  XW2
 Products of Conception
  Antihemophilic Factors
   3027
  Blood
   Platelets 3027
   Red Cells 3027
    Frozen 3027
   White Cells 3027
   Whole 3027
  Factor IX 3027
  Fibrinogen 3027
  Globulin 3027
  Plasma
   Fresh 3027
   Frozen 3027
  Plasma Cryoprecipitate
   3027
  Serum Albumin 3027
 Vein
  4-Factor Prothrombin
   Complex Concentrate
   30283B1
  Central
   Antihemophilic Factors
    30243V
   Blood
    Platelets 30243R
    Red Cells 30243N
     Frozen 30243P
    White Cells 30243Q
    Whole 30243H
   Bone Marrow 30243G
   Factor IX 30243W
   Fibrinogen 30243T
   Globulin 30243S
   Hematopoietic Stem/
    Progenitor Cells (HSPC),
    Genetically Modified
    30243C0
   Pathogen Reduced
    Cryoprecipitated Fibrinogen
    Complex 30243D1
   Plasma
    Fresh 30243L
    Frozen 30243K
   Plasma Cryoprecipitate
    30243M
   Serum Albumin 30243J
   Stem Cells
    Cord Blood 30243X
    Embryonic 30243AZ
    Hematopoietic 30243Y
    T-cell Depleted
     Hematopoietic
     30243U
  Peripheral
   Antihemophilic Factors
    30233V
   Blood
    Platelets 30233R
    Red Cells 30233N
     Frozen 30233P
    White Cells 30233Q
    Whole 30233H
   Bone Marrow 30233G
   Factor IX 30233W
   Fibrinogen 30233T
   Globulin 30233S

Transfusion (continued)
 Vein (continued)
  Peripheral (continued)
   Hematopoietic Stem/
    Progenitor Cells (HSPC),
    Genetically Modified
    30233C0
   Pathogen Reduced
    Cryoprecipitated Fibrinogen
    Complex 30233D1
   Plasma
    Fresh 30233L
    Frozen 30233K
   Plasma Cryoprecipitate 30233M
   Serum Albumin 30233J
   Stem Cells
    Cord Blood 30233X
    Embryonic 30233AZ
    Hematopoietic 30233Y
    T-cell Depleted
     Hematopoietic 30233U
Transplant
 see Transplantation
Transplantation
 Bone marrow
  see Transfusion, Circulatory 302
 Esophagus 0DY50Z
 Face 0WY20Z
 Hand
  Left 0XYK0Z
  Right 0XYJ0Z
 Heart 02YA0Z
 Hematopoietic cell
  see Transfusion, Circulatory 302
 Intestine
  Large 0DYE0Z
  Small 0DY80Z
 Kidney
  Left 0TY10Z
  Right 0TY00Z
 Liver 0FY00Z
 Lung
  Bilateral 0BYM0Z
  Left 0BYL0Z
  Lower Lobe
   Left 0BYJ0Z
   Right 0BYF0Z
  Middle Lobe, Right 0BYD0Z
  Right 0BYK0Z
  Upper Lobe
   Left 0BYG0Z
   Right 0BYC0Z
 Lung Lingula 0BYH0Z
 Ovary
  Left 0UY10Z
  Right 0UY00Z
 Pancreas 0FYG0Z
 Penis 0VYS0Z
 Products of Conception 10Y0
 Scrotum 0VY50Z
 Spleen 07YP0Z
 Stem cell
  see Transfusion, Circulatory 302
 Stomach 0DY60Z
 Thymus 07YM0Z
 Uterus 0UY90Z
Transposition
 see Bypass
 see Reposition
 see Transfer
Transversalis fascia
 use Subcutaneous Tissue and Fascia,
  Trunk
Transverse acetabular ligament
 use Bursa and Ligament, Hip,
  Left
 use Bursa and Ligament, Hip,
  Right
Transverse (cutaneous) cervical
 nerve
 use Nerve, Cervical Plexus

Transverse facial artery
  use Artery, Temporal, Left
  use Artery, Temporal, Right
Transverse foramen
  use Cervical Vertebra
Transverse humeral ligament
  use Bursa and Ligament, Shoulder, Left
  use Bursa and Ligament, Shoulder, Right
Transverse ligament of atlas
  use Bursa and Ligament, Head and Neck
Transverse process
  use Cervical Vertebra
  use Thoracic Vertebra
  use Lumbar Vertebra
Transverse Rectus Abdominis Myocutaneous Flap
  Replacement
    Bilateral 0HRV076
    Left 0HRU076
    Right 0HRT076
  Transfer
    Left 0KXL
    Right 0KXK
Transverse scapular ligament
  use Bursa and Ligament, Shoulder, Left
  use Bursa and Ligament, Shoulder, Right
Transverse thoracis muscle
  use Muscle, Thorax, Left
  use Muscle, Thorax, Right
Transversospinalis muscle
  use Muscle, Trunk, Left
  use Muscle, Trunk, Right
Transversus abdominis muscle
  use Muscle, Abdomen, Left
  use Muscle, Abdomen, Right
Trapezium bone
  use Carpal, Left
  use Carpal, Right
Trapezius muscle
  use Muscle, Trunk, Left
  use Muscle, Trunk, Right
Trapezoid bone
  use Carpal, Left
  use Carpal, Right
Triceps brachii muscle
  use Muscle, Upper Arm, Left
  use Muscle, Upper Arm, Right
Tricuspid annulus
  use Valve, Tricuspid
Trifacial nerve
  use Nerve, Trigeminal
Trifecta™ Valve (aortic)
  use Zooplastic Tissue in Heart and Great Vessels
Trigone of bladder
  use Bladder
TriGuard 3™ CEPD (cerebral embolic protection device)
  X2A6325
Trilaciclib XW0
Trimming, excisional
  see Excision
Triquetral bone
  use Carpal, Left
  use Carpal, Right
Trochanteric bursa
  use Bursa and Ligament, Hip, Left
  use Bursa and Ligament, Hip, Right
TUMT (Transurethral microwave thermotherapy of prostate)
  0V507ZZ
TUNA (transurethral needle ablation of prostate)
  0V507ZZ

Tunneled central venous catheter
  use Vascular Access Device Tunneled in Subcutaneous Tissue and Fascia
Tunneled spinal (intrathecal) catheter
  use Infusion Device
Turbinectomy
  see Excision, Ear, Nose, Sinus 09B
  see Resection, Ear, Nose, Sinus 09T
Turbinoplasty
  see Repair, Ear, Nose, Sinus 09Q
  see Replacement, Ear, Nose, Sinus 09R
  see Supplement, Ear, Nose, Sinus 09U
Turbinotomy
  see Division, Ear, Nose, Sinus 098
  see Drainage, Ear, Nose, Sinus 099
TURP (transurethral resection of prostate)
  see Excision, Prostate 0VB0
  see Resection, Prostate 0VT0
Twelfth cranial nerve
  use Nerve, Hypoglossal
Two lead pacemaker
  use Pacemaker, Dual Chamber in 0JH
Tympanic cavity
  use Ear, Middle, Left
  use Ear, Middle, Right
Tympanic nerve
  use Nerve, Glossopharyngeal
Tympanic part of temoporal bone
  use Bone, Temporal, Left
  use Bone, Temporal, Right
Tympanogram
  see Hearing Assessment, Diagnostic Audiology F13
Tympanoplasty
  see Repair, Ear, Nose, Sinus 09Q
  see Replacement, Ear, Nose, Sinus 09R
  see Supplement, Ear, Nose, Sinus 09U
Tympanosympathectomy
  see Excision, Nerve, Head and Neck Sympathetic 01BK
Tympanotomy
  see Drainage, Ear, Nose, Sinus 099
TYRX Antibacterial Envelope
  use Anti-infective Envelope

U

Ulnar collateral carpal ligament
  use Bursa and Ligament, Wrist, Left
  use Bursa and Ligament, Wrist, Right
Ulnar collateral ligament
  use Bursa and Ligament, Elbow, Left
  use Bursa and Ligament, Elbow, Right
Ulnar notch
  use Radius, Left
  use Radius, Right
Ulnar vein
  use Vein, Brachial, Left
  use Vein, Brachial, Right
Ultrafiltration
  Hemodialysis
    see Performance, Urinary 5A1D
  Therapeutic plasmapheresis
    see Pheresis, Circulatory 6A55
Ultraflex™ Precision Colonic Stent System
  use Intraluminal Device
ULTRAPRO Hernia System (UHS)
  use Synthetic Substitute

ULTRAPRO Partially Absorbable Lightweight Mesh
  use Synthetic Substitute
ULTRAPRO Plug
  use Synthetic Substitute
Ultrasonic osteogenic stimulator
  use Bone Growth Stimulator in Head and Facial Bones
  use Bone Growth Stimulator in Lower Bones
  use Bone Growth Stimulator in Upper Bones
Ultrasonography
  Abdomen BW40ZZZ
  Abdomen and Pelvis BW41ZZZ
  Abdominal Wall BH49ZZZ
  Aorta
    Abdominal, Intravascular B440ZZ3
    Thoracic, Intravascular B340ZZ3
  Appendix BD48ZZZ
  Artery
    Brachiocephalic-Subclavian, Right, Intravascular B341ZZ3
    Celiac and Mesenteric, Intravascular B44KZZ3
    Common Carotid
      Bilateral, Intravascular B345ZZ3
      Left, Intravascular B344ZZ3
      Right, Intravascular B343ZZ3
    Coronary
      Multiple B241YZZ
        Intravascular B241ZZ3
        Transesophageal B241ZZ4
      Single B240YZZ
        Intravascular B240ZZ3
        Transesophageal B240ZZ4
    Femoral, Intravascular B44LZZ3
    Inferior Mesenteric, Intravascular B445ZZ3
    Internal Carotid
      Bilateral, Intravascular B348ZZ3
      Left, Intravascular B347ZZ3
      Right, Intravascular B346ZZ3
    Intra-Abdominal, Other, Intravascular B44BZZ3
    Intracranial, Intravascular B34RZZ3
    Lower Extremity
      Bilateral, Intravascular B44HZZ3
      Left, Intravascular B44GZZ3
      Right, Intravascular B44FZZ3
    Mesenteric and Celiac, Intravascular B44KZZ3
    Ophthalmic, Intravascular B34VZZ3
    Penile, Intravascular B44NZZ3
    Pulmonary
      Left, Intravascular B34TZZ3
      Right, Intravascular B34SZZ3
    Renal
      Bilateral, Intravascular B448ZZ3
      Left, Intravascular B447ZZ3
      Right, Intravascular B446ZZ3
    Subclavian, Left, Intravascular B342ZZ3
    Superior Mesenteric, Intravascular B444ZZ3
    Upper Extremity
      Bilateral, Intravascular B34KZZ3
      Left, Intravascular B34JZZ3
      Right, Intravascular B34HZZ3

Ultrasonography *(continued)*
  Bile Duct BF40ZZZ
  Bile Duct and Gallbladder BF43ZZZ
  Bladder BT40ZZZ
    and Kidney BT4JZZZ
  Brain B040ZZZ
  Breast
    Bilateral BH42ZZZ
    Left BH41ZZZ
    Right BH40ZZZ
  Chest Wall BH4BZZZ
  Coccyx BR4FZZZ
  Connective Tissue
    Lower Extremity BL41ZZZ
    Upper Extremity BL40ZZZ
  Duodenum BD49ZZZ
  Elbow
    Left, Densitometry BP4HZZ1
    Right, Densitometry BP4GZZ1
  Esophagus BD41ZZZ
  Extremity
    Lower BH48ZZZ
    Upper BH47ZZZ
  Eye
    Bilateral B847ZZZ
    Left B846ZZZ
    Right B845ZZZ
  Fallopian Tube
    Bilateral BU42
    Left BU41
    Right BU40
  Fetal Umbilical Cord BY47ZZZ
  Fetus
    First Trimester, Multiple Gestation BY4BZZZ
    Second Trimester, Multiple Gestation BY4DZZZ
    Single
      First Trimester BY49ZZZ
      Second Trimester BY4CZZZ
      Third Trimester BY4FZZZ
    Third Trimester, Multiple Gestation BY4GZZZ
  Gallbladder BF42ZZZ
  Gallbladder and Bile Duct BF43ZZZ
  Gastrointestinal Tract BD47ZZZ
  Gland
    Adrenal
      Bilateral BG42ZZZ
      Left BG41ZZZ
      Right BG40ZZZ
    Parathyroid BG43ZZZ
    Thyroid BG44ZZZ
  Hand
    Left, Densitometry BP4PZZ1
    Right, Densitometry BP4NZZ1
  Head and Neck BH4CZZZ
  Heart
    Left B245YZZ
      Intravascular B245ZZ3
      Transesophageal B245ZZ4
    Pediatric B24DYZZ
      Intravascular B24DZZ3
      Transesophageal B24DZZ4
    Right B244YZZ
      Intravascular B244ZZ3
      Transesophageal B244ZZ4
    Right and Left B246YZZ
      Intravascular B246ZZ3
      Transesophageal B246ZZ4
  Heart with Aorta B24BYZZ
    Intravascular B24BZZ3
    Transesophageal B24BZZ4
  Hepatobiliary System, All BF4CZZZ
  Hip
    Bilateral BQ42ZZZ

Ultrasonography (continued)
Hip (continued)
  Left BQ41ZZZ
  Right BQ40ZZZ
Kidney
  and Bladder BT4JZZZ
  Bilateral BT43ZZZ
  Left BT42ZZZ
  Right BT41ZZZ
  Transplant BT49ZZZ
Knee
  Bilateral BQ49ZZZ
  Left BQ48ZZZ
  Right BQ47ZZZ
Liver BF45ZZZ
Liver and Spleen BF46ZZZ
Mediastinum BB4CZZZ
Neck BW4FZZZ
Ovary
  Bilateral BU45
  Left BU44
  Right BU43
Ovary and Uterus BU4C
Pancreas BF47ZZZ
Pelvic Region BW4GZZZ
Pelvis and Abdomen BW41ZZZ
Penis BV4BZZZ
Pericardium B24CYZZ
  Intravascular B24CZZ3
  Transesophageal B24CZZ4
Placenta BY48ZZZ
Pleura BB4BZZZ
Prostate and Seminal Vesicle
  BV49ZZZ
Rectum BD4CZZZ
Sacrum BR4FZZZ
Scrotum BV44ZZZ
Seminal Vesicle and Prostate
  BV49ZZZ
Shoulder
  Left, Densitometry BP49ZZ1
  Right, Densitometry BP48ZZ1
Spinal Cord B04BZZZ
Spine
  Cervical BR40ZZZ
  Lumbar BR49ZZZ
  Thoracic BR47ZZZ
Spleen and Liver BF46ZZZ
Stomach BD42ZZZ
Tendon
  Lower Extremity BL43ZZZ
  Upper Extremity BL42ZZZ
Ureter
  Bilateral BT48ZZZ
  Left BT47ZZZ
  Right BT46ZZZ
Urethra BT45ZZZ
Uterus BU46
Uterus and Ovary BU4C
Vein
  Jugular
    Left, Intravascular
      B544ZZ3
    Right, Intravascular B543ZZ3
  Lower Extremity
    Bilateral, Intravascular
      B54DZZ3
    Left, Intravascular B54CZZ3
    Right, Intravascular B54BZZ3
  Portal, Intravascular B54TZZ3
  Renal
    Bilateral, Intravascular
      B54LZZ3
    Left, Intravascular
      B54KZZ3
    Right, Intravascular B54JZZ3
  Spanchnic, Intravascular
    B54TZZ3
  Subclavian
    Left, Intravascular B547ZZ3
    Right, Intravascular B546ZZ3

Ultrasonography (continued)
Vein (continued)
  Upper Extremity
    Bilateral, Intravascular
      B54PZZ3
    Left, Intravascular B54NZZ3
    Right, Intravascular
      B54MZZ3
  Vena Cava
    Inferior, Intravascular B549ZZ3
    Superior, Intravascular
      B548ZZ3
  Wrist
    Left, Densitometry BP4MZZ1
    Right, Densitometry BP4LZZ1
Ultrasound bone healing system
  use Bone Growth Stimulator in
    Head and Facial Bones
  use Bone Growth Stimulator in
    Lower Bones
  use Bone Growth Stimulator in
    Upper Bones
Ultrasound Therapy
  Heart 6A75
  No Qualifier 6A75
  Vessels
    Head and Neck 6A75
    Other 6A75
    Peripheral 6A75
Ultraviolet Light Therapy, Skin
  6A80
Umbilical artery
  use Artery, Internal Iliac, Left
  use Artery, Internal Iliac, Right
  use Artery, Lower
Uniplanar external fixator
  use External Fixation Device,
    Monoplanar in 0PH
  use External Fixation Device,
    Monoplanar in 0PS
  use External Fixation Device,
    Monoplanar in 0QH
  use External Fixation Device,
    Monoplanar in 0QS
Upper GI series
  see Fluoroscopy, Gastrointestinal,
    Upper BD15
Ureteral orifice
  use Ureter
  use Ureter, Left
  use Ureter, Right
  use Ureters, Bilateral
Ureterectomy
  see Excision, Urinary System
    0TB
  see Resection, Urinary System
    0TT
Ureterocolostomy
  see Bypass, Urinary System 0T1
Ureterocystostomy
  see Bypass, Urinary System 0T1
Ureteroenterostomy
  see Bypass, Urinary System 0T1
Ureteroileostomy
  see Bypass, Urinary System 0T1
Ureterolithotomy
  see Extirpation, Urinary System
    0TC
Ureterolysis
  see Release, Urinary System 0TN
Ureteroneocystostomy
  see Bypass, Urinary System 0T1
  see Reposition, Urinary System
    0TS
Ureteropelvic junction (UPJ)
  use Kidney Pelvis, Left
  use Kidney Pelvis, Right
Ureteropexy
  see Repair, Urinary System 0TQ
  see Reposition, Urinary System
    0TS

Ureteroplasty
  see Repair, Urinary System 0TQ
  see Replacement, Urinary System
    0TR
  see Supplement, Urinary System
    0TU
Ureteroplication
  see Restriction, Urinary
    System 0TV
Ureteropyelography
  see Fluoroscopy, Urinary System
    BT1
Ureterorrhaphy
  see Repair, Urinary System 0TQ
Ureteroscopy 0TJ98ZZ
Ureterostomy
  see Bypass, Urinary System 0T1
  see Drainage, Urinary
    System 0T9
Ureterotomy
  see Drainage, Urinary
    System 0T9
Ureteroureterostomy
  see Bypass, Urinary System 0T1
Ureterovesical orifice
  use Ureter
  use Ureters, Bilateral
  use Ureter, Left
  use Ureter, Right
Urethral catheterization, indwelling
  0T9B70Z
Urethrectomy
  see Excision, Urethra 0TBD
  see Resection, Urethra 0TTD
Urethrolithotomy
  see Extirpation, Urethra 0TCD
Urethrolysis
  see Release, Urethra 0TND
Urethropexy
  see Repair, Urethra 0TQD
  see Reposition, Urethra 0TSD
Urethroplasty
  see Repair, Urethra 0TQD
  see Replacement, Urethra 0TRD
  see Supplement, Urethra 0TUD
Urethrorrhaphy
  see Repair, Urethra 0TQD
Urethroscopy 0TJD8ZZ
Urethrotomy
  see Drainage, Urethra 0T9D
Uridine Triacetate XW0DX82
**Urinary incontinence stimulator
  lead**
  use Stimulator Lead in Urinary
    System
Urography
  see Fluoroscopy, Urinary System
    BT1
Ustekinumab
  use Other New Technology
    Therapeutic Substance
Uterine Artery
  use Artery, Internal Iliac, Left
  use Artery, Internal Iliac, Right
**Uterine artery embolization
  (UAE)**
  see Occlusion, Lower
    Arteries 04L
Uterine cornu
  use Uterus
Uterine tube
  use Fallopian Tube, Left
  use Fallopian Tube, Right
Uterine vein
  use Vein, Hypogastric, Left
  use Vein, Hypogastric, Right
Uvulectomy
  see Excision, Uvula 0CBN
  see Resection, Uvula 0CTN
Uvulorrhaphy
  see Repair, Uvula 0CQN

Uvulotomy
  see Drainage, Uvula 0C9N

V
V-Wave Interatrial Shunt System
  use Synthetic Substitute
Vabomere™
  use Meropenem-vaboractam Anti-
    infective
Vaccination
  see Introduction of Serum, Toxoid,
    and Vaccine
Vacuum extraction, obstetric
  10D07Z6
Vaginal artery
  use Artery, Internal Iliac, Left
  use Artery, Internal Iliac, Right
Vaginal pessary
  use Intraluminal Device, Pessary
    in Female Reproductive
    System
Vaginal vein
  use Vein, Hypogastric, Left
  use Vein, Hypogastric, Right
Vaginectomy
  see Excision, Vagina 0UBG
  see Resection, Vagina
    0UTG
Vaginofixation
  see Repair, Vagina 0UQG
  see Reposition, Vagina 0USG
Vaginoplasty
  see Repair, Vagina 0UQG
  see Supplement, Vagina 0UUG
Vaginorrhaphy
  see Repair, Vagina 0UQG
Vaginoscopy 0UJH8ZZ
Vaginotomy
  see Drainage, Female Reproductive
    System 0U9
Vagotomy
  see Division, Nerve, Vagus 008Q
Valiant Thoracic Stent Graft
  use Intraluminal Device
Valvotomy, valvulotomy
  see Division, Heart and Great
    Vessels 028
  see Release, Heart and Great Vessels
    02N
Valvuloplasty
  see Repair, Heart and Great Vessels
    02Q
  see Replacement, Heart and Great
    Vessels 02R
  see Supplement, Heart and Great
    Vessels 02U
Valvuloplasty, Alfieri Stitch
  see Restriction, Valve, Mitral 02VG
Vascular Access Device
  Totally Implantable
    Insertion of device in
      Abdomen 0JH8
      Chest 0JH6
      Lower Arm
        Left 0JHH
        Right 0JHG
      Lower Leg
        Left 0JHP
        Right 0JHN
      Upper Arm
        Left 0JHF
        Right 0JHD
      Upper Leg
        Left 0JHM
        Right 0JHL
    Removal of device from
      Lower Extremity 0JPW
      Trunk 0JPT
      Upper Extremity 0JPV
    Revision of device in

Vascular Access Device (continued)
  Totally Implantable (continued)
    Lower Extremity 0JWW
    Trunk 0JWT
    Upper Extremity 0JWV
  Tunneled
    Insertion of device in
      Abdomen 0JH8
      Chest 0JH6
      Lower Arm
        Left 0JHH
        Right 0JHG
      Lower Leg
        Left 0JHP
        Right 0JHN
      Upper Arm
        Left 0JHF
        Right 0JHD
      Upper Leg
        Left 0JHM
        Right 0JHL
    Removal of device from
      Lower Extremity 0JPW
      Trunk 0JPT
      Upper Extremity 0JPV
    Revision of device in
      Lower Extremity 0JWW
      Trunk 0JWT
      Upper Extremity 0JWV

Vasectomy
  see Excision, Male Reproductive
    System 0VB
Vasography
  see Fluoroscopy, Male Reproductive
    System BV1
  see Plain Radiography, Male
    Reproductive System BV0
Vasoligation
  see Occlusion, Male Reproductive
    System 0VL
Vasorrhaphy
  see Repair, Male Reproductive
    System 0VQ
Vasostomy
  see Bypass, Male Reproductive
    System 0V1
Vasotomy
  Drainage
    see Drainage, Male Reproductive
      System 0V9
    see Occlusion, Male
      Reproductive System 0VL
  With ligation
Vasovasostomy
  see Repair, Male Reproductive
    System 0VQ
Vastus intermedius muscle
  use Muscle, Upper Leg, Left
  use Muscle, Upper Leg, Right
Vastus lateralis muscle
  use Muscle, Upper Leg, Left
  use Muscle, Upper Leg, Right
Vastus medialis muscle
  use Muscle, Upper Leg, Left
  use Muscle, Upper Leg, Right
VCG (vectorcardiogram)
  see Measurement, Cardiac
    4A02
Vectra® Vascular Access Graft
  use Vascular Access Device,
    Tunneled in Subcutaneous Tissue
    and Fascia
Veklury use Remdesivir
  Anti-infective
Venclexta®
  use Venetoclax Antineoplastic
Venetoclax Antineoplastic
  XW0DXR5
Venectomy
  see Excision, Lower Veins 06B
  see Excision, Upper Veins 05B

Venography
  see Fluoroscopy, Veins B51
  see Plain Radiography, Veins B50
Venorrhaphy
  see Repair, Lower Veins 06Q
  see Repair, Upper Veins 05Q
Venotripsy
  see Occlusion, Lower Veins 06L
  see Occlusion, Upper Veins 05L
Ventricular fold
  use Larynx
Ventriculoatriostomy
  see Bypass, Central Nervous System
    and Cranial Nerves 001
Ventriculocisternostomy
  see Bypass, Central Nervous System
    and Cranial Nerves 001
Ventriculogram, cardiac
  Combined left and right heart
    see Fluoroscopy, Heart, Right and
      Left B216
  Left ventricle
    see Fluoroscopy, Heart, Left
      B215
  Right ventricle
    see Fluoroscopy, Heart, Right
      B214
Ventriculopuncture, through
  previously implanted
  catheter 8C01X6J
Ventriculoscopy 00J04ZZ
Ventriculostomy
  External drainage
    see Drainage, Cerebral Ventricle
      0096
  Internal shunt
    see Bypass, Cerebral Ventricle
      0016
Ventriculovenostomy
  see Bypass, Cerebral Ventricle
    0016
Ventrio™ Hernia Patch
  use Synthetic Substitute
VEP (visual evoked potential)
  4A07X0Z
Vermiform appendix
  use Appendix
Vermilion border
  use Lip, Lower
  use Lip, Upper
Versa
  use Pacemaker, Dual Chamber
    in 0JH
Version, obstetric
  External 10S0XZZ
  Internal 10S07ZZ
Vertebral arch
  use Vertebra, Cervical
  use Vertebra, Lumbar
  use Vertebra, Thoracic
Vertebral body
  use Cervical Vertebra
  use Thoracic Vertebra
  use Lumbar Vertebra
Vertebral canal
  use Spinal Canal
Vertebral foramen
  use Vertebra, Cervical
  use Vertebra, Lumbar
  use Vertebra, Thoracic
Vertebral lamina
  use Vertebra, Cervical
  use Vertebra, Lumbar
  use Vertebra, Thoracic
Vertebral pedicle
  use Vertebra, Cervical
  use Vertebra, Lumbar
  use Vertebra, Thoracic
Vesical vein
  use Vein, Hypogastric, Left
  use Vein, Hypogastric, Right

Vesicotomy
  see Drainage, Urinary System 0T9
Vesiculectomy
  see Excision, Male Reproductive
    System 0VB
  see Resection, Male Reproductive
    System 0VT
Vesiculogram, seminal
  see Plain Radiography, Male
    Reproductive System BV0
Vesiculotomy
  see Drainage, Male Reproductive
    System 0V9
Vestibular (Scarpa's) ganglion
  use Nerve, Acoustic
Vestibular Assessment F15Z
Vestibular nerve
  use Nerve, Acoustic
Vestibular Treatment F0C
Vestibulocochlear nerve
  use Nerve, Acoustic
VH-IVUS (virtual histology
  intravascular ultrasound)
  see Ultrasonography, Heart B24
Virchow's (supraclavicular) lymph
  node
  use Lymphatic, Neck, Left
  use Lymphatic, Neck, Right
Virtuoso (II) (DR) (VR)
  use Defibrillator Generator
    in 0JH
Vistogard®
  use Uridine Triacetate
Vitrectomy
  see Excision, Eye 08B
  see Resection, Eye 08T
Vitreous body
  use Vitreous, Left
  use Vitreous, Right
Viva (XT)(S)
  use Cardiac Resynchronization
    Defibrillator Pulse Generator in
    0JH
Vocal fold
  use Vocal Cord, Left
  use Vocal Cord, Right
Vocational
  Assessment
  Retraining
    see Activities of Daily Living
      Assessment, Rehabilitation
      F02
    see Activities of Daily Living
      Treatment, Rehabilitation
      F08
Volar (palmar) digital vein
  use Vein, Hand, Left
  use Vein, Hand, Right
Volar (palmar) metacarpal
  vein
  use Vein, Hand, Left
  use Vein, Hand, Right
Vomer bone
  use Septum, Nasal
Vomer of nasal septum
  use Bone, Nasal
Voraxaze
  Glucarpidase
Vulvectomy
  see Excision, Female Reproductive
    System 0UB
  see Resection, Female Reproductive
    System 0UT
VYXEOS™
  use Cytarabine and Daunorubicin
    Liposome Antineoplastic

W

WALLSTENT® Endoprosthesis
  use Intraluminal Device

Washing
  see Irrigation
WavelinQ EndoAVF system
  Radial Artery, Left 031C
  Radial Artery, Right 031B
  Ulnar Artery, Left 031A
  Ulnar Artery, Right 0319
Wedge resection, pulmonary
  see Excision, Respiratory System
    0BB
Whole Blood Nucleic Acid-base
  Microbial Detection XXE5XM5
Window
  see Drainage
Wiring, dental 2W31X9Z

X

X-ray
  see Plain Radiography
X-STOP® Spacer
  use Spinal Stabilization Device,
    Interspinous Process in 0RH
  use Spinal Stabilization Device,
    Interspinous Process in 0SH
Xact Carotid Stent System
  use Intraluminal Device
XENLETA™
  use Lefamulin Anti-infective
Xenograft
  use Zooplastic Tissue in Heart and
    Great Vessels
XIENCE Everolimus Eluting
  Coronary Stent System
  use Intraluminal Device,
    Drug-eluting in Heart and
    Great Vessels
Xiphoid process
  use Sternum
XLIF® System
  use Interbody Fusion Device in
    Lower Joints
XOSPATA®
  use Gilteritinib Antineoplastic

Y

Yescarta®
  use Axicabtagene Ciloleucel
    Immunotherapy
Yoga Therapy 8E0ZXY4

Z

Z-plasty, skin for scar contracture
  see Release, Skin and Breast
    0HN
Zenith AAA Endovascular
  Graft
  use Intraluminal Device
Zenith® Fenestrated AAA
  Endovascular Graft
  use Intraluminal Device, Branched
    or Fenestrated, One or Two
    Arteries in 04V
  use Intraluminal Device, Branched
    or Fenestrated, Three or More
    Arteries in 04V
Zenith Flex® AAA Endovascular
  Graft
  use Intraluminal Device
Zenith TX2® TAA Endovascular
  Graft
  use Intraluminal Device
Zenith® Renu™ AAA Ancillary
  Graft
  use Intraluminal Device
ZEPZELCA™ use Lurbinectedin
ZERBAXA®
  use Ceftolozane/Tazobactam
    Anti-infective

Zilver® PTX® (paclitaxel) Drug-Eluting Peripheral Stent
  use Intraluminal Device, Drug-eluting in Lower Arteries
  use Intraluminal Device, Drug-eluting in Upper Arteries

Zimmer® NexGen® LPS Mobile Bearing Knee
  use Synthetic Substitute

Zimmer® NexGen® LPS-Flex Mobile Knee
  use Synthetic Substitute

ZINPLAVA™
  use Bezlotoxumab Monoclonal AntibodyZonule of Zinn

Zonule of Zinn
  use Lens, Left
  use Lens, Right

Zooplastic Tissue, Rapid Deployment Technique, Replacement X2RF

Zotarolimus-eluting coronary stent
  use Intraluminal Device, Drug-eluting in Heart and Great Vessels

ZULRESSO™
  use Brexanolone

Zygomatic process of frontal bone
  use Bone, Frontal

Zygomatic process of temporal bone
  use Bone, Temporal, Left
  use Bone, Temporal, Right

Zygomaticus muscle
  use Muscle, Facial

Zyvox
  use Oxazolidinones

Within each section of ICD-10-PCS the characters have different meanings. The seven character meanings for the Medical and Surgical section are illustrated here through the procedure example of *Percutaneous needle core biopsy of the right kidney.*

Section	Body System	Root Operation	Body Part	Approach	Device	Qualifier
Med/Surg	Urinary	Excision	Kidney, Right	Percutaneous	None	Diagnostic
0	T	B	0	3	Z	X

Section (Character 1)

All Medical and Surgical procedure codes have a first character value of 0.

Body System (Character 2)

The alphanumeric character for the body system is placed in the second position. The following are the body systems applicable to the Medical and Surgical section.

Character Value	Character Value Description
0	Central Nervous System and Cranial Nerves
1	Peripheral Nervous System
2	Heart and Great Vessels
3	Upper Arteries
4	Lower Arteries
5	Upper Veins
6	Lower Veins
7	Lymphatic and Hemic Systems
8	Eye
9	Ear, Nose, Sinus
B	Respiratory System
C	Mouth and Throat
D	Gastrointestinal System
F	Hepatobiliary System and Pancreas
G	Endocrine System
H	Skin and Breast
J	Subcutaneous Tissue and Fascia
K	Muscles
L	Tendons
M	Bursae and Ligaments
N	Head and Facial Bones
P	Upper Bones
Q	Lower Bones
R	Upper Joints
S	Lower Joints
T	Urinary System
U	Female Reproductive System
V	Male Reproductive System
W	Anatomical Regions, General
X	Anatomical Regions, Upper Extremities
Y	Anatomical Regions, Lower Extremities

Root Operations (Character 3)

The alphanumeric character value for root operations is placed in the third position. Listed below are the root operations applicable to the Medical and Surgical section with their associated meaning.

Character Value	Root Operation	Root Operation Definition
0	Alteration	Modifying the anatomic structure of a body part without affecting the function of the body part
1	Bypass	Altering the route of passage of the contents of a tubular body part
2	Change	Taking out or off a device from a body part and putting back an identical or similar device in or on the same body part without cutting or puncturing the skin or a mucous membrane
3	Control	Stopping, or attempting to stop, postprocedural or other acute bleeding
4	Creation	Making a new genital structure that does not take over the function of a body part
5	Destruction	Physical eradication of all or a portion of a body part by the direct use of energy, force, or a destructive agent
6	Detachment	Cutting off all or a portion of the upper or lower extremities
7	Dilation	Expanding an orifice or the lumen of a tubular body part
8	Division	Cutting into a body part, without draining fluids and/or gases from the body part, in order to separate or transect a body part
9	Drainage	Taking or letting out fluids and/or gases from a body part
B	Excision	Cutting out or off, without replacement, a portion of a body part
C	Extirpation	Taking or cutting out solid matter from a body part
D	Extraction	Pulling or stripping out or off all or a portion of a body part by the use of force
F	Fragmentation	Breaking solid matter in a body part into pieces
G	Fusion	Joining together portions of an articular body part rendering the articular body part immobile
H	Insertion	Putting in a nonbiological appliance that monitors, assists, performs, or prevents a physiological function but does not physically take the place of a body part
J	Inspection	Visually and/or manually exploring a body part
K	Map	Locating the route of passage of electrical impulses and/or locating functional areas in a body part
L	Occlusion	Completely closing an orifice or the lumen of a tubular body part
M	Reattachment	Putting back in or on all or a portion of a separated body part to its normal location or other suitable location
N	Release	Freeing a body part from an abnormal physical constraint by cutting or by the use of force
P	Removal	Taking out or off a device from a body part
Q	Repair	Restoring, to the extent possible, a body part to its normal anatomic structure and function
R	Replacement	Putting in or on biological or synthetic material that physically takes the place and/or function of all or a portion of a body part
S	Reposition	Moving to its normal location, or other suitable location, all or a portion of a body part
T	Resection	Cutting out or off, without replacement, all of a body part
V	Restriction	Partially closing an orifice or the lumen of a tubular body part
W	Revision	Correcting, to the extent possible, a portion of a malfunctioning device or the position of a displaced device
U	Supplement	Putting in or on biological or synthetic material that physically reinforces and/or augments the function of a portion of a body part
X	Transfer	Moving, without taking out, all or a portion of a body part to another location to take over the function of all or a portion of a body part
Y	Transplantation	Putting in or on all or a portion of a living body part taken from another individual or animal to physically take the place and/or function of all or a portion of a similar body part

Body Part (Character 4)

For each body system the applicable body part character values will be available for procedure code construction. An example of a body part for this section is the Large Intestines.

Approach (Character 5)

The approach is the technique used to reach the procedure site. The following are the approach character values for the Medical and Surgical section with the associated definitions.

Character Value	Approach	Approach Definition
0	Open	Cutting through the skin or mucous membrane and any other body layers necessary to expose the site of the procedure
3	Percutaneous	Entry, by puncture or minor incision, of instrumentation through the skin or mucous membrane and any other body layers necessary to reach the site of the procedure
4	Percutaneous Endoscopic	Entry, by puncture or minor incision, of instrumentation through the skin or mucous membrane and any other body layers necessary to reach and visualize the site of the procedure
7	Via Natural or Artificial Opening	Entry of instrumentation through a natural or artificial external opening to reach the site of the procedure
8	Via Natural or Artificial Opening Endoscopic	Entry of instrumentation through a natural or artificial external opening to reach and visualize the site of the procedure
F	Via Natural or Artificial Opening Percutaneous Endoscopic	Entry of instrumentation through a natural or artificial external opening to reach and visualize the site of the procedure, and entry, by puncture or minor incision, of instrumentation through the skin or mucous membrane and any other body layers necessary to aid in the performance of the procedure
X	External	Procedures performed directly on the skin or mucous membrane and procedures performed indirectly by the application of external force through the skin or mucous membrane

Device (Character 6)

Depending on the procedure performed there may or may not be a device used. There are several types of devices included in the Medical and Surgical section that fall into one of the four following categories.

- Electronic Appliances
- Grafts and Prostheses
- Implants
- Simple or Mechanical Appliances

When a device is not utilized during the procedure, the character value of Z should be reported.

If a coder is unsure of which option to select for the device utilized during the procedure, Appendix E can be used to guide the selection. For example, if the coder is in Table 02R (replacement of heart and great vessels) the coder can locate the device categories in Appendix E (Autologous Tissue Substitute, Zooplastic Tissue, Synthetic Substitute, and Nonautologous Tissue Substitue). For each of these categories brand name devices and other devices are listed. The coder should select the category in which the device utilized during the procedure is listed.

Qualifier (Character 7)

The qualifier represents an additional attribute for the procedure when applicable. In the preceding example of *Percutaneous needle core biopsy of the right kidney*, the qualifier of X was used to report that the biopsy procedure was diagnostic in nature. If there is no qualifier for a procedure, the Z character value should be reported.

Important Definitions for the Medical and Surgical Section

Medical Surgical Root Operation	Qualifier	Definition
Detachment of Upper and Lower Extremities (0X6 and 0Y6) Arms and Legs	1 – High	Amputation at the proximal portion of the shaft of the humerus or femur
	2 – Mid	Amputation at the middle portion of the shaft of the humerus or femur
	3 – Low	Amputation at the distal portion of the shaft of the humerus or femur
Detachment of Upper and Lower Extremities (0X6 and 0Y6) Fingers, Thumbs, and Toes	0 – Complete	Amputation at the metacarpophalangeal/metatarsal-phalangeal joint
	1 – High	Amputation anywhere along the proximal phalanx
	2 – Mid	Amputation through the proximal interphalangeal joint or anywhere along the middle phalanx
	3 – Low	Amputation through the distal interphalangeal joint or anywhere along the distal phalanx
Transplantation	0 – Allogeneic	Being genetically different although belonging to or obtained from the same species*
	1 – Syngeneic	Genetically identical or closely related, so as to allow tissue transplant; immunologically compatible*
	2 – Zooplastic	Surgical transfer of tissue from an animal to a human*

*Taken from The Free Dictionary by Farlex at www.thefreedictionary.com

Official Coding Guidelines for the Medical and Surgical Section

Medical and Surgical Section Guidelines (section 0)

B2. Body System

General guidelines

B2.1a The procedure codes in Anatomical Regions, General, Anatomical Regions, Upper Extremities and Anatomical Regions, Lower Extremities can be used when the procedure is performed on an anatomical region rather than a specific body part, or on the rare occasion when no information is available to support assignment of a code to a specific body part.

Examples: Chest tube drainage of the pleural cavity is coded to the root operation Drainage found in the body system Anatomical Regions, General. Suture repair of the abdominal wall is coded to the root operation Repair in the body system Anatomical Regions, General. Amputation of the foot is coded to the root operation Detachment in the body system Anatomical Regions, Lower Extremities.

B2.1b Where the general body part values "upper" and "lower" are provided as an option in the Upper Arteries, Lower Arteries, Upper Veins, Lower Veins, Muscles and Tendons body systems, "upper" or "lower" specifies body parts located above or below the diaphragm respectively.

Example: Vein body parts above the diaphragm are found in the Upper Veins body system; vein body parts below the diaphragm are found in the Lower Veins body system.

B3. Root Operation

General guidelines

B3.1a In order to determine the appropriate root operation, the full definition of the root operation as contained in the PCS Tables must be applied.

B3.1b Components of a procedure specified in the root operation definition or explanation as integral to that root operation are not coded separately. Procedural steps necessary to reach the operative site and close the operative site, including anastomosis of a tubular body part, are also not coded separately.

Examples: Resection of a joint as part of a joint replacement procedure is included in the root operation definition of Replacement and is not coded separately. Laparotomy performed to reach the site of an open liver biopsy is not coded separately. In a resection of sigmoid colon with anastomosis of descending colon to rectum, the anastomosis is not coded separately.

Multiple procedures

B3.2 During the same operative episode, multiple procedures are coded if:

a. The same root operation is performed on different body parts as defined by distinct values of the body part character.

   Examples: Diagnostic excision of liver and pancreas are coded separately. Excision of lesion in the ascending colon and excision of lesion in the transverse colon are coded separately.

b. The same root operation is repeated at different body sites that are included in the same body part value.

   Examples: Excision of the sartorius muscle and excision of the gracilis muscle are both included in the upper leg muscle body part value, and multiple procedures are coded. Extraction of multiple toenails are coded separately.

c. Multiple root operations with distinct objectives are performed on the same body part.

   Example: Destruction of sigmoid lesion and bypass of sigmoid colon are coded separately.

d. The intended root operation is attempted using one approach but is converted to a different approach.

   Example: Laparoscopic cholecystectomy converted to an open cholecystectomy is coded as percutaneous endoscopic Inspection and open Resection.

Discontinued or incomplete procedures

B3.3 If the intended procedure is discontinued or otherwise not complete, code the procedure to the root operation performed. If a procedure is discontinued before any other root operation is performed, code the root operation Inspection of the body part or anatomical region inspected.

Example: A planned aortic valve replacement procedure is discontinued after the initial thoracotomy and before any incision is made in the heart muscle, when the patient becomes hemodynamically unstable. This procedure is coded as an open Inspection of the mediastinum.

Biopsy procedures

B3.4a Biopsy procedures are coded using the root operations Excision, Extraction, or Drainage and the qualifier Diagnostic.

Examples: Fine needle aspiration biopsy of lung is coded to the root operation Drainage with the qualifier Diagnostic. Biopsy of bone marrow is coded to the root operation Extraction with the qualifier Diagnostic. Lymph node sampling for biopsy is coded to the root operation Excision with the qualifier Diagnostic.

Biopsy followed by more definitive treatment

B3.4b If a diagnostic Excision, Extraction, or Drainage procedure (biopsy) is followed by a more definitive procedure, such as Destruction, Excision or Resection at the same procedure site, both the biopsy and the more definitive treatment are coded.

Example: Biopsy of breast followed by partial mastectomy at the same procedure site, both the biopsy and the partial mastectomy procedure are coded.

Overlapping body layers

B3.5 If root operations Excision, Extraction, Repair or Inspection are performed on overlapping layers of the musculoskeletal system, the body part specifying the deepest layer is coded.

Example: Excisional debridement that includes skin and subcutaneous tissue and muscle is coded to the muscle body part.

Bypass procedures

B3.6a Bypass procedures are coded by identifying the body part bypassed "from" and the body part bypassed "to." The fourth character body part specifies the body part bypassed from, and the qualifier specifies the body part bypassed to.

Example: Bypass from stomach to jejunum, stomach is the body part and jejunum is the qualifier.

B3.6b Coronary artery bypass procedures are coded differently than other bypass procedures as described in the previous guideline. Rather than identifying the body part bypassed from, the body part identifies the number of coronary artery sites bypassed to, and the qualifier specifies the vessel bypassed from.

Example: Aortocoronary artery bypass of the left anterior descending coronary artery and the obtuse marginal coronary artery is classified in the body part axis of classification as two coronary arteries and the qualifier specifies the aorta as the body part bypassed from.

B3.6c If multiple coronary arteries are bypassed, a separate procedure is coded for each coronary artery that uses a different device and/or qualifier.

Example: Aortocoronary artery bypass and internal mammary coronary artery bypass are coded separately.

Control vs. more definitive root operations

B3.7 The root operation Control is defined as, "Stopping, or attempting to stop, postprocedural or other acute bleeding." Control is the root operation coded when the procedure performed to achieve hemostasis, beyond what would be considered integral to a procedure, utilizes techniques (e.g. cautery, application of substances or pressure, suturing or ligation or clipping of bleeding points at the site) that are not described by a more specific root operation definition, such as Bypass, Detachment, Excision, Extraction, Reposition, Replacement, or Resection. If a more specific root operation definition applies to the procedure performed, then the more specific root operation is coded instead of Control.

Examples: Silver nitrate cautery to treat acute nasal bleeding is coded to the root operation Control. Liquid embolization of the right internal iliac artery to treat acute hematoma by stopping blood flow is coded to the root operation Occlusion. Suctioning of residual blood to achieve hemostasis during a transbronchial cryobiopsy is considered integral to the cryobiopsy procedure and is not coded separately.

Excision vs. Resection

B3.8 PCS contains specific body parts for anatomical subdivisions of a body part, such as lobes of the lungs or liver and regions of the intestine. Resection of the specific body part is coded whenever all of the body part is cut out or off, rather than coding Excision of a less specific body part.

Example: Left upper lung lobectomy is coded to Resection of Upper Lung Lobe, Left rather than Excision of Lung, Left.

Excision for graft

B3.9 If an autograft is obtained from a different procedure site in order to complete the objective of the procedure, a separate procedure is coded, except when the seventh character qualifier value in the ICD-10-PCS table fully specifies the site from which the autograft was obtained.

Examples: Coronary bypass with excision of saphenous vein graft, excision of saphenous vein is coded separately. Replacement of breast with autologous deep inferior epigastric artery perforator (DIEP) flap, excision of the DIEP flap is not coded separately. The seventh character qualifier value Deep Inferior Epigastric Artery Perforator Flap in the Replacement table fully specifies the site of the autograft harvest.

Fusion procedures of the spine

B3.10a The body part coded for a spinal vertebral joint(s) rendered immobile by a spinal fusion procedure is classified by the level of the spine (e.g. thoracic). There are distinct body part values for a single vertebral joint and for multiple vertebral joints at each spinal level.

Example: Body part values specify Lumbar Vertebral Joint, Lumbar Vertebral Joints, 2 or More and Lumbosacral Vertebral Joint.

B3.10b If multiple vertebral joints are fused, a separate procedure is coded for each vertebral joint that uses a different device and/or qualifier.

Example: Fusion of lumbar vertebral joint, posterior approach, anterior column and fusion of lumbar vertebral joint, posterior approach, posterior column are coded separately.

B3.10c Combinations of devices and materials are often used on a vertebral joint to render the joint immobile. When combinations of devices are used on the same vertebral joint, the device value coded for the procedure is as follows:

- If an interbody fusion device is used to render the joint immobile (containing bone graft or bone graft substitute), the procedure is coded with the device value Interbody Fusion Device
- If bone graft is the only device used to render the joint immobile, the procedure is coded with the device value Nonautologous Tissue Substitute or Autologous Tissue Substitute
- If a mixture of autologous and nonautologous bone graft (with or without biological or synthetic extenders or binders) is used to render the joint immobile, code the procedure with the device value Autologous Tissue Substitute

Examples: Fusion of a vertebral joint using a cage style interbody fusion device containing morsellized bone graft is coded to the device Interbody Fusion Device. Fusion of a vertebral joint using a bone dowel interbody fusion device made of cadaver bone and packed with a mixture of local morsellized bone and demineralized bone matrix is coded to the device Interbody Fusion Device. Fusion of a vertebral joint using both autologous bone graft and bone bank bone graft is coded to the device Autologous Tissue Substitute.

Inspection procedures

B3.11a Inspection of a body part(s) performed in order to achieve the objective of a procedure is not coded separately.

Example: Fiberoptic bronchoscopy performed for irrigation of bronchus, only the irrigation procedure is coded.

B3.11b If multiple tubular body parts are inspected, the most distal body part inspected is coded. If multiple non-tubular body parts in a region are inspected, the body part that specifies the entire area inspected is coded.

Examples: Cystoureteroscopy with inspection of bladder and ureters is coded to the ureter body part value. Exploratory laparotomy with general inspection of abdominal contents is coded to the peritoneal cavity body part value.

B3.11c When both an Inspection procedure and another procedure are performed on the same body part during the same episode, if the Inspection procedure is performed using a different approach than the other procedure, the Inspection procedure is coded separately.

Example: Endoscopic Inspection of the duodenum is coded separately when open Excision of the duodenum is performed during the same procedural episode.

Occlusion vs. Restriction for vessel embolization procedures

B3.12 If the objective of an embolization procedure is to completely close a vessel, the root operation Occlusion is coded. If the objective of an embolization procedure is to narrow the lumen of a vessel, the root operation Restriction is coded.

Examples: Tumor embolization is coded to the root operation Occlusion, because the objective of the procedure is to cut off the blood supply to the vessel. Embolization of a cerebral aneurysm is coded to the root operation Restriction, because the objective of the procedure is not to close off the vessel entirely, but to narrow the lumen of the vessel at the site of the aneurysm where it is abnormally wide.

Release procedures

B3.13 In the root operation Release, the body part value coded is the body part being freed and not the tissue being manipulated or cut to free the body part.

Example: Lysis of intestinal adhesions is coded to the specific intestine body part value.

Release vs. Division

B3.14 If the sole objective of the procedure is freeing a body part without cutting the body part, the root operation is Release. If the sole objective of the procedure is separating or transecting a body part, the root operation is Division.

Example: Freeing a nerve root from surrounding scar tissue to relieve pain is coded to the root operation Release. Severing a nerve root to relieve pain is coded to the root operation Division.

Reposition for fracture treatment

B3.15 Reduction of a displaced fracture is coded to the root operation Reposition and the application of a cast or splint in conjunction with the Reposition procedure is not coded separately. Treatment of a nondisplaced fracture is coded to the procedure performed.

Examples: Putting a pin in a nondisplaced fracture is coded to the root operation Insertion. Casting of a nondisplaced fracture is coded to the root operation Immobilization in the Placement section.

Transplantation vs. Administration

B3.16 Putting in a mature and functioning living body part taken from another individual or animal is coded to the root operation Transplantation. Putting in autologous or nonautologous cells is coded to the Administration section.

Example: Putting in autologous or nonautologous bone marrow, pancreatic islet cells or stem cells is coded to the Administration section.

Transfer procedures using multiple tissue layers

B3.17 The root operation Transfer contains qualifiers that can be used to specify when a transfer flap is composed of more than one tissue layer, such as a musculocutaneous flap. For procedures involving transfer of multiple tissue layers including skin, subcutaneous tissue, fascia or muscle, the procedure is coded to the body part value that describes the deepest tissue layer in the flap, and the qualifier can be used to describe the other tissue layer(s) in the transfer flap.

Example: A musculocutaneous flap transfer is coded to the appropriate body part value in the body system Muscles, and the qualifier is used to describe the additional tissue layer(s) in the transfer flap.

Excision/Resection followed by replacement

B3.18 If an Excision or Resection of a body part is followed by a Replacement procedure, code both procedures to identify each distinct objective, except when the Excision or Resection is considered integral and preparatory for the Replacement procedure.

Examples: Mastectomy followed by reconstruction, both Resection and Replacement of the breast are coded to fully capture the distinct objectives of the procedures performed. Maxillectomy with obturator reconstruction, both Excision and Replacement of the maxilla are coded to fully capture the distinct objectives of the procedures performed. Excisional debridement of tendon with skin graft, both the Excision of the tendon and the Replacement of the skin with a graft are coded to fully capture the distinct objectives of the procedures performed. Esophagectomy followed by reconstruction with colonic interposition, both the Resection and the Transfer of the large intestine to function as the esophagus are coded to fully capture the distinct objectives of the procedures performed.

Examples: Resection of a joint as part of a joint replacement procedure is considered integral and preparatory for the Replacement of the joint and the Resection is not coded separately. Resection of a valve as part of a valve replacement procedure is considered integral and preparatory for the valve Replacement and the Resection is not coded separately.

B4. Body Part

General guidelines

B4.1a If a procedure is performed on a portion of a body part that does not have a separate body part value, code the body part value corresponding to the whole body part.

Example: A procedure performed on the alveolar process of the mandible is coded to the mandible body part.

B4.1b If the prefix "peri" is combined with a body part to identify the site of the procedure, and the site of the procedure is not further specified, then the procedure is coded to the body part named. This guideline applies only when a more specific body part value is not available.

Examples: A procedure site identified as perirenal is coded to the kidney body part when the site of the procedure is not further specified.

A procedure site described in the documentation as peri-urethral tissue, and the documentation also indicates that it is the vulvar tissue and not the urethral tissue that is the site of the procedure, then the procedure is coded to the vulva body part. A procedure site documented as involving the periosteum is coded to the corresponding bone body part.

B4.1c If a procedure is performed on a continuous section of a tubular body part, code the body part value corresponding to the anatomically most proximal (closest to the heart) portion of the tubular body part.

Examples: A procedure performed on a continuous section of artery from the femoral artery to the external iliac artery with the point of entry at the femoral artery is coded to the external iliac body part. A procedure performed on a continuous section of artery from the femoral artery to the external iliac artery with the point of entry at the external iliac artery is also coded to the external iliac artery body part.

Branches of body parts

B4.2 Where a specific branch of a body part does not have its own body part value in PCS, the body part is typically coded to the closest proximal branch that has a specific body part value. In the cardiovascular body systems, if a general body part is available in the correct root operation table, and coding to a proximal branch would require assigning a code in a different body system, the procedure is coded using the general body part value.

Examples: A procedure performed on the mandibular branch of the trigeminal nerve is coded to the trigeminal nerve body part value. Occlusion of the bronchial artery is coded to the body part value Upper Artery in the body system Upper Arteries, and not to the body part value Thoracic Aorta, Descending in the body system Heart and Great Vessels.

Bilateral body part values

B4.3 Bilateral body part values are available for a limited number of body parts. If the identical procedure is performed on contralateral body parts, and a bilateral body part value exists for that body part, a single procedure is coded using the bilateral body part value. If no bilateral body part value exists, each procedure is coded separately using the appropriate body part value.

Examples: The identical procedure performed on both fallopian tubes is coded once using the body part value Fallopian Tube, Bilateral. The identical procedure performed on both knee joints is coded twice using the body part values Knee Joint, Right and Knee Joint, Left.

Coronary arteries

B4.4 The coronary arteries are classified as a single body part that is further specified by number of arteries treated. One procedure code specifying multiple arteries is used when the same procedure is performed, including the same device and qualifier values.

Examples: Angioplasty of two distinct coronary arteries with placement of two stents is coded as Dilation of Coronary Artery, Two Arteries, with Two Intraluminal Devices. Angioplasty of two distinct coronary arteries, one with stent placed and one without, is coded separately as Dilation of Coronary Artery, One Artery with Intraluminal Device, and Dilation of Coronary Artery, One Artery with no device.

Tendons, ligaments, bursae and fascia near a joint

B4.5 Procedures performed on tendons, ligaments, bursae and fascia supporting a joint are coded to the body part in the respective body system that is the focus of the procedure. Procedures performed on joint structures themselves are coded to the body part in the joint body systems.

Examples: Repair of the anterior cruciate ligament of the knee is coded to the knee bursae and ligament body part in the Bursae and Ligaments body system. Knee arthroscopy with shaving of articular cartilage is coded to the knee joint body part in the Lower Joints body system.

Skin, subcutaneous tissue and fascia overlying a joint

B4.6 If a procedure is performed on the skin, subcutaneous tissue or fascia overlying a joint, the procedure is coded to the following body part:

- Shoulder is coded to Upper Arm
- Elbow is coded to Lower Arm
- Wrist is coded to Lower Arm
- Hip is coded to Upper Leg
- Knee is coded to Lower Leg
- Ankle is coded to Foot

Fingers and toes

B4.7 If a body system does not contain a separate body part value for fingers, procedures performed on the fingers are coded to the body part value for the hand. If a body system does not contain a separate body part value for toes, procedures performed on the toes are coded to the body part value for the foot.

Example: Excision of finger muscle is coded to one of the hand muscle body part values in the Muscles body system.

Upper and lower intestinal tract

B4.8 In the Gastrointestinal body system, the general body part values Upper Intestinal Tract and Lower Intestinal Tract are provided as an option for the root operations such as Change, Insertion, Inspection, Removal and Revision. Upper Intestinal Tract includes the portion of the gastrointestinal tract from the esophagus down to and including the duodenum, and Lower Intestinal Tract includes the portion of the gastrointestinal tract from the jejunum down to and including the rectum and anus.

Example: In the root operation Change table, change of a device in the jejunum is coded using the body part Lower Intestinal Tract.

B5. Approach

Open approach with percutaneous endoscopic assistance

B5.2a Procedures performed using the open approach with percutaneous endoscopic assistance are coded to the approach Open.

Example: Laparoscopic-assisted sigmoidectomy is coded to the approach Open.

Percutaneous endoscopic approach with extension of incision

B5.2b Procedures performed using the percutaneous endoscopic approach, with incision or extension of an incision to assist in the removal of all or a portion of a body part or to anastomose a tubular body part to complete the procedure, are coded to the approach value Percutaneous Endoscopic.

Examples: Laparoscopic sigmoid colectomy with extension of stapling port for removal of specimen and direct anastomosis is coded to the approach value Percutaneous Endoscopic. Laparoscopic nephrectomy with midline incision for removing the resected kidney is coded to the approach value Percutaneous Endoscopic. Robotic-assisted laparoscopic prostatectomy with extension of incision for removal of the resected prostate is coded to the approach value Percutaneous Endoscopic.

External approach

B5.3a Procedures performed within an orifice on structures that are visible without the aid of any instrumentation are coded to the approach External.

Example: Resection of tonsils is coded to the approach External.

B5.3b Procedures performed indirectly by the application of external force through the intervening body layers are coded to the approach External.

Example: Closed reduction of fracture is coded to the approach External.

Percutaneous procedure via device

B5.4 Procedures performed percutaneously via a device placed for the procedure are coded to the approach Percutaneous.

Example: Fragmentation of kidney stone performed via percutaneous nephrostomy is coded to the approach Percutaneous.

B6. Device

General guidelines

B6.1a A device is coded only if a device remains after the procedure is completed. If no device remains, the device value No Device is coded. In limited root operations, the classification provides the qualifier values Temporary and Intraoperative, for specific procedures involving clinically significant devices, where the purpose of the device is to be utilized for a brief duration during the procedure or current inpatient stay. If a device that is intended to remain after the procedure is completed requires removal before the end of the operative episode in which it was inserted (for example, the device size is inadequate or a complication occurs), both the insertion and removal of the device should be coded.

B6.1b Materials such as sutures, ligatures, radiological markers and temporary post-operative wound drains are considered integral to the performance of a procedure and are not coded as devices.

B6.1c Procedures performed on a device only and not on a body part are specified in the root operations Change, Irrigation, Removal and Revision, and are coded to the procedure performed.

Example: Irrigation of percutaneous nephrostomy tube is coded to the root operation Irrigation of indwelling device in the Administration section.

Drainage device

B6.2 A separate procedure to put in a drainage device is coded to the root operation Drainage with the device value Drainage Device.

Medial Views of Cerebrum

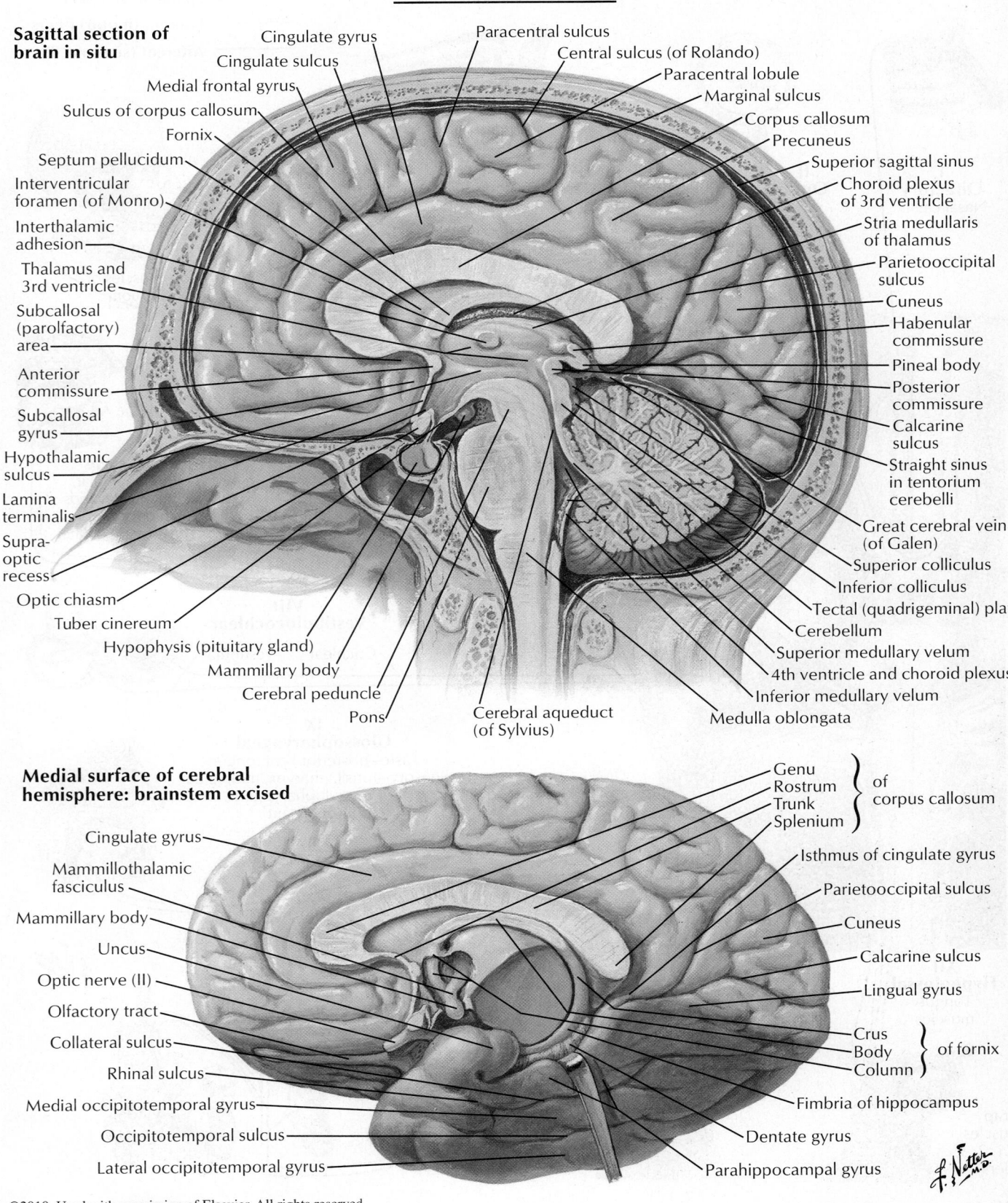

Sagittal section of brain in situ

Cingulate gyrus
Cingulate sulcus
Medial frontal gyrus
Sulcus of corpus callosum
Fornix
Septum pellucidum
Interventricular foramen (of Monro)
Interthalamic adhesion
Thalamus and 3rd ventricle
Subcallosal (parolfactory) area
Anterior commissure
Subcallosal gyrus
Hypothalamic sulcus
Lamina terminalis
Supra-optic recess
Optic chiasm
Tuber cinereum
Hypophysis (pituitary gland)
Mammillary body
Cerebral peduncle
Pons
Cerebral aqueduct (of Sylvius)

Paracentral sulcus
Central sulcus (of Rolando)
Paracentral lobule
Marginal sulcus
Corpus callosum
Precuneus
Superior sagittal sinus
Choroid plexus of 3rd ventricle
Stria medullaris of thalamus
Parietooccipital sulcus
Cuneus
Habenular commissure
Pineal body
Posterior commissure
Calcarine sulcus
Straight sinus in tentorium cerebelli
Great cerebral vein (of Galen)
Superior colliculus
Inferior colliculus
Tectal (quadrigeminal) plate
Cerebellum
Superior medullary velum
4th ventricle and choroid plexus
Inferior medullary velum
Medulla oblongata

Medial surface of cerebral hemisphere: brainstem excised

Cingulate gyrus
Mammillothalamic fasciculus
Mammillary body
Uncus
Optic nerve (II)
Olfactory tract
Collateral sulcus
Rhinal sulcus
Medial occipitotemporal gyrus
Occipitotemporal sulcus
Lateral occipitotemporal gyrus

Genu
Rostrum
Trunk
Splenium
} of corpus callosum

Isthmus of cingulate gyrus
Parietooccipital sulcus
Cuneus
Calcarine sulcus
Lingual gyrus
Crus
Body
Column
} of fornix
Fimbria of hippocampus
Dentate gyrus
Parahippocampal gyrus

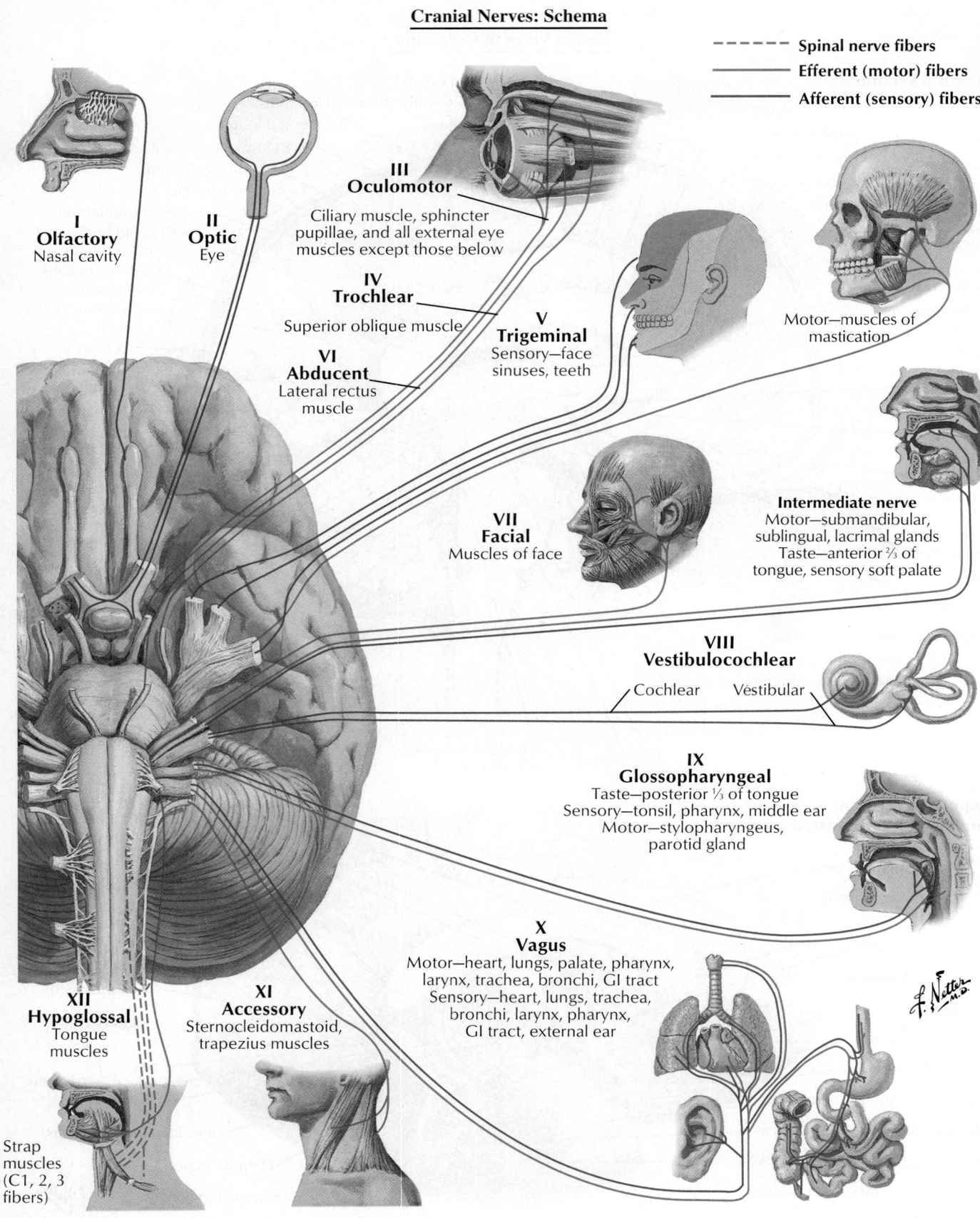

Cranial Nerves: Schema

- - - - - Spinal nerve fibers
——— Efferent (motor) fibers
——— Afferent (sensory) fibers

I Olfactory
Nasal cavity

II Optic
Eye

III Oculomotor
Ciliary muscle, sphincter pupillae, and all external eye muscles except those below

IV Trochlear
Superior oblique muscle

V Trigeminal
Sensory—face sinuses, teeth

VI Abducent
Lateral rectus muscle

Motor—muscles of mastication

VII Facial
Muscles of face

Intermediate nerve
Motor—submandibular, sublingual, lacrimal glands
Taste—anterior ⅔ of tongue, sensory soft palate

VIII Vestibulocochlear
Cochlear   Vestibular

IX Glossopharyngeal
Taste—posterior ⅓ of tongue
Sensory—tonsil, pharynx, middle ear
Motor—stylopharyngeus, parotid gland

X Vagus
Motor—heart, lungs, palate, pharynx, larynx, trachea, bronchi, GI tract
Sensory—heart, lungs, trachea, bronchi, larynx, pharynx, GI tract, external ear

XII Hypoglossal
Tongue muscles

XI Accessory
Sternocleidomastoid, trapezius muscles

Strap muscles (C1, 2, 3 fibers)

F. Netter M.D.

Section 0 **Medical and Surgical**
Body System 0 **Central Nervous System and Cranial Nerves**
Operation 1 **Bypass:** Altering the route of passage of the contents of a tubular body part

Body Part (4th)	Approach (5th)	Device (6th)	Qualifier (7th)
6 Cerebral Ventricle	0 Open 3 Percutaneous 4 Percutaneous Endoscopic	7 Autologous Tissue Substitute J Synthetic Substitute K Nonautologous Tissue Substitute	0 Nasopharynx 1 Mastoid Sinus 2 Atrium 3 Blood Vessel 4 Pleural Cavity 5 Intestine 6 Peritoneal Cavity 7 Urinary Tract 8 Bone Marrow A Subgaleal Space B Cerebral Cisterns
6 Cerebral Ventricle	0 Open 3 Percutaneous 4 Percutaneous Endoscopic	Z No Device	B Cerebral Cisterns
U Spinal Canal	0 Open 3 Percutaneous 4 Percutaneous Endoscopic	7 Autologous Tissue Substitute J Synthetic Substitute K Nonautologous Tissue Substitute	2 Atrium 4 Pleural Cavity 6 Peritoneal Cavity 7 Urinary Tract 9 Fallopian Tube

Section 0 **Medical and Surgical**
Body System 0 **Central Nervous System and Cranial Nerves**
Operation 2 **Change:** Taking out or off a device from a body part and putting back an identical or similar device in or on the same body part without cutting or puncturing the skin or a mucous membrane

Body Part (4th)	Approach (5th)	Device (6th)	Qualifier (7th)
0 Brain E Cranial Nerve U Spinal Canal	X External	0 Drainage Device Y Other Device	Z No Qualifier

Section	0	Medical and Surgical
Body System	0	Central Nervous System and Cranial Nerves
Operation	5	Destruction: Physical eradication of all or a portion of a body part by the direct use of energy, force, or a destructive agent

Body Part (4th)	Approach (5th)	Device (6th)	Qualifier (7th)
0 Brain 1 Cerebral Meninges 2 Dura Mater 6 Cerebral Ventricle 7 Cerebral Hemisphere 8 Basal Ganglia 9 Thalamus A Hypothalamus B Pons C Cerebellum D Medulla Oblongata F Olfactory Nerve G Optic Nerve H Oculomotor Nerve J Trochlear Nerve K Trigeminal Nerve L Abducens Nerve M Facial Nerve N Acoustic Nerve P Glossopharyngeal Nerve Q Vagus Nerve R Accessory Nerve S Hypoglossal Nerve T Spinal Meninges W Cervical Spinal Cord X Thoracic Spinal Cord Y Lumbar Spinal Cord	0 Open 3 Percutaneous 4 Percutaneous Endoscopic	Z No Device	Z No Qualifier

Section	0	Medical and Surgical
Body System	0	Central Nervous System and Cranial Nerves
Operation	7	Dilation: Expanding an orifice or the lumen of a tubular body part

Body Part (4th)	Approach (5th)	Device (6th)	Qualifier (7th)
6 Cerebral Ventricle	0 Open 3 Percutaneous 4 Percutaneous Endoscopic	Z No Device	Z No Qualifie

Section   0   **Medical and Surgical**
Body System   0   **Central Nervous System and Cranial Nerves**
Operation   8   **Division:** Cutting into a body part, without draining fluids and/or gases from the body part, in order to separate or transect a body part

Body Part (4ᵗʰ)	Approach (5ᵗʰ)	Device (6ᵗʰ)	Qualifier (7ᵗʰ)
0 Brain	0 Open	Z No Device	Z No Qualifier
7 Cerebral Hemisphere	3 Percutaneous		
8 Basal Ganglia	4 Percutaneous Endoscopic		
F Olfactory Nerve			
G Optic Nerve			
H Oculomotor Nerve			
J Trochlear Nerve			
K Trigeminal Nerve			
L Abducens Nerve			
M Facial Nerve			
N Acoustic Nerve			
P Glossopharyngeal Nerve			
Q Vagus Nerve			
R Accessory Nerve			
S Hypoglossal Nerve			
W Cervical Spinal Cord			
X Thoracic Spinal Cord			
Y Lumbar Spinal Cord			

Section 0 **Medical and Surgical**
Body System 0 **Central Nervous System and Cranial Nerves**
Operation 9 **Drainage:** Taking or letting out fluids and/or gases from a body part

Body Part (4th)	Approach (5th)	Device (6th)	Qualifier (7th)
0 Brain 1 Cerebral Meninges 2 Dura Mater 3 Epidural Space, Intracranial 4 Subdural Space, Intracranial 5 Subarachnoid Space, Intracranial 6 Cerebral Ventricle 7 Cerebral Hemisphere 8 Basal Ganglia 9 Thalamus A Hypothalamus B Pons C Cerebellum D Medulla Oblongata F Olfactory Nerve G Optic Nerve H Oculomotor Nerve J Trochlear Nerve K Trigeminal Nerve L Abducens Nerve M Facial Nerve N Acoustic Nerve P Glossopharyngeal Nerve Q Vagus Nerve R Accessory Nerve S Hypoglossal Nerve T Spinal Meninges U Spinal Canal W Cervical Spinal Cord X Thoracic Spinal Cord Y Lumbar Spinal Cord	0 Open 3 Percutaneous 4 Percutaneous Endoscopic	0 Drainage Device	Z No Qualifier
0 Brain 1 Cerebral Meninges 2 Dura Mater 3 Epidural Space, Intracranial 4 Subdural Space, Intracranial 5 Subarachnoid Space, Intracranial 6 Cerebral Ventricle 7 Cerebral Hemisphere 8 Basal Ganglia 9 Thalamus A Hypothalamus B Pons C Cerebellum D Medulla Oblongata F Olfactory Nerve G Optic Nerve H Oculomotor Nerve J Trochlear Nerve K Trigeminal Nerve L Abducens Nerve M Facial Nerve N Acoustic Nerve P Glossopharyngeal Nerve Q Vagus Nerve R Accessory Nerve S Hypoglossal Nerve T Spinal Meninges U Spinal Canal W Cervical Spinal Cord X Thoracic Spinal Cord Y Lumbar Spinal Cord	0 Open 3 Percutaneous 4 Percutaneous Endoscopic	Z No Device	X Diagnostic Z No Qualifier

Section	0	Medical and Surgical
Body System	0	Central Nervous System and Cranial Nerves
Operation	B	**Excision:** Cutting out or off, without replacement, a portion of a body part

Body Part (4th)	Approach (5th)	Device (6th)	Qualifier (7th)
0 Brain **1** Cerebral Meninges **2** Dura Mater **6** Cerebral Ventricle **7** Cerebral Hemisphere **8** Basal Ganglia **9** Thalamus **A** Hypothalamus **B** Pons **C** Cerebellum **D** Medulla Oblongata **F** Olfactory Nerve **G** Optic Nerve **H** Oculomotor Nerve **J** Trochlear Nerve **K** Trigeminal Nerve **L** Abducens Nerve **M** Facial Nerve **N** Acoustic Nerve **P** Glossopharyngeal Nerve **Q** Vagus Nerve **R** Accessory Nerve **S** Hypoglossal Nerve **T** Spinal Meninges **W** Cervical Spinal Cord **X** Thoracic Spinal Cord **Y** Lumbar Spinal Cord	**0** Open **3** Percutaneous **4** Percutaneous Endoscopic	**Z** No Device	**X** Diagnostic **Z** No Qualifier

Section	0	**Medical and Surgical**
Body System	0	**Central Nervous System and Cranial Nerves**
Operation	C	**Extirpation:** Taking or cutting out solid matter from a body part

Body Part (4th)	Approach (5th)	Device (6th)	Qualifier (7th)
0 Brain 1 Cerebral Meninges 2 Dura Mater 3 Epidural Space, Intracranial 4 Subdural Space, Intracranial 5 Subarachnoid Space, Intracranial 6 Cerebral Ventricle 7 Cerebral Hemisphere 8 Basal Ganglia 9 Thalamus A Hypothalamus B Pons C Cerebellum D Medulla Oblongata F Olfactory Nerve G Optic Nerve H Oculomotor Nerve J Trochlear Nerve K Trigeminal Nerve L Abducens Nerve M Facial Nerve N Acoustic Nerve P Glossopharyngeal Nerve Q Vagus Nerve R Accessory Nerve S Hypoglossal Nerve T Spinal Meninges U Spinal Canal W Cervical Spinal Cord X Thoracic Spinal Cord Y Lumbar Spinal Cord	0 Open 3 Percutaneous 4 Percutaneous Endoscopic	Z No Device	Z No Qualifier

Section	0	Medical and Surgical
Body System	0	Central Nervous System and Cranial Nerves
Operation	D	Extraction: Pulling or stripping out or off all or a portion of a body part by the use of force

Body Part (4th)	Approach (5th)	Device (6th)	Qualifier (7th)
0 Brain 1 Cerebral Meninges 2 Dura Mater 7 Cerebral Hemisphere F Olfactory Nerve G Optic Nerve H Oculomotor Nerve J Trochlear Nerve K Trigeminal Nerve L Abducens Nerve M Facial Nerve N Acoustic Nerve P Glossopharyngeal Nerve Q Vagus Nerve R Accessory Nerve S Hypoglossal Nerve T Spinal Meninges	0 Open 3 Percutaneous 4 Percutaneous Endoscopic	Z No Device	Z No Qualifier

Section	0	Medical and Surgical
Body System	0	Central Nervous System and Cranial Nerves
Operation	F	Fragmentation: Breaking solid matter in a body part into pieces

Body Part (4th)	Approach (5th)	Device (6th)	Qualifier (7th)
3 Epidural Space, Intracranial 4 Subdural Space, Intracranial 5 Subarachnoid Space, Intracranial 6 Cerebral Ventricle U Spinal Canal	0 Open 3 Percutaneous 4 Percutaneous Endoscopic X External	Z No Device	Z No Qualifier

Section	0	Medical and Surgical
Body System	0	Central Nervous System and Cranial Nerves
Operation	H	Insertion: Putting in a nonbiological appliance that monitors, assists, performs, or prevents a physiological function but does not physically take the place of a body part

Body Part (4th)	Approach (5th)	Device (6th)	Qualifier (7th)
0 Brain	0 Open	1 Radioactive Element 2 Monitoring Device 3 Infusion Device 4 Radioactive Element, Cesium-131 Collagen Implant M Neurostimulator Lead Y Other Device	Z No Qualifier
0 Brain	3 Percutaneous 4 Percutaneous Endoscopic	1 Radioactive Element 2 Monitoring Device 3 Infusion Device M Neurostimulator Lead Y Other Device	Z No Qualifier
6 Cerebral Ventricle E Cranial Nerve U Spinal Canal V Spinal Cord	0 Open 3 Percutaneous 4 Percutaneous Endoscopic	1 Radioactive Element 2 Monitoring Device 3 Infusion Device M Neurostimulator Lead Y Other Device	Z No Qualifier

Section	0	Medical and Surgical
Body System	0	Central Nervous System and Cranial Nerves
Operation	J	**Inspection:** Visually and/or manually exploring a body part

Body Part (4th)	Approach (5th)	Device (6th)	Qualifier (7th)
0 Brain **E** Cranial Nerve **U** Spinal Canal **V** Spinal Cord	**0** Open **3** Percutaneous **4** Percutaneous Endoscopic	**Z** No Device	**Z** No Qualifier

Section	0	Medical and Surgical
Body System	0	Central Nervous System and Cranial Nerves
Operation	K	**Map:** Locating the route of passage of electrical impulses and/or locating functional areas in a body part

Body Part (4th)	Approach (5th)	Device (6th)	Qualifier (7th)
0 Brain **7** Cerebral Hemisphere **8** Basal Ganglia **9** Thalamus **A** Hypothalamus **B** Pons **C** Cerebellum **D** Medulla Oblongata	**0** Open **3** Percutaneous **4** Percutaneous Endoscopic	**Z** No Device	**Z** No Qualifier

Section	0	Medical and Surgical
Body System	0	Central Nervous System and Cranial Nerves
Operation	N	**Release:** Freeing a body part from an abnormal physical constraint by cutting or by the use of force

Body Part (4th)	Approach (5th)	Device (6th)	Qualifier (7th)
0 Brain **1** Cerebral Meninges **2** Dura Mater **6** Cerebral Ventricle **7** Cerebral Hemisphere **8** Basal Ganglia **9** Thalamus **A** Hypothalamus **B** Pons **C** Cerebellum **D** Medulla Oblongata **F** Olfactory Nerve **G** Optic Nerve **H** Oculomotor Nerve **J** Trochlear Nerve **K** Trigeminal Nerve **L** Abducens Nerve **M** Facial Nerve **N** Acoustic Nerve **P** Glossopharyngeal Nerve **Q** Vagus Nerve **R** Accessory Nerve **S** Hypoglossal Nerve **T** Spinal Meninges **W** Cervical Spinal Cord **X** Thoracic Spinal Cord **Y** Lumbar Spinal Cord	**0** Open **3** Percutaneous **4** Percutaneous Endoscopic	**Z** No Device	**Z** No Qualifier

Section	0	Medical and Surgical
Body System	0	Central Nervous System and Cranial Nerves
Operation	P	Removal: Taking out or off a device from a body part

Body Part (4th)	Approach (5th)	Device (6th)	Qualifier (7th)
0 Brain **V** Spinal Cord	**0** Open **3** Percutaneous **4** Percutaneous Endoscopic	**0** Drainage Device **2** Monitoring Device **3** Infusion Device **7** Autologous Tissue Substitute **J** Synthetic Substitute **K** Nonautologous Tissue Substitute **M** Neurostimulator Lead **Y** Other Device	**Z** No Qualifier
0 Brain **V** Spinal Cord	**X** External	**0** Drainage Device **2** Monitoring Device **3** Infusion Device **M** Neurostimulator Lead	**Z** No Qualifier
6 Cerebral Ventricle **U** Spinal Canal	**0** Open **3** Percutaneous **4** Percutaneous Endoscopic	**0** Drainage Device **2** Monitoring Device **3** Infusion Device **J** Synthetic Substitute **M** Neurostimulator Lead **Y** Other Device	**Z** No Qualifier
6 Cerebral Ventricle **U** Spinal Canal	**X** External	**0** Drainage Device **2** Monitoring Device **3** Infusion Device **M** Neurostimulator Lead	**Z** No Qualifier
E Cranial Nerve	**0** Open **3** Percutaneous **4** Percutaneous Endoscopic	**0** Drainage Device **2** Monitoring Device **3** Infusion Device **7** Autologous Tissue Substitute **M** Neurostimulator Lead **Y** Other Device	**Z** No Qualifier
E Cranial Nerve	**X** External	**0** Drainage Device **2** Monitoring Device **3** Infusion Device **M** Neurostimulator Lead	**Z** No Qualifier

Section	0	Medical and Surgical
Body System	0	Central Nervous System and Cranial Nerves
Operation	Q	**Repair:** Restoring, to the extent possible, a body part to its normal anatomic structure and function

Body Part (4th)	Approach (5th)	Device (6th)	Qualifier (7th)
0 Brain	0 Open	Z No Device	Z No Qualifier
1 Cerebral Meninges	3 Percutaneous		
2 Dura Mater	4 Percutaneous Endoscopic		
6 Cerebral Ventricle			
7 Cerebral Hemisphere			
8 Basal Ganglia			
9 Thalamus			
A Hypothalamus			
B Pons			
C Cerebellum			
D Medulla Oblongata			
F Olfactory Nerve			
G Optic Nerve			
H Oculomotor Nerve			
J Trochlear Nerve			
K Trigeminal Nerve			
L Abducens Nerve			
M Facial Nerve			
N Acoustic Nerve			
P Glossopharyngeal Nerve			
Q Vagus Nerve			
R Accessory Nerve			
S Hypoglossal Nerve			
T Spinal Meninges			
W Cervical Spinal Cord			
X Thoracic Spinal Cord			
Y Lumbar Spinal Cord			

Section	0	Medical and Surgical
Body System	0	Central Nervous System and Cranial Nerves
Operation	R	**Replacement:** Putting in or on biological or synthetic material that physically takes the place and/or function of all or a portion of a body part

Body Part (4th)	Approach (5th)	Device (6th)	Qualifier (7th)
1 Cerebral Meninges 2 Dura Mater 6 Cerebral Ventricle F Olfactory Nerve G Optic Nerve H Oculomotor Nerve J Trochlear Nerve K Trigeminal Nerve L Abducens Nerve M Facial Nerve N Acoustic Nerve P Glossopharyngeal Nerve Q Vagus Nerve R Accessory Nerve S Hypoglossal Nerve T Spinal Meninges	0 Open 4 Percutaneous Endoscopic	7 Autologous Tissue Substitute J Synthetic Substitute K Nonautologous Tissue Substitute	Z No Qualifier

Section	0	Medical and Surgical
Body System	0	Central Nervous System and Cranial Nerves
Operation	S	**Reposition:** Moving to its normal location, or other suitable location, all or a portion of a body part

Body Part (4th)	Approach (5th)	Device (6th)	Qualifier (7th)
F Olfactory Nerve G Optic Nerve H Oculomotor Nerve J Trochlear Nerve K Trigeminal Nerve L Abducens Nerve M Facial Nerve N Acoustic Nerve P Glossopharyngeal Nerve Q Vagus Nerve R Accessory Nerve S Hypoglossal Nerve W Cervical Spinal Cord X Thoracic Spinal Cord Y Lumbar Spinal Cord	0 Open 3 Percutaneous 4 Percutaneous Endoscopic	Z No Device	Z No Qualifier

Section	0	Medical and Surgical
Body System	0	Central Nervous System and Cranial Nerves
Operation	T	Resection: Cutting out or off, without replacement, all of a body part

Body Part (4th)	Approach (5th)	Device (6th)	Qualifier (7th)
7 Cerebral Hemisphere	0 Open 3 Percutaneous 4 Percutaneous Endoscopic	Z No Device	Z No Qualifier

Section	0	Medical and Surgical
Body System	0	Central Nervous System and Cranial Nerves
Operation	U	Supplement: Putting in or on biological or synthetic material that physically reinforces and/or augments the function of a portion of a body part

Body Part (4th)	Approach (5th)	Device (6th)	Qualifier (7th)
1 Cerebral Meninges 2 Dura Mater 6 Cerebral Ventricle F Olfactory Nerve G Optic Nerve H Oculomotor Nerve J Trochlear Nerve K Trigeminal Nerve L Abducens Nerve M Facial Nerve N Acoustic Nerve P Glossopharyngeal Nerve Q Vagus Nerve R Accessory Nerve S Hypoglossal Nerve T Spinal Meninges	0 Open 3 Percutaneous 4 Percutaneous Endoscopic	7 Autologous Tissue Substitute J Synthetic Substitute K Nonautologous Tissue Substitute	Z No Qualifier

Section   **0**   **Medical and Surgical**
Body System   **0**   **Central Nervous System and Cranial Nerves**
Operation   **W**   **Revision:** Correcting, to the extent possible, a portion of a malfunctioning device or the position of a displaced device

Body Part (4th)	Approach (5th)	Device (6th)	Qualifier (7th)
0 Brain V Spinal Cord	0 Open 3 Percutaneous 4 Percutaneous Endoscopic	0 Drainage Device 2 Monitoring Device 3 Infusion Device 7 Autologous Tissue Substitute J Synthetic Substitute K Nonautologous Tissue Substitute M Neurostimulator Lead Y Other Device	Z No Qualifier
0 Brain V Spinal Cord	X External	0 Drainage Device 2 Monitoring Device 3 Infusion Device 7 Autologous Tissue Substitute J Synthetic Substitute K Nonautologous Tissue Substitute M Neurostimulator Lead	Z No Qualifier
6 Cerebral Ventricle U Spinal Canal	0 Open 3 Percutaneous 4 Percutaneous Endoscopic	0 Drainage Device 2 Monitoring Device 3 Infusion Device J Synthetic Substitute M Neurostimulator Lead Y Other Device	Z No Qualifier
6 Cerebral Ventricle U Spinal Canal	X External	0 Drainage Device 2 Monitoring Device 3 Infusion Device J Synthetic Substitute M Neurostimulator Lead	Z No Qualifier
E Cranial Nerve	0 Open 3 Percutaneous 4 Percutaneous Endoscopic	0 Drainage Device 2 Monitoring Device 3 Infusion Device 7 Autologous Tissue Substitute M Neurostimulator Lead Y Other Device	Z No Qualifier
E Cranial Nerve	X External	0 Drainage Device 2 Monitoring Device 3 Infusion Device 7 Autologous Tissue Substitute M Neurostimulator Lead	Z No Qualifier

Section   **0**   **Medical and Surgical**
Body System   **0**   **Central Nervous System and Cranial Nerves**
Operation   **X**   **Transfer:** Moving, without taking out, all or a portion of a body part to another location to take over the function of all or a portion of a body part

Body Part (4th)	Approach (5th)	Device (6th)	Qualifier (7th)
F Olfactory Nerve G Optic Nerve H Oculomotor Nerve J Trochlear Nerve K Trigeminal Nerve L Abducens Nerve M Facial Nerve N Acoustic Nerve P Glossopharyngeal Nerve Q Vagus Nerve R Accessory Nerve S Hypoglossal Nerve	0 Open 4 Percutaneous Endoscopic	Z No Device	F Olfactory Nerve G Optic Nerve H Oculomotor Nerve J Trochlear Nerve K Trigeminal Nerve L Abducens Nerve M Facial Nerve N Acoustic Nerve P Glossopharyngeal Nerve Q Vagus Nerve R Accessory Nerve S Hypoglossal Nerve

001 – Central Nervous System and Cranial Nerves, Bypass

Review Coding Guideline B3.6a

0016070 Bypass Cerebral Ventricle to Nasopharynx with Autologous Tissue Substitute, Open Approach

0016071 Bypass Cerebral Ventricle to Mastoid Sinus with Autologous Tissue Substitute, Open Approach

0016072 Bypass Cerebral Ventricle to Atrium with Autologous Tissue Substitute, Open Approach

0016073 Bypass Cerebral Ventricle to Blood Vessel with Autologous Tissue Substitute, Open Approach

0016074 Bypass Cerebral Ventricle to Pleural Cavity with Autologous Tissue Substitute, Open Approach

0016075 Bypass Cerebral Ventricle to Intestine with Autologous Tissue Substitute, Open Approach

0016076 Bypass Cerebral Ventricle to Peritoneal Cavity with Autologous Tissue Substitute, Open Approach

0016077 Bypass Cerebral Ventricle to Urinary Tract with Autologous Tissue Substitute, Open Approach

0016078 Bypass Cerebral Ventricle to Bone Marrow with Autologous Tissue Substitute, Open Approach

001607A Bypass Cerebral Ventricle to Subgaleal Space with Autologous Tissue Substitute, Open Approach

001607B Bypass Cerebral Ventricle to Cerebral Cisterns with Autologous Tissue Substitute, Open Approach

00160J0 Bypass Cerebral Ventricle to Nasopharynx with Synthetic Substitute, Open Approach

00160J1 Bypass Cerebral Ventricle to Mastoid Sinus with Synthetic Substitute, Open Approach

00160J2 Bypass Cerebral Ventricle to Atrium with Synthetic Substitute, Open Approach

00160J3 Bypass Cerebral Ventricle to Blood Vessel with Synthetic Substitute, Open Approach

00160J4 Bypass Cerebral Ventricle to Pleural Cavity with Synthetic Substitute, Open Approach

00160J5 Bypass Cerebral Ventricle to Intestine with Synthetic Substitute, Open Approach

00160J6 Bypass Cerebral Ventricle to Peritoneal Cavity with Synthetic Substitute, Open Approach

00160J7 Bypass Cerebral Ventricle to Urinary Tract with Synthetic Substitute, Open Approach

00160J8 Bypass Cerebral Ventricle to Bone Marrow with Synthetic Substitute, Open Approach

00160JA Bypass Cerebral Ventricle to Subgaleal Space with Synthetic Substitute, Open Approach

00160JB Bypass Cerebral Ventricle to Cerebral Cisterns with Synthetic Substitute, Open Approach

00160K0 Bypass Cerebral Ventricle to Nasopharynx with Nonautologous Tissue Substitute, Open Approach

00160K1 Bypass Cerebral Ventricle to Mastoid Sinus with Nonautologous Tissue Substitute, Open Approach

00160K2 Bypass Cerebral Ventricle to Atrium with Nonautologous Tissue Substitute, Open Approach

00160K3 Bypass Cerebral Ventricle to Blood Vessel with Nonautologous Tissue Substitute, Open Approach

00160K4 Bypass Cerebral Ventricle to Pleural Cavity with Nonautologous Tissue Substitute, Open Approach

00160K5 Bypass Cerebral Ventricle to Intestine with Nonautologous Tissue Substitute, Open Approach

00160K6 Bypass Cerebral Ventricle to Peritoneal Cavity with Nonautologous Tissue Substitute, Open Approach

00160K7 Bypass Cerebral Ventricle to Urinary Tract with Nonautologous Tissue Substitute, Open Approach

00160K8 Bypass Cerebral Ventricle to Bone Marrow with Nonautologous Tissue Substitute, Open Approach

00160KA Bypass Cerebral Ventricle to Subgaleal Space with Nonautologous Tissue Substitute, Open Approach

00160KB Bypass Cerebral Ventricle to Cerebral Cisterns with Nonautologous Tissue Substitute, Open Approach

00160ZB Bypass Cerebral Ventricle to Cerebral Cisterns, Open Approach

0016370 Bypass Cerebral Ventricle to Nasopharynx with Autologous Tissue Substitute, Percutaneous Approach

0016371 Bypass Cerebral Ventricle to Mastoid Sinus with Autologous Tissue Substitute, Percutaneous Approach

0016372 Bypass Cerebral Ventricle to Atrium with Autologous Tissue Substitute, Percutaneous Approach

0016373 Bypass Cerebral Ventricle to Blood Vessel with Autologous Tissue Substitute, Percutaneous Approach

0016374 Bypass Cerebral Ventricle to Pleural Cavity with Autologous Tissue Substitute, Percutaneous Approach

0016375 Bypass Cerebral Ventricle to Intestine with Autologous Tissue Substitute, Percutaneous Approach

0016376 Bypass Cerebral Ventricle to Peritoneal Cavity with Autologous Tissue Substitute, Percutaneous Approach

0016377 Bypass Cerebral Ventricle to Urinary Tract with Autologous Tissue Substitute, Percutaneous Approach

0016378 Bypass Cerebral Ventricle to Bone Marrow with Autologous Tissue Substitute, Percutaneous Approach

001637A Bypass Cerebral Ventricle to Subgaleal Space with Autologous Tissue Substitute, Percutaneous Approach

001637B Bypass Cerebral Ventricle to Cerebral Cisterns with Autologous Tissue Substitute, Percutaneous Approach

00163J0 Bypass Cerebral Ventricle to Nasopharynx with Synthetic Substitute, Percutaneous Approach

00163J1 Bypass Cerebral Ventricle to Mastoid Sinus with Synthetic Substitute, Percutaneous Approach

00163J2 Bypass Cerebral Ventricle to Atrium with Synthetic Substitute, Percutaneous Approach

00163J3 Bypass Cerebral Ventricle to Blood Vessel with Synthetic Substitute, Percutaneous Approach

00163J4 Bypass Cerebral Ventricle to Pleural Cavity with Synthetic Substitute, Percutaneous Approach

00163J5 Bypass Cerebral Ventricle to Intestine with Synthetic Substitute, Percutaneous Approach

00163J6 Bypass Cerebral Ventricle to Peritoneal Cavity with Synthetic Substitute, Percutaneous Approach

AHA CC: 2Q, 2013, 36-37; 2Q, 2021, 19-20

00163J7 Bypass Cerebral Ventricle to Urinary Tract with Synthetic Substitute, Percutaneous Approach

00163J8 Bypass Cerebral Ventricle to Bone Marrow with Synthetic Substitute, Percutaneous Approach

00163JA Bypass Cerebral Ventricle to Subgaleal Space with Synthetic Substitute, Percutaneous Approach

AHA CC: 4Q, 2019, 22

00163JB Bypass Cerebral Ventricle to Cerebral Cisterns with Synthetic Substitute, Percutaneous Approach

00163K0 Bypass Cerebral Ventricle to Nasopharynx with Nonautologous Tissue Substitute, Percutaneous Approach

00163K1 Bypass Cerebral Ventricle to Mastoid Sinus with Nonautologous Tissue Substitute, Percutaneous Approach

00163K2 Bypass Cerebral Ventricle to Atrium with Nonautologous Tissue Substitute, Percutaneous Approach

00163K3 Bypass Cerebral Ventricle to Blood Vessel with Nonautologous Tissue Substitute, Percutaneous Approach

00163K4 Bypass Cerebral Ventricle to Pleural Cavity with Nonautologous Tissue Substitute, Percutaneous Approach

00163K5 Bypass Cerebral Ventricle to Intestine with Nonautologous Tissue Substitute, Percutaneous Approach

00163K6 Bypass Cerebral Ventricle to Peritoneal Cavity with Nonautologous Tissue Substitute, Percutaneous Approach

00163K7 Bypass Cerebral Ventricle to Urinary Tract with Nonautologous Tissue Substitute, Percutaneous Approach

00163K8 Bypass Cerebral Ventricle to Bone Marrow with Nonautologous Tissue Substitute, Percutaneous Approach

00163KA Bypass Cerebral Ventricle to Subgaleal Space with Nonautologous Tissue Substitute, Percutaneous Approach

00163KB Bypass Cerebral Ventricle to Cerebral Cisterns with Nonautologous Tissue Substitute, Percutaneous Approach

00163ZB Bypass Cerebral Ventricle to Cerebral Cisterns, Percutaneous Approach

0016470 Bypass Cerebral Ventricle to Nasopharynx with Autologous Tissue Substitute, Percutaneous Endoscopic Approach

0016471 Bypass Cerebral Ventricle to Mastoid Sinus with Autologous Tissue Substitute, Percutaneous Endoscopic Approach

0016472 Bypass Cerebral Ventricle to Atrium with Autologous Tissue Substitute, Percutaneous Endoscopic Approach

♀ Female-only ♂ Male-only ▲ Limited Coverage ● Non-OR ▮ HAC-associated procedure ▲ Non-covered procedures ➕ Cluster

0016473	Bypass Cerebral Ventricle to Blood Vessel with Autologous Tissue Substitute, Percutaneous Endoscopic Approach
0016474	Bypass Cerebral Ventricle to Pleural Cavity with Autologous Tissue Substitute, Percutaneous Endoscopic Approach
0016475	Bypass Cerebral Ventricle to Intestine with Autologous Tissue Substitute, Percutaneous Endoscopic Approach
0016476	Bypass Cerebral Ventricle to Peritoneal Cavity with Autologous Tissue Substitute, Percutaneous Endoscopic Approach
0016477	Bypass Cerebral Ventricle to Urinary Tract with Autologous Tissue Substitute, Percutaneous Endoscopic Approach
0016478	Bypass Cerebral Ventricle to Bone Marrow with Autologous Tissue Substitute, Percutaneous Endoscopic Approach
001647A	Bypass Cerebral Ventricle to Subgaleal Space with Autologous Tissue Substitute, Percutaneous Endoscopic Approach
001647B	Bypass Cerebral Ventricle to Cerebral Cisterns with Autologous Tissue Substitute, Percutaneous Endoscopic Approach
00164J0	Bypass Cerebral Ventricle to Nasopharynx with Synthetic Substitute, Percutaneous Endoscopic Approach
00164J1	Bypass Cerebral Ventricle to Mastoid Sinus with Synthetic Substitute, Percutaneous Endoscopic Approach
00164J2	Bypass Cerebral Ventricle to Atrium with Synthetic Substitute, Percutaneous Endoscopic Approach
00164J3	Bypass Cerebral Ventricle to Blood Vessel with Synthetic Substitute, Percutaneous Endoscopic Approach
00164J4	Bypass Cerebral Ventricle to Pleural Cavity with Synthetic Substitute, Percutaneous Endoscopic Approach
00164J5	Bypass Cerebral Ventricle to Intestine with Synthetic Substitute, Percutaneous Endoscopic Approach
00164J6	Bypass Cerebral Ventricle to Peritoneal Cavity with Synthetic Substitute, Percutaneous Endoscopic Approach
00164J7	Bypass Cerebral Ventricle to Urinary Tract with Synthetic Substitute, Percutaneous Endoscopic Approach
00164J8	Bypass Cerebral Ventricle to Bone Marrow with Synthetic Substitute, Percutaneous Endoscopic Approach
00164JA	Bypass Cerebral Ventricle to Subgaleal Space with Synthetic Substitute, Percutaneous Endoscopic Approach
00164JB	Bypass Cerebral Ventricle to Cerebral Cisterns with Synthetic Substitute, Percutaneous Endoscopic Approach
00164K0	Bypass Cerebral Ventricle to Nasopharynx with Nonautologous Tissue Substitute, Percutaneous Endoscopic Approach
00164K1	Bypass Cerebral Ventricle to Mastoid Sinus with Nonautologous Tissue Substitute, Percutaneous Endoscopic Approach
00164K2	Bypass Cerebral Ventricle to Atrium with Nonautologous Tissue Substitute, Percutaneous Endoscopic Approach
00164K3	Bypass Cerebral Ventricle to Blood Vessel with Nonautologous Tissue Substitute, Percutaneous Endoscopic Approach
00164K4	Bypass Cerebral Ventricle to Pleural Cavity with Nonautologous Tissue Substitute, Percutaneous Endoscopic Approach
00164K5	Bypass Cerebral Ventricle to Intestine with Nonautologous Tissue Substitute, Percutaneous Endoscopic Approach
00164K6	Bypass Cerebral Ventricle to Peritoneal Cavity with Nonautologous Tissue Substitute, Percutaneous Endoscopic Approach
00164K7	Bypass Cerebral Ventricle to Urinary Tract with Nonautologous Tissue Substitute, Percutaneous Endoscopic Approach
00164K8	Bypass Cerebral Ventricle to Bone Marrow with Nonautologous Tissue Substitute, Percutaneous Endoscopic Approach
00164KA	Bypass Cerebral Ventricle to Subgaleal Space with Nonautologous Tissue Substitute, Percutaneous Endoscopic Approach
00164KB	Bypass Cerebral Ventricle to Cerebral Cisterns with Nonautologous Tissue Substitute, Percutaneous Endoscopic Approach
00164ZB	Bypass Cerebral Ventricle to Cerebral Cisterns, Percutaneous Endoscopic Approach
001U072	Bypass Spinal Canal to Atrium with Autologous Tissue Substitute, Open Approach
001U074	Bypass Spinal Canal to Pleural Cavity with Autologous Tissue Substitute, Open Approach
001U076	Bypass Spinal Canal to Peritoneal Cavity with Autologous Tissue Substitute, Open Approach
001U077	Bypass Spinal Canal to Urinary Tract with Autologous Tissue Substitute, Open Approach
001U079	Bypass Spinal Canal to Fallopian Tube with Autologous Tissue Substitute, Open Approach
001U0J2	Bypass Spinal Canal to Atrium with Synthetic Substitute, Open Approach *AHA CC: 4Q, 2018, 86*
001U0J4	Bypass Spinal Canal to Pleural Cavity with Synthetic Substitute, Open Approach
001U0J6	Bypass Spinal Canal to Peritoneal Cavity with Synthetic Substitute, Open Approach
001U0J7	Bypass Spinal Canal to Urinary Tract with Synthetic Substitute, Open Approach
001U0J9	Bypass Spinal Canal to Fallopian Tube with Synthetic Substitute, Open Approach
001U0K2	Bypass Spinal Canal to Atrium with Nonautologous Tissue Substitute, Open Approach
001U0K4	Bypass Spinal Canal to Pleural Cavity with Nonautologous Tissue Substitute, Open Approach
001U0K6	Bypass Spinal Canal to Peritoneal Cavity with Nonautologous Tissue Substitute, Open Approach
001U0K7	Bypass Spinal Canal to Urinary Tract with Nonautologous Tissue Substitute, Open Approach
001U0K9	Bypass Spinal Canal to Fallopian Tube with Nonautologous Tissue Substitute, Open Approach
001U372	Bypass Spinal Canal to Atrium with Autologous Tissue Substitute, Percutaneous Approach
001U374	Bypass Spinal Canal to Pleural Cavity with Autologous Tissue Substitute, Percutaneous Approach
001U376	Bypass Spinal Canal to Peritoneal Cavity with Autologous Tissue Substitute, Percutaneous Approach
001U377	Bypass Spinal Canal to Urinary Tract with Autologous Tissue Substitute, Percutaneous Approach
001U379	Bypass Spinal Canal to Fallopian Tube with Autologous Tissue Substitute, Percutaneous Approach
001U3J2	Bypass Spinal Canal to Atrium with Synthetic Substitute, Percutaneous Approach
001U3J4	Bypass Spinal Canal to Pleural Cavity with Synthetic Substitute, Percutaneous Approach
001U3J6	Bypass Spinal Canal to Peritoneal Cavity with Synthetic Substitute, Percutaneous Approach
001U3J7	Bypass Spinal Canal to Urinary Tract with Synthetic Substitute, Percutaneous Approach
001U3J9	Bypass Spinal Canal to Fallopian Tube with Synthetic Substitute, Percutaneous Approach
001U3K2	Bypass Spinal Canal to Atrium with Nonautologous Tissue Substitute, Percutaneous Approach
001U3K4	Bypass Spinal Canal to Pleural Cavity with Nonautologous Tissue Substitute, Percutaneous Approach
001U3K6	Bypass Spinal Canal to Peritoneal Cavity with Nonautologous Tissue Substitute, Percutaneous Approach
001U3K7	Bypass Spinal Canal to Urinary Tract with Nonautologous Tissue Substitute, Percutaneous Approach
001U3K9	Bypass Spinal Canal to Fallopian Tube with Nonautologous Tissue Substitute, Percutaneous Approach
001U472	Bypass Spinal Canal to Atrium with Autologous Tissue Substitute, Percutaneous Endoscopic Approach
001U474	Bypass Spinal Canal to Pleural Cavity with Autologous Tissue Substitute, Percutaneous Endoscopic Approach
001U476	Bypass Spinal Canal to Peritoneal Cavity with Autologous Tissue Substitute, Percutaneous Endoscopic Approach
001U477	Bypass Spinal Canal to Urinary Tract with Autologous Tissue Substitute, Percutaneous Endoscopic Approach
001U479	Bypass Spinal Canal to Fallopian Tube with Autologous Tissue Substitute, Percutaneous Endoscopic Approach
001U4J2	Bypass Spinal Canal to Atrium with Synthetic Substitute, Percutaneous Endoscopic Approach
001U4J4	Bypass Spinal Canal to Pleural Cavity with Synthetic Substitute, Percutaneous Endoscopic Approach
001U4J6	Bypass Spinal Canal to Peritoneal Cavity with Synthetic Substitute, Percutaneous Endoscopic Approach

001U4J7 Bypass Spinal Canal to Urinary Tract with Synthetic Substitute, Percutaneous Endoscopic Approach	**001U4K4** Bypass Spinal Canal to Pleural Cavity with Nonautologous Tissue Substitute, Percutaneous Endoscopic Approach	**001U4K7** Bypass Spinal Canal to Urinary Tract with Nonautologous Tissue Substitute, Percutaneous Endoscopic Approach
001U4J9 Bypass Spinal Canal to Fallopian Tube with Synthetic Substitute, Percutaneous Endoscopic Approach	**001U4K6** Bypass Spinal Canal to Peritoneal Cavity with Nonautologous Tissue Substitute, Percutaneous Endoscopic Approach	**001U4K9** Bypass Spinal Canal to Fallopian Tube with Nonautologous Tissue Substitute, Percutaneous Endoscopic Approach
001U4K2 Bypass Spinal Canal to Atrium with Nonautologous Tissue Substitute, Percutaneous Endoscopic Approach		

002 – Central Nervous System and Cranial Nerves, Change

Review Coding Guideline B6.1c

0020X0Z Change Drainage Device in Brain, External Approach	**002EX0Z** Change Drainage Device in Cranial Nerve, External Approach	**002UX0Z** Change Drainage Device in Spinal Canal, External Approach
0020XYZ Change Other Device in Brain, External Approach	**002EXYZ** Change Other Device in Cranial Nerve, External Approach	**002UXYZ** Change Other Device in Spinal Canal, External Approach

005 – Central Nervous System and Cranial Nerves, Destruction

00500ZZ Destruction of Brain, Open Approach	**005C3ZZ** Destruction of Cerebellum, Percutaneous Approach	**005N3ZZ** Destruction of Acoustic Nerve, Percutaneous Approach
00503ZZ Destruction of Brain, Percutaneous Approach	**005C4ZZ** Destruction of Cerebellum, Percutaneous Endoscopic Approach	**005N4ZZ** Destruction of Acoustic Nerve, Percutaneous Endoscopic Approach
00504ZZ Destruction of Brain, Percutaneous Endoscopic Approach	**005D0ZZ** Destruction of Medulla Oblongata, Open Approach	**005P0ZZ** Destruction of Glossopharyngeal Nerve, Open Approach
00510ZZ Destruction of Cerebral Meninges, Open Approach	**005D3ZZ** Destruction of Medulla Oblongata, Percutaneous Approach	**005P3ZZ** Destruction of Glossopharyngeal Nerve, Percutaneous Approach
00513ZZ Destruction of Cerebral Meninges, Percutaneous Approach	**005D4ZZ** Destruction of Medulla Oblongata, Percutaneous Endoscopic Approach	**005P4ZZ** Destruction of Glossopharyngeal Nerve, Percutaneous Endoscopic Approach
00514ZZ Destruction of Cerebral Meninges, Percutaneous Endoscopic Approach	**005F0ZZ** Destruction of Olfactory Nerve, Open Approach	**005Q0ZZ** Destruction of Vagus Nerve, Open Approach
00520ZZ Destruction of Dura Mater, Open Approach	**005F3ZZ** Destruction of Olfactory Nerve, Percutaneous Approach	**005Q3ZZ** Destruction of Vagus Nerve, Percutaneous Approach
00523ZZ Destruction of Dura Mater, Percutaneous Approach	**005F4ZZ** Destruction of Olfactory Nerve, Percutaneous Endoscopic Approach	**005Q4ZZ** Destruction of Vagus Nerve, Percutaneous Endoscopic Approach
00524ZZ Destruction of Dura Mater, Percutaneous Endoscopic Approach	**005G0ZZ** Destruction of Optic Nerve, Open Approach	**005R0ZZ** Destruction of Accessory Nerve, Open Approach
00560ZZ Destruction of Cerebral Ventricle, Open Approach	**005G3ZZ** Destruction of Optic Nerve, Percutaneous Approach	**005R3ZZ** Destruction of Accessory Nerve, Percutaneous Approach
00563ZZ Destruction of Cerebral Ventricle, Percutaneous Approach	**005G4ZZ** Destruction of Optic Nerve, Percutaneous Endoscopic Approach	**005R4ZZ** Destruction of Accessory Nerve, Percutaneous Endoscopic Approach
00564ZZ Destruction of Cerebral Ventricle, Percutaneous Endoscopic Approach	**005H0ZZ** Destruction of Oculomotor Nerve, Open Approach	**005S0ZZ** Destruction of Hypoglossal Nerve, Open Approach
00570ZZ Destruction of Cerebral Hemisphere, Open Approach	**005H3ZZ** Destruction of Oculomotor Nerve, Percutaneous Approach	**005S3ZZ** Destruction of Hypoglossal Nerve, Percutaneous Approach
00573ZZ Destruction of Cerebral Hemisphere, Percutaneous Approach	**005H4ZZ** Destruction of Oculomotor Nerve, Percutaneous Endoscopic Approach	**005S4ZZ** Destruction of Hypoglossal Nerve, Percutaneous Endoscopic Approach
00574ZZ Destruction of Cerebral Hemisphere, Percutaneous Endoscopic Approach	**005J0ZZ** Destruction of Trochlear Nerve, Open Approach	**005T0ZZ** Destruction of Spinal Meninges, Open Approach
00580ZZ Destruction of Basal Ganglia, Open Approach	**005J3ZZ** Destruction of Trochlear Nerve, Percutaneous Approach	**005T3ZZ** Destruction of Spinal Meninges, Percutaneous Approach
00583ZZ Destruction of Basal Ganglia, Percutaneous Approach	**005J4ZZ** Destruction of Trochlear Nerve, Percutaneous Endoscopic Approach	**005T4ZZ** Destruction of Spinal Meninges, Percutaneous Endoscopic Approach
00584ZZ Destruction of Basal Ganglia, Percutaneous Endoscopic Approach	**005K0ZZ** Destruction of Trigeminal Nerve, Open Approach	**005W0ZZ** Destruction of Cervical Spinal Cord, Open Approach
00590ZZ Destruction of Thalamus, Open Approach	**005K3ZZ** Destruction of Trigeminal Nerve, Percutaneous Approach	*AHA CC: 2Q, 2021, 17-18*
00593ZZ Destruction of Thalamus, Percutaneous Approach	**005K4ZZ** Destruction of Trigeminal Nerve, Percutaneous Endoscopic Approach	**005W3ZZ** Destruction of Cervical Spinal Cord, Percutaneous Approach
00594ZZ Destruction of Thalamus, Percutaneous Endoscopic Approach	**005L0ZZ** Destruction of Abducens Nerve, Open Approach	**005W4ZZ** Destruction of Cervical Spinal Cord, Percutaneous Endoscopic Approach
005A0ZZ Destruction of Hypothalamus, Open Approach	**005L3ZZ** Destruction of Abducens Nerve, Percutaneous Approach	**005X0ZZ** Destruction of Thoracic Spinal Cord, Open Approach
005A3ZZ Destruction of Hypothalamus, Percutaneous Approach	**005L4ZZ** Destruction of Abducens Nerve, Percutaneous Endoscopic Approach	*AHA CC: 2Q, 2021, 17-18*
005A4ZZ Destruction of Hypothalamus, Percutaneous Endoscopic Approach	**005M0ZZ** Destruction of Facial Nerve, Open Approach	**005X3ZZ** Destruction of Thoracic Spinal Cord, Percutaneous Approach
005B0ZZ Destruction of Pons, Open Approach	**005M3ZZ** Destruction of Facial Nerve, Percutaneous Approach	**005X4ZZ** Destruction of Thoracic Spinal Cord, Percutaneous Endoscopic Approach
005B3ZZ Destruction of Pons, Percutaneous Approach	**005M4ZZ** Destruction of Facial Nerve, Percutaneous Endoscopic Approach	**005Y0ZZ** Destruction of Lumbar Spinal Cord, Open Approach
005B4ZZ Destruction of Pons, Percutaneous Endoscopic Approach	**005N0ZZ** Destruction of Acoustic Nerve, Open Approach	**005Y3ZZ** Destruction of Lumbar Spinal Cord, Percutaneous Approach
005C0ZZ Destruction of Cerebellum, Open Approach		**005Y4ZZ** Destruction of Lumbar Spinal Cord, Percutaneous Endoscopic Approach

♀ Female-only   ♂ Male-only   ▲ Limited Coverage   ● Non-OR   HAC HAC-associated procedure   ▲ Non-covered procedures   ✚ Cluster

007 – Central Nervous System and Cranial Nerves, Dilation

00760ZZ	Dilation of Cerebral Ventricle, Open Approach	
00763ZZ	Dilation of Cerebral Ventricle, Percutaneous Approach	
00764ZZ	Dilation of Cerebral Ventricle, Percutaneous Endoscopic Approach	
	AHA CC: 4Q, 2017, 40-41	

008 – Central Nervous System and Cranial Nerves, Division

Review Coding Guideline B3.14

00800ZZ	Division of Brain, Open Approach
00803ZZ	Division of Brain, Percutaneous Approach
00804ZZ	Division of Brain, Percutaneous Endoscopic Approach
00870ZZ	Division of Cerebral Hemisphere, Open Approach
00873ZZ	Division of Cerebral Hemisphere, Percutaneous Approach
00874ZZ	Division of Cerebral Hemisphere, Percutaneous Endoscopic Approach
00880ZZ	Division of Basal Ganglia, Open Approach
00883ZZ	Division of Basal Ganglia, Percutaneous Approach
00884ZZ	Division of Basal Ganglia, Percutaneous Endoscopic Approach
008F0ZZ	Division of Olfactory Nerve, Open Approach
008F3ZZ	Division of Olfactory Nerve, Percutaneous Approach
008F4ZZ	Division of Olfactory Nerve, Percutaneous Endoscopic Approach
008G0ZZ	Division of Optic Nerve, Open Approach
008G3ZZ	Division of Optic Nerve, Percutaneous Approach
008G4ZZ	Division of Optic Nerve, Percutaneous Endoscopic Approach
008H0ZZ	Division of Oculomotor Nerve, Open Approach
008H3ZZ	Division of Oculomotor Nerve, Percutaneous Approach
008H4ZZ	Division of Oculomotor Nerve, Percutaneous Endoscopic Approach
008J0ZZ	Division of Trochlear Nerve, Open Approach
008J3ZZ	Division of Trochlear Nerve, Percutaneous Approach
008J4ZZ	Division of Trochlear Nerve, Percutaneous Endoscopic Approach
008K0ZZ	Division of Trigeminal Nerve, Open Approach
008K3ZZ	Division of Trigeminal Nerve, Percutaneous Approach
008K4ZZ	Division of Trigeminal Nerve, Percutaneous Endoscopic Approach
008L0ZZ	Division of Abducens Nerve, Open Approach
008L3ZZ	Division of Abducens Nerve, Percutaneous Approach
008L4ZZ	Division of Abducens Nerve, Percutaneous Endoscopic Approach
008M0ZZ	Division of Facial Nerve, Open Approach
008M3ZZ	Division of Facial Nerve, Percutaneous Approach
008M4ZZ	Division of Facial Nerve, Percutaneous Endoscopic Approach
008N0ZZ	Division of Acoustic Nerve, Open Approach
008N3ZZ	Division of Acoustic Nerve, Percutaneous Approach
008N4ZZ	Division of Acoustic Nerve, Percutaneous Endoscopic Approach
008P0ZZ	Division of Glossopharyngeal Nerve, Open Approach
008P3ZZ	Division of Glossopharyngeal Nerve, Percutaneous Approach
008P4ZZ	Division of Glossopharyngeal Nerve, Percutaneous Endoscopic Approach
008Q0ZZ	Division of Vagus Nerve, Open Approach
008Q3ZZ	Division of Vagus Nerve, Percutaneous Approach
008Q4ZZ	Division of Vagus Nerve, Percutaneous Endoscopic Approach
008R0ZZ	Division of Accessory Nerve, Open Approach
008R3ZZ	Division of Accessory Nerve, Percutaneous Approach
008R4ZZ	Division of Accessory Nerve, Percutaneous Endoscopic Approach
008S0ZZ	Division of Hypoglossal Nerve, Open Approach
008S3ZZ	Division of Hypoglossal Nerve, Percutaneous Approach
008S4ZZ	Division of Hypoglossal Nerve, Percutaneous Endoscopic Approach
008W0ZZ	Division of Cervical Spinal Cord, Open Approach
008W3ZZ	Division of Cervical Spinal Cord, Percutaneous Approach
008W4ZZ	Division of Cervical Spinal Cord, Percutaneous Endoscopic Approach
008X0ZZ	Division of Thoracic Spinal Cord, Open Approach
008X3ZZ	Division of Thoracic Spinal Cord, Percutaneous Approach
008X4ZZ	Division of Thoracic Spinal Cord, Percutaneous Endoscopic Approach
008Y0ZZ	Division of Lumbar Spinal Cord, Open Approach
008Y3ZZ	Division of Lumbar Spinal Cord, Percutaneous Approach
008Y4ZZ	Division of Lumbar Spinal Cord, Percutaneous Endoscopic Approach

009 – Central Nervous System and Cranial Nerves, Drainage

Review Coding Guidelines B3.4a and B3.4b

Review Coding Guideline B6.2

009000Z	Drainage of Brain with Drainage Device, Open Approach
00900ZX	Drainage of Brain, Open Approach, Diagnostic
00900ZZ	Drainage of Brain, Open Approach
009030Z	Drainage of Brain with Drainage Device, Percutaneous Approach
00903ZX	Drainage of Brain, Percutaneous Approach, Diagnostic
00903ZZ	Drainage of Brain, Percutaneous Approach
009040Z	Drainage of Brain with Drainage Device, Percutaneous Endoscopic Approach
00904ZX	Drainage of Brain, Percutaneous Endoscopic Approach, Diagnostic
00904ZZ	Drainage of Brain, Percutaneous Endoscopic Approach
009100Z	Drainage of Cerebral Meninges with Drainage Device, Open Approach
00910ZX	Drainage of Cerebral Meninges, Open Approach, Diagnostic
00910ZZ	Drainage of Cerebral Meninges, Open Approach
009130Z	Drainage of Cerebral Meninges with Drainage Device, Percutaneous Approach
00913ZX	Drainage of Cerebral Meninges, Percutaneous Approach, Diagnostic
00913ZZ	Drainage of Cerebral Meninges, Percutaneous Approach
009140Z	Drainage of Cerebral Meninges with Drainage Device, Percutaneous Endoscopic Approach
00914ZX	Drainage of Cerebral Meninges, Percutaneous Endoscopic Approach, Diagnostic
00914ZZ	Drainage of Cerebral Meninges, Percutaneous Endoscopic Approach
009200Z	Drainage of Dura Mater with Drainage Device, Open Approach
00920ZX	Drainage of Dura Mater, Open Approach, Diagnostic
00920ZZ	Drainage of Dura Mater, Open Approach
009230Z	Drainage of Dura Mater with Drainage Device, Percutaneous Approach
00923ZX	Drainage of Dura Mater, Percutaneous Approach, Diagnostic
00923ZZ	Drainage of Dura Mater, Percutaneous Approach
009240Z	Drainage of Dura Mater with Drainage Device, Percutaneous Endoscopic Approach
00924ZX	Drainage of Dura Mater, Percutaneous Endoscopic Approach, Diagnostic
00924ZZ	Drainage of Dura Mater, Percutaneous Endoscopic Approach
009300Z	Drainage of Intracranial Epidural Space with Drainage Device, Open Approach
00930ZX	Drainage of Intracranial Epidural Space, Open Approach, Diagnostic
00930ZZ	Drainage of Intracranial Epidural Space, Open Approach
009330Z	Drainage of Intracranial Epidural Space with Drainage Device, Percutaneous Approach

---

♀ Female-only   ♂ Male-only   ▲ Limited Coverage   ● Non-OR   🅷🅰🅲 HAC-associated procedure   ▲ Non-covered procedures   ➕ Cluster

00933ZX Drainage of Intracranial Epidural Space, Percutaneous Approach, Diagnostic

00933ZZ Drainage of Intracranial Epidural Space, Percutaneous Approach

009340Z Drainage of Intracranial Epidural Space with Drainage Device, Percutaneous Endoscopic Approach

00934ZX Drainage of Intracranial Epidural Space, Percutaneous Endoscopic Approach, Diagnostic

00934ZZ Drainage of Intracranial Epidural Space, Percutaneous Endoscopic Approach

009400Z Drainage of Intracranial Subdural Space with Drainage Device, Open Approach

00940ZX Drainage of Intracranial Subdural Space, Open Approach, Diagnostic

00940ZZ Drainage of Intracranial Subdural Space, Open Approach

009430Z Drainage of Intracranial Subdural Space with Drainage Device, Percutaneous Approach
AHA CC: 3Q, 2015, 11-12

00943ZX Drainage of Intracranial Subdural Space, Percutaneous Approach, Diagnostic

00943ZZ Drainage of Intracranial Subdural Space, Percutaneous Approach

009440Z Drainage of Intracranial Subdural Space with Drainage Device, Percutaneous Endoscopic Approach

00944ZX Drainage of Intracranial Subdural Space, Percutaneous Endoscopic Approach, Diagnostic

00944ZZ Drainage of Intracranial Subdural Space, Percutaneous Endoscopic Approach

009500Z Drainage of Intracranial Subarachnoid Space with Drainage Device, Open Approach

00950ZX Drainage of Intracranial Subarachnoid Space, Open Approach, Diagnostic

00950ZZ Drainage of Intracranial Subarachnoid Space, Open Approach

009530Z Drainage of Intracranial Subarachnoid Space with Drainage Device, Percutaneous Approach

00953ZX Drainage of Intracranial Subarachnoid Space, Percutaneous Approach, Diagnostic

00953ZZ Drainage of Intracranial Subarachnoid Space, Percutaneous Approach

009540Z Drainage of Intracranial Subarachnoid Space with Drainage Device, Percutaneous Endoscopic Approach

00954ZX Drainage of Intracranial Subarachnoid Space, Percutaneous Endoscopic Approach, Diagnostic

00954ZZ Drainage of Intracranial Subarachnoid Space, Percutaneous Endoscopic Approach

009600Z Drainage of Cerebral Ventricle with Drainage Device, Open Approach

00960ZX Drainage of Cerebral Ventricle, Open Approach, Diagnostic

00960ZZ Drainage of Cerebral Ventricle, Open Approach

009630Z Drainage of Cerebral Ventricle with Drainage Device, Percutaneous Approach
AHA CC: 3Q, 2015, 12-13

00963ZX Drainage of Cerebral Ventricle, Percutaneous Approach, Diagnostic

00963ZZ Drainage of Cerebral Ventricle, Percutaneous Approach

009640Z Drainage of Cerebral Ventricle with Drainage Device, Percutaneous Endoscopic Approach

00964ZX Drainage of Cerebral Ventricle, Percutaneous Endoscopic Approach, Diagnostic

00964ZZ Drainage of Cerebral Ventricle, Percutaneous Endoscopic Approach

009700Z Drainage of Cerebral Hemisphere with Drainage Device, Open Approach

00970ZX Drainage of Cerebral Hemisphere, Open Approach, Diagnostic

00970ZZ Drainage of Cerebral Hemisphere, Open Approach

009730Z Drainage of Cerebral Hemisphere with Drainage Device, Percutaneous Approach

00973ZX Drainage of Cerebral Hemisphere, Percutaneous Approach, Diagnostic

00973ZZ Drainage of Cerebral Hemisphere, Percutaneous Approach

009740Z Drainage of Cerebral Hemisphere with Drainage Device, Percutaneous Endoscopic Approach

00974ZX Drainage of Cerebral Hemisphere, Percutaneous Endoscopic Approach, Diagnostic

00974ZZ Drainage of Cerebral Hemisphere, Percutaneous Endoscopic Approach

009800Z Drainage of Basal Ganglia with Drainage Device, Open Approach

00980ZX Drainage of Basal Ganglia, Open Approach, Diagnostic

00980ZZ Drainage of Basal Ganglia, Open Approach

009830Z Drainage of Basal Ganglia with Drainage Device, Percutaneous Approach

00983ZX Drainage of Basal Ganglia, Percutaneous Approach, Diagnostic

00983ZZ Drainage of Basal Ganglia, Percutaneous Approach

009840Z Drainage of Basal Ganglia with Drainage Device, Percutaneous Endoscopic Approach

00984ZX Drainage of Basal Ganglia, Percutaneous Endoscopic Approach, Diagnostic

00984ZZ Drainage of Basal Ganglia, Percutaneous Endoscopic Approach

009900Z Drainage of Thalamus with Drainage Device, Open Approach

00990ZX Drainage of Thalamus, Open Approach, Diagnostic

00990ZZ Drainage of Thalamus, Open Approach

009930Z Drainage of Thalamus with Drainage Device, Percutaneous Approach

00993ZX Drainage of Thalamus, Percutaneous Approach, Diagnostic

00993ZZ Drainage of Thalamus, Percutaneous Approach

009940Z Drainage of Thalamus with Drainage Device, Percutaneous Endoscopic Approach

00994ZX Drainage of Thalamus, Percutaneous Endoscopic Approach, Diagnostic

00994ZZ Drainage of Thalamus, Percutaneous Endoscopic Approach

009A00Z Drainage of Hypothalamus with Drainage Device, Open Approach

009A0ZX Drainage of Hypothalamus, Open Approach, Diagnostic

009A0ZZ Drainage of Hypothalamus, Open Approach

009A30Z Drainage of Hypothalamus with Drainage Device, Percutaneous Approach

009A3ZX Drainage of Hypothalamus, Percutaneous Approach, Diagnostic

009A3ZZ Drainage of Hypothalamus, Percutaneous Approach

009A40Z Drainage of Hypothalamus with Drainage Device, Percutaneous Endoscopic Approach

009A4ZX Drainage of Hypothalamus, Percutaneous Endoscopic Approach, Diagnostic

009A4ZZ Drainage of Hypothalamus, Percutaneous Endoscopic Approach

009B00Z Drainage of Pons with Drainage Device, Open Approach

009B0ZX Drainage of Pons, Open Approach, Diagnostic

009B0ZZ Drainage of Pons, Open Approach

009B30Z Drainage of Pons with Drainage Device, Percutaneous Approach

009B3ZX Drainage of Pons, Percutaneous Approach, Diagnostic

009B3ZZ Drainage of Pons, Percutaneous Approach

009B40Z Drainage of Pons with Drainage Device, Percutaneous Endoscopic Approach

009B4ZX Drainage of Pons, Percutaneous Endoscopic Approach, Diagnostic

009B4ZZ Drainage of Pons, Percutaneous Endoscopic Approach

009C00Z Drainage of Cerebellum with Drainage Device, Open Approach

009C0ZX Drainage of Cerebellum, Open Approach, Diagnostic

009C0ZZ Drainage of Cerebellum, Open Approach

009C30Z Drainage of Cerebellum with Drainage Device, Percutaneous Approach

009C3ZX Drainage of Cerebellum, Percutaneous Approach, Diagnostic

009C3ZZ Drainage of Cerebellum, Percutaneous Approach

009C40Z Drainage of Cerebellum with Drainage Device, Percutaneous Endoscopic Approach

009C4ZX Drainage of Cerebellum, Percutaneous Endoscopic Approach, Diagnostic

009C4ZZ Drainage of Cerebellum, Percutaneous Endoscopic Approach

009D00Z Drainage of Medulla Oblongata with Drainage Device, Open Approach

009D0ZX Drainage of Medulla Oblongata, Open Approach, Diagnostic

009D0ZZ Drainage of Medulla Oblongata, Open Approach

009D30Z Drainage of Medulla Oblongata with Drainage Device, Percutaneous Approach

009D3ZX Drainage of Medulla Oblongata, Percutaneous Approach, Diagnostic

009D3ZZ Drainage of Medulla Oblongata, Percutaneous Approach

009D40Z Drainage of Medulla Oblongata with Drainage Device, Percutaneous Endoscopic Approach

009D4ZX Drainage of Medulla Oblongata, Percutaneous Endoscopic Approach, Diagnostic

009D4ZZ Drainage of Medulla Oblongata, Percutaneous Endoscopic Approach

009F00Z Drainage of Olfactory Nerve with Drainage Device, Open Approach

009F0ZX Drainage of Olfactory Nerve, Open Approach, Diagnostic

009F0ZZ Drainage of Olfactory Nerve, Open Approach

009F30Z Drainage of Olfactory Nerve with Drainage Device, Percutaneous Approach

♀ Female-only   ♂ Male-only   ▲ Limited Coverage   ● Non-OR   ▦ HAC-associated procedure   ▲ Non-covered procedures   ✚ Cluster

009F3ZX Drainage of Olfactory Nerve, Percutaneous Approach, Diagnostic
009F3ZZ Drainage of Olfactory Nerve, Percutaneous Approach
009F40Z Drainage of Olfactory Nerve with Drainage Device, Percutaneous Endoscopic Approach
009F4ZX Drainage of Olfactory Nerve, Percutaneous Endoscopic Approach, Diagnostic
009F4ZZ Drainage of Olfactory Nerve, Percutaneous Endoscopic Approach
009G00Z Drainage of Optic Nerve with Drainage Device, Open Approach
009G0ZX Drainage of Optic Nerve, Open Approach, Diagnostic
009G0ZZ Drainage of Optic Nerve, Open Approach
009G30Z Drainage of Optic Nerve with Drainage Device, Percutaneous Approach
009G3ZX Drainage of Optic Nerve, Percutaneous Approach, Diagnostic
009G3ZZ Drainage of Optic Nerve, Percutaneous Approach
009G40Z Drainage of Optic Nerve with Drainage Device, Percutaneous Endoscopic Approach
009G4ZX Drainage of Optic Nerve, Percutaneous Endoscopic Approach, Diagnostic
009G4ZZ Drainage of Optic Nerve, Percutaneous Endoscopic Approach
009H00Z Drainage of Oculomotor Nerve with Drainage Device, Open Approach
009H0ZX Drainage of Oculomotor Nerve, Open Approach, Diagnostic
009H0ZZ Drainage of Oculomotor Nerve, Open Approach
009H30Z Drainage of Oculomotor Nerve with Drainage Device, Percutaneous Approach
009H3ZX Drainage of Oculomotor Nerve, Percutaneous Approach, Diagnostic
009H3ZZ Drainage of Oculomotor Nerve, Percutaneous Approach
009H40Z Drainage of Oculomotor Nerve with Drainage Device, Percutaneous Endoscopic Approach
009H4ZX Drainage of Oculomotor Nerve, Percutaneous Endoscopic Approach, Diagnostic
009H4ZZ Drainage of Oculomotor Nerve, Percutaneous Endoscopic Approach
009J00Z Drainage of Trochlear Nerve with Drainage Device, Open Approach
009J0ZX Drainage of Trochlear Nerve, Open Approach, Diagnostic
009J0ZZ Drainage of Trochlear Nerve, Open Approach
009J30Z Drainage of Trochlear Nerve with Drainage Device, Percutaneous Approach
009J3ZX Drainage of Trochlear Nerve, Percutaneous Approach, Diagnostic
009J3ZZ Drainage of Trochlear Nerve, Percutaneous Approach
009J40Z Drainage of Trochlear Nerve with Drainage Device, Percutaneous Endoscopic Approach
009J4ZX Drainage of Trochlear Nerve, Percutaneous Endoscopic Approach, Diagnostic
009J4ZZ Drainage of Trochlear Nerve, Percutaneous Endoscopic Approach
009K00Z Drainage of Trigeminal Nerve with Drainage Device, Open Approach
009K0ZX Drainage of Trigeminal Nerve, Open Approach, Diagnostic

009K0ZZ Drainage of Trigeminal Nerve, Open Approach
009K30Z Drainage of Trigeminal Nerve with Drainage Device, Percutaneous Approach
009K3ZX Drainage of Trigeminal Nerve, Percutaneous Approach, Diagnostic
009K3ZZ Drainage of Trigeminal Nerve, Percutaneous Approach
009K40Z Drainage of Trigeminal Nerve with Drainage Device, Percutaneous Endoscopic Approach
009K4ZX Drainage of Trigeminal Nerve, Percutaneous Endoscopic Approach, Diagnostic
009K4ZZ Drainage of Trigeminal Nerve, Percutaneous Endoscopic Approach
009L00Z Drainage of Abducens Nerve with Drainage Device, Open Approach
009L0ZX Drainage of Abducens Nerve, Open Approach, Diagnostic
009L0ZZ Drainage of Abducens Nerve, Open Approach
009L30Z Drainage of Abducens Nerve with Drainage Device, Percutaneous Approach
009L3ZX Drainage of Abducens Nerve, Percutaneous Approach, Diagnostic
009L3ZZ Drainage of Abducens Nerve, Percutaneous Approach
009L40Z Drainage of Abducens Nerve with Drainage Device, Percutaneous Endoscopic Approach
009L4ZX Drainage of Abducens Nerve, Percutaneous Endoscopic Approach, Diagnostic
009L4ZZ Drainage of Abducens Nerve, Percutaneous Endoscopic Approach
009M00Z Drainage of Facial Nerve with Drainage Device, Open Approach
009M0ZX Drainage of Facial Nerve, Open Approach, Diagnostic
009M0ZZ Drainage of Facial Nerve, Open Approach
009M30Z Drainage of Facial Nerve with Drainage Device, Percutaneous Approach
009M3ZX Drainage of Facial Nerve, Percutaneous Approach, Diagnostic
009M3ZZ Drainage of Facial Nerve, Percutaneous Approach
009M40Z Drainage of Facial Nerve with Drainage Device, Percutaneous Endoscopic Approach
009M4ZX Drainage of Facial Nerve, Percutaneous Endoscopic Approach, Diagnostic
009M4ZZ Drainage of Facial Nerve, Percutaneous Endoscopic Approach
009N00Z Drainage of Acoustic Nerve with Drainage Device, Open Approach
009N0ZX Drainage of Acoustic Nerve, Open Approach, Diagnostic
009N0ZZ Drainage of Acoustic Nerve, Open Approach
009N30Z Drainage of Acoustic Nerve with Drainage Device, Percutaneous Approach
009N3ZX Drainage of Acoustic Nerve, Percutaneous Approach, Diagnostic
009N3ZZ Drainage of Acoustic Nerve, Percutaneous Approach
009N40Z Drainage of Acoustic Nerve with Drainage Device, Percutaneous Endoscopic Approach
009N4ZX Drainage of Acoustic Nerve, Percutaneous Endoscopic Approach, Diagnostic

009N4ZZ Drainage of Acoustic Nerve, Percutaneous Endoscopic Approach
009P00Z Drainage of Glossopharyngeal Nerve with Drainage Device, Open Approach
009P0ZX Drainage of Glossopharyngeal Nerve, Open Approach, Diagnostic
009P0ZZ Drainage of Glossopharyngeal Nerve, Open Approach
009P30Z Drainage of Glossopharyngeal Nerve with Drainage Device, Percutaneous Approach
009P3ZX Drainage of Glossopharyngeal Nerve, Percutaneous Approach, Diagnostic
009P3ZZ Drainage of Glossopharyngeal Nerve, Percutaneous Approach
009P40Z Drainage of Glossopharyngeal Nerve with Drainage Device, Percutaneous Endoscopic Approach
009P4ZX Drainage of Glossopharyngeal Nerve, Percutaneous Endoscopic Approach, Diagnostic
009P4ZZ Drainage of Glossopharyngeal Nerve, Percutaneous Endoscopic Approach
009Q00Z Drainage of Vagus Nerve with Drainage Device, Open Approach
009Q0ZX Drainage of Vagus Nerve, Open Approach, Diagnostic
009Q0ZZ Drainage of Vagus Nerve, Open Approach
009Q30Z Drainage of Vagus Nerve with Drainage Device, Percutaneous Approach
009Q3ZX Drainage of Vagus Nerve, Percutaneous Approach, Diagnostic
009Q3ZZ Drainage of Vagus Nerve, Percutaneous Approach
009Q40Z Drainage of Vagus Nerve with Drainage Device, Percutaneous Endoscopic Approach
009Q4ZX Drainage of Vagus Nerve, Percutaneous Endoscopic Approach, Diagnostic
009Q4ZZ Drainage of Vagus Nerve, Percutaneous Endoscopic Approach
009R00Z Drainage of Accessory Nerve with Drainage Device, Open Approach
009R0ZX Drainage of Accessory Nerve, Open Approach, Diagnostic
009R0ZZ Drainage of Accessory Nerve, Open Approach
009R30Z Drainage of Accessory Nerve with Drainage Device, Percutaneous Approach
009R3ZX Drainage of Accessory Nerve, Percutaneous Approach, Diagnostic
009R3ZZ Drainage of Accessory Nerve, Percutaneous Approach
009R40Z Drainage of Accessory Nerve with Drainage Device, Percutaneous Endoscopic Approach
009R4ZX Drainage of Accessory Nerve, Percutaneous Endoscopic Approach, Diagnostic
009R4ZZ Drainage of Accessory Nerve, Percutaneous Endoscopic Approach
009S00Z Drainage of Hypoglossal Nerve with Drainage Device, Open Approach
009S0ZX Drainage of Hypoglossal Nerve, Open Approach, Diagnostic
009S0ZZ Drainage of Hypoglossal Nerve, Open Approach
009S30Z Drainage of Hypoglossal Nerve with Drainage Device, Percutaneous Approach
009S3ZX Drainage of Hypoglossal Nerve, Percutaneous Approach, Diagnostic
009S3ZZ Drainage of Hypoglossal Nerve, Percutaneous Approach

009S40Z Drainage of Hypoglossal Nerve with Drainage Device, Percutaneous Endoscopic Approach

009S4ZX Drainage of Hypoglossal Nerve, Percutaneous Endoscopic Approach, Diagnostic

009S4ZZ Drainage of Hypoglossal Nerve, Percutaneous Endoscopic Approach

009T00Z Drainage of Spinal Meninges with Drainage Device, Open Approach

009T0ZX Drainage of Spinal Meninges, Open Approach, Diagnostic

009T0ZZ Drainage of Spinal Meninges, Open Approach

009T30Z Drainage of Spinal Meninges with Drainage Device, Percutaneous Approach

009T3ZX Drainage of Spinal Meninges, Percutaneous Approach, Diagnostic

009T3ZZ Drainage of Spinal Meninges, Percutaneous Approach

009T40Z Drainage of Spinal Meninges with Drainage Device, Percutaneous Endoscopic Approach

009T4ZX Drainage of Spinal Meninges, Percutaneous Endoscopic Approach, Diagnostic

009T4ZZ Drainage of Spinal Meninges, Percutaneous Endoscopic Approach

009U00Z Drainage of Spinal Canal with Drainage Device, Open Approach
AHA CC: 4Q, 2018, 85

009U0ZX Drainage of Spinal Canal, Open Approach, Diagnostic

009U0ZZ Drainage of Spinal Canal, Open Approach

009U30Z Drainage of Spinal Canal with Drainage Device, Percutaneous Approach

009U3ZX Drainage of Spinal Canal, Percutaneous Approach, Diagnostic
AHA CC: 1Q, 2014, 8

009U3ZZ Drainage of Spinal Canal, Percutaneous Approach

009U40Z Drainage of Spinal Canal with Drainage Device, Percutaneous Endoscopic Approach

009U4ZX Drainage of Spinal Canal, Percutaneous Endoscopic Approach, Diagnostic

009U4ZZ Drainage of Spinal Canal, Percutaneous Endoscopic Approach

009W00Z Drainage of Cervical Spinal Cord with Drainage Device, Open Approach
AHA CC: 2Q, 2015, 30

009W0ZX Drainage of Cervical Spinal Cord, Open Approach, Diagnostic

009W0ZZ Drainage of Cervical Spinal Cord, Open Approach

009W30Z Drainage of Cervical Spinal Cord with Drainage Device, Percutaneous Approach

009W3ZX Drainage of Cervical Spinal Cord, Percutaneous Approach, Diagnostic

009W3ZZ Drainage of Cervical Spinal Cord, Percutaneous Approach

009W40Z Drainage of Cervical Spinal Cord with Drainage Device, Percutaneous Endoscopic Approach

009W4ZX Drainage of Cervical Spinal Cord, Percutaneous Endoscopic Approach, Diagnostic

009W4ZZ Drainage of Cervical Spinal Cord, Percutaneous Endoscopic Approach

009X00Z Drainage of Thoracic Spinal Cord with Drainage Device, Open Approach

009X0ZX Drainage of Thoracic Spinal Cord, Open Approach, Diagnostic

009X0ZZ Drainage of Thoracic Spinal Cord, Open Approach

009X30Z Drainage of Thoracic Spinal Cord with Drainage Device, Percutaneous Approach

009X3ZX Drainage of Thoracic Spinal Cord, Percutaneous Approach, Diagnostic

009X3ZZ Drainage of Thoracic Spinal Cord, Percutaneous Approach

009X40Z Drainage of Thoracic Spinal Cord with Drainage Device, Percutaneous Endoscopic Approach

009X4ZX Drainage of Thoracic Spinal Cord, Percutaneous Endoscopic Approach, Diagnostic

009X4ZZ Drainage of Thoracic Spinal Cord, Percutaneous Endoscopic Approach

009Y00Z Drainage of Lumbar Spinal Cord with Drainage Device, Open Approach

009Y0ZX Drainage of Lumbar Spinal Cord, Open Approach, Diagnostic

009Y0ZZ Drainage of Lumbar Spinal Cord, Open Approach

009Y30Z Drainage of Lumbar Spinal Cord with Drainage Device, Percutaneous Approach

009Y3ZX Drainage of Lumbar Spinal Cord, Percutaneous Approach, Diagnostic

009Y3ZZ Drainage of Lumbar Spinal Cord, Percutaneous Approach

009Y40Z Drainage of Lumbar Spinal Cord with Drainage Device, Percutaneous Endoscopic Approach

009Y4ZX Drainage of Lumbar Spinal Cord, Percutaneous Endoscopic Approach, Diagnostic

009Y4ZZ Drainage of Lumbar Spinal Cord, Percutaneous Endoscopic Approach

00B – Central Nervous System and Cranial Nerves, Excision

Review Coding Guidelines B3.4a and B3.4b

Review Coding Guideline B3.8

Review Coding Guideline B3.18

00B00ZX Excision of Brain, Open Approach, Diagnostic
AHA CC: 1Q, 2015, 12-13

00B00ZZ Excision of Brain, Open Approach

00B03ZX Excision of Brain, Percutaneous Approach, Diagnostic

00B03ZZ Excision of Brain, Percutaneous Approach

00B04ZX Excision of Brain, Percutaneous Endoscopic Approach, Diagnostic

00B04ZZ Excision of Brain, Percutaneous Endoscopic Approach

00B10ZX Excision of Cerebral Meninges, Open Approach, Diagnostic

00B10ZZ Excision of Cerebral Meninges, Open Approach

00B13ZX Excision of Cerebral Meninges, Percutaneous Approach, Diagnostic

00B13ZZ Excision of Cerebral Meninges, Percutaneous Approach

00B14ZX Excision of Cerebral Meninges, Percutaneous Endoscopic Approach, Diagnostic

00B14ZZ Excision of Cerebral Meninges, Percutaneous Endoscopic Approach

00B20ZX Excision of Dura Mater, Open Approach, Diagnostic

00B20ZZ Excision of Dura Mater, Open Approach

00B23ZX Excision of Dura Mater, Percutaneous Approach, Diagnostic

00B23ZZ Excision of Dura Mater, Percutaneous Approach

00B24ZX Excision of Dura Mater, Percutaneous Endoscopic Approach, Diagnostic

00B24ZZ Excision of Dura Mater, Percutaneous Endoscopic Approach

00B60ZX Excision of Cerebral Ventricle, Open Approach, Diagnostic

00B60ZZ Excision of Cerebral Ventricle, Open Approach

00B63ZX Excision of Cerebral Ventricle, Percutaneous Approach, Diagnostic

00B63ZZ Excision of Cerebral Ventricle, Percutaneous Approach

00B64ZX Excision of Cerebral Ventricle, Percutaneous Endoscopic Approach, Diagnostic

00B64ZZ Excision of Cerebral Ventricle, Percutaneous Endoscopic Approach

00B70ZX Excision of Cerebral Hemisphere, Open Approach, Diagnostic

00B70ZZ Excision of Cerebral Hemisphere, Open Approach
AHA CC: 4Q, 2014, 34-35; 2Q, 2016, 18

00B73ZX Excision of Cerebral Hemisphere, Percutaneous Approach, Diagnostic

00B73ZZ Excision of Cerebral Hemisphere, Percutaneous Approach

00B74ZX Excision of Cerebral Hemisphere, Percutaneous Endoscopic Approach, Diagnostic

00B74ZZ Excision of Cerebral Hemisphere, Percutaneous Endoscopic Approach

00B80ZX Excision of Basal Ganglia, Open Approach, Diagnostic

00B80ZZ Excision of Basal Ganglia, Open Approach

00B83ZX Excision of Basal Ganglia, Percutaneous Approach, Diagnostic

00B83ZZ Excision of Basal Ganglia, Percutaneous Approach

00B84ZX Excision of Basal Ganglia, Percutaneous Endoscopic Approach, Diagnostic

00B84ZZ Excision of Basal Ganglia, Percutaneous Endoscopic Approach

00B90ZX Excision of Thalamus, Open Approach, Diagnostic

00B90ZZ Excision of Thalamus, Open Approach

00B93ZX Excision of Thalamus, Percutaneous Approach, Diagnostic

00B93ZZ Excision of Thalamus, Percutaneous Approach

00B94ZX Excision of Thalamus, Percutaneous Endoscopic Approach, Diagnostic

♀ Female-only   ♂ Male-only   ▲ Limited Coverage   ● Non-OR   🅷🅰🅲 HAC-associated procedure   ▲ Non-covered procedures   ✚ Cluster

00B94ZZ	Excision of Thalamus, Percutaneous Endoscopic Approach
00BA0ZX	Excision of Hypothalamus, Open Approach, Diagnostic
00BA0ZZ	Excision of Hypothalamus, Open Approach
00BA3ZX	Excision of Hypothalamus, Percutaneous Approach, Diagnostic
00BA3ZZ	Excision of Hypothalamus, Percutaneous Approach
00BA4ZX	Excision of Hypothalamus, Percutaneous Endoscopic Approach, Diagnostic
00BA4ZZ	Excision of Hypothalamus, Percutaneous Endoscopic Approach
00BB0ZX	Excision of Pons, Open Approach, Diagnostic
00BB0ZZ	Excision of Pons, Open Approach
00BB3ZX	Excision of Pons, Percutaneous Approach, Diagnostic
00BB3ZZ	Excision of Pons, Percutaneous Approach
00BB4ZX	Excision of Pons, Percutaneous Endoscopic Approach, Diagnostic
00BB4ZZ	Excision of Pons, Percutaneous Endoscopic Approach
00BC0ZX	Excision of Cerebellum, Open Approach, Diagnostic
00BC0ZZ	Excision of Cerebellum, Open Approach
00BC3ZX	Excision of Cerebellum, Percutaneous Approach, Diagnostic
00BC3ZZ	Excision of Cerebellum, Percutaneous Approach
00BC4ZX	Excision of Cerebellum, Percutaneous Endoscopic Approach, Diagnostic
00BC4ZZ	Excision of Cerebellum, Percutaneous Endoscopic Approach
00BD0ZX	Excision of Medulla Oblongata, Open Approach, Diagnostic
00BD0ZZ	Excision of Medulla Oblongata, Open Approach
00BD3ZX	Excision of Medulla Oblongata, Percutaneous Approach, Diagnostic
00BD3ZZ	Excision of Medulla Oblongata, Percutaneous Approach
00BD4ZX	Excision of Medulla Oblongata, Percutaneous Endoscopic Approach, Diagnostic
00BD4ZZ	Excision of Medulla Oblongata, Percutaneous Endoscopic Approach
00BF0ZX	Excision of Olfactory Nerve, Open Approach, Diagnostic
00BF0ZZ	Excision of Olfactory Nerve, Open Approach
00BF3ZX	Excision of Olfactory Nerve, Percutaneous Approach, Diagnostic
00BF3ZZ	Excision of Olfactory Nerve, Percutaneous Approach
00BF4ZX	Excision of Olfactory Nerve, Percutaneous Endoscopic Approach, Diagnostic
00BF4ZZ	Excision of Olfactory Nerve, Percutaneous Endoscopic Approach
00BG0ZX	Excision of Optic Nerve, Open Approach, Diagnostic
00BG0ZZ	Excision of Optic Nerve, Open Approach
00BG3ZX	Excision of Optic Nerve, Percutaneous Approach, Diagnostic
00BG3ZZ	Excision of Optic Nerve, Percutaneous Approach
00BG4ZX	Excision of Optic Nerve, Percutaneous Endoscopic Approach, Diagnostic
00BG4ZZ	Excision of Optic Nerve, Percutaneous Endoscopic Approach

00BH0ZX	Excision of Oculomotor Nerve, Open Approach, Diagnostic
00BH0ZZ	Excision of Oculomotor Nerve, Open Approach
00BH3ZX	Excision of Oculomotor Nerve, Percutaneous Approach, Diagnostic
00BH3ZZ	Excision of Oculomotor Nerve, Percutaneous Approach
00BH4ZX	Excision of Oculomotor Nerve, Percutaneous Endoscopic Approach, Diagnostic
00BH4ZZ	Excision of Oculomotor Nerve, Percutaneous Endoscopic Approach
00BJ0ZX	Excision of Trochlear Nerve, Open Approach, Diagnostic
00BJ0ZZ	Excision of Trochlear Nerve, Open Approach
00BJ3ZX	Excision of Trochlear Nerve, Percutaneous Approach, Diagnostic
00BJ3ZZ	Excision of Trochlear Nerve, Percutaneous Approach
00BJ4ZX	Excision of Trochlear Nerve, Percutaneous Endoscopic Approach, Diagnostic
00BJ4ZZ	Excision of Trochlear Nerve, Percutaneous Endoscopic Approach
00BK0ZX	Excision of Trigeminal Nerve, Open Approach, Diagnostic
00BK0ZZ	Excision of Trigeminal Nerve, Open Approach
00BK3ZX	Excision of Trigeminal Nerve, Percutaneous Approach, Diagnostic
00BK3ZZ	Excision of Trigeminal Nerve, Percutaneous Approach
00BK4ZX	Excision of Trigeminal Nerve, Percutaneous Endoscopic Approach, Diagnostic
00BK4ZZ	Excision of Trigeminal Nerve, Percutaneous Endoscopic Approach
00BL0ZX	Excision of Abducens Nerve, Open Approach, Diagnostic
00BL0ZZ	Excision of Abducens Nerve, Open Approach
00BL3ZX	Excision of Abducens Nerve, Percutaneous Approach, Diagnostic
00BL3ZZ	Excision of Abducens Nerve, Percutaneous Approach
00BL4ZX	Excision of Abducens Nerve, Percutaneous Endoscopic Approach, Diagnostic
00BL4ZZ	Excision of Abducens Nerve, Percutaneous Endoscopic Approach
00BM0ZX	Excision of Facial Nerve, Open Approach, Diagnostic
00BM0ZZ	Excision of Facial Nerve, Open Approach
	AHA CC: 2Q, 2016, 12-14
00BM3ZX	Excision of Facial Nerve, Percutaneous Approach, Diagnostic
00BM3ZZ	Excision of Facial Nerve, Percutaneous Approach
00BM4ZX	Excision of Facial Nerve, Percutaneous Endoscopic Approach, Diagnostic
00BM4ZZ	Excision of Facial Nerve, Percutaneous Endoscopic Approach
00BN0ZX	Excision of Acoustic Nerve, Open Approach, Diagnostic
00BN0ZZ	Excision of Acoustic Nerve, Open Approach
00BN3ZX	Excision of Acoustic Nerve, Percutaneous Approach, Diagnostic
00BN3ZZ	Excision of Acoustic Nerve, Percutaneous Approach
00BN4ZX	Excision of Acoustic Nerve, Percutaneous Endoscopic Approach, Diagnostic

00BN4ZZ	Excision of Acoustic Nerve, Percutaneous Endoscopic Approach
00BP0ZX	Excision of Glossopharyngeal Nerve, Open Approach, Diagnostic
00BP0ZZ	Excision of Glossopharyngeal Nerve, Open Approach
00BP3ZX	Excision of Glossopharyngeal Nerve, Percutaneous Approach, Diagnostic
00BP3ZZ	Excision of Glossopharyngeal Nerve, Percutaneous Approach
00BP4ZX	Excision of Glossopharyngeal Nerve, Percutaneous Endoscopic Approach, Diagnostic
00BP4ZZ	Excision of Glossopharyngeal Nerve, Percutaneous Endoscopic Approach
00BQ0ZX	Excision of Vagus Nerve, Open Approach, Diagnostic
00BQ0ZZ	Excision of Vagus Nerve, Open Approach
00BQ3ZX	Excision of Vagus Nerve, Percutaneous Approach, Diagnostic
00BQ3ZZ	Excision of Vagus Nerve, Percutaneous Approach
00BQ4ZX	Excision of Vagus Nerve, Percutaneous Endoscopic Approach, Diagnostic
00BQ4ZZ	Excision of Vagus Nerve, Percutaneous Endoscopic Approach
00BR0ZX	Excision of Accessory Nerve, Open Approach, Diagnostic
00BR0ZZ	Excision of Accessory Nerve, Open Approach
	AHA CC: 2Q, 2016, 12-14
00BR3ZX	Excision of Accessory Nerve, Percutaneous Approach, Diagnostic
00BR3ZZ	Excision of Accessory Nerve, Percutaneous Approach
00BR4ZX	Excision of Accessory Nerve, Percutaneous Endoscopic Approach, Diagnostic
00BR4ZZ	Excision of Accessory Nerve, Percutaneous Endoscopic Approach
00BS0ZX	Excision of Hypoglossal Nerve, Open Approach, Diagnostic
00BS0ZZ	Excision of Hypoglossal Nerve, Open Approach
	AHA CC: 2Q, 2016, 12-14
00BS3ZX	Excision of Hypoglossal Nerve, Percutaneous Approach, Diagnostic
00BS3ZZ	Excision of Hypoglossal Nerve, Percutaneous Approach
00BS4ZX	Excision of Hypoglossal Nerve, Percutaneous Endoscopic Approach, Diagnostic
00BS4ZZ	Excision of Hypoglossal Nerve, Percutaneous Endoscopic Approach
00BT0ZX	Excision of Spinal Meninges, Open Approach, Diagnostic
00BT0ZZ	Excision of Spinal Meninges, Open Approach
00BT3ZX	Excision of Spinal Meninges, Percutaneous Approach, Diagnostic
00BT3ZZ	Excision of Spinal Meninges, Percutaneous Approach
00BT4ZX	Excision of Spinal Meninges, Percutaneous Endoscopic Approach, Diagnostic
00BT4ZZ	Excision of Spinal Meninges, Percutaneous Endoscopic Approach
00BW0ZX	Excision of Cervical Spinal Cord, Open Approach, Diagnostic
00BW0ZZ	Excision of Cervical Spinal Cord, Open Approach
00BW3ZX	Excision of Cervical Spinal Cord, Percutaneous Approach, Diagnostic
00BW3ZZ	Excision of Cervical Spinal Cord, Percutaneous Approach

00BW4ZX	Excision of Cervical Spinal Cord, Percutaneous Endoscopic Approach, Diagnostic	**00BX3ZZ**	Excision of Thoracic Spinal Cord, Percutaneous Approach	**00BY3ZX**	Excision of Lumbar Spinal Cord, Percutaneous Approach, Diagnostic
00BW4ZZ	Excision of Cervical Spinal Cord, Percutaneous Endoscopic Approach	**00BX4ZX**	Excision of Thoracic Spinal Cord, Percutaneous Endoscopic Approach, Diagnostic	**00BY3ZZ**	Excision of Lumbar Spinal Cord, Percutaneous Approach
00BX0ZX	Excision of Thoracic Spinal Cord, Open Approach, Diagnostic	**00BX4ZZ**	Excision of Thoracic Spinal Cord, Percutaneous Endoscopic Approach	**00BY4ZX**	Excision of Lumbar Spinal Cord, Percutaneous Endoscopic Approach, Diagnostic
00BX0ZZ	Excision of Thoracic Spinal Cord, Open Approach	**00BY0ZX**	Excision of Lumbar Spinal Cord, Open Approach, Diagnostic	**00BY4ZZ**	Excision of Lumbar Spinal Cord, Percutaneous Endoscopic Approach
00BX3ZX	Excision of Thoracic Spinal Cord, Percutaneous Approach, Diagnostic	**00BY0ZZ**	Excision of Lumbar Spinal Cord, Open Approach		
			AHA CC: 3Q, 2014, 24		

00C – Central Nervous System and Cranial Nerves, Extirpation

00C00ZZ	Extirpation of Matter from Brain, Open Approach	**00C73ZZ**	Extirpation of Matter from Cerebral Hemisphere, Percutaneous Approach	**00CH0ZZ**	Extirpation of Matter from Oculomotor Nerve, Open Approach
	AHA CC: 1Q, 2015, 12-13; 4Q, 2016, 27-28	**00C74ZZ**	Extirpation of Matter from Cerebral Hemisphere, Percutaneous Endoscopic Approach	**00CH3ZZ**	Extirpation of Matter from Oculomotor Nerve, Percutaneous Approach
00C03ZZ	Extirpation of Matter from Brain, Percutaneous Approach		*AHA CC: 3Q, 2015, 13*	**00CH4ZZ**	Extirpation of Matter from Oculomotor Nerve, Percutaneous Endoscopic Approach
00C04ZZ	Extirpation of Matter from Brain, Percutaneous Endoscopic Approach	**00C80ZZ**	Extirpation of Matter from Basal Ganglia, Open Approach	**00CJ0ZZ**	Extirpation of Matter from Trochlear Nerve, Open Approach
	AHA CC: 2Q, 2019, 36-37	**00C83ZZ**	Extirpation of Matter from Basal Ganglia, Percutaneous Approach	**00CJ3ZZ**	Extirpation of Matter from Trochlear Nerve, Percutaneous Approach
00C10ZZ	Extirpation of Matter from Cerebral Meninges, Open Approach	**00C84ZZ**	Extirpation of Matter from Basal Ganglia, Percutaneous Endoscopic Approach	**00CJ4ZZ**	Extirpation of Matter from Trochlear Nerve, Percutaneous Endoscopic Approach
00C13ZZ	Extirpation of Matter from Cerebral Meninges, Percutaneous Approach	**00C90ZZ**	Extirpation of Matter from Thalamus, Open Approach	**00CK0ZZ**	Extirpation of Matter from Trigeminal Nerve, Open Approach
00C14ZZ	Extirpation of Matter from Cerebral Meninges, Percutaneous Endoscopic Approach	**00C93ZZ**	Extirpation of Matter from Thalamus, Percutaneous Approach	**00CK3ZZ**	Extirpation of Matter from Trigeminal Nerve, Percutaneous Approach
00C20ZZ	Extirpation of Matter from Dura Mater, Open Approach	**00C94ZZ**	Extirpation of Matter from Thalamus, Percutaneous Endoscopic Approach	**00CK4ZZ**	Extirpation of Matter from Trigeminal Nerve, Percutaneous Endoscopic Approach
00C23ZZ	Extirpation of Matter from Dura Mater, Percutaneous Approach	**00CA0ZZ**	Extirpation of Matter from Hypothalamus, Open Approach	**00CL0ZZ**	Extirpation of Matter from Abducens Nerve, Open Approach
00C24ZZ	Extirpation of Matter from Dura Mater, Percutaneous Endoscopic Approach	**00CA3ZZ**	Extirpation of Matter from Hypothalamus, Percutaneous Approach	**00CL3ZZ**	Extirpation of Matter from Abducens Nerve, Percutaneous Approach
00C30ZZ	Extirpation of Matter from Intracranial Epidural Space, Open Approach	**00CA4ZZ**	Extirpation of Matter from Hypothalamus, Percutaneous Endoscopic Approach	**00CL4ZZ**	Extirpation of Matter from Abducens Nerve, Percutaneous Endoscopic Approach
00C33ZZ	Extirpation of Matter from Intracranial Epidural Space, Percutaneous Approach	**00CB0ZZ**	Extirpation of Matter from Pons, Open Approach	**00CM0ZZ**	Extirpation of Matter from Facial Nerve, Open Approach
00C34ZZ	Extirpation of Matter from Intracranial Epidural Space, Percutaneous Endoscopic Approach	**00CB3ZZ**	Extirpation of Matter from Pons, Percutaneous Approach	**00CM3ZZ**	Extirpation of Matter from Facial Nerve, Percutaneous Approach
00C40ZZ	Extirpation of Matter from Intracranial Subdural Space, Open Approach	**00CB4ZZ**	Extirpation of Matter from Pons, Percutaneous Endoscopic Approach	**00CM4ZZ**	Extirpation of Matter from Facial Nerve, Percutaneous Endoscopic Approach
	AHA CC: 3Q, 2015, 10-11; 2Q, 2016, 29; 3Q, 2019, 4-5	**00CC0ZZ**	Extirpation of Matter from Cerebellum, Open Approach	**00CN0ZZ**	Extirpation of Matter from Acoustic Nerve, Open Approach
00C43ZZ	Extirpation of Matter from Intracranial Subdural Space, Percutaneous Approach	**00CC3ZZ**	Extirpation of Matter from Cerebellum, Percutaneous Approach	**00CN3ZZ**	Extirpation of Matter from Acoustic Nerve, Percutaneous Approach
00C44ZZ	Extirpation of Matter from Intracranial Subdural Space, Percutaneous Endoscopic Approach	**00CC4ZZ**	Extirpation of Matter from Cerebellum, Percutaneous Endoscopic Approach	**00CN4ZZ**	Extirpation of Matter from Acoustic Nerve, Percutaneous Endoscopic Approach
00C50ZZ	Extirpation of Matter from Intracranial Subarachnoid Space, Open Approach	**00CD0ZZ**	Extirpation of Matter from Medulla Oblongata, Open Approach	**00CP0ZZ**	Extirpation of Matter from Glossopharyngeal Nerve, Open Approach
00C53ZZ	Extirpation of Matter from Intracranial Subarachnoid Space, Percutaneous Approach	**00CD3ZZ**	Extirpation of Matter from Medulla Oblongata, Percutaneous Approach	**00CP3ZZ**	Extirpation of Matter from Glossopharyngeal Nerve, Percutaneous Approach
00C54ZZ	Extirpation of Matter from Intracranial Subarachnoid Space, Percutaneous Endoscopic Approach	**00CD4ZZ**	Extirpation of Matter from Medulla Oblongata, Percutaneous Endoscopic Approach	**00CP4ZZ**	Extirpation of Matter from Glossopharyngeal Nerve, Percutaneous Endoscopic Approach
00C60ZZ	Extirpation of Matter from Cerebral Ventricle, Open Approach	**00CF0ZZ**	Extirpation of Matter from Olfactory Nerve, Open Approach	**00CQ0ZZ**	Extirpation of Matter from Vagus Nerve, Open Approach
00C63ZZ	Extirpation of Matter from Cerebral Ventricle, Percutaneous Approach	**00CF3ZZ**	Extirpation of Matter from Olfactory Nerve, Percutaneous Approach	**00CQ3ZZ**	Extirpation of Matter from Vagus Nerve, Percutaneous Approach
00C64ZZ	Extirpation of Matter from Cerebral Ventricle, Percutaneous Endoscopic Approach	**00CF4ZZ**	Extirpation of Matter from Olfactory Nerve, Percutaneous Endoscopic Approach	**00CQ4ZZ**	Extirpation of Matter from Vagus Nerve, Percutaneous Endoscopic Approach
00C70ZZ	Extirpation of Matter from Cerebral Hemisphere, Open Approach	**00CG0ZZ**	Extirpation of Matter from Optic Nerve, Open Approach	**00CR0ZZ**	Extirpation of Matter from Accessory Nerve, Open Approach
		00CG3ZZ	Extirpation of Matter from Optic Nerve, Percutaneous Approach		
		00CG4ZZ	Extirpation of Matter from Optic Nerve, Percutaneous Endoscopic Approach		

♀ Female-only   ♂ Male-only   ▲ Limited Coverage   ● Non-OR   ⬛ HAC-associated procedure   ▲ Non-covered procedures   ➕ Cluster

00CR3ZZ	Extirpation of Matter from Accessory Nerve, Percutaneous Approach
00CR4ZZ	Extirpation of Matter from Accessory Nerve, Percutaneous Endoscopic Approach
00CS0ZZ	Extirpation of Matter from Hypoglossal Nerve, Open Approach
00CS3ZZ	Extirpation of Matter from Hypoglossal Nerve, Percutaneous Approach
00CS4ZZ	Extirpation of Matter from Hypoglossal Nerve, Percutaneous Endoscopic Approach
00CT0ZZ	Extirpation of Matter from Spinal Meninges, Open Approach
00CT3ZZ	Extirpation of Matter from Spinal Meninges, Percutaneous Approach

00CT4ZZ	Extirpation of Matter from Spinal Meninges, Percutaneous Endoscopic Approach
00CU0ZZ	Extirpation of Matter from Spinal Canal, Open Approach
	AHA CC: 4Q, 2017, 48
00CU3ZZ	Extirpation of Matter from Spinal Canal, Percutaneous Approach
00CU4ZZ	Extirpation of Matter from Spinal Canal, Percutaneous Endoscopic Approach
00CW0ZZ	Extirpation of Matter from Cervical Spinal Cord, Open Approach
00CW3ZZ	Extirpation of Matter from Cervical Spinal Cord, Percutaneous Approach
00CW4ZZ	Extirpation of Matter from Cervical Spinal Cord, Percutaneous Endoscopic Approach

00CX0ZZ	Extirpation of Matter from Thoracic Spinal Cord, Open Approach
00CX3ZZ	Extirpation of Matter from Thoracic Spinal Cord, Percutaneous Approach
00CX4ZZ	Extirpation of Matter from Thoracic Spinal Cord, Percutaneous Endoscopic Approach
00CY0ZZ	Extirpation of Matter from Lumbar Spinal Cord, Open Approach
00CY3ZZ	Extirpation of Matter from Lumbar Spinal Cord, Percutaneous Approach
00CY4ZZ	Extirpation of Matter from Lumbar Spinal Cord, Percutaneous Endoscopic Approach

00D – Central Nervous System and Cranial Nerves, Extraction

00D00ZZ	Extraction of Brain, Open Approach
00D03ZZ	Extraction of Brain, Percutaneous Approach
00D04ZZ	Extraction of Brain, Percutaneous Endoscopic Approach
00D10ZZ	Extraction of Cerebral Meninges, Open Approach
00D13ZZ	Extraction of Cerebral Meninges, Percutaneous Approach
00D14ZZ	Extraction of Cerebral Meninges, Percutaneous Endoscopic Approach
00D20ZZ	Extraction of Dura Mater, Open Approach
	AHA CC: 3Q, 2015, 13-14
00D23ZZ	Extraction of Dura Mater, Percutaneous Approach
00D24ZZ	Extraction of Dura Mater, Percutaneous Endoscopic Approach
00D70ZZ	Extraction of Cerebral Hemisphere, Open Approach
00D73ZZ	Extraction of Cerebral Hemisphere, Percutaneous Approach
00D74ZZ	Extraction of Cerebral Hemisphere, Percutaneous Endoscopic Approach
00DF0ZZ	Extraction of Olfactory Nerve, Open Approach
00DF3ZZ	Extraction of Olfactory Nerve, Percutaneous Approach
00DF4ZZ	Extraction of Olfactory Nerve, Percutaneous Endoscopic Approach
00DG0ZZ	Extraction of Optic Nerve, Open Approach
00DG3ZZ	Extraction of Optic Nerve, Percutaneous Approach

00DG4ZZ	Extraction of Optic Nerve, Percutaneous Endoscopic Approach
00DH0ZZ	Extraction of Oculomotor Nerve, Open Approach
00DH3ZZ	Extraction of Oculomotor Nerve, Percutaneous Approach
00DH4ZZ	Extraction of Oculomotor Nerve, Percutaneous Endoscopic Approach
00DJ0ZZ	Extraction of Trochlear Nerve, Open Approach
00DJ3ZZ	Extraction of Trochlear Nerve, Percutaneous Approach
00DJ4ZZ	Extraction of Trochlear Nerve, Percutaneous Endoscopic Approach
00DK0ZZ	Extraction of Trigeminal Nerve, Open Approach
00DK3ZZ	Extraction of Trigeminal Nerve, Percutaneous Approach
00DK4ZZ	Extraction of Trigeminal Nerve, Percutaneous Endoscopic Approach
00DL0ZZ	Extraction of Abducens Nerve, Open Approach
00DL3ZZ	Extraction of Abducens Nerve, Percutaneous Approach
00DL4ZZ	Extraction of Abducens Nerve, Percutaneous Endoscopic Approach
00DM0ZZ	Extraction of Facial Nerve, Open Approach
00DM3ZZ	Extraction of Facial Nerve, Percutaneous Approach
00DM4ZZ	Extraction of Facial Nerve, Percutaneous Endoscopic Approach
00DN0ZZ	Extraction of Acoustic Nerve, Open Approach

00DN3ZZ	Extraction of Acoustic Nerve, Percutaneous Approach
00DN4ZZ	Extraction of Acoustic Nerve, Percutaneous Endoscopic Approach
00DP0ZZ	Extraction of Glossopharyngeal Nerve, Open Approach
00DP3ZZ	Extraction of Glossopharyngeal Nerve, Percutaneous Approach
00DP4ZZ	Extraction of Glossopharyngeal Nerve, Percutaneous Endoscopic Approach
00DQ0ZZ	Extraction of Vagus Nerve, Open Approach
00DQ3ZZ	Extraction of Vagus Nerve, Percutaneous Approach
00DQ4ZZ	Extraction of Vagus Nerve, Percutaneous Endoscopic Approach
00DR0ZZ	Extraction of Accessory Nerve, Open Approach
00DR3ZZ	Extraction of Accessory Nerve, Percutaneous Approach
00DR4ZZ	Extraction of Accessory Nerve, Percutaneous Endoscopic Approach
00DS0ZZ	Extraction of Hypoglossal Nerve, Open Approach
00DS3ZZ	Extraction of Hypoglossal Nerve, Percutaneous Approach
00DS4ZZ	Extraction of Hypoglossal Nerve, Percutaneous Endoscopic Approach
00DT0ZZ	Extraction of Spinal Meninges, Open Approach
00DT3ZZ	Extraction of Spinal Meninges, Percutaneous Approach
00DT4ZZ	Extraction of Spinal Meninges, Percutaneous Endoscopic Approach

00F – Central Nervous System and Cranial Nerves, Fragmentation

00F30ZZ	Fragmentation in Intracranial Epidural Space, Open Approach
00F33ZZ	Fragmentation in Intracranial Epidural Space, Percutaneous Approach
00F34ZZ	Fragmentation in Intracranial Epidural Space, Percutaneous Endoscopic Approach
▲ 00F3XZZ	Fragmentation in Intracranial Epidural Space, External Approach
00F40ZZ	Fragmentation in Intracranial Subdural Space, Open Approach
00F43ZZ	Fragmentation in Intracranial Subdural Space, Percutaneous Approach
00F44ZZ	Fragmentation in Intracranial Subdural Space, Percutaneous Endoscopic Approach

▲ 00F4XZZ	Fragmentation in Intracranial Subdural Space, External Approach
00F50ZZ	Fragmentation in Intracranial Subarachnoid Space, Open Approach
00F53ZZ	Fragmentation in Intracranial Subarachnoid Space, Percutaneous Approach
00F54ZZ	Fragmentation in Intracranial Subarachnoid Space, Percutaneous Endoscopic Approach
▲ 00F5XZZ	Fragmentation in Intracranial Subarachnoid Space, External Approach
00F60ZZ	Fragmentation in Cerebral Ventricle, Open Approach

00F63ZZ	Fragmentation in Cerebral Ventricle, Percutaneous Approach
00F64ZZ	Fragmentation in Cerebral Ventricle, Percutaneous Endoscopic Approach
▲ 00F6XZZ	Fragmentation in Cerebral Ventricle, External Approach
00FU0ZZ	Fragmentation in Spinal Canal, Open Approach
00FU3ZZ	Fragmentation in Spinal Canal, Percutaneous Approach
00FU4ZZ	Fragmentation in Spinal Canal, Percutaneous Endoscopic Approach
00FUXZZ	Fragmentation in Spinal Canal, External Approach

♀ Female-only   ♂ Male-only   ▲ Limited Coverage   ● Non-OR   🅷🅰🅲 HAC-associated procedure   ▲ Non-covered procedures   ✚ Cluster   **125**

00H001Z Insertion of Radioactive Element into Brain, Open Approach

00H002Z Insertion of Monitoring Device into Brain, Open Approach

00H003Z Insertion of Infusion Device into Brain, Open Approach

● **00H004Z** Insertion of Radioactive Element, Cesium-131 Collagen Implant into Brain, Open Approach

00H00MZ Insertion of Neurostimulator Lead into Brain, Open Approach

00H00YZ Insertion of Other Device into Brain, Open Approach

00H031Z Insertion of Radioactive Element into Brain, Percutaneous Approach

00H032Z Insertion of Monitoring Device into Brain, Percutaneous Approach

00H033Z Insertion of Infusion Device into Brain, Percutaneous Approach

00H03MZ Insertion of Neurostimulator Lead into Brain, Percutaneous Approach

00H03YZ Insertion of Other Device into Brain, Percutaneous Approach

00H041Z Insertion of Radioactive Element into Brain, Percutaneous Endoscopic Approach

00H042Z Insertion of Monitoring Device into Brain, Percutaneous Endoscopic Approach

00H043Z Insertion of Infusion Device into Brain, Percutaneous Endoscopic Approach

00H04MZ Insertion of Neurostimulator Lead into Brain, Percutaneous Endoscopic Approach

00H04YZ Insertion of Other Device into Brain, Percutaneous Endoscopic Approach

00H601Z Insertion of Radioactive Element into Cerebral Ventricle, Open Approach

00H602Z Insertion of Monitoring Device into Cerebral Ventricle, Open Approach

00H603Z Insertion of Infusion Device into Cerebral Ventricle, Open Approach

00H60MZ Insertion of Neurostimulator Lead into Cerebral Ventricle, Open Approach

00H60YZ Insertion of Other Device into Cerebral Ventricle, Open Approach

00H631Z Insertion of Radioactive Element into Cerebral Ventricle, Percutaneous Approach

00H632Z Insertion of Monitoring Device into Cerebral Ventricle, Percutaneous Approach

00H633Z Insertion of Infusion Device into Cerebral Ventricle, Percutaneous Approach
AHA CC: 2Q, 2020, 15-16

00H63MZ Insertion of Neurostimulator Lead into Cerebral Ventricle, Percutaneous Approach

00H63YZ Insertion of Other Device into Cerebral Ventricle, Percutaneous Approach

00H641Z Insertion of Radioactive Element into Cerebral Ventricle, Percutaneous Endoscopic Approach

00H642Z Insertion of Monitoring Device into Cerebral Ventricle, Percutaneous Endoscopic Approach

00H643Z Insertion of Infusion Device into Cerebral Ventricle, Percutaneous Endoscopic Approach

00H64MZ Insertion of Neurostimulator Lead into Cerebral Ventricle, Percutaneous Endoscopic Approach

00H64YZ Insertion of Other Device into Cerebral Ventricle, Percutaneous Endoscopic Approach

00HE01Z Insertion of Radioactive Element into Cranial Nerve, Open Approach

00HE02Z Insertion of Monitoring Device into Cranial Nerve, Open Approach

00HE03Z Insertion of Infusion Device into Cranial Nerve, Open Approach

00HE0MZ Insertion of Neurostimulator Lead into Cranial Nerve, Open Approach

00HE0YZ Insertion of Other Device into Cranial Nerve, Open Approach

00HE31Z Insertion of Radioactive Element into Cranial Nerve, Percutaneous Approach

00HE32Z Insertion of Monitoring Device into Cranial Nerve, Percutaneous Approach

00HE33Z Insertion of Infusion Device into Cranial Nerve, Percutaneous Approach

00HE3MZ Insertion of Neurostimulator Lead into Cranial Nerve, Percutaneous Approach

00HE3YZ Insertion of Other Device into Cranial Nerve, Percutaneous Approach

00HE41Z Insertion of Radioactive Element into Cranial Nerve, Percutaneous Endoscopic Approach

00HE42Z Insertion of Monitoring Device into Cranial Nerve, Percutaneous Endoscopic Approach

00HE43Z Insertion of Infusion Device into Cranial Nerve, Percutaneous Endoscopic Approach

00HE4MZ Insertion of Neurostimulator Lead into Cranial Nerve, Percutaneous Endoscopic Approach

00HE4YZ Insertion of Other Device into Cranial Nerve, Percutaneous Endoscopic Approach

00HU01Z Insertion of Radioactive Element into Spinal Canal, Open Approach

00HU02Z Insertion of Monitoring Device into Spinal Canal, Open Approach

00HU03Z Insertion of Infusion Device into Spinal Canal, Open Approach
AHA CC: 2Q, 2020, 16-17

00HU0MZ Insertion of Neurostimulator Lead into Spinal Canal, Open Approach

⊞ Lead device when reported with an Insertion of a stimulator generator (6th character B-E) into the chest or abdomen subcutaneous tissue and fascia. *See table 0JH to construct the Insertion code.*

00HU0YZ Insertion of Other Device into Spinal Canal, Open Approach

00HU31Z Insertion of Radioactive Element into Spinal Canal, Percutaneous Approach

00HU32Z Insertion of Monitoring Device into Spinal Canal, Percutaneous Approach

00HU33Z Insertion of Infusion Device into Spinal Canal, Percutaneous Approach
AHA CC: 3Q, 2014, 19-20

00HU3MZ Insertion of Neurostimulator Lead into Spinal Canal, Percutaneous Approach

⊞ Lead device when reported with an Insertion of a stimulator generator (6th character B-E) into the chest or abdomen subcutaneous tissue and fascia. *See table 0JH to construct the Insertion code.*

00HU3YZ Insertion of Other Device into Spinal Canal, Percutaneous Approach

00HU41Z Insertion of Radioactive Element into Spinal Canal, Percutaneous Endoscopic Approach

00HU42Z Insertion of Monitoring Device into Spinal Canal, Percutaneous Endoscopic Approach

00HU43Z Insertion of Infusion Device into Spinal Canal, Percutaneous Endoscopic Approach

00HU4MZ Insertion of Neurostimulator Lead into Spinal Canal, Percutaneous Endoscopic Approach

⊞ Lead device when reported with an Insertion of a stimulator generator (6th character B-E) into the chest or abdomen subcutaneous tissue and fascia. *See table 0JH to construct the Insertion code.*

00HU4YZ Insertion of Other Device into Spinal Canal, Percutaneous Endoscopic Approach

00HV01Z Insertion of Radioactive Element into Spinal Cord, Open Approach

00HV02Z Insertion of Monitoring Device into Spinal Cord, Open Approach

00HV03Z Insertion of Infusion Device into Spinal Cord, Open Approach

00HV0MZ Insertion of Neurostimulator Lead into Spinal Cord, Open Approach

⊞ Lead device when reported with an Insertion of a stimulator generator (6th character B-E) into the chest or abdomen subcutaneous tissue and fascia. *See table 0JH to construct the Insertion code.*

00HV0YZ Insertion of Other Device into Spinal Cord, Open Approach

00HV31Z Insertion of Radioactive Element into Spinal Cord, Percutaneous Approach

00HV32Z Insertion of Monitoring Device into Spinal Cord, Percutaneous Approach

00HV33Z Insertion of Infusion Device into Spinal Cord, Percutaneous Approach

00HV3MZ Insertion of Neurostimulator Lead into Spinal Cord, Percutaneous Approach

⊞ Lead device when reported with an Insertion of a stimulator generator (6th character B-E) into the chest or abdomen subcutaneous tissue and fascia. *See table 0JH to construct the Insertion code.*

00HV3YZ Insertion of Other Device into Spinal Cord, Percutaneous Approach

00HV41Z Insertion of Radioactive Element into Spinal Cord, Percutaneous Endoscopic Approach

00HV42Z Insertion of Monitoring Device into Spinal Cord, Percutaneous Endoscopic Approach

00HV43Z Insertion of Infusion Device into Spinal Cord, Percutaneous Endoscopic Approach

00HV4MZ Insertion of Neurostimulator Lead into Spinal Cord, Percutaneous Endoscopic Approach

⊞ Lead device when reported with an Insertion of a stimulator generator (6th character B-E) into the chest or abdomen subcutaneous tissue and fascia. *See table 0JH to construct the Insertion code.*

00HV4YZ Insertion of Other Device into Spinal Cord, Percutaneous Endoscopic Approach

♀ Female-only   ♂ Male-only   ▲ Limited Coverage   ● Non-OR   HAC HAC-associated procedure   ▲ Non-covered procedures   ⊞ Cluster

00J – Central Nervous System and Cranial Nerves, Inspection

Review Coding Guidelines B3.11a, B3.11b and B3.11c

00J00ZZ	Inspection of Brain, Open Approach
	AHA CC: 2Q, 2019, 36-37
00J03ZZ	Inspection of Brain, Percutaneous Approach
00J04ZZ	Inspection of Brain, Percutaneous Endoscopic Approach
	AHA CC: 2Q, 2021, 19-20
00JE0ZZ	Inspection of Cranial Nerve, Open Approach
00JE3ZZ	Inspection of Cranial Nerve, Percutaneous Approach
00JE4ZZ	Inspection of Cranial Nerve, Percutaneous Endoscopic Approach
00JU0ZZ	Inspection of Spinal Canal, Open Approach
00JU3ZZ	Inspection of Spinal Canal, Percutaneous Approach
	AHA CC: 1Q, 2017, 50
00JU4ZZ	Inspection of Spinal Canal, Percutaneous Endoscopic Approach
00JV0ZZ	Inspection of Spinal Cord, Open Approach
00JV3ZZ	Inspection of Spinal Cord, Percutaneous Approach
00JV4ZZ	Inspection of Spinal Cord, Percutaneous Endoscopic Approach

00K – Central Nervous System and Cranial Nerves, Map

00K00ZZ	Map Brain, Open Approach
00K03ZZ	Map Brain, Percutaneous Approach
00K04ZZ	Map Brain, Percutaneous Endoscopic Approach
00K70ZZ	Map Cerebral Hemisphere, Open Approach
00K73ZZ	Map Cerebral Hemisphere, Percutaneous Approach
00K74ZZ	Map Cerebral Hemisphere, Percutaneous Endoscopic Approach
00K80ZZ	Map Basal Ganglia, Open Approach
00K83ZZ	Map Basal Ganglia, Percutaneous Approach
00K84ZZ	Map Basal Ganglia, Percutaneous Endoscopic Approach
00K90ZZ	Map Thalamus, Open Approach
00K93ZZ	Map Thalamus, Percutaneous Approach
00K94ZZ	Map Thalamus, Percutaneous Endoscopic Approach
00KA0ZZ	Map Hypothalamus, Open Approach
00KA3ZZ	Map Hypothalamus, Percutaneous Approach
00KA4ZZ	Map Hypothalamus, Percutaneous Endoscopic Approach
00KB0ZZ	Map Pons, Open Approach
00KB3ZZ	Map Pons, Percutaneous Approach
00KB4ZZ	Map Pons, Percutaneous Endoscopic Approach
00KC0ZZ	Map Cerebellum, Open Approach
00KC3ZZ	Map Cerebellum, Percutaneous Approach
00KC4ZZ	Map Cerebellum, Percutaneous Endoscopic Approach
00KD0ZZ	Map Medulla Oblongata, Open Approach
00KD3ZZ	Map Medulla Oblongata, Percutaneous Approach
00KD4ZZ	Map Medulla Oblongata, Percutaneous Endoscopic Approach

00N – Central Nervous System and Cranial Nerves, Release

Review Coding Guideline B3.13

Review Coding Guideline B3.14

00N00ZZ	Release Brain, Open Approach
	AHA CC: 2Q, 2016, 29
00N03ZZ	Release Brain, Percutaneous Approach
00N04ZZ	Release Brain, Percutaneous Endoscopic Approach
00N10ZZ	Release Cerebral Meninges, Open Approach
00N13ZZ	Release Cerebral Meninges, Percutaneous Approach
00N14ZZ	Release Cerebral Meninges, Percutaneous Endoscopic Approach
00N20ZZ	Release Dura Mater, Open Approach
00N23ZZ	Release Dura Mater, Percutaneous Approach
00N24ZZ	Release Dura Mater, Percutaneous Endoscopic Approach
00N60ZZ	Release Cerebral Ventricle, Open Approach
00N63ZZ	Release Cerebral Ventricle, Percutaneous Approach
00N64ZZ	Release Cerebral Ventricle, Percutaneous Endoscopic Approach
00N70ZZ	Release Cerebral Hemisphere, Open Approach
	AHA CC: 3Q, 2018, 30
00N73ZZ	Release Cerebral Hemisphere, Percutaneous Approach
00N74ZZ	Release Cerebral Hemisphere, Percutaneous Endoscopic Approach
00N80ZZ	Release Basal Ganglia, Open Approach
00N83ZZ	Release Basal Ganglia, Percutaneous Approach
00N84ZZ	Release Basal Ganglia, Percutaneous Endoscopic Approach
00N90ZZ	Release Thalamus, Open Approach
00N93ZZ	Release Thalamus, Percutaneous Approach
00N94ZZ	Release Thalamus, Percutaneous Endoscopic Approach
00NA0ZZ	Release Hypothalamus, Open Approach
00NA3ZZ	Release Hypothalamus, Percutaneous Approach
00NA4ZZ	Release Hypothalamus, Percutaneous Endoscopic Approach
00NB0ZZ	Release Pons, Open Approach
00NB3ZZ	Release Pons, Percutaneous Approach
00NB4ZZ	Release Pons, Percutaneous Endoscopic Approach
00NC0ZZ	Release Cerebellum, Open Approach
	AHA CC: 3Q, 2017, 10-11
00NC3ZZ	Release Cerebellum, Percutaneous Approach
00NC4ZZ	Release Cerebellum, Percutaneous Endoscopic Approach
00ND0ZZ	Release Medulla Oblongata, Open Approach
00ND3ZZ	Release Medulla Oblongata, Percutaneous Approach
00ND4ZZ	Release Medulla Oblongata, Percutaneous Endoscopic Approach
00NF0ZZ	Release Olfactory Nerve, Open Approach
00NF3ZZ	Release Olfactory Nerve, Percutaneous Approach
00NF4ZZ	Release Olfactory Nerve, Percutaneous Endoscopic Approach
00NG0ZZ	Release Optic Nerve, Open Approach
00NG3ZZ	Release Optic Nerve, Percutaneous Approach
00NG4ZZ	Release Optic Nerve, Percutaneous Endoscopic Approach
00NH0ZZ	Release Oculomotor Nerve, Open Approach
00NH3ZZ	Release Oculomotor Nerve, Percutaneous Approach
00NH4ZZ	Release Oculomotor Nerve, Percutaneous Endoscopic Approach
00NJ0ZZ	Release Trochlear Nerve, Open Approach
00NJ3ZZ	Release Trochlear Nerve, Percutaneous Approach
00NJ4ZZ	Release Trochlear Nerve, Percutaneous Endoscopic Approach
00NK0ZZ	Release Trigeminal Nerve, Open Approach
00NK3ZZ	Release Trigeminal Nerve, Percutaneous Approach
00NK4ZZ	Release Trigeminal Nerve, Percutaneous Endoscopic Approach
00NL0ZZ	Release Abducens Nerve, Open Approach
00NL3ZZ	Release Abducens Nerve, Percutaneous Approach
00NL4ZZ	Release Abducens Nerve, Percutaneous Endoscopic Approach
00NM0ZZ	Release Facial Nerve, Open Approach
00NM3ZZ	Release Facial Nerve, Percutaneous Approach
00NM4ZZ	Release Facial Nerve, Percutaneous Endoscopic Approach
	AHA CC: 4Q, 2018, 10
00NN0ZZ	Release Acoustic Nerve, Open Approach
00NN3ZZ	Release Acoustic Nerve, Percutaneous Approach
00NN4ZZ	Release Acoustic Nerve, Percutaneous Endoscopic Approach
00NP0ZZ	Release Glossopharyngeal Nerve, Open Approach
00NP3ZZ	Release Glossopharyngeal Nerve, Percutaneous Approach
00NP4ZZ	Release Glossopharyngeal Nerve, Percutaneous Endoscopic Approach

00NQ0ZZ	Release Vagus Nerve, Open Approach	
00NQ3ZZ	Release Vagus Nerve, Percutaneous Approach	
00NQ4ZZ	Release Vagus Nerve, Percutaneous Endoscopic Approach	
00NR0ZZ	Release Accessory Nerve, Open Approach	
00NR3ZZ	Release Accessory Nerve, Percutaneous Approach	
00NR4ZZ	Release Accessory Nerve, Percutaneous Endoscopic Approach	
00NS0ZZ	Release Hypoglossal Nerve, Open Approach	
00NS3ZZ	Release Hypoglossal Nerve, Percutaneous Approach	

00NS4ZZ	Release Hypoglossal Nerve, Percutaneous Endoscopic Approach
00NT0ZZ	Release Spinal Meninges, Open Approach
00NT3ZZ	Release Spinal Meninges, Percutaneous Approach
00NT4ZZ	Release Spinal Meninges, Percutaneous Endoscopic Approach
00NW0ZZ	Release Cervical Spinal Cord, Open Approach

AHA CC: 2Q, 2015, 20-22; 2Q, 2017, 23-24

00NW3ZZ	Release Cervical Spinal Cord, Percutaneous Approach

AHA CC: 2Q, 2019, 19-20

00NW4ZZ	Release Cervical Spinal Cord, Percutaneous Endoscopic Approach

00NX0ZZ	Release Thoracic Spinal Cord, Open Approach
00NX3ZZ	Release Thoracic Spinal Cord, Percutaneous Approach
00NX4ZZ	Release Thoracic Spinal Cord, Percutaneous Endoscopic Approach
00NY0ZZ	Release Lumbar Spinal Cord, Open Approach

AHA CC: 3Q, 2014, 24; 1Q, 2019, 28-29

00NY3ZZ	Release Lumbar Spinal Cord, Percutaneous Approach
00NY4ZZ	Release Lumbar Spinal Cord, Percutaneous Endoscopic Approach

00P – Central Nervous System and Cranial Nerves, Removal

Review Coding Guideline B6.1c

00P000Z	Removal of Drainage Device from Brain, Open Approach
00P002Z	Removal of Monitoring Device from Brain, Open Approach
00P003Z	Removal of Infusion Device from Brain, Open Approach
00P007Z	Removal of Autologous Tissue Substitute from Brain, Open Approach
00P00JZ	Removal of Synthetic Substitute from Brain, Open Approach
00P00KZ	Removal of Nonautologous Tissue Substitute from Brain, Open Approach
00P00MZ	Removal of Neurostimulator Lead from Brain, Open Approach
00P00YZ	Removal of Other Device from Brain, Open Approach
00P030Z	Removal of Drainage Device from Brain, Percutaneous Approach
00P032Z	Removal of Monitoring Device from Brain, Percutaneous Approach
00P033Z	Removal of Infusion Device from Brain, Percutaneous Approach
00P037Z	Removal of Autologous Tissue Substitute from Brain, Percutaneous Approach
00P03JZ	Removal of Synthetic Substitute from Brain, Percutaneous Approach
00P03KZ	Removal of Nonautologous Tissue Substitute from Brain, Percutaneous Approach
00P03MZ	Removal of Neurostimulator Lead from Brain, Percutaneous Approach
00P03YZ	Removal of Other Device from Brain, Percutaneous Approach
00P040Z	Removal of Drainage Device from Brain, Percutaneous Endoscopic Approach
00P042Z	Removal of Monitoring Device from Brain, Percutaneous Endoscopic Approach
00P043Z	Removal of Infusion Device from Brain, Percutaneous Endoscopic Approach
00P047Z	Removal of Autologous Tissue Substitute from Brain, Percutaneous Endoscopic Approach
00P04JZ	Removal of Synthetic Substitute from Brain, Percutaneous Endoscopic Approach
00P04KZ	Removal of Nonautologous Tissue Substitute from Brain, Percutaneous Endoscopic Approach
00P04MZ	Removal of Neurostimulator Lead from Brain, Percutaneous Endoscopic Approach

00P04YZ	Removal of Other Device from Brain, Percutaneous Endoscopic Approach
00P0X0Z	Removal of Drainage Device from Brain, External Approach
00P0X2Z	Removal of Monitoring Device from Brain, External Approach
00P0X3Z	Removal of Infusion Device from Brain, External Approach
00P0XMZ	Removal of Neurostimulator Lead from Brain, External Approach
00P600Z	Removal of Drainage Device from Cerebral Ventricle, Open Approach
00P602Z	Removal of Monitoring Device from Cerebral Ventricle, Open Approach
00P603Z	Removal of Infusion Device from Cerebral Ventricle, Open Approach
00P60JZ	Removal of Synthetic Substitute from Cerebral Ventricle, Open Approach
00P60MZ	Removal of Neurostimulator Lead from Cerebral Ventricle, Open Approach
00P60YZ	Removal of Other Device from Cerebral Ventricle, Open Approach
00P630Z	Removal of Drainage Device from Cerebral Ventricle, Percutaneous Approach
00P632Z	Removal of Monitoring Device from Cerebral Ventricle, Percutaneous Approach
00P633Z	Removal of Infusion Device from Cerebral Ventricle, Percutaneous Approach
00P63JZ	Removal of Synthetic Substitute from Cerebral Ventricle, Percutaneous Approach
00P63MZ	Removal of Neurostimulator Lead from Cerebral Ventricle, Percutaneous Approach
00P63YZ	Removal of Other Device from Cerebral Ventricle, Percutaneous Approach
00P640Z	Removal of Drainage Device from Cerebral Ventricle, Percutaneous Endoscopic Approach
00P642Z	Removal of Monitoring Device from Cerebral Ventricle, Percutaneous Endoscopic Approach
00P643Z	Removal of Infusion Device from Cerebral Ventricle, Percutaneous Endoscopic Approach
00P64JZ	Removal of Synthetic Substitute from Cerebral Ventricle, Percutaneous Endoscopic Approach

00P64MZ	Removal of Neurostimulator Lead from Cerebral Ventricle, Percutaneous Endoscopic Approach
00P64YZ	Removal of Other Device from Cerebral Ventricle, Percutaneous Endoscopic Approach
00P6X0Z	Removal of Drainage Device from Cerebral Ventricle, External Approach
00P6X2Z	Removal of Monitoring Device from Cerebral Ventricle, External Approach
00P6X3Z	Removal of Infusion Device from Cerebral Ventricle, External Approach
00P6XMZ	Removal of Neurostimulator Lead from Cerebral Ventricle, External Approach
00PE00Z	Removal of Drainage Device from Cranial Nerve, Open Approach
00PE02Z	Removal of Monitoring Device from Cranial Nerve, Open Approach
00PE03Z	Removal of Infusion Device from Cranial Nerve, Open Approach
00PE07Z	Removal of Autologous Tissue Substitute from Cranial Nerve, Open Approach
00PE0MZ	Removal of Neurostimulator Lead from Cranial Nerve, Open Approach
00PE0YZ	Removal of Other Device from Cranial Nerve, Open Approach
00PE30Z	Removal of Drainage Device from Cranial Nerve, Percutaneous Approach
00PE32Z	Removal of Monitoring Device from Cranial Nerve, Percutaneous Approach
00PE33Z	Removal of Infusion Device from Cranial Nerve, Percutaneous Approach
00PE37Z	Removal of Autologous Tissue Substitute from Cranial Nerve, Percutaneous Approach
00PE3MZ	Removal of Neurostimulator Lead from Cranial Nerve, Percutaneous Approach
00PE3YZ	Removal of Other Device from Cranial Nerve, Percutaneous Approach
00PE40Z	Removal of Drainage Device from Cranial Nerve, Percutaneous Endoscopic Approach
00PE42Z	Removal of Monitoring Device from Cranial Nerve, Percutaneous Endoscopic Approach
00PE43Z	Removal of Infusion Device from Cranial Nerve, Percutaneous Endoscopic Approach
00PE47Z	Removal of Autologous Tissue Substitute from Cranial Nerve, Percutaneous Endoscopic Approach
00PE4MZ	Removal of Neurostimulator Lead from Cranial Nerve, Percutaneous Endoscopic Approach

♀ Female-only   ♂ Male-only   ▲ Limited Coverage   ● Non-OR   HAC HAC-associated procedure   ▲ Non-covered procedures   ✛ Cluster

00PE4YZ	Removal of Other Device from Cranial Nerve, Percutaneous Endoscopic Approach
00PEX0Z	Removal of Drainage Device from Cranial Nerve, External Approach
00PEX2Z	Removal of Monitoring Device from Cranial Nerve, External Approach
00PEX3Z	Removal of Infusion Device from Cranial Nerve, External Approach
00PEXMZ	Removal of Neurostimulator Lead from Cranial Nerve, External Approach
00PU00Z	Removal of Drainage Device from Spinal Canal, Open Approach
00PU02Z	Removal of Monitoring Device from Spinal Canal, Open Approach
00PU03Z	Removal of Infusion Device from Spinal Canal, Open Approach
	AHA CC: 3Q, 2014, 19-20
00PU0JZ	Removal of Synthetic Substitute from Spinal Canal, Open Approach
00PU0MZ	Removal of Neurostimulator Lead from Spinal Canal, Open Approach
00PU0YZ	Removal of Other Device from Spinal Canal, Open Approach
00PU30Z	Removal of Drainage Device from Spinal Canal, Percutaneous Approach
00PU32Z	Removal of Monitoring Device from Spinal Canal, Percutaneous Approach
00PU33Z	Removal of Infusion Device from Spinal Canal, Percutaneous Approach
00PU3JZ	Removal of Synthetic Substitute from Spinal Canal, Percutaneous Approach
00PU3MZ	Removal of Neurostimulator Lead from Spinal Canal, Percutaneous Approach
00PU3YZ	Removal of Other Device from Spinal Canal, Percutaneous Approach
00PU40Z	Removal of Drainage Device from Spinal Canal, Percutaneous Endoscopic Approach
00PU42Z	Removal of Monitoring Device from Spinal Canal, Percutaneous Endoscopic Approach
00PU43Z	Removal of Infusion Device from Spinal Canal, Percutaneous Endoscopic Approach
00PU4JZ	Removal of Synthetic Substitute from Spinal Canal, Percutaneous Endoscopic Approach
00PU4MZ	Removal of Neurostimulator Lead from Spinal Canal, Percutaneous Endoscopic Approach
00PU4YZ	Removal of Other Device from Spinal Canal, Percutaneous Endoscopic Approach
00PUX0Z	Removal of Drainage Device from Spinal Canal, External Approach
00PUX2Z	Removal of Monitoring Device from Spinal Canal, External Approach
00PUX3Z	Removal of Infusion Device from Spinal Canal, External Approach
00PUXMZ	Removal of Neurostimulator Lead from Spinal Canal, External Approach
00PV00Z	Removal of Drainage Device from Spinal Cord, Open Approach
00PV02Z	Removal of Monitoring Device from Spinal Cord, Open Approach
00PV03Z	Removal of Infusion Device from Spinal Cord, Open Approach
00PV07Z	Removal of Autologous Tissue Substitute from Spinal Cord, Open Approach
00PV0JZ	Removal of Synthetic Substitute from Spinal Cord, Open Approach
00PV0KZ	Removal of Nonautologous Tissue Substitute from Spinal Cord, Open Approach
00PV0MZ	Removal of Neurostimulator Lead from Spinal Cord, Open Approach
00PV0YZ	Removal of Other Device from Spinal Cord, Open Approach
00PV30Z	Removal of Drainage Device from Spinal Cord, Percutaneous Approach
00PV32Z	Removal of Monitoring Device from Spinal Cord, Percutaneous Approach
00PV33Z	Removal of Infusion Device from Spinal Cord, Percutaneous Approach
00PV37Z	Removal of Autologous Tissue Substitute from Spinal Cord, Percutaneous Approach
00PV3JZ	Removal of Synthetic Substitute from Spinal Cord, Percutaneous Approach
00PV3KZ	Removal of Nonautologous Tissue Substitute from Spinal Cord, Percutaneous Approach
00PV3MZ	Removal of Neurostimulator Lead from Spinal Cord, Percutaneous Approach
00PV3YZ	Removal of Other Device from Spinal Cord, Percutaneous Approach
00PV40Z	Removal of Drainage Device from Spinal Cord, Percutaneous Endoscopic Approach
00PV42Z	Removal of Monitoring Device from Spinal Cord, Percutaneous Endoscopic Approach
00PV43Z	Removal of Infusion Device from Spinal Cord, Percutaneous Endoscopic Approach
00PV47Z	Removal of Autologous Tissue Substitute from Spinal Cord, Percutaneous Endoscopic Approach
00PV4JZ	Removal of Synthetic Substitute from Spinal Cord, Percutaneous Endoscopic Approach
00PV4KZ	Removal of Nonautologous Tissue Substitute from Spinal Cord, Percutaneous Endoscopic Approach
00PV4MZ	Removal of Neurostimulator Lead from Spinal Cord, Percutaneous Endoscopic Approach
00PV4YZ	Removal of Other Device from Spinal Cord, Percutaneous Endoscopic Approach
00PVX0Z	Removal of Drainage Device from Spinal Cord, External Approach
00PVX2Z	Removal of Monitoring Device from Spinal Cord, External Approach
00PVX3Z	Removal of Infusion Device from Spinal Cord, External Approach
00PVXMZ	Removal of Neurostimulator Lead from Spinal Cord, External Approach

00Q – Central Nervous System and Cranial Nerves, Repair

00Q00ZZ	Repair Brain, Open Approach
00Q03ZZ	Repair Brain, Percutaneous Approach
00Q04ZZ	Repair Brain, Percutaneous Endoscopic Approach
00Q10ZZ	Repair Cerebral Meninges, Open Approach
00Q13ZZ	Repair Cerebral Meninges, Percutaneous Approach
00Q14ZZ	Repair Cerebral Meninges, Percutaneous Endoscopic Approach
00Q20ZZ	Repair Dura Mater, Open Approach
	AHA CC: 3Q, 2013, 25; 3Q, 2014, 7-8
00Q23ZZ	Repair Dura Mater, Percutaneous Approach
00Q24ZZ	Repair Dura Mater, Percutaneous Endoscopic Approach
00Q60ZZ	Repair Cerebral Ventricle, Open Approach
00Q63ZZ	Repair Cerebral Ventricle, Percutaneous Approach
00Q64ZZ	Repair Cerebral Ventricle, Percutaneous Endoscopic Approach
00Q70ZZ	Repair Cerebral Hemisphere, Open Approach
00Q73ZZ	Repair Cerebral Hemisphere, Percutaneous Approach
00Q74ZZ	Repair Cerebral Hemisphere, Percutaneous Endoscopic Approach
00Q80ZZ	Repair Basal Ganglia, Open Approach
00Q83ZZ	Repair Basal Ganglia, Percutaneous Approach
00Q84ZZ	Repair Basal Ganglia, Percutaneous Endoscopic Approach
00Q90ZZ	Repair Thalamus, Open Approach
00Q93ZZ	Repair Thalamus, Percutaneous Approach
00Q94ZZ	Repair Thalamus, Percutaneous Endoscopic Approach
00QA0ZZ	Repair Hypothalamus, Open Approach
00QA3ZZ	Repair Hypothalamus, Percutaneous Approach
00QA4ZZ	Repair Hypothalamus, Percutaneous Endoscopic Approach
00QB0ZZ	Repair Pons, Open Approach
00QB3ZZ	Repair Pons, Percutaneous Approach
00QB4ZZ	Repair Pons, Percutaneous Endoscopic Approach
00QC0ZZ	Repair Cerebellum, Open Approach
00QC3ZZ	Repair Cerebellum, Percutaneous Approach
00QC4ZZ	Repair Cerebellum, Percutaneous Endoscopic Approach
00QD0ZZ	Repair Medulla Oblongata, Open Approach
00QD3ZZ	Repair Medulla Oblongata, Percutaneous Approach
00QD4ZZ	Repair Medulla Oblongata, Percutaneous Endoscopic Approach
00QF0ZZ	Repair Olfactory Nerve, Open Approach
00QF3ZZ	Repair Olfactory Nerve, Percutaneous Approach
00QF4ZZ	Repair Olfactory Nerve, Percutaneous Endoscopic Approach
00QG0ZZ	Repair Optic Nerve, Open Approach
00QG3ZZ	Repair Optic Nerve, Percutaneous Approach
00QG4ZZ	Repair Optic Nerve, Percutaneous Endoscopic Approach
00QH0ZZ	Repair Oculomotor Nerve, Open Approach
00QH3ZZ	Repair Oculomotor Nerve, Percutaneous Approach
00QH4ZZ	Repair Oculomotor Nerve, Percutaneous Endoscopic Approach
00QJ0ZZ	Repair Trochlear Nerve, Open Approach
00QJ3ZZ	Repair Trochlear Nerve, Percutaneous Approach
00QJ4ZZ	Repair Trochlear Nerve, Percutaneous Endoscopic Approach
00QK0ZZ	Repair Trigeminal Nerve, Open Approach

00QK3ZZ Repair Trigeminal Nerve, Percutaneous Approach
00QK4ZZ Repair Trigeminal Nerve, Percutaneous Endoscopic Approach
00QL0ZZ Repair Abducens Nerve, Open Approach
00QL3ZZ Repair Abducens Nerve, Percutaneous Approach
00QL4ZZ Repair Abducens Nerve, Percutaneous Endoscopic Approach
00QM0ZZ Repair Facial Nerve, Open Approach
00QM3ZZ Repair Facial Nerve, Percutaneous Approach
00QM4ZZ Repair Facial Nerve, Percutaneous Endoscopic Approach
00QN0ZZ Repair Acoustic Nerve, Open Approach
00QN3ZZ Repair Acoustic Nerve, Percutaneous Approach
00QN4ZZ Repair Acoustic Nerve, Percutaneous Endoscopic Approach
00QP0ZZ Repair Glossopharyngeal Nerve, Open Approach

00QP3ZZ Repair Glossopharyngeal Nerve, Percutaneous Approach
00QP4ZZ Repair Glossopharyngeal Nerve, Percutaneous Endoscopic Approach
00QQ0ZZ Repair Vagus Nerve, Open Approach
00QQ3ZZ Repair Vagus Nerve, Percutaneous Approach
00QQ4ZZ Repair Vagus Nerve, Percutaneous Endoscopic Approach
00QR0ZZ Repair Accessory Nerve, Open Approach
00QR3ZZ Repair Accessory Nerve, Percutaneous Approach
00QR4ZZ Repair Accessory Nerve, Percutaneous Endoscopic Approach
00QS0ZZ Repair Hypoglossal Nerve, Open Approach
00QS3ZZ Repair Hypoglossal Nerve, Percutaneous Approach
00QS4ZZ Repair Hypoglossal Nerve, Percutaneous Endoscopic Approach
00QT0ZZ Repair Spinal Meninges, Open Approach

00QT3ZZ Repair Spinal Meninges, Percutaneous Approach
00QT4ZZ Repair Spinal Meninges, Percutaneous Endoscopic Approach
00QW0ZZ Repair Cervical Spinal Cord, Open Approach
00QW3ZZ Repair Cervical Spinal Cord, Percutaneous Approach
00QW4ZZ Repair Cervical Spinal Cord, Percutaneous Endoscopic Approach
00QX0ZZ Repair Thoracic Spinal Cord, Open Approach
00QX3ZZ Repair Thoracic Spinal Cord, Percutaneous Approach
00QX4ZZ Repair Thoracic Spinal Cord, Percutaneous Endoscopic Approach
00QY0ZZ Repair Lumbar Spinal Cord, Open Approach
00QY3ZZ Repair Lumbar Spinal Cord, Percutaneous Approach
00QY4ZZ Repair Lumbar Spinal Cord, Percutaneous Endoscopic Approach

00R – Central Nervous System and Cranial Nerves, Replacement

Review Coding Guideline B3.18

00R107Z Replacement of Cerebral Meninges with Autologous Tissue Substitute, Open Approach
00R10JZ Replacement of Cerebral Meninges with Synthetic Substitute, Open Approach
00R10KZ Replacement of Cerebral Meninges with Nonautologous Tissue Substitute, Open Approach
00R147Z Replacement of Cerebral Meninges with Autologous Tissue Substitute, Percutaneous Endoscopic Approach
00R14JZ Replacement of Cerebral Meninges with Synthetic Substitute, Percutaneous Endoscopic Approach
00R14KZ Replacement of Cerebral Meninges with Nonautologous Tissue Substitute, Percutaneous Endoscopic Approach
00R207Z Replacement of Dura Mater with Autologous Tissue Substitute, Open Approach
00R20JZ Replacement of Dura Mater with Synthetic Substitute, Open Approach
00R20KZ Replacement of Dura Mater with Nonautologous Tissue Substitute, Open Approach
00R247Z Replacement of Dura Mater with Autologous Tissue Substitute, Percutaneous Endoscopic Approach
00R24JZ Replacement of Dura Mater with Synthetic Substitute, Percutaneous Endoscopic Approach
00R24KZ Replacement of Dura Mater with Nonautologous Tissue Substitute, Percutaneous Endoscopic Approach
00R607Z Replacement of Cerebral Ventricle with Autologous Tissue Substitute, Open Approach
00R60JZ Replacement of Cerebral Ventricle with Synthetic Substitute, Open Approach
00R60KZ Replacement of Cerebral Ventricle with Nonautologous Tissue Substitute, Open Approach
00R647Z Replacement of Cerebral Ventricle with Autologous Tissue Substitute, Percutaneous Endoscopic Approach

00R64JZ Replacement of Cerebral Ventricle with Synthetic Substitute, Percutaneous Endoscopic Approach
00R64KZ Replacement of Cerebral Ventricle with Nonautologous Tissue Substitute, Percutaneous Endoscopic Approach
00RF07Z Replacement of Olfactory Nerve with Autologous Tissue Substitute, Open Approach
00RF0JZ Replacement of Olfactory Nerve with Synthetic Substitute, Open Approach
00RF0KZ Replacement of Olfactory Nerve with Nonautologous Tissue Substitute, Open Approach
00RF47Z Replacement of Olfactory Nerve with Autologous Tissue Substitute, Percutaneous Endoscopic Approach
00RF4JZ Replacement of Olfactory Nerve with Synthetic Substitute, Percutaneous Endoscopic Approach
00RF4KZ Replacement of Olfactory Nerve with Nonautologous Tissue Substitute, Percutaneous Endoscopic Approach
00RG07Z Replacement of Optic Nerve with Autologous Tissue Substitute, Open Approach
00RG0JZ Replacement of Optic Nerve with Synthetic Substitute, Open Approach
00RG0KZ Replacement of Optic Nerve with Nonautologous Tissue Substitute, Open Approach
00RG47Z Replacement of Optic Nerve with Autologous Tissue Substitute, Percutaneous Endoscopic Approach
00RG4JZ Replacement of Optic Nerve with Synthetic Substitute, Percutaneous Endoscopic Approach
00RG4KZ Replacement of Optic Nerve with Nonautologous Tissue Substitute, Percutaneous Endoscopic Approach
00RH07Z Replacement of Oculomotor Nerve with Autologous Tissue Substitute, Open Approach
00RH0JZ Replacement of Oculomotor Nerve with Synthetic Substitute, Open Approach

00RH0KZ Replacement of Oculomotor Nerve with Nonautologous Tissue Substitute, Open Approach
00RH47Z Replacement of Oculomotor Nerve with Autologous Tissue Substitute, Percutaneous Endoscopic Approach
00RH4JZ Replacement of Oculomotor Nerve with Synthetic Substitute, Percutaneous Endoscopic Approach
00RH4KZ Replacement of Oculomotor Nerve with Nonautologous Tissue Substitute, Percutaneous Endoscopic Approach
00RJ07Z Replacement of Trochlear Nerve with Autologous Tissue Substitute, Open Approach
00RJ0JZ Replacement of Trochlear Nerve with Synthetic Substitute, Open Approach
00RJ0KZ Replacement of Trochlear Nerve with Nonautologous Tissue Substitute, Open Approach
00RJ47Z Replacement of Trochlear Nerve with Autologous Tissue Substitute, Percutaneous Endoscopic Approach
00RJ4JZ Replacement of Trochlear Nerve with Synthetic Substitute, Percutaneous Endoscopic Approach
00RJ4KZ Replacement of Trochlear Nerve with Nonautologous Tissue Substitute, Percutaneous Endoscopic Approach
00RK07Z Replacement of Trigeminal Nerve with Autologous Tissue Substitute, Open Approach
00RK0JZ Replacement of Trigeminal Nerve with Synthetic Substitute, Open Approach
00RK0KZ Replacement of Trigeminal Nerve with Nonautologous Tissue Substitute, Open Approach
00RK47Z Replacement of Trigeminal Nerve with Autologous Tissue Substitute, Percutaneous Endoscopic Approach
00RK4JZ Replacement of Trigeminal Nerve with Synthetic Substitute, Percut
00RK4KZ Replacement of Trigeminal Nerve with Nonautologous Tissue Substitute, Percutaneous Endoscopic Approach
00RL07Z Replacement of Abducens Nerve with Autologous Tissue Substitute, Open Approach

♀ Female-only   ♂ Male-only   ▲ Limited Coverage   ● Non-OR   HAC HAC-associated procedure   ▲ Non-covered procedures   ✚ Cluster

00RL0JZ	Replacement of Abducens Nerve with Synthetic Substitute, Open Approach
00RL0KZ	Replacement of Abducens Nerve with Nonautologous Tissue Substitute, Open Approach
00RL47Z	Replacement of Abducens Nerve with Autologous Tissue Substitute, Percutaneous Endoscopic Approach
00RL4JZ	Replacement of Abducens Nerve with Synthetic Substitute, Percutaneous Endoscopic Approach
00RL4KZ	Replacement of Abducens Nerve with Nonautologous Tissue Substitute, Percutaneous Endoscopic Approach
00RM07Z	Replacement of Facial Nerve with Autologous Tissue Substitute, Open Approach
00RM0JZ	Replacement of Facial Nerve with Synthetic Substitute, Open Approach
00RM0KZ	Replacement of Facial Nerve with Nonautologous Tissue Substitute, Open Approach
00RM47Z	Replacement of Facial Nerve with Autologous Tissue Substitute, Percutaneous Endoscopic Approach
00RM4JZ	Replacement of Facial Nerve with Synthetic Substitute, Percutaneous Endoscopic Approach
00RM4KZ	Replacement of Facial Nerve with Nonautologous Tissue Substitute, Percutaneous Endoscopic Approach
00RN07Z	Replacement of Acoustic Nerve with Autologous Tissue Substitute, Open Approach
00RN0JZ	Replacement of Acoustic Nerve with Synthetic Substitute, Open Approach
00RN0KZ	Replacement of Acoustic Nerve with Nonautologous Tissue Substitute, Open Approach
00RN47Z	Replacement of Acoustic Nerve with Autologous Tissue Substitute, Percutaneous Endoscopic Approach
00RN4JZ	Replacement of Acoustic Nerve with Synthetic Substitute, Percutaneous Endoscopic Approach

00RN4KZ	Replacement of Acoustic Nerve with Nonautologous Tissue Substitute, Percutaneous Endoscopic Approach
00RP07Z	Replacement of Glossopharyngeal Nerve with Autologous Tissue Substitute, Open Approach
00RP0JZ	Replacement of Glossopharyngeal Nerve with Synthetic Substitute, Open Approach
00RP0KZ	Replacement of Glossopharyngeal Nerve with Nonautologous Tissue Substitute, Open Approach
00RP47Z	Replacement of Glossopharyngeal Nerve with Autologous Tissue Substitute, Percutaneous Endoscopic Approach
00RP4JZ	Replacement of Glossopharyngeal Nerve with Synthetic Substitute, Percutaneous Endoscopic Approach
00RP4KZ	Replacement of Glossopharyngeal Nerve with Nonautologous Tissue Substitute, Percutaneous Endoscopic Approach
00RQ07Z	Replacement of Vagus Nerve with Autologous Tissue Substitute, Open Approach
00RQ0JZ	Replacement of Vagus Nerve with Synthetic Substitute, Open Approach
00RQ0KZ	Replacement of Vagus Nerve with Nonautologous Tissue Substitute, Open Approach
00RQ47Z	Replacement of Vagus Nerve with Autologous Tissue Substitute, Percutaneous Endoscopic Approach
00RQ4JZ	Replacement of Vagus Nerve with Synthetic Substitute, Percutaneous Endoscopic Approach
00RQ4KZ	Replacement of Vagus Nerve with Nonautologous Tissue Substitute, Percutaneous Endoscopic Approach
00RR07Z	Replacement of Accessory Nerve with Autologous Tissue Substitute, Open Approach
00RR0JZ	Replacement of Accessory Nerve with Synthetic Substitute, Open Approach

00RR0KZ	Replacement of Accessory Nerve with Nonautologous Tissue Substitute, Open Approach
00RR47Z	Replacement of Accessory Nerve with Autologous Tissue Substitute, Percutaneous Endoscopic Approach
00RR4JZ	Replacement of Accessory Nerve with Synthetic Substitute, Percutaneous Endoscopic Approach
00RR4KZ	Replacement of Accessory Nerve with Nonautologous Tissue Substitute, Percutaneous Endoscopic Approach
00RS07Z	Replacement of Hypoglossal Nerve with Autologous Tissue Substitute, Open Approach
00RS0JZ	Replacement of Hypoglossal Nerve with Synthetic Substitute, Open Approach
00RS0KZ	Replacement of Hypoglossal Nerve with Nonautologous Tissue Substitute, Open Approach
00RS47Z	Replacement of Hypoglossal Nerve with Autologous Tissue Substitute, Percutaneous Endoscopic Approach
00RS4JZ	Replacement of Hypoglossal Nerve with Synthetic Substitute, Percutaneous Endoscopic Approach
00RS4KZ	Replacement of Hypoglossal Nerve with Nonautologous Tissue Substitute, Percutaneous Endoscopic Approach
00RT07Z	Replacement of Spinal Meninges with Autologous Tissue Substitute, Open Approach
00RT0JZ	Replacement of Spinal Meninges with Synthetic Substitute, Open Approach
00RT0KZ	Replacement of Spinal Meninges with Nonautologous Tissue Substitute, Open Approach
00RT47Z	Replacement of Spinal Meninges with Autologous Tissue Substitute, Percutaneous Endoscopic Approach
00RT4JZ	Replacement of Spinal Meninges with Synthetic Substitute, Percutaneous Endoscopic Approach
00RT4KZ	Replacement of Spinal Meninges with Nonautologous Tissue Substitute, Percutaneous Endoscopic Approach

00S – Central Nervous System and Cranial Nerves, Reposition

00SF0ZZ	Reposition Olfactory Nerve, Open Approach
00SF3ZZ	Reposition Olfactory Nerve, Percutaneous Approach
00SF4ZZ	Reposition Olfactory Nerve, Percutaneous Endoscopic Approach
00SG0ZZ	Reposition Optic Nerve, Open Approach
00SG3ZZ	Reposition Optic Nerve, Percutaneous Approach
00SG4ZZ	Reposition Optic Nerve, Percutaneous Endoscopic Approach
00SH0ZZ	Reposition Oculomotor Nerve, Open Approach
00SH3ZZ	Reposition Oculomotor Nerve, Percutaneous Approach
00SH4ZZ	Reposition Oculomotor Nerve, Percutaneous Endoscopic Approach
00SJ0ZZ	Reposition Trochlear Nerve, Open Approach
00SJ3ZZ	Reposition Trochlear Nerve, Percutaneous Approach
00SJ4ZZ	Reposition Trochlear Nerve, Percutaneous Endoscopic Approach
00SK0ZZ	Reposition Trigeminal Nerve, Open Approach

00SK3ZZ	Reposition Trigeminal Nerve, Percutaneous Approach
00SK4ZZ	Reposition Trigeminal Nerve, Percutaneous Endoscopic Approach
00SL0ZZ	Reposition Abducens Nerve, Open Approach
00SL3ZZ	Reposition Abducens Nerve, Percutaneous Approach
00SL4ZZ	Reposition Abducens Nerve, Percutaneous Endoscopic Approach
00SM0ZZ	Reposition Facial Nerve, Open Approach *AHA CC: 4Q, 2014, 35*
00SM3ZZ	Reposition Facial Nerve, Percutaneous Approach
00SM4ZZ	Reposition Facial Nerve, Percutaneous Endoscopic Approach
00SN0ZZ	Reposition Acoustic Nerve, Open Approach
00SN3ZZ	Reposition Acoustic Nerve, Percutaneous Approach
00SN4ZZ	Reposition Acoustic Nerve, Percutaneous Endoscopic Approach
00SP0ZZ	Reposition Glossopharyngeal Nerve, Open Approach

00SP3ZZ	Reposition Glossopharyngeal Nerve, Percutaneous Approach
00SP4ZZ	Reposition Glossopharyngeal Nerve, Percutaneous Endoscopic Approach
00SQ0ZZ	Reposition Vagus Nerve, Open Approach
00SQ3ZZ	Reposition Vagus Nerve, Percutaneous Approach
00SQ4ZZ	Reposition Vagus Nerve, Percutaneous Endoscopic Approach
00SR0ZZ	Reposition Accessory Nerve, Open Approach
00SR3ZZ	Reposition Accessory Nerve, Percutaneous Approach
00SR4ZZ	Reposition Accessory Nerve, Percutaneous Endoscopic Approach
00SS0ZZ	Reposition Hypoglossal Nerve, Open Approach
00SS3ZZ	Reposition Hypoglossal Nerve, Percutaneous Approach
00SS4ZZ	Reposition Hypoglossal Nerve, Percutaneous Endoscopic Approach
00SW0ZZ	Reposition Cervical Spinal Cord, Open Approach

00SW3ZZ Reposition Cervical Spinal Cord, Percutaneous Approach	**00SX3ZZ** Reposition Thoracic Spinal Cord, Percutaneous Approach	**00SY3ZZ** Reposition Lumbar Spinal Cord, Percutaneous Approach
00SW4ZZ Reposition Cervical Spinal Cord, Percutaneous Endoscopic Approach	**00SX4ZZ** Reposition Thoracic Spinal Cord, Percutaneous Endoscopic Approach	**00SY4ZZ** Reposition Lumbar Spinal Cord, Percutaneous Endoscopic Approach
00SX0ZZ Reposition Thoracic Spinal Cord, Open Approach	**00SY0ZZ** Reposition Lumbar Spinal Cord, Open Approach	

00T – Central Nervous System and Cranial Nerves, Resection

Review Coding Guideline B3.8

Review Coding Guideline B3.18

00T70ZZ Resection of Cerebral Hemisphere, Open Approach	**00T73ZZ** Resection of Cerebral Hemisphere, Percutaneous Approach	**00T74ZZ** Resection of Cerebral Hemisphere, Percutaneous Endoscopic Approach

00U – Central Nervous System and Cranial Nerves, Supplement

00U107Z Supplement Cerebral Meninges with Autologous Tissue Substitute, Open Approach	**00U60KZ** Supplement Cerebral Ventricle with Nonautologous Tissue Substitute, Open Approach	**00UG3JZ** Supplement Optic Nerve with Synthetic Substitute, Percutaneous Approach
00U10JZ Supplement Cerebral Meninges with Synthetic Substitute, Open Approach	**00U637Z** Supplement Cerebral Ventricle with Autologous Tissue Substitute, Percutaneous Approach	**00UG3KZ** Supplement Optic Nerve with Nonautologous Tissue Substitute, Percutaneous Approach
00U10KZ Supplement Cerebral Meninges with Nonautologous Tissue Substitute, Open Approach	**00U63JZ** Supplement Cerebral Ventricle with Synthetic Substitute, Percutaneous Approach	**00UG47Z** Supplement Optic Nerve with Autologous Tissue Substitute, Percutaneous Endoscopic Approach
00U137Z Supplement Cerebral Meninges with Autologous Tissue Substitute, Percutaneous Approach	**00U63KZ** Supplement Cerebral Ventricle with Nonautologous Tissue Substitute, Percutaneous Approach	**00UG4JZ** Supplement Optic Nerve with Synthetic Substitute, Percutaneous Endoscopic Approach
00U13JZ Supplement Cerebral Meninges with Synthetic Substitute, Percutaneous Approach	**00U647Z** Supplement Cerebral Ventricle with Autologous Tissue Substitute, Percutaneous Endoscopic Approach	**00UG4KZ** Supplement Optic Nerve with Nonautologous Tissue Substitute, Percutaneous Endoscopic Approach
00U13KZ Supplement Cerebral Meninges with Nonautologous Tissue Substitute, Percutaneous Approach	**00U64JZ** Supplement Cerebral Ventricle with Synthetic Substitute, Percutaneous Endoscopic Approach	**00UH07Z** Supplement Oculomotor Nerve with Autologous Tissue Substitute, Open Approach
00U147Z Supplement Cerebral Meninges with Autologous Tissue Substitute, Percutaneous Endoscopic Approach	**00U64KZ** Supplement Cerebral Ventricle with Nonautologous Tissue Substitute, Percutaneous Endoscopic Approach	**00UH0JZ** Supplement Oculomotor Nerve with Synthetic Substitute, Open Approach
00U14JZ Supplement Cerebral Meninges with Synthetic Substitute, Percutaneous Endoscopic Approach	**00UF07Z** Supplement Olfactory Nerve with Autologous Tissue Substitute, Open Approach	**00UH0KZ** Supplement Oculomotor Nerve with Nonautologous Tissue Substitute, Open Approach
00U14KZ Supplement Cerebral Meninges with Nonautologous Tissue Substitute, Percutaneous Endoscopic Approach	**00UF0JZ** Supplement Olfactory Nerve with Synthetic Substitute, Open Approach	**00UH37Z** Supplement Oculomotor Nerve with Autologous Tissue Substitute, Percutaneous Approach
00U207Z Supplement Dura Mater with Autologous Tissue Substitute, Open Approach	**00UF0KZ** Supplement Olfactory Nerve with Nonautologous Tissue Substitute, Open Approach	**00UH3JZ** Supplement Oculomotor Nerve with Synthetic Substitute, Percutaneous Approach
00U20JZ Supplement Dura Mater with Synthetic Substitute, Open Approach	**00UF37Z** Supplement Olfactory Nerve with Autologous Tissue Substitute, Percutaneous Approach	**00UH3KZ** Supplement Oculomotor Nerve with Nonautologous Tissue Substitute, Percutaneous Approach
00U20KZ Supplement Dura Mater with Nonautologous Tissue Substitute, Open Approach *AHA CC: 3Q, 2017, 10-11; 1Q, 2018, 9*	**00UF3JZ** Supplement Olfactory Nerve with Synthetic Substitute, Percutaneous Approach	**00UH47Z** Supplement Oculomotor Nerve with Autologous Tissue Substitute, Percutaneous Endoscopic Approach
00U237Z Supplement Dura Mater with Autologous Tissue Substitute, Percutaneous Approach	**00UF3KZ** Supplement Olfactory Nerve with Nonautologous Tissue Substitute, Percutaneous Approach	**00UH4JZ** Supplement Oculomotor Nerve with Synthetic Substitute, Percutaneous Endoscopic Approach
00U23JZ Supplement Dura Mater with Synthetic Substitute, Percutaneous Approach	**00UF47Z** Supplement Olfactory Nerve with Autologous Tissue Substitute, Percutaneous Endoscopic Approach	**00UH4KZ** Supplement Oculomotor Nerve with Nonautologous Tissue Substitute, Percutaneous Endoscopic Approach
00U23KZ Supplement Dura Mater with Nonautologous Tissue Substitute, Percutaneous Approach	**00UF4JZ** Supplement Olfactory Nerve with Synthetic Substitute, Percutaneous Endoscopic Approach	**00UJ07Z** Supplement Trochlear Nerve with Autologous Tissue Substitute, Open Approach
00U247Z Supplement Dura Mater with Autologous Tissue Substitute, Percutaneous Endoscopic Approach	**00UF4KZ** Supplement Olfactory Nerve with Nonautologous Tissue Substitute, Percutaneous Endoscopic Approach	**00UJ0JZ** Supplement Trochlear Nerve with Synthetic Substitute, Open Approach
00U24JZ Supplement Dura Mater with Synthetic Substitute, Percutaneous Endoscopic Approach	**00UG07Z** Supplement Optic Nerve with Autologous Tissue Substitute, Open Approach	**00UJ0KZ** Supplement Trochlear Nerve with Nonautologous Tissue Substitute, Open Approach
00U24KZ Supplement Dura Mater with Nonautologous Tissue Substitute, Percutaneous Endoscopic Approach	**00UG0JZ** Supplement Optic Nerve with Synthetic Substitute, Open Approach	**00UJ37Z** Supplement Trochlear Nerve with Autologous Tissue Substitute, Percutaneous Approach
00U607Z Supplement Cerebral Ventricle with Autologous Tissue Substitute, Open Approach	**00UG0KZ** Supplement Optic Nerve with Nonautologous Tissue Substitute, Open Approach	**00UJ3JZ** Supplement Trochlear Nerve with Synthetic Substitute, Percutaneous Approach
00U60JZ Supplement Cerebral Ventricle with Synthetic Substitute, Open Approach	**00UG37Z** Supplement Optic Nerve with Autologous Tissue Substitute, Percutaneous Approach	**00UJ3KZ** Supplement Trochlear Nerve with Nonautologous Tissue Substitute, Percutaneous Approach

♀ Female-only   ♂ Male-only   ▲ Limited Coverage   ● Non-OR   HAC HAC-associated procedure   ▲ Non-covered procedures   ✚ Cluster

00UJ47Z Supplement Trochlear Nerve with Autologous Tissue Substitute, Percutaneous Endoscopic Approach

00UJ4JZ Supplement Trochlear Nerve with Synthetic Substitute, Percutaneous Endoscopic Approach

00UJ4KZ Supplement Trochlear Nerve with Nonautologous Tissue Substitute, Percutaneous Endoscopic Approach

00UK07Z Supplement Trigeminal Nerve with Autologous Tissue Substitute, Open Approach

00UK0JZ Supplement Trigeminal Nerve with Synthetic Substitute, Open Approach

00UK0KZ Supplement Trigeminal Nerve with Nonautologous Tissue Substitute, Open Approach

00UK37Z Supplement Trigeminal Nerve with Autologous Tissue Substitute, Percutaneous Approach

00UK3JZ Supplement Trigeminal Nerve with Synthetic Substitute, Percutaneous Approach

00UK3KZ Supplement Trigeminal Nerve with Nonautologous Tissue Substitute, Percutaneous Approach

00UK47Z Supplement Trigeminal Nerve with Autologous Tissue Substitute, Percutaneous Endoscopic Approach

00UK4JZ Supplement Trigeminal Nerve with Synthetic Substitute, Percutaneous Endoscopic Approach

00UK4KZ Supplement Trigeminal Nerve with Nonautologous Tissue Substitute, Percutaneous Endoscopic Approach

00UL07Z Supplement Abducens Nerve with Autologous Tissue Substitute, Open Approach

00UL0JZ Supplement Abducens Nerve with Synthetic Substitute, Open Approach

00UL0KZ Supplement Abducens Nerve with Nonautologous Tissue Substitute, Open Approach

00UL37Z Supplement Abducens Nerve with Autologous Tissue Substitute, Percutaneous Approach

00UL3JZ Supplement Abducens Nerve with Synthetic Substitute, Percutaneous Approach

00UL3KZ Supplement Abducens Nerve with Nonautologous Tissue Substitute, Percutaneous Approach

00UL47Z Supplement Abducens Nerve with Autologous Tissue Substitute, Percutaneous Endoscopic Approach

00UL4JZ Supplement Abducens Nerve with Synthetic Substitute, Percutaneous Endoscopic Approach

00UL4KZ Supplement Abducens Nerve with Nonautologous Tissue Substitute, Percutaneous Endoscopic Approach

00UM07Z Supplement Facial Nerve with Autologous Tissue Substitute, Open Approach

00UM0JZ Supplement Facial Nerve with Synthetic Substitute, Open Approach

00UM0KZ Supplement Facial Nerve with Nonautologous Tissue Substitute, Open Approach

00UM37Z Supplement Facial Nerve with Autologous Tissue Substitute, Percutaneous Approach

00UM3JZ Supplement Facial Nerve with Synthetic Substitute, Percutaneous Approach

00UM3KZ Supplement Facial Nerve with Nonautologous Tissue Substitute, Percutaneous Approach

00UM47Z Supplement Facial Nerve with Autologous Tissue Substitute, Percutaneous Endoscopic Approach

00UM4JZ Supplement Facial Nerve with Synthetic Substitute, Percutaneous Endoscopic Approach

00UM4KZ Supplement Facial Nerve with Nonautologous Tissue Substitute, Percutaneous Endoscopic Approach

00UN07Z Supplement Acoustic Nerve with Autologous Tissue Substitute, Open Approach

00UN0JZ Supplement Acoustic Nerve with Synthetic Substitute, Open Approach

00UN0KZ Supplement Acoustic Nerve with Nonautologous Tissue Substitute, Open Approach

00UN37Z Supplement Acoustic Nerve with Autologous Tissue Substitute, Percutaneous Approach

00UN3JZ Supplement Acoustic Nerve with Synthetic Substitute, Percutaneous Approach

00UN3KZ Supplement Acoustic Nerve with Nonautologous Tissue Substitute, Percutaneous Approach

00UN47Z Supplement Acoustic Nerve with Autologous Tissue Substitute, Percutaneous Endoscopic Approach

00UN4JZ Supplement Acoustic Nerve with Synthetic Substitute, Percutaneous Endoscopic Approach

00UN4KZ Supplement Acoustic Nerve with Nonautologous Tissue Substitute, Percutaneous Endoscopic Approach

00UP07Z Supplement Glossopharyngeal Nerve with Autologous Tissue Substitute, Open Approach

00UP0JZ Supplement Glossopharyngeal Nerve with Synthetic Substitute, Open Approach

00UP0KZ Supplement Glossopharyngeal Nerve with Nonautologous Tissue Substitute, Open Approach

00UP37Z Supplement Glossopharyngeal Nerve with Autologous Tissue Substitute, Percutaneous Approach

00UP3JZ Supplement Glossopharyngeal Nerve with Synthetic Substitute, Percutaneous Approach

00UP3KZ Supplement Glossopharyngeal Nerve with Nonautologous Tissue Substitute, Percutaneous Approach

00UP47Z Supplement Glossopharyngeal Nerve with Autologous Tissue Substitute, Percutaneous Endoscopic Approach

00UP4JZ Supplement Glossopharyngeal Nerve with Synthetic Substitute, Percutaneous Endoscopic Approach

00UP4KZ Supplement Glossopharyngeal Nerve with Nonautologous Tissue Substitute, Percutaneous Endoscopic Approach

00UQ07Z Supplement Vagus Nerve with Autologous Tissue Substitute, Open Approach

00UQ0JZ Supplement Vagus Nerve with Synthetic Substitute, Open Approach

00UQ0KZ Supplement Vagus Nerve with Nonautologous Tissue Substitute, Open Approach

00UQ37Z Supplement Vagus Nerve with Autologous Tissue Substitute, Percutaneous Approach

00UQ3JZ Supplement Vagus Nerve with Synthetic Substitute, Percutaneous Approach

00UQ3KZ Supplement Vagus Nerve with Nonautologous Tissue Substitute, Percutaneous Approach

00UQ47Z Supplement Vagus Nerve with Autologous Tissue Substitute, Percutaneous Endoscopic Approach

00UQ4JZ Supplement Vagus Nerve with Synthetic Substitute, Percutaneous Endoscopic Approach

00UQ4KZ Supplement Vagus Nerve with Nonautologous Tissue Substitute, Percutaneous Endoscopic Approach

00UR07Z Supplement Accessory Nerve with Autologous Tissue Substitute, Open Approach

00UR0JZ Supplement Accessory Nerve with Synthetic Substitute, Open Approach

00UR0KZ Supplement Accessory Nerve with Nonautologous Tissue Substitute, Open Approach

00UR37Z Supplement Accessory Nerve with Autologous Tissue Substitute, Percutaneous Approach

00UR3JZ Supplement Accessory Nerve with Synthetic Substitute, Percutaneous Approach

00UR3KZ Supplement Accessory Nerve with Nonautologous Tissue Substitute, Percutaneous Approach

00UR47Z Supplement Accessory Nerve with Autologous Tissue Substitute, Percutaneous Endoscopic Approach

00UR4JZ Supplement Accessory Nerve with Synthetic Substitute, Percutaneous Endoscopic Approach

00UR4KZ Supplement Accessory Nerve with Nonautologous Tissue Substitute, Percutaneous Endoscopic Approach

00US07Z Supplement Hypoglossal Nerve with Autologous Tissue Substitute, Open Approach

00US0JZ Supplement Hypoglossal Nerve with Synthetic Substitute, Open Approach

00US0KZ Supplement Hypoglossal Nerve with Nonautologous Tissue Substitute, Open Approach

00US37Z Supplement Hypoglossal Nerve with Autologous Tissue Substitute, Percutaneous Approach

00US3JZ Supplement Hypoglossal Nerve with Synthetic Substitute, Percutaneous Approach

00US3KZ Supplement Hypoglossal Nerve with Nonautologous Tissue Substitute, Percutaneous Approach

00US47Z Supplement Hypoglossal Nerve with Autologous Tissue Substitute, Percutaneous Endoscopic Approach

00US4JZ Supplement Hypoglossal Nerve with Synthetic Substitute, Percutaneous Endoscopic Approach

00US4KZ Supplement Hypoglossal Nerve with Nonautologous Tissue Substitute, Percutaneous Endoscopic Approach

00UT07Z Supplement Spinal Meninges with Autologous Tissue Substitute, Open Approach

00UT0JZ Supplement Spinal Meninges with Synthetic Substitute, Open Approach

00UT0KZ Supplement Spinal Meninges with Nonautologous Tissue Substitute, Open Approach

AHA CC: 3Q, 2014, 24

♀ Female-only   ♂ Male-only   ▲ Limited Coverage   ● Non-OR   HAC HAC-associated procedure   ▲ Non-covered procedures   ✚ Cluster

00UT37Z Supplement Spinal Meninges with Autologous Tissue Substitute, Percutaneous Approach

00UT3JZ Supplement Spinal Meninges with Synthetic Substitute, Percutaneous Approach

00UT3KZ Supplement Spinal Meninges with Nonautologous Tissue Substitute, Percutaneous Approach

00UT47Z Supplement Spinal Meninges with Autologous Tissue Substitute, Percutaneous Endoscopic Approach

00UT4JZ Supplement Spinal Meninges with Synthetic Substitute, Percutaneous Endoscopic Approach

00UT4KZ Supplement Spinal Meninges with Nonautologous Tissue Substitute, Percutaneous Endoscopic Approach

00W – Central Nervous System and Cranial Nerves, Revision

Review Coding Guideline B6.1c

00W000Z Revision of Drainage Device in Brain, Open Approach

00W002Z Revision of Monitoring Device in Brain, Open Approach

00W003Z Revision of Infusion Device in Brain, Open Approach

00W007Z Revision of Autologous Tissue Substitute in Brain, Open Approach

00W00JZ Revision of Synthetic Substitute in Brain, Open Approach

00W00KZ Revision of Nonautologous Tissue Substitute in Brain, Open Approach

00W00MZ Revision of Neurostimulator Lead in Brain, Open Approach

00W00YZ Revision of Other Device in Brain, Open Approach

00W030Z Revision of Drainage Device in Brain, Percutaneous Approach

00W032Z Revision of Monitoring Device in Brain, Percutaneous Approach

00W033Z Revision of Infusion Device in Brain, Percutaneous Approach

00W037Z Revision of Autologous Tissue Substitute in Brain, Percutaneous Approach

00W03JZ Revision of Synthetic Substitute in Brain, Percutaneous Approach

00W03KZ Revision of Nonautologous Tissue Substitute in Brain, Percutaneous Approach

00W03MZ Revision of Neurostimulator Lead in Brain, Percutaneous Approach

00W03YZ Revision of Other Device in Brain, Percutaneous Approach

00W040Z Revision of Drainage Device in Brain, Percutaneous Endoscopic Approach

00W042Z Revision of Monitoring Device in Brain, Percutaneous Endoscopic Approach

00W043Z Revision of Infusion Device in Brain, Percutaneous Endoscopic Approach

00W047Z Revision of Autologous Tissue Substitute in Brain, Percutaneous Endoscopic Approach

00W04JZ Revision of Synthetic Substitute in Brain, Percutaneous Endoscopic Approach

00W04KZ Revision of Nonautologous Tissue Substitute in Brain, Percutaneous Endoscopic Approach

00W04MZ Revision of Neurostimulator Lead in Brain, Percutaneous Endoscopic Approach

00W04YZ Revision of Other Device in Brain, Percutaneous Endoscopic Approach

00W0X0Z Revision of Drainage Device in Brain, External Approach

00W0X2Z Revision of Monitoring Device in Brain, External Approach

00W0X3Z Revision of Infusion Device in Brain, External Approach

00W0X7Z Revision of Autologous Tissue Substitute in Brain, External Approach

00W0XJZ Revision of Synthetic Substitute in Brain, External Approach

00W0XKZ Revision of Nonautologous Tissue Substitute in Brain, External Approach

00W0XMZ Revision of Neurostimulator Lead in Brain, External Approach

00W600Z Revision of Drainage Device in Cerebral Ventricle, Open Approach

00W602Z Revision of Monitoring Device in Cerebral Ventricle, Open Approach

00W603Z Revision of Infusion Device in Cerebral Ventricle, Open Approach

00W60JZ Revision of Synthetic Substitute in Cerebral Ventricle, Open Approach

00W60MZ Revision of Neurostimulator Lead in Cerebral Ventricle, Open Approach

00W60YZ Revision of Other Device in Cerebral Ventricle, Open Approach

00W630Z Revision of Drainage Device in Cerebral Ventricle, Percutaneous Approach

00W632Z Revision of Monitoring Device in Cerebral Ventricle, Percutaneous Approach

00W633Z Revision of Infusion Device in Cerebral Ventricle, Percutaneous Approach

00W63JZ Revision of Synthetic Substitute in Cerebral Ventricle, Percutaneous Approach

00W63MZ Revision of Neurostimulator Lead in Cerebral Ventricle, Percutaneous Approach

00W63YZ Revision of Other Device in Cerebral Ventricle, Percutaneous Approach

00W640Z Revision of Drainage Device in Cerebral Ventricle, Percutaneous Endoscopic Approach

00W642Z Revision of Monitoring Device in Cerebral Ventricle, Percutaneous Endoscopic Approach

00W643Z Revision of Infusion Device in Cerebral Ventricle, Percutaneous Endoscopic Approach

00W64JZ Revision of Synthetic Substitute in Cerebral Ventricle, Percutaneous Endoscopic Approach

00W64MZ Revision of Neurostimulator Lead in Cerebral Ventricle, Percutaneous Endoscopic Approach

00W64YZ Revision of Other Device in Cerebral Ventricle, Percutaneous Endoscopic Approach

00W6X0Z Revision of Drainage Device in Cerebral Ventricle, External Approach

00W6X2Z Revision of Monitoring Device in Cerebral Ventricle, External Approach

00W6X3Z Revision of Infusion Device in Cerebral Ventricle, External Approach

00W6XJZ Revision of Synthetic Substitute in Cerebral Ventricle, External Approach

00W6XMZ Revision of Neurostimulator Lead in Cerebral Ventricle, External Approach

00WE00Z Revision of Drainage Device in Cranial Nerve, Open Approach

00WE02Z Revision of Monitoring Device in Cranial Nerve, Open Approach

00WE03Z Revision of Infusion Device in Cranial Nerve, Open Approach

00WE07Z Revision of Autologous Tissue Substitute in Cranial Nerve, Open Approach

00WE0MZ Revision of Neurostimulator Lead in Cranial Nerve, Open Approach

00WE0YZ Revision of Other Device in Cranial Nerve, Open Approach

00WE30Z Revision of Drainage Device in Cranial Nerve, Percutaneous Approach

00WE32Z Revision of Monitoring Device in Cranial Nerve, Percutaneous Approach

00WE33Z Revision of Infusion Device in Cranial Nerve, Percutaneous Approach

00WE37Z Revision of Autologous Tissue Substitute in Cranial Nerve, Percutaneous Approach

00WE3MZ Revision of Neurostimulator Lead in Cranial Nerve, Percutaneous Approach

00WE3YZ Revision of Other Device in Cranial Nerve, Percutaneous Approach

00WE40Z Revision of Drainage Device in Cranial Nerve, Percutaneous Endoscopic Approach

00WE42Z Revision of Monitoring Device in Cranial Nerve, Percutaneous Endoscopic Approach

00WE43Z Revision of Infusion Device in Cranial Nerve, Percutaneous Endoscopic Approach

00WE47Z Revision of Autologous Tissue Substitute in Cranial Nerve, Percutaneous Endoscopic Approach

00WE4MZ Revision of Neurostimulator Lead in Cranial Nerve, Percutaneous Endoscopic Approach

00WE4YZ Revision of Other Device in Cranial Nerve, Percutaneous Endoscopic Approach

00WEX0Z Revision of Drainage Device in Cranial Nerve, External Approach

00WEX2Z Revision of Monitoring Device in Cranial Nerve, External Approach

00WEX3Z Revision of Infusion Device in Cranial Nerve, External Approach

00WEX7Z Revision of Autologous Tissue Substitute in Cranial Nerve, External Approach

00WEXMZ Revision of Neurostimulator Lead in Cranial Nerve, External Approach

00WU00Z Revision of Drainage Device in Spinal Canal, Open Approach

00WU02Z Revision of Monitoring Device in Spinal Canal, Open Approach

00WU03Z Revision of Infusion Device in Spinal Canal, Open Approach

00WU0JZ Revision of Synthetic Substitute in Spinal Canal, Open Approach

00WU0MZ Revision of Neurostimulator Lead in Spinal Canal, Open Approach

00WU0YZ Revision of Other Device in Spinal Canal, Open Approach

♀ Female-only   ♂ Male-only   ▲ Limited Coverage   ● Non-OR   HAC HAC-associated procedure   ▲ Non-covered procedures   ✚ Cluster

00WU30Z	Revision of Drainage Device in Spinal Canal, Percutaneous Approach
00WU32Z	Revision of Monitoring Device in Spinal Canal, Percutaneous Approach
00WU33Z	Revision of Infusion Device in Spinal Canal, Percutaneous Approach
00WU3JZ	Revision of Synthetic Substitute in Spinal Canal, Percutaneous Approach
00WU3MZ	Revision of Neurostimulator Lead in Spinal Canal, Percutaneous Approach
00WU3YZ	Revision of Other Device in Spinal Canal, Percutaneous Approach
00WU40Z	Revision of Drainage Device in Spinal Canal, Percutaneous Endoscopic Approach
00WU42Z	Revision of Monitoring Device in Spinal Canal, Percutaneous Endoscopic Approach
00WU43Z	Revision of Infusion Device in Spinal Canal, Percutaneous Endoscopic Approach
00WU4JZ	Revision of Synthetic Substitute in Spinal Canal, Percutaneous Endoscopic Approach
00WU4MZ	Revision of Neurostimulator Lead in Spinal Canal, Percutaneous Endoscopic Approach
00WU4YZ	Revision of Other Device in Spinal Canal, Percutaneous Endoscopic Approach
00WUX0Z	Revision of Drainage Device in Spinal Canal, External Approach
00WUX2Z	Revision of Monitoring Device in Spinal Canal, External Approach
00WUX3Z	Revision of Infusion Device in Spinal Canal, External Approach
00WUXJZ	Revision of Synthetic Substitute in Spinal Canal, External Approach
00WUXMZ	Revision of Neurostimulator Lead in Spinal Canal, External Approach

00WV00Z	Revision of Drainage Device in Spinal Cord, Open Approach
00WV02Z	Revision of Monitoring Device in Spinal Cord, Open Approach
00WV03Z	Revision of Infusion Device in Spinal Cord, Open Approach
00WV07Z	Revision of Autologous Tissue Substitute in Spinal Cord, Open Approach
00WV0JZ	Revision of Synthetic Substitute in Spinal Cord, Open Approach
00WV0KZ	Revision of Nonautologous Tissue Substitute in Spinal Cord, Open Approach
00WV0MZ	Revision of Neurostimulator Lead in Spinal Cord, Open Approach
00WV0YZ	Revision of Other Device in Spinal Cord, Open Approach
00WV30Z	Revision of Drainage Device in Spinal Cord, Percutaneous Approach
00WV32Z	Revision of Monitoring Device in Spinal Cord, Percutaneous Approach
00WV33Z	Revision of Infusion Device in Spinal Cord, Percutaneous Approach
00WV37Z	Revision of Autologous Tissue Substitute in Spinal Cord, Percutaneous Approach
00WV3JZ	Revision of Synthetic Substitute in Spinal Cord, Percutaneous Approach
00WV3KZ	Revision of Nonautologous Tissue Substitute in Spinal Cord, Percutaneous Approach
00WV3MZ	Revision of Neurostimulator Lead in Spinal Cord, Percutaneous Approach
00WV3YZ	Revision of Other Device in Spinal Cord, Percutaneous Approach
00WV40Z	Revision of Drainage Device in Spinal Cord, Percutaneous Endoscopic Approach

00WV42Z	Revision of Monitoring Device in Spinal Cord, Percutaneous Endoscopic Approach
00WV43Z	Revision of Infusion Device in Spinal Cord, Percutaneous Endoscopic Approach
00WV47Z	Revision of Autologous Tissue Substitute in Spinal Cord, Percutaneous Endoscopic Approach
00WV4JZ	Revision of Synthetic Substitute in Spinal Cord, Percutaneous Endoscopic Approach
00WV4KZ	Revision of Nonautologous Tissue Substitute in Spinal Cord, Percutaneous Endoscopic Approach
00WV4MZ	Revision of Neurostimulator Lead in Spinal Cord, Percutaneous Endoscopic Approach
00WV4YZ	Revision of Other Device in Spinal Cord, Percutaneous Endoscopic Approach
00WVX0Z	Revision of Drainage Device in Spinal Cord, External Approach
00WVX2Z	Revision of Monitoring Device in Spinal Cord, External Approach
00WVX3Z	Revision of Infusion Device in Spinal Cord, External Approach
00WVX7Z	Revision of Autologous Tissue Substitute in Spinal Cord, External Approach
00WVXJZ	Revision of Synthetic Substitute in Spinal Cord, External Approach
00WVXKZ	Revision of Nonautologous Tissue Substitute in Spinal Cord, External Approach
00WVXMZ	Revision of Neurostimulator Lead in Spinal Cord, External Approach

00X – Central Nervous System and Cranial Nerves, Transfer

00XF0ZF	Transfer Olfactory Nerve to Olfactory Nerve, Open Approach
00XF0ZG	Transfer Olfactory Nerve to Optic Nerve, Open Approach
00XF0ZH	Transfer Olfactory Nerve to Oculomotor Nerve, Open Approach
00XF0ZJ	Transfer Olfactory Nerve to Trochlear Nerve, Open Approach
00XF0ZK	Transfer Olfactory Nerve to Trigeminal Nerve, Open Approach
00XF0ZL	Transfer Olfactory Nerve to Abducens Nerve, Open Approach
00XF0ZM	Transfer Olfactory Nerve to Facial Nerve, Open Approach
00XF0ZN	Transfer Olfactory Nerve to Acoustic Nerve, Open Approach
00XF0ZP	Transfer Olfactory Nerve to Glossopharyngeal Nerve, Open Approach
00XF0ZQ	Transfer Olfactory Nerve to Vagus Nerve, Open Approach
00XF0ZR	Transfer Olfactory Nerve to Accessory Nerve, Open Approach
00XF0ZS	Transfer Olfactory Nerve to Hypoglossal Nerve, Open Approach
00XF4ZF	Transfer Olfactory Nerve to Olfactory Nerve, Percutaneous Endoscopic Approach
00XF4ZG	Transfer Olfactory Nerve to Optic Nerve, Percutaneous Endoscopic Approach

00XF4ZH	Transfer Olfactory Nerve to Oculomotor Nerve, Percutaneous Endoscopic Approach
00XF4ZJ	Transfer Olfactory Nerve to Trochlear Nerve, Percutaneous Endoscopic Approach
00XF4ZK	Transfer Olfactory Nerve to Trigeminal Nerve, Percutaneous Endoscopic Approach
00XF4ZL	Transfer Olfactory Nerve to Abducens Nerve, Percutaneous Endoscopic Approach
00XF4ZM	Transfer Olfactory Nerve to Facial Nerve, Percutaneous Endoscopic Approach
00XF4ZN	Transfer Olfactory Nerve to Acoustic Nerve, Percutaneous Endoscopic Approach
00XF4ZP	Transfer Olfactory Nerve to Glossopharyngeal Nerve, Percutaneous Endoscopic Approach
00XF4ZQ	Transfer Olfactory Nerve to Vagus Nerve, Percutaneous Endoscopic Approach
00XF4ZR	Transfer Olfactory Nerve to Accessory Nerve, Percutaneous Endoscopic Approach
00XF4ZS	Transfer Olfactory Nerve to Hypoglossal Nerve, Percutaneous Endoscopic Approach
00XG0ZF	Transfer Optic Nerve to Olfactory Nerve, Open Approach

00XG0ZG	Transfer Optic Nerve to Optic Nerve, Open Approach
00XG0ZH	Transfer Optic Nerve to Oculomotor Nerve, Open Approach
00XG0ZJ	Transfer Optic Nerve to Trochlear Nerve, Open Approach
00XG0ZK	Transfer Optic Nerve to Trigeminal Nerve, Open Approach
00XG0ZL	Transfer Optic Nerve to Abducens Nerve, Open Approach
00XG0ZM	Transfer Optic Nerve to Facial Nerve, Open Approach
00XG0ZN	Transfer Optic Nerve to Acoustic Nerve, Open Approach
00XG0ZP	Transfer Optic Nerve to Glossopharyngeal Nerve, Open Approach
00XG0ZQ	Transfer Optic Nerve to Vagus Nerve, Open Approach
00XG0ZR	Transfer Optic Nerve to Accessory Nerve, Open Approach
00XG0ZS	Transfer Optic Nerve to Hypoglossal Nerve, Open Approach
00XG4ZF	Transfer Optic Nerve to Olfactory Nerve, Percutaneous Endoscopic Approach
00XG4ZG	Transfer Optic Nerve to Optic Nerve, Percutaneous Endoscopic Approach
00XG4ZH	Transfer Optic Nerve to Oculomotor Nerve, Percutaneous Endoscopic Approach

00XG4ZJ Transfer Optic Nerve to Trochlear Nerve, Percutaneous Endoscopic Approach

00XG4ZK Transfer Optic Nerve to Trigeminal Nerve, Percutaneous Endoscopic Approach

00XG4ZL Transfer Optic Nerve to Abducens Nerve, Percutaneous Endoscopic Approach

00XG4ZM Transfer Optic Nerve to Facial Nerve, Percutaneous Endoscopic Approach

00XG4ZN Transfer Optic Nerve to Acoustic Nerve, Percutaneous Endoscopic Approach

00XG4ZP Transfer Optic Nerve to Glossopharyngeal Nerve, Percutaneous Endoscopic Approach

00XG4ZQ Transfer Optic Nerve to Vagus Nerve, Percutaneous Endoscopic Approach

00XG4ZR Transfer Optic Nerve to Accessory Nerve, Percutaneous Endoscopic Approach

00XG4ZS Transfer Optic Nerve to Hypoglossal Nerve, Percutaneous Endoscopic Approach

00XH0ZF Transfer Oculomotor Nerve to Olfactory Nerve, Open Approach

00XH0ZG Transfer Oculomotor Nerve to Optic Nerve, Open Approach

00XH0ZH Transfer Oculomotor Nerve to Oculomotor Nerve, Open Approach

00XH0ZJ Transfer Oculomotor Nerve to Trochlear Nerve, Open Approach

00XH0ZK Transfer Oculomotor Nerve to Trigeminal Nerve, Open Approach

00XH0ZL Transfer Oculomotor Nerve to Abducens Nerve, Open Approach

00XH0ZM Transfer Oculomotor Nerve to Facial Nerve, Open Approach

00XH0ZN Transfer Oculomotor Nerve to Acoustic Nerve, Open Approach

00XH0ZP Transfer Oculomotor Nerve to Glossopharyngeal Nerve, Open Approach

00XH0ZQ Transfer Oculomotor Nerve to Vagus Nerve, Open Approach

00XH0ZR Transfer Oculomotor Nerve to Accessory Nerve, Open Approach

00XH0ZS Transfer Oculomotor Nerve to Hypoglossal Nerve, Open Approach

00XH4ZF Transfer Oculomotor Nerve to Olfactory Nerve, Percutaneous Endoscopic Approach

00XH4ZG Transfer Oculomotor Nerve to Optic Nerve, Percutaneous Endoscopic Approach

00XH4ZH Transfer Oculomotor Nerve to Oculomotor Nerve, Percutaneous Endoscopic Approach

00XH4ZJ Transfer Oculomotor Nerve to Trochlear Nerve, Percutaneous Endoscopic Approach

00XH4ZK Transfer Oculomotor Nerve to Trigeminal Nerve, Percutaneous Endoscopic Approach

00XH4ZL Transfer Oculomotor Nerve to Abducens Nerve, Percutaneous Endoscopic Approach

00XH4ZM Transfer Oculomotor Nerve to Facial Nerve, Percutaneous Endoscopic Approach

00XH4ZN Transfer Oculomotor Nerve to Acoustic Nerve, Percutaneous Endoscopic Approach

00XH4ZP Transfer Oculomotor Nerve to Glossopharyngeal Nerve, Percutaneous Endoscopic Approach

00XH4ZQ Transfer Oculomotor Nerve to Vagus Nerve, Percutaneous Endoscopic Approach

00XH4ZR Transfer Oculomotor Nerve to Accessory Nerve, Percutaneous Endoscopic Approach

00XH4ZS Transfer Oculomotor Nerve to Hypoglossal Nerve, Percutaneous Endoscopic Approach

00XJ0ZF Transfer Trochlear Nerve to Olfactory Nerve, Open Approach

00XJ0ZG Transfer Trochlear Nerve to Optic Nerve, Open Approach

00XJ0ZH Transfer Trochlear Nerve to Oculomotor Nerve, Open Approach

00XJ0ZJ Transfer Trochlear Nerve to Trochlear Nerve, Open Approach

00XJ0ZK Transfer Trochlear Nerve to Trigeminal Nerve, Open Approach

00XJ0ZL Transfer Trochlear Nerve to Abducens Nerve, Open Approach

00XJ0ZM Transfer Trochlear Nerve to Facial Nerve, Open Approach

00XJ0ZN Transfer Trochlear Nerve to Acoustic Nerve, Open Approach

00XJ0ZP Transfer Trochlear Nerve to Glossopharyngeal Nerve, Open Approach

00XJ0ZQ Transfer Trochlear Nerve to Vagus Nerve, Open Approach

00XJ0ZR Transfer Trochlear Nerve to Accessory Nerve, Open Approach

00XJ0ZS Transfer Trochlear Nerve to Hypoglossal Nerve, Open Approach

00XJ4ZF Transfer Trochlear Nerve to Olfactory Nerve, Percutaneous Endoscopic Approach

00XJ4ZG Transfer Trochlear Nerve to Optic Nerve, Percutaneous Endoscopic Approach

00XJ4ZH Transfer Trochlear Nerve to Oculomotor Nerve, Percutaneous Endoscopic Approach

00XJ4ZJ Transfer Trochlear Nerve to Trochlear Nerve, Percutaneous Endoscopic Approach

00XJ4ZK Transfer Trochlear Nerve to Trigeminal Nerve, Percutaneous Endoscopic Approach

00XJ4ZL Transfer Trochlear Nerve to Abducens Nerve, Percutaneous Endoscopic Approach

00XJ4ZM Transfer Trochlear Nerve to Facial Nerve, Percutaneous Endoscopic Approach

00XJ4ZN Transfer Trochlear Nerve to Acoustic Nerve, Percutaneous Endoscopic Approach

00XJ4ZP Transfer Trochlear Nerve to Glossopharyngeal Nerve, Percutaneous Endoscopic Approach

00XJ4ZQ Transfer Trochlear Nerve to Vagus Nerve, Percutaneous Endoscopic Approach

00XJ4ZR Transfer Trochlear Nerve to Accessory Nerve, Percutaneous Endoscopic Approach

00XJ4ZS Transfer Trochlear Nerve to Hypoglossal Nerve, Percutaneous Endoscopic Approach

00XK0ZF Transfer Trigeminal Nerve to Olfactory Nerve, Open Approach

00XK0ZG Transfer Trigeminal Nerve to Optic Nerve, Open Approach

00XK0ZH Transfer Trigeminal Nerve to Oculomotor Nerve, Open Approach

00XK0ZJ Transfer Trigeminal Nerve to Trochlear Nerve, Open Approach

00XK0ZK Transfer Trigeminal Nerve to Trigeminal Nerve, Open Approach

00XK0ZL Transfer Trigeminal Nerve to Abducens Nerve, Open Approach

00XK0ZM Transfer Trigeminal Nerve to Facial Nerve, Open Approach

00XK0ZN Transfer Trigeminal Nerve to Acoustic Nerve, Open Approach

00XK0ZP Transfer Trigeminal Nerve to Glossopharyngeal Nerve, Open Approach

00XK0ZQ Transfer Trigeminal Nerve to Vagus Nerve, Open Approach

00XK0ZR Transfer Trigeminal Nerve to Accessory Nerve, Open Approach

00XK0ZS Transfer Trigeminal Nerve to Hypoglossal Nerve, Open Approach

00XK4ZF Transfer Trigeminal Nerve to Olfactory Nerve, Percutaneous Endoscopic Approach

00XK4ZG Transfer Trigeminal Nerve to Optic Nerve, Percutaneous Endoscopic Approach

00XK4ZH Transfer Trigeminal Nerve to Oculomotor Nerve, Percutaneous Endoscopic Approach

00XK4ZJ Transfer Trigeminal Nerve to Trochlear Nerve, Percutaneous Endoscopic Approach

00XK4ZK Transfer Trigeminal Nerve to Trigeminal Nerve, Percutaneous Endoscopic Approach

00XK4ZL Transfer Trigeminal Nerve to Abducens Nerve, Percutaneous Endoscopic Approach

00XK4ZM Transfer Trigeminal Nerve to Facial Nerve, Percutaneous Endoscopic Approach

00XK4ZN Transfer Trigeminal Nerve to Acoustic Nerve, Percutaneous Endoscopic Approach

00XK4ZP Transfer Trigeminal Nerve to Glossopharyngeal Nerve, Percutaneous Endoscopic Approach

00XK4ZQ Transfer Trigeminal Nerve to Vagus Nerve, Percutaneous Endoscopic Approach

00XK4ZR Transfer Trigeminal Nerve to Accessory Nerve, Percutaneous Endoscopic Approach

00XK4ZS Transfer Trigeminal Nerve to Hypoglossal Nerve, Percutaneous Endoscopic Approach

00XL0ZF Transfer Abducens Nerve to Olfactory Nerve, Open Approach

00XL0ZG Transfer Abducens Nerve to Optic Nerve, Open Approach

00XL0ZH Transfer Abducens Nerve to Oculomotor Nerve, Open Approach

00XL0ZJ Transfer Abducens Nerve to Trochlear Nerve, Open Approach

00XL0ZK Transfer Abducens Nerve to Trigeminal Nerve, Open Approach

00XL0ZL Transfer Abducens Nerve to Abducens Nerve, Open Approach

00XL0ZM Transfer Abducens Nerve to Facial Nerve, Open Approach

00XL0ZN Transfer Abducens Nerve to Acoustic Nerve, Open Approach

00XL0ZP Transfer Abducens Nerve to Glossopharyngeal Nerve, Open Approach

00XL0ZQ Transfer Abducens Nerve to Vagus Nerve, Open Approach

♀ Female-only   ♂ Male-only   ▲ Limited Coverage   ● Non-OR   HAC HAC-associated procedure   ▲ Non-covered procedures   ✚ Cluster

00XL0ZR	Transfer Abducens Nerve to Accessory Nerve, Open Approach
00XL0ZS	Transfer Abducens Nerve to Hypoglossal Nerve, Open Approach
00XL4ZF	Transfer Abducens Nerve to Olfactory Nerve, Percutaneous Endoscopic Approach
00XL4ZG	Transfer Abducens Nerve to Optic Nerve, Percutaneous Endoscopic Approach
00XL4ZH	Transfer Abducens Nerve to Oculomotor Nerve, Percutaneous Endoscopic Approach
00XL4ZJ	Transfer Abducens Nerve to Trochlear Nerve, Percutaneous Endoscopic Approach
00XL4ZK	Transfer Abducens Nerve to Trigeminal Nerve, Percutaneous Endoscopic Approach
00XL4ZL	Transfer Abducens Nerve to Abducens Nerve, Percutaneous Endoscopic Approach
00XL4ZM	Transfer Abducens Nerve to Facial Nerve, Percutaneous Endoscopic Approach
00XL4ZN	Transfer Abducens Nerve to Acoustic Nerve, Percutaneous Endoscopic Approach
00XL4ZP	Transfer Abducens Nerve to Glossopharyngeal Nerve, Percutaneous Endoscopic Approach
00XL4ZQ	Transfer Abducens Nerve to Vagus Nerve, Percutaneous Endoscopic Approach
00XL4ZR	Transfer Abducens Nerve to Accessory Nerve, Percutaneous Endoscopic Approach
00XL4ZS	Transfer Abducens Nerve to Hypoglossal Nerve, Percutaneous Endoscopic Approach
00XM0ZF	Transfer Facial Nerve to Olfactory Nerve, Open Approach
00XM0ZG	Transfer Facial Nerve to Optic Nerve, Open Approach
00XM0ZH	Transfer Facial Nerve to Oculomotor Nerve, Open Approach
00XM0ZJ	Transfer Facial Nerve to Trochlear Nerve, Open Approach
00XM0ZK	Transfer Facial Nerve to Trigeminal Nerve, Open Approach
00XM0ZL	Transfer Facial Nerve to Abducens Nerve, Open Approach
00XM0ZM	Transfer Facial Nerve to Facial Nerve, Open Approach
00XM0ZN	Transfer Facial Nerve to Acoustic Nerve, Open Approach
00XM0ZP	Transfer Facial Nerve to Glossopharyngeal Nerve, Open Approach
00XM0ZQ	Transfer Facial Nerve to Vagus Nerve, Open Approach
00XM0ZR	Transfer Facial Nerve to Accessory Nerve, Open Approach
00XM0ZS	Transfer Facial Nerve to Hypoglossal Nerve, Open Approach
00XM4ZF	Transfer Facial Nerve to Olfactory Nerve, Percutaneous Endoscopic Approach
00XM4ZG	Transfer Facial Nerve to Optic Nerve, Percutaneous Endoscopic Approach
00XM4ZH	Transfer Facial Nerve to Oculomotor Nerve, Percutaneous Endoscopic Approach
00XM4ZJ	Transfer Facial Nerve to Trochlear Nerve, Percutaneous Endoscopic Approach

00XM4ZK	Transfer Facial Nerve to Trigeminal Nerve, Percutaneous Endoscopic Approach
00XM4ZL	Transfer Facial Nerve to Abducens Nerve, Percutaneous Endoscopic Approach
00XM4ZM	Transfer Facial Nerve to Facial Nerve, Percutaneous Endoscopic Approach
00XM4ZN	Transfer Facial Nerve to Acoustic Nerve, Percutaneous Endoscopic Approach
00XM4ZP	Transfer Facial Nerve to Glossopharyngeal Nerve, Percutaneous Endoscopic Approach
00XM4ZQ	Transfer Facial Nerve to Vagus Nerve, Percutaneous Endoscopic Approach
00XM4ZR	Transfer Facial Nerve to Accessory Nerve, Percutaneous Endoscopic Approach
00XM4ZS	Transfer Facial Nerve to Hypoglossal Nerve, Percutaneous Endoscopic Approach
00XN0ZF	Transfer Acoustic Nerve to Olfactory Nerve, Open Approach
00XN0ZG	Transfer Acoustic Nerve to Optic Nerve, Open Approach
00XN0ZH	Transfer Acoustic Nerve to Oculomotor Nerve, Open Approach
00XN0ZJ	Transfer Acoustic Nerve to Trochlear Nerve, Open Approach
00XN0ZK	Transfer Acoustic Nerve to Trigeminal Nerve, Open Approach
00XN0ZL	Transfer Acoustic Nerve to Abducens Nerve, Open Approach
00XN0ZM	Transfer Acoustic Nerve to Facial Nerve, Open Approach
00XN0ZN	Transfer Acoustic Nerve to Acoustic Nerve, Open Approach
00XN0ZP	Transfer Acoustic Nerve to Glossopharyngeal Nerve, Open Approach
00XN0ZQ	Transfer Acoustic Nerve to Vagus Nerve, Open Approach
00XN0ZR	Transfer Acoustic Nerve to Accessory Nerve, Open Approach
00XN0ZS	Transfer Acoustic Nerve to Hypoglossal Nerve, Open Approach
00XN4ZF	Transfer Acoustic Nerve to Olfactory Nerve, Percutaneous Endoscopic Approach
00XN4ZG	Transfer Acoustic Nerve to Optic Nerve, Percutaneous Endoscopic Approach
00XN4ZH	Transfer Acoustic Nerve to Oculomotor Nerve, Percutaneous Endoscopic Approach
00XN4ZJ	Transfer Acoustic Nerve to Trochlear Nerve, Percutaneous Endoscopic Approach
00XN4ZK	Transfer Acoustic Nerve to Trigeminal Nerve, Percutaneous Endoscopic Approach
00XN4ZL	Transfer Acoustic Nerve to Abducens Nerve, Percutaneous Endoscopic Approach
00XN4ZM	Transfer Acoustic Nerve to Facial Nerve, Percutaneous Endoscopic Approach
00XN4ZN	Transfer Acoustic Nerve to Acoustic Nerve, Percutaneous Endoscopic Approach
00XN4ZP	Transfer Acoustic Nerve to Glossopharyngeal Nerve, Percutaneous Endoscopic Approach
00XN4ZQ	Transfer Acoustic Nerve to Vagus Nerve, Percutaneous Endoscopic Approach

00XN4ZR	Transfer Acoustic Nerve to Accessory Nerve, Percutaneous Endoscopic Approach
00XN4ZS	Transfer Acoustic Nerve to Hypoglossal Nerve, Percutaneous Endoscopic Approach
00XP0ZF	Transfer Glossopharyngeal Nerve to Olfactory Nerve, Open Approach
00XP0ZG	Transfer Glossopharyngeal Nerve to Optic Nerve, Open Approach
00XP0ZH	Transfer Glossopharyngeal Nerve to Oculomotor Nerve, Open Approach
00XP0ZJ	Transfer Glossopharyngeal Nerve to Trochlear Nerve, Open Approach
00XP0ZK	Transfer Glossopharyngeal Nerve to Trigeminal Nerve, Open Approach
00XP0ZL	Transfer Glossopharyngeal Nerve to Abducens Nerve, Open Approach
00XP0ZM	Transfer Glossopharyngeal Nerve to Facial Nerve, Open Approach
00XP0ZN	Transfer Glossopharyngeal Nerve to Acoustic Nerve, Open Approach
00XP0ZP	Transfer Glossopharyngeal Nerve to Glossopharyngeal Nerve, Open Approach
00XP0ZQ	Transfer Glossopharyngeal Nerve to Vagus Nerve, Open Approach
00XP0ZR	Transfer Glossopharyngeal Nerve to Accessory Nerve, Open Approach
00XP0ZS	Transfer Glossopharyngeal Nerve to Hypoglossal Nerve, Open Approach
00XP4ZF	Transfer Glossopharyngeal Nerve to Olfactory Nerve, Percutaneous Endoscopic Approach
00XP4ZG	Transfer Glossopharyngeal Nerve to Optic Nerve, Percutaneous Endoscopic Approach
00XP4ZH	Transfer Glossopharyngeal Nerve to Oculomotor Nerve, Percutaneous Endoscopic Approach
00XP4ZJ	Transfer Glossopharyngeal Nerve to Trochlear Nerve, Percutaneous Endoscopic Approach
00XP4ZK	Transfer Glossopharyngeal Nerve to Trigeminal Nerve, Percutaneous Endoscopic Approach
00XP4ZL	Transfer Glossopharyngeal Nerve to Abducens Nerve, Percutaneous Endoscopic Approach
00XP4ZM	Transfer Glossopharyngeal Nerve to Facial Nerve, Percutaneous Endoscopic Approach
00XP4ZN	Transfer Glossopharyngeal Nerve to Acoustic Nerve, Percutaneous Endoscopic Approach
00XP4ZP	Transfer Glossopharyngeal Nerve to Glossopharyngeal Nerve, Percutaneous Endoscopic Approach
00XP4ZQ	Transfer Glossopharyngeal Nerve to Vagus Nerve, Percutaneous Endoscopic Approach
00XP4ZR	Transfer Glossopharyngeal Nerve to Accessory Nerve, Percutaneous Endoscopic Approach
00XP4ZS	Transfer Glossopharyngeal Nerve to Hypoglossal Nerve, Percutaneous Endoscopic Approach
00XQ0ZF	Transfer Vagus Nerve to Olfactory Nerve, Open Approach
00XQ0ZG	Transfer Vagus Nerve to Optic Nerve, Open Approach
00XQ0ZH	Transfer Vagus Nerve to Oculomotor Nerve, Open Approach
00XQ0ZJ	Transfer Vagus Nerve to Trochlear Nerve, Open Approach
00XQ0ZK	Transfer Vagus Nerve to Trigeminal Nerve, Open Approach

---

♀ Female-only ♂ Male-only ▲ Limited Coverage ● Non-OR ▬ HAC-associated procedure ▲ Non-covered procedures ✚ Cluster

00XQ0ZL Transfer Vagus Nerve to Abducens Nerve, Open Approach

00XQ0ZM Transfer Vagus Nerve to Facial Nerve, Open Approach

00XQ0ZN Transfer Vagus Nerve to Acoustic Nerve, Open Approach

00XQ0ZP Transfer Vagus Nerve to Glossopharyngeal Nerve, Open Approach

00XQ0ZQ Transfer Vagus Nerve to Vagus Nerve, Open Approach

00XQ0ZR Transfer Vagus Nerve to Accessory Nerve, Open Approach

00XQ0ZS Transfer Vagus Nerve to Hypoglossal Nerve, Open Approach

00XQ4ZF Transfer Vagus Nerve to Olfactory Nerve, Percutaneous Endoscopic Approach

00XQ4ZG Transfer Vagus Nerve to Optic Nerve, Percutaneous Endoscopic Approach

00XQ4ZH Transfer Vagus Nerve to Oculomotor Nerve, Percutaneous Endoscopic Approach

00XQ4ZJ Transfer Vagus Nerve to Trochlear Nerve, Percutaneous Endoscopic Approach

00XQ4ZK Transfer Vagus Nerve to Trigeminal Nerve, Percutaneous Endoscopic Approach

00XQ4ZL Transfer Vagus Nerve to Abducens Nerve, Percutaneous Endoscopic Approach

00XQ4ZM Transfer Vagus Nerve to Facial Nerve, Percutaneous Endoscopic Approach

00XQ4ZN Transfer Vagus Nerve to Acoustic Nerve, Percutaneous Endoscopic Approach

00XQ4ZP Transfer Vagus Nerve to Glossopharyngeal Nerve, Percutaneous Endoscopic Approach

00XQ4ZQ Transfer Vagus Nerve to Vagus Nerve, Percutaneous Endoscopic Approach

00XQ4ZR Transfer Vagus Nerve to Accessory Nerve, Percutaneous Endoscopic Approach

00XQ4ZS Transfer Vagus Nerve to Hypoglossal Nerve, Percutaneous Endoscopic Approach

00XR0ZF Transfer Accessory Nerve to Olfactory Nerve, Open Approach

00XR0ZG Transfer Accessory Nerve to Optic Nerve, Open Approach

00XR0ZH Transfer Accessory Nerve to Oculomotor Nerve, Open Approach

00XR0ZJ Transfer Accessory Nerve to Trochlear Nerve, Open Approach

00XR0ZK Transfer Accessory Nerve to Trigeminal Nerve, Open Approach

00XR0ZL Transfer Accessory Nerve to Abducens Nerve, Open Approach

00XR0ZM Transfer Accessory Nerve to Facial Nerve, Open Approach

00XR0ZN Transfer Accessory Nerve to Acoustic Nerve, Open Approach

00XR0ZP Transfer Accessory Nerve to Glossopharyngeal Nerve, Open Approach

00XR0ZQ Transfer Accessory Nerve to Vagus Nerve, Open Approach

00XR0ZR Transfer Accessory Nerve to Accessory Nerve, Open Approach

00XR0ZS Transfer Accessory Nerve to Hypoglossal Nerve, Open Approach

00XR4ZF Transfer Accessory Nerve to Olfactory Nerve, Percutaneous Endoscopic Approach

00XR4ZG Transfer Accessory Nerve to Optic Nerve, Percutaneous Endoscopic Approach

00XR4ZH Transfer Accessory Nerve to Oculomotor Nerve, Percutaneous Endoscopic Approach

00XR4ZJ Transfer Accessory Nerve to Trochlear Nerve, Percutaneous Endoscopic Approach

00XR4ZK Transfer Accessory Nerve to Trigeminal Nerve, Percutaneous Endoscopic Approach

00XR4ZL Transfer Accessory Nerve to Abducens Nerve, Percutaneous Endoscopic Approach

00XR4ZM Transfer Accessory Nerve to Facial Nerve, Percutaneous Endoscopic Approach

00XR4ZN Transfer Accessory Nerve to Acoustic Nerve, Percutaneous Endoscopic Approach

00XR4ZP Transfer Accessory Nerve to Glossopharyngeal Nerve, Percutaneous Endoscopic Approach

00XR4ZQ Transfer Accessory Nerve to Vagus Nerve, Percutaneous Endoscopic Approach

00XR4ZR Transfer Accessory Nerve to Accessory Nerve, Percutaneous Endoscopic Approach

00XR4ZS Transfer Accessory Nerve to Hypoglossal Nerve, Percutaneous Endoscopic Approach

00XS0ZF Transfer Hypoglossal Nerve to Olfactory Nerve, Open Approach

00XS0ZG Transfer Hypoglossal Nerve to Optic Nerve, Open Approach

00XS0ZH Transfer Hypoglossal Nerve to Oculomotor Nerve, Open Approach

00XS0ZJ Transfer Hypoglossal Nerve to Trochlear Nerve, Open Approach

00XS0ZK Transfer Hypoglossal Nerve to Trigeminal Nerve, Open Approach

00XS0ZL Transfer Hypoglossal Nerve to Abducens Nerve, Open Approach

00XS0ZM Transfer Hypoglossal Nerve to Facial Nerve, Open Approach

00XS0ZN Transfer Hypoglossal Nerve to Acoustic Nerve, Open Approach

00XS0ZP Transfer Hypoglossal Nerve to Glossopharyngeal Nerve, Open Approach

00XS0ZQ Transfer Hypoglossal Nerve to Vagus Nerve, Open Approach

00XS0ZR Transfer Hypoglossal Nerve to Accessory Nerve, Open Approach

00XS0ZS Transfer Hypoglossal Nerve to Hypoglossal Nerve, Open Approach

00XS4ZF Transfer Hypoglossal Nerve to Olfactory Nerve, Percutaneous Endoscopic Approach

00XS4ZG Transfer Hypoglossal Nerve to Optic Nerve, Percutaneous Endoscopic Approach

00XS4ZH Transfer Hypoglossal Nerve to Oculomotor Nerve, Percutaneous Endoscopic Approach

00XS4ZJ Transfer Hypoglossal Nerve to Trochlear Nerve, Percutaneous Endoscopic Approach

00XS4ZK Transfer Hypoglossal Nerve to Trigeminal Nerve, Percutaneous Endoscopic Approach

00XS4ZL Transfer Hypoglossal Nerve to Abducens Nerve, Percutaneous Endoscopic Approach

00XS4ZM Transfer Hypoglossal Nerve to Facial Nerve, Percutaneous Endoscopic Approach

00XS4ZN Transfer Hypoglossal Nerve to Acoustic Nerve, Percutaneous Endoscopic Approach

00XS4ZP Transfer Hypoglossal Nerve to Glossopharyngeal Nerve, Percutaneous Endoscopic Approach

00XS4ZQ Transfer Hypoglossal Nerve to Vagus Nerve, Percutaneous Endoscopic Approach

♀ Female-only   ♂ Male-only   ▲ Limited Coverage   ● Non-OR   ◨ HAC-associated procedure   ▲ Non-covered procedures   ✚ Cluster

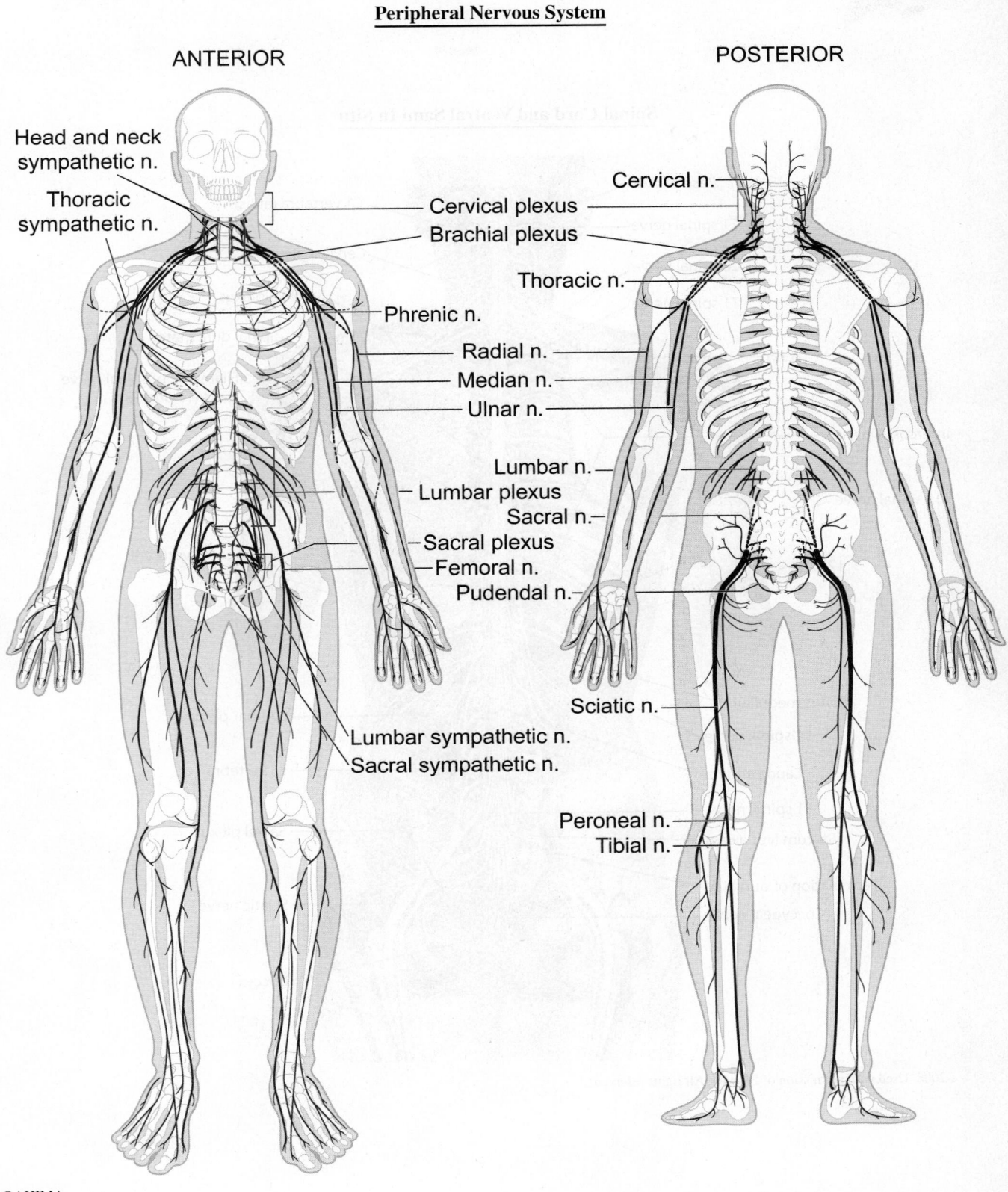

Peripheral Nervous System

ANTERIOR

POSTERIOR

Head and neck sympathetic n.

Thoracic sympathetic n.

Cervical n.

Cervical plexus

Brachial plexus

Thoracic n.

Phrenic n.

Radial n.

Median n.

Ulnar n.

Lumbar n.

Lumbar plexus

Sacral n.

Sacral plexus

Femoral n.

Pudendal n.

Sciatic n.

Lumbar sympathetic n.

Sacral sympathetic n.

Peroneal n.

Tibial n.

©AHIMA

Spinal Cord and Ventral Sami In Situ

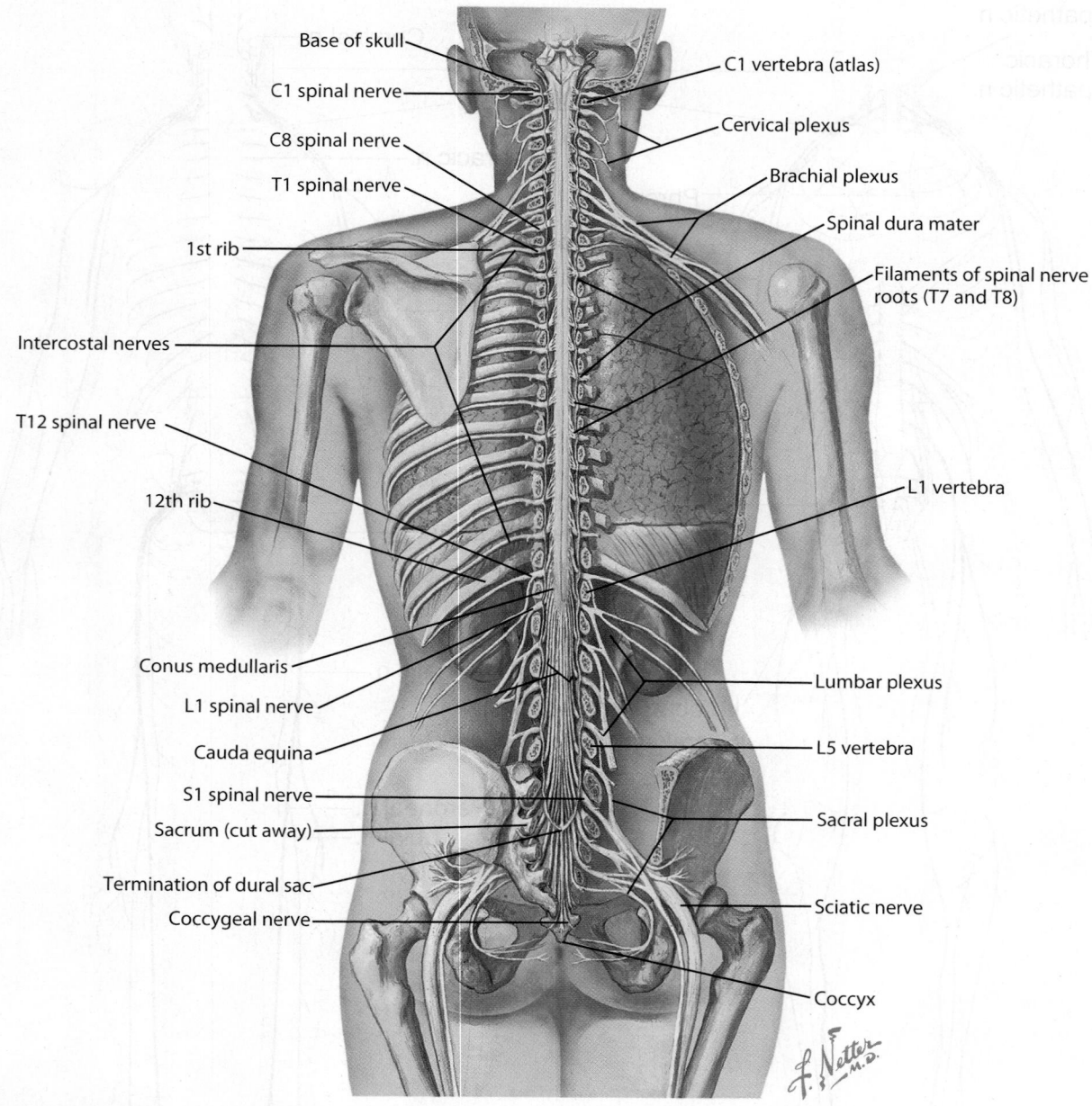

Base of skull

C1 spinal nerve

C8 spinal nerve

T1 spinal nerve

1st rib

Intercostal nerves

T12 spinal nerve

12th rib

Conus medullaris

L1 spinal nerve

Cauda equina

S1 spinal nerve

Sacrum (cut away)

Termination of dural sac

Coccygeal nerve

C1 vertebra (atlas)

Cervical plexus

Brachial plexus

Spinal dura mater

Filaments of spinal nerve roots (T7 and T8)

L1 vertebra

Lumbar plexus

L5 vertebra

Sacral plexus

Sciatic nerve

Coccyx

Peripheral Nervous System Tables 012–01X

Section	0	Medical and Surgical
Body System	1	Peripheral Nervous System
Operation	2	**Change:** Taking out or off a device from a body part and putting back an identical or similar device in or on the same body part without cutting or puncturing the skin or a mucous membrane

Body Part (4th)	Approach (5th)	Device (6th)	Qualifier (7th)
Y Peripheral Nerve	**X** External	**0** Drainage Device **Y** Other Device	**Z** No Qualifier

Section	0	Medical and Surgical
Body System	1	Peripheral Nervous System
Operation	5	**Destruction:** Physical eradication of all or a portion of a body part by the direct use of energy, force, or a destructive agent

Body Part (4th)	Approach (5th)	Device (6th)	Qualifier (7th)
0 Cervical Plexus **1** Cervical Nerve **2** Phrenic Nerve **3** Brachial Plexus **4** Ulnar Nerve **5** Median Nerve **6** Radial Nerve **8** Thoracic Nerve **9** Lumbar Plexus **A** Lumbosacral Plexus **B** Lumbar Nerve **C** Pudendal Nerve **D** Femoral Nerve **F** Sciatic Nerve **G** Tibial Nerve **H** Peroneal Nerve **K** Head and Neck Sympathetic Nerve **L** Thoracic Sympathetic Nerve **M** Abdominal Sympathetic Nerve **N** Lumbar Sympathetic Nerve **P** Sacral Sympathetic Nerve **Q** Sacral Plexus **R** Sacral Nerve	**0** Open **3** Percutaneous **4** Percutaneous Endoscopic	**Z** No Device	**Z** No Qualifier

Section	0	Medical and Surgical
Body System	1	Peripheral Nervous System
Operation	8	**Division:** Cutting into a body part, without draining fluids and/or gases from the body part, in order to separate or transect a body part

Body Part (4th)	Approach (5th)	Device (6th)	Qualifier (7th)
0 Cervical Plexus	**0** Open	**Z** No Device	**Z** No Qualifier
1 Cervical Nerve	**3** Percutaneous		
2 Phrenic Nerve	**4** Percutaneous Endoscopic		
3 Brachial Plexus			
4 Ulnar Nerve			
5 Median Nerve			
6 Radial Nerve			
8 Thoracic Nerve			
9 Lumbar Plexus			
A Lumbosacral Plexus			
B Lumbar Nerve			
C Pudendal Nerve			
D Femoral Nerve			
F Sciatic Nerve			
G Tibial Nerve			
H Peroneal Nerve			
K Head and Neck Sympathetic Nerve			
L Thoracic Sympathetic Nerve			
M Abdominal Sympathetic Nerve			
N Lumbar Sympathetic Nerve			
P Sacral Sympathetic Nerve			
Q Sacral Plexus			
R Sacral Nerve			

Section	0	Medical and Surgical
Body System	1	Peripheral Nervous System
Operation	9	**Drainage:** Taking or letting out fluids and/or gases from a body part

Body Part (4th)	Approach (5th)	Device (6th)	Qualifier (7th)
0 Cervical Plexus 1 Cervical Nerve 2 Phrenic Nerve 3 Brachial Plexus 4 Ulnar Nerve 5 Median Nerve 6 Radial Nerve 8 Thoracic Nerve 9 Lumbar Plexus A Lumbosacral Plexus B Lumbar Nerve C Pudendal Nerve D Femoral Nerve F Sciatic Nerve G Tibial Nerve H Peroneal Nerve K Head and Neck Sympathetic Nerve L Thoracic Sympathetic Nerve M Abdominal Sympathetic Nerve N Lumbar Sympathetic Nerve P Sacral Sympathetic Nerve Q Sacral Plexus R Sacral Nerve	0 Open 3 Percutaneous 4 Percutaneous Endoscopic	0 Drainage Device	Z No Qualifier
0 Cervical Plexus 1 Cervical Nerve 2 Phrenic Nerve 3 Brachial Plexus 4 Ulnar Nerve 5 Median Nerve 6 Radial Nerve 8 Thoracic Nerve 9 Lumbar Plexus A Lumbosacral Plexus B Lumbar Nerve C Pudendal Nerve D Femoral Nerve F Sciatic Nerve G Tibial Nerve H Peroneal Nerve K Head and Neck Sympathetic Nerve L Thoracic Sympathetic Nerve M Abdominal Sympathetic Nerve N Lumbar Sympathetic Nerve P Sacral Sympathetic Nerve Q Sacral Plexus R Sacral Nerve	0 Open 3 Percutaneous 4 Percutaneous Endoscopic	Z No Device	X Diagnostic Z No Qualifier

Section	0	Medical and Surgical
Body System	1	Peripheral Nervous System
Operation	B	Excision: Cutting out or off, without replacement, a portion of a body part

Body Part (4th)	Approach (5th)	Device (6th)	Qualifier (7th)
0 Cervical Plexus 1 Cervical Nerve 2 Phrenic Nerve 3 Brachial Plexus 4 Ulnar Nerve 5 Median Nerve 6 Radial Nerve 8 Thoracic Nerve 9 Lumbar Plexus A Lumbosacral Plexus B Lumbar Nerve C Pudendal Nerve D Femoral Nerve F Sciatic Nerve G Tibial Nerve H Peroneal Nerve K Head and Neck Sympathetic Nerve L Thoracic Sympathetic Nerve M Abdominal Sympathetic Nerve N Lumbar Sympathetic Nerve P Sacral Sympathetic Nerve Q Sacral Plexus R Sacral Nerve	0 Open 3 Percutaneous 4 Percutaneous Endoscopic	Z No Device	X Diagnostic Z No Qualifier

Section	0	Medical and Surgical
Body System	1	Peripheral Nervous System
Operation	C	Extirpation: Taking or cutting out solid matter from a body part

Body Part (4th)	Approach (5th)	Device (6th)	Qualifier (7th)
0 Cervical Plexus 1 Cervical Nerve 2 Phrenic Nerve 3 Brachial Plexus 4 Ulnar Nerve 5 Median Nerve 6 Radial Nerve 8 Thoracic Nerve 9 Lumbar Plexus A Lumbosacral Plexus B Lumbar Nerve C Pudendal Nerve D Femoral Nerve F Sciatic Nerve G Tibial Nerve H Peroneal Nerve K Head and Neck Sympathetic Nerve L Thoracic Sympathetic Nerve M Abdominal Sympathetic Nerve N Lumbar Sympathetic Nerve P Sacral Sympathetic Nerve Q Sacral Plexus R Sacral Nerve	0 Open 3 Percutaneous 4 Percutaneous Endoscopic	Z No Device	Z No Qualifier

Section 0 **Medical and Surgical**
Body System 1 **Peripheral Nervous System**
Operation D **Extraction:** Pulling or stripping out or off all or a portion of a body part by the use of force

Body Part (4th)	Approach (5th)	Device (6th)	Qualifier (7th)
0 Cervical Plexus 1 Cervical Nerve 2 Phrenic Nerve 3 Brachial Plexus 4 Ulnar Nerve 5 Median Nerve 6 Radial Nerve 8 Thoracic Nerve 9 Lumbar Plexus A Lumbosacral Plexus B Lumbar Nerve C Pudendal Nerve D Femoral Nerve F Sciatic Nerve G Tibial Nerve H Peroneal Nerve K Head and Neck Sympathetic Nerve L Thoracic Sympathetic Nerve M Abdominal Sympathetic Nerve N Lumbar Sympathetic Nerve P Sacral Sympathetic Nerve Q Sacral Plexus R Sacral Nerve	0 Open 3 Percutaneous 4 Percutaneous Endoscopic	Z No Device	Z No Qualifier

Section 0 **Medical and Surgical**
Body System 1 **Peripheral Nervous System**
Operation H **Insertion:** Putting in a nonbiological appliance that monitors, assists, performs, or prevents a physiological function but does not physically take the place of a body part

Body Part (4th)	Approach (5th)	Device (6th)	Qualifier (7th)
Y Peripheral Nerve	0 Open 3 Percutaneous 4 Percutaneous Endoscopic	1 Radioactive Element 2 Monitoring Device M Neurostimulator Lead Y Other Device	Z No Qualifier

Section 0 **Medical and Surgical**
Body System 1 **Peripheral Nervous System**
Operation J **Inspection:** Visually and/or manually exploring a body part

Body Part (4th)	Approach (5th)	Device (6th)	Qualifier (7th)
Y Peripheral Nerve	0 Open 3 Percutaneous 4 Percutaneous Endoscopic	Z No Device	Z No Qualifier

Section	0	Medical and Surgical
Body System	1	Peripheral Nervous System
Operation	N	**Release:** Freeing a body part from an abnormal physical constraint by cutting or by the use of force

Body Part (4th)	Approach (5th)	Device (6th)	Qualifier (7th)
0 Cervical Plexus 1 Cervical Nerve 2 Phrenic Nerve 3 Brachial Plexus 4 Ulnar Nerve 5 Median Nerve 6 Radial Nerve 8 Thoracic Nerve 9 Lumbar Plexus A Lumbosacral Plexus B Lumbar Nerve C Pudendal Nerve D Femoral Nerve F Sciatic Nerve G Tibial Nerve H Peroneal Nerve K Head and Neck Sympathetic Nerve L Thoracic Sympathetic Nerve M Abdominal Sympathetic Nerve N Lumbar Sympathetic Nerve P Sacral Sympathetic Nerve Q Sacral Plexus R Sacral Nerve	0 Open 3 Percutaneous 4 Percutaneous Endoscopic	Z No Device	Z No Qualifier

Section	0	Medical and Surgical
Body System	1	Peripheral Nervous System
Operation	P	**Removal:** Taking out or off a device from a body part

Body Part (4th)	Approach (5th)	Device (6th)	Qualifier (7th)
Y Peripheral Nerve	0 Open 3 Percutaneous 4 Percutaneous Endoscopic	0 Drainage Device 2 Monitoring Device 7 Autologous Tissue Substitute M Neurostimulator Lead Y Other Device	Z No Qualifier
Y Peripheral Nerve	X External	0 Drainage Device 2 Monitoring Device M Neurostimulator Lead	Z No Qualifier

Section	0	Medical and Surgical
Body System	1	Peripheral Nervous System
Operation	Q	**Repair:** Restoring, to the extent possible, a body part to its normal anatomic structure and function

Body Part (4th)	Approach (5th)	Device (6th)	Qualifier (7th)
0 Cervical Plexus 1 Cervical Nerve 2 Phrenic Nerve 3 Brachial Plexus 4 Ulnar Nerve 5 Median Nerve 6 Radial Nerve 8 Thoracic Nerve 9 Lumbar Plexus A Lumbosacral Plexus B Lumbar Nerve C Pudendal Nerve D Femoral Nerve F Sciatic Nerve G Tibial Nerve H Peroneal Nerve K Head and Neck Sympathetic Nerve L Thoracic Sympathetic Nerve M Abdominal Sympathetic Nerve N Lumbar Sympathetic Nerve P Sacral Sympathetic Nerve Q Sacral Plexus R Sacral Nerve	0 Open 3 Percutaneous 4 Percutaneous Endoscopic	Z No Device	Z No Qualifier

Section	0	Medical and Surgical
Body System	1	Peripheral Nervous System
Operation	R	**Replacement:** Putting in or on biological or synthetic material that physically takes the place and/or function of all or a portion of a body part

Body Part (4th)	Approach (5th)	Device (6th)	Qualifier (7th)
1 Cervical Nerve 2 Phrenic Nerve 4 Ulnar Nerve 5 Median Nerve 6 Radial Nerve 8 Thoracic Nerve B Lumbar Nerve C Pudendal Nerve D Femoral Nerve F Sciatic Nerve G Tibial Nerve H Peroneal Nerve R Sacral Nerve	0 Open 4 Percutaneous Endoscopic	7 Autologous Tissue Substitute J Synthetic Substitute K Nonautologous Tissue Substitute	Z No Qualifier

Section	0	Medical and Surgical
Body System	1	Peripheral Nervous System
Operation	S	**Reposition:** Moving to its normal location, or other suitable location, all or a portion of a body part

Body Part (4th)	Approach (5th)	Device (6th)	Qualifier (7th)
0 Cervical Plexus 1 Cervical Nerve 2 Phrenic Nerve 3 Brachial Plexus 4 Ulnar Nerve 5 Median Nerve 6 Radial Nerve 8 Thoracic Nerve 9 Lumbar Plexus A Lumbosacral Plexus B Lumbar Nerve C Pudendal Nerve D Femoral Nerve F Sciatic Nerve G Tibial Nerve H Peroneal Nerve Q Sacral Plexus R Sacral Nerve	0 Open 3 Percutaneous 4 Percutaneous Endoscopic	Z No Device	Z No Qualifier

Section	0	Medical and Surgical
Body System	1	Peripheral Nervous System
Operation	U	**Supplement:** Putting in or on biological or synthetic material that physically reinforces and/or augments the function of a portion of a body part

Body Part (4th)	Approach (5th)	Device (6th)	Qualifier (7th)
1 Cervical Nerve 2 Phrenic Nerve 4 Ulnar Nerve 5 Median Nerve 6 Radial Nerve 8 Thoracic Nerve B Lumbar Nerve C Pudendal Nerve D Femoral Nerve F Sciatic Nerve G Tibial Nerve H Peroneal Nerve R Sacral Nerve	0 Open 3 Percutaneous 4 Percutaneous Endoscopic	7 Autologous Tissue Substitute J Synthetic Substitute K Nonautologous Tissue Substitute	Z No Qualifier

Section	0	Medical and Surgical
Body System	1	Peripheral Nervous System
Operation	W	**Revision:** Correcting, to the extent possible, a portion of a malfunctioning device or the position of a displaced device

Body Part (4th)	Approach (5th)	Device (6th)	Qualifier (7th)
Y Peripheral Nerve	0 Open 3 Percutaneous 4 Percutaneous Endoscopic	0 Drainage Device 2 Monitoring Device 7 Autologous Tissue Substitute M Neurostimulator Lead Y Other Device	Z No Qualifier
Y Peripheral Nerve	X External	0 Drainage Device 2 Monitoring Device 7 Autologous Tissue Substitute M Neurostimulator Lead	Z No Qualifier

Section	0	Medical and Surgical
Body System	1	Peripheral Nervous System
Operation	X	**Transfer:** Moving, without taking out, all or a portion of a body part to another location to take over the function of all or a portion of a body part

Body Part (4th)	Approach (5th)	Device (6th)	Qualifier (7th)
1 Cervical Nerve 2 Phrenic Nerve	0 Open 4 Percutaneous Endoscopic	Z No Device	1 Cervical Nerve 2 Phrenic Nerve
4 Ulnar Nerve 5 Median Nerve 6 Radial Nerve	0 Open 4 Percutaneous Endoscopic	Z No Device	4 Ulnar Nerve 5 Median Nerve 6 Radial Nerve
8 Thoracic Nerve	0 Open 4 Percutaneous Endoscopic	Z No Device	8 Thoracic Nerve
B Lumbar Nerve C Pudendal Nerve	0 Open 4 Percutaneous Endoscopic	Z No Device	B Lumbar Nerve C Perineal Nerve
D Femoral Nerve F Sciatic Nerve G Tibial Nerve H Peroneal Nerve	0 Open 4 Percutaneous Endoscopic	Z No Device	D Femoral Nerve F Sciatic Nerve G Tibial Nerve H Peroneal Nerve

Peripheral Nervous System Code Listing 012–01X

012 – Peripheral Nervous System, Change

Review Coding Guideline B6.1c

012YX0Z Change Drainage Device in Peripheral Nerve, External Approach

012YXYZ Change Other Device in Peripheral Nerve, External Approach

015 – Peripheral Nervous System, Destruction

01500ZZ Destruction of Cervical Plexus, Open Approach

01503ZZ Destruction of Cervical Plexus, Percutaneous Approach

01504ZZ Destruction of Cervical Plexus, Percutaneous Endoscopic Approach

01510ZZ Destruction of Cervical Nerve, Open Approach

01513ZZ Destruction of Cervical Nerve, Percutaneous Approach

01514ZZ Destruction of Cervical Nerve, Percutaneous Endoscopic Approach

01520ZZ Destruction of Phrenic Nerve, Open Approach

01523ZZ Destruction of Phrenic Nerve, Percutaneous Approach

01524ZZ Destruction of Phrenic Nerve, Percutaneous Endoscopic Approach

01530ZZ Destruction of Brachial Plexus, Open Approach

01533ZZ Destruction of Brachial Plexus, Percutaneous Approach

01534ZZ Destruction of Brachial Plexus, Percutaneous Endoscopic Approach

01540ZZ Destruction of Ulnar Nerve, Open Approach

01543ZZ Destruction of Ulnar Nerve, Percutaneous Approach

01544ZZ Destruction of Ulnar Nerve, Percutaneous Endoscopic Approach

01550ZZ Destruction of Median Nerve, Open Approach

01553ZZ Destruction of Median Nerve, Percutaneous Approach

01554ZZ Destruction of Median Nerve, Percutaneous Endoscopic Approach

01560ZZ Destruction of Radial Nerve, Open Approach

01563ZZ Destruction of Radial Nerve, Percutaneous Approach

01564ZZ Destruction of Radial Nerve, Percutaneous Endoscopic Approach

01580ZZ Destruction of Thoracic Nerve, Open Approach

01583ZZ Destruction of Thoracic Nerve, Percutaneous Approach

01584ZZ Destruction of Thoracic Nerve, Percutaneous Endoscopic Approach

01590ZZ Destruction of Lumbar Plexus, Open Approach

01593ZZ Destruction of Lumbar Plexus, Percutaneous Approach

01594ZZ Destruction of Lumbar Plexus, Percutaneous Endoscopic Approach

015A0ZZ Destruction of Lumbosacral Plexus, Open Approach

015A3ZZ Destruction of Lumbosacral Plexus, Percutaneous Approach

015A4ZZ Destruction of Lumbosacral Plexus, Percutaneous Endoscopic Approach

015B0ZZ Destruction of Lumbar Nerve, Open Approach

015B3ZZ Destruction of Lumbar Nerve, Percutaneous Approach

015B4ZZ Destruction of Lumbar Nerve, Percutaneous Endoscopic Approach

015C0ZZ Destruction of Pudendal Nerve, Open Approach

015C3ZZ Destruction of Pudendal Nerve, Percutaneous Approach

015C4ZZ Destruction of Pudendal Nerve, Percutaneous Endoscopic Approach

015D0ZZ Destruction of Femoral Nerve, Open Approach

015D3ZZ Destruction of Femoral Nerve, Percutaneous Approach

015D4ZZ Destruction of Femoral Nerve, Percutaneous Endoscopic Approach

015F0ZZ Destruction of Sciatic Nerve, Open Approach

015F3ZZ Destruction of Sciatic Nerve, Percutaneous Approach

015F4ZZ Destruction of Sciatic Nerve, Percutaneous Endoscopic Approach

015G0ZZ Destruction of Tibial Nerve, Open Approach

015G3ZZ Destruction of Tibial Nerve, Percutaneous Approach

015G4ZZ Destruction of Tibial Nerve, Percutaneous Endoscopic Approach

015H0ZZ Destruction of Peroneal Nerve, Open Approach

015H3ZZ Destruction of Peroneal Nerve, Percutaneous Approach

015H4ZZ Destruction of Peroneal Nerve, Percutaneous Endoscopic Approach

015K0ZZ Destruction of Head and Neck Sympathetic Nerve, Open Approach

015K3ZZ Destruction of Head and Neck Sympathetic Nerve, Percutaneous Approach

015K4ZZ Destruction of Head and Neck Sympathetic Nerve, Percutaneous Endoscopic Approach

015L0ZZ Destruction of Thoracic Sympathetic Nerve, Open Approach

015L3ZZ Destruction of Thoracic Sympathetic Nerve, Percutaneous Approach

015L4ZZ Destruction of Thoracic Sympathetic Nerve, Percutaneous Endoscopic Approach

015M0ZZ Destruction of Abdominal Sympathetic Nerve, Open Approach

015M3ZZ Destruction of Abdominal Sympathetic Nerve, Percutaneous Approach

015M4ZZ Destruction of Abdominal Sympathetic Nerve, Percutaneous Endoscopic Approach

015N0ZZ Destruction of Lumbar Sympathetic Nerve, Open Approach

015N3ZZ Destruction of Lumbar Sympathetic Nerve, Percutaneous Approach

015N4ZZ Destruction of Lumbar Sympathetic Nerve, Percutaneous Endoscopic Approach

015P0ZZ Destruction of Sacral Sympathetic Nerve, Open Approach

015P3ZZ Destruction of Sacral Sympathetic Nerve, Percutaneous Approach

015P4ZZ Destruction of Sacral Sympathetic Nerve, Percutaneous Endoscopic Approach

015Q0ZZ Destruction of Sacral Plexus, Open Approach

015Q3ZZ Destruction of Sacral Plexus, Percutaneous Approach

015Q4ZZ Destruction of Sacral Plexus, Percutaneous Endoscopic Approach

015R0ZZ Destruction of Sacral Nerve, Open Approach

015R3ZZ Destruction of Sacral Nerve, Percutaneous Approach

015R4ZZ Destruction of Sacral Nerve, Percutaneous Endoscopic Approach

018 – Peripheral Nervous System, Division

Review Coding Guideline B3.14

01800ZZ Division of Cervical Plexus, Open Approach

01803ZZ Division of Cervical Plexus, Percutaneous Approach

01804ZZ Division of Cervical Plexus, Percutaneous Endoscopic Approach

01810ZZ Division of Cervical Nerve, Open Approach

01813ZZ Division of Cervical Nerve, Percutaneous Approach

01814ZZ Division of Cervical Nerve, Percutaneous Endoscopic Approach

01820ZZ Division of Phrenic Nerve, Open Approach

01823ZZ Division of Phrenic Nerve, Percutaneous Approach

01824ZZ Division of Phrenic Nerve, Percutaneous Endoscopic Approach

01830ZZ Division of Brachial Plexus, Open Approach

01833ZZ Division of Brachial Plexus, Percutaneous Approach

01834ZZ Division of Brachial Plexus, Percutaneous Endoscopic Approach

01840ZZ Division of Ulnar Nerve, Open Approach

01843ZZ Division of Ulnar Nerve, Percutaneous Approach

01844ZZ Division of Ulnar Nerve, Percutaneous Endoscopic Approach

01850ZZ Division of Median Nerve, Open Approach

01853ZZ Division of Median Nerve, Percutaneous Approach

01854ZZ Division of Median Nerve, Percutaneous Endoscopic Approach

♀ Female-only   ♂ Male-only   ▲ Limited Coverage   ● Non-OR   ᴴᴬᶜ HAC-associated procedure   ▲ Non-covered procedures   ✚ Cluster

01860ZZ	Division of Radial Nerve, Open Approach
01863ZZ	Division of Radial Nerve, Percutaneous Approach
01864ZZ	Division of Radial Nerve, Percutaneous Endoscopic Approach
01880ZZ	Division of Thoracic Nerve, Open Approach
01883ZZ	Division of Thoracic Nerve, Percutaneous Approach
01884ZZ	Division of Thoracic Nerve, Percutaneous Endoscopic Approach
01890ZZ	Division of Lumbar Plexus, Open Approach
01893ZZ	Division of Lumbar Plexus, Percutaneous Approach
01894ZZ	Division of Lumbar Plexus, Percutaneous Endoscopic Approach
018A0ZZ	Division of Lumbosacral Plexus, Open Approach
018A3ZZ	Division of Lumbosacral Plexus, Percutaneous Approach
018A4ZZ	Division of Lumbosacral Plexus, Percutaneous Endoscopic Approach
018B0ZZ	Division of Lumbar Nerve, Open Approach
018B3ZZ	Division of Lumbar Nerve, Percutaneous Approach
018B4ZZ	Division of Lumbar Nerve, Percutaneous Endoscopic Approach
018C0ZZ	Division of Pudendal Nerve, Open Approach
018C3ZZ	Division of Pudendal Nerve, Percutaneous Approach
018C4ZZ	Division of Pudendal Nerve, Percutaneous Endoscopic Approach

018D0ZZ	Division of Femoral Nerve, Open Approach
018D3ZZ	Division of Femoral Nerve, Percutaneous Approach
018D4ZZ	Division of Femoral Nerve, Percutaneous Endoscopic Approach
018F0ZZ	Division of Sciatic Nerve, Open Approach
018F3ZZ	Division of Sciatic Nerve, Percutaneous Approach
018F4ZZ	Division of Sciatic Nerve, Percutaneous Endoscopic Approach
018G0ZZ	Division of Tibial Nerve, Open Approach
018G3ZZ	Division of Tibial Nerve, Percutaneous Approach
018G4ZZ	Division of Tibial Nerve, Percutaneous Endoscopic Approach
018H0ZZ	Division of Peroneal Nerve, Open Approach
018H3ZZ	Division of Peroneal Nerve, Percutaneous Approach
018H4ZZ	Division of Peroneal Nerve, Percutaneous Endoscopic Approach
018K0ZZ	Division of Head and Neck Sympathetic Nerve, Open Approach
018K3ZZ	Division of Head and Neck Sympathetic Nerve, Percutaneous Approach
018K4ZZ	Division of Head and Neck Sympathetic Nerve, Percutaneous Endoscopic Approach
018L0ZZ	Division of Thoracic Sympathetic Nerve, Open Approach
018L3ZZ	Division of Thoracic Sympathetic Nerve, Percutaneous Approach

018L4ZZ	Division of Thoracic Sympathetic Nerve, Percutaneous Endoscopic Approach
018M0ZZ	Division of Abdominal Sympathetic Nerve, Open Approach
018M3ZZ	Division of Abdominal Sympathetic Nerve, Percutaneous Approach
018M4ZZ	Division of Abdominal Sympathetic Nerve, Percutaneous Endoscopic Approach
018N0ZZ	Division of Lumbar Sympathetic Nerve, Open Approach
018N3ZZ	Division of Lumbar Sympathetic Nerve, Percutaneous Approach
018N4ZZ	Division of Lumbar Sympathetic Nerve, Percutaneous Endoscopic Approach
018P0ZZ	Division of Sacral Sympathetic Nerve, Open Approach
018P3ZZ	Division of Sacral Sympathetic Nerve, Percutaneous Approach
018P4ZZ	Division of Sacral Sympathetic Nerve, Percutaneous Endoscopic Approach
018Q0ZZ	Division of Sacral Plexus, Open Approach
018Q3ZZ	Division of Sacral Plexus, Percutaneous Approach
018Q4ZZ	Division of Sacral Plexus, Percutaneous Endoscopic Approach
018R0ZZ	Division of Sacral Nerve, Open Approach
018R3ZZ	Division of Sacral Nerve, Percutaneous Approach
018R4ZZ	Division of Sacral Nerve, Percutaneous Endoscopic Approach

019 – Peripheral Nervous System, Drainage

Review Coding Guidelines B3.4a and B3.4b

Review Coding Guideline B6.2

019000Z	Drainage of Cervical Plexus with Drainage Device, Open Approach
01900ZX	Drainage of Cervical Plexus, Open Approach, Diagnostic
01900ZZ	Drainage of Cervical Plexus, Open Approach
019030Z	Drainage of Cervical Plexus with Drainage Device, Percutaneous Approach
01903ZX	Drainage of Cervical Plexus, Percutaneous Approach, Diagnostic
01903ZZ	Drainage of Cervical Plexus, Percutaneous Approach
019040Z	Drainage of Cervical Plexus with Drainage Device, Percutaneous Endoscopic Approach
01904ZX	Drainage of Cervical Plexus, Percutaneous Endoscopic Approach, Diagnostic
01904ZZ	Drainage of Cervical Plexus, Percutaneous Endoscopic Approach
019100Z	Drainage of Cervical Nerve with Drainage Device, Open Approach
01910ZX	Drainage of Cervical Nerve, Open Approach, Diagnostic
01910ZZ	Drainage of Cervical Nerve, Open Approach
019130Z	Drainage of Cervical Nerve with Drainage Device, Percutaneous Approach
01913ZX	Drainage of Cervical Nerve, Percutaneous Approach, Diagnostic

01913ZZ	Drainage of Cervical Nerve, Percutaneous Approach
019140Z	Drainage of Cervical Nerve with Drainage Device, Percutaneous Endoscopic Approach
01914ZX	Drainage of Cervical Nerve, Percutaneous Endoscopic Approach, Diagnostic
01914ZZ	Drainage of Cervical Nerve, Percutaneous Endoscopic Approach
019200Z	Drainage of Phrenic Nerve with Drainage Device, Open Approach
01920ZX	Drainage of Phrenic Nerve, Open Approach, Diagnostic
01920ZZ	Drainage of Phrenic Nerve, Open Approach
019230Z	Drainage of Phrenic Nerve with Drainage Device, Percutaneous Approach
01923ZX	Drainage of Phrenic Nerve, Percutaneous Approach, Diagnostic
01923ZZ	Drainage of Phrenic Nerve, Percutaneous Approach
019240Z	Drainage of Phrenic Nerve with Drainage Device, Percutaneous Endoscopic Approach
01924ZX	Drainage of Phrenic Nerve, Percutaneous Endoscopic Approach, Diagnostic
01924ZZ	Drainage of Phrenic Nerve, Percutaneous Endoscopic Approach
019300Z	Drainage of Brachial Plexus with Drainage Device, Open Approach

01930ZX	Drainage of Brachial Plexus, Open Approach, Diagnostic
01930ZZ	Drainage of Brachial Plexus, Open Approach
019330Z	Drainage of Brachial Plexus with Drainage Device, Percutaneous Approach
01933ZX	Drainage of Brachial Plexus, Percutaneous Approach, Diagnostic
01933ZZ	Drainage of Brachial Plexus, Percutaneous Approach
019340Z	Drainage of Brachial Plexus with Drainage Device, Percutaneous Endoscopic Approach
01934ZX	Drainage of Brachial Plexus, Percutaneous Endoscopic Approach, Diagnostic
01934ZZ	Drainage of Brachial Plexus, Percutaneous Endoscopic Approach
019400Z	Drainage of Ulnar Nerve with Drainage Device, Open Approach
01940ZX	Drainage of Ulnar Nerve, Open Approach, Diagnostic
01940ZZ	Drainage of Ulnar Nerve, Open Approach
019430Z	Drainage of Ulnar Nerve with Drainage Device, Percutaneous Approach
01943ZX	Drainage of Ulnar Nerve, Percutaneous Approach, Diagnostic
01943ZZ	Drainage of Ulnar Nerve, Percutaneous Approach

019440Z	Drainage of Ulnar Nerve with Drainage Device, Percutaneous Endoscopic Approach
01944ZX	Drainage of Ulnar Nerve, Percutaneous Endoscopic Approach, Diagnostic
01944ZZ	Drainage of Ulnar Nerve, Percutaneous Endoscopic Approach
019500Z	Drainage of Median Nerve with Drainage Device, Open Approach
01950ZX	Drainage of Median Nerve, Open Approach, Diagnostic
01950ZZ	Drainage of Median Nerve, Open Approach
019530Z	Drainage of Median Nerve with Drainage Device, Percutaneous Approach
01953ZX	Drainage of Median Nerve, Percutaneous Approach, Diagnostic
01953ZZ	Drainage of Median Nerve, Percutaneous Approach
019540Z	Drainage of Median Nerve with Drainage Device, Percutaneous Endoscopic Approach
01954ZX	Drainage of Median Nerve, Percutaneous Endoscopic Approach, Diagnostic
01954ZZ	Drainage of Median Nerve, Percutaneous Endoscopic Approach
019600Z	Drainage of Radial Nerve with Drainage Device, Open Approach
01960ZX	Drainage of Radial Nerve, Open Approach, Diagnostic
01960ZZ	Drainage of Radial Nerve, Open Approach
019630Z	Drainage of Radial Nerve with Drainage Device, Percutaneous Approach
01963ZX	Drainage of Radial Nerve, Percutaneous Approach, Diagnostic
01963ZZ	Drainage of Radial Nerve, Percutaneous Approach
019640Z	Drainage of Radial Nerve with Drainage Device, Percutaneous Endoscopic Approach
01964ZX	Drainage of Radial Nerve, Percutaneous Endoscopic Approach, Diagnostic
01964ZZ	Drainage of Radial Nerve, Percutaneous Endoscopic Approach
019800Z	Drainage of Thoracic Nerve with Drainage Device, Open Approach
01980ZX	Drainage of Thoracic Nerve, Open Approach, Diagnostic
01980ZZ	Drainage of Thoracic Nerve, Open Approach
019830Z	Drainage of Thoracic Nerve with Drainage Device, Percutaneous Approach
01983ZX	Drainage of Thoracic Nerve, Percutaneous Approach, Diagnostic
01983ZZ	Drainage of Thoracic Nerve, Percutaneous Approach
019840Z	Drainage of Thoracic Nerve with Drainage Device, Percutaneous Endoscopic Approach
01984ZX	Drainage of Thoracic Nerve, Percutaneous Endoscopic Approach, Diagnostic
01984ZZ	Drainage of Thoracic Nerve, Percutaneous Endoscopic Approach
019900Z	Drainage of Lumbar Plexus with Drainage Device, Open Approach
01990ZX	Drainage of Lumbar Plexus, Open Approach, Diagnostic
01990ZZ	Drainage of Lumbar Plexus, Open Approach
019930Z	Drainage of Lumbar Plexus with Drainage Device, Percutaneous Approach
01993ZX	Drainage of Lumbar Plexus, Percutaneous Approach, Diagnostic
01993ZZ	Drainage of Lumbar Plexus, Percutaneous Approach
019940Z	Drainage of Lumbar Plexus with Drainage Device, Percutaneous Endoscopic Approach
01994ZX	Drainage of Lumbar Plexus, Percutaneous Endoscopic Approach, Diagnostic
01994ZZ	Drainage of Lumbar Plexus, Percutaneous Endoscopic Approach
019A00Z	Drainage of Lumbosacral Plexus with Drainage Device, Open Approach
019A0ZX	Drainage of Lumbosacral Plexus, Open Approach, Diagnostic
019A0ZZ	Drainage of Lumbosacral Plexus, Open Approach
019A30Z	Drainage of Lumbosacral Plexus with Drainage Device, Percutaneous Approach
019A3ZX	Drainage of Lumbosacral Plexus, Percutaneous Approach, Diagnostic
019A3ZZ	Drainage of Lumbosacral Plexus, Percutaneous Approach
019A40Z	Drainage of Lumbosacral Plexus with Drainage Device, Percutaneous Endoscopic Approach
019A4ZX	Drainage of Lumbosacral Plexus, Percutaneous Endoscopic Approach, Diagnostic
019A4ZZ	Drainage of Lumbosacral Plexus, Percutaneous Endoscopic Approach
019B00Z	Drainage of Lumbar Nerve with Drainage Device, Open Approach
019B0ZX	Drainage of Lumbar Nerve, Open Approach, Diagnostic
019B0ZZ	Drainage of Lumbar Nerve, Open Approach
019B30Z	Drainage of Lumbar Nerve with Drainage Device, Percutaneous Approach
019B3ZX	Drainage of Lumbar Nerve, Percutaneous Approach, Diagnostic
019B3ZZ	Drainage of Lumbar Nerve, Percutaneous Approach
019B40Z	Drainage of Lumbar Nerve with Drainage Device, Percutaneous Endoscopic Approach
019B4ZX	Drainage of Lumbar Nerve, Percutaneous Endoscopic Approach, Diagnostic
019B4ZZ	Drainage of Lumbar Nerve, Percutaneous Endoscopic Approach
019C00Z	Drainage of Pudendal Nerve with Drainage Device, Open Approach
019C0ZX	Drainage of Pudendal Nerve, Open Approach, Diagnostic
019C0ZZ	Drainage of Pudendal Nerve, Open Approach
019C30Z	Drainage of Pudendal Nerve with Drainage Device, Percutaneous Approach
019C3ZX	Drainage of Pudendal Nerve, Percutaneous Approach, Diagnostic
019C3ZZ	Drainage of Pudendal Nerve, Percutaneous Approach
019C40Z	Drainage of Pudendal Nerve with Drainage Device, Percutaneous Endoscopic Approach
019C4ZX	Drainage of Pudendal Nerve, Percutaneous Endoscopic Approach, Diagnostic
019C4ZZ	Drainage of Pudendal Nerve, Percutaneous Endoscopic Approach
019D00Z	Drainage of Femoral Nerve with Drainage Device, Open Approach
019D0ZX	Drainage of Femoral Nerve, Open Approach, Diagnostic
019D0ZZ	Drainage of Femoral Nerve, Open Approach
019D30Z	Drainage of Femoral Nerve with Drainage Device, Percutaneous Approach
019D3ZX	Drainage of Femoral Nerve, Percutaneous Approach, Diagnostic
019D3ZZ	Drainage of Femoral Nerve, Percutaneous Approach
019D40Z	Drainage of Femoral Nerve with Drainage Device, Percutaneous Endoscopic Approach
019D4ZX	Drainage of Femoral Nerve, Percutaneous Endoscopic Approach, Diagnostic
019D4ZZ	Drainage of Femoral Nerve, Percutaneous Endoscopic Approach
019F00Z	Drainage of Sciatic Nerve with Drainage Device, Open Approach
019F0ZX	Drainage of Sciatic Nerve, Open Approach, Diagnostic
019F0ZZ	Drainage of Sciatic Nerve, Open Approach
019F30Z	Drainage of Sciatic Nerve with Drainage Device, Percutaneous Approach
019F3ZX	Drainage of Sciatic Nerve, Percutaneous Approach, Diagnostic
019F3ZZ	Drainage of Sciatic Nerve, Percutaneous Approach
019F40Z	Drainage of Sciatic Nerve with Drainage Device, Percutaneous Endoscopic Approach
019F4ZX	Drainage of Sciatic Nerve, Percutaneous Endoscopic Approach, Diagnostic
019F4ZZ	Drainage of Sciatic Nerve, Percutaneous Endoscopic Approach
019G00Z	Drainage of Tibial Nerve with Drainage Device, Open Approach
019G0ZX	Drainage of Tibial Nerve, Open Approach, Diagnostic
019G0ZZ	Drainage of Tibial Nerve, Open Approach
019G30Z	Drainage of Tibial Nerve with Drainage Device, Percutaneous Approach
019G3ZX	Drainage of Tibial Nerve, Percutaneous Approach, Diagnostic
019G3ZZ	Drainage of Tibial Nerve, Percutaneous Approach
019G40Z	Drainage of Tibial Nerve with Drainage Device, Percutaneous Endoscopic Approach
019G4ZX	Drainage of Tibial Nerve, Percutaneous Endoscopic Approach, Diagnostic
019G4ZZ	Drainage of Tibial Nerve, Percutaneous Endoscopic Approach
019H00Z	Drainage of Peroneal Nerve with Drainage Device, Open Approach
019H0ZX	Drainage of Peroneal Nerve, Open Approach, Diagnostic
019H0ZZ	Drainage of Peroneal Nerve, Open Approach
019H30Z	Drainage of Peroneal Nerve with Drainage Device, Percutaneous Approach
019H3ZX	Drainage of Peroneal Nerve, Percutaneous Approach, Diagnostic
019H3ZZ	Drainage of Peroneal Nerve, Percutaneous Approach
019H40Z	Drainage of Peroneal Nerve with Drainage Device, Percutaneous Endoscopic Approach
019H4ZX	Drainage of Peroneal Nerve, Percutaneous Endoscopic Approach, Diagnostic

♀ Female-only   ♂ Male-only   ▲ Limited Coverage   ● Non-OR   ▦ HAC-associated procedure   ▲ Non-covered procedures   ✚ Cluster

019H4ZZ	Drainage of Peroneal Nerve, Percutaneous Endoscopic Approach
019K00Z	Drainage of Head and Neck Sympathetic Nerve with Drainage Device, Open Approach
019K0ZX	Drainage of Head and Neck Sympathetic Nerve, Open Approach, Diagnostic
019K0ZZ	Drainage of Head and Neck Sympathetic Nerve, Open Approach
019K30Z	Drainage of Head and Neck Sympathetic Nerve with Drainage Device, Percutaneous Approach
019K3ZX	Drainage of Head and Neck Sympathetic Nerve, Percutaneous Approach, Diagnostic
019K3ZZ	Drainage of Head and Neck Sympathetic Nerve, Percutaneous Approach
019K40Z	Drainage of Head and Neck Sympathetic Nerve with Drainage Device, Percutaneous Endoscopic Approach
019K4ZX	Drainage of Head and Neck Sympathetic Nerve, Percutaneous Endoscopic Approach, Diagnostic
019K4ZZ	Drainage of Head and Neck Sympathetic Nerve, Percutaneous Endoscopic Approach
019L00Z	Drainage of Thoracic Sympathetic Nerve with Drainage Device, Open Approach
019L0ZX	Drainage of Thoracic Sympathetic Nerve, Open Approach, Diagnostic
019L0ZZ	Drainage of Thoracic Sympathetic Nerve, Open Approach
019L30Z	Drainage of Thoracic Sympathetic Nerve with Drainage Device, Percutaneous Approach
019L3ZX	Drainage of Thoracic Sympathetic Nerve, Percutaneous Approach, Diagnostic
019L3ZZ	Drainage of Thoracic Sympathetic Nerve, Percutaneous Approach
019L40Z	Drainage of Thoracic Sympathetic Nerve with Drainage Device, Percutaneous Endoscopic Approach
019L4ZX	Drainage of Thoracic Sympathetic Nerve, Percutaneous Endoscopic Approach, Diagnostic
019L4ZZ	Drainage of Thoracic Sympathetic Nerve, Percutaneous Endoscopic Approach
019M00Z	Drainage of Abdominal Sympathetic Nerve with Drainage Device, Open Approach
019M0ZX	Drainage of Abdominal Sympathetic Nerve, Open Approach, Diagnostic
019M0ZZ	Drainage of Abdominal Sympathetic Nerve, Open Approach
019M30Z	Drainage of Abdominal Sympathetic Nerve with Drainage Device, Percutaneous Approach
019M3ZX	Drainage of Abdominal Sympathetic Nerve, Percutaneous Approach, Diagnostic
019M3ZZ	Drainage of Abdominal Sympathetic Nerve, Percutaneous Approach
019M40Z	Drainage of Abdominal Sympathetic Nerve with Drainage Device, Percutaneous Endoscopic Approach
019M4ZX	Drainage of Abdominal Sympathetic Nerve, Percutaneous Endoscopic Approach, Diagnostic
019M4ZZ	Drainage of Abdominal Sympathetic Nerve, Percutaneous Endoscopic Approach
019N00Z	Drainage of Lumbar Sympathetic Nerve with Drainage Device, Open Approach
019N0ZX	Drainage of Lumbar Sympathetic Nerve, Open Approach, Diagnostic
019N0ZZ	Drainage of Lumbar Sympathetic Nerve, Open Approach
019N30Z	Drainage of Lumbar Sympathetic Nerve with Drainage Device, Percutaneous Approach
019N3ZX	Drainage of Lumbar Sympathetic Nerve, Percutaneous Approach, Diagnostic
019N3ZZ	Drainage of Lumbar Sympathetic Nerve, Percutaneous Approach
019N40Z	Drainage of Lumbar Sympathetic Nerve with Drainage Device, Percutaneous Endoscopic Approach
019N4ZX	Drainage of Lumbar Sympathetic Nerve, Percutaneous Endoscopic Approach, Diagnostic
019N4ZZ	Drainage of Lumbar Sympathetic Nerve, Percutaneous Endoscopic Approach
019P00Z	Drainage of Sacral Sympathetic Nerve with Drainage Device, Open Approach
019P0ZX	Drainage of Sacral Sympathetic Nerve, Open Approach, Diagnostic
019P0ZZ	Drainage of Sacral Sympathetic Nerve, Open Approach
019P30Z	Drainage of Sacral Sympathetic Nerve with Drainage Device, Percutaneous Approach
019P3ZX	Drainage of Sacral Sympathetic Nerve, Percutaneous Approach, Diagnostic
019P3ZZ	Drainage of Sacral Sympathetic Nerve, Percutaneous Approach
019P40Z	Drainage of Sacral Sympathetic Nerve with Drainage Device, Percutaneous Endoscopic Approach
019P4ZX	Drainage of Sacral Sympathetic Nerve, Percutaneous Endoscopic Approach, Diagnostic
019P4ZZ	Drainage of Sacral Sympathetic Nerve, Percutaneous Endoscopic Approach
019Q00Z	Drainage of Sacral Plexus with Drainage Device, Open Approach
019Q0ZX	Drainage of Sacral Plexus, Open Approach, Diagnostic
019Q0ZZ	Drainage of Sacral Plexus, Open Approach
019Q30Z	Drainage of Sacral Plexus with Drainage Device, Percutaneous Approach
019Q3ZX	Drainage of Sacral Plexus, Percutaneous Approach, Diagnostic
019Q3ZZ	Drainage of Sacral Plexus, Percutaneous Approach
019Q40Z	Drainage of Sacral Plexus with Drainage Device, Percutaneous Endoscopic Approach
019Q4ZX	Drainage of Sacral Plexus, Percutaneous Endoscopic Approach, Diagnostic
019Q4ZZ	Drainage of Sacral Plexus, Percutaneous Endoscopic Approach
019R00Z	Drainage of Sacral Nerve with Drainage Device, Open Approach
019R0ZX	Drainage of Sacral Nerve, Open Approach, Diagnostic
019R0ZZ	Drainage of Sacral Nerve, Open Approach
019R30Z	Drainage of Sacral Nerve with Drainage Device, Percutaneous Approach
019R3ZX	Drainage of Sacral Nerve, Percutaneous Approach, Diagnostic
019R3ZZ	Drainage of Sacral Nerve, Percutaneous Approach
019R40Z	Drainage of Sacral Nerve with Drainage Device, Percutaneous Endoscopic Approach
019R4ZX	Drainage of Sacral Nerve, Percutaneous Endoscopic Approach, Diagnostic
019R4ZZ	Drainage of Sacral Nerve, Percutaneous Endoscopic Approach

01B – Peripheral Nervous System, Excision

Review Coding Guidelines B3.4a and B3.4b

Review Coding Guideline B3.8

Review Coding Guideline B3.18

01B00ZX	Excision of Cervical Plexus, Open Approach, Diagnostic
01B00ZZ	Excision of Cervical Plexus, Open Approach
01B03ZX	Excision of Cervical Plexus, Percutaneous Approach, Diagnostic
01B03ZZ	Excision of Cervical Plexus, Percutaneous Approach
01B04ZX	Excision of Cervical Plexus, Percutaneous Endoscopic Approach, Diagnostic
01B04ZZ	Excision of Cervical Plexus, Percutaneous Endoscopic Approach
01B10ZX	Excision of Cervical Nerve, Open Approach, Diagnostic
01B10ZZ	Excision of Cervical Nerve, Open Approach
01B13ZX	Excision of Cervical Nerve, Percutaneous Approach, Diagnostic
01B13ZZ	Excision of Cervical Nerve, Percutaneous Approach
01B14ZX	Excision of Cervical Nerve, Percutaneous Endoscopic Approach, Diagnostic
01B14ZZ	Excision of Cervical Nerve, Percutaneous Endoscopic Approach
01B20ZX	Excision of Phrenic Nerve, Open Approach, Diagnostic
01B20ZZ	Excision of Phrenic Nerve, Open Approach
01B23ZX	Excision of Phrenic Nerve, Percutaneous Approach, Diagnostic
01B23ZZ	Excision of Phrenic Nerve, Percutaneous Approach
01B24ZX	Excision of Phrenic Nerve, Percutaneous Endoscopic Approach, Diagnostic
01B24ZZ	Excision of Phrenic Nerve, Percutaneous Endoscopic Approach
01B30ZX	Excision of Brachial Plexus, Open Approach, Diagnostic
01B30ZZ	Excision of Brachial Plexus, Open Approach
01B33ZX	Excision of Brachial Plexus, Percutaneous Approach, Diagnostic

01B33ZZ Excision of Brachial Plexus, Percutaneous Approach

01B34ZX Excision of Brachial Plexus, Percutaneous Endoscopic Approach, Diagnostic

01B34ZZ Excision of Brachial Plexus, Percutaneous Endoscopic Approach

01B40ZX Excision of Ulnar Nerve, Open Approach, Diagnostic

01B40ZZ Excision of Ulnar Nerve, Open Approach

01B43ZX Excision of Ulnar Nerve, Percutaneous Approach, Diagnostic

01B43ZZ Excision of Ulnar Nerve, Percutaneous Approach

01B44ZX Excision of Ulnar Nerve, Percutaneous Endoscopic Approach, Diagnostic

01B44ZZ Excision of Ulnar Nerve, Percutaneous Endoscopic Approach

01B50ZX Excision of Median Nerve, Open Approach, Diagnostic

01B50ZZ Excision of Median Nerve, Open Approach

01B53ZX Excision of Median Nerve, Percutaneous Approach, Diagnostic

01B53ZZ Excision of Median Nerve, Percutaneous Approach

01B54ZX Excision of Median Nerve, Percutaneous Endoscopic Approach, Diagnostic

01B54ZZ Excision of Median Nerve, Percutaneous Endoscopic Approach

01B60ZX Excision of Radial Nerve, Open Approach, Diagnostic

01B60ZZ Excision of Radial Nerve, Open Approach

01B63ZX Excision of Radial Nerve, Percutaneous Approach, Diagnostic

01B63ZZ Excision of Radial Nerve, Percutaneous Approach

01B64ZX Excision of Radial Nerve, Percutaneous Endoscopic Approach, Diagnostic

01B64ZZ Excision of Radial Nerve, Percutaneous Endoscopic Approach

01B80ZX Excision of Thoracic Nerve, Open Approach, Diagnostic

01B80ZZ Excision of Thoracic Nerve, Open Approach

01B83ZX Excision of Thoracic Nerve, Percutaneous Approach, Diagnostic

01B83ZZ Excision of Thoracic Nerve, Percutaneous Approach

01B84ZX Excision of Thoracic Nerve, Percutaneous Endoscopic Approach, Diagnostic

01B84ZZ Excision of Thoracic Nerve, Percutaneous Endoscopic Approach

01B90ZX Excision of Lumbar Plexus, Open Approach, Diagnostic

01B90ZZ Excision of Lumbar Plexus, Open Approach

01B93ZX Excision of Lumbar Plexus, Percutaneous Approach, Diagnostic

01B93ZZ Excision of Lumbar Plexus, Percutaneous Approach

01B94ZX Excision of Lumbar Plexus, Percutaneous Endoscopic Approach, Diagnostic

01B94ZZ Excision of Lumbar Plexus, Percutaneous Endoscopic Approach

01BA0ZX Excision of Lumbosacral Plexus, Open Approach, Diagnostic

01BA0ZZ Excision of Lumbosacral Plexus, Open Approach

01BA3ZX Excision of Lumbosacral Plexus, Percutaneous Approach, Diagnostic

01BA3ZZ Excision of Lumbosacral Plexus, Percutaneous Approach

01BA4ZX Excision of Lumbosacral Plexus, Percutaneous Endoscopic Approach, Diagnostic

01BA4ZZ Excision of Lumbosacral Plexus, Percutaneous Endoscopic Approach

01BB0ZX Excision of Lumbar Nerve, Open Approach, Diagnostic

01BB0ZZ Excision of Lumbar Nerve, Open Approach

01BB3ZX Excision of Lumbar Nerve, Percutaneous Approach, Diagnostic

01BB3ZZ Excision of Lumbar Nerve, Percutaneous Approach

01BB4ZX Excision of Lumbar Nerve, Percutaneous Endoscopic Approach, Diagnostic

01BB4ZZ Excision of Lumbar Nerve, Percutaneous Endoscopic Approach

01BC0ZX Excision of Pudendal Nerve, Open Approach, Diagnostic

01BC0ZZ Excision of Pudendal Nerve, Open Approach

01BC3ZX Excision of Pudendal Nerve, Percutaneous Approach, Diagnostic

01BC3ZZ Excision of Pudendal Nerve, Percutaneous Approach

01BC4ZX Excision of Pudendal Nerve, Percutaneous Endoscopic Approach, Diagnostic

01BC4ZZ Excision of Pudendal Nerve, Percutaneous Endoscopic Approach

01BD0ZX Excision of Femoral Nerve, Open Approach, Diagnostic

01BD0ZZ Excision of Femoral Nerve, Open Approach

01BD3ZX Excision of Femoral Nerve, Percutaneous Approach, Diagnostic

01BD3ZZ Excision of Femoral Nerve, Percutaneous Approach

01BD4ZX Excision of Femoral Nerve, Percutaneous Endoscopic Approach, Diagnostic

01BD4ZZ Excision of Femoral Nerve, Percutaneous Endoscopic Approach

01BF0ZX Excision of Sciatic Nerve, Open Approach, Diagnostic

01BF0ZZ Excision of Sciatic Nerve, Open Approach

01BF3ZX Excision of Sciatic Nerve, Percutaneous Approach, Diagnostic

01BF3ZZ Excision of Sciatic Nerve, Percutaneous Approach

01BF4ZX Excision of Sciatic Nerve, Percutaneous Endoscopic Approach, Diagnostic

01BF4ZZ Excision of Sciatic Nerve, Percutaneous Endoscopic Approach

01BG0ZX Excision of Tibial Nerve, Open Approach, Diagnostic

01BG0ZZ Excision of Tibial Nerve, Open Approach

01BG3ZX Excision of Tibial Nerve, Percutaneous Approach, Diagnostic

01BG3ZZ Excision of Tibial Nerve, Percutaneous Approach

01BG4ZX Excision of Tibial Nerve, Percutaneous Endoscopic Approach, Diagnostic

01BG4ZZ Excision of Tibial Nerve, Percutaneous Endoscopic Approach

01BH0ZX Excision of Peroneal Nerve, Open Approach, Diagnostic

01BH0ZZ Excision of Peroneal Nerve, Open Approach

01BH3ZX Excision of Peroneal Nerve, Percutaneous Approach, Diagnostic

01BH3ZZ Excision of Peroneal Nerve, Percutaneous Approach

01BH4ZX Excision of Peroneal Nerve, Percutaneous Endoscopic Approach, Diagnostic

01BH4ZZ Excision of Peroneal Nerve, Percutaneous Endoscopic Approach

01BK0ZX Excision of Head and Neck Sympathetic Nerve, Open Approach, Diagnostic

01BK0ZZ Excision of Head and Neck Sympathetic Nerve, Open Approach

01BK3ZX Excision of Head and Neck Sympathetic Nerve, Percutaneous Approach, Diagnostic

01BK3ZZ Excision of Head and Neck Sympathetic Nerve, Percutaneous Approach

01BK4ZX Excision of Head and Neck Sympathetic Nerve, Percutaneous Endoscopic Approach, Diagnostic

01BK4ZZ Excision of Head and Neck Sympathetic Nerve, Percutaneous Endoscopic Approach

01BL0ZX Excision of Thoracic Sympathetic Nerve, Open Approach, Diagnostic

01BL0ZZ Excision of Thoracic Sympathetic Nerve, Open Approach

AHA CC: 2Q, 2017, 19-20

01BL3ZX Excision of Thoracic Sympathetic Nerve, Percutaneous Approach, Diagnostic

01BL3ZZ Excision of Thoracic Sympathetic Nerve, Percutaneous Approach

01BL4ZX Excision of Thoracic Sympathetic Nerve, Percutaneous Endoscopic Approach, Diagnostic

01BL4ZZ Excision of Thoracic Sympathetic Nerve, Percutaneous Endoscopic Approach

01BM0ZX Excision of Abdominal Sympathetic Nerve, Open Approach, Diagnostic

01BM0ZZ Excision of Abdominal Sympathetic Nerve, Open Approach

01BM3ZX Excision of Abdominal Sympathetic Nerve, Percutaneous Approach, Diagnostic

01BM3ZZ Excision of Abdominal Sympathetic Nerve, Percutaneous Approach

01BM4ZX Excision of Abdominal Sympathetic Nerve, Percutaneous Endoscopic Approach, Diagnostic

01BM4ZZ Excision of Abdominal Sympathetic Nerve, Percutaneous Endoscopic Approach

01BN0ZX Excision of Lumbar Sympathetic Nerve, Open Approach, Diagnostic

01BN0ZZ Excision of Lumbar Sympathetic Nerve, Open Approach

01BN3ZX Excision of Lumbar Sympathetic Nerve, Percutaneous Approach, Diagnostic

01BN3ZZ Excision of Lumbar Sympathetic Nerve, Percutaneous Approach

01BN4ZX Excision of Lumbar Sympathetic Nerve, Percutaneous Endoscopic Approach, Diagnostic

01BN4ZZ Excision of Lumbar Sympathetic Nerve, Percutaneous Endoscopic Approach

01BP0ZX Excision of Sacral Sympathetic Nerve, Open Approach, Diagnostic

01BP0ZZ Excision of Sacral Sympathetic Nerve, Open Approach

01BP3ZX Excision of Sacral Sympathetic Nerve, Percutaneous Approach, Diagnostic

01BP3ZZ Excision of Sacral Sympathetic Nerve, Percutaneous Approach

01BP4ZX Excision of Sacral Sympathetic Nerve, Percutaneous Endoscopic Approach, Diagnostic

01BP4ZZ Excision of Sacral Sympathetic Nerve, Percutaneous Endoscopic Approach

♀ Female-only   ♂ Male-only   ▲ Limited Coverage   ● Non-OR   HAC HAC-associated procedure   ▲ Non-covered procedures   ✚ Cluster

01BQ0ZX Excision of Sacral Plexus, Open Approach, Diagnostic
01BQ0ZZ Excision of Sacral Plexus, Open Approach
01BQ3ZX Excision of Sacral Plexus, Percutaneous Approach, Diagnostic
01BQ3ZZ Excision of Sacral Plexus, Percutaneous Approach

01BQ4ZX Excision of Sacral Plexus, Percutaneous Endoscopic Approach, Diagnostic
01BQ4ZZ Excision of Sacral Plexus, Percutaneous Endoscopic Approach
01BR0ZX Excision of Sacral Nerve, Open Approach, Diagnostic
01BR0ZZ Excision of Sacral Nerve, Open Approach

01BR3ZX Excision of Sacral Nerve, Percutaneous Approach, Diagnostic
01BR3ZZ Excision of Sacral Nerve, Percutaneous Approach
01BR4ZX Excision of Sacral Nerve, Percutaneous Endoscopic Approach, Diagnostic
01BR4ZZ Excision of Sacral Nerve, Percutaneous Endoscopic Approach

01C – Peripheral Nervous System, Extirpation

01C00ZZ Extirpation of Matter from Cervical Plexus, Open Approach
01C03ZZ Extirpation of Matter from Cervical Plexus, Percutaneous Approach
01C04ZZ Extirpation of Matter from Cervical Plexus, Percutaneous Endoscopic Approach
01C10ZZ Extirpation of Matter from Cervical Nerve, Open Approach
01C13ZZ Extirpation of Matter from Cervical Nerve, Percutaneous Approach
01C14ZZ Extirpation of Matter from Cervical Nerve, Percutaneous Endoscopic Approach
01C20ZZ Extirpation of Matter from Phrenic Nerve, Open Approach
01C23ZZ Extirpation of Matter from Phrenic Nerve, Percutaneous Approach
01C24ZZ Extirpation of Matter from Phrenic Nerve, Percutaneous Endoscopic Approach
01C30ZZ Extirpation of Matter from Brachial Plexus, Open Approach
01C33ZZ Extirpation of Matter from Brachial Plexus, Percutaneous Approach
01C34ZZ Extirpation of Matter from Brachial Plexus, Percutaneous Endoscopic Approach
01C40ZZ Extirpation of Matter from Ulnar Nerve, Open Approach
01C43ZZ Extirpation of Matter from Ulnar Nerve, Percutaneous Approach
01C44ZZ Extirpation of Matter from Ulnar Nerve, Percutaneous Endoscopic Approach
01C50ZZ Extirpation of Matter from Median Nerve, Open Approach
01C53ZZ Extirpation of Matter from Median Nerve, Percutaneous Approach
01C54ZZ Extirpation of Matter from Median Nerve, Percutaneous Endoscopic Approach
01C60ZZ Extirpation of Matter from Radial Nerve, Open Approach
01C63ZZ Extirpation of Matter from Radial Nerve, Percutaneous Approach
01C64ZZ Extirpation of Matter from Radial Nerve, Percutaneous Endoscopic Approach
01C80ZZ Extirpation of Matter from Thoracic Nerve, Open Approach
01C83ZZ Extirpation of Matter from Thoracic Nerve, Percutaneous Approach
01C84ZZ Extirpation of Matter from Thoracic Nerve, Percutaneous Endoscopic Approach

01C90ZZ Extirpation of Matter from Lumbar Plexus, Open Approach
01C93ZZ Extirpation of Matter from Lumbar Plexus, Percutaneous Approach
01C94ZZ Extirpation of Matter from Lumbar Plexus, Percutaneous Endoscopic Approach
01CA0ZZ Extirpation of Matter from Lumbosacral Plexus, Open Approach
01CA3ZZ Extirpation of Matter from Lumbosacral Plexus, Percutaneous Approach
01CA4ZZ Extirpation of Matter from Lumbosacral Plexus, Percutaneous Endoscopic Approach
01CB0ZZ Extirpation of Matter from Lumbar Nerve, Open Approach
01CB3ZZ Extirpation of Matter from Lumbar Nerve, Percutaneous Approach
01CB4ZZ Extirpation of Matter from Lumbar Nerve, Percutaneous Endoscopic Approach
01CC0ZZ Extirpation of Matter from Pudendal Nerve, Open Approach
01CC3ZZ Extirpation of Matter from Pudendal Nerve, Percutaneous Approach
01CC4ZZ Extirpation of Matter from Pudendal Nerve, Percutaneous Endoscopic Approach
01CD0ZZ Extirpation of Matter from Femoral Nerve, Open Approach
01CD3ZZ Extirpation of Matter from Femoral Nerve, Percutaneous Approach
01CD4ZZ Extirpation of Matter from Femoral Nerve, Percutaneous Endoscopic Approach
01CF0ZZ Extirpation of Matter from Sciatic Nerve, Open Approach
01CF3ZZ Extirpation of Matter from Sciatic Nerve, Percutaneous Approach
01CF4ZZ Extirpation of Matter from Sciatic Nerve, Percutaneous Endoscopic Approach
01CG0ZZ Extirpation of Matter from Tibial Nerve, Open Approach
01CG3ZZ Extirpation of Matter from Tibial Nerve, Percutaneous Approach
01CG4ZZ Extirpation of Matter from Tibial Nerve, Percutaneous Endoscopic Approach
01CH0ZZ Extirpation of Matter from Peroneal Nerve, Open Approach
01CH3ZZ Extirpation of Matter from Peroneal Nerve, Percutaneous Approach
01CH4ZZ Extirpation of Matter from Peroneal Nerve, Percutaneous Endoscopic Approach

01CK0ZZ Extirpation of Matter from Head and Neck Sympathetic Nerve, Open Approach
01CK3ZZ Extirpation of Matter from Head and Neck Sympathetic Nerve, Percutaneous Approach
01CK4ZZ Extirpation of Matter from Head and Neck Sympathetic Nerve, Percutaneous Endoscopic Approach
01CL0ZZ Extirpation of Matter from Thoracic Sympathetic Nerve, Open Approach
01CL3ZZ Extirpation of Matter from Thoracic Sympathetic Nerve, Percutaneous Approach
01CL4ZZ Extirpation of Matter from Thoracic Sympathetic Nerve, Percutaneous Endoscopic Approach
01CM0ZZ Extirpation of Matter from Abdominal Sympathetic Nerve, Open Approach
01CM3ZZ Extirpation of Matter from Abdominal Sympathetic Nerve, Percutaneous Approach
01CM4ZZ Extirpation of Matter from Abdominal Sympathetic Nerve, Percutaneous Endoscopic Approach
01CN0ZZ Extirpation of Matter from Lumbar Sympathetic Nerve, Open Approach
01CN3ZZ Extirpation of Matter from Lumbar Sympathetic Nerve, Percutaneous Approach
01CN4ZZ Extirpation of Matter from Lumbar Sympathetic Nerve, Percutaneous Endoscopic Approach
01CP0ZZ Extirpation of Matter from Sacral Sympathetic Nerve, Open Approach
01CP3ZZ Extirpation of Matter from Sacral Sympathetic Nerve, Percutaneous Approach
01CP4ZZ Extirpation of Matter from Sacral Sympathetic Nerve, Percutaneous Endoscopic Approach
01CQ0ZZ Extirpation of Matter from Sacral Plexus, Open Approach
01CQ3ZZ Extirpation of Matter from Sacral Plexus, Percutaneous Approach
01CQ4ZZ Extirpation of Matter from Sacral Plexus, Percutaneous Endoscopic Approach
01CR0ZZ Extirpation of Matter from Sacral Nerve, Open Approach
01CR3ZZ Extirpation of Matter from Sacral Nerve, Percutaneous Approach
01CR4ZZ Extirpation of Matter from Sacral Nerve, Percutaneous Endoscopic Approach

01D – Peripheral Nervous System, Extraction

01D00ZZ Extraction of Cervical Plexus, Open Approach
01D03ZZ Extraction of Cervical Plexus, Percutaneous Approach
01D04ZZ Extraction of Cervical Plexus, Percutaneous Endoscopic Approach

01D10ZZ Extraction of Cervical Nerve, Open Approach
01D13ZZ Extraction of Cervical Nerve, Percutaneous Approach
01D14ZZ Extraction of Cervical Nerve, Percutaneous Endoscopic Approach

01D20ZZ Extraction of Phrenic Nerve, Open Approach
01D23ZZ Extraction of Phrenic Nerve, Percutaneous Approach
01D24ZZ Extraction of Phrenic Nerve, Percutaneous Endoscopic Approach

♀ Female-only   ♂ Male-only   ▲ Limited Coverage   ● Non-OR   🄷🄰🄲 HAC-associated procedure   ▲ Non-covered procedures   ➕ Cluster

01D30ZZ	Extraction of Brachial Plexus, Open Approach	**01DB0ZZ**	Extraction of Lumbar Nerve, Open Approach	**01DK4ZZ**	Extraction of Head and Neck Sympathetic Nerve, Percutaneous Endoscopic Approach
01D33ZZ	Extraction of Brachial Plexus, Percutaneous Approach	**01DB3ZZ**	Extraction of Lumbar Nerve, Percutaneous Approach	**01DL0ZZ**	Extraction of Thoracic Sympathetic Nerve, Open Approach
01D34ZZ	Extraction of Brachial Plexus, Percutaneous Endoscopic Approach	**01DB4ZZ**	Extraction of Lumbar Nerve, Percutaneous Endoscopic Approach	**01DL3ZZ**	Extraction of Thoracic Sympathetic Nerve, Percutaneous Approach
01D40ZZ	Extraction of Ulnar Nerve, Open Approach	**01DC0ZZ**	Extraction of Pudendal Nerve, Open Approach	**01DL4ZZ**	Extraction of Thoracic Sympathetic Nerve, Percutaneous Endoscopic Approach
01D43ZZ	Extraction of Ulnar Nerve, Percutaneous Approach	**01DC3ZZ**	Extraction of Pudendal Nerve, Percutaneous Approach	**01DM0ZZ**	Extraction of Abdominal Sympathetic Nerve, Open Approach
01D44ZZ	Extraction of Ulnar Nerve, Percutaneous Endoscopic Approach	**01DC4ZZ**	Extraction of Pudendal Nerve, Percutaneous Endoscopic Approach	**01DM3ZZ**	Extraction of Abdominal Sympathetic Nerve, Percutaneous Approach
01D50ZZ	Extraction of Median Nerve, Open Approach	**01DD0ZZ**	Extraction of Femoral Nerve, Open Approach	**01DM4ZZ**	Extraction of Abdominal Sympathetic Nerve, Percutaneous Endoscopic Approach
01D53ZZ	Extraction of Median Nerve, Percutaneous Approach	**01DD3ZZ**	Extraction of Femoral Nerve, Percutaneous Approach	**01DN0ZZ**	Extraction of Lumbar Sympathetic Nerve, Open Approach
01D54ZZ	Extraction of Median Nerve, Percutaneous Endoscopic Approach	**01DD4ZZ**	Extraction of Femoral Nerve, Percutaneous Endoscopic Approach	**01DN3ZZ**	Extraction of Lumbar Sympathetic Nerve, Percutaneous Approach
01D60ZZ	Extraction of Radial Nerve, Open Approach	**01DF0ZZ**	Extraction of Sciatic Nerve, Open Approach	**01DN4ZZ**	Extraction of Lumbar Sympathetic Nerve, Percutaneous Endoscopic Approach
01D63ZZ	Extraction of Radial Nerve, Percutaneous Approach	**01DF3ZZ**	Extraction of Sciatic Nerve, Percutaneous Approach	**01DP0ZZ**	Extraction of Sacral Sympathetic Nerve, Open Approach
01D64ZZ	Extraction of Radial Nerve, Percutaneous Endoscopic Approach	**01DF4ZZ**	Extraction of Sciatic Nerve, Percutaneous Endoscopic Approach	**01DP3ZZ**	Extraction of Sacral Sympathetic Nerve, Percutaneous Approach
01D80ZZ	Extraction of Thoracic Nerve, Open Approach	**01DG0ZZ**	Extraction of Tibial Nerve, Open Approach	**01DP4ZZ**	Extraction of Sacral Sympathetic Nerve, Percutaneous Endoscopic Approach
01D83ZZ	Extraction of Thoracic Nerve, Percutaneous Approach	**01DG3ZZ**	Extraction of Tibial Nerve, Percutaneous Approach	**01DQ0ZZ**	Extraction of Sacral Plexus, Open Approach
01D84ZZ	Extraction of Thoracic Nerve, Percutaneous Endoscopic Approach	**01DG4ZZ**	Extraction of Tibial Nerve, Percutaneous Endoscopic Approach	**01DQ3ZZ**	Extraction of Sacral Plexus, Percutaneous Approach
01D90ZZ	Extraction of Lumbar Plexus, Open Approach	**01DH0ZZ**	Extraction of Peroneal Nerve, Open Approach	**01DQ4ZZ**	Extraction of Sacral Plexus, Percutaneous Endoscopic Approach
01D93ZZ	Extraction of Lumbar Plexus, Percutaneous Approach	**01DH3ZZ**	Extraction of Peroneal Nerve, Percutaneous Approach	**01DR0ZZ**	Extraction of Sacral Nerve, Open Approach
01D94ZZ	Extraction of Lumbar Plexus, Percutaneous Endoscopic Approach	**01DH4ZZ**	Extraction of Peroneal Nerve, Percutaneous Endoscopic Approach	**01DR3ZZ**	Extraction of Sacral Nerve, Percutaneous Approach
01DA0ZZ	Extraction of Lumbosacral Plexus, Open Approach	**01DK0ZZ**	Extraction of Head and Neck Sympathetic Nerve, Open Approach	**01DR4ZZ**	Extraction of Sacral Nerve, Percutaneous Endoscopic Approach
01DA3ZZ	Extraction of Lumbosacral Plexus, Percutaneous Approach	**01DK3ZZ**	Extraction of Head and Neck Sympathetic Nerve, Percutaneous Approach		
01DA4ZZ	Extraction of Lumbosacral Plexus, Percutaneous Endoscopic Approach				

01H – Peripheral Nervous System, Insertion

01HY01Z	Insertion of Radioactive Element into Peripheral Nerve, Open Approach	**01HY32Z**	Insertion of Monitoring Device into Peripheral Nerve, Percutaneous Approach	**01HY42Z**	Insertion of Monitoring Device into Peripheral Nerve, Percutaneous Endoscopic Approach
01HY02Z	Insertion of Monitoring Device into Peripheral Nerve, Open Approach	**01HY3MZ**	Insertion of Neurostimulator Lead into Peripheral Nerve, Percutaneous Approach	**01HY4MZ**	Insertion of Neurostimulator Lead into Peripheral Nerve, Percutaneous Endoscopic Approach
01HY0MZ	Insertion of Neurostimulator Lead into Peripheral Nerve, Open Approach	**01HY3YZ**	Insertion of Other Device into Peripheral Nerve, Percutaneous Approach	**01HY4YZ**	Insertion of Other Device into Peripheral Nerve, Percutaneous Endoscopic Approach
01HY0YZ	Insertion of Other Device into Peripheral Nerve, Open Approach	**01HY41Z**	Insertion of Radioactive Element into Peripheral Nerve, Percutaneous Endoscopic Approach		
01HY31Z	Insertion of Radioactive Element into Peripheral Nerve, Percutaneous Approach				

01J – Peripheral Nervous System, Inspection

Review Coding Guidelines B3.11a, B3.11b and B3.11c

01JY0ZZ	Inspection of Peripheral Nerve, Open Approach	**01JY3ZZ**	Inspection of Peripheral Nerve, Percutaneous Approach	**01JY4ZZ**	Inspection of Peripheral Nerve, Percutaneous Endoscopic Approach

01N – Peripheral Nervous System, Release

Review Coding Guideline B3.13

Review Coding Guideline B3.14

01N00ZZ	Release Cervical Plexus, Open Approach	**01N10ZZ**	Release Cervical Nerve, Open Approach	**01N14ZZ**	Release Cervical Nerve, Percutaneous Endoscopic Approach
01N03ZZ	Release Cervical Plexus, Percutaneous Approach		*AHA CC: 2Q, 2016, 17*	**01N20ZZ**	Release Phrenic Nerve, Open Approach
01N04ZZ	Release Cervical Plexus, Percutaneous Endoscopic Approach	**01N13ZZ**	Release Cervical Nerve, Percutaneous Approach	**01N23ZZ**	Release Phrenic Nerve, Percutaneous Approach

♀ Female-only   ♂ Male-only   ▲ Limited Coverage   ● Non-OR   HAC HAC-associated procedure   ▲ Non-covered procedures   ✚ Cluster

01N24ZZ	Release Phrenic Nerve, Percutaneous Endoscopic Approach	**01NA3ZZ**	Release Lumbosacral Plexus, Percutaneous Approach
01N30ZZ	Release Brachial Plexus, Open Approach	**01NA4ZZ**	Release Lumbosacral Plexus, Percutaneous Endoscopic Approach

01N24ZZ Release Phrenic Nerve, Percutaneous Endoscopic Approach

01N30ZZ Release Brachial Plexus, Open Approach
AHA CC: 2Q, 2016, 23

01N33ZZ Release Brachial Plexus, Percutaneous Approach

01N34ZZ Release Brachial Plexus, Percutaneous Endoscopic Approach

01N40ZZ Release Ulnar Nerve, Open Approach

01N43ZZ Release Ulnar Nerve, Percutaneous Approach

01N44ZZ Release Ulnar Nerve, Percutaneous Endoscopic Approach

01N50ZZ Release Median Nerve, Open Approach
AHA CC: 3Q, 2014, 33-34

01N53ZZ Release Median Nerve, Percutaneous Approach

01N54ZZ Release Median Nerve, Percutaneous Endoscopic Approach

01N60ZZ Release Radial Nerve, Open Approach

01N63ZZ Release Radial Nerve, Percutaneous Approach

01N64ZZ Release Radial Nerve, Percutaneous Endoscopic Approach

01N80ZZ Release Thoracic Nerve, Open Approach

01N83ZZ Release Thoracic Nerve, Percutaneous Approach

01N84ZZ Release Thoracic Nerve, Percutaneous Endoscopic Approach

01N90ZZ Release Lumbar Plexus, Open Approach

01N93ZZ Release Lumbar Plexus, Percutaneous Approach

01N94ZZ Release Lumbar Plexus, Percutaneous Endoscopic Approach

01NA0ZZ Release Lumbosacral Plexus, Open Approach

01NA3ZZ Release Lumbosacral Plexus, Percutaneous Approach

01NA4ZZ Release Lumbosacral Plexus, Percutaneous Endoscopic Approach

01NB0ZZ Release Lumbar Nerve, Open Approach
AHA CC: 2Q, 2015, 34; 2Q, 2016, 16; 2Q, 2018, 22-23; 1Q, 2019, 28-29

01NB3ZZ Release Lumbar Nerve, Percutaneous Approach

01NB4ZZ Release Lumbar Nerve, Percutaneous Endoscopic Approach

01NC0ZZ Release Pudendal Nerve, Open Approach

01NC3ZZ Release Pudendal Nerve, Percutaneous Approach

01NC4ZZ Release Pudendal Nerve, Percutaneous Endoscopic Approach

01ND0ZZ Release Femoral Nerve, Open Approach

01ND3ZZ Release Femoral Nerve, Percutaneous Approach

01ND4ZZ Release Femoral Nerve, Percutaneous Endoscopic Approach

01NF0ZZ Release Sciatic Nerve, Open Approach

01NF3ZZ Release Sciatic Nerve, Percutaneous Approach

01NF4ZZ Release Sciatic Nerve, Percutaneous Endoscopic Approach

01NG0ZZ Release Tibial Nerve, Open Approach

01NG3ZZ Release Tibial Nerve, Percutaneous Approach

01NG4ZZ Release Tibial Nerve, Percutaneous Endoscopic Approach

01NH0ZZ Release Peroneal Nerve, Open Approach

01NH3ZZ Release Peroneal Nerve, Percutaneous Approach

01NH4ZZ Release Peroneal Nerve, Percutaneous Endoscopic Approach

01NK0ZZ Release Head and Neck Sympathetic Nerve, Open Approach

01NK3ZZ Release Head and Neck Sympathetic Nerve, Percutaneous Approach

01NK4ZZ Release Head and Neck Sympathetic Nerve, Percutaneous Endoscopic Approach

01NL0ZZ Release Thoracic Sympathetic Nerve, Open Approach

01NL3ZZ Release Thoracic Sympathetic Nerve, Percutaneous Approach

01NL4ZZ Release Thoracic Sympathetic Nerve, Percutaneous Endoscopic Approach

01NM0ZZ Release Abdominal Sympathetic Nerve, Open Approach

01NM3ZZ Release Abdominal Sympathetic Nerve, Percutaneous Approach

01NM4ZZ Release Abdominal Sympathetic Nerve, Percutaneous Endoscopic Approach

01NN0ZZ Release Lumbar Sympathetic Nerve, Open Approach

01NN3ZZ Release Lumbar Sympathetic Nerve, Percutaneous Approach

01NN4ZZ Release Lumbar Sympathetic Nerve, Percutaneous Endoscopic Approach

01NP0ZZ Release Sacral Sympathetic Nerve, Open Approach

01NP3ZZ Release Sacral Sympathetic Nerve, Percutaneous Approach

01NP4ZZ Release Sacral Sympathetic Nerve, Percutaneous Endoscopic Approach

01NQ0ZZ Release Sacral Plexus, Open Approach

01NQ3ZZ Release Sacral Plexus, Percutaneous Approach

01NQ4ZZ Release Sacral Plexus, Percutaneous Endoscopic Approach

01NR0ZZ Release Sacral Nerve, Open Approach
AHA CC: 1Q, 2019, 28-29

01NR3ZZ Release Sacral Nerve, Percutaneous Approach

01NR4ZZ Release Sacral Nerve, Percutaneous Endoscopic Approach

01P – Peripheral Nervous System, Removal

Review Coding Guideline B6.1c

01PY00Z Removal of Drainage Device from Peripheral Nerve, Open Approach

01PY02Z Removal of Monitoring Device from Peripheral Nerve, Open Approach

01PY07Z Removal of Autologous Tissue Substitute from Peripheral Nerve, Open Approach

01PY0MZ Removal of Neurostimulator Lead from Peripheral Nerve, Open Approach

01PY0YZ Removal of Other Device from Peripheral Nerve, Open Approach

01PY30Z Removal of Drainage Device from Peripheral Nerve, Percutaneous Approach

01PY32Z Removal of Monitoring Device from Peripheral Nerve, Percutaneous Approach

01PY37Z Removal of Autologous Tissue Substitute from Peripheral Nerve, Percutaneous Approach

01PY3MZ Removal of Neurostimulator Lead from Peripheral Nerve, Percutaneous Approach

01PY3YZ Removal of Other Device from Peripheral Nerve, Percutaneous Approach

01PY40Z Removal of Drainage Device from Peripheral Nerve, Percutaneous Endoscopic Approach

01PY42Z Removal of Monitoring Device from Peripheral Nerve, Percutaneous Endoscopic Approach

01PY47Z Removal of Autologous Tissue Substitute from Peripheral Nerve, Percutaneous Endoscopic Approach

01PY4MZ Removal of Neurostimulator Lead from Peripheral Nerve, Percutaneous Endoscopic Approach

01PY4YZ Removal of Other Device from Peripheral Nerve, Percutaneous Endoscopic Approach

01PYX0Z Removal of Drainage Device from Peripheral Nerve, External Approach

01PYX2Z Removal of Monitoring Device from Peripheral Nerve, External Approach

01PYXMZ Removal of Neurostimulator Lead from Peripheral Nerve, External Approach

01Q – Peripheral Nervous System, Repair

01Q00ZZ Repair Cervical Plexus, Open Approach

01Q03ZZ Repair Cervical Plexus, Percutaneous Approach

01Q04ZZ Repair Cervical Plexus, Percutaneous Endoscopic Approach

01Q10ZZ Repair Cervical Nerve, Open Approach

01Q13ZZ Repair Cervical Nerve, Percutaneous Approach

01Q14ZZ Repair Cervical Nerve, Percutaneous Endoscopic Approach

01Q20ZZ Repair Phrenic Nerve, Open Approach

01Q23ZZ Repair Phrenic Nerve, Percutaneous Approach

01Q24ZZ Repair Phrenic Nerve, Percutaneous Endoscopic Approach

01Q30ZZ Repair Brachial Plexus, Open Approach

01Q33ZZ Repair Brachial Plexus, Percutaneous Approach

01Q34ZZ Repair Brachial Plexus, Percutaneous Endoscopic Approach

01Q40ZZ Repair Ulnar Nerve, Open Approach

01Q43ZZ Repair Ulnar Nerve, Percutaneous Approach

01Q44ZZ Repair Ulnar Nerve, Percutaneous Endoscopic Approach

01Q50ZZ Repair Median Nerve, Open Approach

01Q53ZZ Repair Median Nerve, Percutaneous Approach

01Q54ZZ Repair Median Nerve, Percutaneous Endoscopic Approach

♀ Female-only ♂ Male-only ▲ Limited Coverage ● Non-OR ▨ HAC-associated procedure ▲ Non-covered procedures ➕ Cluster

01Q60ZZ Repair Radial Nerve, Open Approach	01QD0ZZ Repair Femoral Nerve, Open Approach	01QL4ZZ Repair Thoracic Sympathetic Nerve, Percutaneous Endoscopic Approach
01Q63ZZ Repair Radial Nerve, Percutaneous Approach	01QD3ZZ Repair Femoral Nerve, Percutaneous Approach	01QM0ZZ Repair Abdominal Sympathetic Nerve, Open Approach
01Q64ZZ Repair Radial Nerve, Percutaneous Endoscopic Approach	01QD4ZZ Repair Femoral Nerve, Percutaneous Endoscopic Approach	01QM3ZZ Repair Abdominal Sympathetic Nerve, Percutaneous Approach
01Q80ZZ Repair Thoracic Nerve, Open Approach	01QF0ZZ Repair Sciatic Nerve, Open Approach	01QM4ZZ Repair Abdominal Sympathetic Nerve, Percutaneous Endoscopic Approach
01Q83ZZ Repair Thoracic Nerve, Percutaneous Approach	01QF3ZZ Repair Sciatic Nerve, Percutaneous Approach	01QN0ZZ Repair Lumbar Sympathetic Nerve, Open Approach
01Q84ZZ Repair Thoracic Nerve, Percutaneous Endoscopic Approach	01QF4ZZ Repair Sciatic Nerve, Percutaneous Endoscopic Approach	01QN3ZZ Repair Lumbar Sympathetic Nerve, Percutaneous Approach
01Q90ZZ Repair Lumbar Plexus, Open Approach	01QG0ZZ Repair Tibial Nerve, Open Approach	01QN4ZZ Repair Lumbar Sympathetic Nerve, Percutaneous Endoscopic Approach
01Q93ZZ Repair Lumbar Plexus, Percutaneous Approach	01QG3ZZ Repair Tibial Nerve, Percutaneous Approach	01QP0ZZ Repair Sacral Sympathetic Nerve, Open Approach
01Q94ZZ Repair Lumbar Plexus, Percutaneous Endoscopic Approach	01QG4ZZ Repair Tibial Nerve, Percutaneous Endoscopic Approach	01QP3ZZ Repair Sacral Sympathetic Nerve, Percutaneous Approach
01QA0ZZ Repair Lumbosacral Plexus, Open Approach	01QH0ZZ Repair Peroneal Nerve, Open Approach	01QP4ZZ Repair Sacral Sympathetic Nerve, Percutaneous Endoscopic Approach
01QA3ZZ Repair Lumbosacral Plexus, Percutaneous Approach	01QH3ZZ Repair Peroneal Nerve, Percutaneous Approach	01QQ0ZZ Repair Sacral Plexus, Open Approach
01QA4ZZ Repair Lumbosacral Plexus, Percutaneous Endoscopic Approach	01QH4ZZ Repair Peroneal Nerve, Percutaneous Endoscopic Approach	01QQ3ZZ Repair Sacral Plexus, Percutaneous Approach
01QB0ZZ Repair Lumbar Nerve, Open Approach	01QK0ZZ Repair Head and Neck Sympathetic Nerve, Open Approach	01QQ4ZZ Repair Sacral Plexus, Percutaneous Endoscopic Approach
01QB3ZZ Repair Lumbar Nerve, Percutaneous Approach	01QK3ZZ Repair Head and Neck Sympathetic Nerve, Percutaneous Approach	01QR0ZZ Repair Sacral Nerve, Open Approach
01QB4ZZ Repair Lumbar Nerve, Percutaneous Endoscopic Approach	01QK4ZZ Repair Head and Neck Sympathetic Nerve, Percutaneous Endoscopic Approach	01QR3ZZ Repair Sacral Nerve, Percutaneous Approach
01QC0ZZ Repair Pudendal Nerve, Open Approach	01QL0ZZ Repair Thoracic Sympathetic Nerve, Open Approach	01QR4ZZ Repair Sacral Nerve, Percutaneous Endoscopic Approach
01QC3ZZ Repair Pudendal Nerve, Percutaneous Approach	01QL3ZZ Repair Thoracic Sympathetic Nerve, Percutaneous Approach	
01QC4ZZ Repair Pudendal Nerve, Percutaneous Endoscopic Approach		

01R – Peripheral Nervous System, Replacement

Review Coding Guideline B3.18

01R107Z Replacement of Cervical Nerve with Autologous Tissue Substitute, Open Approach	01R40KZ Replacement of Ulnar Nerve with Nonautologous Tissue Substitute, Open Approach	01R64JZ Replacement of Radial Nerve with Synthetic Substitute, Percutaneous Endoscopic Approach
01R10JZ Replacement of Cervical Nerve with Synthetic Substitute, Open Approach	01R447Z Replacement of Ulnar Nerve with Autologous Tissue Substitute, Percutaneous Endoscopic Approach	01R64KZ Replacement of Radial Nerve with Nonautologous Tissue Substitute, Percutaneous Endoscopic Approach
01R10KZ Replacement of Cervical Nerve with Nonautologous Tissue Substitute, Open Approach	01R44JZ Replacement of Ulnar Nerve with Synthetic Substitute, Percutaneous Endoscopic Approach	01R807Z Replacement of Thoracic Nerve with Autologous Tissue Substitute, Open Approach
01R147Z Replacement of Cervical Nerve with Autologous Tissue Substitute, Percutaneous Endoscopic Approach	01R44KZ Replacement of Ulnar Nerve with Nonautologous Tissue Substitute, Percutaneous Endoscopic Approach	01R80JZ Replacement of Thoracic Nerve with Synthetic Substitute, Open Approach
01R14JZ Replacement of Cervical Nerve with Synthetic Substitute, Percutaneous Endoscopic Approach	01R507Z Replacement of Median Nerve with Autologous Tissue Substitute, Open Approach	01R80KZ Replacement of Thoracic Nerve with Nonautologous Tissue Substitute, Open Approach
01R14KZ Replacement of Cervical Nerve with Nonautologous Tissue Substitute, Percutaneous Endoscopic Approach	01R50JZ Replacement of Median Nerve with Synthetic Substitute, Open Approach	01R847Z Replacement of Thoracic Nerve with Autologous Tissue Substitute, Percutaneous Endoscopic Approach
01R207Z Replacement of Phrenic Nerve with Autologous Tissue Substitute, Open Approach	01R50KZ Replacement of Median Nerve with Nonautologous Tissue Substitute, Open Approach	01R84JZ Replacement of Thoracic Nerve with Synthetic Substitute, Percutaneous Endoscopic Approach
01R20JZ Replacement of Phrenic Nerve with Synthetic Substitute, Open Approach	01R547Z Replacement of Median Nerve with Autologous Tissue Substitute, Percutaneous Endoscopic Approach	01R84KZ Replacement of Thoracic Nerve with Nonautologous Tissue Substitute, Percutaneous Endoscopic Approach
01R20KZ Replacement of Phrenic Nerve with Nonautologous Tissue Substitute, Open Approach	01R54JZ Replacement of Median Nerve with Synthetic Substitute, Percutaneous Endoscopic Approach	01RB07Z Replacement of Lumbar Nerve with Autologous Tissue Substitute, Open Approach
01R247Z Replacement of Phrenic Nerve with Autologous Tissue Substitute, Percutaneous Endoscopic Approach	01R54KZ Replacement of Median Nerve with Nonautologous Tissue Substitute, Percutaneous Endoscopic Approach	01RB0JZ Replacement of Lumbar Nerve with Synthetic Substitute, Open Approach
01R24JZ Replacement of Phrenic Nerve with Synthetic Substitute, Percutaneous Endoscopic Approach	01R607Z Replacement of Radial Nerve with Autologous Tissue Substitute, Open Approach	01RB0KZ Replacement of Lumbar Nerve with Nonautologous Tissue Substitute, Open Approach
01R24KZ Replacement of Phrenic Nerve with Nonautologous Tissue Substitute, Percutaneous Endoscopic Approach	01R60JZ Replacement of Radial Nerve with Synthetic Substitute, Open Approach	01RB47Z Replacement of Lumbar Nerve with Autologous Tissue Substitute, Percutaneous Endoscopic Approach
01R407Z Replacement of Ulnar Nerve with Autologous Tissue Substitute, Open Approach	01R60KZ Replacement of Radial Nerve with Nonautologous Tissue Substitute, Open Approach	01RB4JZ Replacement of Lumbar Nerve with Synthetic Substitute, Percutaneous Endoscopic Approach
01R40JZ Replacement of Ulnar Nerve with Synthetic Substitute, Open Approach	01R647Z Replacement of Radial Nerve with Autologous Tissue Substitute, Percutaneous Endoscopic Approach	01RB4KZ Replacement of Lumbar Nerve with Nonautologous Tissue Substitute, Percutaneous Endoscopic Approach

♀ Female-only   ♂ Male-only   ▲ Limited Coverage   ● Non-OR   HAC HAC-associated procedure   ▲ Non-covered procedures   ✚ Cluster

01RC07Z Replacement of Pudendal Nerve with Autologous Tissue Substitute, Open Approach

01RC0JZ Replacement of Pudendal Nerve with Synthetic Substitute, Open Approach

01RC0KZ Replacement of Pudendal Nerve with Nonautologous Tissue Substitute, Open Approach

01RC47Z Replacement of Pudendal Nerve with Autologous Tissue Substitute, Percutaneous Endoscopic Approach

01RC4JZ Replacement of Pudendal Nerve with Synthetic Substitute, Percutaneous Endoscopic Approach

01RC4KZ Replacement of Pudendal Nerve with Nonautologous Tissue Substitute, Percutaneous Endoscopic Approach

01RD07Z Replacement of Femoral Nerve with Autologous Tissue Substitute, Open Approach

01RD0JZ Replacement of Femoral Nerve with Synthetic Substitute, Open Approach

01RD0KZ Replacement of Femoral Nerve with Nonautologous Tissue Substitute, Open Approach

01RD47Z Replacement of Femoral Nerve with Autologous Tissue Substitute, Percutaneous Endoscopic Approach

01RD4JZ Replacement of Femoral Nerve with Synthetic Substitute, Percutaneous Endoscopic Approach

01RD4KZ Replacement of Femoral Nerve with Nonautologous Tissue Substitute, Percutaneous Endoscopic Approach

01RF07Z Replacement of Sciatic Nerve with Autologous Tissue Substitute, Open Approach

01RF0JZ Replacement of Sciatic Nerve with Synthetic Substitute, Open Approach

01RF0KZ Replacement of Sciatic Nerve with Nonautologous Tissue Substitute, Open Approach

01RF47Z Replacement of Sciatic Nerve with Autologous Tissue Substitute, Percutaneous Endoscopic Approach

01RF4JZ Replacement of Sciatic Nerve with Synthetic Substitute, Percutaneous Endoscopic Approach

01RF4KZ Replacement of Sciatic Nerve with Nonautologous Tissue Substitute, Percutaneous Endoscopic Approach

01RG07Z Replacement of Tibial Nerve with Autologous Tissue Substitute, Open Approach

01RG0JZ Replacement of Tibial Nerve with Synthetic Substitute, Open Approach

01RG0KZ Replacement of Tibial Nerve with Nonautologous Tissue Substitute, Open Approach

01RG47Z Replacement of Tibial Nerve with Autologous Tissue Substitute, Percutaneous Endoscopic Approach

01RG4JZ Replacement of Tibial Nerve with Synthetic Substitute, Percutaneous Endoscopic Approach

01RG4KZ Replacement of Tibial Nerve with Nonautologous Tissue Substitute, Percutaneous Endoscopic Approach

01RH07Z Replacement of Peroneal Nerve with Autologous Tissue Substitute, Open Approach

01RH0JZ Replacement of Peroneal Nerve with Synthetic Substitute, Open Approach

01RH0KZ Replacement of Peroneal Nerve with Nonautologous Tissue Substitute, Open Approach

01RH47Z Replacement of Peroneal Nerve with Autologous Tissue Substitute, Percutaneous Endoscopic Approach

01RH4JZ Replacement of Peroneal Nerve with Synthetic Substitute, Percutaneous Endoscopic Approach

01RH4KZ Replacement of Peroneal Nerve with Nonautologous Tissue Substitute, Percutaneous Endoscopic Approach

01RR07Z Replacement of Sacral Nerve with Autologous Tissue Substitute, Open Approach

01RR0JZ Replacement of Sacral Nerve with Synthetic Substitute, Open Approach

01RR0KZ Replacement of Sacral Nerve with Nonautologous Tissue Substitute, Open Approach

01RR47Z Replacement of Sacral Nerve with Autologous Tissue Substitute, Percutaneous Endoscopic Approach

01RR4JZ Replacement of Sacral Nerve with Synthetic Substitute, Percutaneous Endoscopic Approach

01RR4KZ Replacement of Sacral Nerve with Nonautologous Tissue Substitute, Percutaneous Endoscopic Approach

01S – Peripheral Nervous System, Reposition

01S00ZZ Reposition Cervical Plexus, Open Approach

01S03ZZ Reposition Cervical Plexus, Percutaneous Approach

01S04ZZ Reposition Cervical Plexus, Percutaneous Endoscopic Approach

01S10ZZ Reposition Cervical Nerve, Open Approach

01S13ZZ Reposition Cervical Nerve, Percutaneous Approach

01S14ZZ Reposition Cervical Nerve, Percutaneous Endoscopic Approach

01S20ZZ Reposition Phrenic Nerve, Open Approach

01S23ZZ Reposition Phrenic Nerve, Percutaneous Approach

01S24ZZ Reposition Phrenic Nerve, Percutaneous Endoscopic Approach

01S30ZZ Reposition Brachial Plexus, Open Approach

01S33ZZ Reposition Brachial Plexus, Percutaneous Approach

01S34ZZ Reposition Brachial Plexus, Percutaneous Endoscopic Approach

01S40ZZ Reposition Ulnar Nerve, Open Approach

01S43ZZ Reposition Ulnar Nerve, Percutaneous Approach

01S44ZZ Reposition Ulnar Nerve, Percutaneous Endoscopic Approach

01S50ZZ Reposition Median Nerve, Open Approach

01S53ZZ Reposition Median Nerve, Percutaneous Approach

01S54ZZ Reposition Median Nerve, Percutaneous Endoscopic Approach

01S60ZZ Reposition Radial Nerve, Open Approach

01S63ZZ Reposition Radial Nerve, Percutaneous Approach

01S64ZZ Reposition Radial Nerve, Percutaneous Endoscopic Approach

01S80ZZ Reposition Thoracic Nerve, Open Approach

01S83ZZ Reposition Thoracic Nerve, Percutaneous Approach

01S84ZZ Reposition Thoracic Nerve, Percutaneous Endoscopic Approach

01S90ZZ Reposition Lumbar Plexus, Open Approach

01S93ZZ Reposition Lumbar Plexus, Percutaneous Approach

01S94ZZ Reposition Lumbar Plexus, Percutaneous Endoscopic Approach

01SA0ZZ Reposition Lumbosacral Plexus, Open Approach

01SA3ZZ Reposition Lumbosacral Plexus, Percutaneous Approach

01SA4ZZ Reposition Lumbosacral Plexus, Percutaneous Endoscopic Approach

01SB0ZZ Reposition Lumbar Nerve, Open Approach

01SB3ZZ Reposition Lumbar Nerve, Percutaneous Approach

01SB4ZZ Reposition Lumbar Nerve, Percutaneous Endoscopic Approach

01SC0ZZ Reposition Pudendal Nerve, Open Approach

01SC3ZZ Reposition Pudendal Nerve, Percutaneous Approach

01SC4ZZ Reposition Pudendal Nerve, Percutaneous Endoscopic Approach

01SD0ZZ Reposition Femoral Nerve, Open Approach

01SD3ZZ Reposition Femoral Nerve, Percutaneous Approach

01SD4ZZ Reposition Femoral Nerve, Percutaneous Endoscopic Approach

01SF0ZZ Reposition Sciatic Nerve, Open Approach

01SF3ZZ Reposition Sciatic Nerve, Percutaneous Approach

01SF4ZZ Reposition Sciatic Nerve, Percutaneous Endoscopic Approach

01SG0ZZ Reposition Tibial Nerve, Open Approach

01SG3ZZ Reposition Tibial Nerve, Percutaneous Approach

01SG4ZZ Reposition Tibial Nerve, Percutaneous Endoscopic Approach

01SH0ZZ Reposition Peroneal Nerve, Open Approach

01SH3ZZ Reposition Peroneal Nerve, Percutaneous Approach

01SH4ZZ Reposition Peroneal Nerve, Percutaneous Endoscopic Approach

01SQ0ZZ Reposition Sacral Plexus, Open Approach

01SQ3ZZ Reposition Sacral Plexus, Percutaneous Approach

01SQ4ZZ Reposition Sacral Plexus, Percutaneous Endoscopic Approach

01SR0ZZ Reposition Sacral Nerve, Open Approach

01SR3ZZ Reposition Sacral Nerve, Percutaneous Approach

01SR4ZZ Reposition Sacral Nerve, Percutaneous Endoscopic Approach

01U107Z Supplement Cervical Nerve with Autologous Tissue Substitute, Open Approach

01U10JZ Supplement Cervical Nerve with Synthetic Substitute, Open Approach

01U10KZ Supplement Cervical Nerve with Nonautologous Tissue Substitute, Open Approach

01U137Z Supplement Cervical Nerve with Autologous Tissue Substitute, Percutaneous Approach

01U13JZ Supplement Cervical Nerve with Synthetic Substitute, Percutaneous Approach

01U13KZ Supplement Cervical Nerve with Nonautologous Tissue Substitute, Percutaneous Approach

01U147Z Supplement Cervical Nerve with Autologous Tissue Substitute, Percutaneous Endoscopic Approach

01U14JZ Supplement Cervical Nerve with Synthetic Substitute, Percutaneous Endoscopic Approach

01U14KZ Supplement Cervical Nerve with Nonautologous Tissue Substitute, Percutaneous Endoscopic Approach

01U207Z Supplement Phrenic Nerve with Autologous Tissue Substitute, Open Approach

01U20JZ Supplement Phrenic Nerve with Synthetic Substitute, Open Approach

01U20KZ Supplement Phrenic Nerve with Nonautologous Tissue Substitute, Open Approach

01U237Z Supplement Phrenic Nerve with Autologous Tissue Substitute, Percutaneous Approach

01U23JZ Supplement Phrenic Nerve with Synthetic Substitute, Percutaneous Approach

01U23KZ Supplement Phrenic Nerve with Nonautologous Tissue Substitute, Percutaneous Approach

01U247Z Supplement Phrenic Nerve with Autologous Tissue Substitute, Percutaneous Endoscopic Approach

01U24JZ Supplement Phrenic Nerve with Synthetic Substitute, Percutaneous Endoscopic Approach

01U24KZ Supplement Phrenic Nerve with Nonautologous Tissue Substitute, Percutaneous Endoscopic Approach

01U407Z Supplement Ulnar Nerve with Autologous Tissue Substitute, Open Approach

01U40JZ Supplement Ulnar Nerve with Synthetic Substitute, Open Approach

01U40KZ Supplement Ulnar Nerve with Nonautologous Tissue Substitute, Open Approach

01U437Z Supplement Ulnar Nerve with Autologous Tissue Substitute, Percutaneous Approach

01U43JZ Supplement Ulnar Nerve with Synthetic Substitute, Percutaneous Approach

01U43KZ Supplement Ulnar Nerve with Nonautologous Tissue Substitute, Percutaneous Approach

01U447Z Supplement Ulnar Nerve with Autologous Tissue Substitute, Percutaneous Endoscopic Approach

01U44JZ Supplement Ulnar Nerve with Synthetic Substitute, Percutaneous Endoscopic Approach

01U44KZ Supplement Ulnar Nerve with Nonautologous Tissue Substitute, Percutaneous Endoscopic Approach

01U507Z Supplement Median Nerve with Autologous Tissue Substitute, Open Approach

01U50JZ Supplement Median Nerve with Synthetic Substitute, Open Approach

01U50KZ Supplement Median Nerve with Nonautologous Tissue Substitute, Open Approach

AHA CC: 4Q, 2017, 62

01U537Z Supplement Median Nerve with Autologous Tissue Substitute, Percutaneous Approach

01U53JZ Supplement Median Nerve with Synthetic Substitute, Percutaneous Approach

01U53KZ Supplement Median Nerve with Nonautologous Tissue Substitute, Percutaneous Approach

01U547Z Supplement Median Nerve with Autologous Tissue Substitute, Percutaneous Endoscopic Approach

01U54JZ Supplement Median Nerve with Synthetic Substitute, Percutaneous Endoscopic Approach

01U54KZ Supplement Median Nerve with Nonautologous Tissue Substitute, Percutaneous Endoscopic Approach

01U607Z Supplement Radial Nerve with Autologous Tissue Substitute, Open Approach

01U60JZ Supplement Radial Nerve with Synthetic Substitute, Open Approach

01U60KZ Supplement Radial Nerve with Nonautologous Tissue Substitute, Open Approach

01U637Z Supplement Radial Nerve with Autologous Tissue Substitute, Percutaneous Approach

01U63JZ Supplement Radial Nerve with Synthetic Substitute, Percutaneous Approach

01U63KZ Supplement Radial Nerve with Nonautologous Tissue Substitute, Percutaneous Approach

01U647Z Supplement Radial Nerve with Autologous Tissue Substitute, Percutaneous Endoscopic Approach

01U64JZ Supplement Radial Nerve with Synthetic Substitute, Percutaneous Endoscopic Approach

01U64KZ Supplement Radial Nerve with Nonautologous Tissue Substitute, Percutaneous Endoscopic Approach

01U807Z Supplement Thoracic Nerve with Autologous Tissue Substitute, Open Approach

01U80JZ Supplement Thoracic Nerve with Synthetic Substitute, Open Approach

01U80KZ Supplement Thoracic Nerve with Nonautologous Tissue Substitute, Open Approach

AHA CC: 3Q, 2019, 32-33

01U837Z Supplement Thoracic Nerve with Autologous Tissue Substitute, Percutaneous Approach

01U83JZ Supplement Thoracic Nerve with Synthetic Substitute, Percutaneous Approach

01U83KZ Supplement Thoracic Nerve with Nonautologous Tissue Substitute, Percutaneous Approach

01U847Z Supplement Thoracic Nerve with Autologous Tissue Substitute, Percutaneous Endoscopic Approach

01U84JZ Supplement Thoracic Nerve with Synthetic Substitute, Percutaneous Endoscopic Approach

01U84KZ Supplement Thoracic Nerve with Nonautologous Tissue Substitute, Percutaneous Endoscopic Approach

01UB07Z Supplement Lumbar Nerve with Autologous Tissue Substitute, Open Approach

01UB0JZ Supplement Lumbar Nerve with Synthetic Substitute, Open Approach

01UB0KZ Supplement Lumbar Nerve with Nonautologous Tissue Substitute, Open Approach

01UB37Z Supplement Lumbar Nerve with Autologous Tissue Substitute, Percutaneous Approach

01UB3JZ Supplement Lumbar Nerve with Synthetic Substitute, Percutaneous Approach

01UB3KZ Supplement Lumbar Nerve with Nonautologous Tissue Substitute, Percutaneous Approach

01UB47Z Supplement Lumbar Nerve with Autologous Tissue Substitute, Percutaneous Endoscopic Approach

01UB4JZ Supplement Lumbar Nerve with Synthetic Substitute, Percutaneous Endoscopic Approach

01UB4KZ Supplement Lumbar Nerve with Nonautologous Tissue Substitute, Percutaneous Endoscopic Approach

01UC07Z Supplement Pudendal Nerve with Autologous Tissue Substitute, Open Approach

01UC0JZ Supplement Pudendal Nerve with Synthetic Substitute, Open Approach

01UC0KZ Supplement Pudendal Nerve with Nonautologous Tissue Substitute, Open Approach

01UC37Z Supplement Pudendal Nerve with Autologous Tissue Substitute, Percutaneous Approach

01UC3JZ Supplement Pudendal Nerve with Synthetic Substitute, Percutaneous Approach

01UC3KZ Supplement Pudendal Nerve with Nonautologous Tissue Substitute, Percutaneous Approach

01UC47Z Supplement Pudendal Nerve with Autologous Tissue Substitute, Percutaneous Endoscopic Approach

01UC4JZ Supplement Pudendal Nerve with Synthetic Substitute, Percutaneous Endoscopic Approach

01UC4KZ Supplement Pudendal Nerve with Nonautologous Tissue Substitute, Percutaneous Endoscopic Approach

01UD07Z Supplement Femoral Nerve with Autologous Tissue Substitute, Open Approach

01UD0JZ Supplement Femoral Nerve with Synthetic Substitute, Open Approach

01UD0KZ Supplement Femoral Nerve with Nonautologous Tissue Substitute, Open Approach

♀ Female-only   ♂ Male-only   ▲ Limited Coverage   ● Non-OR   ▦ HAC-associated procedure   ▲ Non-covered procedures   ✚ Cluster

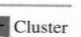

01UD37Z	Supplement Femoral Nerve with Autologous Tissue Substitute, Percutaneous Approach
01UD3JZ	Supplement Femoral Nerve with Synthetic Substitute, Percutaneous Approach
01UD3KZ	Supplement Femoral Nerve with Nonautologous Tissue Substitute, Percutaneous Approach
01UD47Z	Supplement Femoral Nerve with Autologous Tissue Substitute, Percutaneous Endoscopic Approach
01UD4JZ	Supplement Femoral Nerve with Synthetic Substitute, Percutaneous Endoscopic Approach
01UD4KZ	Supplement Femoral Nerve with Nonautologous Tissue Substitute, Percutaneous Endoscopic Approach
01UF07Z	Supplement Sciatic Nerve with Autologous Tissue Substitute, Open Approach
01UF0JZ	Supplement Sciatic Nerve with Synthetic Substitute, Open Approach
01UF0KZ	Supplement Sciatic Nerve with Nonautologous Tissue Substitute, Open Approach
01UF37Z	Supplement Sciatic Nerve with Autologous Tissue Substitute, Percutaneous Approach
01UF3JZ	Supplement Sciatic Nerve with Synthetic Substitute, Percutaneous Approach
01UF3KZ	Supplement Sciatic Nerve with Nonautologous Tissue Substitute, Percutaneous Approach
01UF47Z	Supplement Sciatic Nerve with Autologous Tissue Substitute, Percutaneous Endoscopic Approach
01UF4JZ	Supplement Sciatic Nerve with Synthetic Substitute, Percutaneous Endoscopic Approach
01UF4KZ	Supplement Sciatic Nerve with Nonautologous Tissue Substitute, Percutaneous Endoscopic Approach
01UG07Z	Supplement Tibial Nerve with Autologous Tissue Substitute, Open Approach
01UG0JZ	Supplement Tibial Nerve with Synthetic Substitute, Open Approach
01UG0KZ	Supplement Tibial Nerve with Nonautologous Tissue Substitute, Open Approach
01UG37Z	Supplement Tibial Nerve with Autologous Tissue Substitute, Percutaneous Approach
01UG3JZ	Supplement Tibial Nerve with Synthetic Substitute, Percutaneous Approach
01UG3KZ	Supplement Tibial Nerve with Nonautologous Tissue Substitute, Percutaneous Approach
01UG47Z	Supplement Tibial Nerve with Autologous Tissue Substitute, Percutaneous Endoscopic Approach
01UG4JZ	Supplement Tibial Nerve with Synthetic Substitute, Percutaneous Endoscopic Approach
01UG4KZ	Supplement Tibial Nerve with Nonautologous Tissue Substitute, Percutaneous Endoscopic Approach
01UH07Z	Supplement Peroneal Nerve with Autologous Tissue Substitute, Open Approach
01UH0JZ	Supplement Peroneal Nerve with Synthetic Substitute, Open Approach
01UH0KZ	Supplement Peroneal Nerve with Nonautologous Tissue Substitute, Open Approach
01UH37Z	Supplement Peroneal Nerve with Autologous Tissue Substitute, Percutaneous Approach
01UH3JZ	Supplement Peroneal Nerve with Synthetic Substitute, Percutaneous Approach
01UH3KZ	Supplement Peroneal Nerve with Nonautologous Tissue Substitute, Percutaneous Approach
01UH47Z	Supplement Peroneal Nerve with Autologous Tissue Substitute, Percutaneous Endoscopic Approach
01UH4JZ	Supplement Peroneal Nerve with Synthetic Substitute, Percutaneous Endoscopic Approach
01UH4KZ	Supplement Peroneal Nerve with Nonautologous Tissue Substitute, Percutaneous Endoscopic Approach
01UR07Z	Supplement Sacral Nerve with Autologous Tissue Substitute, Open Approach
01UR0JZ	Supplement Sacral Nerve with Synthetic Substitute, Open Approach
01UR0KZ	Supplement Sacral Nerve with Nonautologous Tissue Substitute, Open Approach
01UR37Z	Supplement Sacral Nerve with Autologous Tissue Substitute, Percutaneous Approach
01UR3JZ	Supplement Sacral Nerve with Synthetic Substitute, Percutaneous Approach
01UR3KZ	Supplement Sacral Nerve with Nonautologous Tissue Substitute, Percutaneous Approach
01UR47Z	Supplement Sacral Nerve with Autologous Tissue Substitute, Percutaneous Endoscopic Approach
01UR4JZ	Supplement Sacral Nerve with Synthetic Substitute, Percutaneous Endoscopic Approach
01UR4KZ	Supplement Sacral Nerve with Nonautologous Tissue Substitute, Percutaneous Endoscopic Approach

01W – Peripheral Nervous System, Revision

Review Coding Guideline B6.1c

01WY00Z	Revision of Drainage Device in Peripheral Nerve, Open Approach
01WY02Z	Revision of Monitoring Device in Peripheral Nerve, Open Approach
01WY07Z	Revision of Autologous Tissue Substitute in Peripheral Nerve, Open Approach
01WY0MZ	Revision of Neurostimulator Lead in Peripheral Nerve, Open Approach
01WY0YZ	Revision of Other Device in Peripheral Nerve, Open Approach
01WY30Z	Revision of Drainage Device in Peripheral Nerve, Percutaneous Approach
01WY32Z	Revision of Monitoring Device in Peripheral Nerve, Percutaneous Approach
01WY37Z	Revision of Autologous Tissue Substitute in Peripheral Nerve, Percutaneous Approach
01WY3MZ	Revision of Neurostimulator Lead in Peripheral Nerve, Percutaneous Approach
01WY3YZ	Revision of Other Device in Peripheral Nerve, Percutaneous Approach
01WY40Z	Revision of Drainage Device in Peripheral Nerve, Percutaneous Endoscopic Approach
01WY42Z	Revision of Monitoring Device in Peripheral Nerve, Percutaneous Endoscopic Approach
01WY47Z	Revision of Autologous Tissue Substitute in Peripheral Nerve, Percutaneous Endoscopic Approach
01WY4MZ	Revision of Neurostimulator Lead in Peripheral Nerve, Percutaneous Endoscopic Approach
01WY4YZ	Revision of Other Device in Peripheral Nerve, Percutaneous Endoscopic Approach
01WYX0Z	Revision of Drainage Device in Peripheral Nerve, External Approach
01WYX2Z	Revision of Monitoring Device in Peripheral Nerve, External Approach
01WYX7Z	Revision of Autologous Tissue Substitute in Peripheral Nerve, External Approach
01WYXMZ	Revision of Neurostimulator Lead in Peripheral Nerve, External Approach

01X – Peripheral Nervous System, Transfer

01X10Z1	Transfer Cervical Nerve to Cervical Nerve, Open Approach
01X10Z2	Transfer Cervical Nerve to Phrenic Nerve, Open Approach
01X14Z1	Transfer Cervical Nerve to Cervical Nerve, Percutaneous Endoscopic Approach
01X14Z2	Transfer Cervical Nerve to Phrenic Nerve, Percutaneous Endoscopic Approach
01X20Z1	Transfer Phrenic Nerve to Cervical Nerve, Open Approach
01X20Z2	Transfer Phrenic Nerve to Phrenic Nerve, Open Approach
01X24Z1	Transfer Phrenic Nerve to Cervical Nerve, Percutaneous Endoscopic Approach
01X24Z2	Transfer Phrenic Nerve to Phrenic Nerve, Percutaneous Endoscopic Approach
01X40Z4	Transfer Ulnar Nerve to Ulnar Nerve, Open Approach
01X40Z5	Transfer Ulnar Nerve to Median Nerve, Open Approach
01X40Z6	Transfer Ulnar Nerve to Radial Nerve, Open Approach
01X44Z4	Transfer Ulnar Nerve to Ulnar Nerve, Percutaneous Endoscopic Approach
01X44Z5	Transfer Ulnar Nerve to Median Nerve, Percutaneous Endoscopic Approach

01X44Z6	Transfer Ulnar Nerve to Radial Nerve, Percutaneous Endoscopic Approach
01X50Z4	Transfer Median Nerve to Ulnar Nerve, Open Approach
01X50Z5	Transfer Median Nerve to Median Nerve, Open Approach
01X50Z6	Transfer Median Nerve to Radial Nerve, Open Approach
01X54Z4	Transfer Median Nerve to Ulnar Nerve, Percutaneous Endoscopic Approach
01X54Z5	Transfer Median Nerve to Median Nerve, Percutaneous Endoscopic Approach
01X54Z6	Transfer Median Nerve to Radial Nerve, Percutaneous Endoscopic Approach
01X60Z4	Transfer Radial Nerve to Ulnar Nerve, Open Approach
01X60Z5	Transfer Radial Nerve to Median Nerve, Open Approach
01X60Z6	Transfer Radial Nerve to Radial Nerve, Open Approach
01X64Z4	Transfer Radial Nerve to Ulnar Nerve, Percutaneous Endoscopic Approach
01X64Z5	Transfer Radial Nerve to Median Nerve, Percutaneous Endoscopic Approach
01X64Z6	Transfer Radial Nerve to Radial Nerve, Percutaneous Endoscopic Approach
01X80Z8	Transfer Thoracic Nerve to Thoracic Nerve, Open Approach
01X84Z8	Transfer Thoracic Nerve to Thoracic Nerve, Percutaneous Endoscopic Approach
01XB0ZB	Transfer Lumbar Nerve to Lumbar Nerve, Open Approach
01XB0ZC	Transfer Lumbar Nerve to Perineal Nerve, Open Approach
01XB4ZB	Transfer Lumbar Nerve to Lumbar Nerve, Percutaneous Endoscopic Approach
01XB4ZC	Transfer Lumbar Nerve to Perineal Nerve, Percutaneous Endoscopic Approach

01XC0ZB	Transfer Pudendal Nerve to Lumbar Nerve, Open Approach
01XC0ZC	Transfer Pudendal Nerve to Perineal Nerve, Open Approach
01XC4ZB	Transfer Pudendal Nerve to Lumbar Nerve, Percutaneous Endoscopic Approach
01XC4ZC	Transfer Pudendal Nerve to Perineal Nerve, Percutaneous Endoscopic Approach
01XD0ZD	Transfer Femoral Nerve to Femoral Nerve, Open Approach
01XD0ZF	Transfer Femoral Nerve to Sciatic Nerve, Open Approach
01XD0ZG	Transfer Femoral Nerve to Tibial Nerve, Open Approach
01XD0ZH	Transfer Femoral Nerve to Peroneal Nerve, Open Approach
01XD4ZD	Transfer Femoral Nerve to Femoral Nerve, Percutaneous Endoscopic Approach
01XD4ZF	Transfer Femoral Nerve to Sciatic Nerve, Percutaneous Endoscopic Approach
01XD4ZG	Transfer Femoral Nerve to Tibial Nerve, Percutaneous Endoscopic Approach
01XD4ZH	Transfer Femoral Nerve to Peroneal Nerve, Percutaneous Endoscopic Approach
01XF0ZD	Transfer Sciatic Nerve to Femoral Nerve, Open Approach
01XF0ZF	Transfer Sciatic Nerve to Sciatic Nerve, Open Approach
01XF0ZG	Transfer Sciatic Nerve to Tibial Nerve, Open Approach
01XF0ZH	Transfer Sciatic Nerve to Peroneal Nerve, Open Approach
01XF4ZD	Transfer Sciatic Nerve to Femoral Nerve, Percutaneous Endoscopic Approach
01XF4ZF	Transfer Sciatic Nerve to Sciatic Nerve, Percutaneous Endoscopic Approach

01XF4ZG	Transfer Sciatic Nerve to Tibial Nerve, Percutaneous Endoscopic Approach
01XF4ZH	Transfer Sciatic Nerve to Peroneal Nerve, Percutaneous Endoscopic Approach
01XG0ZD	Transfer Tibial Nerve to Femoral Nerve, Open Approach
01XG0ZF	Transfer Tibial Nerve to Sciatic Nerve, Open Approach
01XG0ZG	Transfer Tibial Nerve to Tibial Nerve, Open Approach
01XG0ZH	Transfer Tibial Nerve to Peroneal Nerve, Open Approach
01XG4ZD	Transfer Tibial Nerve to Femoral Nerve, Percutaneous Endoscopic Approach
01XG4ZF	Transfer Tibial Nerve to Sciatic Nerve, Percutaneous Endoscopic Approach
01XG4ZG	Transfer Tibial Nerve to Tibial Nerve, Percutaneous Endoscopic Approach
01XG4ZH	Transfer Tibial Nerve to Peroneal Nerve, Percutaneous Endoscopic Approach
01XH0ZD	Transfer Peroneal Nerve to Femoral Nerve, Open Approach
01XH0ZF	Transfer Peroneal Nerve to Sciatic Nerve, Open Approach
01XH0ZG	Transfer Peroneal Nerve to Tibial Nerve, Open Approach
01XH0ZH	Transfer Peroneal Nerve to Peroneal Nerve, Open Approach
01XH4ZD	Transfer Peroneal Nerve to Femoral Nerve, Percutaneous Endoscopic Approach
01XH4ZF	Transfer Peroneal Nerve to Sciatic Nerve, Percutaneous Endoscopic Approach
01XH4ZG	Transfer Peroneal Nerve to Tibial Nerve, Percutaneous Endoscopic Approach
01XH4ZH	Transfer Peroneal Nerve to Peroneal Nerve, Percutaneous Endoscopic Approach

♀ Female-only   ♂ Male-only   ▲ Limited Coverage   ● Non-OR   ⬛ HAC-associated procedure   ▲ Non-covered procedures   ✚ Cluster

Atria, Ventricles and Interventricular Septum

Mitral valve { Posterior cusp
Anterior cusp

Right superior pulmonary vein

Aortic sinus (of Valsalva)

Ascending aorta

Aortic valve { Left semilunar cusp
Posterior semilunar (non-coronary) cusp

Superior vena cava

Membranous septum { Atrioventricular part
Interventricular part

Pulmonary trunk

Anterior cusp of mitral valve

Left atrium

Left auricle (atrial appendage)

Left pulmonary veins

Openings of coronary arteries

Ascending aorta

Right auricle (atrial appendage)

Aortic valve { Left semilunar cusp
Right semilunar cusp

Supraventricular crest

Outflow to pulmonary trunk

Conus arteriosus

Right anterior papillary muscle (cut)

Right ventricle

Right atrium

Tricuspid valve { Anterior cusp (retracted)
Septal cusp
Posterior cusp

Right ventricle

Right anterior papillary muscle (cut)

Right posterior papillary muscle

Muscular part of interventricular septum

Left ventricle

Left posterior papillary muscle

Left anterior papillary muscle

Left ventricle

Septomarginal trabecula (moderator band)

Septal (medial) papillary muscle

Plane of section

F. Netter m.d.

Arteries and Veins of the Heart; Arteries and Cardiac Veins

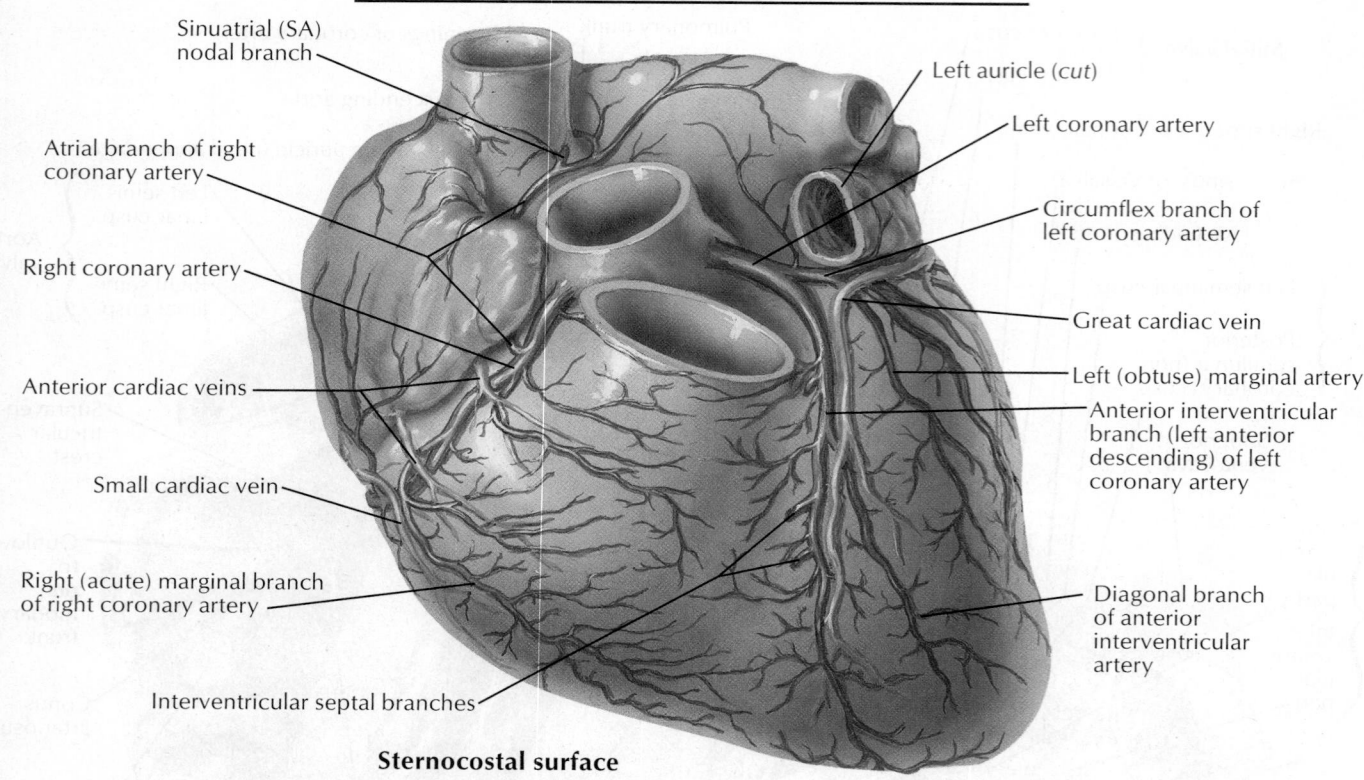

Sinuatrial (SA) nodal branch

Atrial branch of right coronary artery

Right coronary artery

Anterior cardiac veins

Small cardiac vein

Right (acute) marginal branch of right coronary artery

Interventricular septal branches

Left auricle (*cut*)

Left coronary artery

Circumflex branch of left coronary artery

Great cardiac vein

Left (obtuse) marginal artery

Anterior interventricular branch (left anterior descending) of left coronary artery

Diagonal branch of anterior interventricular artery

Sternocostal surface

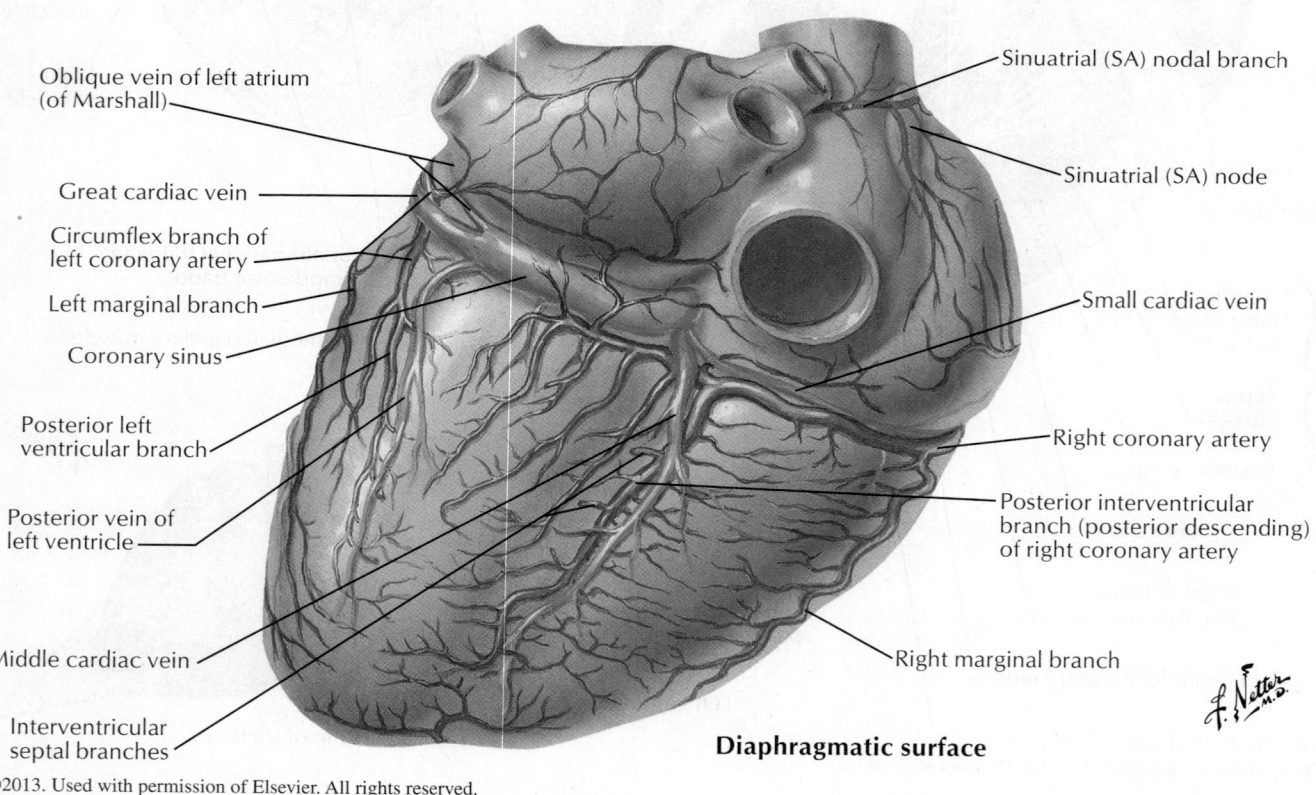

Oblique vein of left atrium (of Marshall)

Great cardiac vein

Circumflex branch of left coronary artery

Left marginal branch

Coronary sinus

Posterior left ventricular branch

Posterior vein of left ventricle

Middle cardiac vein

Interventricular septal branches

Sinuatrial (SA) nodal branch

Sinuatrial (SA) node

Small cardiac vein

Right coronary artery

Posterior interventricular branch (posterior descending) of right coronary artery

Right marginal branch

Diaphragmatic surface

Right Coronary Artery – Segmental Replacement

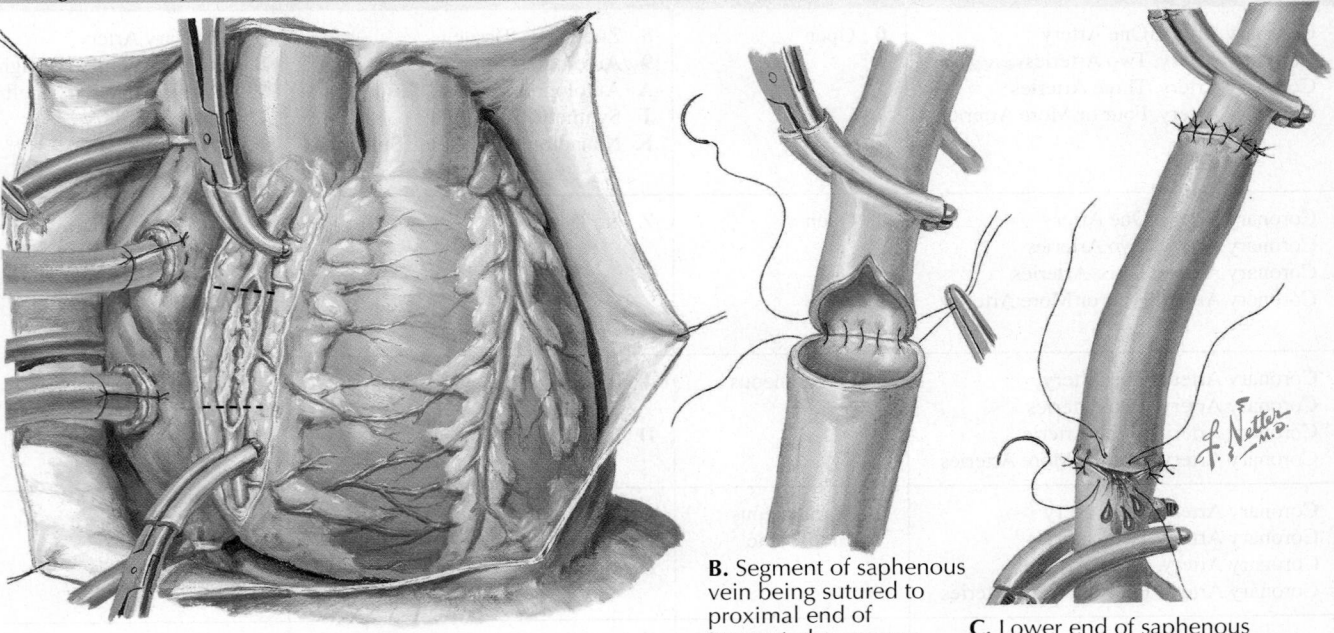

A. Diseased segment of right coronary artery widely exposed, clamped, and incised; portion between broken lines to be excised

B. Segment of saphenous vein being sutured to proximal end of transected coronary artery

C. Lower end of saphenous graft sutured to distal portion of artery; blood and air allowed to escape by loosening distal clamp prior to final closure

Right coronary-artery bypass

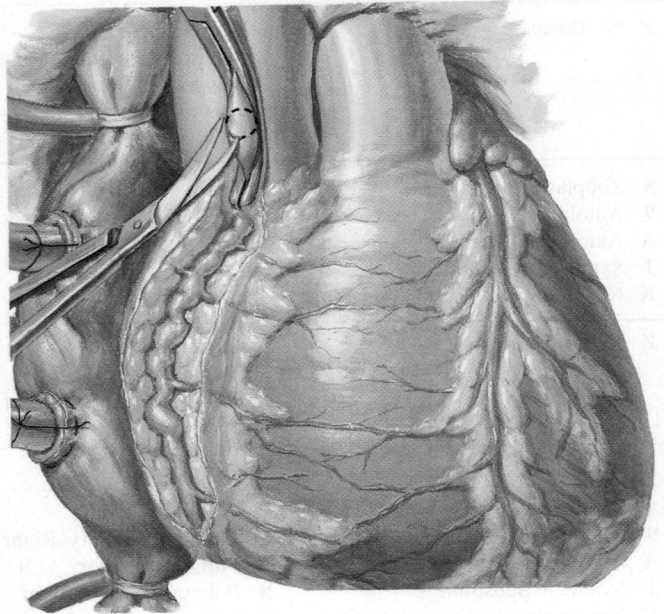

A'. Small area of aorta longitudinally isolated by clamp above right coronary orifice, and ostium created therein

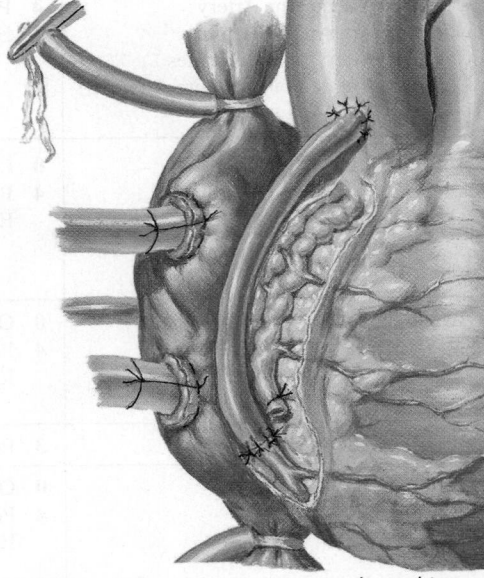

B'. Segment of saphenous vein implanted into new aortic ostium and anastomosed to end of divided right coronary artery distal to diseased area; proximal end of artery ligated

Medical and Surgical, Heart and Great Vessels

Heart and Great Vessels Tables 021–02Y

Section	0	Medical and Surgical
Body System	2	Heart and Great Vessels
Operation	1	**Bypass:** Altering the route of passage of the contents of a tubular body part

Body Part (4ᵗʰ)	Approach (5ᵗʰ)	Device (6ᵗʰ)	Qualifier (7ᵗʰ)
0 Coronary Artery, One Artery 1 Coronary Artery, Two Arteries 2 Coronary Artery, Three Arteries 3 Coronary Artery, Four or More Arteries	0 Open	8 Zooplastic Tissue 9 Autologous Venous Tissue A Autologous Arterial Tissue J Synthetic Substitute K Nonautologous Tissue Substitute	3 Coronary Artery 8 Internal Mammary, Right 9 Internal Mammary, Left C Thoracic Artery F Abdominal Artery W Aorta
0 Coronary Artery, One Artery 1 Coronary Artery, Two Arteries 2 Coronary Artery, Three Arteries 3 Coronary Artery, Four or More Arteries	0 Open	Z No Device	3 Coronary Artery 8 Internal Mammary, Right 9 Internal Mammary, Left C Thoracic Artery F Abdominal Artery
0 Coronary Artery, One Artery 1 Coronary Artery, Two Arteries 2 Coronary Artery, Three Arteries 3 Coronary Artery, Four or More Arteries	3 Percutaneous	4 Intraluminal Device, Drug-eluting D Intraluminal Device	4 Coronary Vein
0 Coronary Artery, One Artery 1 Coronary Artery, Two Arteries 2 Coronary Artery, Three Arteries 3 Coronary Artery, Four or More Arteries	4 Percutaneous Endoscopic	4 Intraluminal Device, Drug-eluting D Intraluminal Device	4 Coronary Vein
0 Coronary Artery, One Artery 1 Coronary Artery, Two Arteries 2 Coronary Artery, Three Arteries 3 Coronary Artery, Four or More Arteries	4 Percutaneous Endoscopic	8 Zooplastic Tissue 9 Autologous Venous Tissue A Autologous Arterial Tissue J Synthetic Substitute K Nonautologous Tissue Substitute	3 Coronary Artery 8 Internal Mammary, Right 9 Internal Mammary, Left C Thoracic Artery F Abdominal Artery W Aorta
0 Coronary Artery, One Artery 1 Coronary Artery, Two Arteries 2 Coronary Artery, Three Arteries 3 Coronary Artery, Four or More Arteries	4 Percutaneous Endoscopic	Z No Device	3 Coronary Artery 8 Internal Mammary, Right 9 Internal Mammary, Left C Thoracic Artery F Abdominal Artery
6 Atrium, Right	0 Open 4 Percutaneous Endoscopic	8 Zooplastic Tissue 9 Autologous Venous Tissue A Autologous Arterial Tissue J Synthetic Substitute K Nonautologous Tissue Substitute	P Pulmonary Trunk Q Pulmonary Artery, Right R Pulmonary Artery, Left
6 Atrium, Right	0 Open 4 Percutaneous Endoscopic	Z No Device	7 Atrium, Left P Pulmonary Trunk Q Pulmonary Artery, Right R Pulmonary Artery, Left
6 Atrium, Right	3 Percutaneous	Z No Device	7 Atrium, Left
7 Atrium, Left	0 Open 4 Percutaneous Endoscopic	8 Zooplastic Tissue 9 Autologous Venous Tissue A Autologous Arterial Tissue J Synthetic Substitute K Nonautologous Tissue Substitute Z No Device	P Pulmonary Trunk Q Pulmonary Artery, Right R Pulmonary Artery, Left S Pulmonary Vein, Right T Pulmonary Vein, Left U Pulmonary Vein, Confluence
7 Atrium	3 Percutaneous	J Synthetic Substitute	6 Atrium, Right

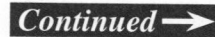

Continued →

Section	0	Medical and Surgical
Body System	2	Heart and Great Vessels
Operation	1	Bypass: Altering the route of passage of the contents of a tubular body part

Body Part (4th)	Approach (5th)	Device (6th)	Qualifier (7th)
K Ventricle, Right L Ventricle, Left	0 Open 4 Percutaneous Endoscopic	8 Zooplastic Tissue 9 Autologous Venous Tissue A Autologous Arterial Tissue J Synthetic Substitute K Nonautologous Tissue Substitute	P Pulmonary Trunk Q Pulmonary Artery, Right R Pulmonary Artery, Left
K Ventricle, Right L Ventricle, Left	0 Open 4 Percutaneous Endoscopic	Z No Device	5 Coronary Circulation 8 Internal Mammary, Right 9 Internal Mammary, Left C Thoracic Artery F Abdominal Artery P Pulmonary Trunk Q Pulmonary Artery, Right R Pulmonary Artery, Left W Aorta
P Pulmonary Trunk Q Right Pulmonary Artery R Left Pulmonary Artery	0 Open 4 Percutaneous Endoscopic	8 Zooplastic Tissue 9 Autologous Venous Tissue A Autologous Arterial Tissue J Synthetic Substitute K Nonautologous Tissue Substitute Z No Device	A Innominate Artery B Subclavin D Carotid
V Superior Vena Cava	0 Open 4 Percutaneous Endoscopic	8 Zooplastic Tissue 9 Autologous Venous Tissue A Autologous Arterial Tissue J Synthetic Substitute K Nonautologous Tissue Substitute Z No Device	P Pulmonary Trunk Q Pulmonary Artery, Right R Pulmonary Artery, Left S Pulmonary Vein, Right T Pulmonary Vein, Left U Pulmonary Vein, Confluence
W Thoracic Aorta, Descending	0 Open	8 Zooplastic Tissue 9 Autologous Venous Tissue A Autologous Arterial Tissue J Synthetic Substitute K Nonautologous Tissue Substitute	A Innominate Artery B Subclavian D Carotid F Abdominal Artery G Axillary Artery H Brachial Artery P Pulmonary Trunk Q Pulmonary Artery, Right R Pulmonary Artery, Left V Lower Extremity Artery
W Thoracic Aorta, Descending	0 Open	Z No Device	A Innominate Artery B Subclavian D Carotid P Pulmonary Trunk Q Pulmonary Artery, Right R Pulmonary Artery, Left
W Thoracic Aorta, Descending	4 Percutaneous Endoscopic	8 Zooplastic Tissue 9 Autologous Venous Tissue A Autologous Arterial Tissue J Synthetic Substitute K Nonautologous Tissue Substitute Z No Device	A Innominate Artery B Subclavian D Carotid P Pulmonary Trunk Q Pulmonary Artery, Right R Pulmonary Artery, Left
X Thoracic Aorta, Ascending/Arch	0 Open 4 Percutaneous Endoscopic	8 Zooplastic Tissue 9 Autologous Venous Tissue A Autologous Arterial Tissue J Synthetic Substitute K Nonautologous Tissue Substitute Z No Device	A Innominate Artery B Subclavian D Carotid P Pulmonary Trunk Q Pulmonary Artery, Right R Pulmonary Artery, Left

Section	0	Medical and Surgical
Body System	2	Heart and Great Vessels
Operation	4	Creation: Putting in or on biological or synthetic material to form a new body part that to the extent possible replicates the anatomic structure or function of an absent body part

Body Part (4th)	Approach (5th)	Device (6th)	Qualifier (7th)
F Aortic Valve	0 Open	7 Autologous Tissue Substitute 8 Zooplastic Tissue J Synthetic Substitute K Nonautologous Tissue Substitute	J Truncal Valve
G Mitral Valve J Tricuspid Valve	0 Open	7 Autologous Tissue Substitute 8 Zooplastic Tissue J Synthetic Substitute K Nonautologous Tissue Substitute	2 Common Atrioventricular Valve

Section	0	Medical and Surgical
Body System	2	Heart and Great Vessels
Operation	5	Destruction: Physical eradication of all or a portion of a body part by the direct use of energy, force, or a destructive agent

Body Part (4th)	Approach (5th)	Device (6th)	Qualifier (7th)
4 Coronary Vein 5 Atrial Septum 6 Atrium, Right 8 Conduction Mechanism 9 Chordae Tendineae D Papillary Muscle F Aortic Valve G Mitral Valve H Pulmonary Valve J Tricuspid Valve K Ventricle, Right L Ventricle, Left M Ventricular Septum N Pericardium P Pulmonary Trunk Q Pulmonary Artery, Right R Pulmonary Artery, Left S Pulmonary Vein, Right T Pulmonary Vein, Left V Superior Vena Cava W Thoracic Aorta, Descending X Thoracic Aorta, Ascending/Arch	0 Open 3 Percutaneous 4 Percutaneous Endoscopic	Z No Device	Z No Qualifier
7 Atrium, Left	0 Open 3 Percutaneous 4 Percutaneous Endoscopic	Z No Device	K Left Atrial Appendage Z No Qualifier

Section	0	Medical and Surgical
Body System	2	Heart and Great Vessels
Operation	7	Dilation: Expanding an orifice or the lumen of a tubular body part

Body Part (4th)	Approach (5th)	Device (6th)	Qualifier (7th)
0 Coronary Artery, One Artery 1 Coronary Artery, Two Arteries 2 Coronary Artery, Three Arteries 3 Coronary Artery, Four or More Arteries	0 Open 3 Percutaneous 4 Percutaneous Endoscopic	4 Intraluminal Device, Drug-eluting 5 Intraluminal Device, Drug-eluting, Two 6 Intraluminal Device, Drug-eluting, Three 7 Intraluminal Device, Drug-eluting, Four or More D Intraluminal Device E Intraluminal Devices, Two F Intraluminal Devices, Three G Intraluminal Devices, Four or More T Intraluminal Device, Radioactive Z No Device	6 Bifurcation Z No Qualifier

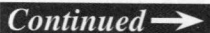

Continued →

Section	0	Medical and Surgical
Body System	2	Heart and Great Vessels
Operation	7	**Dilation:** Expanding an orifice or the lumen of a tubular body part

Body Part (4th)	Approach (5th)	Device (6th)	Qualifier (7th)
F Aortic Valve G Mitral Valve H Pulmonary Valve J Tricuspid Valve K Ventricle, Right L Ventricle, Left P Pulmonary Trunk Q Pulmonary Artery, Right S Pulmonary Vein, Right T Pulmonary Vein, Left V Superior Vena Cava W Thoracic Aorta, Descending X Thoracic Aorta, Ascending/Arch	0 Open 3 Percutaneous 4 Percutaneous Endoscopic	4 Intraluminal Device, Drug-eluting D Intraluminal Device Z No Device	Z No Qualifier
R Pulmonary Artery, Left	0 Open 3 Percutaneous 4 Percutaneous Endoscopic	4 Intraluminal Device, Drug-eluting D Intraluminal Device Z No Device	T Ductus Arteriosus Z No Qualifier

Section	0	Medical and Surgical
Body System	2	Heart and Great Vessels
Operation	8	**Division:** Cutting into a body part, without draining fluids and/or gases from the body part, in order to separate or transect a body part

Body Part (4th)	Approach (5th)	Device (6th)	Qualifier (7th)
8 Conduction Mechanism 9 Chordae Tendineae D Papillary Muscle	0 Open 3 Percutaneous 4 Percutaneous Endoscopic	Z No Device	Z No Qualifier

Section	0	Medical and Surgical
Body System	2	Heart and Great Vessels
Operation	B	**Excision:** Cutting out or off, without replacement, a portion of a body part

Body Part (4th)	Approach (5th)	Device (6th)	Qualifier (7th)
4 Coronary Vein 5 Atrial Septum 6 Atrium, Right 8 Conduction Mechanism 9 Chordae Tendineae D Papillary Muscle F Aortic Valve G Mitral Valve H Pulmonary Valve J Tricuspid Valve K Ventricle, Right L Ventricle, Left M Ventricular Septum N Pericardium P Pulmonary Trunk Q Pulmonary Artery, Right R Pulmonary Artery, Left S Pulmonary Vein, Right T Pulmonary Vein, Left V Superior Vena Cava W Thoracic Aorta, Descending X Thoracic Aorta, Ascending/Arch	0 Open 3 Percutaneous 4 Percutaneous Endoscopic	Z No Device	X Diagnostic Z No Qualifier
7 Atrium, Left	0 Open 3 Percutaneous 4 Percutaneous Endoscopic	Z No Device	K Left Atrial Appendage X Diagnostic Z No Qualifier

Section	0	Medical and Surgical
Body System	2	Heart and Great Vessels
Operation	C	Extirpation: Taking or cutting out solid matter from a body part

Body Part (4th)	Approach (5th)	Device (6th)	Qualifier (7th)
0 Coronary Artery, One Artery 1 Coronary Artery, Two Arteries 2 Coronary Artery, Three Arteries 3 Coronary Artery, Four or More Arteries	0 Open 4 Percutaneous Endoscopic	Z No Device	6 Bifurcation Z No Qualifier
0 Coronary Artery, One Artery 1 Coronary Artery, Two Arteries 2 Coronary Artery, Three Arteries 3 Coronary Artery, Four or More Arteries	3 Percutaneous	Z No Device	6 Bifurcation 7 Orbital Atherectomy Technique Z No Qualifier
4 Coronary Vein 5 Atrial Septum 6 Atrium, Right 7 Atrium, Left 8 Conduction Mechanism 9 Chordae Tendineae D Papillary Muscle F Aortic Valve G Mitral Valve H Pulmonary Valve J Tricuspid Valve K Ventricle, Right L Ventricle, Left M Ventricular Septum N Pericardium P Pulmonary Trunk Q Pulmonary Artery, Right R Pulmonary Artery, Left S Pulmonary Vein, Right T Pulmonary Vein, Left V Superior Vena Cava W Thoracic Aorta, Descending X Thoracic Aorta, Ascending/Arch	0 Open 3 Percutaneous 4 Percutaneous Endoscopic	Z No Device	Z No Qualifier

Section	0	Medical and Surgical
Body System	2	Heart and Great Vessels
Operation	F	Fragmentation: Breaking solid matter in a body part into pieces

Body Part (4th)	Approach (5th)	Device (6th)	Qualifier (7th)
0 Coronary Artery, One Artery 1 Coronary Artery, Two Arteries 2 Coronary Artery, Three Arteries 3 Coronary Artery, Four or More Arteries	3 Percutaneous	Z No Device	Z No Qualifier
N Pericardium	0 Open 3 Percutaneous 4 Percutaneous Endoscopic X External	Z No Device	Z No Qualifier
P Pulmonary Trunk Q Pulmonary Artery, Right R Pulmonary Artery, Left S Pulmonary Vein, Right T Pulmonary Vein, Left	3 Percutaneous	Z No Device	0 Ultrasonic Z No Qualifier

Section   0   **Medical and Surgical**
Body System   2   **Heart and Great Vessels**
Operation   H   **Insertion:** Putting in a nonbiological appliance that monitors, assists, performs, or prevents a physiological function but does not physically take the place of a body part

Body Part (4ᵗʰ)	Approach (5ᵗʰ)	Device (6ᵗʰ)	Qualifier (7ᵗʰ)
0 Coronary Artery, One Artery 1 Coronary Artery, Two Arteries 2 Coronary Artery, Three Arteries 3 Coronary Artery, Four or More Arteries	0 Open 3 Percutaneous 4 Percutaneous Endoscopic	D Intraluminal Device Y Other Device	Z No Qualifier
4 Coronary Vein 6 Atrium, Right 7 Atrium, Left K Ventricle, Right L Ventricle, Left	0 Open 3 Percutaneous 4 Percutaneous Endoscopic	0 Monitoring Device, Pressure Sensor 2 Monitoring Device 3 Infusion Device D Intraluminal Device J Cardiac Lead, Pacemaker K Cardiac Lead, Defibrillator M Cardiac Lead N Intracardiac Pacemaker Y Other Device	Z No Qualifier
A Heart	0 Open 3 Percutaneous 4 Percutaneous Endoscopic	Q Implantable Heart Assist System Y Other Device	Z No Qualifier
A Heart	0 Open 3 Percutaneous 4 Percutaneous Endoscopic	R Short-term External Heart Assist System	J Intraoperative S Biventricular Z No Qualifier
N Pericardium	0 Open 3 Percutaneous 4 Percutaneous Endoscopic	0 Monitoring Device, Pressure Sensor 2 Monitoring Device J Cardiac Lead, Pacemaker K Cardiac Lead, Defibrillator M Cardiac Lead Y Other Device	Z No Qualifier
P Pulmonary Trunk Q Pulmonary Artery, Right R Pulmonary Artery, Left S Pulmonary Vein, Right T Pulmonary Vein, Left V Superior Vena Cava W Thoracic Aorta, Descending	0 Open 3 Percutaneous 4 Percutaneous Endoscopic	0 Monitoring Device, Pressure Sensor 2 Monitoring Device 3 Infusion Device D Intraluminal Device Y Other Device	Z No Qualifier
X Thoracic Aorta, Ascending/Arch	0 Open 3 Percutaneous 4 Percutaneous Endoscopic	0 Monitoring Device, Pressure Sensor 2 Monitoring Device 3 Infusion Device D Intraluminal Device	Z No Qualifier

Section   0   **Medical and Surgical**
Body System   2   **Heart and Great Vessels**
Operation   J   **Inspection:** Visually and/or manually exploring a body part

Body Part (4ᵗʰ)	Approach (5ᵗʰ)	Device (6ᵗʰ)	Qualifier (7ᵗʰ)
A Heart Y Great Vessel	0 Open 3 Percutaneous 4 Percutaneous Endoscopic	Z No Device	Z No Qualifier

Section	0	Medical and Surgical
Body System	2	Heart and Great Vessels
Operation	K	Map: Locating the route of passage of electrical impulses and/or locating functional areas in a body part

Body Part (4th)	Approach (5th)	Device (6th)	Qualifier (7th)
8 Conduction Mechanism	0 Open 3 Percutaneous 4 Percutaneous Endoscopic	Z No Device	Z No Qualifier

Section	0	Medical and Surgical
Body System	2	Heart and Great Vessels
Operation	L	Occlusion: Completely closing an orifice or the lumen of a tubular body part

Body Part (4th)	Approach (5th)	Device (6th)	Qualifier (7th)
7 Atrium, Left	0 Open 3 Percutaneous 4 Percutaneous Endoscopic	C Extraluminal Device D Intraluminal Device Z No Device	K Left Atrial Appendage
H Pulmonary Valve P Pulmonary Trunk Q Pulmonary Artery, Right S Pulmonary Vein, Right T Pulmonary Vein, Left V Superior Vena Cava	0 Open 3 Percutaneous 4 Percutaneous Endoscopic	C Extraluminal Device D Intraluminal Device Z No Device	Z No Qualifier
R Pulmonary Artery, Left	0 Open 3 Percutaneous 4 Percutaneous Endoscopic	C Extraluminal Device D Intraluminal Device Z No Device	T Ductus Arteriosus Z No Qualifier
W Thoracic Aorta, Descending	3 Percutaneous	D Intraluminal Device	J Temporary

Section	0	Medical and Surgical
Body System	2	Heart and Great Vessels
Operation	N	Release: Freeing a body part from an abnormal physical constraint by cutting or by the use of force

Body Part (4th)	Approach (5th)	Device (6th)	Qualifier (7th)
0 Coronary Artery, One Artery 1 Coronary Artery, Two Arteries 2 Coronary Artery, Three Arteries 3 Coronary Artery, Four or More Arteries 4 Coronary Vein 5 Atrial Septum 6 Atrium, Right 7 Atrium, Left 8 Conduction Mechanism 9 Chordae Tendineae D Papillary Muscle F Aortic Valve G Mitral Valve H Pulmonary Valve J Tricuspid Valve K Ventricle, Right L Ventricle, Left M Ventricular Septum N Pericardium P Pulmonary Trunk Q Pulmonary Artery, Right R Pulmonary Artery, Left S Pulmonary Vein, Right T Pulmonary Vein, Left V Superior Vena Cava W Thoracic Aorta, Descending X Thoracic Aorta, Ascending/ Arch	0 Open 3 Percutaneous 4 Percutaneous Endoscopic	Z No Device	Z No Qualifier

Section	0	Medical and Surgical
Body System	2	Heart and Great Vessels
Operation	P	**Removal:** Taking out or off a device from a body part

Body Part (4th)	Approach (5th)	Device (6th)	Qualifier (7th)
A Heart	**0** Open **3** Percutaneous **4** Percutaneous Endoscopic	**2** Monitoring Device **3** Infusion Device **7** Autologous Tissue Substitute **8** Zooplastic Tissue **C** Extraluminal Device **D** Intraluminal Device **J** Synthetic Substitute **K** Nonautologous Tissue Substitute **M** Cardiac Lead **N** Intracardiac Pacemaker **Q** Implantable Heart Assist System **Y** Other Device	**Z** No Qualifier
A Heart	**0** Open **3** Percutaneous **4** Percutaneous Endoscopic	**R** Short-term External Heart Assist System	**S** Biventricular **Z** No Qualifier
A Heart	**X** External	**2** Monitoring Device **3** Infusion Device **D** Intraluminal Device **M** Cardiac Lead	**Z** No Qualifier
Y Great Vessel	**0** Open **3** Percutaneous **4** Percutaneous Endoscopic	**2** Monitoring Device **3** Infusion Device **7** Autologous Tissue Substitute **8** Zooplastic Tissue **C** Extraluminal Device **D** Intraluminal Device **J** Synthetic Substitute **K** Nonautologous Tissue Substitute **Y** Other Device	**Z** No Qualifier
Y Great Vessel	**X** External	**2** Monitoring Device **3** Infusion Device **D** Intraluminal Device	**Z** No Qualifier

Body Part (4th)	Approach (5th)	Device (6th)	Qualifier (7th)
0 Coronary Artery, One Artery **1** Coronary Artery, Two Arteries **2** Coronary Artery, Three Arteries **3** Coronary Artery, Four or More Arteries **4** Coronary Vein **5** Atrial Septum **6** Atrium, Right **7** Atrium, Left **8** Conduction Mechanism **9** Chordae Tendineae **A** Heart **B** Heart, Right **C** Heart, Left **D** Papillary Muscle **H** Pulmonary Valve **K** Ventricle, Right **L** Ventricle, Left **M** Ventricular Septum **N** Pericardium **P** Pulmonary Trunk **Q** Pulmonary Artery, Right **R** Pulmonary Artery, Left **S** Pulmonary Vein, Right **T** Pulmonary Vein, Left **V** Superior Vena Cava **W** Thoracic Aorta, Descending **X** Thoracic Aorta, Ascending/Arch	**0** Open **3** Percutaneous **4** Percutaneous Endoscopic	**Z** No Device	**Z** No Qualifier
F Aortic Valve	**0** Open **3** Percutaneous **4** Percutaneous Endoscopic	**Z** No Device	**J** Truncal Valve **Z** No Qualifier
G Mitral Valve	**0** Open **3** Percutaneous **4** Percutaneous Endoscopic	**Z** No Device	**E** Atrioventricular Valve, Left **Z** No Qualifier
J Tricuspid Valve	**0** Open **3** Percutaneous **4** Percutaneous Endoscopic	**Z** No Device	**G** Atrioventricular Valve, Right **Z** No Qualifier

Section	0	Medical and Surgical
Body System	2	Heart and Great Vessels
Operation	R	Replacement: Putting in or on biological or synthetic material that physically takes the place and/or function of all or a portion of a body part

Body Part (4th)	Approach (5th)	Device (6th)	Qualifier (7th)
5 Atrial Septum 6 Atrium, Right 7 Atrium, Left 9 Chordae Tendineae D Papillary Muscle K Ventricle, Right L Ventricle, Left M Ventricular Septum N Pericardium P Pulmonary Trunk Q Pulmonary Artery, Right R Pulmonary Artery, Left S Pulmonary Vein, Right T Pulmonary Vein, Left V Superior Vena Cava W Thoracic Aorta, Descending X Thoracic Aorta, Ascending/Arch	0 Open 4 Percutaneous Endoscopic	7 Autologous Tissue Substitute 8 Zooplastic Tissue J Synthetic Substitute K Nonautologous Tissue Substitute	Z No Qualifier
A Heart	0 Open	L Biologic with Synthetic Substitute, Autoregulated Electrohydraulic M Synthetic Substitute, Pneumatic	Z No Qualifier
F Aortic Valve G Mitral Valve J Tricuspid Valve	0 Open 4 Percutaneous Endoscopic	7 Autologous Tissue Substitute 8 Zooplastic Tissue J Synthetic Substitute K Nonautologous Tissue Substitute	Z No Qualifier
F Aortic Valve G Mitral Valve J Tricuspid Valve	3 Percutaneous	7 Autologous Tissue Substitute 8 Zooplastic Tissue J Synthetic Substitute K Nonautologous Tissue Substitute	H Transapical Z No Qualifier
H Pulmonary Valve	0 Open 4 Percutaneous Endoscopic	7 Autologous Tissue Substitute 8 Zooplastic Tissue J Synthetic Substitute K Nonautologous Tissue Substitute	Z No Qualifier
H Pulmonary Valve	3 Percutaneous	7 Autologous Tissue Substitute J Synthetic Substitute K Nonautologous Tissue Substitute	H Transapical Z No Qualifier
H Pulmonary Valve	3 Percutaneous	8 Zooplastic Tissue	H Transapical L In Existing Conduit M Native Site Z No Qualifier

Section	0	Medical and Surgical
Body System	2	Heart and Great Vessels
Operation	S	Reposition: Moving to its normal location, or other suitable location, all or a portion of a body part

Body Part (4th)	Approach (5th)	Device (6th)	Qualifier (7th)
0 Coronary Artery, One Artery 1 Coronary Artery, Two Arteries P Pulmonary Trunk Q Pulmonary Artery, Right R Pulmonary Artery, Left S Pulmonary Vein, Right T Pulmonary Vein, Left V Superior Vena Cava W Thoracic Aorta, Descending X Thoracic Aorta, Ascending/Arch	0 Open	Z No Device	Z No Qualifier

Section	0	Medical and Surgical
Body System	2	Heart and Great Vessels
Operation	T	**Resection:** Cutting out or off, without replacement, all of a body part

Body Part (4th)	Approach (5th)	Device (6th)	Qualifier (7th)
5 Atrial Septum 8 Conduction Mechanism 9 Chordae Tendineae D Papillary Muscle H Pulmonary Valve M Ventricular Septum N Pericardium	0 Open 3 Percutaneous 4 Percutaneous Endoscopic	Z No Device	Z No Qualifier

Section	0	Medical and Surgical
Body System	2	Heart and Great Vessels
Operation	U	**Supplement:** Putting in or on biological or synthetic material that physically reinforces and/or augments the function of a portion of a body part

Body Part (4th)	Approach (5th)	Device (6th)	Qualifier (7th)
0 Coronary Artery, One Artery 1 Coronary Artery, Two Arteries 2 Coronary Artery, Three Arteries 3 Coronary Artery, Four or More Arteries 5 Atrial Septum 6 Atrium, Right 7 Atrium, Left 9 Chordae Tendineae A Heart D Papillary Muscle H Pulmonary Valve K Ventricle, Right L Ventricle, Left M Ventricular Septum N Pericardium P Pulmonary Trunk Q Pulmonary Artery, Right R Pulmonary Artery, Left S Pulmonary Vein, Right T Pulmonary Vein, Left V Superior Vena Cava W Thoracic Aorta, Descending X Thoracic Aorta, Ascending/Arch	0 Open 3 Percutaneous 4 Percutaneous Endoscopic	7 Autologous Tissue Substitute 8 Zooplastic Tissue J Synthetic Substitute K Nonautologous Tissue Substitute	Z No Qualifier
F Aortic Valve	0 Open 3 Percutaneous 4 Percutaneous Endoscopic	7 Autologous Tissue Substitute 8 Zooplastic Tissue J Synthetic Substitute K Nonautologous Tissue Substitute	J Truncal Valve Z No Qualifier
G Mitral Valve	0 Open 4 Percutaneous Endoscopic	7 Autologous Tissue Substitute 8 Zooplastic Tissue J Synthetic Substitute K Nonautologous Tissue Substitute	E Atrioventricular Valve, Left Z No Qualifier
G Mitral Valve	3 Percutaneous	7 Autologous Tissue Substitute 8 Zooplastic Tissue K Nonautologous Tissue Substitute	E Atrioventricular Valve, Left Z No Qualifier
G Mitral Valve	3 Percutaneous	J Synthetic Substitute	E Atrioventricular Valve, Left H Transapical Z No Qualifier
J Tricuspid Valve	0 Open 3 Percutaneous 4 Percutaneous Endoscopic	7 Autologous Tissue Substitute 8 Zooplastic Tissue J Synthetic Substitute K Nonautologous Tissue Substitute	G Atrioventricular Valve, Right Z No Qualifier

Section   **0**   **Medical and Surgical**
Body System   **2**   **Heart and Great Vessels**
Operation   **V**   **Restriction:** Partially closing an orifice or the lumen of a tubular body part

Body Part (4th)	Approach (5th)	Device (6th)	Qualifier (7th)
A Heart	0 Open 3 Percutaneous 4 Percutaneous Endoscopic	C Extraluminal Device Z No Device	Z No Qualifier
G Mitral Valve	0 Open 3 Percutaneous 4 Percutaneous Endoscopic	Z No Device	Z No Qualifier
L Ventricle, Left P Pulmonary Trunk Q Pulmonary Artery, Right S Pulmonary Vein, Right T Pulmonary Vein, Left V Superior Vena Cava	0 Open 3 Percutaneous 4 Percutaneous Endoscopic	C Extraluminal Device D Intraluminal Device Z No Device	Z No Qualifier
R Pulmonary Artery, Left	0 Open 3 Percutaneous 4 Percutaneous Endoscopic	C Extraluminal Device D Intraluminal Device Z No Device	T Ductus Arteriosus Z No Qualifier

W Thoracic Aorta, Descending
X Thoracic Aorta, Ascending/
   Arch
	0 Open
	3 Percutaneous
	4 Percutaneous Endoscopic
		C Extraluminal Device
		D Intraluminal Device
		E Intraluminal Device, Branched or
		   Fenestrated, One or Two Arteries
		F Intraluminal Device, Branched or
		   Fenestrated, Three or More Arteries
		Z No Device
			Z No Qualifier

Section   **0**   **Medical and Surgical**
Body System   **2**   **Heart and Great Vessels**
Operation   **W**   **Revision:** Correcting, to the extent possible, a portion of a malfunctioning device or the position of a displaced device

Body Part (4th)	Approach (5th)	Device (6th)	Qualifier (7th)
5 Atrial Septum M Ventricular Septum	0 Open 4 Percutaneous Endoscopic	J Synthetic Substitute	Z No Qualifier
A Heart	0 Open 3 Percutaneous 4 Percutaneous Endoscopic	2 Monitoring Device 3 Infusion Device 7 Autologous Tissue Substitute 8 Zooplastic Tissue C Extraluminal Device D Intraluminal Device J Synthetic Substitute K Nonautologous Tissue Substitute M Cardiac Lead N Intracardiac Pacemaker Q Implantable Heart Assist System Y Other Device	Z No Qualifier
A Heart	0 Open 3 Percutaneous 4 Percutaneous Endoscopic	R Short-term External Heart Assist System	S Biventricular Z No Qualifier
A Heart	X External	2 Monitoring Device 3 Infusion Device 7 Autologous Tissue Substitute 8 Zooplastic Tissue C Extraluminal Device D Intraluminal Device J Synthetic Substitute K Nonautologous Tissue Substitute M Cardiac Lead N Intracardiac Pacemaker Q Implantable Heart Assist System	Z No Qualifier
A Heart	X External	R Short-term External Heart Assist System	S Biventricular Z No Qualifier

Continued →

Section	0	Medical and Surgical
Body System	2	Heart and Great Vessels
Operation	W	**Revision:** Correcting, to the extent possible, a portion of a malfunctioning device or the position of a displaced device

Body Part (4th)	Approach (5th)	Device (6th)	Qualifier (7th)
F Aortic Valve G Mitral Valve H Pulmonary Valve J Tricuspid Valve	0 Open 3 Percutaneous 4 Percutaneous Endoscopic	7 Autologous Tissue Substitute 8 Zooplastic Tissue J Synthetic Substitute K Nonautologous Tissue Substitute	Z No Qualifier
Y Great Vessel	0 Open 3 Percutaneous 4 Percutaneous Endoscopic	2 Monitoring Device 3 Infusion Device 7 Autologous Tissue Substitute 8 Zooplastic Tissue C Extraluminal Device D Intraluminal Device J Synthetic Substitute K Nonautologous Tissue Substitute Y Other Device	Z No Qualifier
Y Great Vessel	X External	2 Monitoring Device 3 Infusion Device 7 Autologous Tissue Substitute 8 Zooplastic Tissue C Extraluminal Device D Intraluminal Device J Synthetic Substitute K Nonautologous Tissue Substitute	Z No Qualifier

Section	0	Medical and Surgical
Body System	2	Heart and Great Vessels
Operation	Y	**Transplantation:** Putting in or on all or a portion of a living body part taken from another individual or animal to physically take the place and/or function of all or a portion of a similar body part

Body Part (4th)	Approach (5th)	Device (6th)	Qualifier (7th)
A Heart	0 Open	Z No Device	0 Allogeneic 1 Syngeneic 2 Zooplastic

Heart and Great Vessels Code Listing 021–02Y

021 – Heart and Great Vessels, Bypass

Review Coding Guideline B3.6a

For Bypass procedures involving the coronary arteries, review Coding Guidelines B3.6b and B3.6c

For Bypass procedures involving the coronary arteries, review Coding Guideline B4.4

0210083 Bypass Coronary Artery, One Artery from Coronary Artery with Zooplastic Tissue, Open Approach
HAC When reported with secondary diagnosis code J98.51 or J98.59

0210088 Bypass Coronary Artery, One Artery from Right Internal Mammary with Zooplastic Tissue, Open Approach
HAC When reported with secondary diagnosis code J98.51 or J98.59

0210089 Bypass Coronary Artery, One Artery from Left Internal Mammary with Zooplastic Tissue, Open Approach
HAC When reported with secondary diagnosis code J98.51 or J98.59

021008C Bypass Coronary Artery, One Artery from Thoracic Artery with Zooplastic Tissue, Open Approach
HAC When reported with secondary diagnosis code J98.51 or J98.59

021008F Bypass Coronary Artery, One Artery from Abdominal Artery with Zooplastic Tissue, Open Approach
HAC When reported with secondary diagnosis code J98.51 or J98.59

021008W Bypass Coronary Artery, One Artery from Aorta with Zooplastic Tissue, Open Approach
HAC When reported with secondary diagnosis code J98.51 or J98.59

0210093 Bypass Coronary Artery, One Artery from Coronary Artery with Autologous Venous Tissue, Open Approach
HAC When reported with secondary diagnosis code J98.51 or J98.59

0210098 Bypass Coronary Artery, One Artery from Right Internal Mammary with Autologous Venous Tissue, Open Approach
HAC When reported with secondary diagnosis code J98.51 or J98.59
AHA CC: 3Q, 2018, 8-9

0210099 Bypass Coronary Artery, One Artery from Left Internal Mammary with Autologous Venous Tissue, Open Approach
HAC When reported with secondary diagnosis code J98.51 or J98.59

021009C Bypass Coronary Artery, One Artery from Thoracic Artery with Autologous Venous Tissue, Open Approach
HAC When reported with secondary diagnosis code J98.51 or J98.59

021009F Bypass Coronary Artery, One Artery from Abdominal Artery with Autologous Venous Tissue, Open Approach
HAC When reported with secondary diagnosis code J98.51 or J98.59

021009W Bypass Coronary Artery, One Artery from Aorta with Autologous Venous Tissue, Open Approach
HAC When reported with secondary diagnosis code J98.51 or J98.59
AHA CC: 1Q, 2014, 10-11

♀ Female-only   ♂ Male-only   ▲ Limited Coverage   ● Non-OR   HAC HAC-associated procedure   ▲ Non-covered procedures   ✚ Cluster

02100A3 Bypass Coronary Artery, One Artery from Coronary Artery with Autologous Arterial Tissue, Open Approach
- ᴴᴬᶜ When reported with secondary diagnosis code J98.51 or J98.59

02100A8 Bypass Coronary Artery, One Artery from Right Internal Mammary with Autologous Arterial Tissue, Open Approach
- ᴴᴬᶜ When reported with secondary diagnosis code J98.51 or J98.59

02100A9 Bypass Coronary Artery, One Artery from Left Internal Mammary with Autologous Arterial Tissue, Open Approach
- ᴴᴬᶜ When reported with secondary diagnosis code J98.51 or J98.59

02100AC Bypass Coronary Artery, One Artery from Thoracic Artery with Autologous Arterial Tissue, Open Approach
- ᴴᴬᶜ When reported with secondary diagnosis code J98.51 or J98.59

02100AF Bypass Coronary Artery, One Artery from Abdominal Artery with Autologous Arterial Tissue, Open Approach
- ᴴᴬᶜ When reported with secondary diagnosis code J98.51 or J98.59

02100AW Bypass Coronary Artery, One Artery from Aorta with Autologous Arterial Tissue, Open Approach
- ᴴᴬᶜ When reported with secondary diagnosis code J98.51 or J98.59
- *AHA CC: 4Q, 2016, 83-84*

02100J3 Bypass Coronary Artery, One Artery from Coronary Artery with Synthetic Substitute, Open Approach
- ᴴᴬᶜ When reported with secondary diagnosis code J98.51 or J98.59

02100J8 Bypass Coronary Artery, One Artery from Right Internal Mammary with Synthetic Substitute, Open Approach
- ᴴᴬᶜ When reported with secondary diagnosis code J98.51 or J98.59

02100J9 Bypass Coronary Artery, One Artery from Left Internal Mammary with Synthetic Substitute, Open Approach
- ᴴᴬᶜ When reported with secondary diagnosis code J98.51 or J98.59

02100JC Bypass Coronary Artery, One Artery from Thoracic Artery with Synthetic Substitute, Open Approach
- ᴴᴬᶜ When reported with secondary diagnosis code J98.51 or J98.59

02100JF Bypass Coronary Artery, One Artery from Abdominal Artery with Synthetic Substitute, Open Approach
- ᴴᴬᶜ When reported with secondary diagnosis code J98.51 or J98.59

02100JW Bypass Coronary Artery, One Artery from Aorta with Synthetic Substitute, Open Approach
- ᴴᴬᶜ When reported with secondary diagnosis code J98.51 or J98.59

02100K3 Bypass Coronary Artery, One Artery from Coronary Artery with Nonautologous Tissue Substitute, Open Approach
- ᴴᴬᶜ When reported with secondary diagnosis code J98.51 or J98.59

02100K8 Bypass Coronary Artery, One Artery from Right Internal Mammary with Nonautologous Tissue Substitute, Open Approach
- ᴴᴬᶜ When reported with secondary diagnosis code J98.51 or J98.59

02100K9 Bypass Coronary Artery, One Artery from Left Internal Mammary with Nonautologous Tissue Substitute, Open Approach
- ᴴᴬᶜ When reported with secondary diagnosis code J98.51 or J98.59

02100KC Bypass Coronary Artery, One Artery from Thoracic Artery with Nonautologous Tissue Substitute, Open Approach
- ᴴᴬᶜ When reported with secondary diagnosis code J98.51 or J98.59

02100KF Bypass Coronary Artery, One Artery from Abdominal Artery with Nonautologous Tissue Substitute, Open Approach
- ᴴᴬᶜ When reported with secondary diagnosis code J98.51 or J98.59

02100KW Bypass Coronary Artery, One Artery from Aorta with Nonautologous Tissue Substitute, Open Approach
- ᴴᴬᶜ When reported with secondary diagnosis code J98.51 or J98.59

02100Z3 Bypass Coronary Artery, One Artery from Coronary Artery, Open Approach
- ᴴᴬᶜ When reported with secondary diagnosis code J98.51 or J98.59

02100Z8 Bypass Coronary Artery, One Artery from Right Internal Mammary, Open Approach
- ᴴᴬᶜ When reported with secondary diagnosis code J98.51 or J98.59

02100Z9 Bypass Coronary Artery, One Artery from Left Internal Mammary, Open Approach
- ᴴᴬᶜ When reported with secondary diagnosis code J98.51 or J98.59
- *AHA CC: 3Q, 2014, 8, 20-21; 1Q, 2016, 27-28; 4Q, 2016, 83-84*

02100ZC Bypass Coronary Artery, One Artery from Thoracic Artery, Open Approach
- ᴴᴬᶜ When reported with secondary diagnosis code J98.51 or J98.59

02100ZF Bypass Coronary Artery, One Artery from Abdominal Artery, Open Approach
- ᴴᴬᶜ When reported with secondary diagnosis code J98.51 or J98.59

0210344 Bypass Coronary Artery, One Artery from Coronary Vein with Drug-eluting Intraluminal Device, Percutaneous Approach

02103D4 Bypass Coronary Artery, One Artery from Coronary Vein with Intraluminal Device, Percutaneous Approach

0210444 Bypass Coronary Artery, One Artery from Coronary Vein with Drug-eluting Intraluminal Device, Percutaneous Endoscopic Approach

0210483 Bypass Coronary Artery, One Artery from Coronary Artery with Zooplastic Tissue, Percutaneous Endoscopic Approach
- ᴴᴬᶜ When reported with secondary diagnosis code J98.51 or J98.59

0210488 Bypass Coronary Artery, One Artery from Right Internal Mammary with Zooplastic Tissue, Percutaneous Endoscopic Approach
- ᴴᴬᶜ When reported with secondary diagnosis code J98.51 or J98.59

0210489 Bypass Coronary Artery, One Artery from Left Internal Mammary with Zooplastic Tissue, Percutaneous Endoscopic Approach
- ᴴᴬᶜ When reported with secondary diagnosis code J98.51 or J98.59

021048C Bypass Coronary Artery, One Artery from Thoracic Artery with Zooplastic Tissue, Percutaneous Endoscopic Approach
- ᴴᴬᶜ When reported with secondary diagnosis code J98.51 or J98.59

021048F Bypass Coronary Artery, One Artery from Abdominal Artery with Zooplastic Tissue, Percutaneous Endoscopic Approach
- ᴴᴬᶜ When reported with secondary diagnosis code J98.51 or J98.59

021048W Bypass Coronary Artery, One Artery from Aorta with Zooplastic Tissue, Percutaneous Endoscopic Approach
- ᴴᴬᶜ When reported with secondary diagnosis code J98.51 or J98.59

0210493 Bypass Coronary Artery, One Artery from Coronary Artery with Autologous Venous Tissue, Percutaneous Endoscopic Approach
- ᴴᴬᶜ When reported with secondary diagnosis code J98.51 or J98.59

0210498 Bypass Coronary Artery, One Artery from Right Internal Mammary with Autologous Venous Tissue, Percutaneous Endoscopic Approach
- ᴴᴬᶜ When reported with secondary diagnosis code J98.51 or J98.59

0210499 Bypass Coronary Artery, One Artery from Left Internal Mammary with Autologous Venous Tissue, Percutaneous Endoscopic Approach
- ᴴᴬᶜ When reported with secondary diagnosis code J98.51 or J98.59

021049C Bypass Coronary Artery, One Artery from Thoracic Artery with Autologous Venous Tissue, Percutaneous Endoscopic Approach
- ᴴᴬᶜ When reported with secondary diagnosis code J98.51 or J98.59

021049F Bypass Coronary Artery, One Artery from Abdominal Artery with Autologous Venous Tissue, Percutaneous Endoscopic Approach
- ᴴᴬᶜ When reported with secondary diagnosis code J98.51 or J98.59

021049W Bypass Coronary Artery, One Artery from Aorta with Autologous Venous Tissue, Percutaneous Endoscopic Approach
- ᴴᴬᶜ When reported with secondary diagnosis code J98.51 or J98.59

02104A3 Bypass Coronary Artery, One Artery from Coronary Artery with Autologous Arterial Tissue, Percutaneous Endoscopic Approach
- ᴴᴬᶜ When reported with secondary diagnosis code J98.51 or J98.59

02104A8 Bypass Coronary Artery, One Artery from Right Internal Mammary with Autologous Arterial Tissue, Percutaneous Endoscopic Approach
- ᴴᴬᶜ When reported with secondary diagnosis code J98.51 or J98.59

02104A9 Bypass Coronary Artery, One Artery from Left Internal Mammary with Autologous Arterial Tissue, Percutaneous Endoscopic Approach
- ᴴᴬᶜ When reported with secondary diagnosis code J98.51 or J98.59

02104AC Bypass Coronary Artery, One Artery from Thoracic Artery with Autologous Arterial Tissue, Percutaneous Endoscopic Approach
- ᴴᴬᶜ When reported with secondary diagnosis code J98.51 or J98.59

02104AF Bypass Coronary Artery, One Artery from Abdominal Artery with Autologous Arterial Tissue, Percutaneous Endoscopic Approach

HAC When reported with secondary diagnosis code J98.51 or J98.59

02104AW Bypass Coronary Artery, One Artery from Aorta with Autologous Arterial Tissue, Percutaneous Endoscopic Approach

HAC When reported with secondary diagnosis code J98.51 or J98.59

02104D4 Bypass Coronary Artery, One Artery from Coronary Vein with Intraluminal Device, Percutaneous Endoscopic Approach

HAC When reported with secondary diagnosis code J98.51 or J98.59

02104J3 Bypass Coronary Artery, One Artery from Coronary Artery with Synthetic Substitute, Percutaneous Endoscopic Approach

HAC When reported with secondary diagnosis code J98.51 or J98.59

02104J8 Bypass Coronary Artery, One Artery from Right Internal Mammary with Synthetic Substitute, Percutaneous Endoscopic Approach

HAC When reported with secondary diagnosis code J98.51 or J98.59

02104J9 Bypass Coronary Artery, One Artery from Left Internal Mammary with Synthetic Substitute, Percutaneous Endoscopic Approach

HAC When reported with secondary diagnosis code J98.51 or J98.59

02104JC Bypass Coronary Artery, One Artery from Thoracic Artery with Synthetic Substitute, Percutaneous Endoscopic Approach

HAC When reported with secondary diagnosis code J98.51 or J98.59

02104JF Bypass Coronary Artery, One Artery from Abdominal Artery with Synthetic Substitute, Percutaneous Endoscopic Approach

HAC When reported with secondary diagnosis code J98.51 or J98.59

02104JW Bypass Coronary Artery, One Artery from Aorta with Synthetic Substitute, Percutaneous Endoscopic Approach

HAC When reported with secondary diagnosis code J98.51 or J98.59

02104K3 Bypass Coronary Artery, One Artery from Coronary Artery with Nonautologous Tissue Substitute, Percutaneous Endoscopic Approach

HAC When reported with secondary diagnosis code J98.51 or J98.59

02104K8 Bypass Coronary Artery, One Artery from Right Internal Mammary with Nonautologous Tissue Substitute, Percutaneous Endoscopic Approach

HAC When reported with secondary diagnosis code J98.51 or J98.59

02104K9 Bypass Coronary Artery, One Artery from Left Internal Mammary with Nonautologous Tissue Substitute, Percutaneous Endoscopic Approach

HAC When reported with secondary diagnosis code J98.51 or J98.59

02104KC Bypass Coronary Artery, One Artery from Thoracic Artery with Nonautologous Tissue Substitute, Percutaneous Endoscopic Approach

HAC When reported with secondary diagnosis code J98.51 or J98.59

02104KF Bypass Coronary Artery, One Artery from Abdominal Artery with Nonautologous Tissue Substitute, Percutaneous Endoscopic Approach

HAC When reported with secondary diagnosis code J98.51 or J98.59

02104KW Bypass Coronary Artery, One Artery from Aorta with Nonautologous Tissue Substitute, Percutaneous Endoscopic Approach

HAC When reported with secondary diagnosis code J98.51 or J98.59

02104Z3 Bypass Coronary Artery, One Artery from Coronary Artery, Percutaneous Endoscopic Approach

HAC When reported with secondary diagnosis code J98.51 or J98.59

02104Z8 Bypass Coronary Artery, One Artery from Right Internal Mammary, Percutaneous Endoscopic Approach

HAC When reported with secondary diagnosis code J98.51 or J98.59

02104Z9 Bypass Coronary Artery, One Artery from Left Internal Mammary, Percutaneous Endoscopic Approach

HAC When reported with secondary diagnosis code J98.51 or J98.59

02104ZC Bypass Coronary Artery, One Artery from Thoracic Artery, Percutaneous Endoscopic Approach

HAC When reported with secondary diagnosis code J98.51 or J98.59

02104ZF Bypass Coronary Artery, One Artery from Abdominal Artery, Percutaneous Endoscopic Approach

HAC When reported with secondary diagnosis code J98.51 or J98.59

0211083 Bypass Coronary Artery, Two Arteries from Coronary Artery with Zooplastic Tissue, Open Approach

HAC When reported with secondary diagnosis code J98.51 or J98.59

0211088 Bypass Coronary Artery, Two Arteries from Right Internal Mammary with Zooplastic Tissue, Open Approach

HAC When reported with secondary diagnosis code J98.51 or J98.59

0211089 Bypass Coronary Artery, Two Arteries from Left Internal Mammary with Zooplastic Tissue, Open Approach

HAC When reported with secondary diagnosis code J98.51 or J98.59

021108C Bypass Coronary Artery, Two Arteries from Thoracic Artery with Zooplastic Tissue, Open Approach

HAC When reported with secondary diagnosis code J98.51 or J98.59

021108F Bypass Coronary Artery, Two Arteries from Abdominal Artery with Zooplastic Tissue, Open Approach

HAC When reported with secondary diagnosis code J98.51 or J98.59

021108W Bypass Coronary Artery, Two Arteries from Aorta with Zooplastic Tissue, Open Approach

HAC When reported with secondary diagnosis code J98.51 or J98.59

0211093 Bypass Coronary Artery, Two Arteries from Coronary Artery with Autologous Venous Tissue, Open Approach

HAC When reported with secondary diagnosis code J98.51 or J98.59

0211098 Bypass Coronary Artery, Two Arteries from Right Internal Mammary with Autologous Venous Tissue, Open Approach

HAC When reported with secondary diagnosis code J98.51 or J98.59

0211099 Bypass Coronary Artery, Two Arteries from Left Internal Mammary with Autologous Venous Tissue, Open Approach

HAC When reported with secondary diagnosis code J98.51 or J98.59

021109C Bypass Coronary Artery, Two Arteries from Thoracic Artery with Autologous Venous Tissue, Open Approach

HAC When reported with secondary diagnosis code J98.51 or J98.59

021109F Bypass Coronary Artery, Two Arteries from Abdominal Artery with Autologous Venous Tissue, Open Approach

HAC When reported with secondary diagnosis code J98.51 or J98.59

021109W Bypass Coronary Artery, Two Arteries from Aorta with Autologous Venous Tissue, Open Approach

HAC When reported with secondary diagnosis code J98.51 or J98.59

AHA CC: 3Q, 2014, 20-21; 4Q, 2016, 83-84

02110A3 Bypass Coronary Artery, Two Arteries from Coronary Artery with Autologous Arterial Tissue, Open Approach

HAC When reported with secondary diagnosis code J98.51 or J98.59

02110A8 Bypass Coronary Artery, Two Arteries from Right Internal Mammary with Autologous Arterial Tissue, Open Approach

HAC When reported with secondary diagnosis code J98.51 or J98.59

02110A9 Bypass Coronary Artery, Two Arteries from Left Internal Mammary with Autologous Arterial Tissue, Open Approach

HAC When reported with secondary diagnosis code J98.51 or J98.59

02110AC Bypass Coronary Artery, Two Arteries from Thoracic Artery with Autologous Arterial Tissue, Open Approach

HAC When reported with secondary diagnosis code J98.51 or J98.59

02110AF Bypass Coronary Artery, Two Arteries from Abdominal Artery with Autologous Arterial Tissue, Open Approach

HAC When reported with secondary diagnosis code J98.51 or J98.59

02110AW Bypass Coronary Artery, Two Arteries from Aorta with Autologous Arterial Tissue, Open Approach

HAC When reported with secondary diagnosis code J98.51 or J98.59

02110J3 Bypass Coronary Artery, Two Arteries from Coronary Artery with Synthetic Substitute, Open Approach

HAC When reported with secondary diagnosis code J98.51 or J98.59

02110J8 Bypass Coronary Artery, Two Arteries from Right Internal Mammary with Synthetic Substitute, Open Approach

HAC When reported with secondary diagnosis code J98.51 or J98.59

♀ Female-only   ♂ Male-only   ▲ Limited Coverage   ● Non-OR   HAC HAC-associated procedure   ▲ Non-covered procedures   ✚ Cluster

02110J9 Bypass Coronary Artery, Two Arteries from Left Internal Mammary with Synthetic Substitute, Open Approach
▪ HAC When reported with secondary diagnosis code J98.51 or J98.59

02110JC Bypass Coronary Artery, Two Arteries from Thoracic Artery with Synthetic Substitute, Open Approach
▪ HAC When reported with secondary diagnosis code J98.51 or J98.59

02110JF Bypass Coronary Artery, Two Arteries from Abdominal Artery with Synthetic Substitute, Open Approach
▪ HAC When reported with secondary diagnosis code J98.51 or J98.59

02110JW Bypass Coronary Artery, Two Arteries from Aorta with Synthetic Substitute, Open Approach
▪ HAC When reported with secondary diagnosis code J98.51 or J98.59

02110K3 Bypass Coronary Artery, Two Arteries from Coronary Artery with Nonautologous Tissue Substitute, Open Approach
▪ HAC When reported with secondary diagnosis code J98.51 or J98.59

02110K8 Bypass Coronary Artery, Two Arteries from Right Internal Mammary with Nonautologous Tissue Substitute, Open Approach
▪ HAC When reported with secondary diagnosis code J98.51 or J98.59

02110K9 Bypass Coronary Artery, Two Arteries from Left Internal Mammary with Nonautologous Tissue Substitute, Open Approach
▪ HAC When reported with secondary diagnosis code J98.51 or J98.59

02110KC Bypass Coronary Artery, Two Arteries from Thoracic Artery with Nonautologous Tissue Substitute, Open Approach
▪ HAC When reported with secondary diagnosis code J98.51 or J98.59

02110KF Bypass Coronary Artery, Two Arteries from Abdominal Artery with Nonautologous Tissue Substitute, Open Approach
▪ HAC When reported with secondary diagnosis code J98.51 or J98.59

02110KW Bypass Coronary Artery, Two Arteries from Aorta with Nonautologous Tissue Substitute, Open Approach
▪ HAC When reported with secondary diagnosis code J98.51 or J98.59

02110Z3 Bypass Coronary Artery, Two Arteries from Coronary Artery, Open Approach
▪ HAC When reported with secondary diagnosis code J98.51 or J98.59

02110Z8 Bypass Coronary Artery, Two Arteries from Right Internal Mammary, Open Approach
▪ HAC When reported with secondary diagnosis code J98.51 or J98.59

02110Z9 Bypass Coronary Artery, Two Arteries from Left Internal Mammary, Open Approach
▪ HAC When reported with secondary diagnosis code J98.51 or J98.59

02110ZC Bypass Coronary Artery, Two Arteries from Thoracic Artery, Open Approach
▪ HAC When reported with secondary diagnosis code J98.51 or J98.59

02110ZF Bypass Coronary Artery, Two Arteries from Abdominal Artery, Open Approach
▪ HAC When reported with secondary diagnosis code J98.51 or J98.59

0211344 Bypass Coronary Artery, Two Arteries from Coronary Vein with Drug-eluting Intraluminal Device, Percutaneous Approach

02113D4 Bypass Coronary Artery, Two Arteries from Coronary Vein with Intraluminal Device, Percutaneous Approach

0211444 Bypass Coronary Artery, Two Arteries from Coronary Vein with Drug-eluting Intraluminal Device, Percutaneous Endoscopic Approach
▪ HAC When reported with secondary diagnosis code J98.51 or J98.59

0211483 Bypass Coronary Artery, Two Arteries from Coronary Artery with Zooplastic Tissue, Percutaneous Endoscopic Approach
▪ HAC When reported with secondary diagnosis code J98.51 or J98.59

0211488 Bypass Coronary Artery, Two Arteries from Right Internal Mammary with Zooplastic Tissue, Percutaneous Endoscopic Approach
▪ HAC When reported with secondary diagnosis code J98.51 or J98.59

0211489 Bypass Coronary Artery, Two Arteries from Left Internal Mammary with Zooplastic Tissue, Percutaneous Endoscopic Approach
▪ HAC When reported with secondary diagnosis code J98.51 or J98.59

021148C Bypass Coronary Artery, Two Arteries from Thoracic Artery with Zooplastic Tissue, Percutaneous Endoscopic Approach
▪ HAC When reported with secondary diagnosis code J98.51 or J98.59

021148F Bypass Coronary Artery, Two Arteries from Abdominal Artery with Zooplastic Tissue, Percutaneous Endoscopic Approach
▪ HAC When reported with secondary diagnosis code J98.51 or J98.59

021148W Bypass Coronary Artery, Two Arteries from Aorta with Zooplastic Tissue, Percutaneous Endoscopic Approach
▪ HAC When reported with secondary diagnosis code J98.51 or J98.59

0211493 Bypass Coronary Artery, Two Arteries from Coronary Artery with Autologous Venous Tissue, Percutaneous Endoscopic Approach
▪ HAC When reported with secondary diagnosis code J98.51 or J98.59

0211498 Bypass Coronary Artery, Two Arteries from Right Internal Mammary with Autologous Venous Tissue, Percutaneous Endoscopic Approach
▪ HAC When reported with secondary diagnosis code J98.51 or J98.59

0211499 Bypass Coronary Artery, Two Arteries from Left Internal Mammary with Autologous Venous Tissue, Percutaneous Endoscopic Approach
▪ HAC When reported with secondary diagnosis code J98.51 or J98.59

021149C Bypass Coronary Artery, Two Arteries from Thoracic Artery with Autologous Venous Tissue, Percutaneous Endoscopic Approach
▪ HAC When reported with secondary diagnosis code J98.51 or J98.59

021149F Bypass Coronary Artery, Two Arteries from Abdominal Artery with Autologous Venous Tissue, Percutaneous Endoscopic Approach
▪ HAC When reported with secondary diagnosis code J98.51 or J98.59

021149W Bypass Coronary Artery, Two Arteries from Aorta with Autologous Venous Tissue, Percutaneous Endoscopic Approach
▪ HAC When reported with secondary diagnosis code J98.51 or J98.59

02114A3 Bypass Coronary Artery, Two Arteries from Coronary Artery with Autologous Arterial Tissue, Percutaneous Endoscopic Approach
▪ HAC When reported with secondary diagnosis code J98.51 or J98.59

02114A8 Bypass Coronary Artery, Two Arteries from Right Internal Mammary with Autologous Arterial Tissue, Percutaneous Endoscopic Approach
▪ HAC When reported with secondary diagnosis code J98.51 or J98.59

02114A9 Bypass Coronary Artery, Two Arteries from Left Internal Mammary with Autologous Arterial Tissue, Percutaneous Endoscopic Approach
▪ HAC When reported with secondary diagnosis code J98.51 or J98.59

02114AC Bypass Coronary Artery, Two Arteries from Thoracic Artery with Autologous Arterial Tissue, Percutaneous Endoscopic Approach
▪ HAC When reported with secondary diagnosis code J98.51 or J98.59

02114AF Bypass Coronary Artery, Two Arteries from Abdominal Artery with Autologous Arterial Tissue, Percutaneous Endoscopic Approach
▪ HAC When reported with secondary diagnosis code J98.51 or J98.59

02114AW Bypass Coronary Artery, Two Arteries from Aorta with Autologous Arterial Tissue, Percutaneous Endoscopic Approach
▪ HAC When reported with secondary diagnosis code J98.51 or J98.59

02114D4 Bypass Coronary Artery, Two Arteries from Coronary Vein with Intraluminal Device, Percutaneous Endoscopic Approach

02114J3 Bypass Coronary Artery, Two Arteries from Coronary Artery with Synthetic Substitute, Percutaneous Endoscopic Approach
▪ HAC When reported with secondary diagnosis code J98.51 or J98.59

02114J8 Bypass Coronary Artery, Two Arteries from Right Internal Mammary with Synthetic Substitute, Percutaneous Endoscopic Approach
▪ HAC When reported with secondary diagnosis code J98.51 or J98.59

02114J9 Bypass Coronary Artery, Two Arteries from Left Internal Mammary with Synthetic Substitute, Percutaneous Endoscopic Approach
▪ HAC When reported with secondary diagnosis code J98.51 or J98.59

02114JC Bypass Coronary Artery, Two Arteries from Thoracic Artery with Synthetic Substitute, Percutaneous Endoscopic Approach
▪ HAC When reported with secondary diagnosis code J98.51 or J98.59

02114JF Bypass Coronary Artery, Two Arteries from Abdominal Artery with Synthetic Substitute, Percutaneous Endoscopic Approach
HAC When reported with secondary diagnosis code J98.51 or J98.59

02114JW Bypass Coronary Artery, Two Arteries from Aorta with Synthetic Substitute, Percutaneous Endoscopic Approach
HAC When reported with secondary diagnosis code J98.51 or J98.59

02114K3 Bypass Coronary Artery, Two Arteries from Coronary Artery with Nonautologous Tissue Substitute, Percutaneous Endoscopic Approach
HAC When reported with secondary diagnosis code J98.51 or J98.59

02114K8 Bypass Coronary Artery, Two Arteries from Right Internal Mammary with Nonautologous Tissue Substitute, Percutaneous Endoscopic Approach
HAC When reported with secondary diagnosis code J98.51 or J98.59

02114K9 Bypass Coronary Artery, Two Arteries from Left Internal Mammary with Nonautologous Tissue Substitute, Percutaneous Endoscopic Approach
HAC When reported with secondary diagnosis code J98.51 or J98.59

02114KC Bypass Coronary Artery, Two Arteries from Thoracic Artery with Nonautologous Tissue Substitute, Percutaneous Endoscopic Approach
HAC When reported with secondary diagnosis code J98.51 or J98.59

02114KF Bypass Coronary Artery, Two Arteries from Abdominal Artery with Nonautologous Tissue Substitute, Percutaneous Endoscopic Approach
HAC When reported with secondary diagnosis code J98.51 or J98.59

02114KW Bypass Coronary Artery, Two Arteries from Aorta with Nonautologous Tissue Substitute, Percutaneous Endoscopic Approach
HAC When reported with secondary diagnosis code J98.51 or J98.59

02114Z3 Bypass Coronary Artery, Two Arteries from Coronary Artery, Percutaneous Endoscopic Approach
HAC When reported with secondary diagnosis code J98.51 or J98.59

02114Z8 Bypass Coronary Artery, Two Arteries from Right Internal Mammary, Percutaneous Endoscopic Approach
HAC When reported with secondary diagnosis code J98.51 or J98.59

02114Z9 Bypass Coronary Artery, Two Arteries from Left Internal Mammary, Percutaneous Endoscopic Approach
HAC When reported with secondary diagnosis code J98.51 or J98.59

02114ZC Bypass Coronary Artery, Two Arteries from Thoracic Artery, Percutaneous Endoscopic Approach
HAC When reported with secondary diagnosis code J98.51 or J98.59

02114ZF Bypass Coronary Artery, Two Arteries from Abdominal Artery, Percutaneous Endoscopic Approach
HAC When reported with secondary diagnosis code J98.51 or J98.59

0212083 Bypass Coronary Artery, Three Arteries from Coronary Artery with Zooplastic Tissue, Open Approach
HAC When reported with secondary diagnosis code J98.51 or J98.59

0212088 Bypass Coronary Artery, Three Arteries from Right Internal Mammary with Zooplastic Tissue, Open Approach
HAC When reported with secondary diagnosis code J98.51 or J98.59

0212089 Bypass Coronary Artery, Three Arteries from Left Internal Mammary with Zooplastic Tissue, Open Approach
HAC When reported with secondary diagnosis code J98.51 or J98.59

021208C Bypass Coronary Artery, Three Arteries from Thoracic Artery with Zooplastic Tissue, Open Approach
HAC When reported with secondary diagnosis code J98.51 or J98.59

021208F Bypass Coronary Artery, Three Arteries from Abdominal Artery with Zooplastic Tissue, Open Approach
HAC When reported with secondary diagnosis code J98.51 or J98.59

021208W Bypass Coronary Artery, Three Arteries from Aorta with Zooplastic Tissue, Open Approach
HAC When reported with secondary diagnosis code J98.51 or J98.59

0212093 Bypass Coronary Artery, Three Arteries from Coronary Artery with Autologous Venous Tissue, Open Approach
HAC When reported with secondary diagnosis code J98.51 or J98.59

0212098 Bypass Coronary Artery, Three Arteries from Right Internal Mammary with Autologous Venous Tissue, Open Approach
HAC When reported with secondary diagnosis code J98.51 or J98.59

0212099 Bypass Coronary Artery, Three Arteries from Left Internal Mammary with Autologous Venous Tissue, Open Approach
HAC When reported with secondary diagnosis code J98.51 or J98.59

021209C Bypass Coronary Artery, Three Arteries from Thoracic Artery with Autologous Venous Tissue, Open Approach
HAC When reported with secondary diagnosis code J98.51 or J98.59

021209F Bypass Coronary Artery, Three Arteries from Abdominal Artery with Autologous Venous Tissue, Open Approach
HAC When reported with secondary diagnosis code J98.51 or J98.59

021209W Bypass Coronary Artery, Three Arteries from Aorta with Autologous Venous Tissue, Open Approach
HAC When reported with secondary diagnosis code J98.51 or J98.59
AHA CC: 1Q, 2016, 27-28

02120A3 Bypass Coronary Artery, Three Arteries from Coronary Artery with Autologous Arterial Tissue, Open Approach
HAC When reported with secondary diagnosis code J98.51 or J98.59

02120A8 Bypass Coronary Artery, Three Arteries from Right Internal Mammary with Autologous Arterial Tissue, Open Approach
HAC When reported with secondary diagnosis code J98.51 or J98.59

02120A9 Bypass Coronary Artery, Three Arteries from Left Internal Mammary with Autologous Arterial Tissue, Open Approach
HAC When reported with secondary diagnosis code J98.51 or J98.59

02120AC Bypass Coronary Artery, Three Arteries from Thoracic Artery with Autologous Arterial Tissue, Open Approach
HAC When reported with secondary diagnosis code J98.51 or J98.59

02120AF Bypass Coronary Artery, Three Arteries from Abdominal Artery with Autologous Arterial Tissue, Open Approach
HAC When reported with secondary diagnosis code J98.51 or J98.59

02120AW Bypass Coronary Artery, Three Arteries from Aorta with Autologous Arterial Tissue, Open Approach
HAC When reported with secondary diagnosis code J98.51 or J98.59

02120J3 Bypass Coronary Artery, Three Arteries from Coronary Artery with Synthetic Substitute, Open Approach
HAC When reported with secondary diagnosis code J98.51 or J98.59

02120J8 Bypass Coronary Artery, Three Arteries from Right Internal Mammary with Synthetic Substitute, Open Approach
HAC When reported with secondary diagnosis code J98.51 or J98.59

02120J9 Bypass Coronary Artery, Three Arteries from Left Internal Mammary with Synthetic Substitute, Open Approach
HAC When reported with secondary diagnosis code J98.51 or J98.59

02120JC Bypass Coronary Artery, Three Arteries from Thoracic Artery with Synthetic Substitute, Open Approach
HAC When reported with secondary diagnosis code J98.51 or J98.59

02120JF Bypass Coronary Artery, Three Arteries from Abdominal Artery with Synthetic Substitute, Open Approach
HAC When reported with secondary diagnosis code J98.51 or J98.59

02120JW Bypass Coronary Artery, Three Arteries from Aorta with Synthetic Substitute, Open Approach
HAC When reported with secondary diagnosis code J98.51 or J98.59

02120K3 Bypass Coronary Artery, Three Arteries from Coronary Artery with Nonautologous Tissue Substitute, Open Approach
HAC When reported with secondary diagnosis code J98.51 or J98.59

02120K8 Bypass Coronary Artery, Three Arteries from Right Internal Mammary with Nonautologous Tissue Substitute, Open Approach
HAC When reported with secondary diagnosis code J98.51 or J98.59

02120K9 Bypass Coronary Artery, Three Arteries from Left Internal Mammary with Nonautologous Tissue Substitute, Open Approach
HAC When reported with secondary diagnosis code J98.51 or J98.59

02120KC Bypass Coronary Artery, Three Arteries from Thoracic Artery with Nonautologous Tissue Substitute, Open Approach
HAC When reported with secondary diagnosis code J98.51 or J98.59

02120KF Bypass Coronary Artery, Three Arteries from Abdominal Artery with Nonautologous Tissue Substitute, Open Approach
HAC When reported with secondary diagnosis code J98.51 or J98.59

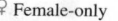

♀ Female-only   ♂ Male-only   ▲ Limited Coverage   ● Non-OR   HAC HAC-associated procedure   ▲ Non-covered procedures   ✚ Cluster

02120KW Bypass Coronary Artery, Three Arteries from Aorta with Nonautologous Tissue Substitute, Open Approach
HAC When reported with secondary diagnosis code J98.51 or J98.59

02120Z3 Bypass Coronary Artery, Three Arteries from Coronary Artery, Open Approach
HAC When reported with secondary diagnosis code J98.51 or J98.59

02120Z8 Bypass Coronary Artery, Three Arteries from Right Internal Mammary, Open Approach
HAC When reported with secondary diagnosis code J98.51 or J98.59

02120Z9 Bypass Coronary Artery, Three Arteries from Left Internal Mammary, Open Approach
HAC When reported with secondary diagnosis code J98.51 or J98.59

02120ZC Bypass Coronary Artery, Three Arteries from Thoracic Artery, Open Approach
HAC When reported with secondary diagnosis code J98.51 or J98.59

02120ZF Bypass Coronary Artery, Three Arteries from Abdominal Artery, Open Approach
HAC When reported with secondary diagnosis code J98.51 or J98.59

0212344 Bypass Coronary Artery, Three Arteries from Coronary Vein with Drug-eluting Intraluminal Device, Percutaneous Approach

02123D4 Bypass Coronary Artery, Three Arteries from Coronary Vein with Intraluminal Device, Percutaneous Approach

0212444 Bypass Coronary Artery, Three from Coronary Vein with Drug-eluting Intraluminal Device, Percutaneous Endoscopic Approach

0212483 Bypass Coronary Artery, Three Arteries from Coronary Artery with Zooplastic Tissue, Percutaneous Endoscopic Approach
HAC When reported with secondary diagnosis code J98.51 or J98.59

0212488 Bypass Coronary Artery, Three Arteries from Right Internal Mammary with Zooplastic Tissue, Percutaneous Endoscopic Approach
HAC When reported with secondary diagnosis code J98.51 or J98.59

0212489 Bypass Coronary Artery, Three Arteries from Left Internal Mammary with Zooplastic Tissue, Percutaneous Endoscopic Approach
HAC When reported with secondary diagnosis code J98.51 or J98.59

021248C Bypass Coronary Artery, Three Arteries from Thoracic Artery with Zooplastic Tissue, Percutaneous Endoscopic Approach
HAC When reported with secondary diagnosis code J98.51 or J98.59

021248F Bypass Coronary Artery, Three Arteries from Abdominal Artery with Zooplastic Tissue, Percutaneous Endoscopic Approach
HAC When reported with secondary diagnosis code J98.51 or J98.59

021248W Bypass Coronary Artery, Three Arteries from Aorta with Zooplastic Tissue, Percutaneous Endoscopic Approach
HAC When reported with secondary diagnosis code J98.51 or J98.59

0212493 Bypass Coronary Artery, Three Arteries from Coronary Artery with Autologous Venous Tissue, Percutaneous Endoscopic Approach
HAC When reported with secondary diagnosis code J98.51 or J98.59

0212498 Bypass Coronary Artery, Three Arteries from Right Internal Mammary with Autologous Venous Tissue, Percutaneous Endoscopic Approach
HAC When reported with secondary diagnosis code J98.51 or J98.59

0212499 Bypass Coronary Artery, Three Arteries from Left Internal Mammary with Autologous Venous Tissue, Percutaneous Endoscopic Approach
HAC When reported with secondary diagnosis code J98.51 or J98.59

021249C Bypass Coronary Artery, Three Arteries from Thoracic Artery with Autologous Venous Tissue, Percutaneous Endoscopic Approach
HAC When reported with secondary diagnosis code J98.51 or J98.59

021249F Bypass Coronary Artery, Three Arteries from Abdominal Artery with Autologous Venous Tissue, Percutaneous Endoscopic Approach
HAC When reported with secondary diagnosis code J98.51 or J98.59

021249W Bypass Coronary Artery, Three Arteries from Aorta with Autologous Venous Tissue, Percutaneous Endoscopic Approach
HAC When reported with secondary diagnosis code J98.51 or J98.59

02124A3 Bypass Coronary Artery, Three Arteries from Coronary Artery with Autologous Arterial Tissue, Percutaneous Endoscopic Approach
HAC When reported with secondary diagnosis code J98.51 or J98.59

02124A8 Bypass Coronary Artery, Three Arteries from Right Internal Mammary with Autologous Arterial Tissue, Percutaneous Endoscopic Approach
HAC When reported with secondary diagnosis code J98.51 or J98.59

02124A9 Bypass Coronary Artery, Three Arteries from Left Internal Mammary with Autologous Arterial Tissue, Percutaneous Endoscopic Approach
HAC When reported with secondary diagnosis code J98.51 or J98.59

02124AC Bypass Coronary Artery, Three Arteries from Thoracic Artery with Autologous Arterial Tissue, Percutaneous Endoscopic Approach
HAC When reported with secondary diagnosis code J98.51 or J98.59

02124AF Bypass Coronary Artery, Three Arteries from Abdominal Artery with Autologous Arterial Tissue, Percutaneous Endoscopic Approach
HAC When reported with secondary diagnosis code J98.51 or J98.59

02124AW Bypass Coronary Artery, Three Arteries from Aorta with Autologous Arterial Tissue, Percutaneous Endoscopic Approach
HAC When reported with secondary diagnosis code J98.51 or J98.59

02124D4 Bypass Coronary Artery, Three Arteries from Coronary Vein with Intraluminal Device, Percutaneous Endoscopic Approach
HAC When reported with secondary diagnosis code J98.51 or J98.59

02124J3 Bypass Coronary Artery, Three Arteries from Coronary Artery with Synthetic Substitute, Percutaneous Endoscopic Approach
HAC When reported with secondary diagnosis code J98.51 or J98.59

02124J8 Bypass Coronary Artery, Three Arteries from Right Internal Mammary with Synthetic Substitute, Percutaneous Endoscopic Approach
HAC When reported with secondary diagnosis code J98.51 or J98.59

02124J9 Bypass Coronary Artery, Three Arteries from Left Internal Mammary with Synthetic Substitute, Percutaneous Endoscopic Approach
HAC When reported with secondary diagnosis code J98.51 or J98.59

02124JC Bypass Coronary Artery, Three Arteries from Thoracic Artery with Synthetic Substitute, Percutaneous Endoscopic Approach
HAC When reported with secondary diagnosis code J98.51 or J98.59

02124JF Bypass Coronary Artery, Three Arteries from Abdominal Artery with Synthetic Substitute, Percutaneous Endoscopic Approach
HAC When reported with secondary diagnosis code J98.51 or J98.59

02124JW Bypass Coronary Artery, Three Arteries from Aorta with Synthetic Substitute, Percutaneous Endoscopic Approach
HAC When reported with secondary diagnosis code J98.51 or J98.59

02124K3 Bypass Coronary Artery, Three Arteries from Coronary Artery with Nonautologous Tissue Substitute, Percutaneous Endoscopic Approach
HAC When reported with secondary diagnosis code J98.51 or J98.59

02124K8 Bypass Coronary Artery, Three Arteries from Right Internal Mammary with Nonautologous Tissue Substitute, Percutaneous Endoscopic Approach
HAC When reported with secondary diagnosis code J98.51 or J98.59

02124K9 Bypass Coronary Artery, Three Arteries from Left Internal Mammary with Nonautologous Tissue Substitute, Percutaneous Endoscopic Approach
HAC When reported with secondary diagnosis code J98.51 or J98.59

02124KC Bypass Coronary Artery, Three Arteries from Thoracic Artery with Nonautologous Tissue Substitute, Percutaneous Endoscopic Approach
HAC When reported with secondary diagnosis code J98.51 or J98.59

02124KF Bypass Coronary Artery, Three Arteries from Abdominal Artery with Nonautologous Tissue Substitute, Percutaneous Endoscopic Approach
HAC When reported with secondary diagnosis code J98.51 or J98.59

02124KW Bypass Coronary Artery, Three Arteries from Aorta with Nonautologous Tissue Substitute, Percutaneous Endoscopic Approach
HAC When reported with secondary diagnosis code J98.51 or J98.59

♀ Female-only   ♂ Male-only   ▲ Limited Coverage   ● Non-OR   HAC HAC-associated procedure   ▲ Non-covered procedures   + Cluster

02124Z3 Bypass Coronary Artery, Three Arteries from Coronary Artery, Percutaneous Endoscopic Approach
- HAC When reported with secondary diagnosis code J98.51 or J98.59

02124Z8 Bypass Coronary Artery, Three Arteries from Right Internal Mammary, Percutaneous Endoscopic Approach
- HAC When reported with secondary diagnosis code J98.51 or J98.59

02124Z9 Bypass Coronary Artery, Three Arteries from Left Internal Mammary, Percutaneous Endoscopic Approach
- HAC When reported with secondary diagnosis code J98.51 or J98.59

02124ZC Bypass Coronary Artery, Three Arteries from Thoracic Artery, Percutaneous Endoscopic Approach
- HAC When reported with secondary diagnosis code J98.51 or J98.59

02124ZF Bypass Coronary Artery, Three Arteries from Abdominal Artery, Percutaneous Endoscopic Approach
- HAC When reported with secondary diagnosis code J98.51 or J98.59

0213083 Bypass Coronary Artery, Four or More Arteries from Coronary Artery with Zooplastic Tissue, Open Approach
- HAC When reported with secondary diagnosis code J98.51 or J98.59

0213088 Bypass Coronary Artery, Four or More Arteries from Right Internal Mammary with Zooplastic Tissue, Open Approach
- HAC When reported with secondary diagnosis code J98.51 or J98.59

0213089 Bypass Coronary Artery, Four or More Arteries from Left Internal Mammary with Zooplastic Tissue, Open Approach
- HAC When reported with secondary diagnosis code J98.51 or J98.59

021308C Bypass Coronary Artery, Four or More Arteries from Thoracic Artery with Zooplastic Tissue, Open Approach
- HAC When reported with secondary diagnosis code J98.51 or J98.59

021308F Bypass Coronary Artery, Four or More Arteries from Abdominal Artery with Zooplastic Tissue, Open Approach
- HAC When reported with secondary diagnosis code J98.51 or J98.59

021308W Bypass Coronary Artery, Four or More Arteries from Aorta with Zooplastic Tissue, Open Approach
- HAC When reported with secondary diagnosis code J98.51 or J98.59

0213093 Bypass Coronary Artery, Four or More Arteries from Coronary Artery with Autologous Venous Tissue, Open Approach
- HAC When reported with secondary diagnosis code J98.51 or J98.59

0213098 Bypass Coronary Artery, Four or More Arteries from Right Internal Mammary with Autologous Venous Tissue, Open Approach
- HAC When reported with secondary diagnosis code J98.51 or J98.59

0213099 Bypass Coronary Artery, Four or More Arteries from Left Internal Mammary with Autologous Venous Tissue, Open Approach
- HAC When reported with secondary diagnosis code J98.51 or J98.59

021309C Bypass Coronary Artery, Four or More Arteries from Thoracic Artery with Autologous Venous Tissue, Open Approach
- HAC When reported with secondary diagnosis code J98.51 or J98.59

021309F Bypass Coronary Artery, Four or More Arteries from Abdominal Artery with Autologous Venous Tissue, Open Approach
- HAC When reported with secondary diagnosis code J98.51 or J98.59

021309W Bypass Coronary Artery, Four or More Arteries from Aorta with Autologous Venous Tissue, Open Approach
- HAC When reported with secondary diagnosis code J98.51 or J98.59

02130A3 Bypass Coronary Artery, Four or More Arteries from Coronary Artery with Autologous Arterial Tissue, Open Approach
- HAC When reported with secondary diagnosis code J98.51 or J98.59

02130A8 Bypass Coronary Artery, Four or More Arteries from Right Internal Mammary with Autologous Arterial Tissue, Open Approach
- HAC When reported with secondary diagnosis code J98.51 or J98.59

02130A9 Bypass Coronary Artery, Four or More Arteries from Left Internal Mammary with Autologous Arterial Tissue, Open Approach
- HAC When reported with secondary diagnosis code J98.51 or J98.59

02130AC Bypass Coronary Artery, Four or More Arteries from Thoracic Artery with Autologous Arterial Tissue, Open Approach
- HAC When reported with secondary diagnosis code J98.51 or J98.59

02130AF Bypass Coronary Artery, Four or More Arteries from Abdominal Artery with Autologous Arterial Tissue, Open Approach
- HAC When reported with secondary diagnosis code J98.51 or J98.59

02130AW Bypass Coronary Artery, Four or More Arteries from Aorta with Autologous Arterial Tissue, Open Approach
- HAC When reported with secondary diagnosis code J98.51 or J98.59

02130J3 Bypass Coronary Artery, Four or More Arteries from Coronary Artery with Synthetic Substitute, Open Approach
- HAC When reported with secondary diagnosis code J98.51 or J98.59

02130J8 Bypass Coronary Artery, Four or More Arteries from Right Internal Mammary with Synthetic Substitute, Open Approach
- HAC When reported with secondary diagnosis code J98.51 or J98.59

02130J9 Bypass Coronary Artery, Four or More Arteries from Left Internal Mammary with Synthetic Substitute, Open Approach
- HAC When reported with secondary diagnosis code J98.51 or J98.59

02130JC Bypass Coronary Artery, Four or More Arteries from Thoracic Artery with Synthetic Substitute, Open Approach
- HAC When reported with secondary diagnosis code J98.51 or J98.59

02130JF Bypass Coronary Artery, Four or More Arteries from Abdominal Artery with Synthetic Substitute, Open Approach
- HAC When reported with secondary diagnosis code J98.51 or J98.59

02130JW Bypass Coronary Artery, Four or More Arteries from Aorta with Synthetic Substitute, Open Approach
- HAC When reported with secondary diagnosis code J98.51 or J98.59

02130K3 Bypass Coronary Artery, Four or More Arteries from Coronary Artery with Nonautologous Tissue Substitute, Open Approach
- HAC When reported with secondary diagnosis code J98.51 or J98.59

02130K8 Bypass Coronary Artery, Four or More Arteries from Right Internal Mammary with Nonautologous Tissue Substitute, Open Approach
- HAC When reported with secondary diagnosis code J98.51 or J98.59

02130K9 Bypass Coronary Artery, Four or More Arteries from Left Internal Mammary with Nonautologous Tissue Substitute, Open Approach
- HAC When reported with secondary diagnosis code J98.51 or J98.59

02130KC Bypass Coronary Artery, Four or More Arteries from Thoracic Artery with Nonautologous Tissue Substitute, Open Approach
- HAC When reported with secondary diagnosis code J98.51 or J98.59

02130KF Bypass Coronary Artery, Four or More Arteries from Abdominal Artery with Nonautologous Tissue Substitute, Open Approach
- HAC When reported with secondary diagnosis code J98.51 or J98.59

02130KW Bypass Coronary Artery, Four or More Arteries from Aorta with Nonautologous Tissue Substitute, Open Approach
- HAC When reported with secondary diagnosis code J98.51 or J98.59

02130Z3 Bypass Coronary Artery, Four or More Arteries from Coronary Artery, Open Approach
- HAC When reported with secondary diagnosis code J98.51 or J98.59

02130Z8 Bypass Coronary Artery, Four or More Arteries from Right Internal Mammary, Open Approach
- HAC When reported with secondary diagnosis code J98.51 or J98.59

02130Z9 Bypass Coronary Artery, Four or More Arteries from Left Internal Mammary, Open Approach
- HAC When reported with secondary diagnosis code J98.51 or J98.59

02130ZC Bypass Coronary Artery, Four or More Arteries from Thoracic Artery, Open Approach
- HAC When reported with secondary diagnosis code J98.51 or J98.59

02130ZF Bypass Coronary Artery, Four or More Arteries from Abdominal Artery, Open Approach
- HAC When reported with secondary diagnosis code J98.51 or J98.59

0213344 Bypass Coronary Artery, Four or More Arteries from Coronary Vein with Drug-eluting Intraluminal Device, Percutaneous Approach
- HAC When reported with secondary diagnosis code J98.51 or J98.59

02133D4 Bypass Coronary Artery, Four or More Arteries from Coronary Vein with Intraluminal Device, Percutaneous Approach
HAC When reported with secondary diagnosis code J98.51 or J98.59

0213444 Bypass Coronary Artery, Four or More Arteries from Coronary Vein with Drug-eluting Intraluminal Device, Percutaneous Endoscopic Approach
HAC When reported with secondary diagnosis code J98.51 or J98.59

0213483 Bypass Coronary Artery, Four or More Arteries from Coronary Artery with Zooplastic Tissue, Percutaneous Endoscopic Approach
HAC When reported with secondary diagnosis code J98.51 or J98.59

0213488 Bypass Coronary Artery, Four or More Arteries from Right Internal Mammary with Zooplastic Tissue, Percutaneous Endoscopic Approach
HAC When reported with secondary diagnosis code J98.51 or J98.59

0213489 Bypass Coronary Artery, Four or More Arteries from Left Internal Mammary with Zooplastic Tissue, Percutaneous Endoscopic Approach
HAC When reported with secondary diagnosis code J98.51 or J98.59

021348C Bypass Coronary Artery, Four or More Arteries from Thoracic Artery with Zooplastic Tissue, Percutaneous Endoscopic Approach
HAC When reported with secondary diagnosis code J98.51 or J98.59

021348F Bypass Coronary Artery, Four or More Arteries from Abdominal Artery with Zooplastic Tissue, Percutaneous Endoscopic Approach
HAC When reported with secondary diagnosis code J98.51 or J98.59

021348W Bypass Coronary Artery, Four or More Arteries from Aorta with Zooplastic Tissue, Percutaneous Endoscopic Approach
HAC When reported with secondary diagnosis code J98.51 or J98.59

0213493 Bypass Coronary Artery, Four or More Arteries from Coronary Artery with Autologous Venous Tissue, Percutaneous Endoscopic Approach
HAC When reported with secondary diagnosis code J98.51 or J98.59

0213498 Bypass Coronary Artery, Four or More Arteries from Right Internal Mammary with Autologous Venous Tissue, Percutaneous Endoscopic Approach
HAC When reported with secondary diagnosis code J98.51 or J98.59

0213499 Bypass Coronary Artery, Four or More Arteries from Left Internal Mammary with Autologous Venous Tissue, Percutaneous Endoscopic Approach
HAC When reported with secondary diagnosis code J98.51 or J98.59

021349C Bypass Coronary Artery, Four or More Arteries from Thoracic Artery with Autologous Venous Tissue, Percutaneous Endoscopic Approach
HAC When reported with secondary diagnosis code J98.51 or J98.59

021349F Bypass Coronary Artery, Four or More Arteries from Abdominal Artery with Autologous Venous Tissue, Percutaneous Endoscopic Approach
HAC When reported with secondary diagnosis code J98.51 or J98.59

021349W Bypass Coronary Artery, Four or More Arteries from Aorta with Autologous Venous Tissue, Percutaneous Endoscopic Approach
HAC When reported with secondary diagnosis code J98.51 or J98.59

02134A3 Bypass Coronary Artery, Four or More Arteries from Coronary Artery with Autologous Arterial Tissue, Percutaneous Endoscopic Approach
HAC When reported with secondary diagnosis code J98.51 or J98.59

02134A8 Bypass Coronary Artery, Four or More Arteries from Right Internal Mammary with Autologous Arterial Tissue, Percutaneous Endoscopic Approach
HAC When reported with secondary diagnosis code J98.51 or J98.59

02134A9 Bypass Coronary Artery, Four or More Arteries from Left Internal Mammary with Autologous Arterial Tissue, Percutaneous Endoscopic Approach
HAC When reported with secondary diagnosis code J98.51 or J98.59

02134AC Bypass Coronary Artery, Four or More Arteries from Thoracic Artery with Autologous Arterial Tissue, Percutaneous Endoscopic Approach
HAC When reported with secondary diagnosis code J98.51 or J98.59

02134AF Bypass Coronary Artery, Four or More Arteries from Abdominal Artery with Autologous Arterial Tissue, Percutaneous Endoscopic Approach
HAC When reported with secondary diagnosis code J98.51 or J98.59

02134AW Bypass Coronary Artery, Four or More Arteries from Aorta with Autologous Arterial Tissue, Percutaneous Endoscopic Approach
HAC When reported with secondary diagnosis code J98.51 or J98.59

02134D4 Bypass Coronary Artery, Four or More Arteries from Coronary Vein with Intraluminal Device, Percutaneous Endoscopic Approach
HAC When reported with secondary diagnosis code J98.51 or J98.59

02134J3 Bypass Coronary Artery, Four or More Arteries from Coronary Artery with Synthetic Substitute, Percutaneous Endoscopic Approach
HAC When reported with secondary diagnosis code J98.51 or J98.59

02134J8 Bypass Coronary Artery, Four or More Arteries from Right Internal Mammary with Synthetic Substitute, Percutaneous Endoscopic Approach
HAC When reported with secondary diagnosis code J98.51 or J98.59

02134J9 Bypass Coronary Artery, Four or More Arteries from Left Internal Mammary with Synthetic Substitute, Percutaneous Endoscopic Approach
HAC When reported with secondary diagnosis code J98.51 or J98.59

02134JC Bypass Coronary Artery, Four or More Arteries from Thoracic Artery with Synthetic Substitute, Percutaneous Endoscopic Approach
HAC When reported with secondary diagnosis code J98.51 or J98.59

02134JF Bypass Coronary Artery, Four or More Arteries from Abdominal Artery with Synthetic Substitute, Percutaneous Endoscopic Approach
HAC When reported with secondary diagnosis code J98.51 or J98.59

02134JW Bypass Coronary Artery, Four or More Arteries from Aorta with Synthetic Substitute, Percutaneous Endoscopic Approach
HAC When reported with secondary diagnosis code J98.51 or J98.59

02134K3 Bypass Coronary Artery, Four or More Arteries from Coronary Artery with Nonautologous Tissue Substitute, Percutaneous Endoscopic Approach
HAC When reported with secondary diagnosis code J98.51 or J98.59

02134K8 Bypass Coronary Artery, Four or More Arteries from Right Internal Mammary with Nonautologous Tissue Substitute, Percutaneous Endoscopic Approach
HAC When reported with secondary diagnosis code J98.51 or J98.59

02134K9 Bypass Coronary Artery, Four or More Arteries from Left Internal Mammary with Nonautologous Tissue Substitute, Percutaneous Endoscopic Approach
HAC When reported with secondary diagnosis code J98.51 or J98.59

02134KC Bypass Coronary Artery, Four or More Arteries from Thoracic Artery with Nonautologous Tissue Substitute, Percutaneous Endoscopic Approach
HAC When reported with secondary diagnosis code J98.51 or J98.59

02134KF Bypass Coronary Artery, Four or More Arteries from Abdominal Artery with Nonautologous Tissue Substitute, Percutaneous Endoscopic Approach
HAC When reported with secondary diagnosis code J98.51 or J98.59

02134KW Bypass Coronary Artery, Four or More Arteries from Aorta with Nonautologous Tissue Substitute, Percutaneous Endoscopic Approach
HAC When reported with secondary diagnosis code J98.51 or J98.59

02134Z3 Bypass Coronary Artery, Four or More Arteries from Coronary Artery, Percutaneous Endoscopic Approach
HAC When reported with secondary diagnosis code J98.51 or J98.59

02134Z8 Bypass Coronary Artery, Four or More Arteries from Right Internal Mammary, Percutaneous Endoscopic Approach
HAC When reported with secondary diagnosis code J98.51 or J98.59

02134Z9 Bypass Coronary Artery, Four or More Arteries from Left Internal Mammary, Percutaneous Endoscopic Approach
HAC When reported with secondary diagnosis code J98.51 or J98.59

02134ZC Bypass Coronary Artery, Four or More Arteries from Thoracic Artery, Percutaneous Endoscopic Approach
HAC When reported with secondary diagnosis code J98.51 or J98.59

♀ Female-only   ♂ Male-only   ▲ Limited Coverage   ● Non-OR   HAC HAC-associated procedure   ▲ Non-covered procedures   ✚ Cluster   185

Medical and Surgical, Heart and Great Vessels Code Listings

02134ZF Bypass Coronary Artery, Four or More Arteries from Abdominal Artery, Percutaneous Endoscopic Approach

[HAC] When reported with secondary diagnosis code J98.51 or J98.59

021608P Bypass Right Atrium to Pulmonary Trunk with Zooplastic Tissue, Open Approach

021608Q Bypass Right Atrium to Right Pulmonary Artery with Zooplastic Tissue, Open Approach

021608R Bypass Right Atrium to Left Pulmonary Artery with Zooplastic Tissue, Open Approach

021609P Bypass Right Atrium to Pulmonary Trunk with Autologous Venous Tissue, Open Approach

021609Q Bypass Right Atrium to Right Pulmonary Artery with Autologous Venous Tissue, Open Approach

021609R Bypass Right Atrium to Left Pulmonary Artery with Autologous Venous Tissue, Open Approach

02160AP Bypass Right Atrium to Pulmonary Trunk with Autologous Arterial Tissue, Open Approach

02160AQ Bypass Right Atrium to Right Pulmonary Artery with Autologous Arterial Tissue, Open Approach

02160AR Bypass Right Atrium to Left Pulmonary Artery with Autologous Arterial Tissue, Open Approach

02160JP Bypass Right Atrium to Pulmonary Trunk with Synthetic Substitute, Open Approach

02160JQ Bypass Right Atrium to Right Pulmonary Artery with Synthetic Substitute, Open Approach

AHA CC: 3Q, 2014, 29

02160JR Bypass Right Atrium to Left Pulmonary Artery with Synthetic Substitute, Open Approach

02160KP Bypass Right Atrium to Pulmonary Trunk with Nonautologous Tissue Substitute, Open Approach

02160KQ Bypass Right Atrium to Right Pulmonary Artery with Nonautologous Tissue Substitute, Open Approach

02160KR Bypass Right Atrium to Left Pulmonary Artery with Nonautologous Tissue Substitute, Open Approach

02160Z7 Bypass Right Atrium to Left Atrium, Open Approach

02160ZP Bypass Right Atrium to Pulmonary Trunk, Open Approach

02160ZQ Bypass Right Atrium to Right Pulmonary Artery, Open Approach

02160ZR Bypass Right Atrium to Left Pulmonary Artery, Open Approach

02163Z7 Bypass Right Atrium to Left Atrium, Percutaneous Approach

AHA CC: 4Q, 2017, 56

021648P Bypass Right Atrium to Pulmonary Trunk with Zooplastic Tissue, Percutaneous Endoscopic Approach

021648Q Bypass Right Atrium to Right Pulmonary Artery with Zooplastic Tissue, Percutaneous Endoscopic Approach

021648R Bypass Right Atrium to Left Pulmonary Artery with Zooplastic Tissue, Percutaneous Endoscopic Approach

021649P Bypass Right Atrium to Pulmonary Trunk with Autologous Venous Tissue, Percutaneous Endoscopic Approach

021649Q Bypass Right Atrium to Right Pulmonary Artery with Autologous Venous Tissue, Percutaneous Endoscopic Approach

021649R Bypass Right Atrium to Left Pulmonary Artery with Autologous Venous Tissue, Percutaneous Endoscopic Approach

02164AP Bypass Right Atrium to Pulmonary Trunk with Autologous Arterial Tissue, Percutaneous Endoscopic Approach

02164AQ Bypass Right Atrium to Right Pulmonary Artery with Autologous Arterial Tissue, Percutaneous Endoscopic Approach

02164AR Bypass Right Atrium to Left Pulmonary Artery with Autologous Arterial Tissue, Percutaneous Endoscopic Approach

02164JP Bypass Right Atrium to Pulmonary Trunk with Synthetic Substitute, Percutaneous Endoscopic Approach

02164JQ Bypass Right Atrium to Right Pulmonary Artery with Synthetic Substitute, Percutaneous Endoscopic Approach

02164JR Bypass Right Atrium to Left Pulmonary Artery with Synthetic Substitute, Percutaneous Endoscopic Approach

02164KP Bypass Right Atrium to Pulmonary Trunk with Nonautologous Tissue Substitute, Percutaneous Endoscopic Approach

02164KQ Bypass Right Atrium to Right Pulmonary Artery with Nonautologous Tissue Substitute, Percutaneous Endoscopic Approach

02164KR Bypass Right Atrium to Left Pulmonary Artery with Nonautologous Tissue Substitute, Percutaneous Endoscopic Approach

02164Z7 Bypass Right Atrium to Left Atrium, Percutaneous Endoscopic Approach

02164ZP Bypass Right Atrium to Pulmonary Trunk, Percutaneous Endoscopic Approach

02164ZQ Bypass Right Atrium to Right Pulmonary Artery, Percutaneous Endoscopic Approach

02164ZR Bypass Right Atrium to Left Pulmonary Artery, Percutaneous Endoscopic Approach

021708P Bypass Left Atrium to Pulmonary Trunk with Zooplastic Tissue, Open Approach

021708Q Bypass Left Atrium to Right Pulmonary Artery with Zooplastic Tissue, Open Approach

021708R Bypass Left Atrium to Left Pulmonary Artery with Zooplastic Tissue, Open Approach

021708S Bypass Left Atrium to Right Pulmonary Vein with Zooplastic Tissue, Open Approach

021708T Bypass Left Atrium to Left Pulmonary Vein with Zooplastic Tissue, Open Approach

021708U Bypass Left Atrium to Pulmonary Vein Confluence with Zooplastic Tissue, Open Approach

021709P Bypass Left Atrium to Pulmonary Trunk with Autologous Venous Tissue, Open Approach

021709Q Bypass Left Atrium to Right Pulmonary Artery with Autologous Venous Tissue, Open Approach

021709R Bypass Left Atrium to Left Pulmonary Artery with Autologous Venous Tissue, Open Approach

021709S Bypass Left Atrium to Right Pulmonary Vein with Autologous Venous Tissue, Open Approach

021709T Bypass Left Atrium to Left Pulmonary Vein with Autologous Venous Tissue, Open Approach

021709U Bypass Left Atrium to Pulmonary Vein Confluence with Autologous Venous Tissue, Open Approach

02170AP Bypass Left Atrium to Pulmonary Trunk with Autologous Arterial Tissue, Open Approach

02170AQ Bypass Left Atrium to Right Pulmonary Artery with Autologous Arterial Tissue, Open Approach

02170AR Bypass Left Atrium to Left Pulmonary Artery with Autologous Arterial Tissue, Open Approach

02170AS Bypass Left Atrium to Right Pulmonary Vein with Autologous Arterial Tissue, Open Approach

02170AT Bypass Left Atrium to Left Pulmonary Vein with Autologous Arterial Tissue, Open Approach

02170AU Bypass Left Atrium to Pulmonary Vein Confluence with Autologous Arterial Tissue, Open Approach

02170JP Bypass Left Atrium to Pulmonary Trunk with Synthetic Substitute, Open Approach

02170JQ Bypass Left Atrium to Right Pulmonary Artery with Synthetic Substitute, Open Approach

02170JR Bypass Left Atrium to Left Pulmonary Artery with Synthetic Substitute, Open Approach

02170JS Bypass Left Atrium to Right Pulmonary Vein with Synthetic Substitute, Open Approach

02170JT Bypass Left Atrium to Left Pulmonary Vein with Synthetic Substitute, Open Approach

02170JU Bypass Left Atrium to Pulmonary Vein Confluence with Synthetic Substitute, Open Approach

02170KP Bypass Left Atrium to Pulmonary Trunk with Nonautologous Tissue Substitute, Open Approach

02170KQ Bypass Left Atrium to Right Pulmonary Artery with Nonautologous Tissue Substitute, Open Approach

02170KR Bypass Left Atrium to Left Pulmonary Artery with Nonautologous Tissue Substitute, Open Approach

02170KS Bypass Left Atrium to Right Pulmonary Vein with Nonautologous Tissue Substitute, Open Approach

02170KT Bypass Left Atrium to Left Pulmonary Vein with Nonautologous Tissue Substitute, Open Approach

02170KU Bypass Left Atrium to Pulmonary Vein Confluence with Nonautologous Tissue Substitute, Open Approach

02170ZP Bypass Left Atrium to Pulmonary Trunk, Open Approach

02170ZQ Bypass Left Atrium to Right Pulmonary Artery, Open Approach

02170ZR Bypass Left Atrium to Left Pulmonary Artery, Open Approach

02170ZS Bypass Left Atrium to Right Pulmonary Vein, Open Approach

02170ZT Bypass Left Atrium to Left Pulmonary Vein, Open Approach

02170ZU Bypass Left Atrium to Pulmonary Vein Confluence, Open Approach

AHA CC: 4Q, 2016, 108-109

♀ Female-only   ♂ Male-only   ▲ Limited Coverage   ● Non-OR   [HAC] HAC-associated procedure   ▲ Non-covered procedures   ✚ Cluster

02173J6	Bypass Left Atrium to Right Atrium with Synthetic Substitute, Percutaneous Approach
	AHA CC: 4Q, 2020, 44-45
021748P	Bypass Left Atrium to Pulmonary Trunk with Zooplastic Tissue, Percutaneous Endoscopic Approach
021748Q	Bypass Left Atrium to Right Pulmonary Artery with Zooplastic Tissue, Percutaneous Endoscopic Approach
021748R	Bypass Left Atrium to Left Pulmonary Artery with Zooplastic Tissue, Percutaneous Endoscopic Approach
021748S	Bypass Left Atrium to Right Pulmonary Vein with Zooplastic Tissue, Percutaneous Endoscopic Approach
021748T	Bypass Left Atrium to Left Pulmonary Vein with Zooplastic Tissue, Percutaneous Endoscopic Approach
021748U	Bypass Left Atrium to Pulmonary Vein Confluence with Zooplastic Tissue, Percutaneous Endoscopic Approach
021749P	Bypass Left Atrium to Pulmonary Trunk with Autologous Venous Tissue, Percutaneous Endoscopic Approach
021749Q	Bypass Left Atrium to Right Pulmonary Artery with Autologous Venous Tissue, Percutaneous Endoscopic Approach
021749R	Bypass Left Atrium to Left Pulmonary Artery with Autologous Venous Tissue, Percutaneous Endoscopic Approach
021749S	Bypass Left Atrium to Right Pulmonary Vein with Autologous Venous Tissue, Percutaneous Endoscopic Approach
021749T	Bypass Left Atrium to Left Pulmonary Vein with Autologous Venous Tissue, Percutaneous Endoscopic Approach
021749U	Bypass Left Atrium to Pulmonary Vein Confluence with Autologous Venous Tissue, Percutaneous Endoscopic Approach
02174AP	Bypass Left Atrium to Pulmonary Trunk with Autologous Arterial Tissue, Percutaneous Endoscopic Approach
02174AQ	Bypass Left Atrium to Right Pulmonary Artery with Autologous Arterial Tissue, Percutaneous Endoscopic Approach
02174AR	Bypass Left Atrium to Left Pulmonary Artery with Autologous Arterial Tissue, Percutaneous Endoscopic Approach
02174AS	Bypass Left Atrium to Right Pulmonary Vein with Autologous Arterial Tissue, Percutaneous Endoscopic Approach
02174AT	Bypass Left Atrium to Left Pulmonary Vein with Autologous Arterial Tissue, Percutaneous Endoscopic Approach
02174AU	Bypass Left Atrium to Pulmonary Vein Confluence with Autologous Arterial Tissue, Percutaneous Endoscopic Approach
02174JP	Bypass Left Atrium to Pulmonary Trunk with Synthetic Substitute, Percutaneous Endoscopic Approach
02174JQ	Bypass Left Atrium to Right Pulmonary Artery with Synthetic Substitute, Percutaneous Endoscopic Approach
02174JR	Bypass Left Atrium to Left Pulmonary Artery with Synthetic Substitute, Percutaneous Endoscopic Approach
02174JS	Bypass Left Atrium to Right Pulmonary Vein with Synthetic Substitute, Percutaneous Endoscopic Approach
02174JT	Bypass Left Atrium to Left Pulmonary Vein with Synthetic Substitute, Percutaneous Endoscopic Approach

02174JU	Bypass Left Atrium to Pulmonary Vein Confluence with Synthetic Substitute, Percutaneous Endoscopic Approach
02174KP	Bypass Left Atrium to Pulmonary Trunk with Nonautologous Tissue Substitute, Percutaneous Endoscopic Approach
02174KQ	Bypass Left Atrium to Right Pulmonary Artery with Nonautologous Tissue Substitute, Percutaneous Endoscopic Approach
02174KR	Bypass Left Atrium to Left Pulmonary Artery with Nonautologous Tissue Substitute, Percutaneous Endoscopic Approach
02174KS	Bypass Left Atrium to Right Pulmonary Vein with Nonautologous Tissue Substitute, Percutaneous Endoscopic Approach
02174KT	Bypass Left Atrium to Left Pulmonary Vein with Nonautologous Tissue Substitute, Percutaneous Endoscopic Approach
02174KU	Bypass Left Atrium to Pulmonary Vein Confluence with Nonautologous Tissue Substitute, Percutaneous Endoscopic Approach
02174ZP	Bypass Left Atrium to Pulmonary Trunk, Percutaneous Endoscopic Approach
02174ZQ	Bypass Left Atrium to Right Pulmonary Artery, Percutaneous Endoscopic Approach
02174ZR	Bypass Left Atrium to Left Pulmonary Artery, Percutaneous Endoscopic Approach
02174ZS	Bypass Left Atrium to Right Pulmonary Vein, Percutaneous Endoscopic Approach
02174ZT	Bypass Left Atrium to Left Pulmonary Vein, Percutaneous Endoscopic Approach
02174ZU	Bypass Left Atrium to Pulmonary Vein Confluence, Percutaneous Endoscopic Approach
021K08P	Bypass Right Ventricle to Pulmonary Trunk with Zooplastic Tissue, Open Approach
021K08Q	Bypass Right Ventricle to Right Pulmonary Artery with Zooplastic Tissue, Open Approach
021K08R	Bypass Right Ventricle to Left Pulmonary Artery with Zooplastic Tissue, Open Approach
021K09P	Bypass Right Ventricle to Pulmonary Trunk with Autologous Venous Tissue, Open Approach
021K09Q	Bypass Right Ventricle to Right Pulmonary Artery with Autologous Venous Tissue, Open Approach
021K09R	Bypass Right Ventricle to Left Pulmonary Artery with Autologous Venous Tissue, Open Approach
021K0AP	Bypass Right Ventricle to Pulmonary Trunk with Autologous Arterial Tissue, Open Approach
021K0AQ	Bypass Right Ventricle to Right Pulmonary Artery with Autologous Arterial Tissue, Open Approach
021K0AR	Bypass Right Ventricle to Left Pulmonary Artery with Autologous Arterial Tissue, Open Approach
021K0JP	Bypass Right Ventricle to Pulmonary Trunk with Synthetic Substitute, Open Approach
	AHA CC: 1Q, 2017, 19-20; 1Q, 2020, 24-25

021K0JQ	Bypass Right Ventricle to Right Pulmonary Artery with Synthetic Substitute, Open Approach
	AHA CC: 3Q, 2014, 30
021K0JR	Bypass Right Ventricle to Left Pulmonary Artery with Synthetic Substitute, Open Approach
021K0KP	Bypass Right Ventricle to Pulmonary Trunk with Nonautologous Tissue Substitute, Open Approach
	AHA CC: 3Q, 2015, 16-17; 4Q, 2015, 22-23, 25
021K0KQ	Bypass Right Ventricle to Right Pulmonary Artery with Nonautologous Tissue Substitute, Open Approach
021K0KR	Bypass Right Ventricle to Left Pulmonary Artery with Nonautologous Tissue Substitute, Open Approach
021K0Z5	Bypass Right Ventricle to Coronary Circulation, Open Approach
021K0Z8	Bypass Right Ventricle to Right Internal Mammary, Open Approach
021K0Z9	Bypass Right Ventricle to Left Internal Mammary, Open Approach
021K0ZC	Bypass Right Ventricle to Thoracic Artery, Open Approach
021K0ZF	Bypass Right Ventricle to Abdominal Artery, Open Approach
021K0ZP	Bypass Right Ventricle to Pulmonary Trunk, Open Approach
021K0ZQ	Bypass Right Ventricle to Right Pulmonary Artery, Open Approach
021K0ZR	Bypass Right Ventricle to Left Pulmonary Artery, Open Approach
021K0ZW	Bypass Right Ventricle to Aorta, Open Approach
021K48P	Bypass Right Ventricle to Pulmonary Trunk with Zooplastic Tissue, Percutaneous Endoscopic Approach
021K48Q	Bypass Right Ventricle to Right Pulmonary Artery with Zooplastic Tissue, Percutaneous Endoscopic Approach
021K48R	Bypass Right Ventricle to Left Pulmonary Artery with Zooplastic Tissue, Percutaneous Endoscopic Approach
021K49P	Bypass Right Ventricle to Pulmonary Trunk with Autologous Venous Tissue, Percutaneous Endoscopic Approach
021K49Q	Bypass Right Ventricle to Right Pulmonary Artery with Autologous Venous Tissue, Percutaneous Endoscopic Approach
021K49R	Bypass Right Ventricle to Left Pulmonary Artery with Autologous Venous Tissue, Percutaneous Endoscopic Approach
021K4AP	Bypass Right Ventricle to Pulmonary Trunk with Autologous Arterial Tissue, Percutaneous Endoscopic Approach
021K4AQ	Bypass Right Ventricle to Right Pulmonary Artery with Autologous Arterial Tissue, Percutaneous Endoscopic Approach
021K4AR	Bypass Right Ventricle to Left Pulmonary Artery with Autologous Arterial Tissue, Percutaneous Endoscopic Approach
021K4JP	Bypass Right Ventricle to Pulmonary Trunk with Synthetic Substitute, Percutaneous Endoscopic Approach
021K4JQ	Bypass Right Ventricle to Right Pulmonary Artery with Synthetic Substitute, Percutaneous Endoscopic Approach

---

♀ Female-only   ♂ Male-only   ▲ Limited Coverage   ● Non-OR   ⬛ HAC-associated procedure   ▲ Non-covered procedures   ✚ Cluster

021K4JR Bypass Right Ventricle to Left Pulmonary Artery with Synthetic Substitute, Percutaneous Endoscopic Approach

021K4KP Bypass Right Ventricle to Pulmonary Trunk with Nonautologous Tissue Substitute, Percutaneous Endoscopic Approach

021K4KQ Bypass Right Ventricle to Right Pulmonary Artery with Nonautologous Tissue Substitute, Percutaneous Endoscopic Approach

021K4KR Bypass Right Ventricle to Left Pulmonary Artery with Nonautologous Tissue Substitute, Percutaneous Endoscopic Approach

021K4Z5 Bypass Right Ventricle to Coronary Circulation, Percutaneous Endoscopic Approach

021K4Z8 Bypass Right Ventricle to Right Internal Mammary, Percutaneous Endoscopic Approach

021K4Z9 Bypass Right Ventricle to Left Internal Mammary, Percutaneous Endoscopic Approach

021K4ZC Bypass Right Ventricle to Thoracic Artery, Percutaneous Endoscopic Approach

021K4ZF Bypass Right Ventricle to Abdominal Artery, Percutaneous Endoscopic Approach

021K4ZP Bypass Right Ventricle to Pulmonary Trunk, Percutaneous Endoscopic Approach

021K4ZQ Bypass Right Ventricle to Right Pulmonary Artery, Percutaneous Endoscopic Approach

021K4ZR Bypass Right Ventricle to Left Pulmonary Artery, Percutaneous Endoscopic Approach

021K4ZW Bypass Right Ventricle to Aorta, Percutaneous Endoscopic Approach

021L08P Bypass Left Ventricle to Pulmonary Trunk with Zooplastic Tissue, Open Approach

021L08Q Bypass Left Ventricle to Right Pulmonary Artery with Zooplastic Tissue, Open Approach

021L08R Bypass Left Ventricle to Left Pulmonary Artery with Zooplastic Tissue, Open Approach

021L09P Bypass Left Ventricle to Pulmonary Trunk with Autologous Venous Tissue, Open Approach

021L09Q Bypass Left Ventricle to Right Pulmonary Artery with Autologous Venous Tissue, Open Approach

021L09R Bypass Left Ventricle to Left Pulmonary Artery with Autologous Venous Tissue, Open Approach

021L0AP Bypass Left Ventricle to Pulmonary Trunk with Autologous Arterial Tissue, Open Approach

021L0AQ Bypass Left Ventricle to Right Pulmonary Artery with Autologous Arterial Tissue, Open Approach

021L0AR Bypass Left Ventricle to Left Pulmonary Artery with Autologous Arterial Tissue, Open Approach

021L0JP Bypass Left Ventricle to Pulmonary Trunk with Synthetic Substitute, Open Approach

021L0JQ Bypass Left Ventricle to Right Pulmonary Artery with Synthetic Substitute, Open Approach

021L0JR Bypass Left Ventricle to Left Pulmonary Artery with Synthetic Substitute, Open Approach

021L0KP Bypass Left Ventricle to Pulmonary Trunk with Nonautologous Tissue Substitute, Open Approach

021L0KQ Bypass Left Ventricle to Right Pulmonary Artery with Nonautologous Tissue Substitute, Open Approach

021L0KR Bypass Left Ventricle to Left Pulmonary Artery with Nonautologous Tissue Substitute, Open Approach

021L0Z5 Bypass Left Ventricle to Coronary Circulation, Open Approach

021L0Z8 Bypass Left Ventricle to Right Internal Mammary, Open Approach

021L0Z9 Bypass Left Ventricle to Left Internal Mammary, Open Approach

021L0ZC Bypass Left Ventricle to Thoracic Artery, Open Approach

021L0ZF Bypass Left Ventricle to Abdominal Artery, Open Approach

021L0ZP Bypass Left Ventricle to Pulmonary Trunk, Open Approach

021L0ZQ Bypass Left Ventricle to Right Pulmonary Artery, Open Approach

021L0ZR Bypass Left Ventricle to Left Pulmonary Artery, Open Approach

021L0ZW Bypass Left Ventricle to Aorta, Open Approach

021L48P Bypass Left Ventricle to Pulmonary Trunk with Zooplastic Tissue, Percutaneous Endoscopic Approach

021L48Q Bypass Left Ventricle to Right Pulmonary Artery with Zooplastic Tissue, Percutaneous Endoscopic Approach

021L48R Bypass Left Ventricle to Left Pulmonary Artery with Zooplastic Tissue, Percutaneous Endoscopic Approach

021L49P Bypass Left Ventricle to Pulmonary Trunk with Autologous Venous Tissue, Percutaneous Endoscopic Approach

021L49Q Bypass Left Ventricle to Right Pulmonary Artery with Autologous Venous Tissue, Percutaneous Endoscopic Approach

021L49R Bypass Left Ventricle to Left Pulmonary Artery with Autologous Venous Tissue, Percutaneous Endoscopic Approach

021L4AP Bypass Left Ventricle to Pulmonary Trunk with Autologous Arterial Tissue, Percutaneous Endoscopic Approach

021L4AQ Bypass Left Ventricle to Right Pulmonary Artery with Autologous Arterial Tissue, Percutaneous Endoscopic Approach

021L4AR Bypass Left Ventricle to Left Pulmonary Artery with Autologous Arterial Tissue, Percutaneous Endoscopic Approach

021L4JP Bypass Left Ventricle to Pulmonary Trunk with Synthetic Substitute, Percutaneous Endoscopic Approach

021L4JQ Bypass Left Ventricle to Right Pulmonary Artery with Synthetic Substitute, Percutaneous Endoscopic Approach

021L4JR Bypass Left Ventricle to Left Pulmonary Artery with Synthetic Substitute, Percutaneous Endoscopic Approach

021L4KP Bypass Left Ventricle to Pulmonary Trunk with Nonautologous Tissue Substitute, Percutaneous Endoscopic Approach

021L4KQ Bypass Left Ventricle to Right Pulmonary Artery with Nonautologous Tissue Substitute, Percutaneous Endoscopic Approach

021L4KR Bypass Left Ventricle to Left Pulmonary Artery with Nonautologous Tissue Substitute, Percutaneous Endoscopic Approach

021L4Z5 Bypass Left Ventricle to Coronary Circulation, Percutaneous Endoscopic Approach

021L4Z8 Bypass Left Ventricle to Right Internal Mammary, Percutaneous Endoscopic Approach

021L4Z9 Bypass Left Ventricle to Left Internal Mammary, Percutaneous Endoscopic Approach

021L4ZC Bypass Left Ventricle to Thoracic Artery, Percutaneous Endoscopic Approach

021L4ZF Bypass Left Ventricle to Abdominal Artery, Percutaneous Endoscopic Approach

021L4ZP Bypass Left Ventricle to Pulmonary Trunk, Percutaneous Endoscopic Approach

021L4ZQ Bypass Left Ventricle to Right Pulmonary Artery, Percutaneous Endoscopic Approach

021L4ZR Bypass Left Ventricle to Left Pulmonary Artery, Percutaneous Endoscopic Approach

021L4ZW Bypass Left Ventricle to Aorta, Percutaneous Endoscopic Approach

021P08A Bypass Pulmonary Trunk from Innominate Artery with Zooplastic Tissue, Open Approach

021P08B Bypass Pulmonary Trunk from Subclavian with Zooplastic Tissue, Open Approach

021P08D Bypass Pulmonary Trunk from Carotid with Zooplastic Tissue, Open Approach

021P09A Bypass Pulmonary Trunk from Innominate Artery with Autologous Venous Tissue, Open Approach

021P09B Bypass Pulmonary Trunk from Subclavian with Autologous Venous Tissue, Open Approach

021P09D Bypass Pulmonary Trunk from Carotid with Autologous Venous Tissue, Open Approach

021P0AA Bypass Pulmonary Trunk from Innominate Artery with Autologous Arterial Tissue, Open Approach

021P0AB Bypass Pulmonary Trunk from Subclavian with Autologous Arterial Tissue, Open Approach

021P0AD Bypass Pulmonary Trunk from Carotid with Autologous Arterial Tissue, Open Approach

021P0JA Bypass Pulmonary Trunk from Innominate Artery with Synthetic Substitute, Open Approach

021P0JB Bypass Pulmonary Trunk from Subclavian with Synthetic Substitute, Open Approach

021P0JD Bypass Pulmonary Trunk from Carotid with Synthetic Substitute, Open Approach

021P0KA Bypass Pulmonary Trunk from Innominate Artery with Nonautologous Tissue Substitute, Open Approach

021P0KB Bypass Pulmonary Trunk from Subclavian with Nonautologous Tissue Substitute, Open Approach

021P0KD Bypass Pulmonary Trunk from Carotid with Nonautologous Tissue Substitute, Open Approach

021P0ZA Bypass Pulmonary Trunk from Innominate Artery with No Device, Open Approach

021P0ZB Bypass Pulmonary Trunk from Subclavian with No Device, Open Approach

021P0ZD Bypass Pulmonary Trunk from Carotid with No Device, Open Approach

021P48A Bypass Pulmonary Trunk from Innominate Artery with Zooplastic Tissue, Percutaneous Endoscopic Approach

021P48B Bypass Pulmonary Trunk from Subclavian with Zooplastic Tissue, Percutaneous Endoscopic Approach

021P48D Bypass Pulmonary Trunk from Carotid with Zooplastic Tissue, Percutaneous Endoscopic Approach

021P49A Bypass Pulmonary Trunk from Innominate Artery with Autologous Venous Tissue, Percutaneous Endoscopic Approach

021P49B Bypass Pulmonary Trunk from Subclavian with Autologous Venous Tissue, Percutaneous Endoscopic Approach

021P49D Bypass Pulmonary Trunk from Carotid with Autologous Venous Tissue, Percutaneous Endoscopic Approach

021P4AA Bypass Pulmonary Trunk from Innominate Artery with Autologous Arterial Tissue, Percutaneous Endoscopic Approach

021P4AB Bypass Pulmonary Trunk from Subclavian with Autologous Arterial Tissue, Percutaneous Endoscopic Approach

021P4AD Bypass Pulmonary Trunk from Carotid with Autologous Arterial Tissue, Percutaneous Endoscopic Approach

021P4JA Bypass Pulmonary Trunk from Innominate Artery with Synthetic Substitute, Percutaneous Endoscopic Approach

021P4JB Bypass Pulmonary Trunk from Subclavian with Synthetic Substitute, Percutaneous Endoscopic Approach

021P4JD Bypass Pulmonary Trunk from Carotid with Synthetic Substitute, Percutaneous Endoscopic Approach

021P4KA Bypass Pulmonary Trunk from Innominate Artery with Nonautologous Tissue Substitute, Percutaneos Endoscopic Approach

021P4KB Bypass Pulmonary Trunk from Subclavian with Nonautologous Tissue Substitute, Percutaneous Endoscopic Approach

021P4KD Bypass Pulmonary Trunk from Carotid with Nonautologous Tissue Substitute, Percutaneous Endoscopic Approach

021P4ZA Bypass Pulmonary Trunk from Innominate Artery with No Device, Percutaneous Endoscopic Approach

021P4ZB Bypass Pulmonary Trunk from Subclavian with No Device, Percutaneous Endoscopic Approach

021P4ZD Bypass Pulmonary Trunk from Carotid with No Device, Percutaneous Endoscopic Approach

021Q08A Bypass Right Pulmonary Artery from Innominate Artery with Zooplastic Tissue, Open Approach

021Q08B Bypass Right Pulmonary Artery from Subclavian with Zooplastic Tissue, Open Approach

021Q08D Bypass Right Pulmonary Artery from Carotid with Zooplastic Tissue, Open Approach

021Q09A Bypass Right Pulmonary Artery from Innominate Artery with Autologous Venous Tissue, Open Approach

021Q09B Bypass Right Pulmonary Artery from Subclavian with Autologous Venous Tissue, Open Approach

021Q09D Bypass Right Pulmonary Artery from Carotid with Autologous Venous Tissue, Open Approach

021Q0AA Bypass Right Pulmonary Artery from Innominate Artery with Autologous Arterial Tissue, Open Approach

021Q0AB Bypass Right Pulmonary Artery from Subclavian with Autologous Arterial Tissue, Open Approach

021Q0AD Bypass Right Pulmonary Artery from Carotid with Autologous Arterial Tissue, Open Approach

021Q0JA Bypass Right Pulmonary Artery from Innominate Artery with Synthetic Substitute, Open Approach

021Q0JB Bypass Right Pulmonary Artery from Subclavian with Synthetic Substitute, Open Approach

021Q0JD Bypass Right Pulmonary Artery from Carotid with Synthetic Substitute, Open Approach

021Q0KA Bypass Right Pulmonary Artery from Innominate Artery with Nonautologous Tissue Substitute, Open Approach

021Q0KB Bypass Right Pulmonary Artery from Subclavian with Nonautologous Tissue Substitute, Open Approach

021Q0KD Bypass Right Pulmonary Artery from Carotid with Nonautologous Tissue Substitute, Open Approach

021Q0ZA Bypass Right Pulmonary Artery from Innominate Artery with No Device, Open Approach

021Q0ZB Bypass Right Pulmonary Artery from Subclavian with No Device, Open Approach

021Q0ZD Bypass Right Pulmonary Artery from Carotid with No Device, Open Approach

021Q48A Bypass Right Pulmonary Artery from Innominate Artery with Zooplastic Tissue, Percutaneous Endoscopic Approach

021Q48B Bypass Right Pulmonary Artery from Subclavian with Zooplastic Tissue, Percutaneous Endoscopic Approach

021Q48D Bypass Right Pulmonary Artery from Carotid with Zooplastic Tissue, Percutaneous Endoscopic Approach

021Q49A Bypass Right Pulmonary Artery from Innominate Artery with Autologous Venous Tissue, Percutaneous Endoscopic Approach

021Q49B Bypass Right Pulmonary Artery from Subclavian with Autologous Venous Tissue, Percutaneous Endoscopic Approach

021Q49D Bypass Right Pulmonary Artery from Carotid with Autologous Venous Tissue, Percutaneous Endoscopic Approach

021Q4AA Bypass Right Pulmonary Artery from Innominate Artery with Autologous Arterial Tissue, Percutaneous Endoscopic Approach

021Q4AB Bypass Right Pulmonary Artery from Subclavian with Autologous Arterial Tissue, Percutaneous Endoscopic Approach

021Q4AD Bypass Right Pulmonary Artery from Carotid with Autologous Arterial Tissue, Percutaneous Endoscopic Approach

021Q4JA Bypass Right Pulmonary Artery from Innominate Artery with Synthetic Substitute, Percutaneous Endoscopic Approach

021Q4JB Bypass Right Pulmonary Artery from Subclavian with Synthetic Substitute, Percutaneous Endoscopic Approach

021Q4JD Bypass Right Pulmonary Artery from Carotid with Synthetic Substitute, Percutaneous Endoscopic Approach

021Q4KA Bypass Right Pulmonary Artery from Innominate Artery with Nonautologous Tissue Substitute, Percutaneous Endoscopic Approach

021Q4KB Bypass Right Pulmonary Artery from Subclavian with Nonautologous Tissue Substitute, Percutaneous Endoscopic Approach

021Q4KD Bypass Right Pulmonary Artery from Carotid with Nonautologous Tissue Substitute, Percutaneous Endoscopic Approach

021Q4ZA Bypass Right Pulmonary Artery from Innominate Artery with No Device, Percutaneous Endoscopic Approach

021Q4ZB Bypass Right Pulmonary Artery from Subclavian with No Device, Percutaneous Endoscopic Approach

021Q4ZD Bypass Right Pulmonary Artery from Carotid with No Device, Percutaneous Endoscopic Approach

021R08A Bypass Left Pulmonary Artery from Innominate Artery with Zooplastic Tissue, Open Approach

021R08B Bypass Left Pulmonary Artery from Subclavian with Zooplastic Tissue, Open Approach

021R08D Bypass Left Pulmonary Artery from Carotid with Zooplastic Tissue, Open Approach

021R09A Bypass Left Pulmonary Artery from Innominate Artery with Autologous Venous Tissue, Open Approach

021R09B Bypass Left Pulmonary Artery from Subclavian with Autologous Venous Tissue, Open Approach

021R09D Bypass Left Pulmonary Artery from Carotid with Autologous Venous Tissue, Open Approach

021R0AA Bypass Left Pulmonary Artery from Innominate Artery with Autologous Arterial Tissue, Open Approach

021R0AB Bypass Left Pulmonary Artery from Subclavian with Autologous Arterial Tissue, Open Approach

021R0AD Bypass Left Pulmonary Artery from Carotid with Autologous Arterial Tissue, Open Approach

021R0JA Bypass Left Pulmonary Artery from Innominate Artery with Synthetic Substitute, Open Approach

---

♀ Female-only   ♂ Male-only   ▲ Limited Coverage   ● Non-OR   🅗🅐🅒 HAC-associated procedure   ▲ Non-covered procedures   ✚ Cluster

021R0JB Bypass Left Pulmonary Artery from Subclavian with Synthetic Substitute, Open Approach

021R0JD Bypass Left Pulmonary Artery from Carotid with Synthetic Substitute, Open Approach

021R0KA Bypass Left Pulmonary Artery from Innominate Artery with Nonautologous Tissue Substitute, Open Approach

021R0KB Bypass Left Pulmonary Artery from Subclavian with Nonautologous Tissue Substitute, Open Approach

021R0KD Bypass Left Pulmonary Artery from Carotid with Nonautologous Tissue Substitute, Open Approach

021R0ZA Bypass Left Pulmonary Artery from Innominate Artery with No Device, Open Approach

021R0ZB Bypass Left Pulmonary Artery from Subclavian with No Device, Open Approach

021R0ZD Bypass Left Pulmonary Artery from Carotid with No Device, Open Approach

021R48A Bypass Left Pulmonary Artery from Innominate Artery with Zooplastic Tissue, Percutaneous Endoscopic Approach

021R48B Bypass Left Pulmonary Artery from Subclavian with Zooplastic Tissue, Percutaneous Endoscopic Approach

021R48D Bypass Left Pulmonary Artery from Carotid with Zooplastic Tissue, Percutaneous Endoscopic Approach

021R49A Bypass Left Pulmonary Artery from Innominate Artery with Autologous Venous Tissue, Percutaneous Endoscopic Approach

021R49B Bypass Left Pulmonary Artery from Subclavian with Autologous Venous Tissue, Percutaneous Endoscopic Approach

021R49D Bypass Left Pulmonary Artery from Carotid with Autologous Venous Tissue, Percutaneous Endoscopic Approach

021R4AA Bypass Left Pulmonary Artery from Innominate Artery with Autologous Arterial Tissue, Percutaneous Endoscopic Approach

021R4AB Bypass Left Pulmonary Artery from Subclavian with Autologous Arterial Tissue, Percutaneous Endoscopic Approach

021R4AD Bypass Left Pulmonary Artery from Carotid with Autologous Arterial Tissue, Percutaneous Endoscopic Approach

021R4JA Bypass Left Pulmonary Artery from Innominate Artery with Synthetic Substitute, Percutaneous Endoscopic Approach

021R4JB Bypass Left Pulmonary Artery from Subclavian with Synthetic Substitute, Percutaneous Endoscopic Approach

021R4JD Bypass Left Pulmonary Artery from Carotid with Synthetic Substitute, Percutaneous Endoscopic Approach

021R4KA Bypass Left Pulmonary Artery from Innominate Artery with Nonautologous Tissue Substitute, Percutaneous Endoscopic Approach

021R4KB Bypass Left Pulmonary Artery from Subclavian with Nonautologous Tissue Substitute, Percutaneous Endoscopic Approach

021R4KD Bypass Left Pulmonary Artery from Carotid with Nonautologous Tissue Substitute, Percutaneous Endoscopic Approach

021R4ZA Bypass Left Pulmonary Artery from Innominate Artery with No Device, Percutaneous Endoscopic Approach

021R4ZB Bypass Left Pulmonary Artery from Subclavian with No Device, Percutaneous Endoscopic Approach

021R4ZD Bypass Left Pulmonary Artery from Carotid with No Device, Percutaneous Endoscopic Approach

021V08P Bypass Superior Vena Cava to Pulmonary Trunk with Zooplastic Tissue, Open Approach

021V08Q Bypass Superior Vena Cava to Right Pulmonary Artery with Zooplastic Tissue, Open Approach

021V08R Bypass Superior Vena Cava to Left Pulmonary Artery with Zooplastic Tissue, Open Approach

021V08S Bypass Superior Vena Cava to Right Pulmonary Vein with Zooplastic Tissue, Open Approach
AHA CC: 4Q, 2016, 145

021V08T Bypass Superior Vena Cava to Left Pulmonary Vein with Zooplastic Tissue, Open Approach

021V08U Bypass Superior Vena Cava to Pulmonary Vein Confluence with Zooplastic Tissue, Open Approach

021V09P Bypass Superior Vena Cava to Pulmonary Trunk with Autologous Venous Tissue, Open Approach

021V09Q Bypass Superior Vena Cava to Right Pulmonary Artery with Autologous Venous Tissue, Open Approach

021V09R Bypass Superior Vena Cava to Left Pulmonary Artery with Autologous Venous Tissue, Open Approach

021V09S Bypass Superior Vena Cava to Right Pulmonary Vein with Autologous Venous Tissue, Open Approach
AHA CC: 4Q, 2016, 144

021V09T Bypass Superior Vena Cava to Left Pulmonary Vein with Autologous Venous Tissue, Open Approach

021V09U Bypass Superior Vena Cava to Pulmonary Vein Confluence with Autologous Venous Tissue, Open Approach

021V0AP Bypass Superior Vena Cava to Pulmonary Trunk with Autologous Arterial Tissue, Open Approach

021V0AQ Bypass Superior Vena Cava to Right Pulmonary Artery with Autologous Arterial Tissue, Open Approach

021V0AR Bypass Superior Vena Cava to Left Pulmonary Artery with Autologous Arterial Tissue, Open Approach

021V0AS Bypass Superior Vena Cava to Right Pulmonary Vein with Autologous Arterial Tissue, Open Approach

021V0AT Bypass Superior Vena Cava to Left Pulmonary Vein with Autologous Arterial Tissue, Open Approach

021V0AU Bypass Superior Vena Cava to Pulmonary Vein Confluence with Autologous Arterial Tissue, Open Approach

021V0JP Bypass Superior Vena Cava to Pulmonary Trunk with Synthetic Substitute, Open Approach

021V0JQ Bypass Superior Vena Cava to Right Pulmonary Artery with Synthetic Substitute, Open Approach

021V0JR Bypass Superior Vena Cava to Left Pulmonary Artery with Synthetic Substitute, Open Approach

021V0JS Bypass Superior Vena Cava to Right Pulmonary Vein with Synthetic Substitute, Open Approach

021V0JT Bypass Superior Vena Cava to Left Pulmonary Vein with Synthetic Substitute, Open Approach

021V0JU Bypass Superior Vena Cava to Pulmonary Vein Confluence with Synthetic Substitute, Open Approach

021V0KP Bypass Superior Vena Cava to Pulmonary Trunk with Nonautologous Tissue Substitute, Open Approach

021V0KQ Bypass Superior Vena Cava to Right Pulmonary Artery with Nonautologous Tissue Substitute, Open Approach

021V0KR Bypass Superior Vena Cava to Left Pulmonary Artery with Nonautologous Tissue Substitute, Open Approach

021V0KS Bypass Superior Vena Cava to Right Pulmonary Vein with Nonautologous Tissue Substitute, Open Approach

021V0KT Bypass Superior Vena Cava to Left Pulmonary Vein with Nonautologous Tissue Substitute, Open Approach

021V0KU Bypass Superior Vena Cava to Pulmonary Vein Confluence with Nonautologous Tissue Substitute, Open Approach

021V0ZP Bypass Superior Vena Cava to Pulmonary Trunk, Open Approach

021V0ZQ Bypass Superior Vena Cava to Right Pulmonary Artery, Open Approach

021V0ZR Bypass Superior Vena Cava to Left Pulmonary Artery, Open Approach

021V0ZS Bypass Superior Vena Cava to Right Pulmonary Vein, Open Approach

021V0ZT Bypass Superior Vena Cava to Left Pulmonary Vein, Open Approach

021V0ZU Bypass Superior Vena Cava to Pulmonary Vein Confluence, Open Approach

021V48P Bypass Superior Vena Cava to Pulmonary Trunk with Zooplastic Tissue, Percutaneous Endoscopic Approach

021V48Q Bypass Superior Vena Cava to Right Pulmonary Artery with Zooplastic Tissue, Percutaneous Endoscopic Approach

021V48R Bypass Superior Vena Cava to Left Pulmonary Artery with Zooplastic Tissue, Percutaneous Endoscopic Approach

021V48S Bypass Superior Vena Cava to Right Pulmonary Vein with Zooplastic Tissue, Percutaneous Endoscopic Approach

021V48T Bypass Superior Vena Cava to Left Pulmonary Vein with Zooplastic Tissue, Percutaneous Endoscopic Approach

021V48U Bypass Superior Vena Cava to Pulmonary Vein Confluence with Zooplastic Tissue, Percutaneous Endoscopic Approach

021V49P Bypass Superior Vena Cava to Pulmonary Trunk with Autologous Venous Tissue, Percutaneous Endoscopic Approach

♀ Female-only   ♂ Male-only   ▲ Limited Coverage   ● Non-OR   ▨ HAC-associated procedure   ▲ Non-covered procedures   ✚ Cluster

021V49Q Bypass Superior Vena Cava to Right Pulmonary Artery with Autologous Venous Tissue, Percutaneous Endoscopic Approach

021V49R Bypass Superior Vena Cava to Left Pulmonary Artery with Autologous Venous Tissue, Percutaneous Endoscopic Approach

021V49S Bypass Superior Vena Cava to Right Pulmonary Vein with Autologous Venous Tissue, Percutaneous Endoscopic Approach

021V49T Bypass Superior Vena Cava to Left Pulmonary Vein with Autologous Venous Tissue, Percutaneous Endoscopic Approach

021V49U Bypass Superior Vena Cava to Pulmonary Vein Confluence with Autologous Venous Tissue, Percutaneous Endoscopic Approach

021V4AP Bypass Superior Vena Cava to Pulmonary Trunk with Autologous Arterial Tissue, Percutaneous Endoscopic Approach

021V4AQ Bypass Superior Vena Cava to Right Pulmonary Artery with Autologous Arterial Tissue, Percutaneous Endoscopic Approach

021V4AR Bypass Superior Vena Cava to Left Pulmonary Artery with Autologous Arterial Tissue, Percutaneous Endoscopic Approach

021V4AS Bypass Superior Vena Cava to Right Pulmonary Vein with Autologous Arterial Tissue, Percutaneous Endoscopic Approach

021V4AT Bypass Superior Vena Cava to Left Pulmonary Vein with Autologous Arterial Tissue, Percutaneous Endoscopic Approach

021V4AU Bypass Superior Vena Cava to Pulmonary Vein Confluence with Autologous Arterial Tissue, Percutaneous Endoscopic Approach

021V4JP Bypass Superior Vena Cava to Pulmonary Trunk with Synthetic Substitute, Percutaneous Endoscopic Approach

021V4JQ Bypass Superior Vena Cava to Right Pulmonary Artery with Synthetic Substitute, Percutaneous Endoscopic Approach

021V4JR Bypass Superior Vena Cava to Left Pulmonary Artery with Synthetic Substitute, Percutaneous Endoscopic Approach

021V4JS Bypass Superior Vena Cava to Right Pulmonary Vein with Synthetic Substitute, Percutaneous Endoscopic Approach

021V4JT Bypass Superior Vena Cava to Left Pulmonary Vein with Synthetic Substitute, Percutaneous Endoscopic Approach

021V4JU Bypass Superior Vena Cava to Pulmonary Vein Confluence with Synthetic Substitute, Percutaneous Endoscopic Approach

021V4KP Bypass Superior Vena Cava to Pulmonary Trunk with Nonautologous Tissue Substitute, Percutaneous Endoscopic Approach

021V4KQ Bypass Superior Vena Cava to Right Pulmonary Artery with Nonautologous Tissue Substitute, Percutaneous Endoscopic Approach

021V4KR Bypass Superior Vena Cava to Left Pulmonary Artery with Nonautologous Tissue Substitute, Percutaneous Endoscopic Approach

021V4KS Bypass Superior Vena Cava to Right Pulmonary Vein with Nonautologous Tissue Substitute, Percutaneous Endoscopic Approach

021V4KT Bypass Superior Vena Cava to Left Pulmonary Vein with Nonautologous Tissue Substitute, Percutaneous Endoscopic Approach

021V4KU Bypass Superior Vena Cava to Pulmonary Vein Confluence with Nonautologous Tissue Substitute, Percutaneous Endoscopic Approach

021V4ZP Bypass Superior Vena Cava to Pulmonary Trunk, Percutaneous Endoscopic Approach

021V4ZQ Bypass Superior Vena Cava to Right Pulmonary Artery, Percutaneous Endoscopic Approach

021V4ZR Bypass Superior Vena Cava to Left Pulmonary Artery, Percutaneous Endoscopic Approach

021V4ZS Bypass Superior Vena Cava to Right Pulmonary Vein, Percutaneous Endoscopic Approach

021V4ZT Bypass Superior Vena Cava to Left Pulmonary Vein, Percutaneous Endoscopic Approach

021V4ZU Bypass Superior Vena Cava to Pulmonary Vein Confluence, Percutaneous Endoscopic Approach

021W08A Bypass Thoracic Aorta, Descending to Innominate Artery with Zooplastic Tissue, Open Approach

021W08B Bypass Thoracic Aorta, Descending to Subclavian with Zooplastic Tissue, Open Approach

021W08D Bypass Thoracic Aorta, Descending to Carotid with Zooplastic Tissue, Open Approach

021W08F Bypass Thoracic Aorta, Descending to Abdominal Artery with Zooplastic Tissue, Open Approach

021W08G Bypass Thoracic Aorta, Descending to Axillary Artery with Zooplastic Tissue, Open Approach

021W08H Bypass Thoracic Aorta, Descending to Brachial Artery with Zooplastic Tissue, Open Approach

021W08P Bypass Thoracic Aorta, Descending to Pulmonary Trunk with Zooplastic Tissue, Open Approach

021W08Q Bypass Thoracic Aorta, Descending to Right Pulmonary Artery with Zooplastic Tissue, Open Approach

021W08R Bypass Thoracic Aorta, Descending to Left Pulmonary Artery with Zooplastic Tissue, Open Approach

021W08V Bypass Thoracic Aorta, Descending to Lower Extremity Artery with Zooplastic Tissue, Open Approach

021W09A Bypass Thoracic Aorta, Descending to Innominate Artery with Autologous Venous Tissue, Open Approach

021W09B Bypass Thoracic Aorta, Descending to Subclavian with Autologous Venous Tissue, Open Approach

021W09D Bypass Thoracic Aorta, Descending to Carotid with Autologous Venous Tissue, Open Approach

021W09F Bypass Thoracic Aorta, Descending to Abdominal Artery with Autologous Venous Tissue, Open Approach

021W09G Bypass Thoracic Aorta, Descending to Axillary Artery with Autologous Venous Tissue, Open Approach

021W09H Bypass Thoracic Aorta, Descending to Brachial Artery with Autologous Venous Tissue, Open Approach

021W09P Bypass Thoracic Aorta, Descending to Pulmonary Trunk with Autologous Venous Tissue, Open Approach

021W09Q Bypass Thoracic Aorta, Descending to Right Pulmonary Artery with Autologous Venous Tissue, Open Approach

021W09R Bypass Thoracic Aorta, Descending to Left Pulmonary Artery with Autologous Venous Tissue, Open Approach

021W09V Bypass Thoracic Aorta, Descending to Lower Extremity Artery with Autologous Venous Tissue, Open Approach

021W0AA Bypass Thoracic Aorta, Descending to Innominate Artery with Autologous Arterial Tissue, Open Approach

021W0AB Bypass Thoracic Aorta, Descending to Subclavian with Autologous Arterial Tissue, Open Approach

021W0AD Bypass Thoracic Aorta, Descending to Carotid with Autologous Arterial Tissue, Open Approach

021W0AF Bypass Thoracic Aorta, Descending to Abdominal Artery with Autologous Arterial Tissue, Open Approach

021W0AG Bypass Thoracic Aorta, Descending to Axillary Artery with Autologous Arterial Tissue, Open Approach

021W0AH Bypass Thoracic Aorta, Descending to Brachial Artery with Autologous Arterial Tissue, Open Approach

021W0AP Bypass Thoracic Aorta, Descending to Pulmonary Trunk with Autologous Arterial Tissue, Open Approach

021W0AQ Bypass Thoracic Aorta, Descending to Right Pulmonary Artery with Autologous Arterial Tissue, Open Approach

021W0AR Bypass Thoracic Aorta, Descending to Left Pulmonary Artery with Autologous Arterial Tissue, Open Approach

021W0AV Bypass Thoracic Aorta, Descending to Lower Extremity Artery with Autologous Arterial Tissue, Open Approach

021W0JA Bypass Thoracic Aorta, Descending to Innominate Artery with Synthetic Substitute, Open Approach

021W0JB Bypass Thoracic Aorta, Descending to Subclavian with Synthetic Substitute, Open Approach

021W0JD Bypass Thoracic Aorta, Descending to Carotid with Synthetic Substitute, Open Approach

021W0JF Bypass Thoracic Aorta, Descending to Abdominal Artery with Synthetic Substitute, Open Approach

021W0JG Bypass Thoracic Aorta, Descending to Axillary Artery with Synthetic Substitute, Open Approach

021W0JH Bypass Thoracic Aorta, Descending to Brachial Artery with Synthetic Substitute, Open Approach

021W0JP Bypass Thoracic Aorta, Descending to Pulmonary Trunk with Synthetic Substitute, Open Approach

021W0JQ Bypass Thoracic Aorta, Descending to Right Pulmonary Artery with Synthetic Substitute, Open Approach
AHA CC: 3Q, 2014, 3

021W0JR Bypass Thoracic Aorta, Descending to Left Pulmonary Artery with Synthetic Substitute, Open Approach

021W0JV Bypass Thoracic Aorta, Descending to Lower Extremity Artery with Synthetic Substitute, Open Approach
AHA CC: 4Q, 2018, 46

021W0KA Bypass Thoracic Aorta, Descending to Innominate Artery with Nonautologous Tissue Substitute, Open Approach

021W0KB Bypass Thoracic Aorta, Descending to Subclavian with Nonautologous Tissue Substitute, Open Approach

021W0KD Bypass Thoracic Aorta, Descending to Carotid with Nonautologous Tissue Substitute, Open Approach

021W0KF Bypass Thoracic Aorta, Descending to Abdominal Artery with Nonautologous Tissue Substitute, Open Approach

021W0KG Bypass Thoracic Aorta, Descending to Axillary Artery with Nonautologous Tissue Substitute, Open Approach

021W0KH Bypass Thoracic Aorta, Descending to Brachial Artery with Nonautologous Tissue Substitute, Open Approach

021W0KP Bypass Thoracic Aorta, Descending to Pulmonary Trunk with Nonautologous Tissue Substitute, Open Approach

021W0KQ Bypass Thoracic Aorta, Descending to Right Pulmonary Artery with Nonautologous Tissue Substitute, Open Approach

021W0KR Bypass Thoracic Aorta, Descending to Left Pulmonary Artery with Nonautologous Tissue Substitute, Open Approach

021W0KV Bypass Thoracic Aorta, Descending to Lower Extremity Artery with Nonautologous Tissue Substitute, Open Approach

021W0ZA Bypass Thoracic Aorta, Descending to Innominate Artery, Open Approach

021W0ZB Bypass Thoracic Aorta, Descending to Subclavian, Open Approach

021W0ZD Bypass Thoracic Aorta, Descending to Carotid, Open Approach

021W0ZP Bypass Thoracic Aorta, Descending to Pulmonary Trunk, Open Approach

021W0ZQ Bypass Thoracic Aorta, Descending to Right Pulmonary Artery, Open Approach

021W0ZR Bypass Thoracic Aorta, Descending to Left Pulmonary Artery, Open Approach

021W48A Bypass Thoracic Aorta, Descending to Innominate Artery with Zooplastic Tissue, Percutaneous Endoscopic Approach

021W48B Bypass Thoracic Aorta, Descending to Subclavian with Zooplastic Tissue, Percutaneous Endoscopic Approach

021W48D Bypass Thoracic Aorta, Descending to Carotid with Zooplastic Tissue, Percutaneous Endoscopic Approach

021W48P Bypass Thoracic Aorta, Descending to Pulmonary Trunk with Zooplastic Tissue, Percutaneous Endoscopic Approach

021W48Q Bypass Thoracic Aorta, Descending to Right Pulmonary Artery with Zooplastic Tissue, Percutaneous Endoscopic Approach

021W48R Bypass Thoracic Aorta, Descending to Left Pulmonary Artery with Zooplastic Tissue, Percutaneous Endoscopic Approach

021W49A Bypass Thoracic Aorta, Descending to Innominate Artery with Autologous Venous Tissue, Percutaneous Endoscopic Approach

021W49B Bypass Thoracic Aorta, Descending to Subclavian with Autologous Venous Tissue, Percutaneous Endoscopic Approach

021W49D Bypass Thoracic Aorta, Descending to Carotid with Autologous Venous Tissue, Percutaneous Endoscopic Approach

021W49P Bypass Thoracic Aorta, Descending to Pulmonary Trunk with Autologous Venous Tissue, Percutaneous Endoscopic Approach

021W49Q Bypass Thoracic Aorta, Descending to Right Pulmonary Artery with Autologous Venous Tissue, Percutaneous Endoscopic Approach

021W49R Bypass Thoracic Aorta, Descending to Left Pulmonary Artery with Autologous Venous Tissue, Percutaneous Endoscopic Approach

021W4AA Bypass Thoracic Aorta, Descending to Innominate Artery with Autologous Arterial Tissue, Percutaneous Endoscopic Approach

021W4AB Bypass Thoracic Aorta, Descending to Subclavian with Autologous Arterial Tissue, Percutaneous Endoscopic Approach

021W4AD Bypass Thoracic Aorta , Descending to Carotid with Autologous Arterial Tissue, Percutaneous Endoscopic Approach

021W4AP Bypass Thoracic Aorta, Descending to Pulmonary Trunk with Autologous Arterial Tissue, Percutaneous Endoscopic Approach

021W4AQ Bypass Thoracic Aorta, Descending to Right Pulmonary Artery with Autologous Arterial Tissue, Percutaneous Endoscopic Approach

021W4AR Bypass Thoracic Aorta, Descending to Left Pulmonary Artery with Autologous Arterial Tissue, Percutaneous Endoscopic Approach

021W4JA Bypass Thoracic Aorta, Descending to Innominate Artery with Synthetic Substitute, Percutaneous Endoscopic Approach

021W4JB Bypass Thoracic Aorta, Descending to Subclavian with Synthetic Substitute, Percutaneous Endoscopic Approach

021W4JD Bypass Thoracic Aorta, Descending to Carotid with Synthetic Substitute, Percutaneous Endoscopic Approach

021W4JP Bypass Thoracic Aorta, Descending to Pulmonary Trunk with Synthetic Substitute, Percutaneous Endoscopic Approach

021W4JQ Bypass Thoracic Aorta, Descending to Right Pulmonary Artery with Synthetic Substitute, Percutaneous Endoscopic Approach

021W4JR Bypass Thoracic Aorta, Descending to Left Pulmonary Artery with Synthetic Substitute, Percutaneous Endoscopic Approach

021W4KA Bypass Thoracic Aorta, Descending to Innominate Artery with Nonautologous Tissue Substitute, Percutaneous Endoscopic Approach

021W4KB Bypass Thoracic Aorta, Descending to Subclavian with Nonautologous Tissue Substitute, Percutaneous Endoscopic Approach

021W4KD Bypass Thoracic Aorta, Descending to Carotid with Nonautologous Tissue Substitute, Percutaneous Endoscopic Approach

021W4KP Bypass Thoracic Aorta, Descending to Pulmonary Trunk with Nonautologous Tissue Substitute, Percutaneous Endoscopic Approach

021W4KQ Bypass Thoracic Aorta, Descending to Right Pulmonary Artery with Nonautologous Tissue Substitute, Percutaneous Endoscopic Approach

021W4KR Bypass Thoracic Aorta, Descending to Left Pulmonary Artery with Nonautologous Tissue Substitute, Percutaneous Endoscopic Approach

021W4ZA Bypass Thoracic Aorta, Descending to Innominate Artery, Percutaneous Endoscopic Approach

021W4ZB Bypass Thoracic Aorta, Descending to Subclavian, Percutaneous Endoscopic Approach

021W4ZD Bypass Thoracic Aorta, Descending to Carotid, Percutaneous Endoscopic Approach

021W4ZP Bypass Thoracic Aorta, Descending to Pulmonary Trunk, Percutaneous Endoscopic Approach

021W4ZQ Bypass Thoracic Aorta, Descending to Right Pulmonary Artery, Percutaneous Endoscopic Approach

021W4ZR Bypass Thoracic Aorta, Descending to Left Pulmonary Artery, Percutaneous Endoscopic Approach

021X08A Bypass Thoracic Aorta, Ascending/Arch to Innominate Artery with Zooplastic Tissue, Open Approach

021X08B Bypass Thoracic Aorta, Ascending/Arch to Subclavian with Zooplastic Tissue, Open Approach

021X08D Bypass Thoracic Aorta, Ascending/Arch to Carotid with Zooplastic Tissue, Open Approach

021X08P Bypass Thoracic Aorta, Ascending/Arch to Pulmonary Trunk with Zooplastic Tissue, Open Approach

021X08Q Bypass Thoracic Aorta, Ascending/Arch to Right Pulmonary Artery with Zooplastic Tissue, Open Approach

021X08R Bypass Thoracic Aorta, Ascending/Arch to Left Pulmonary Artery with Zooplastic Tissue, Open Approach

021X09A Bypass Thoracic Aorta, Ascending/Arch to Innominate Artery with Autologous Venous Tissue, Open Approach

021X09B Bypass Thoracic Aorta, Ascending/Arch to Subclavian with Autologous Venous Tissue, Open Approach

021X09D Bypass Thoracic Aorta, Ascending/Arch to Carotid with Autologous Venous Tissue, Open Approach

021X09P Bypass Thoracic Aorta, Ascending/Arch to Pulmonary Trunk with Autologous Venous Tissue, Open Approach

021X09Q Bypass Thoracic Aorta, Ascending/Arch to Right Pulmonary Artery with Autologous Venous Tissue, Open Approach

021X09R Bypass Thoracic Aorta, Ascending/Arch to Left Pulmonary Artery with Autologous Venous Tissue, Open Approach

021X0AA Bypass Thoracic Aorta, Ascending/Arch to Innominate Artery with Autologous Arterial Tissue, Open Approach

021X0AB Bypass Thoracic Aorta, Ascending/ Arch to Subclavian with Autologous Arterial Tissue, Open Approach

021X0AD Bypass Thoracic Aorta, Ascending/ Arch to Carotid with Autologous Arterial Tissue, Open Approach

021X0AP Bypass Thoracic Aorta, Ascending/Arch to Pulmonary Trunk with Autologous Arterial Tissue, Open Approach

021X0AQ Bypass Thoracic Aorta, Ascending/ Arch to Right Pulmonary Artery with Autologous Arterial Tissue, Open Approach

021X0AR Bypass Thoracic Aorta, Ascending/Arch to Left Pulmonary Artery with Autologous Arterial Tissue, Open Approach

021X0JA Bypass Thoracic Aorta, Ascending/ Arch to Innominate Artery with Synthetic Substitute, Open Approach
AHA CC: 3Q, 2019, 30-31; 4Q, 2019, 23; 1Q, 2020, 37

021X0JB Bypass Thoracic Aorta, Ascending/ Arch to Subclavian with Synthetic Substitute, Open Approach

021X0JD Bypass Thoracic Aorta, Ascending/ Arch to Carotid with Synthetic Substitute, Open Approach
AHA CC: 3Q, 2019, 30-31

021X0JP Bypass Thoracic Aorta, Ascending/ Arch to Pulmonary Trunk with Synthetic Substitute, Open Approach

021X0JQ Bypass Thoracic Aorta, Ascending/ Arch to Right Pulmonary Artery with Synthetic Substitute, Open Approach

021X0JR Bypass Thoracic Aorta, Ascending/ Arch to Left Pulmonary Artery with Synthetic Substitute, Open Approach

021X0KA Bypass Thoracic Aorta, Ascending/ Arch to Innominate Artery with Nonautologous Tissue Substitute, Open Approach

021X0KB Bypass Thoracic Aorta, Ascending/ Arch to Subclavian with Nonautologous Tissue Substitute, Open Approach

021X0KD Bypass Thoracic Aorta, Ascending/ Arch to Carotid with Nonautologous Tissue Substitute, Open Approach

021X0KP Bypass Thoracic Aorta, Ascending/ Arch to Pulmonary Trunk with Nonautologous Tissue Substitute, Open Approach

021X0KQ Bypass Thoracic Aorta, Ascending/ Arch to Right Pulmonary Artery with Nonautologous Tissue Substitute, Open Approach

021X0KR Bypass Thoracic Aorta, Ascending/ Arch to Left Pulmonary Artery with Nonautologous Tissue Substitute, Open Approach

021X0ZA Bypass Thoracic Aorta, Ascending/Arch to Innominate Artery, Open Approach

021X0ZB Bypass Thoracic Aorta, Ascending/ Arch to Subclavian, Open Approach

021X0ZD Bypass Thoracic Aorta, Ascending/ Arch to Carotid, Open Approach

021X0ZP Bypass Thoracic Aorta, Ascending/ Arch to Pulmonary Trunk, Open Approach

021X0ZQ Bypass Thoracic Aorta, Ascending/Arch to Right Pulmonary Artery, Open Approach

021X0ZR Bypass Thoracic Aorta, Ascending/ Arch to Left Pulmonary Artery, Open Approach

021X48A Bypass Thoracic Aorta, Ascending/ Arch to Innominate Artery with Zooplastic Tissue, Percutaneous Endoscopic Approach

021X48B Bypass Thoracic Aorta, Ascending/ Arch to Subclavian with Zooplastic Tissue, Percutaneous Endoscopic Approach

021X48D Bypass Thoracic Aorta, Ascending/ Arch to Carotid with Zooplastic Tissue, Percutaneous Endoscopic Approach

021X48P Bypass Thoracic Aorta, Ascending/Arch to Pulmonary Trunk with Zooplastic Tissue, Percutaneous Endoscopic Approach

021X48Q Bypass Thoracic Aorta, Ascending/ Arch to Right Pulmonary Artery with Zooplastic Tissue, Percutaneous Endoscopic Approach

021X48R Bypass Thoracic Aorta, Ascending/ Arch to Left Pulmonary Artery with Zooplastic Tissue, Percutaneous Endoscopic Approach

021X49A Bypass Thoracic Aorta, Ascending/ Arch to Innominate Artery with Autologous Venous Tissue, Percutaneous Endoscopic Approach

021X49B Bypass Thoracic Aorta, Ascending/ Arch to Subclavian with Autologous Venous Tissue, Percutaneous Endoscopic Approach

021X49D Bypass Thoracic Aorta, Ascending/ Arch to Carotid with Autologous Venous Tissue, Percutaneous Endoscopic Approach

021X49P Bypass Thoracic Aorta, Ascending/ Arch to Pulmonary Trunk with Autologous Venous Tissue, Percutaneous Endoscopic Approach

021X49Q Bypass Thoracic Aorta, Ascending/ Arch to Right Pulmonary Artery with Autologous Venous Tissue, Percutaneous Endoscopic Approach

021X49R Bypass Thoracic Aorta, Ascending/ Arch to Left Pulmonary Artery with Autologous Venous Tissue, Percutaneous Endoscopic Approach

021X4AA Bypass Thoracic Aorta, Ascending/ Arch to Innominate Artery with Autologous Arterial Tissue, Percutaneous Endoscopic Approach

021X4AB Bypass Thoracic Aorta, Ascending/ Arch to Subclavian with Autologous Arterial Tissue, Percutaneous Endoscopic Approach

021X4AD Bypass Thoracic Aorta, Ascending/ Arch to Carotid with Autologous Arterial Tissue, Percutaneous Endoscopic Approach

021X4AP Bypass Thoracic Aorta, Ascending/ Arch to Pulmonary Trunk with Autologous Arterial Tissue, Percutaneous Endoscopic Approach

021X4AQ Bypass Thoracic Aorta, Ascending/ Arch to Right Pulmonary Artery with Autologous Arterial Tissue, Percutaneous Endoscopic Approach

021X4AR Bypass Thoracic Aorta, Ascending/ Arch to Left Pulmonary Artery with Autologous Arterial Tissue, Percutaneous Endoscopic Approach

021X4JA Bypass Thoracic Aorta, Ascending/ Arch to Innominate Artery with Synthetic Substitute, Percutaneous Endoscopic Approach

021X4JB Bypass Thoracic Aorta, Ascending/ Arch to Subclavian with Synthetic Substitute, Percutaneous Endoscopic Approach

021X4JD Bypass Thoracic Aorta, Ascending/ Arch to Carotid with Synthetic Substitute, Percutaneous Endoscopic Approach

021X4JP Bypass Thoracic Aorta, Ascending/ Arch to Pulmonary Trunk with Synthetic Substitute, Percutaneous Endoscopic Approach

021X4JQ Bypass Thoracic Aorta, Ascending/ Arch to Right Pulmonary Artery with Synthetic Substitute, Percutaneous Endoscopic Approach

021X4JR Bypass Thoracic Aorta, Ascending/ Arch to Left Pulmonary Artery with Synthetic Substitute, Percutaneous Endoscopic Approach

021X4KA Bypass Thoracic Aorta, Ascending/ Arch to Innominate Artery with Nonautologous Tissue Substitute, Percutaneous Endoscopic Approach

021X4KB Bypass Thoracic Aorta, Ascending/ Arch to Subclavian with Nonautologous

021X4KD Bypass Thoracic Aorta, Ascending/ Arch to Carotid with Nonautologous Tissue Substitute, Percutaneous Endoscopic Approach

021X4KP Bypass Thoracic Aorta, Ascending/ Arch to Pulmonary Trunk with Nonautologous Tissue Substitute, Percutaneous Endoscopic Approach

021X4KQ Bypass Thoracic Aorta, Ascending/ Arch to Right Pulmonary Artery with Nonautologous Tissue Substitute, Percutaneous Endoscopic Approach

021X4KR Bypass Thoracic Aorta, Ascending/ Arch to Left Pulmonary Artery with Nonautologous Tissue Substitute, Percutaneous Endoscopic Approach

021X4ZA Bypass Thoracic Aorta, Ascending/ Arch to Innominate Artery, Percutaneous Endoscopic Approach

021X4ZB Bypass Thoracic Aorta, Ascending/ Arch to Subclavian, Percutaneous Endoscopic Approach

021X4ZD Bypass Thoracic Aorta, Ascending/ Arch to Carotid, Percutaneous Endoscopic Approach

021X4ZP Bypass Thoracic Aorta, Ascending/ Arch to Pulmonary Trunk, Percutaneous Endoscopic Approach

021X4ZQ Bypass Thoracic Aorta, Ascending/ Arch to Right Pulmonary Artery, Percutaneous Endoscopic Approach

021X4ZR Bypass Thoracic Aorta, Ascending/ Arch to Left Pulmonary Artery, Percutaneous Endoscopic Approach

024 – Heart and Great Vessels, Creation

024F07J Creation of Aortic Valve from Truncal Valve using Autologous Tissue Substitute, Open Approach

024F08J Creation of Aortic Valve from Truncal Valve using Zooplastic Tissue, Open Approach

024F0JJ Creation of Aortic Valve from Truncal Valve using Synthetic Substitute, Open Approach

024F0KJ Creation of Aortic Valve from Truncal Valve using Nonautologous Tissue Substitute, Open Approach	**024G0J2** Creation of Mitral Valve from Common Atrioventricular Valve using Synthetic Substitute, Open Approach	**024J082** Creation of Tricuspid Valve from Common Atrioventricular Valve using Zooplastic Tissue, Open Approach
024G072 Creation of Mitral Valve from Common Atrioventricular Valve using Autologous Tissue Substitute, Open Approach	**024G0K2** Creation of Mitral Valve from Common Atrioventricular Valve using Nonautologous Tissue Substitute, Open Approach	**024J0J2** Creation of Tricuspid Valve from Common Atrioventricular Valve using Synthetic Substitute, Open Approach
024G082 Creation of Mitral Valve from Common Atrioventricular Valve using Zooplastic Tissue, Open Approach	**024J072** Creation of Tricuspid Valve from Common Atrioventricular Valve using Autologous Tissue Substitute, Open Approach	**024J0K2** Creation of Tricuspid Valve from Common Atrioventricular Valve using Nonautologous Tissue Substitute, Open Approach

025 – Heart and Great Vessels, Destruction

02540ZZ Destruction of Coronary Vein, Open Approach	**025D4ZZ** Destruction of Papillary Muscle, Percutaneous Endoscopic Approach	**025P0ZZ** Destruction of Pulmonary Trunk, Open Approach
02543ZZ Destruction of Coronary Vein, Percutaneous Approach	**025F0ZZ** Destruction of Aortic Valve, Open Approach	**025P3ZZ** Destruction of Pulmonary Trunk, Percutaneous Approach
02544ZZ Destruction of Coronary Vein, Percutaneous Endoscopic Approach	**025F3ZZ** Destruction of Aortic Valve, Percutaneous Approach	**025P4ZZ** Destruction of Pulmonary Trunk, Percutaneous Endoscopic Approach
02550ZZ Destruction of Atrial Septum, Open Approach	**025F4ZZ** Destruction of Aortic Valve, Percutaneous Endoscopic Approach	**025Q0ZZ** Destruction of Right Pulmonary Artery, Open Approach
02553ZZ Destruction of Atrial Septum, Percutaneous Approach	**025G0ZZ** Destruction of Mitral Valve, Open Approach	**025Q3ZZ** Destruction of Right Pulmonary Artery, Percutaneous Approach
02554ZZ Destruction of Atrial Septum, Percutaneous Endoscopic Approach	**025G3ZZ** Destruction of Mitral Valve, Percutaneous Approach	**025Q4ZZ** Destruction of Right Pulmonary Artery, Percutaneous Endoscopic Approach
02560ZZ Destruction of Right Atrium, Open Approach	**025G4ZZ** Destruction of Mitral Valve, Percutaneous Endoscopic Approach	**025R0ZZ** Destruction of Left Pulmonary Artery, Open Approach
02563ZZ Destruction of Right Atrium, Percutaneous Approach	**025H0ZZ** Destruction of Pulmonary Valve, Open Approach	**025R3ZZ** Destruction of Left Pulmonary Artery, Percutaneous Approach
02564ZZ Destruction of Right Atrium, Percutaneous Endoscopic Approach	**025H3ZZ** Destruction of Pulmonary Valve, Percutaneous Approach	**025R4ZZ** Destruction of Left Pulmonary Artery, Percutaneous Endoscopic Approach
●**02570ZK** Destruction of Left Atrial Appendage, Open Approach *AHA CC: 3Q, 2014, 20-21*	**025H4ZZ** Destruction of Pulmonary Valve, Percutaneous Endoscopic Approach	**025S0ZZ** Destruction of Right Pulmonary Vein, Open Approach
02570ZZ Destruction of Left Atrium, Open Approach	**025J0ZZ** Destruction of Tricuspid Valve, Open Approach	**025S3ZZ** Destruction of Right Pulmonary Vein, Percutaneous Approach
●**02573ZK** Destruction of Left Atrial Appendage, Percutaneous Approach	**025J3ZZ** Destruction of Tricuspid Valve, Percutaneous Approach	**025S4ZZ** Destruction of Right Pulmonary Vein, Percutaneous Endoscopic Approach
02573ZZ Destruction of Left Atrium, Percutaneous Approach	**025J4ZZ** Destruction of Tricuspid Valve, Percutaneous Endoscopic Approach	**025T0ZZ** Destruction of Left Pulmonary Vein, Open Approach
●**02574ZK** Destruction of Left Atrial Appendage, Percutaneous Endoscopic Approach	**025K0ZZ** Destruction of Right Ventricle, Open Approach	**025T3ZZ** Destruction of Left Pulmonary Vein, Percutaneous Approach
02574ZZ Destruction of Left Atrium, Percutaneous Endoscopic Approach	**025K3ZZ** Destruction of Right Ventricle, Percutaneous Approach	**025T4ZZ** Destruction of Left Pulmonary Vein, Percutaneous Endoscopic Approach
02580ZZ Destruction of Conduction Mechanism, Open Approach *AHA CC: 3Q, 2016, 44*	**025K4ZZ** Destruction of Right Ventricle, Percutaneous Endoscopic Approach	**025V0ZZ** Destruction of Superior Vena Cava, Open Approach
02583ZZ Destruction of Conduction Mechanism, Percutaneous Approach *AHA CC: 3Q, 2014, 19; 4Q, 2014, 47-48;* *3Q, 2016, 43-44; 1Q, 2020, 32-33*	**025L0ZZ** Destruction of Left Ventricle, Open Approach	**025V3ZZ** Destruction of Superior Vena Cava, Percutaneous Approach
	025L3ZZ Destruction of Left Ventricle, Percutaneous Approach	**025V4ZZ** Destruction of Superior Vena Cava, Percutaneous Endoscopic Approach
02584ZZ Destruction of Conduction Mechanism, Percutaneous Endoscopic Approach *AHA CC: 1Q, 2020, 32-33*	**025L4ZZ** Destruction of Left Ventricle, Percutaneous Endoscopic Approach	**025W0ZZ** Destruction of Thoracic Aorta, Descending, Open Approach
02590ZZ Destruction of Chordae Tendineae, Open Approach	**025M0ZZ** Destruction of Ventricular Septum, Open Approach	**025W3ZZ** Destruction of Thoracic Aorta, Descending, Percutaneous Approach
02593ZZ Destruction of Chordae Tendineae, Percutaneous Approach	**025M3ZZ** Destruction of Ventricular Septum, Percutaneous Approach *AHA CC: 3Q, 2018, 27*	**025W4ZZ** Destruction of Thoracic Aorta, Descending, Percutaneous Endoscopic Approach
02594ZZ Destruction of Chordae Tendineae, Percutaneous Endoscopic Approach	**025M4ZZ** Destruction of Ventricular Septum, Percutaneous Endoscopic Approach	**025X0ZZ** Destruction of Thoracic Aorta, Ascending/Arch, Open Approach
025D0ZZ Destruction of Papillary Muscle, Open Approach	**025N0ZZ** Destruction of Pericardium, Open Approach *AHA CC: 2Q, 2016, 17-18*	**025X3ZZ** Destruction of Thoracic Aorta, Ascending/Arch, Percutaneous Approach
025D3ZZ Destruction of Papillary Muscle, Percutaneous Approach	**025N3ZZ** Destruction of Pericardium, Percutaneous Approach	**025X4ZZ** Destruction of Thoracic Aorta, Ascending/Arch, Percutaneous Endoscopic Approach
	025N4ZZ Destruction of Pericardium, Percutaneous Endoscopic Approach	

027 – Heart and Great Vessels, Dilation

For Dilation procedures involving the coronary arteries, Review Coding Guideline B4.4

0270046 Dilation of Coronary Artery, One Artery, Bifurcation, with Drug-eluting Intraluminal Device, Open Approach	**0270056** Dilation of Coronary Artery, One Artery, Bifurcation, with Two Drug-eluting Intraluminal Devices, Open Approach	**0270066** Dilation of Coronary Artery, One Artery, Bifurcation, with Three Drug-eluting Intraluminal Devices, Open Approach
027004Z Dilation of Coronary Artery, One Artery with Drug-eluting Intraluminal Device, Open Approach	**027005Z** Dilation of Coronary Artery, One Artery with Two Drug-eluting Intraluminal Devices, Open Approach	**027006Z** Dilation of Coronary Artery, One Artery with Three Drug-eluting Intraluminal Devices, Open Approach

♀ Female-only   ♂ Male-only   ▲ Limited Coverage   ● Non-OR   HAC HAC-associated procedure   ▲ Non-covered procedures   ✚ Cluster

0270076 Dilation of Coronary Artery, One Artery, Bifurcation, with Four or More Drug-eluting Intraluminal Devices, Open Approach

027007Z Dilation of Coronary Artery, One Artery with Four or More Drug-eluting Intraluminal Devices, Open Approach

02700D6 Dilation of Coronary Artery, One Artery, Bifurcation, with Intraluminal Device, Open Approach

02700DZ Dilation of Coronary Artery, One Artery with Intraluminal Device, Open Approach

02700E6 Dilation of Coronary Artery, One Artery, Bifurcation, with Two Intraluminal Devices, Open Approach

02700EZ Dilation of Coronary Artery, One Artery with Two Intraluminal Devices, Open Approach

02700F6 Dilation of Coronary Artery, One Artery, Bifurcation, with Three Intraluminal Devices, Open Approach

02700FZ Dilation of Coronary Artery, One Artery with Three Intraluminal Devices, Open Approach

02700G6 Dilation of Coronary Artery, One Artery, Bifurcation, with Four or More Intraluminal Devices, Open Approach

02700GZ Dilation of Coronary Artery, One Artery with Four or More Intraluminal Devices, Open Approach

02700T6 Dilation of Coronary Artery, One Artery, Bifurcation, with Radioactive Intraluminal Device, Open Approach

02700TZ Dilation of Coronary Artery, One Artery with Radioactive Intraluminal Device, Open Approach

02700Z6 Dilation of Coronary Artery, One Artery, Bifurcation, Open Approach

02700ZZ Dilation of Coronary Artery, One Artery, Open Approach

0270346 Dilation of Coronary Artery, One Artery, Bifurcation, with Drug-eluting Intraluminal Device, Percutaneous Approach
AHA CC: 2Q, 2015, 4-5; 4Q, 2016, 88

027034Z Dilation of Coronary Artery, One Artery with Drug-eluting Intraluminal Device, Percutaneous Approach
AHA CC: 2Q, 2014, 4; 2Q, 2015, 3-4; 4Q, 2015, 13-14; 4Q, 2019, 39-40

0270356 Dilation of Coronary Artery, One Artery, Bifurcation, with Two Drug-eluting Intraluminal Devices, Percutaneous Approach

027035Z Dilation of Coronary Artery, One Artery with Two Drug-eluting Intraluminal Devices, Percutaneous Approach

0270366 Dilation of Coronary Artery, One Artery, Bifurcation, with Three Drug-eluting Intraluminal Devices, Percutaneous Approach

027036Z Dilation of Coronary Artery, One Artery with Three Drug-eluting Intraluminal Devices, Percutaneous Approach

0270376 Dilation of Coronary Artery, One Artery, Bifurcation, with Four or More Drug-eluting Intraluminal Devices, Percutaneous Approach

027037Z Dilation of Coronary Artery, One Artery with Four or More Drug-eluting Intraluminal Devices, Percutaneous Approach
AHA CC: 4Q, 2016, 85-86

02703D6 Dilation of Coronary Artery, One Artery, Bifurcation, with Intraluminal Device, Percutaneous Approach

02703DZ Dilation of Coronary Artery, One Artery with Intraluminal Device, Percutaneous Approach
AHA CC: 2Q, 2015, 4

02703E6 Dilation of Coronary Artery, One Artery, Bifurcation, with Two Intraluminal Devices, Percutaneous Approach

02703EZ Dilation of Coronary Artery, One Artery with Two Intraluminal Devices, Percutaneous Approach
AHA CC: 4Q, 2016, 84-85

02703F6 Dilation of Coronary Artery, One Artery, Bifurcation, with Three Intraluminal Devices, Percutaneous Approach

02703FZ Dilation of Coronary Artery, One Artery with Three Intraluminal Devices, Percutaneous Approach

02703G6 Dilation of Coronary Artery, One Artery, Bifurcation, with Four or More Intraluminal Devices, Percutaneous Approach

02703GZ Dilation of Coronary Artery, One Artery with Four or More Intraluminal Devices, Percutaneous Approach

02703T6 Dilation of Coronary Artery, One Artery, Bifurcation, with Radioactive Intraluminal Device, Percutaneous Approach

02703TZ Dilation of Coronary Artery, One Artery with Radioactive Intraluminal Device, Percutaneous Approach

02703Z6 Dilation of Coronary Artery, One Artery, Bifurcation, Percutaneous Approach

02703ZZ Dilation of Coronary Artery, One Artery, Percutaneous Approach
AHA CC: 3Q, 2015, 10; 4Q, 2016, 88; 3Q, 2018, 7-8

0270446 Dilation of Coronary Artery, One Artery, Bifurcation, with Drug-eluting Intraluminal Device, Percutaneous Endoscopic Approach

027044Z Dilation of Coronary Artery, One Artery with Drug-eluting Intraluminal Device, Percutaneous Endoscopic Approach

0270456 Dilation of Coronary Artery, One Artery, Bifurcation, with Two Drug-eluting Intraluminal Devices, Percutaneous Endoscopic Approach

027045Z Dilation of Coronary Artery, One Artery with Two Drug-eluting Intraluminal Devices, Percutaneous Endoscopic Approach

0270466 Dilation of Coronary Artery, One Artery, Bifurcation, with Three Drug-eluting Intraluminal Devices, Percutaneous Endoscopic Approach

027046Z Dilation of Coronary Artery, One Artery with Three Drug-eluting Intraluminal Devices, Percutaneous Endoscopic Approach

0270476 Dilation of Coronary Artery, One Artery, Bifurcation, with Four or More Drug-eluting Intraluminal Devices, Percutaneous Endoscopic Approach

027047Z Dilation of Coronary Artery, One Artery with Four or More Drug-eluting Intraluminal Devices, Percutaneous Endoscopic Approach

02704D6 Dilation of Coronary Artery, One Artery, Bifurcation, with Intraluminal Device, Percutaneous Endoscopic Approach

02704DZ Dilation of Coronary Artery, One Artery with Intraluminal Device, Percutaneous Endoscopic Approach

02704E6 Dilation of Coronary Artery, One Artery, Bifurcation, with Two Intraluminal Devices, Percutaneous Endoscopic Approach

02704EZ Dilation of Coronary Artery, One Artery with Two Intraluminal Devices, Percutaneous Endoscopic Approach

02704F6 Dilation of Coronary Artery, One Artery, Bifurcation, with Three Intraluminal Devices, Percutaneous Endoscopic Approach

02704FZ Dilation of Coronary Artery, One Artery with Three Intraluminal Devices, Percutaneous Endoscopic Approach

02704G6 Dilation of Coronary Artery, One Artery, Bifurcation, with Four or More Intraluminal Devices, Percutaneous Endoscopic Approach

02704GZ Dilation of Coronary Artery, One Artery with Four or More Intraluminal Devices, Percutaneous Endoscopic Approach

02704T6 Dilation of Coronary Artery, One Artery, Bifurcation, with Radioactive Intraluminal Device, Percutaneous Endoscopic Approach

02704TZ Dilation of Coronary Artery, One Artery with Radioactive Intraluminal Device, Percutaneous Endoscopic Approach

02704Z6 Dilation of Coronary Artery, One Artery, Bifurcation, Percutaneous Endoscopic Approach

02704ZZ Dilation of Coronary Artery, One Artery, Percutaneous Endoscopic Approach

0271046 Dilation of Coronary Artery, Two Arteries, Bifurcation, with Drug-eluting Intraluminal Device, Open Approach

027104Z Dilation of Coronary Artery, Two Arteries with Drug-eluting Intraluminal Device, Open Approach

0271056 Dilation of Coronary Artery, Two Arteries, Bifurcation, with Two Drug-eluting Intraluminal Devices, Open Approach

027105Z Dilation of Coronary Artery, Two Arteries with Two Drug-eluting Intraluminal Devices, Open Approach

0271066 Dilation of Coronary Artery, Two Arteries, Bifurcation, with Three Drug-eluting Intraluminal Devices, Open Approach

027106Z Dilation of Coronary Artery, Two Arteries with Three Drug-eluting Intraluminal Devices, Open Approach

0271076 Dilation of Coronary Artery, Two Arteries, Bifurcation, with Four or More Drug-eluting Intraluminal Devices, Open Approach

027107Z Dilation of Coronary Artery, Two Arteries with Four or More Drug-eluting Intraluminal Devices, Open Approach

02710D6 Dilation of Coronary Artery, Two Arteries, Bifurcation, with Intraluminal Device, Open Approach

02710DZ Dilation of Coronary Artery, Two Arteries with Intraluminal Device, Open Approach

02710E6 Dilation of Coronary Artery, Two Arteries, Bifurcation, with Two Intraluminal Devices, Open Approach

02710EZ Dilation of Coronary Artery, Two Arteries with Two Intraluminal Devices, Open Approach

02710F6 Dilation of Coronary Artery, Two Arteries, Bifurcation, with Three Intraluminal Devices, Open Approach

02710FZ Dilation of Coronary Artery, Two Arteries with Three Intraluminal Devices, Open Approach

02710G6 Dilation of Coronary Artery, Two Arteries, Bifurcation, with Four or More Intraluminal Devices, Open Approach

02710GZ Dilation of Coronary Artery, Two Arteries with Four or More Intraluminal Devices, Open Approach

02710T6 Dilation of Coronary Artery, Two Arteries, Bifurcation, with Radioactive Intraluminal Device, Open Approach

02710TZ Dilation of Coronary Artery, Two Arteries with Radioactive Intraluminal Device, Open Approach

02710Z6 Dilation of Coronary Artery, Two Arteries, Bifurcation, Open Approach

02710ZZ Dilation of Coronary Artery, Two Arteries, Open Approach

0271346 Dilation of Coronary Artery, Two Arteries, Bifurcation, with Drug-eluting Intraluminal Device, Percutaneous Approach

027134Z Dilation of Coronary Artery, Two Arteries with Drug-eluting Intraluminal Device, Percutaneous Approach
AHA CC: 2Q, 2015, 5

0271356 Dilation of Coronary Artery, Two Arteries, Bifurcation, with Two Drug-eluting Intraluminal Devices, Percutaneous Approach
AHA CC: 4Q, 2016, 87

027135Z Dilation of Coronary Artery, Two Arteries with Two Drug-eluting Intraluminal Devices, Percutaneous Approach

0271366 Dilation of Coronary Artery, Two Arteries, Bifurcation, with Three Drug-eluting Intraluminal Devices, Percutaneous Approach

027136Z Dilation of Coronary Artery, Two Arteries with Three Drug-eluting Intraluminal Devices, Percutaneous Approach
AHA CC: 4Q, 2016, 84-85

0271376 Dilation of Coronary Artery, Two Arteries, Bifurcation, with Four or More Drug-eluting Intraluminal Devices, Percutaneous Approach

027137Z Dilation of Coronary Artery, Two Arteries with Four or More Drug-eluting Intraluminal Devices, Percutaneous Approach

02713D6 Dilation of Coronary Artery, Two Arteries, Bifurcation, with Intraluminal Device, Percutaneous Approach

02713DZ Dilation of Coronary Artery, Two Arteries with Intraluminal Device, Percutaneous Approach

02713E6 Dilation of Coronary Artery, Two Arteries, Bifurcation, with Two Intraluminal Devices, Percutaneous Approach

02713EZ Dilation of Coronary Artery, Two Arteries with Two Intraluminal Devices, Percutaneous Approach

02713F6 Dilation of Coronary Artery, Two Arteries, Bifurcation, with Three Intraluminal Devices, Percutaneous Approach

02713FZ Dilation of Coronary Artery, Two Arteries with Three Intraluminal Devices, Percutaneous Approach

02713G6 Dilation of Coronary Artery, Two Arteries, Bifurcation, with Four or More Intraluminal Devices, Percutaneous Approach

02713GZ Dilation of Coronary Artery, Two Arteries with Four or More Intraluminal Devices, Percutaneous Approach

02713T6 Dilation of Coronary Artery, Two Arteries, Bifurcation, with Radioactive Intraluminal Device, Percutaneous Approach

02713TZ Dilation of Coronary Artery, Two Arteries with Radioactive Intraluminal Device, Percutaneous Approach

02713Z6 Dilation of Coronary Artery, Two Arteries, Bifurcation, Percutaneous Approach

02713ZZ Dilation of Coronary Artery, Two Arteries, Percutaneous Approach

0271446 Dilation of Coronary Artery, Two Arteries, Bifurcation, with Drug-eluting Intraluminal Device, Percutaneous Endoscopic Approach

027144Z Dilation of Coronary Artery, Two Arteries with Drug-eluting Intraluminal Device, Percutaneous Endoscopic Approach

0271456 Dilation of Coronary Artery, Two Arteries, Bifurcation, with Two Drug-eluting Intraluminal Devices, Percutaneous Endoscopic Approach

027145Z Dilation of Coronary Artery, Two Arteries with Two Drug-eluting Intraluminal Devices, Percutaneous Endoscopic Approach

0271466 Dilation of Coronary Artery, Two Arteries, Bifurcation, with Three Drug-eluting Intraluminal Devices, Percutaneous Endoscopic Approach

027146Z Dilation of Coronary Artery, Two Arteries with Three Drug-eluting Intraluminal Devices, Percutaneous Endoscopic Approach

0271476 Dilation of Coronary Artery, Two Arteries, Bifurcation, with Four or More Drug-eluting Intraluminal Devices, Percutaneous Endoscopic Approach

027147Z Dilation of Coronary Artery, Two Arteries with Four or More Drug-eluting Intraluminal Devices, Percutaneous Endoscopic Approach

02714D6 Dilation of Coronary Artery, Two Arteries, Bifurcation, with Intraluminal Device, Percutaneous Endoscopic Approach

02714DZ Dilation of Coronary Artery, Two Arteries with Intraluminal Device, Percutaneous Endoscopic Approach

02714E6 Dilation of Coronary Artery, Two Arteries, Bifurcation, with Two Intraluminal Devices, Percutaneous Endoscopic Approach

02714EZ Dilation of Coronary Artery, Two Arteries with Two Intraluminal Devices, Percutaneous Endoscopic Approach

02714F6 Dilation of Coronary Artery, Two Arteries, Bifurcation, with Three Intraluminal Devices, Percutaneous Endoscopic Approach

02714FZ Dilation of Coronary Artery, Two Arteries with Three Intraluminal Devices, Percutaneous Endoscopic Approach

02714G6 Dilation of Coronary Artery, Two Arteries, Bifurcation, with Four or More Intraluminal Devices, Percutaneous Endoscopic Approach

02714GZ Dilation of Coronary Artery, Two Arteries with Four or More Intraluminal Devices, Percutaneous Endoscopic Approach

02714T6 Dilation of Coronary Artery, Two Arteries, Bifurcation, with Radioactive Intraluminal Device, Percutaneous Endoscopic Approach

02714TZ Dilation of Coronary Artery, Two Arteries with Radioactive Intraluminal Device, Percutaneous Endoscopic Approach

02714Z6 Dilation of Coronary Artery, Two Arteries, Bifurcation, Percutaneous Endoscopic Approach

02714ZZ Dilation of Coronary Artery, Two Arteries, Percutaneous Endoscopic Approach

0272046 Dilation of Coronary Artery, Three Arteries, Bifurcation, with Drug-eluting Intraluminal Device, Open Approach

027204Z Dilation of Coronary Artery, Three Arteries with Drug-eluting Intraluminal Device, Open Approach

0272056 Dilation of Coronary Artery, Three Arteries, Bifurcation, with Two Drug-eluting Intraluminal Devices, Open Approach

027205Z Dilation of Coronary Artery, Three Arteries with Two Drug-eluting Intraluminal Devices, Open Approach

0272066 Dilation of Coronary Artery, Three Arteries, Bifurcation, with Three Drug-eluting Intraluminal Devices, Open Approach

027206Z Dilation of Coronary Artery, Three Arteries with Three Drug-eluting Intraluminal Devices, Open Approach

0272076 Dilation of Coronary Artery, Three Arteries, Bifurcation, with Four or More Drug-eluting Intraluminal Devices, Open Approach

027207Z Dilation of Coronary Artery, Three Arteries with Four or More Drug-eluting Intraluminal Devices, Open Approach

02720D6 Dilation of Coronary Artery, Three Arteries, Bifurcation, with Intraluminal Device, Open Approach

02720DZ Dilation of Coronary Artery, Three Arteries with Intraluminal Device, Open Approach

02720E6 Dilation of Coronary Artery, Three Arteries, Bifurcation, with Two Intraluminal Devices, Open Approach

02720EZ Dilation of Coronary Artery, Three Arteries with Two Intraluminal Devices, Open Approach

02720F6 Dilation of Coronary Artery, Three Arteries, Bifurcation, with Three Intraluminal Devices, Open Approach

02720FZ Dilation of Coronary Artery, Three Arteries with Three Intraluminal Devices, Open Approach

02720G6 Dilation of Coronary Artery, Three Arteries, Bifurcation, with Four or More Intraluminal Devices, Open Approach

02720GZ Dilation of Coronary Artery, Three Arteries with Four or More Intraluminal Devices, Open Approach

02720T6 Dilation of Coronary Artery, Three Arteries, Bifurcation, with Radioactive Intraluminal Device, Open Approach

02720TZ Dilation of Coronary Artery, Three Arteries with Radioactive Intraluminal Device, Open Approach

02720Z6 Dilation of Coronary Artery, Three Arteries, Bifurcation, Open Approach

02720ZZ Dilation of Coronary Artery, Three Arteries, Open Approach

0272346 Dilation of Coronary Artery, Three Arteries, Bifurcation, with Drug-eluting Intraluminal Device, Percutaneous Approach

027234Z Dilation of Coronary Artery, Three Arteries with Drug-eluting Intraluminal Device, Percutaneous Approach
AHA CC: 2Q, 2015, 3

0272356 Dilation of Coronary Artery, Three Arteries, Bifurcation, with Two Drug-eluting Intraluminal Devices, Percutaneous Approach

027235Z Dilation of Coronary Artery, Three Arteries with Two Drug-eluting Intraluminal Devices, Percutaneous Approach

0272366 Dilation of Coronary Artery, Three Arteries, Bifurcation, with Three Drug-eluting Intraluminal Devices, Percutaneous Approach

027236Z Dilation of Coronary Artery, Three Arteries with Three Drug-eluting Intraluminal Devices, Percutaneous Approach

0272376 Dilation of Coronary Artery, Three Arteries, Bifurcation, with Four or More Drug-eluting Intraluminal Devices, Percutaneous Approach

027237Z Dilation of Coronary Artery, Three Arteries with Four or More Drug-eluting Intraluminal Devices, Percutaneous Approach

02723D6 Dilation of Coronary Artery, Three Arteries, Bifurcation, with Intraluminal Device, Percutaneous Approach

02723DZ Dilation of Coronary Artery, Three Arteries with Intraluminal Device, Percutaneous Approach

02723E6 Dilation of Coronary Artery, Three Arteries, Bifurcation, with Two Intraluminal Devices, Percutaneous Approach

02723EZ Dilation of Coronary Artery, Three Arteries with Two Intraluminal Devices, Percutaneous Approach

02723F6 Dilation of Coronary Artery, Three Arteries, Bifurcation, with Three Intraluminal Devices, Percutaneous Approach

02723FZ Dilation of Coronary Artery, Three Arteries with Three Intraluminal Devices, Percutaneous Approach

02723G6 Dilation of Coronary Artery, Three Arteries, Bifurcation, with Four or More Intraluminal Devices, Percutaneous Approach

02723GZ Dilation of Coronary Artery, Three Arteries with Four or More Intraluminal Devices, Percutaneous Approach

02723T6 Dilation of Coronary Artery, Three Arteries, Bifurcation, with Radioactive Intraluminal Device, Percutaneous Approach

02723TZ Dilation of Coronary Artery, Three Arteries with Radioactive Intraluminal Device, Percutaneous Approach

02723Z6 Dilation of Coronary Artery, Three Arteries, Bifurcation, Percutaneous Approach

02723ZZ Dilation of Coronary Artery, Three Arteries, Percutaneous Approach

0272446 Dilation of Coronary Artery, Three Arteries, Bifurcation, with Drug-eluting Intraluminal Device, Percutaneous Endoscopic Approach

027244Z Dilation of Coronary Artery, Three Arteries with Drug-eluting Intraluminal Device, Percutaneous Endoscopic Approach

0272456 Dilation of Coronary Artery, Three Arteries, Bifurcation, with Two Drug-eluting Intraluminal Devices, Percutaneous Endoscopic Approach

027245Z Dilation of Coronary Artery, Three Arteries with Two Drug-eluting Intraluminal Devices, Percutaneous Endoscopic Approach

0272466 Dilation of Coronary Artery, Three Arteries, Bifurcation, with Three Drug-eluting Intraluminal Devices, Percutaneous Endoscopic Approach

027246Z Dilation of Coronary Artery, Three Arteries with Three Drug-eluting Intraluminal Devices, Percutaneous Endoscopic Approach

0272476 Dilation of Coronary Artery, Three Arteries, Bifurcation, with Four or More Drug-eluting Intraluminal Devices, Percutaneous Endoscopic Approach

027247Z Dilation of Coronary Artery, Three Arteries with Four or More Drug-eluting Intraluminal Devices, Percutaneous Endoscopic Approach

02724D6 Dilation of Coronary Artery, Three Arteries, Bifurcation, with Intraluminal Device, Percutaneous Endoscopic Approach

02724DZ Dilation of Coronary Artery, Three Arteries with Intraluminal Device, Percutaneous Endoscopic Approach

02724E6 Dilation of Coronary Artery, Three Arteries, Bifurcation, with Two Intraluminal Devices, Percutaneous Endoscopic Approach

02724EZ Dilation of Coronary Artery, Three Arteries with Two Intraluminal Devices, Percutaneous Endoscopic Approach

02724F6 Dilation of Coronary Artery, Three Arteries, Bifurcation, with Three Intraluminal Devices, Percutaneous Endoscopic Approach

02724FZ Dilation of Coronary Artery, Three Arteries with Three Intraluminal Devices, Percutaneous Endoscopic Approach

02724G6 Dilation of Coronary Artery, Three Arteries, Bifurcation, with Four or More Intraluminal Devices, Percutaneous Endoscopic Approach

02724GZ Dilation of Coronary Artery, Three Arteries with Four or More Intraluminal Devices, Percutaneous Endoscopic Approach

02724T6 Dilation of Coronary Artery, Three Arteries, Bifurcation, with Radioactive Intraluminal Device, Percutaneous Endoscopic Approach

02724TZ Dilation of Coronary Artery, Three Arteries with Radioactive Intraluminal Device, Percutaneous Endoscopic Approach

02724Z6 Dilation of Coronary Artery, Three Arteries, Bifurcation, Percutaneous Endoscopic Approach

02724ZZ Dilation of Coronary Artery, Three Arteries, Percutaneous Endoscopic Approach

0273046 Dilation of Coronary Artery, Four or More Arteries, Bifurcation, with Drug-eluting Intraluminal Device, Open Approach

027304Z Dilation of Coronary Artery, Four or More Arteries with Drug-eluting Intraluminal Device, Open Approach

0273056 Dilation of Coronary Artery, Four or More Arteries, Bifurcation, with Two Drug-eluting Intraluminal Devices, Open Approach

027305Z Dilation of Coronary Artery, Four or More Arteries with Two Drug-eluting Intraluminal Devices, Open Approach

0273066 Dilation of Coronary Artery, Four or More Arteries, Bifurcation, with Three Drug-eluting Intraluminal Devices, Open Approach

027306Z Dilation of Coronary Artery, Four or More Arteries with Three Drug-eluting Intraluminal Devices, Open Approach

0273076 Dilation of Coronary Artery, Four or More Arteries, Bifurcation, with Four or More Drug-eluting Intraluminal Devices, Open Approach

027307Z Dilation of Coronary Artery, Four or More Arteries with Four or More Drug-eluting Intraluminal Devices, Open Approach

02730D6 Dilation of Coronary Artery, Four or More Arteries, Bifurcation, with Intraluminal Device, Open Approach

02730DZ Dilation of Coronary Artery, Four or More Arteries with Intraluminal Device, Open Approach

02730E6 Dilation of Coronary Artery, Four or More Arteries, Bifurcation, with Two Intraluminal Devices, Open Approach

02730EZ Dilation of Coronary Artery, Four or More Arteries with Two Intraluminal Devices, Open Approach

02730F6 Dilation of Coronary Artery, Four or More Arteries, Bifurcation, with Three Intraluminal Devices, Open Approach

02730FZ Dilation of Coronary Artery, Four or More Arteries with Three Intraluminal Devices, Open Approach

02730G6 Dilation of Coronary Artery, Four or More Arteries, Bifurcation, with Four or More Intraluminal Devices, Open Approach

02730GZ Dilation of Coronary Artery, Four or More Arteries with Four or More Intraluminal Devices, Open Approach

02730T6 Dilation of Coronary Artery, Four or More Arteries, Bifurcation, with Radioactive Intraluminal Device, Open Approach

02730TZ Dilation of Coronary Artery, Four or More Arteries with Radioactive Intraluminal Device, Open Approach

02730Z6 Dilation of Coronary Artery, Four or More Arteries, Bifurcation, Open Approach

02730ZZ Dilation of Coronary Artery, Four or More Arteries, Open Approach

0273346 Dilation of Coronary Artery, Four or More Arteries, Bifurcation, with Drug-eluting Intraluminal Device, Percutaneous Approach

027334Z Dilation of Coronary Artery, Four or More Arteries with Drug-eluting Intraluminal Device, Percutaneous Approach

0273356 Dilation of Coronary Artery, Four or More Arteries, Bifurcation, with Two Drug-eluting Intraluminal Devices, Percutaneous Approach

027335Z Dilation of Coronary Artery, Four or More Arteries with Two Drug-eluting Intraluminal Devices, Percutaneous Approach

0273366 Dilation of Coronary Artery, Four or More Arteries, Bifurcation, with Three Drug-eluting Intraluminal Devices, Percutaneous Approach

027336Z Dilation of Coronary Artery, Four or More Arteries with Three Drug-eluting Intraluminal Devices, Percutaneous Approach

0273376 Dilation of Coronary Artery, Four or More Arteries, Bifurcation, with Four or More Drug-eluting Intraluminal Devices, Percutaneous Approach

027337Z Dilation of Coronary Artery, Four or More Arteries with Four or More Drug-eluting Intraluminal Devices, Percutaneous Approach

02733D6 Dilation of Coronary Artery, Four or More Arteries, Bifurcation, with Intraluminal Device, Percutaneous Approach

02733DZ Dilation of Coronary Artery, Four or More Arteries with Intraluminal Device, Percutaneous Approach

02733E6 Dilation of Coronary Artery, Four or More Arteries, Bifurcation, with Two Intraluminal Devices, Percutaneous Approach

02733EZ Dilation of Coronary Artery, Four or More Arteries with Two Intraluminal Devices, Percutaneous Approach

02733F6 Dilation of Coronary Artery, Four or More Arteries, Bifurcation, with Three Intraluminal Devices, Percutaneous Approach

02733FZ Dilation of Coronary Artery, Four or More Arteries with Three Intraluminal Devices, Percutaneous Approach

02733G6 Dilation of Coronary Artery, Four or More Arteries, Bifurcation, with Four or More Intraluminal Devices, Percutaneous Approach

02733GZ Dilation of Coronary Artery, Four or More Arteries with Four or More Intraluminal Devices, Percutaneous Approach

02733T6 Dilation of Coronary Artery, Four or More Arteries, Bifurcation, with Radioactive Intraluminal Device, Percutaneous Approach

02733TZ Dilation of Coronary Artery, Four or More Arteries with Radioactive Intraluminal Device, Percutaneous Approach

02733Z6 Dilation of Coronary Artery, Four or More Arteries, Bifurcation, Percutaneous Approach

02733ZZ Dilation of Coronary Artery, Four or More Arteries, Percutaneous Approach

0273446 Dilation of Coronary Artery, Four or More Arteries, Bifurcation, with Drug-eluting Intraluminal Device, Percutaneous Endoscopic Approach

027344Z Dilation of Coronary Artery, Four or More Arteries with Drug-eluting Intraluminal Device, Percutaneous Endoscopic Approach

0273456 Dilation of Coronary Artery, Four or More Arteries, Bifurcation, with Two Drug-eluting Intraluminal Devices, Percutaneous Endoscopic Approach

027345Z Dilation of Coronary Artery, Four or More Arteries with Two Drug-eluting Intraluminal Devices, Percutaneous Endoscopic Approach

0273466 Dilation of Coronary Artery, Four or More Arteries, Bifurcation, with Three Drug-eluting Intraluminal Devices, Percutaneous Endoscopic Approach

027346Z Dilation of Coronary Artery, Four or More Arteries with Three Drug-eluting Intraluminal Devices, Percutaneous Endoscopic Approach

0273476 Dilation of Coronary Artery, Four or More Arteries, Bifurcation, with Four or More Drug-eluting Intraluminal Devices, Percutaneous Endoscopic Approach

027347Z Dilation of Coronary Artery, Four or More Arteries with Four or More Drug-eluting Intraluminal Devices, Percutaneous Endoscopic Approach

02734D6 Dilation of Coronary Artery, Four or More Arteries, Bifurcation, with Intraluminal Device, Percutaneous Endoscopic Approach

02734DZ Dilation of Coronary Artery, Four or More Arteries with Intraluminal Device, Percutaneous Endoscopic Approach

02734E6 Dilation of Coronary Artery, Four or More Arteries, Bifurcation, with Two Intraluminal Devices, Percutaneous Endoscopic Approach

02734EZ Dilation of Coronary Artery, Four or More Arteries with Two Intraluminal Devices, Percutaneous Endoscopic Approach

02734F6 Dilation of Coronary Artery, Four or More Arteries, Bifurcation, with Three Intraluminal Devices, Percutaneous Endoscopic Approach

02734FZ Dilation of Coronary Artery, Four or More Arteries with Three Intraluminal Devices, Percutaneous Endoscopic Approach

02734G6 Dilation of Coronary Artery, Four or More Arteries, Bifurcation, with Four or More Intraluminal Devices, Percutaneous Endoscopic Approach

02734GZ Dilation of Coronary Artery, Four or More Arteries with Four or More Intraluminal Devices, Percutaneous Endoscopic Approach

02734T6 Dilation of Coronary Artery, Four or More Arteries, Bifurcation, with Radioactive Intraluminal Device, Percutaneous Endoscopic Approach

02734TZ Dilation of Coronary Artery, Four or More Arteries with Radioactive Intraluminal Device, Percutaneous Endoscopic Approach

02734Z6 Dilation of Coronary Artery, Four or More Arteries, Bifurcation, Percutaneous Endoscopic Approach

02734ZZ Dilation of Coronary Artery, Four or More Arteries, Percutaneous Endoscopic Approach

027F04Z Dilation of Aortic Valve with Drug-eluting Intraluminal Device, Open Approach

027F0DZ Dilation of Aortic Valve with Intraluminal Device, Open Approach

027F0ZZ Dilation of Aortic Valve, Open Approach

027F34Z Dilation of Aortic Valve with Drug-eluting Intraluminal Device, Percutaneous Approach

027F3DZ Dilation of Aortic Valve with Intraluminal Device, Percutaneous Approach

027F3ZZ Dilation of Aortic Valve, Percutaneous Approach

027F44Z Dilation of Aortic Valve with Drug-eluting Intraluminal Device, Percutaneous Endoscopic Approach

027F4DZ Dilation of Aortic Valve with Intraluminal Device, Percutaneous Endoscopic Approach

027F4ZZ Dilation of Aortic Valve, Percutaneous Endoscopic Approach

027G04Z Dilation of Mitral Valve with Drug-eluting Intraluminal Device, Open Approach

027G0DZ Dilation of Mitral Valve with Intraluminal Device, Open Approach

027G0ZZ Dilation of Mitral Valve, Open Approach

027G34Z Dilation of Mitral Valve with Drug-eluting Intraluminal Device, Percutaneous Approach

027G3DZ Dilation of Mitral Valve with Intraluminal Device, Percutaneous Approach

027G3ZZ Dilation of Mitral Valve, Percutaneous Approach

027G44Z Dilation of Mitral Valve with Drug-eluting Intraluminal Device, Percutaneous Endoscopic Approach

027G4DZ Dilation of Mitral Valve with Intraluminal Device, Percutaneous Endoscopic Approach

027G4ZZ Dilation of Mitral Valve, Percutaneous Endoscopic Approach

027H04Z Dilation of Pulmonary Valve with Drug-eluting Intraluminal Device, Open Approach

027H0DZ Dilation of Pulmonary Valve with Intraluminal Device, Open Approach

027H0ZZ Dilation of Pulmonary Valve, Open Approach

AHA CC: 1Q, 2016, 16-17

027H34Z Dilation of Pulmonary Valve with Drug-eluting Intraluminal Device, Percutaneous Approach

027H3DZ Dilation of Pulmonary Valve with Intraluminal Device, Percutaneous Approach

027H3ZZ Dilation of Pulmonary Valve, Percutaneous Approach

027H44Z Dilation of Pulmonary Valve with Drug-eluting Intraluminal Device, Percutaneous Endoscopic Approach

027H4DZ Dilation of Pulmonary Valve with Intraluminal Device, Percutaneous Endoscopic Approach

027H4ZZ Dilation of Pulmonary Valve, Percutaneous Endoscopic Approach

027J04Z Dilation of Tricuspid Valve with Drug-eluting Intraluminal Device, Open Approach

♀ Female-only   ♂ Male-only   ▲ Limited Coverage   ● Non-OR   ᴴᴬᶜ HAC-associated procedure   ▲ Non-covered procedures   ✚ Cluster

027J0DZ Dilation of Tricuspid Valve with Intraluminal Device, Open Approach

027J0ZZ Dilation of Tricuspid Valve, Open Approach

027J34Z Dilation of Tricuspid Valve with Drug-eluting Intraluminal Device, Percutaneous Approach

027J3DZ Dilation of Tricuspid Valve with Intraluminal Device, Percutaneous Approach

027J3ZZ Dilation of Tricuspid Valve, Percutaneous Approach

027J44Z Dilation of Tricuspid Valve with Drug-eluting Intraluminal Device, Percutaneous Endoscopic Approach

027J4DZ Dilation of Tricuspid Valve with Intraluminal Device, Percutaneous Endoscopic Approach

027J4ZZ Dilation of Tricuspid Valve, Percutaneous Endoscopic Approach

027K04Z Dilation of Right Ventricle with Drug-eluting Intraluminal Device, Open Approach

027K0DZ Dilation of Right Ventricle with Intraluminal Device, Open Approach

027K0ZZ Dilation of Right Ventricle, Open Approach

027K34Z Dilation of Right Ventricle with Drug-eluting Intraluminal Device, Percutaneous Approach

027K3DZ Dilation of Right Ventricle with Intraluminal Device, Percutaneous Approach

027K3ZZ Dilation of Right Ventricle, Percutaneous Approach

027K44Z Dilation of Right Ventricle with Drug-eluting Intraluminal Device, Percutaneous Endoscopic Approach

027K4DZ Dilation of Right Ventricle with Intraluminal Device, Percutaneous Endoscopic Approach

027K4ZZ Dilation of Right Ventricle, Percutaneous Endoscopic Approach

027L04Z Dilation of Left Ventricle with Drug-eluting Intraluminal Device, Open Approach

027L0DZ Dilation of Left Ventricle with Intraluminal Device, Open Approach

027L0ZZ Dilation of Left Ventricle, Open Approach

AHA CC: 4Q, 2017, 33

027L34Z Dilation of Left Ventricle with Drug-eluting Intraluminal Device, Percutaneous Approach

027L3DZ Dilation of Left Ventricle with Intraluminal Device, Percutaneous Approach

027L3ZZ Dilation of Left Ventricle, Percutaneous Approach

027L44Z Dilation of Left Ventricle with Drug-eluting Intraluminal Device, Percutaneous Endoscopic Approach

027L4DZ Dilation of Left Ventricle with Intraluminal Device, Percutaneous Endoscopic Approach

027L4ZZ Dilation of Left Ventricle, Percutaneous Endoscopic Approach

027P04Z Dilation of Pulmonary Trunk with Drug-eluting Intraluminal Device, Open Approach

027P0DZ Dilation of Pulmonary Trunk with Intraluminal Device, Open Approach

027P0ZZ Dilation of Pulmonary Trunk, Open Approach

027P34Z Dilation of Pulmonary Trunk with Drug-eluting Intraluminal Device, Percutaneous Approach

027P3DZ Dilation of Pulmonary Trunk with Intraluminal Device, Percutaneous Approach

027P3ZZ Dilation of Pulmonary Trunk, Percutaneous Approach

027P44Z Dilation of Pulmonary Trunk with Drug-eluting Intraluminal Device, Percutaneous Endoscopic Approach

027P4DZ Dilation of Pulmonary Trunk with Intraluminal Device, Percutaneous Endoscopic Approach

027P4ZZ Dilation of Pulmonary Trunk, Percutaneous Endoscopic Approach

027Q04Z Dilation of Right Pulmonary Artery with Drug-eluting Intraluminal Device, Open Approach

027Q0DZ Dilation of Right Pulmonary Artery with Intraluminal Device, Open Approach

AHA CC: 3Q, 2015, 16-17

027Q0ZZ Dilation of Right Pulmonary Artery, Open Approach

027Q34Z Dilation of Right Pulmonary Artery with Drug-eluting Intraluminal Device, Percutaneous Approach

027Q3DZ Dilation of Right Pulmonary Artery with Intraluminal Device, Percutaneous Approach

027Q3ZZ Dilation of Right Pulmonary Artery, Percutaneous Approach

027Q44Z Dilation of Right Pulmonary Artery with Drug-eluting Intraluminal Device, Percutaneous Endoscopic Approach

027Q4DZ Dilation of Right Pulmonary Artery with Intraluminal Device, Percutaneous Endoscopic Approach

027Q4ZZ Dilation of Right Pulmonary Artery, Percutaneous Endoscopic Approach

027R04T Dilation of Ductus Arteriosus with Drug-eluting Intraluminal Device, Open Approach

027R04Z Dilation of Left Pulmonary Artery with Drug-eluting Intraluminal Device, Open Approach

027R0DT Dilation of Ductus Arteriosus with Intraluminal Device, Open Approach

027R0DZ Dilation of Left Pulmonary Artery with Intraluminal Device, Open Approach

027R0ZT Dilation of Ductus Arteriosus, Open Approach

027R0ZZ Dilation of Left Pulmonary Artery, Open Approach

027R34T Dilation of Ductus Arteriosus with Drug-eluting Intraluminal Device, Percutaneous Approach

027R34Z Dilation of Left Pulmonary Artery with Drug-eluting Intraluminal Device, Percutaneous Approach

027R3DT Dilation of Ductus Arteriosus with Intraluminal Device, Percutaneous Approach

027R3DZ Dilation of Left Pulmonary Artery with Intraluminal Device, Percutaneous Approach

027R3ZT Dilation of Ductus Arteriosus, Percutaneous Approach

027R3ZZ Dilation of Left Pulmonary Artery, Percutaneous Approach

027R44T Dilation of Ductus Arteriosus with Drug-eluting Intraluminal Device, Percutaneous Endoscopic Approach

027R44Z Dilation of Left Pulmonary Artery with Drug-eluting Intraluminal Device, Percutaneous Endoscopic Approach

027R4DT Dilation of Ductus Arteriosus with Intraluminal Device, Percutaneous Endoscopic Approach

027R4DZ Dilation of Left Pulmonary Artery with Intraluminal Device, Percutaneous Endoscopic Approach

027R4ZT Dilation of Ductus Arteriosus, Percutaneous Endoscopic Approach

027R4ZZ Dilation of Left Pulmonary Artery, Percutaneous Endoscopic Approach

027S04Z Dilation of Right Pulmonary Vein with Drug-eluting Intraluminal Device, Open Approach

027S0DZ Dilation of Right Pulmonary Vein with Intraluminal Device, Open Approach

027S0ZZ Dilation of Right Pulmonary Vein, Open Approach

027S34Z Dilation of Right Pulmonary Vein with Drug-eluting Intraluminal Device, Percutaneous Approach

027S3DZ Dilation of Right Pulmonary Vein with Intraluminal Device, Percutaneous Approach

027S3ZZ Dilation of Right Pulmonary Vein, Percutaneous Approach

027S44Z Dilation of Right Pulmonary Vein with Drug-eluting Intraluminal Device, Percutaneous Endoscopic Approach

027S4DZ Dilation of Right Pulmonary Vein with Intraluminal Device, Percutaneous Endoscopic Approach

027S4ZZ Dilation of Right Pulmonary Vein, Percutaneous Endoscopic Approach

027T04Z Dilation of Left Pulmonary Vein with Drug-eluting Intraluminal Device, Open Approach

027T0DZ Dilation of Left Pulmonary Vein with Intraluminal Device, Open Approach

027T0ZZ Dilation of Left Pulmonary Vein, Open Approach

027T34Z Dilation of Left Pulmonary Vein with Drug-eluting Intraluminal Device, Percutaneous Approach

027T3DZ Dilation of Left Pulmonary Vein with Intraluminal Device, Percutaneous Approach

027T3ZZ Dilation of Left Pulmonary Vein, Percutaneous Approach

027T44Z Dilation of Left Pulmonary Vein with Drug-eluting Intraluminal Device, Percutaneous Endoscopic Approach

027T4DZ Dilation of Left Pulmonary Vein with Intraluminal Device, Percutaneous Endoscopic Approach

027T4ZZ Dilation of Left Pulmonary Vein, Percutaneous Endoscopic Approach

027V04Z Dilation of Superior Vena Cava with Drug-eluting Intraluminal Device, Open Approach

027V0DZ Dilation of Superior Vena Cava with Intraluminal Device, Open Approach

027V0ZZ Dilation of Superior Vena Cava, Open Approach

027V34Z Dilation of Superior Vena Cava with Drug-eluting Intraluminal Device, Percutaneous Approach

027V3DZ Dilation of Superior Vena Cava with Intraluminal Device, Percutaneous Approach

027V3ZZ Dilation of Superior Vena Cava, Percutaneous Approach

AHA CC: 3Q, 2018, 10

027V44Z Dilation of Superior Vena Cava with Drug-eluting Intraluminal Device, Percutaneous Endoscopic Approach

027V4DZ Dilation of Superior Vena Cava with Intraluminal Device, Percutaneous Endoscopic Approach	**027W3ZZ** Dilation of Thoracic Aorta, Descending, Percutaneous Approach	**027X34Z** Dilation of Thoracic Aorta, Ascending/Arch with Drug-eluting Intraluminal Device, Percutaneous Approach
027V4ZZ Dilation of Superior Vena Cava, Percutaneous Endoscopic Approach	**027W44Z** Dilation of Thoracic Aorta, Descending with Drug-eluting Intraluminal Device, Percutaneous Endoscopic Approach	**027X3DZ** Dilation of Thoracic Aorta, Ascending/Arch with Intraluminal Device, Percutaneous Approach
027W04Z Dilation of Thoracic Aorta, Descending with Drug-eluting Intraluminal Device, Open Approach	**027W4DZ** Dilation of Thoracic Aorta, Descending with Intraluminal Device, Percutaneous Endoscopic Approach	**027X3ZZ** Dilation of Thoracic Aorta, Ascending/Arch, Percutaneous Approach
027W0DZ Dilation of Thoracic Aorta, Descending with Intraluminal Device, Open Approach	**027W4ZZ** Dilation of Thoracic Aorta, Descending, Percutaneous Endoscopic Approach	**027X44Z** Dilation of Thoracic Aorta, Ascending/Arch with Drug-eluting Intraluminal Device, Percutaneous Endoscopic Approach
027W0ZZ Dilation of Thoracic Aorta, Descending, Open Approach	**027X04Z** Dilation of Thoracic Aorta, Ascending/Arch with Drug-eluting Intraluminal Device, Open Approach	**027X4DZ** Dilation of Thoracic Aorta, Ascending/Arch with Intraluminal Device, Percutaneous Endoscopic Approach
027W34Z Dilation of Thoracic Aorta, Descending with Drug-eluting Intraluminal Device, Percutaneous Approach	**027X0DZ** Dilation of Thoracic Aorta, Ascending/Arch with Intraluminal Device, Open Approach	**027X4ZZ** Dilation of Thoracic Aorta, Ascending/Arch, Percutaneous Endoscopic Approach
027W3DZ Dilation of Thoracic Aorta, Descending with Intraluminal Device, Percutaneous Approach	**027X0ZZ** Dilation of Thoracic Aorta, Ascending/Arch, Open Approach	

028 – Heart and Great Vessels, Division

Review Coding Guideline B3.14

02850ZZ Division of Atrial Septum, Open Approach	**02883ZZ** Division of Conduction Mechanism, Percutaneous Approach	**02894ZZ** Division of Chordae Tendineae, Percutaneous Endoscopic Approach
02853ZZ Division of Atrial Septum, Percutaneous Approach	**02884ZZ** Division of Conduction Mechanism, Percutaneous Endoscopic Approach	**028D0ZZ** Division of Papillary Muscle, Open Approach
02854ZZ Division of Atrial Septum, Percutaneous Endoscopic Approach	**02890ZZ** Division of Chordae Tendineae, Open Approach	**028D3ZZ** Division of Papillary Muscle, Percutaneous Approach
02880ZZ Division of Conduction Mechanism, Open Approach	**02893ZZ** Division of Chordae Tendineae, Percutaneous Approach	**028D4ZZ** Division of Papillary Muscle, Percutaneous Endoscopic Approach

02B – Heart and Great Vessels, Excision

Review Coding Guidelines B3.4a and B3.4b

Review Coding Guideline B3.8

Review Coding Guideline B3.18

02B40ZX Excision of Coronary Vein, Open Approach, Diagnostic	**02B64ZZ** Excision of Right Atrium, Percutaneous Endoscopic Approach	**02B93ZX** Excision of Chordae Tendineae, Percutaneous Approach, Diagnostic
02B40ZZ Excision of Coronary Vein, Open Approach	● **02B70ZK** Excision of Left Atrial Appendage, Open Approach	**02B93ZZ** Excision of Chordae Tendineae, Percutaneous Approach
02B43ZX Excision of Coronary Vein, Percutaneous Approach, Diagnostic	**02B70ZX** Excision of Left Atrium, Open Approach, Diagnostic	**02B94ZX** Excision of Chordae Tendineae, Percutaneous Endoscopic Approach, Diagnostic
02B43ZZ Excision of Coronary Vein, Percutaneous Approach	**02B70ZZ** Excision of Left Atrium, Open Approach	**02B94ZZ** Excision of Chordae Tendineae, Percutaneous Endoscopic Approach
02B44ZX Excision of Coronary Vein, Percutaneous Endoscopic Approach, Diagnostic	● **02B73ZK** Excision of Left Atrial Appendage, Percutaneous Approach	**02BD0ZX** Excision of Papillary Muscle, Open Approach, Diagnostic
02B44ZZ Excision of Coronary Vein, Percutaneous Endoscopic Approach	**02B73ZX** Excision of Left Atrium, Percutaneous Approach, Diagnostic	**02BD0ZZ** Excision of Papillary Muscle, Open Approach
02B50ZX Excision of Atrial Septum, Open Approach, Diagnostic	**02B73ZZ** Excision of Left Atrium, Percutaneous Approach	**02BD3ZX** Excision of Papillary Muscle, Percutaneous Approach, Diagnostic
02B50ZZ Excision of Atrial Septum, Open Approach	● **02B74ZK** Excision of Left Atrial Appendage, Percutaneous Endoscopic Approach	**02BD3ZZ** Excision of Papillary Muscle, Percutaneous Approach
02B53ZX Excision of Atrial Septum, Percutaneous Approach, Diagnostic	**02B74ZX** Excision of Left Atrium, Percutaneous Endoscopic Approach, Diagnostic	**02BD4ZX** Excision of Papillary Muscle, Percutaneous Endoscopic Approach, Diagnostic
02B53ZZ Excision of Atrial Septum, Percutaneous Approach	**02B74ZZ** Excision of Left Atrium, Percutaneous Endoscopic Approach	**02BD4ZZ** Excision of Papillary Muscle, Percutaneous Endoscopic Approach
02B54ZX Excision of Atrial Septum, Percutaneous Endoscopic Approach, Diagnostic	**02B80ZX** Excision of Conduction Mechanism, Open Approach, Diagnostic	**02BF0ZX** Excision of Aortic Valve, Open Approach, Diagnostic
02B54ZZ Excision of Atrial Septum, Percutaneous Endoscopic Approach	**02B80ZZ** Excision of Conduction Mechanism, Open Approach	**02BF0ZZ** Excision of Aortic Valve, Open Approach
02B60ZX Excision of Right Atrium, Open Approach, Diagnostic	**02B83ZX** Excision of Conduction Mechanism, Percutaneous Approach, Diagnostic	**02BF3ZX** Excision of Aortic Valve, Percutaneous Approach, Diagnostic
02B60ZZ Excision of Right Atrium, Open Approach	**02B83ZZ** Excision of Conduction Mechanism, Percutaneous Approach	**02BF3ZZ** Excision of Aortic Valve, Percutaneous Approach
02B63ZX Excision of Right Atrium, Percutaneous Approach, Diagnostic	**02B84ZX** Excision of Conduction Mechanism, Percutaneous Endoscopic Approach, Diagnostic	**02BF4ZX** Excision of Aortic Valve, Percutaneous Endoscopic Approach, Diagnostic
02B63ZZ Excision of Right Atrium, Percutaneous Approach	**02B84ZZ** Excision of Conduction Mechanism, Percutaneous Endoscopic Approach	**02BF4ZZ** Excision of Aortic Valve, Percutaneous Endoscopic Approach
02B64ZX Excision of Right Atrium, Percutaneous Endoscopic Approach, Diagnostic	**02B90ZX** Excision of Chordae Tendineae, Open Approach, Diagnostic	**02BG0ZX** Excision of Mitral Valve, Open Approach, Diagnostic
	02B90ZZ Excision of Chordae Tendineae, Open Approach	

♀ Female-only ♂ Male-only ▲ Limited Coverage ● Non-OR [HAC] HAC-associated procedure ▲ Non-covered procedures ✚ Cluster

02BG0ZZ	Excision of Mitral Valve, Open Approach *AHA CC: 2Q, 2015, 23-24*	**02BM0ZZ**	Excision of Ventricular Septum, Open Approach	**02BS3ZX**	Excision of Right Pulmonary Vein, Percutaneous Approach, Diagnostic
02BG3ZX	Excision of Mitral Valve, Percutaneous Approach, Diagnostic	**02BM3ZX**	Excision of Ventricular Septum, Percutaneous Approach, Diagnostic	**02BS3ZZ**	Excision of Right Pulmonary Vein, Percutaneous Approach
02BG3ZZ	Excision of Mitral Valve, Percutaneous Approach	**02BM3ZZ**	Excision of Ventricular Septum, Percutaneous Approach	**02BS4ZX**	Excision of Right Pulmonary Vein, Percutaneous Endoscopic Approach, Diagnostic
02BG4ZX	Excision of Mitral Valve, Percutaneous Endoscopic Approach, Diagnostic	**02BM4ZX**	Excision of Ventricular Septum, Percutaneous Endoscopic Approach, Diagnostic	**02BS4ZZ**	Excision of Right Pulmonary Vein, Percutaneous Endoscopic Approach
02BG4ZZ	Excision of Mitral Valve, Percutaneous Endoscopic Approach	**02BM4ZZ**	Excision of Ventricular Septum, Percutaneous Endoscopic Approach	**02BT0ZX**	Excision of Left Pulmonary Vein, Open Approach, Diagnostic
02BH0ZX	Excision of Pulmonary Valve, Open Approach, Diagnostic	**02BN0ZX**	Excision of Pericardium, Open Approach, Diagnostic	**02BT0ZZ**	Excision of Left Pulmonary Vein, Open Approach
02BH0ZZ	Excision of Pulmonary Valve, Open Approach	**02BN0ZZ**	Excision of Pericardium, Open Approach *AHA CC: 2Q, 2019, 20-21*	**02BT3ZX**	Excision of Left Pulmonary Vein, Percutaneous Approach, Diagnostic
02BH3ZX	Excision of Pulmonary Valve, Percutaneous Approach, Diagnostic	**02BN3ZX**	Excision of Pericardium, Percutaneous Approach, Diagnostic	**02BT3ZZ**	Excision of Left Pulmonary Vein, Percutaneous Approach
02BH3ZZ	Excision of Pulmonary Valve, Percutaneous Approach	**02BN3ZZ**	Excision of Pericardium, Percutaneous Approach	**02BT4ZX**	Excision of Left Pulmonary Vein, Percutaneous Endoscopic Approach, Diagnostic
02BH4ZX	Excision of Pulmonary Valve, Percutaneous Endoscopic Approach, Diagnostic	**02BN4ZX**	Excision of Pericardium, Percutaneous Endoscopic Approach, Diagnostic	**02BT4ZZ**	Excision of Left Pulmonary Vein, Percutaneous Endoscopic Approach
02BH4ZZ	Excision of Pulmonary Valve, Percutaneous Endoscopic Approach	**02BN4ZZ**	Excision of Pericardium, Percutaneous Endoscopic Approach	**02BV0ZX**	Excision of Superior Vena Cava, Open Approach, Diagnostic
02BJ0ZX	Excision of Tricuspid Valve, Open Approach, Diagnostic	**02BP0ZX**	Excision of Pulmonary Trunk, Open Approach, Diagnostic	**02BV0ZZ**	Excision of Superior Vena Cava, Open Approach
02BJ0ZZ	Excision of Tricuspid Valve, Open Approach	**02BP0ZZ**	Excision of Pulmonary Trunk, Open Approach	**02BV3ZX**	Excision of Superior Vena Cava, Percutaneous Approach, Diagnostic
02BJ3ZX	Excision of Tricuspid Valve, Percutaneous Approach, Diagnostic	**02BP3ZX**	Excision of Pulmonary Trunk, Percutaneous Approach, Diagnostic	**02BV3ZZ**	Excision of Superior Vena Cava, Percutaneous Approach
02BJ3ZZ	Excision of Tricuspid Valve, Percutaneous Approach	**02BP3ZZ**	Excision of Pulmonary Trunk, Percutaneous Approach	**02BV4ZX**	Excision of Superior Vena Cava, Percutaneous Endoscopic Approach, Diagnostic
02BJ4ZX	Excision of Tricuspid Valve, Percutaneous Endoscopic Approach, Diagnostic	**02BP4ZX**	Excision of Pulmonary Trunk, Percutaneous Endoscopic Approach, Diagnostic	**02BV4ZZ**	Excision of Superior Vena Cava, Percutaneous Endoscopic Approach
02BJ4ZZ	Excision of Tricuspid Valve, Percutaneous Endoscopic Approach	**02BP4ZZ**	Excision of Pulmonary Trunk, Percutaneous Endoscopic Approach	**02BW0ZX**	Excision of Thoracic Aorta, Descending, Open Approach, Diagnostic
02BK0ZX	Excision of Right Ventricle, Open Approach, Diagnostic	**02BQ0ZX**	Excision of Right Pulmonary Artery, Open Approach, Diagnostic	**02BW0ZZ**	Excision of Thoracic Aorta, Descending, Open Approach
▲ **02BK0ZZ**	Excision of Right Ventricle, Open Approach	**02BQ0ZZ**	Excision of Right Pulmonary Artery, Open Approach	**02BW3ZX**	Excision of Thoracic Aorta, Descending, Percutaneous Approach, Diagnostic
02BK3ZX	Excision of Right Ventricle, Percutaneous Approach, Diagnostic *AHA CC: 3Q, 2019, 32*	**02BQ3ZX**	Excision of Right Pulmonary Artery, Percutaneous Approach, Diagnostic	**02BW3ZZ**	Excision of Thoracic Aorta, Descending, Percutaneous Approach
▲ **02BK3ZZ**	Excision of Right Ventricle, Percutaneous Approach	**02BQ3ZZ**	Excision of Right Pulmonary Artery, Percutaneous Approach	**02BW4ZX**	Excision of Thoracic Aorta, Descending, Percutaneous Endoscopic Approach, Diagnostic
02BK4ZX	Excision of Right Ventricle, Percutaneous Endoscopic Approach, Diagnostic	**02BQ4ZX**	Excision of Right Pulmonary Artery, Percutaneous Endoscopic Approach, Diagnostic	**02BW4ZZ**	Excision of Thoracic Aorta, Descending, Percutaneous Endoscopic Approach
▲ **02BK4ZZ**	Excision of Right Ventricle, Percutaneous Endoscopic Approach	**02BQ4ZZ**	Excision of Right Pulmonary Artery, Percutaneous Endoscopic Approach	**02BX0ZX**	Excision of Thoracic Aorta, Ascending/Arch, Open Approach, Diagnostic
02BL0ZX	Excision of Left Ventricle, Open Approach, Diagnostic	**02BR0ZX**	Excision of Left Pulmonary Artery, Open Approach, Diagnostic	**02BX0ZZ**	Excision of Thoracic Aorta, Ascending/Arch, Open Approach
▲ **02BL0ZZ**	Excision of Left Ventricle, Open Approach	**02BR0ZZ**	Excision of Left Pulmonary Artery, Open Approach	**02BX3ZX**	Excision of Thoracic Aorta, Ascending/Arch, Percutaneous Approach, Diagnostic
02BL3ZX	Excision of Left Ventricle, Percutaneous Approach, Diagnostic	**02BR3ZX**	Excision of Left Pulmonary Artery, Percutaneous Approach, Diagnostic	**02BX3ZZ**	Excision of Thoracic Aorta, Ascending/Arch, Percutaneous Approach
▲ **02BL3ZZ**	Excision of Left Ventricle, Percutaneous Approach	**02BR3ZZ**	Excision of Left Pulmonary Artery, Percutaneous Approach	**02BX4ZX**	Excision of Thoracic Aorta, Ascending/Arch, Percutaneous Endoscopic Approach, Diagnostic
02BL4ZX	Excision of Left Ventricle, Percutaneous Endoscopic Approach, Diagnostic	**02BR4ZX**	Excision of Left Pulmonary Artery, Percutaneous Endoscopic Approach, Diagnostic	**02BX4ZZ**	Excision of Thoracic Aorta, Ascending/Arch, Percutaneous Endoscopic Approach
▲ **02BL4ZZ**	Excision of Left Ventricle, Percutaneous Endoscopic Approach	**02BR4ZZ**	Excision of Left Pulmonary Artery, Percutaneous Endoscopic Approach		
02BM0ZX	Excision of Ventricular Septum, Open Approach, Diagnostic	**02BS0ZX**	Excision of Right Pulmonary Vein, Open Approach, Diagnostic		
		02BS0ZZ	Excision of Right Pulmonary Vein, Open Approach		

02C – Heart and Great Vessels, Extirpation

For Extirpation procedures involving coronary arteries, Review Coding Guideline B4.4

02C00Z6	Extirpation of Matter from Coronary Artery, One Artery, Bifurcation, Open Approach	**02C00ZZ**	Extirpation of Matter from Coronary Artery, One Artery, Open Approach	**02C03Z6**	Extirpation of Matter from Coronary Artery, One Artery, Bifurcation, Percutaneous Approach

♀ Female-only   ♂ Male-only   ▲ Limited Coverage   ● Non-OR   HAC HAC-associated procedure   ▲ Non-covered procedures   ✚ Cluster   **201**

02C03Z7 Extirpation of Matter from Coronary Artery, One Artery, Orbital Atherectomy Technique, Percutaneous Approach

02C03ZZ Extirpation of Matter from Coronary Artery, One Artery, Percutaneous Approach

02C04Z6 Extirpation of Matter from Coronary Artery, One Artery, Bifurcation, Percutaneous Endoscopic Approach

02C04ZZ Extirpation of Matter from Coronary Artery, One Artery, Percutaneous Endoscopic Approach

02C10Z6 Extirpation of Matter from Coronary Artery, Two Arteries, Bifurcation, Open Approach

02C10ZZ Extirpation of Matter from Coronary Artery, Two Arteries, Open Approach

02C13Z6 Extirpation of Matter from Coronary Artery, Two Arteries, Bifurcation, Percutaneous Approach

02C13Z7 Extirpation of Matter from Coronary Artery, Two Arteries, Orbital Atherectomy Technique, Percutaneous Approach

02C13ZZ Extirpation of Matter from Coronary Artery, Two Arteries, Percutaneous Approach

02C14Z6 Extirpation of Matter from Coronary Artery, Two Arteries, Bifurcation, Percutaneous Endoscopic Approach

02C14ZZ Extirpation of Matter from Coronary Artery, Two Arteries, Percutaneous Endoscopic Approach

02C20Z6 Extirpation of Matter from Coronary Artery, Three Arteries, Bifurcation, Open Approach

02C20ZZ Extirpation of Matter from Coronary Artery, Three Arteries, Open Approach

02C23Z6 Extirpation of Matter from Coronary Artery, Three Arteries, Bifurcation, Percutaneous Approach

02C23Z7 Extirpation of Matter from Coronary Artery, Three Arteries, Orbital Atherectomy Technique, Percutaneous Approach

02C23ZZ Extirpation of Matter from Coronary Artery, Three Arteries, Percutaneous Approach

02C24Z6 Extirpation of Matter from Coronary Artery, Three Arteries, Bifurcation, Percutaneous Endoscopic Approach

02C24ZZ Extirpation of Matter from Coronary Artery, Three Arteries, Percutaneous Endoscopic Approach

02C30Z6 Extirpation of Matter from Coronary Artery, Four or More Arteries, Bifurcation, Open Approach

02C30ZZ Extirpation of Matter from Coronary Artery, Four or More Arteries, Open Approach

02C33Z6 Extirpation of Matter from Coronary Artery, Four or More Arteries, Bifurcation, Percutaneous Approach

02C33Z7 Extirpation of Matter from Coronary Artery, Four or More Arteries, Orbital Atherectomy Technique, Percutaneous Approach

02C33ZZ Extirpation of Matter from Coronary Artery, Four or More Arteries, Percutaneous Approach

02C34Z6 Extirpation of Matter from Coronary Artery, Four or More Arteries, Bifurcation, Percutaneous Endoscopic Approach

02C34ZZ Extirpation of Matter from Coronary Artery, Four or More Arteries, Percutaneous Endoscopic Approach

02C40ZZ Extirpation of Matter from Coronary Vein, Open Approach

02C43ZZ Extirpation of Matter from Coronary Vein, Percutaneous Approach

02C44ZZ Extirpation of Matter from Coronary Vein, Percutaneous Endoscopic Approach

02C50ZZ Extirpation of Matter from Atrial Septum, Open Approach

02C53ZZ Extirpation of Matter from Atrial Septum, Percutaneous Approach

02C54ZZ Extirpation of Matter from Atrial Septum, Percutaneous Endoscopic Approach

02C60ZZ Extirpation of Matter from Right Atrium, Open Approach

02C63ZZ Extirpation of Matter from Right Atrium, Percutaneous Approach

02C64ZZ Extirpation of Matter from Right Atrium, Percutaneous Endoscopic Approach

02C70ZZ Extirpation of Matter from Left Atrium, Open Approach

02C73ZZ Extirpation of Matter from Left Atrium, Percutaneous Approach

02C74ZZ Extirpation of Matter from Left Atrium, Percutaneous Endoscopic Approach

02C80ZZ Extirpation of Matter from Conduction Mechanism, Open Approach

02C83ZZ Extirpation of Matter from Conduction Mechanism, Percutaneous Approach

02C84ZZ Extirpation of Matter from Conduction Mechanism, Percutaneous Endoscopic Approach

02C90ZZ Extirpation of Matter from Chordae Tendineae, Open Approach

02C93ZZ Extirpation of Matter from Chordae Tendineae, Percutaneous Approach

02C94ZZ Extirpation of Matter from Chordae Tendineae, Percutaneous Endoscopic Approach

02CD0ZZ Extirpation of Matter from Papillary Muscle, Open Approach

02CD3ZZ Extirpation of Matter from Papillary Muscle, Percutaneous Approach

02CD4ZZ Extirpation of Matter from Papillary Muscle, Percutaneous Endoscopic Approach

02CF0ZZ Extirpation of Matter from Aortic Valve, Open Approach

02CF3ZZ Extirpation of Matter from Aortic Valve, Percutaneous Approach

02CF4ZZ Extirpation of Matter from Aortic Valve, Percutaneous Endoscopic Approach

02CG0ZZ Extirpation of Matter from Mitral Valve, Open Approach

AHA CC: 2Q, 2016, 24-25

02CG3ZZ Extirpation of Matter from Mitral Valve, Percutaneous Approach

02CG4ZZ Extirpation of Matter from Mitral Valve, Percutaneous Endoscopic Approach

02CH0ZZ Extirpation of Matter from Pulmonary Valve, Open Approach

02CH3ZZ Extirpation of Matter from Pulmonary Valve, Percutaneous Approach

02CH4ZZ Extirpation of Matter from Pulmonary Valve, Percutaneous Endoscopic Approach

02CJ0ZZ Extirpation of Matter from Tricuspid Valve, Open Approach

02CJ3ZZ Extirpation of Matter from Tricuspid Valve, Percutaneous Approach

02CJ4ZZ Extirpation of Matter from Tricuspid Valve, Percutaneous Endoscopic Approach

02CK0ZZ Extirpation of Matter from Right Ventricle, Open Approach

02CK3ZZ Extirpation of Matter from Right Ventricle, Percutaneous Approach

02CK4ZZ Extirpation of Matter from Right Ventricle, Percutaneous Endoscopic Approach

02CL0ZZ Extirpation of Matter from Left Ventricle, Open Approach

02CL3ZZ Extirpation of Matter from Left Ventricle, Percutaneous Approach

02CL4ZZ Extirpation of Matter from Left Ventricle, Percutaneous Endoscopic Approach

02CM0ZZ Extirpation of Matter from Ventricular Septum, Open Approach

02CM3ZZ Extirpation of Matter from Ventricular Septum, Percutaneous Approach

02CM4ZZ Extirpation of Matter from Ventricular Septum, Percutaneous Endoscopic Approach

02CN0ZZ Extirpation of Matter from Pericardium, Open Approach

02CN3ZZ Extirpation of Matter from Pericardium, Percutaneous Approach

02CN4ZZ Extirpation of Matter from Pericardium, Percutaneous Endoscopic Approach

02CP0ZZ Extirpation of Matter from Pulmonary Trunk, Open Approach

02CP3ZZ Extirpation of Matter from Pulmonary Trunk, Percutaneous Approach

02CP4ZZ Extirpation of Matter from Pulmonary Trunk, Percutaneous Endoscopic Approach

02CQ0ZZ Extirpation of Matter from Right Pulmonary Artery, Open Approach

02CQ3ZZ Extirpation of Matter from Right Pulmonary Artery, Percutaneous Approach

02CQ4ZZ Extirpation of Matter from Right Pulmonary Artery, Percutaneous Endoscopic Approach

02CR0ZZ Extirpation of Matter from Left Pulmonary Artery, Open Approach

02CR3ZZ Extirpation of Matter from Left Pulmonary Artery, Percutaneous Approach

02CR4ZZ Extirpation of Matter from Left Pulmonary Artery, Percutaneous Endoscopic Approach

02CS0ZZ Extirpation of Matter from Right Pulmonary Vein, Open Approach

02CS3ZZ Extirpation of Matter from Right Pulmonary Vein, Percutaneous Approach

02CS4ZZ Extirpation of Matter from Right Pulmonary Vein, Percutaneous Endoscopic Approach

02CT0ZZ Extirpation of Matter from Left Pulmonary Vein, Open Approach

02CT3ZZ Extirpation of Matter from Left Pulmonary Vein, Percutaneous Approach

02CT4ZZ Extirpation of Matter from Left Pulmonary Vein, Percutaneous Endoscopic Approach

02CV0ZZ Extirpation of Matter from Superior Vena Cava, Open Approach

02CV3ZZ Extirpation of Matter from Superior Vena Cava, Percutaneous Approach

02CV4ZZ Extirpation of Matter from Superior Vena Cava, Percutaneous Endoscopic Approach

♀ Female-only ♂ Male-only ▲ Limited Coverage ● Non-OR HAC HAC-associated procedure ▲ Non-covered procedures ✚ Cluster

02CW0ZZ Extirpation of Matter from Thoracic Aorta, Descending, Open Approach

02CW3ZZ Extirpation of Matter from Thoracic Aorta, Descending, Percutaneous Approach

02CW4ZZ Extirpation of Matter from Thoracic Aorta, Descending, Percutaneous Endoscopic Approach

02CX0ZZ Extirpation of Matter from Thoracic Aorta, Ascending/Arch, Open Approach

02CX3ZZ Extirpation of Matter from Thoracic Aorta, Ascending/Arch, Percutaneous Approach

02CX4ZZ Extirpation of Matter from Thoracic Aorta, Ascending/Arch, Percutaneous Endoscopic Approach

02F – Heart and Great Vessels, Fragmentation

02F03ZZ Fragmentation in Coronary Artery, One Artery, Percutaneous Approach

▲ **02F13ZZ** Fragmentation in Coronary Artery, Two Arteries, Percutaneous Approach

02F23ZZ Fragmentation in Coronary Artery, Three Arteries, Percutaneous Approach

02F33ZZ Fragmentation in Coronary Artery, Four or More Arteries, Percutaneous Approach

02FN0ZZ Fragmentation in Pericardium, Open Approach

02FN3ZZ Fragmentation in Pericardium, Percutaneous Approach

02FN4ZZ Fragmentation in Pericardium, Percutaneous Endoscopic Approach

▲ **02FNXZZ** Fragmentation in Pericardium, External Approach

02FP3Z0 Fragmentation of Pulmonary Trunk, Percutaneous Approach, Ultrasonic

02FP3ZZ Fragmentation of Pulmonary Trunk, Percutaneous Approach

02FQ3Z0 Fragmentation of Right Pulmonary Artery, Percutaneous Approach, Ultrasonic

02FQ3ZZ Fragmentation of Right Pulmonary Artery, Percutaneous Approach

02FR3Z0 Fragmentation of Left Pulmonary Artery, Percutaneous Approach, Ultrasonic

02FR3ZZ Fragmentation of Left Pulmonary Artery, Percutaneous Approach

02FS3Z0 Fragmentation of Right Pulmonary Vein, Percutaneous Approach, Ultrasonic

02FS3ZZ Fragmentation of Right Pulmonary Vein, Percutaneous Approach

02FT3Z0 Fragmentation of Left Pulmonary Vein, Percutaneous Approach, Ultrasonic

02FT3ZZ Fragmentation of Left Pulmonary Vein, Percutaneous Approach

02H – Heart and Great Vessels, Insertion

02H00DZ Insertion of Intraluminal Device into Coronary Artery, One Artery, Open Approach

02H00YZ Insertion of Other Device into Coronary Artery, One Artery, Open Approach

02H03DZ Insertion of Intraluminal Device into Coronary Artery, One Artery, Percutaneous Approach

02H03YZ Insertion of Other Device into Coronary Artery, One Artery, Percutaneous Approach

02H04DZ Insertion of Intraluminal Device into Coronary Artery, One Artery, Percutaneous Endoscopic Approach

02H04YZ Insertion of Other Device into Coronary Artery, One Artery, Percutaneous Endoscopic Approach

02H10DZ Insertion of Intraluminal Device into Coronary Artery, Two Arteries, Open Approach

02H10YZ Insertion of Other Device into Coronary Artery, Two Arteries, Open Approach

02H13DZ Insertion of Intraluminal Device into Coronary Artery, Two Arteries, Percutaneous Approach
AHA CC: 4Q, 2019, 24

02H13YZ Insertion of Other Device into Coronary Artery, Two Arteries, Percutaneous Approach

02H14DZ Insertion of Intraluminal Device into Coronary Artery, Two Arteries, Percutaneous Endoscopic Approach

02H14YZ Insertion of Other Device into Coronary Artery, Two Arteries, Percutaneous Endoscopic Approach

02H20DZ Insertion of Intraluminal Device into Coronary Artery, Three Arteries, Open Approach

02H20YZ Insertion of Other Device into Coronary Artery, Three Arteries, Open Approach

02H23DZ Insertion of Intraluminal Device into Coronary Artery, Three Arteries, Percutaneous Approach

02H23YZ Insertion of Other Device into Coronary Artery, Three Arteries, Percutaneous Approach

02H24DZ Insertion of Intraluminal Device into Coronary Artery, Three Arteries, Percutaneous Endoscopic Approach

02H24YZ Insertion of Other Device into Coronary Artery, Three Arteries, Percutaneous Endoscopic Approach

02H30DZ Insertion of Intraluminal Device into Coronary Artery, Four or More Arteries, Open Approach

02H30YZ Insertion of Other Device into Coronary Artery, Four or More Arteries, Open Approach

02H33DZ Insertion of Intraluminal Device into Coronary Artery, Four or More Arteries, Percutaneous Approach

02H33YZ Insertion of Other Device into Coronary Artery, Four or More Arteries, Percutaneous Approach

02H34DZ Insertion of Intraluminal Device into Coronary Artery, Four or More Arteries, Percutaneous Endoscopic Approach

02H34YZ Insertion of Other Device into Coronary Artery, Four or More Arteries, Percutaneous Endoscopic Approach

02H400Z Insertion of Pressure Sensor Monitoring Device into Coronary Vein, Open Approach

02H402Z Insertion of Monitoring Device into Coronary Vein, Open Approach

02H403Z Insertion of Infusion Device into Coronary Vein, Open Approach

02H40DZ Insertion of Intraluminal Device into Coronary Vein, Open Approach

● **02H40JZ** Insertion of Pacemaker Lead into Coronary Vein, Open Approach

➕ Pacemaker lead is part of pacemaker cluster for MS-DRG assignment when reported with pacemaker device code. *See table 0JH to construct pacemaker device Insertion code.*

02H40KZ Insertion of Defibrillator Lead into Coronary Vein, Open Approach

➕ Lead device when reported with an Insertion of a cardiac resynchronization defibrillator device (6th character 9) into the chest or abdomen subcutaneous tissue and fascia. *See table 0JH to construct the Insertion code.*

● **02H40MZ** Insertion of Cardiac Lead into Coronary Vein, Open Approach

➕ Pacemaker lead is part of pacemaker cluster for MS-DRG assignment when reported with pacemaker device code. *See table 0JH to construct pacemaker device Insertion code.*

02H40NZ Insertion of Intracardiac Pacemaker into Coronary Vein, Open Approach

02H40YZ Insertion of Other Device into Coronary Vein, Open Approach

02H430Z Insertion of Pressure Sensor Monitoring Device into Coronary Vein, Percutaneous Approach

02H432Z Insertion of Monitoring Device into Coronary Vein, Percutaneous Approach

02H433Z Insertion of Infusion Device into Coronary Vein, Percutaneous Approach

02H43DZ Insertion of Intraluminal Device into Coronary Vein, Percutaneous Approach

● **02H43JZ** Insertion of Pacemaker Lead into Coronary Vein, Percutaneous Approach

➕ Pacemaker lead is part of pacemaker cluster for MS-DRG assignment when reported with pacemaker device code. *See table 0JH to construct pacemaker device Insertion code.*

➕ Lead device when reported with an Insertion of a cardiac resynchronization defibrillator device (6th character 9) into the chest or abdomen subcutaneous tissue and fascia. *See table 0JH to construct the Insertion code.*

HAC With a secondary diagnosis code of K68.11, T81.40XA, T81.41XA, T81.42XA, T81.43XA, T81.44XA, T82.6XXA, T82.7XXA

02H43KZ Insertion of Defibrillator Lead into Coronary Vein, Percutaneous Approach

HAC With a secondary diagnosis code of K68.11, T81.40XA, T81.41XA, T81.42XA, T81.43XA, T81.44XA, T82.6XXA, T82.7XXA

● **02H43MZ** Insertion of Cardiac Lead into Coronary Vein, Percutaneous Approach

➕ Pacemaker lead is part of pacemaker cluster for MS-DRG assignment when reported with pacemaker device code. *See table 0JH to construct pacemaker device Insertion code.*

♀ Female-only   ♂ Male-only   ▲ Limited Coverage   ● Non-OR   HAC HAC-associated procedure   ▲ Non-covered procedures   ➕ Cluster

+ Lead device when reported with an Insertion of a cardiac resynchronization defibrillator device (6th character 9) into the chest or abdomen subcutaneous tissue and fascia. *See table 0JH to construct the Insertion code.*

HAC With a secondary diagnosis code of K68.11, T81.40XA, T81.41XA, T81.42XA, T81.43XA, T81.44XA, T82.6XXA, T82.7XXA

02H43NZ Insertion of Intracardiac Pacemaker into Coronary Vein, Percutaneous Approach

● **02H43YZ** Insertion of Other Device into Coronary Vein, Percutaneous Approach

02H440Z Insertion of Pressure Sensor Monitoring Device into Coronary Vein, Percutaneous Endoscopic Approach

02H442Z Insertion of Monitoring Device into Coronary Vein, Percutaneous Endoscopic Approach

02H443Z Insertion of Infusion Device into Coronary Vein, Percutaneous Endoscopic Approach

02H44DZ Insertion of Intraluminal Device into Coronary Vein, Percutaneous Endoscopic Approach

● **02H44JZ** Insertion of Pacemaker Lead into Coronary Vein, Percutaneous Endoscopic Approach

+ Pacemaker lead is part of pacemaker cluster for MS-DRG assignment when reported with pacemaker device code. *See table 0JH to construct pacemaker device Insertion code.*

02H44KZ Insertion of Defibrillator Lead into Coronary Vein, Percutaneous Endoscopic Approach

+ Lead device when reported with an Insertion of a cardiac resynchronization defibrillator device (6th character 9) into the chest or abdomen subcutaneous tissue and fascia. *See table 0JH to construct the Insertion code.*

● **02H44MZ** Insertion of Cardiac Lead into Coronary Vein, Percutaneous Endoscopic Approach

+ Pacemaker lead is part of pacemaker cluster for MS-DRG assignment when reported with pacemaker device code. *See table 0JH to construct pacemaker device Insertion code.*

02H44NZ Insertion of Intracardiac Pacemaker into Coronary Vein, Percutaneous Endoscopic Approach

02H44YZ Insertion of Other Device into Coronary Vein, Percutaneous Endoscopic Approach

02H600Z Insertion of Pressure Sensor Monitoring Device into Right Atrium, Open Approach

02H602Z Insertion of Monitoring Device into Right Atrium, Open Approach

02H603Z Insertion of Infusion Device into Right Atrium, Open Approach

02H60DZ Insertion of Intraluminal Device into Right Atrium, Open Approach

● **02H60JZ** Insertion of Pacemaker Lead into Right Atrium, Open Approach

+ Pacemaker lead is part of pacemaker cluster for MS-DRG assignment when reported with pacemaker device code. *See table 0JH to construct pacemaker device Insertion code.*

02H60KZ Insertion of Defibrillator Lead into Right Atrium, Open Approach

+ Lead device when reported with an Insertion of a defibrillator generator (6th character 8 or 9) into the chest or abdomen subcutaneous tissue and fascia. *See table 0JH to construct the Insertion code.*

● **02H60MZ** Insertion of Cardiac Lead into Right Atrium, Open Approach

+ Pacemaker lead is part of pacemaker cluster for MS-DRG assignment when reported with pacemaker device code. *See table 0JH to construct pacemaker device Insertion code.*

+ Lead device when reported with an Insertion of contractility modulation device (6th character A) into the chest or abdomen subcutaneous tissue and fascia. *See table 0JH to construct the Insertion code.*

02H60NZ Insertion of Intracardiac Pacemaker into Right Atrium, Open Approach

02H60YZ Insertion of Other Device into Right Atrium, Open Approach

02H630Z Insertion of Pressure Sensor Monitoring Device into Right Atrium, Percutaneous Approach

02H632Z Insertion of Monitoring Device into Right Atrium, Percutaneous Approach

02H633Z Insertion of Infusion Device into Right Atrium, Percutaneous Approach

HAC When reported with secondary diagnosis code J95.811

AHA CC: 2Q, 2016, 15-16; 2Q, 2017, 24-26

02H63DZ Insertion of Intraluminal Device into Right Atrium, Percutaneous Approach

● **02H63JZ** Insertion of Pacemaker Lead into Right Atrium, Percutaneous Approach

HAC With a secondary diagnosis code of K68.11, T81.40XA, T81.41XA, T81.42XA, T81.43XA, T81.44XA, T82.6XXA, T82.7XXA

+ Pacemaker lead is part of pacemaker cluster for MS-DRG assignment when reported with pacemaker device code. *See table 0JH to construct pacemaker device Insertion code.*

02H63KZ Insertion of Defibrillator Lead into Right Atrium, Percutaneous Approach

+ Lead device when reported with an Insertion of a defibrillator generator (6th character 8 or 9) into the chest or abdomen subcutaneous tissue and fascia. *See table 0JH to construct the Insertion code.*

AHA CC: 2Q, 2018, 19

● **02H63MZ** Insertion of Cardiac Lead into Right Atrium, Percutaneous Approach

+ Pacemaker lead is part of pacemaker cluster for MS-DRG assignment when reported with pacemaker device code. *See table 0JH to construct pacemaker device Insertion code.*

+ Lead device when reported with an Insertion of contractility modulation device (6th character A) into the chest or abdomen subcutaneous tissue and fascia. *See table 0JH to construct the Insertion code.*

HAC With a secondary diagnosis code of K68.11, T81.40XA, T81.41XA, T81.42XA, T81.43XA, T81.44XA, T82.6XXA, T82.7XXA

02H63NZ Insertion of Intracardiac Pacemaker into Right Atrium, Percutaneous Approach

02H63YZ Insertion of Other Device into Right Atrium, Percutaneous Approach

02H640Z Insertion of Pressure Sensor Monitoring Device into Right Atrium, Percutaneous Endoscopic Approach

02H642Z Insertion of Monitoring Device into Right Atrium, Percutaneous Endoscopic Approach

02H643Z Insertion of Infusion Device into Right Atrium, Percutaneous Endoscopic Approach

02H64DZ Insertion of Intraluminal Device into Right Atrium, Percutaneous Endoscopic Approach

● **02H64JZ** Insertion of Pacemaker Lead into Right Atrium, Percutaneous Endoscopic Approach

+ Pacemaker lead is part of pacemaker cluster for MS-DRG assignment when reported with pacemaker device code. *See table 0JH to construct pacemaker device Insertion code.*

02H64KZ Insertion of Defibrillator Lead into Right Atrium, Percutaneous Endoscopic Approach

+ Lead device when reported with an Insertion of a defibrillator generator (6th character 8 or 9) into the chest or abdomen subcutaneous tissue and fascia. *See table 0JH to construct the Insertion code.*

● **02H64MZ** Insertion of Cardiac Lead into Right Atrium, Percutaneous Endoscopic Approach

+ Pacemaker lead is part of pacemaker cluster for MS-DRG assignment when reported with pacemaker device code. *See table 0JH to construct pacemaker device Insertion code.*

+ Lead device when reported with an Insertion of contractility modulation device (6th character A) into the chest or abdomen subcutaneous tissue and fascia. *See table 0JH to construct the Insertion code.*

02H64NZ Insertion of Intracardiac Pacemaker into Right Atrium, Percutaneous Endoscopic Approach

02H64YZ Insertion of Other Device into Right Atrium, Percutaneous Endoscopic Approach

02H700Z Insertion of Pressure Sensor Monitoring Device into Left Atrium, Open Approach

02H702Z Insertion of Monitoring Device into Left Atrium, Open Approach

02H703Z Insertion of Infusion Device into Left Atrium, Open Approach

02H70DZ Insertion of Intraluminal Device into Left Atrium, Open Approach

● **02H70JZ** Insertion of Pacemaker Lead into Left Atrium, Open Approach

+ Pacemaker lead is part of pacemaker cluster for MS-DRG assignment when reported with pacemaker device code. *See table 0JH to construct pacemaker device Insertion code.*

02H70KZ Insertion of Defibrillator Lead into Left Atrium, Open Approach

+ Lead device when reported with an Insertion of a defibrillator generator (6th character 8 or 9) into the chest or abdomen subcutaneous tissue and fascia. *See table 0JH to construct the Insertion code.*

● **02H70MZ** Insertion of Cardiac Lead into Left Atrium, Open Approach

♀ Female-only   ♂ Male-only   ▲ Limited Coverage   ● Non-OR   HAC HAC-associated procedure   ▲ Non-covered procedures   + Cluster

⊕ Pacemaker lead is part of pacemaker cluster for MS-DRG assignment when reported with pacemaker device code. *See table 0JH to construct pacemaker device Insertion code.*

02H70NZ Insertion of Intracardiac Pacemaker into Left Atrium, Open Approach

02H70YZ Insertion of Other Device into Left Atrium, Open Approach

02H730Z Insertion of Pressure Sensor Monitoring Device into Left Atrium, Percutaneous Approach

02H732Z Insertion of Monitoring Device into Left Atrium, Percutaneous Approach

02H733Z Insertion of Infusion Device into Left Atrium, Percutaneous Approach

02H73DZ Insertion of Intraluminal Device into Left Atrium, Percutaneous Approach

AHA CC: 4Q, 2017, 104-105

● **02H73JZ** Insertion of Pacemaker Lead into Left Atrium, Percutaneous Approach

HAC With a secondary diagnosis code of K68.11, T81.40XA, T81.41XA, T81.42XA, T81.43XA, T81.44XA, T82.6XXA, T82.7XXA

⊕ Pacemaker lead is part of pacemaker cluster for MS-DRG assignment when reported with pacemaker device code. *See table 0JH to construct pacemaker device Insertion code.*

02H73KZ Insertion of Defibrillator Lead into Left Atrium, Percutaneous Approach

⊕ Lead device when reported with an Insertion of a defibrillator generator (6th character 8 or 9) into the chest or abdomen subcutaneous tissue and fascia. *See table 0JH to construct the Insertion code.*

● **02H73MZ** Insertion of Cardiac Lead into Left Atrium, Percutaneous Approach

HAC With a secondary diagnosis code of K68.11, T81.40XA, T81.41XA, T81.42XA, T81.43XA, T81.44XA, T82.6XXA, T82.7XXA

02H73NZ Insertion of Intracardiac Pacemaker into Left Atrium, Percutaneous Approach

02H73YZ Insertion of Other Device into Left Atrium, Percutaneous Approach

02H740Z Insertion of Pressure Sensor Monitoring Device into Left Atrium, Percutaneous Endoscopic Approach

02H742Z Insertion of Monitoring Device into Left Atrium, Percutaneous Endoscopic Approach

02H743Z Insertion of Infusion Device into Left Atrium, Percutaneous Endoscopic Approach

02H74DZ Insertion of Intraluminal Device into Left Atrium, Percutaneous Endoscopic Approach

● **02H74JZ** Insertion of Pacemaker Lead into Left Atrium, Percutaneous Endoscopic Approach

⊕ Pacemaker lead is part of pacemaker cluster for MS-DRG assignment when reported with pacemaker device code. *See table 0JH to construct pacemaker device Insertion code.*

02H74KZ Insertion of Defibrillator Lead into Left Atrium, Percutaneous Endoscopic Approach

⊕ Lead device when reported with an Insertion of a defibrillator generator (6th character 8 or 9) into the chest or abdomen subcutaneous tissue and fascia. *See table 0JH to construct the Insertion code.*

● **02H74MZ** Insertion of Cardiac Lead into Left Atrium, Percutaneous Endoscopic Approach

⊕ Pacemaker lead is part of pacemaker cluster for MS-DRG assignment when reported with pacemaker device code. *See table 0JH to construct pacemaker device Insertion code.*

02H74NZ Insertion of Intracardiac Pacemaker into Left Atrium, Percutaneous Endoscopic Approach

02H74YZ Insertion of Other Device into Left Atrium, Percutaneous Endoscopic Approach

▲ **02HA0QZ** Insertion of Implantable Heart Assist System into Heart, Open Approach

AHA CC: 1Q, 2019, 24

02HA0RJ Insertion of Short-term External Heart Assist System into Heart, Intraoperative, Open Approach

02HA0RS Insertion of Biventricular Short-term External Heart Assist System into Heart, Open Approach

⊕ Heart assist system replacement when reported with a removal of an external heart assist system (6th character R) from the heart. *See table 02P to construct the Removal code.*

02HA0RZ Insertion of Short-term External Heart Assist System into Heart, Open Approach

⊕ Heart assist system replacement when reported with a removal of an external heart assist system (6th character R) from the heart. *See table 02P to construct the Removal code.*

02HA0YZ Insertion of Other Device into Heart, Open Approach

▲ **02HA3QZ** Insertion of Implantable Heart Assist System into Heart, Percutaneous Approach

02HA3RJ Insertion of Short-term External Heart Assist System into Heart, Intraoperative, Percutaneous Approach

AHA CC: 4Q, 2017, 43-44

02HA3RS Insertion of Biventricular Short-term External Heart Assist System into Heart, Percutaneous Approach

⊕ Heart assist system replacement when reported with a removal of an external heart assist system (6th character R) from the heart. *See table 02P to construct the Removal code.*

AHA CC: 4Q, 2016, 138-139

02HA3RZ Insertion of Short-term External Heart Assist System into Heart, Percutaneous Approach

⊕ Heart assist system replacement when reported with a removal of an external heart assist system (6th character R) from the heart. *See table 02P to construct the Removal code.*

AHA CC: 1Q, 2017, 11-12; 4Q, 2017, 44-45

02HA3YZ Insertion of Other Device into Heart, Percutaneous Approach

▲ **02HA4QZ** Insertion of Implantable Heart Assist System into Heart, Percutaneous Endoscopic Approach

02HA4RJ Insertion of Short-term External Heart Assist System into Heart, Intraoperative, Percutaneous Endoscopic Approach

02HA4RS Insertion of Biventricular Short-term External Heart Assist System into Heart, Percutaneous Endoscopic Approach

⊕ Heart assist system replacement when reported with a removal of an external heart assist system (6th character R) from the heart. *See table 02P to construct the Removal code.*

02HA4RZ Insertion of Short-term External Heart Assist System into Heart, Percutaneous Endoscopic Approach

⊕ Heart assist system replacement when reported with a removal of an external heart assist system (6th character R) from the heart. *See table 02P to construct the Removal code.*

02HA4YZ Insertion of Other Device into Heart, Percutaneous Endoscopic Approach

02HK00Z Insertion of Pressure Sensor Monitoring Device into Right Ventricle, Open Approach

02HK02Z Insertion of Monitoring Device into Right Ventricle, Open Approach

02HK03Z Insertion of Infusion Device into Right Ventricle, Open Approach

02HK0DZ Insertion of Intraluminal Device into Right Ventricle, Open Approach

● **02HK0JZ** Insertion of Pacemaker Lead into Right Ventricle, Open Approach

⊕ Pacemaker lead is part of pacemaker cluster for MS-DRG assignment when reported with pacemaker device code. *See table 0JH to construct pacemaker device Insertion code.*

02HK0KZ Insertion of Defibrillator Lead into Right Ventricle, Open Approach

⊕ Lead device when reported with an Insertion of a defibrillator generator (6th character 8 or 9) into the chest or abdomen subcutaneous tissue and fascia. *See table 0JH to construct the Insertion code.*

● **02HK0MZ** Insertion of Cardiac Lead into Right Ventricle, Open Approach

⊕ Pacemaker lead is part of pacemaker cluster for MS-DRG assignment when reported with pacemaker device code. *See table 0JH to construct pacemaker device Insertion code.*

⊕ Lead device when reported with an Insertion of contractility modulation device (6th character A) into the chest or abdomen subcutaneous tissue and fascia. *See table 0JH to construct the Insertion code.*

02HK0NZ Insertion of Intracardiac Pacemaker into Right Ventricle, Open Approach

02HK0YZ Insertion of Other Device into Right Ventricle, Open Approach

02HK30Z Insertion of Pressure Sensor Monitoring Device into Right Ventricle, Percutaneous Approach

● **02HK32Z** Insertion of Monitoring Device into Right Ventricle, Percutaneous Approach

02HK33Z Insertion of Infusion Device into Right Ventricle, Percutaneous Approach

HAC When reported with secondary diagnosis code J95.811

02HK3DZ Insertion of Intraluminal Device into Right Ventricle, Percutaneous Approach

AHA CC: 2Q, 2015, 31-32

● **02HK3JZ** Insertion of Pacemaker Lead into Right Ventricle, Percutaneous Approach

HAC With a secondary diagnosis code of K68.11, T81.40XA, T81.41XA, T81.42XA, T81.43XA, T81.44XA, T82.6XXA, T82.7XXA

+   Pacemaker lead is part of pacemaker cluster for MS-DRG assignment when reported with pacemaker device code. *See table 0JH to construct pacemaker device Insertion code.*

02HK3KZ   Insertion of Defibrillator Lead into Right Ventricle, Percutaneous Approach

+   Lead device when reported with an Insertion of a defibrillator generator (6th character 8 or 9) into the chest or abdomen subcutaneous tissue and fascia. *See table 0JH to construct the Insertion code.*

● **02HK3MZ**   Insertion of Cardiac Lead into Right Ventricle, Percutaneous Approach

+   Pacemaker lead is part of pacemaker cluster for MS-DRG assignment when reported with pacemaker device code. *See table 0JH to construct pacemaker device Insertion code.*

+   Lead device when reported with an Insertion of contractility modulation device (6th character A) into the chest or abdomen subcutaneous tissue and fascia. *See table 0JH to construct the Insertion code.*

02HK3NZ   Insertion of Intracardiac Pacemaker into Right Ventricle, Percutaneous Approach

02HK3YZ   Insertion of Other Device into Right Ventricle, Percutaneous Approach

02HK40Z   Insertion of Pressure Sensor Monitoring Device into Right Ventricle, Percutaneous Endoscopic Approach

02HK42Z   Insertion of Monitoring Device into Right Ventricle, Percutaneous Endoscopic Approach

02HK43Z   Insertion of Infusion Device into Right Ventricle, Percutaneous Endoscopic Approach

02HK4DZ   Insertion of Intraluminal Device into Right Ventricle, Percutaneous Endoscopic Approach

● **02HK4JZ**   Insertion of Pacemaker Lead into Right Ventricle, Percutaneous Endoscopic Approach

+   Pacemaker lead is part of pacemaker cluster for MS-DRG assignment when reported with pacemaker device code. *See table 0JH to construct pacemaker device Insertion code.*

02HK4KZ   Insertion of Defibrillator Lead into Right Ventricle, Percutaneous Endoscopic Approach

+   Lead device when reported with an Insertion of a defibrillator generator (6th character 8 or 9) into the chest or abdomen subcutaneous tissue and fascia. *See table 0JH to construct the Insertion code.*

● **02HK4MZ**   Insertion of Cardiac Lead into Right Ventricle, Percutaneous Endoscopic Approach

+   Pacemaker lead is part of pacemaker cluster for MS-DRG assignment when reported with pacemaker device code. *See table 0JH to construct pacemaker device Insertion code.*

+   Lead device when reported with an Insertion of contractility modulation device (6th character A) into the chest or abdomen subcutaneous tissue and fascia. *See table 0JH to construct the Insertion code.*

02HK4NZ   Insertion of Intracardiac Pacemaker into Right Ventricle, Percutaneous Endoscopic Approach

02HK4YZ   Insertion of Other Device into Right Ventricle, Percutaneous Endoscopic Approach

02HL00Z   Insertion of Pressure Sensor Monitoring Device into Left Ventricle, Open Approach

02HL02Z   Insertion of Monitoring Device into Left Ventricle, Open Approach

02HL03Z   Insertion of Infusion Device into Left Ventricle, Open Approach

02HL0DZ   Insertion of Intraluminal Device into Left Ventricle, Open Approach

AHA CC: 3Q, 2019, 19-20

● **02HL0JZ**   Insertion of Pacemaker Lead into Left Ventricle, Open Approach

+   Pacemaker lead is part of pacemaker cluster for MS-DRG assignment when reported with pacemaker device code. *See table 0JH to construct pacemaker device Insertion code.*

02HL0KZ   Insertion of Defibrillator Lead into Left Ventricle, Open Approach

+   Lead device when reported with an Insertion of a defibrillator generator (6th character 8 or 9) into the chest or abdomen subcutaneous tissue and fascia. *See table 0JH to construct the Insertion code.*

● **02HL0MZ**   Insertion of Cardiac Lead into Left Ventricle, Open Approach

+   Pacemaker lead is part of pacemaker cluster for MS-DRG assignment when reported with pacemaker device code. *See table 0JH to construct pacemaker device Insertion code.*

02HL0NZ   Insertion of Intracardiac Pacemaker into Left Ventricle, Open Approach

02HL0YZ   Insertion of Other Device into Left Ventricle, Open Approach

02HL30Z   Insertion of Pressure Sensor Monitoring Device into Left Ventricle, Percutaneous Approach

02HL32Z   Insertion of Monitoring Device into Left Ventricle, Percutaneous Approach

02HL33Z   Insertion of Infusion Device into Left Ventricle, Percutaneous Approach

02HL3DZ   Insertion of Intraluminal Device into Left Ventricle, Percutaneous Approach

● **02HL3JZ**   Insertion of Pacemaker Lead into Left Ventricle, Percutaneous Approach

AHA CC: 3Q, 2019, 23

HAC   With a secondary diagnosis code of K68.11, T81.40XA, T81.41XA, T81.42XA, T81.43XA, T81.44XA, T82.6XXA, T82.7XXA

+   Pacemaker lead is part of pacemaker cluster for MS-DRG assignment when reported with pacemaker device code. *See table 0JH to construct pacemaker device Insertion code.*

02HL3KZ   Insertion of Defibrillator Lead into Left Ventricle, Percutaneous Approach

+   Lead device when reported with an Insertion of a defibrillator generator (6th character 8 or 9) into the chest or abdomen subcutaneous tissue and fascia. *See table 0JH to construct the Insertion code.*

● **02HL3MZ**   Insertion of Cardiac Lead into Left Ventricle, Percutaneous Approach

+   Pacemaker lead is part of pacemaker cluster for MS-DRG assignment when reported with pacemaker device code. *See table 0JH to construct pacemaker device Insertion code.*

02HL3NZ   Insertion of Intracardiac Pacemaker into Left Ventricle, Percutaneous Approach

02HL3YZ   Insertion of Other Device into Left Ventricle, Percutaneous Approach

02HL40Z   Insertion of Pressure Sensor Monitoring Device into Left Ventricle, Percutaneous Endoscopic Approach

02HL42Z   Insertion of Monitoring Device into Left Ventricle, Percutaneous Endoscopic Approach

02HL43Z   Insertion of Infusion Device into Left Ventricle, Percutaneous Endoscopic Approach

02HL4DZ   Insertion of Intraluminal Device into Left Ventricle, Percutaneous Endoscopic Approach

● **02HL4JZ**   Insertion of Pacemaker Lead into Left Ventricle, Percutaneous Endoscopic Approach

+   Pacemaker lead is part of pacemaker cluster for MS-DRG assignment when reported with pacemaker device code. *See table 0JH to construct pacemaker device Insertion code.*

02HL4KZ   Insertion of Defibrillator Lead into Left Ventricle, Percutaneous Endoscopic Approach

+   Lead device when reported with an Insertion of defibrillator generator (6th character 8 or 9) into the chest or abdomen subcutaneous tissue and fascia. *See table 0JH to construct the Insertion code.*

● **02HL4MZ**   Insertion of Cardiac Lead into Left Ventricle, Percutaneous Endoscopic Approach

+   Pacemaker lead is part of pacemaker cluster for MS-DRG assignment when reported with pacemaker device code. *See table 0JH to construct pacemaker device Insertion code.*

02HL4NZ   Insertion of Intracardiac Pacemaker into Left Ventricle, Percutaneous Endoscopic Approach

02HL4YZ   Insertion of Other Device into Left Ventricle, Percutaneous Endoscopic Approach

02HN00Z   Insertion of Pressure Sensor Monitoring Device into Pericardium, Open Approach

02HN02Z   Insertion of Monitoring Device into Pericardium, Open Approach

● **02HN0JZ**   Insertion of Pacemaker Lead into Pericardium, Open Approach

HAC   With a secondary diagnosis code of K68.11, T81.40XA, T81.41XA, T81.42XA, T81.43XA, T81.44XA, T82.6XXA, T82.7XXA

+   Pacemaker lead is part of pacemaker cluster for MS-DRG assignment when reported with pacemaker device code. *See table 0JH to construct pacemaker device Insertion code.*

+   Lead device when reported with an Insertion of a cardiac resynchronization defibrillator device (6th character 9) into the chest or abdomen subcutaneous tissue and fascia. *See table 0JH to construct the Insertion code.*

♀ Female-only   ♂ Male-only   ▲ Limited Coverage   ● Non-OR   **HAC** HAC-associated procedure   ▲ Non-covered procedures   **+** Cluster

02HN0KZ Insertion of Defibrillator Lead into Pericardium, Open Approach

+ Lead device when reported with an Insertion of a cardiac resynchronization defibrillator device (6th character 9) into the chest or abdomen subcutaneous tissue and fascia. *See table 0JH to construct the Insertion code.*

● **02HN0MZ** Insertion of Cardiac Lead into Pericardium, Open Approach

HAC With a secondary diagnosis code of K68.11, T81.40XA, T81.41XA, T81.42XA, T81.43XA, T81.44XA, T82.6XXA, T82.7XXA

+ Pacemaker lead is part of pacemaker cluster for MS-DRG assignment when reported with pacemaker device code. *See table 0JH to construct pacemaker device Insertion code.*

+ Lead device when reported with an Insertion of a cardiac resynchronization defibrillator device (6th character 9) into the chest or abdomen subcutaneous tissue and fascia. *See table 0JH to construct the Insertion code.*

02HN0YZ Insertion of Other Device into Pericardium, Open Approach

02HN30Z Insertion of Pressure Sensor Monitoring Device into Pericardium, Percutaneous Approach

02HN32Z Insertion of Monitoring Device into Pericardium, Percutaneous Approach

● **02HN3JZ** Insertion of Pacemaker Lead into Pericardium, Percutaneous Approach

HAC With a secondary diagnosis code of K68.11, T81.40XA, T81.41XA, T81.42XA, T81.43XA, T81.44XA, T82.6XXA, T82.7XXA

+ Pacemaker lead is part of pacemaker cluster for MS-DRG assignment when reported with pacemaker device code. *See table 0JH to construct pacemaker device Insertion code.*

+ Lead device when reported with an Insertion of a cardiac resynchronization defibrillator device (6th character 9) into the chest or abdomen subcutaneous tissue and fascia. *See table 0JH to construct the Insertion code.*

02HN3KZ Insertion of Defibrillator Lead into Pericardium, Percutaneous Approach

+ Lead device when reported with an Insertion of a cardiac resynchronization defibrillator device (6th character 9) into the chest or abdomen subcutaneous tissue and fascia. *See table 0JH to construct the Insertion code.*

● **02HN3MZ** Insertion of Cardiac Lead into Pericardium, Percutaneous Approach

HAC With a secondary diagnosis code of K68.11, T81.40XA, T81.41XA, T81.42XA, T81.43XA, T81.44XA, T82.6XXA, T82.7XXA

+ Pacemaker lead is part of pacemaker cluster for MS-DRG assignment when reported with pacemaker device code. *See table 0JH to construct pacemaker device Insertion code.*

+ Lead device when reported with an Insertion of a cardiac resynchronization defibrillator device (6th character 9) into the chest or abdomen subcutaneous tissue and fascia. *See table 0JH to construct the Insertion code.*

02HN3YZ Insertion of Other Device into Pericardium, Percutaneous Approach

02HN40Z Insertion of Pressure Sensor Monitoring Device into Pericardium, Percutaneous Endoscopic Approach

02HN42Z Insertion of Monitoring Device into Pericardium, Percutaneous Endoscopic Approach

● **02HN4JZ** Insertion of Pacemaker Lead into Pericardium, Percutaneous Endoscopic Approach

HAC With a secondary diagnosis code of K68.11, T81.40XA, T81.41XA, T81.42XA, T81.43XA, T81.44XA, T82.6XXA, T82.7XXA

+ Pacemaker lead is part of pacemaker cluster for MS-DRG assignment when reported with pacemaker device code. *See table 0JH to construct pacemaker device Insertion code.*

+ Lead device when reported with an Insertion of a cardiac resynchronization defibrillator device (6th character 9) into the chest or abdomen subcutaneous tissue and fascia. *See table 0JH to construct the Insertion code.*

02HN4KZ Insertion of Defibrillator Lead into Pericardium, Percutaneous Endoscopic Approach

+ Lead device when reported with an Insertion of a cardiac resynchronization defibrillator device (6th character 9) into the chest or abdomen subcutaneous tissue and fascia. *See table 0JH to construct the Insertion code.*

● **02HN4MZ** Insertion of Cardiac Lead into Pericardium, Percutaneous Endoscopic Approach

HAC With a secondary diagnosis code of K68.11, T81.40XA, T81.41XA, T81.42XA, T81.43XA, T81.44XA, T82.6XXA, T82.7XXA

+ Pacemaker lead is part of pacemaker cluster for MS-DRG assignment when reported with pacemaker device code. *See table 0JH to construct pacemaker device Insertion code.*

+ Lead device when reported with an Insertion of a cardiac resynchronization defibrillator device (6th character 9) into the chest or abdomen subcutaneous tissue and fascia. *See table 0JH to construct the Insertion code.*

02HN4YZ Insertion of Other Device into Pericardium, Percutaneous Endoscopic Approach

02HP00Z Insertion of Pressure Sensor Monitoring Device into Pulmonary Trunk, Open Approach

02HP02Z Insertion of Monitoring Device into Pulmonary Trunk, Open Approach

02HP03Z Insertion of Infusion Device into Pulmonary Trunk, Open Approach

02HP0DZ Insertion of Intraluminal Device into Pulmonary Trunk, Open Approach

02HP0YZ Insertion of Other Device into Pulmonary Trunk, Open Approach

02HP30Z Insertion of Pressure Sensor Monitoring Device into Pulmonary Trunk, Percutaneous Approach

02HP32Z Insertion of Monitoring Device into Pulmonary Trunk, Percutaneous Approach

AHA CC: 3Q, 2015, 35

02HP33Z Insertion of Infusion Device into Pulmonary Trunk, Percutaneous Approach

02HP3DZ Insertion of Intraluminal Device into Pulmonary Trunk, Percutaneous Approach

02HP3YZ Insertion of Other Device into Pulmonary Trunk, Percutaneous Approach

02HP40Z Insertion of Pressure Sensor Monitoring Device into Pulmonary Trunk, Percutaneous Endoscopic Approach

02HP42Z Insertion of Monitoring Device into Pulmonary Trunk, Percutaneous Endoscopic Approach

02HP43Z Insertion of Infusion Device into Pulmonary Trunk, Percutaneous Endoscopic Approach

02HP4DZ Insertion of Intraluminal Device into Pulmonary Trunk, Percutaneous Endoscopic Approach

02HP4YZ Insertion of Other Device into Pulmonary Trunk, Percutaneous Endoscopic Approach

02HQ00Z Insertion of Pressure Sensor Monitoring Device into Right Pulmonary Artery, Open Approach

02HQ02Z Insertion of Monitoring Device into Right Pulmonary Artery, Open Approach

02HQ03Z Insertion of Infusion Device into Right Pulmonary Artery, Open Approach

02HQ0DZ Insertion of Intraluminal Device into Right Pulmonary Artery, Open Approach

02HQ0YZ Insertion of Other Device into Right Pulmonary Artery, Open Approach

02HQ30Z Insertion of Pressure Sensor Monitoring Device into Right Pulmonary Artery, Percutaneous Approach

02HQ32Z Insertion of Monitoring Device into Right Pulmonary Artery, Percutaneous Approach

02HQ33Z Insertion of Infusion Device into Right Pulmonary Artery, Percutaneous Approach

02HQ3DZ Insertion of Intraluminal Device into Right Pulmonary Artery, Percutaneous Approach

02HQ3YZ Insertion of Other Device into Right Pulmonary Artery, Percutaneous Approach

02HQ40Z Insertion of Pressure Sensor Monitoring Device into Right Pulmonary Artery, Percutaneous Endoscopic Approach

02HQ42Z Insertion of Monitoring Device into Right Pulmonary Artery, Percutaneous Endoscopic Approach

02HQ43Z Insertion of Infusion Device into Right Pulmonary Artery, Percutaneous Endoscopic Approach

02HQ4DZ Insertion of Intraluminal Device into Right Pulmonary Artery, Percutaneous Endoscopic Approach

02HQ4YZ Insertion of Other Device into Right Pulmonary Artery, Percutaneous Endoscopic Approach

02HR00Z Insertion of Pressure Sensor Monitoring Device into Left Pulmonary Artery, Open Approach

02HR02Z Insertion of Monitoring Device into Left Pulmonary Artery, Open Approach

---

♀ Female-only   ♂ Male-only   ▲ Limited Coverage   ● Non-OR   HAC HAC-associated procedure   ▲ Non-covered procedures   + Cluster

02HR03Z	Insertion of Infusion Device into Left Pulmonary Artery, Open Approach
02HR0DZ	Insertion of Intraluminal Device into Left Pulmonary Artery, Open Approach
02HR0YZ	Insertion of Other Device into Left Pulmonary Artery, Open Approach
02HR30Z	Insertion of Pressure Sensor Monitoring Device into Left Pulmonary Artery, Percutaneous Approach
02HR32Z	Insertion of Monitoring Device into Left Pulmonary Artery, Percutaneous Approach
02HR33Z	Insertion of Infusion Device into Left Pulmonary Artery, Percutaneous Approach
02HR3DZ	Insertion of Intraluminal Device into Left Pulmonary Artery, Percutaneous Approach
02HR3YZ	Insertion of Other Device into Left Pulmonary Artery, Percutaneous Approach
02HR40Z	Insertion of Pressure Sensor Monitoring Device into Left Pulmonary Artery, Percutaneous Endoscopic Approach
02HR42Z	Insertion of Monitoring Device into Left Pulmonary Artery, Percutaneous Endoscopic Approach
02HR43Z	Insertion of Infusion Device into Left Pulmonary Artery, Percutaneous Endoscopic Approach
02HR4DZ	Insertion of Intraluminal Device into Left Pulmonary Artery, Percutaneous Endoscopic Approach
02HR4YZ	Insertion of Other Device into Left Pulmonary Artery, Percutaneous Endoscopic Approach
02HS00Z	Insertion of Pressure Sensor Monitoring Device into Right Pulmonary Vein, Open Approach
02HS02Z	Insertion of Monitoring Device into Right Pulmonary Vein, Open Approach
02HS03Z	Insertion of Infusion Device into Right Pulmonary Vein, Open Approach
02HS0DZ	Insertion of Intraluminal Device into Right Pulmonary Vein, Open Approach
02HS0YZ	Insertion of Other Device into Right Pulmonary Vein, Open Approach
02HS30Z	Insertion of Pressure Sensor Monitoring Device into Right Pulmonary Vein, Percutaneous Approach
02HS32Z	Insertion of Monitoring Device into Right Pulmonary Vein, Percutaneous Approach
02HS33Z	Insertion of Infusion Device into Right Pulmonary Vein, Percutaneous Approach
HAC	When reported with secondary diagnosis code J95.811
02HS3DZ	Insertion of Intraluminal Device into Right Pulmonary Vein, Percutaneous Approach
02HS3YZ	Insertion of Other Device into Right Pulmonary Vein, Percutaneous Approach
02HS40Z	Insertion of Pressure Sensor Monitoring Device into Right Pulmonary Vein, Percutaneous Endoscopic Approach
02HS42Z	Insertion of Monitoring Device into Right Pulmonary Vein, Percutaneous Endoscopic Approach
02HS43Z	Insertion of Infusion Device into Right Pulmonary Vein, Percutaneous Endoscopic Approach
HAC	When reported with secondary diagnosis code J95.811
02HS4DZ	Insertion of Intraluminal Device into Right Pulmonary Vein, Percutaneous Endoscopic Approach
02HS4YZ	Insertion of Other Device into Right Pulmonary Vein, Percutaneous Endoscopic Approach
02HT00Z	Insertion of Pressure Sensor Monitoring Device into Left Pulmonary Vein, Open Approach
02HT02Z	Insertion of Monitoring Device into Left Pulmonary Vein, Open Approach
02HT03Z	Insertion of Infusion Device into Left Pulmonary Vein, Open Approach
02HT0DZ	Insertion of Intraluminal Device into Left Pulmonary Vein, Open Approach
02HT0YZ	Insertion of Other Device into Left Pulmonary Vein, Open Approach
02HT30Z	Insertion of Pressure Sensor Monitoring Device into Left Pulmonary Vein, Percutaneous Approach
02HT32Z	Insertion of Monitoring Device into Left Pulmonary Vein, Percutaneous Approach
02HT33Z	Insertion of Infusion Device into Left Pulmonary Vein, Percutaneous Approach
HAC	When reported with secondary diagnosis code J95.811
02HT3DZ	Insertion of Intraluminal Device into Left Pulmonary Vein, Percutaneous Approach
02HT3YZ	Insertion of Other Device into Left Pulmonary Vein, Percutaneous Approach
02HT40Z	Insertion of Pressure Sensor Monitoring Device into Left Pulmonary Vein, Percutaneous Endoscopic Approach
02HT42Z	Insertion of Monitoring Device into Left Pulmonary Vein, Percutaneous Endoscopic Approach
02HT43Z	Insertion of Infusion Device into Left Pulmonary Vein, Percutaneous Endoscopic Approach
HAC	When reported with secondary diagnosis code J95.811
02HT4DZ	Insertion of Intraluminal Device into Left Pulmonary Vein, Percutaneous Endoscopic Approach
02HT4YZ	Insertion of Other Device into Left Pulmonary Vein, Percutaneous Endoscopic Approach
02HV00Z	Insertion of Pressure Sensor Monitoring Device into Superior Vena Cava, Open Approach
02HV02Z	Insertion of Monitoring Device into Superior Vena Cava, Open Approach
02HV03Z	Insertion of Infusion Device into Superior Vena Cava, Open Approach
02HV0DZ	Insertion of Intraluminal Device into Superior Vena Cava, Open Approach
02HV0YZ	Insertion of Other Device into Superior Vena Cava, Open Approach
02HV30Z	Insertion of Pressure Sensor Monitoring Device into Superior Vena Cava, Percutaneous Approach
02HV32Z	Insertion of Monitoring Device into Superior Vena Cava, Percutaneous Approach
02HV33Z	Insertion of Infusion Device into Superior Vena Cava, Percutaneous Approach
HAC	When reported with secondary diagnosis code J95.811
	AHA CC: 3Q, 2013, 18; 2Q, 2015, 33-34; 4Q, 2015, 14-15, 28-32; 4Q, 2017, 63-64
02HV3DZ	Insertion of Intraluminal Device into Superior Vena Cava, Percutaneous Approach
02HV3YZ	Insertion of Other Device into Superior Vena Cava, Percutaneous Approach
02HV40Z	Insertion of Pressure Sensor Monitoring Device into Superior Vena Cava, Percutaneous Endoscopic Approach
02HV42Z	Insertion of Monitoring Device into Superior Vena Cava, Percutaneous Endoscopic Approach
02HV43Z	Insertion of Infusion Device into Superior Vena Cava, Percutaneous Endoscopic Approach
HAC	When reported with secondary diagnosis code J95.811
02HV4DZ	Insertion of Intraluminal Device into Superior Vena Cava, Percutaneous Endoscopic Approach
02HV4YZ	Insertion of Other Device into Superior Vena Cava, Percutaneous Endoscopic Approach
02HW00Z	Insertion of Pressure Sensor Monitoring Device into Thoracic Aorta, Descending, Open Approach
02HW02Z	Insertion of Monitoring Device into Thoracic Aorta, Descending, Open Approach
02HW03Z	Insertion of Infusion Device into Thoracic Aorta, Descending, Open Approach
02HW0DZ	Insertion of Intraluminal Device into Thoracic Aorta, Descending, Open Approach
02HW0YZ	Insertion of Other Device into Thoracic Aorta, Descending, Open Approach
02HW30Z	Insertion of Pressure Sensor Monitoring Device into Thoracic Aorta, Descending, Percutaneous Approach
02HW32Z	Insertion of Monitoring Device into Thoracic Aorta, Descending, Percutaneous Approach
02HW33Z	Insertion of Infusion Device into Thoracic Aorta, Descending, Percutaneous Approach
02HW3DZ	Insertion of Intraluminal Device into Thoracic Aorta, Descending, Percutaneous Approach
02HW3YZ	Insertion of Other Device into Thoracic Aorta, Descending, Percutaneous Approach
02HW40Z	Insertion of Pressure Sensor Monitoring Device into Thoracic Aorta, Descending, Percutaneous Endoscopic Approach
02HW42Z	Insertion of Monitoring Device into Thoracic Aorta, Descending, Percutaneous Endoscopic Approach
02HW43Z	Insertion of Infusion Device into Thoracic Aorta, Descending, Percutaneous Endoscopic Approach
02HW4DZ	Insertion of Intraluminal Device into Thoracic Aorta, Descending, Percutaneous Endoscopic Approach
02HW4YZ	Insertion of Other Device into Thoracic Aorta, Descending, Percutaneous Endoscopic Approach

♀ Female-only   ♂ Male-only   ▲ Limited Coverage   ● Non-OR   HAC HAC-associated procedure   ▲ Non-covered procedures   ✛ Cluster

02HX00Z	Insertion of Pressure Sensor Monitoring Device into Thoracic Aorta, Ascending/Arch, Open Approach	02HX30Z	Insertion of Pressure Sensor Monitoring Device into Thoracic Aorta, Ascending/Arch, Percutaneous Approach	02HX40Z	Insertion of Pressure Sensor Monitoring Device into Thoracic Aorta, Ascending/Arch, Percutaneous Endoscopic Approach
02HX02Z	Insertion of Monitoring Device into Thoracic Aorta, Ascending/Arch, Open Approach	02HX32Z	Insertion of Monitoring Device into Thoracic Aorta, Ascending/Arch, Percutaneous Approach	02HX42Z	Insertion of Monitoring Device into Thoracic Aorta, Ascending/Arch, Percutaneous Endoscopic Approach
02HX03Z	Insertion of Infusion Device into Thoracic Aorta, Ascending/Arch, Open Approach	02HX33Z	Insertion of Infusion Device into Thoracic Aorta, Ascending/Arch, Percutaneous Approach	02HX43Z	Insertion of Infusion Device into Thoracic Aorta, Ascending/Arch, Percutaneous Endoscopic Approach
02HX0DZ	Insertion of Intraluminal Device into Thoracic Aorta, Ascending/Arch, Open Approach	02HX3DZ	Insertion of Intraluminal Device into Thoracic Aorta, Ascending/Arch, Percutaneous Approach	02HX4DZ	Insertion of Intraluminal Device into Thoracic Aorta, Ascending/Arch, Percutaneous Endoscopic Approach

02J – Heart and Great Vessels, Inspection

Review Coding Guidelines B3.11a, B3.11b and B3.11c

02JA0ZZ	Inspection of Heart, Open Approach	02JA4ZZ	Inspection of Heart, Percutaneous Endoscopic Approach	02JY3ZZ	Inspection of Great Vessel, Percutaneous Approach
02JA3ZZ	Inspection of Heart, Percutaneous Approach	02JY0ZZ	Inspection of Great Vessel, Open Approach	02JY4ZZ	Inspection of Great Vessel, Percutaneous Endoscopic Approach
	AHA CC: 3Q, 2015, 9				

02K – Heart and Great Vessels, Map

02K80ZZ	Map Conduction Mechanism, Open Approach	● 02K83ZZ	Map Conduction Mechanism, Percutaneous Approach	● 02K84ZZ	Map Conduction Mechanism, Percutaneous Endoscopic Approach

02L – Heart and Great Vessels, Occlusion

02L70CK	Occlusion of Left Atrial Appendage with Extraluminal Device, Open Approach	02LH4ZZ	Occlusion of Pulmonary Valve, Percutaneous Endoscopic Approach	02LQ4DZ	Occlusion of Right Pulmonary Artery with Intraluminal Device, Percutaneous Endoscopic Approach
	AHA CC: 3Q, 2014, 20-21	02LP0CZ	Occlusion of Pulmonary Trunk with Extraluminal Device, Open Approach	02LQ4ZZ	Occlusion of Right Pulmonary Artery, Percutaneous Endoscopic Approach
02L70DK	Occlusion of Left Atrial Appendage with Intraluminal Device, Open Approach	02LP0DZ	Occlusion of Pulmonary Trunk with Extraluminal Device, Open Approach	02LR0CT	Occlusion of Ductus Arteriosus with Extraluminal Device, Open Approach
02L70ZK	Occlusion of Left Atrial Appendage, Open Approach	02LP0ZZ	Occlusion of Pulmonary Trunk, Open Approach	02LR0CZ	Occlusion of Left Pulmonary Artery with Extraluminal Device, Open Approach
02L73CK	Occlusion of Left Atrial Appendage with Extraluminal Device, Percutaneous Approach	02LP3CZ	Occlusion of Pulmonary Trunk with Extraluminal Device, Percutaneous Approach	02LR0DT	Occlusion of Ductus Arteriosus with Intraluminal Device, Open Approach
02L73DK	Occlusion of Left Atrial Appendage with Intraluminal Device, Percutaneous Approach	02LP3DZ	Occlusion of Pulmonary Trunk with Intraluminal Device, Percutaneous Approach	02LR0DZ	Occlusion of Left Pulmonary Artery with Intraluminal Device, Open Approach
	AHA CC: 4Q, 2018, 94	02LP3ZZ	Occlusion of Pulmonary Trunk, Percutaneous Approach	02LR0ZT	Occlusion of Ductus Arteriosus, Open Approach
02L73ZK	Occlusion of Left Atrial Appendage, Percutaneous Approach	02LP4CZ	Occlusion of Pulmonary Trunk with Extraluminal Device, Percutaneous Endoscopic Approach		*AHA CC: 4Q, 2015, 23-24*
02L74CK	Occlusion of Left Atrial Appendage with Extraluminal Device, Percutaneous Endoscopic Approach	02LP4DZ	Occlusion of Pulmonary Trunk with Intraluminal Device, Percutaneous Endoscopic Approach	02LR0ZZ	Occlusion of Left Pulmonary Artery, Open Approach
02L74DK	Occlusion of Left Atrial Appendage with Intraluminal Device, Percutaneous Endoscopic Approach	02LP4ZZ	Occlusion of Pulmonary Trunk, Percutaneous Endoscopic Approach	02LR3CT	Occlusion of Ductus Arteriosus with Extraluminal Device, Percutaneous Approach
02L74ZK	Occlusion of Left Atrial Appendage, Percutaneous Endoscopic Approach	02LQ0CZ	Occlusion of Right Pulmonary Artery with Extraluminal Device, Open Approach	02LR3CZ	Occlusion of Left Pulmonary Artery with Extraluminal Device, Percutaneous Approach
02LH0CZ	Occlusion of Pulmonary Valve with Extraluminal Device, Open Approach	02LQ0DZ	Occlusion of Right Pulmonary Artery with Intraluminal Device, Open Approach	02LR3DT	Occlusion of Ductus Arteriosus with Intraluminal Device, Percutaneous Approach
02LH0DZ	Occlusion of Pulmonary Valve with Intraluminal Device, Open Approach	02LQ0ZZ	Occlusion of Right Pulmonary Artery, Open Approach	02LR3DZ	Occlusion of Left Pulmonary Artery with Intraluminal Device, Percutaneous Approach
02LH0ZZ	Occlusion of Pulmonary Valve, Open Approach	02LQ3CZ	Occlusion of Right Pulmonary Artery with Extraluminal Device, Percutaneous Approach	02LR3ZT	Occlusion of Ductus Arteriosus, Percutaneous Approach
02LH3CZ	Occlusion of Pulmonary Valve with Extraluminal Device, Percutaneous Approach	02LQ3DZ	Occlusion of Right Pulmonary Artery with Intraluminal Device, Percutaneous Approach	02LR3ZZ	Occlusion of Left Pulmonary Artery, Percutaneous Approach
02LH3DZ	Occlusion of Pulmonary Valve with Intraluminal Device, Percutaneous Approach		*AHA CC: 4Q, 2017, 34*	02LR4CT	Occlusion of Ductus Arteriosus with Extraluminal Device, Percutaneous Endoscopic Approach
02LH3ZZ	Occlusion of Pulmonary Valve, Percutaneous Approach	02LQ3ZZ	Occlusion of Right Pulmonary Artery, Percutaneous Approach	02LR4CZ	Occlusion of Left Pulmonary Artery with Extraluminal Device, Percutaneous Endoscopic Approach
02LH4CZ	Occlusion of Pulmonary Valve with Extraluminal Device, Percutaneous Endoscopic Approach	02LQ4CZ	Occlusion of Right Pulmonary Artery with Extraluminal Device, Percutaneous Endoscopic Approach	02LR4DT	Occlusion of Ductus Arteriosus with Intraluminal Device, Percutaneous Endoscopic Approach
02LH4DZ	Occlusion of Pulmonary Valve with Intraluminal Device, Percutaneous Endoscopic Approach				

02LR4DZ	Occlusion of Left Pulmonary Artery with Intraluminal Device, Percutaneous Endoscopic Approach	
02LR4ZT	Occlusion of Ductus Arteriosus, Percutaneous Endoscopic Approach	
02LR4ZZ	Occlusion of Left Pulmonary Artery, Percutaneous Endoscopic Approach	
02LS0CZ	Occlusion of Right Pulmonary Vein with Extraluminal Device, Open Approach	
02LS0DZ	Occlusion of Right Pulmonary Vein with Intraluminal Device, Open Approach	
02LS0ZZ	Occlusion of Right Pulmonary Vein, Open Approach	
02LS3CZ	Occlusion of Right Pulmonary Vein with Extraluminal Device, Percutaneous Approach	
02LS3DZ	Occlusion of Right Pulmonary Vein with Intraluminal Device, Percutaneous Approach	
	AHA CC: 2Q, 2016, 26; 4Q, 2017, 34	
02LS3ZZ	Occlusion of Right Pulmonary Vein, Percutaneous Approach	
02LS4CZ	Occlusion of Right Pulmonary Vein with Extraluminal Device, Percutaneous Endoscopic Approach	

02LS4DZ	Occlusion of Right Pulmonary Vein with Intraluminal Device, Percutaneous Endoscopic Approach
02LS4ZZ	Occlusion of Right Pulmonary Vein, Percutaneous Endoscopic Approach
02LT0CZ	Occlusion of Left Pulmonary Vein with Extraluminal Device, Open Approach
02LT0DZ	Occlusion of Left Pulmonary Vein with Intraluminal Device, Open Approach
02LT0ZZ	Occlusion of Left Pulmonary Vein, Open Approach
02LT3CZ	Occlusion of Left Pulmonary Vein with Extraluminal Device, Percutaneous Approach
02LT3DZ	Occlusion of Left Pulmonary Vein with Intraluminal Device, Percutaneous Approach
02LT3ZZ	Occlusion of Left Pulmonary Vein, Percutaneous Approach
02LT4CZ	Occlusion of Left Pulmonary Vein with Extraluminal Device, Percutaneous Endoscopic Approach
02LT4DZ	Occlusion of Left Pulmonary Vein with Intraluminal Device, Percutaneous Endoscopic Approach
02LT4ZZ	Occlusion of Left Pulmonary Vein, Percutaneous Endoscopic Approach

02LV0CZ	Occlusion of Superior Vena Cava with Extraluminal Device, Open Approach
02LV0DZ	Occlusion of Superior Vena Cava with Intraluminal Device, Open Approach
02LV0ZZ	Occlusion of Superior Vena Cava, Open Approach
02LV3CZ	Occlusion of Superior Vena Cava with Extraluminal Device, Percutaneous Approach
02LV3DZ	Occlusion of Superior Vena Cava with Intraluminal Device, Percutaneous Approach
02LV3ZZ	Occlusion of Superior Vena Cava, Percutaneous Approach
02LV4CZ	Occlusion of Superior Vena Cava with Extraluminal Device, Percutaneous Endoscopic Approach
02LV4DZ	Occlusion of Superior Vena Cava with Intraluminal Device, Percutaneous Endoscopic Approach
02LV4ZZ	Occlusion of Superior Vena Cava, Percutaneous Endoscopic Approach
02LW3DJ	Occlusion of Thoracic Aorta, Descending with Intraluminal Device, Temporary, Percutaneous Approach

02N – Heart and Great Vessels, Release

Review Coding Guideline B3.13

Review Coding Guideline B3.14

02N00ZZ	Release Coronary Artery, One Artery, Open Approach	
	AHA CC: 2Q, 2019, 13-14	
02N03ZZ	Release Coronary Artery, One Artery, Percutaneous Approach	
02N04ZZ	Release Coronary Artery, One Artery, Percutaneous Endoscopic Approach	
02N10ZZ	Release Coronary Artery, Two Arteries, Open Approach	
02N13ZZ	Release Coronary Artery, Two Arteries, Percutaneous Approach	
02N14ZZ	Release Coronary Artery, Two Arteries, Percutaneous Endoscopic Approach	
02N20ZZ	Release Coronary Artery, Three Arteries, Open Approach	
02N23ZT	Release Coronary Artery, Three Arteries, Percutaneous Approach	
02N24ZZ	Release Coronary Artery, Three Arteries, Percutaneous Endoscopic Approach	
02N30ZZ	Release Coronary Artery, Four or More Arteries, Open Approach	
02N33ZZ	Release Coronary Artery, Four or More Arteries, Percutaneous Approach	
02N34ZZ	Release Coronary Artery, Four or More Arteries, Percutaneous Endoscopic Approach	
02N40ZZ	Release Coronary Vein, Open Approach	
02N43ZZ	Release Coronary Vein, Percutaneous Approach	
02N44ZZ	Release Coronary Vein, Percutaneous Endoscopic Approach	
02N50ZZ	Release Atrial Septum, Open Approach	
02N53ZZ	Release Atrial Septum, Percutaneous Approach	
02N54ZZ	Release Atrial Septum, Percutaneous Endoscopic Approach	
02N60ZZ	Release Right Atrium, Open Approach	
02N63ZZ	Release Right Atrium, Percutaneous Approach	
02N64ZZ	Release Right Atrium, Percutaneous Endoscopic Approach	

02N70ZZ	Release Left Atrium, Open Approach
02N73ZZ	Release Left Atrium, Percutaneous Approach
02N74ZZ	Release Left Atrium, Percutaneous Endoscopic Approach
02N80ZZ	Release Conduction Mechanism, Open Approach
02N83ZZ	Release Conduction Mechanism, Percutaneous Approach
02N84ZZ	Release Conduction Mechanism, Percutaneous Endoscopic Approach
02N90ZZ	Release Chordae Tendineae, Open Approach
02N93ZZ	Release Chordae Tendineae, Percutaneous Approach
02N94ZZ	Release Chordae Tendineae, Percutaneous Endoscopic Approach
02ND0ZZ	Release Papillary Muscle, Open Approach
02ND3ZZ	Release Papillary Muscle, Percutaneous Approach
02ND4ZZ	Release Papillary Muscle, Percutaneous Endoscopic Approach
02NF0ZZ	Release Aortic Valve, Open Approach
02NF3ZZ	Release Aortic Valve, Percutaneous Approach
02NF4ZZ	Release Aortic Valve, Percutaneous Endoscopic Approach
02NG0ZZ	Release Mitral Valve, Open Approach
02NG3ZZ	Release Mitral Valve, Percutaneous Approach
02NG4ZZ	Release Mitral Valve, Percutaneous Endoscopic Approach
02NH0ZZ	Release Pulmonary Valve, Open Approach
02NH3ZZ	Release Pulmonary Valve, Percutaneous Approach
02NH4ZZ	Release Pulmonary Valve, Percutaneous Endoscopic Approach
02NJ0ZZ	Release Tricuspid Valve, Open Approach

02NJ3ZZ	Release Tricuspid Valve, Percutaneous Approach	
02NJ4ZZ	Release Tricuspid Valve, Percutaneous Endoscopic Approach	
02NK0ZZ	Release Right Ventricle, Open Approach	
	AHA CC: 3Q, 2014, 16-17	
02NK3ZZ	Release Right Ventricle, Percutaneous Approach	
02NK4ZZ	Release Right Ventricle, Percutaneous Endoscopic Approach	
02NL0ZZ	Release Left Ventricle, Open Approach	
02NL3ZZ	Release Left Ventricle, Percutaneous Approach	
02NL4ZZ	Release Left Ventricle, Percutaneous Endoscopic Approach	
02NM0ZZ	Release Ventricular Septum, Open Approach	
02NM3ZZ	Release Ventricular Septum, Percutaneous Approach	
02NM4ZZ	Release Ventricular Septum, Percutaneous Endoscopic Approach	
02NN0ZZ	Release Pericardium, Open Approach	
	AHA CC: 2Q, 2019, 20-21	
02NN3ZZ	Release Pericardium, Percutaneous Approach	
02NN4ZZ	Release Pericardium, Percutaneous Endoscopic Approach	
02NP0ZZ	Release Pulmonary Trunk, Open Approach	
02NP3ZZ	Release Pulmonary Trunk, Percutaneous Approach	
02NP4ZZ	Release Pulmonary Trunk, Percutaneous Endoscopic Approach	
02NQ0ZZ	Release Right Pulmonary Artery, Open Approach	
02NQ3ZZ	Release Right Pulmonary Artery, Percutaneous Approach	
02NQ4ZZ	Release Right Pulmonary Artery, Percutaneous Endoscopic Approach	
02NR0ZZ	Release Left Pulmonary Artery, Open Approach	

02NR3ZZ Release Left Pulmonary Artery, Percutaneous Approach
02NR4ZZ Release Left Pulmonary Artery, Percutaneous Endoscopic Approach
02NS0ZZ Release Right Pulmonary Vein, Open Approach
02NS3ZZ Release Right Pulmonary Vein, Percutaneous Approach
02NS4ZZ Release Right Pulmonary Vein, Percutaneous Endoscopic Approach
02NT0ZZ Release Left Pulmonary Vein, Open Approach

02NT3ZZ Release Left Pulmonary Vein, Percutaneous Approach
02NT4ZZ Release Left Pulmonary Vein, Percutaneous Endoscopic Approach
02NV0ZZ Release Superior Vena Cava, Open Approach
02NV3ZZ Release Superior Vena Cava, Percutaneous Approach
02NV4ZZ Release Superior Vena Cava, Percutaneous Endoscopic Approach
02NW0ZZ Release Thoracic Aorta, Descending, Open Approach

02NW3ZZ Release Thoracic Aorta, Descending, Percutaneous Approach
02NW4ZZ Release Thoracic Aorta, Descending, Percutaneous Endoscopic Approach
02NX0ZZ Release Thoracic Aorta, Ascending/Arch, Open Approach
02NX3ZZ Release Thoracic Aorta, Ascending/Arch, Percutaneous Approach
02NX4ZZ Release Thoracic Aorta, Ascending/Arch, Percutaneous Endoscopic Approach

02P – Heart and Great Vessels, Removal

Review Coding Guideline B6.1c

02PA02Z Removal of Monitoring Device from Heart, Open Approach
02PA03Z Removal of Infusion Device from Heart, Open Approach
02PA07Z Removal of Autologous Tissue Substitute from Heart, Open Approach
02PA08Z Removal of Zooplastic Tissue from Heart, Open Approach
02PA0CZ Removal of Extraluminal Device from Heart, Open Approach
02PA0DZ Removal of Intraluminal Device from Heart, Open Approach
02PA0JZ Removal of Synthetic Substitute from Heart, Open Approach
02PA0KZ Removal of Nonautologous Tissue Substitute from Heart, Open Approach
02PA0MZ Removal of Cardiac Lead from Heart, Open Approach
  HAC With a secondary diagnosis code of K68.11, T81.40XA, T81.41XA, T81.42XA, T81.43XA, T81.44XA, T82.6XXA, T82.7XXA
02PA0NZ Removal of Intracardiac Pacemaker from Heart, Open Approach
02PA0QZ Removal of Implantable Heart Assist System from Heart, Open Approach
  AHA CC: 1Q, 2019, 24
02PA0RS Removal of Biventricular Short-term External Heart Assist System from Heart, Open Approach
02PA0RZ Removal of Short-term External Heart Assist System from Heart, Open Approach
  AHA CC: 1Q, 2017, 13-14
02PA0YZ Removal of Other Device from Heart, Open Approach
02PA32Z Removal of Monitoring Device from Heart, Percutaneous Approach
02PA33Z Removal of Infusion Device from Heart, Percutaneous Approach
02PA37Z Removal of Autologous Tissue Substitute from Heart, Percutaneous Approach
02PA38Z Removal of Zooplastic Tissue from Heart, Percutaneous Approach
02PA3CZ Removal of Extraluminal Device from Heart, Percutaneous Approach
02PA3DZ Removal of Intraluminal Device from Heart, Percutaneous Approach
  AHA CC: 4Q, 2017, 104-105
02PA3JZ Removal of Synthetic Substitute from Heart, Percutaneous Approach
02PA3KZ Removal of Nonautologous Tissue Substitute from Heart, Percutaneous Approach
02PA3MZ Removal of Cardiac Lead from Heart, Percutaneous Approach
  AHA CC: 3Q, 2015, 33

  HAC With a secondary diagnosis code of K68.11, T81.40XA, T81.41XA, T81.42XA, T81.43XA, T81.44XA, T82.6XXA, T82.7XXA
02PA3NZ Removal of Intracardiac Pacemaker from Heart, Percutaneous Approach
  AHA CC: 4Q, 2016, 96-97
02PA3QZ Removal of Implantable Heart Assist System from Heart, Percutaneous Approach
02PA3RS Removal of Biventricular Short-term External Heart Assist System from Heart, Percutaneous Approach
02PA3RZ Removal of Short-term External Heart Assist System from Heart, Percutaneous Approach
  AHA CC: 4Q, 2016, 139; 1Q, 2017, 11-12; 4Q, 2017, 44-45; 4Q, 2018, 54
02PA3YZ Removal of Other Device from Heart, Percutaneous Approach
02PA42Z Removal of Monitoring Device from Heart, Percutaneous Endoscopic Approach
02PA43Z Removal of Infusion Device from Heart, Percutaneous Endoscopic Approach
02PA47Z Removal of Autologous Tissue Substitute from Heart, Percutaneous Endoscopic Approach
02PA48Z Removal of Zooplastic Tissue from Heart, Percutaneous Endoscopic Approach
02PA4CZ Removal of Extraluminal Device from Heart, Percutaneous Endoscopic Approach
02PA4DZ Removal of Intraluminal Device from Heart, Percutaneous Endoscopic Approach
02PA4JZ Removal of Synthetic Substitute from Heart, Percutaneous Endoscopic Approach
02PA4KZ Removal of Nonautologous Tissue Substitute from Heart, Percutaneous Endoscopic Approach
02PA4MZ Removal of Cardiac Lead from Heart, Percutaneous Endoscopic Approach
  HAC With a secondary diagnosis code of K68.11, T81.40XA, T81.41XA, T81.42XA, T81.43XA, T81.44XA, T82.6XXA, T82.7XXA
02PA4NZ Removal of Intracardiac Pacemaker from Heart, Percutaneous Endoscopic Approach
02PA4QZ Removal of Implantable Heart Assist System from Heart, Percutaneous Endoscopic Approach

02PA4RS Removal of Biventricular Short-term External Heart Assist System from Heart, Percutaneous Endoscopic Approach
02PA4RZ Removal of Short-term External Heart Assist System from Heart, Percutaneous Endoscopic Approach
02PA4YZ Removal of Other Device from Heart, Percutaneous Endoscopic Approach
02PAX2Z Removal of Monitoring Device from Heart, External Approach
02PAX3Z Removal of Infusion Device from Heart, External Approach
02PAXDZ Removal of Intraluminal Device from Heart, External Approach
02PAXMZ Removal of Cardiac Lead from Heart, External Approach
  HAC With a secondary diagnosis code of K68.11, T81.40XA, T81.41XA, T81.42XA, T81.43XA, T81.44XA, T82.6XXA, T82.7XXA
02PY02Z Removal of Monitoring Device from Great Vessel, Open Approach
02PY03Z Removal of Infusion Device from Great Vessel, Open Approach
02PY07Z Removal of Autologous Tissue Substitute from Great Vessel, Open Approach
02PY08Z Removal of Zooplastic Tissue from Great Vessel, Open Approach
02PY0CZ Removal of Extraluminal Device from Great Vessel, Open Approach
02PY0DZ Removal of Intraluminal Device from Great Vessel, Open Approach
02PY0JZ Removal of Synthetic Substitute from Great Vessel, Open Approach
02PY0KZ Removal of Nonautologous Tissue Substitute from Great Vessel, Open Approach
02PY0YZ Removal of Other Device from Great Vessel, Open Approach
02PY32Z Removal of Monitoring Device from Great Vessel, Percutaneous Approach
02PY33Z Removal of Infusion Device from Great Vessel, Percutaneous Approach
  AHA CC: 4Q, 2015, 31-32; 2Q, 2016, 15-16; 2Q, 2017, 24-26
02PY37Z Removal of Autologous Tissue Substitute from Great Vessel, Percutaneous Approach
02PY38Z Removal of Zooplastic Tissue from Great Vessel, Percutaneous Approach
02PY3CZ Removal of Extraluminal Device from Great Vessel, Percutaneous Approach
02PY3DZ Removal of Intraluminal Device from Great Vessel, Percutaneous Approach
02PY3JZ Removal of Synthetic Substitute from Great Vessel, Percutaneous Approach
  AHA CC: 4Q, 2018, 85

02PY3KZ	Removal of Nonautologous Tissue Substitute from Great Vessel, Percutaneous Approach	
02PY3YZ	Removal of Other Device from Great Vessel, Percutaneous Approach	
02PY42Z	Removal of Monitoring Device from Great Vessel, Percutaneous Endoscopic Approach	
02PY43Z	Removal of Infusion Device from Great Vessel, Percutaneous Endoscopic Approach	
02PY47Z	Removal of Autologous Tissue Substitute from Great Vessel, Percutaneous Endoscopic Approach	

02PY48Z	Removal of Zooplastic Tissue from Great Vessel, Percutaneous Endoscopic Approach
02PY4CZ	Removal of Extraluminal Device from Great Vessel, Percutaneous Endoscopic Approach
02PY4DZ	Removal of Intraluminal Device from Great Vessel, Percutaneous Endoscopic Approach
02PY4JZ	Removal of Synthetic Substitute from Great Vessel, Percutaneous Endoscopic Approach
02PY4KZ	Removal of Nonautologous Tissue Substitute from Great Vessel, Percutaneous Endoscopic Approach

02PY4YZ	Removal of Other Device from Great Vessel, Percutaneous Endoscopic Approach
02PYX2Z	Removal of Monitoring Device from Great Vessel, External Approach
02PYX3Z	Removal of Infusion Device from Great Vessel, External Approach
	AHA CC: 3Q, 2016, 19
02PYXDZ	Removal of Intraluminal Device from Great Vessel, External Approach

02Q – Heart and Great Vessels, Repair

For Repair of coronary arteries, Review Coding Guideline B4.4

02Q00ZZ	Repair Coronary Artery, One Artery, Open Approach
02Q03ZZ	Repair Coronary Artery, One Artery, Percutaneous Approach
02Q04ZZ	Repair Coronary Artery, One Artery, Percutaneous Endoscopic Approach
02Q10ZZ	Repair Coronary Artery, Two Arteries, Open Approach
02Q13ZZ	Repair Coronary Artery, Two Arteries, Percutaneous Approach
02Q14ZZ	Repair Coronary Artery, Two Arteries, Percutaneous Endoscopic Approach
02Q20ZZ	Repair Coronary Artery, Three Arteries, Open Approach
02Q23ZZ	Repair Coronary Artery, Three Arteries, Percutaneous Approach
02Q24ZZ	Repair Coronary Artery, Three Arteries, Percutaneous Endoscopic Approach
02Q30ZZ	Repair Coronary Artery, Four or More Arteries, Open Approach
02Q33ZZ	Repair Coronary Artery, Four or More Arteries, Percutaneous Approach
02Q34ZZ	Repair Coronary Artery, Four or More Arteries, Percutaneous Endoscopic Approach
02Q40ZZ	Repair Coronary Vein, Open Approach
02Q43ZZ	Repair Coronary Vein, Percutaneous Approach
02Q44ZZ	Repair Coronary Vein, Percutaneous Endoscopic Approach
02Q50ZZ	Repair Atrial Septum, Open Approach
	AHA CC: 4Q, 2015, 23-24
02Q53ZZ	Repair Atrial Septum, Percutaneous Approach
02Q54ZZ	Repair Atrial Septum, Percutaneous Endoscopic Approach
02Q60ZZ	Repair Right Atrium, Open Approach
02Q63ZZ	Repair Right Atrium, Percutaneous Approach
02Q64ZZ	Repair Right Atrium, Percutaneous Endoscopic Approach
02Q70ZZ	Repair Left Atrium, Open Approach
02Q73ZZ	Repair Left Atrium, Percutaneous Approach
02Q74ZZ	Repair Left Atrium, Percutaneous Endoscopic Approach
02Q80ZZ	Repair Conduction Mechanism, Open Approach
02Q83ZZ	Repair Conduction Mechanism, Percutaneous Approach
02Q84ZZ	Repair Conduction Mechanism, Percutaneous Endoscopic Approach
02Q90ZZ	Repair Chordae Tendineae, Open Approach

02Q93ZZ	Repair Chordae Tendineae, Percutaneous Approach
02Q94ZZ	Repair Chordae Tendineae, Percutaneous Endoscopic Approach
02QA0ZZ	Repair Heart, Open Approach
02QA3ZZ	Repair Heart, Percutaneous Approach
02QA4ZZ	Repair Heart, Percutaneous Endoscopic Approach
02QB0ZZ	Repair Right Heart, Open Approach
02QB3ZZ	Repair Right Heart, Percutaneous Approach
02QB4ZZ	Repair Right Heart, Percutaneous Endoscopic Approach
02QC0ZZ	Repair Left Heart, Open Approach
02QC3ZZ	Repair Left Heart, Percutaneous Approach
02QC4ZZ	Repair Left Heart, Percutaneous Endoscopic Approach
02QD0ZZ	Repair Papillary Muscle, Open Approach
02QD3ZZ	Repair Papillary Muscle, Percutaneous Approach
02QD4ZZ	Repair Papillary Muscle, Percutaneous Endoscopic Approach
02QF0ZJ	Repair Aortic Valve created from Truncal Valve, Open Approach
02QF0ZZ	Repair Aortic Valve, Open Approach
02QF3ZJ	Repair Aortic Valve created from Truncal Valve, Percutaneous Approach
02QF3ZZ	Repair Aortic Valve, Percutaneous Approach
02QF4ZJ	Repair Aortic Valve created from Truncal Valve, Percutaneous Endoscopic Approach
02QF4ZZ	Repair Aortic Valve, Percutaneous Endoscopic Approach
02QG0ZE	Repair Mitral Valve created from Left Atrioventricular Valve, Open Approach
02QG0ZZ	Repair Mitral Valve, Open Approach
02QG3ZE	Repair Mitral Valve created from Left Atrioventricular Valve, Percutaneous Approach
02QG3ZZ	Repair Mitral Valve, Percutaneous Approach
02QG4ZE	Repair Mitral Valve created from Left Atrioventricular Valve, Percutaneous Endoscopic Approach
02QG4ZZ	Repair Mitral Valve, Percutaneous Endoscopic Approach
02QH0ZZ	Repair Pulmonary Valve, Open Approach
02QH3ZZ	Repair Pulmonary Valve, Percutaneous Approach
02QH4ZZ	Repair Pulmonary Valve, Percutaneous Endoscopic Approach

02QJ0ZG	Repair Tricuspid Valve created from Right Atrioventricular Valve, Open Approach
02QJ0ZZ	Repair Tricuspid Valve, Open Approach
02QJ3ZG	Repair Tricuspid Valve created from Right Atrioventricular Valve, Percutaneous Approach
02QJ3ZZ	Repair Tricuspid Valve, Percutaneous Approach
02QJ4ZG	Repair Tricuspid Valve created from Right Atrioventricular Valve, Percutaneous Endoscopic Approach
02QJ4ZZ	Repair Tricuspid Valve, Percutaneous Endoscopic Approach
02QK0ZZ	Repair Right Ventricle, Open Approach
02QK3ZZ	Repair Right Ventricle, Percutaneous Approach
02QK4ZZ	Repair Right Ventricle, Percutaneous Endoscopic Approach
02QL0ZZ	Repair Left Ventricle, Open Approach
02QL3ZZ	Repair Left Ventricle, Percutaneous Approach
02QL4ZZ	Repair Left Ventricle, Percutaneous Endoscopic Approach
02QM0ZZ	Repair Ventricular Septum, Open Approach
02QM3ZZ	Repair Ventricular Septum, Percutaneous Approach
02QM4ZZ	Repair Ventricular Septum, Percutaneous Endoscopic Approach
02QN0ZZ	Repair Pericardium, Open Approach
02QN3ZZ	Repair Pericardium, Percutaneous Approach
02QN4ZZ	Repair Pericardium, Percutaneous Endoscopic Approach
02QP0ZZ	Repair Pulmonary Trunk, Open Approach
02QP3ZZ	Repair Pulmonary Trunk, Percutaneous Approach
02QP4ZZ	Repair Pulmonary Trunk, Percutaneous Endoscopic Approach
02QQ0ZZ	Repair Right Pulmonary Artery, Open Approach
02QQ3ZZ	Repair Right Pulmonary Artery, Percutaneous Approach
02QQ4ZZ	Repair Right Pulmonary Artery, Percutaneous Endoscopic Approach
02QR0ZZ	Repair Left Pulmonary Artery, Open Approach
02QR3ZZ	Repair Left Pulmonary Artery, Percutaneous Approach
02QR4ZZ	Repair Left Pulmonary Artery, Percutaneous Endoscopic Approach
02QS0ZZ	Repair Right Pulmonary Vein, Open Approach
	AHA CC: 1Q, 2017, 18-19

♀ Female-only   ♂ Male-only   ▲ Limited Coverage   ● Non-OR   HAC HAC-associated procedure   ▲ Non-covered procedures   ➕ Cluster

02QS3ZZ	Repair Right Pulmonary Vein, Percutaneous Approach	
02QS4ZZ	Repair Right Pulmonary Vein, Percutaneous Endoscopic Approach	
02QT0ZZ	Repair Left Pulmonary Vein, Open Approach	
	AHA CC: 1Q, 2017, 18-19	
02QT3ZZ	Repair Left Pulmonary Vein, Percutaneous Approach	
02QT4ZZ	Repair Left Pulmonary Vein, Percutaneous Endoscopic Approach	

02QV0ZZ	Repair Superior Vena Cava, Open Approach
02QV3ZZ	Repair Superior Vena Cava, Percutaneous Approach
02QV4ZZ	Repair Superior Vena Cava, Percutaneous Endoscopic Approach
02QW0ZZ	Repair Thoracic Aorta, Descending, Open Approach
	AHA CC: 3Q, 2015, 16
02QW3ZZ	Repair Thoracic Aorta, Descending, Percutaneous Approach

02QW4ZZ	Repair Thoracic Aorta, Descending, Percutaneous Endoscopic Approach
02QX0ZZ	Repair Thoracic Aorta, Ascending/ Arch, Open Approach
02QX3ZZ	Repair Thoracic Aorta, Ascending/ Arch, Percutaneous Approach
02QX4ZZ	Repair Thoracic Aorta, Ascending/ Arch, Percutaneous Endoscopic Approach

02R – Heart and Great Vessels, Replacement

Review Coding Guideline B3.18

02R507Z	Replacement of Atrial Septum with Autologous Tissue Substitute, Open Approach
02R508Z	Replacement of Atrial Septum with Zooplastic Tissue, Open Approach
02R50JZ	Replacement of Atrial Septum with Synthetic Substitute, Open Approach
02R50KZ	Replacement of Atrial Septum with Nonautologous Tissue Substitute, Open Approach
02R547Z	Replacement of Atrial Septum with Autologous Tissue Substitute, Percutaneous Endoscopic Approach
02R548Z	Replacement of Atrial Septum with Zooplastic Tissue, Percutaneous Endoscopic Approach
02R54JZ	Replacement of Atrial Septum with Synthetic Substitute, Percutaneous Endoscopic Approach
02R54KZ	Replacement of Atrial Septum with Nonautologous Tissue Substitute, Percutaneous Endoscopic Approach
02R607Z	Replacement of Right Atrium with Autologous Tissue Substitute, Open Approach
02R608Z	Replacement of Right Atrium with Zooplastic Tissue, Open Approach
02R60JZ	Replacement of Right Atrium with Synthetic Substitute, Open Approach
02R60KZ	Replacement of Right Atrium with Nonautologous Tissue Substitute, Open Approach
02R647Z	Replacement of Right Atrium with Autologous Tissue Substitute, Percutaneous Endoscopic Approach
02R648Z	Replacement of Right Atrium with Zooplastic Tissue, Percutaneous Endoscopic Approach
02R64JZ	Replacement of Right Atrium with Synthetic Substitute, Percutaneous Endoscopic Approach
02R64KZ	Replacement of Right Atrium with Nonautologous Tissue Substitute, Percutaneous Endoscopic Approach
02R707Z	Replacement of Left Atrium with Autologous Tissue Substitute, Open Approach
02R708Z	Replacement of Left Atrium with Zooplastic Tissue, Open Approach
02R70JZ	Replacement of Left Atrium with Synthetic Substitute, Open Approach
02R70KZ	Replacement of Left Atrium with Nonautologous Tissue Substitute, Open Approach
02R747Z	Replacement of Left Atrium with Autologous Tissue Substitute, Percutaneous Endoscopic Approach

02R748Z	Replacement of Left Atrium with Zooplastic Tissue, Percutaneous Endoscopic Approach
02R74JZ	Replacement of Left Atrium with Synthetic Substitute, Percutaneous Endoscopic Approach
02R74KZ	Replacement of Left Atrium with Nonautologous Tissue Substitute, Percutaneous Endoscopic Approach
02R907Z	Replacement of Chordae Tendineae with Autologous Tissue Substitute, Open Approach
02R908Z	Replacement of Chordae Tendineae with Zooplastic Tissue, Open Approach
02R90JZ	Replacement of Chordae Tendineae with Synthetic Substitute, Open Approach
02R90KZ	Replacement of Chordae Tendineae with Nonautologous Tissue Substitute, Open Approach
02R947Z	Replacement of Chordae Tendineae with Autologous Tissue Substitute, Percutaneous Endoscopic Approach
02R948Z	Replacement of Chordae Tendineae with Zooplastic Tissue, Percutaneous Endoscopic Approach
02R94JZ	Replacement of Chordae Tendineae with Synthetic Substitute, Percutaneous Endoscopic Approach
02R94KZ	Replacement of Chordae Tendineae with Nonautologous Tissue Substitute, Percutaneous Endoscopic Approach
02RA0LZ	Replacement of Heart with Biologic and Synthetic Substitute, Autoregulated Electrohydraulic, Open Approach
02RA0MZ	Replacement of Heart with Synthetic Substitute, Pneumatic, Open Approach
02RD07Z	Replacement of Papillary Muscle with Autologous Tissue Substitute, Open Approach
02RD08Z	Replacement of Papillary Muscle with Zooplastic Tissue, Open Approach
02RD0JZ	Replacement of Papillary Muscle with Synthetic Substitute, Open Approach
02RD0KZ	Replacement of Papillary Muscle with Nonautologous Tissue Substitute, Open Approach
02RD47Z	Replacement of Papillary Muscle with Autologous Tissue Substitute, Percutaneous Endoscopic Approach
02RD48Z	Replacement of Papillary Muscle with Zooplastic Tissue, Percutaneous Endoscopic Approach
02RD4JZ	Replacement of Papillary Muscle with Synthetic Substitute, Percutaneous Endoscopic Approach

02RD4KZ	Replacement of Papillary Muscle with Nonautologous Tissue Substitute, Percutaneous Endoscopic Approach
02RF07Z	Replacement of Aortic Valve with Autologous Tissue Substitute, Open Approach
02RF08Z	Replacement of Aortic Valve with Zooplastic Tissue, Open Approach
02RF0JZ	Replacement of Aortic Valve with Synthetic Substitute, Open Approach
02RF0KZ	Replacement of Aortic Valve with Nonautologous Tissue Substitute, Open Approach
02RF37H	Replacement of Aortic Valve with Autologous Tissue Substitute, Transapical, Percutaneous Approach
02RF37Z	Replacement of Aortic Valve with Autologous Tissue Substitute, Percutaneous Approach
02RF38H	Replacement of Aortic Valve with Zooplastic Tissue, Transapical, Percutaneous Approach
02RF38Z	Replacement of Aortic Valve with Zooplastic Tissue, Percutaneous Approach
	AHA CC: 1Q, 2019, 31-32
02RF3JH	Replacement of Aortic Valve with Synthetic Substitute, Transapical, Percutaneous Approach
02RF3JZ	Replacement of Aortic Valve with Synthetic Substitute, Percutaneous Approach
	AHA CC: 4Q, 2019, 24
02RF3KH	Replacement of Aortic Valve with Nonautologous Tissue Substitute, Transapical, Percutaneous Approach
02RF3KZ	Replacement of Aortic Valve with Nonautologous Tissue Substitute, Percutaneous Approach
02RF47Z	Replacement of Aortic Valve with Autologous Tissue Substitute, Percutaneous Endoscopic Approach
02RF48Z	Replacement of Aortic Valve with Zooplastic Tissue, Percutaneous Endoscopic Approach
02RF4JZ	Replacement of Aortic Valve with Synthetic Substitute, Percutaneous Endoscopic Approach
02RF4KZ	Replacement of Aortic Valve with Nonautologous Tissue Substitute, Percutaneous Endoscopic Approach
02RG07Z	Replacement of Mitral Valve with Autologous Tissue Substitute, Open Approach
02RG08Z	Replacement of Mitral Valve with Zooplastic Tissue, Open Approach
	AHA CC: 3Q, 2019, 23-24
02RG0JZ	Replacement of Mitral Valve with Synthetic Substitute, Open Approach

02RG0KZ Replacement of Mitral Valve with Nonautologous Tissue Substitute, Open Approach

02RG37H Replacement of Mitral Valve with Autologous Tissue Substitute, Transapical, Percutaneous Approach

02RG37Z Replacement of Mitral Valve with Autologous Tissue Substitute, Percutaneous Approach

02RG38H Replacement of Mitral Valve with Zooplastic Tissue, Transapical, Percutaneous Approach

02RG38Z Replacement of Mitral Valve with Zooplastic Tissue, Percutaneous Approach

02RG3JH Replacement of Mitral Valve with Synthetic Substitute, Transapical, Percutaneous Approach

02RG3JZ Replacement of Mitral Valve with Synthetic Substitute, Percutaneous Approach

02RG3KH Replacement of Mitral Valve with Nonautologous Tissue Substitute, Transapical, Percutaneous Approach

02RG3KZ Replacement of Mitral Valve with Nonautologous Tissue Substitute, Percutaneous Approach

02RG47Z Replacement of Mitral Valve with Autologous Tissue Substitute, Percutaneous Endoscopic Approach

02RG48Z Replacement of Mitral Valve with Zooplastic Tissue, Percutaneous Endoscopic Approach

02RG4JZ Replacement of Mitral Valve with Synthetic Substitute, Percutaneous Endoscopic Approach

02RG4KZ Replacement of Mitral Valve with Nonautologous Tissue Substitute, Percutaneous Endoscopic Approach

02RH07Z Replacement of Pulmonary Valve with Autologous Tissue Substitute, Open Approach

02RH08Z Replacement of Pulmonary Valve with Zooplastic Tissue, Open Approach

02RH0JZ Replacement of Pulmonary Valve with Synthetic Substitute, Open Approach

02RH0KZ Replacement of Pulmonary Valve with Nonautologous Tissue Substitute, Open Approach

02RH37H Replacement of Pulmonary Valve with Autologous Tissue Substitute, Transapical, Percutaneous Approach

02RH37Z Replacement of Pulmonary Valve with Autologous Tissue Substitute, Percutaneous Approach

02RH38H Replacement of Pulmonary Valve with Zooplastic Tissue, Transapical, Percutaneous Approach

02RH38L Replacement of Pulmonary Valve with Zooplastic Tissue, In Existing Conduit, Percutaneous Approach

02RH38M Replacement of Pulmonary Valve with Zooplastic Tissue, Native Site, Percutaneous Approach

02RH38Z Replacement of Pulmonary Valve with Zooplastic Tissue, Percutaneous Approach

02RH3JH Replacement of Pulmonary Valve with Synthetic Substitute, Transapical, Percutaneous Approach

02RH3JZ Replacement of Pulmonary Valve with Synthetic Substitute, Percutaneous Approach

02RH3KH Replacement of Pulmonary Valve with Nonautologous Tissue Substitute, Transapical, Percutaneous Approach

02RH3KZ Replacement of Pulmonary Valve with Nonautologous Tissue Substitute, Percutaneous Approach

02RH47Z Replacement of Pulmonary Valve with Autologous Tissue Substitute, Percutaneous Endoscopic Approach

02RH48Z Replacement of Pulmonary Valve with Zooplastic Tissue, Percutaneous Endoscopic Approach

02RH4JZ Replacement of Pulmonary Valve with Synthetic Substitute, Percutaneous Endoscopic Approach

02RH4KZ Replacement of Pulmonary Valve with Nonautologous Tissue Substitute, Percutaneous Endoscopic Approach

02RJ07Z Replacement of Tricuspid Valve with Autologous Tissue Substitute, Open Approach

02RJ08Z Replacement of Tricuspid Valve with Zooplastic Tissue, Open Approach

02RJ0JZ Replacement of Tricuspid Valve with Synthetic Substitute, Open Approach

02RJ0KZ Replacement of Tricuspid Valve with Nonautologous Tissue Substitute, Open Approach

02RJ37H Replacement of Tricuspid Valve with Autologous Tissue Substitute, Transapical, Percutaneous Approach

02RJ37Z Replacement of Tricuspid Valve with Autologous Tissue Substitute, Percutaneous Approach

02RJ38H Replacement of Tricuspid Valve with Zooplastic Tissue, Transapical, Percutaneous Approach

02RJ38Z Replacement of Tricuspid Valve with Zooplastic Tissue, Percutaneous Approach

02RJ3JH Replacement of Tricuspid Valve with Synthetic Substitute, Transapical, Percutaneous Approach

02RJ3JZ Replacement of Tricuspid Valve with Synthetic Substitute, Percutaneous Approach
AHA CC: 4Q, 2017, 56

02RJ3KH Replacement of Tricuspid Valve with Nonautologous Tissue Substitute, Transapical, Percutaneous Approach

02RJ3KZ Replacement of Tricuspid Valve with Nonautologous Tissue Substitute, Percutaneous Approach

02RJ47Z Replacement of Tricuspid Valve with Autologous Tissue Substitute, Percutaneous Endoscopic Approach

02RJ48Z Replacement of Tricuspid Valve with Zooplastic Tissue, Percutaneous Endoscopic Approach
AHA CC: 3Q, 2016, 32

02RJ4JZ Replacement of Tricuspid Valve with Synthetic Substitute, Percutaneous Endoscopic Approach

02RJ4KZ Replacement of Tricuspid Valve with Nonautologous Tissue Substitute, Percutaneous Endoscopic Approach

02RK07Z Replacement of Right Ventricle with Autologous Tissue Substitute, Open Approach

02RK08Z Replacement of Right Ventricle with Zooplastic Tissue, Open Approach

02RK0JZ Replacement of Right Ventricle with Synthetic Substitute, Open Approach
▲ *When reported with 02RL0JZ and diagnosis code Z00.6*
+ Biventricular heart replacement (artificial heart) when reported with 02RL0JZ.
AHA CC: 1Q, 2017, 13-14

02RK0KZ Replacement of Right Ventricle with Nonautologous Tissue Substitute, Open Approach

02RK47Z Replacement of Right Ventricle with Autologous Tissue Substitute, Percutaneous Endoscopic Approach

02RK48Z Replacement of Right Ventricle with Zooplastic Tissue, Percutaneous Endoscopic Approach

02RK4JZ Replacement of Right Ventricle with Synthetic Substitute, Percutaneous Endoscopic Approach

02RK4KZ Replacement of Right Ventricle with Nonautologous Tissue Substitute, Percutaneous Endoscopic Approach

02RL07Z Replacement of Left Ventricle with Autologous Tissue Substitute, Open Approach

02RL08Z Replacement of Left Ventricle with Zooplastic Tissue, Open Approach

02RL0JZ Replacement of Left Ventricle with Synthetic Substitute, Open Approach
▲ *When reported with 02RK0JZ and diagnosis code Z00.6*
+ Biventricular heart replacement (artificial heart) when reported with 02RK0JZ.
AHA CC: 1Q, 2017, 13-14

02RL0KZ Replacement of Left Ventricle with Nonautologous Tissue Substitute, Open Approach

02RL47Z Replacement of Left Ventricle with Autologous Tissue Substitute, Percutaneous Endoscopic Approach

02RL48Z Replacement of Left Ventricle with Zooplastic Tissue, Percutaneous Endoscopic Approach

02RL4JZ Replacement of Left Ventricle with Synthetic Substitute, Percutaneous Endoscopic Approach

02RL4KZ Replacement of Left Ventricle with Nonautologous Tissue Substitute, Percutaneous Endoscopic Approach

02RM07Z Replacement of Ventricular Septum with Autologous Tissue Substitute, Open Approach

02RM08Z Replacement of Ventricular Septum with Zooplastic Tissue, Open Approach

02RM0JZ Replacement of Ventricular Septum with Synthetic Substitute, Open Approach

02RM0KZ Replacement of Ventricular Septum with Nonautologous Tissue Substitute, Open Approach

02RM47Z Replacement of Ventricular Septum with Autologous Tissue Substitute, Percutaneous Endoscopic Approach

02RM48Z Replacement of Ventricular Septum with Zooplastic Tissue, Percutaneous Endoscopic Approach

02RM4JZ Replacement of Ventricular Septum with Synthetic Substitute, Percutaneous Endoscopic Approach

02RM4KZ Replacement of Ventricular Septum with Nonautologous Tissue Substitute, Percutaneous Endoscopic Approach

02RN07Z Replacement of Pericardium with Autologous Tissue Substitute, Open Approach

02RN08Z Replacement of Pericardium with Zooplastic Tissue, Open Approach

02RN0JZ Replacement of Pericardium with Synthetic Substitute, Open Approach

02RN0KZ Replacement of Pericardium with Nonautologous Tissue Substitute, Open Approach

♀ Female-only ♂ Male-only ▲ Limited Coverage ● Non-OR ■HAC HAC-associated procedure ▲ Non-covered procedures + Cluster

02RN47Z Replacement of Pericardium with Autologous Tissue Substitute, Percutaneous Endoscopic Approach

02RN48Z Replacement of Pericardium with Zooplastic Tissue, Percutaneous Endoscopic Approach

02RN4JZ Replacement of Pericardium with Synthetic Substitute, Percutaneous Endoscopic Approach

02RN4KZ Replacement of Pericardium with Nonautologous Tissue Substitute, Percutaneous Endoscopic Approach

02RP07Z Replacement of Pulmonary Trunk with Autologous Tissue Substitute, Open Approach

02RP08Z Replacement of Pulmonary Trunk with Zooplastic Tissue, Open Approach

02RP0JZ Replacement of Pulmonary Trunk with Synthetic Substitute, Open Approach

02RP0KZ Replacement of Pulmonary Trunk with Nonautologous Tissue Substitute, Open Approach

02RP47Z Replacement of Pulmonary Trunk with Autologous Tissue Substitute, Percutaneous Endoscopic Approach

02RP48Z Replacement of Pulmonary Trunk with Zooplastic Tissue, Percutaneous Endoscopic Approach

02RP4JZ Replacement of Pulmonary Trunk with Synthetic Substitute, Percutaneous Endoscopic Approach

02RP4KZ Replacement of Pulmonary Trunk with Nonautologous Tissue Substitute, Percutaneous Endoscopic Approach

02RQ07Z Replacement of Right Pulmonary Artery with Autologous Tissue Substitute, Open Approach

02RQ08Z Replacement of Right Pulmonary Artery with Zooplastic Tissue, Open Approach

02RQ0JZ Replacement of Right Pulmonary Artery with Synthetic Substitute, Open Approach

02RQ0KZ Replacement of Right Pulmonary Artery with Nonautologous Tissue Substitute, Open Approach

02RQ47Z Replacement of Right Pulmonary Artery with Autologous Tissue Substitute, Percutaneous Endoscopic Approach

02RQ48Z Replacement of Right Pulmonary Artery with Zooplastic Tissue, Percutaneous Endoscopic Approach

02RQ4JZ Replacement of Right Pulmonary Artery with Synthetic Substitute, Percutaneous Endoscopic Approach

02RQ4KZ Replacement of Right Pulmonary Artery with Nonautologous Tissue Substitute, Percutaneous Endoscopic Approach

02RR07Z Replacement of Left Pulmonary Artery with Autologous Tissue Substitute, Open Approach

02RR08Z Replacement of Left Pulmonary Artery with Zooplastic Tissue, Open Approach

02RR0JZ Replacement of Left Pulmonary Artery with Synthetic Substitute, Open Approach

02RR0KZ Replacement of Left Pulmonary Artery with Nonautologous Tissue Substitute, Open Approach

02RR47Z Replacement of Left Pulmonary Artery with Autologous Tissue Substitute, Percutaneous Endoscopic Approach

02RR48Z Replacement of Left Pulmonary Artery with Zooplastic Tissue, Percutaneous Endoscopic Approach

02RR4JZ Replacement of Left Pulmonary Artery with Synthetic Substitute, Percutaneous Endoscopic Approach

02RR4KZ Replacement of Left Pulmonary Artery with Nonautologous Tissue Substitute, Percutaneous Endoscopic Approach

02RS07Z Replacement of Right Pulmonary Vein with Autologous Tissue Substitute, Open Approach

02RS08Z Replacement of Right Pulmonary Vein with Zooplastic Tissue, Open Approach

02RS0JZ Replacement of Right Pulmonary Vein with Synthetic Substitute, Open Approach

02RS0KZ Replacement of Right Pulmonary Vein with Nonautologous Tissue Substitute, Open Approach

02RS47Z Replacement of Right Pulmonary Vein with Autologous Tissue Substitute, Percutaneous Endoscopic Approach

02RS48Z Replacement of Right Pulmonary Vein with Zooplastic Tissue, Percutaneous Endoscopic Approach

02RS4JZ Replacement of Right Pulmonary Vein with Synthetic Substitute, Percutaneous Endoscopic Approach

02RS4KZ Replacement of Right Pulmonary Vein with Nonautologous Tissue Substitute, Percutaneous Endoscopic Approach

02RT07Z Replacement of Left Pulmonary Vein with Autologous Tissue Substitute, Open Approach

02RT08Z Replacement of Left Pulmonary Vein with Zooplastic Tissue, Open Approach

02RT0JZ Replacement of Left Pulmonary Vein with Synthetic Substitute, Open Approach

02RT0KZ Replacement of Left Pulmonary Vein with Nonautologous Tissue Substitute, Open Approach

02RT47Z Replacement of Left Pulmonary Vein with Autologous Tissue Substitute, Percutaneous Endoscopic Approach

02RT48Z Replacement of Left Pulmonary Vein with Zooplastic Tissue, Percutaneous Endoscopic Approach

02RT4JZ Replacement of Left Pulmonary Vein with Synthetic Substitute, Percutaneous Endoscopic Approach

02RT4KZ Replacement of Left Pulmonary Vein with Nonautologous Tissue Substitute, Percutaneous Endoscopic Approach

02RV07Z Replacement of Superior Vena Cava with Autologous Tissue Substitute, Open Approach

02RV08Z Replacement of Superior Vena Cava with Zooplastic Tissue, Open Approach

02RV0JZ Replacement of Superior Vena Cava with Synthetic Substitute, Open Approach

02RV0KZ Replacement of Superior Vena Cava with Nonautologous Tissue Substitute, Open Approach

02RV47Z Replacement of Superior Vena Cava with Autologous Tissue Substitute, Percutaneous Endoscopic Approach

02RV48Z Replacement of Superior Vena Cava with Zooplastic Tissue, Percutaneous Endoscopic Approach

02RV4JZ Replacement of Superior Vena Cava with Synthetic Substitute, Percutaneous Endoscopic Approach

02RV4KZ Replacement of Superior Vena Cava with Nonautologous Tissue Substitute, Percutaneous Endoscopic Approach

02RW07Z Replacement of Thoracic Aorta, Descending with Autologous Tissue Substitute, Open Approach

02RW08Z Replacement of Thoracic Aorta, Descending with Zooplastic Tissue, Open Approach

02RW0JZ Replacement of Thoracic Aorta, Descending with Synthetic Substitute, Open Approach

02RW0KZ Replacement of Thoracic Aorta, Descending with Nonautologous Tissue Substitute, Open Approach
AHA CC: 1Q, 2014, 10-11

02RW47Z Replacement of Thoracic Aorta, Descending with Autologous Tissue Substitute, Percutaneous Endoscopic Approach

02RW48Z Replacement of Thoracic Aorta, Descending with Zooplastic Tissue, Percutaneous Endoscopic Approach

02RW4JZ Replacement of Thoracic Aorta, Descending with Synthetic Substitute, Percutaneous Endoscopic Approach

02RW4KZ Replacement of Thoracic Aorta, Descending with Nonautologous Tissue Substitute, Percutaneous Endoscopic Approach

02RX07Z Replacement of Thoracic Aorta, Ascending/Arch with Autologous Tissue Substitute, Open Approach

02RX08Z Replacement of Thoracic Aorta, Ascending/Arch with Zooplastic Tissue, Open Approach

02RX0JZ Replacement of Thoracic Aorta, Ascending/Arch with Synthetic Substitute, Open Approach
AHA CC: 3Q, 2019, 24; 1Q, 2020, 25-26

02RX0KZ Replacement of Thoracic Aorta, Ascending/Arch with Nonautologous Tissue Substitute, Open Approach

02RX47Z Replacement of Thoracic Aorta, Ascending/Arch with Autologous Tissue Substitute, Percutaneous Endoscopic Approach

02RX48Z Replacement of Thoracic Aorta, Ascending/Arch with Zooplastic Tissue, Percutaneous Endoscopic Approach

02RX4JZ Replacement of Thoracic Aorta, Ascending/Arch with Synthetic Substitute, Percutaneous Endoscopic Approach

02RX4KZ Replacement of Thoracic Aorta, Ascending/Arch with Nonautologous Tissue Substitute, Percutaneous Endoscopic Approach

02S – Heart and Great Vessels, Reposition

02S00ZZ Reposition Coronary Artery, One Artery, Open Approach

02S10ZZ Reposition Coronary Artery, Two Arteries, Open Approach
AHA CC: 4Q, 2016, 103-104

02SP0ZZ Reposition Pulmonary Trunk, Open Approach
AHA CC: 4Q, 2015, 23-24; 4Q, 2016, 103-104

02SQ0ZZ Reposition Right Pulmonary Artery, Open Approach

02SR0ZZ Reposition Left Pulmonary Artery, Open Approach

02SS0ZZ Reposition Right Pulmonary Vein, Open Approach

♀ Female-only   ♂ Male-only   ▲ Limited Coverage   ● Non-OR   HAC HAC-associated procedure   ▲ Non-covered procedures   ✚ Cluster

02ST0ZZ	Reposition Left Pulmonary Vein, Open Approach	
02SV0ZZ	Reposition Superior Vena Cava, Open Approach	

02SW0ZZ	Reposition Thoracic Aorta, Descending, Open Approach
	AHA CC: 4Q, 2015, 23-24

02SX0ZZ	Reposition Thoracic Aorta, Ascending/ Arch, Open Approach
	AHA CC: 4Q, 2016, 103-104

02T – Heart and Great Vessels, Resection

Review Coding Guideline B3.8

Review Coding Guideline B3.18

02T50ZZ	Resection of Atrial Septum, Open Approach	**02T93ZZ**	Resection of Chordae Tendineae, Percutaneous Approach	**02TH4ZZ**	Resection of Pulmonary Valve, Percutaneous Endoscopic Approach
02T53ZZ	Resection of Atrial Septum, Percutaneous Approach	**02T94ZZ**	Resection of Chordae Tendineae, Percutaneous Endoscopic Approach	**02TM0ZZ**	Resection of Ventricular Septum, Open Approach
02T54ZZ	Resection of Atrial Septum, Percutaneous Endoscopic Approach	**02TD0ZZ**	Resection of Papillary Muscle, Open Approach	**02TM3ZZ**	Resection of Ventricular Septum, Percutaneous Approach
02T80ZZ	Resection of Conduction Mechanism, Open Approach	**02TD3ZZ**	Resection of Papillary Muscle, Percutaneous Approach	**02TM4ZZ**	Resection of Ventricular Septum, Percutaneous Endoscopic Approach
02T83ZZ	Resection of Conduction Mechanism, Percutaneous Approach	**02TD4ZZ**	Resection of Papillary Muscle, Percutaneous Endoscopic Approach	**02TN0ZZ**	Resection of Pericardium, Open Approach
02T84ZZ	Resection of Conduction Mechanism, Percutaneous Endoscopic Approach	**02TH0ZZ**	Resection of Pulmonary Valve, Open Approach	**02TN3ZZ**	Resection of Pericardium, Percutaneous Approach
02T90ZZ	Resection of Chordae Tendineae, Open Approach	**02TH3ZZ**	Resection of Pulmonary Valve, Percutaneous Approach	**02TN4ZZ**	Resection of Pericardium, Percutaneous Endoscopic Approach

02U – Heart and Great Vessels, Supplement

02U007Z	Supplement Coronary Artery, One Artery with Autologous Tissue Substitute, Open Approach	**02U10KZ**	Supplement Coronary Artery, Two Arteries with Nonautologous Tissue Substitute, Open Approach	**02U23JZ**	Supplement Coronary Artery, Three Arteries with Synthetic Substitute, Percutaneous Approach
02U008Z	Supplement Coronary Artery, One Artery with Zooplastic Tissue, Open Approach	**02U137Z**	Supplement Coronary Artery, Two Arteries with Autologous Tissue Substitute, Percutaneous Approach	**02U23KZ**	Supplement Coronary Artery, Three Arteries with Nonautologous Tissue Substitute, Percutaneous Approach
02U00JZ	Supplement Coronary Artery, One Artery with Synthetic Substitute, Open Approach	**02U138Z**	Supplement Coronary Artery, Two Arteries with Zooplastic Tissue, Percutaneous Approach	**02U247Z**	Supplement Coronary Artery, Three Arteries with Autologous Tissue Substitute, Percutaneous Endoscopic Approach
02U00KZ	Supplement Coronary Artery, One Artery with Nonautologous Tissue Substitute, Open Approach	**02U13JZ**	Supplement Coronary Artery, Two Arteries with Synthetic Substitute, Percutaneous Approach	**02U248Z**	Supplement Coronary Artery, Three Arteries with Zooplastic Tissue, Percutaneous Endoscopic Approach
02U037Z	Supplement Coronary Artery, One Artery with Autologous Tissue Substitute, Percutaneous Approach	**02U13KZ**	Supplement Coronary Artery, Two Arteries with Nonautologous Tissue Substitute, Percutaneous Approach	**02U24JZ**	Supplement Coronary Artery, Three Arteries with Synthetic Substitute, Percutaneous Endoscopic Approach
02U038Z	Supplement Coronary Artery, One Artery with Zooplastic Tissue, Percutaneous Approach	**02U147Z**	Supplement Coronary Artery, Two Arteries with Autologous Tissue Substitute, Percutaneous Endoscopic Approach	**02U24KZ**	Supplement Coronary Artery, Three Arteries with Nonautologous Tissue Substitute, Percutaneous Endoscopic Approach
02U03JZ	Supplement Coronary Artery, One Artery with Synthetic Substitute, Percutaneous Approach *AHA CC: 4Q, 2019, 25-26*	**02U148Z**	Supplement Coronary Artery, Two Arteries with Zooplastic Tissue, Percutaneous Endoscopic Approach	**02U307Z**	Supplement Coronary Artery, Four or More Arteries with Autologous Tissue Substitute, Open Approach
02U03KZ	Supplement Coronary Artery, One Artery with Nonautologous Tissue Substitute, Percutaneous Approach	**02U14JZ**	Supplement Coronary Artery, Two Arteries with Synthetic Substitute, Percutaneous Endoscopic Approach	**02U308Z**	Supplement Coronary Artery, Four or More Arteries with Zooplastic Tissue, Open Approach
02U047Z	Supplement Coronary Artery, One Artery with Autologous Tissue Substitute, Percutaneous Endoscopic Approach	**02U14KZ**	Supplement Coronary Artery, Two Arteries with Nonautologous Tissue Substitute, Percutaneous Endoscopic Approach	**02U30JZ**	Supplement Coronary Artery, Four or More Arteries with Synthetic Substitute, Open Approach
02U048Z	Supplement Coronary Artery, One Artery with Zooplastic Tissue, Percutaneous Endoscopic Approach	**02U207Z**	Supplement Coronary Artery, Three Arteries with Autologous Tissue Substitute, Open Approach	**02U30KZ**	Supplement Coronary Artery, Four or More Arteries with Nonautologous Tissue Substitute, Open Approach
02U04JZ	Supplement Coronary Artery, One Artery with Synthetic Substitute, Percutaneous Endoscopic Approach	**02U208Z**	Supplement Coronary Artery, Three Arteries with Zooplastic Tissue, Open Approach	**02U337Z**	Supplement Coronary Artery, Four or More Arteries with Autologous Tissue Substitute, Percutaneous Approach
02U04KZ	Supplement Coronary Artery, One Artery with Nonautologous Tissue Substitute, Percutaneous Endoscopic Approach	**02U20JZ**	Supplement Coronary Artery, Three Arteries with Synthetic Substitute, Open Approach	**02U338Z**	Supplement Coronary Artery, Four or More Arteries with Zooplastic Tissue, Percutaneous Approach
02U107Z	Supplement Coronary Artery, Two Arteries with Autologous Tissue Substitute, Open Approach	**02U20KZ**	Supplement Coronary Artery, Three Arteries with Nonautologous Tissue Substitute, Open Approach	**02U33JZ**	Supplement Coronary Artery, Four or More Arteries with Synthetic Substitute, Percutaneous Approach
02U108Z	Supplement Coronary Artery, Two Arteries with Zooplastic Tissue, Open Approach	**02U237Z**	Supplement Coronary Artery, Three Arteries with Autologous Tissue Substitute, Percutaneous Approach	**02U33KZ**	Supplement Coronary Artery, Four or More Arteries with Nonautologous Tissue Substitute, Percutaneous Approach
02U10JZ	Supplement Coronary Artery, Two Arteries with Synthetic Substitute, Open Approach	**02U238Z**	Supplement Coronary Artery, Three Arteries with Zooplastic Tissue, Percutaneous Approach	**02U347Z**	Supplement Coronary Artery, Four or More Arteries with Autologous Tissue Substitute, Percutaneous Endoscopic Approach

♀ Female-only   ♂ Male-only   ▲ Limited Coverage   ● Non-OR   **HAC** HAC-associated procedure   ▲ Non-covered procedures   ✚ Cluster

02U348Z	Supplement Coronary Artery, Four or More Arteries with Zooplastic Tissue, Percutaneous Endoscopic Approach
02U34JZ	Supplement Coronary Artery, Four or More Arteries with Synthetic Substitute, Percutaneous Endoscopic Approach
02U34KZ	Supplement Coronary Artery, Four or More Arteries with Nonautologous Tissue Substitute, Percutaneous Endoscopic Approach
02U507Z	Supplement Atrial Septum with Autologous Tissue Substitute, Open Approach
02U508Z	Supplement Atrial Septum with Zooplastic Tissue, Open Approach
02U50JZ	Supplement Atrial Septum with Synthetic Substitute, Open Approach
02U50KZ	Supplement Atrial Septum with Nonautologous Tissue Substitute, Open Approach
02U537Z	Supplement Atrial Septum with Autologous Tissue Substitute, Percutaneous Approach
02U538Z	Supplement Atrial Septum with Zooplastic Tissue, Percutaneous Approach
02U53JZ	Supplement Atrial Septum with Synthetic Substitute, Percutaneous Approach
02U53KZ	Supplement Atrial Septum with Nonautologous Tissue Substitute, Percutaneous Approach
02U547Z	Supplement Atrial Septum with Autologous Tissue Substitute, Percutaneous Endoscopic Approach
02U548Z	Supplement Atrial Septum with Zooplastic Tissue, Percutaneous Endoscopic Approach
02U54JZ	Supplement Atrial Septum with Synthetic Substitute, Percutaneous Endoscopic Approach
02U54KZ	Supplement Atrial Septum with Nonautologous Tissue Substitute, Percutaneous Endoscopic Approach
02U607Z	Supplement Right Atrium with Autologous Tissue Substitute, Open Approach
	AHA CC: 3Q, 2017, 7-8
02U608Z	Supplement Right Atrium with Zooplastic Tissue, Open Approach
02U60JZ	Supplement Right Atrium with Synthetic Substitute, Open Approach
02U60KZ	Supplement Right Atrium with Nonautologous Tissue Substitute, Open Approach
02U637Z	Supplement Right Atrium with Autologous Tissue Substitute, Percutaneous Approach
02U638Z	Supplement Right Atrium with Zooplastic Tissue, Percutaneous Approach
02U63JZ	Supplement Right Atrium with Synthetic Substitute, Percutaneous Approach
02U63KZ	Supplement Right Atrium with Nonautologous Tissue Substitute, Percutaneous Approach
02U647Z	Supplement Right Atrium with Autologous Tissue Substitute, Percutaneous Endoscopic Approach
02U648Z	Supplement Right Atrium with Zooplastic Tissue, Percutaneous Endoscopic Approach
02U64JZ	Supplement Right Atrium with Synthetic Substitute, Percutaneous Endoscopic Approach

02U64KZ	Supplement Right Atrium with Nonautologous Tissue Substitute, Percutaneous Endoscopic Approach
02U707Z	Supplement Left Atrium with Autologous Tissue Substitute, Open Approach
	AHA CC: 3Q, 2017, 7-8
02U708Z	Supplement Left Atrium with Zooplastic Tissue, Open Approach
02U70JZ	Supplement Left Atrium with Synthetic Substitute, Open Approach
02U70KZ	Supplement Left Atrium with Nonautologous Tissue Substitute, Open Approach
02U737Z	Supplement Left Atrium with Autologous Tissue Substitute, Percutaneous Approach
02U738Z	Supplement Left Atrium with Zooplastic Tissue, Percutaneous Approach
● **02U73JZ**	Supplement Left Atrium with Synthetic Substitute, Percutaneous Approach
02U73KZ	Supplement Left Atrium with Nonautologous Tissue Substitute, Percutaneous Approach
02U747Z	Supplement Left Atrium with Autologous Tissue Substitute, Percutaneous Endoscopic Approach
02U748Z	Supplement Left Atrium with Zooplastic Tissue, Percutaneous Endoscopic Approach
● **02U74JZ**	Supplement Left Atrium with Synthetic Substitute, Percutaneous Endoscopic Approach
02U74KZ	Supplement Left Atrium with Nonautologous Tissue Substitute, Percutaneous Endoscopic Approach
02U907Z	Supplement Chordae Tendineae with Autologous Tissue Substitute, Open Approach
02U908Z	Supplement Chordae Tendineae with Zooplastic Tissue, Open Approach
02U90JZ	Supplement Chordae Tendineae with Synthetic Substitute, Open Approach
02U90KZ	Supplement Chordae Tendineae with Nonautologous Tissue Substitute, Open Approach
02U937Z	Supplement Chordae Tendineae with Autologous Tissue Substitute, Percutaneous Approach
02U938Z	Supplement Chordae Tendineae with Zooplastic Tissue, Percutaneous Approach
02U93JZ	Supplement Chordae Tendineae with Synthetic Substitute, Percutaneous Approach
02U93KZ	Supplement Chordae Tendineae with Nonautologous Tissue Substitute, Percutaneous Approach
02U947Z	Supplement Chordae Tendineae with Autologous Tissue Substitute, Percutaneous Endoscopic Approach
02U948Z	Supplement Chordae Tendineae with Zooplastic Tissue, Percutaneous Endoscopic Approach
02U94JZ	Supplement Chordae Tendineae with Synthetic Substitute, Percutaneous Endoscopic Approach
02U94KZ	Supplement Chordae Tendineae with Nonautologous Tissue Substitute, Percutaneous Endoscopic Approach
02UA07Z	Supplement Heart with Autologous Tissue Substitute, Open Approach
02UA08Z	Supplement Heart with Zooplastic Tissue, Open Approach

02UA0JZ	Supplement Heart with Synthetic Substitute, Open Approach
02UA0KZ	Supplement Heart with Nonautologous Tissue Substitute, Open Approach
02UA37Z	Supplement Heart with Autologous Tissue Substitute, Percutaneous Approach
02UA38Z	Supplement Heart with Zooplastic Tissue, Percutaneous Approach
02UA3JZ	Supplement Heart with Synthetic Substitute, Percutaneous Approach
02UA3KZ	Supplement Heart with Nonautologous Tissue Substitute, Percutaneous Approach
02UA47Z	Supplement Heart with Autologous Tissue Substitute, Percutaneous Endoscopic Approach
02UA48Z	Supplement Heart with Zooplastic Tissue, Percutaneous Endoscopic Approach
02UA4JZ	Supplement Heart with Synthetic Substitute, Percutaneous Endoscopic Approach
02UA4KZ	Supplement Heart with Nonautologous Tissue Substitute, Percutaneous Endoscopic Approach
02UD07Z	Supplement Papillary Muscle with Autologous Tissue Substitute, Open Approach
02UD08Z	Supplement Papillary Muscle with Zooplastic Tissue, Open Approach
02UD0JZ	Supplement Papillary Muscle with Synthetic Substitute, Open Approach
02UD0KZ	Supplement Papillary Muscle with Nonautologous Tissue Substitute, Open Approach
02UD37Z	Supplement Papillary Muscle with Autologous Tissue Substitute, Percutaneous Approach
02UD38Z	Supplement Papillary Muscle with Zooplastic Tissue, Percutaneous Approach
02UD3JZ	Supplement Papillary Muscle with Synthetic Substitute, Percutaneous Approach
02UD3KZ	Supplement Papillary Muscle with Nonautologous Tissue Substitute, Percutaneous Approach
02UD47Z	Supplement Papillary Muscle with Autologous Tissue Substitute, Percutaneous Endoscopic Approach
02UD48Z	Supplement Papillary Muscle with Zooplastic Tissue, Percutaneous Endoscopic Approach
02UD4JZ	Supplement Papillary Muscle with Synthetic Substitute, Percutaneous Endoscopic Approach
02UD4KZ	Supplement Papillary Muscle with Nonautologous Tissue Substitute, Percutaneous Endoscopic Approach
02UF07J	Supplement Aortic Valve created from Truncal Valve with Autologous Tissue Substitute, Open Approach
02UF07Z	Supplement Aortic Valve with Autologous Tissue Substitute, Open Approach
02UF08J	Supplement Aortic Valve created from Truncal Valve with Zooplastic Tissue, Open Approach
02UF08Z	Supplement Aortic Valve with Zooplastic Tissue, Open Approach
	AHA CC: 4Q, 2015, 25
02UF0JJ	Supplement Aortic Valve created from Truncal Valve with Synthetic Substitute, Open Approach
02UF0JZ	Supplement Aortic Valve with Synthetic Substitute, Open Approach

02UF0KJ Supplement Aortic Valve created from Truncal Valve with Nonautologous Tissue Substitute, Open Approach

02UF0KZ Supplement Aortic Valve with Nonautologous Tissue Substitute, Open Approach

02UF37J Supplement Aortic Valve created from Truncal Valve with Autologous Tissue Substitute, Percutaneous Approach

02UF37Z Supplement Aortic Valve with Autologous Tissue Substitute, Percutaneous Approach

02UF38J Supplement Aortic Valve created from Truncal Valve with Zooplastic Tissue, Percutaneous Approach

02UF38Z Supplement Aortic Valve with Zooplastic Tissue, Percutaneous Approach

02UF3JJ Supplement Aortic Valve created from Truncal Valve with Synthetic Substitute, Percutaneous Approach

02UF3JZ Supplement Aortic Valve with Synthetic Substitute, Percutaneous Approach

02UF3KJ Supplement Aortic Valve created from Truncal Valve with Nonautologous Tissue Substitute, Percutaneous Approach

02UF3KZ Supplement Aortic Valve with Nonautologous Tissue Substitute, Percutaneous Approach

02UF47J Supplement Aortic Valve created from Truncal Valve with Autologous Tissue Substitute, Percutaneous Endoscopic Approach

02UF47Z Supplement Aortic Valve with Autologous Tissue Substitute, Percutaneous Endoscopic Approach

02UF48J Supplement Aortic Valve created from Truncal Valve with Zooplastic Tissue, Percutaneous Endoscopic Approach

02UF48Z Supplement Aortic Valve with Zooplastic Tissue, Percutaneous Endoscopic Approach

02UF4JJ Supplement Aortic Valve created from Truncal Valve with Synthetic Substitute, Percutaneous Endoscopic Approach

02UF4JZ Supplement Aortic Valve with Synthetic Substitute, Percutaneous Endoscopic Approach

02UF4KJ Supplement Aortic Valve created from Truncal Valve with Nonautologous Tissue Substitute, Percutaneous Endoscopic Approach

02UF4KZ Supplement Aortic Valve with Nonautologous Tissue Substitute, Percutaneous Endoscopic Approach

02UG07E Supplement Mitral Valve created from Left Atrioventricular Valve with Autologous Tissue Substitute, Open Approach

02UG07Z Supplement Mitral Valve with Autologous Tissue Substitute, Open Approach

02UG08E Supplement Mitral Valve created from Left Atrioventricular Valve with Zooplastic Tissue, Open Approach

02UG08Z Supplement Mitral Valve with Zooplastic Tissue, Open Approach
AHA CC: 4Q, 2017, 36

02UG0JE Supplement Mitral Valve created from Left Atrioventricular Valve with Synthetic Substitute, Open Approach

02UG0JZ Supplement Mitral Valve with Synthetic Substitute, Open Approach
AHA CC: 2Q, 2015, 23-24

02UG0KE Supplement Mitral Valve created from Left Atrioventricular Valve with Nonautologous Tissue Substitute, Open Approach

02UG0KZ Supplement Mitral Valve with Nonautologous Tissue Substitute, Open Approach

02UG37E Supplement Mitral Valve created from Left Atrioventricular Valve with Autologous Tissue Substitute, Percutaneous Approach

02UG37Z Supplement Mitral Valve with Autologous Tissue Substitute, Percutaneous Approach

02UG38E Supplement Mitral Valve created from Left Atrioventricular Valve with Zooplastic Tissue, Percutaneous Approach

02UG38Z Supplement Mitral Valve with Zooplastic Tissue, Percutaneous Approach

02UG3JE Supplement Mitral Valve created from Left Atrioventricular Valve with Synthetic Substitute, Percutaneous Approach

02UG3JH Supplement Mitral Valve with Synthetic Substitute, Transapical, Percutaneous Approach
AHA CC: 4Q, 2020, 52

02UG3JZ Supplement Mitral Valve with Synthetic Substitute, Percutaneous Approach

02UG3KE Supplement Mitral Valve created from Left Atrioventricular Valve with Nonautologous Tissue Substitute, Percutaneous Approach

02UG3KZ Supplement Mitral Valve with Nonautologous Tissue Substitute, Percutaneous Approach

02UG47E Supplement Mitral Valve created from Left Atrioventricular Valve with Autologous Tissue Substitute, Percutaneous Endoscopic Approach

02UG47Z Supplement Mitral Valve with Autologous Tissue Substitute, Percutaneous Endoscopic Approach

02UG48E Supplement Mitral Valve created from Left Atrioventricular Valve with Zooplastic Tissue, Percutaneous Endoscopic Approach

02UG48Z Supplement Mitral Valve with Zooplastic Tissue, Percutaneous Endoscopic Approach

02UG4JE Supplement Mitral Valve created from Left Atrioventricular Valve with Synthetic Substitute, Percutaneous Endoscopic Approach

02UG4JZ Supplement Mitral Valve with Synthetic Substitute, Percutaneous Endoscopic Approach

02UG4KE Supplement Mitral Valve created from Left Atrioventricular Valve with Nonautologous Tissue Substitute, Percutaneous Endoscopic Approach

02UG4KZ Supplement Mitral Valve with Nonautologous Tissue Substitute, Percutaneous Endoscopic Approach

02UH07Z Supplement Pulmonary Valve with Autologous Tissue Substitute, Open Approach

02UH08Z Supplement Pulmonary Valve with Zooplastic Tissue, Open Approach

02UH0JZ Supplement Pulmonary Valve with Synthetic Substitute, Open Approach

02UH0KZ Supplement Pulmonary Valve with Nonautologous Tissue Substitute, Open Approach

02UH37Z Supplement Pulmonary Valve with Autologous Tissue Substitute, Percutaneous Approach

02UH38Z Supplement Pulmonary Valve with Zooplastic Tissue, Percutaneous Approach

02UH3JZ Supplement Pulmonary Valve with Synthetic Substitute, Percutaneous Approach

02UH3KZ Supplement Pulmonary Valve with Nonautologous Tissue Substitute, Percutaneous Approach

02UH47Z Supplement Pulmonary Valve with Autologous Tissue Substitute, Percutaneous Endoscopic Approach

02UH48Z Supplement Pulmonary Valve with Zooplastic Tissue, Percutaneous Endoscopic Approach

02UH4JZ Supplement Pulmonary Valve with Synthetic Substitute, Percutaneous Endoscopic Approach

02UH4KZ Supplement Pulmonary Valve with Nonautologous Tissue Substitute, Percutaneous Endoscopic Approach

02UJ07G Supplement Tricuspid Valve created from Right Atrioventricular Valve with Autologous Tissue Substitute, Open Approach

02UJ07Z Supplement Tricuspid Valve with Autologous Tissue Substitute, Open Approach

02UJ08G Supplement Tricuspid Valve created from Right Atrioventricular Valve with Zooplastic Tissue, Open Approach

02UJ08Z Supplement Tricuspid Valve with Zooplastic Tissue, Open Approach

02UJ0JG Supplement Tricuspid Valve created from Right Atrioventricular Valve with Synthetic Substitute, Open Approach

02UJ0JZ Supplement Tricuspid Valve with Synthetic Substitute, Open Approach

02UJ0KG Supplement Tricuspid Valve created from Right Atrioventricular Valve with Nonautologous Tissue Substitute, Open Approach

02UJ0KZ Supplement Tricuspid Valve with Nonautologous Tissue Substitute, Open Approach

02UJ37G Supplement Tricuspid Valve created from Right Atrioventricular Valve with Autologous Tissue Substitute, Percutaneous Approach

02UJ37Z Supplement Tricuspid Valve with Autologous Tissue Substitute, Percutaneous Approach

02UJ38G Supplement Tricuspid Valve created from Right Atrioventricular Valve with Zooplastic Tissue, Percutaneous Approach

02UJ38Z Supplement Tricuspid Valve with Zooplastic Tissue, Percutaneous Approach

02UJ3JG Supplement Tricuspid Valve created from Right Atrioventricular Valve with Synthetic Substitute, Percutaneous Approach

02UJ3JZ Supplement Tricuspid Valve with Synthetic Substitute, Percutaneous Approach

02UJ3KG Supplement Tricuspid Valve created from Right Atrioventricular Valve with Nonautologous Tissue Substitute, Percutaneous Approach

02UJ3KZ Supplement Tricuspid Valve with Nonautologous Tissue Substitute, Percutaneous Approach

♀ Female-only   ♂ Male-only   ▲ Limited Coverage   ● Non-OR   ᴴᴬᶜ HAC-associated procedure   ▲ Non-covered procedures   ✚ Cluster

02UJ47G Supplement Tricuspid Valve created from Right Atrioventricular Valve with Autologous Tissue Substitute, Percutaneous Endoscopic Approach

02UJ47Z Supplement Tricuspid Valve with Autologous Tissue Substitute, Percutaneous Endoscopic Approach

02UJ48G Supplement Tricuspid Valve created from Right Atrioventricular Valve with Zooplastic Tissue, Percutaneous Endoscopic Approach

02UJ48Z Supplement Tricuspid Valve with Zooplastic Tissue, Percutaneous Endoscopic Approach

02UJ4JG Supplement Tricuspid Valve created from Right Atrioventricular Valve with Synthetic Substitute, Percutaneous Endoscopic Approach

02UJ4JZ Supplement Tricuspid Valve with Synthetic Substitute, Percutaneous Endoscopic Approach

02UJ4KG Supplement Tricuspid Valve created from Right Atrioventricular Valve with Nonautologous Tissue Substitute, Percutaneous Endoscopic Approach

02UJ4KZ Supplement Tricuspid Valve with Nonautologous Tissue Substitute, Percutaneous Endoscopic Approach

02UK07Z Supplement Right Ventricle with Autologous Tissue Substitute, Open Approach

02UK08Z Supplement Right Ventricle with Zooplastic Tissue, Open Approach

02UK0JZ Supplement Right Ventricle with Synthetic Substitute, Open Approach

02UK0KZ Supplement Right Ventricle with Nonautologous Tissue Substitute, Open Approach

02UK37Z Supplement Right Ventricle with Autologous Tissue Substitute, Percutaneous Approach

02UK38Z Supplement Right Ventricle with Zooplastic Tissue, Percutaneous Approach

02UK3JZ Supplement Right Ventricle with Synthetic Substitute, Percutaneous Approach

02UK3KZ Supplement Right Ventricle with Nonautologous Tissue Substitute, Percutaneous Approach

02UK47Z Supplement Right Ventricle with Autologous Tissue Substitute, Percutaneous Endoscopic Approach

02UK48Z Supplement Right Ventricle with Zooplastic Tissue, Percutaneous Endoscopic Approach

02UK4JZ Supplement Right Ventricle with Synthetic Substitute, Percutaneous Endoscopic Approach

02UK4KZ Supplement Right Ventricle with Nonautologous Tissue Substitute, Percutaneous Endoscopic Approach

02UL07Z Supplement Left Ventricle with Autologous Tissue Substitute, Open Approach

02UL08Z Supplement Left Ventricle with Zooplastic Tissue, Open Approach

02UL0JZ Supplement Left Ventricle with Synthetic Substitute, Open Approach

02UL0KZ Supplement Left Ventricle with Nonautologous Tissue Substitute, Open Approach

02UL37Z Supplement Left Ventricle with Autologous Tissue Substitute, Percutaneous Approach

02UL38Z Supplement Left Ventricle with Zooplastic Tissue, Percutaneous Approach

02UL3JZ Supplement Left Ventricle with Synthetic Substitute, Percutaneous Approach

02UL3KZ Supplement Left Ventricle with Nonautologous Tissue Substitute, Percutaneous Approach

02UL47Z Supplement Left Ventricle with Autologous Tissue Substitute, Percutaneous Endoscopic Approach

02UL48Z Supplement Left Ventricle with Zooplastic Tissue, Percutaneous Endoscopic Approach

02UL4JZ Supplement Left Ventricle with Synthetic Substitute, Percutaneous Endoscopic Approach

02UL4KZ Supplement Left Ventricle with Nonautologous Tissue Substitute, Percutaneous Endoscopic Approach

02UM07Z Supplement Ventricular Septum with Autologous Tissue Substitute, Open Approach

02UM08Z Supplement Ventricular Septum with Zooplastic Tissue, Open Approach

AHA CC: 4Q, 2015, 25

02UM0JZ Supplement Ventricular Septum with Synthetic Substitute, Open Approach

AHA CC: 3Q, 2014, 16-17; 4Q, 2015, 22-23

02UM0KZ Supplement Ventricular Septum with Nonautologous Tissue Substitute, Open Approach

02UM37Z Supplement Ventricular Septum with Autologous Tissue Substitute, Percutaneous Approach

02UM38Z Supplement Ventricular Septum with Zooplastic Tissue, Percutaneous Approach

02UM3JZ Supplement Ventricular Septum with Synthetic Substitute, Percutaneous Approach

02UM3KZ Supplement Ventricular Septum with Nonautologous Tissue Substitute, Percutaneous Approach

02UM47Z Supplement Ventricular Septum with Autologous Tissue Substitute, Percutaneous Endoscopic Approach

02UM48Z Supplement Ventricular Septum with Zooplastic Tissue, Percutaneous Endoscopic Approach

02UM4JZ Supplement Ventricular Septum with Synthetic Substitute, Percutaneous Endoscopic Approach

02UM4KZ Supplement Ventricular Septum with Nonautologous Tissue Substitute, Percutaneous Endoscopic Approach

02UN07Z Supplement Pericardium with Autologous Tissue Substitute, Open Approach

02UN08Z Supplement Pericardium with Zooplastic Tissue, Open Approach

02UN0JZ Supplement Pericardium with Synthetic Substitute, Open Approach

02UN0KZ Supplement Pericardium with Nonautologous Tissue Substitute, Open Approach

02UN37Z Supplement Pericardium with Autologous Tissue Substitute, Percutaneous Approach

02UN38Z Supplement Pericardium with Zooplastic Tissue, Percutaneous Approach

02UN3JZ Supplement Pericardium with Synthetic Substitute, Percutaneous Approach

02UN3KZ Supplement Pericardium with Nonautologous Tissue Substitute, Percutaneous Approach

02UN47Z Supplement Pericardium with Autologous Tissue Substitute, Percutaneous Endoscopic Approach

02UN48Z Supplement Pericardium with Zooplastic Tissue, Percutaneous Endoscopic Approach

02UN4JZ Supplement Pericardium with Synthetic Substitute, Percutaneous Endoscopic Approach

02UN4KZ Supplement Pericardium with Nonautologous Tissue Substitute, Percutaneous Endoscopic Approach

02UP07Z Supplement Pulmonary Trunk with Autologous Tissue Substitute, Open Approach

AHA CC: 2Q, 2016, 23-24

02UP08Z Supplement Pulmonary Trunk with Zooplastic Tissue, Open Approach

AHA CC: 1Q, 2020, 24-25

02UP0JZ Supplement Pulmonary Trunk with Synthetic Substitute, Open Approach

02UP0KZ Supplement Pulmonary Trunk with Nonautologous Tissue Substitute, Open Approach

02UP37Z Supplement Pulmonary Trunk with Autologous Tissue Substitute, Percutaneous Approach

02UP38Z Supplement Pulmonary Trunk with Zooplastic Tissue, Percutaneous Approach

02UP3JZ Supplement Pulmonary Trunk with Synthetic Substitute, Percutaneous Approach

02UP3KZ Supplement Pulmonary Trunk with Nonautologous Tissue Substitute, Percutaneous Approach

02UP47Z Supplement Pulmonary Trunk with Autologous Tissue Substitute, Percutaneous Endoscopic Approach

02UP48Z Supplement Pulmonary Trunk with Zooplastic Tissue, Percutaneous Endoscopic Approach

02UP4JZ Supplement Pulmonary Trunk with Synthetic Substitute, Percutaneous Endoscopic Approach

02UP4KZ Supplement Pulmonary Trunk with Nonautologous Tissue Substitute, Percutaneous Endoscopic Approach

02UQ07Z Supplement Right Pulmonary Artery with Autologous Tissue Substitute, Open Approach

02UQ08Z Supplement Right Pulmonary Artery with Zooplastic Tissue, Open Approach

02UQ0JZ Supplement Right Pulmonary Artery with Synthetic Substitute, Open Approach

02UQ0KZ Supplement Right Pulmonary Artery with Nonautologous Tissue Substitute, Open Approach

AHA CC: 3Q, 2015, 16-17

02UQ37Z Supplement Right Pulmonary Artery with Autologous Tissue Substitute, Percutaneous Approach

02UQ38Z Supplement Right Pulmonary Artery with Zooplastic Tissue, Percutaneous Approach

02UQ3JZ Supplement Right Pulmonary Artery with Synthetic Substitute, Percutaneous Approach

02UQ3KZ Supplement Right Pulmonary Artery with Nonautologous Tissue Substitute, Percutaneous Approach

02UQ47Z Supplement Right Pulmonary Artery with Autologous Tissue Substitute, Percutaneous Endoscopic Approach

02UQ48Z Supplement Right Pulmonary Artery with Zooplastic Tissue, Percutaneous Endoscopic Approach

02UQ4JZ Supplement Right Pulmonary Artery with Synthetic Substitute, Percutaneous Endoscopic Approach

02UQ4KZ Supplement Right Pulmonary Artery with Nonautologous Tissue Substitute, Percutaneous Endoscopic Approach

02UR07Z Supplement Left Pulmonary Artery with Autologous Tissue Substitute, Open Approach
AHA CC: 2Q, 2016, 23-24

02UR08Z Supplement Left Pulmonary Artery with Zooplastic Tissue, Open Approach

02UR0JZ Supplement Left Pulmonary Artery with Synthetic Substitute, Open Approach

02UR0KZ Supplement Left Pulmonary Artery with Nonautologous Tissue Substitute, Open Approach
AHA CC: 3Q, 2015, 16-17

02UR37Z Supplement Left Pulmonary Artery with Autologous Tissue Substitute, Percutaneous Approach

02UR38Z Supplement Left Pulmonary Artery with Zooplastic Tissue, Percutaneous Approach

02UR3JZ Supplement Left Pulmonary Artery with Synthetic Substitute, Percutaneous Approach

02UR3KZ Supplement Left Pulmonary Artery with Nonautologous Tissue Substitute, Percutaneous Approach

02UR47Z Supplement Left Pulmonary Artery with Autologous Tissue Substitute, Percutaneous Endoscopic Approach

02UR48Z Supplement Left Pulmonary Artery with Zooplastic Tissue, Percutaneous Endoscopic Approach

02UR4JZ Supplement Left Pulmonary Artery with Synthetic Substitute, Percutaneous Endoscopic Approach

02UR4KZ Supplement Left Pulmonary Artery with Nonautologous Tissue Substitute, Percutaneous Endoscopic Approach

02US07Z Supplement Right Pulmonary Vein with Autologous Tissue Substitute, Open Approach

02US08Z Supplement Right Pulmonary Vein with Zooplastic Tissue, Open Approach

02US0JZ Supplement Right Pulmonary Vein with Synthetic Substitute, Open Approach

02US0KZ Supplement Right Pulmonary Vein with Nonautologous Tissue Substitute, Open Approach

02US37Z Supplement Right Pulmonary Vein with Autologous Tissue Substitute, Percutaneous Approach

02US38Z Supplement Right Pulmonary Vein with Zooplastic Tissue, Percutaneous Approach

02US3JZ Supplement Right Pulmonary Vein with Synthetic Substitute, Percutaneous Approach

02US3KZ Supplement Right Pulmonary Vein with Nonautologous Tissue Substitute, Percutaneous Approach

02US47Z Supplement Right Pulmonary Vein with Autologous Tissue Substitute, Percutaneous Endoscopic Approach

02US48Z Supplement Right Pulmonary Vein with Zooplastic Tissue, Percutaneous Endoscopic Approach

02US4JZ Supplement Right Pulmonary Vein with Synthetic Substitute, Percutaneous Endoscopic Approach

02US4KZ Supplement Right Pulmonary Vein with Nonautologous Tissue Substitute, Percutaneous Endoscopic Approach

02UT07Z Supplement Left Pulmonary Vein with Autologous Tissue Substitute, Open Approach

02UT08Z Supplement Left Pulmonary Vein with Zooplastic Tissue, Open Approach

02UT0JZ Supplement Left Pulmonary Vein with Synthetic Substitute, Open Approach

02UT0KZ Supplement Left Pulmonary Vein with Nonautologous Tissue Substitute, Open Approach

02UT37Z Supplement Left Pulmonary Vein with Autologous Tissue Substitute, Percutaneous Approach

02UT38Z Supplement Left Pulmonary Vein with Zooplastic Tissue, Percutaneous Approach

02UT3JZ Supplement Left Pulmonary Vein with Synthetic Substitute, Percutaneous Approach

02UT3KZ Supplement Left Pulmonary Vein with Nonautologous Tissue Substitute, Percutaneous Approach

02UT47Z Supplement Left Pulmonary Vein with Autologous Tissue Substitute, Percutaneous Endoscopic Approach

02UT48Z Supplement Left Pulmonary Vein with Zooplastic Tissue, Percutaneous Endoscopic Approach

02UT4JZ Supplement Left Pulmonary Vein with Synthetic Substitute, Percutaneous Endoscopic Approach

02UT4KZ Supplement Left Pulmonary Vein with Nonautologous Tissue Substitute, Percutaneous Endoscopic Approach

02UV07Z Supplement Superior Vena Cava with Autologous Tissue Substitute, Open Approach

02UV08Z Supplement Superior Vena Cava with Zooplastic Tissue, Open Approach

02UV0JZ Supplement Superior Vena Cava with Synthetic Substitute, Open Approach

02UV0KZ Supplement Superior Vena Cava with Nonautologous Tissue Substitute, Open Approach

02UV37Z Supplement Superior Vena Cava with Autologous Tissue Substitute, Percutaneous Approach

02UV38Z Supplement Superior Vena Cava with Zooplastic Tissue, Percutaneous Approach

02UV3JZ Supplement Superior Vena Cava with Synthetic Substitute, Percutaneous Approach

02UV3KZ Supplement Superior Vena Cava with Nonautologous Tissue Substitute, Percutaneous Approach

02UV47Z Supplement Superior Vena Cava with Autologous Tissue Substitute, Percutaneous Endoscopic Approach

02UV48Z Supplement Superior Vena Cava with Zooplastic Tissue, Percutaneous Endoscopic Approach

02UV4JZ Supplement Superior Vena Cava with Synthetic Substitute, Percutaneous Endoscopic Approach

02UV4KZ Supplement Superior Vena Cava with Nonautologous Tissue Substitute, Percutaneous Endoscopic Approach

02UW07Z Supplement Thoracic Aorta, Descending with Autologous Tissue Substitute, Open Approach
AHA CC: 4Q, 2015, 23-24

02UW08Z Supplement Thoracic Aorta, Descending with Zooplastic Tissue, Open Approach

02UW0JZ Supplement Thoracic Aorta, Descending with Synthetic Substitute, Open Approach
AHA CC: 2Q, 2016, 26-27

02UW0KZ Supplement Thoracic Aorta, Descending with Nonautologous Tissue Substitute, Open Approach

02UW37Z Supplement Thoracic Aorta, Descending with Autologous Tissue Substitute, Percutaneous Approach

02UW38Z Supplement Thoracic Aorta, Descending with Zooplastic Tissue, Percutaneous Approach

02UW3JZ Supplement Thoracic Aorta, Descending with Synthetic Substitute, Percutaneous Approach

02UW3KZ Supplement Thoracic Aorta, Descending with Nonautologous Tissue Substitute, Percutaneous Approach

02UW47Z Supplement Thoracic Aorta, Descending with Autologous Tissue Substitute, Percutaneous Endoscopic Approach

02UW48Z Supplement Thoracic Aorta, Descending with Zooplastic Tissue, Percutaneous Endoscopic Approach

02UW4JZ Supplement Thoracic Aorta, Descending with Synthetic Substitute, Percutaneous Endoscopic Approach

02UW4KZ Supplement Thoracic Aorta, Descending with Nonautologous Tissue Substitute, Percutaneous Endoscopic Approach

02UX07Z Supplement Thoracic Aorta, Ascending/Arch with Autologous Tissue Substitute, Open Approach

02UX08Z Supplement Thoracic Aorta, Ascending/Arch with Zooplastic Tissue, Open Approach

02UX0JZ Supplement Thoracic Aorta, Ascending/Arch with Synthetic Substitute, Open Approach

02UX0KZ Supplement Thoracic Aorta, Ascending/Arch with Nonautologous Tissue Substitute, Open Approach
AHA CC: 1Q, 2017, 19-20

02UX37Z Supplement Thoracic Aorta, Ascending/Arch with Autologous Tissue Substitute, Percutaneous Approach

02UX38Z Supplement Thoracic Aorta, Ascending/Arch with Zooplastic Tissue, Percutaneous Approach

02UX3JZ Supplement Thoracic Aorta, Ascending/Arch with Synthetic Substitute, Percutaneous Approach

02UX3KZ Supplement Thoracic Aorta, Ascending/Arch with Nonautologous Tissue Substitute, Percutaneous Approach

02UX47Z Supplement Thoracic Aorta, Ascending/Arch with Autologous Tissue Substitute, Percutaneous Endoscopic Approach

♀ Female-only　　♂ Male-only　　▲ Limited Coverage　　● Non-OR　　▨ HAC-associated procedure　　▲ Non-covered procedures　　✚ Cluster

02UX48Z Supplement Thoracic Aorta, Ascending/Arch with Zooplastic Tissue, Percutaneous Endoscopic Approach

02UX4JZ Supplement Thoracic Aorta, Ascending/Arch with Synthetic Substitute, Percutaneous Endoscopic Approach

02UX4KZ Supplement Thoracic Aorta, Ascending/Arch with Nonautologous Tissue Substitute, Percutaneous Endoscopic Approach

02V – Heart and Great Vessels, Restriction

02VA0CZ Restriction of Heart with Extraluminal Device, Open Approach
02VA0ZZ Restriction of Heart, Open Approach
02VA3CZ Restriction of Heart with Extraluminal Device, Percutaneous Approach
02VA3ZZ Restriction of Heart, Percutaneous Approach
02VA4CZ Restriction of Heart with Extraluminal Device, Percutaneous Endoscopic Approach
02VA4ZZ Restriction of Heart, Percutaneous Endoscopic Approach
02VG0ZZ Restriction of Mitral Valve, Open Approach
    AHA CC: 4Q, 2017, 36
02VG3ZZ Restriction of Mitral Valve, Percutaneous Approach
02VG4ZZ Restriction of Mitral Valve, Percutaneous Endoscopic Approach
02VL0CZ Restriction of Left Ventricle with Extraluminal Device, Open Approach
02VL0DZ Restriction of Left Ventricle with Intraluminal Device, Open Approach
02VL0ZZ Restriction of Left Ventricle, Open Approach
02VL3CZ Restriction of Left Ventricle with Extraluminal Device, Percutaneous Approach
02VL3DZ Restriction of Left Ventricle with Intraluminal Device, Percutaneous Approach
02VL3ZZ Restriction of Left Ventricle, Percutaneous Approach
02VL4CZ Restriction of Left Ventricle with Extraluminal Device, Percutaneous Endoscopic Approach
02VL4DZ Restriction of Left Ventricle with Intraluminal Device, Percutaneous Endoscopic Approach
02VL4ZZ Restriction of Left Ventricle, Percutaneous Endoscopic Approach
02VP0CZ Restriction of Pulmonary Trunk with Extraluminal Device, Open Approach
02VP0DZ Restriction of Pulmonary Trunk with Intraluminal Device, Open Approach
02VP0ZZ Restriction of Pulmonary Trunk, Open Approach
02VP3CZ Restriction of Pulmonary Trunk with Extraluminal Device, Percutaneous Approach
02VP3DZ Restriction of Pulmonary Trunk with Intraluminal Device, Percutaneous Approach
02VP3ZZ Restriction of Pulmonary Trunk, Percutaneous Approach
02VP4CZ Restriction of Pulmonary Trunk with Extraluminal Device, Percutaneous Endoscopic Approach
02VP4DZ Restriction of Pulmonary Trunk with Intraluminal Device, Percutaneous Endoscopic Approach
02VP4ZZ Restriction of Pulmonary Trunk, Percutaneous Endoscopic Approach
02VQ0CZ Restriction of Right Pulmonary Artery with Extraluminal Device, Open Approach
02VQ0DZ Restriction of Right Pulmonary Artery with Intraluminal Device, Open Approach

02VQ0ZZ Restriction of Right Pulmonary Artery, Open Approach
02VQ3CZ Restriction of Right Pulmonary Artery with Extraluminal Device, Percutaneous Approach
02VQ3DZ Restriction of Right Pulmonary Artery with Intraluminal Device, Percutaneous Approach
02VQ3ZZ Restriction of Right Pulmonary Artery, Percutaneous Approach
02VQ4CZ Restriction of Right Pulmonary Artery with Extraluminal Device, Percutaneous Endoscopic Approach
02VQ4DZ Restriction of Right Pulmonary Artery with Intraluminal Device, Percutaneous Endoscopic Approach
02VQ4ZZ Restriction of Right Pulmonary Artery, Percutaneous Endoscopic Approach
02VR0CT Restriction of Ductus Arteriosus with Extraluminal Device, Open Approach
02VR0CZ Restriction of Left Pulmonary Artery with Extraluminal Device, Open Approach
02VR0DT Restriction of Ductus Arteriosus with Intraluminal Device, Open Approach
02VR0DZ Restriction of Left Pulmonary Artery with Intraluminal Device, Open Approach
02VR0ZT Restriction of Ductus Arteriosus, Open Approach
02VR0ZZ Restriction of Left Pulmonary Artery, Open Approach
02VR3CT Restriction of Ductus Arteriosus with Extraluminal Device, Percutaneous Approach
02VR3CZ Restriction of Left Pulmonary Artery with Extraluminal Device, Percutaneous Approach
02VR3DT Restriction of Ductus Arteriosus with Intraluminal Device, Percutaneous Approach
02VR3DZ Restriction of Left Pulmonary Artery with Intraluminal Device, Percutaneous Approach
02VR3ZT Restriction of Ductus Arteriosus, Percutaneous Approach
02VR3ZZ Restriction of Left Pulmonary Artery, Percutaneous Approach
02VR4CT Restriction of Ductus Arteriosus with Extraluminal Device, Percutaneous Endoscopic Approach
02VR4CZ Restriction of Left Pulmonary Artery with Extraluminal Device, Percutaneous Endoscopic Approach
02VR4DT Restriction of Ductus Arteriosus with Intraluminal Device, Percutaneous Endoscopic Approach
02VR4DZ Restriction of Left Pulmonary Artery with Intraluminal Device, Percutaneous Endoscopic Approach
02VR4ZT Restriction of Ductus Arteriosus, Percutaneous Endoscopic Approach
02VR4ZZ Restriction of Left Pulmonary Artery, Percutaneous Endoscopic Approach
02VS0CZ Restriction of Right Pulmonary Vein with Extraluminal Device, Open Approach

02VS0DZ Restriction of Right Pulmonary Vein with Intraluminal Device, Open Approach
02VS0ZZ Restriction of Right Pulmonary Vein, Open Approach
02VS3CZ Restriction of Right Pulmonary Vein with Extraluminal Device, Percutaneous Approach
02VS3DZ Restriction of Right Pulmonary Vein with Intraluminal Device, Percutaneous Approach
02VS3ZZ Restriction of Right Pulmonary Vein, Percutaneous Approach
02VS4CZ Restriction of Right Pulmonary Vein with Extraluminal Device, Percutaneous Endoscopic Approach
02VS4DZ Restriction of Right Pulmonary Vein with Intraluminal Device, Percutaneous Endoscopic Approach
02VS4ZZ Restriction of Right Pulmonary Vein, Percutaneous Endoscopic Approach
02VT0CZ Restriction of Left Pulmonary Vein with Extraluminal Device, Open Approach
02VT0DZ Restriction of Left Pulmonary Vein with Intraluminal Device, Open Approach
02VT0ZZ Restriction of Left Pulmonary Vein, Open Approach
02VT3CZ Restriction of Left Pulmonary Vein with Extraluminal Device, Percutaneous Approach
02VT3DZ Restriction of Left Pulmonary Vein with Intraluminal Device, Percutaneous Approach
02VT3ZZ Restriction of Left Pulmonary Vein, Percutaneous Approach
02VT4CZ Restriction of Left Pulmonary Vein with Extraluminal Device, Percutaneous Endoscopic Approach
02VT4DZ Restriction of Left Pulmonary Vein with Intraluminal Device, Percutaneous Endoscopic Approach
02VT4ZZ Restriction of Left Pulmonary Vein, Percutaneous Endoscopic Approach
02VV0CZ Restriction of Superior Vena Cava with Extraluminal Device, Open Approach
02VV0DZ Restriction of Superior Vena Cava with Intraluminal Device, Open Approach
02VV0ZZ Restriction of Superior Vena Cava, Open Approach
02VV3CZ Restriction of Superior Vena Cava with Extraluminal Device, Percutaneous Approach
02VV3DZ Restriction of Superior Vena Cava with Intraluminal Device, Percutaneous Approach
02VV3ZZ Restriction of Superior Vena Cava, Percutaneous Approach
02VV4CZ Restriction of Superior Vena Cava with Extraluminal Device, Percutaneous Endoscopic Approach
02VV4DZ Restriction of Superior Vena Cava with Intraluminal Device, Percutaneous Endoscopic Approach
02VV4ZZ Restriction of Superior Vena Cava, Percutaneous Endoscopic Approach
02VW0CZ Restriction of Thoracic Aorta, Descending with Extraluminal Device, Open Approach

02VW0DZ Restriction of Thoracic Aorta, Descending with Intraluminal Device, Open Approach
AHA CC: 1Q, 2020, 25-26

02VW0EZ Restriction of Thoracic Aorta, Descending with Branched or Fenestrated Intraluminal Device, One or Two Arteries, Open Approach

02VW0FZ Restriction of Thoracic Aorta, Descending with Branched or Fenestrated Intraluminal Device, Three or More Arteries, Open Approach

02VW0ZZ Restriction of Thoracic Aorta, Descending, Open Approach

02VW3CZ Restriction of Thoracic Aorta, Descending with Extraluminal Device, Percutaneous Approach

02VW3DZ Restriction of Thoracic Aorta, Descending with Intraluminal Device, Percutaneous Approach
AHA CC: 4Q, 2016, 92-93

02VW3EZ Restriction of Thoracic Aorta, Descending with Branched or Fenestrated Intraluminal Device, One or Two Arteries, Percutaneous Approach

02VW3FZ Restriction of Thoracic Aorta, Descending with Branched or Fenestrated Intraluminal Device, Three or More Arteries, Percutaneous Approach

02VW3ZZ Restriction of Thoracic Aorta, Descending, Percutaneous Approach

02VW4CZ Restriction of Thoracic Aorta, Descending with Extraluminal Device, Percutaneous Endoscopic Approach

02VW4DZ Restriction of Thoracic Aorta, Descending with Intraluminal Device, Percutaneous Endoscopic Approach

02VW4EZ Restriction of Thoracic Aorta, Descending with Branched or Fenestrated Intraluminal Device, One or Two Arteries, Percutaneous Endoscopic Approach

02VW4FZ Restriction of Thoracic Aorta, Descending with Branched or Fenestrated Intraluminal Device, Three or More Arteries, Percutaneous Endoscopic Approach

02VW4ZZ Restriction of Thoracic Aorta, Descending, Percutaneous Endoscopic Approach

02VX0CZ Restriction of Thoracic Aorta, Ascending/Arch with Extraluminal Device, Open Approach

02VX0DZ Restriction of Thoracic Aorta, Ascending/Arch with Intraluminal Device, Open Approach

02VX0EZ Restriction of Thoracic Aorta, Ascending/Arch with Branched or Fenestrated Intraluminal Device, One or Two Arteries, Open Approach

02VX0FZ Restriction of Thoracic Aorta, Ascending/Arch with Branched or Fenestrated Intraluminal Device, Three or More Arteries, Open Approach

02VX0ZZ Restriction of Thoracic Aorta, Ascending/Arch, Open Approach

02VX3CZ Restriction of Thoracic Aorta, Ascending/Arch with Extraluminal Device, Percutaneous Approach

02VX3DZ Restriction of Thoracic Aorta, Ascending/Arch with Intraluminal Device, Percutaneous Approach

02VX3EZ Restriction of Thoracic Aorta, Ascending/Arch with Branched or Fenestrated Intraluminal Device, One or Two Arteries, Percutaneous Approach

02VX3FZ Restriction of Thoracic Aorta, Ascending/Arch with Branched or Fenestrated Intraluminal Device, Three or More Arteries, Percutaneous Approach

02VX3ZZ Restriction of Thoracic Aorta, Ascending/Arch, Percutaneous Approach

02VX4CZ Restriction of Thoracic Aorta, Ascending/Arch with Extraluminal Device, Percutaneous Endoscopic Approach

02VX4DZ Restriction of Thoracic Aorta, Ascending/Arch with Intraluminal Device, Percutaneous Endoscopic Approach

02VX4EZ Restriction of Thoracic Aorta, Ascending/Arch with Branched or Fenestrated Intraluminal Device, One or Two Arteries, Percutaneous Endoscopic Approach

02VX4FZ Restriction of Thoracic Aorta, Ascending/Arch with Branched or Fenestrated Intraluminal Device, Three or More Arteries, Percutaneous Endoscopic Approach

02VX4ZZ Restriction of Thoracic Aorta, Ascending/Arch, Percutaneous Endoscopic Approach

02W – Heart and Great Vessels, Revision

Review Coding Guideline B6.1c

02W50JZ Revision of Synthetic Substitute in Atrial Septum, Open Approach

02W54JZ Revision of Synthetic Substitute in Atrial Septum, Percutaneous Endoscopic Approach

02WA02Z Revision of Monitoring Device in Heart, Open Approach

02WA03Z Revision of Infusion Device in Heart, Open Approach

02WA07Z Revision of Autologous Tissue Substitute in Heart, Open Approach

02WA08Z Revision of Zooplastic Tissue in Heart, Open Approach

02WA0CZ Revision of Extraluminal Device in Heart, Open Approach

02WA0DZ Revision of Intraluminal Device in Heart, Open Approach

▲ **02WA0JZ** Revision of Synthetic Substitute in Heart, Open Approach

02WA0KZ Revision of Nonautologous Tissue Substitute in Heart, Open Approach

02WA0MZ Revision of Cardiac Lead in Heart, Open Approach
HAC With a secondary diagnosis code of K68.11, T81.40XA, T81.41XA, T81.42XA, T81.43XA, T81.44XA, T82.6XXA, T82.7XXA

02WA0NZ Revision of Intracardiac Pacemaker in Heart, Open Approach

▲ **02WA0QZ** Revision of Implantable Heart Assist System in Heart, Open Approach

➕ Heart assist system replacement when reported with a removal of an external heart assist system (6th character R) from the heart. *See table 02P to construct the Removal code.*

02WA0RS Revision of Biventricular Short-term External Heart Assist System in Heart, Open Approach

02WA0RZ Revision of Short-term External Heart Assist System in Heart, Open Approach

➕ Heart assist system replacement when reported with a removal of an external heart assist system (6th character R) from the heart. *See table 02P to construct the Removal code.*

02WA0YZ Revision of Other Device in Heart, Open Approach

02WA32Z Revision of Monitoring Device in Heart, Percutaneous Approach

02WA33Z Revision of Infusion Device in Heart, Percutaneous Approach

02WA37Z Revision of Autologous Tissue Substitute in Heart, Percutaneous Approach

02WA38Z Revision of Zooplastic Tissue in Heart, Percutaneous Approach

02WA3CZ Revision of Extraluminal Device in Heart, Percutaneous Approach

02WA3DZ Revision of Intraluminal Device in Heart, Percutaneous Approach

02WA3JZ Revision of Synthetic Substitute in Heart, Percutaneous Approach
AHA CC: 3Q, 2014, 31-32

02WA3KZ Revision of Nonautologous Tissue Substitute in Heart, Percutaneous Approach

02WA3MZ Revision of Cardiac Lead in Heart, Percutaneous Approach
AHA CC: 3Q, 2015, 32
HAC With a secondary diagnosis code of K68.11, T81.40XA, T81.41XA, T81.42XA, T81.43XA, T81.44XA, T82.6XXA, T82.7XXA

02WA3NZ Revision of Intracardiac Pacemaker in Heart, Percutaneous Approach
AHA CC: 4Q, 2016, 96

▲ **02WA3QZ** Revision of Implantable Heart Assist System in Heart, Percutaneous Approach

➕ Heart assist system replacement when reported with a removal of an external heart assist system (6th character R) from the heart. *See table 02P to construct the Removal code.*

02WA3RS Revision of Biventricular Short-term External Heart Assist System in Heart, Percutaneous Approach

02WA3RZ Revision of Short-term External Heart Assist System in Heart, Percutaneous Approach

➕ Heart assist system replacement when reported with a removal of an external heart assist system (6th character R) from the heart. *See table 02P to construct the Removal code.*

02WA3YZ Revision of Other Device in Heart, Percutaneous Approach

♀ Female-only   ♂ Male-only   ▲ Limited Coverage   ● Non-OR   HAC HAC-associated procedure   ▲ Non-covered procedures   ➕ Cluster

02WA42Z Revision of Monitoring Device in Heart, Percutaneous Endoscopic Approach

02WA43Z Revision of Infusion Device in Heart, Percutaneous Endoscopic Approach

02WA47Z Revision of Autologous Tissue Substitute in Heart, Percutaneous Endoscopic Approach

02WA48Z Revision of Zooplastic Tissue in Heart, Percutaneous Endoscopic Approach

02WA4CZ Revision of Extraluminal Device in Heart, Percutaneous Endoscopic Approach

02WA4DZ Revision of Intraluminal Device in Heart, Percutaneous Endoscopic Approach

02WA4JZ Revision of Synthetic Substitute in Heart, Percutaneous Endoscopic Approach

02WA4KZ Revision of Nonautologous Tissue Substitute in Heart, Percutaneous Endoscopic Approach

02WA4MZ Revision of Cardiac Lead in Heart, Percutaneous Endoscopic Approach

HAC With a secondary diagnosis code of K68.11, T81.40XA, T81.41XA, T81.42XA, T81.43XA, T81.44XA, T82.6XXA, T82.7XXA

02WA4NZ Revision of Intracardiac Pacemaker in Heart, Percutaneous Endoscopic Approach

▲ **02WA4QZ** Revision of Implantable Heart Assist System in Heart, Percutaneous Endoscopic Approach

➕ Heart assist system replacement when reported with a removal of an external heart assist system (6th character R) from the heart. *See table 02P to construct the Removal code.*

02WA4RS Revision of Biventricular Short-term External Heart Assist System in Heart, Percutaneous Endoscopic Approach

02WA4RZ Revision of Short-term External Heart Assist System in Heart, Percutaneous Endoscopic Approach

➕ Heart assist system replacement when reported with a removal of an external heart assist system (6th character R) from the heart. *See table 02P to construct the Removal code.*

02WA4YZ Revision of Other Device in Heart, Percutaneous Endoscopic Approach

02WAX2Z Revision of Monitoring Device in Heart, External Approach

02WAX3Z Revision of Infusion Device in Heart, External Approach

02WAX7Z Revision of Autologous Tissue Substitute in Heart, External Approach

02WAX8Z Revision of Zooplastic Tissue in Heart, External Approach

02WAXCZ Revision of Extraluminal Device in Heart, External Approach

02WAXDZ Revision of Intraluminal Device in Heart, External Approach

02WAXJZ Revision of Synthetic Substitute in Heart, External Approach

02WAXKZ Revision of Nonautologous Tissue Substitute in Heart, External Approach

02WAXMZ Revision of Cardiac Lead in Heart, External Approach

02WAXNZ Revision of Intracardiac Pacemaker in Heart, External Approach

02WAXQZ Revision of Implantable Heart Assist System in Heart, External Approach

02WAXRS Revision of Biventricular Short-term External Heart Assist System in Heart, External Approach

02WAXRZ Revision of Short-term External Heart Assist System in Heart, External Approach

AHA CC: 1Q, 2018, 17

02WF07Z Revision of Autologous Tissue Substitute in Aortic Valve, Open Approach

02WF08Z Revision of Zooplastic Tissue in Aortic Valve, Open Approach

02WF0JZ Revision of Synthetic Substitute in Aortic Valve, Open Approach

02WF0KZ Revision of Nonautologous Tissue Substitute in Aortic Valve, Open Approach

02WF37Z Revision of Autologous Tissue Substitute in Aortic Valve, Percutaneous Approach

02WF38Z Revision of Zooplastic Tissue in Aortic Valve, Percutaneous Approach

02WF3JZ Revision of Synthetic Substitute in Aortic Valve, Percutaneous Approach

02WF3KZ Revision of Nonautologous Tissue Substitute in Aortic Valve, Percutaneous Approach

02WF47Z Revision of Autologous Tissue Substitute in Aortic Valve, Percutaneous Endoscopic Approach

02WF48Z Revision of Zooplastic Tissue in Aortic Valve, Percutaneous Endoscopic Approach

02WF4JZ Revision of Synthetic Substitute in Aortic Valve, Percutaneous Endoscopic Approach

02WF4KZ Revision of Nonautologous Tissue Substitute in Aortic Valve, Percutaneous Endoscopic Approach

02WG07Z Revision of Autologous Tissue Substitute in Mitral Valve, Open Approach

02WG08Z Revision of Zooplastic Tissue in Mitral Valve, Open Approach

02WG0JZ Revision of Synthetic Substitute in Mitral Valve, Open Approach

02WG0KZ Revision of Nonautologous Tissue Substitute in Mitral Valve, Open Approach

02WG37Z Revision of Autologous Tissue Substitute in Mitral Valve, Percutaneous Approach

02WG38Z Revision of Zooplastic Tissue in Mitral Valve, Percutaneous Approach

02WG3JZ Revision of Synthetic Substitute in Mitral Valve, Percutaneous Approach

02WG3KZ Revision of Nonautologous Tissue Substitute in Mitral Valve, Percutaneous Approach

02WG47Z Revision of Autologous Tissue Substitute in Mitral Valve, Percutaneous Endoscopic Approach

02WG48Z Revision of Zooplastic Tissue in Mitral Valve, Percutaneous Endoscopic Approach

02WG4JZ Revision of Synthetic Substitute in Mitral Valve, Percutaneous Endoscopic Approach

02WG4KZ Revision of Nonautologous Tissue Substitute in Mitral Valve, Percutaneous Endoscopic Approach

02WH07Z Revision of Autologous Tissue Substitute in Pulmonary Valve, Open Approach

02WH08Z Revision of Zooplastic Tissue in Pulmonary Valve, Open Approach

02WH0JZ Revision of Synthetic Substitute in Pulmonary Valve, Open Approach

02WH0KZ Revision of Nonautologous Tissue Substitute in Pulmonary Valve, Open Approach

02WH37Z Revision of Autologous Tissue Substitute in Pulmonary Valve, Percutaneous Approach

02WH38Z Revision of Zooplastic Tissue in Pulmonary Valve, Percutaneous Approach

02WH3JZ Revision of Synthetic Substitute in Pulmonary Valve, Percutaneous Approach

02WH3KZ Revision of Nonautologous Tissue Substitute in Pulmonary Valve, Percutaneous Approach

02WH47Z Revision of Autologous Tissue Substitute in Pulmonary Valve, Percutaneous Endoscopic Approach

02WH48Z Revision of Zooplastic Tissue in Pulmonary Valve, Percutaneous Endoscopic Approach

02WH4JZ Revision of Synthetic Substitute in Pulmonary Valve, Percutaneous Endoscopic Approach

02WH4KZ Revision of Nonautologous Tissue Substitute in Pulmonary Valve, Percutaneous Endoscopic Approach

02WJ07Z Revision of Autologous Tissue Substitute in Tricuspid Valve, Open Approach

02WJ08Z Revision of Zooplastic Tissue in Tricuspid Valve, Open Approach

02WJ0JZ Revision of Synthetic Substitute in Tricuspid Valve, Open Approach

02WJ0KZ Revision of Nonautologous Tissue Substitute in Tricuspid Valve, Open Approach

02WJ37Z Revision of Autologous Tissue Substitute in Tricuspid Valve, Percutaneous Approach

02WJ38Z Revision of Zooplastic Tissue in Tricuspid Valve, Percutaneous Approach

02WJ3JZ Revision of Synthetic Substitute in Tricuspid Valve, Percutaneous Approach

02WJ3KZ Revision of Nonautologous Tissue Substitute in Tricuspid Valve, Percutaneous Approach

02WJ47Z Revision of Autologous Tissue Substitute in Tricuspid Valve, Percutaneous Endoscopic Approach

02WJ48Z Revision of Zooplastic Tissue in Tricuspid Valve, Percutaneous Endoscopic Approach

02WJ4JZ Revision of Synthetic Substitute in Tricuspid Valve, Percutaneous Endoscopic Approach

02WJ4KZ Revision of Nonautologous Tissue Substitute in Tricuspid Valve, Percutaneous Endoscopic Approach

02WM0JZ Revision of Synthetic Substitute in Ventricular Septum, Open Approach

02WM4JZ Revision of Synthetic Substitute in Ventricular Septum, Percutaneous Endoscopic Approach

02WY02Z Revision of Monitoring Device in Great Vessel, Open Approach

02WY03Z Revision of Infusion Device in Great Vessel, Open Approach

02WY07Z Revision of Autologous Tissue Substitute in Great Vessel, Open Approach

02WY08Z Revision of Zooplastic Tissue in Great Vessel, Open Approach

02WY0CZ	Revision of Extraluminal Device in Great Vessel, Open Approach
02WY0DZ	Revision of Intraluminal Device in Great Vessel, Open Approach
02WY0JZ	Revision of Synthetic Substitute in Great Vessel, Open Approach
02WY0KZ	Revision of Nonautologous Tissue Substitute in Great Vessel, Open Approach
02WY0YZ	Revision of Other Device in Great Vessel, Open Approach
02WY32Z	Revision of Monitoring Device in Great Vessel, Percutaneous Approach
02WY33Z	Revision of Infusion Device in Great Vessel, Percutaneous Approach
	AHA CC: 3Q, 2018, 9-10
02WY37Z	Revision of Autologous Tissue Substitute in Great Vessel, Percutaneous Approach
02WY38Z	Revision of Zooplastic Tissue in Great Vessel, Percutaneous Approach
02WY3CZ	Revision of Extraluminal Device in Great Vessel, Percutaneous Approach
02WY3DZ	Revision of Intraluminal Device in Great Vessel, Percutaneous Approach

02WY3JZ	Revision of Synthetic Substitute in Great Vessel, Percutaneous Approach
02WY3KZ	Revision of Nonautologous Tissue Substitute in Great Vessel, Percutaneous Approach
02WY3YZ	Revision of Other Device in Great Vessel, Percutaneous Approach
02WY42Z	Revision of Monitoring Device in Great Vessel, Percutaneous Endoscopic Approach
02WY43Z	Revision of Infusion Device in Great Vessel, Percutaneous Endoscopic Approach
02WY47Z	Revision of Autologous Tissue Substitute in Great Vessel, Percutaneous Endoscopic Approach
02WY48Z	Revision of Zooplastic Tissue in Great Vessel, Percutaneous Endoscopic Approach
02WY4CZ	Revision of Extraluminal Device in Great Vessel, Percutaneous Endoscopic Approach
02WY4DZ	Revision of Intraluminal Device in Great Vessel, Percutaneous Endoscopic Approach

02WY4JZ	Revision of Synthetic Substitute in Great Vessel, Percutaneous Endoscopic Approach
02WY4KZ	Revision of Nonautologous Tissue Substitute in Great Vessel, Percutaneous Endoscopic Approach
02WY4YZ	Revision of Other Device in Great Vessel, Percutaneous Endoscopic Approach
02WYX2Z	Revision of Monitoring Device in Great Vessel, External Approach
02WYX3Z	Revision of Infusion Device in Great Vessel, External Approach
02WYX7Z	Revision of Autologous Tissue Substitute in Great Vessel, External Approach
02WYX8Z	Revision of Zooplastic Tissue in Great Vessel, External Approach
02WYXCZ	Revision of Extraluminal Device in Great Vessel, External Approach
02WYXDZ	Revision of Intraluminal Device in Great Vessel, External Approach
02WYXJZ	Revision of Synthetic Substitute in Great Vessel, External Approach
02WYXKZ	Revision of Nonautologous Tissue Substitute in Great Vessel, External Approach

02Y – Heart and Great Vessels, Transplantation

Review Coding Guideline B3.16

▲ **02YA0Z0** Transplantation of Heart, Allogeneic, Open Approach
AHA CC: 3Q, 2013, 18-19

▲ **02YA0Z1** Transplantation of Heart, Syngeneic, Open Approach

▲ **02YA0Z2** Transplantation of Heart, Zooplastic, Open Approach

 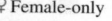

Arteries

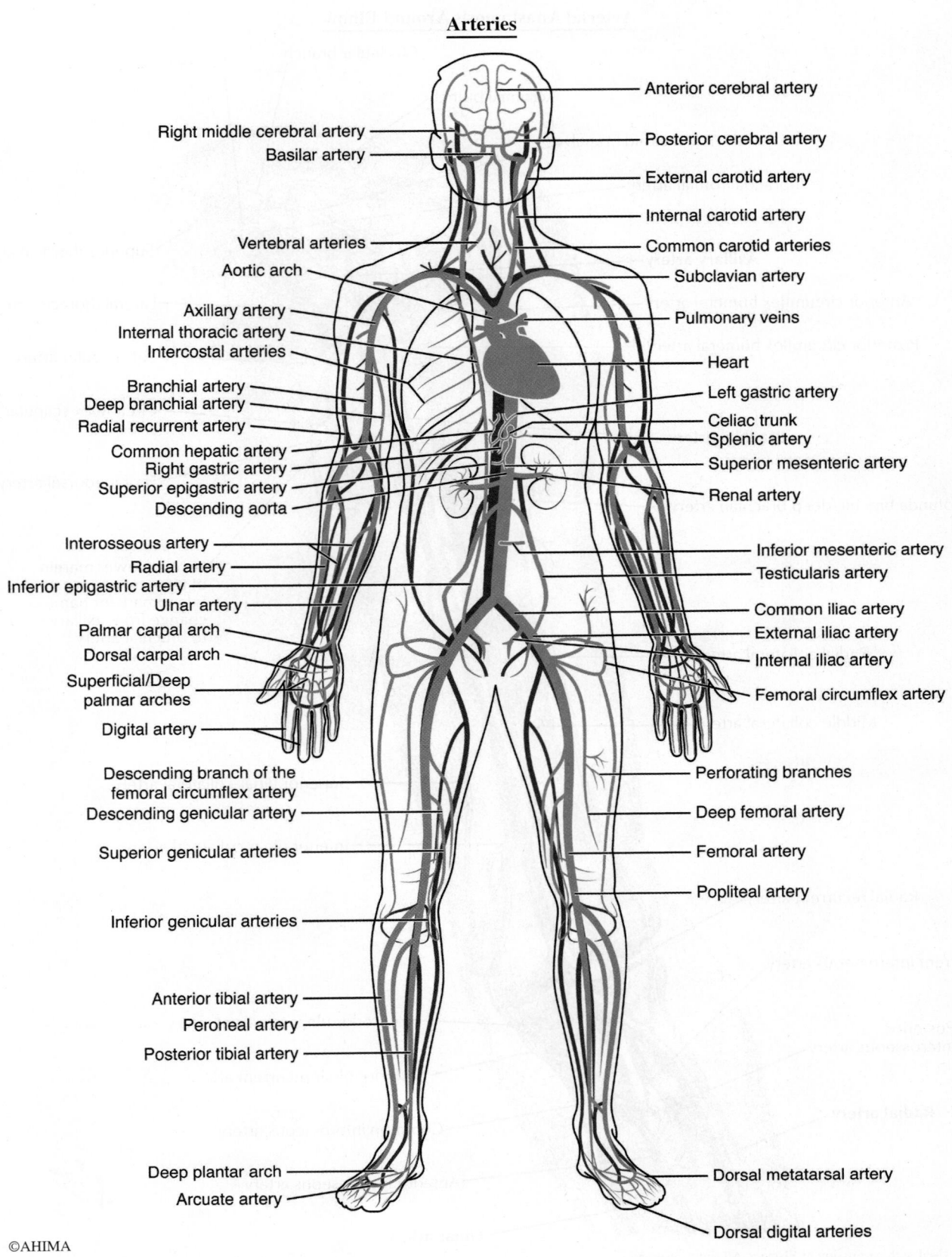

Anterior cerebral artery

Right middle cerebral artery

Posterior cerebral artery

Basilar artery

External carotid artery

Internal carotid artery

Vertebral arteries

Common carotid arteries

Aortic arch

Subclavian artery

Axillary artery

Pulmonary veins

Internal thoracic artery

Intercostal arteries

Heart

Branchial artery

Left gastric artery

Deep branchial artery

Celiac trunk

Radial recurrent artery

Splenic artery

Common hepatic artery

Superior mesenteric artery

Right gastric artery

Superior epigastric artery

Renal artery

Descending aorta

Interosseous artery

Inferior mesenteric artery

Radial artery

Testicularis artery

Inferior epigastric artery

Common iliac artery

Ulnar artery

External iliac artery

Palmar carpal arch

Internal iliac artery

Dorsal carpal arch

Femoral circumflex artery

Superficial/Deep
palmar arches

Digital artery

Descending branch of the
femoral circumflex artery

Perforating branches

Descending genicular artery

Deep femoral artery

Superior genicular arteries

Femoral artery

Popliteal artery

Inferior genicular arteries

Anterior tibial artery

Peroneal artery

Posterior tibial artery

Deep plantar arch

Dorsal metatarsal artery

Arcuate artery

Dorsal digital arteries

©AHIMA

Arterial Anastomosis Around Elbow

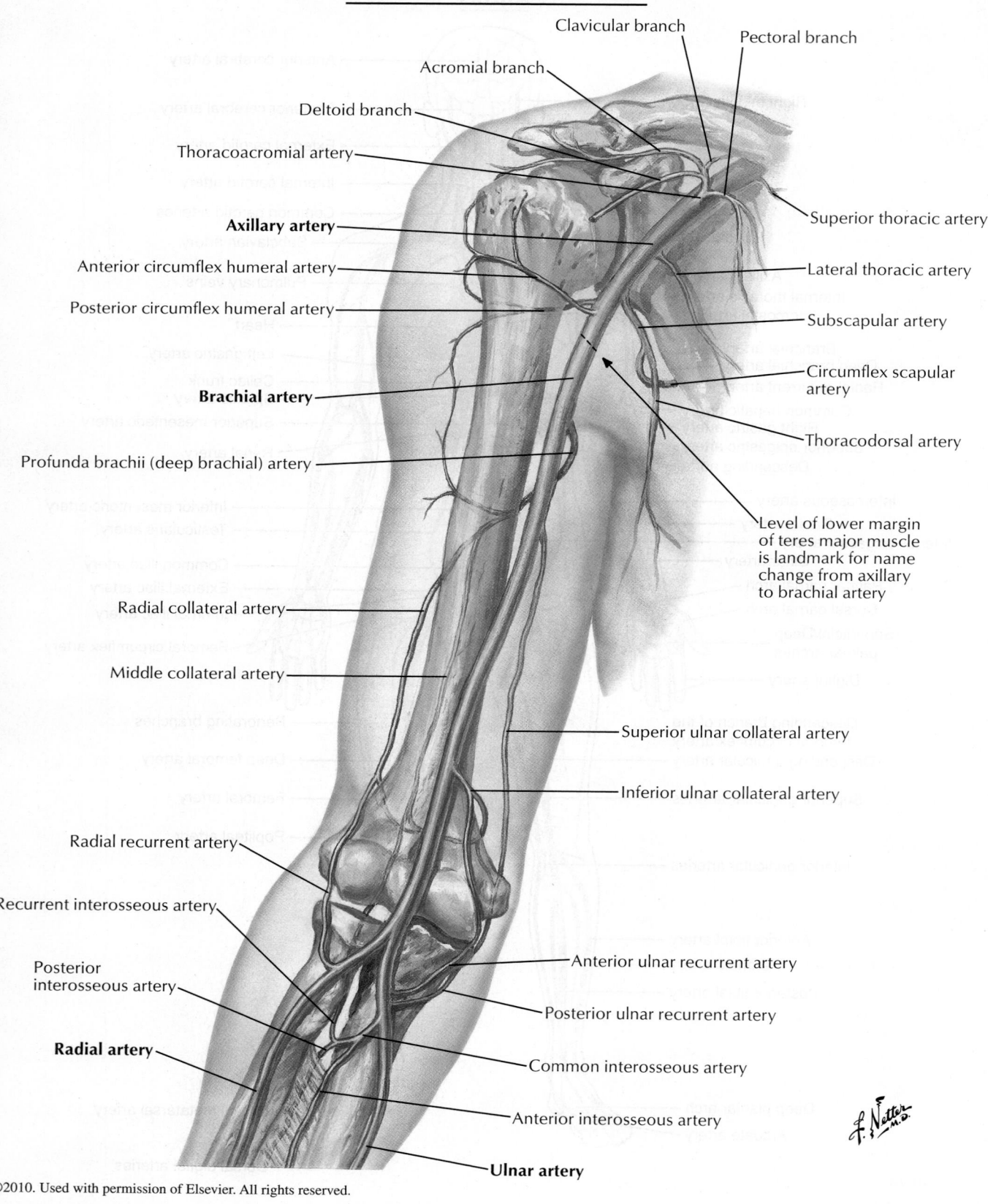

Clavicular branch

Pectoral branch

Acromial branch

Deltoid branch

Thoracoacromial artery

Superior thoracic artery

Axillary artery

Lateral thoracic artery

Anterior circumflex humeral artery

Posterior circumflex humeral artery

Subscapular artery

Circumflex scapular artery

Brachial artery

Thoracodorsal artery

Profunda brachii (deep brachial) artery

Level of lower margin of teres major muscle is landmark for name change from axillary to brachial artery

Radial collateral artery

Middle collateral artery

Superior ulnar collateral artery

Inferior ulnar collateral artery

Radial recurrent artery

Recurrent interosseous artery

Posterior interosseous artery

Anterior ulnar recurrent artery

Posterior ulnar recurrent artery

Radial artery

Common interosseous artery

Anterior interosseous artery

Ulnar artery

Section   **0**   **Medical and Surgical**
Body System   **3**   **Upper Arteries**
Operation   **1**   **Bypass:** Altering the route of passage of the contents of a tubular body part

Body Part (4th)	Approach (5th)	Device (6th)	Qualifier (7th)
2 Innominate Artery	0 Open	9 Autologous Venous Tissue A Autologous Arterial Tissue J Synthetic Substitute K Nonautologous Tissue Substitute Z No Device	0 Upper Arm Artery, Right 1 Upper Arm Artery, Left 2 Upper Arm Artery, Bilateral 3 Lower Arm Artery, Right 4 Lower Arm Artery, Left 5 Lower Arm Artery, Bilateral 6 Upper Leg Artery, Right 7 Upper Leg Artery, Left 8 Upper Leg Artery, Bilateral 9 Lower Leg Artery, Right B Lower Leg Artery, Left C Lower Leg Artery, Bilateral D Upper Arm Vein F Lower Arm Vein J Extracranial Artery, Right K Extracranial Artery, Left W Lower Extremity Vein
3 Subclavian Artery, Right 4 Subclavian Artery, Left	0 Open	9 Autologous Venous Tissue A Autologous Arterial Tissue J Synthetic Substitute K Nonautologous Tissue Substitute Z No Device	0 Upper Arm Artery, Right 1 Upper Arm Artery, Left 2 Upper Arm Artery, Bilateral 3 Lower Arm Artery, Right 4 Lower Arm Artery, Left 5 Lower Arm Artery, Bilateral 6 Upper Leg Artery, Right 7 Upper Leg Artery, Left 8 Upper Leg Artery, Bilateral 9 Lower Leg Artery, Right B Lower Leg Artery, Left C Lower Leg Artery, Bilateral D Upper Arm Vein F Lower Arm Vein J Extracranial Artery, Right K Extracranial Artery, Left M Pulmonary Artery, Right N Pulmonary Artery, Left W Lower Extremity Vein
5 Axillary Artery, Right 6 Axillary Artery, Left	0 Open	9 Autologous Venous Tissue A Autologous Arterial Tissue J Synthetic Substitute K Nonautologous Tissue Substitute Z No Device	0 Upper Arm Artery, Right 1 Upper Arm Artery, Left 2 Upper Arm Artery, Bilateral 3 Lower Arm Artery, Right 4 Lower Arm Artery, Left 5 Lower Arm Artery, Bilateral 6 Upper Leg Artery, Right 7 Upper Leg Artery, Left 8 Upper Leg Artery, Bilateral 9 Lower Leg Artery, Right B Lower Leg Artery, Left C Lower Leg Artery, Bilateral D Upper Arm Vein F Lower Arm Vein J Extracranial Artery, Right K Extracranial Artery, Left T Abdominal Artery V Superior Vena Cava W Lower Extremity Vein

Continued →

031

Section 0 Medical and Surgical
Body System 3 Upper Arteries
Operation 1 Bypass: Altering the route of passage of the contents of a tubular body part

031 Continued

Body Part (4th)	Approach (5th)	Device (6th)	Qualifier (7th)
7 Brachial Artery, Right	0 Open	9 Autologous Venous Tissue A Autologous Arterial Tissue J Synthetic Substitute K Nonautologous Tissue Substitute Z No Device	0 Upper Arm Artery, Right 3 Lower Arm Artery, Right D Upper Arm Vein F Lower Arm Vein V Superior Vena Cava W Lower Extremity Vein
7 Brachial Artery, Right	3 Percutaneous	Z No Device	F Lower Arm Vein
8 Brachial Artery, Left	0 Open	9 Autologous Venous Tissue A Autologous Arterial Tissue J Synthetic Substitute K Nonautologous Tissue Substitute Z No Device	1 Upper Arm Artery, Left 4 Lower Arm Artery, Left D Upper Arm Vein F Lower Arm Vein V Superior Vena Cava W Lower Extremity Vein
8 Brachial Artery, Left	3 Percutaneous	Z No Device	F Lower Arm Vein
9 Ulnar Artery, Right B Radial Artery, Right	0 Open	9 Autologous Venous Tissue A Autologous Arterial Tissue J Synthetic Substitute K Nonautologous Tissue Substitute Z No Device	3 Lower Arm Artery, Right F Lower Arm Vein
9 Ulnar Artery, Right B Radial Artery, Right	3 Percutaneous	Z No Device	F Lower Arm Vein
A Ulnar Artery, Left C Radial Artery, Left	0 Open	9 Autologous Venous Tissue A Autologous Arterial Tissue J Synthetic Substitute K Nonautologous Tissue Substitute Z No Device	4 Lower Arm Artery, Left F Lower Arm Vein
A Ulnar Artery, Left C Radial Artery, Left	3 Percutaneous	Z No Device	F Lower Arm Vein
G Intracranial Artery S Temporal Artery, Right T Temporal Artery, Left	0 Open	9 Autologous Venous Tissue A Autologous Arterial Tissue J Synthetic Substitute K Nonautologous Tissue Substitute Z No Device	G Intracranial Artery
H Common Carotid Artery, Right J Common Carotid Artery, Left	0 Open	9 Autologous Venous Tissue A Autologous Arterial Tissue J Synthetic Substitute K Nonautologous Tissue Substitute Z No Device	G Intracranial Artery J Extracranial Artery, Right K Extracranial Artery, Left Y Upper Artery
K Internal Carotid Artery, Right L Internal Carotid Artery, Left M External Carotid Artery, Right N External Carotid Artery, Left	0 Open	9 Autologous Venous Tissue A Autologous Arterial Tissue J Synthetic Substitute K Nonautologous Tissue Substitute Z No Device	J Extracranial Artery, Right K Extracranial Artery, Left

Section	0	Medical and Surgical
Body System	3	Upper Arteries
Operation	5	**Destruction:** Physical eradication of all or a portion of a body part by the direct use of energy, force, or a destructive agent

Body Part (4th)	Approach (5th)	Device (6th)	Qualifier (7th)
0 Internal Mammary Artery, Right 1 Internal Mammary Artery, Left 2 Innominate Artery 3 Subclavian Artery, Right 4 Subclavian Artery, Left 5 Axillary Artery, Right 6 Axillary Artery, Left 7 Brachial Artery, Right 8 Brachial Artery, Left 9 Ulnar Artery, Right A Ulnar Artery, Left B Radial Artery, Right C Radial Artery, Left D Hand Artery, Right F Hand Artery, Left G Intracranial Artery H Common Carotid Artery, Right J Common Carotid Artery, Left K Internal Carotid Artery, Right L Internal Carotid Artery, Left M External Carotid Artery, Right N External Carotid Artery, Left P Vertebral Artery, Right Q Vertebral Artery, Left R Face Artery S Temporal Artery, Right T Temporal Artery, Left U Thyroid Artery, Right V Thyroid Artery, Left Y Upper Artery	0 Open 3 Percutaneous 4 Percutaneous Endoscopic	Z No Device	Z No Qualifier

Section   0   **Medical and Surgical**
Body System   3   **Upper Arteries**
Operation   7   **Dilation:** Expanding an orifice or the lumen of a tubular body part

Body Part (4ᵗʰ)	Approach (5ᵗʰ)	Device (6ᵗʰ)	Qualifier (7ᵗʰ)
0 Internal Mammary Artery, Right 1 Internal Mammary Artery, Left 2 Innominate Artery 3 Subclavian Artery, Right 4 Subclavian Artery, Left 5 Axillary Artery, Right 6 Axillary Artery, Left 7 Brachial Artery, Right 8 Brachial Artery, Left 9 Ulnar Artery, Right A Ulnar Artery, Left B Radial Artery, Right C Radial Artery, Left	0 Open 3 Percutaneous 4 Percutaneous Endoscopic	4 Intraluminal Device, Drug-eluting 5 Intraluminal Device, Drug-eluting, Two 6 Intraluminal Device, Drug-eluting, Three 7 Intraluminal Device, Drug-eluting, Four or More E Intraluminal Devices, Two F Intraluminal Devices, Three G Intraluminal Devices, Four or More	Z No Qualifier
0 Internal Mammary Artery, Right 1 Internal Mammary Artery, Left 2 Innominate Artery 3 Subclavian Artery, Right 4 Subclavian Artery, Left 5 Axillary Artery, Right 6 Axillary Artery, Left 7 Brachial Artery, Right 8 Brachial Artery, Left 9 Ulnar Artery, Right A Ulnar Artery, Left B Radial Artery, Right C Radial Artery, Left	0 Open 3 Percutaneous 4 Percutaneous Endoscopic	D Intraluminal Device Z No Device	1 Drug-Coated Balloon Z No Qualifier
D Hand Artery, Right F Hand Artery, Left G Intracranial Artery H Common Carotid Artery, Right J Common Carotid Artery, Left K Internal Carotid Artery, Right L Internal Carotid Artery, Left M External Carotid Artery, Right N External Carotid Artery, Left P Vertebral Artery, Right Q Vertebral Artery, Left R Face Artery S Temporal Artery, Right T Temporal Artery, Left U Thyroid Artery, Right V Thyroid Artery, Left Y Upper Artery	0 Open 3 Percutaneous 4 Percutaneous Endoscopic	4 Intraluminal Device, Drug-eluting 5 Intraluminal Device, Drug-eluting, Two 6 Intraluminal Device, Drug-eluting, Three 7 Intraluminal Device, Drug-eluting, Four or More D Intraluminal Device E Intraluminal Device, Two F Intraluminal Device, Three G Intraluminal Device, Four or More Z No Device	Z No Qualifier

Section	0	Medical and Surgical
Body System	3	Upper Arteries
Operation	9	**Drainage:** Taking or letting out fluids and/or gases from a body part

Body Part (4th)	Approach (5th)	Device (6th)	Qualifier (7th)
0 Internal Mammary Artery, Right 1 Internal Mammary Artery, Left 2 Innominate Artery 3 Subclavian Artery, Right 4 Subclavian Artery, Left 5 Axillary Artery, Right 6 Axillary Artery, Left 7 Brachial Artery, Right 8 Brachial Artery, Left 9 Ulnar Artery, Right A Ulnar Artery, Left B Radial Artery, Right C Radial Artery, Left D Hand Artery, Right F Hand Artery, Left G Intracranial Artery H Common Carotid Artery, Right J Common Carotid Artery, Left K Internal Carotid Artery, Right L Internal Carotid Artery, Left M External Carotid Artery, Right N External Carotid Artery, Left P Vertebral Artery, Right Q Vertebral Artery, Left R Face Artery S Temporal Artery, Right T Temporal Artery, Left U Thyroid Artery, Right V Thyroid Artery, Left Y Upper Artery	0 Open 3 Percutaneous 4 Percutaneous Endoscopic	0 Drainage Device	Z No Qualifier
0 Internal Mammary Artery, Right 1 Internal Mammary Artery, Left 2 Innominate Artery 3 Subclavian Artery, Right 4 Subclavian Artery, Left 5 Axillary Artery, Right 6 Axillary Artery, Left 7 Brachial Artery, Right 8 Brachial Artery, Left 9 Ulnar Artery, Right A Ulnar Artery, Left B Radial Artery, Right C Radial Artery, Left D Hand Artery, Right F Hand Artery, Left G Intracranial Artery H Common Carotid Artery, Right J Common Carotid Artery, Left K Internal Carotid Artery, Right L Internal Carotid Artery, Left M External Carotid Artery, Right N External Carotid Artery, Left P Vertebral Artery, Right Q Vertebral Artery, Left R Face Artery S Temporal Artery, Right T Temporal Artery, Left U Thyroid Artery, Right V Thyroid Artery, Left Y Upper Artery	0 Open 3 Percutaneous 4 Percutaneous Endoscopic	Z No Device	X Diagnostic Z No Qualifier

Section	0	Medical and Surgical
Body System	3	Upper Arteries
Operation	B	Excision: Cutting out or off, without replacement, a portion of a body part

Body Part (4th)	Approach (5th)	Device (6th)	Qualifier (7th)
0 Internal Mammary Artery, Right 1 Internal Mammary Artery, Left 2 Innominate Artery 3 Subclavian Artery, Right 4 Subclavian Artery, Left 5 Axillary Artery, Right 6 Axillary Artery, Left 7 Brachial Artery, Right 8 Brachial Artery, Left 9 Ulnar Artery, Right A Ulnar Artery, Left B Radial Artery, Right C Radial Artery, Left D Hand Artery, Right F Hand Artery, Left G Intracranial Artery H Common Carotid Artery, Right J Common Carotid Artery, Left K Internal Carotid Artery, Right L Internal Carotid Artery, Left M External Carotid Artery, Right N External Carotid Artery, Left P Vertebral Artery, Right Q Vertebral Artery, Left R Face Artery S Temporal Artery, Right T Temporal Artery, Left U Thyroid Artery, Right V Thyroid Artery, Left Y Upper Artery	0 Open 3 Percutaneous 4 Percutaneous Endoscopic	Z No Device	X Diagnostic Z No Qualifier

Section	0	Medical and Surgical
Body System	3	Upper Arteries
Operation	C	Extirpation: Taking or cutting out solid matter from a body part

Body Part (4th)	Approach (5th)	Device (6th)	Qualifier (7th)
0 Internal Mammary Artery, Right 1 Internal Mammary Artery, Left 2 Innominate Artery 3 Subclavian Artery, Right 4 Subclavian Artery, Left 5 Axillary Artery, Right 6 Axillary Artery, Left 7 Brachial Artery, Right 8 Brachial Artery, Left 9 Ulnar Artery, Right A Ulnar Artery, Left B Radial Artery, Right C Radial Artery, Left D Hand Artery, Right F Hand Artery, Left R Face Artery S Temporal Artery, Right T Temporal Artery, Left U Thyroid Artery, Right V Thyroid Artery, Left Y Upper Artery	0 Open 3 Percutaneous 4 Percutaneous Endoscopic	Z No Device	Z No Qualifier

Continued →

Section	0	Medical and Surgical
Body System	3	Upper Arteries
Operation	C	**Extirpation:** Taking or cutting out solid matter from a body part

Body Part (4ᵗʰ)	Approach (5ᵗʰ)	Device (6ᵗʰ)	Qualifier (7ᵗʰ)
G Intracranial Artery H Common Carotid Artery, Right J Common Carotid Artery, Left K Internal Carotid Artery, Right L Internal Carotid Artery, Left M External Carotid Artery, Right N External Carotid Artery, Left P Vertebral Artery, Right Q Vertebral Artery, Left	0 Open 4 Percutaneous Endoscopic	Z No Device	Z No Qualifier
G Intracranial Artery H Common Carotid Artery, Right J Common Carotid Artery, Left K Internal Carotid Artery, Right L Internal Carotid Artery, Left M External Carotid Artery, Right N External Carotid Artery, Left P Vertebral Artery, Right Q Vertebral Artery, Left	3 Percutaneous	Z No Device	7 Stent Retriever Z No Qualifier

Section	0	Medical and Surgical
Body System	3	Upper Arteries
Operation	F	**Fragmentation:** Breaking solid matter in a body part into pieces

Body Part (4ᵗʰ)	Approach (5ᵗʰ)	Device (6ᵗʰ)	Qualifier (7ᵗʰ)
2 Innominate Artery 3 Subclavian Artery, Right 4 Subclavian Artery, Left 5 Axillary Artery, Right 6 Axillary Artery, Left 7 Brachial Artery, Right 8 Brachial Artery, Left 9 Ulnar Artery, Right A Ulnar Artery, Left B Radial Artery, Right C Radial Artery, Left G Intracranial Artery Y Upper Artery	3 Percutaneous	Z No Device	0 Ultrasonic Z No Qualifier

Section	0	Medical and Surgical
Body System	3	Upper Arteries
Operation	H	**Insertion:** Putting in a nonbiological appliance that monitors, assists, performs, or prevents a physiological function but does not physically take the place of a body part

Body Part (4th)	Approach (5th)	Device (6th)	Qualifier (7th)
0 Internal Mammary Artery, Right 1 Internal Mammary Artery, Left 2 Innominate Artery 3 Subclavian Artery, Right 4 Subclavian Artery, Left 5 Axillary Artery, Right 6 Axillary Artery, Left 7 Brachial Artery, Right 8 Brachial Artery, Left 9 Ulnar Artery, Right A Ulnar Artery, Left B Radial Artery, Right C Radial Artery, Left D Hand Artery, Right F Hand Artery, Left G Intracranial Artery H Common Carotid Artery, Right J Common Carotid Artery, Left M External Carotid Artery, Right N External Carotid Artery, Left P Vertebral Artery, Right Q Vertebral Artery, Left R Face Artery S Temporal Artery, Right T Temporal Artery, Left U Thyroid Artery, Right V Thyroid Artery, Left	0 Open 3 Percutaneous 4 Percutaneous Endoscopic	3 Infusion Device D Intraluminal Device	Z No Qualifier
K Internal Carotid Artery, Right L Internal Carotid Artery, Left	0 Open 3 Percutaneous 4 Percutaneous Endoscopic	3 Infusion Device D Intraluminal Device M Stimulator Lead	Z No Qualifier
Y Upper Artery	0 Open 3 Percutaneous 4 Percutaneous Endoscopic	2 Monitoring Device 3 Infusion Device D Intraluminal Device Y Other Device	Z No Qualifier

Section	0	Medical and Surgical
Body System	3	Upper Arteries
Operation	J	**Inspection:** Visually and/or manually exploring a body part

Body Part (4th)	Approach (5th)	Device (6th)	Qualifier (7th)
Y Upper Artery	0 Open 3 Percutaneous 4 Percutaneous Endoscopic X External	Z No Device	Z No Qualifier

Section	0	Medical and Surgical
Body System	3	Upper Arteries
Operation	L	Occlusion: Completely closing an orifice or the lumen of a tubular body part

Body Part (4ᵗʰ)	Approach (5ᵗʰ)	Device (6ᵗʰ)	Qualifier (7ᵗʰ)
0 Internal Mammary Artery, Right 1 Internal Mammary Artery, Left 2 Innominate Artery 3 Subclavian Artery, Right 4 Subclavian Artery, Left 5 Axillary Artery, Right 6 Axillary Artery, Left 7 Brachial Artery, Right 8 Brachial Artery, Left 9 Ulnar Artery, Right A Ulnar Artery, Left B Radial Artery, Right C Radial Artery, Left D Hand Artery, Right F Hand Artery, Left R Face Artery S Temporal Artery, Right T Temporal Artery, Left U Thyroid Artery, Right V Thyroid Artery, Left Y Upper Artery	0 Open 3 Percutaneous 4 Percutaneous Endoscopic	C Extraluminal Device D Intraluminal Device Z No Device	Z No Qualifier
G Intracranial Artery H Common Carotid Artery, Right J Common Carotid Artery, Left K Internal Carotid Artery, Right L Internal Carotid Artery, Left M External Carotid Artery, Right N External Carotid Artery, Left P Vertebral Artery, Right Q Vertebral Artery, Left	0 Open 3 Percutaneous 4 Percutaneous Endoscopic	B Intraluminal Device, Bioactive C Extraluminal Device D Intraluminal Device Z No Device	Z No Qualifier

Section	0	Medical and Surgical
Body System	3	Upper Arteries
Operation	N	**Release:** Freeing a body part from an abnormal physical constraint by cutting or by the use of force

Body Part (4th)	Approach (5th)	Device (6th)	Qualifier (7th)
0 Internal Mammary Artery, Right 1 Internal Mammary Artery, Left 2 Innominate Artery 3 Subclavian Artery, Right 4 Subclavian Artery, Left 5 Axillary Artery, Right 6 Axillary Artery, Left 7 Brachial Artery, Right 8 Brachial Artery, Left 9 Ulnar Artery, Right A Ulnar Artery, Left B Radial Artery, Right C Radial Artery, Left D Hand Artery, Right F Hand Artery, Left G Intracranial Artery H Common Carotid Artery, Right J Common Carotid Artery, Left K Internal Carotid Artery, Right L Internal Carotid Artery, Left M External Carotid Artery, Right N External Carotid Artery, Left P Vertebral Artery, Right Q Vertebral Artery, Left R Face Artery S Temporal Artery, Right T Temporal Artery, Left U Thyroid Artery, Right V Thyroid Artery, Left Y Upper Artery	0 Open 3 Percutaneous 4 Percutaneous Endoscopic	Z No Device	Z No Qualifier

Section	0	Medical and Surgical
Body System	3	Upper Arteries
Operation	P	**Removal:** Taking out or off a device from a body part

Body Part (4th)	Approach (5th)	Device (6th)	Qualifier (7th)
Y Upper Artery	0 Open 3 Percutaneous 4 Percutaneous Endoscopic	0 Drainage Device 2 Monitoring Device 3 Infusion Device 7 Autologous Tissue Substitute C Extraluminal Device D Intraluminal Device J Synthetic Substitute K Nonautologous Tissue Substitute M Stimulator Lead Y Other Device	Z No Qualifier
Y Upper Artery	X External	0 Drainage Device 2 Monitoring Device 3 Infusion Device D Intraluminal Device M Stimulator Lead	Z No Qualifier

Section	0	Medical and Surgical
Body System	3	Upper Arteries
Operation	Q	**Repair:** Restoring, to the extent possible, a body part to its normal anatomic structure and function

Body Part (4th)	Approach (5th)	Device (6th)	Qualifier (7th)
0 Internal Mammary Artery, Right **1** Internal Mammary Artery, Left **2** Innominate Artery **3** Subclavian Artery, Right **4** Subclavian Artery, Left **5** Axillary Artery, Right **6** Axillary Artery, Left **7** Brachial Artery, Right **8** Brachial Artery, Left **9** Ulnar Artery, Right **A** Ulnar Artery, Left **B** Radial Artery, Right **C** Radial Artery, Left **D** Hand Artery, Right **F** Hand Artery, Left **G** Intracranial Artery **H** Common Carotid Artery, Right **J** Common Carotid Artery, Left **K** Internal Carotid Artery, Right **L** Internal Carotid Artery, Left **M** External Carotid Artery, Right **N** External Carotid Artery, Left **P** Vertebral Artery, Right **Q** Vertebral Artery, Left **R** Face Artery **S** Temporal Artery, Right **T** Temporal Artery, Left **U** Thyroid Artery, Right **V** Thyroid Artery, Left **Y** Upper Artery	**0** Open **3** Percutaneous **4** Percutaneous Endoscopic	**Z** No Device	**Z** No Qualifier

Section	0	Medical and Surgical
Body System	3	Upper Arteries
Operation	R	**Replacement:** Putting in or on biological or synthetic material that physically takes the place and/or function of all or a portion of a body part

Body Part (4th)	Approach (5th)	Device (6th)	Qualifier (7th)
0 Internal Mammary Artery, Right **1** Internal Mammary Artery, Left **2** Innominate Artery **3** Subclavian Artery, Right **4** Subclavian Artery, Left **5** Axillary Artery, Right **6** Axillary Artery, Left **7** Brachial Artery, Right **8** Brachial Artery, Left **9** Ulnar Artery, Right **A** Ulnar Artery, Left **B** Radial Artery, Right **C** Radial Artery, Left **D** Hand Artery, Right **F** Hand Artery, Left **G** Intracranial Artery **H** Common Carotid Artery, Right **J** Common Carotid Artery, Left **K** Internal Carotid Artery, Right **L** Internal Carotid Artery, Left **M** External Carotid Artery, Right **N** External Carotid Artery, Left **P** Vertebral Artery, Right **Q** Vertebral Artery, Left **R** Face Artery **S** Temporal Artery, Right **T** Temporal Artery, Left **U** Thyroid Artery, Right **V** Thyroid Artery, Left **Y** Upper Artery	**0** Open **4** Percutaneous Endoscopic	**7** Autologous Tissue Substitute **J** Synthetic Substitute **K** Nonautologous Tissue Substitute	**Z** No Qualifier

Section	0	Medical and Surgical
Body System	3	Upper Arteries
Operation	S	**Reposition:** Moving to its normal location, or other suitable location, all or a portion of a body part

Body Part (4ᵗʰ)	Approach (5ᵗʰ)	Device (6ᵗʰ)	Qualifier (7ᵗʰ)
0 Internal Mammary Artery, Right 1 Internal Mammary Artery, Left 2 Innominate Artery 3 Subclavian Artery, Right 4 Subclavian Artery, Left 5 Axillary Artery, Right 6 Axillary Artery, Left 7 Brachial Artery, Right 8 Brachial Artery, Left 9 Ulnar Artery, Right A Ulnar Artery, Left B Radial Artery, Right C Radial Artery, Left D Hand Artery, Right F Hand Artery, Left G Intracranial Artery H Common Carotid Artery, Right J Common Carotid Artery, Left K Internal Carotid Artery, Right L Internal Carotid Artery, Left M External Carotid Artery, Right N External Carotid Artery, Left P Vertebral Artery, Right Q Vertebral Artery, Left R Face Artery S Temporal Artery, Right T Temporal Artery, Left U Thyroid Artery, Right V Thyroid Artery, Left Y Upper Artery	0 Open 3 Percutaneous 4 Percutaneous Endoscopic	Z No Device	Z No Qualifier

Section   0   **Medical and Surgical**
Body System   3   **Upper Arteries**
Operation   U   **Supplement:** Putting in or on biological or synthetic material that physically reinforces and/or augments the function of a portion of a body part

Body Part (4ᵗʰ)	Approach (5ᵗʰ)	Device (6ᵗʰ)	Qualifier (7ᵗʰ)
0 Internal Mammary Artery, Right	0 Open	7 Autologous Tissue Substitute	Z No Qualifier
1 Internal Mammary Artery, Left	3 Percutaneous	J Synthetic Substitute	
2 Innominate Artery	4 Percutaneous Endoscopic	K Nonautologous Tissue Substitute	
3 Subclavian Artery, Right			
4 Subclavian Artery, Left			
5 Axillary Artery, Right			
6 Axillary Artery, Left			
7 Brachial Artery, Right			
8 Brachial Artery, Left			
9 Ulnar Artery, Right			
A Ulnar Artery, Left			
B Radial Artery, Right			
C Radial Artery, Left			
D Hand Artery, Right			
F Hand Artery, Left			
G Intracranial Artery			
H Common Carotid Artery, Right			
J Common Carotid Artery, Left			
K Internal Carotid Artery, Right			
L Internal Carotid Artery, Left			
M External Carotid Artery, Right			
N External Carotid Artery, Left			
P Vertebral Artery, Right			
Q Vertebral Artery, Left			
R Face Artery			
S Temporal Artery, Right			
T Temporal Artery, Left			
U Thyroid Artery, Right			
V Thyroid Artery, Left			
Y Upper Artery			

Section   0   **Medical and Surgical**
Body System   3   **Upper Arteries**
Operation   V   **Restriction:** Partially closing an orifice or the lumen of a tubular body part

Body Part (4ᵗʰ)	Approach (5ᵗʰ)	Device (6ᵗʰ)	Qualifier (7ᵗʰ)
0 Internal Mammary Artery, Right	0 Open	C Extraluminal Device	Z No Qualifier
1 Internal Mammary Artery, Left	3 Percutaneous	D Intraluminal Device	
2 Innominate Artery	4 Percutaneous Endoscopic	Z No Device	
3 Subclavian Artery, Right			
4 Subclavian Artery, Left			
5 Axillary Artery, Right			
6 Axillary Artery, Left			
7 Brachial Artery, Right			
8 Brachial Artery, Left			
9 Ulnar Artery, Right			
A Ulnar Artery, Left			
B Radial Artery, Right			
C Radial Artery, Left			
D Hand Artery, Right			
F Hand Artery, Left			
R Face Artery			
S Temporal Artery, Right			
T Temporal Artery, Left			
U Thyroid Artery, Right			
V Thyroid Artery, Left			
Y Upper Artery			

Continued →

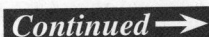

Section 0 Medical and Surgical
Body System 3 Upper Arteries
Operation V Restriction: Partially closing an orifice or the lumen of a tubular body part

Body Part (4th)	Approach (5th)	Device (6th)	Qualifier (7th)
G Intracranial Artery H Common Carotid Artery, Right J Common Carotid Artery, Left K Internal Carotid Artery, Right L Internal Carotid Artery, Left M External Carotid Artery, Right N External Carotid Artery, Left P Vertebral Artery, Right Q Vertebral Artery, Left	0 Open 3 Percutaneous 4 Percutaneous Endoscopic	B Intraluminal Device, Bioactive C Extraluminal Device D Intraluminal Device H Intraluminal Device, Flow Diverter Z No Device	Z No Qualifier

Section 0 Medical and Surgical
Body System 3 Upper Arteries
Operation W Revision: Correcting, to the extent possible, a portion of a malfunctioning device or the position of a displaced device

Body Part (4th)	Approach (5th)	Device (6th)	Qualifier (7th)
Y Upper Artery	0 Open 3 Percutaneous 4 Percutaneous Endoscopic	0 Drainage Device 2 Monitoring Device 3 Infusion Device 7 Autologous Tissue Substitute C Extraluminal Device D Intraluminal Device J Synthetic Substitute K Nonautologous Tissue Substitute M Stimulator Lead Y Other Device	Z No Qualifier
Y Upper Artery	X External	0 Drainage Device 2 Monitoring Device 3 Infusion Device 7 Autologous Tissue Substitute C Extraluminal Device D Intraluminal Device J Synthetic Substitute K Nonautologous Tissue Substitute M Neurostimulator Lead	Z No Qualifier

Upper Arteries Code Listing 031–03W

031 – Upper Arteries, Bypass

Review Coding Guideline B3.6a

0312090 Bypass Innominate Artery to Right Upper Arm Artery with Autologous Venous Tissue, Open Approach	0312097 Bypass Innominate Artery to Left Upper Leg Artery with Autologous Venous Tissue, Open Approach	031209J Bypass Innominate Artery to Right Extracranial Artery with Autologous Venous Tissue, Open Approach
0312091 Bypass Innominate Artery to Left Upper Arm Artery with Autologous Venous Tissue, Open Approach	0312098 Bypass Innominate Artery to Bilateral Upper Leg Artery with Autologous Venous Tissue, Open Approach	031209K Bypass Innominate Artery to Left Extracranial Artery with Autologous Venous Tissue, Open Approach
0312092 Bypass Innominate Artery to Bilateral Upper Arm Artery with Autologous Venous Tissue, Open Approach	0312099 Bypass Innominate Artery to Right Lower Leg Artery with Autologous Venous Tissue, Open Approach	031209W Bypass Innominate Artery to Lower Extremity Vein with Autologous Venous Tissue, Open Approach
0312093 Bypass Innominate Artery to Right Lower Arm Artery with Autologous Venous Tissue, Open Approach	031209B Bypass Innominate Artery to Left Lower Leg Artery with Autologous Venous Tissue, Open Approach	03120A0 Bypass Innominate Artery to Right Upper Arm Artery with Autologous Arterial Tissue, Open Approach
0312094 Bypass Innominate Artery to Left Lower Arm Artery with Autologous Venous Tissue, Open Approach	031209C Bypass Innominate Artery to Bilateral Lower Leg Artery with Autologous Venous Tissue, Open Approach	03120A1 Bypass Innominate Artery to Left Upper Arm Artery with Autologous Arterial Tissue, Open Approach
0312095 Bypass Innominate Artery to Bilateral Lower Arm Artery with Autologous Venous Tissue, Open Approach	031209D Bypass Innominate Artery to Upper Arm Vein with Autologous Venous Tissue, Open Approach	03120A2 Bypass Innominate Artery to Bilateral Upper Arm Artery with Autologous Arterial Tissue, Open Approach
0312096 Bypass Innominate Artery to Right Upper Leg Artery with Autologous Venous Tissue, Open Approach	031209F Bypass Innominate Artery to Lower Arm Vein with Autologous Venous Tissue, Open Approach	03120A3 Bypass Innominate Artery to Right Lower Arm Artery with Autologous Arterial Tissue, Open Approach

03120A4 Bypass Innominate Artery to Left Lower Arm Artery with Autologous Arterial Tissue, Open Approach

03120A5 Bypass Innominate Artery to Bilateral Lower Arm Artery with Autologous Arterial Tissue, Open Approach

03120A6 Bypass Innominate Artery to Right Upper Leg Artery with Autologous Arterial Tissue, Open Approach

03120A7 Bypass Innominate Artery to Left Upper Leg Artery with Autologous Arterial Tissue, Open Approach

03120A8 Bypass Innominate Artery to Bilateral Upper Leg Artery with Autologous Arterial Tissue, Open Approach

03120A9 Bypass Innominate Artery to Right Lower Leg Artery with Autologous Arterial Tissue, Open Approach

03120AB Bypass Innominate Artery to Left Lower Leg Artery with Autologous Arterial Tissue, Open Approach

03120AC Bypass Innominate Artery to Bilateral Lower Leg Artery with Autologous Arterial Tissue, Open Approach

03120AD Bypass Innominate Artery to Upper Arm Vein with Autologous Arterial Tissue, Open Approach

03120AF Bypass Innominate Artery to Lower Arm Vein with Autologous Arterial Tissue, Open Approach

03120AJ Bypass Innominate Artery to Right Extracranial Artery with Autologous Arterial Tissue, Open Approach

03120AK Bypass Innominate Artery to Left Extracranial Artery with Autologous Arterial Tissue, Open Approach

03120AW Bypass Innominate Artery to Lower Extremity Vein with Autologous Arterial Tissue, Open Approach

03120J0 Bypass Innominate Artery to Right Upper Arm Artery with Synthetic Substitute, Open Approach

03120J1 Bypass Innominate Artery to Left Upper Arm Artery with Synthetic Substitute, Open Approach

03120J2 Bypass Innominate Artery to Bilateral Upper Arm Artery with Synthetic Substitute, Open Approach

03120J3 Bypass Innominate Artery to Right Lower Arm Artery with Synthetic Substitute, Open Approach

03120J4 Bypass Innominate Artery to Left Lower Arm Artery with Synthetic Substitute, Open Approach

03120J5 Bypass Innominate Artery to Bilateral Lower Arm Artery with Synthetic Substitute, Open Approach

03120J6 Bypass Innominate Artery to Right Upper Leg Artery with Synthetic Substitute, Open Approach

03120J7 Bypass Innominate Artery to Left Upper Leg Artery with Synthetic Substitute, Open Approach

03120J8 Bypass Innominate Artery to Bilateral Upper Leg Artery with Synthetic Substitute, Open Approach

03120J9 Bypass Innominate Artery to Right Lower Leg Artery with Synthetic Substitute, Open Approach

03120JB Bypass Innominate Artery to Left Lower Leg Artery with Synthetic Substitute, Open Approach

03120JC Bypass Innominate Artery to Bilateral Lower Leg Artery with Synthetic Substitute, Open Approach

03120JD Bypass Innominate Artery to Upper Arm Vein with Synthetic Substitute, Open Approach

03120JF Bypass Innominate Artery to Lower Arm Vein with Synthetic Substitute, Open Approach

03120JJ Bypass Innominate Artery to Right Extracranial Artery with Synthetic Substitute, Open Approach

03120JK Bypass Innominate Artery to Left Extracranial Artery with Synthetic Substitute, Open Approach

03120JW Bypass Innominate Artery to Lower Extremity Vein with Synthetic Substitute, Open Approach

03120K0 Bypass Innominate Artery to Right Upper Arm Artery with Nonautologous Tissue Substitute, Open Approach

03120K1 Bypass Innominate Artery to Left Upper Arm Artery with Nonautologous Tissue Substitute, Open Approach

03120K2 Bypass Innominate Artery to Bilateral Upper Arm Artery with Nonautologous Tissue Substitute, Open Approach

03120K3 Bypass Innominate Artery to Right Lower Arm Artery with Nonautologous Tissue Substitute, Open Approach

03120K4 Bypass Innominate Artery to Left Lower Arm Artery with Nonautologous Tissue Substitute, Open Approach

03120K5 Bypass Innominate Artery to Bilateral Lower Arm Artery with Nonautologous Tissue Substitute, Open Approach

03120K6 Bypass Innominate Artery to Right Upper Leg Artery with Nonautologous Tissue Substitute, Open Approach

03120K7 Bypass Innominate Artery to Left Upper Leg Artery with Nonautologous Tissue Substitute, Open Approach

03120K8 Bypass Innominate Artery to Bilateral Upper Leg Artery with Nonautologous Tissue Substitute, Open Approach

03120K9 Bypass Innominate Artery to Right Lower Leg Artery with Nonautologous Tissue Substitute, Open Approach

03120KB Bypass Innominate Artery to Left Lower Leg Artery with Nonautologous Tissue Substitute, Open Approach

03120KC Bypass Innominate Artery to Bilateral Lower Leg Artery with Nonautologous Tissue Substitute, Open Approach

03120KD Bypass Innominate Artery to Upper Arm Vein with Nonautologous Tissue Substitute, Open Approach

03120KF Bypass Innominate Artery to Lower Arm Vein with Nonautologous Tissue Substitute, Open Approach

03120KJ Bypass Innominate Artery to Right Extracranial Artery with Nonautologous Tissue Substitute, Open Approach

03120KK Bypass Innominate Artery to Left Extracranial Artery with Nonautologous Tissue Substitute, Open Approach

03120KW Bypass Innominate Artery to Lower Extremity Vein with Nonautologous Tissue Substitute, Open Approach

03120Z0 Bypass Innominate Artery to Right Upper Arm Artery, Open Approach

03120Z1 Bypass Innominate Artery to Left Upper Arm Artery, Open Approach

03120Z2 Bypass Innominate Artery to Bilateral Upper Arm Artery, Open Approach

03120Z3 Bypass Innominate Artery to Right Lower Arm Artery, Open Approach

03120Z4 Bypass Innominate Artery to Left Lower Arm Artery, Open Approach

03120Z5 Bypass Innominate Artery to Bilateral Lower Arm Artery, Open Approach

03120Z6 Bypass Innominate Artery to Right Upper Leg Artery, Open Approach

03120Z7 Bypass Innominate Artery to Left Upper Leg Artery, Open Approach

03120Z8 Bypass Innominate Artery to Bilateral Upper Leg Artery, Open Approach

03120Z9 Bypass Innominate Artery to Right Lower Leg Artery, Open Approach

03120ZB Bypass Innominate Artery to Left Lower Leg Artery, Open Approach

03120ZC Bypass Innominate Artery to Bilateral Lower Leg Artery, Open Approach

03120ZD Bypass Innominate Artery to Upper Arm Vein, Open Approach

03120ZF Bypass Innominate Artery to Lower Arm Vein, Open Approach

03120ZJ Bypass Innominate Artery to Right Extracranial Artery, Open Approach

03120ZK Bypass Innominate Artery to Left Extracranial Artery, Open Approach

03120ZW Bypass Innominate Artery to Lower Extremity Vein, Open Approach

0313090 Bypass Right Subclavian Artery to Right Upper Arm Artery with Autologous Venous Tissue, Open Approach

0313091 Bypass Right Subclavian Artery to Left Upper Arm Artery with Autologous Venous Tissue, Open Approach

0313092 Bypass Right Subclavian Artery to Bilateral Upper Arm Artery with Autologous Venous Tissue, Open Approach

0313093 Bypass Right Subclavian Artery to Right Lower Arm Artery with Autologous Venous Tissue, Open Approach

0313094 Bypass Right Subclavian Artery to Left Lower Arm Artery with Autologous Venous Tissue, Open Approach

0313095 Bypass Right Subclavian Artery to Bilateral Lower Arm Artery with Autologous Venous Tissue, Open Approach

0313096 Bypass Right Subclavian Artery to Right Upper Leg Artery with Autologous Venous Tissue, Open Approach

0313097 Bypass Right Subclavian Artery to Left Upper Leg Artery with Autologous Venous Tissue, Open Approach

0313098 Bypass Right Subclavian Artery to Bilateral Upper Leg Artery with Autologous Venous Tissue, Open Approach

0313099 Bypass Right Subclavian Artery to Right Lower Leg Artery with Autologous Venous Tissue, Open Approach

031309B Bypass Right Subclavian Artery to Left Lower Leg Artery with Autologous Venous Tissue, Open Approach

031309C Bypass Right Subclavian Artery to Bilateral Lower Leg Artery with Autologous Venous Tissue, Open Approach

031309D Bypass Right Subclavian Artery to Upper Arm Vein with Autologous Venous Tissue, Open Approach

031309F Bypass Right Subclavian Artery to Lower Arm Vein with Autologous Venous Tissue, Open Approach

031309J Bypass Right Subclavian Artery to Right Extracranial Artery with Autologous Venous Tissue, Open Approach

031309K Bypass Right Subclavian Artery to Left Extracranial Artery with Autologous Venous Tissue, Open Approach

031309M Bypass Right Subclavian Artery to Right Pulmonary Artery with Autologous Venous Tissue, Open Approach

031309N Bypass Right Subclavian Artery to Left Pulmonary Artery with Autologous Venous Tissue, Open Approach

031309W Bypass Right Subclavian Artery to Lower Extremity Vein with Autologous Venous Tissue, Open Approach

03130A0 Bypass Right Subclavian Artery to Right Upper Arm Artery with Autologous Arterial Tissue, Open Approach

03130A1 Bypass Right Subclavian Artery to Left Upper Arm Artery with Autologous Arterial Tissue, Open Approach

03130A2 Bypass Right Subclavian Artery to Bilateral Upper Arm Artery with Autologous Arterial Tissue, Open Approach

03130A3 Bypass Right Subclavian Artery to Right Lower Arm Artery with Autologous Arterial Tissue, Open Approach

03130A4 Bypass Right Subclavian Artery to Left Lower Arm Artery with Autologous Arterial Tissue, Open Approach

03130A5 Bypass Right Subclavian Artery to Bilateral Lower Arm Artery with Autologous Arterial Tissue, Open Approach

03130A6 Bypass Right Subclavian Artery to Right Upper Leg Artery with Autologous Arterial Tissue, Open Approach

03130A7 Bypass Right Subclavian Artery to Left Upper Leg Artery with Autologous Arterial Tissue, Open Approach

03130A8 Bypass Right Subclavian Artery to Bilateral Upper Leg Artery with Autologous Arterial Tissue, Open Approach

03130A9 Bypass Right Subclavian Artery to Right Lower Leg Artery with Autologous Arterial Tissue, Open Approach

03130AB Bypass Right Subclavian Artery to Left Lower Leg Artery with Autologous Arterial Tissue, Open Approach

03130AC Bypass Right Subclavian Artery to Bilateral Lower Leg Artery with Autologous Arterial Tissue, Open Approach

03130AD Bypass Right Subclavian Artery to Upper Arm Vein with Autologous Arterial Tissue, Open Approach

03130AF Bypass Right Subclavian Artery to Lower Arm Vein with Autologous Arterial Tissue, Open Approach

03130AJ Bypass Right Subclavian Artery to Right Extracranial Artery with Autologous Arterial Tissue, Open Approach

03130AK Bypass Right Subclavian Artery to Left Extracranial Artery with Autologous Arterial Tissue, Open Approach

03130AM Bypass Right Subclavian Artery to Right Pulmonary Artery with Autologous Arterial Tissue, Open Approach

03130AN Bypass Right Subclavian Artery to Left Pulmonary Artery with Autologous Arterial Tissue, Open Approach

03130AW Bypass Right Subclavian Artery to Lower Extremity Vein with Autologous Arterial Tissue, Open Approach

03130J0 Bypass Right Subclavian Artery to Right Upper Arm Artery with Synthetic Substitute, Open Approach

03130J1 Bypass Right Subclavian Artery to Left Upper Arm Artery with Synthetic Substitute, Open Approach

03130J2 Bypass Right Subclavian Artery to Bilateral Upper Arm Artery with Synthetic Substitute, Open Approach

03130J3 Bypass Right Subclavian Artery to Right Lower Arm Artery with Synthetic Substitute, Open Approach

03130J4 Bypass Right Subclavian Artery to Left Lower Arm Artery with Synthetic Substitute, Open Approach

03130J5 Bypass Right Subclavian Artery to Bilateral Lower Arm Artery with Synthetic Substitute, Open Approach

03130J6 Bypass Right Subclavian Artery to Right Upper Leg Artery with Synthetic Substitute, Open Approach

03130J7 Bypass Right Subclavian Artery to Left Upper Leg Artery with Synthetic Substitute, Open Approach

03130J8 Bypass Right Subclavian Artery to Bilateral Upper Leg Artery with Synthetic Substitute, Open Approach

03130J9 Bypass Right Subclavian Artery to Right Lower Leg Artery with Synthetic Substitute, Open Approach

03130JB Bypass Right Subclavian Artery to Left Lower Leg Artery with Synthetic Substitute, Open Approach

03130JC Bypass Right Subclavian Artery to Bilateral Lower Leg Artery with Synthetic Substitute, Open Approach

03130JD Bypass Right Subclavian Artery to Upper Arm Vein with Synthetic Substitute, Open Approach

03130JF Bypass Right Subclavian Artery to Lower Arm Vein with Synthetic Substitute, Open Approach

03130JJ Bypass Right Subclavian Artery to Right Extracranial Artery with Synthetic Substitute, Open Approach

03130JK Bypass Right Subclavian Artery to Left Extracranial Artery with Synthetic Substitute, Open Approach

03130JM Bypass Right Subclavian Artery to Right Pulmonary Artery with Synthetic Substitute, Open Approach

03130JN Bypass Right Subclavian Artery to Left Pulmonary Artery with Synthetic Substitute, Open Approach

03130JW Bypass Right Subclavian Artery to Lower Extremity Vein with Synthetic Substitute, Open Approach

03130K0 Bypass Right Subclavian Artery to Right Upper Arm Artery with Nonautologous Tissue Substitute, Open Approach

03130K1 Bypass Right Subclavian Artery to Left Upper Arm Artery with Nonautologous Tissue Substitute, Open Approach

03130K2 Bypass Right Subclavian Artery to Bilateral Upper Arm Artery with Nonautologous Tissue Substitute, Open Approach

03130K3 Bypass Right Subclavian Artery to Right Lower Arm Artery with Nonautologous Tissue Substitute, Open Approach

03130K4 Bypass Right Subclavian Artery to Left Lower Arm Artery with Nonautologous Tissue Substitute, Open Approach

03130K5 Bypass Right Subclavian Artery to Bilateral Lower Arm Artery with Nonautologous Tissue Substitute, Open Approach

03130K6 Bypass Right Subclavian Artery to Right Upper Leg Artery with Nonautologous Tissue Substitute, Open Approach

03130K7 Bypass Right Subclavian Artery to Left Upper Leg Artery with Nonautologous Tissue Substitute, Open Approach

03130K8 Bypass Right Subclavian Artery to Bilateral Upper Leg Artery with Nonautologous Tissue Substitute, Open Approach

03130K9 Bypass Right Subclavian Artery to Right Lower Leg Artery with Nonautologous Tissue Substitute, Open Approach

03130KB Bypass Right Subclavian Artery to Left Lower Leg Artery with Nonautologous Tissue Substitute, Open Approach

03130KC Bypass Right Subclavian Artery to Bilateral Lower Leg Artery with Nonautologous Tissue Substitute, Open Approach

03130KD Bypass Right Subclavian Artery to Upper Arm Vein with Nonautologous Tissue Substitute, Open Approach

03130KF Bypass Right Subclavian Artery to Lower Arm Vein with Nonautologous Tissue Substitute, Open Approach

03130KJ Bypass Right Subclavian Artery to Right Extracranial Artery with Nonautologous Tissue Substitute, Open Approach

03130KK Bypass Right Subclavian Artery to Left Extracranial Artery with Nonautologous Tissue Substitute, Open Approach

03130KM Bypass Right Subclavian Artery to Right Pulmonary Artery with Nonautologous Tissue Substitute, Open Approach

03130KN Bypass Right Subclavian Artery to Left Pulmonary Artery with Nonautologous Tissue Substitute, Open Approach

03130KW Bypass Right Subclavian Artery to Lower Extremity Vein with Nonautologous Tissue Substitute, Open Approach

03130Z0 Bypass Right Subclavian Artery to Right Upper Arm Artery, Open Approach

03130Z1 Bypass Right Subclavian Artery to Left Upper Arm Artery, Open Approach

03130Z2 Bypass Right Subclavian Artery to Bilateral Upper Arm Artery, Open Approach

03130Z3 Bypass Right Subclavian Artery to Right Lower Arm Artery, Open Approach

03130Z4 Bypass Right Subclavian Artery to Left Lower Arm Artery, Open Approach

03130Z5 Bypass Right Subclavian Artery to Bilateral Lower Arm Artery, Open Approach

03130Z6 Bypass Right Subclavian Artery to Right Upper Leg Artery, Open Approach

03130Z7 Bypass Right Subclavian Artery to Left Upper Leg Artery, Open Approach

♀ Female-only   ♂ Male-only   ▲ Limited Coverage   ● Non-OR   HAC HAC-associated procedure   ▲ Non-covered procedures   ✚ Cluster

03130Z8	Bypass Right Subclavian Artery to Bilateral Upper Leg Artery, Open Approach
03130Z9	Bypass Right Subclavian Artery to Right Lower Leg Artery, Open Approach
03130ZB	Bypass Right Subclavian Artery to Left Lower Leg Artery, Open Approach
03130ZC	Bypass Right Subclavian Artery to Bilateral Lower Leg Artery, Open Approach
03130ZD	Bypass Right Subclavian Artery to Upper Arm Vein, Open Approach
03130ZF	Bypass Right Subclavian Artery to Lower Arm Vein, Open Approach
03130ZJ	Bypass Right Subclavian Artery to Right Extracranial Artery, Open Approach
03130ZK	Bypass Right Subclavian Artery to Left Extracranial Artery, Open Approach
03130ZM	Bypass Right Subclavian Artery to Right Pulmonary Artery, Open Approach
03130ZN	Bypass Right Subclavian Artery to Left Pulmonary Artery, Open Approach
03130ZW	Bypass Right Subclavian Artery to Lower Extremity Vein, Open Approach
0314090	Bypass Left Subclavian Artery to Right Upper Arm Artery with Autologous Venous Tissue, Open Approach
0314091	Bypass Left Subclavian Artery to Left Upper Arm Artery with Autologous Venous Tissue, Open Approach
0314092	Bypass Left Subclavian Artery to Bilateral Upper Arm Artery with Autologous Venous Tissue, Open Approach
0314093	Bypass Left Subclavian Artery to Right Lower Arm Artery with Autologous Venous Tissue, Open Approach
0314094	Bypass Left Subclavian Artery to Left Lower Arm Artery with Autologous Venous Tissue, Open Approach
0314095	Bypass Left Subclavian Artery to Bilateral Lower Arm Artery with Autologous Venous Tissue, Open Approach
0314096	Bypass Left Subclavian Artery to Right Upper Leg Artery with Autologous Venous Tissue, Open Approach
0314097	Bypass Left Subclavian Artery to Left Upper Leg Artery with Autologous Venous Tissue, Open Approach
0314098	Bypass Left Subclavian Artery to Bilateral Upper Leg Artery with Autologous Venous Tissue, Open Approach
0314099	Bypass Left Subclavian Artery to Right Lower Leg Artery with Autologous Venous Tissue, Open Approach
031409B	Bypass Left Subclavian Artery to Left Lower Leg Artery with Autologous Venous Tissue, Open Approach
031409C	Bypass Left Subclavian Artery to Bilateral Lower Leg Artery with Autologous Venous Tissue, Open Approach
031409D	Bypass Left Subclavian Artery to Upper Arm Vein with Autologous Venous Tissue, Open Approach
031409F	Bypass Left Subclavian Artery to Lower Arm Vein with Autologous Venous Tissue, Open Approach
031409J	Bypass Left Subclavian Artery to Right Extracranial Artery with Autologous Venous Tissue, Open Approach
031409K	Bypass Left Subclavian Artery to Left Extracranial Artery with Autologous Venous Tissue, Open Approach
031409M	Bypass Left Subclavian Artery to Right Pulmonary Artery with Autologous Venous Tissue, Open Approach
031409N	Bypass Left Subclavian Artery to Left Pulmonary Artery with Autologous Venous Tissue, Open Approach
031409W	Bypass Left Subclavian Artery to Lower Extremity Vein with Autologous Venous Tissue, Open Approach
03140A0	Bypass Left Subclavian Artery to Right Upper Arm Artery with Autologous Arterial Tissue, Open Approach
03140A1	Bypass Left Subclavian Artery to Left Upper Arm Artery with Autologous Arterial Tissue, Open Approach
03140A2	Bypass Left Subclavian Artery to Bilateral Upper Arm Artery with Autologous Arterial Tissue, Open Approach
03140A3	Bypass Left Subclavian Artery to Right Lower Arm Artery with Autologous Arterial Tissue, Open Approach
03140A4	Bypass Left Subclavian Artery to Left Lower Arm Artery with Autologous Arterial Tissue, Open Approach
03140A5	Bypass Left Subclavian Artery to Bilateral Lower Arm Artery with Autologous Arterial Tissue, Open Approach
03140A6	Bypass Left Subclavian Artery to Right Upper Leg Artery with Autologous Arterial Tissue, Open Approach
03140A7	Bypass Left Subclavian Artery to Left Upper Leg Artery with Autologous Arterial Tissue, Open Approach
03140A8	Bypass Left Subclavian Artery to Bilateral Upper Leg Artery with Autologous Arterial Tissue, Open Approach
03140A9	Bypass Left Subclavian Artery to Right Lower Leg Artery with Autologous Arterial Tissue, Open Approach
03140AB	Bypass Left Subclavian Artery to Left Lower Leg Artery with Autologous Arterial Tissue, Open Approach
03140AC	Bypass Left Subclavian Artery to Bilateral Lower Leg Artery with Autologous Arterial Tissue, Open Approach
03140AD	Bypass Left Subclavian Artery to Upper Arm Vein with Autologous Arterial Tissue, Open Approach
03140AF	Bypass Left Subclavian Artery to Lower Arm Vein with Autologous Arterial Tissue, Open Approach
03140AJ	Bypass Left Subclavian Artery to Right Extracranial Artery with Autologous Arterial Tissue, Open Approach
03140AK	Bypass Left Subclavian Artery to Left Extracranial Artery with Autologous Arterial Tissue, Open Approach
03140AM	Bypass Left Subclavian Artery to Right Pulmonary Artery with Autologous Arterial Tissue, Open Approach
03140AN	Bypass Left Subclavian Artery to Left Pulmonary Artery with Autologous Arterial Tissue, Open Approach
03140AW	Bypass Left Subclavian Artery to Lower Extremity Vein with Autologous Arterial Tissue, Open Approach
03140J0	Bypass Left Subclavian Artery to Right Upper Arm Artery with Synthetic Substitute, Open Approach
03140J1	Bypass Left Subclavian Artery to Left Upper Arm Artery with Synthetic Substitute, Open Approach
03140J2	Bypass Left Subclavian Artery to Bilateral Upper Arm Artery with Synthetic Substitute, Open Approach
03140J3	Bypass Left Subclavian Artery to Right Lower Arm Artery with Synthetic Substitute, Open Approach
03140J4	Bypass Left Subclavian Artery to Left Lower Arm Artery with Synthetic Substitute, Open Approach
03140J5	Bypass Left Subclavian Artery to Bilateral Lower Arm Artery with Synthetic Substitute, Open Approach
03140J6	Bypass Left Subclavian Artery to Right Upper Leg Artery with Synthetic Substitute, Open Approach
03140J7	Bypass Left Subclavian Artery to Left Upper Leg Artery with Synthetic Substitute, Open Approach
03140J8	Bypass Left Subclavian Artery to Bilateral Upper Leg Artery with Synthetic Substitute, Open Approach
03140J9	Bypass Left Subclavian Artery to Right Lower Leg Artery with Synthetic Substitute, Open Approach
03140JB	Bypass Left Subclavian Artery to Left Lower Leg Artery with Synthetic Substitute, Open Approach
03140JC	Bypass Left Subclavian Artery to Bilateral Lower Leg Artery with Synthetic Substitute, Open Approach
03140JD	Bypass Left Subclavian Artery to Upper Arm Vein with Synthetic Substitute, Open Approach
03140JF	Bypass Left Subclavian Artery to Lower Arm Vein with Synthetic Substitute, Open Approach
03140JJ	Bypass Left Subclavian Artery to Right Extracranial Artery with Synthetic Substitute, Open Approach
03140JK	Bypass Left Subclavian Artery to Left Extracranial Artery with Synthetic Substitute, Open Approach
03140JM	Bypass Left Subclavian Artery to Right Pulmonary Artery with Synthetic Substitute, Open Approach
03140JN	Bypass Left Subclavian Artery to Left Pulmonary Artery with Synthetic Substitute, Open Approach
03140JW	Bypass Left Subclavian Artery to Lower Extremity Vein with Synthetic Substitute, Open Approach
03140K0	Bypass Left Subclavian Artery to Right Upper Arm Artery with Nonautologous Tissue Substitute, Open Approach
03140K1	Bypass Left Subclavian Artery to Left Upper Arm Artery with Nonautologous Tissue Substitute, Open Approach
03140K2	Bypass Left Subclavian Artery to Bilateral Upper Arm Artery with Nonautologous Tissue Substitute, Open Approach
03140K3	Bypass Left Subclavian Artery to Right Lower Arm Artery with Nonautologous Tissue Substitute, Open Approach
03140K4	Bypass Left Subclavian Artery to Left Lower Arm Artery with Nonautologous Tissue Substitute, Open Approach
03140K5	Bypass Left Subclavian Artery to Bilateral Lower Arm Artery with Nonautologous Tissue Substitute, Open Approach

03140K6 Bypass Left Subclavian Artery to Right Upper Leg Artery with Nonautologous Tissue Substitute, Open Approach

03140K7 Bypass Left Subclavian Artery to Left Upper Leg Artery with Nonautologous Tissue Substitute, Open Approach

03140K8 Bypass Left Subclavian Artery to Bilateral Upper Leg Artery with Nonautologous Tissue Substitute, Open Approach

03140K9 Bypass Left Subclavian Artery to Right Lower Leg Artery with Nonautologous Tissue Substitute, Open Approach

03140KB Bypass Left Subclavian Artery to Left Lower Leg Artery with Nonautologous Tissue Substitute, Open Approach

03140KC Bypass Left Subclavian Artery to Bilateral Lower Leg Artery with Nonautologous Tissue Substitute, Open Approach

03140KD Bypass Left Subclavian Artery to Upper Arm Vein with Nonautologous Tissue Substitute, Open Approach

03140KF Bypass Left Subclavian Artery to Lower Arm Vein with Nonautologous Tissue Substitute, Open Approach

03140KJ Bypass Left Subclavian Artery to Right Extracranial Artery with Nonautologous Tissue Substitute, Open Approach

03140KK Bypass Left Subclavian Artery to Left Extracranial Artery with Nonautologous Tissue Substitute, Open Approach

03140KM Bypass Left Subclavian Artery to Right Pulmonary Artery with Nonautologous Tissue Substitute, Open Approach

03140KN Bypass Left Subclavian Artery to Left Pulmonary Artery with Nonautologous Tissue Substitute, Open Approach

03140KW Bypass Left Subclavian Artery to Lower Extremity Vein with Nonautologous Tissue Substitute, Open Approach

03140Z0 Bypass Left Subclavian Artery to Right Upper Arm Artery, Open Approach

03140Z1 Bypass Left Subclavian Artery to Left Upper Arm Artery, Open Approach

03140Z2 Bypass Left Subclavian Artery to Bilateral Upper Arm Artery, Open Approach

03140Z3 Bypass Left Subclavian Artery to Right Lower Arm Artery, Open Approach

03140Z4 Bypass Left Subclavian Artery to Left Lower Arm Artery, Open Approach

03140Z5 Bypass Left Subclavian Artery to Bilateral Lower Arm Artery, Open Approach

03140Z6 Bypass Left Subclavian Artery to Right Upper Leg Artery, Open Approach

03140Z7 Bypass Left Subclavian Artery to Left Upper Leg Artery, Open Approach

03140Z8 Bypass Left Subclavian Artery to Bilateral Upper Leg Artery, Open Approach

03140Z9 Bypass Left Subclavian Artery to Right Lower Leg Artery, Open Approach

03140ZB Bypass Left Subclavian Artery to Left Lower Leg Artery, Open Approach

03140ZC Bypass Left Subclavian Artery to Bilateral Lower Leg Artery, Open Approach

03140ZD Bypass Left Subclavian Artery to Upper Arm Vein, Open Approach

03140ZF Bypass Left Subclavian Artery to Lower Arm Vein, Open Approach

03140ZJ Bypass Left Subclavian Artery to Right Extracranial Artery, Open Approach

03140ZK Bypass Left Subclavian Artery to Left Extracranial Artery, Open Approach

03140ZM Bypass Left Subclavian Artery to Right Pulmonary Artery, Open Approach

03140ZN Bypass Left Subclavian Artery to Left Pulmonary Artery, Open Approach

03140ZW Bypass Left Subclavian Artery to Lower Extremity Vein, Open Approach

0315090 Bypass Right Axillary Artery to Right Upper Arm Artery with Autologous Venous Tissue, Open Approach

0315091 Bypass Right Axillary Artery to Left Upper Arm Artery with Autologous Venous Tissue, Open Approach

0315092 Bypass Right Axillary Artery to Bilateral Upper Arm Artery with Autologous Venous Tissue, Open Approach

0315093 Bypass Right Axillary Artery to Right Lower Arm Artery with Autologous Venous Tissue, Open Approach

0315094 Bypass Right Axillary Artery to Left Lower Arm Artery with Autologous Venous Tissue, Open Approach

0315095 Bypass Right Axillary Artery to Bilateral Lower Arm Artery with Autologous Venous Tissue, Open Approach

0315096 Bypass Right Axillary Artery to Right Upper Leg Artery with Autologous Venous Tissue, Open Approach

0315097 Bypass Right Axillary Artery to Left Upper Leg Artery with Autologous Venous Tissue, Open Approach

0315098 Bypass Right Axillary Artery to Bilateral Upper Leg Artery with Autologous Venous Tissue, Open Approach

0315099 Bypass Right Axillary Artery to Right Lower Leg Artery with Autologous Venous Tissue, Open Approach

031509B Bypass Right Axillary Artery to Left Lower Leg Artery with Autologous Venous Tissue, Open Approach

031509C Bypass Right Axillary Artery to Bilateral Lower Leg Artery with Autologous Venous Tissue, Open Approach

031509D Bypass Right Axillary Artery to Upper Arm Vein with Autologous Venous Tissue, Open Approach

031509F Bypass Right Axillary Artery to Lower Arm Vein with Autologous Venous Tissue, Open Approach

031509J Bypass Right Axillary Artery to Right Extracranial Artery with Autologous Venous Tissue, Open Approach

031509K Bypass Right Axillary Artery to Left Extracranial Artery with Autologous Venous Tissue, Open Approach

031509T Bypass Right Axillary Artery to Abdominal Artery with Autologous Venous Tissue, Open Approach

031509V Bypass Right Axillary Artery to Superior Vena Cava with Autologous Venous Tissue, Open Approach

031509W Bypass Right Axillary Artery to Lower Extremity Vein with Autologous Venous Tissue, Open Approach

03150A0 Bypass Right Axillary Artery to Right Upper Arm Artery with Autologous Arterial Tissue, Open Approach

03150A1 Bypass Right Axillary Artery to Left Upper Arm Artery with Autologous Arterial Tissue, Open Approach

03150A2 Bypass Right Axillary Artery to Bilateral Upper Arm Artery with Autologous Arterial Tissue, Open Approach

03150A3 Bypass Right Axillary Artery to Right Lower Arm Artery with Autologous Arterial Tissue, Open Approach

03150A4 Bypass Right Axillary Artery to Left Lower Arm Artery with Autologous Arterial Tissue, Open Approach

03150A5 Bypass Right Axillary Artery to Bilateral Lower Arm Artery with Autologous Arterial Tissue, Open Approach

03150A6 Bypass Right Axillary Artery to Right Upper Leg Artery with Autologous Arterial Tissue, Open Approach

03150A7 Bypass Right Axillary Artery to Left Upper Leg Artery with Autologous Arterial Tissue, Open Approach

03150A8 Bypass Right Axillary Artery to Bilateral Upper Leg Artery with Autologous Arterial Tissue, Open Approach

03150A9 Bypass Right Axillary Artery to Right Lower Leg Artery with Autologous Arterial Tissue, Open Approach

03150AB Bypass Right Axillary Artery to Left Lower Leg Artery with Autologous Arterial Tissue, Open Approach

03150AC Bypass Right Axillary Artery to Bilateral Lower Leg Artery with Autologous Arterial Tissue, Open Approach

03150AD Bypass Right Axillary Artery to Upper Arm Vein with Autologous Arterial Tissue, Open Approach

03150AF Bypass Right Axillary Artery to Lower Arm Vein with Autologous Arterial Tissue, Open Approach

03150AJ Bypass Right Axillary Artery to Right Extracranial Artery with Autologous Arterial Tissue, Open Approach

03150AK Bypass Right Axillary Artery to Left Extracranial Artery with Autologous Arterial Tissue, Open Approach

03150AT Bypass Right Axillary Artery to Abdominal Artery with Autologous Arterial Tissue, Open Approach

03150AV Bypass Right Axillary Artery to Superior Vena Cava with Autologous Arterial Tissue, Open Approach

03150AW Bypass Right Axillary Artery to Lower Extremity Vein with Autologous Arterial Tissue, Open Approach

03150J0 Bypass Right Axillary Artery to Right Upper Arm Artery with Synthetic Substitute, Open Approach

03150J1 Bypass Right Axillary Artery to Left Upper Arm Artery with Synthetic Substitute, Open Approach

03150J2 Bypass Right Axillary Artery to Bilateral Upper Arm Artery with Synthetic Substitute, Open Approach

03150J3 Bypass Right Axillary Artery to Right Lower Arm Artery with Synthetic Substitute, Open Approach

03150J4 Bypass Right Axillary Artery to Left Lower Arm Artery with Synthetic Substitute, Open Approach

03150J5 Bypass Right Axillary Artery to Bilateral Lower Arm Artery with Synthetic Substitute, Open Approach

♀ Female-only   ♂ Male-only   ▲ Limited Coverage   ● Non-OR   ▣ HAC-associated procedure   ▲ Non-covered procedures   ✚ Cluster

03150J6   Bypass Right Axillary Artery to Right Upper Leg Artery with Synthetic Substitute, Open Approach

03150J7   Bypass Right Axillary Artery to Left Upper Leg Artery with Synthetic Substitute, Open Approach

03150J8   Bypass Right Axillary Artery to Bilateral Upper Leg Artery with Synthetic Substitute, Open Approach

03150J9   Bypass Right Axillary Artery to Right Lower Leg Artery with Synthetic Substitute, Open Approach

03150JB   Bypass Right Axillary Artery to Left Lower Leg Artery with Synthetic Substitute, Open Approach

03150JC   Bypass Right Axillary Artery to Bilateral Lower Leg Artery with Synthetic Substitute, Open Approach

03150JD   Bypass Right Axillary Artery to Upper Arm Vein with Synthetic Substitute, Open Approach

03150JF   Bypass Right Axillary Artery to Lower Arm Vein with Synthetic Substitute, Open Approach

03150JJ   Bypass Right Axillary Artery to Right Extracranial Artery with Synthetic Substitute, Open Approach

03150JK   Bypass Right Axillary Artery to Left Extracranial Artery with Synthetic Substitute, Open Approach

03150JT   Bypass Right Axillary Artery to Abdominal Artery with Synthetic Substitute, Open Approach

03150JV   Bypass Right Axillary Artery to Superior Vena Cava with Synthetic Substitute, Open Approach

03150JW   Bypass Right Axillary Artery to Lower Extremity Vein with Synthetic Substitute, Open Approach

03150K0   Bypass Right Axillary Artery to Right Upper Arm Artery with Nonautologous Tissue Substitute, Open Approach

03150K1   Bypass Right Axillary Artery to Left Upper Arm Artery with Nonautologous Tissue Substitute, Open Approach

03150K2   Bypass Right Axillary Artery to Bilateral Upper Arm Artery with Nonautologous Tissue Substitute, Open Approach

03150K3   Bypass Right Axillary Artery to Right Lower Arm Artery with Nonautologous Tissue Substitute, Open Approach

03150K4   Bypass Right Axillary Artery to Left Lower Arm Artery with Nonautologous Tissue Substitute, Open Approach

03150K5   Bypass Right Axillary Artery to Bilateral Lower Arm Artery with Nonautologous Tissue Substitute, Open Approach

03150K6   Bypass Right Axillary Artery to Right Upper Leg Artery with Nonautologous Tissue Substitute, Open Approach

03150K7   Bypass Right Axillary Artery to Left Upper Leg Artery with Nonautologous Tissue Substitute, Open Approach

03150K8   Bypass Right Axillary Artery to Bilateral Upper Leg Artery with Nonautologous Tissue Substitute, Open Approach

03150K9   Bypass Right Axillary Artery to Right Lower Leg Artery with Nonautologous Tissue Substitute, Open Approach

03150KB   Bypass Right Axillary Artery to Left Lower Leg Artery with Nonautologous Tissue Substitute, Open Approach

03150KC   Bypass Right Axillary Artery to Bilateral Lower Leg Artery with Nonautologous Tissue Substitute, Open Approach

03150KD   Bypass Right Axillary Artery to Upper Arm Vein with Nonautologous Tissue Substitute, Open Approach

03150KF   Bypass Right Axillary Artery to Lower Arm Vein with Nonautologous Tissue Substitute, Open Approach

03150KJ   Bypass Right Axillary Artery to Right Extracranial Artery with Nonautologous Tissue Substitute, Open Approach

03150KK   Bypass Right Axillary Artery to Left Extracranial Artery with Nonautologous Tissue Substitute, Open Approach

03150KT   Bypass Right Axillary Artery to Abdominal Artery with Nonautologous Tissue Substitute, Open Approach

03150KV   Bypass Right Axillary Artery to Superior Vena Cava with Nonautologous Tissue Substitute, Open Approach

03150KW   Bypass Right Axillary Artery to Lower Extremity Vein with Nonautologous Tissue Substitute, Open Approach

03150Z0   Bypass Right Axillary Artery to Right Upper Arm Artery, Open Approach

03150Z1   Bypass Right Axillary Artery to Left Upper Arm Artery, Open Approach

03150Z2   Bypass Right Axillary Artery to Bilateral Upper Arm Artery, Open Approach

03150Z3   Bypass Right Axillary Artery to Right Lower Arm Artery, Open Approach

03150Z4   Bypass Right Axillary Artery to Left Lower Arm Artery, Open Approach

03150Z5   Bypass Right Axillary Artery to Bilateral Lower Arm Artery, Open Approach

03150Z6   Bypass Right Axillary Artery to Right Upper Leg Artery, Open Approach

03150Z7   Bypass Right Axillary Artery to Left Upper Leg Artery, Open Approach

03150Z8   Bypass Right Axillary Artery to Bilateral Upper Leg Artery, Open Approach

03150Z9   Bypass Right Axillary Artery to Right Lower Leg Artery, Open Approach

03150ZB   Bypass Right Axillary Artery to Left Lower Leg Artery, Open Approach

03150ZC   Bypass Right Axillary Artery to Bilateral Lower Leg Artery, Open Approach

03150ZD   Bypass Right Axillary Artery to Upper Arm Vein, Open Approach

03150ZF   Bypass Right Axillary Artery to Lower Arm Vein, Open Approach

03150ZJ   Bypass Right Axillary Artery to Right Extracranial Artery, Open Approach

03150ZK   Bypass Right Axillary Artery to Left Extracranial Artery, Open Approach

03150ZT   Bypass Right Axillary Artery to Abdominal Artery, Open Approach

03150ZV   Bypass Right Axillary Artery to Superior Vena Cava, Open Approach

03150ZW   Bypass Right Axillary Artery to Lower Extremity Vein, Open Approach

0316090   Bypass Left Axillary Artery to Right Upper Arm Artery with Autologous Venous Tissue, Open Approach

0316091   Bypass Left Axillary Artery to Left Upper Arm Artery with Autologous Venous Tissue, Open Approach

0316092   Bypass Left Axillary Artery to Bilateral Upper Arm Artery with Autologous Venous Tissue, Open Approach

0316093   Bypass Left Axillary Artery to Right Lower Arm Artery with Autologous Venous Tissue, Open Approach

0316094   Bypass Left Axillary Artery to Left Lower Arm Artery with Autologous Venous Tissue, Open Approach

0316095   Bypass Left Axillary Artery to Bilateral Lower Arm Artery with Autologous Venous Tissue, Open Approach

0316096   Bypass Left Axillary Artery to Right Upper Leg Artery with Autologous Venous Tissue, Open Approach

0316097   Bypass Left Axillary Artery to Left Upper Leg Artery with Autologous Venous Tissue, Open Approach

0316098   Bypass Left Axillary Artery to Bilateral Upper Leg Artery with Autologous Venous Tissue, Open Approach

0316099   Bypass Left Axillary Artery to Right Lower Leg Artery with Autologous Venous Tissue, Open Approach

031609B   Bypass Left Axillary Artery to Left Lower Leg Artery with Autologous Venous Tissue, Open Approach

031609C   Bypass Left Axillary Artery to Bilateral Lower Leg Artery with Autologous Venous Tissue, Open Approach

031609D   Bypass Left Axillary Artery to Upper Arm Vein with Autologous Venous Tissue, Open Approach

031609F   Bypass Left Axillary Artery to Lower Arm Vein with Autologous Venous Tissue, Open Approach

031609J   Bypass Left Axillary Artery to Right Extracranial Artery with Autologous Venous Tissue, Open Approach

031609K   Bypass Left Axillary Artery to Left Extracranial Artery with Autologous Venous Tissue, Open Approach

031609T   Bypass Left Axillary Artery to Abdominal Artery with Autologous Venous Tissue, Open Approach

031609V   Bypass Left Axillary Artery to Superior Vena Cava with Autologous Venous Tissue, Open Approach

031609W   Bypass Left Axillary Artery to Lower Extremity Vein with Autologous Venous Tissue, Open Approach

03160A0   Bypass Left Axillary Artery to Right Upper Arm Artery with Autologous Arterial Tissue, Open Approach

03160A1   Bypass Left Axillary Artery to Left Upper Arm Artery with Autologous Arterial Tissue, Open Approach

03160A2   Bypass Left Axillary Artery to Bilateral Upper Arm Artery with Autologous Arterial Tissue, Open Approach

03160A3   Bypass Left Axillary Artery to Right Lower Arm Artery with Autologous Arterial Tissue, Open Approach

03160A4   Bypass Left Axillary Artery to Left Lower Arm Artery with Autologous Arterial Tissue, Open Approach

03160A5   Bypass Left Axillary Artery to Bilateral Lower Arm Artery with Autologous Arterial Tissue, Open Approach

03160A6   Bypass Left Axillary Artery to Right Upper Leg Artery with Autologous Arterial Tissue, Open Approach

03160A7   Bypass Left Axillary Artery to Left Upper Leg Artery with Autologous Arterial Tissue, Open Approach

03160A8 Bypass Left Axillary Artery to Bilateral Upper Leg Artery with Autologous Arterial Tissue, Open Approach

03160A9 Bypass Left Axillary Artery to Right Lower Leg Artery with Autologous Arterial Tissue, Open Approach

03160AB Bypass Left Axillary Artery to Left Lower Leg Artery with Autologous Arterial Tissue, Open Approach

03160AC Bypass Left Axillary Artery to Bilateral Lower Leg Artery with Autologous Arterial Tissue, Open Approach

03160AD Bypass Left Axillary Artery to Upper Arm Vein with Autologous Arterial Tissue, Open Approach

03160AF Bypass Left Axillary Artery to Lower Arm Vein with Autologous Arterial Tissue, Open Approach

03160AJ Bypass Left Axillary Artery to Right Extracranial Artery with Autologous Arterial Tissue, Open Approach

03160AK Bypass Left Axillary Artery to Left Extracranial Artery with Autologous Arterial Tissue, Open Approach

03160AT Bypass Left Axillary Artery to Abdominal Artery with Autologous Arterial Tissue, Open Approach

03160AV Bypass Left Axillary Artery to Superior Vena Cava with Autologous Arterial Tissue, Open Approach

03160AW Bypass Left Axillary Artery to Lower Extremity Vein with Autologous Arterial Tissue, Open Approach

03160J0 Bypass Left Axillary Artery to Right Upper Arm Artery with Synthetic Substitute, Open Approach

03160J1 Bypass Left Axillary Artery to Left Upper Arm Artery with Synthetic Substitute, Open Approach

03160J2 Bypass Left Axillary Artery to Bilateral Upper Arm Artery with Synthetic Substitute, Open Approach

03160J3 Bypass Left Axillary Artery to Right Lower Arm Artery with Synthetic Substitute, Open Approach

03160J4 Bypass Left Axillary Artery to Left Lower Arm Artery with Synthetic Substitute, Open Approach

03160J5 Bypass Left Axillary Artery to Bilateral Lower Arm Artery with Synthetic Substitute, Open Approach

03160J6 Bypass Left Axillary Artery to Right Upper Leg Artery with Synthetic Substitute, Open Approach

03160J7 Bypass Left Axillary Artery to Left Upper Leg Artery with Synthetic Substitute, Open Approach

03160J8 Bypass Left Axillary Artery to Bilateral Upper Leg Artery with Synthetic Substitute, Open Approach

03160J9 Bypass Left Axillary Artery to Right Lower Leg Artery with Synthetic Substitute, Open Approach

03160JB Bypass Left Axillary Artery to Left Lower Leg Artery with Synthetic Substitute, Open Approach

03160JC Bypass Left Axillary Artery to Bilateral Lower Leg Artery with Synthetic Substitute, Open Approach

03160JD Bypass Left Axillary Artery to Upper Arm Vein with Synthetic Substitute, Open Approach

03160JF Bypass Left Axillary Artery to Lower Arm Vein with Synthetic Substitute, Open Approach

03160JJ Bypass Left Axillary Artery to Right Extracranial Artery with Synthetic Substitute, Open Approach

03160JK Bypass Left Axillary Artery to Left Extracranial Artery with Synthetic Substitute, Open Approach

03160JT Bypass Left Axillary Artery to Abdominal Artery with Synthetic Substitute, Open Approach

03160JV Bypass Left Axillary Artery to Superior Vena Cava with Synthetic Substitute, Open Approach

03160JW Bypass Left Axillary Artery to Lower Extremity Vein with Synthetic Substitute, Open Approach

03160K0 Bypass Left Axillary Artery to Right Upper Arm Artery with Nonautologous Tissue Substitute, Open Approach

03160K1 Bypass Left Axillary Artery to Left Upper Arm Artery with Nonautologous Tissue Substitute, Open Approach

03160K2 Bypass Left Axillary Artery to Bilateral Upper Arm Artery with Nonautologous Tissue Substitute, Open Approach

03160K3 Bypass Left Axillary Artery to Right Lower Arm Artery with Nonautologous Tissue Substitute, Open Approach

03160K4 Bypass Left Axillary Artery to Left Lower Arm Artery with Nonautologous Tissue Substitute, Open Approach

03160K5 Bypass Left Axillary Artery to Bilateral Lower Arm Artery with Nonautologous Tissue Substitute, Open Approach

03160K6 Bypass Left Axillary Artery to Right Upper Leg Artery with Nonautologous Tissue Substitute, Open Approach

03160K7 Bypass Left Axillary Artery to Left Upper Leg Artery with Nonautologous Tissue Substitute, Open Approach

03160K8 Bypass Left Axillary Artery to Bilateral Upper Leg Artery with Nonautologous Tissue Substitute, Open Approach

03160K9 Bypass Left Axillary Artery to Right Lower Leg Artery with Nonautologous Tissue Substitute, Open Approach

03160KB Bypass Left Axillary Artery to Left Lower Leg Artery with Nonautologous Tissue Substitute, Open Approach

03160KC Bypass Left Axillary Artery to Bilateral Lower Leg Artery with Nonautologous Tissue Substitute, Open Approach

03160KD Bypass Left Axillary Artery to Upper Arm Vein with Nonautologous Tissue Substitute, Open Approach

03160KF Bypass Left Axillary Artery to Lower Arm Vein with Nonautologous Tissue Substitute, Open Approach

03160KJ Bypass Left Axillary Artery to Right Extracranial Artery with Nonautologous Tissue Substitute, Open Approach

03160KK Bypass Left Axillary Artery to Left Extracranial Artery with Nonautologous Tissue Substitute, Open Approach

03160KT Bypass Left Axillary Artery to Abdominal Artery with Nonautologous Tissue Substitute, Open Approach

03160KV Bypass Left Axillary Artery to Superior Vena Cava with Nonautologous Tissue Substitute, Open Approach

03160KW Bypass Left Axillary Artery to Lower Extremity Vein with Nonautologous Tissue Substitute, Open Approach

03160Z0 Bypass Left Axillary Artery to Right Upper Arm Artery, Open Approach

03160Z1 Bypass Left Axillary Artery to Left Upper Arm Artery, Open Approach

03160Z2 Bypass Left Axillary Artery to Bilateral Upper Arm Artery, Open Approach

03160Z3 Bypass Left Axillary Artery to Right Lower Arm Artery, Open Approach

03160Z4 Bypass Left Axillary Artery to Left Lower Arm Artery, Open Approach

03160Z5 Bypass Left Axillary Artery to Bilateral Lower Arm Artery, Open Approach

03160Z6 Bypass Left Axillary Artery to Right Upper Leg Artery, Open Approach

03160Z7 Bypass Left Axillary Artery to Left Upper Leg Artery, Open Approach

03160Z8 Bypass Left Axillary Artery to Bilateral Upper Leg Artery, Open Approach

03160Z9 Bypass Left Axillary Artery to Right Lower Leg Artery, Open Approach

03160ZB Bypass Left Axillary Artery to Left Lower Leg Artery, Open Approach

03160ZC Bypass Left Axillary Artery to Bilateral Lower Leg Artery, Open Approach

03160ZD Bypass Left Axillary Artery to Upper Arm Vein, Open Approach

03160ZF Bypass Left Axillary Artery to Lower Arm Vein, Open Approach

03160ZJ Bypass Left Axillary Artery to Right Extracranial Artery, Open Approach

03160ZK Bypass Left Axillary Artery to Left Extracranial Artery, Open Approach

03160ZT Bypass Left Axillary Artery to Abdominal Artery, Open Approach

03160ZV Bypass Left Axillary Artery to Superior Vena Cava, Open Approach

03160ZW Bypass Left Axillary Artery to Lower Extremity Vein, Open Approach

0317090 Bypass Right Brachial Artery to Right Upper Arm Artery with Autologous Venous Tissue, Open Approach

0317093 Bypass Right Brachial Artery to Right Lower Arm Artery with Autologous Venous Tissue, Open Approach

031709D Bypass Right Brachial Artery to Upper Arm Vein with Autologous Venous Tissue, Open Approach

031709F Bypass Right Brachial Artery to Lower Arm Vein with Autologous Venous Tissue, Open Approach

031709V Bypass Right Brachial Artery to Superior Vena Cava with Autologous Venous Tissue, Open Approach

031709W Bypass Right Brachial Artery to Lower Extremity Vein with Autologous Venous Tissue, Open Approach

03170A0 Bypass Right Brachial Artery to Right Upper Arm Artery with Autologous Arterial Tissue, Open Approach

03170A3 Bypass Right Brachial Artery to Right Lower Arm Artery with Autologous Arterial Tissue, Open Approach

03170AD Bypass Right Brachial Artery to Upper Arm Vein with Autologous Arterial Tissue, Open Approach

03170AF Bypass Right Brachial Artery to Lower Arm Vein with Autologous Arterial Tissue, Open Approach

03170AV Bypass Right Brachial Artery to Superior Vena Cava with Autologous Arterial Tissue, Open Approach

03170AW Bypass Right Brachial Artery to Lower Extremity Vein with Autologous Arterial Tissue, Open Approach

03170J0 Bypass Right Brachial Artery to Right Upper Arm Artery with Synthetic Substitute, Open Approach

0317OJ3	Bypass Right Brachial Artery to Right Lower Arm Artery with Synthetic Substitute, Open Approach
0317OJD	Bypass Right Brachial Artery to Upper Arm Vein with Synthetic Substitute, Open Approach
0317OJF	Bypass Right Brachial Artery to Lower Arm Vein with Synthetic Substitute, Open Approach
0317OJV	Bypass Right Brachial Artery to Superior Vena Cava with Synthetic Substitute, Open Approach
0317OJW	Bypass Right Brachial Artery to Lower Extremity Vein with Synthetic Substitute, Open Approach
0317OK0	Bypass Right Brachial Artery to Right Upper Arm Artery with Nonautologous Tissue Substitute, Open Approach
0317OK3	Bypass Right Brachial Artery to Right Lower Arm Artery with Nonautologous Tissue Substitute, Open Approach
0317OKD	Bypass Right Brachial Artery to Upper Arm Vein with Nonautologous Tissue Substitute, Open Approach
0317OKF	Bypass Right Brachial Artery to Lower Arm Vein with Nonautologous Tissue Substitute, Open Approach
0317OKV	Bypass Right Brachial Artery to Superior Vena Cava with Nonautologous Tissue Substitute, Open Approach
0317OKW	Bypass Right Brachial Artery to Lower Extremity Vein with Nonautologous Tissue Substitute, Open Approach
0317OZ0	Bypass Right Brachial Artery to Right Upper Arm Artery, Open Approach
0317OZ3	Bypass Right Brachial Artery to Right Lower Arm Artery, Open Approach
0317OZD	Bypass Right Brachial Artery to Upper Arm Vein, Open Approach
	AHA CC: 4Q, 2013, 125-126
0317OZF	Bypass Right Brachial Artery to Lower Arm Vein, Open Approach
0317OZV	Bypass Right Brachial Artery to Superior Vena Cava, Open Approach
0317OZW	Bypass Right Brachial Artery to Lower Extremity Vein, Open Approach
03173ZF	Bypass Right Brachial Artery to Lower Arm Vein, Percutaneous Approach
0318091	Bypass Left Brachial Artery to Left Upper Arm Artery with Autologous Venous Tissue, Open Approach
0318094	Bypass Left Brachial Artery to Left Lower Arm Artery with Autologous Venous Tissue, Open Approach
031809D	Bypass Left Brachial Artery to Upper Arm Vein with Autologous Venous Tissue, Open Approach
031809F	Bypass Left Brachial Artery to Lower Arm Vein with Autologous Venous Tissue, Open Approach
031809V	Bypass Left Brachial Artery to Superior Vena Cava with Autologous Venous Tissue, Open Approach
031809W	Bypass Left Brachial Artery to Lower Extremity Vein with Autologous Venous Tissue, Open Approach
03180A1	Bypass Left Brachial Artery to Left Upper Arm Artery with Autologous Arterial Tissue, Open Approach
03180A4	Bypass Left Brachial Artery to Left Lower Arm Artery with Autologous Arterial Tissue, Open Approach
03180AD	Bypass Left Brachial Artery to Upper Arm Vein with Autologous Arterial Tissue, Open Approach
03180AF	Bypass Left Brachial Artery to Lower Arm Vein with Autologous Arterial Tissue, Open Approach
03180AV	Bypass Left Brachial Artery to Superior Vena Cava with Autologous Arterial Tissue, Open Approach
03180AW	Bypass Left Brachial Artery to Lower Extremity Vein with Autologous Arterial Tissue, Open Approach
03180J1	Bypass Left Brachial Artery to Left Upper Arm Artery with Synthetic Substitute, Open Approach
03180J4	Bypass Left Brachial Artery to Left Lower Arm Artery with Synthetic Substitute, Open Approach
03180JD	Bypass Left Brachial Artery to Upper Arm Vein with Synthetic Substitute, Open Approach
	AHA CC: 3Q, 2016, 37-38
03180JF	Bypass Left Brachial Artery to Lower Arm Vein with Synthetic Substitute, Open Approach
03180JV	Bypass Left Brachial Artery to Superior Vena Cava with Synthetic Substitute, Open Approach
03180JW	Bypass Left Brachial Artery to Lower Extremity Vein with Synthetic Substitute, Open Approach
03180K1	Bypass Left Brachial Artery to Left Upper Arm Artery with Nonautologous Tissue Substitute, Open Approach
03180K4	Bypass Left Brachial Artery to Left Lower Arm Artery with Nonautologous Tissue Substitute, Open Approach
03180KD	Bypass Left Brachial Artery to Upper Arm Vein with Nonautologous Tissue Substitute, Open Approach
03180KF	Bypass Left Brachial Artery to Lower Arm Vein with Nonautologous Tissue Substitute, Open Approach
03180KV	Bypass Left Brachial Artery to Superior Vena Cava with Nonautologous Tissue Substitute, Open Approach
03180KW	Bypass Left Brachial Artery to Lower Extremity Vein with Nonautologous Tissue Substitute, Open Approach
03180Z1	Bypass Left Brachial Artery to Left Upper Arm Artery, Open Approach
03180Z4	Bypass Left Brachial Artery to Left Lower Arm Artery, Open Approach
03180ZD	Bypass Left Brachial Artery to Upper Arm Vein, Open Approach
03180ZF	Bypass Left Brachial Artery to Lower Arm Vein, Open Approach
03180ZV	Bypass Left Brachial Artery to Superior Vena Cava, Open Approach
03180ZW	Bypass Left Brachial Artery to Lower Extremity Vein, Open Approach
03183ZF	Bypass Left Brachial Artery to Lower Arm Vein, Percutaneous Approach
0319093	Bypass Right Ulnar Artery to Right Lower Arm Artery with Autologous Venous Tissue, Open Approach
031909F	Bypass Right Ulnar Artery to Lower Arm Vein with Autologous Venous Tissue, Open Approach
03190A3	Bypass Right Ulnar Artery to Right Lower Arm Artery with Autologous Arterial Tissue, Open Approach
03190AF	Bypass Right Ulnar Artery to Lower Arm Vein with Autologous Arterial Tissue, Open Approach
03190J3	Bypass Right Ulnar Artery to Right Lower Arm Artery with Synthetic Substitute, Open Approach
03190JF	Bypass Right Ulnar Artery to Lower Arm Vein with Synthetic Substitute, Open Approach
03190K3	Bypass Right Ulnar Artery to Right Lower Arm Artery with Nonautologous Tissue Substitute, Open Approach
03190KF	Bypass Right Ulnar Artery to Lower Arm Vein with Nonautologous Tissue Substitute, Open Approach
03190Z3	Bypass Right Ulnar Artery to Right Lower Arm Artery, Open Approach
03190ZF	Bypass Right Ulnar Artery to Lower Arm Vein, Open Approach
03193ZF	Bypass Right Ulnar Artery to Lower Arm Vein, Percutaneous Approach
031A094	Bypass Left Ulnar Artery to Left Lower Arm Artery with Autologous Venous Tissue, Open Approach
031A09F	Bypass Left Ulnar Artery to Lower Arm Vein with Autologous Venous Tissue, Open Approach
031A0A4	Bypass Left Ulnar Artery to Left Lower Arm Artery with Autologous Arterial Tissue, Open Approach
031A0AF	Bypass Left Ulnar Artery to Lower Arm Vein with Autologous Arterial Tissue, Open Approach
031A0J4	Bypass Left Ulnar Artery to Left Lower Arm Artery with Synthetic Substitute, Open Approach
031A0JF	Bypass Left Ulnar Artery to Lower Arm Vein with Synthetic Substitute, Open Approach
031A0K4	Bypass Left Ulnar Artery to Left Lower Arm Artery with Nonautologous Tissue Substitute, Open Approach
031A0KF	Bypass Left Ulnar Artery to Lower Arm Vein with Nonautologous Tissue Substitute, Open Approach
031A0Z4	Bypass Left Ulnar Artery to Left Lower Arm Artery, Open Approach
031A0ZF	Bypass Left Ulnar Artery to Lower Arm Vein, Open Approach
031A3ZF	Bypass Left Ulnar Artery to Lower Arm Vein, Percutaneous Approach
031B093	Bypass Right Radial Artery to Right Lower Arm Artery with Autologous Venous Tissue, Open Approach
031B09F	Bypass Right Radial Artery to Lower Arm Vein with Autologous Venous Tissue, Open Approach
031B0A3	Bypass Right Radial Artery to Right Lower Arm Artery with Autologous Arterial Tissue, Open Approach
031B0AF	Bypass Right Radial Artery to Lower Arm Vein with Autologous Arterial Tissue, Open Approach
031B0J3	Bypass Right Radial Artery to Right Lower Arm Artery with Synthetic Substitute, Open Approach
031B0JF	Bypass Right Radial Artery to Lower Arm Vein with Synthetic Substitute, Open Approach
031B0K3	Bypass Right Radial Artery to Right Lower Arm Artery with Nonautologous Tissue Substitute, Open Approach
031B0KF	Bypass Right Radial Artery to Lower Arm Vein with Nonautologous Tissue Substitute, Open Approach
031B0Z3	Bypass Right Radial Artery to Right Lower Arm Artery, Open Approach
031B0ZF	Bypass Right Radial Artery to Lower Arm Vein, Open Approach
031B3ZF	Bypass Right Radial Artery to Lower Arm Vein, Percutaneous Approach

031C094 Bypass Left Radial Artery to Left Lower Arm Artery with Autologous Venous Tissue, Open Approach

031C09F Bypass Left Radial Artery to Lower Arm Vein with Autologous Venous Tissue, Open Approach

031C0A4 Bypass Left Radial Artery to Left Lower Arm Artery with Autologous Arterial Tissue, Open Approach

031C0AF Bypass Left Radial Artery to Lower Arm Vein with Autologous Arterial Tissue, Open Approach

031C0J4 Bypass Left Radial Artery to Left Lower Arm Artery with Synthetic Substitute, Open Approach

031C0JF Bypass Left Radial Artery to Lower Arm Vein with Synthetic Substitute, Open Approach

031C0K4 Bypass Left Radial Artery to Left Lower Arm Artery with Nonautologous Tissue Substitute, Open Approach

031C0KF Bypass Left Radial Artery to Lower Arm Vein with Nonautologous Tissue Substitute, Open Approach

031C0Z4 Bypass Left Radial Artery to Left Lower Arm Artery, Open Approach

031C0ZF Bypass Left Radial Artery to Lower Arm Vein, Open Approach
AHA CC: 1Q, 2013, 27-28

031C3ZF Bypass Left Radial Artery to Lower Arm Vein, Percutaneous Approach

031G09G Bypass Intracranial Artery to Intracranial Artery with Autologous Venous Tissue, Open Approach

031G0AG Bypass Intracranial Artery to Intracranial Artery with Autologous Arterial Tissue, Open Approach

031G0JG Bypass Intracranial Artery to Intracranial Artery with Synthetic Substitute, Open Approach

031G0KG Bypass Intracranial Artery to Intracranial Artery with Nonautologous Tissue Substitute, Open Approach

031G0ZG Bypass Intracranial Artery to Intracranial Artery, Open Approach

031H09G Bypass Right Common Carotid Artery to Intracranial Artery with Autologous Venous Tissue, Open Approach

031H09J Bypass Right Common Carotid Artery to Right Extracranial Artery with Autologous Venous Tissue, Open Approach

031H09K Bypass Right Common Carotid Artery to Left Extracranial Artery with Autologous Venous Tissue, Open Approach

031H09Y Bypass Right Common Carotid Artery to Upper Artery with Autologous Venous Tissue, Open Approach

031H0AG Bypass Right Common Carotid Artery to Intracranial Artery with Autologous Arterial Tissue, Open Approach

031H0AJ Bypass Right Common Carotid Artery to Right Extracranial Artery with Autologous Arterial Tissue, Open Approach

031H0AK Bypass Right Common Carotid Artery to Left Extracranial Artery with Autologous Arterial Tissue, Open Approach

031H0AY Bypass Right Common Carotid Artery to Upper Artery with Autologous Arterial Tissue, Open Approach

031H0JG Bypass Right Common Carotid Artery to Intracranial Artery with Synthetic Substitute, Open Approach

031H0JJ Bypass Right Common Carotid Artery to Right Extracranial Artery with Synthetic Substitute, Open Approach

031H0JK Bypass Right Common Carotid Artery to Left Extracranial Artery with Synthetic Substitute, Open Approach

031H0JY Bypass Right Common Carotid Artery to Upper Artery with Synthetic Substitute, Open Approach

031H0KG Bypass Right Common Carotid Artery to Intracranial Artery with Nonautologous Tissue Substitute, Open Approach

031H0KJ Bypass Right Common Carotid Artery to Right Extracranial Artery with Nonautologous Tissue Substitute, Open Approach

031H0KK Bypass Right Common Carotid Artery to Left Extracranial Artery with Nonautologous Tissue Substitute, Open Approach

031H0KY Bypass Right Common Carotid Artery to Upper Artery with Nonautologous Tissue Substitute, Open Approach

031H0ZG Bypass Right Common Carotid Artery to Intracranial Artery, Open Approach

031H0ZJ Bypass Right Common Carotid Artery to Right Extracranial Artery, Open Approach

031H0ZK Bypass Right Common Carotid Artery to Left Extracranial Artery, Open Approach

031H0ZY Bypass Right Common Carotid Artery to Upper Artery, Open Approach

031J09G Bypass Left Common Carotid Artery to Intracranial Artery with Autologous Venous Tissue, Open Approach

031J09J Bypass Left Common Carotid Artery to Right Extracranial Artery with Autologous Venous Tissue, Open Approach

031J09K Bypass Left Common Carotid Artery to Left Extracranial Artery with Autologous Venous Tissue, Open Approach

031J09Y Bypass Left Common Carotid Artery to Upper Artery with Autologous Venous Tissue, Open Approach

031J0AG Bypass Left Common Carotid Artery to Intracranial Artery with Autologous Arterial Tissue, Open Approach

031J0AJ Bypass Left Common Carotid Artery to Right Extracranial Artery with Autologous Arterial Tissue, Open Approach

031J0AK Bypass Left Common Carotid Artery to Left Extracranial Artery with Autologous Arterial Tissue, Open Approach

031J0AY Bypass Left Common Carotid Artery to Upper Artery with Autologous Arterial Tissue, Open Approach

031J0JG Bypass Left Common Carotid Artery to Intracranial Artery with Synthetic Substitute, Open Approach

031J0JJ Bypass Left Common Carotid Artery to Right Extracranial Artery with Synthetic Substitute, Open Approach
AHA CC: 4Q, 2017, 65

031J0JK Bypass Left Common Carotid Artery to Left Extracranial Artery with Synthetic Substitute, Open Approach

031J0JY Bypass Left Common Carotid Artery to Upper Artery with Synthetic Substitute, Open Approach

031J0KG Bypass Left Common Carotid Artery to Intracranial Artery with Nonautologous Tissue Substitute, Open Approach

031J0KJ Bypass Left Common Carotid Artery to Right Extracranial Artery with Nonautologous Tissue Substitute, Open Approach

031J0KK Bypass Left Common Carotid Artery to Left Extracranial Artery with Nonautologous Tissue Substitute, Open Approach

031J0KY Bypass Left Common Carotid Artery to Upper Artery with Nonautologous Tissue Substitute, Open Approach

031J0ZG Bypass Left Common Carotid Artery to Intracranial Artery, Open Approach

031J0ZJ Bypass Left Common Carotid Artery to Right Extracranial Artery, Open Approach

031J0ZK Bypass Left Common Carotid Artery to Left Extracranial Artery, Open Approach
AHA CC: 2Q, 2017, 22

031J0ZY Bypass Left Common Carotid Artery to Upper Artery, Open Approach

031K09J Bypass Right Internal Carotid Artery to Right Extracranial Artery with Autologous Venous Tissue, Open Approach

031K09K Bypass Right Internal Carotid Artery to Left Extracranial Artery with Autologous Venous Tissue, Open Approach

031K0AJ Bypass Right Internal Carotid Artery to Right Extracranial Artery with Autologous Arterial Tissue, Open Approach

031K0AK Bypass Right Internal Carotid Artery to Left Extracranial Artery with Autologous Arterial Tissue, Open Approach

031K0JJ Bypass Right Internal Carotid Artery to Right Extracranial Artery with Synthetic Substitute, Open Approach

031K0JK Bypass Right Internal Carotid Artery to Left Extracranial Artery with Synthetic Substitute, Open Approach

031K0KJ Bypass Right Internal Carotid Artery to Right Extracranial Artery with Nonautologous Tissue Substitute, Open Approach

031K0KK Bypass Right Internal Carotid Artery to Left Extracranial Artery with Nonautologous Tissue Substitute, Open Approach

031K0ZJ Bypass Right Internal Carotid Artery to Right Extracranial Artery, Open Approach

031K0ZK Bypass Right Internal Carotid Artery to Left Extracranial Artery, Open Approach

031L09J Bypass Left Internal Carotid Artery to Right Extracranial Artery with Autologous Venous Tissue, Open Approach

031L09K Bypass Left Internal Carotid Artery to Left Extracranial Artery with Autologous Venous Tissue, Open Approach

031L0AJ Bypass Left Internal Carotid Artery to Right Extracranial Artery with Autologous Arterial Tissue, Open Approach

031L0AK Bypass Left Internal Carotid Artery to Left Extracranial Artery with Autologous Arterial Tissue, Open Approach

♀ Female-only ♂ Male-only ▲ Limited Coverage ● Non-OR ▪ HAC-associated procedure ▲ Non-covered procedures ✛ Cluster

031L0JJ Bypass Left Internal Carotid Artery to Right Extracranial Artery with Synthetic Substitute, Open Approach

031L0JK Bypass Left Internal Carotid Artery to Left Extracranial Artery with Synthetic Substitute, Open Approach

031L0KJ Bypass Left Internal Carotid Artery to Right Extracranial Artery with Nonautologous Tissue Substitute, Open Approach

031L0KK Bypass Left Internal Carotid Artery to Left Extracranial Artery with Nonautologous Tissue Substitute, Open Approach

031L0ZJ Bypass Left Internal Carotid Artery to Right Extracranial Artery, Open Approach

031L0ZK Bypass Left Internal Carotid Artery to Left Extracranial Artery, Open Approach

031M09J Bypass Right External Carotid Artery to Right Extracranial Artery with Autologous Venous Tissue, Open Approach

031M09K Bypass Right External Carotid Artery to Left Extracranial Artery with Autologous Venous Tissue, Open Approach

031M0AJ Bypass Right External Carotid Artery to Right Extracranial Artery with Autologous Arterial Tissue, Open Approach

031M0AK Bypass Right External Carotid Artery to Left Extracranial Artery with Autologous Arterial Tissue, Open Approach

031M0JJ Bypass Right External Carotid Artery to Right Extracranial Artery with Synthetic Substitute, Open Approach

031M0JK Bypass Right External Carotid Artery to Left Extracranial Artery with Synthetic Substitute, Open Approach

031M0KJ Bypass Right External Carotid Artery to Right Extracranial Artery with Nonautologous Tissue Substitute, Open Approach

031M0KK Bypass Right External Carotid Artery to Left Extracranial Artery with Nonautologous Tissue Substitute, Open Approach

031M0ZJ Bypass Right External Carotid Artery to Right Extracranial Artery, Open Approach

031M0ZK Bypass Right External Carotid Artery to Left Extracranial Artery, Open Approach

031N09J Bypass Left External Carotid Artery to Right Extracranial Artery with Autologous Venous Tissue, Open Approach

031N09K Bypass Left External Carotid Artery to Left Extracranial Artery with Autologous Venous Tissue, Open Approach

031N0AJ Bypass Left External Carotid Artery to Right Extracranial Artery with Autologous Arterial Tissue, Open Approach

031N0AK Bypass Left External Carotid Artery to Left Extracranial Artery with Autologous Arterial Tissue, Open Approach

031N0JJ Bypass Left External Carotid Artery to Right Extracranial Artery with Synthetic Substitute, Open Approach

031N0JK Bypass Left External Carotid Artery to Left Extracranial Artery with Synthetic Substitute, Open Approach

031N0KJ Bypass Left External Carotid Artery to Right Extracranial Artery with Nonautologous Tissue Substitute, Open Approach

031N0KK Bypass Left External Carotid Artery to Left Extracranial Artery with Nonautologous Tissue Substitute, Open Approach

031N0ZJ Bypass Left External Carotid Artery to Right Extracranial Artery, Open Approach

031N0ZK Bypass Left External Carotid Artery to Left Extracranial Artery, Open Approach

031S09G Bypass Right Temporal Artery to Intracranial Artery with Autologous Venous Tissue, Open Approach

031S0AG Bypass Right Temporal Artery to Intracranial Artery with Autologous Arterial Tissue, Open Approach

031S0JG Bypass Right Temporal Artery to Intracranial Artery with Synthetic Substitute, Open Approach

031S0KG Bypass Right Temporal Artery to Intracranial Artery with Nonautologous Tissue Substitute, Open Approach

031S0ZG Bypass Right Temporal Artery to Intracranial Artery, Open Approach

031T09G Bypass Left Temporal Artery to Intracranial Artery with Autologous Venous Tissue, Open Approach

031T0AG Bypass Left Temporal Artery to Intracranial Artery with Autologous Arterial Tissue, Open Approach

031T0JG Bypass Left Temporal Artery to Intracranial Artery with Synthetic Substitute, Open Approach

031T0KG Bypass Left Temporal Artery to Intracranial Artery with Nonautologous Tissue Substitute, Open Approach

031T0ZG Bypass Left Temporal Artery to Intracranial Artery, Open Approach

035 – Upper Arteries, Destruction

03500ZZ Destruction of Right Internal Mammary Artery, Open Approach

03503ZZ Destruction of Right Internal Mammary Artery, Percutaneous Approach

03504ZZ Destruction of Right Internal Mammary Artery, Percutaneous Endoscopic Approach

03510ZZ Destruction of Left Internal Mammary Artery, Open Approach

03513ZZ Destruction of Left Internal Mammary Artery, Percutaneous Approach

03514ZZ Destruction of Left Internal Mammary Artery, Percutaneous Endoscopic Approach

03520ZZ Destruction of Innominate Artery, Open Approach

03523ZZ Destruction of Innominate Artery, Percutaneous Approach

03524ZZ Destruction of Innominate Artery, Percutaneous Endoscopic Approach

03530ZZ Destruction of Right Subclavian Artery, Open Approach

03533ZZ Destruction of Right Subclavian Artery, Percutaneous Approach

03534ZZ Destruction of Right Subclavian Artery, Percutaneous Endoscopic Approach

03540ZZ Destruction of Left Subclavian Artery, Open Approach

03543ZZ Destruction of Left Subclavian Artery, Percutaneous Approach

03544ZZ Destruction of Left Subclavian Artery, Percutaneous Endoscopic Approach

03550ZZ Destruction of Right Axillary Artery, Open Approach

03553ZZ Destruction of Right Axillary Artery, Percutaneous Approach

03554ZZ Destruction of Right Axillary Artery, Percutaneous Endoscopic Approach

03560ZZ Destruction of Left Axillary Artery, Open Approach

03563ZZ Destruction of Left Axillary Artery, Percutaneous Approach

03564ZZ Destruction of Left Axillary Artery, Percutaneous Endoscopic Approach

03570ZZ Destruction of Right Brachial Artery, Open Approach

03573ZZ Destruction of Right Brachial Artery, Percutaneous Approach

03574ZZ Destruction of Right Brachial Artery, Percutaneous Endoscopic Approach

03580ZZ Destruction of Left Brachial Artery, Open Approach

03583ZZ Destruction of Left Brachial Artery, Percutaneous Approach

03584ZZ Destruction of Left Brachial Artery, Percutaneous Endoscopic Approach

03590ZZ Destruction of Right Ulnar Artery, Open Approach

03593ZZ Destruction of Right Ulnar Artery, Percutaneous Approach

03594ZZ Destruction of Right Ulnar Artery, Percutaneous Endoscopic Approach

035A0ZZ Destruction of Left Ulnar Artery, Open Approach

035A3ZZ Destruction of Left Ulnar Artery, Percutaneous Approach

035A4ZZ Destruction of Left Ulnar Artery, Percutaneous Endoscopic Approach

035B0ZZ Destruction of Right Radial Artery, Open Approach

035B3ZZ Destruction of Right Radial Artery, Percutaneous Approach

035B4ZZ Destruction of Right Radial Artery, Percutaneous Endoscopic Approach

035C0ZZ Destruction of Left Radial Artery, Open Approach

035C3ZZ Destruction of Left Radial Artery, Percutaneous Approach

035C4ZZ Destruction of Left Radial Artery, Percutaneous Endoscopic Approach

035D0ZZ Destruction of Right Hand Artery, Open Approach

035D3ZZ Destruction of Right Hand Artery, Percutaneous Approach

035D4ZZ Destruction of Right Hand Artery, Percutaneous Endoscopic Approach

035F0ZZ Destruction of Left Hand Artery, Open Approach

035F3ZZ Destruction of Left Hand Artery, Percutaneous Approach

035F4ZZ Destruction of Left Hand Artery, Percutaneous Endoscopic Approach

035G0ZZ Destruction of Intracranial Artery, Open Approach

035G3ZZ Destruction of Intracranial Artery, Percutaneous Approach

035G4ZZ Destruction of Intracranial Artery, Percutaneous Endoscopic Approach

035H0ZZ Destruction of Right Common Carotid Artery, Open Approach

035H3ZZ Destruction of Right Common Carotid Artery, Percutaneous Approach

035H4ZZ Destruction of Right Common Carotid Artery, Percutaneous Endoscopic Approach

035J0ZZ Destruction of Left Common Carotid Artery, Open Approach

035J3ZZ Destruction of Left Common Carotid Artery, Percutaneous Approach

035J4ZZ Destruction of Left Common Carotid Artery, Percutaneous Endoscopic Approach

035K0ZZ Destruction of Right Internal Carotid Artery, Open Approach

035K3ZZ Destruction of Right Internal Carotid Artery, Percutaneous Approach

035K4ZZ Destruction of Right Internal Carotid Artery, Percutaneous Endoscopic Approach

035L0ZZ Destruction of Left Internal Carotid Artery, Open Approach

035L3ZZ Destruction of Left Internal Carotid Artery, Percutaneous Approach

035L4ZZ Destruction of Left Internal Carotid Artery, Percutaneous Endoscopic Approach

035M0ZZ Destruction of Right External Carotid Artery, Open Approach

035M3ZZ Destruction of Right External Carotid Artery, Percutaneous Approach

035M4ZZ Destruction of Right External Carotid Artery, Percutaneous Endoscopic Approach

035N0ZZ Destruction of Left External Carotid Artery, Open Approach

035N3ZZ Destruction of Left External Carotid Artery, Percutaneous Approach

035N4ZZ Destruction of Left External Carotid Artery, Percutaneous Endoscopic Approach

035P0ZZ Destruction of Right Vertebral Artery, Open Approach

035P3ZZ Destruction of Right Vertebral Artery, Percutaneous Approach

035P4ZZ Destruction of Right Vertebral Artery, Percutaneous Endoscopic Approach

035Q0ZZ Destruction of Left Vertebral Artery, Open Approach

035Q3ZZ Destruction of Left Vertebral Artery, Percutaneous Approach

035Q4ZZ Destruction of Left Vertebral Artery, Percutaneous Endoscopic Approach

035R0ZZ Destruction of Face Artery, Open Approach

035R3ZZ Destruction of Face Artery, Percutaneous Approach

035R4ZZ Destruction of Face Artery, Percutaneous Endoscopic Approach

035S0ZZ Destruction of Right Temporal Artery, Open Approach

035S3ZZ Destruction of Right Temporal Artery, Percutaneous Approach

035S4ZZ Destruction of Right Temporal Artery, Percutaneous Endoscopic Approach

035T0ZZ Destruction of Left Temporal Artery, Open Approach

035T3ZZ Destruction of Left Temporal Artery, Percutaneous Approach

035T4ZZ Destruction of Left Temporal Artery, Percutaneous Endoscopic Approach

035U0ZZ Destruction of Right Thyroid Artery, Open Approach

035U3ZZ Destruction of Right Thyroid Artery, Percutaneous Approach

035U4ZZ Destruction of Right Thyroid Artery, Percutaneous Endoscopic Approach

035V0ZZ Destruction of Left Thyroid Artery, Open Approach

035V3ZZ Destruction of Left Thyroid Artery, Percutaneous Approach

035V4ZZ Destruction of Left Thyroid Artery, Percutaneous Endoscopic Approach

035Y0ZZ Destruction of Upper Artery, Open Approach

035Y3ZZ Destruction of Upper Artery, Percutaneous Approach

035Y4ZZ Destruction of Upper Artery, Percutaneous Endoscopic Approach

037 – Upper Arteries, Dilation

037004Z Dilation of Right Internal Mammary Artery with Drug-eluting Intraluminal Device, Open Approach

037005Z Dilation of Right Internal Mammary Artery with Two Drug-eluting Intraluminal Devices, Open Approach

037006Z Dilation of Right Internal Mammary Artery with Three Drug-eluting Intraluminal Devices, Open Approach

037007Z Dilation of Right Internal Mammary Artery with Four or More Drug-eluting Intraluminal Devices, Open Approach

03700D1 Dilation of Right Internal Mammary Artery with Intraluminal Device, using Drug-Coated Balloon, Open Approach

03700DZ Dilation of Right Internal Mammary Artery with Intraluminal Device, Open Approach

03700EZ Dilation of Right Internal Mammary Artery with Two Intraluminal Devices, Open Approach

03700FZ Dilation of Right Internal Mammary Artery with Three Intraluminal Devices, Open Approach

03700GZ Dilation of Right Internal Mammary Artery with Four or More Intraluminal Devices, Open Approach

03700Z1 Dilation of Right Internal Mammary Artery using Drug-Coated Balloon, Open Approach

03700ZZ Dilation of Right Internal Mammary Artery, Open Approach

037034Z Dilation of Right Internal Mammary Artery with Drug-eluting Intraluminal Device, Percutaneous Approach

037035Z Dilation of Right Internal Mammary Artery with Two Drug-eluting Intraluminal Devices, Percutaneous Approach

037036Z Dilation of Right Internal Mammary Artery with Three Drug-eluting Intraluminal Devices, Percutaneous Approach

037037Z Dilation of Right Internal Mammary Artery with Four or More Drug-eluting Intraluminal Devices, Percutaneous Approach

03703D1 Dilation of Right Internal Mammary Artery with Intraluminal Device, using Drug-Coated Balloon, Percutaneous Approach

03703DZ Dilation of Right Internal Mammary Artery with Intraluminal Device, Percutaneous Approach

03703EZ Dilation of Right Internal Mammary Artery with Two Intraluminal Devices, Percutaneous Approach

03703FZ Dilation of Right Internal Mammary Artery with Three Intraluminal Devices, Percutaneous Approach

03703GZ Dilation of Right Internal Mammary Artery with Four or More Intraluminal Devices, Percutaneous Approach

03703Z1 Dilation of Right Internal Mammary Artery using Drug-Coated Balloon, Percutaneous Approach

03703ZZ Dilation of Right Internal Mammary Artery, Percutaneous Approach

037044Z Dilation of Right Internal Mammary Artery with Drug-eluting Intraluminal Device, Percutaneous Endoscopic Approach

037045Z Dilation of Right Internal Mammary Artery with Two Drug-eluting Intraluminal Devices, Percutaneous Endoscopic Approach

037046Z Dilation of Right Internal Mammary Artery with Three Drug-eluting Intraluminal Devices, Percutaneous Endoscopic Approach

037047Z Dilation of Right Internal Mammary Artery with Four or More Drug-eluting Intraluminal Devices, Percutaneous Endoscopic Approach

03704D1 Dilation of Right Internal Mammary Artery with Intraluminal Device, using Drug-Coated Balloon, Percutaneous Endoscopic Approach

03704DZ Dilation of Right Internal Mammary Artery with Intraluminal Device, Percutaneous Endoscopic Approach

03704EZ Dilation of Right Internal Mammary Artery with Two Intraluminal Devices, Percutaneous Endoscopic Approach

03704FZ Dilation of Right Internal Mammary Artery with Three Intraluminal Devices, Percutaneous Endoscopic Approach

03704GZ Dilation of Right Internal Mammary Artery with Four or More Intraluminal Devices, Percutaneous Endoscopic Approach

03704Z1 Dilation of Right Internal Mammary Artery using Drug-Coated Balloon, Percutaneous Endoscopic Approach

03704ZZ Dilation of Right Internal Mammary Artery, Percutaneous Endoscopic Approach

037104Z Dilation of Left Internal Mammary Artery with Drug-eluting Intraluminal Device, Open Approach

037105Z Dilation of Left Internal Mammary Artery with Two Drug-eluting Intraluminal Devices, Open Approach

037106Z Dilation of Left Internal Mammary Artery with Three Drug-eluting Intraluminal Devices, Open Approach

037107Z Dilation of Left Internal Mammary Artery with Four or More Drug-eluting Intraluminal Devices, Open Approach

♀ Female-only   ♂ Male-only   ▲ Limited Coverage   ● Non-OR   HAC HAC-associated procedure   ▲ Non-covered procedures   ✚ Cluster

03710D1 Dilation of Left Internal Mammary Artery with Intraluminal Device, using Drug-Coated Balloon, Open Approach

03710DZ Dilation of Left Internal Mammary Artery with Intraluminal Device, Open Approach

03710EZ Dilation of Left Internal Mammary Artery with Two Intraluminal Devices, Open Approach

03710FZ Dilation of Left Internal Mammary Artery with Three Intraluminal Devices, Open Approach

03710GZ Dilation of Left Internal Mammary Artery with Four or More Intraluminal Devices, Open Approach

03710Z1 Dilation of Left Internal Mammary Artery using Drug-Coated Balloon, Open Approach

03710ZZ Dilation of Left Internal Mammary Artery, Open Approach

037134Z Dilation of Left Internal Mammary Artery with Drug-eluting Intraluminal Device, Percutaneous Approach

037135Z Dilation of Left Internal Mammary Artery with Two Drug-eluting Intraluminal Devices, Percutaneous Approach

037136Z Dilation of Left Internal Mammary Artery with Three Drug-eluting Intraluminal Devices, Percutaneous Approach

037137Z Dilation of Left Internal Mammary Artery with Four or More Drug-eluting Intraluminal Devices, Percutaneous Approach

03713D1 Dilation of Left Internal Mammary Artery with Intraluminal Device, using Drug-Coated Balloon, Percutaneous Approach

03713DZ Dilation of Left Internal Mammary Artery with Intraluminal Device, Percutaneous Approach

03713EZ Dilation of Left Internal Mammary Artery with Two Intraluminal Devices, Percutaneous Approach

03713FZ Dilation of Left Internal Mammary Artery with Three Intraluminal Devices, Percutaneous Approach

03713GZ Dilation of Left Internal Mammary Artery with Four or More Intraluminal Devices, Percutaneous Approach

03713Z1 Dilation of Left Internal Mammary Artery using Drug-Coated Balloon, Percutaneous Approach

03713ZZ Dilation of Left Internal Mammary Artery, Percutaneous Approach

037144Z Dilation of Left Internal Mammary Artery with Drug-eluting Intraluminal Device, Percutaneous Endoscopic Approach

037145Z Dilation of Left Internal Mammary Artery with Two Drug-eluting Intraluminal Devices, Percutaneous Endoscopic Approach

037146Z Dilation of Left Internal Mammary Artery with Three Drug-eluting Intraluminal Devices, Percutaneous Endoscopic Approach

037147Z Dilation of Left Internal Mammary Artery with Four or More Drug-eluting Intraluminal Devices, Percutaneous Endoscopic Approach

03714D1 Dilation of Left Internal Mammary Artery with Intraluminal Device, using Drug-Coated Balloon, Percutaneous Endoscopic Approach

03714DZ Dilation of Left Internal Mammary Artery with Intraluminal Device, Percutaneous Endoscopic Approach

03714EZ Dilation of Left Internal Mammary Artery with Two Intraluminal Devices, Percutaneous Endoscopic Approach

03714FZ Dilation of Left Internal Mammary Artery with Three Intraluminal Devices, Percutaneous Endoscopic Approach

03714GZ Dilation of Left Internal Mammary Artery with Four or More Intraluminal Devices, Percutaneous Endoscopic Approach

03714Z1 Dilation of Left Internal Mammary Artery using Drug-Coated Balloon, Percutaneous Endoscopic Approach

03714ZZ Dilation of Left Internal Mammary Artery, Percutaneous Endoscopic Approach

037204Z Dilation of Innominate Artery with Drug-eluting Intraluminal Device, Open Approach

037205Z Dilation of Innominate Artery with Two Drug-eluting Intraluminal Devices, Open Approach

037206Z Dilation of Innominate Artery with Three Drug-eluting Intraluminal Devices, Open Approach

037207Z Dilation of Innominate Artery with Four or More Drug-eluting Intraluminal Devices, Open Approach

03720D1 Dilation of Innominate Artery with Intraluminal Device, using Drug-Coated Balloon, Open Approach

03720DZ Dilation of Innominate Artery with Intraluminal Device, Open Approach

03720EZ Dilation of Innominate Artery with Two Intraluminal Devices, Open Approach

03720FZ Dilation of Innominate Artery with Three Intraluminal Devices, Open Approach

03720GZ Dilation of Innominate Artery with Four or More Intraluminal Devices, Open Approach

03720Z1 Dilation of Innominate Artery using Drug-Coated Balloon, Open Approach

03720ZZ Dilation of Innominate Artery, Open Approach

037234Z Dilation of Innominate Artery with Drug-eluting Intraluminal Device, Percutaneous Approach

037235Z Dilation of Innominate Artery with Two Drug-eluting Intraluminal Devices, Percutaneous Approach

037236Z Dilation of Innominate Artery with Three Drug-eluting Intraluminal Devices, Percutaneous Approach

037237Z Dilation of Innominate Artery with Four or More Drug-eluting Intraluminal Devices, Percutaneous Approach

03723D1 Dilation of Innominate Artery with Intraluminal Device, using Drug-Coated Balloon, Percutaneous Approach

03723DZ Dilation of Innominate Artery with Intraluminal Device, Percutaneous Approach

03723EZ Dilation of Innominate Artery with Two Intraluminal Devices, Percutaneous Approach

03723FZ Dilation of Innominate Artery with Three Intraluminal Devices, Percutaneous Approach

03723GZ Dilation of Innominate Artery with Four or More Intraluminal Devices, Percutaneous Approach

03723Z1 Dilation of Innominate Artery using Drug-Coated Balloon, Percutaneous Approach

03723ZZ Dilation of Innominate Artery, Percutaneous Approach

037244Z Dilation of Innominate Artery with Drug-eluting Intraluminal Device, Percutaneous Endoscopic Approach

037245Z Dilation of Innominate Artery with Two Drug-eluting Intraluminal Devices, Percutaneous Endoscopic Approach

037246Z Dilation of Innominate Artery with Three Drug-eluting Intraluminal Devices, Percutaneous Endoscopic Approach

037247Z Dilation of Innominate Artery with Four or More Drug-eluting Intraluminal Devices, Percutaneous Endoscopic Approach

03724D1 Dilation of Innominate Artery with Intraluminal Device, using Drug-Coated Balloon, Percutaneous Endoscopic Approach

03724DZ Dilation of Innominate Artery with Intraluminal Device, Percutaneous Endoscopic Approach

03724EZ Dilation of Innominate Artery with Two Intraluminal Devices, Percutaneous Endoscopic Approach

03724FZ Dilation of Innominate Artery with Three Intraluminal Devices, Percutaneous Endoscopic Approach

03724GZ Dilation of Innominate Artery with Four or More Intraluminal Devices, Percutaneous Endoscopic Approach

03724Z1 Dilation of Innominate Artery using Drug-Coated Balloon, Percutaneous Endoscopic Approach

03724ZZ Dilation of Innominate Artery, Percutaneous Endoscopic Approach

037304Z Dilation of Right Subclavian Artery with Drug-eluting Intraluminal Device, Open Approach

037305Z Dilation of Right Subclavian Artery with Two Drug-eluting Intraluminal Devices, Open Approach

037306Z Dilation of Right Subclavian Artery with Three Drug-eluting Intraluminal Devices, Open Approach

037307Z Dilation of Right Subclavian Artery with Four or More Drug-eluting Intraluminal Devices, Open Approach

03730D1 Dilation of Right Subclavian Artery with Intraluminal Device, using Drug-Coated Balloon, Open Approach

03730DZ Dilation of Right Subclavian Artery with Intraluminal Device, Open Approach

03730EZ Dilation of Right Subclavian Artery with Two Intraluminal Devices, Open Approach

03730FZ Dilation of Right Subclavian Artery with Three Intraluminal Devices, Open Approach

03730GZ Dilation of Right Subclavian Artery with Four or More Intraluminal Devices, Open Approach

03730Z1 Dilation of Right Subclavian Artery using Drug-Coated Balloon, Open Approach

03730ZZ Dilation of Right Subclavian Artery, Open Approach

037334Z Dilation of Right Subclavian Artery with Drug-eluting Intraluminal Device, Percutaneous Approach

037335Z Dilation of Right Subclavian Artery with Two Drug-eluting Intraluminal Devices, Percutaneous Approach

037336Z Dilation of Right Subclavian Artery with Three Drug-eluting Intraluminal Devices, Percutaneous Approach

037337Z Dilation of Right Subclavian Artery with Four or More Drug-eluting Intraluminal Devices, Percutaneous Approach

03733D1 Dilation of Right Subclavian Artery with Intraluminal Device, using Drug-Coated Balloon, Percutaneous Approach

03733DZ Dilation of Right Subclavian Artery with Intraluminal Device, Percutaneous Approach

03733EZ Dilation of Right Subclavian Artery with Two Intraluminal Devices, Percutaneous Approach

03733FZ Dilation of Right Subclavian Artery with Three Intraluminal Devices, Percutaneous Approach

03733GZ Dilation of Right Subclavian Artery with Four or More Intraluminal Devices, Percutaneous Approach

03733Z1 Dilation of Right Subclavian Artery using Drug-Coated Balloon, Percutaneous Approach

03733ZZ Dilation of Right Subclavian Artery, Percutaneous Approach

037344Z Dilation of Right Subclavian Artery with Drug-eluting Intraluminal Device, Percutaneous Endoscopic Approach

037345Z Dilation of Right Subclavian Artery with Two Drug-eluting Intraluminal Devices, Percutaneous Endoscopic Approach

037346Z Dilation of Right Subclavian Artery with Three Drug-eluting Intraluminal Devices, Percutaneous Endoscopic Approach

037347Z Dilation of Right Subclavian Artery with Four or More Drug-eluting Intraluminal Devices, Percutaneous Endoscopic Approach

03734D1 Dilation of Right Subclavian Artery with Intraluminal Device, using Drug-Coated Balloon, Percutaneous Endoscopic Approach

03734DZ Dilation of Right Subclavian Artery with Intraluminal Device, Percutaneous Endoscopic Approach

03734EZ Dilation of Right Subclavian Artery with Two Intraluminal Devices, Percutaneous Endoscopic Approach

03734FZ Dilation of Right Subclavian Artery with Three Intraluminal Devices, Percutaneous Endoscopic Approach

03734GZ Dilation of Right Subclavian Artery with Four or More Intraluminal Devices, Percutaneous Endoscopic Approach

03734Z1 Dilation of Right Subclavian Artery using Drug-Coated Balloon, Percutaneous Endoscopic Approach

03734ZZ Dilation of Right Subclavian Artery, Percutaneous Endoscopic Approach

037404Z Dilation of Left Subclavian Artery with Drug-eluting Intraluminal Device, Open Approach

037405Z Dilation of Left Subclavian Artery with Two Drug-eluting Intraluminal Devices, Open Approach

037406Z Dilation of Left Subclavian Artery with Three Drug-eluting Intraluminal Devices, Open Approach

037407Z Dilation of Left Subclavian Artery with Four or More Drug-eluting Intraluminal Devices, Open Approach

03740D1 Dilation of Left Subclavian Artery with Intraluminal Device, using Drug-Coated Balloon, Open Approach

03740DZ Dilation of Left Subclavian Artery with Intraluminal Device, Open Approach

03740EZ Dilation of Left Subclavian Artery with Two Intraluminal Devices, Open Approach

03740FZ Dilation of Left Subclavian Artery with Three Intraluminal Devices, Open Approach

03740GZ Dilation of Left Subclavian Artery with Four or More Intraluminal Devices, Open Approach

03740Z1 Dilation of Left Subclavian Artery using Drug-Coated Balloon, Open Approach

03740ZZ Dilation of Left Subclavian Artery, Open Approach

037434Z Dilation of Left Subclavian Artery with Drug-eluting Intraluminal Device, Percutaneous Approach

037435Z Dilation of Left Subclavian Artery with Two Drug-eluting Intraluminal Devices, Percutaneous Approach

037436Z Dilation of Left Subclavian Artery with Three Drug-eluting Intraluminal Devices, Percutaneous Approach

037437Z Dilation of Left Subclavian Artery with Four or More Drug-eluting Intraluminal Devices, Percutaneous Approach

03743D1 Dilation of Left Subclavian Artery with Intraluminal Device, using Drug-Coated Balloon, Percutaneous Approach

03743DZ Dilation of Left Subclavian Artery with Intraluminal Device, Percutaneous Approach

03743EZ Dilation of Left Subclavian Artery with Two Intraluminal Devices, Percutaneous Approach

03743FZ Dilation of Left Subclavian Artery with Three Intraluminal Devices, Percutaneous Approach

03743GZ Dilation of Left Subclavian Artery with Four or More Intraluminal Devices, Percutaneous Approach

03743Z1 Dilation of Left Subclavian Artery using Drug-Coated Balloon, Percutaneous Approach

03743ZZ Dilation of Left Subclavian Artery, Percutaneous Approach

037444Z Dilation of Left Subclavian Artery with Drug-eluting Intraluminal Device, Percutaneous Endoscopic Approach

037445Z Dilation of Left Subclavian Artery with Two Drug-eluting Intraluminal Devices, Percutaneous Endoscopic Approach

037446Z Dilation of Left Subclavian Artery with Three Drug-eluting Intraluminal Devices, Percutaneous Endoscopic Approach

037447Z Dilation of Left Subclavian Artery with Four or More Drug-eluting Intraluminal Devices, Percutaneous Endoscopic Approach

03744D1 Dilation of Left Subclavian Artery with Intraluminal Device, using Drug-Coated Balloon, Percutaneous Endoscopic Approach

03744DZ Dilation of Left Subclavian Artery with Intraluminal Device, Percutaneous Endoscopic Approach

03744EZ Dilation of Left Subclavian Artery with Two Intraluminal Devices, Percutaneous Endoscopic Approach

03744FZ Dilation of Left Subclavian Artery with Three Intraluminal Devices, Percutaneous Endoscopic Approach

03744GZ Dilation of Left Subclavian Artery with Four or More Intraluminal Devices, Percutaneous Endoscopic Approach

03744Z1 Dilation of Left Subclavian Artery using Drug-Coated Balloon, Percutaneous Endoscopic Approach

03744ZZ Dilation of Left Subclavian Artery, Percutaneous Endoscopic Approach

037504Z Dilation of Right Axillary Artery with Drug-eluting Intraluminal Device, Open Approach

037505Z Dilation of Right Axillary Artery with Two Drug-eluting Intraluminal Devices, Open Approach

037506Z Dilation of Right Axillary Artery with Three Drug-eluting Intraluminal Devices, Open Approach

037507Z Dilation of Right Axillary Artery with Four or More Drug-eluting Intraluminal Devices, Open Approach

03750D1 Dilation of Right Axillary Artery with Intraluminal Device, using Drug-Coated Balloon, Open Approach

03750DZ Dilation of Right Axillary Artery with Intraluminal Device, Open Approach

03750EZ Dilation of Right Axillary Artery with Two Intraluminal Devices, Open Approach

03750FZ Dilation of Right Axillary Artery with Three Intraluminal Devices, Open Approach

03750GZ Dilation of Right Axillary Artery with Four or More Intraluminal Devices, Open Approach

03750Z1 Dilation of Right Axillary Artery using Drug-Coated Balloon, Open Approach

03750ZZ Dilation of Right Axillary Artery, Open Approach

037534Z Dilation of Right Axillary Artery with Drug-eluting Intraluminal Device, Percutaneous Approach

037535Z Dilation of Right Axillary Artery with Two Drug-eluting Intraluminal Devices, Percutaneous Approach

037536Z Dilation of Right Axillary Artery with Three Drug-eluting Intraluminal Devices, Percutaneous Approach

037537Z Dilation of Right Axillary Artery with Four or More Drug-eluting Intraluminal Devices, Percutaneous Approach

03753D1 Dilation of Right Axillary Artery with Intraluminal Device, using Drug-Coated Balloon, Percutaneous Approach

03753DZ Dilation of Right Axillary Artery with Intraluminal Device, Percutaneous Approach

03753EZ Dilation of Right Axillary Artery with Two Intraluminal Devices, Percutaneous Approach

03753FZ Dilation of Right Axillary Artery with Three Intraluminal Devices, Percutaneous Approach

03753GZ Dilation of Right Axillary Artery with Four or More Intraluminal Devices, Percutaneous Approach

03753Z1	Dilation of Right Axillary Artery using Drug-Coated Balloon, Percutaneous Approach
03753ZZ	Dilation of Right Axillary Artery, Percutaneous Approach
037544Z	Dilation of Right Axillary Artery with Drug-eluting Intraluminal Device, Percutaneous Endoscopic Approach
037545Z	Dilation of Right Axillary Artery with Two Drug-eluting Intraluminal Devices, Percutaneous Endoscopic Approach
037546Z	Dilation of Right Axillary Artery with Three Drug-eluting Intraluminal Devices, Percutaneous Endoscopic Approach
037547Z	Dilation of Right Axillary Artery with Four or More Drug-eluting Intraluminal Devices, Percutaneous Endoscopic Approach
03754D1	Dilation of Right Axillary Artery with Intraluminal Device, using Drug-Coated Balloon, Percutaneous Endoscopic Approach
03754DZ	Dilation of Right Axillary Artery with Intraluminal Device, Percutaneous Endoscopic Approach
03754EZ	Dilation of Right Axillary Artery with Two Intraluminal Devices, Percutaneous Endoscopic Approach
03754FZ	Dilation of Right Axillary Artery with Three Intraluminal Devices, Percutaneous Endoscopic Approach
03754GZ	Dilation of Right Axillary Artery with Four or More Intraluminal Devices, Percutaneous Endoscopic Approach
03754Z1	Dilation of Right Axillary Artery using Drug-Coated Balloon, Percutaneous Endoscopic Approach
03754ZZ	Dilation of Right Axillary Artery, Percutaneous Endoscopic Approach
037604Z	Dilation of Left Axillary Artery with Drug-eluting Intraluminal Device, Open Approach
037605Z	Dilation of Left Axillary Artery with Two Drug-eluting Intraluminal Devices, Open Approach
037606Z	Dilation of Left Axillary Artery with Three Drug-eluting Intraluminal Devices, Open Approach
037607Z	Dilation of Left Axillary Artery with Four or More Drug-eluting Intraluminal Devices, Open Approach
03760D1	Dilation of Left Axillary Artery with Intraluminal Device, using Drug-Coated Balloon, Open Approach
03760DZ	Dilation of Left Axillary Artery with Intraluminal Device, Open Approach
03760EZ	Dilation of Left Axillary Artery with Two Intraluminal Devices, Open Approach
03760FZ	Dilation of Left Axillary Artery with Three Intraluminal Devices, Open Approach
03760GZ	Dilation of Left Axillary Artery with Four or More Intraluminal Devices, Open Approach
03760Z1	Dilation of Left Axillary Artery using Drug-Coated Balloon, Open Approach
03760ZZ	Dilation of Left Axillary Artery, Open Approach
037634Z	Dilation of Left Axillary Artery with Drug-eluting Intraluminal Device, Percutaneous Approach
037635Z	Dilation of Left Axillary Artery with Two Drug-eluting Intraluminal Devices, Percutaneous Approach
037636Z	Dilation of Left Axillary Artery with Three Drug-eluting Intraluminal Devices, Percutaneous Approach
037637Z	Dilation of Left Axillary Artery with Four or More Drug-eluting Intraluminal Devices, Percutaneous Approach
03763D1	Dilation of Left Axillary Artery with Intraluminal Device, using Drug-Coated Balloon, Percutaneous Approach
03763DZ	Dilation of Left Axillary Artery with Intraluminal Device, Percutaneous Approach
03763EZ	Dilation of Left Axillary Artery with Two Intraluminal Devices, Percutaneous Approach
03763FZ	Dilation of Left Axillary Artery with Three Intraluminal Devices, Percutaneous Approach
03763GZ	Dilation of Left Axillary Artery with Four or More Intraluminal Devices, Percutaneous Approach
03763Z1	Dilation of Left Axillary Artery using Drug-Coated Balloon, Percutaneous Approach
03763ZZ	Dilation of Left Axillary Artery, Percutaneous Approach
037644Z	Dilation of Left Axillary Artery with Drug-eluting Intraluminal Device, Percutaneous Endoscopic Approach
037645Z	Dilation of Left Axillary Artery with Two Drug-eluting Intraluminal Devices, Percutaneous Endoscopic Approach
037646Z	Dilation of Left Axillary Artery with Three Drug-eluting Intraluminal Devices, Percutaneous Endoscopic Approach
037647Z	Dilation of Left Axillary Artery with Four or More Drug-eluting Intraluminal Devices, Percutaneous Endoscopic Approach
03764D1	Dilation of Left Axillary Artery with Intraluminal Device, using Drug-Coated Balloon, Percutaneous Endoscopic Approach
03764DZ	Dilation of Left Axillary Artery with Intraluminal Device, Percutaneous Endoscopic Approach
03764EZ	Dilation of Left Axillary Artery with Two Intraluminal Devices, Percutaneous Endoscopic Approach
03764FZ	Dilation of Left Axillary Artery with Three Intraluminal Devices, Percutaneous Endoscopic Approach
03764GZ	Dilation of Left Axillary Artery with Four or More Intraluminal Devices, Percutaneous Endoscopic Approach
03764Z1	Dilation of Left Axillary Artery using Drug-Coated Balloon, Percutaneous Endoscopic Approach
03764ZZ	Dilation of Left Axillary Artery, Percutaneous Endoscopic Approach
037704Z	Dilation of Right Brachial Artery with Drug-eluting Intraluminal Device, Open Approach
037705Z	Dilation of Right Brachial Artery with Two Drug-eluting Intraluminal Devices, Open Approach
037706Z	Dilation of Right Brachial Artery with Three Drug-eluting Intraluminal Devices, Open Approach
037707Z	Dilation of Right Brachial Artery with Four or More Drug-eluting Intraluminal Devices, Open Approach
03770D1	Dilation of Right Brachial Artery with Intraluminal Device, using Drug-Coated Balloon, Open Approach
03770DZ	Dilation of Right Brachial Artery with Intraluminal Device, Open Approach
03770EZ	Dilation of Right Brachial Artery with Two Intraluminal Devices, Open Approach
03770FZ	Dilation of Right Brachial Artery with Three Intraluminal Devices, Open Approach
03770GZ	Dilation of Right Brachial Artery with Four or More Intraluminal Devices, Open Approach
03770Z1	Dilation of Right Brachial Artery using Drug-Coated Balloon, Open Approach
03770ZZ	Dilation of Right Brachial Artery, Open Approach
037734Z	Dilation of Right Brachial Artery with Drug-eluting Intraluminal Device, Percutaneous Approach
037735Z	Dilation of Right Brachial Artery with Two Drug-eluting Intraluminal Devices, Percutaneous Approach
037736Z	Dilation of Right Brachial Artery with Three Drug-eluting Intraluminal Devices, Percutaneous Approach
037737Z	Dilation of Right Brachial Artery with Four or More Drug-eluting Intraluminal Devices, Percutaneous Approach
03773D1	Dilation of Right Brachial Artery with Intraluminal Device, using Drug-Coated Balloon, Percutaneous Approach
03773DZ	Dilation of Right Brachial Artery with Intraluminal Device, Percutaneous Approach
03773EZ	Dilation of Right Brachial Artery with Two Intraluminal Devices, Percutaneous Approach
03773FZ	Dilation of Right Brachial Artery with Three Intraluminal Devices, Percutaneous Approach
03773GZ	Dilation of Right Brachial Artery with Four or More Intraluminal Devices, Percutaneous Approach
03773Z1	Dilation of Right Brachial Artery using Drug-Coated Balloon, Percutaneous Approach
03773ZZ	Dilation of Right Brachial Artery, Percutaneous Approach
037744Z	Dilation of Right Brachial Artery with Drug-eluting Intraluminal Device, Percutaneous Endoscopic Approach
037745Z	Dilation of Right Brachial Artery with Two Drug-eluting Intraluminal Devices, Percutaneous Endoscopic Approach
037746Z	Dilation of Right Brachial Artery with Three Drug-eluting Intraluminal Devices, Percutaneous Endoscopic Approach
037747Z	Dilation of Right Brachial Artery with Four or More Drug-eluting Intraluminal Devices, Percutaneous Endoscopic Approach
03774D1	Dilation of Right Brachial Artery with Intraluminal Device, using Drug-Coated Balloon, Percutaneous Endoscopic Approach
03774DZ	Dilation of Right Brachial Artery with Intraluminal Device, Percutaneous Endoscopic Approach

03774EZ Dilation of Right Brachial Artery with Two Intraluminal Devices, Percutaneous Endoscopic Approach

03774FZ Dilation of Right Brachial Artery with Three Intraluminal Devices, Percutaneous Endoscopic Approach

03774GZ Dilation of Right Brachial Artery with Four or More Intraluminal Devices, Percutaneous Endoscopic Approach

03774Z1 Dilation of Right Brachial Artery using Drug-Coated Balloon, Percutaneous Endoscopic Approach

03774ZZ Dilation of Right Brachial Artery, Percutaneous Endoscopic Approach

037804Z Dilation of Left Brachial Artery with Drug-eluting Intraluminal Device, Open Approach

037805Z Dilation of Left Brachial Artery with Two Drug-eluting Intraluminal Devices, Open Approach

037806Z Dilation of Left Brachial Artery with Three Drug-eluting Intraluminal Devices, Open Approach

037807Z Dilation of Left Brachial Artery with Four or More Drug-eluting Intraluminal Devices, Open Approach

03780D1 Dilation of Left Brachial Artery with Intraluminal Device, using Drug-Coated Balloon, Open Approach

03780DZ Dilation of Left Brachial Artery with Intraluminal Device, Open Approach

03780EZ Dilation of Left Brachial Artery with Two Intraluminal Devices, Open Approach

03780FZ Dilation of Left Brachial Artery with Three Intraluminal Devices, Open Approach

03780GZ Dilation of Left Brachial Artery with Four or More Intraluminal Devices, Open Approach

03780Z1 Dilation of Left Brachial Artery using Drug-Coated Balloon, Open Approach

03780ZZ Dilation of Left Brachial Artery, Open Approach

037834Z Dilation of Left Brachial Artery with Drug-eluting Intraluminal Device, Percutaneous Approach

037835Z Dilation of Left Brachial Artery with Two Drug-eluting Intraluminal Devices, Percutaneous Approach

037836Z Dilation of Left Brachial Artery with Three Drug-eluting Intraluminal Devices, Percutaneous Approach

037837Z Dilation of Left Brachial Artery with Four or More Drug-eluting Intraluminal Devices, Percutaneous Approach

03783D1 Dilation of Left Brachial Artery with Intraluminal Device, using Drug-Coated Balloon, Percutaneous Approach

03783DZ Dilation of Left Brachial Artery with Intraluminal Device, Percutaneous Approach

03783EZ Dilation of Left Brachial Artery with Two Intraluminal Devices, Percutaneous Approach

03783FZ Dilation of Left Brachial Artery with Three Intraluminal Devices, Percutaneous Approach

03783GZ Dilation of Left Brachial Artery with Four or More Intraluminal Devices, Percutaneous Approach

03783Z1 Dilation of Left Brachial Artery using Drug-Coated Balloon, Percutaneous Approach

03783ZZ Dilation of Left Brachial Artery, Percutaneous Approach

037844Z Dilation of Left Brachial Artery with Drug-eluting Intraluminal Device, Percutaneous Endoscopic Approach

037845Z Dilation of Left Brachial Artery with Two Drug-eluting Intraluminal Devices, Percutaneous Endoscopic Approach

037846Z Dilation of Left Brachial Artery with Three Drug-eluting Intraluminal Devices, Percutaneous Endoscopic Approach

037847Z Dilation of Left Brachial Artery with Four or More Drug-eluting Intraluminal Devices, Percutaneous Endoscopic Approach

03784D1 Dilation of Left Brachial Artery with Intraluminal Device, using Drug-Coated Balloon, Percutaneous Endoscopic Approach

03784DZ Dilation of Left Brachial Artery with Intraluminal Device, Percutaneous Endoscopic Approach

03784EZ Dilation of Left Brachial Artery with Two Intraluminal Devices, Percutaneous Endoscopic Approach

03784FZ Dilation of Left Brachial Artery with Three Intraluminal Devices, Percutaneous Endoscopic Approach

03784GZ Dilation of Left Brachial Artery with Four or More Intraluminal Devices, Percutaneous Endoscopic Approach

03784Z1 Dilation of Left Brachial Artery using Drug-Coated Balloon, Percutaneous Endoscopic Approach

03784ZZ Dilation of Left Brachial Artery, Percutaneous Endoscopic Approach

037904Z Dilation of Right Ulnar Artery with Drug-eluting Intraluminal Device, Open Approach

037905Z Dilation of Right Ulnar Artery with Two Drug-eluting Intraluminal Devices, Open Approach

037906Z Dilation of Right Ulnar Artery with Three Drug-eluting Intraluminal Devices, Open Approach

037907Z Dilation of Right Ulnar Artery with Four or More Drug-eluting Intraluminal Devices, Open Approach

03790D1 Dilation of Right Ulnar Artery with Intraluminal Device, using Drug-Coated Balloon, Open Approach

03790DZ Dilation of Right Ulnar Artery with Intraluminal Device, Open Approach

03790EZ Dilation of Right Ulnar Artery with Two Intraluminal Devices, Open Approach

03790FZ Dilation of Right Ulnar Artery with Three Intraluminal Devices, Open Approach

03790GZ Dilation of Right Ulnar Artery with Four or More Intraluminal Devices, Open Approach

03790Z1 Dilation of Right Ulnar Artery using Drug-Coated Balloon, Open Approach

03790ZZ Dilation of Right Ulnar Artery, Open Approach

037934Z Dilation of Right Ulnar Artery with Drug-eluting Intraluminal Device, Percutaneous Approach

037935Z Dilation of Right Ulnar Artery with Two Drug-eluting Intraluminal Devices, Percutaneous Approach

037936Z Dilation of Right Ulnar Artery with Three Drug-eluting Intraluminal Devices, Percutaneous Approach

037937Z Dilation of Right Ulnar Artery with Four or More Drug-eluting Intraluminal Devices, Percutaneous Approach

03793D1 Dilation of Right Ulnar Artery with Intraluminal Device, using Drug-Coated Balloon, Percutaneous Approach

03793DZ Dilation of Right Ulnar Artery with Intraluminal Device, Percutaneous Approach

03793EZ Dilation of Right Ulnar Artery with Two Intraluminal Devices, Percutaneous Approach

03793FZ Dilation of Right Ulnar Artery with Three Intraluminal Devices, Percutaneous Approach

03793GZ Dilation of Right Ulnar Artery with Four or More Intraluminal Devices, Percutaneous Approach

03793Z1 Dilation of Right Ulnar Artery using Drug-Coated Balloon, Percutaneous Approach

03793ZZ Dilation of Right Ulnar Artery, Percutaneous Approach

037944Z Dilation of Right Ulnar Artery with Drug-eluting Intraluminal Device, Percutaneous Endoscopic Approach

037945Z Dilation of Right Ulnar Artery with Two Drug-eluting Intraluminal Devices, Percutaneous Endoscopic Approach

037946Z Dilation of Right Ulnar Artery with Three Drug-eluting Intraluminal Devices, Percutaneous Endoscopic Approach

037947Z Dilation of Right Ulnar Artery with Four or More Drug-eluting Intraluminal Devices, Percutaneous Endoscopic Approach

03794D1 Dilation of Right Ulnar Artery with Intraluminal Device, using Drug-Coated Balloon, Percutaneous Endoscopic Approach

03794DZ Dilation of Right Ulnar Artery with Intraluminal Device, Percutaneous Endoscopic Approach

03794EZ Dilation of Right Ulnar Artery with Two Intraluminal Devices, Percutaneous Endoscopic Approach

03794FZ Dilation of Right Ulnar Artery with Three Intraluminal Devices, Percutaneous Endoscopic Approach

03794GZ Dilation of Right Ulnar Artery with Four or More Intraluminal Devices, Percutaneous Endoscopic Approach

03794Z1 Dilation of Right Ulnar Artery using Drug-Coated Balloon, Percutaneous Endoscopic Approach

03794ZZ Dilation of Right Ulnar Artery, Percutaneous Endoscopic Approach

037A04Z Dilation of Left Ulnar Artery with Drug-eluting Intraluminal Device, Open Approach

037A05Z Dilation of Left Ulnar Artery with Two Drug-eluting Intraluminal Devices, Open Approach

037A06Z Dilation of Left Ulnar Artery with Three Drug-eluting Intraluminal Devices, Open Approach

037A07Z Dilation of Left Ulnar Artery with Four or More Drug-eluting Intraluminal Devices, Open Approach

037A0D1 Dilation of Left Ulnar Artery with Intraluminal Device, using Drug-Coated Balloon, Open Approach

♀ Female-only   ♂ Male-only   ▲ Limited Coverage   ● Non-OR   **HAC** HAC-associated procedure   ▲ Non-covered procedures   ➕ Cluster

037A0DZ Dilation of Left Ulnar Artery with Intraluminal Device, Open Approach
037A0EZ Dilation of Left Ulnar Artery with Two Intraluminal Devices, Open Approach
037A0FZ Dilation of Left Ulnar Artery with Three Intraluminal Devices, Open Approach
037A0GZ Dilation of Left Ulnar Artery with Four or More Intraluminal Devices, Open Approach
037A0Z1 Dilation of Left Ulnar Artery using Drug-Coated Balloon, Open Approach
037A0ZZ Dilation of Left Ulnar Artery, Open Approach
037A34Z Dilation of Left Ulnar Artery with Drug-eluting Intraluminal Device, Percutaneous Approach
037A35Z Dilation of Left Ulnar Artery with Two Drug-eluting Intraluminal Devices, Percutaneous Approach
037A36Z Dilation of Left Ulnar Artery with Three Drug-eluting Intraluminal Devices, Percutaneous Approach
037A37Z Dilation of Left Ulnar Artery with Four or More Drug-eluting Intraluminal Devices, Percutaneous Approach
037A3D1 Dilation of Left Ulnar Artery with Intraluminal Device, using Drug-Coated Balloon, Percutaneous Approach
037A3DZ Dilation of Left Ulnar Artery with Intraluminal Device, Percutaneous Approach
037A3EZ Dilation of Left Ulnar Artery with Two Intraluminal Devices, Percutaneous Approach
037A3FZ Dilation of Left Ulnar Artery with Three Intraluminal Devices, Percutaneous Approach
037A3GZ Dilation of Left Ulnar Artery with Four or More Intraluminal Devices, Percutaneous Approach
037A3Z1 Dilation of Left Ulnar Artery using Drug-Coated Balloon, Percutaneous Approach
037A3ZZ Dilation of Left Ulnar Artery, Percutaneous Approach
037A44Z Dilation of Left Ulnar Artery with Drug-eluting Intraluminal Device, Percutaneous Endoscopic Approach
037A45Z Dilation of Left Ulnar Artery with Two Drug-eluting Intraluminal Devices, Percutaneous Endoscopic Approach
037A46Z Dilation of Left Ulnar Artery with Three Drug-eluting Intraluminal Devices, Percutaneous Endoscopic Approach
037A47Z Dilation of Left Ulnar Artery with Four or More Drug-eluting Intraluminal Devices, Percutaneous Endoscopic Approach
037A4D1 Dilation of Left Ulnar Artery with Intraluminal Device, using Drug-Coated Balloon, Percutaneous Endoscopic Approach
037A4DZ Dilation of Left Ulnar Artery with Intraluminal Device, Percutaneous Endoscopic Approach
037A4EZ Dilation of Left Ulnar Artery with Two Intraluminal Devices, Percutaneous Endoscopic Approach
037A4FZ Dilation of Left Ulnar Artery with Three Intraluminal Devices, Percutaneous Endoscopic Approach
037A4GZ Dilation of Left Ulnar Artery with Four or More Intraluminal Devices, Percutaneous Endoscopic Approach

037A4Z1 Dilation of Left Ulnar Artery using Drug-Coated Balloon, Percutaneous Endoscopic Approach
037A4ZZ Dilation of Left Ulnar Artery, Percutaneous Endoscopic Approach
037B04Z Dilation of Right Radial Artery with Drug-eluting Intraluminal Device, Open Approach
037B05Z Dilation of Right Radial Artery with Two Drug-eluting Intraluminal Devices, Open Approach
037B06Z Dilation of Right Radial Artery with Three Drug-eluting Intraluminal Devices, Open Approach
037B07Z Dilation of Right Radial Artery with Four or More Drug-eluting Intraluminal Devices, Open Approach
037B0D1 Dilation of Right Radial Artery with Intraluminal Device, using Drug-Coated Balloon, Open Approach
037B0DZ Dilation of Right Radial Artery with Intraluminal Device, Open Approach
037B0EZ Dilation of Right Radial Artery with Two Intraluminal Devices, Open Approach
037B0FZ Dilation of Right Radial Artery with Three Intraluminal Devices, Open Approach
037B0GZ Dilation of Right Radial Artery with Four or More Intraluminal Devices, Open Approach
037B0Z1 Dilation of Right Radial Artery using Drug-Coated Balloon, Open Approach
037B0ZZ Dilation of Right Radial Artery, Open Approach
037B34Z Dilation of Right Radial Artery with Drug-eluting Intraluminal Device, Percutaneous Approach
037B35Z Dilation of Right Radial Artery with Two Drug-eluting Intraluminal Devices, Percutaneous Approach
037B36Z Dilation of Right Radial Artery with Three Drug-eluting Intraluminal Devices, Percutaneous Approach
037B37Z Dilation of Right Radial Artery with Four or More Drug-eluting Intraluminal Devices, Percutaneous Approach
037B3D1 Dilation of Right Radial Artery with Intraluminal Device, using Drug-Coated Balloon, Percutaneous Approach
037B3DZ Dilation of Right Radial Artery with Intraluminal Device, Percutaneous Approach
037B3EZ Dilation of Right Radial Artery with Two Intraluminal Devices, Percutaneous Approach
037B3FZ Dilation of Right Radial Artery with Three Intraluminal Devices, Percutaneous Approach
037B3GZ Dilation of Right Radial Artery with Four or More Intraluminal Devices, Percutaneous Approach
037B3Z1 Dilation of Right Radial Artery using Drug-Coated Balloon, Percutaneous Approach
037B3ZZ Dilation of Right Radial Artery, Percutaneous Approach
037B44Z Dilation of Right Radial Artery with Drug-eluting Intraluminal Device, Percutaneous Endoscopic Approach
037B45Z Dilation of Right Radial Artery with Two Drug-eluting Intraluminal Devices, Percutaneous Endoscopic Approach
037B46Z Dilation of Right Radial Artery with Three Drug-eluting Intraluminal Devices, Percutaneous Endoscopic Approach

037B47Z Dilation of Right Radial Artery with Four or More Drug-eluting Intraluminal Devices, Percutaneous Endoscopic Approach
037B4D1 Dilation of Right Radial Artery with Intraluminal Device, using Drug-Coated Balloon, Percutaneous Endoscopic Approach
037B4DZ Dilation of Right Radial Artery with Intraluminal Device, Percutaneous Endoscopic Approach
037B4EZ Dilation of Right Radial Artery with Two Intraluminal Devices, Percutaneous Endoscopic Approach
037B4FZ Dilation of Right Radial Artery with Three Intraluminal Devices, Percutaneous Endoscopic Approach
037B4GZ Dilation of Right Radial Artery with Four or More Intraluminal Devices, Percutaneous Endoscopic Approach
037B4Z1 Dilation of Right Radial Artery using Drug-Coated Balloon, Percutaneous Endoscopic Approach
037B4ZZ Dilation of Right Radial Artery, Percutaneous Endoscopic Approach
037C04Z Dilation of Left Radial Artery with Drug-eluting Intraluminal Device, Open Approach
037C05Z Dilation of Left Radial Artery with Two Drug-eluting Intraluminal Devices, Open Approach
037C06Z Dilation of Left Radial Artery with Three Drug-eluting Intraluminal Devices, Open Approach
037C07Z Dilation of Left Radial Artery with Four or More Drug-eluting Intraluminal Devices, Open Approach
037C0D1 Dilation of Left Radial Artery with Intraluminal Device, using Drug-Coated Balloon, Open Approach
037C0DZ Dilation of Left Radial Artery with Intraluminal Device, Open Approach
037C0EZ Dilation of Left Radial Artery with Two Intraluminal Devices, Open Approach
037C0FZ Dilation of Left Radial Artery with Three Intraluminal Devices, Open Approach
037C0GZ Dilation of Left Radial Artery with Four or More Intraluminal Devices, Open Approach
037C0Z1 Dilation of Left Radial Artery using Drug-Coated Balloon, Open Approach
037C0ZZ Dilation of Left Radial Artery, Open Approach
037C34Z Dilation of Left Radial Artery with Drug-eluting Intraluminal Device, Percutaneous Approach
037C35Z Dilation of Left Radial Artery with Two Drug-eluting Intraluminal Devices, Percutaneous Approach
037C36Z Dilation of Left Radial Artery with Three Drug-eluting Intraluminal Devices, Percutaneous Approach
037C37Z Dilation of Left Radial Artery with Four or More Drug-eluting Intraluminal Devices, Percutaneous Approach
037C3D1 Dilation of Left Radial Artery with Intraluminal Device, using Drug-Coated Balloon, Percutaneous Approach
037C3DZ Dilation of Left Radial Artery with Intraluminal Device, Percutaneous Approach
037C3EZ Dilation of Left Radial Artery with Two Intraluminal Devices, Percutaneous Approach

037C3FZ Dilation of Left Radial Artery with Three Intraluminal Devices, Percutaneous Approach

037C3GZ Dilation of Left Radial Artery with Four or More Intraluminal Devices, Percutaneous Approach

037C3Z1 Dilation of Left Radial Artery using Drug-Coated Balloon, Percutaneous Approach

037C3ZZ Dilation of Left Radial Artery, Percutaneous Approach

037C44Z Dilation of Left Radial Artery with Drug-eluting Intraluminal Device, Percutaneous Endoscopic Approach

037C45Z Dilation of Left Radial Artery with Two Drug-eluting Intraluminal Devices, Percutaneous Endoscopic Approach

037C46Z Dilation of Left Radial Artery with Three Drug-eluting Intraluminal Devices, Percutaneous Endoscopic Approach

037C47Z Dilation of Left Radial Artery with Four or More Drug-eluting Intraluminal Devices, Percutaneous Endoscopic Approach

037C4D1 Dilation of Left Radial Artery with Intraluminal Device, using Drug-Coated Balloon, Percutaneous Endoscopic Approach

037C4DZ Dilation of Left Radial Artery with Intraluminal Device, Percutaneous Endoscopic Approach

037C4EZ Dilation of Left Radial Artery with Two Intraluminal Devices, Percutaneous Endoscopic Approach

037C4FZ Dilation of Left Radial Artery with Three Intraluminal Devices, Percutaneous Endoscopic Approach

037C4GZ Dilation of Left Radial Artery with Four or More Intraluminal Devices, Percutaneous Endoscopic Approach

037C4Z1 Dilation of Left Radial Artery using Drug-Coated Balloon, Percutaneous Endoscopic Approach

037C4ZZ Dilation of Left Radial Artery, Percutaneous Endoscopic Approach

037D04Z Dilation of Right Hand Artery with Drug-eluting Intraluminal Device, Open Approach

037D05Z Dilation of Right Hand Artery with Two Drug-eluting Intraluminal Devices, Open Approach

037D06Z Dilation of Right Hand Artery with Three Drug-eluting Intraluminal Devices, Open Approach

037D07Z Dilation of Right Hand Artery with Four or More Drug-eluting Intraluminal Devices, Open Approach

037D0DZ Dilation of Right Hand Artery with Intraluminal Device, Open Approach

037D0EZ Dilation of Right Hand Artery with Two Intraluminal Devices, Open Approach

037D0FZ Dilation of Right Hand Artery with Three Intraluminal Devices, Open Approach

037D0GZ Dilation of Right Hand Artery with Four or More Intraluminal Devices, Open Approach

037D0ZZ Dilation of Right Hand Artery, Open Approach

037D34Z Dilation of Right Hand Artery with Drug-eluting Intraluminal Device, Percutaneous Approach

037D35Z Dilation of Right Hand Artery with Two Drug-eluting Intraluminal Devices, Percutaneous Approach

037D36Z Dilation of Right Hand Artery with Three Drug-eluting Intraluminal Devices, Percutaneous Approach

037D37Z Dilation of Right Hand Artery with Four or More Drug-eluting Intraluminal Devices, Percutaneous Approach

037D3DZ Dilation of Right Hand Artery with Intraluminal Device, Percutaneous Approach

037D3EZ Dilation of Right Hand Artery with Two Intraluminal Devices, Percutaneous Approach

037D3FZ Dilation of Right Hand Artery with Three Intraluminal Devices, Percutaneous Approach

037D3GZ Dilation of Right Hand Artery with Four or More Intraluminal Devices, Percutaneous Approach

037D3ZZ Dilation of Right Hand Artery, Percutaneous Approach

037D44Z Dilation of Right Hand Artery with Drug-eluting Intraluminal Device, Percutaneous Endoscopic Approach

037D45Z Dilation of Right Hand Artery with Two Drug-eluting Intraluminal Devices, Percutaneous Endoscopic Approach

037D46Z Dilation of Right Hand Artery with Three Drug-eluting Intraluminal Devices, Percutaneous Endoscopic Approach

037D47Z Dilation of Right Hand Artery with Four or More Drug-eluting Intraluminal Devices, Percutaneous Endoscopic Approach

037D4DZ Dilation of Right Hand Artery with Intraluminal Device, Percutaneous Endoscopic Approach

037D4EZ Dilation of Right Hand Artery with Two Intraluminal Devices, Percutaneous Endoscopic Approach

037D4FZ Dilation of Right Hand Artery with Three Intraluminal Devices, Percutaneous Endoscopic Approach

037D4GZ Dilation of Right Hand Artery with Four or More Intraluminal Devices, Percutaneous Endoscopic Approach

037D4ZZ Dilation of Right Hand Artery, Percutaneous Endoscopic Approach

037F04Z Dilation of Left Hand Artery with Drug-eluting Intraluminal Device, Open Approach

037F05Z Dilation of Left Hand Artery with Two Drug-eluting Intraluminal Devices, Open Approach

037F06Z Dilation of Left Hand Artery with Three Drug-eluting Intraluminal Devices, Open Approach

037F07Z Dilation of Left Hand Artery with Four or More Drug-eluting Intraluminal Devices, Open Approach

037F0DZ Dilation of Left Hand Artery with Intraluminal Device, Open Approach

037F0EZ Dilation of Left Hand Artery with Two Intraluminal Devices, Open Approach

037F0FZ Dilation of Left Hand Artery with Three Intraluminal Devices, Open Approach

037F0GZ Dilation of Left Hand Artery with Four or More Intraluminal Devices, Open Approach

037F0ZZ Dilation of Left Hand Artery, Open Approach

037F34Z Dilation of Left Hand Artery with Drug-eluting Intraluminal Device, Percutaneous Approach

037F35Z Dilation of Left Hand Artery with Two Drug-eluting Intraluminal Devices, Percutaneous Approach

037F36Z Dilation of Left Hand Artery with Three Drug-eluting Intraluminal Devices, Percutaneous Approach

037F37Z Dilation of Left Hand Artery with Four or More Drug-eluting Intraluminal Devices, Percutaneous Approach

037F3DZ Dilation of Left Hand Artery with Intraluminal Device, Percutaneous Approach

037F3EZ Dilation of Left Hand Artery with Two Intraluminal Devices, Percutaneous Approach

037F3FZ Dilation of Left Hand Artery with Three Intraluminal Devices, Percutaneous Approach

037F3GZ Dilation of Left Hand Artery with Four or More Intraluminal Devices, Percutaneous Approach

037F3ZZ Dilation of Left Hand Artery, Percutaneous Approach

037F44Z Dilation of Left Hand Artery with Drug-eluting Intraluminal Device, Percutaneous Endoscopic Approach

037F45Z Dilation of Left Hand Artery with Two Drug-eluting Intraluminal Devices, Percutaneous Endoscopic Approach

037F46Z Dilation of Left Hand Artery with Three Drug-eluting Intraluminal Devices, Percutaneous Endoscopic Approach

037F47Z Dilation of Left Hand Artery with Four or More Drug-eluting Intraluminal Devices, Percutaneous Endoscopic Approach

037F4DZ Dilation of Left Hand Artery with Intraluminal Device, Percutaneous Endoscopic Approach

037F4EZ Dilation of Left Hand Artery with Two Intraluminal Devices, Percutaneous Endoscopic Approach

037F4FZ Dilation of Left Hand Artery with Three Intraluminal Devices, Percutaneous Endoscopic Approach

037F4GZ Dilation of Left Hand Artery with Four or More Intraluminal Devices, Percutaneous Endoscopic Approach

037F4ZZ Dilation of Left Hand Artery, Percutaneous Endoscopic Approach

037G04Z Dilation of Intracranial Artery with Drug-eluting Intraluminal Device, Open Approach

037G05Z Dilation of Intracranial Artery with Two Drug-eluting Intraluminal Devices, Open Approach

037G06Z Dilation of Intracranial Artery with Three Drug-eluting Intraluminal Devices, Open Approach

037G07Z Dilation of Intracranial Artery with Four or More Drug-eluting Intraluminal Devices, Open Approach

037G0DZ Dilation of Intracranial Artery with Intraluminal Device, Open Approach

037G0EZ Dilation of Intracranial Artery with Two Intraluminal Devices, Open Approach

037G0FZ Dilation of Intracranial Artery with Three Intraluminal Devices, Open Approach

037G0GZ Dilation of Intracranial Artery with Four or More Intraluminal Devices, Open Approach

037G0ZZ Dilation of Intracranial Artery, Open Approach

♀ Female-only   ♂ Male-only   ▲ Limited Coverage   ● Non-OR   **HAC** HAC-associated procedure   ▲ Non-covered procedures   ✚ Cluster

037G34Z Dilation of Intracranial Artery with Drug-eluting Intraluminal Device, Percutaneous Approach

037G35Z Dilation of Intracranial Artery with Two Drug-eluting Intraluminal Devices, Percutaneous Approach

037G36Z Dilation of Intracranial Artery with Three Drug-eluting Intraluminal Devices, Percutaneous Approach

037G37Z Dilation of Intracranial Artery with Four or More Drug-eluting Intraluminal Devices, Percutaneous Approach

037G3DZ Dilation of Intracranial Artery with Intraluminal Device, Percutaneous Approach

037G3EZ Dilation of Intracranial Artery with Two Intraluminal Devices, Percutaneous Approach

037G3FZ Dilation of Intracranial Artery with Three Intraluminal Devices, Percutaneous Approach

037G3GZ Dilation of Intracranial Artery with Four or More Intraluminal Devices, Percutaneous Approach

▲ **037G3ZZ** Dilation of Intracranial Artery, Percutaneous Approach

037G44Z Dilation of Intracranial Artery with Drug-eluting Intraluminal Device, Percutaneous Endoscopic Approach

037G45Z Dilation of Intracranial Artery with Two Drug-eluting Intraluminal Devices, Percutaneous Endoscopic Approach

037G46Z Dilation of Intracranial Artery with Three Drug-eluting Intraluminal Devices, Percutaneous Endoscopic Approach

037G47Z Dilation of Intracranial Artery with Four or More Drug-eluting Intraluminal Devices, Percutaneous Endoscopic Approach

037G4DZ Dilation of Intracranial Artery with Intraluminal Device, Percutaneous Endoscopic Approach

037G4EZ Dilation of Intracranial Artery with Two Intraluminal Devices, Percutaneous Endoscopic Approach

037G4FZ Dilation of Intracranial Artery with Three Intraluminal Devices, Percutaneous Endoscopic Approach

037G4GZ Dilation of Intracranial Artery with Four or More Intraluminal Devices, Percutaneous Endoscopic Approach

▲ **037G4ZZ** Dilation of Intracranial Artery, Percutaneous Endoscopic Approach

037H04Z Dilation of Right Common Carotid Artery with Drug-eluting Intraluminal Device, Open Approach

037H05Z Dilation of Right Common Carotid Artery with Two Drug-eluting Intraluminal Devices, Open Approach

037H06Z Dilation of Right Common Carotid Artery with Three Drug-eluting Intraluminal Devices, Open Approach

037H07Z Dilation of Right Common Carotid Artery with Four or More Drug-eluting Intraluminal Devices, Open Approach

037H0DZ Dilation of Right Common Carotid Artery with Intraluminal Device, Open Approach

037H0EZ Dilation of Right Common Carotid Artery with Two Intraluminal Devices, Open Approach

037H0FZ Dilation of Right Common Carotid Artery with Three Intraluminal Devices, Open Approach

037H0GZ Dilation of Right Common Carotid Artery with Four or More Intraluminal Devices, Open Approach

037H0ZZ Dilation of Right Common Carotid Artery, Open Approach

037H34Z Dilation of Right Common Carotid Artery with Drug-eluting Intraluminal Device, Percutaneous Approach

037H35Z Dilation of Right Common Carotid Artery with Two Drug-eluting Intraluminal Devices, Percutaneous Approach

037H36Z Dilation of Right Common Carotid Artery with Three Drug-eluting Intraluminal Devices, Percutaneous Approach

037H37Z Dilation of Right Common Carotid Artery with Four or More Drug-eluting Intraluminal Devices, Percutaneous Approach

037H3DZ Dilation of Right Common Carotid Artery with Intraluminal Device, Percutaneous Approach

037H3EZ Dilation of Right Common Carotid Artery with Two Intraluminal Devices, Percutaneous Approach

037H3FZ Dilation of Right Common Carotid Artery with Three Intraluminal Devices, Percutaneous Approach

037H3GZ Dilation of Right Common Carotid Artery with Four or More Intraluminal Devices, Percutaneous Approach

037H3ZZ Dilation of Right Common Carotid Artery, Percutaneous Approach

037H44Z Dilation of Right Common Carotid Artery with Drug-eluting Intraluminal Device, Percutaneous Endoscopic Approach

037H45Z Dilation of Right Common Carotid Artery with Two Drug-eluting Intraluminal Devices, Percutaneous Endoscopic Approach

037H46Z Dilation of Right Common Carotid Artery with Three Drug-eluting Intraluminal Devices, Percutaneous Endoscopic Approach

037H47Z Dilation of Right Common Carotid Artery with Four or More Drug-eluting Intraluminal Devices, Percutaneous Endoscopic Approach

037H4DZ Dilation of Right Common Carotid Artery with Intraluminal Device, Percutaneous Endoscopic Approach

037H4EZ Dilation of Right Common Carotid Artery with Two Intraluminal Devices, Percutaneous Endoscopic Approach

037H4FZ Dilation of Right Common Carotid Artery with Three Intraluminal Devices, Percutaneous Endoscopic Approach

037H4GZ Dilation of Right Common Carotid Artery with Four or More Intraluminal Devices, Percutaneous Endoscopic Approach

037H4ZZ Dilation of Right Common Carotid Artery, Percutaneous Endoscopic Approach

037J04Z Dilation of Left Common Carotid Artery with Drug-eluting Intraluminal Device, Open Approach

037J05Z Dilation of Left Common Carotid Artery with Two Drug-eluting Intraluminal Devices, Open Approach

037J06Z Dilation of Left Common Carotid Artery with Three Drug-eluting Intraluminal Devices, Open Approach

037J07Z Dilation of Left Common Carotid Artery with Four or More Drug-eluting Intraluminal Devices, Open Approach

037J0DZ Dilation of Left Common Carotid Artery with Intraluminal Device, Open Approach

037J0EZ Dilation of Left Common Carotid Artery with Two Intraluminal Devices, Open Approach

037J0FZ Dilation of Left Common Carotid Artery with Three Intraluminal Devices, Open Approach

037J0GZ Dilation of Left Common Carotid Artery with Four or More Intraluminal Devices, Open Approach

037J0ZZ Dilation of Left Common Carotid Artery, Open Approach

037J34Z Dilation of Left Common Carotid Artery with Drug-eluting Intraluminal Device, Percutaneous Approach

037J35Z Dilation of Left Common Carotid Artery with Two Drug-eluting Intraluminal Devices, Percutaneous Approach

037J36Z Dilation of Left Common Carotid Artery with Three Drug-eluting Intraluminal Devices, Percutaneous Approach

037J37Z Dilation of Left Common Carotid Artery with Four or More Drug-eluting Intraluminal Devices, Percutaneous Approach

037J3DZ Dilation of Left Common Carotid Artery with Intraluminal Device, Percutaneous Approach

037J3EZ Dilation of Left Common Carotid Artery with Two Intraluminal Devices, Percutaneous Approach

037J3FZ Dilation of Left Common Carotid Artery with Three Intraluminal Devices, Percutaneous Approach

037J3GZ Dilation of Left Common Carotid Artery with Four or More Intraluminal Devices, Percutaneous Approach

037J3ZZ Dilation of Left Common Carotid Artery, Percutaneous Approach

037J44Z Dilation of Left Common Carotid Artery with Drug-eluting Intraluminal Device, Percutaneous Endoscopic Approach

037J45Z Dilation of Left Common Carotid Artery with Two Drug-eluting Intraluminal Devices, Percutaneous Endoscopic Approach

037J46Z Dilation of Left Common Carotid Artery with Three Drug-eluting Intraluminal Devices, Percutaneous Endoscopic Approach

037J47Z Dilation of Left Common Carotid Artery with Four or More Drug-eluting Intraluminal Devices, Percutaneous Endoscopic Approach

037J4DZ Dilation of Left Common Carotid Artery with Intraluminal Device, Percutaneous Endoscopic Approach

037J4EZ Dilation of Left Common Carotid Artery with Two Intraluminal Devices, Percutaneous Endoscopic Approach

037J4FZ Dilation of Left Common Carotid Artery with Three Intraluminal Devices, Percutaneous Endoscopic Approach

037J4GZ Dilation of Left Common Carotid Artery with Four or More Intraluminal Devices, Percutaneous Endoscopic Approach

037J4ZZ Dilation of Left Common Carotid Artery, Percutaneous Endoscopic Approach

037K04Z Dilation of Right Internal Carotid Artery with Drug-eluting Intraluminal Device, Open Approach

037K05Z Dilation of Right Internal Carotid Artery with Two Drug-eluting Intraluminal Devices, Open Approach

037K06Z Dilation of Right Internal Carotid Artery with Three Drug-eluting Intraluminal Devices, Open Approach

037K07Z Dilation of Right Internal Carotid Artery with Four or More Drug-eluting Intraluminal Devices, Open Approach

037K0DZ Dilation of Right Internal Carotid Artery with Intraluminal Device, Open Approach

037K0EZ Dilation of Right Internal Carotid Artery with Two Intraluminal Devices, Open Approach

037K0FZ Dilation of Right Internal Carotid Artery with Three Intraluminal Devices, Open Approach

037K0GZ Dilation of Right Internal Carotid Artery with Four or More Intraluminal Devices, Open Approach

037K0ZZ Dilation of Right Internal Carotid Artery, Open Approach

037K34Z Dilation of Right Internal Carotid Artery with Drug-eluting Intraluminal Device, Percutaneous Approach

037K35Z Dilation of Right Internal Carotid Artery with Two Drug-eluting Intraluminal Devices, Percutaneous Approach

037K36Z Dilation of Right Internal Carotid Artery with Three Drug-eluting Intraluminal Devices, Percutaneous Approach

037K37Z Dilation of Right Internal Carotid Artery with Four or More Drug-eluting Intraluminal Devices, Percutaneous Approach

037K3DZ Dilation of Right Internal Carotid Artery with Intraluminal Device, Percutaneous Approach
AHA CC: 3Q, 2019, 29-30

037K3EZ Dilation of Right Internal Carotid Artery with Two Intraluminal Devices, Percutaneous Approach

037K3FZ Dilation of Right Internal Carotid Artery with Three Intraluminal Devices, Percutaneous Approach

037K3GZ Dilation of Right Internal Carotid Artery with Four or More Intraluminal Devices, Percutaneous Approach

037K3ZZ Dilation of Right Internal Carotid Artery, Percutaneous Approach

037K44Z Dilation of Right Internal Carotid Artery with Drug-eluting Intraluminal Device, Percutaneous Endoscopic Approach

037K45Z Dilation of Right Internal Carotid Artery with Two Drug-eluting Intraluminal Devices, Percutaneous Endoscopic Approach

037K46Z Dilation of Right Internal Carotid Artery with Three Drug-eluting Intraluminal Devices, Percutaneous Endoscopic Approach

037K47Z Dilation of Right Internal Carotid Artery with Four or More Drug-eluting Intraluminal Devices, Percutaneous Endoscopic Approach

037K4DZ Dilation of Right Internal Carotid Artery with Intraluminal Device, Percutaneous Endoscopic Approach

037K4EZ Dilation of Right Internal Carotid Artery with Two Intraluminal Devices, Percutaneous Endoscopic Approach

037K4FZ Dilation of Right Internal Carotid Artery with Three Intraluminal Devices, Percutaneous Endoscopic Approach

037K4GZ Dilation of Right Internal Carotid Artery with Four or More Intraluminal Devices, Percutaneous Endoscopic Approach

037K4ZZ Dilation of Right Internal Carotid Artery, Percutaneous Endoscopic Approach

037L04Z Dilation of Left Internal Carotid Artery with Drug-eluting Intraluminal Device, Open Approach

037L05Z Dilation of Left Internal Carotid Artery with Two Drug-eluting Intraluminal Devices, Open Approach

037L06Z Dilation of Left Internal Carotid Artery with Three Drug-eluting Intraluminal Devices, Open Approach

037L07Z Dilation of Left Internal Carotid Artery with Four or More Drug-eluting Intraluminal Devices, Open Approach

037L0DZ Dilation of Left Internal Carotid Artery with Intraluminal Device, Open Approach

037L0EZ Dilation of Left Internal Carotid Artery with Two Intraluminal Devices, Open Approach

037L0FZ Dilation of Left Internal Carotid Artery with Three Intraluminal Devices, Open Approach

037L0GZ Dilation of Left Internal Carotid Artery with Four or More Intraluminal Devices, Open Approach

037L0ZZ Dilation of Left Internal Carotid Artery, Open Approach

037L34Z Dilation of Left Internal Carotid Artery with Drug-eluting Intraluminal Device, Percutaneous Approach

037L35Z Dilation of Left Internal Carotid Artery with Two Drug-eluting Intraluminal Devices, Percutaneous Approach

037L36Z Dilation of Left Internal Carotid Artery with Three Drug-eluting Intraluminal Devices, Percutaneous Approach

037L37Z Dilation of Left Internal Carotid Artery with Four or More Drug-eluting Intraluminal Devices, Percutaneous Approach

037L3DZ Dilation of Left Internal Carotid Artery with Intraluminal Device, Percutaneous Approach

037L3EZ Dilation of Left Internal Carotid Artery with Two Intraluminal Devices, Percutaneous Approach

037L3FZ Dilation of Left Internal Carotid Artery with Three Intraluminal Devices, Percutaneous Approach

037L3GZ Dilation of Left Internal Carotid Artery with Four or More Intraluminal Devices, Percutaneous Approach

037L3ZZ Dilation of Left Internal Carotid Artery, Percutaneous Approach

037L44Z Dilation of Left Internal Carotid Artery with Drug-eluting Intraluminal Device, Percutaneous Endoscopic Approach

037L45Z Dilation of Left Internal Carotid Artery with Two Drug-eluting Intraluminal Devices, Percutaneous Endoscopic Approach

037L46Z Dilation of Left Internal Carotid Artery with Three Drug-eluting Intraluminal Devices, Percutaneous Endoscopic Approach

037L47Z Dilation of Left Internal Carotid Artery with Four or More Drug-eluting Intraluminal Devices, Percutaneous Endoscopic Approach

037L4DZ Dilation of Left Internal Carotid Artery with Intraluminal Device, Percutaneous Endoscopic Approach

037L4EZ Dilation of Left Internal Carotid Artery with Two Intraluminal Devices, Percutaneous Endoscopic Approach

037L4FZ Dilation of Left Internal Carotid Artery with Three Intraluminal Devices, Percutaneous Endoscopic Approach

037L4GZ Dilation of Left Internal Carotid Artery with Four or More Intraluminal Devices, Percutaneous Endoscopic Approach

037L4ZZ Dilation of Left Internal Carotid Artery, Percutaneous Endoscopic Approach

037M04Z Dilation of Right External Carotid Artery with Drug-eluting Intraluminal Device, Open Approach

037M05Z Dilation of Right External Carotid Artery with Two Drug-eluting Intraluminal Devices, Open Approach

037M06Z Dilation of Right External Carotid Artery with Three Drug-eluting Intraluminal Devices, Open Approach

037M07Z Dilation of Right External Carotid Artery with Four or More Drug-eluting Intraluminal Devices, Open Approach

037M0DZ Dilation of Right External Carotid Artery with Intraluminal Device, Open Approach

037M0EZ Dilation of Right External Carotid Artery with Two Intraluminal Devices, Open Approach

037M0FZ Dilation of Right External Carotid Artery with Three Intraluminal Devices, Open Approach

037M0GZ Dilation of Right External Carotid Artery with Four or More Intraluminal Devices, Open Approach

037M0ZZ Dilation of Right External Carotid Artery, Open Approach

037M34Z Dilation of Right External Carotid Artery with Drug-eluting Intraluminal Device, Percutaneous Approach

037M35Z Dilation of Right External Carotid Artery with Two Drug-eluting Intraluminal Devices, Percutaneous Approach

037M36Z Dilation of Right External Carotid Artery with Three Drug-eluting Intraluminal Devices, Percutaneous Approach

037M37Z Dilation of Right External Carotid Artery with Four or More Drug-eluting Intraluminal Devices, Percutaneous Approach

037M3DZ Dilation of Right External Carotid Artery with Intraluminal Device, Percutaneous Approach

037M3EZ Dilation of Right External Carotid Artery with Two Intraluminal Devices, Percutaneous Approach

037M3FZ Dilation of Right External Carotid Artery with Three Intraluminal Devices, Percutaneous Approach

037M3GZ Dilation of Right External Carotid Artery with Four or More Intraluminal Devices, Percutaneous Approach

♀ Female-only ♂ Male-only ▲ Limited Coverage ● Non-OR ᴴᴬᶜ HAC-associated procedure ▲ Non-covered procedures ✚ Cluster

37M3ZZ Dilation of Right External Carotid Artery, Percutaneous Approach

37M44Z Dilation of Right External Carotid Artery with Drug-eluting Intraluminal Device, Percutaneous Endoscopic Approach

37M45Z Dilation of Right External Carotid Artery with Two Drug-eluting Intraluminal Devices, Percutaneous Endoscopic Approach

37M46Z Dilation of Right External Carotid Artery with Three Drug-eluting Intraluminal Devices, Percutaneous Endoscopic Approach

37M47Z Dilation of Right External Carotid Artery with Four or More Drug-eluting Intraluminal Devices, Percutaneous Endoscopic Approach

37M4DZ Dilation of Right External Carotid Artery with Intraluminal Device, Percutaneous Endoscopic Approach

37M4EZ Dilation of Right External Carotid Artery with Two Intraluminal Devices, Percutaneous Endoscopic Approach

37M4FZ Dilation of Right External Carotid Artery with Three Intraluminal Devices, Percutaneous Endoscopic Approach

37M4GZ Dilation of Right External Carotid Artery with Four or More Intraluminal Devices, Percutaneous Endoscopic Approach

37M4ZZ Dilation of Right External Carotid Artery, Percutaneous Endoscopic Approach

37N04Z Dilation of Left External Carotid Artery with Drug-eluting Intraluminal Device, Open Approach

37N05Z Dilation of Left External Carotid Artery with Two Drug-eluting Intraluminal Devices, Open Approach

37N06Z Dilation of Left External Carotid Artery with Three Drug-eluting Intraluminal Devices, Open Approach

37N07Z Dilation of Left External Carotid Artery with Four or More Drug-eluting Intraluminal Devices, Open Approach

37N0DZ Dilation of Left External Carotid Artery with Intraluminal Device, Open Approach

37N0EZ Dilation of Left External Carotid Artery with Two Intraluminal Devices, Open Approach

37N0FZ Dilation of Left External Carotid Artery with Three Intraluminal Devices, Open Approach

37N0GZ Dilation of Left External Carotid Artery with Four or More Intraluminal Devices, Open Approach

37N0ZZ Dilation of Left External Carotid Artery, Open Approach

37N34Z Dilation of Left External Carotid Artery with Drug-eluting Intraluminal Device, Percutaneous Approach

37N35Z Dilation of Left External Carotid Artery with Two Drug-eluting Intraluminal Devices, Percutaneous Approach

37N36Z Dilation of Left External Carotid Artery with Three Drug-eluting Intraluminal Devices, Percutaneous Approach

37N37Z Dilation of Left External Carotid Artery with Four or More Drug-eluting Intraluminal Devices, Percutaneous Approach

37N3DZ Dilation of Left External Carotid Artery with Intraluminal Device, Percutaneous Approach

037N3EZ Dilation of Left External Carotid Artery with Two Intraluminal Devices, Percutaneous Approach

037N3FZ Dilation of Left External Carotid Artery with Three Intraluminal Devices, Percutaneous Approach

037N3GZ Dilation of Left External Carotid Artery with Four or More Intraluminal Devices, Percutaneous Approach

037N3ZZ Dilation of Left External Carotid Artery, Percutaneous Approach

037N44Z Dilation of Left External Carotid Artery with Drug-eluting Intraluminal Device, Percutaneous Endoscopic Approach

037N45Z Dilation of Left External Carotid Artery with Two Drug-eluting Intraluminal Devices, Percutaneous Endoscopic Approach

037N46Z Dilation of Left External Carotid Artery with Three Drug-eluting Intraluminal Devices, Percutaneous Endoscopic Approach

037N47Z Dilation of Left External Carotid Artery with Four or More Drug-eluting Intraluminal Devices, Percutaneous Endoscopic Approach

037N4DZ Dilation of Left External Carotid Artery with Intraluminal Device, Percutaneous Endoscopic Approach

037N4EZ Dilation of Left External Carotid Artery with Two Intraluminal Devices, Percutaneous Endoscopic Approach

037N4FZ Dilation of Left External Carotid Artery with Three Intraluminal Devices, Percutaneous Endoscopic Approach

037N4GZ Dilation of Left External Carotid Artery with Four or More Intraluminal Devices, Percutaneous Endoscopic Approach

037N4ZZ Dilation of Left External Carotid Artery, Percutaneous Endoscopic Approach

037P04Z Dilation of Right Vertebral Artery with Drug-eluting Intraluminal Device, Open Approach

037P05Z Dilation of Right Vertebral Artery with Two Drug-eluting Intraluminal Devices, Open Approach

037P06Z Dilation of Right Vertebral Artery with Three Drug-eluting Intraluminal Devices, Open Approach

037P07Z Dilation of Right Vertebral Artery with Four or More Drug-eluting Intraluminal Devices, Open Approach

037P0DZ Dilation of Right Vertebral Artery with Intraluminal Device, Open Approach

037P0EZ Dilation of Right Vertebral Artery with Two Intraluminal Devices, Open Approach

037P0FZ Dilation of Right Vertebral Artery with Three Intraluminal Devices, Open Approach

037P0GZ Dilation of Right Vertebral Artery with Four or More Intraluminal Devices, Open Approach

037P0ZZ Dilation of Right Vertebral Artery, Open Approach

037P34Z Dilation of Right Vertebral Artery with Drug-eluting Intraluminal Device, Percutaneous Approach

037P35Z Dilation of Right Vertebral Artery with Two Drug-eluting Intraluminal Devices, Percutaneous Approach

037P36Z Dilation of Right Vertebral Artery with Three Drug-eluting Intraluminal Devices, Percutaneous Approach

037P37Z Dilation of Right Vertebral Artery with Four or More Drug-eluting Intraluminal Devices, Percutaneous Approach

037P3DZ Dilation of Right Vertebral Artery with Intraluminal Device, Percutaneous Approach

037P3EZ Dilation of Right Vertebral Artery with Two Intraluminal Devices, Percutaneous Approach

037P3FZ Dilation of Right Vertebral Artery with Three Intraluminal Devices, Percutaneous Approach

037P3GZ Dilation of Right Vertebral Artery with Four or More Intraluminal Devices, Percutaneous Approach

037P3ZZ Dilation of Right Vertebral Artery, Percutaneous Approach

037P44Z Dilation of Right Vertebral Artery with Drug-eluting Intraluminal Device, Percutaneous Endoscopic Approach

037P45Z Dilation of Right Vertebral Artery with Two Drug-eluting Intraluminal Devices, Percutaneous Endoscopic Approach

037P46Z Dilation of Right Vertebral Artery with Three Drug-eluting Intraluminal Devices, Percutaneous Endoscopic Approach

037P47Z Dilation of Right Vertebral Artery with Four or More Drug-eluting Intraluminal Devices, Percutaneous Endoscopic Approach

037P4DZ Dilation of Right Vertebral Artery with Intraluminal Device, Percutaneous Endoscopic Approach

037P4EZ Dilation of Right Vertebral Artery with Two Intraluminal Devices, Percutaneous Endoscopic Approach

037P4FZ Dilation of Right Vertebral Artery with Three Intraluminal Devices, Percutaneous Endoscopic Approach

037P4GZ Dilation of Right Vertebral Artery with Four or More Intraluminal Devices, Percutaneous Endoscopic Approach

037P4ZZ Dilation of Right Vertebral Artery, Percutaneous Endoscopic Approach

037Q04Z Dilation of Left Vertebral Artery with Drug-eluting Intraluminal Device, Open Approach

037Q05Z Dilation of Left Vertebral Artery with Two Drug-eluting Intraluminal Devices, Open Approach

037Q06Z Dilation of Left Vertebral Artery with Three Drug-eluting Intraluminal Devices, Open Approach

037Q07Z Dilation of Left Vertebral Artery with Four or More Drug-eluting Intraluminal Devices, Open Approach

037Q0DZ Dilation of Left Vertebral Artery with Intraluminal Device, Open Approach

037Q0EZ Dilation of Left Vertebral Artery with Two Intraluminal Devices, Open Approach

037Q0FZ Dilation of Left Vertebral Artery with Three Intraluminal Devices, Open Approach

037Q0GZ Dilation of Left Vertebral Artery with Four or More Intraluminal Devices, Open Approach

037Q0ZZ Dilation of Left Vertebral Artery, Open Approach

037Q34Z Dilation of Left Vertebral Artery with Drug-eluting Intraluminal Device, Percutaneous Approach

037Q35Z Dilation of Left Vertebral Artery with Two Drug-eluting Intraluminal Devices, Percutaneous Approach

037Q36Z Dilation of Left Vertebral Artery with Three Drug-eluting Intraluminal Devices, Percutaneous Approach

037Q37Z Dilation of Left Vertebral Artery with Four or More Drug-eluting Intraluminal Devices, Percutaneous Approach

037Q3DZ Dilation of Left Vertebral Artery with Intraluminal Device, Percutaneous Approach

037Q3EZ Dilation of Left Vertebral Artery with Two Intraluminal Devices, Percutaneous Approach

037Q3FZ Dilation of Left Vertebral Artery with Three Intraluminal Devices, Percutaneous Approach

037Q3GZ Dilation of Left Vertebral Artery with Four or More Intraluminal Devices, Percutaneous Approach

037Q3ZZ Dilation of Left Vertebral Artery, Percutaneous Approach

037Q44Z Dilation of Left Vertebral Artery with Drug-eluting Intraluminal Device, Percutaneous Endoscopic Approach

037Q45Z Dilation of Left Vertebral Artery with Two Drug-eluting Intraluminal Devices, Percutaneous Endoscopic Approach

037Q46Z Dilation of Left Vertebral Artery with Three Drug-eluting Intraluminal Devices, Percutaneous Endoscopic Approach

037Q47Z Dilation of Left Vertebral Artery with Four or More Drug-eluting Intraluminal Devices, Percutaneous Endoscopic Approach

037Q4DZ Dilation of Left Vertebral Artery with Intraluminal Device, Percutaneous Endoscopic Approach

037Q4EZ Dilation of Left Vertebral Artery with Two Intraluminal Devices, Percutaneous Endoscopic Approach

037Q4FZ Dilation of Left Vertebral Artery with Three Intraluminal Devices, Percutaneous Endoscopic Approach

037Q4GZ Dilation of Left Vertebral Artery with Four or More Intraluminal Devices, Percutaneous Endoscopic Approach

037Q4ZZ Dilation of Left Vertebral Artery, Percutaneous Endoscopic Approach

037R04Z Dilation of Face Artery with Drug-eluting Intraluminal Device, Open Approach

037R05Z Dilation of Face Artery with Two Drug-eluting Intraluminal Devices, Open Approach

037R06Z Dilation of Face Artery with Three Drug-eluting Intraluminal Devices, Open Approach

037R07Z Dilation of Face Artery with Four or More Drug-eluting Intraluminal Devices, Open Approach

037R0DZ Dilation of Face Artery with Intraluminal Device, Open Approach

037R0EZ Dilation of Face Artery with Two Intraluminal Devices, Open Approach

037R0FZ Dilation of Face Artery with Three Intraluminal Devices, Open Approach

037R0GZ Dilation of Face Artery with Four or More Intraluminal Devices, Open Approach

037R0ZZ Dilation of Face Artery, Open Approach

037R34Z Dilation of Face Artery with Drug-eluting Intraluminal Device, Percutaneous Approach

037R35Z Dilation of Face Artery with Two Drug-eluting Intraluminal Devices, Percutaneous Approach

037R36Z Dilation of Face Artery with Three Drug-eluting Intraluminal Devices, Percutaneous Approach

037R37Z Dilation of Face Artery with Four or More Drug-eluting Intraluminal Devices, Percutaneous Approach

037R3DZ Dilation of Face Artery with Intraluminal Device, Percutaneous Approach

037R3EZ Dilation of Face Artery with Two Intraluminal Devices, Percutaneous Approach

037R3FZ Dilation of Face Artery with Three Intraluminal Devices, Percutaneous Approach

037R3GZ Dilation of Face Artery with Four or More Intraluminal Devices, Percutaneous Approach

037R3ZZ Dilation of Face Artery, Percutaneous Approach

037R44Z Dilation of Face Artery with Drug-eluting Intraluminal Device, Percutaneous Endoscopic Approach

037R45Z Dilation of Face Artery with Two Drug-eluting Intraluminal Devices, Percutaneous Endoscopic Approach

037R46Z Dilation of Face Artery with Three Drug-eluting Intraluminal Devices, Percutaneous Endoscopic Approach

037R47Z Dilation of Face Artery with Four or More Drug-eluting Intraluminal Devices, Percutaneous Endoscopic Approach

037R4DZ Dilation of Face Artery with Intraluminal Device, Percutaneous Endoscopic Approach

037R4EZ Dilation of Face Artery with Two Intraluminal Devices, Percutaneous Endoscopic Approach

037R4FZ Dilation of Face Artery with Three Intraluminal Devices, Percutaneous Endoscopic Approach

037R4GZ Dilation of Face Artery with Four or More Intraluminal Devices, Percutaneous Endoscopic Approach

037R4ZZ Dilation of Face Artery, Percutaneous Endoscopic Approach

037S04Z Dilation of Right Temporal Artery with Drug-eluting Intraluminal Device, Open Approach

037S05Z Dilation of Right Temporal Artery with Two Drug-eluting Intraluminal Devices, Open Approach

037S06Z Dilation of Right Temporal Artery with Three Drug-eluting Intraluminal Devices, Open Approach

037S07Z Dilation of Right Temporal Artery with Four or More Drug-eluting Intraluminal Devices, Open Approach

037S0DZ Dilation of Right Temporal Artery with Intraluminal Device, Open Approach

037S0EZ Dilation of Right Temporal Artery with Two Intraluminal Devices, Open Approach

037S0FZ Dilation of Right Temporal Artery with Three Intraluminal Devices, Open Approach

037S0GZ Dilation of Right Temporal Artery with Four or More Intraluminal Devices, Open Approach

037S0ZZ Dilation of Right Temporal Artery, Open Approach

037S34Z Dilation of Right Temporal Artery with Drug-eluting Intraluminal Device, Percutaneous Approach

037S35Z Dilation of Right Temporal Artery with Two Drug-eluting Intraluminal Devices, Percutaneous Approach

037S36Z Dilation of Right Temporal Artery with Three Drug-eluting Intraluminal Devices, Percutaneous Approach

037S37Z Dilation of Right Temporal Artery with Four or More Drug-eluting Intraluminal Devices, Percutaneous Approach

037S3DZ Dilation of Right Temporal Artery with Intraluminal Device, Percutaneous Approach

037S3EZ Dilation of Right Temporal Artery with Two Intraluminal Devices, Percutaneous Approach

037S3FZ Dilation of Right Temporal Artery with Three Intraluminal Devices, Percutaneous Approach

037S3GZ Dilation of Right Temporal Artery with Four or More Intraluminal Devices, Percutaneous Approach

037S3ZZ Dilation of Right Temporal Artery, Percutaneous Approach

037S44Z Dilation of Right Temporal Artery with Drug-eluting Intraluminal Device, Percutaneous Endoscopic Approach

037S45Z Dilation of Right Temporal Artery with Two Drug-eluting Intraluminal Devices, Percutaneous Endoscopic Approach

037S46Z Dilation of Right Temporal Artery with Three Drug-eluting Intraluminal Devices, Percutaneous Endoscopic Approach

037S47Z Dilation of Right Temporal Artery with Four or More Drug-eluting Intraluminal Devices, Percutaneous Endoscopic Approach

037S4DZ Dilation of Right Temporal Artery with Intraluminal Device, Percutaneous Endoscopic Approach

037S4EZ Dilation of Right Temporal Artery with Two Intraluminal Devices, Percutaneous Endoscopic Approach

037S4FZ Dilation of Right Temporal Artery with Three Intraluminal Devices, Percutaneous Endoscopic Approach

037S4GZ Dilation of Right Temporal Artery with Four or More Intraluminal Devices, Percutaneous Endoscopic Approach

037S4ZZ Dilation of Right Temporal Artery, Percutaneous Endoscopic Approach

037T04Z Dilation of Left Temporal Artery with Drug-eluting Intraluminal Device, Open Approach

037T05Z Dilation of Left Temporal Artery with Two Drug-eluting Intraluminal Devices, Open Approach

037T06Z Dilation of Left Temporal Artery with Three Drug-eluting Intraluminal Devices, Open Approach

037T07Z Dilation of Left Temporal Artery with Four or More Drug-eluting Intraluminal Devices, Open Approach

037T0DZ Dilation of Left Temporal Artery with Intraluminal Device, Open Approach

037T0EZ Dilation of Left Temporal Artery with Two Intraluminal Devices, Open Approach

♀ Female-only   ♂ Male-only   ▲ Limited Coverage   ● Non-OR   ▧ HAC-associated procedure   ▲ Non-covered procedures   ✛ Cluster

37T0FZ Dilation of Left Temporal Artery with Three Intraluminal Devices, Open Approach

37T0GZ Dilation of Left Temporal Artery with Four or More Intraluminal Devices, Open Approach

37T0ZZ Dilation of Left Temporal Artery, Open Approach

37T34Z Dilation of Left Temporal Artery with Drug-eluting Intraluminal Device, Percutaneous Approach

37T35Z Dilation of Left Temporal Artery with Two Drug-eluting Intraluminal Devices, Percutaneous Approach

37T36Z Dilation of Left Temporal Artery with Three Drug-eluting Intraluminal Devices, Percutaneous Approach

37T37Z Dilation of Left Temporal Artery with Four or More Drug-eluting Intraluminal Devices, Percutaneous Approach

37T3DZ Dilation of Left Temporal Artery with Intraluminal Device, Percutaneous Approach

37T3EZ Dilation of Left Temporal Artery with Two Intraluminal Devices, Percutaneous Approach

37T3FZ Dilation of Left Temporal Artery with Three Intraluminal Devices, Percutaneous Approach

37T3GZ Dilation of Left Temporal Artery with Four or More Intraluminal Devices, Percutaneous Approach

37T3ZZ Dilation of Left Temporal Artery, Percutaneous Approach

37T44Z Dilation of Left Temporal Artery with Drug-eluting Intraluminal Device, Percutaneous Endoscopic Approach

37T45Z Dilation of Left Temporal Artery with Two Drug-eluting Intraluminal Devices, Percutaneous Endoscopic Approach

37T46Z Dilation of Left Temporal Artery with Three Drug-eluting Intraluminal Devices, Percutaneous Endoscopic Approach

37T47Z Dilation of Left Temporal Artery with Four or More Drug-eluting Intraluminal Devices, Percutaneous Endoscopic Approach

37T4DZ Dilation of Left Temporal Artery with Intraluminal Device, Percutaneous Endoscopic Approach

37T4EZ Dilation of Left Temporal Artery with Two Intraluminal Devices, Percutaneous Endoscopic Approach

37T4FZ Dilation of Left Temporal Artery with Three Intraluminal Devices, Percutaneous Endoscopic Approach

37T4GZ Dilation of Left Temporal Artery with Four or More Intraluminal Devices, Percutaneous Endoscopic Approach

37T4ZZ Dilation of Left Temporal Artery, Percutaneous Endoscopic Approach

37U04Z Dilation of Right Thyroid Artery with Drug-eluting Intraluminal Device, Open Approach

37U05Z Dilation of Right Thyroid Artery with Two Drug-eluting Intraluminal Devices, Open Approach

37U06Z Dilation of Right Thyroid Artery with Three Drug-eluting Intraluminal Devices, Open Approach

37U07Z Dilation of Right Thyroid Artery with Four or More Drug-eluting Intraluminal Devices, Open Approach

37U0DZ Dilation of Right Thyroid Artery with Intraluminal Device, Open Approach

037U0EZ Dilation of Right Thyroid Artery with Two Intraluminal Devices, Open Approach

037U0FZ Dilation of Right Thyroid Artery with Three Intraluminal Devices, Open Approach

037U0GZ Dilation of Right Thyroid Artery with Four or More Intraluminal Devices, Open Approach

037U0ZZ Dilation of Right Thyroid Artery, Open Approach

037U34Z Dilation of Right Thyroid Artery with Drug-eluting Intraluminal Device, Percutaneous Approach

037U35Z Dilation of Right Thyroid Artery with Two Drug-eluting Intraluminal Devices, Percutaneous Approach

037U36Z Dilation of Right Thyroid Artery with Three Drug-eluting Intraluminal Devices, Percutaneous Approach

037U37Z Dilation of Right Thyroid Artery with Four or More Drug-eluting Intraluminal Devices, Percutaneous Approach

037U3DZ Dilation of Right Thyroid Artery with Intraluminal Device, Percutaneous Approach

037U3EZ Dilation of Right Thyroid Artery with Two Intraluminal Devices, Percutaneous Approach

037U3FZ Dilation of Right Thyroid Artery with Three Intraluminal Devices, Percutaneous Approach

037U3GZ Dilation of Right Thyroid Artery with Four or More Intraluminal Devices, Percutaneous Approach

037U3ZZ Dilation of Right Thyroid Artery, Percutaneous Approach

037U44Z Dilation of Right Thyroid Artery with Drug-eluting Intraluminal Device, Percutaneous Endoscopic Approach

037U45Z Dilation of Right Thyroid Artery with Two Drug-eluting Intraluminal Devices, Percutaneous Endoscopic Approach

037U46Z Dilation of Right Thyroid Artery with Three Drug-eluting Intraluminal Devices, Percutaneous Endoscopic Approach

037U47Z Dilation of Right Thyroid Artery with Four or More Drug-eluting Intraluminal Devices, Percutaneous Endoscopic Approach

037U4DZ Dilation of Right Thyroid Artery with Intraluminal Device, Percutaneous Endoscopic Approach

037U4EZ Dilation of Right Thyroid Artery with Two Intraluminal Devices, Percutaneous Endoscopic Approach

037U4FZ Dilation of Right Thyroid Artery with Three Intraluminal Devices, Percutaneous Endoscopic Approach

037U4GZ Dilation of Right Thyroid Artery with Four or More Intraluminal Devices, Percutaneous Endoscopic Approach

037U4ZZ Dilation of Right Thyroid Artery, Percutaneous Endoscopic Approach

037V04Z Dilation of Left Thyroid Artery with Drug-eluting Intraluminal Device, Open Approach

037V05Z Dilation of Left Thyroid Artery with Two Drug-eluting Intraluminal Devices, Open Approach

037V06Z Dilation of Left Thyroid Artery with Three Drug-eluting Intraluminal Devices, Open Approach

037V07Z Dilation of Left Thyroid Artery with Four or More Drug-eluting Intraluminal Devices, Open Approach

037V0DZ Dilation of Left Thyroid Artery with Intraluminal Device, Open Approach

037V0EZ Dilation of Left Thyroid Artery with Two Intraluminal Devices, Open Approach

037V0FZ Dilation of Left Thyroid Artery with Three Intraluminal Devices, Open Approach

037V0GZ Dilation of Left Thyroid Artery with Four or More Intraluminal Devices, Open Approach

037V0ZZ Dilation of Left Thyroid Artery, Open Approach

037V34Z Dilation of Left Thyroid Artery with Drug-eluting Intraluminal Device, Percutaneous Approach

037V35Z Dilation of Left Thyroid Artery with Two Drug-eluting Intraluminal Devices, Percutaneous Approach

037V36Z Dilation of Left Thyroid Artery with Three Drug-eluting Intraluminal Devices, Percutaneous Approach

037V37Z Dilation of Left Thyroid Artery with Four or More Drug-eluting Intraluminal Devices, Percutaneous Approach

037V3DZ Dilation of Left Thyroid Artery with Intraluminal Device, Percutaneous Approach

037V3EZ Dilation of Left Thyroid Artery with Two Intraluminal Devices, Percutaneous Approach

037V3FZ Dilation of Left Thyroid Artery with Three Intraluminal Devices, Percutaneous Approach

037V3GZ Dilation of Left Thyroid Artery with Four or More Intraluminal Devices, Percutaneous Approach

037V3ZZ Dilation of Left Thyroid Artery, Percutaneous Approach

037V44Z Dilation of Left Thyroid Artery with Drug-eluting Intraluminal Device, Percutaneous Endoscopic Approach

037V45Z Dilation of Left Thyroid Artery with Two Drug-eluting Intraluminal Devices, Percutaneous Endoscopic Approach

037V46Z Dilation of Left Thyroid Artery with Three Drug-eluting Intraluminal Devices, Percutaneous Endoscopic Approach

037V47Z Dilation of Left Thyroid Artery with Four or More Drug-eluting Intraluminal Devices, Percutaneous Endoscopic Approach

037V4DZ Dilation of Left Thyroid Artery with Intraluminal Device, Percutaneous Endoscopic Approach

037V4EZ Dilation of Left Thyroid Artery with Two Intraluminal Devices, Percutaneous Endoscopic Approach

037V4FZ Dilation of Left Thyroid Artery with Three Intraluminal Devices, Percutaneous Endoscopic Approach

037V4GZ Dilation of Left Thyroid Artery with Four or More Intraluminal Devices, Percutaneous Endoscopic Approach

037V4ZZ Dilation of Left Thyroid Artery, Percutaneous Endoscopic Approach

037Y04Z Dilation of Upper Artery with Drug-eluting Intraluminal Device, Open Approach

037Y05Z Dilation of Upper Artery with Two Drug-eluting Intraluminal Devices, Open Approach	**037Y35Z** Dilation of Upper Artery with Two Drug-eluting Intraluminal Devices, Percutaneous Approach	**037Y45Z** Dilation of Upper Artery with Two Drug-eluting Intraluminal Devices, Percutaneous Endoscopic Approach
037Y06Z Dilation of Upper Artery with Three Drug-eluting Intraluminal Devices, Open Approach	**037Y36Z** Dilation of Upper Artery with Three Drug-eluting Intraluminal Devices, Percutaneous Approach	**037Y46Z** Dilation of Upper Artery with Three Drug-eluting Intraluminal Devices, Percutaneous Endoscopic Approach
037Y07Z Dilation of Upper Artery with Four or More Drug-eluting Intraluminal Devices, Open Approach	**037Y37Z** Dilation of Upper Artery with Four or More Drug-eluting Intraluminal Devices, Percutaneous Approach	**037Y47Z** Dilation of Upper Artery with Four or More Drug-eluting Intraluminal Devices, Percutaneous Endoscopic Approach
037Y0DZ Dilation of Upper Artery with Intraluminal Device, Open Approach	**037Y3DZ** Dilation of Upper Artery with Intraluminal Device, Percutaneous Approach	**037Y4DZ** Dilation of Upper Artery with Intraluminal Device, Percutaneous Endoscopic Approach
037Y0EZ Dilation of Upper Artery with Two Intraluminal Devices, Open Approach	**037Y3EZ** Dilation of Upper Artery with Two Intraluminal Devices, Percutaneous Approach	**037Y4EZ** Dilation of Upper Artery with Two Intraluminal Devices, Percutaneous Endoscopic Approach
037Y0FZ Dilation of Upper Artery with Three Intraluminal Devices, Open Approach	**037Y3FZ** Dilation of Upper Artery with Three Intraluminal Devices, Percutaneous Approach	**037Y4FZ** Dilation of Upper Artery with Three Intraluminal Devices, Percutaneous Endoscopic Approach
037Y0GZ Dilation of Upper Artery with Four or More Intraluminal Devices, Open Approach	**037Y3GZ** Dilation of Upper Artery with Four or More Intraluminal Devices, Percutaneous Approach	**037Y4GZ** Dilation of Upper Artery with Four or More Intraluminal Devices, Percutaneous Endoscopic Approach
037Y0ZZ Dilation of Upper Artery, Open Approach	**037Y3ZZ** Dilation of Upper Artery, Percutaneous Approach	**037Y4ZZ** Dilation of Upper Artery, Percutaneous Endoscopic Approach
037Y34Z Dilation of Upper Artery with Drug-eluting Intraluminal Device, Percutaneous Approach	**037Y44Z** Dilation of Upper Artery with Drug-eluting Intraluminal Device, Percutaneous Endoscopic Approach	

039 – Upper Arteries, Drainage

Review Coding Guidelines B3.4a and B3.4b

Review Coding Guideline B6.2

039000Z Drainage of Right Internal Mammary Artery with Drainage Device, Open Approach	**03914ZX** Drainage of Left Internal Mammary Artery, Percutaneous Endoscopic Approach, Diagnostic	**03934ZX** Drainage of Right Subclavian Artery, Percutaneous Endoscopic Approach, Diagnostic
03900ZX Drainage of Right Internal Mammary Artery, Open Approach, Diagnostic	**03914ZZ** Drainage of Left Internal Mammary Artery, Percutaneous Endoscopic Approach	**03934ZZ** Drainage of Right Subclavian Artery, Percutaneous Endoscopic Approach
03900ZZ Drainage of Right Internal Mammary Artery, Open Approach	**039200Z** Drainage of Innominate Artery with Drainage Device, Open Approach	**039400Z** Drainage of Left Subclavian Artery with Drainage Device, Open Approach
039030Z Drainage of Right Internal Mammary Artery with Drainage Device, Percutaneous Approach	**03920ZX** Drainage of Innominate Artery, Open Approach, Diagnostic	**03940ZX** Drainage of Left Subclavian Artery, Open Approach, Diagnostic
03903ZX Drainage of Right Internal Mammary Artery, Percutaneous Approach, Diagnostic	**03920ZZ** Drainage of Innominate Artery, Open Approach	**03940ZZ** Drainage of Left Subclavian Artery, Open Approach
03903ZZ Drainage of Right Internal Mammary Artery, Percutaneous Approach	**039230Z** Drainage of Innominate Artery with Drainage Device, Percutaneous Approach	**039430Z** Drainage of Left Subclavian Artery with Drainage Device, Percutaneous Approach
039040Z Drainage of Right Internal Mammary Artery with Drainage Device, Percutaneous Endoscopic Approach	**03923ZX** Drainage of Innominate Artery, Percutaneous Approach, Diagnostic	**03943ZX** Drainage of Left Subclavian Artery, Percutaneous Approach, Diagnostic
03904ZX Drainage of Right Internal Mammary Artery, Percutaneous Endoscopic Approach, Diagnostic	**03923ZZ** Drainage of Innominate Artery, Percutaneous Approach	**03943ZZ** Drainage of Left Subclavian Artery, Percutaneous Approach
03904ZZ Drainage of Right Internal Mammary Artery, Percutaneous Endoscopic Approach	**039240Z** Drainage of Innominate Artery with Drainage Device, Percutaneous Endoscopic Approach	**039440Z** Drainage of Left Subclavian Artery with Drainage Device, Percutaneous Endoscopic Approach
039100Z Drainage of Left Internal Mammary Artery with Drainage Device, Open Approach	**03924ZX** Drainage of Innominate Artery, Percutaneous Endoscopic Approach, Diagnostic	**03944ZX** Drainage of Left Subclavian Artery, Percutaneous Endoscopic Approach, Diagnostic
03910ZX Drainage of Left Internal Mammary Artery, Open Approach, Diagnostic	**03924ZZ** Drainage of Innominate Artery, Percutaneous Endoscopic Approach	**03944ZZ** Drainage of Left Subclavian Artery, Percutaneous Endoscopic Approach
03910ZZ Drainage of Left Internal Mammary Artery, Open Approach	**039300Z** Drainage of Right Subclavian Artery with Drainage Device, Open Approach	**039500Z** Drainage of Right Axillary Artery with Drainage Device, Open Approach
039130Z Drainage of Left Internal Mammary Artery with Drainage Device, Percutaneous Approach	**03930ZX** Drainage of Right Subclavian Artery, Open Approach, Diagnostic	**03950ZX** Drainage of Right Axillary Artery, Open Approach, Diagnostic
03913ZX Drainage of Left Internal Mammary Artery, Percutaneous Approach, Diagnostic	**03930ZZ** Drainage of Right Subclavian Artery, Open Approach	**03950ZZ** Drainage of Right Axillary Artery, Open Approach
03913ZZ Drainage of Left Internal Mammary Artery, Percutaneous Approach	**039330Z** Drainage of Right Subclavian Artery with Drainage Device, Percutaneous Approach	**039530Z** Drainage of Right Axillary Artery with Drainage Device, Percutaneous Approach
039140Z Drainage of Left Internal Mammary Artery with Drainage Device, Percutaneous Endoscopic Approach	**03933ZX** Drainage of Right Subclavian Artery, Percutaneous Approach, Diagnostic	**03953ZX** Drainage of Right Axillary Artery, Percutaneous Approach, Diagnostic
	03933ZZ Drainage of Right Subclavian Artery, Percutaneous Approach	**03953ZZ** Drainage of Right Axillary Artery, Percutaneous Approach
	039340Z Drainage of Right Subclavian Artery with Drainage Device, Percutaneous Endoscopic Approach	**039540Z** Drainage of Right Axillary Artery with Drainage Device, Percutaneous Endoscopic Approach

♀ Female-only   ♂ Male-only   ▲ Limited Coverage   ● Non-OR   🔲 HAC-associated procedure   ▲ Non-covered procedures   ➕ Cluster

03954ZX Drainage of Right Axillary Artery, Percutaneous Endoscopic Approach, Diagnostic

03954ZZ Drainage of Right Axillary Artery, Percutaneous Endoscopic Approach

039600Z Drainage of Left Axillary Artery with Drainage Device, Open Approach

03960ZX Drainage of Left Axillary Artery, Open Approach, Diagnostic

03960ZZ Drainage of Left Axillary Artery, Open Approach

039630Z Drainage of Left Axillary Artery with Drainage Device, Percutaneous Approach

03963ZX Drainage of Left Axillary Artery, Percutaneous Approach, Diagnostic

03963ZZ Drainage of Left Axillary Artery, Percutaneous Approach

039640Z Drainage of Left Axillary Artery with Drainage Device, Percutaneous Endoscopic Approach

03964ZX Drainage of Left Axillary Artery, Percutaneous Endoscopic Approach, Diagnostic

03964ZZ Drainage of Left Axillary Artery, Percutaneous Endoscopic Approach

039700Z Drainage of Right Brachial Artery with Drainage Device, Open Approach

03970ZX Drainage of Right Brachial Artery, Open Approach, Diagnostic

03970ZZ Drainage of Right Brachial Artery, Open Approach

039730Z Drainage of Right Brachial Artery with Drainage Device, Percutaneous Approach

03973ZX Drainage of Right Brachial Artery, Percutaneous Approach, Diagnostic

03973ZZ Drainage of Right Brachial Artery, Percutaneous Approach

039740Z Drainage of Right Brachial Artery with Drainage Device, Percutaneous Endoscopic Approach

03974ZX Drainage of Right Brachial Artery, Percutaneous Endoscopic Approach, Diagnostic

03974ZZ Drainage of Right Brachial Artery, Percutaneous Endoscopic Approach

039800Z Drainage of Left Brachial Artery with Drainage Device, Open Approach

03980ZX Drainage of Left Brachial Artery, Open Approach, Diagnostic

03980ZZ Drainage of Left Brachial Artery, Open Approach

039830Z Drainage of Left Brachial Artery with Drainage Device, Percutaneous Approach

03983ZX Drainage of Left Brachial Artery, Percutaneous Approach, Diagnostic

03983ZZ Drainage of Left Brachial Artery, Percutaneous Approach

039840Z Drainage of Left Brachial Artery with Drainage Device, Percutaneous Endoscopic Approach

03984ZX Drainage of Left Brachial Artery, Percutaneous Endoscopic Approach, Diagnostic

03984ZZ Drainage of Left Brachial Artery, Percutaneous Endoscopic Approach

039900Z Drainage of Right Ulnar Artery with Drainage Device, Open Approach

03990ZX Drainage of Right Ulnar Artery, Open Approach, Diagnostic

03990ZZ Drainage of Right Ulnar Artery, Open Approach

039930Z Drainage of Right Ulnar Artery with Drainage Device, Percutaneous Approach

03993ZX Drainage of Right Ulnar Artery, Percutaneous Approach, Diagnostic

03993ZZ Drainage of Right Ulnar Artery, Percutaneous Approach

039940Z Drainage of Right Ulnar Artery with Drainage Device, Percutaneous Endoscopic Approach

03994ZX Drainage of Right Ulnar Artery, Percutaneous Endoscopic Approach, Diagnostic

03994ZZ Drainage of Right Ulnar Artery, Percutaneous Endoscopic Approach

039A00Z Drainage of Left Ulnar Artery with Drainage Device, Open Approach

039A0ZX Drainage of Left Ulnar Artery, Open Approach, Diagnostic

039A0ZZ Drainage of Left Ulnar Artery, Open Approach

039A30Z Drainage of Left Ulnar Artery with Drainage Device, Percutaneous Approach

039A3ZX Drainage of Left Ulnar Artery, Percutaneous Approach, Diagnostic

039A3ZZ Drainage of Left Ulnar Artery, Percutaneous Approach

039A40Z Drainage of Left Ulnar Artery with Drainage Device, Percutaneous Endoscopic Approach

039A4ZX Drainage of Left Ulnar Artery, Percutaneous Endoscopic Approach, Diagnostic

039A4ZZ Drainage of Left Ulnar Artery, Percutaneous Endoscopic Approach

039B00Z Drainage of Right Radial Artery with Drainage Device, Open Approach

039B0ZX Drainage of Right Radial Artery, Open Approach, Diagnostic

039B0ZZ Drainage of Right Radial Artery, Open Approach

039B30Z Drainage of Right Radial Artery with Drainage Device, Percutaneous Approach

039B3ZX Drainage of Right Radial Artery, Percutaneous Approach, Diagnostic

039B3ZZ Drainage of Right Radial Artery, Percutaneous Approach

039B40Z Drainage of Right Radial Artery with Drainage Device, Percutaneous Endoscopic Approach

039B4ZX Drainage of Right Radial Artery, Percutaneous Endoscopic Approach, Diagnostic

039B4ZZ Drainage of Right Radial Artery, Percutaneous Endoscopic Approach

039C00Z Drainage of Left Radial Artery with Drainage Device, Open Approach

039C0ZX Drainage of Left Radial Artery, Open Approach, Diagnostic

039C0ZZ Drainage of Left Radial Artery, Open Approach

039C30Z Drainage of Left Radial Artery with Drainage Device, Percutaneous Approach

039C3ZX Drainage of Left Radial Artery, Percutaneous Approach, Diagnostic

039C3ZZ Drainage of Left Radial Artery, Percutaneous Approach

039C40Z Drainage of Left Radial Artery with Drainage Device, Percutaneous Endoscopic Approach

039C4ZX Drainage of Left Radial Artery, Percutaneous Endoscopic Approach, Diagnostic

039C4ZZ Drainage of Left Radial Artery, Percutaneous Endoscopic Approach

039D00Z Drainage of Right Hand Artery with Drainage Device, Open Approach

039D0ZX Drainage of Right Hand Artery, Open Approach, Diagnostic

039D0ZZ Drainage of Right Hand Artery, Open Approach

039D30Z Drainage of Right Hand Artery with Drainage Device, Percutaneous Approach

039D3ZX Drainage of Right Hand Artery, Percutaneous Approach, Diagnostic

039D3ZZ Drainage of Right Hand Artery, Percutaneous Approach

039D40Z Drainage of Right Hand Artery with Drainage Device, Percutaneous Endoscopic Approach

039D4ZX Drainage of Right Hand Artery, Percutaneous Endoscopic Approach, Diagnostic

039D4ZZ Drainage of Right Hand Artery, Percutaneous Endoscopic Approach

039F00Z Drainage of Left Hand Artery with Drainage Device, Open Approach

039F0ZX Drainage of Left Hand Artery, Open Approach, Diagnostic

039F0ZZ Drainage of Left Hand Artery, Open Approach

039F30Z Drainage of Left Hand Artery with Drainage Device, Percutaneous Approach

039F3ZX Drainage of Left Hand Artery, Percutaneous Approach, Diagnostic

039F3ZZ Drainage of Left Hand Artery, Percutaneous Approach

039F40Z Drainage of Left Hand Artery with Drainage Device, Percutaneous Endoscopic Approach

039F4ZX Drainage of Left Hand Artery, Percutaneous Endoscopic Approach, Diagnostic

039F4ZZ Drainage of Left Hand Artery, Percutaneous Endoscopic Approach

039G00Z Drainage of Intracranial Artery with Drainage Device, Open Approach

039G0ZX Drainage of Intracranial Artery, Open Approach, Diagnostic

039G0ZZ Drainage of Intracranial Artery, Open Approach

039G30Z Drainage of Intracranial Artery with Drainage Device, Percutaneous Approach

039G3ZX Drainage of Intracranial Artery, Percutaneous Approach, Diagnostic

039G3ZZ Drainage of Intracranial Artery, Percutaneous Approach

039G40Z Drainage of Intracranial Artery with Drainage Device, Percutaneous Endoscopic Approach

039G4ZX Drainage of Intracranial Artery, Percutaneous Endoscopic Approach, Diagnostic

039G4ZZ Drainage of Intracranial Artery, Percutaneous Endoscopic Approach

039H00Z Drainage of Right Common Carotid Artery with Drainage Device, Open Approach

039H0ZX Drainage of Right Common Carotid Artery, Open Approach, Diagnostic

039H0ZZ Drainage of Right Common Carotid Artery, Open Approach

039H30Z Drainage of Right Common Carotid Artery with Drainage Device, Percutaneous Approach

039H3ZX Drainage of Right Common Carotid Artery, Percutaneous Approach, Diagnostic

039H3ZZ Drainage of Right Common Carotid Artery, Percutaneous Approach

039H40Z Drainage of Right Common Carotid Artery with Drainage Device, Percutaneous Endoscopic Approach

039H4ZX Drainage of Right Common Carotid Artery, Percutaneous Endoscopic Approach, Diagnostic

039H4ZZ Drainage of Right Common Carotid Artery, Percutaneous Endoscopic Approach

039J00Z Drainage of Left Common Carotid Artery with Drainage Device, Open Approach

039J0ZX Drainage of Left Common Carotid Artery, Open Approach, Diagnostic

039J0ZZ Drainage of Left Common Carotid Artery, Open Approach

039J30Z Drainage of Left Common Carotid Artery with Drainage Device, Percutaneous Approach

039J3ZX Drainage of Left Common Carotid Artery, Percutaneous Approach, Diagnostic

039J3ZZ Drainage of Left Common Carotid Artery, Percutaneous Approach

039J40Z Drainage of Left Common Carotid Artery with Drainage Device, Percutaneous Endoscopic Approach

039J4ZX Drainage of Left Common Carotid Artery, Percutaneous Endoscopic Approach, Diagnostic

039J4ZZ Drainage of Left Common Carotid Artery, Percutaneous Endoscopic Approach

039K00Z Drainage of Right Internal Carotid Artery with Drainage Device, Open Approach

039K0ZX Drainage of Right Internal Carotid Artery, Open Approach, Diagnostic

039K0ZZ Drainage of Right Internal Carotid Artery, Open Approach

039K30Z Drainage of Right Internal Carotid Artery with Drainage Device, Percutaneous Approach

039K3ZX Drainage of Right Internal Carotid Artery, Percutaneous Approach, Diagnostic

039K3ZZ Drainage of Right Internal Carotid Artery, Percutaneous Approach

039K40Z Drainage of Right Internal Carotid Artery with Drainage Device, Percutaneous Endoscopic Approach

039K4ZX Drainage of Right Internal Carotid Artery, Percutaneous Endoscopic Approach, Diagnostic

039K4ZZ Drainage of Right Internal Carotid Artery, Percutaneous Endoscopic Approach

039L00Z Drainage of Left Internal Carotid Artery with Drainage Device, Open Approach

039L0ZX Drainage of Left Internal Carotid Artery, Open Approach, Diagnostic

039L0ZZ Drainage of Left Internal Carotid Artery, Open Approach

039L30Z Drainage of Left Internal Carotid Artery with Drainage Device, Percutaneous Approach

039L3ZX Drainage of Left Internal Carotid Artery, Percutaneous Approach, Diagnostic

039L3ZZ Drainage of Left Internal Carotid Artery, Percutaneous Approach

039L40Z Drainage of Left Internal Carotid Artery with Drainage Device, Percutaneous Endoscopic Approach

039L4ZX Drainage of Left Internal Carotid Artery, Percutaneous Endoscopic Approach, Diagnostic

039L4ZZ Drainage of Left Internal Carotid Artery, Percutaneous Endoscopic Approach

039M00Z Drainage of Right External Carotid Artery with Drainage Device, Open Approach

039M0ZX Drainage of Right External Carotid Artery, Open Approach, Diagnostic

039M0ZZ Drainage of Right External Carotid Artery, Open Approach

039M30Z Drainage of Right External Carotid Artery with Drainage Device, Percutaneous Approach

039M3ZX Drainage of Right External Carotid Artery, Percutaneous Approach, Diagnostic

039M3ZZ Drainage of Right External Carotid Artery, Percutaneous Approach

039M40Z Drainage of Right External Carotid Artery with Drainage Device, Percutaneous Endoscopic Approach

039M4ZX Drainage of Right External Carotid Artery, Percutaneous Endoscopic Approach, Diagnostic

039M4ZZ Drainage of Right External Carotid Artery, Percutaneous Endoscopic Approach

039N00Z Drainage of Left External Carotid Artery with Drainage Device, Open Approach

039N0ZX Drainage of Left External Carotid Artery, Open Approach, Diagnostic

039N0ZZ Drainage of Left External Carotid Artery, Open Approach

039N30Z Drainage of Left External Carotid Artery with Drainage Device, Percutaneous Approach

039N3ZX Drainage of Left External Carotid Artery, Percutaneous Approach, Diagnostic

039N3ZZ Drainage of Left External Carotid Artery, Percutaneous Approach

039N40Z Drainage of Left External Carotid Artery with Drainage Device, Percutaneous Endoscopic Approach

039N4ZX Drainage of Left External Carotid Artery, Percutaneous Endoscopic Approach, Diagnostic

039N4ZZ Drainage of Left External Carotid Artery, Percutaneous Endoscopic Approach

039P00Z Drainage of Right Vertebral Artery with Drainage Device, Open Approach

039P0ZX Drainage of Right Vertebral Artery, Open Approach, Diagnostic

039P0ZZ Drainage of Right Vertebral Artery, Open Approach

039P30Z Drainage of Right Vertebral Artery with Drainage Device, Percutaneous Approach

039P3ZX Drainage of Right Vertebral Artery, Percutaneous Approach, Diagnostic

039P3ZZ Drainage of Right Vertebral Artery, Percutaneous Approach

039P40Z Drainage of Right Vertebral Artery with Drainage Device, Percutaneous Endoscopic Approach

039P4ZX Drainage of Right Vertebral Artery, Percutaneous Endoscopic Approach, Diagnostic

039P4ZZ Drainage of Right Vertebral Artery, Percutaneous Endoscopic Approach

039Q00Z Drainage of Left Vertebral Artery with Drainage Device, Open Approach

039Q0ZX Drainage of Left Vertebral Artery, Open Approach, Diagnostic

039Q0ZZ Drainage of Left Vertebral Artery, Open Approach

039Q30Z Drainage of Left Vertebral Artery with Drainage Device, Percutaneous Approach

039Q3ZX Drainage of Left Vertebral Artery, Percutaneous Approach, Diagnostic

039Q3ZZ Drainage of Left Vertebral Artery, Percutaneous Approach

039Q40Z Drainage of Left Vertebral Artery with Drainage Device, Percutaneous Endoscopic Approach

039Q4ZX Drainage of Left Vertebral Artery, Percutaneous Endoscopic Approach, Diagnostic

039Q4ZZ Drainage of Left Vertebral Artery, Percutaneous Endoscopic Approach

039R00Z Drainage of Face Artery with Drainage Device, Open Approach

039R0ZX Drainage of Face Artery, Open Approach, Diagnostic

039R0ZZ Drainage of Face Artery, Open Approach

039R30Z Drainage of Face Artery with Drainage Device, Percutaneous Approach

039R3ZX Drainage of Face Artery, Percutaneous Approach, Diagnostic

039R3ZZ Drainage of Face Artery, Percutaneous Approach

039R40Z Drainage of Face Artery with Drainage Device, Percutaneous Endoscopic Approach

039R4ZX Drainage of Face Artery, Percutaneous Endoscopic Approach, Diagnostic

039R4ZZ Drainage of Face Artery, Percutaneous Endoscopic Approach

039S00Z Drainage of Right Temporal Artery with Drainage Device, Open Approach

039S0ZX Drainage of Right Temporal Artery, Open Approach, Diagnostic

039S0ZZ Drainage of Right Temporal Artery, Open Approach

039S30Z Drainage of Right Temporal Artery with Drainage Device, Percutaneous Approach

039S3ZX Drainage of Right Temporal Artery, Percutaneous Approach, Diagnostic

039S3ZZ Drainage of Right Temporal Artery, Percutaneous Approach

039S40Z Drainage of Right Temporal Artery with Drainage Device, Percutaneous Endoscopic Approach

039S4ZX Drainage of Right Temporal Artery, Percutaneous Endoscopic Approach, Diagnostic

039S4ZZ Drainage of Right Temporal Artery, Percutaneous Endoscopic Approach

039T00Z Drainage of Left Temporal Artery with Drainage Device, Open Approach

039T0ZX Drainage of Left Temporal Artery, Open Approach, Diagnostic

039T0ZZ Drainage of Left Temporal Artery, Open Approach

039T30Z Drainage of Left Temporal Artery with Drainage Device, Percutaneous Approach

039T3ZX Drainage of Left Temporal Artery, Percutaneous Approach, Diagnostic

039T3ZZ Drainage of Left Temporal Artery, Percutaneous Approach

039T40Z Drainage of Left Temporal Artery with Drainage Device, Percutaneous Endoscopic Approach

♀ Female-only   ♂ Male-only   ▲ Limited Coverage   ● Non-OR   HAC HAC-associated procedure   ▲ Non-covered procedures   ✚ Cluster

039T4ZX Drainage of Left Temporal Artery, Percutaneous Endoscopic Approach, Diagnostic

039T4ZZ Drainage of Left Temporal Artery, Percutaneous Endoscopic Approach

039U00Z Drainage of Right Thyroid Artery with Drainage Device, Open Approach

039U0ZX Drainage of Right Thyroid Artery, Open Approach, Diagnostic

039U0ZZ Drainage of Right Thyroid Artery, Open Approach

039U30Z Drainage of Right Thyroid Artery with Drainage Device, Percutaneous Approach

039U3ZX Drainage of Right Thyroid Artery, Percutaneous Approach, Diagnostic

039U3ZZ Drainage of Right Thyroid Artery, Percutaneous Approach

039U40Z Drainage of Right Thyroid Artery with Drainage Device, Percutaneous Endoscopic Approach

039U4ZX Drainage of Right Thyroid Artery, Percutaneous Endoscopic Approach, Diagnostic

039U4ZZ Drainage of Right Thyroid Artery, Percutaneous Endoscopic Approach

039V00Z Drainage of Left Thyroid Artery with Drainage Device, Open Approach

039V0ZX Drainage of Left Thyroid Artery, Open Approach, Diagnostic

039V0ZZ Drainage of Left Thyroid Artery, Open Approach

039V30Z Drainage of Left Thyroid Artery with Drainage Device, Percutaneous Approach

039V3ZX Drainage of Left Thyroid Artery, Percutaneous Approach, Diagnostic

039V3ZZ Drainage of Left Thyroid Artery, Percutaneous Approach

039V40Z Drainage of Left Thyroid Artery with Drainage Device, Percutaneous Endoscopic Approach

039V4ZX Drainage of Left Thyroid Artery, Percutaneous Endoscopic Approach, Diagnostic

039V4ZZ Drainage of Left Thyroid Artery, Percutaneous Endoscopic Approach

039Y00Z Drainage of Upper Artery with Drainage Device, Open Approach

039Y0ZX Drainage of Upper Artery, Open Approach, Diagnostic

039Y0ZZ Drainage of Upper Artery, Open Approach

039Y30Z Drainage of Upper Artery with Drainage Device, Percutaneous Approach

039Y3ZX Drainage of Upper Artery, Percutaneous Approach, Diagnostic

039Y3ZZ Drainage of Upper Artery, Percutaneous Approach

039Y40Z Drainage of Upper Artery with Drainage Device, Percutaneous Endoscopic Approach

039Y4ZX Drainage of Upper Artery, Percutaneous Endoscopic Approach, Diagnostic

039Y4ZZ Drainage of Upper Artery, Percutaneous Endoscopic Approach

03B – Upper Arteries, Excision

Review Coding Guidelines B3.4a and B3.4b

Review Coding Guideline B3.8

Review Coding Guideline B3.18

03B00ZX Excision of Right Internal Mammary Artery, Open Approach, Diagnostic

03B00ZZ Excision of Right Internal Mammary Artery, Open Approach

03B03ZX Excision of Right Internal Mammary Artery, Percutaneous Approach, Diagnostic

03B03ZZ Excision of Right Internal Mammary Artery, Percutaneous Approach

03B04ZX Excision of Right Internal Mammary Artery, Percutaneous Endoscopic Approach, Diagnostic

03B04ZZ Excision of Right Internal Mammary Artery, Percutaneous Endoscopic Approach

03B10ZX Excision of Left Internal Mammary Artery, Open Approach, Diagnostic

03B10ZZ Excision of Left Internal Mammary Artery, Open Approach

03B13ZX Excision of Left Internal Mammary Artery, Percutaneous Approach, Diagnostic

03B13ZZ Excision of Left Internal Mammary Artery, Percutaneous Approach

03B14ZX Excision of Left Internal Mammary Artery, Percutaneous Endoscopic Approach, Diagnostic

03B14ZZ Excision of Left Internal Mammary Artery, Percutaneous Endoscopic Approach

03B20ZX Excision of Innominate Artery, Open Approach, Diagnostic

03B20ZZ Excision of Innominate Artery, Open Approach

03B23ZX Excision of Innominate Artery, Percutaneous Approach, Diagnostic

03B23ZZ Excision of Innominate Artery, Percutaneous Approach

03B24ZX Excision of Innominate Artery, Percutaneous Endoscopic Approach, Diagnostic

03B24ZZ Excision of Innominate Artery, Percutaneous Endoscopic Approach

03B30ZX Excision of Right Subclavian Artery, Open Approach, Diagnostic

03B30ZZ Excision of Right Subclavian Artery, Open Approach

03B33ZX Excision of Right Subclavian Artery, Percutaneous Approach, Diagnostic

03B33ZZ Excision of Right Subclavian Artery, Percutaneous Approach

03B34ZX Excision of Right Subclavian Artery, Percutaneous Endoscopic Approach, Diagnostic

03B34ZZ Excision of Right Subclavian Artery, Percutaneous Endoscopic Approach

03B40ZX Excision of Left Subclavian Artery, Open Approach, Diagnostic

03B40ZZ Excision of Left Subclavian Artery, Open Approach

03B43ZX Excision of Left Subclavian Artery, Percutaneous Approach, Diagnostic

03B43ZZ Excision of Left Subclavian Artery, Percutaneous Approach

03B44ZX Excision of Left Subclavian Artery, Percutaneous Endoscopic Approach, Diagnostic

03B44ZZ Excision of Left Subclavian Artery, Percutaneous Endoscopic Approach

03B50ZX Excision of Right Axillary Artery, Open Approach, Diagnostic

03B50ZZ Excision of Right Axillary Artery, Open Approach

03B53ZX Excision of Right Axillary Artery, Percutaneous Approach, Diagnostic

03B53ZZ Excision of Right Axillary Artery, Percutaneous Approach

03B54ZX Excision of Right Axillary Artery, Percutaneous Endoscopic Approach, Diagnostic

03B54ZZ Excision of Right Axillary Artery, Percutaneous Endoscopic Approach

03B60ZX Excision of Left Axillary Artery, Open Approach, Diagnostic

03B60ZZ Excision of Left Axillary Artery, Open Approach

03B63ZX Excision of Left Axillary Artery, Percutaneous Approach, Diagnostic

03B63ZZ Excision of Left Axillary Artery, Percutaneous Approach

03B64ZX Excision of Left Axillary Artery, Percutaneous Endoscopic Approach, Diagnostic

03B64ZZ Excision of Left Axillary Artery, Percutaneous Endoscopic Approach

03B70ZX Excision of Right Brachial Artery, Open Approach, Diagnostic

03B70ZZ Excision of Right Brachial Artery, Open Approach

03B73ZX Excision of Right Brachial Artery, Percutaneous Approach, Diagnostic

03B73ZZ Excision of Right Brachial Artery, Percutaneous Approach

03B74ZX Excision of Right Brachial Artery, Percutaneous Endoscopic Approach, Diagnostic

03B74ZZ Excision of Right Brachial Artery, Percutaneous Endoscopic Approach

03B80ZX Excision of Left Brachial Artery, Open Approach, Diagnostic

03B80ZZ Excision of Left Brachial Artery, Open Approach

03B83ZX Excision of Left Brachial Artery, Percutaneous Approach, Diagnostic

03B83ZZ Excision of Left Brachial Artery, Percutaneous Approach

03B84ZX Excision of Left Brachial Artery, Percutaneous Endoscopic Approach, Diagnostic

03B84ZZ Excision of Left Brachial Artery, Percutaneous Endoscopic Approach

03B90ZX Excision of Right Ulnar Artery, Open Approach, Diagnostic

03B90ZZ Excision of Right Ulnar Artery, Open Approach

03B93ZX Excision of Right Ulnar Artery, Percutaneous Approach, Diagnostic

03B93ZZ Excision of Right Ulnar Artery, Percutaneous Approach

03B94ZX Excision of Right Ulnar Artery, Percutaneous Endoscopic Approach, Diagnostic

03B94ZZ Excision of Right Ulnar Artery, Percutaneous Endoscopic Approach

03BA0ZX Excision of Left Ulnar Artery, Open Approach, Diagnostic

03BA0ZZ Excision of Left Ulnar Artery, Open Approach

03BA3ZX Excision of Left Ulnar Artery, Percutaneous Approach, Diagnostic

03BA3ZZ Excision of Left Ulnar Artery, Percutaneous Approach

03BA4ZX Excision of Left Ulnar Artery, Percutaneous Endoscopic Approach, Diagnostic

03BA4ZZ Excision of Left Ulnar Artery, Percutaneous Endoscopic Approach

03BB0ZX Excision of Right Radial Artery, Open Approach, Diagnostic

03BB0ZZ Excision of Right Radial Artery, Open Approach

03BB3ZX Excision of Right Radial Artery, Percutaneous Approach, Diagnostic

03BB3ZZ Excision of Right Radial Artery, Percutaneous Approach

03BB4ZX Excision of Right Radial Artery, Percutaneous Endoscopic Approach, Diagnostic

03BB4ZZ Excision of Right Radial Artery, Percutaneous Endoscopic Approach

03BC0ZX Excision of Left Radial Artery, Open Approach, Diagnostic

03BC0ZZ Excision of Left Radial Artery, Open Approach

03BC3ZX Excision of Left Radial Artery, Percutaneous Approach, Diagnostic

03BC3ZZ Excision of Left Radial Artery, Percutaneous Approach

03BC4ZX Excision of Left Radial Artery, Percutaneous Endoscopic Approach, Diagnostic

03BC4ZZ Excision of Left Radial Artery, Percutaneous Endoscopic Approach

03BD0ZX Excision of Right Hand Artery, Open Approach, Diagnostic

03BD0ZZ Excision of Right Hand Artery, Open Approach

03BD3ZX Excision of Right Hand Artery, Percutaneous Approach, Diagnostic

03BD3ZZ Excision of Right Hand Artery, Percutaneous Approach

03BD4ZX Excision of Right Hand Artery, Percutaneous Endoscopic Approach, Diagnostic

03BD4ZZ Excision of Right Hand Artery, Percutaneous Endoscopic Approach

03BF0ZX Excision of Left Hand Artery, Open Approach, Diagnostic

03BF0ZZ Excision of Left Hand Artery, Open Approach

03BF3ZX Excision of Left Hand Artery, Percutaneous Approach, Diagnostic

03BF3ZZ Excision of Left Hand Artery, Percutaneous Approach

03BF4ZX Excision of Left Hand Artery, Percutaneous Endoscopic Approach, Diagnostic

03BF4ZZ Excision of Left Hand Artery, Percutaneous Endoscopic Approach

03BG0ZX Excision of Intracranial Artery, Open Approach, Diagnostic

03BG0ZZ Excision of Intracranial Artery, Open Approach

03BG3ZX Excision of Intracranial Artery, Percutaneous Approach, Diagnostic

03BG3ZZ Excision of Intracranial Artery, Percutaneous Approach

03BG4ZX Excision of Intracranial Artery, Percutaneous Endoscopic Approach, Diagnostic

03BG4ZZ Excision of Intracranial Artery, Percutaneous Endoscopic Approach

03BH0ZX Excision of Right Common Carotid Artery, Open Approach, Diagnostic

03BH0ZZ Excision of Right Common Carotid Artery, Open Approach

03BH3ZX Excision of Right Common Carotid Artery, Percutaneous Approach, Diagnostic

03BH3ZZ Excision of Right Common Carotid Artery, Percutaneous Approach

03BH4ZX Excision of Right Common Carotid Artery, Percutaneous Endoscopic Approach, Diagnostic

03BH4ZZ Excision of Right Common Carotid Artery, Percutaneous Endoscopic Approach

03BJ0ZX Excision of Left Common Carotid Artery, Open Approach, Diagnostic

03BJ0ZZ Excision of Left Common Carotid Artery, Open Approach

03BJ3ZX Excision of Left Common Carotid Artery, Percutaneous Approach, Diagnostic

03BJ3ZZ Excision of Left Common Carotid Artery, Percutaneous Approach

03BJ4ZX Excision of Left Common Carotid Artery, Percutaneous Endoscopic Approach, Diagnostic

03BJ4ZZ Excision of Left Common Carotid Artery, Percutaneous Endoscopic Approach

03BK0ZX Excision of Right Internal Carotid Artery, Open Approach, Diagnostic

03BK0ZZ Excision of Right Internal Carotid Artery, Open Approach

03BK3ZX Excision of Right Internal Carotid Artery, Percutaneous Approach, Diagnostic

03BK3ZZ Excision of Right Internal Carotid Artery, Percutaneous Approach

03BK4ZX Excision of Right Internal Carotid Artery, Percutaneous Endoscopic Approach, Diagnostic

03BK4ZZ Excision of Right Internal Carotid Artery, Percutaneous Endoscopic Approach

03BL0ZX Excision of Left Internal Carotid Artery, Open Approach, Diagnostic

03BL0ZZ Excision of Left Internal Carotid Artery, Open Approach

03BL3ZX Excision of Left Internal Carotid Artery, Percutaneous Approach, Diagnostic

03BL3ZZ Excision of Left Internal Carotid Artery, Percutaneous Approach

03BL4ZX Excision of Left Internal Carotid Artery, Percutaneous Endoscopic Approach, Diagnostic

03BL4ZZ Excision of Left Internal Carotid Artery, Percutaneous Endoscopic Approach

03BM0ZX Excision of Right External Carotid Artery, Open Approach, Diagnostic

03BM0ZZ Excision of Right External Carotid Artery, Open Approach

03BM3ZX Excision of Right External Carotid Artery, Percutaneous Approach, Diagnostic

03BM3ZZ Excision of Right External Carotid Artery, Percutaneous Approach

03BM4ZX Excision of Right External Carotid Artery, Percutaneous Endoscopic Approach, Diagnostic

03BM4ZZ Excision of Right External Carotid Artery, Percutaneous Endoscopic Approach

03BN0ZX Excision of Left External Carotid Artery, Open Approach, Diagnostic

03BN0ZZ Excision of Left External Carotid Artery, Open Approach

AHA CC: 2Q, 2016, 12-14

03BN3ZX Excision of Left External Carotid Artery, Percutaneous Approach, Diagnostic

03BN3ZZ Excision of Left External Carotid Artery, Percutaneous Approach

03BN4ZX Excision of Left External Carotid Artery, Percutaneous Endoscopic Approach, Diagnostic

03BN4ZZ Excision of Left External Carotid Artery, Percutaneous Endoscopic Approach

03BP0ZX Excision of Right Vertebral Artery, Open Approach, Diagnostic

03BP0ZZ Excision of Right Vertebral Artery, Open Approach

03BP3ZX Excision of Right Vertebral Artery, Percutaneous Approach, Diagnostic

03BP3ZZ Excision of Right Vertebral Artery, Percutaneous Approach

03BP4ZX Excision of Right Vertebral Artery, Percutaneous Endoscopic Approach, Diagnostic

03BP4ZZ Excision of Right Vertebral Artery, Percutaneous Endoscopic Approach

03BQ0ZX Excision of Left Vertebral Artery, Open Approach, Diagnostic

03BQ0ZZ Excision of Left Vertebral Artery, Open Approach

03BQ3ZX Excision of Left Vertebral Artery, Percutaneous Approach, Diagnostic

03BQ3ZZ Excision of Left Vertebral Artery, Percutaneous Approach

03BQ4ZX Excision of Left Vertebral Artery, Percutaneous Endoscopic Approach, Diagnostic

03BQ4ZZ Excision of Left Vertebral Artery, Percutaneous Endoscopic Approach

03BR0ZX Excision of Face Artery, Open Approach, Diagnostic

03BR0ZZ Excision of Face Artery, Open Approach

03BR3ZX Excision of Face Artery, Percutaneous Approach, Diagnostic

03BR3ZZ Excision of Face Artery, Percutaneous Approach

03BR4ZX Excision of Face Artery, Percutaneous Endoscopic Approach, Diagnostic

03BR4ZZ Excision of Face Artery, Percutaneous Endoscopic Approach

03BS0ZX Excision of Right Temporal Artery, Open Approach, Diagnostic

03BS0ZZ Excision of Right Temporal Artery, Open Approach

03BS3ZX Excision of Right Temporal Artery, Percutaneous Approach, Diagnostic

03BS3ZZ Excision of Right Temporal Artery, Percutaneous Approach

03BS4ZX Excision of Right Temporal Artery, Percutaneous Endoscopic Approach, Diagnostic

03BS4ZZ Excision of Right Temporal Artery, Percutaneous Endoscopic Approach

03BT0ZX Excision of Left Temporal Artery, Open Approach, Diagnostic

♀ Female-only   ♂ Male-only   ▲ Limited Coverage   ● Non-OR   HAC HAC-associated procedure   ▲ Non-covered procedures   ✛ Cluster

03BT0ZZ Excision of Left Temporal Artery, Open Approach

03BT3ZX Excision of Left Temporal Artery, Percutaneous Approach, Diagnostic

03BT3ZZ Excision of Left Temporal Artery, Percutaneous Approach

03BT4ZX Excision of Left Temporal Artery, Percutaneous Endoscopic Approach, Diagnostic

03BT4ZZ Excision of Left Temporal Artery, Percutaneous Endoscopic Approach

03BU0ZX Excision of Right Thyroid Artery, Open Approach, Diagnostic

03BU0ZZ Excision of Right Thyroid Artery, Open Approach

03BU3ZX Excision of Right Thyroid Artery, Percutaneous Approach, Diagnostic

03BU3ZZ Excision of Right Thyroid Artery, Percutaneous Approach

03BU4ZX Excision of Right Thyroid Artery, Percutaneous Endoscopic Approach, Diagnostic

03BU4ZZ Excision of Right Thyroid Artery, Percutaneous Endoscopic Approach

03BV0ZX Excision of Left Thyroid Artery, Open Approach, Diagnostic

03BV0ZZ Excision of Left Thyroid Artery, Open Approach

03BV3ZX Excision of Left Thyroid Artery, Percutaneous Approach, Diagnostic

03BV3ZZ Excision of Left Thyroid Artery, Percutaneous Approach

03BV4ZX Excision of Left Thyroid Artery, Percutaneous Endoscopic Approach, Diagnostic

03BV4ZZ Excision of Left Thyroid Artery, Percutaneous Endoscopic Approach

03BY0ZX Excision of Upper Artery, Open Approach, Diagnostic

03BY0ZZ Excision of Upper Artery, Open Approach

03BY3ZX Excision of Upper Artery, Percutaneous Approach, Diagnostic

03BY3ZZ Excision of Upper Artery, Percutaneous Approach

03BY4ZX Excision of Upper Artery, Percutaneous Endoscopic Approach, Diagnostic

03BY4ZZ Excision of Upper Artery, Percutaneous Endoscopic Approach

03C – Upper Arteries, Extirpation

03C00ZZ Extirpation of Matter from Right Internal Mammary Artery, Open Approach

03C03ZZ Extirpation of Matter from Right Internal Mammary Artery, Percutaneous Approach

03C04ZZ Extirpation of Matter from Right Internal Mammary Artery, Percutaneous Endoscopic Approach

03C10ZZ Extirpation of Matter from Left Internal Mammary Artery, Open Approach

03C13ZZ Extirpation of Matter from Left Internal Mammary Artery, Percutaneous Approach

03C14ZZ Extirpation of Matter from Left Internal Mammary Artery, Percutaneous Endoscopic Approach

03C20ZZ Extirpation of Matter from Innominate Artery, Open Approach

03C23ZZ Extirpation of Matter from Innominate Artery, Percutaneous Approach

03C24ZZ Extirpation of Matter from Innominate Artery, Percutaneous Endoscopic Approach

03C30ZZ Extirpation of Matter from Right Subclavian Artery, Open Approach

03C33ZZ Extirpation of Matter from Right Subclavian Artery, Percutaneous Approach

03C34ZZ Extirpation of Matter from Right Subclavian Artery, Percutaneous Endoscopic Approach

03C40ZZ Extirpation of Matter from Left Subclavian Artery, Open Approach

03C43ZZ Extirpation of Matter from Left Subclavian Artery, Percutaneous Approach

03C44ZZ Extirpation of Matter from Left Subclavian Artery, Percutaneous Endoscopic Approach

03C50ZZ Extirpation of Matter from Right Axillary Artery, Open Approach

03C53ZZ Extirpation of Matter from Right Axillary Artery, Percutaneous Approach

03C54ZZ Extirpation of Matter from Right Axillary Artery, Percutaneous Endoscopic Approach

03C60ZZ Extirpation of Matter from Left Axillary Artery, Open Approach

03C63ZZ Extirpation of Matter from Left Axillary Artery, Percutaneous Approach

03C64ZZ Extirpation of Matter from Left Axillary Artery, Percutaneous Endoscopic Approach

03C70ZZ Extirpation of Matter from Right Brachial Artery, Open Approach

AHA CC: 3Q, 2020, 38-40

03C73ZZ Extirpation of Matter from Right Brachial Artery, Percutaneous Approach

03C74ZZ Extirpation of Matter from Right Brachial Artery, Percutaneous Endoscopic Approach

03C80ZZ Extirpation of Matter from Left Brachial Artery, Open Approach

03C83ZZ Extirpation of Matter from Left Brachial Artery, Percutaneous Approach

03C84ZZ Extirpation of Matter from Left Brachial Artery, Percutaneous Endoscopic Approach

03C90ZZ Extirpation of Matter from Right Ulnar Artery, Open Approach

03C93ZZ Extirpation of Matter from Right Ulnar Artery, Percutaneous Approach

03C94ZZ Extirpation of Matter from Right Ulnar Artery, Percutaneous Endoscopic Approach

03CA0ZZ Extirpation of Matter from Left Ulnar Artery, Open Approach

03CA3ZZ Extirpation of Matter from Left Ulnar Artery, Percutaneous Approach

03CA4ZZ Extirpation of Matter from Left Ulnar Artery, Percutaneous Endoscopic Approach

03CB0ZZ Extirpation of Matter from Right Radial Artery, Open Approach

03CB3ZZ Extirpation of Matter from Right Radial Artery, Percutaneous Approach

03CB4ZZ Extirpation of Matter from Right Radial Artery, Percutaneous Endoscopic Approach

03CC0ZZ Extirpation of Matter from Left Radial Artery, Open Approach

03CC3ZZ Extirpation of Matter from Left Radial Artery, Percutaneous Approach

03CC4ZZ Extirpation of Matter from Left Radial Artery, Percutaneous Endoscopic Approach

03CD0ZZ Extirpation of Matter from Right Hand Artery, Open Approach

03CD3ZZ Extirpation of Matter from Right Hand Artery, Percutaneous Approach

03CD4ZZ Extirpation of Matter from Right Hand Artery, Percutaneous Endoscopic Approach

03CF0ZZ Extirpation of Matter from Left Hand Artery, Open Approach

03CF3ZZ Extirpation of Matter from Left Hand Artery, Percutaneous Approach

03CF4ZZ Extirpation of Matter from Left Hand Artery, Percutaneous Endoscopic Approach

03CG0ZZ Extirpation of Matter from Intracranial Artery, Open Approach

03CG3Z7 Extirpation of Matter from Intracranial Artery using Stent Retriever, Percutaneous Approach

03CG3ZZ Extirpation of Matter from Intracranial Artery, Percutaneous Approach

03CG4ZZ Extirpation of Matter from Intracranial Artery, Percutaneous Endoscopic Approach

03CH0ZZ Extirpation of Matter from Right Common Carotid Artery, Open Approach

03CH3Z7 Extirpation of Matter from Right Common Carotid Artery using Stent Retriever, Percutaneous Approach

03CH3ZZ Extirpation of Matter from Right Common Carotid Artery, Percutaneous Approach

03CH4ZZ Extirpation of Matter from Right Common Carotid Artery, Percutaneous Endoscopic Approach

03CJ0ZZ Extirpation of Matter from Left Common Carotid Artery, Open Approach

03CJ3Z7 Extirpation of Matter from Left Common Carotid Artery using Stent Retriever, Percutaneous Approach

03CJ3ZZ Extirpation of Matter from Left Common Carotid Artery, Percutaneous Approach

03CJ4ZZ Extirpation of Matter from Left Common Carotid Artery, Percutaneous Endoscopic Approach

03CK0ZZ Extirpation of Matter from Right Internal Carotid Artery, Open Approach

AHA CC: 2Q, 2016, 11-12

03CK3Z7 Extirpation of Matter from Right Internal Carotid Artery using Stent Retriever, Percutaneous Approach

03CK3ZZ Extirpation of Matter from Right Internal Carotid Artery, Percutaneous Approach

03CK4ZZ Extirpation of Matter from Right Internal Carotid Artery, Percutaneous Endoscopic Approach

03CL0ZZ Extirpation of Matter from Left Internal Carotid Artery, Open Approach

AHA CC: 2Q, 2021, 13

03CL3Z7 Extirpation of Matter from Left Internal Carotid Artery using Stent Retriever, Percutaneous Approach

03CL3ZZ Extirpation of Matter from Left Internal Carotid Artery, Percutaneous Approach

03CL4ZZ Extirpation of Matter from Left Internal Carotid Artery, Percutaneous Endoscopic Approach

03CM0ZZ Extirpation of Matter from Right External Carotid Artery, Open Approach

03CM3Z7 Extirpation of Matter from Right External Carotid Artery using Stent Retriever, Percutaneous Approach

03CM3ZZ Extirpation of Matter from Right External Carotid Artery, Percutaneous Approach

03CM4ZZ Extirpation of Matter from Right External Carotid Artery, Percutaneous Endoscopic Approach

03CN0ZZ Extirpation of Matter from Left External Carotid Artery, Open Approach
AHA CC: 4Q, 2017, 65

03CN3Z7 Extirpation of Matter from Left External Carotid Artery using Stent Retriever, Percutaneous Approach

03CN3ZZ Extirpation of Matter from Left External Carotid Artery, Percutaneous Approach

03CN4ZZ Extirpation of Matter from Left External Carotid Artery, Percutaneous Endoscopic Approach

03CP0ZZ Extirpation of Matter from Right Vertebral Artery, Open Approach

03CP3Z7 Extirpation of Matter from Right Vertebral Artery using Stent Retriever, Percutaneous Approach

03CP3ZZ Extirpation of Matter from Right Vertebral Artery, Percutaneous Approach

03CP4ZZ Extirpation of Matter from Right Vertebral Artery, Percutaneous Endoscopic Approach

03CQ0ZZ Extirpation of Matter from Left Vertebral Artery, Open Approach

03CQ3Z7 Extirpation of Matter from Left Vertebral Artery using Stent Retriever, Percutaneous Approach

03CQ3ZZ Extirpation of Matter from Left Vertebral Artery, Percutaneous Approach

03CQ4ZZ Extirpation of Matter from Left Vertebral Artery, Percutaneous Endoscopic Approach

03CR0ZZ Extirpation of Matter from Face Artery, Open Approach

03CR3ZZ Extirpation of Matter from Face Artery, Percutaneous Approach

03CR4ZZ Extirpation of Matter from Face Artery, Percutaneous Endoscopic Approach

03CS0ZZ Extirpation of Matter from Right Temporal Artery, Open Approach

03CS3ZZ Extirpation of Matter from Right Temporal Artery, Percutaneous Approach

03CS4ZZ Extirpation of Matter from Right Temporal Artery, Percutaneous Endoscopic Approach

03CT0ZZ Extirpation of Matter from Left Temporal Artery, Open Approach

03CT3ZZ Extirpation of Matter from Left Temporal Artery, Percutaneous Approach

03CT4ZZ Extirpation of Matter from Left Temporal Artery, Percutaneous Endoscopic Approach

03CU0ZZ Extirpation of Matter from Right Thyroid Artery, Open Approach

03CU3ZZ Extirpation of Matter from Right Thyroid Artery, Percutaneous Approach

03CU4ZZ Extirpation of Matter from Right Thyroid Artery, Percutaneous Endoscopic Approach

03CV0ZZ Extirpation of Matter from Left Thyroid Artery, Open Approach

03CV3ZZ Extirpation of Matter from Left Thyroid Artery, Percutaneous Approach

03CV4ZZ Extirpation of Matter from Left Thyroid Artery, Percutaneous Endoscopic Approach

03CY0ZZ Extirpation of Matter from Upper Artery, Open Approach

03CY3ZZ Extirpation of Matter from Upper Artery, Percutaneous Approach

03CY4ZZ Extirpation of Matter from Upper Artery, Percutaneous Endoscopic Approach

03F – Upper Arteries, Fragmentation

03F23Z0 Fragmentation of Innominate Artery, Percutaneous Approach, Ultrasonic

03F23ZZ Fragmentation of Innominate Artery, Percutaneous Approach

03F33Z0 Fragmentation of Right Subclavian Artery, Percutaneous Approach, Ultrasonic

03F33ZZ Fragmentation of Right Subclavian Artery, Percutaneous Approach

03F43Z0 Fragmentation of Left Subclavian Artery, Percutaneous Approach, Ultrasonic

03F43ZZ Fragmentation of Left Subclavian Artery, Percutaneous Approach

03F53Z0 Fragmentation of Right Axillary Artery, Percutaneous Approach, Ultrasonic

03F53ZZ Fragmentation of Right Axillary Artery, Percutaneous Approach

03F63Z0 Fragmentation of Left Axillary Artery, Percutaneous Approach, Ultrasonic

03F63ZZ Fragmentation of Left Axillary Artery, Percutaneous Approach

03F73Z0 Fragmentation of Right Brachial Artery, Percutaneous Approach, Ultrasonic

03F73ZZ Fragmentation of Right Brachial Artery, Percutaneous Approach

03F83Z0 Fragmentation of Left Brachial Artery, Percutaneous Approach, Ultrasonic

03F83ZZ Fragmentation of Left Brachial Artery, Percutaneous Approach

03F93Z0 Fragmentation of Right Ulnar Artery, Percutaneous Approach, Ultrasonic

03F93ZZ Fragmentation of Right Ulnar Artery, Percutaneous Approach

03FA3Z0 Fragmentation of Left Ulnar Artery, Percutaneous Approach, Ultrasonic

03FA3ZZ Fragmentation of Left Ulnar Artery, Percutaneous Approach

03FB3Z0 Fragmentation of Right Radial Artery, Percutaneous Approach, Ultrasonic

03FB3ZZ Fragmentation of Right Radial Artery, Percutaneous Approach

03FC3Z0 Fragmentation of Left Radial Artery, Percutaneous Approach, Ultrasonic

03FC3ZZ Fragmentation of Left Radial Artery, Percutaneous Approach

03FG3Z0 Fragmentation of Intracranial Artery, Percutaneous Approach, Ultrasonic

03FG3ZZ Fragmentation of Intracranial Artery, Percutaneous Approach

03FY3Z0 Fragmentation of Upper Artery, Percutaneous Approach, Ultrasonic

03FY3ZZ Fragmentation of Upper Artery, Percutaneous Approach

03H – Upper Arteries, Insertion

03H003Z Insertion of Infusion Device into Right Internal Mammary Artery, Open Approach

03H00DZ Insertion of Intraluminal Device into Right Internal Mammary Artery, Open Approach

03H033Z Insertion of Infusion Device into Right Internal Mammary Artery, Percutaneous Approach

03H03DZ Insertion of Intraluminal Device into Right Internal Mammary Artery, Percutaneous Approach

03H043Z Insertion of Infusion Device into Right Internal Mammary Artery, Percutaneous Endoscopic Approach

03H04DZ Insertion of Intraluminal Device into Right Internal Mammary Artery, Percutaneous Endoscopic Approach

03H103Z Insertion of Infusion Device into Left Internal Mammary Artery, Open Approach

03H10DZ Insertion of Intraluminal Device into Left Internal Mammary Artery, Open Approach

03H133Z Insertion of Infusion Device into Left Internal Mammary Artery, Percutaneous Approach

03H13DZ Insertion of Intraluminal Device into Left Internal Mammary Artery, Percutaneous Approach

03H143Z Insertion of Infusion Device into Left Internal Mammary Artery, Percutaneous Endoscopic Approach

03H14DZ Insertion of Intraluminal Device into Left Internal Mammary Artery, Percutaneous Endoscopic Approach

03H203Z Insertion of Infusion Device into Innominate Artery, Open Approach

03H20DZ Insertion of Intraluminal Device into Innominate Artery, Open Approach

03H233Z Insertion of Infusion Device into Innominate Artery, Percutaneous Approach

03H23DZ Insertion of Intraluminal Device into Innominate Artery, Percutaneous Approach

03H243Z Insertion of Infusion Device into Innominate Artery, Percutaneous Endoscopic Approach

03H24DZ Insertion of Intraluminal Device into Innominate Artery, Percutaneous Endoscopic Approach

03H303Z Insertion of Infusion Device into Right Subclavian Artery, Open Approach

03H30DZ Insertion of Intraluminal Device into Right Subclavian Artery, Open Approach

03H333Z Insertion of Infusion Device into Right Subclavian Artery, Percutaneous Approach

03H33DZ Insertion of Intraluminal Device into Right Subclavian Artery, Percutaneous Approach

03H343Z Insertion of Infusion Device into Right Subclavian Artery, Percutaneous Endoscopic Approach

03H34DZ Insertion of Intraluminal Device into Right Subclavian Artery, Percutaneous Endoscopic Approach

03H403Z Insertion of Infusion Device into Left Subclavian Artery, Open Approach

03H40DZ Insertion of Intraluminal Device into Left Subclavian Artery, Open Approach

AHA CC: 1Q, 2020, 25-27

03H433Z Insertion of Infusion Device into Left Subclavian Artery, Percutaneous Approach

03H43DZ Insertion of Intraluminal Device into Left Subclavian Artery, Percutaneous Approach

03H443Z Insertion of Infusion Device into Left Subclavian Artery, Percutaneous Endoscopic Approach

03H44DZ Insertion of Intraluminal Device into Left Subclavian Artery, Percutaneous Endoscopic Approach

03H503Z Insertion of Infusion Device into Right Axillary Artery, Open Approach

03H50DZ Insertion of Intraluminal Device into Right Axillary Artery, Open Approach

03H533Z Insertion of Infusion Device into Right Axillary Artery, Percutaneous Approach

03H53DZ Insertion of Intraluminal Device into Right Axillary Artery, Percutaneous Approach

03H543Z Insertion of Infusion Device into Right Axillary Artery, Percutaneous Endoscopic Approach

03H54DZ Insertion of Intraluminal Device into Right Axillary Artery, Percutaneous Endoscopic Approach

03H603Z Insertion of Infusion Device into Left Axillary Artery, Open Approach

03H60DZ Insertion of Intraluminal Device into Left Axillary Artery, Open Approach

03H633Z Insertion of Infusion Device into Left Axillary Artery, Percutaneous Approach

03H63DZ Insertion of Intraluminal Device into Left Axillary Artery, Percutaneous Approach

03H643Z Insertion of Infusion Device into Left Axillary Artery, Percutaneous Endoscopic Approach

03H64DZ Insertion of Intraluminal Device into Left Axillary Artery, Percutaneous Endoscopic Approach

03H703Z Insertion of Infusion Device into Right Brachial Artery, Open Approach

03H70DZ Insertion of Intraluminal Device into Right Brachial Artery, Open Approach

03H733Z Insertion of Infusion Device into Right Brachial Artery, Percutaneous Approach

03H73DZ Insertion of Intraluminal Device into Right Brachial Artery, Percutaneous Approach

03H743Z Insertion of Infusion Device into Right Brachial Artery, Percutaneous Endoscopic Approach

03H74DZ Insertion of Intraluminal Device into Right Brachial Artery, Percutaneous Endoscopic Approach

03H803Z Insertion of Infusion Device into Left Brachial Artery, Open Approach

03H80DZ Insertion of Intraluminal Device into Left Brachial Artery, Open Approach

03H833Z Insertion of Infusion Device into Left Brachial Artery, Percutaneous Approach

03H83DZ Insertion of Intraluminal Device into Left Brachial Artery, Percutaneous Approach

03H843Z Insertion of Infusion Device into Left Brachial Artery, Percutaneous Endoscopic Approach

03H84DZ Insertion of Intraluminal Device into Left Brachial Artery, Percutaneous Endoscopic Approach

03H903Z Insertion of Infusion Device into Right Ulnar Artery, Open Approach

03H90DZ Insertion of Intraluminal Device into Right Ulnar Artery, Open Approach

03H933Z Insertion of Infusion Device into Right Ulnar Artery, Percutaneous Approach

03H93DZ Insertion of Intraluminal Device into Right Ulnar Artery, Percutaneous Approach

03H943Z Insertion of Infusion Device into Right Ulnar Artery, Percutaneous Endoscopic Approach

03H94DZ Insertion of Intraluminal Device into Right Ulnar Artery, Percutaneous Endoscopic Approach

03HA03Z Insertion of Infusion Device into Left Ulnar Artery, Open Approach

03HA0DZ Insertion of Intraluminal Device into Left Ulnar Artery, Open Approach

03HA33Z Insertion of Infusion Device into Left Ulnar Artery, Percutaneous Approach

03HA3DZ Insertion of Intraluminal Device into Left Ulnar Artery, Percutaneous Approach

03HA43Z Insertion of Infusion Device into Left Ulnar Artery, Percutaneous Endoscopic Approach

03HA4DZ Insertion of Intraluminal Device into Left Ulnar Artery, Percutaneous Endoscopic Approach

03HB03Z Insertion of Infusion Device into Right Radial Artery, Open Approach

03HB0DZ Insertion of Intraluminal Device into Right Radial Artery, Open Approach

03HB33Z Insertion of Infusion Device into Right Radial Artery, Percutaneous Approach

03HB3DZ Insertion of Intraluminal Device into Right Radial Artery, Percutaneous Approach

03HB43Z Insertion of Infusion Device into Right Radial Artery, Percutaneous Endoscopic Approach

03HB4DZ Insertion of Intraluminal Device into Right Radial Artery, Percutaneous Endoscopic Approach

03HC03Z Insertion of Infusion Device into Left Radial Artery, Open Approach

03HC0DZ Insertion of Intraluminal Device into Left Radial Artery, Open Approach

03HC33Z Insertion of Infusion Device into Left Radial Artery, Percutaneous Approach

03HC3DZ Insertion of Intraluminal Device into Left Radial Artery, Percutaneous Approach

03HC43Z Insertion of Infusion Device into Left Radial Artery, Percutaneous Endoscopic Approach

03HC4DZ Insertion of Intraluminal Device into Left Radial Artery, Percutaneous Endoscopic Approach

03HD03Z Insertion of Infusion Device into Right Hand Artery, Open Approach

03HD0DZ Insertion of Intraluminal Device into Right Hand Artery, Open Approach

03HD33Z Insertion of Infusion Device into Right Hand Artery, Percutaneous Approach

03HD3DZ Insertion of Intraluminal Device into Right Hand Artery, Percutaneous Approach

03HD43Z Insertion of Infusion Device into Right Hand Artery, Percutaneous Endoscopic Approach

03HD4DZ Insertion of Intraluminal Device into Right Hand Artery, Percutaneous Endoscopic Approach

03HF03Z Insertion of Infusion Device into Left Hand Artery, Open Approach

03HF0DZ Insertion of Intraluminal Device into Left Hand Artery, Open Approach

03HF33Z Insertion of Infusion Device into Left Hand Artery, Percutaneous Approach

03HF3DZ Insertion of Intraluminal Device into Left Hand Artery, Percutaneous Approach

03HF43Z Insertion of Infusion Device into Left Hand Artery, Percutaneous Endoscopic Approach

03HF4DZ Insertion of Intraluminal Device into Left Hand Artery, Percutaneous Endoscopic Approach

03HG03Z Insertion of Infusion Device into Intracranial Artery, Open Approach

03HG0DZ Insertion of Intraluminal Device into Intracranial Artery, Open Approach

03HG33Z Insertion of Infusion Device into Intracranial Artery, Percutaneous Approach

03HG3DZ Insertion of Intraluminal Device into Intracranial Artery, Percutaneous Approach

03HG43Z Insertion of Infusion Device into Intracranial Artery, Percutaneous Endoscopic Approach

03HG4DZ Insertion of Intraluminal Device into Intracranial Artery, Percutaneous Endoscopic Approach

03HH03Z Insertion of Infusion Device into Right Common Carotid Artery, Open Approach

03HH0DZ Insertion of Intraluminal Device into Right Common Carotid Artery, Open Approach

03HH33Z Insertion of Infusion Device into Right Common Carotid Artery, Percutaneous Approach

03HH3DZ Insertion of Intraluminal Device into Right Common Carotid Artery, Percutaneous Approach

03HH43Z Insertion of Infusion Device into Right Common Carotid Artery, Percutaneous Endoscopic Approach

03HH4DZ Insertion of Intraluminal Device into Right Common Carotid Artery, Percutaneous Endoscopic Approach

03HJ03Z Insertion of Infusion Device into Left Common Carotid Artery, Open Approach

03HJ0DZ Insertion of Intraluminal Device into Left Common Carotid Artery, Open Approach

03HJ33Z Insertion of Infusion Device into Left Common Carotid Artery, Percutaneous Approach

03HJ3DZ Insertion of Intraluminal Device into Left Common Carotid Artery, Percutaneous Approach

03HJ43Z Insertion of Infusion Device into Left Common Carotid Artery, Percutaneous Endoscopic Approach

03HJ4DZ Insertion of Intraluminal Device into Left Common Carotid Artery, Percutaneous Endoscopic Approach

03HK03Z Insertion of Infusion Device into Right Internal Carotid Artery, Open Approach

03HK0DZ Insertion of Intraluminal Device into Right Internal Carotid Artery, Open Approach

03HK0MZ Insertion of Stimulator Lead into Right Internal Carotid Artery, Open Approach

03HK33Z Insertion of Infusion Device into Right Internal Carotid Artery, Percutaneous Approach

03HK3DZ Insertion of Intraluminal Device into Right Internal Carotid Artery, Percutaneous Approach

03HK3MZ Insertion of Stimulator Lead into Right Internal Carotid Artery, Percutaneous Approach

03HK43Z Insertion of Infusion Device into Right Internal Carotid Artery, Percutaneous Endoscopic Approach

03HK4DZ Insertion of Intraluminal Device into Right Internal Carotid Artery, Percutaneous Endoscopic Approach

03HK4MZ Insertion of Stimulator Lead into Right Internal Carotid Artery, Percutaneous Endoscopic Approach

03HL03Z Insertion of Infusion Device into Left Internal Carotid Artery, Open Approach

03HL0DZ Insertion of Intraluminal Device into Left Internal Carotid Artery, Open Approach

03HL0MZ Insertion of Stimulator Lead into Left Internal Carotid Artery, Open Approach

03HL33Z Insertion of Infusion Device into Left Internal Carotid Artery, Percutaneous Approach

03HL3DZ Insertion of Intraluminal Device into Left Internal Carotid Artery, Percutaneous Approach

03HL3MZ Insertion of Stimulator Lead into Left Internal Carotid Artery, Percutaneous Approach

03HL43Z Insertion of Infusion Device into Left Internal Carotid Artery, Percutaneous Endoscopic Approach

03HL4DZ Insertion of Intraluminal Device into Left Internal Carotid Artery, Percutaneous Endoscopic Approach

03HL4MZ Insertion of Stimulator Lead into Left Internal Carotid Artery, Percutaneous Endoscopic Approach

03HM03Z Insertion of Infusion Device into Right External Carotid Artery, Open Approach

03HM0DZ Insertion of Intraluminal Device into Right External Carotid Artery, Open Approach

03HM33Z Insertion of Infusion Device into Right External Carotid Artery, Percutaneous Approach

03HM3DZ Insertion of Intraluminal Device into Right External Carotid Artery, Percutaneous Approach

03HM43Z Insertion of Infusion Device into Right External Carotid Artery, Percutaneous Endoscopic Approach

03HM4DZ Insertion of Intraluminal Device into Right External Carotid Artery, Percutaneous Endoscopic Approach

03HN03Z Insertion of Infusion Device into Left External Carotid Artery, Open Approach

03HN0DZ Insertion of Intraluminal Device into Left External Carotid Artery, Open Approach

03HN33Z Insertion of Infusion Device into Left External Carotid Artery, Percutaneous Approach

03HN3DZ Insertion of Intraluminal Device into Left External Carotid Artery, Percutaneous Approach

03HN43Z Insertion of Infusion Device into Left External Carotid Artery, Percutaneous Endoscopic Approach

03HN4DZ Insertion of Intraluminal Device into Left External Carotid Artery, Percutaneous Endoscopic Approach

03HP03Z Insertion of Infusion Device into Right Vertebral Artery, Open Approach

03HP0DZ Insertion of Intraluminal Device into Right Vertebral Artery, Open Approach

03HP33Z Insertion of Infusion Device into Right Vertebral Artery, Percutaneous Approach

03HP3DZ Insertion of Intraluminal Device into Right Vertebral Artery, Percutaneous Approach

03HP43Z Insertion of Infusion Device into Right Vertebral Artery, Percutaneous Endoscopic Approach

03HP4DZ Insertion of Intraluminal Device into Right Vertebral Artery, Percutaneous Endoscopic Approach

03HQ03Z Insertion of Infusion Device into Left Vertebral Artery, Open Approach

03HQ0DZ Insertion of Intraluminal Device into Left Vertebral Artery, Open Approach

03HQ33Z Insertion of Infusion Device into Left Vertebral Artery, Percutaneous Approach

03HQ3DZ Insertion of Intraluminal Device into Left Vertebral Artery, Percutaneous Approach

03HQ43Z Insertion of Infusion Device into Left Vertebral Artery, Percutaneous Endoscopic Approach

03HQ4DZ Insertion of Intraluminal Device into Left Vertebral Artery, Percutaneous Endoscopic Approach

03HR03Z Insertion of Infusion Device into Face Artery, Open Approach

03HR0DZ Insertion of Intraluminal Device into Face Artery, Open Approach

03HR33Z Insertion of Infusion Device into Face Artery, Percutaneous Approach

03HR3DZ Insertion of Intraluminal Device into Face Artery, Percutaneous Approach

03HR43Z Insertion of Infusion Device into Face Artery, Percutaneous Endoscopic Approach

03HR4DZ Insertion of Intraluminal Device into Face Artery, Percutaneous Endoscopic Approach

03HS03Z Insertion of Infusion Device into Right Temporal Artery, Open Approach

03HS0DZ Insertion of Intraluminal Device into Right Temporal Artery, Open Approach

03HS33Z Insertion of Infusion Device into Right Temporal Artery, Percutaneous Approach

03HS3DZ Insertion of Intraluminal Device into Right Temporal Artery, Percutaneous Approach

03HS43Z Insertion of Infusion Device into Right Temporal Artery, Percutaneous Endoscopic Approach

03HS4DZ Insertion of Intraluminal Device into Right Temporal Artery, Percutaneous Endoscopic Approach

03HT03Z Insertion of Infusion Device into Left Temporal Artery, Open Approach

03HT0DZ Insertion of Intraluminal Device into Left Temporal Artery, Open Approach

03HT33Z Insertion of Infusion Device into Left Temporal Artery, Percutaneous Approach

03HT3DZ Insertion of Intraluminal Device into Left Temporal Artery, Percutaneous Approach

03HT43Z Insertion of Infusion Device into Left Temporal Artery, Percutaneous Endoscopic Approach

03HT4DZ Insertion of Intraluminal Device into Left Temporal Artery, Percutaneous Endoscopic Approach

03HU03Z Insertion of Infusion Device into Right Thyroid Artery, Open Approach

03HU0DZ Insertion of Intraluminal Device into Right Thyroid Artery, Open Approach

03HU33Z Insertion of Infusion Device into Right Thyroid Artery, Percutaneous Approach

03HU3DZ Insertion of Intraluminal Device into Right Thyroid Artery, Percutaneous Approach

03HU43Z Insertion of Infusion Device into Right Thyroid Artery, Percutaneous Endoscopic Approach

03HU4DZ Insertion of Intraluminal Device into Right Thyroid Artery, Percutaneous Endoscopic Approach

03HV03Z Insertion of Infusion Device into Left Thyroid Artery, Open Approach

03HV0DZ Insertion of Intraluminal Device into Left Thyroid Artery, Open Approach

03HV33Z Insertion of Infusion Device into Left Thyroid Artery, Percutaneous Approach

03HV3DZ Insertion of Intraluminal Device into Left Thyroid Artery, Percutaneous Approach

03HV43Z Insertion of Infusion Device into Left Thyroid Artery, Percutaneous Endoscopic Approach

03HV4DZ Insertion of Intraluminal Device into Left Thyroid Artery, Percutaneous Endoscopic Approach

03HY02Z Insertion of Monitoring Device into Upper Artery, Open Approach

03HY03Z Insertion of Infusion Device into Upper Artery, Open Approach

03HY0DZ Insertion of Intraluminal Device into Upper Artery, Open Approach

03HY0YZ Insertion of Other Device into Upper Artery, Open Approach

03HY32Z Insertion of Monitoring Device into Upper Artery, Percutaneous Approach

AHA CC: 2Q, 2016, 32-33

03HY33Z Insertion of Infusion Device into Upper Artery, Percutaneous Approach

03HY3DZ Insertion of Intraluminal Device into Upper Artery, Percutaneous Approach

03HY3YZ Insertion of Other Device into Upper Artery, Percutaneous Approach

03HY42Z Insertion of Monitoring Device into Upper Artery, Percutaneous Endoscopic Approach

03HY43Z Insertion of Infusion Device into Upper Artery, Percutaneous Endoscopic Approach

03HY4DZ Insertion of Intraluminal Device into Upper Artery, Percutaneous Endoscopic Approach

03HY4YZ Insertion of Other Device into Upper Artery, Percutaneous Endoscopic Approach

♀ Female-only   ♂ Male-only   ▲ Limited Coverage   ● Non-OR   ▦ HAC-associated procedure   ▲ Non-covered procedures   ✚ Cluster

Review Coding Guidelines B3.11a, B3.11b and B3.11c

03JY0ZZ Inspection of Upper Artery, Open Approach
AHA CC: 1Q, 2015, 29

03JY3ZZ Inspection of Upper Artery, Percutaneous Approach
AHA CC: 1Q, 2021, 16-17

03JY4ZZ Inspection of Upper Artery, Percutaneous Endoscopic Approach

03JYXZZ Inspection of Upper Artery, External Approach

03L – Upper Arteries, Occlusion

Review Coding Guideline B3.12

03L00CZ Occlusion of Right Internal Mammary Artery with Extraluminal Device, Open Approach

03L00DZ Occlusion of Right Internal Mammary Artery with Intraluminal Device, Open Approach

03L00ZZ Occlusion of Right Internal Mammary Artery, Open Approach

03L03CZ Occlusion of Right Internal Mammary Artery with Extraluminal Device, Percutaneous Approach

03L03DZ Occlusion of Right Internal Mammary Artery with Intraluminal Device, Percutaneous Approach

03L03ZZ Occlusion of Right Internal Mammary Artery, Percutaneous Approach

03L04CZ Occlusion of Right Internal Mammary Artery with Extraluminal Device, Percutaneous Endoscopic Approach

03L04DZ Occlusion of Right Internal Mammary Artery with Intraluminal Device, Percutaneous Endoscopic Approach

03L04ZZ Occlusion of Right Internal Mammary Artery, Percutaneous Endoscopic Approach

03L10CZ Occlusion of Left Internal Mammary Artery with Extraluminal Device, Open Approach

03L10DZ Occlusion of Left Internal Mammary Artery with Intraluminal Device, Open Approach

03L10ZZ Occlusion of Left Internal Mammary Artery, Open Approach

03L13CZ Occlusion of Left Internal Mammary Artery with Extraluminal Device, Percutaneous Approach

03L13DZ Occlusion of Left Internal Mammary Artery with Intraluminal Device, Percutaneous Approach

03L13ZZ Occlusion of Left Internal Mammary Artery, Percutaneous Approach

03L14CZ Occlusion of Left Internal Mammary Artery with Extraluminal Device, Percutaneous Endoscopic Approach

03L14DZ Occlusion of Left Internal Mammary Artery with Intraluminal Device, Percutaneous Endoscopic Approach

03L14ZZ Occlusion of Left Internal Mammary Artery, Percutaneous Endoscopic Approach

03L20CZ Occlusion of Innominate Artery with Extraluminal Device, Open Approach

03L20DZ Occlusion of Innominate Artery with Intraluminal Device, Open Approach

03L20ZZ Occlusion of Innominate Artery, Open Approach

03L23CZ Occlusion of Innominate Artery with Extraluminal Device, Percutaneous Approach

03L23DZ Occlusion of Innominate Artery with Intraluminal Device, Percutaneous Approach

03L23ZZ Occlusion of Innominate Artery, Percutaneous Approach

03L24CZ Occlusion of Innominate Artery with Extraluminal Device, Percutaneous Endoscopic Approach

03L24DZ Occlusion of Innominate Artery with Intraluminal Device, Percutaneous Endoscopic Approach

03L24ZZ Occlusion of Innominate Artery, Percutaneous Endoscopic Approach

03L30CZ Occlusion of Right Subclavian Artery with Extraluminal Device, Open Approach

03L30DZ Occlusion of Right Subclavian Artery with Intraluminal Device, Open Approach

03L30ZZ Occlusion of Right Subclavian Artery, Open Approach

03L33CZ Occlusion of Right Subclavian Artery with Extraluminal Device, Percutaneous Approach

03L33DZ Occlusion of Right Subclavian Artery with Intraluminal Device, Percutaneous Approach

03L33ZZ Occlusion of Right Subclavian Artery, Percutaneous Approach

03L34CZ Occlusion of Right Subclavian Artery with Extraluminal Device, Percutaneous Endoscopic Approach

03L34DZ Occlusion of Right Subclavian Artery with Intraluminal Device, Percutaneous Endoscopic Approach

03L34ZZ Occlusion of Right Subclavian Artery, Percutaneous Endoscopic Approach

03L40CZ Occlusion of Left Subclavian Artery with Extraluminal Device, Open Approach

03L40DZ Occlusion of Left Subclavian Artery with Intraluminal Device, Open Approach

03L40ZZ Occlusion of Left Subclavian Artery, Open Approach

03L43CZ Occlusion of Left Subclavian Artery with Extraluminal Device, Percutaneous Approach

03L43DZ Occlusion of Left Subclavian Artery with Intraluminal Device, Percutaneous Approach

03L43ZZ Occlusion of Left Subclavian Artery, Percutaneous Approach

03L44CZ Occlusion of Left Subclavian Artery with Extraluminal Device, Percutaneous Endoscopic Approach

03L44DZ Occlusion of Left Subclavian Artery with Intraluminal Device, Percutaneous Endoscopic Approach

03L44ZZ Occlusion of Left Subclavian Artery, Percutaneous Endoscopic Approach

03L50CZ Occlusion of Right Axillary Artery with Extraluminal Device, Open Approach

03L50DZ Occlusion of Right Axillary Artery with Intraluminal Device, Open Approach

03L50ZZ Occlusion of Right Axillary Artery, Open Approach

03L53CZ Occlusion of Right Axillary Artery with Extraluminal Device, Percutaneous Approach

03L53DZ Occlusion of Right Axillary Artery with Intraluminal Device, Percutaneous Approach

03L53ZZ Occlusion of Right Axillary Artery, Percutaneous Approach

03L54CZ Occlusion of Right Axillary Artery with Extraluminal Device, Percutaneous Endoscopic Approach

03L54DZ Occlusion of Right Axillary Artery with Intraluminal Device, Percutaneous Endoscopic Approach

03L54ZZ Occlusion of Right Axillary Artery, Percutaneous Endoscopic Approach

03L60CZ Occlusion of Left Axillary Artery with Extraluminal Device, Open Approach

03L60DZ Occlusion of Left Axillary Artery with Intraluminal Device, Open Approach

03L60ZZ Occlusion of Left Axillary Artery, Open Approach

03L63CZ Occlusion of Left Axillary Artery with Extraluminal Device, Percutaneous Approach

03L63DZ Occlusion of Left Axillary Artery with Intraluminal Device, Percutaneous Approach

03L63ZZ Occlusion of Left Axillary Artery, Percutaneous Approach

03L64CZ Occlusion of Left Axillary Artery with Extraluminal Device, Percutaneous Endoscopic Approach

03L64DZ Occlusion of Left Axillary Artery with Intraluminal Device, Percutaneous Endoscopic Approach

03L64ZZ Occlusion of Left Axillary Artery, Percutaneous Endoscopic Approach

03L70CZ Occlusion of Right Brachial Artery with Extraluminal Device, Open Approach

03L70DZ Occlusion of Right Brachial Artery with Intraluminal Device, Open Approach

03L70ZZ Occlusion of Right Brachial Artery, Open Approach

03L73CZ Occlusion of Right Brachial Artery with Extraluminal Device, Percutaneous Approach

03L73DZ Occlusion of Right Brachial Artery with Intraluminal Device, Percutaneous Approach

03L73ZZ Occlusion of Right Brachial Artery, Percutaneous Approach

03L74CZ Occlusion of Right Brachial Artery with Extraluminal Device, Percutaneous Endoscopic Approach

03L74DZ Occlusion of Right Brachial Artery with Intraluminal Device, Percutaneous Endoscopic Approach

03L74ZZ Occlusion of Right Brachial Artery, Percutaneous Endoscopic Approach

03L80CZ Occlusion of Left Brachial Artery with Extraluminal Device, Open Approach

03L80DZ Occlusion of Left Brachial Artery with Intraluminal Device, Open Approach

03L80ZZ Occlusion of Left Brachial Artery, Open Approach

03L83CZ Occlusion of Left Brachial Artery with Extraluminal Device, Percutaneous Approach

03L83DZ Occlusion of Left Brachial Artery with Intraluminal Device, Percutaneous Approach

03L83ZZ Occlusion of Left Brachial Artery, Percutaneous Approach

03L84CZ Occlusion of Left Brachial Artery with Extraluminal Device, Percutaneous Endoscopic Approach

03L84DZ Occlusion of Left Brachial Artery with Intraluminal Device, Percutaneous Endoscopic Approach

03L84ZZ Occlusion of Left Brachial Artery, Percutaneous Endoscopic Approach

03L90CZ Occlusion of Right Ulnar Artery with Extraluminal Device, Open Approach

03L90DZ Occlusion of Right Ulnar Artery with Intraluminal Device, Open Approach

03L90ZZ Occlusion of Right Ulnar Artery, Open Approach

03L93CZ Occlusion of Right Ulnar Artery with Extraluminal Device, Percutaneous Approach

03L93DZ Occlusion of Right Ulnar Artery with Intraluminal Device, Percutaneous Approach

03L93ZZ Occlusion of Right Ulnar Artery, Percutaneous Approach

03L94CZ Occlusion of Right Ulnar Artery with Extraluminal Device, Percutaneous Endoscopic Approach

03L94DZ Occlusion of Right Ulnar Artery with Intraluminal Device, Percutaneous Endoscopic Approach

03L94ZZ Occlusion of Right Ulnar Artery, Percutaneous Endoscopic Approach

03LA0CZ Occlusion of Left Ulnar Artery with Extraluminal Device, Open Approach

03LA0DZ Occlusion of Left Ulnar Artery with Intraluminal Device, Open Approach

03LA0ZZ Occlusion of Left Ulnar Artery, Open Approach

03LA3CZ Occlusion of Left Ulnar Artery with Extraluminal Device, Percutaneous Approach

03LA3DZ Occlusion of Left Ulnar Artery with Intraluminal Device, Percutaneous Approach

03LA3ZZ Occlusion of Left Ulnar Artery, Percutaneous Approach

03LA4CZ Occlusion of Left Ulnar Artery with Extraluminal Device, Percutaneous Endoscopic Approach

03LA4DZ Occlusion of Left Ulnar Artery with Intraluminal Device, Percutaneous Endoscopic Approach

03LA4ZZ Occlusion of Left Ulnar Artery, Percutaneous Endoscopic Approach

03LB0CZ Occlusion of Right Radial Artery with Extraluminal Device, Open Approach

03LB0DZ Occlusion of Right Radial Artery with Intraluminal Device, Open Approach

03LB0ZZ Occlusion of Right Radial Artery, Open Approach

03LB3CZ Occlusion of Right Radial Artery with Extraluminal Device, Percutaneous Approach

03LB3DZ Occlusion of Right Radial Artery with Intraluminal Device, Percutaneous Approach

03LB3ZZ Occlusion of Right Radial Artery, Percutaneous Approach

03LB4CZ Occlusion of Right Radial Artery with Extraluminal Device, Percutaneous Endoscopic Approach

03LB4DZ Occlusion of Right Radial Artery with Intraluminal Device, Percutaneous Endoscopic Approach

03LB4ZZ Occlusion of Right Radial Artery, Percutaneous Endoscopic Approach

03LC0CZ Occlusion of Left Radial Artery with Extraluminal Device, Open Approach

03LC0DZ Occlusion of Left Radial Artery with Intraluminal Device, Open Approach

03LC0ZZ Occlusion of Left Radial Artery, Open Approach

03LC3CZ Occlusion of Left Radial Artery with Extraluminal Device, Percutaneous Approach

03LC3DZ Occlusion of Left Radial Artery with Intraluminal Device, Percutaneous Approach

03LC3ZZ Occlusion of Left Radial Artery, Percutaneous Approach

03LC4CZ Occlusion of Left Radial Artery with Extraluminal Device, Percutaneous Endoscopic Approach

03LC4DZ Occlusion of Left Radial Artery with Intraluminal Device, Percutaneous Endoscopic Approach

03LC4ZZ Occlusion of Left Radial Artery, Percutaneous Endoscopic Approach

03LD0CZ Occlusion of Right Hand Artery with Extraluminal Device, Open Approach

03LD0DZ Occlusion of Right Hand Artery with Intraluminal Device, Open Approach

03LD0ZZ Occlusion of Right Hand Artery, Open Approach

03LD3CZ Occlusion of Right Hand Artery with Extraluminal Device, Percutaneous Approach

03LD3DZ Occlusion of Right Hand Artery with Intraluminal Device, Percutaneous Approach

03LD3ZZ Occlusion of Right Hand Artery, Percutaneous Approach

03LD4CZ Occlusion of Right Hand Artery with Extraluminal Device, Percutaneous Endoscopic Approach

03LD4DZ Occlusion of Right Hand Artery with Intraluminal Device, Percutaneous Endoscopic Approach

03LD4ZZ Occlusion of Right Hand Artery, Percutaneous Endoscopic Approach

03LF0CZ Occlusion of Left Hand Artery with Extraluminal Device, Open Approach

03LF0DZ Occlusion of Left Hand Artery with Intraluminal Device, Open Approach

03LF0ZZ Occlusion of Left Hand Artery, Open Approach

03LF3CZ Occlusion of Left Hand Artery with Extraluminal Device, Percutaneous Approach

03LF3DZ Occlusion of Left Hand Artery with Intraluminal Device, Percutaneous Approach

03LF3ZZ Occlusion of Left Hand Artery, Percutaneous Approach

03LF4CZ Occlusion of Left Hand Artery with Extraluminal Device, Percutaneous Endoscopic Approach

03LF4DZ Occlusion of Left Hand Artery with Intraluminal Device, Percutaneous Endoscopic Approach

03LF4ZZ Occlusion of Left Hand Artery, Percutaneous Endoscopic Approach

03LG0BZ Occlusion of Intracranial Artery with Bioactive Intraluminal Device, Open Approach

03LG0CZ Occlusion of Intracranial Artery with Extraluminal Device, Open Approach

AHA CC: 2Q, 2016, 30

03LG0DZ Occlusion of Intracranial Artery with Intraluminal Device, Open Approach

03LG0ZZ Occlusion of Intracranial Artery, Open Approach

03LG3BZ Occlusion of Intracranial Artery with Bioactive Intraluminal Device, Percutaneous Approach

03LG3CZ Occlusion of Intracranial Artery with Extraluminal Device, Percutaneous Approach

03LG3DZ Occlusion of Intracranial Artery with Intraluminal Device, Percutaneous Approach

AHA CC: 4Q, 2014, 37

03LG3ZZ Occlusion of Intracranial Artery, Percutaneous Approach

03LG4BZ Occlusion of Intracranial Artery with Bioactive Intraluminal Device, Percutaneous Endoscopic Approach

03LG4CZ Occlusion of Intracranial Artery with Extraluminal Device, Percutaneous Endoscopic Approach

03LG4DZ Occlusion of Intracranial Artery with Intraluminal Device, Percutaneous Endoscopic Approach

03LG4ZZ Occlusion of Intracranial Artery, Percutaneous Endoscopic Approach

03LH0BZ Occlusion of Right Common Carotid Artery with Bioactive Intraluminal Device, Open Approach

03LH0CZ Occlusion of Right Common Carotid Artery with Extraluminal Device, Open Approach

03LH0DZ Occlusion of Right Common Carotid Artery with Intraluminal Device, Open Approach

03LH0ZZ Occlusion of Right Common Carotid Artery, Open Approach

03LH3BZ Occlusion of Right Common Carotid Artery with Bioactive Intraluminal Device, Percutaneous Approach

03LH3CZ Occlusion of Right Common Carotid Artery with Extraluminal Device, Percutaneous Approach

03LH3DZ Occlusion of Right Common Carotid Artery with Intraluminal Device, Percutaneous Approach

03LH3ZZ Occlusion of Right Common Carotid Artery, Percutaneous Approach

03LH4BZ Occlusion of Right Common Carotid Artery with Bioactive Intraluminal Device, Percutaneous Endoscopic Approach

03LH4CZ Occlusion of Right Common Carotid Artery with Extraluminal Device, Percutaneous Endoscopic Approach

03LH4DZ Occlusion of Right Common Carotid Artery with Intraluminal Device, Percutaneous Endoscopic Approach

♀ Female-only   ♂ Male-only   ▲ Limited Coverage   ● Non-OR   HAC HAC-associated procedure   ▲ Non-covered procedures   ✚ Cluster

03LH4ZZ Occlusion of Right Common Carotid Artery, Percutaneous Endoscopic Approach

03LJ0BZ Occlusion of Left Common Carotid Artery with Bioactive Intraluminal Device, Open Approach

03LJ0CZ Occlusion of Left Common Carotid Artery with Extraluminal Device, Open Approach

03LJ0DZ Occlusion of Left Common Carotid Artery with Intraluminal Device, Open Approach

03LJ0ZZ Occlusion of Left Common Carotid Artery, Open Approach

03LJ3BZ Occlusion of Left Common Carotid Artery with Bioactive Intraluminal Device, Percutaneous Approach

03LJ3CZ Occlusion of Left Common Carotid Artery with Extraluminal Device, Percutaneous Approach

03LJ3DZ Occlusion of Left Common Carotid Artery with Intraluminal Device, Percutaneous Approach

03LJ3ZZ Occlusion of Left Common Carotid Artery, Percutaneous Approach

03LJ4BZ Occlusion of Left Common Carotid Artery with Bioactive Intraluminal Device, Percutaneous Endoscopic Approach

03LJ4CZ Occlusion of Left Common Carotid Artery with Extraluminal Device, Percutaneous Endoscopic Approach

03LJ4DZ Occlusion of Left Common Carotid Artery with Intraluminal Device, Percutaneous Endoscopic Approach

03LJ4ZZ Occlusion of Left Common Carotid Artery, Percutaneous Endoscopic Approach

03LK0BZ Occlusion of Right Internal Carotid Artery with Bioactive Intraluminal Device, Open Approach

03LK0CZ Occlusion of Right Internal Carotid Artery with Extraluminal Device, Open Approach

03LK0DZ Occlusion of Right Internal Carotid Artery with Intraluminal Device, Open Approach

03LK0ZZ Occlusion of Right Internal Carotid Artery, Open Approach

03LK3BZ Occlusion of Right Internal Carotid Artery with Bioactive Intraluminal Device, Percutaneous Approach

03LK3CZ Occlusion of Right Internal Carotid Artery with Extraluminal Device, Percutaneous Approach

03LK3DZ Occlusion of Right Internal Carotid Artery with Intraluminal Device, Percutaneous Approach

03LK3ZZ Occlusion of Right Internal Carotid Artery, Percutaneous Approach

03LK4BZ Occlusion of Right Internal Carotid Artery with Bioactive Intraluminal Device, Percutaneous Endoscopic Approach

03LK4CZ Occlusion of Right Internal Carotid Artery with Extraluminal Device, Percutaneous Endoscopic Approach

03LK4DZ Occlusion of Right Internal Carotid Artery with Intraluminal Device, Percutaneous Endoscopic Approach

03LK4ZZ Occlusion of Right Internal Carotid Artery, Percutaneous Endoscopic Approach

03LL0BZ Occlusion of Left Internal Carotid Artery with Bioactive Intraluminal Device, Open Approach

03LL0CZ Occlusion of Left Internal Carotid Artery with Extraluminal Device, Open Approach

03LL0DZ Occlusion of Left Internal Carotid Artery with Intraluminal Device, Open Approach

03LL0ZZ Occlusion of Left Internal Carotid Artery, Open Approach
AHA CC: 2Q, 2021, 13

03LL3BZ Occlusion of Left Internal Carotid Artery with Bioactive Intraluminal Device, Percutaneous Approach

03LL3CZ Occlusion of Left Internal Carotid Artery with Extraluminal Device, Percutaneous Approach

03LL3DZ Occlusion of Left Internal Carotid Artery with Intraluminal Device, Percutaneous Approach

03LL3ZZ Occlusion of Left Internal Carotid Artery, Percutaneous Approach

03LL4BZ Occlusion of Left Internal Carotid Artery with Bioactive Intraluminal Device, Percutaneous Endoscopic Approach

03LL4CZ Occlusion of Left Internal Carotid Artery with Extraluminal Device, Percutaneous Endoscopic Approach

03LL4DZ Occlusion of Left Internal Carotid Artery with Intraluminal Device, Percutaneous Endoscopic Approach

03LL4ZZ Occlusion of Left Internal Carotid Artery, Percutaneous Endoscopic Approach

03LM0BZ Occlusion of Right External Carotid Artery with Bioactive Intraluminal Device, Open Approach

03LM0CZ Occlusion of Right External Carotid Artery with Extraluminal Device, Open Approach

03LM0DZ Occlusion of Right External Carotid Artery with Intraluminal Device, Open Approach

03LM0ZZ Occlusion of Right External Carotid Artery, Open Approach

03LM3BZ Occlusion of Right External Carotid Artery with Bioactive Intraluminal Device, Percutaneous Approach

03LM3CZ Occlusion of Right External Carotid Artery with Extraluminal Device, Percutaneous Approach

03LM3DZ Occlusion of Right External Carotid Artery with Intraluminal Device, Percutaneous Approach

03LM3ZZ Occlusion of Right External Carotid Artery, Percutaneous Approach

03LM4BZ Occlusion of Right External Carotid Artery with Bioactive Intraluminal Device, Percutaneous Endoscopic Approach

03LM4CZ Occlusion of Right External Carotid Artery with Extraluminal Device, Percutaneous Endoscopic Approach

03LM4DZ Occlusion of Right External Carotid Artery with Intraluminal Device, Percutaneous Endoscopic Approach

03LM4ZZ Occlusion of Right External Carotid Artery, Percutaneous Endoscopic Approach

03LN0BZ Occlusion of Left External Carotid Artery with Bioactive Intraluminal Device, Open Approach

03LN0CZ Occlusion of Left External Carotid Artery with Extraluminal Device, Open Approach

03LN0DZ Occlusion of Left External Carotid Artery with Intraluminal Device, Open Approach

03LN0ZZ Occlusion of Left External Carotid Artery, Open Approach

03LN3BZ Occlusion of Left External Carotid Artery with Bioactive Intraluminal Device, Percutaneous Approach

03LN3CZ Occlusion of Left External Carotid Artery with Extraluminal Device, Percutaneous Approach

03LN3DZ Occlusion of Left External Carotid Artery with Intraluminal Device, Percutaneous Approach

03LN3ZZ Occlusion of Left External Carotid Artery, Percutaneous Approach

03LN4BZ Occlusion of Left External Carotid Artery with Bioactive Intraluminal Device, Percutaneous Endoscopic Approach

03LN4CZ Occlusion of Left External Carotid Artery with Extraluminal Device, Percutaneous Endoscopic Approach

03LN4DZ Occlusion of Left External Carotid Artery with Intraluminal Device, Percutaneous Endoscopic Approach

03LN4ZZ Occlusion of Left External Carotid Artery, Percutaneous Endoscopic Approach

03LP0BZ Occlusion of Right Vertebral Artery with Bioactive Intraluminal Device, Open Approach

03LP0CZ Occlusion of Right Vertebral Artery with Extraluminal Device, Open Approach

03LP0DZ Occlusion of Right Vertebral Artery with Intraluminal Device, Open Approach

03LP0ZZ Occlusion of Right Vertebral Artery, Open Approach

03LP3BZ Occlusion of Right Vertebral Artery with Bioactive Intraluminal Device, Percutaneous Approach

03LP3CZ Occlusion of Right Vertebral Artery with Extraluminal Device, Percutaneous Approach

03LP3DZ Occlusion of Right Vertebral Artery with Intraluminal Device, Percutaneous Approach

03LP3ZZ Occlusion of Right Vertebral Artery, Percutaneous Approach

03LP4BZ Occlusion of Right Vertebral Artery with Bioactive Intraluminal Device, Percutaneous Endoscopic Approach

03LP4CZ Occlusion of Right Vertebral Artery with Extraluminal Device, Percutaneous Endoscopic Approach

03LP4DZ Occlusion of Right Vertebral Artery with Intraluminal Device, Percutaneous Endoscopic Approach

03LP4ZZ Occlusion of Right Vertebral Artery, Percutaneous Endoscopic Approach

03LQ0BZ Occlusion of Left Vertebral Artery with Bioactive Intraluminal Device, Open Approach

03LQ0CZ Occlusion of Left Vertebral Artery with Extraluminal Device, Open Approach

03LQ0DZ Occlusion of Left Vertebral Artery with Intraluminal Device, Open Approach

03LQ0ZZ Occlusion of Left Vertebral Artery, Open Approach

03LQ3BZ Occlusion of Left Vertebral Artery with Bioactive Intraluminal Device, Percutaneous Approach

03LQ3CZ Occlusion of Left Vertebral Artery with Extraluminal Device, Percutaneous Approach

03LQ3DZ Occlusion of Left Vertebral Artery with Intraluminal Device, Percutaneous Approach

03LQ3ZZ Occlusion of Left Vertebral Artery, Percutaneous Approach

03LQ4BZ Occlusion of Left Vertebral Artery with Bioactive Intraluminal Device, Percutaneous Endoscopic Approach

03LQ4CZ Occlusion of Left Vertebral Artery with Extraluminal Device, Percutaneous Endoscopic Approach

03LQ4DZ Occlusion of Left Vertebral Artery with Intraluminal Device, Percutaneous Endoscopic Approach

03LQ4ZZ Occlusion of Left Vertebral Artery, Percutaneous Endoscopic Approach

03LR0CZ Occlusion of Face Artery with Extraluminal Device, Open Approach

03LR0DZ Occlusion of Face Artery with Intraluminal Device, Open Approach

03LR0ZZ Occlusion of Face Artery, Open Approach

03LR3CZ Occlusion of Face Artery with Extraluminal Device, Percutaneous Approach

03LR3DZ Occlusion of Face Artery with Intraluminal Device, Percutaneous Approach

03LR3ZZ Occlusion of Face Artery, Percutaneous Approach

03LR4CZ Occlusion of Face Artery with Extraluminal Device, Percutaneous Endoscopic Approach

03LR4DZ Occlusion of Face Artery with Intraluminal Device, Percutaneous Endoscopic Approach

03LR4ZZ Occlusion of Face Artery, Percutaneous Endoscopic Approach

03LS0CZ Occlusion of Right Temporal Artery with Extraluminal Device, Open Approach

03LS0DZ Occlusion of Right Temporal Artery with Intraluminal Device, Open Approach

03LS0ZZ Occlusion of Right Temporal Artery, Open Approach

03LS3CZ Occlusion of Right Temporal Artery with Extraluminal Device, Percutaneous Approach

03LS3DZ Occlusion of Right Temporal Artery with Intraluminal Device, Percutaneous Approach

03LS3ZZ Occlusion of Right Temporal Artery, Percutaneous Approach

03LS4CZ Occlusion of Right Temporal Artery with Extraluminal Device, Percutaneous Endoscopic Approach

03LS4DZ Occlusion of Right Temporal Artery with Intraluminal Device, Percutaneous Endoscopic Approach

03LS4ZZ Occlusion of Right Temporal Artery, Percutaneous Endoscopic Approach

03LT0CZ Occlusion of Left Temporal Artery with Extraluminal Device, Open Approach

03LT0DZ Occlusion of Left Temporal Artery with Intraluminal Device, Open Approach

03LT0ZZ Occlusion of Left Temporal Artery, Open Approach

03LT3CZ Occlusion of Left Temporal Artery with Extraluminal Device, Percutaneous Approach

03LT3DZ Occlusion of Left Temporal Artery with Intraluminal Device, Percutaneous Approach

03LT3ZZ Occlusion of Left Temporal Artery, Percutaneous Approach

03LT4CZ Occlusion of Left Temporal Artery with Extraluminal Device, Percutaneous Endoscopic Approach

03LT4DZ Occlusion of Left Temporal Artery with Intraluminal Device, Percutaneous Endoscopic Approach

03LT4ZZ Occlusion of Left Temporal Artery, Percutaneous Endoscopic Approach

03LU0CZ Occlusion of Right Thyroid Artery with Extraluminal Device, Open Approach

03LU0DZ Occlusion of Right Thyroid Artery with Intraluminal Device, Open Approach

03LU0ZZ Occlusion of Right Thyroid Artery, Open Approach

03LU3CZ Occlusion of Right Thyroid Artery with Extraluminal Device, Percutaneous Approach

03LU3DZ Occlusion of Right Thyroid Artery with Intraluminal Device, Percutaneous Approach

03LU3ZZ Occlusion of Right Thyroid Artery, Percutaneous Approach

03LU4CZ Occlusion of Right Thyroid Artery with Extraluminal Device, Percutaneous Endoscopic Approach

03LU4DZ Occlusion of Right Thyroid Artery with Intraluminal Device, Percutaneous Endoscopic Approach

03LU4ZZ Occlusion of Right Thyroid Artery, Percutaneous Endoscopic Approach

03LV0CZ Occlusion of Left Thyroid Artery with Extraluminal Device, Open Approach

03LV0DZ Occlusion of Left Thyroid Artery with Intraluminal Device, Open Approach

03LV0ZZ Occlusion of Left Thyroid Artery, Open Approach

03LV3CZ Occlusion of Left Thyroid Artery with Extraluminal Device, Percutaneous Approach

03LV3DZ Occlusion of Left Thyroid Artery with Intraluminal Device, Percutaneous Approach

03LV3ZZ Occlusion of Left Thyroid Artery, Percutaneous Approach

03LV4CZ Occlusion of Left Thyroid Artery with Extraluminal Device, Percutaneous Endoscopic Approach

03LV4DZ Occlusion of Left Thyroid Artery with Intraluminal Device, Percutaneous Endoscopic Approach

03LV4ZZ Occlusion of Left Thyroid Artery, Percutaneous Endoscopic Approach

03LY0CZ Occlusion of Upper Artery with Extraluminal Device, Open Approach

03LY0DZ Occlusion of Upper Artery with Intraluminal Device, Open Approach

03LY0ZZ Occlusion of Upper Artery, Open Approach

03LY3CZ Occlusion of Upper Artery with Extraluminal Device, Percutaneous Approach

03LY3DZ Occlusion of Upper Artery with Intraluminal Device, Percutaneous Approach

03LY3ZZ Occlusion of Upper Artery, Percutaneous Approach

03LY4CZ Occlusion of Upper Artery with Extraluminal Device, Percutaneous Endoscopic Approach

03LY4DZ Occlusion of Upper Artery with Intraluminal Device, Percutaneous Endoscopic Approach

03LY4ZZ Occlusion of Upper Artery, Percutaneous Endoscopic Approach

03N – Upper Arteries, Release

Review Coding Guidelines B3.13 and B3.14

03N00ZZ Release Right Internal Mammary Artery, Open Approach

03N03ZZ Release Right Internal Mammary Artery, Percutaneous Approach

03N04ZZ Release Right Internal Mammary Artery, Percutaneous Endoscopic Approach

03N10ZZ Release Left Internal Mammary Artery, Open Approach

03N13ZZ Release Left Internal Mammary Artery, Percutaneous Approach

03N14ZZ Release Left Internal Mammary Artery, Percutaneous Endoscopic Approach

03N20ZZ Release Innominate Artery, Open Approach

03N23ZZ Release Innominate Artery, Percutaneous Approach

03N24ZZ Release Innominate Artery, Percutaneous Endoscopic Approach

03N30ZZ Release Right Subclavian Artery, Open Approach

03N33ZZ Release Right Subclavian Artery, Percutaneous Approach

03N34ZZ Release Right Subclavian Artery, Percutaneous Endoscopic Approach

03N40ZZ Release Left Subclavian Artery, Open Approach

03N43ZZ Release Left Subclavian Artery, Percutaneous Approach

03N44ZZ Release Left Subclavian Artery, Percutaneous Endoscopic Approach

03N50ZZ Release Right Axillary Artery, Open Approach

03N53ZZ Release Right Axillary Artery, Percutaneous Approach

03N54ZZ Release Right Axillary Artery, Percutaneous Endoscopic Approach

03N60ZZ Release Left Axillary Artery, Open Approach

03N63ZZ Release Left Axillary Artery, Percutaneous Approach

03N64ZZ Release Left Axillary Artery, Percutaneous Endoscopic Approach

03N70ZZ Release Right Brachial Artery, Open Approach

03N73ZZ Release Right Brachial Artery, Percutaneous Approach

03N74ZZ Release Right Brachial Artery, Percutaneous Endoscopic Approach

03N80ZZ Release Left Brachial Artery, Open Approach

03N83ZZ Release Left Brachial Artery, Percutaneous Approach

03N84ZZ Release Left Brachial Artery, Percutaneous Endoscopic Approach

03N90ZZ Release Right Ulnar Artery, Open Approach

03N93ZZ Release Right Ulnar Artery, Percutaneous Approach

♀ Female-only   ♂ Male-only   ▲ Limited Coverage   ● Non-OR   HAC HAC-associated procedure   ▲ Non-covered procedures   ✚ Cluster

03N94ZZ	Release Right Ulnar Artery, Percutaneous Endoscopic Approach	03NH4ZZ	Release Right Common Carotid Artery, Percutaneous Endoscopic Approach	03NP4ZZ	Release Right Vertebral Artery, Percutaneous Endoscopic Approach
03NA0ZZ	Release Left Ulnar Artery, Open Approach	03NJ0ZZ	Release Left Common Carotid Artery, Open Approach	03NQ0ZZ	Release Left Vertebral Artery, Open Approach
03NA3ZZ	Release Left Ulnar Artery, Percutaneous Approach	03NJ3ZZ	Release Left Common Carotid Artery, Percutaneous Approach	03NQ3ZZ	Release Left Vertebral Artery, Percutaneous Approach
03NA4ZZ	Release Left Ulnar Artery, Percutaneous Endoscopic Approach	03NJ4ZZ	Release Left Common Carotid Artery, Percutaneous Endoscopic Approach	03NQ4ZZ	Release Left Vertebral Artery, Percutaneous Endoscopic Approach
03NB0ZZ	Release Right Radial Artery, Open Approach	03NK0ZZ	Release Right Internal Carotid Artery, Open Approach	03NR0ZZ	Release Face Artery, Open Approach
03NB3ZZ	Release Right Radial Artery, Percutaneous Approach	03NK3ZZ	Release Right Internal Carotid Artery, Percutaneous Approach	03NR3ZZ	Release Face Artery, Percutaneous Approach
03NB4ZZ	Release Right Radial Artery, Percutaneous Endoscopic Approach	03NK4ZZ	Release Right Internal Carotid Artery, Percutaneous Endoscopic Approach	03NR4ZZ	Release Face Artery, Percutaneous Endoscopic Approach
03NC0ZZ	Release Left Radial Artery, Open Approach	03NL0ZZ	Release Left Internal Carotid Artery, Open Approach	03NS0ZZ	Release Right Temporal Artery, Open Approach
03NC3ZZ	Release Left Radial Artery, Percutaneous Approach	03NL3ZZ	Release Left Internal Carotid Artery, Percutaneous Approach	03NS3ZZ	Release Right Temporal Artery, Percutaneous Approach
03NC4ZZ	Release Left Radial Artery, Percutaneous Endoscopic Approach	03NL4ZZ	Release Left Internal Carotid Artery, Percutaneous Endoscopic Approach	03NS4ZZ	Release Right Temporal Artery, Percutaneous Endoscopic Approach
03ND0ZZ	Release Right Hand Artery, Open Approach	03NM0ZZ	Release Right External Carotid Artery, Open Approach	03NT0ZZ	Release Left Temporal Artery, Open Approach
03ND3ZZ	Release Right Hand Artery, Percutaneous Approach	03NM3ZZ	Release Right External Carotid Artery, Percutaneous Approach	03NT3ZZ	Release Left Temporal Artery, Percutaneous Approach
03ND4ZZ	Release Right Hand Artery, Percutaneous Endoscopic Approach	03NM4ZZ	Release Right External Carotid Artery, Percutaneous Endoscopic Approach	03NT4ZZ	Release Left Temporal Artery, Percutaneous Endoscopic Approach
03NF0ZZ	Release Left Hand Artery, Open Approach	03NN0ZZ	Release Left External Carotid Artery, Open Approach	03NU0ZZ	Release Right Thyroid Artery, Open Approach
03NF3ZZ	Release Left Hand Artery, Percutaneous Approach	03NN3ZZ	Release Left External Carotid Artery, Percutaneous Approach	03NU3ZZ	Release Right Thyroid Artery, Percutaneous Approach
03NF4ZZ	Release Left Hand Artery, Percutaneous Endoscopic Approach	03NN4ZZ	Release Left External Carotid Artery, Percutaneous Endoscopic Approach	03NU4ZZ	Release Right Thyroid Artery, Percutaneous Endoscopic Approach
03NG0ZZ	Release Intracranial Artery, Open Approach	03NP0ZZ	Release Right Vertebral Artery, Open Approach	03NV0ZZ	Release Left Thyroid Artery, Open Approach
03NG3ZZ	Release Intracranial Artery, Percutaneous Approach	03NP3ZZ	Release Right Vertebral Artery, Percutaneous Approach	03NV3ZZ	Release Left Thyroid Artery, Percutaneous Approach
03NG4ZZ	Release Intracranial Artery, Percutaneous Endoscopic Approach			03NV4ZZ	Release Left Thyroid Artery, Percutaneous Endoscopic Approach
03NH0ZZ	Release Right Common Carotid Artery, Open Approach			03NY0ZZ	Release Upper Artery, Open Approach
03NH3ZZ	Release Right Common Carotid Artery, Percutaneous Approach			03NY3ZZ	Release Upper Artery, Percutaneous Approach
				03NY4ZZ	Release Upper Artery, Percutaneous Endoscopic Approach

03P – Upper Arteries, Removal

Review Coding Guideline B6.1c

03PY00Z	Removal of Drainage Device from Upper Artery, Open Approach	03PY37Z	Removal of Autologous Tissue Substitute from Upper Artery, Percutaneous Approach	03PY4CZ	Removal of Extraluminal Device from Upper Artery, Percutaneous Endoscopic Approach
03PY02Z	Removal of Monitoring Device from Upper Artery, Open Approach	03PY3CZ	Removal of Extraluminal Device from Upper Artery, Percutaneous Approach	03PY4DZ	Removal of Intraluminal Device from Upper Artery, Percutaneous Endoscopic Approach
03PY03Z	Removal of Infusion Device from Upper Artery, Open Approach	03PY3DZ	Removal of Intraluminal Device from Upper Artery, Percutaneous Approach	03PY4JZ	Removal of Synthetic Substitute from Upper Artery, Percutaneous Endoscopic Approach
03PY07Z	Removal of Autologous Tissue Substitute from Upper Artery, Open Approach	03PY3JZ	Removal of Synthetic Substitute from Upper Artery, Percutaneous Approach	03PY4KZ	Removal of Nonautologous Tissue Substitute from Upper Artery, Percutaneous Endoscopic Approach
03PY0CZ	Removal of Extraluminal Device from Upper Artery, Open Approach	03PY3KZ	Removal of Nonautologous Tissue Substitute from Upper Artery, Percutaneous Approach	03PY4MZ	Removal of Stimulator Lead from Upper Artery, Percutaneous Endoscopic Approach
03PY0DZ	Removal of Intraluminal Device from Upper Artery, Open Approach	03PY3MZ	Removal of Stimulator Lead from Upper Artery, Percutaneous Approach	03PY4YZ	Removal of Other Device from Upper Artery, Percutaneous Endoscopic Approach
03PY0JZ	Removal of Synthetic Substitute from Upper Artery, Open Approach	03PY3YZ	Removal of Other Device from Upper Artery, Percutaneous Approach	03PYX0Z	Removal of Drainage Device from Upper Artery, External Approach
03PY0KZ	Removal of Nonautologous Tissue Substitute from Upper Artery, Open Approach	03PY40Z	Removal of Drainage Device from Upper Artery, Percutaneous Endoscopic Approach	03PYX2Z	Removal of Monitoring Device from Upper Artery, External Approach
03PY0MZ	Removal of Stimulator Lead from Upper Artery, Open Approach	03PY42Z	Removal of Monitoring Device from Upper Artery, Percutaneous Endoscopic Approach	03PYX3Z	Removal of Infusion Device from Upper Artery, External Approach
03PY0YZ	Removal of Other Device from Upper Artery, Open Approach	03PY43Z	Removal of Infusion Device from Upper Artery, Percutaneous Endoscopic Approach	03PYXDZ	Removal of Intraluminal Device from Upper Artery, External Approach
03PY30Z	Removal of Drainage Device from Upper Artery, Percutaneous Approach	03PY47Z	Removal of Autologous Tissue Substitute from Upper Artery, Percutaneous Endoscopic Approach	03PYXMZ	Removal of Stimulator Lead from Upper Artery, External Approach
03PY32Z	Removal of Monitoring Device from Upper Artery, Percutaneous Approach				
03PY33Z	Removal of Infusion Device from Upper Artery, Percutaneous Approach				

03Q – Upper Arteries, Repair

03Q00ZZ	Repair Right Internal Mammary Artery, Open Approach	03Q94ZZ	Repair Right Ulnar Artery, Percutaneous Endoscopic Approach	03QL4ZZ	Repair Left Internal Carotid Artery, Percutaneous Endoscopic Approach
03Q03ZZ	Repair Right Internal Mammary Artery, Percutaneous Approach	03QA0ZZ	Repair Left Ulnar Artery, Open Approach	03QM0ZZ	Repair Right External Carotid Artery, Open Approach
03Q04ZZ	Repair Right Internal Mammary Artery, Percutaneous Endoscopic Approach	03QA3ZZ	Repair Left Ulnar Artery, Percutaneous Approach	03QM3ZZ	Repair Right External Carotid Artery, Percutaneous Approach
03Q10ZZ	Repair Left Internal Mammary Artery, Open Approach	03QA4ZZ	Repair Left Ulnar Artery, Percutaneous Endoscopic Approach	03QM4ZZ	Repair Right External Carotid Artery, Percutaneous Endoscopic Approach
03Q13ZZ	Repair Left Internal Mammary Artery, Percutaneous Approach	03QB0ZZ	Repair Right Radial Artery, Open Approach	03QN0ZZ	Repair Left External Carotid Artery, Open Approach
03Q14ZZ	Repair Left Internal Mammary Artery, Percutaneous Endoscopic Approach	03QB3ZZ	Repair Right Radial Artery, Percutaneous Approach	03QN3ZZ	Repair Left External Carotid Artery, Percutaneous Approach
03Q20ZZ	Repair Innominate Artery, Open Approach	03QB4ZZ	Repair Right Radial Artery, Percutaneous Endoscopic Approach	03QN4ZZ	Repair Left External Carotid Artery, Percutaneous Endoscopic Approach
03Q23ZZ	Repair Innominate Artery, Percutaneous Approach	03QC0ZZ	Repair Left Radial Artery, Open Approach	03QP0ZZ	Repair Right Vertebral Artery, Open Approach
03Q24ZZ	Repair Innominate Artery, Percutaneous Endoscopic Approach	03QC3ZZ	Repair Left Radial Artery, Percutaneous Approach	03QP3ZZ	Repair Right Vertebral Artery, Percutaneous Approach
03Q30ZZ	Repair Right Subclavian Artery, Open Approach	03QC4ZZ	Repair Left Radial Artery, Percutaneous Endoscopic Approach	03QP4ZZ	Repair Right Vertebral Artery, Percutaneous Endoscopic Approach
03Q33ZZ	Repair Right Subclavian Artery, Percutaneous Approach	03QD0ZZ	Repair Right Hand Artery, Open Approach	03QQ0ZZ	Repair Left Vertebral Artery, Open Approach
03Q34ZZ	Repair Right Subclavian Artery, Percutaneous Endoscopic Approach	03QD3ZZ	Repair Right Hand Artery, Percutaneous Approach	03QQ3ZZ	Repair Left Vertebral Artery, Percutaneous Approach
03Q40ZZ	Repair Left Subclavian Artery, Open Approach	03QD4ZZ	Repair Right Hand Artery, Percutaneous Endoscopic Approach	03QQ4ZZ	Repair Left Vertebral Artery, Percutaneous Endoscopic Approach
03Q43ZZ	Repair Left Subclavian Artery, Percutaneous Approach	03QF0ZZ	Repair Left Hand Artery, Open Approach	03QR0ZZ	Repair Face Artery, Open Approach
03Q44ZZ	Repair Left Subclavian Artery, Percutaneous Endoscopic Approach	03QF3ZZ	Repair Left Hand Artery, Percutaneous Approach	03QR3ZZ	Repair Face Artery, Percutaneous Approach
03Q50ZZ	Repair Right Axillary Artery, Open Approach	03QF4ZZ	Repair Left Hand Artery, Percutaneous Endoscopic Approach	03QR4ZZ	Repair Face Artery, Percutaneous Endoscopic Approach
03Q53ZZ	Repair Right Axillary Artery, Percutaneous Approach	03QG0ZZ	Repair Intracranial Artery, Open Approach	03QS0ZZ	Repair Right Temporal Artery, Open Approach
03Q54ZZ	Repair Right Axillary Artery, Percutaneous Endoscopic Approach	03QG3ZZ	Repair Intracranial Artery, Percutaneous Approach	03QS3ZZ	Repair Right Temporal Artery, Percutaneous Approach
03Q60ZZ	Repair Left Axillary Artery, Open Approach	03QG4ZZ	Repair Intracranial Artery, Percutaneous Endoscopic Approach	03QS4ZZ	Repair Right Temporal Artery, Percutaneous Endoscopic Approach
03Q63ZZ	Repair Left Axillary Artery, Percutaneous Approach	03QH0ZZ	Repair Right Common Carotid Artery, Open Approach	03QT0ZZ	Repair Left Temporal Artery, Open Approach
03Q64ZZ	Repair Left Axillary Artery, Percutaneous Endoscopic Approach	*AHA CC: 1Q, 2017, 31-32*		03QT3ZZ	Repair Left Temporal Artery, Percutaneous Approach
03Q70ZZ	Repair Right Brachial Artery, Open Approach	03QH3ZZ	Repair Right Common Carotid Artery, Percutaneous Approach	03QT4ZZ	Repair Left Temporal Artery, Percutaneous Endoscopic Approach
03Q73ZZ	Repair Right Brachial Artery, Percutaneous Approach	03QH4ZZ	Repair Right Common Carotid Artery, Percutaneous Endoscopic Approach	03QU0ZZ	Repair Right Thyroid Artery, Open Approach
03Q74ZZ	Repair Right Brachial Artery, Percutaneous Endoscopic Approach	03QJ0ZZ	Repair Left Common Carotid Artery, Open Approach	03QU3ZZ	Repair Right Thyroid Artery, Percutaneous Approach
03Q80ZZ	Repair Left Brachial Artery, Open Approach	03QJ3ZZ	Repair Left Common Carotid Artery, Percutaneous Approach	03QU4ZZ	Repair Right Thyroid Artery, Percutaneous Endoscopic Approach
03Q83ZZ	Repair Left Brachial Artery, Percutaneous Approach	03QJ4ZZ	Repair Left Common Carotid Artery, Percutaneous Endoscopic Approach	03QV0ZZ	Repair Left Thyroid Artery, Open Approach
03Q84ZZ	Repair Left Brachial Artery, Percutaneous Endoscopic Approach	03QK0ZZ	Repair Right Internal Carotid Artery, Open Approach	03QV3ZZ	Repair Left Thyroid Artery, Percutaneous Approach
03Q80ZZ	Repair Left Brachial Artery, Open Approach	03QK3ZZ	Repair Right Internal Carotid Artery, Percutaneous Approach	03QV4ZZ	Repair Left Thyroid Artery, Percutaneous Endoscopic Approach
03Q90ZZ	Repair Right Ulnar Artery, Open Approach	03QK4ZZ	Repair Right Internal Carotid Artery, Percutaneous Endoscopic Approach	03QY0ZZ	Repair Upper Artery, Open Approach
03Q93ZZ	Repair Right Ulnar Artery, Percutaneous Approach	03QL0ZZ	Repair Left Internal Carotid Artery, Open Approach	03QY3ZZ	Repair Upper Artery, Percutaneous Approach
		03QL3ZZ	Repair Left Internal Carotid Artery, Percutaneous Approach	03QY4ZZ	Repair Upper Artery, Percutaneous Endoscopic Approach

03R – Upper Arteries, Replacement

Review Coding Guideline B3.18

03R007Z	Replacement of Right Internal Mammary Artery with Autologous Tissue Substitute, Open Approach	03R00KZ	Replacement of Right Internal Mammary Artery with Nonautologous Tissue Substitute, Open Approach	03R04JZ	Replacement of Right Internal Mammary Artery with Synthetic Substitute, Percutaneous Endoscopic Approach
03R00JZ	Replacement of Right Internal Mammary Artery with Synthetic Substitute, Open Approach	03R047Z	Replacement of Right Internal Mammary Artery with Autologous Tissue Substitute, Percutaneous Endoscopic Approach	03R04KZ	Replacement of Right Internal Mammary Artery with Nonautologous Tissue Substitute, Percutaneous Endoscopic Approach

♀ Female-only   ♂ Male-only   ▲ Limited Coverage   ● Non-OR   HAC HAC-associated procedure   ▲ Non-covered procedures   ✚ Cluster

03R107Z Replacement of Left Internal Mammary Artery with Autologous Tissue Substitute, Open Approach

03R10JZ Replacement of Left Internal Mammary Artery with Synthetic Substitute, Open Approach

03R10KZ Replacement of Left Internal Mammary Artery with Nonautologous Tissue Substitute, Open Approach

03R147Z Replacement of Left Internal Mammary Artery with Autologous Tissue Substitute, Percutaneous Endoscopic Approach

03R14JZ Replacement of Left Internal Mammary Artery with Synthetic Substitute, Percutaneous Endoscopic Approach

03R14KZ Replacement of Left Internal Mammary Artery with Nonautologous Tissue Substitute, Percutaneous Endoscopic Approach

03R207Z Replacement of Innominate Artery with Autologous Tissue Substitute, Open Approach

03R20JZ Replacement of Innominate Artery with Synthetic Substitute, Open Approach

03R20KZ Replacement of Innominate Artery with Nonautologous Tissue Substitute, Open Approach

03R247Z Replacement of Innominate Artery with Autologous Tissue Substitute, Percutaneous Endoscopic Approach

03R24JZ Replacement of Innominate Artery with Synthetic Substitute, Percutaneous Endoscopic Approach

03R24KZ Replacement of Innominate Artery with Nonautologous Tissue Substitute, Percutaneous Endoscopic Approach

03R307Z Replacement of Right Subclavian Artery with Autologous Tissue Substitute, Open Approach

03R30JZ Replacement of Right Subclavian Artery with Synthetic Substitute, Open Approach

03R30KZ Replacement of Right Subclavian Artery with Nonautologous Tissue Substitute, Open Approach

03R347Z Replacement of Right Subclavian Artery with Autologous Tissue Substitute, Percutaneous Endoscopic Approach

03R34JZ Replacement of Right Subclavian Artery with Synthetic Substitute, Percutaneous Endoscopic Approach

03R34KZ Replacement of Right Subclavian Artery with Nonautologous Tissue Substitute, Percutaneous Endoscopic Approach

03R407Z Replacement of Left Subclavian Artery with Autologous Tissue Substitute, Open Approach

03R40JZ Replacement of Left Subclavian Artery with Synthetic Substitute, Open Approach

03R40KZ Replacement of Left Subclavian Artery with Nonautologous Tissue Substitute, Open Approach

03R447Z Replacement of Left Subclavian Artery with Autologous Tissue Substitute, Percutaneous Endoscopic Approach

03R44JZ Replacement of Left Subclavian Artery with Synthetic Substitute, Percutaneous Endoscopic Approach

03R44KZ Replacement of Left Subclavian Artery with Nonautologous Tissue Substitute, Percutaneous Endoscopic Approach

03R507Z Replacement of Right Axillary Artery with Autologous Tissue Substitute, Open Approach

03R50JZ Replacement of Right Axillary Artery with Synthetic Substitute, Open Approach

03R50KZ Replacement of Right Axillary Artery with Nonautologous Tissue Substitute, Open Approach

03R547Z Replacement of Right Axillary Artery with Autologous Tissue Substitute, Percutaneous Endoscopic Approach

03R54JZ Replacement of Right Axillary Artery with Synthetic Substitute, Percutaneous Endoscopic Approach

03R54KZ Replacement of Right Axillary Artery with Nonautologous Tissue Substitute, Percutaneous Endoscopic Approach

03R607Z Replacement of Left Axillary Artery with Autologous Tissue Substitute, Open Approach

03R60JZ Replacement of Left Axillary Artery with Synthetic Substitute, Open Approach

03R60KZ Replacement of Left Axillary Artery with Nonautologous Tissue Substitute, Open Approach

03R647Z Replacement of Left Axillary Artery with Autologous Tissue Substitute, Percutaneous Endoscopic Approach

03R64JZ Replacement of Left Axillary Artery with Synthetic Substitute, Percutaneous Endoscopic Approach

03R64KZ Replacement of Left Axillary Artery with Nonautologous Tissue Substitute, Percutaneous Endoscopic Approach

03R707Z Replacement of Right Brachial Artery with Autologous Tissue Substitute, Open Approach

03R70JZ Replacement of Right Brachial Artery with Synthetic Substitute, Open Approach

03R70KZ Replacement of Right Brachial Artery with Nonautologous Tissue Substitute, Open Approach

03R747Z Replacement of Right Brachial Artery with Autologous Tissue Substitute, Percutaneous Endoscopic Approach

03R74JZ Replacement of Right Brachial Artery with Synthetic Substitute, Percutaneous Endoscopic Approach

03R74KZ Replacement of Right Brachial Artery with Nonautologous Tissue Substitute, Percutaneous Endoscopic Approach

03R807Z Replacement of Left Brachial Artery with Autologous Tissue Substitute, Open Approach

03R80JZ Replacement of Left Brachial Artery with Synthetic Substitute, Open Approach

03R80KZ Replacement of Left Brachial Artery with Nonautologous Tissue Substitute, Open Approach

03R847Z Replacement of Left Brachial Artery with Autologous Tissue Substitute, Percutaneous Endoscopic Approach

03R84JZ Replacement of Left Brachial Artery with Synthetic Substitute, Percutaneous Endoscopic Approach

03R84KZ Replacement of Left Brachial Artery with Nonautologous Tissue Substitute, Percutaneous Endoscopic Approach

03R907Z Replacement of Right Ulnar Artery with Autologous Tissue Substitute, Open Approach

03R90JZ Replacement of Right Ulnar Artery with Synthetic Substitute, Open Approach

03R90KZ Replacement of Right Ulnar Artery with Nonautologous Tissue Substitute, Open Approach

03R947Z Replacement of Right Ulnar Artery with Autologous Tissue Substitute, Percutaneous Endoscopic Approach

03R94JZ Replacement of Right Ulnar Artery with Synthetic Substitute, Percutaneous Endoscopic Approach

03R94KZ Replacement of Right Ulnar Artery with Nonautologous Tissue Substitute, Percutaneous Endoscopic Approach

03RA07Z Replacement of Left Ulnar Artery with Autologous Tissue Substitute, Open Approach

03RA0JZ Replacement of Left Ulnar Artery with Synthetic Substitute, Open Approach

03RA0KZ Replacement of Left Ulnar Artery with Nonautologous Tissue Substitute, Open Approach

03RA47Z Replacement of Left Ulnar Artery with Autologous Tissue Substitute, Percutaneous Endoscopic Approach

03RA4JZ Replacement of Left Ulnar Artery with Synthetic Substitute, Percutaneous Endoscopic Approach

03RA4KZ Replacement of Left Ulnar Artery with Nonautologous Tissue Substitute, Percutaneous Endoscopic Approach

03RB07Z Replacement of Right Radial Artery with Autologous Tissue Substitute, Open Approach

03RB0JZ Replacement of Right Radial Artery with Synthetic Substitute, Open Approach

03RB0KZ Replacement of Right Radial Artery with Nonautologous Tissue Substitute, Open Approach

03RB47Z Replacement of Right Radial Artery with Autologous Tissue Substitute, Percutaneous Endoscopic Approach

03RB4JZ Replacement of Right Radial Artery with Synthetic Substitute, Percutaneous Endoscopic Approach

03RB4KZ Replacement of Right Radial Artery with Nonautologous Tissue Substitute, Percutaneous Endoscopic Approach

03RC07Z Replacement of Left Radial Artery with Autologous Tissue Substitute, Open Approach

03RC0JZ Replacement of Left Radial Artery with Synthetic Substitute, Open Approach

03RC0KZ Replacement of Left Radial Artery with Nonautologous Tissue Substitute, Open Approach

03RC47Z Replacement of Left Radial Artery with Autologous Tissue Substitute, Percutaneous Endoscopic Approach

03RC4JZ Replacement of Left Radial Artery with Synthetic Substitute, Percutaneous Endoscopic Approach

03RC4KZ Replacement of Left Radial Artery with Nonautologous Tissue Substitute, Percutaneous Endoscopic Approach

03RD07Z Replacement of Right Hand Artery with Autologous Tissue Substitute, Open Approach

03RD0JZ Replacement of Right Hand Artery with Synthetic Substitute, Open Approach

03RD0KZ Replacement of Right Hand Artery with Nonautologous Tissue Substitute, Open Approach

03RD47Z Replacement of Right Hand Artery with Autologous Tissue Substitute, Percutaneous Endoscopic Approach

03RD4JZ Replacement of Right Hand Artery with Synthetic Substitute, Percutaneous Endoscopic Approach

03RD4KZ Replacement of Right Hand Artery with Nonautologous Tissue Substitute, Percutaneous Endoscopic Approach

03RF07Z Replacement of Left Hand Artery with Autologous Tissue Substitute, Open Approach

03RF0JZ Replacement of Left Hand Artery with Synthetic Substitute, Open Approach

03RF0KZ Replacement of Left Hand Artery with Nonautologous Tissue Substitute, Open Approach

03RF47Z Replacement of Left Hand Artery with Autologous Tissue Substitute, Percutaneous Endoscopic Approach

03RF4JZ Replacement of Left Hand Artery with Synthetic Substitute, Percutaneous Endoscopic Approach

03RF4KZ Replacement of Left Hand Artery with Nonautologous Tissue Substitute, Percutaneous Endoscopic Approach

03RG07Z Replacement of Intracranial Artery with Autologous Tissue Substitute, Open Approach

03RG0JZ Replacement of Intracranial Artery with Synthetic Substitute, Open Approach

03RG0KZ Replacement of Intracranial Artery with Nonautologous Tissue Substitute, Open Approach

03RG47Z Replacement of Intracranial Artery with Autologous Tissue Substitute, Percutaneous Endoscopic Approach

03RG4JZ Replacement of Intracranial Artery with Synthetic Substitute, Percutaneous Endoscopic Approach

03RG4KZ Replacement of Intracranial Artery with Nonautologous Tissue Substitute, Percutaneous Endoscopic Approach

03RH07Z Replacement of Right Common Carotid Artery with Autologous Tissue Substitute, Open Approach

03RH0JZ Replacement of Right Common Carotid Artery with Synthetic Substitute, Open Approach

03RH0KZ Replacement of Right Common Carotid Artery with Nonautologous Tissue Substitute, Open Approach

03RH47Z Replacement of Right Common Carotid Artery with Autologous Tissue Substitute, Percutaneous Endoscopic Approach

03RH4JZ Replacement of Right Common Carotid Artery with Synthetic Substitute, Percutaneous Endoscopic Approach

03RH4KZ Replacement of Right Common Carotid Artery with Nonautologous Tissue Substitute, Percutaneous Endoscopic Approach

03RJ07Z Replacement of Left Common Carotid Artery with Autologous Tissue Substitute, Open Approach

03RJ0JZ Replacement of Left Common Carotid Artery with Synthetic Substitute, Open Approach

03RJ0KZ Replacement of Left Common Carotid Artery with Nonautologous Tissue Substitute, Open Approach

03RJ47Z Replacement of Left Common Carotid Artery with Autologous Tissue Substitute, Percutaneous Endoscopic Approach

03RJ4JZ Replacement of Left Common Carotid Artery with Synthetic Substitute, Percutaneous Endoscopic Approach

03RJ4KZ Replacement of Left Common Carotid Artery with Nonautologous Tissue Substitute, Percutaneous Endoscopic Approach

03RK07Z Replacement of Right Internal Carotid Artery with Autologous Tissue Substitute, Open Approach

03RK0JZ Replacement of Right Internal Carotid Artery with Synthetic Substitute, Open Approach

03RK0KZ Replacement of Right Internal Carotid Artery with Nonautologous Tissue Substitute, Open Approach

03RK47Z Replacement of Right Internal Carotid Artery with Autologous Tissue Substitute, Percutaneous Endoscopic Approach

03RK4JZ Replacement of Right Internal Carotid Artery with Synthetic Substitute, Percutaneous Endoscopic Approach

03RK4KZ Replacement of Right Internal Carotid Artery with Nonautologous Tissue Substitute, Percutaneous Endoscopic Approach

03RL07Z Replacement of Left Internal Carotid Artery with Autologous Tissue Substitute, Open Approach

03RL0JZ Replacement of Left Internal Carotid Artery with Synthetic Substitute, Open Approach

03RL0KZ Replacement of Left Internal Carotid Artery with Nonautologous Tissue Substitute, Open Approach

03RL47Z Replacement of Left Internal Carotid Artery with Autologous Tissue Substitute, Percutaneous Endoscopic Approach

03RL4JZ Replacement of Left Internal Carotid Artery with Synthetic Substitute, Percutaneous Endoscopic Approach

03RL4KZ Replacement of Left Internal Carotid Artery with Nonautologous Tissue Substitute, Percutaneous Endoscopic Approach

03RM07Z Replacement of Right External Carotid Artery with Autologous Tissue Substitute, Open Approach

03RM0JZ Replacement of Right External Carotid Artery with Synthetic Substitute, Open Approach

03RM0KZ Replacement of Right External Carotid Artery with Nonautologous Tissue Substitute, Open Approach

03RM47Z Replacement of Right External Carotid Artery with Autologous Tissue Substitute, Percutaneous Endoscopic Approach

03RM4JZ Replacement of Right External Carotid Artery with Synthetic Substitute, Percutaneous Endoscopic Approach

03RM4KZ Replacement of Right External Carotid Artery with Nonautologous Tissue Substitute, Percutaneous Endoscopic Approach

03RN07Z Replacement of Left External Carotid Artery with Autologous Tissue Substitute, Open Approach

03RN0JZ Replacement of Left External Carotid Artery with Synthetic Substitute, Open Approach

03RN0KZ Replacement of Left External Carotid Artery with Nonautologous Tissue Substitute, Open Approach

03RN47Z Replacement of Left External Carotid Artery with Autologous Tissue Substitute, Percutaneous Endoscopic Approach

03RN4JZ Replacement of Left External Carotid Artery with Synthetic Substitute, Percutaneous Endoscopic Approach

03RN4KZ Replacement of Left External Carotid Artery with Nonautologous Tissue Substitute, Percutaneous Endoscopic Approach

03RP07Z Replacement of Right Vertebral Artery with Autologous Tissue Substitute, Open Approach

03RP0JZ Replacement of Right Vertebral Artery with Synthetic Substitute, Open Approach

03RP0KZ Replacement of Right Vertebral Artery with Nonautologous Tissue Substitute, Open Approach

03RP47Z Replacement of Right Vertebral Artery with Autologous Tissue Substitute, Percutaneous Endoscopic Approach

03RP4JZ Replacement of Right Vertebral Artery with Synthetic Substitute, Percutaneous Endoscopic Approach

03RP4KZ Replacement of Right Vertebral Artery with Nonautologous Tissue Substitute, Percutaneous Endoscopic Approach

03RQ07Z Replacement of Left Vertebral Artery with Autologous Tissue Substitute, Open Approach

03RQ0JZ Replacement of Left Vertebral Artery with Synthetic Substitute, Open Approach

03RQ0KZ Replacement of Left Vertebral Artery with Nonautologous Tissue Substitute, Open Approach

03RQ47Z Replacement of Left Vertebral Artery with Autologous Tissue Substitute, Percutaneous Endoscopic Approach

03RQ4JZ Replacement of Left Vertebral Artery with Synthetic Substitute, Percutaneous Endoscopic Approach

03RQ4KZ Replacement of Left Vertebral Artery with Nonautologous Tissue Substitute, Percutaneous Endoscopic Approach

03RR07Z Replacement of Face Artery with Autologous Tissue Substitute, Open Approach

03RR0JZ Replacement of Face Artery with Synthetic Substitute, Open Approach

03RR0KZ Replacement of Face Artery with Nonautologous Tissue Substitute, Open Approach

03RR47Z Replacement of Face Artery with Autologous Tissue Substitute, Percutaneous Endoscopic Approach

03RR4JZ Replacement of Face Artery with Synthetic Substitute, Percutaneous Endoscopic Approach

03RR4KZ Replacement of Face Artery with Nonautologous Tissue Substitute, Percutaneous Endoscopic Approach

03RS07Z Replacement of Right Temporal Artery with Autologous Tissue Substitute, Open Approach

03RS0JZ Replacement of Right Temporal Artery with Synthetic Substitute, Open Approach

♀ Female-only ♂ Male-only ▲ Limited Coverage ● Non-OR ▥ HAC-associated procedure ▲ Non-covered procedures ✚ Cluster

03RS0KZ Replacement of Right Temporal Artery with Nonautologous Tissue Substitute, Open Approach

03RS47Z Replacement of Right Temporal Artery with Autologous Tissue Substitute, Percutaneous Endoscopic Approach

03RS4JZ Replacement of Right Temporal Artery with Synthetic Substitute, Percutaneous Endoscopic Approach

03RS4KZ Replacement of Right Temporal Artery with Nonautologous Tissue Substitute, Percutaneous Endoscopic Approach

03RT07Z Replacement of Left Temporal Artery with Autologous Tissue Substitute, Open Approach

03RT0JZ Replacement of Left Temporal Artery with Synthetic Substitute, Open Approach

03RT0KZ Replacement of Left Temporal Artery with Nonautologous Tissue Substitute, Open Approach

03RT47Z Replacement of Left Temporal Artery with Autologous Tissue Substitute, Percutaneous Endoscopic Approach

03RT4JZ Replacement of Left Temporal Artery with Synthetic Substitute, Percutaneous Endoscopic Approach

03RT4KZ Replacement of Left Temporal Artery with Nonautologous Tissue Substitute, Percutaneous Endoscopic Approach

03RU07Z Replacement of Right Thyroid Artery with Autologous Tissue Substitute, Open Approach

03RU0JZ Replacement of Right Thyroid Artery with Synthetic Substitute, Open Approach

03RU0KZ Replacement of Right Thyroid Artery with Nonautologous Tissue Substitute, Open Approach

03RU47Z Replacement of Right Thyroid Artery with Autologous Tissue Substitute, Percutaneous Endoscopic Approach

03RU4JZ Replacement of Right Thyroid Artery with Synthetic Substitute, Percutaneous Endoscopic Approach

03RU4KZ Replacement of Right Thyroid Artery with Nonautologous Tissue Substitute, Percutaneous Endoscopic Approach

03RV07Z Replacement of Left Thyroid Artery with Autologous Tissue Substitute, Open Approach

03RV0JZ Replacement of Left Thyroid Artery with Synthetic Substitute, Open Approach

03RV0KZ Replacement of Left Thyroid Artery with Nonautologous Tissue Substitute, Open Approach

03RV47Z Replacement of Left Thyroid Artery with Autologous Tissue Substitute, Percutaneous Endoscopic Approach

03RV4JZ Replacement of Left Thyroid Artery with Synthetic Substitute, Percutaneous Endoscopic Approach

03RV4KZ Replacement of Left Thyroid Artery with Nonautologous Tissue Substitute, Percutaneous Endoscopic Approach

03RY07Z Replacement of Upper Artery with Autologous Tissue Substitute, Open Approach

03RY0JZ Replacement of Upper Artery with Synthetic Substitute, Open Approach

03RY0KZ Replacement of Upper Artery with Nonautologous Tissue Substitute, Open Approach

03RY47Z Replacement of Upper Artery with Autologous Tissue Substitute, Percutaneous Endoscopic Approach

03RY4JZ Replacement of Upper Artery with Synthetic Substitute, Percutaneous Endoscopic Approach

03RY4KZ Replacement of Upper Artery with Nonautologous Tissue Substitute, Percutaneous Endoscopic Approach

03S – Upper Arteries, Reposition

03S00ZZ Reposition Right Internal Mammary Artery, Open Approach

03S03ZZ Reposition Right Internal Mammary Artery, Percutaneous Approach

03S04ZZ Reposition Right Internal Mammary Artery, Percutaneous Endoscopic Approach

03S10ZZ Reposition Left Internal Mammary Artery, Open Approach

03S13ZZ Reposition Left Internal Mammary Artery, Percutaneous Approach

03S14ZZ Reposition Left Internal Mammary Artery, Percutaneous Endoscopic Approach

03S20ZZ Reposition Innominate Artery, Open Approach

03S23ZZ Reposition Innominate Artery, Percutaneous Approach

03S24ZZ Reposition Innominate Artery, Percutaneous Endoscopic Approach

03S30ZZ Reposition Right Subclavian Artery, Open Approach

03S33ZZ Reposition Right Subclavian Artery, Percutaneous Approach

03S34ZZ Reposition Right Subclavian Artery, Percutaneous Endoscopic Approach

03S40ZZ Reposition Left Subclavian Artery, Open Approach

03S43ZZ Reposition Left Subclavian Artery, Percutaneous Approach

03S44ZZ Reposition Left Subclavian Artery, Percutaneous Endoscopic Approach

03S50ZZ Reposition Right Axillary Artery, Open Approach

03S53ZZ Reposition Right Axillary Artery, Percutaneous Approach

03S54ZZ Reposition Right Axillary Artery, Percutaneous Endoscopic Approach

03S60ZZ Reposition Left Axillary Artery, Open Approach

03S63ZZ Reposition Left Axillary Artery, Percutaneous Approach

03S64ZZ Reposition Left Axillary Artery, Percutaneous Endoscopic Approach

03S70ZZ Reposition Right Brachial Artery, Open Approach

03S73ZZ Reposition Right Brachial Artery, Percutaneous Approach

03S74ZZ Reposition Right Brachial Artery, Percutaneous Endoscopic Approach

03S80ZZ Reposition Left Brachial Artery, Open Approach

03S83ZZ Reposition Left Brachial Artery, Percutaneous Approach

03S84ZZ Reposition Left Brachial Artery, Percutaneous Endoscopic Approach

03S90ZZ Reposition Right Ulnar Artery, Open Approach

03S93ZZ Reposition Right Ulnar Artery, Percutaneous Approach

03S94ZZ Reposition Right Ulnar Artery, Percutaneous Endoscopic Approach

03SA0ZZ Reposition Left Ulnar Artery, Open Approach

03SA3ZZ Reposition Left Ulnar Artery, Percutaneous Approach

03SA4ZZ Reposition Left Ulnar Artery, Percutaneous Endoscopic Approach

03SB0ZZ Reposition Right Radial Artery, Open Approach

03SB3ZZ Reposition Right Radial Artery, Percutaneous Approach

03SB4ZZ Reposition Right Radial Artery, Percutaneous Endoscopic Approach

03SC0ZZ Reposition Left Radial Artery, Open Approach

03SC3ZZ Reposition Left Radial Artery, Percutaneous Approach

03SC4ZZ Reposition Left Radial Artery, Percutaneous Endoscopic Approach

03SD0ZZ Reposition Right Hand Artery, Open Approach

03SD3ZZ Reposition Right Hand Artery, Percutaneous Approach

03SD4ZZ Reposition Right Hand Artery, Percutaneous Endoscopic Approach

03SF0ZZ Reposition Left Hand Artery, Open Approach

03SF3ZZ Reposition Left Hand Artery, Percutaneous Approach

03SF4ZZ Reposition Left Hand Artery, Percutaneous Endoscopic Approach

03SG0ZZ Reposition Intracranial Artery, Open Approach

03SG3ZZ Reposition Intracranial Artery, Percutaneous Approach

03SG4ZZ Reposition Intracranial Artery, Percutaneous Endoscopic Approach

03SH0ZZ Reposition Right Common Carotid Artery, Open Approach

03SH3ZZ Reposition Right Common Carotid Artery, Percutaneous Approach

03SH4ZZ Reposition Right Common Carotid Artery, Percutaneous Endoscopic Approach

03SJ0ZZ Reposition Left Common Carotid Artery, Open Approach

03SJ3ZZ Reposition Left Common Carotid Artery, Percutaneous Approach

03SJ4ZZ Reposition Left Common Carotid Artery, Percutaneous Endoscopic Approach

03SK0ZZ Reposition Right Internal Carotid Artery, Open Approach

03SK3ZZ Reposition Right Internal Carotid Artery, Percutaneous Approach

03SK4ZZ Reposition Right Internal Carotid Artery, Percutaneous Endoscopic Approach

03SL0ZZ Reposition Left Internal Carotid Artery, Open Approach

03SL3ZZ Reposition Left Internal Carotid Artery, Percutaneous Approach

03SL4ZZ Reposition Left Internal Carotid Artery, Percutaneous Endoscopic Approach

03SM0ZZ Reposition Right External Carotid Artery, Open Approach

03SM3ZZ Reposition Right External Carotid Artery, Percutaneous Approach

03SM4ZZ Reposition Right External Carotid Artery, Percutaneous Endoscopic Approach

03SN0ZZ	Reposition Left External Carotid Artery, Open Approach
03SN3ZZ	Reposition Left External Carotid Artery, Percutaneous Approach
03SN4ZZ	Reposition Left External Carotid Artery, Percutaneous Endoscopic Approach
03SP0ZZ	Reposition Right Vertebral Artery, Open Approach
03SP3ZZ	Reposition Right Vertebral Artery, Percutaneous Approach
03SP4ZZ	Reposition Right Vertebral Artery, Percutaneous Endoscopic Approach
03SQ0ZZ	Reposition Left Vertebral Artery, Open Approach
03SQ3ZZ	Reposition Left Vertebral Artery, Percutaneous Approach
03SQ4ZZ	Reposition Left Vertebral Artery, Percutaneous Endoscopic Approach

03SR0ZZ	Reposition Face Artery, Open Approach
03SR3ZZ	Reposition Face Artery, Percutaneous Approach
03SR4ZZ	Reposition Face Artery, Percutaneous Endoscopic Approach
03SS0ZZ	Reposition Right Temporal Artery, Open Approach
	AHA CC: 3Q, 2015, 27-28
03SS3ZZ	Reposition Right Temporal Artery, Percutaneous Approach
03SS4ZZ	Reposition Right Temporal Artery, Percutaneous Endoscopic Approach
03ST0ZZ	Reposition Left Temporal Artery, Open Approach
03ST3ZZ	Reposition Left Temporal Artery, Percutaneous Approach
03ST4ZZ	Reposition Left Temporal Artery, Percutaneous Endoscopic Approach

03SU0ZZ	Reposition Right Thyroid Artery, Open Approach
03SU3ZZ	Reposition Right Thyroid Artery, Percutaneous Approach
03SU4ZZ	Reposition Right Thyroid Artery, Percutaneous Endoscopic Approach
03SV0ZZ	Reposition Left Thyroid Artery, Open Approach
03SV3ZZ	Reposition Left Thyroid Artery, Percutaneous Approach
03SV4ZZ	Reposition Left Thyroid Artery, Percutaneous Endoscopic Approach
03SY0ZZ	Reposition Upper Artery, Open Approach
03SY3ZZ	Reposition Upper Artery, Percutaneous Approach
03SY4ZZ	Reposition Upper Artery, Percutaneous Endoscopic Approach

03U – Upper Arteries, Supplement

03U007Z	Supplement Right Internal Mammary Artery with Autologous Tissue Substitute, Open Approach
03U00JZ	Supplement Right Internal Mammary Artery with Synthetic Substitute, Open Approach
03U00KZ	Supplement Right Internal Mammary Artery with Nonautologous Tissue Substitute, Open Approach
03U037Z	Supplement Right Internal Mammary Artery with Autologous Tissue Substitute, Percutaneous Approach
03U03JZ	Supplement Right Internal Mammary Artery with Synthetic Substitute, Percutaneous Approach
03U03KZ	Supplement Right Internal Mammary Artery with Nonautologous Tissue Substitute, Percutaneous Approach
03U047Z	Supplement Right Internal Mammary Artery with Autologous Tissue Substitute, Percutaneous Endoscopic Approach
03U04JZ	Supplement Right Internal Mammary Artery with Synthetic Substitute, Percutaneous Endoscopic Approach
03U04KZ	Supplement Right Internal Mammary Artery with Nonautologous Tissue Substitute, Percutaneous Endoscopic Approach
03U107Z	Supplement Left Internal Mammary Artery with Autologous Tissue Substitute, Open Approach
03U10JZ	Supplement Left Internal Mammary Artery with Synthetic Substitute, Open Approach
03U10KZ	Supplement Left Internal Mammary Artery with Nonautologous Tissue Substitute, Open Approach
03U137Z	Supplement Left Internal Mammary Artery with Autologous Tissue Substitute, Percutaneous Approach
03U13JZ	Supplement Left Internal Mammary Artery with Synthetic Substitute, Percutaneous Approach
03U13KZ	Supplement Left Internal Mammary Artery with Nonautologous Tissue Substitute, Percutaneous Approach
03U147Z	Supplement Left Internal Mammary Artery with Autologous Tissue Substitute, Percutaneous Endoscopic Approach
03U14JZ	Supplement Left Internal Mammary Artery with Synthetic Substitute, Percutaneous Endoscopic Approach

03U14KZ	Supplement Left Internal Mammary Artery with Nonautologous Tissue Substitute, Percutaneous Endoscopic Approach
03U207Z	Supplement Innominate Artery with Autologous Tissue Substitute, Open Approach
03U20JZ	Supplement Innominate Artery with Synthetic Substitute, Open Approach
03U20KZ	Supplement Innominate Artery with Nonautologous Tissue Substitute, Open Approach
03U237Z	Supplement Innominate Artery with Autologous Tissue Substitute, Percutaneous Approach
03U23JZ	Supplement Innominate Artery with Synthetic Substitute, Percutaneous Approach
03U23KZ	Supplement Innominate Artery with Nonautologous Tissue Substitute, Percutaneous Approach
03U247Z	Supplement Innominate Artery with Autologous Tissue Substitute, Percutaneous Endoscopic Approach
03U24JZ	Supplement Innominate Artery with Synthetic Substitute, Percutaneous Endoscopic Approach
03U24KZ	Supplement Innominate Artery with Nonautologous Tissue Substitute, Percutaneous Endoscopic Approach
03U307Z	Supplement Right Subclavian Artery with Autologous Tissue Substitute, Open Approach
03U30JZ	Supplement Right Subclavian Artery with Synthetic Substitute, Open Approach
03U30KZ	Supplement Right Subclavian Artery with Nonautologous Tissue Substitute, Open Approach
03U337Z	Supplement Right Subclavian Artery with Autologous Tissue Substitute, Percutaneous Approach
03U33JZ	Supplement Right Subclavian Artery with Synthetic Substitute, Percutaneous Approach
03U33KZ	Supplement Right Subclavian Artery with Nonautologous Tissue Substitute, Percutaneous Approach
03U347Z	Supplement Right Subclavian Artery with Autologous Tissue Substitute, Percutaneous Endoscopic Approach
03U34JZ	Supplement Right Subclavian Artery with Synthetic Substitute, Percutaneous Endoscopic Approach

03U34KZ	Supplement Right Subclavian Artery with Nonautologous Tissue Substitute, Percutaneous Endoscopic Approach
03U407Z	Supplement Left Subclavian Artery with Autologous Tissue Substitute, Open Approach
03U40JZ	Supplement Left Subclavian Artery with Synthetic Substitute, Open Approach
03U40KZ	Supplement Left Subclavian Artery with Nonautologous Tissue Substitute, Open Approach
03U437Z	Supplement Left Subclavian Artery with Autologous Tissue Substitute, Percutaneous Approach
03U43JZ	Supplement Left Subclavian Artery with Synthetic Substitute, Percutaneous Approach
03U43KZ	Supplement Left Subclavian Artery with Nonautologous Tissue Substitute, Percutaneous Approach
03U447Z	Supplement Left Subclavian Artery with Autologous Tissue Substitute, Percutaneous Endoscopic Approach
03U44JZ	Supplement Left Subclavian Artery with Synthetic Substitute, Percutaneous Endoscopic Approach
03U44KZ	Supplement Left Subclavian Artery with Nonautologous Tissue Substitute, Percutaneous Endoscopic Approach
03U507Z	Supplement Right Axillary Artery with Autologous Tissue Substitute, Open Approach
03U50JZ	Supplement Right Axillary Artery with Synthetic Substitute, Open Approach
03U50KZ	Supplement Right Axillary Artery with Nonautologous Tissue Substitute, Open Approach
03U537Z	Supplement Right Axillary Artery with Autologous Tissue Substitute, Percutaneous Approach
03U53JZ	Supplement Right Axillary Artery with Synthetic Substitute, Percutaneous Approach
03U53KZ	Supplement Right Axillary Artery with Nonautologous Tissue Substitute, Percutaneous Approach
03U547Z	Supplement Right Axillary Artery with Autologous Tissue Substitute, Percutaneous Endoscopic Approach
03U54JZ	Supplement Right Axillary Artery with Synthetic Substitute, Percutaneous Endoscopic Approach

♀ Female-only   ♂ Male-only   ▲ Limited Coverage   ● Non-OR   ▉ HAC-associated procedure   ▲ Non-covered procedures   ✚ Cluster

03U54KZ Supplement Right Axillary Artery with Nonautologous Tissue Substitute, Percutaneous Endoscopic Approach

03U607Z Supplement Left Axillary Artery with Autologous Tissue Substitute, Open Approach

03U60JZ Supplement Left Axillary Artery with Synthetic Substitute, Open Approach

03U60KZ Supplement Left Axillary Artery with Nonautologous Tissue Substitute, Open Approach

03U637Z Supplement Left Axillary Artery with Autologous Tissue Substitute, Percutaneous Approach

03U63JZ Supplement Left Axillary Artery with Synthetic Substitute, Percutaneous Approach

03U63KZ Supplement Left Axillary Artery with Nonautologous Tissue Substitute, Percutaneous Approach

03U647Z Supplement Left Axillary Artery with Autologous Tissue Substitute, Percutaneous Endoscopic Approach

03U64JZ Supplement Left Axillary Artery with Synthetic Substitute, Percutaneous Endoscopic Approach

03U64KZ Supplement Left Axillary Artery with Nonautologous Tissue Substitute, Percutaneous Endoscopic Approach

03U707Z Supplement Right Brachial Artery with Autologous Tissue Substitute, Open Approach

03U70JZ Supplement Right Brachial Artery with Synthetic Substitute, Open Approach

03U70KZ Supplement Right Brachial Artery with Nonautologous Tissue Substitute, Open Approach

03U737Z Supplement Right Brachial Artery with Autologous Tissue Substitute, Percutaneous Approach

03U73JZ Supplement Right Brachial Artery with Synthetic Substitute, Percutaneous Approach

03U73KZ Supplement Right Brachial Artery with Nonautologous Tissue Substitute, Percutaneous Approach

03U747Z Supplement Right Brachial Artery with Autologous Tissue Substitute, Percutaneous Endoscopic Approach

03U74JZ Supplement Right Brachial Artery with Synthetic Substitute, Percutaneous Endoscopic Approach

03U74KZ Supplement Right Brachial Artery with Nonautologous Tissue Substitute, Percutaneous Endoscopic Approach

03U807Z Supplement Left Brachial Artery with Autologous Tissue Substitute, Open Approach

03U80JZ Supplement Left Brachial Artery with Synthetic Substitute, Open Approach

03U80KZ Supplement Left Brachial Artery with Nonautologous Tissue Substitute, Open Approach

03U837Z Supplement Left Brachial Artery with Autologous Tissue Substitute, Percutaneous Approach

03U83JZ Supplement Left Brachial Artery with Synthetic Substitute, Percutaneous Approach

03U83KZ Supplement Left Brachial Artery with Nonautologous Tissue Substitute, Percutaneous Approach

03U847Z Supplement Left Brachial Artery with Autologous Tissue Substitute, Percutaneous Endoscopic Approach

03U84JZ Supplement Left Brachial Artery with Synthetic Substitute, Percutaneous Endoscopic Approach

03U84KZ Supplement Left Brachial Artery with Nonautologous Tissue Substitute, Percutaneous Endoscopic Approach

03U907Z Supplement Right Ulnar Artery with Autologous Tissue Substitute, Open Approach

03U90JZ Supplement Right Ulnar Artery with Synthetic Substitute, Open Approach

03U90KZ Supplement Right Ulnar Artery with Nonautologous Tissue Substitute, Open Approach

03U937Z Supplement Right Ulnar Artery with Autologous Tissue Substitute, Percutaneous Approach

03U93JZ Supplement Right Ulnar Artery with Synthetic Substitute, Percutaneous Approach

03U93KZ Supplement Right Ulnar Artery with Nonautologous Tissue Substitute, Percutaneous Approach

03U947Z Supplement Right Ulnar Artery with Autologous Tissue Substitute, Percutaneous Endoscopic Approach

03U94JZ Supplement Right Ulnar Artery with Synthetic Substitute, Percutaneous Endoscopic Approach

03U94KZ Supplement Right Ulnar Artery with Nonautologous Tissue Substitute, Percutaneous Endoscopic Approach

03UA07Z Supplement Left Ulnar Artery with Autologous Tissue Substitute, Open Approach

03UA0JZ Supplement Left Ulnar Artery with Synthetic Substitute, Open Approach

03UA0KZ Supplement Left Ulnar Artery with Nonautologous Tissue Substitute, Open Approach

03UA37Z Supplement Left Ulnar Artery with Autologous Tissue Substitute, Percutaneous Approach

03UA3JZ Supplement Left Ulnar Artery with Synthetic Substitute, Percutaneous Approach

03UA3KZ Supplement Left Ulnar Artery with Nonautologous Tissue Substitute, Percutaneous Approach

03UA47Z Supplement Left Ulnar Artery with Autologous Tissue Substitute, Percutaneous Endoscopic Approach

03UA4JZ Supplement Left Ulnar Artery with Synthetic Substitute, Percutaneous Endoscopic Approach

03UA4KZ Supplement Left Ulnar Artery with Nonautologous Tissue Substitute, Percutaneous Endoscopic Approach

03UB07Z Supplement Right Radial Artery with Autologous Tissue Substitute, Open Approach

03UB0JZ Supplement Right Radial Artery with Synthetic Substitute, Open Approach

03UB0KZ Supplement Right Radial Artery with Nonautologous Tissue Substitute, Open Approach

03UB37Z Supplement Right Radial Artery with Autologous Tissue Substitute, Percutaneous Approach

03UB3JZ Supplement Right Radial Artery with Synthetic Substitute, Percutaneous Approach

03UB3KZ Supplement Right Radial Artery with Nonautologous Tissue Substitute, Percutaneous Approach

03UB47Z Supplement Right Radial Artery with Autologous Tissue Substitute, Percutaneous Endoscopic Approach

03UB4JZ Supplement Right Radial Artery with Synthetic Substitute, Percutaneous Endoscopic Approach

03UB4KZ Supplement Right Radial Artery with Nonautologous Tissue Substitute, Percutaneous Endoscopic Approach

03UC07Z Supplement Left Radial Artery with Autologous Tissue Substitute, Open Approach

03UC0JZ Supplement Left Radial Artery with Synthetic Substitute, Open Approach

03UC0KZ Supplement Left Radial Artery with Nonautologous Tissue Substitute, Open Approach

03UC37Z Supplement Left Radial Artery with Autologous Tissue Substitute, Percutaneous Approach

03UC3JZ Supplement Left Radial Artery with Synthetic Substitute, Percutaneous Approach

03UC3KZ Supplement Left Radial Artery with Nonautologous Tissue Substitute, Percutaneous Approach

03UC47Z Supplement Left Radial Artery with Autologous Tissue Substitute, Percutaneous Endoscopic Approach

03UC4JZ Supplement Left Radial Artery with Synthetic Substitute, Percutaneous Endoscopic Approach

03UC4KZ Supplement Left Radial Artery with Nonautologous Tissue Substitute, Percutaneous Endoscopic Approach

03UD07Z Supplement Right Hand Artery with Autologous Tissue Substitute, Open Approach

03UD0JZ Supplement Right Hand Artery with Synthetic Substitute, Open Approach

03UD0KZ Supplement Right Hand Artery with Nonautologous Tissue Substitute, Open Approach

03UD37Z Supplement Right Hand Artery with Autologous Tissue Substitute, Percutaneous Approach

03UD3JZ Supplement Right Hand Artery with Synthetic Substitute, Percutaneous Approach

03UD3KZ Supplement Right Hand Artery with Nonautologous Tissue Substitute, Percutaneous Approach

03UD47Z Supplement Right Hand Artery with Autologous Tissue Substitute, Percutaneous Endoscopic Approach

03UD4JZ Supplement Right Hand Artery with Synthetic Substitute, Percutaneous Endoscopic Approach

03UD4KZ Supplement Right Hand Artery with Nonautologous Tissue Substitute, Percutaneous Endoscopic Approach

03UF07Z Supplement Left Hand Artery with Autologous Tissue Substitute, Open Approach

03UF0JZ Supplement Left Hand Artery with Synthetic Substitute, Open Approach

03UF0KZ Supplement Left Hand Artery with Nonautologous Tissue Substitute, Open Approach

03UF37Z Supplement Left Hand Artery with Autologous Tissue Substitute, Percutaneous Approach

03UF3JZ Supplement Left Hand Artery with Synthetic Substitute, Percutaneous Approach

03UF3KZ Supplement Left Hand Artery with Nonautologous Tissue Substitute, Percutaneous Approach

03UF47Z Supplement Left Hand Artery with Autologous Tissue Substitute, Percutaneous Endoscopic Approach

03UF4JZ Supplement Left Hand Artery with Synthetic Substitute, Percutaneous Endoscopic Approach

03UF4KZ Supplement Left Hand Artery with Nonautologous Tissue Substitute, Percutaneous Endoscopic Approach

03UG07Z Supplement Intracranial Artery with Autologous Tissue Substitute, Open Approach

03UG0JZ Supplement Intracranial Artery with Synthetic Substitute, Open Approach

03UG0KZ Supplement Intracranial Artery with Nonautologous Tissue Substitute, Open Approach

03UG37Z Supplement Intracranial Artery with Autologous Tissue Substitute, Percutaneous Approach

03UG3JZ Supplement Intracranial Artery with Synthetic Substitute, Percutaneous Approach

03UG3KZ Supplement Intracranial Artery with Nonautologous Tissue Substitute, Percutaneous Approach

03UG47Z Supplement Intracranial Artery with Autologous Tissue Substitute, Percutaneous Endoscopic Approach

03UG4JZ Supplement Intracranial Artery with Synthetic Substitute, Percutaneous Endoscopic Approach

03UG4KZ Supplement Intracranial Artery with Nonautologous Tissue Substitute, Percutaneous Endoscopic Approach

03UH07Z Supplement Right Common Carotid Artery with Autologous Tissue Substitute, Open Approach

03UH0JZ Supplement Right Common Carotid Artery with Synthetic Substitute, Open Approach

03UH0KZ Supplement Right Common Carotid Artery with Nonautologous Tissue Substitute, Open Approach

03UH37Z Supplement Right Common Carotid Artery with Autologous Tissue Substitute, Percutaneous Approach

03UH3JZ Supplement Right Common Carotid Artery with Synthetic Substitute, Percutaneous Approach

03UH3KZ Supplement Right Common Carotid Artery with Nonautologous Tissue Substitute, Percutaneous Approach

03UH47Z Supplement Right Common Carotid Artery with Autologous Tissue Substitute, Percutaneous Endoscopic Approach

03UH4JZ Supplement Right Common Carotid Artery with Synthetic Substitute, Percutaneous Endoscopic Approach

03UH4KZ Supplement Right Common Carotid Artery with Nonautologous Tissue Substitute, Percutaneous Endoscopic Approach

03UJ07Z Supplement Left Common Carotid Artery with Autologous Tissue Substitute, Open Approach

03UJ0JZ Supplement Left Common Carotid Artery with Synthetic Substitute, Open Approach

03UJ0KZ Supplement Left Common Carotid Artery with Nonautologous Tissue Substitute, Open Approach

03UJ37Z Supplement Left Common Carotid Artery with Autologous Tissue Substitute, Percutaneous Approach

03UJ3JZ Supplement Left Common Carotid Artery with Synthetic Substitute, Percutaneous Approach

03UJ3KZ Supplement Left Common Carotid Artery with Nonautologous Tissue Substitute, Percutaneous Approach

03UJ47Z Supplement Left Common Carotid Artery with Autologous Tissue Substitute, Percutaneous Endoscopic Approach

03UJ4JZ Supplement Left Common Carotid Artery with Synthetic Substitute, Percutaneous Endoscopic Approach

03UJ4KZ Supplement Left Common Carotid Artery with Nonautologous Tissue Substitute, Percutaneous Endoscopic Approach

03UK07Z Supplement Right Internal Carotid Artery with Autologous Tissue Substitute, Open Approach

03UK0JZ Supplement Right Internal Carotid Artery with Synthetic Substitute, Open Approach

AHA CC: 2Q, 2016, 11-12

03UK0KZ Supplement Right Internal Carotid Artery with Nonautologous Tissue Substitute, Open Approach

03UK37Z Supplement Right Internal Carotid Artery with Autologous Tissue Substitute, Percutaneous Approach

03UK3JZ Supplement Right Internal Carotid Artery with Synthetic Substitute, Percutaneous Approach

03UK3KZ Supplement Right Internal Carotid Artery with Nonautologous Tissue Substitute, Percutaneous Approach

03UK47Z Supplement Right Internal Carotid Artery with Autologous Tissue Substitute, Percutaneous Endoscopic Approach

03UK4JZ Supplement Right Internal Carotid Artery with Synthetic Substitute, Percutaneous Endoscopic Approach

03UK4KZ Supplement Right Internal Carotid Artery with Nonautologous Tissue Substitute, Percutaneous Endoscopic Approach

03UL07Z Supplement Left Internal Carotid Artery with Autologous Tissue Substitute, Open Approach

03UL0JZ Supplement Left Internal Carotid Artery with Synthetic Substitute, Open Approach

03UL0KZ Supplement Left Internal Carotid Artery with Nonautologous Tissue Substitute, Open Approach

03UL37Z Supplement Left Internal Carotid Artery with Autologous Tissue Substitute, Percutaneous Approach

03UL3JZ Supplement Left Internal Carotid Artery with Synthetic Substitute, Percutaneous Approach

03UL3KZ Supplement Left Internal Carotid Artery with Nonautologous Tissue Substitute, Percutaneous Approach

03UL47Z Supplement Left Internal Carotid Artery with Autologous Tissue Substitute, Percutaneous Endoscopic Approach

03UL4JZ Supplement Left Internal Carotid Artery with Synthetic Substitute, Percutaneous Endoscopic Approach

03UL4KZ Supplement Left Internal Carotid Artery with Nonautologous Tissue

Substitute, Percutaneous Endoscopic Approach

03UM07Z Supplement Right External Carotid Artery with Autologous Tissue Substitute, Open Approach

03UM0JZ Supplement Right External Carotid Artery with Synthetic Substitute, Open Approach

03UM0KZ Supplement Right External Carotid Artery with Nonautologous Tissue Substitute, Open Approach

03UM37Z Supplement Right External Carotid Artery with Autologous Tissue Substitute, Percutaneous Approach

03UM3JZ Supplement Right External Carotid Artery with Synthetic Substitute, Percutaneous Approach

03UM3KZ Supplement Right External Carotid Artery with Nonautologous Tissue Substitute, Percutaneous Approach

03UM47Z Supplement Right External Carotid Artery with Autologous Tissue Substitute, Percutaneous Endoscopic Approach

03UM4JZ Supplement Right External Carotid Artery with Synthetic Substitute, Percutaneous Endoscopic Approach

03UM4KZ Supplement Right External Carotid Artery with Nonautologous Tissue Substitute, Percutaneous Endoscopic Approach

03UN07Z Supplement Left External Carotid Artery with Autologous Tissue Substitute, Open Approach

03UN0JZ Supplement Left External Carotid Artery with Synthetic Substitute, Open Approach

03UN0KZ Supplement Left External Carotid Artery with Nonautologous Tissue Substitute, Open Approach

03UN37Z Supplement Left External Carotid Artery with Autologous Tissue Substitute, Percutaneous Approach

03UN3JZ Supplement Left External Carotid Artery with Synthetic Substitute, Percutaneous Approach

03UN3KZ Supplement Left External Carotid Artery with Nonautologous Tissue Substitute, Percutaneous Approach

03UN47Z Supplement Left External Carotid Artery with Autologous Tissue Substitute, Percutaneous Endoscopic Approach

03UN4JZ Supplement Left External Carotid Artery with Synthetic Substitute, Percutaneous Endoscopic Approach

03UN4KZ Supplement Left External Carotid Artery with Nonautologous Tissue Substitute, Percutaneous Endoscopic Approach

03UP07Z Supplement Right Vertebral Artery with Autologous Tissue Substitute, Open Approach

03UP0JZ Supplement Right Vertebral Artery with Synthetic Substitute, Open Approach

03UP0KZ Supplement Right Vertebral Artery with Nonautologous Tissue Substitute, Open Approach

03UP37Z Supplement Right Vertebral Artery with Autologous Tissue Substitute, Percutaneous Approach

03UP3JZ Supplement Right Vertebral Artery with Synthetic Substitute, Percutaneous Approach

03UP3KZ | Supplement Right Vertebral Artery with Nonautologous Tissue Substitute, Percutaneous Approach

03UP47Z | Supplement Right Vertebral Artery with Autologous Tissue Substitute, Percutaneous Endoscopic Approach

03UP4JZ | Supplement Right Vertebral Artery with Synthetic Substitute, Percutaneous Endoscopic Approach

03UP4KZ | Supplement Right Vertebral Artery with Nonautologous Tissue Substitute, Percutaneous Endoscopic Approach

03UQ07Z | Supplement Left Vertebral Artery with Autologous Tissue Substitute, Open Approach

03UQ0JZ | Supplement Left Vertebral Artery with Synthetic Substitute, Open Approach

03UQ0KZ | Supplement Left Vertebral Artery with Nonautologous Tissue Substitute, Open Approach

03UQ37Z | Supplement Left Vertebral Artery with Autologous Tissue Substitute, Percutaneous Approach

03UQ3JZ | Supplement Left Vertebral Artery with Synthetic Substitute, Percutaneous Approach

03UQ3KZ | Supplement Left Vertebral Artery with Nonautologous Tissue Substitute, Percutaneous Approach

03UQ47Z | Supplement Left Vertebral Artery with Autologous Tissue Substitute, Percutaneous Endoscopic Approach

03UQ4JZ | Supplement Left Vertebral Artery with Synthetic Substitute, Percutaneous Endoscopic Approach

03UQ4KZ | Supplement Left Vertebral Artery with Nonautologous Tissue Substitute, Percutaneous Endoscopic Approach

03UR07Z | Supplement Face Artery with Autologous Tissue Substitute, Open Approach

03UR0JZ | Supplement Face Artery with Synthetic Substitute, Open Approach

03UR0KZ | Supplement Face Artery with Nonautologous Tissue Substitute, Open Approach

03UR37Z | Supplement Face Artery with Autologous Tissue Substitute, Percutaneous Approach

03UR3JZ | Supplement Face Artery with Synthetic Substitute, Percutaneous Approach

03UR3KZ | Supplement Face Artery with Nonautologous Tissue Substitute, Percutaneous Approach

03UR47Z | Supplement Face Artery with Autologous Tissue Substitute, Percutaneous Endoscopic Approach

03UR4JZ | Supplement Face Artery with Synthetic Substitute, Percutaneous Endoscopic Approach

03UR4KZ | Supplement Face Artery with Nonautologous Tissue Substitute, Percutaneous Endoscopic Approach

03US07Z | Supplement Right Temporal Artery with Autologous Tissue Substitute, Open Approach

03US0JZ | Supplement Right Temporal Artery with Synthetic Substitute, Open Approach

03US0KZ | Supplement Right Temporal Artery with Nonautologous Tissue Substitute, Open Approach

03US37Z | Supplement Right Temporal Artery with Autologous Tissue Substitute, Percutaneous Approach

03US3JZ | Supplement Right Temporal Artery with Synthetic Substitute, Percutaneous Approach

03US3KZ | Supplement Right Temporal Artery with Nonautologous Tissue Substitute, Percutaneous Approach

03US47Z | Supplement Right Temporal Artery with Autologous Tissue Substitute, Percutaneous Endoscopic Approach

03US4JZ | Supplement Right Temporal Artery with Synthetic Substitute, Percutaneous Endoscopic Approach

03US4KZ | Supplement Right Temporal Artery with Nonautologous Tissue Substitute, Percutaneous Endoscopic Approach

03UT07Z | Supplement Left Temporal Artery with Autologous Tissue Substitute, Open Approach

03UT0JZ | Supplement Left Temporal Artery with Synthetic Substitute, Open Approach

03UT0KZ | Supplement Left Temporal Artery with Nonautologous Tissue Substitute, Open Approach

03UT37Z | Supplement Left Temporal Artery with Autologous Tissue Substitute, Percutaneous Approach

03UT3JZ | Supplement Left Temporal Artery with Synthetic Substitute, Percutaneous Approach

03UT3KZ | Supplement Left Temporal Artery with Nonautologous Tissue Substitute, Percutaneous Approach

03UT47Z | Supplement Left Temporal Artery with Autologous Tissue Substitute, Percutaneous Endoscopic Approach

03UT4JZ | Supplement Left Temporal Artery with Synthetic Substitute, Percutaneous Endoscopic Approach

03UT4KZ | Supplement Left Temporal Artery with Nonautologous Tissue Substitute, Percutaneous Endoscopic Approach

03UU07Z | Supplement Right Thyroid Artery with Autologous Tissue Substitute, Open Approach

03UU0JZ | Supplement Right Thyroid Artery with Synthetic Substitute, Open Approach

03UU0KZ | Supplement Right Thyroid Artery with Nonautologous Tissue Substitute, Open Approach

03UU37Z | Supplement Right Thyroid Artery with Autologous Tissue Substitute, Percutaneous Approach

03UU3JZ | Supplement Right Thyroid Artery with Synthetic Substitute, Percutaneous Approach

03UU3KZ | Supplement Right Thyroid Artery with Nonautologous Tissue Substitute, Percutaneous Approach

03UU47Z | Supplement Right Thyroid Artery with Autologous Tissue Substitute, Percutaneous Endoscopic Approach

03UU4JZ | Supplement Right Thyroid Artery with Synthetic Substitute, Percutaneous Endoscopic Approach

03UU4KZ | Supplement Right Thyroid Artery with Nonautologous Tissue Substitute, Percutaneous Endoscopic Approach

03UV07Z | Supplement Left Thyroid Artery with Autologous Tissue Substitute, Open Approach

03UV0JZ | Supplement Left Thyroid Artery with Synthetic Substitute, Open Approach

03UV0KZ | Supplement Left Thyroid Artery with Nonautologous Tissue Substitute, Open Approach

03UV37Z | Supplement Left Thyroid Artery with Autologous Tissue Substitute, Percutaneous Approach

03UV3JZ | Supplement Left Thyroid Artery with Synthetic Substitute, Percutaneous Approach

03UV3KZ | Supplement Left Thyroid Artery with Nonautologous Tissue Substitute, Percutaneous Approach

03UV47Z | Supplement Left Thyroid Artery with Autologous Tissue Substitute, Percutaneous Endoscopic Approach

03UV4JZ | Supplement Left Thyroid Artery with Synthetic Substitute, Percutaneous Endoscopic Approach

03UV4KZ | Supplement Left Thyroid Artery with Nonautologous Tissue Substitute, Percutaneous Endoscopic Approach

03UY07Z | Supplement Upper Artery with Autologous Tissue Substitute, Open Approach

03UY0JZ | Supplement Upper Artery with Synthetic Substitute, Open Approach

03UY0KZ | Supplement Upper Artery with Nonautologous Tissue Substitute, Open Approach

03UY37Z | Supplement Upper Artery with Autologous Tissue Substitute, Percutaneous Approach

03UY3JZ | Supplement Upper Artery with Synthetic Substitute, Percutaneous Approach

03UY3KZ | Supplement Upper Artery with Nonautologous Tissue Substitute, Percutaneous Approach

03UY47Z | Supplement Upper Artery with Autologous Tissue Substitute, Percutaneous Endoscopic Approach

03UY4JZ | Supplement Upper Artery with Synthetic Substitute, Percutaneous Endoscopic Approach

03UY4KZ | Supplement Upper Artery with Nonautologous Tissue Substitute, Percutaneous Endoscopic Approach

03V – Upper Arteries, Restriction

Review Coding Guideline B3.12

03V00CZ | Restriction of Right Internal Mammary Artery with Extraluminal Device, Open Approach

03V00DZ | Restriction of Right Internal Mammary Artery with Intraluminal Device, Open Approach

03V00ZZ | Restriction of Right Internal Mammary Artery, Open Approach

03V03CZ | Restriction of Right Internal Mammary Artery with Extraluminal Device, Percutaneous Approach

03V03DZ | Restriction of Right Internal Mammary Artery with Intraluminal Device, Percutaneous Approach

03V03ZZ | Restriction of Right Internal Mammary Artery, Percutaneous Approach

♀ Female-only   ♂ Male-only   ▲ Limited Coverage   ● Non-OR   ▥ HAC HAC-associated procedure   ▲ Non-covered procedures   ✚ Cluster   283

Medical and Surgical, Upper Arteries Code Listings

03V04CZ Restriction of Right Internal Mammary Artery with Extraluminal Device, Percutaneous Endoscopic Approach

03V04DZ Restriction of Right Internal Mammary Artery with Intraluminal Device, Percutaneous Endoscopic Approach

03V04ZZ Restriction of Right Internal Mammary Artery, Percutaneous Endoscopic Approach

03V10CZ Restriction of Left Internal Mammary Artery with Extraluminal Device, Open Approach

03V10DZ Restriction of Left Internal Mammary Artery with Intraluminal Device, Open Approach

03V10ZZ Restriction of Left Internal Mammary Artery, Open Approach

03V13CZ Restriction of Left Internal Mammary Artery with Extraluminal Device, Percutaneous Approach

03V13DZ Restriction of Left Internal Mammary Artery with Intraluminal Device, Percutaneous Approach

03V13ZZ Restriction of Left Internal Mammary Artery, Percutaneous Approach

03V14CZ Restriction of Left Internal Mammary Artery with Extraluminal Device, Percutaneous Endoscopic Approach

03V14DZ Restriction of Left Internal Mammary Artery with Intraluminal Device, Percutaneous Endoscopic Approach

03V14ZZ Restriction of Left Internal Mammary Artery, Percutaneous Endoscopic Approach

03V20CZ Restriction of Innominate Artery with Extraluminal Device, Open Approach

03V20DZ Restriction of Innominate Artery with Intraluminal Device, Open Approach

03V20ZZ Restriction of Innominate Artery, Open Approach

03V23CZ Restriction of Innominate Artery with Extraluminal Device, Percutaneous Approach

03V23DZ Restriction of Innominate Artery with Intraluminal Device, Percutaneous Approach

03V23ZZ Restriction of Innominate Artery, Percutaneous Approach

03V24CZ Restriction of Innominate Artery with Extraluminal Device, Percutaneous Endoscopic Approach

03V24DZ Restriction of Innominate Artery with Intraluminal Device, Percutaneous Endoscopic Approach

03V24ZZ Restriction of Innominate Artery, Percutaneous Endoscopic Approach

03V30CZ Restriction of Right Subclavian Artery with Extraluminal Device, Open Approach

03V30DZ Restriction of Right Subclavian Artery with Intraluminal Device, Open Approach

03V30ZZ Restriction of Right Subclavian Artery, Open Approach

03V33CZ Restriction of Right Subclavian Artery with Extraluminal Device, Percutaneous Approach

03V33DZ Restriction of Right Subclavian Artery with Intraluminal Device, Percutaneous Approach

03V33ZZ Restriction of Right Subclavian Artery, Percutaneous Approach

03V34CZ Restriction of Right Subclavian Artery with Extraluminal Device, Percutaneous Endoscopic Approach

03V34DZ Restriction of Right Subclavian Artery with Intraluminal Device, Percutaneous Endoscopic Approach

03V34ZZ Restriction of Right Subclavian Artery, Percutaneous Endoscopic Approach

03V40CZ Restriction of Left Subclavian Artery with Extraluminal Device, Open Approach

03V40DZ Restriction of Left Subclavian Artery with Intraluminal Device, Open Approach

03V40ZZ Restriction of Left Subclavian Artery, Open Approach

03V43CZ Restriction of Left Subclavian Artery with Extraluminal Device, Percutaneous Approach

03V43DZ Restriction of Left Subclavian Artery with Intraluminal Device, Percutaneous Approach

03V43ZZ Restriction of Left Subclavian Artery, Percutaneous Approach

03V44CZ Restriction of Left Subclavian Artery with Extraluminal Device, Percutaneous Endoscopic Approach

03V44DZ Restriction of Left Subclavian Artery with Intraluminal Device, Percutaneous Endoscopic Approach

03V44ZZ Restriction of Left Subclavian Artery, Percutaneous Endoscopic Approach

03V50CZ Restriction of Right Axillary Artery with Extraluminal Device, Open Approach

03V50DZ Restriction of Right Axillary Artery with Intraluminal Device, Open Approach

03V50ZZ Restriction of Right Axillary Artery, Open Approach

03V53CZ Restriction of Right Axillary Artery with Extraluminal Device, Percutaneous Approach

03V53DZ Restriction of Right Axillary Artery with Intraluminal Device, Percutaneous Approach

03V53ZZ Restriction of Right Axillary Artery, Percutaneous Approach

03V54CZ Restriction of Right Axillary Artery with Extraluminal Device, Percutaneous Endoscopic Approach

03V54DZ Restriction of Right Axillary Artery with Intraluminal Device, Percutaneous Endoscopic Approach

03V54ZZ Restriction of Right Axillary Artery, Percutaneous Endoscopic Approach

03V60CZ Restriction of Left Axillary Artery with Extraluminal Device, Open Approach

03V60DZ Restriction of Left Axillary Artery with Intraluminal Device, Open Approach

03V60ZZ Restriction of Left Axillary Artery, Open Approach

03V63CZ Restriction of Left Axillary Artery with Extraluminal Device, Percutaneous Approach

03V63DZ Restriction of Left Axillary Artery with Intraluminal Device, Percutaneous Approach

03V63ZZ Restriction of Left Axillary Artery, Percutaneous Approach

03V64CZ Restriction of Left Axillary Artery with Extraluminal Device, Percutaneous Endoscopic Approach

03V64DZ Restriction of Left Axillary Artery with Intraluminal Device, Percutaneous Endoscopic Approach

03V64ZZ Restriction of Left Axillary Artery, Percutaneous Endoscopic Approach

03V70CZ Restriction of Right Brachial Artery with Extraluminal Device, Open Approach

03V70DZ Restriction of Right Brachial Artery with Intraluminal Device, Open Approach

03V70ZZ Restriction of Right Brachial Artery, Open Approach

03V73CZ Restriction of Right Brachial Artery with Extraluminal Device, Percutaneous Approach

03V73DZ Restriction of Right Brachial Artery with Intraluminal Device, Percutaneous Approach

03V73ZZ Restriction of Right Brachial Artery, Percutaneous Approach

03V74CZ Restriction of Right Brachial Artery with Extraluminal Device, Percutaneous Endoscopic Approach

03V74DZ Restriction of Right Brachial Artery with Intraluminal Device, Percutaneous Endoscopic Approach

03V74ZZ Restriction of Right Brachial Artery, Percutaneous Endoscopic Approach

03V80CZ Restriction of Left Brachial Artery with Extraluminal Device, Open Approach

03V80DZ Restriction of Left Brachial Artery with Intraluminal Device, Open Approach

03V80ZZ Restriction of Left Brachial Artery, Open Approach

03V83CZ Restriction of Left Brachial Artery with Extraluminal Device, Percutaneous Approach

03V83DZ Restriction of Left Brachial Artery with Intraluminal Device, Percutaneous Approach

03V83ZZ Restriction of Left Brachial Artery, Percutaneous Approach

03V84CZ Restriction of Left Brachial Artery with Extraluminal Device, Percutaneous Endoscopic Approach

03V84DZ Restriction of Left Brachial Artery with Intraluminal Device, Percutaneous Endoscopic Approach

03V84ZZ Restriction of Left Brachial Artery, Percutaneous Endoscopic Approach

03V90CZ Restriction of Right Ulnar Artery with Extraluminal Device, Open Approach

03V90DZ Restriction of Right Ulnar Artery with Intraluminal Device, Open Approach

03V90ZZ Restriction of Right Ulnar Artery, Open Approach

03V93CZ Restriction of Right Ulnar Artery with Extraluminal Device, Percutaneous Approach

03V93DZ Restriction of Right Ulnar Artery with Intraluminal Device, Percutaneous Approach

03V93ZZ Restriction of Right Ulnar Artery, Percutaneous Approach

03V94CZ Restriction of Right Ulnar Artery with Extraluminal Device, Percutaneous Endoscopic Approach

03V94DZ Restriction of Right Ulnar Artery with Intraluminal Device, Percutaneous Endoscopic Approach

03V94ZZ Restriction of Right Ulnar Artery, Percutaneous Endoscopic Approach

♀ Female-only   ♂ Male-only   ▲ Limited Coverage   ● Non-OR   HAC HAC-associated procedure   ▲ Non-covered procedures   ✚ Cluster

03VA0CZ Restriction of Left Ulnar Artery with Extraluminal Device, Open Approach

03VA0DZ Restriction of Left Ulnar Artery with Intraluminal Device, Open Approach

03VA0ZZ Restriction of Left Ulnar Artery, Open Approach

03VA3CZ Restriction of Left Ulnar Artery with Extraluminal Device, Percutaneous Approach

03VA3DZ Restriction of Left Ulnar Artery with Intraluminal Device, Percutaneous Approach

03VA3ZZ Restriction of Left Ulnar Artery, Percutaneous Approach

03VA4CZ Restriction of Left Ulnar Artery with Extraluminal Device, Percutaneous Endoscopic Approach

03VA4DZ Restriction of Left Ulnar Artery with Intraluminal Device, Percutaneous Endoscopic Approach

03VA4ZZ Restriction of Left Ulnar Artery, Percutaneous Endoscopic Approach

03VB0CZ Restriction of Right Radial Artery with Extraluminal Device, Open Approach

03VB0DZ Restriction of Right Radial Artery with Intraluminal Device, Open Approach

03VB0ZZ Restriction of Right Radial Artery, Open Approach

03VB3CZ Restriction of Right Radial Artery with Extraluminal Device, Percutaneous Approach

03VB3DZ Restriction of Right Radial Artery with Intraluminal Device, Percutaneous Approach

03VB3ZZ Restriction of Right Radial Artery, Percutaneous Approach

03VB4CZ Restriction of Right Radial Artery with Extraluminal Device, Percutaneous Endoscopic Approach

03VB4DZ Restriction of Right Radial Artery with Intraluminal Device, Percutaneous Endoscopic Approach

03VB4ZZ Restriction of Right Radial Artery, Percutaneous Endoscopic Approach

03VC0CZ Restriction of Left Radial Artery with Extraluminal Device, Open Approach

03VC0DZ Restriction of Left Radial Artery with Intraluminal Device, Open Approach

03VC0ZZ Restriction of Left Radial Artery, Open Approach

03VC3CZ Restriction of Left Radial Artery with Extraluminal Device, Percutaneous Approach

03VC3DZ Restriction of Left Radial Artery with Intraluminal Device, Percutaneous Approach

03VC3ZZ Restriction of Left Radial Artery, Percutaneous Approach

03VC4CZ Restriction of Left Radial Artery with Extraluminal Device, Percutaneous Endoscopic Approach

03VC4DZ Restriction of Left Radial Artery with Intraluminal Device, Percutaneous Endoscopic Approach

03VC4ZZ Restriction of Left Radial Artery, Percutaneous Endoscopic Approach

03VD0CZ Restriction of Right Hand Artery with Extraluminal Device, Open Approach

03VD0DZ Restriction of Right Hand Artery with Intraluminal Device, Open Approach

03VD0ZZ Restriction of Right Hand Artery, Open Approach

03VD3CZ Restriction of Right Hand Artery with Extraluminal Device, Percutaneous Approach

03VD3DZ Restriction of Right Hand Artery with Intraluminal Device, Percutaneous Approach

03VD3ZZ Restriction of Right Hand Artery, Percutaneous Approach

03VD4CZ Restriction of Right Hand Artery with Extraluminal Device, Percutaneous Endoscopic Approach

03VD4DZ Restriction of Right Hand Artery with Intraluminal Device, Percutaneous Endoscopic Approach

03VD4ZZ Restriction of Right Hand Artery, Percutaneous Endoscopic Approach

03VF0CZ Restriction of Left Hand Artery with Extraluminal Device, Open Approach

03VF0DZ Restriction of Left Hand Artery with Intraluminal Device, Open Approach

03VF0ZZ Restriction of Left Hand Artery, Open Approach

03VF3CZ Restriction of Left Hand Artery with Extraluminal Device, Percutaneous Approach

03VF3DZ Restriction of Left Hand Artery with Intraluminal Device, Percutaneous Approach

03VF3ZZ Restriction of Left Hand Artery, Percutaneous Approach

03VF4CZ Restriction of Left Hand Artery with Extraluminal Device, Percutaneous Endoscopic Approach

03VF4DZ Restriction of Left Hand Artery with Intraluminal Device, Percutaneous Endoscopic Approach

03VF4ZZ Restriction of Left Hand Artery, Percutaneous Endoscopic Approach

03VG0BZ Restriction of Intracranial Artery with Bioactive Intraluminal Device, Open Approach

03VG0CZ Restriction of Intracranial Artery with Extraluminal Device, Open Approach
AHA CC: 1Q, 2019, 22

03VG0DZ Restriction of Intracranial Artery with Intraluminal Device, Open Approach

03VG0HZ Restriction of Intracranial Artery with Intraluminal Device, Flow Diverter, Open Approach

03VG0ZZ Restriction of Intracranial Artery, Open Approach

03VG0HZ Restriction of Intracranial Artery with Intraluminal Device, Flow Diverter, Open Approach

03VG3BZ Restriction of Intracranial Artery with Bioactive Intraluminal Device, Percutaneous Approach

03VG3CZ Restriction of Intracranial Artery with Extraluminal Device, Percutaneous Approach

03VG3DZ Restriction of Intracranial Artery with Intraluminal Device, Percutaneous Approach
AHA CC: 1Q, 2016, 19-20

03VG3HZ Restriction of Intracranial Artery with Intraluminal Device, Flow Diverter, Percutaneous Approach

03VG3ZZ Restriction of Intracranial Artery, Percutaneous Approach

03VG4BZ Restriction of Intracranial Artery with Bioactive Intraluminal Device, Percutaneous Endoscopic Approach

03VG4CZ Restriction of Intracranial Artery with Extraluminal Device, Percutaneous Endoscopic Approach

03VG4DZ Restriction of Intracranial Artery with Intraluminal Device, Percutaneous Endoscopic Approach

03VG4HZ Restriction of Intracranial Artery with Intraluminal Device, Flow Diverter, Percutaneous Endoscopic Approach

03VG4ZZ Restriction of Intracranial Artery, Percutaneous Endoscopic Approach

03VH0BZ Restriction of Right Common Carotid Artery with Bioactive Intraluminal Device, Open Approach

03VH0CZ Restriction of Right Common Carotid Artery with Extraluminal Device, Open Approach

03VH0DZ Restriction of Right Common Carotid Artery with Intraluminal Device, Open Approach

03VH0HZ Restriction of Right Common Carotid Artery with Intraluminal Device, Flow Diverter, Open Approach

03VH0ZZ Restriction of Right Common Carotid Artery, Open Approach

03VH3BZ Restriction of Right Common Carotid Artery with Bioactive Intraluminal Device, Percutaneous Approach

03VH3CZ Restriction of Right Common Carotid Artery with Extraluminal Device, Percutaneous Approach

03VH3DZ Restriction of Right Common Carotid Artery with Intraluminal Device, Percutaneous Approach

03VH3HZ Restriction of Right Common Carotid Artery with Intraluminal Device, Flow Diverter, Percutaneous Approach

03VH3ZZ Restriction of Right Common Carotid Artery, Percutaneous Approach

03VH4BZ Restriction of Right Common Carotid Artery with Bioactive Intraluminal Device, Percutaneous Endoscopic Approach

03VH4CZ Restriction of Right Common Carotid Artery with Extraluminal Device, Percutaneous Endoscopic Approach

03VH4DZ Restriction of Right Common Carotid Artery with Intraluminal Device, Percutaneous Endoscopic Approach

03VH4HZ Restriction of Right Common Carotid Artery with Intraluminal Device, Flow Diverter, Percutaneous Endoscopic Approach

03VH4ZZ Restriction of Right Common Carotid Artery, Percutaneous Endoscopic Approach

03VJ0BZ Restriction of Left Common Carotid Artery with Bioactive Intraluminal Device, Open Approach

03VJ0CZ Restriction of Left Common Carotid Artery with Extraluminal Device, Open Approach

03VJ0DZ Restriction of Left Common Carotid Artery with Intraluminal Device, Open Approach

03VJ0HZ Restriction of Left Common Carotid Artery with Intraluminal Device, Flow Diverter, Open Approach

03VJ0ZZ Restriction of Left Common Carotid Artery, Open Approach

03VJ3BZ Restriction of Left Common Carotid Artery with Bioactive Intraluminal Device, Percutaneous Approach

03VJ3CZ Restriction of Left Common Carotid Artery with Extraluminal Device, Percutaneous Approach

03VJ3DZ Restriction of Left Common Carotid Artery with Intraluminal Device, Percutaneous Approach

♀ Female-only   ♂ Male-only   ▲ Limited Coverage   ● Non-OR   **HAC** HAC-associated procedure   ▲ Non-covered procedures   ✚ Cluster

03VJ3HZ Restriction of Left Common Carotid Artery with Intraluminal Device, Flow Diverter, Percutaneous Approach

03VJ3ZZ Restriction of Left Common Carotid Artery, Percutaneous Approach

03VJ4BZ Restriction of Left Common Carotid Artery with Bioactive Intraluminal Device, Percutaneous Endoscopic Approach

03VJ4CZ Restriction of Left Common Carotid Artery with Extraluminal Device, Percutaneous Endoscopic Approach

03VJ4DZ Restriction of Left Common Carotid Artery with Intraluminal Device, Percutaneous Endoscopic Approach

03VJ4HZ Restriction of Left Common Carotid Artery with Intraluminal Device, Flow Diverter, Percutaneous Endoscopic Approach

03VJ4ZZ Restriction of Left Common Carotid Artery, Percutaneous Endoscopic Approach

03VK0BZ Restriction of Right Internal Carotid Artery with Bioactive Intraluminal Device, Open Approach

03VK0CZ Restriction of Right Internal Carotid Artery with Extraluminal Device, Open Approach

03VK0DZ Restriction of Right Internal Carotid Artery with Intraluminal Device, Open Approach

03VK0HZ Restriction of Right Internal Carotid Artery with Intraluminal Device, Flow Diverter, Open Approach

03VK0ZZ Restriction of Right Internal Carotid Artery, Open Approach

03VK3BZ Restriction of Right Internal Carotid Artery with Bioactive Intraluminal Device, Percutaneous Approach

03VK3CZ Restriction of Right Internal Carotid Artery with Extraluminal Device, Percutaneous Approach

03VK3DZ Restriction of Right Internal Carotid Artery with Intraluminal Device, Percutaneous Approach

03VK3HZ Restriction of Right Internal Carotid Artery with Intraluminal Device, Flow Diverter, Percutaneous Approach

03VK3ZZ Restriction of Right Internal Carotid Artery, Percutaneous Approach

03VK4BZ Restriction of Right Internal Carotid Artery with Bioactive Intraluminal Device, Percutaneous Endoscopic Approach

03VK4CZ Restriction of Right Internal Carotid Artery with Extraluminal Device, Percutaneous Endoscopic Approach

03VK4DZ Restriction of Right Internal Carotid Artery with Intraluminal Device, Percutaneous Endoscopic Approach

03VK4HZ Restriction of Right Internal Carotid Artery with Intraluminal Device, Flow Diverter, Percutaneous Endoscopic Approach

03VK4ZZ Restriction of Right Internal Carotid Artery, Percutaneous Endoscopic Approach

03VL0BZ Restriction of Left Internal Carotid Artery with Bioactive Intraluminal Device, Open Approach

03VL0CZ Restriction of Left Internal Carotid Artery with Extraluminal Device, Open Approach

03VL0DZ Restriction of Left Internal Carotid Artery with Intraluminal Device, Open Approach

03VL0HZ Restriction of Left Internal Carotid Artery with Intraluminal Device, Flow Diverter, Open Approach

03VL0ZZ Restriction of Left Internal Carotid Artery, Open Approach

03VL3BZ Restriction of Left Internal Carotid Artery with Bioactive Intraluminal Device, Percutaneous Approach

03VL3CZ Restriction of Left Internal Carotid Artery with Extraluminal Device, Percutaneous Approach

03VL3DZ Restriction of Left Internal Carotid Artery with Intraluminal Device, Percutaneous Approach

03VL3HZ Restriction of Left Internal Carotid Artery with Intraluminal Device, Flow Diverter, Percutaneous Approach

03VL3ZZ Restriction of Left Internal Carotid Artery, Percutaneous Approach

03VL4BZ Restriction of Left Internal Carotid Artery with Bioactive Intraluminal Device, Percutaneous Endoscopic Approach

03VL4CZ Restriction of Left Internal Carotid Artery with Extraluminal Device, Percutaneous Endoscopic Approach

03VL4DZ Restriction of Left Internal Carotid Artery with Intraluminal Device, Percutaneous Endoscopic Approach

03VL4HZ Restriction of Left Internal Carotid Artery with Intraluminal Device, Flow Diverter, Percutaneous Endoscopic Approach

03VL4ZZ Restriction of Left Internal Carotid Artery, Percutaneous Endoscopic Approach

03VM0BZ Restriction of Right External Carotid Artery with Bioactive Intraluminal Device, Open Approach

03VM0CZ Restriction of Right External Carotid Artery with Extraluminal Device, Open Approach

03VM0DZ Restriction of Right External Carotid Artery with Intraluminal Device, Open Approach

03VM0HZ Restriction of Right External Carotid Artery with Intraluminal Device, Flow Diverter, Open Approach

03VM0ZZ Restriction of Right External Carotid Artery, Open Approach

03VM3BZ Restriction of Right External Carotid Artery with Bioactive Intraluminal Device, Percutaneous Approach

03VM3CZ Restriction of Right External Carotid Artery with Extraluminal Device, Percutaneous Approach

03VM3DZ Restriction of Right External Carotid Artery with Intraluminal Device, Percutaneous Approach

AHA CC: 4Q, 2016, 26

03VM3HZ Restriction of Right External Carotid Artery with Intraluminal Device, Flow Diverter, Percutaneous Approach

03VM3ZZ Restriction of Right External Carotid Artery, Percutaneous Approach

03VM4BZ Restriction of Right External Carotid Artery with Bioactive Intraluminal Device, Percutaneous Endoscopic Approach

03VM4CZ Restriction of Right External Carotid Artery with Extraluminal Device, Percutaneous Endoscopic Approach

03VM4DZ Restriction of Right External Carotid Artery with Intraluminal Device, Percutaneous Endoscopic Approach

03VM4HZ Restriction of Right External Carotid Artery with Intraluminal Device, Flow Diverter, Percutaneous Endoscopic Approach

03VM4ZZ Restriction of Right External Carotid Artery, Percutaneous Endoscopic Approach

03VN0BZ Restriction of Left External Carotid Artery with Bioactive Intraluminal Device, Open Approach

03VN0CZ Restriction of Left External Carotid Artery with Extraluminal Device, Open Approach

03VN0DZ Restriction of Left External Carotid Artery with Intraluminal Device, Open Approach

03VN0HZ Restriction of Left External Carotid Artery with Intraluminal Device, Flow Diverter, Open Approach

03VN0ZZ Restriction of Left External Carotid Artery, Open Approach

03VN3BZ Restriction of Left External Carotid Artery with Bioactive Intraluminal Device, Percutaneous Approach

03VN3CZ Restriction of Left External Carotid Artery with Extraluminal Device, Percutaneous Approach

03VN3DZ Restriction of Left External Carotid Artery with Intraluminal Device, Percutaneous Approach

03VN3HZ Restriction of Left External Carotid Artery with Intraluminal Device, Flow Diverter, Percutaneous Approach

03VN3ZZ Restriction of Left External Carotid Artery, Percutaneous Approach

03VN4BZ Restriction of Left External Carotid Artery with Bioactive Intraluminal Device, Percutaneous Endoscopic Approach

03VN4CZ Restriction of Left External Carotid Artery with Extraluminal Device, Percutaneous Endoscopic Approach

03VN4DZ Restriction of Left External Carotid Artery with Intraluminal Device, Percutaneous Endoscopic Approach

03VN4HZ Restriction of Left External Carotid Artery with Intraluminal Device, Flow Diverter, Percutaneous Endoscopic Approach

03VN4ZZ Restriction of Left External Carotid Artery, Percutaneous Endoscopic Approach

03VP0BZ Restriction of Right Vertebral Artery with Bioactive Intraluminal Device, Open Approach

03VP0CZ Restriction of Right Vertebral Artery with Extraluminal Device, Open Approach

03VP0DZ Restriction of Right Vertebral Artery with Intraluminal Device, Open Approach

03VP0HZ Restriction of Right Vertebral Artery with Intraluminal Device, Flow Diverter, Open Approach

03VP0ZZ Restriction of Right Vertebral Artery, Open Approach

03VP3BZ Restriction of Right Vertebral Artery with Bioactive Intraluminal Device, Percutaneous Approach

03VP3CZ Restriction of Right Vertebral Artery with Extraluminal Device, Percutaneous Approach

♀ Female-only   ♂ Male-only   ▲ Limited Coverage   ● Non-OR   HAC HAC-associated procedure   ▲ Non-covered procedures   + Cluster

03VP3DZ	Restriction of Right Vertebral Artery with Intraluminal Device, Percutaneous Approach
03VP3HZ	Restriction of Right Vertebral Artery with Intraluminal Device, Flow Diverter, Percutaneous Approach
03VP3ZZ	Restriction of Right Vertebral Artery, Percutaneous Approach
03VP4BZ	Restriction of Right Vertebral Artery with Bioactive Intraluminal Device, Percutaneous Endoscopic Approach
03VP4CZ	Restriction of Right Vertebral Artery with Extraluminal Device, Percutaneous Endoscopic Approach
03VP4DZ	Restriction of Right Vertebral Artery with Intraluminal Device, Percutaneous Endoscopic Approach
03VP4HZ	Restriction of Right Vertebral Artery with Intraluminal Device, Flow Diverter, Percutaneous Endoscopic Approach
03VP4ZZ	Restriction of Right Vertebral Artery, Percutaneous Endoscopic Approach
03VQ0BZ	Restriction of Left Vertebral Artery with Bioactive Intraluminal Device, Open Approach
03VQ0CZ	Restriction of Left Vertebral Artery with Extraluminal Device, Open Approach
03VQ0DZ	Restriction of Left Vertebral Artery with Intraluminal Device, Open Approach
03VQ0HZ	Restriction of Left Vertebral Artery with Intraluminal Device, Flow Diverter, Open Approach
03VQ0ZZ	Restriction of Left Vertebral Artery, Open Approach
03VQ3BZ	Restriction of Left Vertebral Artery with Bioactive Intraluminal Device, Percutaneous Approach
03VQ3CZ	Restriction of Left Vertebral Artery with Extraluminal Device, Percutaneous Approach
03VQ3DZ	Restriction of Left Vertebral Artery with Intraluminal Device, Percutaneous Approach
03VQ3HZ	Restriction of Left Vertebral Artery with Intraluminal Device, Flow Diverter, Percutaneous Approach
03VQ3ZZ	Restriction of Left Vertebral Artery, Percutaneous Approach
03VQ4BZ	Restriction of Left Vertebral Artery with Bioactive Intraluminal Device, Percutaneous Endoscopic Approach
03VQ4CZ	Restriction of Left Vertebral Artery with Extraluminal Device, Percutaneous Endoscopic Approach
03VQ4DZ	Restriction of Left Vertebral Artery with Intraluminal Device, Percutaneous Endoscopic Approach
03VQ4HZ	Restriction of Left Vertebral Artery with Intraluminal Device, Flow Diverter, Percutaneous Endoscopic Approach
03VQ4ZZ	Restriction of Left Vertebral Artery, Percutaneous Endoscopic Approach
03VR0CZ	Restriction of Face Artery with Extraluminal Device, Open Approach
03VR0DZ	Restriction of Face Artery with Intraluminal Device, Open Approach
03VR0ZZ	Restriction of Face Artery, Open Approach
03VR3CZ	Restriction of Face Artery with Extraluminal Device, Percutaneous Approach
03VR3DZ	Restriction of Face Artery with Intraluminal Device, Percutaneous Approach
03VR3ZZ	Restriction of Face Artery, Percutaneous Approach
03VR4CZ	Restriction of Face Artery with Extraluminal Device, Percutaneous Endoscopic Approach
03VR4DZ	Restriction of Face Artery with Intraluminal Device, Percutaneous Endoscopic Approach
03VR4ZZ	Restriction of Face Artery, Percutaneous Endoscopic Approach
03VS0CZ	Restriction of Right Temporal Artery with Extraluminal Device, Open Approach
03VS0DZ	Restriction of Right Temporal Artery with Intraluminal Device, Open Approach
03VS0ZZ	Restriction of Right Temporal Artery, Open Approach
03VS3CZ	Restriction of Right Temporal Artery with Extraluminal Device, Percutaneous Approach
03VS3DZ	Restriction of Right Temporal Artery with Intraluminal Device, Percutaneous Approach
03VS3ZZ	Restriction of Right Temporal Artery, Percutaneous Approach
03VS4CZ	Restriction of Right Temporal Artery with Extraluminal Device, Percutaneous Endoscopic Approach
03VS4DZ	Restriction of Right Temporal Artery with Intraluminal Device, Percutaneous Endoscopic Approach
03VS4ZZ	Restriction of Right Temporal Artery, Percutaneous Endoscopic Approach
03VT0CZ	Restriction of Left Temporal Artery with Extraluminal Device, Open Approach
03VT0DZ	Restriction of Left Temporal Artery with Intraluminal Device, Open Approach
03VT0ZZ	Restriction of Left Temporal Artery, Open Approach
03VT3CZ	Restriction of Left Temporal Artery with Extraluminal Device, Percutaneous Approach
03VT3DZ	Restriction of Left Temporal Artery with Intraluminal Device, Percutaneous Approach
03VT3ZZ	Restriction of Left Temporal Artery, Percutaneous Approach
03VT4CZ	Restriction of Left Temporal Artery with Extraluminal Device, Percutaneous Endoscopic Approach
03VT4DZ	Restriction of Left Temporal Artery with Intraluminal Device, Percutaneous Endoscopic Approach
03VT4ZZ	Restriction of Left Temporal Artery, Percutaneous Endoscopic Approach
03VU0CZ	Restriction of Right Thyroid Artery with Extraluminal Device, Open Approach
03VU0DZ	Restriction of Right Thyroid Artery with Intraluminal Device, Open Approach
03VU0ZZ	Restriction of Right Thyroid Artery, Open Approach
03VU3CZ	Restriction of Right Thyroid Artery with Extraluminal Device, Percutaneous Approach
03VU3DZ	Restriction of Right Thyroid Artery with Intraluminal Device, Percutaneous Approach
03VU3ZZ	Restriction of Right Thyroid Artery, Percutaneous Approach
03VU4CZ	Restriction of Right Thyroid Artery with Extraluminal Device, Percutaneous Endoscopic Approach
03VU4DZ	Restriction of Right Thyroid Artery with Intraluminal Device, Percutaneous Endoscopic Approach
03VU4ZZ	Restriction of Right Thyroid Artery, Percutaneous Endoscopic Approach
03VV0CZ	Restriction of Left Thyroid Artery with Extraluminal Device, Open Approach
03VV0DZ	Restriction of Left Thyroid Artery with Intraluminal Device, Open Approach
03VV0ZZ	Restriction of Left Thyroid Artery, Open Approach
03VV3CZ	Restriction of Left Thyroid Artery with Extraluminal Device, Percutaneous Approach
03VV3DZ	Restriction of Left Thyroid Artery with Intraluminal Device, Percutaneous Approach
03VV3ZZ	Restriction of Left Thyroid Artery, Percutaneous Approach
03VV4CZ	Restriction of Left Thyroid Artery with Extraluminal Device, Percutaneous Endoscopic Approach
03VV4DZ	Restriction of Left Thyroid Artery with Intraluminal Device, Percutaneous Endoscopic Approach
03VV4ZZ	Restriction of Left Thyroid Artery, Percutaneous Endoscopic Approach
03VY0CZ	Restriction of Upper Artery with Extraluminal Device, Open Approach
03VY0DZ	Restriction of Upper Artery with Intraluminal Device, Open Approach
03VY0ZZ	Restriction of Upper Artery, Open Approach
03VY3CZ	Restriction of Upper Artery with Extraluminal Device, Percutaneous Approach
03VY3DZ	Restriction of Upper Artery with Intraluminal Device, Percutaneous Approach
03VY3ZZ	Restriction of Upper Artery, Percutaneous Approach
03VY4CZ	Restriction of Upper Artery with Extraluminal Device, Percutaneous Endoscopic Approach
03VY4DZ	Restriction of Upper Artery with Intraluminal Device, Percutaneous Endoscopic Approach
03VY4ZZ	Restriction of Upper Artery, Percutaneous Endoscopic Approach

03W – Upper Arteries, Revision

Review Coding Guideline B6.1c

03WY00Z	Revision of Drainage Device in Upper Artery, Open Approach
03WY02Z	Revision of Monitoring Device in Upper Artery, Open Approach
03WY03Z	Revision of Infusion Device in Upper Artery, Open Approach

03WY07Z	Revision of Autologous Tissue Substitute in Upper Artery, Open Approach
03WY0CZ	Revision of Extraluminal Device in Upper Artery, Open Approach
03WY0DZ	Revision of Intraluminal Device in Upper Artery, Open Approach
03WY0JZ	Revision of Synthetic Substitute in Upper Artery, Open Approach
	AHA CC: 3Q, 2016, 39-40
03WY0KZ	Revision of Nonautologous Tissue Substitute in Upper Artery, Open Approach
03WY0MZ	Revision of Stimulator Lead in Upper Artery, Open Approach
03WY0YZ	Revision of Other Device in Upper Artery, Open Approach
03WY30Z	Revision of Drainage Device in Upper Artery, Percutaneous Approach
03WY32Z	Revision of Monitoring Device in Upper Artery, Percutaneous Approach
03WY33Z	Revision of Infusion Device in Upper Artery, Percutaneous Approach
03WY37Z	Revision of Autologous Tissue Substitute in Upper Artery, Percutaneous Approach
03WY3CZ	Revision of Extraluminal Device in Upper Artery, Percutaneous Approach
03WY3DZ	Revision of Intraluminal Device in Upper Artery, Percutaneous Approach
	AHA CC: 1Q, 2015, 32-33

03WY3JZ	Revision of Synthetic Substitute in Upper Artery, Percutaneous Approach
03WY3KZ	Revision of Nonautologous Tissue Substitute in Upper Artery, Percutaneous Approach
03WY3MZ	Revision of Stimulator Lead in Upper Artery, Percutaneous Approach
03WY3YZ	Revision of Other Device in Upper Artery, Percutaneous Approach
03WY40Z	Revision of Drainage Device in Upper Artery, Percutaneous Endoscopic Approach
03WY42Z	Revision of Monitoring Device in Upper Artery, Percutaneous Endoscopic Approach
03WY43Z	Revision of Infusion Device in Upper Artery, Percutaneous Endoscopic Approach
03WY47Z	Revision of Autologous Tissue Substitute in Upper Artery, Percutaneous Endoscopic Approach
03WY4CZ	Revision of Extraluminal Device in Upper Artery, Percutaneous Endoscopic Approach
03WY4DZ	Revision of Intraluminal Device in Upper Artery, Percutaneous Endoscopic Approach
03WY4JZ	Revision of Synthetic Substitute in Upper Artery, Percutaneous Endoscopic Approach

03WY4KZ	Revision of Nonautologous Tissue Substitute in Upper Artery, Percutaneous Endoscopic Approach
03WY4MZ	Revision of Stimulator Lead in Upper Artery, Percutaneous Endoscopic Approach
03WY4YZ	Revision of Other Device in Upper Artery, Percutaneous Endoscopic Approach
03WYX0Z	Revision of Drainage Device in Upper Artery, External Approach
03WYX2Z	Revision of Monitoring Device in Upper Artery, External Approach
03WYX3Z	Revision of Infusion Device in Upper Artery, External Approach
03WYX7Z	Revision of Autologous Tissue Substitute in Upper Artery, External Approach
03WYXCZ	Revision of Extraluminal Device in Upper Artery, External Approach
03WYXDZ	Revision of Intraluminal Device in Upper Artery, External Approach
03WYXJZ	Revision of Synthetic Substitute in Upper Artery, External Approach
03WYXKZ	Revision of Nonautologous Tissue Substitute in Upper Artery, External Approach
03WYXMZ	Revision of Stimulator Lead in Upper Artery, External Approach

♀ Female-only ♂ Male-only ▲ Limited Coverage ● Non-OR HAC HAC-associated procedure ▲ Non-covered procedures ✚ Cluster

Arteries

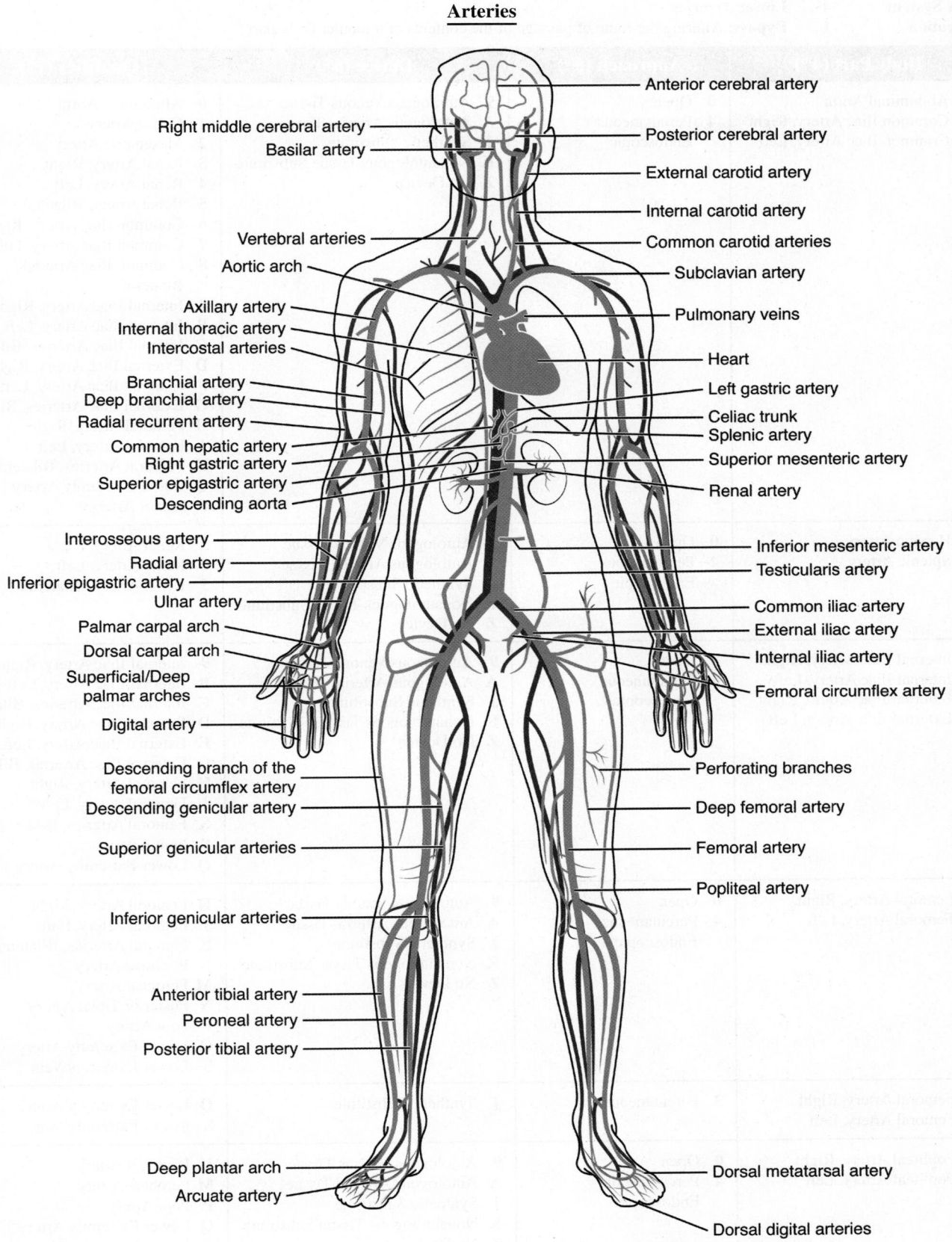

Anterior cerebral artery

Right middle cerebral artery

Posterior cerebral artery

Basilar artery

External carotid artery

Internal carotid artery

Vertebral arteries

Common carotid arteries

Aortic arch

Subclavian artery

Axillary artery

Pulmonary veins

Internal thoracic artery

Intercostal arteries

Heart

Branchial artery

Left gastric artery

Deep branchial artery

Celiac trunk

Radial recurrent artery

Splenic artery

Common hepatic artery

Superior mesenteric artery

Right gastric artery

Renal artery

Superior epigastric artery

Descending aorta

Interosseous artery

Inferior mesenteric artery

Radial artery

Testicularis artery

Inferior epigastric artery

Common iliac artery

Ulnar artery

External iliac artery

Palmar carpal arch

Internal iliac artery

Dorsal carpal arch

Femoral circumflex artery

Superficial/Deep
palmar arches

Digital artery

Descending branch of the
femoral circumflex artery

Perforating branches

Descending genicular artery

Deep femoral artery

Superior genicular arteries

Femoral artery

Popliteal artery

Inferior genicular arteries

Anterior tibial artery

Peroneal artery

Posterior tibial artery

Deep plantar arch

Dorsal metatarsal artery

Arcuate artery

Dorsal digital arteries

©AHIMA

Section 0 **Medical and Surgical**
Body System 4 **Lower Arteries**
Operation 1 **Bypass:** Altering the route of passage of the contents of a tubular body part

Body Part (4th)	Approach (5th)	Device (6th)	Qualifier (7th)
0 Abdominal Aorta C Common Iliac Artery, Right D Common Iliac Artery, Left	0 Open 4 Percutaneous Endoscopic	9 Autologous Venous Tissue A Autologous Arterial Tissue J Synthetic Substitute K Nonautologous Tissue Substitute Z No Device	0 Abdominal Aorta 1 Celiac Artery 2 Mesenteric Artery 3 Renal Artery, Right 4 Renal Artery, Left 5 Renal Artery, Bilateral 6 Common Iliac Artery, Right 7 Common Iliac Artery, Left 8 Common Iliac Arteries, Bilateral 9 Internal Iliac Artery, Right B Internal Iliac Artery, Left C Internal Iliac Arteries, Bilateral D External Iliac Artery, Right F External Iliac Artery, Left G External Iliac Arteries, Bilateral H Femoral Artery, Right J Femoral Artery, Left K Femoral Arteries, Bilateral Q Lower Extremity Artery R Lower Artery
3 Hepatic Artery 4 Splenic Artery	0 Open 4 Percutaneous Endoscopic	9 Autologous Venous Tissue A Autologous Arterial Tissue J Synthetic Substitute K Nonautologous Tissue Substitute Z No Device	3 Renal Artery, Right 4 Renal Artery, Left 5 Renal Artery, Bilateral
E Internal Iliac Artery, Right F Internal Iliac Artery, Left H External Iliac Artery, Right J External Iliac Artery, Left	0 Open 4 Percutaneous Endoscopic	9 Autologous Venous Tissue A Autologous Arterial Tissue J Synthetic Substitute K Nonautologous Tissue Substitute Z No Device	9 Internal Iliac Artery, Right B Internal Iliac Artery, Left C Internal Iliac Arteries, Bilateral D External Iliac Artery, Right F External Iliac Artery, Left G External Iliac Arteries, Bilateral H Femoral Artery, Right J Femoral Artery, Left K Femoral Arteries, Bilateral P Foot Artery Q Lower Extremity Artery
K Femoral Artery, Right L Femoral Artery, Left	0 Open 4 Percutaneous Endoscopic	9 Autologous Venous Tissue A Autologous Arterial Tissue J Synthetic Substitute K Nonautologous Tissue Substitute Z No Device	H Femoral Artery, Right J Femoral Artery, Left K Femoral Arteries, Bilateral L Popliteal Artery M Peroneal Artery N Posterior Tibial Artery P Foot Artery Q Lower Extremity Artery S Lower Extremity Vein
K Femoral Artery, Right L Femoral Artery, Left	3 Percutaneous	J Synthetic Substitute	Q Lower Extremity Artery S Lower Extremity Vein
M Popliteal Artery, Right N Popliteal Artery, Left	0 Open 4 Percutaneous Endoscopic	9 Autologous Venous Tissue A Autologous Arterial Tissue J Synthetic Substitute K Nonautologous Tissue Substitute Z No Device	L Popliteal Artery M Peroneal Artery P Foot Artery Q Lower Extremity Artery S Lower Extremity Vein

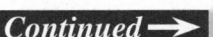

Continued →

Section	0	Medical and Surgical					
Body System	4	Lower Arteries					
Operation	1	**Bypass:** Altering the route of passage of the contents of a tubular body part					

Body Part (4th)	Approach (5th)	Device (6th)	Qualifier (7th)
M Popliteal Artery, Right N Popliteal Artery, Left	3 Percutaneous	J Synthetic Substitute	Q Lower Extremity Artery S Lower Extremity Vein
P Anterior Tibial Artery, Right Q Anterior Tibial Artery, Left R Posterior Tibial Artery, Right S Posterior Tibial Artery, Left	0 Open 3 Percutaneous 4 Percutaneous Endoscopic	J Synthetic Substitute	Q Lower Extremity Artery S Lower Extremity Vein
T Peroneal Artery, Right U Peroneal Artery, Left V Foot Artery, Right W Foot Artery, Left	0 Open 4 Percutaneous Endoscopic	9 Autologous Venous Tissue A Autologous Arterial Tissue J Synthetic Substitute K Nonautologous Tissue Substitute Z No Device	P Foot Artery Q Lower Extremity Artery S Lower Extremity Vein
T Peroneal Artery, Right U Peroneal Artery, Left V Foot Artery, Right W Foot Artery, Left	3 Percutaneous	J Synthetic Substitute	Q Lower Extremity Artery S Lower Extremity Vein

Section	0	Medical and Surgical
Body System	4	Lower Arteries
Operation	5	**Destruction:** Physical eradication of all or a portion of a body part by the direct use of energy, force, or a destructive agent

Body Part (4th)	Approach (5th)	Device (6th)	Qualifier (7th)
0 Abdominal Aorta 1 Celiac Artery 2 Gastric Artery 3 Hepatic Artery 4 Splenic Artery 5 Superior Mesenteric Artery 6 Colic Artery, Right 7 Colic Artery, Left 8 Colic Artery, Middle 9 Renal Artery, Right A Renal Artery, Left B Inferior Mesenteric Artery C Common Iliac Artery, Right D Common Iliac Artery, Left E Internal Iliac Artery, Right F Internal Iliac Artery, Left H External Iliac Artery, Right J External Iliac Artery, Left K Femoral Artery, Right L Femoral Artery, Left M Popliteal Artery, Right N Popliteal Artery, Left P Anterior Tibial Artery, Right Q Anterior Tibial Artery, Left R Posterior Tibial Artery, Right S Posterior Tibial Artery, Left T Peroneal Artery, Right U Peroneal Artery, Left V Foot Artery, Right W Foot Artery, Left Y Lower Artery	0 Open 3 Percutaneous 4 Percutaneous Endoscopic	Z No Device	Z No Qualifier

Section	0	Medical and Surgical
Body System	4	Lower Arteries
Operation	7	**Dilation:** Expanding an orifice or the lumen of a tubular body part

Body Part (4th)	Approach (5th)	Device (6th)	Qualifier (7th)
0 Abdominal Aorta **1** Celiac Artery **2** Gastric Artery **3** Hepatic Artery **4** Splenic Artery **5** Superior Mesenteric Artery **6** Colic Artery, Right **7** Colic Artery, Left **8** Colic Artery, Middle **9** Renal Artery, Right **A** Renal Artery, Left **B** Inferior Mesenteric Artery **C** Common Iliac Artery, Right **D** Common Iliac Artery, Left **E** Internal Iliac Artery, Right **F** Internal Iliac Artery, Left **H** External Iliac Artery, Right **J** External Iliac Artery, Left **K** Femoral Artery, Right **L** Femoral Artery, Left **M** Popliteal Artery, Right **N** Popliteal Artery, Left **P** Anterior Tibial Artery, Right **Q** Anterior Tibial Artery, Left **R** Posterior Tibial Artery, Right **S** Posterior Tibial Artery, Left **T** Peroneal Artery, Right **U** Peroneal Artery, Left **V** Foot Artery, Right **W** Foot Artery, Left **Y** Lower Artery	**0** Open **3** Percutaneous **4** Percutaneous Endoscopic	**4** Intraluminal Device, Drug-eluting **D** Intraluminal Device **Z** No Device	**1** Drug-Coated Balloon **Z** No Qualifier
0 Abdominal Aorta **1** Celiac Artery **2** Gastric Artery **3** Hepatic Artery **4** Splenic Artery **5** Superior Mesenteric Artery **6** Colic Artery, Right **7** Colic Artery, Left **8** Colic Artery, Middle **9** Renal Artery, Right **A** Renal Artery, Left **B** Inferior Mesenteric Artery **C** Common Iliac Artery, Right **D** Common Iliac Artery, Left **E** Internal Iliac Artery, Right **F** Internal Iliac Artery, Left **H** External Iliac Artery, Right **J** External Iliac Artery, Left **K** Femoral Artery, Right **L** Femoral Artery, Left **M** Popliteal Artery, Right **N** Popliteal Artery, Left **P** Anterior Tibial Artery, Right **Q** Anterior Tibial Artery, Left **R** Posterior Tibial Artery, Right **S** Posterior Tibial Artery, Left **T** Peroneal Artery, Right **U** Peroneal Artery, Left **V** Foot Artery, Right **W** Foot Artery, Left **Y** Lower Artery	**0** Open **3** Percutaneous **4** Percutaneous Endoscopic	**5** Intraluminal Device, Drug-eluting, Two **6** Intraluminal Device, Drug-eluting, Three **7** Intraluminal Device, Drug-eluting, Four or More **E** Intraluminal Devices, Two **F** Intraluminal Devices, Three **G** Intraluminal Devices, Four or More	**Z** No Qualifier

Section	0	Medical and Surgical
Body System	4	Lower Arteries
Operation	9	Drainage: Taking or letting out fluids and/or gases from a body part

Body Part (4ᵗʰ)	Approach (5ᵗʰ)	Device (6ᵗʰ)	Qualifier (7ᵗʰ)
0 Abdominal Aorta 1 Celiac Artery 2 Gastric Artery 3 Hepatic Artery 4 Splenic Artery 5 Superior Mesenteric Artery 6 Colic Artery, Right 7 Colic Artery, Left 8 Colic Artery, Middle 9 Renal Artery, Right A Renal Artery, Left B Inferior Mesenteric Artery C Common Iliac Artery, Right D Common Iliac Artery, Left E Internal Iliac Artery, Right F Internal Iliac Artery, Left H External Iliac Artery, Right J External Iliac Artery, Left K Femoral Artery, Right L Femoral Artery, Left M Popliteal Artery, Right N Popliteal Artery, Left P Anterior Tibial Artery, Right Q Anterior Tibial Artery, Left R Posterior Tibial Artery, Right S Posterior Tibial Artery, Left T Peroneal Artery, Right U Peroneal Artery, Left V Foot Artery, Right W Foot Artery, Left Y Lower Artery	0 Open 3 Percutaneous 4 Percutaneous Endoscopic	0 Drainage Device	Z No Qualifier
0 Abdominal Aorta 1 Celiac Artery 2 Gastric Artery 3 Hepatic Artery 4 Splenic Artery 5 Superior Mesenteric Artery 6 Colic Artery, Right 7 Colic Artery, Left 8 Colic Artery, Middle 9 Renal Artery, Right A Renal Artery, Left B Inferior Mesenteric Artery C Common Iliac Artery, Right D Common Iliac Artery, Left E Internal Iliac Artery, Right F Internal Iliac Artery, Left H External Iliac Artery, Right J External Iliac Artery, Left K Femoral Artery, Right L Femoral Artery, Left M Popliteal Artery, Right N Popliteal Artery, Left P Anterior Tibial Artery, Right Q Anterior Tibial Artery, Left R Posterior Tibial Artery, Right S Posterior Tibial Artery, Left T Peroneal Artery, Right U Peroneal Artery, Left V Foot Artery, Right W Foot Artery, Left Y Lower Artery	0 Open 3 Percutaneous 4 Percutaneous Endoscopic	Z No Device	X Diagnostic Z No Qualifier

Section	0	Medical and Surgical
Body System	4	Lower Arteries
Operation	B	**Excision:** Cutting out or off, without replacement, a portion of a body part

Body Part (4th)	Approach (5th)	Device (6th)	Qualifier (7th)
0 Abdominal Aorta **1** Celiac Artery **2** Gastric Artery **3** Hepatic Artery **4** Splenic Artery **5** Superior Mesenteric Artery **6** Colic Artery, Right **7** Colic Artery, Left **8** Colic Artery, Middle **9** Renal Artery, Right **A** Renal Artery, Left **B** Inferior Mesenteric Artery **C** Common Iliac Artery, Right **D** Common Iliac Artery, Left **E** Internal Iliac Artery, Right **F** Internal Iliac Artery, Left **H** External Iliac Artery, Right **J** External Iliac Artery, Left **K** Femoral Artery, Right **L** Femoral Artery, Left **M** Popliteal Artery, Right **N** Popliteal Artery, Left **P** Anterior Tibial Artery, Right **Q** Anterior Tibial Artery, Left **R** Posterior Tibial Artery, Right **S** Posterior Tibial Artery, Left **T** Peroneal Artery, Right **U** Peroneal Artery, Left **V** Foot Artery, Right **W** Foot Artery, Left **Y** Lower Artery	**0** Open **3** Percutaneous **4** Percutaneous Endoscopic	**Z** No Device	**X** Diagnostic **Z** No Qualifier

Section	0	Medical and Surgical
Body System	4	Lower Arteries
Operation	C	Extirpation: Taking or cutting out solid matter from a body part

Body Part (4th)	Approach (5th)	Device (6th)	Qualifier (7th)
0 Abdominal Aorta 1 Celiac Artery 2 Gastric Artery 3 Hepatic Artery 4 Splenic Artery 5 Superior Mesenteric Artery 6 Colic Artery, Right 7 Colic Artery, Left 8 Colic Artery, Middle 9 Renal Artery, Right A Renal Artery, Left B Inferior Mesenteric Artery C Common Iliac Artery, Right D Common Iliac Artery, Left E Internal Iliac Artery, Right F Internal Iliac Artery, Left H External Iliac Artery, Right J External Iliac Artery, Left K Femoral Artery, Right L Femoral Artery, Left M Popliteal Artery, Right N Popliteal Artery, Left P Anterior Tibial Artery, Right Q Anterior Tibial Artery, Left R Posterior Tibial Artery, Right S Posterior Tibial Artery, Left T Peroneal Artery, Right U Peroneal Artery, Left V Foot Artery, Right W Foot Artery, Left Y Lower Artery	0 Open 3 Percutaneous 4 Percutaneous Endoscopic	Z No Device	Z No Qualifier

Section	0	Medical and Surgical
Body System	4	Lower Arteries
Operation	F	Fragmentation: Breaking solid matter in a body part into pieces

Body Part (4th)	Approach (5th)	Device (6th)	Qualifier (7th)
C Common Iliac Artery, Right D Common Iliac Artery, Left E Internal Iliac Artery, Right F Internal Iliac Artery, Left H External Iliac Artery, Right J External Iliac Artery, Left K Femoral Artery, Right L Femoral Artery, Left M Popliteal Artery, Right N Popliteal Artery, Left P Anterior Tibial Artery, Right Q Anterior Tibial Artery, Left R Posterior Tibial Artery, Right S Posterior Tibial Artery, Left T Peroneal Artery, Right U Peroneal Artery, Left Y Lower Artery	3 Percutaneous	Z No Device	0 Ultrasonic Z No Qualifier

Section	**0**	**Medical and Surgical**
Body System	**4**	**Lower Arteries**
Operation	**H**	**Insertion:** Putting in a nonbiological appliance that monitors, assists, performs, or prevents a physiological function but does not physically take the place of a body part

Body Part (4th)	Approach (5th)	Device (6th)	Qualifier (7th)
0 Abdominal Aorta	**0** Open **3** Percutaneous **4** Percutaneous Endoscopic	**2** Monitoring Device **3** Infusion Device **D** Intraluminal Device	**Z** No Qualifier
1 Celiac Artery **2** Gastric Artery **3** Hepatic Artery **4** Splenic Artery **5** Superior Mesenteric Artery **6** Colic Artery, Right **7** Colic Artery, Left **8** Colic Artery, Middle **9** Renal Artery, Right **A** Renal Artery, Left **B** Inferior Mesenteric Artery **C** Common Iliac Artery, Right **D** Common Iliac Artery, Left **E** Internal Iliac Artery, Right **F** Internal Iliac Artery, Left **H** External Iliac Artery, Right **J** External Iliac Artery, Left **K** Femoral Artery, Right **L** Femoral Artery, Left **M** Popliteal Artery, Right **N** Popliteal Artery, Left **P** Anterior Tibial Artery, Right **Q** Anterior Tibial Artery, Left **R** Posterior Tibial Artery, Right **S** Posterior Tibial Artery, Left **T** Peroneal Artery, Right **U** Peroneal Artery, Left **V** Foot Artery, Right **W** Foot Artery, Left	**0** Open **3** Percutaneous **4** Percutaneous Endoscopic	**3** Infusion Device **D** Intraluminal Device	**Z** No Qualifier
Y Lower Artery	**0** Open **3** Percutaneous **4** Percutaneous Endoscopic	**2** Monitoring Device **3** Infusion Device **D** Intraluminal Device **Y** Other Device	**Z** No Qualifier

Section	**0**	**Medical and Surgical**
Body System	**4**	**Lower Arteries**
Operation	**J**	**Inspection:** Visually and/or manually exploring a body part

Body Part (4th)	Approach (5th)	Device (6th)	Qualifier (7th)
Y Lower Artery	**0** Open **3** Percutaneous **4** Percutaneous Endoscopic **X** External	**Z** No Device	**Z** No Qualifier

Section	0	**Medical and Surgical**
Body System	4	**Lower Arteries**
Operation	L	**Occlusion:** Completely closing an orifice or the lumen of a tubular body part

Body Part (4th)	Approach (5th)	Device (6th)	Qualifier (7th)
0 Abdominal Aorta	**0** Open **4** Percutaneous Endoscopic	**C** Extraluminal Device **D** Intraluminal Device **Z** No Device	**Z** No Qualifier
0 Abdominal Aorta	**3** Percutaneous	**C** Extraluminal Device **Z** No Device	**Z** No Qualifier
0 Abdominal Aorta	**3** Percutaneous	**D** Intraluminal Device	**J** Temporary **Z** No Qualifier
1 Celiac Artery **2** Gastric Artery **3** Hepatic Artery **4** Splenic Artery **5** Superior Mesenteric Artery **6** Colic Artery, Right **7** Colic Artery, Left **8** Colic Artery, Middle **9** Renal Artery, Right **A** Renal Artery, Left **B** Inferior Mesenteric Artery **C** Common Iliac Artery, Right **D** Common Iliac Artery, Left **H** External Iliac Artery, Right **J** External Iliac Artery, Left **K** Femoral Artery, Right **L** Femoral Artery, Left **M** Popliteal Artery, Right **N** Popliteal Artery, Left **P** Anterior Tibial Artery, Right **Q** Anterior Tibial Artery, Left **R** Posterior Tibial Artery, Right **S** Posterior Tibial Artery, Left **T** Peroneal Artery, Right **U** Peroneal Artery, Left **V** Foot Artery, Right **W** Foot Artery, Left **Y** Lower Artery	**0** Open **3** Percutaneous **4** Percutaneous Endoscopic	**C** Extraluminal Device **D** Intraluminal Device **Z** No Device	**Z** No Qualifier
E Internal Iliac Artery, Right	**0** Open **3** Percutaneous **4** Percutaneous Endoscopic	**C** Extraluminal Device **D** Intraluminal Device **Z** No Device	**T** Uterine Artery, Right **Z** No Qualifier
F Internal Iliac Artery, Left	**0** Open **3** Percutaneous **4** Percutaneous Endoscopic	**C** Extraluminal Device **D** Intraluminal Device **Z** No Device	**U** Uterine Artery, Left **Z** No Qualifier

Section   0   **Medical and Surgical**
Body System   4   **Lower Arteries**
Operation   N   **Release:** Freeing a body part from an abnormal physical constraint by cutting or by the use of force

Body Part (4th)	Approach (5th)	Device (6th)	Qualifier (7th)
0 Abdominal Aorta **1** Celiac Artery **2** Gastric Artery **3** Hepatic Artery **4** Splenic Artery **5** Superior Mesenteric Artery **6** Colic Artery, Right **7** Colic Artery, Left **8** Colic Artery, Middle **9** Renal Artery, Right **A** Renal Artery, Left **B** Inferior Mesenteric Artery **C** Common Iliac Artery, Right **D** Common Iliac Artery, Left **E** Internal Iliac Artery, Right **F** Internal Iliac Artery, Left **H** External Iliac Artery, Right **J** External Iliac Artery, Left **K** Femoral Artery, Right **L** Femoral Artery, Left **M** Popliteal Artery, Right **N** Popliteal Artery, Left **P** Anterior Tibial Artery, Right **Q** Anterior Tibial Artery, Left **R** Posterior Tibial Artery, Right **S** Posterior Tibial Artery, Left **T** Peroneal Artery, Right **U** Peroneal Artery, Left **V** Foot Artery, Right **W** Foot Artery, Left **Y** Lower Artery	**0** Open **3** Percutaneous **4** Percutaneous Endoscopic	**Z** No Device	**Z** No Qualifier

Section   0   **Medical and Surgical**
Body System   4   **Lower Arteries**
Operation   P   **Removal:** Taking out or off a device from a body part

Body Part (4th)	Approach (5th)	Device (6th)	Qualifier (7th)
Y Lower Artery	**0** Open **3** Percutaneous **4** Percutaneous Endoscopic	**0** Drainage Device **2** Monitoring Device **3** Infusion Device **7** Autologous Tissue Substitute **C** Extraluminal Device **D** Intraluminal Device **J** Synthetic Substitute **K** Nonautologous Tissue Substitute **Y** Other Device	**Z** No Qualifier
Y Lower Artery	**X** External	**0** Drainage Device **1** Radioactive Element **2** Monitoring Device **3** Infusion Device **D** Intraluminal Device	**Z** No Qualifier

Section	0	**Medical and Surgical**
Body System	4	**Lower Arteries**
Operation	Q	**Repair:** Restoring, to the extent possible, a body part to its normal anatomic structure and function

Body Part (4ᵗʰ)	Approach (5ᵗʰ)	Device (6ᵗʰ)	Qualifier (7ᵗʰ)
0 Abdominal Aorta	0 Open	Z No Device	Z No Qualifier
1 Celiac Artery	3 Percutaneous		
2 Gastric Artery	4 Percutaneous		
3 Hepatic Artery	Endoscopic		
4 Splenic Artery			
5 Superior Mesenteric Artery			
6 Colic Artery, Right			
7 Colic Artery, Left			
8 Colic Artery, Middle			
9 Renal Artery, Right			
A Renal Artery, Left			
B Inferior Mesenteric Artery			
C Common Iliac Artery, Right			
D Common Iliac Artery, Left			
E Internal Iliac Artery, Right			
F Internal Iliac Artery, Left			
H External Iliac Artery, Right			
J External Iliac Artery, Left			
K Femoral Artery, Right			
L Femoral Artery, Left			
M Popliteal Artery, Right			
N Popliteal Artery, Left			
P Anterior Tibial Artery, Right			
Q Anterior Tibial Artery, Left			
R Posterior Tibial Artery, Right			
S Posterior Tibial Artery, Left			
T Peroneal Artery, Right			
U Peroneal Artery, Left			
V Foot Artery, Right			
W Foot Artery, Left			
Y Lower Artery			

Section	0	Medical and Surgical
Body System	4	Lower Arteries
Operation	R	**Replacement:** Putting in or on biological or synthetic material that physically takes the place and/or function of all or a portion of a body part

Body Part (4th)	Approach (5th)	Device (6th)	Qualifier (7th)
0 Abdominal Aorta	0 Open	7 Autologous Tissue Substitute	Z No Qualifier
1 Celiac Artery	4 Percutaneous Endoscopic	J Synthetic Substitute	
2 Gastric Artery		K Nonautologous Tissue Substitute	
3 Hepatic Artery			
4 Splenic Artery			
5 Superior Mesenteric Artery			
6 Colic Artery, Right			
7 Colic Artery, Left			
8 Colic Artery, Middle			
9 Renal Artery, Right			
A Renal Artery, Left			
B Inferior Mesenteric Artery			
C Common Iliac Artery, Right			
D Common Iliac Artery, Left			
E Internal Iliac Artery, Right			
F Internal Iliac Artery, Left			
H External Iliac Artery, Right			
J External Iliac Artery, Left			
K Femoral Artery, Right			
L Femoral Artery, Left			
M Popliteal Artery, Right			
N Popliteal Artery, Left			
P Anterior Tibial Artery, Right			
Q Anterior Tibial Artery, Left			
R Posterior Tibial Artery, Right			
S Posterior Tibial Artery, Left			
T Peroneal Artery, Right			
U Peroneal Artery, Left			
V Foot Artery, Right			
W Foot Artery, Left			
Y Lower Artery			

Section	0	Medical and Surgical
Body System	4	Lower Arteries
Operation	S	**Reposition:** Moving to its normal location, or other suitable location, all or a portion of a body part

Body Part (4th)	Approach (5th)	Device (6th)	Qualifier (7th)
0 Abdominal Aorta **1** Celiac Artery **2** Gastric Artery **3** Hepatic Artery **4** Splenic Artery **5** Superior Mesenteric Artery **6** Colic Artery, Right **7** Colic Artery, Left **8** Colic Artery, Middle **9** Renal Artery, Right **A** Renal Artery, Left **B** Inferior Mesenteric Artery **C** Common Iliac Artery, Right **D** Common Iliac Artery, Left **E** Internal Iliac Artery, Right **F** Internal Iliac Artery, Left **H** External Iliac Artery, Right **J** External Iliac Artery, Left **K** Femoral Artery, Right **L** Femoral Artery, Left **M** Popliteal Artery, Right **N** Popliteal Artery, Left **P** Anterior Tibial Artery, Right **Q** Anterior Tibial Artery, Left **R** Posterior Tibial Artery, Right **S** Posterior Tibial Artery, Left **T** Peroneal Artery, Right **U** Peroneal Artery, Left **V** Foot Artery, Right **W** Foot Artery, Left **Y** Lower Artery	**0** Open **3** Percutaneous **4** Percutaneous Endoscopic	**Z** No Device	**Z** No Qualifier

Section   0   **Medical and Surgical**
Body System   4   **Lower Arteries**
Operation   U   **Supplement:** Putting in or on biological or synthetic material that physically reinforces and/or augments the function
                                  of a portion of a body part

Body Part (4th)	Approach (5th)	Device (6th)	Qualifier (7th)
0 Abdominal Aorta 1 Celiac Artery 2 Gastric Artery 3 Hepatic Artery 4 Splenic Artery 5 Superior Mesenteric Artery 6 Colic Artery, Right 7 Colic Artery, Left 8 Colic Artery, Middle 9 Renal Artery, Right A Renal Artery, Left B Inferior Mesenteric Artery C Common Iliac Artery, Right D Common Iliac Artery, Left E Internal Iliac Artery, Right F Internal Iliac Artery, Left H External Iliac Artery, Right J External Iliac Artery, Left K Femoral Artery, Right L Femoral Artery, Left M Popliteal Artery, Right N Popliteal Artery, Left P Anterior Tibial Artery, Right Q Anterior Tibial Artery, Left R Posterior Tibial Artery, Right S Posterior Tibial Artery, Left T Peroneal Artery, Right U Peroneal Artery, Left V Foot Artery, Right W Foot Artery, Left Y Lower Artery	0 Open 3 Percutaneous 4 Percutaneous Endoscopic	7 Autologous Tissue Substitute J Synthetic Substitute K Nonautologous Tissue Substitute	Z No Qualifier

Section   0   **Medical and Surgical**
Body System   4   **Lower Arteries**
Operation   V   **Restriction:** Partially closing an orifice or the lumen of a tubular body part

Body Part (4th)	Approach (5th)	Device (6th)	Qualifier (7th)

0 Abdominal Aorta	0 Open
	3 Percutaneous
	4 Percutaneous Endoscopic
		C Extraluminal Device
		E Intraluminal Device,
		   Branched or Fenestrated,
		   One or Two Arteries
		F Intraluminal Device,
		   Branched or Fenestrated,
		   Three or More Arteries
		Z No Device
			Z No Qualifier

0 Abdominal Aorta	0 Open 3 Percutaneous 4 Percutaneous Endoscopic	D Intraluminal Device	J Temporary Z No Qualifier

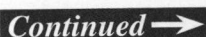
Continued →

Section	0	Medical and Surgical		04V Continued
Body System	4	Lower Arteries		
Operation	V	Restriction: Partially closing an orifice or the lumen of a tubular body part		

Body Part (4th)	Approach (5th)	Device (6th)	Qualifier (7th)
1 Celiac Artery 2 Gastric Artery 3 Hepatic Artery 4 Splenic Artery 5 Superior Mesenteric Artery 6 Colic Artery, Right 7 Colic Artery, Left 8 Colic Artery, Middle 9 Renal Artery, Right A Renal Artery, Left B Inferior Mesenteric Artery E Internal Iliac Artery, Right F Internal Iliac Artery, Left H External Iliac Artery, Right J External Iliac Artery, Left K Femoral Artery, Right L Femoral Artery, Left M Popliteal Artery, Right N Popliteal Artery, Left P Anterior Tibial Artery, Right Q Anterior Tibial Artery, Left R Posterior Tibial Artery, Right S Posterior Tibial Artery, Left T Peroneal Artery, Right U Peroneal Artery, Left V Foot Artery, Right W Foot Artery, Left Y Lower Artery	0 Open 3 Percutaneous 4 Percutaneous Endoscopic	C Extraluminal Device D Intraluminal Device Z No Device	Z No Qualifier
C Common Iliac Artery, Right D Common Iliac Artery, Left	0 Open 3 Percutaneous 4 Percutaneous Endoscopic	C Extraluminal Device D Intraluminal Device E Intraluminal Device, Branched or Fenestrated, One or Two Arteries Z No Device	Z No Qualifier

Section	0	Medical and Surgical
Body System	4	Lower Arteries
Operation	W	Revision: Correcting, to the extent possible, a portion of a malfunctioning device or the position of a displaced device

Body Part (4th)	Approach (5th)	Device (6th)	Qualifier (7th)
Y Lower Artery	0 Open 3 Percutaneous 4 Percutaneous Endoscopic	0 Drainage Device 2 Monitoring Device 3 Infusion Device 7 Autologous Tissue Substitute C Extraluminal Device D Intraluminal Device J Synthetic Substitute K Nonautologous Tissue Substitute Y Other Device	Z No Qualifier
Y Lower Artery	X External	0 Drainage Device 2 Monitoring Device 3 Infusion Device 7 Autologous Tissue Substitute C Extraluminal Device D Intraluminal Device J Synthetic Substitute K Nonautologus Tissue Substitute	Z No Qualifier

Review Coding Guideline B3.6a

0410090 Bypass Abdominal Aorta to Abdominal Aorta with Autologous Venous Tissue, Open Approach

0410091 Bypass Abdominal Aorta to Celiac Artery with Autologous Venous Tissue, Open Approach

0410092 Bypass Abdominal Aorta to Mesenteric Artery with Autologous Venous Tissue, Open Approach

0410093 Bypass Abdominal Aorta to Right Renal Artery with Autologous Venous Tissue, Open Approach

0410094 Bypass Abdominal Aorta to Left Renal Artery with Autologous Venous Tissue, Open Approach

0410095 Bypass Abdominal Aorta to Bilateral Renal Artery with Autologous Venous Tissue, Open Approach

0410096 Bypass Abdominal Aorta to Right Common Iliac Artery with Autologous Venous Tissue, Open Approach

0410097 Bypass Abdominal Aorta to Left Common Iliac Artery with Autologous Venous Tissue, Open Approach

0410098 Bypass Abdominal Aorta to Bilateral Common Iliac Arteries with Autologous Venous Tissue, Open Approach

0410099 Bypass Abdominal Aorta to Right Internal Iliac Artery with Autologous Venous Tissue, Open Approach

041009B Bypass Abdominal Aorta to Left Internal Iliac Artery with Autologous Venous Tissue, Open Approach

041009C Bypass Abdominal Aorta to Bilateral Internal Iliac Arteries with Autologous Venous Tissue, Open Approach

041009D Bypass Abdominal Aorta to Right External Iliac Artery with Autologous Venous Tissue, Open Approach

041009F Bypass Abdominal Aorta to Left External Iliac Artery with Autologous Venous Tissue, Open Approach

041009G Bypass Abdominal Aorta to Bilateral External Iliac Arteries with Autologous Venous Tissue, Open Approach

041009H Bypass Abdominal Aorta to Right Femoral Artery with Autologous Venous Tissue, Open Approach

041009J Bypass Abdominal Aorta to Left Femoral Artery with Autologous Venous Tissue, Open Approach

041009K Bypass Abdominal Aorta to Bilateral Femoral Arteries with Autologous Venous Tissue, Open Approach

041009Q Bypass Abdominal Aorta to Lower Extremity Artery with Autologous Venous Tissue, Open Approach

041009R Bypass Abdominal Aorta to Lower Artery with Autologous Venous Tissue, Open Approach

04100A0 Bypass Abdominal Aorta to Abdominal Aorta with Autologous Arterial Tissue, Open Approach

04100A1 Bypass Abdominal Aorta to Celiac Artery with Autologous Arterial Tissue, Open Approach

04100A2 Bypass Abdominal Aorta to Mesenteric Artery with Autologous Arterial Tissue, Open Approach

04100A3 Bypass Abdominal Aorta to Right Renal Artery with Autologous Arterial Tissue, Open Approach

04100A4 Bypass Abdominal Aorta to Left Renal Artery with Autologous Arterial Tissue, Open Approach

04100A5 Bypass Abdominal Aorta to Bilateral Renal Artery with Autologous Arterial Tissue, Open Approach

04100A6 Bypass Abdominal Aorta to Right Common Iliac Artery with Autologous Arterial Tissue, Open Approach

04100A7 Bypass Abdominal Aorta to Left Common Iliac Artery with Autologous Arterial Tissue, Open Approach

04100A8 Bypass Abdominal Aorta to Bilateral Common Iliac Arteries with Autologous Arterial Tissue, Open Approach

04100A9 Bypass Abdominal Aorta to Right Internal Iliac Artery with Autologous Arterial Tissue, Open Approach

04100AB Bypass Abdominal Aorta to Left Internal Iliac Artery with Autologous Arterial Tissue, Open Approach

04100AC Bypass Abdominal Aorta to Bilateral Internal Iliac Arteries with Autologous Arterial Tissue, Open Approach

04100AD Bypass Abdominal Aorta to Right External Iliac Artery with Autologous Arterial Tissue, Open Approach

04100AF Bypass Abdominal Aorta to Left External Iliac Artery with Autologous Arterial Tissue, Open Approach

04100AG Bypass Abdominal Aorta to Bilateral External Iliac Arteries with Autologous Arterial Tissue, Open Approach

04100AH Bypass Abdominal Aorta to Right Femoral Artery with Autologous Arterial Tissue, Open Approach

04100AJ Bypass Abdominal Aorta to Left Femoral Artery with Autologous Arterial Tissue, Open Approach

04100AK Bypass Abdominal Aorta to Bilateral Femoral Arteries with Autologous Arterial Tissue, Open Approach

04100AQ Bypass Abdominal Aorta to Lower Extremity Artery with Autologous Arterial Tissue, Open Approach

04100AR Bypass Abdominal Aorta to Lower Artery with Autologous Arterial Tissue, Open Approach

04100J0 Bypass Abdominal Aorta to Abdominal Aorta with Synthetic Substitute, Open Approach

04100J1 Bypass Abdominal Aorta to Celiac Artery with Synthetic Substitute, Open Approach

04100J2 Bypass Abdominal Aorta to Mesenteric Artery with Synthetic Substitute, Open Approach

04100J3 Bypass Abdominal Aorta to Right Renal Artery with Synthetic Substitute, Open Approach

04100J4 Bypass Abdominal Aorta to Left Renal Artery with Synthetic Substitute, Open Approach

04100J5 Bypass Abdominal Aorta to Bilateral Renal Artery with Synthetic Substitute, Open Approach

04100J6 Bypass Abdominal Aorta to Right Common Iliac Artery with Synthetic Substitute, Open Approach

04100J7 Bypass Abdominal Aorta to Left Common Iliac Artery with Synthetic Substitute, Open Approach

04100J8 Bypass Abdominal Aorta to Bilateral Common Iliac Arteries with Synthetic Substitute, Open Approach

04100J9 Bypass Abdominal Aorta to Right Internal Iliac Artery with Synthetic Substitute, Open Approach

04100JB Bypass Abdominal Aorta to Left Internal Iliac Artery with Synthetic Substitute, Open Approach

04100JC Bypass Abdominal Aorta to Bilateral Internal Iliac Arteries with Synthetic Substitute, Open Approach

04100JD Bypass Abdominal Aorta to Right External Iliac Artery with Synthetic Substitute, Open Approach

04100JF Bypass Abdominal Aorta to Left External Iliac Artery with Synthetic Substitute, Open Approach

04100JG Bypass Abdominal Aorta to Bilateral External Iliac Arteries with Synthetic Substitute, Open Approach

04100JH Bypass Abdominal Aorta to Right Femoral Artery with Synthetic Substitute, Open Approach

04100JJ Bypass Abdominal Aorta to Left Femoral Artery with Synthetic Substitute, Open Approach

04100JK Bypass Abdominal Aorta to Bilateral Femoral Arteries with Synthetic Substitute, Open Approach

04100JQ Bypass Abdominal Aorta to Lower Extremity Artery with Synthetic Substitute, Open Approach

04100JR Bypass Abdominal Aorta to Lower Artery with Synthetic Substitute, Open Approach

04100K0 Bypass Abdominal Aorta to Abdominal Aorta with Nonautologous Tissue Substitute, Open Approach

04100K1 Bypass Abdominal Aorta to Celiac Artery with Nonautologous Tissue Substitute, Open Approach

04100K2 Bypass Abdominal Aorta to Mesenteric Artery with Nonautologous Tissue Substitute, Open Approach

04100K3 Bypass Abdominal Aorta to Right Renal Artery with Nonautologous Tissue Substitute, Open Approach

04100K4 Bypass Abdominal Aorta to Left Renal Artery with Nonautologous Tissue Substitute, Open Approach

04100K5 Bypass Abdominal Aorta to Bilateral Renal Artery with Nonautologous Tissue Substitute, Open Approach

04100K6 Bypass Abdominal Aorta to Right Common Iliac Artery with Nonautologous Tissue Substitute, Open Approach

04100K7 Bypass Abdominal Aorta to Left Common Iliac Artery with Nonautologous Tissue Substitute, Open Approach

04100K8 Bypass Abdominal Aorta to Bilateral Common Iliac Arteries with Nonautologous Tissue Substitute, Open Approach

04100K9 Bypass Abdominal Aorta to Right Internal Iliac Artery with Nonautologous Tissue Substitute, Open Approach

04100KB Bypass Abdominal Aorta to Left Internal Iliac Artery with Nonautologous Tissue Substitute, Open Approach

04100KC Bypass Abdominal Aorta to Bilateral Internal Iliac Arteries with Nonautologous Tissue Substitute, Open Approach

04100KD Bypass Abdominal Aorta to Right External Iliac Artery with Nonautologous Tissue Substitute, Open Approach

04100KF Bypass Abdominal Aorta to Left External Iliac Artery with Nonautologous Tissue Substitute, Open Approach

04100KG Bypass Abdominal Aorta to Bilateral External Iliac Arteries with Nonautologous Tissue Substitute, Open Approach

04100KH Bypass Abdominal Aorta to Right Femoral Artery with Nonautologous Tissue Substitute, Open Approach

04100KJ Bypass Abdominal Aorta to Left Femoral Artery with Nonautologous Tissue Substitute, Open Approach

04100KK Bypass Abdominal Aorta to Bilateral Femoral Arteries with Nonautologous Tissue Substitute, Open Approach

04100KQ Bypass Abdominal Aorta to Lower Extremity Artery with Nonautologous Tissue Substitute, Open Approach

04100KR Bypass Abdominal Aorta to Lower Artery with Nonautologous Tissue Substitute, Open Approach

04100Z0 Bypass Abdominal Aorta to Abdominal Aorta, Open Approach

04100Z1 Bypass Abdominal Aorta to Celiac Artery, Open Approach

04100Z2 Bypass Abdominal Aorta to Mesenteric Artery, Open Approach

04100Z3 Bypass Abdominal Aorta to Right Renal Artery, Open Approach
AHA CC: 3Q, 2015, 28

04100Z4 Bypass Abdominal Aorta to Left Renal Artery, Open Approach

04100Z5 Bypass Abdominal Aorta to Bilateral Renal Artery, Open Approach

04100Z6 Bypass Abdominal Aorta to Right Common Iliac Artery, Open Approach

04100Z7 Bypass Abdominal Aorta to Left Common Iliac Artery, Open Approach

04100Z8 Bypass Abdominal Aorta to Bilateral Common Iliac Arteries, Open Approach

04100Z9 Bypass Abdominal Aorta to Right Internal Iliac Artery, Open Approach

04100ZB Bypass Abdominal Aorta to Left Internal Iliac Artery, Open Approach

04100ZC Bypass Abdominal Aorta to Bilateral Internal Iliac Arteries, Open Approach

04100ZD Bypass Abdominal Aorta to Right External Iliac Artery, Open Approach

04100ZF Bypass Abdominal Aorta to Left External Iliac Artery, Open Approach

04100ZG Bypass Abdominal Aorta to Bilateral External Iliac Arteries, Open Approach

04100ZH Bypass Abdominal Aorta to Right Femoral Artery, Open Approach

04100ZJ Bypass Abdominal Aorta to Left Femoral Artery, Open Approach

04100ZK Bypass Abdominal Aorta to Bilateral Femoral Arteries, Open Approach

04100ZQ Bypass Abdominal Aorta to Lower Extremity Artery, Open Approach

04100ZR Bypass Abdominal Aorta to Lower Artery, Open Approach

0410490 Bypass Abdominal Aorta to Abdominal Aorta with Autologous Venous Tissue, Percutaneous Endoscopic Approach

0410491 Bypass Abdominal Aorta to Celiac Artery with Autologous Venous Tissue, Percutaneous Endoscopic Approach

0410492 Bypass Abdominal Aorta to Mesenteric Artery with Autologous Venous Tissue, Percutaneous Endoscopic Approach

0410493 Bypass Abdominal Aorta to Right Renal Artery with Autologous Venous Tissue, Percutaneous Endoscopic Approach

0410494 Bypass Abdominal Aorta to Left Renal Artery with Autologous Venous Tissue, Percutaneous Endoscopic Approach

0410495 Bypass Abdominal Aorta to Bilateral Renal Artery with Autologous Venous Tissue, Percutaneous Endoscopic Approach

0410496 Bypass Abdominal Aorta to Right Common Iliac Artery with Autologous Venous Tissue, Percutaneous Endoscopic Approach

0410497 Bypass Abdominal Aorta to Left Common Iliac Artery with Autologous Venous Tissue, Percutaneous Endoscopic Approach

0410498 Bypass Abdominal Aorta to Bilateral Common Iliac Arteries with Autologous Venous Tissue, Percutaneous Endoscopic Approach

0410499 Bypass Abdominal Aorta to Right Internal Iliac Artery with Autologous Venous Tissue, Percutaneous Endoscopic Approach

041049B Bypass Abdominal Aorta to Left Internal Iliac Artery with Autologous Venous Tissue, Percutaneous Endoscopic Approach

041049C Bypass Abdominal Aorta to Bilateral Internal Iliac Arteries with Autologous Venous Tissue, Percutaneous Endoscopic Approach

041049D Bypass Abdominal Aorta to Right External Iliac Artery with Autologous Venous Tissue, Percutaneous Endoscopic Approach

041049F Bypass Abdominal Aorta to Left External Iliac Artery with Autologous Venous Tissue, Percutaneous Endoscopic Approach

041049G Bypass Abdominal Aorta to Bilateral External Iliac Arteries with Autologous Venous Tissue, Percutaneous Endoscopic Approach

041049H Bypass Abdominal Aorta to Right Femoral Artery with Autologous Venous Tissue, Percutaneous Endoscopic Approach

041049J Bypass Abdominal Aorta to Left Femoral Artery with Autologous Venous Tissue, Percutaneous Endoscopic Approach

041049K Bypass Abdominal Aorta to Bilateral Femoral Arteries with Autologous Venous Tissue, Percutaneous Endoscopic Approach

041049Q Bypass Abdominal Aorta to Lower Extremity Artery with Autologous Venous Tissue, Percutaneous Endoscopic Approach

041049R Bypass Abdominal Aorta to Lower Artery with Autologous Venous Tissue, Percutaneous Endoscopic Approach

04104A0 Bypass Abdominal Aorta to Abdominal Aorta with Autologous Arterial Tissue, Percutaneous Endoscopic Approach

04104A1 Bypass Abdominal Aorta to Celiac Artery with Autologous Arterial Tissue, Percutaneous Endoscopic Approach

04104A2 Bypass Abdominal Aorta to Mesenteric Artery with Autologous Arterial Tissue, Percutaneous Endoscopic Approach

04104A3 Bypass Abdominal Aorta to Right Renal Artery with Autologous Arterial Tissue, Percutaneous Endoscopic Approach

04104A4 Bypass Abdominal Aorta to Left Renal Artery with Autologous Arterial Tissue, Percutaneous Endoscopic Approach

04104A5 Bypass Abdominal Aorta to Bilateral Renal Artery with Autologous Arterial Tissue, Percutaneous Endoscopic Approach

04104A6 Bypass Abdominal Aorta to Right Common Iliac Artery with Autologous Arterial Tissue, Percutaneous Endoscopic Approach

04104A7 Bypass Abdominal Aorta to Left Common Iliac Artery with Autologous Arterial Tissue, Percutaneous Endoscopic Approach

04104A8 Bypass Abdominal Aorta to Bilateral Common Iliac Arteries with Autologous Arterial Tissue, Percutaneous Endoscopic Approach

04104A9 Bypass Abdominal Aorta to Right Internal Iliac Artery with Autologous Arterial Tissue, Percutaneous Endoscopic Approach

04104AB Bypass Abdominal Aorta to Left Internal Iliac Artery with Autologous Arterial Tissue, Percutaneous Endoscopic Approach

04104AC Bypass Abdominal Aorta to Bilateral Internal Iliac Arteries with Autologous Arterial Tissue, Percutaneous Endoscopic Approach

04104AD Bypass Abdominal Aorta to Right External Iliac Artery with Autologous Arterial Tissue, Percutaneous Endoscopic Approach

04104AF Bypass Abdominal Aorta to Left External Iliac Artery with Autologous Arterial Tissue, Percutaneous Endoscopic Approach

04104AG Bypass Abdominal Aorta to Bilateral External Iliac Arteries with Autologous Arterial Tissue, Percutaneous Endoscopic Approach

04104AH Bypass Abdominal Aorta to Right Femoral Artery with Autologous Arterial Tissue, Percutaneous Endoscopic Approach

04104AJ Bypass Abdominal Aorta to Left Femoral Artery with Autologous Arterial Tissue, Percutaneous Endoscopic Approach

04104AK Bypass Abdominal Aorta to Bilateral Femoral Arteries with Autologous Arterial Tissue, Percutaneous Endoscopic Approach

04104AQ Bypass Abdominal Aorta to Lower Extremity Artery with Autologous Arterial Tissue, Percutaneous Endoscopic Approach

♀ Female-only   ♂ Male-only   ▲ Limited Coverage   ● Non-OR   ᴴᴬᶜ HAC-associated procedure   ▲ Non-covered procedure

04104AR   Bypass Abdominal Aorta to Lower Artery with Autologous Arterial Tissue, Percutaneous Endoscopic Approach
04104J0   Bypass Abdominal Aorta to Abdominal Aorta with Synthetic Substitute, Percutaneous Endoscopic Approach
04104J1   Bypass Abdominal Aorta to Celiac Artery with Synthetic Substitute, Percutaneous Endoscopic Approach
04104J2   Bypass Abdominal Aorta to Mesenteric Artery with Synthetic Substitute, Percutaneous Endoscopic Approach
04104J3   Bypass Abdominal Aorta to Right Renal Artery with Synthetic Substitute, Percutaneous Endoscopic Approach
04104J4   Bypass Abdominal Aorta to Left Renal Artery with Synthetic Substitute, Percutaneous Endoscopic Approach
04104J5   Bypass Abdominal Aorta to Bilateral Renal Artery with Synthetic Substitute, Percutaneous Endoscopic Approach
04104J6   Bypass Abdominal Aorta to Right Common Iliac Artery with Synthetic Substitute, Percutaneous Endoscopic Approach
04104J7   Bypass Abdominal Aorta to Left Common Iliac Artery with Synthetic Substitute, Percutaneous Endoscopic Approach
04104J8   Bypass Abdominal Aorta to Bilateral Common Iliac Arteries with Synthetic Substitute, Percutaneous Endoscopic Approach
04104J9   Bypass Abdominal Aorta to Right Internal Iliac Artery with Synthetic Substitute, Percutaneous Endoscopic Approach
04104JB   Bypass Abdominal Aorta to Left Internal Iliac Artery with Synthetic Substitute, Percutaneous Endoscopic Approach
04104JC   Bypass Abdominal Aorta to Bilateral Internal Iliac Arteries with Synthetic Substitute, Percutaneous Endoscopic Approach
04104JD   Bypass Abdominal Aorta to Right External Iliac Artery with Synthetic Substitute, Percutaneous Endoscopic Approach
04104JF   Bypass Abdominal Aorta to Left External Iliac Artery with Synthetic Substitute, Percutaneous Endoscopic Approach
04104JG   Bypass Abdominal Aorta to Bilateral External Iliac Arteries with Synthetic Substitute, Percutaneous Endoscopic Approach
04104JH   Bypass Abdominal Aorta to Right Femoral Artery with Synthetic Substitute, Percutaneous Endoscopic Approach
04104JJ   Bypass Abdominal Aorta to Left Femoral Artery with Synthetic Substitute, Percutaneous Endoscopic Approach
04104JK   Bypass Abdominal Aorta to Bilateral Femoral Arteries with Synthetic Substitute, Percutaneous Endoscopic Approach
04104JQ   Bypass Abdominal Aorta to Lower Extremity Artery with Synthetic Substitute, Percutaneous Endoscopic Approach
04104JR   Bypass Abdominal Aorta to Lower Artery with Synthetic Substitute, Percutaneous Endoscopic Approach

04104K0   Bypass Abdominal Aorta to Abdominal Aorta with Nonautologous Tissue Substitute, Percutaneous Endoscopic Approach
04104K1   Bypass Abdominal Aorta to Celiac Artery with Nonautologous Tissue Substitute, Percutaneous Endoscopic Approach
04104K2   Bypass Abdominal Aorta to Mesenteric Artery with Nonautologous Tissue Substitute, Percutaneous Endoscopic Approach
04104K3   Bypass Abdominal Aorta to Right Renal Artery with Nonautologous Tissue Substitute, Percutaneous Endoscopic Approach
04104K4   Bypass Abdominal Aorta to Left Renal Artery with Nonautologous Tissue Substitute, Percutaneous Endoscopic Approach
04104K5   Bypass Abdominal Aorta to Bilateral Renal Artery with Nonautologous Tissue Substitute, Percutaneous Endoscopic Approach
04104K6   Bypass Abdominal Aorta to Right Common Iliac Artery with Nonautologous Tissue Substitute, Percutaneous Endoscopic Approach
04104K7   Bypass Abdominal Aorta to Left Common Iliac Artery with Nonautologous Tissue Substitute, Percutaneous Endoscopic Approach
04104K8   Bypass Abdominal Aorta to Bilateral Common Iliac Arteries with Nonautologous Tissue Substitute, Percutaneous Endoscopic Approach
04104K9   Bypass Abdominal Aorta to Right Internal Iliac Artery with Nonautologous Tissue Substitute, Percutaneous Endoscopic Approach
04104KB   Bypass Abdominal Aorta to Left Internal Iliac Artery with Nonautologous Tissue Substitute, Percutaneous Endoscopic Approach
04104KC   Bypass Abdominal Aorta to Bilateral Internal Iliac Arteries with Nonautologous Tissue Substitute, Percutaneous Endoscopic Approach
04104KD   Bypass Abdominal Aorta to Right External Iliac Artery with Nonautologous Tissue Substitute, Percutaneous Endoscopic Approach
04104KF   Bypass Abdominal Aorta to Left External Iliac Artery with Nonautologous Tissue Substitute, Percutaneous Endoscopic Approach
04104KG   Bypass Abdominal Aorta to Bilateral External Iliac Arteries with Nonautologous Tissue Substitute, Percutaneous Endoscopic Approach
04104KH   Bypass Abdominal Aorta to Right Femoral Artery with Nonautologous Tissue Substitute, Percutaneous Endoscopic Approach
04104KJ   Bypass Abdominal Aorta to Left Femoral Artery with Nonautologous Tissue Substitute, Percutaneous Endoscopic Approach
04104KK   Bypass Abdominal Aorta to Bilateral Femoral Arteries with Nonautologous Tissue Substitute, Percutaneous Endoscopic Approach
04104KQ   Bypass Abdominal Aorta to Lower Extremity Artery with Nonautologous Tissue Substitute, Percutaneous Endoscopic Approach

04104KR   Bypass Abdominal Aorta to Lower Artery with Nonautologous Tissue Substitute, Percutaneous Endoscopic Approach
04104Z0   Bypass Abdominal Aorta to Abdominal Aorta, Percutaneous Endoscopic Approach
04104Z1   Bypass Abdominal Aorta to Celiac Artery, Percutaneous Endoscopic Approach
04104Z2   Bypass Abdominal Aorta to Mesenteric Artery, Percutaneous Endoscopic Approach
04104Z3   Bypass Abdominal Aorta to Right Renal Artery, Percutaneous Endoscopic Approach
04104Z4   Bypass Abdominal Aorta to Left Renal Artery, Percutaneous Endoscopic Approach
04104Z5   Bypass Abdominal Aorta to Bilateral Renal Artery, Percutaneous Endoscopic Approach
04104Z6   Bypass Abdominal Aorta to Right Common Iliac Artery, Percutaneous Endoscopic Approach
04104Z7   Bypass Abdominal Aorta to Left Common Iliac Artery, Percutaneous Endoscopic Approach
04104Z8   Bypass Abdominal Aorta to Bilateral Common Iliac Arteries, Percutaneous Endoscopic Approach
04104Z9   Bypass Abdominal Aorta to Right Internal Iliac Artery, Percutaneous Endoscopic Approach
04104ZB   Bypass Abdominal Aorta to Left Internal Iliac Artery, Percutaneous Endoscopic Approach
04104ZC   Bypass Abdominal Aorta to Bilateral Internal Iliac Arteries, Percutaneous Endoscopic Approach
04104ZD   Bypass Abdominal Aorta to Right External Iliac Artery, Percutaneous Endoscopic Approach
04104ZF   Bypass Abdominal Aorta to Left External Iliac Artery, Percutaneous Endoscopic Approach
04104ZG   Bypass Abdominal Aorta to Bilateral External Iliac Arteries, Percutaneous Endoscopic Approach
04104ZH   Bypass Abdominal Aorta to Right Femoral Artery, Percutaneous Endoscopic Approach
04104ZJ   Bypass Abdominal Aorta to Left Femoral Artery, Percutaneous Endoscopic Approach
04104ZK   Bypass Abdominal Aorta to Bilateral Femoral Arteries, Percutaneous Endoscopic Approach
04104ZQ   Bypass Abdominal Aorta to Lower Extremity Artery, Percutaneous Endoscopic Approach
04104ZR   Bypass Abdominal Aorta to Lower Artery, Percutaneous Endoscopic Approach
0413093   Bypass Hepatic Artery to Right Renal Artery with Autologous Venous Tissue, Open Approach
0413094   Bypass Hepatic Artery to Left Renal Artery with Autologous Venous Tissue, Open Approach
0413095   Bypass Hepatic Artery to Bilateral Renal Artery with Autologous Venous Tissue, Open Approach
04130A3   Bypass Hepatic Artery to Right Renal Artery with Autologous Arterial Tissue, Open Approach

04130A4 Bypass Hepatic Artery to Left Renal Artery with Autologous Arterial Tissue, Open Approach

04130A5 Bypass Hepatic Artery to Bilateral Renal Artery with Autologous Arterial Tissue, Open Approach

04130J3 Bypass Hepatic Artery to Right Renal Artery with Synthetic Substitute, Open Approach

04130J4 Bypass Hepatic Artery to Left Renal Artery with Synthetic Substitute, Open Approach

04130J5 Bypass Hepatic Artery to Bilateral Renal Artery with Synthetic Substitute, Open Approach

04130K3 Bypass Hepatic Artery to Right Renal Artery with Nonautologous Tissue Substitute, Open Approach

04130K4 Bypass Hepatic Artery to Left Renal Artery with Nonautologous Tissue Substitute, Open Approach

04130K5 Bypass Hepatic Artery to Bilateral Renal Artery with Nonautologous Tissue Substitute, Open Approach

04130Z3 Bypass Hepatic Artery to Right Renal Artery, Open Approach
AHA CC: 4Q, 2017, 47

04130Z4 Bypass Hepatic Artery to Left Renal Artery, Open Approach

04130Z5 Bypass Hepatic Artery to Bilateral Renal Artery, Open Approach

0413493 Bypass Hepatic Artery to Right Renal Artery with Autologous Venous Tissue, Percutaneous Endoscopic Approach

0413494 Bypass Hepatic Artery to Left Renal Artery with Autologous Venous Tissue, Percutaneous Endoscopic Approach

0413495 Bypass Hepatic Artery to Bilateral Renal Artery with Autologous Venous Tissue, Percutaneous Endoscopic Approach

04134A3 Bypass Hepatic Artery to Right Renal Artery with Autologous Arterial Tissue, Percutaneous Endoscopic Approach

04134A4 Bypass Hepatic Artery to Left Renal Artery with Autologous Arterial Tissue, Percutaneous Endoscopic Approach

04134A5 Bypass Hepatic Artery to Bilateral Renal Artery with Autologous Arterial Tissue, Percutaneous Endoscopic Approach

04134J3 Bypass Hepatic Artery to Right Renal Artery with Synthetic Substitute, Percutaneous Endoscopic Approach

04134J4 Bypass Hepatic Artery to Left Renal Artery with Synthetic Substitute, Percutaneous Endoscopic Approach

04134J5 Bypass Hepatic Artery to Bilateral Renal Artery with Synthetic Substitute, Percutaneous Endoscopic Approach

04134K3 Bypass Hepatic Artery to Right Renal Artery with Nonautologous Tissue Substitute, Percutaneous Endoscopic Approach

04134K4 Bypass Hepatic Artery to Left Renal Artery with Nonautologous Tissue Substitute, Percutaneous Endoscopic Approach

04134K5 Bypass Hepatic Artery to Bilateral Renal Artery with Nonautologous Tissue Substitute, Percutaneous Endoscopic Approach

04134Z3 Bypass Hepatic Artery to Right Renal Artery, Percutaneous Endoscopic Approach

04134Z4 Bypass Hepatic Artery to Left Renal Artery, Percutaneous Endoscopic Approach

04134Z5 Bypass Hepatic Artery to Bilateral Renal Artery, Percutaneous Endoscopic Approach

0414093 Bypass Splenic Artery to Right Renal Artery with Autologous Venous Tissue, Open Approach

0414094 Bypass Splenic Artery to Left Renal Artery with Autologous Venous Tissue, Open Approach

0414095 Bypass Splenic Artery to Bilateral Renal Artery with Autologous Venous Tissue, Open Approach

04140A3 Bypass Splenic Artery to Right Renal Artery with Autologous Arterial Tissue, Open Approach

04140A4 Bypass Splenic Artery to Left Renal Artery with Autologous Arterial Tissue, Open Approach

04140A5 Bypass Splenic Artery to Bilateral Renal Artery with Autologous Arterial Tissue, Open Approach

04140J3 Bypass Splenic Artery to Right Renal Artery with Synthetic Substitute, Open Approach

04140J4 Bypass Splenic Artery to Left Renal Artery with Synthetic Substitute, Open Approach

04140J5 Bypass Splenic Artery to Bilateral Renal Artery with Synthetic Substitute, Open Approach

04140K3 Bypass Splenic Artery to Right Renal Artery with Nonautologous Tissue Substitute, Open Approach

04140K4 Bypass Splenic Artery to Left Renal Artery with Nonautologous Tissue Substitute, Open Approach

04140K5 Bypass Splenic Artery to Bilateral Renal Artery with Nonautologous Tissue Substitute, Open Approach

04140Z3 Bypass Splenic Artery to Right Renal Artery, Open Approach

04140Z4 Bypass Splenic Artery to Left Renal Artery, Open Approach
AHA CC: 3Q, 2015, 28; 4Q, 2017, 47

04140Z5 Bypass Splenic Artery to Bilateral Renal Artery, Open Approach

0414493 Bypass Splenic Artery to Right Renal Artery with Autologous Venous Tissue, Percutaneous Endoscopic Approach

0414494 Bypass Splenic Artery to Left Renal Artery with Autologous Venous Tissue, Percutaneous Endoscopic Approach

0414495 Bypass Splenic Artery to Bilateral Renal Artery with Autologous Venous Tissue, Percutaneous Endoscopic Approach

04144A3 Bypass Splenic Artery to Right Renal Artery with Autologous Arterial Tissue, Percutaneous Endoscopic Approach

04144A4 Bypass Splenic Artery to Left Renal Artery with Autologous Arterial Tissue, Percutaneous Endoscopic Approach

04144A5 Bypass Splenic Artery to Bilateral Renal Artery with Autologous Arterial Tissue, Percutaneous Endoscopic Approach

04144J3 Bypass Splenic Artery to Right Renal Artery with Synthetic Substitute, Percutaneous Endoscopic Approach

04144J4 Bypass Splenic Artery to Left Renal Artery with Synthetic Substitute, Percutaneous Endoscopic Approach

04144J5 Bypass Splenic Artery to Bilateral Renal Artery with Synthetic Substitute, Percutaneous Endoscopic Approach

04144K3 Bypass Splenic Artery to Right Renal Artery with Nonautologous Tissue Substitute, Percutaneous Endoscopic Approach

04144K4 Bypass Splenic Artery to Left Renal Artery with Nonautologous Tissue Substitute, Percutaneous Endoscopic Approach

04144K5 Bypass Splenic Artery to Bilateral Renal Artery with Nonautologous Tissue Substitute, Percutaneous Endoscopic Approach

04144Z3 Bypass Splenic Artery to Right Renal Artery, Percutaneous Endoscopic Approach

04144Z4 Bypass Splenic Artery to Left Renal Artery, Percutaneous Endoscopic Approach

04144Z5 Bypass Splenic Artery to Bilateral Renal Artery, Percutaneous Endoscopic Approach

041C090 Bypass Right Common Iliac Artery to Abdominal Aorta with Autologous Venous Tissue, Open Approach

041C091 Bypass Right Common Iliac Artery to Celiac Artery with Autologous Venous Tissue, Open Approach

041C092 Bypass Right Common Iliac Artery to Mesenteric Artery with Autologous Venous Tissue, Open Approach

041C093 Bypass Right Common Iliac Artery to Right Renal Artery with Autologous Venous Tissue, Open Approach

041C094 Bypass Right Common Iliac Artery to Left Renal Artery with Autologous Venous Tissue, Open Approach

041C095 Bypass Right Common Iliac Artery to Bilateral Renal Artery with Autologous Venous Tissue, Open Approach

041C096 Bypass Right Common Iliac Artery to Right Common Iliac Artery with Autologous Venous Tissue, Open Approach

041C097 Bypass Right Common Iliac Artery to Left Common Iliac Artery with Autologous Venous Tissue, Open Approach

041C098 Bypass Right Common Iliac Artery to Bilateral Common Iliac Arteries with Autologous Venous Tissue, Open Approach

041C099 Bypass Right Common Iliac Artery to Right Internal Iliac Artery with Autologous Venous Tissue, Open Approach

041C09B Bypass Right Common Iliac Artery to Left Internal Iliac Artery with Autologous Venous Tissue, Open Approach

041C09C Bypass Right Common Iliac Artery to Bilateral Internal Iliac Arteries with Autologous Venous Tissue, Open Approach

041C09D Bypass Right Common Iliac Artery to Right External Iliac Artery with Autologous Venous Tissue, Open Approach

041C09F Bypass Right Common Iliac Artery to Left External Iliac Artery with Autologous Venous Tissue, Open Approach

041C09G Bypass Right Common Iliac Artery to Bilateral External Iliac Arteries with Autologous Venous Tissue, Open Approach

041C09H Bypass Right Common Iliac Artery to Right Femoral Artery with Autologous Venous Tissue, Open Approach

041C09J Bypass Right Common Iliac Artery to Left Femoral Artery with Autologous Venous Tissue, Open Approach

041C09K Bypass Right Common Iliac Artery to Bilateral Femoral Arteries with Autologous Venous Tissue, Open Approach

041C09Q Bypass Right Common Iliac Artery to Lower Extremity Artery with Autologous Venous Tissue, Open Approach

041C09R Bypass Right Common Iliac Artery to Lower Artery with Autologous Venous Tissue, Open Approach

041C0A0 Bypass Right Common Iliac Artery to Abdominal Aorta with Autologous Arterial Tissue, Open Approach

041C0A1 Bypass Right Common Iliac Artery to Celiac Artery with Autologous Arterial Tissue, Open Approach

041C0A2 Bypass Right Common Iliac Artery to Mesenteric Artery with Autologous Arterial Tissue, Open Approach

041C0A3 Bypass Right Common Iliac Artery to Right Renal Artery with Autologous Arterial Tissue, Open Approach

041C0A4 Bypass Right Common Iliac Artery to Left Renal Artery with Autologous Arterial Tissue, Open Approach

041C0A5 Bypass Right Common Iliac Artery to Bilateral Renal Artery with Autologous Arterial Tissue, Open Approach

041C0A6 Bypass Right Common Iliac Artery to Right Common Iliac Artery with Autologous Arterial Tissue, Open Approach

041C0A7 Bypass Right Common Iliac Artery to Left Common Iliac Artery with Autologous Arterial Tissue, Open Approach

041C0A8 Bypass Right Common Iliac Artery to Bilateral Common Iliac Arteries with Autologous Arterial Tissue, Open Approach

041C0A9 Bypass Right Common Iliac Artery to Right Internal Iliac Artery with Autologous Arterial Tissue, Open Approach

041C0AB Bypass Right Common Iliac Artery to Left Internal Iliac Artery with Autologous Arterial Tissue, Open Approach

041C0AC Bypass Right Common Iliac Artery to Bilateral Internal Iliac Arteries with Autologous Arterial Tissue, Open Approach

041C0AD Bypass Right Common Iliac Artery to Right External Iliac Artery with Autologous Arterial Tissue, Open Approach

041C0AF Bypass Right Common Iliac Artery to Left External Iliac Artery with Autologous Arterial Tissue, Open Approach

041C0AG Bypass Right Common Iliac Artery to Bilateral External Iliac Arteries with Autologous Arterial Tissue, Open Approach

041C0AH Bypass Right Common Iliac Artery to Right Femoral Artery with Autologous Arterial Tissue, Open Approach

041C0AJ Bypass Right Common Iliac Artery to Left Femoral Artery with Autologous Arterial Tissue, Open Approach

041C0AK Bypass Right Common Iliac Artery to Bilateral Femoral Arteries with Autologous Arterial Tissue, Open Approach

041C0AQ Bypass Right Common Iliac Artery to Lower Extremity Artery with Autologous Arterial Tissue, Open Approach

041C0AR Bypass Right Common Iliac Artery to Lower Artery with Autologous Arterial Tissue, Open Approach

041C0J0 Bypass Right Common Iliac Artery to Abdominal Aorta with Synthetic Substitute, Open Approach

041C0J1 Bypass Right Common Iliac Artery to Celiac Artery with Synthetic Substitute, Open Approach

041C0J2 Bypass Right Common Iliac Artery to Mesenteric Artery with Synthetic Substitute, Open Approach
AHA CC: 3Q, 2017, 16

041C0J3 Bypass Right Common Iliac Artery to Right Renal Artery with Synthetic Substitute, Open Approach

041C0J4 Bypass Right Common Iliac Artery to Left Renal Artery with Synthetic Substitute, Open Approach

041C0J5 Bypass Right Common Iliac Artery to Bilateral Renal Artery with Synthetic Substitute, Open Approach
AHA CC: 3Q, 2017, 16

041C0J6 Bypass Right Common Iliac Artery to Right Common Iliac Artery with Synthetic Substitute, Open Approach

041C0J7 Bypass Right Common Iliac Artery to Left Common Iliac Artery with Synthetic Substitute, Open Approach

041C0J8 Bypass Right Common Iliac Artery to Bilateral Common Iliac Arteries with Synthetic Substitute, Open Approach

041C0J9 Bypass Right Common Iliac Artery to Right Internal Iliac Artery with Synthetic Substitute, Open Approach

041C0JB Bypass Right Common Iliac Artery to Left Internal Iliac Artery with Synthetic Substitute, Open Approach

041C0JC Bypass Right Common Iliac Artery to Bilateral Internal Iliac Arteries with Synthetic Substitute, Open Approach

041C0JD Bypass Right Common Iliac Artery to Right External Iliac Artery with Synthetic Substitute, Open Approach

041C0JF Bypass Right Common Iliac Artery to Left External Iliac Artery with Synthetic Substitute, Open Approach

041C0JG Bypass Right Common Iliac Artery to Bilateral External Iliac Arteries with Synthetic Substitute, Open Approach

041C0JH Bypass Right Common Iliac Artery to Right Femoral Artery with Synthetic Substitute, Open Approach

041C0JJ Bypass Right Common Iliac Artery to Left Femoral Artery with Synthetic Substitute, Open Approach

041C0JK Bypass Right Common Iliac Artery to Bilateral Femoral Arteries with Synthetic Substitute, Open Approach

041C0JQ Bypass Right Common Iliac Artery to Lower Extremity Artery with Synthetic Substitute, Open Approach

041C0JR Bypass Right Common Iliac Artery to Lower Artery with Synthetic Substitute, Open Approach

041C0K0 Bypass Right Common Iliac Artery to Abdominal Aorta with Nonautologous Tissue Substitute, Open Approach

041C0K1 Bypass Right Common Iliac Artery to Celiac Artery with Nonautologous Tissue Substitute, Open Approach

041C0K2 Bypass Right Common Iliac Artery to Mesenteric Artery with Nonautologous Tissue Substitute, Open Approach

041C0K3 Bypass Right Common Iliac Artery to Right Renal Artery with Nonautologous Tissue Substitute, Open Approach

041C0K4 Bypass Right Common Iliac Artery to Left Renal Artery with Nonautologous Tissue Substitute, Open Approach

041C0K5 Bypass Right Common Iliac Artery to Bilateral Renal Artery with Nonautologous Tissue Substitute, Open Approach

041C0K6 Bypass Right Common Iliac Artery to Right Common Iliac Artery with Nonautologous Tissue Substitute, Open Approach

041C0K7 Bypass Right Common Iliac Artery to Left Common Iliac Artery with Nonautologous Tissue Substitute, Open Approach

041C0K8 Bypass Right Common Iliac Artery to Bilateral Common Iliac Arteries with Nonautologous Tissue Substitute, Open Approach

041C0K9 Bypass Right Common Iliac Artery to Right Internal Iliac Artery with Nonautologous Tissue Substitute, Open Approach

041C0KB Bypass Right Common Iliac Artery to Left Internal Iliac Artery with Nonautologous Tissue Substitute, Open Approach

041C0KC Bypass Right Common Iliac Artery to Bilateral Internal Iliac Arteries with Nonautologous Tissue Substitute, Open Approach

041C0KD Bypass Right Common Iliac Artery to Right External Iliac Artery with Nonautologous Tissue Substitute, Open Approach

041C0KF Bypass Right Common Iliac Artery to Left External Iliac Artery with Nonautologous Tissue Substitute, Open Approach

041C0KG Bypass Right Common Iliac Artery to Bilateral External Iliac Arteries with Nonautologous Tissue Substitute, Open Approach

041C0KH Bypass Right Common Iliac Artery to Right Femoral Artery with Nonautologous Tissue Substitute, Open Approach

041C0KJ Bypass Right Common Iliac Artery to Left Femoral Artery with Nonautologous Tissue Substitute, Open Approach

041C0KK Bypass Right Common Iliac Artery to Bilateral Femoral Arteries with Nonautologous Tissue Substitute, Open Approach

041C0KQ Bypass Right Common Iliac Artery to Lower Extremity Artery with Nonautologous Tissue Substitute, Open Approach

041C0KR Bypass Right Common Iliac Artery to Lower Artery with Nonautologous Tissue Substitute, Open Approach

041C0Z0 Bypass Right Common Iliac Artery to Abdominal Aorta, Open Approach

041C0Z1 Bypass Right Common Iliac Artery to Celiac Artery, Open Approach

041C0Z2 Bypass Right Common Iliac Artery to Mesenteric Artery, Open Approach

041C0Z3 Bypass Right Common Iliac Artery to Right Renal Artery, Open Approach

041C0Z4 Bypass Right Common Iliac Artery to Left Renal Artery, Open Approach

041C0Z5 Bypass Right Common Iliac Artery to Bilateral Renal Artery, Open Approach

041C0Z6 Bypass Right Common Iliac Artery to Right Common Iliac Artery, Open Approach

041C0Z7 Bypass Right Common Iliac Artery to Left Common Iliac Artery, Open Approach

041C0Z8 Bypass Right Common Iliac Artery to Bilateral Common Iliac Arteries, Open Approach

041C0Z9 Bypass Right Common Iliac Artery to Right Internal Iliac Artery, Open Approach

041C0ZB Bypass Right Common Iliac Artery to Left Internal Iliac Artery, Open Approach

041C0ZC Bypass Right Common Iliac Artery to Bilateral Internal Iliac Arteries, Open Approach

041C0ZD Bypass Right Common Iliac Artery to Right External Iliac Artery, Open Approach

041C0ZF Bypass Right Common Iliac Artery to Left External Iliac Artery, Open Approach

041C0ZG Bypass Right Common Iliac Artery to Bilateral External Iliac Arteries, Open Approach

041C0ZH Bypass Right Common Iliac Artery to Right Femoral Artery, Open Approach

041C0ZJ Bypass Right Common Iliac Artery to Left Femoral Artery, Open Approach

041C0ZK Bypass Right Common Iliac Artery to Bilateral Femoral Arteries, Open Approach

041C0ZQ Bypass Right Common Iliac Artery to Lower Extremity Artery, Open Approach

041C0ZR Bypass Right Common Iliac Artery to Lower Artery, Open Approach

041C490 Bypass Right Common Iliac Artery to Abdominal Aorta with Autologous Venous Tissue, Percutaneous Endoscopic Approach

041C491 Bypass Right Common Iliac Artery to Celiac Artery with Autologous Venous Tissue, Percutaneous Endoscopic Approach

041C492 Bypass Right Common Iliac Artery to Mesenteric Artery with Autologous Venous Tissue, Percutaneous Endoscopic Approach

041C493 Bypass Right Common Iliac Artery to Right Renal Artery with Autologous Venous Tissue, Percutaneous Endoscopic Approach

041C494 Bypass Right Common Iliac Artery to Left Renal Artery with Autologous Venous Tissue, Percutaneous Endoscopic Approach

041C495 Bypass Right Common Iliac Artery to Bilateral Renal Artery with Autologous Venous Tissue, Percutaneous Endoscopic Approach

041C496 Bypass Right Common Iliac Artery to Right Common Iliac Artery with Autologous Venous Tissue, Percutaneous Endoscopic Approach

041C497 Bypass Right Common Iliac Artery to Left Common Iliac Artery with Autologous Venous Tissue, Percutaneous Endoscopic Approach

041C498 Bypass Right Common Iliac Artery to Bilateral Common Iliac Arteries with Autologous Venous Tissue, Percutaneous Endoscopic Approach

041C499 Bypass Right Common Iliac Artery to Right Internal Iliac Artery with Autologous Venous Tissue, Percutaneous Endoscopic Approach

041C49B Bypass Right Common Iliac Artery to Left Internal Iliac Artery with Autologous Venous Tissue, Percutaneous Endoscopic Approach

041C49C Bypass Right Common Iliac Artery to Bilateral Internal Iliac Arteries with Autologous Venous Tissue, Percutaneous Endoscopic Approach

041C49D Bypass Right Common Iliac Artery to Right External Iliac Artery with Autologous Venous Tissue, Percutaneous Endoscopic Approach

041C49F Bypass Right Common Iliac Artery to Left External Iliac Artery with Autologous Venous Tissue, Percutaneous Endoscopic Approach

041C49G Bypass Right Common Iliac Artery to Bilateral External Iliac Arteries with Autologous Venous Tissue, Percutaneous Endoscopic Approach

041C49H Bypass Right Common Iliac Artery to Right Femoral Artery with Autologous Venous Tissue, Percutaneous Endoscopic Approach

041C49J Bypass Right Common Iliac Artery to Left Femoral Artery with Autologous Venous Tissue, Percutaneous Endoscopic Approach

041C49K Bypass Right Common Iliac Artery to Bilateral Femoral Arteries with Autologous Venous Tissue, Percutaneous Endoscopic Approach

041C49Q Bypass Right Common Iliac Artery to Lower Extremity Artery with Autologous Venous Tissue, Percutaneous Endoscopic Approach

041C49R Bypass Right Common Iliac Artery to Lower Artery with Autologous Venous Tissue, Percutaneous Endoscopic Approach

041C4A0 Bypass Right Common Iliac Artery to Abdominal Aorta with Autologous Arterial Tissue, Percutaneous Endoscopic Approach

041C4A1 Bypass Right Common Iliac Artery to Celiac Artery with Autologous Arterial Tissue, Percutaneous Endoscopic Approach

041C4A2 Bypass Right Common Iliac Artery to Mesenteric Artery with Autologous Arterial Tissue, Percutaneous Endoscopic Approach

041C4A3 Bypass Right Common Iliac Artery to Right Renal Artery with Autologous Arterial Tissue, Percutaneous Endoscopic Approach

041C4A4 Bypass Right Common Iliac Artery to Left Renal Artery with Autologous Arterial Tissue, Percutaneous Endoscopic Approach

041C4A5 Bypass Right Common Iliac Artery to Bilateral Renal Artery with Autologous Arterial Tissue, Percutaneous Endoscopic Approach

041C4A6 Bypass Right Common Iliac Artery to Right Common Iliac Artery with Autologous Arterial Tissue, Percutaneous Endoscopic Approach

041C4A7 Bypass Right Common Iliac Artery to Left Common Iliac Artery with Autologous Arterial Tissue, Percutaneous Endoscopic Approach

041C4A8 Bypass Right Common Iliac Artery to Bilateral Common Iliac Arteries with Autologous Arterial Tissue, Percutaneous Endoscopic Approach

041C4A9 Bypass Right Common Iliac Artery to Right Internal Iliac Artery with Autologous Arterial Tissue, Percutaneous Endoscopic Approach

041C4AB Bypass Right Common Iliac Artery to Left Internal Iliac Artery with Autologous Arterial Tissue, Percutaneous Endoscopic Approach

041C4AC Bypass Right Common Iliac Artery to Bilateral Internal Iliac Arteries with Autologous Arterial Tissue, Percutaneous Endoscopic Approach

041C4AD Bypass Right Common Iliac Artery to Right External Iliac Artery with Autologous Arterial Tissue, Percutaneous Endoscopic Approach

041C4AF Bypass Right Common Iliac Artery to Left External Iliac Artery with Autologous Arterial Tissue, Percutaneous Endoscopic Approach

041C4AG Bypass Right Common Iliac Artery to Bilateral External Iliac Arteries with Autologous Arterial Tissue, Percutaneous Endoscopic Approach

041C4AH Bypass Right Common Iliac Artery to Right Femoral Artery with Autologous Arterial Tissue, Percutaneous Endoscopic Approach

041C4AJ Bypass Right Common Iliac Artery to Left Femoral Artery with Autologous Arterial Tissue, Percutaneous Endoscopic Approach

041C4AK Bypass Right Common Iliac Artery to Bilateral Femoral Arteries with Autologous Arterial Tissue, Percutaneous Endoscopic Approach

041C4AQ Bypass Right Common Iliac Artery to Lower Extremity Artery with Autologous Arterial Tissue, Percutaneous Endoscopic Approach

041C4AR Bypass Right Common Iliac Artery to Lower Artery with Autologous Arterial Tissue, Percutaneous Endoscopic Approach

041C4J0 Bypass Right Common Iliac Artery to Abdominal Aorta with Synthetic Substitute, Percutaneous Endoscopic Approach

041C4J1 Bypass Right Common Iliac Artery to Celiac Artery with Synthetic Substitute, Percutaneous Endoscopic Approach

041C4J2 Bypass Right Common Iliac Artery to Mesenteric Artery with Synthetic Substitute, Percutaneous Endoscopic Approach

041C4J3 Bypass Right Common Iliac Artery to Right Renal Artery with Synthetic Substitute, Percutaneous Endoscopic Approach

041C4J4 Bypass Right Common Iliac Artery to Left Renal Artery with Synthetic Substitute, Percutaneous Endoscopic Approach

041C4J5 Bypass Right Common Iliac Artery to Bilateral Renal Artery with Synthetic Substitute, Percutaneous Endoscopic Approach

041C4J6 Bypass Right Common Iliac Artery to Right Common Iliac Artery with Synthetic Substitute, Percutaneous Endoscopic Approach

041C4J7 Bypass Right Common Iliac Artery to Left Common Iliac Artery with Synthetic Substitute, Percutaneous Endoscopic Approach

041C4J8 Bypass Right Common Iliac Artery to Bilateral Common Iliac Arteries with Synthetic Substitute, Percutaneous Endoscopic Approach

041C4J9 Bypass Right Common Iliac Artery to Right Internal Iliac Artery with Synthetic Substitute, Percutaneous Endoscopic Approach

041C4JB Bypass Right Common Iliac Artery to Left Internal Iliac Artery with Synthetic Substitute, Percutaneous Endoscopic Approach

041C4JC Bypass Right Common Iliac Artery to Bilateral Internal Iliac Arteries with Synthetic Substitute, Percutaneous Endoscopic Approach

041C4JD Bypass Right Common Iliac Artery to Right External Iliac Artery with Synthetic Substitute, Percutaneous Endoscopic Approach

041C4JF Bypass Right Common Iliac Artery to Left External Iliac Artery with Synthetic Substitute, Percutaneous Endoscopic Approach

041C4JG Bypass Right Common Iliac Artery to Bilateral External Iliac Arteries with Synthetic Substitute, Percutaneous Endoscopic Approach

041C4JH Bypass Right Common Iliac Artery to Right Femoral Artery with Synthetic Substitute, Percutaneous Endoscopic Approach

041C4JJ Bypass Right Common Iliac Artery to Left Femoral Artery with Synthetic Substitute, Percutaneous Endoscopic Approach

041C4JK Bypass Right Common Iliac Artery to Bilateral Femoral Arteries with Synthetic Substitute, Percutaneous Endoscopic Approach

041C4JQ Bypass Right Common Iliac Artery to Lower Extremity Artery with Synthetic Substitute, Percutaneous Endoscopic Approach

041C4JR Bypass Right Common Iliac Artery to Lower Artery with Synthetic Substitute, Percutaneous Endoscopic Approach

041C4K0 Bypass Right Common Iliac Artery to Abdominal Aorta with Nonautologous Tissue Substitute, Percutaneous Endoscopic Approach

041C4K1 Bypass Right Common Iliac Artery to Celiac Artery with Nonautologous Tissue Substitute, Percutaneous Endoscopic Approach

041C4K2 Bypass Right Common Iliac Artery to Mesenteric Artery with Nonautologous Tissue Substitute, Percutaneous Endoscopic Approach

041C4K3 Bypass Right Common Iliac Artery to Right Renal Artery with Nonautologous Tissue Substitute, Percutaneous Endoscopic Approach

041C4K4 Bypass Right Common Iliac Artery to Left Renal Artery with Nonautologous Tissue Substitute, Percutaneous Endoscopic Approach

041C4K5 Bypass Right Common Iliac Artery to Bilateral Renal Artery with Nonautologous Tissue Substitute, Percutaneous Endoscopic Approach

041C4K6 Bypass Right Common Iliac Artery to Right Common Iliac Artery with Nonautologous Tissue Substitute, Percutaneous Endoscopic Approach

041C4K7 Bypass Right Common Iliac Artery to Left Common Iliac Artery with Nonautologous Tissue Substitute, Percutaneous Endoscopic Approach

041C4K8 Bypass Right Common Iliac Artery to Bilateral Common Iliac Arteries with Nonautologous Tissue Substitute, Percutaneous Endoscopic Approach

041C4K9 Bypass Right Common Iliac Artery to Right Internal Iliac Artery with Nonautologous Tissue Substitute, Percutaneous Endoscopic Approach

041C4KB Bypass Right Common Iliac Artery to Left Internal Iliac Artery with Nonautologous Tissue Substitute, Percutaneous Endoscopic Approach

041C4KC Bypass Right Common Iliac Artery to Bilateral Internal Iliac Arteries with Nonautologous Tissue Substitute, Percutaneous Endoscopic Approach

041C4KD Bypass Right Common Iliac Artery to Right External Iliac Artery with Nonautologous Tissue Substitute, Percutaneous Endoscopic Approach

041C4KF Bypass Right Common Iliac Artery to Left External Iliac Artery with Nonautologous Tissue Substitute, Percutaneous Endoscopic Approach

041C4KG Bypass Right Common Iliac Artery to Bilateral External Iliac Arteries with Nonautologous Tissue Substitute, Percutaneous Endoscopic Approach

041C4KH Bypass Right Common Iliac Artery to Right Femoral Artery with Nonautologous Tissue Substitute, Percutaneous Endoscopic Approach

041C4KJ Bypass Right Common Iliac Artery to Left Femoral Artery with Nonautologous Tissue Substitute, Percutaneous Endoscopic Approach

041C4KK Bypass Right Common Iliac Artery to Bilateral Femoral Arteries with Nonautologous Tissue Substitute, Percutaneous Endoscopic Approach

041C4KQ Bypass Right Common Iliac Artery to Lower Extremity Artery with Nonautologous Tissue Substitute, Percutaneous Endoscopic Approach

041C4KR Bypass Right Common Iliac Artery to Lower Artery with Nonautologous Tissue Substitute, Percutaneous Endoscopic Approach

041C4Z0 Bypass Right Common Iliac Artery to Abdominal Aorta, Percutaneous Endoscopic Approach

041C4Z1 Bypass Right Common Iliac Artery to Celiac Artery, Percutaneous Endoscopic Approach

041C4Z2 Bypass Right Common Iliac Artery to Mesenteric Artery, Percutaneous Endoscopic Approach

041C4Z3 Bypass Right Common Iliac Artery to Right Renal Artery, Percutaneous Endoscopic Approach

041C4Z4 Bypass Right Common Iliac Artery to Left Renal Artery, Percutaneous Endoscopic Approach

041C4Z5 Bypass Right Common Iliac Artery to Bilateral Renal Artery, Percutaneous Endoscopic Approach

041C4Z6 Bypass Right Common Iliac Artery to Right Common Iliac Artery, Percutaneous Endoscopic Approach

041C4Z7 Bypass Right Common Iliac Artery to Left Common Iliac Artery, Percutaneous Endoscopic Approach

041C4Z8 Bypass Right Common Iliac Artery to Bilateral Common Iliac Arteries, Percutaneous Endoscopic Approach

041C4Z9 Bypass Right Common Iliac Artery to Right Internal Iliac Artery, Percutaneous Endoscopic Approach

041C4ZB Bypass Right Common Iliac Artery to Left Internal Iliac Artery, Percutaneous Endoscopic Approach

041C4ZC Bypass Right Common Iliac Artery to Bilateral Internal Iliac Arteries, Percutaneous Endoscopic Approach

041C4ZD Bypass Right Common Iliac Artery to Right External Iliac Artery, Percutaneous Endoscopic Approach

041C4ZF Bypass Right Common Iliac Artery to Left External Iliac Artery, Percutaneous Endoscopic Approach

041C4ZG Bypass Right Common Iliac Artery to Bilateral External Iliac Arteries, Percutaneous Endoscopic Approach

041C4ZH Bypass Right Common Iliac Artery to Right Femoral Artery, Percutaneous Endoscopic Approach

041C4ZJ Bypass Right Common Iliac Artery to Left Femoral Artery, Percutaneous Endoscopic Approach

041C4ZK Bypass Right Common Iliac Artery to Bilateral Femoral Arteries, Percutaneous Endoscopic Approach

041C4ZQ Bypass Right Common Iliac Artery to Lower Extremity Artery, Percutaneous Endoscopic Approach

041C4ZR Bypass Right Common Iliac Artery to Lower Artery, Percutaneous Endoscopic Approach

041D090 Bypass Left Common Iliac Artery to Abdominal Aorta with Autologous Venous Tissue, Open Approach

041D091 Bypass Left Common Iliac Artery to Celiac Artery with Autologous Venous Tissue, Open Approach

041D092 Bypass Left Common Iliac Artery to Mesenteric Artery with Autologous Venous Tissue, Open Approach

041D093 Bypass Left Common Iliac Artery to Right Renal Artery with Autologous Venous Tissue, Open Approach

041D094 Bypass Left Common Iliac Artery to Left Renal Artery with Autologous Venous Tissue, Open Approach

041D095 Bypass Left Common Iliac Artery to Bilateral Renal Artery with Autologous Venous Tissue, Open Approach

041D096 Bypass Left Common Iliac Artery to Right Common Iliac Artery with Autologous Venous Tissue, Open Approach

041D097 Bypass Left Common Iliac Artery to Left Common Iliac Artery with Autologous Venous Tissue, Open Approach

041D098 Bypass Left Common Iliac Artery to Bilateral Common Iliac Arteries with Autologous Venous Tissue, Open Approach

041D099 Bypass Left Common Iliac Artery to Right Internal Iliac Artery with Autologous Venous Tissue, Open Approach

041D09B Bypass Left Common Iliac Artery to Left Internal Iliac Artery with Autologous Venous Tissue, Open Approach

041D09C Bypass Left Common Iliac Artery to Bilateral Internal Iliac Arteries with Autologous Venous Tissue, Open Approach

041D09D Bypass Left Common Iliac Artery to Right External Iliac Artery with Autologous Venous Tissue, Open Approach

041D09F Bypass Left Common Iliac Artery to Left External Iliac Artery with Autologous Venous Tissue, Open Approach

041D09G Bypass Left Common Iliac Artery to Bilateral External Iliac Arteries with Autologous Venous Tissue, Open Approach

041D09H Bypass Left Common Iliac Artery to Right Femoral Artery with Autologous Venous Tissue, Open Approach

041D09J Bypass Left Common Iliac Artery to Left Femoral Artery with Autologous Venous Tissue, Open Approach

041D09K Bypass Left Common Iliac Artery to Bilateral Femoral Arteries with Autologous Venous Tissue, Open Approach

041D09Q Bypass Left Common Iliac Artery to Lower Extremity Artery with Autologous Venous Tissue, Open Approach

041D09R Bypass Left Common Iliac Artery to Lower Artery with Autologous Venous Tissue, Open Approach

041D0A0 Bypass Left Common Iliac Artery to Abdominal Aorta with Autologous Arterial Tissue, Open Approach

041D0A1 Bypass Left Common Iliac Artery to Celiac Artery with Autologous Arterial Tissue, Open Approach

041D0A2 Bypass Left Common Iliac Artery to Mesenteric Artery with Autologous Arterial Tissue, Open Approach

041D0A3 Bypass Left Common Iliac Artery to Right Renal Artery with Autologous Arterial Tissue, Open Approach

041D0A4 Bypass Left Common Iliac Artery to Left Renal Artery with Autologous Arterial Tissue, Open Approach

041D0A5 Bypass Left Common Iliac Artery to Bilateral Renal Artery with Autologous Arterial Tissue, Open Approach

041D0A6 Bypass Left Common Iliac Artery to Right Common Iliac Artery with Autologous Arterial Tissue, Open Approach

041D0A7 Bypass Left Common Iliac Artery to Left Common Iliac Artery with Autologous Arterial Tissue, Open Approach

041D0A8 Bypass Left Common Iliac Artery to Bilateral Common Iliac Arteries with Autologous Arterial Tissue, Open Approach

041D0A9 Bypass Left Common Iliac Artery to Right Internal Iliac Artery with Autologous Arterial Tissue, Open Approach

041D0AB Bypass Left Common Iliac Artery to Left Internal Iliac Artery with Autologous Arterial Tissue, Open Approach

041D0AC Bypass Left Common Iliac Artery to Bilateral Internal Iliac Arteries with Autologous Arterial Tissue, Open Approach

041D0AD Bypass Left Common Iliac Artery to Right External Iliac Artery with Autologous Arterial Tissue, Open Approach

041D0AF Bypass Left Common Iliac Artery to Left External Iliac Artery with Autologous Arterial Tissue, Open Approach

041D0AG Bypass Left Common Iliac Artery to Bilateral External Iliac Arteries with Autologous Arterial Tissue, Open Approach

041D0AH Bypass Left Common Iliac Artery to Right Femoral Artery with Autologous Arterial Tissue, Open Approach

041D0AJ Bypass Left Common Iliac Artery to Left Femoral Artery with Autologous Arterial Tissue, Open Approach

041D0AK Bypass Left Common Iliac Artery to Bilateral Femoral Arteries with Autologous Arterial Tissue, Open Approach

041D0AQ Bypass Left Common Iliac Artery to Lower Extremity Artery with Autologous Arterial Tissue, Open Approach

041D0AR Bypass Left Common Iliac Artery to Lower Artery with Autologous Arterial Tissue, Open Approach

041D0J0 Bypass Left Common Iliac Artery to Abdominal Aorta with Synthetic Substitute, Open Approach

041D0J1 Bypass Left Common Iliac Artery to Celiac Artery with Synthetic Substitute, Open Approach

041D0J2 Bypass Left Common Iliac Artery to Mesenteric Artery with Synthetic Substitute, Open Approach

041D0J3 Bypass Left Common Iliac Artery to Right Renal Artery with Synthetic Substitute, Open Approach

041D0J4 Bypass Left Common Iliac Artery to Left Renal Artery with Synthetic Substitute, Open Approach

041D0J5 Bypass Left Common Iliac Artery to Bilateral Renal Artery with Synthetic Substitute, Open Approach

041D0J6 Bypass Left Common Iliac Artery to Right Common Iliac Artery with Synthetic Substitute, Open Approach

041D0J7 Bypass Left Common Iliac Artery to Left Common Iliac Artery with Synthetic Substitute, Open Approach

041D0J8 Bypass Left Common Iliac Artery to Bilateral Common Iliac Arteries with Synthetic Substitute, Open Approach

041D0J9 Bypass Left Common Iliac Artery to Right Internal Iliac Artery with Synthetic Substitute, Open Approach

041D0JB Bypass Left Common Iliac Artery to Left Internal Iliac Artery with Synthetic Substitute, Open Approach

041D0JC Bypass Left Common Iliac Artery to Bilateral Internal Iliac Arteries with Synthetic Substitute, Open Approach

041D0JD Bypass Left Common Iliac Artery to Right External Iliac Artery with Synthetic Substitute, Open Approach

041D0JF Bypass Left Common Iliac Artery to Left External Iliac Artery with Synthetic Substitute, Open Approach

041D0JG Bypass Left Common Iliac Artery to Bilateral External Iliac Arteries with Synthetic Substitute, Open Approach

041D0JH Bypass Left Common Iliac Artery to Right Femoral Artery with Synthetic Substitute, Open Approach

041D0JJ Bypass Left Common Iliac Artery to Left Femoral Artery with Synthetic Substitute, Open Approach

041D0JK Bypass Left Common Iliac Artery to Bilateral Femoral Arteries with Synthetic Substitute, Open Approach

041D0JQ Bypass Left Common Iliac Artery to Lower Extremity Artery with Synthetic Substitute, Open Approach

041D0JR Bypass Left Common Iliac Artery to Lower Artery with Synthetic Substitute, Open Approach

041D0K0 Bypass Left Common Iliac Artery to Abdominal Aorta with Nonautologous Tissue Substitute, Open Approach

041D0K1 Bypass Left Common Iliac Artery to Celiac Artery with Nonautologous Tissue Substitute, Open Approach

041D0K2 Bypass Left Common Iliac Artery to Mesenteric Artery with Nonautologous Tissue Substitute, Open Approach

041D0K3 Bypass Left Common Iliac Artery to Right Renal Artery with Nonautologous Tissue Substitute, Open Approach

041D0K4 Bypass Left Common Iliac Artery to Left Renal Artery with Nonautologous Tissue Substitute, Open Approach

041D0K5 Bypass Left Common Iliac Artery to Bilateral Renal Artery with Nonautologous Tissue Substitute, Open Approach

041D0K6 Bypass Left Common Iliac Artery to Right Common Iliac Artery with Nonautologous Tissue Substitute, Open Approach

041D0K7 Bypass Left Common Iliac Artery to Left Common Iliac Artery with Nonautologous Tissue Substitute, Open Approach

041D0K8 Bypass Left Common Iliac Artery to Bilateral Common Iliac Arteries with Nonautologous Tissue Substitute, Open Approach

041D0K9 Bypass Left Common Iliac Artery to Right Internal Iliac Artery with Nonautologous Tissue Substitute, Open Approach

041D0KB Bypass Left Common Iliac Artery to Left Internal Iliac Artery with Nonautologous Tissue Substitute, Open Approach

041D0KC Bypass Left Common Iliac Artery to Bilateral Internal Iliac Arteries with Nonautologous Tissue Substitute, Open Approach

♀ Female-only   ♂ Male-only   ▲ Limited Coverage   ● Non-OR   **HAC** HAC-associated procedure   ▲ Non-covered procedures   ✚ Cluster

041D0KD Bypass Left Common Iliac Artery to Right External Iliac Artery with Nonautologous Tissue Substitute, Open Approach

041D0KF Bypass Left Common Iliac Artery to Left External Iliac Artery with Nonautologous Tissue Substitute, Open Approach

041D0KG Bypass Left Common Iliac Artery to Bilateral External Iliac Arteries with Nonautologous Tissue Substitute, Open Approach

041D0KH Bypass Left Common Iliac Artery to Right Femoral Artery with Nonautologous Tissue Substitute, Open Approach

041D0KJ Bypass Left Common Iliac Artery to Left Femoral Artery with Nonautologous Tissue Substitute, Open Approach

041D0KK Bypass Left Common Iliac Artery to Bilateral Femoral Arteries with Nonautologous Tissue Substitute, Open Approach

041D0KQ Bypass Left Common Iliac Artery to Lower Extremity Artery with Nonautologous Tissue Substitute, Open Approach

041D0KR Bypass Left Common Iliac Artery to Lower Artery with Nonautologous Tissue Substitute, Open Approach

041D0Z0 Bypass Left Common Iliac Artery to Abdominal Aorta, Open Approach

041D0Z1 Bypass Left Common Iliac Artery to Celiac Artery, Open Approach

041D0Z2 Bypass Left Common Iliac Artery to Mesenteric Artery, Open Approach

041D0Z3 Bypass Left Common Iliac Artery to Right Renal Artery, Open Approach

041D0Z4 Bypass Left Common Iliac Artery to Left Renal Artery, Open Approach

041D0Z5 Bypass Left Common Iliac Artery to Bilateral Renal Artery, Open Approach

041D0Z6 Bypass Left Common Iliac Artery to Right Common Iliac Artery, Open Approach

041D0Z7 Bypass Left Common Iliac Artery to Left Common Iliac Artery, Open Approach

041D0Z8 Bypass Left Common Iliac Artery to Bilateral Common Iliac Arteries, Open Approach

041D0Z9 Bypass Left Common Iliac Artery to Right Internal Iliac Artery, Open Approach

041D0ZB Bypass Left Common Iliac Artery to Left Internal Iliac Artery, Open Approach

041D0ZC Bypass Left Common Iliac Artery to Bilateral Internal Iliac Arteries, Open Approach

041D0ZD Bypass Left Common Iliac Artery to Right External Iliac Artery, Open Approach

041D0ZF Bypass Left Common Iliac Artery to Left External Iliac Artery, Open Approach

041D0ZG Bypass Left Common Iliac Artery to Bilateral External Iliac Arteries, Open Approach

041D0ZH Bypass Left Common Iliac Artery to Right Femoral Artery, Open Approach

041D0ZJ Bypass Left Common Iliac Artery to Left Femoral Artery, Open Approach

041D0ZK Bypass Left Common Iliac Artery to Bilateral Femoral Arteries, Open Approach

041D0ZQ Bypass Left Common Iliac Artery to Lower Extremity Artery, Open Approach

041D0ZR Bypass Left Common Iliac Artery to Lower Artery, Open Approach

041D490 Bypass Left Common Iliac Artery to Abdominal Aorta with Autologous Venous Tissue, Percutaneous Endoscopic Approach

041D491 Bypass Left Common Iliac Artery to Celiac Artery with Autologous Venous Tissue, Percutaneous Endoscopic Approach

041D492 Bypass Left Common Iliac Artery to Mesenteric Artery with Autologous Venous Tissue, Percutaneous Endoscopic Approach

041D493 Bypass Left Common Iliac Artery to Right Renal Artery with Autologous Venous Tissue, Percutaneous Endoscopic Approach

041D494 Bypass Left Common Iliac Artery to Left Renal Artery with Autologous Venous Tissue, Percutaneous Endoscopic Approach

041D495 Bypass Left Common Iliac Artery to Bilateral Renal Artery with Autologous Venous Tissue, Percutaneous Endoscopic Approach

041D496 Bypass Left Common Iliac Artery to Right Common Iliac Artery with Autologous Venous Tissue, Percutaneous Endoscopic Approach

041D497 Bypass Left Common Iliac Artery to Left Common Iliac Artery with Autologous Venous Tissue, Percutaneous Endoscopic Approach

041D498 Bypass Left Common Iliac Artery to Bilateral Common Iliac Arteries with Autologous Venous Tissue, Percutaneous Endoscopic Approach

041D499 Bypass Left Common Iliac Artery to Right Internal Iliac Artery with Autologous Venous Tissue, Percutaneous Endoscopic Approach

041D49B Bypass Left Common Iliac Artery to Left Internal Iliac Artery with Autologous Venous Tissue, Percutaneous Endoscopic Approach

041D49C Bypass Left Common Iliac Artery to Bilateral Internal Iliac Arteries with Autologous Venous Tissue, Percutaneous Endoscopic Approach

041D49D Bypass Left Common Iliac Artery to Right External Iliac Artery with Autologous Venous Tissue, Percutaneous Endoscopic Approach

041D49F Bypass Left Common Iliac Artery to Left External Iliac Artery with Autologous Venous Tissue, Percutaneous Endoscopic Approach

041D49G Bypass Left Common Iliac Artery to Bilateral External Iliac Arteries with Autologous Venous Tissue, Percutaneous Endoscopic Approach

041D49H Bypass Left Common Iliac Artery to Right Femoral Artery with Autologous Venous Tissue, Percutaneous Endoscopic Approach

041D49J Bypass Left Common Iliac Artery to Left Femoral Artery with Autologous Venous Tissue, Percutaneous Endoscopic Approach

041D49K Bypass Left Common Iliac Artery to Bilateral Femoral Arteries with Autologous Venous Tissue, Percutaneous Endoscopic Approach

041D49Q Bypass Left Common Iliac Artery to Lower Extremity Artery with Autologous Venous Tissue, Percutaneous Endoscopic Approach

041D49R Bypass Left Common Iliac Artery to Lower Artery with Autologous Venous Tissue, Percutaneous Endoscopic Approach

041D4A0 Bypass Left Common Iliac Artery to Abdominal Aorta with Autologous Arterial Tissue, Percutaneous Endoscopic Approach

041D4A1 Bypass Left Common Iliac Artery to Celiac Artery with Autologous Arterial Tissue, Percutaneous Endoscopic Approach

041D4A2 Bypass Left Common Iliac Artery to Mesenteric Artery with Autologous Arterial Tissue, Percutaneous Endoscopic Approach

041D4A3 Bypass Left Common Iliac Artery to Right Renal Artery with Autologous Arterial Tissue, Percutaneous Endoscopic Approach

041D4A4 Bypass Left Common Iliac Artery to Left Renal Artery with Autologous Arterial Tissue, Percutaneous Endoscopic Approach

041D4A5 Bypass Left Common Iliac Artery to Bilateral Renal Artery with Autologous Arterial Tissue, Percutaneous Endoscopic Approach

041D4A6 Bypass Left Common Iliac Artery to Right Common Iliac Artery with Autologous Arterial Tissue, Percutaneous Endoscopic Approach

041D4A7 Bypass Left Common Iliac Artery to Left Common Iliac Artery with Autologous Arterial Tissue, Percutaneous Endoscopic Approach

041D4A8 Bypass Left Common Iliac Artery to Bilateral Common Iliac Arteries with Autologous Arterial Tissue, Percutaneous Endoscopic Approach

041D4A9 Bypass Left Common Iliac Artery to Right Internal Iliac Artery with Autologous Arterial Tissue, Percutaneous Endoscopic Approach

041D4AB Bypass Left Common Iliac Artery to Left Internal Iliac Artery with Autologous Arterial Tissue, Percutaneous Endoscopic Approach

041D4AC Bypass Left Common Iliac Artery to Bilateral Internal Iliac Arteries with Autologous Arterial Tissue, Percutaneous Endoscopic Approach

041D4AD Bypass Left Common Iliac Artery to Right External Iliac Artery with Autologous Arterial Tissue, Percutaneous Endoscopic Approach

041D4AF Bypass Left Common Iliac Artery to Left External Iliac Artery with Autologous Arterial Tissue, Percutaneous Endoscopic Approach

041D4AG Bypass Left Common Iliac Artery to Bilateral External Iliac Arteries with Autologous Arterial Tissue, Percutaneous Endoscopic Approach

041D4AH Bypass Left Common Iliac Artery to Right Femoral Artery with Autologous Arterial Tissue, Percutaneous Endoscopic Approach

041D4AJ Bypass Left Common Iliac Artery to Left Femoral Artery with Autologous Arterial Tissue, Percutaneous Endoscopic Approach

041D4AK Bypass Left Common Iliac Artery to Bilateral Femoral Arteries with Autologous Arterial Tissue, Percutaneous Endoscopic Approach

041D4AQ Bypass Left Common Iliac Artery to Lower Extremity Artery with Autologous Arterial Tissue, Percutaneous Endoscopic Approach

041D4AR Bypass Left Common Iliac Artery to Lower Artery with Autologous Arterial Tissue, Percutaneous Endoscopic Approach

041D4J0 Bypass Left Common Iliac Artery to Abdominal Aorta with Synthetic Substitute, Percutaneous Endoscopic Approach

041D4J1 Bypass Left Common Iliac Artery to Celiac Artery with Synthetic Substitute, Percutaneous Endoscopic Approach

041D4J2 Bypass Left Common Iliac Artery to Mesenteric Artery with Synthetic Substitute, Percutaneous Endoscopic Approach

041D4J3 Bypass Left Common Iliac Artery to Right Renal Artery with Synthetic Substitute, Percutaneous Endoscopic Approach

041D4J4 Bypass Left Common Iliac Artery to Left Renal Artery with Synthetic Substitute, Percutaneous Endoscopic Approach

041D4J5 Bypass Left Common Iliac Artery to Bilateral Renal Artery with Synthetic Substitute, Percutaneous Endoscopic Approach

041D4J6 Bypass Left Common Iliac Artery to Right Common Iliac Artery with Synthetic Substitute, Percutaneous Endoscopic Approach

041D4J7 Bypass Left Common Iliac Artery to Left Common Iliac Artery with Synthetic Substitute, Percutaneous Endoscopic Approach

041D4J8 Bypass Left Common Iliac Artery to Bilateral Common Iliac Arteries with Synthetic Substitute, Percutaneous Endoscopic Approach

041D4J9 Bypass Left Common Iliac Artery to Right Internal Iliac Artery with Synthetic Substitute, Percutaneous Endoscopic Approach

041D4JB Bypass Left Common Iliac Artery to Left Internal Iliac Artery with Synthetic Substitute, Percutaneous Endoscopic Approach

041D4JC Bypass Left Common Iliac Artery to Bilateral Internal Iliac Arteries with Synthetic Substitute, Percutaneous Endoscopic Approach

041D4JD Bypass Left Common Iliac Artery to Right External Iliac Artery with Synthetic Substitute, Percutaneous Endoscopic Approach

041D4JF Bypass Left Common Iliac Artery to Left External Iliac Artery with Synthetic Substitute, Percutaneous Endoscopic Approach

041D4JG Bypass Left Common Iliac Artery to Bilateral External Iliac Arteries with Synthetic Substitute, Percutaneous Endoscopic Approach

041D4JH Bypass Left Common Iliac Artery to Right Femoral Artery with Synthetic Substitute, Percutaneous Endoscopic Approach

041D4JJ Bypass Left Common Iliac Artery to Left Femoral Artery with Synthetic Substitute, Percutaneous Endoscopic Approach

041D4JK Bypass Left Common Iliac Artery to Bilateral Femoral Arteries with Synthetic Substitute, Percutaneous Endoscopic Approach

041D4JQ Bypass Left Common Iliac Artery to Lower Extremity Artery with Synthetic Substitute, Percutaneous Endoscopic Approach

041D4JR Bypass Left Common Iliac Artery to Lower Artery with Synthetic Substitute, Percutaneous Endoscopic Approach

041D4K0 Bypass Left Common Iliac Artery to Abdominal Aorta with Nonautologous Tissue Substitute, Percutaneous Endoscopic Approach

041D4K1 Bypass Left Common Iliac Artery to Celiac Artery with Nonautologous Tissue Substitute, Percutaneous Endoscopic Approach

041D4K2 Bypass Left Common Iliac Artery to Mesenteric Artery with Nonautologous Tissue Substitute, Percutaneous Endoscopic Approach

041D4K3 Bypass Left Common Iliac Artery to Right Renal Artery with Nonautologous Tissue Substitute, Percutaneous Endoscopic Approach

041D4K4 Bypass Left Common Iliac Artery to Left Renal Artery with Nonautologous Tissue Substitute, Percutaneous Endoscopic Approach

041D4K5 Bypass Left Common Iliac Artery to Bilateral Renal Artery with Nonautologous Tissue Substitute, Percutaneous Endoscopic Approach

041D4K6 Bypass Left Common Iliac Artery to Right Common Iliac Artery with Nonautologous Tissue Substitute, Percutaneous Endoscopic Approach

041D4K7 Bypass Left Common Iliac Artery to Left Common Iliac Artery with Nonautologous Tissue Substitute, Percutaneous Endoscopic Approach

041D4K8 Bypass Left Common Iliac Artery to Bilateral Common Iliac Arteries with Nonautologous Tissue Substitute, Percutaneous Endoscopic Approach

041D4K9 Bypass Left Common Iliac Artery to Right Internal Iliac Artery with Nonautologous Tissue Substitute, Percutaneous Endoscopic Approach

041D4KB Bypass Left Common Iliac Artery to Left Internal Iliac Artery with Nonautologous Tissue Substitute, Percutaneous Endoscopic Approach

041D4KC Bypass Left Common Iliac Artery to Bilateral Internal Iliac Arteries with Nonautologous Tissue Substitute, Percutaneous Endoscopic Approach

041D4KD Bypass Left Common Iliac Artery to Right External Iliac Artery with Nonautologous Tissue Substitute, Percutaneous Endoscopic Approach

041D4KF Bypass Left Common Iliac Artery to Left External Iliac Artery with Nonautologous Tissue Substitute, Percutaneous Endoscopic Approach

041D4KG Bypass Left Common Iliac Artery to Bilateral External Iliac Arteries with Nonautologous Tissue Substitute, Percutaneous Endoscopic Approach

041D4KH Bypass Left Common Iliac Artery to Right Femoral Artery with Nonautologous Tissue Substitute, Percutaneous Endoscopic Approach

041D4KJ Bypass Left Common Iliac Artery to Left Femoral Artery with Nonautologous Tissue Substitute, Percutaneous Endoscopic Approach

041D4KK Bypass Left Common Iliac Artery to Bilateral Femoral Arteries with Nonautologous Tissue Substitute, Percutaneous Endoscopic Approach

041D4KQ Bypass Left Common Iliac Artery to Lower Extremity Artery with Nonautologous Tissue Substitute, Percutaneous Endoscopic Approach

041D4KR Bypass Left Common Iliac Artery to Lower Artery with Nonautologous Tissue Substitute, Percutaneous Endoscopic Approach

041D4Z0 Bypass Left Common Iliac Artery to Abdominal Aorta, Percutaneous Endoscopic Approach

041D4Z1 Bypass Left Common Iliac Artery to Celiac Artery, Percutaneous Endoscopic Approach

041D4Z2 Bypass Left Common Iliac Artery to Mesenteric Artery, Percutaneous Endoscopic Approach

041D4Z3 Bypass Left Common Iliac Artery to Right Renal Artery, Percutaneous Endoscopic Approach

041D4Z4 Bypass Left Common Iliac Artery to Left Renal Artery, Percutaneous Endoscopic Approach

041D4Z5 Bypass Left Common Iliac Artery to Bilateral Renal Artery, Percutaneous Endoscopic Approach

041D4Z6 Bypass Left Common Iliac Artery to Right Common Iliac Artery, Percutaneous Endoscopic Approach

041D4Z7 Bypass Left Common Iliac Artery to Left Common Iliac Artery, Percutaneous Endoscopic Approach

041D4Z8 Bypass Left Common Iliac Artery to Bilateral Common Iliac Arteries, Percutaneous Endoscopic Approach

041D4Z9 Bypass Left Common Iliac Artery to Right Internal Iliac Artery, Percutaneous Endoscopic Approach

041D4ZB Bypass Left Common Iliac Artery to Left Internal Iliac Artery, Percutaneous Endoscopic Approach

041D4ZC Bypass Left Common Iliac Artery to Bilateral Internal Iliac Arteries, Percutaneous Endoscopic Approach

041D4ZD Bypass Left Common Iliac Artery to Right External Iliac Artery, Percutaneous Endoscopic Approach

041D4ZF Bypass Left Common Iliac Artery to Left External Iliac Artery, Percutaneous Endoscopic Approach

041D4ZG Bypass Left Common Iliac Artery to Bilateral External Iliac Arteries, Percutaneous Endoscopic Approach

041D4ZH Bypass Left Common Iliac Artery to Right Femoral Artery, Percutaneous Endoscopic Approach

♀ Female-only ♂ Male-only ▲ Limited Coverage ● Non-OR ▦ HAC-associated procedure ▲ Non-covered procedures ✚ Cluster

041D4ZJ	Bypass Left Common Iliac Artery to Left Femoral Artery, Percutaneous Endoscopic Approach	

041D4ZJ Bypass Left Common Iliac Artery to Left Femoral Artery, Percutaneous Endoscopic Approach

041D4ZK Bypass Left Common Iliac Artery to Bilateral Femoral Arteries, Percutaneous Endoscopic Approach

041D4ZQ Bypass Left Common Iliac Artery to Lower Extremity Artery, Percutaneous Endoscopic Approach

041D4ZR Bypass Left Common Iliac Artery to Lower Artery, Percutaneous Endoscopic Approach

041E099 Bypass Right Internal Iliac Artery to Right Internal Iliac Artery with Autologous Venous Tissue, Open Approach

041E09B Bypass Right Internal Iliac Artery to Left Internal Iliac Artery with Autologous Venous Tissue, Open Approach

041E09C Bypass Right Internal Iliac Artery to Bilateral Internal Iliac Arteries with Autologous Venous Tissue, Open Approach

041E09D Bypass Right Internal Iliac Artery to Right External Iliac Artery with Autologous Venous Tissue, Open Approach

041E09F Bypass Right Internal Iliac Artery to Left External Iliac Artery with Autologous Venous Tissue, Open Approach

041E09G Bypass Right Internal Iliac Artery to Bilateral External Iliac Arteries with Autologous Venous Tissue, Open Approach

041E09H Bypass Right Internal Iliac Artery to Right Femoral Artery with Autologous Venous Tissue, Open Approach

041E09J Bypass Right Internal Iliac Artery to Left Femoral Artery with Autologous Venous Tissue, Open Approach

041E09K Bypass Right Internal Iliac Artery to Bilateral Femoral Arteries with Autologous Venous Tissue, Open Approach

041E09P Bypass Right Internal Iliac Artery to Foot Artery with Autologous Venous Tissue, Open Approach

041E09Q Bypass Right Internal Iliac Artery to Lower Extremity Artery with Autologous Venous Tissue, Open Approach

041E0A9 Bypass Right Internal Iliac Artery to Right Internal Iliac Artery with Autologous Arterial Tissue, Open Approach

041E0AB Bypass Right Internal Iliac Artery to Left Internal Iliac Artery with Autologous Arterial Tissue, Open Approach

041E0AC Bypass Right Internal Iliac Artery to Bilateral Internal Iliac Arteries with Autologous Arterial Tissue, Open Approach

041E0AD Bypass Right Internal Iliac Artery to Right External Iliac Artery with Autologous Arterial Tissue, Open Approach

041E0AF Bypass Right Internal Iliac Artery to Left External Iliac Artery with Autologous Arterial Tissue, Open Approach

041E0AG Bypass Right Internal Iliac Artery to Bilateral External Iliac Arteries with Autologous Arterial Tissue, Open Approach

041E0AH Bypass Right Internal Iliac Artery to Right Femoral Artery with Autologous Arterial Tissue, Open Approach

041E0AJ Bypass Right Internal Iliac Artery to Left Femoral Artery with Autologous Arterial Tissue, Open Approach

041E0AK Bypass Right Internal Iliac Artery to Bilateral Femoral Arteries with Autologous Arterial Tissue, Open Approach

041E0AP Bypass Right Internal Iliac Artery to Foot Artery with Autologous Arterial Tissue, Open Approach

041E0AQ Bypass Right Internal Iliac Artery to Lower Extremity Artery with Autologous Arterial Tissue, Open Approach

041E0J9 Bypass Right Internal Iliac Artery to Right Internal Iliac Artery with Synthetic Substitute, Open Approach

041E0JB Bypass Right Internal Iliac Artery to Left Internal Iliac Artery with Synthetic Substitute, Open Approach

041E0JC Bypass Right Internal Iliac Artery to Bilateral Internal Iliac Arteries with Synthetic Substitute, Open Approach

041E0JD Bypass Right Internal Iliac Artery to Right External Iliac Artery with Synthetic Substitute, Open Approach

041E0JF Bypass Right Internal Iliac Artery to Left External Iliac Artery with Synthetic Substitute, Open Approach

041E0JG Bypass Right Internal Iliac Artery to Bilateral External Iliac Arteries with Synthetic Substitute, Open Approach

041E0JH Bypass Right Internal Iliac Artery to Right Femoral Artery with Synthetic Substitute, Open Approach

041E0JJ Bypass Right Internal Iliac Artery to Left Femoral Artery with Synthetic Substitute, Open Approach

041E0JK Bypass Right Internal Iliac Artery to Bilateral Femoral Arteries with Synthetic Substitute, Open Approach

041E0JP Bypass Right Internal Iliac Artery to Foot Artery with Synthetic Substitute, Open Approach

041E0JQ Bypass Right Internal Iliac Artery to Lower Extremity Artery with Synthetic Substitute, Open Approach

041E0K9 Bypass Right Internal Iliac Artery to Right Internal Iliac Artery with Nonautologous Tissue Substitute, Open Approach

041E0KB Bypass Right Internal Iliac Artery to Left Internal Iliac Artery with Nonautologous Tissue Substitute, Open Approach

041E0KC Bypass Right Internal Iliac Artery to Bilateral Internal Iliac Arteries with Nonautologous Tissue Substitute, Open Approach

041E0KD Bypass Right Internal Iliac Artery to Right External Iliac Artery with Nonautologous Tissue Substitute, Open Approach

041E0KF Bypass Right Internal Iliac Artery to Left External Iliac Artery with Nonautologous Tissue Substitute, Open Approach

041E0KG Bypass Right Internal Iliac Artery to Bilateral External Iliac Arteries with Nonautologous Tissue Substitute, Open Approach

041E0KH Bypass Right Internal Iliac Artery to Right Femoral Artery with Nonautologous Tissue Substitute, Open Approach

041E0KJ Bypass Right Internal Iliac Artery to Left Femoral Artery with Nonautologous Tissue Substitute, Open Approach

041E0KK Bypass Right Internal Iliac Artery to Bilateral Femoral Arteries with Nonautologous Tissue Substitute, Open Approach

041E0KP Bypass Right Internal Iliac Artery to Foot Artery with Nonautologous Tissue Substitute, Open Approach

041E0KQ Bypass Right Internal Iliac Artery to Lower Extremity Artery with Nonautologous Tissue Substitute, Open Approach

041E0Z9 Bypass Right Internal Iliac Artery to Right Internal Iliac Artery, Open Approach

041E0ZB Bypass Right Internal Iliac Artery to Left Internal Iliac Artery, Open Approach

041E0ZC Bypass Right Internal Iliac Artery to Bilateral Internal Iliac Arteries, Open Approach

041E0ZD Bypass Right Internal Iliac Artery to Right External Iliac Artery, Open Approach

041E0ZF Bypass Right Internal Iliac Artery to Left External Iliac Artery, Open Approach

041E0ZG Bypass Right Internal Iliac Artery to Bilateral External Iliac Arteries, Open Approach

041E0ZH Bypass Right Internal Iliac Artery to Right Femoral Artery, Open Approach

041E0ZJ Bypass Right Internal Iliac Artery to Left Femoral Artery, Open Approach

041E0ZK Bypass Right Internal Iliac Artery to Bilateral Femoral Arteries, Open Approach

041E0ZP Bypass Right Internal Iliac Artery to Foot Artery, Open Approach

041E0ZQ Bypass Right Internal Iliac Artery to Lower Extremity Artery, Open Approach

041E499 Bypass Right Internal Iliac Artery to Right Internal Iliac Artery with Autologous Venous Tissue, Percutaneous Endoscopic Approach

041E49B Bypass Right Internal Iliac Artery to Left Internal Iliac Artery with Autologous Venous Tissue, Percutaneous Endoscopic Approach

041E49C Bypass Right Internal Iliac Artery to Bilateral Internal Iliac Arteries with Autologous Venous Tissue, Percutaneous Endoscopic Approach

041E49D Bypass Right Internal Iliac Artery to Right External Iliac Artery with Autologous Venous Tissue, Percutaneous Endoscopic Approach

041E49F Bypass Right Internal Iliac Artery to Left External Iliac Artery with Autologous Venous Tissue, Percutaneous Endoscopic Approach

041E49G Bypass Right Internal Iliac Artery to Bilateral External Iliac Arteries with Autologous Venous Tissue, Percutaneous Endoscopic Approach

041E49H Bypass Right Internal Iliac Artery to Right Femoral Artery with Autologous Venous Tissue, Percutaneous Endoscopic Approach

041E49J Bypass Right Internal Iliac Artery to Left Femoral Artery with Autologous Venous Tissue, Percutaneous Endoscopic Approach

041E49K Bypass Right Internal Iliac Artery to Bilateral Femoral Arteries with Autologous Venous Tissue, Percutaneous Endoscopic Approach

041E49P Bypass Right Internal Iliac Artery to Foot Artery with Autologous Venous Tissue, Percutaneous Endoscopic Approach

041E49Q Bypass Right Internal Iliac Artery to Lower Extremity Artery with Autologous Venous Tissue, Percutaneous Endoscopic Approach

041E4A9 Bypass Right Internal Iliac Artery to Right Internal Iliac Artery with Autologous Arterial Tissue, Percutaneous Endoscopic Approach

041E4AB Bypass Right Internal Iliac Artery to Left Internal Iliac Artery with Autologous Arterial Tissue, Percutaneous Endoscopic Approach

041E4AC Bypass Right Internal Iliac Artery to Bilateral Internal Iliac Arteries with Autologous Arterial Tissue, Percutaneous Endoscopic Approach

041E4AD Bypass Right Internal Iliac Artery to Right External Iliac Artery with Autologous Arterial Tissue, Percutaneous Endoscopic Approach

041E4AF Bypass Right Internal Iliac Artery to Left External Iliac Artery with Autologous Arterial Tissue, Percutaneous Endoscopic Approach

041E4AG Bypass Right Internal Iliac Artery to Bilateral External Iliac Arteries with Autologous Arterial Tissue, Percutaneous Endoscopic Approach

041E4AH Bypass Right Internal Iliac Artery to Right Femoral Artery with Autologous Arterial Tissue, Percutaneous Endoscopic Approach

041E4AJ Bypass Right Internal Iliac Artery to Left Femoral Artery with Autologous Arterial Tissue, Percutaneous Endoscopic Approach

041E4AK Bypass Right Internal Iliac Artery to Bilateral Femoral Arteries with Autologous Arterial Tissue, Percutaneous Endoscopic Approach

041E4AP Bypass Right Internal Iliac Artery to Foot Artery with Autologous Arterial Tissue, Percutaneous Endoscopic Approach

041E4AQ Bypass Right Internal Iliac Artery to Lower Extremity Artery with Autologous Arterial Tissue, Percutaneous Endoscopic Approach

041E4J9 Bypass Right Internal Iliac Artery to Right Internal Iliac Artery with Synthetic Substitute, Percutaneous Endoscopic Approach

041E4JB Bypass Right Internal Iliac Artery to Left Internal Iliac Artery with Synthetic Substitute, Percutaneous Endoscopic Approach

041E4JC Bypass Right Internal Iliac Artery to Bilateral Internal Iliac Arteries with Synthetic Substitute, Percutaneous Endoscopic Approach

041E4JD Bypass Right Internal Iliac Artery to Right External Iliac Artery with Synthetic Substitute, Percutaneous Endoscopic Approach

041E4JF Bypass Right Internal Iliac Artery to Left External Iliac Artery with Synthetic Substitute, Percutaneous Endoscopic Approach

041E4JG Bypass Right Internal Iliac Artery to Bilateral External Iliac Arteries with Synthetic Substitute, Percutaneous Endoscopic Approach

041E4JH Bypass Right Internal Iliac Artery to Right Femoral Artery with Synthetic Substitute, Percutaneous Endoscopic Approach

041E4JJ Bypass Right Internal Iliac Artery to Left Femoral Artery with Synthetic Substitute, Percutaneous Endoscopic Approach

041E4JK Bypass Right Internal Iliac Artery to Bilateral Femoral Arteries with Synthetic Substitute, Percutaneous Endoscopic Approach

041E4JP Bypass Right Internal Iliac Artery to Foot Artery with Synthetic Substitute, Percutaneous Endoscopic Approach

041E4JQ Bypass Right Internal Iliac Artery to Lower Extremity Artery with Synthetic Substitute, Percutaneous Endoscopic Approach

041E4K9 Bypass Right Internal Iliac Artery to Right Internal Iliac Artery with Nonautologous Tissue Substitute, Percutaneous Endoscopic Approach

041E4KB Bypass Right Internal Iliac Artery to Left Internal Iliac Artery with Nonautologous Tissue Substitute, Percutaneous Endoscopic Approach

041E4KC Bypass Right Internal Iliac Artery to Bilateral Internal Iliac Arteries with Nonautologous Tissue Substitute, Percutaneous Endoscopic Approach

041E4KD Bypass Right Internal Iliac Artery to Right External Iliac Artery with Nonautologous Tissue Substitute, Percutaneous Endoscopic Approach

041E4KF Bypass Right Internal Iliac Artery to Left External Iliac Artery with Nonautologous Tissue Substitute, Percutaneous Endoscopic Approach

041E4KG Bypass Right Internal Iliac Artery to Bilateral External Iliac Arteries with Nonautologous Tissue Substitute, Percutaneous Endoscopic Approach

041E4KH Bypass Right Internal Iliac Artery to Right Femoral Artery with Nonautologous Tissue Substitute, Percutaneous Endoscopic Approach

041E4KJ Bypass Right Internal Iliac Artery to Left Femoral Artery with Nonautologous Tissue Substitute, Percutaneous Endoscopic Approach

041E4KK Bypass Right Internal Iliac Artery to Bilateral Femoral Arteries with Nonautologous Tissue Substitute, Percutaneous Endoscopic Approach

041E4KP Bypass Right Internal Iliac Artery to Foot Artery with Nonautologous Tissue Substitute, Percutaneous Endoscopic Approach

041E4KQ Bypass Right Internal Iliac Artery to Lower Extremity Artery with Nonautologous Tissue Substitute, Percutaneous Endoscopic Approach

041E4Z9 Bypass Right Internal Iliac Artery to Right Internal Iliac Artery, Percutaneous Endoscopic Approach

041E4ZB Bypass Right Internal Iliac Artery to Left Internal Iliac Artery, Percutaneous Endoscopic Approach

041E4ZC Bypass Right Internal Iliac Artery to Bilateral Internal Iliac Arteries, Percutaneous Endoscopic Approach

041E4ZD Bypass Right Internal Iliac Artery to Right External Iliac Artery, Percutaneous Endoscopic Approach

041E4ZF Bypass Right Internal Iliac Artery to Left External Iliac Artery, Percutaneous Endoscopic Approach

041E4ZG Bypass Right Internal Iliac Artery to Bilateral External Iliac Arteries, Percutaneous Endoscopic Approach

041E4ZH Bypass Right Internal Iliac Artery to Right Femoral Artery, Percutaneous Endoscopic Approach

041E4ZJ Bypass Right Internal Iliac Artery to Left Femoral Artery, Percutaneous Endoscopic Approach

041E4ZK Bypass Right Internal Iliac Artery to Bilateral Femoral Arteries, Percutaneous Endoscopic Approach

041E4ZP Bypass Right Internal Iliac Artery to Foot Artery, Percutaneous Endoscopic Approach

041E4ZQ Bypass Right Internal Iliac Artery to Lower Extremity Artery, Percutaneous Endoscopic Approach

041F099 Bypass Left Internal Iliac Artery to Right Internal Iliac Artery with Autologous Venous Tissue, Open Approach

041F09B Bypass Left Internal Iliac Artery to Left Internal Iliac Artery with Autologous Venous Tissue, Open Approach

041F09C Bypass Left Internal Iliac Artery to Bilateral Internal Iliac Arteries with Autologous Venous Tissue, Open Approach

041F09D Bypass Left Internal Iliac Artery to Right External Iliac Artery with Autologous Venous Tissue, Open Approach

041F09F Bypass Left Internal Iliac Artery to Left External Iliac Artery with Autologous Venous Tissue, Open Approach

041F09G Bypass Left Internal Iliac Artery to Bilateral External Iliac Arteries with Autologous Venous Tissue, Open Approach

041F09H Bypass Left Internal Iliac Artery to Right Femoral Artery with Autologous Venous Tissue, Open Approach

041F09J Bypass Left Internal Iliac Artery to Left Femoral Artery with Autologous Venous Tissue, Open Approach

041F09K Bypass Left Internal Iliac Artery to Bilateral Femoral Arteries with Autologous Venous Tissue, Open Approach

041F09P Bypass Left Internal Iliac Artery to Foot Artery with Autologous Venous Tissue, Open Approach

041F09Q Bypass Left Internal Iliac Artery to Lower Extremity Artery with Autologous Venous Tissue, Open Approach

♀ Female-only   ♂ Male-only   ▲ Limited Coverage   ● Non-OR   ▨ HAC-associated procedure   ▲ Non-covered procedures   ✚ Cluster

041F0A9 Bypass Left Internal Iliac Artery to Right Internal Iliac Artery with Autologous Arterial Tissue, Open Approach

041F0AB Bypass Left Internal Iliac Artery to Left Internal Iliac Artery with Autologous Arterial Tissue, Open Approach

041F0AC Bypass Left Internal Iliac Artery to Bilateral Internal Iliac Arteries with Autologous Arterial Tissue, Open Approach

041F0AD Bypass Left Internal Iliac Artery to Right External Iliac Artery with Autologous Arterial Tissue, Open Approach

041F0AF Bypass Left Internal Iliac Artery to Left External Iliac Artery with Autologous Arterial Tissue, Open Approach

041F0AG Bypass Left Internal Iliac Artery to Bilateral External Iliac Arteries with Autologous Arterial Tissue, Open Approach

041F0AH Bypass Left Internal Iliac Artery to Right Femoral Artery with Autologous Arterial Tissue, Open Approach

041F0AJ Bypass Left Internal Iliac Artery to Left Femoral Artery with Autologous Arterial Tissue, Open Approach

041F0AK Bypass Left Internal Iliac Artery to Bilateral Femoral Arteries with Autologous Arterial Tissue, Open Approach

041F0AP Bypass Left Internal Iliac Artery to Foot Artery with Autologous Arterial Tissue, Open Approach

041F0AQ Bypass Left Internal Iliac Artery to Lower Extremity Artery with Autologous Arterial Tissue, Open Approach

041F0J9 Bypass Left Internal Iliac Artery to Right Internal Iliac Artery with Synthetic Substitute, Open Approach

041F0JB Bypass Left Internal Iliac Artery to Left Internal Iliac Artery with Synthetic Substitute, Open Approach

041F0JC Bypass Left Internal Iliac Artery to Bilateral Internal Iliac Arteries with Synthetic Substitute, Open Approach

041F0JD Bypass Left Internal Iliac Artery to Right External Iliac Artery with Synthetic Substitute, Open Approach

041F0JF Bypass Left Internal Iliac Artery to Left External Iliac Artery with Synthetic Substitute, Open Approach

041F0JG Bypass Left Internal Iliac Artery to Bilateral External Iliac Arteries with Synthetic Substitute, Open Approach

041F0JH Bypass Left Internal Iliac Artery to Right Femoral Artery with Synthetic Substitute, Open Approach

041F0JJ Bypass Left Internal Iliac Artery to Left Femoral Artery with Synthetic Substitute, Open Approach

041F0JK Bypass Left Internal Iliac Artery to Bilateral Femoral Arteries with Synthetic Substitute, Open Approach

041F0JP Bypass Left Internal Iliac Artery to Foot Artery with Synthetic Substitute, Open Approach

041F0JQ Bypass Left Internal Iliac Artery to Lower Extremity Artery with Synthetic Substitute, Open Approach

041F0K9 Bypass Left Internal Iliac Artery to Right Internal Iliac Artery with Nonautologous Tissue Substitute, Open Approach

041F0KB Bypass Left Internal Iliac Artery to Left Internal Iliac Artery with Nonautologous Tissue Substitute, Open Approach

041F0KC Bypass Left Internal Iliac Artery to Bilateral Internal Iliac Arteries with Nonautologous Tissue Substitute, Open Approach

041F0KD Bypass Left Internal Iliac Artery to Right External Iliac Artery with Nonautologous Tissue Substitute, Open Approach

041F0KF Bypass Left Internal Iliac Artery to Left External Iliac Artery with Nonautologous Tissue Substitute, Open Approach

041F0KG Bypass Left Internal Iliac Artery to Bilateral External Iliac Arteries with Nonautologous Tissue Substitute, Open Approach

041F0KH Bypass Left Internal Iliac Artery to Right Femoral Artery with Nonautologous Tissue Substitute, Open Approach

041F0KJ Bypass Left Internal Iliac Artery to Left Femoral Artery with Nonautologous Tissue Substitute, Open Approach

041F0KK Bypass Left Internal Iliac Artery to Bilateral Femoral Arteries with Nonautologous Tissue Substitute, Open Approach

041F0KP Bypass Left Internal Iliac Artery to Foot Artery with Nonautologous Tissue Substitute, Open Approach

041F0KQ Bypass Left Internal Iliac Artery to Lower Extremity Artery with Nonautologous Tissue Substitute, Open Approach

041F0Z9 Bypass Left Internal Iliac Artery to Right Internal Iliac Artery, Open Approach

041F0ZB Bypass Left Internal Iliac Artery to Left Internal Iliac Artery, Open Approach

041F0ZC Bypass Left Internal Iliac Artery to Bilateral Internal Iliac Arteries, Open Approach

041F0ZD Bypass Left Internal Iliac Artery to Right External Iliac Artery, Open Approach

041F0ZF Bypass Left Internal Iliac Artery to Left External Iliac Artery, Open Approach

041F0ZG Bypass Left Internal Iliac Artery to Bilateral External Iliac Arteries, Open Approach

041F0ZH Bypass Left Internal Iliac Artery to Right Femoral Artery, Open Approach

041F0ZJ Bypass Left Internal Iliac Artery to Left Femoral Artery, Open Approach

041F0ZK Bypass Left Internal Iliac Artery to Bilateral Femoral Arteries, Open Approach

041F0ZP Bypass Left Internal Iliac Artery to Foot Artery, Open Approach

041F0ZQ Bypass Left Internal Iliac Artery to Lower Extremity Artery, Open Approach

041F499 Bypass Left Internal Iliac Artery to Right Internal Iliac Artery with Autologous Venous Tissue, Percutaneous Endoscopic Approach

041F49B Bypass Left Internal Iliac Artery to Left Internal Iliac Artery with Autologous Venous Tissue, Percutaneous Endoscopic Approach

041F49C Bypass Left Internal Iliac Artery to Bilateral Internal Iliac Arteries with Autologous Venous Tissue, Percutaneous Endoscopic Approach

041F49D Bypass Left Internal Iliac Artery to Right External Iliac Artery with Autologous Venous Tissue, Percutaneous Endoscopic Approach

041F49F Bypass Left Internal Iliac Artery to Left External Iliac Artery with Autologous Venous Tissue, Percutaneous Endoscopic Approach

041F49G Bypass Left Internal Iliac Artery to Bilateral External Iliac Arteries with Autologous Venous Tissue, Percutaneous Endoscopic Approach

041F49H Bypass Left Internal Iliac Artery to Right Femoral Artery with Autologous Venous Tissue, Percutaneous Endoscopic Approach

041F49J Bypass Left Internal Iliac Artery to Left Femoral Artery with Autologous Venous Tissue, Percutaneous Endoscopic Approach

041F49K Bypass Left Internal Iliac Artery to Bilateral Femoral Arteries with Autologous Venous Tissue, Percutaneous Endoscopic Approach

041F49P Bypass Left Internal Iliac Artery to Foot Artery with Autologous Venous Tissue, Percutaneous Endoscopic Approach

041F49Q Bypass Left Internal Iliac Artery to Lower Extremity Artery with Autologous Venous Tissue, Percutaneous Endoscopic Approach

041F4A9 Bypass Left Internal Iliac Artery to Right Internal Iliac Artery with Autologous Arterial Tissue, Percutaneous Endoscopic Approach

041F4AB Bypass Left Internal Iliac Artery to Left Internal Iliac Artery with Autologous Arterial Tissue, Percutaneous Endoscopic Approach

041F4AC Bypass Left Internal Iliac Artery to Bilateral Internal Iliac Arteries with Autologous Arterial Tissue, Percutaneous Endoscopic Approach

041F4AD Bypass Left Internal Iliac Artery to Right External Iliac Artery with Autologous Arterial Tissue, Percutaneous Endoscopic Approach

041F4AF Bypass Left Internal Iliac Artery to Left External Iliac Artery with Autologous Arterial Tissue, Percutaneous Endoscopic Approach

041F4AG Bypass Left Internal Iliac Artery to Bilateral External Iliac Arteries with Autologous Arterial Tissue, Percutaneous Endoscopic Approach

041F4AH Bypass Left Internal Iliac Artery to Right Femoral Artery with Autologous Arterial Tissue, Percutaneous Endoscopic Approach

041F4AJ Bypass Left Internal Iliac Artery to Left Femoral Artery with Autologous Arterial Tissue, Percutaneous Endoscopic Approach

041F4AK Bypass Left Internal Iliac Artery to Bilateral Femoral Arteries with Autologous Arterial Tissue, Percutaneous Endoscopic Approach

041F4AP Bypass Left Internal Iliac Artery to Foot Artery with Autologous Arterial Tissue, Percutaneous Endoscopic Approach

---

♀ Female-only   ♂ Male-only   ▲ Limited Coverage   ● Non-OR   ▨ HAC-associated procedure   ▲ Non-covered procedures   ✚ Cluster

041F4AQ Bypass Left Internal Iliac Artery to Lower Extremity Artery with Autologous Arterial Tissue, Percutaneous Endoscopic Approach

041F4J9 Bypass Left Internal Iliac Artery to Right Internal Iliac Artery with Synthetic Substitute, Percutaneous Endoscopic Approach

041F4JB Bypass Left Internal Iliac Artery to Left Internal Iliac Artery with Synthetic Substitute, Percutaneous Endoscopic Approach

041F4JC Bypass Left Internal Iliac Artery to Bilateral Internal Iliac Arteries with Synthetic Substitute, Percutaneous Endoscopic Approach

041F4JD Bypass Left Internal Iliac Artery to Right External Iliac Artery with Synthetic Substitute, Percutaneous Endoscopic Approach

041F4JF Bypass Left Internal Iliac Artery to Left External Iliac Artery with Synthetic Substitute, Percutaneous Endoscopic Approach

041F4JG Bypass Left Internal Iliac Artery to Bilateral External Iliac Arteries with Synthetic Substitute, Percutaneous Endoscopic Approach

041F4JH Bypass Left Internal Iliac Artery to Right Femoral Artery with Synthetic Substitute, Percutaneous Endoscopic Approach

041F4JJ Bypass Left Internal Iliac Artery to Left Femoral Artery with Synthetic Substitute, Percutaneous Endoscopic Approach

041F4JK Bypass Left Internal Iliac Artery to Bilateral Femoral Arteries with Synthetic Substitute, Percutaneous Endoscopic Approach

041F4JP Bypass Left Internal Iliac Artery to Foot Artery with Synthetic Substitute, Percutaneous Endoscopic Approach

041F4JQ Bypass Left Internal Iliac Artery to Lower Extremity Artery with Synthetic Substitute, Percutaneous Endoscopic Approach

041F4K9 Bypass Left Internal Iliac Artery to Right Internal Iliac Artery with Nonautologous Tissue Substitute, Percutaneous Endoscopic Approach

041F4KB Bypass Left Internal Iliac Artery to Left Internal Iliac Artery with Nonautologous Tissue Substitute, Percutaneous Endoscopic Approach

041F4KC Bypass Left Internal Iliac Artery to Bilateral Internal Iliac Arteries with Nonautologous Tissue Substitute, Percutaneous Endoscopic Approach

041F4KD Bypass Left Internal Iliac Artery to Right External Iliac Artery with Nonautologous Tissue Substitute, Percutaneous Endoscopic Approach

041F4KF Bypass Left Internal Iliac Artery to Left External Iliac Artery with Nonautologous Tissue Substitute, Percutaneous Endoscopic Approach

041F4KG Bypass Left Internal Iliac Artery to Bilateral External Iliac Arteries with Nonautologous Tissue Substitute, Percutaneous Endoscopic Approach

041F4KH Bypass Left Internal Iliac Artery to Right Femoral Artery with Nonautologous Tissue Substitute, Percutaneous Endoscopic Approach

041F4KJ Bypass Left Internal Iliac Artery to Left Femoral Artery with Nonautologous Tissue Substitute, Percutaneous Endoscopic Approach

041F4KK Bypass Left Internal Iliac Artery to Bilateral Femoral Arteries with Nonautologous Tissue Substitute, Percutaneous Endoscopic Approach

041F4KP Bypass Left Internal Iliac Artery to Foot Artery with Nonautologous Tissue Substitute, Percutaneous Endoscopic Approach

041F4KQ Bypass Left Internal Iliac Artery to Lower Extremity Artery with Nonautologous Tissue Substitute, Percutaneous Endoscopic Approach

041F4Z9 Bypass Left Internal Iliac Artery to Right Internal Iliac Artery, Percutaneous Endoscopic Approach

041F4ZB Bypass Left Internal Iliac Artery to Left Internal Iliac Artery, Percutaneous Endoscopic Approach

041F4ZC Bypass Left Internal Iliac Artery to Bilateral Internal Iliac Arteries, Percutaneous Endoscopic Approach

041F4ZD Bypass Left Internal Iliac Artery to Right External Iliac Artery, Percutaneous Endoscopic Approach

041F4ZF Bypass Left Internal Iliac Artery to Left External Iliac Artery, Percutaneous Endoscopic Approach

041F4ZG Bypass Left Internal Iliac Artery to Bilateral External Iliac Arteries, Percutaneous Endoscopic Approach

041F4ZH Bypass Left Internal Iliac Artery to Right Femoral Artery, Percutaneous Endoscopic Approach

041F4ZJ Bypass Left Internal Iliac Artery to Left Femoral Artery, Percutaneous Endoscopic Approach

041F4ZK Bypass Left Internal Iliac Artery to Bilateral Femoral Arteries, Percutaneous Endoscopic Approach

041F4ZP Bypass Left Internal Iliac Artery to Foot Artery, Percutaneous Endoscopic Approach

041F4ZQ Bypass Left Internal Iliac Artery to Lower Extremity Artery, Percutaneous Endoscopic Approach

041H099 Bypass Right External Iliac Artery to Right Internal Iliac Artery with Autologous Venous Tissue, Open Approach

041H09B Bypass Right External Iliac Artery to Left Internal Iliac Artery with Autologous Venous Tissue, Open Approach

041H09C Bypass Right External Iliac Artery to Bilateral Internal Iliac Arteries with Autologous Venous Tissue, Open Approach

041H09D Bypass Right External Iliac Artery to Right External Iliac Artery with Autologous Venous Tissue, Open Approach

041H09F Bypass Right External Iliac Artery to Left External Iliac Artery with Autologous Venous Tissue, Open Approach

041H09G Bypass Right External Iliac Artery to Bilateral External Iliac Arteries with Autologous Venous Tissue, Open Approach

041H09H Bypass Right External Iliac Artery to Right Femoral Artery with Autologous Venous Tissue, Open Approach

041H09J Bypass Right External Iliac Artery to Left Femoral Artery with Autologous Venous Tissue, Open Approach

041H09K Bypass Right External Iliac Artery to Bilateral Femoral Arteries with Autologous Venous Tissue, Open Approach

041H09P Bypass Right External Iliac Artery to Foot Artery with Autologous Venous Tissue, Open Approach

041H09Q Bypass Right External Iliac Artery to Lower Extremity Artery with Autologous Venous Tissue, Open Approach

041H0A9 Bypass Right External Iliac Artery to Right Internal Iliac Artery with Autologous Arterial Tissue, Open Approach

041H0AB Bypass Right External Iliac Artery to Left Internal Iliac Artery with Autologous Arterial Tissue, Open Approach

041H0AC Bypass Right External Iliac Artery to Bilateral Internal Iliac Arteries with Autologous Arterial Tissue, Open Approach

041H0AD Bypass Right External Iliac Artery to Right Internal Iliac Artery with Autologous Arterial Tissue, Open Approach

041H0AF Bypass Right External Iliac Artery to Left External Iliac Artery with Autologous Arterial Tissue, Open Approach

041H0AG Bypass Right External Iliac Artery to Bilateral External Iliac Arteries with Autologous Arterial Tissue, Open Approach

041H0AH Bypass Right External Iliac Artery to Right Femoral Artery with Autologous Arterial Tissue, Open Approach

041H0AJ Bypass Right External Iliac Artery to Left Femoral Artery with Autologous Arterial Tissue, Open Approach

041H0AK Bypass Right External Iliac Artery to Bilateral Femoral Arteries with Autologous Arterial Tissue, Open Approach

041H0AP Bypass Right External Iliac Artery to Foot Artery with Autologous Arterial Tissue, Open Approach

041H0AQ Bypass Right External Iliac Artery to Lower Extremity Artery with Autologous Arterial Tissue, Open Approach

041H0J9 Bypass Right External Iliac Artery to Right Internal Iliac Artery with Synthetic Substitute, Open Approach

041H0JB Bypass Right External Iliac Artery to Left Internal Iliac Artery with Synthetic Substitute, Open Approach

041H0JC Bypass Right External Iliac Artery to Bilateral Internal Iliac Arteries with Synthetic Substitute, Open Approach

041H0JD Bypass Right External Iliac Artery to Right External Iliac Artery with Synthetic Substitute, Open Approach

041H0JF Bypass Right External Iliac Artery to Left External Iliac Artery with Synthetic Substitute, Open Approach

041H0JG Bypass Right External Iliac Artery to Bilateral External Iliac Arteries with Synthetic Substitute, Open Approach

041H0JH Bypass Right External Iliac Artery to Right Femoral Artery with Synthetic Substitute, Open Approach

041H0JJ Bypass Right External Iliac Artery to Left Femoral Artery with Synthetic Substitute, Open Approach

041H0JK Bypass Right External Iliac Artery to Bilateral Femoral Arteries with Synthetic Substitute, Open Approach

041H0JP Bypass Right External Iliac Artery to Foot Artery with Synthetic Substitute, Open Approach

041H0JQ Bypass Right External Iliac Artery to Lower Extremity Artery with Synthetic Substitute, Open Approach

041H0K9 Bypass Right External Iliac Artery to Right Internal Iliac Artery with Nonautologous Tissue Substitute, Open Approach

041H0KB Bypass Right External Iliac Artery to Left Internal Iliac Artery with Nonautologous Tissue Substitute, Open Approach

041H0KC Bypass Right External Iliac Artery to Bilateral Internal Iliac Arteries with Nonautologous Tissue Substitute, Open Approach

041H0KD Bypass Right External Iliac Artery to Right External Iliac Artery with Nonautologous Tissue Substitute, Open Approach

041H0KF Bypass Right External Iliac Artery to Left External Iliac Artery with Nonautologous Tissue Substitute, Open Approach

041H0KG Bypass Right External Iliac Artery to Bilateral External Iliac Arteries with Nonautologous Tissue Substitute, Open Approach

041H0KH Bypass Right External Iliac Artery to Right Femoral Artery with Nonautologous Tissue Substitute, Open Approach

041H0KJ Bypass Right External Iliac Artery to Left Femoral Artery with Nonautologous Tissue Substitute, Open Approach

041H0KK Bypass Right External Iliac Artery to Bilateral Femoral Arteries with Nonautologous Tissue Substitute, Open Approach

041H0KP Bypass Right External Iliac Artery to Foot Artery with Nonautologous Tissue Substitute, Open Approach

041H0KQ Bypass Right External Iliac Artery to Lower Extremity Artery with Nonautologous Tissue Substitute, Open Approach

041H0Z9 Bypass Right External Iliac Artery to Right Internal Iliac Artery, Open Approach

041H0ZB Bypass Right External Iliac Artery to Left Internal Iliac Artery, Open Approach

041H0ZC Bypass Right External Iliac Artery to Bilateral Internal Iliac Arteries, Open Approach

041H0ZD Bypass Right External Iliac Artery to Right External Iliac Artery, Open Approach

041H0ZF Bypass Right External Iliac Artery to Left External Iliac Artery, Open Approach

041H0ZG Bypass Right External Iliac Artery to Bilateral External Iliac Arteries, Open Approach

041H0ZH Bypass Right External Iliac Artery to Right Femoral Artery, Open Approach

041H0ZJ Bypass Right External Iliac Artery to Left Femoral Artery, Open Approach

041H0ZK Bypass Right External Iliac Artery to Bilateral Femoral Arteries, Open Approach

041H0ZP Bypass Right External Iliac Artery to Foot Artery, Open Approach

041H0ZQ Bypass Right External Iliac Artery to Lower Extremity Artery, Open Approach

041H499 Bypass Right External Iliac Artery to Right Internal Iliac Artery with Autologous Venous Tissue, Percutaneous Endoscopic Approach

041H49B Bypass Right External Iliac Artery to Left Internal Iliac Artery with Autologous Venous Tissue, Percutaneous Endoscopic Approach

041H49C Bypass Right External Iliac Artery to Bilateral Internal Iliac Arteries with Autologous Venous Tissue, Percutaneous Endoscopic Approach

041H49D Bypass Right External Iliac Artery to Right External Iliac Artery with Autologous Venous Tissue, Percutaneous Endoscopic Approach

041H49F Bypass Right External Iliac Artery to Left External Iliac Artery with Autologous Venous Tissue, Percutaneous Endoscopic Approach

041H49G Bypass Right External Iliac Artery to Bilateral External Iliac Arteries with Autologous Venous Tissue, Percutaneous Endoscopic Approach

041H49H Bypass Right External Iliac Artery to Right Femoral Artery with Autologous Venous Tissue, Percutaneous Endoscopic Approach

041H49J Bypass Right External Iliac Artery to Left Femoral Artery with Autologous Venous Tissue, Percutaneous Endoscopic Approach

041H49K Bypass Right External Iliac Artery to Bilateral Femoral Arteries with Autologous Venous Tissue, Percutaneous Endoscopic Approach

041H49P Bypass Right External Iliac Artery to Foot Artery with Autologous Venous Tissue, Percutaneous Endoscopic Approach

041H49Q Bypass Right External Iliac Artery to Lower Extremity Artery with Autologous Venous Tissue, Percutaneous Endoscopic Approach

041H4A9 Bypass Right External Iliac Artery to Right Internal Iliac Artery with Autologous Arterial Tissue, Percutaneous Endoscopic Approach

041H4AB Bypass Right External Iliac Artery to Left Internal Iliac Artery with Autologous Arterial Tissue, Percutaneous Endoscopic Approach

041H4AC Bypass Right External Iliac Artery to Bilateral Internal Iliac Arteries with Autologous Arterial Tissue, Percutaneous Endoscopic Approach

041H4AD Bypass Right External Iliac Artery to Right External Iliac Artery with Autologous Arterial Tissue, Percutaneous Endoscopic Approach

041H4AF Bypass Right External Iliac Artery to Left External Iliac Artery with Autologous Arterial Tissue, Percutaneous Endoscopic Approach

041H4AG Bypass Right External Iliac Artery to Bilateral External Iliac Arteries with Autologous Arterial Tissue, Percutaneous Endoscopic Approach

041H4AH Bypass Right External Iliac Artery to Right Femoral Artery with Autologous Arterial Tissue, Percutaneous Endoscopic Approach

041H4AJ Bypass Right External Iliac Artery to Left Femoral Artery with Autologous Arterial Tissue, Percutaneous Endoscopic Approach

041H4AK Bypass Right External Iliac Artery to Bilateral Femoral Arteries with Autologous Arterial Tissue, Percutaneous Endoscopic Approach

041H4AP Bypass Right External Iliac Artery to Foot Artery with Autologous Arterial Tissue, Percutaneous Endoscopic Approach

041H4AQ Bypass Right External Iliac Artery to Lower Extremity Artery with Autologous Arterial Tissue, Percutaneous Endoscopic Approach

041H4J9 Bypass Right External Iliac Artery to Right Internal Iliac Artery with Synthetic Substitute, Percutaneous Endoscopic Approach

041H4JB Bypass Right External Iliac Artery to Left Internal Iliac Artery with Synthetic Substitute, Percutaneous Endoscopic Approach

041H4JC Bypass Right External Iliac Artery to Bilateral Internal Iliac Arteries with Synthetic Substitute, Percutaneous Endoscopic Approach

041H4JD Bypass Right External Iliac Artery to Right External Iliac Artery with Synthetic Substitute, Percutaneous Endoscopic Approach

041H4JF Bypass Right External Iliac Artery to Left External Iliac Artery with Synthetic Substitute, Percutaneous Endoscopic Approach

041H4JG Bypass Right External Iliac Artery to Bilateral External Iliac Arteries with Synthetic Substitute, Percutaneous Endoscopic Approach

041H4JH Bypass Right External Iliac Artery to Right Femoral Artery with Synthetic Substitute, Percutaneous Endoscopic Approach

041H4JJ Bypass Right External Iliac Artery to Left Femoral Artery with Synthetic Substitute, Percutaneous Endoscopic Approach

041H4JK Bypass Right External Iliac Artery to Bilateral Femoral Arteries with Synthetic Substitute, Percutaneous Endoscopic Approach

041H4JP Bypass Right External Iliac Artery to Foot Artery with Synthetic Substitute, Percutaneous Endoscopic Approach

041H4JQ Bypass Right External Iliac Artery to Lower Extremity Artery with Synthetic Substitute, Percutaneous Endoscopic Approach

041H4K9 Bypass Right External Iliac Artery to Right Internal Iliac Artery with Nonautologous Tissue Substitute, Percutaneous Endoscopic Approach

041H4KB Bypass Right External Iliac Artery to Left Internal Iliac Artery with Nonautologous Tissue Substitute, Percutaneous Endoscopic Approach

041H4KC Bypass Right External Iliac Artery to Bilateral Internal Iliac Arteries with Nonautologous Tissue Substitute, Percutaneous Endoscopic Approach

041H4KD Bypass Right External Iliac Artery to Right External Iliac Artery with Nonautologous Tissue Substitute, Percutaneous Endoscopic Approach

041H4KF Bypass Right External Iliac Artery to Left External Iliac Artery with Nonautologous Tissue Substitute, Percutaneous Endoscopic Approach

041H4KG Bypass Right External Iliac Artery to Bilateral External Iliac Arteries with Nonautologous Tissue Substitute, Percutaneous Endoscopic Approach

041H4KH Bypass Right External Iliac Artery to Right Femoral Artery with Nonautologous Tissue Substitute, Percutaneous Endoscopic Approach

041H4KJ Bypass Right External Iliac Artery to Left Femoral Artery with Nonautologous Tissue Substitute, Percutaneous Endoscopic Approach

041H4KK Bypass Right External Iliac Artery to Bilateral Femoral Arteries with Nonautologous Tissue Substitute, Percutaneous Endoscopic Approach

041H4KP Bypass Right External Iliac Artery to Foot Artery with Nonautologous Tissue Substitute, Percutaneous Endoscopic Approach

041H4KQ Bypass Right External Iliac Artery to Lower Extremity Artery with Nonautologous Tissue Substitute, Percutaneous Endoscopic Approach

041H4Z9 Bypass Right External Iliac Artery to Right Internal Iliac Artery, Percutaneous Endoscopic Approach

041H4ZB Bypass Right External Iliac Artery to Left Internal Iliac Artery, Percutaneous Endoscopic Approach

041H4ZC Bypass Right External Iliac Artery to Bilateral Internal Iliac Arteries, Percutaneous Endoscopic Approach

041H4ZD Bypass Right External Iliac Artery to Right External Iliac Artery, Percutaneous Endoscopic Approach

041H4ZF Bypass Right External Iliac Artery to Left External Iliac Artery, Percutaneous Endoscopic Approach

041H4ZG Bypass Right External Iliac Artery to Bilateral External Iliac Arteries, Percutaneous Endoscopic Approach

041H4ZH Bypass Right External Iliac Artery to Right Femoral Artery, Percutaneous Endoscopic Approach

041H4ZJ Bypass Right External Iliac Artery to Left Femoral Artery, Percutaneous Endoscopic Approach

041H4ZK Bypass Right External Iliac Artery to Bilateral Femoral Arteries, Percutaneous Endoscopic Approach

041H4ZP Bypass Right External Iliac Artery to Foot Artery, Percutaneous Endoscopic Approach

041H4ZQ Bypass Right External Iliac Artery to Lower Extremity Artery, Percutaneous Endoscopic Approach

041J099 Bypass Left External Iliac Artery to Right Internal Iliac Artery with Autologous Venous Tissue, Open Approach

041J09B Bypass Left External Iliac Artery to Left Internal Iliac Artery with Autologous Venous Tissue, Open Approach

041J09C Bypass Left External Iliac Artery to Bilateral Internal Iliac Arteries with Autologous Venous Tissue, Open Approach

041J09D Bypass Left External Iliac Artery to Right External Iliac Artery with Autologous Venous Tissue, Open Approach

041J09F Bypass Left External Iliac Artery to Left External Iliac Artery with Autologous Venous Tissue, Open Approach

041J09G Bypass Left External Iliac Artery to Bilateral External Iliac Arteries with Autologous Venous Tissue, Open Approach

041J09H Bypass Left External Iliac Artery to Right Femoral Artery with Autologous Venous Tissue, Open Approach

041J09J Bypass Left External Iliac Artery to Left Femoral Artery with Autologous Venous Tissue, Open Approach

041J09K Bypass Left External Iliac Artery to Bilateral Femoral Arteries with Autologous Venous Tissue, Open Approach

041J09P Bypass Left External Iliac Artery to Foot Artery with Autologous Venous Tissue, Open Approach

041J09Q Bypass Left External Iliac Artery to Lower Extremity Artery with Autologous Venous Tissue, Open Approach

041J0A9 Bypass Left External Iliac Artery to Right Internal Iliac Artery with Autologous Arterial Tissue, Open Approach

041J0AB Bypass Left External Iliac Artery to Left Internal Iliac Artery with Autologous Arterial Tissue, Open Approach

041J0AC Bypass Left External Iliac Artery to Bilateral Internal Iliac Arteries with Autologous Arterial Tissue, Open Approach

041J0AD Bypass Left External Iliac Artery to Right External Iliac Artery with Autologous Arterial Tissue, Open Approach

041J0AF Bypass Left External Iliac Artery to Left External Iliac Artery with Autologous Arterial Tissue, Open Approach

041J0AG Bypass Left External Iliac Artery to Bilateral External Iliac Arteries with Autologous Arterial Tissue, Open Approach

041J0AH Bypass Left External Iliac Artery to Right Femoral Artery with Autologous Arterial Tissue, Open Approach

041J0AJ Bypass Left External Iliac Artery to Left Femoral Artery with Autologous Arterial Tissue, Open Approach

041J0AK Bypass Left External Iliac Artery to Bilateral Femoral Arteries with Autologous Arterial Tissue, Open Approach

041J0AP Bypass Left External Iliac Artery to Foot Artery with Autologous Arterial Tissue, Open Approach

041J0AQ Bypass Left External Iliac Artery to Lower Extremity Artery with Autologous Arterial Tissue, Open Approach

041J0J9 Bypass Left External Iliac Artery to Right Internal Iliac Artery with Synthetic Substitute, Open Approach

041J0JB Bypass Left External Iliac Artery to Left Internal Iliac Artery with Synthetic Substitute, Open Approach

041J0JC Bypass Left External Iliac Artery to Bilateral Internal Iliac Arteries with Synthetic Substitute, Open Approach

041J0JD Bypass Left External Iliac Artery to Right External Iliac Artery with Synthetic Substitute, Open Approach

041J0JF Bypass Left External Iliac Artery to Left External Iliac Artery with Synthetic Substitute, Open Approach

041J0JG Bypass Left External Iliac Artery to Bilateral External Iliac Arteries with Synthetic Substitute, Open Approach

041J0JH Bypass Left External Iliac Artery to Right Femoral Artery with Synthetic Substitute, Open Approach

041J0JJ Bypass Left External Iliac Artery to Left Femoral Artery with Synthetic Substitute, Open Approach

041J0JK Bypass Left External Iliac Artery to Bilateral Femoral Arteries with Synthetic Substitute, Open Approach

041J0JP Bypass Left External Iliac Artery to Foot Artery with Synthetic Substitute, Open Approach

041J0JQ Bypass Left External Iliac Artery to Lower Extremity Artery with Synthetic Substitute, Open Approach

041J0K9 Bypass Left External Iliac Artery to Right Internal Iliac Artery with Nonautologous Tissue Substitute, Open Approach

041J0KB Bypass Left External Iliac Artery to Left Internal Iliac Artery with Nonautologous Tissue Substitute, Open Approach

041J0KC Bypass Left External Iliac Artery to Bilateral Internal Iliac Arteries with Nonautologous Tissue Substitute, Open Approach

041J0KD Bypass Left External Iliac Artery to Right External Iliac Artery with Nonautologous Tissue Substitute, Open Approach

041J0KF Bypass Left External Iliac Artery to Left External Iliac Artery with Nonautologous Tissue Substitute, Open Approach

041J0KG Bypass Left External Iliac Artery to Bilateral External Iliac Arteries with Nonautologous Tissue Substitute, Open Approach

041J0KH Bypass Left External Iliac Artery to Right Femoral Artery with Nonautologous Tissue Substitute, Open Approach

041J0KJ Bypass Left External Iliac Artery to Left Femoral Artery with Nonautologous Tissue Substitute, Open Approach

041J0KK Bypass Left External Iliac Artery to Bilateral Femoral Arteries with Nonautologous Tissue Substitute, Open Approach

041J0KP Bypass Left External Iliac Artery to Foot Artery with Nonautologous Tissue Substitute, Open Approach

041J0KQ Bypass Left External Iliac Artery to Lower Extremity Artery with Nonautologous Tissue Substitute, Open Approach

041J0Z9 Bypass Left External Iliac Artery to Right Internal Iliac Artery, Open Approach

♀ Female-only   ♂ Male-only   ▲ Limited Coverage   ● Non-OR   ▆ HAC-associated procedure   ▲ Non-covered procedures   ✚ Cluster

041J0ZB Bypass Left External Iliac Artery to Left Internal Iliac Artery, Open Approach

041J0ZC Bypass Left External Iliac Artery to Bilateral Internal Iliac Arteries, Open Approach

041J0ZD Bypass Left External Iliac Artery to Right External Iliac Artery, Open Approach

041J0ZF Bypass Left External Iliac Artery to Left External Iliac Artery, Open Approach

041J0ZG Bypass Left External Iliac Artery to Bilateral External Iliac Arteries, Open Approach

041J0ZH Bypass Left External Iliac Artery to Right Femoral Artery, Open Approach

041J0ZJ Bypass Left External Iliac Artery to Left Femoral Artery, Open Approach

041J0ZK Bypass Left External Iliac Artery to Bilateral Femoral Arteries, Open Approach

041J0ZP Bypass Left External Iliac Artery to Foot Artery, Open Approach

041J0ZQ Bypass Left External Iliac Artery to Lower Extremity Artery, Open Approach

041J499 Bypass Left External Iliac Artery to Right Internal Iliac Artery with Autologous Venous Tissue, Percutaneous Endoscopic Approach

041J49B Bypass Left External Iliac Artery to Left Internal Iliac Artery with Autologous Venous Tissue, Percutaneous Endoscopic Approach

041J49C Bypass Left External Iliac Artery to Bilateral Internal Iliac Arteries with Autologous Venous Tissue, Percutaneous Endoscopic Approach

041J49D Bypass Left External Iliac Artery to Right External Iliac Artery with Autologous Venous Tissue, Percutaneous Endoscopic Approach

041J49F Bypass Left External Iliac Artery to Left External Iliac Artery with Autologous Venous Tissue, Percutaneous Endoscopic Approach

041J49G Bypass Left External Iliac Artery to Bilateral External Iliac Arteries with Autologous Venous Tissue, Percutaneous Endoscopic Approach

041J49H Bypass Left External Iliac Artery to Right Femoral Artery with Autologous Venous Tissue, Percutaneous Endoscopic Approach

041J49J Bypass Left External Iliac Artery to Left Femoral Artery with Autologous Venous Tissue, Percutaneous Endoscopic Approach

041J49K Bypass Left External Iliac Artery to Bilateral Femoral Arteries with Autologous Venous Tissue, Percutaneous Endoscopic Approach

041J49P Bypass Left External Iliac Artery to Foot Artery with Autologous Venous Tissue, Percutaneous Endoscopic Approach

041J49Q Bypass Left External Iliac Artery to Lower Extremity Artery with Autologous Venous Tissue, Percutaneous Endoscopic Approach

041J4A9 Bypass Left External Iliac Artery to Right Internal Iliac Artery with Autologous Arterial Tissue, Percutaneous Endoscopic Approach

041J4AB Bypass Left External Iliac Artery to Left Internal Iliac Artery with Autologous Arterial Tissue, Percutaneous Endoscopic Approach

041J4AC Bypass Left External Iliac Artery to Bilateral Internal Iliac Arteries with Autologous Arterial Tissue, Percutaneous Endoscopic Approach

041J4AD Bypass Left External Iliac Artery to Right External Iliac Artery with Autologous Arterial Tissue, Percutaneous Endoscopic Approach

041J4AF Bypass Left External Iliac Artery to Left External Iliac Artery with Autologous Arterial Tissue, Percutaneous Endoscopic Approach

041J4AG Bypass Left External Iliac Artery to Bilateral External Iliac Arteries with Autologous Arterial Tissue, Percutaneous Endoscopic Approach

041J4AH Bypass Left External Iliac Artery to Right Femoral Artery with Autologous Arterial Tissue, Percutaneous Endoscopic Approach

041J4AJ Bypass Left External Iliac Artery to Left Femoral Artery with Autologous Arterial Tissue, Percutaneous Endoscopic Approach

041J4AK Bypass Left External Iliac Artery to Bilateral Femoral Arteries with Autologous Arterial Tissue, Percutaneous Endoscopic Approach

041J4AP Bypass Left External Iliac Artery to Foot Artery with Autologous Arterial Tissue, Percutaneous Endoscopic Approach

041J4AQ Bypass Left External Iliac Artery to Lower Extremity Artery with Autologous Arterial Tissue, Percutaneous Endoscopic Approach

041J4J9 Bypass Left External Iliac Artery to Right Internal Iliac Artery with Synthetic Substitute, Percutaneous Endoscopic Approach

041J4JB Bypass Left External Iliac Artery to Left Internal Iliac Artery with Synthetic Substitute, Percutaneous Endoscopic Approach

041J4JC Bypass Left External Iliac Artery to Bilateral Internal Iliac Arteries with Synthetic Substitute, Percutaneous Endoscopic Approach

041J4JD Bypass Left External Iliac Artery to Right External Iliac Artery with Synthetic Substitute, Percutaneous Endoscopic Approach

041J4JF Bypass Left External Iliac Artery to Left External Iliac Artery with Synthetic Substitute, Percutaneous Endoscopic Approach

041J4JG Bypass Left External Iliac Artery to Bilateral External Iliac Arteries with Synthetic Substitute, Percutaneous Endoscopic Approach

041J4JH Bypass Left External Iliac Artery to Right Femoral Artery with Synthetic Substitute, Percutaneous Endoscopic Approach

041J4JJ Bypass Left External Iliac Artery to Left Femoral Artery with Synthetic Substitute, Percutaneous Endoscopic Approach

041J4JK Bypass Left External Iliac Artery to Bilateral Femoral Arteries with Synthetic Substitute, Percutaneous Endoscopic Approach

041J4JP Bypass Left External Iliac Artery to Foot Artery with Synthetic Substitute, Percutaneous Endoscopic Approach

041J4JQ Bypass Left External Iliac Artery to Lower Extremity Artery with Synthetic Substitute, Percutaneous Endoscopic Approach

041J4K9 Bypass Left External Iliac Artery to Right Internal Iliac Artery with Nonautologous Tissue Substitute, Percutaneous Endoscopic Approach

041J4KB Bypass Left External Iliac Artery to Left Internal Iliac Artery with Nonautologous Tissue Substitute, Percutaneous Endoscopic Approach

041J4KC Bypass Left External Iliac Artery to Bilateral Internal Iliac Arteries with Nonautologous Tissue Substitute, Percutaneous Endoscopic Approach

041J4KD Bypass Left External Iliac Artery to Right External Iliac Artery with Nonautologous Tissue Substitute, Percutaneous Endoscopic Approach

041J4KF Bypass Left External Iliac Artery to Left External Iliac Artery with Nonautologous Tissue Substitute, Percutaneous Endoscopic Approach

041J4KG Bypass Left External Iliac Artery to Bilateral External Iliac Arteries with Nonautologous Tissue Substitute, Percutaneous Endoscopic Approach

041J4KH Bypass Left External Iliac Artery to Right Femoral Artery with Nonautologous Tissue Substitute, Percutaneous Endoscopic Approach

041J4KJ Bypass Left External Iliac Artery to Left Femoral Artery with Nonautologous Tissue Substitute, Percutaneous Endoscopic Approach

041J4KK Bypass Left External Iliac Artery to Bilateral Femoral Arteries with Nonautologous Tissue Substitute, Percutaneous Endoscopic Approach

041J4KP Bypass Left External Iliac Artery to Foot Artery with Nonautologous Tissue Substitute, Percutaneous Endoscopic Approach

041J4KQ Bypass Left External Iliac Artery to Lower Extremity Artery with Nonautologous Tissue Substitute, Percutaneous Endoscopic Approach

041J4Z9 Bypass Left External Iliac Artery to Right Internal Iliac Artery, Percutaneous Endoscopic Approach

041J4ZB Bypass Left External Iliac Artery to Left Internal Iliac Artery, Percutaneous Endoscopic Approach

041J4ZC Bypass Left External Iliac Artery to Bilateral Internal Iliac Arteries, Percutaneous Endoscopic Approach

041J4ZD Bypass Left External Iliac Artery to Right External Iliac Artery, Percutaneous Endoscopic Approach

041J4ZF Bypass Left External Iliac Artery to Left External Iliac Artery, Percutaneous Endoscopic Approach

041J4ZG Bypass Left External Iliac Artery to Bilateral External Iliac Arteries, Percutaneous Endoscopic Approach

041J4ZH Bypass Left External Iliac Artery to Right Femoral Artery, Percutaneous Endoscopic Approach

041J4ZJ Bypass Left External Iliac Artery to Left Femoral Artery, Percutaneous Endoscopic Approach

041J4ZK Bypass Left External Iliac Artery to Bilateral Femoral Arteries, Percutaneous Endoscopic Approach

041J4ZP Bypass Left External Iliac Artery to Foot Artery, Percutaneous Endoscopic Approach

041J4ZQ Bypass Left External Iliac Artery to Lower Extremity Artery, Percutaneous Endoscopic Approach

041K09H Bypass Right Femoral Artery to Right Femoral Artery with Autologous Venous Tissue, Open Approach

041K09J Bypass Right Femoral Artery to Left Femoral Artery with Autologous Venous Tissue, Open Approach

041K09K Bypass Right Femoral Artery to Bilateral Femoral Arteries with Autologous Venous Tissue, Open Approach

041K09L Bypass Right Femoral Artery to Popliteal Artery with Autologous Venous Tissue, Open Approach

041K09M Bypass Right Femoral Artery to Peroneal Artery with Autologous Venous Tissue, Open Approach

041K09N Bypass Right Femoral Artery to Posterior Tibial Artery with Autologous Venous Tissue, Open Approach

AHA CC: 3Q, 2017, 5-6

041K09P Bypass Right Femoral Artery to Foot Artery with Autologous Venous Tissue, Open Approach

041K09Q Bypass Right Femoral Artery to Lower Extremity Artery with Autologous Venous Tissue, Open Approach

041K09S Bypass Right Femoral Artery to Lower Extremity Vein with Autologous Venous Tissue, Open Approach

041K0AH Bypass Right Femoral Artery to Right Femoral Artery with Autologous Arterial Tissue, Open Approach

041K0AJ Bypass Right Femoral Artery to Left Femoral Artery with Autologous Arterial Tissue, Open Approach

041K0AK Bypass Right Femoral Artery to Bilateral Femoral Arteries with Autologous Arterial Tissue, Open Approach

041K0AL Bypass Right Femoral Artery to Popliteal Artery with Autologous Arterial Tissue, Open Approach

041K0AM Bypass Right Femoral Artery to Peroneal Artery with Autologous Arterial Tissue, Open Approach

041K0AN Bypass Right Femoral Artery to Posterior Tibial Artery with Autologous Arterial Tissue, Open Approach

041K0AP Bypass Right Femoral Artery to Foot Artery with Autologous Arterial Tissue, Open Approach

041K0AQ Bypass Right Femoral Artery to Lower Extremity Artery with Autologous Arterial Tissue, Open Approach

041K0AS Bypass Right Femoral Artery to Lower Extremity Vein with Autologous Arterial Tissue, Open Approach

041K0JH Bypass Right Femoral Artery to Right Femoral Artery with Synthetic Substitute, Open Approach

041K0JJ Bypass Right Femoral Artery to Left Femoral Artery with Synthetic Substitute, Open Approach

041K0JK Bypass Right Femoral Artery to Bilateral Femoral Arteries with Synthetic Substitute, Open Approach

041K0JL Bypass Right Femoral Artery to Popliteal Artery with Synthetic Substitute, Open Approach

AHA CC: 3Q, 2018, 25

041K0JM Bypass Right Femoral Artery to Peroneal Artery with Synthetic Substitute, Open Approach

041K0JN Bypass Right Femoral Artery to Posterior Tibial Artery with Synthetic Substitute, Open Approach

AHA CC: 2Q, 2016, 18-19; 3Q, 2017, 5-6

041K0JP Bypass Right Femoral Artery to Foot Artery with Synthetic Substitute, Open Approach

041K0JQ Bypass Right Femoral Artery to Lower Extremity Artery with Synthetic Substitute, Open Approach

041K0JS Bypass Right Femoral Artery to Lower Extremity Vein with Synthetic Substitute, Open Approach

041K0KH Bypass Right Femoral Artery to Right Femoral Artery with Nonautologous Tissue Substitute, Open Approach

041K0KJ Bypass Right Femoral Artery to Left Femoral Artery with Nonautologous Tissue Substitute, Open Approach

041K0KK Bypass Right Femoral Artery to Bilateral Femoral Arteries with Nonautologous Tissue Substitute, Open Approach

041K0KL Bypass Right Femoral Artery to Popliteal Artery with Nonautologous Tissue Substitute, Open Approach

041K0KM Bypass Right Femoral Artery to Peroneal Artery with Nonautologous Tissue Substitute, Open Approach

041K0KN Bypass Right Femoral Artery to Posterior Tibial Artery with Nonautologous Tissue Substitute, Open Approach

041K0KP Bypass Right Femoral Artery to Foot Artery with Nonautologous Tissue Substitute, Open Approach

041K0KQ Bypass Right Femoral Artery to Lower Extremity Artery with Nonautologous Tissue Substitute, Open Approach

041K0KS Bypass Right Femoral Artery to Lower Extremity Vein with Nonautologous Tissue Substitute, Open Approach

041K0ZH Bypass Right Femoral Artery to Right Femoral Artery, Open Approach

041K0ZJ Bypass Right Femoral Artery to Left Femoral Artery, Open Approach

041K0ZK Bypass Right Femoral Artery to Bilateral Femoral Arteries, Open Approach

041K0ZL Bypass Right Femoral Artery to Popliteal Artery, Open Approach

041K0ZM Bypass Right Femoral Artery to Peroneal Artery, Open Approach

041K0ZN Bypass Right Femoral Artery to Posterior Tibial Artery, Open Approach

041K0ZP Bypass Right Femoral Artery to Foot Artery, Open Approach

041K0ZQ Bypass Right Femoral Artery to Lower Extremity Artery, Open Approach

041K0ZS Bypass Right Femoral Artery to Lower Extremity Vein, Open Approach

041K3JQ Bypass Right Femoral Artery to Lower Extremity Artery with Synthetic Substitute, Percutaneous Approach

041K3JS Bypass Right Femoral Artery to Lower Extremity Vein with Synthetic Substitute, Percutaneous Approach

041K49H Bypass Right Femoral Artery to Right Femoral Artery with Autologous Venous Tissue, Percutaneous Endoscopic Approach

041K49J Bypass Right Femoral Artery to Left Femoral Artery with Autologous Venous Tissue, Percutaneous Endoscopic Approach

041K49K Bypass Right Femoral Artery to Bilateral Femoral Arteries with Autologous Venous Tissue, Percutaneous Endoscopic Approach

041K49L Bypass Right Femoral Artery to Popliteal Artery with Autologous Venous Tissue, Percutaneous Endoscopic Approach

041K49M Bypass Right Femoral Artery to Peroneal Artery with Autologous Venous Tissue, Percutaneous Endoscopic Approach

041K49N Bypass Right Femoral Artery to Posterior Tibial Artery with Autologous Venous Tissue, Percutaneous Endoscopic Approach

041K49P Bypass Right Femoral Artery to Foot Artery with Autologous Venous Tissue, Percutaneous Endoscopic Approach

041K49Q Bypass Right Femoral Artery to Lower Extremity Artery with Autologous Venous Tissue, Percutaneous Endoscopic Approach

041K49S Bypass Right Femoral Artery to Lower Extremity Vein with Autologous Venous Tissue, Percutaneous Endoscopic Approach

041K4AH Bypass Right Femoral Artery to Right Femoral Artery with Autologous Arterial Tissue, Percutaneous Endoscopic Approach

041K4AJ Bypass Right Femoral Artery to Left Femoral Artery with Autologous Arterial Tissue, Percutaneous Endoscopic Approach

041K4AK Bypass Right Femoral Artery to Bilateral Femoral Arteries with Autologous Arterial Tissue, Percutaneous Endoscopic Approach

041K4AL Bypass Right Femoral Artery to Popliteal Artery with Autologous Arterial Tissue, Percutaneous Endoscopic Approach

041K4AM Bypass Right Femoral Artery to Peroneal Artery with Autologous Arterial Tissue, Percutaneous Endoscopic Approach

041K4AN Bypass Right Femoral Artery to Posterior Tibial Artery with Autologous Arterial Tissue, Percutaneous Endoscopic Approach

041K4AP Bypass Right Femoral Artery to Foot Artery with Autologous Arterial Tissue, Percutaneous Endoscopic Approach

041K4AQ Bypass Right Femoral Artery to Lower Extremity Artery with Autologous Arterial Tissue, Percutaneous Endoscopic Approach

041K4AS Bypass Right Femoral Artery to Lower Extremity Vein with Autologous Arterial Tissue, Percutaneous Endoscopic Approach

041K4JH Bypass Right Femoral Artery to Right Femoral Artery with Synthetic Substitute, Percutaneous Endoscopic Approach

♀ Female-only   ♂ Male-only   ▲ Limited Coverage   ● Non-OR   ⬛ HAC-associated procedure   ▲ Non-covered procedures   ✚ Cluster

041K4JJ Bypass Right Femoral Artery to Left Femoral Artery with Synthetic Substitute, Percutaneous Endoscopic Approach

041K4JK Bypass Right Femoral Artery to Bilateral Femoral Arteries with Synthetic Substitute, Percutaneous Endoscopic Approach

041K4JL Bypass Right Femoral Artery to Popliteal Artery with Synthetic Substitute, Percutaneous Endoscopic Approach

041K4JM Bypass Right Femoral Artery to Peroneal Artery with Synthetic Substitute, Percutaneous Endoscopic Approach

041K4JN Bypass Right Femoral Artery to Posterior Tibial Artery with Synthetic Substitute, Percutaneous Endoscopic Approach

041K4JP Bypass Right Femoral Artery to Foot Artery with Synthetic Substitute, Percutaneous Endoscopic Approach

041K4JQ Bypass Right Femoral Artery to Lower Extremity Artery with Synthetic Substitute, Percutaneous Endoscopic Approach

041K4JS Bypass Right Femoral Artery to Lower Extremity Vein with Synthetic Substitute, Percutaneous Endoscopic Approach

041K4KH Bypass Right Femoral Artery to Right Femoral Artery with Nonautologous Tissue Substitute, Percutaneous Endoscopic Approach

041K4KJ Bypass Right Femoral Artery to Left Femoral Artery with Nonautologous Tissue Substitute, Percutaneous Endoscopic Approach

041K4KK Bypass Right Femoral Artery to Bilateral Femoral Arteries with Nonautologous Tissue Substitute, Percutaneous Endoscopic Approach

041K4KL Bypass Right Femoral Artery to Popliteal Artery with Nonautologous Tissue Substitute, Percutaneous Endoscopic Approach

041K4KM Bypass Right Femoral Artery to Peroneal Artery with Nonautologous Tissue Substitute, Percutaneous Endoscopic Approach

041K4KN Bypass Right Femoral Artery to Posterior Tibial Artery with Nonautologous Tissue Substitute, Percutaneous Endoscopic Approach

041K4KP Bypass Right Femoral Artery to Foot Artery with Nonautologous Tissue Substitute, Percutaneous Endoscopic Approach

041K4KQ Bypass Right Femoral Artery to Lower Extremity Artery with Nonautologous Tissue Substitute, Percutaneous Endoscopic Approach

041K4KS Bypass Right Femoral Artery to Lower Extremity Vein with Nonautologous Tissue Substitute, Percutaneous Endoscopic Approach

041K4ZH Bypass Right Femoral Artery to Right Femoral Artery, Percutaneous Endoscopic Approach

041K4ZJ Bypass Right Femoral Artery to Left Femoral Artery, Percutaneous Endoscopic Approach

041K4ZK Bypass Right Femoral Artery to Bilateral Femoral Arteries, Percutaneous Endoscopic Approach

041K4ZL Bypass Right Femoral Artery to Popliteal Artery, Percutaneous Endoscopic Approach

041K4ZM Bypass Right Femoral Artery to Peroneal Artery, Percutaneous Endoscopic Approach

041K4ZN Bypass Right Femoral Artery to Posterior Tibial Artery, Percutaneous Endoscopic Approach

041K4ZP Bypass Right Femoral Artery to Foot Artery, Percutaneous Endoscopic Approach

041K4ZQ Bypass Right Femoral Artery to Lower Extremity Artery, Percutaneous Endoscopic Approach

041K4ZS Bypass Right Femoral Artery to Lower Extremity Vein, Percutaneous Endoscopic Approach

041L09H Bypass Left Femoral Artery to Right Femoral Artery with Autologous Venous Tissue, Open Approach

041L09J Bypass Left Femoral Artery to Left Femoral Artery with Autologous Venous Tissue, Open Approach

041L09K Bypass Left Femoral Artery to Bilateral Femoral Arteries with Autologous Venous Tissue, Open Approach

041L09L Bypass Left Femoral Artery to Popliteal Artery with Autologous Venous Tissue, Open Approach

041L09M Bypass Left Femoral Artery to Peroneal Artery with Autologous Venous Tissue, Open Approach

041L09N Bypass Left Femoral Artery to Posterior Tibial Artery with Autologous Venous Tissue, Open Approach

041L09P Bypass Left Femoral Artery to Foot Artery with Autologous Venous Tissue, Open Approach

041L09Q Bypass Left Femoral Artery to Lower Extremity Artery with Autologous Venous Tissue, Open Approach

041L09S Bypass Left Femoral Artery to Lower Extremity Vein with Autologous Venous Tissue, Open Approach

041L0AH Bypass Left Femoral Artery to Right Femoral Artery with Autologous Arterial Tissue, Open Approach

041L0AJ Bypass Left Femoral Artery to Left Femoral Artery with Autologous Arterial Tissue, Open Approach

041L0AK Bypass Left Femoral Artery to Bilateral Femoral Arteries with Autologous Arterial Tissue, Open Approach

041L0AL Bypass Left Femoral Artery to Popliteal Artery with Autologous Arterial Tissue, Open Approach

041L0AM Bypass Left Femoral Artery to Peroneal Artery with Autologous Arterial Tissue, Open Approach

041L0AN Bypass Left Femoral Artery to Posterior Tibial Artery with Autologous Arterial Tissue, Open Approach

041L0AP Bypass Left Femoral Artery to Foot Artery with Autologous Arterial Tissue, Open Approach

041L0AQ Bypass Left Femoral Artery to Lower Extremity Artery with Autologous Arterial Tissue, Open Approach

041L0AS Bypass Left Femoral Artery to Lower Extremity Vein with Autologous Arterial Tissue, Open Approach

041L0JH Bypass Left Femoral Artery to Right Femoral Artery with Synthetic Substitute, Open Approach

041L0JJ Bypass Left Femoral Artery to Left Femoral Artery with Synthetic Substitute, Open Approach

041L0JK Bypass Left Femoral Artery to Bilateral Femoral Arteries with Synthetic Substitute, Open Approach

041L0JL Bypass Left Femoral Artery to Popliteal Artery with Synthetic Substitute, Open Approach

041L0JM Bypass Left Femoral Artery to Peroneal Artery with Synthetic Substitute, Open Approach

041L0JN Bypass Left Femoral Artery to Posterior Tibial Artery with Synthetic Substitute, Open Approach

041L0JP Bypass Left Femoral Artery to Foot Artery with Synthetic Substitute, Open Approach

041L0JQ Bypass Left Femoral Artery to Lower Extremity Artery with Synthetic Substitute, Open Approach

041L0JS Bypass Left Femoral Artery to Lower Extremity Vein with Synthetic Substitute, Open Approach

041L0KH Bypass Left Femoral Artery to Right Femoral Artery with Nonautologous Tissue Substitute, Open Approach

041L0KJ Bypass Left Femoral Artery to Left Femoral Artery with Nonautologous Tissue Substitute, Open Approach

041L0KK Bypass Left Femoral Artery to Bilateral Femoral Arteries with Nonautologous Tissue Substitute, Open Approach

041L0KL Bypass Left Femoral Artery to Popliteal Artery with Nonautologous Tissue Substitute, Open Approach

041L0KM Bypass Left Femoral Artery to Peroneal Artery with Nonautologous Tissue Substitute, Open Approach

041L0KN Bypass Left Femoral Artery to Posterior Tibial Artery with Nonautologous Tissue Substitute, Open Approach

041L0KP Bypass Left Femoral Artery to Foot Artery with Nonautologous Tissue Substitute, Open Approach

041L0KQ Bypass Left Femoral Artery to Lower Extremity Artery with Nonautologous Tissue Substitute, Open Approach

041L0KS Bypass Left Femoral Artery to Lower Extremity Vein with Nonautologous Tissue Substitute, Open Approach

041L0ZH Bypass Left Femoral Artery to Right Femoral Artery, Open Approach

041L0ZJ Bypass Left Femoral Artery to Left Femoral Artery, Open Approach

041L0ZK Bypass Left Femoral Artery to Bilateral Femoral Arteries, Open Approach

041L0ZL Bypass Left Femoral Artery to Popliteal Artery, Open Approach

041L0ZM Bypass Left Femoral Artery to Peroneal Artery, Open Approach

041L0ZN Bypass Left Femoral Artery to Posterior Tibial Artery, Open Approach

041L0ZP Bypass Left Femoral Artery to Foot Artery, Open Approach

041L0ZQ Bypass Left Femoral Artery to Lower Extremity Artery, Open Approach

041L0ZS Bypass Left Femoral Artery to Lower Extremity Vein, Open Approach

041L3JQ Bypass Left Femoral Artery to Lower Extremity Artery with Synthetic Substitute, Percutaneous Approach

---

♀ Female-only   ♂ Male-only   ▲ Limited Coverage   ● Non-OR   ▥ HAC-associated procedure   ▲ Non-covered procedures   ✚ Cluster

041L3JS Bypass Left Femoral Artery to Lower Extremity Vein with Synthetic Substitute, Percutaneous Approach

041L49H Bypass Left Femoral Artery to Right Femoral Artery with Autologous Venous Tissue, Percutaneous Endoscopic Approach

041L49J Bypass Left Femoral Artery to Left Femoral Artery with Autologous Venous Tissue, Percutaneous Endoscopic Approach

041L49K Bypass Left Femoral Artery to Bilateral Femoral Arteries with Autologous Venous Tissue, Percutaneous Endoscopic Approach

041L49L Bypass Left Femoral Artery to Popliteal Artery with Autologous Venous Tissue, Percutaneous Endoscopic Approach

041L49M Bypass Left Femoral Artery to Peroneal Artery with Autologous Venous Tissue, Percutaneous Endoscopic Approach

041L49N Bypass Left Femoral Artery to Posterior Tibial Artery with Autologous Venous Tissue, Percutaneous Endoscopic Approach

041L49P Bypass Left Femoral Artery to Foot Artery with Autologous Venous Tissue, Percutaneous Endoscopic Approach

041L49Q Bypass Left Femoral Artery to Lower Extremity Artery with Autologous Venous Tissue, Percutaneous Endoscopic Approach

041L49S Bypass Left Femoral Artery to Lower Extremity Vein with Autologous Venous Tissue, Percutaneous Endoscopic Approach

041L4AH Bypass Left Femoral Artery to Right Femoral Artery with Autologous Arterial Tissue, Percutaneous Endoscopic Approach

041L4AJ Bypass Left Femoral Artery to Left Femoral Artery with Autologous Arterial Tissue, Percutaneous Endoscopic Approach

041L4AK Bypass Left Femoral Artery to Bilateral Femoral Arteries with Autologous Arterial Tissue, Percutaneous Endoscopic Approach

041L4AL Bypass Left Femoral Artery to Popliteal Artery with Autologous Arterial Tissue, Percutaneous Endoscopic Approach

041L4AM Bypass Left Femoral Artery to Peroneal Artery with Autologous Arterial Tissue, Percutaneous Endoscopic Approach

041L4AN Bypass Left Femoral Artery to Posterior Tibial Artery with Autologous Arterial Tissue, Percutaneous Endoscopic Approach

041L4AP Bypass Left Femoral Artery to Foot Artery with Autologous Arterial Tissue, Percutaneous Endoscopic Approach

041L4AQ Bypass Left Femoral Artery to Lower Extremity Artery with Autologous Arterial Tissue, Percutaneous Endoscopic Approach

041L4AS Bypass Left Femoral Artery to Lower Extremity Vein with Autologous Arterial Tissue, Percutaneous Endoscopic Approach

041L4JH Bypass Left Femoral Artery to Right Femoral Artery with Synthetic Substitute, Percutaneous Endoscopic Approach

041L4JJ Bypass Left Femoral Artery to Left Femoral Artery with Synthetic Substitute, Percutaneous Endoscopic Approach

041L4JK Bypass Left Femoral Artery to Bilateral Femoral Arteries with Synthetic Substitute, Percutaneous Endoscopic Approach

041L4JL Bypass Left Femoral Artery to Popliteal Artery with Synthetic Substitute, Percutaneous Endoscopic Approach

041L4JM Bypass Left Femoral Artery to Peroneal Artery with Synthetic Substitute, Percutaneous Endoscopic Approach

041L4JN Bypass Left Femoral Artery to Posterior Tibial Artery with Synthetic Substitute, Percutaneous Endoscopic Approach

041L4JP Bypass Left Femoral Artery to Foot Artery with Synthetic Substitute, Percutaneous Endoscopic Approach

041L4JQ Bypass Left Femoral Artery to Lower Extremity Artery with Synthetic Substitute, Percutaneous Endoscopic Approach

041L4JS Bypass Left Femoral Artery to Lower Extremity Vein with Synthetic Substitute, Percutaneous Endoscopic Approach

041L4KH Bypass Left Femoral Artery to Right Femoral Artery with Nonautologous Tissue Substitute, Percutaneous Endoscopic Approach

041L4KJ Bypass Left Femoral Artery to Left Femoral Artery with Nonautologous Tissue Substitute, Percutaneous Endoscopic Approach

041L4KK Bypass Left Femoral Artery to Bilateral Femoral Arteries with Nonautologous Tissue Substitute, Percutaneous Endoscopic Approach

041L4KL Bypass Left Femoral Artery to Popliteal Artery with Nonautologous Tissue Substitute, Percutaneous Endoscopic Approach

041L4KM Bypass Left Femoral Artery to Peroneal Artery with Nonautologous Tissue Substitute, Percutaneous Endoscopic Approach

041L4KN Bypass Left Femoral Artery to Posterior Tibial Artery with Nonautologous Tissue Substitute, Percutaneous Endoscopic Approach

041L4KP Bypass Left Femoral Artery to Foot Artery with Nonautologous Tissue Substitute, Percutaneous Endoscopic Approach

041L4KQ Bypass Left Femoral Artery to Lower Extremity Artery with Nonautologous Tissue Substitute, Percutaneous Endoscopic Approach

041L4KS Bypass Left Femoral Artery to Lower Extremity Vein with Nonautologous Tissue Substitute, Percutaneous Endoscopic Approach

041L4ZH Bypass Left Femoral Artery to Right Femoral Artery, Percutaneous Endoscopic Approach

041L4ZJ Bypass Left Femoral Artery to Left Femoral Artery, Percutaneous Endoscopic Approach

041L4ZK Bypass Left Femoral Artery to Bilateral Femoral Arteries, Percutaneous Endoscopic Approach

041L4ZL Bypass Left Femoral Artery to Popliteal Artery, Percutaneous Endoscopic Approach

041L4ZM Bypass Left Femoral Artery to Peroneal Artery, Percutaneous Endoscopic Approach

041L4ZN Bypass Left Femoral Artery to Posterior Tibial Artery, Percutaneous Endoscopic Approach

041L4ZP Bypass Left Femoral Artery to Foot Artery, Percutaneous Endoscopic Approach

041L4ZQ Bypass Left Femoral Artery to Lower Extremity Artery, Percutaneous Endoscopic Approach

041L4ZS Bypass Left Femoral Artery to Lower Extremity Vein, Percutaneous Endoscopic Approach

041M09L Bypass Right Popliteal Artery to Popliteal Artery with Autologous Venous Tissue, Open Approach

041M09M Bypass Right Popliteal Artery to Peroneal Artery with Autologous Venous Tissue, Open Approach

041M09P Bypass Right Popliteal Artery to Foot Artery with Autologous Venous Tissue Open Approach

AHA CC: 1Q, 2017, 32-33

041M09Q Bypass Right Popliteal Artery to Lower Extremity Artery with Autologous Venous Tissue, Open Approach

041M09S Bypass Right Popliteal Artery to Lower Extremity Vein with Autologous Venous Tissue, Open Approach

041M0AL Bypass Right Popliteal Artery to Popliteal Artery with Autologous Arterial Tissue, Open Approach

041M0AM Bypass Right Popliteal Artery to Peroneal Artery with Autologous Arterial Tissue, Open Approach

041M0AP Bypass Right Popliteal Artery to Foot Artery with Autologous Arterial Tissue, Open Approach

041M0AQ Bypass Right Popliteal Artery to Lower Extremity Artery with Autologous Arterial Tissue, Open Approach

041M0AS Bypass Right Popliteal Artery to Lower Extremity Vein with Autologous Arterial Tissue, Open Approach

041M0JL Bypass Right Popliteal Artery to Popliteal Artery with Synthetic Substitute, Open Approach

041M0JM Bypass Right Popliteal Artery to Peroneal Artery with Synthetic Substitute, Open Approach

041M0JP Bypass Right Popliteal Artery to Foot Artery with Synthetic Substitute, Open Approach

041M0JQ Bypass Right Popliteal Artery to Lower Extremity Artery with Synthetic Substitute, Open Approach

041M0JS Bypass Right Popliteal Artery to Lower Extremity Vein with Synthetic Substitute, Open Approach

041M0KL Bypass Right Popliteal Artery to Popliteal Artery with Nonautologous Tissue Substitute, Open Approach

041M0KM Bypass Right Popliteal Artery to Peroneal Artery with Nonautologous Tissue Substitute, Open Approach

♀ Female-only ♂ Male-only ▲ Limited Coverage ● Non-OR ▧ HAC-associated procedure ▲ Non-covered procedures ✚ Cluster

041M0KP Bypass Right Popliteal Artery to Foot Artery with Nonautologous Tissue Substitute, Open Approach

041M0KQ Bypass Right Popliteal Artery to Lower Extremity Artery with Nonautologous Tissue Substitute, Open Approach

041M0KS Bypass Right Popliteal Artery to Lower Extremity Vein with Nonautologous Tissue Substitute, Open Approach

041M0ZL Bypass Right Popliteal Artery to Popliteal Artery, Open Approach

041M0ZM Bypass Right Popliteal Artery to Peroneal Artery, Open Approach

041M0ZP Bypass Right Popliteal Artery to Foot Artery, Open Approach

041M0ZQ Bypass Right Popliteal Artery to Lower Extremity Artery, Open Approach

041M0ZS Bypass Right Popliteal Artery to Lower Extremity Vein, Open Approach

041M3JQ Bypass Right Popliteal Artery to Lower Extremity Artery with Synthetic Substitute, Percutaneous Approach

041M3JS Bypass Right Popliteal Artery to Lower Extremity Vein with Synthetic Substitute, Percutaneous Approach

041M49L Bypass Right Popliteal Artery to Popliteal Artery with Autologous Venous Tissue, Percutaneous Endoscopic Approach

041M49M Bypass Right Popliteal Artery to Peroneal Artery with Autologous Venous Tissue, Percutaneous Endoscopic Approach

041M49P Bypass Right Popliteal Artery to Foot Artery with Autologous Venous Tissue, Percutaneous Endoscopic Approach

041M49Q Bypass Right Popliteal Artery to Lower Extremity Artery with Autologous Venous Tissue, Percutaneous Endoscopic Approach

041M49S Bypass Right Popliteal Artery to Lower Extremity Vein with Autologous Venous Tissue, Percutaneous Endoscopic Approach

041M4AL Bypass Right Popliteal Artery to Popliteal Artery with Autologous Arterial Tissue, Percutaneous Endoscopic Approach

041M4AM Bypass Right Popliteal Artery to Peroneal Artery with Autologous Arterial Tissue, Percutaneous Endoscopic Approach

041M4AP Bypass Right Popliteal Artery to Foot Artery with Autologous Arterial Tissue, Percutaneous Endoscopic Approach

041M4AQ Bypass Right Popliteal Artery to Lower Extremity Artery with Autologous Arterial Tissue, Percutaneous Endoscopic Approach

041M4AS Bypass Right Popliteal Artery to Lower Extremity Vein with Autologous Arterial Tissue, Percutaneous Endoscopic Approach

041M4JL Bypass Right Popliteal Artery to Popliteal Artery with Synthetic Substitute, Percutaneous Endoscopic Approach

041M4JM Bypass Right Popliteal Artery to Peroneal Artery with Synthetic Substitute, Percutaneous Endoscopic Approach

041M4JP Bypass Right Popliteal Artery to Foot Artery with Synthetic Substitute, Percutaneous Endoscopic Approach

041M4JQ Bypass Right Popliteal Artery to Lower Extremity Artery with Synthetic Substitute, Percutaneous Endoscopic Approach

041M4JS Bypass Right Popliteal Artery to Lower Extremity Vein with Synthetic Substitute, Percutaneous Endoscopic Approach

041M4KL Bypass Right Popliteal Artery to Popliteal Artery with Nonautologous Tissue Substitute, Percutaneous Endoscopic Approach

041M4KM Bypass Right Popliteal Artery to Peroneal Artery with Nonautologous Tissue Substitute, Percutaneous Endoscopic Approach

041M4KP Bypass Right Popliteal Artery to Foot Artery with Nonautologous Tissue Substitute, Percutaneous Endoscopic Approach

041M4KQ Bypass Right Popliteal Artery to Lower Extremity Artery with Nonautologous Tissue Substitute, Percutaneous Endoscopic Approach

041M4KS Bypass Right Popliteal Artery to Lower Extremity Vein with Nonautologous Tissue Substitute, Percutaneous Endoscopic Approach

041M4ZL Bypass Right Popliteal Artery to Popliteal Artery, Percutaneous Endoscopic Approach

041M4ZM Bypass Right Popliteal Artery to Peroneal Artery, Percutaneous Endoscopic Approach

041M4ZP Bypass Right Popliteal Artery to Foot Artery, Percutaneous Endoscopic Approach

041M4ZQ Bypass Right Popliteal Artery to Lower Extremity Artery, Percutaneous Endoscopic Approach

041M4ZS Bypass Right Popliteal Artery to Lower Extremity Vein, Percutaneous Endoscopic Approach

041N09L Bypass Left Popliteal Artery to Popliteal Artery with Autologous Venous Tissue, Open Approach

041N09M Bypass Left Popliteal Artery to Peroneal Artery with Autologous Venous Tissue, Open Approach

041N09P Bypass Left Popliteal Artery to Foot Artery with Autologous Venous Tissue, Open Approach

041N09Q Bypass Left Popliteal Artery to Lower Extremity Artery with Autologous Venous Tissue, Open Approach

041N09S Bypass Left Popliteal Artery to Lower Extremity Vein with Autologous Venous Tissue, Open Approach

041N0AL Bypass Left Popliteal Artery to Popliteal Artery with Autologous Arterial Tissue, Open Approach

041N0AM Bypass Left Popliteal Artery to Peroneal Artery with Autologous Arterial Tissue, Open Approach

041N0AP Bypass Left Popliteal Artery to Foot Artery with Autologous Arterial Tissue, Open Approach

041N0AQ Bypass Left Popliteal Artery to Lower Extremity Artery with Autologous Arterial Tissue, Open Approach

041N0AS Bypass Left Popliteal Artery to Lower Extremity Vein with Autologous Arterial Tissue, Open Approach

041N0JL Bypass Left Popliteal Artery to Popliteal Artery with Synthetic Substitute, Open Approach

041N0JM Bypass Left Popliteal Artery to Peroneal Artery with Synthetic Substitute, Open Approach

041N0JP Bypass Left Popliteal Artery to Foot Artery with Synthetic Substitute, Open Approach

041N0JQ Bypass Left Popliteal Artery to Lower Extremity Artery with Synthetic Substitute, Open Approach

041N0JS Bypass Left Popliteal Artery to Lower Extremity Vein with Synthetic Substitute, Open Approach

041N0KL Bypass Left Popliteal Artery to Popliteal Artery with Nonautologous Tissue Substitute, Open Approach

041N0KM Bypass Left Popliteal Artery to Peroneal Artery with Nonautologous Tissue Substitute, Open Approach

041N0KP Bypass Left Popliteal Artery to Foot Artery with Nonautologous Tissue Substitute, Open Approach

041N0KQ Bypass Left Popliteal Artery to Lower Extremity Artery with Nonautologous Tissue Substitute, Open Approach

041N0KS Bypass Left Popliteal Artery to Lower Extremity Vein with Nonautologous Tissue Substitute, Open Approach

041N0ZL Bypass Left Popliteal Artery to Popliteal Artery, Open Approach

041N0ZM Bypass Left Popliteal Artery to Peroneal Artery, Open Approach

041N0ZP Bypass Left Popliteal Artery to Foot Artery, Open Approach

041N0ZQ Bypass Left Popliteal Artery to Lower Extremity Artery, Open Approach

041N0ZS Bypass Left Popliteal Artery to Lower Extremity Vein, Open Approach

041N3JQ Bypass Left Popliteal Artery to Lower Extremity Artery with Synthetic Substitute, Percutaneous Approach

041N3JS Bypass Left Popliteal Artery to Lower Extremity Vein with Synthetic Substitute, Percutaneous Approach

041N49L Bypass Left Popliteal Artery to Popliteal Artery with Autologous Venous Tissue, Percutaneous Endoscopic Approach

041N49M Bypass Left Popliteal Artery to Peroneal Artery with Autologous Venous Tissue, Percutaneous Endoscopic Approach

041N49P Bypass Left Popliteal Artery to Foot Artery with Autologous Venous Tissue, Percutaneous Endoscopic Approach

041N49Q Bypass Left Popliteal Artery to Lower Extremity Artery with Autologous Venous Tissue, Percutaneous Endoscopic Approach

041N49S Bypass Left Popliteal Artery to Lower Extremity Vein with Autologous Venous Tissue, Percutaneous Endoscopic Approach

041N4AL Bypass Left Popliteal Artery to Popliteal Artery with Autologous Arterial Tissue, Percutaneous Endoscopic Approach

041N4AM Bypass Left Popliteal Artery to Peroneal Artery with Autologous Arterial Tissue, Percutaneous Endoscopic Approach

041N4AP Bypass Left Popliteal Artery to Foot Artery with Autologous Arterial Tissue, Percutaneous Endoscopic Approach

041N4AQ Bypass Left Popliteal Artery to Lower Extremity Artery with Autologous Arterial Tissue, Percutaneous Endoscopic Approach

041N4AS Bypass Left Popliteal Artery to Lower Extremity Vein with Autologous Arterial Tissue, Percutaneous Endoscopic Approach

041N4JL Bypass Left Popliteal Artery to Popliteal Artery with Synthetic Substitute, Percutaneous Endoscopic Approach

041N4JM Bypass Left Popliteal Artery to Peroneal Artery with Synthetic Substitute, Percutaneous Endoscopic Approach

041N4JP Bypass Left Popliteal Artery to Foot Artery with Synthetic Substitute, Percutaneous Endoscopic Approach

041N4JQ Bypass Left Popliteal Artery to Lower Extremity Artery with Synthetic Substitute, Percutaneous Endoscopic Approach

041N4JS Bypass Left Popliteal Artery to Lower Extremity Vein with Synthetic Substitute, Percutaneous Endoscopic Approach

041N4KL Bypass Left Popliteal Artery to Popliteal Artery with Nonautologous Tissue Substitute, Percutaneous Endoscopic Approach

041N4KM Bypass Left Popliteal Artery to Peroneal Artery with Nonautologous Tissue Substitute, Percutaneous Endoscopic Approach

041N4KP Bypass Left Popliteal Artery to Foot Artery with Nonautologous Tissue Substitute, Percutaneous Endoscopic Approach

041N4KQ Bypass Left Popliteal Artery to Lower Extremity Artery with Nonautologous Tissue Substitute, Percutaneous Endoscopic Approach

041N4KS Bypass Left Popliteal Artery to Lower Extremity Vein with Nonautologous Tissue Substitute, Percutaneous Endoscopic Approach

041N4ZL Bypass Left Popliteal Artery to Popliteal Artery, Percutaneous Endoscopic Approach

041N4ZM Bypass Left Popliteal Artery to Peroneal Artery, Percutaneous Endoscopic Approach

041N4ZP Bypass Left Popliteal Artery to Foot Artery, Percutaneous Endoscopic Approach

041N4ZQ Bypass Left Popliteal Artery to Lower Extremity Artery, Percutaneous Endoscopic Approach

041N4ZS Bypass Left Popliteal Artery to Lower Extremity Vein, Percutaneous Endoscopic Approach

041P0JQ Bypass Right Anterior Tibial Artery to Lower Extremity Artery with Synthetic Substitute, Open Approach

041P0JS Bypass Right Anterior Tibial Artery to Lower Extremity Vein with Synthetic Substitute, Open Approach

041P3JQ Bypass Right Anterior Tibial Artery to Lower Extremity Artery with Synthetic Substitute, Percutaneous Approach

041P3JS Bypass Right Anterior Tibial Artery to Lower Extremity Vein with Synthetic Substitute, Percutaneous Approach

041P4JQ Bypass Right Anterior Tibial Artery to Lower Extremity Artery with Synthetic Substitute, Percutaneous Endoscopic Approach

041P4JS Bypass Right Anterior Tibial Artery to Lower Extremity Vein with Synthetic Substitute, Percutaneous Endoscopic Approach

041Q0JQ Bypass Left Anterior Tibial Artery to Lower Extremity Artery with Synthetic Substitute, Open Approach

041Q0JS Bypass Left Anterior Tibial Artery to Lower Extremity Vein with Synthetic Substitute, Open Approach

041Q3JQ Bypass Left Anterior Tibial Artery to Lower Extremity Artery with Synthetic Substitute, Percutaneous Approach

041Q3JS Bypass Left Anterior Tibial Artery to Lower Extremity Vein with Synthetic Substitute, Percutaneous Approach

041Q4JQ Bypass Left Anterior Tibial Artery to Lower Extremity Artery with Synthetic Substitute, Percutaneous Endoscopic Approach

041Q4JS Bypass Left Anterior Tibial Artery to Lower Extremity Vein with Synthetic Substitute, Percutaneous Endoscopic Approach

041R0JQ Bypass Right Posterior Tibial Artery to Lower Extremity Artery with Synthetic Substitute, Open Approach

041R0JS Bypass Right Posterior Tibial Artery to Lower Extremity Vein with Synthetic Substitute, Open Approach

041R3JQ Bypass Right Posterior Tibial Artery to Lower Extremity Artery with Synthetic Substitute, Percutaneous Approach

041R3JS Bypass Right Posterior Tibial Artery to Lower Extremity Vein with Synthetic Substitute, Percutaneous Approach

041R4JQ Bypass Right Posterior Tibial Artery to Lower Extremity Artery with Synthetic Substitute, Percutaneous Endoscopic Approach

041R4JS Bypass Right Posterior Tibial Artery to Lower Extremity Vein with Synthetic Substitute, Percutaneous Endoscopic Approach

041S0JQ Bypass Left Posterior Tibial Artery to Lower Extremity Artery with Synthetic Substitute, Open Approach

041S0JS Bypass Left Posterior Tibial Artery to Lower Extremity Vein with Synthetic Substitute, Open Approach

041S3JQ Bypass Left Posterior Tibial Artery to Lower Extremity Artery with Synthetic Substitute, Percutaneous Approach

041S3JS Bypass Left Posterior Tibial Artery to Lower Extremity Vein with Synthetic Substitute, Percutaneous Approach

041S4JQ Bypass Left Posterior Tibial Artery to Lower Extremity Artery with Synthetic Substitute, Percutaneous Endoscopic Approach

041S4JS Bypass Left Posterior Tibial Artery to Lower Extremity Vein with Synthetic Substitute, Percutaneous Endoscopic Approach

041T09P Bypass Right Peroneal Artery to Foot Artery with Autologous Venous Tissue, Open Approach

041T09Q Bypass Right Peroneal Artery to Lower Extremity Artery with Autologous Venous Tissue, Open Approach

041T09S Bypass Right Peroneal Artery to Lower Extremity Vein with Autologous Venous Tissue, Open Approach

041T0AP Bypass Right Peroneal Artery to Foot Artery with Autologous Arterial Tissue, Open Approach

041T0AQ Bypass Right Peroneal Artery to Lower Extremity Artery with Autologous Arterial Tissue, Open Approach

041T0AS Bypass Right Peroneal Artery to Lower Extremity Vein with Autologous Arterial Tissue, Open Approach

041T0JP Bypass Right Peroneal Artery to Foot Artery with Synthetic Substitute, Open Approach

041T0JQ Bypass Right Peroneal Artery to Lower Extremity Artery with Synthetic Substitute, Open Approach

041T0JS Bypass Right Peroneal Artery to Lower Extremity Vein with Synthetic Substitute, Open Approach

041T0KP Bypass Right Peroneal Artery to Foot Artery with Nonautologous Tissue Substitute, Open Approach

041T0KQ Bypass Right Peroneal Artery to Lower Extremity Artery with Nonautologous Tissue Substitute, Open Approach

041T0KS Bypass Right Peroneal Artery to Lower Extremity Vein with Nonautologous Tissue Substitute, Open Approach

041T0ZP Bypass Right Peroneal Artery to Foot Artery, Open Approach

041T0ZQ Bypass Right Peroneal Artery to Lower Extremity Artery, Open Approach

041T0ZS Bypass Right Peroneal Artery to Lower Extremity Vein, Open Approach

041T3JQ Bypass Right Peroneal Artery to Lower Extremity Artery with Synthetic Substitute, Percutaneous Approach

041T3JS Bypass Right Peroneal Artery to Lower Extremity Vein with Synthetic Substitute, Percutaneous Approach

041T49P Bypass Right Peroneal Artery to Foot Artery with Autologous Venous Tissue, Percutaneous Endoscopic Approach

041T49Q Bypass Right Peroneal Artery to Lower Extremity Artery with Autologous Venous Tissue, Percutaneous Endoscopic Approach

041T49S Bypass Right Peroneal Artery to Lower Extremity Vein with Autologous Venous Tissue, Percutaneous Endoscopic Approach

041T4AP Bypass Right Peroneal Artery to Foot Artery with Autologous Arterial Tissue, Percutaneous Endoscopic Approach

041T4AQ Bypass Right Peroneal Artery to Lower Extremity Artery with Autologous Arterial Tissue, Percutaneous Endoscopic Approach

041T4AS Bypass Right Peroneal Artery to Lower Extremity Vein with Autologous Arterial Tissue, Percutaneous Endoscopic Approach

041T4JP Bypass Right Peroneal Artery to Foot Artery with Synthetic Substitute, Percutaneous Endoscopic Approach

041T4JQ Bypass Right Peroneal Artery to Lower Extremity Artery with Synthetic Substitute, Percutaneous Endoscopic Approach

♀ Female-only ♂ Male-only ▲ Limited Coverage ● Non-OR ᴴᴬᶜ HAC-associated procedure ▲ Non-covered procedures ✛ Cluster

041T4JS Bypass Right Peroneal Artery to Lower Extremity Vein with Synthetic Substitute, Percutaneous Endoscopic Approach

041T4KP Bypass Right Peroneal Artery to Foot Artery with Nonautologous Tissue Substitute, Percutaneous Endoscopic Approach

041T4KQ Bypass Right Peroneal Artery to Lower Extremity Artery with Nonautologous Tissue Substitute, Percutaneous Endoscopic Approach

041T4KS Bypass Right Peroneal Artery to Lower Extremity Vein with Nonautologous Tissue Substitute, Percutaneous Endoscopic Approach

041T4ZP Bypass Right Peroneal Artery to Foot Artery, Percutaneous Endoscopic Approach

041T4ZQ Bypass Right Peroneal Artery to Lower Extremity Artery, Percutaneous Endoscopic Approach

041T4ZS Bypass Right Peroneal Artery to Lower Extremity Vein, Percutaneous Endoscopic Approach

041U09P Bypass Left Peroneal Artery to Foot Artery with Autologous Venous Tissue, Open Approach

041U09Q Bypass Left Peroneal Artery to Lower Extremity Artery with Autologous Venous Tissue, Open Approach

041U09S Bypass Left Peroneal Artery to Lower Extremity Vein with Autologous Venous Tissue, Open Approach

041U0AP Bypass Left Peroneal Artery to Foot Artery with Autologous Arterial Tissue, Open Approach

041U0AQ Bypass Left Peroneal Artery to Lower Extremity Artery with Autologous Arterial Tissue, Open Approach

041U0AS Bypass Left Peroneal Artery to Lower Extremity Vein with Autologous Arterial Tissue, Open Approach

041U0JP Bypass Left Peroneal Artery to Foot Artery with Synthetic Substitute, Open Approach

041U0JQ Bypass Left Peroneal Artery to Lower Extremity Artery with Synthetic Substitute, Open Approach

041U0JS Bypass Left Peroneal Artery to Lower Extremity Vein with Synthetic Substitute, Open Approach

041U0KP Bypass Left Peroneal Artery to Foot Artery with Nonautologous Tissue Substitute, Open Approach

041U0KQ Bypass Left Peroneal Artery to Lower Extremity Artery with Nonautologous Tissue Substitute, Open Approach

041U0KS Bypass Left Peroneal Artery to Lower Extremity Vein with Nonautologous Tissue Substitute, Open Approach

041U0ZP Bypass Left Peroneal Artery to Foot Artery, Open Approach

041U0ZQ Bypass Left Peroneal Artery to Lower Extremity Artery, Open Approach

041U0ZS Bypass Left Peroneal Artery to Lower Extremity Vein, Open Approach

041U3JQ Bypass Left Peroneal Artery to Lower Extremity Artery with Synthetic Substitute, Percutaneous Approach

041U3JS Bypass Left Peroneal Artery to Lower Extremity Vein with Synthetic Substitute, Percutaneous Approach

041U49P Bypass Left Peroneal Artery to Foot Artery with Autologous Venous Tissue, Percutaneous Endoscopic Approach

041U49Q Bypass Left Peroneal Artery to Lower Extremity Artery with Autologous Venous Tissue, Percutaneous Endoscopic Approach

041U49S Bypass Left Peroneal Artery to Lower Extremity Vein with Autologous Venous Tissue, Percutaneous Endoscopic Approach

041U4AP Bypass Left Peroneal Artery to Foot Artery with Autologous Arterial Tissue, Percutaneous Endoscopic Approach

041U4AQ Bypass Left Peroneal Artery to Lower Extremity Artery with Autologous Arterial Tissue, Percutaneous Endoscopic Approach

041U4AS Bypass Left Peroneal Artery to Lower Extremity Vein with Autologous Arterial Tissue, Percutaneous Endoscopic Approach

041U4JP Bypass Left Peroneal Artery to Foot Artery with Synthetic Substitute, Percutaneous Endoscopic Approach

041U4JQ Bypass Left Peroneal Artery to Lower Extremity Artery with Synthetic Substitute, Percutaneous Endoscopic Approach

041U4JS Bypass Left Peroneal Artery to Lower Extremity Vein with Synthetic Substitute, Percutaneous Endoscopic Approach

041U4KP Bypass Left Peroneal Artery to Foot Artery with Nonautologous Tissue Substitute, Percutaneous Endoscopic Approach

041U4KQ Bypass Left Peroneal Artery to Lower Extremity Artery with Nonautologous Tissue Substitute, Percutaneous Endoscopic Approach

041U4KS Bypass Left Peroneal Artery to Lower Extremity Vein with Nonautologous Tissue Substitute, Percutaneous Endoscopic Approach

041U4ZP Bypass Left Peroneal Artery to Foot Artery, Percutaneous Endoscopic Approach

041U4ZQ Bypass Left Peroneal Artery to Lower Extremity Artery, Percutaneous Endoscopic Approach

041U4ZS Bypass Left Peroneal Artery to Lower Extremity Vein, Percutaneous Endoscopic Approach

041V09P Bypass Right Foot Artery to Foot Artery with Autologous Venous Tissue, Open Approach

041V09Q Bypass Right Foot Artery to Lower Extremity Artery with Autologous Venous Tissue, Open Approach

041V09S Bypass Right Foot Artery to Lower Extremity Vein with Autologous Venous Tissue, Open Approach

041V0AP Bypass Right Foot Artery to Foot Artery with Autologous Arterial Tissue, Open Approach

041V0AQ Bypass Right Foot Artery to Lower Extremity Artery with Autologous Arterial Tissue, Open Approach

041V0AS Bypass Right Foot Artery to Lower Extremity Vein with Autologous Arterial Tissue, Open Approach

041V0JP Bypass Right Foot Artery to Foot Artery with Synthetic Substitute, Open Approach

041V0JQ Bypass Right Foot Artery to Lower Extremity Artery with Synthetic Substitute, Open Approach

041V0JS Bypass Right Foot Artery to Lower Extremity Vein with Synthetic Substitute, Open Approach

041V0KP Bypass Right Foot Artery to Foot Artery with Nonautologous Tissue Substitute, Open Approach

041V0KQ Bypass Right Foot Artery to Lower Extremity Artery with Nonautologous Tissue Substitute, Open Approach

041V0KS Bypass Right Foot Artery to Lower Extremity Vein with Nonautologous Tissue Substitute, Open Approach

041V0ZP Bypass Right Foot Artery to Foot Artery, Open Approach

041V0ZQ Bypass Right Foot Artery to Lower Extremity Artery, Open Approach

041V0ZS Bypass Right Foot Artery to Lower Extremity Vein, Open Approach

041V3JQ Bypass Right Foot Artery to Lower Extremity Artery with Synthetic Substitute, Percutaneous Approach

041V3JS Bypass Right Foot Artery to Lower Extremity Vein with Synthetic Substitute, Percutaneous Approach

041V49P Bypass Right Foot Artery to Foot Artery with Autologous Venous Tissue, Percutaneous Endoscopic Approach

041V49Q Bypass Right Foot Artery to Lower Extremity Artery with Autologous Venous Tissue, Percutaneous Endoscopic Approach

041V49S Bypass Right Foot Artery to Lower Extremity Vein with Autologous Venous Tissue, Percutaneous Endoscopic Approach

041V4AP Bypass Right Foot Artery to Foot Artery with Autologous Arterial Tissue, Percutaneous Endoscopic Approach

041V4AQ Bypass Right Foot Artery to Lower Extremity Artery with Autologous Arterial Tissue, Percutaneous Endoscopic Approach

041V4AS Bypass Right Foot Artery to Lower Extremity Vein with Autologous Arterial Tissue, Percutaneous Endoscopic Approach

041V4JP Bypass Right Foot Artery to Foot Artery with Synthetic Substitute, Percutaneous Endoscopic Approach

041V4JQ Bypass Right Foot Artery to Lower Extremity Artery with Synthetic Substitute, Percutaneous Endoscopic Approach

041V4JS Bypass Right Foot Artery to Lower Extremity Vein with Synthetic Substitute, Percutaneous Endoscopic Approach

041V4KP Bypass Right Foot Artery to Foot Artery with Nonautologous Tissue Substitute, Percutaneous Endoscopic Approach

041V4KQ Bypass Right Foot Artery to Lower Extremity Artery with Nonautologous Tissue Substitute, Percutaneous Endoscopic Approach

041V4KS Bypass Right Foot Artery to Lower Extremity Vein with Nonautologous Tissue Substitute, Percutaneous Endoscopic Approach

041V4ZP Bypass Right Foot Artery to Foot Artery, Percutaneous Endoscopic Approach

041V4ZQ Bypass Right Foot Artery to Lower Extremity Artery, Percutaneous Endoscopic Approach

041V4ZS Bypass Right Foot Artery to Lower Extremity Vein, Percutaneous Endoscopic Approach

041W09P Bypass Left Foot Artery to Foot Artery with Autologous Venous Tissue, Open Approach

041W09Q Bypass Left Foot Artery to Lower Extremity Artery with Autologous Venous Tissue, Open Approach

041W09S Bypass Left Foot Artery to Lower Extremity Vein with Autologous Venous Tissue, Open Approach

041W0AP Bypass Left Foot Artery to Foot Artery with Autologous Arterial Tissue, Open Approach

041W0AQ Bypass Left Foot Artery to Lower Extremity Artery with Autologous Arterial Tissue, Open Approach

041W0AS Bypass Left Foot Artery to Lower Extremity Vein with Autologous Arterial Tissue, Open Approach

041W0JP Bypass Left Foot Artery to Foot Artery with Synthetic Substitute, Open Approach

041W0JQ Bypass Left Foot Artery to Lower Extremity Artery with Synthetic Substitute, Open Approach

041W0JS Bypass Left Foot Artery to Lower Extremity Vein with Synthetic Substitute, Open Approach

041W0KP Bypass Left Foot Artery to Foot Artery with Nonautologous Tissue Substitute, Open Approach

041W0KQ Bypass Left Foot Artery to Lower Extremity Artery with Nonautologous Tissue Substitute, Open Approach

041W0KS Bypass Left Foot Artery to Lower Extremity Vein with Nonautologous Tissue Substitute, Open Approach

041W0ZP Bypass Left Foot Artery to Foot Artery, Open Approach

041W0ZQ Bypass Left Foot Artery to Lower Extremity Artery, Open Approach

041W0ZS Bypass Left Foot Artery to Lower Extremity Vein, Open Approach

041W3JQ Bypass Left Foot Artery to Lower Extremity Artery with Synthetic Substitute, Percutaneous Approach

041W3JS Bypass Left Foot Artery to Lower Extremity Vein with Synthetic Substitute, Percutaneous Approach

041W49P Bypass Left Foot Artery to Foot Artery with Autologous Venous Tissue, Percutaneous Endoscopic Approach

041W49Q Bypass Left Foot Artery to Lower Extremity Artery with Autologous Venous Tissue, Percutaneous Endoscopic Approach

041W49S Bypass Left Foot Artery to Lower Extremity Vein with Autologous Venous Tissue, Percutaneous Endoscopic Approach

041W4AP Bypass Left Foot Artery to Foot Artery with Autologous Arterial Tissue, Percutaneous Endoscopic Approach

041W4AQ Bypass Left Foot Artery to Lower Extremity Artery with Autologous Arterial Tissue, Percutaneous Endoscopic Approach

041W4AS Bypass Left Foot Artery to Lower Extremity Vein with Autologous Arterial Tissue, Percutaneous Endoscopic Approach

041W4JP Bypass Left Foot Artery to Foot Artery with Synthetic Substitute, Percutaneous Endoscopic Approach

041W4JQ Bypass Left Foot Artery to Lower Extremity Artery with Synthetic Substitute, Percutaneous Endoscopic Approach

041W4JS Bypass Left Foot Artery to Lower Extremity Vein with Synthetic Substitute, Percutaneous Endoscopic Approach

041W4KP Bypass Left Foot Artery to Foot Artery with Nonautologous Tissue Substitute, Percutaneous Endoscopic Approach

041W4KQ Bypass Left Foot Artery to Lower Extremity Artery with Nonautologous Tissue Substitute, Percutaneous Endoscopic Approach

041W4KS Bypass Left Foot Artery to Lower Extremity Vein with Nonautologous Tissue Substitute, Percutaneous Endoscopic Approach

041W4ZP Bypass Left Foot Artery to Foot Artery, Percutaneous Endoscopic Approach

041W4ZQ Bypass Left Foot Artery to Lower Extremity Artery, Percutaneous Endoscopic Approach

041W4ZS Bypass Left Foot Artery to Lower Extremity Vein, Percutaneous Endoscopic Approach

045 – Lower Arteries, Destruction

04500ZZ Destruction of Abdominal Aorta, Open Approach

04503ZZ Destruction of Abdominal Aorta, Percutaneous Approach

04504ZZ Destruction of Abdominal Aorta, Percutaneous Endoscopic Approach

04510ZZ Destruction of Celiac Artery, Open Approach

04513ZZ Destruction of Celiac Artery, Percutaneous Approach

04514ZZ Destruction of Celiac Artery, Percutaneous Endoscopic Approach

04520ZZ Destruction of Gastric Artery, Open Approach

04523ZZ Destruction of Gastric Artery, Percutaneous Approach

04524ZZ Destruction of Gastric Artery, Percutaneous Endoscopic Approach

04530ZZ Destruction of Hepatic Artery, Open Approach

04533ZZ Destruction of Hepatic Artery, Percutaneous Approach

04534ZZ Destruction of Hepatic Artery, Percutaneous Endoscopic Approach

04540ZZ Destruction of Splenic Artery, Open Approach

04543ZZ Destruction of Splenic Artery, Percutaneous Approach

04544ZZ Destruction of Splenic Artery, Percutaneous Endoscopic Approach

04550ZZ Destruction of Superior Mesenteric Artery, Open Approach

04553ZZ Destruction of Superior Mesenteric Artery, Percutaneous Approach

04554ZZ Destruction of Superior Mesenteric Artery, Percutaneous Endoscopic Approach

04560ZZ Destruction of Right Colic Artery, Open Approach

04563ZZ Destruction of Right Colic Artery, Percutaneous Approach

04564ZZ Destruction of Right Colic Artery, Percutaneous Endoscopic Approach

04570ZZ Destruction of Left Colic Artery, Open Approach

04573ZZ Destruction of Left Colic Artery, Percutaneous Approach

04574ZZ Destruction of Left Colic Artery, Percutaneous Endoscopic Approach

04580ZZ Destruction of Middle Colic Artery, Open Approach

04583ZZ Destruction of Middle Colic Artery, Percutaneous Approach

04584ZZ Destruction of Middle Colic Artery, Percutaneous Endoscopic Approach

04590ZZ Destruction of Right Renal Artery, Open Approach

04593ZZ Destruction of Right Renal Artery, Percutaneous Approach

04594ZZ Destruction of Right Renal Artery, Percutaneous Endoscopic Approach

045A0ZZ Destruction of Left Renal Artery, Open Approach

045A3ZZ Destruction of Left Renal Artery, Percutaneous Approach

045A4ZZ Destruction of Left Renal Artery, Percutaneous Endoscopic Approach

045B0ZZ Destruction of Inferior Mesenteric Artery, Open Approach

045B3ZZ Destruction of Inferior Mesenteric Artery, Percutaneous Approach

045B4ZZ Destruction of Inferior Mesenteric Artery, Percutaneous Endoscopic Approach

045C0ZZ Destruction of Right Common Iliac Artery, Open Approach

045C3ZZ Destruction of Right Common Iliac Artery, Percutaneous Approach

045C4ZZ Destruction of Right Common Iliac Artery, Percutaneous Endoscopic Approach

045D0ZZ Destruction of Left Common Iliac Artery, Open Approach

045D3ZZ Destruction of Left Common Iliac Artery, Percutaneous Approach

045D4ZZ Destruction of Left Common Iliac Artery, Percutaneous Endoscopic Approach

045E0ZZ Destruction of Right Internal Iliac Artery, Open Approach

045E3ZZ Destruction of Right Internal Iliac Artery, Percutaneous Approach

045E4ZZ Destruction of Right Internal Iliac Artery, Percutaneous Endoscopic Approach

045F0ZZ Destruction of Left Internal Iliac Artery, Open Approach

045F3ZZ Destruction of Left Internal Iliac Artery, Percutaneous Approach

045F4ZZ Destruction of Left Internal Iliac Artery, Percutaneous Endoscopic Approach

045H0ZZ Destruction of Right External Iliac Artery, Open Approach

045H3ZZ Destruction of Right External Iliac Artery, Percutaneous Approach

045H4ZZ Destruction of Right External Iliac Artery, Percutaneous Endoscopic Approach

045J0ZZ Destruction of Left External Iliac Artery, Open Approach

♀ Female-only   ♂ Male-only   ▲ Limited Coverage   ● Non-OR   ■ HAC-associated procedure   ▲ Non-covered procedures   ✚ Cluster

045J3ZZ Destruction of Left External Iliac Artery, Percutaneous Approach

045J4ZZ Destruction of Left External Iliac Artery, Percutaneous Endoscopic Approach

045K0ZZ Destruction of Right Femoral Artery, Open Approach

045K3ZZ Destruction of Right Femoral Artery, Percutaneous Approach

045K4ZZ Destruction of Right Femoral Artery, Percutaneous Endoscopic Approach

045L0ZZ Destruction of Left Femoral Artery, Open Approach

045L3ZZ Destruction of Left Femoral Artery, Percutaneous Approach

045L4ZZ Destruction of Left Femoral Artery, Percutaneous Endoscopic Approach

045M0ZZ Destruction of Right Popliteal Artery, Open Approach

045M3ZZ Destruction of Right Popliteal Artery, Percutaneous Approach

045M4ZZ Destruction of Right Popliteal Artery, Percutaneous Endoscopic Approach

045N0ZZ Destruction of Left Popliteal Artery, Open Approach

045N3ZZ Destruction of Left Popliteal Artery, Percutaneous Approach

045N4ZZ Destruction of Left Popliteal Artery, Percutaneous Endoscopic Approach

045P0ZZ Destruction of Right Anterior Tibial Artery, Open Approach

045P3ZZ Destruction of Right Anterior Tibial Artery, Percutaneous Approach

045P4ZZ Destruction of Right Anterior Tibial Artery, Percutaneous Endoscopic Approach

045Q0ZZ Destruction of Left Anterior Tibial Artery, Open Approach

045Q3ZZ Destruction of Left Anterior Tibial Artery, Percutaneous Approach

045Q4ZZ Destruction of Left Anterior Tibial Artery, Percutaneous Endoscopic Approach

045R0ZZ Destruction of Right Posterior Tibial Artery, Open Approach

045R3ZZ Destruction of Right Posterior Tibial Artery, Percutaneous Approach

045R4ZZ Destruction of Right Posterior Tibial Artery, Percutaneous Endoscopic Approach

045S0ZZ Destruction of Left Posterior Tibial Artery, Open Approach

045S3ZZ Destruction of Left Posterior Tibial Artery, Percutaneous Approach

045S4ZZ Destruction of Left Posterior Tibial Artery, Percutaneous Endoscopic Approach

045T0ZZ Destruction of Right Peroneal Artery, Open Approach

045T3ZZ Destruction of Right Peroneal Artery, Percutaneous Approach

045T4ZZ Destruction of Right Peroneal Artery, Percutaneous Endoscopic Approach

045U0ZZ Destruction of Left Peroneal Artery, Open Approach

045U3ZZ Destruction of Left Peroneal Artery, Percutaneous Approach

045U4ZZ Destruction of Left Peroneal Artery, Percutaneous Endoscopic Approach

045V0ZZ Destruction of Right Foot Artery, Open Approach

045V3ZZ Destruction of Right Foot Artery, Percutaneous Approach

045V4ZZ Destruction of Right Foot Artery, Percutaneous Endoscopic Approach

045W0ZZ Destruction of Left Foot Artery, Open Approach

045W3ZZ Destruction of Left Foot Artery, Percutaneous Approach

045W4ZZ Destruction of Left Foot Artery, Percutaneous Endoscopic Approach

045Y0ZZ Destruction of Lower Artery, Open Approach

045Y3ZZ Destruction of Lower Artery, Percutaneous Approach

045Y4ZZ Destruction of Lower Artery, Percutaneous Endoscopic Approach

047 – Lower Arteries, Dilation

0470041 Dilation of Abdominal Aorta with Drug-eluting Intraluminal Device, using Drug-Coated Balloon, Open Approach

047004Z Dilation of Abdominal Aorta with Drug-eluting Intraluminal Device, Open Approach

047005Z Dilation of Abdominal Aorta with Two Drug-eluting Intraluminal Devices, Open Approach

047006Z Dilation of Abdominal Aorta with Three Drug-eluting Intraluminal Devices, Open Approach

047007Z Dilation of Abdominal Aorta with Four or More Drug-eluting Intraluminal Devices, Open Approach

04700D1 Dilation of Abdominal Aorta with Intraluminal Device, using Drug-Coated Balloon, Open Approach

04700DZ Dilation of Abdominal Aorta with Intraluminal Device, Open Approach

04700EZ Dilation of Abdominal Aorta with Two Intraluminal Devices, Open Approach

04700FZ Dilation of Abdominal Aorta with Three Intraluminal Devices, Open Approach

04700GZ Dilation of Abdominal Aorta with Four or More Intraluminal Devices, Open Approach

04700Z1 Dilation of Abdominal Aorta using Drug-Coated Balloon, Open Approach

04700ZZ Dilation of Abdominal Aorta, Open Approach

0470341 Dilation of Abdominal Aorta with Drug-eluting Intraluminal Device, using Drug-Coated Balloon, Percutaneous Approach

047034Z Dilation of Abdominal Aorta with Drug-eluting Intraluminal Device, Percutaneous Approach

047035Z Dilation of Abdominal Aorta with Two Drug-eluting Intraluminal Devices, Percutaneous Approach

047036Z Dilation of Abdominal Aorta with Three Drug-eluting Intraluminal Devices, Percutaneous Approach

047037Z Dilation of Abdominal Aorta with Four or More Drug-eluting Intraluminal Devices, Percutaneous Approach

04703D1 Dilation of Abdominal Aorta with Intraluminal Device, using Drug-Coated Balloon, Percutaneous Approach

04703DZ Dilation of Abdominal Aorta with Intraluminal Device, Percutaneous Approach

04703EZ Dilation of Abdominal Aorta with Two Intraluminal Devices, Percutaneous Approach

04703FZ Dilation of Abdominal Aorta with Three Intraluminal Devices, Percutaneous Approach

04703GZ Dilation of Abdominal Aorta with Four or More Intraluminal Devices, Percutaneous Approach

04703Z1 Dilation of Abdominal Aorta using Drug-Coated Balloon, Percutaneous Approach

04703ZZ Dilation of Abdominal Aorta, Percutaneous Approach

0470341 Dilation of Abdominal Aorta with Drug-eluting Intraluminal Device, using Drug-Coated Balloon, Percutaneous Endoscopic Approach

047044Z Dilation of Abdominal Aorta with Drug-eluting Intraluminal Device, Percutaneous Endoscopic Approach

047045Z Dilation of Abdominal Aorta with Two Drug-eluting Intraluminal Devices, Percutaneous Endoscopic Approach

047046Z Dilation of Abdominal Aorta with Three Drug-eluting Intraluminal Devices, Percutaneous Endoscopic Approach

047047Z Dilation of Abdominal Aorta with Four or More Drug-eluting Intraluminal Devices, Percutaneous Endoscopic Approach

04704D1 Dilation of Abdominal Aorta with Intraluminal Device, using Drug-Coated Balloon, Percutaneous Endoscopic Approach

04704DZ Dilation of Abdominal Aorta with Intraluminal Device, Percutaneous Endoscopic Approach

04704EZ Dilation of Abdominal Aorta with Two Intraluminal Devices, Percutaneous Endoscopic Approach

04704FZ Dilation of Abdominal Aorta with Three Intraluminal Devices, Percutaneous Endoscopic Approach

04704GZ Dilation of Abdominal Aorta with Four or More Intraluminal Devices, Percutaneous Endoscopic Approach

04704Z1 Dilation of Abdominal Aorta using Drug-Coated Balloon, Percutaneous Endoscopic Approach

04704ZZ Dilation of Abdominal Aorta, Percutaneous Endoscopic Approach

0471041 Dilation of Celiac Artery with Drug-eluting Intraluminal Device, using Drug-Coated Balloon, Open Approach

047104Z Dilation of Celiac Artery with Drug-eluting Intraluminal Device, Open Approach

047105Z Dilation of Celiac Artery with Two Drug-eluting Intraluminal Devices, Open Approach

047106Z Dilation of Celiac Artery with Three Drug-eluting Intraluminal Devices, Open Approach

047107Z Dilation of Celiac Artery with Four or More Drug-eluting Intraluminal Devices, Open Approach

04710D1 Dilation of Celiac Artery with Intraluminal Device, using Drug-Coated Balloon, Open Approach

04710DZ Dilation of Celiac Artery with Intraluminal Device, Open Approach

04710EZ Dilation of Celiac Artery with Two Intraluminal Devices, Open Approach

04710FZ Dilation of Celiac Artery with Three Intraluminal Devices, Open Approach

04710GZ Dilation of Celiac Artery with Four or More Intraluminal Devices, Open Approach

04710Z1 Dilation of Celiac Artery using Drug-Coated Balloon, Open Approach

04710ZZ Dilation of Celiac Artery, Open Approach

0471341 Dilation of Celiac Artery with Drug-eluting Intraluminal Device, using Drug-Coated Balloon, Percutaneous Approach

047134Z Dilation of Celiac Artery with Drug-eluting Intraluminal Device, Percutaneous Approach

047135Z Dilation of Celiac Artery with Two Drug-eluting Intraluminal Devices, Percutaneous Approach

047136Z Dilation of Celiac Artery with Three Drug-eluting Intraluminal Devices, Percutaneous Approach

047137Z Dilation of Celiac Artery with Four or More Drug-eluting Intraluminal Devices, Percutaneous Approach

04713D1 Dilation of Celiac Artery with Intraluminal Device, using Drug-Coated Balloon, Percutaneous Approach

04713DZ Dilation of Celiac Artery with Intraluminal Device, Percutaneous Approach

04713EZ Dilation of Celiac Artery with Two Intraluminal Devices, Percutaneous Approach

04713FZ Dilation of Celiac Artery with Three Intraluminal Devices, Percutaneous Approach

04713GZ Dilation of Celiac Artery with Four or More Intraluminal Devices, Percutaneous Approach

04713Z1 Dilation of Celiac Artery using Drug-Coated Balloon, Percutaneous Approach

04713ZZ Dilation of Celiac Artery, Percutaneous Approach

0471441 Dilation of Celiac Artery with Drug-eluting Intraluminal Device, using Drug-Coated Balloon, Percutaneous Endoscopic Approach

047144Z Dilation of Celiac Artery with Drug-eluting Intraluminal Device, Percutaneous Endoscopic Approach

047145Z Dilation of Celiac Artery with Two Drug-eluting Intraluminal Devices, Percutaneous Endoscopic Approach

047146Z Dilation of Celiac Artery with Three Drug-eluting Intraluminal Devices, Percutaneous Endoscopic Approach

047147Z Dilation of Celiac Artery with Four or More Drug-eluting Intraluminal Devices, Percutaneous Endoscopic Approach

04714D1 Dilation of Celiac Artery with Intraluminal Device, using Drug-Coated Balloon, Percutaneous Endoscopic Approach

04714DZ Dilation of Celiac Artery with Intraluminal Device, Percutaneous Endoscopic Approach

04714EZ Dilation of Celiac Artery with Two Intraluminal Devices, Percutaneous Endoscopic Approach

04714FZ Dilation of Celiac Artery with Three Intraluminal Devices, Percutaneous Endoscopic Approach

04714GZ Dilation of Celiac Artery with Four or More Intraluminal Devices, Percutaneous Endoscopic Approach

04714Z1 Dilation of Celiac Artery using Drug-Coated Balloon, Percutaneous Endoscopic Approach

04714ZZ Dilation of Celiac Artery, Percutaneous Endoscopic Approach

0472041 Dilation of Gastric Artery with Drug-eluting Intraluminal Device, using Drug-Coated Balloon, Open Approach

047204Z Dilation of Gastric Artery with Drug-eluting Intraluminal Device, Open Approach

047205Z Dilation of Gastric Artery with Two Drug-eluting Intraluminal Devices, Open Approach

047206Z Dilation of Gastric Artery with Three Drug-eluting Intraluminal Devices, Open Approach

047207Z Dilation of Gastric Artery with Four or More Drug-eluting Intraluminal Devices, Open Approach

04720D1 Dilation of Gastric Artery with Intraluminal Device, using Drug-Coated Balloon, Open Approach

04720DZ Dilation of Gastric Artery with Intraluminal Device, Open Approach

04720EZ Dilation of Gastric Artery with Two Intraluminal Devices, Open Approach

04720FZ Dilation of Gastric Artery with Three Intraluminal Devices, Open Approach

04720GZ Dilation of Gastric Artery with Four or More Intraluminal Devices, Open Approach

04720Z1 Dilation of Gastric Artery using Drug-Coated Balloon, Open Approach

04720ZZ Dilation of Gastric Artery, Open Approach

0472341 Dilation of Gastric Artery with Drug-eluting Intraluminal Device, using Drug-Coated Balloon, Percutaneous Approach

047234Z Dilation of Gastric Artery with Drug-eluting Intraluminal Device, Percutaneous Approach

047235Z Dilation of Gastric Artery with Two Drug-eluting Intraluminal Devices, Percutaneous Approach

047236Z Dilation of Gastric Artery with Three Drug-eluting Intraluminal Devices, Percutaneous Approach

047237Z Dilation of Gastric Artery with Four or More Drug-eluting Intraluminal Devices, Percutaneous Approach

04723D1 Dilation of Gastric Artery with Intraluminal Device, using Drug-Coated Balloon, Percutaneous Approach

04723DZ Dilation of Gastric Artery with Intraluminal Device, Percutaneous Approach

04723EZ Dilation of Gastric Artery with Two Intraluminal Devices, Percutaneous Approach

04723FZ Dilation of Gastric Artery with Three Intraluminal Devices, Percutaneous Approach

04723GZ Dilation of Gastric Artery with Four or More Intraluminal Devices, Percutaneous Approach

04723Z1 Dilation of Gastric Artery using Drug-Coated Balloon, Percutaneous Approach

04723ZZ Dilation of Gastric Artery, Percutaneous Approach

0472441 Dilation of Gastric Artery with Drug-eluting Intraluminal Device, using Drug-Coated Balloon, Percutaneous Endoscopic Approach

047244Z Dilation of Gastric Artery with Drug-eluting Intraluminal Device, Percutaneous Endoscopic Approach

047245Z Dilation of Gastric Artery with Two Drug-eluting Intraluminal Devices, Percutaneous Endoscopic Approach

047246Z Dilation of Gastric Artery with Three Drug-eluting Intraluminal Devices, Percutaneous Endoscopic Approach

047247Z Dilation of Gastric Artery with Four or More Drug-eluting Intraluminal Devices, Percutaneous Endoscopic Approach

04724D1 Dilation of Gastric Artery with Intraluminal Device, using Drug-Coated Balloon, Percutaneous Endoscopic Approach

04724DZ Dilation of Gastric Artery with Intraluminal Device, Percutaneous Endoscopic Approach

04724EZ Dilation of Gastric Artery with Two Intraluminal Devices, Percutaneous Endoscopic Approach

04724FZ Dilation of Gastric Artery with Three Intraluminal Devices, Percutaneous Endoscopic Approach

04724GZ Dilation of Gastric Artery with Four or More Intraluminal Devices, Percutaneous Endoscopic Approach

04724Z1 Dilation of Gastric Artery using Drug-Coated Balloon, Percutaneous Endoscopic Approach

04724ZZ Dilation of Gastric Artery, Percutaneous Endoscopic Approach

0473041 Dilation of Hepatic Artery with Drug-eluting Intraluminal Device, using Drug-Coated Balloon, Open Approach

047304Z Dilation of Hepatic Artery with Drug-eluting Intraluminal Device, Open Approach

047305Z Dilation of Hepatic Artery with Two Drug-eluting Intraluminal Devices, Open Approach

047306Z Dilation of Hepatic Artery with Three Drug-eluting Intraluminal Devices, Open Approach

047307Z Dilation of Hepatic Artery with Four or More Drug-eluting Intraluminal Devices, Open Approach

04730D1 Dilation of Hepatic Artery with Intraluminal Device, using Drug-Coated Balloon, Open Approach

04730DZ Dilation of Hepatic Artery with Intraluminal Device, Open Approach

04730EZ Dilation of Hepatic Artery with Two Intraluminal Devices, Open Approach

04730FZ Dilation of Hepatic Artery with Three Intraluminal Devices, Open Approach

04730GZ Dilation of Hepatic Artery with Four or More Intraluminal Devices, Open Approach

04730Z1 Dilation of Hepatic Artery using Drug-Coated Balloon, Open Approach

04730ZZ Dilation of Hepatic Artery, Open Approach

 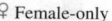

0473341 Dilation of Hepatic Artery with Drug-eluting Intraluminal Device, using Drug-Coated Balloon, Percutaneous Approach

047334Z Dilation of Hepatic Artery with Drug-eluting Intraluminal Device, Percutaneous Approach

047335Z Dilation of Hepatic Artery with Two Drug-eluting Intraluminal Devices, Percutaneous Approach

047336Z Dilation of Hepatic Artery with Three Drug-eluting Intraluminal Devices, Percutaneous Approach

047337Z Dilation of Hepatic Artery with Four or More Drug-eluting Intraluminal Devices, Percutaneous Approach

04733D1 Dilation of Hepatic Artery with Intraluminal Device, using Drug-Coated Balloon, Percutaneous Approach

04733DZ Dilation of Hepatic Artery with Intraluminal Device, Percutaneous Approach

04733EZ Dilation of Hepatic Artery with Two Intraluminal Devices, Percutaneous Approach

04733FZ Dilation of Hepatic Artery with Three Intraluminal Devices, Percutaneous Approach

04733GZ Dilation of Hepatic Artery with Four or More Intraluminal Devices, Percutaneous Approach

04733Z1 Dilation of Hepatic Artery using Drug-Coated Balloon, Percutaneous Approach

04733ZZ Dilation of Hepatic Artery, Percutaneous Approach

0473441 Dilation of Hepatic Artery with Drug-eluting Intraluminal Device, using Drug-Coated Balloon, Percutaneous Endoscopic Approach

047344Z Dilation of Hepatic Artery with Drug-eluting Intraluminal Device, Percutaneous Endoscopic Approach

047345Z Dilation of Hepatic Artery with Two Drug-eluting Intraluminal Devices, Percutaneous Endoscopic Approach

047346Z Dilation of Hepatic Artery with Three Drug-eluting Intraluminal Devices, Percutaneous Endoscopic Approach

047347Z Dilation of Hepatic Artery with Four or More Drug-eluting Intraluminal Devices, Percutaneous Endoscopic Approach

04734D1 Dilation of Hepatic Artery with Intraluminal Device, using Drug-Coated Balloon, Percutaneous Endoscopic Approach

04734DZ Dilation of Hepatic Artery with Intraluminal Device, Percutaneous Endoscopic Approach

04734EZ Dilation of Hepatic Artery with Two Intraluminal Devices, Percutaneous Endoscopic Approach

04734FZ Dilation of Hepatic Artery with Three Intraluminal Devices, Percutaneous Endoscopic Approach

04734GZ Dilation of Hepatic Artery with Four or More Intraluminal Devices, Percutaneous Endoscopic Approach

04734Z1 Dilation of Hepatic Artery using Drug-Coated Balloon, Percutaneous Endoscopic Approach

04734ZZ Dilation of Hepatic Artery, Percutaneous Endoscopic Approach

0474041 Dilation of Splenic Artery with Drug-eluting Intraluminal Device, using Drug-Coated Balloon, Open Approach

047404Z Dilation of Splenic Artery with Drug-eluting Intraluminal Device, Open Approach

047405Z Dilation of Splenic Artery with Two Drug-eluting Intraluminal Devices, Open Approach

047406Z Dilation of Splenic Artery with Three Drug-eluting Intraluminal Devices, Open Approach

047407Z Dilation of Splenic Artery with Four or More Drug-eluting Intraluminal Devices, Open Approach

04740D1 Dilation of Splenic Artery with Intraluminal Device, using Drug-Coated Balloon, Open Approach

04740DZ Dilation of Splenic Artery with Intraluminal Device, Open Approach

04740EZ Dilation of Splenic Artery with Two Intraluminal Devices, Open Approach

04740FZ Dilation of Splenic Artery with Three Intraluminal Devices, Open Approach

04740GZ Dilation of Splenic Artery with Four or More Intraluminal Devices, Open Approach

04740Z1 Dilation of Splenic Artery using Drug-Coated Balloon, Open Approach

04740ZZ Dilation of Splenic Artery, Open Approach

0474341 Dilation of Splenic Artery with Drug-eluting Intraluminal Device, using Drug-Coated Balloon, Percutaneous Approach

047434Z Dilation of Splenic Artery with Drug-eluting Intraluminal Device, Percutaneous Approach

047435Z Dilation of Splenic Artery with Two Drug-eluting Intraluminal Devices, Percutaneous Approach

047436Z Dilation of Splenic Artery with Three Drug-eluting Intraluminal Devices, Percutaneous Approach

047437Z Dilation of Splenic Artery with Four or More Drug-eluting Intraluminal Devices, Percutaneous Approach

04743D1 Dilation of Splenic Artery with Intraluminal Device, using Drug-Coated Balloon, Percutaneous Approach

04743DZ Dilation of Splenic Artery with Intraluminal Device, Percutaneous Approach

04743EZ Dilation of Splenic Artery with Two Intraluminal Devices, Percutaneous Approach

04743FZ Dilation of Splenic Artery with Three Intraluminal Devices, Percutaneous Approach

04743GZ Dilation of Splenic Artery with Four or More Intraluminal Devices, Percutaneous Approach

04743Z1 Dilation of Splenic Artery using Drug-Coated Balloon, Percutaneous Approach

04743ZZ Dilation of Splenic Artery, Percutaneous Approach

0474441 Dilation of Splenic Artery with Drug-eluting Intraluminal Device, using Drug-Coated Balloon, Percutaneous Endoscopic Approach

047444Z Dilation of Splenic Artery with Drug-eluting Intraluminal Device, Percutaneous Endoscopic Approach

047445Z Dilation of Splenic Artery with Two Drug-eluting Intraluminal Devices, Percutaneous Endoscopic Approach

047446Z Dilation of Splenic Artery with Three Drug-eluting Intraluminal Devices, Percutaneous Endoscopic Approach

047447Z Dilation of Splenic Artery with Four or More Drug-eluting Intraluminal Devices, Percutaneous Endoscopic Approach

04744D1 Dilation of Splenic Artery with Intraluminal Device, using Drug-Coated Balloon, Percutaneous Endoscopic Approach

04744DZ Dilation of Splenic Artery with Intraluminal Device, Percutaneous Endoscopic Approach

04744EZ Dilation of Splenic Artery with Two Intraluminal Devices, Percutaneous Endoscopic Approach

04744FZ Dilation of Splenic Artery with Three Intraluminal Devices, Percutaneous Endoscopic Approach

04744GZ Dilation of Splenic Artery with Four or More Intraluminal Devices, Percutaneous Endoscopic Approach

04744Z1 Dilation of Splenic Artery using Drug-Coated Balloon, Percutaneous Endoscopic Approach

04744ZZ Dilation of Splenic Artery, Percutaneous Endoscopic Approach

0475041 Dilation of Superior Mesenteric Artery with Drug-eluting Intraluminal Device, using Drug-Coated Balloon, Open Approach

047504Z Dilation of Superior Mesenteric Artery with Drug-eluting Intraluminal Device, Open Approach

047505Z Dilation of Superior Mesenteric Artery with Two Drug-eluting Intraluminal Devices, Open Approach

047506Z Dilation of Superior Mesenteric Artery with Three Drug-eluting Intraluminal Devices, Open Approach

047507Z Dilation of Superior Mesenteric Artery with Four or More Drug-eluting Intraluminal Devices, Open Approach

04750D1 Dilation of Superior Mesenteric Artery with Intraluminal Device, using Drug-Coated Balloon, Open Approach

04750DZ Dilation of Superior Mesenteric Artery with Intraluminal Device, Open Approach

04750EZ Dilation of Superior Mesenteric Artery with Two Intraluminal Devices, Open Approach

04750FZ Dilation of Superior Mesenteric Artery with Three Intraluminal Devices, Open Approach

04750GZ Dilation of Superior Mesenteric Artery with Four or More Intraluminal Devices, Open Approach

04750Z1 Dilation of Superior Mesenteric Artery using Drug-Coated Balloon, Open Approach

04750ZZ Dilation of Superior Mesenteric Artery, Open Approach

0475341 Dilation of Superior Mesenteric Artery with Drug-eluting Intraluminal Device, using Drug-Coated Balloon, Percutaneous Approach

047534Z Dilation of Superior Mesenteric Artery with Drug-eluting Intraluminal Device, Percutaneous Approach

047535Z Dilation of Superior Mesenteric Artery with Two Drug-eluting Intraluminal Devices, Percutaneous Approach

047536Z Dilation of Superior Mesenteric Artery with Three Drug-eluting Intraluminal Devices, Percutaneous Approach

047537Z Dilation of Superior Mesenteric Artery with Four or More Drug-eluting Intraluminal Devices, Percutaneous Approach

04753D1 Dilation of Superior Mesenteric Artery with Intraluminal Device, using Drug-Coated Balloon, Percutaneous Approach

04753DZ Dilation of Superior Mesenteric Artery with Intraluminal Device, Percutaneous Approach

04753EZ Dilation of Superior Mesenteric Artery with Two Intraluminal Devices, Percutaneous Approach

04753FZ Dilation of Superior Mesenteric Artery with Three Intraluminal Devices, Percutaneous Approach

04753GZ Dilation of Superior Mesenteric Artery with Four or More Intraluminal Devices, Percutaneous Approach

04753Z1 Dilation of Superior Mesenteric Artery using Drug-Coated Balloon, Percutaneous Approach

04753ZZ Dilation of Superior Mesenteric Artery, Percutaneous Approach

0475441 Dilation of Superior Mesenteric Artery with Drug-eluting Intraluminal Device, using Drug-Coated Balloon, Percutaneous Endoscopic Approach

047544Z Dilation of Superior Mesenteric Artery with Drug-eluting Intraluminal Device, Percutaneous Endoscopic Approach

047545Z Dilation of Superior Mesenteric Artery with Two Drug-eluting Intraluminal Devices, Percutaneous Endoscopic Approach

047546Z Dilation of Superior Mesenteric Artery with Three Drug-eluting Intraluminal Devices, Percutaneous Endoscopic Approach

047547Z Dilation of Superior Mesenteric Artery with Four or More Drug-eluting Intraluminal Devices, Percutaneous Endoscopic Approach

04754D1 Dilation of Superior Mesenteric Artery with Intraluminal Device, using Drug-Coated Balloon, Percutaneous Endoscopic Approach

04754DZ Dilation of Superior Mesenteric Artery with Intraluminal Device, Percutaneous Endoscopic Approach

04754EZ Dilation of Superior Mesenteric Artery with Two Intraluminal Devices, Percutaneous Endoscopic Approach

04754FZ Dilation of Superior Mesenteric Artery with Three Intraluminal Devices, Percutaneous Endoscopic Approach

04754GZ Dilation of Superior Mesenteric Artery with Four or More Intraluminal Devices, Percutaneous Endoscopic Approach

04754Z1 Dilation of Superior Mesenteric Artery using Drug-Coated Balloon, Percutaneous Endoscopic Approach

04754ZZ Dilation of Superior Mesenteric Artery, Percutaneous Endoscopic Approach

0476041 Dilation of Right Colic Artery with Drug-eluting Intraluminal Device, using Drug-Coated Balloon, Open Approach

047604Z Dilation of Right Colic Artery with Drug-eluting Intraluminal Device, Open Approach

047605Z Dilation of Right Colic Artery with Two Drug-eluting Intraluminal Devices, Open Approach

047606Z Dilation of Right Colic Artery with Three Drug-eluting Intraluminal Devices, Open Approach

047607Z Dilation of Right Colic Artery with Four or More Drug-eluting Intraluminal Devices, Open Approach

04760D1 Dilation of Right Colic Artery with Intraluminal Device, using Drug-Coated Balloon, Open Approach

04760DZ Dilation of Right Colic Artery with Intraluminal Device, Open Approach

04760EZ Dilation of Right Colic Artery with Two Intraluminal Devices, Open Approach

04760FZ Dilation of Right Colic Artery with Three Intraluminal Devices, Open Approach

04760GZ Dilation of Right Colic Artery with Four or More Intraluminal Devices, Open Approach

04760Z1 Dilation of Right Colic Artery using Drug-Coated Balloon, Open Approach

04760ZZ Dilation of Right Colic Artery, Open Approach

0476341 Dilation of Right Colic Artery with Drug-eluting Intraluminal Device, using Drug-Coated Balloon, Percutaneous Approach

047634Z Dilation of Right Colic Artery with Drug-eluting Intraluminal Device, Percutaneous Approach

047635Z Dilation of Right Colic Artery with Two Drug-eluting Intraluminal Devices, Percutaneous Approach

047636Z Dilation of Right Colic Artery with Three Drug-eluting Intraluminal Devices, Percutaneous Approach

047637Z Dilation of Right Colic Artery with Four or More Drug-eluting Intraluminal Devices, Percutaneous Approach

04763D1 Dilation of Right Colic Artery with Intraluminal Device, using Drug-Coated Balloon, Percutaneous Approach

04763DZ Dilation of Right Colic Artery with Intraluminal Device, Percutaneous Approach

04763EZ Dilation of Right Colic Artery with Two Intraluminal Devices, Percutaneous Approach

04763FZ Dilation of Right Colic Artery with Three Intraluminal Devices, Percutaneous Approach

04763GZ Dilation of Right Colic Artery with Four or More Intraluminal Devices, Percutaneous Approach

04763Z1 Dilation of Right Colic Artery using Drug-Coated Balloon, Percutaneous Approach

04763ZZ Dilation of Right Colic Artery, Percutaneous Approach

0476441 Dilation of Right Colic Artery with Drug-eluting Intraluminal Device, using Drug-Coated Balloon, Percutaneous Endoscopic Approach

047644Z Dilation of Right Colic Artery with Drug-eluting Intraluminal Device, Percutaneous Endoscopic Approach

047645Z Dilation of Right Colic Artery with Two Drug-eluting Intraluminal Devices, Percutaneous Endoscopic Approach

047646Z Dilation of Right Colic Artery with Three Drug-eluting Intraluminal Devices, Percutaneous Endoscopic Approach

047647Z Dilation of Right Colic Artery with Four or More Drug-eluting Intraluminal Devices, Percutaneous Endoscopic Approach

04764D1 Dilation of Right Colic Artery with Intraluminal Device, using Drug-Coated Balloon, Percutaneous Endoscopic Approach

04764DZ Dilation of Right Colic Artery with Intraluminal Device, Percutaneous Endoscopic Approach

04764EZ Dilation of Right Colic Artery with Two Intraluminal Devices, Percutaneous Endoscopic Approach

04764FZ Dilation of Right Colic Artery with Three Intraluminal Devices, Percutaneous Endoscopic Approach

04764GZ Dilation of Right Colic Artery with Four or More Intraluminal Devices, Percutaneous Endoscopic Approach

04764Z1 Dilation of Right Colic Artery using Drug-Coated Balloon, Percutaneous Endoscopic Approach

04764ZZ Dilation of Right Colic Artery, Percutaneous Endoscopic Approach

0477041 Dilation of Left Colic Artery with Drug-eluting Intraluminal Device, using Drug-Coated Balloon, Open Approach

047704Z Dilation of Left Colic Artery with Drug-eluting Intraluminal Device, Open Approach

047705Z Dilation of Left Colic Artery with Two Drug-eluting Intraluminal Devices, Open Approach

047706Z Dilation of Left Colic Artery with Three Drug-eluting Intraluminal Devices, Open Approach

047707Z Dilation of Left Colic Artery with Four or More Drug-eluting Intraluminal Devices, Open Approach

04770D1 Dilation of Left Colic Artery with Intraluminal Device, using Drug-Coated Balloon, Open Approach

04770DZ Dilation of Left Colic Artery with Intraluminal Device, Open Approach

04770EZ Dilation of Left Colic Artery with Two Intraluminal Devices, Open Approach

04770FZ Dilation of Left Colic Artery with Three Intraluminal Devices, Open Approach

04770GZ Dilation of Left Colic Artery with Four or More Intraluminal Devices, Open Approach

04770Z1 Dilation of Left Colic Artery using Drug-Coated Balloon, Open Approach

04770ZZ Dilation of Left Colic Artery, Open Approach

0477341 Dilation of Left Colic Artery with Drug-eluting Intraluminal Device, using Drug-Coated Balloon, Percutaneous Approach

047734Z Dilation of Left Colic Artery with Drug-eluting Intraluminal Device, Percutaneous Approach

047735Z Dilation of Left Colic Artery with Two Drug-eluting Intraluminal Devices, Percutaneous Approach

047736Z Dilation of Left Colic Artery with Three Drug-eluting Intraluminal Devices, Percutaneous Approach

047737Z Dilation of Left Colic Artery with Four or More Drug-eluting Intraluminal Devices, Percutaneous Approach

04773D1 Dilation of Left Colic Artery with Intraluminal Device, using Drug-Coated Balloon, Percutaneous Approach

04773DZ Dilation of Left Colic Artery with Intraluminal Device, Percutaneous Approach

04773EZ Dilation of Left Colic Artery with Two Intraluminal Devices, Percutaneous Approach

04773FZ Dilation of Left Colic Artery with Three Intraluminal Devices, Percutaneous Approach

04773GZ Dilation of Left Colic Artery with Four or More Intraluminal Devices, Percutaneous Approach

04773Z1 Dilation of Left Colic Artery using Drug-Coated Balloon, Percutaneous Approach

04773ZZ Dilation of Left Colic Artery, Percutaneous Approach

0477441 Dilation of Left Colic Artery with Drug-eluting Intraluminal Device, using Drug-Coated Balloon, Percutaneous Endoscopic Approach

047744Z Dilation of Left Colic Artery with Drug-eluting Intraluminal Device, Percutaneous Endoscopic Approach

047745Z Dilation of Left Colic Artery with Two Drug-eluting Intraluminal Devices, Percutaneous Endoscopic Approach

047746Z Dilation of Left Colic Artery with Three Drug-eluting Intraluminal Devices, Percutaneous Endoscopic Approach

047747Z Dilation of Left Colic Artery with Four or More Drug-eluting Intraluminal Devices, Percutaneous Endoscopic Approach

04774D1 Dilation of Left Colic Artery with Intraluminal Device, using Drug-Coated Balloon, Percutaneous Endoscopic Approach

04774DZ Dilation of Left Colic Artery with Intraluminal Device, Percutaneous Endoscopic Approach

04774EZ Dilation of Left Colic Artery with Two Intraluminal Devices, Percutaneous Endoscopic Approach

04774FZ Dilation of Left Colic Artery with Three Intraluminal Devices, Percutaneous Endoscopic Approach

04774GZ Dilation of Left Colic Artery with Four or More Intraluminal Devices, Percutaneous Endoscopic Approach

04774Z1 Dilation of Left Colic Artery using Drug-Coated Balloon, Percutaneous Endoscopic Approach

04774ZZ Dilation of Left Colic Artery, Percutaneous Endoscopic Approach

0478041 Dilation of Middle Colic Artery with Drug-eluting Intraluminal Device, using Drug-Coated Balloon, Open Approach

047804Z Dilation of Middle Colic Artery with Drug-eluting Intraluminal Device, Open Approach

047805Z Dilation of Middle Colic Artery with Two Drug-eluting Intraluminal Devices, Open Approach

047806Z Dilation of Middle Colic Artery with Three Drug-eluting Intraluminal Devices, Open Approach

047807Z Dilation of Middle Colic Artery with Four or More Drug-eluting Intraluminal Devices, Open Approach

04780D1 Dilation of Middle Colic Artery with Intraluminal Device, using Drug-Coated Balloon, Open Approach

04780DZ Dilation of Middle Colic Artery with Intraluminal Device, Open Approach

04780EZ Dilation of Middle Colic Artery with Two Intraluminal Devices, Open Approach

04780FZ Dilation of Middle Colic Artery with Three Intraluminal Devices, Open Approach

04780GZ Dilation of Middle Colic Artery with Four or More Intraluminal Devices, Open Approach

04780Z1 Dilation of Middle Colic Artery using Drug-Coated Balloon, Open Approach

04780ZZ Dilation of Middle Colic Artery, Open Approach

0478341 Dilation of Middle Colic Artery with Drug-eluting Intraluminal Device, using Drug-Coated Balloon, Percutaneous Approach

047834Z Dilation of Middle Colic Artery with Drug-eluting Intraluminal Device, Percutaneous Approach

047835Z Dilation of Middle Colic Artery with Two Drug-eluting Intraluminal Devices, Percutaneous Approach

047836Z Dilation of Middle Colic Artery with Three Drug-eluting Intraluminal Devices, Percutaneous Approach

047837Z Dilation of Middle Colic Artery with Four or More Drug-eluting Intraluminal Devices, Percutaneous Approach

04783D1 Dilation of Middle Colic Artery with Intraluminal Device, using Drug-Coated Balloon, Percutaneous Approach

04783DZ Dilation of Middle Colic Artery with Intraluminal Device, Percutaneous Approach

04783EZ Dilation of Middle Colic Artery with Two Intraluminal Devices, Percutaneous Approach

04783FZ Dilation of Middle Colic Artery with Three Intraluminal Devices, Percutaneous Approach

04783GZ Dilation of Middle Colic Artery with Four or More Intraluminal Devices, Percutaneous Approach

04783Z1 Dilation of Middle Colic Artery using Drug-Coated Balloon, Percutaneous Approach

04783ZZ Dilation of Middle Colic Artery, Percutaneous Approach

0478441 Dilation of Middle Colic Artery with Drug-eluting Intraluminal Device, using Drug-Coated Balloon, Percutaneous Endoscopic Approach

047844Z Dilation of Middle Colic Artery with Drug-eluting Intraluminal Device, Percutaneous Endoscopic Approach

047845Z Dilation of Middle Colic Artery with Two Drug-eluting Intraluminal Devices, Percutaneous Endoscopic Approach

047846Z Dilation of Middle Colic Artery with Three Drug-eluting Intraluminal Devices, Percutaneous Endoscopic Approach

047847Z Dilation of Middle Colic Artery with Four or More Drug-eluting Intraluminal Devices, Percutaneous Endoscopic Approach

04784D1 Dilation of Middle Colic Artery with Intraluminal Device, using Drug-Coated Balloon, Percutaneous Endoscopic Approach

04784DZ Dilation of Middle Colic Artery with Intraluminal Device, Percutaneous Endoscopic Approach

04784EZ Dilation of Middle Colic Artery with Two Intraluminal Devices, Percutaneous Endoscopic Approach

04784FZ Dilation of Middle Colic Artery with Three Intraluminal Devices, Percutaneous Endoscopic Approach

04784GZ Dilation of Middle Colic Artery with Four or More Intraluminal Devices, Percutaneous Endoscopic Approach

04784Z1 Dilation of Middle Colic Artery using Drug-Coated Balloon, Percutaneous Endoscopic Approach

04784ZZ Dilation of Middle Colic Artery, Percutaneous Endoscopic Approach

0479041 Dilation of Right Renal Artery with Drug-eluting Intraluminal Device, using Drug-Coated Balloon, Open Approach

047904Z Dilation of Right Renal Artery with Drug-eluting Intraluminal Device, Open Approach

047905Z Dilation of Right Renal Artery with Two Drug-eluting Intraluminal Devices, Open Approach

047906Z Dilation of Right Renal Artery with Three Drug-eluting Intraluminal Devices, Open Approach

047907Z Dilation of Right Renal Artery with Four or More Drug-eluting Intraluminal Devices, Open Approach

04790D1 Dilation of Right Renal Artery with Intraluminal Device, using Drug-Coated Balloon, Open Approach

04790DZ Dilation of Right Renal Artery with Intraluminal Device, Open Approach

04790EZ Dilation of Right Renal Artery with Two Intraluminal Devices, Open Approach

04790FZ Dilation of Right Renal Artery with Three Intraluminal Devices, Open Approach

04790GZ Dilation of Right Renal Artery with Four or More Intraluminal Devices, Open Approach

04790Z1 Dilation of Right Renal Artery using Drug-Coated Balloon, Open Approach

04790ZZ Dilation of Right Renal Artery, Open Approach

0479341 Dilation of Right Renal Artery with Drug-eluting Intraluminal Device, using Drug-Coated Balloon, Percutaneous Approach

047934Z Dilation of Right Renal Artery with Drug-eluting Intraluminal Device, Percutaneous Approach

047935Z Dilation of Right Renal Artery with Two Drug-eluting Intraluminal Devices, Percutaneous Approach

047936Z Dilation of Right Renal Artery with Three Drug-eluting Intraluminal Devices, Percutaneous Approach

047937Z Dilation of Right Renal Artery with Four or More Drug-eluting Intraluminal Devices, Percutaneous Approach

04793D1 Dilation of Right Renal Artery with Intraluminal Device, using Drug-Coated Balloon, Percutaneous Approach

04793DZ Dilation of Right Renal Artery with Intraluminal Device, Percutaneous Approach

04793EZ Dilation of Right Renal Artery with Two Intraluminal Devices, Percutaneous Approach

04793FZ Dilation of Right Renal Artery with Three Intraluminal Devices, Percutaneous Approach

04793GZ Dilation of Right Renal Artery with Four or More Intraluminal Devices, Percutaneous Approach

04793Z1 Dilation of Right Renal Artery using Drug-Coated Balloon, Percutaneous Approach

04793ZZ Dilation of Right Renal Artery, Percutaneous Approach

0479441 Dilation of Right Renal Artery with Drug-eluting Intraluminal Device, using Drug-Coated Balloon, Percutaneous Endoscopic Approach

047944Z Dilation of Right Renal Artery with Drug-eluting Intraluminal Device, Percutaneous Endoscopic Approach

047945Z Dilation of Right Renal Artery with Two Drug-eluting Intraluminal Devices, Percutaneous Endoscopic Approach

047946Z Dilation of Right Renal Artery with Three Drug-eluting Intraluminal Devices, Percutaneous Endoscopic Approach

047947Z Dilation of Right Renal Artery with Four or More Drug-eluting Intraluminal Devices, Percutaneous Endoscopic Approach

04794D1 Dilation of Right Renal Artery with Intraluminal Device, using Drug-Coated Balloon, Percutaneous Endoscopic Approach

04794DZ Dilation of Right Renal Artery with Intraluminal Device, Percutaneous Endoscopic Approach

04794EZ Dilation of Right Renal Artery with Two Intraluminal Devices, Percutaneous Endoscopic Approach

04794FZ Dilation of Right Renal Artery with Three Intraluminal Devices, Percutaneous Endoscopic Approach

04794GZ Dilation of Right Renal Artery with Four or More Intraluminal Devices, Percutaneous Endoscopic Approach

04794Z1 Dilation of Right Renal Artery using Drug-Coated Balloon, Percutaneous Endoscopic Approach

04794ZZ Dilation of Right Renal Artery, Percutaneous Endoscopic Approach

047A041 Dilation of Left Renal Artery with Drug-eluting Intraluminal Device, using Drug-Coated Balloon, Open Approach

047A04Z Dilation of Left Renal Artery with Drug-eluting Intraluminal Device, Open Approach

047A05Z Dilation of Left Renal Artery with Two Drug-eluting Intraluminal Devices, Open Approach

047A06Z Dilation of Left Renal Artery with Three Drug-eluting Intraluminal Devices, Open Approach

047A07Z Dilation of Left Renal Artery with Four or More Drug-eluting Intraluminal Devices, Open Approach

047A0D1 Dilation of Left Renal Artery with Intraluminal Device, using Drug-Coated Balloon, Open Approach

047A0DZ Dilation of Left Renal Artery with Intraluminal Device, Open Approach

047A0EZ Dilation of Left Renal Artery with Two Intraluminal Devices, Open Approach

047A0FZ Dilation of Left Renal Artery with Three Intraluminal Devices, Open Approach

047A0GZ Dilation of Left Renal Artery with Four or More Intraluminal Devices, Open Approach

047A0Z1 Dilation of Left Renal Artery using Drug-Coated Balloon, Open Approach

047A0ZZ Dilation of Left Renal Artery, Open Approach

047A341 Dilation of Left Renal Artery with Drug-eluting Intraluminal Device, using Drug-Coated Balloon, Percutaneous Approach

047A34Z Dilation of Left Renal Artery with Drug-eluting Intraluminal Device, Percutaneous Approach

047A35Z Dilation of Left Renal Artery with Two Drug-eluting Intraluminal Devices, Percutaneous Approach

047A36Z Dilation of Left Renal Artery with Three Drug-eluting Intraluminal Devices, Percutaneous Approach

047A37Z Dilation of Left Renal Artery with Four or More Drug-eluting Intraluminal Devices, Percutaneous Approach

047A3D1 Dilation of Left Renal Artery with Intraluminal Device, using Drug-Coated Balloon, Percutaneous Approach

047A3DZ Dilation of Left Renal Artery with Intraluminal Device, Percutaneous Approach

047A3EZ Dilation of Left Renal Artery with Two Intraluminal Devices, Percutaneous Approach

047A3FZ Dilation of Left Renal Artery with Three Intraluminal Devices, Percutaneous Approach

047A3GZ Dilation of Left Renal Artery with Four or More Intraluminal Devices, Percutaneous Approach

047A3Z1 Dilation of Left Renal Artery using Drug-Coated Balloon, Percutaneous Approach

047A3ZZ Dilation of Left Renal Artery, Percutaneous Approach

047A441 Dilation of Left Renal Artery with Drug-eluting Intraluminal Device, using Drug-Coated Balloon, Percutaneous Endoscopic Approach

047A44Z Dilation of Left Renal Artery with Drug-eluting Intraluminal Device, Percutaneous Endoscopic Approach

047A45Z Dilation of Left Renal Artery with Two Drug-eluting Intraluminal Devices, Percutaneous Endoscopic Approach

047A46Z Dilation of Left Renal Artery with Three Drug-eluting Intraluminal Devices, Percutaneous Endoscopic Approach

047A47Z Dilation of Left Renal Artery with Four or More Drug-eluting Intraluminal Devices, Percutaneous Endoscopic Approach

047A4D1 Dilation of Left Renal Artery with Intraluminal Device, using Drug-Coated Balloon, Percutaneous Endoscopic Approach

047A4DZ Dilation of Left Renal Artery with Intraluminal Device, Percutaneous Endoscopic Approach

047A4EZ Dilation of Left Renal Artery with Two Intraluminal Devices, Percutaneous Endoscopic Approach

047A4FZ Dilation of Left Renal Artery with Three Intraluminal Devices, Percutaneous Endoscopic Approach

047A4GZ Dilation of Left Renal Artery with Four or More Intraluminal Devices, Percutaneous Endoscopic Approach

047A4Z1 Dilation of Left Renal Artery using Drug-Coated Balloon, Percutaneous Endoscopic Approach

047A4ZZ Dilation of Left Renal Artery, Percutaneous Endoscopic Approach

047B041 Dilation of Inferior Mesenteric Artery with Drug-eluting Intraluminal Device, using Drug-Coated Balloon, Open Approach

047B04Z Dilation of Inferior Mesenteric Artery with Drug-eluting Intraluminal Device, Open Approach

047B05Z Dilation of Inferior Mesenteric Artery with Two Drug-eluting Intraluminal Devices, Open Approach

047B06Z Dilation of Inferior Mesenteric Artery with Three Drug-eluting Intraluminal Devices, Open Approach

047B07Z Dilation of Inferior Mesenteric Artery with Four or More Drug-eluting Intraluminal Devices, Open Approach

047B0D1 Dilation of Inferior Mesenteric Artery with Intraluminal Device, using Drug-Coated Balloon, Open Approach

047B0DZ Dilation of Inferior Mesenteric Artery with Intraluminal Device, Open Approach

047B0EZ Dilation of Inferior Mesenteric Artery with Two Intraluminal Devices, Open Approach

047B0FZ Dilation of Inferior Mesenteric Artery with Three Intraluminal Devices, Open Approach

047B0GZ Dilation of Inferior Mesenteric Artery with Four or More Intraluminal Devices, Open Approach

047B0Z1 Dilation of Inferior Mesenteric Artery using Drug-Coated Balloon, Open Approach

047B0ZZ Dilation of Inferior Mesenteric Artery, Open Approach

047B341 Dilation of Inferior Mesenteric Artery with Drug-eluting Intraluminal Device, using Drug-Coated Balloon, Percutaneous Approach

047B34Z Dilation of Inferior Mesenteric Artery with Drug-eluting Intraluminal Device, Percutaneous Approach

047B35Z Dilation of Inferior Mesenteric Artery with Two Drug-eluting Intraluminal Devices, Percutaneous Approach

047B36Z Dilation of Inferior Mesenteric Artery with Three Drug-eluting Intraluminal Devices, Percutaneous Approach

047B37Z Dilation of Inferior Mesenteric Artery with Four or More Drug-eluting Intraluminal Devices, Percutaneous Approach

047B3D1 Dilation of Inferior Mesenteric Artery with Intraluminal Device, using Drug-Coated Balloon, Percutaneous Approach

047B3DZ Dilation of Inferior Mesenteric Artery with Intraluminal Device, Percutaneous Approach

047B3EZ Dilation of Inferior Mesenteric Artery with Two Intraluminal Devices, Percutaneous Approach

047B3FZ Dilation of Inferior Mesenteric Artery with Three Intraluminal Devices, Percutaneous Approach

047B3GZ Dilation of Inferior Mesenteric Artery with Four or More Intraluminal Devices, Percutaneous Approach

047B3Z1 Dilation of Inferior Mesenteric Artery using Drug-Coated Balloon, Percutaneous Approach

047B3ZZ Dilation of Inferior Mesenteric Artery, Percutaneous Approach

047B441 Dilation of Inferior Mesenteric Artery with Drug-eluting Intraluminal Device, using Drug-Coated Balloon, Percutaneous Endoscopic Approach

047B44Z Dilation of Inferior Mesenteric Artery with Drug-eluting Intraluminal Device, Percutaneous Endoscopic Approach

047B45Z Dilation of Inferior Mesenteric Artery with Two Drug-eluting Intraluminal Devices, Percutaneous Endoscopic Approach

047B46Z Dilation of Inferior Mesenteric Artery with Three Drug-eluting Intraluminal Devices, Percutaneous Endoscopic Approach

047B47Z Dilation of Inferior Mesenteric Artery with Four or More Drug-eluting Intraluminal Devices, Percutaneous Endoscopic Approach

047B4D1 Dilation of Inferior Mesenteric Artery with Intraluminal Device, using Drug-Coated Balloon, Percutaneous Endoscopic Approach

047B4DZ Dilation of Inferior Mesenteric Artery with Intraluminal Device, Percutaneous Endoscopic Approach

047B4EZ Dilation of Inferior Mesenteric Artery with Two Intraluminal Devices, Percutaneous Endoscopic Approach

047B4FZ Dilation of Inferior Mesenteric Artery with Three Intraluminal Devices, Percutaneous Endoscopic Approach

047B4GZ Dilation of Inferior Mesenteric Artery with Four or More Intraluminal Devices, Percutaneous Endoscopic Approach

047B4Z1 Dilation of Inferior Mesenteric Artery using Drug-Coated Balloon, Percutaneous Endoscopic Approach

047B4ZZ Dilation of Inferior Mesenteric Artery, Percutaneous Endoscopic Approach

047C041 Dilation of Right Common Iliac Artery with Drug-eluting Intraluminal Device, using Drug-Coated Balloon, Open Approach

047C04Z Dilation of Right Common Iliac Artery with Drug-eluting Intraluminal Device, Open Approach

047C05Z Dilation of Right Common Iliac Artery with Two Drug-eluting Intraluminal Devices, Open Approach

047C06Z Dilation of Right Common Iliac Artery with Three Drug-eluting Intraluminal Devices, Open Approach

047C07Z Dilation of Right Common Iliac Artery with Four or More Drug-eluting Intraluminal Devices, Open Approach

047C0D1 Dilation of Right Common Iliac Artery with Intraluminal Device, using Drug-Coated Balloon, Open Approach

047C0DZ Dilation of Right Common Iliac Artery with Intraluminal Device, Open Approach

047C0EZ Dilation of Right Common Iliac Artery with Two Intraluminal Devices, Open Approach

047C0FZ Dilation of Right Common Iliac Artery with Three Intraluminal Devices, Open Approach

047C0GZ Dilation of Right Common Iliac Artery with Four or More Intraluminal Devices, Open Approach

047C0Z1 Dilation of Right Common Iliac Artery using Drug-Coated Balloon, Open Approach

047C0ZZ Dilation of Right Common Iliac Artery, Open Approach

047C341 Dilation of Right Common Iliac Artery with Drug-eluting Intraluminal Device, using Drug-Coated Balloon, Percutaneous Approach

047C34Z Dilation of Right Common Iliac Artery with Drug-eluting Intraluminal Device, Percutaneous Approach

047C35Z Dilation of Right Common Iliac Artery with Two Drug-eluting Intraluminal Devices, Percutaneous Approach

047C36Z Dilation of Right Common Iliac Artery with Three Drug-eluting Intraluminal Devices, Percutaneous Approach

047C37Z Dilation of Right Common Iliac Artery with Four or More Drug-eluting Intraluminal Devices, Percutaneous Approach

047C3D1 Dilation of Right Common Iliac Artery with Intraluminal Device, using Drug-Coated Balloon, Percutaneous Approach

047C3DZ Dilation of Right Common Iliac Artery with Intraluminal Device, Percutaneous Approach

047C3EZ Dilation of Right Common Iliac Artery with Two Intraluminal Devices, Percutaneous Approach

047C3FZ Dilation of Right Common Iliac Artery with Three Intraluminal Devices, Percutaneous Approach

047C3GZ Dilation of Right Common Iliac Artery with Four or More Intraluminal Devices, Percutaneous Approach

047C3Z1 Dilation of Right Common Iliac Artery using Drug-Coated Balloon, Percutaneous Approach

047C3ZZ Dilation of Right Common Iliac Artery, Percutaneous Approach

047C441 Dilation of Right Common Iliac Artery with Drug-eluting Intraluminal Device, using Drug-Coated Balloon, Percutaneous Endoscopic Approach

047C44Z Dilation of Right Common Iliac Artery with Drug-eluting Intraluminal Device, Percutaneous Endoscopic Approach

047C45Z Dilation of Right Common Iliac Artery with Two Drug-eluting Intraluminal Devices, Percutaneous Endoscopic Approach

047C46Z Dilation of Right Common Iliac Artery with Three Drug-eluting Intraluminal Devices, Percutaneous Endoscopic Approach

047C47Z Dilation of Right Common Iliac Artery with Four or More Drug-eluting Intraluminal Devices, Percutaneous Endoscopic Approach

047C4D1 Dilation of Right Common Iliac Artery with Intraluminal Device, using Drug-Coated Balloon, Percutaneous Endoscopic Approach

047C4DZ Dilation of Right Common Iliac Artery with Intraluminal Device, Percutaneous Endoscopic Approach

047C4EZ Dilation of Right Common Iliac Artery with Two Intraluminal Devices, Percutaneous Endoscopic Approach

047C4FZ Dilation of Right Common Iliac Artery with Three Intraluminal Devices, Percutaneous Endoscopic Approach

047C4GZ Dilation of Right Common Iliac Artery with Four or More Intraluminal Devices, Percutaneous Endoscopic Approach

047C4Z1 Dilation of Right Common Iliac Artery using Drug-Coated Balloon, Percutaneous Endoscopic Approach

047C4ZZ Dilation of Right Common Iliac Artery, Percutaneous Endoscopic Approach

047D041 Dilation of Left Common Iliac Artery with Drug-eluting Intraluminal Device, using Drug-Coated Balloon, Open Approach

047D04Z Dilation of Left Common Iliac Artery with Drug-eluting Intraluminal Device, Open Approach

047D05Z Dilation of Left Common Iliac Artery with Two Drug-eluting Intraluminal Devices, Open Approach

047D06Z Dilation of Left Common Iliac Artery with Three Drug-eluting Intraluminal Devices, Open Approach

047D07Z Dilation of Left Common Iliac Artery with Four or More Drug-eluting Intraluminal Devices, Open Approach

047D0D1 Dilation of Left Common Iliac Artery with Intraluminal Device, using Drug-Coated Balloon, Open Approach

047D0DZ Dilation of Left Common Iliac Artery with Intraluminal Device, Open Approach

047D0EZ Dilation of Left Common Iliac Artery with Two Intraluminal Devices, Open Approach

047D0FZ Dilation of Left Common Iliac Artery with Three Intraluminal Devices, Open Approach

047D0GZ Dilation of Left Common Iliac Artery with Four or More Intraluminal Devices, Open Approach

047D0Z1 Dilation of Left Common Iliac Artery using Drug-Coated Balloon, Open Approach

047D0ZZ Dilation of Left Common Iliac Artery, Open Approach

047D341 Dilation of Left Common Iliac Artery with Drug-eluting Intraluminal Device, using Drug-Coated Balloon, Percutaneous Approach

047D34Z Dilation of Left Common Iliac Artery with Drug-eluting Intraluminal Device, Percutaneous Approach

047D35Z Dilation of Left Common Iliac Artery with Two Drug-eluting Intraluminal Devices, Percutaneous Approach

047D36Z Dilation of Left Common Iliac Artery with Three Drug-eluting Intraluminal Devices, Percutaneous Approach

047D37Z Dilation of Left Common Iliac Artery with Four or More Drug-eluting Intraluminal Devices, Percutaneous Approach

047D3D1 Dilation of Left Common Iliac Artery with Intraluminal Device, using Drug-Coated Balloon, Percutaneous Approach

047D3DZ Dilation of Left Common Iliac Artery with Intraluminal Device, Percutaneous Approach

047D3EZ Dilation of Left Common Iliac Artery with Two Intraluminal Devices, Percutaneous Approach

047D3FZ Dilation of Left Common Iliac Artery with Three Intraluminal Devices, Percutaneous Approach

047D3GZ Dilation of Left Common Iliac Artery with Four or More Intraluminal Devices, Percutaneous Approach

047D3Z1 Dilation of Left Common Iliac Artery using Drug-Coated Balloon, Percutaneous Approach

047D3ZZ Dilation of Left Common Iliac Artery, Percutaneous Approach

047D441 Dilation of Left Common Iliac Artery with Drug-eluting Intraluminal Device, using Drug-Coated Balloon, Percutaneous Endoscopic Approach

047D44Z Dilation of Left Common Iliac Artery with Drug-eluting Intraluminal Device, Percutaneous Endoscopic Approach

047D45Z Dilation of Left Common Iliac Artery with Two Drug-eluting Intraluminal Devices, Percutaneous Endoscopic Approach

047D46Z Dilation of Left Common Iliac Artery with Three Drug-eluting Intraluminal Devices, Percutaneous Endoscopic Approach

047D47Z Dilation of Left Common Iliac Artery with Four or More Drug-eluting Intraluminal Devices, Percutaneous Endoscopic Approach

047D4D1 Dilation of Left Common Iliac Artery with Intraluminal Device, using Drug-Coated Balloon, Percutaneous Endoscopic Approach

047D4DZ Dilation of Left Common Iliac Artery with Intraluminal Device, Percutaneous Endoscopic Approach

047D4EZ Dilation of Left Common Iliac Artery with Two Intraluminal Devices, Percutaneous Endoscopic Approach

047D4FZ Dilation of Left Common Iliac Artery with Three Intraluminal Devices, Percutaneous Endoscopic Approach

047D4GZ Dilation of Left Common Iliac Artery with Four or More Intraluminal Devices, Percutaneous Endoscopic Approach

047D4Z1 Dilation of Left Common Iliac Artery using Drug-Coated Balloon, Percutaneous Endoscopic Approach

047D4ZZ Dilation of Left Common Iliac Artery, Percutaneous Endoscopic Approach

047E041 Dilation of Right Internal Iliac Artery with Drug-eluting Intraluminal Device, using Drug-Coated Balloon, Open Approach

047E04Z Dilation of Right Internal Iliac Artery with Drug-eluting Intraluminal Device, Open Approach

047E05Z Dilation of Right Internal Iliac Artery with Two Drug-eluting Intraluminal Devices, Open Approach

047E06Z Dilation of Right Internal Iliac Artery with Three Drug-eluting Intraluminal Devices, Open Approach

047E07Z Dilation of Right Internal Iliac Artery with Four or More Drug-eluting Intraluminal Devices, Open Approach

047E0D1 Dilation of Right Internal Iliac Artery with Intraluminal Device, using Drug-Coated Balloon, Open Approach

047E0DZ Dilation of Right Internal Iliac Artery with Intraluminal Device, Open Approach

047E0EZ Dilation of Right Internal Iliac Artery with Two Intraluminal Devices, Open Approach

047E0FZ Dilation of Right Internal Iliac Artery with Three Intraluminal Devices, Open Approach

047E0GZ Dilation of Right Internal Iliac Artery with Four or More Intraluminal Devices, Open Approach

047E0Z1 Dilation of Right Internal Iliac Artery using Drug-Coated Balloon, Open Approach

047E0ZZ Dilation of Right Internal Iliac Artery, Open Approach

047E341 Dilation of Right Internal Iliac Artery with Drug-eluting Intraluminal Device, using Drug-Coated Balloon, Percutaneous Approach

047E34Z Dilation of Right Internal Iliac Artery with Drug-eluting Intraluminal Device, Percutaneous Approach

047E35Z Dilation of Right Internal Iliac Artery with Two Drug-eluting Intraluminal Devices, Percutaneous Approach

047E36Z Dilation of Right Internal Iliac Artery with Three Drug-eluting Intraluminal Devices, Percutaneous Approach

047E37Z Dilation of Right Internal Iliac Artery with Four or More Drug-eluting Intraluminal Devices, Percutaneous Approach

047E3D1 Dilation of Right Internal Iliac Artery with Intraluminal Device, using Drug-Coated Balloon, Percutaneous Approach

047E3DZ Dilation of Right Internal Iliac Artery with Intraluminal Device, Percutaneous Approach

047E3EZ Dilation of Right Internal Iliac Artery with Two Intraluminal Devices, Percutaneous Approach

047E3FZ Dilation of Right Internal Iliac Artery with Three Intraluminal Devices, Percutaneous Approach

047E3GZ Dilation of Right Internal Iliac Artery with Four or More Intraluminal Devices, Percutaneous Approach

047E3Z1 Dilation of Right Internal Iliac Artery using Drug-Coated Balloon, Percutaneous Approach

047E3ZZ Dilation of Right Internal Iliac Artery, Percutaneous Approach

047E441 Dilation of Right Internal Iliac Artery with Drug-eluting Intraluminal Device, using Drug-Coated Balloon, Percutaneous Endoscopic Approach

047E44Z Dilation of Right Internal Iliac Artery with Drug-eluting Intraluminal Device, Percutaneous Endoscopic Approach

047E45Z Dilation of Right Internal Iliac Artery with Two Drug-eluting Intraluminal Devices, Percutaneous Endoscopic Approach

047E46Z Dilation of Right Internal Iliac Artery with Three Drug-eluting Intraluminal Devices, Percutaneous Endoscopic Approach

047E47Z Dilation of Right Internal Iliac Artery with Four or More Drug-eluting Intraluminal Devices, Percutaneous Endoscopic Approach

047E4D1 Dilation of Right Internal Iliac Artery with Intraluminal Device, using Drug-Coated Balloon, Percutaneous Endoscopic Approach

047E4DZ Dilation of Right Internal Iliac Artery with Intraluminal Device, Percutaneous Endoscopic Approach

047E4EZ Dilation of Right Internal Iliac Artery with Two Intraluminal Devices, Percutaneous Endoscopic Approach

047E4FZ Dilation of Right Internal Iliac Artery with Three Intraluminal Devices, Percutaneous Endoscopic Approach

047E4GZ Dilation of Right Internal Iliac Artery with Four or More Intraluminal Devices, Percutaneous Endoscopic Approach

047E4Z1 Dilation of Right Internal Iliac Artery using Drug-Coated Balloon, Percutaneous Endoscopic Approach

047E4ZZ Dilation of Right Internal Iliac Artery, Percutaneous Endoscopic Approach

047F041 Dilation of Left Internal Iliac Artery with Drug-eluting Intraluminal Device, using Drug-Coated Balloon, Open Approach

047F04Z Dilation of Left Internal Iliac Artery with Drug-eluting Intraluminal Device, Open Approach

047F05Z Dilation of Left Internal Iliac Artery with Two Drug-eluting Intraluminal Devices, Open Approach

047F06Z Dilation of Left Internal Iliac Artery with Three Drug-eluting Intraluminal Devices, Open Approach

047F07Z Dilation of Left Internal Iliac Artery with Four or More Drug-eluting Intraluminal Devices, Open Approach

047F0D1 Dilation of Left Internal Iliac Artery with Intraluminal Device, using Drug-Coated Balloon, Open Approach

047F0DZ Dilation of Left Internal Iliac Artery with Intraluminal Device, Open Approach

047F0EZ Dilation of Left Internal Iliac Artery with Two Intraluminal Devices, Open Approach

047F0FZ Dilation of Left Internal Iliac Artery with Three Intraluminal Devices, Open Approach

047F0GZ Dilation of Left Internal Iliac Artery with Four or More Intraluminal Devices, Open Approach

047F0Z1 Dilation of Left Internal Iliac Artery using Drug-Coated Balloon, Open Approach

047F0ZZ Dilation of Left Internal Iliac Artery, Open Approach

047F341 Dilation of Left Internal Iliac Artery with Drug-eluting Intraluminal Device, using Drug-Coated Balloon, Percutaneous Approach

047F34Z Dilation of Left Internal Iliac Artery with Drug-eluting Intraluminal Device, Percutaneous Approach

047F35Z Dilation of Left Internal Iliac Artery with Two Drug-eluting Intraluminal Devices, Percutaneous Approach

047F36Z Dilation of Left Internal Iliac Artery with Three Drug-eluting Intraluminal Devices, Percutaneous Approach

047F37Z Dilation of Left Internal Iliac Artery with Four or More Drug-eluting Intraluminal Devices, Percutaneous Approach

♀ Female-only   ♂ Male-only   ▲ Limited Coverage   ● Non-OR   ⬛ HAC-associated procedure   ▲ Non-covered procedures   ✚ Cluster

047F3D1 Dilation of Left Internal Iliac Artery with Intraluminal Device, using Drug-Coated Balloon, Percutaneous Approach

047F3DZ Dilation of Left Internal Iliac Artery with Intraluminal Device, Percutaneous Approach

047F3EZ Dilation of Left Internal Iliac Artery with Two Intraluminal Devices, Percutaneous Approach

047F3FZ Dilation of Left Internal Iliac Artery with Three Intraluminal Devices, Percutaneous Approach

047F3GZ Dilation of Left Internal Iliac Artery with Four or More Intraluminal Devices, Percutaneous Approach

047F3Z1 Dilation of Left Internal Iliac Artery using Drug-Coated Balloon, Percutaneous Approach

047F3ZZ Dilation of Left Internal Iliac Artery, Percutaneous Approach

047F441 Dilation of Left Internal Iliac Artery with Drug-eluting Intraluminal Device, using Drug-Coated Balloon, Percutaneous Endoscopic Approach

047F44Z Dilation of Left Internal Iliac Artery with Drug-eluting Intraluminal Device, Percutaneous Endoscopic Approach

047F45Z Dilation of Left Internal Iliac Artery with Two Drug-eluting Intraluminal Devices, Percutaneous Endoscopic Approach

047F46Z Dilation of Left Internal Iliac Artery with Three Drug-eluting Intraluminal Devices, Percutaneous Endoscopic Approach

047F47Z Dilation of Left Internal Iliac Artery with Four or More Drug-eluting Intraluminal Devices, Percutaneous Endoscopic Approach

047F4D1 Dilation of Left Internal Iliac Artery with Intraluminal Device, using Drug-Coated Balloon, Percutaneous Endoscopic Approach

047F4DZ Dilation of Left Internal Iliac Artery with Intraluminal Device, Percutaneous Endoscopic Approach

047F4EZ Dilation of Left Internal Iliac Artery with Two Intraluminal Devices, Percutaneous Endoscopic Approach

047F4FZ Dilation of Left Internal Iliac Artery with Three Intraluminal Devices, Percutaneous Endoscopic Approach

047F4GZ Dilation of Left Internal Iliac Artery with Four or More Intraluminal Devices, Percutaneous Endoscopic Approach

047F4Z1 Dilation of Left Internal Iliac Artery using Drug-Coated Balloon, Percutaneous Endoscopic Approach

047F4ZZ Dilation of Left Internal Iliac Artery, Percutaneous Endoscopic Approach

047H041 Dilation of Right External Iliac Artery with Drug-eluting Intraluminal Device, using Drug-Coated Balloon, Open Approach

047H04Z Dilation of Right External Iliac Artery with Drug-eluting Intraluminal Device, Open Approach

047H05Z Dilation of Right External Iliac Artery with Two Drug-eluting Intraluminal Devices, Open Approach

047H06Z Dilation of Right External Iliac Artery with Three Drug-eluting Intraluminal Devices, Open Approach

047H07Z Dilation of Right External Iliac Artery with Four or More Drug-eluting Intraluminal Devices, Open Approach

047H0D1 Dilation of Right External Iliac Artery with Intraluminal Device, using Drug-Coated Balloon, Open Approach

047H0DZ Dilation of Right External Iliac Artery with Intraluminal Device, Open Approach

047H0EZ Dilation of Right External Iliac Artery with Two Intraluminal Devices, Open Approach

047H0FZ Dilation of Right External Iliac Artery with Three Intraluminal Devices, Open Approach

047H0GZ Dilation of Right External Iliac Artery with Four or More Intraluminal Devices, Open Approach

047H0Z1 Dilation of Right External Iliac Artery using Drug-Coated Balloon, Open Approach

047H0ZZ Dilation of Right External Iliac Artery, Open Approach

047H341 Dilation of Right External Iliac Artery with Drug-eluting Intraluminal Device, using Drug-Coated Balloon, Percutaneous Approach

047H34Z Dilation of Right External Iliac Artery with Drug-eluting Intraluminal Device, Percutaneous Approach

047H35Z Dilation of Right External Iliac Artery with Two Drug-eluting Intraluminal Devices, Percutaneous Approach

047H36Z Dilation of Right External Iliac Artery with Three Drug-eluting Intraluminal Devices, Percutaneous Approach

047H37Z Dilation of Right External Iliac Artery with Four or More Drug-eluting Intraluminal Devices, Percutaneous Approach

047H3D1 Dilation of Right External Iliac Artery with Intraluminal Device, using Drug-Coated Balloon, Percutaneous Approach

047H3DZ Dilation of Right External Iliac Artery with Intraluminal Device, Percutaneous Approach

047H3EZ Dilation of Right External Iliac Artery with Two Intraluminal Devices, Percutaneous Approach

047H3FZ Dilation of Right External Iliac Artery with Three Intraluminal Devices, Percutaneous Approach

047H3GZ Dilation of Right External Iliac Artery with Four or More Intraluminal Devices, Percutaneous Approach

047H3Z1 Dilation of Right External Iliac Artery using Drug-Coated Balloon, Percutaneous Approach

AHA CC: 4Q, 2020, 50-51

047H3ZZ Dilation of Right External Iliac Artery, Percutaneous Approach

047H441 Dilation of Right External Iliac Artery with Drug-eluting Intraluminal Device, using Drug-Coated Balloon, Percutaneous Endoscopic Approach

047H44Z Dilation of Right External Iliac Artery with Drug-eluting Intraluminal Device, Percutaneous Endoscopic Approach

047H45Z Dilation of Right External Iliac Artery with Two Drug-eluting Intraluminal Devices, Percutaneous Endoscopic Approach

047H46Z Dilation of Right External Iliac Artery with Three Drug-eluting Intraluminal Devices, Percutaneous Endoscopic Approach

047H47Z Dilation of Right External Iliac Artery with Four or More Drug-eluting Intraluminal Devices, Percutaneous Endoscopic Approach

047H4D1 Dilation of Right External Iliac Artery with Intraluminal Device, using Drug-Coated Balloon, Percutaneous Endoscopic Approach

047H4DZ Dilation of Right External Iliac Artery with Intraluminal Device, Percutaneous Endoscopic Approach

047H4EZ Dilation of Right External Iliac Artery with Two Intraluminal Devices, Percutaneous Endoscopic Approach

047H4FZ Dilation of Right External Iliac Artery with Three Intraluminal Devices, Percutaneous Endoscopic Approach

047H4GZ Dilation of Right External Iliac Artery with Four or More Intraluminal Devices, Percutaneous Endoscopic Approach

047H4Z1 Dilation of Right External Iliac Artery using Drug-Coated Balloon, Percutaneous Endoscopic Approach

047H4ZZ Dilation of Right External Iliac Artery, Percutaneous Endoscopic Approach

047J041 Dilation of Left External Iliac Artery with Drug-eluting Intraluminal Device, using Drug-Coated Balloon, Open Approach

047J04Z Dilation of Left External Iliac Artery with Drug-eluting Intraluminal Device, Open Approach

047J05Z Dilation of Left External Iliac Artery with Two Drug-eluting Intraluminal Devices, Open Approach

047J06Z Dilation of Left External Iliac Artery with Three Drug-eluting Intraluminal Devices, Open Approach

047J07Z Dilation of Left External Iliac Artery with Four or More Drug-eluting Intraluminal Devices, Open Approach

047J0D1 Dilation of Left External Iliac Artery with Intraluminal Device, using Drug-Coated Balloon, Open Approach

047J0DZ Dilation of Left External Iliac Artery with Intraluminal Device, Open Approach

047J0EZ Dilation of Left External Iliac Artery with Two Intraluminal Devices, Open Approach

047J0FZ Dilation of Left External Iliac Artery with Three Intraluminal Devices, Open Approach

047J0GZ Dilation of Left External Iliac Artery with Four or More Intraluminal Devices, Open Approach

047J0Z1 Dilation of Left External Iliac Artery using Drug-Coated Balloon, Open Approach

047J0ZZ Dilation of Left External Iliac Artery, Open Approach

047J341 Dilation of Left External Iliac Artery with Drug-eluting Intraluminal Device, using Drug-Coated Balloon, Percutaneous Approach

047J34Z Dilation of Left External Iliac Artery with Drug-eluting Intraluminal Device, Percutaneous Approach

047J35Z Dilation of Left External Iliac Artery with Two Drug-eluting Intraluminal Devices, Percutaneous Approach

047J36Z Dilation of Left External Iliac Artery with Three Drug-eluting Intraluminal Devices, Percutaneous Approach

047J37Z Dilation of Left External Iliac Artery with Four or More Drug-eluting Intraluminal Devices, Percutaneous Approach

047J3D1 Dilation of Left External Iliac Artery with Intraluminal Device, using Drug-Coated Balloon, Percutaneous Approach

047J3DZ Dilation of Left External Iliac Artery with Intraluminal Device, Percutaneous Approach

047J3EZ Dilation of Left External Iliac Artery with Two Intraluminal Devices, Percutaneous Approach

047J3FZ Dilation of Left External Iliac Artery with Three Intraluminal Devices, Percutaneous Approach

047J3GZ Dilation of Left External Iliac Artery with Four or More Intraluminal Devices, Percutaneous Approach

047J3Z1 Dilation of Left External Iliac Artery using Drug-Coated Balloon, Percutaneous Approach

047J3ZZ Dilation of Left External Iliac Artery, Percutaneous Approach

047J441 Dilation of Left External Iliac Artery with Drug-eluting Intraluminal Device, using Drug-Coated Balloon, Percutaneous Endoscopic Approach

047J44Z Dilation of Left External Iliac Artery with Drug-eluting Intraluminal Device, Percutaneous Endoscopic Approach

047J45Z Dilation of Left External Iliac Artery with Two Drug-eluting Intraluminal Devices, Percutaneous Endoscopic Approach

047J46Z Dilation of Left External Iliac Artery with Three Drug-eluting Intraluminal Devices, Percutaneous Endoscopic Approach

047J47Z Dilation of Left External Iliac Artery with Four or More Drug-eluting Intraluminal Devices, Percutaneous Endoscopic Approach

047J4D1 Dilation of Left External Iliac Artery with Intraluminal Device, using Drug-Coated Balloon, Percutaneous Endoscopic Approach

047J4DZ Dilation of Left External Iliac Artery with Intraluminal Device, Percutaneous Endoscopic Approach

047J4EZ Dilation of Left External Iliac Artery with Two Intraluminal Devices, Percutaneous Endoscopic Approach

047J4FZ Dilation of Left External Iliac Artery with Three Intraluminal Devices, Percutaneous Endoscopic Approach

047J4GZ Dilation of Left External Iliac Artery with Four or More Intraluminal Devices, Percutaneous Endoscopic Approach

047J4Z1 Dilation of Left External Iliac Artery using Drug-Coated Balloon, Percutaneous Endoscopic Approach

047J4ZZ Dilation of Left External Iliac Artery, Percutaneous Endoscopic Approach

047K041 Dilation of Right Femoral Artery with Drug-eluting Intraluminal Device, using Drug-Coated Balloon, Open Approach

047K04Z Dilation of Right Femoral Artery with Drug-eluting Intraluminal Device, Open Approach

047K05Z Dilation of Right Femoral Artery with Two Drug-eluting Intraluminal Devices, Open Approach

047K06Z Dilation of Right Femoral Artery with Three Drug-eluting Intraluminal Devices, Open Approach

047K07Z Dilation of Right Femoral Artery with Four or More Drug-eluting Intraluminal Devices, Open Approach

047K0D1 Dilation of Right Femoral Artery with Intraluminal Device, using Drug-Coated Balloon, Open Approach

047K0DZ Dilation of Right Femoral Artery with Intraluminal Device, Open Approach

047K0EZ Dilation of Right Femoral Artery with Two Intraluminal Devices, Open Approach

047K0FZ Dilation of Right Femoral Artery with Three Intraluminal Devices, Open Approach

047K0GZ Dilation of Right Femoral Artery with Four or More Intraluminal Devices, Open Approach

047K0Z1 Dilation of Right Femoral Artery using Drug-Coated Balloon, Open Approach

047K0ZZ Dilation of Right Femoral Artery, Open Approach

047K341 Dilation of Right Femoral Artery with Drug-eluting Intraluminal Device, using Drug-Coated Balloon, Percutaneous Approach

047K34Z Dilation of Right Femoral Artery with Drug-eluting Intraluminal Device, Percutaneous Approach

047K35Z Dilation of Right Femoral Artery with Two Drug-eluting Intraluminal Devices, Percutaneous Approach

047K36Z Dilation of Right Femoral Artery with Three Drug-eluting Intraluminal Devices, Percutaneous Approach

047K37Z Dilation of Right Femoral Artery with Four or More Drug-eluting Intraluminal Devices, Percutaneous Approach

047K3D1 Dilation of Right Femoral Artery with Intraluminal Device, using Drug-Coated Balloon, Percutaneous Approach
AHA CC: 4Q, 2015, 7,15

047K3DZ Dilation of Right Femoral Artery with Intraluminal Device, Percutaneous Approach

047K3EZ Dilation of Right Femoral Artery with Two Intraluminal Devices, Percutaneous Approach

047K3FZ Dilation of Right Femoral Artery with Three Intraluminal Devices, Percutaneous Approach

047K3GZ Dilation of Right Femoral Artery with Four or More Intraluminal Devices, Percutaneous Approach

047K3Z1 Dilation of Right Femoral Artery using Drug-Coated Balloon, Percutaneous Approach
AHA CC: 4Q, 2020, 50-51

047K3ZZ Dilation of Right Femoral Artery, Percutaneous Approach

047K441 Dilation of Right Femoral Artery with Drug-eluting Intraluminal Device, using Drug-Coated Balloon, Percutaneous Endoscopic Approach

047K44Z Dilation of Right Femoral Artery with Drug-eluting Intraluminal Device, Percutaneous Endoscopic Approach

047K45Z Dilation of Right Femoral Artery with Two Drug-eluting Intraluminal Devices, Percutaneous Endoscopic Approach

047K46Z Dilation of Right Femoral Artery with Three Drug-eluting Intraluminal Devices, Percutaneous Endoscopic Approach

047K47Z Dilation of Right Femoral Artery with Four or More Drug-eluting Intraluminal Devices, Percutaneous Endoscopic Approach

047K4D1 Dilation of Right Femoral Artery with Intraluminal Device, using Drug-Coated Balloon, Percutaneous Endoscopic Approach

047K4DZ Dilation of Right Femoral Artery with Intraluminal Device, Percutaneous Endoscopic Approach

047K4EZ Dilation of Right Femoral Artery with Two Intraluminal Devices, Percutaneous Endoscopic Approach

047K4FZ Dilation of Right Femoral Artery with Three Intraluminal Devices, Percutaneous Endoscopic Approach

047K4GZ Dilation of Right Femoral Artery with Four or More Intraluminal Devices, Percutaneous Endoscopic Approach

047K4Z1 Dilation of Right Femoral Artery using Drug-Coated Balloon, Percutaneous Endoscopic Approach

047K4ZZ Dilation of Right Femoral Artery, Percutaneous Endoscopic Approach

047L041 Dilation of Left Femoral Artery with Drug-eluting Intraluminal Device, using Drug-Coated Balloon, Open Approach

047L04Z Dilation of Left Femoral Artery with Drug-eluting Intraluminal Device, Open Approach

047L05Z Dilation of Left Femoral Artery with Two Drug-eluting Intraluminal Devices, Open Approach

047L06Z Dilation of Left Femoral Artery with Three Drug-eluting Intraluminal Devices, Open Approach

047L07Z Dilation of Left Femoral Artery with Four or More Drug-eluting Intraluminal Devices, Open Approach

047L0D1 Dilation of Left Femoral Artery with Intraluminal Device, using Drug-Coated Balloon, Open Approach

047L0DZ Dilation of Left Femoral Artery with Intraluminal Device, Open Approach

047L0EZ Dilation of Left Femoral Artery with Two Intraluminal Devices, Open Approach

047L0FZ Dilation of Left Femoral Artery with Three Intraluminal Devices, Open Approach

047L0GZ Dilation of Left Femoral Artery with Four or More Intraluminal Devices, Open Approach

047L0Z1 Dilation of Left Femoral Artery using Drug-Coated Balloon, Open Approach

047L0ZZ Dilation of Left Femoral Artery, Open Approach

047L341 Dilation of Left Femoral Artery with Drug-eluting Intraluminal Device, using Drug-Coated Balloon, Percutaneous Approach

047L34Z Dilation of Left Femoral Artery with Drug-eluting Intraluminal Device, Percutaneous Approach

047L35Z Dilation of Left Femoral Artery with Two Drug-eluting Intraluminal Devices, Percutaneous Approach

047L36Z Dilation of Left Femoral Artery with Three Drug-eluting Intraluminal Devices, Percutaneous Approach

♀ Female-only   ♂ Male-only   ▲ Limited Coverage   ● Non-OR   ▬ HAC-associated procedure   ▲ Non-covered procedures   ➕ Cluster

047L37Z Dilation of Left Femoral Artery with Four or More Drug-eluting Intraluminal Devices, Percutaneous Approach

047L3D1 Dilation of Left Femoral Artery with Intraluminal Device, using Drug-Coated Balloon, Percutaneous Approach

047L3DZ Dilation of Left Femoral Artery with Intraluminal Device, Percutaneous Approach

047L3EZ Dilation of Left Femoral Artery with Two Intraluminal Devices, Percutaneous Approach

047L3FZ Dilation of Left Femoral Artery with Three Intraluminal Devices, Percutaneous Approach

047L3GZ Dilation of Left Femoral Artery with Four or More Intraluminal Devices, Percutaneous Approach

047L3Z1 Dilation of Left Femoral Artery using Drug-Coated Balloon, Percutaneous Approach

AHA CC: 4Q, 2015, 15

047L3ZZ Dilation of Left Femoral Artery, Percutaneous Approach

047L441 Dilation of Left Femoral Artery with Drug-eluting Intraluminal Device, using Drug-Coated Balloon, Percutaneous Endoscopic Approach

047L44Z Dilation of Left Femoral Artery with Drug-eluting Intraluminal Device, Percutaneous Endoscopic Approach

047L45Z Dilation of Left Femoral Artery with Two Drug-eluting Intraluminal Devices, Percutaneous Endoscopic Approach

047L46Z Dilation of Left Femoral Artery with Three Drug-eluting Intraluminal Devices, Percutaneous Endoscopic Approach

047L47Z Dilation of Left Femoral Artery with Four or More Drug-eluting Intraluminal Devices, Percutaneous Endoscopic Approach

047L4D1 Dilation of Left Femoral Artery with Intraluminal Device, using Drug-Coated Balloon, Percutaneous Endoscopic Approach

047L4DZ Dilation of Left Femoral Artery with Intraluminal Device, Percutaneous Endoscopic Approach

047L4EZ Dilation of Left Femoral Artery with Two Intraluminal Devices, Percutaneous Endoscopic Approach

047L4FZ Dilation of Left Femoral Artery with Three Intraluminal Devices, Percutaneous Endoscopic Approach

047L4GZ Dilation of Left Femoral Artery with Four or More Intraluminal Devices, Percutaneous Endoscopic Approach

047L4Z1 Dilation of Left Femoral Artery using Drug-Coated Balloon, Percutaneous Endoscopic Approach

047L4ZZ Dilation of Left Femoral Artery, Percutaneous Endoscopic Approach

047M041 Dilation of Right Popliteal Artery with Drug-eluting Intraluminal Device, using Drug-Coated Balloon, Open Approach

047M04Z Dilation of Right Popliteal Artery with Drug-eluting Intraluminal Device, Open Approach

047M05Z Dilation of Right Popliteal Artery with Two Drug-eluting Intraluminal Devices, Open Approach

047M06Z Dilation of Right Popliteal Artery with Three Drug-eluting Intraluminal Devices, Open Approach

047M07Z Dilation of Right Popliteal Artery with Four or More Drug-eluting Intraluminal Devices, Open Approach

047M0D1 Dilation of Right Popliteal Artery with Intraluminal Device, using Drug-Coated Balloon, Open Approach

047M0DZ Dilation of Right Popliteal Artery with Intraluminal Device, Open Approach

047M0EZ Dilation of Right Popliteal Artery with Two Intraluminal Devices, Open Approach

047M0FZ Dilation of Right Popliteal Artery with Three Intraluminal Devices, Open Approach

047M0GZ Dilation of Right Popliteal Artery with Four or More Intraluminal Devices, Open Approach

047M0Z1 Dilation of Right Popliteal Artery using Drug-Coated Balloon, Open Approach

047M0ZZ Dilation of Right Popliteal Artery, Open Approach

047M341 Dilation of Right Popliteal Artery with Drug-eluting Intraluminal Device, using Drug-Coated Balloon, Percutaneous Approach

047M34Z Dilation of Right Popliteal Artery with Drug-eluting Intraluminal Device, Percutaneous Approach

047M35Z Dilation of Right Popliteal Artery with Two Drug-eluting Intraluminal Devices, Percutaneous Approach

047M36Z Dilation of Right Popliteal Artery with Three Drug-eluting Intraluminal Devices, Percutaneous Approach

047M37Z Dilation of Right Popliteal Artery with Four or More Drug-eluting Intraluminal Devices, Percutaneous Approach

047M3D1 Dilation of Right Popliteal Artery with Intraluminal Device, using Drug-Coated Balloon, Percutaneous Approach

047M3DZ Dilation of Right Popliteal Artery with Intraluminal Device, Percutaneous Approach

047M3EZ Dilation of Right Popliteal Artery with Two Intraluminal Devices, Percutaneous Approach

047M3FZ Dilation of Right Popliteal Artery with Three Intraluminal Devices, Percutaneous Approach

047M3GZ Dilation of Right Popliteal Artery with Four or More Intraluminal Devices, Percutaneous Approach

047M3Z1 Dilation of Right Popliteal Artery using Drug-Coated Balloon, Percutaneous Approach

047M3ZZ Dilation of Right Popliteal Artery, Percutaneous Approach

047M441 Dilation of Right Popliteal Artery with Drug-eluting Intraluminal Device, using Drug-Coated Balloon, Percutaneous Endoscopic Approach

047M44Z Dilation of Right Popliteal Artery with Drug-eluting Intraluminal Device, Percutaneous Endoscopic Approach

047M45Z Dilation of Right Popliteal Artery with Two Drug-eluting Intraluminal Devices, Percutaneous Endoscopic Approach

047M46Z Dilation of Right Popliteal Artery with Three Drug-eluting Intraluminal Devices, Percutaneous Endoscopic Approach

047M47Z Dilation of Right Popliteal Artery with Four or More Drug-eluting Intraluminal Devices, Percutaneous Endoscopic Approach

047M4D1 Dilation of Right Popliteal Artery with Intraluminal Device, using Drug-Coated Balloon, Percutaneous Endoscopic Approach

047M4DZ Dilation of Right Popliteal Artery with Intraluminal Device, Percutaneous Endoscopic Approach

047M4EZ Dilation of Right Popliteal Artery with Two Intraluminal Devices, Percutaneous Endoscopic Approach

047M4FZ Dilation of Right Popliteal Artery with Three Intraluminal Devices, Percutaneous Endoscopic Approach

047M4GZ Dilation of Right Popliteal Artery with Four or More Intraluminal Devices, Percutaneous Endoscopic Approach

047M4Z1 Dilation of Right Popliteal Artery using Drug-Coated Balloon, Percutaneous Endoscopic Approach

047M4ZZ Dilation of Right Popliteal Artery, Percutaneous Endoscopic Approach

047N041 Dilation of Left Popliteal Artery with Drug-eluting Intraluminal Device, using Drug-Coated Balloon, Open Approach

047N04Z Dilation of Left Popliteal Artery with Drug-eluting Intraluminal Device, Open Approach

047N05Z Dilation of Left Popliteal Artery with Two Drug-eluting Intraluminal Devices, Open Approach

047N06Z Dilation of Left Popliteal Artery with Three Drug-eluting Intraluminal Devices, Open Approach

047N07Z Dilation of Left Popliteal Artery with Four or More Drug-eluting Intraluminal Devices, Open Approach

047N0D1 Dilation of Left Popliteal Artery with Intraluminal Device, using Drug-Coated Balloon, Open Approach

047N0DZ Dilation of Left Popliteal Artery with Intraluminal Device, Open Approach

047N0EZ Dilation of Left Popliteal Artery with Two Intraluminal Devices, Open Approach

047N0FZ Dilation of Left Popliteal Artery with Three Intraluminal Devices, Open Approach

047N0GZ Dilation of Left Popliteal Artery with Four or More Intraluminal Devices, Open Approach

047N0Z1 Dilation of Left Popliteal Artery using Drug-Coated Balloon, Open Approach

047N0ZZ Dilation of Left Popliteal Artery, Open Approach

047N341 Dilation of Left Popliteal Artery with Drug-eluting Intraluminal Device, using Drug-Coated Balloon, Percutaneous Approach

047N34Z Dilation of Left Popliteal Artery with Drug-eluting Intraluminal Device, Percutaneous Approach

047N35Z Dilation of Left Popliteal Artery with Two Drug-eluting Intraluminal Devices, Percutaneous Approach

047N36Z Dilation of Left Popliteal Artery with Three Drug-eluting Intraluminal Devices, Percutaneous Approach

047N37Z Dilation of Left Popliteal Artery with Four or More Drug-eluting Intraluminal Devices, Percutaneous Approach

047N3D1 Dilation of Left Popliteal Artery with Intraluminal Device, using Drug-Coated Balloon, Percutaneous Approach

047N3DZ Dilation of Left Popliteal Artery with Intraluminal Device, Percutaneous Approach

047N3EZ Dilation of Left Popliteal Artery with Two Intraluminal Devices, Percutaneous Approach

047N3FZ Dilation of Left Popliteal Artery with Three Intraluminal Devices, Percutaneous Approach

047N3GZ Dilation of Left Popliteal Artery with Four or More Intraluminal Devices, Percutaneous Approach

047N3Z1 Dilation of Left Popliteal Artery using Drug-Coated Balloon, Percutaneous Approach

047N3ZZ Dilation of Left Popliteal Artery, Percutaneous Approach

047N441 Dilation of Left Popliteal Artery with Drug-eluting Intraluminal Device, using Drug-Coated Balloon, Percutaneous Endoscopic Approach

047N44Z Dilation of Left Popliteal Artery with Drug-eluting Intraluminal Device, Percutaneous Endoscopic Approach

047N45Z Dilation of Left Popliteal Artery with Two Drug-eluting Intraluminal Devices, Percutaneous Endoscopic Approach

047N46Z Dilation of Left Popliteal Artery with Three Drug-eluting Intraluminal Devices, Percutaneous Endoscopic Approach

047N47Z Dilation of Left Popliteal Artery with Four or More Drug-eluting Intraluminal Devices, Percutaneous Endoscopic Approach

047N4D1 Dilation of Left Popliteal Artery with Intraluminal Device, using Drug-Coated Balloon, Percutaneous Endoscopic Approach

047N4DZ Dilation of Left Popliteal Artery with Intraluminal Device, Percutaneous Endoscopic Approach

047N4EZ Dilation of Left Popliteal Artery with Two Intraluminal Devices, Percutaneous Endoscopic Approach

047N4FZ Dilation of Left Popliteal Artery with Three Intraluminal Devices, Percutaneous Endoscopic Approach

047N4GZ Dilation of Left Popliteal Artery with Four or More Intraluminal Devices, Percutaneous Endoscopic Approach

047N4Z1 Dilation of Left Popliteal Artery using Drug-Coated Balloon, Percutaneous Endoscopic Approach

047N4ZZ Dilation of Left Popliteal Artery, Percutaneous Endoscopic Approach

047P041 Dilation of Right Anterior Tibial Artery with Drug-eluting Intraluminal Device, using Drug-Coated Balloon, Open Approach

047P04Z Dilation of Right Anterior Tibial Artery with Drug-eluting Intraluminal Device, Open Approach

047P05Z Dilation of Right Anterior Tibial Artery with Two Drug-eluting Intraluminal Devices, Open Approach

047P06Z Dilation of Right Anterior Tibial Artery with Three Drug-eluting Intraluminal Devices, Open Approach

047P07Z Dilation of Right Anterior Tibial Artery with Four or More Drug-eluting Intraluminal Devices, Open Approach

047P0D1 Dilation of Right Anterior Tibial Artery with Intraluminal Device, using Drug-Coated Balloon, Open Approach

047P0DZ Dilation of Right Anterior Tibial Artery with Intraluminal Device, Open Approach

047P0EZ Dilation of Right Anterior Tibial Artery with Two Intraluminal Devices, Open Approach

047P0FZ Dilation of Right Anterior Tibial Artery with Three Intraluminal Devices, Open Approach

047P0GZ Dilation of Right Anterior Tibial Artery with Four or More Intraluminal Devices, Open Approach

047P0Z1 Dilation of Right Anterior Tibial Artery using Drug-Coated Balloon, Open Approach

047P0ZZ Dilation of Right Anterior Tibial Artery, Open Approach

047P341 Dilation of Right Anterior Tibial Artery with Drug-eluting Intraluminal Device, using Drug-Coated Balloon, Percutaneous Approach

047P34Z Dilation of Right Anterior Tibial Artery with Drug-eluting Intraluminal Device, Percutaneous Approach

047P35Z Dilation of Right Anterior Tibial Artery with Two Drug-eluting Intraluminal Devices, Percutaneous Approach

047P36Z Dilation of Right Anterior Tibial Artery with Three Drug-eluting Intraluminal Devices, Percutaneous Approach

047P37Z Dilation of Right Anterior Tibial Artery with Four or More Drug-eluting Intraluminal Devices, Percutaneous Approach

047P3D1 Dilation of Right Anterior Tibial Artery with Intraluminal Device, using Drug-Coated Balloon, Percutaneous Approach

047P3DZ Dilation of Right Anterior Tibial Artery with Intraluminal Device, Percutaneous Approach

047P3EZ Dilation of Right Anterior Tibial Artery with Two Intraluminal Devices, Percutaneous Approach

047P3FZ Dilation of Right Anterior Tibial Artery with Three Intraluminal Devices, Percutaneous Approach

047P3GZ Dilation of Right Anterior Tibial Artery with Four or More Intraluminal Devices, Percutaneous Approach

047P3Z1 Dilation of Right Anterior Tibial Artery using Drug-Coated Balloon, Percutaneous Approach

047P3ZZ Dilation of Right Anterior Tibial Artery, Percutaneous Approach

047P441 Dilation of Right Anterior Tibial Artery with Drug-eluting Intraluminal Device, using Drug-Coated Balloon, Percutaneous Endoscopic Approach

047P44Z Dilation of Right Anterior Tibial Artery with Drug-eluting Intraluminal Device, Percutaneous Endoscopic Approach

047P45Z Dilation of Right Anterior Tibial Artery with Two Drug-eluting Intraluminal Devices, Percutaneous Endoscopic Approach

047P46Z Dilation of Right Anterior Tibial Artery with Three Drug-eluting Intraluminal Devices, Percutaneous Endoscopic Approach

047P47Z Dilation of Right Anterior Tibial Artery with Four or More Drug-eluting Intraluminal Devices, Percutaneous Endoscopic Approach

047P4D1 Dilation of Right Anterior Tibial Artery with Intraluminal Device, using Drug-Coated Balloon, Percutaneous Endoscopic Approach

047P4DZ Dilation of Right Anterior Tibial Artery with Intraluminal Device, Percutaneous Endoscopic Approach

047P4EZ Dilation of Right Anterior Tibial Artery with Two Intraluminal Devices, Percutaneous Endoscopic Approach

047P4FZ Dilation of Right Anterior Tibial Artery with Three Intraluminal Devices, Percutaneous Endoscopic Approach

047P4GZ Dilation of Right Anterior Tibial Artery with Four or More Intraluminal Devices, Percutaneous Endoscopic Approach

047P4Z1 Dilation of Right Anterior Tibial Artery using Drug-Coated Balloon, Percutaneous Endoscopic Approach

047P4ZZ Dilation of Right Anterior Tibial Artery, Percutaneous Endoscopic Approach

047Q041 Dilation of Left Anterior Tibial Artery with Drug-eluting Intraluminal Device, using Drug-Coated Balloon, Open Approach

047Q04Z Dilation of Left Anterior Tibial Artery with Drug-eluting Intraluminal Device, Open Approach

047Q05Z Dilation of Left Anterior Tibial Artery with Two Drug-eluting Intraluminal Devices, Open Approach

047Q06Z Dilation of Left Anterior Tibial Artery with Three Drug-eluting Intraluminal Devices, Open Approach

047Q07Z Dilation of Left Anterior Tibial Artery with Four or More Drug-eluting Intraluminal Devices, Open Approach

047Q0D1 Dilation of Left Anterior Tibial Artery with Intraluminal Device, using Drug-Coated Balloon, Open Approach

047Q0DZ Dilation of Left Anterior Tibial Artery with Intraluminal Device, Open Approach

047Q0EZ Dilation of Left Anterior Tibial Artery with Two Intraluminal Devices, Open Approach

047Q0FZ Dilation of Left Anterior Tibial Artery with Three Intraluminal Devices, Open Approach

047Q0GZ Dilation of Left Anterior Tibial Artery with Four or More Intraluminal Devices, Open Approach

047Q0Z1 Dilation of Left Anterior Tibial Artery using Drug-Coated Balloon, Open Approach

047Q0ZZ Dilation of Left Anterior Tibial Artery, Open Approach

047Q341 Dilation of Left Anterior Tibial Artery with Drug-eluting Intraluminal Device, using Drug-Coated Balloon, Percutaneous Approach

047Q34Z Dilation of Left Anterior Tibial Artery with Drug-eluting Intraluminal Device, Percutaneous Approach

047Q35Z Dilation of Left Anterior Tibial Artery with Two Drug-eluting Intraluminal Devices, Percutaneous Approach

047Q36Z Dilation of Left Anterior Tibial Artery with Three Drug-eluting Intraluminal Devices, Percutaneous Approach

♀ Female-only   ♂ Male-only   ▲ Limited Coverage   ● Non-OR   HAC HAC-associated procedure   ▲ Non-covered procedures   ✚ Cluster

047Q37Z	Dilation of Left Anterior Tibial Artery with Four or More Drug-eluting Intraluminal Devices, Percutaneous Approach
047Q3D1	Dilation of Left Anterior Tibial Artery with Intraluminal Device, using Drug-Coated Balloon, Percutaneous Approach
047Q3DZ	Dilation of Left Anterior Tibial Artery with Intraluminal Device, Percutaneous Approach
047Q3EZ	Dilation of Left Anterior Tibial Artery with Two Intraluminal Devices, Percutaneous Approach
047Q3FZ	Dilation of Left Anterior Tibial Artery with Three Intraluminal Devices, Percutaneous Approach
047Q3GZ	Dilation of Left Anterior Tibial Artery with Four or More Intraluminal Devices, Percutaneous Approach
047Q3Z1	Dilation of Left Anterior Tibial Artery using Drug-Coated Balloon, Percutaneous Approach
047Q3ZZ	Dilation of Left Anterior Tibial Artery, Percutaneous Approach
047Q441	Dilation of Left Anterior Tibial Artery with Drug-eluting Intraluminal Device, using Drug-Coated Balloon, Percutaneous Endoscopic Approach
047Q44Z	Dilation of Left Anterior Tibial Artery with Drug-eluting Intraluminal Device, Percutaneous Endoscopic Approach
047Q45Z	Dilation of Left Anterior Tibial Artery with Two Drug-eluting Intraluminal Devices, Percutaneous Endoscopic Approach
047Q46Z	Dilation of Left Anterior Tibial Artery with Three Drug-eluting Intraluminal Devices, Percutaneous Endoscopic Approach
047Q47Z	Dilation of Left Anterior Tibial Artery with Four or More Drug-eluting Intraluminal Devices, Percutaneous Endoscopic Approach
047Q4D1	Dilation of Left Anterior Tibial Artery with Intraluminal Device, using Drug-Coated Balloon, Percutaneous Endoscopic Approach
047Q4DZ	Dilation of Left Anterior Tibial Artery with Intraluminal Device, Percutaneous Endoscopic Approach
047Q4EZ	Dilation of Left Anterior Tibial Artery with Two Intraluminal Devices, Percutaneous Endoscopic Approach
047Q4FZ	Dilation of Left Anterior Tibial Artery with Three Intraluminal Devices, Percutaneous Endoscopic Approach
047Q4GZ	Dilation of Left Anterior Tibial Artery with Four or More Intraluminal Devices, Percutaneous Endoscopic Approach
047Q4Z1	Dilation of Left Anterior Tibial Artery using Drug-Coated Balloon, Percutaneous Endoscopic Approach
047Q4ZZ	Dilation of Left Anterior Tibial Artery, Percutaneous Endoscopic Approach
047R041	Dilation of Right Posterior Tibial Artery with Drug-eluting Intraluminal Device, using Drug-Coated Balloon, Open Approach
047R04Z	Dilation of Right Posterior Tibial Artery with Drug-eluting Intraluminal Device, Open Approach
047R05Z	Dilation of Right Posterior Tibial Artery with Two Drug-eluting Intraluminal Devices, Open Approach
047R06Z	Dilation of Right Posterior Tibial Artery with Three Drug-eluting Intraluminal Devices, Open Approach
047R07Z	Dilation of Right Posterior Tibial Artery with Four or More Drug-eluting Intraluminal Devices, Open Approach
047R0D1	Dilation of Right Posterior Tibial Artery with Intraluminal Device, using Drug-Coated Balloon, Open Approach
047R0DZ	Dilation of Right Posterior Tibial Artery with Intraluminal Device, Open Approach
047R0EZ	Dilation of Right Posterior Tibial Artery with Two Intraluminal Devices, Open Approach
047R0FZ	Dilation of Right Posterior Tibial Artery with Three Intraluminal Devices, Open Approach
047R0GZ	Dilation of Right Posterior Tibial Artery with Four or More Intraluminal Devices, Open Approach
047R0Z1	Dilation of Right Posterior Tibial Artery using Drug-Coated Balloon, Open Approach
047R0ZZ	Dilation of Right Posterior Tibial Artery, Open Approach
047R341	Dilation of Right Posterior Tibial Artery with Drug-eluting Intraluminal Device, using Drug-Coated Balloon, Percutaneous Approach
047R34Z	Dilation of Right Posterior Tibial Artery with Drug-eluting Intraluminal Device, Percutaneous Approach
047R35Z	Dilation of Right Posterior Tibial Artery with Two Drug-eluting Intraluminal Devices, Percutaneous Approach
047R36Z	Dilation of Right Posterior Tibial Artery with Three Drug-eluting Intraluminal Devices, Percutaneous Approach
047R37Z	Dilation of Right Posterior Tibial Artery with Four or More Drug-eluting Intraluminal Devices, Percutaneous Approach
047R3D1	Dilation of Right Posterior Tibial Artery with Intraluminal Device, using Drug-Coated Balloon, Percutaneous Approach
047R3DZ	Dilation of Right Posterior Tibial Artery with Intraluminal Device, Percutaneous Approach
047R3EZ	Dilation of Right Posterior Tibial Artery with Two Intraluminal Devices, Percutaneous Approach
047R3FZ	Dilation of Right Posterior Tibial Artery with Three Intraluminal Devices, Percutaneous Approach
047R3GZ	Dilation of Right Posterior Tibial Artery with Four or More Intraluminal Devices, Percutaneous Approach
047R3Z1	Dilation of Right Posterior Tibial Artery using Drug-Coated Balloon, Percutaneous Approach
047R3ZZ	Dilation of Right Posterior Tibial Artery, Percutaneous Approach
047R441	Dilation of Right Posterior Tibial Artery with Drug-eluting Intraluminal Device, using Drug-Coated Balloon, Percutaneous Endoscopic Approach
047R44Z	Dilation of Right Posterior Tibial Artery with Drug-eluting Intraluminal Device, Percutaneous Endoscopic Approach
047R45Z	Dilation of Right Posterior Tibial Artery with Two Drug-eluting Intraluminal Devices, Percutaneous Endoscopic Approach
047R46Z	Dilation of Right Posterior Tibial Artery with Three Drug-eluting Intraluminal Devices, Percutaneous Endoscopic Approach
047R47Z	Dilation of Right Posterior Tibial Artery with Four or More Drug-eluting Intraluminal Devices, Percutaneous Endoscopic Approach
047R4D1	Dilation of Right Posterior Tibial Artery with Intraluminal Device, using Drug-Coated Balloon, Percutaneous Endoscopic Approach
047R4DZ	Dilation of Right Posterior Tibial Artery with Intraluminal Device, Percutaneous Endoscopic Approach
047R4EZ	Dilation of Right Posterior Tibial Artery with Two Intraluminal Devices, Percutaneous Endoscopic Approach
047R4FZ	Dilation of Right Posterior Tibial Artery with Three Intraluminal Devices, Percutaneous Endoscopic Approach
047R4GZ	Dilation of Right Posterior Tibial Artery with Four or More Intraluminal Devices, Percutaneous Endoscopic Approach
047R4Z1	Dilation of Right Posterior Tibial Artery using Drug-Coated Balloon, Percutaneous Endoscopic Approach
047R4ZZ	Dilation of Right Posterior Tibial Artery, Percutaneous Endoscopic Approach
047S041	Dilation of Left Posterior Tibial Artery with Drug-eluting Intraluminal Device, using Drug-Coated Balloon, Open Approach
047S04Z	Dilation of Left Posterior Tibial Artery with Drug-eluting Intraluminal Device, Open Approach
047S05Z	Dilation of Left Posterior Tibial Artery with Two Drug-eluting Intraluminal Devices, Open Approach
047S06Z	Dilation of Left Posterior Tibial Artery with Three Drug-eluting Intraluminal Devices, Open Approach
047S07Z	Dilation of Left Posterior Tibial Artery with Four or More Drug-eluting Intraluminal Devices, Open Approach
047S0D1	Dilation of Left Posterior Tibial Artery with Intraluminal Device, using Drug-Coated Balloon, Open Approach
047S0DZ	Dilation of Left Posterior Tibial Artery with Intraluminal Device, Open Approach
047S0EZ	Dilation of Left Posterior Tibial Artery with Two Intraluminal Devices, Open Approach
047S0FZ	Dilation of Left Posterior Tibial Artery with Three Intraluminal Devices, Open Approach
047S0GZ	Dilation of Left Posterior Tibial Artery with Four or More Intraluminal Devices, Open Approach
047S0Z1	Dilation of Left Posterior Tibial Artery using Drug-Coated Balloon, Open Approach
047S0ZZ	Dilation of Left Posterior Tibial Artery, Open Approach
047S341	Dilation of Left Posterior Tibial Artery with Drug-eluting Intraluminal Device, using Drug-Coated Balloon, Percutaneous Approach

047S34Z Dilation of Left Posterior Tibial Artery with Drug-eluting Intraluminal Device, Percutaneous Approach

047S35Z Dilation of Left Posterior Tibial Artery with Two Drug-eluting Intraluminal Devices, Percutaneous Approach

047S36Z Dilation of Left Posterior Tibial Artery with Three Drug-eluting Intraluminal Devices, Percutaneous Approach

047S37Z Dilation of Left Posterior Tibial Artery with Four or More Drug-eluting Intraluminal Devices, Percutaneous Approach

047S3D1 Dilation of Left Posterior Tibial Artery with Intraluminal Device, using Drug-Coated Balloon, Percutaneous Approach

047S3DZ Dilation of Left Posterior Tibial Artery with Intraluminal Device, Percutaneous Approach

047S3EZ Dilation of Left Posterior Tibial Artery with Two Intraluminal Devices, Percutaneous Approach

047S3FZ Dilation of Left Posterior Tibial Artery with Three Intraluminal Devices, Percutaneous Approach

047S3GZ Dilation of Left Posterior Tibial Artery with Four or More Intraluminal Devices, Percutaneous Approach

047S3Z1 Dilation of Left Posterior Tibial Artery using Drug-Coated Balloon, Percutaneous Approach

047S3ZZ Dilation of Left Posterior Tibial Artery, Percutaneous Approach

047S441 Dilation of Left Posterior Tibial Artery with Drug-eluting Intraluminal Device, using Drug-Coated Balloon, Percutaneous Endoscopic Approach

047S44Z Dilation of Left Posterior Tibial Artery with Drug-eluting Intraluminal Device, Percutaneous Endoscopic Approach

047S45Z Dilation of Left Posterior Tibial Artery with Two Drug-eluting Intraluminal Devices, Percutaneous Endoscopic Approach

047S46Z Dilation of Left Posterior Tibial Artery with Three Drug-eluting Intraluminal Devices, Percutaneous Endoscopic Approach

047S47Z Dilation of Left Posterior Tibial Artery with Four or More Drug-eluting Intraluminal Devices, Percutaneous Endoscopic Approach

047S4D1 Dilation of Left Posterior Tibial Artery with Intraluminal Device, using Drug-Coated Balloon, Percutaneous Endoscopic Approach

047S4DZ Dilation of Left Posterior Tibial Artery with Intraluminal Device, Percutaneous Endoscopic Approach

047S4EZ Dilation of Left Posterior Tibial Artery with Two Intraluminal Devices, Percutaneous Endoscopic Approach

047S4FZ Dilation of Left Posterior Tibial Artery with Three Intraluminal Devices, Percutaneous Endoscopic Approach

047S4GZ Dilation of Left Posterior Tibial Artery with Four or More Intraluminal Devices, Percutaneous Endoscopic Approach

047S4Z1 Dilation of Left Posterior Tibial Artery using Drug-Coated Balloon, Percutaneous Endoscopic Approach

047S4ZZ Dilation of Left Posterior Tibial Artery, Percutaneous Endoscopic Approach

047T041 Dilation of Right Peroneal Artery with Drug-eluting Intraluminal Device, using Drug-Coated Balloon, Open Approach

047T04Z Dilation of Right Peroneal Artery with Drug-eluting Intraluminal Device, Open Approach

047T05Z Dilation of Right Peroneal Artery with Two Drug-eluting Intraluminal Devices, Open Approach

047T06Z Dilation of Right Peroneal Artery with Three Drug-eluting Intraluminal Devices, Open Approach

047T07Z Dilation of Right Peroneal Artery with Four or More Drug-eluting Intraluminal Devices, Open Approach

047T0D1 Dilation of Right Peroneal Artery with Intraluminal Device, using Drug-Coated Balloon, Open Approach

047T0DZ Dilation of Right Peroneal Artery with Intraluminal Device, Open Approach

047T0EZ Dilation of Right Peroneal Artery with Two Intraluminal Devices, Open Approach

047T0FZ Dilation of Right Peroneal Artery with Three Intraluminal Devices, Open Approach

047T0GZ Dilation of Right Peroneal Artery with Four or More Intraluminal Devices, Open Approach

047T0Z1 Dilation of Right Peroneal Artery using Drug-Coated Balloon, Open Approach

047T0ZZ Dilation of Right Peroneal Artery, Open Approach

047T341 Dilation of Right Peroneal Artery with Drug-eluting Intraluminal Device, using Drug-Coated Balloon, Percutaneous Approach

047T34Z Dilation of Right Peroneal Artery with Drug-eluting Intraluminal Device, Percutaneous Approach

047T35Z Dilation of Right Peroneal Artery with Two Drug-eluting Intraluminal Devices, Percutaneous Approach

047T36Z Dilation of Right Peroneal Artery with Three Drug-eluting Intraluminal Devices, Percutaneous Approach

047T37Z Dilation of Right Peroneal Artery with Four or More Drug-eluting Intraluminal Devices, Percutaneous Approach

047T3D1 Dilation of Right Peroneal Artery with Intraluminal Device, using Drug-Coated Balloon, Percutaneous Approach

047T3DZ Dilation of Right Peroneal Artery with Intraluminal Device, Percutaneous Approach

047T3EZ Dilation of Right Peroneal Artery with Two Intraluminal Devices, Percutaneous Approach

047T3FZ Dilation of Right Peroneal Artery with Three Intraluminal Devices, Percutaneous Approach

047T3GZ Dilation of Right Peroneal Artery with Four or More Intraluminal Devices, Percutaneous Approach

047T3Z1 Dilation of Right Peroneal Artery using Drug-Coated Balloon, Percutaneous Approach

047T3ZZ Dilation of Right Peroneal Artery, Percutaneous Approach

047T441 Dilation of Right Peroneal Artery with Drug-eluting Intraluminal Device, using Drug-Coated Balloon, Percutaneous Endoscopic Approach

047T44Z Dilation of Right Peroneal Artery with Drug-eluting Intraluminal Device, Percutaneous Endoscopic Approach

047T45Z Dilation of Right Peroneal Artery with Two Drug-eluting Intraluminal Devices, Percutaneous Endoscopic Approach

047T46Z Dilation of Right Peroneal Artery with Three Drug-eluting Intraluminal Devices, Percutaneous Endoscopic Approach

047T47Z Dilation of Right Peroneal Artery with Four or More Drug-eluting Intraluminal Devices, Percutaneous Endoscopic Approach

047T4D1 Dilation of Right Peroneal Artery with Intraluminal Device, using Drug-Coated Balloon, Percutaneous Endoscopic Approach

047T4DZ Dilation of Right Peroneal Artery with Intraluminal Device, Percutaneous Endoscopic Approach

047T4EZ Dilation of Right Peroneal Artery with Two Intraluminal Devices, Percutaneous Endoscopic Approach

047T4FZ Dilation of Right Peroneal Artery with Three Intraluminal Devices, Percutaneous Endoscopic Approach

047T4GZ Dilation of Right Peroneal Artery with Four or More Intraluminal Devices, Percutaneous Endoscopic Approach

047T4Z1 Dilation of Right Peroneal Artery using Drug-Coated Balloon, Percutaneous Endoscopic Approach

047T4ZZ Dilation of Right Peroneal Artery, Percutaneous Endoscopic Approach

047U041 Dilation of Left Peroneal Artery with Drug-eluting Intraluminal Device, using Drug-Coated Balloon, Open Approach

047U04Z Dilation of Left Peroneal Artery with Drug-eluting Intraluminal Device, Open Approach

047U05Z Dilation of Left Peroneal Artery with Two Drug-eluting Intraluminal Devices, Open Approach

047U06Z Dilation of Left Peroneal Artery with Three Drug-eluting Intraluminal Devices, Open Approach

047U07Z Dilation of Left Peroneal Artery with Four or More Drug-eluting Intraluminal Devices, Open Approach

047U0D1 Dilation of Left Peroneal Artery with Intraluminal Device, using Drug-Coated Balloon, Open Approach

047U0DZ Dilation of Left Peroneal Artery with Intraluminal Device, Open Approach

047U0EZ Dilation of Left Peroneal Artery with Two Intraluminal Devices, Open Approach

047U0FZ Dilation of Left Peroneal Artery with Three Intraluminal Devices, Open Approach

047U0GZ Dilation of Left Peroneal Artery with Four or More Intraluminal Devices, Open Approach

047U0Z1 Dilation of Left Peroneal Artery using Drug-Coated Balloon, Open Approach

047U0ZZ Dilation of Left Peroneal Artery, Open Approach

047U341 Dilation of Left Peroneal Artery with Drug-eluting Intraluminal Device, using Drug-Coated Balloon, Percutaneous Approach

047U34Z Dilation of Left Peroneal Artery with Drug-eluting Intraluminal Device, Percutaneous Approach

---

♀ Female-only   ♂ Male-only   ▲ Limited Coverage   ● Non-OR   ▆ HAC-associated procedure   ▲ Non-covered procedures   ✚ Cluster

047U35Z Dilation of Left Peroneal Artery with Two Drug-eluting Intraluminal Devices, Percutaneous Approach

047U36Z Dilation of Left Peroneal Artery with Three Drug-eluting Intraluminal Devices, Percutaneous Approach

047U37Z Dilation of Left Peroneal Artery with Four or More Drug-eluting Intraluminal Devices, Percutaneous Approach

047U3D1 Dilation of Left Peroneal Artery with Intraluminal Device, using Drug-Coated Balloon, Percutaneous Approach

047U3DZ Dilation of Left Peroneal Artery with Intraluminal Device, Percutaneous Approach

047U3EZ Dilation of Left Peroneal Artery with Two Intraluminal Devices, Percutaneous Approach

047U3FZ Dilation of Left Peroneal Artery with Three Intraluminal Devices, Percutaneous Approach

047U3GZ Dilation of Left Peroneal Artery with Four or More Intraluminal Devices, Percutaneous Approach

047U3Z1 Dilation of Left Peroneal Artery using Drug-Coated Balloon, Percutaneous Approach

047U3ZZ Dilation of Left Peroneal Artery, Percutaneous Approach

047U441 Dilation of Left Peroneal Artery with Drug-eluting Intraluminal Device, using Drug-Coated Balloon, Percutaneous Endoscopic Approach

047U44Z Dilation of Left Peroneal Artery with Drug-eluting Intraluminal Device, Percutaneous Endoscopic Approach

047U45Z Dilation of Left Peroneal Artery with Two Drug-eluting Intraluminal Devices, Percutaneous Endoscopic Approach

047U46Z Dilation of Left Peroneal Artery with Three Drug-eluting Intraluminal Devices, Percutaneous Endoscopic Approach

047U47Z Dilation of Left Peroneal Artery with Four or More Drug-eluting Intraluminal Devices, Percutaneous Endoscopic Approach

047U4D1 Dilation of Left Peroneal Artery with Intraluminal Device, using Drug-Coated Balloon, Percutaneous Endoscopic Approach

047U4DZ Dilation of Left Peroneal Artery with Intraluminal Device, Percutaneous Endoscopic Approach

047U4EZ Dilation of Left Peroneal Artery with Two Intraluminal Devices, Percutaneous Endoscopic Approach

047U4FZ Dilation of Left Peroneal Artery with Three Intraluminal Devices, Percutaneous Endoscopic Approach

047U4GZ Dilation of Left Peroneal Artery with Four or More Intraluminal Devices, Percutaneous Endoscopic Approach

047U4Z1 Dilation of Left Peroneal Artery using Drug-Coated Balloon, Percutaneous Endoscopic Approach

047U4ZZ Dilation of Left Peroneal Artery, Percutaneous Endoscopic Approach

047V041 Dilation of Right Foot Artery with Drug-eluting Intraluminal Device, using Drug-Coated Balloon, Open Approach

047V04Z Dilation of Right Foot Artery with Drug-eluting Intraluminal Device, Open Approach

047V05Z Dilation of Right Foot Artery with Two Drug-eluting Intraluminal Devices, Open Approach

047V06Z Dilation of Right Foot Artery with Three Drug-eluting Intraluminal Devices, Open Approach

047V07Z Dilation of Right Foot Artery with Four or More Drug-eluting Intraluminal Devices, Open Approach

047V0D1 Dilation of Right Foot Artery with Intraluminal Device, using Drug-Coated Balloon, Open Approach

047V0DZ Dilation of Right Foot Artery with Intraluminal Device, Open Approach

047V0EZ Dilation of Right Foot Artery with Two Intraluminal Devices, Open Approach

047V0FZ Dilation of Right Foot Artery with Three Intraluminal Devices, Open Approach

047V0GZ Dilation of Right Foot Artery with Four or More Intraluminal Devices, Open Approach

047V0Z1 Dilation of Right Foot Artery using Drug-Coated Balloon, Open Approach

047V0ZZ Dilation of Right Foot Artery, Open Approach

047V341 Dilation of Right Foot Artery with Drug-eluting Intraluminal Device, using Drug-Coated Balloon, Percutaneous Approach

047V34Z Dilation of Right Foot Artery with Drug-eluting Intraluminal Device, Percutaneous Approach

047V35Z Dilation of Right Foot Artery with Two Drug-eluting Intraluminal Devices, Percutaneous Approach

047V36Z Dilation of Right Foot Artery with Three Drug-eluting Intraluminal Devices, Percutaneous Approach

047V37Z Dilation of Right Foot Artery with Four or More Drug-eluting Intraluminal Devices, Percutaneous Approach

047V3D1 Dilation of Right Foot Artery with Intraluminal Device, using Drug-Coated Balloon, Percutaneous Approach

047V3DZ Dilation of Right Foot Artery with Intraluminal Device, Percutaneous Approach

047V3EZ Dilation of Right Foot Artery with Two Intraluminal Devices, Percutaneous Approach

047V3FZ Dilation of Right Foot Artery with Three Intraluminal Devices, Percutaneous Approach

047V3GZ Dilation of Right Foot Artery with Four or More Intraluminal Devices, Percutaneous Approach

047V3Z1 Dilation of Right Foot Artery using Drug-Coated Balloon, Percutaneous Approach

047V3ZZ Dilation of Right Foot Artery, Percutaneous Approach

047V441 Dilation of Right Foot Artery with Drug-eluting Intraluminal Device, using Drug-Coated Balloon, Percutaneous Endoscopic Approach

047V44Z Dilation of Right Foot Artery with Drug-eluting Intraluminal Device, Percutaneous Endoscopic Approach

047V45Z Dilation of Right Foot Artery with Two Drug-eluting Intraluminal Devices, Percutaneous Endoscopic Approach

047V46Z Dilation of Right Foot Artery with Three Drug-eluting Intraluminal Devices, Percutaneous Endoscopic Approach

047V47Z Dilation of Right Foot Artery with Four or More Drug-eluting Intraluminal Devices, Percutaneous Endoscopic Approach

047V4D1 Dilation of Right Foot Artery with Intraluminal Device, using Drug-Coated Balloon, Percutaneous Endoscopic Approach

047V4DZ Dilation of Right Foot Artery with Intraluminal Device, Percutaneous Endoscopic Approach

047V4EZ Dilation of Right Foot Artery with Two Intraluminal Devices, Percutaneous Endoscopic Approach

047V4FZ Dilation of Right Foot Artery with Three Intraluminal Devices, Percutaneous Endoscopic Approach

047V4GZ Dilation of Right Foot Artery with Four or More Intraluminal Devices, Percutaneous Endoscopic Approach

047V4Z1 Dilation of Right Foot Artery using Drug-Coated Balloon, Percutaneous Endoscopic Approach

047V4ZZ Dilation of Right Foot Artery, Percutaneous Endoscopic Approach

047W041 Dilation of Left Foot Artery with Drug-eluting Intraluminal Device, using Drug-Coated Balloon, Open Approach

047W04Z Dilation of Left Foot Artery with Drug-eluting Intraluminal Device, Open Approach

047W05Z Dilation of Left Foot Artery with Two Drug-eluting Intraluminal Devices, Open Approach

047W06Z Dilation of Left Foot Artery with Three Drug-eluting Intraluminal Devices, Open Approach

047W07Z Dilation of Left Foot Artery with Four or More Drug-eluting Intraluminal Devices, Open Approach

047W0D1 Dilation of Left Foot Artery with Intraluminal Device, using Drug-Coated Balloon, Open Approach

047W0DZ Dilation of Left Foot Artery with Intraluminal Device, Open Approach

047W0EZ Dilation of Left Foot Artery with Two Intraluminal Devices, Open Approach

047W0FZ Dilation of Left Foot Artery with Three Intraluminal Devices, Open Approach

047W0GZ Dilation of Left Foot Artery with Four or More Intraluminal Devices, Open Approach

047W0Z1 Dilation of Left Foot Artery using Drug-Coated Balloon, Open Approach

047W0ZZ Dilation of Left Foot Artery, Open Approach

047W341 Dilation of Left Foot Artery with Drug-eluting Intraluminal Device, using Drug-Coated Balloon, Percutaneous Approach

047W34Z Dilation of Left Foot Artery with Drug-eluting Intraluminal Device, Percutaneous Approach

047W35Z Dilation of Left Foot Artery with Two Drug-eluting Intraluminal Devices, Percutaneous Approach

047W36Z Dilation of Left Foot Artery with Three Drug-eluting Intraluminal Devices, Percutaneous Approach

047W37Z Dilation of Left Foot Artery with Four or More Drug-eluting Intraluminal Devices, Percutaneous Approach

♀ Female-only   ♂ Male-only   ▲ Limited Coverage   ● Non-OR   ▥ HAC-associated procedure   ▲ Non-covered procedures   ➕ Cluster

047W3D1 Dilation of Left Foot Artery with Intraluminal Device, using Drug-Coated Balloon, Percutaneous Approach

047W3DZ Dilation of Left Foot Artery with Intraluminal Device, Percutaneous Approach

047W3EZ Dilation of Left Foot Artery with Two Intraluminal Devices, Percutaneous Approach

047W3FZ Dilation of Left Foot Artery with Three Intraluminal Devices, Percutaneous Approach

047W3GZ Dilation of Left Foot Artery with Four or More Intraluminal Devices, Percutaneous Approach

047W3Z1 Dilation of Left Foot Artery using Drug-Coated Balloon, Percutaneous Approach

047W3ZZ Dilation of Left Foot Artery, Percutaneous Approach

047W441 Dilation of Left Foot Artery with Drug-eluting Intraluminal Device, using Drug-Coated Balloon, Percutaneous Endoscopic Approach

047W44Z Dilation of Left Foot Artery with Drug-eluting Intraluminal Device, Percutaneous Endoscopic Approach

047W45Z Dilation of Left Foot Artery with Two Drug-eluting Intraluminal Devices, Percutaneous Endoscopic Approach

047W46Z Dilation of Left Foot Artery with Three Drug-eluting Intraluminal Devices, Percutaneous Endoscopic Approach

047W47Z Dilation of Left Foot Artery with Four or More Drug-eluting Intraluminal Devices, Percutaneous Endoscopic Approach

047W4D1 Dilation of Left Foot Artery with Intraluminal Device, using Drug-Coated Balloon, Percutaneous Endoscopic Approach

047W4DZ Dilation of Left Foot Artery with Intraluminal Device, Percutaneous Endoscopic Approach

047W4EZ Dilation of Left Foot Artery with Two Intraluminal Devices, Percutaneous Endoscopic Approach

047W4FZ Dilation of Left Foot Artery with Three Intraluminal Devices, Percutaneous Endoscopic Approach

047W4GZ Dilation of Left Foot Artery with Four or More Intraluminal Devices, Percutaneous Endoscopic Approach

047W4Z1 Dilation of Left Foot Artery using Drug-Coated Balloon, Percutaneous Endoscopic Approach

047W4ZZ Dilation of Left Foot Artery, Percutaneous Endoscopic Approach

047Y041 Dilation of Lower Artery with Drug-eluting Intraluminal Device, using Drug-Coated Balloon, Open Approach

047Y04Z Dilation of Lower Artery with Drug-eluting Intraluminal Device, Open Approach

047Y05Z Dilation of Lower Artery with Two Drug-eluting Intraluminal Devices, Open Approach

047Y06Z Dilation of Lower Artery with Three Drug-eluting Intraluminal Devices, Open Approach

047Y07Z Dilation of Lower Artery with Four or More Drug-eluting Intraluminal Devices, Open Approach

047Y0D1 Dilation of Lower Artery with Intraluminal Device, using Drug-Coated Balloon, Open Approach

047Y0DZ Dilation of Lower Artery with Intraluminal Device, Open Approach

047Y0EZ Dilation of Lower Artery with Two Intraluminal Devices, Open Approach

047Y0FZ Dilation of Lower Artery with Three Intraluminal Devices, Open Approach

047Y0GZ Dilation of Lower Artery with Four or More Intraluminal Devices, Open Approach

047Y0Z1 Dilation of Lower Artery using Drug-Coated Balloon, Open Approach

047Y0ZZ Dilation of Lower Artery, Open Approach

047Y341 Dilation of Lower Artery with Drug-eluting Intraluminal Device, using Drug-Coated Balloon, Percutaneous Approach

047Y34Z Dilation of Lower Artery with Drug-eluting Intraluminal Device, Percutaneous Approach

047Y35Z Dilation of Lower Artery with Two Drug-eluting Intraluminal Devices, Percutaneous Approach

047Y36Z Dilation of Lower Artery with Three Drug-eluting Intraluminal Devices, Percutaneous Approach

047Y37Z Dilation of Lower Artery with Four or More Drug-eluting Intraluminal Devices, Percutaneous Approach

047Y3D1 Dilation of Lower Artery with Intraluminal Device, using Drug-Coated Balloon, Percutaneous Approach

047Y3DZ Dilation of Lower Artery with Intraluminal Device, Percutaneous Approach

047Y3EZ Dilation of Lower Artery with Two Intraluminal Devices, Percutaneous Approach

047Y3FZ Dilation of Lower Artery with Three Intraluminal Devices, Percutaneous Approach

047Y3GZ Dilation of Lower Artery with Four or More Intraluminal Devices, Percutaneous Approach

047Y3Z1 Dilation of Lower Artery using Drug-Coated Balloon, Percutaneous Approach

047Y3ZZ Dilation of Lower Artery, Percutaneous Approach

047Y441 Dilation of Lower Artery with Drug-eluting Intraluminal Device, using Drug-Coated Balloon, Percutaneous Endoscopic Approach

047Y44Z Dilation of Lower Artery with Drug-eluting Intraluminal Device, Percutaneous Endoscopic Approach

047Y45Z Dilation of Lower Artery with Two Drug-eluting Intraluminal Devices, Percutaneous Endoscopic Approach

047Y46Z Dilation of Lower Artery with Three Drug-eluting Intraluminal Devices, Percutaneous Endoscopic Approach

047Y47Z Dilation of Lower Artery with Four or More Drug-eluting Intraluminal Devices, Percutaneous Endoscopic Approach

047Y4D1 Dilation of Lower Artery with Intraluminal Device, using Drug-Coated Balloon, Percutaneous Endoscopic Approach

047Y4DZ Dilation of Lower Artery with Intraluminal Device, Percutaneous Endoscopic Approach

047Y4EZ Dilation of Lower Artery with Two Intraluminal Devices, Percutaneous Endoscopic Approach

047Y4FZ Dilation of Lower Artery with Three Intraluminal Devices, Percutaneous Endoscopic Approach

047Y4GZ Dilation of Lower Artery with Four or More Intraluminal Devices, Percutaneous Endoscopic Approach

047Y4Z1 Dilation of Lower Artery using Drug-Coated Balloon, Percutaneous Endoscopic Approach

047Y4ZZ Dilation of Lower Artery, Percutaneous Endoscopic Approach

049 – Lower Arteries, Drainage

Review Coding Guidelines B3.4a and B3.4b

Review Coding Guideline B6.2

049000Z Drainage of Abdominal Aorta with Drainage Device, Open Approach

04900ZX Drainage of Abdominal Aorta, Open Approach, Diagnostic

04900ZZ Drainage of Abdominal Aorta, Open Approach

049030Z Drainage of Abdominal Aorta with Drainage Device, Percutaneous Approach

04903ZX Drainage of Abdominal Aorta, Percutaneous Approach, Diagnostic

04903ZZ Drainage of Abdominal Aorta, Percutaneous Approach

049040Z Drainage of Abdominal Aorta with Drainage Device, Percutaneous Endoscopic Approach

04904ZX Drainage of Abdominal Aorta, Percutaneous Endoscopic Approach, Diagnostic

04904ZZ Drainage of Abdominal Aorta, Percutaneous Endoscopic Approach

049100Z Drainage of Celiac Artery with Drainage Device, Open Approach

04910ZX Drainage of Celiac Artery, Open Approach, Diagnostic

04910ZZ Drainage of Celiac Artery, Open Approach

049130Z Drainage of Celiac Artery with Drainage Device, Percutaneous Approach

04913ZX Drainage of Celiac Artery, Percutaneous Approach, Diagnostic

04913ZZ Drainage of Celiac Artery, Percutaneous Approach

049140Z Drainage of Celiac Artery with Drainage Device, Percutaneous Endoscopic Approach

♀ Female-only   ♂ Male-only   ▲ Limited Coverage   ● Non-OR   ▦ HAC-associated procedure   ▲ Non-covered procedures   ✚ Cluster

04914ZX Drainage of Celiac Artery, Percutaneous Endoscopic Approach, Diagnostic

04914ZZ Drainage of Celiac Artery, Percutaneous Endoscopic Approach

049200Z Drainage of Gastric Artery with Drainage Device, Open Approach

04920ZX Drainage of Gastric Artery, Open Approach, Diagnostic

04920ZZ Drainage of Gastric Artery, Open Approach

049230Z Drainage of Gastric Artery with Drainage Device, Percutaneous Approach

04923ZX Drainage of Gastric Artery, Percutaneous Approach, Diagnostic

04923ZZ Drainage of Gastric Artery, Percutaneous Approach

049240Z Drainage of Gastric Artery with Drainage Device, Percutaneous Endoscopic Approach

04924ZX Drainage of Gastric Artery, Percutaneous Endoscopic Approach, Diagnostic

04924ZZ Drainage of Gastric Artery, Percutaneous Endoscopic Approach

049300Z Drainage of Hepatic Artery with Drainage Device, Open Approach

04930ZX Drainage of Hepatic Artery, Open Approach, Diagnostic

04930ZZ Drainage of Hepatic Artery, Open Approach

049330Z Drainage of Hepatic Artery with Drainage Device, Percutaneous Approach

04933ZX Drainage of Hepatic Artery, Percutaneous Approach, Diagnostic

04933ZZ Drainage of Hepatic Artery, Percutaneous Approach

049340Z Drainage of Hepatic Artery with Drainage Device, Percutaneous Endoscopic Approach

04934ZX Drainage of Hepatic Artery, Percutaneous Endoscopic Approach, Diagnostic

04934ZZ Drainage of Hepatic Artery, Percutaneous Endoscopic Approach

049400Z Drainage of Splenic Artery with Drainage Device, Open Approach

04940ZX Drainage of Splenic Artery, Open Approach, Diagnostic

04940ZZ Drainage of Splenic Artery, Open Approach

049430Z Drainage of Splenic Artery with Drainage Device, Percutaneous Approach

04943ZX Drainage of Splenic Artery, Percutaneous Approach, Diagnostic

04943ZZ Drainage of Splenic Artery, Percutaneous Approach

049440Z Drainage of Splenic Artery with Drainage Device, Percutaneous Endoscopic Approach

04944ZX Drainage of Splenic Artery, Percutaneous Endoscopic Approach, Diagnostic

04944ZZ Drainage of Splenic Artery, Percutaneous Endoscopic Approach

049500Z Drainage of Superior Mesenteric Artery with Drainage Device, Open Approach

04950ZX Drainage of Superior Mesenteric Artery, Open Approach, Diagnostic

04950ZZ Drainage of Superior Mesenteric Artery, Open Approach

049530Z Drainage of Superior Mesenteric Artery with Drainage Device, Percutaneous Approach

04953ZX Drainage of Superior Mesenteric Artery, Percutaneous Approach, Diagnostic

04953ZZ Drainage of Superior Mesenteric Artery, Percutaneous Approach

049540Z Drainage of Superior Mesenteric Artery with Drainage Device, Percutaneous Endoscopic Approach

04954ZX Drainage of Superior Mesenteric Artery, Percutaneous Endoscopic Approach, Diagnostic

04954ZZ Drainage of Superior Mesenteric Artery, Percutaneous Endoscopic Approach

049600Z Drainage of Right Colic Artery with Drainage Device, Open Approach

04960ZX Drainage of Right Colic Artery, Open Approach, Diagnostic

04960ZZ Drainage of Right Colic Artery, Open Approach

049630Z Drainage of Right Colic Artery with Drainage Device, Percutaneous Approach

04963ZX Drainage of Right Colic Artery, Percutaneous Approach, Diagnostic

04963ZZ Drainage of Right Colic Artery, Percutaneous Approach

049640Z Drainage of Right Colic Artery with Drainage Device, Percutaneous Endoscopic Approach

04964ZX Drainage of Right Colic Artery, Percutaneous Endoscopic Approach, Diagnostic

04964ZZ Drainage of Right Colic Artery, Percutaneous Endoscopic Approach

049700Z Drainage of Left Colic Artery with Drainage Device, Open Approach

04970ZX Drainage of Left Colic Artery, Open Approach, Diagnostic

04970ZZ Drainage of Left Colic Artery, Open Approach

049730Z Drainage of Left Colic Artery with Drainage Device, Percutaneous Approach

04973ZX Drainage of Left Colic Artery, Percutaneous Approach, Diagnostic

04973ZZ Drainage of Left Colic Artery, Percutaneous Approach

049740Z Drainage of Left Colic Artery with Drainage Device, Percutaneous Endoscopic Approach

04974ZX Drainage of Left Colic Artery, Percutaneous Endoscopic Approach, Diagnostic

04974ZZ Drainage of Left Colic Artery, Percutaneous Endoscopic Approach

049800Z Drainage of Middle Colic Artery with Drainage Device, Open Approach

04980ZX Drainage of Middle Colic Artery, Open Approach, Diagnostic

04980ZZ Drainage of Middle Colic Artery, Open Approach

049830Z Drainage of Middle Colic Artery with Drainage Device, Percutaneous Approach

04983ZX Drainage of Middle Colic Artery, Percutaneous Approach, Diagnostic

04983ZZ Drainage of Middle Colic Artery, Percutaneous Approach

049840Z Drainage of Middle Colic Artery with Drainage Device, Percutaneous Endoscopic Approach

04984ZX Drainage of Middle Colic Artery, Percutaneous Endoscopic Approach, Diagnostic

04984ZZ Drainage of Middle Colic Artery, Percutaneous Endoscopic Approach

049900Z Drainage of Right Renal Artery with Drainage Device, Open Approach

04990ZX Drainage of Right Renal Artery, Open Approach, Diagnostic

04990ZZ Drainage of Right Renal Artery, Open Approach

049930Z Drainage of Right Renal Artery with Drainage Device, Percutaneous Approach

04993ZX Drainage of Right Renal Artery, Percutaneous Approach, Diagnostic

04993ZZ Drainage of Right Renal Artery, Percutaneous Approach

049940Z Drainage of Right Renal Artery with Drainage Device, Percutaneous Endoscopic Approach

04994ZX Drainage of Right Renal Artery, Percutaneous Endoscopic Approach, Diagnostic

04994ZZ Drainage of Right Renal Artery, Percutaneous Endoscopic Approach

049A00Z Drainage of Left Renal Artery with Drainage Device, Open Approach

049A0ZX Drainage of Left Renal Artery, Open Approach, Diagnostic

049A0ZZ Drainage of Left Renal Artery, Open Approach

049A30Z Drainage of Left Renal Artery with Drainage Device, Percutaneous Approach

049A3ZX Drainage of Left Renal Artery, Percutaneous Approach, Diagnostic

049A3ZZ Drainage of Left Renal Artery, Percutaneous Approach

049A40Z Drainage of Left Renal Artery with Drainage Device, Percutaneous Endoscopic Approach

049A4ZX Drainage of Left Renal Artery, Percutaneous Endoscopic Approach, Diagnostic

049A4ZZ Drainage of Left Renal Artery, Percutaneous Endoscopic Approach

049B00Z Drainage of Inferior Mesenteric Artery with Drainage Device, Open Approach

049B0ZX Drainage of Inferior Mesenteric Artery, Open Approach, Diagnostic

049B0ZZ Drainage of Inferior Mesenteric Artery, Open Approach

049B30Z Drainage of Inferior Mesenteric Artery with Drainage Device, Percutaneous Approach

049B3ZX Drainage of Inferior Mesenteric Artery, Percutaneous Approach, Diagnostic

049B3ZZ Drainage of Inferior Mesenteric Artery, Percutaneous Approach

049B40Z Drainage of Inferior Mesenteric Artery with Drainage Device, Percutaneous Endoscopic Approach

049B4ZX Drainage of Inferior Mesenteric Artery, Percutaneous Endoscopic Approach, Diagnostic

049B4ZZ Drainage of Inferior Mesenteric Artery, Percutaneous Endoscopic Approach

049C00Z Drainage of Right Common Iliac Artery with Drainage Device, Open Approach

049C0ZX Drainage of Right Common Iliac Artery, Open Approach, Diagnostic

049C0ZZ Drainage of Right Common Iliac Artery, Open Approach

049C30Z Drainage of Right Common Iliac Artery with Drainage Device, Percutaneous Approach

049C3ZX Drainage of Right Common Iliac Artery, Percutaneous Approach, Diagnostic

049C3ZZ Drainage of Right Common Iliac Artery, Percutaneous Approach

049C40Z Drainage of Right Common Iliac Artery with Drainage Device, Percutaneous Endoscopic Approach

049C4ZX Drainage of Right Common Iliac Artery, Percutaneous Endoscopic Approach, Diagnostic

049C4ZZ Drainage of Right Common Iliac Artery, Percutaneous Endoscopic Approach

049D00Z Drainage of Left Common Iliac Artery with Drainage Device, Open Approach

049D0ZX Drainage of Left Common Iliac Artery, Open Approach, Diagnostic

049D0ZZ Drainage of Left Common Iliac Artery, Open Approach

049D30Z Drainage of Left Common Iliac Artery with Drainage Device, Percutaneous Approach

049D3ZX Drainage of Left Common Iliac Artery, Percutaneous Approach, Diagnostic

049D3ZZ Drainage of Left Common Iliac Artery, Percutaneous Approach

049D40Z Drainage of Left Common Iliac Artery with Drainage Device, Percutaneous Endoscopic Approach

049D4ZX Drainage of Left Common Iliac Artery, Percutaneous Endoscopic Approach, Diagnostic

049D4ZZ Drainage of Left Common Iliac Artery, Percutaneous Endoscopic Approach

049E00Z Drainage of Right Internal Iliac Artery with Drainage Device, Open Approach

049E0ZX Drainage of Right Internal Iliac Artery, Open Approach, Diagnostic

049E0ZZ Drainage of Right Internal Iliac Artery, Open Approach

049E30Z Drainage of Right Internal Iliac Artery with Drainage Device, Percutaneous Approach

049E3ZX Drainage of Right Internal Iliac Artery, Percutaneous Approach, Diagnostic

049E3ZZ Drainage of Right Internal Iliac Artery, Percutaneous Approach

049E40Z Drainage of Right Internal Iliac Artery with Drainage Device, Percutaneous Endoscopic Approach

049E4ZX Drainage of Right Internal Iliac Artery, Percutaneous Endoscopic Approach, Diagnostic

049E4ZZ Drainage of Right Internal Iliac Artery, Percutaneous Endoscopic Approach

049F00Z Drainage of Left Internal Iliac Artery with Drainage Device, Open Approach

049F0ZX Drainage of Left Internal Iliac Artery, Open Approach, Diagnostic

049F0ZZ Drainage of Left Internal Iliac Artery, Open Approach

049F30Z Drainage of Left Internal Iliac Artery with Drainage Device, Percutaneous Approach

049F3ZX Drainage of Left Internal Iliac Artery, Percutaneous Approach, Diagnostic

049F3ZZ Drainage of Left Internal Iliac Artery, Percutaneous Approach

049F40Z Drainage of Left Internal Iliac Artery with Drainage Device, Percutaneous Endoscopic Approach

049F4ZX Drainage of Left Internal Iliac Artery, Percutaneous Endoscopic Approach, Diagnostic

049F4ZZ Drainage of Left Internal Iliac Artery, Percutaneous Endoscopic Approach

049H00Z Drainage of Right External Iliac Artery with Drainage Device, Open Approach

049H0ZX Drainage of Right External Iliac Artery, Open Approach, Diagnostic

049H0ZZ Drainage of Right External Iliac Artery, Open Approach

049H30Z Drainage of Right External Iliac Artery with Drainage Device, Percutaneous Approach

049H3ZX Drainage of Right External Iliac Artery, Percutaneous Approach, Diagnostic

049H3ZZ Drainage of Right External Iliac Artery, Percutaneous Approach

049H40Z Drainage of Right External Iliac Artery with Drainage Device, Percutaneous Endoscopic Approach

049H4ZX Drainage of Right External Iliac Artery, Percutaneous Endoscopic Approach, Diagnostic

049H4ZZ Drainage of Right External Iliac Artery, Percutaneous Endoscopic Approach

049J00Z Drainage of Left External Iliac Artery with Drainage Device, Open Approach

049J0ZX Drainage of Left External Iliac Artery, Open Approach, Diagnostic

049J0ZZ Drainage of Left External Iliac Artery, Open Approach

049J30Z Drainage of Left External Iliac Artery with Drainage Device, Percutaneous Approach

049J3ZX Drainage of Left External Iliac Artery, Percutaneous Approach, Diagnostic

049J3ZZ Drainage of Left External Iliac Artery, Percutaneous Approach

049J40Z Drainage of Left External Iliac Artery with Drainage Device, Percutaneous Endoscopic Approach

049J4ZX Drainage of Left External Iliac Artery, Percutaneous Endoscopic Approach, Diagnostic

049J4ZZ Drainage of Left External Iliac Artery, Percutaneous Endoscopic Approach

049K00Z Drainage of Right Femoral Artery with Drainage Device, Open Approach

049K0ZX Drainage of Right Femoral Artery, Open Approach, Diagnostic

049K0ZZ Drainage of Right Femoral Artery, Open Approach

049K30Z Drainage of Right Femoral Artery with Drainage Device, Percutaneous Approach

049K3ZX Drainage of Right Femoral Artery, Percutaneous Approach, Diagnostic

049K3ZZ Drainage of Right Femoral Artery, Percutaneous Approach

049K40Z Drainage of Right Femoral Artery with Drainage Device, Percutaneous Endoscopic Approach

049K4ZX Drainage of Right Femoral Artery, Percutaneous Endoscopic Approach, Diagnostic

049K4ZZ Drainage of Right Femoral Artery, Percutaneous Endoscopic Approach

049L00Z Drainage of Left Femoral Artery with Drainage Device, Open Approach

049L0ZX Drainage of Left Femoral Artery, Open Approach, Diagnostic

049L0ZZ Drainage of Left Femoral Artery, Open Approach

049L30Z Drainage of Left Femoral Artery with Drainage Device, Percutaneous Approach

049L3ZX Drainage of Left Femoral Artery, Percutaneous Approach, Diagnostic

049L3ZZ Drainage of Left Femoral Artery, Percutaneous Approach

049L40Z Drainage of Left Femoral Artery with Drainage Device, Percutaneous Endoscopic Approach

049L4ZX Drainage of Left Femoral Artery, Percutaneous Endoscopic Approach, Diagnostic

049L4ZZ Drainage of Left Femoral Artery, Percutaneous Endoscopic Approach

049M00Z Drainage of Right Popliteal Artery with Drainage Device, Open Approach

049M0ZX Drainage of Right Popliteal Artery, Open Approach, Diagnostic

049M0ZZ Drainage of Right Popliteal Artery, Open Approach

049M30Z Drainage of Right Popliteal Artery with Drainage Device, Percutaneous Approach

049M3ZX Drainage of Right Popliteal Artery, Percutaneous Approach, Diagnostic

049M3ZZ Drainage of Right Popliteal Artery, Percutaneous Approach

049M40Z Drainage of Right Popliteal Artery with Drainage Device, Percutaneous Endoscopic Approach

049M4ZX Drainage of Right Popliteal Artery, Percutaneous Endoscopic Approach, Diagnostic

049M4ZZ Drainage of Right Popliteal Artery, Percutaneous Endoscopic Approach

049N00Z Drainage of Left Popliteal Artery with Drainage Device, Open Approach

049N0ZX Drainage of Left Popliteal Artery, Open Approach, Diagnostic

049N0ZZ Drainage of Left Popliteal Artery, Open Approach

049N30Z Drainage of Left Popliteal Artery with Drainage Device, Percutaneous Approach

049N3ZX Drainage of Left Popliteal Artery, Percutaneous Approach, Diagnostic

049N3ZZ Drainage of Left Popliteal Artery, Percutaneous Approach

049N40Z Drainage of Left Popliteal Artery with Drainage Device, Percutaneous Endoscopic Approach

049N4ZX Drainage of Left Popliteal Artery, Percutaneous Endoscopic Approach, Diagnostic

049N4ZZ Drainage of Left Popliteal Artery, Percutaneous Endoscopic Approach

049P00Z Drainage of Right Anterior Tibial Artery with Drainage Device, Open Approach

049P0ZX Drainage of Right Anterior Tibial Artery, Open Approach, Diagnostic

049P0ZZ Drainage of Right Anterior Tibial Artery, Open Approach

049P30Z Drainage of Right Anterior Tibial Artery with Drainage Device, Percutaneous Approach

049P3ZX Drainage of Right Anterior Tibial Artery, Percutaneous Approach, Diagnostic

049P3ZZ Drainage of Right Anterior Tibial Artery, Percutaneous Approach

049P40Z Drainage of Right Anterior Tibial Artery with Drainage Device, Percutaneous Endoscopic Approach

♀ Female-only   ♂ Male-only   ▲ Limited Coverage   ● Non-OR   ᴴᴬᶜ HAC-associated procedure   ▲ Non-covered procedures   ✚ Cluster

049P4ZX Drainage of Right Anterior Tibial Artery, Percutaneous Endoscopic Approach, Diagnostic

049P4ZZ Drainage of Right Anterior Tibial Artery, Percutaneous Endoscopic Approach

049Q00Z Drainage of Left Anterior Tibial Artery with Drainage Device, Open Approach

049Q0ZX Drainage of Left Anterior Tibial Artery, Open Approach, Diagnostic

049Q0ZZ Drainage of Left Anterior Tibial Artery, Open Approach

049Q30Z Drainage of Left Anterior Tibial Artery with Drainage Device, Percutaneous Approach

049Q3ZX Drainage of Left Anterior Tibial Artery, Percutaneous Approach, Diagnostic

049Q3ZZ Drainage of Left Anterior Tibial Artery, Percutaneous Approach

049Q40Z Drainage of Left Anterior Tibial Artery with Drainage Device, Percutaneous Endoscopic Approach

049Q4ZX Drainage of Left Anterior Tibial Artery, Percutaneous Endoscopic Approach, Diagnostic

049Q4ZZ Drainage of Left Anterior Tibial Artery, Percutaneous Endoscopic Approach

049R00Z Drainage of Right Posterior Tibial Artery with Drainage Device, Open Approach

049R0ZX Drainage of Right Posterior Tibial Artery, Open Approach, Diagnostic

049R0ZZ Drainage of Right Posterior Tibial Artery, Open Approach

049R30Z Drainage of Right Posterior Tibial Artery with Drainage Device, Percutaneous Approach

049R3ZX Drainage of Right Posterior Tibial Artery, Percutaneous Approach, Diagnostic

049R3ZZ Drainage of Right Posterior Tibial Artery, Percutaneous Approach

049R40Z Drainage of Right Posterior Tibial Artery with Drainage Device, Percutaneous Endoscopic Approach

049R4ZX Drainage of Right Posterior Tibial Artery, Percutaneous Endoscopic Approach, Diagnostic

049R4ZZ Drainage of Right Posterior Tibial Artery, Percutaneous Endoscopic Approach

049S00Z Drainage of Left Posterior Tibial Artery with Drainage Device, Open Approach

049S0ZX Drainage of Left Posterior Tibial Artery, Open Approach, Diagnostic

049S0ZZ Drainage of Left Posterior Tibial Artery, Open Approach

049S30Z Drainage of Left Posterior Tibial Artery with Drainage Device, Percutaneous Approach

049S3ZX Drainage of Left Posterior Tibial Artery, Percutaneous Approach, Diagnostic

049S3ZZ Drainage of Left Posterior Tibial Artery, Percutaneous Approach

049S40Z Drainage of Left Posterior Tibial Artery with Drainage Device, Percutaneous Endoscopic Approach

049S4ZX Drainage of Left Posterior Tibial Artery, Percutaneous Endoscopic Approach, Diagnostic

049S4ZZ Drainage of Left Posterior Tibial Artery, Percutaneous Endoscopic Approach

049T00Z Drainage of Right Peroneal Artery with Drainage Device, Open Approach

049T0ZX Drainage of Right Peroneal Artery, Open Approach, Diagnostic

049T0ZZ Drainage of Right Peroneal Artery, Open Approach

049T30Z Drainage of Right Peroneal Artery with Drainage Device, Percutaneous Approach

049T3ZX Drainage of Right Peroneal Artery, Percutaneous Approach, Diagnostic

049T3ZZ Drainage of Right Peroneal Artery, Percutaneous Approach

049T40Z Drainage of Right Peroneal Artery with Drainage Device, Percutaneous Endoscopic Approach

049T4ZX Drainage of Right Peroneal Artery, Percutaneous Endoscopic Approach, Diagnostic

049T4ZZ Drainage of Right Peroneal Artery, Percutaneous Endoscopic Approach

049U00Z Drainage of Left Peroneal Artery with Drainage Device, Open Approach

049U0ZX Drainage of Left Peroneal Artery, Open Approach, Diagnostic

049U0ZZ Drainage of Left Peroneal Artery, Open Approach

049U30Z Drainage of Left Peroneal Artery with Drainage Device, Percutaneous Approach

049U3ZX Drainage of Left Peroneal Artery, Percutaneous Approach, Diagnostic

049U3ZZ Drainage of Left Peroneal Artery, Percutaneous Approach

049U40Z Drainage of Left Peroneal Artery with Drainage Device, Percutaneous Endoscopic Approach

049U4ZX Drainage of Left Peroneal Artery, Percutaneous Endoscopic Approach, Diagnostic

049U4ZZ Drainage of Left Peroneal Artery, Percutaneous Endoscopic Approach

049V00Z Drainage of Right Foot Artery with Drainage Device, Open Approach

049V0ZX Drainage of Right Foot Artery, Open Approach, Diagnostic

049V0ZZ Drainage of Right Foot Artery, Open Approach

049V30Z Drainage of Right Foot Artery with Drainage Device, Percutaneous Approach

049V3ZX Drainage of Right Foot Artery, Percutaneous Approach, Diagnostic

049V3ZZ Drainage of Right Foot Artery, Percutaneous Approach

049V40Z Drainage of Right Foot Artery with Drainage Device, Percutaneous Endoscopic Approach

049V4ZX Drainage of Right Foot Artery, Percutaneous Endoscopic Approach, Diagnostic

049V4ZZ Drainage of Right Foot Artery, Percutaneous Endoscopic Approach

049W00Z Drainage of Left Foot Artery with Drainage Device, Open Approach

049W0ZX Drainage of Left Foot Artery, Open Approach, Diagnostic

049W0ZZ Drainage of Left Foot Artery, Open Approach

049W30Z Drainage of Left Foot Artery with Drainage Device, Percutaneous Approach

049W3ZX Drainage of Left Foot Artery, Percutaneous Approach, Diagnostic

049W3ZZ Drainage of Left Foot Artery, Percutaneous Approach

049W40Z Drainage of Left Foot Artery with Drainage Device, Percutaneous Endoscopic Approach

049W4ZX Drainage of Left Foot Artery, Percutaneous Endoscopic Approach, Diagnostic

049W4ZZ Drainage of Left Foot Artery, Percutaneous Endoscopic Approach

049Y00Z Drainage of Lower Artery with Drainage Device, Open Approach

049Y0ZX Drainage of Lower Artery, Open Approach, Diagnostic

049Y0ZZ Drainage of Lower Artery, Open Approach

049Y30Z Drainage of Lower Artery with Drainage Device, Percutaneous Approach

049Y3ZX Drainage of Lower Artery, Percutaneous Approach, Diagnostic

049Y3ZZ Drainage of Lower Artery, Percutaneous Approach

049Y40Z Drainage of Lower Artery with Drainage Device, Percutaneous Endoscopic Approach

049Y4ZX Drainage of Lower Artery, Percutaneous Endoscopic Approach, Diagnostic

049Y4ZZ Drainage of Lower Artery, Percutaneous Endoscopic Approach

04B – Lower Arteries, Excision

Review Coding Guidelines B3.4a and B3.4b

Review Coding Guideline B3.8

Review Coding Guideline B3.18

04B00ZX Excision of Abdominal Aorta, Open Approach, Diagnostic

04B00ZZ Excision of Abdominal Aorta, Open Approach

04B03ZX Excision of Abdominal Aorta, Percutaneous Approach, Diagnostic

04B03ZZ Excision of Abdominal Aorta, Percutaneous Approach

04B04ZX Excision of Abdominal Aorta, Percutaneous Endoscopic Approach, Diagnostic

04B04ZZ Excision of Abdominal Aorta, Percutaneous Endoscopic Approach

04B10ZX Excision of Celiac Artery, Open Approach, Diagnostic

04B10ZZ Excision of Celiac Artery, Open Approach

04B13ZX Excision of Celiac Artery, Percutaneous Approach, Diagnostic

04B13ZZ Excision of Celiac Artery, Percutaneous Approach

04B14ZX Excision of Celiac Artery, Percutaneous Endoscopic Approach, Diagnostic

04B14ZZ Excision of Celiac Artery, Percutaneous Endoscopic Approach

04B20ZX Excision of Gastric Artery, Open Approach, Diagnostic

04B20ZZ Excision of Gastric Artery, Open Approach

04B23ZX Excision of Gastric Artery, Percutaneous Approach, Diagnostic

04B23ZZ Excision of Gastric Artery, Percutaneous Approach

04B24ZX Excision of Gastric Artery, Percutaneous Endoscopic Approach, Diagnostic

04B24ZZ Excision of Gastric Artery, Percutaneous Endoscopic Approach

04B30ZX Excision of Hepatic Artery, Open Approach, Diagnostic

04B30ZZ Excision of Hepatic Artery, Open Approach

04B33ZX Excision of Hepatic Artery, Percutaneous Approach, Diagnostic

04B33ZZ Excision of Hepatic Artery, Percutaneous Approach

04B34ZX Excision of Hepatic Artery, Percutaneous Endoscopic Approach, Diagnostic

04B34ZZ Excision of Hepatic Artery, Percutaneous Endoscopic Approach

04B40ZX Excision of Splenic Artery, Open Approach, Diagnostic

04B40ZZ Excision of Splenic Artery, Open Approach

04B43ZX Excision of Splenic Artery, Percutaneous Approach, Diagnostic

04B43ZZ Excision of Splenic Artery, Percutaneous Approach

04B44ZX Excision of Splenic Artery, Percutaneous Endoscopic Approach, Diagnostic

04B44ZZ Excision of Splenic Artery, Percutaneous Endoscopic Approach

04B50ZX Excision of Superior Mesenteric Artery, Open Approach, Diagnostic

04B50ZZ Excision of Superior Mesenteric Artery, Open Approach

04B53ZX Excision of Superior Mesenteric Artery, Percutaneous Approach, Diagnostic

04B53ZZ Excision of Superior Mesenteric Artery, Percutaneous Approach

04B54ZX Excision of Superior Mesenteric Artery, Percutaneous Endoscopic Approach, Diagnostic

04B54ZZ Excision of Superior Mesenteric Artery, Percutaneous Endoscopic Approach

04B60ZX Excision of Right Colic Artery, Open Approach, Diagnostic

04B60ZZ Excision of Right Colic Artery, Open Approach

04B63ZX Excision of Right Colic Artery, Percutaneous Approach, Diagnostic

04B63ZZ Excision of Right Colic Artery, Percutaneous Approach

04B64ZX Excision of Right Colic Artery, Percutaneous Endoscopic Approach, Diagnostic

04B64ZZ Excision of Right Colic Artery, Percutaneous Endoscopic Approach

04B70ZX Excision of Left Colic Artery, Open Approach, Diagnostic

04B70ZZ Excision of Left Colic Artery, Open Approach

04B73ZX Excision of Left Colic Artery, Percutaneous Approach, Diagnostic

04B73ZZ Excision of Left Colic Artery, Percutaneous Approach

04B74ZX Excision of Left Colic Artery, Percutaneous Endoscopic Approach, Diagnostic

04B74ZZ Excision of Left Colic Artery, Percutaneous Endoscopic Approach

04B80ZX Excision of Middle Colic Artery, Open Approach, Diagnostic

04B80ZZ Excision of Middle Colic Artery, Open Approach

04B83ZX Excision of Middle Colic Artery, Percutaneous Approach, Diagnostic

04B83ZZ Excision of Middle Colic Artery, Percutaneous Approach

04B84ZX Excision of Middle Colic Artery, Percutaneous Endoscopic Approach, Diagnostic

04B84ZZ Excision of Middle Colic Artery, Percutaneous Endoscopic Approach

04B90ZX Excision of Right Renal Artery, Open Approach, Diagnostic

04B90ZZ Excision of Right Renal Artery, Open Approach

04B93ZX Excision of Right Renal Artery, Percutaneous Approach, Diagnostic

04B93ZZ Excision of Right Renal Artery, Percutaneous Approach

04B94ZX Excision of Right Renal Artery, Percutaneous Endoscopic Approach, Diagnostic

04B94ZZ Excision of Right Renal Artery, Percutaneous Endoscopic Approach

04BA0ZX Excision of Left Renal Artery, Open Approach, Diagnostic

04BA0ZZ Excision of Left Renal Artery, Open Approach

04BA3ZX Excision of Left Renal Artery, Percutaneous Approach, Diagnostic

04BA3ZZ Excision of Left Renal Artery, Percutaneous Approach

04BA4ZX Excision of Left Renal Artery, Percutaneous Endoscopic Approach, Diagnostic

04BA4ZZ Excision of Left Renal Artery, Percutaneous Endoscopic Approach

04BB0ZX Excision of Inferior Mesenteric Artery, Open Approach, Diagnostic

04BB0ZZ Excision of Inferior Mesenteric Artery, Open Approach

04BB3ZX Excision of Inferior Mesenteric Artery, Percutaneous Approach, Diagnostic

04BB3ZZ Excision of Inferior Mesenteric Artery, Percutaneous Approach

04BB4ZX Excision of Inferior Mesenteric Artery, Percutaneous Endoscopic Approach, Diagnostic

04BB4ZZ Excision of Inferior Mesenteric Artery, Percutaneous Endoscopic Approach

04BC0ZX Excision of Right Common Iliac Artery, Open Approach, Diagnostic

04BC0ZZ Excision of Right Common Iliac Artery, Open Approach

04BC3ZX Excision of Right Common Iliac Artery, Percutaneous Approach, Diagnostic

04BC3ZZ Excision of Right Common Iliac Artery, Percutaneous Approach

04BC4ZX Excision of Right Common Iliac Artery, Percutaneous Endoscopic Approach, Diagnostic

04BC4ZZ Excision of Right Common Iliac Artery, Percutaneous Endoscopic Approach

04BD0ZX Excision of Left Common Iliac Artery, Open Approach, Diagnostic

04BD0ZZ Excision of Left Common Iliac Artery, Open Approach

04BD3ZX Excision of Left Common Iliac Artery, Percutaneous Approach, Diagnostic

04BD3ZZ Excision of Left Common Iliac Artery, Percutaneous Approach

04BD4ZX Excision of Left Common Iliac Artery, Percutaneous Endoscopic Approach, Diagnostic

04BD4ZZ Excision of Left Common Iliac Artery, Percutaneous Endoscopic Approach

04BE0ZX Excision of Right Internal Iliac Artery, Open Approach, Diagnostic

04BE0ZZ Excision of Right Internal Iliac Artery, Open Approach

04BE3ZX Excision of Right Internal Iliac Artery, Percutaneous Approach, Diagnostic

04BE3ZZ Excision of Right Internal Iliac Artery, Percutaneous Approach

04BE4ZX Excision of Right Internal Iliac Artery, Percutaneous Endoscopic Approach, Diagnostic

04BE4ZZ Excision of Right Internal Iliac Artery, Percutaneous Endoscopic Approach

04BF0ZX Excision of Left Internal Iliac Artery, Open Approach, Diagnostic

04BF0ZZ Excision of Left Internal Iliac Artery, Open Approach

04BF3ZX Excision of Left Internal Iliac Artery, Percutaneous Approach, Diagnostic

04BF3ZZ Excision of Left Internal Iliac Artery, Percutaneous Approach

04BF4ZX Excision of Left Internal Iliac Artery, Percutaneous Endoscopic Approach, Diagnostic

04BF4ZZ Excision of Left Internal Iliac Artery, Percutaneous Endoscopic Approach

04BH0ZX Excision of Right External Iliac Artery, Open Approach, Diagnostic

04BH0ZZ Excision of Right External Iliac Artery, Open Approach

04BH3ZX Excision of Right External Iliac Artery, Percutaneous Approach, Diagnostic

04BH3ZZ Excision of Right External Iliac Artery, Percutaneous Approach

04BH4ZX Excision of Right External Iliac Artery, Percutaneous Endoscopic Approach, Diagnostic

04BH4ZZ Excision of Right External Iliac Artery, Percutaneous Endoscopic Approach

04BJ0ZX Excision of Left External Iliac Artery, Open Approach, Diagnostic

04BJ0ZZ Excision of Left External Iliac Artery, Open Approach

04BJ3ZX Excision of Left External Iliac Artery, Percutaneous Approach, Diagnostic

04BJ3ZZ Excision of Left External Iliac Artery, Percutaneous Approach

04BJ4ZX Excision of Left External Iliac Artery, Percutaneous Endoscopic Approach, Diagnostic

04BJ4ZZ Excision of Left External Iliac Artery, Percutaneous Endoscopic Approach

04BK0ZX Excision of Right Femoral Artery, Open Approach, Diagnostic

04BL4ZZ Excision of Left Femoral Artery, Percutaneous Endoscopic Approach

04BM0ZX Excision of Right Popliteal Artery, Open Approach, Diagnostic

04BM0ZZ Excision of Right Popliteal Artery, Open Approach

04BM3ZX Excision of Right Popliteal Artery, Percutaneous Approach, Diagnostic

04BM3ZZ Excision of Right Popliteal Artery, Percutaneous Approach

04BM4ZX Excision of Right Popliteal Artery, Percutaneous Endoscopic Approach, Diagnostic

♀ Female-only   ♂ Male-only   ▲ Limited Coverage   ● Non-OR   HAC HAC-associated procedure   ▲ Non-covered procedures   ✚ Cluster

04BM4ZZ Excision of Right Popliteal Artery, Percutaneous Endoscopic Approach

04BN0ZX Excision of Left Popliteal Artery, Open Approach, Diagnostic

04BN0ZZ Excision of Left Popliteal Artery, Open Approach

04BN3ZX Excision of Left Popliteal Artery, Percutaneous Approach, Diagnostic

04BN3ZZ Excision of Left Popliteal Artery, Percutaneous Approach

04BN4ZX Excision of Left Popliteal Artery, Percutaneous Endoscopic Approach, Diagnostic

04BN4ZZ Excision of Left Popliteal Artery, Percutaneous Endoscopic Approach

04BP0ZX Excision of Right Anterior Tibial Artery, Open Approach, Diagnostic

04BP0ZZ Excision of Right Anterior Tibial Artery, Open Approach

04BP3ZX Excision of Right Anterior Tibial Artery, Percutaneous Approach, Diagnostic

04BP3ZZ Excision of Right Anterior Tibial Artery, Percutaneous Approach

04BP4ZX Excision of Right Anterior Tibial Artery, Percutaneous Endoscopic Approach, Diagnostic

04BP4ZZ Excision of Right Anterior Tibial Artery, Percutaneous Endoscopic Approach

04BQ0ZX Excision of Left Anterior Tibial Artery, Open Approach, Diagnostic

04BQ0ZZ Excision of Left Anterior Tibial Artery, Open Approach

04BQ3ZX Excision of Left Anterior Tibial Artery, Percutaneous Approach, Diagnostic

04BQ3ZZ Excision of Left Anterior Tibial Artery, Percutaneous Approach

04BQ4ZX Excision of Left Anterior Tibial Artery, Percutaneous Endoscopic Approach, Diagnostic

04BQ4ZZ Excision of Left Anterior Tibial Artery, Percutaneous Endoscopic Approach

04BR0ZX Excision of Right Posterior Tibial Artery, Open Approach, Diagnostic

04BR0ZZ Excision of Right Posterior Tibial Artery, Open Approach

04BR3ZX Excision of Right Posterior Tibial Artery, Percutaneous Approach, Diagnostic

04BR3ZZ Excision of Right Posterior Tibial Artery, Percutaneous Approach

04BR4ZX Excision of Right Posterior Tibial Artery, Percutaneous Endoscopic Approach, Diagnostic

04BR4ZZ Excision of Right Posterior Tibial Artery, Percutaneous Endoscopic Approach

04BS0ZX Excision of Left Posterior Tibial Artery, Open Approach, Diagnostic

04BS0ZZ Excision of Left Posterior Tibial Artery, Open Approach

04BS3ZX Excision of Left Posterior Tibial Artery, Percutaneous Approach, Diagnostic

04BS3ZZ Excision of Left Posterior Tibial Artery, Percutaneous Approach

04BS4ZX Excision of Left Posterior Tibial Artery, Percutaneous Endoscopic Approach, Diagnostic

04BS4ZZ Excision of Left Posterior Tibial Artery, Percutaneous Endoscopic Approach

04BT0ZX Excision of Right Peroneal Artery, Open Approach, Diagnostic

04BT0ZZ Excision of Right Peroneal Artery, Open Approach

04BT3ZX Excision of Right Peroneal Artery, Percutaneous Approach, Diagnostic

04BT3ZZ Excision of Right Peroneal Artery, Percutaneous Approach

04BT4ZX Excision of Right Peroneal Artery, Percutaneous Endoscopic Approach, Diagnostic

04BT4ZZ Excision of Right Peroneal Artery, Percutaneous Endoscopic Approach

04BU0ZX Excision of Left Peroneal Artery, Open Approach, Diagnostic

04BU0ZZ Excision of Left Peroneal Artery, Open Approach

04BU3ZX Excision of Left Peroneal Artery, Percutaneous Approach, Diagnostic

04BU3ZZ Excision of Left Peroneal Artery, Percutaneous Approach

04BU4ZX Excision of Left Peroneal Artery, Percutaneous Endoscopic Approach, Diagnostic

04BU4ZZ Excision of Left Peroneal Artery, Percutaneous Endoscopic Approach

04BV0ZX Excision of Right Foot Artery, Open Approach, Diagnostic

04BV0ZZ Excision of Right Foot Artery, Open Approach

04BV3ZX Excision of Right Foot Artery, Percutaneous Approach, Diagnostic

04BV3ZZ Excision of Right Foot Artery, Percutaneous Approach

04BV4ZX Excision of Right Foot Artery, Percutaneous Endoscopic Approach, Diagnostic

04BV4ZZ Excision of Right Foot Artery, Percutaneous Endoscopic Approach

04BW0ZX Excision of Left Foot Artery, Open Approach, Diagnostic

04BW0ZZ Excision of Left Foot Artery, Open Approach

04BW3ZX Excision of Left Foot Artery, Percutaneous Approach, Diagnostic

04BW3ZZ Excision of Left Foot Artery, Percutaneous Approach

04BW4ZX Excision of Left Foot Artery, Percutaneous Endoscopic Approach, Diagnostic

04BW4ZZ Excision of Left Foot Artery, Percutaneous Endoscopic Approach

04BY0ZX Excision of Lower Artery, Open Approach, Diagnostic

04BY0ZZ Excision of Lower Artery, Open Approach

04BY3ZX Excision of Lower Artery, Percutaneous Approach, Diagnostic

04BY3ZZ Excision of Lower Artery, Percutaneous Approach

04BY4ZX Excision of Lower Artery, Percutaneous Endoscopic Approach, Diagnostic

04BY4ZZ Excision of Lower Artery, Percutaneous Endoscopic Approach

04C – Lower Arteries, Extirpation

04C00ZZ Extirpation of Matter from Abdominal Aorta, Open Approach

04C03ZZ Extirpation of Matter from Abdominal Aorta, Percutaneous Approach

04C04ZZ Extirpation of Matter from Abdominal Aorta, Percutaneous Endoscopic Approach

04C10ZZ Extirpation of Matter from Celiac Artery, Open Approach

04C13ZZ Extirpation of Matter from Celiac Artery, Percutaneous Approach

04C14ZZ Extirpation of Matter from Celiac Artery, Percutaneous Endoscopic Approach

04C20ZZ Extirpation of Matter from Gastric Artery, Open Approach

04C23ZZ Extirpation of Matter from Gastric Artery, Percutaneous Approach

04C24ZZ Extirpation of Matter from Gastric Artery, Percutaneous Endoscopic Approach

04C30ZZ Extirpation of Matter from Hepatic Artery, Open Approach

04C33ZZ Extirpation of Matter from Hepatic Artery, Percutaneous Approach

04C34ZZ Extirpation of Matter from Hepatic Artery, Percutaneous Endoscopic Approach

04C40ZZ Extirpation of Matter from Splenic Artery, Open Approach

04C43ZZ Extirpation of Matter from Splenic Artery, Percutaneous Approach

04C44ZZ Extirpation of Matter from Splenic Artery, Percutaneous Endoscopic Approach

04C50ZZ Extirpation of Matter from Superior Mesenteric Artery, Open Approach

04C53ZZ Extirpation of Matter from Superior Mesenteric Artery, Percutaneous Approach

04C54ZZ Extirpation of Matter from Superior Mesenteric Artery, Percutaneous Endoscopic Approach

04C60ZZ Extirpation of Matter from Right Colic Artery, Open Approach

04C63ZZ Extirpation of Matter from Right Colic Artery, Percutaneous Approach

04C64ZZ Extirpation of Matter from Right Colic Artery, Percutaneous Endoscopic Approach

04C70ZZ Extirpation of Matter from Left Colic Artery, Open Approach

04C73ZZ Extirpation of Matter from Left Colic Artery, Percutaneous Approach

04C74ZZ Extirpation of Matter from Left Colic Artery, Percutaneous Endoscopic Approach

04C80ZZ Extirpation of Matter from Middle Colic Artery, Open Approach

04C83ZZ Extirpation of Matter from Middle Colic Artery, Percutaneous Approach

04C84ZZ Extirpation of Matter from Middle Colic Artery, Percutaneous Endoscopic Approach

04C90ZZ Extirpation of Matter from Right Renal Artery, Open Approach

04C93ZZ Extirpation of Matter from Right Renal Artery, Percutaneous Approach

04C94ZZ Extirpation of Matter from Right Renal Artery, Percutaneous Endoscopic Approach

04CA0ZZ Extirpation of Matter from Left Renal Artery, Open Approach

04CA3ZZ Extirpation of Matter from Left Renal Artery, Percutaneous Approach

04CA4ZZ Extirpation of Matter from Left Renal Artery, Percutaneous Endoscopic Approach

04CB0ZZ Extirpation of Matter from Inferior Mesenteric Artery, Open Approach

04CB3ZZ Extirpation of Matter from Inferior Mesenteric Artery, Percutaneous Approach

04CB4ZZ Extirpation of Matter from Inferior Mesenteric Artery, Percutaneous Endoscopic Approach

04CC0ZZ Extirpation of Matter from Right Common Iliac Artery, Open Approach

04CC3ZZ Extirpation of Matter from Right Common Iliac Artery, Percutaneous Approach

04CC4ZZ Extirpation of Matter from Right Common Iliac Artery, Percutaneous Endoscopic Approach

04CD0ZZ Extirpation of Matter from Left Common Iliac Artery, Open Approach

04CD3ZZ Extirpation of Matter from Left Common Iliac Artery, Percutaneous Approach

04CD4ZZ Extirpation of Matter from Left Common Iliac Artery, Percutaneous Endoscopic Approach

04CE0ZZ Extirpation of Matter from Right Internal Iliac Artery, Open Approach

04CE3ZZ Extirpation of Matter from Right Internal Iliac Artery, Percutaneous Approach

04CE4ZZ Extirpation of Matter from Right Internal Iliac Artery, Percutaneous Endoscopic Approach

04CF0ZZ Extirpation of Matter from Left Internal Iliac Artery, Open Approach

04CF3ZZ Extirpation of Matter from Left Internal Iliac Artery, Percutaneous Approach

04CF4ZZ Extirpation of Matter from Left Internal Iliac Artery, Percutaneous Endoscopic Approach

04CH0ZZ Extirpation of Matter from Right External Iliac Artery, Open Approach
AHA CC: 1Q, 2021, 15-16

04CH3ZZ Extirpation of Matter from Right External Iliac Artery, Percutaneous Approach

04CH4ZZ Extirpation of Matter from Right External Iliac Artery, Percutaneous Endoscopic Approach

04CJ0ZZ Extirpation of Matter from Left External Iliac Artery, Open Approach
AHA CC: 1Q, 2016, 31; 1Q, 2021, 15-16

04CJ3ZZ Extirpation of Matter from Left External Iliac Artery, Percutaneous Approach

04CJ4ZZ Extirpation of Matter from Left External Iliac Artery, Percutaneous Endoscopic Approach

04CK0ZZ Extirpation of Matter from Right Femoral Artery, Open Approach

04CK3ZZ Extirpation of Matter from Right Femoral Artery, Percutaneous Approach

04CK4ZZ Extirpation of Matter from Right Femoral Artery, Percutaneous Endoscopic Approach

04CL0ZZ Extirpation of Matter from Left Femoral Artery, Open Approach

04CL3ZZ Extirpation of Matter from Left Femoral Artery, Percutaneous Approach
AHA CC: 1Q, 2015, 36

04CL4ZZ Extirpation of Matter from Left Femoral Artery, Percutaneous Endoscopic Approach

04CM0ZZ Extirpation of Matter from Right Popliteal Artery, Open Approach

04CM3ZZ Extirpation of Matter from Right Popliteal Artery, Percutaneous Approach

04CM4ZZ Extirpation of Matter from Right Popliteal Artery, Percutaneous Endoscopic Approach

04CN0ZZ Extirpation of Matter from Left Popliteal Artery, Open Approach

04CN3ZZ Extirpation of Matter from Left Popliteal Artery, Percutaneous Approach

04CN4ZZ Extirpation of Matter from Left Popliteal Artery, Percutaneous Endoscopic Approach

04CP0ZZ Extirpation of Matter from Right Anterior Tibial Artery, Open Approach

04CP3ZZ Extirpation of Matter from Right Anterior Tibial Artery, Percutaneous Approach

04CP4ZZ Extirpation of Matter from Right Anterior Tibial Artery, Percutaneous Endoscopic Approach

04CQ0ZZ Extirpation of Matter from Left Anterior Tibial Artery, Open Approach

04CQ3ZZ Extirpation of Matter from Left Anterior Tibial Artery, Percutaneous Approach

04CQ4ZZ Extirpation of Matter from Left Anterior Tibial Artery, Percutaneous Endoscopic Approach

04CR0ZZ Extirpation of Matter from Right Posterior Tibial Artery, Open Approach

04CR3ZZ Extirpation of Matter from Right Posterior Tibial Artery, Percutaneous Approach

04CR4ZZ Extirpation of Matter from Right Posterior Tibial Artery, Percutaneous Endoscopic Approach

04CS0ZZ Extirpation of Matter from Left Posterior Tibial Artery, Open Approach

04CS3ZZ Extirpation of Matter from Left Posterior Tibial Artery, Percutaneous Approach

04CS4ZZ Extirpation of Matter from Left Posterior Tibial Artery, Percutaneous Endoscopic Approach

04CT0ZZ Extirpation of Matter from Right Peroneal Artery, Open Approach

04CT3ZZ Extirpation of Matter from Right Peroneal Artery, Percutaneous Approach

04CT4ZZ Extirpation of Matter from Right Peroneal Artery, Percutaneous Endoscopic Approach

04CU0ZZ Extirpation of Matter from Left Peroneal Artery, Open Approach

04CU3ZZ Extirpation of Matter from Left Peroneal Artery, Percutaneous Approach

04CU4ZZ Extirpation of Matter from Left Peroneal Artery, Percutaneous Endoscopic Approach

04CV0ZZ Extirpation of Matter from Right Foot Artery, Open Approach

04CV3ZZ Extirpation of Matter from Right Foot Artery, Percutaneous Approach

04CV4ZZ Extirpation of Matter from Right Foot Artery, Percutaneous Endoscopic Approach

04CW0ZZ Extirpation of Matter from Left Foot Artery, Open Approach

04CW3ZZ Extirpation of Matter from Left Foot Artery, Percutaneous Approach

04CW4ZZ Extirpation of Matter from Left Foot Artery, Percutaneous Endoscopic Approach

04CY0ZZ Extirpation of Matter from Lower Artery, Open Approach

04CY3ZZ Extirpation of Matter from Lower Artery, Percutaneous Approach

04CY4ZZ Extirpation of Matter from Lower Artery, Percutaneous Endoscopic Approach

04F – Lower Arteries, Fragmentation

04FC3Z0 Fragmentation of Right Common Iliac Artery, Percutaneous Approach, Ultrasonic

04FC3ZZ Fragmentation of Right Common Iliac Artery, Percutaneous Approach
AHA CC: 4Q, 2020, 51-52

04FD3Z0 Fragmentation of Left Common Iliac Artery, Percutaneous Approach, Ultrasonic

04FD3ZZ Fragmentation of Left Common Iliac Artery, Percutaneous Approach

04FE3Z0 Fragmentation of Right Internal Iliac Artery, Percutaneous Approach, Ultrasonic

04FE3ZZ Fragmentation of Right Internal Iliac Artery, Percutaneous Approach

04FF3Z0 Fragmentation of Left Internal Iliac Artery, Percutaneous Approach, Ultrasonic

04FF3ZZ Fragmentation of Left Internal Iliac Artery, Percutaneous Approach

04FH3Z0 Fragmentation of Right External Iliac Artery, Percutaneous Approach, Ultrasonic

04FH3ZZ Fragmentation of Right External Iliac Artery, Percutaneous Approach
AHA CC: 4Q, 2020, 50-52

04FJ3Z0 Fragmentation of Left External Iliac Artery, Percutaneous Approach, Ultrasonic

04FJ3ZZ Fragmentation of Left External Iliac Artery, Percutaneous Approach

04FK3Z0 Fragmentation of Right Femoral Artery, Percutaneous Approach, Ultrasonic

04FK3ZZ Fragmentation of Right Femoral Artery, Percutaneous Approach
AHA CC: 4Q, 2020, 50-51

04FL3Z0 Fragmentation of Left Femoral Artery, Percutaneous Approach, Ultrasonic

04FL3ZZ Fragmentation of Left Femoral Artery, Percutaneous Approach

04FM3Z0 Fragmentation of Right Popliteal Artery, Percutaneous Approach, Ultrasonic

04FM3ZZ Fragmentation of Right Popliteal Artery, Percutaneous Approach

04FN3Z0 Fragmentation of Left Popliteal Artery, Percutaneous Approach, Ultrasonic

04FN3ZZ Fragmentation of Left Popliteal Artery, Percutaneous Approach

04FP3Z0 Fragmentation of Right Anterior Tibial Artery, Percutaneous Approach, Ultrasonic

04FP3ZZ Fragmentation of Right Anterior Tibial Artery, Percutaneous Approach

04FQ3Z0 Fragmentation of Left Anterior Tibial Artery, Percutaneous Approach, Ultrasonic

04FQ3ZZ Fragmentation of Left Anterior Tibial Artery, Percutaneous Approach

♀ Female-only   ♂ Male-only   ▲ Limited Coverage   ● Non-OR   ᴴᴬᶜ HAC-associated procedure   ▲ Non-covered procedures   ✚ Cluster

04FR3Z0 Fragmentation of Right Posterior Tibial Artery, Percutaneous Approach, Ultrasonic

04FR3ZZ Fragmentation of Right Posterior Tibial Artery, Percutaneous Approach

04FS3Z0 Fragmentation of Left Posterior Tibial Artery, Percutaneous Approach, Ultrasonic

04FS3ZZ Fragmentation of Left Posterior Tibial Artery, Percutaneous Approach

04FT3Z0 Fragmentation of Right Peroneal Artery, Percutaneous Approach, Ultrasonic

04FT3ZZ Fragmentation of Right Peroneal Artery, Percutaneous Approach

04FU3Z0 Fragmentation of Left Peroneal Artery, Percutaneous Approach, Ultrasonic

04FU3ZZ Fragmentation of Left Peroneal Artery, Percutaneous Approach

04FY3Z0 Fragmentation of Lower Artery, Percutaneous Approach, Ultrasonic

04FY3ZZ Fragmentation of Lower Artery, Percutaneous Approach

04H – Lower Arteries, Insertion

04H002Z Insertion of Monitoring Device into Abdominal Aorta, Open Approach

04H003Z Insertion of Infusion Device into Abdominal Aorta, Open Approach

04H00DZ Insertion of Intraluminal Device into Abdominal Aorta, Open Approach

04H032Z Insertion of Monitoring Device into Abdominal Aorta, Percutaneous Approach

04H033Z Insertion of Infusion Device into Abdominal Aorta, Percutaneous Approach

04H03DZ Insertion of Intraluminal Device into Abdominal Aorta, Percutaneous Approach

04H042Z Insertion of Monitoring Device into Abdominal Aorta, Percutaneous Endoscopic Approach

04H043Z Insertion of Infusion Device into Abdominal Aorta, Percutaneous Endoscopic Approach

04H04DZ Insertion of Intraluminal Device into Abdominal Aorta, Percutaneous Endoscopic Approach

04H103Z Insertion of Infusion Device into Celiac Artery, Open Approach

04H10DZ Insertion of Intraluminal Device into Celiac Artery, Open Approach

04H133Z Insertion of Infusion Device into Celiac Artery, Percutaneous Approach

04H13DZ Insertion of Intraluminal Device into Celiac Artery, Percutaneous Approach
AHA CC: 1Q, 2019, 23

04H143Z Insertion of Infusion Device into Celiac Artery, Percutaneous Endoscopic Approach

04H14DZ Insertion of Intraluminal Device into Celiac Artery, Percutaneous Endoscopic Approach

04H203Z Insertion of Infusion Device into Gastric Artery, Open Approach

04H20DZ Insertion of Intraluminal Device into Gastric Artery, Open Approach

04H233Z Insertion of Infusion Device into Gastric Artery, Percutaneous Approach

04H23DZ Insertion of Intraluminal Device into Gastric Artery, Percutaneous Approach

04H243Z Insertion of Infusion Device into Gastric Artery, Percutaneous Endoscopic Approach

04H24DZ Insertion of Intraluminal Device into Gastric Artery, Percutaneous Endoscopic Approach

04H303Z Insertion of Infusion Device into Hepatic Artery, Open Approach

04H30DZ Insertion of Intraluminal Device into Hepatic Artery, Open Approach

04H333Z Insertion of Infusion Device into Hepatic Artery, Percutaneous Approach

04H33DZ Insertion of Intraluminal Device into Hepatic Artery, Percutaneous Approach

04H343Z Insertion of Infusion Device into Hepatic Artery, Percutaneous Endoscopic Approach

04H34DZ Insertion of Intraluminal Device into Hepatic Artery, Percutaneous Endoscopic Approach

04H403Z Insertion of Infusion Device into Splenic Artery, Open Approach

04H40DZ Insertion of Intraluminal Device into Splenic Artery, Open Approach

04H433Z Insertion of Infusion Device into Splenic Artery, Percutaneous Approach

04H43DZ Insertion of Intraluminal Device into Splenic Artery, Percutaneous Approach

04H443Z Insertion of Infusion Device into Splenic Artery, Percutaneous Endoscopic Approach

04H44DZ Insertion of Intraluminal Device into Splenic Artery, Percutaneous Endoscopic Approach

04H503Z Insertion of Infusion Device into Superior Mesenteric Artery, Open Approach

04H50DZ Insertion of Intraluminal Device into Superior Mesenteric Artery, Open Approach

04H533Z Insertion of Infusion Device into Superior Mesenteric Artery, Percutaneous Approach

04H53DZ Insertion of Intraluminal Device into Superior Mesenteric Artery, Percutaneous Approach
AHA CC: 1Q, 2019, 23

04H543Z Insertion of Infusion Device into Superior Mesenteric Artery, Percutaneous Endoscopic Approach

04H54DZ Insertion of Intraluminal Device into Superior Mesenteric Artery, Percutaneous Endoscopic Approach

04H603Z Insertion of Infusion Device into Right Colic Artery, Open Approach

04H60DZ Insertion of Intraluminal Device into Right Colic Artery, Open Approach

04H633Z Insertion of Infusion Device into Right Colic Artery, Percutaneous Approach

04H63DZ Insertion of Intraluminal Device into Right Colic Artery, Percutaneous Approach

04H643Z Insertion of Infusion Device into Right Colic Artery, Percutaneous Endoscopic Approach

04H64DZ Insertion of Intraluminal Device into Right Colic Artery, Percutaneous Endoscopic Approach

04H703Z Insertion of Infusion Device into Left Colic Artery, Open Approach

04H70DZ Insertion of Intraluminal Device into Left Colic Artery, Open Approach

04H733Z Insertion of Infusion Device into Left Colic Artery, Percutaneous Approach

04H73DZ Insertion of Intraluminal Device into Left Colic Artery, Percutaneous Approach

04H743Z Insertion of Infusion Device into Left Colic Artery, Percutaneous Endoscopic Approach

04H74DZ Insertion of Intraluminal Device into Left Colic Artery, Percutaneous Endoscopic Approach

04H803Z Insertion of Infusion Device into Middle Colic Artery, Open Approach

04H80DZ Insertion of Intraluminal Device into Middle Colic Artery, Open Approach

04H833Z Insertion of Infusion Device into Middle Colic Artery, Percutaneous Approach

04H83DZ Insertion of Intraluminal Device into Middle Colic Artery, Percutaneous Approach

04H843Z Insertion of Infusion Device into Middle Colic Artery, Percutaneous Endoscopic Approach

04H84DZ Insertion of Intraluminal Device into Middle Colic Artery, Percutaneous Endoscopic Approach

04H903Z Insertion of Infusion Device into Right Renal Artery, Open Approach

04H90DZ Insertion of Intraluminal Device into Right Renal Artery, Open Approach

04H933Z Insertion of Infusion Device into Right Renal Artery, Percutaneous Approach

04H93DZ Insertion of Intraluminal Device into Right Renal Artery, Percutaneous Approach
AHA CC: 1Q, 2019, 23

04H943Z Insertion of Infusion Device into Right Renal Artery, Percutaneous Endoscopic Approach

04H94DZ Insertion of Intraluminal Device into Right Renal Artery, Percutaneous Endoscopic Approach

04HA03Z Insertion of Infusion Device into Left Renal Artery, Open Approach

04HA0DZ Insertion of Intraluminal Device into Left Renal Artery, Open Approach

04HA33Z Insertion of Infusion Device into Left Renal Artery, Percutaneous Approach

04HA3DZ Insertion of Intraluminal Device into Left Renal Artery, Percutaneous Approach
AHA CC: 1Q, 2019, 23

04HA43Z Insertion of Infusion Device into Left Renal Artery, Percutaneous Endoscopic Approach

04HA4DZ Insertion of Intraluminal Device into Left Renal Artery, Percutaneous Endoscopic Approach

04HB03Z Insertion of Infusion Device into Inferior Mesenteric Artery, Open Approach

04HB0DZ Insertion of Intraluminal Device into Inferior Mesenteric Artery, Open Approach

04HB33Z Insertion of Infusion Device into Inferior Mesenteric Artery, Percutaneous Approach

04HB3DZ Insertion of Intraluminal Device into Inferior Mesenteric Artery, Percutaneous Approach

04HB43Z Insertion of Infusion Device into Inferior Mesenteric Artery, Percutaneous Endoscopic Approach

04HB4DZ Insertion of Intraluminal Device into Inferior Mesenteric Artery, Percutaneous Endoscopic Approach

04HC03Z Insertion of Infusion Device into Right Common Iliac Artery, Open Approach

04HC0DZ Insertion of Intraluminal Device into Right Common Iliac Artery, Open Approach

04HC33Z Insertion of Infusion Device into Right Common Iliac Artery, Percutaneous Approach

04HC3DZ Insertion of Intraluminal Device into Right Common Iliac Artery, Percutaneous Approach

04HC43Z Insertion of Infusion Device into Right Common Iliac Artery, Percutaneous Endoscopic Approach

04HC4DZ Insertion of Intraluminal Device into Right Common Iliac Artery, Percutaneous Endoscopic Approach

04HD03Z Insertion of Infusion Device into Left Common Iliac Artery, Open Approach

04HD0DZ Insertion of Intraluminal Device into Left Common Iliac Artery, Open Approach

04HD33Z Insertion of Infusion Device into Left Common Iliac Artery, Percutaneous Approach

04HD3DZ Insertion of Intraluminal Device into Left Common Iliac Artery, Percutaneous Approach

04HD43Z Insertion of Infusion Device into Left Common Iliac Artery, Percutaneous Endoscopic Approach

04HD4DZ Insertion of Intraluminal Device into Left Common Iliac Artery, Percutaneous Endoscopic Approach

04HE03Z Insertion of Infusion Device into Right Internal Iliac Artery, Open Approach

04HE0DZ Insertion of Intraluminal Device into Right Internal Iliac Artery, Open Approach

04HE33Z Insertion of Infusion Device into Right Internal Iliac Artery, Percutaneous Approach

04HE3DZ Insertion of Intraluminal Device into Right Internal Iliac Artery, Percutaneous Approach

04HE43Z Insertion of Infusion Device into Right Internal Iliac Artery, Percutaneous Endoscopic Approach

04HE4DZ Insertion of Intraluminal Device into Right Internal Iliac Artery, Percutaneous Endoscopic Approach

04HF03Z Insertion of Infusion Device into Left Internal Iliac Artery, Open Approach

04HF0DZ Insertion of Intraluminal Device into Left Internal Iliac Artery, Open Approach

04HF33Z Insertion of Infusion Device into Left Internal Iliac Artery, Percutaneous Approach

04HF3DZ Insertion of Intraluminal Device into Left Internal Iliac Artery, Percutaneous Approach

04HF43Z Insertion of Infusion Device into Left Internal Iliac Artery, Percutaneous Endoscopic Approach

04HF4DZ Insertion of Intraluminal Device into Left Internal Iliac Artery, Percutaneous Endoscopic Approach

04HH03Z Insertion of Infusion Device into Right External Iliac Artery, Open Approach

04HH0DZ Insertion of Intraluminal Device into Right External Iliac Artery, Open Approach

04HH33Z Insertion of Infusion Device into Right External Iliac Artery, Percutaneous Approach

04HH3DZ Insertion of Intraluminal Device into Right External Iliac Artery, Percutaneous Approach

04HH43Z Insertion of Infusion Device into Right External Iliac Artery, Percutaneous Endoscopic Approach

04HH4DZ Insertion of Intraluminal Device into Right External Iliac Artery, Percutaneous Endoscopic Approach

04HJ03Z Insertion of Infusion Device into Left External Iliac Artery, Open Approach

04HJ0DZ Insertion of Intraluminal Device into Left External Iliac Artery, Open Approach

04HJ33Z Insertion of Infusion Device into Left External Iliac Artery, Percutaneous Approach

04HJ3DZ Insertion of Intraluminal Device into Left External Iliac Artery, Percutaneous Approach

04HJ43Z Insertion of Infusion Device into Left External Iliac Artery, Percutaneous Endoscopic Approach

04HJ4DZ Insertion of Intraluminal Device into Left External Iliac Artery, Percutaneous Endoscopic Approach

04HK03Z Insertion of Infusion Device into Right Femoral Artery, Open Approach

04HK0DZ Insertion of Intraluminal Device into Right Femoral Artery, Open Approach

04HK33Z Insertion of Infusion Device into Right Femoral Artery, Percutaneous Approach

04HK3DZ Insertion of Intraluminal Device into Right Femoral Artery, Percutaneous Approach

04HK43Z Insertion of Infusion Device into Right Femoral Artery, Percutaneous Endoscopic Approach

04HK4DZ Insertion of Intraluminal Device into Right Femoral Artery, Percutaneous Endoscopic Approach

04HL03Z Insertion of Infusion Device into Left Femoral Artery, Open Approach

04HL0DZ Insertion of Intraluminal Device into Left Femoral Artery, Open Approach

04HL33Z Insertion of Infusion Device into Left Femoral Artery, Percutaneous Approach

04HL3DZ Insertion of Intraluminal Device into Left Femoral Artery, Percutaneous Approach

04HL43Z Insertion of Infusion Device into Left Femoral Artery, Percutaneous Endoscopic Approach

04HL4DZ Insertion of Intraluminal Device into Left Femoral Artery, Percutaneous Endoscopic Approach

04HM03Z Insertion of Infusion Device into Right Popliteal Artery, Open Approach

04HM0DZ Insertion of Intraluminal Device into Right Popliteal Artery, Open Approach

04HM33Z Insertion of Infusion Device into Right Popliteal Artery, Percutaneous Approach

04HM3DZ Insertion of Intraluminal Device into Right Popliteal Artery, Percutaneous Approach

04HM43Z Insertion of Infusion Device into Right Popliteal Artery, Percutaneous Endoscopic Approach

04HM4DZ Insertion of Intraluminal Device into Right Popliteal Artery, Percutaneous Endoscopic Approach

04HN03Z Insertion of Infusion Device into Left Popliteal Artery, Open Approach

04HN0DZ Insertion of Intraluminal Device into Left Popliteal Artery, Open Approach

04HN33Z Insertion of Infusion Device into Left Popliteal Artery, Percutaneous Approach

04HN3DZ Insertion of Intraluminal Device into Left Popliteal Artery, Percutaneous Approach

04HN43Z Insertion of Infusion Device into Left Popliteal Artery, Percutaneous Endoscopic Approach

04HN4DZ Insertion of Intraluminal Device into Left Popliteal Artery, Percutaneous Endoscopic Approach

04HP03Z Insertion of Infusion Device into Right Anterior Tibial Artery, Open Approach

04HP0DZ Insertion of Intraluminal Device into Right Anterior Tibial Artery, Open Approach

04HP33Z Insertion of Infusion Device into Right Anterior Tibial Artery, Percutaneous Approach

04HP3DZ Insertion of Intraluminal Device into Right Anterior Tibial Artery, Percutaneous Approach

04HP43Z Insertion of Infusion Device into Right Anterior Tibial Artery, Percutaneous Endoscopic Approach

04HP4DZ Insertion of Intraluminal Device into Right Anterior Tibial Artery, Percutaneous Endoscopic Approach

04HQ03Z Insertion of Infusion Device into Left Anterior Tibial Artery, Open Approach

04HQ0DZ Insertion of Intraluminal Device into Left Anterior Tibial Artery, Open Approach

04HQ33Z Insertion of Infusion Device into Left Anterior Tibial Artery, Percutaneous Approach

04HQ3DZ Insertion of Intraluminal Device into Left Anterior Tibial Artery, Percutaneous Approach

04HQ43Z Insertion of Infusion Device into Left Anterior Tibial Artery, Percutaneous Endoscopic Approach

04HQ4DZ Insertion of Intraluminal Device into Left Anterior Tibial Artery, Percutaneous Endoscopic Approach

04HR03Z Insertion of Infusion Device into Right Posterior Tibial Artery, Open Approach

04HR0DZ Insertion of Intraluminal Device into Right Posterior Tibial Artery, Open Approach

04HR33Z Insertion of Infusion Device into Right Posterior Tibial Artery, Percutaneous Approach

04HR3DZ Insertion of Intraluminal Device into Right Posterior Tibial Artery, Percutaneous Approach

04HR43Z Insertion of Infusion Device into Right Posterior Tibial Artery, Percutaneous Endoscopic Approach

04HR4DZ Insertion of Intraluminal Device into Right Posterior Tibial Artery, Percutaneous Endoscopic Approach

04HS03Z Insertion of Infusion Device into Left Posterior Tibial Artery, Open Approach

04HS0DZ Insertion of Intraluminal Device into Left Posterior Tibial Artery, Open Approach

♀ Female-only ♂ Male-only ▲ Limited Coverage ● Non-OR ⬛ HAC-associated procedure ▲ Non-covered procedures ✚ Cluster

04HS33Z Insertion of Infusion Device into Left Posterior Tibial Artery, Percutaneous Approach

04HS3DZ Insertion of Intraluminal Device into Left Posterior Tibial Artery, Percutaneous Approach

04HS43Z Insertion of Infusion Device into Left Posterior Tibial Artery, Percutaneous Endoscopic Approach

04HS4DZ Insertion of Intraluminal Device into Left Posterior Tibial Artery, Percutaneous Endoscopic Approach

04HT03Z Insertion of Infusion Device into Right Peroneal Artery, Open Approach

04HT0DZ Insertion of Intraluminal Device into Right Peroneal Artery, Open Approach

04HT33Z Insertion of Infusion Device into Right Peroneal Artery, Percutaneous Approach

04HT3DZ Insertion of Intraluminal Device into Right Peroneal Artery, Percutaneous Approach

04HT43Z Insertion of Infusion Device into Right Peroneal Artery, Percutaneous Endoscopic Approach

04HT4DZ Insertion of Intraluminal Device into Right Peroneal Artery, Percutaneous Endoscopic Approach

04HU03Z Insertion of Infusion Device into Left Peroneal Artery, Open Approach

04HU0DZ Insertion of Intraluminal Device into Left Peroneal Artery, Open Approach

04HU33Z Insertion of Infusion Device into Left Peroneal Artery, Percutaneous Approach

04HU3DZ Insertion of Intraluminal Device into Left Peroneal Artery, Percutaneous Approach

04HU43Z Insertion of Infusion Device into Left Peroneal Artery, Percutaneous Endoscopic Approach

04HU4DZ Insertion of Intraluminal Device into Left Peroneal Artery, Percutaneous Endoscopic Approach

04HV03Z Insertion of Infusion Device into Right Foot Artery, Open Approach

04HV0DZ Insertion of Intraluminal Device into Right Foot Artery, Open Approach

04HV33Z Insertion of Infusion Device into Right Foot Artery, Percutaneous Approach

04HV3DZ Insertion of Intraluminal Device into Right Foot Artery, Percutaneous Approach

04HV43Z Insertion of Infusion Device into Right Foot Artery, Percutaneous Endoscopic Approach

04HV4DZ Insertion of Intraluminal Device into Right Foot Artery, Percutaneous Endoscopic Approach

04HW03Z Insertion of Infusion Device into Left Foot Artery, Open Approach

04HW0DZ Insertion of Intraluminal Device into Left Foot Artery, Open Approach

04HW33Z Insertion of Infusion Device into Left Foot Artery, Percutaneous Approach

04HW3DZ Insertion of Intraluminal Device into Left Foot Artery, Percutaneous Approach

04HW43Z Insertion of Infusion Device into Left Foot Artery, Percutaneous Endoscopic Approach

04HW4DZ Insertion of Intraluminal Device into Left Foot Artery, Percutaneous Endoscopic Approach

04HY02Z Insertion of Monitoring Device into Lower Artery, Open Approach

04HY03Z Insertion of Infusion Device into Lower Artery, Open Approach

04HY0DZ Insertion of Intraluminal Device into Lower Artery, Open Approach

04HY0YZ Insertion of Other Device into Lower Artery, Open Approach

04HY32Z Insertion of Monitoring Device into Lower Artery, Percutaneous Approach
AHA CC: 1Q, 2017, 30

04HY33Z Insertion of Infusion Device into Lower Artery, Percutaneous Approach
AHA CC: 3Q, 2019, 20-21

04HY3DZ Insertion of Intraluminal Device into Lower Artery, Percutaneous Approach

04HY3YZ Insertion of Other Device into Lower Artery, Percutaneous Approach

04HY42Z Insertion of Monitoring Device into Lower Artery, Percutaneous Endoscopic Approach

04HY43Z Insertion of Infusion Device into Lower Artery, Percutaneous Endoscopic Approach

04HY4DZ Insertion of Intraluminal Device into Lower Artery, Percutaneous Endoscopic Approach

04HY4YZ Insertion of Other Device into Lower Artery, Percutaneous Endoscopic Approach

04J – Lower Arteries, Inspection

Review Coding Guidelines B3.11a, B3.11b and B3.11c

04JY0ZZ Inspection of Lower Artery, Open Approach

04JY3ZZ Inspection of Lower Artery, Percutaneous Approach

04JY4ZZ Inspection of Lower Artery, Percutaneous Endoscopic Approach

04JYXZZ Inspection of Lower Artery, External Approach

04L – Lower Arteries, Occlusion

Review Coding Guideline B3.12

04L00CZ Occlusion of Abdominal Aorta with Extraluminal Device, Open Approach

04L00DZ Occlusion of Abdominal Aorta with Intraluminal Device, Open Approach

04L00ZZ Occlusion of Abdominal Aorta, Open Approach

04L03CZ Occlusion of Abdominal Aorta with Extraluminal Device, Percutaneous Approach

04L03DJ Occlusion of Abdominal Aorta with Intraluminal Device, Temporary, Percutaneous Approach

04L03DZ Occlusion of Abdominal Aorta with Intraluminal Device, Percutaneous Approach

04L03ZZ Occlusion of Abdominal Aorta, Percutaneous Approach

04L04CZ Occlusion of Abdominal Aorta with Extraluminal Device, Percutaneous Endoscopic Approach

04L04DZ Occlusion of Abdominal Aorta with Intraluminal Device, Percutaneous Endoscopic Approach

04L04ZZ Occlusion of Abdominal Aorta, Percutaneous Endoscopic Approach

04L10CZ Occlusion of Celiac Artery with Extraluminal Device, Open Approach

04L10DZ Occlusion of Celiac Artery with Intraluminal Device, Open Approach

04L10ZZ Occlusion of Celiac Artery, Open Approach

04L13CZ Occlusion of Celiac Artery with Extraluminal Device, Percutaneous Approach

04L13DZ Occlusion of Celiac Artery with Intraluminal Device, Percutaneous Approach

04L13ZZ Occlusion of Celiac Artery, Percutaneous Approach

04L14CZ Occlusion of Celiac Artery with Extraluminal Device, Percutaneous Endoscopic Approach

04L14DZ Occlusion of Celiac Artery with Intraluminal Device, Percutaneous Endoscopic Approach

04L14ZZ Occlusion of Celiac Artery, Percutaneous Endoscopic Approach

04L20CZ Occlusion of Gastric Artery with Extraluminal Device, Open Approach

04L20DZ Occlusion of Gastric Artery with Intraluminal Device, Open Approach

04L20ZZ Occlusion of Gastric Artery, Open Approach

04L23CZ Occlusion of Gastric Artery with Extraluminal Device, Percutaneous Approach

04L23DZ Occlusion of Gastric Artery with Intraluminal Device, Percutaneous Approach

04L23ZZ Occlusion of Gastric Artery, Percutaneous Approach

04L24CZ Occlusion of Gastric Artery with Extraluminal Device, Percutaneous Endoscopic Approach

04L24DZ Occlusion of Gastric Artery with Intraluminal Device, Percutaneous Endoscopic Approach

04L24ZZ Occlusion of Gastric Artery, Percutaneous Endoscopic Approach
AHA CC: 3Q, 2020, 43

04L30CZ Occlusion of Hepatic Artery with Extraluminal Device, Open Approach

04L30DZ Occlusion of Hepatic Artery with Intraluminal Device, Open Approach

04L30ZZ Occlusion of Hepatic Artery, Open Approach

04L33CZ Occlusion of Hepatic Artery with Extraluminal Device, Percutaneous Approach

04L33DZ Occlusion of Hepatic Artery with Intraluminal Device, Percutaneous Approach
AHA CC: 3Q, 2014, 26-27

04L33ZZ Occlusion of Hepatic Artery, Percutaneous Approach

04L34CZ Occlusion of Hepatic Artery with Extraluminal Device, Percutaneous Endoscopic Approach

04L34DZ Occlusion of Hepatic Artery with Intraluminal Device, Percutaneous Endoscopic Approach

04L34ZZ Occlusion of Hepatic Artery, Percutaneous Endoscopic Approach

04L40CZ Occlusion of Splenic Artery with Extraluminal Device, Open Approach

04L40DZ Occlusion of Splenic Artery with Intraluminal Device, Open Approach

04L40ZZ Occlusion of Splenic Artery, Open Approach

04L43CZ Occlusion of Splenic Artery with Extraluminal Device, Percutaneous Approach

04L43DZ Occlusion of Splenic Artery with Intraluminal Device, Percutaneous Approach

04L43ZZ Occlusion of Splenic Artery, Percutaneous Approach

04L44CZ Occlusion of Splenic Artery with Extraluminal Device, Percutaneous Endoscopic Approach

04L44DZ Occlusion of Splenic Artery with Intraluminal Device, Percutaneous Endoscopic Approach

04L44ZZ Occlusion of Splenic Artery, Percutaneous Endoscopic Approach

04L50CZ Occlusion of Superior Mesenteric Artery with Extraluminal Device, Open Approach

04L50DZ Occlusion of Superior Mesenteric Artery with Intraluminal Device, Open Approach

04L50ZZ Occlusion of Superior Mesenteric Artery, Open Approach

04L53CZ Occlusion of Superior Mesenteric Artery with Extraluminal Device, Percutaneous Approach

04L53DZ Occlusion of Superior Mesenteric Artery with Intraluminal Device, Percutaneous Approach

04L53ZZ Occlusion of Superior Mesenteric Artery, Percutaneous Approach

04L54CZ Occlusion of Superior Mesenteric Artery with Extraluminal Device, Percutaneous Endoscopic Approach

04L54DZ Occlusion of Superior Mesenteric Artery with Intraluminal Device, Percutaneous Endoscopic Approach

04L54ZZ Occlusion of Superior Mesenteric Artery, Percutaneous Endoscopic Approach

04L60CZ Occlusion of Right Colic Artery with Extraluminal Device, Open Approach

04L60DZ Occlusion of Right Colic Artery with Intraluminal Device, Open Approach

04L60ZZ Occlusion of Right Colic Artery, Open Approach

04L63CZ Occlusion of Right Colic Artery with Extraluminal Device, Percutaneous Approach

04L63DZ Occlusion of Right Colic Artery with Intraluminal Device, Percutaneous Approach

04L63ZZ Occlusion of Right Colic Artery, Percutaneous Approach

04L64CZ Occlusion of Right Colic Artery with Extraluminal Device, Percutaneous Endoscopic Approach

04L64DZ Occlusion of Right Colic Artery with Intraluminal Device, Percutaneous Endoscopic Approach

04L64ZZ Occlusion of Right Colic Artery, Percutaneous Endoscopic Approach

04L70CZ Occlusion of Left Colic Artery with Extraluminal Device, Open Approach

04L70DZ Occlusion of Left Colic Artery with Intraluminal Device, Open Approach

04L70ZZ Occlusion of Left Colic Artery, Open Approach

04L73CZ Occlusion of Left Colic Artery with Extraluminal Device, Percutaneous Approach

04L73DZ Occlusion of Left Colic Artery with Intraluminal Device, Percutaneous Approach
AHA CC: 1Q, 2014, 24

04L73ZZ Occlusion of Left Colic Artery, Percutaneous Approach

04L74CZ Occlusion of Left Colic Artery with Extraluminal Device, Percutaneous Endoscopic Approach

04L74DZ Occlusion of Left Colic Artery with Intraluminal Device, Percutaneous Endoscopic Approach

04L74ZZ Occlusion of Left Colic Artery, Percutaneous Endoscopic Approach

04L80CZ Occlusion of Middle Colic Artery with Extraluminal Device, Open Approach

04L80DZ Occlusion of Middle Colic Artery with Intraluminal Device, Open Approach

04L80ZZ Occlusion of Middle Colic Artery, Open Approach

04L83CZ Occlusion of Middle Colic Artery with Extraluminal Device, Percutaneous Approach

04L83DZ Occlusion of Middle Colic Artery with Intraluminal Device, Percutaneous Approach

04L83ZZ Occlusion of Middle Colic Artery, Percutaneous Approach

04L84CZ Occlusion of Middle Colic Artery with Extraluminal Device, Percutaneous Endoscopic Approach

04L84DZ Occlusion of Middle Colic Artery with Intraluminal Device, Percutaneous Endoscopic Approach

04L84ZZ Occlusion of Middle Colic Artery, Percutaneous Endoscopic Approach

04L90CZ Occlusion of Right Renal Artery with Extraluminal Device, Open Approach

04L90DZ Occlusion of Right Renal Artery with Intraluminal Device, Open Approach

04L90ZZ Occlusion of Right Renal Artery, Open Approach

04L93CZ Occlusion of Right Renal Artery with Extraluminal Device, Percutaneous Approach

04L93DZ Occlusion of Right Renal Artery with Intraluminal Device, Percutaneous Approach

04L93ZZ Occlusion of Right Renal Artery, Percutaneous Approach

04L94CZ Occlusion of Right Renal Artery with Extraluminal Device, Percutaneous Endoscopic Approach

04L94DZ Occlusion of Right Renal Artery with Intraluminal Device, Percutaneous Endoscopic Approach

04L94ZZ Occlusion of Right Renal Artery, Percutaneous Endoscopic Approach

04LA0CZ Occlusion of Left Renal Artery with Extraluminal Device, Open Approach

04LA0DZ Occlusion of Left Renal Artery with Intraluminal Device, Open Approach

04LA0ZZ Occlusion of Left Renal Artery, Open Approach

04LA3CZ Occlusion of Left Renal Artery with Extraluminal Device, Percutaneous Approach

04LA3DZ Occlusion of Left Renal Artery with Intraluminal Device, Percutaneous Approach

04LA3ZZ Occlusion of Left Renal Artery, Percutaneous Approach

04LA4CZ Occlusion of Left Renal Artery with Extraluminal Device, Percutaneous Endoscopic Approach

04LA4DZ Occlusion of Left Renal Artery with Intraluminal Device, Percutaneous Endoscopic Approach

04LA4ZZ Occlusion of Left Renal Artery, Percutaneous Endoscopic Approach

04LB0CZ Occlusion of Inferior Mesenteric Artery with Extraluminal Device, Open Approach

04LB0DZ Occlusion of Inferior Mesenteric Artery with Intraluminal Device, Open Approach

04LB0ZZ Occlusion of Inferior Mesenteric Artery, Open Approach

04LB3CZ Occlusion of Inferior Mesenteric Artery with Extraluminal Device, Percutaneous Approach

04LB3DZ Occlusion of Inferior Mesenteric Artery with Intraluminal Device, Percutaneous Approach
AHA CC: 1Q, 2014, 24

04LB3ZZ Occlusion of Inferior Mesenteric Artery, Percutaneous Approach

04LB4CZ Occlusion of Inferior Mesenteric Artery with Extraluminal Device, Percutaneous Endoscopic Approach

04LB4DZ Occlusion of Inferior Mesenteric Artery with Intraluminal Device, Percutaneous Endoscopic Approach

04LB4ZZ Occlusion of Inferior Mesenteric Artery, Percutaneous Endoscopic Approach

04LC0CZ Occlusion of Right Common Iliac Artery with Extraluminal Device, Open Approach

04LC0DZ Occlusion of Right Common Iliac Artery with Intraluminal Device, Open Approach

04LC0ZZ Occlusion of Right Common Iliac Artery, Open Approach

04LC3CZ Occlusion of Right Common Iliac Artery with Extraluminal Device, Percutaneous Approach

04LC3DZ Occlusion of Right Common Iliac Artery with Intraluminal Device, Percutaneous Approach

04LC3ZZ Occlusion of Right Common Iliac Artery, Percutaneous Approach

04LC4CZ Occlusion of Right Common Iliac Artery with Extraluminal Device, Percutaneous Endoscopic Approach

04LC4DZ Occlusion of Right Common Iliac Artery with Intraluminal Device, Percutaneous Endoscopic Approach

04LC4ZZ Occlusion of Right Common Iliac Artery, Percutaneous Endoscopic Approach

04LD0CZ Occlusion of Left Common Iliac Artery with Extraluminal Device, Open Approach

♀ Female-only   ♂ Male-only   ▲ Limited Coverage   ● Non-OR   ▥ HAC-associated procedure   ▲ Non-covered procedures   ✛ Cluste

04LD0DZ Occlusion of Left Common Iliac Artery with Intraluminal Device, Open Approach

04LD0ZZ Occlusion of Left Common Iliac Artery, Open Approach

04LD3CZ Occlusion of Left Common Iliac Artery with Extraluminal Device, Percutaneous Approach

04LD3DZ Occlusion of Left Common Iliac Artery with Intraluminal Device, Percutaneous Approach

04LD3ZZ Occlusion of Left Common Iliac Artery, Percutaneous Approach

04LD4CZ Occlusion of Left Common Iliac Artery with Extraluminal Device, Percutaneous Endoscopic Approach

04LD4DZ Occlusion of Left Common Iliac Artery with Intraluminal Device, Percutaneous Endoscopic Approach

04LD4ZZ Occlusion of Left Common Iliac Artery, Percutaneous Endoscopic Approach

04LE0CT Occlusion of Right Uterine Artery with Extraluminal Device, Open Approach

04LE0CZ Occlusion of Right Internal Iliac Artery with Extraluminal Device, Open Approach

04LE0DT Occlusion of Right Uterine Artery with Intraluminal Device, Open Approach

04LE0DZ Occlusion of Right Internal Iliac Artery with Intraluminal Device, Open Approach

♀ **04LE0ZT** Occlusion of Right Uterine Artery, Open Approach

04LE0ZZ Occlusion of Right Internal Iliac Artery, Open Approach

♀ **04LE3CT** Occlusion of Right Uterine Artery with Extraluminal Device, Percutaneous Approach

04LE3CZ Occlusion of Right Internal Iliac Artery with Extraluminal Device, Percutaneous Approach

♀ **04LE3DT** Occlusion of Right Uterine Artery with Intraluminal Device, Percutaneous Approach
AHA CC: 2Q, 2015, 27

04LE3DZ Occlusion of Right Internal Iliac Artery with Intraluminal Device, Percutaneous Approach

♀ **04LE3ZT** Occlusion of Right Uterine Artery, Percutaneous Approach

04LE3ZZ Occlusion of Right Internal Iliac Artery, Percutaneous Approach

♀ **04LE4CT** Occlusion of Right Uterine Artery with Extraluminal Device, Percutaneous Endoscopic Approach

04LE4CZ Occlusion of Right Internal Iliac Artery with Extraluminal Device, Percutaneous Endoscopic Approach

♀ **04LE4DT** Occlusion of Right Uterine Artery with Intraluminal Device, Percutaneous Endoscopic Approach

04LE4DZ Occlusion of Right Internal Iliac Artery with Intraluminal Device, Percutaneous Endoscopic Approach

♀ **04LE4ZT** Occlusion of Right Uterine Artery, Percutaneous Endoscopic Approach

04LE4ZZ Occlusion of Right Internal Iliac Artery, Percutaneous Endoscopic Approach

♀ **04LF0CU** Occlusion of Left Uterine Artery with Extraluminal Device, Open Approach

04LF0CZ Occlusion of Left Internal Iliac Artery with Extraluminal Device, Open Approach

♀ **04LF0DU** Occlusion of Left Uterine Artery with Intraluminal Device, Open Approach

04LF0DZ Occlusion of Left Internal Iliac Artery with Intraluminal Device, Open Approach

♀ **04LF0ZU** Occlusion of Left Uterine Artery, Open Approach

04LF0ZZ Occlusion of Left Internal Iliac Artery, Open Approach

♀ **04LF3CU** Occlusion of Left Uterine Artery with Extraluminal Device, Percutaneous Approach

04LF3CZ Occlusion of Left Internal Iliac Artery with Extraluminal Device, Percutaneous Approach

♀ **04LF3DU** Occlusion of Left Uterine Artery with Intraluminal Device, Percutaneous Approach

04LF3DZ Occlusion of Left Internal Iliac Artery with Intraluminal Device, Percutaneous Approach

♀ **04LF3ZU** Occlusion of Left Uterine Artery, Percutaneous Approach

04LF3ZZ Occlusion of Left Internal Iliac Artery, Percutaneous Approach

♀ **04LF4CU** Occlusion of Left Uterine Artery with Extraluminal Device, Percutaneous Endoscopic Approach

04LF4CZ Occlusion of Left Internal Iliac Artery with Extraluminal Device, Percutaneous Endoscopic Approach

♀ **04LF4DU** Occlusion of Left Uterine Artery with Intraluminal Device, Percutaneous Endoscopic Approach

04LF4DZ Occlusion of Left Internal Iliac Artery with Intraluminal Device, Percutaneous Endoscopic Approach

♀ **04LF4ZU** Occlusion of Left Uterine Artery, Percutaneous Endoscopic Approach

04LF4ZZ Occlusion of Left Internal Iliac Artery, Percutaneous Endoscopic Approach

04LH0CZ Occlusion of Right External Iliac Artery with Extraluminal Device, Open Approach
AHA CC: 2Q, 2018, 18-19

04LH0DZ Occlusion of Right External Iliac Artery with Intraluminal Device, Open Approach

04LH0ZZ Occlusion of Right External Iliac Artery, Open Approach

04LH3CZ Occlusion of Right External Iliac Artery with Extraluminal Device, Percutaneous Approach

04LH3DZ Occlusion of Right External Iliac Artery with Intraluminal Device, Percutaneous Approach

04LH3ZZ Occlusion of Right External Iliac Artery, Percutaneous Approach

04LH4CZ Occlusion of Right External Iliac Artery with Extraluminal Device, Percutaneous Endoscopic Approach

04LH4DZ Occlusion of Right External Iliac Artery with Intraluminal Device, Percutaneous Endoscopic Approach

04LH4ZZ Occlusion of Right External Iliac Artery, Percutaneous Endoscopic Approach

04LJ0CZ Occlusion of Left External Iliac Artery with Extraluminal Device, Open Approach
AHA CC: 2Q, 2018, 18-19

04LJ0DZ Occlusion of Left External Iliac Artery with Intraluminal Device, Open Approach

04LJ0ZZ Occlusion of Left External Iliac Artery, Open Approach

04LJ3CZ Occlusion of Left External Iliac Artery with Extraluminal Device, Percutaneous Approach

04LJ3DZ Occlusion of Left External Iliac Artery with Intraluminal Device, Percutaneous Approach

04LJ3ZZ Occlusion of Left External Iliac Artery, Percutaneous Approach

04LJ4CZ Occlusion of Left External Iliac Artery with Extraluminal Device, Percutaneous Endoscopic Approach

04LJ4DZ Occlusion of Left External Iliac Artery with Intraluminal Device, Percutaneous Endoscopic Approach

04LJ4ZZ Occlusion of Left External Iliac Artery, Percutaneous Endoscopic Approach

04LK0CZ Occlusion of Right Femoral Artery with Extraluminal Device, Open Approach

04LK0DZ Occlusion of Right Femoral Artery with Intraluminal Device, Open Approach

04LK0ZZ Occlusion of Right Femoral Artery, Open Approach

04LK3CZ Occlusion of Right Femoral Artery with Extraluminal Device, Percutaneous Approach

04LK3DZ Occlusion of Right Femoral Artery with Intraluminal Device, Percutaneous Approach

04LK3ZZ Occlusion of Right Femoral Artery, Percutaneous Approach

04LK4CZ Occlusion of Right Femoral Artery with Extraluminal Device, Percutaneous Endoscopic Approach

04LK4DZ Occlusion of Right Femoral Artery with Intraluminal Device, Percutaneous Endoscopic Approach

04LK4ZZ Occlusion of Right Femoral Artery, Percutaneous Endoscopic Approach

04LL0CZ Occlusion of Left Femoral Artery with Extraluminal Device, Open Approach

04LL0DZ Occlusion of Left Femoral Artery with Intraluminal Device, Open Approach

04LL0ZZ Occlusion of Left Femoral Artery, Open Approach

04LL3CZ Occlusion of Left Femoral Artery with Extraluminal Device, Percutaneous Approach

04LL3DZ Occlusion of Left Femoral Artery with Intraluminal Device, Percutaneous Approach

04LL3ZZ Occlusion of Left Femoral Artery, Percutaneous Approach

04LL4CZ Occlusion of Left Femoral Artery with Extraluminal Device, Percutaneous Endoscopic Approach

04LL4DZ Occlusion of Left Femoral Artery with Intraluminal Device, Percutaneous Endoscopic Approach

04LL4ZZ Occlusion of Left Femoral Artery, Percutaneous Endoscopic Approach

04LM0CZ Occlusion of Right Popliteal Artery with Extraluminal Device, Open Approach

04LM0DZ Occlusion of Right Popliteal Artery with Intraluminal Device, Open Approach

04LM0ZZ Occlusion of Right Popliteal Artery, Open Approach

04LM3CZ Occlusion of Right Popliteal Artery with Extraluminal Device, Percutaneous Approach

04LM3DZ Occlusion of Right Popliteal Artery with Intraluminal Device, Percutaneous Approach

04LM3ZZ Occlusion of Right Popliteal Artery, Percutaneous Approach

04LM4CZ Occlusion of Right Popliteal Artery with Extraluminal Device, Percutaneous Endoscopic Approach

04LM4DZ Occlusion of Right Popliteal Artery with Intraluminal Device, Percutaneous Endoscopic Approach

04LM4ZZ Occlusion of Right Popliteal Artery, Percutaneous Endoscopic Approach

04LN0CZ Occlusion of Left Popliteal Artery with Extraluminal Device, Open Approach

04LN0DZ Occlusion of Left Popliteal Artery with Intraluminal Device, Open Approach

04LN0ZZ Occlusion of Left Popliteal Artery, Open Approach

04LN3CZ Occlusion of Left Popliteal Artery with Extraluminal Device, Percutaneous Approach

04LN3DZ Occlusion of Left Popliteal Artery with Intraluminal Device, Percutaneous Approach

04LN3ZZ Occlusion of Left Popliteal Artery, Percutaneous Approach

04LN4CZ Occlusion of Left Popliteal Artery with Extraluminal Device, Percutaneous Endoscopic Approach

04LN4DZ Occlusion of Left Popliteal Artery with Intraluminal Device, Percutaneous Endoscopic Approach

04LN4ZZ Occlusion of Left Popliteal Artery, Percutaneous Endoscopic Approach

04LP0CZ Occlusion of Right Anterior Tibial Artery with Extraluminal Device, Open Approach

04LP0DZ Occlusion of Right Anterior Tibial Artery with Intraluminal Device, Open Approach

04LP0ZZ Occlusion of Right Anterior Tibial Artery, Open Approach

04LP3CZ Occlusion of Right Anterior Tibial Artery with Extraluminal Device, Percutaneous Approach

04LP3DZ Occlusion of Right Anterior Tibial Artery with Intraluminal Device, Percutaneous Approach

04LP3ZZ Occlusion of Right Anterior Tibial Artery, Percutaneous Approach

04LP4CZ Occlusion of Right Anterior Tibial Artery with Extraluminal Device, Percutaneous Endoscopic Approach

04LP4DZ Occlusion of Right Anterior Tibial Artery with Intraluminal Device, Percutaneous Endoscopic Approach

04LP4ZZ Occlusion of Right Anterior Tibial Artery, Percutaneous Endoscopic Approach

04LQ0CZ Occlusion of Left Anterior Tibial Artery with Extraluminal Device, Open Approach

04LQ0DZ Occlusion of Left Anterior Tibial Artery with Intraluminal Device, Open Approach

04LQ0ZZ Occlusion of Left Anterior Tibial Artery, Open Approach

04LQ3CZ Occlusion of Left Anterior Tibial Artery with Extraluminal Device, Percutaneous Approach

04LQ3DZ Occlusion of Left Anterior Tibial Artery with Intraluminal Device, Percutaneous Approach

04LQ3ZZ Occlusion of Left Anterior Tibial Artery, Percutaneous Approach

04LQ4CZ Occlusion of Left Anterior Tibial Artery with Extraluminal Device, Percutaneous Endoscopic Approach

04LQ4DZ Occlusion of Left Anterior Tibial Artery with Intraluminal Device, Percutaneous Endoscopic Approach

04LQ4ZZ Occlusion of Left Anterior Tibial Artery, Percutaneous Endoscopic Approach

04LR0CZ Occlusion of Right Posterior Tibial Artery with Extraluminal Device, Open Approach

04LR0DZ Occlusion of Right Posterior Tibial Artery with Intraluminal Device, Open Approach

04LR0ZZ Occlusion of Right Posterior Tibial Artery, Open Approach

04LR3CZ Occlusion of Right Posterior Tibial Artery with Extraluminal Device, Percutaneous Approach

04LR3DZ Occlusion of Right Posterior Tibial Artery with Intraluminal Device, Percutaneous Approach

04LR3ZZ Occlusion of Right Posterior Tibial Artery, Percutaneous Approach

04LR4CZ Occlusion of Right Posterior Tibial Artery with Extraluminal Device, Percutaneous Endoscopic Approach

04LR4DZ Occlusion of Right Posterior Tibial Artery with Intraluminal Device, Percutaneous Endoscopic Approach

04LR4ZZ Occlusion of Right Posterior Tibial Artery, Percutaneous Endoscopic Approach

04LS0CZ Occlusion of Left Posterior Tibial Artery with Extraluminal Device, Open Approach

04LS0DZ Occlusion of Left Posterior Tibial Artery with Intraluminal Device, Open Approach

04LS0ZZ Occlusion of Left Posterior Tibial Artery, Open Approach

04LS3CZ Occlusion of Left Posterior Tibial Artery with Extraluminal Device, Percutaneous Approach

04LS3DZ Occlusion of Left Posterior Tibial Artery with Intraluminal Device, Percutaneous Approach

04LS3ZZ Occlusion of Left Posterior Tibial Artery, Percutaneous Approach

04LS4CZ Occlusion of Left Posterior Tibial Artery with Extraluminal Device, Percutaneous Endoscopic Approach

04LS4DZ Occlusion of Left Posterior Tibial Artery with Intraluminal Device, Percutaneous Endoscopic Approach

04LS4ZZ Occlusion of Left Posterior Tibial Artery, Percutaneous Endoscopic Approach

04LT0CZ Occlusion of Right Peroneal Artery with Extraluminal Device, Open Approach

04LT0DZ Occlusion of Right Peroneal Artery with Intraluminal Device, Open Approach

04LT0ZZ Occlusion of Right Peroneal Artery, Open Approach

04LT3CZ Occlusion of Right Peroneal Artery with Extraluminal Device, Percutaneous Approach

04LT3DZ Occlusion of Right Peroneal Artery with Intraluminal Device, Percutaneous Approach

04LT3ZZ Occlusion of Right Peroneal Artery, Percutaneous Approach

04LT4CZ Occlusion of Right Peroneal Artery with Extraluminal Device, Percutaneous Endoscopic Approach

04LT4DZ Occlusion of Right Peroneal Artery with Intraluminal Device, Percutaneous Endoscopic Approach

04LT4ZZ Occlusion of Right Peroneal Artery, Percutaneous Endoscopic Approach

04LU0CZ Occlusion of Left Peroneal Artery with Extraluminal Device, Open Approach

04LU0DZ Occlusion of Left Peroneal Artery with Intraluminal Device, Open Approach

04LU0ZZ Occlusion of Left Peroneal Artery, Open Approach

04LU3CZ Occlusion of Left Peroneal Artery with Extraluminal Device, Percutaneous Approach

04LU3DZ Occlusion of Left Peroneal Artery with Intraluminal Device, Percutaneous Approach

04LU3ZZ Occlusion of Left Peroneal Artery, Percutaneous Approach

04LU4CZ Occlusion of Left Peroneal Artery with Extraluminal Device, Percutaneous Endoscopic Approach

04LU4DZ Occlusion of Left Peroneal Artery with Intraluminal Device, Percutaneous Endoscopic Approach

04LU4ZZ Occlusion of Left Peroneal Artery, Percutaneous Endoscopic Approach

04LV0CZ Occlusion of Right Foot Artery with Extraluminal Device, Open Approach

04LV0DZ Occlusion of Right Foot Artery with Intraluminal Device, Open Approach

04LV0ZZ Occlusion of Right Foot Artery, Open Approach

04LV3CZ Occlusion of Right Foot Artery with Extraluminal Device, Percutaneous Approach

04LV3DZ Occlusion of Right Foot Artery with Intraluminal Device, Percutaneous Approach

04LV3ZZ Occlusion of Right Foot Artery, Percutaneous Approach

04LV4CZ Occlusion of Right Foot Artery with Extraluminal Device, Percutaneous Endoscopic Approach

04LV4DZ Occlusion of Right Foot Artery with Intraluminal Device, Percutaneous Endoscopic Approach

04LV4ZZ Occlusion of Right Foot Artery, Percutaneous Endoscopic Approach

04LW0CZ Occlusion of Left Foot Artery with Extraluminal Device, Open Approach

04LW0DZ Occlusion of Left Foot Artery with Intraluminal Device, Open Approach

04LW0ZZ Occlusion of Left Foot Artery, Open Approach

04LW3CZ Occlusion of Left Foot Artery with Extraluminal Device, Percutaneous Approach

04LW3DZ Occlusion of Left Foot Artery with Intraluminal Device, Percutaneous Approach

04LW3ZZ Occlusion of Left Foot Artery, Percutaneous Approach

04LW4CZ Occlusion of Left Foot Artery with Extraluminal Device, Percutaneous Endoscopic Approach

04LW4DZ Occlusion of Left Foot Artery with Intraluminal Device, Percutaneous Endoscopic Approach

04LW4ZZ Occlusion of Left Foot Artery, Percutaneous Endoscopic Approach

04LY0CZ Occlusion of Lower Artery with Extraluminal Device, Open Approach

♀ Female-only   ♂ Male-only   ▲ Limited Coverage   ● Non-OR   HAC HAC-associated procedure   ▲ Non-covered procedures   ✚ Cluster

04LY0DZ Occlusion of Lower Artery with Intraluminal Device, Open Approach

04LY0ZZ Occlusion of Lower Artery, Open Approach

04LY3CZ Occlusion of Lower Artery with Extraluminal Device, Percutaneous Approach

04LY3DZ Occlusion of Lower Artery with Intraluminal Device, Percutaneous Approach

04LY3ZZ Occlusion of Lower Artery, Percutaneous Approach

04LY4CZ Occlusion of Lower Artery with Extraluminal Device, Percutaneous Endoscopic Approach

04LY4DZ Occlusion of Lower Artery with Intraluminal Device, Percutaneous Endoscopic Approach

04LY4ZZ Occlusion of Lower Artery, Percutaneous Endoscopic Approach

04N – Lower Arteries, Release

Review Coding Guidelines B3.13 and B3.14

04N00ZZ Release Abdominal Aorta, Open Approach

04N03ZZ Release Abdominal Aorta, Percutaneous Approach

04N04ZZ Release Abdominal Aorta, Percutaneous Endoscopic Approach

04N10ZZ Release Celiac Artery, Open Approach
AHA CC: 2Q, 2015, 28

04N13ZZ Release Celiac Artery, Percutaneous Approach

04N14ZZ Release Celiac Artery, Percutaneous Endoscopic Approach

04N20ZZ Release Gastric Artery, Open Approach

04N23ZZ Release Gastric Artery, Percutaneous Approach

04N24ZZ Release Gastric Artery, Percutaneous Endoscopic Approach

04N30ZZ Release Hepatic Artery, Open Approach

04N33ZZ Release Hepatic Artery, Percutaneous Approach

04N34ZZ Release Hepatic Artery, Percutaneous Endoscopic Approach

04N40ZZ Release Splenic Artery, Open Approach

04N43ZZ Release Splenic Artery, Percutaneous Approach

04N44ZZ Release Splenic Artery, Percutaneous Endoscopic Approach

04N50ZZ Release Superior Mesenteric Artery, Open Approach

04N53ZZ Release Superior Mesenteric Artery, Percutaneous Approach

04N54ZZ Release Superior Mesenteric Artery, Percutaneous Endoscopic Approach

04N60ZZ Release Right Colic Artery, Open Approach

04N63ZZ Release Right Colic Artery, Percutaneous Approach

04N64ZZ Release Right Colic Artery, Percutaneous Endoscopic Approach

04N70ZZ Release Left Colic Artery, Open Approach

04N73ZZ Release Left Colic Artery, Percutaneous Approach

04N74ZZ Release Left Colic Artery, Percutaneous Endoscopic Approach

04N80ZZ Release Middle Colic Artery, Open Approach

04N83ZZ Release Middle Colic Artery, Percutaneous Approach

04N84ZZ Release Middle Colic Artery, Percutaneous Endoscopic Approach

04N90ZZ Release Right Renal Artery, Open Approach

04N93ZZ Release Right Renal Artery, Percutaneous Approach

04N94ZZ Release Right Renal Artery, Percutaneous Endoscopic Approach

04NA0ZZ Release Left Renal Artery, Open Approach

04NA3ZZ Release Left Renal Artery, Percutaneous Approach

04NA4ZZ Release Left Renal Artery, Percutaneous Endoscopic Approach

04NB0ZZ Release Inferior Mesenteric Artery, Open Approach

04NB3ZZ Release Inferior Mesenteric Artery, Percutaneous Approach

04NB4ZZ Release Inferior Mesenteric Artery, Percutaneous Endoscopic Approach

04NC0ZZ Release Right Common Iliac Artery, Open Approach

04NC3ZZ Release Right Common Iliac Artery, Percutaneous Approach

04NC4ZZ Release Right Common Iliac Artery, Percutaneous Endoscopic Approach

04ND0ZZ Release Left Common Iliac Artery, Open Approach

04ND3ZZ Release Left Common Iliac Artery, Percutaneous Approach

04ND4ZZ Release Left Common Iliac Artery, Percutaneous Endoscopic Approach

04NE0ZZ Release Right Internal Iliac Artery, Open Approach

04NE3ZZ Release Right Internal Iliac Artery, Percutaneous Approach

04NE4ZZ Release Right Internal Iliac Artery, Percutaneous Endoscopic Approach

04NF0ZZ Release Left Internal Iliac Artery, Open Approach

04NF3ZZ Release Left Internal Iliac Artery, Percutaneous Approach

04NF4ZZ Release Left Internal Iliac Artery, Percutaneous Endoscopic Approach

04NH0ZZ Release Right External Iliac Artery, Open Approach

04NH3ZZ Release Right External Iliac Artery, Percutaneous Approach

04NH4ZZ Release Right External Iliac Artery, Percutaneous Endoscopic Approach

04NJ0ZZ Release Left External Iliac Artery, Open Approach

04NJ3ZZ Release Left External Iliac Artery, Percutaneous Approach

04NJ4ZZ Release Left External Iliac Artery, Percutaneous Endoscopic Approach

04NK0ZZ Release Right Femoral Artery, Open Approach

04NK3ZZ Release Right Femoral Artery, Percutaneous Approach

04NK4ZZ Release Right Femoral Artery, Percutaneous Endoscopic Approach

04NL0ZZ Release Left Femoral Artery, Open Approach

04NL3ZZ Release Left Femoral Artery, Percutaneous Approach

04NL4ZZ Release Left Femoral Artery, Percutaneous Endoscopic Approach

04NM0ZZ Release Right Popliteal Artery, Open Approach

04NM3ZZ Release Right Popliteal Artery, Percutaneous Approach

04NM4ZZ Release Right Popliteal Artery, Percutaneous Endoscopic Approach

04NN0ZZ Release Left Popliteal Artery, Open Approach

04NN3ZZ Release Left Popliteal Artery, Percutaneous Approach

04NN4ZZ Release Left Popliteal Artery, Percutaneous Endoscopic Approach

04NP0ZZ Release Right Anterior Tibial Artery, Open Approach

04NP3ZZ Release Right Anterior Tibial Artery, Percutaneous Approach

04NP4ZZ Release Right Anterior Tibial Artery, Percutaneous Endoscopic Approach

04NQ0ZZ Release Left Anterior Tibial Artery, Open Approach

04NQ3ZZ Release Left Anterior Tibial Artery, Percutaneous Approach

04NQ4ZZ Release Left Anterior Tibial Artery, Percutaneous Endoscopic Approach

04NR0ZZ Release Right Posterior Tibial Artery, Open Approach

04NR3ZZ Release Right Posterior Tibial Artery, Percutaneous Approach

04NR4ZZ Release Right Posterior Tibial Artery, Percutaneous Endoscopic Approach

04NS0ZZ Release Left Posterior Tibial Artery, Open Approach

04NS3ZZ Release Left Posterior Tibial Artery, Percutaneous Approach

04NS4ZZ Release Left Posterior Tibial Artery, Percutaneous Endoscopic Approach

04NT0ZZ Release Right Peroneal Artery, Open Approach

04NT3ZZ Release Right Peroneal Artery, Percutaneous Approach

04NT4ZZ Release Right Peroneal Artery, Percutaneous Endoscopic Approach

04NU0ZZ Release Left Peroneal Artery, Open Approach

04NU3ZZ Release Left Peroneal Artery, Percutaneous Approach

04NU4ZZ Release Left Peroneal Artery, Percutaneous Endoscopic Approach

04NV0ZZ Release Right Foot Artery, Open Approach

04NV3ZZ Release Right Foot Artery, Percutaneous Approach

04NV4ZZ Release Right Foot Artery, Percutaneous Endoscopic Approach

04NW0ZZ Release Left Foot Artery, Open Approach

04NW3ZZ Release Left Foot Artery, Percutaneous Approach

04NW4ZZ Release Left Foot Artery, Percutaneous Endoscopic Approach

04NY0ZZ Release Lower Artery, Open Approach

04NY3ZZ Release Lower Artery, Percutaneous Approach

04NY4ZZ Release Lower Artery, Percutaneous Endoscopic Approach

♀ Female-only   ♂ Male-only   ▲ Limited Coverage   ● Non-OR   HAC HAC-associated procedure   ▲ Non-covered procedures   ✚ Cluster

04P – Lower Arteries, Removal

Review Coding Guideline B6.1c

04PY00Z Removal of Drainage Device from Lower Artery, Open Approach

04PY02Z Removal of Monitoring Device from Lower Artery, Open Approach

04PY03Z Removal of Infusion Device from Lower Artery, Open Approach

04PY07Z Removal of Autologous Tissue Substitute from Lower Artery, Open Approach

04PY0CZ Removal of Extraluminal Device from Lower Artery, Open Approach

04PY0DZ Removal of Intraluminal Device from Lower Artery, Open Approach

04PY0JZ Removal of Synthetic Substitute from Lower Artery, Open Approach

04PY0KZ Removal of Nonautologous Tissue Substitute from Lower Artery, Open Approach

04PY0YZ Removal of Other Device from Lower Artery, Open Approach

04PY30Z Removal of Drainage Device from Lower Artery, Percutaneous Approach

04PY32Z Removal of Monitoring Device from Lower Artery, Percutaneous Approach

04PY33Z Removal of Infusion Device from Lower Artery, Percutaneous Approach

AHA CC: 3Q, 2019, 20-21

04PY37Z Removal of Autologous Tissue Substitute from Lower Artery, Percutaneous Approach

04PY3CZ Removal of Extraluminal Device from Lower Artery, Percutaneous Approach

04PY3DZ Removal of Intraluminal Device from Lower Artery, Percutaneous Approach

04PY3JZ Removal of Synthetic Substitute from Lower Artery, Percutaneous Approach

04PY3KZ Removal of Nonautologous Tissue Substitute from Lower Artery, Percutaneous Approach

04PY3YZ Removal of Other Device from Lower Artery, Percutaneous Approach

04PY40Z Removal of Drainage Device from Lower Artery, Percutaneous Endoscopic Approach

04PY42Z Removal of Monitoring Device from Lower Artery, Percutaneous Endoscopic Approach

04PY43Z Removal of Infusion Device from Lower Artery, Percutaneous Endoscopic Approach

04PY47Z Removal of Autologous Tissue Substitute from Lower Artery, Percutaneous Endoscopic Approach

04PY4CZ Removal of Extraluminal Device from Lower Artery, Percutaneous Endoscopic Approach

04PY4DZ Removal of Intraluminal Device from Lower Artery, Percutaneous Endoscopic Approach

04PY4JZ Removal of Synthetic Substitute from Lower Artery, Percutaneous Endoscopic Approach

04PY4KZ Removal of Nonautologous Tissue Substitute from Lower Artery, Percutaneous Endoscopic Approach

04PY4YZ Removal of Other Device from Lower Artery, Percutaneous Endoscopic Approach

04PYX0Z Removal of Drainage Device from Lower Artery, External Approach

04PYX1Z Removal of Radioactive Element from Lower Artery, External Approach

04PYX2Z Removal of Monitoring Device from Lower Artery, External Approach

04PYX3Z Removal of Infusion Device from Lower Artery, External Approach

04PYXDZ Removal of Intraluminal Device from Lower Artery, External Approach

04Q – Lower Arteries, Repair

04Q00ZZ Repair Abdominal Aorta, Open Approach

04Q03ZZ Repair Abdominal Aorta, Percutaneous Approach

04Q04ZZ Repair Abdominal Aorta, Percutaneous Endoscopic Approach

04Q10ZZ Repair Celiac Artery, Open Approach

04Q13ZZ Repair Celiac Artery, Percutaneous Approach

04Q14ZZ Repair Celiac Artery, Percutaneous Endoscopic Approach

04Q20ZZ Repair Gastric Artery, Open Approach

04Q23ZZ Repair Gastric Artery, Percutaneous Approach

04Q24ZZ Repair Gastric Artery, Percutaneous Endoscopic Approach

04Q30ZZ Repair Hepatic Artery, Open Approach

04Q33ZZ Repair Hepatic Artery, Percutaneous Approach

04Q34ZZ Repair Hepatic Artery, Percutaneous Endoscopic Approach

04Q40ZZ Repair Splenic Artery, Open Approach

04Q43ZZ Repair Splenic Artery, Percutaneous Approach

04Q44ZZ Repair Splenic Artery, Percutaneous Endoscopic Approach

04Q50ZZ Repair Superior Mesenteric Artery, Open Approach

04Q53ZZ Repair Superior Mesenteric Artery, Percutaneous Approach

04Q54ZZ Repair Superior Mesenteric Artery, Percutaneous Endoscopic Approach

04Q60ZZ Repair Right Colic Artery, Open Approach

04Q63ZZ Repair Right Colic Artery, Percutaneous Approach

04Q64ZZ Repair Right Colic Artery, Percutaneous Endoscopic Approach

04Q70ZZ Repair Left Colic Artery, Open Approach

04Q73ZZ Repair Left Colic Artery, Percutaneous Approach

04Q74ZZ Repair Left Colic Artery, Percutaneous Endoscopic Approach

04Q80ZZ Repair Middle Colic Artery, Open Approach

04Q83ZZ Repair Middle Colic Artery, Percutaneous Approach

04Q84ZZ Repair Middle Colic Artery, Percutaneous Endoscopic Approach

04Q90ZZ Repair Right Renal Artery, Open Approach

04Q93ZZ Repair Right Renal Artery, Percutaneous Approach

04Q94ZZ Repair Right Renal Artery, Percutaneous Endoscopic Approach

04QA0ZZ Repair Left Renal Artery, Open Approach

04QA3ZZ Repair Left Renal Artery, Percutaneous Approach

04QA4ZZ Repair Left Renal Artery, Percutaneous Endoscopic Approach

04QB0ZZ Repair Inferior Mesenteric Artery, Open Approach

04QB3ZZ Repair Inferior Mesenteric Artery, Percutaneous Approach

04QB4ZZ Repair Inferior Mesenteric Artery, Percutaneous Endoscopic Approach

04QC0ZZ Repair Right Common Iliac Artery, Open Approach

04QC3ZZ Repair Right Common Iliac Artery, Percutaneous Approach

04QC4ZZ Repair Right Common Iliac Artery, Percutaneous Endoscopic Approach

04QD0ZZ Repair Left Common Iliac Artery, Open Approach

04QD3ZZ Repair Left Common Iliac Artery, Percutaneous Approach

04QD4ZZ Repair Left Common Iliac Artery, Percutaneous Endoscopic Approach

04QE0ZZ Repair Right Internal Iliac Artery, Open Approach

04QE3ZZ Repair Right Internal Iliac Artery, Percutaneous Approach

04QE4ZZ Repair Right Internal Iliac Artery, Percutaneous Endoscopic Approach

04QF0ZZ Repair Left Internal Iliac Artery, Open Approach

04QF3ZZ Repair Left Internal Iliac Artery, Percutaneous Approach

04QF4ZZ Repair Left Internal Iliac Artery, Percutaneous Endoscopic Approach

04QH0ZZ Repair Right External Iliac Artery, Open Approach

04QH3ZZ Repair Right External Iliac Artery, Percutaneous Approach

04QH4ZZ Repair Right External Iliac Artery, Percutaneous Endoscopic Approach

04QJ0ZZ Repair Left External Iliac Artery, Open Approach

04QJ3ZZ Repair Left External Iliac Artery, Percutaneous Approach

04QJ4ZZ Repair Left External Iliac Artery, Percutaneous Endoscopic Approach

04QK0ZZ Repair Right Femoral Artery, Open Approach

AHA CC: 1Q, 2014, 21-22

04QK3ZZ Repair Right Femoral Artery, Percutaneous Approach

04QK4ZZ Repair Right Femoral Artery, Percutaneous Endoscopic Approach

04QL0ZZ Repair Left Femoral Artery, Open Approach

04QL3ZZ Repair Left Femoral Artery, Percutaneous Approach

04QL4ZZ Repair Left Femoral Artery, Percutaneous Endoscopic Approach

04QM0ZZ Repair Right Popliteal Artery, Open Approach

04QM3ZZ Repair Right Popliteal Artery, Percutaneous Approach

04QM4ZZ Repair Right Popliteal Artery, Percutaneous Endoscopic Approach

04QN0ZZ Repair Left Popliteal Artery, Open Approach

♀ Female-only ♂ Male-only ▲ Limited Coverage ● Non-OR HAC HAC-associated procedure ▲ Non-covered procedures ✚ Cluster

04QN3ZZ Repair Left Popliteal Artery, Percutaneous Approach
04QN4ZZ Repair Left Popliteal Artery, Percutaneous Endoscopic Approach
04QP0ZZ Repair Right Anterior Tibial Artery, Open Approach
04QP3ZZ Repair Right Anterior Tibial Artery, Percutaneous Approach
04QP4ZZ Repair Right Anterior Tibial Artery, Percutaneous Endoscopic Approach
04QQ0ZZ Repair Left Anterior Tibial Artery, Open Approach
04QQ3ZZ Repair Left Anterior Tibial Artery, Percutaneous Approach
04QQ4ZZ Repair Left Anterior Tibial Artery, Percutaneous Endoscopic Approach
04QR0ZZ Repair Right Posterior Tibial Artery, Open Approach
04QR3ZZ Repair Right Posterior Tibial Artery, Percutaneous Approach

04QR4ZZ Repair Right Posterior Tibial Artery, Percutaneous Endoscopic Approach
04QS0ZZ Repair Left Posterior Tibial Artery, Open Approach
04QS3ZZ Repair Left Posterior Tibial Artery, Percutaneous Approach
04QS4ZZ Repair Left Posterior Tibial Artery, Percutaneous Endoscopic Approach
04QT0ZZ Repair Right Peroneal Artery, Open Approach
04QT3ZZ Repair Right Peroneal Artery, Percutaneous Approach
04QT4ZZ Repair Right Peroneal Artery, Percutaneous Endoscopic Approach
04QU0ZZ Repair Left Peroneal Artery, Open Approach
04QU3ZZ Repair Left Peroneal Artery, Percutaneous Approach

04QU4ZZ Repair Left Peroneal Artery, Percutaneous Endoscopic Approach
04QV0ZZ Repair Right Foot Artery, Open Approach
04QV3ZZ Repair Right Foot Artery, Percutaneous Approach
04QV4ZZ Repair Right Foot Artery, Percutaneous Endoscopic Approach
04QW0ZZ Repair Left Foot Artery, Open Approach
04QW3ZZ Repair Left Foot Artery, Percutaneous Approach
04QW4ZZ Repair Left Foot Artery, Percutaneous Endoscopic Approach
04QY0ZZ Repair Lower Artery, Open Approach
04QY3ZZ Repair Lower Artery, Percutaneous Approach
04QY4ZZ Repair Lower Artery, Percutaneous Endoscopic Approach

04R – Lower Arteries, Replacement

Review Coding Guideline B3.18

04R007Z Replacement of Abdominal Aorta with Autologous Tissue Substitute, Open Approach
04R00JZ Replacement of Abdominal Aorta with Synthetic Substitute, Open Approach
04R00KZ Replacement of Abdominal Aorta with Nonautologous Tissue Substitute, Open Approach
04R047Z Replacement of Abdominal Aorta with Autologous Tissue Substitute, Percutaneous Endoscopic Approach
04R04JZ Replacement of Abdominal Aorta with Synthetic Substitute, Percutaneous Endoscopic Approach
04R04KZ Replacement of Abdominal Aorta with Nonautologous Tissue Substitute, Percutaneous Endoscopic Approach
04R107Z Replacement of Celiac Artery with Autologous Tissue Substitute, Open Approach
04R10JZ Replacement of Celiac Artery with Synthetic Substitute, Open Approach
AHA CC: 2Q, 2015, 28
04R10KZ Replacement of Celiac Artery with Nonautologous Tissue Substitute, Open Approach
04R147Z Replacement of Celiac Artery with Autologous Tissue Substitute, Percutaneous Endoscopic Approach
04R14JZ Replacement of Celiac Artery with Synthetic Substitute, Percutaneous Endoscopic Approach
04R14KZ Replacement of Celiac Artery with Nonautologous Tissue Substitute, Percutaneous Endoscopic Approach
04R207Z Replacement of Gastric Artery with Autologous Tissue Substitute, Open Approach
04R20JZ Replacement of Gastric Artery with Synthetic Substitute, Open Approach
04R20KZ Replacement of Gastric Artery with Nonautologous Tissue Substitute, Open Approach
04R247Z Replacement of Gastric Artery with Autologous Tissue Substitute, Percutaneous Endoscopic Approach
04R24JZ Replacement of Gastric Artery with Synthetic Substitute, Percutaneous Endoscopic Approach

04R24KZ Replacement of Gastric Artery with Nonautologous Tissue Substitute, Percutaneous Endoscopic Approach
04R307Z Replacement of Hepatic Artery with Autologous Tissue Substitute, Open Approach
04R30JZ Replacement of Hepatic Artery with Synthetic Substitute, Open Approach
04R30KZ Replacement of Hepatic Artery with Nonautologous Tissue Substitute, Open Approach
04R347Z Replacement of Hepatic Artery with Autologous Tissue Substitute, Percutaneous Endoscopic Approach
04R34JZ Replacement of Hepatic Artery with Synthetic Substitute, Percutaneous Endoscopic Approach
04R34KZ Replacement of Hepatic Artery with Nonautologous Tissue Substitute, Percutaneous Endoscopic Approach
04R407Z Replacement of Splenic Artery with Autologous Tissue Substitute, Open Approach
04R40JZ Replacement of Splenic Artery with Synthetic Substitute, Open Approach
04R40KZ Replacement of Splenic Artery with Nonautologous Tissue Substitute, Open Approach
04R447Z Replacement of Splenic Artery with Autologous Tissue Substitute, Percutaneous Endoscopic Approach
04R44JZ Replacement of Splenic Artery with Synthetic Substitute, Percutaneous Endoscopic Approach
04R44KZ Replacement of Splenic Artery with Nonautologous Tissue Substitute, Percutaneous Endoscopic Approach
04R507Z Replacement of Superior Mesenteric Artery with Autologous Tissue Substitute, Open Approach
04R50JZ Replacement of Superior Mesenteric Artery with Synthetic Substitute, Open Approach
04R50KZ Replacement of Superior Mesenteric Artery with Nonautologous Tissue Substitute, Open Approach
04R547Z Replacement of Superior Mesenteric Artery with Autologous Tissue Substitute, Percutaneous Endoscopic Approach

04R54JZ Replacement of Superior Mesenteric Artery with Synthetic Substitute, Percutaneous Endoscopic Approach
04R54KZ Replacement of Superior Mesenteric Artery with Nonautologous Tissue Substitute, Percutaneous Endoscopic Approach
04R607Z Replacement of Right Colic Artery with Autologous Tissue Substitute, Open Approach
04R60JZ Replacement of Right Colic Artery with Synthetic Substitute, Open Approach
04R60KZ Replacement of Right Colic Artery with Nonautologous Tissue Substitute, Open Approach
04R647Z Replacement of Right Colic Artery with Autologous Tissue Substitute, Percutaneous Endoscopic Approach
04R64JZ Replacement of Right Colic Artery with Synthetic Substitute, Percutaneous Endoscopic Approach
04R64KZ Replacement of Right Colic Artery with Nonautologous Tissue Substitute, Percutaneous Endoscopic Approach
04R707Z Replacement of Left Colic Artery with Autologous Tissue Substitute, Open Approach
04R70JZ Replacement of Left Colic Artery with Synthetic Substitute, Open Approach
04R70KZ Replacement of Left Colic Artery with Nonautologous Tissue Substitute, Open Approach
04R747Z Replacement of Left Colic Artery with Autologous Tissue Substitute, Percutaneous Endoscopic Approach
04R74JZ Replacement of Left Colic Artery with Synthetic Substitute, Percutaneous Endoscopic Approach
04R74KZ Replacement of Left Colic Artery with Nonautologous Tissue Substitute, Percutaneous Endoscopic Approach
04R807Z Replacement of Middle Colic Artery with Autologous Tissue Substitute, Open Approach
04R80JZ Replacement of Middle Colic Artery with Synthetic Substitute, Open Approach
04R80KZ Replacement of Middle Colic Artery with Nonautologous Tissue Substitute, Open Approach

04R847Z Replacement of Middle Colic Artery with Autologous Tissue Substitute, Percutaneous Endoscopic Approach

04R84JZ Replacement of Middle Colic Artery with Synthetic Substitute, Percutaneous Endoscopic Approach

04R84KZ Replacement of Middle Colic Artery with Nonautologous Tissue Substitute, Percutaneous Endoscopic Approach

04R907Z Replacement of Right Renal Artery with Autologous Tissue Substitute, Open Approach

04R90JZ Replacement of Right Renal Artery with Synthetic Substitute, Open Approach

04R90KZ Replacement of Right Renal Artery with Nonautologous Tissue Substitute, Open Approach

04R947Z Replacement of Right Renal Artery with Autologous Tissue Substitute, Percutaneous Endoscopic Approach

04R94JZ Replacement of Right Renal Artery with Synthetic Substitute, Percutaneous Endoscopic Approach

04R94KZ Replacement of Right Renal Artery with Nonautologous Tissue Substitute, Percutaneous Endoscopic Approach

04RA07Z Replacement of Left Renal Artery with Autologous Tissue Substitute, Open Approach

04RA0JZ Replacement of Left Renal Artery with Synthetic Substitute, Open Approach

04RA0KZ Replacement of Left Renal Artery with Nonautologous Tissue Substitute, Open Approach

04RA47Z Replacement of Left Renal Artery with Autologous Tissue Substitute, Percutaneous Endoscopic Approach

04RA4JZ Replacement of Left Renal Artery with Synthetic Substitute, Percutaneous Endoscopic Approach

04RA4KZ Replacement of Left Renal Artery with Nonautologous Tissue Substitute, Percutaneous Endoscopic Approach

04RB07Z Replacement of Inferior Mesenteric Artery with Autologous Tissue Substitute, Open Approach

04RB0JZ Replacement of Inferior Mesenteric Artery with Synthetic Substitute, Open Approach

04RB0KZ Replacement of Inferior Mesenteric Artery with Nonautologous Tissue Substitute, Open Approach

04RB47Z Replacement of Inferior Mesenteric Artery with Autologous Tissue Substitute, Percutaneous Endoscopic Approach

04RB4JZ Replacement of Inferior Mesenteric Artery with Synthetic Substitute, Percutaneous Endoscopic Approach

04RB4KZ Replacement of Inferior Mesenteric Artery with Nonautologous Tissue Substitute, Percutaneous Endoscopic Approach

04RC07Z Replacement of Right Common Iliac Artery with Autologous Tissue Substitute, Open Approach

04RC0JZ Replacement of Right Common Iliac Artery with Synthetic Substitute, Open Approach

04RC0KZ Replacement of Right Common Iliac Artery with Nonautologous Tissue Substitute, Open Approach

04RC47Z Replacement of Right Common Iliac Artery with Autologous Tissue Substitute, Percutaneous Endoscopic Approach

04RC4JZ Replacement of Right Common Iliac Artery with Synthetic Substitute, Percutaneous Endoscopic Approach

04RC4KZ Replacement of Right Common Iliac Artery with Nonautologous Tissue Substitute, Percutaneous Endoscopic Approach

04RD07Z Replacement of Left Common Iliac Artery with Autologous Tissue Substitute, Open Approach

04RD0JZ Replacement of Left Common Iliac Artery with Synthetic Substitute, Open Approach

04RD0KZ Replacement of Left Common Iliac Artery with Nonautologous Tissue Substitute, Open Approach

04RD47Z Replacement of Left Common Iliac Artery with Autologous Tissue Substitute, Percutaneous Endoscopic Approach

04RD4JZ Replacement of Left Common Iliac Artery with Synthetic Substitute, Percutaneous Endoscopic Approach

04RD4KZ Replacement of Left Common Iliac Artery with Nonautologous Tissue Substitute, Percutaneous Endoscopic Approach

04RE07Z Replacement of Right Internal Iliac Artery with Autologous Tissue Substitute, Open Approach

04RE0JZ Replacement of Right Internal Iliac Artery with Synthetic Substitute, Open Approach

04RE0KZ Replacement of Right Internal Iliac Artery with Nonautologous Tissue Substitute, Open Approach

04RE47Z Replacement of Right Internal Iliac Artery with Autologous Tissue Substitute, Percutaneous Endoscopic Approach

04RE4JZ Replacement of Right Internal Iliac Artery with Synthetic Substitute, Percutaneous Endoscopic Approach

04RE4KZ Replacement of Right Internal Iliac Artery with Nonautologous Tissue Substitute, Percutaneous Endoscopic Approach

04RF07Z Replacement of Left Internal Iliac Artery with Autologous Tissue Substitute, Open Approach

04RF0JZ Replacement of Left Internal Iliac Artery with Synthetic Substitute, Open Approach

04RF0KZ Replacement of Left Internal Iliac Artery with Nonautologous Tissue Substitute, Open Approach

04RF47Z Replacement of Left Internal Iliac Artery with Autologous Tissue Substitute, Percutaneous Endoscopic Approach

04RF4JZ Replacement of Left Internal Iliac Artery with Synthetic Substitute, Percutaneous Endoscopic Approach

04RF4KZ Replacement of Left Internal Iliac Artery with Nonautologous Tissue Substitute, Percutaneous Endoscopic Approach

04RH07Z Replacement of Right External Iliac Artery with Autologous Tissue Substitute, Open Approach

04RH0JZ Replacement of Right External Iliac Artery with Synthetic Substitute, Open Approach

04RH0KZ Replacement of Right External Iliac Artery with Nonautologous Tissue Substitute, Open Approach

04RH47Z Replacement of Right External Iliac Artery with Autologous Tissue Substitute, Percutaneous Endoscopic Approach

04RH4JZ Replacement of Right External Iliac Artery with Synthetic Substitute, Percutaneous Endoscopic Approach

04RH4KZ Replacement of Right External Iliac Artery with Nonautologous Tissue Substitute, Percutaneous Endoscopic Approach

04RJ07Z Replacement of Left External Iliac Artery with Autologous Tissue Substitute, Open Approach

04RJ0JZ Replacement of Left External Iliac Artery with Synthetic Substitute, Open Approach

04RJ0KZ Replacement of Left External Iliac Artery with Nonautologous Tissue Substitute, Open Approach

04RJ47Z Replacement of Left External Iliac Artery with Autologous Tissue Substitute, Percutaneous Endoscopic Approach

04RJ4JZ Replacement of Left External Iliac Artery with Synthetic Substitute, Percutaneous Endoscopic Approach

04RJ4KZ Replacement of Left External Iliac Artery with Nonautologous Tissue Substitute, Percutaneous Endoscopic Approach

04RK07Z Replacement of Right Femoral Artery with Autologous Tissue Substitute, Open Approach

04RK0JZ Replacement of Right Femoral Artery with Synthetic Substitute, Open Approach

04RK0KZ Replacement of Right Femoral Artery with Nonautologous Tissue Substitute, Open Approach

04RK47Z Replacement of Right Femoral Artery with Autologous Tissue Substitute, Percutaneous Endoscopic Approach

04RK4JZ Replacement of Right Femoral Artery with Synthetic Substitute, Percutaneous Endoscopic Approach

04RK4KZ Replacement of Right Femoral Artery with Nonautologous Tissue Substitute, Percutaneous Endoscopic Approach

04RL07Z Replacement of Left Femoral Artery with Autologous Tissue Substitute, Open Approach

04RL0JZ Replacement of Left Femoral Artery with Synthetic Substitute, Open Approach

04RL0KZ Replacement of Left Femoral Artery with Nonautologous Tissue Substitute, Open Approach

04RL47Z Replacement of Left Femoral Artery with Autologous Tissue Substitute, Percutaneous Endoscopic Approach

04RL4JZ Replacement of Left Femoral Artery with Synthetic Substitute, Percutaneous Endoscopic Approach

04RL4KZ Replacement of Left Femoral Artery with Nonautologous Tissue Substitute, Percutaneous Endoscopic Approach

04RM07Z Replacement of Right Popliteal Artery with Autologous Tissue Substitute, Open Approach

04RM0JZ Replacement of Right Popliteal Artery with Synthetic Substitute, Open Approach

04RM0KZ Replacement of Right Popliteal Artery with Nonautologous Tissue Substitute, Open Approach

♀ Female-only   ♂ Male-only   ▲ Limited Coverage   ● Non-OR   ▦ HAC-associated procedure   ▲ Non-covered procedures   ✚ Cluster

04RM47Z Replacement of Right Popliteal Artery with Autologous Tissue Substitute, Percutaneous Endoscopic Approach

04RM4JZ Replacement of Right Popliteal Artery with Synthetic Substitute, Percutaneous Endoscopic Approach

04RM4KZ Replacement of Right Popliteal Artery with Nonautologous Tissue Substitute, Percutaneous Endoscopic Approach

04RN07Z Replacement of Left Popliteal Artery with Autologous Tissue Substitute, Open Approach

04RN0JZ Replacement of Left Popliteal Artery with Synthetic Substitute, Open Approach

04RN0KZ Replacement of Left Popliteal Artery with Nonautologous Tissue Substitute, Open Approach

04RN47Z Replacement of Left Popliteal Artery with Autologous Tissue Substitute, Percutaneous Endoscopic Approach

04RN4JZ Replacement of Left Popliteal Artery with Synthetic Substitute, Percutaneous Endoscopic Approach

04RN4KZ Replacement of Left Popliteal Artery with Nonautologous Tissue Substitute, Percutaneous Endoscopic Approach

04RP07Z Replacement of Right Anterior Tibial Artery with Autologous Tissue Substitute, Open Approach

04RP0JZ Replacement of Right Anterior Tibial Artery with Synthetic Substitute, Open Approach

04RP0KZ Replacement of Right Anterior Tibial Artery with Nonautologous Tissue Substitute, Open Approach

04RP47Z Replacement of Right Anterior Tibial Artery with Autologous Tissue Substitute, Percutaneous Endoscopic Approach

04RP4JZ Replacement of Right Anterior Tibial Artery with Synthetic Substitute, Percutaneous Endoscopic Approach

04RP4KZ Replacement of Right Anterior Tibial Artery with Nonautologous Tissue Substitute, Percutaneous Endoscopic Approach

04RQ07Z Replacement of Left Anterior Tibial Artery with Autologous Tissue Substitute, Open Approach

04RQ0JZ Replacement of Left Anterior Tibial Artery with Synthetic Substitute, Open Approach

04RQ0KZ Replacement of Left Anterior Tibial Artery with Nonautologous Tissue Substitute, Open Approach

04RQ47Z Replacement of Left Anterior Tibial Artery with Autologous Tissue Substitute, Percutaneous Endoscopic Approach

04RQ4JZ Replacement of Left Anterior Tibial Artery with Synthetic Substitute, Percutaneous Endoscopic Approach

04RQ4KZ Replacement of Left Anterior Tibial Artery with Nonautologous Tissue Substitute, Percutaneous Endoscopic Approach

04RR07Z Replacement of Right Posterior Tibial Artery with Autologous Tissue Substitute, Open Approach

04RR0JZ Replacement of Right Posterior Tibial Artery with Synthetic Substitute, Open Approach

04RR0KZ Replacement of Right Posterior Tibial Artery with Nonautologous Tissue Substitute, Open Approach

04RR47Z Replacement of Right Posterior Tibial Artery with Autologous Tissue Substitute, Percutaneous Endoscopic Approach

04RR4JZ Replacement of Right Posterior Tibial Artery with Synthetic Substitute, Percutaneous Endoscopic Approach

04RR4KZ Replacement of Right Posterior Tibial Artery with Nonautologous Tissue Substitute, Percutaneous Endoscopic Approach

04RS07Z Replacement of Left Posterior Tibial Artery with Autologous Tissue Substitute, Open Approach

04RS0JZ Replacement of Left Posterior Tibial Artery with Synthetic Substitute, Open Approach

04RS0KZ Replacement of Left Posterior Tibial Artery with Nonautologous Tissue Substitute, Open Approach

04RS47Z Replacement of Left Posterior Tibial Artery with Autologous Tissue Substitute, Percutaneous Endoscopic Approach

04RS4JZ Replacement of Left Posterior Tibial Artery with Synthetic Substitute, Percutaneous Endoscopic Approach

04RS4KZ Replacement of Left Posterior Tibial Artery with Nonautologous Tissue Substitute, Percutaneous Endoscopic Approach

04RT07Z Replacement of Right Peroneal Artery with Autologous Tissue Substitute, Open Approach

04RT0JZ Replacement of Right Peroneal Artery with Synthetic Substitute, Open Approach

04RT0KZ Replacement of Right Peroneal Artery with Nonautologous Tissue Substitute, Open Approach

04RT47Z Replacement of Right Peroneal Artery with Autologous Tissue Substitute, Percutaneous Endoscopic Approach

04RT4JZ Replacement of Right Peroneal Artery with Synthetic Substitute, Percutaneous Endoscopic Approach

04RT4KZ Replacement of Right Peroneal Artery with Nonautologous Tissue Substitute, Percutaneous Endoscopic Approach

04RU07Z Replacement of Left Peroneal Artery with Autologous Tissue Substitute, Open Approach

04RU0JZ Replacement of Left Peroneal Artery with Synthetic Substitute, Open Approach

04RU0KZ Replacement of Left Peroneal Artery with Nonautologous Tissue Substitute, Open Approach

04RU47Z Replacement of Left Peroneal Artery with Autologous Tissue Substitute, Percutaneous Endoscopic Approach

04RU4JZ Replacement of Left Peroneal Artery with Synthetic Substitute, Percutaneous Endoscopic Approach

04RU4KZ Replacement of Left Peroneal Artery with Nonautologous Tissue Substitute, Percutaneous Endoscopic Approach

04RV07Z Replacement of Right Foot Artery with Autologous Tissue Substitute, Open Approach

04RV0JZ Replacement of Right Foot Artery with Synthetic Substitute, Open Approach

04RV0KZ Replacement of Right Foot Artery with Nonautologous Tissue Substitute, Open Approach

04RV47Z Replacement of Right Foot Artery with Autologous Tissue Substitute, Percutaneous Endoscopic Approach

04RV4JZ Replacement of Right Foot Artery with Synthetic Substitute, Percutaneous Endoscopic Approach

04RV4KZ Replacement of Right Foot Artery with Nonautologous Tissue Substitute, Percutaneous Endoscopic Approach

04RW07Z Replacement of Left Foot Artery with Autologous Tissue Substitute, Open Approach

04RW0JZ Replacement of Left Foot Artery with Synthetic Substitute, Open Approach

04RW0KZ Replacement of Left Foot Artery with Nonautologous Tissue Substitute, Open Approach

04RW47Z Replacement of Left Foot Artery with Autologous Tissue Substitute, Percutaneous Endoscopic Approach

04RW4JZ Replacement of Left Foot Artery with Synthetic Substitute, Percutaneous Endoscopic Approach

04RW4KZ Replacement of Left Foot Artery with Nonautologous Tissue Substitute, Percutaneous Endoscopic Approach

04RY07Z Replacement of Lower Artery with Autologous Tissue Substitute, Open Approach

04RY0JZ Replacement of Lower Artery with Synthetic Substitute, Open Approach

04RY0KZ Replacement of Lower Artery with Nonautologous Tissue Substitute, Open Approach

04RY47Z Replacement of Lower Artery with Autologous Tissue Substitute, Percutaneous Endoscopic Approach

04RY4JZ Replacement of Lower Artery with Synthetic Substitute, Percutaneous Endoscopic Approach

04RY4KZ Replacement of Lower Artery with Nonautologous Tissue Substitute, Percutaneous Endoscopic Approach

04S – Lower Arteries, Reposition

04S00ZZ Reposition Abdominal Aorta, Open Approach

04S03ZZ Reposition Abdominal Aorta, Percutaneous Approach

04S04ZZ Reposition Abdominal Aorta, Percutaneous Endoscopic Approach

04S10ZZ Reposition Celiac Artery, Open Approach

04S13ZZ Reposition Celiac Artery, Percutaneous Approach

04S14ZZ Reposition Celiac Artery, Percutaneous Endoscopic Approach

04S20ZZ Reposition Gastric Artery, Open Approach

04S23ZZ Reposition Gastric Artery, Percutaneous Approach

04S24ZZ Reposition Gastric Artery, Percutaneous Endoscopic Approach

04S30ZZ Reposition Hepatic Artery, Open Approach

04S33ZZ Reposition Hepatic Artery, Percutaneous Approach

04S34ZZ Reposition Hepatic Artery, Percutaneous Endoscopic Approach

04S40ZZ	Reposition Splenic Artery, Open Approach	**04SD0ZZ**	Reposition Left Common Iliac Artery, Open Approach	**04SP3ZZ**	Reposition Right Anterior Tibial Artery, Percutaneous Approach
04S43ZZ	Reposition Splenic Artery, Percutaneous Approach	**04SD3ZZ**	Reposition Left Common Iliac Artery, Percutaneous Approach	**04SP4ZZ**	Reposition Right Anterior Tibial Artery, Percutaneous Endoscopic Approach
04S44ZZ	Reposition Splenic Artery, Percutaneous Endoscopic Approach	**04SD4ZZ**	Reposition Left Common Iliac Artery, Percutaneous Endoscopic Approach	**04SQ0ZZ**	Reposition Left Anterior Tibial Artery, Open Approach
04S50ZZ	Reposition Superior Mesenteric Artery, Open Approach	**04SE0ZZ**	Reposition Right Internal Iliac Artery, Open Approach	**04SQ3ZZ**	Reposition Left Anterior Tibial Artery, Percutaneous Approach
04S53ZZ	Reposition Superior Mesenteric Artery, Percutaneous Approach	**04SE3ZZ**	Reposition Right Internal Iliac Artery, Percutaneous Approach	**04SQ4ZZ**	Reposition Left Anterior Tibial Artery, Percutaneous Endoscopic Approach
04S54ZZ	Reposition Superior Mesenteric Artery, Percutaneous Endoscopic Approach	**04SE4ZZ**	Reposition Right Internal Iliac Artery, Percutaneous Endoscopic Approach	**04SR0ZZ**	Reposition Right Posterior Tibial Artery, Open Approach
04S60ZZ	Reposition Right Colic Artery, Open Approach	**04SF0ZZ**	Reposition Left Internal Iliac Artery, Open Approach	**04SR3ZZ**	Reposition Right Posterior Tibial Artery, Percutaneous Approach
04S63ZZ	Reposition Right Colic Artery, Percutaneous Approach	**04SF3ZZ**	Reposition Left Internal Iliac Artery, Percutaneous Approach	**04SR4ZZ**	Reposition Right Posterior Tibial Artery, Percutaneous Endoscopic Approach
04S64ZZ	Reposition Right Colic Artery, Percutaneous Endoscopic Approach	**04SF4ZZ**	Reposition Left Internal Iliac Artery, Percutaneous Endoscopic Approach	**04SS0ZZ**	Reposition Left Posterior Tibial Artery, Open Approach
04S70ZZ	Reposition Left Colic Artery, Open Approach	**04SH0ZZ**	Reposition Right External Iliac Artery, Open Approach	**04SS3ZZ**	Reposition Left Posterior Tibial Artery, Percutaneous Approach
04S73ZZ	Reposition Left Colic Artery, Percutaneous Approach	**04SH3ZZ**	Reposition Right External Iliac Artery, Percutaneous Approach	**04SS4ZZ**	Reposition Left Posterior Tibial Artery, Percutaneous Endoscopic Approach
04S74ZZ	Reposition Left Colic Artery, Percutaneous Endoscopic Approach	**04SH4ZZ**	Reposition Right External Iliac Artery, Percutaneous Endoscopic Approach	**04ST0ZZ**	Reposition Right Peroneal Artery, Open Approach
04S80ZZ	Reposition Middle Colic Artery, Open Approach	**04SJ0ZZ**	Reposition Left External Iliac Artery, Open Approach	**04ST3ZZ**	Reposition Right Peroneal Artery, Percutaneous Approach
04S83ZZ	Reposition Middle Colic Artery, Percutaneous Approach	**04SJ3ZZ**	Reposition Left External Iliac Artery, Percutaneous Approach	**04ST4ZZ**	Reposition Right Peroneal Artery, Percutaneous Endoscopic Approach
04S84ZZ	Reposition Middle Colic Artery, Percutaneous Endoscopic Approach	**04SJ4ZZ**	Reposition Left External Iliac Artery, Percutaneous Endoscopic Approach	**04SU0ZZ**	Reposition Left Peroneal Artery, Open Approach
04S90ZZ	Reposition Right Renal Artery, Open Approach	**04SK0ZZ**	Reposition Right Femoral Artery, Open Approach	**04SU3ZZ**	Reposition Left Peroneal Artery, Percutaneous Approach
04S93ZZ	Reposition Right Renal Artery, Percutaneous Approach	**04SK3ZZ**	Reposition Right Femoral Artery, Percutaneous Approach	**04SU4ZZ**	Reposition Left Peroneal Artery, Percutaneous Endoscopic Approach
04S94ZZ	Reposition Right Renal Artery, Percutaneous Endoscopic Approach	**04SK4ZZ**	Reposition Right Femoral Artery, Percutaneous Endoscopic Approach	**04SV0ZZ**	Reposition Right Foot Artery, Open Approach
04SA0ZZ	Reposition Left Renal Artery, Open Approach	**04SL0ZZ**	Reposition Left Femoral Artery, Open Approach	**04SV3ZZ**	Reposition Right Foot Artery, Percutaneous Approach
04SA3ZZ	Reposition Left Renal Artery, Percutaneous Approach	**04SL3ZZ**	Reposition Left Femoral Artery, Percutaneous Approach	**04SV4ZZ**	Reposition Right Foot Artery, Percutaneous Endoscopic Approach
04SA4ZZ	Reposition Left Renal Artery, Percutaneous Endoscopic Approach	**04SL4ZZ**	Reposition Left Femoral Artery, Percutaneous Endoscopic Approach	**04SW0ZZ**	Reposition Left Foot Artery, Open Approach
04SB0ZZ	Reposition Inferior Mesenteric Artery, Open Approach	**04SM0ZZ**	Reposition Right Popliteal Artery, Open Approach	**04SW3ZZ**	Reposition Left Foot Artery, Percutaneous Approach
04SB3ZZ	Reposition Inferior Mesenteric Artery, Percutaneous Approach	**04SM3ZZ**	Reposition Right Popliteal Artery, Percutaneous Approach	**04SW4ZZ**	Reposition Left Foot Artery, Percutaneous Endoscopic Approach
04SB4ZZ	Reposition Inferior Mesenteric Artery, Percutaneous Endoscopic Approach	**04SM4ZZ**	Reposition Right Popliteal Artery, Percutaneous Endoscopic Approach	**04SY0ZZ**	Reposition Lower Artery, Open Approach
04SC0ZZ	Reposition Right Common Iliac Artery, Open Approach	**04SN0ZZ**	Reposition Left Popliteal Artery, Open Approach	**04SY3ZZ**	Reposition Lower Artery, Percutaneous Approach
04SC3ZZ	Reposition Right Common Iliac Artery, Percutaneous Approach	**04SN3ZZ**	Reposition Left Popliteal Artery, Percutaneous Approach	**04SY4ZZ**	Reposition Lower Artery, Percutaneous Endoscopic Approach
04SC4ZZ	Reposition Right Common Iliac Artery, Percutaneous Endoscopic Approach	**04SN4ZZ**	Reposition Left Popliteal Artery, Percutaneous Endoscopic Approach		
		04SP0ZZ	Reposition Right Anterior Tibial Artery, Open Approach		

04U – Lower Arteries, Supplement

04U007Z	Supplement Abdominal Aorta with Autologous Tissue Substitute, Open Approach	**04U047Z**	Supplement Abdominal Aorta with Autologous Tissue Substitute, Percutaneous Endoscopic Approach	**04U137Z**	Supplement Celiac Artery with Autologous Tissue Substitute, Percutaneous Approach
04U00JZ	Supplement Abdominal Aorta with Synthetic Substitute, Open Approach	**04U04JZ**	Supplement Abdominal Aorta with Synthetic Substitute, Percutaneous Endoscopic Approach	**04U13JZ**	Supplement Celiac Artery with Synthetic Substitute, Percutaneous Approach
04U00KZ	Supplement Abdominal Aorta with Nonautologous Tissue Substitute, Open Approach	**04U04KZ**	Supplement Abdominal Aorta with Nonautologous Tissue Substitute, Percutaneous Endoscopic Approach	**04U13KZ**	Supplement Celiac Artery with Nonautologous Tissue Substitute, Percutaneous Approach
04U037Z	Supplement Abdominal Aorta with Autologous Tissue Substitute, Percutaneous Approach	**04U107Z**	Supplement Celiac Artery with Autologous Tissue Substitute, Open Approach	**04U147Z**	Supplement Celiac Artery with Autologous Tissue Substitute, Percutaneous Endoscopic Approach
04U03JZ	Supplement Abdominal Aorta with Synthetic Substitute, Percutaneous Approach	**04U10JZ**	Supplement Celiac Artery with Synthetic Substitute, Open Approach	**04U14JZ**	Supplement Celiac Artery with Synthetic Substitute, Percutaneous Endoscopic Approach
04U03KZ	Supplement Abdominal Aorta with Nonautologous Tissue Substitute, Percutaneous Approach	**04U10KZ**	Supplement Celiac Artery with Nonautologous Tissue Substitute, Open Approach	**04U14KZ**	Supplement Celiac Artery with Nonautologous Tissue Substitute, Percutaneous Endoscopic Approach

♀ Female-only   ♂ Male-only   ▲ Limited Coverage   ● Non-OR   🅷🅰🅲 HAC-associated procedure   ▲ Non-covered procedures   ✚ Cluster

04U207Z Supplement Gastric Artery with Autologous Tissue Substitute, Open Approach

04U20JZ Supplement Gastric Artery with Synthetic Substitute, Open Approach

04U20KZ Supplement Gastric Artery with Nonautologous Tissue Substitute, Open Approach

04U237Z Supplement Gastric Artery with Autologous Tissue Substitute, Percutaneous Approach

04U23JZ Supplement Gastric Artery with Synthetic Substitute, Percutaneous Approach

04U23KZ Supplement Gastric Artery with Nonautologous Tissue Substitute, Percutaneous Approach

04U247Z Supplement Gastric Artery with Autologous Tissue Substitute, Percutaneous Endoscopic Approach

04U24JZ Supplement Gastric Artery with Synthetic Substitute, Percutaneous Endoscopic Approach

04U24KZ Supplement Gastric Artery with Nonautologous Tissue Substitute, Percutaneous Endoscopic Approach

04U307Z Supplement Hepatic Artery with Autologous Tissue Substitute, Open Approach

04U30JZ Supplement Hepatic Artery with Synthetic Substitute, Open Approach

04U30KZ Supplement Hepatic Artery with Nonautologous Tissue Substitute, Open Approach

04U337Z Supplement Hepatic Artery with Autologous Tissue Substitute, Percutaneous Approach

04U33JZ Supplement Hepatic Artery with Synthetic Substitute, Percutaneous Approach

04U33KZ Supplement Hepatic Artery with Nonautologous Tissue Substitute, Percutaneous Approach

04U347Z Supplement Hepatic Artery with Autologous Tissue Substitute, Percutaneous Endoscopic Approach

04U34JZ Supplement Hepatic Artery with Synthetic Substitute, Percutaneous Endoscopic Approach

04U34KZ Supplement Hepatic Artery with Nonautologous Tissue Substitute, Percutaneous Endoscopic Approach

04U407Z Supplement Splenic Artery with Autologous Tissue Substitute, Open Approach

04U40JZ Supplement Splenic Artery with Synthetic Substitute, Open Approach

04U40KZ Supplement Splenic Artery with Nonautologous Tissue Substitute, Open Approach

04U437Z Supplement Splenic Artery with Autologous Tissue Substitute, Percutaneous Approach

04U43JZ Supplement Splenic Artery with Synthetic Substitute, Percutaneous Approach

04U43KZ Supplement Splenic Artery with Nonautologous Tissue Substitute, Percutaneous Approach

04U447Z Supplement Splenic Artery with Autologous Tissue Substitute, Percutaneous Endoscopic Approach

04U44JZ Supplement Splenic Artery with Synthetic Substitute, Percutaneous Endoscopic Approach

04U44KZ Supplement Splenic Artery with Nonautologous Tissue Substitute, Percutaneous Endoscopic Approach

04U507Z Supplement Superior Mesenteric Artery with Autologous Tissue Substitute, Open Approach

04U50JZ Supplement Superior Mesenteric Artery with Synthetic Substitute, Open Approach

04U50KZ Supplement Superior Mesenteric Artery with Nonautologous Tissue Substitute, Open Approach

04U537Z Supplement Superior Mesenteric Artery with Autologous Tissue Substitute, Percutaneous Approach

04U53JZ Supplement Superior Mesenteric Artery with Synthetic Substitute, Percutaneous Approach

04U53KZ Supplement Superior Mesenteric Artery with Nonautologous Tissue Substitute, Percutaneous Approach

04U547Z Supplement Superior Mesenteric Artery with Autologous Tissue Substitute, Percutaneous Endoscopic Approach

04U54JZ Supplement Superior Mesenteric Artery with Synthetic Substitute, Percutaneous Endoscopic Approach

04U54KZ Supplement Superior Mesenteric Artery with Nonautologous Tissue Substitute, Percutaneous Endoscopic Approach

04U607Z Supplement Right Colic Artery with Autologous Tissue Substitute, Open Approach

04U60JZ Supplement Right Colic Artery with Synthetic Substitute, Open Approach

04U60KZ Supplement Right Colic Artery with Nonautologous Tissue Substitute, Open Approach

04U637Z Supplement Right Colic Artery with Autologous Tissue Substitute, Percutaneous Approach

04U63JZ Supplement Right Colic Artery with Synthetic Substitute, Percutaneous Approach

04U63KZ Supplement Right Colic Artery with Nonautologous Tissue Substitute, Percutaneous Approach

04U647Z Supplement Right Colic Artery with Autologous Tissue Substitute, Percutaneous Endoscopic Approach

04U64JZ Supplement Right Colic Artery with Synthetic Substitute, Percutaneous Endoscopic Approach

04U64KZ Supplement Right Colic Artery with Nonautologous Tissue Substitute, Percutaneous Endoscopic Approach

04U707Z Supplement Left Colic Artery with Autologous Tissue Substitute, Open Approach

04U70JZ Supplement Left Colic Artery with Synthetic Substitute, Open Approach

04U70KZ Supplement Left Colic Artery with Nonautologous Tissue Substitute, Open Approach

04U737Z Supplement Left Colic Artery with Autologous Tissue Substitute, Percutaneous Approach

04U73JZ Supplement Left Colic Artery with Synthetic Substitute, Percutaneous Approach

04U73KZ Supplement Left Colic Artery with Nonautologous Tissue Substitute, Percutaneous Approach

04U747Z Supplement Left Colic Artery with Autologous Tissue Substitute, Percutaneous Endoscopic Approach

04U74JZ Supplement Left Colic Artery with Synthetic Substitute, Percutaneous Endoscopic Approach

04U74KZ Supplement Left Colic Artery with Nonautologous Tissue Substitute, Percutaneous Endoscopic Approach

04U807Z Supplement Middle Colic Artery with Autologous Tissue Substitute, Open Approach

04U80JZ Supplement Middle Colic Artery with Synthetic Substitute, Open Approach

04U80KZ Supplement Middle Colic Artery with Nonautologous Tissue Substitute, Open Approach

04U837Z Supplement Middle Colic Artery with Autologous Tissue Substitute, Percutaneous Approach

04U83JZ Supplement Middle Colic Artery with Synthetic Substitute, Percutaneous Approach

04U83KZ Supplement Middle Colic Artery with Nonautologous Tissue Substitute, Percutaneous Approach

04U847Z Supplement Middle Colic Artery with Autologous Tissue Substitute, Percutaneous Endoscopic Approach

04U84JZ Supplement Middle Colic Artery with Synthetic Substitute, Percutaneous Endoscopic Approach

04U84KZ Supplement Middle Colic Artery with Nonautologous Tissue Substitute, Percutaneous Endoscopic Approach

04U907Z Supplement Right Renal Artery with Autologous Tissue Substitute, Open Approach

04U90JZ Supplement Right Renal Artery with Synthetic Substitute, Open Approach

04U90KZ Supplement Right Renal Artery with Nonautologous Tissue Substitute, Open Approach

04U937Z Supplement Right Renal Artery with Autologous Tissue Substitute, Percutaneous Approach

04U93JZ Supplement Right Renal Artery with Synthetic Substitute, Percutaneous Approach

04U93KZ Supplement Right Renal Artery with Nonautologous Tissue Substitute, Percutaneous Approach

04U947Z Supplement Right Renal Artery with Autologous Tissue Substitute, Percutaneous Endoscopic Approach

04U94JZ Supplement Right Renal Artery with Synthetic Substitute, Percutaneous Endoscopic Approach

04U94KZ Supplement Right Renal Artery with Nonautologous Tissue Substitute, Percutaneous Endoscopic Approach

04UA07Z Supplement Left Renal Artery with Autologous Tissue Substitute, Open Approach

04UA0JZ Supplement Left Renal Artery with Synthetic Substitute, Open Approach

04UA0KZ Supplement Left Renal Artery with Nonautologous Tissue Substitute, Open Approach

04UA37Z Supplement Left Renal Artery with Autologous Tissue Substitute, Percutaneous Approach

04UA3JZ Supplement Left Renal Artery with Synthetic Substitute, Percutaneous Approach

04UA3KZ Supplement Left Renal Artery with Nonautologous Tissue Substitute, Percutaneous Approach

04UA47Z Supplement Left Renal Artery with Autologous Tissue Substitute, Percutaneous Endoscopic Approach

04UA4JZ Supplement Left Renal Artery with Synthetic Substitute, Percutaneous Endoscopic Approach

04UA4KZ Supplement Left Renal Artery with Nonautologous Tissue Substitute, Percutaneous Endoscopic Approach

04UB07Z Supplement Inferior Mesenteric Artery with Autologous Tissue Substitute, Open Approach

04UB0JZ Supplement Inferior Mesenteric Artery with Synthetic Substitute, Open Approach

04UB0KZ Supplement Inferior Mesenteric Artery with Nonautologous Tissue Substitute, Open Approach

04UB37Z Supplement Inferior Mesenteric Artery with Autologous Tissue Substitute, Percutaneous Approach

04UB3JZ Supplement Inferior Mesenteric Artery with Synthetic Substitute, Percutaneous Approach

04UB3KZ Supplement Inferior Mesenteric Artery with Nonautologous Tissue Substitute, Percutaneous Approach

04UB47Z Supplement Inferior Mesenteric Artery with Autologous Tissue Substitute, Percutaneous Endoscopic Approach

04UB4JZ Supplement Inferior Mesenteric Artery with Synthetic Substitute, Percutaneous Endoscopic Approach

04UB4KZ Supplement Inferior Mesenteric Artery with Nonautologous Tissue Substitute, Percutaneous Endoscopic Approach

04UC07Z Supplement Right Common Iliac Artery with Autologous Tissue Substitute, Open Approach

04UC0JZ Supplement Right Common Iliac Artery with Synthetic Substitute, Open Approach

04UC0KZ Supplement Right Common Iliac Artery with Nonautologous Tissue Substitute, Open Approach

04UC37Z Supplement Right Common Iliac Artery with Autologous Tissue Substitute, Percutaneous Approach

04UC3JZ Supplement Right Common Iliac Artery with Synthetic Substitute, Percutaneous Approach

04UC3KZ Supplement Right Common Iliac Artery with Nonautologous Tissue Substitute, Percutaneous Approach

04UC47Z Supplement Right Common Iliac Artery with Autologous Tissue Substitute, Percutaneous Endoscopic Approach

04UC4JZ Supplement Right Common Iliac Artery with Synthetic Substitute, Percutaneous Endoscopic Approach

04UC4KZ Supplement Right Common Iliac Artery with Nonautologous Tissue Substitute, Percutaneous Endoscopic Approach

04UD07Z Supplement Left Common Iliac Artery with Autologous Tissue Substitute, Open Approach

04UD0JZ Supplement Left Common Iliac Artery with Synthetic Substitute, Open Approach

04UD0KZ Supplement Left Common Iliac Artery with Nonautologous Tissue Substitute, Open Approach

04UD37Z Supplement Left Common Iliac Artery with Autologous Tissue Substitute, Percutaneous Approach

04UD3JZ Supplement Left Common Iliac Artery with Synthetic Substitute, Percutaneous Approach

04UD3KZ Supplement Left Common Iliac Artery with Nonautologous Tissue Substitute, Percutaneous Approach

04UD47Z Supplement Left Common Iliac Artery with Autologous Tissue Substitute, Percutaneous Endoscopic Approach

04UD4JZ Supplement Left Common Iliac Artery with Synthetic Substitute, Percutaneous Endoscopic Approach

04UD4KZ Supplement Left Common Iliac Artery with Nonautologous Tissue Substitute, Percutaneous Endoscopic Approach

04UE07Z Supplement Right Internal Iliac Artery with Autologous Tissue Substitute, Open Approach

04UE0JZ Supplement Right Internal Iliac Artery with Synthetic Substitute, Open Approach

04UE0KZ Supplement Right Internal Iliac Artery with Nonautologous Tissue Substitute, Open Approach

04UE37Z Supplement Right Internal Iliac Artery with Autologous Tissue Substitute, Percutaneous Approach

04UE3JZ Supplement Right Internal Iliac Artery with Synthetic Substitute, Percutaneous Approach

04UE3KZ Supplement Right Internal Iliac Artery with Nonautologous Tissue Substitute, Percutaneous Approach

04UE47Z Supplement Right Internal Iliac Artery with Autologous Tissue Substitute, Percutaneous Endoscopic Approach

04UE4JZ Supplement Right Internal Iliac Artery with Synthetic Substitute, Percutaneous Endoscopic Approach

04UE4KZ Supplement Right Internal Iliac Artery with Nonautologous Tissue Substitute, Percutaneous Endoscopic Approach

04UF07Z Supplement Left Internal Iliac Artery with Autologous Tissue Substitute, Open Approach

04UF0JZ Supplement Left Internal Iliac Artery with Synthetic Substitute, Open Approach

04UF0KZ Supplement Left Internal Iliac Artery with Nonautologous Tissue Substitute, Open Approach

04UF37Z Supplement Left Internal Iliac Artery with Autologous Tissue Substitute, Percutaneous Approach

04UF3JZ Supplement Left Internal Iliac Artery with Synthetic Substitute, Percutaneous Approach

04UF3KZ Supplement Left Internal Iliac Artery with Nonautologous Tissue Substitute, Percutaneous Approach

04UF47Z Supplement Left Internal Iliac Artery with Autologous Tissue Substitute, Percutaneous Endoscopic Approach

04UF4JZ Supplement Left Internal Iliac Artery with Synthetic Substitute, Percutaneous Endoscopic Approach

04UF4KZ Supplement Left Internal Iliac Artery with Nonautologous Tissue Substitute, Percutaneous Endoscopic Approach

04UH07Z Supplement Right External Iliac Artery with Autologous Tissue Substitute, Open Approach

04UH0JZ Supplement Right External Iliac Artery with Synthetic Substitute, Open Approach

04UH0KZ Supplement Right External Iliac Artery with Nonautologous Tissue Substitute, Open Approach

04UH37Z Supplement Right External Iliac Artery with Autologous Tissue Substitute, Percutaneous Approach

04UH3JZ Supplement Right External Iliac Artery with Synthetic Substitute, Percutaneous Approach

04UH3KZ Supplement Right External Iliac Artery with Nonautologous Tissue Substitute, Percutaneous Approach

04UH47Z Supplement Right External Iliac Artery with Autologous Tissue Substitute, Percutaneous Endoscopic Approach

04UH4JZ Supplement Right External Iliac Artery with Synthetic Substitute, Percutaneous Endoscopic Approach

04UH4KZ Supplement Right External Iliac Artery with Nonautologous Tissue Substitute, Percutaneous Endoscopic Approach

04UJ07Z Supplement Left External Iliac Artery with Autologous Tissue Substitute, Open Approach

04UJ0JZ Supplement Left External Iliac Artery with Synthetic Substitute, Open Approach

04UJ0KZ Supplement Left External Iliac Artery with Nonautologous Tissue Substitute, Open Approach

AHA CC: 1Q, 2016, 31

04UJ37Z Supplement Left External Iliac Artery with Autologous Tissue Substitute, Percutaneous Approach

04UJ3JZ Supplement Left External Iliac Artery with Synthetic Substitute, Percutaneous Approach

04UJ3KZ Supplement Left External Iliac Artery with Nonautologous Tissue Substitute, Percutaneous Approach

04UJ47Z Supplement Left External Iliac Artery with Autologous Tissue Substitute, Percutaneous Endoscopic Approach

04UJ4JZ Supplement Left External Iliac Artery with Synthetic Substitute, Percutaneous Endoscopic Approach

04UJ4KZ Supplement Left External Iliac Artery with Nonautologous Tissue Substitute, Percutaneous Endoscopic Approach

04UK07Z Supplement Right Femoral Artery with Autologous Tissue Substitute, Open Approach

04UK0JZ Supplement Right Femoral Artery with Synthetic Substitute, Open Approach

04UK0KZ Supplement Right Femoral Artery with Nonautologous Tissue Substitute, Open Approach

AHA CC: 4Q, 2014, 37-38

04UK37Z Supplement Right Femoral Artery with Autologous Tissue Substitute, Percutaneous Approach

04UK3JZ Supplement Right Femoral Artery with Synthetic Substitute, Percutaneous Approach

AHA CC: 1Q, 2014, 22-23

04UK3KZ Supplement Right Femoral Artery with Nonautologous Tissue Substitute, Percutaneous Approach

04UK47Z Supplement Right Femoral Artery with Autologous Tissue Substitute, Percutaneous Endoscopic Approach

04UK4JZ Supplement Right Femoral Artery with Synthetic Substitute, Percutaneous Endoscopic Approach

04UK4KZ Supplement Right Femoral Artery with Nonautologous Tissue Substitute, Percutaneous Endoscopic Approach

♀ Female-only   ♂ Male-only   ▲ Limited Coverage   ● Non-OR   🔲 HAC-associated procedure   ▲ Non-covered procedures   ✚ Cluster

04UL07Z Supplement Left Femoral Artery with Autologous Tissue Substitute, Open Approach

04UL0JZ Supplement Left Femoral Artery with Synthetic Substitute, Open Approach

04UL0KZ Supplement Left Femoral Artery with Nonautologous Tissue Substitute, Open Approach

04UL37Z Supplement Left Femoral Artery with Autologous Tissue Substitute, Percutaneous Approach

04UL3JZ Supplement Left Femoral Artery with Synthetic Substitute, Percutaneous Approach

04UL3KZ Supplement Left Femoral Artery with Nonautologous Tissue Substitute, Percutaneous Approach

04UL47Z Supplement Left Femoral Artery with Autologous Tissue Substitute, Percutaneous Endoscopic Approach

04UL4JZ Supplement Left Femoral Artery with Synthetic Substitute, Percutaneous Endoscopic Approach

04UL4KZ Supplement Left Femoral Artery with Nonautologous Tissue Substitute, Percutaneous Endoscopic Approach

04UM07Z Supplement Right Popliteal Artery with Autologous Tissue Substitute, Open Approach

04UM0JZ Supplement Right Popliteal Artery with Synthetic Substitute, Open Approach

04UM0KZ Supplement Right Popliteal Artery with Nonautologous Tissue Substitute, Open Approach

04UM37Z Supplement Right Popliteal Artery with Autologous Tissue Substitute, Percutaneous Approach

04UM3JZ Supplement Right Popliteal Artery with Synthetic Substitute, Percutaneous Approach

04UM3KZ Supplement Right Popliteal Artery with Nonautologous Tissue Substitute, Percutaneous Approach

04UM47Z Supplement Right Popliteal Artery with Autologous Tissue Substitute, Percutaneous Endoscopic Approach

04UM4JZ Supplement Right Popliteal Artery with Synthetic Substitute, Percutaneous Endoscopic Approach

04UM4KZ Supplement Right Popliteal Artery with Nonautologous Tissue Substitute, Percutaneous Endoscopic Approach

04UN07Z Supplement Left Popliteal Artery with Autologous Tissue Substitute, Open Approach

04UN0JZ Supplement Left Popliteal Artery with Synthetic Substitute, Open Approach

04UN0KZ Supplement Left Popliteal Artery with Nonautologous Tissue Substitute, Open Approach

04UN37Z Supplement Left Popliteal Artery with Autologous Tissue Substitute, Percutaneous Approach

04UN3JZ Supplement Left Popliteal Artery with Synthetic Substitute, Percutaneous Approach

04UN3KZ Supplement Left Popliteal Artery with Nonautologous Tissue Substitute, Percutaneous Approach

04UN47Z Supplement Left Popliteal Artery with Autologous Tissue Substitute, Percutaneous Endoscopic Approach

04UN4JZ Supplement Left Popliteal Artery with Synthetic Substitute, Percutaneous Endoscopic Approach

04UN4KZ Supplement Left Popliteal Artery with Nonautologous Tissue Substitute, Percutaneous Endoscopic Approach

04UP07Z Supplement Right Anterior Tibial Artery with Autologous Tissue Substitute, Open Approach

04UP0JZ Supplement Right Anterior Tibial Artery with Synthetic Substitute, Open Approach

04UP0KZ Supplement Right Anterior Tibial Artery with Nonautologous Tissue Substitute, Open Approach

04UP37Z Supplement Right Anterior Tibial Artery with Autologous Tissue Substitute, Percutaneous Approach

04UP3JZ Supplement Right Anterior Tibial Artery with Synthetic Substitute, Percutaneous Approach

04UP3KZ Supplement Right Anterior Tibial Artery with Nonautologous Tissue Substitute, Percutaneous Approach

04UP47Z Supplement Right Anterior Tibial Artery with Autologous Tissue Substitute, Percutaneous Endoscopic Approach

04UP4JZ Supplement Right Anterior Tibial Artery with Synthetic Substitute, Percutaneous Endoscopic Approach

04UP4KZ Supplement Right Anterior Tibial Artery with Nonautologous Tissue Substitute, Percutaneous Endoscopic Approach

04UQ07Z Supplement Left Anterior Tibial Artery with Autologous Tissue Substitute, Open Approach

04UQ0JZ Supplement Left Anterior Tibial Artery with Synthetic Substitute, Open Approach

04UQ0KZ Supplement Left Anterior Tibial Artery with Nonautologous Tissue Substitute, Open Approach

04UQ37Z Supplement Left Anterior Tibial Artery with Autologous Tissue Substitute, Percutaneous Approach

04UQ3JZ Supplement Left Anterior Tibial Artery with Synthetic Substitute, Percutaneous Approach

04UQ3KZ Supplement Left Anterior Tibial Artery with Nonautologous Tissue Substitute, Percutaneous Approach

04UQ47Z Supplement Left Anterior Tibial Artery with Autologous Tissue Substitute, Percutaneous Endoscopic Approach

04UQ4JZ Supplement Left Anterior Tibial Artery with Synthetic Substitute, Percutaneous Endoscopic Approach

04UQ4KZ Supplement Left Anterior Tibial Artery with Nonautologous Tissue Substitute, Percutaneous Endoscopic Approach

04UR07Z Supplement Right Posterior Tibial Artery with Autologous Tissue Substitute, Open Approach
AHA CC: 2Q, 2016, 18-19

04UR0JZ Supplement Right Posterior Tibial Artery with Synthetic Substitute, Open Approach

04UR0KZ Supplement Right Posterior Tibial Artery with Nonautologous Tissue Substitute, Open Approach

04UR37Z Supplement Right Posterior Tibial Artery with Autologous Tissue Substitute, Percutaneous Approach

04UR3JZ Supplement Right Posterior Tibial Artery with Synthetic Substitute, Percutaneous Approach

04UR3KZ Supplement Right Posterior Tibial Artery with Nonautologous Tissue Substitute, Percutaneous Approach

04UR47Z Supplement Right Posterior Tibial Artery with Autologous Tissue Substitute, Percutaneous Endoscopic Approach

04UR4JZ Supplement Right Posterior Tibial Artery with Synthetic Substitute, Percutaneous Endoscopic Approach

04UR4KZ Supplement Right Posterior Tibial Artery with Nonautologous Tissue Substitute, Percutaneous Endoscopic Approach

04US07Z Supplement Left Posterior Tibial Artery with Autologous Tissue Substitute, Open Approach

04US0JZ Supplement Left Posterior Tibial Artery with Synthetic Substitute, Open Approach

04US0KZ Supplement Left Posterior Tibial Artery with Nonautologous Tissue Substitute, Open Approach

04US37Z Supplement Left Posterior Tibial Artery with Autologous Tissue Substitute, Percutaneous Approach

04US3JZ Supplement Left Posterior Tibial Artery with Synthetic Substitute, Percutaneous Approach

04US3KZ Supplement Left Posterior Tibial Artery with Nonautologous Tissue Substitute, Percutaneous Approach

04US47Z Supplement Left Posterior Tibial Artery with Autologous Tissue Substitute, Percutaneous Endoscopic Approach

04US4JZ Supplement Left Posterior Tibial Artery with Synthetic Substitute, Percutaneous Endoscopic Approach

04US4KZ Supplement Left Posterior Tibial Artery with Nonautologous Tissue Substitute, Percutaneous Endoscopic Approach

04UT07Z Supplement Right Peroneal Artery with Autologous Tissue Substitute, Open Approach

04UT0JZ Supplement Right Peroneal Artery with Synthetic Substitute, Open Approach

04UT0KZ Supplement Right Peroneal Artery with Nonautologous Tissue Substitute, Open Approach

04UT37Z Supplement Right Peroneal Artery with Autologous Tissue Substitute, Percutaneous Approach

04UT3JZ Supplement Right Peroneal Artery with Synthetic Substitute, Percutaneous Approach

04UT3KZ Supplement Right Peroneal Artery with Nonautologous Tissue Substitute, Percutaneous Approach

04UT47Z Supplement Right Peroneal Artery with Autologous Tissue Substitute, Percutaneous Endoscopic Approach

04UT4JZ Supplement Right Peroneal Artery with Synthetic Substitute, Percutaneous Endoscopic Approach

04UT4KZ Supplement Right Peroneal Artery with Nonautologous Tissue Substitute, Percutaneous Endoscopic Approach

04UU07Z Supplement Left Peroneal Artery with Autologous Tissue Substitute, Open Approach

04UU0JZ Supplement Left Peroneal Artery with Synthetic Substitute, Open Approach

---

♀ Female-only   ♂ Male-only   ▲ Limited Coverage   ● Non-OR   ▣ HAC-associated procedure   ▲ Non-covered procedures   ✚ Cluster

04UU0KZ Supplement Left Peroneal Artery with Nonautologous Tissue Substitute, Open Approach

04UU37Z Supplement Left Peroneal Artery with Autologous Tissue Substitute, Percutaneous Approach

04UU3JZ Supplement Left Peroneal Artery with Synthetic Substitute, Percutaneous Approach

04UU3KZ Supplement Left Peroneal Artery with Nonautologous Tissue Substitute, Percutaneous Approach

04UU47Z Supplement Left Peroneal Artery with Autologous Tissue Substitute, Percutaneous Endoscopic Approach

04UU4JZ Supplement Left Peroneal Artery with Synthetic Substitute, Percutaneous Endoscopic Approach

04UU4KZ Supplement Left Peroneal Artery with Nonautologous Tissue Substitute, Percutaneous Endoscopic Approach

04UV07Z Supplement Right Foot Artery with Autologous Tissue Substitute, Open Approach

04UV0JZ Supplement Right Foot Artery with Synthetic Substitute, Open Approach

04UV0KZ Supplement Right Foot Artery with Nonautologous Tissue Substitute, Open Approach

04UV37Z Supplement Right Foot Artery with Autologous Tissue Substitute, Percutaneous Approach

04UV3JZ Supplement Right Foot Artery with Synthetic Substitute, Percutaneous Approach

04UV3KZ Supplement Right Foot Artery with Nonautologous Tissue Substitute, Percutaneous Approach

04UV47Z Supplement Right Foot Artery with Autologous Tissue Substitute, Percutaneous Endoscopic Approach

04UV4JZ Supplement Right Foot Artery with Synthetic Substitute, Percutaneous Endoscopic Approach

04UV4KZ Supplement Right Foot Artery with Nonautologous Tissue Substitute, Percutaneous Endoscopic Approach

04UW07Z Supplement Left Foot Artery with Autologous Tissue Substitute, Open Approach

04UW0JZ Supplement Left Foot Artery with Synthetic Substitute, Open Approach

04UW0KZ Supplement Left Foot Artery with Nonautologous Tissue Substitute, Open Approach

04UW37Z Supplement Left Foot Artery with Autologous Tissue Substitute, Percutaneous Approach

04UW3JZ Supplement Left Foot Artery with Synthetic Substitute, Percutaneous Approach

04UW3KZ Supplement Left Foot Artery with Nonautologous Tissue Substitute, Percutaneous Approach

04UW47Z Supplement Left Foot Artery with Autologous Tissue Substitute, Percutaneous Endoscopic Approach

04UW4JZ Supplement Left Foot Artery with Synthetic Substitute, Percutaneous Endoscopic Approach

04UW4KZ Supplement Left Foot Artery with Nonautologous Tissue Substitute, Percutaneous Endoscopic Approach

04UY07Z Supplement Lower Artery with Autologous Tissue Substitute, Open Approach

04UY0JZ Supplement Lower Artery with Synthetic Substitute, Open Approach

04UY0KZ Supplement Lower Artery with Nonautologous Tissue Substitute, Open Approach

04UY37Z Supplement Lower Artery with Autologous Tissue Substitute, Percutaneous Approach

04UY3JZ Supplement Lower Artery with Synthetic Substitute, Percutaneous Approach

04UY3KZ Supplement Lower Artery with Nonautologous Tissue Substitute, Percutaneous Approach

04UY47Z Supplement Lower Artery with Autologous Tissue Substitute, Percutaneous Endoscopic Approach

04UY4JZ Supplement Lower Artery with Synthetic Substitute, Percutaneous Endoscopic Approach

04UY4KZ Supplement Lower Artery with Nonautologous Tissue Substitute, Percutaneous Endoscopic Approach

04V – Lower Arteries, Restriction

Review Coding Guideline B3.12

04V00CZ Restriction of Abdominal Aorta with Extraluminal Device, Open Approach

04V00DJ Restriction of Abdominal Aorta with Intraluminal Device, Temporary, Open Approach

04V00DZ Restriction of Abdominal Aorta with Intraluminal Device, Open Approach
AHA CC: 1Q, 2019, 22

04V00EZ Restriction of Abdominal Aorta with Branched or Fenestrated Intraluminal Device, One or Two Arteries, Open Approach

04V00FZ Restriction of Abdominal Aorta with Branched or Fenestrated Intraluminal Device, Three or More Arteries, Open Approach

04V00ZZ Restriction of Abdominal Aorta, Open Approach

04V03CZ Restriction of Abdominal Aorta with Extraluminal Device, Percutaneous Approach

04V03DJ Restriction of Abdominal Aorta with Intraluminal Device, Temporary, Percutaneous Approach

04V03DZ Restriction of Abdominal Aorta with Intraluminal Device, Percutaneous Approach
AHA CC: 1Q, 2014, 9; 3Q, 2016, 39

04V03EZ Restriction of Abdominal Aorta with Branched or Fenestrated Intraluminal Device, One or Two Arteries, Percutaneous Approach

04V03FZ Restriction of Abdominal Aorta with Branched or Fenestrated Intraluminal Device, Three or More Arteries, Percutaneous Approach

04V03ZZ Restriction of Abdominal Aorta, Percutaneous Approach

04V04CZ Restriction of Abdominal Aorta with Extraluminal Device, Percutaneous Endoscopic Approach

04V04DJ Restriction of Abdominal Aorta with Intraluminal Device, Temporary, Percutaneous Endoscopic Approach

04V04DZ Restriction of Abdominal Aorta with Intraluminal Device, Percutaneous Endoscopic Approach

04V04EZ Restriction of Abdominal Aorta with Branched or Fenestrated Intraluminal Device, One or Two Arteries, Percutaneous Endoscopic Approach

04V04FZ Restriction of Abdominal Aorta with Branched or Fenestrated Intraluminal Device, Three or More Arteries, Percutaneous Endoscopic Approach

04V04ZZ Restriction of Abdominal Aorta, Percutaneous Endoscopic Approach

04V10CZ Restriction of Celiac Artery with Extraluminal Device, Open Approach

04V10DZ Restriction of Celiac Artery with Intraluminal Device, Open Approach

04V10ZZ Restriction of Celiac Artery, Open Approach

04V13CZ Restriction of Celiac Artery with Extraluminal Device, Percutaneous Approach

04V13DZ Restriction of Celiac Artery with Intraluminal Device, Percutaneous Approach

04V13ZZ Restriction of Celiac Artery, Percutaneous Approach

04V14CZ Restriction of Celiac Artery with Extraluminal Device, Percutaneous Endoscopic Approach

04V14DZ Restriction of Celiac Artery with Intraluminal Device, Percutaneous Endoscopic Approach

04V14ZZ Restriction of Celiac Artery, Percutaneous Endoscopic Approach

04V20CZ Restriction of Gastric Artery with Extraluminal Device, Open Approach

04V20DZ Restriction of Gastric Artery with Intraluminal Device, Open Approach

04V20ZZ Restriction of Gastric Artery, Open Approach

04V23CZ Restriction of Gastric Artery with Extraluminal Device, Percutaneous Approach

04V23DZ Restriction of Gastric Artery with Intraluminal Device, Percutaneous Approach

04V23ZZ Restriction of Gastric Artery, Percutaneous Approach

04V24CZ Restriction of Gastric Artery with Extraluminal Device, Percutaneous Endoscopic Approach

04V24DZ Restriction of Gastric Artery with Intraluminal Device, Percutaneous Endoscopic Approach

04V24ZZ Restriction of Gastric Artery, Percutaneous Endoscopic Approach

04V30CZ Restriction of Hepatic Artery with Extraluminal Device, Open Approach

04V30DZ Restriction of Hepatic Artery with Intraluminal Device, Open Approach

04V30ZZ Restriction of Hepatic Artery, Open Approach

04V33CZ Restriction of Hepatic Artery with Extraluminal Device, Percutaneous Approach

04V33DZ Restriction of Hepatic Artery with Intraluminal Device, Percutaneous Approach

04V33ZZ Restriction of Hepatic Artery, Percutaneous Approach

04V34CZ Restriction of Hepatic Artery with Extraluminal Device, Percutaneous Endoscopic Approach

04V34DZ Restriction of Hepatic Artery with Intraluminal Device, Percutaneous Endoscopic Approach

04V34ZZ Restriction of Hepatic Artery, Percutaneous Endoscopic Approach

04V40CZ Restriction of Splenic Artery with Extraluminal Device, Open Approach

04V40DZ Restriction of Splenic Artery with Intraluminal Device, Open Approach

04V40ZZ Restriction of Splenic Artery, Open Approach

04V43CZ Restriction of Splenic Artery with Extraluminal Device, Percutaneous Approach

04V43DZ Restriction of Splenic Artery with Intraluminal Device, Percutaneous Approach

04V43ZZ Restriction of Splenic Artery, Percutaneous Approach

04V44CZ Restriction of Splenic Artery with Extraluminal Device, Percutaneous Endoscopic Approach

04V44DZ Restriction of Splenic Artery with Intraluminal Device, Percutaneous Endoscopic Approach

04V44ZZ Restriction of Splenic Artery, Percutaneous Endoscopic Approach

04V50CZ Restriction of Superior Mesenteric Artery with Extraluminal Device, Open Approach

04V50DZ Restriction of Superior Mesenteric Artery with Intraluminal Device, Open Approach

04V50ZZ Restriction of Superior Mesenteric Artery, Open Approach

04V53CZ Restriction of Superior Mesenteric Artery with Extraluminal Device, Percutaneous Approach

04V53DZ Restriction of Superior Mesenteric Artery with Intraluminal Device, Percutaneous Approach

04V53ZZ Restriction of Superior Mesenteric Artery, Percutaneous Approach

04V54CZ Restriction of Superior Mesenteric Artery with Extraluminal Device, Percutaneous Endoscopic Approach

04V54DZ Restriction of Superior Mesenteric Artery with Intraluminal Device, Percutaneous Endoscopic Approach

04V54ZZ Restriction of Superior Mesenteric Artery, Percutaneous Endoscopic Approach

04V60CZ Restriction of Right Colic Artery with Extraluminal Device, Open Approach

04V60DZ Restriction of Right Colic Artery with Intraluminal Device, Open Approach

04V60ZZ Restriction of Right Colic Artery, Open Approach

04V63CZ Restriction of Right Colic Artery with Extraluminal Device, Percutaneous Approach

04V63DZ Restriction of Right Colic Artery with Intraluminal Device, Percutaneous Approach

04V63ZZ Restriction of Right Colic Artery, Percutaneous Approach

04V64CZ Restriction of Right Colic Artery with Extraluminal Device, Percutaneous Endoscopic Approach

04V64DZ Restriction of Right Colic Artery with Intraluminal Device, Percutaneous Endoscopic Approach

04V64ZZ Restriction of Right Colic Artery, Percutaneous Endoscopic Approach

04V70CZ Restriction of Left Colic Artery with Extraluminal Device, Open Approach

04V70DZ Restriction of Left Colic Artery with Intraluminal Device, Open Approach

04V70ZZ Restriction of Left Colic Artery, Open Approach

04V73CZ Restriction of Left Colic Artery with Extraluminal Device, Percutaneous Approach

04V73DZ Restriction of Left Colic Artery with Intraluminal Device, Percutaneous Approach

04V73ZZ Restriction of Left Colic Artery, Percutaneous Approach

04V74CZ Restriction of Left Colic Artery with Extraluminal Device, Percutaneous Endoscopic Approach

04V74DZ Restriction of Left Colic Artery with Intraluminal Device, Percutaneous Endoscopic Approach

04V74ZZ Restriction of Left Colic Artery, Percutaneous Endoscopic Approach

04V80CZ Restriction of Middle Colic Artery with Extraluminal Device, Open Approach

04V80DZ Restriction of Middle Colic Artery with Intraluminal Device, Open Approach

04V80ZZ Restriction of Middle Colic Artery, Open Approach

04V83CZ Restriction of Middle Colic Artery with Extraluminal Device, Percutaneous Approach

04V83DZ Restriction of Middle Colic Artery with Intraluminal Device, Percutaneous Approach

04V83ZZ Restriction of Middle Colic Artery, Percutaneous Approach

04V84CZ Restriction of Middle Colic Artery with Extraluminal Device, Percutaneous Endoscopic Approach

04V84DZ Restriction of Middle Colic Artery with Intraluminal Device, Percutaneous Endoscopic Approach

04V84ZZ Restriction of Middle Colic Artery, Percutaneous Endoscopic Approach

04V90CZ Restriction of Right Renal Artery with Extraluminal Device, Open Approach

04V90DZ Restriction of Right Renal Artery with Intraluminal Device, Open Approach

04V90ZZ Restriction of Right Renal Artery, Open Approach

04V93CZ Restriction of Right Renal Artery with Extraluminal Device, Percutaneous Approach

04V93DZ Restriction of Right Renal Artery with Intraluminal Device, Percutaneous Approach

04V93ZZ Restriction of Right Renal Artery, Percutaneous Approach

04V94CZ Restriction of Right Renal Artery with Extraluminal Device, Percutaneous Endoscopic Approach

04V94DZ Restriction of Right Renal Artery with Intraluminal Device, Percutaneous Endoscopic Approach

04V94ZZ Restriction of Right Renal Artery, Percutaneous Endoscopic Approach

04VA0CZ Restriction of Left Renal Artery with Extraluminal Device, Open Approach

04VA0DZ Restriction of Left Renal Artery with Intraluminal Device, Open Approach

04VA0ZZ Restriction of Left Renal Artery, Open Approach

04VA3CZ Restriction of Left Renal Artery with Extraluminal Device, Percutaneous Approach

04VA3DZ Restriction of Left Renal Artery with Intraluminal Device, Percutaneous Approach

04VA3ZZ Restriction of Left Renal Artery, Percutaneous Approach

04VA4CZ Restriction of Left Renal Artery with Extraluminal Device, Percutaneous Endoscopic Approach

04VA4DZ Restriction of Left Renal Artery with Intraluminal Device, Percutaneous Endoscopic Approach

04VA4ZZ Restriction of Left Renal Artery, Percutaneous Endoscopic Approach

04VB0CZ Restriction of Inferior Mesenteric Artery with Extraluminal Device, Open Approach

04VB0DZ Restriction of Inferior Mesenteric Artery with Intraluminal Device, Open Approach

04VB0ZZ Restriction of Inferior Mesenteric Artery, Open Approach

04VB3CZ Restriction of Inferior Mesenteric Artery with Extraluminal Device, Percutaneous Approach

04VB3DZ Restriction of Inferior Mesenteric Artery with Intraluminal Device, Percutaneous Approach

04VB3ZZ Restriction of Inferior Mesenteric Artery, Percutaneous Approach

04VB4CZ Restriction of Inferior Mesenteric Artery with Extraluminal Device, Percutaneous Endoscopic Approach

04VB4DZ Restriction of Inferior Mesenteric Artery with Intraluminal Device, Percutaneous Endoscopic Approach

04VB4ZZ Restriction of Inferior Mesenteric Artery, Percutaneous Endoscopic Approach

04VC0CZ Restriction of Right Common Iliac Artery with Extraluminal Device, Open Approach

04VC0DZ Restriction of Right Common Iliac Artery with Intraluminal Device, Open Approach

04VC0EZ Restriction of Right Common Iliac Artery with Branched or Fenestrated Intraluminal Device, One or Two Arteries, Open Approach

04VC0ZZ Restriction of Right Common Iliac Artery, Open Approach

04VC3CZ Restriction of Right Common Iliac Artery with Extraluminal Device, Percutaneous Approach

04VC3DZ Restriction of Right Common Iliac Artery with Intraluminal Device, Percutaneous Approach

04VC3EZ Restriction of Right Common Iliac Artery with Branched or Fenestrated Intraluminal Device, One or Two Arteries, Percutaneous Approach
AHA CC: 4Q, 2016, 93-94

04VC3ZZ Restriction of Right Common Iliac Artery, Percutaneous Approach

04VC4CZ Restriction of Right Common Iliac Artery with Extraluminal Device, Percutaneous Endoscopic Approach

04VC4DZ Restriction of Right Common Iliac Artery with Intraluminal Device, Percutaneous Endoscopic Approach

04VC4EZ Restriction of Right Common Iliac Artery with Branched or Fenestrated Intraluminal Device, One or Two Arteries, Percutaneous Endoscopic Approach

04VC4ZZ Restriction of Right Common Iliac Artery, Percutaneous Endoscopic Approach

04VD0CZ Restriction of Left Common Iliac Artery with Extraluminal Device, Open Approach

04VD0DZ Restriction of Left Common Iliac Artery with Intraluminal Device, Open Approach

04VD0EZ Restriction of Left Common Iliac Artery with Branched or Fenestrated Intraluminal Device, One or Two Arteries, Open Approach

04VD0ZZ Restriction of Left Common Iliac Artery, Open Approach

04VD3CZ Restriction of Left Common Iliac Artery with Extraluminal Device, Percutaneous Approach

04VD3DZ Restriction of Left Common Iliac Artery with Intraluminal Device, Percutaneous Approach

04VD3EZ Restriction of Left Common Iliac Artery with Branched or Fenestrated Intraluminal Device, One or Two Arteries, Percutaneous Approach
AHA CC: 4Q, 2016, 93-94

04VD3ZZ Restriction of Left Common Iliac Artery, Percutaneous Approach

04VD4CZ Restriction of Left Common Iliac Artery with Extraluminal Device, Percutaneous Endoscopic Approach

04VD4DZ Restriction of Left Common Iliac Artery with Intraluminal Device, Percutaneous Endoscopic Approach

04VD4EZ Restriction of Left Common Iliac Artery with Branched or Fenestrated Intraluminal Device, One or Two Arteries, Percutaneous Endoscopic Approach

04VD4ZZ Restriction of Left Common Iliac Artery, Percutaneous Endoscopic Approach

04VE0CZ Restriction of Right Internal Iliac Artery with Extraluminal Device, Open Approach

04VE0DZ Restriction of Right Internal Iliac Artery with Intraluminal Device, Open Approach

04VE0ZZ Restriction of Right Internal Iliac Artery, Open Approach

04VE3CZ Restriction of Right Internal Iliac Artery with Extraluminal Device, Percutaneous Approach

04VE3DZ Restriction of Right Internal Iliac Artery with Intraluminal Device, Percutaneous Approach

04VE3ZZ Restriction of Right Internal Iliac Artery, Percutaneous Approach

04VE4CZ Restriction of Right Internal Iliac Artery with Extraluminal Device, Percutaneous Endoscopic Approach

04VE4DZ Restriction of Right Internal Iliac Artery with Intraluminal Device, Percutaneous Endoscopic Approach

04VE4ZZ Restriction of Right Internal Iliac Artery, Percutaneous Endoscopic Approach

04VF0CZ Restriction of Left Internal Iliac Artery with Extraluminal Device, Open Approach

04VF0DZ Restriction of Left Internal Iliac Artery with Intraluminal Device, Open Approach

04VF0ZZ Restriction of Left Internal Iliac Artery, Open Approach

04VF3CZ Restriction of Left Internal Iliac Artery with Extraluminal Device, Percutaneous Approach

04VF3DZ Restriction of Left Internal Iliac Artery with Intraluminal Device, Percutaneous Approach

04VF3ZZ Restriction of Left Internal Iliac Artery, Percutaneous Approach

04VF4CZ Restriction of Left Internal Iliac Artery with Extraluminal Device, Percutaneous Endoscopic Approach

04VF4DZ Restriction of Left Internal Iliac Artery with Intraluminal Device, Percutaneous Endoscopic Approach

04VF4ZZ Restriction of Left Internal Iliac Artery, Percutaneous Endoscopic Approach

04VH0CZ Restriction of Right External Iliac Artery with Extraluminal Device, Open Approach

04VH0DZ Restriction of Right External Iliac Artery with Intraluminal Device, Open Approach

04VH0ZZ Restriction of Right External Iliac Artery, Open Approach

04VH3CZ Restriction of Right External Iliac Artery with Extraluminal Device, Percutaneous Approach

04VH3DZ Restriction of Right External Iliac Artery with Intraluminal Device, Percutaneous Approach

04VH3ZZ Restriction of Right External Iliac Artery, Percutaneous Approach

04VH4CZ Restriction of Right External Iliac Artery with Extraluminal Device, Percutaneous Endoscopic Approach

04VH4DZ Restriction of Right External Iliac Artery with Intraluminal Device, Percutaneous Endoscopic Approach

04VH4ZZ Restriction of Right External Iliac Artery, Percutaneous Endoscopic Approach

04VJ0CZ Restriction of Left External Iliac Artery with Extraluminal Device, Open Approach

04VJ0DZ Restriction of Left External Iliac Artery with Intraluminal Device, Open Approach

04VJ0ZZ Restriction of Left External Iliac Artery, Open Approach

04VJ3CZ Restriction of Left External Iliac Artery with Extraluminal Device, Percutaneous Approach

04VJ3DZ Restriction of Left External Iliac Artery with Intraluminal Device, Percutaneous Approach

04VJ3ZZ Restriction of Left External Iliac Artery, Percutaneous Approach

04VJ4CZ Restriction of Left External Iliac Artery with Extraluminal Device, Percutaneous Endoscopic Approach

04VJ4DZ Restriction of Left External Iliac Artery with Intraluminal Device, Percutaneous Endoscopic Approach

04VJ4ZZ Restriction of Left External Iliac Artery, Percutaneous Endoscopic Approach

04VK0CZ Restriction of Right Femoral Artery with Extraluminal Device, Open Approach

04VK0DZ Restriction of Right Femoral Artery with Intraluminal Device, Open Approach

04VK0ZZ Restriction of Right Femoral Artery, Open Approach

04VK3CZ Restriction of Right Femoral Artery with Extraluminal Device, Percutaneous Approach

04VK3DZ Restriction of Right Femoral Artery with Intraluminal Device, Percutaneous Approach

04VK3ZZ Restriction of Right Femoral Artery, Percutaneous Approach

04VK4CZ Restriction of Right Femoral Artery with Extraluminal Device, Percutaneous Endoscopic Approach

04VK4DZ Restriction of Right Femoral Artery with Intraluminal Device, Percutaneous Endoscopic Approach

04VK4ZZ Restriction of Right Femoral Artery, Percutaneous Endoscopic Approach

04VL0CZ Restriction of Left Femoral Artery with Extraluminal Device, Open Approach

04VL0DZ Restriction of Left Femoral Artery with Intraluminal Device, Open Approach

04VL0ZZ Restriction of Left Femoral Artery, Open Approach

04VL3CZ Restriction of Left Femoral Artery with Extraluminal Device, Percutaneous Approach

04VL3DZ Restriction of Left Femoral Artery with Intraluminal Device, Percutaneous Approach

04VL3ZZ Restriction of Left Femoral Artery, Percutaneous Approach

04VL4CZ Restriction of Left Femoral Artery with Extraluminal Device, Percutaneous Endoscopic Approach

04VL4DZ Restriction of Left Femoral Artery with Intraluminal Device, Percutaneous Endoscopic Approach

04VL4ZZ Restriction of Left Femoral Artery, Percutaneous Endoscopic Approach

04VM0CZ Restriction of Right Popliteal Artery with Extraluminal Device, Open Approach

04VM0DZ Restriction of Right Popliteal Artery with Intraluminal Device, Open Approach

04VM0ZZ Restriction of Right Popliteal Artery, Open Approach

04VM3CZ Restriction of Right Popliteal Artery with Extraluminal Device, Percutaneous Approach

04VM3DZ Restriction of Right Popliteal Artery with Intraluminal Device, Percutaneous Approach

04VM3ZZ Restriction of Right Popliteal Artery, Percutaneous Approach

04VM4CZ Restriction of Right Popliteal Artery with Extraluminal Device, Percutaneous Endoscopic Approach

04VM4DZ Restriction of Right Popliteal Artery with Intraluminal Device, Percutaneous Endoscopic Approach

04VM4ZZ Restriction of Right Popliteal Artery, Percutaneous Endoscopic Approach

♀ Female-only   ♂ Male-only   ▲ Limited Coverage   ● Non-OR   ⬛ HAC-associated procedure   ▲ Non-covered procedures   ✚ Cluster

04VN0CZ	Restriction of Left Popliteal Artery with Extraluminal Device, Open Approach
04VN0DZ	Restriction of Left Popliteal Artery with Intraluminal Device, Open Approach
04VN0ZZ	Restriction of Left Popliteal Artery, Open Approach
04VN3CZ	Restriction of Left Popliteal Artery with Extraluminal Device, Percutaneous Approach
04VN3DZ	Restriction of Left Popliteal Artery with Intraluminal Device, Percutaneous Approach
04VN3ZZ	Restriction of Left Popliteal Artery, Percutaneous Approach
04VN4CZ	Restriction of Left Popliteal Artery with Extraluminal Device, Percutaneous Endoscopic Approach
04VN4DZ	Restriction of Left Popliteal Artery with Intraluminal Device, Percutaneous Endoscopic Approach
04VN4ZZ	Restriction of Left Popliteal Artery, Percutaneous Endoscopic Approach
04VP0CZ	Restriction of Right Anterior Tibial Artery with Extraluminal Device, Open Approach
04VP0DZ	Restriction of Right Anterior Tibial Artery with Intraluminal Device, Open Approach
04VP0ZZ	Restriction of Right Anterior Tibial Artery, Open Approach
04VP3CZ	Restriction of Right Anterior Tibial Artery with Extraluminal Device, Percutaneous Approach
04VP3DZ	Restriction of Right Anterior Tibial Artery with Intraluminal Device, Percutaneous Approach
04VP3ZZ	Restriction of Right Anterior Tibial Artery, Percutaneous Approach
04VP4CZ	Restriction of Right Anterior Tibial Artery with Extraluminal Device, Percutaneous Endoscopic Approach
04VP4DZ	Restriction of Right Anterior Tibial Artery with Intraluminal Device, Percutaneous Endoscopic Approach
04VP4ZZ	Restriction of Right Anterior Tibial Artery, Percutaneous Endoscopic Approach
04VQ0CZ	Restriction of Left Anterior Tibial Artery with Extraluminal Device, Open Approach
04VQ0DZ	Restriction of Left Anterior Tibial Artery with Intraluminal Device, Open Approach
04VQ0ZZ	Restriction of Left Anterior Tibial Artery, Open Approach
04VQ3CZ	Restriction of Left Anterior Tibial Artery with Extraluminal Device, Percutaneous Approach
04VQ3DZ	Restriction of Left Anterior Tibial Artery with Intraluminal Device, Percutaneous Approach
04VQ3ZZ	Restriction of Left Anterior Tibial Artery, Percutaneous Approach
04VQ4CZ	Restriction of Left Anterior Tibial Artery with Extraluminal Device, Percutaneous Endoscopic Approach
04VQ4DZ	Restriction of Left Anterior Tibial Artery with Intraluminal Device, Percutaneous Endoscopic Approach
04VQ4ZZ	Restriction of Left Anterior Tibial Artery, Percutaneous Endoscopic Approach
04VR0CZ	Restriction of Right Posterior Tibial Artery with Extraluminal Device, Open Approach
04VR0DZ	Restriction of Right Posterior Tibial Artery with Intraluminal Device, Open Approach
04VR0ZZ	Restriction of Right Posterior Tibial Artery, Open Approach
04VR3CZ	Restriction of Right Posterior Tibial Artery with Extraluminal Device, Percutaneous Approach
04VR3DZ	Restriction of Right Posterior Tibial Artery with Intraluminal Device, Percutaneous Approach
04VR3ZZ	Restriction of Right Posterior Tibial Artery, Percutaneous Approach
04VR4CZ	Restriction of Right Posterior Tibial Artery with Extraluminal Device, Percutaneous Endoscopic Approach
04VR4DZ	Restriction of Right Posterior Tibial Artery with Intraluminal Device, Percutaneous Endoscopic Approach
04VR4ZZ	Restriction of Right Posterior Tibial Artery, Percutaneous Endoscopic Approach
04VS0CZ	Restriction of Left Posterior Tibial Artery with Extraluminal Device, Open Approach
04VS0DZ	Restriction of Left Posterior Tibial Artery with Intraluminal Device, Open Approach
04VS0ZZ	Restriction of Left Posterior Tibial Artery, Open Approach
04VS3CZ	Restriction of Left Posterior Tibial Artery with Extraluminal Device, Percutaneous Approach
04VS3DZ	Restriction of Left Posterior Tibial Artery with Intraluminal Device, Percutaneous Approach
04VS3ZZ	Restriction of Left Posterior Tibial Artery, Percutaneous Approach
04VS4CZ	Restriction of Left Posterior Tibial Artery with Extraluminal Device, Percutaneous Endoscopic Approach
04VS4DZ	Restriction of Left Posterior Tibial Artery with Intraluminal Device, Percutaneous Endoscopic Approach
04VS4ZZ	Restriction of Left Posterior Tibial Artery, Percutaneous Endoscopic Approach
04VT0CZ	Restriction of Right Peroneal Artery with Extraluminal Device, Open Approach
04VT0DZ	Restriction of Right Peroneal Artery with Intraluminal Device, Open Approach
04VT0ZZ	Restriction of Right Peroneal Artery, Open Approach
04VT3CZ	Restriction of Right Peroneal Artery with Extraluminal Device, Percutaneous Approach
04VT3DZ	Restriction of Right Peroneal Artery with Intraluminal Device, Percutaneous Approach
04VT3ZZ	Restriction of Right Peroneal Artery, Percutaneous Approach
04VT4CZ	Restriction of Right Peroneal Artery with Extraluminal Device, Percutaneous Endoscopic Approach
04VT4DZ	Restriction of Right Peroneal Artery with Intraluminal Device, Percutaneous Endoscopic Approach
04VT4ZZ	Restriction of Right Peroneal Artery, Percutaneous Endoscopic Approach
04VU0CZ	Restriction of Left Peroneal Artery with Extraluminal Device, Open Approach
04VU0DZ	Restriction of Left Peroneal Artery with Intraluminal Device, Open Approach
04VU0ZZ	Restriction of Left Peroneal Artery, Open Approach
04VU3CZ	Restriction of Left Peroneal Artery with Extraluminal Device, Percutaneous Approach
04VU3DZ	Restriction of Left Peroneal Artery with Intraluminal Device, Percutaneous Approach
04VU3ZZ	Restriction of Left Peroneal Artery, Percutaneous Approach
04VU4CZ	Restriction of Left Peroneal Artery with Extraluminal Device, Percutaneous Endoscopic Approach
04VU4DZ	Restriction of Left Peroneal Artery with Intraluminal Device, Percutaneous Endoscopic Approach
04VU4ZZ	Restriction of Left Peroneal Artery, Percutaneous Endoscopic Approach
04VV0CZ	Restriction of Right Foot Artery with Extraluminal Device, Open Approach
04VV0DZ	Restriction of Right Foot Artery with Intraluminal Device, Open Approach
04VV0ZZ	Restriction of Right Foot Artery, Open Approach
04VV3CZ	Restriction of Right Foot Artery with Extraluminal Device, Percutaneous Approach
04VV3DZ	Restriction of Right Foot Artery with Intraluminal Device, Percutaneous Approach
04VV3ZZ	Restriction of Right Foot Artery, Percutaneous Approach
04VV4CZ	Restriction of Right Foot Artery with Extraluminal Device, Percutaneous Endoscopic Approach
04VV4DZ	Restriction of Right Foot Artery with Intraluminal Device, Percutaneous Endoscopic Approach
04VV4ZZ	Restriction of Right Foot Artery, Percutaneous Endoscopic Approach
04VW0CZ	Restriction of Left Foot Artery with Extraluminal Device, Open Approach
04VW0DZ	Restriction of Left Foot Artery with Intraluminal Device, Open Approach
04VW0ZZ	Restriction of Left Foot Artery, Open Approach
04VW3CZ	Restriction of Left Foot Artery with Extraluminal Device, Percutaneous Approach
04VW3DZ	Restriction of Left Foot Artery with Intraluminal Device, Percutaneous Approach
04VW3ZZ	Restriction of Left Foot Artery, Percutaneous Approach
04VW4CZ	Restriction of Left Foot Artery with Extraluminal Device, Percutaneous Endoscopic Approach
04VW4DZ	Restriction of Left Foot Artery with Intraluminal Device, Percutaneous Endoscopic Approach
04VW4ZZ	Restriction of Left Foot Artery, Percutaneous Endoscopic Approach
04VY0CZ	Restriction of Lower Artery with Extraluminal Device, Open Approach
04VY0DZ	Restriction of Lower Artery with Intraluminal Device, Open Approach
04VY0ZZ	Restriction of Lower Artery, Open Approach
04VY3CZ	Restriction of Lower Artery with Extraluminal Device, Percutaneous Approach
04VY3DZ	Restriction of Lower Artery with Intraluminal Device, Percutaneous Approach
04VY3ZZ	Restriction of Lower Artery, Percutaneous Approach

04VY4CZ	Restriction of Lower Artery with Extraluminal Device, Percutaneous Endoscopic Approach
04VY4DZ	Restriction of Lower Artery with Intraluminal Device, Percutaneous Endoscopic Approach
04VY4ZZ	Restriction of Lower Artery, Percutaneous Endoscopic Approach

04W – Lower Arteries, Revision

Review Coding Guideline B6.1c

04WY00Z	Revision of Drainage Device in Lower Artery, Open Approach
04WY02Z	Revision of Monitoring Device in Lower Artery, Open Approach
04WY03Z	Revision of Infusion Device in Lower Artery, Open Approach
04WY07Z	Revision of Autologous Tissue Substitute in Lower Artery, Open Approach
	AHA CC: 1Q, 2015, 36-37
04WY0CZ	Revision of Extraluminal Device in Lower Artery, Open Approach
04WY0DZ	Revision of Intraluminal Device in Lower Artery, Open Approach
04WY0JZ	Revision of Synthetic Substitute in Lower Artery, Open Approach
	AHA CC: 2Q, 2019, 14-15
04WY0KZ	Revision of Nonautologous Tissue Substitute in Lower Artery, Open Approach
04WY0YZ	Revision of Other Device in Lower Artery, Open Approach
04WY30Z	Revision of Drainage Device in Lower Artery, Percutaneous Approach
04WY32Z	Revision of Monitoring Device in Lower Artery, Percutaneous Approach
04WY33Z	Revision of Infusion Device in Lower Artery, Percutaneous Approach
04WY37Z	Revision of Autologous Tissue Substitute in Lower Artery, Percutaneous Approach
	AHA CC: 1Q, 2014, 26

04WY3CZ	Revision of Extraluminal Device in Lower Artery, Percutaneous Approach
04WY3DZ	Revision of Intraluminal Device in Lower Artery, Percutaneous Approach
	AHA CC: 1Q, 2014, 9-10; 3Q, 2020, 6
04WY3JZ	Revision of Synthetic Substitute in Lower Artery, Percutaneous Approach
04WY3KZ	Revision of Nonautologous Tissue Substitute in Lower Artery, Percutaneous Approach
04WY3YZ	Revision of Other Device in Lower Artery, Percutaneous Approach
04WY40Z	Revision of Drainage Device in Lower Artery, Percutaneous Endoscopic Approach
04WY42Z	Revision of Monitoring Device in Lower Artery, Percutaneous Endoscopic Approach
04WY43Z	Revision of Infusion Device in Lower Artery, Percutaneous Endoscopic Approach
04WY47Z	Revision of Autologous Tissue Substitute in Lower Artery, Percutaneous Endoscopic Approach
04WY4CZ	Revision of Extraluminal Device in Lower Artery, Percutaneous Endoscopic Approach
04WY4DZ	Revision of Intraluminal Device in Lower Artery, Percutaneous Endoscopic Approach

04WY4JZ	Revision of Synthetic Substitute in Lower Artery, Percutaneous Endoscopic Approach
04WY4KZ	Revision of Nonautologous Tissue Substitute in Lower Artery, Percutaneous Endoscopic Approach
04WY4YZ	Revision of Other Device in Lower Artery, Percutaneous Endoscopic Approach
04WYX0Z	Revision of Drainage Device in Lower Artery, External Approach
04WYX2Z	Revision of Monitoring Device in Lower Artery, External Approach
04WYX3Z	Revision of Infusion Device in Lower Artery, External Approach
04WYX7Z	Revision of Autologous Tissue Substitute in Lower Artery, External Approach
04WYXCZ	Revision of Extraluminal Device in Lower Artery, External Approach
04WYXDZ	Revision of Intraluminal Device in Lower Artery, External Approach
04WYXJZ	Revision of Synthetic Substitute in Lower Artery, External Approach
04WYXKZ	Revision of Nonautologous Tissue Substitute in Lower Artery, External Approach

Medical and Surgical, Lower Arteries Code Listings

370 ♀ Female-only ♂ Male-only ▲ Limited Coverage ● Non-OR ▥ HAC-associated procedure ▲ Non-covered procedures ✚ Cluster

Veins

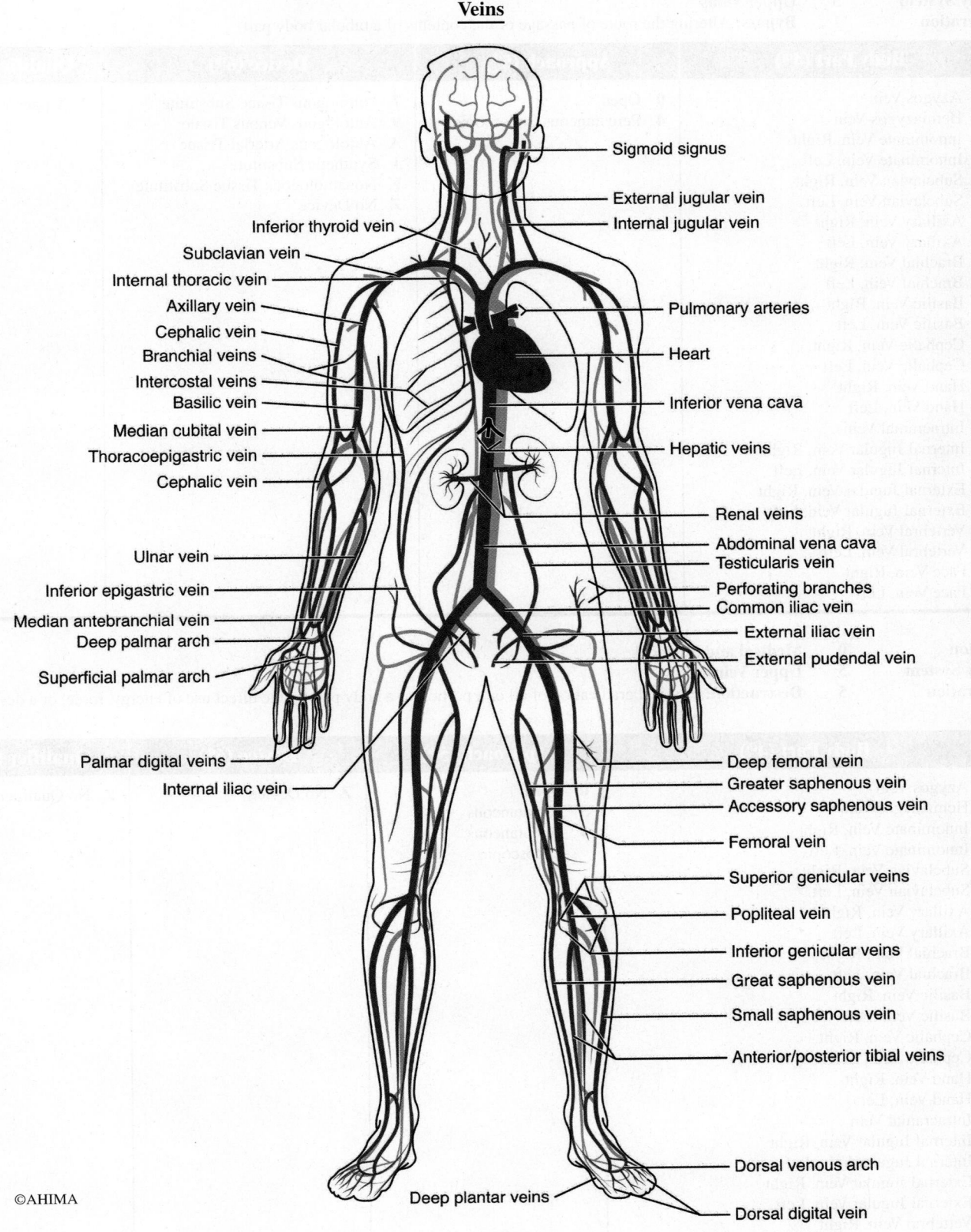

Sigmoid signus

External jugular vein

Internal jugular vein

Inferior thyroid vein

Subclavian vein

Internal thoracic vein

Axillary vein

Cephalic vein

Branchial veins

Intercostal veins

Basilic vein

Median cubital vein

Thoracoepigastric vein

Cephalic vein

Pulmonary arteries

Heart

Inferior vena cava

Hepatic veins

Renal veins

Abdominal vena cava

Testicularis vein

Perforating branches

Common iliac vein

External iliac vein

External pudendal vein

Ulnar vein

Inferior epigastric vein

Median antebranchial vein

Deep palmar arch

Superficial palmar arch

Palmar digital veins

Internal iliac vein

Deep femoral vein

Greater saphenous vein

Accessory saphenous vein

Femoral vein

Superior genicular veins

Popliteal vein

Inferior genicular veins

Great saphenous vein

Small saphenous vein

Anterior/posterior tibial veins

Dorsal venous arch

Deep plantar veins

Dorsal digital vein

©AHIMA

Upper Veins Tables 051–05W

Section	0	Medical and Surgical
Body System	5	Upper Veins
Operation	1	**Bypass:** Altering the route of passage of the contents of a tubular body part

Body Part (4th)	Approach (5th)	Device (6th)	Qualifier (7th)
0 Azygos Vein	0 Open	7 Autologous Tissue Substitute	Y Upper Vein
1 Hemiazygos Vein	4 Percutaneous Endoscopic	9 Autologous Venous Tissue	
3 Innominate Vein, Right		A Autologous Arterial Tissue	
4 Innominate Vein, Left		J Synthetic Substitute	
5 Subclavian Vein, Right		K Nonautologous Tissue Substitute	
6 Subclavian Vein, Left		Z No Device	
7 Axillary Vein, Right			
8 Axillary Vein, Left			
9 Brachial Vein, Right			
A Brachial Vein, Left			
B Basilic Vein, Right			
C Basilic Vein, Left			
D Cephalic Vein, Right			
F Cephalic Vein, Left			
G Hand Vein, Right			
H Hand Vein, Left			
L Intracranial Vein			
M Internal Jugular Vein, Right			
N Internal Jugular Vein, Left			
P External Jugular Vein, Right			
Q External Jugular Vein, Left			
R Vertebral Vein, Right			
S Vertebral Vein, Left			
T Face Vein, Right			
V Face Vein, Left			

Section	0	Medical and Surgical
Body System	5	Upper Veins
Operation	5	**Destruction:** Physical eradication of all or a portion of a body part by the direct use of energy, force, or a destructive agent

Body Part (4th)	Approach (5th)	Device (6th)	Qualifier (7th)
0 Azygos Vein	0 Open	Z No Device	Z No Qualifier
1 Hemiazygos Vein	3 Percutaneous		
3 Innominate Vein, Right	4 Percutaneous Endoscopic		
4 Innominate Vein, Left			
5 Subclavian Vein, Right			
6 Subclavian Vein, Left			
7 Axillary Vein, Right			
8 Axillary Vein, Left			
9 Brachial Vein, Right			
A Brachial Vein, Left			
B Basilic Vein, Right			
C Basilic Vein, Left			
D Cephalic Vein, Right			
F Cephalic Vein, Left			
G Hand Vein, Right			
H Hand Vein, Left			
L Intracranial Vein			
M Internal Jugular Vein, Right			
N Internal Jugular Vein, Left			
P External Jugular Vein, Right			
Q External Jugular Vein, Left			
R Vertebral Vein, Right			
S Vertebral Vein, Left			
T Face Vein, Right			
V Face Vein, Left			
Y Upper Vein			

Section	0	Medical and Surgical
Body System	5	Upper Veins
Operation	7	Dilation: Expanding an orifice or the lumen of a tubular body part

Body Part (4th)	Approach (5th)	Device (6th)	Qualifier (7th)
0 Azygos Vein 1 Hemiazygos Vein G Hand Vein, Right H Hand Vein, Left L Intracranial Vein M Internal Jugular Vein, Right N Internal Jugular Vein, Left P External Jugular Vein, Right Q External Jugular Vein, Left R Vertebral Vein, Right S Vertebral Vein, Left T Face Vein, Right V Face Vein, Left Y Upper Vein	0 Open 3 Percutaneous 4 Percutaneous Endoscopic	D Intraluminal Device Z No Device	Z No Qualifier
3 Innominate Vein, Right 4 Innominate Vein, Left 5 Subclavian Vein, Right 6 Subclavian Vein, Left 7 Axillary Vein, Right 8 Axillary Vein, Left 9 Brachial Vein, Right A Brachial Vein, Left B Basilic Vein, Right C Basilic Vein, Left D Cephalic Vein, Right F Cephalic Vein, Left	0 Open 3 Percutaneous 4 Percutaneous Endoscopic	D Intraluminal Device Z No Device	1 Drug-Coated Balloon Z No Qualifier

Section	0	Medical and Surgical
Body System	5	Upper Veins
Operation	9	Drainage: Taking or letting out fluids and/or gases from a body part

Body Part (4th)	Approach (5th)	Device (6th)	Qualifier (7th)
0 Azygos Vein 1 Hemiazygos Vein 3 Innominate Vein, Right 4 Innominate Vein, Left 5 Subclavian Vein, Right 6 Subclavian Vein, Left 7 Axillary Vein, Right 8 Axillary Vein, Left 9 Brachial Vein, Right A Brachial Vein, Left B Basilic Vein, Right C Basilic Vein, Left D Cephalic Vein, Right F Cephalic Vein, Left G Hand Vein, Right H Hand Vein, Left L Intracranial Vein M Internal Jugular Vein, Right N Internal Jugular Vein, Left P External Jugular Vein, Right Q External Jugular Vein, Left R Vertebral Vein, Right S Vertebral Vein, Left T Face Vein, Right V Face Vein, Left Y Upper Vein	0 Open 3 Percutaneous 4 Percutaneous Endoscopic	0 Drainage Device	Z No Qualifier

Continued →

Section	0	Medical and Surgical
Body System	5	Upper Veins
Operation	9	Drainage: Taking or letting out fluids and/or gases from a body part

Body Part (4th)	Approach (5th)	Device (6th)	Qualifier (7th)
0 Azygos Vein 1 Hemiazygos Vein 3 Innominate Vein, Right 4 Innominate Vein, Left 5 Subclavian Vein, Right 6 Subclavian Vein, Left 7 Axillary Vein, Right 8 Axillary Vein, Left 9 Brachial Vein, Right A Brachial Vein, Left B Basilic Vein, Right C Basilic Vein, Left D Cephalic Vein, Right F Cephalic Vein, Left G Hand Vein, Right H Hand Vein, Left L Intracranial Vein M Internal Jugular Vein, Right N Internal Jugular Vein, Left P External Jugular Vein, Right Q External Jugular Vein, Left R Vertebral Vein, Right S Vertebral Vein, Left T Face Vein, Right V Face Vein, Left Y Upper Vein	0 Open 3 Percutaneous 4 Percutaneous Endoscopic	Z No Device	X Diagnostic Z No Qualifier

Section	0	Medical and Surgical
Body System	5	Upper Veins
Operation	B	Excision: Cutting out or off, without replacement, a portion of a body part

Body Part (4th)	Approach (5th)	Device (6th)	Qualifier (7th)
0 Azygos Vein 1 Hemiazygos Vein 3 Innominate Vein, Right 4 Innominate Vein, Left 5 Subclavian Vein, Right 6 Subclavian Vein, Left 7 Axillary Vein, Right 8 Axillary Vein, Left 9 Brachial Vein, Right A Brachial Vein, Left B Basilic Vein, Right C Basilic Vein, Left D Cephalic Vein, Right F Cephalic Vein, Left G Hand Vein, Right H Hand Vein, Left L Intracranial Vein M Internal Jugular Vein, Right N Internal Jugular Vein, Left P External Jugular Vein, Right Q External Jugular Vein, Left R Vertebral Vein, Right S Vertebral Vein, Left T Face Vein, Right V Face Vein, Left Y Upper Vein	0 Open 3 Percutaneous 4 Percutaneous Endoscopic	Z No Device	X Diagnostic Z No Qualifier

Section   **0**   **Medical and Surgical**
Body System   **5**   **Upper Veins**
Operation   **C**   **Extirpation:** Taking or cutting out solid matter from a body part

Body Part (4ᵗʰ)	Approach (5ᵗʰ)	Device (6ᵗʰ)	Qualifier (7ᵗʰ)
0 Azygos Vein	**0** Open	**Z** No Device	**Z** No Qualifier
1 Hemiazygos Vein	**3** Percutaneous		
3 Innominate Vein, Right	**4** Percutaneous Endoscopic		
4 Innominate Vein, Left			
5 Subclavian Vein, Right			
6 Subclavian Vein, Left			
7 Axillary Vein, Right			
8 Axillary Vein, Left			
9 Brachial Vein, Right			
A Brachial Vein, Left			
B Basilic Vein, Right			
C Basilic Vein, Left			
D Cephalic Vein, Right			
F Cephalic Vein, Left			
G Hand Vein, Right			
H Hand Vein, Left			
L Intracranial Vein			
M Internal Jugular Vein, Right			
N Internal Jugular Vein, Left			
P External Jugular Vein, Right			
Q External Jugular Vein, Left			
R Vertebral Vein, Right			
S Vertebral Vein, Left			
T Face Vein, Right			
V Face Vein, Left			
Y Upper Vein			

Section   **0**   **Medical and Surgical**
Body System   **5**   **Upper Veins**
Operation   **D**   **Extraction:** Pulling or stripping out or off all or a portion of a body part by the use of force

Body Part (4ᵗʰ)	Approach (5ᵗʰ)	Device (6ᵗʰ)	Qualifier (7ᵗʰ)
9 Brachial Vein, Right	**0** Open	**Z** No Device	**Z** No Qualifier
A Brachial Vein, Left	**3** Percutaneous		
B Basilic Vein, Right			
C Basilic Vein, Left			
D Cephalic Vein, Right			
F Cephalic Vein, Left			
G Hand Vein, Right			
H Hand Vein, Left			
Y Upper Vein			

Section   **0**   **Medical and Surgical**
Body System   **5**   **Upper Veins**
Operation   **F**   **Fragmentation:** Breaking solid matter in a body part into pieces

Body Part (4ᵗʰ)	Approach (5ᵗʰ)	Device (6ᵗʰ)	Qualifier (7ᵗʰ)
3 Innominate Vein, Right	**3** Percutaneous	**Z** No Device	**0** Ultrasonic
4 Innominate Vein, Left			**Z** No Qualifier
5 Subclavian Vein, Right			
6 Subclavian Vein, Left			
7 Axillary Vein, Right			
8 Axillary Vein, Left			
9 Brachial Vein, Right			
A Brachial Vein, Left			
B Basilic Vein, Right			
C Basilic Vein, Left			
D Cephalic Vein, Right			
F Cephalic Vein, Left			
Y Upper Vein			

Section	0	Medical and Surgical
Body System	5	Upper Veins
Operation	H	**Insertion:** Putting in a nonbiological appliance that monitors, assists, performs, or prevents a physiological function but does not physically take the place of a body part

Body Part (4th)	Approach (5th)	Device (6th)	Qualifier (7th)
0 Azygos Vein	0 Open 3 Percutaneous 4 Percutaneous Endoscopic	2 Monitoring Device 3 Infusion Device D Intraluminal Device M Neurostimulator Lead	Z No Qualifier
1 Hemiazygos Vein 5 Subclavian Vein, Right 6 Subclavian Vein, Left 7 Axillary Vein, Right 8 Axillary Vein, Left 9 Brachial Vein, Right A Brachial Vein, Left B Basilic Vein, Right C Basilic Vein, Left D Cephalic Vein, Right F Cephalic Vein, Left G Hand Vein, Right H Hand Vein, Left L Intracranial Vein M Internal Jugular Vein, Right N Internal Jugular Vein, Left P External Jugular Vein, Right Q External Jugular Vein, Left R Vertebral Vein, Right S Vertebral Vein, Left T Face Vein, Right V Face Vein, Left	0 Open 3 Percutaneous 4 Percutaneous Endoscopic	3 Infusion Device D Intraluminal Device	Z No Qualifier
3 Innominate Vein, Right 4 Innominate Vein, Left	0 Open 3 Percutaneous 4 Percutaneous Endoscopic	3 Infusion Device D Intraluminal Device M Neurostimulator Lead	Z No Qualifier
Y Upper Vein	0 Open 3 Percutaneous 4 Percutaneous Endoscopic	2 Monitoring Device 3 Infusion Device D Intraluminal Device Y Other Device	Z No Qualifier

Section	0	Medical and Surgical
Body System	5	Upper Veins
Operation	J	**Inspection:** Visually and/or manually exploring a body part

Body Part (4th)	Approach (5th)	Device (6th)	Qualifier (7th)
Y Upper Vein	0 Open 3 Percutaneous 4 Percutaneous Endoscopic X External	Z No Device	Z No Qualifier

Section	0	Medical and Surgical
Body System	5	Upper Veins
Operation	L	Occlusion: Completely closing an orifice or the lumen of a tubular body part

Body Part (4th)	Approach (5th)	Device (6th)	Qualifier (7th)
0 Azygos Vein	0 Open	C Extraluminal Device	Z No Qualifier
1 Hemiazygos Vein	3 Percutaneous	D Intraluminal Device	
3 Innominate Vein, Right	4 Percutaneous Endoscopic	Z No Device	
4 Innominate Vein, Left			
5 Subclavian Vein, Right			
6 Subclavian Vein, Left			
7 Axillary Vein, Right			
8 Axillary Vein, Left			
9 Brachial Vein, Right			
A Brachial Vein, Left			
B Basilic Vein, Right			
C Basilic Vein, Left			
D Cephalic Vein, Right			
F Cephalic Vein, Left			
G Hand Vein, Right			
H Hand Vein, Left			
L Intracranial Vein			
M Internal Jugular Vein, Right			
N Internal Jugular Vein, Left			
P External Jugular Vein, Right			
Q External Jugular Vein, Left			
R Vertebral Vein, Right			
S Vertebral Vein, Left			
T Face Vein, Right			
V Face Vein, Left			
Y Upper Vein			

Section	0	Medical and Surgical
Body System	5	Upper Veins
Operation	N	Release: Freeing a body part from an abnormal physical constraint by cutting or by the use of force

Body Part (4th)	Approach (5th)	Device (6th)	Qualifier (7th)
0 Azygos Vein	0 Open	Z No Device	Z No Qualifier
1 Hemiazygos Vein	3 Percutaneous		
3 Innominate Vein, Right	4 Percutaneous Endoscopic		
4 Innominate Vein, Left			
5 Subclavian Vein, Right			
6 Subclavian Vein, Left			
7 Axillary Vein, Right			
8 Axillary Vein, Left			
9 Brachial Vein, Right			
A Brachial Vein, Left			
B Basilic Vein, Right			
C Basilic Vein, Left			
D Cephalic Vein, Right			
F Cephalic Vein, Left			
G Hand Vein, Right			
H Hand Vein, Left			
L Intracranial Vein			
M Internal Jugular Vein, Right			
N Internal Jugular Vein, Left			
P External Jugular Vein, Right			
Q External Jugular Vein, Left			
R Vertebral Vein, Right			
S Vertebral Vein, Left			
T Face Vein, Right			
V Face Vein, Left			
Y Upper Vein			

Section 0 **Medical and Surgical**
Body System 5 **Upper Veins**
Operation P **Removal:** Taking out or off a device from a body part

Body Part (4th)	Approach (5th)	Device (6th)	Qualifier (7th)
0 Azygos Vein	0 Open 3 Percutaneous 4 Percutaneous Endoscopic X External	2 Monitoring Device M Neurostimulator Lead	Z No Qualifier
3 Innominate Vein, Right 4 Innominate Vein, Left	0 Open 3 Percutaneous 4 Percutaneous Endoscopic X External	M Neurostimulator Lead	Z No Qualifier
Y Upper Vein	0 Open 3 Percutaneous 4 Percutaneous Endoscopic	0 Drainage Device 2 Monitoring Device 3 Infusion Device 7 Autologous Tissue Substitute C Extraluminal Device D Intraluminal Device J Synthetic Substitute K Nonautologous Tissue Substitute Y Other Device	Z No Qualifier
Y Upper Vein	X External	0 Drainage Device 2 Monitoring Device 3 Infusion Device D Intraluminal Device	Z No Qualifier

Section 0 **Medical and Surgical**
Body System 5 **Upper Veins**
Operation Q **Repair:** Restoring, to the extent possible, a body part to its normal anatomic structure and function

Body Part (4th)	Approach (5th)	Device (6th)	Qualifier (7th)
0 Azygos Vein 1 Hemiazygos Vein 3 Innominate Vein, Right 4 Innominate Vein, Left 5 Subclavian Vein, Right 6 Subclavian Vein, Left 7 Axillary Vein, Right 8 Axillary Vein, Left 9 Brachial Vein, Right A Brachial Vein, Left B Basilic Vein, Right C Basilic Vein, Left D Cephalic Vein, Right F Cephalic Vein, Left G Hand Vein, Right H Hand Vein, Left L Intracranial Vein M Internal Jugular Vein, Right N Internal Jugular Vein, Left P External Jugular Vein, Right Q External Jugular Vein, Left R Vertebral Vein, Right S Vertebral Vein, Left T Face Vein, Right V Face Vein, Left Y Upper Vein	0 Open 3 Percutaneous 4 Percutaneous Endoscopic	Z No Device	Z No Qualifier

Section   **0**   **Medical and Surgical**
Body System   **5**   **Upper Veins**
Operation   **R**   **Replacement:** Putting in or on biological or synthetic material that physically takes the place and/or function of all or a portion of a body part

Body Part (4th)	Approach (5th)	Device (6th)	Qualifier (7th)
0 Azygos Vein	0 Open	7 Autologous Tissue Substitute	Z No Qualifier
1 Hemiazygos Vein	4 Percutaneous Endoscopic	J Synthetic Substitute	
3 Innominate Vein, Right		K Nonautologous Tissue Substitute	
4 Innominate Vein, Left			
5 Subclavian Vein, Right			
6 Subclavian Vein, Left			
7 Axillary Vein, Right			
8 Axillary Vein, Left			
9 Brachial Vein, Right			
A Brachial Vein, Left			
B Basilic Vein, Right			
C Basilic Vein, Left			
D Cephalic Vein, Right			
F Cephalic Vein, Left			
G Hand Vein, Right			
H Hand Vein, Left			
L Intracranial Vein			
M Internal Jugular Vein, Right			
N Internal Jugular Vein, Left			
P External Jugular Vein, Right			
Q External Jugular Vein, Left			
R Vertebral Vein, Right			
S Vertebral Vein, Left			
T Face Vein, Right			
V Face Vein, Left			
Y Upper Vein			

Section   **0**   **Medical and Surgical**
Body System   **5**   **Upper Veins**
Operation   **S**   **Reposition:** Moving to its normal location, or other suitable location, all or a portion of a body part

Body Part (4th)	Approach (5th)	Device (6th)	Qualifier (7th)
0 Azygos Vein	0 Open	Z No Device	Z No Qualifier
1 Hemiazygos Vein	3 Percutaneous		
3 Innominate Vein, Right	4 Percutaneous Endoscopic		
4 Innominate Vein, Left			
5 Subclavian Vein, Right			
6 Subclavian Vein, Left			
7 Axillary Vein, Right			
8 Axillary Vein, Left			
9 Brachial Vein, Right			
A Brachial Vein, Left			
B Basilic Vein, Right			
C Basilic Vein, Left			
D Cephalic Vein, Right			
F Cephalic Vein, Left			
G Hand Vein, Right			
H Hand Vein, Left			
L Intracranial Vein			
M Internal Jugular Vein, Right			
N Internal Jugular Vein, Left			
P External Jugular Vein, Right			
Q External Jugular Vein, Left			
R Vertebral Vein, Right			
S Vertebral Vein, Left			
T Face Vein, Right			
V Face Vein, Left			
Y Upper Vein			

Section	0	Medical and Surgical
Body System	5	Upper Veins
Operation	U	Supplement: Putting in or on biological or synthetic material that physically reinforces and/or augments the function of a portion of a body part

Body Part (4th)	Approach (5th)	Device (6th)	Qualifier (7th)
0 Azygos Vein	0 Open	7 Autologous Tissue Substitute	Z No Qualifier
1 Hemiazygos Vein	3 Percutaneous	J Synthetic Substitute	
3 Innominate Vein, Right	4 Percutaneous Endoscopic	K Nonautologous Tissue Substitute	
4 Innominate Vein, Left			
5 Subclavian Vein, Right			
6 Subclavian Vein, Left			
7 Axillary Vein, Right			
8 Axillary Vein, Left			
9 Brachial Vein, Right			
A Brachial Vein, Left			
B Basilic Vein, Right			
C Basilic Vein, Left			
D Cephalic Vein, Right			
F Cephalic Vein, Left			
G Hand Vein, Right			
H Hand Vein, Left			
L Intracranial Vein			
M Internal Jugular Vein, Right			
N Internal Jugular Vein, Left			
P External Jugular Vein, Right			
Q External Jugular Vein, Left			
R Vertebral Vein, Right			
S Vertebral Vein, Left			
T Face Vein, Right			
V Face Vein, Left			
Y Upper Vein			

Section	0	Medical and Surgical
Body System	5	Upper Veins
Operation	V	Restriction: Partially closing an orifice or the lumen of a tubular body part

Body Part (4th)	Approach (5th)	Device (6th)	Qualifier (7th)
0 Azygos Vein	0 Open	C Extraluminal Device	Z No Qualifier
1 Hemiazygos Vein	3 Percutaneous	D Intraluminal Device	
3 Innominate Vein, Right	4 Percutaneous Endoscopic	Z No Device	
4 Innominate Vein, Left			
5 Subclavian Vein, Right			
6 Subclavian Vein, Left			
7 Axillary Vein, Right			
8 Axillary Vein, Left			
9 Brachial Vein, Right			
A Brachial Vein, Left			
B Basilic Vein, Right			
C Basilic Vein, Left			
D Cephalic Vein, Right			
F Cephalic Vein, Left			
G Hand Vein, Right			
H Hand Vein, Left			
L Intracranial Vein			
M Internal Jugular Vein, Right			
N Internal Jugular Vein, Left			
P External Jugular Vein, Right			
Q External Jugular Vein, Left			
R Vertebral Vein, Right			
S Vertebral Vein, Left			
T Face Vein, Right			
V Face Vein, Left			
Y Upper Vein			

Section   **0**   **Medical and Surgical**
Body System   **5**   **Upper Veins**
Operation   **W**   **Revision:** Correcting, to the extent possible, a portion of a malfunctioning device or the position of a displaced device

Body Part (4th)	Approach (5th)	Device (6th)	Qualifier (7th)
0 Azygos Vein	0 Open 3 Percutaneous 4 Percutaneous Endoscopic X External	2 Monitoring Device M Neurostimulator Lead	Z No Qualifier
3 Innominate Vein, Right 4 Innominate Vein, Left	0 Open 3 Percutaneous 4 Percutaneous Endoscopic X External	M Neurostimulator Lead	Z No Qualifier
Y Upper Vein	0 Open 3 Percutaneous 4 Percutaneous Endoscopic	0 Drainage Device 2 Monitoring Device 3 Infusion Device 7 Autologous Tissue Substitute C Extraluminal Device D Intraluminal Device J Synthetic Substitute K Nonautologous Tissue Substitute Y Other Device	Z No Qualifier
Y Upper Vein	X External	0 Drainage Device 2 Monitoring Device 3 Infusion Device 7 Autologous Tissue Substitute C Extraluminal Device D Intraluminal Device J Synthetic Substitute K Nonautologus Tissue Substitute	Z No Qualifier

Upper Veins Code Listing 051–05W

051 – Upper Veins, Bypass

Review Coding Guideline B3.6a

051007Y Bypass Azygos Vein to Upper Vein with Autologous Tissue Substitute, Open Approach

051009Y Bypass Azygos Vein to Upper Vein with Autologous Venous Tissue, Open Approach

05100AY Bypass Azygos Vein to Upper Vein with Autologous Arterial Tissue, Open Approach

05100JY Bypass Azygos Vein to Upper Vein with Synthetic Substitute, Open Approach

05100KY Bypass Azygos Vein to Upper Vein with Nonautologous Tissue Substitute, Open Approach

05100ZY Bypass Azygos Vein to Upper Vein, Open Approach

051047Y Bypass Azygos Vein to Upper Vein with Autologous Tissue Substitute, Percutaneous Endoscopic Approach

051049Y Bypass Azygos Vein to Upper Vein with Autologous Venous Tissue, Percutaneous Endoscopic Approach

05104AY Bypass Azygos Vein to Upper Vein with Autologous Arterial Tissue, Percutaneous Endoscopic Approach

05104JY Bypass Azygos Vein to Upper Vein with Synthetic Substitute, Percutaneous Endoscopic Approach

05104KY Bypass Azygos Vein to Upper Vein with Nonautologous Tissue Substitute, Percutaneous Endoscopic Approach

05104ZY Bypass Azygos Vein to Upper Vein, Percutaneous Endoscopic Approach

051107Y Bypass Hemiazygos Vein to Upper Vein with Autologous Tissue Substitute, Open Approach

051109Y Bypass Hemiazygos Vein to Upper Vein with Autologous Venous Tissue, Open Approach

05110AY Bypass Hemiazygos Vein to Upper Vein with Autologous Arterial Tissue, Open Approach

05110JY Bypass Hemiazygos Vein to Upper Vein with Synthetic Substitute, Open Approach

05110KY Bypass Hemiazygos Vein to Upper Vein with Nonautologous Tissue Substitute, Open Approach

05110ZY Bypass Hemiazygos Vein to Upper Vein, Open Approach

051147Y Bypass Hemiazygos Vein to Upper Vein with Autologous Tissue Substitute, Percutaneous Endoscopic Approach

051149Y Bypass Hemiazygos Vein to Upper Vein with Autologous Venous Tissue, Percutaneous Endoscopic Approach

05114AY Bypass Hemiazygos Vein to Upper Vein with Autologous Arterial Tissue, Percutaneous Endoscopic Approach

05114JY Bypass Hemiazygos Vein to Upper Vein with Synthetic Substitute, Percutaneous Endoscopic Approach

05114KY Bypass Hemiazygos Vein to Upper Vein with Nonautologous Tissue Substitute, Percutaneous Endoscopic Approach

05114ZY Bypass Hemiazygos Vein to Upper Vein, Percutaneous Endoscopic Approach

051307Y Bypass Right Innominate Vein to Upper Vein with Autologous Tissue Substitute, Open Approach

051309Y Bypass Right Innominate Vein to Upper Vein with Autologous Venous Tissue, Open Approach

05130AY Bypass Right Innominate Vein to Upper Vein with Autologous Arterial Tissue, Open Approach

05130JY Bypass Right Innominate Vein to Upper Vein with Synthetic Substitute, Open Approach

05130KY Bypass Right Innominate Vein to Upper Vein with Nonautologous Tissue Substitute, Open Approach

05130ZY Bypass Right Innominate Vein to Upper Vein, Open Approach

051347Y Bypass Right Innominate Vein to Upper Vein with Autologous Tissue Substitute, Percutaneous Endoscopic Approach

051349Y Bypass Right Innominate Vein to Upper Vein with Autologous Venous Tissue, Percutaneous Endoscopic Approach

♀ Female-only   ♂ Male-only   ▲ Limited Coverage   ● Non-OR   HAC HAC-associated procedure   ▲ Non-covered procedures   ✚ Cluster   **381**

05134AY Bypass Right Innominate Vein to Upper Vein with Autologous Arterial Tissue, Percutaneous Endoscopic Approach

05134JY Bypass Right Innominate Vein to Upper Vein with Synthetic Substitute, Percutaneous Endoscopic Approach

05134KY Bypass Right Innominate Vein to Upper Vein with Nonautologous Tissue Substitute, Percutaneous Endoscopic Approach

05134ZY Bypass Right Innominate Vein to Upper Vein, Percutaneous Endoscopic Approach

051407Y Bypass Left Innominate Vein to Upper Vein with Autologous Tissue Substitute, Open Approach

051409Y Bypass Left Innominate Vein to Upper Vein with Autologous Venous Tissue, Open Approach

05140AY Bypass Left Innominate Vein to Upper Vein with Autologous Arterial Tissue, Open Approach

05140JY Bypass Left Innominate Vein to Upper Vein with Synthetic Substitute, Open Approach

05140KY Bypass Left Innominate Vein to Upper Vein with Nonautologous Tissue Substitute, Open Approach

05140ZY Bypass Left Innominate Vein to Upper Vein, Open Approach

051447Y Bypass Left Innominate Vein to Upper Vein with Autologous Tissue Substitute, Percutaneous Endoscopic Approach

051449Y Bypass Left Innominate Vein to Upper Vein with Autologous Venous Tissue, Percutaneous Endoscopic Approach

05144AY Bypass Left Innominate Vein to Upper Vein with Autologous Arterial Tissue, Percutaneous Endoscopic Approach

05144JY Bypass Left Innominate Vein to Upper Vein with Synthetic Substitute, Percutaneous Endoscopic Approach

05144KY Bypass Left Innominate Vein to Upper Vein with Nonautologous Tissue Substitute, Percutaneous Endoscopic Approach

05144ZY Bypass Left Innominate Vein to Upper Vein, Percutaneous Endoscopic Approach

051507Y Bypass Right Subclavian Vein to Upper Vein with Autologous Tissue Substitute, Open Approach

051509Y Bypass Right Subclavian Vein to Upper Vein with Autologous Venous Tissue, Open Approach

05150AY Bypass Right Subclavian Vein to Upper Vein with Autologous Arterial Tissue, Open Approach

05150JY Bypass Right Subclavian Vein to Upper Vein with Synthetic Substitute, Open Approach

05150KY Bypass Right Subclavian Vein to Upper Vein with Nonautologous Tissue Substitute, Open Approach

05150ZY Bypass Right Subclavian Vein to Upper Vein, Open Approach

051547Y Bypass Right Subclavian Vein to Upper Vein with Autologous Tissue Substitute, Percutaneous Endoscopic Approach

051549Y Bypass Right Subclavian Vein to Upper Vein with Autologous Venous Tissue, Percutaneous Endoscopic Approach

05154AY Bypass Right Subclavian Vein to Upper Vein with Autologous Arterial Tissue, Percutaneous Endoscopic Approach

05154JY Bypass Right Subclavian Vein to Upper Vein with Synthetic Substitute, Percutaneous Endoscopic Approach

05154KY Bypass Right Subclavian Vein to Upper Vein with Nonautologous Tissue Substitute, Percutaneous Endoscopic Approach

05154ZY Bypass Right Subclavian Vein to Upper Vein, Percutaneous Endoscopic Approach

051607Y Bypass Left Subclavian Vein to Upper Vein with Autologous Tissue Substitute, Open Approach

051609Y Bypass Left Subclavian Vein to Upper Vein with Autologous Venous Tissue, Open Approach

05160AY Bypass Left Subclavian Vein to Upper Vein with Autologous Arterial Tissue, Open Approach

05160JY Bypass Left Subclavian Vein to Upper Vein with Synthetic Substitute, Open Approach

05160KY Bypass Left Subclavian Vein to Upper Vein with Nonautologous Tissue Substitute, Open Approach

05160ZY Bypass Left Subclavian Vein to Upper Vein, Open Approach

051647Y Bypass Left Subclavian Vein to Upper Vein with Autologous Tissue Substitute, Percutaneous Endoscopic Approach

051649Y Bypass Left Subclavian Vein to Upper Vein with Autologous Venous Tissue, Percutaneous Endoscopic Approach

05164AY Bypass Left Subclavian Vein to Upper Vein with Autologous Arterial Tissue, Percutaneous Endoscopic Approach

05164JY Bypass Left Subclavian Vein to Upper Vein with Synthetic Substitute, Percutaneous Endoscopic Approach

05164KY Bypass Left Subclavian Vein to Upper Vein with Nonautologous Tissue Substitute, Percutaneous Endoscopic Approach

05164ZY Bypass Left Subclavian Vein to Upper Vein, Percutaneous Endoscopic Approach

051707Y Bypass Right Axillary Vein to Upper Vein with Autologous Tissue Substitute, Open Approach

051709Y Bypass Right Axillary Vein to Upper Vein with Autologous Venous Tissue, Open Approach

05170AY Bypass Right Axillary Vein to Upper Vein with Autologous Arterial Tissue, Open Approach

05170JY Bypass Right Axillary Vein to Upper Vein with Synthetic Substitute, Open Approach

05170KY Bypass Right Axillary Vein to Upper Vein with Nonautologous Tissue Substitute, Open Approach

05170ZY Bypass Right Axillary Vein to Upper Vein, Open Approach

051747Y Bypass Right Axillary Vein to Upper Vein with Autologous Tissue Substitute, Percutaneous Endoscopic Approach

051749Y Bypass Right Axillary Vein to Upper Vein with Autologous Venous Tissue, Percutaneous Endoscopic Approach

05174AY Bypass Right Axillary Vein to Upper Vein with Autologous Arterial Tissue, Percutaneous Endoscopic Approach

05174JY Bypass Right Axillary Vein to Upper Vein with Synthetic Substitute, Percutaneous Endoscopic Approach

05174KY Bypass Right Axillary Vein to Upper Vein with Nonautologous Tissue Substitute, Percutaneous Endoscopic Approach

05174ZY Bypass Right Axillary Vein to Upper Vein, Percutaneous Endoscopic Approach

051807Y Bypass Left Axillary Vein to Upper Vein with Autologous Tissue Substitute, Open Approach

051809Y Bypass Left Axillary Vein to Upper Vein with Autologous Venous Tissue, Open Approach

05180AY Bypass Left Axillary Vein to Upper Vein with Autologous Arterial Tissue, Open Approach

05180JY Bypass Left Axillary Vein to Upper Vein with Synthetic Substitute, Open Approach

05180KY Bypass Left Axillary Vein to Upper Vein with Nonautologous Tissue Substitute, Open Approach

05180ZY Bypass Left Axillary Vein to Upper Vein, Open Approach

051847Y Bypass Left Axillary Vein to Upper Vein with Autologous Tissue Substitute, Percutaneous Endoscopic Approach

051849Y Bypass Left Axillary Vein to Upper Vein with Autologous Venous Tissue, Percutaneous Endoscopic Approach

05184AY Bypass Left Axillary Vein to Upper Vein with Autologous Arterial Tissue, Percutaneous Endoscopic Approach

05184JY Bypass Left Axillary Vein to Upper Vein with Synthetic Substitute, Percutaneous Endoscopic Approach

05184KY Bypass Left Axillary Vein to Upper Vein with Nonautologous Tissue Substitute, Percutaneous Endoscopic Approach

05184ZY Bypass Left Axillary Vein to Upper Vein, Percutaneous Endoscopic Approach

051907Y Bypass Right Brachial Vein to Upper Vein with Autologous Tissue Substitute, Open Approach

051909Y Bypass Right Brachial Vein to Upper Vein with Autologous Venous Tissue, Open Approach

05190AY Bypass Right Brachial Vein to Upper Vein with Autologous Arterial Tissue, Open Approach

05190JY Bypass Right Brachial Vein to Upper Vein with Synthetic Substitute, Open Approach

05190KY Bypass Right Brachial Vein to Upper Vein with Nonautologous Tissue Substitute, Open Approach

05190ZY Bypass Right Brachial Vein to Upper Vein, Open Approach

051947Y Bypass Right Brachial Vein to Upper Vein with Autologous Tissue Substitute, Percutaneous Endoscopic Approach

051949Y Bypass Right Brachial Vein to Upper Vein with Autologous Venous Tissue, Percutaneous Endoscopic Approach

05194AY Bypass Right Brachial Vein to Upper Vein with Autologous Arterial Tissue, Percutaneous Endoscopic Approach

05194JY Bypass Right Brachial Vein to Upper Vein with Synthetic Substitute, Percutaneous Endoscopic Approach

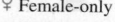 ♀ Female-only   ♂ Male-only   ▲ Limited Coverage   ● Non-OR   🅗🅐🅒 HAC-associated procedure   ▲ Non-covered procedures   ➕ Cluster

05194KY	Bypass Right Brachial Vein to Upper Vein with Nonautologous Tissue Substitute, Percutaneous Endoscopic Approach	
05194ZY	Bypass Right Brachial Vein to Upper Vein, Percutaneous Endoscopic Approach	
051A07Y	Bypass Left Brachial Vein to Upper Vein with Autologous Tissue Substitute, Open Approach	
051A09Y	Bypass Left Brachial Vein to Upper Vein with Autologous Venous Tissue, Open Approach	
051A0AY	Bypass Left Brachial Vein to Upper Vein with Autologous Arterial Tissue, Open Approach	
051A0JY	Bypass Left Brachial Vein to Upper Vein with Synthetic Substitute, Open Approach	
051A0KY	Bypass Left Brachial Vein to Upper Vein with Nonautologous Tissue Substitute, Open Approach	
051A0ZY	Bypass Left Brachial Vein to Upper Vein, Open Approach	
051A47Y	Bypass Left Brachial Vein to Upper Vein with Autologous Tissue Substitute, Percutaneous Endoscopic Approach	
051A49Y	Bypass Left Brachial Vein to Upper Vein with Autologous Venous Tissue, Percutaneous Endoscopic Approach	
051A4AY	Bypass Left Brachial Vein to Upper Vein with Autologous Arterial Tissue, Percutaneous Endoscopic Approach	
051A4JY	Bypass Left Brachial Vein to Upper Vein with Synthetic Substitute, Percutaneous Endoscopic Approach	
051A4KY	Bypass Left Brachial Vein to Upper Vein with Nonautologous Tissue Substitute, Percutaneous Endoscopic Approach	
051A4ZY	Bypass Left Brachial Vein to Upper Vein, Percutaneous Endoscopic Approach	
051B07Y	Bypass Right Basilic Vein to Upper Vein with Autologous Tissue Substitute, Open Approach	
051B09Y	Bypass Right Basilic Vein to Upper Vein with Autologous Venous Tissue, Open Approach	
051B0AY	Bypass Right Basilic Vein to Upper Vein with Autologous Arterial Tissue, Open Approach	
051B0JY	Bypass Right Basilic Vein to Upper Vein with Synthetic Substitute, Open Approach	
051B0KY	Bypass Right Basilic Vein to Upper Vein with Nonautologous Tissue Substitute, Open Approach	
051B0ZY	Bypass Right Basilic Vein to Upper Vein, Open Approach	
051B47Y	Bypass Right Basilic Vein to Upper Vein with Autologous Tissue Substitute, Percutaneous Endoscopic Approach	
051B49Y	Bypass Right Basilic Vein to Upper Vein with Autologous Venous Tissue, Percutaneous Endoscopic Approach	
051B4AY	Bypass Right Basilic Vein to Upper Vein with Autologous Arterial Tissue, Percutaneous Endoscopic Approach	
051B4JY	Bypass Right Basilic Vein to Upper Vein with Synthetic Substitute, Percutaneous Endoscopic Approach	
051B4KY	Bypass Right Basilic Vein to Upper Vein with Nonautologous Tissue Substitute, Percutaneous Endoscopic Approach	

051B4ZY	Bypass Right Basilic Vein to Upper Vein, Percutaneous Endoscopic Approach	
051C07Y	Bypass Left Basilic Vein to Upper Vein with Autologous Tissue Substitute, Open Approach	
051C09Y	Bypass Left Basilic Vein to Upper Vein with Autologous Venous Tissue, Open Approach	
051C0AY	Bypass Left Basilic Vein to Upper Vein with Autologous Arterial Tissue, Open Approach	
051C0JY	Bypass Left Basilic Vein to Upper Vein with Synthetic Substitute, Open Approach	
051C0KY	Bypass Left Basilic Vein to Upper Vein with Nonautologous Tissue Substitute, Open Approach	
051C0ZY	Bypass Left Basilic Vein to Upper Vein, Open Approach	
051C47Y	Bypass Left Basilic Vein to Upper Vein with Autologous Tissue Substitute, Percutaneous Endoscopic Approach	
051C49Y	Bypass Left Basilic Vein to Upper Vein with Autologous Venous Tissue, Percutaneous Endoscopic Approach	
051C4AY	Bypass Left Basilic Vein to Upper Vein with Autologous Arterial Tissue, Percutaneous Endoscopic Approach	
051C4JY	Bypass Left Basilic Vein to Upper Vein with Synthetic Substitute, Percutaneous Endoscopic Approach	
051C4KY	Bypass Left Basilic Vein to Upper Vein with Nonautologous Tissue Substitute, Percutaneous Endoscopic Approach	
051C4ZY	Bypass Left Basilic Vein to Upper Vein, Percutaneous Endoscopic Approach	
051D07Y	Bypass Right Cephalic Vein to Upper Vein with Autologous Tissue Substitute, Open Approach	
051D09Y	Bypass Right Cephalic Vein to Upper Vein with Autologous Venous Tissue, Open Approach	
051D0AY	Bypass Right Cephalic Vein to Upper Vein with Autologous Arterial Tissue, Open Approach	
051D0JY	Bypass Right Cephalic Vein to Upper Vein with Synthetic Substitute, Open Approach	
051D0KY	Bypass Right Cephalic Vein to Upper Vein with Nonautologous Tissue Substitute, Open Approach	
051D0ZY	Bypass Right Cephalic Vein to Upper Vein, Open Approach	
051D47Y	Bypass Right Cephalic Vein to Upper Vein with Autologous Tissue Substitute, Percutaneous Endoscopic Approach	
051D49Y	Bypass Right Cephalic Vein to Upper Vein with Autologous Venous Tissue, Percutaneous Endoscopic Approach	
051D4AY	Bypass Right Cephalic Vein to Upper Vein with Autologous Arterial Tissue, Percutaneous Endoscopic Approach	
051D4JY	Bypass Right Cephalic Vein to Upper Vein with Synthetic Substitute, Percutaneous Endoscopic Approach	
051D4KY	Bypass Right Cephalic Vein to Upper Vein with Nonautologous Tissue Substitute, Percutaneous Endoscopic Approach	
051D4ZY	Bypass Right Cephalic Vein to Upper Vein, Percutaneous Endoscopic Approach	
051F07Y	Bypass Left Cephalic Vein to Upper Vein with Autologous Tissue Substitute, Open Approach	

051F09Y	Bypass Left Cephalic Vein to Upper Vein with Autologous Venous Tissue, Open Approach	
051F0AY	Bypass Left Cephalic Vein to Upper Vein with Autologous Arterial Tissue, Open Approach	
051F0JY	Bypass Left Cephalic Vein to Upper Vein with Synthetic Substitute, Open Approach	
051F0KY	Bypass Left Cephalic Vein to Upper Vein with Nonautologous Tissue Substitute, Open Approach	
051F0ZY	Bypass Left Cephalic Vein to Upper Vein, Open Approach	
051F47Y	Bypass Left Cephalic Vein to Upper Vein with Autologous Tissue Substitute, Percutaneous Endoscopic Approach	
051F49Y	Bypass Left Cephalic Vein to Upper Vein with Autologous Venous Tissue, Percutaneous Endoscopic Approach	
051F4AY	Bypass Left Cephalic Vein to Upper Vein with Autologous Arterial Tissue, Percutaneous Endoscopic Approach	
051F4JY	Bypass Left Cephalic Vein to Upper Vein with Synthetic Substitute, Percutaneous Endoscopic Approach	
051F4KY	Bypass Left Cephalic Vein to Upper Vein with Nonautologous Tissue Substitute, Percutaneous Endoscopic Approach	
051F4ZY	Bypass Left Cephalic Vein to Upper Vein, Percutaneous Endoscopic Approach	
051G07Y	Bypass Right Hand Vein to Upper Vein with Autologous Tissue Substitute, Open Approach	
051G09Y	Bypass Right Hand Vein to Upper Vein with Autologous Venous Tissue, Open Approach	
051G0AY	Bypass Right Hand Vein to Upper Vein with Autologous Arterial Tissue, Open Approach	
051G0JY	Bypass Right Hand Vein to Upper Vein with Synthetic Substitute, Open Approach	
051G0KY	Bypass Right Hand Vein to Upper Vein with Nonautologous Tissue Substitute, Open Approach	
051G0ZY	Bypass Right Hand Vein to Upper Vein, Open Approach	
051G47Y	Bypass Right Hand Vein to Upper Vein with Autologous Tissue Substitute, Percutaneous Endoscopic Approach	
051G49Y	Bypass Right Hand Vein to Upper Vein with Autologous Venous Tissue, Percutaneous Endoscopic Approach	
051G4AY	Bypass Right Hand Vein to Upper Vein with Autologous Arterial Tissue, Percutaneous Endoscopic Approach	
051G4JY	Bypass Right Hand Vein to Upper Vein with Synthetic Substitute, Percutaneous Endoscopic Approach	
051G4KY	Bypass Right Hand Vein to Upper Vein with Nonautologous Tissue Substitute, Percutaneous Endoscopic Approach	
051G4ZY	Bypass Right Hand Vein to Upper Vein, Percutaneous Endoscopic Approach	
051H07Y	Bypass Left Hand Vein to Upper Vein with Autologous Tissue Substitute, Open Approach	
051H09Y	Bypass Left Hand Vein to Upper Vein with Autologous Venous Tissue, Open Approach	
051H0AY	Bypass Left Hand Vein to Upper Vein with Autologous Arterial Tissue, Open Approach	

051H0JY	Bypass Left Hand Vein to Upper Vein with Synthetic Substitute, Open Approach
051H0KY	Bypass Left Hand Vein to Upper Vein with Nonautologous Tissue Substitute, Open Approach
051H0ZY	Bypass Left Hand Vein to Upper Vein, Open Approach
051H47Y	Bypass Left Hand Vein to Upper Vein with Autologous Tissue Substitute, Percutaneous Endoscopic Approach
051H49Y	Bypass Left Hand Vein to Upper Vein with Autologous Venous Tissue, Percutaneous Endoscopic Approach
051H4AY	Bypass Left Hand Vein to Upper Vein with Autologous Arterial Tissue, Percutaneous Endoscopic Approach
051H4JY	Bypass Left Hand Vein to Upper Vein with Synthetic Substitute, Percutaneous Endoscopic Approach
051H4KY	Bypass Left Hand Vein to Upper Vein with Nonautologous Tissue Substitute, Percutaneous Endoscopic Approach
051H4ZY	Bypass Left Hand Vein to Upper Vein, Percutaneous Endoscopic Approach
051L07Y	Bypass Intracranial Vein to Upper Vein with Autologous Tissue Substitute, Open Approach
051L09Y	Bypass Intracranial Vein to Upper Vein with Autologous Venous Tissue, Open Approach
051L0AY	Bypass Intracranial Vein to Upper Vein with Autologous Arterial Tissue, Open Approach
051L0JY	Bypass Intracranial Vein to Upper Vein with Synthetic Substitute, Open Approach
051L0KY	Bypass Intracranial Vein to Upper Vein with Nonautologous Tissue Substitute, Open Approach
051L0ZY	Bypass Intracranial Vein to Upper Vein, Open Approach
051L47Y	Bypass Intracranial Vein to Upper Vein with Autologous Tissue Substitute, Percutaneous Endoscopic Approach
051L49Y	Bypass Intracranial Vein to Upper Vein with Autologous Venous Tissue, Percutaneous Endoscopic Approach
051L4AY	Bypass Intracranial Vein to Upper Vein with Autologous Arterial Tissue, Percutaneous Endoscopic Approach
051L4JY	Bypass Intracranial Vein to Upper Vein with Synthetic Substitute, Percutaneous Endoscopic Approach
051L4KY	Bypass Intracranial Vein to Upper Vein with Nonautologous Tissue Substitute, Percutaneous Endoscopic Approach
051L4ZY	Bypass Intracranial Vein to Upper Vein, Percutaneous Endoscopic Approach
051M07Y	Bypass Right Internal Jugular Vein to Upper Vein with Autologous Tissue Substitute, Open Approach
051M09Y	Bypass Right Internal Jugular Vein to Upper Vein with Autologous Venous Tissue, Open Approach
051M0AY	Bypass Right Internal Jugular Vein to Upper Vein with Autologous Arterial Tissue, Open Approach
051M0JY	Bypass Right Internal Jugular Vein to Upper Vein with Synthetic Substitute, Open Approach
051M0KY	Bypass Right Internal Jugular Vein to Upper Vein with Nonautologous Tissue Substitute, Open Approach
051M0ZY	Bypass Right Internal Jugular Vein to Upper Vein, Open Approach
051M47Y	Bypass Right Internal Jugular Vein to Upper Vein with Autologous Tissue Substitute, Percutaneous Endoscopic Approach
051M49Y	Bypass Right Internal Jugular Vein to Upper Vein with Autologous Venous Tissue, Percutaneous Endoscopic Approach
051M4AY	Bypass Right Internal Jugular Vein to Upper Vein with Autologous Arterial Tissue, Percutaneous Endoscopic Approach
051M4JY	Bypass Right Internal Jugular Vein to Upper Vein with Synthetic Substitute, Percutaneous Endoscopic Approach
051M4KY	Bypass Right Internal Jugular Vein to Upper Vein with Nonautologous Tissue Substitute, Percutaneous Endoscopic Approach
051M4ZY	Bypass Right Internal Jugular Vein to Upper Vein, Percutaneous Endoscopic Approach
051N07Y	Bypass Left Internal Jugular Vein to Upper Vein with Autologous Tissue Substitute, Open Approach
051N09Y	Bypass Left Internal Jugular Vein to Upper Vein with Autologous Venous Tissue, Open Approach
051N0AY	Bypass Left Internal Jugular Vein to Upper Vein with Autologous Arterial Tissue, Open Approach
051N0JY	Bypass Left Internal Jugular Vein to Upper Vein with Synthetic Substitute, Open Approach
051N0KY	Bypass Left Internal Jugular Vein to Upper Vein with Nonautologous Tissue Substitute, Open Approach
051N0ZY	Bypass Left Internal Jugular Vein to Upper Vein, Open Approach
051N47Y	Bypass Left Internal Jugular Vein to Upper Vein with Autologous Tissue Substitute, Percutaneous Endoscopic Approach
051N49Y	Bypass Left Internal Jugular Vein to Upper Vein with Autologous Venous Tissue, Percutaneous Endoscopic Approach
051N4AY	Bypass Left Internal Jugular Vein to Upper Vein with Autologous Arterial Tissue, Percutaneous Endoscopic Approach
051N4JY	Bypass Left Internal Jugular Vein to Upper Vein with Synthetic Substitute, Percutaneous Endoscopic Approach
051N4KY	Bypass Left Internal Jugular Vein to Upper Vein with Nonautologous Tissue Substitute, Percutaneous Endoscopic Approach
051N4ZY	Bypass Left Internal Jugular Vein to Upper Vein, Percutaneous Endoscopic Approach
051P07Y	Bypass Right External Jugular Vein to Upper Vein with Autologous Tissue Substitute, Open Approach
051P09Y	Bypass Right External Jugular Vein to Upper Vein with Autologous Venous Tissue, Open Approach
051P0AY	Bypass Right External Jugular Vein to Upper Vein with Autologous Arterial Tissue, Open Approach
051P0JY	Bypass Right External Jugular Vein to Upper Vein with Synthetic Substitute, Open Approach
051P0KY	Bypass Right External Jugular Vein to Upper Vein with Nonautologous Tissue Substitute, Open Approach
051P0ZY	Bypass Right External Jugular Vein to Upper Vein, Open Approach
051P47Y	Bypass Right External Jugular Vein to Upper Vein with Autologous Tissue Substitute, Percutaneous Endoscopic Approach
051P49Y	Bypass Right External Jugular Vein to Upper Vein with Autologous Venous Tissue, Percutaneous Endoscopic Approach
051P4AY	Bypass Right External Jugular Vein to Upper Vein with Autologous Arterial Tissue, Percutaneous Endoscopic Approach
051P4JY	Bypass Right External Jugular Vein to Upper Vein with Synthetic Substitute, Percutaneous Endoscopic Approach
051P4KY	Bypass Right External Jugular Vein to Upper Vein with Nonautologous Tissue Substitute, Percutaneous Endoscopic Approach
051P4ZY	Bypass Right External Jugular Vein to Upper Vein, Percutaneous Endoscopic Approach
051Q07Y	Bypass Left External Jugular Vein to Upper Vein with Autologous Tissue Substitute, Open Approach
051Q09Y	Bypass Left External Jugular Vein to Upper Vein with Autologous Venous Tissue, Open Approach
051Q0AY	Bypass Left External Jugular Vein to Upper Vein with Autologous Arterial Tissue, Open Approach
051Q0JY	Bypass Left External Jugular Vein to Upper Vein with Synthetic Substitute, Open Approach
051Q0KY	Bypass Left External Jugular Vein to Upper Vein with Nonautologous Tissue Substitute, Open Approach
051Q0ZY	Bypass Left External Jugular Vein to Upper Vein, Open Approach
051Q47Y	Bypass Left External Jugular Vein to Upper Vein with Autologous Tissue Substitute, Percutaneous Endoscopic Approach
051Q49Y	Bypass Left External Jugular Vein to Upper Vein with Autologous Venous Tissue, Percutaneous Endoscopic Approach *AHA CC: 1Q, 2020, 28-29*
051Q4AY	Bypass Left External Jugular Vein to Upper Vein with Autologous Arterial Tissue, Percutaneous Endoscopic Approach
051Q4JY	Bypass Left External Jugular Vein to Upper Vein with Synthetic Substitute, Percutaneous Endoscopic Approach
051Q4KY	Bypass Left External Jugular Vein to Upper Vein with Nonautologous Tissue Substitute, Percutaneous Endoscopic Approach
051Q4ZY	Bypass Left External Jugular Vein to Upper Vein, Percutaneous Endoscopic Approach
051R07Y	Bypass Right Vertebral Vein to Upper Vein with Autologous Tissue Substitute, Open Approach
051R09Y	Bypass Right Vertebral Vein to Upper Vein with Autologous Venous Tissue, Open Approach
051R0AY	Bypass Right Vertebral Vein to Upper Vein with Autologous Arterial Tissue, Open Approach
051R0JY	Bypass Right Vertebral Vein to Upper Vein with Synthetic Substitute, Open Approach

♀ Female-only ♂ Male-only ▲ Limited Coverage ● Non-OR ▨ HAC-associated procedure ▲ Non-covered procedures ✚ Cluster

051R0KY Bypass Right Vertebral Vein to Upper Vein with Nonautologous Tissue Substitute, Open Approach

051R0ZY Bypass Right Vertebral Vein to Upper Vein, Open Approach

051R47Y Bypass Right Vertebral Vein to Upper Vein with Autologous Tissue Substitute, Percutaneous Endoscopic Approach

051R49Y Bypass Right Vertebral Vein to Upper Vein with Autologous Venous Tissue, Percutaneous Endoscopic Approach

051R4AY Bypass Right Vertebral Vein to Upper Vein with Autologous Arterial Tissue, Percutaneous Endoscopic Approach

051R4JY Bypass Right Vertebral Vein to Upper Vein with Synthetic Substitute, Percutaneous Endoscopic Approach

051R4KY Bypass Right Vertebral Vein to Upper Vein with Nonautologous Tissue Substitute, Percutaneous Endoscopic Approach

051R4ZY Bypass Right Vertebral Vein to Upper Vein, Percutaneous Endoscopic Approach

051S07Y Bypass Left Vertebral Vein to Upper Vein with Autologous Tissue Substitute, Open Approach

051S09Y Bypass Left Vertebral Vein to Upper Vein with Autologous Venous Tissue, Open Approach

051S0AY Bypass Left Vertebral Vein to Upper Vein with Autologous Arterial Tissue, Open Approach

051S0JY Bypass Left Vertebral Vein to Upper Vein with Synthetic Substitute, Open Approach

051S0KY Bypass Left Vertebral Vein to Upper Vein with Nonautologous Tissue Substitute, Open Approach

051S0ZY Bypass Left Vertebral Vein to Upper Vein, Open Approach

051S47Y Bypass Left Vertebral Vein to Upper Vein with Autologous Tissue Substitute, Percutaneous Endoscopic Approach

051S49Y Bypass Left Vertebral Vein to Upper Vein with Autologous Venous Tissue, Percutaneous Endoscopic Approach

051S4AY Bypass Left Vertebral Vein to Upper Vein with Autologous Arterial Tissue, Percutaneous Endoscopic Approach

051S4JY Bypass Left Vertebral Vein to Upper Vein with Synthetic Substitute, Percutaneous Endoscopic Approach

051S4KY Bypass Left Vertebral Vein to Upper Vein with Nonautologous Tissue Substitute, Percutaneous Endoscopic Approach

051S4ZY Bypass Left Vertebral Vein to Upper Vein, Percutaneous Endoscopic Approach

051T07Y Bypass Right Face Vein to Upper Vein with Autologous Tissue Substitute, Open Approach

051T09Y Bypass Right Face Vein to Upper Vein with Autologous Venous Tissue, Open Approach

051T0AY Bypass Right Face Vein to Upper Vein with Autologous Arterial Tissue, Open Approach

051T0JY Bypass Right Face Vein to Upper Vein with Synthetic Substitute, Open Approach

051T0KY Bypass Right Face Vein to Upper Vein with Nonautologous Tissue Substitute, Open Approach

051T0ZY Bypass Right Face Vein to Upper Vein, Open Approach

051T47Y Bypass Right Face Vein to Upper Vein with Autologous Tissue Substitute, Percutaneous Endoscopic Approach

051T49Y Bypass Right Face Vein to Upper Vein with Autologous Venous Tissue, Percutaneous Endoscopic Approach

051T4AY Bypass Right Face Vein to Upper Vein with Autologous Arterial Tissue, Percutaneous Endoscopic Approach

051T4JY Bypass Right Face Vein to Upper Vein with Synthetic Substitute, Percutaneous Endoscopic Approach

051T4KY Bypass Right Face Vein to Upper Vein with Nonautologous Tissue Substitute, Percutaneous Endoscopic Approach

051T4ZY Bypass Right Face Vein to Upper Vein, Percutaneous Endoscopic Approach

051V07Y Bypass Left Face Vein to Upper Vein with Autologous Tissue Substitute, Open Approach

051V09Y Bypass Left Face Vein to Upper Vein with Autologous Venous Tissue, Open Approach

051V0AY Bypass Left Face Vein to Upper Vein with Autologous Arterial Tissue, Open Approach

051V0JY Bypass Left Face Vein to Upper Vein with Synthetic Substitute, Open Approach

051V0KY Bypass Left Face Vein to Upper Vein with Nonautologous Tissue Substitute, Open Approach

051V0ZY Bypass Left Face Vein to Upper Vein, Open Approach

051V47Y Bypass Left Face Vein to Upper Vein with Autologous Tissue Substitute, Percutaneous Endoscopic Approach

051V49Y Bypass Left Face Vein to Upper Vein with Autologous Venous Tissue, Percutaneous Endoscopic Approach

051V4AY Bypass Left Face Vein to Upper Vein with Autologous Arterial Tissue, Percutaneous Endoscopic Approach

051V4JY Bypass Left Face Vein to Upper Vein with Synthetic Substitute, Percutaneous Endoscopic Approach

051V4KY Bypass Left Face Vein to Upper Vein with Nonautologous Tissue Substitute, Percutaneous Endoscopic Approach

051V4ZY Bypass Left Face Vein to Upper Vein, Percutaneous Endoscopic Approach

055 – Upper Veins, Destruction

05500ZZ Destruction of Azygos Vein, Open Approach

05503ZZ Destruction of Azygos Vein, Percutaneous Approach

05504ZZ Destruction of Azygos Vein, Percutaneous Endoscopic Approach

05510ZZ Destruction of Hemiazygos Vein, Open Approach

05513ZZ Destruction of Hemiazygos Vein, Percutaneous Approach

05514ZZ Destruction of Hemiazygos Vein, Percutaneous Endoscopic Approach

05530ZZ Destruction of Right Innominate Vein, Open Approach

05533ZZ Destruction of Right Innominate Vein, Percutaneous Approach

05534ZZ Destruction of Right Innominate Vein, Percutaneous Endoscopic Approach

05540ZZ Destruction of Left Innominate Vein, Open Approach

05543ZZ Destruction of Left Innominate Vein, Percutaneous Approach

05544ZZ Destruction of Left Innominate Vein, Percutaneous Endoscopic Approach

05550ZZ Destruction of Right Subclavian Vein, Open Approach

05553ZZ Destruction of Right Subclavian Vein, Percutaneous Approach

05554ZZ Destruction of Right Subclavian Vein, Percutaneous Endoscopic Approach

05560ZZ Destruction of Left Subclavian Vein, Open Approach

05563ZZ Destruction of Left Subclavian Vein, Percutaneous Approach

05564ZZ Destruction of Left Subclavian Vein, Percutaneous Endoscopic Approach

05570ZZ Destruction of Right Axillary Vein, Open Approach

05573ZZ Destruction of Right Axillary Vein, Percutaneous Approach

05574ZZ Destruction of Right Axillary Vein, Percutaneous Endoscopic Approach

05580ZZ Destruction of Left Axillary Vein, Open Approach

05583ZZ Destruction of Left Axillary Vein, Percutaneous Approach

05584ZZ Destruction of Left Axillary Vein, Percutaneous Endoscopic Approach

05590ZZ Destruction of Right Brachial Vein, Open Approach

05593ZZ Destruction of Right Brachial Vein, Percutaneous Approach

05594ZZ Destruction of Right Brachial Vein, Percutaneous Endoscopic Approach

055A0ZZ Destruction of Left Brachial Vein, Open Approach

055A3ZZ Destruction of Left Brachial Vein, Percutaneous Approach

055A4ZZ Destruction of Left Brachial Vein, Percutaneous Endoscopic Approach

055B0ZZ Destruction of Right Basilic Vein, Open Approach

055B3ZZ Destruction of Right Basilic Vein, Percutaneous Approach

055B4ZZ Destruction of Right Basilic Vein, Percutaneous Endoscopic Approach

055C0ZZ Destruction of Left Basilic Vein, Open Approach

055C3ZZ Destruction of Left Basilic Vein, Percutaneous Approach

055C4ZZ Destruction of Left Basilic Vein, Percutaneous Endoscopic Approach

055D0ZZ Destruction of Right Cephalic Vein, Open Approach

055D3ZZ Destruction of Right Cephalic Vein, Percutaneous Approach

055D4ZZ Destruction of Right Cephalic Vein, Percutaneous Endoscopic Approach

055F0ZZ Destruction of Left Cephalic Vein, Open Approach

055F3ZZ Destruction of Left Cephalic Vein, Percutaneous Approach

055F4ZZ Destruction of Left Cephalic Vein, Percutaneous Endoscopic Approach

055G0ZZ Destruction of Right Hand Vein, Open Approach	**055N0ZZ** Destruction of Left Internal Jugular Vein, Open Approach	**055R4ZZ** Destruction of Right Vertebral Vein, Percutaneous Endoscopic Approach
055G3ZZ Destruction of Right Hand Vein, Percutaneous Approach	**055N3ZZ** Destruction of Left Internal Jugular Vein, Percutaneous Approach	**055S0ZZ** Destruction of Left Vertebral Vein, Open Approach
055G4ZZ Destruction of Right Hand Vein, Percutaneous Endoscopic Approach	**055N4ZZ** Destruction of Left Internal Jugular Vein, Percutaneous Endoscopic Approach	**055S3ZZ** Destruction of Left Vertebral Vein, Percutaneous Approach
055H0ZZ Destruction of Left Hand Vein, Open Approach	**055P0ZZ** Destruction of Right External Jugular Vein, Open Approach	**055S4ZZ** Destruction of Left Vertebral Vein, Percutaneous Endoscopic Approach
055H3ZZ Destruction of Left Hand Vein, Percutaneous Approach	**055P3ZZ** Destruction of Right External Jugular Vein, Percutaneous Approach	**055T0ZZ** Destruction of Right Face Vein, Open Approach
055H4ZZ Destruction of Left Hand Vein, Percutaneous Endoscopic Approach	**055P4ZZ** Destruction of Right External Jugular Vein, Percutaneous Endoscopic Approach	**055T3ZZ** Destruction of Right Face Vein, Percutaneous Approach
055L0ZZ Destruction of Intracranial Vein, Open Approach	**055Q0ZZ** Destruction of Left External Jugular Vein, Open Approach	**055T4ZZ** Destruction of Right Face Vein, Percutaneous Endoscopic Approach
055L3ZZ Destruction of Intracranial Vein, Percutaneous Approach	**055Q3ZZ** Destruction of Left External Jugular Vein, Percutaneous Approach	**055V0ZZ** Destruction of Left Face Vein, Open Approach
055L4ZZ Destruction of Intracranial Vein, Percutaneous Endoscopic Approach	**055Q4ZZ** Destruction of Left External Jugular Vein, Percutaneous Endoscopic Approach	**055V3ZZ** Destruction of Left Face Vein, Percutaneous Approach
055M0ZZ Destruction of Right Internal Jugular Vein, Open Approach	**055R0ZZ** Destruction of Right Vertebral Vein, Open Approach	**055V4ZZ** Destruction of Left Face Vein, Percutaneous Endoscopic Approach
055M3ZZ Destruction of Right Internal Jugular Vein, Percutaneous Approach	**055R3ZZ** Destruction of Right Vertebral Vein, Percutaneous Approach	**055Y0ZZ** Destruction of Upper Vein, Open Approach
055M4ZZ Destruction of Right Internal Jugular Vein, Percutaneous Endoscopic Approach		**055Y3ZZ** Destruction of Upper Vein, Percutaneous Approach
		055Y4ZZ Destruction of Upper Vein, Percutaneous Endoscopic Approach

057 – Upper Veins, Dilation

05700DZ Dilation of Azygos Vein with Intraluminal Device, Open Approach	**05733Z1** Dilation of Right Innominate Vein using Drug-Coated Balloon, Percutaneous Approach	**05744Z1** Dilation of Left Innominate Vein using Drug-Coated Balloon, Percutaneous Endoscopic Approach
05700ZZ Dilation of Azygos Vein, Open Approach	**05733ZZ** Dilation of Right Innominate Vein, Percutaneous Approach	**05744ZZ** Dilation of Left Innominate Vein, Percutaneous Endoscopic Approach
05703DZ Dilation of Azygos Vein with Intraluminal Device, Percutaneous Approach	**05734D1** Dilation of Right Innominate Vein with Intraluminal Device, using Drug-Coated Balloon, Percutaneous Endoscopic Approach	**05750D1** Dilation of Right Subclavian Vein with Intraluminal Device, using Drug-Coated Balloon, Open Approach
05703ZZ Dilation of Azygos Vein, Percutaneous Approach	**05734DZ** Dilation of Right Innominate Vein with Intraluminal Device, Percutaneous Endoscopic Approach	**05750DZ** Dilation of Right Subclavian Vein with Intraluminal Device, Open Approach
05704DZ Dilation of Azygos Vein with Intraluminal Device, Percutaneous Endoscopic Approach	**05734Z1** Dilation of Right Innominate Vein using Drug-Coated Balloon, Percutaneous Endoscopic Approach	**05750Z1** Dilation of Right Subclavian Vein using Drug-Coated Balloon, Open Approach
05704ZZ Dilation of Azygos Vein, Percutaneous Endoscopic Approach	**05734ZZ** Dilation of Right Innominate Vein, Percutaneous Endoscopic Approach	**05750ZZ** Dilation of Right Subclavian Vein, Open Approach
05710DZ Dilation of Hemiazygos Vein with Intraluminal Device, Open Approach	**05740D1** Dilation of Left Innominate Vein with Intraluminal Device, using Drug-Coated Balloon, Open Approach	**05753D1** Dilation of Right Subclavian Vein with Intraluminal Device, using Drug-Coated Balloon, Percutaneous Approach
05710ZZ Dilation of Hemiazygos Vein, Open Approach	**05740DZ** Dilation of Left Innominate Vein with Intraluminal Device, Open Approach	**05753DZ** Dilation of Right Subclavian Vein with Intraluminal Device, Percutaneous Approach
05713DZ Dilation of Hemiazygos Vein with Intraluminal Device, Percutaneous Approach	**05740Z1** Dilation of Left Innominate Vein using Drug-Coated Balloon, Open Approach	**05753Z1** Dilation of Right Subclavian Vein using Drug-Coated Balloon, Percutaneous Approach
05713ZZ Dilation of Hemiazygos Vein, Percutaneous Approach	**05740ZZ** Dilation of Left Innominate Vein, Open Approach	**05753ZZ** Dilation of Right Subclavian Vein, Percutaneous Approach
05714DZ Dilation of Hemiazygos Vein with Intraluminal Device, Percutaneous Endoscopic Approach	**05743D1** Dilation of Left Innominate Vein with Intraluminal Device, using Drug-Coated Balloon, Percutaneous Approach	**05754D1** Dilation of Right Subclavian Vein with Intraluminal Device, using Drug-Coated Balloon, Percutaneous Endoscopic Approach
05714ZZ Dilation of Hemiazygos Vein, Percutaneous Endoscopic Approach	**05743DZ** Dilation of Left Innominate Vein with Intraluminal Device, Percutaneous Approach	**05754DZ** Dilation of Right Subclavian Vein with Intraluminal Device, Percutaneous Endoscopic Approach
05730D1 Dilation of Right Innominate Vein with Intraluminal Device, using Drug-Coated Balloon, Open Approach	**05743Z1** Dilation of Left Innominate Vein using Drug-Coated Balloon, Percutaneous Approach	**05754Z1** Dilation of Right Subclavian Vein using Drug-Coated Balloon, Percutaneous Endoscopic Approach
05730DZ Dilation of Right Innominate Vein with Intraluminal Device, Open Approach	**05743ZZ** Dilation of Left Innominate Vein, Percutaneous Approach	**05754ZZ** Dilation of Right Subclavian Vein, Percutaneous Endoscopic Approach
05730Z1 Dilation of Right Innominate Vein using Drug-Coated Balloon, Open Approach	**05744D1** Dilation of Left Innominate Vein with Intraluminal Device, using Drug-Coated Balloon, Percutaneous Endoscopic Approach	**05760D1** Dilation of Left Subclavian Vein with Intraluminal Device, using Drug-Coated Balloon, Open Approach
05730ZZ Dilation of Right Innominate Vein, Open Approach	**05744DZ** Dilation of Left Innominate Vein with Intraluminal Device, Percutaneous Endoscopic Approach	**05760DZ** Dilation of Left Subclavian Vein with Intraluminal Device, Open Approach
05733D1 Dilation of Right Innominate Vein with Intraluminal Device, using Drug-Coated Balloon, Percutaneous Approach		**05760Z1** Dilation of Left Subclavian Vein using Drug-Coated Balloon, Open Approach
05733DZ Dilation of Right Innominate Vein with Intraluminal Device, Percutaneous Approach		**05760ZZ** Dilation of Left Subclavian Vein, Open Approach

AHA CC: 3Q, 2020, 38-40

♀ Female-only   ♂ Male-only   ▲ Limited Coverage   ● Non-OR   **HAC** HAC-associated procedure   ▲ Non-covered procedures   ✚ Cluster

05763D1 Dilation of Left Subclavian Vein with Intraluminal Device, using Drug-Coated Balloon, Percutaneous Approach

05763DZ Dilation of Left Subclavian Vein with Intraluminal Device, Percutaneous Approach

05763Z1 Dilation of Left Subclavian Vein using Drug-Coated Balloon, Percutaneous Approach

05763ZZ Dilation of Left Subclavian Vein, Percutaneous Approach

05764D1 Dilation of Left Subclavian Vein with Intraluminal Device, using Drug-Coated Balloon, Percutaneous Endoscopic Approach

05764DZ Dilation of Left Subclavian Vein with Intraluminal Device, Percutaneous Endoscopic Approach

05764Z1 Dilation of Left Subclavian Vein using Drug-Coated Balloon, Percutaneous Endoscopic Approach

05764ZZ Dilation of Left Subclavian Vein, Percutaneous Endoscopic Approach

05770D1 Dilation of Right Axillary Vein with Intraluminal Device, using Drug-Coated Balloon, Open Approach

05770DZ Dilation of Right Axillary Vein with Intraluminal Device, Open Approach

05770Z1 Dilation of Right Axillary Vein using Drug-Coated Balloon, Open Approach

05770ZZ Dilation of Right Axillary Vein, Open Approach

05773D1 Dilation of Right Axillary Vein with Intraluminal Device, using Drug-Coated Balloon, Percutaneous Approach

05773DZ Dilation of Right Axillary Vein with Intraluminal Device, Percutaneous Approach

05773Z1 Dilation of Right Axillary Vein using Drug-Coated Balloon, Percutaneous Approach

05773ZZ Dilation of Right Axillary Vein, Percutaneous Approach

05774D1 Dilation of Right Axillary Vein with Intraluminal Device, using Drug-Coated Balloon, Percutaneous Endoscopic Approach

05774DZ Dilation of Right Axillary Vein with Intraluminal Device, Percutaneous Endoscopic Approach

05774Z1 Dilation of Right Axillary Vein using Drug-Coated Balloon, Percutaneous Endoscopic Approach

05774ZZ Dilation of Right Axillary Vein, Percutaneous Endoscopic Approach

05780D1 Dilation of Left Axillary Vein with Intraluminal Device, using Drug-Coated Balloon, Open Approach

05780DZ Dilation of Left Axillary Vein with Intraluminal Device, Open Approach

05780Z1 Dilation of Left Axillary Vein using Drug-Coated Balloon, Open Approach

05780ZZ Dilation of Left Axillary Vein, Open Approach

05783D1 Dilation of Left Axillary Vein with Intraluminal Device, using Drug-Coated Balloon, Percutaneous Approach

05783DZ Dilation of Left Axillary Vein with Intraluminal Device, Percutaneous Approach

05783Z1 Dilation of Left Axillary Vein using Drug-Coated Balloon, Percutaneous Approach

05783ZZ Dilation of Left Axillary Vein, Percutaneous Approach

05784D1 Dilation of Left Axillary Vein with Intraluminal Device, using Drug-Coated Balloon, Percutaneous Endoscopic Approach

05784DZ Dilation of Left Axillary Vein with Intraluminal Device, Percutaneous Endoscopic Approach

05784Z1 Dilation of Left Axillary Vein using Drug-Coated Balloon, Percutaneous Endoscopic Approach

05784ZZ Dilation of Left Axillary Vein, Percutaneous Endoscopic Approach

05790D1 Dilation of Right Brachial Vein with Intraluminal Device, using Drug-Coated Balloon, Open Approach

05790DZ Dilation of Right Brachial Vein with Intraluminal Device, Open Approach

05790Z1 Dilation of Right Brachial Vein using Drug-Coated Balloon, Open Approach

05790ZZ Dilation of Right Brachial Vein, Open Approach

05793D1 Dilation of Right Brachial Vein with Intraluminal Device, using Drug-Coated Balloon, Percutaneous Approach

05793DZ Dilation of Right Brachial Vein with Intraluminal Device, Percutaneous Approach

05793Z1 Dilation of Right Brachial Vein using Drug-Coated Balloon, Percutaneous Approach

05793ZZ Dilation of Right Brachial Vein, Percutaneous Approach

05794D1 Dilation of Right Brachial Vein with Intraluminal Device, using Drug-Coated Balloon, Percutaneous Endoscopic Approach

05794DZ Dilation of Right Brachial Vein with Intraluminal Device, Percutaneous Endoscopic Approach

05794Z1 Dilation of Right Brachial Vein using Drug-Coated Balloon, Percutaneous Endoscopic Approach

05794ZZ Dilation of Right Brachial Vein, Percutaneous Endoscopic Approach

057A0D1 Dilation of Left Brachial Vein with Intraluminal Device, using Drug-Coated Balloon, Open Approach

057A0DZ Dilation of Left Brachial Vein with Intraluminal Device, Open Approach

057A0Z1 Dilation of Left Brachial Vein using Drug-Coated Balloon, Open Approach

057A0ZZ Dilation of Left Brachial Vein, Open Approach

057A3D1 Dilation of Left Brachial Vein with Intraluminal Device, using Drug-Coated Balloon, Percutaneous Approach

057A3DZ Dilation of Left Brachial Vein with Intraluminal Device, Percutaneous Approach

057A3Z1 Dilation of Left Brachial Vein using Drug-Coated Balloon, Percutaneous Approach

057A3ZZ Dilation of Left Brachial Vein, Percutaneous Approach

057A4D1 Dilation of Left Brachial Vein with Intraluminal Device, using Drug-Coated Balloon, Percutaneous Endoscopic Approach

057A4DZ Dilation of Left Brachial Vein with Intraluminal Device, Percutaneous Endoscopic Approach

057A4Z1 Dilation of Left Brachial Vein using Drug-Coated Balloon, Percutaneous Endoscopic Approach

057A4ZZ Dilation of Left Brachial Vein, Percutaneous Endoscopic Approach

057B0D1 Dilation of Right Basilic Vein with Intraluminal Device, using Drug-Coated Balloon, Open Approach

057B0DZ Dilation of Right Basilic Vein with Intraluminal Device, Open Approach

057B0Z1 Dilation of Right Basilic Vein using Drug-Coated Balloon, Open Approach

057B0ZZ Dilation of Right Basilic Vein, Open Approach

057B3D1 Dilation of Right Basilic Vein with Intraluminal Device, using Drug-Coated Balloon, Percutaneous Approach

057B3DZ Dilation of Right Basilic Vein with Intraluminal Device, Percutaneous Approach

057B3Z1 Dilation of Right Basilic Vein using Drug-Coated Balloon, Percutaneous Approach

057B3ZZ Dilation of Right Basilic Vein, Percutaneous Approach

057B4D1 Dilation of Right Basilic Vein with Intraluminal Device, using Drug-Coated Balloon, Percutaneous Endoscopic Approach

057B4DZ Dilation of Right Basilic Vein with Intraluminal Device, Percutaneous Endoscopic Approach

057B4Z1 Dilation of Right Basilic Vein using Drug-Coated Balloon, Percutaneous Endoscopic Approach

057B4ZZ Dilation of Right Basilic Vein, Percutaneous Endoscopic Approach

057C0D1 Dilation of Left Basilic Vein with Intraluminal Device, using Drug-Coated Balloon, Open Approach

057C0DZ Dilation of Left Basilic Vein with Intraluminal Device, Open Approach

057C0Z1 Dilation of Left Basilic Vein using Drug-Coated Balloon, Open Approach

057C0ZZ Dilation of Left Basilic Vein, Open Approach

057C3D1 Dilation of Left Basilic Vein with Intraluminal Device, using Drug-Coated Balloon, Percutaneous Approach

057C3DZ Dilation of Left Basilic Vein with Intraluminal Device, Percutaneous Approach

057C3Z1 Dilation of Left Basilic Vein using Drug-Coated Balloon, Percutaneous Approach

057C3ZZ Dilation of Left Basilic Vein, Percutaneous Approach

057C4D1 Dilation of Left Basilic Vein with Intraluminal Device, using Drug-Coated Balloon, Percutaneous Endoscopic Approach

057C4DZ Dilation of Left Basilic Vein with Intraluminal Device, Percutaneous Endoscopic Approach

057C4Z1 Dilation of Left Basilic Vein using Drug-Coated Balloon, Percutaneous Endoscopic Approach

057C4ZZ Dilation of Left Basilic Vein, Percutaneous Endoscopic Approach

057D0D1 Dilation of Right Cephalic Vein with Intraluminal Device, using Drug-Coated Balloon, Open Approach

057D0DZ Dilation of Right Cephalic Vein with Intraluminal Device, Open Approach

057D0Z1 Dilation of Right Cephalic Vein using Drug-Coated Balloon, Open Approach

057D0ZZ Dilation of Right Cephalic Vein, Open Approach

057D3D1 Dilation of Right Cephalic Vein with Intraluminal Device, using Drug-Coated Balloon, Percutaneous Approach

057D3DZ Dilation of Right Cephalic Vein with Intraluminal Device, Percutaneous Approach

057D3Z1 Dilation of Right Cephalic Vein using Drug-Coated Balloon, Percutaneous Approach

057D3ZZ Dilation of Right Cephalic Vein, Percutaneous Approach

057D4D1 Dilation of Right Cephalic Vein with Intraluminal Device, using Drug-Coated Balloon, Percutaneous Endoscopic Approach

057D4DZ Dilation of Right Cephalic Vein with Intraluminal Device, Percutaneous Endoscopic Approach

057D4Z1 Dilation of Right Cephalic Vein using Drug-Coated Balloon, Percutaneous Endoscopic Approach

057D4ZZ Dilation of Right Cephalic Vein, Percutaneous Endoscopic Approach

057F0D1 Dilation of Left Cephalic Vein with Intraluminal Device, using Drug-Coated Balloon, Open Approach

057F0DZ Dilation of Left Cephalic Vein with Intraluminal Device, Open Approach

057F0Z1 Dilation of Left Cephalic Vein using Drug-Coated Balloon, Open Approach

057F0ZZ Dilation of Left Cephalic Vein, Open Approach

057F3D1 Dilation of Left Cephalic Vein with Intraluminal Device, using Drug-Coated Balloon, Percutaneous Approach

057F3DZ Dilation of Left Cephalic Vein with Intraluminal Device, Percutaneous Approach

057F3Z1 Dilation of Left Cephalic Vein using Drug-Coated Balloon, Percutaneous Approach

057F3ZZ Dilation of Left Cephalic Vein, Percutaneous Approach

057F4D1 Dilation of Left Cephalic Vein with Intraluminal Device, using Drug-Coated Balloon, Percutaneous Endoscopic Approach

057F4DZ Dilation of Left Cephalic Vein with Intraluminal Device, Percutaneous Endoscopic Approach

057F4Z1 Dilation of Left Cephalic Vein using Drug-Coated Balloon, Percutaneous Endoscopic Approach

057F4ZZ Dilation of Left Cephalic Vein, Percutaneous Endoscopic Approach

057G0DZ Dilation of Right Hand Vein with Intraluminal Device, Open Approach

057G0ZZ Dilation of Right Hand Vein, Open Approach

057G3DZ Dilation of Right Hand Vein with Intraluminal Device, Percutaneous Approach

057G3ZZ Dilation of Right Hand Vein, Percutaneous Approach

057G4DZ Dilation of Right Hand Vein with Intraluminal Device, Percutaneous Endoscopic Approach

057G4ZZ Dilation of Right Hand Vein, Percutaneous Endoscopic Approach

057H0DZ Dilation of Left Hand Vein with Intraluminal Device, Open Approach

057H0ZZ Dilation of Left Hand Vein, Open Approach

057H3DZ Dilation of Left Hand Vein with Intraluminal Device, Percutaneous Approach

057H3ZZ Dilation of Left Hand Vein, Percutaneous Approach

057H4DZ Dilation of Left Hand Vein with Intraluminal Device, Percutaneous Endoscopic Approach

057H4ZZ Dilation of Left Hand Vein, Percutaneous Endoscopic Approach

057L0DZ Dilation of Intracranial Vein with Intraluminal Device, Open Approach

057L0ZZ Dilation of Intracranial Vein, Open Approach

057L3DZ Dilation of Intracranial Vein with Intraluminal Device, Percutaneous Approach

▲ **057L3ZZ** Dilation of Intracranial Vein, Percutaneous Approach

057L4DZ Dilation of Intracranial Vein with Intraluminal Device, Percutaneous Endoscopic Approach

▲ **057L4ZZ** Dilation of Intracranial Vein, Percutaneous Endoscopic Approach

057M0DZ Dilation of Right Internal Jugular Vein with Intraluminal Device, Open Approach

057M0ZZ Dilation of Right Internal Jugular Vein, Open Approach

057M3DZ Dilation of Right Internal Jugular Vein with Intraluminal Device, Percutaneous Approach

057M3ZZ Dilation of Right Internal Jugular Vein, Percutaneous Approach

057M4DZ Dilation of Right Internal Jugular Vein with Intraluminal Device, Percutaneous Endoscopic Approach

057M4ZZ Dilation of Right Internal Jugular Vein, Percutaneous Endoscopic Approach

057N0DZ Dilation of Left Internal Jugular Vein with Intraluminal Device, Open Approach

057N0ZZ Dilation of Left Internal Jugular Vein, Open Approach

057N3DZ Dilation of Left Internal Jugular Vein with Intraluminal Device, Percutaneous Approach

057N3ZZ Dilation of Left Internal Jugular Vein, Percutaneous Approach

057N4DZ Dilation of Left Internal Jugular Vein with Intraluminal Device, Percutaneous Endoscopic Approach

057N4ZZ Dilation of Left Internal Jugular Vein, Percutaneous Endoscopic Approach

057P0DZ Dilation of Right External Jugular Vein with Intraluminal Device, Open Approach

057P0ZZ Dilation of Right External Jugular Vein, Open Approach

057P3DZ Dilation of Right External Jugular Vein with Intraluminal Device, Percutaneous Approach

057P3ZZ Dilation of Right External Jugular Vein, Percutaneous Approach

057P4DZ Dilation of Right External Jugular Vein with Intraluminal Device, Percutaneous Endoscopic Approach

057P4ZZ Dilation of Right External Jugular Vein, Percutaneous Endoscopic Approach

057Q0DZ Dilation of Left External Jugular Vein with Intraluminal Device, Open Approach

057Q0ZZ Dilation of Left External Jugular Vein, Open Approach

057Q3DZ Dilation of Left External Jugular Vein with Intraluminal Device, Percutaneous Approach

057Q3ZZ Dilation of Left External Jugular Vein, Percutaneous Approach

057Q4DZ Dilation of Left External Jugular Vein with Intraluminal Device, Percutaneous Endoscopic Approach

057Q4ZZ Dilation of Left External Jugular Vein, Percutaneous Endoscopic Approach

057R0DZ Dilation of Right Vertebral Vein with Intraluminal Device, Open Approach

057R0ZZ Dilation of Right Vertebral Vein, Open Approach

057R3DZ Dilation of Right Vertebral Vein with Intraluminal Device, Percutaneous Approach

057R3ZZ Dilation of Right Vertebral Vein, Percutaneous Approach

057R4DZ Dilation of Right Vertebral Vein with Intraluminal Device, Percutaneous Endoscopic Approach

057R4ZZ Dilation of Right Vertebral Vein, Percutaneous Endoscopic Approach

057S0DZ Dilation of Left Vertebral Vein with Intraluminal Device, Open Approach

057S0ZZ Dilation of Left Vertebral Vein, Open Approach

057S3DZ Dilation of Left Vertebral Vein with Intraluminal Device, Percutaneous Approach

057S3ZZ Dilation of Left Vertebral Vein, Percutaneous Approach

057S4DZ Dilation of Left Vertebral Vein with Intraluminal Device, Percutaneous Endoscopic Approach

057S4ZZ Dilation of Left Vertebral Vein, Percutaneous Endoscopic Approach

057T0DZ Dilation of Right Face Vein with Intraluminal Device, Open Approach

057T0ZZ Dilation of Right Face Vein, Open Approach

057T3DZ Dilation of Right Face Vein with Intraluminal Device, Percutaneous Approach

057T3ZZ Dilation of Right Face Vein, Percutaneous Approach

057T4DZ Dilation of Right Face Vein with Intraluminal Device, Percutaneous Endoscopic Approach

057T4ZZ Dilation of Right Face Vein, Percutaneous Endoscopic Approach

057V0DZ Dilation of Left Face Vein with Intraluminal Device, Open Approach

057V0ZZ Dilation of Left Face Vein, Open Approach

057V3DZ Dilation of Left Face Vein with Intraluminal Device, Percutaneous Approach

057V3ZZ Dilation of Left Face Vein, Percutaneous Approach

057V4DZ Dilation of Left Face Vein with Intraluminal Device, Percutaneous Endoscopic Approach

♀ Female-only   ♂ Male-only   ▲ Limited Coverage   ● Non-OR   ▨ HAC-associated procedure   ▲ Non-covered procedures   ✚ Cluster

57V4ZZ Dilation of Left Face Vein, Percutaneous Endoscopic Approach	**057Y3DZ** Dilation of Upper Vein with Intraluminal Device, Percutaneous Approach	**057Y4DZ** Dilation of Upper Vein with Intraluminal Device, Percutaneous Endoscopic Approach
57Y0DZ Dilation of Upper Vein with Intraluminal Device, Open Approach	**057Y3ZZ** Dilation of Upper Vein, Percutaneous Approach	**057Y4ZZ** Dilation of Upper Vein, Percutaneous Endoscopic Approach
57Y0ZZ Dilation of Upper Vein, Open Approach		

059 – Upper Veins, Drainage

Review Coding Guidelines B3.4a and B3.4b

Review Coding Guideline B6.2

059000Z Drainage of Azygos Vein with Drainage Device, Open Approach

05900ZX Drainage of Azygos Vein, Open Approach, Diagnostic

05900ZZ Drainage of Azygos Vein, Open Approach

059030Z Drainage of Azygos Vein with Drainage Device, Percutaneous Approach

05903ZX Drainage of Azygos Vein, Percutaneous Approach, Diagnostic

05903ZZ Drainage of Azygos Vein, Percutaneous Approach

059040Z Drainage of Azygos Vein with Drainage Device, Percutaneous Endoscopic Approach

05904ZX Drainage of Azygos Vein, Percutaneous Endoscopic Approach, Diagnostic

05904ZZ Drainage of Azygos Vein, Percutaneous Endoscopic Approach

059100Z Drainage of Hemiazygos Vein with Drainage Device, Open Approach

05910ZX Drainage of Hemiazygos Vein, Open Approach, Diagnostic

05910ZZ Drainage of Hemiazygos Vein, Open Approach

059130Z Drainage of Hemiazygos Vein with Drainage Device, Percutaneous Approach

05913ZX Drainage of Hemiazygos Vein, Percutaneous Approach, Diagnostic

05913ZZ Drainage of Hemiazygos Vein, Percutaneous Approach

059140Z Drainage of Hemiazygos Vein with Drainage Device, Percutaneous Endoscopic Approach

05914ZX Drainage of Hemiazygos Vein, Percutaneous Endoscopic Approach, Diagnostic

05914ZZ Drainage of Hemiazygos Vein, Percutaneous Endoscopic Approach

059300Z Drainage of Right Innominate Vein with Drainage Device, Open Approach

05930ZX Drainage of Right Innominate Vein, Open Approach, Diagnostic

05930ZZ Drainage of Right Innominate Vein, Open Approach

059330Z Drainage of Right Innominate Vein with Drainage Device, Percutaneous Approach

05933ZX Drainage of Right Innominate Vein, Percutaneous Approach, Diagnostic

05933ZZ Drainage of Right Innominate Vein, Percutaneous Approach

059340Z Drainage of Right Innominate Vein with Drainage Device, Percutaneous Endoscopic Approach

05934ZX Drainage of Right Innominate Vein, Percutaneous Endoscopic Approach, Diagnostic

05934ZZ Drainage of Right Innominate Vein, Percutaneous Endoscopic Approach

059400Z Drainage of Left Innominate Vein with Drainage Device, Open Approach

05940ZX Drainage of Left Innominate Vein, Open Approach, Diagnostic

05940ZZ Drainage of Left Innominate Vein, Open Approach

059430Z Drainage of Left Innominate Vein with Drainage Device, Percutaneous Approach

AHA CC: 3Q, 2018. 7

05943ZX Drainage of Left Innominate Vein, Percutaneous Approach, Diagnostic

05943ZZ Drainage of Left Innominate Vein, Percutaneous Approach

059440Z Drainage of Left Innominate Vein with Drainage Device, Percutaneous Endoscopic Approach

05944ZX Drainage of Left Innominate Vein, Percutaneous Endoscopic Approach, Diagnostic

05944ZZ Drainage of Left Innominate Vein, Percutaneous Endoscopic Approach

059500Z Drainage of Right Subclavian Vein with Drainage Device, Open Approach

05950ZX Drainage of Right Subclavian Vein, Open Approach, Diagnostic

05950ZZ Drainage of Right Subclavian Vein, Open Approach

059530Z Drainage of Right Subclavian Vein with Drainage Device, Percutaneous Approach

05953ZX Drainage of Right Subclavian Vein, Percutaneous Approach, Diagnostic

05953ZZ Drainage of Right Subclavian Vein, Percutaneous Approach

059540Z Drainage of Right Subclavian Vein with Drainage Device, Percutaneous Endoscopic Approach

05954ZX Drainage of Right Subclavian Vein, Percutaneous Endoscopic Approach, Diagnostic

05954ZZ Drainage of Right Subclavian Vein, Percutaneous Endoscopic Approach

059600Z Drainage of Left Subclavian Vein with Drainage Device, Open Approach

05960ZX Drainage of Left Subclavian Vein, Open Approach, Diagnostic

05960ZZ Drainage of Left Subclavian Vein, Open Approach

059630Z Drainage of Left Subclavian Vein with Drainage Device, Percutaneous Approach

05963ZX Drainage of Left Subclavian Vein, Percutaneous Approach, Diagnostic

05963ZZ Drainage of Left Subclavian Vein, Percutaneous Approach

059640Z Drainage of Left Subclavian Vein with Drainage Device, Percutaneous Endoscopic Approach

05964ZX Drainage of Left Subclavian Vein, Percutaneous Endoscopic Approach, Diagnostic

05964ZZ Drainage of Left Subclavian Vein, Percutaneous Endoscopic Approach

059700Z Drainage of Right Axillary Vein with Drainage Device, Open Approach

05970ZX Drainage of Right Axillary Vein, Open Approach, Diagnostic

05970ZZ Drainage of Right Axillary Vein, Open Approach

059730Z Drainage of Right Axillary Vein with Drainage Device, Percutaneous Approach

05973ZX Drainage of Right Axillary Vein, Percutaneous Approach, Diagnostic

05973ZZ Drainage of Right Axillary Vein, Percutaneous Approach

059740Z Drainage of Right Axillary Vein with Drainage Device, Percutaneous Endoscopic Approach

05974ZX Drainage of Right Axillary Vein, Percutaneous Endoscopic Approach, Diagnostic

05974ZZ Drainage of Right Axillary Vein, Percutaneous Endoscopic Approach

059800Z Drainage of Left Axillary Vein with Drainage Device, Open Approach

05980ZX Drainage of Left Axillary Vein, Open Approach, Diagnostic

05980ZZ Drainage of Left Axillary Vein, Open Approach

059830Z Drainage of Left Axillary Vein with Drainage Device, Percutaneous Approach

05983ZX Drainage of Left Axillary Vein, Percutaneous Approach, Diagnostic

05983ZZ Drainage of Left Axillary Vein, Percutaneous Approach

059840Z Drainage of Left Axillary Vein with Drainage Device, Percutaneous Endoscopic Approach

05984ZX Drainage of Left Axillary Vein, Percutaneous Endoscopic Approach, Diagnostic

05984ZZ Drainage of Left Axillary Vein, Percutaneous Endoscopic Approach

059900Z Drainage of Right Brachial Vein with Drainage Device, Open Approach

05990ZX Drainage of Right Brachial Vein, Open Approach, Diagnostic

05990ZZ Drainage of Right Brachial Vein, Open Approach

059930Z Drainage of Right Brachial Vein with Drainage Device, Percutaneous Approach

05993ZX Drainage of Right Brachial Vein, Percutaneous Approach, Diagnostic

05993ZZ Drainage of Right Brachial Vein, Percutaneous Approach

059940Z Drainage of Right Brachial Vein with Drainage Device, Percutaneous Endoscopic Approach

05994ZX Drainage of Right Brachial Vein, Percutaneous Endoscopic Approach, Diagnostic

05994ZZ Drainage of Right Brachial Vein, Percutaneous Endoscopic Approach

059A00Z Drainage of Left Brachial Vein with Drainage Device, Open Approach

♀ Female-only   ♂ Male-only   ▲ Limited Coverage   ● Non-OR   ▧ HAC-associated procedure   ▲ Non-covered procedures   ✚ Cluster   **389**

059A0ZX Drainage of Left Brachial Vein, Open Approach, Diagnostic

059A0ZZ Drainage of Left Brachial Vein, Open Approach

059A30Z Drainage of Left Brachial Vein with Drainage Device, Percutaneous Approach

059A3ZX Drainage of Left Brachial Vein, Percutaneous Approach, Diagnostic

059A3ZZ Drainage of Left Brachial Vein, Percutaneous Approach

059A40Z Drainage of Left Brachial Vein with Drainage Device, Percutaneous Endoscopic Approach

059A4ZX Drainage of Left Brachial Vein, Percutaneous Endoscopic Approach, Diagnostic

059A4ZZ Drainage of Left Brachial Vein, Percutaneous Endoscopic Approach

059B00Z Drainage of Right Basilic Vein with Drainage Device, Open Approach

059B0ZX Drainage of Right Basilic Vein, Open Approach, Diagnostic

059B0ZZ Drainage of Right Basilic Vein, Open Approach

059B30Z Drainage of Right Basilic Vein with Drainage Device, Percutaneous Approach

059B3ZX Drainage of Right Basilic Vein, Percutaneous Approach, Diagnostic

059B3ZZ Drainage of Right Basilic Vein, Percutaneous Approach

059B40Z Drainage of Right Basilic Vein with Drainage Device, Percutaneous Endoscopic Approach

059B4ZX Drainage of Right Basilic Vein, Percutaneous Endoscopic Approach, Diagnostic

059B4ZZ Drainage of Right Basilic Vein, Percutaneous Endoscopic Approach

059C00Z Drainage of Left Basilic Vein with Drainage Device, Open Approach

059C0ZX Drainage of Left Basilic Vein, Open Approach, Diagnostic

059C0ZZ Drainage of Left Basilic Vein, Open Approach

059C30Z Drainage of Left Basilic Vein with Drainage Device, Percutaneous Approach

059C3ZX Drainage of Left Basilic Vein, Percutaneous Approach, Diagnostic

059C3ZZ Drainage of Left Basilic Vein, Percutaneous Approach

059C40Z Drainage of Left Basilic Vein with Drainage Device, Percutaneous Endoscopic Approach

059C4ZX Drainage of Left Basilic Vein, Percutaneous Endoscopic Approach, Diagnostic

059C4ZZ Drainage of Left Basilic Vein, Percutaneous Endoscopic Approach

059D00Z Drainage of Right Cephalic Vein with Drainage Device, Open Approach

059D0ZX Drainage of Right Cephalic Vein, Open Approach, Diagnostic

059D0ZZ Drainage of Right Cephalic Vein, Open Approach

059D30Z Drainage of Right Cephalic Vein with Drainage Device, Percutaneous Approach

059D3ZX Drainage of Right Cephalic Vein, Percutaneous Approach, Diagnostic

059D3ZZ Drainage of Right Cephalic Vein, Percutaneous Approach

059D40Z Drainage of Right Cephalic Vein with Drainage Device, Percutaneous Endoscopic Approach

059D4ZX Drainage of Right Cephalic Vein, Percutaneous Endoscopic Approach, Diagnostic

059D4ZZ Drainage of Right Cephalic Vein, Percutaneous Endoscopic Approach

059F00Z Drainage of Left Cephalic Vein with Drainage Device, Open Approach

059F0ZX Drainage of Left Cephalic Vein, Open Approach, Diagnostic

059F0ZZ Drainage of Left Cephalic Vein, Open Approach

059F30Z Drainage of Left Cephalic Vein with Drainage Device, Percutaneous Approach

059F3ZX Drainage of Left Cephalic Vein, Percutaneous Approach, Diagnostic

059F3ZZ Drainage of Left Cephalic Vein, Percutaneous Approach

059F40Z Drainage of Left Cephalic Vein with Drainage Device, Percutaneous Endoscopic Approach

059F4ZX Drainage of Left Cephalic Vein, Percutaneous Endoscopic Approach, Diagnostic

059F4ZZ Drainage of Left Cephalic Vein, Percutaneous Endoscopic Approach

059G00Z Drainage of Right Hand Vein with Drainage Device, Open Approach

059G0ZX Drainage of Right Hand Vein, Open Approach, Diagnostic

059G0ZZ Drainage of Right Hand Vein, Open Approach

059G30Z Drainage of Right Hand Vein with Drainage Device, Percutaneous Approach

059G3ZX Drainage of Right Hand Vein, Percutaneous Approach, Diagnostic

059G3ZZ Drainage of Right Hand Vein, Percutaneous Approach

059G40Z Drainage of Right Hand Vein with Drainage Device, Percutaneous Endoscopic Approach

059G4ZX Drainage of Right Hand Vein, Percutaneous Endoscopic Approach, Diagnostic

059G4ZZ Drainage of Right Hand Vein, Percutaneous Endoscopic Approach

059H00Z Drainage of Left Hand Vein with Drainage Device, Open Approach

059H0ZX Drainage of Left Hand Vein, Open Approach, Diagnostic

059H0ZZ Drainage of Left Hand Vein, Open Approach

059H30Z Drainage of Left Hand Vein with Drainage Device, Percutaneous Approach

059H3ZX Drainage of Left Hand Vein, Percutaneous Approach, Diagnostic

059H3ZZ Drainage of Left Hand Vein, Percutaneous Approach

059H40Z Drainage of Left Hand Vein with Drainage Device, Percutaneous Endoscopic Approach

059H4ZX Drainage of Left Hand Vein, Percutaneous Endoscopic Approach, Diagnostic

059H4ZZ Drainage of Left Hand Vein, Percutaneous Endoscopic Approach

059L00Z Drainage of Intracranial Vein with Drainage Device, Open Approach

059L0ZX Drainage of Intracranial Vein, Open Approach, Diagnostic

059L0ZZ Drainage of Intracranial Vein, Open Approach

059L30Z Drainage of Intracranial Vein with Drainage Device, Percutaneous Approach

059L3ZX Drainage of Intracranial Vein, Percutaneous Approach, Diagnostic

059L3ZZ Drainage of Intracranial Vein, Percutaneous Approach

059L40Z Drainage of Intracranial Vein with Drainage Device, Percutaneous Endoscopic Approach

059L4ZX Drainage of Intracranial Vein, Percutaneous Endoscopic Approach, Diagnostic

059L4ZZ Drainage of Intracranial Vein, Percutaneous Endoscopic Approach

059M00Z Drainage of Right Internal Jugular Vein with Drainage Device, Open Approach

059M0ZX Drainage of Right Internal Jugular Vein, Open Approach, Diagnostic

059M0ZZ Drainage of Right Internal Jugular Vein, Open Approach

059M30Z Drainage of Right Internal Jugular Vein with Drainage Device, Percutaneous Approach

059M3ZX Drainage of Right Internal Jugular Vein, Percutaneous Approach, Diagnostic

059M3ZZ Drainage of Right Internal Jugular Vein, Percutaneous Approach

059M40Z Drainage of Right Internal Jugular Vein with Drainage Device, Percutaneous Endoscopic Approach

059M4ZX Drainage of Right Internal Jugular Vein, Percutaneous Endoscopic Approach, Diagnostic

059M4ZZ Drainage of Right Internal Jugular Vein, Percutaneous Endoscopic Approach

059N00Z Drainage of Left Internal Jugular Vein with Drainage Device, Open Approach

059N0ZX Drainage of Left Internal Jugular Vein, Open Approach, Diagnostic

059N0ZZ Drainage of Left Internal Jugular Vein, Open Approach

059N30Z Drainage of Left Internal Jugular Vein with Drainage Device, Percutaneous Approach

059N3ZX Drainage of Left Internal Jugular Vein, Percutaneous Approach, Diagnostic

059N3ZZ Drainage of Left Internal Jugular Vein, Percutaneous Approach

059N40Z Drainage of Left Internal Jugular Vein with Drainage Device, Percutaneous Endoscopic Approach

059N4ZX Drainage of Left Internal Jugular Vein, Percutaneous Endoscopic Approach, Diagnostic

059N4ZZ Drainage of Left Internal Jugular Vein, Percutaneous Endoscopic Approach

059P00Z Drainage of Right External Jugular Vein with Drainage Device, Open Approach

059P0ZX Drainage of Right External Jugular Vein, Open Approach, Diagnostic

059P0ZZ Drainage of Right External Jugular Vein, Open Approach

059P30Z Drainage of Right External Jugular Vein with Drainage Device, Percutaneous Approach

059P3ZX Drainage of Right External Jugular Vein, Percutaneous Approach, Diagnostic

059P3ZZ Drainage of Right External Jugular Vein, Percutaneous Approach

059P40Z Drainage of Right External Jugular Vein with Drainage Device, Percutaneous Endoscopic Approach

♀ Female-only   ♂ Male-only   ▲ Limited Coverage   ● Non-OR   HAC HAC-associated procedure   ▲ Non-covered procedures   ✚ Cluster

059P4ZX Drainage of Right External Jugular Vein, Percutaneous Endoscopic Approach, Diagnostic

059P4ZZ Drainage of Right External Jugular Vein, Percutaneous Endoscopic Approach

059Q00Z Drainage of Left External Jugular Vein with Drainage Device, Open Approach

059Q0ZX Drainage of Left External Jugular Vein, Open Approach, Diagnostic

059Q0ZZ Drainage of Left External Jugular Vein, Open Approach

059Q30Z Drainage of Left External Jugular Vein with Drainage Device, Percutaneous Approach

059Q3ZX Drainage of Left External Jugular Vein, Percutaneous Approach, Diagnostic

059Q3ZZ Drainage of Left External Jugular Vein, Percutaneous Approach

059Q40Z Drainage of Left External Jugular Vein with Drainage Device, Percutaneous Endoscopic Approach

059Q4ZX Drainage of Left External Jugular Vein, Percutaneous Endoscopic Approach, Diagnostic

059Q4ZZ Drainage of Left External Jugular Vein, Percutaneous Endoscopic Approach

059R00Z Drainage of Right Vertebral Vein with Drainage Device, Open Approach

059R0ZX Drainage of Right Vertebral Vein, Open Approach, Diagnostic

059R0ZZ Drainage of Right Vertebral Vein, Open Approach

059R30Z Drainage of Right Vertebral Vein with Drainage Device, Percutaneous Approach

059R3ZX Drainage of Right Vertebral Vein, Percutaneous Approach, Diagnostic

059R3ZZ Drainage of Right Vertebral Vein, Percutaneous Approach

059R40Z Drainage of Right Vertebral Vein with Drainage Device, Percutaneous Endoscopic Approach

059R4ZX Drainage of Right Vertebral Vein, Percutaneous Endoscopic Approach, Diagnostic

059R4ZZ Drainage of Right Vertebral Vein, Percutaneous Endoscopic Approach

059S00Z Drainage of Left Vertebral Vein with Drainage Device, Open Approach

059S0ZX Drainage of Left Vertebral Vein, Open Approach, Diagnostic

059S0ZZ Drainage of Left Vertebral Vein, Open Approach

059S30Z Drainage of Left Vertebral Vein with Drainage Device, Percutaneous Approach

059S3ZX Drainage of Left Vertebral Vein, Percutaneous Approach, Diagnostic

059S3ZZ Drainage of Left Vertebral Vein, Percutaneous Approach

059S40Z Drainage of Left Vertebral Vein with Drainage Device, Percutaneous Endoscopic Approach

059S4ZX Drainage of Left Vertebral Vein, Percutaneous Endoscopic Approach, Diagnostic

059S4ZZ Drainage of Left Vertebral Vein, Percutaneous Endoscopic Approach

059T00Z Drainage of Right Face Vein with Drainage Device, Open Approach

059T0ZX Drainage of Right Face Vein, Open Approach, Diagnostic

059T0ZZ Drainage of Right Face Vein, Open Approach

059T30Z Drainage of Right Face Vein with Drainage Device, Percutaneous Approach

059T3ZX Drainage of Right Face Vein, Percutaneous Approach, Diagnostic

059T3ZZ Drainage of Right Face Vein, Percutaneous Approach

059T40Z Drainage of Right Face Vein with Drainage Device, Percutaneous Endoscopic Approach

059T4ZX Drainage of Right Face Vein, Percutaneous Endoscopic Approach, Diagnostic

059T4ZZ Drainage of Right Face Vein, Percutaneous Endoscopic Approach

059V00Z Drainage of Left Face Vein with Drainage Device, Open Approach

059V0ZX Drainage of Left Face Vein, Open Approach, Diagnostic

059V0ZZ Drainage of Left Face Vein, Open Approach

059V30Z Drainage of Left Face Vein with Drainage Device, Percutaneous Approach

059V3ZX Drainage of Left Face Vein, Percutaneous Approach, Diagnostic

059V3ZZ Drainage of Left Face Vein, Percutaneous Approach

059V40Z Drainage of Left Face Vein with Drainage Device, Percutaneous Endoscopic Approach

059V4ZX Drainage of Left Face Vein, Percutaneous Endoscopic Approach, Diagnostic

059V4ZZ Drainage of Left Face Vein, Percutaneous Endoscopic Approach

059Y00Z Drainage of Upper Vein with Drainage Device, Open Approach

059Y0ZX Drainage of Upper Vein, Open Approach, Diagnostic

059Y0ZZ Drainage of Upper Vein, Open Approach

059Y30Z Drainage of Upper Vein with Drainage Device, Percutaneous Approach

059Y3ZX Drainage of Upper Vein, Percutaneous Approach, Diagnostic

059Y3ZZ Drainage of Upper Vein, Percutaneous Approach

059Y40Z Drainage of Upper Vein with Drainage Device, Percutaneous Endoscopic Approach

059Y4ZX Drainage of Upper Vein, Percutaneous Endoscopic Approach, Diagnostic

059Y4ZZ Drainage of Upper Vein, Percutaneous Endoscopic Approach

05B – Upper Veins, Excision

Review Coding Guidelines B3.4a and B3.4b

Review Coding Guideline B3.8

Review Coding Guideline B3.18

05B00ZX Excision of Azygos Vein, Open Approach, Diagnostic

05B00ZZ Excision of Azygos Vein, Open Approach

05B03ZX Excision of Azygos Vein, Percutaneous Approach, Diagnostic

05B03ZZ Excision of Azygos Vein, Percutaneous Approach

05B04ZX Excision of Azygos Vein, Percutaneous Endoscopic Approach, Diagnostic

05B04ZZ Excision of Azygos Vein, Percutaneous Endoscopic Approach

05B10ZX Excision of Hemiazygos Vein, Open Approach, Diagnostic

05B10ZZ Excision of Hemiazygos Vein, Open Approach

05B13ZX Excision of Hemiazygos Vein, Percutaneous Approach, Diagnostic

05B13ZZ Excision of Hemiazygos Vein, Percutaneous Approach

05B14ZX Excision of Hemiazygos Vein, Percutaneous Endoscopic Approach, Diagnostic

05B14ZZ Excision of Hemiazygos Vein, Percutaneous Endoscopic Approach

05B30ZX Excision of Right Innominate Vein, Open Approach, Diagnostic

05B30ZZ Excision of Right Innominate Vein, Open Approach

05B33ZX Excision of Right Innominate Vein, Percutaneous Approach, Diagnostic

05B33ZZ Excision of Right Innominate Vein, Percutaneous Approach

05B34ZX Excision of Right Innominate Vein, Percutaneous Endoscopic Approach, Diagnostic

05B34ZZ Excision of Right Innominate Vein, Percutaneous Endoscopic Approach

05B40ZX Excision of Left Innominate Vein, Open Approach, Diagnostic

05B40ZZ Excision of Left Innominate Vein, Open Approach

05B43ZX Excision of Left Innominate Vein, Percutaneous Approach, Diagnostic

05B43ZZ Excision of Left Innominate Vein, Percutaneous Approach

05B44ZX Excision of Left Innominate Vein, Percutaneous Endoscopic Approach, Diagnostic

05B44ZZ Excision of Left Innominate Vein, Percutaneous Endoscopic Approach

05B50ZX Excision of Right Subclavian Vein, Open Approach, Diagnostic

05B50ZZ Excision of Right Subclavian Vein, Open Approach

05B53ZX Excision of Right Subclavian Vein, Percutaneous Approach, Diagnostic

05B53ZZ Excision of Right Subclavian Vein, Percutaneous Approach

05B54ZX Excision of Right Subclavian Vein, Percutaneous Endoscopic Approach, Diagnostic

05B54ZZ Excision of Right Subclavian Vein, Percutaneous Endoscopic Approach

05B60ZX Excision of Left Subclavian Vein, Open Approach, Diagnostic

05B60ZZ Excision of Left Subclavian Vein, Open Approach

♀ Female-only ♂ Male-only ▲ Limited Coverage ● Non-OR ▥ HAC-associated procedure ▲ Non-covered procedures ✚ Cluster

05B63ZX Excision of Left Subclavian Vein, Percutaneous Approach, Diagnostic

05B63ZZ Excision of Left Subclavian Vein, Percutaneous Approach

05B64ZX Excision of Left Subclavian Vein, Percutaneous Endoscopic Approach, Diagnostic

05B64ZZ Excision of Left Subclavian Vein, Percutaneous Endoscopic Approach

05B70ZX Excision of Right Axillary Vein, Open Approach, Diagnostic

05B70ZZ Excision of Right Axillary Vein, Open Approach

05B73ZX Excision of Right Axillary Vein, Percutaneous Approach, Diagnostic

05B73ZZ Excision of Right Axillary Vein, Percutaneous Approach

05B74ZX Excision of Right Axillary Vein, Percutaneous Endoscopic Approach, Diagnostic

05B74ZZ Excision of Right Axillary Vein, Percutaneous Endoscopic Approach

05B80ZX Excision of Left Axillary Vein, Open Approach, Diagnostic

05B80ZZ Excision of Left Axillary Vein, Open Approach

05B83ZX Excision of Left Axillary Vein, Percutaneous Approach, Diagnostic

05B83ZZ Excision of Left Axillary Vein, Percutaneous Approach

05B84ZX Excision of Left Axillary Vein, Percutaneous Endoscopic Approach, Diagnostic

05B84ZZ Excision of Left Axillary Vein, Percutaneous Endoscopic Approach

05B90ZX Excision of Right Brachial Vein, Open Approach, Diagnostic

05B90ZZ Excision of Right Brachial Vein, Open Approach

05B93ZX Excision of Right Brachial Vein, Percutaneous Approach, Diagnostic

05B93ZZ Excision of Right Brachial Vein, Percutaneous Approach

05B94ZX Excision of Right Brachial Vein, Percutaneous Endoscopic Approach, Diagnostic

05B94ZZ Excision of Right Brachial Vein, Percutaneous Endoscopic Approach

05BA0ZX Excision of Left Brachial Vein, Open Approach, Diagnostic

05BA0ZZ Excision of Left Brachial Vein, Open Approach

05BA3ZX Excision of Left Brachial Vein, Percutaneous Approach, Diagnostic

05BA3ZZ Excision of Left Brachial Vein, Percutaneous Approach

05BA4ZX Excision of Left Brachial Vein, Percutaneous Endoscopic Approach, Diagnostic

05BA4ZZ Excision of Left Brachial Vein, Percutaneous Endoscopic Approach

05BB0ZX Excision of Right Basilic Vein, Open Approach, Diagnostic

05BB0ZZ Excision of Right Basilic Vein, Open Approach

05BB3ZX Excision of Right Basilic Vein, Percutaneous Approach, Diagnostic

05BB3ZZ Excision of Right Basilic Vein, Percutaneous Approach

05BB4ZX Excision of Right Basilic Vein, Percutaneous Endoscopic Approach, Diagnostic

05BB4ZZ Excision of Right Basilic Vein, Percutaneous Endoscopic Approach

05BC0ZX Excision of Left Basilic Vein, Open Approach, Diagnostic

05BC0ZZ Excision of Left Basilic Vein, Open Approach

05BC3ZX Excision of Left Basilic Vein, Percutaneous Approach, Diagnostic

05BC3ZZ Excision of Left Basilic Vein, Percutaneous Approach

05BC4ZX Excision of Left Basilic Vein, Percutaneous Endoscopic Approach, Diagnostic

05BC4ZZ Excision of Left Basilic Vein, Percutaneous Endoscopic Approach

05BD0ZX Excision of Right Cephalic Vein, Open Approach, Diagnostic

05BD0ZZ Excision of Right Cephalic Vein, Open Approach

AHA CC: 3Q, 2020, 40

05BD3ZX Excision of Right Cephalic Vein, Percutaneous Approach, Diagnostic

05BD3ZZ Excision of Right Cephalic Vein, Percutaneous Approach

05BD4ZX Excision of Right Cephalic Vein, Percutaneous Endoscopic Approach, Diagnostic

05BD4ZZ Excision of Right Cephalic Vein, Percutaneous Endoscopic Approach

05BF0ZX Excision of Left Cephalic Vein, Open Approach, Diagnostic

05BF0ZZ Excision of Left Cephalic Vein, Open Approach

05BF3ZX Excision of Left Cephalic Vein, Percutaneous Approach, Diagnostic

05BF3ZZ Excision of Left Cephalic Vein, Percutaneous Approach

05BF4ZX Excision of Left Cephalic Vein, Percutaneous Endoscopic Approach, Diagnostic

05BF4ZZ Excision of Left Cephalic Vein, Percutaneous Endoscopic Approach

05BG0ZX Excision of Right Hand Vein, Open Approach, Diagnostic

05BG0ZZ Excision of Right Hand Vein, Open Approach

05BG3ZX Excision of Right Hand Vein, Percutaneous Approach, Diagnostic

05BG3ZZ Excision of Right Hand Vein, Percutaneous Approach

05BG4ZX Excision of Right Hand Vein, Percutaneous Endoscopic Approach, Diagnostic

05BG4ZZ Excision of Right Hand Vein, Percutaneous Endoscopic Approach

05BH0ZX Excision of Left Hand Vein, Open Approach, Diagnostic

05BH0ZZ Excision of Left Hand Vein, Open Approach

05BH3ZX Excision of Left Hand Vein, Percutaneous Approach, Diagnostic

05BH3ZZ Excision of Left Hand Vein, Percutaneous Approach

05BH4ZX Excision of Left Hand Vein, Percutaneous Endoscopic Approach, Diagnostic

05BH4ZZ Excision of Left Hand Vein, Percutaneous Endoscopic Approach

05BL0ZX Excision of Intracranial Vein, Open Approach, Diagnostic

05BL0ZZ Excision of Intracranial Vein, Open Approach

AHA CC: 1Q, 2020, 24; 2Q, 2021, 15-16

05BL3ZX Excision of Intracranial Vein, Percutaneous Approach, Diagnostic

05BL3ZZ Excision of Intracranial Vein, Percutaneous Approach

05BL4ZX Excision of Intracranial Vein, Percutaneous Endoscopic Approach, Diagnostic

05BL4ZZ Excision of Intracranial Vein, Percutaneous Endoscopic Approach

05BM0ZX Excision of Right Internal Jugular Vein, Open Approach, Diagnostic

05BM0ZZ Excision of Right Internal Jugular Vein, Open Approach

05BM3ZX Excision of Right Internal Jugular Vein, Percutaneous Approach, Diagnostic

05BM3ZZ Excision of Right Internal Jugular Vein, Percutaneous Approach

05BM4ZX Excision of Right Internal Jugular Vein, Percutaneous Endoscopic Approach, Diagnostic

05BM4ZZ Excision of Right Internal Jugular Vein, Percutaneous Endoscopic Approach

05BN0ZX Excision of Left Internal Jugular Vein, Open Approach, Diagnostic

05BN0ZZ Excision of Left Internal Jugular Vein, Open Approach

AHA CC: 2Q, 2016, 12-14

05BN3ZX Excision of Left Internal Jugular Vein, Percutaneous Approach, Diagnostic

05BN3ZZ Excision of Left Internal Jugular Vein, Percutaneous Approach

05BN4ZX Excision of Left Internal Jugular Vein, Percutaneous Endoscopic Approach, Diagnostic

05BN4ZZ Excision of Left Internal Jugular Vein, Percutaneous Endoscopic Approach

05BP0ZX Excision of Right External Jugular Vein, Open Approach, Diagnostic

05BP0ZZ Excision of Right External Jugular Vein, Open Approach

05BP3ZX Excision of Right External Jugular Vein, Percutaneous Approach, Diagnostic

05BP3ZZ Excision of Right External Jugular Vein, Percutaneous Approach

05BP4ZX Excision of Right External Jugular Vein, Percutaneous Endoscopic Approach, Diagnostic

05BP4ZZ Excision of Right External Jugular Vein, Percutaneous Endoscopic Approach

05BQ0ZX Excision of Left External Jugular Vein, Open Approach, Diagnostic

05BQ0ZZ Excision of Left External Jugular Vein, Open Approach

AHA CC: 2Q, 2016, 12-14

05BQ3ZX Excision of Left External Jugular Vein, Percutaneous Approach, Diagnostic

05BQ3ZZ Excision of Left External Jugular Vein, Percutaneous Approach

05BQ4ZX Excision of Left External Jugular Vein, Percutaneous Endoscopic Approach, Diagnostic

05BQ4ZZ Excision of Left External Jugular Vein, Percutaneous Endoscopic Approach

05BR0ZX Excision of Right Vertebral Vein, Open Approach, Diagnostic

05BR0ZZ Excision of Right Vertebral Vein, Open Approach

05BR3ZX Excision of Right Vertebral Vein, Percutaneous Approach, Diagnostic

05BR3ZZ Excision of Right Vertebral Vein, Percutaneous Approach

05BR4ZX Excision of Right Vertebral Vein, Percutaneous Endoscopic Approach, Diagnostic

05BR4ZZ Excision of Right Vertebral Vein, Percutaneous Endoscopic Approach

05BS0ZX Excision of Left Vertebral Vein, Open Approach, Diagnostic

05BS0ZZ Excision of Left Vertebral Vein, Open Approach

05BS3ZX Excision of Left Vertebral Vein, Percutaneous Approach, Diagnostic

♀ Female-only   ♂ Male-only   ▲ Limited Coverage   ● Non-OR   ▣ HAC-associated procedure   ▲ Non-covered procedures   ✚ Cluster

05BS3ZZ Excision of Left Vertebral Vein, Percutaneous Approach
05BS4ZX Excision of Left Vertebral Vein, Percutaneous Endoscopic Approach, Diagnostic
05BS4ZZ Excision of Left Vertebral Vein, Percutaneous Endoscopic Approach
05BT0ZX Excision of Right Face Vein, Open Approach, Diagnostic
05BT0ZZ Excision of Right Face Vein, Open Approach
05BT3ZX Excision of Right Face Vein, Percutaneous Approach, Diagnostic
05BT3ZZ Excision of Right Face Vein, Percutaneous Approach

05BT4ZX Excision of Right Face Vein, Percutaneous Endoscopic Approach, Diagnostic
05BT4ZZ Excision of Right Face Vein, Percutaneous Endoscopic Approach
05BV0ZX Excision of Left Face Vein, Open Approach, Diagnostic
05BV0ZZ Excision of Left Face Vein, Open Approach
05BV3ZX Excision of Left Face Vein, Percutaneous Approach, Diagnostic
05BV3ZZ Excision of Left Face Vein, Percutaneous Approach
05BV4ZX Excision of Left Face Vein, Percutaneous Endoscopic Approach, Diagnostic

05BV4ZZ Excision of Left Face Vein, Percutaneous Endoscopic Approach
05BY0ZX Excision of Upper Vein, Open Approach, Diagnostic
05BY0ZZ Excision of Upper Vein, Open Approach
05BY3ZX Excision of Upper Vein, Percutaneous Approach, Diagnostic
05BY3ZZ Excision of Upper Vein, Percutaneous Approach
05BY4ZX Excision of Upper Vein, Percutaneous Endoscopic Approach, Diagnostic
05BY4ZZ Excision of Upper Vein, Percutaneous Endoscopic Approach

05C – Upper Veins, Extirpation

05C00ZZ Extirpation of Matter from Azygos Vein, Open Approach
05C03ZZ Extirpation of Matter from Azygos Vein, Percutaneous Approach
05C04ZZ Extirpation of Matter from Azygos Vein, Percutaneous Endoscopic Approach
05C10ZZ Extirpation of Matter from Hemiazygos Vein, Open Approach
05C13ZZ Extirpation of Matter from Hemiazygos Vein, Percutaneous Approach
05C14ZZ Extirpation of Matter from Hemiazygos Vein, Percutaneous Endoscopic Approach
05C30ZZ Extirpation of Matter from Right Innominate Vein, Open Approach
05C33ZZ Extirpation of Matter from Right Innominate Vein, Percutaneous Approach
05C34ZZ Extirpation of Matter from Right Innominate Vein, Percutaneous Endoscopic Approach
05C40ZZ Extirpation of Matter from Left Innominate Vein, Open Approach
05C43ZZ Extirpation of Matter from Left Innominate Vein, Percutaneous Approach
05C44ZZ Extirpation of Matter from Left Innominate Vein, Percutaneous Endoscopic Approach
05C50ZZ Extirpation of Matter from Right Subclavian Vein, Open Approach
05C53ZZ Extirpation of Matter from Right Subclavian Vein, Percutaneous Approach
05C54ZZ Extirpation of Matter from Right Subclavian Vein, Percutaneous Endoscopic Approach
05C60ZZ Extirpation of Matter from Left Subclavian Vein, Open Approach
05C63ZZ Extirpation of Matter from Left Subclavian Vein, Percutaneous Approach
05C64ZZ Extirpation of Matter from Left Subclavian Vein, Percutaneous Endoscopic Approach
05C70ZZ Extirpation of Matter from Right Axillary Vein, Open Approach
05C73ZZ Extirpation of Matter from Right Axillary Vein, Percutaneous Approach
05C74ZZ Extirpation of Matter from Right Axillary Vein, Percutaneous Endoscopic Approach
05C80ZZ Extirpation of Matter from Left Axillary Vein, Open Approach
05C83ZZ Extirpation of Matter from Left Axillary Vein, Percutaneous Approach

05C84ZZ Extirpation of Matter from Left Axillary Vein, Percutaneous Endoscopic Approach
05C90ZZ Extirpation of Matter from Right Brachial Vein, Open Approach
05C93ZZ Extirpation of Matter from Right Brachial Vein, Percutaneous Approach
05C94ZZ Extirpation of Matter from Right Brachial Vein, Percutaneous Endoscopic Approach
05CA0ZZ Extirpation of Matter from Left Brachial Vein, Open Approach
05CA3ZZ Extirpation of Matter from Left Brachial Vein, Percutaneous Approach
05CA4ZZ Extirpation of Matter from Left Brachial Vein, Percutaneous Endoscopic Approach
05CB0ZZ Extirpation of Matter from Right Basilic Vein, Open Approach
05CB3ZZ Extirpation of Matter from Right Basilic Vein, Percutaneous Approach
05CB4ZZ Extirpation of Matter from Right Basilic Vein, Percutaneous Endoscopic Approach
05CC0ZZ Extirpation of Matter from Left Basilic Vein, Open Approach
05CC3ZZ Extirpation of Matter from Left Basilic Vein, Percutaneous Approach
05CC4ZZ Extirpation of Matter from Left Basilic Vein, Percutaneous Endoscopic Approach
05CD0ZZ Extirpation of Matter from Right Cephalic Vein, Open Approach
AHA CC: 3Q, 2020, 37-40
05CD3ZZ Extirpation of Matter from Right Cephalic Vein, Percutaneous Approach
05CD4ZZ Extirpation of Matter from Right Cephalic Vein, Percutaneous Endoscopic Approach
05CF0ZZ Extirpation of Matter from Left Cephalic Vein, Open Approach
05CF3ZZ Extirpation of Matter from Left Cephalic Vein, Percutaneous Approach
05CF4ZZ Extirpation of Matter from Left Cephalic Vein, Percutaneous Endoscopic Approach
05CG0ZZ Extirpation of Matter from Right Hand Vein, Open Approach
05CG3ZZ Extirpation of Matter from Right Hand Vein, Percutaneous Approach
05CG4ZZ Extirpation of Matter from Right Hand Vein, Percutaneous Endoscopic Approach
05CH0ZZ Extirpation of Matter from Left Hand Vein, Open Approach
05CH3ZZ Extirpation of Matter from Left Hand Vein, Percutaneous Approach

05CH4ZZ Extirpation of Matter from Left Hand Vein, Percutaneous Endoscopic Approach
05CL0ZZ Extirpation of Matter from Intracranial Vein, Open Approach
05CL3ZZ Extirpation of Matter from Intracranial Vein, Percutaneous Approach
05CL4ZZ Extirpation of Matter from Intracranial Vein, Percutaneous Endoscopic Approach
05CM0ZZ Extirpation of Matter from Right Internal Jugular Vein, Open Approach
05CM3ZZ Extirpation of Matter from Right Internal Jugular Vein, Percutaneous Approach
05CM4ZZ Extirpation of Matter from Right Internal Jugular Vein, Percutaneous Endoscopic Approach
05CN0ZZ Extirpation of Matter from Left Internal Jugular Vein, Open Approach
05CN3ZZ Extirpation of Matter from Left Internal Jugular Vein, Percutaneous Approach
05CN4ZZ Extirpation of Matter from Left Internal Jugular Vein, Percutaneous Endoscopic Approach
05CP0ZZ Extirpation of Matter from Right External Jugular Vein, Open Approach
05CP3ZZ Extirpation of Matter from Right External Jugular Vein, Percutaneous Approach
05CP4ZZ Extirpation of Matter from Right External Jugular Vein, Percutaneous Endoscopic Approach
05CQ0ZZ Extirpation of Matter from Left External Jugular Vein, Open Approach
05CQ3ZZ Extirpation of Matter from Left External Jugular Vein, Percutaneous Approach
05CQ4ZZ Extirpation of Matter from Left External Jugular Vein, Percutaneous Endoscopic Approach
05CR0ZZ Extirpation of Matter from Right Vertebral Vein, Open Approach
05CR3ZZ Extirpation of Matter from Right Vertebral Vein, Percutaneous Approach
05CR4ZZ Extirpation of Matter from Right Vertebral Vein, Percutaneous Endoscopic Approach
05CS0ZZ Extirpation of Matter from Left Vertebral Vein, Open Approach
05CS3ZZ Extirpation of Matter from Left Vertebral Vein, Percutaneous Approach
05CS4ZZ Extirpation of Matter from Left Vertebral Vein, Percutaneous Endoscopic Approach
05CT0ZZ Extirpation of Matter from Right Face Vein, Open Approach

05CT3ZZ Extirpation of Matter from Right Face Vein, Percutaneous Approach

05CT4ZZ Extirpation of Matter from Right Face Vein, Percutaneous Endoscopic Approach

05CV0ZZ Extirpation of Matter from Left Face Vein, Open Approach

05CV3ZZ Extirpation of Matter from Left Face Vein, Percutaneous Approach

05CV4ZZ Extirpation of Matter from Left Face Vein, Percutaneous Endoscopic Approach

05CY0ZZ Extirpation of Matter from Upper Vein, Open Approach

05CY3ZZ Extirpation of Matter from Upper Vein, Percutaneous Approach

05CY4ZZ Extirpation of Matter from Upper Vein, Percutaneous Endoscopic Approach

05D – Upper Veins, Extraction

05D90ZZ Extraction of Right Brachial Vein, Open Approach

05D93ZZ Extraction of Right Brachial Vein, Percutaneous Approach

05DA0ZZ Extraction of Left Brachial Vein, Open Approach

05DA3ZZ Extraction of Left Brachial Vein, Percutaneous Approach

05DB0ZZ Extraction of Right Basilic Vein, Open Approach

05DB3ZZ Extraction of Right Basilic Vein, Percutaneous Approach

05DC0ZZ Extraction of Left Basilic Vein, Open Approach

05DC3ZZ Extraction of Left Basilic Vein, Percutaneous Approach

05DD0ZZ Extraction of Right Cephalic Vein, Open Approach

05DD3ZZ Extraction of Right Cephalic Vein, Percutaneous Approach

05DF0ZZ Extraction of Left Cephalic Vein, Open Approach

05DF3ZZ Extraction of Left Cephalic Vein, Percutaneous Approach

05DG0ZZ Extraction of Right Hand Vein, Open Approach

05DG3ZZ Extraction of Right Hand Vein, Percutaneous Approach

05DH0ZZ Extraction of Left Hand Vein, Open Approach

05DH3ZZ Extraction of Left Hand Vein, Percutaneous Approach

05DY0ZZ Extraction of Upper Vein, Open Approach

05DY3ZZ Extraction of Upper Vein, Percutaneous Approach

05F – Upper Veins, Fragmentation

05F33Z0 Fragmentation of Right Innominate Vein, Percutaneous Approach, Ultrasonic

05F33ZZ Fragmentation of Right Innominate Vein, Percutaneous Approach

05F43Z0 Fragmentation of Left Innominate Vein, Percutaneous Approach, Ultrasonic

05F43ZZ Fragmentation of Left Innominate Vein, Percutaneous Approach

05F53Z0 Fragmentation of Right Subclavian Vein, Percutaneous Approach, Ultrasonic

05F53ZZ Fragmentation of Right Subclavian Vein, Percutaneous Approach

05F63Z0 Fragmentation of Left Subclavian Vein, Percutaneous Approach, Ultrasonic

05F63ZZ Fragmentation of Left Subclavian Vein, Percutaneous Approach

05F73Z0 Fragmentation of Right Axillary Vein, Percutaneous Approach, Ultrasonic

05F73ZZ Fragmentation of Right Axillary Vein, Percutaneous Approach

05F83Z0 Fragmentation of Left Axillary Vein, Percutaneous Approach, Ultrasonic

05F83ZZ Fragmentation of Left Axillary Vein, Percutaneous Approach

05F93Z0 Fragmentation of Right Brachial Vein, Percutaneous Approach, Ultrasonic

05F93ZZ Fragmentation of Right Brachial Vein, Percutaneous Approach

05FA3Z0 Fragmentation of Left Brachial Vein, Percutaneous Approach, Ultrasonic

05FA3ZZ Fragmentation of Left Brachial Vein, Percutaneous Approach

05FB3Z0 Fragmentation of Right Basilic Vein, Percutaneous Approach, Ultrasonic

05FB3ZZ Fragmentation of Right Basilic Vein, Percutaneous Approach

05FC3Z0 Fragmentation of Left Basilic Vein, Percutaneous Approach, Ultrasonic

05FC3ZZ Fragmentation of Left Basilic Vein, Percutaneous Approach

05FD3Z0 Fragmentation of Right Cephalic Vein, Percutaneous Approach, Ultrasonic

05FD3ZZ Fragmentation of Right Cephalic Vein, Percutaneous Approach

05FF3Z0 Fragmentation of Left Cephalic Vein, Percutaneous Approach, Ultrasonic

05FF3ZZ Fragmentation of Left Cephalic Vein, Percutaneous Approach

05FY3Z0 Fragmentation of Upper Vein, Percutaneous Approach, Ultrasonic

05FY3ZZ Fragmentation of Upper Vein, Percutaneous Approach

05H – Upper Veins, Insertion

05H002Z Insertion of Monitoring Device into Azygos Vein, Open Approach

05H003Z Insertion of Infusion Device into Azygos Vein, Open Approach

05H00DZ Insertion of Intraluminal Device into Azygos Vein, Open Approach

05H00MZ Insertion of Neurostimulator Lead into Azygos Vein, Open Approach

➕ Lead device when reported with an Insertion of a stimulator generator (6th character B-E) into the chest or abdomen subcutaneous tissue and fascia. *See table 0JH to construct the Insertion code.*

05H032Z Insertion of Monitoring Device into Azygos Vein, Percutaneous Approach
AHA CC: 4Q, 2016, 98-99

05H033Z Insertion of Infusion Device into Azygos Vein, Percutaneous Approach
HAC When reported with secondary diagnosis code J95.811

05H03DZ Insertion of Intraluminal Device into Azygos Vein, Percutaneous Approach

05H03MZ Insertion of Neurostimulator Lead into Azygos Vein, Percutaneous Approach

➕ Lead device when reported with an Insertion of a stimulator generator (6th character B-E) into the chest or abdomen subcutaneous tissue and fascia. *See table 0JH to construct the Insertion code.*

05H042Z Insertion of Monitoring Device into Azygos Vein, Percutaneous Endoscopic Approach

05H043Z Insertion of Infusion Device into Azygos Vein, Percutaneous Endoscopic Approach
HAC When reported with secondary diagnosis code J95.811

05H04DZ Insertion of Intraluminal Device into Azygos Vein, Percutaneous Endoscopic Approach

05H04MZ Insertion of Neurostimulator Lead into Azygos Vein, Percutaneous Endoscopic Approach

➕ Lead device when reported with an Insertion of a stimulator generator (6th character B-E) into the chest or abdomen subcutaneous tissue and fascia. *See table 0JH to construct the Insertion code.*

05H103Z Insertion of Infusion Device into Hemiazygos Vein, Open Approach

05H10DZ Insertion of Intraluminal Device into Hemiazygos Vein, Open Approach

05H133Z Insertion of Infusion Device into Hemiazygos Vein, Percutaneous Approach
HAC When reported with secondary diagnosis code J95.811

05H13DZ Insertion of Intraluminal Device into Hemiazygos Vein, Percutaneous Approach

05H143Z Insertion of Infusion Device into Hemiazygos Vein, Percutaneous Endoscopic Approach
HAC When reported with secondary diagnosis code J95.811

05H14DZ Insertion of Intraluminal Device into Hemiazygos Vein, Percutaneous Endoscopic Approach

05H303Z Insertion of Infusion Device into Right Innominate Vein, Open Approach

05H30DZ Insertion of Intraluminal Device into Right Innominate Vein, Open Approach

05H30MZ Insertion of Neurostimulator Lead into Right Innominate Vein, Open Approach

➕ Lead device when reported with an Insertion of a stimulator generator (6th character B-E) into the chest or abdomen subcutaneous tissue and fascia. *See table 0JH to construct the Insertion code.*

05H333Z Insertion of Infusion Device into Right Innominate Vein, Percutaneous Approach
HAC When reported with secondary diagnosis code J95.811

♀ Female-only　　♂ Male-only　　▲ Limited Coverage　　● Non-OR　　HAC HAC-associated procedure　　▲ Non-covered procedures　　➕ Cluster

5H33DZ Insertion of Intraluminal Device into Right Innominate Vein, Percutaneous Approach

5H33MZ Insertion of Neurostimulator Lead into Right Innominate Vein, Percutaneous Approach

➕ Lead device when reported with an Insertion of a stimulator generator (6th character B-E) into the chest or abdomen subcutaneous tissue and fascia. *See table 0JH to construct the Insertion code.*

05H343Z Insertion of Infusion Device into Right Innominate Vein, Percutaneous Endoscopic Approach

HAC When reported with secondary diagnosis code J95.811

05H34DZ Insertion of Intraluminal Device into Right Innominate Vein, Percutaneous Endoscopic Approach

05H34MZ Insertion of Neurostimulator Lead into Right Innominate Vein, Percutaneous Endoscopic Approach

➕ Lead device when reported with an Insertion of a stimulator generator (6th character B-E) into the chest or abdomen subcutaneous tissue and fascia. *See table 0JH to construct the Insertion code.*

05H403Z Insertion of Infusion Device into Left Innominate Vein, Open Approach

05H40DZ Insertion of Intraluminal Device into Left Innominate Vein, Open Approach

05H40MZ Insertion of Neurostimulator Lead into Left Innominate Vein, Open Approach

➕ Lead device when reported with an Insertion of a stimulator generator (6th character B-E) into the chest or abdomen subcutaneous tissue and fascia. *See table 0JH to construct the Insertion code.*

05H433Z Insertion of Infusion Device into Left Innominate Vein, Percutaneous Approach

HAC When reported with secondary diagnosis code J95.811

05H43DZ Insertion of Intraluminal Device into Left Innominate Vein, Percutaneous Approach

05H43MZ Insertion of Neurostimulator Lead into Left Innominate Vein, Percutaneous Approach

➕ Lead device when reported with an Insertion of a stimulator generator (6th character B-E) into the chest or abdomen subcutaneous tissue and fascia. *See table 0JH to construct the Insertion code.*
AHA CC: 4Q, 2016, 98-99

05H443Z Insertion of Infusion Device into Left Innominate Vein, Percutaneous Endoscopic Approach

HAC When reported with secondary diagnosis code J95.811

05H44DZ Insertion of Intraluminal Device into Left Innominate Vein, Percutaneous Endoscopic Approach

05H44MZ Insertion of Neurostimulator Lead into Left Innominate Vein, Percutaneous Endoscopic Approach

➕ Lead device when reported with an Insertion of a stimulator generator (6th character B-E) into the chest or abdomen subcutaneous tissue and fascia. *See table 0JH to construct the Insertion code.*

05H503Z Insertion of Infusion Device into Right Subclavian Vein, Open Approach

05H50DZ Insertion of Intraluminal Device into Right Subclavian Vein, Open Approach

● **05H533Z** Insertion of Infusion Device into Right Subclavian Vein, Percutaneous Approach

HAC When reported with secondary diagnosis code J95.811

05H53DZ Insertion of Intraluminal Device into Right Subclavian Vein, Percutaneous Approach

05H543Z Insertion of Infusion Device into Right Subclavian Vein, Percutaneous Endoscopic Approach

HAC When reported with secondary diagnosis code J95.811

05H54DZ Insertion of Intraluminal Device into Right Subclavian Vein, Percutaneous Endoscopic Approach

05H603Z Insertion of Infusion Device into Left Subclavian Vein, Open Approach

05H60DZ Insertion of Intraluminal Device into Left Subclavian Vein, Open Approach

● **05H633Z** Insertion of Infusion Device into Left Subclavian Vein, Percutaneous Approach

HAC When reported with secondary diagnosis code J95.811

05H63DZ Insertion of Intraluminal Device into Left Subclavian Vein, Percutaneous Approach

05H643Z Insertion of Infusion Device into Left Subclavian Vein, Percutaneous Endoscopic Approach

HAC When reported with secondary diagnosis code J95.811

05H64DZ Insertion of Intraluminal Device into Left Subclavian Vein, Percutaneous Endoscopic Approach

05H703Z Insertion of Infusion Device into Right Axillary Vein, Open Approach

05H70DZ Insertion of Intraluminal Device into Right Axillary Vein, Open Approach

05H733Z Insertion of Infusion Device into Right Axillary Vein, Percutaneous Approach

05H73DZ Insertion of Intraluminal Device into Right Axillary Vein, Percutaneous Approach

05H743Z Insertion of Infusion Device into Right Axillary Vein, Percutaneous Endoscopic Approach

05H74DZ Insertion of Intraluminal Device into Right Axillary Vein, Percutaneous Endoscopic Approach

05H803Z Insertion of Infusion Device into Left Axillary Vein, Open Approach

05H80DZ Insertion of Intraluminal Device into Left Axillary Vein, Open Approach

05H833Z Insertion of Infusion Device into Left Axillary Vein, Percutaneous Approach

05H83DZ Insertion of Intraluminal Device into Left Axillary Vein, Percutaneous Approach

05H843Z Insertion of Infusion Device into Left Axillary Vein, Percutaneous Endoscopic Approach

05H84DZ Insertion of Intraluminal Device into Left Axillary Vein, Percutaneous Endoscopic Approach

05H903Z Insertion of Infusion Device into Right Brachial Vein, Open Approach

05H90DZ Insertion of Intraluminal Device into Right Brachial Vein, Open Approach

05H933Z Insertion of Infusion Device into Right Brachial Vein, Percutaneous Approach

05H93DZ Insertion of Intraluminal Device into Right Brachial Vein, Percutaneous Approach

05H943Z Insertion of Infusion Device into Right Brachial Vein, Percutaneous Endoscopic Approach

05H94DZ Insertion of Intraluminal Device into Right Brachial Vein, Percutaneous Endoscopic Approach

05HA03Z Insertion of Infusion Device into Left Brachial Vein, Open Approach

05HA0DZ Insertion of Intraluminal Device into Left Brachial Vein, Open Approach

05HA33Z Insertion of Infusion Device into Left Brachial Vein, Percutaneous Approach

05HA3DZ Insertion of Intraluminal Device into Left Brachial Vein, Percutaneous Approach

05HA43Z Insertion of Infusion Device into Left Brachial Vein, Percutaneous Endoscopic Approach

05HA4DZ Insertion of Intraluminal Device into Left Brachial Vein, Percutaneous Endoscopic Approach

05HB03Z Insertion of Infusion Device into Right Basilic Vein, Open Approach

05HB0DZ Insertion of Intraluminal Device into Right Basilic Vein, Open Approach

05HB33Z Insertion of Infusion Device into Right Basilic Vein, Percutaneous Approach

05HB3DZ Insertion of Intraluminal Device into Right Basilic Vein, Percutaneous Approach

05HB43Z Insertion of Infusion Device into Right Basilic Vein, Percutaneous Endoscopic Approach

05HB4DZ Insertion of Intraluminal Device into Right Basilic Vein, Percutaneous Endoscopic Approach

05HC03Z Insertion of Infusion Device into Left Basilic Vein, Open Approach

05HC0DZ Insertion of Intraluminal Device into Left Basilic Vein, Open Approach

05HC33Z Insertion of Infusion Device into Left Basilic Vein, Percutaneous Approach

05HC3DZ Insertion of Intraluminal Device into Left Basilic Vein, Percutaneous Approach

05HC43Z Insertion of Infusion Device into Left Basilic Vein, Percutaneous Endoscopic Approach

05HC4DZ Insertion of Intraluminal Device into Left Basilic Vein, Percutaneous Endoscopic Approach

05HD03Z Insertion of Infusion Device into Right Cephalic Vein, Open Approach

05HD0DZ Insertion of Intraluminal Device into Right Cephalic Vein, Open Approach

05HD33Z Insertion of Infusion Device into Right Cephalic Vein, Percutaneous Approach

05HD3DZ Insertion of Intraluminal Device into Right Cephalic Vein, Percutaneous Approach

05HD43Z Insertion of Infusion Device into Right Cephalic Vein, Percutaneous Endoscopic Approach

05HD4DZ Insertion of Intraluminal Device into Right Cephalic Vein, Percutaneous Endoscopic Approach

05HF03Z Insertion of Infusion Device into Left Cephalic Vein, Open Approach

Medical and Surgical, Upper Veins Code Listings

♀ Female-only   ♂ Male-only   ▲ Limited Coverage   ● Non-OR   HAC HAC-associated procedure   ▲ Non-covered procedures   ➕ Cluster   **395**

05HF0DZ Insertion of Intraluminal Device into Left Cephalic Vein, Open Approach

05HF33Z Insertion of Infusion Device into Left Cephalic Vein, Percutaneous Approach

05HF3DZ Insertion of Intraluminal Device into Left Cephalic Vein, Percutaneous Approach

05HF43Z Insertion of Infusion Device into Left Cephalic Vein, Percutaneous Endoscopic Approach

05HF4DZ Insertion of Intraluminal Device into Left Cephalic Vein, Percutaneous Endoscopic Approach

05HG03Z Insertion of Infusion Device into Right Hand Vein, Open Approach

05HG0DZ Insertion of Intraluminal Device into Right Hand Vein, Open Approach

05HG33Z Insertion of Infusion Device into Right Hand Vein, Percutaneous Approach

05HG3DZ Insertion of Intraluminal Device into Right Hand Vein, Percutaneous Approach

05HG43Z Insertion of Infusion Device into Right Hand Vein, Percutaneous Endoscopic Approach

05HG4DZ Insertion of Intraluminal Device into Right Hand Vein, Percutaneous Endoscopic Approach

05HH03Z Insertion of Infusion Device into Left Hand Vein, Open Approach

05HH0DZ Insertion of Intraluminal Device into Left Hand Vein, Open Approach

05HH33Z Insertion of Infusion Device into Left Hand Vein, Percutaneous Approach

05HH3DZ Insertion of Intraluminal Device into Left Hand Vein, Percutaneous Approach

05HH43Z Insertion of Infusion Device into Left Hand Vein, Percutaneous Endoscopic Approach

05HH4DZ Insertion of Intraluminal Device into Left Hand Vein, Percutaneous Endoscopic Approach

05HL03Z Insertion of Infusion Device into Intracranial Vein, Open Approach

05HL0DZ Insertion of Intraluminal Device into Intracranial Vein, Open Approach

05HL33Z Insertion of Infusion Device into Intracranial Vein, Percutaneous Approach

05HL3DZ Insertion of Intraluminal Device into Intracranial Vein, Percutaneous Approach

05HL43Z Insertion of Infusion Device into Intracranial Vein, Percutaneous Endoscopic Approach

05HL4DZ Insertion of Intraluminal Device into Intracranial Vein, Percutaneous Endoscopic Approach

05HM03Z Insertion of Infusion Device into Right Internal Jugular Vein, Open Approach

05HM0DZ Insertion of Intraluminal Device into Right Internal Jugular Vein, Open Approach

05HM33Z Insertion of Infusion Device into Right Internal Jugular Vein, Percutaneous Approach

    HAC With secondary diagnosis code J95.811

05HM3DZ Insertion of Intraluminal Device into Right Internal Jugular Vein, Percutaneous Approach

05HM43Z Insertion of Infusion Device into Right Internal Jugular Vein, Percutaneous Endoscopic Approach

05HM4DZ Insertion of Intraluminal Device into Right Internal Jugular Vein, Percutaneous Endoscopic Approach

05HN03Z Insertion of Infusion Device into Left Internal Jugular Vein, Open Approach

05HN0DZ Insertion of Intraluminal Device into Left Internal Jugular Vein, Open Approach

05HN33Z Insertion of Infusion Device into Left Internal Jugular Vein, Percutaneous Approach

    HAC With secondary diagnosis code J95.811

05HN3DZ Insertion of Intraluminal Device into Left Internal Jugular Vein, Percutaneous Approach

05HN43Z Insertion of Infusion Device into Left Internal Jugular Vein, Percutaneous Endoscopic Approach

05HN4DZ Insertion of Intraluminal Device into Left Internal Jugular Vein, Percutaneous Endoscopic Approach

05HP03Z Insertion of Infusion Device into Right External Jugular Vein, Open Approach

05HP0DZ Insertion of Intraluminal Device into Right External Jugular Vein, Open Approach

05HP33Z Insertion of Infusion Device into Right External Jugular Vein, Percutaneous Approach

    HAC With secondary diagnosis code J95.811

05HP3DZ Insertion of Intraluminal Device into Right External Jugular Vein, Percutaneous Approach

05HP43Z Insertion of Infusion Device into Right External Jugular Vein, Percutaneous Endoscopic Approach

05HP4DZ Insertion of Intraluminal Device into Right External Jugular Vein, Percutaneous Endoscopic Approach

05HQ03Z Insertion of Infusion Device into Left External Jugular Vein, Open Approach

05HQ0DZ Insertion of Intraluminal Device into Left External Jugular Vein, Open Approach

05HQ33Z Insertion of Infusion Device into Left External Jugular Vein, Percutaneous Approach

    HAC With secondary diagnosis code J95.811

05HQ3DZ Insertion of Intraluminal Device into Left External Jugular Vein, Percutaneous Approach

05HQ43Z Insertion of Infusion Device into Left External Jugular Vein, Percutaneous Endoscopic Approach

05HQ4DZ Insertion of Intraluminal Device into Left External Jugular Vein, Percutaneous Endoscopic Approach

05HR03Z Insertion of Infusion Device into Right Vertebral Vein, Open Approach

05HR0DZ Insertion of Intraluminal Device into Right Vertebral Vein, Open Approach

05HR33Z Insertion of Infusion Device into Right Vertebral Vein, Percutaneous Approach

05HR3DZ Insertion of Intraluminal Device into Right Vertebral Vein, Percutaneous Approach

05HR43Z Insertion of Infusion Device into Right Vertebral Vein, Percutaneous Endoscopic Approach

05HR4DZ Insertion of Intraluminal Device into Right Vertebral Vein, Percutaneous Endoscopic Approach

05HS03Z Insertion of Infusion Device into Left Vertebral Vein, Open Approach

05HS0DZ Insertion of Intraluminal Device into Left Vertebral Vein, Open Approach

05HS33Z Insertion of Infusion Device into Left Vertebral Vein, Percutaneous Approach

05HS3DZ Insertion of Intraluminal Device into Left Vertebral Vein, Percutaneous Approach

05HS43Z Insertion of Infusion Device into Left Vertebral Vein, Percutaneous Endoscopic Approach

05HS4DZ Insertion of Intraluminal Device into Left Vertebral Vein, Percutaneous Endoscopic Approach

05HT03Z Insertion of Infusion Device into Right Face Vein, Open Approach

05HT0DZ Insertion of Intraluminal Device into Right Face Vein, Open Approach

05HT33Z Insertion of Infusion Device into Right Face Vein, Percutaneous Approach

05HT3DZ Insertion of Intraluminal Device into Right Face Vein, Percutaneous Approach

05HT43Z Insertion of Infusion Device into Right Face Vein, Percutaneous Endoscopic Approach

05HT4DZ Insertion of Intraluminal Device into Right Face Vein, Percutaneous Endoscopic Approach

05HV03Z Insertion of Infusion Device into Left Face Vein, Open Approach

05HV0DZ Insertion of Intraluminal Device into Left Face Vein, Open Approach

05HV33Z Insertion of Infusion Device into Left Face Vein, Percutaneous Approach

05HV3DZ Insertion of Intraluminal Device into Left Face Vein, Percutaneous Approach

05HV43Z Insertion of Infusion Device into Left Face Vein, Percutaneous Endoscopic Approach

05HV4DZ Insertion of Intraluminal Device into Left Face Vein, Percutaneous Endoscopic Approach

05HY02Z Insertion of Monitoring Device into Upper Vein, Open Approach

05HY03Z Insertion of Infusion Device into Upper Vein, Open Approach

05HY0DZ Insertion of Intraluminal Device into Upper Vein, Open Approach

05HY0YZ Insertion of Other Device into Upper Vein, Open Approach

05HY32Z Insertion of Monitoring Device into Upper Vein, Percutaneous Approach

05HY33Z Insertion of Infusion Device into Upper Vein, Percutaneous Approach

05HY3DZ Insertion of Intraluminal Device into Upper Vein, Percutaneous Approach

05HY3YZ Insertion of Other Device into Upper Vein, Percutaneous Approach

05HY42Z Insertion of Monitoring Device into Upper Vein, Percutaneous Endoscopic Approach

05HY43Z Insertion of Infusion Device into Upper Vein, Percutaneous Endoscopic Approach

05HY4DZ Insertion of Intraluminal Device into Upper Vein, Percutaneous Endoscopic Approach

05HY4YZ Insertion of Other Device into Upper Vein, Percutaneous Endoscopic Approach

♀ Female-only   ♂ Male-only   ▲ Limited Coverage   ● Non-OR   HAC HAC-associated procedure   ▲ Non-covered procedures   ✚ Cluster

05J – Upper Veins, Inspection

Review Coding Guidelines B3.11a, B3.11b and B3.11c

05JY0ZZ Inspection of Upper Vein, Open Approach

05JY3ZZ Inspection of Upper Vein, Percutaneous Approach

05JY4ZZ Inspection of Upper Vein, Percutaneous Endoscopic Approach

05JYXZZ Inspection of Upper Vein, External Approach

05L – Upper Veins, Occlusion

Review Coding Guideline B3.12

05L00CZ Occlusion of Azygos Vein with Extraluminal Device, Open Approach

05L00DZ Occlusion of Azygos Vein with Intraluminal Device, Open Approach

05L00ZZ Occlusion of Azygos Vein, Open Approach

05L03CZ Occlusion of Azygos Vein with Extraluminal Device, Percutaneous Approach

05L03DZ Occlusion of Azygos Vein with Intraluminal Device, Percutaneous Approach

05L03ZZ Occlusion of Azygos Vein, Percutaneous Approach

05L04CZ Occlusion of Azygos Vein with Extraluminal Device, Percutaneous Endoscopic Approach

05L04DZ Occlusion of Azygos Vein with Intraluminal Device, Percutaneous Endoscopic Approach

05L04ZZ Occlusion of Azygos Vein, Percutaneous Endoscopic Approach

05L10CZ Occlusion of Hemiazygos Vein with Extraluminal Device, Open Approach

05L10DZ Occlusion of Hemiazygos Vein with Intraluminal Device, Open Approach

05L10ZZ Occlusion of Hemiazygos Vein, Open Approach

05L13CZ Occlusion of Hemiazygos Vein with Extraluminal Device, Percutaneous Approach

05L13DZ Occlusion of Hemiazygos Vein with Intraluminal Device, Percutaneous Approach

05L13ZZ Occlusion of Hemiazygos Vein, Percutaneous Approach

05L14CZ Occlusion of Hemiazygos Vein with Extraluminal Device, Percutaneous Endoscopic Approach

05L14DZ Occlusion of Hemiazygos Vein with Intraluminal Device, Percutaneous Endoscopic Approach

05L14ZZ Occlusion of Hemiazygos Vein, Percutaneous Endoscopic Approach

05L30CZ Occlusion of Right Innominate Vein with Extraluminal Device, Open Approach

05L30DZ Occlusion of Right Innominate Vein with Intraluminal Device, Open Approach

05L30ZZ Occlusion of Right Innominate Vein, Open Approach

05L33CZ Occlusion of Right Innominate Vein with Extraluminal Device, Percutaneous Approach

05L33DZ Occlusion of Right Innominate Vein with Intraluminal Device, Percutaneous Approach

05L33ZZ Occlusion of Right Innominate Vein, Percutaneous Approach

05L34CZ Occlusion of Right Innominate Vein with Extraluminal Device, Percutaneous Endoscopic Approach

05L34DZ Occlusion of Right Innominate Vein with Intraluminal Device, Percutaneous Endoscopic Approach

05L34ZZ Occlusion of Right Innominate Vein, Percutaneous Endoscopic Approach

05L40CZ Occlusion of Left Innominate Vein with Extraluminal Device, Open Approach

05L40DZ Occlusion of Left Innominate Vein with Intraluminal Device, Open Approach

05L40ZZ Occlusion of Left Innominate Vein, Open Approach

05L43CZ Occlusion of Left Innominate Vein with Extraluminal Device, Percutaneous Approach

05L43DZ Occlusion of Left Innominate Vein with Intraluminal Device, Percutaneous Approach

05L43ZZ Occlusion of Left Innominate Vein, Percutaneous Approach

05L44CZ Occlusion of Left Innominate Vein with Extraluminal Device, Percutaneous Endoscopic Approach

05L44DZ Occlusion of Left Innominate Vein with Intraluminal Device, Percutaneous Endoscopic Approach

05L44ZZ Occlusion of Left Innominate Vein, Percutaneous Endoscopic Approach

05L50CZ Occlusion of Right Subclavian Vein with Extraluminal Device, Open Approach

05L50DZ Occlusion of Right Subclavian Vein with Intraluminal Device, Open Approach

05L50ZZ Occlusion of Right Subclavian Vein, Open Approach

05L53CZ Occlusion of Right Subclavian Vein with Extraluminal Device, Percutaneous Approach

05L53DZ Occlusion of Right Subclavian Vein with Intraluminal Device, Percutaneous Approach

05L53ZZ Occlusion of Right Subclavian Vein, Percutaneous Approach

05L54CZ Occlusion of Right Subclavian Vein with Extraluminal Device, Percutaneous Endoscopic Approach

05L54DZ Occlusion of Right Subclavian Vein with Intraluminal Device, Percutaneous Endoscopic Approach

05L54ZZ Occlusion of Right Subclavian Vein, Percutaneous Endoscopic Approach

05L60CZ Occlusion of Left Subclavian Vein with Extraluminal Device, Open Approach

05L60DZ Occlusion of Left Subclavian Vein with Intraluminal Device, Open Approach

05L60ZZ Occlusion of Left Subclavian Vein, Open Approach

05L63CZ Occlusion of Left Subclavian Vein with Extraluminal Device, Percutaneous Approach

05L63DZ Occlusion of Left Subclavian Vein with Intraluminal Device, Percutaneous Approach

05L63ZZ Occlusion of Left Subclavian Vein, Percutaneous Approach

05L64CZ Occlusion of Left Subclavian Vein with Extraluminal Device, Percutaneous Endoscopic Approach

05L64DZ Occlusion of Left Subclavian Vein with Intraluminal Device, Percutaneous Endoscopic Approach

05L64ZZ Occlusion of Left Subclavian Vein, Percutaneous Endoscopic Approach

05L70CZ Occlusion of Right Axillary Vein with Extraluminal Device, Open Approach

05L70DZ Occlusion of Right Axillary Vein with Intraluminal Device, Open Approach

05L70ZZ Occlusion of Right Axillary Vein, Open Approach

05L73CZ Occlusion of Right Axillary Vein with Extraluminal Device, Percutaneous Approach

05L73DZ Occlusion of Right Axillary Vein with Intraluminal Device, Percutaneous Approach

05L73ZZ Occlusion of Right Axillary Vein, Percutaneous Approach

05L74CZ Occlusion of Right Axillary Vein with Extraluminal Device, Percutaneous Endoscopic Approach

05L74DZ Occlusion of Right Axillary Vein with Intraluminal Device, Percutaneous Endoscopic Approach

05L74ZZ Occlusion of Right Axillary Vein, Percutaneous Endoscopic Approach

05L80CZ Occlusion of Left Axillary Vein with Extraluminal Device, Open Approach

05L80DZ Occlusion of Left Axillary Vein with Intraluminal Device, Open Approach

05L80ZZ Occlusion of Left Axillary Vein, Open Approach

05L83CZ Occlusion of Left Axillary Vein with Extraluminal Device, Percutaneous Approach

05L83DZ Occlusion of Left Axillary Vein with Intraluminal Device, Percutaneous Approach

05L83ZZ Occlusion of Left Axillary Vein, Percutaneous Approach

05L84CZ Occlusion of Left Axillary Vein with Extraluminal Device, Percutaneous Endoscopic Approach

05L84DZ Occlusion of Left Axillary Vein with Intraluminal Device, Percutaneous Endoscopic Approach

05L84ZZ Occlusion of Left Axillary Vein, Percutaneous Endoscopic Approach

05L90CZ Occlusion of Right Brachial Vein with Extraluminal Device, Open Approach

05L90DZ Occlusion of Right Brachial Vein with Intraluminal Device, Open Approach

05L90ZZ Occlusion of Right Brachial Vein, Open Approach

05L93CZ Occlusion of Right Brachial Vein with Extraluminal Device, Percutaneous Approach

05L93DZ Occlusion of Right Brachial Vein with Intraluminal Device, Percutaneous Approach

05L93ZZ Occlusion of Right Brachial Vein, Percutaneous Approach

05L94CZ Occlusion of Right Brachial Vein with Extraluminal Device, Percutaneous Endoscopic Approach

05L94DZ Occlusion of Right Brachial Vein with Intraluminal Device, Percutaneous Endoscopic Approach

05L94ZZ Occlusion of Right Brachial Vein, Percutaneous Endoscopic Approach

05LA0CZ Occlusion of Left Brachial Vein with Extraluminal Device, Open Approach

05LA0DZ Occlusion of Left Brachial Vein with Intraluminal Device, Open Approach

05LA0ZZ Occlusion of Left Brachial Vein, Open Approach

05LA3CZ Occlusion of Left Brachial Vein with Extraluminal Device, Percutaneous Approach

05LA3DZ Occlusion of Left Brachial Vein with Intraluminal Device, Percutaneous Approach

05LA3ZZ Occlusion of Left Brachial Vein, Percutaneous Approach

05LA4CZ Occlusion of Left Brachial Vein with Extraluminal Device, Percutaneous Endoscopic Approach

05LA4DZ Occlusion of Left Brachial Vein with Intraluminal Device, Percutaneous Endoscopic Approach

05LA4ZZ Occlusion of Left Brachial Vein, Percutaneous Endoscopic Approach

05LB0CZ Occlusion of Right Basilic Vein with Extraluminal Device, Open Approach

05LB0DZ Occlusion of Right Basilic Vein with Intraluminal Device, Open Approach

05LB0ZZ Occlusion of Right Basilic Vein, Open Approach

05LB3CZ Occlusion of Right Basilic Vein with Extraluminal Device, Percutaneous Approach

05LB3DZ Occlusion of Right Basilic Vein with Intraluminal Device, Percutaneous Approach

05LB3ZZ Occlusion of Right Basilic Vein, Percutaneous Approach

05LB4CZ Occlusion of Right Basilic Vein with Extraluminal Device, Percutaneous Endoscopic Approach

05LB4DZ Occlusion of Right Basilic Vein with Intraluminal Device, Percutaneous Endoscopic Approach

05LB4ZZ Occlusion of Right Basilic Vein, Percutaneous Endoscopic Approach

05LC0CZ Occlusion of Left Basilic Vein with Extraluminal Device, Open Approach

05LC0DZ Occlusion of Left Basilic Vein with Intraluminal Device, Open Approach

05LC0ZZ Occlusion of Left Basilic Vein, Open Approach

05LC3CZ Occlusion of Left Basilic Vein with Extraluminal Device, Percutaneous Approach

05LC3DZ Occlusion of Left Basilic Vein with Intraluminal Device, Percutaneous Approach

05LC3ZZ Occlusion of Left Basilic Vein, Percutaneous Approach

05LC4CZ Occlusion of Left Basilic Vein with Extraluminal Device, Percutaneous Endoscopic Approach

05LC4DZ Occlusion of Left Basilic Vein with Intraluminal Device, Percutaneous Endoscopic Approach

05LC4ZZ Occlusion of Left Basilic Vein, Percutaneous Endoscopic Approach

05LD0CZ Occlusion of Right Cephalic Vein with Extraluminal Device, Open Approach

05LD0DZ Occlusion of Right Cephalic Vein with Intraluminal Device, Open Approach

05LD0ZZ Occlusion of Right Cephalic Vein, Open Approach

05LD3CZ Occlusion of Right Cephalic Vein with Extraluminal Device, Percutaneous Approach

05LD3DZ Occlusion of Right Cephalic Vein with Intraluminal Device, Percutaneous Approach

05LD3ZZ Occlusion of Right Cephalic Vein, Percutaneous Approach

05LD4CZ Occlusion of Right Cephalic Vein with Extraluminal Device, Percutaneous Endoscopic Approach

05LD4DZ Occlusion of Right Cephalic Vein with Intraluminal Device, Percutaneous Endoscopic Approach

05LD4ZZ Occlusion of Right Cephalic Vein, Percutaneous Endoscopic Approach

05LF0CZ Occlusion of Left Cephalic Vein with Extraluminal Device, Open Approach

05LF0DZ Occlusion of Left Cephalic Vein with Intraluminal Device, Open Approach

05LF0ZZ Occlusion of Left Cephalic Vein, Open Approach

05LF3CZ Occlusion of Left Cephalic Vein with Extraluminal Device, Percutaneous Approach

05LF3DZ Occlusion of Left Cephalic Vein with Intraluminal Device, Percutaneous Approach

05LF3ZZ Occlusion of Left Cephalic Vein, Percutaneous Approach

05LF4CZ Occlusion of Left Cephalic Vein with Extraluminal Device, Percutaneous Endoscopic Approach

05LF4DZ Occlusion of Left Cephalic Vein with Intraluminal Device, Percutaneous Endoscopic Approach

05LF4ZZ Occlusion of Left Cephalic Vein, Percutaneous Endoscopic Approach

05LG0CZ Occlusion of Right Hand Vein with Extraluminal Device, Open Approach

05LG0DZ Occlusion of Right Hand Vein with Intraluminal Device, Open Approach

05LG0ZZ Occlusion of Right Hand Vein, Open Approach

05LG3CZ Occlusion of Right Hand Vein with Extraluminal Device, Percutaneous Approach

05LG3DZ Occlusion of Right Hand Vein with Intraluminal Device, Percutaneous Approach

05LG3ZZ Occlusion of Right Hand Vein, Percutaneous Approach

05LG4CZ Occlusion of Right Hand Vein with Extraluminal Device, Percutaneous Endoscopic Approach

05LG4DZ Occlusion of Right Hand Vein with Intraluminal Device, Percutaneous Endoscopic Approach

05LG4ZZ Occlusion of Right Hand Vein, Percutaneous Endoscopic Approach

05LH0CZ Occlusion of Left Hand Vein with Extraluminal Device, Open Approach

05LH0DZ Occlusion of Left Hand Vein with Intraluminal Device, Open Approach

05LH0ZZ Occlusion of Left Hand Vein, Open Approach

05LH3CZ Occlusion of Left Hand Vein with Extraluminal Device, Percutaneous Approach

05LH3DZ Occlusion of Left Hand Vein with Intraluminal Device, Percutaneous Approach

05LH3ZZ Occlusion of Left Hand Vein, Percutaneous Approach

05LH4CZ Occlusion of Left Hand Vein with Extraluminal Device, Percutaneous Endoscopic Approach

05LH4DZ Occlusion of Left Hand Vein with Intraluminal Device, Percutaneous Endoscopic Approach

05LH4ZZ Occlusion of Left Hand Vein, Percutaneous Endoscopic Approach

05LL0CZ Occlusion of Intracranial Vein with Extraluminal Device, Open Approach

05LL0DZ Occlusion of Intracranial Vein with Intraluminal Device, Open Approach

05LL0ZZ Occlusion of Intracranial Vein, Open Approach

05LL3CZ Occlusion of Intracranial Vein with Extraluminal Device, Percutaneous Approach

05LL3DZ Occlusion of Intracranial Vein with Intraluminal Device, Percutaneous Approach

05LL3ZZ Occlusion of Intracranial Vein, Percutaneous Approach

05LL4CZ Occlusion of Intracranial Vein with Extraluminal Device, Percutaneous Endoscopic Approach

05LL4DZ Occlusion of Intracranial Vein with Intraluminal Device, Percutaneous Endoscopic Approach

05LL4ZZ Occlusion of Intracranial Vein, Percutaneous Endoscopic Approach

05LM0CZ Occlusion of Right Internal Jugular Vein with Extraluminal Device, Open Approach

05LM0DZ Occlusion of Right Internal Jugular Vein with Intraluminal Device, Open Approach

05LM0ZZ Occlusion of Right Internal Jugular Vein, Open Approach

05LM3CZ Occlusion of Right Internal Jugular Vein with Extraluminal Device, Percutaneous Approach

05LM3DZ Occlusion of Right Internal Jugular Vein with Intraluminal Device, Percutaneous Approach

05LM3ZZ Occlusion of Right Internal Jugular Vein, Percutaneous Approach

05LM4CZ Occlusion of Right Internal Jugular Vein with Extraluminal Device, Percutaneous Endoscopic Approach

05LM4DZ Occlusion of Right Internal Jugular Vein with Intraluminal Device, Percutaneous Endoscopic Approach

05LM4ZZ Occlusion of Right Internal Jugular Vein, Percutaneous Endoscopic Approach

05LN0CZ Occlusion of Left Internal Jugular Vein with Extraluminal Device, Open Approach

05LN0DZ Occlusion of Left Internal Jugular Vein with Intraluminal Device, Open Approach

05LN0ZZ Occlusion of Left Internal Jugular Vein, Open Approach

05LN3CZ Occlusion of Left Internal Jugular Vein with Extraluminal Device, Percutaneous Approach

05LN3DZ Occlusion of Left Internal Jugular Vein with Intraluminal Device, Percutaneous Approach

05LN3ZZ Occlusion of Left Internal Jugular Vein, Percutaneous Approach

♀ Female-only   ♂ Male-only   ▲ Limited Coverage   ● Non-OR   HAC HAC-associated procedure   ▲ Non-covered procedures   ✚ Cluster

05LN4CZ	Occlusion of Left Internal Jugular Vein with Extraluminal Device, Percutaneous Endoscopic Approach
05LN4DZ	Occlusion of Left Internal Jugular Vein with Intraluminal Device, Percutaneous Endoscopic Approach
05LN4ZZ	Occlusion of Left Internal Jugular Vein, Percutaneous Endoscopic Approach
05LP0CZ	Occlusion of Right External Jugular Vein with Extraluminal Device, Open Approach
05LP0DZ	Occlusion of Right External Jugular Vein with Intraluminal Device, Open Approach
05LP0ZZ	Occlusion of Right External Jugular Vein, Open Approach
05LP3CZ	Occlusion of Right External Jugular Vein with Extraluminal Device, Percutaneous Approach
05LP3DZ	Occlusion of Right External Jugular Vein with Intraluminal Device, Percutaneous Approach
05LP3ZZ	Occlusion of Right External Jugular Vein, Percutaneous Approach
05LP4CZ	Occlusion of Right External Jugular Vein with Extraluminal Device, Percutaneous Endoscopic Approach
05LP4DZ	Occlusion of Right External Jugular Vein with Intraluminal Device, Percutaneous Endoscopic Approach
05LP4ZZ	Occlusion of Right External Jugular Vein, Percutaneous Endoscopic Approach
05LQ0CZ	Occlusion of Left External Jugular Vein with Extraluminal Device, Open Approach
05LQ0DZ	Occlusion of Left External Jugular Vein with Intraluminal Device, Open Approach
05LQ0ZZ	Occlusion of Left External Jugular Vein, Open Approach
05LQ3CZ	Occlusion of Left External Jugular Vein with Extraluminal Device, Percutaneous Approach
05LQ3DZ	Occlusion of Left External Jugular Vein with Intraluminal Device, Percutaneous Approach
05LQ3ZZ	Occlusion of Left External Jugular Vein, Percutaneous Approach
05LQ4CZ	Occlusion of Left External Jugular Vein with Extraluminal Device, Percutaneous Endoscopic Approach
05LQ4DZ	Occlusion of Left External Jugular Vein with Intraluminal Device, Percutaneous Endoscopic Approach
05LQ4ZZ	Occlusion of Left External Jugular Vein, Percutaneous Endoscopic Approach
05LR0CZ	Occlusion of Right Vertebral Vein with Extraluminal Device, Open Approach
05LR0DZ	Occlusion of Right Vertebral Vein with Intraluminal Device, Open Approach
05LR0ZZ	Occlusion of Right Vertebral Vein, Open Approach
05LR3CZ	Occlusion of Right Vertebral Vein with Extraluminal Device, Percutaneous Approach
05LR3DZ	Occlusion of Right Vertebral Vein with Intraluminal Device, Percutaneous Approach
05LR3ZZ	Occlusion of Right Vertebral Vein, Percutaneous Approach
05LR4CZ	Occlusion of Right Vertebral Vein with Extraluminal Device, Percutaneous Endoscopic Approach
05LR4DZ	Occlusion of Right Vertebral Vein with Intraluminal Device, Percutaneous Endoscopic Approach
05LR4ZZ	Occlusion of Right Vertebral Vein, Percutaneous Endoscopic Approach
05LS0CZ	Occlusion of Left Vertebral Vein with Extraluminal Device, Open Approach
05LS0DZ	Occlusion of Left Vertebral Vein with Intraluminal Device, Open Approach
05LS0ZZ	Occlusion of Left Vertebral Vein, Open Approach
05LS3CZ	Occlusion of Left Vertebral Vein with Extraluminal Device, Percutaneous Approach
05LS3DZ	Occlusion of Left Vertebral Vein with Intraluminal Device, Percutaneous Approach
05LS3ZZ	Occlusion of Left Vertebral Vein, Percutaneous Approach
05LS4CZ	Occlusion of Left Vertebral Vein with Extraluminal Device, Percutaneous Endoscopic Approach
05LS4DZ	Occlusion of Left Vertebral Vein with Intraluminal Device, Percutaneous Endoscopic Approach
05LS4ZZ	Occlusion of Left Vertebral Vein, Percutaneous Endoscopic Approach
05LT0CZ	Occlusion of Right Face Vein with Extraluminal Device, Open Approach
05LT0DZ	Occlusion of Right Face Vein with Intraluminal Device, Open Approach
05LT0ZZ	Occlusion of Right Face Vein, Open Approach
05LT3CZ	Occlusion of Right Face Vein with Extraluminal Device, Percutaneous Approach
05LT3DZ	Occlusion of Right Face Vein with Intraluminal Device, Percutaneous Approach
05LT3ZZ	Occlusion of Right Face Vein, Percutaneous Approach
05LT4CZ	Occlusion of Right Face Vein with Extraluminal Device, Percutaneous Endoscopic Approach
05LT4DZ	Occlusion of Right Face Vein with Intraluminal Device, Percutaneous Endoscopic Approach
05LT4ZZ	Occlusion of Right Face Vein, Percutaneous Endoscopic Approach
05LV0CZ	Occlusion of Left Face Vein with Extraluminal Device, Open Approach
05LV0DZ	Occlusion of Left Face Vein with Intraluminal Device, Open Approach
05LV0ZZ	Occlusion of Left Face Vein, Open Approach
05LV3CZ	Occlusion of Left Face Vein with Extraluminal Device, Percutaneous Approach
05LV3DZ	Occlusion of Left Face Vein with Intraluminal Device, Percutaneous Approach
05LV3ZZ	Occlusion of Left Face Vein, Percutaneous Approach
05LV4CZ	Occlusion of Left Face Vein with Extraluminal Device, Percutaneous Endoscopic Approach
05LV4DZ	Occlusion of Left Face Vein with Intraluminal Device, Percutaneous Endoscopic Approach
05LV4ZZ	Occlusion of Left Face Vein, Percutaneous Endoscopic Approach
05LY0CZ	Occlusion of Upper Vein with Extraluminal Device, Open Approach
05LY0DZ	Occlusion of Upper Vein with Intraluminal Device, Open Approach
05LY0ZZ	Occlusion of Upper Vein, Open Approach
05LY3CZ	Occlusion of Upper Vein with Extraluminal Device, Percutaneous Approach
05LY3DZ	Occlusion of Upper Vein with Intraluminal Device, Percutaneous Approach
05LY3ZZ	Occlusion of Upper Vein, Percutaneous Approach
05LY4CZ	Occlusion of Upper Vein with Extraluminal Device, Percutaneous Endoscopic Approach
05LY4DZ	Occlusion of Upper Vein with Intraluminal Device, Percutaneous Endoscopic Approach
05LY4ZZ	Occlusion of Upper Vein, Percutaneous Endoscopic Approach

05N – Upper Veins, Release

Review Coding Guidelines B3.13 and B3.14

05N00ZZ	Release Azygos Vein, Open Approach
05N03ZZ	Release Azygos Vein, Percutaneous Approach
05N04ZZ	Release Azygos Vein, Percutaneous Endoscopic Approach
05N10ZZ	Release Hemiazygos Vein, Open Approach
05N13ZZ	Release Hemiazygos Vein, Percutaneous Approach
05N14ZZ	Release Hemiazygos Vein, Percutaneous Endoscopic Approach
05N30ZZ	Release Right Innominate Vein, Open Approach
05N33ZZ	Release Right Innominate Vein, Percutaneous Approach
05N34ZZ	Release Right Innominate Vein, Percutaneous Endoscopic Approach
05N40ZZ	Release Left Innominate Vein, Open Approach
05N43ZZ	Release Left Innominate Vein, Percutaneous Approach
05N44ZZ	Release Left Innominate Vein, Percutaneous Endoscopic Approach
05N50ZZ	Release Right Subclavian Vein, Open Approach
05N53ZZ	Release Right Subclavian Vein, Percutaneous Approach
05N54ZZ	Release Right Subclavian Vein, Percutaneous Endoscopic Approach
05N60ZZ	Release Left Subclavian Vein, Open Approach
05N63ZZ	Release Left Subclavian Vein, Percutaneous Approach
05N64ZZ	Release Left Subclavian Vein, Percutaneous Endoscopic Approach
05N70ZZ	Release Right Axillary Vein, Open Approach
05N73ZZ	Release Right Axillary Vein, Percutaneous Approach
05N74ZZ	Release Right Axillary Vein, Percutaneous Endoscopic Approach
05N80ZZ	Release Left Axillary Vein, Open Approach

05N83ZZ	Release Left Axillary Vein, Percutaneous Approach
05N84ZZ	Release Left Axillary Vein, Percutaneous Endoscopic Approach
05N90ZZ	Release Right Brachial Vein, Open Approach
05N93ZZ	Release Right Brachial Vein, Percutaneous Approach
05N94ZZ	Release Right Brachial Vein, Percutaneous Endoscopic Approach
05NA0ZZ	Release Left Brachial Vein, Open Approach
05NA3ZZ	Release Left Brachial Vein, Percutaneous Approach
05NA4ZZ	Release Left Brachial Vein, Percutaneous Endoscopic Approach
05NB0ZZ	Release Right Basilic Vein, Open Approach
05NB3ZZ	Release Right Basilic Vein, Percutaneous Approach
05NB4ZZ	Release Right Basilic Vein, Percutaneous Endoscopic Approach
05NC0ZZ	Release Left Basilic Vein, Open Approach
05NC3ZZ	Release Left Basilic Vein, Percutaneous Approach
05NC4ZZ	Release Left Basilic Vein, Percutaneous Endoscopic Approach
05ND0ZZ	Release Right Cephalic Vein, Open Approach
05ND3ZZ	Release Right Cephalic Vein, Percutaneous Approach
05ND4ZZ	Release Right Cephalic Vein, Percutaneous Endoscopic Approach
05NF0ZZ	Release Left Cephalic Vein, Open Approach
05NF3ZZ	Release Left Cephalic Vein, Percutaneous Approach

05NF4ZZ	Release Left Cephalic Vein, Percutaneous Endoscopic Approach
05NG0ZZ	Release Right Hand Vein, Open Approach
05NG3ZZ	Release Right Hand Vein, Percutaneous Approach
05NG4ZZ	Release Right Hand Vein, Percutaneous Endoscopic Approach
05NH0ZZ	Release Left Hand Vein, Open Approach
05NH3ZZ	Release Left Hand Vein, Percutaneous Approach
05NH4ZZ	Release Left Hand Vein, Percutaneous Endoscopic Approach
05NL0ZZ	Release Intracranial Vein, Open Approach
05NL3ZZ	Release Intracranial Vein, Percutaneous Approach
05NL4ZZ	Release Intracranial Vein, Percutaneous Endoscopic Approach
05NM0ZZ	Release Right Internal Jugular Vein, Open Approach
05NM3ZZ	Release Right Internal Jugular Vein, Percutaneous Approach
05NM4ZZ	Release Right Internal Jugular Vein, Percutaneous Endoscopic Approach
05NN0ZZ	Release Left Internal Jugular Vein, Open Approach
05NN3ZZ	Release Left Internal Jugular Vein, Percutaneous Approach
05NN4ZZ	Release Left Internal Jugular Vein, Percutaneous Endoscopic Approach
05NP0ZZ	Release Right External Jugular Vein, Open Approach
05NP3ZZ	Release Right External Jugular Vein, Percutaneous Approach
05NP4ZZ	Release Right External Jugular Vein, Percutaneous Endoscopic Approach

05NQ0ZZ	Release Left External Jugular Vein, Open Approach
05NQ3ZZ	Release Left External Jugular Vein, Percutaneous Approach
05NQ4ZZ	Release Left External Jugular Vein, Percutaneous Endoscopic Approach
05NR0ZZ	Release Right Vertebral Vein, Open Approach
05NR3ZZ	Release Right Vertebral Vein, Percutaneous Approach
05NR4ZZ	Release Right Vertebral Vein, Percutaneous Endoscopic Approach
05NS0ZZ	Release Left Vertebral Vein, Open Approach
05NS3ZZ	Release Left Vertebral Vein, Percutaneous Approach
05NS4ZZ	Release Left Vertebral Vein, Percutaneous Endoscopic Approach
05NT0ZZ	Release Right Face Vein, Open Approach
05NT3ZZ	Release Right Face Vein, Percutaneous Approach
05NT4ZZ	Release Right Face Vein, Percutaneous Endoscopic Approach
05NV0ZZ	Release Left Face Vein, Open Approach
05NV3ZZ	Release Left Face Vein, Percutaneous Approach
05NV4ZZ	Release Left Face Vein, Percutaneous Endoscopic Approach
05NY0ZZ	Release Upper Vein, Open Approach
05NY3ZZ	Release Upper Vein, Percutaneous Approach
05NY4ZZ	Release Upper Vein, Percutaneous Endoscopic Approach

05P – Upper Veins, Removal

Review Coding Guideline B6.1c

05P002Z	Removal of Monitoring Device from Azygos Vein, Open Approach
05P00MZ	Removal of Neurostimulator Lead from Azygos Vein, Open Approach
05P032Z	Removal of Monitoring Device from Azygos Vein, Percutaneous Approach
05P03MZ	Removal of Neurostimulator Lead from Azygos Vein, Percutaneous Approach
05P042Z	Removal of Monitoring Device from Azygos Vein, Percutaneous Endoscopic Approach
05P04MZ	Removal of Neurostimulator Lead from Azygos Vein, Percutaneous Endoscopic Approach
05P0X2Z	Removal of Monitoring Device from Azygos Vein, External Approach
05P0XMZ	Removal of Neurostimulator Lead from Azygos Vein, External Approach
05P30MZ	Removal of Neurostimulator Lead from Right Innominate Vein, Open Approach
05P33MZ	Removal of Neurostimulator Lead from Right Innominate Vein, Percutaneous Approach
05P34MZ	Removal of Neurostimulator Lead from Right Innominate Vein, Percutaneous Endoscopic Approach
05P3XMZ	Removal of Neurostimulator Lead from Right Innominate Vein, External Approach
05P40MZ	Removal of Neurostimulator Lead from Left Innominate Vein, Open Approach

05P43MZ	Removal of Neurostimulator Lead from Left Innominate Vein, Percutaneous Approach
05P44MZ	Removal of Neurostimulator Lead from Left Innominate Vein, Percutaneous Endoscopic Approach
05P4XMZ	Removal of Neurostimulator Lead from Left Innominate Vein, External Approach
05PY00Z	Removal of Drainage Device from Upper Vein, Open Approach
05PY02Z	Removal of Monitoring Device from Upper Vein, Open Approach
05PY03Z	Removal of Infusion Device from Upper Vein, Open Approach
05PY07Z	Removal of Autologous Tissue Substitute from Upper Vein, Open Approach
05PY0CZ	Removal of Extraluminal Device from Upper Vein, Open Approach
05PY0DZ	Removal of Intraluminal Device from Upper Vein, Open Approach
05PY0JZ	Removal of Synthetic Substitute from Upper Vein, Open Approach
05PY0KZ	Removal of Nonautologous Tissue Substitute from Upper Vein, Open Approach
05PY0YZ	Removal of Other Device into Upper Vein, Open Approach
05PY30Z	Removal of Drainage Device from Upper Vein, Percutaneous Approach
05PY32Z	Removal of Monitoring Device from Upper Vein, Percutaneous Approach

05PY33Z	Removal of Infusion Device from Upper Vein, Percutaneous Approach
05PY37Z	Removal of Autologous Tissue Substitute from Upper Vein, Percutaneous Approach
05PY3CZ	Removal of Extraluminal Device from Upper Vein, Percutaneous Approach
05PY3DZ	Removal of Intraluminal Device from Upper Vein, Percutaneous Approach
05PY3JZ	Removal of Synthetic Substitute from Upper Vein, Percutaneous Approach
05PY3KZ	Removal of Nonautologous Tissue Substitute from Upper Vein, Percutaneous Approach
05PY3YZ	Removal of Other Device into Upper Vein, Percutaneous Approach
05PY40Z	Removal of Drainage Device from Upper Vein, Percutaneous Endoscopic Approach
05PY42Z	Removal of Monitoring Device from Upper Vein, Percutaneous Endoscopic Approach
05PY43Z	Removal of Infusion Device from Upper Vein, Percutaneous Endoscopic Approach
05PY47Z	Removal of Autologous Tissue Substitute from Upper Vein, Percutaneous Endoscopic Approach

♀ Female-only   ♂ Male-only   ▲ Limited Coverage   ● Non-OR   HAC HAC-associated procedure   ▲ Non-covered procedures   ✚ Cluster

05PY4CZ	Removal of Extraluminal Device from Upper Vein, Percutaneous Endoscopic Approach
05PY4DZ	Removal of Intraluminal Device from Upper Vein, Percutaneous Endoscopic Approach
05PY4JZ	Removal of Synthetic Substitute from Upper Vein, Percutaneous Endoscopic Approach
05PY4KZ	Removal of Nonautologous Tissue Substitute from Upper Vein, Percutaneous Endoscopic Approach
05PY4YZ	Removal of Other Device into Upper Vein, Percutaneous Endoscopic Approach
05PYX0Z	Removal of Drainage Device from Upper Vein, External Approach
05PYX2Z	Removal of Monitoring Device from Upper Vein, External Approach
05PYX3Z	Removal of Infusion Device from Upper Vein, External Approach
05PYXDZ	Removal of Intraluminal Device from Upper Vein, External Approach

05Q – Upper Veins, Repair

05Q00ZZ	Repair Azygos Vein, Open Approach
05Q03ZZ	Repair Azygos Vein, Percutaneous Approach
05Q04ZZ	Repair Azygos Vein, Percutaneous Endoscopic Approach
05Q10ZZ	Repair Hemiazygos Vein, Open Approach
05Q13ZZ	Repair Hemiazygos Vein, Percutaneous Approach
05Q14ZZ	Repair Hemiazygos Vein, Percutaneous Endoscopic Approach
05Q30ZZ	Repair Right Innominate Vein, Open Approach
05Q33ZZ	Repair Right Innominate Vein, Percutaneous Approach
05Q34ZZ	Repair Right Innominate Vein, Percutaneous Endoscopic Approach
05Q40ZZ	Repair Left Innominate Vein, Open Approach
	AHA CC: 3Q, 2017, 15-16
05Q43ZZ	Repair Left Innominate Vein, Percutaneous Approach
05Q44ZZ	Repair Left Innominate Vein, Percutaneous Endoscopic Approach
05Q50ZZ	Repair Right Subclavian Vein, Open Approach
05Q53ZZ	Repair Right Subclavian Vein, Percutaneous Approach
05Q54ZZ	Repair Right Subclavian Vein, Percutaneous Endoscopic Approach
05Q60ZZ	Repair Left Subclavian Vein, Open Approach
05Q63ZZ	Repair Left Subclavian Vein, Percutaneous Approach
05Q64ZZ	Repair Left Subclavian Vein, Percutaneous Endoscopic Approach
05Q70ZZ	Repair Right Axillary Vein, Open Approach
05Q73ZZ	Repair Right Axillary Vein, Percutaneous Approach
05Q74ZZ	Repair Right Axillary Vein, Percutaneous Endoscopic Approach
05Q80ZZ	Repair Left Axillary Vein, Open Approach
05Q83ZZ	Repair Left Axillary Vein, Percutaneous Approach
05Q84ZZ	Repair Left Axillary Vein, Percutaneous Endoscopic Approach
05Q90ZZ	Repair Right Brachial Vein, Open Approach
05Q93ZZ	Repair Right Brachial Vein, Percutaneous Approach

05Q94ZZ	Repair Right Brachial Vein, Percutaneous Endoscopic Approach
05QA0ZZ	Repair Left Brachial Vein, Open Approach
05QA3ZZ	Repair Left Brachial Vein, Percutaneous Approach
05QA4ZZ	Repair Left Brachial Vein, Percutaneous Endoscopic Approach
05QB0ZZ	Repair Right Basilic Vein, Open Approach
05QB3ZZ	Repair Right Basilic Vein, Percutaneous Approach
05QB4ZZ	Repair Right Basilic Vein, Percutaneous Endoscopic Approach
05QC0ZZ	Repair Left Basilic Vein, Open Approach
05QC3ZZ	Repair Left Basilic Vein, Percutaneous Approach
05QC4ZZ	Repair Left Basilic Vein, Percutaneous Endoscopic Approach
05QD0ZZ	Repair Right Cephalic Vein, Open Approach
05QD3ZZ	Repair Right Cephalic Vein, Percutaneous Approach
05QD4ZZ	Repair Right Cephalic Vein, Percutaneous Endoscopic Approach
05QF0ZZ	Repair Left Cephalic Vein, Open Approach
05QF3ZZ	Repair Left Cephalic Vein, Percutaneous Approach
05QF4ZZ	Repair Left Cephalic Vein, Percutaneous Endoscopic Approach
05QG0ZZ	Repair Right Hand Vein, Open Approach
05QG3ZZ	Repair Right Hand Vein, Percutaneous Approach
05QG4ZZ	Repair Right Hand Vein, Percutaneous Endoscopic Approach
05QH0ZZ	Repair Left Hand Vein, Open Approach
05QH3ZZ	Repair Left Hand Vein, Percutaneous Approach
05QH4ZZ	Repair Left Hand Vein, Percutaneous Endoscopic Approach
05QL0ZZ	Repair Intracranial Vein, Open Approach
05QL3ZZ	Repair Intracranial Vein, Percutaneous Approach
05QL4ZZ	Repair Intracranial Vein, Percutaneous Endoscopic Approach
05QM0ZZ	Repair Right Internal Jugular Vein, Open Approach

05QM3ZZ	Repair Right Internal Jugular Vein, Percutaneous Approach
05QM4ZZ	Repair Right Internal Jugular Vein, Percutaneous Endoscopic Approach
05QN0ZZ	Repair Left Internal Jugular Vein, Open Approach
05QN3ZZ	Repair Left Internal Jugular Vein, Percutaneous Approach
05QN4ZZ	Repair Left Internal Jugular Vein, Percutaneous Endoscopic Approach
05QP0ZZ	Repair Right External Jugular Vein, Open Approach
05QP3ZZ	Repair Right External Jugular Vein, Percutaneous Approach
05QP4ZZ	Repair Right External Jugular Vein, Percutaneous Endoscopic Approach
05QQ0ZZ	Repair Left External Jugular Vein, Open Approach
05QQ3ZZ	Repair Left External Jugular Vein, Percutaneous Approach
05QQ4ZZ	Repair Left External Jugular Vein, Percutaneous Endoscopic Approach
05QR0ZZ	Repair Right Vertebral Vein, Open Approach
05QR3ZZ	Repair Right Vertebral Vein, Percutaneous Approach
05QR4ZZ	Repair Right Vertebral Vein, Percutaneous Endoscopic Approach
05QS0ZZ	Repair Left Vertebral Vein, Open Approach
05QS3ZZ	Repair Left Vertebral Vein, Percutaneous Approach
05QS4ZZ	Repair Left Vertebral Vein, Percutaneous Endoscopic Approach
05QT0ZZ	Repair Right Face Vein, Open Approach
05QT3ZZ	Repair Right Face Vein, Percutaneous Approach
05QT4ZZ	Repair Right Face Vein, Percutaneous Endoscopic Approach
05QV0ZZ	Repair Left Face Vein, Open Approach
05QV3ZZ	Repair Left Face Vein, Percutaneous Approach
05QV4ZZ	Repair Left Face Vein, Percutaneous Endoscopic Approach
05QY0ZZ	Repair Upper Vein, Open Approach
05QY3ZZ	Repair Upper Vein, Percutaneous Approach
05QY4ZZ	Repair Upper Vein, Percutaneous Endoscopic Approach

05R – Upper Veins, Replacement

Review Coding Guideline B3.18

05R007Z	Replacement of Azygos Vein with Autologous Tissue Substitute, Open Approach
05R00JZ	Replacement of Azygos Vein with Synthetic Substitute, Open Approach
05R00KZ	Replacement of Azygos Vein with Nonautologous Tissue Substitute, Open Approach
05R047Z	Replacement of Azygos Vein with Autologous Tissue Substitute, Percutaneous Endoscopic Approach
05R04JZ	Replacement of Azygos Vein with Synthetic Substitute, Percutaneous Endoscopic Approach
05R04KZ	Replacement of Azygos Vein with Nonautologous Tissue Substitute, Percutaneous Endoscopic Approach

05R107Z Replacement of Hemiazygos Vein with Autologous Tissue Substitute, Open Approach

05R10JZ Replacement of Hemiazygos Vein with Synthetic Substitute, Open Approach

05R10KZ Replacement of Hemiazygos Vein with Nonautologous Tissue Substitute, Open Approach

05R147Z Replacement of Hemiazygos Vein with Autologous Tissue Substitute, Percutaneous Endoscopic Approach

05R14JZ Replacement of Hemiazygos Vein with Synthetic Substitute, Percutaneous Endoscopic Approach

05R14KZ Replacement of Hemiazygos Vein with Nonautologous Tissue Substitute, Percutaneous Endoscopic Approach

05R307Z Replacement of Right Innominate Vein with Autologous Tissue Substitute, Open Approach

05R30JZ Replacement of Right Innominate Vein with Synthetic Substitute, Open Approach

05R30KZ Replacement of Right Innominate Vein with Nonautologous Tissue Substitute, Open Approach

05R347Z Replacement of Right Innominate Vein with Autologous Tissue Substitute, Percutaneous Endoscopic Approach

05R34JZ Replacement of Right Innominate Vein with Synthetic Substitute, Percutaneous Endoscopic Approach

05R34KZ Replacement of Right Innominate Vein with Nonautologous Tissue Substitute, Percutaneous Endoscopic Approach

05R407Z Replacement of Left Innominate Vein with Autologous Tissue Substitute, Open Approach

05R40JZ Replacement of Left Innominate Vein with Synthetic Substitute, Open Approach

05R40KZ Replacement of Left Innominate Vein with Nonautologous Tissue Substitute, Open Approach

05R447Z Replacement of Left Innominate Vein with Autologous Tissue Substitute, Percutaneous Endoscopic Approach

05R44JZ Replacement of Left Innominate Vein with Synthetic Substitute, Percutaneous Endoscopic Approach

05R44KZ Replacement of Left Innominate Vein with Nonautologous Tissue Substitute, Percutaneous Endoscopic Approach

05R507Z Replacement of Right Subclavian Vein with Autologous Tissue Substitute, Open Approach

05R50JZ Replacement of Right Subclavian Vein with Synthetic Substitute, Open Approach

05R50KZ Replacement of Right Subclavian Vein with Nonautologous Tissue Substitute, Open Approach

05R547Z Replacement of Right Subclavian Vein with Autologous Tissue Substitute, Percutaneous Endoscopic Approach

05R54JZ Replacement of Right Subclavian Vein with Synthetic Substitute, Percutaneous Endoscopic Approach

05R54KZ Replacement of Right Subclavian Vein with Nonautologous Tissue Substitute, Percutaneous Endoscopic Approach

05R607Z Replacement of Left Subclavian Vein with Autologous Tissue Substitute, Open Approach

05R60JZ Replacement of Left Subclavian Vein with Synthetic Substitute, Open Approach

05R60KZ Replacement of Left Subclavian Vein with Nonautologous Tissue Substitute, Open Approach

05R647Z Replacement of Left Subclavian Vein with Autologous Tissue Substitute, Percutaneous Endoscopic Approach

05R64JZ Replacement of Left Subclavian Vein with Synthetic Substitute, Percutaneous Endoscopic Approach

05R64KZ Replacement of Left Subclavian Vein with Nonautologous Tissue Substitute, Percutaneous Endoscopic Approach

05R707Z Replacement of Right Axillary Vein with Autologous Tissue Substitute, Open Approach

05R70JZ Replacement of Right Axillary Vein with Synthetic Substitute, Open Approach

05R70KZ Replacement of Right Axillary Vein with Nonautologous Tissue Substitute, Open Approach

05R747Z Replacement of Right Axillary Vein with Autologous Tissue Substitute, Percutaneous Endoscopic Approach

05R74JZ Replacement of Right Axillary Vein with Synthetic Substitute, Percutaneous Endoscopic Approach

05R74KZ Replacement of Right Axillary Vein with Nonautologous Tissue Substitute, Percutaneous Endoscopic Approach

05R807Z Replacement of Left Axillary Vein with Autologous Tissue Substitute, Open Approach

05R80JZ Replacement of Left Axillary Vein with Synthetic Substitute, Open Approach

05R80KZ Replacement of Left Axillary Vein with Nonautologous Tissue Substitute, Open Approach

05R847Z Replacement of Left Axillary Vein with Autologous Tissue Substitute, Percutaneous Endoscopic Approach

05R84JZ Replacement of Left Axillary Vein with Synthetic Substitute, Percutaneous Endoscopic Approach

05R84KZ Replacement of Left Axillary Vein with Nonautologous Tissue Substitute, Percutaneous Endoscopic Approach

05R907Z Replacement of Right Brachial Vein with Autologous Tissue Substitute, Open Approach

05R90JZ Replacement of Right Brachial Vein with Synthetic Substitute, Open Approach

05R90KZ Replacement of Right Brachial Vein with Nonautologous Tissue Substitute, Open Approach

05R947Z Replacement of Right Brachial Vein with Autologous Tissue Substitute, Percutaneous Endoscopic Approach

05R94JZ Replacement of Right Brachial Vein with Synthetic Substitute, Percutaneous Endoscopic Approach

05R94KZ Replacement of Right Brachial Vein with Nonautologous Tissue Substitute, Percutaneous Endoscopic Approach

05RA07Z Replacement of Left Brachial Vein with Autologous Tissue Substitute, Open Approach

05RA0JZ Replacement of Left Brachial Vein with Synthetic Substitute, Open Approach

05RA0KZ Replacement of Left Brachial Vein with Nonautologous Tissue Substitute, Open Approach

05RA47Z Replacement of Left Brachial Vein with Autologous Tissue Substitute, Percutaneous Endoscopic Approach

05RA4JZ Replacement of Left Brachial Vein with Synthetic Substitute, Percutaneous Endoscopic Approach

05RA4KZ Replacement of Left Brachial Vein with Nonautologous Tissue Substitute, Percutaneous Endoscopic Approach

05RB07Z Replacement of Right Basilic Vein with Autologous Tissue Substitute, Open Approach

05RB0JZ Replacement of Right Basilic Vein with Synthetic Substitute, Open Approach

05RB0KZ Replacement of Right Basilic Vein with Nonautologous Tissue Substitute, Open Approach

05RB47Z Replacement of Right Basilic Vein with Autologous Tissue Substitute, Percutaneous Endoscopic Approach

05RB4JZ Replacement of Right Basilic Vein with Synthetic Substitute, Percutaneous Endoscopic Approach

05RB4KZ Replacement of Right Basilic Vein with Nonautologous Tissue Substitute, Percutaneous Endoscopic Approach

05RC07Z Replacement of Left Basilic Vein with Autologous Tissue Substitute, Open Approach

05RC0JZ Replacement of Left Basilic Vein with Synthetic Substitute, Open Approach

05RC0KZ Replacement of Left Basilic Vein with Nonautologous Tissue Substitute, Open Approach

05RC47Z Replacement of Left Basilic Vein with Autologous Tissue Substitute, Percutaneous Endoscopic Approach

05RC4JZ Replacement of Left Basilic Vein with Synthetic Substitute, Percutaneous Endoscopic Approach

05RC4KZ Replacement of Left Basilic Vein with Nonautologous Tissue Substitute, Percutaneous Endoscopic Approach

05RD07Z Replacement of Right Cephalic Vein with Autologous Tissue Substitute, Open Approach

05RD0JZ Replacement of Right Cephalic Vein with Synthetic Substitute, Open Approach

05RD0KZ Replacement of Right Cephalic Vein with Nonautologous Tissue Substitute, Open Approach

05RD47Z Replacement of Right Cephalic Vein with Autologous Tissue Substitute, Percutaneous Endoscopic Approach

05RD4JZ Replacement of Right Cephalic Vein with Synthetic Substitute, Percutaneous Endoscopic Approach

05RD4KZ Replacement of Right Cephalic Vein with Nonautologous Tissue Substitute, Percutaneous Endoscopic Approach

05RF07Z Replacement of Left Cephalic Vein with Autologous Tissue Substitute, Open Approach

05RF0JZ Replacement of Left Cephalic Vein with Synthetic Substitute, Open Approach

05RF0KZ Replacement of Left Cephalic Vein with Nonautologous Tissue Substitute, Open Approach

05RF47Z Replacement of Left Cephalic Vein with Autologous Tissue Substitute, Percutaneous Endoscopic Approach

05RF4JZ Replacement of Left Cephalic Vein with Synthetic Substitute, Percutaneous Endoscopic Approach

♀ Female-only   ♂ Male-only   ▲ Limited Coverage   ● Non-OR   HAC HAC-associated procedure   ▲ Non-covered procedures   ✚ Cluster

05RF4KZ Replacement of Left Cephalic Vein with Nonautologous Tissue Substitute, Percutaneous Endoscopic Approach

05RG07Z Replacement of Right Hand Vein with Autologous Tissue Substitute, Open Approach

05RG0JZ Replacement of Right Hand Vein with Synthetic Substitute, Open Approach

05RG0KZ Replacement of Right Hand Vein with Nonautologous Tissue Substitute, Open Approach

05RG47Z Replacement of Right Hand Vein with Autologous Tissue Substitute, Percutaneous Endoscopic Approach

05RG4JZ Replacement of Right Hand Vein with Synthetic Substitute, Percutaneous Endoscopic Approach

05RG4KZ Replacement of Right Hand Vein with Nonautologous Tissue Substitute, Percutaneous Endoscopic Approach

05RH07Z Replacement of Left Hand Vein with Autologous Tissue Substitute, Open Approach

05RH0JZ Replacement of Left Hand Vein with Synthetic Substitute, Open Approach

05RH0KZ Replacement of Left Hand Vein with Nonautologous Tissue Substitute, Open Approach

05RH47Z Replacement of Left Hand Vein with Autologous Tissue Substitute, Percutaneous Endoscopic Approach

05RH4JZ Replacement of Left Hand Vein with Synthetic Substitute, Percutaneous Endoscopic Approach

05RH4KZ Replacement of Left Hand Vein with Nonautologous Tissue Substitute, Percutaneous Endoscopic Approach

05RL07Z Replacement of Intracranial Vein with Autologous Tissue Substitute, Open Approach

05RL0JZ Replacement of Intracranial Vein with Synthetic Substitute, Open Approach

05RL0KZ Replacement of Intracranial Vein with Nonautologous Tissue Substitute, Open Approach

05RL47Z Replacement of Intracranial Vein with Autologous Tissue Substitute, Percutaneous Endoscopic Approach

05RL4JZ Replacement of Intracranial Vein with Synthetic Substitute, Percutaneous Endoscopic Approach

05RL4KZ Replacement of Intracranial Vein with Nonautologous Tissue Substitute, Percutaneous Endoscopic Approach

05RM07Z Replacement of Right Internal Jugular Vein with Autologous Tissue Substitute, Open Approach

05RM0JZ Replacement of Right Internal Jugular Vein with Synthetic Substitute, Open Approach

05RM0KZ Replacement of Right Internal Jugular Vein with Nonautologous Tissue Substitute, Open Approach

05RM47Z Replacement of Right Internal Jugular Vein with Autologous Tissue Substitute, Percutaneous Endoscopic Approach

05RM4JZ Replacement of Right Internal Jugular Vein with Synthetic Substitute, Percutaneous Endoscopic Approach

05RM4KZ Replacement of Right Internal Jugular Vein with Nonautologous Tissue Substitute, Percutaneous Endoscopic Approach

05RN07Z Replacement of Left Internal Jugular Vein with Autologous Tissue Substitute, Open Approach

05RN0JZ Replacement of Left Internal Jugular Vein with Synthetic Substitute, Open Approach

05RN0KZ Replacement of Left Internal Jugular Vein with Nonautologous Tissue Substitute, Open Approach

05RN47Z Replacement of Left Internal Jugular Vein with Autologous Tissue Substitute, Percutaneous Endoscopic Approach

05RN4JZ Replacement of Left Internal Jugular Vein with Synthetic Substitute, Percutaneous Endoscopic Approach

05RN4KZ Replacement of Left Internal Jugular Vein with Nonautologous Tissue Substitute, Percutaneous Endoscopic Approach

05RP07Z Replacement of Right External Jugular Vein with Autologous Tissue Substitute, Open Approach

05RP0JZ Replacement of Right External Jugular Vein with Synthetic Substitute, Open Approach

05RP0KZ Replacement of Right External Jugular Vein with Nonautologous Tissue Substitute, Open Approach

05RP47Z Replacement of Right External Jugular Vein with Autologous Tissue Substitute, Percutaneous Endoscopic Approach

05RP4JZ Replacement of Right External Jugular Vein with Synthetic Substitute, Percutaneous Endoscopic Approach

05RP4KZ Replacement of Right External Jugular Vein with Nonautologous Tissue Substitute, Percutaneous Endoscopic Approach

05RQ07Z Replacement of Left External Jugular Vein with Autologous Tissue Substitute, Open Approach

05RQ0JZ Replacement of Left External Jugular Vein with Synthetic Substitute, Open Approach

05RQ0KZ Replacement of Left External Jugular Vein with Nonautologous Tissue Substitute, Open Approach

05RQ47Z Replacement of Left External Jugular Vein with Autologous Tissue Substitute, Percutaneous Endoscopic Approach

05RQ4JZ Replacement of Left External Jugular Vein with Synthetic Substitute, Percutaneous Endoscopic Approach

05RQ4KZ Replacement of Left External Jugular Vein with Nonautologous Tissue Substitute, Percutaneous Endoscopic Approach

05RR07Z Replacement of Right Vertebral Vein with Autologous Tissue Substitute, Open Approach

05RR0JZ Replacement of Right Vertebral Vein with Synthetic Substitute, Open Approach

05RR0KZ Replacement of Right Vertebral Vein with Nonautologous Tissue Substitute, Open Approach

05RR47Z Replacement of Right Vertebral Vein with Autologous Tissue Substitute, Percutaneous Endoscopic Approach

05RR4JZ Replacement of Right Vertebral Vein with Synthetic Substitute, Percutaneous Endoscopic Approach

05RR4KZ Replacement of Right Vertebral Vein with Nonautologous Tissue Substitute, Percutaneous Endoscopic Approach

05RS07Z Replacement of Left Vertebral Vein with Autologous Tissue Substitute, Open Approach

05RS0JZ Replacement of Left Vertebral Vein with Synthetic Substitute, Open Approach

05RS0KZ Replacement of Left Vertebral Vein with Nonautologous Tissue Substitute, Open Approach

05RS47Z Replacement of Left Vertebral Vein with Autologous Tissue Substitute, Percutaneous Endoscopic Approach

05RS4JZ Replacement of Left Vertebral Vein with Synthetic Substitute, Percutaneous Endoscopic Approach

05RS4KZ Replacement of Left Vertebral Vein with Nonautologous Tissue Substitute, Percutaneous Endoscopic Approach

05RT07Z Replacement of Right Face Vein with Autologous Tissue Substitute, Open Approach

05RT0JZ Replacement of Right Face Vein with Synthetic Substitute, Open Approach

05RT0KZ Replacement of Right Face Vein with Nonautologous Tissue Substitute, Open Approach

05RT47Z Replacement of Right Face Vein with Autologous Tissue Substitute, Percutaneous Endoscopic Approach

05RT4JZ Replacement of Right Face Vein with Synthetic Substitute, Percutaneous Endoscopic Approach

05RT4KZ Replacement of Right Face Vein with Nonautologous Tissue Substitute, Percutaneous Endoscopic Approach

05RV07Z Replacement of Left Face Vein with Autologous Tissue Substitute, Open Approach

05RV0JZ Replacement of Left Face Vein with Synthetic Substitute, Open Approach

05RV0KZ Replacement of Left Face Vein with Nonautologous Tissue Substitute, Open Approach

05RV47Z Replacement of Left Face Vein with Autologous Tissue Substitute, Percutaneous Endoscopic Approach

05RV4JZ Replacement of Left Face Vein with Synthetic Substitute, Percutaneous Endoscopic Approach

05RV4KZ Replacement of Left Face Vein with Nonautologous Tissue Substitute, Percutaneous Endoscopic Approach

05RY07Z Replacement of Upper Vein with Autologous Tissue Substitute, Open Approach

05RY0JZ Replacement of Upper Vein with Synthetic Substitute, Open Approach

05RY0KZ Replacement of Upper Vein with Nonautologous Tissue Substitute, Open Approach

05RY47Z Replacement of Upper Vein with Autologous Tissue Substitute, Percutaneous Endoscopic Approach

05RY4JZ Replacement of Upper Vein with Synthetic Substitute, Percutaneous Endoscopic Approach

05RY4KZ Replacement of Upper Vein with Nonautologous Tissue Substitute, Percutaneous Endoscopic Approach

♀ Female-only   ♂ Male-only   ▲ Limited Coverage   ● Non-OR   HAC HAC-associated procedure   ▲ Non-covered procedures   ✚ Cluster

05S – Upper Veins, Reposition

05S00ZZ Reposition Azygos Vein, Open Approach

05S03ZZ Reposition Azygos Vein, Percutaneous Approach

05S04ZZ Reposition Azygos Vein, Percutaneous Endoscopic Approach

05S10ZZ Reposition Hemiazygos Vein, Open Approach

05S13ZZ Reposition Hemiazygos Vein, Percutaneous Approach

05S14ZZ Reposition Hemiazygos Vein, Percutaneous Endoscopic Approach

05S30ZZ Reposition Right Innominate Vein, Open Approach

05S33ZZ Reposition Right Innominate Vein, Percutaneous Approach

05S34ZZ Reposition Right Innominate Vein, Percutaneous Endoscopic Approach

05S40ZZ Reposition Left Innominate Vein, Open Approach

05S43ZZ Reposition Left Innominate Vein, Percutaneous Approach

05S44ZZ Reposition Left Innominate Vein, Percutaneous Endoscopic Approach

05S50ZZ Reposition Right Subclavian Vein, Open Approach

05S53ZZ Reposition Right Subclavian Vein, Percutaneous Approach

05S54ZZ Reposition Right Subclavian Vein, Percutaneous Endoscopic Approach

05S60ZZ Reposition Left Subclavian Vein, Open Approach

05S63ZZ Reposition Left Subclavian Vein, Percutaneous Approach

05S64ZZ Reposition Left Subclavian Vein, Percutaneous Endoscopic Approach

05S70ZZ Reposition Right Axillary Vein, Open Approach

05S73ZZ Reposition Right Axillary Vein, Percutaneous Approach

05S74ZZ Reposition Right Axillary Vein, Percutaneous Endoscopic Approach

05S80ZZ Reposition Left Axillary Vein, Open Approach

05S83ZZ Reposition Left Axillary Vein, Percutaneous Approach

05S84ZZ Reposition Left Axillary Vein, Percutaneous Endoscopic Approach

05S90ZZ Reposition Right Brachial Vein, Open Approach

05S93ZZ Reposition Right Brachial Vein, Percutaneous Approach

05S94ZZ Reposition Right Brachial Vein, Percutaneous Endoscopic Approach

05SA0ZZ Reposition Left Brachial Vein, Open Approach

05SA3ZZ Reposition Left Brachial Vein, Percutaneous Approach

05SA4ZZ Reposition Left Brachial Vein, Percutaneous Endoscopic Approach

05SB0ZZ Reposition Right Basilic Vein, Open Approach

05SB3ZZ Reposition Right Basilic Vein, Percutaneous Approach

05SB4ZZ Reposition Right Basilic Vein, Percutaneous Endoscopic Approach

05SC0ZZ Reposition Left Basilic Vein, Open Approach

05SC3ZZ Reposition Left Basilic Vein, Percutaneous Approach

05SC4ZZ Reposition Left Basilic Vein, Percutaneous Endoscopic Approach

05SD0ZZ Reposition Right Cephalic Vein, Open Approach
AHA CC: 4Q, 2013, 125-126

05SD3ZZ Reposition Right Cephalic Vein, Percutaneous Approach

05SD4ZZ Reposition Right Cephalic Vein, Percutaneous Endoscopic Approach

05SF0ZZ Reposition Left Cephalic Vein, Open Approach

05SF3ZZ Reposition Left Cephalic Vein, Percutaneous Approach

05SF4ZZ Reposition Left Cephalic Vein, Percutaneous Endoscopic Approach

05SG0ZZ Reposition Right Hand Vein, Open Approach

05SG3ZZ Reposition Right Hand Vein, Percutaneous Approach

05SG4ZZ Reposition Right Hand Vein, Percutaneous Endoscopic Approach

05SH0ZZ Reposition Left Hand Vein, Open Approach

05SH3ZZ Reposition Left Hand Vein, Percutaneous Approach

05SH4ZZ Reposition Left Hand Vein, Percutaneous Endoscopic Approach

05SL0ZZ Reposition Intracranial Vein, Open Approach

05SL3ZZ Reposition Intracranial Vein, Percutaneous Approach

05SL4ZZ Reposition Intracranial Vein, Percutaneous Endoscopic Approach

05SM0ZZ Reposition Right Internal Jugular Vein, Open Approach

05SM3ZZ Reposition Right Internal Jugular Vein, Percutaneous Approach

05SM4ZZ Reposition Right Internal Jugular Vein, Percutaneous Endoscopic Approach

05SN0ZZ Reposition Left Internal Jugular Vein, Open Approach

05SN3ZZ Reposition Left Internal Jugular Vein, Percutaneous Approach

05SN4ZZ Reposition Left Internal Jugular Vein, Percutaneous Endoscopic Approach

05SP0ZZ Reposition Right External Jugular Vein, Open Approach

05SP3ZZ Reposition Right External Jugular Vein, Percutaneous Approach

05SP4ZZ Reposition Right External Jugular Vein, Percutaneous Endoscopic Approach

05SQ0ZZ Reposition Left External Jugular Vein, Open Approach

05SQ3ZZ Reposition Left External Jugular Vein, Percutaneous Approach

05SQ4ZZ Reposition Left External Jugular Vein, Percutaneous Endoscopic Approach

05SR0ZZ Reposition Right Vertebral Vein, Open Approach

05SR3ZZ Reposition Right Vertebral Vein, Percutaneous Approach

05SR4ZZ Reposition Right Vertebral Vein, Percutaneous Endoscopic Approach

05SS0ZZ Reposition Left Vertebral Vein, Open Approach

05SS3ZZ Reposition Left Vertebral Vein, Percutaneous Approach

05SS4ZZ Reposition Left Vertebral Vein, Percutaneous Endoscopic Approach

05ST0ZZ Reposition Right Face Vein, Open Approach

05ST3ZZ Reposition Right Face Vein, Percutaneous Approach

05ST4ZZ Reposition Right Face Vein, Percutaneous Endoscopic Approach

05SV0ZZ Reposition Left Face Vein, Open Approach

05SV3ZZ Reposition Left Face Vein, Percutaneous Approach

05SV4ZZ Reposition Left Face Vein, Percutaneous Endoscopic Approach

05SY0ZZ Reposition Upper Vein, Open Approach

05SY3ZZ Reposition Upper Vein, Percutaneous Approach

05SY4ZZ Reposition Upper Vein, Percutaneous Endoscopic Approach

05U – Upper Veins, Supplement

05U007Z Supplement Azygos Vein with Autologous Tissue Substitute, Open Approach

05U00JZ Supplement Azygos Vein with Synthetic Substitute, Open Approach

05U00KZ Supplement Azygos Vein with Nonautologous Tissue Substitute, Open Approach

05U037Z Supplement Azygos Vein with Autologous Tissue Substitute, Percutaneous Approach

05U03JZ Supplement Azygos Vein with Synthetic Substitute, Percutaneous Approach

05U03KZ Supplement Azygos Vein with Nonautologous Tissue Substitute, Percutaneous Approach

05U047Z Supplement Azygos Vein with Autologous Tissue Substitute, Percutaneous Endoscopic Approach

05U04JZ Supplement Azygos Vein with Synthetic Substitute, Percutaneous Endoscopic Approach

05U04KZ Supplement Azygos Vein with Nonautologous Tissue Substitute, Percutaneous Endoscopic Approach

05U107Z Supplement Hemiazygos Vein with Autologous Tissue Substitute, Open Approach

05U10JZ Supplement Hemiazygos Vein with Synthetic Substitute, Open Approach

05U10KZ Supplement Hemiazygos Vein with Nonautologous Tissue Substitute, Open Approach

05U137Z Supplement Hemiazygos Vein with Autologous Tissue Substitute, Percutaneous Approach

05U13JZ Supplement Hemiazygos Vein with Synthetic Substitute, Percutaneous Approach

05U13KZ Supplement Hemiazygos Vein with Nonautologous Tissue Substitute, Percutaneous Approach

05U147Z Supplement Hemiazygos Vein with Autologous Tissue Substitute, Percutaneous Endoscopic Approach

05U14JZ Supplement Hemiazygos Vein with Synthetic Substitute, Percutaneous Endoscopic Approach

05U14KZ Supplement Hemiazygos Vein with Nonautologous Tissue Substitute, Percutaneous Endoscopic Approach

♀ Female-only   ♂ Male-only   ▲ Limited Coverage   ● Non-OR   HAC HAC-associated procedure   ▲ Non-covered procedures   + Cluster

05U307Z	Supplement Right Innominate Vein with Autologous Tissue Substitute, Open Approach
05U30JZ	Supplement Right Innominate Vein with Synthetic Substitute, Open Approach
05U30KZ	Supplement Right Innominate Vein with Nonautologous Tissue Substitute, Open Approach
05U337Z	Supplement Right Innominate Vein with Autologous Tissue Substitute, Percutaneous Approach
05U33JZ	Supplement Right Innominate Vein with Synthetic Substitute, Percutaneous Approach
05U33KZ	Supplement Right Innominate Vein with Nonautologous Tissue Substitute, Percutaneous Approach
05U347Z	Supplement Right Innominate Vein with Autologous Tissue Substitute, Percutaneous Endoscopic Approach
05U34JZ	Supplement Right Innominate Vein with Synthetic Substitute, Percutaneous Endoscopic Approach
05U34KZ	Supplement Right Innominate Vein with Nonautologous Tissue Substitute, Percutaneous Endoscopic Approach
05U407Z	Supplement Left Innominate Vein with Autologous Tissue Substitute, Open Approach
05U40JZ	Supplement Left Innominate Vein with Synthetic Substitute, Open Approach
05U40KZ	Supplement Left Innominate Vein with Nonautologous Tissue Substitute, Open Approach
05U437Z	Supplement Left Innominate Vein with Autologous Tissue Substitute, Percutaneous Approach
05U43JZ	Supplement Left Innominate Vein with Synthetic Substitute, Percutaneous Approach
05U43KZ	Supplement Left Innominate Vein with Nonautologous Tissue Substitute, Percutaneous Approach
05U447Z	Supplement Left Innominate Vein with Autologous Tissue Substitute, Percutaneous Endoscopic Approach
05U44JZ	Supplement Left Innominate Vein with Synthetic Substitute, Percutaneous Endoscopic Approach
05U44KZ	Supplement Left Innominate Vein with Nonautologous Tissue Substitute, Percutaneous Endoscopic Approach
05U507Z	Supplement Right Subclavian Vein with Autologous Tissue Substitute, Open Approach
05U50JZ	Supplement Right Subclavian Vein with Synthetic Substitute, Open Approach
05U50KZ	Supplement Right Subclavian Vein with Nonautologous Tissue Substitute, Open Approach
05U537Z	Supplement Right Subclavian Vein with Autologous Tissue Substitute, Percutaneous Approach
05U53JZ	Supplement Right Subclavian Vein with Synthetic Substitute, Percutaneous Approach
05U53KZ	Supplement Right Subclavian Vein with Nonautologous Tissue Substitute, Percutaneous Approach
05U547Z	Supplement Right Subclavian Vein with Autologous Tissue Substitute, Percutaneous Endoscopic Approach
05U54JZ	Supplement Right Subclavian Vein with Synthetic Substitute, Percutaneous Endoscopic Approach
05U54KZ	Supplement Right Subclavian Vein with Nonautologous Tissue Substitute, Percutaneous Endoscopic Approach
05U607Z	Supplement Left Subclavian Vein with Autologous Tissue Substitute, Open Approach
05U60JZ	Supplement Left Subclavian Vein with Synthetic Substitute, Open Approach
05U60KZ	Supplement Left Subclavian Vein with Nonautologous Tissue Substitute, Open Approach
05U637Z	Supplement Left Subclavian Vein with Autologous Tissue Substitute, Percutaneous Approach
05U63JZ	Supplement Left Subclavian Vein with Synthetic Substitute, Percutaneous Approach
05U63KZ	Supplement Left Subclavian Vein with Nonautologous Tissue Substitute, Percutaneous Approach
05U647Z	Supplement Left Subclavian Vein with Autologous Tissue Substitute, Percutaneous Endoscopic Approach
05U64JZ	Supplement Left Subclavian Vein with Synthetic Substitute, Percutaneous Endoscopic Approach
05U64KZ	Supplement Left Subclavian Vein with Nonautologous Tissue Substitute, Percutaneous Endoscopic Approach
05U707Z	Supplement Right Axillary Vein with Autologous Tissue Substitute, Open Approach
05U70JZ	Supplement Right Axillary Vein with Synthetic Substitute, Open Approach
05U70KZ	Supplement Right Axillary Vein with Nonautologous Tissue Substitute, Open Approach
05U737Z	Supplement Right Axillary Vein with Autologous Tissue Substitute, Percutaneous Approach
05U73JZ	Supplement Right Axillary Vein with Synthetic Substitute, Percutaneous Approach
05U73KZ	Supplement Right Axillary Vein with Nonautologous Tissue Substitute, Percutaneous Approach
05U747Z	Supplement Right Axillary Vein with Autologous Tissue Substitute, Percutaneous Endoscopic Approach
05U74JZ	Supplement Right Axillary Vein with Synthetic Substitute, Percutaneous Endoscopic Approach
05U74KZ	Supplement Right Axillary Vein with Nonautologous Tissue Substitute, Percutaneous Endoscopic Approach
05U807Z	Supplement Left Axillary Vein with Autologous Tissue Substitute, Open Approach
05U80JZ	Supplement Left Axillary Vein with Synthetic Substitute, Open Approach
05U80KZ	Supplement Left Axillary Vein with Nonautologous Tissue Substitute, Open Approach
05U837Z	Supplement Left Axillary Vein with Autologous Tissue Substitute, Percutaneous Approach
05U83JZ	Supplement Left Axillary Vein with Synthetic Substitute, Percutaneous Approach
05U83KZ	Supplement Left Axillary Vein with Nonautologous Tissue Substitute, Percutaneous Approach
05U847Z	Supplement Left Axillary Vein with Autologous Tissue Substitute, Percutaneous Endoscopic Approach
05U84JZ	Supplement Left Axillary Vein with Synthetic Substitute, Percutaneous Endoscopic Approach
05U84KZ	Supplement Left Axillary Vein with Nonautologous Tissue Substitute, Percutaneous Endoscopic Approach
05U907Z	Supplement Right Brachial Vein with Autologous Tissue Substitute, Open Approach
05U90JZ	Supplement Right Brachial Vein with Synthetic Substitute, Open Approach
05U90KZ	Supplement Right Brachial Vein with Nonautologous Tissue Substitute, Open Approach
05U937Z	Supplement Right Brachial Vein with Autologous Tissue Substitute, Percutaneous Approach
05U93JZ	Supplement Right Brachial Vein with Synthetic Substitute, Percutaneous Approach
05U93KZ	Supplement Right Brachial Vein with Nonautologous Tissue Substitute, Percutaneous Approach
05U947Z	Supplement Right Brachial Vein with Autologous Tissue Substitute, Percutaneous Endoscopic Approach
05U94JZ	Supplement Right Brachial Vein with Synthetic Substitute, Percutaneous Endoscopic Approach
05U94KZ	Supplement Right Brachial Vein with Nonautologous Tissue Substitute, Percutaneous Endoscopic Approach
05UA07Z	Supplement Left Brachial Vein with Autologous Tissue Substitute, Open Approach
05UA0JZ	Supplement Left Brachial Vein with Synthetic Substitute, Open Approach
05UA0KZ	Supplement Left Brachial Vein with Nonautologous Tissue Substitute, Open Approach
05UA37Z	Supplement Left Brachial Vein with Autologous Tissue Substitute, Percutaneous Approach
05UA3JZ	Supplement Left Brachial Vein with Synthetic Substitute, Percutaneous Approach
05UA3KZ	Supplement Left Brachial Vein with Nonautologous Tissue Substitute, Percutaneous Approach
05UA47Z	Supplement Left Brachial Vein with Autologous Tissue Substitute, Percutaneous Endoscopic Approach
05UA4JZ	Supplement Left Brachial Vein with Synthetic Substitute, Percutaneous Endoscopic Approach
05UA4KZ	Supplement Left Brachial Vein with Nonautologous Tissue Substitute, Percutaneous Endoscopic Approach
05UB07Z	Supplement Right Basilic Vein with Autologous Tissue Substitute, Open Approach
05UB0JZ	Supplement Right Basilic Vein with Synthetic Substitute, Open Approach
05UB0KZ	Supplement Right Basilic Vein with Nonautologous Tissue Substitute, Open Approach
05UB37Z	Supplement Right Basilic Vein with Autologous Tissue Substitute, Percutaneous Approach
05UB3JZ	Supplement Right Basilic Vein with Synthetic Substitute, Percutaneous Approach
05UB3KZ	Supplement Right Basilic Vein with Nonautologous Tissue Substitute, Percutaneous Approach

05UB47Z Supplement Right Basilic Vein with Autologous Tissue Substitute, Percutaneous Endoscopic Approach

05UB4JZ Supplement Right Basilic Vein with Synthetic Substitute, Percutaneous Endoscopic Approach

05UB4KZ Supplement Right Basilic Vein with Nonautologous Tissue Substitute, Percutaneous Endoscopic Approach

05UC07Z Supplement Left Basilic Vein with Autologous Tissue Substitute, Open Approach

05UC0JZ Supplement Left Basilic Vein with Synthetic Substitute, Open Approach

05UC0KZ Supplement Left Basilic Vein with Nonautologous Tissue Substitute, Open Approach

05UC37Z Supplement Left Basilic Vein with Autologous Tissue Substitute, Percutaneous Approach

05UC3JZ Supplement Left Basilic Vein with Synthetic Substitute, Percutaneous Approach

05UC3KZ Supplement Left Basilic Vein with Nonautologous Tissue Substitute, Percutaneous Approach

05UC47Z Supplement Left Basilic Vein with Autologous Tissue Substitute, Percutaneous Endoscopic Approach

05UC4JZ Supplement Left Basilic Vein with Synthetic Substitute, Percutaneous Endoscopic Approach

05UC4KZ Supplement Left Basilic Vein with Nonautologous Tissue Substitute, Percutaneous Endoscopic Approach

05UD07Z Supplement Right Cephalic Vein with Autologous Tissue Substitute, Open Approach

05UD0JZ Supplement Right Cephalic Vein with Synthetic Substitute, Open Approach

05UD0KZ Supplement Right Cephalic Vein with Nonautologous Tissue Substitute, Open Approach

05UD37Z Supplement Right Cephalic Vein with Autologous Tissue Substitute, Percutaneous Approach

05UD3JZ Supplement Right Cephalic Vein with Synthetic Substitute, Percutaneous Approach

05UD3KZ Supplement Right Cephalic Vein with Nonautologous Tissue Substitute, Percutaneous Approach

05UD47Z Supplement Right Cephalic Vein with Autologous Tissue Substitute, Percutaneous Endoscopic Approach

05UD4JZ Supplement Right Cephalic Vein with Synthetic Substitute, Percutaneous Endoscopic Approach

05UD4KZ Supplement Right Cephalic Vein with Nonautologous Tissue Substitute, Percutaneous Endoscopic Approach

05UF07Z Supplement Left Cephalic Vein with Autologous Tissue Substitute, Open Approach

05UF0JZ Supplement Left Cephalic Vein with Synthetic Substitute, Open Approach

05UF0KZ Supplement Left Cephalic Vein with Nonautologous Tissue Substitute, Open Approach

05UF37Z Supplement Left Cephalic Vein with Autologous Tissue Substitute, Percutaneous Approach

05UF3JZ Supplement Left Cephalic Vein with Synthetic Substitute, Percutaneous Approach

05UF3KZ Supplement Left Cephalic Vein with Nonautologous Tissue Substitute, Percutaneous Approach

05UF47Z Supplement Left Cephalic Vein with Autologous Tissue Substitute, Percutaneous Endoscopic Approach

05UF4JZ Supplement Left Cephalic Vein with Synthetic Substitute, Percutaneous Endoscopic Approach

05UF4KZ Supplement Left Cephalic Vein with Nonautologous Tissue Substitute, Percutaneous Endoscopic Approach

05UG07Z Supplement Right Hand Vein with Autologous Tissue Substitute, Open Approach

05UG0JZ Supplement Right Hand Vein with Synthetic Substitute, Open Approach

05UG0KZ Supplement Right Hand Vein with Nonautologous Tissue Substitute, Open Approach

05UG37Z Supplement Right Hand Vein with Autologous Tissue Substitute, Percutaneous Approach

05UG3JZ Supplement Right Hand Vein with Synthetic Substitute, Percutaneous Approach

05UG3KZ Supplement Right Hand Vein with Nonautologous Tissue Substitute, Percutaneous Approach

05UG47Z Supplement Right Hand Vein with Autologous Tissue Substitute, Percutaneous Endoscopic Approach

05UG4JZ Supplement Right Hand Vein with Synthetic Substitute, Percutaneous Endoscopic Approach

05UG4KZ Supplement Right Hand Vein with Nonautologous Tissue Substitute, Percutaneous Endoscopic Approach

05UH07Z Supplement Left Hand Vein with Autologous Tissue Substitute, Open Approach

05UH0JZ Supplement Left Hand Vein with Synthetic Substitute, Open Approach

05UH0KZ Supplement Left Hand Vein with Nonautologous Tissue Substitute, Open Approach

05UH37Z Supplement Left Hand Vein with Autologous Tissue Substitute, Percutaneous Approach

05UH3JZ Supplement Left Hand Vein with Synthetic Substitute, Percutaneous Approach

05UH3KZ Supplement Left Hand Vein with Nonautologous Tissue Substitute, Percutaneous Approach

05UH47Z Supplement Left Hand Vein with Autologous Tissue Substitute, Percutaneous Endoscopic Approach

05UH4JZ Supplement Left Hand Vein with Synthetic Substitute, Percutaneous Endoscopic Approach

05UH4KZ Supplement Left Hand Vein with Nonautologous Tissue Substitute, Percutaneous Endoscopic Approach

05UL07Z Supplement Intracranial Vein with Autologous Tissue Substitute, Open Approach

05UL0JZ Supplement Intracranial Vein with Synthetic Substitute, Open Approach

05UL0KZ Supplement Intracranial Vein with Nonautologous Tissue Substitute, Open Approach

05UL37Z Supplement Intracranial Vein with Autologous Tissue Substitute, Percutaneous Approach

05UL3JZ Supplement Intracranial Vein with Synthetic Substitute, Percutaneous Approach

05UL3KZ Supplement Intracranial Vein with Nonautologous Tissue Substitute, Percutaneous Approach

05UL47Z Supplement Intracranial Vein with Autologous Tissue Substitute, Percutaneous Endoscopic Approach

05UL4JZ Supplement Intracranial Vein with Synthetic Substitute, Percutaneous Endoscopic Approach

05UL4KZ Supplement Intracranial Vein with Nonautologous Tissue Substitute, Percutaneous Endoscopic Approach

05UM07Z Supplement Right Internal Jugular Vein with Autologous Tissue Substitute, Open Approach

05UM0JZ Supplement Right Internal Jugular Vein with Synthetic Substitute, Open Approach

05UM0KZ Supplement Right Internal Jugular Vein with Nonautologous Tissue Substitute, Open Approach

05UM37Z Supplement Right Internal Jugular Vein with Autologous Tissue Substitute, Percutaneous Approach

05UM3JZ Supplement Right Internal Jugular Vein with Synthetic Substitute, Percutaneous Approach

05UM3KZ Supplement Right Internal Jugular Vein with Nonautologous Tissue Substitute, Percutaneous Approach

05UM47Z Supplement Right Internal Jugular Vein with Autologous Tissue Substitute, Percutaneous Endoscopic Approach

05UM4JZ Supplement Right Internal Jugular Vein with Synthetic Substitute, Percutaneous Endoscopic Approach

05UM4KZ Supplement Right Internal Jugular Vein with Nonautologous Tissue Substitute, Percutaneous Endoscopic Approach

05UN07Z Supplement Left Internal Jugular Vein with Autologous Tissue Substitute, Open Approach

05UN0JZ Supplement Left Internal Jugular Vein with Synthetic Substitute, Open Approach

05UN0KZ Supplement Left Internal Jugular Vein with Nonautologous Tissue Substitute, Open Approach

05UN37Z Supplement Left Internal Jugular Vein with Autologous Tissue Substitute, Percutaneous Approach

05UN3JZ Supplement Left Internal Jugular Vein with Synthetic Substitute, Percutaneous Approach

05UN3KZ Supplement Left Internal Jugular Vein with Nonautologous Tissue Substitute, Percutaneous Approach

05UN47Z Supplement Left Internal Jugular Vein with Autologous Tissue Substitute, Percutaneous Endoscopic Approach

05UN4JZ Supplement Left Internal Jugular Vein with Synthetic Substitute, Percutaneous Endoscopic Approach

05UN4KZ Supplement Left Internal Jugular Vein with Nonautologous Tissue Substitute, Percutaneous Endoscopic Approach

05UP07Z Supplement Right External Jugular Vein with Autologous Tissue Substitute, Open Approach

05UP0JZ Supplement Right External Jugular Vein with Synthetic Substitute, Open Approach

♀ Female-only   ♂ Male-only   ▲ Limited Coverage   ● Non-OR   ᴴᴬᶜ HAC-associated procedure   ▲ Non-covered procedures   ✚ Cluster

05UP0KZ Supplement Right External Jugular Vein with Nonautologous Tissue Substitute, Open Approach

05UP37Z Supplement Right External Jugular Vein with Autologous Tissue Substitute, Percutaneous Approach

05UP3JZ Supplement Right External Jugular Vein with Synthetic Substitute, Percutaneous Approach

05UP3KZ Supplement Right External Jugular Vein with Nonautologous Tissue Substitute, Percutaneous Approach

05UP47Z Supplement Right External Jugular Vein with Autologous Tissue Substitute, Percutaneous Endoscopic Approach

05UP4JZ Supplement Right External Jugular Vein with Synthetic Substitute, Percutaneous Endoscopic Approach

05UP4KZ Supplement Right External Jugular Vein with Nonautologous Tissue Substitute, Percutaneous Endoscopic Approach

05UQ07Z Supplement Left External Jugular Vein with Autologous Tissue Substitute, Open Approach

05UQ0JZ Supplement Left External Jugular Vein with Synthetic Substitute, Open Approach

05UQ0KZ Supplement Left External Jugular Vein with Nonautologous Tissue Substitute, Open Approach

05UQ37Z Supplement Left External Jugular Vein with Autologous Tissue Substitute, Percutaneous Approach

05UQ3JZ Supplement Left External Jugular Vein with Synthetic Substitute, Percutaneous Approach

05UQ3KZ Supplement Left External Jugular Vein with Nonautologous Tissue Substitute, Percutaneous Approach

05UQ47Z Supplement Left External Jugular Vein with Autologous Tissue Substitute, Percutaneous Endoscopic Approach

05UQ4JZ Supplement Left External Jugular Vein with Synthetic Substitute, Percutaneous Endoscopic Approach

05UQ4KZ Supplement Left External Jugular Vein with Nonautologous Tissue Substitute, Percutaneous Endoscopic Approach

05UR07Z Supplement Right Vertebral Vein with Autologous Tissue Substitute, Open Approach

05UR0JZ Supplement Right Vertebral Vein with Synthetic Substitute, Open Approach

05UR0KZ Supplement Right Vertebral Vein with Nonautologous Tissue Substitute, Open Approach

05UR37Z Supplement Right Vertebral Vein with Autologous Tissue Substitute, Percutaneous Approach

05UR3JZ Supplement Right Vertebral Vein with Synthetic Substitute, Percutaneous Approach

05UR3KZ Supplement Right Vertebral Vein with Nonautologous Tissue Substitute, Percutaneous Approach

05UR47Z Supplement Right Vertebral Vein with Autologous Tissue Substitute, Percutaneous Endoscopic Approach

05UR4JZ Supplement Right Vertebral Vein with Synthetic Substitute, Percutaneous Endoscopic Approach

05UR4KZ Supplement Right Vertebral Vein with Nonautologous Tissue Substitute, Percutaneous Endoscopic Approach

05US07Z Supplement Left Vertebral Vein with Autologous Tissue Substitute, Open Approach

05US0JZ Supplement Left Vertebral Vein with Synthetic Substitute, Open Approach

05US0KZ Supplement Left Vertebral Vein with Nonautologous Tissue Substitute, Open Approach

05US37Z Supplement Left Vertebral Vein with Autologous Tissue Substitute, Percutaneous Approach

05US3JZ Supplement Left Vertebral Vein with Synthetic Substitute, Percutaneous Approach

05US3KZ Supplement Left Vertebral Vein with Nonautologous Tissue Substitute, Percutaneous Approach

05US47Z Supplement Left Vertebral Vein with Autologous Tissue Substitute, Percutaneous Endoscopic Approach

05US4JZ Supplement Left Vertebral Vein with Synthetic Substitute, Percutaneous Endoscopic Approach

05US4KZ Supplement Left Vertebral Vein with Nonautologous Tissue Substitute, Percutaneous Endoscopic Approach

05UT07Z Supplement Right Face Vein with Autologous Tissue Substitute, Open Approach

05UT0JZ Supplement Right Face Vein with Synthetic Substitute, Open Approach

05UT0KZ Supplement Right Face Vein with Nonautologous Tissue Substitute, Open Approach

05UT37Z Supplement Right Face Vein with Autologous Tissue Substitute, Percutaneous Approach

05UT3JZ Supplement Right Face Vein with Synthetic Substitute, Percutaneous Approach

05UT3KZ Supplement Right Face Vein with Nonautologous Tissue Substitute, Percutaneous Approach

05UT47Z Supplement Right Face Vein with Autologous Tissue Substitute, Percutaneous Endoscopic Approach

05UT4JZ Supplement Right Face Vein with Synthetic Substitute, Percutaneous Endoscopic Approach

05UT4KZ Supplement Right Face Vein with Nonautologous Tissue Substitute, Percutaneous Endoscopic Approach

05UV07Z Supplement Left Face Vein with Autologous Tissue Substitute, Open Approach

05UV0JZ Supplement Left Face Vein with Synthetic Substitute, Open Approach

05UV0KZ Supplement Left Face Vein with Nonautologous Tissue Substitute, Open Approach

05UV37Z Supplement Left Face Vein with Autologous Tissue Substitute, Percutaneous Approach

05UV3JZ Supplement Left Face Vein with Synthetic Substitute, Percutaneous Approach

05UV3KZ Supplement Left Face Vein with Nonautologous Tissue Substitute, Percutaneous Approach

05UV47Z Supplement Left Face Vein with Autologous Tissue Substitute, Percutaneous Endoscopic Approach

05UV4JZ Supplement Left Face Vein with Synthetic Substitute, Percutaneous Endoscopic Approach

05UV4KZ Supplement Left Face Vein with Nonautologous Tissue Substitute, Percutaneous Endoscopic Approach

05UY07Z Supplement Upper Vein with Autologous Tissue Substitute, Open Approach

05UY0JZ Supplement Upper Vein with Synthetic Substitute, Open Approach

05UY0KZ Supplement Upper Vein with Nonautologous Tissue Substitute, Open Approach

05UY37Z Supplement Upper Vein with Autologous Tissue Substitute, Percutaneous Approach

05UY3JZ Supplement Upper Vein with Synthetic Substitute, Percutaneous Approach

05UY3KZ Supplement Upper Vein with Nonautologous Tissue Substitute, Percutaneous Approach

05UY47Z Supplement Upper Vein with Autologous Tissue Substitute, Percutaneous Endoscopic Approach

05UY4JZ Supplement Upper Vein with Synthetic Substitute, Percutaneous Endoscopic Approach

05UY4KZ Supplement Upper Vein with Nonautologous Tissue Substitute, Percutaneous Endoscopic Approach

05V – Upper Veins, Restriction

Review Coding Guideline B3.12

05V00CZ Restriction of Azygos Vein with Extraluminal Device, Open Approach

05V00DZ Restriction of Azygos Vein with Intraluminal Device, Open Approach

05V00ZZ Restriction of Azygos Vein, Open Approach

05V03CZ Restriction of Azygos Vein with Extraluminal Device, Percutaneous Approach

05V03DZ Restriction of Azygos Vein with Intraluminal Device, Percutaneous Approach

05V03ZZ Restriction of Azygos Vein, Percutaneous Approach

05V04CZ Restriction of Azygos Vein with Extraluminal Device, Percutaneous Endoscopic Approach

05V04DZ Restriction of Azygos Vein with Intraluminal Device, Percutaneous Endoscopic Approach

05V04ZZ Restriction of Azygos Vein, Percutaneous Endoscopic Approach

05V10CZ Restriction of Hemiazygos Vein with Extraluminal Device, Open Approach

05V10DZ Restriction of Hemiazygos Vein with Intraluminal Device, Open Approach

05V10ZZ	Restriction of Hemiazygos Vein, Open Approach
05V13CZ	Restriction of Hemiazygos Vein with Extraluminal Device, Percutaneous Approach
05V13DZ	Restriction of Hemiazygos Vein with Intraluminal Device, Percutaneous Approach
05V13ZZ	Restriction of Hemiazygos Vein, Percutaneous Approach
05V14CZ	Restriction of Hemiazygos Vein with Extraluminal Device, Percutaneous Endoscopic Approach
05V14DZ	Restriction of Hemiazygos Vein with Intraluminal Device, Percutaneous Endoscopic Approach
05V14ZZ	Restriction of Hemiazygos Vein, Percutaneous Endoscopic Approach
05V30CZ	Restriction of Right Innominate Vein with Extraluminal Device, Open Approach
05V30DZ	Restriction of Right Innominate Vein with Intraluminal Device, Open Approach
05V30ZZ	Restriction of Right Innominate Vein, Open Approach
05V33CZ	Restriction of Right Innominate Vein with Extraluminal Device, Percutaneous Approach
05V33DZ	Restriction of Right Innominate Vein with Intraluminal Device, Percutaneous Approach
05V33ZZ	Restriction of Right Innominate Vein, Percutaneous Approach
05V34CZ	Restriction of Right Innominate Vein with Extraluminal Device, Percutaneous Endoscopic Approach
05V34DZ	Restriction of Right Innominate Vein with Intraluminal Device, Percutaneous Endoscopic Approach
05V34ZZ	Restriction of Right Innominate Vein, Percutaneous Endoscopic Approach
05V40CZ	Restriction of Left Innominate Vein with Extraluminal Device, Open Approach
05V40DZ	Restriction of Left Innominate Vein with Intraluminal Device, Open Approach
05V40ZZ	Restriction of Left Innominate Vein, Open Approach
05V43CZ	Restriction of Left Innominate Vein with Extraluminal Device, Percutaneous Approach
05V43DZ	Restriction of Left Innominate Vein with Intraluminal Device, Percutaneous Approach
05V43ZZ	Restriction of Left Innominate Vein, Percutaneous Approach
05V44CZ	Restriction of Left Innominate Vein with Extraluminal Device, Percutaneous Endoscopic Approach
05V44DZ	Restriction of Left Innominate Vein with Intraluminal Device, Percutaneous Endoscopic Approach
05V44ZZ	Restriction of Left Innominate Vein, Percutaneous Endoscopic Approach
05V50CZ	Restriction of Right Subclavian Vein with Extraluminal Device, Open Approach
05V50DZ	Restriction of Right Subclavian Vein with Intraluminal Device, Open Approach
05V50ZZ	Restriction of Right Subclavian Vein, Open Approach
05V53CZ	Restriction of Right Subclavian Vein with Extraluminal Device, Percutaneous Approach
05V53DZ	Restriction of Right Subclavian Vein with Intraluminal Device, Percutaneous Approach
05V53ZZ	Restriction of Right Subclavian Vein, Percutaneous Approach
05V54CZ	Restriction of Right Subclavian Vein with Extraluminal Device, Percutaneous Endoscopic Approach
05V54DZ	Restriction of Right Subclavian Vein with Intraluminal Device, Percutaneous Endoscopic Approach
05V54ZZ	Restriction of Right Subclavian Vein, Percutaneous Endoscopic Approach
05V60CZ	Restriction of Left Subclavian Vein with Extraluminal Device, Open Approach
05V60DZ	Restriction of Left Subclavian Vein with Intraluminal Device, Open Approach
05V60ZZ	Restriction of Left Subclavian Vein, Open Approach
05V63CZ	Restriction of Left Subclavian Vein with Extraluminal Device, Percutaneous Approach
05V63DZ	Restriction of Left Subclavian Vein with Intraluminal Device, Percutaneous Approach
05V63ZZ	Restriction of Left Subclavian Vein, Percutaneous Approach
05V64CZ	Restriction of Left Subclavian Vein with Extraluminal Device, Percutaneous Endoscopic Approach
05V64DZ	Restriction of Left Subclavian Vein with Intraluminal Device, Percutaneous Endoscopic Approach
05V64ZZ	Restriction of Left Subclavian Vein, Percutaneous Endoscopic Approach
05V70CZ	Restriction of Right Axillary Vein with Extraluminal Device, Open Approach
05V70DZ	Restriction of Right Axillary Vein with Intraluminal Device, Open Approach
05V70ZZ	Restriction of Right Axillary Vein, Open Approach
05V73CZ	Restriction of Right Axillary Vein with Extraluminal Device, Percutaneous Approach
05V73DZ	Restriction of Right Axillary Vein with Intraluminal Device, Percutaneous Approach
05V73ZZ	Restriction of Right Axillary Vein, Percutaneous Approach
05V74CZ	Restriction of Right Axillary Vein with Extraluminal Device, Percutaneous Endoscopic Approach
05V74DZ	Restriction of Right Axillary Vein with Intraluminal Device, Percutaneous Endoscopic Approach
05V74ZZ	Restriction of Right Axillary Vein, Percutaneous Endoscopic Approach
05V80CZ	Restriction of Left Axillary Vein with Extraluminal Device, Open Approach
05V80DZ	Restriction of Left Axillary Vein with Intraluminal Device, Open Approach
05V80ZZ	Restriction of Left Axillary Vein, Open Approach
05V83CZ	Restriction of Left Axillary Vein with Extraluminal Device, Percutaneous Approach
05V83DZ	Restriction of Left Axillary Vein with Intraluminal Device, Percutaneous Approach
05V83ZZ	Restriction of Left Axillary Vein, Percutaneous Approach
05V84CZ	Restriction of Left Axillary Vein with Extraluminal Device, Percutaneous Endoscopic Approach
05V84DZ	Restriction of Left Axillary Vein with Intraluminal Device, Percutaneous Endoscopic Approach
05V84ZZ	Restriction of Left Axillary Vein, Percutaneous Endoscopic Approach
05V90CZ	Restriction of Right Brachial Vein with Extraluminal Device, Open Approach
05V90DZ	Restriction of Right Brachial Vein with Intraluminal Device, Open Approach
05V90ZZ	Restriction of Right Brachial Vein, Open Approach
05V93CZ	Restriction of Right Brachial Vein with Extraluminal Device, Percutaneous Approach
05V93DZ	Restriction of Right Brachial Vein with Intraluminal Device, Percutaneous Approach
05V93ZZ	Restriction of Right Brachial Vein, Percutaneous Approach
05V94CZ	Restriction of Right Brachial Vein with Extraluminal Device, Percutaneous Endoscopic Approach
05V94DZ	Restriction of Right Brachial Vein with Intraluminal Device, Percutaneous Endoscopic Approach
05V94ZZ	Restriction of Right Brachial Vein, Percutaneous Endoscopic Approach
05VA0CZ	Restriction of Left Brachial Vein with Extraluminal Device, Open Approach
05VA0DZ	Restriction of Left Brachial Vein with Intraluminal Device, Open Approach
05VA0ZZ	Restriction of Left Brachial Vein, Open Approach
05VA3CZ	Restriction of Left Brachial Vein with Extraluminal Device, Percutaneous Approach
05VA3DZ	Restriction of Left Brachial Vein with Intraluminal Device, Percutaneous Approach
05VA3ZZ	Restriction of Left Brachial Vein, Percutaneous Approach
05VA4CZ	Restriction of Left Brachial Vein with Extraluminal Device, Percutaneous Endoscopic Approach
05VA4DZ	Restriction of Left Brachial Vein with Intraluminal Device, Percutaneous Endoscopic Approach
05VA4ZZ	Restriction of Left Brachial Vein, Percutaneous Endoscopic Approach
05VB0CZ	Restriction of Right Basilic Vein with Extraluminal Device, Open Approach
05VB0DZ	Restriction of Right Basilic Vein with Intraluminal Device, Open Approach
05VB0ZZ	Restriction of Right Basilic Vein, Open Approach
05VB3CZ	Restriction of Right Basilic Vein with Extraluminal Device, Percutaneous Approach
05VB3DZ	Restriction of Right Basilic Vein with Intraluminal Device, Percutaneous Approach
05VB3ZZ	Restriction of Right Basilic Vein, Percutaneous Approach
05VB4CZ	Restriction of Right Basilic Vein with Extraluminal Device, Percutaneous Endoscopic Approach
05VB4DZ	Restriction of Right Basilic Vein with Intraluminal Device, Percutaneous Endoscopic Approach
05VB4ZZ	Restriction of Right Basilic Vein, Percutaneous Endoscopic Approach

♀ Female-only   ♂ Male-only   ▲ Limited Coverage   ● Non-OR   ▨ HAC-associated procedure   ▲ Non-covered procedures   ✚ Cluster

05VC0CZ Restriction of Left Basilic Vein with Extraluminal Device, Open Approach

05VC0DZ Restriction of Left Basilic Vein with Intraluminal Device, Open Approach

05VC0ZZ Restriction of Left Basilic Vein, Open Approach

05VC3CZ Restriction of Left Basilic Vein with Extraluminal Device, Percutaneous Approach

05VC3DZ Restriction of Left Basilic Vein with Intraluminal Device, Percutaneous Approach

05VC3ZZ Restriction of Left Basilic Vein, Percutaneous Approach

05VC4CZ Restriction of Left Basilic Vein with Extraluminal Device, Percutaneous Endoscopic Approach

05VC4DZ Restriction of Left Basilic Vein with Intraluminal Device, Percutaneous Endoscopic Approach

05VC4ZZ Restriction of Left Basilic Vein, Percutaneous Endoscopic Approach

05VD0CZ Restriction of Right Cephalic Vein with Extraluminal Device, Open Approach

05VD0DZ Restriction of Right Cephalic Vein with Intraluminal Device, Open Approach

05VD0ZZ Restriction of Right Cephalic Vein, Open Approach
AHA CC: 3Q, 2020, 37-38

05VD3CZ Restriction of Right Cephalic Vein with Extraluminal Device, Percutaneous Approach

05VD3DZ Restriction of Right Cephalic Vein with Intraluminal Device, Percutaneous Approach

05VD3ZZ Restriction of Right Cephalic Vein, Percutaneous Approach

05VD4CZ Restriction of Right Cephalic Vein with Extraluminal Device, Percutaneous Endoscopic Approach

05VD4DZ Restriction of Right Cephalic Vein with Intraluminal Device, Percutaneous Endoscopic Approach

05VD4ZZ Restriction of Right Cephalic Vein, Percutaneous Endoscopic Approach

05VF0CZ Restriction of Left Cephalic Vein with Extraluminal Device, Open Approach

05VF0DZ Restriction of Left Cephalic Vein with Intraluminal Device, Open Approach

05VF0ZZ Restriction of Left Cephalic Vein, Open Approach

05VF3CZ Restriction of Left Cephalic Vein with Extraluminal Device, Percutaneous Approach

05VF3DZ Restriction of Left Cephalic Vein with Intraluminal Device, Percutaneous Approach

05VF3ZZ Restriction of Left Cephalic Vein, Percutaneous Approach

05VF4CZ Restriction of Left Cephalic Vein with Extraluminal Device, Percutaneous Endoscopic Approach

05VF4DZ Restriction of Left Cephalic Vein with Intraluminal Device, Percutaneous Endoscopic Approach

05VF4ZZ Restriction of Left Cephalic Vein, Percutaneous Endoscopic Approach

05VG0CZ Restriction of Right Hand Vein with Extraluminal Device, Open Approach

05VG0DZ Restriction of Right Hand Vein with Intraluminal Device, Open Approach

05VG0ZZ Restriction of Right Hand Vein, Open Approach

05VG3CZ Restriction of Right Hand Vein with Extraluminal Device, Percutaneous Approach

05VG3DZ Restriction of Right Hand Vein with Intraluminal Device, Percutaneous Approach

05VG3ZZ Restriction of Right Hand Vein, Percutaneous Approach

05VG4CZ Restriction of Right Hand Vein with Extraluminal Device, Percutaneous Endoscopic Approach

05VG4DZ Restriction of Right Hand Vein with Intraluminal Device, Percutaneous Endoscopic Approach

05VG4ZZ Restriction of Right Hand Vein, Percutaneous Endoscopic Approach

05VH0CZ Restriction of Left Hand Vein with Extraluminal Device, Open Approach

05VH0DZ Restriction of Left Hand Vein with Intraluminal Device, Open Approach

05VH0ZZ Restriction of Left Hand Vein, Open Approach

05VH3CZ Restriction of Left Hand Vein with Extraluminal Device, Percutaneous Approach

05VH3DZ Restriction of Left Hand Vein with Intraluminal Device, Percutaneous Approach

05VH3ZZ Restriction of Left Hand Vein, Percutaneous Approach

05VH4CZ Restriction of Left Hand Vein with Extraluminal Device, Percutaneous Endoscopic Approach

05VH4DZ Restriction of Left Hand Vein with Intraluminal Device, Percutaneous Endoscopic Approach

05VH4ZZ Restriction of Left Hand Vein, Percutaneous Endoscopic Approach

05VL0CZ Restriction of Intracranial Vein with Extraluminal Device, Open Approach

05VL0DZ Restriction of Intracranial Vein with Intraluminal Device, Open Approach

05VL0ZZ Restriction of Intracranial Vein, Open Approach

05VL3CZ Restriction of Intracranial Vein with Extraluminal Device, Percutaneous Approach

05VL3DZ Restriction of Intracranial Vein with Intraluminal Device, Percutaneous Approach

05VL3ZZ Restriction of Intracranial Vein, Percutaneous Approach

05VL4CZ Restriction of Intracranial Vein with Extraluminal Device, Percutaneous Endoscopic Approach

05VL4DZ Restriction of Intracranial Vein with Intraluminal Device, Percutaneous Endoscopic Approach

05VL4ZZ Restriction of Intracranial Vein, Percutaneous Endoscopic Approach

05VM0CZ Restriction of Right Internal Jugular Vein with Extraluminal Device, Open Approach

05VM0DZ Restriction of Right Internal Jugular Vein with Intraluminal Device, Open Approach

05VM0ZZ Restriction of Right Internal Jugular Vein, Open Approach

05VM3CZ Restriction of Right Internal Jugular Vein with Extraluminal Device, Percutaneous Approach

05VM3DZ Restriction of Right Internal Jugular Vein with Intraluminal Device, Percutaneous Approach

05VM3ZZ Restriction of Right Internal Jugular Vein, Percutaneous Approach

05VM4CZ Restriction of Right Internal Jugular Vein with Extraluminal Device, Percutaneous Endoscopic Approach

05VM4DZ Restriction of Right Internal Jugular Vein with Intraluminal Device, Percutaneous Endoscopic Approach

05VM4ZZ Restriction of Right Internal Jugular Vein, Percutaneous Endoscopic Approach

05VN0CZ Restriction of Left Internal Jugular Vein with Extraluminal Device, Open Approach

05VN0DZ Restriction of Left Internal Jugular Vein with Intraluminal Device, Open Approach

05VN0ZZ Restriction of Left Internal Jugular Vein, Open Approach

05VN3CZ Restriction of Left Internal Jugular Vein with Extraluminal Device, Percutaneous Approach

05VN3DZ Restriction of Left Internal Jugular Vein with Intraluminal Device, Percutaneous Approach

05VN3ZZ Restriction of Left Internal Jugular Vein, Percutaneous Approach

05VN4CZ Restriction of Left Internal Jugular Vein with Extraluminal Device, Percutaneous Endoscopic Approach

05VN4DZ Restriction of Left Internal Jugular Vein with Intraluminal Device, Percutaneous Endoscopic Approach

05VN4ZZ Restriction of Left Internal Jugular Vein, Percutaneous Endoscopic Approach

05VP0CZ Restriction of Right External Jugular Vein with Extraluminal Device, Open Approach

05VP0DZ Restriction of Right External Jugular Vein with Intraluminal Device, Open Approach

05VP0ZZ Restriction of Right External Jugular Vein, Open Approach

05VP3CZ Restriction of Right External Jugular Vein with Extraluminal Device, Percutaneous Approach

05VP3DZ Restriction of Right External Jugular Vein with Intraluminal Device, Percutaneous Approach

05VP3ZZ Restriction of Right External Jugular Vein, Percutaneous Approach

05VP4CZ Restriction of Right External Jugular Vein with Extraluminal Device, Percutaneous Endoscopic Approach

05VP4DZ Restriction of Right External Jugular Vein with Intraluminal Device, Percutaneous Endoscopic Approach

05VP4ZZ Restriction of Right External Jugular Vein, Percutaneous Endoscopic Approach

05VQ0CZ Restriction of Left External Jugular Vein with Extraluminal Device, Open Approach

05VQ0DZ Restriction of Left External Jugular Vein with Intraluminal Device, Open Approach

05VQ0ZZ Restriction of Left External Jugular Vein, Open Approach

05VQ3CZ Restriction of Left External Jugular Vein with Extraluminal Device, Percutaneous Approach

05VQ3DZ Restriction of Left External Jugular Vein with Intraluminal Device, Percutaneous Approach

05VQ3ZZ Restriction of Left External Jugular Vein, Percutaneous Approach

05VQ4CZ	Restriction of Left External Jugular Vein with Extraluminal Device, Percutaneous Endoscopic Approach	05VS3DZ	Restriction of Left Vertebral Vein with Intraluminal Device, Percutaneous Approach	05VV3CZ	Restriction of Left Face Vein with Extraluminal Device, Percutaneous Approach
05VQ4DZ	Restriction of Left External Jugular Vein with Intraluminal Device, Percutaneous Endoscopic Approach	05VS3ZZ	Restriction of Left Vertebral Vein, Percutaneous Approach	05VV3DZ	Restriction of Left Face Vein with Intraluminal Device, Percutaneous Approach
05VQ4ZZ	Restriction of Left External Jugular Vein, Percutaneous Endoscopic Approach	05VS4CZ	Restriction of Left Vertebral Vein with Extraluminal Device, Percutaneous Endoscopic Approach	05VV3ZZ	Restriction of Left Face Vein, Percutaneous Approach
05VR0CZ	Restriction of Right Vertebral Vein with Extraluminal Device, Open Approach	05VS4DZ	Restriction of Left Vertebral Vein with Intraluminal Device, Percutaneous Endoscopic Approach	05VV4CZ	Restriction of Left Face Vein with Extraluminal Device, Percutaneous Endoscopic Approach
05VR0DZ	Restriction of Right Vertebral Vein with Intraluminal Device, Open Approach	05VS4ZZ	Restriction of Left Vertebral Vein, Percutaneous Endoscopic Approach	05VV4DZ	Restriction of Left Face Vein with Intraluminal Device, Percutaneous Endoscopic Approach
05VR0ZZ	Restriction of Right Vertebral Vein, Open Approach	05VT0CZ	Restriction of Right Face Vein with Extraluminal Device, Open Approach	05VV4ZZ	Restriction of Left Face Vein, Percutaneous Endoscopic Approach
05VR3CZ	Restriction of Right Vertebral Vein with Extraluminal Device, Percutaneous Approach	05VT0DZ	Restriction of Right Face Vein with Intraluminal Device, Open Approach	05VY0CZ	Restriction of Upper Vein with Extraluminal Device, Open Approach
05VR3DZ	Restriction of Right Vertebral Vein with Intraluminal Device, Percutaneous Approach	05VT0ZZ	Restriction of Right Face Vein, Open Approach	05VY0DZ	Restriction of Upper Vein with Intraluminal Device, Open Approach
05VR3ZZ	Restriction of Right Vertebral Vein, Percutaneous Approach	05VT3CZ	Restriction of Right Face Vein with Extraluminal Device, Percutaneous Approach	05VY0ZZ	Restriction of Upper Vein, Open Approach
05VR4CZ	Restriction of Right Vertebral Vein with Extraluminal Device, Percutaneous Endoscopic Approach	05VT3DZ	Restriction of Right Face Vein with Intraluminal Device, Percutaneous Approach	05VY3CZ	Restriction of Upper Vein with Extraluminal Device, Percutaneous Approach
05VR4DZ	Restriction of Right Vertebral Vein with Intraluminal Device, Percutaneous Endoscopic Approach	05VT3ZZ	Restriction of Right Face Vein, Percutaneous Approach	05VY3DZ	Restriction of Upper Vein with Intraluminal Device, Percutaneous Approach
05VR4ZZ	Restriction of Right Vertebral Vein, Percutaneous Endoscopic Approach	05VT4CZ	Restriction of Right Face Vein with Extraluminal Device, Percutaneous Endoscopic Approach	05VY3ZZ	Restriction of Upper Vein, Percutaneous Approach
05VS0CZ	Restriction of Left Vertebral Vein with Extraluminal Device, Open Approach	05VT4DZ	Restriction of Right Face Vein with Intraluminal Device, Percutaneous Endoscopic Approach	05VY4CZ	Restriction of Upper Vein with Extraluminal Device, Percutaneous Endoscopic Approach
05VS0DZ	Restriction of Left Vertebral Vein with Intraluminal Device, Open Approach	05VT4ZZ	Restriction of Right Face Vein, Percutaneous Endoscopic Approach	05VY4DZ	Restriction of Upper Vein with Intraluminal Device, Percutaneous Endoscopic Approach
05VS0ZZ	Restriction of Left Vertebral Vein, Open Approach	05VV0CZ	Restriction of Left Face Vein with Extraluminal Device, Open Approach	05VY4ZZ	Restriction of Upper Vein, Percutaneous Endoscopic Approach
05VS3CZ	Restriction of Left Vertebral Vein with Extraluminal Device, Percutaneous Approach	05VV0DZ	Restriction of Left Face Vein with Intraluminal Device, Open Approach		
		05VV0ZZ	Restriction of Left Face Vein, Open Approach		

05W – Upper Veins, Revision

Review Coding Guideline B6.1c

05W002Z	Revision of Monitoring Device in Azygos Vein, Open Approach	05W3XMZ	Revision of Neurostimulator Lead in Right Innominate Vein, External Approach	05WY0KZ	Revision of Nonautologous Tissue Substitute in Upper Vein, Open Approach
05W00MZ	Revision of Neurostimulator Lead in Azygos Vein, Open Approach	05W40MZ	Revision of Neurostimulator Lead in Left Innominate Vein, Open Approach	05WY0YZ	Revision of Other Device in Upper Vein, Open Approach
05W032Z	Revision of Monitoring Device in Azygos Vein, Percutaneous Approach	05W43MZ	Revision of Neurostimulator Lead in Left Innominate Vein, Percutaneous Approach	05WY30Z	Revision of Drainage Device in Upper Vein, Percutaneous Approach
05W03MZ	Revision of Neurostimulator Lead in Azygos Vein, Percutaneous Approach	05W44MZ	Revision of Neurostimulator Lead in Left Innominate Vein, Percutaneous Endoscopic Approach	05WY32Z	Revision of Monitoring Device in Upper Vein, Percutaneous Approach
05W042Z	Revision of Monitoring Device in Azygos Vein, Percutaneous Endoscopic Approach	05W4XMZ	Revision of Neurostimulator Lead in Left Innominate Vein, External Approach	05WY33Z	Revision of Infusion Device in Upper Vein, Percutaneous Approach
05W04MZ	Revision of Neurostimulator Lead in Azygos Vein, Percutaneous Endoscopic Approach	05WY00Z	Revision of Drainage Device in Upper Vein, Open Approach	05WY37Z	Revision of Autologous Tissue Substitute in Upper Vein, Percutaneous Approach
05W0X2Z	Revision of Monitoring Device in Azygos Vein, External Approach	05WY02Z	Revision of Monitoring Device in Upper Vein, Open Approach	05WY3CZ	Revision of Extraluminal Device in Upper Vein, Percutaneous Approach
05W0XMZ	Revision of Neurostimulator Lead in Azygos Vein, External Approach	05WY03Z	Revision of Infusion Device in Upper Vein, Open Approach	05WY3DZ	Revision of Intraluminal Device in Upper Vein, Percutaneous Approach
05W30MZ	Revision of Neurostimulator Lead in Right Innominate Vein, Open Approach	05WY07Z	Revision of Autologous Tissue Substitute in Upper Vein, Open Approach	05WY3JZ	Revision of Synthetic Substitute in Upper Vein, Percutaneous Approach
05W33MZ	Revision of Neurostimulator Lead in Right Innominate Vein, Percutaneous Approach	05WY0CZ	Revision of Extraluminal Device in Upper Vein, Open Approach	05WY3KZ	Revision of Nonautologous Tissue Substitute in Upper Vein, Percutaneous Approach
05W34MZ	Revision of Neurostimulator Lead in Right Innominate Vein, Percutaneous Endoscopic Approach	05WY0DZ	Revision of Intraluminal Device in Upper Vein, Open Approach	05WY3YZ	Revision of Other Device in Upper Vein, Percutaneous Approach
		05WY0JZ	Revision of Synthetic Substitute in Upper Vein, Open Approach		

♀ Female-only   ♂ Male-only   ▲ Limited Coverage   ● Non-OR   ᴴᴬᶜ HAC-associated procedure   ▲ Non-covered procedures   ✚ Cluster

05WY40Z	Revision of Drainage Device in Upper Vein, Percutaneous Endoscopic Approach
05WY42Z	Revision of Monitoring Device in Upper Vein, Percutaneous Endoscopic Approach
05WY43Z	Revision of Infusion Device in Upper Vein, Percutaneous Endoscopic Approach
05WY47Z	Revision of Autologous Tissue Substitute in Upper Vein, Percutaneous Endoscopic Approach
05WY4CZ	Revision of Extraluminal Device in Upper Vein, Percutaneous Endoscopic Approach

05WY4DZ	Revision of Intraluminal Device in Upper Vein, Percutaneous Endoscopic Approach
05WY4JZ	Revision of Synthetic Substitute in Upper Vein, Percutaneous Endoscopic Approach
05WY4KZ	Revision of Nonautologous Tissue Substitute in Upper Vein, Percutaneous Endoscopic Approach
05WY4YZ	Revision of Other Device in Upper Vein, Percutaneous Endoscopic Approach
05WYX0Z	Revision of Drainage Device in Upper Vein, External Approach
05WYX2Z	Revision of Monitoring Device in Upper Vein, External Approach

05WYX3Z	Revision of Infusion Device in Upper Vein, External Approach
05WYX7Z	Revision of Autologous Tissue Substitute in Upper Vein, External Approach
05WYXCZ	Revision of Extraluminal Device in Upper Vein, External Approach
05WYXDZ	Revision of Intraluminal Device in Upper Vein, External Approach
05WYXJZ	Revision of Synthetic Substitute in Upper Vein, External Approach
05WYXKZ	Revision of Nonautologous Tissue Substitute in Upper Vein, External Approach

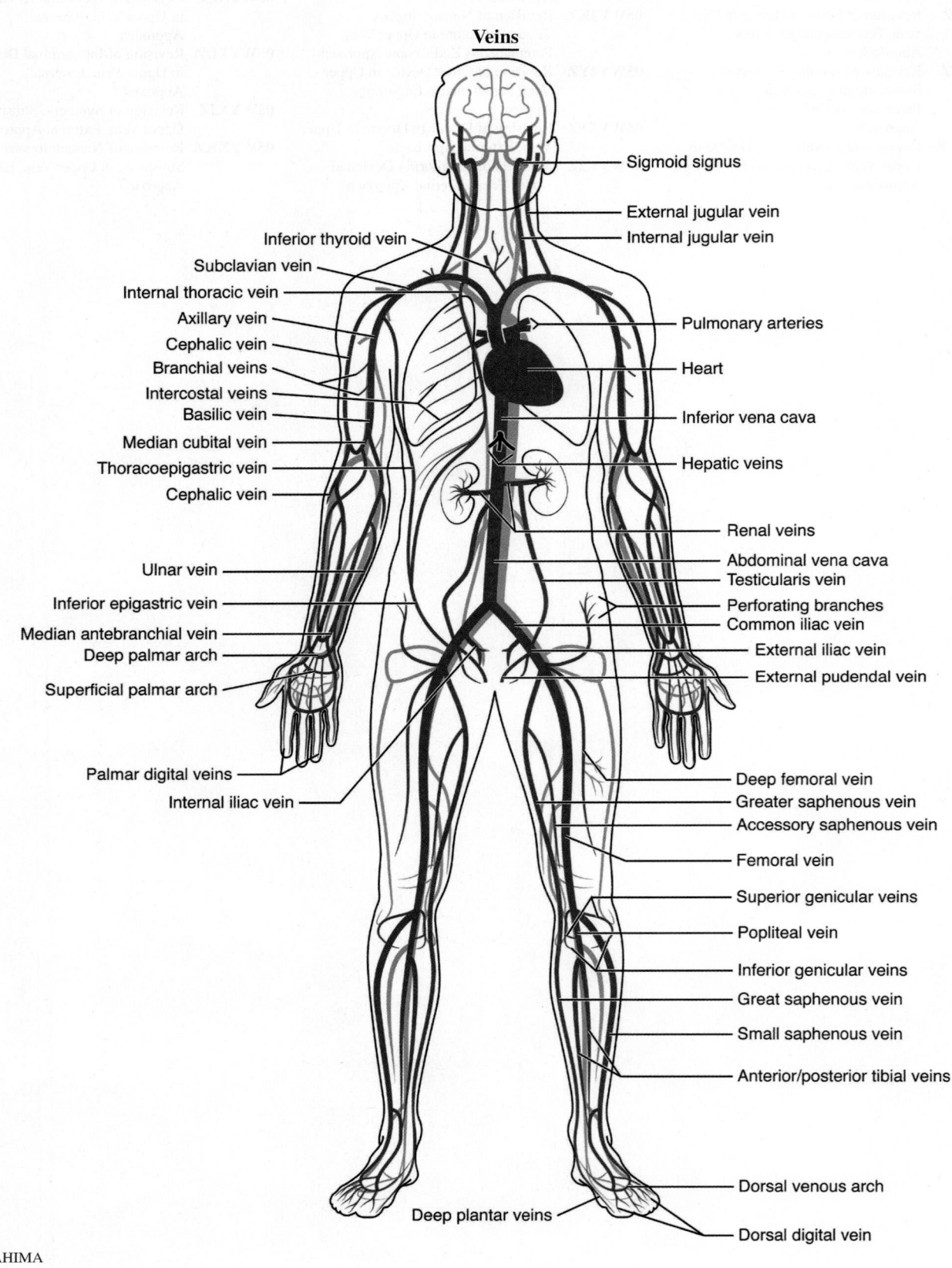

Veins

- Sigmoid signus
- External jugular vein
- Internal jugular vein
- Inferior thyroid vein
- Subclavian vein
- Internal thoracic vein
- Axillary vein
- Cephalic vein
- Branchial veins
- Intercostal veins
- Basilic vein
- Median cubital vein
- Thoracoepigastric vein
- Cephalic vein
- Pulmonary arteries
- Heart
- Inferior vena cava
- Hepatic veins
- Renal veins
- Ulnar vein
- Inferior epigastric vein
- Median antebranchial vein
- Deep palmar arch
- Superficial palmar arch
- Abdominal vena cava
- Testicularis vein
- Perforating branches
- Common iliac vein
- External iliac vein
- External pudendal vein
- Palmar digital veins
- Internal iliac vein
- Deep femoral vein
- Greater saphenous vein
- Accessory saphenous vein
- Femoral vein
- Superior genicular veins
- Popliteal vein
- Inferior genicular veins
- Great saphenous vein
- Small saphenous vein
- Anterior/posterior tibial veins
- Dorsal venous arch
- Deep plantar veins
- Dorsal digital vein

©AHIMA

Lower Veins Tables 061–06W

Section	0	**Medical and Surgical**
Body System	**6**	**Lower Veins**
Operation	**1**	**Bypass:** Altering the route of passage of the contents of a tubular body part

Body Part (4th)	Approach (5th)	Device (6th)	Qualifier (7th)
0 Inferior Vena Cava	**0** Open **4** Percutaneous Endoscopic	**7** Autologous Tissue Substitute **9** Autologous Venous Tissue **A** Autologous Arterial Tissue **J** Synthetic Substitute **K** Nonautologous Tissue Substitute **Z** No Device	**5** Superior Mesenteric Vein **6** Inferior Mesenteric Vein **P** Pulmonary Trunk **Q** Pulmonary Artery, Right **R** Pulmonary Artery, Left **Y** Lower Vein
1 Splenic Vein	**0** Open **4** Percutaneous Endoscopic	**7** Autologous Tissue Substitute **9** Autologous Venous Tissue **A** Autologous Arterial Tissue **J** Synthetic Substitute **K** Nonautologous Tissue Substitute **Z** No Device	**9** Renal Vein, Right **B** Renal Vein, Left **Y** Lower Vein
2 Gastric Vein **3** Esophageal Vein **4** Hepatic Vein **5** Superior Mesenteric Vein **6** Inferior Mesenteric Vein **7** Colic Vein **9** Renal Vein, Right **B** Renal Vein, Left **C** Common Iliac Vein, Right **D** Common Iliac Vein, Left **F** External Iliac Vein, Right **G** External Iliac Vein, Left **H** Hypogastric Vein, Right **J** Hypogastric Vein, Left **M** Femoral Vein, Right **N** Femoral Vein, Left **P** Saphenous Vein, Right **Q** Saphenous Vein, Left **T** Foot Vein, Right **V** Foot Vein, Left	**0** Open **4** Percutaneous Endoscopic	**7** Autologous Tissue Substitute **9** Autologous Venous Tissue **A** Autologous Arterial Tissue **J** Synthetic Substitute **K** Nonautologous Tissue Substitute **Z** No Device	**Y** Lower Vein
8 Portal Vein	**0** Open	**7** Autologous Tissue Substitute **9** Autologous Venous Tissue **A** Autologous Arterial Tissue **J** Synthetic Substitute **K** Nonautologous Tissue Substitute **Z** No Device	**9** Renal Vein, Right **B** Renal Vein, Left **Y** Lower Vein
8 Portal Vein	**3** Percutaneous	**J** Synthetic Substitute	**4** Hepatic Vein **Y** Lower Vein
8 Portal Vein	**4** Percutaneous Endoscopic	**7** Autologous Tissue Substitute **9** Autologous Venous Tissue **A** Autologous Arterial Tissue **K** Nonautologous Tissue Substitute **Z** No Device	**9** Renal Vein, Right **B** Renal Vein, Left **Y** Lower Vein
8 Portal Vein	**4** Percutaneous Endoscopic	**J** Synthetic Substitute	**4** Hepatic Vein **9** Renal Vein, Right **B** Renal Vein, Left **Y** Lower Vein

Section	0	Medical and Surgical
Body System	6	Lower Veins
Operation	5	**Destruction:** Physical eradication of all or a portion of a body part by the direct use of energy, force, or a destructive agent

Body Part (4th)	Approach (5th)	Device (6th)	Qualifier (7th)
0 Inferior Vena Cava	0 Open	Z No Device	Z No Qualifier
1 Splenic Vein	3 Percutaneous		
2 Gastric Vein	4 Percutaneous Endoscopic		
3 Esophageal Vein			
4 Hepatic Vein			
5 Superior Mesenteric Vein			
6 Inferior Mesenteric Vein			
7 Colic Vein			
8 Portal Vein			
9 Renal Vein, Right			
B Renal Vein, Left			
C Common Iliac Vein, Right			
D Common Iliac Vein, Left			
F External Iliac Vein, Right			
G External Iliac Vein, Left			
H Hypogastric Vein, Right			
J Hypogastric Vein, Left			
M Femoral Vein, Right			
N Femoral Vein, Left			
P Saphenous Vein, Right			
Q Saphenous Vein, Left			
T Foot Vein, Right			
V Foot Vein, Left			
Y Lower Vein	0 Open	Z No Device	C Hemorrhoidal Plexus
	3 Percutaneous		Z No Qualifier
	4 Percutaneous Endoscopic		

Section	0	Medical and Surgical
Body System	6	Lower Veins
Operation	7	**Dilation:** Expanding an orifice or the lumen of a tubular body part

Body Part (4th)	Approach (5th)	Device (6th)	Qualifier (7th)
0 Inferior Vena Cava	0 Open	D Intraluminal Device	Z No Qualifier
1 Splenic Vein	3 Percutaneous	Z No Device	
2 Gastric Vein	4 Percutaneous Endoscopic		
3 Esophageal Vein			
4 Hepatic Vein			
5 Superior Mesenteric Vein			
6 Inferior Mesenteric Vein			
7 Colic Vein			
8 Portal Vein			
9 Renal Vein, Right			
B Renal Vein, Left			
C Common Iliac Vein, Right			
D Common Iliac Vein, Left			
F External Iliac Vein, Right			
G External Iliac Vein, Left			
H Hypogastric Vein, Right			
J Hypogastric Vein, Left			
M Femoral Vein, Right			
N Femoral Vein, Left			
P Saphenous Vein, Right			
Q Saphenous Vein, Left			
T Foot Vein, Right			
V Foot Vein, Left			
Y Lower Vein			

Section	0	Medical and Surgical
Body System	6	Lower Veins
Operation	9	Drainage: Taking or letting out fluids and/or gases from a body part

Body Part (4th)	Approach (5th)	Device (6th)	Qualifier (7th)
0 Inferior Vena Cava 1 Splenic Vein 2 Gastric Vein 3 Esophageal Vein 4 Hepatic Vein 5 Superior Mesenteric Vein 6 Inferior Mesenteric Vein 7 Colic Vein 8 Portal Vein 9 Renal Vein, Right B Renal Vein, Left C Common Iliac Vein, Right D Common Iliac Vein, Left F External Iliac Vein, Right G External Iliac Vein, Left H Hypogastric Vein, Right J Hypogastric Vein, Left M Femoral Vein, Right N Femoral Vein, Left P Saphenous Vein, Right Q Saphenous Vein, Left T Foot Vein, Right V Foot Vein, Left Y Lower Vein	0 Open 3 Percutaneous 4 Percutaneous Endoscopic	0 Drainage Device	Z No Qualifier
0 Inferior Vena Cava 1 Splenic Vein 2 Gastric Vein 3 Esophageal Vein 4 Hepatic Vein 5 Superior Mesenteric Vein 6 Inferior Mesenteric Vein 7 Colic Vein 8 Portal Vein 9 Renal Vein, Right B Renal Vein, Left C Common Iliac Vein, Right D Common Iliac Vein, Left F External Iliac Vein, Right G External Iliac Vein, Left H Hypogastric Vein, Right J Hypogastric Vein, Left M Femoral Vein, Right N Femoral Vein, Left P Saphenous Vein, Right Q Saphenous Vein, Left T Foot Vein, Right V Foot Vein, Left Y Lower Vein	0 Open 3 Percutaneous 4 Percutaneous Endoscopic	Z No Device	X Diagnostic Z No Qualifier

Section	0	Medical and Surgical
Body System	6	Lower Veins
Operation	B	Excision: Cutting out or off, without replacement, a portion of a body part

Body Part (4th)	Approach (5th)	Device (6th)	Qualifier (7th)
0 Inferior Vena Cava 1 Splenic Vein 2 Gastric Vein 3 Esophageal Vein 4 Hepatic Vein 5 Superior Mesenteric Vein 6 Inferior Mesenteric Vein 7 Colic Vein 8 Portal Vein 9 Renal Vein, Right B Renal Vein, Left C Common Iliac Vein, Right D Common Iliac Vein, Left F External Iliac Vein, Right G External Iliac Vein, Left H Hypogastric Vein, Right J Hypogastric Vein, Left M Femoral Vein, Right N Femoral Vein, Left P Saphenous Vein, Right Q Saphenous Vein, Left T Foot Vein, Right V Foot Vein, Left	0 Open 3 Percutaneous 4 Percutaneous Endoscopic	Z No Device	X Diagnostic Z No Qualifier
Y Lower Vein	0 Open 3 Percutaneous 4 Percutaneous Endoscopic	Z No Device	C Hemorrhoidal Plexus X Diagnostic Z No Qualifier

Section	0	Medical and Surgical
Body System	6	Lower Veins
Operation	C	Extirpation: Taking or cutting out solid matter from a body part

Body Part (4th)	Approach (5th)	Device (6th)	Qualifier (7th)
0 Inferior Vena Cava 1 Splenic Vein 2 Gastric Vein 3 Esophageal Vein 4 Hepatic Vein 5 Superior Mesenteric Vein 6 Inferior Mesenteric Vein 7 Colic Vein 8 Portal Vein 9 Renal Vein, Right B Renal Vein, Left C Common Iliac Vein, Right D Common Iliac Vein, Left F External Iliac Vein, Right G External Iliac Vein, Left H Hypogastric Vein, Right J Hypogastric Vein, Left M Femoral Vein, Right N Femoral Vein, Left P Saphenous Vein, Right Q Saphenous Vein, Left T Foot Vein, Right V Foot Vein, Left Y Lower Vein	0 Open 3 Percutaneous 4 Percutaneous Endoscopic	Z No Device	Z No Qualifier

Section	0	Medical and Surgical
Body System	6	Lower Veins
Operation	D	Extraction: Pulling or stripping out or off all or a portion of a body part by the use of force

Body Part (4th)	Approach (5th)	Device (6th)	Qualifier (7th)
M Femoral Vein, Right N Femoral Vein, Left P Saphenous Vein, Right Q Saphenous Vein, Left T Foot Vein, Right V Foot Vein, Left Y Lower Vein	0 Open 3 Percutaneous 4 Percutaneous Endoscopic	Z No Device	Z No Qualifier

Section	0	Medical and Surgical
Body System	6	Lower Veins
Operation	F	Fragmentation: Breaking solid matter in a body part into pieces

Body Part (4th)	Approach (5th)	Device (6th)	Qualifier (7th)
C Common Iliac Vein, Right D Common Iliac Vein, Left F External Iliac Vein, Right G External Iliac Vein, Left H Hypogastric Vein, Right J Hypogastric Vein, Left M Femoral Vein, Right N Femoral Vein, Left P Saphenous Vein, Right Q Saphenous Vein, Left Y Lower Vein	3 Percutaneous	Z No Device	0 Ultrasonic Z No Qualifier

Section	0	Medical and Surgical
Body System	6	Lower Veins
Operation	H	Insertion: Putting in a nonbiological appliance that monitors, assists, performs, or prevents a physiological function but does not physically take the place of a body part

Body Part (4th)	Approach (5th)	Device (6th)	Qualifier (7th)
0 Inferior Vena Cava	0 Open 3 Percutaneous	3 Infusion Device	T Via Umbilical Vein Z No Qualifier
0 Inferior Vena Cava	0 Open 3 Percutaneous	D Intraluminal Device	Z No Qualifier
0 Inferior Vena Cava	4 Percutaneous Endoscopic	3 Infusion Device D Intraluminal Device	Z No Qualifier
1 Splenic Vein 2 Gastric Vein 3 Esophageal Vein 4 Hepatic Vein 5 Superior Mesenteric Vein 6 Inferior Mesenteric Vein 7 Colic Vein 8 Portal Vein 9 Renal Vein, Right B Renal Vein, Left C Common Iliac Vein, Right D Common Iliac Vein, Left F External Iliac Vein, Right G External Iliac Vein, Left H Hypogastric Vein, Right J Hypogastric Vein, Left M Femoral Vein, Right N Femoral Vein, Left P Saphenous Vein, Right Q Saphenous Vein, Left T Foot Vein, Right V Foot Vein, Left	0 Open 3 Percutaneous 4 Percutaneous Endoscopic	3 Infusion Device D Intraluminal Device	Z No Qualifier

Continued →

Section	0	Medical and Surgical
Body System	6	Lower Veins
Operation	H	Insertion: Putting in a nonbiological appliance that monitors, assists, performs, or prevents a physiological function but does not physically take the place of a body part

Body Part (4th)	Approach (5th)	Device (6th)	Qualifier (7th)
Y Lower Vein	0 Open 3 Percutaneous 4 Percutaneous Endoscopic	2 Monitoring Device 3 Infusion Device D Intraluminal Device Y Other Device	Z No Qualifier

Section	0	Medical and Surgical
Body System	6	Lower Veins
Operation	J	Inspection: Visually and/or manually exploring a body part

Body Part (4th)	Approach (5th)	Device (6th)	Qualifier (7th)
Y Lower Vein	0 Open 3 Percutaneous 4 Percutaneous Endoscopic X External	Z No Device	Z No Qualifier

Section	0	Medical and Surgical
Body System	6	Lower Veins
Operation	L	Occlusion: Completely closing an orifice or the lumen of a tubular body part

Body Part (4th)	Approach (5th)	Device (6th)	Qualifier (7th)
0 Inferior Vena Cava 1 Splenic Vein 4 Hepatic Vein 5 Superior Mesenteric Vein 6 Inferior Mesenteric Vein 7 Colic Vein 8 Portal Vein 9 Renal Vein, Right B Renal Vein, Left C Common Iliac Vein, Right D Common Iliac Vein, Left F External Iliac Vein, Right G External Iliac Vein, Left H Hypogastric Vein, Right J Hypogastric Vein, Left M Femoral Vein, Right N Femoral Vein, Left P Saphenous Vein, Right Q Saphenous Vein, Left T Foot Vein, Right V Foot Vein, Left	0 Open 3 Percutaneous 4 Percutaneous Endoscopic	C Extraluminal Device D Intraluminal Device Z No Device	Z No Qualifier
2 Gastric Vein 3 Esophageal Vein	0 Open 3 Percutaneous 4 Percutaneous Endoscopic 7 Via Natural or Artificial Opening 8 Via Natural or Artificial Opening Endoscopic	C Extraluminal Device D Intraluminal Device Z No Device	Z No Qualifier
Y Lower Vein	0 Open 3 Percutaneous 4 Percutaneous Endoscopic 7 Via Natural or Artificial Opening 8 Via Natural or Artificial Opening Endoscopic	C Extraluminal Device D Intraluminal Device Z No Device	C Hemorrhoidal Plexus Z No Qualifier

Section	0	Medical and Surgical
Body System	6	Lower Veins
Operation	N	Release: Freeing a body part from an abnormal physical constraint by cutting or by the use of force

Body Part (4th)	Approach (5th)	Device (6th)	Qualifier (7th)
0 Inferior Vena Cava 1 Splenic Vein 2 Gastric Vein 3 Esophageal Vein 4 Hepatic Vein 5 Superior Mesenteric Vein 6 Inferior Mesenteric Vein 7 Colic Vein 8 Portal Vein 9 Renal Vein, Right B Renal Vein, Left C Common Iliac Vein, Right D Common Iliac Vein, Left F External Iliac Vein, Right G External Iliac Vein, Left H Hypogastric Vein, Right J Hypogastric Vein, Left M Femoral Vein, Right N Femoral Vein, Left P Saphenous Vein, Right Q Saphenous Vein, Left T Foot Vein, Right V Foot Vein, Left Y Lower Vein	0 Open 3 Percutaneous 4 Percutaneous Endoscopic	Z No Device	Z No Qualifier

Section	0	Medical and Surgical
Body System	6	Lower Veins
Operation	P	Removal: Taking out or off a device from a body part

Body Part (4th)	Approach (5th)	Device (6th)	Qualifier (7th)
Y Lower Vein	0 Open 3 Percutaneous 4 Percutaneous Endoscopic	0 Drainage Device 2 Monitoring Device 3 Infusion Device 7 Autologous Tissue Substitute C Extraluminal Device D Intraluminal Device J Synthetic Substitute K Nonautologous Tissue Substitute Y Other Device	Z No Qualifier
Y Lower Vein	X External	0 Drainage Device 2 Monitoring Device 3 Infusion Device D Intraluminal Device	Z No Qualifier

Section	0	Medical and Surgical
Body System	6	Lower Veins
Operation	Q	**Repair:** Restoring, to the extent possible, a body part to its normal anatomic structure and function

Body Part (4th)	Approach (5th)	Device (6th)	Qualifier (7th)
0 Inferior Vena Cava 1 Splenic Vein 2 Gastric Vein 3 Esophageal Vein 4 Hepatic Vein 5 Superior Mesenteric Vein 6 Inferior Mesenteric Vein 7 Colic Vein 8 Portal Vein 9 Renal Vein, Right B Renal Vein, Left C Common Iliac Vein, Right D Common Iliac Vein, Left F External Iliac Vein, Right G External Iliac Vein, Left H Hypogastric Vein, Right J Hypogastric Vein, Left M Femoral Vein, Right N Femoral Vein, Left P Saphenous Vein, Right Q Saphenous Vein, Left T Foot Vein, Right V Foot Vein, Left Y Lower Vein	0 Open 3 Percutaneous 4 Percutaneous Endoscopic	Z No Device	Z No Qualifier

Section	0	Medical and Surgical
Body System	6	Lower Veins
Operation	R	**Replacement:** Putting in or on biological or synthetic material that physically takes the place and/or function of all or a portion of a body part

Body Part (4th)	Approach (5th)	Device (6th)	Qualifier (7th)
0 Inferior Vena Cava 1 Splenic Vein 2 Gastric Vein 3 Esophageal Vein 4 Hepatic Vein 5 Superior Mesenteric Vein 6 Inferior Mesenteric Vein 7 Colic Vein 8 Portal Vein 9 Renal Vein, Right B Renal Vein, Left C Common Iliac Vein, Right D Common Iliac Vein, Left F External Iliac Vein, Right G External Iliac Vein, Left H Hypogastric Vein, Right J Hypogastric Vein, Left M Femoral Vein, Right N Femoral Vein, Left P Saphenous Vein, Right Q Saphenous Vein, Left T Foot Vein, Right V Foot Vein, Left Y Lower Vein	0 Open 4 Percutaneous Endoscopic	7 Autologous Tissue Substitute J Synthetic Substitute K Nonautologous Tissue Substitute	Z No Qualifier

Section   0   **Medical and Surgical**
Body System   6   **Lower Veins**
Operation   S   **Reposition:** Moving to its normal location, or other suitable location, all or a portion of a body part

Body Part (4th)	Approach (5th)	Device (6th)	Qualifier (7th)
0 Inferior Vena Cava 1 Splenic Vein 2 Gastric Vein 3 Esophageal Vein 4 Hepatic Vein 5 Superior Mesenteric Vein 6 Inferior Mesenteric Vein 7 Colic Vein 8 Portal Vein 9 Renal Vein, Right B Renal Vein, Left C Common Iliac Vein, Right D Common Iliac Vein, Left F External Iliac Vein, Right G External Iliac Vein, Left H Hypogastric Vein, Right J Hypogastric Vein, Left M Femoral Vein, Right N Femoral Vein, Left P Saphenous Vein, Right Q Saphenous Vein, Left T Foot Vein, Right V Foot Vein, Left Y Lower Vein	0 Open 3 Percutaneous 4 Percutaneous Endoscopic	Z No Device	Z No Qualifier

Section   0   **Medical and Surgical**
Body System   6   **Lower Veins**
Operation   U   **Supplement:** Putting in or on biological or synthetic material that physically reinforces and/or augments the function of a portion of a body part

Body Part (4th)	Approach (5th)	Device (6th)	Qualifier (7th)
0 Inferior Vena Cava 1 Splenic Vein 2 Gastric Vein 3 Esophageal Vein 4 Hepatic Vein 5 Superior Mesenteric Vein 6 Inferior Mesenteric Vein 7 Colic Vein 8 Portal Vein 9 Renal Vein, Right B Renal Vein, Left C Common Iliac Vein, Right D Common Iliac Vein, Left F External Iliac Vein, Right G External Iliac Vein, Left H Hypogastric Vein, Right J Hypogastric Vein, Left M Femoral Vein, Right N Femoral Vein, Left P Saphenous Vein, Right Q Saphenous Vein, Left T Foot Vein, Right V Foot Vein, Left Y Lower Vein	0 Open 3 Percutaneous 4 Percutaneous Endoscopic	7 Autologous Tissue Substitute J Synthetic Substitute K Nonautologous Tissue Substitute	Z No Qualifier

Section	0	Medical and Surgical
Body System	6	Lower Veins
Operation	V	**Restriction:** Partially closing an orifice or the lumen of a tubular body part

Body Part (4th)	Approach (5th)	Device (6th)	Qualifier (7th)
0 Inferior Vena Cava 1 Splenic Vein 2 Gastric Vein 3 Esophageal Vein 4 Hepatic Vein 5 Superior Mesenteric Vein 6 Inferior Mesenteric Vein 7 Colic Vein 8 Portal Vein 9 Renal Vein, Right B Renal Vein, Left C Common Iliac Vein, Right D Common Iliac Vein, Left F External Iliac Vein, Right G External Iliac Vein, Left H Hypogastric Vein, Right J Hypogastric Vein, Left M Femoral Vein, Right N Femoral Vein, Left P Saphenous Vein, Right Q Saphenous Vein, Left T Foot Vein, Right V Foot Vein, Left Y Lower Vein	0 Open 3 Percutaneous 4 Percutaneous Endoscopic	C Extraluminal Device D Intraluminal Device Z No Device	Z No Qualifier

Section	0	Medical and Surgical
Body System	6	Lower Veins
Operation	W	**Revision:** Correcting, to the extent possible, a portion of a malfunctioning device or the position of a displaced device

Body Part (4th)	Approach (5th)	Device (6th)	Qualifier (7th)
Y Lower Vein	0 Open 3 Percutaneous 4 Percutaneous Endoscopic X External	0 Drainage Device 2 Monitoring Device 3 Infusion Device 7 Autologous Tissue Substitute C Extraluminal Device D Intraluminal Device J Synthetic Substitute K Nonautologous Tissue Substitute Y Other Device	Z No Qualifier
Y Lower Vein	X External	0 Drainage Device 2 Monitoring Device 3 Infusion Device 7 Autologous Tissue Substitute C Extraluminal Device D Intraluminal Device J Synthetic Substitute K Nonautologus Tissue Substitute	Z No Qualifier

Lower Veins Code Listing 061–06W

061 – Lower Veins, Bypass

Review Coding Guideline B3.6a

0610075	Bypass Inferior Vena Cava to Superior Mesenteric Vein with Autologous Tissue Substitute, Open Approach
0610076	Bypass Inferior Vena Cava to Inferior Mesenteric Vein with Autologous Tissue Substitute, Open Approach
061007P	Bypass Inferior Vena Cava to Pulmonary Trunk with Autologous Tissue Substitute, Open Approach
061007Q	Bypass Inferior Vena Cava to Right Pulmonary Artery with Autologous Tissue Substitute, Open Approach
061007R	Bypass Inferior Vena Cava to Left Pulmonary Artery with Autologous Tissue Substitute, Open Approach
061007Y	Bypass Inferior Vena Cava to Lower Vein with Autologous Tissue Substitute, Open Approach
0610095	Bypass Inferior Vena Cava to Superior Mesenteric Vein with Autologous Venous Tissue, Open Approach
0610096	Bypass Inferior Vena Cava to Inferior Mesenteric Vein with Autologous Venous Tissue, Open Approach
061009P	Bypass Inferior Vena Cava to Pulmonary Trunk with Autologous Venous Tissue, Open Approach

061009Q Bypass Inferior Vena Cava to Right Pulmonary Artery with Autologous Venous Tissue, Open Approach

061009R Bypass Inferior Vena Cava to Left Pulmonary Artery with Autologous Venous Tissue, Open Approach

061009Y Bypass Inferior Vena Cava to Lower Vein with Autologous Venous Tissue, Open Approach

06100A5 Bypass Inferior Vena Cava to Superior Mesenteric Vein with Autologous Arterial Tissue, Open Approach

06100A6 Bypass Inferior Vena Cava to Inferior Mesenteric Vein with Autologous Arterial Tissue, Open Approach

06100AP Bypass Inferior Vena Cava to Pulmonary Trunk with Autologous Arterial Tissue, Open Approach

06100AQ Bypass Inferior Vena Cava to Right Pulmonary Artery with Autologous Arterial Tissue, Open Approach

06100AR Bypass Inferior Vena Cava to Left Pulmonary Artery with Autologous Arterial Tissue, Open Approach

06100AY Bypass Inferior Vena Cava to Lower Vein with Autologous Arterial Tissue, Open Approach

06100J5 Bypass Inferior Vena Cava to Superior Mesenteric Vein with Synthetic Substitute, Open Approach

06100J6 Bypass Inferior Vena Cava to Inferior Mesenteric Vein with Synthetic Substitute, Open Approach

06100JP Bypass Inferior Vena Cava to Pulmonary Trunk with Synthetic Substitute, Open Approach
AHA CC: 4Q, 2017, 37-38

06100JQ Bypass Inferior Vena Cava to Right Pulmonary Artery with Synthetic Substitute, Open Approach

06100JR Bypass Inferior Vena Cava to Left Pulmonary Artery with Synthetic Substitute, Open Approach

06100JY Bypass Inferior Vena Cava to Lower Vein with Synthetic Substitute, Open Approach

06100K5 Bypass Inferior Vena Cava to Superior Mesenteric Vein with Nonautologous Tissue Substitute, Open Approach

06100K6 Bypass Inferior Vena Cava to Inferior Mesenteric Vein with Nonautologous Tissue Substitute, Open Approach

06100KP Bypass Inferior Vena Cava to Pulmonary Trunk with Nonautologous Tissue Substitute, Open Approach

06100KQ Bypass Inferior Vena Cava to Right Pulmonary Artery with Nonautologous Tissue Substitute, Open Approach

06100KR Bypass Inferior Vena Cava to Left Pulmonary Artery with Nonautologous Tissue Substitute, Open Approach

06100KY Bypass Inferior Vena Cava to Lower Vein with Nonautologous Tissue Substitute, Open Approach

06100Z5 Bypass Inferior Vena Cava to Superior Mesenteric Vein, Open Approach

06100Z6 Bypass Inferior Vena Cava to Inferior Mesenteric Vein, Open Approach

06100ZP Bypass Inferior Vena Cava to Pulmonary Trunk, Open Approach

06100ZQ Bypass Inferior Vena Cava to Right Pulmonary Artery, Open Approach

06100ZR Bypass Inferior Vena Cava to Left Pulmonary Artery, Open Approach

06100ZY Bypass Inferior Vena Cava to Lower Vein, Open Approach

0610475 Bypass Inferior Vena Cava to Superior Mesenteric Vein with Autologous Tissue Substitute, Percutaneous Endoscopic Approach

0610476 Bypass Inferior Vena Cava to Inferior Mesenteric Vein with Autologous Tissue Substitute, Percutaneous Endoscopic Approach

061047P Bypass Inferior Vena Cava to Pulmonary Trunk with Autologous Tissue Substitute, Percutaneous Endoscopic Approach

061047Q Bypass Inferior Vena Cava to Right Pulmonary Artery with Autologous Tissue Substitute, Percutaneous Endoscopic Approach

061047R Bypass Inferior Vena Cava to Left Pulmonary Artery with Autologous Tissue Substitute, Percutaneous Endoscopic Approach

061047Y Bypass Inferior Vena Cava to Lower Vein with Autologous Tissue Substitute, Percutaneous Endoscopic Approach

0610495 Bypass Inferior Vena Cava to Superior Mesenteric Vein with Autologous Venous Tissue, Percutaneous Endoscopic Approach

0610496 Bypass Inferior Vena Cava to Inferior Mesenteric Vein with Autologous Venous Tissue, Percutaneous Endoscopic Approach

061049P Bypass Inferior Vena Cava to Pulmonary Trunk with Autologous Venous Tissue, Percutaneous Endoscopic Approach

061049Q Bypass Inferior Vena Cava to Right Pulmonary Artery with Autologous Venous Tissue, Percutaneous Endoscopic Approach

061049R Bypass Inferior Vena Cava to Left Pulmonary Artery with Autologous Venous Tissue, Percutaneous Endoscopic Approach

061049Y Bypass Inferior Vena Cava to Lower Vein with Autologous Venous Tissue, Percutaneous Endoscopic Approach

06104A5 Bypass Inferior Vena Cava to Superior Mesenteric Vein with Autologous Arterial Tissue, Percutaneous Endoscopic Approach

06104A6 Bypass Inferior Vena Cava to Inferior Mesenteric Vein with Autologous Arterial Tissue, Percutaneous Endoscopic Approach

06104AP Bypass Inferior Vena Cava to Pulmonary Trunk with Autologous Arterial Tissue, Percutaneous Endoscopic Approach

06104AQ Bypass Inferior Vena Cava to Right Pulmonary Artery with Autologous Arterial Tissue, Percutaneous Endoscopic Approach

06104AR Bypass Inferior Vena Cava to Left Pulmonary Artery with Autologous Arterial Tissue, Percutaneous Endoscopic Approach

06104AY Bypass Inferior Vena Cava to Lower Vein with Autologous Arterial Tissue, Percutaneous Endoscopic Approach

06104J5 Bypass Inferior Vena Cava to Superior Mesenteric Vein with Synthetic Substitute, Percutaneous Endoscopic Approach

06104J6 Bypass Inferior Vena Cava to Inferior Mesenteric Vein with Synthetic Substitute, Percutaneous Endoscopic Approach

06104JP Bypass Inferior Vena Cava to Pulmonary Trunk with Synthetic Substitute, Percutaneous Endoscopic Approach

06104JQ Bypass Inferior Vena Cava to Right Pulmonary Artery with Synthetic Substitute, Percutaneous Endoscopic Approach

06104JR Bypass Inferior Vena Cava to Left Pulmonary Artery with Synthetic Substitute, Percutaneous Endoscopic Approach

06104JY Bypass Inferior Vena Cava to Lower Vein with Synthetic Substitute, Percutaneous Endoscopic Approach

06104K5 Bypass Inferior Vena Cava to Superior Mesenteric Vein with Nonautologous Tissue Substitute, Percutaneous Endoscopic Approach

06104K6 Bypass Inferior Vena Cava to Inferior Mesenteric Vein with Nonautologous Tissue Substitute, Percutaneous Endoscopic Approach

06104KP Bypass Inferior Vena Cava to Pulmonary Trunk with Nonautologous Tissue Substitute, Percutaneous Endoscopic Approach

06104KQ Bypass Inferior Vena Cava to Right Pulmonary Artery with Nonautologous Tissue Substitute, Percutaneous Endoscopic Approach

06104KR Bypass Inferior Vena Cava to Left Pulmonary Artery with Nonautologous Tissue Substitute, Percutaneous Endoscopic Approach

06104KY Bypass Inferior Vena Cava to Lower Vein with Nonautologous Tissue Substitute, Percutaneous Endoscopic Approach

06104Z5 Bypass Inferior Vena Cava to Superior Mesenteric Vein, Percutaneous Endoscopic Approach

06104Z6 Bypass Inferior Vena Cava to Inferior Mesenteric Vein, Percutaneous Endoscopic Approach

06104ZP Bypass Inferior Vena Cava to Pulmonary Trunk, Percutaneous Endoscopic Approach

06104ZQ Bypass Inferior Vena Cava to Right Pulmonary Artery, Percutaneous Endoscopic Approach

06104ZR Bypass Inferior Vena Cava to Left Pulmonary Artery, Percutaneous Endoscopic Approach

06104ZY Bypass Inferior Vena Cava to Lower Vein, Percutaneous Endoscopic Approach

0611079 Bypass Splenic Vein to Right Renal Vein with Autologous Tissue Substitute, Open Approach

061107B Bypass Splenic Vein to Left Renal Vein with Autologous Tissue Substitute, Open Approach

061107Y Bypass Splenic Vein to Lower Vein with Autologous Tissue Substitute, Open Approach

0611099 Bypass Splenic Vein to Right Renal Vein with Autologous Venous Tissue, Open Approach

061109B Bypass Splenic Vein to Left Renal Vein with Autologous Venous Tissue, Open Approach

061109Y Bypass Splenic Vein to Lower Vein with Autologous Venous Tissue, Open Approach

06110A9 Bypass Splenic Vein to Right Renal Vein with Autologous Arterial Tissue, Open Approach

06110AB Bypass Splenic Vein to Left Renal Vein with Autologous Arterial Tissue, Open Approach

06110AY Bypass Splenic Vein to Lower Vein with Autologous Arterial Tissue, Open Approach

06110J9 Bypass Splenic Vein to Right Renal Vein with Synthetic Substitute, Open Approach

06110JB Bypass Splenic Vein to Left Renal Vein with Synthetic Substitute, Open Approach

06110JY Bypass Splenic Vein to Lower Vein with Synthetic Substitute, Open Approach

06110K9 Bypass Splenic Vein to Right Renal Vein with Nonautologous Tissue Substitute, Open Approach

06110KB Bypass Splenic Vein to Left Renal Vein with Nonautologous Tissue Substitute, Open Approach

06110KY Bypass Splenic Vein to Lower Vein with Nonautologous Tissue Substitute, Open Approach

06110Z9 Bypass Splenic Vein to Right Renal Vein, Open Approach

06110ZB Bypass Splenic Vein to Left Renal Vein, Open Approach

06110ZY Bypass Splenic Vein to Lower Vein, Open Approach

0611479 Bypass Splenic Vein to Right Renal Vein with Autologous Tissue Substitute, Percutaneous Endoscopic Approach

061147B Bypass Splenic Vein to Left Renal Vein with Autologous Tissue Substitute, Percutaneous Endoscopic Approach

061147Y Bypass Splenic Vein to Lower Vein with Autologous Tissue Substitute, Percutaneous Endoscopic Approach

0611499 Bypass Splenic Vein to Right Renal Vein with Autologous Venous Tissue, Percutaneous Endoscopic Approach

061149B Bypass Splenic Vein to Left Renal Vein with Autologous Venous Tissue, Percutaneous Endoscopic Approach

061149Y Bypass Splenic Vein to Lower Vein with Autologous Venous Tissue, Percutaneous Endoscopic Approach

06114A9 Bypass Splenic Vein to Right Renal Vein with Autologous Arterial Tissue, Percutaneous Endoscopic Approach

06114AB Bypass Splenic Vein to Left Renal Vein with Autologous Arterial Tissue, Percutaneous Endoscopic Approach

06114AY Bypass Splenic Vein to Lower Vein with Autologous Arterial Tissue, Percutaneous Endoscopic Approach

06114J9 Bypass Splenic Vein to Right Renal Vein with Synthetic Substitute, Percutaneous Endoscopic Approach

06114JB Bypass Splenic Vein to Left Renal Vein with Synthetic Substitute, Percutaneous Endoscopic Approach

06114JY Bypass Splenic Vein to Lower Vein with Synthetic Substitute, Percutaneous Endoscopic Approach

06114K9 Bypass Splenic Vein to Right Renal Vein with Nonautologous Tissue Substitute, Percutaneous Endoscopic Approach

06114KB Bypass Splenic Vein to Left Renal Vein with Nonautologous Tissue Substitute, Percutaneous Endoscopic Approach

06114KY Bypass Splenic Vein to Lower Vein with Nonautologous Tissue Substitute, Percutaneous Endoscopic Approach

06114Z9 Bypass Splenic Vein to Right Renal Vein, Percutaneous Endoscopic Approach

06114ZB Bypass Splenic Vein to Left Renal Vein, Percutaneous Endoscopic Approach

06114ZY Bypass Splenic Vein to Lower Vein, Percutaneous Endoscopic Approach

061207Y Bypass Gastric Vein to Lower Vein with Autologous Tissue Substitute, Open Approach

061209Y Bypass Gastric Vein to Lower Vein with Autologous Venous Tissue, Open Approach

06120AY Bypass Gastric Vein to Lower Vein with Autologous Arterial Tissue, Open Approach

06120JY Bypass Gastric Vein to Lower Vein with Synthetic Substitute, Open Approach

06120KY Bypass Gastric Vein to Lower Vein with Nonautologous Tissue Substitute, Open Approach

06120ZY Bypass Gastric Vein to Lower Vein, Open Approach

061247Y Bypass Gastric Vein to Lower Vein with Autologous Tissue Substitute, Percutaneous Endoscopic Approach

061249Y Bypass Gastric Vein to Lower Vein with Autologous Venous Tissue, Percutaneous Endoscopic Approach

06124AY Bypass Gastric Vein to Lower Vein with Autologous Arterial Tissue, Percutaneous Endoscopic Approach

06124JY Bypass Gastric Vein to Lower Vein with Synthetic Substitute, Percutaneous Endoscopic Approach

06124KY Bypass Gastric Vein to Lower Vein with Nonautologous Tissue Substitute, Percutaneous Endoscopic Approach

06124ZY Bypass Gastric Vein to Lower Vein, Percutaneous Endoscopic Approach

061307Y Bypass Esophageal Vein to Lower Vein with Autologous Tissue Substitute, Open Approach

061309Y Bypass Esophageal Vein to Lower Vein with Autologous Venous Tissue, Open Approach

06130AY Bypass Esophageal Vein to Lower Vein with Autologous Arterial Tissue, Open Approach

06130JY Bypass Esophageal Vein to Lower Vein with Synthetic Substitute, Open Approach

06130KY Bypass Esophageal Vein to Lower Vein with Nonautologous Tissue Substitute, Open Approach

06130ZY Bypass Esophageal Vein to Lower Vein, Open Approach

061347Y Bypass Esophageal Vein to Lower Vein with Autologous Tissue Substitute, Percutaneous Endoscopic Approach

061349Y Bypass Esophageal Vein to Lower Vein with Autologous Venous Tissue, Percutaneous Endoscopic Approach

06134AY Bypass Esophageal Vein to Lower Vein with Autologous Arterial Tissue, Percutaneous Endoscopic Approach

06134JY Bypass Esophageal Vein to Lower Vein with Synthetic Substitute, Percutaneous Endoscopic Approach

06134KY Bypass Esophageal Vein to Lower Vein with Nonautologous Tissue Substitute, Percutaneous Endoscopic Approach

06134ZY Bypass Esophageal Vein to Lower Vein, Percutaneous Endoscopic Approach

061407Y Bypass Hepatic Vein to Lower Vein with Autologous Tissue Substitute, Open Approach

061409Y Bypass Hepatic Vein to Lower Vein with Autologous Venous Tissue, Open Approach

06140AY Bypass Hepatic Vein to Lower Vein with Autologous Arterial Tissue, Open Approach

06140JY Bypass Hepatic Vein to Lower Vein with Synthetic Substitute, Open Approach

06140KY Bypass Hepatic Vein to Lower Vein with Nonautologous Tissue Substitute, Open Approach

06140ZY Bypass Hepatic Vein to Lower Vein, Open Approach

061447Y Bypass Hepatic Vein to Lower Vein with Autologous Tissue Substitute, Percutaneous Endoscopic Approach

061449Y Bypass Hepatic Vein to Lower Vein with Autologous Venous Tissue, Percutaneous Endoscopic Approach

06144AY Bypass Hepatic Vein to Lower Vein with Autologous Arterial Tissue, Percutaneous Endoscopic Approach

06144JY Bypass Hepatic Vein to Lower Vein with Synthetic Substitute, Percutaneous Endoscopic Approach

06144KY Bypass Hepatic Vein to Lower Vein with Nonautologous Tissue Substitute, Percutaneous Endoscopic Approach

06144ZY Bypass Hepatic Vein to Lower Vein, Percutaneous Endoscopic Approach

061507Y Bypass Superior Mesenteric Vein to Lower Vein with Autologous Tissue Substitute, Open Approach

061509Y Bypass Superior Mesenteric Vein to Lower Vein with Autologous Venous Tissue, Open Approach

06150AY Bypass Superior Mesenteric Vein to Lower Vein with Autologous Arterial Tissue, Open Approach

06150JY Bypass Superior Mesenteric Vein to Lower Vein with Synthetic Substitute, Open Approach

06150KY Bypass Superior Mesenteric Vein to Lower Vein with Nonautologous Tissue Substitute, Open Approach

06150ZY Bypass Superior Mesenteric Vein to Lower Vein, Open Approach

061547Y Bypass Superior Mesenteric Vein to Lower Vein with Autologous Tissue Substitute, Percutaneous Endoscopic Approach

061549Y Bypass Superior Mesenteric Vein to Lower Vein with Autologous Venous Tissue, Percutaneous Endoscopic Approach

06154AY Bypass Superior Mesenteric Vein to Lower Vein with Autologous Arterial Tissue, Percutaneous Endoscopic Approach

06154JY Bypass Superior Mesenteric Vein to Lower Vein with Synthetic Substitute, Percutaneous Endoscopic Approach

06154KY Bypass Superior Mesenteric Vein to Lower Vein with Nonautologous Tissue Substitute, Percutaneous Endoscopic Approach

06154ZY Bypass Superior Mesenteric Vein to Lower Vein, Percutaneous Endoscopic Approach

061607Y Bypass Inferior Mesenteric Vein to Lower Vein with Autologous Tissue Substitute, Open Approach

♀ Female-only   ♂ Male-only   ▲ Limited Coverage   ● Non-OR   HAC HAC-associated procedure   ▲ Non-covered procedures   ✚ Cluster

061609Y Bypass Inferior Mesenteric Vein to Lower Vein with Autologous Venous Tissue, Open Approach

06160AY Bypass Inferior Mesenteric Vein to Lower Vein with Autologous Arterial Tissue, Open Approach

06160JY Bypass Inferior Mesenteric Vein to Lower Vein with Synthetic Substitute, Open Approach

06160KY Bypass Inferior Mesenteric Vein to Lower Vein with Nonautologous Tissue Substitute, Open Approach

06160ZY Bypass Inferior Mesenteric Vein to Lower Vein, Open Approach

061647Y Bypass Inferior Mesenteric Vein to Lower Vein with Autologous Tissue Substitute, Percutaneous Endoscopic Approach

061649Y Bypass Inferior Mesenteric Vein to Lower Vein with Autologous Venous Tissue, Percutaneous Endoscopic Approach

06164AY Bypass Inferior Mesenteric Vein to Lower Vein with Autologous Arterial Tissue, Percutaneous Endoscopic Approach

06164JY Bypass Inferior Mesenteric Vein to Lower Vein with Synthetic Substitute, Percutaneous Endoscopic Approach

06164KY Bypass Inferior Mesenteric Vein to Lower Vein with Nonautologous Tissue Substitute, Percutaneous Endoscopic Approach

06164ZY Bypass Inferior Mesenteric Vein to Lower Vein, Percutaneous Endoscopic Approach

061707Y Bypass Colic Vein to Lower Vein with Autologous Tissue Substitute, Open Approach

061709Y Bypass Colic Vein to Lower Vein with Autologous Venous Tissue, Open Approach

06170AY Bypass Colic Vein to Lower Vein with Autologous Arterial Tissue, Open Approach

06170JY Bypass Colic Vein to Lower Vein with Synthetic Substitute, Open Approach

06170KY Bypass Colic Vein to Lower Vein with Nonautologous Tissue Substitute, Open Approach

06170ZY Bypass Colic Vein to Lower Vein, Open Approach

061747Y Bypass Colic Vein to Lower Vein with Autologous Tissue Substitute, Percutaneous Endoscopic Approach

061749Y Bypass Colic Vein to Lower Vein with Autologous Venous Tissue, Percutaneous Endoscopic Approach

06174AY Bypass Colic Vein to Lower Vein with Autologous Arterial Tissue, Percutaneous Endoscopic Approach

06174JY Bypass Colic Vein to Lower Vein with Synthetic Substitute, Percutaneous Endoscopic Approach

06174KY Bypass Colic Vein to Lower Vein with Nonautologous Tissue Substitute, Percutaneous Endoscopic Approach

06174ZY Bypass Colic Vein to Lower Vein, Percutaneous Endoscopic Approach

0618079 Bypass Portal Vein to Right Renal Vein with Autologous Tissue Substitute, Open Approach

061807B Bypass Portal Vein to Left Renal Vein with Autologous Tissue Substitute, Open Approach

061807Y Bypass Portal Vein to Lower Vein with Autologous Tissue Substitute, Open Approach

0618099 Bypass Portal Vein to Right Renal Vein with Autologous Venous Tissue, Open Approach

061809B Bypass Portal Vein to Left Renal Vein with Autologous Venous Tissue, Open Approach

061809Y Bypass Portal Vein to Lower Vein with Autologous Venous Tissue, Open Approach

06180A9 Bypass Portal Vein to Right Renal Vein with Autologous Arterial Tissue, Open Approach

06180AB Bypass Portal Vein to Left Renal Vein with Autologous Arterial Tissue, Open Approach

06180AY Bypass Portal Vein to Lower Vein with Autologous Arterial Tissue, Open Approach

06180J9 Bypass Portal Vein to Right Renal Vein with Synthetic Substitute, Open Approach

06180JB Bypass Portal Vein to Left Renal Vein with Synthetic Substitute, Open Approach

06180JY Bypass Portal Vein to Lower Vein with Synthetic Substitute, Open Approach

06180K9 Bypass Portal Vein to Right Renal Vein with Nonautologous Tissue Substitute, Open Approach

06180KB Bypass Portal Vein to Left Renal Vein with Nonautologous Tissue Substitute, Open Approach

06180KY Bypass Portal Vein to Lower Vein with Nonautologous Tissue Substitute, Open Approach

06180Z9 Bypass Portal Vein to Right Renal Vein, Open Approach

06180ZB Bypass Portal Vein to Left Renal Vein, Open Approach

06180ZY Bypass Portal Vein to Lower Vein, Open Approach

06183J4 Bypass Portal Vein to Hepatic Vein with Synthetic Substitute, Percutaneous Approach

06183JY Bypass Portal Vein to Lower Vein with Synthetic Substitute, Percutaneous Approach

06184J4 Bypass Portal Vein to Hepatic Vein with Synthetic Substitute, Percutaneous Endoscopic Approach

0618479 Bypass Portal Vein to Right Renal Vein with Autologous Tissue Substitute, Percutaneous Endoscopic Approach

061847B Bypass Portal Vein to Left Renal Vein with Autologous Tissue Substitute, Percutaneous Endoscopic Approach

061847Y Bypass Portal Vein to Lower Vein with Autologous Tissue Substitute, Percutaneous Endoscopic Approach

0618499 Bypass Portal Vein to Right Renal Vein with Autologous Venous Tissue, Percutaneous Endoscopic Approach

061849B Bypass Portal Vein to Left Renal Vein with Autologous Venous Tissue, Percutaneous Endoscopic Approach

061849Y Bypass Portal Vein to Lower Vein with Autologous Venous Tissue, Percutaneous Endoscopic Approach

06184A9 Bypass Portal Vein to Right Renal Vein with Autologous Arterial Tissue, Percutaneous Endoscopic Approach

06184AB Bypass Portal Vein to Left Renal Vein with Autologous Arterial Tissue, Percutaneous Endoscopic Approach

06184AY Bypass Portal Vein to Lower Vein with Autologous Arterial Tissue, Percutaneous Endoscopic Approach

06184J9 Bypass Portal Vein to Right Renal Vein with Synthetic Substitute, Percutaneous Endoscopic Approach

06184JB Bypass Portal Vein to Left Renal Vein with Synthetic Substitute, Percutaneous Endoscopic Approach

06184JY Bypass Portal Vein to Lower Vein with Synthetic Substitute, Percutaneous Endoscopic Approach

06184K9 Bypass Portal Vein to Right Renal Vein with Nonautologous Tissue Substitute, Percutaneous Endoscopic Approach

06184KB Bypass Portal Vein to Left Renal Vein with Nonautologous Tissue Substitute, Percutaneous Endoscopic Approach

06184KY Bypass Portal Vein to Lower Vein with Nonautologous Tissue Substitute, Percutaneous Endoscopic Approach

06184Z9 Bypass Portal Vein to Right Renal Vein, Percutaneous Endoscopic Approach

06184ZB Bypass Portal Vein to Left Renal Vein, Percutaneous Endoscopic Approach

06184ZY Bypass Portal Vein to Lower Vein, Percutaneous Endoscopic Approach

061907Y Bypass Right Renal Vein to Lower Vein with Autologous Tissue Substitute, Open Approach

061909Y Bypass Right Renal Vein to Lower Vein with Autologous Venous Tissue, Open Approach

06190AY Bypass Right Renal Vein to Lower Vein with Autologous Arterial Tissue, Open Approach

06190JY Bypass Right Renal Vein to Lower Vein with Synthetic Substitute, Open Approach

06190KY Bypass Right Renal Vein to Lower Vein with Nonautologous Tissue Substitute, Open Approach

06190ZY Bypass Right Renal Vein to Lower Vein, Open Approach

061947Y Bypass Right Renal Vein to Lower Vein with Autologous Tissue Substitute, Percutaneous Endoscopic Approach

061949Y Bypass Right Renal Vein to Lower Vein with Autologous Venous Tissue, Percutaneous Endoscopic Approach

06194AY Bypass Right Renal Vein to Lower Vein with Autologous Arterial Tissue, Percutaneous Endoscopic Approach

06194JY Bypass Right Renal Vein to Lower Vein with Synthetic Substitute, Percutaneous Endoscopic Approach

06194KY Bypass Right Renal Vein to Lower Vein with Nonautologous Tissue Substitute, Percutaneous Endoscopic Approach

06194ZY Bypass Right Renal Vein to Lower Vein, Percutaneous Endoscopic Approach

061B07Y Bypass Left Renal Vein to Lower Vein with Autologous Tissue Substitute, Open Approach

061B09Y Bypass Left Renal Vein to Lower Vein with Autologous Venous Tissue, Open Approach

061B0AY Bypass Left Renal Vein to Lower Vein with Autologous Arterial Tissue, Open Approach

061B0JY Bypass Left Renal Vein to Lower Vein with Synthetic Substitute, Open Approach

061B0KY Bypass Left Renal Vein to Lower Vein with Nonautologous Tissue Substitute, Open Approach

061B0ZY Bypass Left Renal Vein to Lower Vein, Open Approach

061B47Y Bypass Left Renal Vein to Lower Vein with Autologous Tissue Substitute, Percutaneous Endoscopic Approach

061B49Y Bypass Left Renal Vein to Lower Vein with Autologous Venous Tissue, Percutaneous Endoscopic Approach

061B4AY Bypass Left Renal Vein to Lower Vein with Autologous Arterial Tissue, Percutaneous Endoscopic Approach

061B4JY Bypass Left Renal Vein to Lower Vein with Synthetic Substitute, Percutaneous Endoscopic Approach

061B4KY Bypass Left Renal Vein to Lower Vein with Nonautologous Tissue Substitute, Percutaneous Endoscopic Approach

061B4ZY Bypass Left Renal Vein to Lower Vein, Percutaneous Endoscopic Approach

061C07Y Bypass Right Common Iliac Vein to Lower Vein with Autologous Tissue Substitute, Open Approach

061C09Y Bypass Right Common Iliac Vein to Lower Vein with Autologous Venous Tissue, Open Approach

061C0AY Bypass Right Common Iliac Vein to Lower Vein with Autologous Arterial Tissue, Open Approach

061C0JY Bypass Right Common Iliac Vein to Lower Vein with Synthetic Substitute, Open Approach

061C0KY Bypass Right Common Iliac Vein to Lower Vein with Nonautologous Tissue Substitute, Open Approach

061C0ZY Bypass Right Common Iliac Vein to Lower Vein, Open Approach

061C47Y Bypass Right Common Iliac Vein to Lower Vein with Autologous Tissue Substitute, Percutaneous Endoscopic Approach

061C49Y Bypass Right Common Iliac Vein to Lower Vein with Autologous Venous Tissue, Percutaneous Endoscopic Approach

061C4AY Bypass Right Common Iliac Vein to Lower Vein with Autologous Arterial Tissue, Percutaneous Endoscopic Approach

061C4JY Bypass Right Common Iliac Vein to Lower Vein with Synthetic Substitute, Percutaneous Endoscopic Approach

061C4KY Bypass Right Common Iliac Vein to Lower Vein with Nonautologous Tissue Substitute, Percutaneous Endoscopic Approach

061C4ZY Bypass Right Common Iliac Vein to Lower Vein, Percutaneous Endoscopic Approach

061D07Y Bypass Left Common Iliac Vein to Lower Vein with Autologous Tissue Substitute, Open Approach

061D09Y Bypass Left Common Iliac Vein to Lower Vein with Autologous Venous Tissue, Open Approach

061D0AY Bypass Left Common Iliac Vein to Lower Vein with Autologous Arterial Tissue, Open Approach

061D0JY Bypass Left Common Iliac Vein to Lower Vein with Synthetic Substitute, Open Approach

061D0KY Bypass Left Common Iliac Vein to Lower Vein with Nonautologous Tissue Substitute, Open Approach

061D0ZY Bypass Left Common Iliac Vein to Lower Vein, Open Approach

061D47Y Bypass Left Common Iliac Vein to Lower Vein with Autologous Tissue Substitute, Percutaneous Endoscopic Approach

061D49Y Bypass Left Common Iliac Vein to Lower Vein with Autologous Venous Tissue, Percutaneous Endoscopic Approach

061D4AY Bypass Left Common Iliac Vein to Lower Vein with Autologous Arterial Tissue, Percutaneous Endoscopic Approach

061D4JY Bypass Left Common Iliac Vein to Lower Vein with Synthetic Substitute, Percutaneous Endoscopic Approach

061D4KY Bypass Left Common Iliac Vein to Lower Vein with Nonautologous Tissue Substitute, Percutaneous Endoscopic Approach

061D4ZY Bypass Left Common Iliac Vein to Lower Vein, Percutaneous Endoscopic Approach

061F07Y Bypass Right External Iliac Vein to Lower Vein with Autologous Tissue Substitute, Open Approach

061F09Y Bypass Right External Iliac Vein to Lower Vein with Autologous Venous Tissue, Open Approach

061F0AY Bypass Right External Iliac Vein to Lower Vein with Autologous Arterial Tissue, Open Approach

061F0JY Bypass Right External Iliac Vein to Lower Vein with Synthetic Substitute, Open Approach

061F0KY Bypass Right External Iliac Vein to Lower Vein with Nonautologous Tissue Substitute, Open Approach

061F0ZY Bypass Right External Iliac Vein to Lower Vein, Open Approach

061F47Y Bypass Right External Iliac Vein to Lower Vein with Autologous Tissue Substitute, Percutaneous Endoscopic Approach

061F49Y Bypass Right External Iliac Vein to Lower Vein with Autologous Venous Tissue, Percutaneous Endoscopic Approach

061F4AY Bypass Right External Iliac Vein to Lower Vein with Autologous Arterial Tissue, Percutaneous Endoscopic Approach

061F4JY Bypass Right External Iliac Vein to Lower Vein with Synthetic Substitute, Percutaneous Endoscopic Approach

061F4KY Bypass Right External Iliac Vein to Lower Vein with Nonautologous Tissue Substitute, Percutaneous Endoscopic Approach

061F4ZY Bypass Right External Iliac Vein to Lower Vein, Percutaneous Endoscopic Approach

061G07Y Bypass Left External Iliac Vein to Lower Vein with Autologous Tissue Substitute, Open Approach

061G09Y Bypass Left External Iliac Vein to Lower Vein with Autologous Venous Tissue, Open Approach

061G0AY Bypass Left External Iliac Vein to Lower Vein with Autologous Arterial Tissue, Open Approach

061G0JY Bypass Left External Iliac Vein to Lower Vein with Synthetic Substitute, Open Approach

061G0KY Bypass Left External Iliac Vein to Lower Vein with Nonautologous Tissue Substitute, Open Approach

061G0ZY Bypass Left External Iliac Vein to Lower Vein, Open Approach

061G47Y Bypass Left External Iliac Vein to Lower Vein with Autologous Tissue Substitute, Percutaneous Endoscopic Approach

061G49Y Bypass Left External Iliac Vein to Lower Vein with Autologous Venous Tissue, Percutaneous Endoscopic Approach

061G4AY Bypass Left External Iliac Vein to Lower Vein with Autologous Arterial Tissue, Percutaneous Endoscopic Approach

061G4JY Bypass Left External Iliac Vein to Lower Vein with Synthetic Substitute, Percutaneous Endoscopic Approach

061G4KY Bypass Left External Iliac Vein to Lower Vein with Nonautologous Tissue Substitute, Percutaneous Endoscopic Approach

061G4ZY Bypass Left External Iliac Vein to Lower Vein, Percutaneous Endoscopic Approach

061H07Y Bypass Right Hypogastric Vein to Lower Vein with Autologous Tissue Substitute, Open Approach

061H09Y Bypass Right Hypogastric Vein to Lower Vein with Autologous Venous Tissue, Open Approach

061H0AY Bypass Right Hypogastric Vein to Lower Vein with Autologous Arterial Tissue, Open Approach

061H0JY Bypass Right Hypogastric Vein to Lower Vein with Synthetic Substitute, Open Approach

061H0KY Bypass Right Hypogastric Vein to Lower Vein with Nonautologous Tissue Substitute, Open Approach

061H0ZY Bypass Right Hypogastric Vein to Lower Vein, Open Approach

061H47Y Bypass Right Hypogastric Vein to Lower Vein with Autologous Tissue Substitute, Percutaneous Endoscopic Approach

061H49Y Bypass Right Hypogastric Vein to Lower Vein with Autologous Venous Tissue, Percutaneous Endoscopic Approach

061H4AY Bypass Right Hypogastric Vein to Lower Vein with Autologous Arterial Tissue, Percutaneous Endoscopic Approach

061H4JY Bypass Right Hypogastric Vein to Lower Vein with Synthetic Substitute, Percutaneous Endoscopic Approach

061H4KY Bypass Right Hypogastric Vein to Lower Vein with Nonautologous Tissue Substitute, Percutaneous Endoscopic Approach

061H4ZY Bypass Right Hypogastric Vein to Lower Vein, Percutaneous Endoscopic Approach

061J07Y Bypass Left Hypogastric Vein to Lower Vein with Autologous Tissue Substitute, Open Approach

061J09Y Bypass Left Hypogastric Vein to Lower Vein with Autologous Venous Tissue, Open Approach

061J0AY Bypass Left Hypogastric Vein to Lower Vein with Autologous Arterial Tissue, Open Approach

♀ Female-only   ♂ Male-only   ▲ Limited Coverage   ● Non-OR   HAC HAC-associated procedure   ▲ Non-covered procedures   ✚ Cluster

061J0JY Bypass Left Hypogastric Vein to Lower Vein with Synthetic Substitute, Open Approach

061J0KY Bypass Left Hypogastric Vein to Lower Vein with Nonautologous Tissue Substitute, Open Approach

061J0ZY Bypass Left Hypogastric Vein to Lower Vein, Open Approach

061J47Y Bypass Left Hypogastric Vein to Lower Vein with Autologous Tissue Substitute, Percutaneous Endoscopic Approach

061J49Y Bypass Left Hypogastric Vein to Lower Vein with Autologous Venous Tissue, Percutaneous Endoscopic Approach

061J4AY Bypass Left Hypogastric Vein to Lower Vein with Autologous Arterial Tissue, Percutaneous Endoscopic Approach

061J4JY Bypass Left Hypogastric Vein to Lower Vein with Synthetic Substitute, Percutaneous Endoscopic Approach

061J4KY Bypass Left Hypogastric Vein to Lower Vein with Nonautologous Tissue Substitute, Percutaneous Endoscopic Approach

061J4ZY Bypass Left Hypogastric Vein to Lower Vein, Percutaneous Endoscopic Approach

061M07Y Bypass Right Femoral Vein to Lower Vein with Autologous Tissue Substitute, Open Approach

061M09Y Bypass Right Femoral Vein to Lower Vein with Autologous Venous Tissue, Open Approach

061M0AY Bypass Right Femoral Vein to Lower Vein with Autologous Arterial Tissue, Open Approach

061M0JY Bypass Right Femoral Vein to Lower Vein with Synthetic Substitute, Open Approach

061M0KY Bypass Right Femoral Vein to Lower Vein with Nonautologous Tissue Substitute, Open Approach

061M0ZY Bypass Right Femoral Vein to Lower Vein, Open Approach

061M47Y Bypass Right Femoral Vein to Lower Vein with Autologous Tissue Substitute, Percutaneous Endoscopic Approach

061M49Y Bypass Right Femoral Vein to Lower Vein with Autologous Venous Tissue, Percutaneous Endoscopic Approach

061M4AY Bypass Right Femoral Vein to Lower Vein with Autologous Arterial Tissue, Percutaneous Endoscopic Approach

061M4JY Bypass Right Femoral Vein to Lower Vein with Synthetic Substitute, Percutaneous Endoscopic Approach

061M4KY Bypass Right Femoral Vein to Lower Vein with Nonautologous Tissue Substitute, Percutaneous Endoscopic Approach

061M4ZY Bypass Right Femoral Vein to Lower Vein, Percutaneous Endoscopic Approach

061N07Y Bypass Left Femoral Vein to Lower Vein with Autologous Tissue Substitute, Open Approach

061N09Y Bypass Left Femoral Vein to Lower Vein with Autologous Venous Tissue, Open Approach

061N0AY Bypass Left Femoral Vein to Lower Vein with Autologous Arterial Tissue, Open Approach

061N0JY Bypass Left Femoral Vein to Lower Vein with Synthetic Substitute, Open Approach

061N0KY Bypass Left Femoral Vein to Lower Vein with Nonautologous Tissue Substitute, Open Approach

061N0ZY Bypass Left Femoral Vein to Lower Vein, Open Approach

061N47Y Bypass Left Femoral Vein to Lower Vein with Autologous Tissue Substitute, Percutaneous Endoscopic Approach

061N49Y Bypass Left Femoral Vein to Lower Vein with Autologous Venous Tissue, Percutaneous Endoscopic Approach

061N4AY Bypass Left Femoral Vein to Lower Vein with Autologous Arterial Tissue, Percutaneous Endoscopic Approach

061N4JY Bypass Left Femoral Vein to Lower Vein with Synthetic Substitute, Percutaneous Endoscopic Approach

061N4KY Bypass Left Femoral Vein to Lower Vein with Nonautologous Tissue Substitute, Percutaneous Endoscopic Approach

061N4ZY Bypass Left Femoral Vein to Lower Vein, Percutaneous Endoscopic Approach

061P07Y Bypass Right Saphenous Vein to Lower Vein with Autologous Tissue Substitute, Open Approach

061P09Y Bypass Right Saphenous Vein to Lower Vein with Autologous Venous Tissue, Open Approach

061P0AY Bypass Right Saphenous Vein to Lower Vein with Autologous Arterial Tissue, Open Approach

061P0JY Bypass Right Saphenous Vein to Lower Vein with Synthetic Substitute, Open Approach

061P0KY Bypass Right Saphenous Vein to Lower Vein with Nonautologous Tissue Substitute, Open Approach

061P0ZY Bypass Right Saphenous Vein to Lower Vein, Open Approach

061P47Y Bypass Right Saphenous Vein to Lower Vein with Autologous Tissue Substitute, Percutaneous Endoscopic Approach

061P49Y Bypass Right Saphenous Vein to Lower Vein with Autologous Venous Tissue, Percutaneous Endoscopic Approach

061P4AY Bypass Right Saphenous Vein to Lower Vein with Autologous Arterial Tissue, Percutaneous Endoscopic Approach

061P4JY Bypass Right Saphenous Vein to Lower Vein with Synthetic Substitute, Percutaneous Endoscopic Approach

061P4KY Bypass Right Saphenous Vein to Lower Vein with Nonautologous Tissue Substitute, Percutaneous Endoscopic Approach

061P4ZY Bypass Right Saphenous Vein to Lower Vein, Percutaneous Endoscopic Approach

061Q07Y Bypass Left Saphenous Vein to Lower Vein with Autologous Tissue Substitute, Open Approach

061Q09Y Bypass Left Saphenous Vein to Lower Vein with Autologous Venous Tissue, Open Approach

061Q0AY Bypass Left Saphenous Vein to Lower Vein with Autologous Arterial Tissue, Open Approach

061Q0JY Bypass Left Saphenous Vein to Lower Vein with Synthetic Substitute, Open Approach

061Q0KY Bypass Left Saphenous Vein to Lower Vein with Nonautologous Tissue Substitute, Open Approach

061Q0ZY Bypass Left Saphenous Vein to Lower Vein, Open Approach

061Q47Y Bypass Left Saphenous Vein to Lower Vein with Autologous Tissue Substitute, Percutaneous Endoscopic Approach

061Q49Y Bypass Left Saphenous Vein to Lower Vein with Autologous Venous Tissue, Percutaneous Endoscopic Approach

061Q4AY Bypass Left Saphenous Vein to Lower Vein with Autologous Arterial Tissue, Percutaneous Endoscopic Approach

061Q4JY Bypass Left Saphenous Vein to Lower Vein with Synthetic Substitute, Percutaneous Endoscopic Approach

061Q4KY Bypass Left Saphenous Vein to Lower Vein with Nonautologous Tissue Substitute, Percutaneous Endoscopic Approach

061Q4ZY Bypass Left Saphenous Vein to Lower Vein, Percutaneous Endoscopic Approach

061T07Y Bypass Right Foot Vein to Lower Vein with Autologous Tissue Substitute, Open Approach

061T09Y Bypass Right Foot Vein to Lower Vein with Autologous Venous Tissue, Open Approach

061T0AY Bypass Right Foot Vein to Lower Vein with Autologous Arterial Tissue, Open Approach

061T0JY Bypass Right Foot Vein to Lower Vein with Synthetic Substitute, Open Approach

061T0KY Bypass Right Foot Vein to Lower Vein with Nonautologous Tissue Substitute, Open Approach

061T0ZY Bypass Right Foot Vein to Lower Vein, Open Approach

061T47Y Bypass Right Foot Vein to Lower Vein with Autologous Tissue Substitute, Percutaneous Endoscopic Approach

061T49Y Bypass Right Foot Vein to Lower Vein with Autologous Venous Tissue, Percutaneous Endoscopic Approach

061T4AY Bypass Right Foot Vein to Lower Vein with Autologous Arterial Tissue, Percutaneous Endoscopic Approach

061T4JY Bypass Right Foot Vein to Lower Vein with Synthetic Substitute, Percutaneous Endoscopic Approach

061T4KY Bypass Right Foot Vein to Lower Vein with Nonautologous Tissue Substitute, Percutaneous Endoscopic Approach

061T4ZY Bypass Right Foot Vein to Lower Vein, Percutaneous Endoscopic Approach

061V07Y Bypass Left Foot Vein to Lower Vein with Autologous Tissue Substitute, Open Approach

061V09Y Bypass Left Foot Vein to Lower Vein with Autologous Venous Tissue, Open Approach

061V0AY Bypass Left Foot Vein to Lower Vein with Autologous Arterial Tissue, Open Approach

061V0JY Bypass Left Foot Vein to Lower Vein with Synthetic Substitute, Open Approach

061V0KY Bypass Left Foot Vein to Lower Vein with Nonautologous Tissue Substitute, Open Approach

061V0ZY Bypass Left Foot Vein to Lower Vein, Open Approach

061V47Y	Bypass Left Foot Vein to Lower Vein with Autologous Tissue Substitute, Percutaneous Endoscopic Approach	061V4AY	Bypass Left Foot Vein to Lower Vein with Autologous Arterial Tissue, Percutaneous Endoscopic Approach	061V4KY	Bypass Left Foot Vein to Lower Vein with Nonautologous Tissue Substitute, Percutaneous Endoscopic Approach
061V49Y	Bypass Left Foot Vein to Lower Vein with Autologous Venous Tissue, Percutaneous Endoscopic Approach	061V4JY	Bypass Left Foot Vein to Lower Vein with Synthetic Substitute, Percutaneous Endoscopic Approach	061V4ZY	Bypass Left Foot Vein to Lower Vein, Percutaneous Endoscopic Approach

065 – Lower Veins, Destruction

06500ZZ	Destruction of Inferior Vena Cava, Open Approach	06583ZZ	Destruction of Portal Vein, Percutaneous Approach	065J4ZZ	Destruction of Left Hypogastric Vein, Percutaneous Endoscopic Approach
06503ZZ	Destruction of Inferior Vena Cava, Percutaneous Approach	06584ZZ	Destruction of Portal Vein, Percutaneous Endoscopic Approach	065M0ZZ	Destruction of Right Femoral Vein, Open Approach
06504ZZ	Destruction of Inferior Vena Cava, Percutaneous Endoscopic Approach	06590ZZ	Destruction of Right Renal Vein, Open Approach	065M3ZZ	Destruction of Right Femoral Vein, Percutaneous Approach
06510ZZ	Destruction of Splenic Vein, Open Approach	06593ZZ	Destruction of Right Renal Vein, Percutaneous Approach	065M4ZZ	Destruction of Right Femoral Vein, Percutaneous Endoscopic Approach
06513ZZ	Destruction of Splenic Vein, Percutaneous Approach	06594ZZ	Destruction of Right Renal Vein, Percutaneous Endoscopic Approach	065N0ZZ	Destruction of Left Femoral Vein, Open Approach
06514ZZ	Destruction of Splenic Vein, Percutaneous Endoscopic Approach	065B0ZZ	Destruction of Left Renal Vein, Open Approach	065N3ZZ	Destruction of Left Femoral Vein, Percutaneous Approach
06520ZZ	Destruction of Gastric Vein, Open Approach	065B3ZZ	Destruction of Left Renal Vein, Percutaneous Approach	065N4ZZ	Destruction of Left Femoral Vein, Percutaneous Endoscopic Approach
06523ZZ	Destruction of Gastric Vein, Percutaneous Approach	065B4ZZ	Destruction of Left Renal Vein, Percutaneous Endoscopic Approach	065P0ZZ	Destruction of Right Saphenous Vein, Open Approach
06524ZZ	Destruction of Gastric Vein, Percutaneous Endoscopic Approach	065C0ZZ	Destruction of Right Common Iliac Vein, Open Approach	065P3ZZ	Destruction of Right Saphenous Vein, Percutaneous Approach
06530ZZ	Destruction of Esophageal Vein, Open Approach	065C3ZZ	Destruction of Right Common Iliac Vein, Percutaneous Approach	065P4ZZ	Destruction of Right Saphenous Vein, Percutaneous Endoscopic Approach
06533ZZ	Destruction of Esophageal Vein, Percutaneous Approach	065C4ZZ	Destruction of Right Common Iliac Vein, Percutaneous Endoscopic Approach	065Q0ZZ	Destruction of Left Saphenous Vein, Open Approach
06534ZZ	Destruction of Esophageal Vein, Percutaneous Endoscopic Approach	065D0ZZ	Destruction of Left Common Iliac Vein, Open Approach	065Q3ZZ	Destruction of Left Saphenous Vein, Percutaneous Approach
06540ZZ	Destruction of Hepatic Vein, Open Approach	065D3ZZ	Destruction of Left Common Iliac Vein, Percutaneous Approach	065Q4ZZ	Destruction of Left Saphenous Vein, Percutaneous Endoscopic Approach
06543ZZ	Destruction of Hepatic Vein, Percutaneous Approach	065D4ZZ	Destruction of Left Common Iliac Vein, Percutaneous Endoscopic Approach	065T0ZZ	Destruction of Right Foot Vein, Open Approach
06544ZZ	Destruction of Hepatic Vein, Percutaneous Endoscopic Approach	065F0ZZ	Destruction of Right External Iliac Vein, Open Approach	065T3ZZ	Destruction of Right Foot Vein, Percutaneous Approach
06550ZZ	Destruction of Superior Mesenteric Vein, Open Approach	065F3ZZ	Destruction of Right External Iliac Vein, Percutaneous Approach	065T4ZZ	Destruction of Right Foot Vein, Percutaneous Endoscopic Approach
06553ZZ	Destruction of Superior Mesenteric Vein, Percutaneous Approach	065F4ZZ	Destruction of Right External Iliac Vein, Percutaneous Endoscopic Approach	065V0ZZ	Destruction of Left Foot Vein, Open Approach
06554ZZ	Destruction of Superior Mesenteric Vein, Percutaneous Endoscopic Approach	065G0ZZ	Destruction of Left External Iliac Vein, Open Approach	065V3ZZ	Destruction of Left Foot Vein, Percutaneous Approach
06560ZZ	Destruction of Inferior Mesenteric Vein, Open Approach	065G3ZZ	Destruction of Left External Iliac Vein, Percutaneous Approach	065V4ZZ	Destruction of Left Foot Vein, Percutaneous Endoscopic Approach
06563ZZ	Destruction of Inferior Mesenteric Vein, Percutaneous Approach	065G4ZZ	Destruction of Left External Iliac Vein, Percutaneous Endoscopic Approach	065Y0ZC	Destruction of Hemorrhoidal Plexus, Open Approach
06564ZZ	Destruction of Inferior Mesenteric Vein, Percutaneous Endoscopic Approach	065H0ZZ	Destruction of Right Hypogastric Vein, Open Approach	065Y0ZZ	Destruction of Lower Vein, Open Approach
06570ZZ	Destruction of Colic Vein, Open Approach	065H3ZZ	Destruction of Right Hypogastric Vein, Percutaneous Approach	065Y3ZC	Destruction of Hemorrhoidal Plexus, Percutaneous Approach
06573ZZ	Destruction of Colic Vein, Percutaneous Approach	065H4ZZ	Destruction of Right Hypogastric Vein, Percutaneous Endoscopic Approach	065Y3ZZ	Destruction of Lower Vein, Percutaneous Approach
06574ZZ	Destruction of Colic Vein, Percutaneous Endoscopic Approach	065J0ZZ	Destruction of Left Hypogastric Vein, Open Approach	065Y4ZC	Destruction of Hemorrhoidal Plexus, Percutaneous Endoscopic Approach
06580ZZ	Destruction of Portal Vein, Open Approach	065J3ZZ	Destruction of Left Hypogastric Vein, Percutaneous Approach	065Y4ZZ	Destruction of Lower Vein, Percutaneous Endoscopic Approach

067 – Lower Veins, Dilation

06700DZ	Dilation of Inferior Vena Cava with Intraluminal Device, Open Approach	06704ZZ	Dilation of Inferior Vena Cava, Percutaneous Endoscopic Approach	06714DZ	Dilation of Splenic Vein with Intraluminal Device, Percutaneous Endoscopic Approach
06700ZZ	Dilation of Inferior Vena Cava, Open Approach	06710DZ	Dilation of Splenic Vein with Intraluminal Device, Open Approach	06714ZZ	Dilation of Splenic Vein, Percutaneous Endoscopic Approach
06703DZ	Dilation of Inferior Vena Cava with Intraluminal Device, Percutaneous Approach	06710ZZ	Dilation of Splenic Vein, Open Approach	06720DZ	Dilation of Gastric Vein with Intraluminal Device, Open Approach
06703ZZ	Dilation of Inferior Vena Cava, Percutaneous Approach	06713DZ	Dilation of Splenic Vein with Intraluminal Device, Percutaneous Approach	06720ZZ	Dilation of Gastric Vein, Open Approach
06704DZ	Dilation of Inferior Vena Cava with Intraluminal Device, Percutaneous Endoscopic Approach	06713ZZ	Dilation of Splenic Vein, Percutaneous Approach	06723DZ	Dilation of Gastric Vein with Intraluminal Device, Percutaneous Approach

♀ Female-only   ♂ Male-only   ▲ Limited Coverage   ● Non-OR   HAC HAC-associated procedure   ▲ Non-covered procedures   ✚ Cluster

06723ZZ Dilation of Gastric Vein, Percutaneous Approach

06724DZ Dilation of Gastric Vein with Intraluminal Device, Percutaneous Endoscopic Approach

06724ZZ Dilation of Gastric Vein, Percutaneous Endoscopic Approach

06730DZ Dilation of Esophageal Vein with Intraluminal Device, Open Approach

06730ZZ Dilation of Esophageal Vein, Open Approach

06733DZ Dilation of Esophageal Vein with Intraluminal Device, Percutaneous Approach

06733ZZ Dilation of Esophageal Vein, Percutaneous Approach

06734DZ Dilation of Esophageal Vein with Intraluminal Device, Percutaneous Endoscopic Approach

06734ZZ Dilation of Esophageal Vein, Percutaneous Endoscopic Approach

06740DZ Dilation of Hepatic Vein with Intraluminal Device, Open Approach

06740ZZ Dilation of Hepatic Vein, Open Approach

06743DZ Dilation of Hepatic Vein with Intraluminal Device, Percutaneous Approach

06743ZZ Dilation of Hepatic Vein, Percutaneous Approach

06744DZ Dilation of Hepatic Vein with Intraluminal Device, Percutaneous Endoscopic Approach

06744ZZ Dilation of Hepatic Vein, Percutaneous Endoscopic Approach

06750DZ Dilation of Superior Mesenteric Vein with Intraluminal Device, Open Approach

06750ZZ Dilation of Superior Mesenteric Vein, Open Approach

06753DZ Dilation of Superior Mesenteric Vein with Intraluminal Device, Percutaneous Approach

06753ZZ Dilation of Superior Mesenteric Vein, Percutaneous Approach

06754DZ Dilation of Superior Mesenteric Vein with Intraluminal Device, Percutaneous Endoscopic Approach

06754ZZ Dilation of Superior Mesenteric Vein, Percutaneous Endoscopic Approach

06760DZ Dilation of Inferior Mesenteric Vein with Intraluminal Device, Open Approach

06760ZZ Dilation of Inferior Mesenteric Vein, Open Approach

06763DZ Dilation of Inferior Mesenteric Vein with Intraluminal Device, Percutaneous Approach

06763ZZ Dilation of Inferior Mesenteric Vein, Percutaneous Approach

06764DZ Dilation of Inferior Mesenteric Vein with Intraluminal Device, Percutaneous Endoscopic Approach

06764ZZ Dilation of Inferior Mesenteric Vein, Percutaneous Endoscopic Approach

06770DZ Dilation of Colic Vein with Intraluminal Device, Open Approach

06770ZZ Dilation of Colic Vein, Open Approach

06773DZ Dilation of Colic Vein with Intraluminal Device, Percutaneous Approach

06773ZZ Dilation of Colic Vein, Percutaneous Approach

06774DZ Dilation of Colic Vein with Intraluminal Device, Percutaneous Endoscopic Approach

06774ZZ Dilation of Colic Vein, Percutaneous Endoscopic Approach

06780DZ Dilation of Portal Vein with Intraluminal Device, Open Approach

06780ZZ Dilation of Portal Vein, Open Approach

06783DZ Dilation of Portal Vein with Intraluminal Device, Percutaneous Approach

06783ZZ Dilation of Portal Vein, Percutaneous Approach

06784DZ Dilation of Portal Vein with Intraluminal Device, Percutaneous Endoscopic Approach

06784ZZ Dilation of Portal Vein, Percutaneous Endoscopic Approach

06790DZ Dilation of Right Renal Vein with Intraluminal Device, Open Approach

06790ZZ Dilation of Right Renal Vein, Open Approach

06793DZ Dilation of Right Renal Vein with Intraluminal Device, Percutaneous Approach

06793ZZ Dilation of Right Renal Vein, Percutaneous Approach

06794DZ Dilation of Right Renal Vein with Intraluminal Device, Percutaneous Endoscopic Approach

06794ZZ Dilation of Right Renal Vein, Percutaneous Endoscopic Approach

067B0DZ Dilation of Left Renal Vein with Intraluminal Device, Open Approach

067B0ZZ Dilation of Left Renal Vein, Open Approach

067B3DZ Dilation of Left Renal Vein with Intraluminal Device, Percutaneous Approach

067B3ZZ Dilation of Left Renal Vein, Percutaneous Approach

067B4DZ Dilation of Left Renal Vein with Intraluminal Device, Percutaneous Endoscopic Approach

067B4ZZ Dilation of Left Renal Vein, Percutaneous Endoscopic Approach

067C0DZ Dilation of Right Common Iliac Vein with Intraluminal Device, Open Approach

067C0ZZ Dilation of Right Common Iliac Vein, Open Approach

067C3DZ Dilation of Right Common Iliac Vein with Intraluminal Device, Percutaneous Approach

067C3ZZ Dilation of Right Common Iliac Vein, Percutaneous Approach

067C4DZ Dilation of Right Common Iliac Vein with Intraluminal Device, Percutaneous Endoscopic Approach

067C4ZZ Dilation of Right Common Iliac Vein, Percutaneous Endoscopic Approach

067D0DZ Dilation of Left Common Iliac Vein with Intraluminal Device, Open Approach

067D0ZZ Dilation of Left Common Iliac Vein, Open Approach

067D3DZ Dilation of Left Common Iliac Vein with Intraluminal Device, Percutaneous Approach

067D3ZZ Dilation of Left Common Iliac Vein, Percutaneous Approach

067D4DZ Dilation of Left Common Iliac Vein with Intraluminal Device, Percutaneous Endoscopic Approach

067D4ZZ Dilation of Left Common Iliac Vein, Percutaneous Endoscopic Approach

067F0DZ Dilation of Right External Iliac Vein with Intraluminal Device, Open Approach

067F0ZZ Dilation of Right External Iliac Vein, Open Approach

067F3DZ Dilation of Right External Iliac Vein with Intraluminal Device, Percutaneous Approach

067F3ZZ Dilation of Right External Iliac Vein, Percutaneous Approach

067F4DZ Dilation of Right External Iliac Vein with Intraluminal Device, Percutaneous Endoscopic Approach

067F4ZZ Dilation of Right External Iliac Vein, Percutaneous Endoscopic Approach

067G0DZ Dilation of Left External Iliac Vein with Intraluminal Device, Open Approach

067G0ZZ Dilation of Left External Iliac Vein, Open Approach

067G3DZ Dilation of Left External Iliac Vein with Intraluminal Device, Percutaneous Approach

067G3ZZ Dilation of Left External Iliac Vein, Percutaneous Approach

067G4DZ Dilation of Left External Iliac Vein with Intraluminal Device, Percutaneous Endoscopic Approach

067G4ZZ Dilation of Left External Iliac Vein, Percutaneous Endoscopic Approach

067H0DZ Dilation of Right Hypogastric Vein with Intraluminal Device, Open Approach

067H0ZZ Dilation of Right Hypogastric Vein, Open Approach

067H3DZ Dilation of Right Hypogastric Vein with Intraluminal Device, Percutaneous Approach

067H3ZZ Dilation of Right Hypogastric Vein, Percutaneous Approach

067H4DZ Dilation of Right Hypogastric Vein with Intraluminal Device, Percutaneous Endoscopic Approach

067H4ZZ Dilation of Right Hypogastric Vein, Percutaneous Endoscopic Approach

067J0DZ Dilation of Left Hypogastric Vein with Intraluminal Device, Open Approach

067J0ZZ Dilation of Left Hypogastric Vein, Open Approach

067J3DZ Dilation of Left Hypogastric Vein with Intraluminal Device, Percutaneous Approach

067J3ZZ Dilation of Left Hypogastric Vein, Percutaneous Approach

067J4DZ Dilation of Left Hypogastric Vein with Intraluminal Device, Percutaneous Endoscopic Approach

067J4ZZ Dilation of Left Hypogastric Vein, Percutaneous Endoscopic Approach

067M0DZ Dilation of Right Femoral Vein with Intraluminal Device, Open Approach

067M0ZZ Dilation of Right Femoral Vein, Open Approach

067M3DZ Dilation of Right Femoral Vein with Intraluminal Device, Percutaneous Approach

067M3ZZ Dilation of Right Femoral Vein, Percutaneous Approach

067M4DZ Dilation of Right Femoral Vein with Intraluminal Device, Percutaneous Endoscopic Approach

067M4ZZ Dilation of Right Femoral Vein, Percutaneous Endoscopic Approach

067N0DZ Dilation of Left Femoral Vein with Intraluminal Device, Open Approach

067N0ZZ Dilation of Left Femoral Vein, Open Approach

067N3DZ Dilation of Left Femoral Vein with Intraluminal Device, Percutaneous Approach

067N3ZZ Dilation of Left Femoral Vein, Percutaneous Approach

067N4DZ Dilation of Left Femoral Vein with Intraluminal Device, Percutaneous Endoscopic Approach

067N4ZZ Dilation of Left Femoral Vein, Percutaneous Endoscopic Approach

067P0DZ Dilation of Right Saphenous Vein with Intraluminal Device, Open Approach

067P0ZZ Dilation of Right Saphenous Vein, Open Approach

067P3DZ Dilation of Right Saphenous Vein with Intraluminal Device, Percutaneous Approach

067P3ZZ Dilation of Right Saphenous Vein, Percutaneous Approach

067P4DZ Dilation of Right Saphenous Vein with Intraluminal Device, Percutaneous Endoscopic Approach

067P4ZZ Dilation of Right Saphenous Vein, Percutaneous Endoscopic Approach

067Q0DZ Dilation of Left Saphenous Vein with Intraluminal Device, Open Approach

067Q0ZZ Dilation of Left Saphenous Vein, Open Approach

067Q3DZ Dilation of Left Saphenous Vein with Intraluminal Device, Percutaneous Approach

067Q3ZZ Dilation of Left Saphenous Vein, Percutaneous Approach

067Q4DZ Dilation of Left Saphenous Vein with Intraluminal Device, Percutaneous Endoscopic Approach

067Q4ZZ Dilation of Left Saphenous Vein, Percutaneous Endoscopic Approach

067T0DZ Dilation of Right Foot Vein with Intraluminal Device, Open Approach

067T0ZZ Dilation of Right Foot Vein, Open Approach

067T3DZ Dilation of Right Foot Vein with Intraluminal Device, Percutaneous Approach

067T3ZZ Dilation of Right Foot Vein, Percutaneous Approach

067T4DZ Dilation of Right Foot Vein with Intraluminal Device, Percutaneous Endoscopic Approach

067T4ZZ Dilation of Right Foot Vein, Percutaneous Endoscopic Approach

067V0DZ Dilation of Left Foot Vein with Intraluminal Device, Open Approach

067V0ZZ Dilation of Left Foot Vein, Open Approach

067V3DZ Dilation of Left Foot Vein with Intraluminal Device, Percutaneous Approach

067V3ZZ Dilation of Left Foot Vein, Percutaneous Approach

067V4DZ Dilation of Left Foot Vein with Intraluminal Device, Percutaneous Endoscopic Approach

067V4ZZ Dilation of Left Foot Vein, Percutaneous Endoscopic Approach

067Y0DZ Dilation of Lower Vein with Intraluminal Device, Open Approach

067Y0ZZ Dilation of Lower Vein, Open Approach

067Y3DZ Dilation of Lower Vein with Intraluminal Device, Percutaneous Approach

067Y3ZZ Dilation of Lower Vein, Percutaneous Approach

067Y4DZ Dilation of Lower Vein with Intraluminal Device, Percutaneous Endoscopic Approach

067Y4ZZ Dilation of Lower Vein, Percutaneous Endoscopic Approach

069 – Lower Veins, Drainage

Review Coding Guidelines B3.4a and B3.4b

Review Coding Guideline B6.2

069000Z Drainage of Inferior Vena Cava with Drainage Device, Open Approach

06900ZX Drainage of Inferior Vena Cava, Open Approach, Diagnostic

06900ZZ Drainage of Inferior Vena Cava, Open Approach

069030Z Drainage of Inferior Vena Cava with Drainage Device, Percutaneous Approach

06903ZX Drainage of Inferior Vena Cava, Percutaneous Approach, Diagnostic

06903ZZ Drainage of Inferior Vena Cava, Percutaneous Approach

069040Z Drainage of Inferior Vena Cava with Drainage Device, Percutaneous Endoscopic Approach

06904ZX Drainage of Inferior Vena Cava, Percutaneous Endoscopic Approach, Diagnostic

06904ZZ Drainage of Inferior Vena Cava, Percutaneous Endoscopic Approach

069100Z Drainage of Splenic Vein with Drainage Device, Open Approach

06910ZX Drainage of Splenic Vein, Open Approach, Diagnostic

06910ZZ Drainage of Splenic Vein, Open Approach

069130Z Drainage of Splenic Vein with Drainage Device, Percutaneous Approach

06913ZX Drainage of Splenic Vein, Percutaneous Approach, Diagnostic

06913ZZ Drainage of Splenic Vein, Percutaneous Approach

069140Z Drainage of Splenic Vein with Drainage Device, Percutaneous Endoscopic Approach

06914ZX Drainage of Splenic Vein, Percutaneous Endoscopic Approach, Diagnostic

06914ZZ Drainage of Splenic Vein, Percutaneous Endoscopic Approach

069200Z Drainage of Gastric Vein with Drainage Device, Open Approach

06920ZX Drainage of Gastric Vein, Open Approach, Diagnostic

06920ZZ Drainage of Gastric Vein, Open Approach

069230Z Drainage of Gastric Vein with Drainage Device, Percutaneous Approach

06923ZX Drainage of Gastric Vein, Percutaneous Approach, Diagnostic

06923ZZ Drainage of Gastric Vein, Percutaneous Approach

069240Z Drainage of Gastric Vein with Drainage Device, Percutaneous Endoscopic Approach

06924ZX Drainage of Gastric Vein, Percutaneous Endoscopic Approach, Diagnostic

06924ZZ Drainage of Gastric Vein, Percutaneous Endoscopic Approach

069300Z Drainage of Esophageal Vein with Drainage Device, Open Approach

06930ZX Drainage of Esophageal Vein, Open Approach, Diagnostic

06930ZZ Drainage of Esophageal Vein, Open Approach

069330Z Drainage of Esophageal Vein with Drainage Device, Percutaneous Approach

06933ZX Drainage of Esophageal Vein, Percutaneous Approach, Diagnostic

06933ZZ Drainage of Esophageal Vein, Percutaneous Approach

069340Z Drainage of Esophageal Vein with Drainage Device, Percutaneous Endoscopic Approach

06934ZX Drainage of Esophageal Vein, Percutaneous Endoscopic Approach, Diagnostic

06934ZZ Drainage of Esophageal Vein, Percutaneous Endoscopic Approach

069400Z Drainage of Hepatic Vein with Drainage Device, Open Approach

06940ZX Drainage of Hepatic Vein, Open Approach, Diagnostic

06940ZZ Drainage of Hepatic Vein, Open Approach

069430Z Drainage of Hepatic Vein with Drainage Device, Percutaneous Approach

06943ZX Drainage of Hepatic Vein, Percutaneous Approach, Diagnostic

06943ZZ Drainage of Hepatic Vein, Percutaneous Approach

069440Z Drainage of Hepatic Vein with Drainage Device, Percutaneous Endoscopic Approach

06944ZX Drainage of Hepatic Vein, Percutaneous Endoscopic Approach, Diagnostic

06944ZZ Drainage of Hepatic Vein, Percutaneous Endoscopic Approach

069500Z Drainage of Superior Mesenteric Vein with Drainage Device, Open Approach

06950ZX Drainage of Superior Mesenteric Vein, Open Approach, Diagnostic

06950ZZ Drainage of Superior Mesenteric Vein, Open Approach

069530Z Drainage of Superior Mesenteric Vein with Drainage Device, Percutaneous Approach

06953ZX Drainage of Superior Mesenteric Vein, Percutaneous Approach, Diagnostic

06953ZZ Drainage of Superior Mesenteric Vein, Percutaneous Approach

069540Z Drainage of Superior Mesenteric Vein with Drainage Device, Percutaneous Endoscopic Approach

06954ZX Drainage of Superior Mesenteric Vein, Percutaneous Endoscopic Approach, Diagnostic

06954ZZ Drainage of Superior Mesenteric Vein, Percutaneous Endoscopic Approach

069600Z Drainage of Inferior Mesenteric Vein with Drainage Device, Open Approach

06960ZX Drainage of Inferior Mesenteric Vein, Open Approach, Diagnostic

06960ZZ Drainage of Inferior Mesenteric Vein, Open Approach

♀ Female-only ♂ Male-only ▲ Limited Coverage ● Non-OR 🅗🅐🅒 HAC-associated procedure ▲ Non-covered procedures ✚ Cluster

069630Z Drainage of Inferior Mesenteric Vein with Drainage Device, Percutaneous Approach

06963ZX Drainage of Inferior Mesenteric Vein, Percutaneous Approach, Diagnostic

06963ZZ Drainage of Inferior Mesenteric Vein, Percutaneous Approach

069640Z Drainage of Inferior Mesenteric Vein with Drainage Device, Percutaneous Endoscopic Approach

06964ZX Drainage of Inferior Mesenteric Vein, Percutaneous Endoscopic Approach, Diagnostic

06964ZZ Drainage of Inferior Mesenteric Vein, Percutaneous Endoscopic Approach

069700Z Drainage of Colic Vein with Drainage Device, Open Approach

06970ZX Drainage of Colic Vein, Open Approach, Diagnostic

06970ZZ Drainage of Colic Vein, Open Approach

069730Z Drainage of Colic Vein with Drainage Device, Percutaneous Approach

06973ZX Drainage of Colic Vein, Percutaneous Approach, Diagnostic

06973ZZ Drainage of Colic Vein, Percutaneous Approach

069740Z Drainage of Colic Vein with Drainage Device, Percutaneous Endoscopic Approach

06974ZX Drainage of Colic Vein, Percutaneous Endoscopic Approach, Diagnostic

06974ZZ Drainage of Colic Vein, Percutaneous Endoscopic Approach

069800Z Drainage of Portal Vein with Drainage Device, Open Approach

06980ZX Drainage of Portal Vein, Open Approach, Diagnostic

06980ZZ Drainage of Portal Vein, Open Approach

069830Z Drainage of Portal Vein with Drainage Device, Percutaneous Approach

06983ZX Drainage of Portal Vein, Percutaneous Approach, Diagnostic

06983ZZ Drainage of Portal Vein, Percutaneous Approach

069840Z Drainage of Portal Vein with Drainage Device, Percutaneous Endoscopic Approach

06984ZX Drainage of Portal Vein, Percutaneous Endoscopic Approach, Diagnostic

06984ZZ Drainage of Portal Vein, Percutaneous Endoscopic Approach

069900Z Drainage of Right Renal Vein with Drainage Device, Open Approach

06990ZX Drainage of Right Renal Vein, Open Approach, Diagnostic

06990ZZ Drainage of Right Renal Vein, Open Approach

069930Z Drainage of Right Renal Vein with Drainage Device, Percutaneous Approach

06993ZX Drainage of Right Renal Vein, Percutaneous Approach, Diagnostic

06993ZZ Drainage of Right Renal Vein, Percutaneous Approach

069940Z Drainage of Right Renal Vein with Drainage Device, Percutaneous Endoscopic Approach

06994ZX Drainage of Right Renal Vein, Percutaneous Endoscopic Approach, Diagnostic

06994ZZ Drainage of Right Renal Vein, Percutaneous Endoscopic Approach

069B00Z Drainage of Left Renal Vein with Drainage Device, Open Approach

069B0ZX Drainage of Left Renal Vein, Open Approach, Diagnostic

069B0ZZ Drainage of Left Renal Vein, Open Approach

069B30Z Drainage of Left Renal Vein with Drainage Device, Percutaneous Approach

069B3ZX Drainage of Left Renal Vein, Percutaneous Approach, Diagnostic

069B3ZZ Drainage of Left Renal Vein, Percutaneous Approach

069B40Z Drainage of Left Renal Vein with Drainage Device, Percutaneous Endoscopic Approach

069B4ZX Drainage of Left Renal Vein, Percutaneous Endoscopic Approach, Diagnostic

069B4ZZ Drainage of Left Renal Vein, Percutaneous Endoscopic Approach

069C00Z Drainage of Right Common Iliac Vein with Drainage Device, Open Approach

069C0ZX Drainage of Right Common Iliac Vein, Open Approach, Diagnostic

069C0ZZ Drainage of Right Common Iliac Vein, Open Approach

069C30Z Drainage of Right Common Iliac Vein with Drainage Device, Percutaneous Approach

069C3ZX Drainage of Right Common Iliac Vein, Percutaneous Approach, Diagnostic

069C3ZZ Drainage of Right Common Iliac Vein, Percutaneous Approach

069C40Z Drainage of Right Common Iliac Vein with Drainage Device, Percutaneous Endoscopic Approach

069C4ZX Drainage of Right Common Iliac Vein, Percutaneous Endoscopic Approach, Diagnostic

069C4ZZ Drainage of Right Common Iliac Vein, Percutaneous Endoscopic Approach

069D00Z Drainage of Left Common Iliac Vein with Drainage Device, Open Approach

069D0ZX Drainage of Left Common Iliac Vein, Open Approach, Diagnostic

069D0ZZ Drainage of Left Common Iliac Vein, Open Approach

069D30Z Drainage of Left Common Iliac Vein with Drainage Device, Percutaneous Approach

069D3ZX Drainage of Left Common Iliac Vein, Percutaneous Approach, Diagnostic

069D3ZZ Drainage of Left Common Iliac Vein, Percutaneous Approach

069D40Z Drainage of Left Common Iliac Vein with Drainage Device, Percutaneous Endoscopic Approach

069D4ZX Drainage of Left Common Iliac Vein, Percutaneous Endoscopic Approach, Diagnostic

069D4ZZ Drainage of Left Common Iliac Vein, Percutaneous Endoscopic Approach

069F00Z Drainage of Right External Iliac Vein with Drainage Device, Open Approach

069F0ZX Drainage of Right External Iliac Vein, Open Approach, Diagnostic

069F0ZZ Drainage of Right External Iliac Vein, Open Approach

069F30Z Drainage of Right External Iliac Vein with Drainage Device, Percutaneous Approach

069F3ZX Drainage of Right External Iliac Vein, Percutaneous Approach, Diagnostic

069F3ZZ Drainage of Right External Iliac Vein, Percutaneous Approach

069F40Z Drainage of Right External Iliac Vein with Drainage Device, Percutaneous Endoscopic Approach

069F4ZX Drainage of Right External Iliac Vein, Percutaneous Endoscopic Approach, Diagnostic

069F4ZZ Drainage of Right External Iliac Vein, Percutaneous Endoscopic Approach

069G00Z Drainage of Left External Iliac Vein with Drainage Device, Open Approach

069G0ZX Drainage of Left External Iliac Vein, Open Approach, Diagnostic

069G0ZZ Drainage of Left External Iliac Vein, Open Approach

069G30Z Drainage of Left External Iliac Vein with Drainage Device, Percutaneous Approach

069G3ZX Drainage of Left External Iliac Vein, Percutaneous Approach, Diagnostic

069G3ZZ Drainage of Left External Iliac Vein, Percutaneous Approach

069G40Z Drainage of Left External Iliac Vein with Drainage Device, Percutaneous Endoscopic Approach

069G4ZX Drainage of Left External Iliac Vein, Percutaneous Endoscopic Approach, Diagnostic

069G4ZZ Drainage of Left External Iliac Vein, Percutaneous Endoscopic Approach

069H00Z Drainage of Right Hypogastric Vein with Drainage Device, Open Approach

069H0ZX Drainage of Right Hypogastric Vein, Open Approach, Diagnostic

069H0ZZ Drainage of Right Hypogastric Vein, Open Approach

069H30Z Drainage of Right Hypogastric Vein with Drainage Device, Percutaneous Approach

069H3ZX Drainage of Right Hypogastric Vein, Percutaneous Approach, Diagnostic

069H3ZZ Drainage of Right Hypogastric Vein, Percutaneous Approach

069H40Z Drainage of Right Hypogastric Vein with Drainage Device, Percutaneous Endoscopic Approach

069H4ZX Drainage of Right Hypogastric Vein, Percutaneous Endoscopic Approach, Diagnostic

069H4ZZ Drainage of Right Hypogastric Vein, Percutaneous Endoscopic Approach

069J00Z Drainage of Left Hypogastric Vein with Drainage Device, Open Approach

069J0ZX Drainage of Left Hypogastric Vein, Open Approach, Diagnostic

069J0ZZ Drainage of Left Hypogastric Vein, Open Approach

069J30Z Drainage of Left Hypogastric Vein with Drainage Device, Percutaneous Approach

069J3ZX Drainage of Left Hypogastric Vein, Percutaneous Approach, Diagnostic

069J3ZZ Drainage of Left Hypogastric Vein, Percutaneous Approach

069J40Z Drainage of Left Hypogastric Vein with Drainage Device, Percutaneous Endoscopic Approach

069J4ZX Drainage of Left Hypogastric Vein, Percutaneous Endoscopic Approach, Diagnostic

069J4ZZ Drainage of Left Hypogastric Vein, Percutaneous Endoscopic Approach

069M00Z Drainage of Right Femoral Vein with Drainage Device, Open Approach

069M0ZX Drainage of Right Femoral Vein, Open Approach, Diagnostic

♀ Female-only   ♂ Male-only   ▲ Limited Coverage   ● Non-OR   ▥ HAC-associated procedure   ▲ Non-covered procedures   ✚ Cluster

Code	Description	Code	Description	Code	Description
069M0ZZ	Drainage of Right Femoral Vein, Open Approach	069P3ZX	Drainage of Right Saphenous Vein, Percutaneous Approach, Diagnostic	069T40Z	Drainage of Right Foot Vein with Drainage Device, Percutaneous Endoscopic Approach
069M30Z	Drainage of Right Femoral Vein with Drainage Device, Percutaneous Approach	069P3ZZ	Drainage of Right Saphenous Vein, Percutaneous Approach	069T4ZX	Drainage of Right Foot Vein, Percutaneous Endoscopic Approach, Diagnostic
069M3ZX	Drainage of Right Femoral Vein, Percutaneous Approach, Diagnostic	069P40Z	Drainage of Right Saphenous Vein with Drainage Device, Percutaneous Endoscopic Approach	069T4ZZ	Drainage of Right Foot Vein, Percutaneous Endoscopic Approach
069M3ZZ	Drainage of Right Femoral Vein, Percutaneous Approach	069P4ZX	Drainage of Right Saphenous Vein, Percutaneous Endoscopic Approach, Diagnostic	069V00Z	Drainage of Left Foot Vein with Drainage Device, Open Approach
069M40Z	Drainage of Right Femoral Vein with Drainage Device, Percutaneous Endoscopic Approach	069P4ZZ	Drainage of Right Saphenous Vein, Percutaneous Endoscopic Approach	069V0ZX	Drainage of Left Foot Vein, Open Approach, Diagnostic
069M4ZX	Drainage of Right Femoral Vein, Percutaneous Endoscopic Approach, Diagnostic	069Q00Z	Drainage of Left Saphenous Vein with Drainage Device, Open Approach	069V0ZZ	Drainage of Left Foot Vein, Open Approach
069M4ZZ	Drainage of Right Femoral Vein, Percutaneous Endoscopic Approach	069Q0ZX	Drainage of Left Saphenous Vein, Open Approach, Diagnostic	069V30Z	Drainage of Left Foot Vein with Drainage Device, Percutaneous Approach
069N00Z	Drainage of Left Femoral Vein with Drainage Device, Open Approach	069Q0ZZ	Drainage of Left Saphenous Vein, Open Approach	069V3ZX	Drainage of Left Foot Vein, Percutaneous Approach, Diagnostic
069N0ZX	Drainage of Left Femoral Vein, Open Approach, Diagnostic	069Q30Z	Drainage of Left Saphenous Vein with Drainage Device, Percutaneous Approach	069V3ZZ	Drainage of Left Foot Vein, Percutaneous Approach
069N0ZZ	Drainage of Left Femoral Vein, Open Approach	069Q3ZX	Drainage of Left Saphenous Vein, Percutaneous Approach, Diagnostic	069V40Z	Drainage of Left Foot Vein with Drainage Device, Percutaneous Endoscopic Approach
069N30Z	Drainage of Left Femoral Vein with Drainage Device, Percutaneous Approach	069Q3ZZ	Drainage of Left Saphenous Vein, Percutaneous Approach	069V4ZX	Drainage of Left Foot Vein, Percutaneous Endoscopic Approach, Diagnostic
069N3ZX	Drainage of Left Femoral Vein, Percutaneous Approach, Diagnostic	069Q40Z	Drainage of Left Saphenous Vein with Drainage Device, Percutaneous Endoscopic Approach	069V4ZZ	Drainage of Left Foot Vein, Percutaneous Endoscopic Approach
069N3ZZ	Drainage of Left Femoral Vein, Percutaneous Approach	069Q4ZX	Drainage of Left Saphenous Vein, Percutaneous Endoscopic Approach, Diagnostic	069Y00Z	Drainage of Lower Vein with Drainage Device, Open Approach
069N40Z	Drainage of Left Femoral Vein with Drainage Device, Percutaneous Endoscopic Approach	069Q4ZZ	Drainage of Left Saphenous Vein, Percutaneous Endoscopic Approach	069Y0ZX	Drainage of Lower Vein, Open Approach, Diagnostic
069N4ZX	Drainage of Left Femoral Vein, Percutaneous Endoscopic Approach, Diagnostic	069T00Z	Drainage of Right Foot Vein with Drainage Device, Open Approach	069Y0ZZ	Drainage of Lower Vein, Open Approach
069N4ZZ	Drainage of Left Femoral Vein, Percutaneous Endoscopic Approach	069T0ZX	Drainage of Right Foot Vein, Open Approach, Diagnostic	069Y30Z	Drainage of Lower Vein with Drainage Device, Percutaneous Approach
069P00Z	Drainage of Right Saphenous Vein with Drainage Device, Open Approach	069T0ZZ	Drainage of Right Foot Vein, Open Approach	069Y3ZX	Drainage of Lower Vein, Percutaneous Approach, Diagnostic
069P0ZX	Drainage of Right Saphenous Vein, Open Approach, Diagnostic	069T30Z	Drainage of Right Foot Vein with Drainage Device, Percutaneous Approach	069Y3ZZ	Drainage of Lower Vein, Percutaneous Approach
069P0ZZ	Drainage of Right Saphenous Vein, Open Approach	069T3ZX	Drainage of Right Foot Vein, Percutaneous Approach, Diagnostic	069Y40Z	Drainage of Lower Vein with Drainage Device, Percutaneous Endoscopic Approach
069P30Z	Drainage of Right Saphenous Vein with Drainage Device, Percutaneous Approach	069T3ZZ	Drainage of Right Foot Vein, Percutaneous Approach	069Y4ZX	Drainage of Lower Vein, Percutaneous Endoscopic Approach, Diagnostic
				069Y4ZZ	Drainage of Lower Vein, Percutaneous Endoscopic Approach

06B – Lower Veins, Excision

Review Coding Guidelines B3.4a and B3.4b

Review Coding Guideline B3.8

Review Coding Guideline B3.18

Code	Description	Code	Description	Code	Description
06B00ZX	Excision of Inferior Vena Cava, Open Approach, Diagnostic	06B13ZZ	Excision of Splenic Vein, Percutaneous Approach	06B30ZZ	Excision of Esophageal Vein, Open Approach
06B00ZZ	Excision of Inferior Vena Cava, Open Approach	06B14ZX	Excision of Splenic Vein, Percutaneous Endoscopic Approach, Diagnostic	06B33ZX	Excision of Esophageal Vein, Percutaneous Approach, Diagnostic
06B03ZX	Excision of Inferior Vena Cava, Percutaneous Approach, Diagnostic	06B14ZZ	Excision of Splenic Vein, Percutaneous Endoscopic Approach	06B33ZZ	Excision of Esophageal Vein, Percutaneous Approach
06B03ZZ	Excision of Inferior Vena Cava, Percutaneous Approach	06B20ZX	Excision of Gastric Vein, Open Approach, Diagnostic	06B34ZX	Excision of Esophageal Vein, Percutaneous Endoscopic Approach, Diagnostic
06B04ZX	Excision of Inferior Vena Cava, Percutaneous Endoscopic Approach, Diagnostic	06B20ZZ	Excision of Gastric Vein, Open Approach	06B34ZZ	Excision of Esophageal Vein, Percutaneous Endoscopic Approach
06B04ZZ	Excision of Inferior Vena Cava, Percutaneous Endoscopic Approach	06B23ZX	Excision of Gastric Vein, Percutaneous Approach, Diagnostic	06B40ZX	Excision of Hepatic Vein, Open Approach, Diagnostic
06B10ZX	Excision of Splenic Vein, Open Approach, Diagnostic	06B23ZZ	Excision of Gastric Vein, Percutaneous Approach	06B40ZZ	Excision of Hepatic Vein, Open Approach
06B10ZZ	Excision of Splenic Vein, Open Approach	06B24ZX	Excision of Gastric Vein, Percutaneous Endoscopic Approach, Diagnostic	06B43ZX	Excision of Hepatic Vein, Percutaneous Approach, Diagnostic
06B13ZX	Excision of Splenic Vein, Percutaneous Approach, Diagnostic	06B24ZZ	Excision of Gastric Vein, Percutaneous Endoscopic Approach	06B43ZZ	Excision of Hepatic Vein, Percutaneous Approach
		06B30ZX	Excision of Esophageal Vein, Open Approach, Diagnostic		

♀ Female-only   ♂ Male-only   ▲ Limited Coverage   ● Non-OR   ▆ HAC-associated procedure   ▲ Non-covered procedures   ✚ Cluster

06B44ZX Excision of Hepatic Vein, Percutaneous Endoscopic Approach, Diagnostic
06B44ZZ Excision of Hepatic Vein, Percutaneous Endoscopic Approach
06B50ZX Excision of Superior Mesenteric Vein, Open Approach, Diagnostic
06B50ZZ Excision of Superior Mesenteric Vein, Open Approach
06B53ZX Excision of Superior Mesenteric Vein, Percutaneous Approach, Diagnostic
06B53ZZ Excision of Superior Mesenteric Vein, Percutaneous Approach
06B54ZX Excision of Superior Mesenteric Vein, Percutaneous Endoscopic Approach, Diagnostic
06B54ZZ Excision of Superior Mesenteric Vein, Percutaneous Endoscopic Approach
06B60ZX Excision of Inferior Mesenteric Vein, Open Approach, Diagnostic
06B60ZZ Excision of Inferior Mesenteric Vein, Open Approach
06B63ZX Excision of Inferior Mesenteric Vein, Percutaneous Approach, Diagnostic
06B63ZZ Excision of Inferior Mesenteric Vein, Percutaneous Approach
06B64ZX Excision of Inferior Mesenteric Vein, Percutaneous Endoscopic Approach, Diagnostic
06B64ZZ Excision of Inferior Mesenteric Vein, Percutaneous Endoscopic Approach
06B70ZX Excision of Colic Vein, Open Approach, Diagnostic
06B70ZZ Excision of Colic Vein, Open Approach
06B73ZX Excision of Colic Vein, Percutaneous Approach, Diagnostic
06B73ZZ Excision of Colic Vein, Percutaneous Approach
06B74ZX Excision of Colic Vein, Percutaneous Endoscopic Approach, Diagnostic
06B74ZZ Excision of Colic Vein, Percutaneous Endoscopic Approach
06B80ZX Excision of Portal Vein, Open Approach, Diagnostic
06B80ZZ Excision of Portal Vein, Open Approach
06B83ZX Excision of Portal Vein, Percutaneous Approach, Diagnostic
06B83ZZ Excision of Portal Vein, Percutaneous Approach
06B84ZX Excision of Portal Vein, Percutaneous Endoscopic Approach, Diagnostic
06B84ZZ Excision of Portal Vein, Percutaneous Endoscopic Approach
06B90ZX Excision of Right Renal Vein, Open Approach, Diagnostic
06B90ZZ Excision of Right Renal Vein, Open Approach
06B93ZX Excision of Right Renal Vein, Percutaneous Approach, Diagnostic
06B93ZZ Excision of Right Renal Vein, Percutaneous Approach
06B94ZX Excision of Right Renal Vein, Percutaneous Endoscopic Approach, Diagnostic
06B94ZZ Excision of Right Renal Vein, Percutaneous Endoscopic Approach
06BB0ZX Excision of Left Renal Vein, Open Approach, Diagnostic
06BB0ZZ Excision of Left Renal Vein, Open Approach
06BB3ZX Excision of Left Renal Vein, Percutaneous Approach, Diagnostic
06BB3ZZ Excision of Left Renal Vein, Percutaneous Approach

06BB4ZX Excision of Left Renal Vein, Percutaneous Endoscopic Approach, Diagnostic
06BB4ZZ Excision of Left Renal Vein, Percutaneous Endoscopic Approach
06BC0ZX Excision of Right Common Iliac Vein, Open Approach, Diagnostic
06BC0ZZ Excision of Right Common Iliac Vein, Open Approach
06BC3ZX Excision of Right Common Iliac Vein, Percutaneous Approach, Diagnostic
06BC3ZZ Excision of Right Common Iliac Vein, Percutaneous Approach
06BC4ZX Excision of Right Common Iliac Vein, Percutaneous Endoscopic Approach, Diagnostic
06BC4ZZ Excision of Right Common Iliac Vein, Percutaneous Endoscopic Approach
06BD0ZX Excision of Left Common Iliac Vein, Open Approach, Diagnostic
06BD0ZZ Excision of Left Common Iliac Vein, Open Approach
06BD3ZX Excision of Left Common Iliac Vein, Percutaneous Approach, Diagnostic
06BD3ZZ Excision of Left Common Iliac Vein, Percutaneous Approach
06BD4ZX Excision of Left Common Iliac Vein, Percutaneous Endoscopic Approach, Diagnostic
06BD4ZZ Excision of Left Common Iliac Vein, Percutaneous Endoscopic Approach
06BF0ZX Excision of Right External Iliac Vein, Open Approach, Diagnostic
06BF0ZZ Excision of Right External Iliac Vein, Open Approach
06BF3ZX Excision of Right External Iliac Vein, Percutaneous Approach, Diagnostic
06BF3ZZ Excision of Right External Iliac Vein, Percutaneous Approach
06BF4ZX Excision of Right External Iliac Vein, Percutaneous Endoscopic Approach, Diagnostic
06BF4ZZ Excision of Right External Iliac Vein, Percutaneous Endoscopic Approach
06BG0ZX Excision of Left External Iliac Vein, Open Approach, Diagnostic
06BG0ZZ Excision of Left External Iliac Vein, Open Approach
06BG3ZX Excision of Left External Iliac Vein, Percutaneous Approach, Diagnostic
06BG3ZZ Excision of Left External Iliac Vein, Percutaneous Approach
06BG4ZX Excision of Left External Iliac Vein, Percutaneous Endoscopic Approach, Diagnostic
06BG4ZZ Excision of Left External Iliac Vein, Percutaneous Endoscopic Approach
06BH0ZX Excision of Right Hypogastric Vein, Open Approach, Diagnostic
06BH0ZZ Excision of Right Hypogastric Vein, Open Approach
06BH3ZX Excision of Right Hypogastric Vein, Percutaneous Approach, Diagnostic
06BH3ZZ Excision of Right Hypogastric Vein, Percutaneous Approach
06BH4ZX Excision of Right Hypogastric Vein, Percutaneous Endoscopic Approach, Diagnostic
06BH4ZZ Excision of Right Hypogastric Vein, Percutaneous Endoscopic Approach
06BJ0ZX Excision of Left Hypogastric Vein, Open Approach, Diagnostic
06BJ0ZZ Excision of Left Hypogastric Vein, Open Approach

06BJ3ZX Excision of Left Hypogastric Vein, Percutaneous Approach, Diagnostic
06BJ3ZZ Excision of Left Hypogastric Vein, Percutaneous Approach
06BJ4ZX Excision of Left Hypogastric Vein, Percutaneous Endoscopic Approach, Diagnostic
06BJ4ZZ Excision of Left Hypogastric Vein, Percutaneous Endoscopic Approach
06BM0ZX Excision of Right Femoral Vein, Open Approach, Diagnostic
06BM0ZZ Excision of Right Femoral Vein, Open Approach
06BM3ZX Excision of Right Femoral Vein, Percutaneous Approach, Diagnostic
06BM3ZZ Excision of Right Femoral Vein, Percutaneous Approach
06BM4ZX Excision of Right Femoral Vein, Percutaneous Endoscopic Approach, Diagnostic
06BM4ZZ Excision of Right Femoral Vein, Percutaneous Endoscopic Approach
06BN0ZX Excision of Left Femoral Vein, Open Approach, Diagnostic
06BN0ZZ Excision of Left Femoral Vein, Open Approach
06BN3ZX Excision of Left Femoral Vein, Percutaneous Approach, Diagnostic
06BN3ZZ Excision of Left Femoral Vein, Percutaneous Approach
06BN4ZX Excision of Left Femoral Vein, Percutaneous Endoscopic Approach, Diagnostic
06BN4ZZ Excision of Left Femoral Vein, Percutaneous Endoscopic Approach
06BP0ZX Excision of Right Saphenous Vein, Open Approach, Diagnostic
06BP0ZZ Excision of Right Saphenous Vein, Open Approach

AHA CC: 1Q, 2014, 10-11; 2Q, 2016, 18-19; 1Q, 2017, 31-32; 3Q, 2017, 5-6

06BP3ZX Excision of Right Saphenous Vein, Percutaneous Approach, Diagnostic
06BP3ZZ Excision of Right Saphenous Vein, Percutaneous Approach
06BP4ZX Excision of Right Saphenous Vein, Percutaneous Endoscopic Approach, Diagnostic
06BP4ZZ Excision of Right Saphenous Vein, Percutaneous Endoscopic Approach

AHA CC: 3Q, 2014, 20-21

06BQ0ZX Excision of Left Saphenous Vein, Open Approach, Diagnostic
06BQ0ZZ Excision of Left Saphenous Vein, Open Approach

AHA CC: 1Q, 2017, 32-33; 1Q, 2020, 28-29

06BQ3ZX Excision of Left Saphenous Vein, Percutaneous Approach, Diagnostic
06BQ3ZZ Excision of Left Saphenous Vein, Percutaneous Approach
06BQ4ZX Excision of Left Saphenous Vein, Percutaneous Endoscopic Approach, Diagnostic
06BQ4ZZ Excision of Left Saphenous Vein, Percutaneous Endoscopic Approach

AHA CC: 3Q, 2014, 20-21; 1Q, 2016, 27-28

06BT0ZX Excision of Right Foot Vein, Open Approach, Diagnostic
06BT0ZZ Excision of Right Foot Vein, Open Approach
06BT3ZX Excision of Right Foot Vein, Percutaneous Approach, Diagnostic
06BT3ZZ Excision of Right Foot Vein, Percutaneous Approach

06BT4ZX Excision of Right Foot Vein, Percutaneous Endoscopic Approach, Diagnostic

06BT4ZZ Excision of Right Foot Vein, Percutaneous Endoscopic Approach

06BV0ZX Excision of Left Foot Vein, Open Approach, Diagnostic

06BV0ZZ Excision of Left Foot Vein, Open Approach

06BV3ZX Excision of Left Foot Vein, Percutaneous Approach, Diagnostic

06BV3ZZ Excision of Left Foot Vein, Percutaneous Approach

06BV4ZX Excision of Left Foot Vein, Percutaneous Endoscopic Approach, Diagnostic

06BV4ZZ Excision of Left Foot Vein, Percutaneous Endoscopic Approach

06BY0ZC Excision of Hemorrhoidal Plexus, Open Approach

06BY0ZX Excision of Lower Vein, Open Approach, Diagnostic

06BY0ZZ Excision of Lower Vein, Open Approach

06BY3ZC Excision of Hemorrhoidal Plexus, Percutaneous Approach

06BY3ZX Excision of Lower Vein, Percutaneous Approach, Diagnostic

06BY3ZZ Excision of Lower Vein, Percutaneous Approach

06BY4ZC Excision of Hemorrhoidal Plexus, Percutaneous Endoscopic Approach

06BY4ZX Excision of Lower Vein, Percutaneous Endoscopic Approach, Diagnostic

06BY4ZZ Excision of Lower Vein, Percutaneous Endoscopic Approach

06C – Lower Veins, Extirpation

06C00ZZ Extirpation of Matter from Inferior Vena Cava, Open Approach

06C03ZZ Extirpation of Matter from Inferior Vena Cava, Percutaneous Approach

06C04ZZ Extirpation of Matter from Inferior Vena Cava, Percutaneous Endoscopic Approach

06C10ZZ Extirpation of Matter from Splenic Vein, Open Approach

06C13ZZ Extirpation of Matter from Splenic Vein, Percutaneous Approach

06C14ZZ Extirpation of Matter from Splenic Vein, Percutaneous Endoscopic Approach

06C20ZZ Extirpation of Matter from Gastric Vein, Open Approach

06C23ZZ Extirpation of Matter from Gastric Vein, Percutaneous Approach

06C24ZZ Extirpation of Matter from Gastric Vein, Percutaneous Endoscopic Approach

06C30ZZ Extirpation of Matter from Esophageal Vein, Open Approach

06C33ZZ Extirpation of Matter from Esophageal Vein, Percutaneous Approach

06C34ZZ Extirpation of Matter from Esophageal Vein, Percutaneous Endoscopic Approach

06C40ZZ Extirpation of Matter from Hepatic Vein, Open Approach

06C43ZZ Extirpation of Matter from Hepatic Vein, Percutaneous Approach

06C44ZZ Extirpation of Matter from Hepatic Vein, Percutaneous Endoscopic Approach

06C50ZZ Extirpation of Matter from Superior Mesenteric Vein, Open Approach

06C53ZZ Extirpation of Matter from Superior Mesenteric Vein, Percutaneous Approach

06C54ZZ Extirpation of Matter from Superior Mesenteric Vein, Percutaneous Endoscopic Approach

06C60ZZ Extirpation of Matter from Inferior Mesenteric Vein, Open Approach

06C63ZZ Extirpation of Matter from Inferior Mesenteric Vein, Percutaneous Approach

06C64ZZ Extirpation of Matter from Inferior Mesenteric Vein, Percutaneous Endoscopic Approach

06C70ZZ Extirpation of Matter from Colic Vein, Open Approach

06C73ZZ Extirpation of Matter from Colic Vein, Percutaneous Approach

06C74ZZ Extirpation of Matter from Colic Vein, Percutaneous Endoscopic Approach

06C80ZZ Extirpation of Matter from Portal Vein, Open Approach

06C83ZZ Extirpation of Matter from Portal Vein, Percutaneous Approach

06C84ZZ Extirpation of Matter from Portal Vein, Percutaneous Endoscopic Approach

06C90ZZ Extirpation of Matter from Right Renal Vein, Open Approach

06C93ZZ Extirpation of Matter from Right Renal Vein, Percutaneous Approach

06C94ZZ Extirpation of Matter from Right Renal Vein, Percutaneous Endoscopic Approach

06CB0ZZ Extirpation of Matter from Left Renal Vein, Open Approach

06CB3ZZ Extirpation of Matter from Left Renal Vein, Percutaneous Approach

06CB4ZZ Extirpation of Matter from Left Renal Vein, Percutaneous Endoscopic Approach

06CC0ZZ Extirpation of Matter from Right Common Iliac Vein, Open Approach

06CC3ZZ Extirpation of Matter from Right Common Iliac Vein, Percutaneous Approach

06CC4ZZ Extirpation of Matter from Right Common Iliac Vein, Percutaneous Endoscopic Approach

06CD0ZZ Extirpation of Matter from Left Common Iliac Vein, Open Approach

06CD3ZZ Extirpation of Matter from Left Common Iliac Vein, Percutaneous Approach

06CD4ZZ Extirpation of Matter from Left Common Iliac Vein, Percutaneous Endoscopic Approach

06CF0ZZ Extirpation of Matter from Right External Iliac Vein, Open Approach

06CF3ZZ Extirpation of Matter from Right External Iliac Vein, Percutaneous Approach

06CF4ZZ Extirpation of Matter from Right External Iliac Vein, Percutaneous Endoscopic Approach

06CG0ZZ Extirpation of Matter from Left External Iliac Vein, Open Approach

06CG3ZZ Extirpation of Matter from Left External Iliac Vein, Percutaneous Approach

06CG4ZZ Extirpation of Matter from Left External Iliac Vein, Percutaneous Endoscopic Approach

06CH0ZZ Extirpation of Matter from Right Hypogastric Vein, Open Approach

06CH3ZZ Extirpation of Matter from Right Hypogastric Vein, Percutaneous Approach

06CH4ZZ Extirpation of Matter from Right Hypogastric Vein, Percutaneous Endoscopic Approach

06CJ0ZZ Extirpation of Matter from Left Hypogastric Vein, Open Approach

06CJ3ZZ Extirpation of Matter from Left Hypogastric Vein, Percutaneous Approach

06CJ4ZZ Extirpation of Matter from Left Hypogastric Vein, Percutaneous Endoscopic Approach

06CM0ZZ Extirpation of Matter from Right Femoral Vein, Open Approach

06CM3ZZ Extirpation of Matter from Right Femoral Vein, Percutaneous Approach

06CM4ZZ Extirpation of Matter from Right Femoral Vein, Percutaneous Endoscopic Approach

06CN0ZZ Extirpation of Matter from Left Femoral Vein, Open Approach

06CN3ZZ Extirpation of Matter from Left Femoral Vein, Percutaneous Approach

06CN4ZZ Extirpation of Matter from Left Femoral Vein, Percutaneous Endoscopic Approach

06CP0ZZ Extirpation of Matter from Right Saphenous Vein, Open Approach

06CP3ZZ Extirpation of Matter from Right Saphenous Vein, Percutaneous Approach

06CP4ZZ Extirpation of Matter from Right Saphenous Vein, Percutaneous Endoscopic Approach

06CQ0ZZ Extirpation of Matter from Left Saphenous Vein, Open Approach

06CQ3ZZ Extirpation of Matter from Left Saphenous Vein, Percutaneous Approach

06CQ4ZZ Extirpation of Matter from Left Saphenous Vein, Percutaneous Endoscopic Approach

06CT0ZZ Extirpation of Matter from Right Foot Vein, Open Approach

06CT3ZZ Extirpation of Matter from Right Foot Vein, Percutaneous Approach

06CT4ZZ Extirpation of Matter from Right Foot Vein, Percutaneous Endoscopic Approach

06CV0ZZ Extirpation of Matter from Left Foot Vein, Open Approach

06CV3ZZ Extirpation of Matter from Left Foot Vein, Percutaneous Approach

06CV4ZZ Extirpation of Matter from Left Foot Vein, Percutaneous Endoscopic Approach

06CY0ZZ Extirpation of Matter from Lower Vein, Open Approach

06CY3ZZ Extirpation of Matter from Lower Vein, Percutaneous Approach

06CY4ZZ Extirpation of Matter from Lower Vein, Percutaneous Endoscopic Approach

♀ Female-only ♂ Male-only ▲ Limited Coverage ● Non-OR ▨ HAC-associated procedure ▲ Non-covered procedures ✚ Cluster

06D – Lower Veins, Extraction

06DM0ZZ Extraction of Right Femoral Vein, Open Approach

06DM3ZZ Extraction of Right Femoral Vein, Percutaneous Approach

06DM4ZZ Extraction of Right Femoral Vein, Percutaneous Endoscopic Approach

06DN0ZZ Extraction of Left Femoral Vein, Open Approach

06DN3ZZ Extraction of Left Femoral Vein, Percutaneous Approach

06DN4ZZ Extraction of Left Femoral Vein, Percutaneous Endoscopic Approach

06DP0ZZ Extraction of Right Saphenous Vein, Open Approach

06DP3ZZ Extraction of Right Saphenous Vein, Percutaneous Approach

06DP4ZZ Extraction of Right Saphenous Vein, Percutaneous Endoscopic Approach

06DQ0ZZ Extraction of Left Saphenous Vein, Open Approach

06DQ3ZZ Extraction of Left Saphenous Vein, Percutaneous Approach

06DQ4ZZ Extraction of Left Saphenous Vein, Percutaneous Endoscopic Approach

06DT0ZZ Extraction of Right Foot Vein, Open Approach

06DT3ZZ Extraction of Right Foot Vein, Percutaneous Approach

06DT4ZZ Extraction of Right Foot Vein, Percutaneous Endoscopic Approach

06DV0ZZ Extraction of Left Foot Vein, Open Approach

06DV3ZZ Extraction of Left Foot Vein, Percutaneous Approach

06DV4ZZ Extraction of Left Foot Vein, Percutaneous Endoscopic Approach

06DY0ZZ Extraction of Lower Vein, Open Approach

06DY3ZZ Extraction of Lower Vein, Percutaneous Approach

06DY4ZZ Extraction of Lower Vein, Percutaneous Endoscopic Approach

06F – Lower Veins, Fragmentation

06FC3Z0 Fragmentation of Right Common Iliac Vein, Percutaneous Approach, Ultrasonic

06FC3ZZ Fragmentation of Right Common Iliac Vein, Percutaneous Approach

06FD3Z0 Fragmentation of Left Common Iliac Vein, Percutaneous Approach, Ultrasonic

06FD3ZZ Fragmentation of Left Common Iliac Vein, Percutaneous Approach

06FF3Z0 Fragmentation of Right External Iliac Vein, Percutaneous Approach, Ultrasonic

06FF3ZZ Fragmentation of Right External Iliac Vein, Percutaneous Approach

06FG3Z0 Fragmentation of Left External Iliac Vein, Percutaneous Approach, Ultrasonic

06FG3ZZ Fragmentation of Left External Iliac Vein, Percutaneous Approach

06FH3Z0 Fragmentation of Right Hypogastric Vein, Percutaneous Approach, Ultrasonic

06FH3ZZ Fragmentation of Right Hypogastric Vein, Percutaneous Approach

06FJ3Z0 Fragmentation of Left Hypogastric Vein, Percutaneous Approach, Ultrasonic

06FJ3ZZ Fragmentation of Left Hypogastric Vein, Percutaneous Approach

06FM3Z0 Fragmentation of Right Femoral Vein, Percutaneous Approach, Ultrasonic

06FM3ZZ Fragmentation of Right Femoral Vein, Percutaneous Approach

06FN3Z0 Fragmentation of Left Femoral Vein, Percutaneous Approach, Ultrasonic

06FN3ZZ Fragmentation of Left Femoral Vein, Percutaneous Approach

06FP3Z0 Fragmentation of Right Saphenous Vein, Percutaneous Approach, Ultrasonic

06FP3ZZ Fragmentation of Right Saphenous Vein, Percutaneous Approach

06FQ3Z0 Fragmentation of Left Saphenous Vein, Percutaneous Approach, Ultrasonic

06FQ3ZZ Fragmentation of Left Saphenous Vein, Percutaneous Approach

06FY3Z0 Fragmentation of Lower Vein, Percutaneous Approach, Ultrasonic

06FY3ZZ Fragmentation of Lower Vein, Percutaneous Approach

06H – Lower Veins, Insertion

06H003T Insertion of Infusion Device, Via Umbilical Vein, into Inferior Vena Cava, Open Approach

06H003Z Insertion of Infusion Device into Inferior Vena Cava, Open Approach

06H00DZ Insertion of Intraluminal Device into Inferior Vena Cava, Open Approach

06H033T Insertion of Infusion Device, Via Umbilical Vein, into Inferior Vena Cava, Percutaneous Approach
AHA CC: 1Q, 2017, 31

06H033Z Insertion of Infusion Device into Inferior Vena Cava, Percutaneous Approach
AHA CC: 3Q, 2013, 18-19

06H03DZ Insertion of Intraluminal Device into Inferior Vena Cava, Percutaneous Approach

06H043Z Insertion of Infusion Device into Inferior Vena Cava, Percutaneous Endoscopic Approach

06H04DZ Insertion of Intraluminal Device into Inferior Vena Cava, Percutaneous Endoscopic Approach

06H103Z Insertion of Infusion Device into Splenic Vein, Open Approach

06H10DZ Insertion of Intraluminal Device into Splenic Vein, Open Approach

06H133Z Insertion of Infusion Device into Splenic Vein, Percutaneous Approach

06H13DZ Insertion of Intraluminal Device into Splenic Vein, Percutaneous Approach

06H143Z Insertion of Infusion Device into Splenic Vein, Percutaneous Endoscopic Approach

06H14DZ Insertion of Intraluminal Device into Splenic Vein, Percutaneous Endoscopic Approach

06H203Z Insertion of Infusion Device into Gastric Vein, Open Approach

06H20DZ Insertion of Intraluminal Device into Gastric Vein, Open Approach

06H233Z Insertion of Infusion Device into Gastric Vein, Percutaneous Approach

06H23DZ Insertion of Intraluminal Device into Gastric Vein, Percutaneous Approach

06H243Z Insertion of Infusion Device into Gastric Vein, Percutaneous Endoscopic Approach

06H24DZ Insertion of Intraluminal Device into Gastric Vein, Percutaneous Endoscopic Approach

06H303Z Insertion of Infusion Device into Esophageal Vein, Open Approach

06H30DZ Insertion of Intraluminal Device into Esophageal Vein, Open Approach

06H333Z Insertion of Infusion Device into Esophageal Vein, Percutaneous Approach

06H33DZ Insertion of Intraluminal Device into Esophageal Vein, Percutaneous Approach

06H343Z Insertion of Infusion Device into Esophageal Vein, Percutaneous Endoscopic Approach

06H34DZ Insertion of Intraluminal Device into Esophageal Vein, Percutaneous Endoscopic Approach

06H403Z Insertion of Infusion Device into Hepatic Vein, Open Approach

06H40DZ Insertion of Intraluminal Device into Hepatic Vein, Open Approach

06H433Z Insertion of Infusion Device into Hepatic Vein, Percutaneous Approach

06H43DZ Insertion of Intraluminal Device into Hepatic Vein, Percutaneous Approach

06H443Z Insertion of Infusion Device into Hepatic Vein, Percutaneous Endoscopic Approach

06H44DZ Insertion of Intraluminal Device into Hepatic Vein, Percutaneous Endoscopic Approach

06H503Z Insertion of Infusion Device into Superior Mesenteric Vein, Open Approach

06H50DZ Insertion of Intraluminal Device into Superior Mesenteric Vein, Open Approach

06H533Z Insertion of Infusion Device into Superior Mesenteric Vein, Percutaneous Approach

06H53DZ Insertion of Intraluminal Device into Superior Mesenteric Vein, Percutaneous Approach

06H543Z Insertion of Infusion Device into Superior Mesenteric Vein, Percutaneous Endoscopic Approach

06H54DZ Insertion of Intraluminal Device into Superior Mesenteric Vein, Percutaneous Endoscopic Approach

06H603Z Insertion of Infusion Device into Inferior Mesenteric Vein, Open Approach

---

♀ Female-only   ♂ Male-only   ▲ Limited Coverage   ● Non-OR   HAC HAC-associated procedure   ▲ Non-covered procedures   ✛ Cluster   **435**

06H60DZ Insertion of Intraluminal Device into Inferior Mesenteric Vein, Open Approach

06H633Z Insertion of Infusion Device into Inferior Mesenteric Vein, Percutaneous Approach

06H63DZ Insertion of Intraluminal Device into Inferior Mesenteric Vein, Percutaneous Approach

06H643Z Insertion of Infusion Device into Inferior Mesenteric Vein, Percutaneous Endoscopic Approach

06H64DZ Insertion of Intraluminal Device into Inferior Mesenteric Vein, Percutaneous Endoscopic Approach

06H703Z Insertion of Infusion Device into Colic Vein, Open Approach

06H70DZ Insertion of Intraluminal Device into Colic Vein, Open Approach

06H733Z Insertion of Infusion Device into Colic Vein, Percutaneous Approach

06H73DZ Insertion of Intraluminal Device into Colic Vein, Percutaneous Approach

06H743Z Insertion of Infusion Device into Colic Vein, Percutaneous Endoscopic Approach

06H74DZ Insertion of Intraluminal Device into Colic Vein, Percutaneous Endoscopic Approach

06H803Z Insertion of Infusion Device into Portal Vein, Open Approach

06H80DZ Insertion of Intraluminal Device into Portal Vein, Open Approach

06H833Z Insertion of Infusion Device into Portal Vein, Percutaneous Approach

06H83DZ Insertion of Intraluminal Device into Portal Vein, Percutaneous Approach

06H843Z Insertion of Infusion Device into Portal Vein, Percutaneous Endoscopic Approach

06H84DZ Insertion of Intraluminal Device into Portal Vein, Percutaneous Endoscopic Approach

06H903Z Insertion of Infusion Device into Right Renal Vein, Open Approach

06H90DZ Insertion of Intraluminal Device into Right Renal Vein, Open Approach

06H933Z Insertion of Infusion Device into Right Renal Vein, Percutaneous Approach

06H93DZ Insertion of Intraluminal Device into Right Renal Vein, Percutaneous Approach

06H943Z Insertion of Infusion Device into Right Renal Vein, Percutaneous Endoscopic Approach

06H94DZ Insertion of Intraluminal Device into Right Renal Vein, Percutaneous Endoscopic Approach

06HB03Z Insertion of Infusion Device into Left Renal Vein, Open Approach

06HB0DZ Insertion of Intraluminal Device into Left Renal Vein, Open Approach

06HB33Z Insertion of Infusion Device into Left Renal Vein, Percutaneous Approach

06HB3DZ Insertion of Intraluminal Device into Left Renal Vein, Percutaneous Approach

06HB43Z Insertion of Infusion Device into Left Renal Vein, Percutaneous Endoscopic Approach

06HB4DZ Insertion of Intraluminal Device into Left Renal Vein, Percutaneous Endoscopic Approach

06HC03Z Insertion of Infusion Device into Right Common Iliac Vein, Open Approach

06HC0DZ Insertion of Intraluminal Device into Right Common Iliac Vein, Open Approach

06HC33Z Insertion of Infusion Device into Right Common Iliac Vein, Percutaneous Approach

06HC3DZ Insertion of Intraluminal Device into Right Common Iliac Vein, Percutaneous Approach

06HC43Z Insertion of Infusion Device into Right Common Iliac Vein, Percutaneous Endoscopic Approach

06HC4DZ Insertion of Intraluminal Device into Right Common Iliac Vein, Percutaneous Endoscopic Approach

06HD03Z Insertion of Infusion Device into Left Common Iliac Vein, Open Approach

06HD0DZ Insertion of Intraluminal Device into Left Common Iliac Vein, Open Approach

06HD33Z Insertion of Infusion Device into Left Common Iliac Vein, Percutaneous Approach

06HD3DZ Insertion of Intraluminal Device into Left Common Iliac Vein, Percutaneous Approach

06HD43Z Insertion of Infusion Device into Left Common Iliac Vein, Percutaneous Endoscopic Approach

06HD4DZ Insertion of Intraluminal Device into Left Common Iliac Vein, Percutaneous Endoscopic Approach

06HF03Z Insertion of Infusion Device into Right External Iliac Vein, Open Approach

06HF0DZ Insertion of Intraluminal Device into Right External Iliac Vein, Open Approach

06HF33Z Insertion of Infusion Device into Right External Iliac Vein, Percutaneous Approach

06HF3DZ Insertion of Intraluminal Device into Right External Iliac Vein, Percutaneous Approach

06HF43Z Insertion of Infusion Device into Right External Iliac Vein, Percutaneous Endoscopic Approach

06HF4DZ Insertion of Intraluminal Device into Right External Iliac Vein, Percutaneous Endoscopic Approach

06HG03Z Insertion of Infusion Device into Left External Iliac Vein, Open Approach

06HG0DZ Insertion of Intraluminal Device into Left External Iliac Vein, Open Approach

06HG33Z Insertion of Infusion Device into Left External Iliac Vein, Percutaneous Approach

06HG3DZ Insertion of Intraluminal Device into Left External Iliac Vein, Percutaneous Approach

06HG43Z Insertion of Infusion Device into Left External Iliac Vein, Percutaneous Endoscopic Approach

06HG4DZ Insertion of Intraluminal Device into Left External Iliac Vein, Percutaneous Endoscopic Approach

06HH03Z Insertion of Infusion Device into Right Hypogastric Vein, Open Approach

06HH0DZ Insertion of Intraluminal Device into Right Hypogastric Vein, Open Approach

06HH33Z Insertion of Infusion Device into Right Hypogastric Vein, Percutaneous Approach

06HH3DZ Insertion of Intraluminal Device into Right Hypogastric Vein, Percutaneous Approach

06HH43Z Insertion of Infusion Device into Right Hypogastric Vein, Percutaneous Endoscopic Approach

06HH4DZ Insertion of Intraluminal Device into Right Hypogastric Vein, Percutaneous Endoscopic Approach

06HJ03Z Insertion of Infusion Device into Left Hypogastric Vein, Open Approach

06HJ0DZ Insertion of Intraluminal Device into Left Hypogastric Vein, Open Approach

06HJ33Z Insertion of Infusion Device into Left Hypogastric Vein, Percutaneous Approach

06HJ3DZ Insertion of Intraluminal Device into Left Hypogastric Vein, Percutaneous Approach

06HJ43Z Insertion of Infusion Device into Left Hypogastric Vein, Percutaneous Endoscopic Approach

06HJ4DZ Insertion of Intraluminal Device into Left Hypogastric Vein, Percutaneous Endoscopic Approach

06HM03Z Insertion of Infusion Device into Right Femoral Vein, Open Approach

06HM0DZ Insertion of Intraluminal Device into Right Femoral Vein, Open Approach

06HM33Z Insertion of Infusion Device into Right Femoral Vein, Percutaneous Approach

06HM3DZ Insertion of Intraluminal Device into Right Femoral Vein, Percutaneous Approach

06HM43Z Insertion of Infusion Device into Right Femoral Vein, Percutaneous Endoscopic Approach

06HM4DZ Insertion of Intraluminal Device into Right Femoral Vein, Percutaneous Endoscopic Approach

06HN03Z Insertion of Infusion Device into Left Femoral Vein, Open Approach

06HN0DZ Insertion of Intraluminal Device into Left Femoral Vein, Open Approach

06HN33Z Insertion of Infusion Device into Left Femoral Vein, Percutaneous Approach

06HN3DZ Insertion of Intraluminal Device into Left Femoral Vein, Percutaneous Approach

06HN43Z Insertion of Infusion Device into Left Femoral Vein, Percutaneous Endoscopic Approach

06HN4DZ Insertion of Intraluminal Device into Left Femoral Vein, Percutaneous Endoscopic Approach

06HP03Z Insertion of Infusion Device into Right Saphenous Vein, Open Approach

06HP0DZ Insertion of Intraluminal Device into Right Saphenous Vein, Open Approach

06HP33Z Insertion of Infusion Device into Right Saphenous Vein, Percutaneous Approach

06HP3DZ Insertion of Intraluminal Device into Right Saphenous Vein, Percutaneous Approach

06HP43Z Insertion of Infusion Device into Right Saphenous Vein, Percutaneous Endoscopic Approach

06HP4DZ Insertion of Intraluminal Device into Right Saphenous Vein, Percutaneous Endoscopic Approach

06HQ03Z Insertion of Infusion Device into Left Saphenous Vein, Open Approach

06HQ0DZ Insertion of Intraluminal Device into Left Saphenous Vein, Open Approach

♀ Female-only ♂ Male-only ▲ Limited Coverage ● Non-OR ▨ HAC-associated procedure ▲ Non-covered procedures ✚ Cluster

06HQ33Z Insertion of Infusion Device into Left Saphenous Vein, Percutaneous Approach

06HQ3DZ Insertion of Intraluminal Device into Left Saphenous Vein, Percutaneous Approach

06HQ43Z Insertion of Infusion Device into Left Saphenous Vein, Percutaneous Endoscopic Approach

06HQ4DZ Insertion of Intraluminal Device into Left Saphenous Vein, Percutaneous Endoscopic Approach

06HT03Z Insertion of Infusion Device into Right Foot Vein, Open Approach

06HT0DZ Insertion of Intraluminal Device into Right Foot Vein, Open Approach

06HT33Z Insertion of Infusion Device into Right Foot Vein, Percutaneous Approach

06HT3DZ Insertion of Intraluminal Device into Right Foot Vein, Percutaneous Approach

06HT43Z Insertion of Infusion Device into Right Foot Vein, Percutaneous Endoscopic Approach

06HT4DZ Insertion of Intraluminal Device into Right Foot Vein, Percutaneous Endoscopic Approach

06HV03Z Insertion of Infusion Device into Left Foot Vein, Open Approach

06HV0DZ Insertion of Intraluminal Device into Left Foot Vein, Open Approach

06HV33Z Insertion of Infusion Device into Left Foot Vein, Percutaneous Approach

06HV3DZ Insertion of Intraluminal Device into Left Foot Vein, Percutaneous Approach

06HV43Z Insertion of Infusion Device into Left Foot Vein, Percutaneous Endoscopic Approach

06HV4DZ Insertion of Intraluminal Device into Left Foot Vein, Percutaneous Endoscopic Approach

06HY02Z Insertion of Monitoring Device into Lower Vein, Open Approach

06HY03Z Insertion of Infusion Device into Lower Vein, Open Approach

06HY0DZ Insertion of Intraluminal Device into Lower Vein, Open Approach

06HY0YZ Insertion of Other Device into Lower Vein, Open Approach

06HY32Z Insertion of Monitoring Device into Lower Vein, Percutaneous Approach

06HY33Z Insertion of Infusion Device into Lower Vein, Percutaneous Approach
AHA CC: 1Q, 2017, 31

06HY3DZ Insertion of Intraluminal Device into Lower Vein, Percutaneous Approach

06HY3YZ Insertion of Other Device into Lower Vein, Percutaneous Approach

06HY42Z Insertion of Monitoring Device into Lower Vein, Percutaneous Endoscopic Approach

06HY43Z Insertion of Infusion Device into Lower Vein, Percutaneous Endoscopic Approach

06HY4DZ Insertion of Intraluminal Device into Lower Vein, Percutaneous Endoscopic Approach

06HY4YZ Insertion of Other Device into Lower Vein, Percutaneous Endoscopic Approach

06J – Lower Veins, Inspection

Review Coding Guidelines B3.11a, B3.11b and B3.11c

06JY0ZZ Inspection of Lower Vein, Open Approach

06JY3ZZ Inspection of Lower Vein, Percutaneous Approach

06JY4ZZ Inspection of Lower Vein, Percutaneous Endoscopic Approach

06JYXZZ Inspection of Lower Vein, External Approach

06L – Lower Veins, Occlusion

Review Coding Guideline B3.12

06L00CZ Occlusion of Inferior Vena Cava with Extraluminal Device, Open Approach

06L00DZ Occlusion of Inferior Vena Cava with Intraluminal Device, Open Approach

06L00ZZ Occlusion of Inferior Vena Cava, Open Approach

06L03CZ Occlusion of Inferior Vena Cava with Extraluminal Device, Percutaneous Approach

06L03DZ Occlusion of Inferior Vena Cava with Intraluminal Device, Percutaneous Approach

06L03ZZ Occlusion of Inferior Vena Cava, Percutaneous Approach

06L04CZ Occlusion of Inferior Vena Cava with Extraluminal Device, Percutaneous Endoscopic Approach

06L04DZ Occlusion of Inferior Vena Cava with Intraluminal Device, Percutaneous Endoscopic Approach

06L04ZZ Occlusion of Inferior Vena Cava, Percutaneous Endoscopic Approach

06L10CZ Occlusion of Splenic Vein with Extraluminal Device, Open Approach

06L10DZ Occlusion of Splenic Vein with Intraluminal Device, Open Approach

06L10ZZ Occlusion of Splenic Vein, Open Approach

06L13CZ Occlusion of Splenic Vein with Extraluminal Device, Percutaneous Approach

06L13DZ Occlusion of Splenic Vein with Intraluminal Device, Percutaneous Approach

06L13ZZ Occlusion of Splenic Vein, Percutaneous Approach

06L14CZ Occlusion of Splenic Vein with Extraluminal Device, Percutaneous Endoscopic Approach

06L14DZ Occlusion of Splenic Vein with Intraluminal Device, Percutaneous Endoscopic Approach

06L14ZZ Occlusion of Splenic Vein, Percutaneous Endoscopic Approach

06L20CZ Occlusion of Gastric Vein with Extraluminal Device, Open Approach

06L20DZ Occlusion of Gastric Vein with Intraluminal Device, Open Approach

06L20ZZ Occlusion of Gastric Vein, Open Approach

06L23CZ Occlusion of Gastric Vein with Extraluminal Device, Percutaneous Approach

06L23DZ Occlusion of Gastric Vein with Intraluminal Device, Percutaneous Approach

06L23ZZ Occlusion of Gastric Vein, Percutaneous Approach

06L24CZ Occlusion of Gastric Vein with Extraluminal Device, Percutaneous Endoscopic Approach

06L24DZ Occlusion of Gastric Vein with Intraluminal Device, Percutaneous Endoscopic Approach

06L24ZZ Occlusion of Gastric Vein, Percutaneous Endoscopic Approach

06L27CZ Occlusion of Gastric Vein with Extraluminal Device, Via Natural or Artificial Opening

06L27DZ Occlusion of Gastric Vein with Intraluminal Device, Via Natural or Artificial Opening

06L27ZZ Occlusion of Gastric Vein, Via Natural or Artificial Opening

06L28CZ Occlusion of Gastric Vein with Extraluminal Device, Via Natural or Artificial Opening Endoscopic

06L28DZ Occlusion of Gastric Vein with Intraluminal Device, Via Natural or Artificial Opening Endoscopic

06L28ZZ Occlusion of Gastric Vein, Via Natural or Artificial Opening Endoscopic

06L30CZ Occlusion of Esophageal Vein with Extraluminal Device, Open Approach

06L30DZ Occlusion of Esophageal Vein with Intraluminal Device, Open Approach

06L30ZZ Occlusion of Esophageal Vein, Open Approach

06L33CZ Occlusion of Esophageal Vein with Extraluminal Device, Percutaneous Approach

06L33DZ Occlusion of Esophageal Vein with Intraluminal Device, Percutaneous Approach

06L33ZZ Occlusion of Esophageal Vein, Percutaneous Approach

06L34CZ Occlusion of Esophageal Vein with Extraluminal Device, Percutaneous Endoscopic Approach
AHA CC: 4Q, 2013, 112-113

06L34DZ Occlusion of Esophageal Vein with Intraluminal Device, Percutaneous Endoscopic Approach

06L34ZZ Occlusion of Esophageal Vein, Percutaneous Endoscopic Approach

♀ Female-only   ♂ Male-only   ▲ Limited Coverage   ● Non-OR   ▦ HAC-associated procedure   ▲ Non-covered procedures   ✚ Cluster   **437**

Medical and Surgical, Lower Veins Code Listings

06L37CZ	Occlusion of Esophageal Vein with Extraluminal Device, Via Natural or Artificial Opening
06L37DZ	Occlusion of Esophageal Vein with Intraluminal Device, Via Natural or Artificial Opening
06L37ZZ	Occlusion of Esophageal Vein, Via Natural or Artificial Opening
06L38CZ	Occlusion of Esophageal Vein with Extraluminal Device, Via Natural or Artificial Opening Endoscopic
	AHA CC: 4Q, 2017, 57-58
06L38DZ	Occlusion of Esophageal Vein with Intraluminal Device, Via Natural or Artificial Opening Endoscopic
06L38ZZ	Occlusion of Esophageal Vein, Via Natural or Artificial Opening Endoscopic
06L40CZ	Occlusion of Hepatic Vein with Extraluminal Device, Open Approach
06L40DZ	Occlusion of Hepatic Vein with Intraluminal Device, Open Approach
06L40ZZ	Occlusion of Hepatic Vein, Open Approach
06L43CZ	Occlusion of Hepatic Vein with Extraluminal Device, Percutaneous Approach
06L43DZ	Occlusion of Hepatic Vein with Intraluminal Device, Percutaneous Approach
06L43ZZ	Occlusion of Hepatic Vein, Percutaneous Approach
06L44CZ	Occlusion of Hepatic Vein with Extraluminal Device, Percutaneous Endoscopic Approach
06L44DZ	Occlusion of Hepatic Vein with Intraluminal Device, Percutaneous Endoscopic Approach
06L44ZZ	Occlusion of Hepatic Vein, Percutaneous Endoscopic Approach
06L50CZ	Occlusion of Superior Mesenteric Vein with Extraluminal Device, Open Approach
06L50DZ	Occlusion of Superior Mesenteric Vein with Intraluminal Device, Open Approach
06L50ZZ	Occlusion of Superior Mesenteric Vein, Open Approach
06L53CZ	Occlusion of Superior Mesenteric Vein with Extraluminal Device, Percutaneous Approach
06L53DZ	Occlusion of Superior Mesenteric Vein with Intraluminal Device, Percutaneous Approach
06L53ZZ	Occlusion of Superior Mesenteric Vein, Percutaneous Approach
06L54CZ	Occlusion of Superior Mesenteric Vein with Extraluminal Device, Percutaneous Endoscopic Approach
06L54DZ	Occlusion of Superior Mesenteric Vein with Intraluminal Device, Percutaneous Endoscopic Approach
06L54ZZ	Occlusion of Superior Mesenteric Vein, Percutaneous Endoscopic Approach
06L60CZ	Occlusion of Inferior Mesenteric Vein with Extraluminal Device, Open Approach
06L60DZ	Occlusion of Inferior Mesenteric Vein with Intraluminal Device, Open Approach
06L60ZZ	Occlusion of Inferior Mesenteric Vein, Open Approach
06L63CZ	Occlusion of Inferior Mesenteric Vein with Extraluminal Device, Percutaneous Approach
06L63DZ	Occlusion of Inferior Mesenteric Vein with Intraluminal Device, Percutaneous Approach
06L63ZZ	Occlusion of Inferior Mesenteric Vein, Percutaneous Approach
06L64CZ	Occlusion of Inferior Mesenteric Vein with Extraluminal Device, Percutaneous Endoscopic Approach
06L64DZ	Occlusion of Inferior Mesenteric Vein with Intraluminal Device, Percutaneous Endoscopic Approach
06L64ZZ	Occlusion of Inferior Mesenteric Vein, Percutaneous Endoscopic Approach
06L70CZ	Occlusion of Colic Vein with Extraluminal Device, Open Approach
06L70DZ	Occlusion of Colic Vein with Intraluminal Device, Open Approach
06L70ZZ	Occlusion of Colic Vein, Open Approach
06L73CZ	Occlusion of Colic Vein with Extraluminal Device, Percutaneous Approach
06L73DZ	Occlusion of Colic Vein with Intraluminal Device, Percutaneous Approach
06L73ZZ	Occlusion of Colic Vein, Percutaneous Approach
06L74CZ	Occlusion of Colic Vein with Extraluminal Device, Percutaneous Endoscopic Approach
06L74DZ	Occlusion of Colic Vein with Intraluminal Device, Percutaneous Endoscopic Approach
06L74ZZ	Occlusion of Colic Vein, Percutaneous Endoscopic Approach
06L80CZ	Occlusion of Portal Vein with Extraluminal Device, Open Approach
06L80DZ	Occlusion of Portal Vein with Intraluminal Device, Open Approach
06L80ZZ	Occlusion of Portal Vein, Open Approach
06L83CZ	Occlusion of Portal Vein with Extraluminal Device, Percutaneous Approach
06L83DZ	Occlusion of Portal Vein with Intraluminal Device, Percutaneous Approach
06L83ZZ	Occlusion of Portal Vein, Percutaneous Approach
06L84CZ	Occlusion of Portal Vein with Extraluminal Device, Percutaneous Endoscopic Approach
06L84DZ	Occlusion of Portal Vein with Intraluminal Device, Percutaneous Endoscopic Approach
06L84ZZ	Occlusion of Portal Vein, Percutaneous Endoscopic Approach
06L90CZ	Occlusion of Right Renal Vein with Extraluminal Device, Open Approach
06L90DZ	Occlusion of Right Renal Vein with Intraluminal Device, Open Approach
06L90ZZ	Occlusion of Right Renal Vein, Open Approach
06L93CZ	Occlusion of Right Renal Vein with Extraluminal Device, Percutaneous Approach
06L93DZ	Occlusion of Right Renal Vein with Intraluminal Device, Percutaneous Approach
06L93ZZ	Occlusion of Right Renal Vein, Percutaneous Approach
06L94CZ	Occlusion of Right Renal Vein with Extraluminal Device, Percutaneous Endoscopic Approach
06L94DZ	Occlusion of Right Renal Vein with Intraluminal Device, Percutaneous Endoscopic Approach
06L94ZZ	Occlusion of Right Renal Vein, Percutaneous Endoscopic Approach
06LB0CZ	Occlusion of Left Renal Vein with Extraluminal Device, Open Approach
06LB0DZ	Occlusion of Left Renal Vein with Intraluminal Device, Open Approach
06LB0ZZ	Occlusion of Left Renal Vein, Open Approach
06LB3CZ	Occlusion of Left Renal Vein with Extraluminal Device, Percutaneous Approach
06LB3DZ	Occlusion of Left Renal Vein with Intraluminal Device, Percutaneous Approach
06LB3ZZ	Occlusion of Left Renal Vein, Percutaneous Approach
06LB4CZ	Occlusion of Left Renal Vein with Extraluminal Device, Percutaneous Endoscopic Approach
06LB4DZ	Occlusion of Left Renal Vein with Intraluminal Device, Percutaneous Endoscopic Approach
06LB4ZZ	Occlusion of Left Renal Vein, Percutaneous Endoscopic Approach
06LC0CZ	Occlusion of Right Common Iliac Vein with Extraluminal Device, Open Approach
06LC0DZ	Occlusion of Right Common Iliac Vein with Intraluminal Device, Open Approach
06LC0ZZ	Occlusion of Right Common Iliac Vein, Open Approach
06LC3CZ	Occlusion of Right Common Iliac Vein with Extraluminal Device, Percutaneous Approach
06LC3DZ	Occlusion of Right Common Iliac Vein with Intraluminal Device, Percutaneous Approach
06LC3ZZ	Occlusion of Right Common Iliac Vein, Percutaneous Approach
06LC4CZ	Occlusion of Right Common Iliac Vein with Extraluminal Device, Percutaneous Endoscopic Approach
06LC4DZ	Occlusion of Right Common Iliac Vein with Intraluminal Device, Percutaneous Endoscopic Approach
06LC4ZZ	Occlusion of Right Common Iliac Vein, Percutaneous Endoscopic Approach
06LD0CZ	Occlusion of Left Common Iliac Vein with Extraluminal Device, Open Approach
06LD0DZ	Occlusion of Left Common Iliac Vein with Intraluminal Device, Open Approach
06LD0ZZ	Occlusion of Left Common Iliac Vein, Open Approach
06LD3CZ	Occlusion of Left Common Iliac Vein with Extraluminal Device, Percutaneous Approach
06LD3DZ	Occlusion of Left Common Iliac Vein with Intraluminal Device, Percutaneous Approach
06LD3ZZ	Occlusion of Left Common Iliac Vein, Percutaneous Approach
06LD4CZ	Occlusion of Left Common Iliac Vein with Extraluminal Device, Percutaneous Endoscopic Approach
06LD4DZ	Occlusion of Left Common Iliac Vein with Intraluminal Device, Percutaneous Endoscopic Approach
06LD4ZZ	Occlusion of Left Common Iliac Vein, Percutaneous Endoscopic Approach

♀ Female-only ♂ Male-only ▲ Limited Coverage ● Non-OR ▪ HAC HAC-associated procedure ▲ Non-covered procedures ✚ Cluster

06LF0CZ Occlusion of Right External Iliac Vein with Extraluminal Device, Open Approach
AHA CC: 2Q, 2018, 18-19

06LF0DZ Occlusion of Right External Iliac Vein with Intraluminal Device, Open Approach

06LF0ZZ Occlusion of Right External Iliac Vein, Open Approach

06LF3CZ Occlusion of Right External Iliac Vein with Extraluminal Device, Percutaneous Approach

06LF3DZ Occlusion of Right External Iliac Vein with Intraluminal Device, Percutaneous Approach

06LF3ZZ Occlusion of Right External Iliac Vein, Percutaneous Approach

06LF4CZ Occlusion of Right External Iliac Vein with Extraluminal Device, Percutaneous Endoscopic Approach

06LF4DZ Occlusion of Right External Iliac Vein with Intraluminal Device, Percutaneous Endoscopic Approach

06LF4ZZ Occlusion of Right External Iliac Vein, Percutaneous Endoscopic Approach

06LG0CZ Occlusion of Left External Iliac Vein with Extraluminal Device, Open Approach
AHA CC: 2Q, 2018, 18-19

06LG0DZ Occlusion of Left External Iliac Vein with Intraluminal Device, Open Approach

06LG0ZZ Occlusion of Left External Iliac Vein, Open Approach

06LG3CZ Occlusion of Left External Iliac Vein with Extraluminal Device, Percutaneous Approach

06LG3DZ Occlusion of Left External Iliac Vein with Intraluminal Device, Percutaneous Approach

06LG3ZZ Occlusion of Left External Iliac Vein, Percutaneous Approach

06LG4CZ Occlusion of Left External Iliac Vein with Extraluminal Device, Percutaneous Endoscopic Approach

06LG4DZ Occlusion of Left External Iliac Vein with Intraluminal Device, Percutaneous Endoscopic Approach

06LG4ZZ Occlusion of Left External Iliac Vein, Percutaneous Endoscopic Approach

06LH0CZ Occlusion of Right Hypogastric Vein with Extraluminal Device, Open Approach

06LH0DZ Occlusion of Right Hypogastric Vein with Intraluminal Device, Open Approach

06LH0ZZ Occlusion of Right Hypogastric Vein, Open Approach

06LH3CZ Occlusion of Right Hypogastric Vein with Extraluminal Device, Percutaneous Approach

06LH3DZ Occlusion of Right Hypogastric Vein with Intraluminal Device, Percutaneous Approach

06LH3ZZ Occlusion of Right Hypogastric Vein, Percutaneous Approach

06LH4CZ Occlusion of Right Hypogastric Vein with Extraluminal Device, Percutaneous Endoscopic Approach

06LH4DZ Occlusion of Right Hypogastric Vein with Intraluminal Device, Percutaneous Endoscopic Approach

06LH4ZZ Occlusion of Right Hypogastric Vein, Percutaneous Endoscopic Approach

06LJ0CZ Occlusion of Left Hypogastric Vein with Extraluminal Device, Open Approach

06LJ0DZ Occlusion of Left Hypogastric Vein with Intraluminal Device, Open Approach

06LJ0ZZ Occlusion of Left Hypogastric Vein, Open Approach

06LJ3CZ Occlusion of Left Hypogastric Vein with Extraluminal Device, Percutaneous Approach

06LJ3DZ Occlusion of Left Hypogastric Vein with Intraluminal Device, Percutaneous Approach

06LJ3ZZ Occlusion of Left Hypogastric Vein, Percutaneous Approach

06LJ4CZ Occlusion of Left Hypogastric Vein with Extraluminal Device, Percutaneous Endoscopic Approach

06LJ4DZ Occlusion of Left Hypogastric Vein with Intraluminal Device, Percutaneous Endoscopic Approach

06LJ4ZZ Occlusion of Left Hypogastric Vein, Percutaneous Endoscopic Approach

06LM0CZ Occlusion of Right Femoral Vein with Extraluminal Device, Open Approach

06LM0DZ Occlusion of Right Femoral Vein with Intraluminal Device, Open Approach

06LM0ZZ Occlusion of Right Femoral Vein, Open Approach

06LM3CZ Occlusion of Right Femoral Vein with Extraluminal Device, Percutaneous Approach

06LM3DZ Occlusion of Right Femoral Vein with Intraluminal Device, Percutaneous Approach

06LM3ZZ Occlusion of Right Femoral Vein, Percutaneous Approach

06LM4CZ Occlusion of Right Femoral Vein with Extraluminal Device, Percutaneous Endoscopic Approach

06LM4DZ Occlusion of Right Femoral Vein with Intraluminal Device, Percutaneous Endoscopic Approach

06LM4ZZ Occlusion of Right Femoral Vein, Percutaneous Endoscopic Approach

06LN0CZ Occlusion of Left Femoral Vein with Extraluminal Device, Open Approach

06LN0DZ Occlusion of Left Femoral Vein with Intraluminal Device, Open Approach

06LN0ZZ Occlusion of Left Femoral Vein, Open Approach

06LN3CZ Occlusion of Left Femoral Vein with Extraluminal Device, Percutaneous Approach

06LN3DZ Occlusion of Left Femoral Vein with Intraluminal Device, Percutaneous Approach

06LN3ZZ Occlusion of Left Femoral Vein, Percutaneous Approach

06LN4CZ Occlusion of Left Femoral Vein with Extraluminal Device, Percutaneous Endoscopic Approach

06LN4DZ Occlusion of Left Femoral Vein with Intraluminal Device, Percutaneous Endoscopic Approach

06LN4ZZ Occlusion of Left Femoral Vein, Percutaneous Endoscopic Approach

06LP0CZ Occlusion of Right Saphenous Vein with Extraluminal Device, Open Approach

06LP0DZ Occlusion of Right Saphenous Vein with Intraluminal Device, Open Approach

06LP0ZZ Occlusion of Right Saphenous Vein, Open Approach

06LP3CZ Occlusion of Right Saphenous Vein with Extraluminal Device, Percutaneous Approach

06LP3DZ Occlusion of Right Saphenous Vein with Intraluminal Device, Percutaneous Approach

06LP3ZZ Occlusion of Right Saphenous Vein, Percutaneous Approach

06LP4CZ Occlusion of Right Saphenous Vein with Extraluminal Device, Percutaneous Endoscopic Approach

06LP4DZ Occlusion of Right Saphenous Vein with Intraluminal Device, Percutaneous Endoscopic Approach

06LP4ZZ Occlusion of Right Saphenous Vein, Percutaneous Endoscopic Approach

06LQ0CZ Occlusion of Left Saphenous Vein with Extraluminal Device, Open Approach

06LQ0DZ Occlusion of Left Saphenous Vein with Intraluminal Device, Open Approach

06LQ0ZZ Occlusion of Left Saphenous Vein, Open Approach

06LQ3CZ Occlusion of Left Saphenous Vein with Extraluminal Device, Percutaneous Approach

06LQ3DZ Occlusion of Left Saphenous Vein with Intraluminal Device, Percutaneous Approach

06LQ3ZZ Occlusion of Left Saphenous Vein, Percutaneous Approach

06LQ4CZ Occlusion of Left Saphenous Vein with Extraluminal Device, Percutaneous Endoscopic Approach

06LQ4DZ Occlusion of Left Saphenous Vein with Intraluminal Device, Percutaneous Endoscopic Approach

06LQ4ZZ Occlusion of Left Saphenous Vein, Percutaneous Endoscopic Approach

06LT0CZ Occlusion of Right Foot Vein with Extraluminal Device, Open Approach

06LT0DZ Occlusion of Right Foot Vein with Intraluminal Device, Open Approach

06LT0ZZ Occlusion of Right Foot Vein, Open Approach

06LT3CZ Occlusion of Right Foot Vein with Extraluminal Device, Percutaneous Approach

06LT3DZ Occlusion of Right Foot Vein with Intraluminal Device, Percutaneous Approach

06LT3ZZ Occlusion of Right Foot Vein, Percutaneous Approach

06LT4CZ Occlusion of Right Foot Vein with Extraluminal Device, Percutaneous Endoscopic Approach

06LT4DZ Occlusion of Right Foot Vein with Intraluminal Device, Percutaneous Endoscopic Approach

06LT4ZZ Occlusion of Right Foot Vein, Percutaneous Endoscopic Approach

06LV0CZ Occlusion of Left Foot Vein with Extraluminal Device, Open Approach

06LV0DZ Occlusion of Left Foot Vein with Intraluminal Device, Open Approach

06LV0ZZ Occlusion of Left Foot Vein, Open Approach

06LV3CZ Occlusion of Left Foot Vein with Extraluminal Device, Percutaneous Approach

06LV3DZ Occlusion of Left Foot Vein with Intraluminal Device, Percutaneous Approach

06LV3ZZ Occlusion of Left Foot Vein, Percutaneous Approach

06LV4CZ Occlusion of Left Foot Vein with Extraluminal Device, Percutaneous Endoscopic Approach

06LV4DZ Occlusion of Left Foot Vein with Intraluminal Device, Percutaneous Endoscopic Approach

06LV4ZZ Occlusion of Left Foot Vein, Percutaneous Endoscopic Approach

06LY0CC Occlusion of Hemorrhoidal Plexus with Extraluminal Device, Open Approach

06LY0CZ Occlusion of Lower Vein with Extraluminal Device, Open Approach

06LY0DC Occlusion of Hemorrhoidal Plexus with Intraluminal Device, Open Approach

06LY0DZ Occlusion of Lower Vein with Intraluminal Device, Open Approach

06LY0ZC Occlusion of Hemorrhoidal Plexus, Open Approach

06LY0ZZ Occlusion of Lower Vein, Open Approach

06LY3CC Occlusion of Hemorrhoidal Plexus with Extraluminal Device, Percutaneous Approach

06LY3CZ Occlusion of Lower Vein with Extraluminal Device, Percutaneous Approach

06LY3DC Occlusion of Hemorrhoidal Plexus with Intraluminal Device, Percutaneous Approach

06LY3DZ Occlusion of Lower Vein with Intraluminal Device, Percutaneous Approach

AHA CC: 3Q, 2020, 44-45

06LY3ZC Occlusion of Hemorrhoidal Plexus, Percutaneous Approach

06LY3ZZ Occlusion of Lower Vein, Percutaneous Approach

06LY4CC Occlusion of Hemorrhoidal Plexus with Extraluminal Device, Percutaneous Endoscopic Approach

06LY4CZ Occlusion of Lower Vein with Extraluminal Device, Percutaneous Endoscopic Approach

06LY4DC Occlusion of Hemorrhoidal Plexus with Intraluminal Device, Percutaneous Endoscopic Approach

06LY4DZ Occlusion of Lower Vein with Intraluminal Device, Percutaneous Endoscopic Approach

06LY4ZC Occlusion of Hemorrhoidal Plexus, Percutaneous Endoscopic Approach

06LY4ZZ Occlusion of Lower Vein, Percutaneous Endoscopic Approach

06LY7CC Occlusion of Hemorrhoidal Plexus with Extraluminal Device, Via Natural or Artificial Opening

06LY7CZ Occlusion of Lower Vein with Extraluminal Device, Via Natural or Artificial Opening

06LY7DC Occlusion of Hemorrhoidal Plexus with Intraluminal Device, Via Natural or Artificial Opening

06LY7DZ Occlusion of Lower Vein with Intraluminal Device, Via Natural or Artificial Opening

06LY7ZC Occlusion of Hemorrhoidal Plexus, Via Natural or Artificial Opening

06LY7ZZ Occlusion of Lower Vein, Via Natural or Artificial Opening

06LY8CC Occlusion of Hemorrhoidal Plexus with Extraluminal Device, Via Natural or Artificial Opening Endoscopic

06LY8CZ Occlusion of Lower Vein with Extraluminal Device, Via Natural or Artificial Opening Endoscopic

06LY8DC Occlusion of Hemorrhoidal Plexus with Intraluminal Device, Via Natural or Artificial Opening Endoscopic

06LY8DZ Occlusion of Lower Vein with Intraluminal Device, Via Natural or Artificial Opening Endoscopic

06LY8ZC Occlusion of Hemorrhoidal Plexus, Via Natural or Artificial Opening Endoscopic

06LY8ZZ Occlusion of Lower Vein, Via Natural or Artificial Opening Endoscopic

06N – Lower Veins, Release

Review Coding Guidelines B3.13 and B3.14

06N00ZZ Release Inferior Vena Cava, Open Approach

06N03ZZ Release Inferior Vena Cava, Percutaneous Approach

06N04ZZ Release Inferior Vena Cava, Percutaneous Endoscopic Approach

06N10ZZ Release Splenic Vein, Open Approach

06N13ZZ Release Splenic Vein, Percutaneous Approach

06N14ZZ Release Splenic Vein, Percutaneous Endoscopic Approach

06N20ZZ Release Gastric Vein, Open Approach

06N23ZZ Release Gastric Vein, Percutaneous Approach

06N24ZZ Release Gastric Vein, Percutaneous Endoscopic Approach

06N30ZZ Release Esophageal Vein, Open Approach

06N33ZZ Release Esophageal Vein, Percutaneous Approach

06N34ZZ Release Esophageal Vein, Percutaneous Endoscopic Approach

06N40ZZ Release Hepatic Vein, Open Approach

06N43ZZ Release Hepatic Vein, Percutaneous Approach

06N44ZZ Release Hepatic Vein, Percutaneous Endoscopic Approach

06N50ZZ Release Superior Mesenteric Vein, Open Approach

06N53ZZ Release Superior Mesenteric Vein, Percutaneous Approach

06N54ZZ Release Superior Mesenteric Vein, Percutaneous Endoscopic Approach

06N60ZZ Release Inferior Mesenteric Vein, Open Approach

06N63ZZ Release Inferior Mesenteric Vein, Percutaneous Approach

06N64ZZ Release Inferior Mesenteric Vein, Percutaneous Endoscopic Approach

06N70ZZ Release Colic Vein, Open Approach

06N73ZZ Release Colic Vein, Percutaneous Approach

06N74ZZ Release Colic Vein, Percutaneous Endoscopic Approach

06N80ZZ Release Portal Vein, Open Approach

06N83ZZ Release Portal Vein, Percutaneous Approach

06N84ZZ Release Portal Vein, Percutaneous Endoscopic Approach

06N90ZZ Release Right Renal Vein, Open Approach

06N93ZZ Release Right Renal Vein, Percutaneous Approach

06N94ZZ Release Right Renal Vein, Percutaneous Endoscopic Approach

06NB0ZZ Release Left Renal Vein, Open Approach

06NB3ZZ Release Left Renal Vein, Percutaneous Approach

06NB4ZZ Release Left Renal Vein, Percutaneous Endoscopic Approach

06NC0ZZ Release Right Common Iliac Vein, Open Approach

06NC3ZZ Release Right Common Iliac Vein, Percutaneous Approach

06NC4ZZ Release Right Common Iliac Vein, Percutaneous Endoscopic Approach

06ND0ZZ Release Left Common Iliac Vein, Open Approach

06ND3ZZ Release Left Common Iliac Vein, Percutaneous Approach

06ND4ZZ Release Left Common Iliac Vein, Percutaneous Endoscopic Approach

06NF0ZZ Release Right External Iliac Vein, Open Approach

06NF3ZZ Release Right External Iliac Vein, Percutaneous Approach

06NF4ZZ Release Right External Iliac Vein, Percutaneous Endoscopic Approach

06NG0ZZ Release Left External Iliac Vein, Open Approach

06NG3ZZ Release Left External Iliac Vein, Percutaneous Approach

06NG4ZZ Release Left External Iliac Vein, Percutaneous Endoscopic Approach

06NH0ZZ Release Right Hypogastric Vein, Open Approach

06NH3ZZ Release Right Hypogastric Vein, Percutaneous Approach

06NH4ZZ Release Right Hypogastric Vein, Percutaneous Endoscopic Approach

06NJ0ZZ Release Left Hypogastric Vein, Open Approach

06NJ3ZZ Release Left Hypogastric Vein, Percutaneous Approach

06NJ4ZZ Release Left Hypogastric Vein, Percutaneous Endoscopic Approach

06NM0ZZ Release Right Femoral Vein, Open Approach

06NM3ZZ Release Right Femoral Vein, Percutaneous Approach

06NM4ZZ Release Right Femoral Vein, Percutaneous Endoscopic Approach

06NN0ZZ Release Left Femoral Vein, Open Approach

06NN3ZZ Release Left Femoral Vein, Percutaneous Approach

06NN4ZZ Release Left Femoral Vein, Percutaneous Endoscopic Approach

06NP0ZZ Release Right Saphenous Vein, Open Approach

06NP3ZZ Release Right Saphenous Vein, Percutaneous Approach

06NP4ZZ Release Right Saphenous Vein, Percutaneous Endoscopic Approach

06NQ0ZZ Release Left Saphenous Vein, Open Approach

06NQ3ZZ Release Left Saphenous Vein, Percutaneous Approach

♀ Female-only   ♂ Male-only   ▲ Limited Coverage   ● Non-OR   HAC HAC-associated procedure   ▲ Non-covered procedures   ✚ Cluste

06NQ4ZZ   Release Left Saphenous Vein, Percutaneous Endoscopic Approach
06NT0ZZ   Release Right Foot Vein, Open Approach
06NT3ZZ   Release Right Foot Vein, Percutaneous Approach

06NT4ZZ   Release Right Foot Vein, Percutaneous Endoscopic Approach
06NV0ZZ   Release Left Foot Vein, Open Approach
06NV3ZZ   Release Left Foot Vein, Percutaneous Approach
06NV4ZZ   Release Left Foot Vein, Percutaneous Endoscopic Approach

06NY0ZZ   Release Lower Vein, Open Approach
06NY3ZZ   Release Lower Vein, Percutaneous Approach
06NY4ZZ   Release Lower Vein, Percutaneous Endoscopic Approach

06P – Lower Veins, Removal

Review Coding Guideline B6.1c

06PY00Z   Removal of Drainage Device from Lower Vein, Open Approach
06PY02Z   Removal of Monitoring Device from Lower Vein, Open Approach
06PY03Z   Removal of Infusion Device from Lower Vein, Open Approach
06PY07Z   Removal of Autologous Tissue Substitute from Lower Vein, Open Approach
06PY0CZ   Removal of Extraluminal Device from Lower Vein, Open Approach
06PY0DZ   Removal of Intraluminal Device from Lower Vein, Open Approach
06PY0JZ   Removal of Synthetic Substitute from Lower Vein, Open Approach
06PY0KZ   Removal of Nonautologous Tissue Substitute from Lower Vein, Open Approach
06PY0YZ   Removal of Other Device from Lower Vein, Open Approach
06PY30Z   Removal of Drainage Device from Lower Vein, Percutaneous Approach
06PY32Z   Removal of Monitoring Device from Lower Vein, Percutaneous Approach
06PY33Z   Removal of Infusion Device from Lower Vein, Percutaneous Approach

06PY37Z   Removal of Autologous Tissue Substitute from Lower Vein, Percutaneous Approach
06PY3CZ   Removal of Extraluminal Device from Lower Vein, Percutaneous Approach
06PY3DZ   Removal of Intraluminal Device from Lower Vein, Percutaneous Approach
06PY3JZ   Removal of Synthetic Substitute from Lower Vein, Percutaneous Approach
06PY3KZ   Removal of Nonautologous Tissue Substitute from Lower Vein, Percutaneous Approach
06PY3YZ   Removal of Other Device from Lower Vein, Percutaneous Approach
06PY40Z   Removal of Drainage Device from Lower Vein, Percutaneous Endoscopic Approach
06PY42Z   Removal of Monitoring Device from Lower Vein, Percutaneous Endoscopic Approach
06PY43Z   Removal of Infusion Device from Lower Vein, Percutaneous Endoscopic Approach
06PY47Z   Removal of Autologous Tissue Substitute from Lower Vein, Percutaneous Endoscopic Approach

06PY4CZ   Removal of Extraluminal Device from Lower Vein, Percutaneous Endoscopic Approach
06PY4DZ   Removal of Intraluminal Device from Lower Vein, Percutaneous Endoscopic Approach
06PY4JZ   Removal of Synthetic Substitute from Lower Vein, Percutaneous Endoscopic Approach
06PY4KZ   Removal of Nonautologous Tissue Substitute from Lower Vein, Percutaneous Endoscopic Approach
06PY4YZ   Removal of Other Device from Lower Vein, Percutaneous Endoscopic Approach
06PYX0Z   Removal of Drainage Device from Lower Vein, External Approach
06PYX2Z   Removal of Monitoring Device from Lower Vein, External Approach
06PYX3Z   Removal of Infusion Device from Lower Vein, External Approach
06PYXDZ   Removal of Intraluminal Device from Lower Vein, External Approach

06Q – Lower Veins, Repair

06Q00ZZ   Repair Inferior Vena Cava, Open Approach
06Q03ZZ   Repair Inferior Vena Cava, Percutaneous Approach
06Q04ZZ   Repair Inferior Vena Cava, Percutaneous Endoscopic Approach
06Q10ZZ   Repair Splenic Vein, Open Approach
06Q13ZZ   Repair Splenic Vein, Percutaneous Approach
06Q14ZZ   Repair Splenic Vein, Percutaneous Endoscopic Approach
06Q20ZZ   Repair Gastric Vein, Open Approach
06Q23ZZ   Repair Gastric Vein, Percutaneous Approach
06Q24ZZ   Repair Gastric Vein, Percutaneous Endoscopic Approach
06Q30ZZ   Repair Esophageal Vein, Open Approach
06Q33ZZ   Repair Esophageal Vein, Percutaneous Approach
06Q34ZZ   Repair Esophageal Vein, Percutaneous Endoscopic Approach
06Q40ZZ   Repair Hepatic Vein, Open Approach
06Q43ZZ   Repair Hepatic Vein, Percutaneous Approach
06Q44ZZ   Repair Hepatic Vein, Percutaneous Endoscopic Approach
06Q50ZZ   Repair Superior Mesenteric Vein, Open Approach
06Q53ZZ   Repair Superior Mesenteric Vein, Percutaneous Approach
06Q54ZZ   Repair Superior Mesenteric Vein, Percutaneous Endoscopic Approach
06Q60ZZ   Repair Inferior Mesenteric Vein, Open Approach

06Q63ZZ   Repair Inferior Mesenteric Vein, Percutaneous Approach
06Q64ZZ   Repair Inferior Mesenteric Vein, Percutaneous Endoscopic Approach
06Q70ZZ   Repair Colic Vein, Open Approach
06Q73ZZ   Repair Colic Vein, Percutaneous Approach
06Q74ZZ   Repair Colic Vein, Percutaneous Endoscopic Approach
06Q80ZZ   Repair Portal Vein, Open Approach
06Q83ZZ   Repair Portal Vein, Percutaneous Approach
06Q84ZZ   Repair Portal Vein, Percutaneous Endoscopic Approach
06Q90ZZ   Repair Right Renal Vein, Open Approach
06Q93ZZ   Repair Right Renal Vein, Percutaneous Approach
06Q94ZZ   Repair Right Renal Vein, Percutaneous Endoscopic Approach
06QB0ZZ   Repair Left Renal Vein, Open Approach
06QB3ZZ   Repair Left Renal Vein, Percutaneous Approach
06QB4ZZ   Repair Left Renal Vein, Percutaneous Endoscopic Approach
06QC0ZZ   Repair Right Common Iliac Vein, Open Approach
06QC3ZZ   Repair Right Common Iliac Vein, Percutaneous Approach
06QC4ZZ   Repair Right Common Iliac Vein, Percutaneous Endoscopic Approach
06QD0ZZ   Repair Left Common Iliac Vein, Open Approach

06QD3ZZ   Repair Left Common Iliac Vein, Percutaneous Approach
06QD4ZZ   Repair Left Common Iliac Vein, Percutaneous Endoscopic Approach
06QF0ZZ   Repair Right External Iliac Vein, Open Approach
06QF3ZZ   Repair Right External Iliac Vein, Percutaneous Approach
06QF4ZZ   Repair Right External Iliac Vein, Percutaneous Endoscopic Approach
06QG0ZZ   Repair Left External Iliac Vein, Open Approach
06QG3ZZ   Repair Left External Iliac Vein, Percutaneous Approach
06QG4ZZ   Repair Left External Iliac Vein, Percutaneous Endoscopic Approach
06QH0ZZ   Repair Right Hypogastric Vein, Open Approach
06QH3ZZ   Repair Right Hypogastric Vein, Percutaneous Approach
06QH4ZZ   Repair Right Hypogastric Vein, Percutaneous Endoscopic Approach
06QJ0ZZ   Repair Left Hypogastric Vein, Open Approach
06QJ3ZZ   Repair Left Hypogastric Vein, Percutaneous Approach
06QJ4ZZ   Repair Left Hypogastric Vein, Percutaneous Endoscopic Approach
06QM0ZZ   Repair Right Femoral Vein, Open Approach
06QM3ZZ   Repair Right Femoral Vein, Percutaneous Approach
06QM4ZZ   Repair Right Femoral Vein, Percutaneous Endoscopic Approach

06QN0ZZ Repair Left Femoral Vein, Open Approach

06QN3ZZ Repair Left Femoral Vein, Percutaneous Approach

06QN4ZZ Repair Left Femoral Vein, Percutaneous Endoscopic Approach

06QP0ZZ Repair Right Saphenous Vein, Open Approach

06QP3ZZ Repair Right Saphenous Vein, Percutaneous Approach

06QP4ZZ Repair Right Saphenous Vein, Percutaneous Endoscopic Approach

06QQ0ZZ Repair Left Saphenous Vein, Open Approach

06QQ3ZZ Repair Left Saphenous Vein, Percutaneous Approach

06QQ4ZZ Repair Left Saphenous Vein, Percutaneous Endoscopic Approach

06QT0ZZ Repair Right Foot Vein, Open Approach

06QT3ZZ Repair Right Foot Vein, Percutaneous Approach

06QT4ZZ Repair Right Foot Vein, Percutaneous Endoscopic Approach

06QV0ZZ Repair Left Foot Vein, Open Approach

06QV3ZZ Repair Left Foot Vein, Percutaneous Approach

06QV4ZZ Repair Left Foot Vein, Percutaneous Endoscopic Approach

06QY0ZZ Repair Lower Vein, Open Approach

06QY3ZZ Repair Lower Vein, Percutaneous Approach

06QY4ZZ Repair Lower Vein, Percutaneous Endoscopic Approach

06R – Lower Veins, Replacement

Review Coding Guideline B3.18

06R007Z Replacement of Inferior Vena Cava with Autologous Tissue Substitute, Open Approach

06R00JZ Replacement of Inferior Vena Cava with Synthetic Substitute, Open Approach

06R00KZ Replacement of Inferior Vena Cava with Nonautologous Tissue Substitute, Open Approach

06R047Z Replacement of Inferior Vena Cava with Autologous Tissue Substitute, Percutaneous Endoscopic Approach

06R04JZ Replacement of Inferior Vena Cava with Synthetic Substitute, Percutaneous Endoscopic Approach

06R04KZ Replacement of Inferior Vena Cava with Nonautologous Tissue Substitute, Percutaneous Endoscopic Approach

06R107Z Replacement of Splenic Vein with Autologous Tissue Substitute, Open Approach

06R10JZ Replacement of Splenic Vein with Synthetic Substitute, Open Approach

06R10KZ Replacement of Splenic Vein with Nonautologous Tissue Substitute, Open Approach

06R147Z Replacement of Splenic Vein with Autologous Tissue Substitute, Percutaneous Endoscopic Approach

06R14JZ Replacement of Splenic Vein with Synthetic Substitute, Percutaneous Endoscopic Approach

06R14KZ Replacement of Splenic Vein with Nonautologous Tissue Substitute, Percutaneous Endoscopic Approach

06R207Z Replacement of Gastric Vein with Autologous Tissue Substitute, Open Approach

06R20JZ Replacement of Gastric Vein with Synthetic Substitute, Open Approach

06R20KZ Replacement of Gastric Vein with Nonautologous Tissue Substitute, Open Approach

06R247Z Replacement of Gastric Vein with Autologous Tissue Substitute, Percutaneous Endoscopic Approach

06R24JZ Replacement of Gastric Vein with Synthetic Substitute, Percutaneous Endoscopic Approach

06R24KZ Replacement of Gastric Vein with Nonautologous Tissue Substitute, Percutaneous Endoscopic Approach

06R307Z Replacement of Esophageal Vein with Autologous Tissue Substitute, Open Approach

06R30JZ Replacement of Esophageal Vein with Synthetic Substitute, Open Approach

06R30KZ Replacement of Esophageal Vein with Nonautologous Tissue Substitute, Open Approach

06R347Z Replacement of Esophageal Vein with Autologous Tissue Substitute, Percutaneous Endoscopic Approach

06R34JZ Replacement of Esophageal Vein with Synthetic Substitute, Percutaneous Endoscopic Approach

06R34KZ Replacement of Esophageal Vein with Nonautologous Tissue Substitute, Percutaneous Endoscopic Approach

06R407Z Replacement of Hepatic Vein with Autologous Tissue Substitute, Open Approach

06R40JZ Replacement of Hepatic Vein with Synthetic Substitute, Open Approach

06R40KZ Replacement of Hepatic Vein with Nonautologous Tissue Substitute, Open Approach

06R447Z Replacement of Hepatic Vein with Autologous Tissue Substitute, Percutaneous Endoscopic Approach

06R44JZ Replacement of Hepatic Vein with Synthetic Substitute, Percutaneous Endoscopic Approach

06R44KZ Replacement of Hepatic Vein with Nonautologous Tissue Substitute, Percutaneous Endoscopic Approach

06R507Z Replacement of Superior Mesenteric Vein with Autologous Tissue Substitute, Open Approach

06R50JZ Replacement of Superior Mesenteric Vein with Synthetic Substitute, Open Approach

06R50KZ Replacement of Superior Mesenteric Vein with Nonautologous Tissue Substitute, Open Approach

06R547Z Replacement of Superior Mesenteric Vein with Autologous Tissue Substitute, Percutaneous Endoscopic Approach

06R54JZ Replacement of Superior Mesenteric Vein with Synthetic Substitute, Percutaneous Endoscopic Approach

06R54KZ Replacement of Superior Mesenteric Vein with Nonautologous Tissue Substitute, Percutaneous Endoscopic Approach

06R607Z Replacement of Inferior Mesenteric Vein with Autologous Tissue Substitute, Open Approach

06R60JZ Replacement of Inferior Mesenteric Vein with Synthetic Substitute, Open Approach

06R60KZ Replacement of Inferior Mesenteric Vein with Nonautologous Tissue Substitute, Open Approach

06R647Z Replacement of Inferior Mesenteric Vein with Autologous Tissue Substitute, Percutaneous Endoscopic Approach

06R64JZ Replacement of Inferior Mesenteric Vein with Synthetic Substitute, Percutaneous Endoscopic Approach

06R64KZ Replacement of Inferior Mesenteric Vein with Nonautologous Tissue Substitute, Percutaneous Endoscopic Approach

06R707Z Replacement of Colic Vein with Autologous Tissue Substitute, Open Approach

06R70JZ Replacement of Colic Vein with Synthetic Substitute, Open Approach

06R70KZ Replacement of Colic Vein with Nonautologous Tissue Substitute, Open Approach

06R747Z Replacement of Colic Vein with Autologous Tissue Substitute, Percutaneous Endoscopic Approach

06R74JZ Replacement of Colic Vein with Synthetic Substitute, Percutaneous Endoscopic Approach

06R74KZ Replacement of Colic Vein with Nonautologous Tissue Substitute, Percutaneous Endoscopic Approach

06R807Z Replacement of Portal Vein with Autologous Tissue Substitute, Open Approach

06R80JZ Replacement of Portal Vein with Synthetic Substitute, Open Approach

06R80KZ Replacement of Portal Vein with Nonautologous Tissue Substitute, Open Approach

06R847Z Replacement of Portal Vein with Autologous Tissue Substitute, Percutaneous Endoscopic Approach

06R84JZ Replacement of Portal Vein with Synthetic Substitute, Percutaneous Endoscopic Approach

06R84KZ Replacement of Portal Vein with Nonautologous Tissue Substitute, Percutaneous Endoscopic Approach

06R907Z Replacement of Right Renal Vein with Autologous Tissue Substitute, Open Approach

06R90JZ Replacement of Right Renal Vein with Synthetic Substitute, Open Approach

06R90KZ Replacement of Right Renal Vein with Nonautologous Tissue Substitute, Open Approach

06R947Z Replacement of Right Renal Vein with Autologous Tissue Substitute, Percutaneous Endoscopic Approach

06R94JZ Replacement of Right Renal Vein with Synthetic Substitute, Percutaneous Endoscopic Approach

06R94KZ Replacement of Right Renal Vein with Nonautologous Tissue Substitute, Percutaneous Endoscopic Approach

♀ Female-only　♂ Male-only　▲ Limited Coverage　● Non-OR　HAC HAC-associated procedure　▲ Non-covered procedures　+ Cluster

06RB07Z Replacement of Left Renal Vein with Autologous Tissue Substitute, Open Approach

06RB0JZ Replacement of Left Renal Vein with Synthetic Substitute, Open Approach

06RB0KZ Replacement of Left Renal Vein with Nonautologous Tissue Substitute, Open Approach

06RB47Z Replacement of Left Renal Vein with Autologous Tissue Substitute, Percutaneous Endoscopic Approach

06RB4JZ Replacement of Left Renal Vein with Synthetic Substitute, Percutaneous Endoscopic Approach

06RB4KZ Replacement of Left Renal Vein with Nonautologous Tissue Substitute, Percutaneous Endoscopic Approach

06RC07Z Replacement of Right Common Iliac Vein with Autologous Tissue Substitute, Open Approach

06RC0JZ Replacement of Right Common Iliac Vein with Synthetic Substitute, Open Approach

06RC0KZ Replacement of Right Common Iliac Vein with Nonautologous Tissue Substitute, Open Approach

06RC47Z Replacement of Right Common Iliac Vein with Autologous Tissue Substitute, Percutaneous Endoscopic Approach

06RC4JZ Replacement of Right Common Iliac Vein with Synthetic Substitute, Percutaneous Endoscopic Approach

06RC4KZ Replacement of Right Common Iliac Vein with Nonautologous Tissue Substitute, Percutaneous Endoscopic Approach

06RD07Z Replacement of Left Common Iliac Vein with Autologous Tissue Substitute, Open Approach

06RD0JZ Replacement of Left Common Iliac Vein with Synthetic Substitute, Open Approach

06RD0KZ Replacement of Left Common Iliac Vein with Nonautologous Tissue Substitute, Open Approach

06RD47Z Replacement of Left Common Iliac Vein with Autologous Tissue Substitute, Percutaneous Endoscopic Approach

06RD4JZ Replacement of Left Common Iliac Vein with Synthetic Substitute, Percutaneous Endoscopic Approach

06RD4KZ Replacement of Left Common Iliac Vein with Nonautologous Tissue Substitute, Percutaneous Endoscopic Approach

06RF07Z Replacement of Right External Iliac Vein with Autologous Tissue Substitute, Open Approach

06RF0JZ Replacement of Right External Iliac Vein with Synthetic Substitute, Open Approach

06RF0KZ Replacement of Right External Iliac Vein with Nonautologous Tissue Substitute, Open Approach

06RF47Z Replacement of Right External Iliac Vein with Autologous Tissue Substitute, Percutaneous Endoscopic Approach

06RF4JZ Replacement of Right External Iliac Vein with Synthetic Substitute, Percutaneous Endoscopic Approach

06RF4KZ Replacement of Right External Iliac Vein with Nonautologous Tissue Substitute, Percutaneous Endoscopic Approach

06RG07Z Replacement of Left External Iliac Vein with Autologous Tissue Substitute, Open Approach

06RG0JZ Replacement of Left External Iliac Vein with Synthetic Substitute, Open Approach

06RG0KZ Replacement of Left External Iliac Vein with Nonautologous Tissue Substitute, Open Approach

06RG47Z Replacement of Left External Iliac Vein with Autologous Tissue Substitute, Percutaneous Endoscopic Approach

06RG4JZ Replacement of Left External Iliac Vein with Synthetic Substitute, Percutaneous Endoscopic Approach

06RG4KZ Replacement of Left External Iliac Vein with Nonautologous Tissue Substitute, Percutaneous Endoscopic Approach

06RH07Z Replacement of Right Hypogastric Vein with Autologous Tissue Substitute, Open Approach

06RH0JZ Replacement of Right Hypogastric Vein with Synthetic Substitute, Open Approach

06RH0KZ Replacement of Right Hypogastric Vein with Nonautologous Tissue Substitute, Open Approach

06RH47Z Replacement of Right Hypogastric Vein with Autologous Tissue Substitute, Percutaneous Endoscopic Approach

06RH4JZ Replacement of Right Hypogastric Vein with Synthetic Substitute, Percutaneous Endoscopic Approach

06RH4KZ Replacement of Right Hypogastric Vein with Nonautologous Tissue Substitute, Percutaneous Endoscopic Approach

06RJ07Z Replacement of Left Hypogastric Vein with Autologous Tissue Substitute, Open Approach

06RJ0JZ Replacement of Left Hypogastric Vein with Synthetic Substitute, Open Approach

06RJ0KZ Replacement of Left Hypogastric Vein with Nonautologous Tissue Substitute, Open Approach

06RJ47Z Replacement of Left Hypogastric Vein with Autologous Tissue Substitute, Percutaneous Endoscopic Approach

06RJ4JZ Replacement of Left Hypogastric Vein with Synthetic Substitute, Percutaneous Endoscopic Approach

06RJ4KZ Replacement of Left Hypogastric Vein with Nonautologous Tissue Substitute, Percutaneous Endoscopic Approach

06RM07Z Replacement of Right Femoral Vein with Autologous Tissue Substitute, Open Approach

06RM0JZ Replacement of Right Femoral Vein with Synthetic Substitute, Open Approach

06RM0KZ Replacement of Right Femoral Vein with Nonautologous Tissue Substitute, Open Approach

06RM47Z Replacement of Right Femoral Vein with Autologous Tissue Substitute, Percutaneous Endoscopic Approach

06RM4JZ Replacement of Right Femoral Vein with Synthetic Substitute, Percutaneous Endoscopic Approach

06RM4KZ Replacement of Right Femoral Vein with Nonautologous Tissue Substitute, Percutaneous Endoscopic Approach

06RN07Z Replacement of Left Femoral Vein with Autologous Tissue Substitute, Open Approach

06RN0JZ Replacement of Left Femoral Vein with Synthetic Substitute, Open Approach

06RN0KZ Replacement of Left Femoral Vein with Nonautologous Tissue Substitute, Open Approach

06RN47Z Replacement of Left Femoral Vein with Autologous Tissue Substitute, Percutaneous Endoscopic Approach

06RN4JZ Replacement of Left Femoral Vein with Synthetic Substitute, Percutaneous Endoscopic Approach

06RN4KZ Replacement of Left Femoral Vein with Nonautologous Tissue Substitute, Percutaneous Endoscopic Approach

06RP07Z Replacement of Right Saphenous Vein with Autologous Tissue Substitute, Open Approach

06RP0JZ Replacement of Right Saphenous Vein with Synthetic Substitute, Open Approach

06RP0KZ Replacement of Right Saphenous Vein with Nonautologous Tissue Substitute, Open Approach

06RP47Z Replacement of Right Saphenous Vein with Autologous Tissue Substitute, Percutaneous Endoscopic Approach

06RP4JZ Replacement of Right Saphenous Vein with Synthetic Substitute, Percutaneous Endoscopic Approach

06RP4KZ Replacement of Right Saphenous Vein with Nonautologous Tissue Substitute, Percutaneous Endoscopic Approach

06RQ07Z Replacement of Left Saphenous Vein with Autologous Tissue Substitute, Open Approach

06RQ0JZ Replacement of Left Saphenous Vein with Synthetic Substitute, Open Approach

06RQ0KZ Replacement of Left Saphenous Vein with Nonautologous Tissue Substitute, Open Approach

06RQ47Z Replacement of Left Saphenous Vein with Autologous Tissue Substitute, Percutaneous Endoscopic Approach

06RQ4JZ Replacement of Left Saphenous Vein with Synthetic Substitute, Percutaneous Endoscopic Approach

06RQ4KZ Replacement of Left Saphenous Vein with Nonautologous Tissue Substitute, Percutaneous Endoscopic Approach

06RT07Z Replacement of Right Foot Vein with Autologous Tissue Substitute, Open Approach

06RT0JZ Replacement of Right Foot Vein with Synthetic Substitute, Open Approach

06RT0KZ Replacement of Right Foot Vein with Nonautologous Tissue Substitute, Open Approach

06RT47Z Replacement of Right Foot Vein with Autologous Tissue Substitute, Percutaneous Endoscopic Approach

06RT4JZ Replacement of Right Foot Vein with Synthetic Substitute, Percutaneous Endoscopic Approach

06RT4KZ Replacement of Right Foot Vein with Nonautologous Tissue Substitute, Percutaneous Endoscopic Approach

06RV07Z Replacement of Left Foot Vein with Autologous Tissue Substitute, Open Approach

06RV0JZ Replacement of Left Foot Vein with Synthetic Substitute, Open Approach	**06RV4KZ** Replacement of Left Foot Vein with Nonautologous Tissue Substitute, Percutaneous Endoscopic Approach	**06RY47Z** Replacement of Lower Vein with Autologous Tissue Substitute, Percutaneous Endoscopic Approach
06RV0KZ Replacement of Left Foot Vein with Nonautologous Tissue Substitute, Open Approach	**06RY07Z** Replacement of Lower Vein with Autologous Tissue Substitute, Open Approach	**06RY4JZ** Replacement of Lower Vein with Synthetic Substitute, Percutaneous Endoscopic Approach
06RV47Z Replacement of Left Foot Vein with Autologous Tissue Substitute, Percutaneous Endoscopic Approach	**06RY0JZ** Replacement of Lower Vein with Synthetic Substitute, Open Approach	**06RY4KZ** Replacement of Lower Vein with Nonautologous Tissue Substitute, Percutaneous Endoscopic Approach
06RV4JZ Replacement of Left Foot Vein with Synthetic Substitute, Percutaneous Endoscopic Approach	**06RY0KZ** Replacement of Lower Vein with Nonautologous Tissue Substitute, Open Approach	

06S – Lower Veins, Reposition

06S00ZZ Reposition Inferior Vena Cava, Open Approach	**06S80ZZ** Reposition Portal Vein, Open Approach	**06SJ0ZZ** Reposition Left Hypogastric Vein, Open Approach
06S03ZZ Reposition Inferior Vena Cava, Percutaneous Approach	**06S83ZZ** Reposition Portal Vein, Percutaneous Approach	**06SJ3ZZ** Reposition Left Hypogastric Vein, Percutaneous Approach
06S04ZZ Reposition Inferior Vena Cava, Percutaneous Endoscopic Approach	**06S84ZZ** Reposition Portal Vein, Percutaneous Endoscopic Approach	**06SJ4ZZ** Reposition Left Hypogastric Vein, Percutaneous Endoscopic Approach
06S10ZZ Reposition Splenic Vein, Open Approach	**06S90ZZ** Reposition Right Renal Vein, Open Approach	**06SM0ZZ** Reposition Right Femoral Vein, Open Approach
06S13ZZ Reposition Splenic Vein, Percutaneous Approach	**06S93ZZ** Reposition Right Renal Vein, Percutaneous Approach	**06SM3ZZ** Reposition Right Femoral Vein, Percutaneous Approach
06S14ZZ Reposition Splenic Vein, Percutaneous Endoscopic Approach	**06S94ZZ** Reposition Right Renal Vein, Percutaneous Endoscopic Approach	**06SM4ZZ** Reposition Right Femoral Vein, Percutaneous Endoscopic Approach
06S20ZZ Reposition Gastric Vein, Open Approach	**06SB0ZZ** Reposition Left Renal Vein, Open Approach	**06SN0ZZ** Reposition Left Femoral Vein, Open Approach
06S23ZZ Reposition Gastric Vein, Percutaneous Approach	**06SB3ZZ** Reposition Left Renal Vein, Percutaneous Approach	**06SN3ZZ** Reposition Left Femoral Vein, Percutaneous Approach
06S24ZZ Reposition Gastric Vein, Percutaneous Endoscopic Approach	**06SB4ZZ** Reposition Left Renal Vein, Percutaneous Endoscopic Approach	**06SN4ZZ** Reposition Left Femoral Vein, Percutaneous Endoscopic Approach
06S30ZZ Reposition Esophageal Vein, Open Approach	**06SC0ZZ** Reposition Right Common Iliac Vein, Open Approach	**06SP0ZZ** Reposition Right Saphenous Vein, Open Approach
06S33ZZ Reposition Esophageal Vein, Percutaneous Approach	**06SC3ZZ** Reposition Right Common Iliac Vein, Percutaneous Approach	**06SP3ZZ** Reposition Right Saphenous Vein, Percutaneous Approach
06S34ZZ Reposition Esophageal Vein, Percutaneous Endoscopic Approach	**06SC4ZZ** Reposition Right Common Iliac Vein, Percutaneous Endoscopic Approach	**06SP4ZZ** Reposition Right Saphenous Vein, Percutaneous Endoscopic Approach
06S40ZZ Reposition Hepatic Vein, Open Approach	**06SD0ZZ** Reposition Left Common Iliac Vein, Open Approach	**06SQ0ZZ** Reposition Left Saphenous Vein, Open Approach
06S43ZZ Reposition Hepatic Vein, Percutaneous Approach	**06SD3ZZ** Reposition Left Common Iliac Vein, Percutaneous Approach	**06SQ3ZZ** Reposition Left Saphenous Vein, Percutaneous Approach
06S44ZZ Reposition Hepatic Vein, Percutaneous Endoscopic Approach	**06SD4ZZ** Reposition Left Common Iliac Vein, Percutaneous Endoscopic Approach	**06SQ4ZZ** Reposition Left Saphenous Vein, Percutaneous Endoscopic Approach
06S50ZZ Reposition Superior Mesenteric Vein, Open Approach	**06SF0ZZ** Reposition Right External Iliac Vein, Open Approach	**06ST0ZZ** Reposition Right Foot Vein, Open Approach
06S53ZZ Reposition Superior Mesenteric Vein, Percutaneous Approach	**06SF3ZZ** Reposition Right External Iliac Vein, Percutaneous Approach	**06ST3ZZ** Reposition Right Foot Vein, Percutaneous Approach
06S54ZZ Reposition Superior Mesenteric Vein, Percutaneous Endoscopic Approach	**06SF4ZZ** Reposition Right External Iliac Vein, Percutaneous Endoscopic Approach	**06ST4ZZ** Reposition Right Foot Vein, Percutaneous Endoscopic Approach
06S60ZZ Reposition Inferior Mesenteric Vein, Open Approach	**06SG0ZZ** Reposition Left External Iliac Vein, Open Approach	**06SV0ZZ** Reposition Left Foot Vein, Open Approach
06S63ZZ Reposition Inferior Mesenteric Vein, Percutaneous Approach	**06SG3ZZ** Reposition Left External Iliac Vein, Percutaneous Approach	**06SV3ZZ** Reposition Left Foot Vein, Percutaneous Approach
06S64ZZ Reposition Inferior Mesenteric Vein, Percutaneous Endoscopic Approach	**06SG4ZZ** Reposition Left External Iliac Vein, Percutaneous Endoscopic Approach	**06SV4ZZ** Reposition Left Foot Vein, Percutaneous Endoscopic Approach
06S70ZZ Reposition Colic Vein, Open Approach	**06SH0ZZ** Reposition Right Hypogastric Vein, Open Approach	**06SY0ZZ** Reposition Lower Vein, Open Approach
06S73ZZ Reposition Colic Vein, Percutaneous Approach	**06SH3ZZ** Reposition Right Hypogastric Vein, Percutaneous Approach	**06SY3ZZ** Reposition Lower Vein, Percutaneous Approach
06S74ZZ Reposition Colic Vein, Percutaneous Endoscopic Approach	**06SH4ZZ** Reposition Right Hypogastric Vein, Percutaneous Endoscopic Approach	**06SY4ZZ** Reposition Lower Vein, Percutaneous Endoscopic Approach

06U – Lower Veins, Supplement

06U007Z Supplement Inferior Vena Cava with Autologous Tissue Substitute, Open Approach	**06U03JZ** Supplement Inferior Vena Cava with Synthetic Substitute, Percutaneous Approach	**06U04JZ** Supplement Inferior Vena Cava with Synthetic Substitute, Percutaneous Endoscopic Approach
06U00JZ Supplement Inferior Vena Cava with Synthetic Substitute, Open Approach	**06U03KZ** Supplement Inferior Vena Cava with Nonautologous Tissue Substitute, Percutaneous Approach	**06U04KZ** Supplement Inferior Vena Cava with Nonautologous Tissue Substitute, Percutaneous Endoscopic Approach
06U00KZ Supplement Inferior Vena Cava with Nonautologous Tissue Substitute, Open Approach		**06U107Z** Supplement Splenic Vein with Autologous Tissue Substitute, Open Approach
06U037Z Supplement Inferior Vena Cava with Autologous Tissue Substitute, Percutaneous Approach	**06U047Z** Supplement Inferior Vena Cava with Autologous Tissue Substitute, Percutaneous Endoscopic Approach	**06U10JZ** Supplement Splenic Vein with Synthetic Substitute, Open Approach

♀ Female-only   ♂ Male-only   ▲ Limited Coverage   ● Non-OR   HAC HAC-associated procedure   ▲ Non-covered procedures   ✚ Cluster

06U10KZ Supplement Splenic Vein with Nonautologous Tissue Substitute, Open Approach

06U137Z Supplement Splenic Vein with Autologous Tissue Substitute, Percutaneous Approach

06U13JZ Supplement Splenic Vein with Synthetic Substitute, Percutaneous Approach

06U13KZ Supplement Splenic Vein with Nonautologous Tissue Substitute, Percutaneous Approach

06U147Z Supplement Splenic Vein with Autologous Tissue Substitute, Percutaneous Endoscopic Approach

06U14JZ Supplement Splenic Vein with Synthetic Substitute, Percutaneous Endoscopic Approach

06U14KZ Supplement Splenic Vein with Nonautologous Tissue Substitute, Percutaneous Endoscopic Approach

06U207Z Supplement Gastric Vein with Autologous Tissue Substitute, Open Approach

06U20JZ Supplement Gastric Vein with Synthetic Substitute, Open Approach

06U20KZ Supplement Gastric Vein with Nonautologous Tissue Substitute, Open Approach

06U237Z Supplement Gastric Vein with Autologous Tissue Substitute, Percutaneous Approach

06U23JZ Supplement Gastric Vein with Synthetic Substitute, Percutaneous Approach

06U23KZ Supplement Gastric Vein with Nonautologous Tissue Substitute, Percutaneous Approach

06U247Z Supplement Gastric Vein with Autologous Tissue Substitute, Percutaneous Endoscopic Approach

06U24JZ Supplement Gastric Vein with Synthetic Substitute, Percutaneous Endoscopic Approach

06U24KZ Supplement Gastric Vein with Nonautologous Tissue Substitute, Percutaneous Endoscopic Approach

06U307Z Supplement Esophageal Vein with Autologous Tissue Substitute, Open Approach

06U30JZ Supplement Esophageal Vein with Synthetic Substitute, Open Approach

06U30KZ Supplement Esophageal Vein with Nonautologous Tissue Substitute, Open Approach

06U337Z Supplement Esophageal Vein with Autologous Tissue Substitute, Percutaneous Approach

06U33JZ Supplement Esophageal Vein with Synthetic Substitute, Percutaneous Approach

06U33KZ Supplement Esophageal Vein with Nonautologous Tissue Substitute, Percutaneous Approach

06U347Z Supplement Esophageal Vein with Autologous Tissue Substitute, Percutaneous Endoscopic Approach

06U34JZ Supplement Esophageal Vein with Synthetic Substitute, Percutaneous Endoscopic Approach

06U34KZ Supplement Esophageal Vein with Nonautologous Tissue Substitute, Percutaneous Endoscopic Approach

06U407Z Supplement Hepatic Vein with Autologous Tissue Substitute, Open Approach

06U40JZ Supplement Hepatic Vein with Synthetic Substitute, Open Approach

06U40KZ Supplement Hepatic Vein with Nonautologous Tissue Substitute, Open Approach

06U437Z Supplement Hepatic Vein with Autologous Tissue Substitute, Percutaneous Approach

06U43JZ Supplement Hepatic Vein with Synthetic Substitute, Percutaneous Approach

06U43KZ Supplement Hepatic Vein with Nonautologous Tissue Substitute, Percutaneous Approach

06U447Z Supplement Hepatic Vein with Autologous Tissue Substitute, Percutaneous Endoscopic Approach

06U44JZ Supplement Hepatic Vein with Synthetic Substitute, Percutaneous Endoscopic Approach

06U44KZ Supplement Hepatic Vein with Nonautologous Tissue Substitute, Percutaneous Endoscopic Approach

06U507Z Supplement Superior Mesenteric Vein with Autologous Tissue Substitute, Open Approach

06U50JZ Supplement Superior Mesenteric Vein with Synthetic Substitute, Open Approach

06U50KZ Supplement Superior Mesenteric Vein with Nonautologous Tissue Substitute, Open Approach

06U537Z Supplement Superior Mesenteric Vein with Autologous Tissue Substitute, Percutaneous Approach

06U53JZ Supplement Superior Mesenteric Vein with Synthetic Substitute, Percutaneous Approach

06U53KZ Supplement Superior Mesenteric Vein with Nonautologous Tissue Substitute, Percutaneous Approach

06U547Z Supplement Superior Mesenteric Vein with Autologous Tissue Substitute, Percutaneous Endoscopic Approach

06U54JZ Supplement Superior Mesenteric Vein with Synthetic Substitute, Percutaneous Endoscopic Approach

06U54KZ Supplement Superior Mesenteric Vein with Nonautologous Tissue Substitute, Percutaneous Endoscopic Approach

06U607Z Supplement Inferior Mesenteric Vein with Autologous Tissue Substitute, Open Approach

06U60JZ Supplement Inferior Mesenteric Vein with Synthetic Substitute, Open Approach

06U60KZ Supplement Inferior Mesenteric Vein with Nonautologous Tissue Substitute, Open Approach

06U637Z Supplement Inferior Mesenteric Vein with Autologous Tissue Substitute, Percutaneous Approach

06U63JZ Supplement Inferior Mesenteric Vein with Synthetic Substitute, Percutaneous Approach

06U63KZ Supplement Inferior Mesenteric Vein with Nonautologous Tissue Substitute, Percutaneous Approach

06U647Z Supplement Inferior Mesenteric Vein with Autologous Tissue Substitute, Percutaneous Endoscopic Approach

06U64JZ Supplement Inferior Mesenteric Vein with Synthetic Substitute, Percutaneous Endoscopic Approach

06U64KZ Supplement Inferior Mesenteric Vein with Nonautologous Tissue Substitute, Percutaneous Endoscopic Approach

06U707Z Supplement Colic Vein with Autologous Tissue Substitute, Open Approach

06U70JZ Supplement Colic Vein with Synthetic Substitute, Open Approach

06U70KZ Supplement Colic Vein with Nonautologous Tissue Substitute, Open Approach

06U737Z Supplement Colic Vein with Autologous Tissue Substitute, Percutaneous Approach

06U73JZ Supplement Colic Vein with Synthetic Substitute, Percutaneous Approach

06U73KZ Supplement Colic Vein with Nonautologous Tissue Substitute, Percutaneous Approach

06U747Z Supplement Colic Vein with Autologous Tissue Substitute, Percutaneous Endoscopic Approach

06U74JZ Supplement Colic Vein with Synthetic Substitute, Percutaneous Endoscopic Approach

06U74KZ Supplement Colic Vein with Nonautologous Tissue Substitute, Percutaneous Endoscopic Approach

06U807Z Supplement Portal Vein with Autologous Tissue Substitute, Open Approach

06U80JZ Supplement Portal Vein with Synthetic Substitute, Open Approach

06U80KZ Supplement Portal Vein with Nonautologous Tissue Substitute, Open Approach

06U837Z Supplement Portal Vein with Autologous Tissue Substitute, Percutaneous Approach

06U83JZ Supplement Portal Vein with Synthetic Substitute, Percutaneous Approach

06U83KZ Supplement Portal Vein with Nonautologous Tissue Substitute, Percutaneous Approach

06U847Z Supplement Portal Vein with Autologous Tissue Substitute, Percutaneous Endoscopic Approach

06U84JZ Supplement Portal Vein with Synthetic Substitute, Percutaneous Endoscopic Approach

06U84KZ Supplement Portal Vein with Nonautologous Tissue Substitute, Percutaneous Endoscopic Approach

06U907Z Supplement Right Renal Vein with Autologous Tissue Substitute, Open Approach

06U90JZ Supplement Right Renal Vein with Synthetic Substitute, Open Approach

06U90KZ Supplement Right Renal Vein with Nonautologous Tissue Substitute, Open Approach

06U937Z Supplement Right Renal Vein with Autologous Tissue Substitute, Percutaneous Approach

06U93JZ Supplement Right Renal Vein with Synthetic Substitute, Percutaneous Approach

06U93KZ Supplement Right Renal Vein with Nonautologous Tissue Substitute, Percutaneous Approach

06U947Z Supplement Right Renal Vein with Autologous Tissue Substitute, Percutaneous Endoscopic Approach

06U94JZ Supplement Right Renal Vein with Synthetic Substitute, Percutaneous Endoscopic Approach

06U94KZ Supplement Right Renal Vein with Nonautologous Tissue Substitute, Percutaneous Endoscopic Approach

06UB07Z Supplement Left Renal Vein with Autologous Tissue Substitute, Open Approach

06UB0JZ Supplement Left Renal Vein with Synthetic Substitute, Open Approach

06UB0KZ Supplement Left Renal Vein with Nonautologous Tissue Substitute, Open Approach

06UB37Z Supplement Left Renal Vein with Autologous Tissue Substitute, Percutaneous Approach

06UB3JZ Supplement Left Renal Vein with Synthetic Substitute, Percutaneous Approach

06UB3KZ Supplement Left Renal Vein with Nonautologous Tissue Substitute, Percutaneous Approach

06UB47Z Supplement Left Renal Vein with Autologous Tissue Substitute, Percutaneous Endoscopic Approach

06UB4JZ Supplement Left Renal Vein with Synthetic Substitute, Percutaneous Endoscopic Approach

06UB4KZ Supplement Left Renal Vein with Nonautologous Tissue Substitute, Percutaneous Endoscopic Approach

06UC07Z Supplement Right Common Iliac Vein with Autologous Tissue Substitute, Open Approach

06UC0JZ Supplement Right Common Iliac Vein with Synthetic Substitute, Open Approach

06UC0KZ Supplement Right Common Iliac Vein with Nonautologous Tissue Substitute, Open Approach

06UC37Z Supplement Right Common Iliac Vein with Autologous Tissue Substitute, Percutaneous Approach

06UC3JZ Supplement Right Common Iliac Vein with Synthetic Substitute, Percutaneous Approach

06UC3KZ Supplement Right Common Iliac Vein with Nonautologous Tissue Substitute, Percutaneous Approach

06UC47Z Supplement Right Common Iliac Vein with Autologous Tissue Substitute, Percutaneous Endoscopic Approach

06UC4JZ Supplement Right Common Iliac Vein with Synthetic Substitute, Percutaneous Endoscopic Approach

06UC4KZ Supplement Right Common Iliac Vein with Nonautologous Tissue Substitute, Percutaneous Endoscopic Approach

06UD07Z Supplement Left Common Iliac Vein with Autologous Tissue Substitute, Open Approach

06UD0JZ Supplement Left Common Iliac Vein with Synthetic Substitute, Open Approach

06UD0KZ Supplement Left Common Iliac Vein with Nonautologous Tissue Substitute, Open Approach

06UD37Z Supplement Left Common Iliac Vein with Autologous Tissue Substitute, Percutaneous Approach

06UD3JZ Supplement Left Common Iliac Vein with Synthetic Substitute, Percutaneous Approach

06UD3KZ Supplement Left Common Iliac Vein with Nonautologous Tissue Substitute, Percutaneous Approach

06UD47Z Supplement Left Common Iliac Vein with Autologous Tissue Substitute, Percutaneous Endoscopic Approach

06UD4JZ Supplement Left Common Iliac Vein with Synthetic Substitute, Percutaneous Endoscopic Approach

06UD4KZ Supplement Left Common Iliac Vein with Nonautologous Tissue Substitute, Percutaneous Endoscopic Approach

06UF07Z Supplement Right External Iliac Vein with Autologous Tissue Substitute, Open Approach

06UF0JZ Supplement Right External Iliac Vein with Synthetic Substitute, Open Approach

06UF0KZ Supplement Right External Iliac Vein with Nonautologous Tissue Substitute, Open Approach

06UF37Z Supplement Right External Iliac Vein with Autologous Tissue Substitute, Percutaneous Approach

06UF3JZ Supplement Right External Iliac Vein with Synthetic Substitute, Percutaneous Approach

06UF3KZ Supplement Right External Iliac Vein with Nonautologous Tissue Substitute, Percutaneous Approach

06UF47Z Supplement Right External Iliac Vein with Autologous Tissue Substitute, Percutaneous Endoscopic Approach

06UF4JZ Supplement Right External Iliac Vein with Synthetic Substitute, Percutaneous Endoscopic Approach

06UF4KZ Supplement Right External Iliac Vein with Nonautologous Tissue Substitute, Percutaneous Endoscopic Approach

06UG07Z Supplement Left External Iliac Vein with Autologous Tissue Substitute, Open Approach

06UG0JZ Supplement Left External Iliac Vein with Synthetic Substitute, Open Approach

06UG0KZ Supplement Left External Iliac Vein with Nonautologous Tissue Substitute, Open Approach

06UG37Z Supplement Left External Iliac Vein with Autologous Tissue Substitute, Percutaneous Approach

06UG3JZ Supplement Left External Iliac Vein with Synthetic Substitute, Percutaneous Approach

06UG3KZ Supplement Left External Iliac Vein with Nonautologous Tissue Substitute, Percutaneous Approach

06UG47Z Supplement Left External Iliac Vein with Autologous Tissue Substitute, Percutaneous Endoscopic Approach

06UG4JZ Supplement Left External Iliac Vein with Synthetic Substitute, Percutaneous Endoscopic Approach

06UG4KZ Supplement Left External Iliac Vein with Nonautologous Tissue Substitute, Percutaneous Endoscopic Approach

06UH07Z Supplement Right Hypogastric Vein with Autologous Tissue Substitute, Open Approach

06UH0JZ Supplement Right Hypogastric Vein with Synthetic Substitute, Open Approach

06UH0KZ Supplement Right Hypogastric Vein with Nonautologous Tissue Substitute, Open Approach

06UH37Z Supplement Right Hypogastric Vein with Autologous Tissue Substitute, Percutaneous Approach

06UH3JZ Supplement Right Hypogastric Vein with Synthetic Substitute, Percutaneous Approach

06UH3KZ Supplement Right Hypogastric Vein with Nonautologous Tissue Substitute, Percutaneous Approach

06UH47Z Supplement Right Hypogastric Vein with Autologous Tissue Substitute, Percutaneous Endoscopic Approach

06UH4JZ Supplement Right Hypogastric Vein with Synthetic Substitute, Percutaneous Endoscopic Approach

06UH4KZ Supplement Right Hypogastric Vein with Nonautologous Tissue Substitute, Percutaneous Endoscopic Approach

06UJ07Z Supplement Left Hypogastric Vein with Autologous Tissue Substitute, Open Approach

06UJ0JZ Supplement Left Hypogastric Vein with Synthetic Substitute, Open Approach

06UJ0KZ Supplement Left Hypogastric Vein with Nonautologous Tissue Substitute, Open Approach

06UJ37Z Supplement Left Hypogastric Vein with Autologous Tissue Substitute, Percutaneous Approach

06UJ3JZ Supplement Left Hypogastric Vein with Synthetic Substitute, Percutaneous Approach

06UJ3KZ Supplement Left Hypogastric Vein with Nonautologous Tissue Substitute, Percutaneous Approach

06UJ47Z Supplement Left Hypogastric Vein with Autologous Tissue Substitute, Percutaneous Endoscopic Approach

06UJ4JZ Supplement Left Hypogastric Vein with Synthetic Substitute, Percutaneous Endoscopic Approach

06UJ4KZ Supplement Left Hypogastric Vein with Nonautologous Tissue Substitute, Percutaneous Endoscopic Approach

06UM07Z Supplement Right Femoral Vein with Autologous Tissue Substitute, Open Approach

06UM0JZ Supplement Right Femoral Vein with Synthetic Substitute, Open Approach

06UM0KZ Supplement Right Femoral Vein with Nonautologous Tissue Substitute, Open Approach

06UM37Z Supplement Right Femoral Vein with Autologous Tissue Substitute, Percutaneous Approach

06UM3JZ Supplement Right Femoral Vein with Synthetic Substitute, Percutaneous Approach

06UM3KZ Supplement Right Femoral Vein with Nonautologous Tissue Substitute, Percutaneous Approach

06UM47Z Supplement Right Femoral Vein with Autologous Tissue Substitute, Percutaneous Endoscopic Approach

06UM4JZ Supplement Right Femoral Vein with Synthetic Substitute, Percutaneous Endoscopic Approach

06UM4KZ Supplement Right Femoral Vein with Nonautologous Tissue Substitute, Percutaneous Endoscopic Approach

06UN07Z Supplement Left Femoral Vein with Autologous Tissue Substitute, Open Approach

06UN0JZ Supplement Left Femoral Vein with Synthetic Substitute, Open Approach

06UN0KZ Supplement Left Femoral Vein with Nonautologous Tissue Substitute, Open Approach

♀ Female-only   ♂ Male-only   ▲ Limited Coverage   ● Non-OR   ⬛ HAC-associated procedure   ▲ Non-covered procedures   ➕ Cluster

06UN37Z Supplement Left Femoral Vein with Autologous Tissue Substitute, Percutaneous Approach

06UN3JZ Supplement Left Femoral Vein with Synthetic Substitute, Percutaneous Approach

06UN3KZ Supplement Left Femoral Vein with Nonautologous Tissue Substitute, Percutaneous Approach

06UN47Z Supplement Left Femoral Vein with Autologous Tissue Substitute, Percutaneous Endoscopic Approach

06UN4JZ Supplement Left Femoral Vein with Synthetic Substitute, Percutaneous Endoscopic Approach

06UN4KZ Supplement Left Femoral Vein with Nonautologous Tissue Substitute, Percutaneous Endoscopic Approach

06UP07Z Supplement Right Saphenous Vein with Autologous Tissue Substitute, Open Approach

06UP0JZ Supplement Right Saphenous Vein with Synthetic Substitute, Open Approach

06UP0KZ Supplement Right Saphenous Vein with Nonautologous Tissue Substitute, Open Approach

06UP37Z Supplement Right Saphenous Vein with Autologous Tissue Substitute, Percutaneous Approach

06UP3JZ Supplement Right Saphenous Vein with Synthetic Substitute, Percutaneous Approach

06UP3KZ Supplement Right Saphenous Vein with Nonautologous Tissue Substitute, Percutaneous Approach

06UP47Z Supplement Right Saphenous Vein with Autologous Tissue Substitute, Percutaneous Endoscopic Approach

06UP4JZ Supplement Right Saphenous Vein with Synthetic Substitute, Percutaneous Endoscopic Approach

06UP4KZ Supplement Right Saphenous Vein with Nonautologous Tissue Substitute, Percutaneous Endoscopic Approach

06UQ07Z Supplement Left Saphenous Vein with Autologous Tissue Substitute, Open Approach

06UQ0JZ Supplement Left Saphenous Vein with Synthetic Substitute, Open Approach

06UQ0KZ Supplement Left Saphenous Vein with Nonautologous Tissue Substitute, Open Approach

06UQ37Z Supplement Left Saphenous Vein with Autologous Tissue Substitute, Percutaneous Approach

06UQ3JZ Supplement Left Saphenous Vein with Synthetic Substitute, Percutaneous Approach

06UQ3KZ Supplement Left Saphenous Vein with Nonautologous Tissue Substitute, Percutaneous Approach

06UQ47Z Supplement Left Saphenous Vein with Autologous Tissue Substitute, Percutaneous Endoscopic Approach

06UQ4JZ Supplement Left Saphenous Vein with Synthetic Substitute, Percutaneous Endoscopic Approach

06UQ4KZ Supplement Left Saphenous Vein with Nonautologous Tissue Substitute, Percutaneous Endoscopic Approach

06UT07Z Supplement Right Foot Vein with Autologous Tissue Substitute, Open Approach

06UT0JZ Supplement Right Foot Vein with Synthetic Substitute, Open Approach

06UT0KZ Supplement Right Foot Vein with Nonautologous Tissue Substitute, Open Approach

06UT37Z Supplement Right Foot Vein with Autologous Tissue Substitute, Percutaneous Approach

06UT3JZ Supplement Right Foot Vein with Synthetic Substitute, Percutaneous Approach

06UT3KZ Supplement Right Foot Vein with Nonautologous Tissue Substitute, Percutaneous Approach

06UT47Z Supplement Right Foot Vein with Autologous Tissue Substitute, Percutaneous Endoscopic Approach

06UT4JZ Supplement Right Foot Vein with Synthetic Substitute, Percutaneous Endoscopic Approach

06UT4KZ Supplement Right Foot Vein with Nonautologous Tissue Substitute, Percutaneous Endoscopic Approach

06UV07Z Supplement Left Foot Vein with Autologous Tissue Substitute, Open Approach

06UV0JZ Supplement Left Foot Vein with Synthetic Substitute, Open Approach

06UV0KZ Supplement Left Foot Vein with Nonautologous Tissue Substitute, Open Approach

06UV37Z Supplement Left Foot Vein with Autologous Tissue Substitute, Percutaneous Approach

06UV3JZ Supplement Left Foot Vein with Synthetic Substitute, Percutaneous Approach

06UV3KZ Supplement Left Foot Vein with Nonautologous Tissue Substitute, Percutaneous Approach

06UV47Z Supplement Left Foot Vein with Autologous Tissue Substitute, Percutaneous Endoscopic Approach

06UV4JZ Supplement Left Foot Vein with Synthetic Substitute, Percutaneous Endoscopic Approach

06UV4KZ Supplement Left Foot Vein with Nonautologous Tissue Substitute, Percutaneous Endoscopic Approach

06UY07Z Supplement Lower Vein with Autologous Tissue Substitute, Open Approach

06UY0JZ Supplement Lower Vein with Synthetic Substitute, Open Approach

06UY0KZ Supplement Lower Vein with Nonautologous Tissue Substitute, Open Approach

06UY37Z Supplement Lower Vein with Autologous Tissue Substitute, Percutaneous Approach

06UY3JZ Supplement Lower Vein with Synthetic Substitute, Percutaneous Approach

06UY3KZ Supplement Lower Vein with Nonautologous Tissue Substitute, Percutaneous Approach

06UY47Z Supplement Lower Vein with Autologous Tissue Substitute, Percutaneous Endoscopic Approach

06UY4JZ Supplement Lower Vein with Synthetic Substitute, Percutaneous Endoscopic Approach

06UY4KZ Supplement Lower Vein with Nonautologous Tissue Substitute, Percutaneous Endoscopic Approach

06V – Lower Veins, Restriction

Review Coding Guideline B3.12

06V00CZ Restriction of Inferior Vena Cava with Extraluminal Device, Open Approach

06V00DZ Restriction of Inferior Vena Cava with Intraluminal Device, Open Approach

06V00ZZ Restriction of Inferior Vena Cava, Open Approach

06V03CZ Restriction of Inferior Vena Cava with Extraluminal Device, Percutaneous Approach

06V03DZ Restriction of Inferior Vena Cava with Intraluminal Device, Percutaneous Approach
AHA CC: 3Q, 2018, 11

06V03ZZ Restriction of Inferior Vena Cava, Percutaneous Approach

06V04CZ Restriction of Inferior Vena Cava with Extraluminal Device, Percutaneous Endoscopic Approach

06V04DZ Restriction of Inferior Vena Cava with Intraluminal Device, Percutaneous Endoscopic Approach

06V04ZZ Restriction of Inferior Vena Cava, Percutaneous Endoscopic Approach

06V10CZ Restriction of Splenic Vein with Extraluminal Device, Open Approach

06V10DZ Restriction of Splenic Vein with Intraluminal Device, Open Approach

06V10ZZ Restriction of Splenic Vein, Open Approach

06V13CZ Restriction of Splenic Vein with Extraluminal Device, Percutaneous Approach

06V13DZ Restriction of Splenic Vein with Intraluminal Device, Percutaneous Approach

06V13ZZ Restriction of Splenic Vein, Percutaneous Approach

06V14CZ Restriction of Splenic Vein with Extraluminal Device, Percutaneous Endoscopic Approach

06V14DZ Restriction of Splenic Vein with Intraluminal Device, Percutaneous Endoscopic Approach

06V14ZZ Restriction of Splenic Vein, Percutaneous Endoscopic Approach

06V20CZ Restriction of Gastric Vein with Extraluminal Device, Open Approach

06V20DZ Restriction of Gastric Vein with Intraluminal Device, Open Approach

06V20ZZ Restriction of Gastric Vein, Open Approach

06V23CZ Restriction of Gastric Vein with Extraluminal Device, Percutaneous Approach

06V23DZ Restriction of Gastric Vein with Intraluminal Device, Percutaneous Approach

06V23ZZ Restriction of Gastric Vein, Percutaneous Approach

06V24CZ Restriction of Gastric Vein with Extraluminal Device, Percutaneous Endoscopic Approach

06V24DZ Restriction of Gastric Vein with Intraluminal Device, Percutaneous Endoscopic Approach

06V24ZZ Restriction of Gastric Vein, Percutaneous Endoscopic Approach

06V30CZ Restriction of Esophageal Vein with Extraluminal Device, Open Approach

06V30DZ Restriction of Esophageal Vein with Intraluminal Device, Open Approach

06V30ZZ Restriction of Esophageal Vein, Open Approach

06V33CZ Restriction of Esophageal Vein with Extraluminal Device, Percutaneous Approach

06V33DZ Restriction of Esophageal Vein with Intraluminal Device, Percutaneous Approach

06V33ZZ Restriction of Esophageal Vein, Percutaneous Approach

06V34CZ Restriction of Esophageal Vein with Extraluminal Device, Percutaneous Endoscopic Approach

06V34DZ Restriction of Esophageal Vein with Intraluminal Device, Percutaneous Endoscopic Approach

06V34ZZ Restriction of Esophageal Vein, Percutaneous Endoscopic Approach

06V40CZ Restriction of Hepatic Vein with Extraluminal Device, Open Approach

06V40DZ Restriction of Hepatic Vein with Intraluminal Device, Open Approach

06V40ZZ Restriction of Hepatic Vein, Open Approach

06V43CZ Restriction of Hepatic Vein with Extraluminal Device, Percutaneous Approach

06V43DZ Restriction of Hepatic Vein with Intraluminal Device, Percutaneous Approach

06V43ZZ Restriction of Hepatic Vein, Percutaneous Approach

06V44CZ Restriction of Hepatic Vein with Extraluminal Device, Percutaneous Endoscopic Approach

06V44DZ Restriction of Hepatic Vein with Intraluminal Device, Percutaneous Endoscopic Approach

06V44ZZ Restriction of Hepatic Vein, Percutaneous Endoscopic Approach

06V50CZ Restriction of Superior Mesenteric Vein with Extraluminal Device, Open Approach

06V50DZ Restriction of Superior Mesenteric Vein with Intraluminal Device, Open Approach

06V50ZZ Restriction of Superior Mesenteric Vein, Open Approach

06V53CZ Restriction of Superior Mesenteric Vein with Extraluminal Device, Percutaneous Approach

06V53DZ Restriction of Superior Mesenteric Vein with Intraluminal Device, Percutaneous Approach

06V53ZZ Restriction of Superior Mesenteric Vein, Percutaneous Approach

06V54CZ Restriction of Superior Mesenteric Vein with Extraluminal Device, Percutaneous Endoscopic Approach

06V54DZ Restriction of Superior Mesenteric Vein with Intraluminal Device, Percutaneous Endoscopic Approach

06V54ZZ Restriction of Superior Mesenteric Vein, Percutaneous Endoscopic Approach

06V60CZ Restriction of Inferior Mesenteric Vein with Extraluminal Device, Open Approach

06V60DZ Restriction of Inferior Mesenteric Vein with Intraluminal Device, Open Approach

06V60ZZ Restriction of Inferior Mesenteric Vein, Open Approach

06V63CZ Restriction of Inferior Mesenteric Vein with Extraluminal Device, Percutaneous Approach

06V63DZ Restriction of Inferior Mesenteric Vein with Intraluminal Device, Percutaneous Approach

06V63ZZ Restriction of Inferior Mesenteric Vein, Percutaneous Approach

06V64CZ Restriction of Inferior Mesenteric Vein with Extraluminal Device, Percutaneous Endoscopic Approach

06V64DZ Restriction of Inferior Mesenteric Vein with Intraluminal Device, Percutaneous Endoscopic Approach

06V64ZZ Restriction of Inferior Mesenteric Vein, Percutaneous Endoscopic Approach

06V70CZ Restriction of Colic Vein with Extraluminal Device, Open Approach

06V70DZ Restriction of Colic Vein with Intraluminal Device, Open Approach

06V70ZZ Restriction of Colic Vein, Open Approach

06V73CZ Restriction of Colic Vein with Extraluminal Device, Percutaneous Approach

06V73DZ Restriction of Colic Vein with Intraluminal Device, Percutaneous Approach

06V73ZZ Restriction of Colic Vein, Percutaneous Approach

06V74CZ Restriction of Colic Vein with Extraluminal Device, Percutaneous Endoscopic Approach

06V74DZ Restriction of Colic Vein with Intraluminal Device, Percutaneous Endoscopic Approach

06V74ZZ Restriction of Colic Vein, Percutaneous Endoscopic Approach

06V80CZ Restriction of Portal Vein with Extraluminal Device, Open Approach

06V80DZ Restriction of Portal Vein with Intraluminal Device, Open Approach

06V80ZZ Restriction of Portal Vein, Open Approach

06V83CZ Restriction of Portal Vein with Extraluminal Device, Percutaneous Approach

06V83DZ Restriction of Portal Vein with Intraluminal Device, Percutaneous Approach

06V83ZZ Restriction of Portal Vein, Percutaneous Approach

06V84CZ Restriction of Portal Vein with Extraluminal Device, Percutaneous Endoscopic Approach

06V84DZ Restriction of Portal Vein with Intraluminal Device, Percutaneous Endoscopic Approach

06V84ZZ Restriction of Portal Vein, Percutaneous Endoscopic Approach

06V90CZ Restriction of Right Renal Vein with Extraluminal Device, Open Approach

06V90DZ Restriction of Right Renal Vein with Intraluminal Device, Open Approach

06V90ZZ Restriction of Right Renal Vein, Open Approach

06V93CZ Restriction of Right Renal Vein with Extraluminal Device, Percutaneous Approach

06V93DZ Restriction of Right Renal Vein with Intraluminal Device, Percutaneous Approach

06V93ZZ Restriction of Right Renal Vein, Percutaneous Approach

06V94CZ Restriction of Right Renal Vein with Extraluminal Device, Percutaneous Endoscopic Approach

06V94DZ Restriction of Right Renal Vein with Intraluminal Device, Percutaneous Endoscopic Approach

06V94ZZ Restriction of Right Renal Vein, Percutaneous Endoscopic Approach

06VB0CZ Restriction of Left Renal Vein with Extraluminal Device, Open Approach

06VB0DZ Restriction of Left Renal Vein with Intraluminal Device, Open Approach

06VB0ZZ Restriction of Left Renal Vein, Open Approach

06VB3CZ Restriction of Left Renal Vein with Extraluminal Device, Percutaneous Approach

06VB3DZ Restriction of Left Renal Vein with Intraluminal Device, Percutaneous Approach

06VB3ZZ Restriction of Left Renal Vein, Percutaneous Approach

06VB4CZ Restriction of Left Renal Vein with Extraluminal Device, Percutaneous Endoscopic Approach

06VB4DZ Restriction of Left Renal Vein with Intraluminal Device, Percutaneous Endoscopic Approach

06VB4ZZ Restriction of Left Renal Vein, Percutaneous Endoscopic Approach

06VC0CZ Restriction of Right Common Iliac Vein with Extraluminal Device, Open Approach

06VC0DZ Restriction of Right Common Iliac Vein with Intraluminal Device, Open Approach

06VC0ZZ Restriction of Right Common Iliac Vein, Open Approach

06VC3CZ Restriction of Right Common Iliac Vein with Extraluminal Device, Percutaneous Approach

06VC3DZ Restriction of Right Common Iliac Vein with Intraluminal Device, Percutaneous Approach

06VC3ZZ Restriction of Right Common Iliac Vein, Percutaneous Approach

06VC4CZ Restriction of Right Common Iliac Vein with Extraluminal Device, Percutaneous Endoscopic Approach

06VC4DZ Restriction of Right Common Iliac Vein with Intraluminal Device, Percutaneous Endoscopic Approach

06VC4ZZ Restriction of Right Common Iliac Vein, Percutaneous Endoscopic Approach

06VD0CZ Restriction of Left Common Iliac Vein with Extraluminal Device, Open Approach

06VD0DZ Restriction of Left Common Iliac Vein with Intraluminal Device, Open Approach

06VD0ZZ Restriction of Left Common Iliac Vein, Open Approach

♀ Female-only   ♂ Male-only   ▲ Limited Coverage   ● Non-OR   ▨ HAC-associated procedure   ▲ Non-covered procedures   ✚ Cluster

06VD3CZ Restriction of Left Common Iliac Vein with Extraluminal Device, Percutaneous Approach

06VD3DZ Restriction of Left Common Iliac Vein with Intraluminal Device, Percutaneous Approach

06VD3ZZ Restriction of Left Common Iliac Vein, Percutaneous Approach

06VD4CZ Restriction of Left Common Iliac Vein with Extraluminal Device, Percutaneous Endoscopic Approach

06VD4DZ Restriction of Left Common Iliac Vein with Intraluminal Device, Percutaneous Endoscopic Approach

06VD4ZZ Restriction of Left Common Iliac Vein, Percutaneous Endoscopic Approach

06VF0CZ Restriction of Right External Iliac Vein with Extraluminal Device, Open Approach

06VF0DZ Restriction of Right External Iliac Vein with Intraluminal Device, Open Approach

06VF0ZZ Restriction of Right External Iliac Vein, Open Approach

06VF3CZ Restriction of Right External Iliac Vein with Extraluminal Device, Percutaneous Approach

06VF3DZ Restriction of Right External Iliac Vein with Intraluminal Device, Percutaneous Approach

06VF3ZZ Restriction of Right External Iliac Vein, Percutaneous Approach

06VF4CZ Restriction of Right External Iliac Vein with Extraluminal Device, Percutaneous Endoscopic Approach

06VF4DZ Restriction of Right External Iliac Vein with Intraluminal Device, Percutaneous Endoscopic Approach

06VF4ZZ Restriction of Right External Iliac Vein, Percutaneous Endoscopic Approach

06VG0CZ Restriction of Left External Iliac Vein with Extraluminal Device, Open Approach

06VG0DZ Restriction of Left External Iliac Vein with Intraluminal Device, Open Approach

06VG0ZZ Restriction of Left External Iliac Vein, Open Approach

06VG3CZ Restriction of Left External Iliac Vein with Extraluminal Device, Percutaneous Approach

06VG3DZ Restriction of Left External Iliac Vein with Intraluminal Device, Percutaneous Approach

06VG3ZZ Restriction of Left External Iliac Vein, Percutaneous Approach

06VG4CZ Restriction of Left External Iliac Vein with Extraluminal Device, Percutaneous Endoscopic Approach

06VG4DZ Restriction of Left External Iliac Vein with Intraluminal Device, Percutaneous Endoscopic Approach

06VG4ZZ Restriction of Left External Iliac Vein, Percutaneous Endoscopic Approach

06VH0CZ Restriction of Right Hypogastric Vein with Extraluminal Device, Open Approach

06VH0DZ Restriction of Right Hypogastric Vein with Intraluminal Device, Open Approach

06VH0ZZ Restriction of Right Hypogastric Vein, Open Approach

06VH3CZ Restriction of Right Hypogastric Vein with Extraluminal Device, Percutaneous Approach

06VH3DZ Restriction of Right Hypogastric Vein with Intraluminal Device, Percutaneous Approach

06VH3ZZ Restriction of Right Hypogastric Vein, Percutaneous Approach

06VH4CZ Restriction of Right Hypogastric Vein with Extraluminal Device, Percutaneous Endoscopic Approach

06VH4DZ Restriction of Right Hypogastric Vein with Intraluminal Device, Percutaneous Endoscopic Approach

06VH4ZZ Restriction of Right Hypogastric Vein, Percutaneous Endoscopic Approach

06VJ0CZ Restriction of Left Hypogastric Vein with Extraluminal Device, Open Approach

06VJ0DZ Restriction of Left Hypogastric Vein with Intraluminal Device, Open Approach

06VJ0ZZ Restriction of Left Hypogastric Vein, Open Approach

06VJ3CZ Restriction of Left Hypogastric Vein with Extraluminal Device, Percutaneous Approach

06VJ3DZ Restriction of Left Hypogastric Vein with Intraluminal Device, Percutaneous Approach

06VJ3ZZ Restriction of Left Hypogastric Vein, Percutaneous Approach

06VJ4CZ Restriction of Left Hypogastric Vein with Extraluminal Device, Percutaneous Endoscopic Approach

06VJ4DZ Restriction of Left Hypogastric Vein with Intraluminal Device, Percutaneous Endoscopic Approach

06VJ4ZZ Restriction of Left Hypogastric Vein, Percutaneous Endoscopic Approach

06VM0CZ Restriction of Right Femoral Vein with Extraluminal Device, Open Approach

06VM0DZ Restriction of Right Femoral Vein with Intraluminal Device, Open Approach

06VM0ZZ Restriction of Right Femoral Vein, Open Approach

06VM3CZ Restriction of Right Femoral Vein with Extraluminal Device, Percutaneous Approach

06VM3DZ Restriction of Right Femoral Vein with Intraluminal Device, Percutaneous Approach

06VM3ZZ Restriction of Right Femoral Vein, Percutaneous Approach

06VM4CZ Restriction of Right Femoral Vein with Extraluminal Device, Percutaneous Endoscopic Approach

06VM4DZ Restriction of Right Femoral Vein with Intraluminal Device, Percutaneous Endoscopic Approach

06VM4ZZ Restriction of Right Femoral Vein, Percutaneous Endoscopic Approach

06VN0CZ Restriction of Left Femoral Vein with Extraluminal Device, Open Approach

06VN0DZ Restriction of Left Femoral Vein with Intraluminal Device, Open Approach

06VN0ZZ Restriction of Left Femoral Vein, Open Approach

06VN3CZ Restriction of Left Femoral Vein with Extraluminal Device, Percutaneous Approach

06VN3DZ Restriction of Left Femoral Vein with Intraluminal Device, Percutaneous Approach

06VN3ZZ Restriction of Left Femoral Vein, Percutaneous Approach

06VN4CZ Restriction of Left Femoral Vein with Extraluminal Device, Percutaneous Endoscopic Approach

06VN4DZ Restriction of Left Femoral Vein with Intraluminal Device, Percutaneous Endoscopic Approach

06VN4ZZ Restriction of Left Femoral Vein, Percutaneous Endoscopic Approach

06VP0CZ Restriction of Right Saphenous Vein with Extraluminal Device, Open Approach

06VP0DZ Restriction of Right Saphenous Vein with Intraluminal Device, Open Approach

06VP0ZZ Restriction of Right Saphenous Vein, Open Approach

06VP3CZ Restriction of Right Saphenous Vein with Extraluminal Device, Percutaneous Approach

06VP3DZ Restriction of Right Saphenous Vein with Intraluminal Device, Percutaneous Approach

06VP3ZZ Restriction of Right Saphenous Vein, Percutaneous Approach

06VP4CZ Restriction of Right Saphenous Vein with Extraluminal Device, Percutaneous Endoscopic Approach

06VP4DZ Restriction of Right Saphenous Vein with Intraluminal Device, Percutaneous Endoscopic Approach

06VP4ZZ Restriction of Right Saphenous Vein, Percutaneous Endoscopic Approach

06VQ0CZ Restriction of Left Saphenous Vein with Extraluminal Device, Open Approach

06VQ0DZ Restriction of Left Saphenous Vein with Intraluminal Device, Open Approach

06VQ0ZZ Restriction of Left Saphenous Vein, Open Approach

06VQ3CZ Restriction of Left Saphenous Vein with Extraluminal Device, Percutaneous Approach

06VQ3DZ Restriction of Left Saphenous Vein with Intraluminal Device, Percutaneous Approach

06VQ3ZZ Restriction of Left Saphenous Vein, Percutaneous Approach

06VQ4CZ Restriction of Left Saphenous Vein with Extraluminal Device, Percutaneous Endoscopic Approach

06VQ4DZ Restriction of Left Saphenous Vein with Intraluminal Device, Percutaneous Endoscopic Approach

06VQ4ZZ Restriction of Left Saphenous Vein, Percutaneous Endoscopic Approach

06VT0CZ Restriction of Right Foot Vein with Extraluminal Device, Open Approach

06VT0DZ Restriction of Right Foot Vein with Intraluminal Device, Open Approach

06VT0ZZ Restriction of Right Foot Vein, Open Approach

06VT3CZ Restriction of Right Foot Vein with Extraluminal Device, Percutaneous Approach

06VT3DZ Restriction of Right Foot Vein with Intraluminal Device, Percutaneous Approach

06VT3ZZ Restriction of Right Foot Vein, Percutaneous Approach

06VT4CZ Restriction of Right Foot Vein with Extraluminal Device, Percutaneous Endoscopic Approach

06VT4DZ	Restriction of Right Foot Vein with Intraluminal Device, Percutaneous Endoscopic Approach
06VT4ZZ	Restriction of Right Foot Vein, Percutaneous Endoscopic Approach
06VV0CZ	Restriction of Left Foot Vein with Extraluminal Device, Open Approach
06VV0DZ	Restriction of Left Foot Vein with Intraluminal Device, Open Approach
06VV0ZZ	Restriction of Left Foot Vein, Open Approach
06VV3CZ	Restriction of Left Foot Vein with Extraluminal Device, Percutaneous Approach
06VV3DZ	Restriction of Left Foot Vein with Intraluminal Device, Percutaneous Approach

06VV3ZZ	Restriction of Left Foot Vein, Percutaneous Approach
06VV4CZ	Restriction of Left Foot Vein with Extraluminal Device, Percutaneous Endoscopic Approach
06VV4DZ	Restriction of Left Foot Vein with Intraluminal Device, Percutaneous Endoscopic Approach
06VV4ZZ	Restriction of Left Foot Vein, Percutaneous Endoscopic Approach
06VY0CZ	Restriction of Lower Vein with Extraluminal Device, Open Approach
06VY0DZ	Restriction of Lower Vein with Intraluminal Device, Open Approach
06VY0ZZ	Restriction of Lower Vein, Open Approach

06VY3CZ	Restriction of Lower Vein with Extraluminal Device, Percutaneous Approach
06VY3DZ	Restriction of Lower Vein with Intraluminal Device, Percutaneous Approach
06VY3ZZ	Restriction of Lower Vein, Percutaneous Approach
06VY4CZ	Restriction of Lower Vein with Extraluminal Device, Percutaneous Endoscopic Approach
06VY4DZ	Restriction of Lower Vein with Intraluminal Device, Percutaneous Endoscopic Approach
06VY4ZZ	Restriction of Lower Vein, Percutaneous Endoscopic Approach

06W – Lower Veins, Revision

Review Coding Guideline B6.1c

06WY00Z	Revision of Drainage Device in Lower Vein, Open Approach
06WY02Z	Revision of Monitoring Device in Lower Vein, Open Approach
06WY03Z	Revision of Infusion Device in Lower Vein, Open Approach
06WY07Z	Revision of Autologous Tissue Substitute in Lower Vein, Open Approach
06WY0CZ	Revision of Extraluminal Device in Lower Vein, Open Approach
06WY0DZ	Revision of Intraluminal Device in Lower Vein, Open Approach
06WY0JZ	Revision of Synthetic Substitute in Lower Vein, Open Approach
06WY0KZ	Revision of Nonautologous Tissue Substitute in Lower Vein, Open Approach
06WY0YZ	Revision of Other Device in Lower Vein, Open Approach
06WY30Z	Revision of Drainage Device in Lower Vein, Percutaneous Approach
06WY32Z	Revision of Monitoring Device in Lower Vein, Percutaneous Approach
06WY33Z	Revision of Infusion Device in Lower Vein, Percutaneous Approach
06WY37Z	Revision of Autologous Tissue Substitute in Lower Vein, Percutaneous Approach

06WY3CZ	Revision of Extraluminal Device in Lower Vein, Percutaneous Approach
06WY3DZ	Revision of Intraluminal Device in Lower Vein, Percutaneous Approach
	AHA CC: 3Q, 2014, 25-26
06WY3JZ	Revision of Synthetic Substitute in Lower Vein, Percutaneous Approach
	AHA CC: 1Q, 2018, 10-11; 2Q, 2019, 39
06WY3KZ	Revision of Nonautologous Tissue Substitute in Lower Vein, Percutaneous Approach
06WY3YZ	Revision of Other Device in Lower Vein, Percutaneous Approach
06WY40Z	Revision of Drainage Device in Lower Vein, Percutaneous Endoscopic Approach
06WY42Z	Revision of Monitoring Device in Lower Vein, Percutaneous Endoscopic Approach
06WY43Z	Revision of Infusion Device in Lower Vein, Percutaneous Endoscopic Approach
06WY47Z	Revision of Autologous Tissue Substitute in Lower Vein, Percutaneous Endoscopic Approach
06WY4CZ	Revision of Extraluminal Device in Lower Vein, Percutaneous Endoscopic Approach

06WY4DZ	Revision of Intraluminal Device in Lower Vein, Percutaneous Endoscopic Approach
06WY4JZ	Revision of Synthetic Substitute in Lower Vein, Percutaneous Endoscopic Approach
06WY4KZ	Revision of Nonautologous Tissue Substitute in Lower Vein, Percutaneous Endoscopic Approach
06WY4YZ	Revision of Other Device in Lower Vein, Percutaneous Endoscopic Approach
06WYX0Z	Revision of Drainage Device in Lower Vein, External Approach
06WYX2Z	Revision of Monitoring Device in Lower Vein, External Approach
06WYX3Z	Revision of Infusion Device in Lower Vein, External Approach
06WYX7Z	Revision of Autologous Tissue Substitute in Lower Vein, External Approach
06WYXCZ	Revision of Extraluminal Device in Lower Vein, External Approach
06WYXDZ	Revision of Intraluminal Device in Lower Vein, External Approach
06WYXJZ	Revision of Synthetic Substitute in Lower Vein, External Approach
06WYXKZ	Revision of Nonautologous Tissue Substitute in Lower Vein, External Approach

Lymph Vessels and Nodes of Head and Neck; Lymphatic Drainage of Mouth and Pharynx

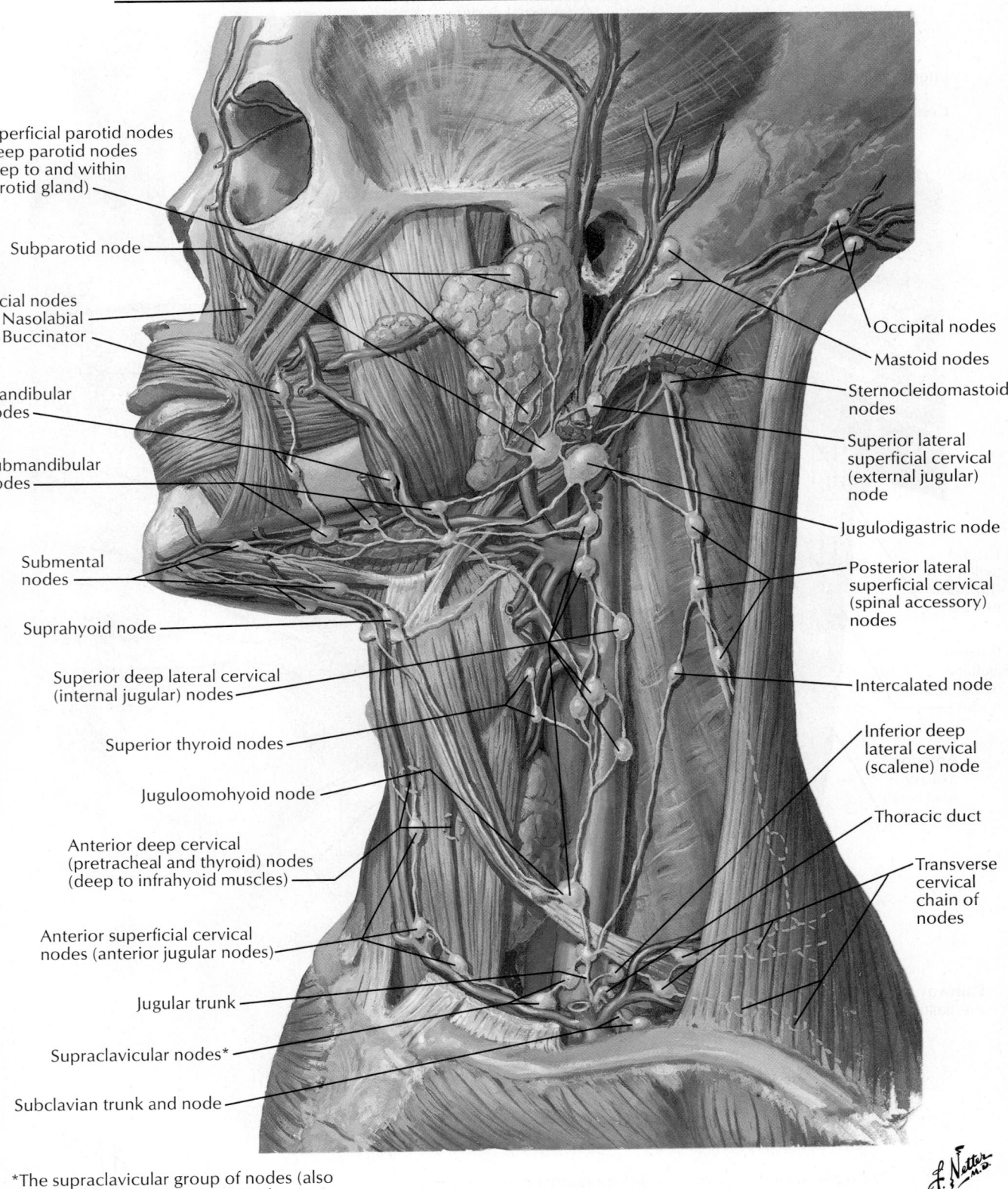

Superficial parotid nodes (deep parotid nodes deep to and within parotid gland)

Subparotid node

Facial nodes
Nasolabial
Buccinator

Mandibular nodes

Submandibular nodes

Submental nodes

Suprahyoid node

Superior deep lateral cervical (internal jugular) nodes

Superior thyroid nodes

Juguloomohyoid node

Anterior deep cervical (pretracheal and thyroid) nodes (deep to infrahyoid muscles)

Anterior superficial cervical nodes (anterior jugular nodes)

Jugular trunk

Supraclavicular nodes*

Subclavian trunk and node

Occipital nodes

Mastoid nodes

Sternocleidomastoid nodes

Superior lateral superficial cervical (external jugular) node

Jugulodigastric node

Posterior lateral superficial cervical (spinal accessory) nodes

Intercalated node

Inferior deep lateral cervical (scalene) node

Thoracic duct

Transverse cervical chain of nodes

*The supraclavicular group of nodes (also known as the lower deep cervical group), especially on the left, are also sometimes referred to as the signal or sentinel lymph nodes of Virchow or Troisier, especially when sufficiently enlarged and palpable. These nodes (or a single node) are so termed because they may be the first recognized presumptive evidence of malignant disease in the viscera.

Lymph Vessels and Nodes of Mammary Gland Lymphatic Drainage

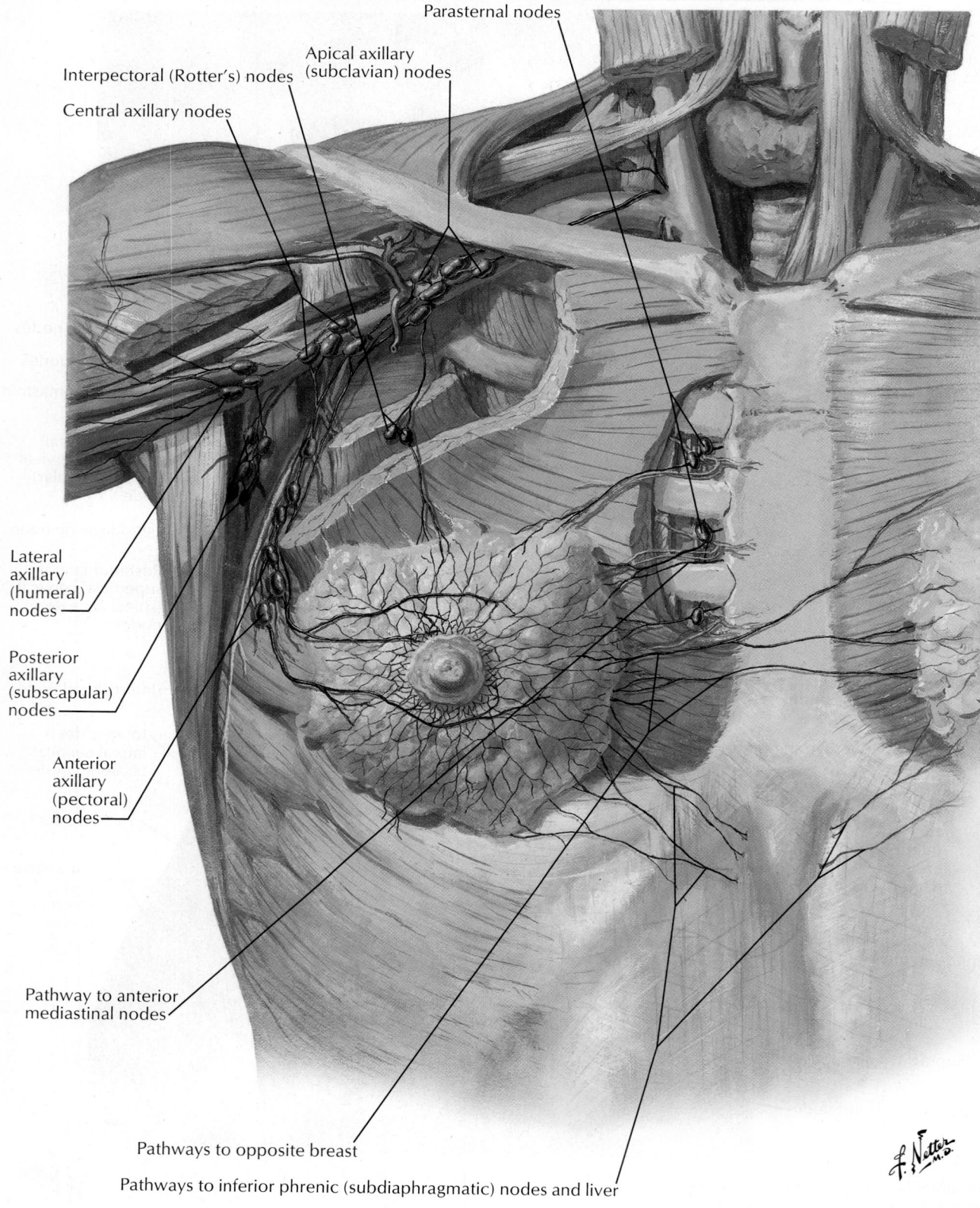

Parasternal nodes

Apical axillary (subclavian) nodes

Interpectoral (Rotter's) nodes

Central axillary nodes

Lateral axillary (humeral) nodes

Posterior axillary (subscapular) nodes

Anterior axillary (pectoral) nodes

Pathway to anterior mediastinal nodes

Pathways to opposite breast

Pathways to inferior phrenic (subdiaphragmatic) nodes and liver

Medical and Surgical, Lymphatic and Hemic System

Section	0	Medical and Surgical
Body System	7	Lymphatic and Hemic Systems
Operation	2	**Change:** Taking out or off a device from a body part and putting back an identical or similar device in or on the same body part without cutting or puncturing the skin or a mucous membrane

Body Part (4th)	Approach (5th)	Device (6th)	Qualifier (7th)
K Thoracic Duct L Cisterna Chyli M Thymus N Lymphatic P Spleen T Bone Marrow	X External	0 Drainage Device Y Other Device	Z No Qualifier

Section	0	Medical and Surgical
Body System	7	Lymphatic and Hemic Systems
Operation	5	**Destruction:** Physical eradication of all or a portion of a body part by the direct use of energy, force, or a destructive agent

Body Part (4th)	Approach (5th)	Device (6th)	Qualifier (7th)
0 Lymphatic, Head 1 Lymphatic, Right Neck 2 Lymphatic, Left Neck 3 Lymphatic, Right Upper Extremity 4 Lymphatic, Left Upper Extremity 5 Lymphatic, Right Axillary 6 Lymphatic, Left Axillary 7 Lymphatic, Thorax 8 Lymphatic, Internal Mammary, Right 9 Lymphatic, Internal Mammary, Left B Lymphatic, Mesenteric C Lymphatic, Pelvis D Lymphatic, Aortic F Lymphatic, Right Lower Extremity G Lymphatic, Left Lower Extremity H Lymphatic, Right Inguinal J Lymphatic, Left Inguinal K Thoracic Duct L Cisterna Chyli M Thymus P Spleen	0 Open 3 Percutaneous 4 Percutaneous Endoscopic	Z No Device	Z No Qualifier

Section	0	Medical and Surgical
Body System	7	Lymphatic and Hemic Systems
Operation	9	**Drainage:** Taking or letting out fluids and/or gases from a body part

Body Part (4th)	Approach (5th)	Device (6th)	Qualifier (7th)
0 Lymphatic, Head 1 Lymphatic, Right Neck 2 Lymphatic, Left Neck 3 Lymphatic, Right Upper Extremity 4 Lymphatic, Left Upper Extremity 5 Lymphatic, Right Axillary 6 Lymphatic, Left Axillary 7 Lymphatic, Thorax 8 Lymphatic, Internal Mammary, Right 9 Lymphatic, Internal Mammary, Left B Lymphatic, Mesenteric C Lymphatic, Pelvis D Lymphatic, Aortic F Lymphatic, Right Lower Extremity G Lymphatic, Left Lower Extremity H Lymphatic, Right Inguinal J Lymphatic, Left Inguinal K Thoracic Duct L Cisterna Chyli	0 Open 3 Percutaneous 4 Percutaneous Endoscopic 8 Via Natural or Artificial Opening Endoscopic	0 Drainage Device	Z No Qualifier
0 Lymphatic, Head 1 Lymphatic, Right Neck 2 Lymphatic, Left Neck 3 Lymphatic, Right Upper Extremity 4 Lymphatic, Left Upper Extremity 5 Lymphatic, Right Axillary 6 Lymphatic, Left Axillary 7 Lymphatic, Thorax 8 Lymphatic, Internal Mammary, Right 9 Lymphatic, Internal Mammary, Left B Lymphatic, Mesenteric C Lymphatic, Pelvis D Lymphatic, Aortic F Lymphatic, Right Lower Extremity G Lymphatic, Left Lower Extremity H Lymphatic, Right Inguinal J Lymphatic, Left Inguinal K Thoracic Duct L Cisterna Chyli	0 Open 3 Percutaneous 4 Percutaneous Endoscopic 8 Via Natural or Artificial Opening Endoscopic	Z No Device	X Diagnostic Z No Qualifier
M Thymus P Spleen T Bone Marrow	0 Open 3 Percutaneous 4 Percutaneous Endoscopic	0 Drainage Device	Z No Qualifier
M Thymus P Spleen T Bone Marrow	0 Open 3 Percutaneous 4 Percutaneous Endoscopic	Z No Device	X No Diagnostic Z No Qualifier

Section	0	Medical and Surgical
Body System	7	Lymphatic and Hemic Systems
Operation	B	Excision: Cutting out or off, without replacement, a portion of a body part

Body Part (4th)	Approach (5th)	Device (6th)	Qualifier (7th)
0 Lymphatic, Head 1 Lymphatic, Right Neck 2 Lymphatic, Left Neck 3 Lymphatic, Right Upper Extremity 4 Lymphatic, Left Upper Extremity 5 Lymphatic, Right Axillary 6 Lymphatic, Left Axillary 7 Lymphatic, Thorax 8 Lymphatic, Internal Mammary, Right 9 Lymphatic, Internal Mammary, Left B Lymphatic, Mesenteric C Lymphatic, Pelvis D Lymphatic, Aortic F Lymphatic, Right Lower Extremity G Lymphatic, Left Lower Extremity H Lymphatic, Right Inguinal J Lymphatic, Left Inguinal K Thoracic Duct L Cisterna Chyli M Thymus P Spleen	0 Open 3 Percutaneous 4 Percutaneous Endoscopic	Z No Device	X Diagnostic Z No Qualifier

Section	0	Medical and Surgical
Body System	7	Lymphatic and Hemic Systems
Operation	C	Extirpation: Taking or cutting out solid matter from a body part

Body Part (4th)	Approach (5th)	Device (6th)	Qualifier (7th)
0 Lymphatic, Head 1 Lymphatic, Right Neck 2 Lymphatic, Left Neck 3 Lymphatic, Right Upper Extremity 4 Lymphatic, Left Upper Extremity 5 Lymphatic, Right Axillary 6 Lymphatic, Left Axillary 7 Lymphatic, Thorax 8 Lymphatic, Internal Mammary, Right 9 Lymphatic, Internal Mammary, Left B Lymphatic, Mesenteric C Lymphatic, Pelvis D Lymphatic, Aortic F Lymphatic, Right Lower Extremity G Lymphatic, Left Lower Extremity H Lymphatic, Right Inguinal J Lymphatic, Left Inguinal K Thoracic Duct L Cisterna Chyli M Thymus P Spleen	0 Open 3 Percutaneous 4 Percutaneous Endoscopic	Z No Device	Z No Qualifier

Section	0	Medical and Surgical
Body System	7	Lymphatic and Hemic Systems
Operation	D	Extraction: Pulling or stripping out or off all or a portion of a body part by the use of force

Body Part (4th)	Approach (5th)	Device (6th)	Qualifier (7th)
0 Lymphatic, Head 1 Lymphatic, Right Neck 2 Lymphatic, Left Neck 3 Lymphatic, Right Upper Extremity 4 Lymphatic, Left Upper Extremity 5 Lymphatic, Right Axillary 6 Lymphatic, Left Axillary 7 Lymphatic, Thorax 8 Lymphatic, Internal Mammary, Right 9 Lymphatic, Internal Mammary, Left B Lymphatic, Mesenteric C Lymphatic, Pelvis D Lymphatic, Aortic F Lymphatic, Right Lower Extremity G Lymphatic, Left Lower Extremity H Lymphatic, Right Inguinal J Lymphatic, Left Inguinal K Thoracic Duct L Cisterna Chyli	3 Percutaneous 4 Percutaneous Endoscopic 8 Via Natural or Artificial Opening Endoscopic	Z No Device	X Diagnostic
M Thymus P Spleen	3 Percutaneous 4 Percutaneous Endoscopic	Z No Device	X No Diagnostic
Q Bone Marrow, Sternum R Bone Marrow, Iliac S Bone Marrow, Vertebral T Bone Marrow	0 Open 3 Percutaneous	Z No Device	X Diagnostic Z No Qualifier

Section	0	Medical and Surgical
Body System	7	Lymphatic and Hemic Systems
Operation	H	Insertion: Putting in a nonbiological appliance that monitors, assists, performs, or prevents a physiological function but does not physically take the place of a body part

Body Part (4th)	Approach (5th)	Device (6th)	Qualifier (7th)
K Thoracic Duct L Cisterna Chyli M Thymus N Lymphatic P Spleen T Bone Marrow	0 Open 3 Percutaneous 4 Percutaneous Endoscopic	1 Radioactive Element 3 Infusion Device Y Other Device	Z No Qualifier

Section	0	Medical and Surgical
Body System	7	Lymphatic and Hemic Systems
Operation	J	Inspection: Visually and/or manually exploring a body part

Body Part (4th)	Approach (5th)	Device (6th)	Qualifier (7th)
K Thoracic Duct L Cisterna Chyli M Thymus T Bone Marrow	0 Open 3 Percutaneous 4 Percutaneous Endoscopic	Z No Device	Z No Qualifier
N Lymphatic	0 Open 3 Percutaneous 4 Percutaneous Endoscopic 8 Via Natural or Artificial Opening Endoscopic X External	Z No Device	Z No Qualifier
P Spleen	0 Open 3 Percutaneous 4 Percutaneous Endoscopic X External	Z No Device	Z No Qualifier

Section	0	Medical and Surgical
Body System	7	Lymphatic and Hemic Systems
Operation	L	**Occlusion:** Completely closing an orifice or the lumen of a tubular body part

Body Part (4th)	Approach (5th)	Device (6th)	Qualifier (7th)
0 Lymphatic, Head 1 Lymphatic, Right Neck 2 Lymphatic, Left Neck 3 Lymphatic, Right Upper Extremity 4 Lymphatic, Left Upper Extremity 5 Lymphatic, Right Axillary 6 Lymphatic, Left Axillary 7 Lymphatic, Thorax 8 Lymphatic, Internal Mammary, Right 9 Lymphatic, Internal Mammary, Left B Lymphatic, Mesenteric C Lymphatic, Pelvis D Lymphatic, Aortic F Lymphatic, Right Lower Extremity G Lymphatic, Left Lower Extremity H Lymphatic, Right Inguinal J Lymphatic, Left Inguinal K Thoracic Duct L Cisterna Chyli	0 Open 3 Percutaneous 4 Percutaneous Endoscopic	C Extraluminal Device D Intraluminal Device Z No Device	Z No Qualifier

Section	0	Medical and Surgical
Body System	7	Lymphatic and Hemic Systems
Operation	N	**Release:** Freeing a body part from an abnormal physical constraint by cutting or by the use of force

Body Part (4th)	Approach (5th)	Device (6th)	Qualifier (7th)
0 Lymphatic, Head 1 Lymphatic, Right Neck 2 Lymphatic, Left Neck 3 Lymphatic, Right Upper Extremity 4 Lymphatic, Left Upper Extremity 5 Lymphatic, Right Axillary 6 Lymphatic, Left Axillary 7 Lymphatic, Thorax 8 Lymphatic, Internal Mammary, Right 9 Lymphatic, Internal Mammary, Left B Lymphatic, Mesenteric C Lymphatic, Pelvis D Lymphatic, Aortic F Lymphatic, Right Lower Extremity G Lymphatic, Left Lower Extremity H Lymphatic, Right Inguinal J Lymphatic, Left Inguinal K Thoracic Duct L Cisterna Chyli M Thymus P Spleen	0 Open 3 Percutaneous 4 Percutaneous Endoscopic	Z No Device	Z No Qualifier

Section	0	Medical and Surgical
Body System	7	Lymphatic and Hemic Systems
Operation	P	**Removal:** Taking out or off a device from a body part

Body Part (4th)	Approach (5th)	Device (6th)	Qualifier (7th)
K Thoracic Duct L Cisterna Chyli N Lymphatic	0 Open 3 Percutaneous 4 Percutaneous Endoscopic	0 Drainage Device 3 Infusion Device 7 Autologous Tissue Substitute C Extraluminal Device D Intraluminal Device J Synthetic Substitute K Nonautologous Tissue Substitute Y Other Device	Z No Qualifier
K Thoracic Duct L Cisterna Chyli N Lymphatic	X External	0 Drainage Device 3 Infusion Device D Intraluminal Device	Z No Qualifier
M Thymus P Spleen	0 Open 3 Percutaneous 4 Percutaneous Endoscopic	0 Drainage Device 3 Infusion Device Y Other Device	Z No Qualifier
M Thymus P Spleen	X External	0 Drainage Device 3 Infusion Device	Z No Qualifier
T Bone Marrow	0 Open 3 Percutaneous 4 Percutaneous Endoscopic X External	0 Drainage Device	Z No Qualifier

Section	0	Medical and Surgical
Body System	7	Lymphatic and Hemic Systems
Operation	Q	**Repair:** Restoring, to the extent possible, a body part to its normal anatomic structure and function

Body Part (4th)	Approach (5th)	Device (6th)	Qualifier (7th)
0 Lymphatic, Head 1 Lymphatic, Right Neck 2 Lymphatic, Left Neck 3 Lymphatic, Right Upper Extremity 4 Lymphatic, Left Upper Extremity 5 Lymphatic, Right Axillary 6 Lymphatic, Left Axillary 7 Lymphatic, Thorax 8 Lymphatic, Internal Mammary, Right 9 Lymphatic, Internal Mammary, Left B Lymphatic, Mesenteric C Lymphatic, Pelvis D Lymphatic, Aortic F Lymphatic, Right Lower Extremity G Lymphatic, Left Lower Extremity H Lymphatic, Right Inguinal J Lymphatic, Left Inguinal K Thoracic Duct L Cisterna Chyli	0 Open 3 Percutaneous 4 Percutaneous Endoscopic 8 Via Natural or Artificial Opening Endoscopic	Z No Device	Z No Qualifier
M Thymus P Spleen	0 Open 3 Percutaneous 4 Percutaneous Endoscopic	Z No Device	Z No Qualifier

458

Section	0	Medical and Surgical
Body System	7	Lymphatic and Hemic Systems
Operation	S	**Reposition:** Moving to its normal location, or other suitable location, all or a portion of a body part

Body Part (4th)	Approach (5th)	Device (6th)	Qualifier (7th)
M Thymus P Spleen	0 Open	Z No Device	Z No Qualifier

Section	0	Medical and Surgical
Body System	7	Lymphatic and Hemic Systems
Operation	T	**Resection:** Cutting out or off, without replacement, all of a body part

Body Part (4th)	Approach (5th)	Device (6th)	Qualifier (7th)
0 Lymphatic, Head 1 Lymphatic, Right Neck 2 Lymphatic, Left Neck 3 Lymphatic, Right Upper Extremity 4 Lymphatic, Left Upper Extremity 5 Lymphatic, Right Axillary 6 Lymphatic, Left Axillary 7 Lymphatic, Thorax 8 Lymphatic, Internal Mammary, Right 9 Lymphatic, Internal Mammary, Left B Lymphatic, Mesenteric C Lymphatic, Pelvis D Lymphatic, Aortic F Lymphatic, Right Lower Extremity G Lymphatic, Left Lower Extremity H Lymphatic, Right Inguinal J Lymphatic, Left Inguinal K Thoracic Duct L Cisterna Chyli M Thymus P Spleen	0 Open 4 Percutaneous Endoscopic	Z No Device	Z No Qualifier

Section	0	Medical and Surgical
Body System	7	Lymphatic and Hemic Systems
Operation	U	**Supplement:** Putting in or on biological or synthetic material that physically reinforces and/or augments the function of a portion of a body part

Body Part (4th)	Approach (5th)	Device (6th)	Qualifier (7th)
0 Lymphatic, Head 1 Lymphatic, Right Neck 2 Lymphatic, Left Neck 3 Lymphatic, Right Upper Extremity 4 Lymphatic, Left Upper Extremity 5 Lymphatic, Right Axillary 6 Lymphatic, Left Axillary 7 Lymphatic, Thorax 8 Lymphatic, Internal Mammary, Right 9 Lymphatic, Internal Mammary, Left B Lymphatic, Mesenteric C Lymphatic, Pelvis D Lymphatic, Aortic F Lymphatic, Right Lower Extremity G Lymphatic, Left Lower Extremity H Lymphatic, Right Inguinal J Lymphatic, Left Inguinal K Thoracic Duct L Cisterna Chyli	0 Open 4 Percutaneous Endoscopic	7 Autologous Tissue Substitute J Synthetic Substitute K Nonautologous Tissue Substitute	Z No Qualifier

Section	0	Medical and Surgical
Body System	7	Lymphatic and Hemic Systems
Operation	V	**Restriction:** Partially closing an orifice or the lumen of a tubular body part

Body Part (4th)	Approach (5th)	Device (6th)	Qualifier (7th)
0 Lymphatic, Head 1 Lymphatic, Right Neck 2 Lymphatic, Left Neck 3 Lymphatic, Right Upper Extremity 4 Lymphatic, Left Upper Extremity 5 Lymphatic, Right Axillary 6 Lymphatic, Left Axillary 7 Lymphatic, Thorax 8 Lymphatic, Internal Mammary, Right 9 Lymphatic, Internal Mammary, Left B Lymphatic, Mesenteric C Lymphatic, Pelvis D Lymphatic, Aortic F Lymphatic, Right Lower Extremity G Lymphatic, Left Lower Extremity H Lymphatic, Right Inguinal J Lymphatic, Left Inguinal K Thoracic Duct L Cisterna Chyli	0 Open 3 Percutaneous 4 Percutaneous Endoscopic	C Extraluminal Device D Intraluminal Device Z No Device	Z No Qualifier

Section	0	Medical and Surgical
Body System	7	Lymphatic and Hemic Systems
Operation	W	**Revision:** Correcting, to the extent possible, a portion of a malfunctioning device or the position of a displaced device

Body Part (4th)	Approach (5th)	Device (6th)	Qualifier (7th)
K Thoracic Duct L Cisterna Chyli N Lymphatic	0 Open 3 Percutaneous 4 Percutaneous Endoscopic	0 Drainage Device 3 Infusion Device 7 Autologous Tissue Substitute C Extraluminal Device D Intraluminal Device J Synthetic Substitute K Nonautologous Tissue Substitute Y Other Device	Z No Qualifier
K Thoracic Duct L Cisterna Chyli N Lymphatic	X External	0 Drainage Device 3 Infusion Device 7 Autologous Tissue Substitute C Extraluminal Device D Intraluminal Device J Synthetic Substitute K Nonautologous Tissue Substitute	Z No Qualifier
M Thymus P Spleen	0 Open 3 Percutaneous 4 Percutaneous Endoscopic	0 Drainage Device 3 Infusion Device Y Other Device	Z No Qualifier
M Thymus P Spleen	X External	0 Drainage Device 3 Infusion Device	Z No Qualifier
T Bone Marrow	0 Open 3 Percutaneous 4 Percutaneous Endoscopic X External	0 Drainage Device	Z No Qualifier

| | | Section | 0 | Medical and Surgical |
| | | Body System | 7 | Lymphatic and Hemic Systems |

Section 0 **Medical and Surgical**
Body System 7 **Lymphatic and Hemic Systems**
Operation Y **Transplantation:** Putting in or on all or a portion of a living body part taken from another individual or animal to physically take the place and/or function of all or a portion of a similar body part

Body Part (4th)	Approach (5th)	Device (6th)	Qualifier (7th)
M Thymus P Spleen	0 Open	Z No Device	0 Allogeneic 1 Syngeneic 2 Zooplastic

Lymphatic and Hemic Systems Code Listing 072–07Y

072 – Lymphatic and Hemic Systems, Change

Review Coding Guideline B6.1c

072KX0Z Change Drainage Device in Thoracic Duct, External Approach
072KXYZ Change Other Device in Thoracic Duct, External Approach
072LX0Z Change Drainage Device in Cisterna Chyli, External Approach
072LXYZ Change Other Device in Cisterna Chyli, External Approach

072MX0Z Change Drainage Device in Thymus, External Approach
072MXYZ Change Other Device in Thymus, External Approach
072NX0Z Change Drainage Device in Lymphatic, External Approach
072NXYZ Change Other Device in Lymphatic, External Approach

072PX0Z Change Drainage Device in Spleen, External Approach
072PXYZ Change Other Device in Spleen, External Approach
072TX0Z Change Drainage Device in Bone Marrow, External Approach
072TXYZ Change Other Device in Bone Marrow, External Approach

075 – Lymphatic and Hemic Systems, Destruction

07500ZZ Destruction of Head Lymphatic, Open Approach
07503ZZ Destruction of Head Lymphatic, Percutaneous Approach
07504ZZ Destruction of Head Lymphatic, Percutaneous Endoscopic Approach
07510ZZ Destruction of Right Neck Lymphatic, Open Approach
07513ZZ Destruction of Right Neck Lymphatic, Percutaneous Approach
07514ZZ Destruction of Right Neck Lymphatic, Percutaneous Endoscopic Approach
07520ZZ Destruction of Left Neck Lymphatic, Open Approach
07523ZZ Destruction of Left Neck Lymphatic, Percutaneous Approach
07524ZZ Destruction of Left Neck Lymphatic, Percutaneous Endoscopic Approach
07530ZZ Destruction of Right Upper Extremity Lymphatic, Open Approach
07533ZZ Destruction of Right Upper Extremity Lymphatic, Percutaneous Approach
07534ZZ Destruction of Right Upper Extremity Lymphatic, Percutaneous Endoscopic Approach
07540ZZ Destruction of Left Upper Extremity Lymphatic, Open Approach
07543ZZ Destruction of Left Upper Extremity Lymphatic, Percutaneous Approach
07544ZZ Destruction of Left Upper Extremity Lymphatic, Percutaneous Endoscopic Approach
07550ZZ Destruction of Right Axillary Lymphatic, Open Approach
07553ZZ Destruction of Right Axillary Lymphatic, Percutaneous Approach
07554ZZ Destruction of Right Axillary Lymphatic, Percutaneous Endoscopic Approach
07560ZZ Destruction of Left Axillary Lymphatic, Open Approach
07563ZZ Destruction of Left Axillary Lymphatic, Percutaneous Approach
07564ZZ Destruction of Left Axillary Lymphatic, Percutaneous Endoscopic Approach

07570ZZ Destruction of Thorax Lymphatic, Open Approach
07573ZZ Destruction of Thorax Lymphatic, Percutaneous Approach
07574ZZ Destruction of Thorax Lymphatic, Percutaneous Endoscopic Approach
07580ZZ Destruction of Right Internal Mammary Lymphatic, Open Approach
07583ZZ Destruction of Right Internal Mammary Lymphatic, Percutaneous Approach
07584ZZ Destruction of Right Internal Mammary Lymphatic, Percutaneous Endoscopic Approach
07590ZZ Destruction of Left Internal Mammary Lymphatic, Open Approach
07593ZZ Destruction of Left Internal Mammary Lymphatic, Percutaneous Approach
07594ZZ Destruction of Left Internal Mammary Lymphatic, Percutaneous Endoscopic Approach
075B0ZZ Destruction of Mesenteric Lymphatic, Open Approach
075B3ZZ Destruction of Mesenteric Lymphatic, Percutaneous Approach
075B4ZZ Destruction of Mesenteric Lymphatic, Percutaneous Endoscopic Approach
075C0ZZ Destruction of Pelvis Lymphatic, Open Approach
075C3ZZ Destruction of Pelvis Lymphatic, Percutaneous Approach
075C4ZZ Destruction of Pelvis Lymphatic, Percutaneous Endoscopic Approach
075D0ZZ Destruction of Aortic Lymphatic, Open Approach
075D3ZZ Destruction of Aortic Lymphatic, Percutaneous Approach
075D4ZZ Destruction of Aortic Lymphatic, Percutaneous Endoscopic Approach
075F0ZZ Destruction of Right Lower Extremity Lymphatic, Open Approach
075F3ZZ Destruction of Right Lower Extremity Lymphatic, Percutaneous Approach

075F4ZZ Destruction of Right Lower Extremity Lymphatic, Percutaneous Endoscopic Approach
075G0ZZ Destruction of Left Lower Extremity Lymphatic, Open Approach
075G3ZZ Destruction of Left Lower Extremity Lymphatic, Percutaneous Approach
075G4ZZ Destruction of Left Lower Extremity Lymphatic, Percutaneous Endoscopic Approach
075H0ZZ Destruction of Right Inguinal Lymphatic, Open Approach
075H3ZZ Destruction of Right Inguinal Lymphatic, Percutaneous Approach
075H4ZZ Destruction of Right Inguinal Lymphatic, Percutaneous Endoscopic Approach
075J0ZZ Destruction of Left Inguinal Lymphatic, Open Approach
075J3ZZ Destruction of Left Inguinal Lymphatic, Percutaneous Approach
075J4ZZ Destruction of Left Inguinal Lymphatic, Percutaneous Endoscopic Approach
075K0ZZ Destruction of Thoracic Duct, Open Approach
075K3ZZ Destruction of Thoracic Duct, Percutaneous Approach
075K4ZZ Destruction of Thoracic Duct, Percutaneous Endoscopic Approach
075L0ZZ Destruction of Cisterna Chyli, Open Approach
075L3ZZ Destruction of Cisterna Chyli, Percutaneous Approach
075L4ZZ Destruction of Cisterna Chyli, Percutaneous Endoscopic Approach
075M0ZZ Destruction of Thymus, Open Approach
075M3ZZ Destruction of Thymus, Percutaneous Approach
075M4ZZ Destruction of Thymus, Percutaneous Endoscopic Approach
075P0ZZ Destruction of Spleen, Open Approach
075P3ZZ Destruction of Spleen, Percutaneous Approach
075P4ZZ Destruction of Spleen, Percutaneous Endoscopic Approach

♀ Female-only   ♂ Male-only   ▲ Limited Coverage   ● Non-OR   ▧ HAC-associated procedure   ▲ Non-covered procedures   ✚ Cluster

Review Coding Guidelines B3.4a and B3.4b

Review Coding Guideline B6.2

079000Z	Drainage of Head Lymphatic with Drainage Device, Open Approach
07900ZX	Drainage of Head Lymphatic, Open Approach, Diagnostic
07900ZZ	Drainage of Head Lymphatic, Open Approach
079030Z	Drainage of Head Lymphatic with Drainage Device, Percutaneous Approach
07903ZX	Drainage of Head Lymphatic, Percutaneous Approach, Diagnostic
07903ZZ	Drainage of Head Lymphatic, Percutaneous Approach
079040Z	Drainage of Head Lymphatic with Drainage Device, Percutaneous Endoscopic Approach
07904ZX	Drainage of Head Lymphatic, Percutaneous Endoscopic Approach, Diagnostic
07904ZZ	Drainage of Head Lymphatic, Percutaneous Endoscopic Approach
079080Z	Drainage of Head Lymphatic with Drainage Device, Via Natural or Artificial Opening Endoscopic
07908ZX	Drainage of Head Lymphatic, Via Natural or Artificial Opening Endoscopic Approach, Diagnostic
07908ZZ	Drainage of Head Lymphatic, Via Natural or Artificial Opening Endoscopic
079100Z	Drainage of Right Neck Lymphatic with Drainage Device, Open Approach
07910ZX	Drainage of Right Neck Lymphatic, Open Approach, Diagnostic
07910ZZ	Drainage of Right Neck Lymphatic, Open Approach
079130Z	Drainage of Right Neck Lymphatic with Drainage Device, Percutaneous Approach
07913ZX	Drainage of Right Neck Lymphatic, Percutaneous Approach, Diagnostic
07913ZZ	Drainage of Right Neck Lymphatic, Percutaneous Approach
079140Z	Drainage of Right Neck Lymphatic with Drainage Device, Percutaneous Endoscopic Approach
07914ZX	Drainage of Right Neck Lymphatic, Percutaneous Endoscopic Approach, Diagnostic
07914ZZ	Drainage of Right Neck Lymphatic, Percutaneous Endoscopic Approach
079180Z	Drainage of Right Neck Lymphatic with Drainage Device, Via Natural or Artificial Opening Endoscopic
07918ZX	Drainage of Right Neck Lymphatic, Via Natural or Artificial Opening Endoscopic Approach, Diagnostic
07918ZZ	Drainage of Right Neck Lymphatic, Via Natural or Artificial Opening Endoscopic
079200Z	Drainage of Left Neck Lymphatic with Drainage Device, Open Approach
07920ZX	Drainage of Left Neck Lymphatic, Open Approach, Diagnostic
07920ZZ	Drainage of Left Neck Lymphatic, Open Approach
079230Z	Drainage of Left Neck Lymphatic with Drainage Device, Percutaneous Approach
07923ZX	Drainage of Left Neck Lymphatic, Percutaneous Approach, Diagnostic
07923ZZ	Drainage of Left Neck Lymphatic, Percutaneous Approach
079240Z	Drainage of Left Neck Lymphatic with Drainage Device, Percutaneous Endoscopic Approach
07924ZX	Drainage of Left Neck Lymphatic, Percutaneous Endoscopic Approach, Diagnostic
07924ZZ	Drainage of Left Neck Lymphatic, Percutaneous Endoscopic Approach
079280Z	Drainage of Left Neck Lymphatic with Drainage Device, Via Natural or Artificial Opening Endoscopic
07928ZX	Drainage of Left Neck Lymphatic, Via Natural or Artificial Opening Endoscopic Approach, Diagnostic
07928ZZ	Drainage of Left Neck Lymphatic, Via Natural or Artificial Opening Endoscopic
079300Z	Drainage of Right Upper Extremity Lymphatic with Drainage Device, Open Approach
07930ZX	Drainage of Right Upper Extremity Lymphatic, Open Approach, Diagnostic
07930ZZ	Drainage of Right Upper Extremity Lymphatic, Open Approach
079330Z	Drainage of Right Upper Extremity Lymphatic with Drainage Device, Percutaneous Approach
07933ZX	Drainage of Right Upper Extremity Lymphatic, Percutaneous Approach, Diagnostic
07933ZZ	Drainage of Right Upper Extremity Lymphatic, Percutaneous Approach
079340Z	Drainage of Right Upper Extremity Lymphatic with Drainage Device, Percutaneous Endoscopic Approach
07934ZX	Drainage of Right Upper Extremity Lymphatic, Percutaneous Endoscopic Approach, Diagnostic
07934ZZ	Drainage of Right Upper Extremity Lymphatic, Percutaneous Endoscopic Approach
079380Z	Drainage of Right Upper Extremity Lymphatic with Drainage Device, Via Natural or Artificial Opening Endoscopic
07938ZX	Drainage of Right Upper Extremity Lymphatic, Via Natural or Artificial Opening Endoscopic Approach, Diagnostic
07938ZZ	Drainage of Right Upper Extremity Lymphatic, Via Natural or Artificial Opening Endoscopic
079400Z	Drainage of Left Upper Extremity Lymphatic with Drainage Device, Open Approach
07940ZX	Drainage of Left Upper Extremity Lymphatic, Open Approach, Diagnostic
07940ZZ	Drainage of Left Upper Extremity Lymphatic, Open Approach
079430Z	Drainage of Left Upper Extremity Lymphatic with Drainage Device, Percutaneous Approach
07943ZX	Drainage of Left Upper Extremity Lymphatic, Percutaneous Approach, Diagnostic
07943ZZ	Drainage of Left Upper Extremity Lymphatic, Percutaneous Approach
079440Z	Drainage of Left Upper Extremity Lymphatic with Drainage Device, Percutaneous Endoscopic Approach
07944ZX	Drainage of Left Upper Extremity Lymphatic, Percutaneous Endoscopic Approach, Diagnostic
07944ZZ	Drainage of Left Upper Extremity Lymphatic, Percutaneous Endoscopic Approach
079480Z	Drainage of Left Upper Extremity Lymphatic with Drainage Device, Via Natural or Artificial Opening Endoscopic
07948ZX	Drainage of Left Upper Extremity Lymphatic, Via Natural or Artificial Opening Endoscopic Approach, Diagnostic
07948ZZ	Drainage of Left Upper Extremity Lymphatic, Via Natural or Artificial Opening Endoscopic
079500Z	Drainage of Right Axillary Lymphatic with Drainage Device, Open Approach
07950ZX	Drainage of Right Axillary Lymphatic, Open Approach, Diagnostic
07950ZZ	Drainage of Right Axillary Lymphatic, Open Approach
079530Z	Drainage of Right Axillary Lymphatic with Drainage Device, Percutaneous Approach
07953ZX	Drainage of Right Axillary Lymphatic, Percutaneous Approach, Diagnostic
07953ZZ	Drainage of Right Axillary Lymphatic, Percutaneous Approach
079540Z	Drainage of Right Axillary Lymphatic with Drainage Device, Percutaneous Endoscopic Approach
07954ZX	Drainage of Right Axillary Lymphatic, Percutaneous Endoscopic Approach, Diagnostic
07954ZZ	Drainage of Right Axillary Lymphatic, Percutaneous Endoscopic Approach
079580Z	Drainage of Right Axillary Lymphatic with Drainage Device, Via Natural or Artificial Opening Endoscopic
07958ZX	Drainage of Right Axillary Lymphatic, Via Natural or Artificial Opening Endoscopic Approach, Diagnostic
07958ZZ	Drainage of Right Axillary Lymphatic, Via Natural or Artificial Opening Endoscopic
079600Z	Drainage of Left Axillary Lymphatic with Drainage Device, Open Approach
07960ZX	Drainage of Left Axillary Lymphatic, Open Approach, Diagnostic
07960ZZ	Drainage of Left Axillary Lymphatic, Open Approach
079630Z	Drainage of Left Axillary Lymphatic with Drainage Device, Percutaneous Approach
07963ZX	Drainage of Left Axillary Lymphatic, Percutaneous Approach, Diagnostic
07963ZZ	Drainage of Left Axillary Lymphatic, Percutaneous Approach
079640Z	Drainage of Left Axillary Lymphatic with Drainage Device, Percutaneous Endoscopic Approach
07964ZX	Drainage of Left Axillary Lymphatic, Percutaneous Endoscopic Approach, Diagnostic
07964ZZ	Drainage of Left Axillary Lymphatic, Percutaneous Endoscopic Approach
079680Z	Drainage of Left Axillary Lymphatic with Drainage Device, Via Natural or Artificial Opening Endoscopic

♀ Female-only   ♂ Male-only   ▲ Limited Coverage   ● Non-OR   ᴴᴬᶜ HAC-associated procedure   ▲ Non-covered procedures   ✚ Cluster

7968ZX	Drainage of Left Axillary Lymphatic, Via Natural or Artificial Opening Endoscopic Approach, Diagnostic
7968ZZ	Drainage of Left Axillary Lymphatic, Via Natural or Artificial Opening Endoscopic
79700Z	Drainage of Thorax Lymphatic with Drainage Device, Open Approach
7970ZX	Drainage of Thorax Lymphatic, Open Approach, Diagnostic
7970ZZ	Drainage of Thorax Lymphatic, Open Approach
79730Z	Drainage of Thorax Lymphatic with Drainage Device, Percutaneous Approach
7973ZX	Drainage of Thorax Lymphatic, Percutaneous Approach, Diagnostic
7973ZZ	Drainage of Thorax Lymphatic, Percutaneous Approach
79740Z	Drainage of Thorax Lymphatic with Drainage Device, Percutaneous Endoscopic Approach
7974ZX	Drainage of Thorax Lymphatic, Percutaneous Endoscopic Approach, Diagnostic
7974ZZ	Drainage of Thorax Lymphatic, Percutaneous Endoscopic Approach
79780Z	Drainage of Thorax Lymphatic with Drainage Device, Via Natural or Artificial Opening Endoscopic
7978ZX	Drainage of Thorax Lymphatic, Via Natural or Artificial Opening Endoscopic Approach, Diagnostic
7978ZZ	Drainage of Thorax Lymphatic, Via Natural or Artificial Opening Endoscopic
079800Z	Drainage of Right Internal Mammary Lymphatic with Drainage Device, Open Approach
07980ZX	Drainage of Right Internal Mammary Lymphatic, Open Approach, Diagnostic
07980ZZ	Drainage of Right Internal Mammary Lymphatic, Open Approach
079830Z	Drainage of Right Internal Mammary Lymphatic with Drainage Device, Percutaneous Approach
07983ZX	Drainage of Right Internal Mammary Lymphatic, Percutaneous Approach, Diagnostic
07983ZZ	Drainage of Right Internal Mammary Lymphatic, Percutaneous Approach
079840Z	Drainage of Right Internal Mammary Lymphatic with Drainage Device, Percutaneous Endoscopic Approach
07984ZX	Drainage of Right Internal Mammary Lymphatic, Percutaneous Endoscopic Approach, Diagnostic
07984ZZ	Drainage of Right Internal Mammary Lymphatic, Percutaneous Endoscopic Approach
079880Z	Drainage of Right Internal Mammary Lymphatic with Drainage Device, Via Natural or Artificial Opening Endoscopic
07988ZX	Drainage of Right Internal Mammary Lymphatic, Via Natural or Artificial Opening Endoscopic Approach, Diagnostic
07988ZZ	Drainage of Right Internal Mammary Lymphatic, Via Natural or Artificial Opening Endoscopic
079900Z	Drainage of Left Internal Mammary Lymphatic with Drainage Device, Open Approach
07990ZX	Drainage of Left Internal Mammary Lymphatic, Open Approach, Diagnostic
07990ZZ	Drainage of Left Internal Mammary Lymphatic, Open Approach
079930Z	Drainage of Left Internal Mammary Lymphatic with Drainage Device, Percutaneous Approach

07993ZX	Drainage of Left Internal Mammary Lymphatic, Percutaneous Approach, Diagnostic
07993ZZ	Drainage of Left Internal Mammary Lymphatic, Percutaneous Approach
079940Z	Drainage of Left Internal Mammary Lymphatic with Drainage Device, Percutaneous Endoscopic Approach
07994ZX	Drainage of Left Internal Mammary Lymphatic, Percutaneous Endoscopic Approach, Diagnostic
07994ZZ	Drainage of Left Internal Mammary Lymphatic, Percutaneous Endoscopic Approach
079980Z	Drainage of Left Internal Mammary Lymphatic with Drainage Device, Via Natural or Artificial Opening Endoscopic
07998ZX	Drainage of Left Internal Mammary Lymphatic, Via Natural or Artificial Opening Endoscopic Approach, Diagnostic
07998ZZ	Drainage of Left Internal Mammary Lymphatic, Via Natural or Artificial Opening Endoscopic
079B00Z	Drainage of Mesenteric Lymphatic with Drainage Device, Open Approach
079B0ZX	Drainage of Mesenteric Lymphatic, Open Approach, Diagnostic
079B0ZZ	Drainage of Mesenteric Lymphatic, Open Approach
079B30Z	Drainage of Mesenteric Lymphatic with Drainage Device, Percutaneous Approach
079B3ZX	Drainage of Mesenteric Lymphatic, Percutaneous Approach, Diagnostic
079B3ZZ	Drainage of Mesenteric Lymphatic, Percutaneous Approach
079B40Z	Drainage of Mesenteric Lymphatic with Drainage Device, Percutaneous Endoscopic Approach
079B4ZX	Drainage of Mesenteric Lymphatic, Percutaneous Endoscopic Approach, Diagnostic
079B4ZZ	Drainage of Mesenteric Lymphatic, Percutaneous Endoscopic Approach
079B80Z	Drainage of Mesenteric Lymphatic with Drainage Device, Via Natural or Artificial Opening Endoscopic
079B8ZX	Drainage of Mesenteric Lymphatic, Via Natural or Artificial Opening Endoscopic Approach, Diagnostic
079B8ZZ	Drainage of Mesenteric Lymphatic, Via Natural or Artificial Opening Endoscopic
079C00Z	Drainage of Pelvis Lymphatic with Drainage Device, Open Approach
079C0ZX	Drainage of Pelvis Lymphatic, Open Approach, Diagnostic
079C0ZZ	Drainage of Pelvis Lymphatic, Open Approach
079C30Z	Drainage of Pelvis Lymphatic with Drainage Device, Percutaneous Approach
079C3ZX	Drainage of Pelvis Lymphatic, Percutaneous Approach, Diagnostic
079C3ZZ	Drainage of Pelvis Lymphatic, Percutaneous Approach
079C40Z	Drainage of Pelvis Lymphatic with Drainage Device, Percutaneous Endoscopic Approach
079C4ZX	Drainage of Pelvis Lymphatic, Percutaneous Endoscopic Approach, Diagnostic
079C4ZZ	Drainage of Pelvis Lymphatic, Percutaneous Endoscopic Approach
079C80Z	Drainage of Pelvis Lymphatic with Drainage Device, Via Natural or Artificial Opening Endoscopic

079C8ZX	Drainage of Pelvis Lymphatic, Via Natural or Artificial Opening Endoscopic Approach, Diagnostic
079C8ZZ	Drainage of Pelvis Lymphatic, Via Natural or Artificial Opening Endoscopic
079D00Z	Drainage of Aortic Lymphatic with Drainage Device, Open Approach
079D0ZX	Drainage of Aortic Lymphatic, Open Approach, Diagnostic
079D0ZZ	Drainage of Aortic Lymphatic, Open Approach
079D30Z	Drainage of Aortic Lymphatic with Drainage Device, Percutaneous Approach
079D3ZX	Drainage of Aortic Lymphatic, Percutaneous Approach, Diagnostic
079D3ZZ	Drainage of Aortic Lymphatic, Percutaneous Approach
079D40Z	Drainage of Aortic Lymphatic with Drainage Device, Percutaneous Endoscopic Approach
079D4ZX	Drainage of Aortic Lymphatic, Percutaneous Endoscopic Approach, Diagnostic
079D4ZZ	Drainage of Aortic Lymphatic, Percutaneous Endoscopic Approach
079D80Z	Drainage of Aortic Lymphatic with Drainage Device, Via Natural or Artificial Opening Endoscopic
079D8ZX	Drainage of Aortic Lymphatic, Via Natural or Artificial Opening Endoscopic Approach, Diagnostic
079D8ZZ	Drainage of Aortic Lymphatic, Via Natural or Artificial Opening Endoscopic
079F00Z	Drainage of Right Lower Extremity Lymphatic with Drainage Device, Open Approach
079F0ZX	Drainage of Right Lower Extremity Lymphatic, Open Approach, Diagnostic
079F0ZZ	Drainage of Right Lower Extremity Lymphatic, Open Approach
079F30Z	Drainage of Right Lower Extremity Lymphatic with Drainage Device, Percutaneous Approach
079F3ZX	Drainage of Right Lower Extremity Lymphatic, Percutaneous Approach, Diagnostic
079F3ZZ	Drainage of Right Lower Extremity Lymphatic, Percutaneous Approach
079F40Z	Drainage of Right Lower Extremity Lymphatic with Drainage Device, Percutaneous Endoscopic Approach
079F4ZX	Drainage of Right Lower Extremity Lymphatic, Percutaneous Endoscopic Approach, Diagnostic
079F4ZZ	Drainage of Right Lower Extremity Lymphatic, Percutaneous Endoscopic Approach
079F80Z	Drainage of Right Lower Extremity Lymphatic with Drainage Device, Via Natural or Artificial Opening Endoscopic
079F8ZX	Drainage of Right Lower Extremity Lymphatic, Via Natural or Artificial Opening Endoscopic Approach, Diagnostic
079F8ZZ	Drainage of Right Lower Extremity Lymphatic, Via Natural or Artificial Opening Endoscopic
079G00Z	Drainage of Left Lower Extremity Lymphatic with Drainage Device, Open Approach
079G0ZX	Drainage of Left Lower Extremity Lymphatic, Open Approach, Diagnostic
079G0ZZ	Drainage of Left Lower Extremity Lymphatic, Open Approach
079G30Z	Drainage of Left Lower Extremity Lymphatic with Drainage Device, Percutaneous Approach

079G3ZX	Drainage of Left Lower Extremity Lymphatic, Percutaneous Approach, Diagnostic
079G3ZZ	Drainage of Left Lower Extremity Lymphatic, Percutaneous Approach
079G40Z	Drainage of Left Lower Extremity Lymphatic with Drainage Device, Percutaneous Endoscopic Approach
079G4ZX	Drainage of Left Lower Extremity Lymphatic, Percutaneous Endoscopic Approach, Diagnostic
079G4ZZ	Drainage of Left Lower Extremity Lymphatic, Percutaneous Endoscopic Approach
079G80Z	Drainage of Left Lower Extremity Lymphatic with Drainage Device, Via Natural or Artificial Opening Endoscopic
079G8ZX	Drainage of Left Lower Extremity Lymphatic, Via Natural or Artificial Opening Endoscopic Approach, Diagnostic
079G8ZZ	Drainage of Left Lower Extremity Lymphatic, Via Natural or Artificial Opening Endoscopic
079H00Z	Drainage of Right Inguinal Lymphatic with Drainage Device, Open Approach
079H0ZX	Drainage of Right Inguinal Lymphatic, Open Approach, Diagnostic
079H0ZZ	Drainage of Right Inguinal Lymphatic, Open Approach
079H30Z	Drainage of Right Inguinal Lymphatic with Drainage Device, Percutaneous Approach
079H3ZX	Drainage of Right Inguinal Lymphatic, Percutaneous Approach, Diagnostic
079H3ZZ	Drainage of Right Inguinal Lymphatic, Percutaneous Approach
079H40Z	Drainage of Right Inguinal Lymphatic with Drainage Device, Percutaneous Endoscopic Approach
079H4ZX	Drainage of Right Inguinal Lymphatic, Percutaneous Endoscopic Approach, Diagnostic
079H4ZZ	Drainage of Right Inguinal Lymphatic, Percutaneous Endoscopic Approach
079H80Z	Drainage of Right Inguinal Lymphatic with Drainage Device, Via Natural or Artificial Opening Endoscopic
079H8ZX	Drainage of Right Inguinal Lymphatic, Via Natural or Artificial Opening Endoscopic Approach, Diagnostic
079H8ZZ	Drainage of Right Inguinal Lymphatic, Via Natural or Artificial Opening Endoscopic
079J00Z	Drainage of Left Inguinal Lymphatic with Drainage Device, Open Approach
079J0ZX	Drainage of Left Inguinal Lymphatic, Open Approach, Diagnostic
079J0ZZ	Drainage of Left Inguinal Lymphatic, Open Approach
079J30Z	Drainage of Left Inguinal Lymphatic with Drainage Device, Percutaneous Approach
079J3ZX	Drainage of Left Inguinal Lymphatic, Percutaneous Approach, Diagnostic
079J3ZZ	Drainage of Left Inguinal Lymphatic, Percutaneous Approach
079J40Z	Drainage of Left Inguinal Lymphatic with Drainage Device, Percutaneous Endoscopic Approach
079J4ZX	Drainage of Left Inguinal Lymphatic, Percutaneous Endoscopic Approach, Diagnostic
079J4ZZ	Drainage of Left Inguinal Lymphatic, Percutaneous Endoscopic Approach
079J80Z	Drainage of Left Inguinal Lymphatic with Drainage Device, Via Natural or Artificial Opening Endoscopic
079J8ZX	Drainage of Left Inguinal Lymphatic, Via Natural or Artificial Opening Endoscopic Approach, Diagnostic
079J8ZZ	Drainage of Left Inguinal Lymphatic, Via Natural or Artificial Opening Endoscopic
079K00Z	Drainage of Thoracic Duct with Drainage Device, Open Approach
079K0ZX	Drainage of Thoracic Duct, Open Approach, Diagnostic
079K0ZZ	Drainage of Thoracic Duct, Open Approach
079K30Z	Drainage of Thoracic Duct with Drainage Device, Percutaneous Approach
079K3ZX	Drainage of Thoracic Duct, Percutaneous Approach, Diagnostic
079K3ZZ	Drainage of Thoracic Duct, Percutaneous Approach
079K40Z	Drainage of Thoracic Duct with Drainage Device, Percutaneous Endoscopic Approach
079K4ZX	Drainage of Thoracic Duct, Percutaneous Endoscopic Approach, Diagnostic
079K4ZZ	Drainage of Thoracic Duct, Percutaneous Endoscopic Approach
079K80Z	Drainage of Thoracic Duct with Drainage Device, Via Natural or Artificial Opening Endoscopic
079K8ZX	Drainage of Thoracic Duct, Via Natural or Artificial Opening Endoscopic Approach, Diagnostic
079K8ZZ	Drainage of Thoracic Duct, Via Natural or Artificial Opening Endoscopic
079L00Z	Drainage of Cisterna Chyli with Drainage Device, Open Approach
079L0ZX	Drainage of Cisterna Chyli, Open Approach, Diagnostic
079L0ZZ	Drainage of Cisterna Chyli, Open Approach
079L30Z	Drainage of Cisterna Chyli with Drainage Device, Percutaneous Approach
079L3ZX	Drainage of Cisterna Chyli, Percutaneous Approach, Diagnostic
079L3ZZ	Drainage of Cisterna Chyli, Percutaneous Approach
079L40Z	Drainage of Cisterna Chyli with Drainage Device, Percutaneous Endoscopic Approach
079L4ZX	Drainage of Cisterna Chyli, Percutaneous Endoscopic Approach, Diagnostic
079L4ZZ	Drainage of Cisterna Chyli, Percutaneous Endoscopic Approach
079L80Z	Drainage of Cisterna Chyli with Drainage Device, Via Natural or Artificial Opening Endoscopic
079L8ZX	Drainage of Cisterna Chyli, Via Natural or Artificial Opening Endoscopic Approach, Diagnostic
079L8ZZ	Drainage of Cisterna Chyli, Via Natural or Artificial Opening Endoscopic
079M00Z	Drainage of Thymus with Drainage Device, Open Approach
079M0ZX	Drainage of Thymus, Open Approach, Diagnostic
079M0ZZ	Drainage of Thymus, Open Approach
079M30Z	Drainage of Thymus with Drainage Device, Percutaneous Approach
079M3ZX	Drainage of Thymus, Percutaneous Approach, Diagnostic
079M3ZZ	Drainage of Thymus, Percutaneous Approach
079M40Z	Drainage of Thymus with Drainage Device, Percutaneous Endoscopic Approach
079M4ZX	Drainage of Thymus, Percutaneous Endoscopic Approach, Diagnostic
079M4ZZ	Drainage of Thymus, Percutaneous Endoscopic Approach
079P00Z	Drainage of Spleen with Drainage Device, Open Approach
079P0ZX	Drainage of Spleen, Open Approach, Diagnostic
079P0ZZ	Drainage of Spleen, Open Approach
079P30Z	Drainage of Spleen with Drainage Device, Percutaneous Approach
079P3ZX	Drainage of Spleen, Percutaneous Approach, Diagnostic
079P3ZZ	Drainage of Spleen, Percutaneous Approach
079P40Z	Drainage of Spleen with Drainage Device, Percutaneous Endoscopic Approach
079P4ZX	Drainage of Spleen, Percutaneous Endoscopic Approach, Diagnostic
079P4ZZ	Drainage of Spleen, Percutaneous Endoscopic Approach
079T00Z	Drainage of Bone Marrow with Drainage Device, Open Approach
079T0ZX	Drainage of Bone Marrow, Open Approach, Diagnostic
079T0ZZ	Drainage of Bone Marrow, Open Approach
079T30Z	Drainage of Bone Marrow with Drainage Device, Percutaneous Approach
079T3ZX	Drainage of Bone Marrow, Percutaneous Approach, Diagnostic
079T3ZZ	Drainage of Bone Marrow, Percutaneous Approach
079T40Z	Drainage of Bone Marrow with Drainage Device, Percutaneous Endoscopic Approach
079T4ZX	Drainage of Bone Marrow, Percutaneous Endoscopic Approach, Diagnostic
079T4ZZ	Drainage of Bone Marrow, Percutaneous Endoscopic Approach

07B – Lymphatic and Hemic Systems, Excision

Review Coding Guidelines B3.4a and B3.4b

Review Coding Guideline B3.8

Review Coding Guideline B3.18

07B00ZX	Excision of Head Lymphatic, Open Approach, Diagnostic
07B00ZZ	Excision of Head Lymphatic, Open Approach
	AHA CC: 1Q, 2019, 6-7
07B03ZX	Excision of Head Lymphatic, Percutaneous Approach, Diagnostic

♀ Female-only   ♂ Male-only   ▲ Limited Coverage   ● Non-OR   HAC HAC-associated procedure   ▲ Non-covered procedures   ✚ Cluster

07B03ZZ	Excision of Head Lymphatic, Percutaneous Approach
07B04ZX	Excision of Head Lymphatic, Percutaneous Endoscopic Approach, Diagnostic
07B04ZZ	Excision of Head Lymphatic, Percutaneous Endoscopic Approach
07B10ZX	Excision of Right Neck Lymphatic, Open Approach, Diagnostic
07B10ZZ	Excision of Right Neck Lymphatic, Open Approach
07B13ZX	Excision of Right Neck Lymphatic, Percutaneous Approach, Diagnostic
07B13ZZ	Excision of Right Neck Lymphatic, Percutaneous Approach
07B14ZX	Excision of Right Neck Lymphatic, Percutaneous Endoscopic Approach, Diagnostic
07B14ZZ	Excision of Right Neck Lymphatic, Percutaneous Endoscopic Approach
07B20ZX	Excision of Left Neck Lymphatic, Open Approach, Diagnostic
07B20ZZ	Excision of Left Neck Lymphatic, Open Approach
07B23ZX	Excision of Left Neck Lymphatic, Percutaneous Approach, Diagnostic
07B23ZZ	Excision of Left Neck Lymphatic, Percutaneous Approach
07B24ZX	Excision of Left Neck Lymphatic, Percutaneous Endoscopic Approach, Diagnostic
07B24ZZ	Excision of Left Neck Lymphatic, Percutaneous Endoscopic Approach
07B30ZX	Excision of Right Upper Extremity Lymphatic, Open Approach, Diagnostic
07B30ZZ	Excision of Right Upper Extremity Lymphatic, Open Approach
07B33ZX	Excision of Right Upper Extremity Lymphatic, Percutaneous Approach, Diagnostic
07B33ZZ	Excision of Right Upper Extremity Lymphatic, Percutaneous Approach
07B34ZX	Excision of Right Upper Extremity Lymphatic, Percutaneous Endoscopic Approach, Diagnostic
07B34ZZ	Excision of Right Upper Extremity Lymphatic, Percutaneous Endoscopic Approach
07B40ZX	Excision of Left Upper Extremity Lymphatic, Open Approach, Diagnostic
07B40ZZ	Excision of Left Upper Extremity Lymphatic, Open Approach
07B43ZX	Excision of Left Upper Extremity Lymphatic, Percutaneous Approach, Diagnostic
07B43ZZ	Excision of Left Upper Extremity Lymphatic, Percutaneous Approach
07B44ZX	Excision of Left Upper Extremity Lymphatic, Percutaneous Endoscopic Approach, Diagnostic
07B44ZZ	Excision of Left Upper Extremity Lymphatic, Percutaneous Endoscopic Approach
07B50ZX	Excision of Right Axillary Lymphatic, Open Approach, Diagnostic
07B50ZZ	Excision of Right Axillary Lymphatic, Open Approach
07B53ZX	Excision of Right Axillary Lymphatic, Percutaneous Approach, Diagnostic
07B53ZZ	Excision of Right Axillary Lymphatic, Percutaneous Approach
07B54ZX	Excision of Right Axillary Lymphatic, Percutaneous Endoscopic Approach, Diagnostic
07B54ZZ	Excision of Right Axillary Lymphatic, Percutaneous Endoscopic Approach

07B60ZX	Excision of Left Axillary Lymphatic, Open Approach, Diagnostic
07B60ZZ	Excision of Left Axillary Lymphatic, Open Approach
07B63ZX	Excision of Left Axillary Lymphatic, Percutaneous Approach, Diagnostic
07B63ZZ	Excision of Left Axillary Lymphatic, Percutaneous Approach
07B64ZX	Excision of Left Axillary Lymphatic, Percutaneous Endoscopic Approach, Diagnostic
07B64ZZ	Excision of Left Axillary Lymphatic, Percutaneous Endoscopic Approach
07B70ZX	Excision of Thorax Lymphatic, Open Approach, Diagnostic
07B70ZZ	Excision of Thorax Lymphatic, Open Approach
07B73ZX	Excision of Thorax Lymphatic, Percutaneous Approach, Diagnostic
07B73ZZ	Excision of Thorax Lymphatic, Percutaneous Approach
07B74ZX	Excision of Thorax Lymphatic, Percutaneous Endoscopic Approach, Diagnostic

AHA CC: 1Q, 2014, 20-21, 26; 3Q, 2014, 10-11

07B74ZZ	Excision of Thorax Lymphatic, Percutaneous Endoscopic Approach
07B80ZX	Excision of Right Internal Mammary Lymphatic, Open Approach, Diagnostic
07B80ZZ	Excision of Right Internal Mammary Lymphatic, Open Approach
07B83ZX	Excision of Right Internal Mammary Lymphatic, Percutaneous Approach, Diagnostic
07B83ZZ	Excision of Right Internal Mammary Lymphatic, Percutaneous Approach
07B84ZX	Excision of Right Internal Mammary Lymphatic, Percutaneous Endoscopic Approach, Diagnostic
07B84ZZ	Excision of Right Internal Mammary Lymphatic, Percutaneous Endoscopic Approach
07B90ZX	Excision of Left Internal Mammary Lymphatic, Open Approach, Diagnostic
07B90ZZ	Excision of Left Internal Mammary Lymphatic, Open Approach
07B93ZX	Excision of Left Internal Mammary Lymphatic, Percutaneous Approach, Diagnostic
07B93ZZ	Excision of Left Internal Mammary Lymphatic, Percutaneous Approach
07B94ZX	Excision of Left Internal Mammary Lymphatic, Percutaneous Endoscopic Approach, Diagnostic
07B94ZZ	Excision of Left Internal Mammary Lymphatic, Percutaneous Endoscopic Approach
07BB0ZX	Excision of Mesenteric Lymphatic, Open Approach, Diagnostic
07BB0ZZ	Excision of Mesenteric Lymphatic, Open Approach
07BB3ZX	Excision of Mesenteric Lymphatic, Percutaneous Approach, Diagnostic
07BB3ZZ	Excision of Mesenteric Lymphatic, Percutaneous Approach
07BB4ZX	Excision of Mesenteric Lymphatic, Percutaneous Endoscopic Approach, Diagnostic
07BB4ZZ	Excision of Mesenteric Lymphatic, Percutaneous Endoscopic Approach
07BC0ZX	Excision of Pelvis Lymphatic, Open Approach, Diagnostic
07BC0ZZ	Excision of Pelvis Lymphatic, Open Approach
07BC3ZX	Excision of Pelvis Lymphatic, Percutaneous Approach, Diagnostic

07BC3ZZ	Excision of Pelvis Lymphatic, Percutaneous Approach
07BC4ZX	Excision of Pelvis Lymphatic, Percutaneous Endoscopic Approach, Diagnostic
07BC4ZZ	Excision of Pelvis Lymphatic, Percutaneous Endoscopic Approach
07BD0ZX	Excision of Aortic Lymphatic, Open Approach, Diagnostic
07BD0ZZ	Excision of Aortic Lymphatic, Open Approach

AHA CC: 1Q, 2019, 6-7

07BD3ZX	Excision of Aortic Lymphatic, Percutaneous Approach, Diagnostic
07BD3ZZ	Excision of Aortic Lymphatic, Percutaneous Approach
07BD4ZX	Excision of Aortic Lymphatic, Percutaneous Endoscopic Approach, Diagnostic
07BD4ZZ	Excision of Aortic Lymphatic, Percutaneous Endoscopic Approach
07BF0ZX	Excision of Right Lower Extremity Lymphatic, Open Approach, Diagnostic
07BF0ZZ	Excision of Right Lower Extremity Lymphatic, Open Approach
07BF3ZX	Excision of Right Lower Extremity Lymphatic, Percutaneous Approach, Diagnostic
07BF3ZZ	Excision of Right Lower Extremity Lymphatic, Percutaneous Approach
07BF4ZX	Excision of Right Lower Extremity Lymphatic, Percutaneous Endoscopic Approach, Diagnostic
07BF4ZZ	Excision of Right Lower Extremity Lymphatic, Percutaneous Endoscopic Approach
07BG0ZX	Excision of Left Lower Extremity Lymphatic, Open Approach, Diagnostic
07BG0ZZ	Excision of Left Lower Extremity Lymphatic, Open Approach
07BG3ZX	Excision of Left Lower Extremity Lymphatic, Percutaneous Approach, Diagnostic
07BG3ZZ	Excision of Left Lower Extremity Lymphatic, Percutaneous Approach
07BG4ZX	Excision of Left Lower Extremity Lymphatic, Percutaneous Endoscopic Approach, Diagnostic
07BG4ZZ	Excision of Left Lower Extremity Lymphatic, Percutaneous Endoscopic Approach
07BH0ZX	Excision of Right Inguinal Lymphatic, Open Approach, Diagnostic
07BH0ZZ	Excision of Right Inguinal Lymphatic, Open Approach
➕	Radical vulvectomy when reported with resection of vulva. *See table 0UT to construct the Resection code.*
07BH3ZX	Excision of Right Inguinal Lymphatic, Percutaneous Approach, Diagnostic
07BH3ZZ	Excision of Right Inguinal Lymphatic, Percutaneous Approach
07BH4ZX	Excision of Right Inguinal Lymphatic, Percutaneous Endoscopic Approach, Diagnostic
07BH4ZZ	Excision of Right Inguinal Lymphatic, Percutaneous Endoscopic Approach
➕	Radical vulvectomy when reported with resection of vulva. *See table 0UT to construct the Resection code.*
07BJ0ZX	Excision of Left Inguinal Lymphatic, Open Approach, Diagnostic
07BJ0ZZ	Excision of Left Inguinal Lymphatic, Open Approach

  ➕ Radical vulvectomy when reported with resection of vulva. *See table 0UT to construct the Resection code.*

07BJ3ZX Excision of Left Inguinal Lymphatic, Percutaneous Approach, Diagnostic

07BJ3ZZ Excision of Left Inguinal Lymphatic, Percutaneous Approach

07BJ4ZX Excision of Left Inguinal Lymphatic, Percutaneous Endoscopic Approach, Diagnostic

07BJ4ZZ Excision of Left Inguinal Lymphatic, Percutaneous Endoscopic Approach

  ➕ Radical vulvectomy when reported with resection of vulva. *See table 0UT to construct the Resection code.*

07BK0ZX Excision of Thoracic Duct, Open Approach, Diagnostic

07BK0ZZ Excision of Thoracic Duct, Open Approach

07BK3ZX Excision of Thoracic Duct, Percutaneous Approach, Diagnostic

07BK3ZZ Excision of Thoracic Duct, Percutaneous Approach

07BK4ZX Excision of Thoracic Duct, Percutaneous Endoscopic Approach, Diagnostic

07BK4ZZ Excision of Thoracic Duct, Percutaneous Endoscopic Approach

07BL0ZX Excision of Cisterna Chyli, Open Approach, Diagnostic

07BL0ZZ Excision of Cisterna Chyli, Open Approach

07BL3ZX Excision of Cisterna Chyli, Percutaneous Approach, Diagnostic

07BL3ZZ Excision of Cisterna Chyli, Percutaneous Approach

07BL4ZX Excision of Cisterna Chyli, Percutaneous Endoscopic Approach, Diagnostic

07BL4ZZ Excision of Cisterna Chyli, Percutaneous Endoscopic Approach

07BM0ZX Excision of Thymus, Open Approach, Diagnostic

07BM0ZZ Excision of Thymus, Open Approach

07BM3ZX Excision of Thymus, Percutaneous Approach, Diagnostic

07BM3ZZ Excision of Thymus, Percutaneous Approach

07BM4ZX Excision of Thymus, Percutaneous Endoscopic Approach, Diagnostic

07BM4ZZ Excision of Thymus, Percutaneous Endoscopic Approach

07BP0ZX Excision of Spleen, Open Approach, Diagnostic

07BP0ZZ Excision of Spleen, Open Approach

07BP3ZX Excision of Spleen, Percutaneous Approach, Diagnostic

07BP3ZZ Excision of Spleen, Percutaneous Approach

07BP4ZX Excision of Spleen, Percutaneous Endoscopic Approach, Diagnostic

07BP4ZZ Excision of Spleen, Percutaneous Endoscopic Approach

07C – Lymphatic and Hemic Systems, Extirpation

07C00ZZ Extirpation of Matter from Head Lymphatic, Open Approach

07C03ZZ Extirpation of Matter from Head Lymphatic, Percutaneous Approach

07C04ZZ Extirpation of Matter from Head Lymphatic, Percutaneous Endoscopic Approach

07C10ZZ Extirpation of Matter from Right Neck Lymphatic, Open Approach

07C13ZZ Extirpation of Matter from Right Neck Lymphatic, Percutaneous Approach

07C14ZZ Extirpation of Matter from Right Neck Lymphatic, Percutaneous Endoscopic Approach

07C20ZZ Extirpation of Matter from Left Neck Lymphatic, Open Approach

07C23ZZ Extirpation of Matter from Left Neck Lymphatic, Percutaneous Approach

07C24ZZ Extirpation of Matter from Left Neck Lymphatic, Percutaneous Endoscopic Approach

07C30ZZ Extirpation of Matter from Right Upper Extremity Lymphatic, Open Approach

07C33ZZ Extirpation of Matter from Right Upper Extremity Lymphatic, Percutaneous Approach

07C34ZZ Extirpation of Matter from Right Upper Extremity Lymphatic, Percutaneous Endoscopic Approach

07C40ZZ Extirpation of Matter from Left Upper Extremity Lymphatic, Open Approach

07C43ZZ Extirpation of Matter from Left Upper Extremity Lymphatic, Percutaneous Approach

07C44ZZ Extirpation of Matter from Left Upper Extremity Lymphatic, Percutaneous Endoscopic Approach

07C50ZZ Extirpation of Matter from Right Axillary Lymphatic, Open Approach

07C53ZZ Extirpation of Matter from Right Axillary Lymphatic, Percutaneous Approach

07C54ZZ Extirpation of Matter from Right Axillary Lymphatic, Percutaneous Endoscopic Approach

07C60ZZ Extirpation of Matter from Left Axillary Lymphatic, Open Approach

07C63ZZ Extirpation of Matter from Left Axillary Lymphatic, Percutaneous Approach

07C64ZZ Extirpation of Matter from Left Axillary Lymphatic, Percutaneous Endoscopic Approach

07C70ZZ Extirpation of Matter from Thorax Lymphatic, Open Approach

07C73ZZ Extirpation of Matter from Thorax Lymphatic, Percutaneous Approach

07C74ZZ Extirpation of Matter from Thorax Lymphatic, Percutaneous Endoscopic Approach

07C80ZZ Extirpation of Matter from Right Internal Mammary Lymphatic, Open Approach

07C83ZZ Extirpation of Matter from Right Internal Mammary Lymphatic, Percutaneous Approach

07C84ZZ Extirpation of Matter from Right Internal Mammary Lymphatic, Percutaneous Endoscopic Approach

07C90ZZ Extirpation of Matter from Left Internal Mammary Lymphatic, Open Approach

07C93ZZ Extirpation of Matter from Left Internal Mammary Lymphatic, Percutaneous Approach

07C94ZZ Extirpation of Matter from Left Internal Mammary Lymphatic, Percutaneous Endoscopic Approach

07CB0ZZ Extirpation of Matter from Mesenteric Lymphatic, Open Approach

07CB3ZZ Extirpation of Matter from Mesenteric Lymphatic, Percutaneous Approach

07CB4ZZ Extirpation of Matter from Mesenteric Lymphatic, Percutaneous Endoscopic Approach

07CC0ZZ Extirpation of Matter from Pelvis Lymphatic, Open Approach

07CC3ZZ Extirpation of Matter from Pelvis Lymphatic, Percutaneous Approach

07CC4ZZ Extirpation of Matter from Pelvis Lymphatic, Percutaneous Endoscopic Approach

07CD0ZZ Extirpation of Matter from Aortic Lymphatic, Open Approach

07CD3ZZ Extirpation of Matter from Aortic Lymphatic, Percutaneous Approach

07CD4ZZ Extirpation of Matter from Aortic Lymphatic, Percutaneous Endoscopic Approach

07CF0ZZ Extirpation of Matter from Right Lower Extremity Lymphatic, Open Approach

07CF3ZZ Extirpation of Matter from Right Lower Extremity Lymphatic, Percutaneous Approach

07CF4ZZ Extirpation of Matter from Right Lower Extremity Lymphatic, Percutaneous Endoscopic Approach

07CG0ZZ Extirpation of Matter from Left Lower Extremity Lymphatic, Open Approach

07CG3ZZ Extirpation of Matter from Left Lower Extremity Lymphatic, Percutaneous Approach

07CG4ZZ Extirpation of Matter from Left Lower Extremity Lymphatic, Percutaneous Endoscopic Approach

07CH0ZZ Extirpation of Matter from Right Inguinal Lymphatic, Open Approach

07CH3ZZ Extirpation of Matter from Right Inguinal Lymphatic, Percutaneous Approach

07CH4ZZ Extirpation of Matter from Right Inguinal Lymphatic, Percutaneous Endoscopic Approach

07CJ0ZZ Extirpation of Matter from Left Inguinal Lymphatic, Open Approach

07CJ3ZZ Extirpation of Matter from Left Inguinal Lymphatic, Percutaneous Approach

07CJ4ZZ Extirpation of Matter from Left Inguinal Lymphatic, Percutaneous Endoscopic Approach

07CK0ZZ Extirpation of Matter from Thoracic Duct, Open Approach

07CK3ZZ Extirpation of Matter from Thoracic Duct, Percutaneous Approach

07CK4ZZ Extirpation of Matter from Thoracic Duct, Percutaneous Endoscopic Approach

07CL0ZZ Extirpation of Matter from Cisterna Chyli, Open Approach

07CL3ZZ Extirpation of Matter from Cisterna Chyli, Percutaneous Approach

07CL4ZZ Extirpation of Matter from Cisterna Chyli, Percutaneous Endoscopic Approach

07CM0ZZ Extirpation of Matter from Thymus, Open Approach

07CM3ZZ Extirpation of Matter from Thymus, Percutaneous Approach

07CM4ZZ Extirpation of Matter from Thymus, Percutaneous Endoscopic Approach

07CP0ZZ Extirpation of Matter from Spleen, Open Approach

07CP3ZZ Extirpation of Matter from Spleen, Percutaneous Approach

07CP4ZZ Extirpation of Matter from Spleen, Percutaneous Endoscopic Approach

♀ Female-only   ♂ Male-only   ▲ Limited Coverage   ● Non-OR   HAC HAC-associated procedure   ▲ Non-covered procedures   ➕ Cluster

Review Coding Guidelines B3.4a and B3.4b

07D03ZX   Extraction of Head Lymphatic, Percutaneous Approach, Diagnostic

07D04ZX   Extraction of Head Lymphatic, Percutaneous Endoscopic Approach, Diagnostic

07D08ZX   Extraction of Head Lymphatic, Via Natural or Artificial Opening Endoscopic, Diagnostic

07D13ZX   Extraction of Right Neck Lymphatic, Percutaneous Approach, Diagnostic

07D14ZX   Extraction of Right Neck Lymphatic, Percutaneous Endoscopic Approach, Diagnostic

07D18ZX   Extraction of Right Neck Lymphatic, Via Natural or Artificial Opening Endoscopic, Diagnostic

07D23ZX   Extraction of Left Neck Lymphatic, Percutaneous Approach, Diagnostic

07D24ZX   Extraction of Left Neck Lymphatic, Percutaneous Endoscopic Approach, Diagnostic

07D28ZX   Extraction of Left Neck Lymphatic, Via Natural or Artificial Opening Endoscopic, Diagnostic

07D33ZX   Extraction of Right Upper Extremity Lymphatic, Percutaneous Approach, Diagnostic

07D34ZX   Extraction of Right Upper Extremity Lymphatic, Percutaneous Endoscopic Approach, Diagnostic

07D38ZX   Extraction of Right Upper Extremity Lymphatic, Via Natural or Artificial Opening Endoscopic, Diagnostic

07D43ZX   Extraction of Left Upper Extremity Lymphatic, Percutaneous Approach, Diagnostic

07D44ZX   Extraction of Left Upper Extremity Lymphatic, Percutaneous Endoscopic Approach, Diagnostic

07D48ZX   Extraction of Left Upper Extremity Lymphatic, Via Natural or Artificial Opening Endoscopic, Diagnostic

07D53ZX   Extraction of Right Axillary Lymphatic, Percutaneous Approach, Diagnostic

07D54ZX   Extraction of Right Axillary Lymphatic, Percutaneous Endoscopic Approach, Diagnostic

07D58ZX   Extraction of Right Axillary Lymphatic, Via Natural or Artificial Opening Endoscopic, Diagnostic

07D63ZX   Extraction of Left Axillary Lymphatic, Percutaneous Approach, Diagnostic

07D64ZX   Extraction of Left Axillary Lymphatic, Percutaneous Endoscopic Approach, Diagnostic

07D68ZX   Extraction of Left Axillary Lymphatic, Via Natural or Artificial Opening Endoscopic, Diagnostic

07D73ZX   Extraction of Thorax Lymphatic, Percutaneous Approach, Diagnostic

07D74ZX   Extraction of Thorax Lymphatic, Percutaneous Endoscopic Approach, Diagnostic

07D78ZX   Extraction of Thorax Lymphatic, Via Natural or Artificial Opening Endoscopic, Diagnostic

07D83ZX   Extraction of Right Internal Mammary Lymphatic, Percutaneous Approach, Diagnostic

07D84ZX   Extraction of Right Internal Mammary Lymphatic, Percutaneous Endoscopic Approach, Diagnostic

07D88ZX   Extraction of Right Internal Mammary Lymphatic, Via Natural or Artificial Opening Endoscopic, Diagnostic

07D93ZX   Extraction of Left Internal Mammary Lymphatic, Percutaneous Approach, Diagnostic

07D94ZX   Extraction of Left Internal Mammary Lymphatic, Percutaneous Endoscopic Approach, Diagnostic

07D98ZX   Extraction of Left Internal Mammary Lymphatic, Via Natural or Artificial Opening Endoscopic, Diagnostic

07DB3ZX   Extraction of Mesenteric Lymphatic, Percutaneous Approach, Diagnostic

07DB4ZX   Extraction of Mesenteric Lymphatic, Percutaneous Endoscopic Approach, Diagnostic

07DB8ZX   Extraction of Mesenteric Lymphatic, Via Natural or Artificial Opening Endoscopic, Diagnostic

07DC3ZX   Extraction of Pelvis Lymphatic, Percutaneous Approach, Diagnostic

07DC4ZX   Extraction of Pelvis Lymphatic, Percutaneous Endoscopic Approach, Diagnostic

07DC8ZX   Extraction of Pelvis Lymphatic, Via Natural or Artificial Opening Endoscopic, Diagnostic

07DD3ZX   Extraction of Aortic Lymphatic, Percutaneous Approach, Diagnostic

07DD4ZX   Extraction of Aortic Lymphatic, Percutaneous Endoscopic Approach, Diagnostic

07DD8ZX   Extraction of Aortic Lymphatic, Via Natural or Artificial Opening Endoscopic, Diagnostic

07DF3ZX   Extraction of Right Lower Extremity Lymphatic, Percutaneous Approach, Diagnostic

07DF4ZX   Extraction of Right Lower Extremity Lymphatic, Percutaneous Endoscopic Approach, Diagnostic

07DF8ZX   Extraction of Right Lower Extremity Lymphatic, Via Natural or Artificial Opening Endoscopic, Diagnostic

07DG3ZX   Extraction of Left Lower Extremity Lymphatic, Percutaneous Approach, Diagnostic

07DG4ZX   Extraction of Left Lower Extremity Lymphatic, Percutaneous Endoscopic Approach, Diagnostic

07DG8ZX   Extraction of Left Lower Extremity Lymphatic, Via Natural or Artificial Opening Endoscopic, Diagnostic

07DH3ZX   Extraction of Right Inguinal Lymphatic, Percutaneous Approach, Diagnostic

07DH4ZX   Extraction of Right Inguinal Lymphatic, Percutaneous Endoscopic Approach, Diagnostic

07DH8ZX   Extraction of Right Inguinal Lymphatic, Via Natural or Artificial Opening Endoscopic, Diagnostic

07DJ3ZX   Extraction of Left Inguinal Lymphatic, Percutaneous Approach, Diagnostic

07DJ4ZX   Extraction of Left Inguinal Lymphatic, Percutaneous Endoscopic Approach, Diagnostic

07DJ8ZX   Extraction of Left Inguinal Lymphatic, Via Natural or Artificial Opening Endoscopic, Diagnostic

07DK3ZX   Extraction of Thoracic Duct, Percutaneous Approach, Diagnostic

07DK4ZX   Extraction of Thoracic Duct, Percutaneous Endoscopic Approach, Diagnostic

07DK8ZX   Extraction of Thoracic Duct, Via Natural or Artificial Opening Endoscopic, Diagnostic

07DL3ZX   Extraction of Cisterna Chyli, Percutaneous Approach, Diagnostic

07DL4ZX   Extraction of Cisterna Chyli, Percutaneous Endoscopic Approach, Diagnostic

07DL8ZX   Extraction of Cisterna Chyli, Via Natural or Artificial Opening Endoscopic, Diagnostic

07DM3ZX   Extraction of Thymus, Percutaneous Approach, Diagnostic

07DM4ZX   Extraction of Thymus, Percutaneous Endoscopic Approach, Diagnostic

07DP3ZX   Extraction of Spleen, Percutaneous Approach, Diagnostic

07DP4ZX   Extraction of Spleen, Percutaneous Endoscopic Approach, Diagnostic

07DQ0ZX   Extraction of Sternum Bone Marrow, Open Approach, Diagnostic

07DQ0ZZ   Extraction of Sternum Bone Marrow, Open Approach

07DQ3ZX   Extraction of Sternum Bone Marrow, Percutaneous Approach, Diagnostic

07DQ3ZZ   Extraction of Sternum Bone Marrow, Percutaneous Approach

07DR0ZX   Extraction of Iliac Bone Marrow, Open Approach, Diagnostic

07DR0ZZ   Extraction of Iliac Bone Marrow, Open Approach

07DR3ZX   Extraction of Iliac Bone Marrow, Percutaneous Approach, Diagnostic

07DR3ZZ   Extraction of Iliac Bone Marrow, Percutaneous Approach

07DS0ZX   Extraction of Vertebral Bone Marrow, Open Approach, Diagnostic

07DS0ZZ   Extraction of Vertebral Bone Marrow, Open Approach

07DS3ZX   Extraction of Vertebral Bone Marrow, Percutaneous Approach, Diagnostic

07DS3ZZ   Extraction of Vertebral Bone Marrow, Percutaneous Approach

07DT0ZX   Extraction of Bone Marrow, Open Approach, Diagnostic

07DT0ZZ   Extraction of Bone Marrow, Open Approach

07DT3ZX   Extraction of Bone Marrow, Percutaneous Approach, Diagnostic

07DT3ZZ   Extraction of Bone Marrow, Percutaneous Approach

07H – Lymphatic and Hemic Systems, Insertion

07HK01Z   Insertion of Radioactive Element into Thoracic Duct, Open Approach

07HK03Z   Insertion of Infusion Device into Thoracic Duct, Open Approach

07HK0YZ   Insertion of Other Device into Thoracic Duct, Open Approach

♀ Female-only   ♂ Male-only   ▲ Limited Coverage   ● Non-OR   ▦ HAC-associated procedure   ▲ Non-covered procedures   ✚ Cluster

07HK31Z Insertion of Radioactive Element into Thoracic Duct, Percutaneous Approach

07HK33Z Insertion of Infusion Device into Thoracic Duct, Percutaneous Approach

07HK3YZ Insertion of Other Device into Thoracic Duct, Percutaneous Approach

07HK41Z Insertion of Radioactive Element into Thoracic Duct, Percutaneous Endoscopic Approach

07HK43Z Insertion of Infusion Device into Thoracic Duct, Percutaneous Endoscopic Approach

07HK4YZ Insertion of Other Device into Thoracic Duct, Percutaneous Endoscopic Approach

07HL01Z Insertion of Radioactive Element into Cisterna Chyli, Open Approach

07HL03Z Insertion of Infusion Device into Cisterna Chyli, Open Approach

07HL0YZ Insertion of Other Device into Cisterna Chyli, Open Approach

07HL31Z Insertion of Radioactive Element into Cisterna Chyli, Percutaneous Approach

07HL33Z Insertion of Infusion Device into Cisterna Chyli, Percutaneous Approach

07HL3YZ Insertion of Other Device into Cisterna Chyli, Percutaneous Approach

07HL41Z Insertion of Radioactive Element into Cisterna Chyli, Percutaneous Endoscopic Approach

07HL43Z Insertion of Infusion Device into Cisterna Chyli, Percutaneous Endoscopic Approach

07HL4YZ Insertion of Other Device into Cisterna Chyli, Percutaneous Endoscopic Approach

07HM01Z Insertion of Radioactive Element into Thymus, Open Approach

07HM03Z Insertion of Infusion Device into Thymus, Open Approach

07HM0YZ Insertion of Other Device into Thymus, Open Approach

07HM31Z Insertion of Radioactive Element into Thymus, Percutaneous Approach

07HM33Z Insertion of Infusion Device into Thymus, Percutaneous Approach

07HM3YZ Insertion of Other Device into Thymus, Percutaneous Approach

07HM41Z Insertion of Radioactive Element into Thymus, Percutaneous Endoscopic Approach

07HM43Z Insertion of Infusion Device into Thymus, Percutaneous Endoscopic Approach

07HM4YZ Insertion of Other Device into Thymus, Percutaneous Endoscopic Approach

07HN01Z Insertion of Radioactive Element into Lymphatic, Open Approach

07HN03Z Insertion of Infusion Device into Lymphatic, Open Approach

07HN0YZ Insertion of Other Device into Lymphatic, Open Approach

07HN31Z Insertion of Radioactive Element into Lymphatic, Percutaneous Approach

07HN33Z Insertion of Infusion Device into Lymphatic, Percutaneous Approach

07HN3YZ Insertion of Other Device into Lymphatic, Percutaneous Approach

07HN41Z Insertion of Radioactive Element into Lymphatic, Percutaneous Endoscopic Approach

07HN43Z Insertion of Infusion Device into Lymphatic, Percutaneous Endoscopic Approach

07HN4YZ Insertion of Other Device into Lymphatic, Percutaneous Endoscopic Approach

07HP01Z Insertion of Radioactive Element into Spleen, Open Approach

07HP03Z Insertion of Infusion Device into Spleen, Open Approach

07HP0YZ Insertion of Other Device into Spleen, Open Approach

07HP31Z Insertion of Radioactive Element into Spleen, Percutaneous Approach

07HP33Z Insertion of Infusion Device into Spleen, Percutaneous Approach

07HP3YZ Insertion of Other Device into Spleen, Percutaneous Approach

07HP41Z Insertion of Radioactive Element into Spleen, Percutaneous Endoscopic Approach

07HP43Z Insertion of Infusion Device into Spleen, Percutaneous Endoscopic Approach

07HP4YZ Insertion of Other Device into Spleen, Percutaneous Endoscopic Approach

07HT01Z Insertion of Radioactive Element into Bone Marrow, Open Approach

07HT03Z Insertion of Infusion Device into Bone Marrow, Open Approach

07HT0YZ Insertion of Other Device into Bone Marrow, Open Approach

07HT31Z Insertion of Radioactive Element into Bone Marrow, Percutaneous Approach

07HT33Z Insertion of Infusion Device into Bone Marrow, Percutaneous Approach

07HT3YZ Insertion of Other Device into Bone Marrow, Percutaneous Approach

07HT41Z Insertion of Radioactive Element into Bone Marrow, Percutaneous Endoscopic Approach

07HT43Z Insertion of Infusion Device into Bone Marrow, Percutaneous Endoscopic Approach

07HT4YZ Insertion of Other Device into Bone Marrow, Percutaneous Endoscopic Approach

07J – Lymphatic and Hemic Systems, Inspection

Review Coding Guidelines B3.11a, B3.11b and B3.11c

07JK0ZZ Inspection of Thoracic Duct, Open Approach

07JK3ZZ Inspection of Thoracic Duct, Percutaneous Approach

07JK4ZZ Inspection of Thoracic Duct, Percutaneous Endoscopic Approach

07JL0ZZ Inspection of Cisterna Chyli, Open Approach

07JL3ZZ Inspection of Cisterna Chyli, Percutaneous Approach

07JL4ZZ Inspection of Cisterna Chyli, Percutaneous Endoscopic Approach

07JM0ZZ Inspection of Thymus, Open Approach

07JM3ZZ Inspection of Thymus, Percutaneous Approach

07JM4ZZ Inspection of Thymus, Percutaneous Endoscopic Approach

07JN0ZZ Inspection of Lymphatic, Open Approach

07JN3ZZ Inspection of Lymphatic, Percutaneous Approach

07JN4ZZ Inspection of Lymphatic, Percutaneous Endoscopic Approach

07JN8ZZ Inspection of Lymphatic, Via Natural or Artificial Opening Endoscopic

07JNXZZ Inspection of Lymphatic, External Approach

07JP0ZZ Inspection of Spleen, Open Approach

07JP3ZZ Inspection of Spleen, Percutaneous Approach

07JP4ZZ Inspection of Spleen, Percutaneous Endoscopic Approach

07JPXZZ Inspection of Spleen, External Approach

07JT0ZZ Inspection of Bone Marrow, Open Approach

07JT3ZZ Inspection of Bone Marrow, Percutaneous Approach

07JT4ZZ Inspection of Bone Marrow, Percutaneous Endoscopic Approach

07L – Lymphatic and Hemic Systems, Occlusion

07L00CZ Occlusion of Head Lymphatic with Extraluminal Device, Open Approach

07L00DZ Occlusion of Head Lymphatic with Intraluminal Device, Open Approach

07L00ZZ Occlusion of Head Lymphatic, Open Approach

07L03CZ Occlusion of Head Lymphatic with Extraluminal Device, Percutaneous Approach

07L03DZ Occlusion of Head Lymphatic with Intraluminal Device, Percutaneous Approach

07L03ZZ Occlusion of Head Lymphatic, Percutaneous Approach

07L04CZ Occlusion of Head Lymphatic with Extraluminal Device, Percutaneous Endoscopic Approach

07L04DZ Occlusion of Head Lymphatic with Intraluminal Device, Percutaneous Endoscopic Approach

07L04ZZ Occlusion of Head Lymphatic, Percutaneous Endoscopic Approach

07L10CZ Occlusion of Right Neck Lymphatic with Extraluminal Device, Open Approach

07L10DZ Occlusion of Right Neck Lymphatic with Intraluminal Device, Open Approach

07L10ZZ Occlusion of Right Neck Lymphatic, Open Approach

07L13CZ Occlusion of Right Neck Lymphatic with Extraluminal Device, Percutaneous Approach

07L13DZ Occlusion of Right Neck Lymphatic with Intraluminal Device, Percutaneous Approach

07L13ZZ Occlusion of Right Neck Lymphatic, Percutaneous Approach

07L14CZ Occlusion of Right Neck Lymphatic with Extraluminal Device, Percutaneous Endoscopic Approach

♀ Female-only   ♂ Male-only   ▲ Limited Coverage   ● Non-OR   ▨ HAC-associated procedure   ▲ Non-covered procedures   ✚ Cluster

07L14DZ Occlusion of Right Neck Lymphatic with Intraluminal Device, Percutaneous Endoscopic Approach

07L14ZZ Occlusion of Right Neck Lymphatic, Percutaneous Endoscopic Approach

07L20CZ Occlusion of Left Neck Lymphatic with Extraluminal Device, Open Approach

07L20DZ Occlusion of Left Neck Lymphatic with Intraluminal Device, Open Approach

07L20ZZ Occlusion of Left Neck Lymphatic, Open Approach

07L23CZ Occlusion of Left Neck Lymphatic with Extraluminal Device, Percutaneous Approach

07L23DZ Occlusion of Left Neck Lymphatic with Intraluminal Device, Percutaneous Approach

07L23ZZ Occlusion of Left Neck Lymphatic, Percutaneous Approach

07L24CZ Occlusion of Left Neck Lymphatic with Extraluminal Device, Percutaneous Endoscopic Approach

07L24DZ Occlusion of Left Neck Lymphatic with Intraluminal Device, Percutaneous Endoscopic Approach

07L24ZZ Occlusion of Left Neck Lymphatic, Percutaneous Endoscopic Approach

07L30CZ Occlusion of Right Upper Extremity Lymphatic with Extraluminal Device, Open Approach

07L30DZ Occlusion of Right Upper Extremity Lymphatic with Intraluminal Device, Open Approach

07L30ZZ Occlusion of Right Upper Extremity Lymphatic, Open Approach

07L33CZ Occlusion of Right Upper Extremity Lymphatic with Extraluminal Device, Percutaneous Approach

07L33DZ Occlusion of Right Upper Extremity Lymphatic with Intraluminal Device, Percutaneous Approach

07L33ZZ Occlusion of Right Upper Extremity Lymphatic, Percutaneous Approach

07L34CZ Occlusion of Right Upper Extremity Lymphatic with Extraluminal Device, Percutaneous Endoscopic Approach

07L34DZ Occlusion of Right Upper Extremity Lymphatic with Intraluminal Device, Percutaneous Endoscopic Approach

07L34ZZ Occlusion of Right Upper Extremity Lymphatic, Percutaneous Endoscopic Approach

07L40CZ Occlusion of Left Upper Extremity Lymphatic with Extraluminal Device, Open Approach

07L40DZ Occlusion of Left Upper Extremity Lymphatic with Intraluminal Device, Open Approach

07L40ZZ Occlusion of Left Upper Extremity Lymphatic, Open Approach

07L43CZ Occlusion of Left Upper Extremity Lymphatic with Extraluminal Device, Percutaneous Approach

07L43DZ Occlusion of Left Upper Extremity Lymphatic with Intraluminal Device, Percutaneous Approach

07L43ZZ Occlusion of Left Upper Extremity Lymphatic, Percutaneous Approach

07L44CZ Occlusion of Left Upper Extremity Lymphatic with Extraluminal Device, Percutaneous Endoscopic Approach

07L44DZ Occlusion of Left Upper Extremity Lymphatic with Intraluminal Device, Percutaneous Endoscopic Approach

07L44ZZ Occlusion of Left Upper Extremity Lymphatic, Percutaneous Endoscopic Approach

07L50CZ Occlusion of Right Axillary Lymphatic with Extraluminal Device, Open Approach

07L50DZ Occlusion of Right Axillary Lymphatic with Intraluminal Device, Open Approach

07L50ZZ Occlusion of Right Axillary Lymphatic, Open Approach

07L53CZ Occlusion of Right Axillary Lymphatic with Extraluminal Device, Percutaneous Approach

07L53DZ Occlusion of Right Axillary Lymphatic with Intraluminal Device, Percutaneous Approach

07L53ZZ Occlusion of Right Axillary Lymphatic, Percutaneous Approach

07L54CZ Occlusion of Right Axillary Lymphatic with Extraluminal Device, Percutaneous Endoscopic Approach

07L54DZ Occlusion of Right Axillary Lymphatic with Intraluminal Device, Percutaneous Endoscopic Approach

07L54ZZ Occlusion of Right Axillary Lymphatic, Percutaneous Endoscopic Approach

07L60CZ Occlusion of Left Axillary Lymphatic with Extraluminal Device, Open Approach

07L60DZ Occlusion of Left Axillary Lymphatic with Intraluminal Device, Open Approach

07L60ZZ Occlusion of Left Axillary Lymphatic, Open Approach

07L63CZ Occlusion of Left Axillary Lymphatic with Extraluminal Device, Percutaneous Approach

07L63DZ Occlusion of Left Axillary Lymphatic with Intraluminal Device, Percutaneous Approach

07L63ZZ Occlusion of Left Axillary Lymphatic, Percutaneous Approach

07L64CZ Occlusion of Left Axillary Lymphatic with Extraluminal Device, Percutaneous Endoscopic Approach

07L64DZ Occlusion of Left Axillary Lymphatic with Intraluminal Device, Percutaneous Endoscopic Approach

07L64ZZ Occlusion of Left Axillary Lymphatic, Percutaneous Endoscopic Approach

07L70CZ Occlusion of Thorax Lymphatic with Extraluminal Device, Open Approach

07L70DZ Occlusion of Thorax Lymphatic with Intraluminal Device, Open Approach

07L70ZZ Occlusion of Thorax Lymphatic, Open Approach

07L73CZ Occlusion of Thorax Lymphatic with Extraluminal Device, Percutaneous Approach

07L73DZ Occlusion of Thorax Lymphatic with Intraluminal Device, Percutaneous Approach

07L73ZZ Occlusion of Thorax Lymphatic, Percutaneous Approach

07L74CZ Occlusion of Thorax Lymphatic with Extraluminal Device, Percutaneous Endoscopic Approach

07L74DZ Occlusion of Thorax Lymphatic with Intraluminal Device, Percutaneous Endoscopic Approach

07L74ZZ Occlusion of Thorax Lymphatic, Percutaneous Endoscopic Approach

07L80CZ Occlusion of Right Internal Mammary Lymphatic with Extraluminal Device, Open Approach

07L80DZ Occlusion of Right Internal Mammary Lymphatic with Intraluminal Device, Open Approach

07L80ZZ Occlusion of Right Internal Mammary Lymphatic, Open Approach

07L83CZ Occlusion of Right Internal Mammary Lymphatic with Extraluminal Device, Percutaneous Approach

07L83DZ Occlusion of Right Internal Mammary Lymphatic with Intraluminal Device, Percutaneous Approach

07L83ZZ Occlusion of Right Internal Mammary Lymphatic, Percutaneous Approach

07L84CZ Occlusion of Right Internal Mammary Lymphatic with Extraluminal Device, Percutaneous Endoscopic Approach

07L84DZ Occlusion of Right Internal Mammary Lymphatic with Intraluminal Device, Percutaneous Endoscopic Approach

07L84ZZ Occlusion of Right Internal Mammary Lymphatic, Percutaneous Endoscopic Approach

07L90CZ Occlusion of Left Internal Mammary Lymphatic with Extraluminal Device, Open Approach

07L90DZ Occlusion of Left Internal Mammary Lymphatic with Intraluminal Device, Open Approach

07L90ZZ Occlusion of Left Internal Mammary Lymphatic, Open Approach

07L93CZ Occlusion of Left Internal Mammary Lymphatic with Extraluminal Device, Percutaneous Approach

07L93DZ Occlusion of Left Internal Mammary Lymphatic with Intraluminal Device, Percutaneous Approach

07L93ZZ Occlusion of Left Internal Mammary Lymphatic, Percutaneous Approach

07L94CZ Occlusion of Left Internal Mammary Lymphatic with Extraluminal Device, Percutaneous Endoscopic Approach

07L94DZ Occlusion of Left Internal Mammary Lymphatic with Intraluminal Device, Percutaneous Endoscopic Approach

07L94ZZ Occlusion of Left Internal Mammary Lymphatic, Percutaneous Endoscopic Approach

07LB0CZ Occlusion of Mesenteric Lymphatic with Extraluminal Device, Open Approach

07LB0DZ Occlusion of Mesenteric Lymphatic with Intraluminal Device, Open Approach

07LB0ZZ Occlusion of Mesenteric Lymphatic, Open Approach

07LB3CZ Occlusion of Mesenteric Lymphatic with Extraluminal Device, Percutaneous Approach

07LB3DZ Occlusion of Mesenteric Lymphatic with Intraluminal Device, Percutaneous Approach

07LB3ZZ Occlusion of Mesenteric Lymphatic, Percutaneous Approach

07LB4CZ Occlusion of Mesenteric Lymphatic with Extraluminal Device, Percutaneous Endoscopic Approach

07LB4DZ Occlusion of Mesenteric Lymphatic with Intraluminal Device, Percutaneous Endoscopic Approach

07LB4ZZ Occlusion of Mesenteric Lymphatic, Percutaneous Endoscopic Approach

07LC0CZ Occlusion of Pelvis Lymphatic with Extraluminal Device, Open Approach

07LC0DZ Occlusion of Pelvis Lymphatic with Intraluminal Device, Open Approach

07LC0ZZ Occlusion of Pelvis Lymphatic, Open Approach

07LC3CZ Occlusion of Pelvis Lymphatic with Extraluminal Device, Percutaneous Approach

07LC3DZ Occlusion of Pelvis Lymphatic with Intraluminal Device, Percutaneous Approach

07LC3ZZ Occlusion of Pelvis Lymphatic, Percutaneous Approach
07LC4CZ Occlusion of Pelvis Lymphatic with Extraluminal Device, Percutaneous Endoscopic Approach
07LC4DZ Occlusion of Pelvis Lymphatic with Intraluminal Device, Percutaneous Endoscopic Approach
07LC4ZZ Occlusion of Pelvis Lymphatic, Percutaneous Endoscopic Approach
07LD0CZ Occlusion of Aortic Lymphatic with Extraluminal Device, Open Approach
07LD0DZ Occlusion of Aortic Lymphatic with Intraluminal Device, Open Approach
07LD0ZZ Occlusion of Aortic Lymphatic, Open Approach
07LD3CZ Occlusion of Aortic Lymphatic with Extraluminal Device, Percutaneous Approach
07LD3DZ Occlusion of Aortic Lymphatic with Intraluminal Device, Percutaneous Approach
07LD3ZZ Occlusion of Aortic Lymphatic, Percutaneous Approach
07LD4CZ Occlusion of Aortic Lymphatic with Extraluminal Device, Percutaneous Endoscopic Approach
07LD4DZ Occlusion of Aortic Lymphatic with Intraluminal Device, Percutaneous Endoscopic Approach
07LD4ZZ Occlusion of Aortic Lymphatic, Percutaneous Endoscopic Approach
07LF0CZ Occlusion of Right Lower Extremity Lymphatic with Extraluminal Device, Open Approach
07LF0DZ Occlusion of Right Lower Extremity Lymphatic with Intraluminal Device, Open Approach
07LF0ZZ Occlusion of Right Lower Extremity Lymphatic, Open Approach
07LF3CZ Occlusion of Right Lower Extremity Lymphatic with Extraluminal Device, Percutaneous Approach
07LF3DZ Occlusion of Right Lower Extremity Lymphatic with Intraluminal Device, Percutaneous Approach
07LF3ZZ Occlusion of Right Lower Extremity Lymphatic, Percutaneous Approach
07LF4CZ Occlusion of Right Lower Extremity Lymphatic with Extraluminal Device, Percutaneous Endoscopic Approach
07LF4DZ Occlusion of Right Lower Extremity Lymphatic with Intraluminal Device, Percutaneous Endoscopic Approach
07LF4ZZ Occlusion of Right Lower Extremity Lymphatic, Percutaneous Endoscopic Approach
07LG0CZ Occlusion of Left Lower Extremity Lymphatic with Extraluminal Device, Open Approach

07LG0DZ Occlusion of Left Lower Extremity Lymphatic with Intraluminal Device, Open Approach
07LG0ZZ Occlusion of Left Lower Extremity Lymphatic, Open Approach
07LG3CZ Occlusion of Left Lower Extremity Lymphatic with Extraluminal Device, Percutaneous Approach
07LG3DZ Occlusion of Left Lower Extremity Lymphatic with Intraluminal Device, Percutaneous Approach
07LG3ZZ Occlusion of Left Lower Extremity Lymphatic, Percutaneous Approach
07LG4CZ Occlusion of Left Lower Extremity Lymphatic with Extraluminal Device, Percutaneous Endoscopic Approach
07LG4DZ Occlusion of Left Lower Extremity Lymphatic with Intraluminal Device, Percutaneous Endoscopic Approach
07LG4ZZ Occlusion of Left Lower Extremity Lymphatic, Percutaneous Endoscopic Approach
07LH0CZ Occlusion of Right Inguinal Lymphatic with Extraluminal Device, Open Approach
07LH0DZ Occlusion of Right Inguinal Lymphatic with Intraluminal Device, Open Approach
07LH0ZZ Occlusion of Right Inguinal Lymphatic, Open Approach
07LH3CZ Occlusion of Right Inguinal Lymphatic with Extraluminal Device, Percutaneous Approach
07LH3DZ Occlusion of Right Inguinal Lymphatic with Intraluminal Device, Percutaneous Approach
07LH3ZZ Occlusion of Right Inguinal Lymphatic, Percutaneous Approach
07LH4CZ Occlusion of Right Inguinal Lymphatic with Extraluminal Device, Percutaneous Endoscopic Approach
07LH4DZ Occlusion of Right Inguinal Lymphatic with Intraluminal Device, Percutaneous Endoscopic Approach
07LH4ZZ Occlusion of Right Inguinal Lymphatic, Percutaneous Endoscopic Approach
07LJ0CZ Occlusion of Left Inguinal Lymphatic with Extraluminal Device, Open Approach
07LJ0DZ Occlusion of Left Inguinal Lymphatic with Intraluminal Device, Open Approach
07LJ0ZZ Occlusion of Left Inguinal Lymphatic, Open Approach
07LJ3CZ Occlusion of Left Inguinal Lymphatic with Extraluminal Device, Percutaneous Approach
07LJ3DZ Occlusion of Left Inguinal Lymphatic with Intraluminal Device, Percutaneous Approach

07LJ3ZZ Occlusion of Left Inguinal Lymphatic, Percutaneous Approach
07LJ4CZ Occlusion of Left Inguinal Lymphatic with Extraluminal Device, Percutaneous Endoscopic Approach
07LJ4DZ Occlusion of Left Inguinal Lymphatic with Intraluminal Device, Percutaneous Endoscopic Approach
07LJ4ZZ Occlusion of Left Inguinal Lymphatic, Percutaneous Endoscopic Approach
07LK0CZ Occlusion of Thoracic Duct with Extraluminal Device, Open Approach
07LK0DZ Occlusion of Thoracic Duct with Intraluminal Device, Open Approach
07LK0ZZ Occlusion of Thoracic Duct, Open Approach
07LK3CZ Occlusion of Thoracic Duct with Extraluminal Device, Percutaneous Approach
07LK3DZ Occlusion of Thoracic Duct with Intraluminal Device, Percutaneous Approach
07LK3ZZ Occlusion of Thoracic Duct, Percutaneous Approach
07LK4CZ Occlusion of Thoracic Duct with Extraluminal Device, Percutaneous Endoscopic Approach
07LK4DZ Occlusion of Thoracic Duct with Intraluminal Device, Percutaneous Endoscopic Approach
07LK4ZZ Occlusion of Thoracic Duct, Percutaneous Endoscopic Approach
07LL0CZ Occlusion of Cisterna Chyli with Extraluminal Device, Open Approach
07LL0DZ Occlusion of Cisterna Chyli with Intraluminal Device, Open Approach
07LL0ZZ Occlusion of Cisterna Chyli, Open Approach
07LL3CZ Occlusion of Cisterna Chyli with Extraluminal Device, Percutaneous Approach
07LL3DZ Occlusion of Cisterna Chyli with Intraluminal Device, Percutaneous Approach
07LL3ZZ Occlusion of Cisterna Chyli, Percutaneous Approach
07LL4CZ Occlusion of Cisterna Chyli with Extraluminal Device, Percutaneous Endoscopic Approach
07LL4DZ Occlusion of Cisterna Chyli with Intraluminal Device, Percutaneous Endoscopic Approach
07LL4ZZ Occlusion of Cisterna Chyli, Percutaneous Endoscopic Approach

07N – Lymphatic and Hemic Systems, Release

Review Coding Guidelines B3.13 and B3.14

07N00ZZ Release Head Lymphatic, Open Approach
07N03ZZ Release Head Lymphatic, Percutaneous Approach
07N04ZZ Release Head Lymphatic, Percutaneous Endoscopic Approach
07N10ZZ Release Right Neck Lymphatic, Open Approach
07N13ZZ Release Right Neck Lymphatic, Percutaneous Approach
07N14ZZ Release Right Neck Lymphatic, Percutaneous Endoscopic Approach

07N20ZZ Release Left Neck Lymphatic, Open Approach
07N23ZZ Release Left Neck Lymphatic, Percutaneous Approach
07N24ZZ Release Left Neck Lymphatic, Percutaneous Endoscopic Approach
07N30ZZ Release Right Upper Extremity Lymphatic, Open Approach
07N33ZZ Release Right Upper Extremity Lymphatic, Percutaneous Approach

07N34ZZ Release Right Upper Extremity Lymphatic, Percutaneous Endoscopic Approach
07N40ZZ Release Left Upper Extremity Lymphatic, Open Approach
07N43ZZ Release Left Upper Extremity Lymphatic, Percutaneous Approach
07N44ZZ Release Left Upper Extremity Lymphatic, Percutaneous Endoscopic Approach
07N50ZZ Release Right Axillary Lymphatic, Open Approach

♀ Female-only   ♂ Male-only   ▲ Limited Coverage   ● Non-OR   HAC HAC-associated procedure   ▲ Non-covered procedures   ✚ Cluster

07N53ZZ	Release Right Axillary Lymphatic, Percutaneous Approach
07N54ZZ	Release Right Axillary Lymphatic, Percutaneous Endoscopic Approach
07N60ZZ	Release Left Axillary Lymphatic, Open Approach
07N63ZZ	Release Left Axillary Lymphatic, Percutaneous Approach
07N64ZZ	Release Left Axillary Lymphatic, Percutaneous Endoscopic Approach
07N70ZZ	Release Thorax Lymphatic, Open Approach
07N73ZZ	Release Thorax Lymphatic, Percutaneous Approach
07N74ZZ	Release Thorax Lymphatic, Percutaneous Endoscopic Approach
07N80ZZ	Release Right Internal Mammary Lymphatic, Open Approach
07N83ZZ	Release Right Internal Mammary Lymphatic, Percutaneous Approach
07N84ZZ	Release Right Internal Mammary Lymphatic, Percutaneous Endoscopic Approach
07N90ZZ	Release Left Internal Mammary Lymphatic, Open Approach
07N93ZZ	Release Left Internal Mammary Lymphatic, Percutaneous Approach
07N94ZZ	Release Left Internal Mammary Lymphatic, Percutaneous Endoscopic Approach
07NB0ZZ	Release Mesenteric Lymphatic, Open Approach
07NB3ZZ	Release Mesenteric Lymphatic, Percutaneous Approach
07NB4ZZ	Release Mesenteric Lymphatic, Percutaneous Endoscopic Approach
07NC0ZZ	Release Pelvis Lymphatic, Open Approach
07NC3ZZ	Release Pelvis Lymphatic, Percutaneous Approach
07NC4ZZ	Release Pelvis Lymphatic, Percutaneous Endoscopic Approach
07ND0ZZ	Release Aortic Lymphatic, Open Approach
07ND3ZZ	Release Aortic Lymphatic, Percutaneous Approach
07ND4ZZ	Release Aortic Lymphatic, Percutaneous Endoscopic Approach
07NF0ZZ	Release Right Lower Extremity Lymphatic, Open Approach
07NF3ZZ	Release Right Lower Extremity Lymphatic, Percutaneous Approach
07NF4ZZ	Release Right Lower Extremity Lymphatic, Percutaneous Endoscopic Approach
07NG0ZZ	Release Left Lower Extremity Lymphatic, Open Approach
07NG3ZZ	Release Left Lower Extremity Lymphatic, Percutaneous Approach
07NG4ZZ	Release Left Lower Extremity Lymphatic, Percutaneous Endoscopic Approach
07NH0ZZ	Release Right Inguinal Lymphatic, Open Approach
07NH3ZZ	Release Right Inguinal Lymphatic, Percutaneous Approach
07NH4ZZ	Release Right Inguinal Lymphatic, Percutaneous Endoscopic Approach
07NJ0ZZ	Release Left Inguinal Lymphatic, Open Approach
07NJ3ZZ	Release Left Inguinal Lymphatic, Percutaneous Approach
07NJ4ZZ	Release Left Inguinal Lymphatic, Percutaneous Endoscopic Approach
07NK0ZZ	Release Thoracic Duct, Open Approach
07NK3ZZ	Release Thoracic Duct, Percutaneous Approach
07NK4ZZ	Release Thoracic Duct, Percutaneous Endoscopic Approach
07NL0ZZ	Release Cisterna Chyli, Open Approach
07NL3ZZ	Release Cisterna Chyli, Percutaneous Approach
07NL4ZZ	Release Cisterna Chyli, Percutaneous Endoscopic Approach
07NM0ZZ	Release Thymus, Open Approach
07NM3ZZ	Release Thymus, Percutaneous Approach
07NM4ZZ	Release Thymus, Percutaneous Endoscopic Approach
07NP0ZZ	Release Spleen, Open Approach
07NP3ZZ	Release Spleen, Percutaneous Approach
07NP4ZZ	Release Spleen, Percutaneous Endoscopic Approach

07P – Lymphatic and Hemic Systems, Removal

Review Coding Guideline B6.1c

07PK00Z	Removal of Drainage Device from Thoracic Duct, Open Approach
07PK03Z	Removal of Infusion Device from Thoracic Duct, Open Approach
07PK07Z	Removal of Autologous Tissue Substitute from Thoracic Duct, Open Approach
07PK0CZ	Removal of Extraluminal Device from Thoracic Duct, Open Approach
07PK0DZ	Removal of Intraluminal Device from Thoracic Duct, Open Approach
07PK0JZ	Removal of Synthetic Substitute from Thoracic Duct, Open Approach
07PK0KZ	Removal of Nonautologous Tissue Substitute from Thoracic Duct, Open Approach
07PK0YZ	Removal of Other Device from Thoracic Duct, Open Approach
07PK30Z	Removal of Drainage Device from Thoracic Duct, Percutaneous Approach
07PK33Z	Removal of Infusion Device from Thoracic Duct, Percutaneous Approach
07PK37Z	Removal of Autologous Tissue Substitute from Thoracic Duct, Percutaneous Approach
07PK3CZ	Removal of Extraluminal Device from Thoracic Duct, Percutaneous Approach
07PK3DZ	Removal of Intraluminal Device from Thoracic Duct, Percutaneous Approach
07PK3JZ	Removal of Synthetic Substitute from Thoracic Duct, Percutaneous Approach
07PK3KZ	Removal of Nonautologous Tissue Substitute from Thoracic Duct, Percutaneous Approach
07PK3YZ	Removal of Other Device from Thoracic Duct, Percutaneous Approach
07PK40Z	Removal of Drainage Device from Thoracic Duct, Percutaneous Endoscopic Approach
07PK43Z	Removal of Infusion Device from Thoracic Duct, Percutaneous Endoscopic Approach
07PK47Z	Removal of Autologous Tissue Substitute from Thoracic Duct, Percutaneous Endoscopic Approach
07PK4CZ	Removal of Extraluminal Device from Thoracic Duct, Percutaneous Endoscopic Approach
07PK4DZ	Removal of Intraluminal Device from Thoracic Duct, Percutaneous Endoscopic Approach
07PK4JZ	Removal of Synthetic Substitute from Thoracic Duct, Percutaneous Endoscopic Approach
07PK4KZ	Removal of Nonautologous Tissue Substitute from Thoracic Duct, Percutaneous Endoscopic Approach
07PK4YZ	Removal of Other Device from Thoracic Duct, Percutaneous Endoscopic Approach
07PKX0Z	Removal of Drainage Device from Thoracic Duct, External Approach
07PKX3Z	Removal of Infusion Device from Thoracic Duct, External Approach
07PKXDZ	Removal of Intraluminal Device from Thoracic Duct, External Approach
07PL00Z	Removal of Drainage Device from Cisterna Chyli, Open Approach
07PL03Z	Removal of Infusion Device from Cisterna Chyli, Open Approach
07PL07Z	Removal of Autologous Tissue Substitute from Cisterna Chyli, Open Approach
07PL0CZ	Removal of Extraluminal Device from Cisterna Chyli, Open Approach
07PL0DZ	Removal of Intraluminal Device from Cisterna Chyli, Open Approach
07PL0JZ	Removal of Synthetic Substitute from Cisterna Chyli, Open Approach
07PL0KZ	Removal of Nonautologous Tissue Substitute from Cisterna Chyli, Open Approach
07PL0YZ	Removal of Other Device from Cisterna Chyli, Open Approach
07PL30Z	Removal of Drainage Device from Cisterna Chyli, Percutaneous Approach
07PL33Z	Removal of Infusion Device from Cisterna Chyli, Percutaneous Approach
07PL37Z	Removal of Autologous Tissue Substitute from Cisterna Chyli, Percutaneous Approach
07PL3CZ	Removal of Extraluminal Device from Cisterna Chyli, Percutaneous Approach
07PL3DZ	Removal of Intraluminal Device from Cisterna Chyli, Percutaneous Approach
07PL3JZ	Removal of Synthetic Substitute from Cisterna Chyli, Percutaneous Approach
07PL3KZ	Removal of Nonautologous Tissue Substitute from Cisterna Chyli, Percutaneous Approach
07PL3YZ	Removal of Other Device from Cisterna Chyli, Percutaneous Approach
07PL40Z	Removal of Drainage Device from Cisterna Chyli, Percutaneous Endoscopic Approach
07PL43Z	Removal of Infusion Device from Cisterna Chyli, Percutaneous Endoscopic Approach
07PL47Z	Removal of Autologous Tissue Substitute from Cisterna Chyli, Percutaneous Endoscopic Approach
07PL4CZ	Removal of Extraluminal Device from Cisterna Chyli, Percutaneous Endoscopic Approach
07PL4DZ	Removal of Intraluminal Device from Cisterna Chyli, Percutaneous Endoscopic Approach

07PL4JZ Removal of Synthetic Substitute from Cisterna Chyli, Percutaneous Endoscopic Approach

07PL4KZ Removal of Nonautologous Tissue Substitute from Cisterna Chyli, Percutaneous Endoscopic Approach

07PL4YZ Removal of Other Device from Cisterna Chyli, Percutaneous Endoscopic Approach

07PLX0Z Removal of Drainage Device from Cisterna Chyli, External Approach

07PLX3Z Removal of Infusion Device from Cisterna Chyli, External Approach

07PLXDZ Removal of Intraluminal Device from Cisterna Chyli, External Approach

07PM00Z Removal of Drainage Device from Thymus, Open Approach

07PM03Z Removal of Infusion Device from Thymus, Open Approach

07PM0YZ Removal of Other Device from Thymus, Open Approach

07PM30Z Removal of Drainage Device from Thymus, Percutaneous Approach

07PM33Z Removal of Infusion Device from Thymus, Percutaneous Approach

07PM3YZ Removal of Other Device from Thymus, Percutaneous Approach

07PM40Z Removal of Drainage Device from Thymus, Percutaneous Endoscopic Approach

07PM43Z Removal of Infusion Device from Thymus, Percutaneous Endoscopic Approach

07PM4YZ Removal of Other Device from Thymus, Percutaneous Endoscopic Approach

07PMX0Z Removal of Drainage Device from Thymus, External Approach

07PMX3Z Removal of Infusion Device from Thymus, External Approach

07PN00Z Removal of Drainage Device from Lymphatic, Open Approach

07PN03Z Removal of Infusion Device from Lymphatic, Open Approach

07PN07Z Removal of Autologous Tissue Substitute from Lymphatic, Open Approach

07PN0CZ Removal of Extraluminal Device from Lymphatic, Open Approach

07PN0DZ Removal of Intraluminal Device from Lymphatic, Open Approach

07PN0JZ Removal of Synthetic Substitute from Lymphatic, Open Approach

07PN0KZ Removal of Nonautologous Tissue Substitute from Lymphatic, Open Approach

07PN0YZ Removal of Other Device from Lymphatic, Open Approach

07PN30Z Removal of Drainage Device from Lymphatic, Percutaneous Approach

07PN33Z Removal of Infusion Device from Lymphatic, Percutaneous Approach

07PN37Z Removal of Autologous Tissue Substitute from Lymphatic, Percutaneous Approach

07PN3CZ Removal of Extraluminal Device from Lymphatic, Percutaneous Approach

07PN3DZ Removal of Intraluminal Device from Lymphatic, Percutaneous Approach

07PN3JZ Removal of Synthetic Substitute from Lymphatic, Percutaneous Approach

07PN3KZ Removal of Nonautologous Tissue Substitute from Lymphatic, Percutaneous Approach

07PN3YZ Removal of Other Device from Lymphatic, Percutaneous Approach

07PN40Z Removal of Drainage Device from Lymphatic, Percutaneous Endoscopic Approach

07PN43Z Removal of Infusion Device from Lymphatic, Percutaneous Endoscopic Approach

07PN47Z Removal of Autologous Tissue Substitute from Lymphatic, Percutaneous Endoscopic Approach

07PN4CZ Removal of Extraluminal Device from Lymphatic, Percutaneous Endoscopic Approach

07PN4DZ Removal of Intraluminal Device from Lymphatic, Percutaneous Endoscopic Approach

07PN4JZ Removal of Synthetic Substitute from Lymphatic, Percutaneous Endoscopic Approach

07PN4KZ Removal of Nonautologous Tissue Substitute from Lymphatic, Percutaneous Endoscopic Approach

07PN4YZ Removal of Other Device from Lymphatic, Percutaneous Endoscopic Approach

07PNX0Z Removal of Drainage Device from Lymphatic, External Approach

07PNX3Z Removal of Infusion Device from Lymphatic, External Approach

07PNXDZ Removal of Intraluminal Device from Lymphatic, External Approach

07PP00Z Removal of Drainage Device from Spleen, Open Approach

07PP03Z Removal of Infusion Device from Spleen, Open Approach

07PP0YZ Removal of Other Device from Spleen, Open Approach

07PP30Z Removal of Drainage Device from Spleen, Percutaneous Approach

07PP33Z Removal of Infusion Device from Spleen, Percutaneous Approach

07PP3YZ Removal of Other Device from Spleen, Percutaneous Approach

07PP40Z Removal of Drainage Device from Spleen, Percutaneous Endoscopic Approach

07PP43Z Removal of Infusion Device from Spleen, Percutaneous Endoscopic Approach

07PP4YZ Removal of Other Device from Spleen, Percutaneous Endoscopic Approach

07PPX0Z Removal of Drainage Device from Spleen, External Approach

07PPX3Z Removal of Infusion Device from Spleen, External Approach

07PT00Z Removal of Drainage Device from Bone Marrow, Open Approach

07PT30Z Removal of Drainage Device from Bone Marrow, Percutaneous Approach

07PT40Z Removal of Drainage Device from Bone Marrow, Percutaneous Endoscopic Approach

07PTX0Z Removal of Drainage Device from Bone Marrow, External Approach

07Q – Lymphatic and Hemic Systems, Repair

07Q00ZZ Repair Head Lymphatic, Open Approach

07Q03ZZ Repair Head Lymphatic, Percutaneous Approach

07Q04ZZ Repair Head Lymphatic, Percutaneous Endoscopic Approach

07Q08ZZ Repair Head Lymphatic, Via Natural or Artificial Opening Endoscopic Approach

07Q10ZZ Repair Right Neck Lymphatic, Open Approach

07Q13ZZ Repair Right Neck Lymphatic, Percutaneous Approach

07Q14ZZ Repair Right Neck Lymphatic, Percutaneous Endoscopic Approach

07Q18ZZ Repair Right Neck Lymphatic, Via Natural or Artificial Opening Endoscopic Approach

07Q20ZZ Repair Left Neck Lymphatic, Open Approach

07Q23ZZ Repair Left Neck Lymphatic, Percutaneous Approach

07Q24ZZ Repair Left Neck Lymphatic, Percutaneous Endoscopic Approach

07Q28ZZ Repair Left Neck Lymphatic, Via Natural or Artificial Opening Endoscopic Approach

07Q30ZZ Repair Right Upper Extremity Lymphatic, Open Approach

07Q33ZZ Repair Right Upper Extremity Lymphatic, Percutaneous Approach

07Q34ZZ Repair Right Upper Extremity Lymphatic, Percutaneous Endoscopic Approach

07Q38ZZ Repair Right Upper Extremity Lymphatic, Via Natural or Artificial Opening Endoscopic Approach

07Q40ZZ Repair Left Upper Extremity Lymphatic, Open Approach

07Q43ZZ Repair Left Upper Extremity Lymphatic, Percutaneous Approach

07Q44ZZ Repair Left Upper Extremity Lymphatic, Percutaneous Endoscopic Approach

07Q48ZZ Repair Left Upper Extremity Lymphatic, Via Natural or Artificial Opening Endoscopic Approach

07Q50ZZ Repair Right Axillary Lymphatic, Open Approach

07Q53ZZ Repair Right Axillary Lymphatic, Percutaneous Approach

07Q54ZZ Repair Right Axillary Lymphatic, Percutaneous Endoscopic Approach

07Q58ZZ Repair Right Axillary Lymphatic, Via Natural or Artificial Opening Endoscopic Approach

07Q60ZZ Repair Left Axillary Lymphatic, Open Approach

AHA CC: 1Q, 2017, 34

07Q63ZZ Repair Left Axillary Lymphatic, Percutaneous Approach

07Q64ZZ Repair Left Axillary Lymphatic, Percutaneous Endoscopic Approach

07Q68ZZ Repair Left Axillary Lymphatic, Via Natural or Artificial Opening Endoscopic Approach

07Q70ZZ Repair Thorax Lymphatic, Open Approach

07Q73ZZ Repair Thorax Lymphatic, Percutaneous Approach

07Q74ZZ Repair Thorax Lymphatic, Percutaneous Endoscopic Approach

07Q78ZZ Repair Thorax Lymphatic, Via Natural or Artificial Opening Endoscopic Approach

07Q80ZZ Repair Right Internal Mammary Lymphatic, Open Approach

07Q83ZZ Repair Right Internal Mammary Lymphatic, Percutaneous Approach

07Q84ZZ Repair Right Internal Mammary Lymphatic, Percutaneous Endoscopic Approach

♀ Female-only   ♂ Male-only   ▲ Limited Coverage   ● Non-OR   🄷🄰🄲 HAC-associated procedure   ▲ Non-covered procedures   ✚ Cluster

07Q88ZZ Repair Right Internal Mammary Lymphatic, Via Natural or Artificial Opening Endoscopic Approach
07Q90ZZ Repair Left Internal Mammary Lymphatic, Open Approach
07Q93ZZ Repair Left Internal Mammary Lymphatic, Percutaneous Approach
07Q94ZZ Repair Left Internal Mammary Lymphatic, Percutaneous Endoscopic Approach
07Q98ZZ Repair Left Internal Mammary Lymphatic, Via Natural or Artificial Opening Endoscopic Approach
07QB0ZZ Repair Mesenteric Lymphatic, Open Approach
07QB3ZZ Repair Mesenteric Lymphatic, Percutaneous Approach
07QB4ZZ Repair Mesenteric Lymphatic, Percutaneous Endoscopic Approach
07QB8ZZ Repair Mesenteric Lymphatic, Via Natural or Artificial Opening Endoscopic Approach
07QC0ZZ Repair Pelvis Lymphatic, Open Approach
07QC3ZZ Repair Pelvis Lymphatic, Percutaneous Approach
07QC4ZZ Repair Pelvis Lymphatic, Percutaneous Endoscopic Approach
07QC8ZZ Repair Pelvis Lymphatic, Via Natural or Artificial Opening Endoscopic Approach
07QD0ZZ Repair Aortic Lymphatic, Open Approach
07QD3ZZ Repair Aortic Lymphatic, Percutaneous Approach

07QD4ZZ Repair Aortic Lymphatic, Percutaneous Endoscopic Approach
07QD8ZZ Repair Aortic Lymphatic, Via Natural or Artificial Opening Endoscopic Approach
07QF0ZZ Repair Right Lower Extremity Lymphatic, Open Approach
07QF3ZZ Repair Right Lower Extremity Lymphatic, Percutaneous Approach
07QF4ZZ Repair Right Lower Extremity Lymphatic, Percutaneous Endoscopic Approach
07QF8ZZ Repair Right Lower Extremity Lymphatic, Via Natural or Artificial Opening Endoscopic Approach
07QG0ZZ Repair Left Lower Extremity Lymphatic, Open Approach
07QG3ZZ Repair Left Lower Extremity Lymphatic, Percutaneous Approach
07QG4ZZ Repair Left Lower Extremity Lymphatic, Percutaneous Endoscopic Approach
07QG8ZZ Repair Left Lower Extremity Lymphatic, Via Natural or Artificial Opening Endoscopic Approach
07QH0ZZ Repair Right Inguinal Lymphatic, Open Approach
07QH3ZZ Repair Right Inguinal Lymphatic, Percutaneous Approach
07QH4ZZ Repair Right Inguinal Lymphatic, Percutaneous Endoscopic Approach
07QH8ZZ Repair Right Inguinal Lymphatic, Via Natural or Artificial Opening Endoscopic Approach

07QJ0ZZ Repair Left Inguinal Lymphatic, Open Approach
07QJ3ZZ Repair Left Inguinal Lymphatic, Percutaneous Approach
07QJ4ZZ Repair Left Inguinal Lymphatic, Percutaneous Endoscopic Approach
07QJ8ZZ Repair Left Inguinal Lymphatic, Via Natural or Artificial Opening Endoscopic Approach
07QK0ZZ Repair Thoracic Duct, Open Approach
07QK3ZZ Repair Thoracic Duct, Percutaneous Approach
07QK4ZZ Repair Thoracic Duct, Percutaneous Endoscopic Approach
07QK8ZZ Repair Thoracic Duct, Via Natural or Artificial Opening Endoscopic Approach
07QL0ZZ Repair Cisterna Chyli, Open Approach
07QL3ZZ Repair Cisterna Chyli, Percutaneous Approach
07QL4ZZ Repair Cisterna Chyli, Percutaneous Endoscopic Approach
07QL8ZZ Repair Cisterna Chyli, Via Natural or Artificial Opening Endoscopic Approach
07QM0ZZ Repair Thymus, Open Approach
07QM3ZZ Repair Thymus, Percutaneous Approach
07QM4ZZ Repair Thymus, Percutaneous Endoscopic Approach
07QP0ZZ Repair Spleen, Open Approach
07QP3ZZ Repair Spleen, Percutaneous Approach
07QP4ZZ Repair Spleen, Percutaneous Endoscopic Approach

07S – Lymphatic and Hemic Systems, Reposition

07SM0ZZ Reposition Thymus, Open Approach

07SP0ZZ Reposition Spleen, Open Approach

07T – Lymphatic and Hemic Systems, Resection

Review Coding Guideline B3.8

Review Coding Guideline B3.18

07T00ZZ Resection of Head Lymphatic, Open Approach
07T04ZZ Resection of Head Lymphatic, Percutaneous Endoscopic Approach
07T10ZZ Resection of Right Neck Lymphatic, Open Approach
AHA CC: 3Q, 2014, 9-10
07T14ZZ Resection of Right Neck Lymphatic, Percutaneous Endoscopic Approach
07T20ZZ Resection of Left Neck Lymphatic, Open Approach
AHA CC: 3Q, 2014, 9-10; 2Q, 2016, 12-14
07T24ZZ Resection of Left Neck Lymphatic, Percutaneous Endoscopic Approach
07T30ZZ Resection of Right Upper Extremity Lymphatic, Open Approach
07T34ZZ Resection of Right Upper Extremity Lymphatic, Percutaneous Endoscopic Approach
07T40ZZ Resection of Left Upper Extremity Lymphatic, Open Approach
07T44ZZ Resection of Left Upper Extremity Lymphatic, Percutaneous Endoscopic Approach
07T50ZZ Resection of Right Axillary Lymphatic, Open Approach
AHA CC: 1Q, 2016, 30
➕ Mastectomy procedure when reported with resection of breast. *See table 0HT to construct the Resection of breast code. See table 0KT to construct the Resection*

of thorax muscle code if applicable. See table 07T to report additional lymph node resections.
07T54ZZ Resection of Right Axillary Lymphatic, Percutaneous Endoscopic Approach
07T60ZZ Resection of Left Axillary Lymphatic, Open Approach
➕ Mastectomy procedure when reported with resection of breast. *See table 0HT to construct the Resection of breast code. See table 0KT to construct the Resection of thorax muscle code if applicable. See table 07T to report additional lymph node resections.*
07T64ZZ Resection of Left Axillary Lymphatic, Percutaneous Endoscopic Approach
07T70ZZ Resection of Thorax Lymphatic, Open Approach
07T74ZZ Resection of Thorax Lymphatic, Percutaneous Endoscopic Approach
07T80ZZ Resection of Right Internal Mammary Lymphatic, Open Approach
07T84ZZ Resection of Right Internal Mammary Lymphatic, Percutaneous Endoscopic Approach
07T90ZZ Resection of Left Internal Mammary Lymphatic, Open Approach
07T94ZZ Resection of Left Internal Mammary Lymphatic, Percutaneous Endoscopic Approach

07TB0ZZ Resection of Mesenteric Lymphatic, Open Approach
07TB4ZZ Resection of Mesenteric Lymphatic, Percutaneous Endoscopic Approach
07TC0ZZ Resection of Pelvis Lymphatic, Open Approach
07TC4ZZ Resection of Pelvis Lymphatic, Percutaneous Endoscopic Approach
07TD0ZZ Resection of Aortic Lymphatic, Open Approach
07TD4ZZ Resection of Aortic Lymphatic, Percutaneous Endoscopic Approach
07TF0ZZ Resection of Right Lower Extremity Lymphatic, Open Approach
07TF4ZZ Resection of Right Lower Extremity Lymphatic, Percutaneous Endoscopic Approach
07TG0ZZ Resection of Left Lower Extremity Lymphatic, Open Approach
07TG4ZZ Resection of Left Lower Extremity Lymphatic, Percutaneous Endoscopic Approach
07TH0ZZ Resection of Right Inguinal Lymphatic, Open Approach
07TH4ZZ Resection of Right Inguinal Lymphatic, Percutaneous Endoscopic Approach
07TJ0ZZ Resection of Left Inguinal Lymphatic, Open Approach
07TJ4ZZ Resection of Left Inguinal Lymphatic, Percutaneous Endoscopic Approach

07TK0ZZ Resection of Thoracic Duct, Open Approach

07TK4ZZ Resection of Thoracic Duct, Percutaneous Endoscopic Approach

07TL0ZZ Resection of Cisterna Chyli, Open Approach

07TL4ZZ Resection of Cisterna Chyli, Percutaneous Endoscopic Approach

07TM0ZZ Resection of Thymus, Open Approach
AHA CC: 3Q, 2014, 16-17

07TM4ZZ Resection of Thymus, Percutaneous Endoscopic Approach

07TP0ZZ Resection of Spleen, Open Approach
AHA CC: 4Q, 2015, 13

07TP4ZZ Resection of Spleen, Percutaneous Endoscopic Approach

07U – Lymphatic and Hemic Systems, Supplement

07U007Z Supplement Head Lymphatic with Autologous Tissue Substitute, Open Approach

07U00JZ Supplement Head Lymphatic with Synthetic Substitute, Open Approach

07U00KZ Supplement Head Lymphatic with Nonautologous Tissue Substitute, Open Approach

07U047Z Supplement Head Lymphatic with Autologous Tissue Substitute, Percutaneous Endoscopic Approach

07U04JZ Supplement Head Lymphatic with Synthetic Substitute, Percutaneous Endoscopic Approach

07U04KZ Supplement Head Lymphatic with Nonautologous Tissue Substitute, Percutaneous Endoscopic Approach

07U107Z Supplement Right Neck Lymphatic with Autologous Tissue Substitute, Open Approach

07U10JZ Supplement Right Neck Lymphatic with Synthetic Substitute, Open Approach

07U10KZ Supplement Right Neck Lymphatic with Nonautologous Tissue Substitute, Open Approach

07U147Z Supplement Right Neck Lymphatic with Autologous Tissue Substitute, Percutaneous Endoscopic Approach

07U14JZ Supplement Right Neck Lymphatic with Synthetic Substitute, Percutaneous Endoscopic Approach

07U14KZ Supplement Right Neck Lymphatic with Nonautologous Tissue Substitute, Percutaneous Endoscopic Approach

07U207Z Supplement Left Neck Lymphatic with Autologous Tissue Substitute, Open Approach

07U20JZ Supplement Left Neck Lymphatic with Synthetic Substitute, Open Approach

07U20KZ Supplement Left Neck Lymphatic with Nonautologous Tissue Substitute, Open Approach

07U247Z Supplement Left Neck Lymphatic with Autologous Tissue Substitute, Percutaneous Endoscopic Approach

07U24JZ Supplement Left Neck Lymphatic with Synthetic Substitute, Percutaneous Endoscopic Approach

07U24KZ Supplement Left Neck Lymphatic with Nonautologous Tissue Substitute, Percutaneous Endoscopic Approach

07U307Z Supplement Right Upper Extremity Lymphatic with Autologous Tissue Substitute, Open Approach

07U30JZ Supplement Right Upper Extremity Lymphatic with Synthetic Substitute, Open Approach

07U30KZ Supplement Right Upper Extremity Lymphatic with Nonautologous Tissue Substitute, Open Approach

07U347Z Supplement Right Upper Extremity Lymphatic with Autologous Tissue Substitute, Percutaneous Endoscopic Approach

07U34JZ Supplement Right Upper Extremity Lymphatic with Synthetic Substitute, Percutaneous Endoscopic Approach

07U34KZ Supplement Right Upper Extremity Lymphatic with Nonautologous Tissue Substitute, Percutaneous Endoscopic Approach

07U407Z Supplement Left Upper Extremity Lymphatic with Autologous Tissue Substitute, Open Approach

07U40JZ Supplement Left Upper Extremity Lymphatic with Synthetic Substitute, Open Approach

07U40KZ Supplement Left Upper Extremity Lymphatic with Nonautologous Tissue Substitute, Open Approach

07U447Z Supplement Left Upper Extremity Lymphatic with Autologous Tissue Substitute, Percutaneous Endoscopic Approach

07U44JZ Supplement Left Upper Extremity Lymphatic with Synthetic Substitute, Percutaneous Endoscopic Approach

07U44KZ Supplement Left Upper Extremity Lymphatic with Nonautologous Tissue Substitute, Percutaneous Endoscopic Approach

07U507Z Supplement Right Axillary Lymphatic with Autologous Tissue Substitute, Open Approach

07U50JZ Supplement Right Axillary Lymphatic with Synthetic Substitute, Open Approach

07U50KZ Supplement Right Axillary Lymphatic with Nonautologous Tissue Substitute, Open Approach

07U547Z Supplement Right Axillary Lymphatic with Autologous Tissue Substitute, Percutaneous Endoscopic Approach

07U54JZ Supplement Right Axillary Lymphatic with Synthetic Substitute, Percutaneous Endoscopic Approach

07U54KZ Supplement Right Axillary Lymphatic with Nonautologous Tissue Substitute, Percutaneous Endoscopic Approach

07U607Z Supplement Left Axillary Lymphatic with Autologous Tissue Substitute, Open Approach

07U60JZ Supplement Left Axillary Lymphatic with Synthetic Substitute, Open Approach

07U60KZ Supplement Left Axillary Lymphatic with Nonautologous Tissue Substitute, Open Approach

07U647Z Supplement Left Axillary Lymphatic with Autologous Tissue Substitute, Percutaneous Endoscopic Approach

07U64JZ Supplement Left Axillary Lymphatic with Synthetic Substitute, Percutaneous Endoscopic Approach

07U64KZ Supplement Left Axillary Lymphatic with Nonautologous Tissue Substitute, Percutaneous Endoscopic Approach

07U707Z Supplement Thorax Lymphatic with Autologous Tissue Substitute, Open Approach

07U70JZ Supplement Thorax Lymphatic with Synthetic Substitute, Open Approach

07U70KZ Supplement Thorax Lymphatic with Nonautologous Tissue Substitute, Open Approach

07U747Z Supplement Thorax Lymphatic with Autologous Tissue Substitute, Percutaneous Endoscopic Approach

07U74JZ Supplement Thorax Lymphatic with Synthetic Substitute, Percutaneous Endoscopic Approach

07U74KZ Supplement Thorax Lymphatic with Nonautologous Tissue Substitute, Percutaneous Endoscopic Approach

07U807Z Supplement Right Internal Mammary Lymphatic with Autologous Tissue Substitute, Open Approach

07U80JZ Supplement Right Internal Mammary Lymphatic with Synthetic Substitute, Open Approach

07U80KZ Supplement Right Internal Mammary Lymphatic with Nonautologous Tissue Substitute, Open Approach

07U847Z Supplement Right Internal Mammary Lymphatic with Autologous Tissue Substitute, Percutaneous Endoscopic Approach

07U84JZ Supplement Right Internal Mammary Lymphatic with Synthetic Substitute, Percutaneous Endoscopic Approach

07U84KZ Supplement Right Internal Mammary Lymphatic with Nonautologous Tissue Substitute, Percutaneous Endoscopic Approach

07U907Z Supplement Left Internal Mammary Lymphatic with Autologous Tissue Substitute, Open Approach

07U90JZ Supplement Left Internal Mammary Lymphatic with Synthetic Substitute, Open Approach

07U90KZ Supplement Left Internal Mammary Lymphatic with Nonautologous Tissue Substitute, Open Approach

07U947Z Supplement Left Internal Mammary Lymphatic with Autologous Tissue Substitute, Percutaneous Endoscopic Approach

07U94JZ Supplement Left Internal Mammary Lymphatic with Synthetic Substitute, Percutaneous Endoscopic Approach

07U94KZ Supplement Left Internal Mammary Lymphatic with Nonautologous Tissue Substitute, Percutaneous Endoscopic Approach

07UB07Z Supplement Mesenteric Lymphatic with Autologous Tissue Substitute, Open Approach

07UB0JZ Supplement Mesenteric Lymphatic with Synthetic Substitute, Open Approach

07UB0KZ Supplement Mesenteric Lymphatic with Nonautologous Tissue Substitute, Open Approach

07UB47Z Supplement Mesenteric Lymphatic with Autologous Tissue Substitute, Percutaneous Endoscopic Approach

07UB4JZ Supplement Mesenteric Lymphatic with Synthetic Substitute, Percutaneous Endoscopic Approach

07UB4KZ Supplement Mesenteric Lymphatic with Nonautologous Tissue Substitute, Percutaneous Endoscopic Approach

♀ Female-only   ♂ Male-only   ▲ Limited Coverage   ● Non-OR   HAC HAC-associated procedure   ▲ Non-covered procedures   ✚ Cluster

07UC07Z Supplement Pelvis Lymphatic with Autologous Tissue Substitute, Open Approach

07UC0JZ Supplement Pelvis Lymphatic with Synthetic Substitute, Open Approach

07UC0KZ Supplement Pelvis Lymphatic with Nonautologous Tissue Substitute, Open Approach

07UC47Z Supplement Pelvis Lymphatic with Autologous Tissue Substitute, Percutaneous Endoscopic Approach

07UC4JZ Supplement Pelvis Lymphatic with Synthetic Substitute, Percutaneous Endoscopic Approach

07UC4KZ Supplement Pelvis Lymphatic with Nonautologous Tissue Substitute, Percutaneous Endoscopic Approach

07UD07Z Supplement Aortic Lymphatic with Autologous Tissue Substitute, Open Approach

07UD0JZ Supplement Aortic Lymphatic with Synthetic Substitute, Open Approach

07UD0KZ Supplement Aortic Lymphatic with Nonautologous Tissue Substitute, Open Approach

07UD47Z Supplement Aortic Lymphatic with Autologous Tissue Substitute, Percutaneous Endoscopic Approach

07UD4JZ Supplement Aortic Lymphatic with Synthetic Substitute, Percutaneous Endoscopic Approach

07UD4KZ Supplement Aortic Lymphatic with Nonautologous Tissue Substitute, Percutaneous Endoscopic Approach

07UF07Z Supplement Right Lower Extremity Lymphatic with Autologous Tissue Substitute, Open Approach

07UF0JZ Supplement Right Lower Extremity Lymphatic with Synthetic Substitute, Open Approach

07UF0KZ Supplement Right Lower Extremity Lymphatic with Nonautologous Tissue Substitute, Open Approach

07UF47Z Supplement Right Lower Extremity Lymphatic with Autologous Tissue Substitute, Percutaneous Endoscopic Approach

07UF4JZ Supplement Right Lower Extremity Lymphatic with Synthetic Substitute, Percutaneous Endoscopic Approach

07UF4KZ Supplement Right Lower Extremity Lymphatic with Nonautologous Tissue Substitute, Percutaneous Endoscopic Approach

07UG07Z Supplement Left Lower Extremity Lymphatic with Autologous Tissue Substitute, Open Approach

07UG0JZ Supplement Left Lower Extremity Lymphatic with Synthetic Substitute, Open Approach

07UG0KZ Supplement Left Lower Extremity Lymphatic with Nonautologous Tissue Substitute, Open Approach

07UG47Z Supplement Left Lower Extremity Lymphatic with Autologous Tissue Substitute, Percutaneous Endoscopic Approach

07UG4JZ Supplement Left Lower Extremity Lymphatic with Synthetic Substitute, Percutaneous Endoscopic Approach

07UG4KZ Supplement Left Lower Extremity Lymphatic with Nonautologous Tissue Substitute, Percutaneous Endoscopic Approach

07UH07Z Supplement Right Inguinal Lymphatic with Autologous Tissue Substitute, Open Approach

07UH0JZ Supplement Right Inguinal Lymphatic with Synthetic Substitute, Open Approach

07UH0KZ Supplement Right Inguinal Lymphatic with Nonautologous Tissue Substitute, Open Approach

07UH47Z Supplement Right Inguinal Lymphatic with Autologous Tissue Substitute, Percutaneous Endoscopic Approach

07UH4JZ Supplement Right Inguinal Lymphatic with Synthetic Substitute, Percutaneous Endoscopic Approach

07UH4KZ Supplement Right Inguinal Lymphatic with Nonautologous Tissue Substitute, Percutaneous Endoscopic Approach

07UJ07Z Supplement Left Inguinal Lymphatic with Autologous Tissue Substitute, Open Approach

07UJ0JZ Supplement Left Inguinal Lymphatic with Synthetic Substitute, Open Approach

07UJ0KZ Supplement Left Inguinal Lymphatic with Nonautologous Tissue Substitute, Open Approach

07UJ47Z Supplement Left Inguinal Lymphatic with Autologous Tissue Substitute, Percutaneous Endoscopic Approach

07UJ4JZ Supplement Left Inguinal Lymphatic with Synthetic Substitute, Percutaneous Endoscopic Approach

07UJ4KZ Supplement Left Inguinal Lymphatic with Nonautologous Tissue Substitute, Percutaneous Endoscopic Approach

07UK07Z Supplement Thoracic Duct with Autologous Tissue Substitute, Open Approach

07UK0JZ Supplement Thoracic Duct with Synthetic Substitute, Open Approach

07UK0KZ Supplement Thoracic Duct with Nonautologous Tissue Substitute, Open Approach

07UK47Z Supplement Thoracic Duct with Autologous Tissue Substitute, Percutaneous Endoscopic Approach

07UK4JZ Supplement Thoracic Duct with Synthetic Substitute, Percutaneous Endoscopic Approach

07UK4KZ Supplement Thoracic Duct with Nonautologous Tissue Substitute, Percutaneous Endoscopic Approach

07UL07Z Supplement Cisterna Chyli with Autologous Tissue Substitute, Open Approach

07UL0JZ Supplement Cisterna Chyli with Synthetic Substitute, Open Approach

07UL0KZ Supplement Cisterna Chyli with Nonautologous Tissue Substitute, Open Approach

07UL47Z Supplement Cisterna Chyli with Autologous Tissue Substitute, Percutaneous Endoscopic Approach

07UL4JZ Supplement Cisterna Chyli with Synthetic Substitute, Percutaneous Endoscopic Approach

07UL4KZ Supplement Cisterna Chyli with Nonautologous Tissue Substitute, Percutaneous Endoscopic Approach

07V – Lymphatic and Hemic Systems, Restriction

07V00CZ Restriction of Head Lymphatic with Extraluminal Device, Open Approach

07V00DZ Restriction of Head Lymphatic with Intraluminal Device, Open Approach

07V00ZZ Restriction of Head Lymphatic, Open Approach

07V03CZ Restriction of Head Lymphatic with Extraluminal Device, Percutaneous Approach

07V03DZ Restriction of Head Lymphatic with Intraluminal Device, Percutaneous Approach

07V03ZZ Restriction of Head Lymphatic, Percutaneous Approach

07V04CZ Restriction of Head Lymphatic with Extraluminal Device, Percutaneous Endoscopic Approach

07V04DZ Restriction of Head Lymphatic with Intraluminal Device, Percutaneous Endoscopic Approach

07V04ZZ Restriction of Head Lymphatic, Percutaneous Endoscopic Approach

07V10CZ Restriction of Right Neck Lymphatic with Extraluminal Device, Open Approach

07V10DZ Restriction of Right Neck Lymphatic with Intraluminal Device, Open Approach

07V10ZZ Restriction of Right Neck Lymphatic, Open Approach

07V13CZ Restriction of Right Neck Lymphatic with Extraluminal Device, Percutaneous Approach

07V13DZ Restriction of Right Neck Lymphatic with Intraluminal Device, Percutaneous Approach

07V13ZZ Restriction of Right Neck Lymphatic, Percutaneous Approach

07V14CZ Restriction of Right Neck Lymphatic with Extraluminal Device, Percutaneous Endoscopic Approach

07V14DZ Restriction of Right Neck Lymphatic with Intraluminal Device, Percutaneous Endoscopic Approach

07V14ZZ Restriction of Right Neck Lymphatic, Percutaneous Endoscopic Approach

07V20CZ Restriction of Left Neck Lymphatic with Extraluminal Device, Open Approach

07V20DZ Restriction of Left Neck Lymphatic with Intraluminal Device, Open Approach

07V20ZZ Restriction of Left Neck Lymphatic, Open Approach

07V23CZ Restriction of Left Neck Lymphatic with Extraluminal Device, Percutaneous Approach

07V23DZ Restriction of Left Neck Lymphatic with Intraluminal Device, Percutaneous Approach

07V23ZZ Restriction of Left Neck Lymphatic, Percutaneous Approach

07V24CZ Restriction of Left Neck Lymphatic with Extraluminal Device, Percutaneous Endoscopic Approach

07V24DZ Restriction of Left Neck Lymphatic with Intraluminal Device, Percutaneous Endoscopic Approach

07V24ZZ Restriction of Left Neck Lymphatic, Percutaneous Endoscopic Approach

07V30CZ Restriction of Right Upper Extremity Lymphatic with Extraluminal Device, Open Approach

07V30DZ Restriction of Right Upper Extremity Lymphatic with Intraluminal Device, Open Approach

07V30ZZ Restriction of Right Upper Extremity Lymphatic, Open Approach

07V33CZ Restriction of Right Upper Extremity Lymphatic with Extraluminal Device, Percutaneous Approach

07V33DZ Restriction of Right Upper Extremity Lymphatic with Intraluminal Device, Percutaneous Approach

07V33ZZ Restriction of Right Upper Extremity Lymphatic, Percutaneous Approach

07V34CZ Restriction of Right Upper Extremity Lymphatic with Extraluminal Device, Percutaneous Endoscopic Approach

07V34DZ Restriction of Right Upper Extremity Lymphatic with Intraluminal Device, Percutaneous Endoscopic Approach

07V34ZZ Restriction of Right Upper Extremity Lymphatic, Percutaneous Endoscopic Approach

07V40CZ Restriction of Left Upper Extremity Lymphatic with Extraluminal Device, Open Approach

07V40DZ Restriction of Left Upper Extremity Lymphatic with Intraluminal Device, Open Approach

07V40ZZ Restriction of Left Upper Extremity Lymphatic, Open Approach

07V43CZ Restriction of Left Upper Extremity Lymphatic with Extraluminal Device, Percutaneous Approach

07V43DZ Restriction of Left Upper Extremity Lymphatic with Intraluminal Device, Percutaneous Approach

07V43ZZ Restriction of Left Upper Extremity Lymphatic, Percutaneous Approach

07V44CZ Restriction of Left Upper Extremity Lymphatic with Extraluminal Device, Percutaneous Endoscopic Approach

07V44DZ Restriction of Left Upper Extremity Lymphatic with Intraluminal Device, Percutaneous Endoscopic Approach

07V44ZZ Restriction of Left Upper Extremity Lymphatic, Percutaneous Endoscopic Approach

07V50CZ Restriction of Right Axillary Lymphatic with Extraluminal Device, Open Approach

07V50DZ Restriction of Right Axillary Lymphatic with Intraluminal Device, Open Approach

07V50ZZ Restriction of Right Axillary Lymphatic, Open Approach

07V53CZ Restriction of Right Axillary Lymphatic with Extraluminal Device, Percutaneous Approach

07V53DZ Restriction of Right Axillary Lymphatic with Intraluminal Device, Percutaneous Approach

07V53ZZ Restriction of Right Axillary Lymphatic, Percutaneous Approach

07V54CZ Restriction of Right Axillary Lymphatic with Extraluminal Device, Percutaneous Endoscopic Approach

07V54DZ Restriction of Right Axillary Lymphatic with Intraluminal Device, Percutaneous Endoscopic Approach

07V54ZZ Restriction of Right Axillary Lymphatic, Percutaneous Endoscopic Approach

07V60CZ Restriction of Left Axillary Lymphatic with Extraluminal Device, Open Approach

07V60DZ Restriction of Left Axillary Lymphatic with Intraluminal Device, Open Approach

07V60ZZ Restriction of Left Axillary Lymphatic, Open Approach

07V63CZ Restriction of Left Axillary Lymphatic with Extraluminal Device, Percutaneous Approach

07V63DZ Restriction of Left Axillary Lymphatic with Intraluminal Device, Percutaneous Approach

07V63ZZ Restriction of Left Axillary Lymphatic, Percutaneous Approach

07V64CZ Restriction of Left Axillary Lymphatic with Extraluminal Device, Percutaneous Endoscopic Approach

07V64DZ Restriction of Left Axillary Lymphatic with Intraluminal Device, Percutaneous Endoscopic Approach

07V64ZZ Restriction of Left Axillary Lymphatic, Percutaneous Endoscopic Approach

07V70CZ Restriction of Thorax Lymphatic with Extraluminal Device, Open Approach

07V70DZ Restriction of Thorax Lymphatic with Intraluminal Device, Open Approach

07V70ZZ Restriction of Thorax Lymphatic, Open Approach

07V73CZ Restriction of Thorax Lymphatic with Extraluminal Device, Percutaneous Approach

07V73DZ Restriction of Thorax Lymphatic with Intraluminal Device, Percutaneous Approach

07V73ZZ Restriction of Thorax Lymphatic, Percutaneous Approach

07V74CZ Restriction of Thorax Lymphatic with Extraluminal Device, Percutaneous Endoscopic Approach

07V74DZ Restriction of Thorax Lymphatic with Intraluminal Device, Percutaneous Endoscopic Approach

07V74ZZ Restriction of Thorax Lymphatic, Percutaneous Endoscopic Approach

07V80CZ Restriction of Right Internal Mammary Lymphatic with Extraluminal Device, Open Approach

07V80DZ Restriction of Right Internal Mammary Lymphatic with Intraluminal Device, Open Approach

07V80ZZ Restriction of Right Internal Mammary Lymphatic, Open Approach

07V83CZ Restriction of Right Internal Mammary Lymphatic with Extraluminal Device, Percutaneous Approach

07V83DZ Restriction of Right Internal Mammary Lymphatic with Intraluminal Device, Percutaneous Approach

07V83ZZ Restriction of Right Internal Mammary Lymphatic, Percutaneous Approach

07V84CZ Restriction of Right Internal Mammary Lymphatic with Extraluminal Device, Percutaneous Endoscopic Approach

07V84DZ Restriction of Right Internal Mammary Lymphatic with Intraluminal Device, Percutaneous Endoscopic Approach

07V84ZZ Restriction of Right Internal Mammary Lymphatic, Percutaneous Endoscopic Approach

07V90CZ Restriction of Left Internal Mammary Lymphatic with Extraluminal Device, Open Approach

07V90DZ Restriction of Left Internal Mammary Lymphatic with Intraluminal Device, Open Approach

07V90ZZ Restriction of Left Internal Mammary Lymphatic, Open Approach

07V93CZ Restriction of Left Internal Mammary Lymphatic with Extraluminal Device, Percutaneous Approach

07V93DZ Restriction of Left Internal Mammary Lymphatic with Intraluminal Device, Percutaneous Approach

07V93ZZ Restriction of Left Internal Mammary Lymphatic, Percutaneous Approach

07V94CZ Restriction of Left Internal Mammary Lymphatic with Extraluminal Device, Percutaneous Endoscopic Approach

07V94DZ Restriction of Left Internal Mammary Lymphatic with Intraluminal Device, Percutaneous Endoscopic Approach

07V94ZZ Restriction of Left Internal Mammary Lymphatic, Percutaneous Endoscopic Approach

07VB0CZ Restriction of Mesenteric Lymphatic with Extraluminal Device, Open Approach

07VB0DZ Restriction of Mesenteric Lymphatic with Intraluminal Device, Open Approach

07VB0ZZ Restriction of Mesenteric Lymphatic, Open Approach

07VB3CZ Restriction of Mesenteric Lymphatic with Extraluminal Device, Percutaneous Approach

07VB3DZ Restriction of Mesenteric Lymphatic with Intraluminal Device, Percutaneous Approach

07VB3ZZ Restriction of Mesenteric Lymphatic, Percutaneous Approach

07VB4CZ Restriction of Mesenteric Lymphatic with Extraluminal Device, Percutaneous Endoscopic Approach

07VB4DZ Restriction of Mesenteric Lymphatic with Intraluminal Device, Percutaneous Endoscopic Approach

07VB4ZZ Restriction of Mesenteric Lymphatic, Percutaneous Endoscopic Approach

07VC0CZ Restriction of Pelvis Lymphatic with Extraluminal Device, Open Approach

07VC0DZ Restriction of Pelvis Lymphatic with Intraluminal Device, Open Approach

07VC0ZZ Restriction of Pelvis Lymphatic, Open Approach

07VC3CZ Restriction of Pelvis Lymphatic with Extraluminal Device, Percutaneous Approach

07VC3DZ Restriction of Pelvis Lymphatic with Intraluminal Device, Percutaneous Approach

07VC3ZZ Restriction of Pelvis Lymphatic, Percutaneous Approach

07VC4CZ Restriction of Pelvis Lymphatic with Extraluminal Device, Percutaneous Endoscopic Approach

07VC4DZ Restriction of Pelvis Lymphatic with Intraluminal Device, Percutaneous Endoscopic Approach

07VC4ZZ Restriction of Pelvis Lymphatic, Percutaneous Endoscopic Approach

07VD0CZ Restriction of Aortic Lymphatic with Extraluminal Device, Open Approach

07VD0DZ Restriction of Aortic Lymphatic with Intraluminal Device, Open Approach

07VD0ZZ Restriction of Aortic Lymphatic, Open Approach

07VD3CZ Restriction of Aortic Lymphatic with Extraluminal Device, Percutaneous Approach

07VD3DZ Restriction of Aortic Lymphatic with Intraluminal Device, Percutaneous Approach

07VD3ZZ Restriction of Aortic Lymphatic, Percutaneous Approach

07VD4CZ Restriction of Aortic Lymphatic with Extraluminal Device, Percutaneous Endoscopic Approach

07VD4DZ Restriction of Aortic Lymphatic with Intraluminal Device, Percutaneous Endoscopic Approach

07VD4ZZ Restriction of Aortic Lymphatic, Percutaneous Endoscopic Approach

07VF0CZ Restriction of Right Lower Extremity Lymphatic with Extraluminal Device, Open Approach

♀ Female-only ♂ Male-only ▲ Limited Coverage ● Non-OR 🅗🅐🅒 HAC-associated procedure ▲ Non-covered procedures ➕ Cluster

07VF0DZ	Restriction of Right Lower Extremity Lymphatic with Intraluminal Device, Open Approach
07VF0ZZ	Restriction of Right Lower Extremity Lymphatic, Open Approach
07VF3CZ	Restriction of Right Lower Extremity Lymphatic with Extraluminal Device, Percutaneous Approach
07VF3DZ	Restriction of Right Lower Extremity Lymphatic with Intraluminal Device, Percutaneous Approach
07VF3ZZ	Restriction of Right Lower Extremity Lymphatic, Percutaneous Approach
07VF4CZ	Restriction of Right Lower Extremity Lymphatic with Extraluminal Device, Percutaneous Endoscopic Approach
07VF4DZ	Restriction of Right Lower Extremity Lymphatic with Intraluminal Device, Percutaneous Endoscopic Approach
07VF4ZZ	Restriction of Right Lower Extremity Lymphatic, Percutaneous Endoscopic Approach
07VG0CZ	Restriction of Left Lower Extremity Lymphatic with Extraluminal Device, Open Approach
07VG0DZ	Restriction of Left Lower Extremity Lymphatic with Intraluminal Device, Open Approach
07VG0ZZ	Restriction of Left Lower Extremity Lymphatic, Open Approach
07VG3CZ	Restriction of Left Lower Extremity Lymphatic with Extraluminal Device, Percutaneous Approach
07VG3DZ	Restriction of Left Lower Extremity Lymphatic with Intraluminal Device, Percutaneous Approach
07VG3ZZ	Restriction of Left Lower Extremity Lymphatic, Percutaneous Approach
07VG4CZ	Restriction of Left Lower Extremity Lymphatic with Extraluminal Device, Percutaneous Endoscopic Approach
07VG4DZ	Restriction of Left Lower Extremity Lymphatic with Intraluminal Device, Percutaneous Endoscopic Approach

07VG4ZZ	Restriction of Left Lower Extremity Lymphatic, Percutaneous Endoscopic Approach
07VH0CZ	Restriction of Right Inguinal Lymphatic with Extraluminal Device, Open Approach
07VH0DZ	Restriction of Right Inguinal Lymphatic with Intraluminal Device, Open Approach
07VH0ZZ	Restriction of Right Inguinal Lymphatic, Open Approach
07VH3CZ	Restriction of Right Inguinal Lymphatic with Extraluminal Device, Percutaneous Approach
07VH3DZ	Restriction of Right Inguinal Lymphatic with Intraluminal Device, Percutaneous Approach
07VH3ZZ	Restriction of Right Inguinal Lymphatic, Percutaneous Approach
07VH4CZ	Restriction of Right Inguinal Lymphatic with Extraluminal Device, Percutaneous Endoscopic Approach
07VH4DZ	Restriction of Right Inguinal Lymphatic with Intraluminal Device, Percutaneous Endoscopic Approach
07VH4ZZ	Restriction of Right Inguinal Lymphatic, Percutaneous Endoscopic Approach
07VJ0CZ	Restriction of Left Inguinal Lymphatic with Extraluminal Device, Open Approach
07VJ0DZ	Restriction of Left Inguinal Lymphatic with Intraluminal Device, Open Approach
07VJ0ZZ	Restriction of Left Inguinal Lymphatic, Open Approach
07VJ3CZ	Restriction of Left Inguinal Lymphatic with Extraluminal Device, Percutaneous Approach
07VJ3DZ	Restriction of Left Inguinal Lymphatic with Intraluminal Device, Percutaneous Approach
07VJ3ZZ	Restriction of Left Inguinal Lymphatic, Percutaneous Approach
07VJ4CZ	Restriction of Left Inguinal Lymphatic with Extraluminal Device, Percutaneous Endoscopic Approach
07VJ4DZ	Restriction of Left Inguinal Lymphatic with Intraluminal Device, Percutaneous Endoscopic Approach

07VJ4ZZ	Restriction of Left Inguinal Lymphatic, Percutaneous Endoscopic Approach
07VK0CZ	Restriction of Thoracic Duct with Extraluminal Device, Open Approach
07VK0DZ	Restriction of Thoracic Duct with Intraluminal Device, Open Approach
07VK0ZZ	Restriction of Thoracic Duct, Open Approach
07VK3CZ	Restriction of Thoracic Duct with Extraluminal Device, Percutaneous Approach
07VK3DZ	Restriction of Thoracic Duct with Intraluminal Device, Percutaneous Approach
07VK3ZZ	Restriction of Thoracic Duct, Percutaneous Approach
07VK4CZ	Restriction of Thoracic Duct with Extraluminal Device, Percutaneous Endoscopic Approach
07VK4DZ	Restriction of Thoracic Duct with Intraluminal Device, Percutaneous Endoscopic Approach
07VK4ZZ	Restriction of Thoracic Duct, Percutaneous Endoscopic Approach
07VL0CZ	Restriction of Cisterna Chyli with Extraluminal Device, Open Approach
07VL0DZ	Restriction of Cisterna Chyli with Intraluminal Device, Open Approach
07VL0ZZ	Restriction of Cisterna Chyli, Open Approach
07VL3CZ	Restriction of Cisterna Chyli with Extraluminal Device, Percutaneous Approach
07VL3DZ	Restriction of Cisterna Chyli with Intraluminal Device, Percutaneous Approach
07VL3ZZ	Restriction of Cisterna Chyli, Percutaneous Approach
07VL4CZ	Restriction of Cisterna Chyli with Extraluminal Device, Percutaneous Endoscopic Approach
07VL4DZ	Restriction of Cisterna Chyli with Intraluminal Device, Percutaneous Endoscopic Approach
07VL4ZZ	Restriction of Cisterna Chyli, Percutaneous Endoscopic Approach

07W – Lymphatic and Hemic Systems, Revision

Review Coding Guideline B6.1c

07WK00Z	Revision of Drainage Device in Thoracic Duct, Open Approach
07WK03Z	Revision of Infusion Device in Thoracic Duct, Open Approach
07WK07Z	Revision of Autologous Tissue Substitute in Thoracic Duct, Open Approach
07WK0CZ	Revision of Extraluminal Device in Thoracic Duct, Open Approach
07WK0DZ	Revision of Intraluminal Device in Thoracic Duct, Open Approach
07WK0JZ	Revision of Synthetic Substitute in Thoracic Duct, Open Approach
07WK0KZ	Revision of Nonautologous Tissue Substitute in Thoracic Duct, Open Approach
07WK0YZ	Revision of Other Device in Thoracic Duct, Open Approach
07WK30Z	Revision of Drainage Device in Thoracic Duct, Percutaneous Approach
07WK33Z	Revision of Infusion Device in Thoracic Duct, Percutaneous Approach
07WK37Z	Revision of Autologous Tissue Substitute in Thoracic Duct, Percutaneous Approach
07WK3CZ	Revision of Extraluminal Device in Thoracic Duct, Percutaneous Approach

07WK3DZ	Revision of Intraluminal Device in Thoracic Duct, Percutaneous Approach
07WK3JZ	Revision of Synthetic Substitute in Thoracic Duct, Percutaneous Approach
07WK3KZ	Revision of Nonautologous Tissue Substitute in Thoracic Duct, Percutaneous Approach
07WK3YZ	Revision of Other Device in Thoracic Duct, Percutaneous Approach
07WK40Z	Revision of Drainage Device in Thoracic Duct, Percutaneous Endoscopic Approach
07WK43Z	Revision of Infusion Device in Thoracic Duct, Percutaneous Endoscopic Approach
07WK47Z	Revision of Autologous Tissue Substitute in Thoracic Duct, Percutaneous Endoscopic Approach
07WK4CZ	Revision of Extraluminal Device in Thoracic Duct, Percutaneous Endoscopic Approach
07WK4DZ	Revision of Intraluminal Device in Thoracic Duct, Percutaneous Endoscopic Approach
07WK4JZ	Revision of Synthetic Substitute in Thoracic Duct, Percutaneous Endoscopic Approach

07WK4KZ	Revision of Nonautologous Tissue Substitute in Thoracic Duct, Percutaneous Endoscopic Approach
07WK4YZ	Revision of Other Device in Thoracic Duct, Percutaneous Endoscopic Approach
07WKX0Z	Revision of Drainage Device in Thoracic Duct, External Approach
07WKX3Z	Revision of Infusion Device in Thoracic Duct, External Approach
07WKX7Z	Revision of Autologous Tissue Substitute in Thoracic Duct, External Approach
07WKXCZ	Revision of Extraluminal Device in Thoracic Duct, External Approach
07WKXDZ	Revision of Intraluminal Device in Thoracic Duct, External Approach
07WKXJZ	Revision of Synthetic Substitute in Thoracic Duct, External Approach
07WKXKZ	Revision of Nonautologous Tissue Substitute in Thoracic Duct, External Approach
07WL00Z	Revision of Drainage Device in Cisterna Chyli, Open Approach
07WL03Z	Revision of Infusion Device in Cisterna Chyli, Open Approach

07WL07Z   Revision of Autologous Tissue Substitute in Cisterna Chyli, Open Approach

07WL0CZ   Revision of Extraluminal Device in Cisterna Chyli, Open Approach

07WL0DZ   Revision of Intraluminal Device in Cisterna Chyli, Open Approach

07WL0JZ   Revision of Synthetic Substitute in Cisterna Chyli, Open Approach

07WL0KZ   Revision of Nonautologous Tissue Substitute in Cisterna Chyli, Open Approach

07WL0YZ   Revision of Other Device in Cisterna Chyli, Open Approach

07WL30Z   Revision of Drainage Device in Cisterna Chyli, Percutaneous Approach

07WL33Z   Revision of Infusion Device in Cisterna Chyli, Percutaneous Approach

07WL37Z   Revision of Autologous Tissue Substitute in Cisterna Chyli, Percutaneous Approach

07WL3CZ   Revision of Extraluminal Device in Cisterna Chyli, Percutaneous Approach

07WL3DZ   Revision of Intraluminal Device in Cisterna Chyli, Percutaneous Approach

07WL3JZ   Revision of Synthetic Substitute in Cisterna Chyli, Percutaneous Approach

07WL3KZ   Revision of Nonautologous Tissue Substitute in Cisterna Chyli, Percutaneous Approach

07WL3YZ   Revision of Other Device in Cisterna Chyli, Percutaneous Approach

07WL40Z   Revision of Drainage Device in Cisterna Chyli, Percutaneous Endoscopic Approach

07WL43Z   Revision of Infusion Device in Cisterna Chyli, Percutaneous Endoscopic Approach

07WL47Z   Revision of Autologous Tissue Substitute in Cisterna Chyli, Percutaneous Endoscopic Approach

07WL4CZ   Revision of Extraluminal Device in Cisterna Chyli, Percutaneous Endoscopic Approach

07WL4DZ   Revision of Intraluminal Device in Cisterna Chyli, Percutaneous Endoscopic Approach

07WL4JZ   Revision of Synthetic Substitute in Cisterna Chyli, Percutaneous Endoscopic Approach

07WL4KZ   Revision of Nonautologous Tissue Substitute in Cisterna Chyli, Percutaneous Endoscopic Approach

07WL4YZ   Revision of Other Device in Cisterna Chyli, Percutaneous Endoscopic Approach

07WLX0Z   Revision of Drainage Device in Cisterna Chyli, External Approach

07WLX3Z   Revision of Infusion Device in Cisterna Chyli, External Approach

07WLX7Z   Revision of Autologous Tissue Substitute in Cisterna Chyli, External Approach

07WLXCZ   Revision of Extraluminal Device in Cisterna Chyli, External Approach

07WLXDZ   Revision of Intraluminal Device in Cisterna Chyli, External Approach

07WLXJZ   Revision of Synthetic Substitute in Cisterna Chyli, External Approach

07WLXKZ   Revision of Nonautologous Tissue Substitute in Cisterna Chyli, External Approach

07WM00Z   Revision of Drainage Device in Thymus, Open Approach

07WM03Z   Revision of Infusion Device in Thymus, Open Approach

07WM0YZ   Revision of Other Device in Thymus, Open Approach

07WM30Z   Revision of Drainage Device in Thymus, Percutaneous Approach

07WM33Z   Revision of Infusion Device in Thymus, Percutaneous Approach

07WM3YZ   Revision of Other Device in Thymus, Percutaneous Approach

07WM40Z   Revision of Drainage Device in Thymus, Percutaneous Endoscopic Approach

07WM43Z   Revision of Infusion Device in Thymus, Percutaneous Endoscopic Approach

07WM4YZ   Revision of Other Device in Thymus, Percutaneous Endoscopic Approach

07WMX0Z   Revision of Drainage Device in Thymus, External Approach

07WMX3Z   Revision of Infusion Device in Thymus, External Approach

07WN00Z   Revision of Drainage Device in Lymphatic, Open Approach

07WN03Z   Revision of Infusion Device in Lymphatic, Open Approach

07WN07Z   Revision of Autologous Tissue Substitute in Lymphatic, Open Approach

07WN0CZ   Revision of Extraluminal Device in Lymphatic, Open Approach

07WN0DZ   Revision of Intraluminal Device in Lymphatic, Open Approach

07WN0JZ   Revision of Synthetic Substitute in Lymphatic, Open Approach

07WN0KZ   Revision of Nonautologous Tissue Substitute in Lymphatic, Open Approach

07WN0YZ   Revision of Other Device in Lymphatic, Open Approach

07WN30Z   Revision of Drainage Device in Lymphatic, Percutaneous Approach

07WN33Z   Revision of Infusion Device in Lymphatic, Percutaneous Approach

07WN37Z   Revision of Autologous Tissue Substitute in Lymphatic, Percutaneous Approach

07WN3CZ   Revision of Extraluminal Device in Lymphatic, Percutaneous Approach

07WN3DZ   Revision of Intraluminal Device in Lymphatic, Percutaneous Approach

07WN3JZ   Revision of Synthetic Substitute in Lymphatic, Percutaneous Approach

07WN3KZ   Revision of Nonautologous Tissue Substitute in Lymphatic, Percutaneous Approach

07WN3YZ   Revision of Other Device in Lymphatic, Percutaneous Approach

07WN40Z   Revision of Drainage Device in Lymphatic, Percutaneous Endoscopic Approach

07WN43Z   Revision of Infusion Device in Lymphatic, Percutaneous Endoscopic Approach

07WN47Z   Revision of Autologous Tissue Substitute in Lymphatic, Percutaneous Endoscopic Approach

07WN4CZ   Revision of Extraluminal Device in Lymphatic, Percutaneous Endoscopic Approach

07WN4DZ   Revision of Intraluminal Device in Lymphatic, Percutaneous Endoscopic Approach

07WN4JZ   Revision of Synthetic Substitute in Lymphatic, Percutaneous Endoscopic Approach

07WN4KZ   Revision of Nonautologous Tissue Substitute in Lymphatic, Percutaneous Endoscopic Approach

07WN4YZ   Revision of Other Device in Lymphatic, Percutaneous Endoscopic Approach

07WNX0Z   Revision of Drainage Device in Lymphatic, External Approach

07WNX3Z   Revision of Infusion Device in Lymphatic, External Approach

07WNX7Z   Revision of Autologous Tissue Substitute in Lymphatic, External Approach

07WNXCZ   Revision of Extraluminal Device in Lymphatic, External Approach

07WNXDZ   Revision of Intraluminal Device in Lymphatic, External Approach

07WNXJZ   Revision of Synthetic Substitute in Lymphatic, External Approach

07WNXKZ   Revision of Nonautologous Tissue Substitute in Lymphatic, External Approach

07WP00Z   Revision of Drainage Device in Spleen, Open Approach

07WP03Z   Revision of Infusion Device in Spleen, Open Approach

07WP0YZ   Revision of Other Device in Spleen, Open Approach

07WP30Z   Revision of Drainage Device in Spleen, Percutaneous Approach

07WP33Z   Revision of Infusion Device in Spleen, Percutaneous Approach

07WP3YZ   Revision of Other Device in Spleen, Percutaneous Approach

07WP40Z   Revision of Drainage Device in Spleen, Percutaneous Endoscopic Approach

07WP43Z   Revision of Infusion Device in Spleen, Percutaneous Endoscopic Approach

07WP4YZ   Revision of Other Device in Spleen, Percutaneous Endoscopic Approach

07WPX0Z   Revision of Drainage Device in Spleen, External Approach

07WPX3Z   Revision of Infusion Device in Spleen, External Approach

07WT00Z   Revision of Drainage Device in Bone Marrow, Open Approach

07WT30Z   Revision of Drainage Device in Bone Marrow, Percutaneous Approach

07WT40Z   Revision of Drainage Device in Bone Marrow, Percutaneous Endoscopic Approach

07WTX0Z   Revision of Drainage Device in Bone Marrow, External Approach

07Y – Lymphatic and Hemic Systems, Transplantation

Review Coding Guideline B3.16

07YM0Z0   Transplantation of Thymus, Allogeneic, Open Approach
AHA CC: 3Q, 2019, 29

07YM0Z1   Transplantation of Thymus, Syngeneic, Open Approach

07YM0Z2   Transplantation of Thymus, Zooplastic, Open Approach

07YP0Z0   Transplantation of Spleen, Allogeneic, Open Approach

07YP0Z1   Transplantation of Spleen, Syngeneic, Open Approach

07YP0Z2   Transplantation of Spleen, Zooplastic, Open Approach

♀ Female-only   ♂ Male-only   ▲ Limited Coverage   ● Non-OR   HAC HAC-associated procedure   ▲ Non-covered procedures   ➕ Cluster

Anatomy of the Eyeball

Horizontal section

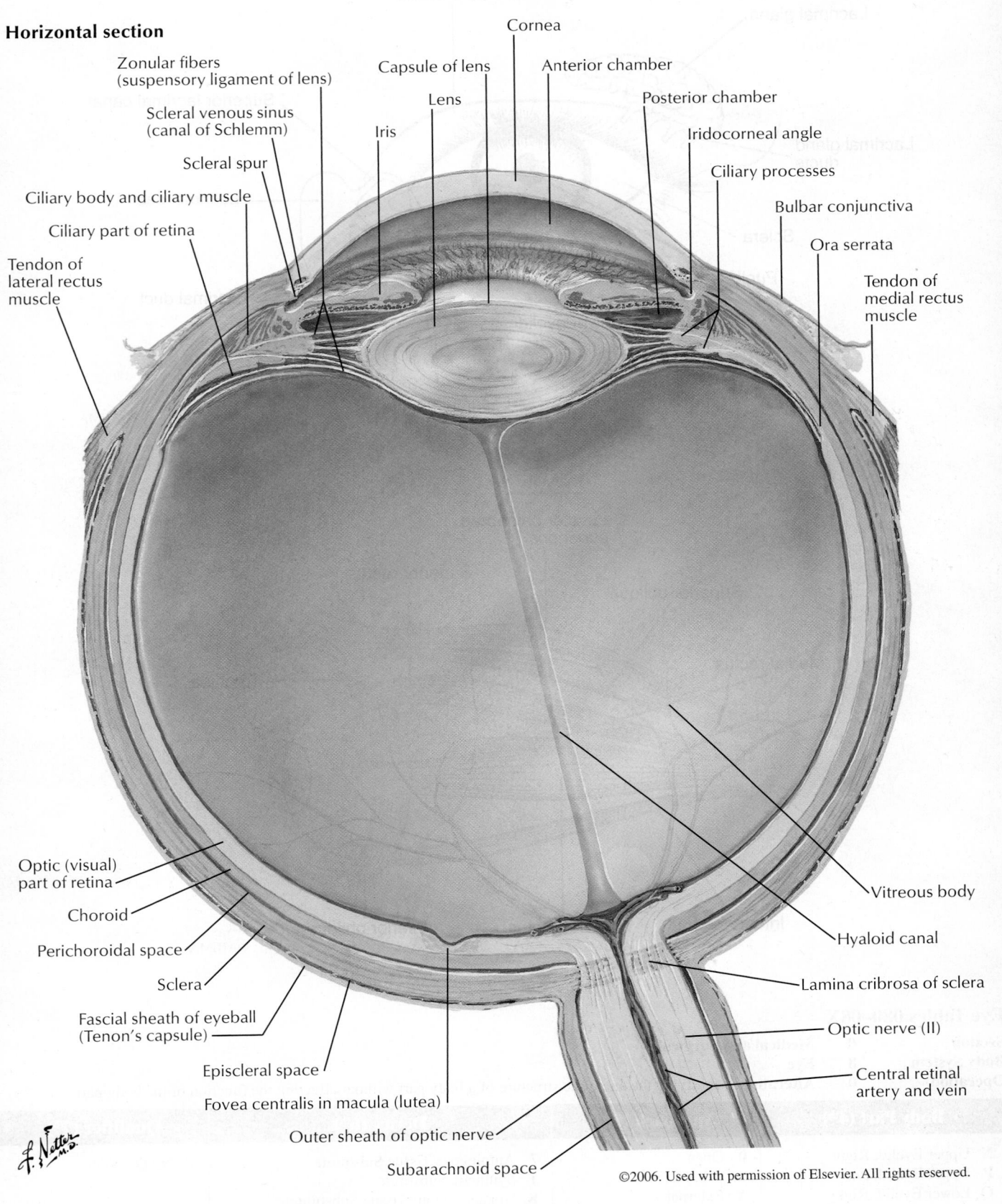

Zonular fibers (suspensory ligament of lens)

Scleral venous sinus (canal of Schlemm)

Scleral spur

Ciliary body and ciliary muscle

Ciliary part of retina

Tendon of lateral rectus muscle

Capsule of lens

Lens

Iris

Cornea

Anterior chamber

Posterior chamber

Iridocorneal angle

Ciliary processes

Bulbar conjunctiva

Ora serrata

Tendon of medial rectus muscle

Optic (visual) part of retina

Choroid

Perichoroidal space

Sclera

Fascial sheath of eyeball (Tenon's capsule)

Episcleral space

Fovea centralis in macula (lutea)

Outer sheath of optic nerve

Subarachnoid space

Vitreous body

Hyaloid canal

Lamina cribrosa of sclera

Optic nerve (II)

Central retinal artery and vein

080

Eyelid

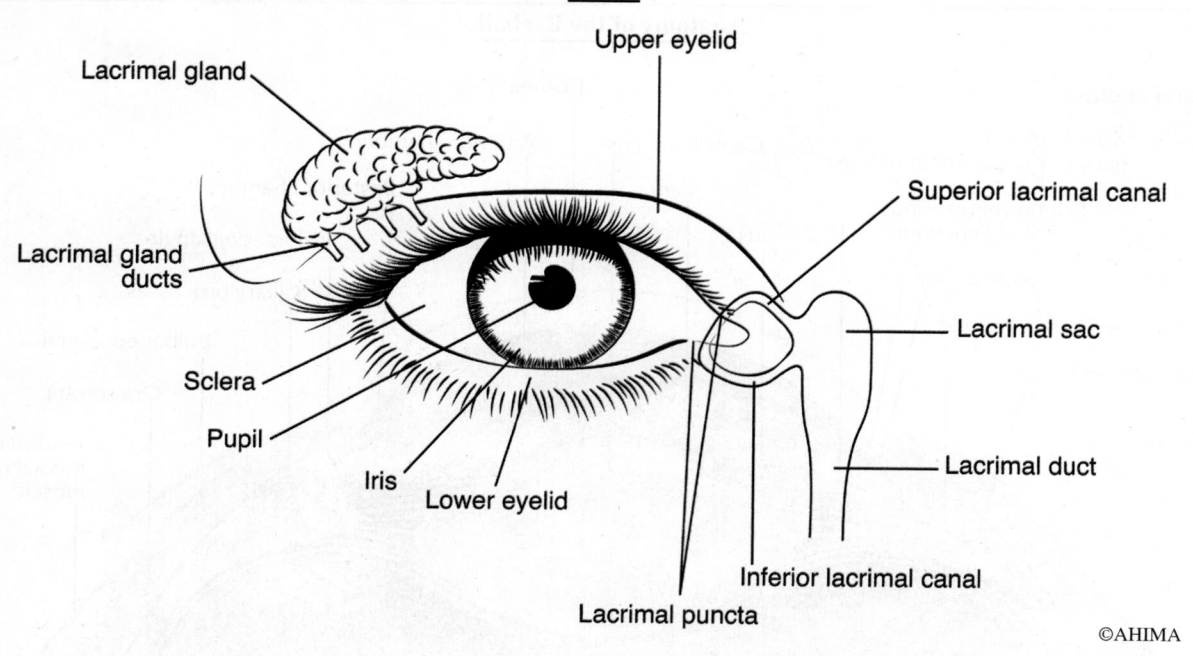

Lacrimal gland

Upper eyelid

Lacrimal gland ducts

Superior lacrimal canal

Sclera

Lacrimal sac

Pupil

Lacrimal duct

Iris

Lower eyelid

Inferior lacrimal canal

Lacrimal puncta

©AHIMA

Eye Muscles

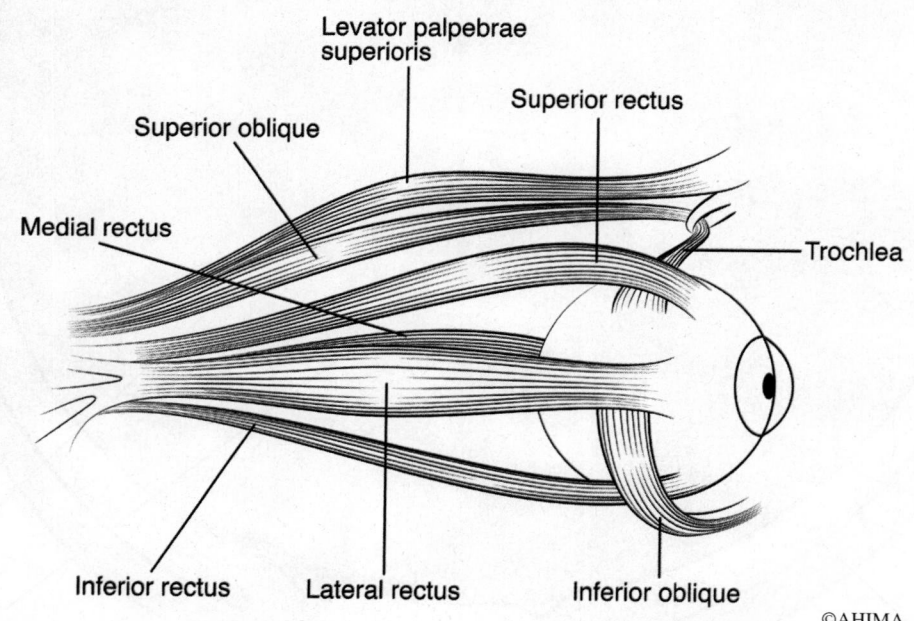

Levator palpebrae superioris

Superior rectus

Superior oblique

Medial rectus

Trochlea

Inferior rectus

Lateral rectus

Inferior oblique

©AHIMA

Eye Tables 080–08X

Section   **0**   **Medical and Surgical**
Body System   **8**   **Eye**
Operation   **0**   **Alteration:** Modifying the anatomic structure of a body part without affecting the function of the body part

Body Part (4ᵗʰ)	Approach (5ᵗʰ)	Device (6ᵗʰ)	Qualifier (7ᵗʰ)
N Upper Eyelid, Right **P** Upper Eyelid, Left **Q** Lower Eyelid, Right **R** Lower Eyelid, Left	**0** Open **3** Percutaneous **X** External	**7** Autologous Tissue Substitute **J** Synthetic Substitute **K** Nonautologous Tissue Substitute **Z** No Device	**Z** No Qualifier

Section   **0**   **Medical and Surgical**
Body System   **8**   **Eye**
Operation   **1**   **Bypass:** Altering the route of passage of the contents of a tubular body part

Body Part (4th)	Approach (5th)	Device (6th)	Qualifier (7th)
2 Anterior Chamber, Right 3 Anterior Chamber, Left	3 Percutaneous	J Synthetic Substitute K Nonautologous Tissue Substitute Z No Device	4 Sclera
X Lacrimal Duct, Right Y Lacrimal Duct, Left	0 Open 3 Percutaneous	J Synthetic Substitute K Nonautologous Tissue Substitute Z No Device	3 Nasal Cavity

Section   **0**   **Medical and Surgical**
Body System   **8**   **Eye**
Operation   **2**   **Change:** Taking out or off a device from a body part and putting back an identical or similar device in or on the same body part without cutting or puncturing the skin or a mucous membrane

Body Part (4th)	Approach (5th)	Device (6th)	Qualifier (7th)
0 Eye, Right 1 Eye, Left	X External	0 Drainage Device Y Other Device	Z No Qualifier

Section   **0**   **Medical and Surgical**
Body System   **8**   **Eye**
Operation   **5**   **Destruction:** Physical eradication of all or a portion of a body part by the direct use of energy, force, or a destructive agent

Body Part (4th)	Approach (5th)	Device (6th)	Qualifier (7th)
0 Eye, Right 1 Eye, Left 6 Sclera, Right 7 Sclera, Left 8 Cornea, Right 9 Cornea, Left S Conjunctiva, Right T Conjunctiva, Left	X External	Z No Device	Z No Qualifier
2 Anterior Chamber, Right 3 Anterior Chamber, Left 4 Vitreous, Right 5 Vitreous, Left C Iris, Right D Iris, Left E Retina, Right F Retina, Left G Retinal Vessel, Right H Retinal Vessel, Left J Lens, Right K Lens, Left	3 Percutaneous	Z No Device	Z No Qualifier
A Choroid, Right B Choroid, Left L Extraocular Muscle, Right M Extraocular Muscle, Left V Lacrimal Gland, Right W Lacrimal Gland, Left	0 Open 3 Percutaneous	Z No Device	Z No Qualifier
N Upper Eyelid, Right P Upper Eyelid, Left Q Lower Eyelid, Right R Lower Eyelid, Left	0 Open 3 Percutaneous X External	Z No Device	Z No Qualifier
X Lacrimal Duct, Right Y Lacrimal Duct, Left	0 Open 3 Percutaneous 7 Via Natural or Artificial Opening 8 Via Natural or Artificial Opening Endoscopic	Z No Device	Z No Qualifier

Section   **0**   **Medical and Surgical**
Body System   **8**   **Eye**
Operation   **7**   **Dilation:** Expanding an orifice or the lumen of a tubular body part

Body Part (4th)	Approach (5th)	Device (6th)	Qualifier (7th)
X Lacrimal Duct, Right Y Lacrimal Duct, Left	0 Open 3 Percutaneous 7 Via Natural or Artificial Opening 8 Via Natural or Artificial Opening Endoscopic	D Intraluminal Device Z No Device	Z No Qualifier

Section   **0**   **Medical and Surgical**
Body System   **8**   **Eye**
Operation   **9**   **Drainage:** Taking or letting out fluids and/or gases from a body part

Body Part (4th)	Approach (5th)	Device (6th)	Qualifier (7th)
0 Eye, Right 1 Eye, Left 6 Sclera, Right 7 Sclera, Left 8 Cornea, Right 9 Cornea, Left S Conjunctiva, Right T Conjunctiva, Left	X External	0 Drainage Device	Z No Qualifier
0 Eye, Right 1 Eye, Left 6 Sclera, Right 7 Sclera, Left 8 Cornea, Right 9 Cornea, Left S Conjunctiva, Right T Conjunctiva, Left	X External	Z No Device	X Diagnostic Z No Qualifier
2 Anterior Chamber, Right 3 Anterior Chamber, Left 4 Vitreous, Right 5 Vitreous, Left C Iris, Right D Iris, Left E Retina, Right F Retina, Left G Retinal Vessel, Right H Retinal Vessel, Left J Lens, Right K Lens, Left	3 Percutaneous	0 Drainage Device	Z No Qualifier
2 Anterior Chamber, Right 3 Anterior Chamber, Left 4 Vitreous, Right 5 Vitreous, Left C Iris, Right D Iris, Left E Retina, Right F Retina, Left G Retinal Vessel, Right H Retinal Vessel, Left J Lens, Right K Lens, Left	3 Percutaneous	Z No Device	X Diagnostic Z No Qualifier
A Choroid, Right B Choroid, Left L Extraocular Muscle, Right M Extraocular Muscle, Left V Lacrimal Gland, Right W Lacrimal Gland, Left	0 Open 3 Percutaneous	0 Drainage Device	Z No Qualifier

Continued →

Section 0 **Medical and Surgical**
Body System 8 **Eye**
Operation 9 **Drainage:** Taking or letting out fluids and/or gases from a body part

Body Part (4th)	Approach (5th)	Device (6th)	Qualifier (7th)
A Choroid, Right B Choroid, Left L Extraocular Muscle, Right M Extraocular Muscle, Left V Lacrimal Gland, Right W Lacrimal Gland, Left	0 Open 3 Percutaneous	Z No Device	X Diagnostic Z No Qualifier
N Upper Eyelid, Right P Upper Eyelid, Left Q Lower Eyelid, Right R Lower Eyelid, Left	0 Open 3 Percutaneous X External	0 Drainage Device	Z No Qualifier
N Upper Eyelid, Right P Upper Eyelid, Left Q Lower Eyelid, Right R Lower Eyelid, Left	0 Open 3 Percutaneous X External	Z No Device	X Diagnostic Z No Qualifier
X Lacrimal Duct, Right Y Lacrimal Duct, Left	0 Open 3 Percutaneous 7 Via Natural or Artificial Opening 8 Via Natural or Artificial Opening Endoscopic	0 Drainage Device	Z No Qualifier
X Lacrimal Duct, Right Y Lacrimal Duct, Left	0 Open 3 Percutaneous 7 Via Natural or Artificial Opening 8 Via Natural or Artificial Opening Endoscopic	Z No Device	X Diagnostic Z No Qualifier

Section 0 **Medical and Surgical**
Body System 8 **Eye**
Operation B **Excision:** Cutting out or off, without replacement, a portion of a body part

Body Part (4th)	Approach (5th)	Device (6th)	Qualifier (7th)
0 Eye, Right 1 Eye, Left N Upper Eyelid, Right P Upper Eyelid, Left Q Lower Eyelid, Right R Lower Eyelid, Left	0 Open 3 Percutaneous X External	Z No Device	X Diagnostic Z No Qualifier
4 Vitreous, Right 5 Vitreous, Left C Iris, Right D Iris, Left E Retina, Right F Retina, Left J Lens, Right K Lens, Left	3 Percutaneous	Z No Device	X Diagnostic Z No Qualifier
6 Sclera, Right 7 Sclera, Left 8 Cornea, Right 9 Cornea, Left S Conjunctiva, Right T Conjunctiva, Left	X External	Z No Device	X Diagnostic Z No Qualifier

Continued →

Section	0	Medical and Surgical
Body System	8	Eye
Operation	B	Excision: Cutting out or off, without replacement, a portion of a body part

Body Part (4th)	Approach (5th)	Device (6th)	Qualifier (7th)
A Choroid, Right B Choroid, Left L Extraocular Muscle, Right M Extraocular Muscle, Left V Lacrimal Gland, Right W Lacrimal Gland, Left	0 Open 3 Percutaneous	Z No Device	X Diagnostic Z No Qualifier
X Lacrimal Duct, Right Y Lacrimal Duct, Left	0 Open 3 Percutaneous 7 Via Natural or Artificial Opening 8 Via Natural or Artificial Opening Endoscopic	Z No Device	X Diagnostic Z No Qualifier

Section	0	Medical and Surgical
Body System	8	Eye
Operation	C	Extirpation: Taking or cutting out solid matter from a body part

Body Part (4th)	Approach (5th)	Device (6th)	Qualifier (7th)
0 Eye, Right 1 Eye, Left 6 Sclera, Right 7 Sclera, Left 8 Cornea, Right 9 Cornea, Left S Conjunctiva, Right T Conjunctiva, Left	X External	Z No Device	Z No Qualifier
2 Anterior Chamber, Right 3 Anterior Chamber, Left 4 Vitreous, Right 5 Vitreous, Left C Iris, Right D Iris, Left E Retina, Right F Retina, Left G Retinal Vessel, Right H Retinal Vessel, Left J Lens, Right K Lens, Left	3 Percutaneous X External	Z No Device	Z No Qualifier
A Choroid, Right B Choroid, Left L Extraocular Muscle, Right M Extraocular Muscle, Left N Upper Eyelid, Right P Upper Eyelid, Left Q Lower Eyelid, Right R Lower Eyelid, Left V Lacrimal Gland, Right W Lacrimal Gland, Left	0 Open 3 Percutaneous X External	Z No Device	Z No Qualifier
X Lacrimal Duct, Right Y Lacrimal Duct, Left	0 Open 3 Percutaneous 7 Via Natural or Artificial Opening 8 Via Natural or Artificial Opening Endoscopic	Z No Device	Z No Qualifier

Section   0   Medical and Surgical
Body System   8   Eye
Operation   D   **Extraction:** Pulling or stripping out or off all or a portion of a body part by the use of force

Body Part (4th)	Approach (5th)	Device (6th)	Qualifier (7th)
8 Cornea, Right 9 Cornea, Left	X External	Z No Device	X Diagnostic Z No Qualifier
J Lens, Right K Lens, Left	3 Percutaneous	Z No Device	Z No Qualifier

Section   0   Medical and Surgical
Body System   8   Eye
Operation   F   **Fragmentation:** Breaking solid matter in a body part into pieces

Body Part (4th)	Approach (5th)	Device (6th)	Qualifier (7th)
4 Vitreous, Right 5 Vitreous, Left	3 Percutaneous X External	Z No Device	Z No Qualifier

Section   0   Medical and Surgical
Body System   8   Eye
Operation   H   **Insertion:** Putting in a nonbiological appliance that monitors, assists, performs, or prevents a physiological function but does not physically take the place of a body part

Body Part (4th)	Approach (5th)	Device (6th)	Qualifier (7th)
0 Eye, Right 1 Eye, Left	0 Open	5 Epiretinal Visual Prosthesis Y Other Device	Z No Qualifier
0 Eye, Right 1 Eye, Left	3 Percutaneous	1 Radioactive Element 3 Infusion Device Y Other Device	Z No Qualifier
0 Eye, Right 1 Eye, Left	7 Via Natural or Artificial Opening 8 Via Natural or Artificial Opening Endoscopic	Y Other Device	Z No Qualifier
0 Eye, Right 1 Eye, Left	X External	1 Radioactive Element 3 Infusion Device	Z No Qualifier

Section   0   Medical and Surgical
Body System   8   Eye
Operation   J   **Inspection:** Visually and/or manually exploring a body part

Body Part (4th)	Approach (5th)	Device (6th)	Qualifier (7th)
0 Eye, Right 1 Eye, Left J Lens, Right K Lens, Left	X External	Z No Device	Z No Qualifier
L Extraocular Muscle, Right M Extraocular Muscle, Left	0 Open X External	Z No Device	Z No Qualifier

Section   0   Medical and Surgical
Body System   8   Eye
Operation   L   **Occlusion:** Completely closing an orifice or the lumen of a tubular body part

Body Part (4th)	Approach (5th)	Device (6th)	Qualifier (7th)
X Lacrimal Duct, Right Y Lacrimal Duct, Left	0 Open 3 Percutaneous	C Extraluminal Device D Intraluminal Device Z No Device	Z No Qualifier
X Lacrimal Duct, Right Y Lacrimal Duct, Left	7 Via Natural or Artificial Opening 8 Via Natural or Artificial Opening Endoscopic	D Intraluminal Device Z No Device	Z No Qualifier

Section   0   **Medical and Surgical**
Body System   8   **Eye**
Operation   M   **Reattachment:** Putting back in or on all or a portion of a separated body part to its normal location or other suitable location

Body Part (4th)	Approach (5th)	Device (6th)	Qualifier (7th)
N Upper Eyelid, Right **P** Upper Eyelid, Left **Q** Lower Eyelid, Right **R** Lower Eyelid, Left	**X** External	**Z** No Device	**Z** No Qualifier

Section   0   **Medical and Surgical**
Body System   8   **Eye**
Operation   N   **Release:** Freeing a body part from an abnormal physical constraint by cutting or by the use of force

Body Part (4th)	Approach (5th)	Device (6th)	Qualifier (7th)
0 Eye, Right **1** Eye, Left **6** Sclera, Right **7** Sclera, Left **8** Cornea, Right **9** Cornea, Left **S** Conjunctiva, Right **T** Conjunctiva, Left	**X** External	**Z** No Device	**Z** No Qualifier
2 Anterior Chamber, Right **3** Anterior Chamber, Left **4** Vitreous, Right **5** Vitreous, Left **C** Iris, Right **D** Iris, Left **E** Retina, Right **F** Retina, Left **G** Retinal Vessel, Right **H** Retinal Vessel, Left **J** Lens, Right **K** Lens, Left	**3** Percutaneous	**Z** No Device	**Z** No Qualifier
A Choroid, Right **B** Choroid, Left **L** Extraocular Muscle, Right **M** Extraocular Muscle, Left **V** Lacrimal Gland, Right **W** Lacrimal Gland, Left	**0** Open **3** Percutaneous	**Z** No Device	**Z** No Qualifier
N Upper Eyelid, Right **P** Upper Eyelid, Left **Q** Lower Eyelid, Right **R** Lower Eyelid, Left	**0** Open **3** Percutaneous **X** External	**Z** No Device	**Z** No Qualifier
X Lacrimal Duct, Right **Y** Lacrimal Duct, Left	**0** Open **3** Percutaneous **7** Via Natural or Artificial Opening **8** Via Natural or Artificial Opening Endoscopic	**Z** No Device	**Z** No Qualifier

Section   0   **Medical and Surgical**
Body System   8   **Eye**
Operation   P   **Removal:** Taking out or off a device from a body part

Body Part (4th)	Approach (5th)	Device (6th)	Qualifier (7th)
0 Eye, Right 1 Eye, Left	0 Open 3 Percutaneous 7 Via Natural or Artificial Opening 8 Via Natural or Artificial Opening Endoscopic	0 Drainage Device 1 Radioactive Element 3 Infusion Device 7 Autologous Tissue Substitute C Extraluminal Device D Intraluminal Device J Synthetic Substitute K Nonautologous Tissue Substitute Y Other Device	Z No Qualifier
0 Eye, Right 1 Eye, Left	X External	0 Drainage Device 1 Radioactive Element 3 Infusion Device 7 Autologous Tissue Substitute C Extraluminal Device D Intraluminal Device J Synthetic Substitute K Nonautologous Tissue Substitute	Z No Qualifier
J Lens, Right K Lens, Left	3 Percutaneous	J Synthetic Substitute Y Other Device	Z No Qualifier
L Extraocular Muscle, Right M Extraocular Muscle, Left	0 Open 3 Percutaneous	0 Drainage Device 7 Autologous Tissue Substitute J Synthetic Substitute K Nonautologous Tissue Substitute Y Other Device	Z No Qualifier

Section   0   **Medical and Surgical**
Body System   8   **Eye**
Operation   Q   **Repair:** Restoring, to the extent possible, a body part to its normal anatomic structure and function

Body Part (4th)	Approach (5th)	Device (6th)	Qualifier (7th)
0 Eye, Right 1 Eye, Left 6 Sclera, Right 7 Sclera, Left 8 Cornea, Right 9 Cornea, Left S Conjunctiva, Right T Conjunctiva, Left	X External	Z No Device	Z No Qualifier
2 Anterior Chamber, Right 3 Anterior Chamber, Left 4 Vitreous, Right 5 Vitreous, Left C Iris, Right D Iris, Left E Retina, Right F Retina, Left G Retinal Vessel, Right H Retinal Vessel, Left J Lens, Right K Lens, Left	3 Percutaneous	Z No Device	Z No Qualifier

Continued →

Section	0	Medical and Surgical
Body System	8	Eye
Operation	Q	Repair: Restoring, to the extent possible, a body part to its normal anatomic structure and function

Body Part (4th)	Approach (5th)	Device (6th)	Qualifier (7th)
A Choroid, Right B Choroid, Left L Extraocular Muscle, Right M Extraocular Muscle, Left V Lacrimal Gland, Right W Lacrimal Gland, Left	0 Open 3 Percutaneous	Z No Device	Z No Qualifier
N Upper Eyelid, Right P Upper Eyelid, Left Q Lower Eyelid, Right R Lower Eyelid, Left	0 Open 3 Percutaneous X External	Z No Device	Z No Qualifier
X Lacrimal Duct, Right Y Lacrimal Duct, Left	0 Open 3 Percutaneous 7 Via Natural or Artificial Opening 8 Via Natural or Artificial Opening Endoscopic	Z No Device	Z No Qualifier

Section	0	Medical and Surgical
Body System	8	Eye
Operation	R	Replacement: Putting in or on biological or synthetic material that physically takes the place and/or function of all or a portion of a body part

Body Part (4th)	Approach (5th)	Device (6th)	Qualifier (7th)
0 Eye, Right 1 Eye, Left A Choroid, Right B Choroid, Left	0 Open 3 Percutaneous	7 Autologous Tissue Substitute J Synthetic Substitute K Nonautologous Tissue Substitute	Z No Qualifier
4 Vitreous, Right 5 Vitreous, Left C Iris, Right D Iris, Left G Retinal Vessel, Right H Retinal Vessel, Left	3 Percutaneous	7 Autologous Tissue Substitute J Synthetic Substitute K Nonautologous Tissue Substitute	Z No Qualifier
6 Sclera, Right 7 Sclera, Left S Conjunctiva, Right T Conjunctiva, Left	X External	7 Autologous Tissue Substitute J Synthetic Substitute K Nonautologous Tissue Substitute	Z No Qualifier
8 Cornea, Right 9 Cornea, Left	3 Percutaneous X External	7 Autologous Tissue Substitute J Synthetic Substitute K Nonautologous Tissue Substitute	Z No Qualifier
J Lens, Right K Lens, Left	3 Percutaneous	0 Synthetic Substitute, Intraocular Telescope 7 Autologous Tissue Substitute J Synthetic Substitute K Nonautologous Tissue Substitute	Z No Qualifier
N Upper Eyelid, Right P Upper Eyelid, Left Q Lower Eyelid, Right R Lower Eyelid, Left	0 Open 3 Percutaneous X External	7 Autologous Tissue Substitute J Synthetic Substitute K Nonautologous Tissue Substitute	Z No Qualifier
X Lacrimal Duct, Right Y Lacrimal Duct, Left	0 Open 3 Percutaneous 7 Via Natural or Artificial Opening 8 Via Natural or Artificial Opening Endoscopic	7 Autologous Tissue Substitute J Synthetic Substitute K Nonautologous Tissue Substitute	Z No Qualifier

Section   0   **Medical and Surgical**
Body System   8   **Eye**
Operation   S   **Reposition:** Moving to its normal location, or other suitable location, all or a portion of a body part

Body Part (4th)	Approach (5th)	Device (6th)	Qualifier (7th)
C Iris, Right D Iris, Left G Retinal Vessel, Right H Retinal Vessel, Left J Lens, Right K Lens, Left	3 Percutaneous	Z No Device	Z No Qualifier
L Extraocular Muscle, Right M Extraocular Muscle, Left V Lacrimal Gland, Right W Lacrimal Gland, Left	0 Open 3 Percutaneous	Z No Device	Z No Qualifier
N Upper Eyelid, Right P Upper Eyelid, Left Q Lower Eyelid, Right R Lower Eyelid, Left	0 Open 3 Percutaneous X External	Z No Device	Z No Qualifier
X Lacrimal Duct, Right Y Lacrimal Duct, Left	0 Open 3 Percutaneous 7 Via Natural or Artificial Opening 8 Via Natural or Artificial Opening Endoscopic	Z No Device	Z No Qualifier

Section   0   **Medical and Surgical**
Body System   8   **Eye**
Operation   T   **Resection:** Cutting out or off, without replacement, all of a body part

Body Part (4th)	Approach (5th)	Device (6th)	Qualifier (7th)
0 Eye, Right 1 Eye, Left 8 Cornea, Right 9 Cornea, Left	X External	Z No Device	Z No Qualifier
4 Vitreous, Right 5 Vitreous, Left C Iris, Right D Iris, Left J Lens, Right K Lens, Left	3 Percutaneous	Z No Device	Z No Qualifier
L Extraocular Muscle, Right M Extraocular Muscle, Left V Lacrimal Gland, Right W Lacrimal Gland, Left	0 Open 3 Percutaneous	Z No Device	Z No Qualifier
N Upper Eyelid, Right P Upper Eyelid, Left Q Lower Eyelid, Right R Lower Eyelid, Left	0 Open X External	Z No Device	Z No Qualifier
X Lacrimal Duct, Right Y Lacrimal Duct, Left	0 Open 3 Percutaneous 7 Via Natural or Artificial Opening 8 Via Natural or Artificial Opening Endoscopic	Z No Device	Z No Qualifier

Section	0	Medical and Surgical
Body System	8	Eye
Operation	U	Supplement: Putting in or on biological or synthetic material that physically reinforces and/or augments the function of a portion of a body part

Body Part (4th)	Approach (5th)	Device (6th)	Qualifier (7th)
0 Eye, Right 1 Eye, Left C Iris, Right D Iris, Left E Retina, Right F Retina, Left G Retinal Vessel, Right H Retinal Vessel, Left L Extraocular Muscle, Right M Extraocular Muscle, Left	0 Open 3 Percutaneous	7 Autologous Tissue Substitute J Synthetic Substitute K Nonautologous Tissue Substitute	Z No Qualifier
8 Cornea, Right 9 Cornea, Left N Upper Eyelid, Right P Upper Eyelid, Left Q Lower Eyelid, Right R Lower Eyelid, Left	0 Open 3 Percutaneous X External	7 Autologous Tissue Substitute J Synthetic Substitute K Nonautologous Tissue Substitute	Z No Qualifier
X Lacrimal Duct, Right Y Lacrimal Duct, Left	0 Open 3 Percutaneous 7 Via Natural or Artificial Opening 8 Via Natural or Artificial Opening Endoscopic	7 Autologous Tissue Substitute J Synthetic Substitute K Nonautologous Tissue Substitute	Z No Qualifier

Section	0	Medical and Surgical
Body System	8	Eye
Operation	V	Restriction: Partially closing an orifice or the lumen of a tubular body part

Body Part (4th)	Approach (5th)	Device (6th)	Qualifier (7th)
X Lacrimal Duct, Right Y Lacrimal Duct, Left	0 Open 3 Percutaneous	C Extraluminal Device D Intraluminal Device Z No Device	Z No Qualifier
X Lacrimal Duct, Right Y Lacrimal Duct, Left	7 Via Natural or Artificial Opening 8 Via Natural or Artificial Opening Endoscopic	D Intraluminal Device Z No Device	Z No Qualifier

Section	0	Medical and Surgical
Body System	8	Eye
Operation	W	Revision: Correcting, to the extent possible, a portion of a malfunctioning device or the position of a displaced device

Body Part (4th)	Approach (5th)	Device (6th)	Qualifier (7th)
0 Eye, Right 1 Eye, Left	0 Open 3 Percutaneous 7 Via Natural or Artificial Opening 8 Via Natural or Artificial Opening Endoscopic	0 Drainage Device 3 Infusion Device 7 Autologous Tissue Substitute C Extraluminal Device D Intraluminal Device J Synthetic Substitute K Nonautologous Tissue Substitute Y Other Device	Z No Qualifier
0 Eye, Right 1 Eye, Left	X External	0 Drainage Device 3 Infusion Device 7 Autologous Tissue Substitute C Extraluminal Device D Intraluminal Device J Synthetic Substitute K Nonautologous Tissue Substitute	Z No Qualifier

Continued →

Section	0	Medical and Surgical	
Body System	8	Eye	
Operation	W	Revision: Correcting, to the extent possible, a portion of a malfunctioning device or the position of a displaced device	

Body Part (4th)	Approach (5th)	Device (6th)	Qualifier (7th)
J Lens, Right K Lens, Left	3 Percutaneous	J Synthetic Substitute Y Other Device	Z No Qualifier
J Lens, Right K Lens, Left	X External	J Synthetic Substitute	Z No Qualifier
L Extraocular Muscle, Right M Extraocular Muscle, Left	0 Open 3 Percutaneous	0 Drainage Device 7 Autologous Tissue Substitute J Synthetic Substitute K Nonautologous Tissue Substitute Y Other Device	Z No Qualifier

Section	0	Medical and Surgical	
Body System	8	Eye	
Operation	X	Transfer: Moving, without taking out, all or a portion of a body part to another location to take over the function of all or a portion of a body part	

Body Part (4th)	Approach (5th)	Device (6th)	Qualifier (7th)
L Extraocular Muscle, Right M Extraocular Muscle, Left	0 Open 3 Percutaneous	Z No Device	Z No Qualifier

Eye Code Listing 080–08X

080 – Eye, Alteration

080N07Z Alteration of Right Upper Eyelid with Autologous Tissue Substitute, Open Approach

080N0JZ Alteration of Right Upper Eyelid with Synthetic Substitute, Open Approach

080N0KZ Alteration of Right Upper Eyelid with Nonautologous Tissue Substitute, Open Approach

080N0ZZ Alteration of Right Upper Eyelid, Open Approach

080N37Z Alteration of Right Upper Eyelid with Autologous Tissue Substitute, Percutaneous Approach

080N3JZ Alteration of Right Upper Eyelid with Synthetic Substitute, Percutaneous Approach

080N3KZ Alteration of Right Upper Eyelid with Nonautologous Tissue Substitute, Percutaneous Approach

080N3ZZ Alteration of Right Upper Eyelid, Percutaneous Approach

080NX7Z Alteration of Right Upper Eyelid with Autologous Tissue Substitute, External Approach

080NXJZ Alteration of Right Upper Eyelid with Synthetic Substitute, External Approach

080NXKZ Alteration of Right Upper Eyelid with Nonautologous Tissue Substitute, External Approach

080NXZZ Alteration of Right Upper Eyelid, External Approach

080P07Z Alteration of Left Upper Eyelid with Autologous Tissue Substitute, Open Approach

080P0JZ Alteration of Left Upper Eyelid with Synthetic Substitute, Open Approach

080P0KZ Alteration of Left Upper Eyelid with Nonautologous Tissue Substitute, Open Approach

080P0ZZ Alteration of Left Upper Eyelid, Open Approach

080P37Z Alteration of Left Upper Eyelid with Autologous Tissue Substitute, Percutaneous Approach

080P3JZ Alteration of Left Upper Eyelid with Synthetic Substitute, Percutaneous Approach

080P3KZ Alteration of Left Upper Eyelid with Nonautologous Tissue Substitute, Percutaneous Approach

080P3ZZ Alteration of Left Upper Eyelid, Percutaneous Approach

080PX7Z Alteration of Left Upper Eyelid with Autologous Tissue Substitute, External Approach

080PXJZ Alteration of Left Upper Eyelid with Synthetic Substitute, External Approach

080PXKZ Alteration of Left Upper Eyelid with Nonautologous Tissue Substitute, External Approach

080PXZZ Alteration of Left Upper Eyelid, External Approach

080Q07Z Alteration of Right Lower Eyelid with Autologous Tissue Substitute, Open Approach

080Q0JZ Alteration of Right Lower Eyelid with Synthetic Substitute, Open Approach

080Q0KZ Alteration of Right Lower Eyelid with Nonautologous Tissue Substitute, Open Approach

080Q0ZZ Alteration of Right Lower Eyelid, Open Approach

080Q37Z Alteration of Right Lower Eyelid with Autologous Tissue Substitute, Percutaneous Approach

080Q3JZ Alteration of Right Lower Eyelid with Synthetic Substitute, Percutaneous Approach

080Q3KZ Alteration of Right Lower Eyelid with Nonautologous Tissue Substitute, Percutaneous Approach

080Q3ZZ Alteration of Right Lower Eyelid, Percutaneous Approach

080QX7Z Alteration of Right Lower Eyelid with Autologous Tissue Substitute, External Approach

080QXJZ Alteration of Right Lower Eyelid with Synthetic Substitute, External Approach

080QXKZ Alteration of Right Lower Eyelid with Nonautologous Tissue Substitute, External Approach

080QXZZ Alteration of Right Lower Eyelid, External Approach

080R07Z Alteration of Left Lower Eyelid with Autologous Tissue Substitute, Open Approach

080R0JZ Alteration of Left Lower Eyelid with Synthetic Substitute, Open Approach

080R0KZ Alteration of Left Lower Eyelid with Nonautologous Tissue Substitute, Open Approach

080R0ZZ Alteration of Left Lower Eyelid, Open Approach

080R37Z Alteration of Left Lower Eyelid with Autologous Tissue Substitute, Percutaneous Approach

080R3JZ Alteration of Left Lower Eyelid with Synthetic Substitute, Percutaneous Approach

080R3KZ Alteration of Left Lower Eyelid with Nonautologous Tissue Substitute, Percutaneous Approach

080R3ZZ Alteration of Left Lower Eyelid, Percutaneous Approach

080RX7Z Alteration of Left Lower Eyelid with Autologous Tissue Substitute, External Approach

080RXJZ Alteration of Left Lower Eyelid with Synthetic Substitute, External Approach	**080RXKZ** Alteration of Left Lower Eyelid with Nonautologous Tissue Substitute, External Approach	**080RXZZ** Alteration of Left Lower Eyelid, External Approach

081 – Eye, Bypass

Review Coding Guideline B3.6a

08123J4 Bypass Right Anterior Chamber to Sclera with Synthetic Substitute, Percutaneous Approach	**081X0J3** Bypass Right Lacrimal Duct to Nasal Cavity with Synthetic Substitute, Open Approach	**081Y0J3** Bypass Left Lacrimal Duct to Nasal Cavity with Synthetic Substitute, Open Approach
08123K4 Bypass Right Anterior Chamber to Sclera with Nonautologous Tissue Substitute, Percutaneous Approach	**081X0K3** Bypass Right Lacrimal Duct to Nasal Cavity with Nonautologous Tissue Substitute, Open Approach	**081Y0K3** Bypass Left Lacrimal Duct to Nasal Cavity with Nonautologous Tissue Substitute, Open Approach
08123Z4 Bypass Right Anterior Chamber to Sclera, Percutaneous Approach	**081X0Z3** Bypass Right Lacrimal Duct to Nasal Cavity, Open Approach	**081Y0Z3** Bypass Left Lacrimal Duct to Nasal Cavity, Open Approach
08133J4 Bypass Left Anterior Chamber to Sclera with Synthetic Substitute, Percutaneous Approach	**081X3J3** Bypass Right Lacrimal Duct to Nasal Cavity with Synthetic Substitute, Percutaneous Approach	**081Y3J3** Bypass Left Lacrimal Duct to Nasal Cavity with Synthetic Substitute, Percutaneous Approach
AHA CC: 1Q, 2019, 27-28	**081X3K3** Bypass Right Lacrimal Duct to Nasal Cavity with Nonautologous Tissue Substitute, Percutaneous Approach	**081Y3K3** Bypass Left Lacrimal Duct to Nasal Cavity with Nonautologous Tissue Substitute, Percutaneous Approach
08133K4 Bypass Left Anterior Chamber to Sclera with Nonautologous Tissue Substitute, Percutaneous Approach		
08133Z4 Bypass Left Anterior Chamber to Sclera, Percutaneous Approach	**081X3Z3** Bypass Right Lacrimal Duct to Nasal Cavity, Percutaneous Approach	**081Y3Z3** Bypass Left Lacrimal Duct to Nasal Cavity, Percutaneous Approach

082 – Eye, Change

Review Coding Guideline B6.1c

0820X0Z Change Drainage Device in Right Eye, External Approach	**0821X0Z** Change Drainage Device in Left Eye, External Approach
0820XYZ Change Other Device in Right Eye, External Approach	**0821XYZ** Change Other Device in Left Eye, External Approach

085 – Eye, Destruction

0850XZZ Destruction of Right Eye, External Approach	**085G3ZZ** Destruction of Right Retinal Vessel, Percutaneous Approach	**085R3ZZ** Destruction of Left Lower Eyelid, Percutaneous Approach
0851XZZ Destruction of Left Eye, External Approach	**085H3ZZ** Destruction of Left Retinal Vessel, Percutaneous Approach	**085RXZZ** Destruction of Left Lower Eyelid, External Approach
08523ZZ Destruction of Right Anterior Chamber, Percutaneous Approach	**085J3ZZ** Destruction of Right Lens, Percutaneous Approach	**085SXZZ** Destruction of Right Conjunctiva, External Approach
08533ZZ Destruction of Left Anterior Chamber, Percutaneous Approach	**085K3ZZ** Destruction of Left Lens, Percutaneous Approach	**085TXZZ** Destruction of Left Conjunctiva, External Approach
08543ZZ Destruction of Right Vitreous, Percutaneous Approach	**085L0ZZ** Destruction of Right Extraocular Muscle, Open Approach	**085V0ZZ** Destruction of Right Lacrimal Gland, Open Approach
08553ZZ Destruction of Left Vitreous, Percutaneous Approach	**085L3ZZ** Destruction of Right Extraocular Muscle, Percutaneous Approach	**085V3ZZ** Destruction of Right Lacrimal Gland, Percutaneous Approach
0856XZZ Destruction of Right Sclera, External Approach	**085M0ZZ** Destruction of Left Extraocular Muscle, Open Approach	**085W0ZZ** Destruction of Left Lacrimal Gland, Open Approach
0857XZZ Destruction of Left Sclera, External Approach	**085M3ZZ** Destruction of Left Extraocular Muscle, Percutaneous Approach	**085W3ZZ** Destruction of Left Lacrimal Gland, Percutaneous Approach
0858XZZ Destruction of Right Cornea, External Approach	**085N0ZZ** Destruction of Right Upper Eyelid, Open Approach	**085X0ZZ** Destruction of Right Lacrimal Duct, Open Approach
0859XZZ Destruction of Left Cornea, External Approach	**085N3ZZ** Destruction of Right Upper Eyelid, Percutaneous Approach	**085X3ZZ** Destruction of Right Lacrimal Duct, Percutaneous Approach
085A0ZZ Destruction of Right Choroid, Open Approach	**085NXZZ** Destruction of Right Upper Eyelid, External Approach	**085X7ZZ** Destruction of Right Lacrimal Duct, Via Natural or Artificial Opening
085A3ZZ Destruction of Right Choroid, Percutaneous Approach	**085P0ZZ** Destruction of Left Upper Eyelid, Open Approach	
085B0ZZ Destruction of Left Choroid, Open Approach	**085P3ZZ** Destruction of Left Upper Eyelid, Percutaneous Approach	**085X8ZZ** Destruction of Right Lacrimal Duct, Via Natural or Artificial Opening Endoscopic
085B3ZZ Destruction of Left Choroid, Percutaneous Approach	**085PXZZ** Destruction of Left Upper Eyelid, External Approach	**085Y0ZZ** Destruction of Left Lacrimal Duct, Open Approach
085C3ZZ Destruction of Right Iris, Percutaneous Approach	**085Q0ZZ** Destruction of Right Lower Eyelid, Open Approach	**085Y3ZZ** Destruction of Left Lacrimal Duct, Percutaneous Approach
085D3ZZ Destruction of Left Iris, Percutaneous Approach	**085Q3ZZ** Destruction of Right Lower Eyelid, Percutaneous Approach	**085Y7ZZ** Destruction of Left Lacrimal Duct, Via Natural or Artificial Opening
085E3ZZ Destruction of Right Retina, Percutaneous Approach	**085QXZZ** Destruction of Right Lower Eyelid, External Approach	**085Y8ZZ** Destruction of Left Lacrimal Duct, Via Natural or Artificial Opening Endoscopic
085F3ZZ Destruction of Left Retina, Percutaneous Approach	**085R0ZZ** Destruction of Left Lower Eyelid, Open Approach	

♀ Female-only   ♂ Male-only   ▲ Limited Coverage   ● Non-OR   **HAC** HAC-associated procedure   ▲ Non-covered procedures   ✛ Cluster

087 – Eye, Dilation

087X0DZ Dilation of Right Lacrimal Duct with Intraluminal Device, Open Approach

087X0ZZ Dilation of Right Lacrimal Duct, Open Approach

087X3DZ Dilation of Right Lacrimal Duct with Intraluminal Device, Percutaneous Approach

087X3ZZ Dilation of Right Lacrimal Duct, Percutaneous Approach

087X7DZ Dilation of Right Lacrimal Duct with Intraluminal Device, Via Natural or Artificial Opening

087X7ZZ Dilation of Right Lacrimal Duct, Via Natural or Artificial Opening

087X8DZ Dilation of Right Lacrimal Duct with Intraluminal Device, Via Natural or Artificial Opening Endoscopic

087X8ZZ Dilation of Right Lacrimal Duct, Via Natural or Artificial Opening Endoscopic

087Y0DZ Dilation of Left Lacrimal Duct with Intraluminal Device, Open Approach

087Y0ZZ Dilation of Left Lacrimal Duct, Open Approach

087Y3DZ Dilation of Left Lacrimal Duct with Intraluminal Device, Percutaneous Approach

087Y3ZZ Dilation of Left Lacrimal Duct, Percutaneous Approach

087Y7DZ Dilation of Left Lacrimal Duct with Intraluminal Device, Via Natural or Artificial Opening

087Y7ZZ Dilation of Left Lacrimal Duct, Via Natural or Artificial Opening

087Y8DZ Dilation of Left Lacrimal Duct with Intraluminal Device, Via Natural or Artificial Opening Endoscopic

087Y8ZZ Dilation of Left Lacrimal Duct, Via Natural or Artificial Opening Endoscopic

089 – Eye, Drainage

Review Coding Guidelines B3.4a and B3.4b

Review Coding Guideline B6.2

0890X0Z Drainage of Right Eye with Drainage Device, External Approach

0890XZX Drainage of Right Eye, External Approach, Diagnostic

0890XZZ Drainage of Right Eye, External Approach

0891X0Z Drainage of Left Eye with Drainage Device, External Approach

0891XZX Drainage of Left Eye, External Approach, Diagnostic

0891XZZ Drainage of Left Eye, External Approach

0899230Z Drainage of Right Anterior Chamber with Drainage Device, Percutaneous Approach

08923ZX Drainage of Right Anterior Chamber, Percutaneous Approach, Diagnostic

08923ZZ Drainage of Right Anterior Chamber, Percutaneous Approach
AHA CC: 2Q, 2016, 21-22

08933030Z Drainage of Left Anterior Chamber with Drainage Device, Percutaneous Approach

08933ZX Drainage of Left Anterior Chamber, Percutaneous Approach, Diagnostic

08933ZZ Drainage of Left Anterior Chamber, Percutaneous Approach

08943030Z Drainage of Right Vitreous with Drainage Device, Percutaneous Approach

08943ZX Drainage of Right Vitreous, Percutaneous Approach, Diagnostic

08943ZZ Drainage of Right Vitreous, Percutaneous Approach

08953030Z Drainage of Left Vitreous with Drainage Device, Percutaneous Approach

08953ZX Drainage of Left Vitreous, Percutaneous Approach, Diagnostic

08953ZZ Drainage of Left Vitreous, Percutaneous Approach

0896X0Z Drainage of Right Sclera with Drainage Device, External Approach

0896XZX Drainage of Right Sclera, External Approach, Diagnostic

0896XZZ Drainage of Right Sclera, External Approach

0897X0Z Drainage of Left Sclera with Drainage Device, External Approach

0897XZX Drainage of Left Sclera, External Approach, Diagnostic

0897XZZ Drainage of Left Sclera, External Approach

0898X0Z Drainage of Right Cornea with Drainage Device, External Approach

0898XZX Drainage of Right Cornea, External Approach, Diagnostic

0898XZZ Drainage of Right Cornea, External Approach

0899X0Z Drainage of Left Cornea with Drainage Device, External Approach

0899XZX Drainage of Left Cornea, External Approach, Diagnostic

0899XZZ Drainage of Left Cornea, External Approach

089A00Z Drainage of Right Choroid with Drainage Device, Open Approach

089A0ZX Drainage of Right Choroid, Open Approach, Diagnostic

089A0ZZ Drainage of Right Choroid, Open Approach

089A30Z Drainage of Right Choroid with Drainage Device, Percutaneous Approach

089A3ZX Drainage of Right Choroid, Percutaneous Approach, Diagnostic

089A3ZZ Drainage of Right Choroid, Percutaneous Approach

089B00Z Drainage of Left Choroid with Drainage Device, Open Approach

089B0ZX Drainage of Left Choroid, Open Approach, Diagnostic

089B0ZZ Drainage of Left Choroid, Open Approach

089B30Z Drainage of Left Choroid with Drainage Device, Percutaneous Approach

089B3ZX Drainage of Left Choroid, Percutaneous Approach, Diagnostic

089B3ZZ Drainage of Left Choroid, Percutaneous Approach

089C30Z Drainage of Right Iris with Drainage Device, Percutaneous Approach

089C3ZX Drainage of Right Iris, Percutaneous Approach, Diagnostic

089C3ZZ Drainage of Right Iris, Percutaneous Approach

089D30Z Drainage of Left Iris with Drainage Device, Percutaneous Approach

089D3ZX Drainage of Left Iris, Percutaneous Approach, Diagnostic

089D3ZZ Drainage of Left Iris, Percutaneous Approach

089E30Z Drainage of Right Retina with Drainage Device, Percutaneous Approach

089E3ZX Drainage of Right Retina, Percutaneous Approach, Diagnostic

089E3ZZ Drainage of Right Retina, Percutaneous Approach

089F30Z Drainage of Left Retina with Drainage Device, Percutaneous Approach

089F3ZX Drainage of Left Retina, Percutaneous Approach, Diagnostic

089F3ZZ Drainage of Left Retina, Percutaneous Approach

089G30Z Drainage of Right Retinal Vessel with Drainage Device, Percutaneous Approach

089G3ZX Drainage of Right Retinal Vessel, Percutaneous Approach, Diagnostic

089G3ZZ Drainage of Right Retinal Vessel, Percutaneous Approach

089H30Z Drainage of Left Retinal Vessel with Drainage Device, Percutaneous Approach

089H3ZX Drainage of Left Retinal Vessel, Percutaneous Approach, Diagnostic

089H3ZZ Drainage of Left Retinal Vessel, Percutaneous Approach

089J30Z Drainage of Right Lens with Drainage Device, Percutaneous Approach

089J3ZX Drainage of Right Lens, Percutaneous Approach, Diagnostic

089J3ZZ Drainage of Right Lens, Percutaneous Approach

089K30Z Drainage of Left Lens with Drainage Device, Percutaneous Approach

089K3ZX Drainage of Left Lens, Percutaneous Approach, Diagnostic

089K3ZZ Drainage of Left Lens, Percutaneous Approach

089L00Z Drainage of Right Extraocular Muscle with Drainage Device, Open Approach

089L0ZX Drainage of Right Extraocular Muscle, Open Approach, Diagnostic

089L0ZZ Drainage of Right Extraocular Muscle, Open Approach

089L30Z Drainage of Right Extraocular Muscle with Drainage Device, Percutaneous Approach

089L3ZX Drainage of Right Extraocular Muscle, Percutaneous Approach, Diagnostic

089L3ZZ Drainage of Right Extraocular Muscle, Percutaneous Approach

089M00Z Drainage of Left Extraocular Muscle with Drainage Device, Open Approach

089M0ZX Drainage of Left Extraocular Muscle, Open Approach, Diagnostic

089M0ZZ Drainage of Left Extraocular Muscle, Open Approach

089M30Z Drainage of Left Extraocular Muscle with Drainage Device, Percutaneous Approach

089M3ZX Drainage of Left Extraocular Muscle, Percutaneous Approach, Diagnostic

089M3ZZ Drainage of Left Extraocular Muscle, Percutaneous Approach

089N00Z Drainage of Right Upper Eyelid with Drainage Device, Open Approach

089N0ZX Drainage of Right Upper Eyelid, Open Approach, Diagnostic

089N0ZZ Drainage of Right Upper Eyelid, Open Approach

089N30Z Drainage of Right Upper Eyelid with Drainage Device, Percutaneous Approach

089N3ZX Drainage of Right Upper Eyelid, Percutaneous Approach, Diagnostic

089N3ZZ Drainage of Right Upper Eyelid, Percutaneous Approach

089NX0Z Drainage of Right Upper Eyelid with Drainage Device, External Approach

089NXZX Drainage of Right Upper Eyelid, External Approach, Diagnostic

089NXZZ Drainage of Right Upper Eyelid, External Approach

089P00Z Drainage of Left Upper Eyelid with Drainage Device, Open Approach

089P0ZX Drainage of Left Upper Eyelid, Open Approach, Diagnostic

089P0ZZ Drainage of Left Upper Eyelid, Open Approach

089P30Z Drainage of Left Upper Eyelid with Drainage Device, Percutaneous Approach

089P3ZX Drainage of Left Upper Eyelid, Percutaneous Approach, Diagnostic

089P3ZZ Drainage of Left Upper Eyelid, Percutaneous Approach

089PX0Z Drainage of Left Upper Eyelid with Drainage Device, External Approach

089PXZX Drainage of Left Upper Eyelid, External Approach, Diagnostic

089PXZZ Drainage of Left Upper Eyelid, External Approach

089Q00Z Drainage of Right Lower Eyelid with Drainage Device, Open Approach

089Q0ZX Drainage of Right Lower Eyelid, Open Approach, Diagnostic

089Q0ZZ Drainage of Right Lower Eyelid, Open Approach

089Q30Z Drainage of Right Lower Eyelid with Drainage Device, Percutaneous Approach

089Q3ZX Drainage of Right Lower Eyelid, Percutaneous Approach, Diagnostic

089Q3ZZ Drainage of Right Lower Eyelid, Percutaneous Approach

089QX0Z Drainage of Right Lower Eyelid with Drainage Device, External Approach

089QXZX Drainage of Right Lower Eyelid, External Approach, Diagnostic

089QXZZ Drainage of Right Lower Eyelid, External Approach

089R00Z Drainage of Left Lower Eyelid with Drainage Device, Open Approach

089R0ZX Drainage of Left Lower Eyelid, Open Approach, Diagnostic

089R0ZZ Drainage of Left Lower Eyelid, Open Approach

089R30Z Drainage of Left Lower Eyelid with Drainage Device, Percutaneous Approach

089R3ZX Drainage of Left Lower Eyelid, Percutaneous Approach, Diagnostic

089R3ZZ Drainage of Left Lower Eyelid, Percutaneous Approach

089RX0Z Drainage of Left Lower Eyelid with Drainage Device, External Approach

089RXZX Drainage of Left Lower Eyelid, External Approach, Diagnostic

089RXZZ Drainage of Left Lower Eyelid, External Approach

089SX0Z Drainage of Right Conjunctiva with Drainage Device, External Approach

089SXZX Drainage of Right Conjunctiva, External Approach, Diagnostic

089SXZZ Drainage of Right Conjunctiva, External Approach

089TX0Z Drainage of Left Conjunctiva with Drainage Device, External Approach

089TXZX Drainage of Left Conjunctiva, External Approach, Diagnostic

089TXZZ Drainage of Left Conjunctiva, External Approach

089V00Z Drainage of Right Lacrimal Gland with Drainage Device, Open Approach

089V0ZX Drainage of Right Lacrimal Gland, Open Approach, Diagnostic

089V0ZZ Drainage of Right Lacrimal Gland, Open Approach

089V30Z Drainage of Right Lacrimal Gland with Drainage Device, Percutaneous Approach

089V3ZX Drainage of Right Lacrimal Gland, Percutaneous Approach, Diagnostic

089V3ZZ Drainage of Right Lacrimal Gland, Percutaneous Approach

089W00Z Drainage of Left Lacrimal Gland with Drainage Device, Open Approach

089W0ZX Drainage of Left Lacrimal Gland, Open Approach, Diagnostic

089W0ZZ Drainage of Left Lacrimal Gland, Open Approach

089W30Z Drainage of Left Lacrimal Gland with Drainage Device, Percutaneous Approach

089W3ZX Drainage of Left Lacrimal Gland, Percutaneous Approach, Diagnostic

089W3ZZ Drainage of Left Lacrimal Gland, Percutaneous Approach

089X00Z Drainage of Right Lacrimal Duct with Drainage Device, Open Approach

089X0ZX Drainage of Right Lacrimal Duct, Open Approach, Diagnostic

089X0ZZ Drainage of Right Lacrimal Duct, Open Approach

089X30Z Drainage of Right Lacrimal Duct with Drainage Device, Percutaneous Approach

089X3ZX Drainage of Right Lacrimal Duct, Percutaneous Approach, Diagnostic

089X3ZZ Drainage of Right Lacrimal Duct, Percutaneous Approach

089X70Z Drainage of Right Lacrimal Duct with Drainage Device, Via Natural or Artificial Opening

089X7ZX Drainage of Right Lacrimal Duct, Via Natural or Artificial Opening, Diagnostic

089X7ZZ Drainage of Right Lacrimal Duct, Via Natural or Artificial Opening

089X80Z Drainage of Right Lacrimal Duct with Drainage Device, Via Natural or Artificial Opening Endoscopic

089X8ZX Drainage of Right Lacrimal Duct, Via Natural or Artificial Opening Endoscopic, Diagnostic

089X8ZZ Drainage of Right Lacrimal Duct, Via Natural or Artificial Opening Endoscopic

089Y00Z Drainage of Left Lacrimal Duct with Drainage Device, Open Approach

089Y0ZX Drainage of Left Lacrimal Duct, Open Approach, Diagnostic

089Y0ZZ Drainage of Left Lacrimal Duct, Open Approach

089Y30Z Drainage of Left Lacrimal Duct with Drainage Device, Percutaneous Approach

089Y3ZX Drainage of Left Lacrimal Duct, Percutaneous Approach, Diagnostic

089Y3ZZ Drainage of Left Lacrimal Duct, Percutaneous Approach

089Y70Z Drainage of Left Lacrimal Duct with Drainage Device, Via Natural or Artificial Opening

089Y7ZX Drainage of Left Lacrimal Duct, Via Natural or Artificial Opening, Diagnostic

089Y7ZZ Drainage of Left Lacrimal Duct, Via Natural or Artificial Opening

089Y80Z Drainage of Left Lacrimal Duct with Drainage Device, Via Natural or Artificial Opening Endoscopic

089Y8ZX Drainage of Left Lacrimal Duct, Via Natural or Artificial Opening Endoscopic, Diagnostic

089Y8ZZ Drainage of Left Lacrimal Duct, Via Natural or Artificial Opening Endoscopic

08B – Eye, Excision

Review Coding Guidelines B3.4a and B3.4b

Review Coding Guideline B3.8

Review Coding Guideline B3.18

08B00ZX Excision of Right Eye, Open Approach, Diagnostic

08B00ZZ Excision of Right Eye, Open Approach

08B03ZX Excision of Right Eye, Percutaneous Approach, Diagnostic

08B03ZZ Excision of Right Eye, Percutaneous Approach

08B0XZX Excision of Right Eye, External Approach, Diagnostic

08B0XZZ Excision of Right Eye, External Approach

08B10ZX Excision of Left Eye, Open Approach, Diagnostic

08B10ZZ Excision of Left Eye, Open Approach

08B13ZX Excision of Left Eye, Percutaneous Approach, Diagnostic

08B13ZZ Excision of Left Eye, Percutaneous Approach

08B1XZX Excision of Left Eye, External Approach, Diagnostic

08B1XZZ Excision of Left Eye, External Approach

08B43ZX Excision of Right Vitreous, Percutaneous Approach, Diagnostic

08B43ZZ Excision of Right Vitreous, Percutaneous Approach

AHA CC: 4Q, 2014, 36-37

♀ Female-only   ♂ Male-only   ▲ Limited Coverage   ● Non-OR   ᴴᴬᶜ HAC-associated procedure   ▲ Non-covered procedures   ✚ Cluste

08B53ZX Excision of Left Vitreous, Percutaneous Approach, Diagnostic

08B53ZZ Excision of Left Vitreous, Percutaneous Approach
AHA CC: 4Q, 2014, 35-36

08B6XZX Excision of Right Sclera, External Approach, Diagnostic

08B6XZZ Excision of Right Sclera, External Approach

08B7XZX Excision of Left Sclera, External Approach, Diagnostic

08B7XZZ Excision of Left Sclera, External Approach

08B8XZX Excision of Right Cornea, External Approach, Diagnostic

08B8XZZ Excision of Right Cornea, External Approach

08B9XZX Excision of Left Cornea, External Approach, Diagnostic

08B9XZZ Excision of Left Cornea, External Approach

08BA0ZX Excision of Right Choroid, Open Approach, Diagnostic

08BA0ZZ Excision of Right Choroid, Open Approach

08BA3ZX Excision of Right Choroid, Percutaneous Approach, Diagnostic

08BA3ZZ Excision of Right Choroid, Percutaneous Approach

08BB0ZX Excision of Left Choroid, Open Approach, Diagnostic

08BB0ZZ Excision of Left Choroid, Open Approach

08BB3ZX Excision of Left Choroid, Percutaneous Approach, Diagnostic

08BB3ZZ Excision of Left Choroid, Percutaneous Approach

08BC3ZX Excision of Right Iris, Percutaneous Approach, Diagnostic

08BC3ZZ Excision of Right Iris, Percutaneous Approach

08BD3ZX Excision of Left Iris, Percutaneous Approach, Diagnostic

08BD3ZZ Excision of Left Iris, Percutaneous Approach

08BE3ZX Excision of Right Retina, Percutaneous Approach, Diagnostic

08BE3ZZ Excision of Right Retina, Percutaneous Approach

08BF3ZX Excision of Left Retina, Percutaneous Approach, Diagnostic

08BF3ZZ Excision of Left Retina, Percutaneous Approach

08BJ3ZX Excision of Right Lens, Percutaneous Approach, Diagnostic

08BJ3ZZ Excision of Right Lens, Percutaneous Approach

08BK3ZX Excision of Left Lens, Percutaneous Approach, Diagnostic

08BK3ZZ Excision of Left Lens, Percutaneous Approach

08BL0ZX Excision of Right Extraocular Muscle, Open Approach, Diagnostic

08BL0ZZ Excision of Right Extraocular Muscle, Open Approach

08BL3ZX Excision of Right Extraocular Muscle, Percutaneous Approach, Diagnostic

08BL3ZZ Excision of Right Extraocular Muscle, Percutaneous Approach

08BM0ZX Excision of Left Extraocular Muscle, Open Approach, Diagnostic

08BM0ZZ Excision of Left Extraocular Muscle, Open Approach

08BM3ZX Excision of Left Extraocular Muscle, Percutaneous Approach, Diagnostic

08BM3ZZ Excision of Left Extraocular Muscle, Percutaneous Approach

08BN0ZX Excision of Right Upper Eyelid, Open Approach, Diagnostic

08BN0ZZ Excision of Right Upper Eyelid, Open Approach

08BN3ZX Excision of Right Upper Eyelid, Percutaneous Approach, Diagnostic

08BN3ZZ Excision of Right Upper Eyelid, Percutaneous Approach

08BNXZX Excision of Right Upper Eyelid, External Approach, Diagnostic

08BNXZZ Excision of Right Upper Eyelid, External Approach

08BP0ZX Excision of Left Upper Eyelid, Open Approach, Diagnostic

08BP0ZZ Excision of Left Upper Eyelid, Open Approach

08BP3ZX Excision of Left Upper Eyelid, Percutaneous Approach, Diagnostic

08BP3ZZ Excision of Left Upper Eyelid, Percutaneous Approach

08BPXZX Excision of Left Upper Eyelid, External Approach, Diagnostic

08BPXZZ Excision of Left Upper Eyelid, External Approach

08BQ0ZX Excision of Right Lower Eyelid, Open Approach, Diagnostic

08BQ0ZZ Excision of Right Lower Eyelid, Open Approach

08BQ3ZX Excision of Right Lower Eyelid, Percutaneous Approach, Diagnostic

08BQ3ZZ Excision of Right Lower Eyelid, Percutaneous Approach

08BQXZX Excision of Right Lower Eyelid, External Approach, Diagnostic

08BQXZZ Excision of Right Lower Eyelid, External Approach

08BR0ZX Excision of Left Lower Eyelid, Open Approach, Diagnostic

08BR0ZZ Excision of Left Lower Eyelid, Open Approach

08BR3ZX Excision of Left Lower Eyelid, Percutaneous Approach, Diagnostic

08BR3ZZ Excision of Left Lower Eyelid, Percutaneous Approach

08BRXZX Excision of Left Lower Eyelid, External Approach, Diagnostic

08BRXZZ Excision of Left Lower Eyelid, External Approach

08BSXZX Excision of Right Conjunctiva, External Approach, Diagnostic

08BSXZZ Excision of Right Conjunctiva, External Approach

08BTXZX Excision of Left Conjunctiva, External Approach, Diagnostic

08BTXZZ Excision of Left Conjunctiva, External Approach

08BV0ZX Excision of Right Lacrimal Gland, Open Approach, Diagnostic

08BV0ZZ Excision of Right Lacrimal Gland, Open Approach

08BV3ZX Excision of Right Lacrimal Gland, Percutaneous Approach, Diagnostic

08BV3ZZ Excision of Right Lacrimal Gland, Percutaneous Approach

08BW0ZX Excision of Left Lacrimal Gland, Open Approach, Diagnostic

08BW0ZZ Excision of Left Lacrimal Gland, Open Approach

08BW3ZX Excision of Left Lacrimal Gland, Percutaneous Approach, Diagnostic

08BW3ZZ Excision of Left Lacrimal Gland, Percutaneous Approach

08BX0ZX Excision of Right Lacrimal Duct, Open Approach, Diagnostic

08BX0ZZ Excision of Right Lacrimal Duct, Open Approach

08BX3ZX Excision of Right Lacrimal Duct, Percutaneous Approach, Diagnostic

08BX3ZZ Excision of Right Lacrimal Duct, Percutaneous Approach

08BX7ZX Excision of Right Lacrimal Duct, Via Natural or Artificial Opening, Diagnostic

08BX7ZZ Excision of Right Lacrimal Duct, Via Natural or Artificial Opening

08BX8ZX Excision of Right Lacrimal Duct, Via Natural or Artificial Opening Endoscopic, Diagnostic

08BX8ZZ Excision of Right Lacrimal Duct, Via Natural or Artificial Opening Endoscopic

08BY0ZX Excision of Left Lacrimal Duct, Open Approach, Diagnostic

08BY0ZZ Excision of Left Lacrimal Duct, Open Approach

08BY3ZX Excision of Left Lacrimal Duct, Percutaneous Approach, Diagnostic

08BY3ZZ Excision of Left Lacrimal Duct, Percutaneous Approach

08BY7ZX Excision of Left Lacrimal Duct, Via Natural or Artificial Opening, Diagnostic

08BY7ZZ Excision of Left Lacrimal Duct, Via Natural or Artificial Opening

08BY8ZX Excision of Left Lacrimal Duct, Via Natural or Artificial Opening Endoscopic, Diagnostic

08BY8ZZ Excision of Left Lacrimal Duct, Via Natural or Artificial Opening Endoscopic

08C – Eye, Extirpation

08C0XZZ Extirpation of Matter from Right Eye, External Approach

08C1XZZ Extirpation of Matter from Left Eye, External Approach

08C23ZZ Extirpation of Matter from Right Anterior Chamber, Percutaneous Approach

08C2XZZ Extirpation of Matter from Right Anterior Chamber, External Approach

08C33ZZ Extirpation of Matter from Left Anterior Chamber, Percutaneous Approach

08C3XZZ Extirpation of Matter from Left Anterior Chamber, External Approach

08C43ZZ Extirpation of Matter from Right Vitreous, Percutaneous Approach

08C4XZZ Extirpation of Matter from Right Vitreous, External Approach

08C53ZZ Extirpation of Matter from Left Vitreous, Percutaneous Approach

08C5XZZ Extirpation of Matter from Left Vitreous, External Approach

08C6XZZ Extirpation of Matter from Right Sclera, External Approach

08C7XZZ Extirpation of Matter from Left Sclera, External Approach

08C8XZZ Extirpation of Matter from Right Cornea, External Approach

♀ Female-only   ♂ Male-only   ▲ Limited Coverage   ● Non-OR   🆁🅰🅼 HAC-associated procedure   ▲ Non-covered procedures   ➕ Cluster

08C9XZZ Extirpation of Matter from Left Cornea, External Approach

08CA0ZZ Extirpation of Matter from Right Choroid, Open Approach

08CA3ZZ Extirpation of Matter from Right Choroid, Percutaneous Approach

08CAXZZ Extirpation of Matter from Right Choroid, External Approach

08CB0ZZ Extirpation of Matter from Left Choroid, Open Approach

08CB3ZZ Extirpation of Matter from Left Choroid, Percutaneous Approach

08CBXZZ Extirpation of Matter from Left Choroid, External Approach

08CC3ZZ Extirpation of Matter from Right Iris, Percutaneous Approach

08CCXZZ Extirpation of Matter from Right Iris, External Approach

08CD3ZZ Extirpation of Matter from Left Iris, Percutaneous Approach

08CDXZZ Extirpation of Matter from Left Iris, External Approach

08CE3ZZ Extirpation of Matter from Right Retina, Percutaneous Approach

08CEXZZ Extirpation of Matter from Right Retina, External Approach

08CF3ZZ Extirpation of Matter from Left Retina, Percutaneous Approach

08CFXZZ Extirpation of Matter from Left Retina, External Approach

08CG3ZZ Extirpation of Matter from Right Retinal Vessel, Percutaneous Approach

08CGXZZ Extirpation of Matter from Right Retinal Vessel, External Approach

08CH3ZZ Extirpation of Matter from Left Retinal Vessel, Percutaneous Approach

08CHXZZ Extirpation of Matter from Left Retinal Vessel, External Approach

08CJ3ZZ Extirpation of Matter from Right Lens, Percutaneous Approach

08CJXZZ Extirpation of Matter from Right Lens, External Approach

08CK3ZZ Extirpation of Matter from Left Lens, Percutaneous Approach

08CKXZZ Extirpation of Matter from Left Lens, External Approach

08CL0ZZ Extirpation of Matter from Right Extraocular Muscle, Open Approach

08CL3ZZ Extirpation of Matter from Right Extraocular Muscle, Percutaneous Approach

08CLXZZ Extirpation of Matter from Right Extraocular Muscle, External Approach

08CM0ZZ Extirpation of Matter from Left Extraocular Muscle, Open Approach

08CM3ZZ Extirpation of Matter from Left Extraocular Muscle, Percutaneous Approach

08CMXZZ Extirpation of Matter from Left Extraocular Muscle, External Approach

08CN0ZZ Extirpation of Matter from Right Upper Eyelid, Open Approach

08CN3ZZ Extirpation of Matter from Right Upper Eyelid, Percutaneous Approach

08CNXZZ Extirpation of Matter from Right Upper Eyelid, External Approach

08CP0ZZ Extirpation of Matter from Left Upper Eyelid, Open Approach

08CP3ZZ Extirpation of Matter from Left Upper Eyelid, Percutaneous Approach

08CPXZZ Extirpation of Matter from Left Upper Eyelid, External Approach

08CQ0ZZ Extirpation of Matter from Right Lower Eyelid, Open Approach

08CQ3ZZ Extirpation of Matter from Right Lower Eyelid, Percutaneous Approach

08CQXZZ Extirpation of Matter from Right Lower Eyelid, External Approach

08CR0ZZ Extirpation of Matter from Left Lower Eyelid, Open Approach

08CR3ZZ Extirpation of Matter from Left Lower Eyelid, Percutaneous Approach

08CRXZZ Extirpation of Matter from Left Lower Eyelid, External Approach

08CSXZZ Extirpation of Matter from Right Conjunctiva, External Approach

08CTXZZ Extirpation of Matter from Left Conjunctiva, External Approach

08CV0ZZ Extirpation of Matter from Right Lacrimal Gland, Open Approach

08CV3ZZ Extirpation of Matter from Right Lacrimal Gland, Percutaneous Approach

08CVXZZ Extirpation of Matter from Right Lacrimal Gland, External Approach

08CW0ZZ Extirpation of Matter from Left Lacrimal Gland, Open Approach

08CW3ZZ Extirpation of Matter from Left Lacrimal Gland, Percutaneous Approach

08CWXZZ Extirpation of Matter from Left Lacrimal Gland, External Approach

08CX0ZZ Extirpation of Matter from Right Lacrimal Duct, Open Approach

08CX3ZZ Extirpation of Matter from Right Lacrimal Duct, Percutaneous Approach

08CX7ZZ Extirpation of Matter from Right Lacrimal Duct, Via Natural or Artificial Opening

08CX8ZZ Extirpation of Matter from Right Lacrimal Duct, Via Natural or Artificial Opening Endoscopic

08CY0ZZ Extirpation of Matter from Left Lacrimal Duct, Open Approach

08CY3ZZ Extirpation of Matter from Left Lacrimal Duct, Percutaneous Approach

08CY7ZZ Extirpation of Matter from Left Lacrimal Duct, Via Natural or Artificial Opening

08CY8ZZ Extirpation of Matter from Left Lacrimal Duct, Via Natural or Artificial Opening Endoscopic

08D – Eye, Extraction

Review Coding Guidelines B3.4a and B3.4b

08D8XZX Extraction of Right Cornea, External Approach, Diagnostic

08D8XZZ Extraction of Right Cornea, External Approach

08D9XZX Extraction of Left Cornea, External Approach, Diagnostic

08D9XZZ Extraction of Left Cornea, External Approach

08DJ3ZZ Extraction of Right Lens, Percutaneous Approach

08DK3ZZ Extraction of Left Lens, Percutaneous Approach

08F – Eye, Fragmentation

08F43ZZ Fragmentation in Right Vitreous, Percutaneous Approach

▲08F4XZZ Fragmentation in Right Vitreous, External Approach

08F53ZZ Fragmentation in Left Vitreous, Percutaneous Approach

▲08F5XZZ Fragmentation in Left Vitreous, External Approach

08H – Eye, Insertion

08H005Z Insertion of Epiretinal Visual Prosthesis into Right Eye, Open Approach

08H00YZ Insertion of Other Device into Right Eye, Open Approach

08H031Z Insertion of Radioactive Element into Right Eye, Percutaneous Approach

08H033Z Insertion of Infusion Device into Right Eye, Percutaneous Approach

08H03YZ Insertion of Other Device into Right Eye, Percutaneous Approach

08H07YZ Insertion of Other Device into Right Eye, Via Natural or Artificial Opening

08H08YZ Insertion of Other Device into Right Eye, Via Natural or Artificial Opening Endoscopic

08H0X1Z Insertion of Radioactive Element into Right Eye, External Approach

08H0X3Z Insertion of Infusion Device into Right Eye, External Approach

08H105Z Insertion of Epiretinal Visual Prosthesis into Left Eye, Open Approach

08H10YZ Insertion of Other Device into Left Eye, Open Approach

08H131Z Insertion of Radioactive Element into Left Eye, Percutaneous Approach

08H133Z Insertion of Infusion Device into Left Eye, Percutaneous Approach

08H13YZ Insertion of Other Device into Left Eye, Percutaneous Approach

08H17YZ Insertion of Other Device into Left Eye, Via Natural or Artificial Opening

08H18YZ Insertion of Other Device into Left Eye, Via Natural or Artificial Opening Endoscopic

08H1X1Z Insertion of Radioactive Element into Left Eye, External Approach

08H1X3Z Insertion of Infusion Device into Left Eye, External Approach

08J – Eye, Inspection

Review Coding Guidelines B3.11a, B3.11b and B3.11c

08J0XZZ Inspection of Right Eye, External Approach
    AHA CC: 1Q, 2015, 35-36

08J1XZZ Inspection of Left Eye, External Approach

08JJXZZ Inspection of Right Lens, External Approach

08JKXZZ Inspection of Left Lens, External Approach

08JL0ZZ Inspection of Right Extraocular Muscle, Open Approach

08JLXZZ Inspection of Right Extraocular Muscle, External Approach

08JM0ZZ Inspection of Left Extraocular Muscle, Open Approach

08JMXZZ Inspection of Left Extraocular Muscle, External Approach

08L – Eye, Occlusion

08LX0CZ Occlusion of Right Lacrimal Duct with Extraluminal Device, Open Approach

08LX0DZ Occlusion of Right Lacrimal Duct with Intraluminal Device, Open Approach

08LX0ZZ Occlusion of Right Lacrimal Duct, Open Approach

08LX3CZ Occlusion of Right Lacrimal Duct with Extraluminal Device, Percutaneous Approach

08LX3DZ Occlusion of Right Lacrimal Duct with Intraluminal Device, Percutaneous Approach

08LX3ZZ Occlusion of Right Lacrimal Duct, Percutaneous Approach

08LX7DZ Occlusion of Right Lacrimal Duct with Intraluminal Device, Via Natural or Artificial Opening

08LX7ZZ Occlusion of Right Lacrimal Duct, Via Natural or Artificial Opening

08LX8DZ Occlusion of Right Lacrimal Duct with Intraluminal Device, Via Natural or Artificial Opening Endoscopic

08LX8ZZ Occlusion of Right Lacrimal Duct, Via Natural or Artificial Opening Endoscopic

08LY0CZ Occlusion of Left Lacrimal Duct with Extraluminal Device, Open Approach

08LY0DZ Occlusion of Left Lacrimal Duct with Intraluminal Device, Open Approach

08LY0ZZ Occlusion of Left Lacrimal Duct, Open Approach

08LY3CZ Occlusion of Left Lacrimal Duct with Extraluminal Device, Percutaneous Approach

08LY3DZ Occlusion of Left Lacrimal Duct with Intraluminal Device, Percutaneous Approach

08LY3ZZ Occlusion of Left Lacrimal Duct, Percutaneous Approach

08LY7DZ Occlusion of Left Lacrimal Duct with Intraluminal Device, Via Natural or Artificial Opening

08LY7ZZ Occlusion of Left Lacrimal Duct, Via Natural or Artificial Opening

08LY8DZ Occlusion of Left Lacrimal Duct with Intraluminal Device, Via Natural or Artificial Opening Endoscopic

08LY8ZZ Occlusion of Left Lacrimal Duct, Via Natural or Artificial Opening Endoscopic

08M – Eye, Reattachment

08MNXZZ Reattachment of Right Upper Eyelid, External Approach

08MPXZZ Reattachment of Left Upper Eyelid, External Approach

08MQXZZ Reattachment of Right Lower Eyelid, External Approach

08MRXZZ Reattachment of Left Lower Eyelid, External Approach

08N – Eye, Release

Review Coding Guidelines B3.13 and B3.14

08N0XZZ Release Right Eye, External Approach

08N1XZZ Release Left Eye, External Approach

08N23ZZ Release Right Anterior Chamber, Percutaneous Approach

08N33ZZ Release Left Anterior Chamber, Percutaneous Approach

08N43ZZ Release Right Vitreous, Percutaneous Approach

08N53ZZ Release Left Vitreous, Percutaneous Approach

08N6XZZ Release Right Sclera, External Approach

08N7XZZ Release Left Sclera, External Approach

08N8XZZ Release Right Cornea, External Approach

08N9XZZ Release Left Cornea, External Approach

08NA0ZZ Release Right Choroid, Open Approach

08NA3ZZ Release Right Choroid, Percutaneous Approach

08NB0ZZ Release Left Choroid, Open Approach

08NB3ZZ Release Left Choroid, Percutaneous Approach

08NC3ZZ Release Right Iris, Percutaneous Approach
    AHA CC: 2Q, 2015, 24-25

08ND3ZZ Release Left Iris, Percutaneous Approach

08NE3ZZ Release Right Retina, Percutaneous Approach

08NF3ZZ Release Left Retina, Percutaneous Approach

08NG3ZZ Release Right Retinal Vessel, Percutaneous Approach

08NH3ZZ Release Left Retinal Vessel, Percutaneous Approach

08NJ3ZZ Release Right Lens, Percutaneous Approach

08NK3ZZ Release Left Lens, Percutaneous Approach

08NL0ZZ Release Right Extraocular Muscle, Open Approach

08NL3ZZ Release Right Extraocular Muscle, Percutaneous Approach

08NM0ZZ Release Left Extraocular Muscle, Open Approach

08NM3ZZ Release Left Extraocular Muscle, Percutaneous Approach

08NN0ZZ Release Right Upper Eyelid, Open Approach

08NN3ZZ Release Right Upper Eyelid, Percutaneous Approach

08NNXZZ Release Right Upper Eyelid, External Approach

08NP0ZZ Release Left Upper Eyelid, Open Approach

08NP3ZZ Release Left Upper Eyelid, Percutaneous Approach

08NPXZZ Release Left Upper Eyelid, External Approach

08NQ0ZZ Release Right Lower Eyelid, Open Approach

08NQ3ZZ Release Right Lower Eyelid, Percutaneous Approach

08NQXZZ Release Right Lower Eyelid, External Approach

08NR0ZZ Release Left Lower Eyelid, Open Approach

08NR3ZZ Release Left Lower Eyelid, Percutaneous Approach

08NRXZZ Release Left Lower Eyelid, External Approach

08NSXZZ Release Right Conjunctiva, External Approach

08NTXZZ Release Left Conjunctiva, External Approach

08NV0ZZ Release Right Lacrimal Gland, Open Approach

08NV3ZZ Release Right Lacrimal Gland, Percutaneous Approach

08NW0ZZ Release Left Lacrimal Gland, Open Approach

08NW3ZZ Release Left Lacrimal Gland, Percutaneous Approach

08NX0ZZ Release Right Lacrimal Duct, Open Approach

08NX3ZZ Release Right Lacrimal Duct, Percutaneous Approach

08NX7ZZ Release Right Lacrimal Duct, Via Natural or Artificial Opening

08NX8ZZ Release Right Lacrimal Duct, Via Natural or Artificial Opening Endoscopic

08NY0ZZ Release Left Lacrimal Duct, Open Approach

08NY3ZZ Release Left Lacrimal Duct, Percutaneous Approach

08NY7ZZ Release Left Lacrimal Duct, Via Natural or Artificial Opening

08NY8ZZ Release Left Lacrimal Duct, Via Natural or Artificial Opening Endoscopic

08P000Z   Removal of Drainage Device from Right Eye, Open Approach

08P001Z   Removal of Radioactive Element from Right Eye, Open Approach

08P003Z   Removal of Infusion Device from Right Eye, Open Approach

08P007Z   Removal of Autologous Tissue Substitute from Right Eye, Open Approach

08P00CZ   Removal of Extraluminal Device from Right Eye, Open Approach

08P00DZ   Removal of Intraluminal Device from Right Eye, Open Approach

08P00JZ   Removal of Synthetic Substitute from Right Eye, Open Approach

08P00KZ   Removal of Nonautologous Tissue Substitute from Right Eye, Open Approach

08P00YZ   Removal of Other Device from Right Eye, Open Approach

08P030Z   Removal of Drainage Device from Right Eye, Percutaneous Approach

08P031Z   Removal of Radioactive Element from Right Eye, Percutaneous Approach

08P033Z   Removal of Infusion Device from Right Eye, Percutaneous Approach

08P037Z   Removal of Autologous Tissue Substitute from Right Eye, Percutaneous Approach

08P03CZ   Removal of Extraluminal Device from Right Eye, Percutaneous Approach

08P03DZ   Removal of Intraluminal Device from Right Eye, Percutaneous Approach

08P03JZ   Removal of Synthetic Substitute from Right Eye, Percutaneous Approach

08P03KZ   Removal of Nonautologous Tissue Substitute from Right Eye, Percutaneous Approach

08P03YZ   Removal of Other Device from Right Eye, Percutaneous Approach

08P070Z   Removal of Drainage Device from Right Eye, Via Natural or Artificial Opening

08P071Z   Removal of Radioactive Element from Right Eye, Via Natural or Artificial Opening

08P073Z   Removal of Infusion Device from Right Eye, Via Natural or Artificial Opening

08P077Z   Removal of Autologous Tissue Substitute from Right Eye, Via Natural or Artificial Opening

08P07CZ   Removal of Extraluminal Device from Right Eye, Via Natural or Artificial Opening

08P07DZ   Removal of Intraluminal Device from Right Eye, Via Natural or Artificial Opening

08P07JZ   Removal of Synthetic Substitute from Right Eye, Via Natural or Artificial Opening

08P07KZ   Removal of Nonautologous Tissue Substitute from Right Eye, Via Natural or Artificial Opening

08P07YZ   Removal of Other Device from Right Eye, Via Natural or Artificial Opening

08P080Z   Removal of Drainage Device from Right Eye, Via Natural or Artificial Opening Endoscopic

08P081Z   Removal of Radioactive Element from Right Eye, Via Natural or Artificial Opening Endoscopic

08P083Z   Removal of Infusion Device from Right Eye, Via Natural or Artificial Opening Endoscopic

08P087Z   Removal of Autologous Tissue Substitute from Right Eye, Via Natural or Artificial Opening Endoscopic

08P08CZ   Removal of Extraluminal Device from Right Eye, Via Natural or Artificial Opening Endoscopic

08P08DZ   Removal of Intraluminal Device from Right Eye, Via Natural or Artificial Opening Endoscopic

08P08JZ   Removal of Synthetic Substitute from Right Eye, Via Natural or Artificial Opening Endoscopic

08P08KZ   Removal of Nonautologous Tissue Substitute from Right Eye, Via Natural or Artificial Opening Endoscopic

08P08YZ   Removal of Other Device from Right Eye, Via Natural or Artificial Opening Endoscopic

08P0X0Z   Removal of Drainage Device from Right Eye, External Approach

08P0X1Z   Removal of Radioactive Element from Right Eye, External Approach

08P0X3Z   Removal of Infusion Device from Right Eye, External Approach

08P0X7Z   Removal of Autologous Tissue Substitute from Right Eye, External Approach

08P0XCZ   Removal of Extraluminal Device from Right Eye, External Approach

08P0XDZ   Removal of Intraluminal Device from Right Eye, External Approach

08P0XJZ   Removal of Synthetic Substitute from Right Eye, External Approach

08P0XKZ   Removal of Nonautologous Tissue Substitute from Right Eye, External Approach

08P100Z   Removal of Drainage Device from Left Eye, Open Approach

08P101Z   Removal of Radioactive Element from Left Eye, Open Approach

08P103Z   Removal of Infusion Device from Left Eye, Open Approach

08P107Z   Removal of Autologous Tissue Substitute from Left Eye, Open Approach

08P10CZ   Removal of Extraluminal Device from Left Eye, Open Approach

08P10DZ   Removal of Intraluminal Device from Left Eye, Open Approach

08P10JZ   Removal of Synthetic Substitute from Left Eye, Open Approach

08P10KZ   Removal of Nonautologous Tissue Substitute from Left Eye, Open Approach

08P10YZ   Removal of Other Device from Left Eye, Open Approach

08P130Z   Removal of Drainage Device from Left Eye, Percutaneous Approach

08P131Z   Removal of Radioactive Element from Left Eye, Percutaneous Approach

08P133Z   Removal of Infusion Device from Left Eye, Percutaneous Approach

08P137Z   Removal of Autologous Tissue Substitute from Left Eye, Percutaneous Approach

08P13CZ   Removal of Extraluminal Device from Left Eye, Percutaneous Approach

08P13DZ   Removal of Intraluminal Device from Left Eye, Percutaneous Approach

08P13JZ   Removal of Synthetic Substitute from Left Eye, Percutaneous Approach

08P13KZ   Removal of Nonautologous Tissue Substitute from Left Eye, Percutaneous Approach

08P13YZ   Removal of Other Device from Left Eye, Percutaneous Approach

08P170Z   Removal of Drainage Device from Left Eye, Via Natural or Artificial Opening

08P171Z   Removal of Radioactive Element from Left Eye, Via Natural or Artificial Opening

08P173Z   Removal of Infusion Device from Left Eye, Via Natural or Artificial Opening

08P177Z   Removal of Autologous Tissue Substitute from Left Eye, Via Natural or Artificial Opening

08P17CZ   Removal of Extraluminal Device from Left Eye, Via Natural or Artificial Opening

08P17DZ   Removal of Intraluminal Device from Left Eye, Via Natural or Artificial Opening

08P17JZ   Removal of Synthetic Substitute from Left Eye, Via Natural or Artificial Opening

08P17KZ   Removal of Nonautologous Tissue Substitute from Left Eye, Via Natural or Artificial Opening

08P17YZ   Removal of Other Device from Left Eye, Via Natural or Artificial Opening

08P180Z   Removal of Drainage Device from Left Eye, Via Natural or Artificial Opening Endoscopic

08P181Z   Removal of Radioactive Element from Left Eye, Via Natural or Artificial Opening Endoscopic

08P183Z   Removal of Infusion Device from Left Eye, Via Natural or Artificial Opening Endoscopic

08P187Z   Removal of Autologous Tissue Substitute from Left Eye, Via Natural or Artificial Opening Endoscopic

08P18CZ   Removal of Extraluminal Device from Left Eye, Via Natural or Artificial Opening Endoscopic

08P18DZ   Removal of Intraluminal Device from Left Eye, Via Natural or Artificial Opening Endoscopic

08P18JZ   Removal of Synthetic Substitute from Left Eye, Via Natural or Artificial Opening Endoscopic

08P18KZ   Removal of Nonautologous Tissue Substitute from Left Eye, Via Natural or Artificial Opening Endoscopic

08P18YZ   Removal of Other Device from Left Eye, Via Natural or Artificial Opening Endoscopic

08P1X0Z   Removal of Drainage Device from Left Eye, External Approach

08P1X1Z   Removal of Radioactive Element from Left Eye, External Approach

08P1X3Z   Removal of Infusion Device from Left Eye, External Approach

08P1X7Z   Removal of Autologous Tissue Substitute from Left Eye, External Approach

08P1XCZ   Removal of Extraluminal Device from Left Eye, External Approach

08P1XDZ   Removal of Intraluminal Device from Left Eye, External Approach

08P1XJZ   Removal of Synthetic Substitute from Left Eye, External Approach

08P1XKZ   Removal of Nonautologous Tissue Substitute from Left Eye, External Approach

08PJ3JZ   Removal of Synthetic Substitute from Right Lens, Percutaneous Approach

♀ Female-only   ♂ Male-only   ▲ Limited Coverage   ● Non-OR   HAC HAC-associated procedure   ▲ Non-covered procedures   ✚ Cluster

08PJ3YZ Removal of Other Device from Right Lens, Percutaneous Approach

08PK3JZ Removal of Synthetic Substitute from Left Lens, Percutaneous Approach

08PK3YZ Removal of Other Device from Left Lens, Percutaneous Approach

08PL00Z Removal of Drainage Device from Right Extraocular Muscle, Open Approach

08PL07Z Removal of Autologous Tissue Substitute from Right Extraocular Muscle, Open Approach

08PL0JZ Removal of Synthetic Substitute from Right Extraocular Muscle, Open Approach

08PL0KZ Removal of Nonautologous Tissue Substitute from Right Extraocular Muscle, Open Approach

08PL0YZ Removal of Other Device from Right Extraocular Muscle, Open Approach

08PL30Z Removal of Drainage Device from Right Extraocular Muscle, Percutaneous Approach

08PL37Z Removal of Autologous Tissue Substitute from Right Extraocular Muscle, Percutaneous Approach

08PL3JZ Removal of Synthetic Substitute from Right Extraocular Muscle, Percutaneous Approach

08PL3KZ Removal of Nonautologous Tissue Substitute from Right Extraocular Muscle, Percutaneous Approach

08PL3YZ Removal of Other Device from Right Extraocular Muscle, Percutaneous Approach

08PM00Z Removal of Drainage Device from Left Extraocular Muscle, Open Approach

08PM07Z Removal of Autologous Tissue Substitute from Left Extraocular Muscle, Open Approach

08PM0JZ Removal of Synthetic Substitute from Left Extraocular Muscle, Open Approach

08PM0KZ Removal of Nonautologous Tissue Substitute from Left Extraocular Muscle, Open Approach

08PM0YZ Removal of Other Device from Left Extraocular Muscle, Open Approach

08PM30Z Removal of Drainage Device from Left Extraocular Muscle, Percutaneous Approach

08PM37Z Removal of Autologous Tissue Substitute from Left Extraocular Muscle, Percutaneous Approach

08PM3JZ Removal of Synthetic Substitute from Left Extraocular Muscle, Percutaneous Approach

08PM3KZ Removal of Nonautologous Tissue Substitute from Left Extraocular Muscle, Percutaneous Approach

08PM3YZ Removal of Other Device from Left Extraocular Muscle, Percutaneous Approach

08Q – Eye, Repair

08Q0XZZ Repair Right Eye, External Approach

08Q1XZZ Repair Left Eye, External Approach

08Q23ZZ Repair Right Anterior Chamber, Percutaneous Approach

08Q33ZZ Repair Left Anterior Chamber, Percutaneous Approach

08Q43ZZ Repair Right Vitreous, Percutaneous Approach

08Q53ZZ Repair Left Vitreous, Percutaneous Approach

08Q6XZZ Repair Right Sclera, External Approach

08Q7XZZ Repair Left Sclera, External Approach
AHA CC: 3Q, 2018, 13

▲ **08Q8XZZ** Repair Right Cornea, External Approach

▲ **08Q9XZZ** Repair Left Cornea, External Approach
AHA CC: 3Q, 2018, 13

08QA0ZZ Repair Right Choroid, Open Approach

08QA3ZZ Repair Right Choroid, Percutaneous Approach

08QB0ZZ Repair Left Choroid, Open Approach

08QB3ZZ Repair Left Choroid, Percutaneous Approach

08QC3ZZ Repair Right Iris, Percutaneous Approach

08QD3ZZ Repair Left Iris, Percutaneous Approach

08QE3ZZ Repair Right Retina, Percutaneous Approach

08QF3ZZ Repair Left Retina, Percutaneous Approach

08QG3ZZ Repair Right Retinal Vessel, Percutaneous Approach

08QH3ZZ Repair Left Retinal Vessel, Percutaneous Approach

08QJ3ZZ Repair Right Lens, Percutaneous Approach

08QK3ZZ Repair Left Lens, Percutaneous Approach

08QL0ZZ Repair Right Extraocular Muscle, Open Approach

08QL3ZZ Repair Right Extraocular Muscle, Percutaneous Approach

08QM0ZZ Repair Left Extraocular Muscle, Open Approach

08QM3ZZ Repair Left Extraocular Muscle, Percutaneous Approach

08QN0ZZ Repair Right Upper Eyelid, Open Approach

08QN3ZZ Repair Right Upper Eyelid, Percutaneous Approach

08QNXZZ Repair Right Upper Eyelid, External Approach

08QP0ZZ Repair Left Upper Eyelid, Open Approach

08QP3ZZ Repair Left Upper Eyelid, Percutaneous Approach

08QPXZZ Repair Left Upper Eyelid, External Approach

08QQ0ZZ Repair Right Lower Eyelid, Open Approach

08QQ3ZZ Repair Right Lower Eyelid, Percutaneous Approach

08QQXZZ Repair Right Lower Eyelid, External Approach

08QR0ZZ Repair Left Lower Eyelid, Open Approach

08QR3ZZ Repair Left Lower Eyelid, Percutaneous Approach

08QRXZZ Repair Left Lower Eyelid, External Approach

08QSXZZ Repair Right Conjunctiva, External Approach

08QTXZZ Repair Left Conjunctiva, External Approach

08QV0ZZ Repair Right Lacrimal Gland, Open Approach

08QV3ZZ Repair Right Lacrimal Gland, Percutaneous Approach

08QW0ZZ Repair Left Lacrimal Gland, Open Approach

08QW3ZZ Repair Left Lacrimal Gland, Percutaneous Approach

08QX0ZZ Repair Right Lacrimal Duct, Open Approach

08QX3ZZ Repair Right Lacrimal Duct, Percutaneous Approach

08QX7ZZ Repair Right Lacrimal Duct, Via Natural or Artificial Opening

08QX8ZZ Repair Right Lacrimal Duct, Via Natural or Artificial Opening Endoscopic

08QY0ZZ Repair Left Lacrimal Duct, Open Approach

08QY3ZZ Repair Left Lacrimal Duct, Percutaneous Approach

08QY7ZZ Repair Left Lacrimal Duct, Via Natural or Artificial Opening

08QY8ZZ Repair Left Lacrimal Duct, Via Natural or Artificial Opening Endoscopic

08R – Eye, Replacement

Review Coding Guideline B3.18

08R007Z Replacement of Right Eye with Autologous Tissue Substitute, Open Approach

08R00JZ Replacement of Right Eye with Synthetic Substitute, Open Approach

08R00KZ Replacement of Right Eye with Nonautologous Tissue Substitute, Open Approach

08R037Z Replacement of Right Eye with Autologous Tissue Substitute, Percutaneous Approach

08R03JZ Replacement of Right Eye with Synthetic Substitute, Percutaneous Approach

08R03KZ Replacement of Right Eye with Nonautologous Tissue Substitute, Percutaneous Approach

08R107Z Replacement of Left Eye with Autologous Tissue Substitute, Open Approach

08R10JZ Replacement of Left Eye with Synthetic Substitute, Open Approach

08R10KZ Replacement of Left Eye with Nonautologous Tissue Substitute, Open Approach

08R137Z Replacement of Left Eye with Autologous Tissue Substitute, Percutaneous Approach

08R13JZ Replacement of Left Eye with Synthetic Substitute, Percutaneous Approach

08R13KZ Replacement of Left Eye with Nonautologous Tissue Substitute, Percutaneous Approach

08R437Z Replacement of Right Vitreous with Autologous Tissue Substitute, Percutaneous Approach

08R43JZ Replacement of Right Vitreous with Synthetic Substitute, Percutaneous Approach

08R43KZ Replacement of Right Vitreous with Nonautologous Tissue Substitute, Percutaneous Approach

08R537Z Replacement of Left Vitreous with Autologous Tissue Substitute, Percutaneous Approach

08R53JZ Replacement of Left Vitreous with Synthetic Substitute, Percutaneous Approach

08R53KZ Replacement of Left Vitreous with Nonautologous Tissue Substitute, Percutaneous Approach

08R6X7Z Replacement of Right Sclera with Autologous Tissue Substitute, External Approach

08R6XJZ Replacement of Right Sclera with Synthetic Substitute, External Approach

08R6XKZ Replacement of Right Sclera with Nonautologous Tissue Substitute, External Approach

08R7X7Z Replacement of Left Sclera with Autologous Tissue Substitute, External Approach

08R7XJZ Replacement of Left Sclera with Synthetic Substitute, External Approach

08R7XKZ Replacement of Left Sclera with Nonautologous Tissue Substitute, External Approach

08R837Z Replacement of Right Cornea with Autologous Tissue Substitute, Percutaneous Approach

08R83JZ Replacement of Right Cornea with Synthetic Substitute, Percutaneous Approach

08R83KZ Replacement of Right Cornea with Nonautologous Tissue Substitute, Percutaneous Approach

08R8X7Z Replacement of Right Cornea with Autologous Tissue Substitute, External Approach

08R8XJZ Replacement of Right Cornea with Synthetic Substitute, External Approach

08R8XKZ Replacement of Right Cornea with Nonautologous Tissue Substitute, External Approach

AHA CC: 2Q, 2015, 24-26

08R937Z Replacement of Left Cornea with Autologous Tissue Substitute, Percutaneous Approach

08R93JZ Replacement of Left Cornea with Synthetic Substitute, Percutaneous Approach

08R93KZ Replacement of Left Cornea with Nonautologous Tissue Substitute, Percutaneous Approach

08R9X7Z Replacement of Left Cornea with Autologous Tissue Substitute, External Approach

08R9XJZ Replacement of Left Cornea with Synthetic Substitute, External Approach

08R9XKZ Replacement of Left Cornea with Nonautologous Tissue Substitute, External Approach

08RA07Z Replacement of Right Choroid with Autologous Tissue Substitute, Open Approach

08RA0JZ Replacement of Right Choroid with Synthetic Substitute, Open Approach

08RA0KZ Replacement of Right Choroid with Nonautologous Tissue Substitute, Open Approach

08RA37Z Replacement of Right Choroid with Autologous Tissue Substitute, Percutaneous Approach

08RA3JZ Replacement of Right Choroid with Synthetic Substitute, Percutaneous Approach

08RA3KZ Replacement of Right Choroid with Nonautologous Tissue Substitute, Percutaneous Approach

08RB07Z Replacement of Left Choroid with Autologous Tissue Substitute, Open Approach

08RB0JZ Replacement of Left Choroid with Synthetic Substitute, Open Approach

08RB0KZ Replacement of Left Choroid with Nonautologous Tissue Substitute, Open Approach

08RB37Z Replacement of Left Choroid with Autologous Tissue Substitute, Percutaneous Approach

08RB3JZ Replacement of Left Choroid with Synthetic Substitute, Percutaneous Approach

08RB3KZ Replacement of Left Choroid with Nonautologous Tissue Substitute, Percutaneous Approach

08RC37Z Replacement of Right Iris with Autologous Tissue Substitute, Percutaneous Approach

08RC3JZ Replacement of Right Iris with Synthetic Substitute, Percutaneous Approach

08RC3KZ Replacement of Right Iris with Nonautologous Tissue Substitute, Percutaneous Approach

08RD37Z Replacement of Left Iris with Autologous Tissue Substitute, Percutaneous Approach

08RD3JZ Replacement of Left Iris with Synthetic Substitute, Percutaneous Approach

08RD3KZ Replacement of Left Iris with Nonautologous Tissue Substitute, Percutaneous Approach

08RG37Z Replacement of Right Retinal Vessel with Autologous Tissue Substitute, Percutaneous Approach

08RG3JZ Replacement of Right Retinal Vessel with Synthetic Substitute, Percutaneous Approach

08RG3KZ Replacement of Right Retinal Vessel with Nonautologous Tissue Substitute, Percutaneous Approach

08RH37Z Replacement of Left Retinal Vessel with Autologous Tissue Substitute, Percutaneous Approach

08RH3JZ Replacement of Left Retinal Vessel with Synthetic Substitute, Percutaneous Approach

08RH3KZ Replacement of Left Retinal Vessel with Nonautologous Tissue Substitute, Percutaneous Approach

08RJ30Z Replacement of Right Lens with Intraocular Telescope, Percutaneous Approach

08RJ37Z Replacement of Right Lens with Autologous Tissue Substitute, Percutaneous Approach

08RJ3JZ Replacement of Right Lens with Synthetic Substitute, Percutaneous Approach

08RJ3KZ Replacement of Right Lens with Nonautologous Tissue Substitute, Percutaneous Approach

08RK30Z Replacement of Left Lens with Intraocular Telescope, Percutaneous Approach

08RK37Z Replacement of Left Lens with Autologous Tissue Substitute, Percutaneous Approach

08RK3JZ Replacement of Left Lens with Synthetic Substitute, Percutaneous Approach

08RK3KZ Replacement of Left Lens with Nonautologous Tissue Substitute, Percutaneous Approach

08RN07Z Replacement of Right Upper Eyelid with Autologous Tissue Substitute, Open Approach

08RN0JZ Replacement of Right Upper Eyelid with Synthetic Substitute, Open Approach

08RN0KZ Replacement of Right Upper Eyelid with Nonautologous Tissue Substitute, Open Approach

08RN37Z Replacement of Right Upper Eyelid with Autologous Tissue Substitute, Percutaneous Approach

08RN3JZ Replacement of Right Upper Eyelid with Synthetic Substitute, Percutaneous Approach

08RN3KZ Replacement of Right Upper Eyelid with Nonautologous Tissue Substitute, Percutaneous Approach

08RNX7Z Replacement of Right Upper Eyelid with Autologous Tissue Substitute, External Approach

08RNXJZ Replacement of Right Upper Eyelid with Synthetic Substitute, External Approach

08RNXKZ Replacement of Right Upper Eyelid with Nonautologous Tissue Substitute, External Approach

08RP07Z Replacement of Left Upper Eyelid with Autologous Tissue Substitute, Open Approach

08RP0JZ Replacement of Left Upper Eyelid with Synthetic Substitute, Open Approach

08RP0KZ Replacement of Left Upper Eyelid with Nonautologous Tissue Substitute, Open Approach

08RP37Z Replacement of Left Upper Eyelid with Autologous Tissue Substitute, Percutaneous Approach

08RP3JZ Replacement of Left Upper Eyelid with Synthetic Substitute, Percutaneous Approach

08RP3KZ Replacement of Left Upper Eyelid with Nonautologous Tissue Substitute, Percutaneous Approach

08RPX7Z Replacement of Left Upper Eyelid with Autologous Tissue Substitute, External Approach

08RPXJZ Replacement of Left Upper Eyelid with Synthetic Substitute, External Approach

08RPXKZ Replacement of Left Upper Eyelid with Nonautologous Tissue Substitute, External Approach

08RQ07Z Replacement of Right Lower Eyelid with Autologous Tissue Substitute, Open Approach

08RQ0JZ Replacement of Right Lower Eyelid with Synthetic Substitute, Open Approach

08RQ0KZ Replacement of Right Lower Eyelid with Nonautologous Tissue Substitute, Open Approach

♀ Female-only   ♂ Male-only   ▲ Limited Coverage   ● Non-OR   ▦ HAC-associated procedure   ▲ Non-covered procedures   ➕ Cluster

08RQ37Z	Replacement of Right Lower Eyelid with Autologous Tissue Substitute, Percutaneous Approach
08RQ3JZ	Replacement of Right Lower Eyelid with Synthetic Substitute, Percutaneous Approach
08RQ3KZ	Replacement of Right Lower Eyelid with Nonautologous Tissue Substitute, Percutaneous Approach
08RQX7Z	Replacement of Right Lower Eyelid with Autologous Tissue Substitute, External Approach
08RQXJZ	Replacement of Right Lower Eyelid with Synthetic Substitute, External Approach
08RQXKZ	Replacement of Right Lower Eyelid with Nonautologous Tissue Substitute, External Approach
08RR07Z	Replacement of Left Lower Eyelid with Autologous Tissue Substitute, Open Approach
08RR0JZ	Replacement of Left Lower Eyelid with Synthetic Substitute, Open Approach
08RR0KZ	Replacement of Left Lower Eyelid with Nonautologous Tissue Substitute, Open Approach
08RR37Z	Replacement of Left Lower Eyelid with Autologous Tissue Substitute, Percutaneous Approach
08RR3JZ	Replacement of Left Lower Eyelid with Synthetic Substitute, Percutaneous Approach
08RR3KZ	Replacement of Left Lower Eyelid with Nonautologous Tissue Substitute, Percutaneous Approach
08RRX7Z	Replacement of Left Lower Eyelid with Autologous Tissue Substitute, External Approach
08RRXJZ	Replacement of Left Lower Eyelid with Synthetic Substitute, External Approach
08RRXKZ	Replacement of Left Lower Eyelid with Nonautologous Tissue Substitute, External Approach

08RSX7Z	Replacement of Right Conjunctiva with Autologous Tissue Substitute, External Approach
08RSXJZ	Replacement of Right Conjunctiva with Synthetic Substitute, External Approach
08RSXKZ	Replacement of Right Conjunctiva with Nonautologous Tissue Substitute, External Approach
08RTX7Z	Replacement of Left Conjunctiva with Autologous Tissue Substitute, External Approach
08RTXJZ	Replacement of Left Conjunctiva with Synthetic Substitute, External Approach
08RTXKZ	Replacement of Left Conjunctiva with Nonautologous Tissue Substitute, External Approach
08RX07Z	Replacement of Right Lacrimal Duct with Autologous Tissue Substitute, Open Approach
08RX0JZ	Replacement of Right Lacrimal Duct with Synthetic Substitute, Open Approach
08RX0KZ	Replacement of Right Lacrimal Duct with Nonautologous Tissue Substitute, Open Approach
08RX37Z	Replacement of Right Lacrimal Duct with Autologous Tissue Substitute, Percutaneous Approach
08RX3JZ	Replacement of Right Lacrimal Duct with Synthetic Substitute, Percutaneous Approach
08RX3KZ	Replacement of Right Lacrimal Duct with Nonautologous Tissue Substitute, Percutaneous Approach
08RX77Z	Replacement of Right Lacrimal Duct with Autologous Tissue Substitute, Via Natural or Artificial Opening
08RX7JZ	Replacement of Right Lacrimal Duct with Synthetic Substitute, Via Natural or Artificial Opening
08RX7KZ	Replacement of Right Lacrimal Duct with Nonautologous Tissue Substitute, Via Natural or Artificial Opening
08RX87Z	Replacement of Right Lacrimal Duct with Autologous Tissue Substitute, Via Natural or Artificial Opening Endoscopic

08RX8JZ	Replacement of Right Lacrimal Duct with Synthetic Substitute, Via Natural or Artificial Opening Endoscopic
08RX8KZ	Replacement of Right Lacrimal Duct with Nonautologous Tissue Substitute, Via Natural or Artificial Opening Endoscopic
08RY07Z	Replacement of Left Lacrimal Duct with Autologous Tissue Substitute, Open Approach
08RY0JZ	Replacement of Left Lacrimal Duct with Synthetic Substitute, Open Approach
08RY0KZ	Replacement of Left Lacrimal Duct with Nonautologous Tissue Substitute, Open Approach
08RY37Z	Replacement of Left Lacrimal Duct with Autologous Tissue Substitute, Percutaneous Approach
08RY3JZ	Replacement of Left Lacrimal Duct with Synthetic Substitute, Percutaneous Approach
08RY3KZ	Replacement of Left Lacrimal Duct with Nonautologous Tissue Substitute, Percutaneous Approach
08RY77Z	Replacement of Left Lacrimal Duct with Autologous Tissue Substitute, Via Natural or Artificial Opening
08RY7JZ	Replacement of Left Lacrimal Duct with Synthetic Substitute, Via Natural or Artificial Opening
08RY7KZ	Replacement of Left Lacrimal Duct with Nonautologous Tissue Substitute, Via Natural or Artificial Opening
08RY87Z	Replacement of Left Lacrimal Duct with Autologous Tissue Substitute, Via Natural or Artificial Opening Endoscopic
08RY8JZ	Replacement of Left Lacrimal Duct with Synthetic Substitute, Via Natural or Artificial Opening Endoscopic
08RY8KZ	Replacement of Left Lacrimal Duct with Nonautologous Tissue Substitute, Via Natural or Artificial Opening Endoscopic

08S – Eye, Reposition

08SC3ZZ	Reposition Right Iris, Percutaneous Approach
08SD3ZZ	Reposition Left Iris, Percutaneous Approach
08SG3ZZ	Reposition Right Retinal Vessel, Percutaneous Approach
08SH3ZZ	Reposition Left Retinal Vessel, Percutaneous Approach
08SJ3ZZ	Reposition Right Lens, Percutaneous Approach
08SK3ZZ	Reposition Left Lens, Percutaneous Approach
08SL0ZZ	Reposition Right Extraocular Muscle, Open Approach
08SL3ZZ	Reposition Right Extraocular Muscle, Percutaneous Approach
08SM0ZZ	Reposition Left Extraocular Muscle, Open Approach
08SM3ZZ	Reposition Left Extraocular Muscle, Percutaneous Approach
08SN0ZZ	Reposition Right Upper Eyelid, Open Approach
08SN3ZZ	Reposition Right Upper Eyelid, Percutaneous Approach

08SNXZZ	Reposition Right Upper Eyelid, External Approach
08SP0ZZ	Reposition Left Upper Eyelid, Open Approach
08SP3ZZ	Reposition Left Upper Eyelid, Percutaneous Approach
08SPXZZ	Reposition Left Upper Eyelid, External Approach
08SQ0ZZ	Reposition Right Lower Eyelid, Open Approach
08SQ3ZZ	Reposition Right Lower Eyelid, Percutaneous Approach
08SQXZZ	Reposition Right Lower Eyelid, External Approach
08SR0ZZ	Reposition Left Lower Eyelid, Open Approach
08SR3ZZ	Reposition Left Lower Eyelid, Percutaneous Approach
08SRXZZ	Reposition Left Lower Eyelid, External Approach
08SV0ZZ	Reposition Right Lacrimal Gland, Open Approach
08SV3ZZ	Reposition Right Lacrimal Gland, Percutaneous Approach

08SW0ZZ	Reposition Left Lacrimal Gland, Open Approach
08SW3ZZ	Reposition Left Lacrimal Gland, Percutaneous Approach
08SX0ZZ	Reposition Right Lacrimal Duct, Open Approach
08SX3ZZ	Reposition Right Lacrimal Duct, Percutaneous Approach
08SX7ZZ	Reposition Right Lacrimal Duct, Via Natural or Artificial Opening
08SX8ZZ	Reposition Right Lacrimal Duct, Via Natural or Artificial Opening Endoscopic
08SY0ZZ	Reposition Left Lacrimal Duct, Open Approach
08SY3ZZ	Reposition Left Lacrimal Duct, Percutaneous Approach
08SY7ZZ	Reposition Left Lacrimal Duct, Via Natural or Artificial Opening
08SY8ZZ	Reposition Left Lacrimal Duct, Via Natural or Artificial Opening Endoscopic

♀ Female-only　　♂ Male-only　　▲ Limited Coverage　　● Non-OR　　HAC HAC-associated procedure　　▲ Non-covered procedures　　✚ Cluster

08T – Eye, Resection

Review Coding Guideline B3.8

Review Coding Guideline B3.18

08T0XZZ Resection of Right Eye, External Approach

08T1XZZ Resection of Left Eye, External Approach
AHA CC: 2Q, 2015, 12-13

08T43ZZ Resection of Right Vitreous, Percutaneous Approach

08T53ZZ Resection of Left Vitreous, Percutaneous Approach

08T8XZZ Resection of Right Cornea, External Approach

08T9XZZ Resection of Left Cornea, External Approach

08TC3ZZ Resection of Right Iris, Percutaneous Approach

08TD3ZZ Resection of Left Iris, Percutaneous Approach

08TJ3ZZ Resection of Right Lens, Percutaneous Approach

08TK3ZZ Resection of Left Lens, Percutaneous Approach

08TL0ZZ Resection of Right Extraocular Muscle, Open Approach

08TL3ZZ Resection of Right Extraocular Muscle, Percutaneous Approach

08TM0ZZ Resection of Left Extraocular Muscle, Open Approach
AHA CC: 2Q, 2015, 12-13

08TM3ZZ Resection of Left Extraocular Muscle, Percutaneous Approach

08TN0ZZ Resection of Right Upper Eyelid, Open Approach

08TNXZZ Resection of Right Upper Eyelid, External Approach

08TP0ZZ Resection of Left Upper Eyelid, Open Approach

08TPXZZ Resection of Left Upper Eyelid, External Approach

08TQ0ZZ Resection of Right Lower Eyelid, Open Approach

08TQXZZ Resection of Right Lower Eyelid, External Approach

08TR0ZZ Resection of Left Lower Eyelid, Open Approach
AHA CC: 2Q, 2015, 12-13

08TRXZZ Resection of Left Lower Eyelid, External Approach

08TV0ZZ Resection of Right Lacrimal Gland, Open Approach

08TV3ZZ Resection of Right Lacrimal Gland, Percutaneous Approach

08TW0ZZ Resection of Left Lacrimal Gland, Open Approach

08TW3ZZ Resection of Left Lacrimal Gland, Percutaneous Approach

08TX0ZZ Resection of Right Lacrimal Duct, Open Approach

08TX3ZZ Resection of Right Lacrimal Duct, Percutaneous Approach

08TX7ZZ Resection of Right Lacrimal Duct, Via Natural or Artificial Opening

08TX8ZZ Resection of Right Lacrimal Duct, Via Natural or Artificial Opening Endoscopic

08TY0ZZ Resection of Left Lacrimal Duct, Open Approach

08TY3ZZ Resection of Left Lacrimal Duct, Percutaneous Approach

08TY7ZZ Resection of Left Lacrimal Duct, Via Natural or Artificial Opening

08TY8ZZ Resection of Left Lacrimal Duct, Via Natural or Artificial Opening Endoscopic

08U – Eye, Supplement

08U007Z Supplement of Right Eye with Autologous Tissue Substitute, Open Approach

08U00JZ Supplement of Right Eye with Synthetic Substitute, Open Approach

08U00KZ Supplement of Right Eye with Nonautologous Tissue Substitute, Open Approach

08U037Z Supplement of Right Eye with Autologous Tissue Substitute, Percutaneous Approach

08U03JZ Supplement of Right Eye with Synthetic Substitute, Percutaneous Approach

08U03KZ Supplement of Right Eye with Nonautologous Tissue Substitute, Percutaneous Approach

08U107Z Supplement of Left Eye with Autologous Tissue Substitute, Open Approach

08U10JZ Supplement of Left Eye with Synthetic Substitute, Open Approach

08U10KZ Supplement of Left Eye with Nonautologous Tissue Substitute, Open Approach

08U137Z Supplement of Left Eye with Autologous Tissue Substitute, Percutaneous Approach

08U13JZ Supplement of Left Eye with Synthetic Substitute, Percutaneous Approach

08U13KZ Supplement of Left Eye with Nonautologous Tissue Substitute, Percutaneous Approach

08U807Z Supplement Right Cornea with Autologous Tissue Substitute, Open Approach

08U80JZ Supplement Right Cornea with Synthetic Substitute, Open Approach

▲ **08U80KZ** Supplement Right Cornea with Nonautologous Tissue Substitute, Open Approach

08U837Z Supplement Right Cornea with Autologous Tissue Substitute, Percutaneous Approach

08U83JZ Supplement Right Cornea with Synthetic Substitute, Percutaneous Approach

▲ **08U83KZ** Supplement Right Cornea with Nonautologous Tissue Substitute, Percutaneous Approach

08U8X7Z Supplement Right Cornea with Autologous Tissue Substitute, External Approach

08U8XJZ Supplement Right Cornea with Synthetic Substitute, External Approach

▲ **08U8XKZ** Supplement Right Cornea with Nonautologous Tissue Substitute, External Approach

08U907Z Supplement Left Cornea with Autologous Tissue Substitute, Open Approach

08U90JZ Supplement Left Cornea with Synthetic Substitute, Open Approach

▲ **08U90KZ** Supplement Left Cornea with Nonautologous Tissue Substitute, Open Approach

08U937Z Supplement Left Cornea with Autologous Tissue Substitute, Percutaneous Approach

08U93JZ Supplement Left Cornea with Synthetic Substitute, Percutaneous Approach

▲ **08U93KZ** Supplement Left Cornea with Nonautologous Tissue Substitute, Percutaneous Approach

08U9X7Z Supplement Left Cornea with Autologous Tissue Substitute, External Approach

08U9XJZ Supplement Left Cornea with Synthetic Substitute, External Approach

▲ **08U9XKZ** Supplement Left Cornea with Nonautologous Tissue Substitute, External Approach
AHA CC: 3Q, 2014, 31

08UC07Z Supplement Right Iris with Autologous Tissue Substitute, Open Approach

08UC0JZ Supplement Right Iris with Synthetic Substitute, Open Approach

08UC0KZ Supplement Right Iris with Nonautologous Tissue Substitute, Open Approach

08UC37Z Supplement Right Iris with Autologous Tissue Substitute, Percutaneous Approach

08UC3JZ Supplement Right Iris with Synthetic Substitute, Percutaneous Approach

08UC3KZ Supplement Right Iris with Nonautologous Tissue Substitute, Percutaneous Approach

08UD07Z Supplement Left Iris with Autologous Tissue Substitute, Open Approach

08UD0JZ Supplement Left Iris with Synthetic Substitute, Open Approach

08UD0KZ Supplement Left Iris with Nonautologous Tissue Substitute, Open Approach

08UD37Z Supplement Left Iris with Autologous Tissue Substitute, Percutaneous Approach

08UD3JZ Supplement Left Iris with Synthetic Substitute, Percutaneous Approach

08UD3KZ Supplement Left Iris with Nonautologous Tissue Substitute, Percutaneous Approach

08UE07Z Supplement Right Retina with Autologous Tissue Substitute, Open Approach

08UE0JZ Supplement Right Retina with Synthetic Substitute, Open Approach

08UE0KZ Supplement Right Retina with Nonautologous Tissue Substitute, Open Approach

08UE37Z Supplement Right Retina with Autologous Tissue Substitute, Percutaneous Approach

08UE3JZ Supplement Right Retina with Synthetic Substitute, Percutaneous Approach

♀ Female-only   ♂ Male-only   ▲ Limited Coverage   ● Non-OR   **HAC** HAC-associated procedure   ▲ Non-covered procedures   ✚ Cluster

08UE3KZ Supplement Right Retina with Nonautologous Tissue Substitute, Percutaneous Approach

08UF07Z Supplement Left Retina with Autologous Tissue Substitute, Open Approach

08UF0JZ Supplement Left Retina with Synthetic Substitute, Open Approach

08UF0KZ Supplement Left Retina with Nonautologous Tissue Substitute, Open Approach

08UF37Z Supplement Left Retina with Autologous Tissue Substitute, Percutaneous Approach

08UF3JZ Supplement Left Retina with Synthetic Substitute, Percutaneous Approach

08UF3KZ Supplement Left Retina with Nonautologous Tissue Substitute, Percutaneous Approach

08UG07Z Supplement Right Retinal Vessel with Autologous Tissue Substitute, Open Approach

08UG0JZ Supplement Right Retinal Vessel with Synthetic Substitute, Open Approach

08UG0KZ Supplement Right Retinal Vessel with Nonautologous Tissue Substitute, Open Approach

08UG37Z Supplement Right Retinal Vessel with Autologous Tissue Substitute, Percutaneous Approach

08UG3JZ Supplement Right Retinal Vessel with Synthetic Substitute, Percutaneous Approach

08UG3KZ Supplement Right Retinal Vessel with Nonautologous Tissue Substitute, Percutaneous Approach

08UH07Z Supplement Left Retinal Vessel with Autologous Tissue Substitute, Open Approach

08UH0JZ Supplement Left Retinal Vessel with Synthetic Substitute, Open Approach

08UH0KZ Supplement Left Retinal Vessel with Nonautologous Tissue Substitute, Open Approach

08UH37Z Supplement Left Retinal Vessel with Autologous Tissue Substitute, Percutaneous Approach

08UH3JZ Supplement Left Retinal Vessel with Synthetic Substitute, Percutaneous Approach

08UH3KZ Supplement Left Retinal Vessel with Nonautologous Tissue Substitute, Percutaneous Approach

08UL07Z Supplement Right Extraocular Muscle with Autologous Tissue Substitute, Open Approach

08UL0JZ Supplement Right Extraocular Muscle with Synthetic Substitute, Open Approach

08UL0KZ Supplement Right Extraocular Muscle with Nonautologous Tissue Substitute, Open Approach

08UL37Z Supplement Right Extraocular Muscle with Autologous Tissue Substitute, Percutaneous Approach

08UL3JZ Supplement Right Extraocular Muscle with Synthetic Substitute, Percutaneous Approach

08UL3KZ Supplement Right Extraocular Muscle with Nonautologous Tissue Substitute, Percutaneous Approach

08UM07Z Supplement Left Extraocular Muscle with Autologous Tissue Substitute, Open Approach

08UM0JZ Supplement Left Extraocular Muscle with Synthetic Substitute, Open Approach

08UM0KZ Supplement Left Extraocular Muscle with Nonautologous Tissue Substitute, Open Approach

08UM37Z Supplement Left Extraocular Muscle with Autologous Tissue Substitute, Percutaneous Approach

08UM3JZ Supplement Left Extraocular Muscle with Synthetic Substitute, Percutaneous Approach

08UM3KZ Supplement Left Extraocular Muscle with Nonautologous Tissue Substitute, Percutaneous Approach

08UN07Z Supplement Right Upper Eyelid with Autologous Tissue Substitute, Open Approach

08UN0JZ Supplement Right Upper Eyelid with Synthetic Substitute, Open Approach

08UN0KZ Supplement Right Upper Eyelid with Nonautologous Tissue Substitute, Open Approach

08UN37Z Supplement Right Upper Eyelid with Autologous Tissue Substitute, Percutaneous Approach

08UN3JZ Supplement Right Upper Eyelid with Synthetic Substitute, Percutaneous Approach

08UN3KZ Supplement Right Upper Eyelid with Nonautologous Tissue Substitute, Percutaneous Approach

08UNX7Z Supplement Right Upper Eyelid with Autologous Tissue Substitute, External Approach

08UNXJZ Supplement Right Upper Eyelid with Synthetic Substitute, External Approach

08UNXKZ Supplement Right Upper Eyelid with Nonautologous Tissue Substitute, External Approach

08UP07Z Supplement Left Upper Eyelid with Autologous Tissue Substitute, Open Approach

08UP0JZ Supplement Left Upper Eyelid with Synthetic Substitute, Open Approach

08UP0KZ Supplement Left Upper Eyelid with Nonautologous Tissue Substitute, Open Approach

08UP37Z Supplement Left Upper Eyelid with Autologous Tissue Substitute, Percutaneous Approach

08UP3JZ Supplement Left Upper Eyelid with Synthetic Substitute, Percutaneous Approach

08UP3KZ Supplement Left Upper Eyelid with Nonautologous Tissue Substitute, Percutaneous Approach

08UPX7Z Supplement Left Upper Eyelid with Autologous Tissue Substitute, External Approach

08UPXJZ Supplement Left Upper Eyelid with Synthetic Substitute, External Approach

08UPXKZ Supplement Left Upper Eyelid with Nonautologous Tissue Substitute, External Approach

08UQ07Z Supplement Right Lower Eyelid with Autologous Tissue Substitute, Open Approach

08UQ0JZ Supplement Right Lower Eyelid with Synthetic Substitute, Open Approach

08UQ0KZ Supplement Right Lower Eyelid with Nonautologous Tissue Substitute, Open Approach

08UQ37Z Supplement Right Lower Eyelid with Autologous Tissue Substitute, Percutaneous Approach

08UQ3JZ Supplement Right Lower Eyelid with Synthetic Substitute, Percutaneous Approach

08UQ3KZ Supplement Right Lower Eyelid with Nonautologous Tissue Substitute, Percutaneous Approach

08UQX7Z Supplement Right Lower Eyelid with Autologous Tissue Substitute, External Approach

08UQXJZ Supplement Right Lower Eyelid with Synthetic Substitute, External Approach

08UQXKZ Supplement Right Lower Eyelid with Nonautologous Tissue Substitute, External Approach

08UR07Z Supplement Left Lower Eyelid with Autologous Tissue Substitute, Open Approach

08UR0JZ Supplement Left Lower Eyelid with Synthetic Substitute, Open Approach

08UR0KZ Supplement Left Lower Eyelid with Nonautologous Tissue Substitute, Open Approach

08UR37Z Supplement Left Lower Eyelid with Autologous Tissue Substitute, Percutaneous Approach

08UR3JZ Supplement Left Lower Eyelid with Synthetic Substitute, Percutaneous Approach

08UR3KZ Supplement Left Lower Eyelid with Nonautologous Tissue Substitute, Percutaneous Approach

08URX7Z Supplement Left Lower Eyelid with Autologous Tissue Substitute, External Approach

08URXJZ Supplement Left Lower Eyelid with Synthetic Substitute, External Approach

08URXKZ Supplement Left Lower Eyelid with Nonautologous Tissue Substitute, External Approach

08UX07Z Supplement Right Lacrimal Duct with Autologous Tissue Substitute, Open Approach

08UX0JZ Supplement Right Lacrimal Duct with Synthetic Substitute, Open Approach

08UX0KZ Supplement Right Lacrimal Duct with Nonautologous Tissue Substitute, Open Approach

08UX37Z Supplement Right Lacrimal Duct with Autologous Tissue Substitute, Percutaneous Approach

08UX3JZ Supplement Right Lacrimal Duct with Synthetic Substitute, Percutaneous Approach

08UX3KZ Supplement Right Lacrimal Duct with Nonautologous Tissue Substitute, Percutaneous Approach

08UX77Z Supplement Right Lacrimal Duct with Autologous Tissue Substitute, Via Natural or Artificial Opening

08UX7JZ Supplement Right Lacrimal Duct with Synthetic Substitute, Via Natural or Artificial Opening

08UX7KZ Supplement Right Lacrimal Duct with Nonautologous Tissue Substitute, Via Natural or Artificial Opening

08UX87Z Supplement Right Lacrimal Duct with Autologous Tissue Substitute, Via Natural or Artificial Opening Endoscopic

08UX8JZ Supplement Right Lacrimal Duct with Synthetic Substitute, Via Natural or Artificial Opening Endoscopic

♀ Female-only ♂ Male-only ▲ Limited Coverage ● Non-OR ᴴᴬᶜ HAC-associated procedure ▲ Non-covered procedures ✚ Cluster

08UX8KZ Supplement Right Lacrimal Duct with Nonautologous Tissue Substitute, Via Natural or Artificial Opening Endoscopic

08UY07Z Supplement Left Lacrimal Duct with Autologous Tissue Substitute, Open Approach

08UY0JZ Supplement Left Lacrimal Duct with Synthetic Substitute, Open Approach

08UY0KZ Supplement Left Lacrimal Duct with Nonautologous Tissue Substitute, Open Approach

08UY37Z Supplement Left Lacrimal Duct with Autologous Tissue Substitute, Percutaneous Approach

08UY3JZ Supplement Left Lacrimal Duct with Synthetic Substitute, Percutaneous Approach

08UY3KZ Supplement Left Lacrimal Duct with Nonautologous Tissue Substitute, Percutaneous Approach

08UY77Z Supplement Left Lacrimal Duct with Autologous Tissue Substitute, Via Natural or Artificial Opening

08UY7JZ Supplement Left Lacrimal Duct with Synthetic Substitute, Via Natural or Artificial Opening

08UY7KZ Supplement Left Lacrimal Duct with Nonautologous Tissue Substitute, Via Natural or Artificial Opening

08UY87Z Supplement Left Lacrimal Duct with Autologous Tissue Substitute, Via Natural or Artificial Opening Endoscopic

08UY8JZ Supplement Left Lacrimal Duct with Synthetic Substitute, Via Natural or Artificial Opening Endoscopic

08UY8KZ Supplement Left Lacrimal Duct with Nonautologous Tissue Substitute, Via Natural or Artificial Opening Endoscopic

08V – Eye, Restriction

08VX0CZ Restriction of Right Lacrimal Duct with Extraluminal Device, Open Approach

08VX0DZ Restriction of Right Lacrimal Duct with Intraluminal Device, Open Approach

08VX0ZZ Restriction of Right Lacrimal Duct, Open Approach

08VX3CZ Restriction of Right Lacrimal Duct with Extraluminal Device, Percutaneous Approach

08VX3DZ Restriction of Right Lacrimal Duct with Intraluminal Device, Percutaneous Approach

08VX3ZZ Restriction of Right Lacrimal Duct, Percutaneous Approach

08VX7DZ Restriction of Right Lacrimal Duct with Intraluminal Device, Via Natural or Artificial Opening

08VX7ZZ Restriction of Right Lacrimal Duct, Via Natural or Artificial Opening

08VX8DZ Restriction of Right Lacrimal Duct with Intraluminal Device, Via Natural or Artificial Opening Endoscopic

08VX8ZZ Restriction of Right Lacrimal Duct, Via Natural or Artificial Opening Endoscopic

08VY0CZ Restriction of Left Lacrimal Duct with Extraluminal Device, Open Approach

08VY0DZ Restriction of Left Lacrimal Duct with Intraluminal Device, Open Approach

08VY0ZZ Restriction of Left Lacrimal Duct, Open Approach

08VY3CZ Restriction of Left Lacrimal Duct with Extraluminal Device, Percutaneous Approach

08VY3DZ Restriction of Left Lacrimal Duct with Intraluminal Device, Percutaneous Approach

08VY3ZZ Restriction of Left Lacrimal Duct, Percutaneous Approach

08VY7DZ Restriction of Left Lacrimal Duct with Intraluminal Device, Via Natural or Artificial Opening

08VY7ZZ Restriction of Left Lacrimal Duct, Via Natural or Artificial Opening

08VY8DZ Restriction of Left Lacrimal Duct with Intraluminal Device, Via Natural or Artificial Opening Endoscopic

08VY8ZZ Restriction of Left Lacrimal Duct, Via Natural or Artificial Opening Endoscopic

08W – Eye, Revision

Review Coding Guideline B6.1c

08W000Z Revision of Drainage Device in Right Eye, Open Approach

08W003Z Revision of Infusion Device in Right Eye, Open Approach

08W007Z Revision of Autologous Tissue Substitute in Right Eye, Open Approach

08W00CZ Revision of Extraluminal Device in Right Eye, Open Approach

08W00DZ Revision of Intraluminal Device in Right Eye, Open Approach

08W00JZ Revision of Synthetic Substitute in Right Eye, Open Approach

08W00KZ Revision of Nonautologous Tissue Substitute in Right Eye, Open Approach

08W00YZ Revision of Other Device in Right Eye, Open Approach

08W030Z Revision of Drainage Device in Right Eye, Percutaneous Approach

08W033Z Revision of Infusion Device in Right Eye, Percutaneous Approach

08W037Z Revision of Autologous Tissue Substitute in Right Eye, Percutaneous Approach

08W03CZ Revision of Extraluminal Device in Right Eye, Percutaneous Approach

08W03DZ Revision of Intraluminal Device in Right Eye, Percutaneous Approach

08W03JZ Revision of Synthetic Substitute in Right Eye, Percutaneous Approach

08W03KZ Revision of Nonautologous Tissue Substitute in Right Eye, Percutaneous Approach

08W03YZ Revision of Other Device in Right Eye, Percutaneous Approach

08W070Z Revision of Drainage Device in Right Eye, Via Natural or Artificial Opening

08W073Z Revision of Infusion Device in Right Eye, Via Natural or Artificial Opening

08W077Z Revision of Autologous Tissue Substitute in Right Eye, Via Natural or Artificial Opening

08W07CZ Revision of Extraluminal Device in Right Eye, Via Natural or Artificial Opening

08W07DZ Revision of Intraluminal Device in Right Eye, Via Natural or Artificial Opening

08W07JZ Revision of Synthetic Substitute in Right Eye, Via Natural or Artificial Opening

08W07KZ Revision of Nonautologous Tissue Substitute in Right Eye, Via Natural or Artificial Opening

08W07YZ Revision of Other Device in Right Eye, Via Natural or Artificial Opening

08W080Z Revision of Drainage Device in Right Eye, Via Natural or Artificial Opening Endoscopic

08W083Z Revision of Infusion Device in Right Eye, Via Natural or Artificial Opening Endoscopic

08W087Z Revision of Autologous Tissue Substitute in Right Eye, Via Natural or Artificial Opening Endoscopic

08W08CZ Revision of Extraluminal Device in Right Eye, Via Natural or Artificial Opening Endoscopic

08W08DZ Revision of Intraluminal Device in Right Eye, Via Natural or Artificial Opening Endoscopic

08W08JZ Revision of Synthetic Substitute in Right Eye, Via Natural or Artificial Opening Endoscopic

08W08KZ Revision of Nonautologous Tissue Substitute in Right Eye, Via Natural or Artificial Opening Endoscopic

08W08YZ Revision of Other Device in Right Eye, Via Natural or Artificial Opening Endoscopic

08W0X0Z Revision of Drainage Device in Right Eye, External Approach

08W0X3Z Revision of Infusion Device in Right Eye, External Approach

08W0X7Z Revision of Autologous Tissue Substitute in Right Eye, External Approach

08W0XCZ Revision of Extraluminal Device in Right Eye, External Approach

08W0XDZ Revision of Intraluminal Device in Right Eye, External Approach

08W0XJZ Revision of Synthetic Substitute in Right Eye, External Approach

08W0XKZ Revision of Nonautologous Tissue Substitute in Right Eye, External Approach

08W100Z Revision of Drainage Device in Left Eye, Open Approach

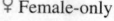

08W103Z Revision of Infusion Device in Left Eye, Open Approach

08W107Z Revision of Autologous Tissue Substitute in Left Eye, Open Approach

08W10CZ Revision of Extraluminal Device in Left Eye, Open Approach

08W10DZ Revision of Intraluminal Device in Left Eye, Open Approach

08W10JZ Revision of Synthetic Substitute in Left Eye, Open Approach

08W10KZ Revision of Nonautologous Tissue Substitute in Left Eye, Open Approach

08W10YZ Revision of Other Device in Left Eye, Open Approach

08W130Z Revision of Drainage Device in Left Eye, Percutaneous Approach

08W133Z Revision of Infusion Device in Left Eye, Percutaneous Approach

08W137Z Revision of Autologous Tissue Substitute in Left Eye, Percutaneous Approach

08W13CZ Revision of Extraluminal Device in Left Eye, Percutaneous Approach

08W13DZ Revision of Intraluminal Device in Left Eye, Percutaneous Approach

08W13JZ Revision of Synthetic Substitute in Left Eye, Percutaneous Approach

08W13KZ Revision of Nonautologous Tissue Substitute in Left Eye, Percutaneous Approach

08W13YZ Revision of Other Device in Left Eye, Percutaneous Approach

08W170Z Revision of Drainage Device in Left Eye, Via Natural or Artificial Opening

08W173Z Revision of Infusion Device in Left Eye, Via Natural or Artificial Opening

08W177Z Revision of Autologous Tissue Substitute in Left Eye, Via Natural or Artificial Opening

08W17CZ Revision of Extraluminal Device in Left Eye, Via Natural or Artificial Opening

08W17DZ Revision of Intraluminal Device in Left Eye, Via Natural or Artificial Opening

08W17JZ Revision of Synthetic Substitute in Left Eye, Via Natural or Artificial Opening

08W17KZ Revision of Nonautologous Tissue Substitute in Left Eye, Via Natural or Artificial Opening

08W17YZ Revision of Other Device in Left Eye, Via Natural or Artificial Opening

08W180Z Revision of Drainage Device in Left Eye, Via Natural or Artificial Opening Endoscopic

08W183Z Revision of Infusion Device in Left Eye, Via Natural or Artificial Opening Endoscopic

08W187Z Revision of Autologous Tissue Substitute in Left Eye, Via Natural or Artificial Opening Endoscopic

08W18CZ Revision of Extraluminal Device in Left Eye, Via Natural or Artificial Opening Endoscopic

08W18DZ Revision of Intraluminal Device in Left Eye, Via Natural or Artificial Opening Endoscopic

08W18JZ Revision of Synthetic Substitute in Left Eye, Via Natural or Artificial Opening Endoscopic

08W18KZ Revision of Nonautologous Tissue Substitute in Left Eye, Via Natural or Artificial Opening Endoscopic

08W18YZ Revision of Other Device in Left Eye, Via Natural or Artificial Opening Endoscopic

08W1X0Z Revision of Drainage Device in Left Eye, External Approach

08W1X3Z Revision of Infusion Device in Left Eye, External Approach

08W1X7Z Revision of Autologous Tissue Substitute in Left Eye, External Approach

08W1XCZ Revision of Extraluminal Device in Left Eye, External Approach

08W1XDZ Revision of Intraluminal Device in Left Eye, External Approach

08W1XJZ Revision of Synthetic Substitute in Left Eye, External Approach

08W1XKZ Revision of Nonautologous Tissue Substitute in Left Eye, External Approach

08WJ3JZ Revision of Synthetic Substitute in Right Lens, Percutaneous Approach

08WJ3YZ Revision of Other Device in Right Lens, Percutaneous Approach

08WJXJZ Revision of Synthetic Substitute in Right Lens, External Approach

08WK3JZ Revision of Synthetic Substitute in Left Lens, Percutaneous Approach

08WK3YZ Revision of Other Device in Left Lens, Percutaneous Approach

08WKXJZ Revision of Synthetic Substitute in Left Lens, External Approach

08WL00Z Revision of Drainage Device in Right Extraocular Muscle, Open Approach

08WL07Z Revision of Autologous Tissue Substitute in Right Extraocular Muscle, Open Approach

08WL0JZ Revision of Synthetic Substitute in Right Extraocular Muscle, Open Approach

08WL0KZ Revision of Nonautologous Tissue Substitute in Right Extraocular Muscle, Open Approach

08WL0YZ Revision of Other Device in Right Extraocular Muscle, Open Approach

08WL30Z Revision of Drainage Device in Right Extraocular Muscle, Percutaneous Approach

08WL37Z Revision of Autologous Tissue Substitute in Right Extraocular Muscle, Percutaneous Approach

08WL3JZ Revision of Synthetic Substitute in Right Extraocular Muscle, Percutaneous Approach

08WL3KZ Revision of Nonautologous Tissue Substitute in Right Extraocular Muscle, Percutaneous Approach

08WL3YZ Revision of Other Device in Right Extraocular Muscle, Percutaneous Approach

08WM00Z Revision of Drainage Device in Left Extraocular Muscle, Open Approach

08WM07Z Revision of Autologous Tissue Substitute in Left Extraocular Muscle, Open Approach

08WM0JZ Revision of Synthetic Substitute in Left Extraocular Muscle, Open Approach

08WM0KZ Revision of Nonautologous Tissue Substitute in Left Extraocular Muscle, Open Approach

08WM0YZ Revision of Other Device in Left Extraocular Muscle, Open Approach

08WM30Z Revision of Drainage Device in Left Extraocular Muscle, Percutaneous Approach

08WM37Z Revision of Autologous Tissue Substitute in Left Extraocular Muscle, Percutaneous Approach

08WM3JZ Revision of Synthetic Substitute in Left Extraocular Muscle, Percutaneous Approach

08WM3KZ Revision of Nonautologous Tissue Substitute in Left Extraocular Muscle, Percutaneous Approach

08WM3YZ Revision of Other Device in Left Extraocular Muscle, Percutaneous Approach

08X – Eye, Transfer

08XL0ZZ Transfer Right Extraocular Muscle, Open Approach

08XL3ZZ Transfer Right Extraocular Muscle, Percutaneous Approach

08XM0ZZ Transfer Left Extraocular Muscle, Open Approach

08XM3ZZ Transfer Left Extraocular Muscle, Percutaneous Approach

Nose and Sinuses

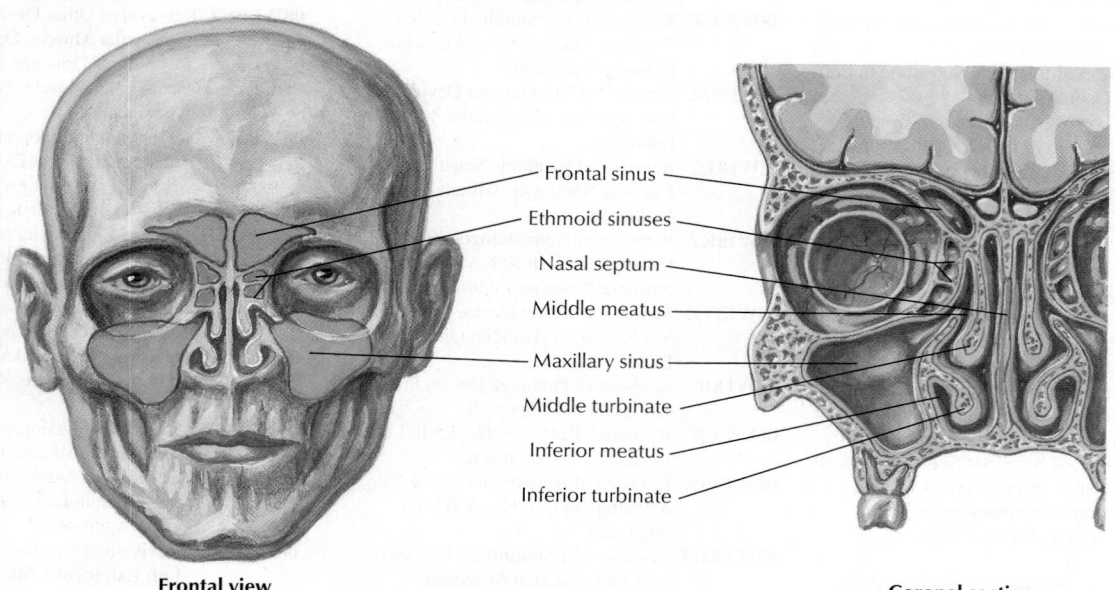

Frontal sinus
Ethmoid sinuses
Nasal septum
Middle meatus
Maxillary sinus
Middle turbinate
Inferior meatus
Inferior turbinate

Frontal view

Coronal section

Anotomy of nasal cavity and sinuses

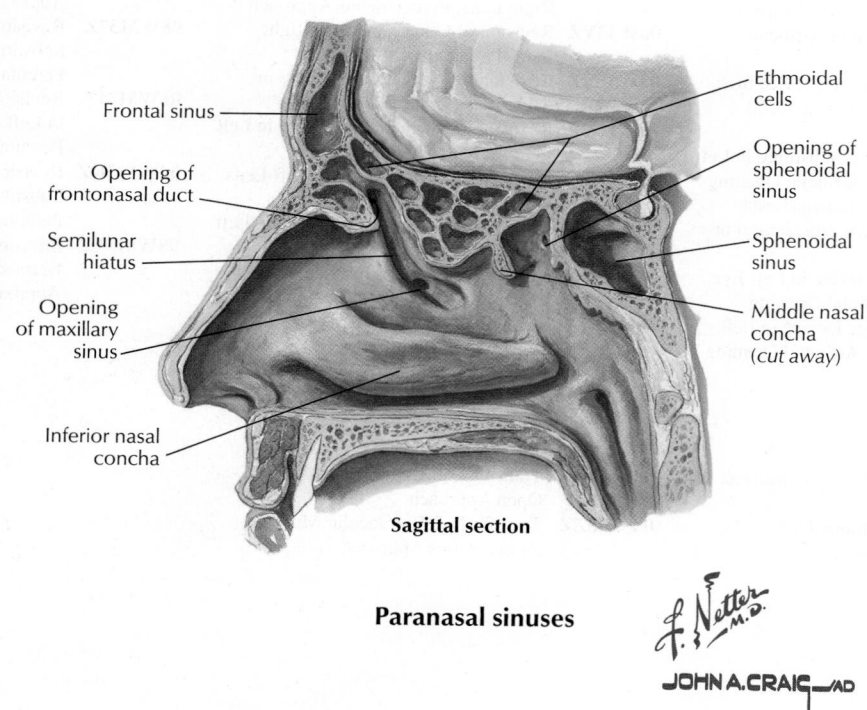

Frontal sinus
Opening of frontonasal duct
Semilunar hiatus
Opening of maxillary sinus
Inferior nasal concha

Ethmoidal cells
Opening of sphenoidal sinus
Sphenoidal sinus
Middle nasal concha (*cut away*)

Sagittal section

Paranasal sinuses

Lateral Wall of Nasal Cavity

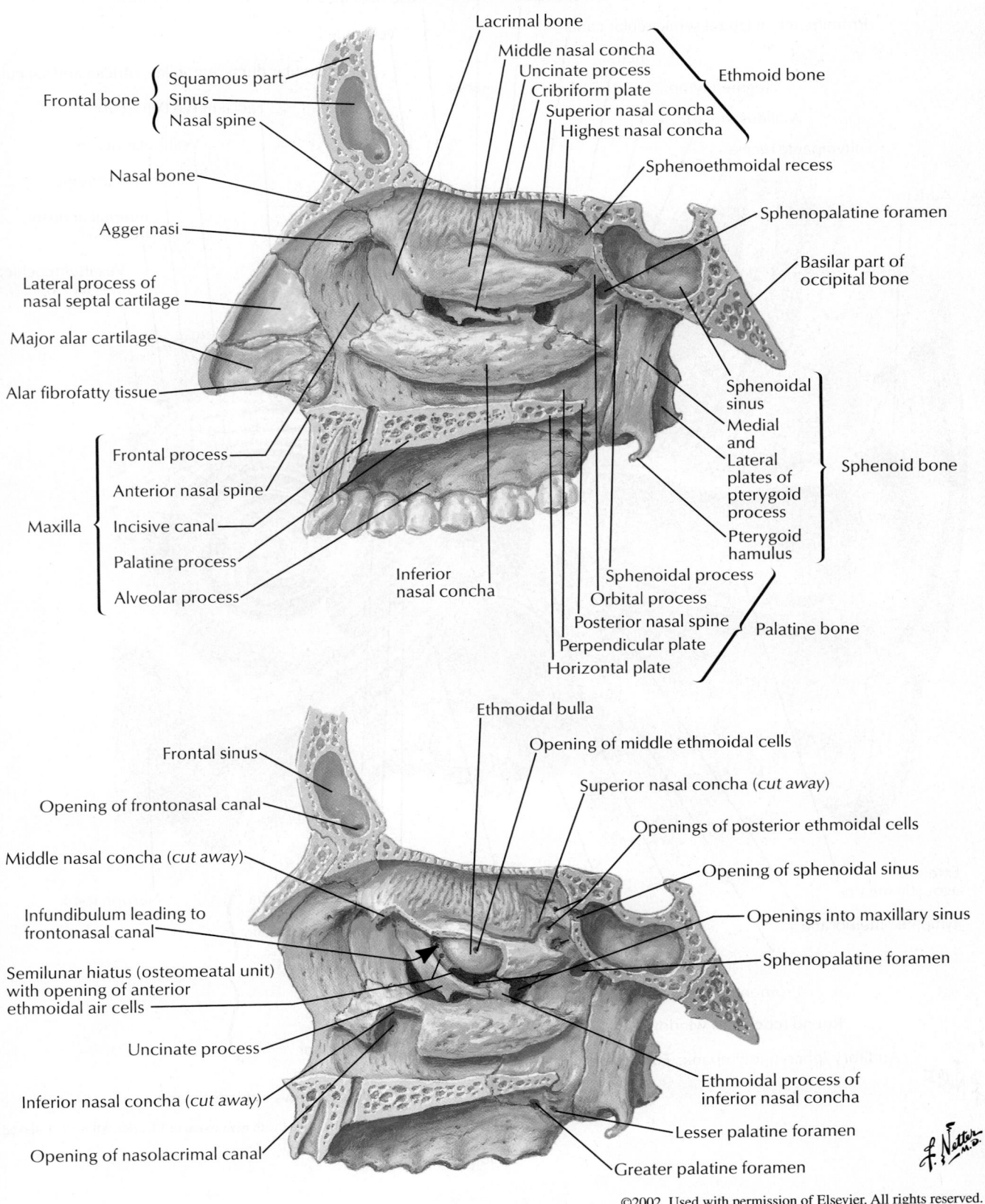

Frontal bone { Squamous part / Sinus / Nasal spine

Lacrimal bone
Middle nasal concha
Uncinate process
Cribriform plate
Superior nasal concha
Highest nasal concha

Ethmoid bone

Nasal bone

Agger nasi

Lateral process of
nasal septal cartilage

Major alar cartilage

Alar fibrofatty tissue

Sphenoethmoidal recess

Sphenopalatine foramen

Basilar part of
occipital bone

Sphenoidal
sinus
Medial
and
Lateral
plates of
pterygoid
process

Sphenoid bone

Pterygoid
hamulus

Maxilla { Frontal process / Anterior nasal spine / Incisive canal / Palatine process / Alveolar process

Inferior
nasal concha

Sphenoidal process
Orbital process
Posterior nasal spine
Perpendicular plate
Horizontal plate

Palatine bone

Ethmoidal bulla
Opening of middle ethmoidal cells

Frontal sinus

Opening of frontonasal canal

Middle nasal concha (cut away)

Infundibulum leading to
frontonasal canal

Semilunar hiatus (osteomeatal unit)
with opening of anterior
ethmoidal air cells

Uncinate process

Inferior nasal concha (cut away)

Opening of nasolacrimal canal

Superior nasal concha (cut away)

Openings of posterior ethmoidal cells

Opening of sphenoidal sinus

Openings into maxillary sinus

Sphenopalatine foramen

Ethmoidal process of
inferior nasal concha

Lesser palatine foramen

Greater palatine foramen

F. Netter M.D.

Pathway of Sound Reception

Frontal section

Facial nerve (VII) (*cut*)

Limbs of stapes

Base of stapes in oval (vestibular) window

Prominence of lateral semicircular canal

Vestibule

Incus

Semicircular ducts, ampullae, utricle, and saccule

Tegmen tympani

Malleus (head)

Facial nerve (VII) (*cut*)

Epitympanic recess

Vestibular nerve

Auricle

Cochlear nerve

Internal acoustic meatus

Vestibulocochlear nerve (VIII)

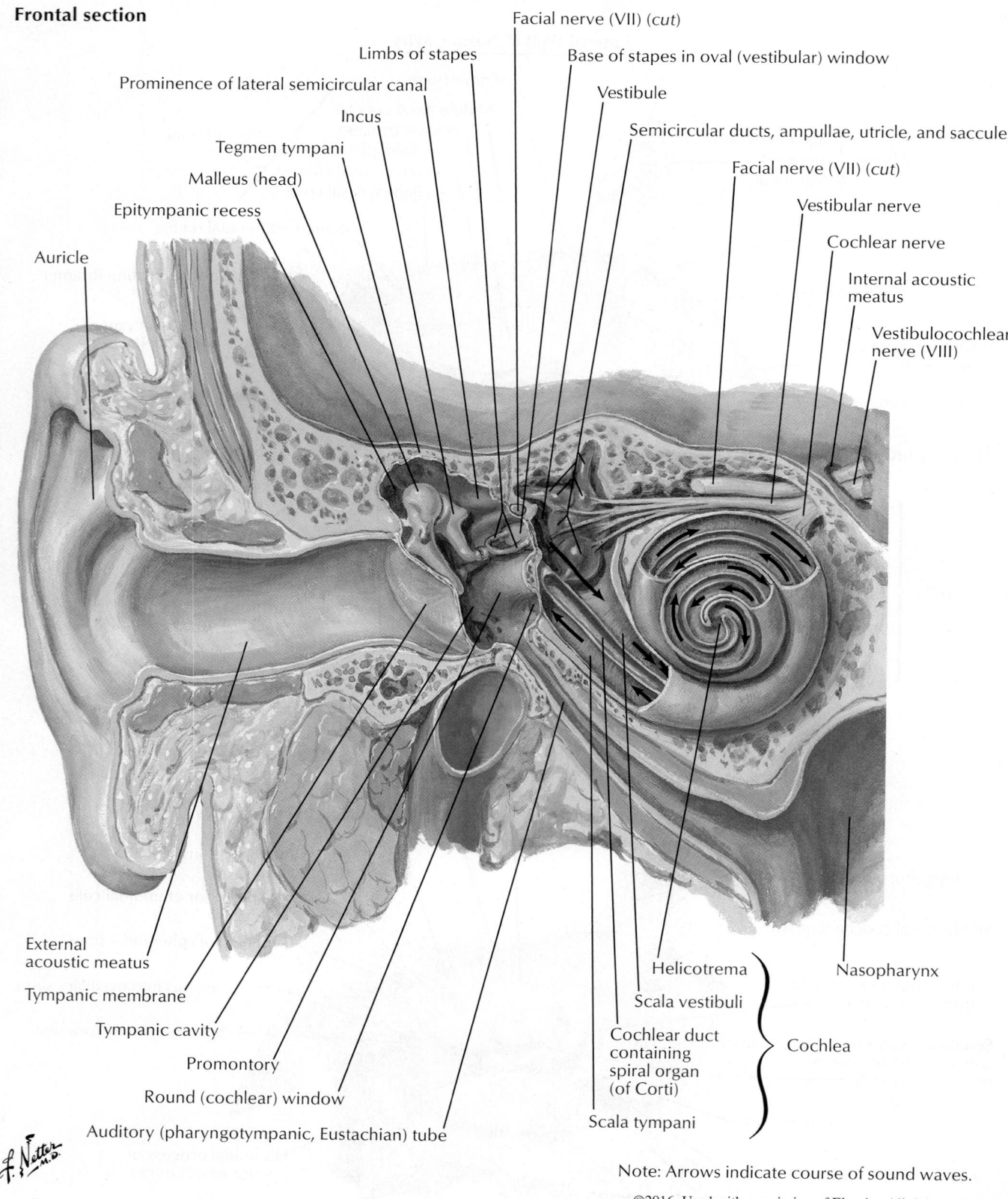

External acoustic meatus

Tympanic membrane

Tympanic cavity

Promontory

Round (cochlear) window

Auditory (pharyngotympanic, Eustachian) tube

Helicotrema

Scala vestibuli

Cochlear duct containing spiral organ (of Corti)

Scala tympani

Nasopharynx

Cochlea

Note: Arrows indicate course of sound waves.

Ear, Nose, Sinus Tables 090–09W

Section	0	Medical and Surgical
Body System	9	Ear, Nose, Sinus
Operation	0	Alteration: Modifying the anatomic structure of a body part without affecting the function of the body part

Body Part (4th)	Approach (5th)	Device (6th)	Qualifier (7th)
0 External Ear, Right 1 External Ear, Left 2 External Ear, Bilateral K Nasal Mucosa and Soft Tissue	0 Open 3 Percutaneous 4 Percutaneous Endoscopic X External	7 Autologous Tissue Substitute J Synthetic Substitute K Nonautologous Tissue Substitute Z No Device	Z No Qualifier

Section	0	Medical and Surgical
Body System	9	Ear, Nose, Sinus
Operation	1	Bypass: Altering the route of passage of the contents of a tubular body part

Body Part (4th)	Approach (5th)	Device (6th)	Qualifier (7th)
D Inner Ear, Right E Inner Ear, Left	0 Open	7 Autologous Tissue Substitute J Synthetic Substitute K Nonautologous Tissue Substitute Z No Device	0 Endolymphatic

Section	0	Medical and Surgical
Body System	9	Ear, Nose, Sinus
Operation	2	Change: Taking out or off a device from a body part and putting back an identical or similar device in or on the same body part without cutting or puncturing the skin or a mucous membrane

Body Part (4th)	Approach (5th)	Device (6th)	Qualifier (7th)
H Ear, Right J Ear, Left K Nasal Mucosa and Soft Tissue Y Sinus	X External	0 Drainage Device Y Other Device	Z No Qualifier

Section	0	Medical and Surgical
Body System	9	Ear, Nose, Sinus
Operation	3	Control: Stopping, or attempting to stop, postprocedural or other acute bleeding

Body Part (4th)	Approach (5th)	Device (6th)	Qualifier (7th)
K Nasal Mucosa and Soft Tissue	7 Via Natural or Artificial Opening 8 Via Natural or Artificial Opening Endoscopic	Z No Device	Z No Qualifier

Section	0	Medical and Surgical
Body System	9	Ear, Nose, Sinus
Operation	5	Destruction: Physical eradication of all or a portion of a body part by the direct use of energy, force, or a destructive agent

Body Part (4th)	Approach (5th)	Device (6th)	Qualifier (7th)
0 External Ear, Right 1 External Ear, Left	0 Open 3 Percutaneous 4 Percutaneous Endoscopic X External	Z No Device	Z No Qualifier
3 External Auditory Canal, Right 4 External Auditory Canal, Left	0 Open 3 Percutaneous 4 Percutaneous Endoscopic 7 Via Natural or Artificial Opening 8 Via Natural or Artificial Opening Endoscopic X External	Z No Device	Z No Qualifier
5 Middle Ear, Right 6 Middle Ear, Left 9 Auditory Ossicle, Right A Auditory Ossicle, Left D Inner Ear, Right E Inner Ear, Left	0 Open 8 Via Natural or Artificial Opening Endoscopic	Z No Device	Z No Qualifier

Continued →

Section	0	Medical and Surgical
Body System	9	Ear, Nose, Sinus
Operation	5	Destruction: Physical eradication of all or a portion of a body part by the direct use of energy, force, or a destructive agent

Body Part (4th)	Approach (5th)	Device (6th)	Qualifier (7th)
7 Tympanic Membrane, Right 8 Tympanic Membrane, Left F Eustachian Tube, Right G Eustachian Tube, Left L Nasal Turbinate N Nasopharynx	0 Open 3 Percutaneous 4 Percutaneous Endoscopic 7 Via Natural or Artificial Opening 8 Via Natural or Artificial Opening Endoscopic	Z No Device	Z No Qualifier
B Mastoid Sinus, Right C Mastoid Sinus, Left M Nasal Septum P Accessory Sinus Q Maxillary Sinus, Right R Maxillary Sinus, Left S Frontal Sinus, Right T Frontal Sinus, Left U Ethmoid Sinus, Right V Ethmoid Sinus, Left W Sphenoid Sinus, Right X Sphenoid Sinus, Left	0 Open 3 Percutaneous 4 Percutaneous Endoscopic 8 Via Natural or Artificial Opening Endoscopic	Z No Device	Z No Qualifier
K Nasal Mucosa and Soft Tissue	0 Open 3 Percutaneous 4 Percutaneous Endoscopic 8 Via Natural or Artificial Opening Endoscopic X External	Z No Device	Z No Qualifier

Section	0	Medical and Surgical
Body System	9	Ear, Nose, Sinus
Operation	7	Dilation: Expanding an orifice or the lumen of a tubular body part

Body Part (4th)	Approach (5th)	Device (6th)	Qualifier (7th)
F Eustachian Tube, Right G Eustachian Tube, Left	0 Open 7 Via Natural or Artificial Opening 8 Via Natural or Artificial Opening Endoscopic	D Intraluminal Device Z No Device	Z No Qualifier
F Eustachian Tube, Right G Eustachian Tube, Left	3 Percutaneous 4 Percutaneous Endoscopic	Z No Device	Z No Qualifier

Section	0	Medical and Surgical
Body System	9	Ear, Nose, Sinus
Operation	8	Division: Cutting into a body part, without draining fluids and/or gases from the body part, in order to separate or transect a body part

Body Part (4th)	Approach (5th)	Device (6th)	Qualifier (7th)
L Nasal Turbinate	0 Open 3 Percutaneous 4 Percutaneous Endoscopic 7 Via Natural or Artificial Opening 8 Via Natural or Artificial Opening Endoscopic	Z No Device	Z No Qualifier

Section	0	Medical and Surgical
Body System	9	Ear, Nose, Sinus
Operation	9	Drainage: Taking or letting out fluids and/or gases from a body part

Body Part (4th)	Approach (5th)	Device (6th)	Qualifier (7th)
0 External Ear, Right 1 External Ear, Left	0 Open 3 Percutaneous 4 Percutaneous Endoscopic X External	0 Drainage Device	Z No Qualifier
0 External Ear, Right 1 External Ear, Left	0 Open 3 Percutaneous 4 Percutaneous Endoscopic X External	Z No Device	X Diagnostic Z No Qualifier

Continued →

Section	0	Medical and Surgical
Body System	9	Ear, Nose, Sinus
Operation	9	Drainage: Taking or letting out fluids and/or gases from a body part

Body Part (4th)	Approach (5th)	Device (6th)	Qualifier (7th)
3 External Auditory Canal, Right 4 External Auditory Canal, Left K Nasal Mucosa and Soft Tissue	0 Open 3 Percutaneous 4 Percutaneous Endoscopic 7 Via Natural or Artificial Opening 8 Via Natural or Artificial Opening Endoscopic X External	0 Drainage Device	Z No Qualifier
3 External Auditory Canal, Right 4 External Auditory Canal, Left K Nasal Mucosa and Soft Tissue	0 Open 3 Percutaneous 4 Percutaneous Endoscopic 7 Via Natural or Artificial Opening 8 Via Natural or Artificial Opening Endoscopic X External	Z No Device	X Diagnostic Z No Qualifier
5 Middle Ear, Right 6 Middle Ear, Left 9 Auditory Ossicle, Right A Auditory Ossicle, Left D Inner Ear, Right E Inner Ear, Left	0 Open 7 Via Natural or Artificial Opening 8 Via Natural or Artificial Opening Endoscopic	0 Drainage Device	Z No Qualifier
5 Middle Ear, Right 6 Middle Ear, Left 9 Auditory Ossicle, Right A Auditory Ossicle, Left D Inner Ear, Right E Inner Ear, Left	0 Open 7 Via Natural or Artificial Opening 8 Via Natural or Artificial Opening Endoscopic	Z No Device	X Diagnostic Z No Qualifier
7 Tympanic Membrane, Right 8 Tympanic Membrane, Left B Mastoid Sinus, Right C Mastoid Sinus, Left F Eustachian Tube, Right G Eustachian Tube, Left L Nasal Turbinate M Nasal Septum N Nasopharynx P Accessory Sinus Q Maxillary Sinus, Right R Maxillary Sinus, Left S Frontal Sinus, Right T Frontal Sinus, Left U Ethmoid Sinus, Right V Ethmoid Sinus, Left W Sphenoid Sinus, Right X Sphenoid Sinus, Left	0 Open 3 Percutaneous 4 Percutaneous Endoscopic 7 Via Natural or Artificial Opening 8 Via Natural or Artificial Opening Endoscopic	0 Drainage Device	Z No Qualifier
7 Tympanic Membrane, Right 8 Tympanic Membrane, Left B Mastoid Sinus, Right C Mastoid Sinus, Left F Eustachian Tube, Right G Eustachian Tube, Left L Nasal Turbinate M Nasal Septum N Nasopharynx P Accessory Sinus Q Maxillary Sinus, Right R Maxillary Sinus, Left S Frontal Sinus, Right T Frontal Sinus, Left U Ethmoid Sinus, Right V Ethmoid Sinus, Left W Sphenoid Sinus, Right X Sphenoid Sinus, Left	0 Open 3 Percutaneous 4 Percutaneous Endoscopic 7 Via Natural or Artificial Opening 8 Via Natural or Artificial Opening Endoscopic	Z No Device	X Diagnostic Z No Qualifier

Section	**0**	**Medical and Surgical**
Body System	**9**	**Ear, Nose, Sinus**
Operation	**B**	**Excision:** Cutting out or off, without replacement, a portion of a body part

Body Part (4th)	Approach (5th)	Device (6th)	Qualifier (7th)
0 External Ear, Right **1** External Ear, Left	**0** Open **3** Percutaneous **4** Percutaneous Endoscopic **X** External	**Z** No Device	**X** Diagnostic **Z** No Qualifier
3 External Auditory Canal, Right **4** External Auditory Canal, Left	**0** Open **3** Percutaneous **4** Percutaneous Endoscopic **7** Via Natural or Artificial Opening **8** Via Natural or Artificial Opening Endoscopic **X** External	**Z** No Device	**X** Diagnostic **Z** No Qualifier
5 Middle Ear, Right **6** Middle Ear, Left **9** Auditory Ossicle, Right **A** Auditory Ossicle, Left **D** Inner Ear, Right **E** Inner Ear, Left	**0** Open **8** Via Natural or Artificial Opening Endoscopic	**Z** No Device	**X** Diagnostic **Z** No Qualifier
7 Tympanic Membrane, Right **8** Tympanic Membrane, Left **F** Eustachian Tube, Right **G** Eustachian Tube, Left **L** Nasal Turbinate **N** Nasopharynx	**0** Open **3** Percutaneous **4** Percutaneous Endoscopic **7** Via Natural or Artificial Opening **8** Via Natural or Artificial Opening Endoscopic	**Z** No Device	**X** Diagnostic **Z** No Qualifier
B Mastoid Sinus, Right **C** Mastoid Sinus, Left **M** Nasal Septum **P** Accessory Sinus **Q** Maxillary Sinus, Right **R** Maxillary Sinus, Left **S** Frontal Sinus, Right **T** Frontal Sinus, Left **U** Ethmoid Sinus, Right **V** Ethmoid Sinus, Left **W** Sphenoid Sinus, Right **X** Sphenoid Sinus, Left	**0** Open **3** Percutaneous **4** Percutaneous Endoscopic **8** Via Natural or Artificial Opening Endoscopic	**Z** No Device	**X** Diagnostic **Z** No Qualifier
K Nasal Mucosa and Soft Tissue	**0** Open **3** Percutaneous **4** Percutaneous Endoscopic **8** Via Natural or Artificial Opening Endoscopic **X** External	**Z** No Device	**X** Diagnostic **Z** No Qualifier

Section   **0**   **Medical and Surgical**
Body System   **9**   **Ear, Nose, Sinus**
Operation   **C**   **Extirpation:** Taking or cutting out solid matter from a body part

Body Part (4ᵗʰ)	Approach (5ᵗʰ)	Device (6ᵗʰ)	Qualifier (7ᵗʰ)
0 External Ear, Right 1 External Ear, Left	0 Open 3 Percutaneous 4 Percutaneous Endoscopic X External	Z No Device	Z No Qualifier
3 External Auditory Canal, Right 4 External Auditory Canal, Left	0 Open 3 Percutaneous 4 Percutaneous Endoscopic 7 Via Natural or Artificial Opening 8 Via Natural or Artificial Opening Endoscopic X External	Z No Device	Z No Qualifier
5 Middle Ear, Right 6 Middle Ear, Left 9 Auditory Ossicle, Right A Auditory Ossicle, Left D Inner Ear, Right E Inner Ear, Left	0 Open 8 Via Natural or Artificial Opening Endoscopic	Z No Device	Z No Qualifier
7 Tympanic Membrane, Right 8 Tympanic Membrane, Left F Eustachian Tube, Right G Eustachian Tube, Left L Nasal Turbinate N Nasopharynx	0 Open 3 Percutaneous 4 Percutaneous Endoscopic 7 Via Natural or Artificial Opening 8 Via Natural or Artificial Opening Endoscopic	Z No Device	Z No Qualifier
B Mastoid Sinus, Right C Mastoid Sinus, Left M Nasal Septum P Accessory Sinus Q Maxillary Sinus, Right R Maxillary Sinus, Left S Frontal Sinus, Right T Frontal Sinus, Left U Ethmoid Sinus, Right V Ethmoid Sinus, Left W Sphenoid Sinus, Right X Sphenoid Sinus, Left	0 Open 3 Percutaneous 4 Percutaneous Endoscopic 8 Via Natural or Artificial Opening Endoscopic	Z No Device	Z No Qualifier
K Nasal Mucosa and Soft Tissue	0 Open 3 Percutaneous 4 Percutaneous Endoscopic 8 Via Natural or Artificial Opening Endoscopic X External	Z No Device	Z No Qualifier

Section   **0**   **Medical and Surgical**
Body System   **9**   **Ear, Nose, Sinus**
Operation   **D**   **Extraction:** Pulling or stripping out or off all or a portion of a body part by the use of force

Body Part (4ᵗʰ)	Approach (5ᵗʰ)	Device (6ᵗʰ)	Qualifier (7ᵗʰ)
7 Tympanic Membrane, Right 8 Tympanic Membrane, Left L Nasal Turbinate	0 Open 3 Percutaneous 4 Percutaneous Endoscopic 7 Via Natural or Artificial Opening 8 Via Natural or Artificial Opening Endoscopic	Z No Device	Z No Qualifier
9 Auditory Ossicle, Right A Auditory Ossicle, Left	0 Open	Z No Device	Z No Qualifier

Continued →

Section 0 **Medical and Surgical**
Body System 9 **Ear, Nose, Sinus**
Operation D **Extraction:** Pulling or stripping out or off all or a portion of a body part by the use of force

Body Part (4th)	Approach (5th)	Device (6th)	Qualifier (7th)
B Mastoid Sinus, Right C Mastoid Sinus, Left M Nasal Septum P Accessory Sinus Q Maxillary Sinus, Right R Maxillary Sinus, Left S Frontal Sinus, Right T Frontal Sinus, Left U Ethmoid Sinus, Right V Ethmoid Sinus, Left W Sphenoid Sinus, Right X Sphenoid Sinus, Left	0 Open 3 Percutaneous 4 Percutaneous Endoscopic	Z No Device	Z No Qualifier

Section 0 **Medical and Surgical**
Body System 9 **Ear, Nose, Sinus**
Operation H **Insertion:** Putting in a nonbiological appliance that monitors, assists, performs, or prevents a physiological function but does not physically take the place of a body part

Body Part (4th)	Approach (5th)	Device (6th)	Qualifier (7th)
D Inner Ear, Right E Inner Ear, Left	0 Open 3 Percutaneous 4 Percutaneous Endoscopic	1 Radioactive Element 4 Hearing Device, Bone Conduction 5 Hearing Device, Single Channel Cochlear Prosthesis 6 Hearing Device, Multiple Channel Cochlear Prosthesis S Hearing Device	Z No Qualifier
H Ear, Right J Ear, Left K Nasal Mucosa and Soft Tissue Y Sinus	0 Open 3 Percutaneous 4 Percutaneous Endoscopic 7 Via Natural or Artificial Opening 8 Via Natural or Artificial Opening Endoscopic	1 Radioactive Element Y Other Device	Z No Qualifier
N Nasopharynx	7 Via Natural or Artificial Opening 8 Via Natural or Artificial Opening Endoscopic	1 Radioactive Element B Intraluminal Device, Airway	Z No Qualifier

Section 0 **Medical and Surgical**
Body System 9 **Ear, Nose, Sinus**
Operation J **Inspection:** Visually and/or manually exploring a body part

Body Part (4th)	Approach (5th)	Device (6th)	Qualifier (7th)
7 Tympanic Membrane, Right 8 Tympanic Membrane, Left H Ear, Right J Ear, Left	0 Open 3 Percutaneous 4 Percutaneous Endoscopic 7 Via Natural or Artificial Opening 8 Via Natural or Artificial Opening Endoscopic X External	Z No Device	Z No Qualifier
D Inner Ear, Right E Inner Ear, Left K Nose Y Sinus	0 Open 3 Percutaneous 4 Percutaneous Endoscopic 8 Via Natural or Artificial Opening Endoscopic X External	Z No Device	Z No Qualifier

Section 0 **Medical and Surgical**
Body System 9 **Ear, Nose, Sinus**
Operation M **Reattachment:** Putting back in or on all or a portion of a separated body part to its normal location or other suitable location

Body Part (4th)	Approach (5th)	Device (6th)	Qualifier (7th)
0 External Ear, Right 1 External Ear, Left K Nasal Mucosa and Soft Tissue	X External	Z No Device	Z No Qualifier

Section 0 **Medical and Surgical**
Body System 9 **Ear, Nose, Sinus**
Operation N **Release:** Freeing a body part from an abnormal physical constraint by cutting or by the use of force

Body Part (4th)	Approach (5th)	Device (6th)	Qualifier (7th)
0 External Ear, Right 1 External Ear, Left	0 Open 3 Percutaneous 4 Percutaneous Endoscopic X External	Z No Device	Z No Qualifier
3 External Auditory Canal, Right 4 External Auditory Canal, Left	0 Open 3 Percutaneous 4 Percutaneous Endoscopic 7 Via Natural or Artificial Opening 8 Via Natural or Artificial Opening Endoscopic X External	Z No Device	Z No Qualifier
5 Middle Ear, Right 6 Middle Ear, Left 9 Auditory Ossicle, Right A Auditory Ossicle, Left D Inner Ear, Right E Inner Ear, Left	0 Open 8 Via Natural or Artificial Opening Endoscopic	Z No Device	Z No Qualifier
7 Tympanic Membrane, Right 8 Tympanic Membrane, Left F Eustachian Tube, Right G Eustachian Tube, Left L Nasal Turbinate N Nasopharynx	0 Open 3 Percutaneous 4 Percutaneous Endoscopic 7 Via Natural or Artificial Opening 8 Via Natural or Artificial Opening Endoscopic	Z No Device	Z No Qualifier
B Mastoid Sinus, Right C Mastoid Sinus, Left M Nasal Septum P Accessory Sinus Q Maxillary Sinus, Right R Maxillary Sinus, Left S Frontal Sinus, Right T Frontal Sinus, Left U Ethmoid Sinus, Right V Ethmoid Sinus, Left W Sphenoid Sinus, Right X Sphenoid Sinus, Left	0 Open 3 Percutaneous 4 Percutaneous Endoscopic 8 Via Natural or Artificial Opening Endoscopic	Z No Device	Z No Qualifier
K Nasal Mucosa and Soft Tissue	0 Open 3 Percutaneous 4 Percutaneous Endoscopic 8 Via Natural or Artificial Opening Endoscopic X External	Z No Device	Z No Qualifier

Section	0	Medical and Surgical
Body System	9	Ear, Nose, Sinus
Operation	P	Removal: Taking out or off a device from a body part

Body Part (4th)	Approach (5th)	Device (6th)	Qualifier (7th)
7 Tympanic Membrane, Right 8 Tympanic Membrane, Left	0 Open 7 Via Natural or Artificial Opening 8 Via Natural or Artificial Opening Endoscopic X External	0 Drainage Device	Z No Qualifier
D Inner Ear, Right E Inner Ear, Left	0 Open 7 Via Natural or Artificial Opening 8 Via Natural or Artificial Opening Endoscopic	S Hearing Device	Z No Qualifier
H Ear, Right J Ear, Left K Nasal Mucosa and Soft Tissue	0 Open 3 Percutaneous 4 Percutaneous Endoscopic 7 Via Natural or Artificial Opening 8 Via Natural or Artificial Opening Endoscopic	0 Drainage Device 7 Autologous Tissue Substitute D Intraluminal Device J Synthetic Substitute K Nonautologous Tissue Substitute Y Other Device	Z No Qualifier
H Ear, Right J Ear, Left K Nasal Mucosa and Soft Tissue	X External	0 Drainage Device 7 Autologous Tissue Substitute D Intraluminal Device J Synthetic Substitute K Nonautologous Tissue Substitute	Z No Qualifier
Y Sinus	0 Open 3 Percutaneous 4 Percutaneous Endoscopic	0 Drainage Device Y Other Device	Z No Qualifier
Y Sinus	7 Via Natural or Artificial Opening 8 Via Natural or Artificial Opening Endoscopic	Y Other Device	Z No Qualifier
Y Sinus	X External	0 Drainage Device	Z No Qualifier

Section	0	Medical and Surgical
Body System	9	Ear, Nose, Sinus
Operation	Q	Repair: Restoring, to the extent possible, a body part to its normal anatomic structure and function

Body Part (4th)	Approach (5th)	Device (6th)	Qualifier (7th)
0 External Ear, Right 1 External Ear, Left 2 External Ear, Bilateral	0 Open 3 Percutaneous 4 Percutaneous Endoscopic X External	Z No Device	Z No Qualifier
3 External Auditory Canal, Right 4 External Auditory Canal, Left F Eustachian Tube, Right G Eustachian Tube, Left	0 Open 3 Percutaneous 4 Percutaneous Endoscopic 7 Via Natural or Artificial Opening 8 Via Natural or Artificial Opening Endoscopic X External	Z No Device	Z No Qualifier
5 Middle Ear, Right 6 Middle Ear, Left 9 Auditory Ossicle, Right A Auditory Ossicle, Left D Inner Ear, Right E Inner Ear, Left	0 Open 8 Via Natural or Artificial Opening Endoscopic	Z No Device	Z No Qualifier
7 Tympanic Membrane, Right 8 Tympanic Membrane, Left L Nasal Turbinate N Nasopharynx	0 Open 3 Percutaneous 4 Percutaneous Endoscopic 7 Via Natural or Artificial Opening 8 Via Natural or Artificial Opening Endoscopic	Z No Device	Z No Qualifier

Continued →

Section   0   **Medical and Surgical**
Body System   9   **Ear, Nose, Sinus**
Operation   Q   **Repair:** Restoring, to the extent possible, a body part to its normal anatomic structure and function

Body Part (4ᵗʰ)	Approach (5ᵗʰ)	Device (6ᵗʰ)	Qualifier (7ᵗʰ)
B Mastoid Sinus, Right C Mastoid Sinus, Left M Nasal Septum P Accessory Sinus Q Maxillary Sinus, Right R Maxillary Sinus, Left S Frontal Sinus, Right T Frontal Sinus, Left U Ethmoid Sinus, Right V Ethmoid Sinus, Left W Sphenoid Sinus, Right X Sphenoid Sinus, Left	0 Open 3 Percutaneous 4 Percutaneous Endoscopic 8 Via Natural or Artificial Opening Endoscopic	Z No Device	Z No Qualifier
K Nasal Mucosa and Soft Tissue	0 Open 3 Percutaneous 4 Percutaneous Endoscopic 8 Via Natural or Artificial Opening Endoscopic X External	Z No Device	Z No Qualifier

Section   0   **Medical and Surgical**
Body System   9   **Ear, Nose, Sinus**
Operation   R   **Replacement:** Putting in or on biological or synthetic material that physically takes the place and/or function of all or a portion of a body part

Body Part (4ᵗʰ)	Approach (5ᵗʰ)	Device (6ᵗʰ)	Qualifier (7ᵗʰ)
0 External Ear, Right 1 External Ear, Left 2 External Ear, Bilateral K Nasal Mucosa and Soft Tissue	0 Open X External	7 Autologous Tissue Substitute J Synthetic Substitute K Nonautologous Tissue Substitute	Z No Qualifier
5 Middle Ear, Right 6 Middle Ear, Left 9 Auditory Ossicle, Right A Auditory Ossicle, Left D Inner Ear, Right E Inner Ear, Left	0 Open	7 Autologous Tissue Substitute J Synthetic Substitute K Nonautologous Tissue Substitute	Z No Qualifier
7 Tympanic Membrane, Right 8 Tympanic Membrane, Left N Nasopharynx	0 Open 7 Via Natural or Artificial Opening 8 Via Natural or Artificial Opening Endoscopic	7 Autologous Tissue Substitute J Synthetic Substitute K Nonautologous Tissue Substitute	Z No Qualifier
L Nasal Turbinate	0 Open 3 Percutaneous 4 Percutaneous Endoscopic 7 Via Natural or Artificial Opening 8 Via Natural or Artificial Opening Endoscopic	7 Autologous Tissue Substitute J Synthetic Substitute K Nonautologous Tissue Substitute	Z No Qualifier
M Nasal Septum	0 Open 3 Percutaneous 4 Percutaneous Endoscopic	7 Autologous Tissue Substitute J Synthetic Substitute K Nonautologous Tissue Substitute	Z No Qualifier

Section	0	Medical and Surgical
Body System	9	Ear, Nose, Sinus
Operation	S	**Reposition:** Moving to its normal location, or other suitable location, all or a portion of a body part

Body Part (4th)	Approach (5th)	Device (6th)	Qualifier (7th)
0 External Ear, Right 1 External Ear, Left 2 External Ear, Bilateral K Nasal Mucosa and Soft Tissue	0 Open 4 Percutaneous Endoscopic X External	Z No Device	Z No Qualifier
7 Tympanic Membrane, Right 8 Tympanic Membrane, Left F Eustachian Tube, Right G Eustachian Tube, Left L Nasal Turbinate	0 Open 4 Percutaneous Endoscopic 7 Via Natural or Artificial Opening 8 Via Natural or Artificial Opening Endoscopic	Z No Device	Z No Qualifier
9 Auditory Ossicle, Right A Auditory Ossicle, Left M Nasal Septum	0 Open 4 Percutaneous Endoscopic	Z No Device	Z No Qualifier

Section	0	Medical and Surgical
Body System	9	Ear, Nose, Sinus
Operation	T	**Resection:** Cutting out or off, without replacement, all of a body part

Body Part (4th)	Approach (5th)	Device (6th)	Qualifier (7th)
0 External Ear, Right 1 External Ear, Left	0 Open 4 Percutaneous Endoscopic X External	Z No Device	Z No Qualifier
5 Middle Ear, Right 6 Middle Ear, Left 9 Auditory Ossicle, Right A Auditory Ossicle, Left D Inner Ear, Right E Inner Ear, Left	0 Open 8 Via Natural or Artificial Opening Endoscopic	Z No Device	Z No Qualifier
7 Tympanic Membrane, Right 8 Tympanic Membrane, Left F Eustachian Tube, Right G Eustachian Tube, Left L Nasal Turbinate N Nasopharynx	0 Open 4 Percutaneous Endoscopic 7 Via Natural or Artificial Opening 8 Via Natural or Artificial Opening Endoscopic	Z No Device	Z No Qualifier
B Mastoid Sinus, Right C Mastoid Sinus, Left M Nasal Septum P Accessory Sinus Q Maxillary Sinus, Right R Maxillary Sinus, Left S Frontal Sinus, Right T Frontal Sinus, Left U Ethmoid Sinus, Right V Ethmoid Sinus, Left W Sphenoid Sinus, Right X Sphenoid Sinus, Left	0 Open 4 Percutaneous Endoscopic 8 Via Natural or Artificial Opening Endoscopic	Z No Device	Z No Qualifier
K Nasal Mucosa and Soft Tissue	0 Open 4 Percutaneous Endoscopic 8 Via Natural or Artificial Opening Endoscopic X External	Z No Device	Z No Qualifier

Section	0	Medical and Surgical
Body System	9	Ear, Nose, Sinus
Operation	U	Supplement: Putting in or on biological or synthetic material that physically reinforces and/or augments the function of a portion of a body part

Body Part (4th)	Approach (5th)	Device (6th)	Qualifier (7th)
0 External Ear, Right 1 External Ear, Left 2 External Ear, Bilateral	0 Open X External	7 Autologous Tissue Substitute J Synthetic Substitute K Nonautologous Tissue Substitute	Z No Qualifier
5 Middle Ear, Right 6 Middle Ear, Left 9 Auditory Ossicle, Right A Auditory Ossicle, Left D Inner Ear, Right E Inner Ear, Left	0 Open 8 Via Natural or Artificial Opening Endoscopic	7 Autologous Tissue Substitute J Synthetic Substitute K Nonautologous Tissue Substitute	Z No Qualifier
7 Tympanic Membrane, Right 8 Tympanic Membrane, Left N Nasopharynx	0 Open 7 Via Natural or Artificial Opening 8 Via Natural or Artificial Opening Endoscopic	7 Autologous Tissue Substitute J Synthetic Substitute K Nonautologous Tissue Substitute	Z No Qualifier
B Mastoid Sinus, Right C Mastoid Sinus, Left L Nasal Turbinate P Accessory Sinus Q Maxillary Sinus, Right R Maxillary Sinus, Left S Frontal Sinus, Right T Frontal Sinus, Left U Ethmoid Sinus, Right V Ethmoid Sinus, Left W Sphenoid Sinus, Right X Sphenoid Sinus, Left	0 Open 3 Percutaneous 4 Percutaneous Endoscopic 7 Via Natural or Artificial Opening 8 Via Natural or Artificial Opening Endoscopic	7 Autologous Tissue Substitute J Synthetic Substitute K Nonautologous Tissue Substitute	Z No Qualifier
K Nasal Mucosa and Soft Tissue	0 Open 8 Via Natural or Artificial Opening Endoscopic X External	7 Autologous Tissue Substitute J Synthetic Substitute K Nonautologous Tissue Substitute	Z No Qualifier
M Nasal Septum	0 Open 3 Percutaneous 4 Percutaneous Endoscopic 8 Via Natural or Artificial Opening Endoscopic	7 Autologous Tissue Substitute J Synthetic Substitute K Nonautologous Tissue Substitute	Z No Qualifier

Section	0	Medical and Surgical
Body System	9	Ear, Nose, Sinus
Operation	W	Revision: Correcting, to the extent possible, a portion of a malfunctioning device or the position of a displaced device

Body Part (4th)	Approach (5th)	Device (6th)	Qualifier (7th)
7 Tympanic Membrane, Right 8 Tympanic Membrane, Left 9 Auditory Ossicle, Right A Auditory Ossicle, Left	0 Open 7 Via Natural or Artificial Opening 8 Via Natural or Artificial Opening Endoscopic	7 Autologous Tissue Substitute J Synthetic Substitute K Nonautologous Tissue Substitute	Z No Qualifier
D Inner Ear, Right E Inner Ear, Left	0 Open 7 Via Natural or Artificial Opening 8 Via Natural or Artificial Opening Endoscopic	S Hearing Device	Z No Qualifier
H Ear, Right J Ear, Left K Nasal Mucosa and Soft Tissue	0 Open 3 Percutaneous 4 Percutaneous Endoscopic 7 Via Natural or Artificial Opening 8 Via Natural or Artificial Opening Endoscopic	0 Drainage Device 7 Autologous Tissue Substitute D Intraluminal Device J Synthetic Substitute K Nonautologous Tissue Substitute Y Other Device	Z No Qualifier

Continued →

Section   **0**   **Medical and Surgical**
Body System   **9**   **Ear, Nose, Sinus**
Operation   **W**   **Revision:** Correcting, to the extent possible, a portion of a malfunctioning device or the position of a displaced device

Body Part (4th)	Approach (5th)	Device (6th)	Qualifier (7th)
H Ear, Right **J** Ear, Left **K** Nasal Mucosa and Soft Tissue	**X** External	**0** Drainage Device **7** Autologous Tissue Substitute **D** Intraluminal Device **J** Synthetic Substitute **K** Nonautologous Tissue Substitute	**Z** No Qualifier
Y Sinus	**0** Open **3** Percutaneous **4** Percutaneous Endoscopic	**0** Drainage Device **Y** Other Device	**Z** No Qualifier
Y Sinus	**7** Via Natural or Artificial Opening **8** Via Natural or Artificial Opening Endoscopic	**Y** Other Device	**Z** No Qualifier
Y Sinus	**X** External	**0** Drainage Device	**Z** No Qualifier

Ear, Nose, Sinus Code Listing 090–09W

090 – Ear, Nose, Sinus, Alteration

090007Z Alteration of Right External Ear with Autologous Tissue Substitute, Open Approach

09000JZ Alteration of Right External Ear with Synthetic Substitute, Open Approach

09000KZ Alteration of Right External Ear with Nonautologous Tissue Substitute, Open Approach

09000ZZ Alteration of Right External Ear, Open Approach

090037Z Alteration of Right External Ear with Autologous Tissue Substitute, Percutaneous Approach

09003JZ Alteration of Right External Ear with Synthetic Substitute, Percutaneous Approach

09003KZ Alteration of Right External Ear with Nonautologous Tissue Substitute, Percutaneous Approach

09003ZZ Alteration of Right External Ear, Percutaneous Approach

090047Z Alteration of Right External Ear with Autologous Tissue Substitute, Percutaneous Endoscopic Approach

09004JZ Alteration of Right External Ear with Synthetic Substitute, Percutaneous Endoscopic Approach

09004KZ Alteration of Right External Ear with Nonautologous Tissue Substitute, Percutaneous Endoscopic Approach

09004ZZ Alteration of Right External Ear, Percutaneous Endoscopic Approach

0900X7Z Alteration of Right External Ear with Autologous Tissue Substitute, External Approach

0900XJZ Alteration of Right External Ear with Synthetic Substitute, External Approach

0900XKZ Alteration of Right External Ear with Nonautologous Tissue Substitute, External Approach

0900XZZ Alteration of Right External Ear, External Approach

090107Z Alteration of Left External Ear with Autologous Tissue Substitute, Open Approach

09010JZ Alteration of Left External Ear with Synthetic Substitute, Open Approach

09010KZ Alteration of Left External Ear with Nonautologous Tissue Substitute, Open Approach

09010ZZ Alteration of Left External Ear, Open Approach

090137Z Alteration of Left External Ear with Autologous Tissue Substitute, Percutaneous Approach

09013JZ Alteration of Left External Ear with Synthetic Substitute, Percutaneous Approach

09013KZ Alteration of Left External Ear with Nonautologous Tissue Substitute, Percutaneous Approach

09013ZZ Alteration of Left External Ear, Percutaneous Approach

090147Z Alteration of Left External Ear with Autologous Tissue Substitute, Percutaneous Endoscopic Approach

09014JZ Alteration of Left External Ear with Synthetic Substitute, Percutaneous Endoscopic Approach

09014KZ Alteration of Left External Ear with Nonautologous Tissue Substitute, Percutaneous Endoscopic Approach

09014ZZ Alteration of Left External Ear, Percutaneous Endoscopic Approach

0901X7Z Alteration of Left External Ear with Autologous Tissue Substitute, External Approach

0901XJZ Alteration of Left External Ear with Synthetic Substitute, External Approach

0901XKZ Alteration of Left External Ear with Nonautologous Tissue Substitute, External Approach

0901XZZ Alteration of Left External Ear, External Approach

090207Z Alteration of Bilateral External Ear with Autologous Tissue Substitute, Open Approach

09020JZ Alteration of Bilateral External Ear with Synthetic Substitute, Open Approach

09020KZ Alteration of Bilateral External Ear with Nonautologous Tissue Substitute, Open Approach

09020ZZ Alteration of Bilateral External Ear, Open Approach

090237Z Alteration of Bilateral External Ear with Autologous Tissue Substitute, Percutaneous Approach

09023JZ Alteration of Bilateral External Ear with Synthetic Substitute, Percutaneous Approach

09023KZ Alteration of Bilateral External Ear with Nonautologous Tissue Substitute, Percutaneous Approach

09023ZZ Alteration of Bilateral External Ear, Percutaneous Approach

090247Z Alteration of Bilateral External Ear with Autologous Tissue Substitute, Percutaneous Endoscopic Approach

09024JZ Alteration of Bilateral External Ear with Synthetic Substitute, Percutaneous Endoscopic Approach

09024KZ Alteration of Bilateral External Ear with Nonautologous Tissue Substitute, Percutaneous Endoscopic Approach

09024ZZ Alteration of Bilateral External Ear, Percutaneous Endoscopic Approach

0902X7Z Alteration of Bilateral External Ear with Autologous Tissue Substitute, External Approach

0902XJZ Alteration of Bilateral External Ear with Synthetic Substitute, External Approach

0902XKZ Alteration of Bilateral External Ear with Nonautologous Tissue Substitute, External Approach

0902XZZ Alteration of Bilateral External Ear, External Approach
090K07Z Alteration of Nasal Mucosa and Soft Tissue with Autologous Tissue Substitute, Open Approach
090K0JZ Alteration of Nasal Mucosa and Soft Tissue with Synthetic Substitute, Open Approach
090K0KZ Alteration of Nasal Mucosa and Soft Tissue with Nonautologous Tissue Substitute, Open Approach
090K0ZZ Alteration of Nasal Mucosa and Soft Tissue, Open Approach
090K37Z Alteration of Nasal Mucosa and Soft Tissue with Autologous Tissue Substitute, Percutaneous Approach

090K3JZ Alteration of Nasal Mucosa and Soft Tissue with Synthetic Substitute, Percutaneous Approach
090K3KZ Alteration of Nasal Mucosa and Soft Tissue with Nonautologous Tissue Substitute, Percutaneous Approach
090K3ZZ Alteration of Nasal Mucosa and Soft Tissue, Percutaneous Approach
090K47Z Alteration of Nasal Mucosa and Soft Tissue with Autologous Tissue Substitute, Percutaneous Endoscopic Approach
090K4JZ Alteration of Nasal Mucosa and Soft Tissue with Synthetic Substitute, Percutaneous Endoscopic Approach
090K4KZ Alteration of Nasal Mucosa and Soft Tissue with Nonautologous Tissue

090K4ZZ Alteration of Nasal Mucosa and Soft Tissue, Percutaneous Endoscopic Approach
090KX7Z Alteration of Nasal Mucosa and Soft Tissue with Autologous Tissue Substitute, External Approach
090KXJZ Alteration of Nasal Mucosa and Soft Tissue with Synthetic Substitute, External Approach
090KXKZ Alteration of Nasal Mucosa and Soft Tissue with Nonautologous Tissue Substitute, External Approach
090KXZZ Alteration of Nasal Mucosa and Soft Tissue, External Approach

(Substitute, Percutaneous Endoscopic Approach)

091 – Ear, Nose, Sinus, Bypass

Review Coding Guideline B3.6a

091D070 Bypass Right Inner Ear to Endolymphatic with Autologous Tissue Substitute, Open Approach
091D0J0 Bypass Right Inner Ear to Endolymphatic with Synthetic Substitute, Open Approach

091D0K0 Bypass Right Inner Ear to Endolymphatic with Nonautologous Tissue Substitute, Open Approach
091D0Z0 Bypass Right Inner Ear to Endolymphatic, Open Approach
091E070 Bypass Left Inner Ear to Endolymphatic with Autologous Tissue Substitute, Open Approach

091E0J0 Bypass Left Inner Ear to Endolymphatic with Synthetic Substitute, Open Approach
091E0K0 Bypass Left Inner Ear to Endolymphatic with Nonautologous Tissue Substitute, Open Approach
091E0Z0 Bypass Left Inner Ear to Endolymphatic, Open Approach

092 – Ear, Nose, Sinus, Change

Review Coding Guideline B6.1c

092HX0Z Change Drainage Device in Right Ear, External Approach
092HXYZ Change Other Device in Right Ear, External Approach
092JX0Z Change Drainage Device in Left Ear, External Approach

092JXYZ Change Other Device in Left Ear, External Approach
092KX0Z Change Drainage Device in Nasal Mucosa and Soft Tissue, External Approach
092KXYZ Change Other Device in Nasal Mucosa and Soft Tissue, External Approach

092YX0Z Change Drainage Device in Sinus, External Approach
092YXYZ Change Other Device in Sinus, External Approach

093 – Ear, Nose, Sinus, Control

Review Coding Guideline B3.7

093K7ZZ Control Bleeding in Nasal Mucosa and Soft Tissue, Via Natural or Artificial Opening

093K8ZZ Control Bleeding in Nasal Mucosa and Soft Tissue, Via Natural or Artificial Opening Endoscopic
AHA CC: 4Q, 2018, 38

095 – Ear, Nose, Sinus, Destruction

09500ZZ Destruction of Right External Ear, Open Approach
09503ZZ Destruction of Right External Ear, Percutaneous Approach
09504ZZ Destruction of Right External Ear, Percutaneous Endoscopic Approach
0950XZZ Destruction of Right External Ear, External Approach
09510ZZ Destruction of Left External Ear, Open Approach
09513ZZ Destruction of Left External Ear, Percutaneous Approach
09514ZZ Destruction of Left External Ear, Percutaneous Endoscopic Approach
0951XZZ Destruction of Left External Ear, External Approach
09530ZZ Destruction of Right External Auditory Canal, Open Approach

09533ZZ Destruction of Right External Auditory Canal, Percutaneous Approach
09534ZZ Destruction of Right External Auditory Canal, Percutaneous Endoscopic Approach
09537ZZ Destruction of Right External Auditory Canal, Via Natural or Artificial Opening
09538ZZ Destruction of Right External Auditory Canal, Via Natural or Artificial Opening Endoscopic
0953XZZ Destruction of Right External Auditory Canal, External Approach
09540ZZ Destruction of Left External Auditory Canal, Open Approach
09543ZZ Destruction of Left External Auditory Canal, Percutaneous Approach

09544ZZ Destruction of Left External Auditory Canal, Percutaneous Endoscopic Approach
09547ZZ Destruction of Left External Auditory Canal, Via Natural or Artificial Opening
09548ZZ Destruction of Left External Auditory Canal, Via Natural or Artificial Opening Endoscopic
0954XZZ Destruction of Left External Auditory Canal, External Approach
09550ZZ Destruction of Right Middle Ear, Open Approach
09558ZZ Destruction of Right Middle Ear, Via Natural or Artificial Opening Endoscopic
09560ZZ Destruction of Left Middle Ear, Open Approach

♀ Female-only   ♂ Male-only   ▲ Limited Coverage   ● Non-OR   ⬛ HAC-associated procedure   ▲ Non-covered procedures   ✚ Cluster

09568ZZ Destruction of Left Middle Ear, Via Natural or Artificial Opening Endoscopic

09570ZZ Destruction of Right Tympanic Membrane, Open Approach

09573ZZ Destruction of Right Tympanic Membrane, Percutaneous Approach

09574ZZ Destruction of Right Tympanic Membrane, Percutaneous Endoscopic Approach

09577ZZ Destruction of Right Tympanic Membrane, Via Natural or Artificial Opening

09578ZZ Destruction of Right Tympanic Membrane, Via Natural or Artificial Opening Endoscopic

09580ZZ Destruction of Left Tympanic Membrane, Open Approach

09583ZZ Destruction of Left Tympanic Membrane, Percutaneous Approach

09584ZZ Destruction of Left Tympanic Membrane, Percutaneous Endoscopic Approach

09587ZZ Destruction of Left Tympanic Membrane, Via Natural or Artificial Opening

09588ZZ Destruction of Left Tympanic Membrane, Via Natural or Artificial Opening Endoscopic

09590ZZ Destruction of Right Auditory Ossicle, Open Approach

09598ZZ Destruction of Right Auditory Ossicle, Via Natural or Artificial Opening Endoscopic

095A0ZZ Destruction of Left Auditory Ossicle, Open Approach

095A8ZZ Destruction of Left Auditory Ossicle, Via Natural or Artificial Opening Endoscopic

095B0ZZ Destruction of Right Mastoid Sinus, Open Approach

095B3ZZ Destruction of Right Mastoid Sinus, Percutaneous Approach

095B4ZZ Destruction of Right Mastoid Sinus, Percutaneous Endoscopic Approach

095B8ZZ Destruction of Right Mastoid Sinus, Via Natural or Artificial Opening Endoscopic

095C0ZZ Destruction of Left Mastoid Sinus, Open Approach

095C3ZZ Destruction of Left Mastoid Sinus, Percutaneous Approach

095C4ZZ Destruction of Left Mastoid Sinus, Percutaneous Endoscopic Approach

095C8ZZ Destruction of Left Mastoid Sinus, Via Natural or Artificial Opening Endoscopic

095D0ZZ Destruction of Right Inner Ear, Open Approach

095D8ZZ Destruction of Right Inner Ear, Via Natural or Artificial Opening Endoscopic

095E0ZZ Destruction of Left Inner Ear, Open Approach

095E8ZZ Destruction of Left Inner Ear, Via Natural or Artificial Opening Endoscopic

095F0ZZ Destruction of Right Eustachian Tube, Open Approach

095F3ZZ Destruction of Right Eustachian Tube, Percutaneous Approach

095F4ZZ Destruction of Right Eustachian Tube, Percutaneous Endoscopic Approach

095F7ZZ Destruction of Right Eustachian Tube, Via Natural or Artificial Opening

095F8ZZ Destruction of Right Eustachian Tube, Via Natural or Artificial Opening Endoscopic

095G0ZZ Destruction of Left Eustachian Tube, Open Approach

095G3ZZ Destruction of Left Eustachian Tube, Percutaneous Approach

095G4ZZ Destruction of Left Eustachian Tube, Percutaneous Endoscopic Approach

095G7ZZ Destruction of Left Eustachian Tube, Via Natural or Artificial Opening

095G8ZZ Destruction of Left Eustachian Tube, Via Natural or Artificial Opening Endoscopic

095K0ZZ Destruction of Nasal Mucosa and Soft Tissue, Open Approach

095K3ZZ Destruction of Nasal Mucosa and Soft Tissue, Percutaneous Approach

095K4ZZ Destruction of Nasal Mucosa and Soft Tissue, Percutaneous Endoscopic Approach

095K8ZZ Destruction of Nasal Mucosa and Soft Tissue, Via Natural or Artificial Opening Endoscopic

095KXZZ Destruction of Nasal Mucosa and Soft Tissue, External Approach

095L0ZZ Destruction of Nasal Turbinate, Open Approach

095L3ZZ Destruction of Nasal Turbinate, Percutaneous Approach

095L4ZZ Destruction of Nasal Turbinate, Percutaneous Endoscopic Approach

095L7ZZ Destruction of Nasal Turbinate, Via Natural or Artificial Opening

095L8ZZ Destruction of Nasal Turbinate, Via Natural or Artificial Opening Endoscopic

095M0ZZ Destruction of Nasal Septum, Open Approach

095M3ZZ Destruction of Nasal Septum, Percutaneous Approach

095M4ZZ Destruction of Nasal Septum, Percutaneous Endoscopic Approach

095M8ZZ Destruction of Nasal Septum, Via Natural or Artificial Opening Endoscopic

095N0ZZ Destruction of Nasopharynx, Open Approach

095N3ZZ Destruction of Nasopharynx, Percutaneous Approach

095N4ZZ Destruction of Nasopharynx, Percutaneous Endoscopic Approach

095N7ZZ Destruction of Nasopharynx, Via Natural or Artificial Opening

095N8ZZ Destruction of Nasopharynx, Via Natural or Artificial Opening Endoscopic

095P0ZZ Destruction of Accessory Sinus, Open Approach

095P3ZZ Destruction of Accessory Sinus, Percutaneous Approach

095P4ZZ Destruction of Accessory Sinus, Percutaneous Endoscopic Approach

095P8ZZ Destruction of Accessory Sinus, Via Natural or Artificial Opening Endoscopic

095Q0ZZ Destruction of Right Maxillary Sinus, Open Approach

095Q3ZZ Destruction of Right Maxillary Sinus, Percutaneous Approach

095Q4ZZ Destruction of Right Maxillary Sinus, Percutaneous Endoscopic Approach

095Q8ZZ Destruction of Right Maxillary Sinus, Via Natural or Artificial Opening Endoscopic

095R0ZZ Destruction of Left Maxillary Sinus, Open Approach

095R3ZZ Destruction of Left Maxillary Sinus, Percutaneous Approach

095R4ZZ Destruction of Left Maxillary Sinus, Percutaneous Endoscopic Approach

095R8ZZ Destruction of Left Maxillary Sinus, Via Natural or Artificial Opening Endoscopic

095S0ZZ Destruction of Right Frontal Sinus, Open Approach

095S3ZZ Destruction of Right Frontal Sinus, Percutaneous Approach

095S4ZZ Destruction of Right Frontal Sinus, Percutaneous Endoscopic Approach

095S8ZZ Destruction of Right Frontal Sinus, Via Natural or Artificial Opening Endoscopic

095T0ZZ Destruction of Left Frontal Sinus, Open Approach

095T3ZZ Destruction of Left Frontal Sinus, Percutaneous Approach

095T4ZZ Destruction of Left Frontal Sinus, Percutaneous Endoscopic Approach

095T8ZZ Destruction of Left Frontal Sinus, Via Natural or Artificial Opening Endoscopic

095U0ZZ Destruction of Right Ethmoid Sinus, Open Approach

095U3ZZ Destruction of Right Ethmoid Sinus, Percutaneous Approach

095U4ZZ Destruction of Right Ethmoid Sinus, Percutaneous Endoscopic Approach

095U8ZZ Destruction of Right Ethmoid Sinus, Via Natural or Artificial Opening Endoscopic

095V0ZZ Destruction of Left Ethmoid Sinus, Open Approach

095V3ZZ Destruction of Left Ethmoid Sinus, Percutaneous Approach

095V4ZZ Destruction of Left Ethmoid Sinus, Percutaneous Endoscopic Approach

095V8ZZ Destruction of Left Ethmoid Sinus, Via Natural or Artificial Opening Endoscopic

095W0ZZ Destruction of Right Sphenoid Sinus, Open Approach

095W3ZZ Destruction of Right Sphenoid Sinus, Percutaneous Approach

095W4ZZ Destruction of Right Sphenoid Sinus, Percutaneous Endoscopic Approach

095W8ZZ Destruction of Right Sphenoid Sinus, Via Natural or Artificial Opening Endoscopic

095X0ZZ Destruction of Left Sphenoid Sinus, Open Approach

095X3ZZ Destruction of Left Sphenoid Sinus, Percutaneous Approach

095X4ZZ Destruction of Left Sphenoid Sinus, Percutaneous Endoscopic Approach

095X8ZZ Destruction of Left Sphenoid Sinus, Via Natural or Artificial Opening Endoscopic

♀ Female-only   ♂ Male-only   ▲ Limited Coverage   ● Non-OR   ▨ HAC-associated procedure   ▲ Non-covered procedures   ✚ Cluster

097 – Ear, Nose, Sinus, Dilation

097F0DZ Dilation of Right Eustachian Tube with Intraluminal Device, Open Approach

097F0ZZ Dilation of Right Eustachian Tube, Open Approach

097F3ZZ Dilation of Right Eustachian Tube, Percutaneous Approach

097F4ZZ Dilation of Right Eustachian Tube, Percutaneous Endoscopic Approach

097F7DZ Dilation of Right Eustachian Tube with Intraluminal Device, Via Natural or Artificial Opening

097F7ZZ Dilation of Right Eustachian Tube, Via Natural or Artificial Opening

097F8DZ Dilation of Right Eustachian Tube with Intraluminal Device, Via Natural or Artificial Opening Endoscopic

097F8ZZ Dilation of Right Eustachian Tube, Via Natural or Artificial Opening Endoscopic

097G0DZ Dilation of Left Eustachian Tube with Intraluminal Device, Open Approach

097G0ZZ Dilation of Left Eustachian Tube, Open Approach

097G3ZZ Dilation of Left Eustachian Tube, Percutaneous Approach

097G4ZZ Dilation of Left Eustachian Tube, Percutaneous Endoscopic Approach

097G7DZ Dilation of Left Eustachian Tube with Intraluminal Device, Via Natural or Artificial Opening

097G7ZZ Dilation of Left Eustachian Tube, Via Natural or Artificial Opening

097G8DZ Dilation of Left Eustachian Tube with Intraluminal Device, Via Natural or Artificial Opening Endoscopic

097G8ZZ Dilation of Left Eustachian Tube, Via Natural or Artificial Opening Endoscopic

098 – Ear, Nose, Sinus, Division

098L0ZZ Division of Nasal Turbinate, Open Approach

098L3ZZ Division of Nasal Turbinate, Percutaneous Approach

098L4ZZ Division of Nasal Turbinate, Percutaneous Endoscopic Approach

098L7ZZ Division of Nasal Turbinate, Via Natural or Artificial Opening

098L8ZZ Division of Nasal Turbinate, Via Natural or Artificial Opening Endoscopic

099 – Ear, Nose, Sinus, Drainage

Review Coding Guidelines B3.4a and B3.4b

Review Coding Guideline B6.2

099000Z Drainage of Right External Ear with Drainage Device, Open Approach

09900ZX Drainage of Right External Ear, Open Approach, Diagnostic

09900ZZ Drainage of Right External Ear, Open Approach

099030Z Drainage of Right External Ear with Drainage Device, Percutaneous Approach

09903ZX Drainage of Right External Ear, Percutaneous Approach, Diagnostic

09903ZZ Drainage of Right External Ear, Percutaneous Approach

099040Z Drainage of Right External Ear with Drainage Device, Percutaneous Endoscopic Approach

09904ZX Drainage of Right External Ear, Percutaneous Endoscopic Approach, Diagnostic

09904ZZ Drainage of Right External Ear, Percutaneous Endoscopic Approach

0990X0Z Drainage of Right External Ear with Drainage Device, External Approach

0990XZX Drainage of Right External Ear, External Approach, Diagnostic

0990XZZ Drainage of Right External Ear, External Approach

099100Z Drainage of Left External Ear with Drainage Device, Open Approach

09910ZX Drainage of Left External Ear, Open Approach, Diagnostic

09910ZZ Drainage of Left External Ear, Open Approach

099130Z Drainage of Left External Ear with Drainage Device, Percutaneous Approach

09913ZX Drainage of Left External Ear, Percutaneous Approach, Diagnostic

09913ZZ Drainage of Left External Ear, Percutaneous Approach

099140Z Drainage of Left External Ear with Drainage Device, Percutaneous Endoscopic Approach

09914ZX Drainage of Left External Ear, Percutaneous Endoscopic Approach, Diagnostic

09914ZZ Drainage of Left External Ear, Percutaneous Endoscopic Approach

0991X0Z Drainage of Left External Ear with Drainage Device, External Approach

0991XZX Drainage of Left External Ear, External Approach, Diagnostic

0991XZZ Drainage of Left External Ear, External Approach

099300Z Drainage of Right External Auditory Canal with Drainage Device, Open Approach

09930ZX Drainage of Right External Auditory Canal, Open Approach, Diagnostic

09930ZZ Drainage of Right External Auditory Canal, Open Approach

099330Z Drainage of Right External Auditory Canal with Drainage Device, Percutaneous Approach

09933ZX Drainage of Right External Auditory Canal, Percutaneous Approach, Diagnostic

09933ZZ Drainage of Right External Auditory Canal, Percutaneous Approach

099340Z Drainage of Right External Auditory Canal with Drainage Device, Percutaneous Endoscopic Approach

09934ZX Drainage of Right External Auditory Canal, Percutaneous Endoscopic Approach, Diagnostic

09934ZZ Drainage of Right External Auditory Canal, Percutaneous Endoscopic Approach

099370Z Drainage of Right External Auditory Canal with Drainage Device, Via Natural or Artificial Opening

09937ZX Drainage of Right External Auditory Canal, Via Natural or Artificial Opening, Diagnostic

09937ZZ Drainage of Right External Auditory Canal, Via Natural or Artificial Opening

099380Z Drainage of Right External Auditory Canal with Drainage Device, Via Natural or Artificial Opening Endoscopic

09938ZX Drainage of Right External Auditory Canal, Via Natural or Artificial Opening Endoscopic, Diagnostic

09938ZZ Drainage of Right External Auditory Canal, Via Natural or Artificial Opening Endoscopic

0993X0Z Drainage of Right External Auditory Canal with Drainage Device, External Approach

0993XZX Drainage of Right External Auditory Canal, External Approach, Diagnostic

0993XZZ Drainage of Right External Auditory Canal, External Approach

099400Z Drainage of Left External Auditory Canal with Drainage Device, Open Approach

09940ZX Drainage of Left External Auditory Canal, Open Approach, Diagnostic

09940ZZ Drainage of Left External Auditory Canal, Open Approach

099430Z Drainage of Left External Auditory Canal with Drainage Device, Percutaneous Approach

09943ZX Drainage of Left External Auditory Canal, Percutaneous Approach, Diagnostic

09943ZZ Drainage of Left External Auditory Canal, Percutaneous Approach

099440Z Drainage of Left External Auditory Canal with Drainage Device, Percutaneous Endoscopic Approach

09944ZX Drainage of Left External Auditory Canal, Percutaneous Endoscopic Approach, Diagnostic

09944ZZ Drainage of Left External Auditory Canal, Percutaneous Endoscopic Approach

099470Z Drainage of Left External Auditory Canal with Drainage Device, Via Natural or Artificial Opening

♀ Female-only   ♂ Male-only   ▲ Limited Coverage   ● Non-OR   HAC HAC-associated procedure   ▲ Non-covered procedures   + Cluster

09947ZX Drainage of Left External Auditory Canal, Via Natural or Artificial Opening, Diagnostic

09947ZZ Drainage of Left External Auditory Canal, Via Natural or Artificial Opening

099480Z Drainage of Left External Auditory Canal with Drainage Device, Via Natural or Artificial Opening Endoscopic

09948ZX Drainage of Left External Auditory Canal, Via Natural or Artificial Opening Endoscopic, Diagnostic

09948ZZ Drainage of Left External Auditory Canal, Via Natural or Artificial Opening Endoscopic

0994X0Z Drainage of Left External Auditory Canal with Drainage Device, External Approach

0994XZX Drainage of Left External Auditory Canal, External Approach, Diagnostic

0994XZZ Drainage of Left External Auditory Canal, External Approach

099500Z Drainage of Right Middle Ear with Drainage Device, Open Approach

09950ZX Drainage of Right Middle Ear, Open Approach, Diagnostic

09950ZZ Drainage of Right Middle Ear, Open Approach

099570Z Drainage of Right Middle Ear with Drainage Device, Via Natural or Artificial Opening

09957ZX Drainage of Right Middle Ear, Via Natural or Artificial Opening, Diagnostic

09957ZZ Drainage of Right Middle Ear, Via Natural or Artificial Opening

099580Z Drainage of Right Middle Ear with Drainage Device, Via Natural or Artificial Opening Endoscopic

09958ZX Drainage of Right Middle Ear, Via Natural or Artificial Opening Endoscopic, Diagnostic

09958ZZ Drainage of Right Middle Ear, Via Natural or Artificial Opening Endoscopic

099600Z Drainage of Left Middle Ear with Drainage Device, Open Approach

09960ZX Drainage of Left Middle Ear, Open Approach, Diagnostic

09960ZZ Drainage of Left Middle Ear, Open Approach

099670Z Drainage of Left Middle Ear with Drainage Device, Via Natural or Artificial Opening

09967ZX Drainage of Left Middle Ear, Via Natural or Artificial Opening, Diagnostic

09967ZZ Drainage of Left Middle Ear, Via Natural or Artificial Opening

099680Z Drainage of Left Middle Ear with Drainage Device, Via Natural or Artificial Opening Endoscopic

09968ZX Drainage of Left Middle Ear, Via Natural or Artificial Opening Endoscopic, Diagnostic

09968ZZ Drainage of Left Middle Ear, Via Natural or Artificial Opening Endoscopic

099700Z Drainage of Right Tympanic Membrane with Drainage Device, Open Approach

09970ZX Drainage of Right Tympanic Membrane, Open Approach, Diagnostic

09970ZZ Drainage of Right Tympanic Membrane, Open Approach

099730Z Drainage of Right Tympanic Membrane with Drainage Device, Percutaneous Approach

09973ZX Drainage of Right Tympanic Membrane, Percutaneous Approach, Diagnostic

09973ZZ Drainage of Right Tympanic Membrane, Percutaneous Approach

099740Z Drainage of Right Tympanic Membrane with Drainage Device, Percutaneous Endoscopic Approach

09974ZX Drainage of Right Tympanic Membrane, Percutaneous Endoscopic Approach, Diagnostic

09974ZZ Drainage of Right Tympanic Membrane, Percutaneous Endoscopic Approach

099770Z Drainage of Right Tympanic Membrane with Drainage Device, Via Natural or Artificial Opening

09977ZX Drainage of Right Tympanic Membrane, Via Natural or Artificial Opening, Diagnostic

09977ZZ Drainage of Right Tympanic Membrane, Via Natural or Artificial Opening

099780Z Drainage of Right Tympanic Membrane with Drainage Device, Via Natural or Artificial Opening Endoscopic

09978ZX Drainage of Right Tympanic Membrane, Via Natural or Artificial Opening Endoscopic, Diagnostic

09978ZZ Drainage of Right Tympanic Membrane, Via Natural or Artificial Opening Endoscopic

099800Z Drainage of Left Tympanic Membrane with Drainage Device, Open Approach

09980ZX Drainage of Left Tympanic Membrane, Open Approach, Diagnostic

09980ZZ Drainage of Left Tympanic Membrane, Open Approach

099830Z Drainage of Left Tympanic Membrane with Drainage Device, Percutaneous Approach

09983ZX Drainage of Left Tympanic Membrane, Percutaneous Approach, Diagnostic

09983ZZ Drainage of Left Tympanic Membrane, Percutaneous Approach

099840Z Drainage of Left Tympanic Membrane with Drainage Device, Percutaneous Endoscopic Approach

09984ZX Drainage of Left Tympanic Membrane, Percutaneous Endoscopic Approach, Diagnostic

09984ZZ Drainage of Left Tympanic Membrane, Percutaneous Endoscopic Approach

099870Z Drainage of Left Tympanic Membrane with Drainage Device, Via Natural or Artificial Opening

09987ZX Drainage of Left Tympanic Membrane, Via Natural or Artificial Opening, Diagnostic

09987ZZ Drainage of Left Tympanic Membrane, Via Natural or Artificial Opening

099880Z Drainage of Left Tympanic Membrane with Drainage Device, Via Natural or Artificial Opening Endoscopic

09988ZX Drainage of Left Tympanic Membrane, Via Natural or Artificial Opening Endoscopic, Diagnostic

09988ZZ Drainage of Left Tympanic Membrane, Via Natural or Artificial Opening Endoscopic

099900Z Drainage of Right Auditory Ossicle with Drainage Device, Open Approach

09990ZX Drainage of Right Auditory Ossicle, Open Approach, Diagnostic

09990ZZ Drainage of Right Auditory Ossicle, Open Approach

099970Z Drainage of Right Auditory Ossicle with Drainage Device, Via Natural or Artificial Opening

09997ZX Drainage of Right Auditory Ossicle, Via Natural or Artificial Opening, Diagnostic

09997ZZ Drainage of Right Auditory Ossicle, Via Natural or Artificial Opening

099980Z Drainage of Right Auditory Ossicle with Drainage Device, Via Natural or Artificial Opening Endoscopic

09998ZX Drainage of Right Auditory Ossicle, Via Natural or Artificial Opening Endoscopic, Diagnostic

09998ZZ Drainage of Right Auditory Ossicle, Via Natural or Artificial Opening Endoscopic

099A00Z Drainage of Left Auditory Ossicle with Drainage Device, Open Approach

099A0ZX Drainage of Left Auditory Ossicle, Open Approach, Diagnostic

099A0ZZ Drainage of Left Auditory Ossicle, Open Approach

099A70Z Drainage of Left Auditory Ossicle with Drainage Device, Via Natural or Artificial Opening

099A7ZX Drainage of Left Auditory Ossicle, Via Natural or Artificial Opening, Diagnostic

099A7ZZ Drainage of Left Auditory Ossicle, Via Natural or Artificial Opening

099A80Z Drainage of Left Auditory Ossicle with Drainage Device, Via Natural or Artificial Opening Endoscopic

099A8ZX Drainage of Left Auditory Ossicle, Via Natural or Artificial Opening Endoscopic, Diagnostic

099A8ZZ Drainage of Left Auditory Ossicle, Via Natural or Artificial Opening Endoscopic

099B00Z Drainage of Right Mastoid Sinus with Drainage Device, Open Approach

099B0ZX Drainage of Right Mastoid Sinus, Open Approach, Diagnostic

099B0ZZ Drainage of Right Mastoid Sinus, Open Approach

099B30Z Drainage of Right Mastoid Sinus with Drainage Device, Percutaneous Approach

099B3ZX Drainage of Right Mastoid Sinus, Percutaneous Approach, Diagnostic

099B3ZZ Drainage of Right Mastoid Sinus, Percutaneous Approach

099B40Z Drainage of Right Mastoid Sinus with Drainage Device, Percutaneous Endoscopic Approach

099B4ZX Drainage of Right Mastoid Sinus, Percutaneous Endoscopic Approach, Diagnostic

099B4ZZ Drainage of Right Mastoid Sinus, Percutaneous Endoscopic Approach

099B70Z Drainage of Right Mastoid Sinus with Drainage Device, Via Natural or Artificial Opening

099B7ZX Drainage of Right Mastoid Sinus, Via Natural or Artificial Opening, Diagnostic

099B7ZZ Drainage of Right Mastoid Sinus, Via Natural or Artificial Opening

099B80Z Drainage of Right Mastoid Sinus with Drainage Device, Via Natural or Artificial Opening Endoscopic

099B8ZX Drainage of Right Mastoid Sinus, Via Natural or Artificial Opening Endoscopic, Diagnostic

099B8ZZ Drainage of Right Mastoid Sinus, Via Natural or Artificial Opening Endoscopic

099C00Z Drainage of Left Mastoid Sinus with Drainage Device, Open Approach

099C0ZX Drainage of Left Mastoid Sinus, Open Approach, Diagnostic

099C0ZZ Drainage of Left Mastoid Sinus, Open Approach

099C30Z Drainage of Left Mastoid Sinus with Drainage Device, Percutaneous Approach

099C3ZX Drainage of Left Mastoid Sinus, Percutaneous Approach, Diagnostic

099C3ZZ Drainage of Left Mastoid Sinus, Percutaneous Approach

099C40Z Drainage of Left Mastoid Sinus with Drainage Device, Percutaneous Endoscopic Approach

099C4ZX Drainage of Left Mastoid Sinus, Percutaneous Endoscopic Approach, Diagnostic

099C4ZZ Drainage of Left Mastoid Sinus, Percutaneous Endoscopic Approach

099C70Z Drainage of Left Mastoid Sinus with Drainage Device, Via Natural or Artificial Opening

099C7ZX Drainage of Left Mastoid Sinus, Via Natural or Artificial Opening, Diagnostic

099C7ZZ Drainage of Left Mastoid Sinus, Via Natural or Artificial Opening

099C80Z Drainage of Left Mastoid Sinus with Drainage Device, Via Natural or Artificial Opening Endoscopic

099C8ZX Drainage of Left Mastoid Sinus, Via Natural or Artificial Opening Endoscopic, Diagnostic

099C8ZZ Drainage of Left Mastoid Sinus, Via Natural or Artificial Opening Endoscopic

099D00Z Drainage of Right Inner Ear with Drainage Device, Open Approach

099D0ZX Drainage of Right Inner Ear, Open Approach, Diagnostic

099D0ZZ Drainage of Right Inner Ear, Open Approach

099D70Z Drainage of Right Inner Ear with Drainage Device, Via Natural or Artificial Opening

099D7ZX Drainage of Right Inner Ear, Via Natural or Artificial Opening, Diagnostic

099D7ZZ Drainage of Right Inner Ear, Via Natural or Artificial Opening

099D80Z Drainage of Right Inner Ear with Drainage Device, Via Natural or Artificial Opening Endoscopic

099D8ZX Drainage of Right Inner Ear, Via Natural or Artificial Opening Endoscopic, Diagnostic

099D8ZZ Drainage of Right Inner Ear, Via Natural or Artificial Opening Endoscopic

099E00Z Drainage of Left Inner Ear with Drainage Device, Open Approach

099E0ZX Drainage of Left Inner Ear, Open Approach, Diagnostic

099E0ZZ Drainage of Left Inner Ear, Open Approach

099E70Z Drainage of Left Inner Ear with Drainage Device, Via Natural or Artificial Opening

099E7ZX Drainage of Left Inner Ear, Via Natural or Artificial Opening, Diagnostic

099E7ZZ Drainage of Left Inner Ear, Via Natural or Artificial Opening

099E80Z Drainage of Left Inner Ear with Drainage Device, Via Natural or Artificial Opening Endoscopic

099E8ZX Drainage of Left Inner Ear, Via Natural or Artificial Opening Endoscopic, Diagnostic

099E8ZZ Drainage of Left Inner Ear, Via Natural or Artificial Opening Endoscopic

099F00Z Drainage of Right Eustachian Tube with Drainage Device, Open Approach

099F0ZX Drainage of Right Eustachian Tube, Open Approach, Diagnostic

099F0ZZ Drainage of Right Eustachian Tube, Open Approach

099F30Z Drainage of Right Eustachian Tube with Drainage Device, Percutaneous Approach

099F3ZX Drainage of Right Eustachian Tube, Percutaneous Approach, Diagnostic

099F3ZZ Drainage of Right Eustachian Tube, Percutaneous Approach

099F40Z Drainage of Right Eustachian Tube with Drainage Device, Percutaneous Endoscopic Approach

099F4ZX Drainage of Right Eustachian Tube, Percutaneous Endoscopic Approach, Diagnostic

099F4ZZ Drainage of Right Eustachian Tube, Percutaneous Endoscopic Approach

099F70Z Drainage of Right Eustachian Tube with Drainage Device, Via Natural or Artificial Opening

099F7ZX Drainage of Right Eustachian Tube, Via Natural or Artificial Opening, Diagnostic

099F7ZZ Drainage of Right Eustachian Tube, Via Natural or Artificial Opening

099F80Z Drainage of Right Eustachian Tube with Drainage Device, Via Natural or Artificial Opening Endoscopic

099F8ZX Drainage of Right Eustachian Tube, Via Natural or Artificial Opening Endoscopic, Diagnostic

099F8ZZ Drainage of Right Eustachian Tube, Via Natural or Artificial Opening Endoscopic

099G00Z Drainage of Left Eustachian Tube with Drainage Device, Open Approach

099G0ZX Drainage of Left Eustachian Tube, Open Approach, Diagnostic

099G0ZZ Drainage of Left Eustachian Tube, Open Approach

099G30Z Drainage of Left Eustachian Tube with Drainage Device, Percutaneous Approach

099G3ZX Drainage of Left Eustachian Tube, Percutaneous Approach, Diagnostic

099G3ZZ Drainage of Left Eustachian Tube, Percutaneous Approach

099G40Z Drainage of Left Eustachian Tube with Drainage Device, Percutaneous Endoscopic Approach

099G4ZX Drainage of Left Eustachian Tube, Percutaneous Endoscopic Approach, Diagnostic

099G4ZZ Drainage of Left Eustachian Tube, Percutaneous Endoscopic Approach

099G70Z Drainage of Left Eustachian Tube with Drainage Device, Via Natural or Artificial Opening

099G7ZX Drainage of Left Eustachian Tube, Via Natural or Artificial Opening, Diagnostic

099G7ZZ Drainage of Left Eustachian Tube, Via Natural or Artificial Opening

099G80Z Drainage of Left Eustachian Tube with Drainage Device, Via Natural or Artificial Opening Endoscopic

099G8ZX Drainage of Left Eustachian Tube, Via Natural or Artificial Opening Endoscopic, Diagnostic

099G8ZZ Drainage of Left Eustachian Tube, Via Natural or Artificial Opening Endoscopic

099K00Z Drainage of Nasal Mucosa and Soft Tissue with Drainage Device, Open Approach

099K0ZX Drainage of Nasal Mucosa and Soft Tissue, Open Approach, Diagnostic

099K0ZZ Drainage of Nasal Mucosa and Soft Tissue, Open Approach

099K30Z Drainage of Nasal Mucosa and Soft Tissue with Drainage Device, Percutaneous Approach

099K3ZX Drainage of Nasal Mucosa and Soft Tissue, Percutaneous Approach, Diagnostic

099K3ZZ Drainage of Nasal Mucosa and Soft Tissue, Percutaneous Approach

099K40Z Drainage of Nasal Mucosa and Soft Tissue with Drainage Device, Percutaneous Endoscopic Approach

099K4ZX Drainage of Nasal Mucosa and Soft Tissue, Percutaneous Endoscopic Approach, Diagnostic

099K4ZZ Drainage of Nasal Mucosa and Soft Tissue, Percutaneous Endoscopic Approach

099K70Z Drainage of Nasal Mucosa and Soft Tissue with Drainage Device, Via Natural or Artificial Opening

099K7ZX Drainage of Nasal Mucosa and Soft Tissue, Via Natural or Artificial Opening, Diagnostic

099K7ZZ Drainage of Nasal Mucosa and Soft Tissue, Via Natural or Artificial Opening

099K80Z Drainage of Nasal Mucosa and Soft Tissue with Drainage Device, Via Natural or Artificial Opening Endoscopic

099K8ZX Drainage of Nasal Mucosa and Soft Tissue, Via Natural or Artificial Opening Endoscopic, Diagnostic

099K8ZZ Drainage of Nasal Mucosa and Soft Tissue, Via Natural or Artificial Opening Endoscopic

099KX0Z Drainage of Nasal Mucosa and Soft Tissue with Drainage Device, External Approach

099KXZX Drainage of Nasal Mucosa and Soft Tissue, External Approach, Diagnostic

099KXZZ Drainage of Nasal Mucosa and Soft Tissue, External Approach

099L00Z Drainage of Nasal Turbinate with Drainage Device, Open Approach

099L0ZX Drainage of Nasal Turbinate, Open Approach, Diagnostic

099L0ZZ Drainage of Nasal Turbinate, Open Approach

099L30Z Drainage of Nasal Turbinate with Drainage Device, Percutaneous Approach

099L3ZX Drainage of Nasal Turbinate, Percutaneous Approach, Diagnostic

099L3ZZ Drainage of Nasal Turbinate, Percutaneous Approach

099L40Z Drainage of Nasal Turbinate with Drainage Device, Percutaneous Endoscopic Approach

099L4ZX Drainage of Nasal Turbinate, Percutaneous Endoscopic Approach, Diagnostic

099L4ZZ Drainage of Nasal Turbinate, Percutaneous Endoscopic Approach

099L70Z Drainage of Nasal Turbinate with Drainage Device, Via Natural or Artificial Opening

099L7ZX Drainage of Nasal Turbinate, Via Natural or Artificial Opening, Diagnostic

099L7ZZ Drainage of Nasal Turbinate, Via Natural or Artificial Opening

099L80Z Drainage of Nasal Turbinate with Drainage Device, Via Natural or Artificial Opening Endoscopic

099L8ZX Drainage of Nasal Turbinate, Via Natural or Artificial Opening Endoscopic, Diagnostic

099L8ZZ Drainage of Nasal Turbinate, Via Natural or Artificial Opening Endoscopic

099M00Z Drainage of Nasal Septum with Drainage Device, Open Approach

099M0ZX Drainage of Nasal Septum, Open Approach, Diagnostic

099M0ZZ Drainage of Nasal Septum, Open Approach

099M30Z Drainage of Nasal Septum with Drainage Device, Percutaneous Approach

099M3ZX Drainage of Nasal Septum, Percutaneous Approach, Diagnostic

099M3ZZ Drainage of Nasal Septum, Percutaneous Approach

099M40Z Drainage of Nasal Septum with Drainage Device, Percutaneous Endoscopic Approach

099M4ZX Drainage of Nasal Septum, Percutaneous Endoscopic Approach, Diagnostic

099M4ZZ Drainage of Nasal Septum, Percutaneous Endoscopic Approach

099M70Z Drainage of Nasal Septum with Drainage Device, Via Natural or Artificial Opening

099M7ZX Drainage of Nasal Septum, Via Natural or Artificial Opening, Diagnostic

099M7ZZ Drainage of Nasal Septum, Via Natural or Artificial Opening

099M80Z Drainage of Nasal Septum with Drainage Device, Via Natural or Artificial Opening Endoscopic

099M8ZX Drainage of Nasal Septum, Via Natural or Artificial Opening Endoscopic, Diagnostic

099M8ZZ Drainage of Nasal Septum, Via Natural or Artificial Opening Endoscopic

099N00Z Drainage of Nasopharynx with Drainage Device, Open Approach

099N0ZX Drainage of Nasopharynx, Open Approach, Diagnostic

099N0ZZ Drainage of Nasopharynx, Open Approach

099N30Z Drainage of Nasopharynx with Drainage Device, Percutaneous Approach

099N3ZX Drainage of Nasopharynx, Percutaneous Approach, Diagnostic

099N3ZZ Drainage of Nasopharynx, Percutaneous Approach

099N40Z Drainage of Nasopharynx with Drainage Device, Percutaneous Endoscopic Approach

099N4ZX Drainage of Nasopharynx, Percutaneous Endoscopic Approach, Diagnostic

099N4ZZ Drainage of Nasopharynx, Percutaneous Endoscopic Approach

099N70Z Drainage of Nasopharynx with Drainage Device, Via Natural or Artificial Opening

099N7ZX Drainage of Nasopharynx, Via Natural or Artificial Opening, Diagnostic

099N7ZZ Drainage of Nasopharynx, Via Natural or Artificial Opening

099N80Z Drainage of Nasopharynx with Drainage Device, Via Natural or Artificial Opening Endoscopic

099N8ZX Drainage of Nasopharynx, Via Natural or Artificial Opening Endoscopic, Diagnostic

099N8ZZ Drainage of Nasopharynx, Via Natural or Artificial Opening Endoscopic

099P00Z Drainage of Accessory Sinus with Drainage Device, Open Approach

099P0ZX Drainage of Accessory Sinus, Open Approach, Diagnostic

099P0ZZ Drainage of Accessory Sinus, Open Approach

099P30Z Drainage of Accessory Sinus with Drainage Device, Percutaneous Approach

099P3ZX Drainage of Accessory Sinus, Percutaneous Approach, Diagnostic

099P3ZZ Drainage of Accessory Sinus, Percutaneous Approach

099P40Z Drainage of Accessory Sinus with Drainage Device, Percutaneous Endoscopic Approach

099P4ZX Drainage of Accessory Sinus, Percutaneous Endoscopic Approach, Diagnostic

099P4ZZ Drainage of Accessory Sinus, Percutaneous Endoscopic Approach

099P70Z Drainage of Accessory Sinus with Drainage Device, Via Natural or Artificial Opening

099P7ZX Drainage of Accessory Sinus, Via Natural or Artificial Opening, Diagnostic

099P7ZZ Drainage of Accessory Sinus, Via Natural or Artificial Opening

099P80Z Drainage of Accessory Sinus with Drainage Device, Via Natural or Artificial Opening Endoscopic

099P8ZX Drainage of Accessory Sinus, Via Natural or Artificial Opening Endoscopic, Diagnostic

099P8ZZ Drainage of Accessory Sinus, Via Natural or Artificial Opening Endoscopic

099Q00Z Drainage of Right Maxillary Sinus with Drainage Device, Open Approach

099Q0ZX Drainage of Right Maxillary Sinus, Open Approach, Diagnostic

099Q0ZZ Drainage of Right Maxillary Sinus, Open Approach

099Q30Z Drainage of Right Maxillary Sinus with Drainage Device, Percutaneous Approach

099Q3ZX Drainage of Right Maxillary Sinus, Percutaneous Approach, Diagnostic

099Q3ZZ Drainage of Right Maxillary Sinus, Percutaneous Approach

099Q40Z Drainage of Right Maxillary Sinus with Drainage Device, Percutaneous Endoscopic Approach

099Q4ZX Drainage of Right Maxillary Sinus, Percutaneous Endoscopic Approach, Diagnostic

099Q4ZZ Drainage of Right Maxillary Sinus, Percutaneous Endoscopic Approach

099Q70Z Drainage of Right Maxillary Sinus with Drainage Device, Via Natural or Artificial Opening

099Q7ZX Drainage of Right Maxillary Sinus, Via Natural or Artificial Opening, Diagnostic

099Q7ZZ Drainage of Right Maxillary Sinus, Via Natural or Artificial Opening

099Q80Z Drainage of Right Maxillary Sinus with Drainage Device, Via Natural or Artificial Opening Endoscopic

099Q8ZX Drainage of Right Maxillary Sinus, Via Natural or Artificial Opening Endoscopic, Diagnostic

099Q8ZZ Drainage of Right Maxillary Sinus, Via Natural or Artificial Opening Endoscopic

099R00Z Drainage of Left Maxillary Sinus with Drainage Device, Open Approach

099R0ZX Drainage of Left Maxillary Sinus, Open Approach, Diagnostic

099R0ZZ Drainage of Left Maxillary Sinus, Open Approach

099R30Z Drainage of Left Maxillary Sinus with Drainage Device, Percutaneous Approach

099R3ZX Drainage of Left Maxillary Sinus, Percutaneous Approach, Diagnostic

099R3ZZ Drainage of Left Maxillary Sinus, Percutaneous Approach

099R40Z Drainage of Left Maxillary Sinus with Drainage Device, Percutaneous Endoscopic Approach

099R4ZX Drainage of Left Maxillary Sinus, Percutaneous Endoscopic Approach, Diagnostic

099R4ZZ Drainage of Left Maxillary Sinus, Percutaneous Endoscopic Approach

099R70Z Drainage of Left Maxillary Sinus with Drainage Device, Via Natural or Artificial Opening

099R7ZX Drainage of Left Maxillary Sinus, Via Natural or Artificial Opening, Diagnostic

099R7ZZ Drainage of Left Maxillary Sinus, Via Natural or Artificial Opening

099R80Z Drainage of Left Maxillary Sinus with Drainage Device, Via Natural or Artificial Opening Endoscopic

099R8ZX Drainage of Left Maxillary Sinus, Via Natural or Artificial Opening Endoscopic, Diagnostic

099R8ZZ Drainage of Left Maxillary Sinus, Via Natural or Artificial Opening Endoscopic

099S00Z Drainage of Right Frontal Sinus with Drainage Device, Open Approach

099S0ZX Drainage of Right Frontal Sinus, Open Approach, Diagnostic

099S0ZZ Drainage of Right Frontal Sinus, Open Approach

099S30Z Drainage of Right Frontal Sinus with Drainage Device, Percutaneous Approach

099S3ZX Drainage of Right Frontal Sinus, Percutaneous Approach, Diagnostic

099S3ZZ Drainage of Right Frontal Sinus, Percutaneous Approach

♀ Female-only   ♂ Male-only   ▲ Limited Coverage   ● Non-OR   HAC HAC-associated procedure   ▲ Non-covered procedures   ✛ Cluster

099S40Z Drainage of Right Frontal Sinus with Drainage Device, Percutaneous Endoscopic Approach

099S4ZX Drainage of Right Frontal Sinus, Percutaneous Endoscopic Approach, Diagnostic

099S4ZZ Drainage of Right Frontal Sinus, Percutaneous Endoscopic Approach

099S70Z Drainage of Right Frontal Sinus with Drainage Device, Via Natural or Artificial Opening

099S7ZX Drainage of Right Frontal Sinus, Via Natural or Artificial Opening, Diagnostic

099S7ZZ Drainage of Right Frontal Sinus, Via Natural or Artificial Opening

099S80Z Drainage of Right Frontal Sinus with Drainage Device, Via Natural or Artificial Opening Endoscopic

099S8ZX Drainage of Right Frontal Sinus, Via Natural or Artificial Opening Endoscopic, Diagnostic

099S8ZZ Drainage of Right Frontal Sinus, Via Natural or Artificial Opening Endoscopic

099T00Z Drainage of Left Frontal Sinus with Drainage Device, Open Approach

099T0ZX Drainage of Left Frontal Sinus, Open Approach, Diagnostic

099T0ZZ Drainage of Left Frontal Sinus, Open Approach

099T30Z Drainage of Left Frontal Sinus with Drainage Device, Percutaneous Approach

099T3ZX Drainage of Left Frontal Sinus, Percutaneous Approach, Diagnostic

099T3ZZ Drainage of Left Frontal Sinus, Percutaneous Approach

099T40Z Drainage of Left Frontal Sinus with Drainage Device, Percutaneous Endoscopic Approach

099T4ZX Drainage of Left Frontal Sinus, Percutaneous Endoscopic Approach, Diagnostic

099T4ZZ Drainage of Left Frontal Sinus, Percutaneous Endoscopic Approach

099T70Z Drainage of Left Frontal Sinus with Drainage Device, Via Natural or Artificial Opening

099T7ZX Drainage of Left Frontal Sinus, Via Natural or Artificial Opening, Diagnostic

099T7ZZ Drainage of Left Frontal Sinus, Via Natural or Artificial Opening

099T80Z Drainage of Left Frontal Sinus with Drainage Device, Via Natural or Artificial Opening Endoscopic

099T8ZX Drainage of Left Frontal Sinus, Via Natural or Artificial Opening Endoscopic, Diagnostic

099T8ZZ Drainage of Left Frontal Sinus, Via Natural or Artificial Opening Endoscopic

099U00Z Drainage of Right Ethmoid Sinus with Drainage Device, Open Approach

099U0ZX Drainage of Right Ethmoid Sinus, Open Approach, Diagnostic

099U0ZZ Drainage of Right Ethmoid Sinus, Open Approach

099U30Z Drainage of Right Ethmoid Sinus with Drainage Device, Percutaneous Approach

099U3ZX Drainage of Right Ethmoid Sinus, Percutaneous Approach, Diagnostic

099U3ZZ Drainage of Right Ethmoid Sinus, Percutaneous Approach

099U40Z Drainage of Right Ethmoid Sinus with Drainage Device, Percutaneous Endoscopic Approach

099U4ZX Drainage of Right Ethmoid Sinus, Percutaneous Endoscopic Approach, Diagnostic

099U4ZZ Drainage of Right Ethmoid Sinus, Percutaneous Endoscopic Approach

099U70Z Drainage of Right Ethmoid Sinus with Drainage Device, Via Natural or Artificial Opening

099U7ZX Drainage of Right Ethmoid Sinus, Via Natural or Artificial Opening, Diagnostic

099U7ZZ Drainage of Right Ethmoid Sinus, Via Natural or Artificial Opening

099U80Z Drainage of Right Ethmoid Sinus with Drainage Device, Via Natural or Artificial Opening Endoscopic

099U8ZX Drainage of Right Ethmoid Sinus, Via Natural or Artificial Opening Endoscopic, Diagnostic

099U8ZZ Drainage of Right Ethmoid Sinus, Via Natural or Artificial Opening Endoscopic

099V00Z Drainage of Left Ethmoid Sinus with Drainage Device, Open Approach

099V0ZX Drainage of Left Ethmoid Sinus, Open Approach, Diagnostic

099V0ZZ Drainage of Left Ethmoid Sinus, Open Approach

099V30Z Drainage of Left Ethmoid Sinus with Drainage Device, Percutaneous Approach

099V3ZX Drainage of Left Ethmoid Sinus, Percutaneous Approach, Diagnostic

099V3ZZ Drainage of Left Ethmoid Sinus, Percutaneous Approach

099V40Z Drainage of Left Ethmoid Sinus with Drainage Device, Percutaneous Endoscopic Approach

099V4ZX Drainage of Left Ethmoid Sinus, Percutaneous Endoscopic Approach, Diagnostic

099V4ZZ Drainage of Left Ethmoid Sinus, Percutaneous Endoscopic Approach

099V70Z Drainage of Left Ethmoid Sinus with Drainage Device, Via Natural or Artificial Opening

099V7ZX Drainage of Left Ethmoid Sinus, Via Natural or Artificial Opening, Diagnostic

099V7ZZ Drainage of Left Ethmoid Sinus, Via Natural or Artificial Opening

099V80Z Drainage of Left Ethmoid Sinus with Drainage Device, Via Natural or Artificial Opening Endoscopic

099V8ZX Drainage of Left Ethmoid Sinus, Via Natural or Artificial Opening Endoscopic, Diagnostic

099V8ZZ Drainage of Left Ethmoid Sinus, Via Natural or Artificial Opening Endoscopic

099W00Z Drainage of Right Sphenoid Sinus with Drainage Device, Open Approach

099W0ZX Drainage of Right Sphenoid Sinus, Open Approach, Diagnostic

099W0ZZ Drainage of Right Sphenoid Sinus, Open Approach

099W30Z Drainage of Right Sphenoid Sinus with Drainage Device, Percutaneous Approach

099W3ZX Drainage of Right Sphenoid Sinus, Percutaneous Approach, Diagnostic

099W3ZZ Drainage of Right Sphenoid Sinus, Percutaneous Approach

099W40Z Drainage of Right Sphenoid Sinus with Drainage Device, Percutaneous Endoscopic Approach

099W4ZX Drainage of Right Sphenoid Sinus, Percutaneous Endoscopic Approach, Diagnostic

099W4ZZ Drainage of Right Sphenoid Sinus, Percutaneous Endoscopic Approach

099W70Z Drainage of Right Sphenoid Sinus with Drainage Device, Via Natural or Artificial Opening

099W7ZX Drainage of Right Sphenoid Sinus, Via Natural or Artificial Opening, Diagnostic

099W7ZZ Drainage of Right Sphenoid Sinus, Via Natural or Artificial Opening

099W80Z Drainage of Right Sphenoid Sinus with Drainage Device, Via Natural or Artificial Opening Endoscopic

099W8ZX Drainage of Right Sphenoid Sinus, Via Natural or Artificial Opening Endoscopic, Diagnostic

099W8ZZ Drainage of Right Sphenoid Sinus, Via Natural or Artificial Opening Endoscopic

099X00Z Drainage of Left Sphenoid Sinus with Drainage Device, Open Approach

099X0ZX Drainage of Left Sphenoid Sinus, Open Approach, Diagnostic

099X0ZZ Drainage of Left Sphenoid Sinus, Open Approach

099X30Z Drainage of Left Sphenoid Sinus with Drainage Device, Percutaneous Approach

099X3ZX Drainage of Left Sphenoid Sinus, Percutaneous Approach, Diagnostic

099X3ZZ Drainage of Left Sphenoid Sinus, Percutaneous Approach

099X40Z Drainage of Left Sphenoid Sinus with Drainage Device, Percutaneous Endoscopic Approach

099X4ZX Drainage of Left Sphenoid Sinus, Percutaneous Endoscopic Approach, Diagnostic

099X4ZZ Drainage of Left Sphenoid Sinus, Percutaneous Endoscopic Approach

099X70Z Drainage of Left Sphenoid Sinus with Drainage Device, Via Natural or Artificial Opening

099X7ZX Drainage of Left Sphenoid Sinus, Via Natural or Artificial Opening, Diagnostic

099X7ZZ Drainage of Left Sphenoid Sinus, Via Natural or Artificial Opening

099X80Z Drainage of Left Sphenoid Sinus with Drainage Device, Via Natural or Artificial Opening Endoscopic

099X8ZX Drainage of Left Sphenoid Sinus, Via Natural or Artificial Opening Endoscopic, Diagnostic

099X8ZZ Drainage of Left Sphenoid Sinus, Via Natural or Artificial Opening Endoscopic

09B – Ear, Nose, Sinus, Excision

Review Coding Guidelines B3.4a and B3.4b

Review Coding Guideline B3.8

Review Coding Guideline B3.18

09B00ZX Excision of Right External Ear, Open Approach, Diagnostic

09B00ZZ Excision of Right External Ear, Open Approach

09B03ZX Excision of Right External Ear, Percutaneous Approach, Diagnostic

09B03ZZ Excision of Right External Ear, Percutaneous Approach

09B04ZX Excision of Right External Ear, Percutaneous Endoscopic Approach, Diagnostic

09B04ZZ Excision of Right External Ear, Percutaneous Endoscopic Approach

09B0XZX Excision of Right External Ear, External Approach, Diagnostic

09B0XZZ Excision of Right External Ear, External Approach

09B10ZX Excision of Left External Ear, Open Approach, Diagnostic

09B10ZZ Excision of Left External Ear, Open Approach

09B13ZX Excision of Left External Ear, Percutaneous Approach, Diagnostic

09B13ZZ Excision of Left External Ear, Percutaneous Approach

09B14ZX Excision of Left External Ear, Percutaneous Endoscopic Approach, Diagnostic

09B14ZZ Excision of Left External Ear, Percutaneous Endoscopic Approach

09B1XZX Excision of Left External Ear, External Approach, Diagnostic

09B1XZZ Excision of Left External Ear, External Approach

09B30ZX Excision of Right External Auditory Canal, Open Approach, Diagnostic

09B30ZZ Excision of Right External Auditory Canal, Open Approach

09B33ZX Excision of Right External Auditory Canal, Percutaneous Approach, Diagnostic

09B33ZZ Excision of Right External Auditory Canal, Percutaneous Approach

09B34ZX Excision of Right External Auditory Canal, Percutaneous Endoscopic Approach, Diagnostic

09B34ZZ Excision of Right External Auditory Canal, Percutaneous Endoscopic Approach

09B37ZX Excision of Right External Auditory Canal, Via Natural or Artificial Opening, Diagnostic

09B37ZZ Excision of Right External Auditory Canal, Via Natural or Artificial Opening

09B38ZX Excision of Right External Auditory Canal, Via Natural or Artificial Opening Endoscopic, Diagnostic

09B38ZZ Excision of Right External Auditory Canal, Via Natural or Artificial Opening Endoscopic

09B3XZX Excision of Right External Auditory Canal, External Approach, Diagnostic

09B3XZZ Excision of Right External Auditory Canal, External Approach

09B40ZX Excision of Left External Auditory Canal, Open Approach, Diagnostic

09B40ZZ Excision of Left External Auditory Canal, Open Approach

09B43ZX Excision of Left External Auditory Canal, Percutaneous Approach, Diagnostic

09B43ZZ Excision of Left External Auditory Canal, Percutaneous Approach

09B44ZX Excision of Left External Auditory Canal, Percutaneous Endoscopic Approach, Diagnostic

09B44ZZ Excision of Left External Auditory Canal, Percutaneous Endoscopic Approach

09B47ZX Excision of Left External Auditory Canal, Via Natural or Artificial Opening, Diagnostic

09B47ZZ Excision of Left External Auditory Canal, Via Natural or Artificial Opening

09B48ZX Excision of Left External Auditory Canal, Via Natural or Artificial Opening Endoscopic, Diagnostic

09B48ZZ Excision of Left External Auditory Canal, Via Natural or Artificial Opening Endoscopic

09B4XZX Excision of Left External Auditory Canal, External Approach, Diagnostic

09B4XZZ Excision of Left External Auditory Canal, External Approach

09B50ZX Excision of Right Middle Ear, Open Approach, Diagnostic

09B50ZZ Excision of Right Middle Ear, Open Approach

09B58ZX Excision of Right Middle Ear, Via Natural or Artificial Opening Endoscopic, Diagnostic

09B58ZZ Excision of Right Middle Ear, Via Natural or Artificial Opening Endoscopic

09B60ZX Excision of Left Middle Ear, Open Approach, Diagnostic

09B60ZZ Excision of Left Middle Ear, Open Approach

09B68ZX Excision of Left Middle Ear, Via Natural or Artificial Opening Endoscopic, Diagnostic

09B68ZZ Excision of Left Middle Ear, Via Natural or Artificial Opening Endoscopic

09B70ZX Excision of Right Tympanic Membrane, Open Approach, Diagnostic

09B70ZZ Excision of Right Tympanic Membrane, Open Approach

09B73ZX Excision of Right Tympanic Membrane, Percutaneous Approach, Diagnostic

09B73ZZ Excision of Right Tympanic Membrane, Percutaneous Approach

09B74ZX Excision of Right Tympanic Membrane, Percutaneous Endoscopic Approach, Diagnostic

09B74ZZ Excision of Right Tympanic Membrane, Percutaneous Endoscopic Approach

09B77ZX Excision of Right Tympanic Membrane, Via Natural or Artificial Opening, Diagnostic

09B77ZZ Excision of Right Tympanic Membrane, Via Natural or Artificial Opening

09B78ZX Excision of Right Tympanic Membrane, Via Natural or Artificial Opening Endoscopic, Diagnostic

09B78ZZ Excision of Right Tympanic Membrane, Via Natural or Artificial Opening Endoscopic

09B80ZX Excision of Left Tympanic Membrane, Open Approach, Diagnostic

09B80ZZ Excision of Left Tympanic Membrane, Open Approach

09B83ZX Excision of Left Tympanic Membrane, Percutaneous Approach, Diagnostic

09B83ZZ Excision of Left Tympanic Membrane, Percutaneous Approach

09B84ZX Excision of Left Tympanic Membrane, Percutaneous Endoscopic Approach, Diagnostic

09B84ZZ Excision of Left Tympanic Membrane, Percutaneous Endoscopic Approach

09B87ZX Excision of Left Tympanic Membrane, Via Natural or Artificial Opening, Diagnostic

09B87ZZ Excision of Left Tympanic Membrane, Via Natural or Artificial Opening

09B88ZX Excision of Left Tympanic Membrane, Via Natural or Artificial Opening Endoscopic, Diagnostic

09B88ZZ Excision of Left Tympanic Membrane, Via Natural or Artificial Opening Endoscopic

09B90ZX Excision of Right Auditory Ossicle, Open Approach, Diagnostic

09B90ZZ Excision of Right Auditory Ossicle, Open Approach

09B98ZX Excision of Right Auditory Ossicle, Via Natural or Artificial Opening Endoscopic, Diagnostic

09B98ZZ Excision of Right Auditory Ossicle, Via Natural or Artificial Opening Endoscopic

09BA0ZX Excision of Left Auditory Ossicle, Open Approach, Diagnostic

09BA0ZZ Excision of Left Auditory Ossicle, Open Approach

09BA8ZX Excision of Left Auditory Ossicle, Via Natural or Artificial Opening Endoscopic, Diagnostic

09BA8ZZ Excision of Left Auditory Ossicle, Via Natural or Artificial Opening Endoscopic

09BB0ZX Excision of Right Mastoid Sinus, Open Approach, Diagnostic

09BB0ZZ Excision of Right Mastoid Sinus, Open Approach

09BB3ZX Excision of Right Mastoid Sinus, Percutaneous Approach, Diagnostic

09BB3ZZ Excision of Right Mastoid Sinus, Percutaneous Approach

09BB4ZX Excision of Right Mastoid Sinus, Percutaneous Endoscopic Approach, Diagnostic

09BB4ZZ Excision of Right Mastoid Sinus, Percutaneous Endoscopic Approach

09BB8ZX Excision of Right Mastoid Sinus, Via Natural or Artificial Opening Endoscopic, Diagnostic

♀ Female-only   ♂ Male-only   ▲ Limited Coverage   ● Non-OR   HAC HAC-associated procedure   ▲ Non-covered procedures   ✚ Cluster

09BB8ZZ Excision of Right Mastoid Sinus, Via Natural or Artificial Opening Endoscopic

09BC0ZX Excision of Left Mastoid Sinus, Open Approach, Diagnostic

09BC0ZZ Excision of Left Mastoid Sinus, Open Approach

09BC3ZX Excision of Left Mastoid Sinus, Percutaneous Approach, Diagnostic

09BC3ZZ Excision of Left Mastoid Sinus, Percutaneous Approach

09BC4ZX Excision of Left Mastoid Sinus, Percutaneous Endoscopic Approach, Diagnostic

09BC4ZZ Excision of Left Mastoid Sinus, Percutaneous Endoscopic Approach

09BC8ZX Excision of Left Mastoid Sinus, Via Natural or Artificial Opening Endoscopic, Diagnostic

09BC8ZZ Excision of Left Mastoid Sinus, Via Natural or Artificial Opening Endoscopic

09BD0ZX Excision of Right Inner Ear, Open Approach, Diagnostic

09BD0ZZ Excision of Right Inner Ear, Open Approach

09BD8ZX Excision of Right Inner Ear, Via Natural or Artificial Opening Endoscopic, Diagnostic

09BD8ZZ Excision of Right Inner Ear, Via Natural or Artificial Opening Endoscopic

09BE0ZX Excision of Left Inner Ear, Open Approach, Diagnostic

09BE0ZZ Excision of Left Inner Ear, Open Approach

09BE8ZX Excision of Left Inner Ear, Via Natural or Artificial Opening Endoscopic, Diagnostic

09BE8ZZ Excision of Left Inner Ear, Via Natural or Artificial Opening Endoscopic

09BF0ZX Excision of Right Eustachian Tube, Open Approach, Diagnostic

09BF0ZZ Excision of Right Eustachian Tube, Open Approach

09BF3ZX Excision of Right Eustachian Tube, Percutaneous Approach, Diagnostic

09BF3ZZ Excision of Right Eustachian Tube, Percutaneous Approach

09BF4ZX Excision of Right Eustachian Tube, Percutaneous Endoscopic Approach, Diagnostic

09BF4ZZ Excision of Right Eustachian Tube, Percutaneous Endoscopic Approach

09BF7ZX Excision of Right Eustachian Tube, Via Natural or Artificial Opening, Diagnostic

09BF7ZZ Excision of Right Eustachian Tube, Via Natural or Artificial Opening

09BF8ZX Excision of Right Eustachian Tube, Via Natural or Artificial Opening Endoscopic, Diagnostic

09BF8ZZ Excision of Right Eustachian Tube, Via Natural or Artificial Opening Endoscopic

09BG0ZX Excision of Left Eustachian Tube, Open Approach, Diagnostic

09BG0ZZ Excision of Left Eustachian Tube, Open Approach

09BG3ZX Excision of Left Eustachian Tube, Percutaneous Approach, Diagnostic

09BG3ZZ Excision of Left Eustachian Tube, Percutaneous Approach

09BG4ZX Excision of Left Eustachian Tube, Percutaneous Endoscopic Approach, Diagnostic

09BG4ZZ Excision of Left Eustachian Tube, Percutaneous Endoscopic Approach

09BG7ZX Excision of Left Eustachian Tube, Via Natural or Artificial Opening, Diagnostic

09BG7ZZ Excision of Left Eustachian Tube, Via Natural or Artificial Opening

09BG8ZX Excision of Left Eustachian Tube, Via Natural or Artificial Opening Endoscopic, Diagnostic

09BG8ZZ Excision of Left Eustachian Tube, Via Natural or Artificial Opening Endoscopic

09BK0ZX Excision of Nasal Mucosa and Soft Tissue, Open Approach, Diagnostic

09BK0ZZ Excision of Nasal Mucosa and Soft Tissue, Open Approach

09BK3ZX Excision of Nasal Mucosa and Soft Tissue, Percutaneous Approach, Diagnostic

09BK3ZZ Excision of Nasal Mucosa and Soft Tissue, Percutaneous Approach

09BK4ZX Excision of Nasal Mucosa and Soft Tissue, Percutaneous Endoscopic Approach, Diagnostic

09BK4ZZ Excision of Nasal Mucosa and Soft Tissue, Percutaneous Endoscopic Approach

09BK8ZX Excision of Nasal Mucosa and Soft Tissue, Via Natural or Artificial Opening Endoscopic, Diagnostic

09BK8ZZ Excision of Nasal Mucosa and Soft Tissue, Via Natural or Artificial Opening Endoscopic

09BKXZX Excision of Nasal Mucosa and Soft Tissue, External Approach, Diagnostic

09BKXZZ Excision of Nasal Mucosa and Soft Tissue, External Approach

09BL0ZX Excision of Nasal Turbinate, Open Approach, Diagnostic

09BL0ZZ Excision of Nasal Turbinate, Open Approach

09BL3ZX Excision of Nasal Turbinate, Percutaneous Approach, Diagnostic

09BL3ZZ Excision of Nasal Turbinate, Percutaneous Approach

09BL4ZX Excision of Nasal Turbinate, Percutaneous Endoscopic Approach, Diagnostic

09BL4ZZ Excision of Nasal Turbinate, Percutaneous Endoscopic Approach

09BL7ZX Excision of Nasal Turbinate, Via Natural or Artificial Opening, Diagnostic

09BL7ZZ Excision of Nasal Turbinate, Via Natural or Artificial Opening

09BL8ZX Excision of Nasal Turbinate, Via Natural or Artificial Opening Endoscopic, Diagnostic

09BL8ZZ Excision of Nasal Turbinate, Via Natural or Artificial Opening Endoscopic

09BM0ZX Excision of Nasal Septum, Open Approach, Diagnostic

09BM0ZZ Excision of Nasal Septum, Open Approach

09BM3ZX Excision of Nasal Septum, Percutaneous Approach, Diagnostic

09BM3ZZ Excision of Nasal Septum, Percutaneous Approach

09BM4ZX Excision of Nasal Septum, Percutaneous Endoscopic Approach, Diagnostic

09BM4ZZ Excision of Nasal Septum, Percutaneous Endoscopic Approach

09BM8ZX Excision of Nasal Septum, Via Natural or Artificial Opening Endoscopic, Diagnostic

09BM8ZZ Excision of Nasal Septum, Via Natural or Artificial Opening Endoscopic

09BN0ZX Excision of Nasopharynx, Open Approach, Diagnostic

09BN0ZZ Excision of Nasopharynx, Open Approach

09BN3ZX Excision of Nasopharynx, Percutaneous Approach, Diagnostic

09BN3ZZ Excision of Nasopharynx, Percutaneous Approach

09BN4ZX Excision of Nasopharynx, Percutaneous Endoscopic Approach, Diagnostic

09BN4ZZ Excision of Nasopharynx, Percutaneous Endoscopic Approach

09BN7ZX Excision of Nasopharynx, Via Natural or Artificial Opening, Diagnostic

09BN7ZZ Excision of Nasopharynx, Via Natural or Artificial Opening

09BN8ZX Excision of Nasopharynx, Via Natural or Artificial Opening Endoscopic, Diagnostic

09BN8ZZ Excision of Nasopharynx, Via Natural or Artificial Opening Endoscopic

09BP0ZX Excision of Accessory Sinus, Open Approach, Diagnostic

09BP0ZZ Excision of Accessory Sinus, Open Approach

09BP3ZX Excision of Accessory Sinus, Percutaneous Approach, Diagnostic

09BP3ZZ Excision of Accessory Sinus, Percutaneous Approach

09BP4ZX Excision of Accessory Sinus, Percutaneous Endoscopic Approach, Diagnostic

09BP4ZZ Excision of Accessory Sinus, Percutaneous Endoscopic Approach

09BP8ZX Excision of Accessory Sinus, Via Natural or Artificial Opening Endoscopic, Diagnostic

09BP8ZZ Excision of Accessory Sinus, Via Natural or Artificial Opening Endoscopic

09BQ0ZX Excision of Right Maxillary Sinus, Open Approach, Diagnostic

09BQ0ZZ Excision of Right Maxillary Sinus, Open Approach

09BQ3ZX Excision of Right Maxillary Sinus, Percutaneous Approach, Diagnostic

09BQ3ZZ Excision of Right Maxillary Sinus, Percutaneous Approach

09BQ4ZX Excision of Right Maxillary Sinus, Percutaneous Endoscopic Approach, Diagnostic

09BQ4ZZ Excision of Right Maxillary Sinus, Percutaneous Endoscopic Approach

09BQ8ZX Excision of Right Maxillary Sinus, Via Natural or Artificial Opening Endoscopic, Diagnostic

09BQ8ZZ Excision of Right Maxillary Sinus, Via Natural or Artificial Opening Endoscopic

09BR0ZX Excision of Left Maxillary Sinus, Open Approach, Diagnostic

09BR0ZZ Excision of Left Maxillary Sinus, Open Approach

09BR3ZX Excision of Left Maxillary Sinus, Percutaneous Approach, Diagnostic

09BR3ZZ Excision of Left Maxillary Sinus, Percutaneous Approach

09BR4ZX Excision of Left Maxillary Sinus, Percutaneous Endoscopic Approach, Diagnostic

09BR4ZZ Excision of Left Maxillary Sinus, Percutaneous Endoscopic Approach

09BR8ZX Excision of Left Maxillary Sinus, Via Natural or Artificial Opening Endoscopic, Diagnostic

09BR8ZZ Excision of Left Maxillary Sinus, Via Natural or Artificial Opening Endoscopic

09BS0ZX Excision of Right Frontal Sinus, Open Approach, Diagnostic

09BS0ZZ Excision of Right Frontal Sinus, Open Approach

09BS3ZX Excision of Right Frontal Sinus, Percutaneous Approach, Diagnostic

09BS3ZZ Excision of Right Frontal Sinus, Percutaneous Approach

09BS4ZX Excision of Right Frontal Sinus, Percutaneous Endoscopic Approach, Diagnostic

09BS4ZZ Excision of Right Frontal Sinus, Percutaneous Endoscopic Approach

09BS8ZX Excision of Right Frontal Sinus, Via Natural or Artificial Opening Endoscopic, Diagnostic

09BS8ZZ Excision of Right Frontal Sinus, Via Natural or Artificial Opening Endoscopic

9BT0ZX Excision of Left Frontal Sinus, Open Approach, Diagnostic

09BT0ZZ Excision of Left Frontal Sinus, Open Approach

09BT3ZX Excision of Left Frontal Sinus, Percutaneous Approach, Diagnostic

09BT3ZZ Excision of Left Frontal Sinus, Percutaneous Approach

09BT4ZX Excision of Left Frontal Sinus, Percutaneous Endoscopic Approach, Diagnostic

09BT4ZZ Excision of Left Frontal Sinus, Percutaneous Endoscopic Approach

09BT8ZX Excision of Left Frontal Sinus, Via Natural or Artificial Opening Endoscopic, Diagnostic

09BT8ZZ Excision of Left Frontal Sinus, Via Natural or Artificial Opening Endoscopic

09BU0ZX Excision of Right Ethmoid Sinus, Open Approach, Diagnostic

09BU0ZZ Excision of Right Ethmoid Sinus, Open Approach

09BU3ZX Excision of Right Ethmoid Sinus, Percutaneous Approach, Diagnostic

09BU3ZZ Excision of Right Ethmoid Sinus, Percutaneous Approach

09BU4ZX Excision of Right Ethmoid Sinus, Percutaneous Endoscopic Approach, Diagnostic

09BU4ZZ Excision of Right Ethmoid Sinus, Percutaneous Endoscopic Approach

09BU8ZX Excision of Right Ethmoid Sinus, Via Natural or Artificial Opening Endoscopic, Diagnostic

09BU8ZZ Excision of Right Ethmoid Sinus, Via Natural or Artificial Opening Endoscopic

09BV0ZX Excision of Left Ethmoid Sinus, Open Approach, Diagnostic

09BV0ZZ Excision of Left Ethmoid Sinus, Open Approach

09BV3ZX Excision of Left Ethmoid Sinus, Percutaneous Approach, Diagnostic

09BV3ZZ Excision of Left Ethmoid Sinus, Percutaneous Approach

09BV4ZX Excision of Left Ethmoid Sinus, Percutaneous Endoscopic Approach, Diagnostic

09BV4ZZ Excision of Left Ethmoid Sinus, Percutaneous Endoscopic Approach

09BV8ZX Excision of Left Ethmoid Sinus, Via Natural or Artificial Opening Endoscopic, Diagnostic

09BV8ZZ Excision of Left Ethmoid Sinus, Via Natural or Artificial Opening Endoscopic

09BW0ZX Excision of Right Sphenoid Sinus, Open Approach, Diagnostic

09BW0ZZ Excision of Right Sphenoid Sinus, Open Approach

09BW3ZX Excision of Right Sphenoid Sinus, Percutaneous Approach, Diagnostic

09BW3ZZ Excision of Right Sphenoid Sinus, Percutaneous Approach

09BW4ZX Excision of Right Sphenoid Sinus, Percutaneous Endoscopic Approach, Diagnostic

09BW4ZZ Excision of Right Sphenoid Sinus, Percutaneous Endoscopic Approach

09BW8ZX Excision of Right Sphenoid Sinus, Via Natural or Artificial Opening Endoscopic, Diagnostic

09BW8ZZ Excision of Right Sphenoid Sinus, Via Natural or Artificial Opening Endoscopic

09BX0ZX Excision of Left Sphenoid Sinus, Open Approach, Diagnostic

09BX0ZZ Excision of Left Sphenoid Sinus, Open Approach

09BX3ZX Excision of Left Sphenoid Sinus, Percutaneous Approach, Diagnostic

09BX3ZZ Excision of Left Sphenoid Sinus, Percutaneous Approach

09BX4ZX Excision of Left Sphenoid Sinus, Percutaneous Endoscopic Approach, Diagnostic

09BX4ZZ Excision of Left Sphenoid Sinus, Percutaneous Endoscopic Approach

09BX8ZX Excision of Left Sphenoid Sinus, Via Natural or Artificial Opening Endoscopic, Diagnostic

09BX8ZZ Excision of Left Sphenoid Sinus, Via Natural or Artificial Opening Endoscopic

09C – Ear, Nose, Sinus, Extirpation

09C00ZZ Extirpation of Matter from Right External Ear, Open Approach

09C03ZZ Extirpation of Matter from Right External Ear, Percutaneous Approach

09C04ZZ Extirpation of Matter from Right External Ear, Percutaneous Endoscopic Approach

09C0XZZ Extirpation of Matter from Right External Ear, External Approach

09C10ZZ Extirpation of Matter from Left External Ear, Open Approach

09C13ZZ Extirpation of Matter from Left External Ear, Percutaneous Approach

09C14ZZ Extirpation of Matter from Left External Ear, Percutaneous Endoscopic Approach

09C1XZZ Extirpation of Matter from Left External Ear, External Approach

09C30ZZ Extirpation of Matter from Right External Auditory Canal, Open Approach

09C33ZZ Extirpation of Matter from Right External Auditory Canal, Percutaneous Approach

09C34ZZ Extirpation of Matter from Right External Auditory Canal, Percutaneous Endoscopic Approach

09C37ZZ Extirpation of Matter from Right External Auditory Canal, Via Natural or Artificial Opening

09C38ZZ Extirpation of Matter from Right External Auditory Canal, Via Natural or Artificial Opening Endoscopic

09C3XZZ Extirpation of Matter from Right External Auditory Canal, External Approach

09C40ZZ Extirpation of Matter from Left External Auditory Canal, Open Approach

09C43ZZ Extirpation of Matter from Left External Auditory Canal, Percutaneous Approach

09C44ZZ Extirpation of Matter from Left External Auditory Canal, Percutaneous Endoscopic Approach

09C47ZZ Extirpation of Matter from Left External Auditory Canal, Via Natural or Artificial Opening

09C48ZZ Extirpation of Matter from Left External Auditory Canal, Via Natural or Artificial Opening Endoscopic

09C4XZZ Extirpation of Matter from Left External Auditory Canal, External Approach

09C50ZZ Extirpation of Matter from Right Middle Ear, Open Approach

09C58ZZ Extirpation of Matter from Right Middle Ear, Via Natural or Artificial Opening Endoscopic

09C60ZZ Extirpation of Matter from Left Middle Ear, Open Approach

09C68ZZ Extirpation of Matter from Left Middle Ear, Via Natural or Artificial Opening Endoscopic

09C70ZZ Extirpation of Matter from Right Tympanic Membrane, Open Approach

09C73ZZ Extirpation of Matter from Right Tympanic Membrane, Percutaneous Approach

09C74ZZ Extirpation of Matter from Right Tympanic Membrane, Percutaneous Endoscopic Approach

09C77ZZ Extirpation of Matter from Right Tympanic Membrane, Via Natural or Artificial Opening

09C78ZZ Extirpation of Matter from Right Tympanic Membrane, Via Natural or Artificial Opening Endoscopic

09C80ZZ Extirpation of Matter from Left Tympanic Membrane, Open Approach

09C83ZZ Extirpation of Matter from Left Tympanic Membrane, Percutaneous Approach

09C84ZZ Extirpation of Matter from Left Tympanic Membrane, Percutaneous Endoscopic Approach

09C87ZZ Extirpation of Matter from Left Tympanic Membrane, Via Natural or Artificial Opening

09C88ZZ Extirpation of Matter from Left Tympanic Membrane, Via Natural or Artificial Opening Endoscopic

♀ Female-only   ♂ Male-only   ▲ Limited Coverage   ● Non-OR   ▦ HAC-associated procedure   ▲ Non-covered procedures   ✚ Cluster

09C90ZZ Extirpation of Matter from Right Auditory Ossicle, Open Approach

09C98ZZ Extirpation of Matter from Right Auditory Ossicle, Via Natural or Artificial Opening Endoscopic

09CA0ZZ Extirpation of Matter from Left Auditory Ossicle, Open Approach

09CA8ZZ Extirpation of Matter from Left Auditory Ossicle, Via Natural or Artificial Opening Endoscopic

09CB0ZZ Extirpation of Matter from Right Mastoid Sinus, Open Approach

09CB3ZZ Extirpation of Matter from Right Mastoid Sinus, Percutaneous Approach

09CB4ZZ Extirpation of Matter from Right Mastoid Sinus, Percutaneous Endoscopic Approach

09CB8ZZ Extirpation of Matter from Right Mastoid Sinus, Via Natural or Artificial Opening Endoscopic

09CC0ZZ Extirpation of Matter from Left Mastoid Sinus, Open Approach

09CC3ZZ Extirpation of Matter from Left Mastoid Sinus, Percutaneous Approach

09CC4ZZ Extirpation of Matter from Left Mastoid Sinus, Percutaneous Endoscopic Approach

09CC8ZZ Extirpation of Matter from Left Mastoid Sinus, Via Natural or Artificial Opening Endoscopic

09CD0ZZ Extirpation of Matter from Right Inner Ear, Open Approach

09CD8ZZ Extirpation of Matter from Right Inner Ear, Via Natural or Artificial Opening Endoscopic

09CE0ZZ Extirpation of Matter from Left Inner Ear, Open Approach

09CE8ZZ Extirpation of Matter from Left Inner Ear, Via Natural or Artificial Opening Endoscopic

09CF0ZZ Extirpation of Matter from Right Eustachian Tube, Open Approach

09CF3ZZ Extirpation of Matter from Right Eustachian Tube, Percutaneous Approach

09CF4ZZ Extirpation of Matter from Right Eustachian Tube, Percutaneous Endoscopic Approach

09CF7ZZ Extirpation of Matter from Right Eustachian Tube, Via Natural or Artificial Opening

09CF8ZZ Extirpation of Matter from Right Eustachian Tube, Via Natural or Artificial Opening Endoscopic

09CG0ZZ Extirpation of Matter from Left Eustachian Tube, Open Approach

09CG3ZZ Extirpation of Matter from Left Eustachian Tube, Percutaneous Approach

09CG4ZZ Extirpation of Matter from Left Eustachian Tube, Percutaneous Endoscopic Approach

09CG7ZZ Extirpation of Matter from Left Eustachian Tube, Via Natural or Artificial Opening

09CG8ZZ Extirpation of Matter from Left Eustachian Tube, Via Natural or Artificial Opening Endoscopic

09CK0ZZ Extirpation of Matter from Nasal Mucosa and Soft Tissue, Open Approach

09CK3ZZ Extirpation of Matter from Nasal Mucosa and Soft Tissue, Percutaneous Approach

09CK4ZZ Extirpation of Matter from Nasal Mucosa and Soft Tissue, Percutaneous Endoscopic Approach

09CK8ZZ Extirpation of Matter from Nasal Mucosa and Soft Tissue, Via Natural or Artificial Opening Endoscopic

09CKXZZ Extirpation of Matter from Nasal Mucosa and Soft Tissue, External Approach

09CL0ZZ Extirpation of Matter from Nasal Turbinate, Open Approach

09CL3ZZ Extirpation of Matter from Nasal Turbinate, Percutaneous Approach

09CL4ZZ Extirpation of Matter from Nasal Turbinate, Percutaneous Endoscopic Approach

09CL7ZZ Extirpation of Matter from Nasal Turbinate, Via Natural or Artificial Opening

09CL8ZZ Extirpation of Matter from Nasal Turbinate, Via Natural or Artificial Opening Endoscopic

09CM0ZZ Extirpation of Matter from Nasal Septum, Open Approach

09CM3ZZ Extirpation of Matter from Nasal Septum, Percutaneous Approach

09CM4ZZ Extirpation of Matter from Nasal Septum, Percutaneous Endoscopic Approach

09CM8ZZ Extirpation of Matter from Nasal Septum, Via Natural or Artificial Opening Endoscopic

09CN0ZZ Extirpation of Matter from Nasopharynx, Open Approach

09CN3ZZ Extirpation of Matter from Nasopharynx, Percutaneous Approach

09CN4ZZ Extirpation of Matter from Nasopharynx, Percutaneous Endoscopic Approach

09CN7ZZ Extirpation of Matter from Nasopharynx, Via Natural or Artificial Opening

09CN8ZZ Extirpation of Matter from Nasopharynx, Via Natural or Artificial Opening Endoscopic

09CP0ZZ Extirpation of Matter from Accessory Sinus, Open Approach

09CP3ZZ Extirpation of Matter from Accessory Sinus, Percutaneous Approach

09CP4ZZ Extirpation of Matter from Accessory Sinus, Percutaneous Endoscopic Approach

09CP8ZZ Extirpation of Matter from Accessory Sinus, Via Natural or Artificial Opening Endoscopic

09CQ0ZZ Extirpation of Matter from Right Maxillary Sinus, Open Approach

09CQ3ZZ Extirpation of Matter from Right Maxillary Sinus, Percutaneous Approach

09CQ4ZZ Extirpation of Matter from Right Maxillary Sinus, Percutaneous Endoscopic Approach

09CQ8ZZ Extirpation of Matter from Right Maxillary Sinus, Via Natural or Artificial Opening Endoscopic

09CR0ZZ Extirpation of Matter from Left Maxillary Sinus, Open Approach

09CR3ZZ Extirpation of Matter from Left Maxillary Sinus, Percutaneous Approach

09CR4ZZ Extirpation of Matter from Left Maxillary Sinus, Percutaneous Endoscopic Approach

09CR8ZZ Extirpation of Matter from Left Maxillary Sinus, Via Natural or Artificial Opening Endoscopic

09CS0ZZ Extirpation of Matter from Right Frontal Sinus, Open Approach

09CS3ZZ Extirpation of Matter from Right Frontal Sinus, Percutaneous Approach

09CS4ZZ Extirpation of Matter from Right Frontal Sinus, Percutaneous Endoscopic Approach

09CS8ZZ Extirpation of Matter from Right Frontal Sinus, Via Natural or Artificial Opening Endoscopic

09CT0ZZ Extirpation of Matter from Left Frontal Sinus, Open Approach

09CT3ZZ Extirpation of Matter from Left Frontal Sinus, Percutaneous Approach

09CT4ZZ Extirpation of Matter from Left Frontal Sinus, Percutaneous Endoscopic Approach

09CT8ZZ Extirpation of Matter from Left Frontal Sinus, Via Natural or Artificial Opening Endoscopic

09CU0ZZ Extirpation of Matter from Right Ethmoid Sinus, Open Approach

09CU3ZZ Extirpation of Matter from Right Ethmoid Sinus, Percutaneous Approach

09CU4ZZ Extirpation of Matter from Right Ethmoid Sinus, Percutaneous Endoscopic Approach

09CU8ZZ Extirpation of Matter from Right Ethmoid Sinus, Via Natural or Artificial Opening Endoscopic

09CV0ZZ Extirpation of Matter from Left Ethmoid Sinus, Open Approach

09CV3ZZ Extirpation of Matter from Left Ethmoid Sinus, Percutaneous Approach

09CV4ZZ Extirpation of Matter from Left Ethmoid Sinus, Percutaneous Endoscopic Approach

09CV8ZZ Extirpation of Matter from Left Ethmoid Sinus, Via Natural or Artificial Opening Endoscopic

09CW0ZZ Extirpation of Matter from Right Sphenoid Sinus, Open Approach

09CW3ZZ Extirpation of Matter from Right Sphenoid Sinus, Percutaneous Approach

09CW4ZZ Extirpation of Matter from Right Sphenoid Sinus, Percutaneous Endoscopic Approach

09CW8ZZ Extirpation of Matter from Right Sphenoid Sinus, Via Natural or Artificial Opening Endoscopic

09CX0ZZ Extirpation of Matter from Left Sphenoid Sinus, Open Approach

09CX3ZZ Extirpation of Matter from Left Sphenoid Sinus, Percutaneous Approach

09CX4ZZ Extirpation of Matter from Left Sphenoid Sinus, Percutaneous Endoscopic Approach

09CX8ZZ Extirpation of Matter from Left Sphenoid Sinus, Via Natural or Artificial Opening Endoscopic

09D – Ear, Nose, Sinus, Extraction

09D70ZZ Extraction of Right Tympanic Membrane, Open Approach

09D73ZZ Extraction of Right Tympanic Membrane, Percutaneous Approach

---

♀ Female-only   ♂ Male-only   ▲ Limited Coverage   ● Non-OR   🅷🅰🅲 HAC-associated procedure   ▲ Non-covered procedures   ➕ Cluster

09D74ZZ	Extraction of Right Tympanic Membrane, Percutaneous Endoscopic Approach	09DC4ZZ	Extraction of Left Mastoid Sinus, Percutaneous Endoscopic Approach	09DS0ZZ	Extraction of Right Frontal Sinus, Open Approach
09D77ZZ	Extraction of Right Tympanic Membrane, Via Natural or Artificial Opening	09DL0ZZ	Extraction of Nasal Turbinate, Open Approach	09DS3ZZ	Extraction of Right Frontal Sinus, Percutaneous Approach
09D78ZZ	Extraction of Right Tympanic Membrane, Via Natural or Artificial Opening Endoscopic	09DL3ZZ	Extraction of Nasal Turbinate, Percutaneous Approach	09DS4ZZ	Extraction of Right Frontal Sinus, Percutaneous Endoscopic Approach
09D80ZZ	Extraction of Left Tympanic Membrane, Open Approach	09DL4ZZ	Extraction of Nasal Turbinate, Percutaneous Endoscopic Approach	09DT0ZZ	Extraction of Left Frontal Sinus, Open Approach
09D83ZZ	Extraction of Left Tympanic Membrane, Percutaneous Approach	09DL7ZZ	Extraction of Nasal Turbinate, Via Natural or Artificial Opening	09DT3ZZ	Extraction of Left Frontal Sinus, Percutaneous Approach
09D84ZZ	Extraction of Left Tympanic Membrane, Percutaneous Endoscopic Approach	09DL8ZZ	Extraction of Nasal Turbinate, Via Natural or Artificial Opening Endoscopic	09DT4ZZ	Extraction of Left Frontal Sinus, Percutaneous Endoscopic Approach
09D87ZZ	Extraction of Left Tympanic Membrane, Via Natural or Artificial Opening	09DM0ZZ	Extraction of Nasal Septum, Open Approach	09DU0ZZ	Extraction of Right Ethmoid Sinus, Open Approach
09D88ZZ	Extraction of Left Tympanic Membrane, Via Natural or Artificial Opening Endoscopic	09DM3ZZ	Extraction of Nasal Septum, Percutaneous Approach	09DU3ZZ	Extraction of Right Ethmoid Sinus, Percutaneous Approach
09D90ZZ	Extraction of Right Auditory Ossicle, Open Approach	09DM4ZZ	Extraction of Nasal Septum, Percutaneous Endoscopic Approach	09DU4ZZ	Extraction of Right Ethmoid Sinus, Percutaneous Endoscopic Approach
09DA0ZZ	Extraction of Left Auditory Ossicle, Open Approach	09DP0ZZ	Extraction of Accessory Sinus, Open Approach	09DV0ZZ	Extraction of Left Ethmoid Sinus, Open Approach
09DB0ZZ	Extraction of Right Mastoid Sinus, Open Approach	09DP3ZZ	Extraction of Accessory Sinus, Percutaneous Approach	09DV3ZZ	Extraction of Left Ethmoid Sinus, Percutaneous Approach
09DB3ZZ	Extraction of Right Mastoid Sinus, Percutaneous Approach	09DP4ZZ	Extraction of Accessory Sinus, Percutaneous Endoscopic Approach	09DV4ZZ	Extraction of Left Ethmoid Sinus, Percutaneous Endoscopic Approach
09DB4ZZ	Extraction of Right Mastoid Sinus, Percutaneous Endoscopic Approach	09DQ0ZZ	Extraction of Right Maxillary Sinus, Open Approach	09DW0ZZ	Extraction of Right Sphenoid Sinus, Open Approach
09DC0ZZ	Extraction of Left Mastoid Sinus, Open Approach	09DQ3ZZ	Extraction of Right Maxillary Sinus, Percutaneous Approach	09DW3ZZ	Extraction of Right Sphenoid Sinus, Percutaneous Approach
09DC3ZZ	Extraction of Left Mastoid Sinus, Percutaneous Approach	09DQ4ZZ	Extraction of Right Maxillary Sinus, Percutaneous Endoscopic Approach	09DW4ZZ	Extraction of Right Sphenoid Sinus, Percutaneous Endoscopic Approach
		09DR0ZZ	Extraction of Left Maxillary Sinus, Open Approach	09DX0ZZ	Extraction of Left Sphenoid Sinus, Open Approach
		09DR3ZZ	Extraction of Left Maxillary Sinus, Percutaneous Approach	09DX3ZZ	Extraction of Left Sphenoid Sinus, Percutaneous Approach
		09DR4ZZ	Extraction of Left Maxillary Sinus, Percutaneous Endoscopic Approach	09DX4ZZ	Extraction of Left Sphenoid Sinus, Percutaneous Endoscopic Approach

09H – Ear, Nose, Sinus, Insertion

09HD01Z	Insertion of Radioactive Element into Right Inner Ear, Open Approach	09HD46Z	Insertion of Multiple Channel Cochlear Prosthesis into Right Inner Ear, Percutaneous Endoscopic Approach	09HE44Z	Insertion of Bone Conduction Hearing Device into Left Inner Ear, Percutaneous Endoscopic Approach
09HD04Z	Insertion of Bone Conduction Hearing Device into Right Inner Ear, Open Approach	09HD4SZ	Insertion of Hearing Device into Right Inner Ear, Percutaneous Endoscopic Approach	09HE45Z	Insertion of Single Channel Cochlear Prosthesis into Left Inner Ear, Percutaneous Endoscopic Approach
09HD05Z	Insertion of Single Channel Cochlear Prosthesis into Right Inner Ear, Open Approach	09HE01Z	Insertion of Radioactive Element into Left Inner Ear, Open Approach	09HE46Z	Insertion of Multiple Channel Cochlear Prosthesis into Left Inner Ear, Percutaneous Endoscopic Approach
09HD06Z	Insertion of Multiple Channel Cochlear Prosthesis into Right Inner Ear, Open Approach	09HE04Z	Insertion of Bone Conduction Hearing Device into Left Inner Ear, Open Approach	09HE4SZ	Insertion of Hearing Device into Left Inner Ear, Percutaneous Endoscopic Approach
09HD0SZ	Insertion of Hearing Device into Right Inner Ear, Open Approach	09HE05Z	Insertion of Single Channel Cochlear Prosthesis into Left Inner Ear, Open Approach	09HH01Z	Insertion of Radioactive Element into Right Ear, Open Approach
09HD31Z	Insertion of Radioactive Element into Right Inner Ear, Percutaneous Approach	09HE06Z	Insertion of Multiple Channel Cochlear Prosthesis into Left Inner Ear, Open Approach	09HH0YZ	Insertion of Other Device into Right Ear, Open Approach
09HD34Z	Insertion of Bone Conduction Hearing Device into Right Inner Ear, Percutaneous Approach	09HE0SZ	Insertion of Hearing Device into Left Inner Ear, Open Approach	09HH31Z	Insertion of Radioactive Element into Right Ear, Percutaneous Approach
09HD35Z	Insertion of Single Channel Cochlear Prosthesis into Right Inner Ear, Percutaneous Approach	09HE31Z	Insertion of Radioactive Element into Left Inner Ear, Percutaneous Approach	09HH3YZ	Insertion of Other Device into Right Ear, Percutaneous Approach
09HD36Z	Insertion of Multiple Channel Cochlear Prosthesis into Right Inner Ear, Percutaneous Approach	09HE34Z	Insertion of Bone Conduction Hearing Device into Left Inner Ear, Percutaneous Approach	09HH41Z	Insertion of Radioactive Element into Right Ear, Percutaneous Endoscopic Approach
09HD3SZ	Insertion of Hearing Device into Right Inner Ear, Percutaneous Approach	09HE35Z	Insertion of Single Channel Cochlear Prosthesis into Left Inner Ear, Percutaneous Approach	09HH4YZ	Insertion of Other Device into Right Ear, Percutaneous Endoscopic Approach
09HD41Z	Insertion of Radioactive Element into Right Inner Ear, Percutaneous Endoscopic Approach	09HE36Z	Insertion of Multiple Channel Cochlear Prosthesis into Left Inner Ear, Percutaneous Approach	09HH71Z	Insertion of Radioactive Element into Right Ear, Via Natural or Artificial Opening
09HD44Z	Insertion of Bone Conduction Hearing Device into Right Inner Ear, Percutaneous Endoscopic Approach	09HE3SZ	Insertion of Hearing Device into Left Inner Ear, Percutaneous Approach	09HH7YZ	Insertion of Other Device into Right Ear, Via Natural or Artificial Opening
09HD45Z	Insertion of Single Channel Cochlear Prosthesis into Right Inner Ear, Percutaneous Endoscopic Approach	09HE41Z	Insertion of Radioactive Element into Left Inner Ear, Percutaneous Endoscopic Approach	09HH81Z	Insertion of Radioactive Element into Right Ear, Via Natural or Artificial Opening Endoscopic
				09HH8YZ	Insertion of Other Device into Right Ear, Via Natural or Artificial Opening Endoscopic

♀ Female-only   ♂ Male-only   ▲ Limited Coverage   ● Non-OR   ⬛ HAC-associated procedure   ▲ Non-covered procedures   ✚ Cluster

09HJ01Z Insertion of Radioactive Element into Left Ear, Open Approach

09HJ0YZ Insertion of Other Device into Left Ear, Open Approach

09HJ31Z Insertion of Radioactive Element into Left Ear, Percutaneous Approach

09HJ3YZ Insertion of Other Device into Left Ear, Percutaneous Approach

09HJ41Z Insertion of Radioactive Element into Left Ear, Percutaneous Endoscopic Approach

09HJ4YZ Insertion of Other Device into Left Ear, Percutaneous Endoscopic Approach

09HJ71Z Insertion of Radioactive Element into Left Ear, Via Natural or Artificial Opening

09HJ7YZ Insertion of Other Device into Left Ear, Via Natural or Artificial Opening

09HJ81Z Insertion of Radioactive Element into Left Ear, Via Natural or Artificial Opening Endoscopic

09HJ8YZ Insertion of Other Device into Left Ear, Via Natural or Artificial Opening Endoscopic

09HK01Z Insertion of Radioactive Element into Nasal Mucosa and Soft Tissue, Open Approach

09HK0YZ Insertion of Other Device into Nasal Mucosa and Soft Tissue, Open Approach

09HK31Z Insertion of Radioactive Element into Nasal Mucosa and Soft Tissue, Percutaneous Approach

09HK3YZ Insertion of Other Device into Nasal Mucosa and Soft Tissue, Percutaneous Approach

09HK41Z Insertion of Radioactive Element into Nasal Mucosa and Soft Tissue, Percutaneous Endoscopic Approach

09HK4YZ Insertion of Other Device into Nasal Mucosa and Soft Tissue, Percutaneous Endoscopic Approach

09HK71Z Insertion of Radioactive Element into Nasal Mucosa and Soft Tissue, Via Natural or Artificial Opening

09HK7YZ Insertion of Other Device into Nasal Mucosa and Soft Tissue, Via Natural or Artificial Opening

09HK81Z Insertion of Radioactive Element into Nasal Mucosa and Soft Tissue, Via Natural or Artificial Opening Endoscopic

09HK8YZ Insertion of Other Device into Nasal Mucosa and Soft Tissue, Via Natural or Artificial Opening Endoscopic

09HN71Z Insertion of Radioactive Element into Nasopharynx, Via Natural or Artificial Opening

09HN7BZ Insertion of Airway into Nasopharynx, Via Natural or Artificial Opening

09HN81Z Insertion of Radioactive Element into Nasopharynx, Via Natural or Artificial Opening Endoscopic

09HN8BZ Insertion of Airway into Nasopharynx, Via Natural or Artificial Opening Endoscopic

09HY01Z Insertion of Radioactive Element into Sinus, Open Approach

09HY0YZ Insertion of Other Device into Sinus, Open Approach

09HY31Z Insertion of Radioactive Element into Sinus, Percutaneous Approach

09HY3YZ Insertion of Other Device into Sinus, Percutaneous Approach

09HY41Z Insertion of Radioactive Element into Sinus, Percutaneous Endoscopic Approach

09HY4YZ Insertion of Other Device into Sinus, Percutaneous Endoscopic Approach

09HY71Z Insertion of Radioactive Element into Sinus, Via Natural or Artificial Opening

09HY7YZ Insertion of Other Device into Sinus, Via Natural or Artificial Opening

09HY81Z Insertion of Radioactive Element into Sinus, Via Natural or Artificial Opening Endoscopic

09HY8YZ Insertion of Other Device into Sinus, Via Natural or Artificial Opening Endoscopic

09J – Ear, Nose, Sinus, Inspection

Review Coding Guidelines B3.11a, B3.11b and B3.11c

09J70ZZ Inspection of Right Tympanic Membrane, Open Approach

09J73ZZ Inspection of Right Tympanic Membrane, Percutaneous Approach

09J74ZZ Inspection of Right Tympanic Membrane, Percutaneous Endoscopic Approach

09J77ZZ Inspection of Right Tympanic Membrane, Via Natural or Artificial Opening

09J78ZZ Inspection of Right Tympanic Membrane, Via Natural or Artificial Opening Endoscopic

09J7XZZ Inspection of Right Tympanic Membrane, External Approach

09J80ZZ Inspection of Left Tympanic Membrane, Open Approach

09J83ZZ Inspection of Left Tympanic Membrane, Percutaneous Approach

09J84ZZ Inspection of Left Tympanic Membrane, Percutaneous Endoscopic Approach

09J87ZZ Inspection of Left Tympanic Membrane, Via Natural or Artificial Opening

09J88ZZ Inspection of Left Tympanic Membrane, Via Natural or Artificial Opening Endoscopic

09J8XZZ Inspection of Left Tympanic Membrane, External Approach

09JD0ZZ Inspection of Right Inner Ear, Open Approach

09JD3ZZ Inspection of Right Inner Ear, Percutaneous Approach

09JD4ZZ Inspection of Right Inner Ear, Percutaneous Endoscopic Approach

09JD8ZZ Inspection of Right Inner Ear, Via Natural or Artificial Opening Endoscopic

09JDXZZ Inspection of Right Inner Ear, External Approach

09JE0ZZ Inspection of Left Inner Ear, Open Approach

09JE3ZZ Inspection of Left Inner Ear, Percutaneous Approach

09JE4ZZ Inspection of Left Inner Ear, Percutaneous Endoscopic Approach

09JE8ZZ Inspection of Left Inner Ear, Via Natural or Artificial Opening Endoscopic

09JEXZZ Inspection of Left Inner Ear, External Approach

09JH0ZZ Inspection of Right Ear, Open Approach

09JH3ZZ Inspection of Right Ear, Percutaneous Approach

09JH4ZZ Inspection of Right Ear, Percutaneous Endoscopic Approach

09JH7ZZ Inspection of Right Ear, Via Natural or Artificial Opening

09JH8ZZ Inspection of Right Ear, Via Natural or Artificial Opening Endoscopic

09JHXZZ Inspection of Right Ear, External Approach

09JJ0ZZ Inspection of Left Ear, Open Approach

09JJ3ZZ Inspection of Left Ear, Percutaneous Approach

09JJ4ZZ Inspection of Left Ear, Percutaneous Endoscopic Approach

09JJ7ZZ Inspection of Left Ear, Via Natural or Artificial Opening

09JJ8ZZ Inspection of Left Ear, Via Natural or Artificial Opening Endoscopic

09JJXZZ Inspection of Left Ear, External Approach

09JK0ZZ Inspection of Nasal Mucosa and Soft Tissue, Open Approach

09JK3ZZ Inspection of Nasal Mucosa and Soft Tissue, Percutaneous Approach

09JK4ZZ Inspection of Nasal Mucosa and Soft Tissue, Percutaneous Endoscopic Approach

09JK8ZZ Inspection of Nasal Mucosa and Soft Tissue, Via Natural or Artificial Opening Endoscopic

09JKXZZ Inspection of Nasal Mucosa and Soft Tissue, External Approach

09JY0ZZ Inspection of Sinus, Open Approach

09JY3ZZ Inspection of Sinus, Percutaneous Approach

09JY4ZZ Inspection of Sinus, Percutaneous Endoscopic Approach

09JY8ZZ Inspection of Sinus, Via Natural or Artificial Opening Endoscopic

09JYXZZ Inspection of Sinus, External Approach

09M – Ear, Nose, Sinus, Reattachment

09M0XZZ Reattachment of Right External Ear, External Approach

09M1XZZ Reattachment of Left External Ear, External Approach

09MKXZZ Reattachment of Nasal Mucosa and Soft Tissue, External Approach

♀ Female-only   ♂ Male-only   ▲ Limited Coverage   ● Non-OR   HAC HAC-associated procedure   ▲ Non-covered procedures   ✚ Cluster

09N – Ear, Nose, Sinus, Release

Review Coding Guidelines B3.13 and B3.14

09N00ZZ	Release Right External Ear, Open Approach
09N03ZZ	Release Right External Ear, Percutaneous Approach
09N04ZZ	Release Right External Ear, Percutaneous Endoscopic Approach
09N0XZZ	Release Right External Ear, External Approach
09N10ZZ	Release Left External Ear, Open Approach
09N13ZZ	Release Left External Ear, Percutaneous Approach
09N14ZZ	Release Left External Ear, Percutaneous Endoscopic Approach
09N1XZZ	Release Left External Ear, External Approach
09N30ZZ	Release Right External Auditory Canal, Open Approach
09N33ZZ	Release Right External Auditory Canal, Percutaneous Approach
09N34ZZ	Release Right External Auditory Canal, Percutaneous Endoscopic Approach
09N37ZZ	Release Right External Auditory Canal, Via Natural or Artificial Opening
09N38ZZ	Release Right External Auditory Canal, Via Natural or Artificial Opening Endoscopic
09N3XZZ	Release Right External Auditory Canal, External Approach
09N40ZZ	Release Left External Auditory Canal, Open Approach
09N43ZZ	Release Left External Auditory Canal, Percutaneous Approach
09N44ZZ	Release Left External Auditory Canal, Percutaneous Endoscopic Approach
09N47ZZ	Release Left External Auditory Canal, Via Natural or Artificial Opening
09N48ZZ	Release Left External Auditory Canal, Via Natural or Artificial Opening Endoscopic
09N4XZZ	Release Left External Auditory Canal, External Approach
09N50ZZ	Release Right Middle Ear, Open Approach
09N58ZZ	Release Right Middle Ear, Via Natural or Artificial Opening Endoscopic
09N60ZZ	Release Left Middle Ear, Open Approach
09N68ZZ	Release Left Middle Ear, Via Natural or Artificial Opening Endoscopic
09N70ZZ	Release Right Tympanic Membrane, Open Approach
09N73ZZ	Release Right Tympanic Membrane, Percutaneous Approach
09N74ZZ	Release Right Tympanic Membrane, Percutaneous Endoscopic Approach
09N77ZZ	Release Right Tympanic Membrane, Via Natural or Artificial Opening
09N78ZZ	Release Right Tympanic Membrane, Via Natural or Artificial Opening Endoscopic
09N80ZZ	Release Left Tympanic Membrane, Open Approach
09N83ZZ	Release Left Tympanic Membrane, Percutaneous Approach
09N84ZZ	Release Left Tympanic Membrane, Percutaneous Endoscopic Approach
09N87ZZ	Release Left Tympanic Membrane, Via Natural or Artificial Opening

09N88ZZ	Release Left Tympanic Membrane, Via Natural or Artificial Opening Endoscopic
09N90ZZ	Release Right Auditory Ossicle, Open Approach
09N98ZZ	Release Right Auditory Ossicle, Via Natural or Artificial Opening Endoscopic
09NA0ZZ	Release Left Auditory Ossicle, Open Approach
09NA8ZZ	Release Left Auditory Ossicle, Via Natural or Artificial Opening Endoscopic
09NB0ZZ	Release Right Mastoid Sinus, Open Approach
09NB3ZZ	Release Right Mastoid Sinus, Percutaneous Approach
09NB4ZZ	Release Right Mastoid Sinus, Percutaneous Endoscopic Approach
09NB8ZZ	Release Right Mastoid Sinus, Via Natural or Artificial Opening Endoscopic
09NC0ZZ	Release Left Mastoid Sinus, Open Approach
09NC3ZZ	Release Left Mastoid Sinus, Percutaneous Approach
09NC4ZZ	Release Left Mastoid Sinus, Percutaneous Endoscopic Approach
09NC8ZZ	Release Left Mastoid Sinus, Via Natural or Artificial Opening Endoscopic
09ND0ZZ	Release Right Inner Ear, Open Approach
09ND8ZZ	Release Right Inner Ear, Via Natural or Artificial Opening Endoscopic
09NE0ZZ	Release Left Inner Ear, Open Approach
09NE8ZZ	Release Left Inner Ear, Via Natural or Artificial Opening Endoscopic
09NF0ZZ	Release Right Eustachian Tube, Open Approach
09NF3ZZ	Release Right Eustachian Tube, Percutaneous Approach
09NF4ZZ	Release Right Eustachian Tube, Percutaneous Endoscopic Approach
09NF7ZZ	Release Right Eustachian Tube, Via Natural or Artificial Opening
09NF8ZZ	Release Right Eustachian Tube, Via Natural or Artificial Opening Endoscopic
09NG0ZZ	Release Left Eustachian Tube, Open Approach
09NG3ZZ	Release Left Eustachian Tube, Percutaneous Approach
09NG4ZZ	Release Left Eustachian Tube, Percutaneous Endoscopic Approach
09NG7ZZ	Release Left Eustachian Tube, Via Natural or Artificial Opening
09NG8ZZ	Release Left Eustachian Tube, Via Natural or Artificial Opening Endoscopic
09NK0ZZ	Release Nasal Mucosa and Soft Tissue, Open Approach
09NK3ZZ	Release Nasal Mucosa and Soft Tissue, Percutaneous Approach
09NK4ZZ	Release Nasal Mucosa and Soft Tissue, Percutaneous Endoscopic Approach
09NK8ZZ	Release Nasal Mucosa and Soft Tissue, Via Natural or Artificial Opening Endoscopic
09NKXZZ	Release Nasal Mucosa and Soft Tissue, External Approach

09NL0ZZ	Release Nasal Turbinate, Open Approach
09NL3ZZ	Release Nasal Turbinate, Percutaneous Approach
09NL4ZZ	Release Nasal Turbinate, Percutaneous Endoscopic Approach
09NL7ZZ	Release Nasal Turbinate, Via Natural or Artificial Opening
09NL8ZZ	Release Nasal Turbinate, Via Natural or Artificial Opening Endoscopic
09NM0ZZ	Release Nasal Septum, Open Approach
09NM3ZZ	Release Nasal Septum, Percutaneous Approach
09NM4ZZ	Release Nasal Septum, Percutaneous Endoscopic Approach
09NM8ZZ	Release Nasal Septum, Via Natural or Artificial Opening Endoscopic
09NN0ZZ	Release Nasopharynx, Open Approach
09NN3ZZ	Release Nasopharynx, Percutaneous Approach
09NN4ZZ	Release Nasopharynx, Percutaneous Endoscopic Approach
09NN7ZZ	Release Nasopharynx, Via Natural or Artificial Opening
09NN8ZZ	Release Nasopharynx, Via Natural or Artificial Opening Endoscopic
09NP0ZZ	Release Accessory Sinus, Open Approach
09NP3ZZ	Release Accessory Sinus, Percutaneous Approach
09NP4ZZ	Release Accessory Sinus, Percutaneous Endoscopic Approach
09NP8ZZ	Release Accessory Sinus, Via Natural or Artificial Opening Endoscopic
09NQ0ZZ	Release Right Maxillary Sinus, Open Approach
09NQ3ZZ	Release Right Maxillary Sinus, Percutaneous Approach
09NQ4ZZ	Release Right Maxillary Sinus, Percutaneous Endoscopic Approach
09NQ8ZZ	Release Right Maxillary Sinus, Via Natural or Artificial Opening Endoscopic
09NR0ZZ	Release Left Maxillary Sinus, Open Approach
09NR3ZZ	Release Left Maxillary Sinus, Percutaneous Approach
09NR4ZZ	Release Left Maxillary Sinus, Percutaneous Endoscopic Approach
09NR8ZZ	Release Left Maxillary Sinus, Via Natural or Artificial Opening Endoscopic
09NS0ZZ	Release Right Frontal Sinus, Open Approach
09NS3ZZ	Release Right Frontal Sinus, Percutaneous Approach
09NS4ZZ	Release Right Frontal Sinus, Percutaneous Endoscopic Approach
09NS8ZZ	Release Right Frontal Sinus, Via Natural or Artificial Opening Endoscopic
09NT0ZZ	Release Left Frontal Sinus, Open Approach
09NT3ZZ	Release Left Frontal Sinus, Percutaneous Approach
09NT4ZZ	Release Left Frontal Sinus, Percutaneous Endoscopic Approach
09NT8ZZ	Release Left Frontal Sinus, Via Natural or Artificial Opening Endoscopic
09NU0ZZ	Release Right Ethmoid Sinus, Open Approach

♀ Female-only   ♂ Male-only   ▲ Limited Coverage   ● Non-OR   🅷🅰🅲 HAC-associated procedure   ▲ Non-covered procedures   ✚ Cluster

09NU3ZZ	Release Right Ethmoid Sinus, Percutaneous Approach
09NU4ZZ	Release Right Ethmoid Sinus, Percutaneous Endoscopic Approach
09NU8ZZ	Release Right Ethmoid Sinus, Via Natural or Artificial Opening Endoscopic
09NV0ZZ	Release Left Ethmoid Sinus, Open Approach
09NV3ZZ	Release Left Ethmoid Sinus, Percutaneous Approach

09NV4ZZ	Release Left Ethmoid Sinus, Percutaneous Endoscopic Approach
09NV8ZZ	Release Left Ethmoid Sinus, Via Natural or Artificial Opening Endoscopic
09NW0ZZ	Release Right Sphenoid Sinus, Open Approach
09NW3ZZ	Release Right Sphenoid Sinus, Percutaneous Approach
09NW4ZZ	Release Right Sphenoid Sinus, Percutaneous Endoscopic Approach

09NW8ZZ	Release Right Sphenoid Sinus, Via Natural or Artificial Opening Endoscopic
09NX0ZZ	Release Left Sphenoid Sinus, Open Approach
09NX3ZZ	Release Left Sphenoid Sinus, Percutaneous Approach
09NX4ZZ	Release Left Sphenoid Sinus, Percutaneous Endoscopic Approach
09NX8ZZ	Release Left Sphenoid Sinus, Via Natural or Artificial Opening Endoscopic

09P – Ear, Nose, Sinus, Removal

Review Coding Guideline B6.1c

09P700Z	Removal of Drainage Device from Right Tympanic Membrane, Open Approach
09P770Z	Removal of Drainage Device from Right Tympanic Membrane, Via Natural or Artificial Opening
09P780Z	Removal of Drainage Device from Right Tympanic Membrane, Via Natural or Artificial Opening Endoscopic
09P7X0Z	Removal of Drainage Device from Right Tympanic Membrane, External Approach
09P800Z	Removal of Drainage Device from Left Tympanic Membrane, Open Approach
09P870Z	Removal of Drainage Device from Left Tympanic Membrane, Via Natural or Artificial Opening
09P880Z	Removal of Drainage Device from Left Tympanic Membrane, Via Natural or Artificial Opening Endoscopic
09P8X0Z	Removal of Drainage Device from Left Tympanic Membrane, External Approach
09PD0SZ	Removal of Hearing Device from Right Inner Ear, Open Approach
09PD7SZ	Removal of Hearing Device from Right Inner Ear, Via Natural or Artificial Opening
09PD8SZ	Removal of Hearing Device from Right Inner Ear, Via Natural or Artificial Opening Endoscopic
09PE0SZ	Removal of Hearing Device from Left Inner Ear, Open Approach
09PE7SZ	Removal of Hearing Device from Left Inner Ear, Via Natural or Artificial Opening
09PE8SZ	Removal of Hearing Device from Left Inner Ear, Via Natural or Artificial Opening Endoscopic
09PH00Z	Removal of Drainage Device from Right Ear, Open Approach
09PH07Z	Removal of Autologous Tissue Substitute from Right Ear, Open Approach
09PH0DZ	Removal of Intraluminal Device from Right Ear, Open Approach
09PH0JZ	Removal of Synthetic Substitute from Right Ear, Open Approach
09PH0KZ	Removal of Nonautologous Tissue Substitute from Right Ear, Open Approach
09PH0YZ	Removal of Other Device from Right Ear, Open Approach
09PH30Z	Removal of Drainage Device from Right Ear, Percutaneous Approach
09PH37Z	Removal of Autologous Tissue Substitute from Right Ear, Percutaneous Approach
09PH3DZ	Removal of Intraluminal Device from Right Ear, Percutaneous Approach

09PH3JZ	Removal of Synthetic Substitute from Right Ear, Percutaneous Approach
09PH3KZ	Removal of Nonautologous Tissue Substitute from Right Ear, Percutaneous Approach
09PH3YZ	Removal of Other Device from Right Ear, Percutaneous Approach
09PH40Z	Removal of Drainage Device from Right Ear, Percutaneous Endoscopic Approach
09PH47Z	Removal of Autologous Tissue Substitute from Right Ear, Percutaneous Endoscopic Approach
09PH4DZ	Removal of Intraluminal Device from Right Ear, Percutaneous Endoscopic Approach
09PH4JZ	Removal of Synthetic Substitute from Right Ear, Percutaneous Endoscopic Approach
09PH4KZ	Removal of Nonautologous Tissue Substitute from Right Ear, Percutaneous Endoscopic Approach
09PH4YZ	Removal of Other Device from Right Ear, Percutaneous Endoscopic Approach
09PH70Z	Removal of Drainage Device from Right Ear, Via Natural or Artificial Opening
09PH77Z	Removal of Autologous Tissue Substitute from Right Ear, Via Natural or Artificial Opening
09PH7DZ	Removal of Intraluminal Device from Right Ear, Via Natural or Artificial Opening
09PH7JZ	Removal of Synthetic Substitute from Right Ear, Via Natural or Artificial Opening
09PH7KZ	Removal of Nonautologous Tissue Substitute from Right Ear, Via Natural or Artificial Opening
09PH7YZ	Removal of Other Device from Right Ear, Via Natural or Artificial Opening
09PH80Z	Removal of Drainage Device from Right Ear, Via Natural or Artificial Opening Endoscopic
09PH87Z	Removal of Autologous Tissue Substitute from Right Ear, Via Natural or Artificial Opening Endoscopic
09PH8DZ	Removal of Intraluminal Device from Right Ear, Via Natural or Artificial Opening Endoscopic
09PH8JZ	Removal of Synthetic Substitute from Right Ear, Via Natural or Artificial Opening Endoscopic
09PH8KZ	Removal of Nonautologous Tissue Substitute from Right Ear, Via Natural or Artificial Opening Endoscopic
09PH8YZ	Removal of Other Device from Right Ear, Via Natural or Artificial Opening Endoscopic

09PHX0Z	Removal of Drainage Device from Right Ear, External Approach
09PHX7Z	Removal of Autologous Tissue Substitute from Right Ear, External Approach
09PHXDZ	Removal of Intraluminal Device from Right Ear, External Approach
09PHXJZ	Removal of Synthetic Substitute from Right Ear, External Approach
09PHXKZ	Removal of Nonautologous Tissue Substitute from Right Ear, External Approach
09PJ00Z	Removal of Drainage Device from Left Ear, Open Approach
09PJ07Z	Removal of Autologous Tissue Substitute from Left Ear, Open Approach
09PJ0DZ	Removal of Intraluminal Device from Left Ear, Open Approach
09PJ0JZ	Removal of Synthetic Substitute from Left Ear, Open Approach
09PJ0KZ	Removal of Nonautologous Tissue Substitute from Left Ear, Open Approach
09PJ0YZ	Removal of Other Device from Left Ear, Open Approach
09PJ30Z	Removal of Drainage Device from Left Ear, Percutaneous Approach
09PJ37Z	Removal of Autologous Tissue Substitute from Left Ear, Percutaneous Approach
09PJ3DZ	Removal of Intraluminal Device from Left Ear, Percutaneous Approach
09PJ3JZ	Removal of Synthetic Substitute from Left Ear, Percutaneous Approach
09PJ3KZ	Removal of Nonautologous Tissue Substitute from Left Ear, Percutaneous Approach
09PJ3YZ	Removal of Other Device from Left Ear, Percutaneous Approach
09PJ40Z	Removal of Drainage Device from Left Ear, Percutaneous Endoscopic Approach
09PJ47Z	Removal of Autologous Tissue Substitute from Left Ear, Percutaneous Endoscopic Approach
09PJ4DZ	Removal of Intraluminal Device from Left Ear, Percutaneous Endoscopic Approach
09PJ4JZ	Removal of Synthetic Substitute from Left Ear, Percutaneous Endoscopic Approach
09PJ4KZ	Removal of Nonautologous Tissue Substitute from Left Ear, Percutaneous Endoscopic Approach
09PJ4YZ	Removal of Other Device from Left Ear, Percutaneous Endoscopic Approach
09PJ70Z	Removal of Drainage Device from Left Ear, Via Natural or Artificial Opening
09PJ77Z	Removal of Autologous Tissue Substitute from Left Ear, Via Natural or Artificial Opening

09PJ7DZ Removal of Intraluminal Device from Left Ear, Via Natural or Artificial Opening

09PJ7JZ Removal of Synthetic Substitute from Left Ear, Via Natural or Artificial Opening

09PJ7KZ Removal of Nonautologous Tissue Substitute from Left Ear, Via Natural or Artificial Opening

09PJ7YZ Removal of Other Device from Left Ear, Via Natural or Artificial Opening

09PJ80Z Removal of Drainage Device from Left Ear, Via Natural or Artificial Opening Endoscopic

09PJ87Z Removal of Autologous Tissue Substitute from Left Ear, Via Natural or Artificial Opening Endoscopic

09PJ8DZ Removal of Intraluminal Device from Left Ear, Via Natural or Artificial Opening Endoscopic

09PJ8JZ Removal of Synthetic Substitute from Left Ear, Via Natural or Artificial Opening Endoscopic

09PJ8KZ Removal of Nonautologous Tissue Substitute from Left Ear, Via Natural or Artificial Opening Endoscopic

09PJ8YZ Removal of Other Device from Left Ear, Via Natural or Artificial Opening Endoscopic

09PJX0Z Removal of Drainage Device from Left Ear, External Approach

09PJX7Z Removal of Autologous Tissue Substitute from Left Ear, External Approach

09PJXDZ Removal of Intraluminal Device from Left Ear, External Approach

09PJXJZ Removal of Synthetic Substitute from Left Ear, External Approach

09PJXKZ Removal of Nonautologous Tissue Substitute from Left Ear, External Approach

09PK00Z Removal of Drainage Device from Nasal Mucosa and Soft Tissue, Open Approach

09PK07Z Removal of Autologous Tissue Substitute from Nasal Mucosa and Soft Tissue, Open Approach

09PK0DZ Removal of Intraluminal Device from Nasal Mucosa and Soft Tissue, Open Approach

09PK0JZ Removal of Synthetic Substitute from Nasal Mucosa and Soft Tissue, Open Approach

09PK0KZ Removal of Nonautologous Tissue Substitute from Nasal Mucosa and Soft Tissue, Open Approach

09PK0YZ Removal of Other Device from Nasal Mucosa and Soft Tissue, Open Approach

09PK30Z Removal of Drainage Device from Nasal Mucosa and Soft Tissue, Percutaneous Approach

09PK37Z Removal of Autologous Tissue Substitute from Nasal Mucosa and Soft Tissue, Percutaneous Approach

09PK3DZ Removal of Intraluminal Device from Nasal Mucosa and Soft Tissue, Percutaneous Approach

09PK3JZ Removal of Synthetic Substitute from Nasal Mucosa and Soft Tissue, Percutaneous Approach

09PK3KZ Removal of Nonautologous Tissue Substitute from Nasal Mucosa and Soft Tissue, Percutaneous Approach

09PK3YZ Removal of Other Device from Nasal Mucosa and Soft Tissue, Percutaneous Approach

09PK40Z Removal of Drainage Device from Nasal Mucosa and Soft Tissue, Percutaneous Endoscopic Approach

09PK47Z Removal of Autologous Tissue Substitute from Nasal Mucosa and Soft Tissue, Percutaneous Endoscopic Approach

09PK4DZ Removal of Intraluminal Device from Nasal Mucosa and Soft Tissue, Percutaneous Endoscopic Approach

09PK4JZ Removal of Synthetic Substitute from Nasal Mucosa and Soft Tissue, Percutaneous Endoscopic Approach

09PK4KZ Removal of Nonautologous Tissue Substitute from Nasal Mucosa and Soft Tissue, Percutaneous Endoscopic Approach

09PK4YZ Removal of Other Device from Nasal Mucosa and Soft Tissue, Percutaneous Endoscopic Approach

09PK70Z Removal of Drainage Device from Nasal Mucosa and Soft Tissue, Via Natural or Artificial Opening

09PK77Z Removal of Autologous Tissue Substitute from Nasal Mucosa and Soft Tissue, Via Natural or Artificial Opening

09PK7DZ Removal of Intraluminal Device from Nasal Mucosa and Soft Tissue, Via Natural or Artificial Opening

09PK7JZ Removal of Synthetic Substitute from Nasal Mucosa and Soft Tissue, Via Natural or Artificial Opening

09PK7KZ Removal of Nonautologous Tissue Substitute from Nasal Mucosa and Soft Tissue, Via Natural or Artificial Opening

09PK7YZ Removal of Other Device from Nasal Mucosa and Soft Tissue, Via Natural or Artificial Opening

09PK80Z Removal of Drainage Device from Nasal Mucosa and Soft Tissue, Via Natural or Artificial Opening Endoscopic

09PK87Z Removal of Autologous Tissue Substitute from Nasal Mucosa and Soft Tissue, Via Natural or Artificial Opening Endoscopic

09PK8DZ Removal of Intraluminal Device from Nasal Mucosa and Soft Tissue, Via Natural or Artificial Opening Endoscopic

09PK8JZ Removal of Synthetic Substitute from Nasal Mucosa and Soft Tissue, Via Natural or Artificial Opening Endoscopic

09PK8KZ Removal of Nonautologous Tissue Substitute from Nasal Mucosa and Soft Tissue, Via Natural or Artificial Opening Endoscopic

09PK8YZ Removal of Other Device from Nasal Mucosa and Soft Tissue, Via Natural or Artificial Opening Endoscopic

09PKX0Z Removal of Drainage Device from Nasal Mucosa and Soft Tissue, External Approach

09PKX7Z Removal of Autologous Tissue Substitute from Nasal Mucosa and Soft Tissue, External Approach

09PKXDZ Removal of Intraluminal Device from Nasal Mucosa and Soft Tissue, External Approach

09PKXJZ Removal of Synthetic Substitute from Nasal Mucosa and Soft Tissue, External Approach

09PKXKZ Removal of Nonautologous Tissue Substitute from Nasal Mucosa and Soft Tissue, External Approach

09PY00Z Removal of Drainage Device from Sinus, Open Approach

09PY0YZ Removal of Other Device from Sinus, Open Approach

09PY30Z Removal of Drainage Device from Sinus, Percutaneous Approach

09PY3YZ Removal of Other Device from Sinus, Percutaneous Approach

09PY40Z Removal of Drainage Device from Sinus, Percutaneous Endoscopic Approach

09PY4YZ Removal of Other Device from Sinus, Percutaneous Endoscopic Approach

09PY7YZ Removal of Other Device from Sinus, Via Natural or Artificial Opening

09PY8YZ Removal of Other Device from Sinus, Via Natural or Artificial Opening Endoscopic

09PYX0Z Removal of Drainage Device from Sinus, External Approach

09Q – Ear, Nose, Sinus, Repair

09Q00ZZ Repair Right External Ear, Open Approach

09Q03ZZ Repair Right External Ear, Percutaneous Approach

09Q04ZZ Repair Right External Ear, Percutaneous Endoscopic Approach

09Q0XZZ Repair Right External Ear, External Approach

09Q10ZZ Repair Left External Ear, Open Approach

09Q13ZZ Repair Left External Ear, Percutaneous Approach

09Q14ZZ Repair Left External Ear, Percutaneous Endoscopic Approach

09Q1XZZ Repair Left External Ear, External Approach

09Q20ZZ Repair Bilateral External Ear, Open Approach

09Q23ZZ Repair Bilateral External Ear, Percutaneous Approach

09Q24ZZ Repair Bilateral External Ear, Percutaneous Endoscopic Approach

09Q2XZZ Repair Bilateral External Ear, External Approach

09Q30ZZ Repair Right External Auditory Canal, Open Approach

09Q33ZZ Repair Right External Auditory Canal, Percutaneous Approach

09Q34ZZ Repair Right External Auditory Canal, Percutaneous Endoscopic Approach

09Q37ZZ Repair Right External Auditory Canal, Via Natural or Artificial Opening

09Q38ZZ Repair Right External Auditory Canal, Via Natural or Artificial Opening Endoscopic

09Q3XZZ	Repair Right External Auditory Canal, External Approach
09Q40ZZ	Repair Left External Auditory Canal, Open Approach
09Q43ZZ	Repair Left External Auditory Canal, Percutaneous Approach
09Q44ZZ	Repair Left External Auditory Canal, Percutaneous Endoscopic Approach
09Q47ZZ	Repair Left External Auditory Canal, Via Natural or Artificial Opening
09Q48ZZ	Repair Left External Auditory Canal, Via Natural or Artificial Opening Endoscopic
09Q4XZZ	Repair Left External Auditory Canal, External Approach
09Q50ZZ	Repair Right Middle Ear, Open Approach
09Q58ZZ	Repair Right Middle Ear, Via Natural or Artificial Opening Endoscopic
09Q60ZZ	Repair Left Middle Ear, Open Approach
09Q68ZZ	Repair Left Middle Ear, Via Natural or Artificial Opening Endoscopic
09Q70ZZ	Repair Right Tympanic Membrane, Open Approach
09Q73ZZ	Repair Right Tympanic Membrane, Percutaneous Approach
09Q74ZZ	Repair Right Tympanic Membrane, Percutaneous Endoscopic Approach
09Q77ZZ	Repair Right Tympanic Membrane, Via Natural or Artificial Opening
09Q78ZZ	Repair Right Tympanic Membrane, Via Natural or Artificial Opening Endoscopic
09Q80ZZ	Repair Left Tympanic Membrane, Open Approach
09Q83ZZ	Repair Left Tympanic Membrane, Percutaneous Approach
09Q84ZZ	Repair Left Tympanic Membrane, Percutaneous Endoscopic Approach
09Q87ZZ	Repair Left Tympanic Membrane, Via Natural or Artificial Opening
09Q88ZZ	Repair Left Tympanic Membrane, Via Natural or Artificial Opening Endoscopic
09Q90ZZ	Repair Right Auditory Ossicle, Open Approach
09Q98ZZ	Repair Right Auditory Ossicle, Via Natural or Artificial Opening Endoscopic
09QA0ZZ	Repair Left Auditory Ossicle, Open Approach
09QA8ZZ	Repair Left Auditory Ossicle, Via Natural or Artificial Opening Endoscopic
09QB0ZZ	Repair Right Mastoid Sinus, Open Approach
09QB3ZZ	Repair Right Mastoid Sinus, Percutaneous Approach
09QB4ZZ	Repair Right Mastoid Sinus, Percutaneous Endoscopic Approach
09QB8ZZ	Repair Right Mastoid Sinus, Via Natural or Artificial Opening Endoscopic
09QC0ZZ	Repair Left Mastoid Sinus, Open Approach
09QC3ZZ	Repair Left Mastoid Sinus, Percutaneous Approach
09QC4ZZ	Repair Left Mastoid Sinus, Percutaneous Endoscopic Approach
09QC8ZZ	Repair Left Mastoid Sinus, Via Natural or Artificial Opening Endoscopic
09QD0ZZ	Repair Right Inner Ear, Open Approach
09QD8ZZ	Repair Right Inner Ear, Via Natural or Artificial Opening Endoscopic
09QE0ZZ	Repair Left Inner Ear, Open Approach
09QE8ZZ	Repair Left Inner Ear, Via Natural or Artificial Opening Endoscopic
09QF0ZZ	Repair Right Eustachian Tube, Open Approach
09QF3ZZ	Repair Right Eustachian Tube, Percutaneous Approach
09QF4ZZ	Repair Right Eustachian Tube, Percutaneous Endoscopic Approach
09QF7ZZ	Repair Right Eustachian Tube, Via Natural or Artificial Opening
09QF8ZZ	Repair Right Eustachian Tube, Via Natural or Artificial Opening Endoscopic
09QFXZZ	Repair Right Eustachian Tube, External Approach
09QG0ZZ	Repair Left Eustachian Tube, Open Approach
09QG3ZZ	Repair Left Eustachian Tube, Percutaneous Approach
09QG4ZZ	Repair Left Eustachian Tube, Percutaneous Endoscopic Approach
09QG7ZZ	Repair Left Eustachian Tube, Via Natural or Artificial Opening
09QG8ZZ	Repair Left Eustachian Tube, Via Natural or Artificial Opening Endoscopic
09QGXZZ	Repair Left Eustachian Tube, External Approach
09QK0ZZ	Repair Nasal Mucosa and Soft Tissue, Open Approach
09QK3ZZ	Repair Nasal Mucosa and Soft Tissue, Percutaneous Approach
09QK4ZZ	Repair Nasal Mucosa and Soft Tissue, Percutaneous Endoscopic Approach
09QK8ZZ	Repair Nasal Mucosa and Soft Tissue, Via Natural or Artificial Opening Endoscopic
09QKXZZ	Repair Nasal Mucosa and Soft Tissue, External Approach
	AHA CC: 4Q, 2014, 20-21
09QL0ZZ	Repair Nasal Turbinate, Open Approach
09QL3ZZ	Repair Nasal Turbinate, Percutaneous Approach
09QL4ZZ	Repair Nasal Turbinate, Percutaneous Endoscopic Approach
09QL7ZZ	Repair Nasal Turbinate, Via Natural or Artificial Opening
09QL8ZZ	Repair Nasal Turbinate, Via Natural or Artificial Opening Endoscopic
09QM0ZZ	Repair Nasal Septum, Open Approach
09QM3ZZ	Repair Nasal Septum, Percutaneous Approach
09QM4ZZ	Repair Nasal Septum, Percutaneous Endoscopic Approach
09QM8ZZ	Repair Nasal Septum, Via Natural or Artificial Opening Endoscopic
09QN0ZZ	Repair Nasopharynx, Open Approach
09QN3ZZ	Repair Nasopharynx, Percutaneous Approach
09QN4ZZ	Repair Nasopharynx, Percutaneous Endoscopic Approach
09QN7ZZ	Repair Nasopharynx, Via Natural or Artificial Opening
09QN8ZZ	Repair Nasopharynx, Via Natural or Artificial Opening Endoscopic
09QP0ZZ	Repair Accessory Sinus, Open Approach
09QP3ZZ	Repair Accessory Sinus, Percutaneous Approach
09QP4ZZ	Repair Accessory Sinus, Percutaneous Endoscopic Approach
09QP8ZZ	Repair Accessory Sinus, Via Natural or Artificial Opening Endoscopic
09QQ0ZZ	Repair Right Maxillary Sinus, Open Approach
09QQ3ZZ	Repair Right Maxillary Sinus, Percutaneous Approach
09QQ4ZZ	Repair Right Maxillary Sinus, Percutaneous Endoscopic Approach
09QQ8ZZ	Repair Right Maxillary Sinus, Via Natural or Artificial Opening Endoscopic
09QR0ZZ	Repair Left Maxillary Sinus, Open Approach
09QR3ZZ	Repair Left Maxillary Sinus, Percutaneous Approach
09QR4ZZ	Repair Left Maxillary Sinus, Percutaneous Endoscopic Approach
09QR8ZZ	Repair Left Maxillary Sinus, Via Natural or Artificial Opening Endoscopic
09QS0ZZ	Repair Right Frontal Sinus, Open Approach
09QS3ZZ	Repair Right Frontal Sinus, Percutaneous Approach
09QS4ZZ	Repair Right Frontal Sinus, Percutaneous Endoscopic Approach
09QS8ZZ	Repair Right Frontal Sinus, Via Natural or Artificial Opening Endoscopic
09QT0ZZ	Repair Left Frontal Sinus, Open Approach
09QT3ZZ	Repair Left Frontal Sinus, Percutaneous Approach
09QT4ZZ	Repair Left Frontal Sinus, Percutaneous Endoscopic Approach
	AHA CC: 4Q, 2013, 114
09QT8ZZ	Repair Left Frontal Sinus, Via Natural or Artificial Opening Endoscopic
09QU0ZZ	Repair Right Ethmoid Sinus, Open Approach
09QU3ZZ	Repair Right Ethmoid Sinus, Percutaneous Approach
09QU4ZZ	Repair Right Ethmoid Sinus, Percutaneous Endoscopic Approach
09QU8ZZ	Repair Right Ethmoid Sinus, Via Natural or Artificial Opening Endoscopic
09QV0ZZ	Repair Left Ethmoid Sinus, Open Approach
09QV3ZZ	Repair Left Ethmoid Sinus, Percutaneous Approach
09QV4ZZ	Repair Left Ethmoid Sinus, Percutaneous Endoscopic Approach
09QV8ZZ	Repair Left Ethmoid Sinus, Via Natural or Artificial Opening Endoscopic
09QW0ZZ	Repair Right Sphenoid Sinus, Open Approach
	AHA CC: 3Q, 2014, 22-23
09QW3ZZ	Repair Right Sphenoid Sinus, Percutaneous Approach
09QW4ZZ	Repair Right Sphenoid Sinus, Percutaneous Endoscopic Approach
09QW8ZZ	Repair Right Sphenoid Sinus, Via Natural or Artificial Opening Endoscopic
09QX0ZZ	Repair Left Sphenoid Sinus, Open Approach
	AHA CC: 3Q, 2014, 22-23
09QX3ZZ	Repair Left Sphenoid Sinus, Percutaneous Approach
09QX4ZZ	Repair Left Sphenoid Sinus, Percutaneous Endoscopic Approach
09QX8ZZ	Repair Left Sphenoid Sinus, Via Natural or Artificial Opening Endoscopic

09R – Ear, Nose, Sinus, Replacement

Review Coding Guideline B3.18

09R007Z Replacement of Right External Ear with Autologous Tissue Substitute, Open Approach

09R00JZ Replacement of Right External Ear with Synthetic Substitute, Open Approach

09R00KZ Replacement of Right External Ear with Nonautologous Tissue Substitute, Open Approach

09R0X7Z Replacement of Right External Ear with Autologous Tissue Substitute, External Approach

09R0XJZ Replacement of Right External Ear with Synthetic Substitute, External Approach

09R0XKZ Replacement of Right External Ear with Nonautologous Tissue Substitute, External Approach

09R107Z Replacement of Left External Ear with Autologous Tissue Substitute, Open Approach

09R10JZ Replacement of Left External Ear with Synthetic Substitute, Open Approach

09R10KZ Replacement of Left External Ear with Nonautologous Tissue Substitute, Open Approach

09R1X7Z Replacement of Left External Ear with Autologous Tissue Substitute, External Approach

09R1XJZ Replacement of Left External Ear with Synthetic Substitute, External Approach

09R1XKZ Replacement of Left External Ear with Nonautologous Tissue Substitute, External Approach

09R207Z Replacement of Bilateral External Ear with Autologous Tissue Substitute, Open Approach

09R20JZ Replacement of Bilateral External Ear with Synthetic Substitute, Open Approach

09R20KZ Replacement of Bilateral External Ear with Nonautologous Tissue Substitute, Open Approach

09R2X7Z Replacement of Bilateral External Ear with Autologous Tissue Substitute, External Approach

09R2XJZ Replacement of Bilateral External Ear with Synthetic Substitute, External Approach

09R2XKZ Replacement of Bilateral External Ear with Nonautologous Tissue Substitute, External Approach

09R507Z Replacement of Right Middle Ear with Autologous Tissue Substitute, Open Approach

09R50JZ Replacement of Right Middle Ear with Synthetic Substitute, Open Approach

09R50KZ Replacement of Right Middle Ear with Nonautologous Tissue Substitute, Open Approach

09R607Z Replacement of Left Middle Ear with Autologous Tissue Substitute, Open Approach

09R60JZ Replacement of Left Middle Ear with Synthetic Substitute, Open Approach

09R60KZ Replacement of Left Middle Ear with Nonautologous Tissue Substitute, Open Approach

09R707Z Replacement of Right Tympanic Membrane with Autologous Tissue Substitute, Open Approach

09R70JZ Replacement of Right Tympanic Membrane with Synthetic Substitute, Open Approach

09R70KZ Replacement of Right Tympanic Membrane with Nonautologous Tissue Substitute, Open Approach

09R777Z Replacement of Right Tympanic Membrane with Autologous Tissue Substitute, Via Natural or Artificial Opening

09R77JZ Replacement of Right Tympanic Membrane with Synthetic Substitute, Via Natural or Artificial Opening

09R77KZ Replacement of Right Tympanic Membrane with Nonautologous Tissue Substitute, Via Natural or Artificial Opening

09R787Z Replacement of Right Tympanic Membrane with Autologous Tissue Substitute, Via Natural or Artificial Opening Endoscopic

09R78JZ Replacement of Right Tympanic Membrane with Synthetic Substitute, Via Natural or Artificial Opening Endoscopic

09R78KZ Replacement of Right Tympanic Membrane with Nonautologous Tissue Substitute, Via Natural or Artificial Opening Endoscopic

09R807Z Replacement of Left Tympanic Membrane with Autologous Tissue Substitute, Open Approach

09R80JZ Replacement of Left Tympanic Membrane with Synthetic Substitute, Open Approach

09R80KZ Replacement of Left Tympanic Membrane with Nonautologous Tissue Substitute, Open Approach

09R877Z Replacement of Left Tympanic Membrane with Autologous Tissue Substitute, Via Natural or Artificial Opening

09R87JZ Replacement of Left Tympanic Membrane with Synthetic Substitute, Via Natural or Artificial Opening

09R87KZ Replacement of Left Tympanic Membrane with Nonautologous Tissue Substitute, Via Natural or Artificial Opening

09R887Z Replacement of Left Tympanic Membrane with Autologous Tissue Substitute, Via Natural or Artificial Opening Endoscopic

09R88JZ Replacement of Left Tympanic Membrane with Synthetic Substitute, Via Natural or Artificial Opening Endoscopic

09R88KZ Replacement of Left Tympanic Membrane with Nonautologous Tissue Substitute, Via Natural or Artificial Opening Endoscopic

09R907Z Replacement of Right Auditory Ossicle with Autologous Tissue Substitute, Open Approach

09R90JZ Replacement of Right Auditory Ossicle with Synthetic Substitute, Open Approach

09R90KZ Replacement of Right Auditory Ossicle with Nonautologous Tissue Substitute, Open Approach

09RA07Z Replacement of Left Auditory Ossicle with Autologous Tissue Substitute, Open Approach

09RA0JZ Replacement of Left Auditory Ossicle with Synthetic Substitute, Open Approach

09RA0KZ Replacement of Left Auditory Ossicle with Nonautologous Tissue Substitute, Open Approach

09RD07Z Replacement of Right Inner Ear with Autologous Tissue Substitute, Open Approach

09RD0JZ Replacement of Right Inner Ear with Synthetic Substitute, Open Approach

09RD0KZ Replacement of Right Inner Ear with Nonautologous Tissue Substitute, Open Approach

09RE07Z Replacement of Left Inner Ear with Autologous Tissue Substitute, Open Approach

09RE0JZ Replacement of Left Inner Ear with Synthetic Substitute, Open Approach

09RE0KZ Replacement of Left Inner Ear with Nonautologous Tissue Substitute, Open Approach

09RK07Z Replacement of Nasal Mucosa and Soft Tissue with Autologous Tissue Substitute, Open Approach

09RK0JZ Replacement of Nasal Mucosa and Soft Tissue with Synthetic Substitute, Open Approach

09RK0KZ Replacement of Nasal Mucosa and Soft Tissue with Nonautologous Tissue Substitute, Open Approach

09RKX7Z Replacement of Nasal Mucosa and Soft Tissue with Autologous Tissue Substitute, External Approach

09RKXJZ Replacement of Nasal Mucosa and Soft Tissue with Synthetic Substitute, External Approach

09RKXKZ Replacement of Nasal Mucosa and Soft Tissue with Nonautologous Tissue Substitute, External Approach

09RL07Z Replacement of Nasal Turbinate with Autologous Tissue Substitute, Open Approach

09RL0JZ Replacement of Nasal Turbinate with Synthetic Substitute, Open Approach

09RL0KZ Replacement of Nasal Turbinate with Nonautologous Tissue Substitute, Open Approach

09RL37Z Replacement of Nasal Turbinate with Autologous Tissue Substitute, Percutaneous Approach

09RL3JZ Replacement of Nasal Turbinate with Synthetic Substitute, Percutaneous Approach

09RL3KZ Replacement of Nasal Turbinate with Nonautologous Tissue Substitute, Percutaneous Approach

09RL47Z Replacement of Nasal Turbinate with Autologous Tissue Substitute, Percutaneous Endoscopic Approach

09RL4JZ Replacement of Nasal Turbinate with Synthetic Substitute, Percutaneous Endoscopic Approach

09RL4KZ Replacement of Nasal Turbinate with Nonautologous Tissue Substitute, Percutaneous Endoscopic Approach

09RL77Z Replacement of Nasal Turbinate with Autologous Tissue Substitute, Via Natural or Artificial Opening

09RL7JZ Replacement of Nasal Turbinate with Synthetic Substitute, Via Natural or Artificial Opening

♀ Female-only   ♂ Male-only   ▲ Limited Coverage   ● Non-OR   HAC HAC-associated procedure   ▲ Non-covered procedures   ✚ Cluster

09RL7KZ Replacement of Nasal Turbinate with Nonautologous Tissue Substitute, Via Natural or Artificial Opening

09RL87Z Replacement of Nasal Turbinate with Autologous Tissue Substitute, Via Natural or Artificial Opening Endoscopic

09RL8JZ Replacement of Nasal Turbinate with Synthetic Substitute, Via Natural or Artificial Opening Endoscopic

09RL8KZ Replacement of Nasal Turbinate with Nonautologous Tissue Substitute, Via Natural or Artificial Opening Endoscopic

09RM07Z Replacement of Nasal Septum with Autologous Tissue Substitute, Open Approach

09RM0JZ Replacement of Nasal Septum with Synthetic Substitute, Open Approach

09RM0KZ Replacement of Nasal Septum with Nonautologous Tissue Substitute, Open Approach

09RM37Z Replacement of Nasal Septum with Autologous Tissue Substitute, Percutaneous Approach

09RM3JZ Replacement of Nasal Septum with Synthetic Substitute, Percutaneous Approach

09RM3KZ Replacement of Nasal Septum with Nonautologous Tissue Substitute, Percutaneous Approach

09RM47Z Replacement of Nasal Septum with Autologous Tissue Substitute, Percutaneous Endoscopic Approach

09RM4JZ Replacement of Nasal Septum with Synthetic Substitute, Percutaneous Endoscopic Approach

09RM4KZ Replacement of Nasal Septum with Nonautologous Tissue Substitute, Percutaneous Endoscopic Approach

09RN07Z Replacement of Nasopharynx with Autologous Tissue Substitute, Open Approach

09RN0JZ Replacement of Nasopharynx with Synthetic Substitute, Open Approach

09RN0KZ Replacement of Nasopharynx with Nonautologous Tissue Substitute, Open Approach

09RN77Z Replacement of Nasopharynx with Autologous Tissue Substitute, Via Natural or Artificial Opening

09RN7JZ Replacement of Nasopharynx with Synthetic Substitute, Via Natural or Artificial Opening

09RN7KZ Replacement of Nasopharynx with Nonautologous Tissue Substitute, Via Natural or Artificial Opening

09RN87Z Replacement of Nasopharynx with Autologous Tissue Substitute, Via Natural or Artificial Opening Endoscopic

09RN8JZ Replacement of Nasopharynx with Synthetic Substitute, Via Natural or Artificial Opening Endoscopic

09RN8KZ Replacement of Nasopharynx with Nonautologous Tissue Substitute, Via Natural or Artificial Opening Endoscopic

09S – Ear, Nose, Sinus, Reposition

09S00ZZ Reposition Right External Ear, Open Approach

09S04ZZ Reposition Right External Ear, Percutaneous Endoscopic Approach

09S0XZZ Reposition Right External Ear, External Approach

09S10ZZ Reposition Left External Ear, Open Approach

09S14ZZ Reposition Left External Ear, Percutaneous Endoscopic Approach

09S1XZZ Reposition Left External Ear, External Approach

09S20ZZ Reposition Bilateral External Ear, Open Approach

09S24ZZ Reposition Bilateral External Ear, Percutaneous Endoscopic Approach

09S2XZZ Reposition Bilateral External Ear, External Approach

09S70ZZ Reposition Right Tympanic Membrane, Open Approach

09S74ZZ Reposition Right Tympanic Membrane, Percutaneous Endoscopic Approach

09S77ZZ Reposition Right Tympanic Membrane, Via Natural or Artificial Opening

09S78ZZ Reposition Right Tympanic Membrane, Via Natural or Artificial Opening Endoscopic

09S80ZZ Reposition Left Tympanic Membrane, Open Approach

09S84ZZ Reposition Left Tympanic Membrane, Percutaneous Endoscopic Approach

09S87ZZ Reposition Left Tympanic Membrane, Via Natural or Artificial Opening

09S88ZZ Reposition Left Tympanic Membrane, Via Natural or Artificial Opening Endoscopic

09S90ZZ Reposition Right Auditory Ossicle, Open Approach

09S94ZZ Reposition Right Auditory Ossicle, Percutaneous Endoscopic Approach

09SA0ZZ Reposition Left Auditory Ossicle, Open Approach

09SA4ZZ Reposition Left Auditory Ossicle, Percutaneous Endoscopic Approach

09SF0ZZ Reposition Right Eustachian Tube, Open Approach

09SF4ZZ Reposition Right Eustachian Tube, Percutaneous Endoscopic Approach

09SF7ZZ Reposition Right Eustachian Tube, Via Natural or Artificial Opening

09SF8ZZ Reposition Right Eustachian Tube, Via Natural or Artificial Opening Endoscopic

09SG0ZZ Reposition Left Eustachian Tube, Open Approach

09SG4ZZ Reposition Left Eustachian Tube, Percutaneous Endoscopic Approach

09SG7ZZ Reposition Left Eustachian Tube, Via Natural or Artificial Opening

09SG8ZZ Reposition Left Eustachian Tube, Via Natural or Artificial Opening Endoscopic

09SK0ZZ Reposition Nasal Mucosa and Soft Tissue, Open Approach

09SK4ZZ Reposition Nasal Mucosa and Soft Tissue, Percutaneous Endoscopic Approach

09SKXZZ Reposition Nasal Mucosa and Soft Tissue, External Approach

09SL0ZZ Reposition Nasal Turbinate, Open Approach

09SL4ZZ Reposition Nasal Turbinate, Percutaneous Endoscopic Approach

09SL7ZZ Reposition Nasal Turbinate, Via Natural or Artificial Opening

09SL8ZZ Reposition Nasal Turbinate, Via Natural or Artificial Opening Endoscopic

09SM0ZZ Reposition Nasal Septum, Open Approach

09SM4ZZ Reposition Nasal Septum, Percutaneous Endoscopic Approach

09T – Ear, Nose, Sinus, Resection

Review Coding Guideline B3.8

Review Coding Guideline B3.18

09T00ZZ Resection of Right External Ear, Open Approach

09T04ZZ Resection of Right External Ear, Percutaneous Endoscopic Approach

09T0XZZ Resection of Right External Ear, External Approach

09T10ZZ Resection of Left External Ear, Open Approach

09T14ZZ Resection of Left External Ear, Percutaneous Endoscopic Approach

09T1XZZ Resection of Left External Ear, External Approach

09T50ZZ Resection of Right Middle Ear, Open Approach

09T58ZZ Resection of Right Middle Ear, Via Natural or Artificial Opening Endoscopic

09T60ZZ Resection of Left Middle Ear, Open Approach

09T68ZZ Resection of Left Middle Ear, Via Natural or Artificial Opening Endoscopic

09T70ZZ Resection of Right Tympanic Membrane, Open Approach

09T74ZZ Resection of Right Tympanic Membrane, Percutaneous Endoscopic Approach

09T77ZZ Resection of Right Tympanic Membrane, Via Natural or Artificial Opening

09T78ZZ Resection of Right Tympanic Membrane, Via Natural or Artificial Opening Endoscopic

09T80ZZ Resection of Left Tympanic Membrane, Open Approach

09T84ZZ Resection of Left Tympanic Membrane, Percutaneous Endoscopic Approach

09T87ZZ Resection of Left Tympanic Membrane, Via Natural or Artificial Opening

09T88ZZ Resection of Left Tympanic Membrane, Via Natural or Artificial Opening Endoscopic

09T90ZZ Resection of Right Auditory Ossicle, Open Approach

09T98ZZ Resection of Right Auditory Ossicle, Via Natural or Artificial Opening Endoscopic

09TA0ZZ Resection of Left Auditory Ossicle, Open Approach

09TA8ZZ Resection of Left Auditory Ossicle, Via Natural or Artificial Opening Endoscopic

09TB0ZZ Resection of Right Mastoid Sinus, Open Approach

09TB4ZZ Resection of Right Mastoid Sinus, Percutaneous Endoscopic Approach

09TB8ZZ Resection of Right Mastoid Sinus, Via Natural or Artificial Opening Endoscopic

09TC0ZZ Resection of Left Mastoid Sinus, Open Approach

09TC4ZZ Resection of Left Mastoid Sinus, Percutaneous Endoscopic Approach

09TC8ZZ Resection of Left Mastoid Sinus, Via Natural or Artificial Opening Endoscopic

09TD0ZZ Resection of Right Inner Ear, Open Approach

09TD8ZZ Resection of Right Inner Ear, Via Natural or Artificial Opening Endoscopic

09TE0ZZ Resection of Left Inner Ear, Open Approach

09TE8ZZ Resection of Left Inner Ear, Via Natural or Artificial Opening Endoscopic

09TF0ZZ Resection of Right Eustachian Tube, Open Approach

09TF4ZZ Resection of Right Eustachian Tube, Percutaneous Endoscopic Approach

09TF7ZZ Resection of Right Eustachian Tube, Via Natural or Artificial Opening

09TF8ZZ Resection of Right Eustachian Tube, Via Natural or Artificial Opening Endoscopic

09TG0ZZ Resection of Left Eustachian Tube, Open Approach

09TG4ZZ Resection of Left Eustachian Tube, Percutaneous Endoscopic Approach

09TG7ZZ Resection of Left Eustachian Tube, Via Natural or Artificial Opening

09TG8ZZ Resection of Left Eustachian Tube, Via Natural or Artificial Opening Endoscopic

09TK0ZZ Resection of Nasal Mucosa and Soft Tissue, Open Approach

09TK4ZZ Resection of Nasal Mucosa and Soft Tissue, Percutaneous Endoscopic Approach

09TK8ZZ Resection of Nasal Mucosa and Soft Tissue, Via Natural or Artificial Opening Endoscopic

09TKXZZ Resection of Nasal Mucosa and Soft Tissue, External Approach

09TL0ZZ Resection of Nasal Turbinate, Open Approach

09TL4ZZ Resection of Nasal Turbinate, Percutaneous Endoscopic Approach

09TL7ZZ Resection of Nasal Turbinate, Via Natural or Artificial Opening

09TL8ZZ Resection of Nasal Turbinate, Via Natural or Artificial Opening Endoscopic

09TM0ZZ Resection of Nasal Septum, Open Approach

09TM4ZZ Resection of Nasal Septum, Percutaneous Endoscopic Approach

09TM8ZZ Resection of Nasal Septum, Via Natural or Artificial Opening Endoscopic

09TN0ZZ Resection of Nasopharynx, Open Approach

09TN4ZZ Resection of Nasopharynx, Percutaneous Endoscopic Approach

09TN7ZZ Resection of Nasopharynx, Via Natural or Artificial Opening

09TN8ZZ Resection of Nasopharynx, Via Natural or Artificial Opening Endoscopic

09TP0ZZ Resection of Accessory Sinus, Open Approach

09TP4ZZ Resection of Accessory Sinus, Percutaneous Endoscopic Approach

09TP8ZZ Resection of Accessory Sinus, Via Natural or Artificial Opening Endoscopic

09TQ0ZZ Resection of Right Maxillary Sinus, Open Approach

09TQ4ZZ Resection of Right Maxillary Sinus, Percutaneous Endoscopic Approach

09TQ8ZZ Resection of Right Maxillary Sinus, Via Natural or Artificial Opening Endoscopic

09TR0ZZ Resection of Left Maxillary Sinus, Open Approach

09TR4ZZ Resection of Left Maxillary Sinus, Percutaneous Endoscopic Approach

09TR8ZZ Resection of Left Maxillary Sinus, Via Natural or Artificial Opening Endoscopic

09TS0ZZ Resection of Right Frontal Sinus, Open Approach

09TS4ZZ Resection of Right Frontal Sinus, Percutaneous Endoscopic Approach

09TS8ZZ Resection of Right Frontal Sinus, Via Natural or Artificial Opening Endoscopic

09TT0ZZ Resection of Left Frontal Sinus, Open Approach

09TT4ZZ Resection of Left Frontal Sinus, Percutaneous Endoscopic Approach

09TT8ZZ Resection of Left Frontal Sinus, Via Natural or Artificial Opening Endoscopic

09TU0ZZ Resection of Right Ethmoid Sinus, Open Approach

09TU4ZZ Resection of Right Ethmoid Sinus, Percutaneous Endoscopic Approach

09TU8ZZ Resection of Right Ethmoid Sinus, Via Natural or Artificial Opening Endoscopic

09TV0ZZ Resection of Left Ethmoid Sinus, Open Approach

09TV4ZZ Resection of Left Ethmoid Sinus, Percutaneous Endoscopic Approach

09TV8ZZ Resection of Left Ethmoid Sinus, Via Natural or Artificial Opening Endoscopic

09TW0ZZ Resection of Right Sphenoid Sinus, Open Approach

09TW4ZZ Resection of Right Sphenoid Sinus, Percutaneous Endoscopic Approach

09TW8ZZ Resection of Right Sphenoid Sinus, Via Natural or Artificial Opening Endoscopic

09TX0ZZ Resection of Left Sphenoid Sinus, Open Approach

09TX4ZZ Resection of Left Sphenoid Sinus, Percutaneous Endoscopic Approach

09TX8ZZ Resection of Left Sphenoid Sinus, Via Natural or Artificial Opening Endoscopic

09U – Ear, Nose, Sinus, Supplement

09U007Z Supplement Right External Ear with Autologous Tissue Substitute, Open Approach

09U00JZ Supplement Right External Ear with Synthetic Substitute, Open Approach

09U00KZ Supplement Right External Ear with Nonautologous Tissue Substitute, Open Approach

09U0X7Z Supplement Right External Ear with Autologous Tissue Substitute, External Approach

09U0XJZ Supplement Right External Ear with Synthetic Substitute, External Approach

09U0XKZ Supplement Right External Ear with Nonautologous Tissue Substitute, External Approach

09U107Z Supplement Left External Ear with Autologous Tissue Substitute, Open Approach

09U10JZ Supplement Left External Ear with Synthetic Substitute, Open Approach

09U10KZ Supplement Left External Ear with Nonautologous Tissue Substitute, Open Approach

09U1X7Z Supplement Left External Ear with Autologous Tissue Substitute, External Approach

09U1XJZ Supplement Left External Ear with Synthetic Substitute, External Approach

09U1XKZ Supplement Left External Ear with Nonautologous Tissue Substitute, External Approach

09U207Z Supplement Bilateral External Ear with Autologous Tissue Substitute, Open Approach

09U20JZ Supplement Bilateral External Ear with Synthetic Substitute, Open Approach

09U20KZ Supplement Bilateral External Ear with Nonautologous Tissue Substitute, Open Approach

09U2X7Z Supplement Bilateral External Ear with Autologous Tissue Substitute, External Approach

09U2XJZ Supplement Bilateral External Ear with Synthetic Substitute, External Approach

09U2XKZ Supplement Bilateral External Ear with Nonautologous Tissue Substitute, External Approach

09U507Z Supplement Right Middle Ear with Autologous Tissue Substitute, Open Approach

09U50JZ Supplement Right Middle Ear with Synthetic Substitute, Open Approach

09U50KZ Supplement Right Middle Ear with Nonautologous Tissue Substitute, Open Approach

09U587Z Supplement Right Middle Ear with Autologous Tissue Substitute, Via Natural or Artificial Opening Endoscopic

09U58JZ Supplement Right Middle Ear with Synthetic Substitute, Via Natural or Artificial Opening Endoscopic

09U58KZ Supplement Right Middle Ear with Nonautologous Tissue Substitute, Via Natural or Artificial Opening Endoscopic

09U607Z Supplement Left Middle Ear with Autologous Tissue Substitute, Open Approach

09U60JZ Supplement Left Middle Ear with Synthetic Substitute, Open Approach

09U60KZ Supplement Left Middle Ear with Nonautologous Tissue Substitute, Open Approach

09U687Z Supplement Left Middle Ear with Autologous Tissue Substitute, Via Natural or Artificial Opening Endoscopic

09U68JZ Supplement Left Middle Ear with Synthetic Substitute, Via Natural or Artificial Opening Endoscopic

♀ Female-only   ♂ Male-only   ▲ Limited Coverage   ● Non-OR   HAC HAC-associated procedure   ▲ Non-covered procedures   ✚ Cluster

09U68KZ Supplement Left Middle Ear with Nonautologous Tissue Substitute, Via Natural or Artificial Opening Endoscopic

09U707Z Supplement Right Tympanic Membrane with Autologous Tissue Substitute, Open Approach

09U70JZ Supplement Right Tympanic Membrane with Synthetic Substitute, Open Approach

09U70KZ Supplement Right Tympanic Membrane with Nonautologous Tissue Substitute, Open Approach

09U777Z Supplement Right Tympanic Membrane with Autologous Tissue Substitute, Via Natural or Artificial Opening

09U77JZ Supplement Right Tympanic Membrane with Synthetic Substitute, Via Natural or Artificial Opening

09U77KZ Supplement Right Tympanic Membrane with Nonautologous Tissue Substitute, Via Natural or Artificial Opening

09U787Z Supplement Right Tympanic Membrane with Autologous Tissue Substitute, Via Natural or Artificial Opening Endoscopic

09U78JZ Supplement Right Tympanic Membrane with Synthetic Substitute, Via Natural or Artificial Opening Endoscopic

09U78KZ Supplement Right Tympanic Membrane with Nonautologous Tissue Substitute, Via Natural or Artificial Opening Endoscopic

09U807Z Supplement Left Tympanic Membrane with Autologous Tissue Substitute, Open Approach

09U80JZ Supplement Left Tympanic Membrane with Synthetic Substitute, Open Approach

09U80KZ Supplement Left Tympanic Membrane with Nonautologous Tissue Substitute, Open Approach

09U877Z Supplement Left Tympanic Membrane with Autologous Tissue Substitute, Via Natural or Artificial Opening

09U87JZ Supplement Left Tympanic Membrane with Synthetic Substitute, Via Natural or Artificial Opening

09U87KZ Supplement Left Tympanic Membrane with Nonautologous Tissue Substitute, Via Natural or Artificial Opening

09U887Z Supplement Left Tympanic Membrane with Autologous Tissue Substitute, Via Natural or Artificial Opening Endoscopic

09U88JZ Supplement Left Tympanic Membrane with Synthetic Substitute, Via Natural or Artificial Opening Endoscopic

09U88KZ Supplement Left Tympanic Membrane with Nonautologous Tissue Substitute, Via Natural or Artificial Opening Endoscopic

09U907Z Supplement Right Auditory Ossicle with Autologous Tissue Substitute, Open Approach

09U90JZ Supplement Right Auditory Ossicle with Synthetic Substitute, Open Approach

09U90KZ Supplement Right Auditory Ossicle with Nonautologous Tissue Substitute, Open Approach

09U987Z Supplement Right Auditory Ossicle with Autologous Tissue Substitute, Via Natural or Artificial Opening Endoscopic

09U98JZ Supplement Right Auditory Ossicle with Synthetic Substitute, Via Natural or Artificial Opening Endoscopic

09U98KZ Supplement Right Auditory Ossicle with Nonautologous Tissue Substitute, Via Natural or Artificial Opening Endoscopic

09UA07Z Supplement Left Auditory Ossicle with Autologous Tissue Substitute, Open Approach

09UA0JZ Supplement Left Auditory Ossicle with Synthetic Substitute, Open Approach

09UA0KZ Supplement Left Auditory Ossicle with Nonautologous Tissue Substitute, Open Approach

09UA87Z Supplement Left Auditory Ossicle with Autologous Tissue Substitute, Via Natural or Artificial Opening Endoscopic

09UA8JZ Supplement Left Auditory Ossicle with Synthetic Substitute, Via Natural or Artificial Opening Endoscopic

09UA8KZ Supplement Left Auditory Ossicle with Nonautologous Tissue Substitute, Via Natural or Artificial Opening Endoscopic

09UB07Z Supplement Right Mastoid Sinus with Autologous Tissue Substitute, Open Approach

09UB0JZ Supplement Right Mastoid Sinus with Synthetic Substitute, Open Approach

09UB0KZ Supplement Right Mastoid Sinus with Nonautologous Tissue Substitute, Open Approach

09UB37Z Supplement Right Mastoid Sinus with Autologous Tissue Substitute, Percutaneous Approach

09UB3JZ Supplement Right Mastoid Sinus with Synthetic Substitute, Percutaneous Approach

09UB3KZ Supplement Right Mastoid Sinus with Nonautologous Tissue Substitute, Percutaneous Approach

09UB47Z Supplement Right Mastoid Sinus with Autologous Tissue Substitute, Percutaneous Endoscopic Approach

09UB4JZ Supplement Right Mastoid Sinus with Synthetic Substitute, Percutaneous Endoscopic Approach

09UB4KZ Supplement Right Mastoid Sinus with Nonautologous Tissue Substitute, Percutaneous Endoscopic Approach

09UB77Z Supplement Right Mastoid Sinus with Autologous Tissue Substitute, Via Natural or Artificial Opening

09UB7JZ Supplement Right Mastoid Sinus with Synthetic Substitute, Via Natural or Artificial Opening

09UB7KZ Supplement Right Mastoid Sinus with Nonautologous Tissue Substitute, Via Natural or Artificial Opening

09UB87Z Supplement Right Mastoid Sinus with Autologous Tissue Substitute, Via Natural or Artificial Opening Endoscopic

09UB8JZ Supplement Right Mastoid Sinus with Synthetic Substitute, Via Natural or Artificial Opening Endoscopic

09UB8KZ Supplement Right Mastoid Sinus with Nonautologous Tissue Substitute, Via Natural or Artificial Opening Endoscopic

09UC07Z Supplement Left Mastoid Sinus with Autologous Tissue Substitute, Open Approach

09UC0JZ Supplement Left Mastoid Sinus with Synthetic Substitute, Open Approach

09UC0KZ Supplement Left Mastoid Sinus with Nonautologous Tissue Substitute, Open Approach

09UC37Z Supplement Left Mastoid Sinus with Autologous Tissue Substitute, Percutaneous Approach

09UC3JZ Supplement Left Mastoid Sinus with Synthetic Substitute, Percutaneous Approach

09UC3KZ Supplement Left Mastoid Sinus with Nonautologous Tissue Substitute, Percutaneous Approach

09UC47Z Supplement Left Mastoid Sinus with Autologous Tissue Substitute, Percutaneous Endoscopic Approach

09UC4JZ Supplement Left Mastoid Sinus with Synthetic Substitute, Percutaneous Endoscopic Approach

09UC4KZ Supplement Left Mastoid Sinus with Nonautologous Tissue Substitute, Percutaneous Endoscopic Approach

09UC77Z Supplement Left Mastoid Sinus with Autologous Tissue Substitute, Via Natural or Artificial Opening

09UC7JZ Supplement Left Mastoid Sinus with Synthetic Substitute, Via Natural or Artificial Opening

09UC7KZ Supplement Left Mastoid Sinus with Nonautologous Tissue Substitute, Via Natural or Artificial Opening

09UC87Z Supplement Left Mastoid Sinus with Autologous Tissue Substitute, Via Natural or Artificial Opening Endoscopic

09UC8JZ Supplement Left Mastoid Sinus with Synthetic Substitute, Via Natural or Artificial Opening Endoscopic

09UC8KZ Supplement Left Mastoid Sinus with Nonautologous Tissue Substitute, Via Natural or Artificial Opening Endoscopic

09UD07Z Supplement Right Inner Ear with Autologous Tissue Substitute, Open Approach

09UD0JZ Supplement Right Inner Ear with Synthetic Substitute, Open Approach

09UD0KZ Supplement Right Inner Ear with Nonautologous Tissue Substitute, Open Approach

09UD87Z Supplement Right Inner Ear with Autologous Tissue Substitute, Via Natural or Artificial Opening Endoscopic

09UD8JZ Supplement Right Inner Ear with Synthetic Substitute, Via Natural or Artificial Opening Endoscopic

09UD8KZ Supplement Right Inner Ear with Nonautologous Tissue Substitute, Via Natural or Artificial Opening Endoscopic

09UE07Z Supplement Left Inner Ear with Autologous Tissue Substitute, Open Approach

09UE0JZ Supplement Left Inner Ear with Synthetic Substitute, Open Approach

09UE0KZ Supplement Left Inner Ear with Nonautologous Tissue Substitute, Open Approach

09UE87Z Supplement Left Inner Ear with Autologous Tissue Substitute, Via Natural or Artificial Opening Endoscopic

09UE8JZ Supplement Left Inner Ear with Synthetic Substitute, Via Natural or Artificial Opening Endoscopic

09UE8KZ Supplement Left Inner Ear with Nonautologous Tissue Substitute, Via Natural or Artificial Opening Endoscopic

09UK07Z Supplement Nasal Mucosa and Soft Tissue with Autologous Tissue Substitute, Open Approach

09UK0JZ Supplement Nasal Mucosa and Soft Tissue with Synthetic Substitute, Open Approach

09UK0KZ Supplement Nasal Mucosa and Soft Tissue with Nonautologous Tissue Substitute, Open Approach

09UK87Z Supplement Nasal Mucosa and Soft Tissue with Autologous Tissue Substitute, Via Natural or Artificial Opening Endoscopic

09UK8JZ Supplement Nasal Mucosa and Soft Tissue with Synthetic Substitute, Via Natural or Artificial Opening Endoscopic

09UK8KZ Supplement Nasal Mucosa and Soft Tissue with Nonautologous Tissue Substitute, Via Natural or Artificial Opening Endoscopic

09UKX7Z Supplement Nasal Mucosa and Soft Tissue with Autologous Tissue Substitute, External Approach

09UKXJZ Supplement Nasal Mucosa and Soft Tissue with Synthetic Substitute, External Approach

09UKXKZ Supplement Nasal Mucosa and Soft Tissue with Nonautologous Tissue Substitute, External Approach

09UL07Z Supplement Nasal Turbinate with Autologous Tissue Substitute, Open Approach

09UL0JZ Supplement Nasal Turbinate with Synthetic Substitute, Open Approach

09UL0KZ Supplement Nasal Turbinate with Nonautologous Tissue Substitute, Open Approach

09UL37Z Supplement Nasal Turbinate with Autologous Tissue Substitute, Percutaneous Approach

09UL3JZ Supplement Nasal Turbinate with Synthetic Substitute, Percutaneous Approach

09UL3KZ Supplement Nasal Turbinate with Nonautologous Tissue Substitute, Percutaneous Approach

09UL47Z Supplement Nasal Turbinate with Autologous Tissue Substitute, Percutaneous Endoscopic Approach

09UL4JZ Supplement Nasal Turbinate with Synthetic Substitute, Percutaneous Endoscopic Approach

09UL4KZ Supplement Nasal Turbinate with Nonautologous Tissue Substitute, Percutaneous Endoscopic Approach

09UL77Z Supplement Nasal Turbinate with Autologous Tissue Substitute, Via Natural or Artificial Opening

09UL7JZ Supplement Nasal Turbinate with Synthetic Substitute, Via Natural or Artificial Opening

09UL7KZ Supplement Nasal Turbinate with Nonautologous Tissue Substitute, Via Natural or Artificial Opening

09UL87Z Supplement Nasal Turbinate with Autologous Tissue Substitute, Via Natural or Artificial Opening Endoscopic

09UL8JZ Supplement Nasal Turbinate with Synthetic Substitute, Via Natural or Artificial Opening Endoscopic

09UL8KZ Supplement Nasal Turbinate with Nonautologous Tissue Substitute, Via Natural or Artificial Opening Endoscopic

09UM07Z Supplement Nasal Septum with Autologous Tissue Substitute, Open Approach

09UM0JZ Supplement Nasal Septum with Synthetic Substitute, Open Approach

09UM0KZ Supplement Nasal Septum with Nonautologous Tissue Substitute, Open Approach

09UM37Z Supplement Nasal Septum with Autologous Tissue Substitute, Percutaneous Approach

09UM3JZ Supplement Nasal Septum with Synthetic Substitute, Percutaneous Approach

09UM3KZ Supplement Nasal Septum with Nonautologous Tissue Substitute, Percutaneous Approach

09UM47Z Supplement Nasal Septum with Autologous Tissue Substitute, Percutaneous Endoscopic Approach

09UM4JZ Supplement Nasal Septum with Synthetic Substitute, Percutaneous Endoscopic Approach

09UM4KZ Supplement Nasal Septum with Nonautologous Tissue Substitute, Percutaneous Endoscopic Approach

09UM87Z Supplement Nasal Septum with Autologous Tissue Substitute, Via Natural or Artificial Opening Endoscopic

09UM8JZ Supplement Nasal Septum with Synthetic Substitute, Via Natural or Artificial Opening Endoscopic

09UM8KZ Supplement Nasal Septum with Nonautologous Tissue Substitute, Via Natural or Artificial Opening Endoscopic

09UN07Z Supplement Nasopharynx with Autologous Tissue Substitute, Open Approach

09UN0JZ Supplement Nasopharynx with Synthetic Substitute, Open Approach

09UN0KZ Supplement Nasopharynx with Nonautologous Tissue Substitute, Open Approach

09UN77Z Supplement Nasopharynx with Autologous Tissue Substitute, Via Natural or Artificial Opening

09UN7JZ Supplement Nasopharynx with Synthetic Substitute, Via Natural or Artificial Opening

09UN7KZ Supplement Nasopharynx with Nonautologous Tissue Substitute, Via Natural or Artificial Opening

09UN87Z Supplement Nasopharynx with Autologous Tissue Substitute, Via Natural or Artificial Opening Endoscopic

09UN8JZ Supplement Nasopharynx with Synthetic Substitute, Via Natural or Artificial Opening Endoscopic

09UN8KZ Supplement Nasopharynx with Nonautologous Tissue Substitute, Via Natural or Artificial Opening Endoscopic

09UP07Z Supplement Accessory Sinus with Autologous Tissue Substitute, Open Approach

09UP0JZ Supplement Accessory Sinus with Synthetic Substitute, Open Approach

09UP0KZ Supplement Accessory Sinus with Nonautologous Tissue Substitute, Open Approach

09UP37Z Supplement Accessory Sinus with Autologous Tissue Substitute, Percutaneous Approach

09UP3JZ Supplement Accessory Sinus with Synthetic Substitute, Percutaneous Approach

09UP3KZ Supplement Accessory Sinus with Nonautologous Tissue Substitute, Percutaneous Approach

09UP47Z Supplement Accessory Sinus with Autologous Tissue Substitute, Percutaneous Endoscopic Approach

09UP4JZ Supplement Accessory Sinus with Synthetic Substitute, Percutaneous Endoscopic Approach

09UP4KZ Supplement Accessory Sinus with Nonautologous Tissue Substitute, Percutaneous Endoscopic Approach

09UP77Z Supplement Accessory Sinus with Autologous Tissue Substitute, Via Natural or Artificial Opening

09UP7JZ Supplement Accessory Sinus with Synthetic Substitute, Via Natural or Artificial Opening

09UP7KZ Supplement Accessory Sinus with Nonautologous Tissue Substitute, Via Natural or Artificial Opening

09UP87Z Supplement Accessory Sinus with Autologous Tissue Substitute, Via Natural or Artificial Opening Endoscopic

09UP8JZ Supplement Accessory Sinus with Synthetic Substitute, Via Natural or Artificial Opening Endoscopic

09UP8KZ Supplement Accessory Sinus with Nonautologous Tissue Substitute, Via Natural or Artificial Opening Endoscopic

09UQ07Z Supplement Right Maxillary Sinus with Autologous Tissue Substitute, Open Approach

09UQ0JZ Supplement Right Maxillary Sinus with Synthetic Substitute, Open Approach

09UQ0KZ Supplement Right Maxillary Sinus with Nonautologous Tissue Substitute, Open Approach

09UQ37Z Supplement Right Maxillary Sinus with Autologous Tissue Substitute, Percutaneous Approach

09UQ3JZ Supplement Right Maxillary Sinus with Synthetic Substitute, Percutaneous Approach

09UQ3KZ Supplement Right Maxillary Sinus with Nonautologous Tissue Substitute, Percutaneous Approach

09UQ47Z Supplement Right Maxillary Sinus with Autologous Tissue Substitute, Percutaneous Endoscopic Approach

09UQ4JZ Supplement Right Maxillary Sinus with Synthetic Substitute, Percutaneous Endoscopic Approach

09UQ4KZ Supplement Right Maxillary Sinus with Nonautologous Tissue Substitute, Percutaneous Endoscopic Approach

09UQ77Z Supplement Right Maxillary Sinus with Autologous Tissue Substitute, Via Natural or Artificial Opening

09UQ7JZ Supplement Right Maxillary Sinus with Synthetic Substitute, Via Natural or Artificial Opening

09UQ7KZ Supplement Right Maxillary Sinus with Nonautologous Tissue Substitute, Via Natural or Artificial Opening

09UQ87Z Supplement Right Maxillary Sinus with Autologous Tissue Substitute, Via Natural or Artificial Opening Endoscopic

♀ Female-only　　♂ Male-only　　▲ Limited Coverage　　● Non-OR　　HAC HAC-associated procedure　　▲ Non-covered procedures　　✚ Cluster

09UQ8JZ	Supplement Right Maxillary Sinus with Synthetic Substitute, Via Natural or Artificial Opening Endoscopic
09UQ8KZ	Supplement Right Maxillary Sinus with Nonautologous Tissue Substitute, Via Natural or Artificial Opening Endoscopic
09UR07Z	Supplement Left Maxillary Sinus with Autologous Tissue Substitute, Open Approach
09UR0JZ	Supplement Left Maxillary Sinus with Synthetic Substitute, Open Approach
09UR0KZ	Supplement Left Maxillary Sinus with Nonautologous Tissue Substitute, Open Approach
09UR37Z	Supplement Left Maxillary Sinus with Autologous Tissue Substitute, Percutaneous Approach
09UR3JZ	Supplement Left Maxillary Sinus with Synthetic Substitute, Percutaneous Approach
09UR3KZ	Supplement Left Maxillary Sinus with Nonautologous Tissue Substitute, Percutaneous Approach
09UR47Z	Supplement Left Maxillary Sinus with Autologous Tissue Substitute, Percutaneous Endoscopic Approach
09UR4JZ	Supplement Left Maxillary Sinus with Synthetic Substitute, Percutaneous Endoscopic Approach
09UR4KZ	Supplement Left Maxillary Sinus with Nonautologous Tissue Substitute, Percutaneous Endoscopic Approach
09UR77Z	Supplement Left Maxillary Sinus with Autologous Tissue Substitute, Via Natural or Artificial Opening
09UR7JZ	Supplement Left Maxillary Sinus with Synthetic Substitute, Via Natural or Artificial Opening
09UR7KZ	Supplement Left Maxillary Sinus with Nonautologous Tissue Substitute, Via Natural or Artificial Opening
09UR87Z	Supplement Left Maxillary Sinus with Autologous Tissue Substitute, Via Natural or Artificial Opening Endoscopic
09UR8JZ	Supplement Left Maxillary Sinus with Synthetic Substitute, Via Natural or Artificial Opening Endoscopic
09UR8KZ	Supplement Left Maxillary Sinus with Nonautologous Tissue Substitute, Via Natural or Artificial Opening Endoscopic
09US07Z	Supplement Right Frontal Sinus with Autologous Tissue Substitute, Open Approach
09US0JZ	Supplement Right Frontal Sinus with Synthetic Substitute, Open Approach
09US0KZ	Supplement Right Frontal Sinus with Nonautologous Tissue Substitute, Open Approach
09US37Z	Supplement Right Frontal Sinus with Autologous Tissue Substitute, Percutaneous Approach
09US3JZ	Supplement Right Frontal Sinus with Synthetic Substitute, Percutaneous Approach
09US3KZ	Supplement Right Frontal Sinus with Nonautologous Tissue Substitute, Percutaneous Approach
09US47Z	Supplement Right Frontal Sinus with Autologous Tissue Substitute, Percutaneous Endoscopic Approach
09US4JZ	Supplement Right Frontal Sinus with Synthetic Substitute, Percutaneous Endoscopic Approach
09US4KZ	Supplement Right Frontal Sinus with Nonautologous Tissue Substitute, Percutaneous Endoscopic Approach
09US77Z	Supplement Right Frontal Sinus with Autologous Tissue Substitute, Via Natural or Artificial Opening
09US7JZ	Supplement Right Frontal Sinus with Synthetic Substitute, Via Natural or Artificial Opening
09US7KZ	Supplement Right Frontal Sinus with Nonautologous Tissue Substitute, Via Natural or Artificial Opening
09US87Z	Supplement Right Frontal Sinus with Autologous Tissue Substitute, Via Natural or Artificial Opening Endoscopic
09US8JZ	Supplement Right Frontal Sinus with Synthetic Substitute, Via Natural or Artificial Opening Endoscopic
09US8KZ	Supplement Right Frontal Sinus with Nonautologous Tissue Substitute, Via Natural or Artificial Opening Endoscopic
09UT07Z	Supplement Left Frontal Sinus with Autologous Tissue Substitute, Open Approach
09UT0JZ	Supplement Left Frontal Sinus with Synthetic Substitute, Open Approach
09UT0KZ	Supplement Left Frontal Sinus with Nonautologous Tissue Substitute, Open Approach
09UT37Z	Supplement Left Frontal Sinus with Autologous Tissue Substitute, Percutaneous Approach
09UT3JZ	Supplement Left Frontal Sinus with Synthetic Substitute, Percutaneous Approach
09UT3KZ	Supplement Left Frontal Sinus with Nonautologous Tissue Substitute, Percutaneous Approach
09UT47Z	Supplement Left Frontal Sinus with Autologous Tissue Substitute, Percutaneous Endoscopic Approach
09UT4JZ	Supplement Left Frontal Sinus with Synthetic Substitute, Percutaneous Endoscopic Approach
09UT4KZ	Supplement Left Frontal Sinus with Nonautologous Tissue Substitute, Percutaneous Endoscopic Approach
09UT77Z	Supplement Left Frontal Sinus with Autologous Tissue Substitute, Via Natural or Artificial Opening
09UT7JZ	Supplement Left Frontal Sinus with Synthetic Substitute, Via Natural or Artificial Opening
09UT7KZ	Supplement Left Frontal Sinus with Nonautologous Tissue Substitute, Via Natural or Artificial Opening
09UT87Z	Supplement Left Frontal Sinus with Autologous Tissue Substitute, Via Natural or Artificial Opening Endoscopic
09UT8JZ	Supplement Left Frontal Sinus with Synthetic Substitute, Via Natural or Artificial Opening Endoscopic
09UT8KZ	Supplement Left Frontal Sinus with Nonautologous Tissue Substitute, Via Natural or Artificial Opening Endoscopic
09UU07Z	Supplement Right Ethmoid Sinus with Autologous Tissue Substitute, Open Approach
09UU0JZ	Supplement Right Ethmoid Sinus with Synthetic Substitute, Open Approach
09UU0KZ	Supplement Right Ethmoid Sinus with Nonautologous Tissue Substitute, Open Approach
09UU37Z	Supplement Right Ethmoid Sinus with Autologous Tissue Substitute, Percutaneous Approach
09UU3JZ	Supplement Right Ethmoid Sinus with Synthetic Substitute, Percutaneous Approach
09UU3KZ	Supplement Right Ethmoid Sinus with Nonautologous Tissue Substitute, Percutaneous Approach
09UU47Z	Supplement Right Ethmoid Sinus with Autologous Tissue Substitute, Percutaneous Endoscopic Approach
09UU4JZ	Supplement Right Ethmoid Sinus with Synthetic Substitute, Percutaneous Endoscopic Approach
09UU4KZ	Supplement Right Ethmoid Sinus with Nonautologous Tissue Substitute, Percutaneous Endoscopic Approach
09UU77Z	Supplement Right Ethmoid Sinus with Autologous Tissue Substitute, Via Natural or Artificial Opening
09UU7JZ	Supplement Right Ethmoid Sinus with Synthetic Substitute, Via Natural or Artificial Opening
09UU7KZ	Supplement Right Ethmoid Sinus with Nonautologous Tissue Substitute, Via Natural or Artificial Opening
09UU87Z	Supplement Right Ethmoid Sinus with Autologous Tissue Substitute, Via Natural or Artificial Opening Endoscopic
09UU8JZ	Supplement Right Ethmoid Sinus with Synthetic Substitute, Via Natural or Artificial Opening Endoscopic
09UU8KZ	Supplement Right Ethmoid Sinus with Nonautologous Tissue Substitute, Via Natural or Artificial Opening Endoscopic
09UV07Z	Supplement Left Ethmoid Sinus with Autologous Tissue Substitute, Open Approach
09UV0JZ	Supplement Left Ethmoid Sinus with Synthetic Substitute, Open Approach
09UV0KZ	Supplement Left Ethmoid Sinus with Nonautologous Tissue Substitute, Open Approach
09UV37Z	Supplement Left Ethmoid Sinus with Autologous Tissue Substitute, Percutaneous Approach
09UV3JZ	Supplement Left Ethmoid Sinus with Synthetic Substitute, Percutaneous Approach
09UV3KZ	Supplement Left Ethmoid Sinus with Nonautologous Tissue Substitute, Percutaneous Approach
09UV47Z	Supplement Left Ethmoid Sinus with Autologous Tissue Substitute, Percutaneous Endoscopic Approach
09UV4JZ	Supplement Left Ethmoid Sinus with Synthetic Substitute, Percutaneous Endoscopic Approach
09UV4KZ	Supplement Left Ethmoid Sinus with Nonautologous Tissue Substitute, Percutaneous Endoscopic Approach
09UV77Z	Supplement Left Ethmoid Sinus with Autologous Tissue Substitute, Via Natural or Artificial Opening
09UV7JZ	Supplement Left Ethmoid Sinus with Synthetic Substitute, Via Natural or Artificial Opening
09UV7KZ	Supplement Left Ethmoid Sinus with Nonautologous Tissue Substitute, Via Natural or Artificial Opening
09UV87Z	Supplement Left Ethmoid Sinus with Autologous Tissue Substitute, Via Natural or Artificial Opening Endoscopic

09UV8JZ Supplement Left Ethmoid Sinus with Synthetic Substitute, Via Natural or Artificial Opening Endoscopic

09UV8KZ Supplement Left Ethmoid Sinus with Nonautologous Tissue Substitute, Via Natural or Artificial Opening Endoscopic

09UW07Z Supplement Right Sphenoid Sinus with Autologous Tissue Substitute, Open Approach

09UW0JZ Supplement Right Sphenoid Sinus with Synthetic Substitute, Open Approach

09UW0KZ Supplement Right Sphenoid Sinus with Nonautologous Tissue Substitute, Open Approach

09UW37Z Supplement Right Sphenoid Sinus with Autologous Tissue Substitute, Percutaneous Approach

09UW3JZ Supplement Right Sphenoid Sinus with Synthetic Substitute, Percutaneous Approach

09UW3KZ Supplement Right Sphenoid Sinus with Nonautologous Tissue Substitute, Percutaneous Approach

09UW47Z Supplement Right Sphenoid Sinus with Autologous Tissue Substitute, Percutaneous Endoscopic Approach

09UW4JZ Supplement Right Sphenoid Sinus with Synthetic Substitute, Percutaneous Endoscopic Approach

09UW4KZ Supplement Right Sphenoid Sinus with Nonautologous Tissue Substitute, Percutaneous Endoscopic Approach

09UW77Z Supplement Right Sphenoid Sinus with Autologous Tissue Substitute, Via Natural or Artificial Opening

09UW7JZ Supplement Right Sphenoid Sinus with Synthetic Substitute, Via Natural or Artificial Opening

09UW7KZ Supplement Right Sphenoid Sinus with Nonautologous Tissue Substitute, Via Natural or Artificial Opening

09UW87Z Supplement Right Sphenoid Sinus with Autologous Tissue Substitute, Via Natural or Artificial Opening Endoscopic

09UW8JZ Supplement Right Sphenoid Sinus with Synthetic Substitute, Via Natural or Artificial Opening Endoscopic

09UW8KZ Supplement Right Sphenoid Sinus with Nonautologous Tissue Substitute, Via Natural or Artificial Opening Endoscopic

09UX07Z Supplement Left Sphenoid Sinus with Autologous Tissue Substitute, Open Approach

09UX0JZ Supplement Left Sphenoid Sinus with Synthetic Substitute, Open Approach

09UX0KZ Supplement Left Sphenoid Sinus with Nonautologous Tissue Substitute, Open Approach

09UX37Z Supplement Left Sphenoid Sinus with Autologous Tissue Substitute, Percutaneous Approach

09UX3JZ Supplement Left Sphenoid Sinus with Synthetic Substitute, Percutaneous Approach

09UX3KZ Supplement Left Sphenoid Sinus with Nonautologous Tissue Substitute, Percutaneous Approach

09UX47Z Supplement Left Sphenoid Sinus with Autologous Tissue Substitute, Percutaneous Endoscopic Approach

09UX4JZ Supplement Left Sphenoid Sinus with Synthetic Substitute, Percutaneous Endoscopic Approach

09UX4KZ Supplement Left Sphenoid Sinus with Nonautologous Tissue Substitute, Percutaneous Endoscopic Approach

09UX77Z Supplement Left Sphenoid Sinus with Autologous Tissue Substitute, Via Natural or Artificial Opening

09UX7JZ Supplement Left Sphenoid Sinus with Synthetic Substitute, Via Natural or Artificial Opening

09UX7KZ Supplement Left Sphenoid Sinus with Nonautologous Tissue Substitute, Via Natural or Artificial Opening

09UX87Z Supplement Left Sphenoid Sinus with Autologous Tissue Substitute, Via Natural or Artificial Opening Endoscopic

09UX8JZ Supplement Left Sphenoid Sinus with Synthetic Substitute, Via Natural or Artificial Opening Endoscopic

09UX8KZ Supplement Left Sphenoid Sinus with Nonautologous Tissue Substitute, Via Natural or Artificial Opening Endoscopic

09W – Ear, Nose, Sinus, Revision

Review Coding Guideline B6.1c

09W707Z Revision of Autologous Tissue Substitute in Right Tympanic Membrane, Open Approach

09W70JZ Revision of Synthetic Substitute in Right Tympanic Membrane, Open Approach

09W70KZ Revision of Nonautologous Tissue Substitute in Right Tympanic Membrane, Open Approach

09W777Z Revision of Autologous Tissue Substitute in Right Tympanic Membrane, Via Natural or Artificial Opening

09W77JZ Revision of Synthetic Substitute in Right Tympanic Membrane, Via Natural or Artificial Opening

09W77KZ Revision of Nonautologous Tissue Substitute in Right Tympanic Membrane, Via Natural or Artificial Opening

09W787Z Revision of Autologous Tissue Substitute in Right Tympanic Membrane, Via Natural or Artificial Opening Endoscopic

09W78JZ Revision of Synthetic Substitute in Right Tympanic Membrane, Via Natural or Artificial Opening Endoscopic

09W78KZ Revision of Nonautologous Tissue Substitute in Right Tympanic Membrane, Via Natural or Artificial Opening Endoscopic

09W807Z Revision of Autologous Tissue Substitute in Left Tympanic Membrane, Open Approach

09W80JZ Revision of Synthetic Substitute in Left Tympanic Membrane, Open Approach

09W80KZ Revision of Nonautologous Tissue Substitute in Left Tympanic Membrane, Open Approach

09W877Z Revision of Autologous Tissue Substitute in Left Tympanic Membrane, Via Natural or Artificial Opening

09W87JZ Revision of Synthetic Substitute in Left Tympanic Membrane, Via Natural or Artificial Opening

09W87KZ Revision of Nonautologous Tissue Substitute in Left Tympanic Membrane, Via Natural or Artificial Opening

09W887Z Revision of Autologous Tissue Substitute in Left Tympanic Membrane, Via Natural or Artificial Opening Endoscopic

09W88JZ Revision of Synthetic Substitute in Left Tympanic Membrane, Via Natural or Artificial Opening Endoscopic

09W88KZ Revision of Nonautologous Tissue Substitute in Left Tympanic Membrane, Via Natural or Artificial Opening Endoscopic

09W907Z Revision of Autologous Tissue Substitute in Right Auditory Ossicle, Open Approach

09W90JZ Revision of Synthetic Substitute in Right Auditory Ossicle, Open Approach

09W90KZ Revision of Nonautologous Tissue Substitute in Right Auditory Ossicle, Open Approach

09W977Z Revision of Autologous Tissue Substitute in Right Auditory Ossicle, Via Natural or Artificial Opening

09W97JZ Revision of Synthetic Substitute in Right Auditory Ossicle, Via Natural or Artificial Opening

09W97KZ Revision of Nonautologous Tissue Substitute in Right Auditory Ossicle, Via Natural or Artificial Opening

09W987Z Revision of Autologous Tissue Substitute in Right Auditory Ossicle, Via Natural or Artificial Opening Endoscopic

09W98JZ Revision of Synthetic Substitute in Right Auditory Ossicle, Via Natural or Artificial Opening Endoscopic

09W98KZ Revision of Nonautologous Tissue Substitute in Right Auditory Ossicle, Via Natural or Artificial Opening Endoscopic

09WA07Z Revision of Autologous Tissue Substitute in Left Auditory Ossicle, Open Approach

09WA0JZ Revision of Synthetic Substitute in Left Auditory Ossicle, Open Approach

09WA0KZ Revision of Nonautologous Tissue Substitute in Left Auditory Ossicle, Open Approach

09WA77Z Revision of Autologous Tissue Substitute in Left Auditory Ossicle, Via Natural or Artificial Opening

09WA7JZ Revision of Synthetic Substitute in Left Auditory Ossicle, Via Natural or Artificial Opening

09WA7KZ Revision of Nonautologous Tissue Substitute in Left Auditory Ossicle, Via Natural or Artificial Opening

09WA87Z Revision of Autologous Tissue Substitute in Left Auditory Ossicle, Via Natural or Artificial Opening Endoscopic

09WA8JZ Revision of Synthetic Substitute in Left Auditory Ossicle, Via Natural or Artificial Opening Endoscopic

09WA8KZ Revision of Nonautologous Tissue Substitute in Left Auditory Ossicle, Via Natural or Artificial Opening Endoscopic

09WD0SZ Revision of Hearing Device in Right Inner Ear, Open Approach

09WD7SZ Revision of Hearing Device in Right Inner Ear, Via Natural or Artificial Opening

09WD8SZ Revision of Hearing Device in Right Inner Ear, Via Natural or Artificial Opening Endoscopic

09WE0SZ Revision of Hearing Device in Left Inner Ear, Open Approach

09WE7SZ Revision of Hearing Device in Left Inner Ear, Via Natural or Artificial Opening

09WE8SZ Revision of Hearing Device in Left Inner Ear, Via Natural or Artificial Opening Endoscopic

09WH00Z Revision of Drainage Device in Right Ear, Open Approach

09WH07Z Revision of Autologous Tissue Substitute in Right Ear, Open Approach

09WH0DZ Revision of Intraluminal Device in Right Ear, Open Approach

09WH0JZ Revision of Synthetic Substitute in Right Ear, Open Approach

09WH0KZ Revision of Nonautologous Tissue Substitute in Right Ear, Open Approach

09WH0YZ Revision of Other Device in Right Ear, Open Approach

09WH30Z Revision of Drainage Device in Right Ear, Percutaneous Approach

09WH37Z Revision of Autologous Tissue Substitute in Right Ear, Percutaneous Approach

09WH3DZ Revision of Intraluminal Device in Right Ear, Percutaneous Approach

09WH3JZ Revision of Synthetic Substitute in Right Ear, Percutaneous Approach

09WH3KZ Revision of Nonautologous Tissue Substitute in Right Ear, Percutaneous Approach

09WH3YZ Revision of Other Device in Right Ear, Percutaneous Approach

09WH40Z Revision of Drainage Device in Right Ear, Percutaneous Endoscopic Approach

09WH47Z Revision of Autologous Tissue Substitute in Right Ear, Percutaneous Endoscopic Approach

09WH4DZ Revision of Intraluminal Device in Right Ear, Percutaneous Endoscopic Approach

09WH4JZ Revision of Synthetic Substitute in Right Ear, Percutaneous Endoscopic Approach

09WH4KZ Revision of Nonautologous Tissue Substitute in Right Ear, Percutaneous Endoscopic Approach

09WH4YZ Revision of Other Device in Right Ear, Percutaneous Endoscopic Approach

09WH70Z Revision of Drainage Device in Right Ear, Via Natural or Artificial Opening

09WH77Z Revision of Autologous Tissue Substitute in Right Ear, Via Natural or Artificial Opening

09WH7DZ Revision of Intraluminal Device in Right Ear, Via Natural or Artificial Opening

09WH7JZ Revision of Synthetic Substitute in Right Ear, Via Natural or Artificial Opening

09WH7KZ Revision of Nonautologous Tissue Substitute in Right Ear, Via Natural or Artificial Opening

09WH7YZ Revision of Other Device in Right Ear, Via Natural or Artificial Opening

09WH80Z Revision of Drainage Device in Right Ear, Via Natural or Artificial Opening Endoscopic

09WH87Z Revision of Autologous Tissue Substitute in Right Ear, Via Natural or Artificial Opening Endoscopic

09WH8DZ Revision of Intraluminal Device in Right Ear, Via Natural or Artificial Opening Endoscopic

09WH8JZ Revision of Synthetic Substitute in Right Ear, Via Natural or Artificial Opening Endoscopic

09WH8KZ Revision of Nonautologous Tissue Substitute in Right Ear, Via Natural or Artificial Opening Endoscopic

09WH8YZ Revision of Other Device in Right Ear, Via Natural or Artificial Opening Endoscopic

09WHX0Z Revision of Drainage Device in Right Ear, External Approach

09WHX7Z Revision of Autologous Tissue Substitute in Right Ear, External Approach

09WHXDZ Revision of Intraluminal Device in Right Ear, External Approach

09WHXJZ Revision of Synthetic Substitute in Right Ear, External Approach

09WHXKZ Revision of Nonautologous Tissue Substitute in Right Ear, External Approach

09WJ00Z Revision of Drainage Device in Left Ear, Open Approach

09WJ07Z Revision of Autologous Tissue Substitute in Left Ear, Open Approach

09WJ0DZ Revision of Intraluminal Device in Left Ear, Open Approach

09WJ0JZ Revision of Synthetic Substitute in Left Ear, Open Approach

09WJ0KZ Revision of Nonautologous Tissue Substitute in Left Ear, Open Approach

09WJ0YZ Revision of Other Device in Left Ear, Open Approach

09WJ30Z Revision of Drainage Device in Left Ear, Percutaneous Approach

09WJ37Z Revision of Autologous Tissue Substitute in Left Ear, Percutaneous Approach

09WJ3DZ Revision of Intraluminal Device in Left Ear, Percutaneous Approach

09WJ3JZ Revision of Synthetic Substitute in Left Ear, Percutaneous Approach

09WJ3KZ Revision of Nonautologous Tissue Substitute in Left Ear, Percutaneous Approach

09WJ3YZ Revision of Other Device in Left Ear, Percutaneous Approach

09WJ40Z Revision of Drainage Device in Left Ear, Percutaneous Endoscopic Approach

09WJ47Z Revision of Autologous Tissue Substitute in Left Ear, Percutaneous Endoscopic Approach

09WJ4DZ Revision of Intraluminal Device in Left Ear, Percutaneous Endoscopic Approach

09WJ4JZ Revision of Synthetic Substitute in Left Ear, Percutaneous Endoscopic Approach

09WJ4KZ Revision of Nonautologous Tissue Substitute in Left Ear, Percutaneous Endoscopic Approach

09WJ4YZ Revision of Other Device in Left Ear, Percutaneous Endoscopic Approach

09WJ70Z Revision of Drainage Device in Left Ear, Via Natural or Artificial Opening

09WJ77Z Revision of Autologous Tissue Substitute in Left Ear, Via Natural or Artificial Opening

09WJ7DZ Revision of Intraluminal Device in Left Ear, Via Natural or Artificial Opening

09WJ7JZ Revision of Synthetic Substitute in Left Ear, Via Natural or Artificial Opening

09WJ7KZ Revision of Nonautologous Tissue Substitute in Left Ear, Via Natural or Artificial Opening

09WJ7YZ Revision of Other Device in Left Ear, Via Natural or Artificial Opening

09WJ80Z Revision of Drainage Device in Left Ear, Via Natural or Artificial Opening Endoscopic

09WJ87Z Revision of Autologous Tissue Substitute in Left Ear, Via Natural or Artificial Opening Endoscopic

09WJ8DZ Revision of Intraluminal Device in Left Ear, Via Natural or Artificial Opening Endoscopic

09WJ8JZ Revision of Synthetic Substitute in Left Ear, Via Natural or Artificial Opening Endoscopic

09WJ8KZ Revision of Nonautologous Tissue Substitute in Left Ear, Via Natural or Artificial Opening Endoscopic

09WJ8YZ Revision of Other Device in Left Ear, Via Natural or Artificial Opening Endoscopic

09WJX0Z Revision of Drainage Device in Left Ear, External Approach

09WJX7Z Revision of Autologous Tissue Substitute in Left Ear, External Approach

09WJXDZ Revision of Intraluminal Device in Left Ear, External Approach

09WJXJZ Revision of Synthetic Substitute in Left Ear, External Approach

09WJXKZ Revision of Nonautologous Tissue Substitute in Left Ear, External Approach

09WK00Z Revision of Drainage Device in Nasal Mucosa and Soft Tissue, Open Approach

09WK07Z Revision of Autologous Tissue Substitute in Nasal Mucosa and Soft Tissue, Open Approach

09WK0DZ Revision of Intraluminal Device in Nasal Mucosa and Soft Tissue, Open Approach

09WK0JZ Revision of Synthetic Substitute in Nasal Mucosa and Soft Tissue, Open Approach

09WK0KZ Revision of Nonautologous Tissue Substitute in Nasal Mucosa and Soft Tissue, Open Approach

09WK0YZ Revision of Other Device in Nasal Mucosa and Soft Tissue, Open Approach

09WK30Z Revision of Drainage Device in Nasal Mucosa and Soft Tissue, Percutaneous Approach

09WK37Z Revision of Autologous Tissue Substitute in Nasal Mucosa and Soft Tissue, Percutaneous Approach

09WK3DZ Revision of Intraluminal Device in Nasal Mucosa and Soft Tissue, Percutaneous Approach

09WK3JZ Revision of Synthetic Substitute in Nasal Mucosa and Soft Tissue, Percutaneous Approach

09WK3KZ Revision of Nonautologous Tissue Substitute in Nasal Mucosa and Soft Tissue, Percutaneous Approach

09WK3YZ Revision of Other Device in Nasal Mucosa and Soft Tissue, Percutaneous Approach

09WK40Z Revision of Drainage Device in Nasal Mucosa and Soft Tissue, Percutaneous Endoscopic Approach

09WK47Z Revision of Autologous Tissue Substitute in Nasal Mucosa and Soft Tissue, Percutaneous Endoscopic Approach

09WK4DZ Revision of Intraluminal Device in Nasal Mucosa and Soft Tissue, Percutaneous Endoscopic Approach

09WK4JZ Revision of Synthetic Substitute in Nasal Mucosa and Soft Tissue, Percutaneous Endoscopic Approach

09WK4KZ Revision of Nonautologous Tissue Substitute in Nasal Mucosa and Soft Tissue, Percutaneous Endoscopic Approach

09WK4YZ Revision of Other Device in Nasal Mucosa and Soft Tissue, Percutaneous Endoscopic Approach

09WK70Z Revision of Drainage Device in Nasal Mucosa and Soft Tissue, Via Natural or Artificial Opening

09WK77Z Revision of Autologous Tissue Substitute in Nasal Mucosa and Soft Tissue, Via Natural or Artificial Opening

09WK7DZ Revision of Intraluminal Device in Nasal Mucosa and Soft Tissue, Via Natural or Artificial Opening

09WK7JZ Revision of Synthetic Substitute in Nasal Mucosa and Soft Tissue, Via Natural or Artificial Opening

09WK7KZ Revision of Nonautologous Tissue Substitute in Nasal Mucosa and Soft Tissue, Via Natural or Artificial Opening

09WK7YZ Revision of Other Device in Nasal Mucosa and Soft Tissue, Via Natural or Artificial Opening

09WK80Z Revision of Drainage Device in Nasal Mucosa and Soft Tissue, Via Natural or Artificial Opening Endoscopic

09WK87Z Revision of Autologous Tissue Substitute in Nasal Mucosa and Soft Tissue, Via Natural or Artificial Opening Endoscopic

09WK8DZ Revision of Intraluminal Device in Nasal Mucosa and Soft Tissue, Via Natural or Artificial Opening Endoscopic

09WK8JZ Revision of Synthetic Substitute in Nasal Mucosa and Soft Tissue, Via Natural or Artificial Opening Endoscopic

09WK8KZ Revision of Nonautologous Tissue Substitute in Nasal Mucosa and Soft Tissue, Via Natural or Artificial Opening Endoscopic

09WK8YZ Revision of Other Device in Nasal Mucosa and Soft Tissue, Via Natural or Artificial Opening Endoscopic

09WKX0Z Revision of Drainage Device in Nasal Mucosa and Soft Tissue, External Approach

09WKX7Z Revision of Autologous Tissue Substitute in Nasal Mucosa and Soft Tissue, External Approach

09WKXDZ Revision of Intraluminal Device in Nasal Mucosa and Soft Tissue, External Approach

09WKXJZ Revision of Synthetic Substitute in Nasal Mucosa and Soft Tissue, External Approach

09WKXKZ Revision of Nonautologous Tissue Substitute in Nasal Mucosa and Soft Tissue, External Approach

09WY00Z Revision of Drainage Device in Sinus, Open Approach

09WY0YZ Revision of Other Device in Sinus, Open Approach

09WY30Z Revision of Drainage Device in Sinus, Percutaneous Approach

09WY3YZ Revision of Other Device in Sinus, Percutaneous Approach

09WY40Z Revision of Drainage Device in Sinus, Percutaneous Endoscopic Approach

09WY4YZ Revision of Other Device in Sinus, Percutaneous Endoscopic Approach

09WY7YZ Revision of Other Device in Sinus, Via Natural or Artificial Opening

09WY8YZ Revision of Other Device in Sinus, Via Natural or Artificial Opening Endoscopic

09WYX0Z Revision of Drainage Device in Sinus, External Approach

♀ Female-only   ♂ Male-only   ▲ Limited Coverage   ● Non-OR   HAC HAC-associated procedure   ▲ Non-covered procedures   ➕ Cluster

Topography of Lungs: Anterior View

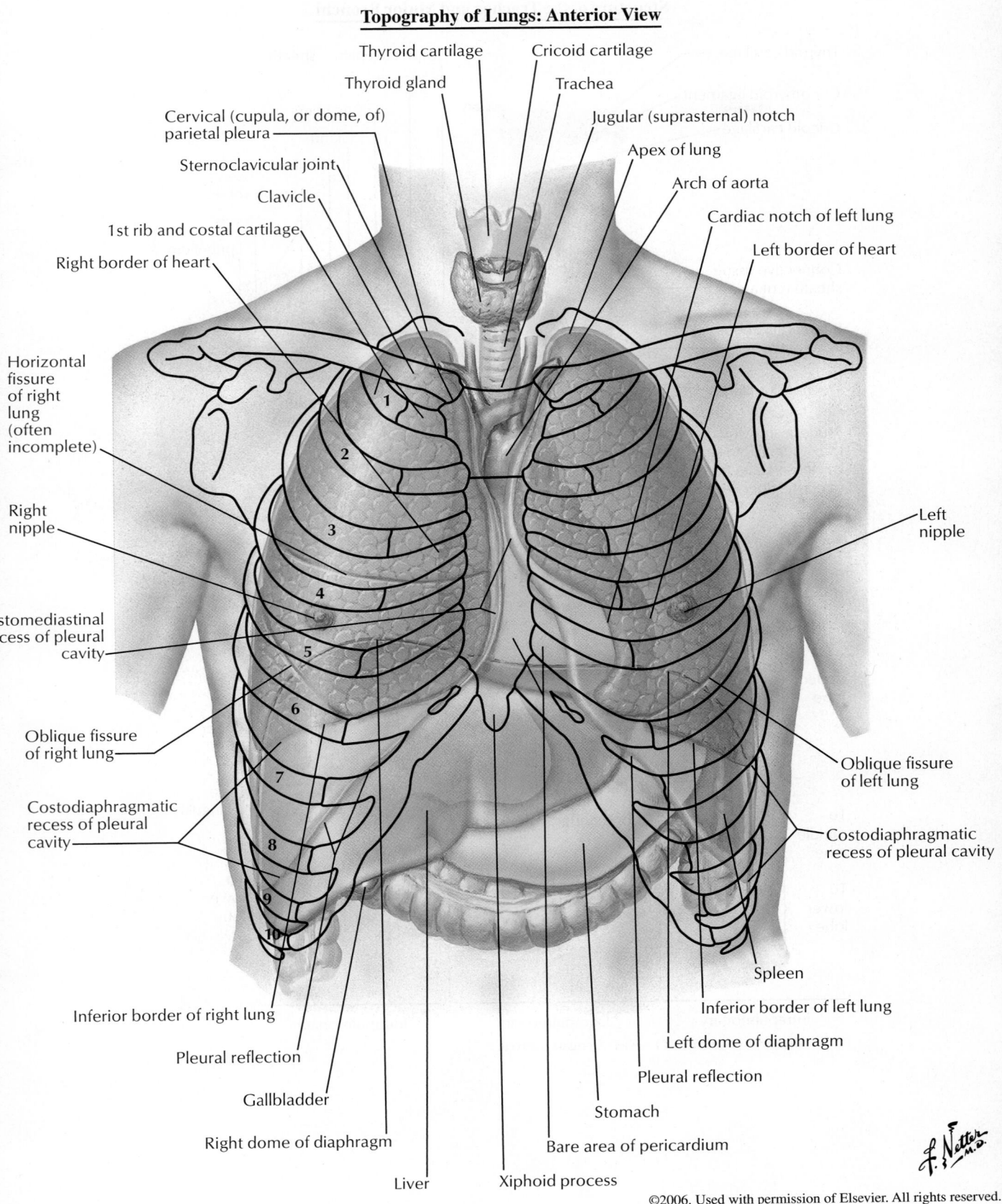

Thyroid cartilage

Cricoid cartilage

Thyroid gland

Trachea

Cervical (cupula, or dome, of) parietal pleura

Jugular (suprasternal) notch

Apex of lung

Sternoclavicular joint

Arch of aorta

Clavicle

Cardiac notch of left lung

1st rib and costal cartilage

Left border of heart

Right border of heart

Horizontal fissure of right lung (often incomplete)

Right nipple

Left nipple

Costomediastinal recess of pleural cavity

Oblique fissure of right lung

Oblique fissure of left lung

Costodiaphragmatic recess of pleural cavity

Costodiaphragmatic recess of pleural cavity

Spleen

Inferior border of right lung

Inferior border of left lung

Pleural reflection

Left dome of diaphragm

Gallbladder

Pleural reflection

Right dome of diaphragm

Stomach

Liver

Bare area of pericardium

Xiphoid process

Structure of the Trachea and Major Bronchi

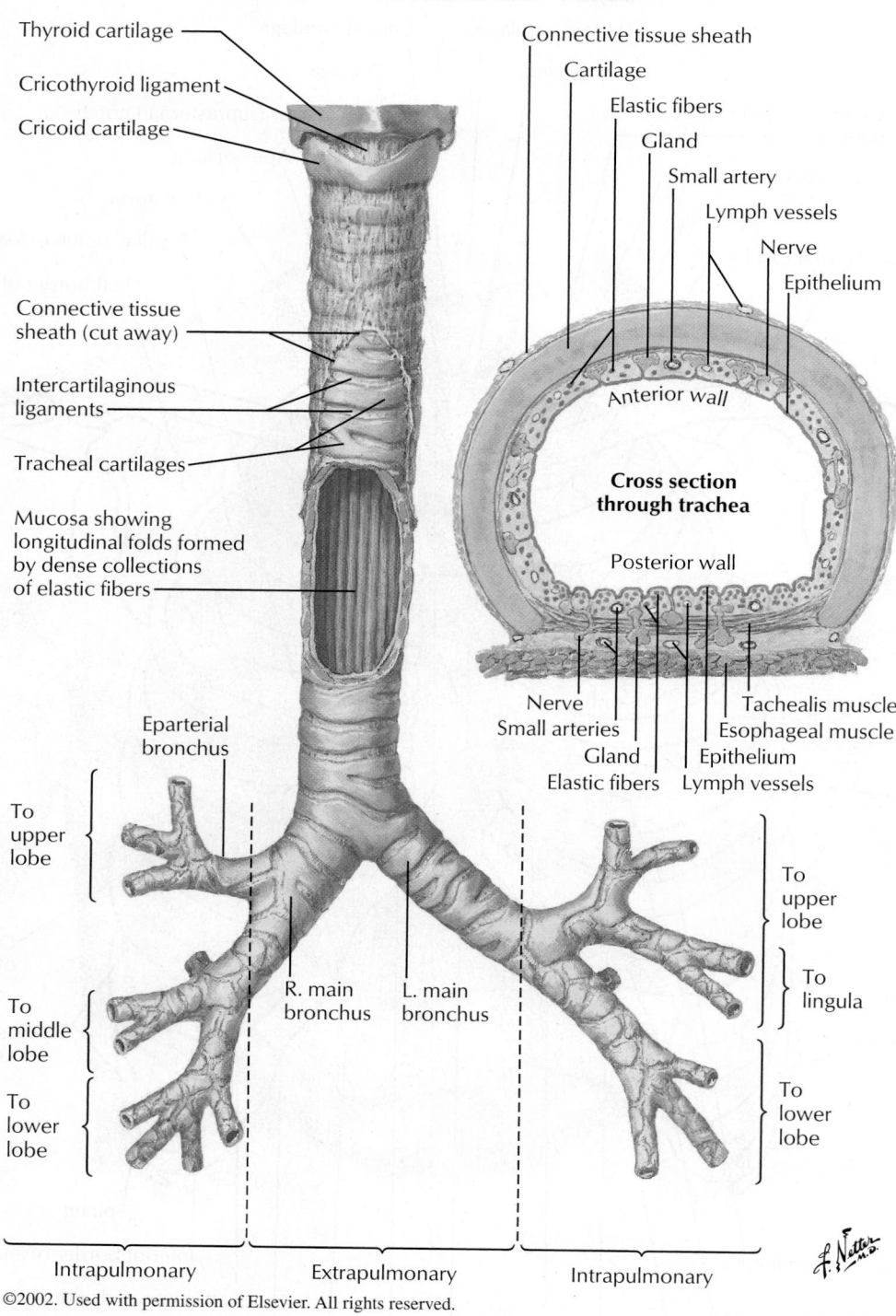

Thyroid cartilage

Cricothyroid ligament

Cricoid cartilage

Connective tissue sheath (cut away)

Intercartilaginous ligaments

Tracheal cartilages

Mucosa showing longitudinal folds formed by dense collections of elastic fibers

Connective tissue sheath

Cartilage

Elastic fibers

Gland

Small artery

Lymph vessels

Nerve

Epithelium

Anterior wall

Cross section through trachea

Posterior wall

Nerve

Small arteries

Gland

Elastic fibers

Tachealis muscle

Esophageal muscle

Epithelium

Lymph vessels

Eparterial bronchus

To upper lobe

To middle lobe

To lower lobe

R. main bronchus

L. main bronchus

To upper lobe

To lingula

To lower lobe

Intrapulmonary

Extrapulmonary

Intrapulmonary

Sublobar Resection and Surgical Lung Biopsy

Segmental resection

Left apical-posterior segment

Intersegmental vein

Segmental bronchus divided and stapled (or oversewn)

Left pulmonary artery

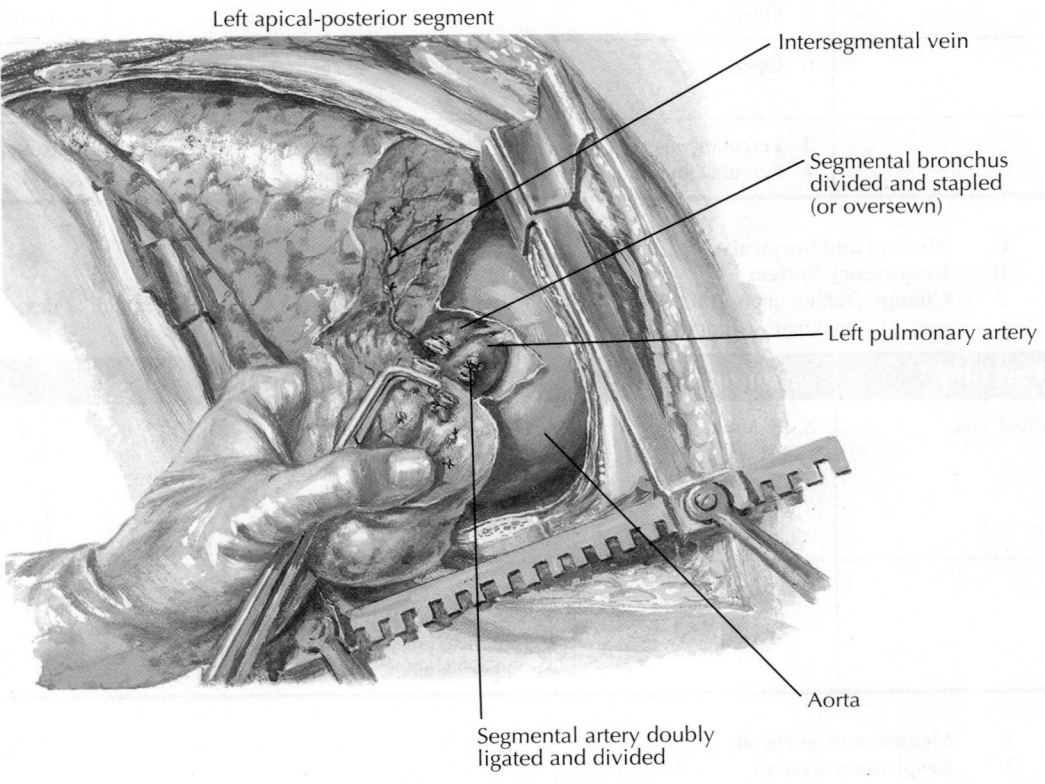

Segmental artery doubly ligated and divided

Aorta

Wedge resection or open lung biopsy

Using stapling-cutting device

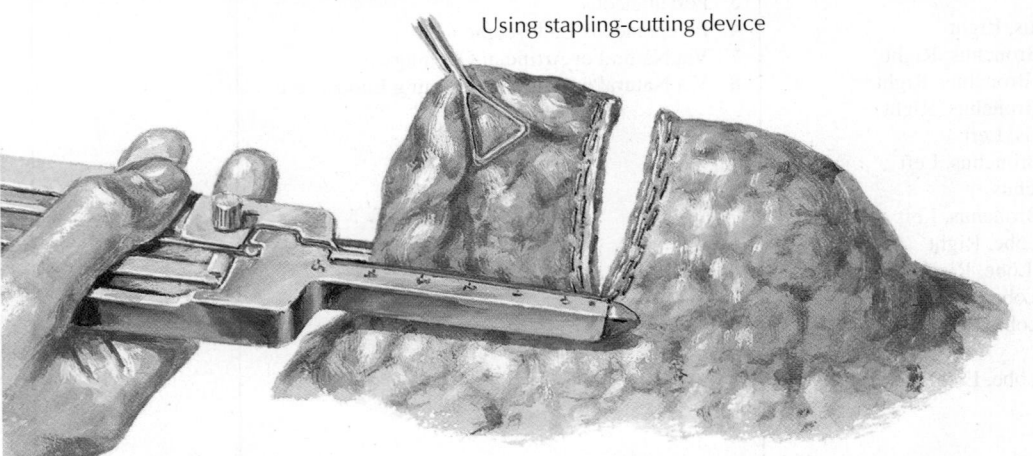

Respiratory System Tables 0B1–0BY

Section	0	Medical and Surgical
Body System	B	Respiratory System
Operation	1	**Bypass:** Altering the route of passage of the contents of a tubular body part

Body Part (4th)	Approach (5th)	Device (6th)	Qualifier (7th)
1 Trachea	0 Open	D Intraluminal Device	6 Esophagus
1 Trachea	0 Open	F Tracheostomy Device Z No Device	4 Cutaneous
1 Trachea	3 Percutaneous 4 Percutaneous Endoscopic	F Tracheostomy Device Z No Device	4 Cutaneous

Section	0	Medical and Surgical
Body System	B	Respiratory System
Operation	2	**Change:** Taking out or off a device from a body part and putting back an identical or similar device in or on the same body part without cutting or puncturing the skin or a mucous membrane

Body Part (4th)	Approach (5th)	Device (6th)	Qualifier (7th)
0 Tracheobronchial Tree K Lung, Right L Lung, Left Q Pleura T Diaphragm	X External	0 Drainage Device Y Other Device	Z No Qualifier
1 Trachea	X External	0 Drainage Device E Intraluminal Device, Endotracheal Airway F Tracheostomy Device Y Other Device	Z No Qualifier

Section	0	Medical and Surgical
Body System	B	Respiratory System
Operation	5	**Destruction:** Physical eradication of all or a portion of a body part by the direct use of energy, force, or a destructive agent

Body Part (4th)	Approach (5th)	Device (6th)	Qualifier (7th)
1 Trachea 2 Carina 3 Main Bronchus, Right 4 Upper Lobe Bronchus, Right 5 Middle Lobe Bronchus, Right 6 Lower Lobe Bronchus, Right 7 Main Bronchus, Left 8 Upper Lobe Bronchus, Left 9 Lingula Bronchus B Lower Lobe Bronchus, Left C Upper Lung Lobe, Right D Middle Lung Lobe, Right F Lower Lung Lobe, Right G Upper Lung Lobe, Left H Lung Lingula J Lower Lung Lobe, Left K Lung, Right L Lung, Left M Lungs, Bilateral	0 Open 3 Percutaneous 4 Percutaneous Endoscopic 7 Via Natural or Artificial Opening 8 Via Natural or Artificial Opening Endoscopic	Z No Device	Z No Qualifier
N Pleura, Right P Pleura, Left T Diaphragm	0 Open 3 Percutaneous 4 Percutaneous Endoscopic	Z No Device	Z No Qualifier

Section   **0**   **Medical and Surgical**
Body System   **B**   **Respiratory System**
Operation   **7**   **Dilation:** Expanding an orifice or the lumen of a tubular body part

Body Part (4th)	Approach (5th)	Device (6th)	Qualifier (7th)
1 Trachea 2 Carina 3 Main Bronchus, Right 4 Upper Lobe Bronchus, Right 5 Middle Lobe Bronchus, Right 6 Lower Lobe Bronchus, Right 7 Main Bronchus, Left 8 Upper Lobe Bronchus, Left 9 Lingula Bronchus B Lower Lobe Bronchus, Left	0 Open 3 Percutaneous 4 Percutaneous Endoscopic 7 Via Natural or Artificial Opening 8 Via Natural or Artificial Opening Endoscopic	D Intraluminal Device Z No Device	Z No Qualifier

Section   **0**   **Medical and Surgical**
Body System   **B**   **Respiratory System**
Operation   **9**   **Drainage:** Taking or letting out fluids and/or gases from a body part

Body Part (4th)	Approach (5th)	Device (6th)	Qualifier (7th)
1 Trachea 2 Carina 3 Main Bronchus, Right 4 Upper Lobe Bronchus, Right 5 Middle Lobe Bronchus, Right 6 Lower Lobe Bronchus, Right 7 Main Bronchus, Left 8 Upper Lobe Bronchus, Left 9 Lingula Bronchus B Lower Lobe Bronchus, Left C Upper Lung Lobe, Right D Middle Lung Lobe, Right F Lower Lung Lobe, Right G Upper Lung Lobe, Left H Lung Lingula J Lower Lung Lobe, Left K Lung, Right L Lung, Left M Lungs, Bilateral	0 Open 3 Percutaneous 4 Percutaneous Endoscopic 7 Via Natural or Artificial Opening 8 Via Natural or Artificial Opening Endoscopic	0 Drainage Device	Z No Qualifier
1 Trachea 2 Carina 3 Main Bronchus, Right 4 Upper Lobe Bronchus, Right 5 Middle Lobe Bronchus, Right 6 Lower Lobe Bronchus, Right 7 Main Bronchus, Left 8 Upper Lobe Bronchus, Left 9 Lingula Bronchus B Lower Lobe Bronchus, Left C Upper Lung Lobe, Right D Middle Lung Lobe, Right F Lower Lung Lobe, Right G Upper Lung Lobe, Left H Lung Lingula J Lower Lung Lobe, Left K Lung, Right L Lung, Left M Lungs, Bilateral	0 Open 3 Percutaneous 4 Percutaneous Endoscopic 7 Via Natural or Artificial Opening 8 Via Natural or Artificial Opening Endoscopic	Z No Device	X Diagnostic Z No Qualifier
N Pleura, Right P Pleura, Left	0 Open 3 Percutaneous 4 Percutaneous Endoscopic 8 Via Natural or Artificial Opening Endoscopic	0 Drainage Device	Z No Qualifier

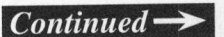
Continued →

Section	0	Medical and Surgical
Body System	B	Respiratory System
Operation	9	Drainage: Taking or letting out fluids and/or gases from a body part

Body Part (4th)	Approach (5th)	Device (6th)	Qualifier (7th)
N Pleura, Right P Pleura, Left	0 Open 3 Percutaneous 4 Percutaneous Endoscopic 8 Via Natural or Artificial Opening Endoscopic	Z No Device	X Diagnostic Z No Qualifier
T Diaphragm	0 Open 3 Percutaneous 4 Percutaneous Endoscopic	0 Drainage Device	Z No Qualifier
T Diaphragm	0 Open 3 Percutaneous 4 Percutaneous Endoscopic	Z No Device	X Diagnostic Z No Qualifier

Section	0	Medical and Surgical
Body System	B	Respiratory System
Operation	B	Excision: Cutting out or off, without replacement, a portion of a body part

Body Part (4th)	Approach (5th)	Device (6th)	Qualifier (7th)
1 Trachea 2 Carina 3 Main Bronchus, Right 4 Upper Lobe Bronchus, Right 5 Middle Lobe Bronchus, Right 6 Lower Lobe Bronchus, Right 7 Main Bronchus, Left 8 Upper Lobe Bronchus, Left 9 Lingula Bronchus B Lower Lobe Bronchus, Left C Upper Lung Lobe, Right D Middle Lung Lobe, Right F Lower Lung Lobe, Right G Upper Lung Lobe, Left H Lung Lingula J Lower Lung Lobe, Left K Lung, Right L Lung, Left M Lungs, Bilateral	0 Open 3 Percutaneous 4 Percutaneous Endoscopic 7 Via Natural or Artificial Opening 8 Via Natural or Artificial Opening Endoscopic	Z No Device	X Diagnostic Z No Qualifier
N Pleura, Right P Pleura, Left	0 Open 3 Percutaneous 4 Percutaneous Endoscopic 8 Via Natural or Artificial Opening Endoscopic	Z No Device	X Diagnostic Z No Qualifier
T Diaphragm	0 Open 3 Percutaneous 4 Percutaneous Endoscopic	Z No Device	X Diagnostic Z No Qualifier

Section   0   **Medical and Surgical**
Body System   B   **Respiratory System**
Operation   C   **Extirpation:** Taking or cutting out solid matter from a body part

Body Part (4th)	Approach (5th)	Device (6th)	Qualifier (7th)
1 Trachea 2 Carina 3 Main Bronchus, Right 4 Upper Lobe Bronchus, Right 5 Middle Lobe Bronchus, Right 6 Lower Lobe Bronchus, Right 7 Main Bronchus, Left 8 Upper Lobe Bronchus, Left 9 Lingula Bronchus B Lower Lobe Bronchus, Left C Upper Lung Lobe, Right D Middle Lung Lobe, Right F Lower Lung Lobe, Right G Upper Lung Lobe, Left H Lung Lingula J Lower Lung Lobe, Left K Lung, Right L Lung, Left M Lungs, Bilateral	0 Open 3 Percutaneous 4 Percutaneous Endoscopic 7 Via Natural or Artificial Opening 8 Via Natural or Artificial Opening Endoscopic	Z No Device	Z No Qualifier
N Pleura, Right P Pleura, Left T Diaphragm	0 Open 3 Percutaneous 4 Percutaneous Endoscopic	Z No Device	Z No Qualifier

Section   0   **Medical and Surgical**
Body System   B   **Respiratory System**
Operation   D   **Extraction:** Pulling or stripping out or off all or a portion of a body part by the use of force

Body Part (4th)	Approach (5th)	Device (6th)	Qualifier (7th)
1 Trachea 2 Carina 3 Main Bronchus, Right 4 Upper Lobe Bronchus, Right 5 Middle Lobe Bronchus, Right 6 Lower Lobe Bronchus, Right 7 Main Bronchus, Left 8 Upper Lobe Bronchus, Left 9 Lingula Bronchus B Lower Lobe Bronchus, Left C Upper Lung Lobe, Right D Middle Lung Lobe, Right F Lower Lung Lobe, Right G Upper Lung Lobe, Left H Lung Lingula J Lower Lung Lobe, Left K Lung, Right L Lung, Left M Lung, Bilateral	4 Percutaneous Endoscopic 8 Via Natural or Artificial Opening Endoscopic	Z No Device	X Diagnostic
N Pleura, Right P Pleura, Left	0 Open 3 Percutaneous 4 Percutaneous Endoscopic	Z No Device	X Diagnostic Z No Qualifier

Section	**0** **Medical and Surgical**
Body System	**B** **Respiratory System**
Operation	**F** **Fragmentation:** Breaking solid matter in a body part into pieces

Body Part (4th)	Approach (5th)	Device (6th)	Qualifier (7th)
1 Trachea 2 Carina 3 Main Bronchus, Right 4 Upper Lobe Bronchus, Right 5 Middle Lobe Bronchus, Right 6 Lower Lobe Bronchus, Right 7 Main Bronchus, Left 8 Upper Lobe Bronchus, Left 9 Lingula Bronchus B Lower Lobe Bronchus, Left	0 Open 3 Percutaneous 4 Percutaneous Endoscopic 7 Via Natural or Artificial Opening 8 Via Natural or Artificial Opening Endoscopic X External	Z No Device	Z No Qualifier

Section	**0** **Medical and Surgical**
Body System	**B** **Respiratory System**
Operation	**H** **Insertion:** Putting in a nonbiological appliance that monitors, assists, performs, or prevents a physiological function but does not physically take the place of a body part

Body Part (4th)	Approach (5th)	Device (6th)	Qualifier (7th)
0 Tracheobronchial Tree	0 Open 3 Percutaneous 4 Percutaneous Endoscopic 7 Via Natural or Artificial Opening 8 Via Natural or Artificial Opening Endoscopic	1 Radioactive Element 2 Monitoring Device 3 Infusion Device D Intraluminal Device Y Other Device	Z No Qualifier
1 Trachea	0 Open	2 Monitoring Device D Intraluminal Device Y Other Device	Z No Qualifier
1 Trachea	3 Percutaneous	D Intraluminal Device E Intraluminal Device, Endotracheal Airway Y Other Device	Z No Qualifier
1 Trachea	4 Percutaneous Endoscopic	D Intraluminal Device Y Other Device	Z No Qualifier
1 Trachea	7 Via Natural or Artificial Opening 8 Via Natural or Artificial Opening Endoscopic	2 Monitoring Device D Intraluminal Device E Intraluminal Device, Endotracheal Airway Y Other Device	Z No Qualifier
3 Main Bronchus, Right 4 Upper Lobe Bronchus, Right 5 Middle Lobe Bronchus, Right 6 Lower Lobe Bronchus, Right 7 Main Bronchus, Left 8 Upper Lobe Bronchus, Left 9 Lingula Bronchus B Lower Lobe Bronchus, Left	0 Open 3 Percutaneous 4 Percutaneous Endoscopic 7 Via Natural or Artificial Opening 8 Via Natural or Artificial Opening Endoscopic	G Intraluminal Device, Endobronchial Valve	Z No Qualifier
K Lung, Right L Lung, Left	0 Open 3 Percutaneous 4 Percutaneous Endoscopic 7 Via Natural or Artificial Opening 8 Via Natural or Artificial Opening Endoscopic	1 Radioactive Element 2 Monitoring Device 3 Infusion Device Y Other Device	Z No Qualifier
Q Pleura	0 Open 3 Percutaneous 4 Percutaneous Endoscopic 7 Via Natural or Artificial Opening 8 Via Natural or Artificial Opening Endoscopic	Y Other Device	Z No Qualifier

Continued →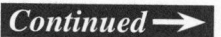

Section 0 **Medical and Surgical**
Body System B **Respiratory System**
Operation H **Insertion:** Putting in a nonbiological appliance that monitors, assists, performs, or prevents a physiological function but does not physically take the place of a body part

Body Part (4th)	Approach (5th)	Device (6th)	Qualifier (7th)
T Diaphragm	0 Open 3 Percutaneous 4 Percutaneous Endoscopic	2 Monitoring Device M Diaphragmatic Pacemaker Lead Y Other Device	Z No Qualifier
T Diaphragm	7 Via Natural or Artificial Opening 8 Via Natural or Artificial Opening Endoscopic	Y Other Device	Z No Qualifier

Section 0 **Medical and Surgical**
Body System B **Respiratory System**
Operation J **Inspection:** Visually and/or manually exploring a body part

Body Part (4th)	Approach (5th)	Device (6th)	Qualifier (7th)
0 Tracheobronchial Tree 1 Trachea K Lung, Right L Lung, Left Q Pleura T Diaphragm	0 Open 3 Percutaneous 4 Percutaneous Endoscopic 7 Via Natural or Artificial Opening 8 Via Natural or Artificial Opening Endoscopic X External	Z No Device	Z No Qualifier

Section 0 **Medical and Surgical**
Body System B **Respiratory System**
Operation L **Occlusion:** Completely closing an orifice or the lumen of a tubular body part

Body Part (4th)	Approach (5th)	Device (6th)	Qualifier (7th)
1 Trachea 2 Carina 3 Main Bronchus, Right 4 Upper Lobe Bronchus, Right 5 Middle Lobe Bronchus, Right 6 Lower Lobe Bronchus, Right 7 Main Bronchus, Left 8 Upper Lobe Bronchus, Left 9 Lingula Bronchus B Lower Lobe Bronchus, Left	0 Open 3 Percutaneous 4 Percutaneous Endoscopic	C Extraluminal Device D Intraluminal Device Z No Device	Z No Qualifier
1 Trachea 2 Carina 3 Main Bronchus, Right 4 Upper Lobe Bronchus, Right 5 Middle Lobe Bronchus, Right 6 Lower Lobe Bronchus, Right 7 Main Bronchus, Left 8 Upper Lobe Bronchus, Left 9 Lingula Bronchus B Lower Lobe Bronchus, Left	7 Via Natural or Artificial Opening 8 Via Natural or Artificial Opening Endoscopic	D Intraluminal Device Z No Device	Z No Qualifier

Section	0	Medical and Surgical
Body System	B	Respiratory System
Operation	M	**Reattachment:** Putting back in or on all or a portion of a separated body part to its normal location or other suitable location

Body Part (4th)	Approach (5th)	Device (6th)	Qualifier (7th)
1 Trachea	**0** Open	**Z** No Device	**Z** No Qualifier
2 Carina			
3 Main Bronchus, Right			
4 Upper Lobe Bronchus, Right			
5 Middle Lobe Bronchus, Right			
6 Lower Lobe Bronchus, Right			
7 Main Bronchus, Left			
8 Upper Lobe Bronchus, Left			
9 Lingula Bronchus			
B Lower Lobe Bronchus, Left			
C Upper Lung Lobe, Right			
D Middle Lung Lobe, Right			
F Lower Lung Lobe, Right			
G Upper Lung Lobe, Left			
H Lung Lingula			
J Lower Lung Lobe, Left			
K Lung, Right			
L Lung, Left			
T Diaphragm			

Section	0	Medical and Surgical
Body System	B	Respiratory System
Operation	N	**Release:** Freeing a body part from an abnormal physical constraint by cutting or by the use of force

Body Part (4th)	Approach (5th)	Device (6th)	Qualifier (7th)
1 Trachea	**0** Open	**Z** No Device	**Z** No Qualifier
2 Carina	**3** Percutaneous		
3 Main Bronchus, Right	**4** Percutaneous Endoscopic		
4 Upper Lobe Bronchus, Right	**7** Via Natural or Artificial Opening		
5 Middle Lobe Bronchus, Right	**8** Via Natural or Artificial Opening Endoscopic		
6 Lower Lobe Bronchus, Right			
7 Main Bronchus, Left			
8 Upper Lobe Bronchus, Left			
9 Lingula Bronchus			
B Lower Lobe Bronchus, Left			
C Upper Lung Lobe, Right			
D Middle Lung Lobe, Right			
F Lower Lung Lobe, Right			
G Upper Lung Lobe, Left			
H Lung Lingula			
J Lower Lung Lobe, Left			
K Lung, Right			
L Lung, Left			
M Lungs, Bilateral			
N Pleura, Right	**0** Open	**Z** No Device	**Z** No Qualifier
P Pleura, Left	**3** Percutaneous		
T Diaphragm	**4** Percutaneous Endoscopic		

Section   **0**   **Medical and Surgical**
Body System   **B**   **Respiratory System**
Operation   **P**   **Removal:** Taking out or off a device from a body part

Body Part (4th)	Approach (5th)	Device (6th)	Qualifier (7th)
0 Tracheobronchial Tree	**0** Open **3** Percutaneous **4** Percutaneous Endoscopic **7** Via Natural or Artificial Opening **8** Via Natural or Artificial Opening Endoscopic	**0** Drainage Device **1** Radioactive Element **2** Monitoring Device **3** Infusion Device **7** Autologous Tissue Substitute **C** Extraluminal Device **D** Intraluminal Device **J** Synthetic Substitute **K** Nonautologous Tissue Substitute **Y** Other Device	**Z** No Qualifier
0 Tracheobronchial Tree	**X** External	**0** Drainage Device **1** Radioactive Element **2** Monitoring Device **3** Infusion Device **D** Intraluminal Device	**Z** No Qualifier
1 Trachea	**0** Open **3** Percutaneous **4** Percutaneous Endoscopic **7** Via Natural or Artificial Opening **8** Via Natural or Artificial Opening Endoscopic	**0** Drainage Device **2** Monitoring Device **7** Autologous Tissue Substitute **C** Extraluminal Device **D** Intraluminal Device **F** Tracheostomy Device **J** Synthetic Substitute **K** Nonautologous Tissue Substitute	**Z** No Qualifier
1 Trachea	**X** External	**0** Drainage Device **2** Monitoring Device **D** Intraluminal Device **F** Tracheostomy Device	**Z** No Qualifier
K Lung, Right **L** Lung, Left	**0** Open **3** Percutaneous **4** Percutaneous Endoscopic **7** Via Natural or Artificial Opening **8** Via Natural or Artificial Opening Endoscopic	**0** Drainage Device **1** Radioactive Element **2** Monitoring Device **3** Infusion Device **Y** Other Device	**Z** No Qualifier
K Lung, Right **L** Lung, Left	**X** External	**0** Drainage Device **1** Radioactive Element **2** Monitoring Device **3** Infusion Device	**Z** No Qualifier
Q Pleura	**0** Open **3** Percutaneous **4** Percutaneous Endoscopic **7** Via Natural or Artificial Opening **8** Via Natural or Artificial Opening Endoscopic	**0** Drainage Device **1** Radioactive Element **2** Monitoring Device **Y** Other Device	**Z** No Qualifier
Q Pleura	**X** External	**0** Drainage Device **1** Radioactive Element **2** Monitoring Device	**Z** No Qualifier
T Diaphragm	**0** Open **3** Percutaneous **4** Percutaneous Endoscopic **7** Via Natural or Artificial Opening **8** Via Natural or Artificial Opening Endoscopic	**0** Drainage Device **2** Monitoring Device **7** Autologous Tissue Substitute **J** Synthetic Substitute **K** Nonautologous Tissue Substitute **M** Diaphragmatic Pacemaker Lead **Y** Other Device	**Z** No Qualifier
T Diaphragm	**X** External	**0** Drainage Device **2** Monitoring Device **M** Diaphragmatic Pacemaker Lead	**Z** No Qualifier

Section	0	Medical and Surgical
Body System	B	Respiratory System
Operation	Q	**Repair:** Restoring, to the extent possible, a body part to its normal anatomic structure and function

Body Part (4th)	Approach (5th)	Device (6th)	Qualifier (7th)
1 Trachea 2 Carina 3 Main Bronchus, Right 4 Upper Lobe Bronchus, Right 5 Middle Lobe Bronchus, Right 6 Lower Lobe Bronchus, Right 7 Main Bronchus, Left 8 Upper Lobe Bronchus, Left 9 Lingula Bronchus B Lower Lobe Bronchus, Left C Upper Lung Lobe, Right D Middle Lung Lobe, Right F Lower Lung Lobe, Right G Upper Lung Lobe, Left H Lung Lingula J Lower Lung Lobe, Left K Lung, Right L Lung, Left M Lungs, Bilateral	0 Open 3 Percutaneous 4 Percutaneous Endoscopic 7 Via Natural or Artificial Opening 8 Via Natural or Artificial Opening Endoscopic	Z No Device	Z No Qualifier
N Pleura, Right P Pleura, Left T Diaphragm	0 Open 3 Percutaneous 4 Percutaneous Endoscopic	Z No Device	Z No Qualifier

Section	0	Medical and Surgical
Body System	B	Respiratory
Operation	R	**Replacement:** Putting in or on biological or synthetic material that physically takes the place and/or function of all or a portion of a body part

Body Part (4th)	Approach (5th)	Device (6th)	Qualifier (7th)
1 Trachea 2 Carina 3 Main Bronchus, Right 4 Upper Lobe Bronchus, Right 5 Middle Lobe Bronchus, Right 6 Lower Lobe Bronchus, Right 7 Main Bronchus, Left 8 Upper Lobe Bronchus, Left 9 Lingula Bronchus B Lower Lobe Bronchus, Left T Diaphragm	0 Open 4 Percutaneous Endoscopic	7 Autologous Tissue Substitute J Synthetic Substitute K Nonautologous Tissue Substitute	Z No Qualifier

Section   **0**   **Medical and Surgical**
Body System   **B**   **Respiratory System**
Operation   **S**   **Reposition:** Moving to its normal location, or other suitable location, all or a portion of a body part

Body Part (4ᵗʰ)	Approach (5ᵗʰ)	Device (6ᵗʰ)	Qualifier (7ᵗʰ)
1 Trachea	**0** Open	**Z** No Device	**Z** No Qualifier
2 Carina			
3 Main Bronchus, Right			
4 Upper Lobe Bronchus, Right			
5 Middle Lobe Bronchus, Right			
6 Lower Lobe Bronchus, Right			
7 Main Bronchus, Left			
8 Upper Lobe Bronchus, Left			
9 Lingula Bronchus			
B Lower Lobe Bronchus, Left			
C Upper Lung Lobe, Right			
D Middle Lung Lobe, Right			
F Lower Lung Lobe, Right			
G Upper Lung Lobe, Left			
H Lung Lingula			
J Lower Lung Lobe, Left			
K Lung, Right			
L Lung, Left			
T Diaphragm			

Section   **0**   **Medical and Surgical**
Body System   **B**   **Respiratory System**
Operation   **T**   **Resection:** Cutting out or off, without replacement, all of a body part

Body Part (4ᵗʰ)	Approach (5ᵗʰ)	Device (6ᵗʰ)	Qualifier (7ᵗʰ)
1 Trachea	**0** Open	**Z** No Device	**Z** No Qualifier
2 Carina	**4** Percutaneous Endoscopic		
3 Main Bronchus, Right			
4 Upper Lobe Bronchus, Right			
5 Middle Lobe Bronchus, Right			
6 Lower Lobe Bronchus, Right			
7 Main Bronchus, Left			
8 Upper Lobe Bronchus, Left			
9 Lingula Bronchus			
B Lower Lobe Bronchus, Left			
C Upper Lung Lobe, Right			
D Middle Lung Lobe, Right			
F Lower Lung Lobe, Right			
G Upper Lung Lobe, Left			
H Lung Lingula			
J Lower Lung Lobe, Left			
K Lung, Right			
L Lung, Left			
M Lungs, Bilateral			
T Diaphragm			

Section	0	Medical and Surgical
Body System	B	Respiratory System
Operation	U	Supplement: Putting in or on biological or synthetic material that physically reinforces and/or augments the function of a portion of a body part

Body Part (4th)	Approach (5th)	Device (6th)	Qualifier (7th)
1 Trachea 2 Carina 3 Main Bronchus, Right 4 Upper Lobe Bronchus, Right 5 Middle Lobe Bronchus, Right 6 Lower Lobe Bronchus, Right 7 Main Bronchus, Left 8 Upper Lobe Bronchus, Left 9 Lingula Bronchus B Lower Lobe Bronchus, Left	0 Open 4 Percutaneous Endoscopic 8 Via Natural or Artificial Opening Endoscopic	7 Autologous Tissue Substitute J Synthetic Substitute K Nonautologous Tissue Substitute	Z No Qualifier
T Diaphragm	0 Open 4 Percutaneous Endoscopic	7 Autologous Tissue Substitute J Synthetic Substitute K Nonautologous Tissue Substitute	Z No Qualifier

Section	0	Medical and Surgical
Body System	B	Respiratory System
Operation	V	Restriction: Partially closing an orifice or the lumen of a tubular body part

Body Part (4th)	Approach (5th)	Device (6th)	Qualifier (7th)
1 Trachea 2 Carina 3 Main Bronchus, Right 4 Upper Lobe Bronchus, Right 5 Middle Lobe Bronchus, Right 6 Lower Lobe Bronchus, Right 7 Main Bronchus, Left 8 Upper Lobe Bronchus, Left 9 Lingula Bronchus B Lower Lobe Bronchus, Left	0 Open 3 Percutaneous 4 Percutaneous Endoscopic	C Extraluminal Device D Intraluminal Device Z No Device	Z No Qualifier
1 Trachea 2 Carina 3 Main Bronchus, Right 4 Upper Lobe Bronchus, Right 5 Middle Lobe Bronchus, Right 6 Lower Lobe Bronchus, Right 7 Main Bronchus, Left 8 Upper Lobe Bronchus, Left 9 Lingula Bronchus B Lower Lobe Bronchus, Left	7 Via Natural or Artificial Opening 8 Via Natural or Artificial Opening Endoscopic	D Intraluminal Device Z No Device	Z No Qualifier

Section	0	Medical and Surgical
Body System	B	Respiratory System
Operation	W	Revision: Correcting, to the extent possible, a portion of a malfunctioning device or the position of a displaced device

Body Part (4th)	Approach (5th)	Device (6th)	Qualifier (7th)
0 Tracheobronchial Tree	0 Open 3 Percutaneous 4 Percutaneous Endoscopic 7 Via Natural or Artificial Opening 8 Via Natural or Artificial Opening Endoscopic	0 Drainage Device 2 Monitoring Device 3 Infusion Device 7 Autologous Tissue Substitute C Extraluminal Device D Intraluminal Device J Synthetic Substitute K Nonautologous Tissue Substitute Y Other Device	Z No Qualifier

Continued →

Section	0	Medical and Surgical
Body System	B	Respiratory System
Operation	W	Revision: Correcting, to the extent possible, a portion of a malfunctioning device or the position of a displaced device

Body Part (4th)	Approach (5th)	Device (6th)	Qualifier (7th)
0 Tracheobronchial Tree	**X** External	**0** Drainage Device **2** Monitoring Device **3** Infusion Device **7** Autologous Tissue Substitute **C** Extraluminal Device **D** Intraluminal Device **J** Synthetic Substitute **K** Nonautologous Tissue Substitute	**Z** No Qualifier
1 Trachea	**0** Open **3** Percutaneous **4** Percutaneous Endoscopic **7** Via Natural or Artificial Opening **8** Via Natural or Artificial Opening Endoscopic **X** External	**0** Drainage Device **2** Monitoring Device **7** Autologous Tissue Substitute **C** Extraluminal Device **D** Intraluminal Device **F** Tracheostomy Device **J** Synthetic Substitute **K** Nonautologous Tissue Substitute	**Z** No Qualifier
K Lung, Right **L** Lung, Left	**0** Open **3** Percutaneous **4** Percutaneous Endoscopic **7** Via Natural or Artificial Opening **8** Via Natural or Artificial Opening Endoscopic	**0** Drainage Device **2** Monitoring Device **3** Infusion Device **Y** Other Device	**Z** No Qualifier
K Lung, Right **L** Lung, Left	**X** External	**0** Drainage Device **2** Monitoring Device **3** Infusion Device	**Z** No Qualifier
Q Pleura	**0** Open **3** Percutaneous **4** Percutaneous Endoscopic **7** Via Natural or Artificial Opening **8** Via Natural or Artificial Opening Endoscopic	**0** Drainage Device **2** Monitoring Device **Y** Other Device	**Z** No Qualifier
Q Pleura	**X** External	**0** Drainage Device **2** Monitoring Device	**Z** No Qualifier
T Diaphragm	**0** Open **3** Percutaneous **4** Percutaneous Endoscopic **7** Via Natural or Artificial Opening **8** Via Natural or Artificial Opening Endoscopic	**0** Drainage Device **2** Monitoring Device **7** Autologous Tissue Substitute **J** Synthetic Substitute **K** Nonautologous Tissue Substitute **M** Diaphragmatic Pacemaker Lead **Y** Other Device	**Z** No Qualifier
T Diaphragm	**X** External	**0** Drainage Device **2** Monitoring Device **7** Autologous Tissue Substitute **J** Synthetic Substitute **K** Nonautologous Tissue Substitute **M** Diaphragmatic Pacemaker Lead	**Z** No Qualifier

Section	0	Medical and Surgical
Body System	B	Respiratory System
Operation	Y	Transplantation: Putting in or on all or a portion of a living body part taken from another individual or animal to physically take the place and/or function of all or a portion of a similar body part

Body Part (4th)	Approach (5th)	Device (6th)	Qualifier (7th)
C Upper Lung Lobe, Right D Middle Lung Lobe, Right F Lower Lung Lobe, Right G Upper Lung Lobe, Left H Lung Lingula J Lower Lung Lobe, Left K Lung, Right L Lung, Left M Lungs, Bilateral	0 Open	Z No Device	0 Allogeneic 1 Syngeneic 2 Zooplastic

Respiratory System Code Listing 0B1–0BY

0B1 – Respiratory System, Bypass

Review Coding Guideline B3.6a

0B110D6 Bypass Trachea to Esophagus with Intraluminal Device, Open Approach	● **0B113F4** Bypass Trachea to Cutaneous with Tracheostomy Device, Percutaneous Approach	**0B114F4** Bypass Trachea to Cutaneous with Tracheostomy Device, Percutaneous Endoscopic Approach
0B110F4 Bypass Trachea to Cutaneous with Tracheostomy Device, Open Approach	● **0B113Z4** Bypass Trachea to Cutaneous, Percutaneous Approach	**0B114Z4** Bypass Trachea to Cutaneous, Percutaneous Endoscopic Approach
0B110Z4 Bypass Trachea to Cutaneous, Open Approach		

0B2 – Respiratory System, Change

Review Coding Guideline B6.1c

0B20X0Z Change Drainage Device in Tracheobronchial Tree, External Approach	**0B21XFZ** Change Tracheostomy Device in Trachea, External Approach	**0B2LXYZ** Change Other Device in Left Lung, External Approach
0B20XYZ Change Other Device in Tracheobronchial Tree, External Approach	**0B21XYZ** Change Other Device in Trachea, External Approach	**0B2QX0Z** Change Drainage Device in Pleura, External Approach
0B21X0Z Change Drainage Device in Trachea, External Approach	**0B2KX0Z** Change Drainage Device in Right Lung, External Approach	**0B2QXYZ** Change Other Device in Pleura, External Approach
0B21XEZ Change Endotracheal Airway in Trachea, External Approach	**0B2KXYZ** Change Other Device in Right Lung, External Approach	**0B2TX0Z** Change Drainage Device in Diaphragm, External Approach
	0B2LX0Z Change Drainage Device in Left Lung, External Approach	**0B2TXYZ** Change Other Device in Diaphragm, External Approach

0B5 – Respiratory System, Destruction

0B510ZZ Destruction of Trachea, Open Approach	**0B538ZZ** Destruction of Right Main Bronchus, Via Natural or Artificial Opening Endoscopic	**0B558ZZ** Destruction of Right Middle Lobe Bronchus, Via Natural or Artificial Opening Endoscopic
0B513ZZ Destruction of Trachea, Percutaneous Approach	**0B540ZZ** Destruction of Right Upper Lobe Bronchus, Open Approach	**0B560ZZ** Destruction of Right Lower Lobe Bronchus, Open Approach
0B514ZZ Destruction of Trachea, Percutaneous Endoscopic Approach	**0B543ZZ** Destruction of Right Upper Lobe Bronchus, Percutaneous Approach	**0B563ZZ** Destruction of Right Lower Lobe Bronchus, Percutaneous Approach
0B517ZZ Destruction of Trachea, Via Natural or Artificial Opening	**0B544ZZ** Destruction of Right Upper Lobe Bronchus, Percutaneous Endoscopic Approach	**0B564ZZ** Destruction of Right Lower Lobe Bronchus, Percutaneous Endoscopic Approach
0B518ZZ Destruction of Trachea, Via Natural or Artificial Opening Endoscopic	**0B547ZZ** Destruction of Right Upper Lobe Bronchus, Via Natural or Artificial Opening	**0B567ZZ** Destruction of Right Lower Lobe Bronchus, Via Natural or Artificial Opening
0B520ZZ Destruction of Carina, Open Approach	**0B548ZZ** Destruction of Right Upper Lobe Bronchus, Via Natural or Artificial Opening Endoscopic	**0B568ZZ** Destruction of Right Lower Lobe Bronchus, Via Natural or Artificial Opening Endoscopic
0B523ZZ Destruction of Carina, Percutaneous Approach	**0B550ZZ** Destruction of Right Middle Lobe Bronchus, Open Approach	**0B570ZZ** Destruction of Left Main Bronchus, Open Approach
0B524ZZ Destruction of Carina, Percutaneous Endoscopic Approach	**0B553ZZ** Destruction of Right Middle Lobe Bronchus, Percutaneous Approach	**0B573ZZ** Destruction of Left Main Bronchus, Percutaneous Approach
0B527ZZ Destruction of Carina, Via Natural or Artificial Opening	**0B554ZZ** Destruction of Right Middle Lobe Bronchus, Percutaneous Endoscopic Approach	**0B574ZZ** Destruction of Left Main Bronchus, Percutaneous Endoscopic Approach
0B528ZZ Destruction of Carina, Via Natural or Artificial Opening Endoscopic	**0B557ZZ** Destruction of Right Middle Lobe Bronchus, Via Natural or Artificial Opening	**0B577ZZ** Destruction of Left Main Bronchus, Via Natural or Artificial Opening
0B530ZZ Destruction of Right Main Bronchus, Open Approach		**0B578ZZ** Destruction of Left Main Bronchus, Via Natural or Artificial Opening Endoscopic
0B533ZZ Destruction of Right Main Bronchus, Percutaneous Approach		
0B534ZZ Destruction of Right Main Bronchus, Percutaneous Endoscopic Approach		
0B537ZZ Destruction of Right Main Bronchus, Via Natural or Artificial Opening		

0B580ZZ Destruction of Left Upper Lobe Bronchus, Open Approach

0B583ZZ Destruction of Left Upper Lobe Bronchus, Percutaneous Approach

0B584ZZ Destruction of Left Upper Lobe Bronchus, Percutaneous Endoscopic Approach

0B587ZZ Destruction of Left Upper Lobe Bronchus, Via Natural or Artificial Opening

0B588ZZ Destruction of Left Upper Lobe Bronchus, Via Natural or Artificial Opening Endoscopic

0B590ZZ Destruction of Lingula Bronchus, Open Approach

0B593ZZ Destruction of Lingula Bronchus, Percutaneous Approach

0B594ZZ Destruction of Lingula Bronchus, Percutaneous Endoscopic Approach

0B597ZZ Destruction of Lingula Bronchus, Via Natural or Artificial Opening

0B598ZZ Destruction of Lingula Bronchus, Via Natural or Artificial Opening Endoscopic

0B5B0ZZ Destruction of Left Lower Lobe Bronchus, Open Approach

0B5B3ZZ Destruction of Left Lower Lobe Bronchus, Percutaneous Approach

0B5B4ZZ Destruction of Left Lower Lobe Bronchus, Percutaneous Endoscopic Approach

0B5B7ZZ Destruction of Left Lower Lobe Bronchus, Via Natural or Artificial Opening

0B5B8ZZ Destruction of Left Lower Lobe Bronchus, Via Natural or Artificial Opening Endoscopic

0B5C0ZZ Destruction of Right Upper Lung Lobe, Open Approach

0B5C3ZZ Destruction of Right Upper Lung Lobe, Percutaneous Approach

0B5C4ZZ Destruction of Right Upper Lung Lobe, Percutaneous Endoscopic Approach

0B5C7ZZ Destruction of Right Upper Lung Lobe, Via Natural or Artificial Opening

0B5C8ZZ Destruction of Right Upper Lung Lobe, Via Natural or Artificial Opening Endoscopic

0B5D0ZZ Destruction of Right Middle Lung Lobe, Open Approach

0B5D3ZZ Destruction of Right Middle Lung Lobe, Percutaneous Approach

0B5D4ZZ Destruction of Right Middle Lung Lobe, Percutaneous Endoscopic Approach

0B5D7ZZ Destruction of Right Middle Lung Lobe, Via Natural or Artificial Opening

0B5D8ZZ Destruction of Right Middle Lung Lobe, Via Natural or Artificial Opening Endoscopic

0B5F0ZZ Destruction of Right Lower Lung Lobe, Open Approach

0B5F3ZZ Destruction of Right Lower Lung Lobe, Percutaneous Approach

0B5F4ZZ Destruction of Right Lower Lung Lobe, Percutaneous Endoscopic Approach

0B5F7ZZ Destruction of Right Lower Lung Lobe, Via Natural or Artificial Opening

0B5F8ZZ Destruction of Right Lower Lung Lobe, Via Natural or Artificial Opening Endoscopic

0B5G0ZZ Destruction of Left Upper Lung Lobe, Open Approach

0B5G3ZZ Destruction of Left Upper Lung Lobe, Percutaneous Approach

0B5G4ZZ Destruction of Left Upper Lung Lobe, Percutaneous Endoscopic Approach

0B5G7ZZ Destruction of Left Upper Lung Lobe, Via Natural or Artificial Opening

0B5G8ZZ Destruction of Left Upper Lung Lobe, Via Natural or Artificial Opening Endoscopic

0B5H0ZZ Destruction of Lung Lingula, Open Approach

0B5H3ZZ Destruction of Lung Lingula, Percutaneous Approach

0B5H4ZZ Destruction of Lung Lingula, Percutaneous Endoscopic Approach

0B5H7ZZ Destruction of Lung Lingula, Via Natural or Artificial Opening

0B5H8ZZ Destruction of Lung Lingula, Via Natural or Artificial Opening Endoscopic

0B5J0ZZ Destruction of Left Lower Lung Lobe, Open Approach

0B5J3ZZ Destruction of Left Lower Lung Lobe, Percutaneous Approach

0B5J4ZZ Destruction of Left Lower Lung Lobe, Percutaneous Endoscopic Approach

0B5J7ZZ Destruction of Left Lower Lung Lobe, Via Natural or Artificial Opening

0B5J8ZZ Destruction of Left Lower Lung Lobe, Via Natural or Artificial Opening Endoscopic

0B5K0ZZ Destruction of Right Lung, Open Approach

0B5K3ZZ Destruction of Right Lung, Percutaneous Approach

0B5K4ZZ Destruction of Right Lung, Percutaneous Endoscopic Approach

0B5K7ZZ Destruction of Right Lung, Via Natural or Artificial Opening

0B5K8ZZ Destruction of Right Lung, Via Natural or Artificial Opening Endoscopic

0B5L0ZZ Destruction of Left Lung, Open Approach

0B5L3ZZ Destruction of Left Lung, Percutaneous Approach

0B5L4ZZ Destruction of Left Lung, Percutaneous Endoscopic Approach

0B5L7ZZ Destruction of Left Lung, Via Natural or Artificial Opening

0B5L8ZZ Destruction of Left Lung, Via Natural or Artificial Opening Endoscopic

0B5M0ZZ Destruction of Bilateral Lungs, Open Approach

0B5M3ZZ Destruction of Bilateral Lungs, Percutaneous Approach

0B5M4ZZ Destruction of Bilateral Lungs, Percutaneous Endoscopic Approach

0B5M7ZZ Destruction of Bilateral Lungs, Via Natural or Artificial Opening

0B5M8ZZ Destruction of Bilateral Lungs, Via Natural or Artificial Opening Endoscopic

0B5N0ZZ Destruction of Right Pleura, Open Approach

0B5N3ZZ Destruction of Right Pleura, Percutaneous Approach

0B5N4ZZ Destruction of Right Pleura, Percutaneous Endoscopic Approach

0B5P0ZZ Destruction of Left Pleura, Open Approach

AHA CC: 2Q, 2016, 17-18

0B5P3ZZ Destruction of Left Pleura, Percutaneous Approach

0B5P4ZZ Destruction of Left Pleura, Percutaneous Endoscopic Approach

0B5T0ZZ Destruction of Diaphragm, Open Approach

0B5T3ZZ Destruction of Diaphragm, Percutaneous Approach

0B5T4ZZ Destruction of Diaphragm, Percutaneous Endoscopic Approach

0B7 – Respiratory System, Dilation

0B710DZ Dilation of Trachea with Intraluminal Device, Open Approach

0B710ZZ Dilation of Trachea, Open Approach

0B713DZ Dilation of Trachea with Intraluminal Device, Percutaneous Approach

0B713ZZ Dilation of Trachea, Percutaneous Approach

0B714DZ Dilation of Trachea with Intraluminal Device, Percutaneous Endoscopic Approach

0B714ZZ Dilation of Trachea, Percutaneous Endoscopic Approach

0B717DZ Dilation of Trachea with Intraluminal Device, Via Natural or Artificial Opening

0B717ZZ Dilation of Trachea, Via Natural or Artificial Opening

0B718DZ Dilation of Trachea with Intraluminal Device, Via Natural or Artificial Opening Endoscopic

0B718ZZ Dilation of Trachea, Via Natural or Artificial Opening Endoscopic

0B720DZ Dilation of Carina with Intraluminal Device, Open Approach

0B720ZZ Dilation of Carina, Open Approach

0B723DZ Dilation of Carina with Intraluminal Device, Percutaneous Approach

0B723ZZ Dilation of Carina, Percutaneous Approach

0B724DZ Dilation of Carina with Intraluminal Device, Percutaneous Endoscopic Approach

0B724ZZ Dilation of Carina, Percutaneous Endoscopic Approach

0B727DZ Dilation of Carina with Intraluminal Device, Via Natural or Artificial Opening

0B727ZZ Dilation of Carina, Via Natural or Artificial Opening

0B728DZ Dilation of Carina with Intraluminal Device, Via Natural or Artificial Opening Endoscopic

0B728ZZ Dilation of Carina, Via Natural or Artificial Opening Endoscopic

0B730DZ Dilation of Right Main Bronchus with Intraluminal Device, Open Approach

0B730ZZ Dilation of Right Main Bronchus, Open Approach

0B733DZ Dilation of Right Main Bronchus with Intraluminal Device, Percutaneous Approach

0B733ZZ Dilation of Right Main Bronchus, Percutaneous Approach

0B734DZ Dilation of Right Main Bronchus with Intraluminal Device, Percutaneous Endoscopic Approach

0B734ZZ Dilation of Right Main Bronchus, Percutaneous Endoscopic Approach

0B737DZ Dilation of Right Main Bronchus with Intraluminal Device, Via Natural or Artificial Opening

0B737ZZ Dilation of Right Main Bronchus, Via Natural or Artificial Opening

0B738DZ Dilation of Right Main Bronchus with Intraluminal Device, Via Natural or Artificial Opening Endoscopic

0B738ZZ   Dilation of Right Main Bronchus, Via Natural or Artificial Opening Endoscopic

0B740DZ   Dilation of Right Upper Lobe Bronchus with Intraluminal Device, Open Approach

0B740ZZ   Dilation of Right Upper Lobe Bronchus, Open Approach

0B743DZ   Dilation of Right Upper Lobe Bronchus with Intraluminal Device, Percutaneous Approach

0B743ZZ   Dilation of Right Upper Lobe Bronchus, Percutaneous Approach

0B744DZ   Dilation of Right Upper Lobe Bronchus with Intraluminal Device, Percutaneous Endoscopic Approach

0B744ZZ   Dilation of Right Upper Lobe Bronchus, Percutaneous Endoscopic Approach

0B747DZ   Dilation of Right Upper Lobe Bronchus with Intraluminal Device, Via Natural or Artificial Opening

0B747ZZ   Dilation of Right Upper Lobe Bronchus, Via Natural or Artificial Opening

0B748DZ   Dilation of Right Upper Lobe Bronchus with Intraluminal Device, Via Natural or Artificial Opening Endoscopic

0B748ZZ   Dilation of Right Upper Lobe Bronchus, Via Natural or Artificial Opening Endoscopic

0B750DZ   Dilation of Right Middle Lobe Bronchus with Intraluminal Device, Open Approach

0B750ZZ   Dilation of Right Middle Lobe Bronchus, Open Approach

0B753DZ   Dilation of Right Middle Lobe Bronchus with Intraluminal Device, Percutaneous Approach

0B753ZZ   Dilation of Right Middle Lobe Bronchus, Percutaneous Approach

0B754DZ   Dilation of Right Middle Lobe Bronchus with Intraluminal Device, Percutaneous Endoscopic Approach

0B754ZZ   Dilation of Right Middle Lobe Bronchus, Percutaneous Endoscopic Approach

0B757DZ   Dilation of Right Middle Lobe Bronchus with Intraluminal Device, Via Natural or Artificial Opening

0B757ZZ   Dilation of Right Middle Lobe Bronchus, Via Natural or Artificial Opening

0B758DZ   Dilation of Right Middle Lobe Bronchus with Intraluminal Device, Via Natural or Artificial Opening Endoscopic

0B758ZZ   Dilation of Right Middle Lobe Bronchus, Via Natural or Artificial Opening Endoscopic

0B760DZ   Dilation of Right Lower Lobe Bronchus with Intraluminal Device, Open Approach

0B760ZZ   Dilation of Right Lower Lobe Bronchus, Open Approach

0B763DZ   Dilation of Right Lower Lobe Bronchus with Intraluminal Device, Percutaneous Approach

0B763ZZ   Dilation of Right Lower Lobe Bronchus, Percutaneous Approach

0B764DZ   Dilation of Right Lower Lobe Bronchus with Intraluminal Device, Percutaneous Endoscopic Approach

0B764ZZ   Dilation of Right Lower Lobe Bronchus, Percutaneous Endoscopic Approach

0B767DZ   Dilation of Right Lower Lobe Bronchus with Intraluminal Device, Via Natural or Artificial Opening

0B767ZZ   Dilation of Right Lower Lobe Bronchus, Via Natural or Artificial Opening

0B768DZ   Dilation of Right Lower Lobe Bronchus with Intraluminal Device, Via Natural or Artificial Opening Endoscopic

0B768ZZ   Dilation of Right Lower Lobe Bronchus, Via Natural or Artificial Opening Endoscopic

0B770DZ   Dilation of Left Main Bronchus with Intraluminal Device, Open Approach

0B770ZZ   Dilation of Left Main Bronchus, Open Approach

0B773DZ   Dilation of Left Main Bronchus with Intraluminal Device, Percutaneous Approach

0B773ZZ   Dilation of Left Main Bronchus, Percutaneous Approach

0B774DZ   Dilation of Left Main Bronchus with Intraluminal Device, Percutaneous Endoscopic Approach

0B774ZZ   Dilation of Left Main Bronchus, Percutaneous Endoscopic Approach

0B777DZ   Dilation of Left Main Bronchus with Intraluminal Device, Via Natural or Artificial Opening

0B777ZZ   Dilation of Left Main Bronchus, Via Natural or Artificial Opening

0B778DZ   Dilation of Left Main Bronchus with Intraluminal Device, Via Natural or Artificial Opening Endoscopic

0B778ZZ   Dilation of Left Main Bronchus, Via Natural or Artificial Opening Endoscopic

0B780DZ   Dilation of Left Upper Lobe Bronchus with Intraluminal Device, Open Approach

0B780ZZ   Dilation of Left Upper Lobe Bronchus, Open Approach

0B783DZ   Dilation of Left Upper Lobe Bronchus with Intraluminal Device, Percutaneous Approach

0B783ZZ   Dilation of Left Upper Lobe Bronchus, Percutaneous Approach

0B784DZ   Dilation of Left Upper Lobe Bronchus with Intraluminal Device, Percutaneous Endoscopic Approach

0B784ZZ   Dilation of Left Upper Lobe Bronchus, Percutaneous Endoscopic Approach

0B787DZ   Dilation of Left Upper Lobe Bronchus with Intraluminal Device, Via Natural or Artificial Opening

0B787ZZ   Dilation of Left Upper Lobe Bronchus, Via Natural or Artificial Opening

0B788DZ   Dilation of Left Upper Lobe Bronchus with Intraluminal Device, Via Natural or Artificial Opening Endoscopic

0B788ZZ   Dilation of Left Upper Lobe Bronchus, Via Natural or Artificial Opening Endoscopic

0B790DZ   Dilation of Lingula Bronchus with Intraluminal Device, Open Approach

0B790ZZ   Dilation of Lingula Bronchus, Open Approach

0B793DZ   Dilation of Lingula Bronchus with Intraluminal Device, Percutaneous Approach

0B793ZZ   Dilation of Lingula Bronchus, Percutaneous Approach

0B794DZ   Dilation of Lingula Bronchus with Intraluminal Device, Percutaneous Endoscopic Approach

0B794ZZ   Dilation of Lingula Bronchus, Percutaneous Endoscopic Approach

0B797DZ   Dilation of Lingula Bronchus with Intraluminal Device, Via Natural or Artificial Opening

0B797ZZ   Dilation of Lingula Bronchus, Via Natural or Artificial Opening

0B798DZ   Dilation of Lingula Bronchus with Intraluminal Device, Via Natural or Artificial Opening Endoscopic

0B798ZZ   Dilation of Lingula Bronchus, Via Natural or Artificial Opening Endoscopic

0B7B0DZ   Dilation of Left Lower Lobe Bronchus with Intraluminal Device, Open Approach

0B7B0ZZ   Dilation of Left Lower Lobe Bronchus, Open Approach

0B7B3DZ   Dilation of Left Lower Lobe Bronchus with Intraluminal Device, Percutaneous Approach

0B7B3ZZ   Dilation of Left Lower Lobe Bronchus, Percutaneous Approach

0B7B4DZ   Dilation of Left Lower Lobe Bronchus with Intraluminal Device, Percutaneous Endoscopic Approach

0B7B4ZZ   Dilation of Left Lower Lobe Bronchus, Percutaneous Endoscopic Approach

0B7B7DZ   Dilation of Left Lower Lobe Bronchus with Intraluminal Device, Via Natural or Artificial Opening

0B7B7ZZ   Dilation of Left Lower Lobe Bronchus, Via Natural or Artificial Opening

0B7B8DZ   Dilation of Left Lower Lobe Bronchus with Intraluminal Device, Via Natural or Artificial Opening Endoscopic

0B7B8ZZ   Dilation of Left Lower Lobe Bronchus, Via Natural or Artificial Opening Endoscopic

0B9 – Respiratory System, Drainage

Review Coding Guidelines B3.4a and B3.4b

Review Coding Guideline B6.2

0B9100Z   Drainage of Trachea with Drainage Device, Open Approach

0B910ZX   Drainage of Trachea, Open Approach, Diagnostic

0B910ZZ   Drainage of Trachea, Open Approach

0B9130Z   Drainage of Trachea with Drainage Device, Percutaneous Approach

0B913ZX   Drainage of Trachea, Percutaneous Approach, Diagnostic

0B913ZZ   Drainage of Trachea, Percutaneous Approach

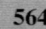 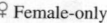 ♀ Female-only   ♂ Male-only   ▲ Limited Coverage   ● Non-OR   HAC HAC-associated procedure   ▲ Non-covered procedures   ✚ Cluster

0B9140Z Drainage of Trachea with Drainage Device, Percutaneous Endoscopic Approach

0B914ZX Drainage of Trachea, Percutaneous Endoscopic Approach, Diagnostic

0B914ZZ Drainage of Trachea, Percutaneous Endoscopic Approach

0B9170Z Drainage of Trachea with Drainage Device, Via Natural or Artificial Opening

0B917ZX Drainage of Trachea, Via Natural or Artificial Opening, Diagnostic

0B917ZZ Drainage of Trachea, Via Natural or Artificial Opening

0B9180Z Drainage of Trachea with Drainage Device, Via Natural or Artificial Opening Endoscopic

0B918ZX Drainage of Trachea, Via Natural or Artificial Opening Endoscopic, Diagnostic

0B918ZZ Drainage of Trachea, Via Natural or Artificial Opening Endoscopic

0B9200Z Drainage of Carina with Drainage Device, Open Approach

0B920ZX Drainage of Carina, Open Approach, Diagnostic

0B920ZZ Drainage of Carina, Open Approach

0B9230Z Drainage of Carina with Drainage Device, Percutaneous Approach

0B923ZX Drainage of Carina, Percutaneous Approach, Diagnostic

0B923ZZ Drainage of Carina, Percutaneous Approach

0B9240Z Drainage of Carina with Drainage Device, Percutaneous Endoscopic Approach

0B924ZX Drainage of Carina, Percutaneous Endoscopic Approach, Diagnostic

0B924ZZ Drainage of Carina, Percutaneous Endoscopic Approach

0B9270Z Drainage of Carina with Drainage Device, Via Natural or Artificial Opening

0B927ZX Drainage of Carina, Via Natural or Artificial Opening, Diagnostic

0B927ZZ Drainage of Carina, Via Natural or Artificial Opening

0B9280Z Drainage of Carina with Drainage Device, Via Natural or Artificial Opening Endoscopic

0B928ZX Drainage of Carina, Via Natural or Artificial Opening Endoscopic, Diagnostic

0B928ZZ Drainage of Carina, Via Natural or Artificial Opening Endoscopic

0B9300Z Drainage of Right Main Bronchus with Drainage Device, Open Approach

0B930ZX Drainage of Right Main Bronchus, Open Approach, Diagnostic

0B930ZZ Drainage of Right Main Bronchus, Open Approach

0B9330Z Drainage of Right Main Bronchus with Drainage Device, Percutaneous Approach

0B933ZX Drainage of Right Main Bronchus, Percutaneous Approach, Diagnostic

0B933ZZ Drainage of Right Main Bronchus, Percutaneous Approach

0B9340Z Drainage of Right Main Bronchus with Drainage Device, Percutaneous Endoscopic Approach

0B934ZX Drainage of Right Main Bronchus, Percutaneous Endoscopic Approach, Diagnostic

0B934ZZ Drainage of Right Main Bronchus, Percutaneous Endoscopic Approach

0B9370Z Drainage of Right Main Bronchus with Drainage Device, Via Natural or Artificial Opening

0B937ZX Drainage of Right Main Bronchus, Via Natural or Artificial Opening, Diagnostic

0B937ZZ Drainage of Right Main Bronchus, Via Natural or Artificial Opening

0B9380Z Drainage of Right Main Bronchus with Drainage Device, Via Natural or Artificial Opening Endoscopic

0B938ZX Drainage of Right Main Bronchus, Via Natural or Artificial Opening Endoscopic, Diagnostic

0B938ZZ Drainage of Right Main Bronchus, Via Natural or Artificial Opening Endoscopic

0B9400Z Drainage of Right Upper Lobe Bronchus with Drainage Device, Open Approach

0B940ZX Drainage of Right Upper Lobe Bronchus, Open Approach, Diagnostic

0B940ZZ Drainage of Right Upper Lobe Bronchus, Open Approach

0B9430Z Drainage of Right Upper Lobe Bronchus with Drainage Device, Percutaneous Approach

0B943ZX Drainage of Right Upper Lobe Bronchus, Percutaneous Approach, Diagnostic

0B943ZZ Drainage of Right Upper Lobe Bronchus, Percutaneous Approach

0B9440Z Drainage of Right Upper Lobe Bronchus with Drainage Device, Percutaneous Endoscopic Approach

0B944ZX Drainage of Right Upper Lobe Bronchus, Percutaneous Endoscopic Approach, Diagnostic

0B944ZZ Drainage of Right Upper Lobe Bronchus, Percutaneous Endoscopic Approach

0B9470Z Drainage of Right Upper Lobe Bronchus with Drainage Device, Via Natural or Artificial Opening

0B947ZX Drainage of Right Upper Lobe Bronchus, Via Natural or Artificial Opening, Diagnostic

0B947ZZ Drainage of Right Upper Lobe Bronchus, Via Natural or Artificial Opening

0B9480Z Drainage of Right Upper Lobe Bronchus with Drainage Device, Via Natural or Artificial Opening Endoscopic

0B948ZX Drainage of Right Upper Lobe Bronchus, Via Natural or Artificial Opening Endoscopic, Diagnostic

AHA CC: 1Q, 2016, 26-27

0B948ZZ Drainage of Right Upper Lobe Bronchus, Via Natural or Artificial Opening Endoscopic

0B9500Z Drainage of Right Middle Lobe Bronchus with Drainage Device, Open Approach

0B950ZX Drainage of Right Middle Lobe Bronchus, Open Approach, Diagnostic

0B950ZZ Drainage of Right Middle Lobe Bronchus, Open Approach

0B9530Z Drainage of Right Middle Lobe Bronchus with Drainage Device, Percutaneous Approach

0B953ZX Drainage of Right Middle Lobe Bronchus, Percutaneous Approach, Diagnostic

0B953ZZ Drainage of Right Middle Lobe Bronchus, Percutaneous Approach

0B9540Z Drainage of Right Middle Lobe Bronchus with Drainage Device, Percutaneous Endoscopic Approach

0B954ZX Drainage of Right Middle Lobe Bronchus, Percutaneous Endoscopic Approach, Diagnostic

0B954ZZ Drainage of Right Middle Lobe Bronchus, Percutaneous Endoscopic Approach

0B9570Z Drainage of Right Middle Lobe Bronchus with Drainage Device, Via Natural or Artificial Opening

0B957ZX Drainage of Right Middle Lobe Bronchus, Via Natural or Artificial Opening, Diagnostic

0B957ZZ Drainage of Right Middle Lobe Bronchus, Via Natural or Artificial Opening

0B9580Z Drainage of Right Middle Lobe Bronchus with Drainage Device, Via Natural or Artificial Opening Endoscopic

0B958ZX Drainage of Right Middle Lobe Bronchus, Via Natural or Artificial Opening Endoscopic, Diagnostic

0B958ZZ Drainage of Right Middle Lobe Bronchus, Via Natural or Artificial Opening Endoscopic

0B9600Z Drainage of Right Lower Lobe Bronchus with Drainage Device, Open Approach

0B960ZX Drainage of Right Lower Lobe Bronchus, Open Approach, Diagnostic

0B960ZZ Drainage of Right Lower Lobe Bronchus, Open Approach

0B9630Z Drainage of Right Lower Lobe Bronchus with Drainage Device, Percutaneous Approach

0B963ZX Drainage of Right Lower Lobe Bronchus, Percutaneous Approach, Diagnostic

0B963ZZ Drainage of Right Lower Lobe Bronchus, Percutaneous Approach

0B9640Z Drainage of Right Lower Lobe Bronchus with Drainage Device, Percutaneous Endoscopic Approach

0B964ZX Drainage of Right Lower Lobe Bronchus, Percutaneous Endoscopic Approach, Diagnostic

0B964ZZ Drainage of Right Lower Lobe Bronchus, Percutaneous Endoscopic Approach

0B9670Z Drainage of Right Lower Lobe Bronchus with Drainage Device, Via Natural or Artificial Opening

0B967ZX Drainage of Right Lower Lobe Bronchus, Via Natural or Artificial Opening, Diagnostic

0B967ZZ Drainage of Right Lower Lobe Bronchus, Via Natural or Artificial Opening

0B9680Z Drainage of Right Lower Lobe Bronchus with Drainage Device, Via Natural or Artificial Opening Endoscopic

0B968ZX Drainage of Right Lower Lobe Bronchus, Via Natural or Artificial Opening Endoscopic, Diagnostic

0B968ZZ Drainage of Right Lower Lobe Bronchus, Via Natural or Artificial Opening Endoscopic

0B9700Z Drainage of Left Main Bronchus with Drainage Device, Open Approach

0B970ZX Drainage of Left Main Bronchus, Open Approach, Diagnostic

0B970ZZ Drainage of Left Main Bronchus, Open Approach

0B9730Z Drainage of Left Main Bronchus with Drainage Device, Percutaneous Approach

0B973ZX Drainage of Left Main Bronchus, Percutaneous Approach, Diagnostic

0B973ZZ Drainage of Left Main Bronchus, Percutaneous Approach

0B9740Z Drainage of Left Main Bronchus with Drainage Device, Percutaneous Endoscopic Approach

0B974ZX Drainage of Left Main Bronchus, Percutaneous Endoscopic Approach, Diagnostic

0B974ZZ Drainage of Left Main Bronchus, Percutaneous Endoscopic Approach

0B9770Z Drainage of Left Main Bronchus with Drainage Device, Via Natural or Artificial Opening

0B977ZX Drainage of Left Main Bronchus, Via Natural or Artificial Opening, Diagnostic

0B977ZZ Drainage of Left Main Bronchus, Via Natural or Artificial Opening

0B9780Z Drainage of Left Main Bronchus with Drainage Device, Via Natural or Artificial Opening Endoscopic

0B978ZX Drainage of Left Main Bronchus, Via Natural or Artificial Opening Endoscopic, Diagnostic

0B978ZZ Drainage of Left Main Bronchus, Via Natural or Artificial Opening Endoscopic

0B9800Z Drainage of Left Upper Lobe Bronchus with Drainage Device, Open Approach

0B980ZX Drainage of Left Upper Lobe Bronchus, Open Approach, Diagnostic

0B980ZZ Drainage of Left Upper Lobe Bronchus, Open Approach

0B9830Z Drainage of Left Upper Lobe Bronchus with Drainage Device, Percutaneous Approach

0B983ZX Drainage of Left Upper Lobe Bronchus, Percutaneous Approach, Diagnostic

0B983ZZ Drainage of Left Upper Lobe Bronchus, Percutaneous Approach

0B9840Z Drainage of Left Upper Lobe Bronchus with Drainage Device, Percutaneous Endoscopic Approach

0B984ZX Drainage of Left Upper Lobe Bronchus, Percutaneous Endoscopic Approach, Diagnostic

0B984ZZ Drainage of Left Upper Lobe Bronchus, Percutaneous Endoscopic Approach

0B9870Z Drainage of Left Upper Lobe Bronchus with Drainage Device, Via Natural or Artificial Opening

0B987ZX Drainage of Left Upper Lobe Bronchus, Via Natural or Artificial Opening, Diagnostic

0B987ZZ Drainage of Left Upper Lobe Bronchus, Via Natural or Artificial Opening

0B9880Z Drainage of Left Upper Lobe Bronchus with Drainage Device, Via Natural or Artificial Opening Endoscopic

0B988ZX Drainage of Left Upper Lobe Bronchus, Via Natural or Artificial Opening Endoscopic, Diagnostic

AHA CC: 1Q, 2016, 27

0B988ZZ Drainage of Left Upper Lobe Bronchus, Via Natural or Artificial Opening Endoscopic

0B9900Z Drainage of Lingula Bronchus with Drainage Device, Open Approach

0B990ZX Drainage of Lingula Bronchus, Open Approach, Diagnostic

0B990ZZ Drainage of Lingula Bronchus, Open Approach

0B9930Z Drainage of Lingula Bronchus with Drainage Device, Percutaneous Approach

0B993ZX Drainage of Lingula Bronchus, Percutaneous Approach, Diagnostic

0B993ZZ Drainage of Lingula Bronchus, Percutaneous Approach

0B9940Z Drainage of Lingula Bronchus with Drainage Device, Percutaneous Endoscopic Approach

0B994ZX Drainage of Lingula Bronchus, Percutaneous Endoscopic Approach, Diagnostic

0B994ZZ Drainage of Lingula Bronchus, Percutaneous Endoscopic Approach

0B9970Z Drainage of Lingula Bronchus with Drainage Device, Via Natural or Artificial Opening

0B997ZX Drainage of Lingula Bronchus, Via Natural or Artificial Opening, Diagnostic

0B997ZZ Drainage of Lingula Bronchus, Via Natural or Artificial Opening

0B9980Z Drainage of Lingula Bronchus with Drainage Device, Via Natural or Artificial Opening Endoscopic

0B998ZX Drainage of Lingula Bronchus, Via Natural or Artificial Opening Endoscopic, Diagnostic

0B998ZZ Drainage of Lingula Bronchus, Via Natural or Artificial Opening Endoscopic

0B9B00Z Drainage of Left Lower Lobe Bronchus with Drainage Device, Open Approach

0B9B0ZX Drainage of Left Lower Lobe Bronchus, Open Approach, Diagnostic

0B9B0ZZ Drainage of Left Lower Lobe Bronchus, Open Approach

0B9B30Z Drainage of Left Lower Lobe Bronchus with Drainage Device, Percutaneous Approach

0B9B3ZX Drainage of Left Lower Lobe Bronchus, Percutaneous Approach, Diagnostic

0B9B3ZZ Drainage of Left Lower Lobe Bronchus, Percutaneous Approach

0B9B40Z Drainage of Left Lower Lobe Bronchus with Drainage Device, Percutaneous Endoscopic Approach

0B9B4ZX Drainage of Left Lower Lobe Bronchus, Percutaneous Endoscopic Approach, Diagnostic

0B9B4ZZ Drainage of Left Lower Lobe Bronchus, Percutaneous Endoscopic Approach

0B9B70Z Drainage of Left Lower Lobe Bronchus with Drainage Device, Via Natural or Artificial Opening

0B9B7ZX Drainage of Left Lower Lobe Bronchus, Via Natural or Artificial Opening, Diagnostic

0B9B7ZZ Drainage of Left Lower Lobe Bronchus, Via Natural or Artificial Opening

0B9B80Z Drainage of Left Lower Lobe Bronchus with Drainage Device, Via Natural or Artificial Opening Endoscopic

0B9B8ZX Drainage of Left Lower Lobe Bronchus, Via Natural or Artificial Opening Endoscopic, Diagnostic

0B9B8ZZ Drainage of Left Lower Lobe Bronchus, Via Natural or Artificial Opening Endoscopic

0B9C00Z Drainage of Right Upper Lung Lobe with Drainage Device, Open Approach

0B9C0ZX Drainage of Right Upper Lung Lobe, Open Approach, Diagnostic

0B9C0ZZ Drainage of Right Upper Lung Lobe, Open Approach

0B9C30Z Drainage of Right Upper Lung Lobe with Drainage Device, Percutaneous Approach

0B9C3ZX Drainage of Right Upper Lung Lobe, Percutaneous Approach, Diagnostic

0B9C3ZZ Drainage of Right Upper Lung Lobe, Percutaneous Approach

0B9C40Z Drainage of Right Upper Lung Lobe with Drainage Device, Percutaneous Endoscopic Approach

0B9C4ZX Drainage of Right Upper Lung Lobe, Percutaneous Endoscopic Approach, Diagnostic

0B9C4ZZ Drainage of Right Upper Lung Lobe, Percutaneous Endoscopic Approach

0B9C70Z Drainage of Right Upper Lung Lobe with Drainage Device, Via Natural or Artificial Opening

0B9C7ZX Drainage of Right Upper Lung Lobe, Via Natural or Artificial Opening, Diagnostic

0B9C7ZZ Drainage of Right Upper Lung Lobe, Via Natural or Artificial Opening

0B9C80Z Drainage of Right Upper Lung Lobe with Drainage Device, Via Natural or Artificial Opening Endoscopic

0B9C8ZX Drainage of Right Upper Lung Lobe, Via Natural or Artificial Opening Endoscopic, Diagnostic

0B9C8ZZ Drainage of Right Upper Lung Lobe, Via Natural or Artificial Opening Endoscopic

0B9D00Z Drainage of Right Middle Lung Lobe with Drainage Device, Open Approach

0B9D0ZX Drainage of Right Middle Lung Lobe, Open Approach, Diagnostic

0B9D0ZZ Drainage of Right Middle Lung Lobe, Open Approach

0B9D30Z Drainage of Right Middle Lung Lobe with Drainage Device, Percutaneous Approach

0B9D3ZX Drainage of Right Middle Lung Lobe, Percutaneous Approach, Diagnostic

0B9D3ZZ Drainage of Right Middle Lung Lobe, Percutaneous Approach

0B9D40Z Drainage of Right Middle Lung Lobe with Drainage Device, Percutaneous Endoscopic Approach

0B9D4ZX Drainage of Right Middle Lung Lobe, Percutaneous Endoscopic Approach, Diagnostic

0B9D4ZZ Drainage of Right Middle Lung Lobe, Percutaneous Endoscopic Approach

0B9D70Z Drainage of Right Middle Lung Lobe with Drainage Device, Via Natural or Artificial Opening

0B9D7ZX Drainage of Right Middle Lung Lobe, Via Natural or Artificial Opening, Diagnostic

0B9D7ZZ Drainage of Right Middle Lung Lobe, Via Natural or Artificial Opening

♀ Female-only   ♂ Male-only   ▲ Limited Coverage   ● Non-OR   🔤 HAC-associated procedure   ▲ Non-covered procedures   ✚ Cluster

0B9D80Z Drainage of Right Middle Lung Lobe with Drainage Device, Via Natural or Artificial Opening Endoscopic

0B9D8ZX Drainage of Right Middle Lung Lobe, Via Natural or Artificial Opening Endoscopic, Diagnostic

0B9D8ZZ Drainage of Right Middle Lung Lobe, Via Natural or Artificial Opening Endoscopic

0B9F00Z Drainage of Right Lower Lung Lobe with Drainage Device, Open Approach

0B9F0ZX Drainage of Right Lower Lung Lobe, Open Approach, Diagnostic

0B9F0ZZ Drainage of Right Lower Lung Lobe, Open Approach

0B9F30Z Drainage of Right Lower Lung Lobe with Drainage Device, Percutaneous Approach

0B9F3ZX Drainage of Right Lower Lung Lobe, Percutaneous Approach, Diagnostic

0B9F3ZZ Drainage of Right Lower Lung Lobe, Percutaneous Approach

0B9F40Z Drainage of Right Lower Lung Lobe with Drainage Device, Percutaneous Endoscopic Approach

0B9F4ZX Drainage of Right Lower Lung Lobe, Percutaneous Endoscopic Approach, Diagnostic

0B9F4ZZ Drainage of Right Lower Lung Lobe, Percutaneous Endoscopic Approach

0B9F70Z Drainage of Right Lower Lung Lobe with Drainage Device, Via Natural or Artificial Opening

0B9F7ZX Drainage of Right Lower Lung Lobe, Via Natural or Artificial Opening, Diagnostic

0B9F7ZZ Drainage of Right Lower Lung Lobe, Via Natural or Artificial Opening

0B9F80Z Drainage of Right Lower Lung Lobe with Drainage Device, Via Natural or Artificial Opening Endoscopic

0B9F8ZX Drainage of Right Lower Lung Lobe, Via Natural or Artificial Opening Endoscopic, Diagnostic

0B9F8ZZ Drainage of Right Lower Lung Lobe, Via Natural or Artificial Opening Endoscopic

0B9G00Z Drainage of Left Upper Lung Lobe with Drainage Device, Open Approach

0B9G0ZX Drainage of Left Upper Lung Lobe, Open Approach, Diagnostic

0B9G0ZZ Drainage of Left Upper Lung Lobe, Open Approach

0B9G30Z Drainage of Left Upper Lung Lobe with Drainage Device, Percutaneous Approach

0B9G3ZX Drainage of Left Upper Lung Lobe, Percutaneous Approach, Diagnostic

0B9G3ZZ Drainage of Left Upper Lung Lobe, Percutaneous Approach

0B9G40Z Drainage of Left Upper Lung Lobe with Drainage Device, Percutaneous Endoscopic Approach

0B9G4ZX Drainage of Left Upper Lung Lobe, Percutaneous Endoscopic Approach, Diagnostic

0B9G4ZZ Drainage of Left Upper Lung Lobe, Percutaneous Endoscopic Approach

0B9G70Z Drainage of Left Upper Lung Lobe with Drainage Device, Via Natural or Artificial Opening

0B9G7ZX Drainage of Left Upper Lung Lobe, Via Natural or Artificial Opening, Diagnostic

0B9G7ZZ Drainage of Left Upper Lung Lobe, Via Natural or Artificial Opening

0B9G80Z Drainage of Left Upper Lung Lobe with Drainage Device, Via Natural or Artificial Opening Endoscopic

0B9G8ZX Drainage of Left Upper Lung Lobe, Via Natural or Artificial Opening Endoscopic, Diagnostic

0B9G8ZZ Drainage of Left Upper Lung Lobe, Via Natural or Artificial Opening Endoscopic

0B9H00Z Drainage of Lung Lingula with Drainage Device, Open Approach

0B9H0ZX Drainage of Lung Lingula, Open Approach, Diagnostic

0B9H0ZZ Drainage of Lung Lingula, Open Approach

0B9H30Z Drainage of Lung Lingula with Drainage Device, Percutaneous Approach

0B9H3ZX Drainage of Lung Lingula, Percutaneous Approach, Diagnostic

0B9H3ZZ Drainage of Lung Lingula, Percutaneous Approach

0B9H40Z Drainage of Lung Lingula with Drainage Device, Percutaneous Endoscopic Approach

0B9H4ZX Drainage of Lung Lingula, Percutaneous Endoscopic Approach, Diagnostic

0B9H4ZZ Drainage of Lung Lingula, Percutaneous Endoscopic Approach

0B9H70Z Drainage of Lung Lingula with Drainage Device, Via Natural or Artificial Opening

0B9H7ZX Drainage of Lung Lingula, Via Natural or Artificial Opening, Diagnostic

0B9H7ZZ Drainage of Lung Lingula, Via Natural or Artificial Opening

0B9H80Z Drainage of Lung Lingula with Drainage Device, Via Natural or Artificial Opening Endoscopic

0B9H8ZX Drainage of Lung Lingula, Via Natural or Artificial Opening Endoscopic, Diagnostic

0B9H8ZZ Drainage of Lung Lingula, Via Natural or Artificial Opening Endoscopic

0B9J00Z Drainage of Left Lower Lung Lobe with Drainage Device, Open Approach

0B9J0ZX Drainage of Left Lower Lung Lobe, Open Approach, Diagnostic

0B9J0ZZ Drainage of Left Lower Lung Lobe, Open Approach

0B9J30Z Drainage of Left Lower Lung Lobe with Drainage Device, Percutaneous Approach

0B9J3ZX Drainage of Left Lower Lung Lobe, Percutaneous Approach, Diagnostic

0B9J3ZZ Drainage of Left Lower Lung Lobe, Percutaneous Approach

0B9J40Z Drainage of Left Lower Lung Lobe with Drainage Device, Percutaneous Endoscopic Approach

0B9J4ZX Drainage of Left Lower Lung Lobe, Percutaneous Endoscopic Approach, Diagnostic

0B9J4ZZ Drainage of Left Lower Lung Lobe, Percutaneous Endoscopic Approach

0B9J70Z Drainage of Left Lower Lung Lobe with Drainage Device, Via Natural or Artificial Opening

0B9J7ZX Drainage of Left Lower Lung Lobe, Via Natural or Artificial Opening, Diagnostic

0B9J7ZZ Drainage of Left Lower Lung Lobe, Via Natural or Artificial Opening

0B9J80Z Drainage of Left Lower Lung Lobe with Drainage Device, Via Natural or Artificial Opening Endoscopic

0B9J8ZX Drainage of Left Lower Lung Lobe, Via Natural or Artificial Opening Endoscopic, Diagnostic

AHA CC: 1Q, 2016, 26-27; 1Q, 2017, 51

0B9J8ZZ Drainage of Left Lower Lung Lobe, Via Natural or Artificial Opening Endoscopic

0B9K00Z Drainage of Right Lung with Drainage Device, Open Approach

0B9K0ZX Drainage of Right Lung, Open Approach, Diagnostic

0B9K0ZZ Drainage of Right Lung, Open Approach

0B9K30Z Drainage of Right Lung with Drainage Device, Percutaneous Approach

0B9K3ZX Drainage of Right Lung, Percutaneous Approach, Diagnostic

0B9K3ZZ Drainage of Right Lung, Percutaneous Approach

0B9K40Z Drainage of Right Lung with Drainage Device, Percutaneous Endoscopic Approach

0B9K4ZX Drainage of Right Lung, Percutaneous Endoscopic Approach, Diagnostic

0B9K4ZZ Drainage of Right Lung, Percutaneous Endoscopic Approach

0B9K70Z Drainage of Right Lung with Drainage Device, Via Natural or Artificial Opening

0B9K7ZX Drainage of Right Lung, Via Natural or Artificial Opening, Diagnostic

0B9K7ZZ Drainage of Right Lung, Via Natural or Artificial Opening

0B9K80Z Drainage of Right Lung with Drainage Device, Via Natural or Artificial Opening Endoscopic

0B9K8ZX Drainage of Right Lung, Via Natural or Artificial Opening Endoscopic, Diagnostic

0B9K8ZZ Drainage of Right Lung, Via Natural or Artificial Opening Endoscopic

0B9L00Z Drainage of Left Lung with Drainage Device, Open Approach

0B9L0ZX Drainage of Left Lung, Open Approach, Diagnostic

0B9L0ZZ Drainage of Left Lung, Open Approach

0B9L30Z Drainage of Left Lung with Drainage Device, Percutaneous Approach

0B9L3ZX Drainage of Left Lung, Percutaneous Approach, Diagnostic

0B9L3ZZ Drainage of Left Lung, Percutaneous Approach

0B9L40Z Drainage of Left Lung with Drainage Device, Percutaneous Endoscopic Approach

0B9L4ZX Drainage of Left Lung, Percutaneous Endoscopic Approach, Diagnostic

0B9L4ZZ Drainage of Left Lung, Percutaneous Endoscopic Approach

0B9L70Z Drainage of Left Lung with Drainage Device, Via Natural or Artificial Opening

0B9L7ZX Drainage of Left Lung, Via Natural or Artificial Opening, Diagnostic

0B9L7ZZ Drainage of Left Lung, Via Natural or Artificial Opening

0B9L80Z Drainage of Left Lung with Drainage Device, Via Natural or Artificial Opening Endoscopic

0B9L8ZX Drainage of Left Lung, Via Natural or Artificial Opening Endoscopic, Diagnostic

0B9L8ZZ Drainage of Left Lung, Via Natural or Artificial Opening Endoscopic

0B9M00Z Drainage of Bilateral Lungs with Drainage Device, Open Approach

0B9M0ZX Drainage of Bilateral Lungs, Open Approach, Diagnostic

0B9M0ZZ Drainage of Bilateral Lungs, Open Approach

0B9M30Z Drainage of Bilateral Lungs with Drainage Device, Percutaneous Approach

0B9M3ZX Drainage of Bilateral Lungs, Percutaneous Approach, Diagnostic

0B9M3ZZ Drainage of Bilateral Lungs, Percutaneous Approach

0B9M40Z Drainage of Bilateral Lungs with Drainage Device, Percutaneous Endoscopic Approach

0B9M4ZX Drainage of Bilateral Lungs, Percutaneous Endoscopic Approach, Diagnostic

0B9M4ZZ Drainage of Bilateral Lungs, Percutaneous Endoscopic Approach

0B9M70Z Drainage of Bilateral Lungs with Drainage Device, Via Natural or Artificial Opening

0B9M7ZX Drainage of Bilateral Lungs, Via Natural or Artificial Opening, Diagnostic

0B9M7ZZ Drainage of Bilateral Lungs, Via Natural or Artificial Opening

0B9M80Z Drainage of Bilateral Lungs with Drainage Device, Via Natural or Artificial Opening Endoscopic

0B9M8ZX Drainage of Bilateral Lungs, Via Natural or Artificial Opening Endoscopic, Diagnostic

0B9M8ZZ Drainage of Bilateral Lungs, Via Natural or Artificial Opening Endoscopic

  AHA CC: 3Q, 2017, 15

0B9N00Z Drainage of Right Pleura with Drainage Device, Open Approach

0B9N0ZX Drainage of Right Pleura, Open Approach, Diagnostic

0B9N0ZZ Drainage of Right Pleura, Open Approach

0B9N30Z Drainage of Right Pleura with Drainage Device, Percutaneous Approach

0B9N3ZX Drainage of Right Pleura, Percutaneous Approach, Diagnostic

0B9N3ZZ Drainage of Right Pleura, Percutaneous Approach

0B9N40Z Drainage of Right Pleura with Drainage Device, Percutaneous Endoscopic Approach

0B9N4ZX Drainage of Right Pleura, Percutaneous Endoscopic Approach, Diagnostic

0B9N4ZZ Drainage of Right Pleura, Percutaneous Endoscopic Approach

0B9N80Z Drainage of Right Pleura with Drainage Device, Via Natural or Artificial Opening Endoscopic

0B9N8ZX Drainage of Right Pleura, Via Natural or Artificial Opening Endoscopic, Diagnostic

0B9N8ZZ Drainage of Right Pleura, Via Natural or Artificial Opening Endoscopic

0B9P00Z Drainage of Left Pleura with Drainage Device, Open Approach

0B9P0ZX Drainage of Left Pleura, Open Approach, Diagnostic

0B9P0ZZ Drainage of Left Pleura, Open Approach

0B9P30Z Drainage of Left Pleura with Drainage Device, Percutaneous Approach

0B9P3ZX Drainage of Left Pleura, Percutaneous Approach, Diagnostic

0B9P3ZZ Drainage of Left Pleura, Percutaneous Approach

0B9P40Z Drainage of Left Pleura with Drainage Device, Percutaneous Endoscopic Approach

0B9P4ZX Drainage of Left Pleura, Percutaneous Endoscopic Approach, Diagnostic

0B9P4ZZ Drainage of Left Pleura, Percutaneous Endoscopic Approach

0B9P80Z Drainage of Left Pleura with Drainage Device, Via Natural or Artificial Opening Endoscopic

0B9P8ZX Drainage of Left Pleura, Via Natural or Artificial Opening Endoscopic, Diagnostic

0B9P8ZZ Drainage of Left Pleura, Via Natural or Artificial Opening Endoscopic

0B9T00Z Drainage of Diaphragm with Drainage Device, Open Approach

0B9T0ZX Drainage of Diaphragm, Open Approach, Diagnostic

0B9T0ZZ Drainage of Diaphragm, Open Approach

0B9T30Z Drainage of Diaphragm with Drainage Device, Percutaneous Approach

0B9T3ZX Drainage of Diaphragm, Percutaneous Approach, Diagnostic

0B9T3ZZ Drainage of Diaphragm, Percutaneous Approach

0B9T40Z Drainage of Diaphragm with Drainage Device, Percutaneous Endoscopic Approach

0B9T4ZX Drainage of Diaphragm, Percutaneous Endoscopic Approach, Diagnostic

0B9T4ZZ Drainage of Diaphragm, Percutaneous Endoscopic Approach

0BB – Respiratory System, Excision

Review Coding Guidelines B3.4a and B3.4b

Review Coding Guideline B3.8

Review Coding Guideline B3.18

0BB10ZX Excision of Trachea, Open Approach, Diagnostic

0BB10ZZ Excision of Trachea, Open Approach
  AHA CC: 1Q, 2015, 15-16

0BB13ZX Excision of Trachea, Percutaneous Approach, Diagnostic

0BB13ZZ Excision of Trachea, Percutaneous Approach

0BB14ZX Excision of Trachea, Percutaneous Endoscopic Approach, Diagnostic

0BB14ZZ Excision of Trachea, Percutaneous Endoscopic Approach

0BB17ZX Excision of Trachea, Via Natural or Artificial Opening, Diagnostic

0BB17ZZ Excision of Trachea, Via Natural or Artificial Opening

0BB18ZX Excision of Trachea, Via Natural or Artificial Opening Endoscopic, Diagnostic

0BB18ZZ Excision of Trachea, Via Natural or Artificial Opening Endoscopic

0BB20ZX Excision of Carina, Open Approach, Diagnostic

0BB20ZZ Excision of Carina, Open Approach

0BB23ZX Excision of Carina, Percutaneous Approach, Diagnostic

0BB23ZZ Excision of Carina, Percutaneous Approach

0BB24ZX Excision of Carina, Percutaneous Endoscopic Approach, Diagnostic

0BB24ZZ Excision of Carina, Percutaneous Endoscopic Approach

0BB27ZX Excision of Carina, Via Natural or Artificial Opening, Diagnostic

0BB27ZZ Excision of Carina, Via Natural or Artificial Opening

0BB28ZX Excision of Carina, Via Natural or Artificial Opening Endoscopic, Diagnostic

0BB28ZZ Excision of Carina, Via Natural or Artificial Opening Endoscopic

0BB30ZX Excision of Right Main Bronchus, Open Approach, Diagnostic

0BB30ZZ Excision of Right Main Bronchus, Open Approach

0BB33ZX Excision of Right Main Bronchus, Percutaneous Approach, Diagnostic

0BB33ZZ Excision of Right Main Bronchus, Percutaneous Approach

0BB34ZX Excision of Right Main Bronchus, Percutaneous Endoscopic Approach, Diagnostic

0BB34ZZ Excision of Right Main Bronchus, Percutaneous Endoscopic Approach

0BB37ZX Excision of Right Main Bronchus, Via Natural or Artificial Opening, Diagnostic

0BB37ZZ Excision of Right Main Bronchus, Via Natural or Artificial Opening

0BB38ZX Excision of Right Main Bronchus, Via Natural or Artificial Opening Endoscopic, Diagnostic

0BB38ZZ Excision of Right Main Bronchus, Via Natural or Artificial Opening Endoscopic

0BB40ZX Excision of Right Upper Lobe Bronchus, Open Approach, Diagnostic

0BB40ZZ Excision of Right Upper Lobe Bronchus, Open Approach

0BB43ZX Excision of Right Upper Lobe Bronchus, Percutaneous Approach, Diagnostic

0BB43ZZ Excision of Right Upper Lobe Bronchus, Percutaneous Approach

0BB44ZX Excision of Right Upper Lobe Bronchus, Percutaneous Endoscopic Approach, Diagnostic

0BB44ZZ Excision of Right Upper Lobe Bronchus, Percutaneous Endoscopic Approach

0BB47ZX Excision of Right Upper Lobe Bronchus, Via Natural or Artificial Opening, Diagnostic

0BB47ZZ Excision of Right Upper Lobe Bronchus, Via Natural or Artificial Opening

0BB48ZX Excision of Right Upper Lobe Bronchus, Via Natural or Artificial Opening Endoscopic, Diagnostic
AHA CC: 1Q, 2016, 26-27

0BB48ZZ Excision of Right Upper Lobe Bronchus, Via Natural or Artificial Opening Endoscopic

0BB50ZX Excision of Right Middle Lobe Bronchus, Open Approach, Diagnostic

0BB50ZZ Excision of Right Middle Lobe Bronchus, Open Approach

0BB53ZX Excision of Right Middle Lobe Bronchus, Percutaneous Approach, Diagnostic

0BB53ZZ Excision of Right Middle Lobe Bronchus, Percutaneous Approach

0BB54ZX Excision of Right Middle Lobe Bronchus, Percutaneous Endoscopic Approach, Diagnostic

0BB54ZZ Excision of Right Middle Lobe Bronchus, Percutaneous Endoscopic Approach

0BB57ZX Excision of Right Middle Lobe Bronchus, Via Natural or Artificial Opening, Diagnostic

0BB57ZZ Excision of Right Middle Lobe Bronchus, Via Natural or Artificial Opening

0BB58ZX Excision of Right Middle Lobe Bronchus, Via Natural or Artificial Opening Endoscopic, Diagnostic

0BB58ZZ Excision of Right Middle Lobe Bronchus, Via Natural or Artificial Opening Endoscopic

0BB60ZX Excision of Right Lower Lobe Bronchus, Open Approach, Diagnostic

0BB60ZZ Excision of Right Lower Lobe Bronchus, Open Approach

0BB63ZX Excision of Right Lower Lobe Bronchus, Percutaneous Approach, Diagnostic

0BB63ZZ Excision of Right Lower Lobe Bronchus, Percutaneous Approach

0BB64ZX Excision of Right Lower Lobe Bronchus, Percutaneous Endoscopic Approach, Diagnostic

0BB64ZZ Excision of Right Lower Lobe Bronchus, Percutaneous Endoscopic Approach

0BB67ZX Excision of Right Lower Lobe Bronchus, Via Natural or Artificial Opening, Diagnostic

0BB67ZZ Excision of Right Lower Lobe Bronchus, Via Natural or Artificial Opening

0BB68ZX Excision of Right Lower Lobe Bronchus, Via Natural or Artificial Opening Endoscopic, Diagnostic

0BB68ZZ Excision of Right Lower Lobe Bronchus, Via Natural or Artificial Opening Endoscopic

0BB70ZX Excision of Left Main Bronchus, Open Approach, Diagnostic

0BB70ZZ Excision of Left Main Bronchus, Open Approach

0BB73ZX Excision of Left Main Bronchus, Percutaneous Approach, Diagnostic

0BB73ZZ Excision of Left Main Bronchus, Percutaneous Approach

0BB74ZX Excision of Left Main Bronchus, Percutaneous Endoscopic Approach, Diagnostic

0BB74ZZ Excision of Left Main Bronchus, Percutaneous Endoscopic Approach

0BB77ZX Excision of Left Main Bronchus, Via Natural or Artificial Opening, Diagnostic

0BB77ZZ Excision of Left Main Bronchus, Via Natural or Artificial Opening

0BB78ZX Excision of Left Main Bronchus, Via Natural or Artificial Opening Endoscopic, Diagnostic

0BB78ZZ Excision of Left Main Bronchus, Via Natural or Artificial Opening Endoscopic

0BB80ZX Excision of Left Upper Lobe Bronchus, Open Approach, Diagnostic

0BB80ZZ Excision of Left Upper Lobe Bronchus, Open Approach

0BB83ZX Excision of Left Upper Lobe Bronchus, Percutaneous Approach, Diagnostic

0BB83ZZ Excision of Left Upper Lobe Bronchus, Percutaneous Approach

0BB84ZX Excision of Left Upper Lobe Bronchus, Percutaneous Endoscopic Approach, Diagnostic

0BB84ZZ Excision of Left Upper Lobe Bronchus, Percutaneous Endoscopic Approach

0BB87ZX Excision of Left Upper Lobe Bronchus, Via Natural or Artificial Opening, Diagnostic

0BB87ZZ Excision of Left Upper Lobe Bronchus, Via Natural or Artificial Opening

0BB88ZX Excision of Left Upper Lobe Bronchus, Via Natural or Artificial Opening Endoscopic, Diagnostic
AHA CC: 1Q, 2016, 27

0BB88ZZ Excision of Left Upper Lobe Bronchus, Via Natural or Artificial Opening Endoscopic

0BB90ZX Excision of Lingula Bronchus, Open Approach, Diagnostic

0BB90ZZ Excision of Lingula Bronchus, Open Approach

0BB93ZX Excision of Lingula Bronchus, Percutaneous Approach, Diagnostic

0BB93ZZ Excision of Lingula Bronchus, Percutaneous Approach

0BB94ZX Excision of Lingula Bronchus, Percutaneous Endoscopic Approach, Diagnostic

0BB94ZZ Excision of Lingula Bronchus, Percutaneous Endoscopic Approach

0BB97ZX Excision of Lingula Bronchus, Via Natural or Artificial Opening, Diagnostic

0BB97ZZ Excision of Lingula Bronchus, Via Natural or Artificial Opening

0BB98ZX Excision of Lingula Bronchus, Via Natural or Artificial Opening Endoscopic, Diagnostic

0BB98ZZ Excision of Lingula Bronchus, Via Natural or Artificial Opening Endoscopic

0BBB0ZX Excision of Left Lower Lobe Bronchus, Open Approach, Diagnostic

0BBB0ZZ Excision of Left Lower Lobe Bronchus, Open Approach

0BBB3ZX Excision of Left Lower Lobe Bronchus, Percutaneous Approach, Diagnostic

0BBB3ZZ Excision of Left Lower Lobe Bronchus, Percutaneous Approach

0BBB4ZX Excision of Left Lower Lobe Bronchus, Percutaneous Endoscopic Approach, Diagnostic

0BBB4ZZ Excision of Left Lower Lobe Bronchus, Percutaneous Endoscopic Approach

0BBB7ZX Excision of Left Lower Lobe Bronchus, Via Natural or Artificial Opening, Diagnostic

0BBB7ZZ Excision of Left Lower Lobe Bronchus, Via Natural or Artificial Opening

0BBB8ZX Excision of Left Lower Lobe Bronchus, Via Natural or Artificial Opening Endoscopic, Diagnostic

0BBB8ZZ Excision of Left Lower Lobe Bronchus, Via Natural or Artificial Opening Endoscopic

0BBC0ZX Excision of Right Upper Lung Lobe, Open Approach, Diagnostic

0BBC0ZZ Excision of Right Upper Lung Lobe, Open Approach

0BBC3ZX Excision of Right Upper Lung Lobe, Percutaneous Approach, Diagnostic

0BBC3ZZ Excision of Right Upper Lung Lobe, Percutaneous Approach

0BBC4ZX Excision of Right Upper Lung Lobe, Percutaneous Endoscopic Approach, Diagnostic

0BBC4ZZ Excision of Right Upper Lung Lobe, Percutaneous Endoscopic Approach

0BBC7ZX Excision of Right Upper Lung Lobe, Via Natural or Artificial Opening, Diagnostic

0BBC7ZZ Excision of Right Upper Lung Lobe, Via Natural or Artificial Opening

0BBC8ZX Excision of Right Upper Lung Lobe, Via Natural or Artificial Opening Endoscopic, Diagnostic
AHA CC: 1Q, 2016, 26-27

0BBC8ZZ Excision of Right Upper Lung Lobe, Via Natural or Artificial Opening Endoscopic

0BBD0ZX Excision of Right Middle Lung Lobe, Open Approach, Diagnostic

0BBD0ZZ Excision of Right Middle Lung Lobe, Open Approach

0BBD3ZX Excision of Right Middle Lung Lobe, Percutaneous Approach, Diagnostic

0BBD3ZZ Excision of Right Middle Lung Lobe, Percutaneous Approach

0BBD4ZX Excision of Right Middle Lung Lobe, Percutaneous Endoscopic Approach, Diagnostic

0BBD4ZZ Excision of Right Middle Lung Lobe, Percutaneous Endoscopic Approach

0BBD7ZX Excision of Right Middle Lung Lobe, Via Natural or Artificial Opening, Diagnostic

0BBD7ZZ Excision of Right Middle Lung Lobe, Via Natural or Artificial Opening

0BBD8ZX Excision of Right Middle Lung Lobe, Via Natural or Artificial Opening Endoscopic, Diagnostic

0BBD8ZZ Excision of Right Middle Lung Lobe, Via Natural or Artificial Opening Endoscopic

0BBF0ZX Excision of Right Lower Lung Lobe, Open Approach, Diagnostic

0BBF0ZZ Excision of Right Lower Lung Lobe, Open Approach

0BBF3ZX Excision of Right Lower Lung Lobe, Percutaneous Approach, Diagnostic

0BBF3ZZ Excision of Right Lower Lung Lobe, Percutaneous Approach

0BBF4ZX Excision of Right Lower Lung Lobe, Percutaneous Endoscopic Approach, Diagnostic

0BBF4ZZ Excision of Right Lower Lung Lobe, Percutaneous Endoscopic Approach

0BBF7ZX Excision of Right Lower Lung Lobe, Via Natural or Artificial Opening, Diagnostic

0BBF7ZZ Excision of Right Lower Lung Lobe, Via Natural or Artificial Opening

0BBF8ZX	Excision of Right Lower Lung Lobe, Via Natural or Artificial Opening Endoscopic, Diagnostic	**0BBJ4ZZ**	Excision of Left Lower Lung Lobe, Percutaneous Endoscopic Approach	**0BBM4ZX**	Excision of Bilateral Lungs, Percutaneous Endoscopic Approach, Diagnostic
0BBF8ZZ	Excision of Right Lower Lung Lobe, Via Natural or Artificial Opening Endoscopic	**0BBJ7ZX**	Excision of Left Lower Lung Lobe, Via Natural or Artificial Opening, Diagnostic	**0BBM4ZZ**	Excision of Bilateral Lungs, Percutaneous Endoscopic Approach
0BBG0ZX	Excision of Left Upper Lung Lobe, Open Approach, Diagnostic	**0BBJ7ZZ**	Excision of Left Lower Lung Lobe, Via Natural or Artificial Opening	**0BBM7ZX**	Excision of Bilateral Lungs, Via Natural or Artificial Opening, Diagnostic
0BBG0ZZ	Excision of Left Upper Lung Lobe, Open Approach	**0BBJ8ZX**	Excision of Left Lower Lung Lobe, Via Natural or Artificial Opening Endoscopic, Diagnostic	**0BBM7ZZ**	Excision of Bilateral Lungs, Via Natural or Artificial Opening
0BBG3ZX	Excision of Left Upper Lung Lobe, Percutaneous Approach, Diagnostic	**0BBJ8ZZ**	Excision of Left Lower Lung Lobe, Via Natural or Artificial Opening Endoscopic	**0BBM8ZX**	Excision of Bilateral Lungs, Via Natural or Artificial Opening Endoscopic, Diagnostic
0BBG3ZZ	Excision of Left Upper Lung Lobe, Percutaneous Approach	**0BBK0ZX**	Excision of Right Lung, Open Approach, Diagnostic	**0BBM8ZZ**	Excision of Bilateral Lungs, Via Natural or Artificial Opening Endoscopic
0BBG4ZX	Excision of Left Upper Lung Lobe, Percutaneous Endoscopic Approach, Diagnostic	**0BBK0ZZ**	Excision of Right Lung, Open Approach	**0BBN0ZX**	Excision of Right Pleura, Open Approach, Diagnostic
0BBG4ZZ	Excision of Left Upper Lung Lobe, Percutaneous Endoscopic Approach	**0BBK3ZX**	Excision of Right Lung, Percutaneous Approach, Diagnostic	**0BBN0ZZ**	Excision of Right Pleura, Open Approach
0BBG7ZX	Excision of Left Upper Lung Lobe, Via Natural or Artificial Opening, Diagnostic	**0BBK3ZZ**	Excision of Right Lung, Percutaneous Approach	**0BBN3ZX**	Excision of Right Pleura, Percutaneous Approach, Diagnostic
0BBG7ZZ	Excision of Left Upper Lung Lobe, Via Natural or Artificial Opening	**0BBK4ZX**	Excision of Right Lung, Percutaneous Endoscopic Approach, Diagnostic	**0BBN3ZZ**	Excision of Right Pleura, Percutaneous Approach
0BBG8ZX	Excision of Left Upper Lung Lobe, Via Natural or Artificial Opening Endoscopic, Diagnostic	**0BBK4ZZ**	Excision of Right Lung, Percutaneous Endoscopic Approach	**0BBN4ZX**	Excision of Right Pleura, Percutaneous Endoscopic Approach, Diagnostic
0BBG8ZZ	Excision of Left Upper Lung Lobe, Via Natural or Artificial Opening Endoscopic	**0BBK7ZX**	Excision of Right Lung, Via Natural or Artificial Opening, Diagnostic	**0BBN4ZZ**	Excision of Right Pleura, Percutaneous Endoscopic Approach
0BBH0ZX	Excision of Lung Lingula, Open Approach, Diagnostic	**0BBK7ZZ**	Excision of Right Lung, Via Natural or Artificial Opening	**0BBN8ZX**	Excision of Right Pleura, Via Natural or Artificial Opening Endoscopic, Diagnostic
0BBH0ZZ	Excision of Lung Lingula, Open Approach	**0BBK8ZX**	Excision of Right Lung, Via Natural or Artificial Opening Endoscopic, Diagnostic	**0BBN8ZZ**	Excision of Right Pleura, Via Natural or Artificial Opening Endoscopic
0BBH3ZX	Excision of Lung Lingula, Percutaneous Approach, Diagnostic	*AHA CC: 1Q, 2014, 20-21*		**0BBP0ZX**	Excision of Left Pleura, Open Approach, Diagnostic
0BBH3ZZ	Excision of Lung Lingula, Percutaneous Approach	**0BBK8ZZ**	Excision of Right Lung, Via Natural or Artificial Opening Endoscopic	**0BBP0ZZ**	Excision of Left Pleura, Open Approach
0BBH4ZX	Excision of Lung Lingula, Percutaneous Endoscopic Approach, Diagnostic	**0BBL0ZX**	Excision of Left Lung, Open Approach, Diagnostic	**0BBP3ZX**	Excision of Left Pleura, Percutaneous Approach, Diagnostic
0BBH4ZZ	Excision of Lung Lingula, Percutaneous Endoscopic Approach	**0BBL0ZZ**	Excision of Left Lung, Open Approach	**0BBP3ZZ**	Excision of Left Pleura, Percutaneous Approach
0BBH7ZX	Excision of Lung Lingula, Via Natural or Artificial Opening, Diagnostic	**0BBL3ZX**	Excision of Left Lung, Percutaneous Approach, Diagnostic	**0BBP4ZX**	Excision of Left Pleura, Percutaneous Endoscopic Approach, Diagnostic
0BBH7ZZ	Excision of Lung Lingula, Via Natural or Artificial Opening	**0BBL3ZZ**	Excision of Left Lung, Percutaneous Approach	**0BBP4ZZ**	Excision of Left Pleura, Percutaneous Endoscopic Approach
0BBH8ZX	Excision of Lung Lingula, Via Natural or Artificial Opening Endoscopic, Diagnostic	**0BBL4ZX**	Excision of Left Lung, Percutaneous Endoscopic Approach, Diagnostic	**0BBP8ZX**	Excision of Left Pleura, Via Natural or Artificial Opening Endoscopic, Diagnostic
0BBH8ZZ	Excision of Lung Lingula, Via Natural or Artificial Opening Endoscopic	**0BBL4ZZ**	Excision of Left Lung, Percutaneous Endoscopic Approach	**0BBP8ZZ**	Excision of Left Pleura, Via Natural or Artificial Opening Endoscopic
0BBJ0ZX	Excision of Left Lower Lung Lobe, Open Approach, Diagnostic	**0BBL7ZX**	Excision of Left Lung, Via Natural or Artificial Opening, Diagnostic	**0BBT0ZX**	Excision of Diaphragm, Open Approach, Diagnostic
0BBJ0ZZ	Excision of Left Lower Lung Lobe, Open Approach	**0BBL7ZZ**	Excision of Left Lung, Via Natural or Artificial Opening	**0BBT0ZZ**	Excision of Diaphragm, Open Approach
0BBJ3ZX	Excision of Left Lower Lung Lobe, Percutaneous Approach, Diagnostic	**0BBL8ZX**	Excision of Left Lung, Via Natural or Artificial Opening Endoscopic, Diagnostic	**0BBT3ZX**	Excision of Diaphragm, Percutaneous Approach, Diagnostic
0BBJ3ZZ	Excision of Left Lower Lung Lobe, Percutaneous Approach	**0BBL8ZZ**	Excision of Left Lung, Via Natural or Artificial Opening Endoscopic	**0BBT3ZZ**	Excision of Diaphragm, Percutaneous Approach
0BBJ4ZX	Excision of Left Lower Lung Lobe, Percutaneous Endoscopic Approach, Diagnostic	**0BBM0ZX**	Excision of Bilateral Lungs, Open Approach, Diagnostic	**0BBT4ZX**	Excision of Diaphragm, Percutaneous Endoscopic Approach, Diagnostic
		0BBM0ZZ	Excision of Bilateral Lungs, Open Approach	**0BBT4ZZ**	Excision of Diaphragm, Percutaneous Endoscopic Approach
		0BBM3ZX	Excision of Bilateral Lungs, Percutaneous Approach, Diagnostic		
		0BBM3ZZ	Excision of Bilateral Lungs, Percutaneous Approach		

0BC – Respiratory System, Extirpation

0BC10ZZ	Extirpation of Matter from Trachea, Open Approach	**0BC20ZZ**	Extirpation of Matter from Carina, Open Approach	**0BC30ZZ**	Extirpation of Matter from Right Main Bronchus, Open Approach
0BC13ZZ	Extirpation of Matter from Trachea, Percutaneous Approach	**0BC23ZZ**	Extirpation of Matter from Carina, Percutaneous Approach	**0BC33ZZ**	Extirpation of Matter from Right Main Bronchus, Percutaneous Approach
0BC14ZZ	Extirpation of Matter from Trachea, Percutaneous Endoscopic Approach	**0BC24ZZ**	Extirpation of Matter from Carina, Percutaneous Endoscopic Approach	**0BC34ZZ**	Extirpation of Matter from Right Main Bronchus, Percutaneous Endoscopic Approach
0BC17ZZ	Extirpation of Matter from Trachea, Via Natural or Artificial Opening	**0BC27ZZ**	Extirpation of Matter from Carina, Via Natural or Artificial Opening	**0BC37ZZ**	Extirpation of Matter from Right Main Bronchus, Via Natural or Artificial Opening
0BC18ZZ	Extirpation of Matter from Trachea, Via Natural or Artificial Opening Endoscopic	**0BC28ZZ**	Extirpation of Matter from Carina, Via Natural or Artificial Opening Endoscopic		

♀ Female-only   ♂ Male-only   ▲ Limited Coverage   ● Non-OR   HAC HAC-associated procedure   ▲ Non-covered procedures   ✛ Cluster

0BC38ZZ Extirpation of Matter from Right Main Bronchus, Via Natural or Artificial Opening Endoscopic

0BC40ZZ Extirpation of Matter from Right Upper Lobe Bronchus, Open Approach

0BC43ZZ Extirpation of Matter from Right Upper Lobe Bronchus, Percutaneous Approach

0BC44ZZ Extirpation of Matter from Right Upper Lobe Bronchus, Percutaneous Endoscopic Approach

0BC47ZZ Extirpation of Matter from Right Upper Lobe Bronchus, Via Natural or Artificial Opening

0BC48ZZ Extirpation of Matter from Right Upper Lobe Bronchus, Via Natural or Artificial Opening Endoscopic

0BC50ZZ Extirpation of Matter from Right Middle Lobe Bronchus, Open Approach

0BC53ZZ Extirpation of Matter from Right Middle Lobe Bronchus, Percutaneous Approach

0BC54ZZ Extirpation of Matter from Right Middle Lobe Bronchus, Percutaneous Endoscopic Approach

0BC57ZZ Extirpation of Matter from Right Middle Lobe Bronchus, Via Natural or Artificial Opening

0BC58ZZ Extirpation of Matter from Right Middle Lobe Bronchus, Via Natural or Artificial Opening Endoscopic
AHA CC: 3Q, 2017, 14-15

0BC60ZZ Extirpation of Matter from Right Lower Lobe Bronchus, Open Approach

0BC63ZZ Extirpation of Matter from Right Lower Lobe Bronchus, Percutaneous Approach

0BC64ZZ Extirpation of Matter from Right Lower Lobe Bronchus, Percutaneous Endoscopic Approach

0BC67ZZ Extirpation of Matter from Right Lower Lobe Bronchus, Via Natural or Artificial Opening

0BC68ZZ Extirpation of Matter from Right Lower Lobe Bronchus, Via Natural or Artificial Opening Endoscopic

0BC70ZZ Extirpation of Matter from Left Main Bronchus, Open Approach

0BC73ZZ Extirpation of Matter from Left Main Bronchus, Percutaneous Approach

0BC74ZZ Extirpation of Matter from Left Main Bronchus, Percutaneous Endoscopic Approach

0BC77ZZ Extirpation of Matter from Left Main Bronchus, Via Natural or Artificial Opening

0BC78ZZ Extirpation of Matter from Left Main Bronchus, Via Natural or Artificial Opening Endoscopic

0BC80ZZ Extirpation of Matter from Left Upper Lobe Bronchus, Open Approach

0BC83ZZ Extirpation of Matter from Left Upper Lobe Bronchus, Percutaneous Approach

0BC84ZZ Extirpation of Matter from Left Upper Lobe Bronchus, Percutaneous Endoscopic Approach

0BC87ZZ Extirpation of Matter from Left Upper Lobe Bronchus, Via Natural or Artificial Opening

0BC88ZZ Extirpation of Matter from Left Upper Lobe Bronchus, Via Natural or Artificial Opening Endoscopic

0BC90ZZ Extirpation of Matter from Lingula Bronchus, Open Approach

0BC93ZZ Extirpation of Matter from Lingula Bronchus, Percutaneous Approach

0BC94ZZ Extirpation of Matter from Lingula Bronchus, Percutaneous Endoscopic Approach

0BC97ZZ Extirpation of Matter from Lingula Bronchus, Via Natural or Artificial Opening

0BC98ZZ Extirpation of Matter from Lingula Bronchus, Via Natural or Artificial Opening Endoscopic

0BCB0ZZ Extirpation of Matter from Left Lower Lobe Bronchus, Open Approach

0BCB3ZZ Extirpation of Matter from Left Lower Lobe Bronchus, Percutaneous Approach

0BCB4ZZ Extirpation of Matter from Left Lower Lobe Bronchus, Percutaneous Endoscopic Approach

0BCB7ZZ Extirpation of Matter from Left Lower Lobe Bronchus, Via Natural or Artificial Opening

0BCB8ZZ Extirpation of Matter from Left Lower Lobe Bronchus, Via Natural or Artificial Opening Endoscopic

0BCC0ZZ Extirpation of Matter from Right Upper Lung Lobe, Open Approach

0BCC3ZZ Extirpation of Matter from Right Upper Lung Lobe, Percutaneous Approach

0BCC4ZZ Extirpation of Matter from Right Upper Lung Lobe, Percutaneous Endoscopic Approach

0BCC7ZZ Extirpation of Matter from Right Upper Lung Lobe, Via Natural or Artificial Opening

0BCC8ZZ Extirpation of Matter from Right Upper Lung Lobe, Via Natural or Artificial Opening Endoscopic

0BCD0ZZ Extirpation of Matter from Right Middle Lung Lobe, Open Approach

0BCD3ZZ Extirpation of Matter from Right Middle Lung Lobe, Percutaneous Approach

0BCD4ZZ Extirpation of Matter from Right Middle Lung Lobe, Percutaneous Endoscopic Approach

0BCD7ZZ Extirpation of Matter from Right Middle Lung Lobe, Via Natural or Artificial Opening

0BCD8ZZ Extirpation of Matter from Right Middle Lung Lobe, Via Natural or Artificial Opening Endoscopic

0BCF0ZZ Extirpation of Matter from Right Lower Lung Lobe, Open Approach

0BCF3ZZ Extirpation of Matter from Right Lower Lung Lobe, Percutaneous Approach

0BCF4ZZ Extirpation of Matter from Right Lower Lung Lobe, Percutaneous Endoscopic Approach

0BCF7ZZ Extirpation of Matter from Right Lower Lung Lobe, Via Natural or Artificial Opening

0BCF8ZZ Extirpation of Matter from Right Lower Lung Lobe, Via Natural or Artificial Opening Endoscopic

0BCG0ZZ Extirpation of Matter from Left Upper Lung Lobe, Open Approach

0BCG3ZZ Extirpation of Matter from Left Upper Lung Lobe, Percutaneous Approach

0BCG4ZZ Extirpation of Matter from Left Upper Lung Lobe, Percutaneous Endoscopic Approach

0BCG7ZZ Extirpation of Matter from Left Upper Lung Lobe, Via Natural or Artificial Opening

0BCG8ZZ Extirpation of Matter from Left Upper Lung Lobe, Via Natural or Artificial Opening Endoscopic

0BCH0ZZ Extirpation of Matter from Lung Lingula, Open Approach

0BCH3ZZ Extirpation of Matter from Lung Lingula, Percutaneous Approach

0BCH4ZZ Extirpation of Matter from Lung Lingula, Percutaneous Endoscopic Approach

0BCH7ZZ Extirpation of Matter from Lung Lingula, Via Natural or Artificial Opening

0BCH8ZZ Extirpation of Matter from Lung Lingula, Via Natural or Artificial Opening Endoscopic

0BCJ0ZZ Extirpation of Matter from Left Lower Lung Lobe, Open Approach

0BCJ3ZZ Extirpation of Matter from Left Lower Lung Lobe, Percutaneous Approach

0BCJ4ZZ Extirpation of Matter from Left Lower Lung Lobe, Percutaneous Endoscopic Approach

0BCJ7ZZ Extirpation of Matter from Left Lower Lung Lobe, Via Natural or Artificial Opening

0BCJ8ZZ Extirpation of Matter from Left Lower Lung Lobe, Via Natural or Artificial Opening Endoscopic

0BCK0ZZ Extirpation of Matter from Right Lung, Open Approach

0BCK3ZZ Extirpation of Matter from Right Lung, Percutaneous Approach

0BCK4ZZ Extirpation of Matter from Right Lung, Percutaneous Endoscopic Approach

0BCK7ZZ Extirpation of Matter from Right Lung, Via Natural or Artificial Opening

0BCK8ZZ Extirpation of Matter from Right Lung, Via Natural or Artificial Opening Endoscopic

0BCL0ZZ Extirpation of Matter from Left Lung, Open Approach

0BCL3ZZ Extirpation of Matter from Left Lung, Percutaneous Approach

0BCL4ZZ Extirpation of Matter from Left Lung, Percutaneous Endoscopic Approach

0BCL7ZZ Extirpation of Matter from Left Lung, Via Natural or Artificial Opening

0BCL8ZZ Extirpation of Matter from Left Lung, Via Natural or Artificial Opening Endoscopic

0BCM0ZZ Extirpation of Matter from Bilateral Lungs, Open Approach

0BCM3ZZ Extirpation of Matter from Bilateral Lungs, Percutaneous Approach

0BCM4ZZ Extirpation of Matter from Bilateral Lungs, Percutaneous Endoscopic Approach

0BCM7ZZ Extirpation of Matter from Bilateral Lungs, Via Natural or Artificial Opening

0BCM8ZZ Extirpation of Matter from Bilateral Lungs, Via Natural or Artificial Opening Endoscopic

0BCN0ZZ Extirpation of Matter from Right Pleura, Open Approach

0BCN3ZZ Extirpation of Matter from Right Pleura, Percutaneous Approach

0BCN4ZZ Extirpation of Matter from Right Pleura, Percutaneous Endoscopic Approach

0BCP0ZZ Extirpation of Matter from Left Pleura, Open Approach

0BCP3ZZ Extirpation of Matter from Left Pleura, Percutaneous Approach

0BCP4ZZ Extirpation of Matter from Left Pleura, Percutaneous Endoscopic Approach

| 0BCT0ZZ | Extirpation of Matter from Diaphragm, Open Approach | 0BCT3ZZ | Extirpation of Matter from Diaphragm, Percutaneous Approach | 0BCT4ZZ | Extirpation of Matter from Diaphragm, Percutaneous Endoscopic Approach |

0BD – Respiratory System, Extraction

Review Coding Guidelines B3.4a and B3.4b

0BD14ZX Extraction of Trachea, Percutaneous Endoscopic Approach, Diagnostic

0BD18ZX Extraction of Trachea, Via Natural or Artificial Opening Endoscopic, Diagnostic

0BD24ZX Extraction of Carina, Percutaneous Endoscopic Approach, Diagnostic

0BD28ZX Extraction of Carina, Via Natural or Artificial Opening Endoscopic, Diagnostic

0BD34ZX Extraction of Right Main Bronchus, Percutaneous Endoscopic Approach, Diagnostic

0BD38ZX Extraction of Right Main Bronchus, Via Natural or Artificial Opening Endoscopic, Diagnostic

0BD44ZX Extraction of Right Upper Lobe Bronchus, Percutaneous Endoscopic Approach, Diagnostic

0BD48ZX Extraction of Right Upper Lobe Bronchus, Via Natural or Artificial Opening Endoscopic, Diagnostic

0BD54ZX Extraction of Right Middle Lobe Bronchus, Percutaneous Endoscopic Approach, Diagnostic

0BD58ZX Extraction of Right Middle Lobe Bronchus, Via Natural or Artificial Opening Endoscopic, Diagnostic

0BD64ZX Extraction of Right Lower Lobe Bronchus, Percutaneous Endoscopic Approach, Diagnostic

0BD68ZX Extraction of Right Lower Lobe Bronchus, Via Natural or Artificial Opening Endoscopic, Diagnostic

0BD74ZX Extraction of Left Main Bronchus, Percutaneous Endoscopic Approach, Diagnostic

0BD78ZX Extraction of Left Main Bronchus, Via Natural or Artificial Opening Endoscopic, Diagnostic

0BD84ZX Extraction of Left Upper Lobe Bronchus, Percutaneous Endoscopic Approach, Diagnostic

0BD88ZX Extraction of Left Upper Lobe Bronchus, Via Natural or Artificial Opening Endoscopic, Diagnostic

0BD94ZX Extraction of Lingula Bronchus, Percutaneous Endoscopic Approach, Diagnostic

0BD98ZX Extraction of Lingula Bronchus, Via Natural or Artificial Opening Endoscopic, Diagnostic

0BDB4ZX Extraction of Left Lower Lobe Bronchus, Percutaneous Endoscopic Approach, Diagnostic

0BDB8ZX Extraction of Left Lower Lobe Bronchus, Via Natural or Artificial Opening Endoscopic, Diagnostic

0BDC4ZX Extraction of Right Upper Lung Lobe, Percutaneous Endoscopic Approach, Diagnostic

0BDC8ZX Extraction of Right Upper Lung Lobe, Via Natural or Artificial Opening Endoscopic, Diagnostic
AHA CC: 3Q, 2020, 40-41

0BDD4ZX Extraction of Right Middle Lung Lobe, Percutaneous Endoscopic Approach, Diagnostic

0BDD8ZX Extraction of Right Middle Lung Lobe, Via Natural or Artificial Opening Endoscopic, Diagnostic
AHA CC: 3Q, 2020, 40-41

0BDF4ZX Extraction of Right Lower Lung Lobe, Percutaneous Endoscopic Approach, Diagnostic

0BDF8ZX Extraction of Right Lower Lung Lobe, Via Natural or Artificial Opening Endoscopic, Diagnostic
AHA CC: 3Q, 2020, 40-41

0BDG4ZX Extraction of Left Upper Lung Lobe, Percutaneous Endoscopic Approach, Diagnostic

0BDG8ZX Extraction of Left Upper Lung Lobe, Via Natural or Artificial Opening Endoscopic, Diagnostic

0BDH4ZX Extraction of Lung Lingula, Percutaneous Endoscopic Approach, Diagnostic

0BDH8ZX Extraction of Lung Lingula, Via Natural or Artificial Opening Endoscopic, Diagnostic

0BDJ4ZX Extraction of Left Lower Lung Lobe, Percutaneous Endoscopic Approach, Diagnostic

0BDJ8ZX Extraction of Left Lower Lung Lobe, Via Natural or Artificial Opening Endoscopic, Diagnostic

0BDK4ZX Extraction of Right Lung, Percutaneous Endoscopic Approach, Diagnostic

0BDK8ZX Extraction of Right Lung, Via Natural or Artificial Opening Endoscopic, Diagnostic

0BDL4ZX Extraction of Left Lung, Percutaneous Endoscopic Approach, Diagnostic

0BDL8ZX Extraction of Left Lung, Via Natural or Artificial Opening Endoscopic, Diagnostic

0BDM4ZX Extraction of Bilateral Lungs, Percutaneous Endoscopic Approach, Diagnostic

0BDM8ZX Extraction of Bilateral Lungs, Via Natural or Artificial Opening Endoscopic, Diagnostic

0BDN0ZX Extraction of Right Pleura, Open Approach, Diagnostic

0BDN0ZZ Extraction of Right Pleura, Open Approach

0BDN3ZX Extraction of Right Pleura, Percutaneous Approach, Diagnostic

0BDN3ZZ Extraction of Right Pleura, Percutaneous Approach

0BDN4ZX Extraction of Right Pleura, Percutaneous Endoscopic Approach, Diagnostic

0BDN4ZZ Extraction of Right Pleura, Percutaneous Endoscopic Approach

0BDP0ZX Extraction of Left Pleura, Open Approach, Diagnostic

0BDP0ZZ Extraction of Left Pleura, Open Approach

0BDP3ZX Extraction of Left Pleura, Percutaneous Approach, Diagnostic

0BDP3ZZ Extraction of Left Pleura, Percutaneous Approach

0BDP4ZX Extraction of Left Pleura, Percutaneous Endoscopic Approach, Diagnostic

0BDP4ZZ Extraction of Left Pleura, Percutaneous Endoscopic Approach

0BF – Respiratory System, Fragmentation

0BF10ZZ Fragmentation in Trachea, Open Approach

0BF13ZZ Fragmentation in Trachea, Percutaneous Approach

0BF14ZZ Fragmentation in Trachea, Percutaneous Endoscopic Approach

0BF17ZZ Fragmentation in Trachea, Via Natural or Artificial Opening

0BF18ZZ Fragmentation in Trachea, Via Natural or Artificial Opening Endoscopic

▲ **0BF1XZZ** Fragmentation in Trachea, External Approach

0BF20ZZ Fragmentation in Carina, Open Approach

0BF23ZZ Fragmentation in Carina, Percutaneous Approach

0BF24ZZ Fragmentation in Carina, Percutaneous Endoscopic Approach

0BF27ZZ Fragmentation in Carina, Via Natural or Artificial Opening

0BF28ZZ Fragmentation in Carina, Via Natural or Artificial Opening Endoscopic

▲ **0BF2XZZ** Fragmentation in Carina, External Approach

0BF30ZZ Fragmentation in Right Main Bronchus, Open Approach

0BF33ZZ Fragmentation in Right Main Bronchus, Percutaneous Approach

0BF34ZZ Fragmentation in Right Main Bronchus, Percutaneous Endoscopic Approach

0BF37ZZ Fragmentation in Right Main Bronchus, Via Natural or Artificial Opening

0BF38ZZ Fragmentation in Right Main Bronchus, Via Natural or Artificial Opening Endoscopic

▲ **0BF3XZZ** Fragmentation in Right Main Bronchus, External Approach

0BF40ZZ Fragmentation in Right Upper Lobe Bronchus, Open Approach

0BF43ZZ Fragmentation in Right Upper Lobe Bronchus, Percutaneous Approach

0BF44ZZ Fragmentation in Right Upper Lobe Bronchus, Percutaneous Endoscopic Approach

0BF47ZZ Fragmentation in Right Upper Lobe Bronchus, Via Natural or Artificial Opening

0BF48ZZ Fragmentation in Right Upper Lobe Bronchus, Via Natural or Artificial Opening Endoscopic

♀ Female-only   ♂ Male-only   ▲ Limited Coverage   ● Non-OR   ⬚ HAC-associated procedure   ▲ Non-covered procedures   ✛ Cluster

0BF4XZZ Fragmentation in Right Upper Lobe Bronchus, External Approach

0BF50ZZ Fragmentation in Right Middle Lobe Bronchus, Open Approach

0BF53ZZ Fragmentation in Right Middle Lobe Bronchus, Percutaneous Approach

0BF54ZZ Fragmentation in Right Middle Lobe Bronchus, Percutaneous Endoscopic Approach

0BF57ZZ Fragmentation in Right Middle Lobe Bronchus, Via Natural or Artificial Opening

0BF58ZZ Fragmentation in Right Middle Lobe Bronchus, Via Natural or Artificial Opening Endoscopic

0BF5XZZ Fragmentation in Right Middle Lobe Bronchus, External Approach

0BF60ZZ Fragmentation in Right Lower Lobe Bronchus, Open Approach

0BF63ZZ Fragmentation in Right Lower Lobe Bronchus, Percutaneous Approach

0BF64ZZ Fragmentation in Right Lower Lobe Bronchus, Percutaneous Endoscopic Approach

0BF67ZZ Fragmentation in Right Lower Lobe Bronchus, Via Natural or Artificial Opening

0BF68ZZ Fragmentation in Right Lower Lobe Bronchus, Via Natural or Artificial Opening Endoscopic

▲ **0BF6XZZ** Fragmentation in Right Lower Lobe Bronchus, External Approach

0BF70ZZ Fragmentation in Left Main Bronchus, Open Approach

0BF73ZZ Fragmentation in Left Main Bronchus, Percutaneous Approach

0BF74ZZ Fragmentation in Left Main Bronchus, Percutaneous Endoscopic Approach

0BF77ZZ Fragmentation in Left Main Bronchus, Via Natural or Artificial Opening

0BF78ZZ Fragmentation in Left Main Bronchus, Via Natural or Artificial Opening Endoscopic

▲ **0BF7XZZ** Fragmentation in Left Main Bronchus, External Approach

0BF80ZZ Fragmentation in Left Upper Lobe Bronchus, Open Approach

0BF83ZZ Fragmentation in Left Upper Lobe Bronchus, Percutaneous Approach

0BF84ZZ Fragmentation in Left Upper Lobe Bronchus, Percutaneous Endoscopic Approach

0BF87ZZ Fragmentation in Left Upper Lobe Bronchus, Via Natural or Artificial Opening

0BF88ZZ Fragmentation in Left Upper Lobe Bronchus, Via Natural or Artificial Opening Endoscopic

▲ **0BF8XZZ** Fragmentation in Left Upper Lobe Bronchus, External Approach

0BF90ZZ Fragmentation in Lingula Bronchus, Open Approach

0BF93ZZ Fragmentation in Lingula Bronchus, Percutaneous Approach

0BF94ZZ Fragmentation in Lingula Bronchus, Percutaneous Endoscopic Approach

0BF97ZZ Fragmentation in Lingula Bronchus, Via Natural or Artificial Opening

0BF98ZZ Fragmentation in Lingula Bronchus, Via Natural or Artificial Opening Endoscopic

▲ **0BF9XZZ** Fragmentation in Lingula Bronchus, External Approach

0BFB0ZZ Fragmentation in Left Lower Lobe Bronchus, Open Approach

0BFB3ZZ Fragmentation in Left Lower Lobe Bronchus, Percutaneous Approach

0BFB4ZZ Fragmentation in Left Lower Lobe Bronchus, Percutaneous Endoscopic Approach

0BFB7ZZ Fragmentation in Left Lower Lobe Bronchus, Via Natural or Artificial Opening

0BFB8ZZ Fragmentation in Left Lower Lobe Bronchus, Via Natural or Artificial Opening Endoscopic

▲ **0BFBXZZ** Fragmentation in Left Lower Lobe Bronchus, External Approach

0BH – Respiratory System, Insertion

0BH001Z Insertion of Radioactive Element into Tracheobronchial Tree, Open Approach

0BH002Z Insertion of Monitoring Device into Tracheobronchial Tree, Open Approach

0BH003Z Insertion of Infusion Device into Tracheobronchial Tree, Open Approach

0BH00DZ Insertion of Intraluminal Device into Tracheobronchial Tree, Open Approach

0BH00YZ Insertion of Other Device into Tracheobronchial Tree, Open Approach

0BH031Z Insertion of Radioactive Element into Tracheobronchial Tree, Percutaneous Approach

0BH032Z Insertion of Monitoring Device into Tracheobronchial Tree, Percutaneous Approach

0BH033Z Insertion of Infusion Device into Tracheobronchial Tree, Percutaneous Approach

0BH03DZ Insertion of Intraluminal Device into Tracheobronchial Tree, Percutaneous Approach

0BH03YZ Insertion of Other Device into Tracheobronchial Tree, Percutaneous Approach

0BH041Z Insertion of Radioactive Element into Tracheobronchial Tree, Percutaneous Endoscopic Approach

0BH042Z Insertion of Monitoring Device into Tracheobronchial Tree, Percutaneous Endoscopic Approach

0BH043Z Insertion of Infusion Device into Tracheobronchial Tree, Percutaneous Endoscopic Approach

0BH04DZ Insertion of Intraluminal Device into Tracheobronchial Tree, Percutaneous Endoscopic Approach

0BH04YZ Insertion of Other Device into Tracheobronchial Tree, Percutaneous Endoscopic Approach

0BH071Z Insertion of Radioactive Element into Tracheobronchial Tree, Via Natural or Artificial Opening

0BH072Z Insertion of Monitoring Device into Tracheobronchial Tree, Via Natural or Artificial Opening

0BH073Z Insertion of Infusion Device into Tracheobronchial Tree, Via Natural or Artificial Opening

0BH07DZ Insertion of Intraluminal Device into Tracheobronchial Tree, Via Natural or Artificial Opening

0BH07YZ Insertion of Other Device into Tracheobronchial Tree, Via Natural or Artificial Opening

0BH081Z Insertion of Radioactive Element into Tracheobronchial Tree, Via Natural or Artificial Opening Endoscopic

0BH082Z Insertion of Monitoring Device into Tracheobronchial Tree, Via Natural or Artificial Opening Endoscopic

0BH083Z Insertion of Infusion Device into Tracheobronchial Tree, Via Natural or Artificial Opening Endoscopic

0BH08DZ Insertion of Intraluminal Device into Tracheobronchial Tree, Via Natural or Artificial Opening Endoscopic

0BH08YZ Insertion of Other Device into Tracheobronchial Tree, Via Natural or Artificial Opening Endoscopic

0BH102Z Insertion of Monitoring Device into Trachea, Open Approach

0BH10DZ Insertion of Intraluminal Device into Trachea, Open Approach

0BH10YZ Insertion of Other Device into Trachea, Open Approach

0BH13DZ Insertion of Intraluminal Device into Trachea, Percutaneous Approach

0BH13EZ Insertion of Endotracheal Airway into Trachea, Percutaneous Approach

0BH13YZ Insertion of Other Device into Trachea, Percutaneous Approach

0BH14DZ Insertion of Intraluminal Device into Trachea, Percutaneous Endoscopic Approach

0BH14YZ Insertion of Other Device into Trachea, Percutaneous Endoscopic Approach

0BH172Z Insertion of Monitoring Device into Trachea, Via Natural or Artificial Opening

0BH17DZ Insertion of Intraluminal Device into Trachea, Via Natural or Artificial Opening

0BH17EZ Insertion of Endotracheal Airway into Trachea, Via Natural or Artificial Opening
AHA CC: 4Q, 2014, 3-15

0BH17YZ Insertion of Other Device into Trachea, Via Natural or Artificial Opening

0BH182Z Insertion of Monitoring Device into Trachea, Via Natural or Artificial Opening Endoscopic

0BH18DZ Insertion of Intraluminal Device into Trachea, Via Natural or Artificial Opening Endoscopic

0BH18EZ Insertion of Endotracheal Airway into Trachea, Via Natural or Artificial Opening Endoscopic
AHA CC: 4Q, 2014, 3-15

0BH18YZ Insertion of Other Device into Trachea, Via Natural or Artificial Opening Endoscopic

0BH30GZ Insertion of Endobronchial Valve into Right Main Bronchus, Open Approach

0BH33GZ Insertion of Endobronchial Valve into Right Main Bronchus, Percutaneous Approach

0BH34GZ Insertion of Endobronchial Valve into Right Main Bronchus, Percutaneous Endoscopic Approach

0BH37GZ Insertion of Endobronchial Valve into Right Main Bronchus, Via Natural or Artificial Opening

0BH38GZ Insertion of Endobronchial Valve into Right Main Bronchus, Via Natural or Artificial Opening Endoscopic

0BH40GZ Insertion of Endobronchial Valve into Right Upper Lobe Bronchus, Open Approach

0BH43GZ Insertion of Endobronchial Valve into Right Upper Lobe Bronchus, Percutaneous Approach

0BH44GZ Insertion of Endobronchial Valve into Right Upper Lobe Bronchus, Percutaneous Endoscopic Approach

0BH47GZ Insertion of Endobronchial Valve into Right Upper Lobe Bronchus, Via Natural or Artificial Opening

0BH48GZ Insertion of Endobronchial Valve into Right Upper Lobe Bronchus, Via Natural or Artificial Opening Endoscopic

0BH50GZ Insertion of Endobronchial Valve into Right Middle Lobe Bronchus, Open Approach

0BH53GZ Insertion of Endobronchial Valve into Right Middle Lobe Bronchus, Percutaneous Approach

0BH54GZ Insertion of Endobronchial Valve into Right Middle Lobe Bronchus, Percutaneous Endoscopic Approach

0BH57GZ Insertion of Endobronchial Valve into Right Middle Lobe Bronchus, Via Natural or Artificial Opening

0BH58GZ Insertion of Endobronchial Valve into Right Middle Lobe Bronchus, Via Natural or Artificial Opening Endoscopic

0BH60GZ Insertion of Endobronchial Valve into Right Lower Lobe Bronchus, Open Approach

0BH63GZ Insertion of Endobronchial Valve into Right Lower Lobe Bronchus, Percutaneous Approach

0BH64GZ Insertion of Endobronchial Valve into Right Lower Lobe Bronchus, Percutaneous Endoscopic Approach

0BH67GZ Insertion of Endobronchial Valve into Right Lower Lobe Bronchus, Via Natural or Artificial Opening

0BH68GZ Insertion of Endobronchial Valve into Right Lower Lobe Bronchus, Via Natural or Artificial Opening Endoscopic

0BH70GZ Insertion of Endobronchial Valve into Left Main Bronchus, Open Approach

0BH73GZ Insertion of Endobronchial Valve into Left Main Bronchus, Percutaneous Approach

0BH74GZ Insertion of Endobronchial Valve into Left Main Bronchus, Percutaneous Endoscopic Approach

0BH77GZ Insertion of Endobronchial Valve into Left Main Bronchus, Via Natural or Artificial Opening

0BH78GZ Insertion of Endobronchial Valve into Left Main Bronchus, Via Natural or Artificial Opening Endoscopic

0BH80GZ Insertion of Endobronchial Valve into Left Upper Lobe Bronchus, Open Approach

0BH83GZ Insertion of Endobronchial Valve into Left Upper Lobe Bronchus, Percutaneous Approach

0BH84GZ Insertion of Endobronchial Valve into Left Upper Lobe Bronchus, Percutaneous Endoscopic Approach

0BH87GZ Insertion of Endobronchial Valve into Left Upper Lobe Bronchus, Via Natural or Artificial Opening

0BH88GZ Insertion of Endobronchial Valve into Left Upper Lobe Bronchus, Via Natural or Artificial Opening Endoscopic

0BH90GZ Insertion of Endobronchial Valve into Lingula Bronchus, Open Approach

0BH93GZ Insertion of Endobronchial Valve into Lingula Bronchus, Percutaneous Approach

0BH94GZ Insertion of Endobronchial Valve into Lingula Bronchus, Percutaneous Endoscopic Approach

0BH97GZ Insertion of Endobronchial Valve into Lingula Bronchus, Via Natural or Artificial Opening

0BH98GZ Insertion of Endobronchial Valve into Lingula Bronchus, Via Natural or Artificial Opening Endoscopic

0BHB0GZ Insertion of Endobronchial Valve into Left Lower Lobe Bronchus, Open Approach

0BHB3GZ Insertion of Endobronchial Valve into Left Lower Lobe Bronchus, Percutaneous Approach

0BHB4GZ Insertion of Endobronchial Valve into Left Lower Lobe Bronchus, Percutaneous Endoscopic Approach

0BHB7GZ Insertion of Endobronchial Valve into Left Lower Lobe Bronchus, Via Natural or Artificial Opening

0BHB8GZ Insertion of Endobronchial Valve into Left Lower Lobe Bronchus, Via Natural or Artificial Opening Endoscopic
AHA CC: 3Q, 2019, 33-34

0BHK01Z Insertion of Radioactive Element into Right Lung, Open Approach

0BHK02Z Insertion of Monitoring Device into Right Lung, Open Approach

0BHK03Z Insertion of Infusion Device into Right Lung, Open Approach

0BHK0YZ Insertion of Other Device into Right Lung, Open Approach

0BHK31Z Insertion of Radioactive Element into Right Lung, Percutaneous Approach

0BHK32Z Insertion of Monitoring Device into Right Lung, Percutaneous Approach

0BHK33Z Insertion of Infusion Device into Right Lung, Percutaneous Approach

0BHK3YZ Insertion of Other Device into Right Lung, Percutaneous Approach

0BHK41Z Insertion of Radioactive Element into Right Lung, Percutaneous Endoscopic Approach

0BHK42Z Insertion of Monitoring Device into Right Lung, Percutaneous Endoscopic Approach

0BHK43Z Insertion of Infusion Device into Right Lung, Percutaneous Endoscopic Approach

0BHK4YZ Insertion of Other Device into Right Lung, Percutaneous Endoscopic Approach

0BHK71Z Insertion of Radioactive Element into Right Lung, Via Natural or Artificial Opening

0BHK72Z Insertion of Monitoring Device into Right Lung, Via Natural or Artificial Opening

0BHK73Z Insertion of Infusion Device into Right Lung, Via Natural or Artificial Opening

0BHK7YZ Insertion of Other Device into Right Lung, Via Natural or Artificial Opening

0BHK81Z Insertion of Radioactive Element into Right Lung, Via Natural or Artificial Opening Endoscopic

0BHK82Z Insertion of Monitoring Device into Right Lung, Via Natural or Artificial Opening Endoscopic

0BHK83Z Insertion of Infusion Device into Right Lung, Via Natural or Artificial Opening Endoscopic

0BHK8YZ Insertion of Other Device into Right Lung, Via Natural or Artificial Opening Endoscopic

0BHL01Z Insertion of Radioactive Element into Left Lung, Open Approach

0BHL02Z Insertion of Monitoring Device into Left Lung, Open Approach

0BHL03Z Insertion of Infusion Device into Left Lung, Open Approach

0BHL0YZ Insertion of Other Device into Left Lung, Open Approach

0BHL31Z Insertion of Radioactive Element into Left Lung, Percutaneous Approach

0BHL32Z Insertion of Monitoring Device into Left Lung, Percutaneous Approach

0BHL33Z Insertion of Infusion Device into Left Lung, Percutaneous Approach

0BHL3YZ Insertion of Other Device into Left Lung, Percutaneous Approach

0BHL41Z Insertion of Radioactive Element into Left Lung, Percutaneous Endoscopic Approach

0BHL42Z Insertion of Monitoring Device into Left Lung, Percutaneous Endoscopic Approach

0BHL43Z Insertion of Infusion Device into Left Lung, Percutaneous Endoscopic Approach

0BHL4YZ Insertion of Other Device into Left Lung, Percutaneous Endoscopic Approach

0BHL71Z Insertion of Radioactive Element into Left Lung, Via Natural or Artificial Opening

0BHL72Z Insertion of Monitoring Device into Left Lung, Via Natural or Artificial Opening

0BHL73Z Insertion of Infusion Device into Left Lung, Via Natural or Artificial Opening

0BHL7YZ Insertion of Other Device into Left Lung, Via Natural or Artificial Opening

0BHL81Z Insertion of Radioactive Element into Left Lung, Via Natural or Artificial Opening Endoscopic

0BHL82Z Insertion of Monitoring Device into Left Lung, Via Natural or Artificial Opening Endoscopic

0BHL83Z Insertion of Infusion Device into Left Lung, Via Natural or Artificial Opening Endoscopic

0BHL8YZ Insertion of Other Device into Left Lung, Via Natural or Artificial Opening Endoscopic

0BHQ0YZ Insertion of Other Device into Pleura, Open Approach

0BHQ3YZ Insertion of Other Device into Pleura, Percutaneous Approach

0BHQ4YZ Insertion of Other Device into Pleura, Percutaneous Endoscopic Approach

0BHQ7YZ Insertion of Other Device into Pleura, Via Natural or Artificial Opening

0BHQ8YZ Insertion of Other Device into Pleura, Via Natural or Artificial Opening Endoscopic

0BHT02Z Insertion of Monitoring Device into Diaphragm, Open Approach

0BHT0MZ Insertion of Diaphragmatic Pacemaker Lead into Diaphragm, Open Approach

0BHT0YZ Insertion of Other Device into Diaphragm, Open Approach

♀ Female-only　　♂ Male-only　　▲ Limited Coverage　　● Non-OR　　HAC HAC-associated procedure　　▲ Non-covered procedures　　✛ Cluster

0BHT32Z Insertion of Monitoring Device into Diaphragm, Percutaneous Approach
0BHT3MZ Insertion of Diaphragmatic Pacemaker Lead into Diaphragm, Percutaneous Approach
0BHT3YZ Insertion of Other Device into Diaphragm, Percutaneous Approach

0BHT42Z Insertion of Monitoring Device into Diaphragm, Percutaneous Endoscopic Approach
0BHT4MZ Insertion of Diaphragmatic Pacemaker Lead into Diaphragm, Percutaneous Endoscopic Approach
0BHT4YZ Insertion of Other Device into Diaphragm, Percutaneous Endoscopic Approach

0BHT7YZ Insertion of Other Device into Diaphragm, Via Natural or Artificial Opening
0BHT8YZ Insertion of Other Device into Diaphragm, Via Natural or Artificial Opening Endoscopic

0BJ – Respiratory System, Inspection

Review Coding Guidelines B3.11a, B3.11b and B3.11c

0BJ00ZZ Inspection of Tracheobronchial Tree, Open Approach
0BJ03ZZ Inspection of Tracheobronchial Tree, Percutaneous Approach
0BJ04ZZ Inspection of Tracheobronchial Tree, Percutaneous Endoscopic Approach
0BJ07ZZ Inspection of Tracheobronchial Tree, Via Natural or Artificial Opening
0BJ08ZZ Inspection of Tracheobronchial Tree, Via Natural or Artificial Opening Endoscopic
0BJ0XZZ Inspection of Tracheobronchial Tree, External Approach
0BJ10ZZ Inspection of Trachea, Open Approach
0BJ13ZZ Inspection of Trachea, Percutaneous Approach
0BJ14ZZ Inspection of Trachea, Percutaneous Endoscopic Approach
0BJ17ZZ Inspection of Trachea, Via Natural or Artificial Opening
0BJ18ZZ Inspection of Trachea, Via Natural or Artificial Opening Endoscopic
0BJ1XZZ Inspection of Trachea, External Approach

0BJK0ZZ Inspection of Right Lung, Open Approach
0BJK3ZZ Inspection of Right Lung, Percutaneous Approach
0BJK4ZZ Inspection of Right Lung, Percutaneous Endoscopic Approach
0BJK7ZZ Inspection of Right Lung, Via Natural or Artificial Opening
0BJK8ZZ Inspection of Right Lung, Via Natural or Artificial Opening Endoscopic
0BJKXZZ Inspection of Right Lung, External Approach
0BJL0ZZ Inspection of Left Lung, Open Approach
0BJL3ZZ Inspection of Left Lung, Percutaneous Approach
0BJL4ZZ Inspection of Left Lung, Percutaneous Endoscopic Approach
0BJL7ZZ Inspection of Left Lung, Via Natural or Artificial Opening
0BJL8ZZ Inspection of Left Lung, Via Natural or Artificial Opening Endoscopic
AHA CC: 1Q, 2014, 20
0BJLXZZ Inspection of Left Lung, External Approach

0BJQ0ZZ Inspection of Pleura, Open Approach
0BJQ3ZZ Inspection of Pleura, Percutaneous Approach
0BJQ4ZZ Inspection of Pleura, Percutaneous Endoscopic Approach
AHA CC: 2Q, 2015, 31
0BJQ7ZZ Inspection of Pleura, Via Natural or Artificial Opening
0BJQ8ZZ Inspection of Pleura, Via Natural or Artificial Opening Endoscopic
0BJQXZZ Inspection of Pleura, External Approach
0BJT0ZZ Inspection of Diaphragm, Open Approach
0BJT3ZZ Inspection of Diaphragm, Percutaneous Approach
0BJT4ZZ Inspection of Diaphragm, Percutaneous Endoscopic Approach
0BJT7ZZ Inspection of Diaphragm, Via Natural or Artificial Opening
0BJT8ZZ Inspection of Diaphragm, Via Natural or Artificial Opening Endoscopic
0BJTXZZ Inspection of Diaphragm, External Approach

0BL – Respiratory System, Occlusion

0BL10CZ Occlusion of Trachea with Extraluminal Device, Open Approach
0BL10DZ Occlusion of Trachea with Intraluminal Device, Open Approach
0BL10ZZ Occlusion of Trachea, Open Approach
0BL13CZ Occlusion of Trachea with Extraluminal Device, Percutaneous Approach
0BL13DZ Occlusion of Trachea with Intraluminal Device, Percutaneous Approach
0BL13ZZ Occlusion of Trachea, Percutaneous Approach
0BL14CZ Occlusion of Trachea with Extraluminal Device, Percutaneous Endoscopic Approach
0BL14DZ Occlusion of Trachea with Intraluminal Device, Percutaneous Endoscopic Approach
0BL14ZZ Occlusion of Trachea, Percutaneous Endoscopic Approach
0BL17DZ Occlusion of Trachea with Intraluminal Device, Via Natural or Artificial Opening
0BL17ZZ Occlusion of Trachea, Via Natural or Artificial Opening
0BL18DZ Occlusion of Trachea with Intraluminal Device, Via Natural or Artificial Opening Endoscopic
0BL18ZZ Occlusion of Trachea, Via Natural or Artificial Opening Endoscopic
0BL20CZ Occlusion of Carina with Extraluminal Device, Open Approach
0BL20DZ Occlusion of Carina with Intraluminal Device, Open Approach

0BL20ZZ Occlusion of Carina, Open Approach
0BL23CZ Occlusion of Carina with Extraluminal Device, Percutaneous Approach
0BL23DZ Occlusion of Carina with Intraluminal Device, Percutaneous Approach
0BL23ZZ Occlusion of Carina, Percutaneous Approach
0BL24CZ Occlusion of Carina with Extraluminal Device, Percutaneous Endoscopic Approach
0BL24DZ Occlusion of Carina with Intraluminal Device, Percutaneous Endoscopic Approach
0BL24ZZ Occlusion of Carina, Percutaneous Endoscopic Approach
0BL27DZ Occlusion of Carina with Intraluminal Device, Via Natural or Artificial Opening
0BL27ZZ Occlusion of Carina, Via Natural or Artificial Opening
0BL28DZ Occlusion of Carina with Intraluminal Device, Via Natural or Artificial Opening Endoscopic
0BL28ZZ Occlusion of Carina, Via Natural or Artificial Opening Endoscopic
0BL30CZ Occlusion of Right Main Bronchus with Extraluminal Device, Open Approach
0BL30DZ Occlusion of Right Main Bronchus with Intraluminal Device, Open Approach
0BL30ZZ Occlusion of Right Main Bronchus, Open Approach

0BL33CZ Occlusion of Right Main Bronchus with Extraluminal Device, Percutaneous Approach
0BL33DZ Occlusion of Right Main Bronchus with Intraluminal Device, Percutaneous Approach
0BL33ZZ Occlusion of Right Main Bronchus, Percutaneous Approach
0BL34CZ Occlusion of Right Main Bronchus with Extraluminal Device, Percutaneous Endoscopic Approach
0BL34DZ Occlusion of Right Main Bronchus with Intraluminal Device, Percutaneous Endoscopic Approach
0BL34ZZ Occlusion of Right Main Bronchus, Percutaneous Endoscopic Approach
0BL37DZ Occlusion of Right Main Bronchus with Intraluminal Device, Via Natural or Artificial Opening
0BL37ZZ Occlusion of Right Main Bronchus, Via Natural or Artificial Opening
0BL38DZ Occlusion of Right Main Bronchus with Intraluminal Device, Via Natural or Artificial Opening Endoscopic
0BL38ZZ Occlusion of Right Main Bronchus, Via Natural or Artificial Opening Endoscopic
0BL40CZ Occlusion of Right Upper Lobe Bronchus with Extraluminal Device, Open Approach
0BL40DZ Occlusion of Right Upper Lobe Bronchus with Intraluminal Device, Open Approach

---

♀ Female-only   ♂ Male-only   ▲ Limited Coverage   ● Non-OR   ▨ HAC-associated procedure   ▲ Non-covered procedures   ✚ Cluster

0BL40ZZ Occlusion of Right Upper Lobe Bronchus, Open Approach

0BL43CZ Occlusion of Right Upper Lobe Bronchus with Extraluminal Device, Percutaneous Approach

0BL43DZ Occlusion of Right Upper Lobe Bronchus with Intraluminal Device, Percutaneous Approach

0BL43ZZ Occlusion of Right Upper Lobe Bronchus, Percutaneous Approach

0BL44CZ Occlusion of Right Upper Lobe Bronchus with Extraluminal Device, Percutaneous Endoscopic Approach

0BL44DZ Occlusion of Right Upper Lobe Bronchus with Intraluminal Device, Percutaneous Endoscopic Approach

0BL44ZZ Occlusion of Right Upper Lobe Bronchus, Percutaneous Endoscopic Approach

0BL47DZ Occlusion of Right Upper Lobe Bronchus with Intraluminal Device, Via Natural or Artificial Opening

0BL47ZZ Occlusion of Right Upper Lobe Bronchus, Via Natural or Artificial Opening

0BL48DZ Occlusion of Right Upper Lobe Bronchus with Intraluminal Device, Via Natural or Artificial Opening Endoscopic

0BL48ZZ Occlusion of Right Upper Lobe Bronchus, Via Natural or Artificial Opening Endoscopic

0BL50CZ Occlusion of Right Middle Lobe Bronchus with Extraluminal Device, Open Approach

0BL50DZ Occlusion of Right Middle Lobe Bronchus with Intraluminal Device, Open Approach

0BL50ZZ Occlusion of Right Middle Lobe Bronchus, Open Approach

0BL53CZ Occlusion of Right Middle Lobe Bronchus with Extraluminal Device, Percutaneous Approach

0BL53DZ Occlusion of Right Middle Lobe Bronchus with Intraluminal Device, Percutaneous Approach

0BL53ZZ Occlusion of Right Middle Lobe Bronchus, Percutaneous Approach

0BL54CZ Occlusion of Right Middle Lobe Bronchus with Extraluminal Device, Percutaneous Endoscopic Approach

0BL54DZ Occlusion of Right Middle Lobe Bronchus with Intraluminal Device, Percutaneous Endoscopic Approach

0BL54ZZ Occlusion of Right Middle Lobe Bronchus, Percutaneous Endoscopic Approach

0BL57DZ Occlusion of Right Middle Lobe Bronchus with Intraluminal Device, Via Natural or Artificial Opening

0BL57ZZ Occlusion of Right Middle Lobe Bronchus, Via Natural or Artificial Opening

0BL58DZ Occlusion of Right Middle Lobe Bronchus with Intraluminal Device, Via Natural or Artificial Opening Endoscopic

0BL58ZZ Occlusion of Right Middle Lobe Bronchus, Via Natural or Artificial Opening Endoscopic

0BL60CZ Occlusion of Right Lower Lobe Bronchus with Extraluminal Device, Open Approach

0BL60DZ Occlusion of Right Lower Lobe Bronchus with Intraluminal Device, Open Approach

0BL60ZZ Occlusion of Right Lower Lobe Bronchus, Open Approach

0BL63CZ Occlusion of Right Lower Lobe Bronchus with Extraluminal Device, Percutaneous Approach

0BL63DZ Occlusion of Right Lower Lobe Bronchus with Intraluminal Device, Percutaneous Approach

0BL63ZZ Occlusion of Right Lower Lobe Bronchus, Percutaneous Approach

0BL64CZ Occlusion of Right Lower Lobe Bronchus with Extraluminal Device, Percutaneous Endoscopic Approach

0BL64DZ Occlusion of Right Lower Lobe Bronchus with Intraluminal Device, Percutaneous Endoscopic Approach

0BL64ZZ Occlusion of Right Lower Lobe Bronchus, Percutaneous Endoscopic Approach

0BL67DZ Occlusion of Right Lower Lobe Bronchus with Intraluminal Device, Via Natural or Artificial Opening

0BL67ZZ Occlusion of Right Lower Lobe Bronchus, Via Natural or Artificial Opening

0BL68DZ Occlusion of Right Lower Lobe Bronchus with Intraluminal Device, Via Natural or Artificial Opening Endoscopic

0BL68ZZ Occlusion of Right Lower Lobe Bronchus, Via Natural or Artificial Opening Endoscopic

0BL70CZ Occlusion of Left Main Bronchus with Extraluminal Device, Open Approach

0BL70DZ Occlusion of Left Main Bronchus with Intraluminal Device, Open Approach

0BL70ZZ Occlusion of Left Main Bronchus, Open Approach

0BL73CZ Occlusion of Left Main Bronchus with Extraluminal Device, Percutaneous Approach

0BL73DZ Occlusion of Left Main Bronchus with Intraluminal Device, Percutaneous Approach

0BL73ZZ Occlusion of Left Main Bronchus, Percutaneous Approach

0BL74CZ Occlusion of Left Main Bronchus with Extraluminal Device, Percutaneous Endoscopic Approach

0BL74DZ Occlusion of Left Main Bronchus with Intraluminal Device, Percutaneous Endoscopic Approach

0BL74ZZ Occlusion of Left Main Bronchus, Percutaneous Endoscopic Approach

0BL77DZ Occlusion of Left Main Bronchus with Intraluminal Device, Via Natural or Artificial Opening

0BL77ZZ Occlusion of Left Main Bronchus, Via Natural or Artificial Opening

0BL78DZ Occlusion of Left Main Bronchus with Intraluminal Device, Via Natural or Artificial Opening Endoscopic

0BL78ZZ Occlusion of Left Main Bronchus, Via Natural or Artificial Opening Endoscopic

0BL80CZ Occlusion of Left Upper Lobe Bronchus with Extraluminal Device, Open Approach

0BL80DZ Occlusion of Left Upper Lobe Bronchus with Intraluminal Device, Open Approach

0BL80ZZ Occlusion of Left Upper Lobe Bronchus, Open Approach

0BL83CZ Occlusion of Left Upper Lobe Bronchus with Extraluminal Device, Percutaneous Approach

0BL83DZ Occlusion of Left Upper Lobe Bronchus with Intraluminal Device, Percutaneous Approach

0BL83ZZ Occlusion of Left Upper Lobe Bronchus, Percutaneous Approach

0BL84CZ Occlusion of Left Upper Lobe Bronchus with Extraluminal Device, Percutaneous Endoscopic Approach

0BL84DZ Occlusion of Left Upper Lobe Bronchus with Intraluminal Device, Percutaneous Endoscopic Approach

0BL84ZZ Occlusion of Left Upper Lobe Bronchus, Percutaneous Endoscopic Approach

0BL87DZ Occlusion of Left Upper Lobe Bronchus with Intraluminal Device, Via Natural or Artificial Opening

0BL87ZZ Occlusion of Left Upper Lobe Bronchus, Via Natural or Artificial Opening

0BL88DZ Occlusion of Left Upper Lobe Bronchus with Intraluminal Device, Via Natural or Artificial Opening Endoscopic

0BL88ZZ Occlusion of Left Upper Lobe Bronchus, Via Natural or Artificial Opening Endoscopic

0BL90CZ Occlusion of Lingula Bronchus with Extraluminal Device, Open Approach

0BL90DZ Occlusion of Lingula Bronchus with Intraluminal Device, Open Approach

0BL90ZZ Occlusion of Lingula Bronchus, Open Approach

0BL93CZ Occlusion of Lingula Bronchus with Extraluminal Device, Percutaneous Approach

0BL93DZ Occlusion of Lingula Bronchus with Intraluminal Device, Percutaneous Approach

0BL93ZZ Occlusion of Lingula Bronchus, Percutaneous Approach

0BL94CZ Occlusion of Lingula Bronchus with Extraluminal Device, Percutaneous Endoscopic Approach

0BL94DZ Occlusion of Lingula Bronchus with Intraluminal Device, Percutaneous Endoscopic Approach

0BL94ZZ Occlusion of Lingula Bronchus, Percutaneous Endoscopic Approach

0BL97DZ Occlusion of Lingula Bronchus with Intraluminal Device, Via Natural or Artificial Opening

0BL97ZZ Occlusion of Lingula Bronchus, Via Natural or Artificial Opening

0BL98DZ Occlusion of Lingula Bronchus with Intraluminal Device, Via Natural or Artificial Opening Endoscopic

0BL98ZZ Occlusion of Lingula Bronchus, Via Natural or Artificial Opening Endoscopic

0BLB0CZ Occlusion of Left Lower Lobe Bronchus with Extraluminal Device, Open Approach

0BLB0DZ Occlusion of Left Lower Lobe Bronchus with Intraluminal Device, Open Approach

0BLB0ZZ Occlusion of Left Lower Lobe Bronchus, Open Approach

0BLB3CZ Occlusion of Left Lower Lobe Bronchus with Extraluminal Device, Percutaneous Approach

♀ Female-only ♂ Male-only ▲ Limited Coverage ● Non-OR HAC HAC-associated procedure ▲ Non-covered procedures ✚ Cluster

0BLB3DZ Occlusion of Left Lower Lobe Bronchus with Intraluminal Device, Percutaneous Approach

0BLB3ZZ Occlusion of Left Lower Lobe Bronchus, Percutaneous Approach

0BLB4CZ Occlusion of Left Lower Lobe Bronchus with Extraluminal Device, Percutaneous Endoscopic Approach

0BLB4DZ Occlusion of Left Lower Lobe Bronchus with Intraluminal Device, Percutaneous Endoscopic Approach

0BLB4ZZ Occlusion of Left Lower Lobe Bronchus, Percutaneous Endoscopic Approach

0BLB7DZ Occlusion of Left Lower Lobe Bronchus with Intraluminal Device, Via Natural or Artificial Opening

0BLB7ZZ Occlusion of Left Lower Lobe Bronchus, Via Natural or Artificial Opening

0BLB8DZ Occlusion of Left Lower Lobe Bronchus with Intraluminal Device, Via Natural or Artificial Opening Endoscopic

0BLB8ZZ Occlusion of Left Lower Lobe Bronchus, Via Natural or Artificial Opening Endoscopic

0BM – Respiratory System, Reattachment

0BM10ZZ Reattachment of Trachea, Open Approach

0BM20ZZ Reattachment of Carina, Open Approach

0BM30ZZ Reattachment of Right Main Bronchus, Open Approach

0BM40ZZ Reattachment of Right Upper Lobe Bronchus, Open Approach

0BM50ZZ Reattachment of Right Middle Lobe Bronchus, Open Approach

0BM60ZZ Reattachment of Right Lower Lobe Bronchus, Open Approach

0BM70ZZ Reattachment of Left Main Bronchus, Open Approach

0BM80ZZ Reattachment of Left Upper Lobe Bronchus, Open Approach

0BM90ZZ Reattachment of Lingula Bronchus, Open Approach

0BMB0ZZ Reattachment of Left Lower Lobe Bronchus, Open Approach

0BMC0ZZ Reattachment of Right Upper Lung Lobe, Open Approach

0BMD0ZZ Reattachment of Right Middle Lung Lobe, Open Approach

0BMF0ZZ Reattachment of Right Lower Lung Lobe, Open Approach

0BMG0ZZ Reattachment of Left Upper Lung Lobe, Open Approach

0BMH0ZZ Reattachment of Lung Lingula, Open Approach

0BMJ0ZZ Reattachment of Left Lower Lung Lobe, Open Approach

0BMK0ZZ Reattachment of Right Lung, Open Approach

0BML0ZZ Reattachment of Left Lung, Open Approach

0BMT0ZZ Reattachment of Diaphragm, Open Approach

0BN – Respiratory System, Release

Review Coding Guidelines B3.13 and B3.14

0BN10ZZ Release Trachea, Open Approach
AHA CC: 3Q, 2015, 15-16

0BN13ZZ Release Trachea, Percutaneous Approach

0BN14ZZ Release Trachea, Percutaneous Endoscopic Approach

0BN17ZZ Release Trachea, Via Natural or Artificial Opening

0BN18ZZ Release Trachea, Via Natural or Artificial Opening Endoscopic

0BN20ZZ Release Carina, Open Approach

0BN23ZZ Release Carina, Percutaneous Approach

0BN24ZZ Release Carina, Percutaneous Endoscopic Approach

0BN27ZZ Release Carina, Via Natural or Artificial Opening

0BN28ZZ Release Carina, Via Natural or Artificial Opening Endoscopic

0BN30ZZ Release Right Main Bronchus, Open Approach

0BN33ZZ Release Right Main Bronchus, Percutaneous Approach

0BN34ZZ Release Right Main Bronchus, Percutaneous Endoscopic Approach

0BN37ZZ Release Right Main Bronchus, Via Natural or Artificial Opening

0BN38ZZ Release Right Main Bronchus, Via Natural or Artificial Opening Endoscopic

0BN40ZZ Release Right Upper Lobe Bronchus, Open Approach

0BN43ZZ Release Right Upper Lobe Bronchus, Percutaneous Approach

0BN44ZZ Release Right Upper Lobe Bronchus, Percutaneous Endoscopic Approach

0BN47ZZ Release Right Upper Lobe Bronchus, Via Natural or Artificial Opening

0BN48ZZ Release Right Upper Lobe Bronchus, Via Natural or Artificial Opening Endoscopic

0BN50ZZ Release Right Middle Lobe Bronchus, Open Approach

0BN53ZZ Release Right Middle Lobe Bronchus, Percutaneous Approach

0BN54ZZ Release Right Middle Lobe Bronchus, Percutaneous Endoscopic Approach

0BN57ZZ Release Right Middle Lobe Bronchus, Via Natural or Artificial Opening

0BN58ZZ Release Right Middle Lobe Bronchus, Via Natural or Artificial Opening Endoscopic

0BN60ZZ Release Right Lower Lobe Bronchus, Open Approach

0BN63ZZ Release Right Lower Lobe Bronchus, Percutaneous Approach

0BN64ZZ Release Right Lower Lobe Bronchus, Percutaneous Endoscopic Approach

0BN67ZZ Release Right Lower Lobe Bronchus, Via Natural or Artificial Opening

0BN68ZZ Release Right Lower Lobe Bronchus, Via Natural or Artificial Opening Endoscopic

0BN70ZZ Release Left Main Bronchus, Open Approach

0BN73ZZ Release Left Main Bronchus, Percutaneous Approach

0BN74ZZ Release Left Main Bronchus, Percutaneous Endoscopic Approach

0BN77ZZ Release Left Main Bronchus, Via Natural or Artificial Opening

0BN78ZZ Release Left Main Bronchus, Via Natural or Artificial Opening Endoscopic

0BN80ZZ Release Left Upper Lobe Bronchus, Open Approach

0BN83ZZ Release Left Upper Lobe Bronchus, Percutaneous Approach

0BN84ZZ Release Left Upper Lobe Bronchus, Percutaneous Endoscopic Approach

0BN87ZZ Release Left Upper Lobe Bronchus, Via Natural or Artificial Opening

0BN88ZZ Release Left Upper Lobe Bronchus, Via Natural or Artificial Opening Endoscopic

0BN90ZZ Release Lingula Bronchus, Open Approach

0BN93ZZ Release Lingula Bronchus, Percutaneous Approach

0BN94ZZ Release Lingula Bronchus, Percutaneous Endoscopic Approach

0BN97ZZ Release Lingula Bronchus, Via Natural or Artificial Opening

0BN98ZZ Release Lingula Bronchus, Via Natural or Artificial Opening Endoscopic

0BNB0ZZ Release Left Lower Lobe Bronchus, Open Approach

0BNB3ZZ Release Left Lower Lobe Bronchus, Percutaneous Approach

0BNB4ZZ Release Left Lower Lobe Bronchus, Percutaneous Endoscopic Approach

0BNB7ZZ Release Left Lower Lobe Bronchus, Via Natural or Artificial Opening

0BNB8ZZ Release Left Lower Lobe Bronchus, Via Natural or Artificial Opening Endoscopic

0BNC0ZZ Release Right Upper Lung Lobe, Open Approach

0BNC3ZZ Release Right Upper Lung Lobe, Percutaneous Approach

0BNC4ZZ Release Right Upper Lung Lobe, Percutaneous Endoscopic Approach

0BNC7ZZ Release Right Upper Lung Lobe, Via Natural or Artificial Opening

0BNC8ZZ Release Right Upper Lung Lobe, Via Natural or Artificial Opening Endoscopic

0BND0ZZ Release Right Middle Lung Lobe, Open Approach

0BND3ZZ Release Right Middle Lung Lobe, Percutaneous Approach

0BND4ZZ Release Right Middle Lung Lobe, Percutaneous Endoscopic Approach

0BND7ZZ Release Right Middle Lung Lobe, Via Natural or Artificial Opening

0BND8ZZ Release Right Middle Lung Lobe, Via Natural or Artificial Opening Endoscopic

0BNF0ZZ Release Right Lower Lung Lobe, Open Approach

0BNF3ZZ Release Right Lower Lung Lobe, Percutaneous Approach

0BNF4ZZ Release Right Lower Lung Lobe, Percutaneous Endoscopic Approach

0BNF7ZZ Release Right Lower Lung Lobe, Via Natural or Artificial Opening

0BNF8ZZ Release Right Lower Lung Lobe, Via Natural or Artificial Opening Endoscopic

0BNG0ZZ Release Left Upper Lung Lobe, Open Approach

0BNG3ZZ Release Left Upper Lung Lobe, Percutaneous Approach

0BNG4ZZ Release Left Upper Lung Lobe, Percutaneous Endoscopic Approach

0BNG7ZZ Release Left Upper Lung Lobe, Via Natural or Artificial Opening

0BNG8ZZ Release Left Upper Lung Lobe, Via Natural or Artificial Opening Endoscopic

0BNH0ZZ Release Lung Lingula, Open Approach

0BNH3ZZ Release Lung Lingula, Percutaneous Approach

0BNH4ZZ Release Lung Lingula, Percutaneous Endoscopic Approach

0BNH7ZZ Release Lung Lingula, Via Natural or Artificial Opening

0BNH8ZZ Release Lung Lingula, Via Natural or Artificial Opening Endoscopic

0BNJ0ZZ Release Left Lower Lung Lobe, Open Approach

0BNJ3ZZ Release Left Lower Lung Lobe, Percutaneous Approach

0BNJ4ZZ Release Left Lower Lung Lobe, Percutaneous Endoscopic Approach

0BNJ7ZZ Release Left Lower Lung Lobe, Via Natural or Artificial Opening

0BNJ8ZZ Release Left Lower Lung Lobe, Via Natural or Artificial Opening Endoscopic

0BNK0ZZ Release Right Lung, Open Approach

0BNK3ZZ Release Right Lung, Percutaneous Approach

0BNK4ZZ Release Right Lung, Percutaneous Endoscopic Approach

0BNK7ZZ Release Right Lung, Via Natural or Artificial Opening

0BNK8ZZ Release Right Lung, Via Natural or Artificial Opening Endoscopic

0BNL0ZZ Release Left Lung, Open Approach
AHA CC: 3Q, 2018, 28

0BNL3ZZ Release Left Lung, Percutaneous Approach

0BNL4ZZ Release Left Lung, Percutaneous Endoscopic Approach

0BNL7ZZ Release Left Lung, Via Natural or Artificial Opening

0BNL8ZZ Release Left Lung, Via Natural or Artificial Opening Endoscopic

0BNM0ZZ Release Bilateral Lungs, Open Approach

0BNM3ZZ Release Bilateral Lungs, Percutaneous Approach

0BNM4ZZ Release Bilateral Lungs, Percutaneous Endoscopic Approach

0BNM7ZZ Release Bilateral Lungs, Via Natural or Artificial Opening

0BNM8ZZ Release Bilateral Lungs, Via Natural or Artificial Opening Endoscopic

0BNN0ZZ Release Right Pleura, Open Approach
AHA CC: 2Q, 2019, 20-21

0BNN3ZZ Release Right Pleura, Percutaneous Approach

0BNN4ZZ Release Right Pleura, Percutaneous Endoscopic Approach

0BNP0ZZ Release Left Pleura, Open Approach

0BNP3ZZ Release Left Pleura, Percutaneous Approach

0BNP4ZZ Release Left Pleura, Percutaneous Endoscopic Approach

0BNT0ZZ Release Diaphragm, Open Approach

0BNT3ZZ Release Diaphragm, Percutaneous Approach

0BNT4ZZ Release Diaphragm, Percutaneous Endoscopic Approach

0BP – Respiratory System, Removal

Review Coding Guideline B6.1c

0BP000Z Removal of Drainage Device from Tracheobronchial Tree, Open Approach

0BP001Z Removal of Radioactive Element from Tracheobronchial Tree, Open Approach

0BP002Z Removal of Monitoring Device from Tracheobronchial Tree, Open Approach

0BP003Z Removal of Infusion Device from Tracheobronchial Tree, Open Approach

0BP007Z Removal of Autologous Tissue Substitute from Tracheobronchial Tree, Open Approach

0BP00CZ Removal of Extraluminal Device from Tracheobronchial Tree, Open Approach

0BP00DZ Removal of Intraluminal Device from Tracheobronchial Tree, Open Approach

0BP00JZ Removal of Synthetic Substitute from Tracheobronchial Tree, Open Approach

0BP00KZ Removal of Nonautologous Tissue Substitute from Tracheobronchial Tree, Open Approach

0BP00YZ Removal of Other Device from Tracheobronchial Tree, Open Approach

0BP030Z Removal of Drainage Device from Tracheobronchial Tree, Percutaneous Approach

0BP031Z Removal of Radioactive Element from Tracheobronchial Tree, Percutaneous Approach

0BP032Z Removal of Monitoring Device from Tracheobronchial Tree, Percutaneous Approach

0BP033Z Removal of Infusion Device from Tracheobronchial Tree, Percutaneous Approach

0BP037Z Removal of Autologous Tissue Substitute from Tracheobronchial Tree, Percutaneous Approach

0BP03CZ Removal of Extraluminal Device from Tracheobronchial Tree, Percutaneous Approach

0BP03DZ Removal of Intraluminal Device from Tracheobronchial Tree, Percutaneous Approach

0BP03JZ Removal of Synthetic Substitute from Tracheobronchial Tree, Percutaneous Approach

0BP03KZ Removal of Nonautologous Tissue Substitute from Tracheobronchial Tree, Percutaneous Approach

0BP03YZ Removal of Other Device from Tracheobronchial Tree, Percutaneous Approach

0BP040Z Removal of Drainage Device from Tracheobronchial Tree, Percutaneous Endoscopic Approach

0BP041Z Removal of Radioactive Element from Tracheobronchial Tree, Percutaneous Endoscopic Approach

0BP042Z Removal of Monitoring Device from Tracheobronchial Tree, Percutaneous Endoscopic Approach

0BP043Z Removal of Infusion Device from Tracheobronchial Tree, Percutaneous Endoscopic Approach

0BP047Z Removal of Autologous Tissue Substitute from Tracheobronchial Tree, Percutaneous Endoscopic Approach

0BP04CZ Removal of Extraluminal Device from Tracheobronchial Tree, Percutaneous Endoscopic Approach

0BP04DZ Removal of Intraluminal Device from Tracheobronchial Tree, Percutaneous Endoscopic Approach

0BP04JZ Removal of Synthetic Substitute from Tracheobronchial Tree, Percutaneous Endoscopic Approach

0BP04KZ Removal of Nonautologous Tissue Substitute from Tracheobronchial Tree, Percutaneous Endoscopic Approach

0BP04YZ Removal of Other Device from Tracheobronchial Tree, Percutaneous Endoscopic Approach

0BP070Z Removal of Drainage Device from Tracheobronchial Tree, Via Natural or Artificial Opening

0BP071Z Removal of Radioactive Element from Tracheobronchial Tree, Via Natural or Artificial Opening

0BP072Z Removal of Monitoring Device from Tracheobronchial Tree, Via Natural or Artificial Opening

0BP073Z Removal of Infusion Device from Tracheobronchial Tree, Via Natural or Artificial Opening

0BP077Z Removal of Autologous Tissue Substitute from Tracheobronchial Tree, Via Natural or Artificial Opening

0BP07CZ Removal of Extraluminal Device from Tracheobronchial Tree, Via Natural or Artificial Opening

0BP07DZ Removal of Intraluminal Device from Tracheobronchial Tree, Via Natural or Artificial Opening

0BP07JZ Removal of Synthetic Substitute from Tracheobronchial Tree, Via Natural or Artificial Opening

0BP07KZ Removal of Nonautologous Tissue Substitute from Tracheobronchial Tree, Via Natural or Artificial Opening

0BP07YZ Removal of Other Device from Tracheobronchial Tree, Via Natural or Artificial Opening

0BP080Z Removal of Drainage Device from Tracheobronchial Tree, Via Natural or Artificial Opening Endoscopic

0BP081Z Removal of Radioactive Element from Tracheobronchial Tree, Via Natural or Artificial Opening Endoscopic

0BP082Z Removal of Monitoring Device from Tracheobronchial Tree, Via Natural or Artificial Opening Endoscopic

0BP083Z Removal of Infusion Device from Tracheobronchial Tree, Via Natural or Artificial Opening Endoscopic

0BP087Z Removal of Autologous Tissue Substitute from Tracheobronchial Tree, Via Natural or Artificial Opening Endoscopic

0BP08CZ Removal of Extraluminal Device from Tracheobronchial Tree, Via Natural or Artificial Opening Endoscopic

♀ Female-only   ♂ Male-only   ▲ Limited Coverage   ● Non-OR   **HAC** HAC-associated procedure   ▲ Non-covered procedures   ✛ Cluster

0BP08DZ Removal of Intraluminal Device from Tracheobronchial Tree, Via Natural or Artificial Opening Endoscopic

0BP08JZ Removal of Synthetic Substitute from Tracheobronchial Tree, Via Natural or Artificial Opening Endoscopic

0BP08KZ Removal of Nonautologous Tissue Substitute from Tracheobronchial Tree, Via Natural or Artificial Opening Endoscopic

0BP08YZ Removal of Other Device from Tracheobronchial Tree, Via Natural or Artificial Opening Endoscopic

0BP0X0Z Removal of Drainage Device from Tracheobronchial Tree, External Approach

0BP0X1Z Removal of Radioactive Element from Tracheobronchial Tree, External Approach

0BP0X2Z Removal of Monitoring Device from Tracheobronchial Tree, External Approach

0BP0X3Z Removal of Infusion Device from Tracheobronchial Tree, External Approach

0BP0XDZ Removal of Intraluminal Device from Tracheobronchial Tree, External Approach

0BP100Z Removal of Drainage Device from Trachea, Open Approach

0BP102Z Removal of Monitoring Device from Trachea, Open Approach

0BP107Z Removal of Autologous Tissue Substitute from Trachea, Open Approach

0BP10CZ Removal of Extraluminal Device from Trachea, Open Approach

0BP10DZ Removal of Intraluminal Device from Trachea, Open Approach

0BP10FZ Removal of Tracheostomy Device from Trachea, Open Approach

0BP10JZ Removal of Synthetic Substitute from Trachea, Open Approach

0BP10KZ Removal of Nonautologous Tissue Substitute from Trachea, Open Approach

0BP130Z Removal of Drainage Device from Trachea, Percutaneous Approach

0BP132Z Removal of Monitoring Device from Trachea, Percutaneous Approach

0BP137Z Removal of Autologous Tissue Substitute from Trachea, Percutaneous Approach

0BP13CZ Removal of Extraluminal Device from Trachea, Percutaneous Approach

0BP13DZ Removal of Intraluminal Device from Trachea, Percutaneous Approach

0BP13FZ Removal of Tracheostomy Device from Trachea, Percutaneous Approach

0BP13JZ Removal of Synthetic Substitute from Trachea, Percutaneous Approach

0BP13KZ Removal of Nonautologous Tissue Substitute from Trachea, Percutaneous Approach

0BP140Z Removal of Drainage Device from Trachea, Percutaneous Endoscopic Approach

0BP142Z Removal of Monitoring Device from Trachea, Percutaneous Endoscopic Approach

0BP147Z Removal of Autologous Tissue Substitute from Trachea, Percutaneous Endoscopic Approach

0BP14CZ Removal of Extraluminal Device from Trachea, Percutaneous Endoscopic Approach

0BP14DZ Removal of Intraluminal Device from Trachea, Percutaneous Endoscopic Approach

0BP14FZ Removal of Tracheostomy Device from Trachea, Percutaneous Endoscopic Approach

0BP14JZ Removal of Synthetic Substitute from Trachea, Percutaneous Endoscopic Approach

0BP14KZ Removal of Nonautologous Tissue Substitute from Trachea, Percutaneous Endoscopic Approach

0BP170Z Removal of Drainage Device from Trachea, Via Natural or Artificial Opening

0BP172Z Removal of Monitoring Device from Trachea, Via Natural or Artificial Opening

0BP177Z Removal of Autologous Tissue Substitute from Trachea, Via Natural or Artificial Opening

0BP17CZ Removal of Extraluminal Device from Trachea, Via Natural or Artificial Opening

0BP17DZ Removal of Intraluminal Device from Trachea, Via Natural or Artificial Opening

0BP17FZ Removal of Tracheostomy Device from Trachea, Via Natural or Artificial Opening

0BP17JZ Removal of Synthetic Substitute from Trachea, Via Natural or Artificial Opening

0BP17KZ Removal of Nonautologous Tissue Substitute from Trachea, Via Natural or Artificial Opening

0BP180Z Removal of Drainage Device from Trachea, Via Natural or Artificial Opening Endoscopic

0BP182Z Removal of Monitoring Device from Trachea, Via Natural or Artificial Opening Endoscopic

0BP187Z Removal of Autologous Tissue Substitute from Trachea, Via Natural or Artificial Opening Endoscopic

0BP18CZ Removal of Extraluminal Device from Trachea, Via Natural or Artificial Opening Endoscopic

0BP18DZ Removal of Intraluminal Device from Trachea, Via Natural or Artificial Opening Endoscopic

0BP18FZ Removal of Tracheostomy Device from Trachea, Via Natural or Artificial Opening Endoscopic

0BP18JZ Removal of Synthetic Substitute from Trachea, Via Natural or Artificial Opening Endoscopic

0BP18KZ Removal of Nonautologous Tissue Substitute from Trachea, Via Natural or Artificial Opening Endoscopic

0BP1X0Z Removal of Drainage Device from Trachea, External Approach

0BP1X2Z Removal of Monitoring Device from Trachea, External Approach

0BP1XDZ Removal of Intraluminal Device from Trachea, External Approach

0BP1XFZ Removal of Tracheostomy Device from Trachea, External Approach

0BPK00Z Removal of Drainage Device from Right Lung, Open Approach

0BPK01Z Removal of Radioactive Element from Right Lung, Open Approach

0BPK02Z Removal of Monitoring Device from Right Lung, Open Approach

0BPK03Z Removal of Infusion Device from Right Lung, Open Approach

0BPK0YZ Removal of Other Device from Right Lung, Open Approach

0BPK30Z Removal of Drainage Device from Right Lung, Percutaneous Approach

0BPK31Z Removal of Radioactive Element from Right Lung, Percutaneous Approach

0BPK32Z Removal of Monitoring Device from Right Lung, Percutaneous Approach

0BPK33Z Removal of Infusion Device from Right Lung, Percutaneous Approach

0BPK3YZ Removal of Other Device from Right Lung, Percutaneous Approach

0BPK40Z Removal of Drainage Device from Right Lung, Percutaneous Endoscopic Approach

0BPK41Z Removal of Radioactive Element from Right Lung, Percutaneous Endoscopic Approach

0BPK42Z Removal of Monitoring Device from Right Lung, Percutaneous Endoscopic Approach

0BPK43Z Removal of Infusion Device from Right Lung, Percutaneous Endoscopic Approach

0BPK4YZ Removal of Other Device from Right Lung, Percutaneous Endoscopic Approach

0BPK70Z Removal of Drainage Device from Right Lung, Via Natural or Artificial Opening

0BPK71Z Removal of Radioactive Element from Right Lung, Via Natural or Artificial Opening

0BPK72Z Removal of Monitoring Device from Right Lung, Via Natural or Artificial Opening

0BPK73Z Removal of Infusion Device from Right Lung, Via Natural or Artificial Opening

0BPK7YZ Removal of Other Device from Right Lung, Via Natural or Artificial Opening

0BPK80Z Removal of Drainage Device from Right Lung, Via Natural or Artificial Opening Endoscopic

0BPK81Z Removal of Radioactive Element from Right Lung, Via Natural or Artificial Opening Endoscopic

0BPK82Z Removal of Monitoring Device from Right Lung, Via Natural or Artificial Opening Endoscopic

0BPK83Z Removal of Infusion Device from Right Lung, Via Natural or Artificial Opening Endoscopic

0BPK8YZ Removal of Other Device from Right Lung, Via Natural or Artificial Opening Endoscopic

0BPKX0Z Removal of Drainage Device from Right Lung, External Approach

0BPKX1Z Removal of Radioactive Element from Right Lung, External Approach

0BPKX2Z Removal of Monitoring Device from Right Lung, External Approach

0BPKX3Z Removal of Infusion Device from Right Lung, External Approach

0BPL00Z Removal of Drainage Device from Left Lung, Open Approach

0BPL01Z Removal of Radioactive Element from Left Lung, Open Approach

0BPL02Z Removal of Monitoring Device from Left Lung, Open Approach

0BPL03Z Removal of Infusion Device from Left Lung, Open Approach

0BPL0YZ Removal of Other Device from Left Lung, Open Approach

0BPL30Z	Removal of Drainage Device from Left Lung, Percutaneous Approach
0BPL31Z	Removal of Radioactive Element from Left Lung, Percutaneous Approach
0BPL32Z	Removal of Monitoring Device from Left Lung, Percutaneous Approach
0BPL33Z	Removal of Infusion Device from Left Lung, Percutaneous Approach
0BPL3YZ	Removal of Other Device from Left Lung, Percutaneous Approach
0BPL40Z	Removal of Drainage Device from Left Lung, Percutaneous Endoscopic Approach
0BPL41Z	Removal of Radioactive Element from Left Lung, Percutaneous Endoscopic Approach
0BPL42Z	Removal of Monitoring Device from Left Lung, Percutaneous Endoscopic Approach
0BPL43Z	Removal of Infusion Device from Left Lung, Percutaneous Endoscopic Approach
0BPL4YZ	Removal of Other Device from Left Lung, Percutaneous Endoscopic Approach
0BPL70Z	Removal of Drainage Device from Left Lung, Via Natural or Artificial Opening
0BPL71Z	Removal of Radioactive Element from Left Lung, Via Natural or Artificial Opening
0BPL72Z	Removal of Monitoring Device from Left Lung, Via Natural or Artificial Opening
0BPL73Z	Removal of Infusion Device from Left Lung, Via Natural or Artificial Opening
0BPL7YZ	Removal of Other Device from Left Lung, Via Natural or Artificial Opening
0BPL80Z	Removal of Drainage Device from Left Lung, Via Natural or Artificial Opening Endoscopic
0BPL81Z	Removal of Radioactive Element from Left Lung, Via Natural or Artificial Opening Endoscopic
0BPL82Z	Removal of Monitoring Device from Left Lung, Via Natural or Artificial Opening Endoscopic
0BPL83Z	Removal of Infusion Device from Left Lung, Via Natural or Artificial Opening Endoscopic
0BPL8YZ	Removal of Other Device from Left Lung, Via Natural or Artificial Opening Endoscopic
0BPLX0Z	Removal of Drainage Device from Left Lung, External Approach
0BPLX1Z	Removal of Radioactive Element from Left Lung, External Approach
0BPLX2Z	Removal of Monitoring Device from Left Lung, External Approach
0BPLX3Z	Removal of Infusion Device from Left Lung, External Approach
0BPQ00Z	Removal of Drainage Device from Pleura, Open Approach
0BPQ01Z	Removal of Radioactive Element from Pleura, Open Approach
0BPQ02Z	Removal of Monitoring Device from Pleura, Open Approach
0BPQ0YZ	Removal of Other Device from Pleura, Open Approach
0BPQ30Z	Removal of Drainage Device from Pleura, Percutaneous Approach
0BPQ31Z	Removal of Radioactive Element from Pleura, Percutaneous Approach
0BPQ32Z	Removal of Monitoring Device from Pleura, Percutaneous Approach
0BPQ3YZ	Removal of Other Device from Pleura, Percutaneous Approach
0BPQ40Z	Removal of Drainage Device from Pleura, Percutaneous Endoscopic Approach
0BPQ41Z	Removal of Radioactive Element from Pleura, Percutaneous Endoscopic Approach
0BPQ42Z	Removal of Monitoring Device from Pleura, Percutaneous Endoscopic Approach
0BPQ4YZ	Removal of Other Device from Pleura, Percutaneous Endoscopic Approach
0BPQ70Z	Removal of Drainage Device from Pleura, Via Natural or Artificial Opening
0BPQ71Z	Removal of Radioactive Element from Pleura, Via Natural or Artificial Opening
0BPQ72Z	Removal of Monitoring Device from Pleura, Via Natural or Artificial Opening
0BPQ7YZ	Removal of Other Device from Pleura, Via Natural or Artificial Opening
0BPQ80Z	Removal of Drainage Device from Pleura, Via Natural or Artificial Opening Endoscopic
0BPQ81Z	Removal of Radioactive Element from Pleura, Via Natural or Artificial Opening Endoscopic
0BPQ82Z	Removal of Monitoring Device from Pleura, Via Natural or Artificial Opening Endoscopic
0BPQ8YZ	Removal of Other Device from Pleura, Via Natural or Artificial Opening Endoscopic
0BPQX0Z	Removal of Drainage Device from Pleura, External Approach
0BPQX1Z	Removal of Radioactive Element from Pleura, External Approach
0BPQX2Z	Removal of Monitoring Device from Pleura, External Approach
0BPT00Z	Removal of Drainage Device from Diaphragm, Open Approach
0BPT02Z	Removal of Monitoring Device from Diaphragm, Open Approach
0BPT07Z	Removal of Autologous Tissue Substitute from Diaphragm, Open Approach
0BPT0JZ	Removal of Synthetic Substitute from Diaphragm, Open Approach
0BPT0KZ	Removal of Nonautologous Tissue Substitute from Diaphragm, Open Approach
0BPT0MZ	Removal of Diaphragmatic Pacemaker Lead from Diaphragm, Open Approach
0BPT0YZ	Removal of Other Device from Diaphragm, Open Approach
0BPT30Z	Removal of Drainage Device from Diaphragm, Percutaneous Approach
0BPT32Z	Removal of Monitoring Device from Diaphragm, Percutaneous Approach
0BPT37Z	Removal of Autologous Tissue Substitute from Diaphragm, Percutaneous Approach
0BPT3JZ	Removal of Synthetic Substitute from Diaphragm, Percutaneous Approach
0BPT3KZ	Removal of Nonautologous Tissue Substitute from Diaphragm, Percutaneous Approach
0BPT3MZ	Removal of Diaphragmatic Pacemaker Lead from Diaphragm, Percutaneous Approach
0BPT3YZ	Removal of Other Device from Diaphragm, Percutaneous Approach
0BPT40Z	Removal of Drainage Device from Diaphragm, Percutaneous Endoscopic Approach
0BPT42Z	Removal of Monitoring Device from Diaphragm, Percutaneous Endoscopic Approach
0BPT47Z	Removal of Autologous Tissue Substitute from Diaphragm, Percutaneous Endoscopic Approach
0BPT4JZ	Removal of Synthetic Substitute from Diaphragm, Percutaneous Endoscopic Approach
0BPT4KZ	Removal of Nonautologous Tissue Substitute from Diaphragm, Percutaneous Endoscopic Approach
0BPT4MZ	Removal of Diaphragmatic Pacemaker Lead from Diaphragm, Percutaneous Endoscopic Approach
0BPT4YZ	Removal of Other Device from Diaphragm, Percutaneous Endoscopic Approach
0BPT70Z	Removal of Drainage Device from Diaphragm, Via Natural or Artificial Opening
0BPT72Z	Removal of Monitoring Device from Diaphragm, Via Natural or Artificial Opening
0BPT77Z	Removal of Autologous Tissue Substitute from Diaphragm, Via Natural or Artificial Opening
0BPT7JZ	Removal of Synthetic Substitute from Diaphragm, Via Natural or Artificial Opening
0BPT7KZ	Removal of Nonautologous Tissue Substitute from Diaphragm, Via Natural or Artificial Opening
0BPT7MZ	Removal of Diaphragmatic Pacemaker Lead from Diaphragm, Via Natural or Artificial Opening
0BPT7YZ	Removal of Other Device from Diaphragm, Via Natural or Artificial Opening
0BPT80Z	Removal of Drainage Device from Diaphragm, Via Natural or Artificial Opening Endoscopic
0BPT82Z	Removal of Monitoring Device from Diaphragm, Via Natural or Artificial Opening Endoscopic
0BPT87Z	Removal of Autologous Tissue Substitute from Diaphragm, Via Natural or Artificial Opening Endoscopic
0BPT8JZ	Removal of Synthetic Substitute from Diaphragm, Via Natural or Artificial Opening Endoscopic
0BPT8KZ	Removal of Nonautologous Tissue Substitute from Diaphragm, Via Natural or Artificial Opening Endoscopic
0BPT8MZ	Removal of Diaphragmatic Pacemaker Lead from Diaphragm, Via Natural or Artificial Opening Endoscopic
0BPT8YZ	Removal of Other Device from Diaphragm, Via Natural or Artificial Opening Endoscopic
0BPTX0Z	Removal of Drainage Device from Diaphragm, External Approach
0BPTX2Z	Removal of Monitoring Device from Diaphragm, External Approach
0BPTXMZ	Removal of Diaphragmatic Pacemaker Lead from Diaphragm, External Approach

♀ Female-only　♂ Male-only　▲ Limited Coverage　● Non-OR　HAC-associated procedure　▲ Non-covered procedures　✛ Cluster

0BQ – Respiratory System, Repair

0BQ10ZZ Repair Trachea, Open Approach

0BQ13ZZ Repair Trachea, Percutaneous Approach

0BQ14ZZ Repair Trachea, Percutaneous Endoscopic Approach

0BQ17ZZ Repair Trachea, Via Natural or Artificial Opening

0BQ18ZZ Repair Trachea, Via Natural or Artificial Opening Endoscopic

0BQ20ZZ Repair Carina, Open Approach

0BQ23ZZ Repair Carina, Percutaneous Approach

0BQ24ZZ Repair Carina, Percutaneous Endoscopic Approach

0BQ27ZZ Repair Carina, Via Natural or Artificial Opening

0BQ28ZZ Repair Carina, Via Natural or Artificial Opening Endoscopic

0BQ30ZZ Repair Right Main Bronchus, Open Approach

0BQ33ZZ Repair Right Main Bronchus, Percutaneous Approach

0BQ34ZZ Repair Right Main Bronchus, Percutaneous Endoscopic Approach

0BQ37ZZ Repair Right Main Bronchus, Via Natural or Artificial Opening

0BQ38ZZ Repair Right Main Bronchus, Via Natural or Artificial Opening Endoscopic

0BQ40ZZ Repair Right Upper Lobe Bronchus, Open Approach

0BQ43ZZ Repair Right Upper Lobe Bronchus, Percutaneous Approach

0BQ44ZZ Repair Right Upper Lobe Bronchus, Percutaneous Endoscopic Approach

0BQ47ZZ Repair Right Upper Lobe Bronchus, Via Natural or Artificial Opening

0BQ48ZZ Repair Right Upper Lobe Bronchus, Via Natural or Artificial Opening Endoscopic

0BQ50ZZ Repair Right Middle Lobe Bronchus, Open Approach

0BQ53ZZ Repair Right Middle Lobe Bronchus, Percutaneous Approach

0BQ54ZZ Repair Right Middle Lobe Bronchus, Percutaneous Endoscopic Approach

0BQ57ZZ Repair Right Middle Lobe Bronchus, Via Natural or Artificial Opening

0BQ58ZZ Repair Right Middle Lobe Bronchus, Via Natural or Artificial Opening Endoscopic

0BQ60ZZ Repair Right Lower Lobe Bronchus, Open Approach

0BQ63ZZ Repair Right Lower Lobe Bronchus, Percutaneous Approach

0BQ64ZZ Repair Right Lower Lobe Bronchus, Percutaneous Endoscopic Approach

0BQ67ZZ Repair Right Lower Lobe Bronchus, Via Natural or Artificial Opening

0BQ68ZZ Repair Right Lower Lobe Bronchus, Via Natural or Artificial Opening Endoscopic

0BQ70ZZ Repair Left Main Bronchus, Open Approach

0BQ73ZZ Repair Left Main Bronchus, Percutaneous Approach

0BQ74ZZ Repair Left Main Bronchus, Percutaneous Endoscopic Approach

0BQ77ZZ Repair Left Main Bronchus, Via Natural or Artificial Opening

0BQ78ZZ Repair Left Main Bronchus, Via Natural or Artificial Opening Endoscopic

0BQ80ZZ Repair Left Upper Lobe Bronchus, Open Approach

0BQ83ZZ Repair Left Upper Lobe Bronchus, Percutaneous Approach

0BQ84ZZ Repair Left Upper Lobe Bronchus, Percutaneous Endoscopic Approach

0BQ87ZZ Repair Left Upper Lobe Bronchus, Via Natural or Artificial Opening

0BQ88ZZ Repair Left Upper Lobe Bronchus, Via Natural or Artificial Opening Endoscopic

0BQ90ZZ Repair Lingula Bronchus, Open Approach

0BQ93ZZ Repair Lingula Bronchus, Percutaneous Approach

0BQ94ZZ Repair Lingula Bronchus, Percutaneous Endoscopic Approach

0BQ97ZZ Repair Lingula Bronchus, Via Natural or Artificial Opening

0BQ98ZZ Repair Lingula Bronchus, Via Natural or Artificial Opening Endoscopic

0BQB0ZZ Repair Left Lower Lobe Bronchus, Open Approach

0BQB3ZZ Repair Left Lower Lobe Bronchus, Percutaneous Approach

0BQB4ZZ Repair Left Lower Lobe Bronchus, Percutaneous Endoscopic Approach

0BQB7ZZ Repair Left Lower Lobe Bronchus, Via Natural or Artificial Opening

0BQB8ZZ Repair Left Lower Lobe Bronchus, Via Natural or Artificial Opening Endoscopic

0BQC0ZZ Repair Right Upper Lung Lobe, Open Approach

0BQC3ZZ Repair Right Upper Lung Lobe, Percutaneous Approach

0BQC4ZZ Repair Right Upper Lung Lobe, Percutaneous Endoscopic Approach

0BQC7ZZ Repair Right Upper Lung Lobe, Via Natural or Artificial Opening

0BQC8ZZ Repair Right Upper Lung Lobe, Via Natural or Artificial Opening Endoscopic

0BQD0ZZ Repair Right Middle Lung Lobe, Open Approach

0BQD3ZZ Repair Right Middle Lung Lobe, Percutaneous Approach

0BQD4ZZ Repair Right Middle Lung Lobe, Percutaneous Endoscopic Approach

0BQD7ZZ Repair Right Middle Lung Lobe, Via Natural or Artificial Opening

0BQD8ZZ Repair Right Middle Lung Lobe, Via Natural or Artificial Opening Endoscopic

0BQF0ZZ Repair Right Lower Lung Lobe, Open Approach

0BQF3ZZ Repair Right Lower Lung Lobe, Percutaneous Approach

0BQF4ZZ Repair Right Lower Lung Lobe, Percutaneous Endoscopic Approach

0BQF7ZZ Repair Right Lower Lung Lobe, Via Natural or Artificial Opening

0BQF8ZZ Repair Right Lower Lung Lobe, Via Natural or Artificial Opening Endoscopic

0BQG0ZZ Repair Left Upper Lung Lobe, Open Approach

0BQG3ZZ Repair Left Upper Lung Lobe, Percutaneous Approach

0BQG4ZZ Repair Left Upper Lung Lobe, Percutaneous Endoscopic Approach

0BQG7ZZ Repair Left Upper Lung Lobe, Via Natural or Artificial Opening

0BQG8ZZ Repair Left Upper Lung Lobe, Via Natural or Artificial Opening Endoscopic

0BQH0ZZ Repair Lung Lingula, Open Approach

0BQH3ZZ Repair Lung Lingula, Percutaneous Approach

0BQH4ZZ Repair Lung Lingula, Percutaneous Endoscopic Approach

0BQH7ZZ Repair Lung Lingula, Via Natural or Artificial Opening

0BQH8ZZ Repair Lung Lingula, Via Natural or Artificial Opening Endoscopic

0BQJ0ZZ Repair Left Lower Lung Lobe, Open Approach

0BQJ3ZZ Repair Left Lower Lung Lobe, Percutaneous Approach

0BQJ4ZZ Repair Left Lower Lung Lobe, Percutaneous Endoscopic Approach

0BQJ7ZZ Repair Left Lower Lung Lobe, Via Natural or Artificial Opening

0BQJ8ZZ Repair Left Lower Lung Lobe, Via Natural or Artificial Opening Endoscopic

0BQK0ZZ Repair Right Lung, Open Approach

0BQK3ZZ Repair Right Lung, Percutaneous Approach

0BQK4ZZ Repair Right Lung, Percutaneous Endoscopic Approach

0BQK7ZZ Repair Right Lung, Via Natural or Artificial Opening

0BQK8ZZ Repair Right Lung, Via Natural or Artificial Opening Endoscopic

0BQL0ZZ Repair Left Lung, Open Approach

0BQL3ZZ Repair Left Lung, Percutaneous Approach

0BQL4ZZ Repair Left Lung, Percutaneous Endoscopic Approach

0BQL7ZZ Repair Left Lung, Via Natural or Artificial Opening

0BQL8ZZ Repair Left Lung, Via Natural or Artificial Opening Endoscopic

0BQM0ZZ Repair Bilateral Lungs, Open Approach

0BQM3ZZ Repair Bilateral Lungs, Percutaneous Approach

0BQM4ZZ Repair Bilateral Lungs, Percutaneous Endoscopic Approach

0BQM7ZZ Repair Bilateral Lungs, Via Natural or Artificial Opening

0BQM8ZZ Repair Bilateral Lungs, Via Natural or Artificial Opening Endoscopic

0BQN0ZZ Repair Right Pleura, Open Approach

0BQN3ZZ Repair Right Pleura, Percutaneous Approach

0BQN4ZZ Repair Right Pleura, Percutaneous Endoscopic Approach

0BQP0ZZ Repair Left Pleura, Open Approach

0BQP3ZZ Repair Left Pleura, Percutaneous Approach

0BQP4ZZ Repair Left Pleura, Percutaneous Endoscopic Approach

0BQT0ZZ Repair Diaphragm, Open Approach

0BQT3ZZ Repair Diaphragm, Percutaneous Approach

0BQT4ZZ Repair Diaphragm, Percutaneous Endoscopic Approach

AHA CC: 3Q, 2020, 41-42

♀ Female-only ♂ Male-only ▲ Limited Coverage ● Non-OR ▦ HAC-associated procedure ▲ Non-covered procedures ✚ Cluster

Review Coding Guideline B3.18

0BR107Z Replacement of Trachea with Autologous Tissue Substitute, Open Approach

0BR10JZ Replacement of Trachea with Synthetic Substitute, Open Approach

0BR10KZ Replacement of Trachea with Nonautologous Tissue Substitute, Open Approach

0BR147Z Replacement of Trachea with Autologous Tissue Substitute, Percutaneous Endoscopic Approach

0BR14JZ Replacement of Trachea with Synthetic Substitute, Percutaneous Endoscopic Approach

0BR14KZ Replacement of Trachea with Nonautologous Tissue Substitute, Percutaneous Endoscopic Approach

0BR207Z Replacement of Carina with Autologous Tissue Substitute, Open Approach

0BR20JZ Replacement of Carina with Synthetic Substitute, Open Approach

0BR20KZ Replacement of Carina with Nonautologous Tissue Substitute, Open Approach

0BR247Z Replacement of Carina with Autologous Tissue Substitute, Percutaneous Endoscopic Approach

0BR24JZ Replacement of Carina with Synthetic Substitute, Percutaneous Endoscopic Approach

0BR24KZ Replacement of Carina with Nonautologous Tissue Substitute, Percutaneous Endoscopic Approach

0BR307Z Replacement of Right Main Bronchus with Autologous Tissue Substitute, Open Approach

0BR30JZ Replacement of Right Main Bronchus with Synthetic Substitute, Open Approach

0BR30KZ Replacement of Right Main Bronchus with Nonautologous Tissue Substitute, Open Approach

0BR347Z Replacement of Right Main Bronchus with Autologous Tissue Substitute, Percutaneous Endoscopic Approach

0BR34JZ Replacement of Right Main Bronchus with Synthetic Substitute, Percutaneous Endoscopic Approach

0BR34KZ Replacement of Right Main Bronchus with Nonautologous Tissue Substitute, Percutaneous Endoscopic Approach

0BR407Z Replacement of Right Upper Lobe Bronchus with Autologous Tissue Substitute, Open Approach

0BR40JZ Replacement of Right Upper Lobe Bronchus with Synthetic Substitute, Open Approach

0BR40KZ Replacement of Right Upper Lobe Bronchus with Nonautologous Tissue Substitute, Open Approach

0BR447Z Replacement of Right Upper Lobe Bronchus with Autologous Tissue Substitute, Percutaneous Endoscopic Approach

0BR44JZ Replacement of Right Upper Lobe Bronchus with Synthetic Substitute, Percutaneous Endoscopic Approach

0BR44KZ Replacement of Right Upper Lobe Bronchus with Nonautologous Tissue Substitute, Percutaneous Endoscopic Approach

0BR507Z Replacement of Right Middle Lobe Bronchus with Autologous Tissue Substitute, Open Approach

0BR50JZ Replacement of Right Middle Lobe Bronchus with Synthetic Substitute, Open Approach

0BR50KZ Replacement of Right Middle Lobe Bronchus with Nonautologous Tissue Substitute, Open Approach

0BR547Z Replacement of Right Middle Lobe Bronchus with Autologous Tissue Substitute, Percutaneous Endoscopic Approach

0BR54JZ Replacement of Right Middle Lobe Bronchus with Synthetic Substitute, Percutaneous Endoscopic Approach

0BR54KZ Replacement of Right Middle Lobe Bronchus with Nonautologous Tissue Substitute, Percutaneous Endoscopic Approach

0BR607Z Replacement of Right Lower Lobe Bronchus with Autologous Tissue Substitute, Open Approach

0BR60JZ Replacement of Right Lower Lobe Bronchus with Synthetic Substitute, Open Approach

0BR60KZ Replacement of Right Lower Lobe Bronchus with Nonautologous Tissue Substitute, Open Approach

0BR647Z Replacement of Right Lower Lobe Bronchus with Autologous Tissue Substitute, Percutaneous Endoscopic Approach

0BR64JZ Replacement of Right Lower Lobe Bronchus with Synthetic Substitute, Percutaneous Endoscopic Approach

0BR64KZ Replacement of Right Lower Lobe Bronchus with Nonautologous Tissue Substitute, Percutaneous Endoscopic Approach

0BR707Z Replacement of Left Main Bronchus with Autologous Tissue Substitute, Open Approach

0BR70JZ Replacement of Left Main Bronchus with Synthetic Substitute, Open Approach

0BR70ZZ Replacement of Left Main Bronchus with Nonautologous Tissue Substitute, Open Approach

0BR747Z Replacement of Left Main Bronchus with Autologous Tissue Substitute, Percutaneous Endoscopic Approach

0BR74JZ Replacement of Left Main Bronchus with Synthetic Substitute, Percutaneous Endoscopic Approach

0BR74ZZ Replacement of Left Main Bronchus with Nonautologous Tissue Substitute, Percutaneous Endoscopic Approach

0BR807Z Replacement of Left Upper Lobe Bronchus with Autologous Tissue Substitute, Open Approach

0BR80JZ Replacement of Left Upper Lobe Bronchus with Synthetic Substitute, Open Approach

0BR80ZZ Replacement of Left Upper Lobe Bronchus with Nonautologous Tissue Substitute, Open Approach

0BR847Z Replacement of Left Upper Lobe Bronchus with Autologous Tissue Substitute, Percutaneous Endoscopic Approach

0BR84JZ Replacement of Left Upper Lobe Bronchus with Synthetic Substitute, Percutaneous Endoscopic Approach

0BR84KZ Replacement of Left Upper Lobe Bronchus with Nonautologous Tissue Substitute, Percutaneous Endoscopic Approach

0BR907Z Replacement of Lingula Bronchus with Autologous Tissue Substitute, Open Approach

0BR90JZ Replacement of Lingula Bronchus with Synthetic Substitute, Open Approach

0BR90KZ Replacement of Lingula Bronchus with Nonautologous Tissue Substitute, Open Approach

0BR947Z Replacement of Lingula Bronchus with Autologous Tissue Substitute, Percutaneous Endoscopic Approach

0BR94JZ Replacement of Lingula Bronchus with Synthetic Substitute, Percutaneous Endoscopic Approach

0BR94KZ Replacement of Lingula Bronchus with Nonautologous Tissue Substitute, Percutaneous Endoscopic Approach

0BRB07Z Replacement of Left Lower Lobe Bronchus with Autologous Tissue Substitute, Open Approach

0BRB0JZ Replacement of Left Lower Lobe Bronchus with Synthetic Substitute, Open Approach

0BRB0KZ Replacement of Left Lower Lobe Bronchus with Nonautologous Tissue Substitute, Open Approach

0BRB47Z Replacement of Left Lower Lobe Bronchus with Autologous Tissue Substitute, Percutaneous Endoscopic Approach

0BRB4JZ Replacement of Left Lower Lobe Bronchus with Synthetic Substitute, Percutaneous Endoscopic Approach

0BRB4KZ Replacement of Left Lower Lobe Bronchus with Nonautologous Tissue Substitute, Percutaneous Endoscopic Approach

0BRT07Z Replacement of Diaphragm with Autologous Tissue Substitute, Open Approach

0BRT0JZ Replacement of Diaphragm with Synthetic Substitute, Open Approach

0BRT0KZ Replacement of Diaphragm with Nonautologous Tissue Substitute, Open Approach

0BRT47Z Replacement of Diaphragm with Autologous Tissue Substitute, Percutaneous Endoscopic Approach

0BRT4JZ Replacement of Diaphragm with Synthetic Substitute, Percutaneous Endoscopic Approach

0BRT4KZ Replacement of Diaphragm with Nonautologous Tissue Substitute, Percutaneous Endoscopic Approach

0BS – Respiratory System, Reposition

0BS10ZZ	Reposition Trachea, Open Approach
0BS20ZZ	Reposition Carina, Open Approach
0BS30ZZ	Reposition Right Main Bronchus, Open Approach
0BS40ZZ	Reposition Right Upper Lobe Bronchus, Open Approach
0BS50ZZ	Reposition Right Middle Lobe Bronchus, Open Approach
0BS60ZZ	Reposition Right Lower Lobe Bronchus, Open Approach
0BS70ZZ	Reposition Left Main Bronchus, Open Approach
0BS80ZZ	Reposition Left Upper Lobe Bronchus, Open Approach
0BS90ZZ	Reposition Lingula Bronchus, Open Approach
0BSB0ZZ	Reposition Left Lower Lobe Bronchus, Open Approach
0BSC0ZZ	Reposition Right Upper Lung Lobe, Open Approach
0BSD0ZZ	Reposition Right Middle Lung Lobe, Open Approach
0BSF0ZZ	Reposition Right Lower Lung Lobe, Open Approach
0BSG0ZZ	Reposition Left Upper Lung Lobe, Open Approach
0BSH0ZZ	Reposition Lung Lingula, Open Approach
0BSJ0ZZ	Reposition Left Lower Lung Lobe, Open Approach
0BSK0ZZ	Reposition Right Lung, Open Approach
0BSL0ZZ	Reposition Left Lung, Open Approach
0BST0ZZ	Reposition Diaphragm, Open Approach

0BT – Respiratory System, Resection

Review Coding Guideline B3.8

Review Coding Guideline B3.18

0BT10ZZ	Resection of Trachea, Open Approach
0BT14ZZ	Resection of Trachea, Percutaneous Endoscopic Approach
0BT20ZZ	Resection of Carina, Open Approach
0BT24ZZ	Resection of Carina, Percutaneous Endoscopic Approach
0BT30ZZ	Resection of Right Main Bronchus, Open Approach
0BT34ZZ	Resection of Right Main Bronchus, Percutaneous Endoscopic Approach
0BT40ZZ	Resection of Right Upper Lobe Bronchus, Open Approach
0BT44ZZ	Resection of Right Upper Lobe Bronchus, Percutaneous Endoscopic Approach
0BT50ZZ	Resection of Right Middle Lobe Bronchus, Open Approach
0BT54ZZ	Resection of Right Middle Lobe Bronchus, Percutaneous Endoscopic Approach
0BT60ZZ	Resection of Right Lower Lobe Bronchus, Open Approach
0BT64ZZ	Resection of Right Lower Lobe Bronchus, Percutaneous Endoscopic Approach
0BT70ZZ	Resection of Left Main Bronchus, Open Approach
0BT74ZZ	Resection of Left Main Bronchus, Percutaneous Endoscopic Approach
0BT80ZZ	Resection of Left Upper Lobe Bronchus, Open Approach
0BT84ZZ	Resection of Left Upper Lobe Bronchus, Percutaneous Endoscopic Approach
0BT90ZZ	Resection of Lingula Bronchus, Open Approach
0BT94ZZ	Resection of Lingula Bronchus, Percutaneous Endoscopic Approach
0BTB0ZZ	Resection of Left Lower Lobe Bronchus, Open Approach
0BTB4ZZ	Resection of Left Lower Lobe Bronchus, Percutaneous Endoscopic Approach
0BTC0ZZ	Resection of Right Upper Lung Lobe, Open Approach
0BTC4ZZ	Resection of Right Upper Lung Lobe, Percutaneous Endoscopic Approach
0BTD0ZZ	Resection of Right Middle Lung Lobe, Open Approach
0BTD4ZZ	Resection of Right Middle Lung Lobe, Percutaneous Endoscopic Approach
0BTF0ZZ	Resection of Right Lower Lung Lobe, Open Approach
0BTF4ZZ	Resection of Right Lower Lung Lobe, Percutaneous Endoscopic Approach
0BTG0ZZ	Resection of Left Upper Lung Lobe, Open Approach
0BTG4ZZ	Resection of Left Upper Lung Lobe, Percutaneous Endoscopic Approach
0BTH0ZZ	Resection of Lung Lingula, Open Approach
0BTH4ZZ	Resection of Lung Lingula, Percutaneous Endoscopic Approach
0BTJ0ZZ	Resection of Left Lower Lung Lobe, Open Approach
0BTJ4ZZ	Resection of Left Lower Lung Lobe, Percutaneous Endoscopic Approach
0BTK0ZZ	Resection of Right Lung, Open Approach
0BTK4ZZ	Resection of Right Lung, Percutaneous Endoscopic Approach
0BTL0ZZ	Resection of Left Lung, Open Approach
0BTL4ZZ	Resection of Left Lung, Percutaneous Endoscopic Approach
0BTM0ZZ	Resection of Bilateral Lungs, Open Approach
0BTM4ZZ	Resection of Bilateral Lungs, Percutaneous Endoscopic Approach
0BTT0ZZ	Resection of Diaphragm, Open Approach
0BTT4ZZ	Resection of Diaphragm, Percutaneous Endoscopic Approach

0BU – Respiratory System, Supplement

0BU107Z	Supplement Trachea with Autologous Tissue Substitute, Open Approach
0BU10JZ	Supplement Trachea with Synthetic Substitute, Open Approach
0BU10KZ	Supplement Trachea with Nonautologous Tissue Substitute, Open Approach
0BU147Z	Supplement Trachea with Autologous Tissue Substitute, Percutaneous Endoscopic Approach
0BU14JZ	Supplement Trachea with Synthetic Substitute, Percutaneous Endoscopic Approach
0BU14KZ	Supplement Trachea with Nonautologous Tissue Substitute, Percutaneous Endoscopic Approach
0BU187Z	Supplement Trachea with Autologous Tissue Substitute, Via Natural or Artificial Opening Endoscopic
0BU18JZ	Supplement Trachea with Synthetic Substitute, Via Natural or Artificial Opening Endoscopic

AHA CC: 3Q, 2020, 43-44

0BU18KZ	Supplement Trachea with Nonautologous Tissue Substitute, Via Natural or Artificial Opening Endoscopic
0BU207Z	Supplement Carina with Autologous Tissue Substitute, Open Approach
0BU20JZ	Supplement Carina with Synthetic Substitute, Open Approach
0BU20KZ	Supplement Carina with Nonautologous Tissue Substitute, Open Approach
0BU247Z	Supplement Carina with Autologous Tissue Substitute, Percutaneous Endoscopic Approach
0BU24JZ	Supplement Carina with Synthetic Substitute, Percutaneous Endoscopic Approach
0BU24KZ	Supplement Carina with Nonautologous Tissue Substitute, Percutaneous Endoscopic Approach
0BU287Z	Supplement Carina with Autologous Tissue Substitute, Via Natural or Artificial Opening Endoscopic
0BU28JZ	Supplement Carina with Synthetic Substitute, Via Natural or Artificial Opening Endoscopic
0BU28KZ	Supplement Carina with Nonautologous Tissue Substitute, Via Natural or Artificial Opening Endoscopic
0BU307Z	Supplement Right Main Bronchus with Autologous Tissue Substitute, Open Approach

AHA CC: 1Q, 2015, 28-29

0BU30JZ	Supplement Right Main Bronchus with Synthetic Substitute, Open Approach
0BU30KZ	Supplement Right Main Bronchus with Nonautologous Tissue Substitute, Open Approach
0BU347Z	Supplement Right Main Bronchus with Autologous Tissue Substitute, Percutaneous Endoscopic Approach
0BU34JZ	Supplement Right Main Bronchus with Synthetic Substitute, Percutaneous Endoscopic Approach

0BU34KZ   Supplement Right Main Bronchus with Nonautologous Tissue Substitute, Percutaneous Endoscopic Approach

0BU387Z   Supplement Right Main Bronchus with Autologous Tissue Substitute, Via Natural or Artificial Opening Endoscopic

0BU38JZ   Supplement Right Main Bronchus with Synthetic Substitute, Via Natural or Artificial Opening Endoscopic

0BU38KZ   Supplement Right Main Bronchus with Nonautologous Tissue Substitute, Via Natural or Artificial Opening Endoscopic

0BU407Z   Supplement Right Upper Lobe Bronchus with Autologous Tissue Substitute, Open Approach

0BU40JZ   Supplement Right Upper Lobe Bronchus with Synthetic Substitute, Open Approach

0BU40KZ   Supplement Right Upper Lobe Bronchus with Nonautologous Tissue Substitute, Open Approach

0BU447Z   Supplement Right Upper Lobe Bronchus with Autologous Tissue Substitute, Percutaneous Endoscopic Approach

0BU44JZ   Supplement Right Upper Lobe Bronchus with Synthetic Substitute, Percutaneous Endoscopic Approach

0BU44KZ   Supplement Right Upper Lobe Bronchus with Nonautologous Tissue Substitute, Percutaneous Endoscopic Approach

0BU487Z   Supplement Right Upper Lobe Bronchus with Autologous Tissue Substitute, Via Natural or Artificial Opening Endoscopic

0BU48JZ   Supplement Right Upper Lobe Bronchus with Synthetic Substitute, Via Natural or Artificial Opening Endoscopic

0BU48KZ   Supplement Right Upper Lobe Bronchus with Nonautologous Tissue Substitute, Via Natural or Artificial Opening Endoscopic

0BU507Z   Supplement Right Middle Lobe Bronchus with Autologous Tissue Substitute, Open Approach

0BU50JZ   Supplement Right Middle Lobe Bronchus with Synthetic Substitute, Open Approach

0BU50KZ   Supplement Right Middle Lobe Bronchus with Nonautologous Tissue Substitute, Open Approach

0BU547Z   Supplement Right Middle Lobe Bronchus with Autologous Tissue Substitute, Percutaneous Endoscopic Approach

0BU54JZ   Supplement Right Middle Lobe Bronchus with Synthetic Substitute, Percutaneous Endoscopic Approach

0BU54KZ   Supplement Right Middle Lobe Bronchus with Nonautologous Tissue Substitute, Percutaneous Endoscopic Approach

0BU587Z   Supplement Right Middle Lobe Bronchus with Autologous Tissue Substitute, Via Natural or Artificial Opening Endoscopic

0BU58JZ   Supplement Right Middle Lobe Bronchus with Synthetic Substitute, Via Natural or Artificial Opening Endoscopic

0BU58KZ   Supplement Right Middle Lobe Bronchus with Nonautologous Tissue Substitute, Via Natural or Artificial Opening Endoscopic

0BU607Z   Supplement Right Lower Lobe Bronchus with Autologous Tissue Substitute, Open Approach

0BU60JZ   Supplement Right Lower Lobe Bronchus with Synthetic Substitute, Open Approach

0BU60KZ   Supplement Right Lower Lobe Bronchus with Nonautologous Tissue Substitute, Open Approach

0BU647Z   Supplement Right Lower Lobe Bronchus with Autologous Tissue Substitute, Percutaneous Endoscopic Approach

0BU64JZ   Supplement Right Lower Lobe Bronchus with Synthetic Substitute, Percutaneous Endoscopic Approach

0BU64KZ   Supplement Right Lower Lobe Bronchus with Nonautologous Tissue Substitute, Percutaneous Endoscopic Approach

0BU687Z   Supplement Right Lower Lobe Bronchus with Autologous Tissue Substitute, Via Natural or Artificial Opening Endoscopic

0BU68JZ   Supplement Right Lower Lobe Bronchus with Synthetic Substitute, Via Natural or Artificial Opening Endoscopic

0BU68KZ   Supplement Right Lower Lobe Bronchus with Nonautologous Tissue Substitute, Via Natural or Artificial Opening Endoscopic

0BU707Z   Supplement Left Main Bronchus with Autologous Tissue Substitute, Open Approach

0BU70JZ   Supplement Left Main Bronchus with Synthetic Substitute, Open Approach

0BU70KZ   Supplement Left Main Bronchus with Nonautologous Tissue Substitute, Open Approach

0BU747Z   Supplement Left Main Bronchus with Autologous Tissue Substitute, Percutaneous Endoscopic Approach

0BU74JZ   Supplement Left Main Bronchus with Synthetic Substitute, Percutaneous Endoscopic Approach

0BU74KZ   Supplement Left Main Bronchus with Nonautologous Tissue Substitute, Percutaneous Endoscopic Approach

0BU787Z   Supplement Left Main Bronchus with Autologous Tissue Substitute, Via Natural or Artificial Opening Endoscopic

0BU78JZ   Supplement Left Main Bronchus with Synthetic Substitute, Via Natural or Artificial Opening Endoscopic

0BU78KZ   Supplement Left Main Bronchus with Nonautologous Tissue Substitute, Via Natural or Artificial Opening Endoscopic

0BU807Z   Supplement Left Upper Lobe Bronchus with Autologous Tissue Substitute, Open Approach

0BU80JZ   Supplement Left Upper Lobe Bronchus with Synthetic Substitute, Open Approach

0BU80KZ   Supplement Left Upper Lobe Bronchus with Nonautologous Tissue Substitute, Open Approach

0BU847Z   Supplement Left Upper Lobe Bronchus with Autologous Tissue Substitute, Percutaneous Endoscopic Approach

0BU84JZ   Supplement Left Upper Lobe Bronchus with Synthetic Substitute, Percutaneous Endoscopic Approach

0BU84KZ   Supplement Left Upper Lobe Bronchus with Nonautologous Tissue Substitute, Percutaneous Endoscopic Approach

0BU887Z   Supplement Left Upper Lobe Bronchus with Autologous Tissue Substitute, Via Natural or Artificial Opening Endoscopic

0BU88JZ   Supplement Left Upper Lobe Bronchus with Synthetic Substitute, Via Natural or Artificial Opening Endoscopic

0BU88KZ   Supplement Left Upper Lobe Bronchus with Nonautologous Tissue Substitute, Via Natural or Artificial Opening Endoscopic

0BU907Z   Supplement Lingula Bronchus with Autologous Tissue Substitute, Open Approach

0BU90JZ   Supplement Lingula Bronchus with Synthetic Substitute, Open Approach

0BU90KZ   Supplement Lingula Bronchus with Nonautologous Tissue Substitute, Open Approach

0BU947Z   Supplement Lingula Bronchus with Autologous Tissue Substitute, Percutaneous Endoscopic Approach

0BU94JZ   Supplement Lingula Bronchus with Synthetic Substitute, Percutaneous Endoscopic Approach

0BU94KZ   Supplement Lingula Bronchus with Nonautologous Tissue Substitute, Percutaneous Endoscopic Approach

0BU987Z   Supplement Lingula Bronchus with Autologous Tissue Substitute, Via Natural or Artificial Opening Endoscopic

0BU98JZ   Supplement Lingula Bronchus with Synthetic Substitute, Via Natural or Artificial Opening Endoscopic

0BU98KZ   Supplement Lingula Bronchus with Nonautologous Tissue Substitute, Via Natural or Artificial Opening Endoscopic

0BUB07Z   Supplement Left Lower Lobe Bronchus with Autologous Tissue Substitute, Open Approach

0BUB0JZ   Supplement Left Lower Lobe Bronchus with Synthetic Substitute, Open Approach

0BUB0KZ   Supplement Left Lower Lobe Bronchus with Nonautologous Tissue Substitute, Open Approach

0BUB47Z   Supplement Left Lower Lobe Bronchus with Autologous Tissue Substitute, Percutaneous Endoscopic Approach

0BUB4JZ   Supplement Left Lower Lobe Bronchus with Synthetic Substitute, Percutaneous Endoscopic Approach

0BUB4KZ   Supplement Left Lower Lobe Bronchus with Nonautologous Tissue Substitute, Percutaneous Endoscopic Approach

0BUB87Z   Supplement Left Lower Lobe Bronchus with Autologous Tissue Substitute, Via Natural or Artificial Opening Endoscopic

0BUB8JZ   Supplement Left Lower Lobe Bronchus with Synthetic Substitute, Via Natural or Artificial Opening Endoscopic

0BUB8KZ   Supplement Left Lower Lobe Bronchus with Nonautologous Tissue Substitute, Via Natural or Artificial Opening Endoscopic

♀ Female-only   ♂ Male-only   ▲ Limited Coverage   ● Non-OR   HAC HAC-associated procedure   ▲ Non-covered procedures   ✛ Cluster

0BUT07Z Supplement Diaphragm with Autologous Tissue Substitute, Open Approach

0BUT0JZ Supplement Diaphragm with Synthetic Substitute, Open Approach

0BUT0KZ Supplement Diaphragm with Nonautologous Tissue Substitute, Open Approach

0BUT47Z Supplement Diaphragm with Autologous Tissue Substitute, Percutaneous Endoscopic Approach

0BUT4JZ Supplement Diaphragm with Synthetic Substitute, Percutaneous Endoscopic Approach

0BUT4KZ Supplement Diaphragm with Nonautologous Tissue Substitute, Percutaneous Endoscopic Approach

0BV – Respiratory System, Restriction

0BV10CZ Restriction of Trachea with Extraluminal Device, Open Approach

0BV10DZ Restriction of Trachea with Intraluminal Device, Open Approach

0BV10ZZ Restriction of Trachea, Open Approach

0BV13CZ Restriction of Trachea with Extraluminal Device, Percutaneous Approach

0BV13DZ Restriction of Trachea with Intraluminal Device, Percutaneous Approach

0BV13ZZ Restriction of Trachea, Percutaneous Approach

0BV14CZ Restriction of Trachea with Extraluminal Device, Percutaneous Endoscopic Approach

0BV14DZ Restriction of Trachea with Intraluminal Device, Percutaneous Endoscopic Approach

0BV14ZZ Restriction of Trachea, Percutaneous Endoscopic Approach

0BV17DZ Restriction of Trachea with Intraluminal Device, Via Natural or Artificial Opening

0BV17ZZ Restriction of Trachea, Via Natural or Artificial Opening

0BV18DZ Restriction of Trachea with Intraluminal Device, Via Natural or Artificial Opening Endoscopic

0BV18ZZ Restriction of Trachea, Via Natural or Artificial Opening Endoscopic

0BV20CZ Restriction of Carina with Extraluminal Device, Open Approach

0BV20DZ Restriction of Carina with Intraluminal Device, Open Approach

0BV20ZZ Restriction of Carina, Open Approach

0BV23CZ Restriction of Carina with Extraluminal Device, Percutaneous Approach

0BV23DZ Restriction of Carina with Intraluminal Device, Percutaneous Approach

0BV23ZZ Restriction of Carina, Percutaneous Approach

0BV24CZ Restriction of Carina with Extraluminal Device, Percutaneous Endoscopic Approach

0BV24DZ Restriction of Carina with Intraluminal Device, Percutaneous Endoscopic Approach

0BV24ZZ Restriction of Carina, Percutaneous Endoscopic Approach

0BV27DZ Restriction of Carina with Intraluminal Device, Via Natural or Artificial Opening

0BV27ZZ Restriction of Carina, Via Natural or Artificial Opening

0BV28DZ Restriction of Carina with Intraluminal Device, Via Natural or Artificial Opening Endoscopic

0BV28ZZ Restriction of Carina, Via Natural or Artificial Opening Endoscopic

0BV30CZ Restriction of Right Main Bronchus with Extraluminal Device, Open Approach

0BV30DZ Restriction of Right Main Bronchus with Intraluminal Device, Open Approach

0BV30ZZ Restriction of Right Main Bronchus, Open Approach

0BV33CZ Restriction of Right Main Bronchus with Extraluminal Device, Percutaneous Approach

0BV33DZ Restriction of Right Main Bronchus with Intraluminal Device, Percutaneous Approach

0BV33ZZ Restriction of Right Main Bronchus, Percutaneous Approach

0BV34CZ Restriction of Right Main Bronchus with Extraluminal Device, Percutaneous Endoscopic Approach

0BV34DZ Restriction of Right Main Bronchus with Intraluminal Device, Percutaneous Endoscopic Approach

0BV34ZZ Restriction of Right Main Bronchus, Percutaneous Endoscopic Approach

0BV37DZ Restriction of Right Main Bronchus with Intraluminal Device, Via Natural or Artificial Opening

0BV37ZZ Restriction of Right Main Bronchus, Via Natural or Artificial Opening

0BV38DZ Restriction of Right Main Bronchus with Intraluminal Device, Via Natural or Artificial Opening Endoscopic

0BV38ZZ Restriction of Right Main Bronchus, Via Natural or Artificial Opening Endoscopic

0BV40CZ Restriction of Right Upper Lobe Bronchus with Extraluminal Device, Open Approach

0BV40DZ Restriction of Right Upper Lobe Bronchus with Intraluminal Device, Open Approach

0BV40ZZ Restriction of Right Upper Lobe Bronchus, Open Approach

0BV43CZ Restriction of Right Upper Lobe Bronchus with Extraluminal Device, Percutaneous Approach

0BV43DZ Restriction of Right Upper Lobe Bronchus with Intraluminal Device, Percutaneous Approach

0BV43ZZ Restriction of Right Upper Lobe Bronchus, Percutaneous Approach

0BV44CZ Restriction of Right Upper Lobe Bronchus with Extraluminal Device, Percutaneous Endoscopic Approach

0BV44DZ Restriction of Right Upper Lobe Bronchus with Intraluminal Device, Percutaneous Endoscopic Approach

0BV44ZZ Restriction of Right Upper Lobe Bronchus, Percutaneous Endoscopic Approach

0BV47DZ Restriction of Right Upper Lobe Bronchus with Intraluminal Device, Via Natural or Artificial Opening

0BV47ZZ Restriction of Right Upper Lobe Bronchus, Via Natural or Artificial Opening

0BV48DZ Restriction of Right Upper Lobe Bronchus with Intraluminal Device, Via Natural or Artificial Opening Endoscopic

0BV48ZZ Restriction of Right Upper Lobe Bronchus, Via Natural or Artificial Opening Endoscopic

0BV50CZ Restriction of Right Middle Lobe Bronchus with Extraluminal Device, Open Approach

0BV50DZ Restriction of Right Middle Lobe Bronchus with Intraluminal Device, Open Approach

0BV50ZZ Restriction of Right Middle Lobe Bronchus, Open Approach

0BV53CZ Restriction of Right Middle Lobe Bronchus with Extraluminal Device, Percutaneous Approach

0BV53DZ Restriction of Right Middle Lobe Bronchus with Intraluminal Device, Percutaneous Approach

0BV53ZZ Restriction of Right Middle Lobe Bronchus, Percutaneous Approach

0BV54CZ Restriction of Right Middle Lobe Bronchus with Extraluminal Device, Percutaneous Endoscopic Approach

0BV54DZ Restriction of Right Middle Lobe Bronchus with Intraluminal Device, Percutaneous Endoscopic Approach

0BV54ZZ Restriction of Right Middle Lobe Bronchus, Percutaneous Endoscopic Approach

0BV57DZ Restriction of Right Middle Lobe Bronchus with Intraluminal Device, Via Natural or Artificial Opening

0BV57ZZ Restriction of Right Middle Lobe Bronchus, Via Natural or Artificial Opening

0BV58DZ Restriction of Right Middle Lobe Bronchus with Intraluminal Device, Via Natural or Artificial Opening Endoscopic

0BV58ZZ Restriction of Right Middle Lobe Bronchus, Via Natural or Artificial Opening Endoscopic

0BV60CZ Restriction of Right Lower Lobe Bronchus with Extraluminal Device, Open Approach

0BV60DZ Restriction of Right Lower Lobe Bronchus with Intraluminal Device, Open Approach

0BV60ZZ Restriction of Right Lower Lobe Bronchus, Open Approach

0BV63CZ Restriction of Right Lower Lobe Bronchus with Extraluminal Device, Percutaneous Approach

0BV63DZ Restriction of Right Lower Lobe Bronchus with Intraluminal Device, Percutaneous Approach

0BV63ZZ Restriction of Right Lower Lobe Bronchus, Percutaneous Approach

0BV64CZ Restriction of Right Lower Lobe Bronchus with Extraluminal Device, Percutaneous Endoscopic Approach

0BV64DZ Restriction of Right Lower Lobe Bronchus with Intraluminal Device, Percutaneous Endoscopic Approach

0BV64ZZ Restriction of Right Lower Lobe Bronchus, Percutaneous Endoscopic Approach

0BV67DZ	Restriction of Right Lower Lobe Bronchus with Intraluminal Device, Via Natural or Artificial Opening	
0BV67ZZ	Restriction of Right Lower Lobe Bronchus, Via Natural or Artificial Opening	
0BV68DZ	Restriction of Right Lower Lobe Bronchus with Intraluminal Device, Via Natural or Artificial Opening Endoscopic	
0BV68ZZ	Restriction of Right Lower Lobe Bronchus, Via Natural or Artificial Opening Endoscopic	
0BV70CZ	Restriction of Left Main Bronchus with Extraluminal Device, Open Approach	
0BV70DZ	Restriction of Left Main Bronchus with Intraluminal Device, Open Approach	
0BV70ZZ	Restriction of Left Main Bronchus, Open Approach	
0BV73CZ	Restriction of Left Main Bronchus with Extraluminal Device, Percutaneous Approach	
0BV73DZ	Restriction of Left Main Bronchus with Intraluminal Device, Percutaneous Approach	
0BV73ZZ	Restriction of Left Main Bronchus, Percutaneous Approach	
0BV74CZ	Restriction of Left Main Bronchus with Extraluminal Device, Percutaneous Endoscopic Approach	
0BV74DZ	Restriction of Left Main Bronchus with Intraluminal Device, Percutaneous Endoscopic Approach	
0BV74ZZ	Restriction of Left Main Bronchus, Percutaneous Endoscopic Approach	
0BV77DZ	Restriction of Left Main Bronchus with Intraluminal Device, Via Natural or Artificial Opening	
0BV77ZZ	Restriction of Left Main Bronchus, Via Natural or Artificial Opening	
0BV78DZ	Restriction of Left Main Bronchus with Intraluminal Device, Via Natural or Artificial Opening Endoscopic	
0BV78ZZ	Restriction of Left Main Bronchus, Via Natural or Artificial Opening Endoscopic	
0BV80CZ	Restriction of Left Upper Lobe Bronchus with Extraluminal Device, Open Approach	
0BV80DZ	Restriction of Left Upper Lobe Bronchus with Intraluminal Device, Open Approach	

0BV80ZZ	Restriction of Left Upper Lobe Bronchus, Open Approach
0BV83CZ	Restriction of Left Upper Lobe Bronchus with Extraluminal Device, Percutaneous Approach
0BV83DZ	Restriction of Left Upper Lobe Bronchus with Intraluminal Device, Percutaneous Approach
0BV83ZZ	Restriction of Left Upper Lobe Bronchus, Percutaneous Approach
0BV84CZ	Restriction of Left Upper Lobe Bronchus with Extraluminal Device, Percutaneous Endoscopic Approach
0BV84DZ	Restriction of Left Upper Lobe Bronchus with Intraluminal Device, Percutaneous Endoscopic Approach
0BV84ZZ	Restriction of Left Upper Lobe Bronchus, Percutaneous Endoscopic Approach
0BV87DZ	Restriction of Left Upper Lobe Bronchus with Intraluminal Device, Via Natural or Artificial Opening
0BV87ZZ	Restriction of Left Upper Lobe Bronchus, Via Natural or Artificial Opening
0BV88DZ	Restriction of Left Upper Lobe Bronchus with Intraluminal Device, Via Natural or Artificial Opening Endoscopic
0BV88ZZ	Restriction of Left Upper Lobe Bronchus, Via Natural or Artificial Opening Endoscopic
0BV90CZ	Restriction of Lingula Bronchus with Extraluminal Device, Open Approach
0BV90DZ	Restriction of Lingula Bronchus with Intraluminal Device, Open Approach
0BV90ZZ	Restriction of Lingula Bronchus, Open Approach
0BV93CZ	Restriction of Lingula Bronchus with Extraluminal Device, Percutaneous Approach
0BV93DZ	Restriction of Lingula Bronchus with Intraluminal Device, Percutaneous Approach
0BV93ZZ	Restriction of Lingula Bronchus, Percutaneous Approach
0BV94CZ	Restriction of Lingula Bronchus with Extraluminal Device, Percutaneous Endoscopic Approach
0BV94DZ	Restriction of Lingula Bronchus with Intraluminal Device, Percutaneous Endoscopic Approach

0BV94ZZ	Restriction of Lingula Bronchus, Percutaneous Endoscopic Approach
0BV97DZ	Restriction of Lingula Bronchus with Intraluminal Device, Via Natural or Artificial Opening
0BV97ZZ	Restriction of Lingula Bronchus, Via Natural or Artificial Opening
0BV98DZ	Restriction of Lingula Bronchus with Intraluminal Device, Via Natural or Artificial Opening Endoscopic
0BV98ZZ	Restriction of Lingula Bronchus, Via Natural or Artificial Opening Endoscopic
0BVB0CZ	Restriction of Left Lower Lobe Bronchus with Extraluminal Device, Open Approach
0BVB0DZ	Restriction of Left Lower Lobe Bronchus with Intraluminal Device, Open Approach
0BVB0ZZ	Restriction of Left Lower Lobe Bronchus, Open Approach
0BVB3CZ	Restriction of Left Lower Lobe Bronchus with Extraluminal Device, Percutaneous Approach
0BVB3DZ	Restriction of Left Lower Lobe Bronchus with Intraluminal Device, Percutaneous Approach
0BVB3ZZ	Restriction of Left Lower Lobe Bronchus, Percutaneous Approach
0BVB4CZ	Restriction of Left Lower Lobe Bronchus with Extraluminal Device, Percutaneous Endoscopic Approach
0BVB4DZ	Restriction of Left Lower Lobe Bronchus with Intraluminal Device, Percutaneous Endoscopic Approach
0BVB4ZZ	Restriction of Left Lower Lobe Bronchus, Percutaneous Endoscopic Approach
0BVB7DZ	Restriction of Left Lower Lobe Bronchus with Intraluminal Device, Via Natural or Artificial Opening
0BVB7ZZ	Restriction of Left Lower Lobe Bronchus, Via Natural or Artificial Opening
0BVB8DZ	Restriction of Left Lower Lobe Bronchus with Intraluminal Device, Via Natural or Artificial Opening Endoscopic
0BVB8ZZ	Restriction of Left Lower Lobe Bronchus, Via Natural or Artificial Opening Endoscopic

0BW – Respiratory System, Revision

Review Coding Guideline B6.1c

0BW000Z	Revision of Drainage Device in Tracheobronchial Tree, Open Approach
0BW002Z	Revision of Monitoring Device in Tracheobronchial Tree, Open Approach
0BW003Z	Revision of Infusion Device in Tracheobronchial Tree, Open Approach
0BW007Z	Revision of Autologous Tissue Substitute in Tracheobronchial Tree, Open Approach
0BW00CZ	Revision of Extraluminal Device in Tracheobronchial Tree, Open Approach
0BW00DZ	Revision of Intraluminal Device in Tracheobronchial Tree, Open Approach
0BW00JZ	Revision of Synthetic Substitute in Tracheobronchial Tree, Open Approach
0BW00KZ	Revision of Nonautologous Tissue Substitute in Tracheobronchial Tree, Open Approach

0BW00YZ	Revision of Other Device in Tracheobronchial Tree, Open Approach
0BW030Z	Revision of Drainage Device in Tracheobronchial Tree, Percutaneous Approach
0BW032Z	Revision of Monitoring Device in Tracheobronchial Tree, Percutaneous Approach
0BW033Z	Revision of Infusion Device in Tracheobronchial Tree, Percutaneous Approach
0BW037Z	Revision of Autologous Tissue Substitute in Tracheobronchial Tree, Percutaneous Approach
0BW03CZ	Revision of Extraluminal Device in Tracheobronchial Tree, Percutaneous Approach

0BW03DZ	Revision of Intraluminal Device in Tracheobronchial Tree, Percutaneous Approach
0BW03JZ	Revision of Synthetic Substitute in Tracheobronchial Tree, Percutaneous Approach
0BW03KZ	Revision of Nonautologous Tissue Substitute in Tracheobronchial Tree, Percutaneous Approach
0BW03YZ	Revision of Other Device in Tracheobronchial Tree, Percutaneous Approach
0BW040Z	Revision of Drainage Device in Tracheobronchial Tree, Percutaneous Endoscopic Approach
0BW042Z	Revision of Monitoring Device in Tracheobronchial Tree, Percutaneous Endoscopic Approach

♀ Female-only   ♂ Male-only   ▲ Limited Coverage   ● Non-OR   ▦ HAC-associated procedure   ▲ Non-covered procedures   ✚ Cluster

0BW043Z Revision of Infusion Device in Tracheobronchial Tree, Percutaneous Endoscopic Approach

0BW047Z Revision of Autologous Tissue Substitute in Tracheobronchial Tree, Percutaneous Endoscopic Approach

0BW04CZ Revision of Extraluminal Device in Tracheobronchial Tree, Percutaneous Endoscopic Approach

0BW04DZ Revision of Intraluminal Device in Tracheobronchial Tree, Percutaneous Endoscopic Approach

0BW04JZ Revision of Synthetic Substitute in Tracheobronchial Tree, Percutaneous Endoscopic Approach

0BW04KZ Revision of Nonautologous Tissue Substitute in Tracheobronchial Tree, Percutaneous Endoscopic Approach

0BW04YZ Revision of Other Device in Tracheobronchial Tree, Percutaneous Endoscopic Approach

0BW070Z Revision of Drainage Device in Tracheobronchial Tree, Via Natural or Artificial Opening

0BW072Z Revision of Monitoring Device in Tracheobronchial Tree, Via Natural or Artificial Opening

0BW073Z Revision of Infusion Device in Tracheobronchial Tree, Via Natural or Artificial Opening

0BW077Z Revision of Autologous Tissue Substitute in Tracheobronchial Tree, Via Natural or Artificial Opening

0BW07CZ Revision of Extraluminal Device in Tracheobronchial Tree, Via Natural or Artificial Opening

0BW07DZ Revision of Intraluminal Device in Tracheobronchial Tree, Via Natural or Artificial Opening

0BW07JZ Revision of Synthetic Substitute in Tracheobronchial Tree, Via Natural or Artificial Opening

0BW07KZ Revision of Nonautologous Tissue Substitute in Tracheobronchial Tree, Via Natural or Artificial Opening

0BW07YZ Revision of Other Device in Tracheobronchial Tree, Via Natural or Artificial Opening

0BW080Z Revision of Drainage Device in Tracheobronchial Tree, Via Natural or Artificial Opening Endoscopic

0BW082Z Revision of Monitoring Device in Tracheobronchial Tree, Via Natural or Artificial Opening Endoscopic

0BW083Z Revision of Infusion Device in Tracheobronchial Tree, Via Natural or Artificial Opening Endoscopic

0BW087Z Revision of Autologous Tissue Substitute in Tracheobronchial Tree, Via Natural or Artificial Opening Endoscopic

0BW08CZ Revision of Extraluminal Device in Tracheobronchial Tree, Via Natural or Artificial Opening Endoscopic

0BW08DZ Revision of Intraluminal Device in Tracheobronchial Tree, Via Natural or Artificial Opening Endoscopic

0BW08JZ Revision of Synthetic Substitute in Tracheobronchial Tree, Via Natural or Artificial Opening Endoscopic

0BW08KZ Revision of Nonautologous Tissue Substitute in Tracheobronchial Tree, Via Natural or Artificial Opening Endoscopic

0BW08YZ Revision of Other Device in Tracheobronchial Tree, Via Natural or Artificial Opening Endoscopic

0BW0X0Z Revision of Drainage Device in Tracheobronchial Tree, External Approach

0BW0X2Z Revision of Monitoring Device in Tracheobronchial Tree, External Approach

0BW0X3Z Revision of Infusion Device in Tracheobronchial Tree, External Approach

0BW0X7Z Revision of Autologous Tissue Substitute in Tracheobronchial Tree, External Approach

0BW0XCZ Revision of Extraluminal Device in Tracheobronchial Tree, External Approach

0BW0XDZ Revision of Intraluminal Device in Tracheobronchial Tree, External Approach

0BW0XJZ Revision of Synthetic Substitute in Tracheobronchial Tree, External Approach

0BW0XKZ Revision of Nonautologous Tissue Substitute in Tracheobronchial Tree, External Approach

0BW100Z Revision of Drainage Device in Trachea, Open Approach

0BW102Z Revision of Monitoring Device in Trachea, Open Approach

0BW107Z Revision of Autologous Tissue Substitute in Trachea, Open Approach

0BW10CZ Revision of Extraluminal Device in Trachea, Open Approach

0BW10DZ Revision of Intraluminal Device in Trachea, Open Approach

0BW10FZ Revision of Tracheostomy Device in Trachea, Open Approach

0BW10JZ Revision of Synthetic Substitute in Trachea, Open Approach

0BW10KZ Revision of Nonautologous Tissue Substitute in Trachea, Open Approach

0BW130Z Revision of Drainage Device in Trachea, Percutaneous Approach

0BW132Z Revision of Monitoring Device in Trachea, Percutaneous Approach

0BW137Z Revision of Autologous Tissue Substitute in Trachea, Percutaneous Approach

0BW13CZ Revision of Extraluminal Device in Trachea, Percutaneous Approach

0BW13DZ Revision of Intraluminal Device in Trachea, Percutaneous Approach

0BW13FZ Revision of Tracheostomy Device in Trachea, Percutaneous Approach

0BW13JZ Revision of Synthetic Substitute in Trachea, Percutaneous Approach

0BW13KZ Revision of Nonautologous Tissue Substitute in Trachea, Percutaneous Approach

0BW140Z Revision of Drainage Device in Trachea, Percutaneous Endoscopic Approach

0BW142Z Revision of Monitoring Device in Trachea, Percutaneous Endoscopic Approach

0BW147Z Revision of Autologous Tissue Substitute in Trachea, Percutaneous Endoscopic Approach

0BW14CZ Revision of Extraluminal Device in Trachea, Percutaneous Endoscopic Approach

0BW14DZ Revision of Intraluminal Device in Trachea, Percutaneous Endoscopic Approach

0BW14FZ Revision of Tracheostomy Device in Trachea, Percutaneous Endoscopic Approach

0BW14JZ Revision of Synthetic Substitute in Trachea, Percutaneous Endoscopic Approach

0BW14KZ Revision of Nonautologous Tissue Substitute in Trachea, Percutaneous Endoscopic Approach

0BW170Z Revision of Drainage Device in Trachea, Via Natural or Artificial Opening

0BW172Z Revision of Monitoring Device in Trachea, Via Natural or Artificial Opening

0BW177Z Revision of Autologous Tissue Substitute in Trachea, Via Natural or Artificial Opening

0BW17CZ Revision of Extraluminal Device in Trachea, Via Natural or Artificial Opening

0BW17DZ Revision of Intraluminal Device in Trachea, Via Natural or Artificial Opening

0BW17FZ Revision of Tracheostomy Device in Trachea, Via Natural or Artificial Opening

0BW17JZ Revision of Synthetic Substitute in Trachea, Via Natural or Artificial Opening

0BW17KZ Revision of Nonautologous Tissue Substitute in Trachea, Via Natural or Artificial Opening

0BW180Z Revision of Drainage Device in Trachea, Via Natural or Artificial Opening Endoscopic

0BW182Z Revision of Monitoring Device in Trachea, Via Natural or Artificial Opening Endoscopic

0BW187Z Revision of Autologous Tissue Substitute in Trachea, Via Natural or Artificial Opening Endoscopic

0BW18CZ Revision of Extraluminal Device in Trachea, Via Natural or Artificial Opening Endoscopic

0BW18DZ Revision of Intraluminal Device in Trachea, Via Natural or Artificial Opening Endoscopic

0BW18FZ Revision of Tracheostomy Device in Trachea, Via Natural or Artificial Opening Endoscopic

0BW18JZ Revision of Synthetic Substitute in Trachea, Via Natural or Artificial Opening Endoscopic

0BW18KZ Revision of Nonautologous Tissue Substitute in Trachea, Via Natural or Artificial Opening Endoscopic

0BW1X0Z Revision of Drainage Device in Trachea, External Approach

0BW1X2Z Revision of Monitoring Device in Trachea, External Approach

0BW1X7Z Revision of Autologous Tissue Substitute in Trachea, External Approach

0BW1XCZ Revision of Extraluminal Device in Trachea, External Approach

0BW1XDZ Revision of Intraluminal Device in Trachea, External Approach

0BW1XFZ Revision of Tracheostomy Device in Trachea, External Approach

0BW1XJZ Revision of Synthetic Substitute in Trachea, External Approach

0BW1XKZ Revision of Nonautologous Tissue Substitute in Trachea, External Approach

0BWK00Z Revision of Drainage Device in Right Lung, Open Approach

0BWK02Z Revision of Monitoring Device in Right Lung, Open Approach

♀ Female-only   ♂ Male-only   ▲ Limited Coverage   ● Non-OR   ▦ HAC-associated procedure   ▲ Non-covered procedures   ✚ Cluster

0BWK03Z	Revision of Infusion Device in Right Lung, Open Approach
0BWK0YZ	Revision of Other Device in Right Lung, Open Approach
0BWK30Z	Revision of Drainage Device in Right Lung, Percutaneous Approach
0BWK32Z	Revision of Monitoring Device in Right Lung, Percutaneous Approach
0BWK33Z	Revision of Infusion Device in Right Lung, Percutaneous Approach
0BWK3YZ	Revision of Other Device in Right Lung, Percutaneous Approach
0BWK40Z	Revision of Drainage Device in Right Lung, Percutaneous Endoscopic Approach
0BWK42Z	Revision of Monitoring Device in Right Lung, Percutaneous Endoscopic Approach
0BWK43Z	Revision of Infusion Device in Right Lung, Percutaneous Endoscopic Approach
0BWK4YZ	Revision of Other Device in Right Lung, Percutaneous Endoscopic Approach
0BWK70Z	Revision of Drainage Device in Right Lung, Via Natural or Artificial Opening
0BWK72Z	Revision of Monitoring Device in Right Lung, Via Natural or Artificial Opening
0BWK73Z	Revision of Infusion Device in Right Lung, Via Natural or Artificial Opening
0BWK7YZ	Revision of Other Device in Right Lung, Via Natural or Artificial Opening
0BWK80Z	Revision of Drainage Device in Right Lung, Via Natural or Artificial Opening Endoscopic
0BWK82Z	Revision of Monitoring Device in Right Lung, Via Natural or Artificial Opening Endoscopic
0BWK83Z	Revision of Infusion Device in Right Lung, Via Natural or Artificial Opening Endoscopic
0BWK8YZ	Revision of Other Device in Right Lung, Via Natural or Artificial Opening Endoscopic
0BWKX0Z	Revision of Drainage Device in Right Lung, External Approach
0BWKX2Z	Revision of Monitoring Device in Right Lung, External Approach
0BWKX3Z	Revision of Infusion Device in Right Lung, External Approach
0BWL00Z	Revision of Drainage Device in Left Lung, Open Approach
0BWL02Z	Revision of Monitoring Device in Left Lung, Open Approach
0BWL03Z	Revision of Infusion Device in Left Lung, Open Approach
0BWL0YZ	Revision of Other Device in Left Lung, Open Approach
0BWL30Z	Revision of Drainage Device in Left Lung, Percutaneous Approach
0BWL32Z	Revision of Monitoring Device in Left Lung, Percutaneous Approach
0BWL33Z	Revision of Infusion Device in Left Lung, Percutaneous Approach
0BWL3YZ	Revision of Other Device in Left Lung, Percutaneous Approach
0BWL40Z	Revision of Drainage Device in Left Lung, Percutaneous Endoscopic Approach
0BWL42Z	Revision of Monitoring Device in Left Lung, Percutaneous Endoscopic Approach
0BWL43Z	Revision of Infusion Device in Left Lung, Percutaneous Endoscopic Approach
0BWL4YZ	Revision of Other Device in Left Lung, Percutaneous Endoscopic Approach
0BWL70Z	Revision of Drainage Device in Left Lung, Via Natural or Artificial Opening
0BWL72Z	Revision of Monitoring Device in Left Lung, Via Natural or Artificial Opening
0BWL73Z	Revision of Infusion Device in Left Lung, Via Natural or Artificial Opening
0BWL7YZ	Revision of Other Device in Left Lung, Via Natural or Artificial Opening
0BWL80Z	Revision of Drainage Device in Left Lung, Via Natural or Artificial Opening Endoscopic
0BWL82Z	Revision of Monitoring Device in Left Lung, Via Natural or Artificial Opening Endoscopic
0BWL83Z	Revision of Infusion Device in Left Lung, Via Natural or Artificial Opening Endoscopic
0BWL8YZ	Revision of Other Device in Left Lung, Via Natural or Artificial Opening Endoscopic
0BWLX0Z	Revision of Drainage Device in Left Lung, External Approach
0BWLX2Z	Revision of Monitoring Device in Left Lung, External Approach
0BWLX3Z	Revision of Infusion Device in Left Lung, External Approach
0BWQ00Z	Revision of Drainage Device in Pleura, Open Approach
0BWQ02Z	Revision of Monitoring Device in Pleura, Open Approach
0BWQ0YZ	Revision of Other Device in Pleura, Open Approach
0BWQ30Z	Revision of Drainage Device in Pleura, Percutaneous Approach
0BWQ32Z	Revision of Monitoring Device in Pleura, Percutaneous Approach
0BWQ3YZ	Revision of Other Device in Pleura, Percutaneous Approach
0BWQ40Z	Revision of Drainage Device in Pleura, Percutaneous Endoscopic Approach
0BWQ42Z	Revision of Monitoring Device in Pleura, Percutaneous Endoscopic Approach
0BWQ4YZ	Revision of Other Device in Pleura, Percutaneous Endoscopic Approach
0BWQ70Z	Revision of Drainage Device in Pleura, Via Natural or Artificial Opening
0BWQ72Z	Revision of Monitoring Device in Pleura, Via Natural or Artificial Opening
0BWQ7YZ	Revision of Other Device in Pleura, Via Natural or Artificial Opening
0BWQ80Z	Revision of Drainage Device in Pleura, Via Natural or Artificial Opening Endoscopic
0BWQ82Z	Revision of Monitoring Device in Pleura, Via Natural or Artificial Opening Endoscopic
0BWQ8YZ	Revision of Other Device in Pleura, Via Natural or Artificial Opening Endoscopic
0BWQX0Z	Revision of Drainage Device in Pleura, External Approach
0BWQX2Z	Revision of Monitoring Device in Pleura, External Approach
0BWT00Z	Revision of Drainage Device in Diaphragm, Open Approach
0BWT02Z	Revision of Monitoring Device in Diaphragm, Open Approach
0BWT07Z	Revision of Autologous Tissue Substitute in Diaphragm, Open Approach
0BWT0JZ	Revision of Synthetic Substitute in Diaphragm, Open Approach
0BWT0KZ	Revision of Nonautologous Tissue Substitute in Diaphragm, Open Approach
0BWT0MZ	Revision of Diaphragmatic Pacemaker Lead in Diaphragm, Open Approach
0BWT0YZ	Revision of Other Device in Diaphragm, Open Approach
0BWT30Z	Revision of Drainage Device in Diaphragm, Percutaneous Approach
0BWT32Z	Revision of Monitoring Device in Diaphragm, Percutaneous Approach
0BWT37Z	Revision of Autologous Tissue Substitute in Diaphragm, Percutaneous Approach
0BWT3JZ	Revision of Synthetic Substitute in Diaphragm, Percutaneous Approach
0BWT3KZ	Revision of Nonautologous Tissue Substitute in Diaphragm, Percutaneous Approach
0BWT3MZ	Revision of Diaphragmatic Pacemaker Lead in Diaphragm, Percutaneous Approach
0BWT3YZ	Revision of Other Device in Diaphragm, Percutaneous Approach
0BWT40Z	Revision of Drainage Device in Diaphragm, Percutaneous Endoscopic Approach
0BWT42Z	Revision of Monitoring Device in Diaphragm, Percutaneous Endoscopic Approach
0BWT47Z	Revision of Autologous Tissue Substitute in Diaphragm, Percutaneous Endoscopic Approach
0BWT4JZ	Revision of Synthetic Substitute in Diaphragm, Percutaneous Endoscopic Approach
0BWT4KZ	Revision of Nonautologous Tissue Substitute in Diaphragm, Percutaneous Endoscopic Approach
0BWT4MZ	Revision of Diaphragmatic Pacemaker Lead in Diaphragm, Percutaneous Endoscopic Approach
0BWT4YZ	Revision of Other Device in Diaphragm, Percutaneous Endoscopic Approach
0BWT70Z	Revision of Drainage Device in Diaphragm, Via Natural or Artificial Opening
0BWT72Z	Revision of Monitoring Device in Diaphragm, Via Natural or Artificial Opening
0BWT77Z	Revision of Autologous Tissue Substitute in Diaphragm, Via Natural or Artificial Opening
0BWT7JZ	Revision of Synthetic Substitute in Diaphragm, Via Natural or Artificial Opening
0BWT7KZ	Revision of Nonautologous Tissue Substitute in Diaphragm, Via Natural or Artificial Opening
0BWT7MZ	Revision of Diaphragmatic Pacemaker Lead in Diaphragm, Via Natural or Artificial Opening

♀ Female-only   ♂ Male-only   ▲ Limited Coverage   ● Non-OR   ⬛ HAC-associated procedure   ▲ Non-covered procedures   ✚ Cluster

0BWT7YZ	Revision of Other Device in Diaphragm, Via Natural or Artificial Opening	0BWT8KZ	Revision of Nonautologous Tissue Substitute in Diaphragm, Via Natural or Artificial Opening Endoscopic	0BWTX7Z	Revision of Autologous Tissue Substitute in Diaphragm, External Approach
0BWT80Z	Revision of Drainage Device in Diaphragm, Via Natural or Artificial Opening Endoscopic	0BWT8MZ	Revision of Diaphragmatic Pacemaker Lead in Diaphragm, Via Natural or Artificial Opening Endoscopic	0BWTXJZ	Revision of Synthetic Substitute in Diaphragm, External Approach
0BWT82Z	Revision of Monitoring Device in Diaphragm, Via Natural or Artificial Opening Endoscopic	0BWT8YZ	Revision of Other Device in Diaphragm, Via Natural or Artificial Opening Endoscopic	0BWTXKZ	Revision of Nonautologous Tissue Substitute in Diaphragm, External Approach
0BWT87Z	Revision of Autologous Tissue Substitute in Diaphragm, Via Natural or Artificial Opening Endoscopic	0BWTX0Z	Revision of Drainage Device in Diaphragm, External Approach	0BWTXMZ	Revision of Diaphragmatic Pacemaker Lead in Diaphragm, External Approach
0BWT8JZ	Revision of Synthetic Substitute in Diaphragm, Via Natural or Artificial Opening Endoscopic	0BWTX2Z	Revision of Monitoring Device in Diaphragm, External Approach		

0BY – Respiratory System, Transplantation

Review Coding Guideline B3.16

0BYC0Z0	Transplantation of Right Upper Lung Lobe, Allogeneic, Open Approach	▲ 0BYG0Z0	Transplantation of Left Upper Lung Lobe, Allogeneic, Open Approach	▲ 0BYK0Z0	Transplantation of Right Lung, Allogeneic, Open Approach
0BYC0Z1	Transplantation of Right Upper Lung Lobe, Syngeneic, Open Approach	▲ 0BYG0Z1	Transplantation of Left Upper Lung Lobe, Syngeneic, Open Approach	▲ 0BYK0Z1	Transplantation of Right Lung, Syngeneic, Open Approach
0BYC0Z2	Transplantation of Right Upper Lung Lobe, Zooplastic, Open Approach	▲ 0BYG0Z2	Transplantation of Left Upper Lung Lobe, Zooplastic, Open Approach	▲ 0BYK0Z2	Transplantation of Right Lung, Zooplastic, Open Approach
0BYD0Z0	Transplantation of Right Middle Lung Lobe, Allogeneic, Open Approach	▲ 0BYH0Z0	Transplantation of Lung Lingula, Allogeneic, Open Approach	▲ 0BYL0Z0	Transplantation of Left Lung, Allogeneic, Open Approach
0BYD0Z1	Transplantation of Right Middle Lung Lobe, Syngeneic, Open Approach	▲ 0BYH0Z1	Transplantation of Lung Lingula, Syngeneic, Open Approach	▲ 0BYL0Z1	Transplantation of Left Lung, Syngeneic, Open Approach
0BYD0Z2	Transplantation of Right Middle Lung Lobe, Zooplastic, Open Approach	▲ 0BYH0Z2	Transplantation of Lung Lingula, Zooplastic, Open Approach	▲ 0BYL0Z2	Transplantation of Left Lung, Zooplastic, Open Approach
0BYF0Z0	Transplantation of Right Lower Lung Lobe, Allogeneic, Open Approach	▲ 0BYJ0Z0	Transplantation of Left Lower Lung Lobe, Allogeneic, Open Approach	▲ 0BYM0Z0	Transplantation of Bilateral Lungs, Allogeneic, Open Approach
0BYF0Z1	Transplantation of Right Lower Lung Lobe, Syngeneic, Open Approach	▲ 0BYJ0Z1	Transplantation of Left Lower Lung Lobe, Syngeneic, Open Approach	▲ 0BYM0Z1	Transplantation of Bilateral Lungs, Syngeneic, Open Approach
0BYF0Z2	Transplantation of Right Lower Lung Lobe, Zooplastic, Open Approach	▲ 0BYJ0Z2	Transplantation of Left Lower Lung Lobe, Zooplastic, Open Approach	▲ 0BYM0Z2	Transplantation of Bilateral Lungs, Zooplastic, Open Approach

Oral Cavity

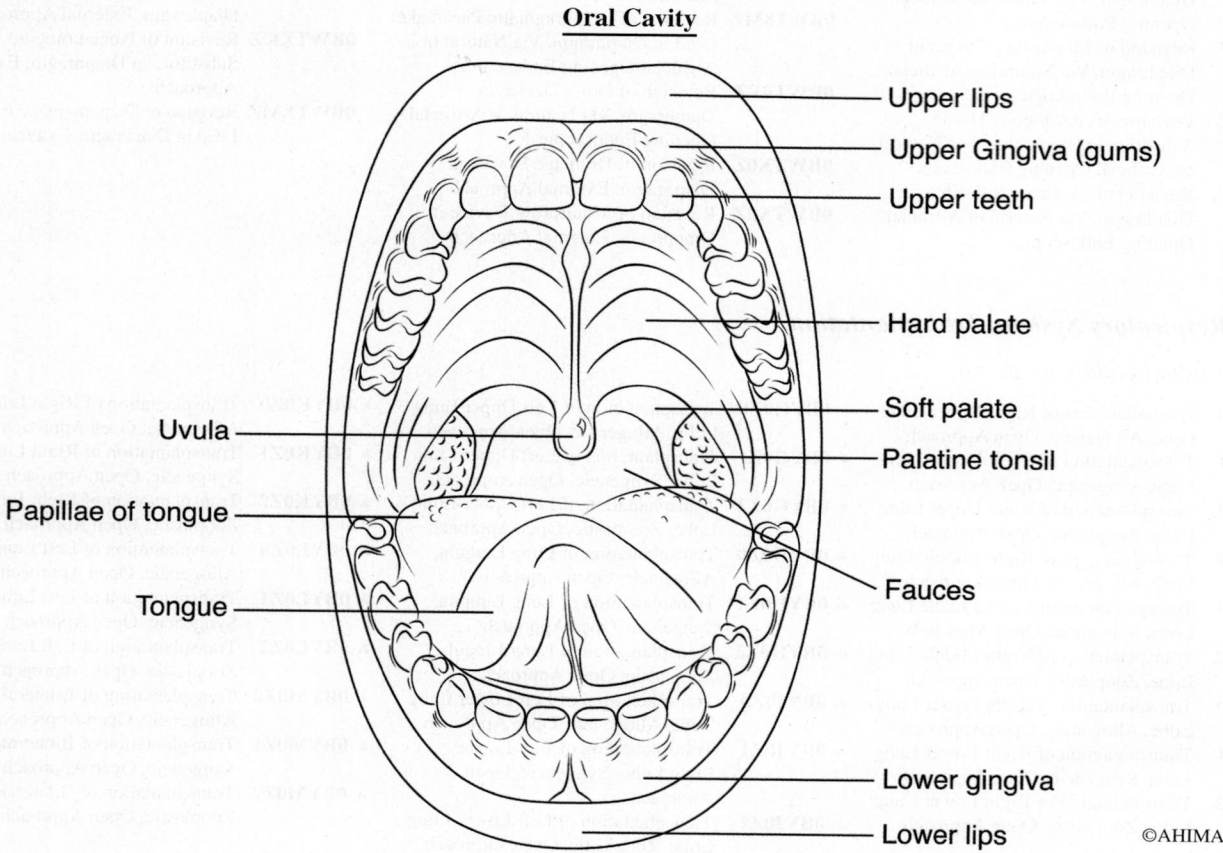

Upper lips

Upper Gingiva (gums)

Upper teeth

Hard palate

Soft palate

Palatine tonsil

Uvula

Papillae of tongue

Fauces

Tongue

Lower gingiva

Lower lips

©AHIMA

Glands of the Oral Cavity

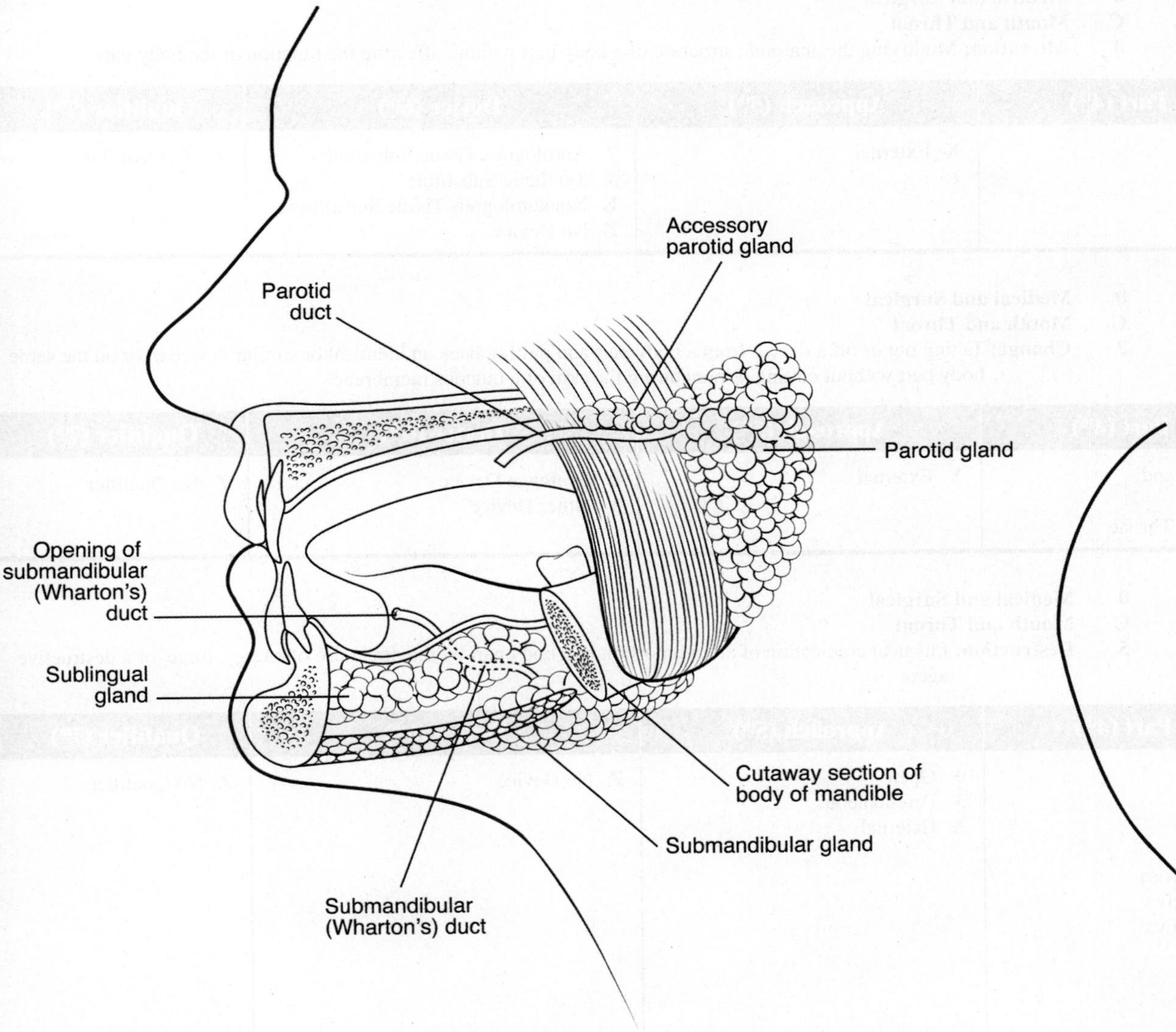

Accessory
parotid gland

Parotid
duct

Parotid gland

Opening of
submandibular
(Wharton's)
duct

Sublingual
gland

Cutaway section of
body of mandible

Submandibular gland

Submandibular
(Wharton's) duct

©AHIMA

Throat

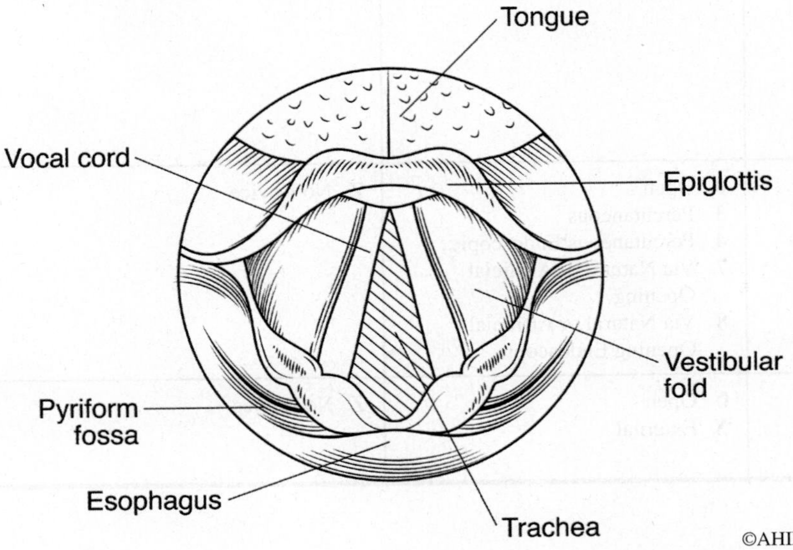

Tongue

Vocal cord

Epiglottis

Vestibular
fold

Pyriform
fossa

Esophagus

Trachea

©AHIMA

Mouth and Throat Tables 0C0–0CX

Section	0	Medical and Surgical
Body System	C	Mouth and Throat
Operation	0	Alteration: Modifying the anatomic structure of a body part without affecting the function of the body part

Body Part (4th)	Approach (5th)	Device (6th)	Qualifier (7th)
0 Upper Lip **1** Lower Lip	**X** External	**7** Autologous Tissue Substitute **J** Synthetic Substitute **K** Nonautologous Tissue Substitute **Z** No Device	**Z** No Qualifier

Section	0	Medical and Surgical
Body System	C	Mouth and Throat
Operation	2	Change: Taking out or off a device from a body part and putting back an identical or similar device in or on the same body part without cutting or puncturing the skin or a mucous membrane

Body Part (4th)	Approach (5th)	Device (6th)	Qualifier (7th)
A Salivary Gland **S** Larynx **Y** Mouth and Throat	**X** External	**0** Drainage Device **Y** Other Device	**Z** No Qualifier

Section	0	Medical and Surgical
Body System	C	Mouth and Throat
Operation	5	Destruction: Physical eradication of all or a portion of a body part by the direct use of energy, force, or a destructive agent

Body Part (4th)	Approach (5th)	Device (6th)	Qualifier (7th)
0 Upper Lip **1** Lower Lip **2** Hard Palate **3** Soft Palate **4** Buccal Mucosa **5** Upper Gingiva **6** Lower Gingiva **7** Tongue **N** Uvula **P** Tonsils **Q** Adenoids	**0** Open **3** Percutaneous **X** External	**Z** No Device	**Z** No Qualifier
8 Parotid Gland, Right **9** Parotid Gland, Left **B** Parotid Duct, Right **C** Parotid Duct, Left **D** Sublingual Gland, Right **F** Sublingual Gland, Left **G** Submaxillary Gland, Right **H** Submaxillary Gland, Left **J** Minor Salivary Gland	**0** Open **3** Percutaneous	**Z** No Device	**Z** No Qualifier
M Pharynx **R** Epiglottis **S** Larynx **T** Vocal Cord, Right **V** Vocal Cord, Left	**0** Open **3** Percutaneous **4** Percutaneous Endoscopic **7** Via Natural or Artificial Opening **8** Via Natural or Artificial Opening Endoscopic	**Z** No Device	**Z** No Qualifier
W Upper Tooth **X** Lower Tooth	**0** Open **X** External	**Z** No Device	**0** Single **1** Multiple **2** All

Section	0	Medical and Surgical
Body System	C	Mouth and Throat
Operation	7	Dilation: Expanding an orifice or the lumen of a tubular body part

Body Part (4th)	Approach (5th)	Device (6th)	Qualifier (7th)
B Parotid Duct, Right C Parotid Duct, Left	0 Open 3 Percutaneous 7 Via Natural or Artificial Opening	D Intraluminal Device Z No Device	Z No Qualifier
M Pharynx	7 Via Natural or Artificial Opening 8 Via Natural or Artificial Opening Endoscopic	D Intraluminal Device Z No Device	Z No Qualifier
S Larynx	0 Open 3 Percutaneous 4 Percutaneous Endoscopic 7 Via Natural or Artificial Opening 8 Via Natural or Artificial Opening Endoscopic	D Intraluminal Device Z No Device	Z No Qualifier

Section	0	Medical and Surgical
Body System	C	Mouth and Throat
Operation	9	Drainage: Taking or letting out fluids and/or gases from a body part

Body Part (4th)	Approach (5th)	Device (6th)	Qualifier (7th)
0 Upper Lip 1 Lower Lip 2 Hard Palate 3 Soft Palate 4 Buccal Mucosa 5 Upper Gingiva 6 Lower Gingiva 7 Tongue N Uvula P Tonsils Q Adenoids	0 Open 3 Percutaneous X External	0 Drainage Device	Z No Qualifier
0 Upper Lip 1 Lower Lip 2 Hard Palate 3 Soft Palate 4 Buccal Mucosa 5 Upper Gingiva 6 Lower Gingiva 7 Tongue N Uvula P Tonsils Q Adenoids	0 Open 3 Percutaneous X External	Z No Device	X Diagnostic Z No Qualifier
8 Parotid Gland, Right 9 Parotid Gland, Left B Parotid Duct, Right C Parotid Duct, Left D Sublingual Gland, Right F Sublingual Gland, Left G Submaxillary Gland, Right H Submaxillary Gland, Left J Minor Salivary Gland	0 Open 3 Percutaneous	0 Drainage Device	Z No Qualifier
8 Parotid Gland, Right 9 Parotid Gland, Left B Parotid Duct, Right C Parotid Duct, Left D Sublingual Gland, Right F Sublingual Gland, Left G Submaxillary Gland, Right H Submaxillary Gland, Left J Minor Salivary Gland	0 Open 3 Percutaneous	Z No Device	X Diagnostic Z No Qualifier

Continued →

Section	0	Medical and Surgical
Body System	C	Mouth and Throat
Operation	9	Drainage: Taking or letting out fluids and/or gases from a body part

Body Part (4th)	Approach (5th)	Device (6th)	Qualifier (7th)
M Pharynx R Epiglottis S Larynx T Vocal Cord, Right V Vocal Cord, Left	0 Open 3 Percutaneous 4 Percutaneous Endoscopic 7 Via Natural or Artificial Opening 8 Via Natural or Artificial Opening Endoscopic	0 Drainage Device	Z No Qualifier
M Pharynx R Epiglottis S Larynx T Vocal Cord, Right V Vocal Cord, Left	0 Open 3 Percutaneous 4 Percutaneous Endoscopic 7 Via Natural or Artificial Opening 8 Via Natural or Artificial Opening Endoscopic	Z No Device	X Diagnostic Z No Qualifier
W Upper Tooth X Lower Tooth	0 Open X External	0 Drainage Device Z No Device	0 Single 1 Multiple 2 All

Section	0	Medical and Surgical
Body System	C	Mouth and Throat
Operation	B	Excision: Cutting out or off, without replacement, a portion of a body part

Body Part (4th)	Approach (5th)	Device (6th)	Qualifier (7th)
0 Upper Lip 1 Lower Lip 2 Hard Palate 3 Soft Palate 4 Buccal Mucosa 5 Upper Gingiva 6 Lower Gingiva 7 Tongue N Uvula P Tonsils Q Adenoids	0 Open 3 Percutaneous X External	Z No Device	X Diagnostic Z No Qualifier
8 Parotid Gland, Right 9 Parotid Gland, Left B Parotid Duct, Right C Parotid Duct, Left D Sublingual Gland, Right F Sublingual Gland, Left G Submaxillary Gland, Right H Submaxillary Gland, Left J Minor Salivary Gland	0 Open 3 Percutaneous	Z No Device	X Diagnostic Z No Qualifier
M Pharynx R Epiglottis S Larynx T Vocal Cord, Right V Vocal Cord, Left	0 Open 3 Percutaneous 4 Percutaneous Endoscopic 7 Via Natural or Artificial Opening 8 Via Natural or Artificial Opening Endoscopic	Z No Device	X Diagnostic Z No Qualifier
W Upper Tooth X Lower Tooth	0 Open X External	Z No Device	0 Single 1 Multiple 2 All

Section	0	Medical and Surgical
Body System	C	Mouth and Throat
Operation	C	Extirpation: Taking or cutting out solid matter from a body part

Body Part (4th)	Approach (5th)	Device (6th)	Qualifier (7th)
0 Upper Lip 1 Lower Lip 2 Hard Palate 3 Soft Palate 4 Buccal Mucosa 5 Upper Gingiva 6 Lower Gingiva 7 Tongue N Uvula P Tonsils Q Adenoids	0 Open 3 Percutaneous X External	Z No Device	Z No Qualifier
8 Parotid Gland, Right 9 Parotid Gland, Left B Parotid Duct, Right C Parotid Duct, Left D Sublingual Gland, Right F Sublingual Gland, Left G Submaxillary Gland, Right H Submaxillary Gland, Left J Minor Salivary Gland	0 Open 3 Percutaneous	Z No Device	Z No Qualifier
M Pharynx R Epiglottis S Larynx T Vocal Cord, Right V Vocal Cord, Left	0 Open 3 Percutaneous 4 Percutaneous Endoscopic 7 Via Natural or Artificial Opening 8 Via Natural or Artificial Opening Endoscopic	Z No Device	Z No Qualifier
W Upper Tooth X Lower Tooth	0 Open X External	Z No Device	0 Single 1 Multiple 2 All

Section	0	Medical and Surgical
Body System	C	Mouth and Throat
Operation	D	**Extraction:** Pulling or stripping out or off all or a portion of a body part by the use of force

Body Part (4th)	Approach (5th)	Device (6th)	Qualifier (7th)
T Vocal Cord, Right V Vocal Cord, Left	0 Open 3 Percutaneous 4 Percutaneous Endoscopic 7 Via Natural or Artificial Opening 8 Via Natural or Artificial Opening Endoscopic	Z No Device	Z No Qualifier
W Upper Tooth X Lower Tooth	X External	Z No Device	0 Single 1 Multiple 2 All

Section	0	Medical and Surgical
Body System	C	Mouth and Throat
Operation	F	**Fragmentation:** Breaking solid matter in a body part into pieces

Body Part (4th)	Approach (5th)	Device (6th)	Qualifier (7th)
B Parotid Duct, Right C Parotid Duct, Left	0 Open 3 Percutaneous 7 Via Natural or Artificial Opening X External	Z No Device	Z No Qualifier

Section	0	Medical and Surgical
Body System	C	Mouth and Throat
Operation	H	**Insertion:** Putting in a nonbiological appliance that monitors, assists, performs, or prevents a physiological function but does not physically take the place of a body part

Body Part (4th)	Approach (5th)	Device (6th)	Qualifier (7th)
7 Tongue	0 Open 3 Percutaneous X External	1 Radioactive Element	Z No Qualifier
A Salivary Gland S Larynx	0 Open 3 Percutaneous 7 Via Natural or Artificial Opening 8 Via Natural or Artificial Opening Endoscopic	1 Radioactive Element Y Other Device	Z No Qualifier
Y Mouth and Throat	0 Open 3 Percutaneous	1 Radioactive Element Y Other Device	Z No Qualifier
Y Mouth and Throat	7 Via Natural or Artificial Opening 8 Via Natural or Artificial Opening Endoscopic	1 Radioactive Element B Intraluminal Device, Airway Y Other Device	Z No Qualifier

Section	0	Medical and Surgical
Body System	C	Mouth and Throat
Operation	J	Inspection: Visually and/or manually exploring a body part

Body Part (4th)	Approach (5th)	Device (6th)	Qualifier (7th)
A SalivaryGland	0 Open 3 Percutaneous X External	Z No Device	Z No Qualifier
S Larynx Y Mouth and Throat	0 Open 3 Percutaneous 4 Percutaneous Endoscopic 7 Via Natural or Artificial Opening 8 Via Natural or Artificial Opening Endoscopic X External	Z No Device	Z No Qualifier

Section	0	Medical and Surgical
Body System	C	Mouth and Throat
Operation	L	Occlusion: Completely closing an orifice or the lumen of a tubular body part

Body Part (4th)	Approach (5th)	Device (6th)	Qualifier (7th)
B Parotid Duct, Right C Parotid Duct, Left	0 Open 3 Percutaneous 4 Percutaneous Endoscopic	C Extraluminal Device D Intraluminal Device Z No Device	Z No Qualifier
B Parotid Duct, Right C Parotid Duct, Left	7 Via Natural or Artificial Opening 8 Via Natural or Artificial Opening Endoscopic	D Intraluminal Device Z No Device	Z No Qualifier

Section	0	Medical and Surgical
Body System	C	Mouth and Throat
Operation	M	Reattachment: Putting back in or on all or a portion of a separated body part to its normal location or other suitable location

Body Part (4th)	Approach (5th)	Device (6th)	Qualifier (7th)
0 Upper Lip 1 Lower Lip 3 Soft Palate 7 Tongue N Uvula	0 Open	Z No Device	Z No Qualifier
W Upper Tooth X Lower Tooth	0 Open X External	Z No Device	0 Single 1 Multiple 2 All

Section 0 **Medical and Surgical**
Body System C **Mouth and Throat**
Operation N **Release:** Freeing a body part from an abnormal physical constraint by cutting or by the use of force

Body Part (4th)	Approach (5th)	Device (6th)	Qualifier (7th)
0 Upper Lip 1 Lower Lip 2 Hard Palate 3 Soft Palate 4 Buccal Mucosa 5 Upper Gingiva 6 Lower Gingiva 7 Tongue N Uvula P Tonsils Q Adenoids	0 Open 3 Percutaneous X External	Z No Device	Z No Qualifier
8 Parotid Gland, Right 9 Parotid Gland, Left B Parotid Duct, Right C Parotid Duct, Left D Sublingual Gland, Right F Sublingual Gland, Left G Submaxillary Gland, Right H Submaxillary Gland, Left J Minor Salivary Gland	0 Open 3 Percutaneous	Z No Device	Z No Qualifier
M Pharynx R Epiglottis S Larynx T Vocal Cord, Right V Vocal Cord, Left	0 Open 3 Percutaneous 4 Percutaneous Endoscopic 7 Via Natural or Artificial Opening 8 Via Natural or Artificial Opening Endoscopic	Z No Device	Z No Qualifier
W Upper Tooth X Lower Tooth	0 Open X External	Z No Device	0 Single 1 Multiple 2 All

Section 0 **Medical and Surgical**
Body System C **Mouth and Throat**
Operation P **Removal:** Taking out or off a device from a body part

Body Part (4th)	Approach (5th)	Device (6th)	Qualifier (7th)
A Salivary Gland	0 Open 3 Percutaneous	0 Drainage Device C Extraluminal Device Y Other Device	Z No Qualifier
A Salivary Gland	7 Via Natural or Artificial Opening 8 Via Natural or Artificial Opening Endoscopic	Y Other Device	Z No Qualifier
S Larynx	0 Open 3 Percutaneous 7 Via Natural or Artificial Opening 8 Via Natural or Artificial Opening Endoscopic	0 Drainage Device 7 Autologous Tissue Substitute D Intraluminal Device J Synthetic Substitute K Nonautologous Tissue Substitute Y Other Device	Z No Qualifier
S Larynx	X External	0 Drainage Device 7 Autologous Tissue Substitute D Intraluminal Device J Synthetic Substitute K Nonautologous Tissue Substitute	Z No Qualifier

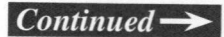
Continued →

Section	0	Medical and Surgical
Body System	C	Mouth and Throat
Operation	P	Removal: Taking out or off a device from a body part

Body Part (4th)	Approach (5th)	Device (6th)	Qualifier (7th)
Y Mouth and Throat	0 Open 3 Percutaneous 7 Via Natural or Artificial Opening 8 Via Natural or Artificial Opening Endoscopic	0 Drainage Device 1 Radioactive Element 7 Autologous Tissue Substitute D Intraluminal Device J Synthetic Substitute K Nonautologous Tissue Substitute Y Other Device	Z No Qualifier
Y Mouth and Throat	X External	0 Drainage Device 1 Radioactive Element 7 Autologous Tissue Substitute D Intraluminal Device J Synthetic Substitute K Nonautologous Tissue Substitute	Z No Qualifier

Section	0	Medical and Surgical
Body System	C	Mouth and Throat
Operation	Q	Repair: Restoring, to the extent possible, a body part to its normal anatomic structure and function

Body Part (4th)	Approach (5th)	Device (6th)	Qualifier (7th)
0 Upper Lip 1 Lower Lip 2 Hard Palate 3 Soft Palate 4 Buccal Mucosa 5 Upper Gingiva 6 Lower Gingiva 7 Tongue N Uvula P Tonsils Q Adenoids	0 Open 3 Percutaneous X External	Z No Device	Z No Qualifier
8 Parotid Gland, Right 9 Parotid Gland, Left B Parotid Duct, Right C Parotid Duct, Left D Sublingual Gland, Right F Sublingual Gland, Left G Submaxillary Gland, Right H Submaxillary Gland, Left J Minor Salivary Gland	0 Open 3 Percutaneous	Z No Device	Z No Qualifier
M Pharynx R Epiglottis S Larynx T Vocal Cord, Right V Vocal Cord, Left	0 Open 3 Percutaneous 4 Percutaneous Endoscopic 7 Via Natural or Artificial Opening 8 Via Natural or Artificial Opening Endoscopic	Z No Device	Z No Qualifier
W Upper Tooth X Lower Tooth	0 Open X External	Z No Device	0 Single 1 Multiple 2 All

Section	0	Medical and Surgical
Body System	C	Mouth and Throat
Operation	R	**Replacement:** Putting in or on biological or synthetic material that physically takes the place and/or function of all or a portion of a body part

Body Part (4th)	Approach (5th)	Device (6th)	Qualifier (7th)
0 Upper Lip 1 Lower Lip 2 Hard Palate 3 Soft Palate 4 Buccal Mucosa 5 Upper Gingiva 6 Lower Gingiva 7 Tongue N Uvula	0 Open 3 Percutaneous X External	7 Autologous Tissue Substitute J Synthetic Substitute K Nonautologous Tissue Substitute	Z No Qualifier
B Parotid Duct, Right C Parotid Duct, Left	0 Open 3 Percutaneous	7 Autologous Tissue Substitute J Synthetic Substitute K Nonautologous Tissue Substitute	Z No Qualifier
M Pharynx R Epiglottis S Larynx T Vocal Cord, Right V Vocal Cord, Left	0 Open 7 Via Natural or Artificial Opening 8 Via Natural or Artificial Opening Endoscopic	7 Autologous Tissue Substitute J Synthetic Substitute K Nonautologous Tissue Substitute	Z No Qualifier
W Upper Tooth X Lower Tooth	0 Open X External	7 Autologous Tissue Substitute J Synthetic Substitute K Nonautologous Tissue Substitute	0 Single 1 Multiple 2 All

Section	0	Medical and Surgical
Body System	C	Mouth and Throat
Operation	S	**Reposition:** Moving to its normal location, or other suitable location, all or a portion of a body part

Body Part (4th)	Approach (5th)	Device (6th)	Qualifier (7th)
0 Upper Lip 1 Lower Lip 2 Hard Palate 3 Soft Palate 7 Tongue N Uvula	0 Open X External	Z No Device	Z No Qualifier
B Parotid Duct, Right C Parotid Duct, Left	0 Open 3 Percutaneous	Z No Device	Z No Qualifier
R Epiglottis T Vocal Cord, Right V Vocal Cord, Left	0 Open 7 Via Natural or Artificial Opening 8 Via Natural or Artificial Opening Endoscopic	Z No Device	Z No Qualifier
W Upper Tooth X Lower Tooth	0 Open X External	5 External Fixation Device Z No Device	0 Single 1 Multiple 2 All

Section   0   **Medical and Surgical**
Body System   C   **Mouth and Throat**
Operation   T   **Resection:** Cutting out or off, without replacement, all of a body part

Body Part (4ᵗʰ)	Approach (5ᵗʰ)	Device (6ᵗʰ)	Qualifier (7ᵗʰ)
0 Upper Lip 1 Lower Lip 2 Hard Palate 3 Soft Palate 7 Tongue N Uvula P Tonsils Q Adenoids	0 Open X External	Z No Device	Z No Qualifier
8 Parotid Gland, Right 9 Parotid Gland, Left B Parotid Duct, Right C Parotid Duct, Left D Sublingual Gland, Right F Sublingual Gland, Left G Submaxillary Gland, Right H Submaxillary Gland, Left J Minor Salivary Gland	0 Open	Z No Device	Z No Qualifier
M Pharynx R Epiglottis S Larynx T Vocal Cord, Right V Vocal Cord, Left	0 Open 4 Percutaneous Endoscopic 7 Via Natural or Artificial Opening 8 Via Natural or Artificial Opening Endoscopic	Z No Device	Z No Qualifier
W Upper Tooth X Lower Tooth	0 Open	Z No Device	0 Single 1 Multiple 2 All

Section   0   **Medical and Surgical**
Body System   C   **Mouth and Throat**
Operation   U   **Supplement:** Putting in or on biological or synthetic material that physically reinforces and/or augments the function of a portion of a body part

Body Part (4ᵗʰ)	Approach (5ᵗʰ)	Device (6ᵗʰ)	Qualifier (7ᵗʰ)
0 Upper Lip 1 Lower Lip 2 Hard Palate 3 Soft Palate 4 Buccal Mucosa 5 Upper Gingiva 6 Lower Gingiva 7 Tongue N Uvula	0 Open 3 Percutaneous X External	7 Autologous Tissue Substitute J Synthetic Substitute K Nonautologous Tissue Substitute	Z No Qualifier
M Pharynx R Epiglottis S Larynx T Vocal Cord, Right V Vocal Cord, Left	0 Open 7 Via Natural or Artificial Opening 8 Via Natural or Artificial Opening Endoscopic	7 Autologous Tissue Substitute J Synthetic Substitute K Nonautologous Tissue Substitute	Z No Qualifier

Section	0	Medical and Surgical
Body System	C	Mouth and Throat
Operation	V	Restriction: Partially closing an orifice or the lumen of a tubular body part

Body Part (4th)	Approach (5th)	Device (6th)	Qualifier (7th)
B Parotid Duct, Right C Parotid Duct, Left	0 Open 3 Percutaneous	C Extraluminal Device D Intraluminal Device Z No Device	Z No Qualifier
B Parotid Duct, Right C Parotid Duct, Left	7 Via Natural or Artificial Opening 8 Via Natural or Artificial Opening Endoscopic	D Intraluminal Device Z No Device	Z No Qualifier

Section	0	Medical and Surgical
Body System	C	Mouth and Throat
Operation	W	Revision: Correcting, to the extent possible, a portion of a malfunctioning device or the position of a displaced device

Body Part (4th)	Approach (5th)	Device (6th)	Qualifier (7th)
A Salivary Gland	0 Open 3 Percutaneous	0 Drainage Device C Extraluminal Device Y Other Device	Z No Qualifier
A Salivary Gland	7 Via Natural or Artificial Opening 8 Via Natural or Artificial Opening Endoscopic	Y Other Device	Z No Qualifier
A Salivary Gland	X External	0 Drainage Device C Extraluminal Device	Z No Qualifier
S Larynx	0 Open 3 Percutaneous 7 Via Natural or Artificial Opening 8 Via Natural or Artificial Opening Endoscopic	0 Drainage Device 7 Autologous Tissue Substitute D Intraluminal Device J Synthetic Substitute K Nonautologous Tissue Substitute Y Other Device	Z No Qualifier
S Larynx	X External	0 Drainage Device 7 Autologous Tissue Substitute D Intraluminal Device J Synthetic Substitute K Nonautologous Tissue Substitute	Z No Qualifier
Y Mouth and Throat	0 Open 3 Percutaneous 7 Via Natural or Artificial Opening 8 Via Natural or Artificial Opening Endoscopic	0 Drainage Device 1 Radioactive Element 7 Autologous Tissue Substitute D Intraluminal Device J Synthetic Substitute K Nonautologous Tissue Substitute Y Other Device	Z No Qualifier
Y Mouth and Throat	X External	0 Drainage Device 1 Radioactive Element 7 Autologous Tissue Substitute D Intraluminal Device J Synthetic Substitute K Nonautologous Tissue Substitute	Z No Qualifier

Section	0	Medical and Surgical
Body System	C	Mouth and Throat
Operation	X	**Transfer:** Moving, without taking out, all or a portion of a body part to another location to take over the function of all or a portion of a body part

Body Part (4th)	Approach (5th)	Device (6th)	Qualifier (7th)
0 Upper Lip 1 Lower Lip 3 Soft Palate 4 Buccal Mucosa 5 Upper Gingiva 6 Lower Gingiva 7 Tongue	0 Open X External	Z No Device	Z No Qualifier

Mouth and Throat Code Listing 0C0–0CX

0C0 – Mouth and Throat, Alteration

0C00X7Z Alteration of Upper Lip with Autologous Tissue Substitute, External Approach

0C00XJZ Alteration of Upper Lip with Synthetic Substitute, External Approach

0C00XKZ Alteration of Upper Lip with Nonautologous Tissue Substitute, External Approach

0C00XZZ Alteration of Upper Lip, External Approach

0C01X7Z Alteration of Lower Lip with Autologous Tissue Substitute, External Approach

0C01XJZ Alteration of Lower Lip with Synthetic Substitute, External Approach

0C01XKZ Alteration of Lower Lip with Nonautologous Tissue Substitute, External Approach

0C01XZZ Alteration of Lower Lip, External Approach

0C2 – Mouth and Throat, Change

Review Coding Guideline B6.1c

0C2AX0Z Change Drainage Device in Salivary Gland, External Approach

0C2AXYZ Change Other Device in Salivary Gland, External Approach

0C2SX0Z Change Drainage Device in Larynx, External Approach

0C2SXYZ Change Other Device in Larynx, External Approach

0C2YX0Z Change Drainage Device in Mouth and Throat, External Approach

0C2YXYZ Change Other Device in Mouth and Throat, External Approach

0C5 – Mouth and Throat, Destruction

0C500ZZ Destruction of Upper Lip, Open Approach

0C503ZZ Destruction of Upper Lip, Percutaneous Approach

0C50XZZ Destruction of Upper Lip, External Approach

0C510ZZ Destruction of Lower Lip, Open Approach

0C513ZZ Destruction of Lower Lip, Percutaneous Approach

0C51XZZ Destruction of Lower Lip, External Approach

0C520ZZ Destruction of Hard Palate, Open Approach

0C523ZZ Destruction of Hard Palate, Percutaneous Approach

0C52XZZ Destruction of Hard Palate, External Approach

0C530ZZ Destruction of Soft Palate, Open Approach

0C533ZZ Destruction of Soft Palate, Percutaneous Approach

0C53XZZ Destruction of Soft Palate, External Approach

0C540ZZ Destruction of Buccal Mucosa, Open Approach

0C543ZZ Destruction of Buccal Mucosa, Percutaneous Approach

0C54XZZ Destruction of Buccal Mucosa, External Approach

0C550ZZ Destruction of Upper Gingiva, Open Approach

0C553ZZ Destruction of Upper Gingiva, Percutaneous Approach

0C55XZZ Destruction of Upper Gingiva, External Approach

0C560ZZ Destruction of Lower Gingiva, Open Approach

0C563ZZ Destruction of Lower Gingiva, Percutaneous Approach

0C56XZZ Destruction of Lower Gingiva, External Approach

0C570ZZ Destruction of Tongue, Open Approach

0C573ZZ Destruction of Tongue, Percutaneous Approach

0C57XZZ Destruction of Tongue, External Approach

0C580ZZ Destruction of Right Parotid Gland, Open Approach

0C583ZZ Destruction of Right Parotid Gland, Percutaneous Approach

0C590ZZ Destruction of Left Parotid Gland, Open Approach

0C593ZZ Destruction of Left Parotid Gland, Percutaneous Approach

0C5B0ZZ Destruction of Right Parotid Duct, Open Approach

0C5B3ZZ Destruction of Right Parotid Duct, Percutaneous Approach

0C5C0ZZ Destruction of Left Parotid Duct, Open Approach

0C5C3ZZ Destruction of Left Parotid Duct, Percutaneous Approach

0C5D0ZZ Destruction of Right Sublingual Gland, Open Approach

0C5D3ZZ Destruction of Right Sublingual Gland, Percutaneous Approach

0C5F0ZZ Destruction of Left Sublingual Gland, Open Approach

0C5F3ZZ Destruction of Left Sublingual Gland, Percutaneous Approach

0C5G0ZZ Destruction of Right Submaxillary Gland, Open Approach

0C5G3ZZ Destruction of Right Submaxillary Gland, Percutaneous Approach

0C5H0ZZ Destruction of Left Submaxillary Gland, Open Approach

0C5H3ZZ Destruction of Left Submaxillary Gland, Percutaneous Approach

0C5J0ZZ Destruction of Minor Salivary Gland, Open Approach

0C5J3ZZ Destruction of Minor Salivary Gland, Percutaneous Approach

0C5M0ZZ Destruction of Pharynx, Open Approach

0C5M3ZZ Destruction of Pharynx, Percutaneous Approach

0C5M4ZZ Destruction of Pharynx, Percutaneous Endoscopic Approach

0C5M7ZZ Destruction of Pharynx, Via Natural or Artificial Opening

0C5M8ZZ Destruction of Pharynx, Via Natural or Artificial Opening Endoscopic

0C5N0ZZ Destruction of Uvula, Open Approach

0C5N3ZZ Destruction of Uvula, Percutaneous Approach

0C5NXZZ Destruction of Uvula, External Approach

0C5P0ZZ Destruction of Tonsils, Open Approach

0C5P3ZZ Destruction of Tonsils, Percutaneous Approach

0C5PXZZ Destruction of Tonsils, External Approach

0C5Q0ZZ Destruction of Adenoids, Open Approach

0C5Q3ZZ Destruction of Adenoids, Percutaneous Approach

0C5QXZZ Destruction of Adenoids, External Approach
0C5R0ZZ Destruction of Epiglottis, Open Approach
0C5R3ZZ Destruction of Epiglottis, Percutaneous Approach
0C5R4ZZ Destruction of Epiglottis, Percutaneous Endoscopic Approach
0C5R7ZZ Destruction of Epiglottis, Via Natural or Artificial Opening
0C5R8ZZ Destruction of Epiglottis, Via Natural or Artificial Opening Endoscopic
0C5S0ZZ Destruction of Larynx, Open Approach
0C5S3ZZ Destruction of Larynx, Percutaneous Approach
0C5S4ZZ Destruction of Larynx, Percutaneous Endoscopic Approach
0C5S7ZZ Destruction of Larynx, Via Natural or Artificial Opening
0C5S8ZZ Destruction of Larynx, Via Natural or Artificial Opening Endoscopic
0C5T0ZZ Destruction of Right Vocal Cord, Open Approach
0C5T3ZZ Destruction of Right Vocal Cord, Percutaneous Approach
0C5T4ZZ Destruction of Right Vocal Cord, Percutaneous Endoscopic Approach
0C5T7ZZ Destruction of Right Vocal Cord, Via Natural or Artificial Opening
0C5T8ZZ Destruction of Right Vocal Cord, Via Natural or Artificial Opening Endoscopic
0C5V0ZZ Destruction of Left Vocal Cord, Open Approach
0C5V3ZZ Destruction of Left Vocal Cord, Percutaneous Approach
0C5V4ZZ Destruction of Left Vocal Cord, Percutaneous Endoscopic Approach
0C5V7ZZ Destruction of Left Vocal Cord, Via Natural or Artificial Opening
0C5V8ZZ Destruction of Left Vocal Cord, Via Natural or Artificial Opening Endoscopic
0C5W0Z0 Destruction of Upper Tooth, Single, Open Approach
0C5W0Z1 Destruction of Upper Tooth, Multiple, Open Approach
0C5W0Z2 Destruction of Upper Tooth, All, Open Approach
0C5WXZ0 Destruction of Upper Tooth, Single, External Approach
0C5WXZ1 Destruction of Upper Tooth, Multiple, External Approach
0C5WXZ2 Destruction of Upper Tooth, All, External Approach
0C5X0Z0 Destruction of Lower Tooth, Single, Open Approach
0C5X0Z1 Destruction of Lower Tooth, Multiple, Open Approach
0C5X0Z2 Destruction of Lower Tooth, All, Open Approach
0C5XXZ0 Destruction of Lower Tooth, Single, External Approach
0C5XXZ1 Destruction of Lower Tooth, Multiple, External Approach
0C5XXZ2 Destruction of Lower Tooth, All, External Approach

0C7 – Mouth and Throat, Dilation

0C7B0DZ Dilation of Right Parotid Duct with Intraluminal Device, Open Approach
0C7B0ZZ Dilation of Right Parotid Duct, Open Approach
0C7B3DZ Dilation of Right Parotid Duct with Intraluminal Device, Percutaneous Approach
0C7B3ZZ Dilation of Right Parotid Duct, Percutaneous Approach
0C7B7DZ Dilation of Right Parotid Duct with Intraluminal Device, Via Natural or Artificial Opening
0C7B7ZZ Dilation of Right Parotid Duct, Via Natural or Artificial Opening
0C7C0DZ Dilation of Left Parotid Duct with Intraluminal Device, Open Approach
0C7C0ZZ Dilation of Left Parotid Duct, Open Approach
0C7C3DZ Dilation of Left Parotid Duct with Intraluminal Device, Percutaneous Approach
0C7C3ZZ Dilation of Left Parotid Duct, Percutaneous Approach
0C7C7DZ Dilation of Left Parotid Duct with Intraluminal Device, Via Natural or Artificial Opening
0C7C7ZZ Dilation of Left Parotid Duct, Via Natural or Artificial Opening
0C7M7DZ Dilation of Pharynx with Intraluminal Device, Via Natural or Artificial Opening
0C7M7ZZ Dilation of Pharynx, Via Natural or Artificial Opening
0C7M8DZ Dilation of Pharynx with Intraluminal Device, Via Natural or Artificial Opening Endoscopic
0C7M8ZZ Dilation of Pharynx, Via Natural or Artificial Opening Endoscopic
0C7S0DZ Dilation of Larynx with Intraluminal Device, Open Approach
0C7S0ZZ Dilation of Larynx, Open Approach
0C7S3DZ Dilation of Larynx with Intraluminal Device, Percutaneous Approach
0C7S3ZZ Dilation of Larynx, Percutaneous Approach
0C7S4DZ Dilation of Larynx with Intraluminal Device, Percutaneous Endoscopic Approach
0C7S4ZZ Dilation of Larynx, Percutaneous Endoscopic Approach
0C7S7DZ Dilation of Larynx with Intraluminal Device, Via Natural or Artificial Opening
0C7S7ZZ Dilation of Larynx, Via Natural or Artificial Opening
0C7S8DZ Dilation of Larynx with Intraluminal Device, Via Natural or Artificial Opening Endoscopic
0C7S8ZZ Dilation of Larynx, Via Natural or Artificial Opening Endoscopic

0C9 – Mouth and Throat, Drainage

Review Coding Guidelines B3.4a and B3.4b

Review Coding Guideline B6.2

0C9000Z Drainage of Upper Lip with Drainage Device, Open Approach
0C900ZX Drainage of Upper Lip, Open Approach, Diagnostic
0C900ZZ Drainage of Upper Lip, Open Approach
0C9030Z Drainage of Upper Lip with Drainage Device, Percutaneous Approach
0C903ZX Drainage of Upper Lip, Percutaneous Approach, Diagnostic
0C903ZZ Drainage of Upper Lip, Percutaneous Approach
0C90X0Z Drainage of Upper Lip with Drainage Device, External Approach
0C90XZX Drainage of Upper Lip, External Approach, Diagnostic
0C90XZZ Drainage of Upper Lip, External Approach
0C9100Z Drainage of Lower Lip with Drainage Device, Open Approach
0C910ZX Drainage of Lower Lip, Open Approach, Diagnostic
0C910ZZ Drainage of Lower Lip, Open Approach
0C9130Z Drainage of Lower Lip with Drainage Device, Percutaneous Approach
0C913ZX Drainage of Lower Lip, Percutaneous Approach, Diagnostic
0C913ZZ Drainage of Lower Lip, Percutaneous Approach
0C91X0Z Drainage of Lower Lip with Drainage Device, External Approach
0C91XZX Drainage of Lower Lip, External Approach, Diagnostic
0C91XZZ Drainage of Lower Lip, External Approach
0C9200Z Drainage of Hard Palate with Drainage Device, Open Approach
0C920ZX Drainage of Hard Palate, Open Approach, Diagnostic
0C920ZZ Drainage of Hard Palate, Open Approach
0C9230Z Drainage of Hard Palate with Drainage Device, Percutaneous Approach
0C923ZX Drainage of Hard Palate, Percutaneous Approach, Diagnostic
0C923ZZ Drainage of Hard Palate, Percutaneous Approach
0C92X0Z Drainage of Hard Palate with Drainage Device, External Approach
0C92XZX Drainage of Hard Palate, External Approach, Diagnostic
0C92XZZ Drainage of Hard Palate, External Approach
0C9300Z Drainage of Soft Palate with Drainage Device, Open Approach
0C930ZX Drainage of Soft Palate, Open Approach, Diagnostic
0C930ZZ Drainage of Soft Palate, Open Approach
0C9330Z Drainage of Soft Palate with Drainage Device, Percutaneous Approach
0C933ZX Drainage of Soft Palate, Percutaneous Approach, Diagnostic
0C933ZZ Drainage of Soft Palate, Percutaneous Approach

♀ Female-only ♂ Male-only ▲ Limited Coverage ● Non-OR ▥ HAC-associated procedure ▲ Non-covered procedures ✛ Cluster

0C93X0Z Drainage of Soft Palate with Drainage Device, External Approach

0C93XZX Drainage of Soft Palate, External Approach, Diagnostic

0C93XZZ Drainage of Soft Palate, External Approach

0C9400Z Drainage of Buccal Mucosa with Drainage Device, Open Approach

0C940ZX Drainage of Buccal Mucosa, Open Approach, Diagnostic

0C940ZZ Drainage of Buccal Mucosa, Open Approach

0C9430Z Drainage of Buccal Mucosa with Drainage Device, Percutaneous Approach

0C943ZX Drainage of Buccal Mucosa, Percutaneous Approach, Diagnostic

0C943ZZ Drainage of Buccal Mucosa, Percutaneous Approach

0C94X0Z Drainage of Buccal Mucosa with Drainage Device, External Approach

0C94XZX Drainage of Buccal Mucosa, External Approach, Diagnostic

0C94XZZ Drainage of Buccal Mucosa, External Approach

0C9500Z Drainage of Upper Gingiva with Drainage Device, Open Approach

0C950ZX Drainage of Upper Gingiva, Open Approach, Diagnostic

0C950ZZ Drainage of Upper Gingiva, Open Approach

0C9530Z Drainage of Upper Gingiva with Drainage Device, Percutaneous Approach

0C953ZX Drainage of Upper Gingiva, Percutaneous Approach, Diagnostic

0C953ZZ Drainage of Upper Gingiva, Percutaneous Approach

0C95X0Z Drainage of Upper Gingiva with Drainage Device, External Approach

0C95XZX Drainage of Upper Gingiva, External Approach, Diagnostic

0C95XZZ Drainage of Upper Gingiva, External Approach

0C9600Z Drainage of Lower Gingiva with Drainage Device, Open Approach

0C960ZX Drainage of Lower Gingiva, Open Approach, Diagnostic

0C960ZZ Drainage of Lower Gingiva, Open Approach

0C9630Z Drainage of Lower Gingiva with Drainage Device, Percutaneous Approach

0C963ZX Drainage of Lower Gingiva, Percutaneous Approach, Diagnostic

0C963ZZ Drainage of Lower Gingiva, Percutaneous Approach

0C96X0Z Drainage of Lower Gingiva with Drainage Device, External Approach

0C96XZX Drainage of Lower Gingiva, External Approach, Diagnostic

0C96XZZ Drainage of Lower Gingiva, External Approach

0C9700Z Drainage of Tongue with Drainage Device, Open Approach

0C970ZX Drainage of Tongue, Open Approach, Diagnostic

0C970ZZ Drainage of Tongue, Open Approach

0C9730Z Drainage of Tongue with Drainage Device, Percutaneous Approach

0C973ZX Drainage of Tongue, Percutaneous Approach, Diagnostic

0C973ZZ Drainage of Tongue, Percutaneous Approach

0C97X0Z Drainage of Tongue with Drainage Device, External Approach

0C97XZX Drainage of Tongue, External Approach, Diagnostic

0C97XZZ Drainage of Tongue, External Approach

0C9800Z Drainage of Right Parotid Gland with Drainage Device, Open Approach

0C980ZX Drainage of Right Parotid Gland, Open Approach, Diagnostic

0C980ZZ Drainage of Right Parotid Gland, Open Approach

0C9830Z Drainage of Right Parotid Gland with Drainage Device, Percutaneous Approach

0C983ZX Drainage of Right Parotid Gland, Percutaneous Approach, Diagnostic

0C983ZZ Drainage of Right Parotid Gland, Percutaneous Approach

0C9900Z Drainage of Left Parotid Gland with Drainage Device, Open Approach

0C990ZX Drainage of Left Parotid Gland, Open Approach, Diagnostic

0C990ZZ Drainage of Left Parotid Gland, Open Approach

0C9930Z Drainage of Left Parotid Gland with Drainage Device, Percutaneous Approach

0C993ZX Drainage of Left Parotid Gland, Percutaneous Approach, Diagnostic

0C993ZZ Drainage of Left Parotid Gland, Percutaneous Approach

0C9B00Z Drainage of Right Parotid Duct with Drainage Device, Open Approach

0C9B0ZX Drainage of Right Parotid Duct, Open Approach, Diagnostic

0C9B0ZZ Drainage of Right Parotid Duct, Open Approach

0C9B30Z Drainage of Right Parotid Duct with Drainage Device, Percutaneous Approach

0C9B3ZX Drainage of Right Parotid Duct, Percutaneous Approach, Diagnostic

0C9B3ZZ Drainage of Right Parotid Duct, Percutaneous Approach

0C9C00Z Drainage of Left Parotid Duct with Drainage Device, Open Approach

0C9C0ZX Drainage of Left Parotid Duct, Open Approach, Diagnostic

0C9C0ZZ Drainage of Left Parotid Duct, Open Approach

0C9C30Z Drainage of Left Parotid Duct with Drainage Device, Percutaneous Approach

0C9C3ZX Drainage of Left Parotid Duct, Percutaneous Approach, Diagnostic

0C9C3ZZ Drainage of Left Parotid Duct, Percutaneous Approach

0C9D00Z Drainage of Right Sublingual Gland with Drainage Device, Open Approach

0C9D0ZX Drainage of Right Sublingual Gland, Open Approach, Diagnostic

0C9D0ZZ Drainage of Right Sublingual Gland, Open Approach

0C9D30Z Drainage of Right Sublingual Gland with Drainage Device, Percutaneous Approach

0C9D3ZX Drainage of Right Sublingual Gland, Percutaneous Approach, Diagnostic

0C9D3ZZ Drainage of Right Sublingual Gland, Percutaneous Approach

0C9F00Z Drainage of Left Sublingual Gland with Drainage Device, Open Approach

0C9F0ZX Drainage of Left Sublingual Gland, Open Approach, Diagnostic

0C9F0ZZ Drainage of Left Sublingual Gland, Open Approach

0C9F30Z Drainage of Left Sublingual Gland with Drainage Device, Percutaneous Approach

0C9F3ZX Drainage of Left Sublingual Gland, Percutaneous Approach, Diagnostic

0C9F3ZZ Drainage of Left Sublingual Gland, Percutaneous Approach

0C9G00Z Drainage of Right Submaxillary Gland with Drainage Device, Open Approach

0C9G0ZX Drainage of Right Submaxillary Gland, Open Approach, Diagnostic

0C9G0ZZ Drainage of Right Submaxillary Gland, Open Approach

0C9G30Z Drainage of Right Submaxillary Gland with Drainage Device, Percutaneous Approach

0C9G3ZX Drainage of Right Submaxillary Gland, Percutaneous Approach, Diagnostic

0C9G3ZZ Drainage of Right Submaxillary Gland, Percutaneous Approach

0C9H00Z Drainage of Left Submaxillary Gland with Drainage Device, Open Approach

0C9H0ZX Drainage of Left Submaxillary Gland, Open Approach, Diagnostic

0C9H0ZZ Drainage of Left Submaxillary Gland, Open Approach

0C9H30Z Drainage of Left Submaxillary Gland with Drainage Device, Percutaneous Approach

0C9H3ZX Drainage of Left Submaxillary Gland, Percutaneous Approach, Diagnostic

0C9H3ZZ Drainage of Left Submaxillary Gland, Percutaneous Approach

0C9J00Z Drainage of Minor Salivary Gland with Drainage Device, Open Approach

0C9J0ZX Drainage of Minor Salivary Gland, Open Approach, Diagnostic

0C9J0ZZ Drainage of Minor Salivary Gland, Open Approach

0C9J30Z Drainage of Minor Salivary Gland with Drainage Device, Percutaneous Approach

0C9J3ZX Drainage of Minor Salivary Gland, Percutaneous Approach, Diagnostic

0C9J3ZZ Drainage of Minor Salivary Gland, Percutaneous Approach

0C9M00Z Drainage of Pharynx with Drainage Device, Open Approach

0C9M0ZX Drainage of Pharynx, Open Approach, Diagnostic

0C9M0ZZ Drainage of Pharynx, Open Approach

0C9M30Z Drainage of Pharynx with Drainage Device, Percutaneous Approach

0C9M3ZX Drainage of Pharynx, Percutaneous Approach, Diagnostic

0C9M3ZZ Drainage of Pharynx, Percutaneous Approach

0C9M40Z Drainage of Pharynx with Drainage Device, Percutaneous Endoscopic Approach

0C9M4ZX Drainage of Pharynx, Percutaneous Endoscopic Approach, Diagnostic

0C9M4ZZ Drainage of Pharynx, Percutaneous Endoscopic Approach

0C9M70Z Drainage of Pharynx with Drainage Device, Via Natural or Artificial Opening

0C9M7ZX Drainage of Pharynx, Via Natural or Artificial Opening, Diagnostic

0C9M7ZZ Drainage of Pharynx, Via Natural or Artificial Opening

0C9M80Z Drainage of Pharynx with Drainage Device, Via Natural or Artificial Opening Endoscopic

0C9M8ZX Drainage of Pharynx, Via Natural or Artificial Opening Endoscopic, Diagnostic

0C9M8ZZ Drainage of Pharynx, Via Natural or Artificial Opening Endoscopic

0C9N00Z Drainage of Uvula with Drainage Device, Open Approach

0C9N0ZX Drainage of Uvula, Open Approach, Diagnostic

0C9N0ZZ Drainage of Uvula, Open Approach

0C9N30Z Drainage of Uvula with Drainage Device, Percutaneous Approach

0C9N3ZX Drainage of Uvula, Percutaneous Approach, Diagnostic

0C9N3ZZ Drainage of Uvula, Percutaneous Approach

0C9NX0Z Drainage of Uvula with Drainage Device, External Approach

0C9NXZX Drainage of Uvula, External Approach, Diagnostic

0C9NXZZ Drainage of Uvula, External Approach

0C9P00Z Drainage of Tonsils with Drainage Device, Open Approach

0C9P0ZX Drainage of Tonsils, Open Approach, Diagnostic

0C9P0ZZ Drainage of Tonsils, Open Approach

0C9P30Z Drainage of Tonsils with Drainage Device, Percutaneous Approach

0C9P3ZX Drainage of Tonsils, Percutaneous Approach, Diagnostic

0C9P3ZZ Drainage of Tonsils, Percutaneous Approach

0C9PX0Z Drainage of Tonsils with Drainage Device, External Approach

0C9PXZX Drainage of Tonsils, External Approach, Diagnostic

0C9PXZZ Drainage of Tonsils, External Approach

0C9Q00Z Drainage of Adenoids with Drainage Device, Open Approach

0C9Q0ZX Drainage of Adenoids, Open Approach, Diagnostic

0C9Q0ZZ Drainage of Adenoids, Open Approach

0C9Q30Z Drainage of Adenoids with Drainage Device, Percutaneous Approach

0C9Q3ZX Drainage of Adenoids, Percutaneous Approach, Diagnostic

0C9Q3ZZ Drainage of Adenoids, Percutaneous Approach

0C9QX0Z Drainage of Adenoids with Drainage Device, External Approach

0C9QXZX Drainage of Adenoids, External Approach, Diagnostic

0C9QXZZ Drainage of Adenoids, External Approach

0C9R00Z Drainage of Epiglottis with Drainage Device, Open Approach

0C9R0ZX Drainage of Epiglottis, Open Approach, Diagnostic

0C9R0ZZ Drainage of Epiglottis, Open Approach

0C9R30Z Drainage of Epiglottis with Drainage Device, Percutaneous Approach

0C9R3ZX Drainage of Epiglottis, Percutaneous Approach, Diagnostic

0C9R3ZZ Drainage of Epiglottis, Percutaneous Approach

0C9R40Z Drainage of Epiglottis with Drainage Device, Percutaneous Endoscopic Approach

0C9R4ZX Drainage of Epiglottis, Percutaneous Endoscopic Approach, Diagnostic

0C9R4ZZ Drainage of Epiglottis, Percutaneous Endoscopic Approach

0C9R70Z Drainage of Epiglottis with Drainage Device, Via Natural or Artificial Opening

0C9R7ZX Drainage of Epiglottis, Via Natural or Artificial Opening, Diagnostic

0C9R7ZZ Drainage of Epiglottis, Via Natural or Artificial Opening

0C9R80Z Drainage of Epiglottis with Drainage Device, Via Natural or Artificial Opening Endoscopic

0C9R8ZX Drainage of Epiglottis, Via Natural or Artificial Opening Endoscopic, Diagnostic

0C9R8ZZ Drainage of Epiglottis, Via Natural or Artificial Opening Endoscopic

0C9S00Z Drainage of Larynx with Drainage Device, Open Approach

0C9S0ZX Drainage of Larynx, Open Approach, Diagnostic

0C9S0ZZ Drainage of Larynx, Open Approach

0C9S30Z Drainage of Larynx with Drainage Device, Percutaneous Approach

0C9S3ZX Drainage of Larynx, Percutaneous Approach, Diagnostic

0C9S3ZZ Drainage of Larynx, Percutaneous Approach

0C9S40Z Drainage of Larynx with Drainage Device, Percutaneous Endoscopic Approach

0C9S4ZX Drainage of Larynx, Percutaneous Endoscopic Approach, Diagnostic

0C9S4ZZ Drainage of Larynx, Percutaneous Endoscopic Approach

0C9S70Z Drainage of Larynx with Drainage Device, Via Natural or Artificial Opening

0C9S7ZX Drainage of Larynx, Via Natural or Artificial Opening, Diagnostic

0C9S7ZZ Drainage of Larynx, Via Natural or Artificial Opening

0C9S80Z Drainage of Larynx with Drainage Device, Via Natural or Artificial Opening Endoscopic

0C9S8ZX Drainage of Larynx, Via Natural or Artificial Opening Endoscopic, Diagnostic

0C9S8ZZ Drainage of Larynx, Via Natural or Artificial Opening Endoscopic

0C9T00Z Drainage of Right Vocal Cord with Drainage Device, Open Approach

0C9T0ZX Drainage of Right Vocal Cord, Open Approach, Diagnostic

0C9T0ZZ Drainage of Right Vocal Cord, Open Approach

0C9T30Z Drainage of Right Vocal Cord with Drainage Device, Percutaneous Approach

0C9T3ZX Drainage of Right Vocal Cord, Percutaneous Approach, Diagnostic

0C9T3ZZ Drainage of Right Vocal Cord, Percutaneous Approach

0C9T40Z Drainage of Right Vocal Cord with Drainage Device, Percutaneous Endoscopic Approach

0C9T4ZX Drainage of Right Vocal Cord, Percutaneous Endoscopic Approach, Diagnostic

0C9T4ZZ Drainage of Right Vocal Cord, Percutaneous Endoscopic Approach

0C9T70Z Drainage of Right Vocal Cord with Drainage Device, Via Natural or Artificial Opening

0C9T7ZX Drainage of Right Vocal Cord, Via Natural or Artificial Opening, Diagnostic

0C9T7ZZ Drainage of Right Vocal Cord, Via Natural or Artificial Opening

0C9T80Z Drainage of Right Vocal Cord with Drainage Device, Via Natural or Artificial Opening Endoscopic

0C9T8ZX Drainage of Right Vocal Cord, Via Natural or Artificial Opening Endoscopic, Diagnostic

0C9T8ZZ Drainage of Right Vocal Cord, Via Natural or Artificial Opening Endoscopic

0C9V00Z Drainage of Left Vocal Cord with Drainage Device, Open Approach

0C9V0ZX Drainage of Left Vocal Cord, Open Approach, Diagnostic

0C9V0ZZ Drainage of Left Vocal Cord, Open Approach

0C9V30Z Drainage of Left Vocal Cord with Drainage Device, Percutaneous Approach

0C9V3ZX Drainage of Left Vocal Cord, Percutaneous Approach, Diagnostic

0C9V3ZZ Drainage of Left Vocal Cord, Percutaneous Approach

0C9V40Z Drainage of Left Vocal Cord with Drainage Device, Percutaneous Endoscopic Approach

0C9V4ZX Drainage of Left Vocal Cord, Percutaneous Endoscopic Approach, Diagnostic

0C9V4ZZ Drainage of Left Vocal Cord, Percutaneous Endoscopic Approach

0C9V70Z Drainage of Left Vocal Cord with Drainage Device, Via Natural or Artificial Opening

0C9V7ZX Drainage of Left Vocal Cord, Via Natural or Artificial Opening, Diagnostic

0C9V7ZZ Drainage of Left Vocal Cord, Via Natural or Artificial Opening

0C9V80Z Drainage of Left Vocal Cord with Drainage Device, Via Natural or Artificial Opening Endoscopic

0C9V8ZX Drainage of Left Vocal Cord, Via Natural or Artificial Opening Endoscopic, Diagnostic

0C9V8ZZ Drainage of Left Vocal Cord, Via Natural or Artificial Opening Endoscopic

0C9W000 Drainage of Upper Tooth with Drainage Device, Open Approach, Single

0C9W001 Drainage of Upper Tooth with Drainage Device, Open Approach, Multiple

0C9W002 Drainage of Upper Tooth with Drainage Device, Open Approach, All

0C9W0Z0 Drainage of Upper Tooth, Open Approach, Single

0C9W0Z1 Drainage of Upper Tooth, Open Approach, Multiple

0C9W0Z2 Drainage of Upper Tooth, Open Approach, All

0C9WX00 Drainage of Upper Tooth with Drainage Device, External Approach, Single

0C9WX01 Drainage of Upper Tooth with Drainage Device, External Approach, Multiple

0C9WX02 Drainage of Upper Tooth with Drainage Device, External Approach, All

0C9WXZ0 Drainage of Upper Tooth, External Approach, Single

0C9WXZ1 Drainage of Upper Tooth, External Approach, Multiple

0C9WXZ2 Drainage of Upper Tooth, External Approach, All

0C9X000 Drainage of Lower Tooth with Drainage Device, Open Approach, Single

0C9X001 Drainage of Lower Tooth with Drainage Device, Open Approach, Multiple

0C9X002 Drainage of Lower Tooth with Drainage Device, Open Approach, All

♀ Female-only   ♂ Male-only   ▲ Limited Coverage   ● Non-OR   HAC HAC-associated procedure   ▲ Non-covered procedures   ✚ Cluster

0C9X0Z0	Drainage of Lower Tooth, Open Approach, Single	0C9XX01	Drainage of Lower Tooth with Drainage Device, External Approach, Multiple	0C9XXZ1	Drainage of Lower Tooth, External Approach, Multiple
0C9X0Z1	Drainage of Lower Tooth, Open Approach, Multiple	0C9XX02	Drainage of Lower Tooth with Drainage Device, External Approach, All	0C9XXZ2	Drainage of Lower Tooth, External Approach, All
0C9X0Z2	Drainage of Lower Tooth, Open Approach, All				
0C9XX00	Drainage of Lower Tooth with Drainage Device, External Approach, Single	0C9XXZ0	Drainage of Lower Tooth, External Approach, Single		

0CB – Mouth and Throat, Excision

Review Coding Guidelines B3.4a and B3.4b

Review Coding Guideline B3.8

Review Coding Guideline B3.18

0CB00ZX	Excision of Upper Lip, Open Approach, Diagnostic	0CB50ZX	Excision of Upper Gingiva, Open Approach, Diagnostic	0CBB3ZZ	Excision of Right Parotid Duct, Percutaneous Approach
0CB00ZZ	Excision of Upper Lip, Open Approach	0CB50ZZ	Excision of Upper Gingiva, Open Approach	0CBC0ZX	Excision of Left Parotid Duct, Open Approach, Diagnostic
0CB03ZX	Excision of Upper Lip, Percutaneous Approach, Diagnostic	0CB53ZX	Excision of Upper Gingiva, Percutaneous Approach, Diagnostic	0CBC0ZZ	Excision of Left Parotid Duct, Open Approach
0CB03ZZ	Excision of Upper Lip, Percutaneous Approach	0CB53ZZ	Excision of Upper Gingiva, Percutaneous Approach	0CBC3ZX	Excision of Left Parotid Duct, Percutaneous Approach, Diagnostic
0CB0XZX	Excision of Upper Lip, External Approach, Diagnostic	0CB5XZX	Excision of Upper Gingiva, External Approach, Diagnostic	0CBC3ZZ	Excision of Left Parotid Duct, Percutaneous Approach
0CB0XZZ	Excision of Upper Lip, External Approach	0CB5XZZ	Excision of Upper Gingiva, External Approach	0CBD0ZX	Excision of Right Sublingual Gland, Open Approach, Diagnostic
0CB10ZX	Excision of Lower Lip, Open Approach, Diagnostic	0CB60ZX	Excision of Lower Gingiva, Open Approach, Diagnostic	0CBD0ZZ	Excision of Right Sublingual Gland, Open Approach
0CB10ZZ	Excision of Lower Lip, Open Approach	0CB60ZZ	Excision of Lower Gingiva, Open Approach	0CBD3ZX	Excision of Right Sublingual Gland, Percutaneous Approach, Diagnostic
0CB13ZX	Excision of Lower Lip, Percutaneous Approach, Diagnostic	0CB63ZX	Excision of Lower Gingiva, Percutaneous Approach, Diagnostic	0CBD3ZZ	Excision of Right Sublingual Gland, Percutaneous Approach
0CB13ZZ	Excision of Lower Lip, Percutaneous Approach	0CB63ZZ	Excision of Lower Gingiva, Percutaneous Approach	0CBF0ZX	Excision of Left Sublingual Gland, Open Approach, Diagnostic
0CB1XZX	Excision of Lower Lip, External Approach, Diagnostic	0CB6XZX	Excision of Lower Gingiva, External Approach, Diagnostic	0CBF0ZZ	Excision of Left Sublingual Gland, Open Approach
0CB1XZZ	Excision of Lower Lip, External Approach	0CB6XZZ	Excision of Lower Gingiva, External Approach	0CBF3ZX	Excision of Left Sublingual Gland, Percutaneous Approach, Diagnostic
0CB20ZX	Excision of Hard Palate, Open Approach, Diagnostic	0CB70ZX	Excision of Tongue, Open Approach, Diagnostic	0CBF3ZZ	Excision of Left Sublingual Gland, Percutaneous Approach
0CB20ZZ	Excision of Hard Palate, Open Approach	0CB70ZZ	Excision of Tongue, Open Approach	0CBG0ZX	Excision of Right Submaxillary Gland, Open Approach, Diagnostic
0CB23ZX	Excision of Hard Palate, Percutaneous Approach, Diagnostic	0CB73ZX	Excision of Tongue, Percutaneous Approach, Diagnostic	0CBG0ZZ	Excision of Right Submaxillary Gland, Open Approach
0CB23ZZ	Excision of Hard Palate, Percutaneous Approach	0CB73ZZ	Excision of Tongue, Percutaneous Approach	0CBG3ZX	Excision of Right Submaxillary Gland, Percutaneous Approach, Diagnostic
0CB2XZX	Excision of Hard Palate, External Approach, Diagnostic	0CB7XZX	Excision of Tongue, External Approach, Diagnostic	0CBG3ZZ	Excision of Right Submaxillary Gland, Percutaneous Approach
0CB2XZZ	Excision of Hard Palate, External Approach	0CB7XZZ	Excision of Tongue, External Approach	0CBH0ZX	Excision of Left Submaxillary Gland, Open Approach, Diagnostic
0CB30ZX	Excision of Soft Palate, Open Approach, Diagnostic	0CB80ZX	Excision of Right Parotid Gland, Open Approach, Diagnostic	0CBH0ZZ	Excision of Left Submaxillary Gland, Open Approach
0CB30ZZ	Excision of Soft Palate, Open Approach	0CB80ZZ	Excision of Right Parotid Gland, Open Approach	0CBH3ZX	Excision of Left Submaxillary Gland, Percutaneous Approach, Diagnostic
0CB33ZX	Excision of Soft Palate, Percutaneous Approach, Diagnostic	*AHA CC: 3Q, 2014, 21-22*		0CBH3ZZ	Excision of Left Submaxillary Gland, Percutaneous Approach
0CB33ZZ	Excision of Soft Palate, Percutaneous Approach	0CB83ZX	Excision of Right Parotid Gland, Percutaneous Approach, Diagnostic	0CBJ0ZX	Excision of Minor Salivary Gland, Open Approach, Diagnostic
0CB3XZX	Excision of Soft Palate, External Approach, Diagnostic	0CB83ZZ	Excision of Right Parotid Gland, Percutaneous Approach	0CBJ0ZZ	Excision of Minor Salivary Gland, Open Approach
0CB3XZZ	Excision of Soft Palate, External Approach	0CB90ZX	Excision of Left Parotid Gland, Open Approach, Diagnostic	0CBJ3ZX	Excision of Minor Salivary Gland, Percutaneous Approach, Diagnostic
0CB40ZX	Excision of Buccal Mucosa, Open Approach, Diagnostic	0CB90ZZ	Excision of Left Parotid Gland, Open Approach	0CBJ3ZZ	Excision of Minor Salivary Gland, Percutaneous Approach
0CB40ZZ	Excision of Buccal Mucosa, Open Approach	0CB93ZX	Excision of Left Parotid Gland, Percutaneous Approach, Diagnostic	0CBM0ZX	Excision of Pharynx, Open Approach, Diagnostic
0CB43ZX	Excision of Buccal Mucosa, Percutaneous Approach, Diagnostic	0CB93ZZ	Excision of Left Parotid Gland, Percutaneous Approach	0CBM0ZZ	Excision of Pharynx, Open Approach
0CB43ZZ	Excision of Buccal Mucosa, Percutaneous Approach	0CBB0ZX	Excision of Right Parotid Duct, Open Approach, Diagnostic	0CBM3ZX	Excision of Pharynx, Percutaneous Approach, Diagnostic
0CB4XZX	Excision of Buccal Mucosa, External Approach, Diagnostic	0CBB0ZZ	Excision of Right Parotid Duct, Open Approach	0CBM3ZZ	Excision of Pharynx, Percutaneous Approach
0CB4XZZ	Excision of Buccal Mucosa, External Approach	0CBB3ZX	Excision of Right Parotid Duct, Percutaneous Approach, Diagnostic		

0CBM4ZX Excision of Pharynx, Percutaneous Endoscopic Approach, Diagnostic
0CBM4ZZ Excision of Pharynx, Percutaneous Endoscopic Approach
0CBM7ZX Excision of Pharynx, Via Natural or Artificial Opening, Diagnostic
0CBM7ZZ Excision of Pharynx, Via Natural or Artificial Opening
0CBM8ZX Excision of Pharynx, Via Natural or Artificial Opening Endoscopic, Diagnostic
AHA CC: 2Q, 2016, 20
0CBM8ZZ Excision of Pharynx, Via Natural or Artificial Opening Endoscopic
AHA CC: 3Q, 2016, 28-29
0CBN0ZX Excision of Uvula, Open Approach, Diagnostic
0CBN0ZZ Excision of Uvula, Open Approach
0CBN3ZX Excision of Uvula, Percutaneous Approach, Diagnostic
0CBN3ZZ Excision of Uvula, Percutaneous Approach
0CBNXZX Excision of Uvula, External Approach, Diagnostic
0CBNXZZ Excision of Uvula, External Approach
0CBP0ZX Excision of Tonsils, Open Approach, Diagnostic
0CBP0ZZ Excision of Tonsils, Open Approach
0CBP3ZX Excision of Tonsils, Percutaneous Approach, Diagnostic
0CBP3ZZ Excision of Tonsils, Percutaneous Approach
0CBPXZX Excision of Tonsils, External Approach, Diagnostic
0CBPXZZ Excision of Tonsils, External Approach
0CBQ0ZX Excision of Adenoids, Open Approach, Diagnostic
0CBQ0ZZ Excision of Adenoids, Open Approach
0CBQ3ZX Excision of Adenoids, Percutaneous Approach, Diagnostic
0CBQ3ZZ Excision of Adenoids, Percutaneous Approach
0CBQXZX Excision of Adenoids, External Approach, Diagnostic
0CBQXZZ Excision of Adenoids, External Approach
0CBR0ZX Excision of Epiglottis, Open Approach, Diagnostic
0CBR0ZZ Excision of Epiglottis, Open Approach
0CBR3ZX Excision of Epiglottis, Percutaneous Approach, Diagnostic
0CBR3ZZ Excision of Epiglottis, Percutaneous Approach

0CBR4ZX Excision of Epiglottis, Percutaneous Endoscopic Approach, Diagnostic
0CBR4ZZ Excision of Epiglottis, Percutaneous Endoscopic Approach
0CBR7ZX Excision of Epiglottis, Via Natural or Artificial Opening, Diagnostic
0CBR7ZZ Excision of Epiglottis, Via Natural or Artificial Opening
0CBR8ZX Excision of Epiglottis, Via Natural or Artificial Opening Endoscopic, Diagnostic
0CBR8ZZ Excision of Epiglottis, Via Natural or Artificial Opening Endoscopic
0CBS0ZX Excision of Larynx, Open Approach, Diagnostic
0CBS0ZZ Excision of Larynx, Open Approach
0CBS3ZX Excision of Larynx, Percutaneous Approach, Diagnostic
0CBS3ZZ Excision of Larynx, Percutaneous Approach
0CBS4ZX Excision of Larynx, Percutaneous Endoscopic Approach, Diagnostic
0CBS4ZZ Excision of Larynx, Percutaneous Endoscopic Approach
0CBS7ZX Excision of Larynx, Via Natural or Artificial Opening, Diagnostic
0CBS7ZZ Excision of Larynx, Via Natural or Artificial Opening
0CBS8ZX Excision of Larynx, Via Natural or Artificial Opening Endoscopic, Diagnostic
0CBS8ZZ Excision of Larynx, Via Natural or Artificial Opening Endoscopic
0CBT0ZX Excision of Right Vocal Cord, Open Approach, Diagnostic
0CBT0ZZ Excision of Right Vocal Cord, Open Approach
0CBT3ZX Excision of Right Vocal Cord, Percutaneous Approach, Diagnostic
0CBT3ZZ Excision of Right Vocal Cord, Percutaneous Approach
0CBT4ZX Excision of Right Vocal Cord, Percutaneous Endoscopic Approach, Diagnostic
0CBT4ZZ Excision of Right Vocal Cord, Percutaneous Endoscopic Approach
0CBT7ZX Excision of Right Vocal Cord, Via Natural or Artificial Opening, Diagnostic
0CBT7ZZ Excision of Right Vocal Cord, Via Natural or Artificial Opening
0CBT8ZX Excision of Right Vocal Cord, Via Natural or Artificial Opening Endoscopic, Diagnostic

0CBT8ZZ Excision of Right Vocal Cord, Via Natural or Artificial Opening Endoscopic
0CBV0ZX Excision of Left Vocal Cord, Open Approach, Diagnostic
0CBV0ZZ Excision of Left Vocal Cord, Open Approach
0CBV3ZX Excision of Left Vocal Cord, Percutaneous Approach, Diagnostic
0CBV3ZZ Excision of Left Vocal Cord, Percutaneous Approach
0CBV4ZX Excision of Left Vocal Cord, Percutaneous Endoscopic Approach, Diagnostic
0CBV4ZZ Excision of Left Vocal Cord, Percutaneous Endoscopic Approach
0CBV7ZX Excision of Left Vocal Cord, Via Natural or Artificial Opening, Diagnostic
0CBV7ZZ Excision of Left Vocal Cord, Via Natural or Artificial Opening
0CBV8ZX Excision of Left Vocal Cord, Via Natural or Artificial Opening Endoscopic, Diagnostic
0CBV8ZZ Excision of Left Vocal Cord, Via Natural or Artificial Opening Endoscopic
0CBW0Z0 Excision of Upper Tooth, Open Approach, Single
0CBW0Z1 Excision of Upper Tooth, Open Approach, Multiple
0CBW0Z2 Excision of Upper Tooth, Open Approach, All
0CBWXZ0 Excision of Upper Tooth, External Approach, Single
0CBWXZ1 Excision of Upper Tooth, External Approach, Multiple
0CBWXZ2 Excision of Upper Tooth, External Approach, All
0CBX0Z0 Excision of Lower Tooth, Open Approach, Single
0CBX0Z1 Excision of Lower Tooth, Open Approach, Multiple
0CBX0Z2 Excision of Lower Tooth, Open Approach, All
0CBXXZ0 Excision of Lower Tooth, External Approach, Single
0CBXXZ1 Excision of Lower Tooth, External Approach, Multiple
0CBXXZ2 Excision of Lower Tooth, External Approach, All

0CC – Mouth and Throat, Extirpation

0CC00ZZ Extirpation of Matter from Upper Lip, Open Approach
0CC03ZZ Extirpation of Matter from Upper Lip, Percutaneous Approach
0CC0XZZ Extirpation of Matter from Upper Lip, External Approach
0CC10ZZ Extirpation of Matter from Lower Lip, Open Approach
0CC13ZZ Extirpation of Matter from Lower Lip, Percutaneous Approach
0CC1XZZ Extirpation of Matter from Lower Lip, External Approach
0CC20ZZ Extirpation of Matter from Hard Palate, Open Approach
0CC23ZZ Extirpation of Matter from Hard Palate, Percutaneous Approach
0CC2XZZ Extirpation of Matter from Hard Palate, External Approach

0CC30ZZ Extirpation of Matter from Soft Palate, Open Approach
0CC33ZZ Extirpation of Matter from Soft Palate, Percutaneous Approach
0CC3XZZ Extirpation of Matter from Soft Palate, External Approach
0CC40ZZ Extirpation of Matter from Buccal Mucosa, Open Approach
0CC43ZZ Extirpation of Matter from Buccal Mucosa, Percutaneous Approach
0CC4XZZ Extirpation of Matter from Buccal Mucosa, External Approach
0CC50ZZ Extirpation of Matter from Upper Gingiva, Open Approach
0CC53ZZ Extirpation of Matter from Upper Gingiva, Percutaneous Approach
0CC5XZZ Extirpation of Matter from Upper Gingiva, External Approach

0CC60ZZ Extirpation of Matter from Lower Gingiva, Open Approach
0CC63ZZ Extirpation of Matter from Lower Gingiva, Percutaneous Approach
0CC6XZZ Extirpation of Matter from Lower Gingiva, External Approach
0CC70ZZ Extirpation of Matter from Tongue, Open Approach
0CC73ZZ Extirpation of Matter from Tongue, Percutaneous Approach
0CC7XZZ Extirpation of Matter from Tongue, External Approach
0CC80ZZ Extirpation of Matter from Right Parotid Gland, Open Approach
0CC83ZZ Extirpation of Matter from Right Parotid Gland, Percutaneous Approach
0CC90ZZ Extirpation of Matter from Left Parotid Gland, Open Approach

♀ Female-only   ♂ Male-only   ▲ Limited Coverage   ● Non-OR   ▨ HAC-associated procedure   ▲ Non-covered procedures   ➕ Cluster

CC93ZZ	Extirpation of Matter from Left Parotid Gland, Percutaneous Approach	
CCB0ZZ	Extirpation of Matter from Right Parotid Duct, Open Approach	
CCB3ZZ	Extirpation of Matter from Right Parotid Duct, Percutaneous Approach	
CCC0ZZ	Extirpation of Matter from Left Parotid Duct, Open Approach	
CCC3ZZ	Extirpation of Matter from Left Parotid Duct, Percutaneous Approach	
CCD0ZZ	Extirpation of Matter from Right Sublingual Gland, Open Approach	
CCD3ZZ	Extirpation of Matter from Right Sublingual Gland, Percutaneous Approach	
CCF0ZZ	Extirpation of Matter from Left Sublingual Gland, Open Approach	
CCF3ZZ	Extirpation of Matter from Left Sublingual Gland, Percutaneous Approach	
0CCG0ZZ	Extirpation of Matter from Right Submaxillary Gland, Open Approach	
0CCG3ZZ	Extirpation of Matter from Right Submaxillary Gland, Percutaneous Approach	
0CCH0ZZ	Extirpation of Matter from Left Submaxillary Gland, Open Approach	
0CCH3ZZ	Extirpation of Matter from Left Submaxillary Gland, Percutaneous Approach	

AHA CC: 2Q, 2016, 20

0CCJ0ZZ	Extirpation of Matter from Minor Salivary Gland, Open Approach
0CCJ3ZZ	Extirpation of Matter from Minor Salivary Gland, Percutaneous Approach
0CCM0ZZ	Extirpation of Matter from Pharynx, Open Approach
0CCM3ZZ	Extirpation of Matter from Pharynx, Percutaneous Approach
0CCM4ZZ	Extirpation of Matter from Pharynx, Percutaneous Endoscopic Approach
0CCM7ZZ	Extirpation of Matter from Pharynx, Via Natural or Artificial Opening
0CCM8ZZ	Extirpation of Matter from Pharynx, Via Natural or Artificial Opening Endoscopic

0CCN0ZZ	Extirpation of Matter from Uvula, Open Approach
0CCN3ZZ	Extirpation of Matter from Uvula, Percutaneous Approach
0CCNXZZ	Extirpation of Matter from Uvula, External Approach
0CCP0ZZ	Extirpation of Matter from Tonsils, Open Approach
0CCP3ZZ	Extirpation of Matter from Tonsils, Percutaneous Approach
0CCPXZZ	Extirpation of Matter from Tonsils, External Approach
0CCQ0ZZ	Extirpation of Matter from Adenoids, Open Approach
0CCQ3ZZ	Extirpation of Matter from Adenoids, Percutaneous Approach
0CCQXZZ	Extirpation of Matter from Adenoids, External Approach
0CCR0ZZ	Extirpation of Matter from Epiglottis, Open Approach
0CCR3ZZ	Extirpation of Matter from Epiglottis, Percutaneous Approach
0CCR4ZZ	Extirpation of Matter from Epiglottis, Percutaneous Endoscopic Approach
0CCR7ZZ	Extirpation of Matter from Epiglottis, Via Natural or Artificial Opening
0CCR8ZZ	Extirpation of Matter from Epiglottis, Via Natural or Artificial Opening Endoscopic
0CCS0ZZ	Extirpation of Matter from Larynx, Open Approach
0CCS3ZZ	Extirpation of Matter from Larynx, Percutaneous Approach
0CCS4ZZ	Extirpation of Matter from Larynx, Percutaneous Endoscopic Approach
0CCS7ZZ	Extirpation of Matter from Larynx, Via Natural or Artificial Opening
0CCS8ZZ	Extirpation of Matter from Larynx, Via Natural or Artificial Opening Endoscopic
0CCT0ZZ	Extirpation of Matter from Right Vocal Cord, Open Approach
0CCT3ZZ	Extirpation of Matter from Right Vocal Cord, Percutaneous Approach
0CCT4ZZ	Extirpation of Matter from Right Vocal Cord, Percutaneous Endoscopic Approach

0CCT7ZZ	Extirpation of Matter from Right Vocal Cord, Via Natural or Artificial Opening
0CCT8ZZ	Extirpation of Matter from Right Vocal Cord, Via Natural or Artificial Opening Endoscopic
0CCV0ZZ	Extirpation of Matter from Left Vocal Cord, Open Approach
0CCV3ZZ	Extirpation of Matter from Left Vocal Cord, Percutaneous Approach
0CCV4ZZ	Extirpation of Matter from Left Vocal Cord, Percutaneous Endoscopic Approach
0CCV7ZZ	Extirpation of Matter from Left Vocal Cord, Via Natural or Artificial Opening
0CCV8ZZ	Extirpation of Matter from Left Vocal Cord, Via Natural or Artificial Opening Endoscopic
0CCW0Z0	Extirpation of Matter from Upper Tooth, Single, Open Approach
0CCW0Z1	Extirpation of Matter from Upper Tooth, Multiple, Open Approach
0CCW0Z2	Extirpation of Matter from Upper Tooth, All, Open Approach
0CCWXZ0	Extirpation of Matter from Upper Tooth, Single, External Approach
0CCWXZ1	Extirpation of Matter from Upper Tooth, Multiple, External Approach
0CCWXZ2	Extirpation of Matter from Upper Tooth, All, External Approach
0CCX0Z0	Extirpation of Matter from Lower Tooth, Single, Open Approach
0CCX0Z1	Extirpation of Matter from Lower Tooth, Multiple, Open Approach
0CCX0Z2	Extirpation of Matter from Lower Tooth, All, Open Approach
0CCXXZ0	Extirpation of Matter from Lower Tooth, Single, External Approach
0CCXXZ1	Extirpation of Matter from Lower Tooth, Multiple, External Approach
0CCXXZ2	Extirpation of Matter from Lower Tooth, All, External Approach

0CD – Mouth and Throat, Extraction

0CDT0ZZ	Extraction of Right Vocal Cord, Open Approach
0CDT3ZZ	Extraction of Right Vocal Cord, Percutaneous Approach
0CDT4ZZ	Extraction of Right Vocal Cord, Percutaneous Endoscopic Approach
0CDT7ZZ	Extraction of Right Vocal Cord, Via Natural or Artificial Opening
0CDT8ZZ	Extraction of Right Vocal Cord, Via Natural or Artificial Opening Endoscopic

0CDV0ZZ	Extraction of Left Vocal Cord, Open Approach
0CDV3ZZ	Extraction of Left Vocal Cord, Percutaneous Approach
0CDV4ZZ	Extraction of Left Vocal Cord, Percutaneous Endoscopic Approach
0CDV7ZZ	Extraction of Left Vocal Cord, Via Natural or Artificial Opening
0CDV8ZZ	Extraction of Left Vocal Cord, Via Natural or Artificial Opening Endoscopic

0CDWXZ0	Extraction of Upper Tooth, Single, External Approach
0CDWXZ1	Extraction of Upper Tooth, Multiple, External Approach
0CDWXZ2	Extraction of Upper Tooth, All, External Approach
0CDXXZ0	Extraction of Lower Tooth, Single, External Approach
0CDXXZ1	Extraction of Lower Tooth, Multiple, External Approach
0CDXXZ2	Extraction of Lower Tooth, All, External Approach

0CF – Mouth and Throat, Fragmentation

0CFB0ZZ	Fragmentation in Right Parotid Duct, Open Approach
0CFB3ZZ	Fragmentation in Right Parotid Duct, Percutaneous Approach
0CFB7ZZ	Fragmentation in Right Parotid Duct, Via Natural or Artificial Opening

▲ **0CFBXZZ**	Fragmentation in Right Parotid Duct, External Approach
0CFC0ZZ	Fragmentation in Left Parotid Duct, Open Approach
0CFC3ZZ	Fragmentation in Left Parotid Duct, Percutaneous Approach

0CFC7ZZ	Fragmentation in Left Parotid Duct, Via Natural or Artificial Opening
▲ **0CFCXZZ**	Fragmentation in Left Parotid Duct, External Approach

0CH – Mouth and Throat, Insertion

0CH701Z	Insertion of Radioactive Element into Tongue, Open Approach
0CH731Z	Insertion of Radioactive Element into Tongue, Percutaneous Approach
0CH7X1Z	Insertion of Radioactive Element into Tongue, External Approach

---

♀ Female-only ♂ Male-only ▲ Limited Coverage ● Non-OR **HAC** HAC-associated procedure ▲ Non-covered procedures + Cluster

0CHA01Z Insertion of Radioactive Element into Salivary Gland, Open Approach	**0CHS01Z** Insertion of Radioactive Element into Larynx, Open Approach	**0CHY31Z** Insertion of Radioactive Element into Mouth and Throat, Percutaneous Approach
0CHA0YZ Insertion of Other Device into Salivary Gland, Open Approach	**0CHS0YZ** Insertion of Other Device into Larynx, Open Approach	**0CHY3YZ** Insertion of Other Device into Mouth and Throat, Percutaneous Approach
0CHA31Z Insertion of Radioactive Element into Salivary Gland, Percutaneous Approach	**0CHS31Z** Insertion of Radioactive Element into Larynx, Percutaneous Approach	**0CHY71Z** Insertion of Radioactive Element into Mouth and Throat, Via Natural or Artificial Opening
0CHA3YZ Insertion of Other Device into Salivary Gland, Percutaneous Approach	**0CHS3YZ** Insertion of Other Device into Larynx, Percutaneous Approach	**0CHY7BZ** Insertion of Airway into Mouth and Throat, Via Natural or Artificial Opening
0CHA71Z Insertion of Radioactive Element into Salivary Gland, Via Natural or Artificial Opening	**0CHS71Z** Insertion of Radioactive Element into Larynx, Via Natural or Artificial Opening	**0CHY7YZ** Insertion of Other Device into Mouth and Throat, Via Natural or Artificial Opening
0CHA7YZ Insertion of Other Device into Salivary Gland, Via Natural or Artificial Opening	**0CHS7YZ** Insertion of Other Device into Larynx, Via Natural or Artificial Opening	**0CHY81Z** Insertion of Radioactive Element into Mouth and Throat, Via Natural or Artificial Opening Endoscopic
0CHA81Z Insertion of Radioactive Element into Salivary Gland, Via Natural or Artificial Opening Endoscopic	**0CHS81Z** Insertion of Radioactive Element into Larynx, Via Natural or Artificial Opening Endoscopic	**0CHY8BZ** Insertion of Airway into Mouth and Throat, Via Natural or Artificial Opening Endoscopic
0CHA8YZ Insertion of Other Device into Salivary Gland, Via Natural or Artificial Opening Endoscopic	**0CHS8YZ** Insertion of Other Device into Larynx, Via Natural or Artificial Opening Endoscopic	**0CHY8YZ** Insertion of Other Device into Mouth and Throat, Via Natural or Artificial Opening Endoscopic
	0CHY01Z Insertion of Radioactive Element into Mouth and Throat, Open Approach	
	0CHY0YZ Insertion of Other Device into Mouth and Throat, Open Approach	

0CJ – Mouth and Throat, Inspection

Review Coding Guidelines B3.11a, B3.11b and B3.11c

0CJA0ZZ Inspection of Salivary Gland, Open Approach	**0CJS4ZZ** Inspection of Larynx, Percutaneous Endoscopic Approach	**0CJY3ZZ** Inspection of Mouth and Throat, Percutaneous Approach
0CJA3ZZ Inspection of Salivary Gland, Percutaneous Approach	**0CJS7ZZ** Inspection of Larynx, Via Natural or Artificial Opening	**0CJY4ZZ** Inspection of Mouth and Throat, Percutaneous Endoscopic Approach
0CJAXZZ Inspection of Salivary Gland, External Approach	**0CJS8ZZ** Inspection of Larynx, Via Natural or Artificial Opening Endoscopic	**0CJY7ZZ** Inspection of Mouth and Throat, Via Natural or Artificial Opening
0CJS0ZZ Inspection of Larynx, Open Approach	**0CJSXZZ** Inspection of Larynx, External Approach	**0CJY8ZZ** Inspection of Mouth and Throat, Via Natural or Artificial Opening Endoscopic
0CJS3ZZ Inspection of Larynx, Percutaneous Approach	**0CJY0ZZ** Inspection of Mouth and Throat, Open Approach	**0CJYXZZ** Inspection of Mouth and Throat, External Approach

0CL – Mouth and Throat, Occlusion

0CLB0CZ Occlusion of Right Parotid Duct with Extraluminal Device, Open Approach	**0CLB7DZ** Occlusion of Right Parotid Duct with Intraluminal Device, Via Natural or Artificial Opening	**0CLC3ZZ** Occlusion of Left Parotid Duct, Percutaneous Approach
0CLB0DZ Occlusion of Right Parotid Duct with Intraluminal Device, Open Approach	**0CLB7ZZ** Occlusion of Right Parotid Duct, Via Natural or Artificial Opening	**0CLC4CZ** Occlusion of Left Parotid Duct with Extraluminal Device, Percutaneous Endoscopic Approach
0CLB0ZZ Occlusion of Right Parotid Duct, Open Approach	**0CLB8DZ** Occlusion of Right Parotid Duct with Intraluminal Device, Via Natural or Artificial Opening Endoscopic	**0CLC4DZ** Occlusion of Left Parotid Duct with Intraluminal Device, Percutaneous Endoscopic Approach
0CLB3CZ Occlusion of Right Parotid Duct with Extraluminal Device, Percutaneous Approach	**0CLB8ZZ** Occlusion of Right Parotid Duct, Via Natural or Artificial Opening Endoscopic	**0CLC4ZZ** Occlusion of Left Parotid Duct, Percutaneous Endoscopic Approach
0CLB3DZ Occlusion of Right Parotid Duct with Intraluminal Device, Percutaneous Approach	**0CLC0CZ** Occlusion of Left Parotid Duct with Extraluminal Device, Open Approach	**0CLC7DZ** Occlusion of Left Parotid Duct with Intraluminal Device, Via Natural or Artificial Opening
0CLB3ZZ Occlusion of Right Parotid Duct, Percutaneous Approach	**0CLC0DZ** Occlusion of Left Parotid Duct with Intraluminal Device, Open Approach	**0CLC7ZZ** Occlusion of Left Parotid Duct, Via Natural or Artificial Opening
0CLB4CZ Occlusion of Right Parotid Duct with Extraluminal Device, Percutaneous Endoscopic Approach	**0CLC0ZZ** Occlusion of Left Parotid Duct, Open Approach	**0CLC8DZ** Occlusion of Left Parotid Duct with Intraluminal Device, Via Natural or Artificial Opening Endoscopic
0CLB4DZ Occlusion of Right Parotid Duct with Intraluminal Device, Percutaneous Endoscopic Approach	**0CLC3CZ** Occlusion of Left Parotid Duct with Extraluminal Device, Percutaneous Approach	**0CLC8ZZ** Occlusion of Left Parotid Duct, Via Natural or Artificial Opening Endoscopic
0CLB4ZZ Occlusion of Right Parotid Duct, Percutaneous Endoscopic Approach	**0CLC3DZ** Occlusion of Left Parotid Duct with Intraluminal Device, Percutaneous Approach	

0CM – Mouth and Throat, Reattachment

0CM00ZZ Reattachment of Upper Lip, Open Approach	**0CMN0ZZ** Reattachment of Uvula, Open Approach	**0CMWXZ0** Reattachment of Upper Tooth, Single, External Approach
0CM10ZZ Reattachment of Lower Lip, Open Approach	**0CMW0Z0** Reattachment of Upper Tooth, Single, Open Approach	**0CMWXZ1** Reattachment of Upper Tooth, Multiple, External Approach
0CM30ZZ Reattachment of Soft Palate, Open Approach	**0CMW0Z1** Reattachment of Upper Tooth, Multiple, Open Approach	**0CMWXZ2** Reattachment of Upper Tooth, All, External Approach
0CM70ZZ Reattachment of Tongue, Open Approach	**0CMW0Z2** Reattachment of Upper Tooth, All, Open Approach	**0CMX0Z0** Reattachment of Lower Tooth, Single, Open Approach

0CMX0Z1	Reattachment of Lower Tooth, Multiple, Open Approach	
0CMX0Z2	Reattachment of Lower Tooth, All, Open Approach	
0CMXXZ0	Reattachment of Lower Tooth, Single, External Approach	
0CMXXZ1	Reattachment of Lower Tooth, Multiple, External Approach	
0CMXXZ2	Reattachment of Lower Tooth, All, External Approach	

0CN – Mouth and Throat, Release

Review Coding Guidelines B3.13 and B3.14

0CN00ZZ	Release Upper Lip, Open Approach
0CN03ZZ	Release Upper Lip, Percutaneous Approach
0CN0XZZ	Release Upper Lip, External Approach
0CN10ZZ	Release Lower Lip, Open Approach
0CN13ZZ	Release Lower Lip, Percutaneous Approach
0CN1XZZ	Release Lower Lip, External Approach
0CN20ZZ	Release Hard Palate, Open Approach
0CN23ZZ	Release Hard Palate, Percutaneous Approach
0CN2XZZ	Release Hard Palate, External Approach
0CN30ZZ	Release Soft Palate, Open Approach
0CN33ZZ	Release Soft Palate, Percutaneous Approach
0CN3XZZ	Release Soft Palate, External Approach
0CN40ZZ	Release Buccal Mucosa, Open Approach
0CN43ZZ	Release Buccal Mucosa, Percutaneous Approach
0CN4XZZ	Release Buccal Mucosa, External Approach
0CN50ZZ	Release Upper Gingiva, Open Approach
0CN53ZZ	Release Upper Gingiva, Percutaneous Approach
0CN5XZZ	Release Upper Gingiva, External Approach
0CN60ZZ	Release Lower Gingiva, Open Approach
0CN63ZZ	Release Lower Gingiva, Percutaneous Approach
0CN6XZZ	Release Lower Gingiva, External Approach
0CN70ZZ	Release Tongue, Open Approach
0CN73ZZ	Release Tongue, Percutaneous Approach
0CN7XZZ	Release Tongue, External Approach
0CN80ZZ	Release Right Parotid Gland, Open Approach
0CN83ZZ	Release Right Parotid Gland, Percutaneous Approach
0CN90ZZ	Release Left Parotid Gland, Open Approach
0CN93ZZ	Release Left Parotid Gland, Percutaneous Approach
0CNB0ZZ	Release Right Parotid Duct, Open Approach
0CNB3ZZ	Release Right Parotid Duct, Percutaneous Approach
0CNC0ZZ	Release Left Parotid Duct, Open Approach
0CNC3ZZ	Release Left Parotid Duct, Percutaneous Approach
0CND0ZZ	Release Right Sublingual Gland, Open Approach
0CND3ZZ	Release Right Sublingual Gland, Percutaneous Approach
0CNF0ZZ	Release Left Sublingual Gland, Open Approach
0CNF3ZZ	Release Left Sublingual Gland, Percutaneous Approach
0CNG0ZZ	Release Right Submaxillary Gland, Open Approach
0CNG3ZZ	Release Right Submaxillary Gland, Percutaneous Approach
0CNH0ZZ	Release Left Submaxillary Gland, Open Approach
0CNH3ZZ	Release Left Submaxillary Gland, Percutaneous Approach
0CNJ0ZZ	Release Minor Salivary Gland, Open Approach
0CNJ3ZZ	Release Minor Salivary Gland, Percutaneous Approach
0CNM0ZZ	Release Pharynx, Open Approach
0CNM3ZZ	Release Pharynx, Percutaneous Approach
0CNM4ZZ	Release Pharynx, Percutaneous Endoscopic Approach
0CNM7ZZ	Release Pharynx, Via Natural or Artificial Opening
0CNM8ZZ	Release Pharynx, Via Natural or Artificial Opening Endoscopic
0CNN0ZZ	Release Uvula, Open Approach
0CNN3ZZ	Release Uvula, Percutaneous Approach
0CNNXZZ	Release Uvula, External Approach
0CNP0ZZ	Release Tonsils, Open Approach
0CNP3ZZ	Release Tonsils, Percutaneous Approach
0CNPXZZ	Release Tonsils, External Approach
0CNQ0ZZ	Release Adenoids, Open Approach
0CNQ3ZZ	Release Adenoids, Percutaneous Approach
0CNQXZZ	Release Adenoids, External Approach
0CNR0ZZ	Release Epiglottis, Open Approach
0CNR3ZZ	Release Epiglottis, Percutaneous Approach
0CNR4ZZ	Release Epiglottis, Percutaneous Endoscopic Approach
0CNR7ZZ	Release Epiglottis, Via Natural or Artificial Opening
0CNR8ZZ	Release Epiglottis, Via Natural or Artificial Opening Endoscopic
0CNS0ZZ	Release Larynx, Open Approach
0CNS3ZZ	Release Larynx, Percutaneous Approach
0CNS4ZZ	Release Larynx, Percutaneous Endoscopic Approach
0CNS7ZZ	Release Larynx, Via Natural or Artificial Opening
0CNS8ZZ	Release Larynx, Via Natural or Artificial Opening Endoscopic
0CNT0ZZ	Release Right Vocal Cord, Open Approach
0CNT3ZZ	Release Right Vocal Cord, Percutaneous Approach
0CNT4ZZ	Release Right Vocal Cord, Percutaneous Endoscopic Approach
0CNT7ZZ	Release Right Vocal Cord, Via Natural or Artificial Opening
0CNT8ZZ	Release Right Vocal Cord, Via Natural or Artificial Opening Endoscopic
0CNV0ZZ	Release Left Vocal Cord, Open Approach
0CNV3ZZ	Release Left Vocal Cord, Percutaneous Approach
0CNV4ZZ	Release Left Vocal Cord, Percutaneous Endoscopic Approach
0CNV7ZZ	Release Left Vocal Cord, Via Natural or Artificial Opening
0CNV8ZZ	Release Left Vocal Cord, Via Natural or Artificial Opening Endoscopic
0CNW0Z0	Release Upper Tooth, Single, Open Approach
0CNW0Z1	Release Upper Tooth, Multiple, Open Approach
0CNW0Z2	Release Upper Tooth, All, Open Approach
0CNWXZ0	Release Upper Tooth, Single, External Approach
0CNWXZ1	Release Upper Tooth, Multiple, External Approach
0CNWXZ2	Release Upper Tooth, All, External Approach
0CNX0Z0	Release Lower Tooth, Single, Open Approach
0CNX0Z1	Release Lower Tooth, Multiple, Open Approach
0CNX0Z2	Release Lower Tooth, All, Open Approach
0CNXXZ0	Release Lower Tooth, Single, External Approach
0CNXXZ1	Release Lower Tooth, Multiple, External Approach
0CNXXZ2	Release Lower Tooth, All, External Approach

0CP – Mouth and Throat, Removal

Review Coding Guideline B6.1c

0CPA00Z	Removal of Drainage Device from Salivary Gland, Open Approach
0CPA0CZ	Removal of Extraluminal Device from Salivary Gland, Open Approach
0CPA0YZ	Removal of Other Device from Salivary Gland, Open Approach
0CPA30Z	Removal of Drainage Device from Salivary Gland, Percutaneous Approach
0CPA3CZ	Removal of Extraluminal Device from Salivary Gland, Percutaneous Approach
0CPA3YZ	Removal of Other Device from Salivary Gland, Percutaneous Approach
0CPA7YZ	Removal of Other Device from Salivary Gland, Via Natural or Artificial Opening
0CPA8YZ	Removal of Other Device from Salivary Gland, Via Natural or Artificial Opening Endoscopic
0CPS00Z	Removal of Drainage Device from Larynx, Open Approach
0CPS07Z	Removal of Autologous Tissue Substitute from Larynx, Open Approach

0CPS0DZ   Removal of Intraluminal Device from Larynx, Open Approach
0CPS0JZ   Removal of Synthetic Substitute from Larynx, Open Approach
0CPS0KZ   Removal of Nonautologous Tissue Substitute from Larynx, Open Approach
0CPS0YZ   Removal of Other Device from Larynx, Open Approach
0CPS30Z   Removal of Drainage Device from Larynx, Percutaneous Approach
0CPS37Z   Removal of Autologous Tissue Substitute from Larynx, Percutaneous Approach
0CPS3DZ   Removal of Intraluminal Device from Larynx, Percutaneous Approach
0CPS3JZ   Removal of Synthetic Substitute from Larynx, Percutaneous Approach
0CPS3KZ   Removal of Nonautologous Tissue Substitute from Larynx, Percutaneous Approach
0CPS3YZ   Removal of Other Device from Larynx, Percutaneous Approach
0CPS70Z   Removal of Drainage Device from Larynx, Via Natural or Artificial Opening
0CPS77Z   Removal of Autologous Tissue Substitute from Larynx, Via Natural or Artificial Opening
0CPS7DZ   Removal of Intraluminal Device from Larynx, Via Natural or Artificial Opening
0CPS7JZ   Removal of Synthetic Substitute from Larynx, Via Natural or Artificial Opening
0CPS7KZ   Removal of Nonautologous Tissue Substitute from Larynx, Via Natural or Artificial Opening
0CPS7YZ   Removal of Other Device from Larynx, Via Natural or Artificial Opening
0CPS80Z   Removal of Drainage Device from Larynx, Via Natural or Artificial Opening Endoscopic
0CPS87Z   Removal of Autologous Tissue Substitute from Larynx, Via Natural or Artificial Opening Endoscopic
0CPS8DZ   Removal of Intraluminal Device from Larynx, Via Natural or Artificial Opening Endoscopic
0CPS8JZ   Removal of Synthetic Substitute from Larynx, Via Natural or Artificial Opening Endoscopic
0CPS8KZ   Removal of Nonautologous Tissue Substitute from Larynx, Via Natural or Artificial Opening Endoscopic

0CPS8YZ   Removal of Other Device from Larynx, Via Natural or Artificial Opening Endoscopic
0CPSX0Z   Removal of Drainage Device from Larynx, External Approach
0CPSX7Z   Removal of Autologous Tissue Substitute from Larynx, External Approach
0CPSXDZ   Removal of Intraluminal Device from Larynx, External Approach
0CPSXJZ   Removal of Synthetic Substitute from Larynx, External Approach
0CPSXKZ   Removal of Nonautologous Tissue Substitute from Larynx, External Approach
0CPY00Z   Removal of Drainage Device from Mouth and Throat, Open Approach
0CPY01Z   Removal of Radioactive Element from Mouth and Throat, Open Approach
0CPY07Z   Removal of Autologous Tissue Substitute from Mouth and Throat, Open Approach
0CPY0DZ   Removal of Intraluminal Device from Mouth and Throat, Open Approach
0CPY0JZ   Removal of Synthetic Substitute from Mouth and Throat, Open Approach
0CPY0KZ   Removal of Nonautologous Tissue Substitute from Mouth and Throat, Open Approach
0CPY0YZ   Removal of Other Device from Mouth and Throat, Open Approach
0CPY30Z   Removal of Drainage Device from Mouth and Throat, Percutaneous Approach
0CPY31Z   Removal of Radioactive Element from Mouth and Throat, Percutaneous Approach
0CPY37Z   Removal of Autologous Tissue Substitute from Mouth and Throat, Percutaneous Approach
0CPY3DZ   Removal of Intraluminal Device from Mouth and Throat, Percutaneous Approach
0CPY3JZ   Removal of Synthetic Substitute from Mouth and Throat, Percutaneous Approach
0CPY3KZ   Removal of Nonautologous Tissue Substitute from Mouth and Throat, Percutaneous Approach
0CPY3YZ   Removal of Other Device from Mouth and Throat, Percutaneous Approach
0CPY70Z   Removal of Drainage Device from Mouth and Throat, Via Natural or Artificial Opening

0CPY71Z   Removal of Radioactive Element from Mouth and Throat, Via Natural or Artificial Opening
0CPY77Z   Removal of Autologous Tissue Substitute from Mouth and Throat, Via Natural or Artificial Opening
0CPY7DZ   Removal of Intraluminal Device from Mouth and Throat, Via Natural or Artificial Opening
0CPY7JZ   Removal of Synthetic Substitute from Mouth and Throat, Via Natural or Artificial Opening
0CPY7KZ   Removal of Nonautologous Tissue Substitute from Mouth and Throat, Via Natural or Artificial Opening
0CPY7YZ   Removal of Other Device from Mouth and Throat, Via Natural or Artificial Opening
0CPY80Z   Removal of Drainage Device from Mouth and Throat, Via Natural or Artificial Opening Endoscopic
0CPY81Z   Removal of Radioactive Element from Mouth and Throat, Via Natural or Artificial Opening Endoscopic
0CPY87Z   Removal of Autologous Tissue Substitute from Mouth and Throat, Via Natural or Artificial Opening Endoscopic
0CPY8DZ   Removal of Intraluminal Device from Mouth and Throat, Via Natural or Artificial Opening Endoscopic
0CPY8JZ   Removal of Synthetic Substitute from Mouth and Throat, Via Natural or Artificial Opening Endoscopic
0CPY8KZ   Removal of Nonautologous Tissue Substitute from Mouth and Throat, Via Natural or Artificial Opening Endoscopic
0CPY8YZ   Removal of Other Device from Mouth and Throat, Via Natural or Artificial Opening Endoscopic
0CPYX0Z   Removal of Drainage Device from Mouth and Throat, External Approach
0CPYX1Z   Removal of Radioactive Element from Mouth and Throat, External Approach
0CPYX7Z   Removal of Autologous Tissue Substitute from Mouth and Throat, External Approach
0CPYXDZ   Removal of Intraluminal Device from Mouth and Throat, External Approach
0CPYXJZ   Removal of Synthetic Substitute from Mouth and Throat, External Approach
0CPYXKZ   Removal of Nonautologous Tissue Substitute from Mouth and Throat, External Approach

0CQ – Mouth and Throat, Repair

0CQ00ZZ   Repair Upper Lip, Open Approach
0CQ03ZZ   Repair Upper Lip, Percutaneous Approach
0CQ0XZZ   Repair Upper Lip, External Approach
0CQ10ZZ   Repair Lower Lip, Open Approach
0CQ13ZZ   Repair Lower Lip, Percutaneous Approach
0CQ1XZZ   Repair Lower Lip, External Approach
0CQ20ZZ   Repair Hard Palate, Open Approach
0CQ23ZZ   Repair Hard Palate, Percutaneous Approach
0CQ2XZZ   Repair Hard Palate, External Approach
0CQ30ZZ   Repair Soft Palate, Open Approach
0CQ33ZZ   Repair Soft Palate, Percutaneous Approach
0CQ3XZZ   Repair Soft Palate, External Approach
0CQ40ZZ   Repair Buccal Mucosa, Open Approach

0CQ43ZZ   Repair Buccal Mucosa, Percutaneous Approach
0CQ4XZZ   Repair Buccal Mucosa, External Approach
0CQ50ZZ   Repair Upper Gingiva, Open Approach
AHA CC: 1Q, 2017, 20-21
0CQ53ZZ   Repair Upper Gingiva, Percutaneous Approach
0CQ5XZZ   Repair Upper Gingiva, External Approach
0CQ60ZZ   Repair Lower Gingiva, Open Approach
0CQ63ZZ   Repair Lower Gingiva, Percutaneous Approach
0CQ6XZZ   Repair Lower Gingiva, External Approach
0CQ70ZZ   Repair Tongue, Open Approach
0CQ73ZZ   Repair Tongue, Percutaneous Approach

0CQ7XZZ   Repair Tongue, External Approach
0CQ80ZZ   Repair Right Parotid Gland, Open Approach
0CQ83ZZ   Repair Right Parotid Gland, Percutaneous Approach
0CQ90ZZ   Repair Left Parotid Gland, Open Approach
0CQ93ZZ   Repair Left Parotid Gland, Percutaneous Approach
0CQB0ZZ   Repair Right Parotid Duct, Open Approach
0CQB3ZZ   Repair Right Parotid Duct, Percutaneous Approach
0CQC0ZZ   Repair Left Parotid Duct, Open Approach
0CQC3ZZ   Repair Left Parotid Duct, Percutaneous Approach

♀ Female-only   ♂ Male-only   ▲ Limited Coverage   ● Non-OR   **HAC** HAC-associated procedure   ▲ Non-covered procedures   ✚ Cluster

0CQD0ZZ	Repair Right Sublingual Gland, Open Approach
0CQD3ZZ	Repair Right Sublingual Gland, Percutaneous Approach
0CQF0ZZ	Repair Left Sublingual Gland, Open Approach
0CQF3ZZ	Repair Left Sublingual Gland, Percutaneous Approach
0CQG0ZZ	Repair Right Submaxillary Gland, Open Approach
0CQG3ZZ	Repair Right Submaxillary Gland, Percutaneous Approach
0CQH0ZZ	Repair Left Submaxillary Gland, Open Approach
0CQH3ZZ	Repair Left Submaxillary Gland, Percutaneous Approach
0CQJ0ZZ	Repair Minor Salivary Gland, Open Approach
0CQJ3ZZ	Repair Minor Salivary Gland, Percutaneous Approach
0CQM0ZZ	Repair Pharynx, Open Approach
0CQM3ZZ	Repair Pharynx, Percutaneous Approach
0CQM4ZZ	Repair Pharynx, Percutaneous Endoscopic Approach
0CQM7ZZ	Repair Pharynx, Via Natural or Artificial Opening
0CQM8ZZ	Repair Pharynx, Via Natural or Artificial Opening Endoscopic
0CQN0ZZ	Repair Uvula, Open Approach
0CQN3ZZ	Repair Uvula, Percutaneous Approach
0CQNXZZ	Repair Uvula, External Approach
0CQP0ZZ	Repair Tonsils, Open Approach
0CQP3ZZ	Repair Tonsils, Percutaneous Approach

0CQPXZZ	Repair Tonsils, External Approach
0CQQ0ZZ	Repair Adenoids, Open Approach
0CQQ3ZZ	Repair Adenoids, Percutaneous Approach
0CQQXZZ	Repair Adenoids, External Approach
0CQR0ZZ	Repair Epiglottis, Open Approach
0CQR3ZZ	Repair Epiglottis, Percutaneous Approach
0CQR4ZZ	Repair Epiglottis, Percutaneous Endoscopic Approach
0CQR7ZZ	Repair Epiglottis, Via Natural or Artificial Opening
0CQR8ZZ	Repair Epiglottis, Via Natural or Artificial Opening Endoscopic
0CQS0ZZ	Repair Larynx, Open Approach
0CQS3ZZ	Repair Larynx, Percutaneous Approach
0CQS4ZZ	Repair Larynx, Percutaneous Endoscopic Approach
0CQS7ZZ	Repair Larynx, Via Natural or Artificial Opening
0CQS8ZZ	Repair Larynx, Via Natural or Artificial Opening Endoscopic
0CQT0ZZ	Repair Right Vocal Cord, Open Approach
0CQT3ZZ	Repair Right Vocal Cord, Percutaneous Approach
0CQT4ZZ	Repair Right Vocal Cord, Percutaneous Endoscopic Approach
0CQT7ZZ	Repair Right Vocal Cord, Via Natural or Artificial Opening
0CQT8ZZ	Repair Right Vocal Cord, Via Natural or Artificial Opening Endoscopic
0CQV0ZZ	Repair Left Vocal Cord, Open Approach

0CQV3ZZ	Repair Left Vocal Cord, Percutaneous Approach
0CQV4ZZ	Repair Left Vocal Cord, Percutaneous Endoscopic Approach
0CQV7ZZ	Repair Left Vocal Cord, Via Natural or Artificial Opening
0CQV8ZZ	Repair Left Vocal Cord, Via Natural or Artificial Opening Endoscopic
0CQW0Z0	Repair of Upper Tooth, Single, Open Approach
0CQW0Z1	Repair of Upper Tooth, Multiple, Open Approach
0CQW0Z2	Repair of Upper Tooth, All, Open Approach
0CQWXZ0	Repair of Upper Tooth, Single, External Approach
0CQWXZ1	Repair of Upper Tooth, Multiple, External Approach
0CQWXZ2	Repair of Upper Tooth, All, External Approach
0CQX0Z0	Repair of Lower Tooth, Single, Open Approach
0CQX0Z1	Repair of Lower Tooth, Multiple, Open Approach
0CQX0Z2	Repair of Lower Tooth, All, Open Approach
0CQXXZ0	Repair of Lower Tooth, Single, External Approach
0CQXXZ1	Repair of Lower Tooth, Multiple, External Approach
0CQXXZ2	Repair of Lower Tooth, All, External Approach

0CR – Mouth and Throat, Replacement

Review Coding Guideline B3.18

0CR007Z	Replacement of Upper Lip with Autologous Tissue Substitute, Open Approach
0CR00JZ	Replacement of Upper Lip with Synthetic Substitute, Open Approach
0CR00KZ	Replacement of Upper Lip with Nonautologous Tissue Substitute, Open Approach
0CR037Z	Replacement of Upper Lip with Autologous Tissue Substitute, Percutaneous Approach
0CR03JZ	Replacement of Upper Lip with Synthetic Substitute, Percutaneous Approach
0CR03KZ	Replacement of Upper Lip with Nonautologous Tissue Substitute, Percutaneous Approach
0CR0X7Z	Replacement of Upper Lip with Autologous Tissue Substitute, External Approach
0CR0XJZ	Replacement of Upper Lip with Synthetic Substitute, External Approach
0CR0XKZ	Replacement of Upper Lip with Nonautologous Tissue Substitute, External Approach
0CR107Z	Replacement of Lower Lip with Autologous Tissue Substitute, Open Approach
0CR10JZ	Replacement of Lower Lip with Synthetic Substitute, Open Approach
0CR10KZ	Replacement of Lower Lip with Nonautologous Tissue Substitute, Open Approach
0CR137Z	Replacement of Lower Lip with Autologous Tissue Substitute, Percutaneous Approach

0CR13JZ	Replacement of Lower Lip with Synthetic Substitute, Percutaneous Approach
0CR13KZ	Replacement of Lower Lip with Nonautologous Tissue Substitute, Percutaneous Approach
0CR1X7Z	Replacement of Lower Lip with Autologous Tissue Substitute, External Approach
0CR1XJZ	Replacement of Lower Lip with Synthetic Substitute, External Approach
0CR1XKZ	Replacement of Lower Lip with Nonautologous Tissue Substitute, External Approach
0CR207Z	Replacement of Hard Palate with Autologous Tissue Substitute, Open Approach
0CR20JZ	Replacement of Hard Palate with Synthetic Substitute, Open Approach
0CR20KZ	Replacement of Hard Palate with Nonautologous Tissue Substitute, Open Approach
0CR237Z	Replacement of Hard Palate with Autologous Tissue Substitute, Percutaneous Approach
0CR23JZ	Replacement of Hard Palate with Synthetic Substitute, Percutaneous Approach
0CR23KZ	Replacement of Hard Palate with Nonautologous Tissue Substitute, Percutaneous Approach
0CR2X7Z	Replacement of Hard Palate with Autologous Tissue Substitute, External Approach
0CR2XJZ	Replacement of Hard Palate with Synthetic Substitute, External Approach

0CR2XKZ	Replacement of Hard Palate with Nonautologous Tissue Substitute, External Approach
0CR307Z	Replacement of Soft Palate with Autologous Tissue Substitute, Open Approach
0CR30JZ	Replacement of Soft Palate with Synthetic Substitute, Open Approach
0CR30KZ	Replacement of Soft Palate with Nonautologous Tissue Substitute, Open Approach
0CR337Z	Replacement of Soft Palate with Autologous Tissue Substitute, Percutaneous Approach
0CR33JZ	Replacement of Soft Palate with Synthetic Substitute, Percutaneous Approach
0CR33KZ	Replacement of Soft Palate with Nonautologous Tissue Substitute, Percutaneous Approach
0CR3X7Z	Replacement of Soft Palate with Autologous Tissue Substitute, External Approach
0CR3XJZ	Replacement of Soft Palate with Synthetic Substitute, External Approach
	AHA CC: 3Q, 2014, 25
0CR3XKZ	Replacement of Soft Palate with Nonautologous Tissue Substitute, External Approach
0CR407Z	Replacement of Buccal Mucosa with Autologous Tissue Substitute, Open Approach
0CR40JZ	Replacement of Buccal Mucosa with Synthetic Substitute, Open Approach
0CR40KZ	Replacement of Buccal Mucosa with Nonautologous Tissue Substitute, Open Approach

0CR437Z Replacement of Buccal Mucosa with Autologous Tissue Substitute, Percutaneous Approach

0CR43JZ Replacement of Buccal Mucosa with Synthetic Substitute, Percutaneous Approach

0CR43KZ Replacement of Buccal Mucosa with Nonautologous Tissue Substitute, Percutaneous Approach

0CR4X7Z Replacement of Buccal Mucosa with Autologous Tissue Substitute, External Approach

0CR4XJZ Replacement of Buccal Mucosa with Synthetic Substitute, External Approach

0CR4XKZ Replacement of Buccal Mucosa with Nonautologous Tissue Substitute, External Approach
AHA CC: 2Q, 2014, 5-6

0CR507Z Replacement of Upper Gingiva with Autologous Tissue Substitute, Open Approach

0CR50JZ Replacement of Upper Gingiva with Synthetic Substitute, Open Approach

0CR50KZ Replacement of Upper Gingiva with Nonautologous Tissue Substitute, Open Approach

0CR537Z Replacement of Upper Gingiva with Autologous Tissue Substitute, Percutaneous Approach

0CR53JZ Replacement of Upper Gingiva with Synthetic Substitute, Percutaneous Approach

0CR53KZ Replacement of Upper Gingiva with Nonautologous Tissue Substitute, Percutaneous Approach

0CR5X7Z Replacement of Upper Gingiva with Autologous Tissue Substitute, External Approach

0CR5XJZ Replacement of Upper Gingiva with Synthetic Substitute, External Approach

0CR5XKZ Replacement of Upper Gingiva with Nonautologous Tissue Substitute, External Approach

0CR607Z Replacement of Lower Gingiva with Autologous Tissue Substitute, Open Approach

0CR60JZ Replacement of Lower Gingiva with Synthetic Substitute, Open Approach

0CR60KZ Replacement of Lower Gingiva with Nonautologous Tissue Substitute, Open Approach

0CR637Z Replacement of Lower Gingiva with Autologous Tissue Substitute, Percutaneous Approach

0CR63JZ Replacement of Lower Gingiva with Synthetic Substitute, Percutaneous Approach

0CR63KZ Replacement of Lower Gingiva with Nonautologous Tissue Substitute, Percutaneous Approach

0CR6X7Z Replacement of Lower Gingiva with Autologous Tissue Substitute, External Approach

0CR6XJZ Replacement of Lower Gingiva with Synthetic Substitute, External Approach

0CR6XKZ Replacement of Lower Gingiva with Nonautologous Tissue Substitute, External Approach

0CR707Z Replacement of Tongue with Autologous Tissue Substitute, Open Approach

0CR70JZ Replacement of Tongue with Synthetic Substitute, Open Approach

0CR70KZ Replacement of Tongue with Nonautologous Tissue Substitute, Open Approach

0CR737Z Replacement of Tongue with Autologous Tissue Substitute, Percutaneous Approach

0CR73JZ Replacement of Tongue with Synthetic Substitute, Percutaneous Approach

0CR73KZ Replacement of Tongue with Nonautologous Tissue Substitute, Percutaneous Approach

0CR7X7Z Replacement of Tongue with Autologous Tissue Substitute, External Approach

0CR7XJZ Replacement of Tongue with Synthetic Substitute, External Approach

0CR7XKZ Replacement of Tongue with Nonautologous Tissue Substitute, External Approach

0CRB07Z Replacement of Right Parotid Duct with Autologous Tissue Substitute, Open Approach

0CRB0JZ Replacement of Right Parotid Duct with Synthetic Substitute, Open Approach

0CRB0KZ Replacement of Right Parotid Duct with Nonautologous Tissue Substitute, Open Approach

0CRB37Z Replacement of Right Parotid Duct with Autologous Tissue Substitute, Percutaneous Approach

0CRB3JZ Replacement of Right Parotid Duct with Synthetic Substitute, Percutaneous Approach

0CRB3KZ Replacement of Right Parotid Duct with Nonautologous Tissue Substitute, Percutaneous Approach

0CRC07Z Replacement of Left Parotid Duct with Autologous Tissue Substitute, Open Approach

0CRC0JZ Replacement of Left Parotid Duct with Synthetic Substitute, Open Approach

0CRC0KZ Replacement of Left Parotid Duct with Nonautologous Tissue Substitute, Open Approach

0CRC37Z Replacement of Left Parotid Duct with Autologous Tissue Substitute, Percutaneous Approach

0CRC3JZ Replacement of Left Parotid Duct with Synthetic Substitute, Percutaneous Approach

0CRC3KZ Replacement of Left Parotid Duct with Nonautologous Tissue Substitute, Percutaneous Approach

0CRM07Z Replacement of Pharynx with Autologous Tissue Substitute, Open Approach

0CRM0JZ Replacement of Pharynx with Synthetic Substitute, Open Approach

0CRM0KZ Replacement of Pharynx with Nonautologous Tissue Substitute, Open Approach

0CRM77Z Replacement of Pharynx with Autologous Tissue Substitute, Via Natural or Artificial Opening

0CRM7JZ Replacement of Pharynx with Synthetic Substitute, Via Natural or Artificial Opening

0CRM7KZ Replacement of Pharynx with Nonautologous Tissue Substitute, Via Natural or Artificial Opening

0CRM87Z Replacement of Pharynx with Autologous Tissue Substitute, Via Natural or Artificial Opening Endoscopic

0CRM8JZ Replacement of Pharynx with Synthetic Substitute, Via Natural or Artificial Opening Endoscopic

0CRM8KZ Replacement of Pharynx with Nonautologous Tissue Substitute, Via Natural or Artificial Opening Endoscopic

0CRN07Z Replacement of Uvula with Autologous Tissue Substitute, Open Approach

0CRN0JZ Replacement of Uvula with Synthetic Substitute, Open Approach

0CRN0KZ Replacement of Uvula with Nonautologous Tissue Substitute, Open Approach

0CRN37Z Replacement of Uvula with Autologous Tissue Substitute, Percutaneous Approach

0CRN3JZ Replacement of Uvula with Synthetic Substitute, Percutaneous Approach

0CRN3KZ Replacement of Uvula with Nonautologous Tissue Substitute, Percutaneous Approach

0CRNX7Z Replacement of Uvula with Autologous Tissue Substitute, External Approach

0CRNXJZ Replacement of Uvula with Synthetic Substitute, External Approach

0CRNXKZ Replacement of Uvula with Nonautologous Tissue Substitute, External Approach

0CRR07Z Replacement of Epiglottis with Autologous Tissue Substitute, Open Approach

0CRR0JZ Replacement of Epiglottis with Synthetic Substitute, Open Approach

0CRR0KZ Replacement of Epiglottis with Nonautologous Tissue Substitute, Open Approach

0CRR77Z Replacement of Epiglottis with Autologous Tissue Substitute, Via Natural or Artificial Opening

0CRR7JZ Replacement of Epiglottis with Synthetic Substitute, Via Natural or Artificial Opening

0CRR7KZ Replacement of Epiglottis with Nonautologous Tissue Substitute, Via Natural or Artificial Opening

0CRR87Z Replacement of Epiglottis with Autologous Tissue Substitute, Via Natural or Artificial Opening Endoscopic

0CRR8JZ Replacement of Epiglottis with Synthetic Substitute, Via Natural or Artificial Opening Endoscopic

0CRR8KZ Replacement of Epiglottis with Nonautologous Tissue Substitute, Via Natural or Artificial Opening Endoscopic

0CRS07Z Replacement of Larynx with Autologous Tissue Substitute, Open Approach

0CRS0JZ Replacement of Larynx with Synthetic Substitute, Open Approach

0CRS0KZ Replacement of Larynx with Nonautologous Tissue Substitute, Open Approach

0CRS77Z Replacement of Larynx with Autologous Tissue Substitute, Via Natural or Artificial Opening

0CRS7JZ Replacement of Larynx with Synthetic Substitute, Via Natural or Artificial Opening

0CRS7KZ Replacement of Larynx with Nonautologous Tissue Substitute, Via Natural or Artificial Opening

♀ Female-only   ♂ Male-only   ▲ Limited Coverage   ● Non-OR   ⬛ HAC-associated procedure   ▲ Non-covered procedures   ✚ Cluster

CRS87Z Replacement of Larynx with Autologous Tissue Substitute, Via Natural or Artificial Opening Endoscopic

CRS8JZ Replacement of Larynx with Synthetic Substitute, Via Natural or Artificial Opening Endoscopic

CRS8KZ Replacement of Larynx with Nonautologous Tissue Substitute, Via Natural or Artificial Opening Endoscopic

CRT07Z Replacement of Right Vocal Cord with Autologous Tissue Substitute, Open Approach

CRT0JZ Replacement of Right Vocal Cord with Synthetic Substitute, Open Approach

CRT0KZ Replacement of Right Vocal Cord with Nonautologous Tissue Substitute, Open Approach

CRT77Z Replacement of Right Vocal Cord with Autologous Tissue Substitute, Via Natural or Artificial Opening

0CRT7JZ Replacement of Right Vocal Cord with Synthetic Substitute, Via Natural or Artificial Opening

0CRT7KZ Replacement of Right Vocal Cord with Nonautologous Tissue Substitute, Via Natural or Artificial Opening

0CRT87Z Replacement of Right Vocal Cord with Autologous Tissue Substitute, Via Natural or Artificial Opening Endoscopic

0CRT8JZ Replacement of Right Vocal Cord with Synthetic Substitute, Via Natural or Artificial Opening Endoscopic

0CRT8KZ Replacement of Right Vocal Cord with Nonautologous Tissue Substitute, Via Natural or Artificial Opening Endoscopic

0CRV07Z Replacement of Left Vocal Cord with Autologous Tissue Substitute, Open Approach

0CRV0JZ Replacement of Left Vocal Cord with Synthetic Substitute, Open Approach

0CRV0KZ Replacement of Left Vocal Cord with Nonautologous Tissue Substitute, Open Approach

0CRV77Z Replacement of Left Vocal Cord with Autologous Tissue Substitute, Via Natural or Artificial Opening

0CRV7JZ Replacement of Left Vocal Cord with Synthetic Substitute, Via Natural or Artificial Opening

0CRV7KZ Replacement of Left Vocal Cord with Nonautologous Tissue Substitute, Via Natural or Artificial Opening

0CRV87Z Replacement of Left Vocal Cord with Autologous Tissue Substitute, Via Natural or Artificial Opening Endoscopic

0CRV8JZ Replacement of Left Vocal Cord with Synthetic Substitute, Via Natural or Artificial Opening Endoscopic

0CRV8KZ Replacement of Left Vocal Cord with Nonautologous Tissue Substitute, Via Natural or Artificial Opening Endoscopic

0CRW070 Replacement of Upper Tooth, Single, with Autologous Tissue Substitute, Open Approach

0CRW071 Replacement of Upper Tooth, Multiple, with Autologous Tissue Substitute, Open Approach

0CRW072 Replacement of Upper Tooth, All, with Autologous Tissue Substitute, Open Approach

0CRW0J0 Replacement of Upper Tooth, Single, with Synthetic Substitute, Open Approach

0CRW0J1 Replacement of Upper Tooth, Multiple, with Synthetic Substitute, Open Approach

0CRW0J2 Replacement of Upper Tooth, All, with Synthetic Substitute, Open Approach

0CRW0K0 Replacement of Upper Tooth, Single, with Nonautologous Tissue Substitute, Open Approach

0CRW0K1 Replacement of Upper Tooth, Multiple, with Nonautologous Tissue Substitute, Open Approach

0CRW0K2 Replacement of Upper Tooth, All, with Nonautologous Tissue Substitute, Open Approach

0CRWX70 Replacement of Upper Tooth, Single, with Autologous Tissue Substitute, External Approach

0CRWX71 Replacement of Upper Tooth, Multiple, with Autologous Tissue Substitute, External Approach

0CRWX72 Replacement of Upper Tooth, All, with Autologous Tissue Substitute, External Approach

0CRWXJ0 Replacement of Upper Tooth, Single, with Synthetic Substitute, External Approach

0CRWXJ1 Replacement of Upper Tooth, Multiple, with Synthetic Substitute, External Approach

0CRWXJ2 Replacement of Upper Tooth, All, with Synthetic Substitute, External Approach

0CRWXK0 Replacement of Upper Tooth, Single, with Nonautologous Tissue Substitute, External Approach

0CRWXK1 Replacement of Upper Tooth, Multiple, with Nonautologous Tissue Substitute, External Approach

0CRWXK2 Replacement of Upper Tooth, All, with Nonautologous Tissue Substitute, External Approach

0CRX070 Replacement of Lower Tooth, Single, with Autologous Tissue Substitute, Open Approach

0CRX071 Replacement of Lower Tooth, Multiple, with Autologous Tissue Substitute, Open Approach

0CRX072 Replacement of Lower Tooth, All, with Autologous Tissue Substitute, Open Approach

0CRX0J0 Replacement of Lower Tooth, Single, with Synthetic Substitute, Open Approach

0CRX0J1 Replacement of Lower Tooth, Multiple, with Synthetic Substitute, Open Approach

0CRX0J2 Replacement of Lower Tooth, All, with Synthetic Substitute, Open Approach

0CRX0K0 Replacement of Lower Tooth, Single, with Nonautologous Tissue Substitute, Open Approach

0CRX0K1 Replacement of Lower Tooth, Multiple, with Nonautologous Tissue Substitute, Open Approach

0CRX0K2 Replacement of Lower Tooth, All, with Nonautologous Tissue Substitute, Open Approach

0CRXX70 Replacement of Lower Tooth, Single, with Autologous Tissue Substitute, External Approach

0CRXX71 Replacement of Lower Tooth, Multiple, with Autologous Tissue Substitute, External Approach

0CRXX72 Replacement of Lower Tooth, All, with Autologous Tissue Substitute, External Approach

0CRXXJ0 Replacement of Lower Tooth, Single, with Synthetic Substitute, External Approach

0CRXXJ1 Replacement of Lower Tooth, Multiple, with Synthetic Substitute, External Approach

0CRXXJ2 Replacement of Lower Tooth, All, with Synthetic Substitute, External Approach

0CRXXK0 Replacement of Lower Tooth, Single, with Nonautologous Tissue Substitute, External Approach

0CRXXK1 Replacement of Lower Tooth, Multiple, with Nonautologous Tissue Substitute, External Approach

0CRXXK2 Replacement of Lower Tooth, All, with Nonautologous Tissue Substitute, External Approach

0CS – Mouth and Throat, Reposition

0CS00ZZ Reposition Upper Lip, Open Approach

0CS0XZZ Reposition Upper Lip, External Approach

0CS10ZZ Reposition Lower Lip, Open Approach

0CS1XZZ Reposition Lower Lip, External Approach

0CS20ZZ Reposition Hard Palate, Open Approach

0CS2XZZ Reposition Hard Palate, External Approach

0CS30ZZ Reposition Soft Palate, Open Approach

0CS3XZZ Reposition Soft Palate, External Approach

0CS70ZZ Reposition Tongue, Open Approach

0CS7XZZ Reposition Tongue, External Approach

0CSB0ZZ Reposition Right Parotid Duct, Open Approach

0CSB3ZZ Reposition Right Parotid Duct, Percutaneous Approach

0CSC0ZZ Reposition Left Parotid Duct, Open Approach

0CSC3ZZ Reposition Left Parotid Duct, Percutaneous Approach

0CSN0ZZ Reposition Uvula, Open Approach

0CSNXZZ Reposition Uvula, External Approach

0CSR0ZZ Reposition Epiglottis, Open Approach

0CSR7ZZ Reposition Epiglottis, Via Natural or Artificial Opening

0CSR8ZZ Reposition Epiglottis, Via Natural or Artificial Opening Endoscopic
AHA CC: 3Q, 2016, 28-29

0CST0ZZ Reposition Right Vocal Cord, Open Approach

0CST7ZZ Reposition Right Vocal Cord, Via Natural or Artificial Opening

0CST8ZZ Reposition Right Vocal Cord, Via Natural or Artificial Opening Endoscopic

0CSV0ZZ	Reposition Left Vocal Cord, Open Approach	0CSWX50	Reposition Upper Tooth, Single, with External Fixation Device, External Approach	0CSX0Z0	Reposition Lower Tooth, Single, Open Approach
0CSV7ZZ	Reposition Left Vocal Cord, Via Natural or Artificial Opening	0CSWX51	Reposition Upper Tooth, Multiple, with External Fixation Device, External Approach	0CSX0Z1	Reposition Lower Tooth, Multiple, Open Approach
0CSV8ZZ	Reposition Left Vocal Cord, Via Natural or Artificial Opening Endoscopic	0CSWX52	Reposition Upper Tooth, All, with External Fixation Device, External Approach	0CSX0Z2	Reposition Lower Tooth, All, Open Approach
0CSW050	Reposition Upper Tooth with External Fixation Device, Single, Open Approach	0CSWXZ0	Reposition Upper Tooth, Single, External Approach	0CSXX50	Reposition Lower Tooth, Single, with External Fixation Device, External Approach
0CSW051	Reposition Upper Tooth with External Fixation Device, Multiple, Open Approach	0CSWXZ1	Reposition Upper Tooth, Multiple, External Approach	0CSXX51	Reposition Lower Tooth, Multiple, with External Fixation Device, External Approach
0CSW052	Reposition Upper Tooth with External Fixation Device, All, Open Approach	0CSWXZ2	Reposition Upper Tooth, All, External Approach	0CSXX52	Reposition Lower Tooth, All, with External Fixation Device, External Approach
0CSW0Z0	Reposition Upper Tooth, Single, Open Approach	0CSX050	Reposition Lower Tooth with External Fixation Device, Single, Open Approach	0CSXXZ0	Reposition Lower Tooth, Single, External Approach
0CSW0Z1	Reposition Upper Tooth, Multiple, Open Approach	0CSX051	Reposition Lower Tooth with External Fixation Device, Multiple, Open Approach	0CSXXZ1	Reposition Lower Tooth, Multiple, External Approach
0CSW0Z2	Reposition Upper Tooth, All, Open Approach	0CSX052	Reposition Lower Tooth with External Fixation Device, All, Open Approach	0CSXXZ2	Reposition Lower Tooth, All, External Approach

0CT – Mouth and Throat, Resection

Review Coding Guideline B3.8

Review Coding Guideline B3.18

0CT00ZZ	Resection of Upper Lip, Open Approach	0CTH0ZZ	Resection of Left Submaxillary Gland, Open Approach	0CTS8ZZ	Resection of Larynx, Via Natural or Artificial Opening Endoscopic
0CT0XZZ	Resection of Upper Lip, External Approach	0CTJ0ZZ	Resection of Minor Salivary Gland, Open Approach	0CTT0ZZ	Resection of Right Vocal Cord, Open Approach
0CT10ZZ	Resection of Lower Lip, Open Approach	0CTM0ZZ	Resection of Pharynx, Open Approach	0CTT4ZZ	Resection of Right Vocal Cord, Percutaneous Endoscopic Approach
0CT1XZZ	Resection of Lower Lip, External Approach	0CTM4ZZ	Resection of Pharynx, Percutaneous Endoscopic Approach	0CTT7ZZ	Resection of Right Vocal Cord, Via Natural or Artificial Opening
0CT20ZZ	Resection of Hard Palate, Open Approach	0CTM7ZZ	Resection of Pharynx, Via Natural or Artificial Opening	0CTT8ZZ	Resection of Right Vocal Cord, Via Natural or Artificial Opening Endoscopic
0CT2XZZ	Resection of Hard Palate, External Approach	0CTM8ZZ	Resection of Pharynx, Via Natural or Artificial Opening Endoscopic	0CTV0ZZ	Resection of Left Vocal Cord, Open Approach
0CT30ZZ	Resection of Soft Palate, Open Approach	0CTN0ZZ	Resection of Uvula, Open Approach	0CTV4ZZ	Resection of Left Vocal Cord, Percutaneous Endoscopic Approach
0CT3XZZ	Resection of Soft Palate, External Approach	0CTNXZZ	Resection of Uvula, External Approach	0CTV7ZZ	Resection of Left Vocal Cord, Via Natural or Artificial Opening
0CT70ZZ	Resection of Tongue, Open Approach	0CTP0ZZ	Resection of Tonsils, Open Approach	0CTV8ZZ	Resection of Left Vocal Cord, Via Natural or Artificial Opening Endoscopic
0CT7XZZ	Resection of Tongue, External Approach	0CTPXZZ	Resection of Tonsils, External Approach	0CTW0Z0	Resection of Upper Tooth, Single, Open Approach
0CT80ZZ	Resection of Right Parotid Gland, Open Approach	0CTQ0ZZ	Resection of Adenoids, Open Approach	0CTW0Z1	Resection of Upper Tooth, Multiple, Open Approach
0CT90ZZ	Resection of Left Parotid Gland, Open Approach	0CTQXZZ	Resection of Adenoids, External Approach	*AHA CC: 3Q, 2014, 23-24*	
AHA CC: 2Q, 2016, 12-14		0CTR0ZZ	Resection of Epiglottis, Open Approach	0CTW0Z2	Resection of Upper Tooth, All, Open Approach
0CTB0ZZ	Resection of Right Parotid Duct, Open Approach	0CTR4ZZ	Resection of Epiglottis, Percutaneous Endoscopic Approach	0CTX0Z0	Resection of Lower Tooth, Single, Open Approach
0CTC0ZZ	Resection of Left Parotid Duct, Open Approach	0CTR7ZZ	Resection of Epiglottis, Via Natural or Artificial Opening	0CTX0Z1	Resection of Lower Tooth, Multiple, Open Approach
0CTD0ZZ	Resection of Right Sublingual Gland, Open Approach	0CTR8ZZ	Resection of Epiglottis, Via Natural or Artificial Opening Endoscopic	*AHA CC: 3Q, 2014, 23-24*	
0CTF0ZZ	Resection of Left Sublingual Gland, Open Approach	0CTS0ZZ	Resection of Larynx, Open Approach	0CTX0Z2	Resection of Lower Tooth, All, Open Approach
0CTG0ZZ	Resection of Right Submaxillary Gland, Open Approach	0CTS4ZZ	Resection of Larynx, Percutaneous Endoscopic Approach		
		0CTS7ZZ	Resection of Larynx, Via Natural or Artificial Opening		

0CU – Mouth and Throat, Supplement

0CU007Z	Supplement Upper Lip with Autologous Tissue Substitute, Open Approach	0CU03JZ	Supplement Upper Lip with Synthetic Substitute, Percutaneous Approach	0CU0XKZ	Supplement Upper Lip with Nonautologous Tissue Substitute, External Approach
0CU00JZ	Supplement Upper Lip with Synthetic Substitute, Open Approach	0CU03KZ	Supplement Upper Lip with Nonautologous Tissue Substitute, Percutaneous Approach	0CU107Z	Supplement Lower Lip with Autologous Tissue Substitute, Open Approach
0CU00KZ	Supplement Upper Lip with Nonautologous Tissue Substitute, Open Approach	0CU0X7Z	Supplement Upper Lip with Autologous Tissue Substitute, External Approach	0CU10JZ	Supplement Lower Lip with Synthetic Substitute, Open Approach
0CU037Z	Supplement Upper Lip with Autologous Tissue Substitute, Percutaneous Approach	0CU0XJZ	Supplement Upper Lip with Synthetic Substitute, External Approach	0CU10KZ	Supplement Lower Lip with Nonautologous Tissue Substitute, Open Approach

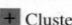

0CU137Z Supplement Lower Lip with Autologous Tissue Substitute, Percutaneous Approach

0CU13JZ Supplement Lower Lip with Synthetic Substitute, Percutaneous Approach

0CU13KZ Supplement Lower Lip with Nonautologous Tissue Substitute, Percutaneous Approach

0CU1X7Z Supplement Lower Lip with Autologous Tissue Substitute, External Approach

0CU1XJZ Supplement Lower Lip with Synthetic Substitute, External Approach

0CU1XKZ Supplement Lower Lip with Nonautologous Tissue Substitute, External Approach

0CU207Z Supplement Hard Palate with Autologous Tissue Substitute, Open Approach

0CU20JZ Supplement Hard Palate with Synthetic Substitute, Open Approach

0CU20KZ Supplement Hard Palate with Nonautologous Tissue Substitute, Open Approach

0CU237Z Supplement Hard Palate with Autologous Tissue Substitute, Percutaneous Approach

0CU23JZ Supplement Hard Palate with Synthetic Substitute, Percutaneous Approach

0CU23KZ Supplement Hard Palate with Nonautologous Tissue Substitute, Percutaneous Approach

0CU2X7Z Supplement Hard Palate with Autologous Tissue Substitute, External Approach

0CU2XJZ Supplement Hard Palate with Synthetic Substitute, External Approach

0CU2XKZ Supplement Hard Palate with Nonautologous Tissue Substitute, External Approach

0CU307Z Supplement Soft Palate with Autologous Tissue Substitute, Open Approach

0CU30JZ Supplement Soft Palate with Synthetic Substitute, Open Approach

0CU30KZ Supplement Soft Palate with Nonautologous Tissue Substitute, Open Approach

0CU337Z Supplement Soft Palate with Autologous Tissue Substitute, Percutaneous Approach

0CU33JZ Supplement Soft Palate with Synthetic Substitute, Percutaneous Approach

0CU33KZ Supplement Soft Palate with Nonautologous Tissue Substitute, Percutaneous Approach

0CU3X7Z Supplement Soft Palate with Autologous Tissue Substitute, External Approach

0CU3XJZ Supplement Soft Palate with Synthetic Substitute, External Approach

0CU3XKZ Supplement Soft Palate with Nonautologous Tissue Substitute, External Approach

0CU407Z Supplement Buccal Mucosa with Autologous Tissue Substitute, Open Approach

0CU40JZ Supplement Buccal Mucosa with Synthetic Substitute, Open Approach

0CU40KZ Supplement Buccal Mucosa with Nonautologous Tissue Substitute, Open Approach

0CU437Z Supplement Buccal Mucosa with Autologous Tissue Substitute, Percutaneous Approach

0CU43JZ Supplement Buccal Mucosa with Synthetic Substitute, Percutaneous Approach

0CU43KZ Supplement Buccal Mucosa with Nonautologous Tissue Substitute, Percutaneous Approach

0CU4X7Z Supplement Buccal Mucosa with Autologous Tissue Substitute, External Approach

0CU4XJZ Supplement Buccal Mucosa with Synthetic Substitute, External Approach

0CU4XKZ Supplement Buccal Mucosa with Nonautologous Tissue Substitute, External Approach

0CU507Z Supplement Upper Gingiva with Autologous Tissue Substitute, Open Approach

0CU50JZ Supplement Upper Gingiva with Synthetic Substitute, Open Approach

0CU50KZ Supplement Upper Gingiva with Nonautologous Tissue Substitute, Open Approach

0CU537Z Supplement Upper Gingiva with Autologous Tissue Substitute, Percutaneous Approach

0CU53JZ Supplement Upper Gingiva with Synthetic Substitute, Percutaneous Approach

0CU53KZ Supplement Upper Gingiva with Nonautologous Tissue Substitute, Percutaneous Approach

0CU5X7Z Supplement Upper Gingiva with Autologous Tissue Substitute, External Approach

0CU5XJZ Supplement Upper Gingiva with Synthetic Substitute, External Approach

0CU5XKZ Supplement Upper Gingiva with Nonautologous Tissue Substitute, External Approach

0CU607Z Supplement Lower Gingiva with Autologous Tissue Substitute, Open Approach

0CU60JZ Supplement Lower Gingiva with Synthetic Substitute, Open Approach

0CU60KZ Supplement Lower Gingiva with Nonautologous Tissue Substitute, Open Approach

0CU637Z Supplement Lower Gingiva with Autologous Tissue Substitute, Percutaneous Approach

0CU63JZ Supplement Lower Gingiva with Synthetic Substitute, Percutaneous Approach

0CU63KZ Supplement Lower Gingiva with Nonautologous Tissue Substitute, Percutaneous Approach

0CU6X7Z Supplement Lower Gingiva with Autologous Tissue Substitute, External Approach

0CU6XJZ Supplement Lower Gingiva with Synthetic Substitute, External Approach

0CU6XKZ Supplement Lower Gingiva with Nonautologous Tissue Substitute, External Approach

0CU707Z Supplement Tongue with Autologous Tissue Substitute, Open Approach

0CU70JZ Supplement Tongue with Synthetic Substitute, Open Approach

0CU70KZ Supplement Tongue with Nonautologous Tissue Substitute, Open Approach

0CU737Z Supplement Tongue with Autologous Tissue Substitute, Percutaneous Approach

0CU73JZ Supplement Tongue with Synthetic Substitute, Percutaneous Approach

0CU73KZ Supplement Tongue with Nonautologous Tissue Substitute, Percutaneous Approach

0CU7X7Z Supplement Tongue with Autologous Tissue Substitute, External Approach

0CU7XJZ Supplement Tongue with Synthetic Substitute, External Approach

0CU7XKZ Supplement Tongue with Nonautologous Tissue Substitute, External Approach

0CUM07Z Supplement Pharynx with Autologous Tissue Substitute, Open Approach

0CUM0JZ Supplement Pharynx with Synthetic Substitute, Open Approach

0CUM0KZ Supplement Pharynx with Nonautologous Tissue Substitute, Open Approach

0CUM77Z Supplement Pharynx with Autologous Tissue Substitute, Via Natural or Artificial Opening

0CUM7JZ Supplement Pharynx with Synthetic Substitute, Via Natural or Artificial Opening

0CUM7KZ Supplement Pharynx with Nonautologous Tissue Substitute, Via Natural or Artificial Opening

0CUM87Z Supplement Pharynx with Autologous Tissue Substitute, Via Natural or Artificial Opening Endoscopic

0CUM8JZ Supplement Pharynx with Synthetic Substitute, Via Natural or Artificial Opening Endoscopic

0CUM8KZ Supplement Pharynx with Nonautologous Tissue Substitute, Via Natural or Artificial Opening Endoscopic

0CUN07Z Supplement Uvula with Autologous Tissue Substitute, Open Approach

0CUN0JZ Supplement Uvula with Synthetic Substitute, Open Approach

0CUN0KZ Supplement Uvula with Nonautologous Tissue Substitute, Open Approach

0CUN37Z Supplement Uvula with Autologous Tissue Substitute, Percutaneous Approach

0CUN3JZ Supplement Uvula with Synthetic Substitute, Percutaneous Approach

0CUN3KZ Supplement Uvula with Nonautologous Tissue Substitute, Percutaneous Approach

0CUNX7Z Supplement Uvula with Autologous Tissue Substitute, External Approach

0CUNXJZ Supplement Uvula with Synthetic Substitute, External Approach

0CUNXKZ Supplement Uvula with Nonautologous Tissue Substitute, External Approach

0CUR07Z Supplement Epiglottis with Autologous Tissue Substitute, Open Approach

0CUR0JZ Supplement Epiglottis with Synthetic Substitute, Open Approach

0CUR0KZ Supplement Epiglottis with Nonautologous Tissue Substitute, Open Approach

0CUR77Z Supplement Epiglottis with Autologous Tissue Substitute, Via Natural or Artificial Opening

0CUR7JZ Supplement Epiglottis with Synthetic Substitute, Via Natural or Artificial Opening

0CUR7KZ Supplement Epiglottis with Nonautologous Tissue Substitute, Via Natural or Artificial Opening

0CUR87Z	Supplement Epiglottis with Autologous Tissue Substitute, Via Natural or Artificial Opening Endoscopic	**0CUS8JZ**	Supplement Larynx with Synthetic Substitute, Via Natural or Artificial Opening Endoscopic	**0CUT8KZ**	Supplement Right Vocal Cord with Nonautologous Tissue Substitute, Via Natural or Artificial Opening Endoscopic
0CUR8JZ	Supplement Epiglottis with Synthetic Substitute, Via Natural or Artificial Opening Endoscopic	**0CUS8KZ**	Supplement Larynx with Nonautologous Tissue Substitute, Via Natural or Artificial Opening Endoscopic	**0CUV07Z**	Supplement Left Vocal Cord with Autologous Tissue Substitute, Open Approach
0CUR8KZ	Supplement Epiglottis with Nonautologous Tissue Substitute, Via Natural or Artificial Opening Endoscopic	**0CUT07Z**	Supplement Right Vocal Cord with Autologous Tissue Substitute, Open Approach	**0CUV0JZ**	Supplement Left Vocal Cord with Synthetic Substitute, Open Approach
0CUS07Z	Supplement Larynx with Autologous Tissue Substitute, Open Approach	**0CUT0JZ**	Supplement Right Vocal Cord with Synthetic Substitute, Open Approach	**0CUV0KZ**	Supplement Left Vocal Cord with Nonautologous Tissue Substitute, Open Approach
0CUS0JZ	Supplement Larynx with Synthetic Substitute, Open Approach	**0CUT0KZ**	Supplement Right Vocal Cord with Nonautologous Tissue Substitute, Open Approach	**0CUV77Z**	Supplement Left Vocal Cord with Autologous Tissue Substitute, Via Natural or Artificial Opening
0CUS0KZ	Supplement Larynx with Nonautologous Tissue Substitute, Open Approach	**0CUT77Z**	Supplement Right Vocal Cord with Autologous Tissue Substitute, Via Natural or Artificial Opening	**0CUV7JZ**	Supplement Left Vocal Cord with Synthetic Substitute, Via Natural or Artificial Opening
0CUS77Z	Supplement Larynx with Autologous Tissue Substitute, Via Natural or Artificial Opening	**0CUT7JZ**	Supplement Right Vocal Cord with Synthetic Substitute, Via Natural or Artificial Opening	**0CUV7KZ**	Supplement Left Vocal Cord with Nonautologous Tissue Substitute, Via Natural or Artificial Opening
0CUS7JZ	Supplement Larynx with Synthetic Substitute, Via Natural or Artificial Opening	**0CUT7KZ**	Supplement Right Vocal Cord with Nonautologous Tissue Substitute, Via Natural or Artificial Opening	**0CUV87Z**	Supplement Left Vocal Cord with Autologous Tissue Substitute, Via Natural or Artificial Opening Endoscopic
0CUS7KZ	Supplement Larynx with Nonautologous Tissue Substitute, Via Natural or Artificial Opening	**0CUT87Z**	Supplement Right Vocal Cord with Autologous Tissue Substitute, Via Natural or Artificial Opening Endoscopic	**0CUV8JZ**	Supplement Left Vocal Cord with Synthetic Substitute, Via Natural or Artificial Opening Endoscopic
0CUS87Z	Supplement Larynx with Autologous Tissue Substitute, Via Natural or Artificial Opening Endoscopic	**0CUT8JZ**	Supplement Right Vocal Cord with Synthetic Substitute, Via Natural or Artificial Opening Endoscopic	**0CUV8KZ**	Supplement Left Vocal Cord with Nonautologous Tissue Substitute, Via Natural or Artificial Opening Endoscopic

0CV – Mouth and Throat, Restriction

0CVB0CZ	Restriction of Right Parotid Duct with Extraluminal Device, Open Approach	**0CVB7ZZ**	Restriction of Right Parotid Duct, Via Natural or Artificial Opening	**0CVC3DZ**	Restriction of Left Parotid Duct with Intraluminal Device, Percutaneous Approach
0CVB0DZ	Restriction of Right Parotid Duct with Intraluminal Device, Open Approach	**0CVB8DZ**	Restriction of Right Parotid Duct with Intraluminal Device, Via Natural or Artificial Opening Endoscopic	**0CVC3ZZ**	Restriction of Left Parotid Duct, Percutaneous Approach
0CVB0ZZ	Restriction of Right Parotid Duct, Open Approach	**0CVB8ZZ**	Restriction of Right Parotid Duct, Via Natural or Artificial Opening Endoscopic	**0CVC7DZ**	Restriction of Left Parotid Duct with Intraluminal Device, Via Natural or Artificial Opening
0CVB3CZ	Restriction of Right Parotid Duct with Extraluminal Device, Percutaneous Approach	**0CVC0CZ**	Restriction of Left Parotid Duct with Extraluminal Device, Open Approach	**0CVC7ZZ**	Restriction of Left Parotid Duct, Via Natural or Artificial Opening
0CVB3DZ	Restriction of Right Parotid Duct with Intraluminal Device, Percutaneous Approach	**0CVC0DZ**	Restriction of Left Parotid Duct with Intraluminal Device, Open Approach	**0CVC8DZ**	Restriction of Left Parotid Duct with Intraluminal Device, Via Natural or Artificial Opening Endoscopic
0CVB3ZZ	Restriction of Right Parotid Duct, Percutaneous Approach	**0CVC0ZZ**	Restriction of Left Parotid Duct, Open Approach	**0CVC8ZZ**	Restriction of Left Parotid Duct, Via Natural or Artificial Opening Endoscopic
0CVB7DZ	Restriction of Right Parotid Duct with Intraluminal Device, Via Natural or Artificial Opening	**0CVC3CZ**	Restriction of Left Parotid Duct with Extraluminal Device, Percutaneous Approach		

0CW – Mouth and Throat, Revision

Review Coding Guideline B6.1c

0CWA00Z	Revision of Drainage Device in Salivary Gland, Open Approach	**0CWAX0Z**	Revision of Drainage Device in Salivary Gland, External Approach	**0CWS37Z**	Revision of Autologous Tissue Substitute in Larynx, Percutaneous Approach
0CWA0CZ	Revision of Extraluminal Device in Salivary Gland, Open Approach	**0CWAXCZ**	Revision of Extraluminal Device in Salivary Gland, External Approach	**0CWS3DZ**	Revision of Intraluminal Device in Larynx, Percutaneous Approach
0CWA0YZ	Revision of Other Device in Salivary Gland, Open Approach	**0CWS00Z**	Revision of Drainage Device in Larynx, Open Approach	**0CWS3JZ**	Revision of Synthetic Substitute in Larynx, Percutaneous Approach
0CWA30Z	Revision of Drainage Device in Salivary Gland, Percutaneous Approach	**0CWS07Z**	Revision of Autologous Tissue Substitute in Larynx, Open Approach	**0CWS3KZ**	Revision of Nonautologous Tissue Substitute in Larynx, Percutaneous Approach
0CWA3CZ	Revision of Extraluminal Device in Salivary Gland, Percutaneous Approach	**0CWS0DZ**	Revision of Intraluminal Device in Larynx, Open Approach	**0CWS3YZ**	Revision of Other Device in Larynx, Percutaneous Approach
0CWA3YZ	Revision of Other Device in Salivary Gland, Percutaneous Approach	**0CWS0JZ**	Revision of Synthetic Substitute in Larynx, Open Approach	**0CWS70Z**	Revision of Drainage Device in Larynx, Via Natural or Artificial Opening
0CWA7YZ	Revision of Other Device in Salivary Gland, Via Natural or Artificial Opening	**0CWS0KZ**	Revision of Nonautologous Tissue Substitute in Larynx, Open Approach	**0CWS77Z**	Revision of Autologous Tissue Substitute in Larynx, Via Natural or Artificial Opening
0CWA8YZ	Revision of Other Device in Salivary Gland, Via Natural or Artificial Opening Endoscopic	**0CWS0YZ**	Revision of Other Device in Larynx, Open Approach	**0CWS7DZ**	Revision of Intraluminal Device in Larynx, Via Natural or Artificial Opening
		0CWS30Z	Revision of Drainage Device in Larynx, Percutaneous Approach		

♀ Female-only   ♂ Male-only   ▲ Limited Coverage   ● Non-OR   HAC HAC-associated procedure   ▲ Non-covered procedures   ✚ Cluster

0CWS7JZ	Revision of Synthetic Substitute in Larynx, Via Natural or Artificial Opening
0CWS7KZ	Revision of Nonautologous Tissue Substitute in Larynx, Via Natural or Artificial Opening
0CWS7YZ	Revision of Other Device in Larynx, Via Natural or Artificial Opening
0CWS80Z	Revision of Drainage Device in Larynx, Via Natural or Artificial Opening Endoscopic
0CWS87Z	Revision of Autologous Tissue Substitute in Larynx, Via Natural or Artificial Opening Endoscopic
0CWS8DZ	Revision of Intraluminal Device in Larynx, Via Natural or Artificial Opening Endoscopic
0CWS8JZ	Revision of Synthetic Substitute in Larynx, Via Natural or Artificial Opening Endoscopic
0CWS8KZ	Revision of Nonautologous Tissue Substitute in Larynx, Via Natural or Artificial Opening Endoscopic
0CWS8YZ	Revision of Other Device in Larynx, Via Natural or Artificial Opening Endoscopic
0CWSX0Z	Revision of Drainage Device in Larynx, External Approach
0CWSX7Z	Revision of Autologous Tissue Substitute in Larynx, External Approach
0CWSXDZ	Revision of Intraluminal Device in Larynx, External Approach
0CWSXJZ	Revision of Synthetic Substitute in Larynx, External Approach
0CWSXKZ	Revision of Nonautologous Tissue Substitute in Larynx, External Approach
0CWY00Z	Revision of Drainage Device in Mouth and Throat, Open Approach
0CWY01Z	Revision of Radioactive Element in Mouth and Throat, Open Approach
0CWY07Z	Revision of Autologous Tissue Substitute in Mouth and Throat, Open Approach
0CWY0DZ	Revision of Intraluminal Device in Mouth and Throat, Open Approach
0CWY0JZ	Revision of Synthetic Substitute in Mouth and Throat, Open Approach
0CWY0KZ	Revision of Nonautologous Tissue Substitute in Mouth and Throat, Open Approach
0CWY0YZ	Revision of Other Device in Mouth and Throat, Open Approach
0CWY30Z	Revision of Drainage Device in Mouth and Throat, Percutaneous Approach
0CWY31Z	Revision of Radioactive Element in Mouth and Throat, Percutaneous Approach
0CWY37Z	Revision of Autologous Tissue Substitute in Mouth and Throat, Percutaneous Approach
0CWY3DZ	Revision of Intraluminal Device in Mouth and Throat, Percutaneous Approach
0CWY3JZ	Revision of Synthetic Substitute in Mouth and Throat, Percutaneous Approach
0CWY3KZ	Revision of Nonautologous Tissue Substitute in Mouth and Throat, Percutaneous Approach
0CWY3YZ	Revision of Other Device in Mouth and Throat, Percutaneous Approach
0CWY70Z	Revision of Drainage Device in Mouth and Throat, Via Natural or Artificial Opening
0CWY71Z	Revision of Radioactive Element in Mouth and Throat, Via Natural or Artificial Opening
0CWY77Z	Revision of Autologous Tissue Substitute in Mouth and Throat, Via Natural or Artificial Opening
0CWY7DZ	Revision of Intraluminal Device in Mouth and Throat, Via Natural or Artificial Opening
0CWY7JZ	Revision of Synthetic Substitute in Mouth and Throat, Via Natural or Artificial Opening
0CWY7KZ	Revision of Nonautologous Tissue Substitute in Mouth and Throat, Via Natural or Artificial Opening
0CWY7YZ	Revision of Other Device in Mouth and Throat, Via Natural or Artificial Opening
0CWY80Z	Revision of Drainage Device in Mouth and Throat, Via Natural or Artificial Opening Endoscopic
0CWY81Z	Revision of Radioactive Element in Mouth and Throat, Via Natural or Artificial Opening Endoscopic
0CWY87Z	Revision of Autologous Tissue Substitute in Mouth and Throat, Via Natural or Artificial Opening Endoscopic
0CWY8DZ	Revision of Intraluminal Device in Mouth and Throat, Via Natural or Artificial Opening Endoscopic
0CWY8JZ	Revision of Synthetic Substitute in Mouth and Throat, Via Natural or Artificial Opening Endoscopic
0CWY8KZ	Revision of Nonautologous Tissue Substitute in Mouth and Throat, Via Natural or Artificial Opening Endoscopic
0CWY8YZ	Revision of Other Device in Mouth and Throat, Via Natural or Artificial Opening Endoscopic
0CWYX0Z	Revision of Drainage Device in Mouth and Throat, External Approach
0CWYX1Z	Revision of Radioactive Element in Mouth and Throat, External Approach
0CWYX7Z	Revision of Autologous Tissue Substitute in Mouth and Throat, External Approach
0CWYXDZ	Revision of Intraluminal Device in Mouth and Throat, External Approach
0CWYXJZ	Revision of Synthetic Substitute in Mouth and Throat, External Approach
0CWYXKZ	Revision of Nonautologous Tissue Substitute in Mouth and Throat, External Approach

0CX – Mouth and Throat, Transfer

0CX00ZZ	Transfer Upper Lip, Open Approach
0CX0XZZ	Transfer Upper Lip, External Approach
0CX10ZZ	Transfer Lower Lip, Open Approach
0CX1XZZ	Transfer Lower Lip, External Approach
0CX30ZZ	Transfer Soft Palate, Open Approach
0CX3XZZ	Transfer Soft Palate, External Approach
0CX40ZZ	Transfer Buccal Mucosa, Open Approach
0CX4XZZ	Transfer Buccal Mucosa, External Approach
0CX50ZZ	Transfer Upper Gingiva, Open Approach
0CX5XZZ	Transfer Upper Gingiva, External Approach
0CX60ZZ	Transfer Lower Gingiva, Open Approach
0CX6XZZ	Transfer Lower Gingiva, External Approach
0CX70ZZ	Transfer Tongue, Open Approach
0CX7XZZ	Transfer Tongue, External Approach

♀ Female-only   ♂ Male-only   ▲ Limited Coverage   ● Non-OR   HAC HAC-associated procedure   ▲ Non-covered procedures   ✚ Cluster

Gastrointestinal System: Organization

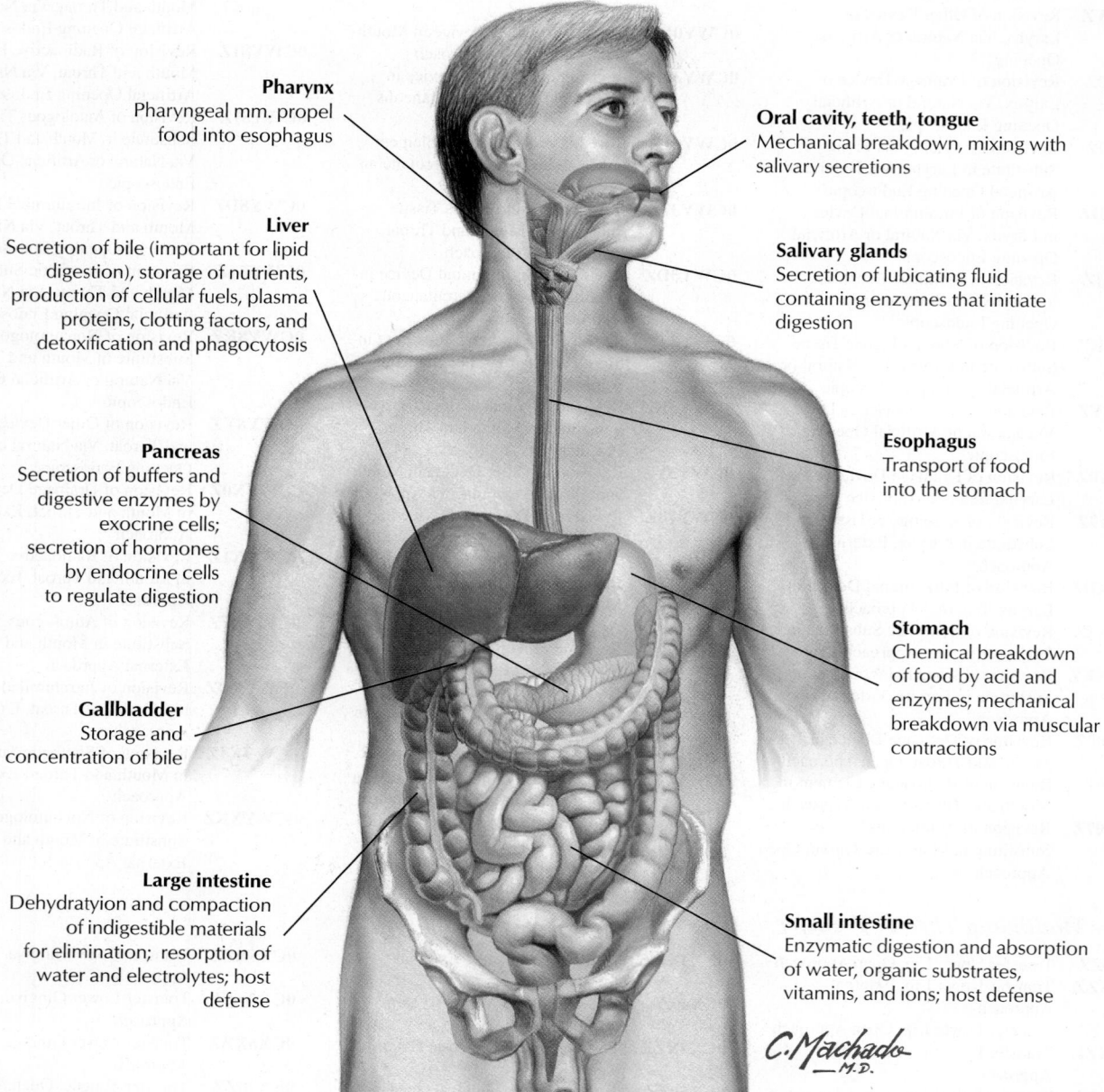

Pharynx
Pharyngeal mm. propel food into esophagus

Oral cavity, teeth, tongue
Mechanical breakdown, mixing with salivary secretions

Liver
Secretion of bile (important for lipid digestion), storage of nutrients, production of cellular fuels, plasma proteins, clotting factors, and detoxification and phagocytosis

Salivary glands
Secretion of lubicating fluid containing enzymes that initiate digestion

Pancreas
Secretion of buffers and digestive enzymes by exocrine cells; secretion of hormones by endocrine cells to regulate digestion

Esophagus
Transport of food into the stomach

Gallbladder
Storage and concentration of bile

Stomach
Chemical breakdown of food by acid and enzymes; mechanical breakdown via muscular contractions

Large intestine
Dehydratyion and compaction of indigestible materials for elimination; resorption of water and electrolytes; host defense

Small intestine
Enzymatic digestion and absorption of water, organic substrates, vitamins, and ions; host defense

C. Machado
—M.D.

Stomach, Liver, Gallbladder

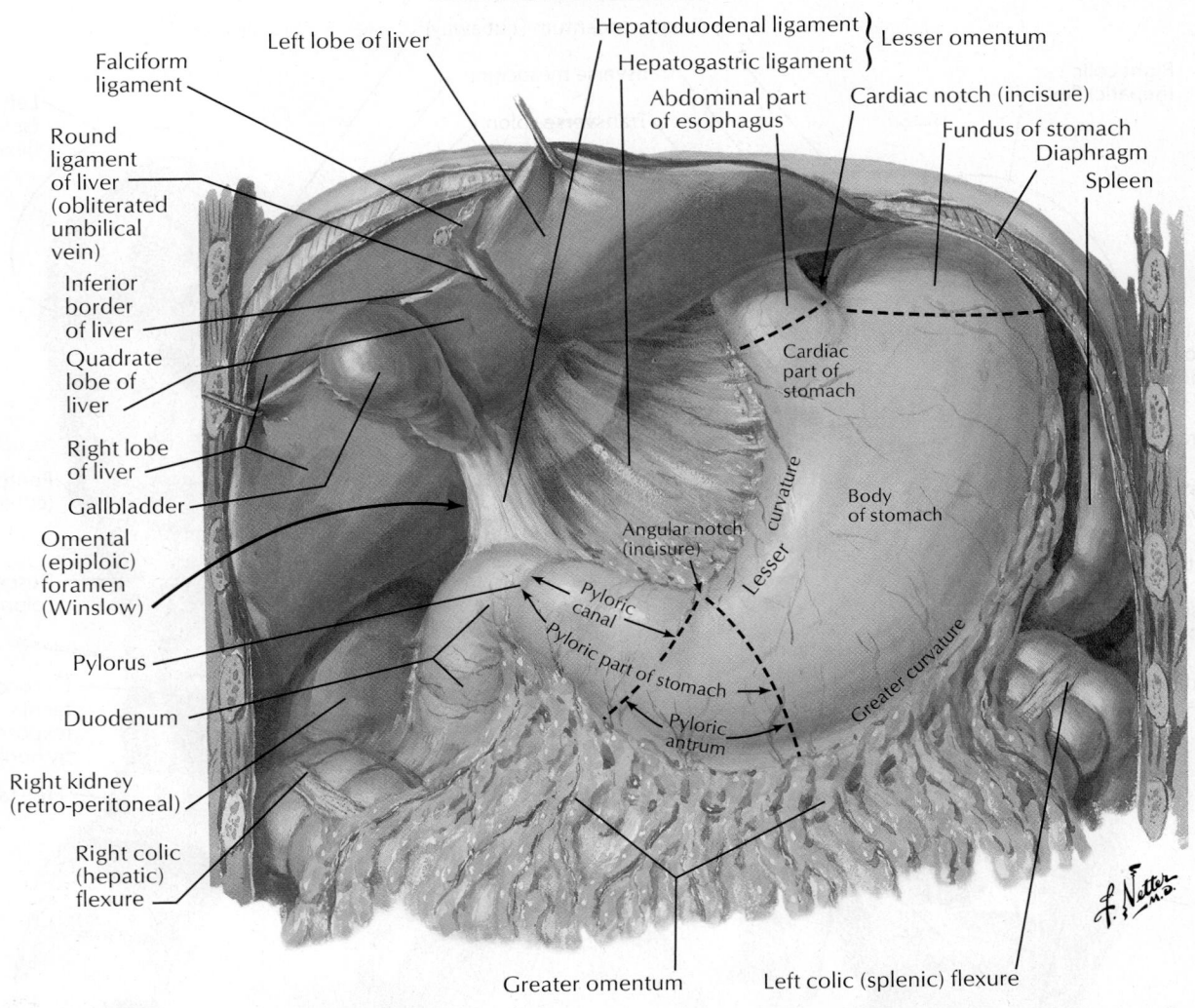

Falciform ligament

Left lobe of liver

Hepatoduodenal ligament

Hepatogastric ligament

} Lesser omentum

Abdominal part of esophagus

Cardiac notch (incisure)

Fundus of stomach
Diaphragm
Spleen

Round ligament of liver (obliterated umbilical vein)

Inferior border of liver

Quadrate lobe of liver

Right lobe of liver

Gallbladder

Omental (epiploic) foramen (Winslow)

Pylorus

Duodenum

Right kidney (retro-peritoneal)

Right colic (hepatic) flexure

Cardiac part of stomach

Body of stomach

Angular notch (incisure)

Lesser curvature

Pyloric canal

Pyloric part of stomach

Pyloric antrum

Greater curvature

Greater omentum

Left colic (splenic) flexure

©2006. Used with permission of Elsevier. All rights reserved.

Medical and Surgical, Gastrointestinal System

Large Intestine Structure of Colon

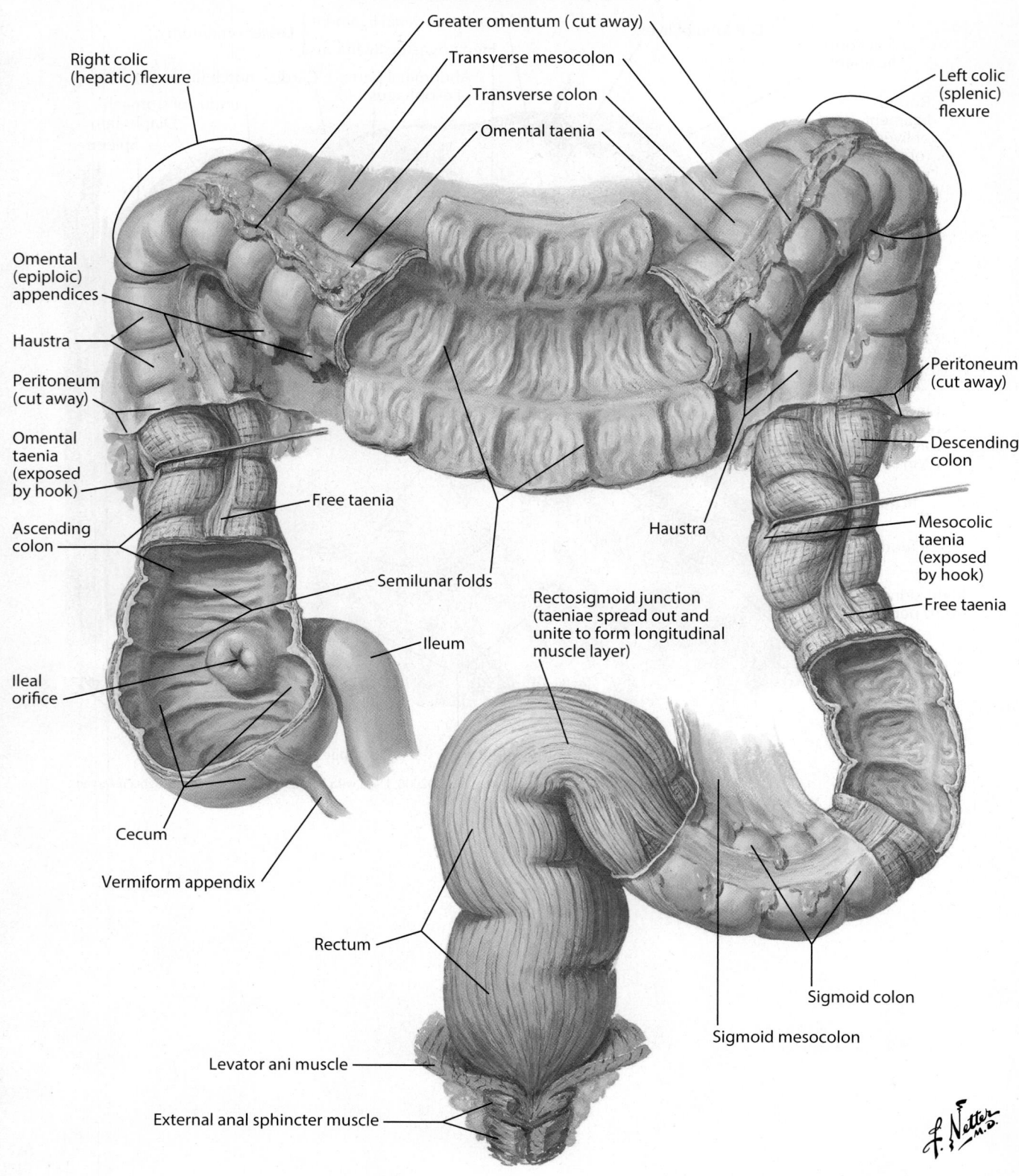

Greater omentum (cut away)

Transverse mesocolon

Transverse colon

Omental taenia

Right colic (hepatic) flexure

Left colic (splenic) flexure

Omental (epiploic) appendices

Haustra

Peritoneum (cut away)

Omental taenia (exposed by hook)

Ascending colon

Free taenia

Semilunar folds

Ileum

Peritoneum (cut away)

Descending colon

Haustra

Mesocolic taenia (exposed by hook)

Free taenia

Rectosigmoid junction (taeniae spread out and unite to form longitudinal muscle layer)

Ileal orifice

Cecum

Vermiform appendix

Rectum

Sigmoid colon

Sigmoid mesocolon

Levator ani muscle

External anal sphincter muscle

Treatment of Morbid Obesity

Gastric stapling (vertical banded gastroplasty)

Esophagus

Stomach pouch

Band

Gastric bypass (Roux-en-Y)

Stomach pouch

Oversewn staple lines

End-to-side type anastomosis
between the gastric pouch
and the Roux-en-Y limb

Duodenum

Bypassed portion of the stomach

Jejunum

C. Machado
_M.D._

Sleeve gastrectomy

Laparoscopic adjustable gastric banding

Adjustable band

Stomach

Skin

Subcutaneous
port (reservoir)

Rectus abdominis muscle

K. Marzejon

Gastrointestinal System Tables 0D1–0DY

Section	0	Medical and Surgical
Body System	D	Gastrointestinal System
Operation	1	**Bypass:** Altering the route of passage of the contents of a tubular body part

Body Part (4ᵗʰ)	Approach (5ᵗʰ)	Device (6ᵗʰ)	Qualifier (7ᵗʰ)
1 Esophagus, Upper 2 Esophagus, Middle 3 Esophagus, Lower 5 Esophagus	0 Open 4 Percutaneous Endoscopic 8 Via Natural or Artificial Opening Endoscopic	7 Autologous Tissue Substitute J Synthetic Substitute K Nonautologous Tissue Substitute Z No Device	4 Cutaneous 6 Stomach 9 Duodenum A Jejunum B Ileum
1 Esophagus, Upper 2 Esophagus, Middle 3 Esophagus, Lower 5 Esophagus	3 Percutaneous	J Synthetic Substitute	4 Cutaneous
6 Stomach 9 Duodenum	0 Open 4 Percutaneous Endoscopic 8 Via Natural or Artificial Opening Endoscopic	7 Autologous Tissue Substitute J Synthetic Substitute K Nonautologous Tissue Substitute Z No Device	4 Cutaneous 9 Duodenum A Jejunum B Ileum L Transverse Colon
6 Stomach 9 Duodenum	3 Percutaneous	J Synthetic Substitute	4 Cutaneous
8 Small Intestine	0 Open 4 Percutaneous Endoscopic 8 Via Natural or Artificial Opening Endoscopic	7 Autologous Tissue Substitute J Synthetic Substitute K Nonautologous Tissue Z No Device	4 Cutaneous 8 Small Intestine H Cecum K Ascending Colon L Transverse Colon M Descending Colon N Sigmoid Colon P Rectum Q Anus
A Jejunum	0 Open 4 Percutaneous Endoscopic 8 Via Natural or Artificial Opening Endoscopic	7 Autologous Tissue Substitute J Synthetic Substitute K Nonautologous Tissue Substitute Z No Device	4 Cutaneous A Jejunum B Ileum H Cecum K Ascending Colon L Transverse Colon M Descending Colon N Sigmoid Colon P Rectum Q Anus
A Jejunum	3 Percutaneous	J Synthetic Substitute	4 Cutaneous
B Ileum	0 Open 4 Percutaneous Endoscopic 8 Via Natural or Artificial Opening Endoscopic	7 Autologous Tissue Substitute J Synthetic Substitute K Nonautologous Tissue Substitute Z No Device	4 Cutaneous B Ileum H Cecum K Ascending Colon L Transverse Colon M Descending Colon N Sigmoid Colon P Rectum Q Anus
B Ileum	3 Percutaneous	J Synthetic Substitute	4 Cutaneous
E Large Intestine	0 Open 4 Percutaneous Endoscopic 8 Via Natural or Artificial Opening Endoscopic	7 Autologous Tissue Substitute J Synthetic Substitute K Nonautologous Tissue Z No Device	4 Cutaneous E Large Intestine P Rectum

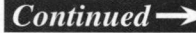
Continued →

Section   **0**   **Medical and Surgical**
Body System   **D**   **Gastrointestinal System**
Operation   **1**   **Bypass:** Altering the route of passage of the contents of a tubular body part

Body Part (4th)	Approach (5th)	Device (6th)	Qualifier (7th)
H Cecum	**0** Open **4** Percutaneous Endoscopic **8** Via Natural or Artificial Opening Endoscopic	**7** Autologous Tissue Substitute **J** Synthetic Substitute **K** Nonautologous Tissue Substitute **Z** No Device	**4** Cutaneous **H** Cecum **K** Ascending Colon **L** Transverse Colon **M** Descending Colon **N** Sigmoid Colon **P** Rectum
H Cecum	**3** Percutaneous	**J** Synthetic Substitute	**4** Cutaneous
K Ascending Colon	**0** Open **4** Percutaneous Endoscopic **8** Via Natural or Artificial Opening Endoscopic	**7** Autologous Tissue Substitute **J** Synthetic Substitute **K** Nonautologous Tissue Substitute **Z** No Device	**4** Cutaneous **K** Ascending Colon **L** Transverse Colon **M** Descending Colon **N** Sigmoid Colon **P** Rectum
K Ascending Colon	**3** Percutaneous	**J** Synthetic Substitute	**4** Cutaneous
L Transverse Colon	**0** Open **4** Percutaneous Endoscopic **8** Via Natural or Artificial Opening Endoscopic	**7** Autologous Tissue Substitute **J** Synthetic Substitute **K** Nonautologous Tissue Substitute **Z** No Device	**4** Cutaneous **L** Transverse Colon **M** Descending Colon **N** Sigmoid Colon **P** Rectum
L Transverse Colon	**3** Percutaneous	**J** Synthetic Substitute	**4** Cutaneous
M Descending Colon	**0** Open **4** Percutaneous Endoscopic **8** Via Natural or Artificial Opening Endoscopic	**7** Autologous Tissue Substitute **J** Synthetic Substitute **K** Nonautologous Tissue Substitute **Z** No Device	**4** Cutaneous **M** Descending Colon **N** Sigmoid Colon **P** Rectum
M Descending Colon	**3** Percutaneous	**J** Synthetic Substitute	**4** Cutaneous
N Sigmoid Colon	**0** Open **4** Percutaneous Endoscopic **8** Via Natural or Artificial Opening Endoscopic	**7** Autologous Tissue Substitute **J** Synthetic Substitute **K** Nonautologous Tissue Substitute **Z** No Device	**4** Cutaneous **N** Sigmoid Colon **P** Rectum
N Sigmoid Colon	**3** Percutaneous	**J** Synthetic Substitute	**4** Cutaneous

Section   **0**   **Medical and Surgical**
Body System   **D**   **Gastrointestinal System**
Operation   **2**   **Change:** Taking out or off a device from a body part and putting back an identical or similar device in or on the same body part without cutting or puncturing the skin or a mucous membrane

Body Part (4th)	Approach (5th)	Device (6th)	Qualifier (7th)
0 Upper Intestinal Tract **D** Lower Intestinal Tract	**X** External	**0** Drainage Device **U** Feeding Device **Y** Other Device	**Z** No Qualifier
U Omentum **V** Mesentery **W** Peritoneum	**X** External	**0** Drainage Device **Y** Other Device	**Z** No Qualifier

Section 0 Medical and Surgical
Body System D Gastrointestinal System
Operation 5 Destruction: Physical eradication of all or a portion of a body part by the direct use of energy, force, or a destructive agent

Body Part (4th)	Approach (5th)	Device (6th)	Qualifier (7th)
1 Esophagus, Upper 2 Esophagus, Middle 3 Esophagus, Lower 4 Esophagogastric Junction 5 Esophagus 6 Stomach 7 Stomach, Pylorus 8 Small Intestine 9 Duodenum A Jejunum B Ileum C Ileocecal Valve E Large Intestine F Large Intestine, Right G Large Intestine, Left H Cecum J Appendix K Ascending Colon L Transverse Colon M Descending Colon N Sigmoid Colon P Rectum	0 Open 3 Percutaneous 4 Percutaneous Endoscopic 7 Via Natural or Artificial Opening 8 Via Natural or Artificial Opening Endoscopic	Z No Device	Z No Qualifier
Q Anus	0 Open 3 Percutaneous 4 Percutaneous Endoscopic 7 Via Natural or Artificial Opening 8 Via Natural or Artificial Opening Endoscopic X External	Z No Device	Z No Qualifier
R Anal Sphincter U Omentum V Mesentery W Peritoneum	0 Open 3 Percutaneous 4 Percutaneous Endoscopic	Z No Device	Z No Qualifier

Section   **0**   **Medical and Surgical**
Body System   **D**   **Gastrointestinal System**
Operation   **7**   **Dilation:** Expanding an orifice or the lumen of a tubular body part

Body Part (4ᵗʰ)	Approach (5ᵗʰ)	Device (6ᵗʰ)	Qualifier (7ᵗʰ)
1 Esophagus, Upper 2 Esophagus, Middle 3 Esophagus, Lower 4 Esophagogastric Junction 5 Esophagus 6 Stomach 7 Stomach, Pylorus 8 Small Intestine 9 Duodenum A Jejunum B Ileum C Ileocecal Valve E Large Intestine F Large Intestine, Right G Large Intestine, Left H Cecum K Ascending Colon L Transverse Colon M Descending Colon N Sigmoid Colon P Rectum Q Anus	0 Open 3 Percutaneous 4 Percutaneous Endoscopic 7 Via Natural or Artificial Opening 8 Via Natural or Artificial Opening Endoscopic	D Intraluminal Device Z No Device	Z No Qualifier

Section   **0**   **Medical and Surgical**
Body System   **D**   **Gastrointestinal System**
Operation   **8**   **Division:** Cutting into a body part, without draining fluids and/or gases from the body part, in order to separate or transect a body part

Body Part (4ᵗʰ)	Approach (5ᵗʰ)	Device (6ᵗʰ)	Qualifier (7ᵗʰ)
4 Esophagogastric Junction 7 Stomach, Pylorus	0 Open 3 Percutaneous 4 Percutaneous Endoscopic 7 Via Natural or Artificial Opening 8 Via Natural or Artificial Opening Endoscopic	Z No Device	Z No Qualifier
R Anal Sphincter	0 Open 3 Percutaneous	Z No Device	Z No Qualifier

Section	0	**Medical and Surgical**
Body System	D	**Gastrointestinal System**
Operation	9	**Drainage:** Taking or letting out fluids and/or gases from a body part

Body Part (4th)	Approach (5th)	Device (6th)	Qualifier (7th)
1 Esophagus, Upper 2 Esophagus, Middle 3 Esophagus, Lower 4 Esophagogastric Junction 5 Esophagus 6 Stomach 7 Stomach, Pylorus 8 Small Intestine 9 Duodenum A Jejunum B Ileum C Ileocecal Valve E Large Intestine F Large Intestine, Right G Large Intestine, Left H Cecum J Appendix K Ascending Colon L Transverse Colon M Descending Colon N Sigmoid Colon P Rectum	0 Open 3 Percutaneous 4 Percutaneous Endoscopic 7 Via Natural or Artificial Opening 8 Via Natural or Artificial Opening Endoscopic	0 Drainage Device	Z No Qualifier
1 Esophagus, Upper 2 Esophagus, Middle 3 Esophagus, Lower 4 Esophagogastric Junction 5 Esophagus 6 Stomach 7 Stomach, Pylorus 8 Small Intestine 9 Duodenum A Jejunum B Ileum C Ileocecal Valve E Large Intestine F Large Intestine, Right G Large Intestine, Left H Cecum J Appendix K Ascending Colon L Transverse Colon M Descending Colon N Sigmoid Colon P Rectum	0 Open 3 Percutaneous 4 Percutaneous Endoscopic 7 Via Natural or Artificial Opening 8 Via Natural or Artificial Opening Endoscopic	Z No Device	X Diagnostic Z No Qualifier

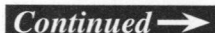

Continued →

Section   **0**   **Medical and Surgical**
Body System   **D**   **Gastrointestinal System**
Operation   **9**   **Drainage:** Taking or letting out fluids and/or gases from a body part

Body Part (4ᵗʰ)	Approach (5ᵗʰ)	Device (6ᵗʰ)	Qualifier (7ᵗʰ)
Q Anus	0 Open 3 Percutaneous 4 Percutaneous Endoscopic 7 Via Natural or Artificial Opening 8 Via Natural or Artificial Opening Endoscopic X External	0 Drainage Device	Z No Qualifier
Q Anus	0 Open 3 Percutaneous 4 Percutaneous Endoscopic 7 Via Natural or Artificial Opening 8 Via Natural or Artificial Opening Endoscopic X External	Z No Device	X Diagnostic Z No Qualifier
R Anal Sphincter U Omentum V Mesentery W Peritoneum	0 Open 3 Percutaneous 4 Percutaneous Endoscopic	0 Drainage Device	Z No Qualifier
R Anal Sphincter U Omentum V Mesentery W Peritoneum	0 Open 3 Percutaneous 4 Percutaneous Endoscopic	Z No Device	X Diagnostic Z No Qualifier

Section   **0**   **Medical and Surgical**
Body System   **D**   **Gastrointestinal System**
Operation   **B**   **Excision:** Cutting out or off, without replacement, a portion of a body part

Body Part (4ᵗʰ)	Approach (5ᵗʰ)	Device (6ᵗʰ)	Qualifier (7ᵗʰ)
1 Esophagus, Upper 2 Esophagus, Middle 3 Esophagus, Lower 4 Esophagogastric Junction 5 Esophagus 7 Stomach, Pylorus 8 Small Intestine 9 Duodenum A Jejunum B Ileum C Ileocecal Valve E Large Intestine F Large Intestine, Right H Cecum J Appendix K Ascending Colon P Rectum	0 Open 3 Percutaneous 4 Percutaneous Endoscopic 7 Via Natural or Artificial Opening 8 Via Natural or Artificial Opening Endoscopic	Z No Device	X Diagnostic Z No Qualifier
6 Stomach	0 Open 3 Percutaneous 4 Percutaneous Endoscopic 7 Via Natural or Artificial Opening 8 Via Natural or Artificial Opening Endoscopic	Z No Device	3 Vertical X Diagnostic Z No Qualifier
G Large Intestine, Left L Transverse Colon M Descending Colon N Sigmoid Colon	0 Open 3 Percutaneous 4 Percutaneous Endoscopic 7 Via Natural or Artificial Opening 8 Via Natural or Artificial Opening Endoscopic	Z No Device	X Diagnostic Z No Qualifier

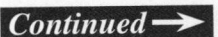
Continued →

Section	0	Medical and Surgical
Body System	D	Gastrointestinal System
Operation	B	Excision: Cutting out or off, without replacement, a portion of a body part

Body Part (4th)	Approach (5th)	Device (6th)	Qualifier (7th)
G Large Intestine, Left L Transverse Colon M Descending Colon N Sigmoid Colon	F Via Natural or Artificial Opening With Percutaneous Endoscopic Assistance	Z No Device	Z No Qualifier
Q Anus	0 Open 3 Percutaneous 4 Percutaneous Endoscopic 7 Via Natural or Artificial Opening 8 Via Natural or Artificial Opening Endoscopic X External	Z No Device	X Diagnostic Z No Qualifier
R Anal Sphincter U Omentum V Mesentery W Peritoneum	0 Open 3 Percutaneous 4 Percutaneous Endoscopic	Z No Device	X Diagnostic Z No Qualifier

Section	0	Medical and Surgical
Body System	D	Gastrointestinal System
Operation	C	Extirpation: Taking or cutting out solid matter from a body part

Body Part (4th)	Approach (5th)	Device (6th)	Qualifier (7th)
1 Esophagus, Upper 2 Esophagus, Middle 3 Esophagus, Lower 4 Esophagogastric Junction 5 Esophagus 6 Stomach 7 Stomach, Pylorus 8 Small Intestine 9 Duodenum A Jejunum B Ileum C Ileocecal Valve E Large Intestine F Large Intestine, Right G Large Intestine, Left H Cecum J Appendix K Ascending Colon L Transverse Colon M Descending Colon N Sigmoid Colon P Rectum	0 Open 3 Percutaneous 4 Percutaneous Endoscopic 7 Via Natural or Artificial Opening 8 Via Natural or Artificial Opening Endoscopic	Z No Device	Z No Qualifier
Q Anus	0 Open 3 Percutaneous 4 Percutaneous Endoscopic 7 Via Natural or Artificial Opening 8 Via Natural or Artificial Opening Endoscopic X External	Z No Device	Z No Qualifier
R Anal Sphincter U Omentum V Mesentery W Peritoneum	0 Open 3 Percutaneous 4 Percutaneous Endoscopic	Z No Device	Z No Qualifier

Section	0	Medical and Surgical
Body System	D	Gastrointestinal System
Operation	D	Extraction: Pulling or stripping out or off all or a portion of a body part by the use of force

Body Part (4th)	Approach (5th)	Device (6th)	Qualifier (7th)
1 Esophagus, Upper 2 Esophagus, Middle 3 Esophagus, Lower 4 Esophagogastric Junction 5 Esophagus 6 Stomach 7 Stomach, Pylorus 8 Small Intestine 9 Duodenum A Jejunum B Ileum C Ileocecal Valve E Large Intestine F Large Intestine, Right G Large Intestine, Left H Cecum J Appendix K Ascending Colon L Transverse Colon M Descending Colon N Sigmoid Colon P Rectum	3 Percutaneous 4 Percutaneous Endoscopic 8 Via Natural or Artificial Opening Endoscopic	Z No Device	X Diagnostic
Q Anus	3 Percutaneous 4 Percutaneous Endoscopic 8 Via Natural or Artificial Opening Endoscopic X External	Z No Device	X Diagnostic

Section	0	Medical and Surgical
Body System	D	Gastrointestinal System
Operation	F	Fragmentation: Breaking solid matter in a body part into pieces

Body Part (4th)	Approach (5th)	Device (6th)	Qualifier (7th)
5 Esophagus 6 Stomach 8 Small Intestine 9 Duodenum A Jejunum B Ileum E Large Intestine F Large Intestine, Right G Large Intestine, Left H Cecum J Appendix K Ascending Colon L Transverse Colon M Descending Colon N Sigmoid Colon P Rectum Q Anus	0 Open 3 Percutaneous 4 Percutaneous Endoscopic 7 Via Natural or Artificial Opening 8 Via Natural or Artificial Opening Endoscopic X External	Z No Device	Z No Qualifier

Section   0   **Medical and Surgical**
Body System   D   **Gastrointestinal System**
Operation   H   **Insertion:** Putting in a nonbiological appliance that monitors, assists, performs, or prevents a physiological function but does not physically take the place of a body part

Body Part (4th)	Approach (5th)	Device (6th)	Qualifier (7th)
0 Upper Intestinal Tract **D** Lower Intestinal Tract	**0** Open **3** Percutaneous **4** Percutaneous Endoscopic **7** Via Natural or Artificial Opening **8** Via Natural or Artificial Opening Endoscopic	**Y** Other Device	**Z** No Qualifier
5 Esophagus	**0** Open **3** Percutaneous **4** Percutaneous Endoscopic	**1** Radioactive Element **2** Monitoring Device **3** Infusion Device **D** Intraluminal Device **U** Feeding Device **Y** Other Device	**Z** No Qualifier
5 Esophagus	**7** Via Natural or Artificial Opening **8** Via Natural or Artificial Opening Endoscopic	**1** Radioactive Element **2** Monitoring Device **3** Infusion Device **B** Intraluminal Device, Airway **D** Intraluminal Device **U** Feeding Device **Y** Other Device	**Z** No Qualifier
6 Stomach	**0** Open **3** Percutaneous **4** Percutaneous Endoscopic	**1** Radioactive Element **2** Monitoring Device **3** Infusion Device **D** Intraluminal Device **M** Stimulator Lead **U** Feeding Device **Y** Other Device	**Z** No Qualifier
6 Stomach	**7** Via Natural or Artificial Opening **8** Via Natural or Artificial Opening Endoscopic	**1** Radioactive Element **2** Monitoring Device **3** Infusion Device **D** Intraluminal Device **U** Feeding Device **Y** Other Device	**Z** No Qualifier
8 Small Intestine **9** Duodenum **A** Jejunum **B** Ileum	**0** Open **3** Percutaneous **4** Percutaneous Endoscopic **7** Via Natural or Artificial Opening **8** Via Natural or Artificial Opening Endoscopic	**1** Radioactive Element **2** Monitoring Device **3** Infusion Device **D** Intraluminal Device **U** Feeding Device	**Z** No Qualifier
E Large Intestine **P** Rectum	**0** Open **3** Percutaneous **4** Percutaneous Endoscopic **7** Via Natural or Artificial Opening **8** Via Natural or Artificial Opening Endoscopic	**1** Radioactive Element **D** Intraluminal Device	**Z** No Qualifier
Q Anus	**0** Open **3** Percutaneous **4** Percutaneous Endoscopic	**D** Intraluminal Device **L** Artificial Sphincter	**Z** No Qualifier
Q Anus	**7** Via Natural or Artificial Opening **8** Via Natural or Artificial Opening Endoscopic	**D** Intraluminal Device	**Z** No Qualifier
R Anal Sphincter	**0** Open **3** Percutaneous **4** Percutaneous Endoscopic	**M** Stimulator Lead	**Z** No Qualifier

Section	0	Medical and Surgical
Body System	D	Gastrointestinal System
Operation	J	Inspection: Visually and/or manually exploring a body part

Body Part (4th)	Approach (5th)	Device (6th)	Qualifier (7th)
0 Upper Intestinal Tract 6 Stomach D Lower Intestinal Tract	0 Open 3 Percutaneous 4 Percutaneous Endoscopic 7 Via Natural or Artificial Opening 8 Via Natural or Artificial Opening Endoscopic X External	Z No Device	Z No Qualifier
U Omentum V Mesentery W Peritoneum	0 Open 3 Percutaneous 4 Percutaneous Endoscopic X External	Z No Device	Z No Qualifier

Section	0	Medical and Surgical
Body System	D	Gastrointestinal System
Operation	L	Occlusion: Completely closing an orifice or the lumen of a tubular body part

Body Part (4th)	Approach (5th)	Device (6th)	Qualifier (7th)
1 Esophagus, Upper 2 Esophagus, Middle 3 Esophagus, Lower 4 Esophagogastric Junction 5 Esophagus 6 Stomach 7 Stomach, Pylorus 8 Small Intestine 9 Duodenum A Jejunum B Ileum C Ileocecal Valve E Large Intestine F Large Intestine, Right G Large Intestine, Left H Cecum K Ascending Colon L Transverse Colon M Descending Colon N Sigmoid Colon P Rectum	0 Open 3 Percutaneous 4 Percutaneous Endoscopic	C Extraluminal Device D Intraluminal Device Z No Device	Z No Qualifier
1 Esophagus, Upper 2 Esophagus, Middle 3 Esophagus, Lower 4 Esophagogastric Junction 5 Esophagus 6 Stomach 7 Stomach, Pylorus 8 Small Intestine 9 Duodenum A Jejunum B Ileum C Ileocecal Valve E Large Intestine F Large Intestine, Right G Large Intestine, Left H Cecum K Ascending Colon L Transverse Colon M Descending Colon N Sigmoid Colon P Rectum	7 Via Natural or Artificial Opening 8 Via Natural or Artificial Opening Endoscopic	D Intraluminal Device Z No Device	Z No Qualifier

Continued →

Section	0	Medical and Surgical
Body System	D	Gastrointestinal System
Operation	L	**Occlusion:** Completely closing an orifice or the lumen of a tubular body part

Body Part (4th)	Approach (5th)	Device (6th)	Qualifier (7th)
Q Anus	0 Open 3 Percutaneous 4 Percutaneous Endoscopic X External	C Extraluminal Device D Intraluminal Device Z No Device	Z No Qualifier
Q Anus	7 Via Natural or Artificial Opening 8 Via Natural or Artificial Opening Endoscopic	D Intraluminal Device Z No Device	Z No Qualifier

Section	0	Medical and Surgical
Body System	D	Gastrointestinal System
Operation	M	**Reattachment:** Putting back in or on all or a portion of a separated body part to its normal location or other suitable location

Body Part (4th)	Approach (5th)	Device (6th)	Qualifier (7th)
5 Esophagus 6 Stomach 8 Small Intestine 9 Duodenum A Jejunum B Ileum E Large Intestine F Large Intestine, Right G Large Intestine, Left H Cecum K Ascending Colon L Transverse Colon M Descending Colon N Sigmoid Colon P Rectum	0 Open 4 Percutaneous Endoscopic	Z No Device	Z No Qualifier

Section	0	Medical and Surgical
Body System	D	Gastrointestinal System
Operation	N	**Release:** Freeing a body part from an abnormal physical constraint by cutting or by the use of force

Body Part (4th)	Approach (5th)	Device (6th)	Qualifier (7th)
1 Esophagus, Upper 2 Esophagus, Middle 3 Esophagus, Lower 4 Esophagogastric Junction 5 Esophagus 6 Stomach 7 Stomach, Pylorus 8 Small Intestine 9 Duodenum A Jejunum B Ileum C Ileocecal Valve E Large Intestine F Large Intestine, Right G Large Intestine, Left H Cecum J Appendix K Ascending Colon L Transverse Colon M Descending Colon N Sigmoid Colon P Rectum	0 Open 3 Percutaneous 4 Percutaneous Endoscopic 7 Via Natural or Artificial Opening 8 Via Natural or Artificial Opening Endoscopic	Z No Device	Z No Qualifier

Continued →

Section	0	Medical and Surgical
Body System	D	Gastrointestinal System
Operation	N	Release: Freeing a body part from an abnormal physical constraint by cutting or by the use of force

Body Part (4th)	Approach (5th)	Device (6th)	Qualifier (7th)
Q Anus	**0** Open **3** Percutaneous **4** Percutaneous Endoscopic **7** Via Natural or Artificial Opening **8** Via Natural or Artificial Opening Endoscopic **X** External	**Z** No Device	**Z** No Qualifier
R Anal Sphincter **U** Omentum **V** Mesentery **W** Peritoneum	**0** Open **3** Percutaneous **4** Percutaneous Endoscopic	**Z** No Device	**Z** No Qualifier

Section	0	Medical and Surgical
Body System	D	Gastrointestinal System
Operation	P	Removal: Taking out or off a device from a body part

Body Part (4th)	Approach (5th)	Device (6th)	Qualifier (7th)
0 Upper Intestinal Tract **D** Lower Intestinal Tract	**0** Open **3** Percutaneous **4** Percutaneous Endoscopic **7** Via Natural or Artificial Opening **8** Via Natural or Artificial Opening Endoscopic	**0** Drainage Device **2** Monitoring Device **3** Infusion Device **7** Autologous Tissue Substitute **C** Extraluminal Device **D** Intraluminal Device **J** Synthetic Substitute **K** Nonautologous Tissue Substitute **U** Feeding Device **Y** Other Device	**Z** No Qualifier
0 Upper Intestinal Tract **D** Lower Intestinal Tract	**X** External	**0** Drainage Device **2** Monitoring Device **3** Infusion Device **D** Intraluminal Device **U** Feeding Device	**Z** No Qualifier
5 Esophagus	**0** Open **3** Percutaneous **4** Percutaneous Endoscopic	**1** Radioactive Element **2** Monitoring Device **3** Infusion Device **U** Feeding Device **Y** Other Device	**Z** No Qualifier
5 Esophagus	**7** Via Natural or Artificial Opening **8** Via Natural or Artificial Opening Endoscopic	**1** Radioactive Element **D** Intraluminal Device **Y** Other Device	**Z** No Qualifier
5 Esophagus	**X** External	**1** Radioactive Element **2** Monitoring Device **3** Infusion Device **D** Intraluminal Device **U** Feeding Device	**Z** No Qualifier

Continued →

	Section	0	**Medical and Surgical**
	Body System	D	**Gastrointestinal System**
	Operation	P	**Removal:** Taking out or off a device from a body part

Body Part (4th)	Approach (5th)	Device (6th)	Qualifier (7th)
6 Stomach	**0** Open **3** Percutaneous **4** Percutaneous Endoscopic	**0** Drainage Device **2** Monitoring Device **3** Infusion Device **7** Autologous Tissue Substitute **C** Extraluminal Device **D** Intraluminal Device **J** Synthetic Substitute **K** Nonautologous Tissue Substitute **M** Stimulator Lead **U** Feeding Device **Y** Other Device	**Z** No Qualifier
6 Stomach	**7** Via Natural or Artificial Opening **8** Via Natural or Artificial Opening Endoscopic	**0** Drainage Device **2** Monitoring Device **3** Infusion Device **7** Autologous Tissue Substitute **C** Extraluminal Device **D** Intraluminal Device **J** Synthetic Substitute **K** Nonautologous Tissue Substitute **U** Feeding Device **Y** Other Device	**Z** No Qualifier
6 Stomach	**X** External	**0** Drainage Device **2** Monitoring Device **3** Infusion Device **D** Intraluminal Device **U** Feeding Device	**Z** No Qualifier
P Rectum	**0** Open **3** Percutaneous **4** Percutaneous Endoscopic **7** Via Natural or Artificial Opening **8** Via Natural or Artificial Opening Endoscopic **X** External	**1** Radioactive Element	**Z** No Qualifier
Q Anus	**0** Open **3** Percutaneous **4** Percutaneous Endoscopic **7** Via Natural or Artificial Opening **8** Via Natural or Artificial Opening Endoscopic	**L** Artificial Sphincter	**Z** No Qualifier
R Anal Sphincter	**0** Open **3** Percutaneous **4** Percutaneous Endoscopic	**M** Stimulator Lead	**Z** No Qualifier
U Omentum **V** Mesentery **W** Peritoneum	**0** Open **3** Percutaneous **4** Percutaneous Endoscopic	**0** Drainage Device **1** Radioactive Element **7** Autologous Tissue Substitute **J** Synthetic Substitute **K** Nonautologous Tissue Substitute	**Z** No Qualifier

Section   0   **Medical and Surgical**
Body System   D   **Gastrointestinal System**
Operation   Q   **Repair:** Restoring, to the extent possible, a body part to its normal anatomic structure and function

Body Part (4ᵗʰ)	Approach (5ᵗʰ)	Device (6ᵗʰ)	Qualifier (7ᵗʰ)
1 Esophagus, Upper 2 Esophagus, Middle 3 Esophagus, Lower 4 Esophagogastric Junction 5 Esophagus 6 Stomach 7 Stomach, Pylorus 8 Small Intestine 9 Duodenum A Jejunum B Ileum C Ileocecal Valve E Large Intestine F Large Intestine, Right G Large Intestine, Left H Cecum J Appendix K Ascending Colon L Transverse Colon M Descending Colon N Sigmoid Colon P Rectum	0 Open 3 Percutaneous 4 Percutaneous Endoscopic 7 Via Natural or Artificial Opening 8 Via Natural or Artificial Opening Endoscopic	Z No Device	Z No Qualifier
Q Anus	0 Open 3 Percutaneous 4 Percutaneous Endoscopic 7 Via Natural or Artificial Opening 8 Via Natural or Artificial Opening Endoscopic X External	Z No Device	Z No Qualifier
R Anal Sphincter U Omentum V Mesentery W Peritoneum	0 Open 3 Percutaneous 4 Percutaneous Endoscopic	Z No Device	Z No Qualifier

Section   0   **Medical and Surgical**
Body System   D   **Gastrointestinal System**
Operation   R   **Replacement:** Putting in or on biological or synthetic material that physically takes the place and/or function of all or a portion of a body part

Body Part (4ᵗʰ)	Approach (5ᵗʰ)	Device (6ᵗʰ)	Qualifier (7ᵗʰ)
5 Esophagus	0 Open 4 Percutaneous Endoscopic 7 Via Natural or Artificial Opening 8 Via Natural or Artificial Opening Endoscopic	7 Autologous Tissue Substitute J Synthetic Substitute K Nonautologous Tissue Substitute	Z No Qualifier
R Anal Sphincter U Omentum V Mesentery W Peritoneum	0 Open 4 Percutaneous Endoscopic	7 Autologous Tissue Substitute J Synthetic Substitute K Nonautologous Tissue Substitute	Z No Qualifier

Section	0	Medical and Surgical
Body System	D	Gastrointestinal System
Operation	S	Reposition: Moving to its normal location, or other suitable location, all or a portion of a body part

Body Part (4th)	Approach (5th)	Device (6th)	Qualifier (7th)
5 Esophagus 6 Stomach 9 Duodenum A Jejunum B Ileum H Cecum K Ascending Colon L Transverse Colon M Descending Colon N Sigmoid Colon P Rectum Q Anus	0 Open 4 Percutaneous Endoscopic 7 Via Natural or Artificial Opening 8 Via Natural or Artificial Opening Endoscopic X External	Z No Device	Z No Qualifier
8 Small Intestine E Large Intestine	0 Open 4 Percutaneous Endoscopic 7 Via Natural or Artificial Opening 8 Via Natural or Artificial Opening Endoscopic	Z No Device	Z No Qualifier

Section	0	Medical and Surgical
Body System	D	Gastrointestinal System
Operation	T	Resection: Cutting out or off, without replacement, all of a body part

Body Part (4th)	Approach (5th)	Device (6th)	Qualifier (7th)
1 Esophagus, Upper 2 Esophagus, Middle 3 Esophagus, Lower 4 Esophagogastric Junction 5 Esophagus 6 Stomach 7 Stomach, Pylorus 8 Small Intestine 9 Duodenum A Jejunum B Ileum C Ileocecal Valve E Large Intestine F Large Intestine, Right H Cecum J Appendix K Ascending Colon P Rectum Q Anus	0 Open 4 Percutaneous Endoscopic 7 Via Natural or Artificial Opening 8 Via Natural or Artificial Opening Endoscopic	Z No Device	Z No Qualifier
G Large Intestine, Left L Transverse Colon M Descending Colon N Sigmoid Colon	0 Open 4 Percutaneous Endoscopic 7 Via Natural or Artificial Opening 8 Via Natural or Artificial Opening Endoscopic F Via Natural or Artificial Opening With Percutaneous Endoscopic Assistance	Z No Device	Z No Qualifier
R Anal Sphincter U Omentum	0 Open 4 Percutaneous Endoscopic	Z No Device	Z No Qualifier

Section	0	Medical and Surgical
Body System	D	Gastrointestinal System
Operation	U	Supplement: Putting in or on biological or synthetic material that physically reinforces and/or augments the function of a portion of a body part

Body Part (4th)	Approach (5th)	Device (6th)	Qualifier (7th)
1 Esophagus, Upper 2 Esophagus, Middle 3 Esophagus, Lower 4 Esophagogastric Junction 5 Esophagus 6 Stomach 7 Stomach, Pylorus 8 Small Intestine 9 Duodenum A Jejunum B Ileum C Ileocecal Valve E Large Intestine F Large Intestine, Right G Large Intestine, Left H Cecum K Ascending Colon L Transverse Colon M Descending Colon N Sigmoid Colon P Rectum	0 Open 4 Percutaneous Endoscopic 7 Via Natural or Artificial Opening 8 Via Natural or Artificial Opening Endoscopic	7 Autologous Tissue Substitute J Synthetic Substitute K Nonautologous Tissue Substitute	Z No Qualifier
Q Anus	0 Open 4 Percutaneous Endoscopic 7 Via Natural or Artificial Opening 8 Via Natural or Artificial Opening Endoscopic X External	7 Autologous Tissue Substitute J Synthetic Substitute K Nonautologous Tissue Substitute	Z No Qualifier
R Anal Sphincter U Omentum V Mesentery W Peritoneum	0 Open 4 Percutaneous Endoscopic	7 Autologous Tissue Substitute J Synthetic Substitute K Nonautologous Tissue Substitute	Z No Qualifier

Section	0	Medical and Surgical
Body System	D	Gastrointestinal System
Operation	V	Restriction: Partially closing an orifice or the lumen of a tubular body part

Body Part (4th)	Approach (5th)	Device (6th)	Qualifier (7th)
1 Esophagus, Upper 2 Esophagus, Middle 3 Esophagus, Lower 4 Esophagogastric Junction 5 Esophagus 6 Stomach 7 Stomach, Pylorus 8 Small Intestine 9 Duodenum A Jejunum B Ileum C Ileocecal Valve E Large Intestine F Large Intestine, Right G Large Intestine, Left H Cecum K Ascending Colon L Transverse Colon M Descending Colon N Sigmoid Colon P Rectum	0 Open 3 Percutaneous 4 Percutaneous Endoscopic	C Extraluminal Device D Intraluminal Device Z No Device	Z No Qualifier

Continued →

Section	0	Medical and Surgical
Body System	D	Gastrointestinal System
Operation	V	Restriction: Partially closing an orifice or the lumen of a tubular body part

Body Part (4th)	Approach (5th)	Device (6th)	Qualifier (7th)
1 Esophagus, Upper 2 Esophagus, Middle 3 Esophagus, Lower 4 Esophagogastric Junction 5 Esophagus 6 Stomach 7 Stomach, Pylorus 8 Small Intestine 9 Duodenum A Jejunum B Ileum C Ileocecal Valve E Large Intestine F Large Intestine, Right G Large Intestine, Left H Cecum K Ascending Colon L Transverse Colon M Descending Colon N Sigmoid Colon P Rectum	7 Via Natural or Artificial Opening 8 Via Natural or Artificial Opening Endoscopic	D Intraluminal Device Z No Device	Z No Qualifier
Q Anus	0 Open 3 Percutaneous 4 Percutaneous Endoscopic X External	C Extraluminal Device D Intraluminal Device Z No Device	Z No Qualifier
Q Anus	7 Via Natural or Artificial Opening 8 Via Natural or Artificial Opening Endoscopic	D Intraluminal Device Z No Device	Z No Qualifier

Section	0	Medical and Surgical
Body System	D	Gastrointestinal System
Operation	W	Revision: Correcting, to the extent possible, a portion of a malfunctioning device or the position of a displaced device

Body Part (4th)	Approach (5th)	Device (6th)	Qualifier (7th)
0 Upper Intestinal Tract D Lower Intestinal Tract	0 Open 3 Percutaneous 4 Percutaneous Endoscopic 7 Via Natural or Artificial Opening 8 Via Natural or Artificial Opening Endoscopic	0 Drainage Device 2 Monitoring Device 3 Infusion Device 7 Autologous Tissue Substitute C Extraluminal Device D Intraluminal Device J Synthetic Substitute K Nonautologous Tissue Substitute U Feeding Device Y Other Device	Z No Qualifier
0 Upper Intestinal Tract D Lower Intestinal Tract	X External	0 Drainage Device 2 Monitoring Device 3 Infusion Device 7 Autologous Tissue Substitute C Extraluminal Device D Intraluminal Device J Synthetic Substitute K Nonautologous Tissue Substitute U Feeding Device	Z No Qualifier

Continued →

Section	0	Medical and Surgical
Body System	D	Gastrointestinal System
Operation	W	Revision: Correcting, to the extent possible, a portion of a malfunctioning device or the position of a displaced device

Body Part (4th)	Approach (5th)	Device (6th)	Qualifier (7th)
5 Esophagus	0 Open 3 Percutaneous 4 Percutaneous Endoscopic	Y Other Device	Z No Qualifier
5 Esophagus	7 Via Natural or Artificial Opening 8 Via Natural or Artificial Opening Endoscopic	D Intraluminal Device Y Other Device	Z No Qualifier
5 Esophagus	X External	D Intraluminal Device	Z No Qualifier
6 Stomach	0 Open 3 Percutaneous 4 Percutaneous Endoscopic	0 Drainage Device 2 Monitoring Device 3 Infusion Device 7 Autologous Tissue Substitute C Extraluminal Device D Intraluminal Device J Synthetic Substitute K Nonautologous Tissue Substitute M Stimulator Lead U Feeding Device Y Other Device	Z No Qualifier
6 Stomach	7 Via Natural or Artificial Opening 8 Via Natural or Artificial Opening Endoscopic	0 Drainage Device 2 Monitoring Device 3 Infusion Device 7 Autologous Tissue Substitute C Extraluminal Device D Intraluminal Device J Synthetic Substitute K Nonautologous Tissue Substitute U Feeding Device Y Other Device	Z No Qualifier
6 Stomach	X External	0 Drainage Device 2 Monitoring Device 3 Infusion Device 7 Autologous Tissue Substitute C Extraluminal Device D Intraluminal Device J Synthetic Substitute K Nonautologous Tissue Substitute U Feeding Device	Z No Qualifier
8 Small Intestine E Large Intestine	0 Open 4 Percutaneous Endoscopic 7 Via Natural or Artificial Opening 8 Via Natural or Artificial Opening Endoscopic	7 Autologous Tissue Substitute J Synthetic Substitute K Nonautologous Tissue Substitute	Z No Qualifier
Q Anus	0 Open 3 Percutaneous 4 Percutaneous Endoscopic 7 Via Natural or Artificial Opening 8 Via Natural or Artificial Opening Endoscopic	L Artificial Sphincter	Z No Qualifier
R Anal Sphincter	0 Open 3 Percutaneous 4 Percutaneous Endoscopic	M Stimulator Lead	Z No Qualifier
U Omentum V Mesentery W Peritoneum	0 Open 3 Percutaneous 4 Percutaneous Endoscopic	0 Drainage Device 7 Autologous Tissue Substitute J Synthetic Substitute K Nonautologous Tissue Substitute	Z No Qualifier

Section	0	**Medical and Surgical**
Body System	D	**Gastrointestinal System**
Operation	X	**Transfer:** Moving, without taking out, all or a portion of a body part to another location to take over the function of all portion of a body part

Body Part (4th)	Approach (5th)	Device (6th)	Qualifier (7th)
6 Stomach 8 Small Intestine	0 Open 4 Percutaneous Endoscopic	Z No Device	5 Esophagus
E Large Intestine	0 Open 4 Percutaneous Endoscopic	Z No Device	5 Esophagus 7 Vagina

Section	0	**Medical and Surgical**
Body System	D	**Gastrointestinal System**
Operation	Y	**Transplantation:** Putting in or on all or a portion of a living body part taken from another individual or animal to physically take the place and/or function of all or a portion of a similar body part

Body Part (4th)	Approach (5th)	Device (6th)	Qualifier (7th)
5 Esophagus 6 Stomach 8 Small Intestine E Large Intestine	0 Open	Z No Device	0 Allogeneic 1 Syngeneic 2 Zooplastic

Gastrointestinal System Code Listing 0D1–0DY

Review Coding Guideline B4.8

0D1 – Gastrointestinal System, Bypass

Review Coding Guideline B3.6a

0D11074 Bypass Upper Esophagus to Cutaneous with Autologous Tissue Substitute, Open Approach

0D11076 Bypass Upper Esophagus to Stomach with Autologous Tissue Substitute, Open Approach

0D11079 Bypass Upper Esophagus to Duodenum with Autologous Tissue Substitute, Open Approach

0D1107A Bypass Upper Esophagus to Jejunum with Autologous Tissue Substitute, Open Approach

0D1107B Bypass Upper Esophagus to Ileum with Autologous Tissue Substitute, Open Approach

0D110J4 Bypass Upper Esophagus to Cutaneous with Synthetic Substitute, Open Approach

0D110J6 Bypass Upper Esophagus to Stomach with Synthetic Substitute, Open Approach

0D110J9 Bypass Upper Esophagus to Duodenum with Synthetic Substitute, Open Approach

0D110JA Bypass Upper Esophagus to Jejunum with Synthetic Substitute, Open Approach

0D110JB Bypass Upper Esophagus to Ileum with Synthetic Substitute, Open Approach

0D110K4 Bypass Upper Esophagus to Cutaneous with Nonautologous Tissue Substitute, Open Approach

0D110K6 Bypass Upper Esophagus to Stomach with Nonautologous Tissue Substitute, Open Approach

0D110K9 Bypass Upper Esophagus to Duodenum with Nonautologous Tissue Substitute, Open Approach

0D110KA Bypass Upper Esophagus to Jejunum with Nonautologous Tissue Substitute, Open Approach

0D110KB Bypass Upper Esophagus to Ileum with Nonautologous Tissue Substitute, Open Approach

0D110Z4 Bypass Upper Esophagus to Cutaneous, Open Approach

0D110Z6 Bypass Upper Esophagus to Stomach, Open Approach

0D110Z9 Bypass Upper Esophagus to Duodenum, Open Approach

0D110ZA Bypass Upper Esophagus to Jejunum, Open Approach

0D110ZB Bypass Upper Esophagus to Ileum, Open Approach

0D113J4 Bypass Upper Esophagus to Cutaneous with Synthetic Substitute, Percutaneous Approach

0D11474 Bypass Upper Esophagus to Cutaneous with Autologous Tissue Substitute, Percutaneous Endoscopic Approach

0D11476 Bypass Upper Esophagus to Stomach with Autologous Tissue Substitute, Percutaneous Endoscopic Approach

0D11479 Bypass Upper Esophagus to Duodenum with Autologous Tissue Substitute, Percutaneous Endoscopic Approach

0D1147A Bypass Upper Esophagus to Jejunum with Autologous Tissue Substitute, Percutaneous Endoscopic Approach

0D1147B Bypass Upper Esophagus to Ileum with Autologous Tissue Substitute, Percutaneous Endoscopic Approach

0D114J4 Bypass Upper Esophagus to Cutaneous with Synthetic Substitute, Percutaneous Endoscopic Approach

0D114J6 Bypass Upper Esophagus to Stomach with Synthetic Substitute, Percutaneous Endoscopic Approach

0D114J9 Bypass Upper Esophagus to Duodenum with Synthetic Substitute, Percutaneous Endoscopic Approach

0D114JA Bypass Upper Esophagus to Jejunum with Synthetic Substitute, Percutaneous Endoscopic Approach

0D114JB Bypass Upper Esophagus to Ileum with Synthetic Substitute, Percutaneous Endoscopic Approach

0D114K4 Bypass Upper Esophagus to Cutaneous with Nonautologous Tissue Substitute, Percutaneous Endoscopic Approach

0D114K6 Bypass Upper Esophagus to Stomach with Nonautologous Tissue Substitute, Percutaneous Endoscopic Approach

0D114K9 Bypass Upper Esophagus to Duodenum with Nonautologous Tissue Substitute, Percutaneous Endoscopic Approach

0D114KA Bypass Upper Esophagus to Jejunum with Nonautologous Tissue Substitute, Percutaneous Endoscopic Approach

0D114KB Bypass Upper Esophagus to Ileum with Nonautologous Tissue Substitute, Percutaneous Endoscopic Approach

0D114Z4 Bypass Upper Esophagus to Cutaneous, Percutaneous Endoscopic Approach

0D114Z6 Bypass Upper Esophagus to Stomach, Percutaneous Endoscopic Approach

0D114Z9 Bypass Upper Esophagus to Duodenum, Percutaneous Endoscopic Approach

0D114ZA Bypass Upper Esophagus to Jejunum, Percutaneous Endoscopic Approach

0D114ZB Bypass Upper Esophagus to Ileum, Percutaneous Endoscopic Approach

0D11874 Bypass Upper Esophagus to Cutaneous with Autologous Tissue Substitute, Via Natural or Artificial Opening Endoscopic

0D11876 Bypass Upper Esophagus to Stomach with Autologous Tissue Substitute, Via Natural or Artificial Opening Endoscopic

0D11879 Bypass Upper Esophagus to Duodenum with Autologous Tissue Substitute, Via Natural or Artificial Opening Endoscopic

0D1187A Bypass Upper Esophagus to Jejunum with Autologous Tissue Substitute, Via Natural or Artificial Opening Endoscopic

0D1187B Bypass Upper Esophagus to Ileum with Autologous Tissue Substitute, Via Natural or Artificial Opening Endoscopic

0D118J4 Bypass Upper Esophagus to Cutaneous with Synthetic Substitute, Via Natural or Artificial Opening Endoscopic

0D118J6 Bypass Upper Esophagus to Stomach with Synthetic Substitute, Via Natural or Artificial Opening Endoscopic

0D118J9 Bypass Upper Esophagus to Duodenum with Synthetic Substitute, Via Natural or Artificial Opening Endoscopic

0D118JA Bypass Upper Esophagus to Jejunum with Synthetic Substitute, Via Natural or Artificial Opening Endoscopic

0D118JB Bypass Upper Esophagus to Ileum with Synthetic Substitute, Via Natural or Artificial Opening Endoscopic

0D118K4 Bypass Upper Esophagus to Cutaneous with Nonautologous Tissue Substitute, Via Natural or Artificial Opening Endoscopic

0D118K6 Bypass Upper Esophagus to Stomach with Nonautologous Tissue Substitute, Via Natural or Artificial Opening Endoscopic

0D118K9 Bypass Upper Esophagus to Duodenum with Nonautologous Tissue Substitute, Via Natural or Artificial Opening Endoscopic

0D118KA Bypass Upper Esophagus to Jejunum with Nonautologous Tissue Substitute, Via Natural or Artificial Opening Endoscopic

0D118KB Bypass Upper Esophagus to Ileum with Nonautologous Tissue Substitute, Via Natural or Artificial Opening Endoscopic

0D118Z4 Bypass Upper Esophagus to Cutaneous, Via Natural or Artificial Opening Endoscopic

0D118Z6 Bypass Upper Esophagus to Stomach, Via Natural or Artificial Opening Endoscopic

0D118Z9 Bypass Upper Esophagus to Duodenum, Via Natural or Artificial Opening Endoscopic

0D118ZA Bypass Upper Esophagus to Jejunum, Via Natural or Artificial Opening Endoscopic

0D118ZB Bypass Upper Esophagus to Ileum, Via Natural or Artificial Opening Endoscopic

0D12074 Bypass Middle Esophagus to Cutaneous with Autologous Tissue Substitute, Open Approach

0D12076 Bypass Middle Esophagus to Stomach with Autologous Tissue Substitute, Open Approach

0D12079 Bypass Middle Esophagus to Duodenum with Autologous Tissue Substitute, Open Approach

0D1207A Bypass Middle Esophagus to Jejunum with Autologous Tissue Substitute, Open Approach

0D1207B Bypass Middle Esophagus to Ileum with Autologous Tissue Substitute, Open Approach

0D120J4 Bypass Middle Esophagus to Cutaneous with Synthetic Substitute, Open Approach

0D120J6 Bypass Middle Esophagus to Stomach with Synthetic Substitute, Open Approach

0D120J9 Bypass Middle Esophagus to Duodenum with Synthetic Substitute, Open Approach

0D120JA Bypass Middle Esophagus to Jejunum with Synthetic Substitute, Open Approach

0D120JB Bypass Middle Esophagus to Ileum with Synthetic Substitute, Open Approach

0D120K4 Bypass Middle Esophagus to Cutaneous with Nonautologous Tissue Substitute, Open Approach

0D120K6 Bypass Middle Esophagus to Stomach with Nonautologous Tissue Substitute, Open Approach

0D120K9 Bypass Middle Esophagus to Duodenum with Nonautologous Tissue Substitute, Open Approach

0D120KA Bypass Middle Esophagus to Jejunum with Nonautologous Tissue Substitute, Open Approach

0D120KB Bypass Middle Esophagus to Ileum with Nonautologous Tissue Substitute, Open Approach

0D120Z4 Bypass Middle Esophagus to Cutaneous, Open Approach

0D120Z6 Bypass Middle Esophagus to Stomach, Open Approach

0D120Z9 Bypass Middle Esophagus to Duodenum, Open Approach

0D120ZA Bypass Middle Esophagus to Jejunum, Open Approach

0D120ZB Bypass Middle Esophagus to Ileum, Open Approach

0D123J4 Bypass Middle Esophagus to Cutaneous with Synthetic Substitute, Percutaneous Approach

0D12474 Bypass Middle Esophagus to Cutaneous with Autologous Tissue Substitute, Percutaneous Endoscopic Approach

0D12476 Bypass Middle Esophagus to Stomach with Autologous Tissue Substitute, Percutaneous Endoscopic Approach

0D12479 Bypass Middle Esophagus to Duodenum with Autologous Tissue Substitute, Percutaneous Endoscopic Approach

0D1247A Bypass Middle Esophagus to Jejunum with Autologous Tissue Substitute, Percutaneous Endoscopic Approach

0D1247B Bypass Middle Esophagus to Ileum with Autologous Tissue Substitute, Percutaneous Endoscopic Approach

0D124J4 Bypass Middle Esophagus to Cutaneous with Synthetic Substitute, Percutaneous Endoscopic Approach

0D124J6 Bypass Middle Esophagus to Stomach with Synthetic Substitute, Percutaneous Endoscopic Approach

0D124J9 Bypass Middle Esophagus to Duodenum with Synthetic Substitute, Percutaneous Endoscopic Approach

0D124JA Bypass Middle Esophagus to Jejunum with Synthetic Substitute, Percutaneous Endoscopic Approach

0D124JB Bypass Middle Esophagus to Ileum with Synthetic Substitute, Percutaneous Endoscopic Approach

0D124K4 Bypass Middle Esophagus to Cutaneous with Nonautologous Tissue Substitute, Percutaneous Endoscopic Approach

0D124K6 Bypass Middle Esophagus to Stomach with Nonautologous Tissue Substitute, Percutaneous Endoscopic Approach

0D124K9 Bypass Middle Esophagus to Duodenum with Nonautologous Tissue Substitute, Percutaneous Endoscopic Approach

0D124KA Bypass Middle Esophagus to Jejunum with Nonautologous Tissue Substitute, Percutaneous Endoscopic Approach

0D124KB Bypass Middle Esophagus to Ileum with Nonautologous Tissue Substitute, Percutaneous Endoscopic Approach

0D124Z4 Bypass Middle Esophagus to Cutaneous, Percutaneous Endoscopic Approach

0D124Z6 Bypass Middle Esophagus to Stomach, Percutaneous Endoscopic Approach

0D124Z9 Bypass Middle Esophagus to Duodenum, Percutaneous Endoscopic Approach

0D124ZA Bypass Middle Esophagus to Jejunum, Percutaneous Endoscopic Approach

0D124ZB Bypass Middle Esophagus to Ileum, Percutaneous Endoscopic Approach

0D12874 Bypass Middle Esophagus to Cutaneous with Autologous Tissue Substitute, Via Natural or Artificial Opening Endoscopic

0D12876 Bypass Middle Esophagus to Stomach with Autologous Tissue Substitute, Via Natural or Artificial Opening Endoscopic

0D12879 Bypass Middle Esophagus to Duodenum with Autologous Tissue Substitute, Via Natural or Artificial Opening Endoscopic

0D1287A Bypass Middle Esophagus to Jejunum with Autologous Tissue Substitute, Via Natural or Artificial Opening Endoscopic

0D1287B Bypass Middle Esophagus to Ileum with Autologous Tissue Substitute, Via Natural or Artificial Opening Endoscopic

0D128J4 Bypass Middle Esophagus to Cutaneous with Synthetic Substitute, Via Natural or Artificial Opening Endoscopic

0D128J6 Bypass Middle Esophagus to Stomach with Synthetic Substitute, Via Natural or Artificial Opening Endoscopic

0D128J9 Bypass Middle Esophagus to Duodenum with Synthetic Substitute, Via Natural or Artificial Opening Endoscopic

0D128JA Bypass Middle Esophagus to Jejunum with Synthetic Substitute, Via Natural or Artificial Opening Endoscopic

0D128JB Bypass Middle Esophagus to Ileum with Synthetic Substitute, Via Natural or Artificial Opening Endoscopic

0D128K4 Bypass Middle Esophagus to Cutaneous with Nonautologous Tissue Substitute, Via Natural or Artificial Opening Endoscopic

0D128K6 Bypass Middle Esophagus to Stomach with Nonautologous Tissue Substitute, Via Natural or Artificial Opening Endoscopic

0D128K9 Bypass Middle Esophagus to Duodenum with Nonautologous Tissue Substitute, Via Natural or Artificial Opening Endoscopic

0D128KA Bypass Middle Esophagus to Jejunum with Nonautologous Tissue Substitute, Via Natural or Artificial Opening Endoscopic

0D128KB Bypass Middle Esophagus to Ileum with Nonautologous Tissue Substitute, Via Natural or Artificial Opening Endoscopic

0D128Z4 Bypass Middle Esophagus to Cutaneous, Via Natural or Artificial Opening Endoscopic

0D128Z6 Bypass Middle Esophagus to Stomach, Via Natural or Artificial Opening Endoscopic

0D128Z9 Bypass Middle Esophagus to Duodenum, Via Natural or Artificial Opening Endoscopic

0D128ZA Bypass Middle Esophagus to Jejunum, Via Natural or Artificial Opening Endoscopic

0D128ZB Bypass Middle Esophagus to Ileum, Via Natural or Artificial Opening Endoscopic

0D13074 Bypass Lower Esophagus to Cutaneous with Autologous Tissue Substitute, Open Approach

0D13076 Bypass Lower Esophagus to Stomach with Autologous Tissue Substitute, Open Approach

0D13079 Bypass Lower Esophagus to Duodenum with Autologous Tissue Substitute, Open Approach

0D1307A Bypass Lower Esophagus to Jejunum with Autologous Tissue Substitute, Open Approach

0D1307B Bypass Lower Esophagus to Ileum with Autologous Tissue Substitute, Open Approach

0D130J4 Bypass Lower Esophagus to Cutaneous with Synthetic Substitute, Open Approach

0D130J6 Bypass Lower Esophagus to Stomach with Synthetic Substitute, Open Approach

0D130J9 Bypass Lower Esophagus to Duodenum with Synthetic Substitute, Open Approach

0D130JA Bypass Lower Esophagus to Jejunum with Synthetic Substitute, Open Approach

0D130JB Bypass Lower Esophagus to Ileum with Synthetic Substitute, Open Approach

0D130K4 Bypass Lower Esophagus to Cutaneous with Nonautologous Tissue Substitute, Open Approach

0D130K6 Bypass Lower Esophagus to Stomach with Nonautologous Tissue Substitute, Open Approach

0D130K9 Bypass Lower Esophagus to Duodenum with Nonautologous Tissue Substitute, Open Approach

0D130KA Bypass Lower Esophagus to Jejunum with Nonautologous Tissue Substitute, Open Approach

0D130KB Bypass Lower Esophagus to Ileum with Nonautologous Tissue Substitute, Open Approach

0D130Z4 Bypass Lower Esophagus to Cutaneous, Open Approach

0D130Z6 Bypass Lower Esophagus to Stomach, Open Approach

0D130Z9 Bypass Lower Esophagus to Duodenum, Open Approach

0D130ZA Bypass Lower Esophagus to Jejunum, Open Approach

0D130ZB Bypass Lower Esophagus to Ileum, Open Approach

0D133J4 Bypass Lower Esophagus to Cutaneous with Synthetic Substitute, Percutaneous Approach

0D13474 Bypass Lower Esophagus to Cutaneous with Autologous Tissue Substitute, Percutaneous Endoscopic Approach

0D13476 Bypass Lower Esophagus to Stomach with Autologous Tissue Substitute, Percutaneous Endoscopic Approach

0D13479 Bypass Lower Esophagus to Duodenum with Autologous Tissue Substitute, Percutaneous Endoscopic Approach

0D1347A Bypass Lower Esophagus to Jejunum with Autologous Tissue Substitute, Percutaneous Endoscopic Approach

0D1347B Bypass Lower Esophagus to Ileum with Autologous Tissue Substitute, Percutaneous Endoscopic Approach

0D134J4 Bypass Lower Esophagus to Cutaneous with Synthetic Substitute, Percutaneous Endoscopic Approach

0D134J6 Bypass Lower Esophagus to Stomach with Synthetic Substitute, Percutaneous Endoscopic Approach

0D134J9 Bypass Lower Esophagus to Duodenum with Synthetic Substitute, Percutaneous Endoscopic Approach

0D134JA Bypass Lower Esophagus to Jejunum with Synthetic Substitute, Percutaneous Endoscopic Approach

0D134JB Bypass Lower Esophagus to Ileum with Synthetic Substitute, Percutaneous Endoscopic Approach

0D134K4 Bypass Lower Esophagus to Cutaneous with Nonautologous Tissue Substitute, Percutaneous Endoscopic Approach

0D134K6 Bypass Lower Esophagus to Stomach with Nonautologous Tissue Substitute, Percutaneous Endoscopic Approach

0D134K9 Bypass Lower Esophagus to Duodenum with Nonautologous Tissue Substitute, Percutaneous Endoscopic Approach

0D134KA Bypass Lower Esophagus to Jejunum with Nonautologous Tissue Substitute, Percutaneous Endoscopic Approach

0D134KB Bypass Lower Esophagus to Ileum with Nonautologous Tissue Substitute, Percutaneous Endoscopic Approach

0D134Z4 Bypass Lower Esophagus to Cutaneous, Percutaneous Endoscopic Approach

0D134Z6 Bypass Lower Esophagus to Stomach, Percutaneous Endoscopic Approach

0D134Z9 Bypass Lower Esophagus to Duodenum, Percutaneous Endoscopic Approach

0D134ZA Bypass Lower Esophagus to Jejunum, Percutaneous Endoscopic Approach

0D134ZB Bypass Lower Esophagus to Ileum, Percutaneous Endoscopic Approach

0D13874 Bypass Lower Esophagus to Cutaneous with Autologous Tissue Substitute, Via Natural or Artificial Opening Endoscopic

0D13876 Bypass Lower Esophagus to Stomach with Autologous Tissue Substitute, Via Natural or Artificial Opening Endoscopic

0D13879 Bypass Lower Esophagus to Duodenum with Autologous Tissue Substitute, Via Natural or Artificial Opening Endoscopic

0D1387A Bypass Lower Esophagus to Jejunum with Autologous Tissue Substitute, Via Natural or Artificial Opening Endoscopic

0D1387B Bypass Lower Esophagus to Ileum with Autologous Tissue Substitute, Via Natural or Artificial Opening Endoscopic

0D138J4 Bypass Lower Esophagus to Cutaneous with Synthetic Substitute, Via Natural or Artificial Opening Endoscopic

0D138J6 Bypass Lower Esophagus to Stomach with Synthetic Substitute, Via Natural or Artificial Opening Endoscopic

0D138J9 Bypass Lower Esophagus to Duodenum with Synthetic Substitute, Via Natural or Artificial Opening Endoscopic

0D138JA Bypass Lower Esophagus to Jejunum with Synthetic Substitute, Via Natural or Artificial Opening Endoscopic

0D138JB Bypass Lower Esophagus to Ileum with Synthetic Substitute, Via Natural or Artificial Opening Endoscopic

0D138K4 Bypass Lower Esophagus to Cutaneous with Nonautologous Tissue Substitute, Via Natural or Artificial Opening Endoscopic

0D138K6 Bypass Lower Esophagus to Stomach with Nonautologous Tissue Substitute, Via Natural or Artificial Opening Endoscopic

0D138K9 Bypass Lower Esophagus to Duodenum with Nonautologous Tissue Substitute, Via Natural or Artificial Opening Endoscopic

0D138KA Bypass Lower Esophagus to Jejunum with Nonautologous Tissue Substitute, Via Natural or Artificial Opening Endoscopic

0D138KB Bypass Lower Esophagus to Ileum with Nonautologous Tissue Substitute, Via Natural or Artificial Opening Endoscopic

0D138Z4 Bypass Lower Esophagus to Cutaneous, Via Natural or Artificial Opening Endoscopic

0D138Z6 Bypass Lower Esophagus to Stomach, Via Natural or Artificial Opening Endoscopic

0D138Z9 Bypass Lower Esophagus to Duodenum Via Natural or Artificial Opening Endoscopic

0D138ZA Bypass Lower Esophagus to Jejunum, Via Natural or Artificial Opening Endoscopic

0D138ZB Bypass Lower Esophagus to Ileum, Via Natural or Artificial Opening Endoscopic

0D15074 Bypass Esophagus to Cutaneous with Autologous Tissue Substitute, Open Approach

0D15076 Bypass Esophagus to Stomach with Autologous Tissue Substitute, Open Approach

0D15079 Bypass Esophagus to Duodenum with Autologous Tissue Substitute, Open Approach

0D1507A Bypass Esophagus to Jejunum with Autologous Tissue Substitute, Open Approach

0D1507B Bypass Esophagus to Ileum with Autologous Tissue Substitute, Open Approach

0D150J4 Bypass Esophagus to Cutaneous with Synthetic Substitute, Open Approach

0D150J6 Bypass Esophagus to Stomach with Synthetic Substitute, Open Approach

0D150J9 Bypass Esophagus to Duodenum with Synthetic Substitute, Open Approach

0D150JA Bypass Esophagus to Jejunum with Synthetic Substitute, Open Approach

0D150JB Bypass Esophagus to Ileum with Synthetic Substitute, Open Approach

♀ Female-only   ♂ Male-only   ▲ Limited Coverage   ● Non-OR   ▨ HAC-associated procedure   ▲ Non-covered procedures   ✛ Cluster

0D150K4 Bypass Esophagus to Cutaneous with Nonautologous Tissue Substitute, Open Approach

0D150K6 Bypass Esophagus to Stomach with Nonautologous Tissue Substitute, Open Approach

0D150K9 Bypass Esophagus to Duodenum with Nonautologous Tissue Substitute, Open Approach

0D150KA Bypass Esophagus to Jejunum with Nonautologous Tissue Substitute, Open Approach

0D150KB Bypass Esophagus to Ileum with Nonautologous Tissue Substitute, Open Approach

0D150Z4 Bypass Esophagus to Cutaneous, Open Approach

0D150Z6 Bypass Esophagus to Stomach, Open Approach

0D150Z9 Bypass Esophagus to Duodenum, Open Approach

0D150ZA Bypass Esophagus to Jejunum, Open Approach

0D150ZB Bypass Esophagus to Ileum, Open Approach

0D153J4 Bypass Esophagus to Cutaneous with Synthetic Substitute, Percutaneous Approach

0D15474 Bypass Esophagus to Cutaneous with Autologous Tissue Substitute, Percutaneous Endoscopic Approach

0D15476 Bypass Esophagus to Stomach with Autologous Tissue Substitute, Percutaneous Endoscopic Approach

0D15479 Bypass Esophagus to Duodenum with Autologous Tissue Substitute, Percutaneous Endoscopic Approach

0D1547A Bypass Esophagus to Jejunum with Autologous Tissue Substitute, Percutaneous Endoscopic Approach

0D1547B Bypass Esophagus to Ileum with Autologous Tissue Substitute, Percutaneous Endoscopic Approach

0D154J4 Bypass Esophagus to Cutaneous with Synthetic Substitute, Percutaneous Endoscopic Approach

0D154J6 Bypass Esophagus to Stomach with Synthetic Substitute, Percutaneous Endoscopic Approach

0D154J9 Bypass Esophagus to Duodenum with Synthetic Substitute, Percutaneous Endoscopic Approach

0D154JA Bypass Esophagus to Jejunum with Synthetic Substitute, Percutaneous Endoscopic Approach

0D154JB Bypass Esophagus to Ileum with Synthetic Substitute, Percutaneous Endoscopic Approach

0D154K4 Bypass Esophagus to Cutaneous with Nonautologous Tissue Substitute, Percutaneous Endoscopic Approach

0D154K6 Bypass Esophagus to Stomach with Nonautologous Tissue Substitute, Percutaneous Endoscopic Approach

0D154K9 Bypass Esophagus to Duodenum with Nonautologous Tissue Substitute, Percutaneous Endoscopic Approach

0D154KA Bypass Esophagus to Jejunum with Nonautologous Tissue Substitute, Percutaneous Endoscopic Approach

0D154KB Bypass Esophagus to Ileum with Nonautologous Tissue Substitute, Percutaneous Endoscopic Approach

0D154Z4 Bypass Esophagus to Cutaneous, Percutaneous Endoscopic Approach

0D154Z6 Bypass Esophagus to Stomach, Percutaneous Endoscopic Approach

0D154Z9 Bypass Esophagus to Duodenum, Percutaneous Endoscopic Approach

0D154ZA Bypass Esophagus to Jejunum, Percutaneous Endoscopic Approach

0D154ZB Bypass Esophagus to Ileum, Percutaneous Endoscopic Approach

0D15874 Bypass Esophagus to Cutaneous with Autologous Tissue Substitute, Via Natural or Artificial Opening Endoscopic

0D15876 Bypass Esophagus to Stomach with Autologous Tissue Substitute, Via Natural or Artificial Opening Endoscopic

0D15879 Bypass Esophagus to Duodenum with Autologous Tissue Substitute, Via Natural or Artificial Opening Endoscopic

0D1587A Bypass Esophagus to Jejunum with Autologous Tissue Substitute, Via Natural or Artificial Opening Endoscopic

0D1587B Bypass Esophagus to Ileum with Autologous Tissue Substitute, Via Natural or Artificial Opening Endoscopic

0D158J4 Bypass Esophagus to Cutaneous with Synthetic Substitute, Via Natural or Artificial Opening Endoscopic

0D158J6 Bypass Esophagus to Stomach with Synthetic Substitute, Via Natural or Artificial Opening Endoscopic

0D158J9 Bypass Esophagus to Duodenum with Synthetic Substitute, Via Natural or Artificial Opening Endoscopic

0D158JA Bypass Esophagus to Jejunum with Synthetic Substitute, Via Natural or Artificial Opening Endoscopic

0D158JB Bypass Esophagus to Ileum with Synthetic Substitute, Via Natural or Artificial Opening Endoscopic

0D158K4 Bypass Esophagus to Cutaneous with Nonautologous Tissue Substitute, Via Natural or Artificial Opening Endoscopic

0D158K6 Bypass Esophagus to Stomach with Nonautologous Tissue Substitute, Via Natural or Artificial Opening Endoscopic

0D158K9 Bypass Esophagus to Duodenum with Nonautologous Tissue Substitute, Via Natural or Artificial Opening Endoscopic

0D158KA Bypass Esophagus to Jejunum with Nonautologous Tissue Substitute, Via Natural or Artificial Opening Endoscopic

0D158KB Bypass Esophagus to Ileum with Nonautologous Tissue Substitute, Via Natural or Artificial Opening Endoscopic

0D158Z4 Bypass Esophagus to Cutaneous, Via Natural or Artificial Opening Endoscopic

0D158Z6 Bypass Esophagus to Stomach, Via Natural or Artificial Opening Endoscopic

0D158Z9 Bypass Esophagus to Duodenum, Via Natural or Artificial Opening Endoscopic

0D158ZA Bypass Esophagus to Jejunum, Via Natural or Artificial Opening Endoscopic

0D158ZB Bypass Esophagus to Ileum, Via Natural or Artificial Opening Endoscopic

0D16074 Bypass Stomach to Cutaneous with Autologous Tissue Substitute, Open Approach

0D16079 Bypass Stomach to Duodenum with Autologous Tissue Substitute, Open Approach

HAC When reported with principal diagnosis code E66.01 and secondary diagnosis code K68.11, K95.01, K95.81, T81.40XA, T81.41XA, T81.42XA, T81.43XA, T81.44XA or T81.49XA

0D1607A Bypass Stomach to Jejunum with Autologous Tissue Substitute, Open Approach

HAC When reported with principal diagnosis E66.01 and secondary diagnosis code K68.11, K95.01, K95.81, T81.40XA, T81.41XA, T81.42XA, T81.43XA, T81.44XA or T81.49XA

0D1607B Bypass Stomach to Ileum with Autologous Tissue Substitute, Open Approach

HAC When reported with principal diagnosis code E66.01 and secondary diagnosis code K68.11, K95.01, K95.81, T81.40XA, T81.41XA, T81.42XA, T81.43XA, T81.44XA or T81.49XA

0D1607L Bypass Stomach to Transverse Colon with Autologous Tissue Substitute, Open Approach

HAC When reported with principal diagnosis code E66.01 and secondary diagnosis code K68.11, K95.01, K95.81, T81.40XA, T81.41XA, T81.42XA, T81.43XA, T81.44XA or T81.49XA

0D160J4 Bypass Stomach to Cutaneous with Synthetic Substitute, Open Approach

0D160J9 Bypass Stomach to Duodenum with Synthetic Substitute, Open Approach

HAC When reported with principal diagnosis code E66.01 and secondary diagnosis code K68.11, K95.01, K95.81, T81.40XA, T81.41XA, T81.42XA, T81.43XA, T81.44XA or T81.49XA

0D160JA Bypass Stomach to Jejunum with Synthetic Substitute, Open Approach

HAC When reported with principal diagnosis code E66.01 and secondary diagnosis code K68.11, K95.01, K95.81, T81.40XA, T81.41XA, T81.42XA, T81.43XA, T81.44XA or T81.49XA

0D160JB Bypass Stomach to Ileum with Synthetic Substitute, Open Approach

HAC When reported with principal diagnosis code E66.01 and secondary diagnosis code K68.11, K95.01, K95.81, T81.40XA, T81.41XA, T81.42XA, T81.43XA, T81.44XA or T81.49XA

0D160JL Bypass Stomach to Transverse Colon with Synthetic Substitute, Open Approach

HAC When reported with principal diagnosis code E66.01 and secondary diagnosis code K68.11, K95.01, K95.81, T81.40XA, T81.41XA, T81.42XA, T81.43XA, T81.44XA or T81.49XA

0D160K4 Bypass Stomach to Cutaneous with Nonautologous Tissue Substitute, Open Approach

0D160K9 Bypass Stomach to Duodenum with Nonautologous Tissue Substitute, Open Approach

HAC When reported with principal diagnosis code E66.01 and secondary diagnosis code K68.11, K95.01, K95.81, T81.40XA, T81.41XA, T81.42XA, T81.43XA, T81.44XA or T81.49XA

0D160KA Bypass Stomach to Jejunum with Nonautologous Tissue Substitute, Open Approach
HAC When reported with principal diagnosis code E66.01 and secondary diagnosis code K68.11, K95.01, K95.81, T81.40XA, T81.41XA, T81.42XA, T81.43XA, T81.44XA or T81.49XA

0D160KB Bypass Stomach to Ileum with Nonautologous Tissue Substitute, Open Approach
HAC When reported with principal diagnosis code E66.01 and secondary diagnosis code K68.11, K95.01, K95.81, T81.40XA, T81.41XA, T81.42XA, T81.43XA, T81.44XA or T81.49XA

0D160KL Bypass Stomach to Transverse Colon with Nonautologous Tissue Substitute, Open Approach
HAC When reported with principal diagnosis code E66.01 and secondary diagnosis code K68.11, K95.01, K95.81, T81.40XA, T81.41XA, T81.42XA, T81.43XA, T81.44XA or T81.49XA

0D160Z4 Bypass Stomach to Cutaneous, Open Approach

0D160Z9 Bypass Stomach to Duodenum, Open Approach
HAC When reported with principal diagnosis code E66.01 and secondary diagnosis code K68.11, K95.01, K95.81, T81.40XA, T81.41XA, T81.42XA, T81.43XA, T81.44XA or T81.49XA

0D160ZA Bypass Stomach to Jejunum, Open Approach
HAC When reported with principal diagnosis code E66.01 and secondary diagnosis code K68.11, K95.01, K95.81, T81.40XA, T81.41XA, T81.42XA, T81.43XA, T81.44XA or T81.49XA
AHA CC: 2Q, 2017, 17-18

0D160ZB Bypass Stomach to Ileum, Open Approach
HAC When reported with principal diagnosis code E66.01 and secondary diagnosis code K68.11, K95.01, K95.81, T81.40XA, T81.41XA, T81.42XA, T81.43XA, T81.44XA or T81.49XA

0D160ZL Bypass Stomach to Transverse Colon, Open Approach
HAC When reported with principal diagnosis code E66.01 and secondary diagnosis code K68.11, K95.01, K95.81, T81.40XA, T81.41XA, T81.42XA, T81.43XA, T81.44XA or T81.49XA

0D163J4 Bypass Stomach to Cutaneous with Synthetic Substitute, Percutaneous Approach

0D16474 Bypass Stomach to Cutaneous with Autologous Tissue Substitute, Percutaneous Endoscopic Approach

0D16479 Bypass Stomach to Duodenum with Autologous Tissue Substitute, Percutaneous Endoscopic Approach
HAC When reported with principal diagnosis code E66.01 and secondary diagnosis code K68.11, K95.01, K95.81, T81.40XA, T81.41XA, T81.42XA, T81.43XA, T81.44XA or T81.49XA

0D1647A Bypass Stomach to Jejunum with Autologous Tissue Substitute, Percutaneous Endoscopic Approach
HAC When reported with principal diagnosis code E66.01 and secondary diagnosis code K68.11, K95.01, K95.81, T81.40XA, T81.41XA, T81.42XA, T81.43XA, T81.44XA or T81.49XA

0D1647B Bypass Stomach to Ileum with Autologous Tissue Substitute, Percutaneous Endoscopic Approach
HAC When reported with principal diagnosis code E66.01 and secondary diagnosis code K68.11, K95.01, K95.81, T81.40XA, T81.41XA, T81.42XA, T81.43XA, T81.44XA or T81.49XA

0D1647L Bypass Stomach to Transverse Colon with Autologous Tissue Substitute, Percutaneous Endoscopic Approach
HAC When reported with principal diagnosis code E66.01 and secondary diagnosis code K68.11, K95.01, K95.81, T81.40XA, T81.41XA, T81.42XA, T81.43XA, T81.44XA or T81.49XA

0D164J4 Bypass Stomach to Cutaneous with Synthetic Substitute, Percutaneous Endoscopic Approach

0D164J9 Bypass Stomach to Duodenum with Synthetic Substitute, Percutaneous Endoscopic Approach
HAC When reported with principal diagnosis code E66.01 and secondary diagnosis code K68.11, K95.01, K95.81, T81.40XA, T81.41XA, T81.42XA, T81.43XA, T81.44XA or T81.49XA

0D164JA Bypass Stomach to Jejunum with Synthetic Substitute, Percutaneous Endoscopic Approach
HAC When reported with principal diagnosis code E66.01 and secondary diagnosis code K68.11, K95.01, K95.81, T81.40XA, T81.41XA, T81.42XA, T81.43XA, T81.44XA or T81.49XA

0D164JB Bypass Stomach to Ileum with Synthetic Substitute, Percutaneous Endoscopic Approach
HAC When reported with principal diagnosis code E66.01 and secondary diagnosis code K68.11, K95.01, K95.81, T81.40XA, T81.41XA, T81.42XA, T81.43XA, T81.44XA or T81.49XA

0D164JL Bypass Stomach to Transverse Colon with Synthetic Substitute, Percutaneous Endoscopic Approach
HAC When reported with principal diagnosis code E66.01 and secondary diagnosis code K68.11, K95.01, K95.81, T81.40XA, T81.41XA, T81.42XA, T81.43XA, T81.44XA or T81.49XA

0D164K4 Bypass Stomach to Cutaneous with Nonautologous Tissue Substitute, Percutaneous Endoscopic Approach

0D164K9 Bypass Stomach to Duodenum with Nonautologous Tissue Substitute, Percutaneous Endoscopic Approach
HAC When reported with principal diagnosis code E66.01 and secondary diagnosis code K68.11, K95.01, K95.81, T81.40XA, T81.41XA, T81.42XA, T81.43XA, T81.44XA or T81.49XA

0D164KA Bypass Stomach to Jejunum with Nonautologous Tissue Substitute, Percutaneous Endoscopic Approach
HAC When reported with principal diagnosis code E66.01 and secondary diagnosis code K68.11, K95.01, K95.81, T81.40XA, T81.41XA, T81.42XA, T81.43XA, T81.44XA or T81.49XA

0D164KB Bypass Stomach to Ileum with Nonautologous Tissue Substitute, Percutaneous Endoscopic Approach
HAC When reported with principal diagnosis code E66.01 and secondary diagnosis code K68.11, K95.01, K95.81,

T81.40XA, T81.41XA, T81.42XA, T81.43XA, T81.44XA or T81.49XA

0D164KL Bypass Stomach to Transverse Colon with Nonautologous Tissue Substitute, Percutaneous Endoscopic Approach
HAC When reported with principal diagnosis code E66.01 and secondary diagnosis code K68.11, K95.01, K95.81, T81.40XA, T81.41XA, T81.42XA, T81.43XA, T81.44XA or T81.49XA

0D164Z4 Bypass Stomach to Cutaneous, Percutaneous Endoscopic Approach

0D164Z9 Bypass Stomach to Duodenum, Percutaneous Endoscopic Approach
HAC When reported with principal diagnosis code E66.01 and secondary diagnosis code K68.11, K95.01, K95.81, T81.40XA, T81.41XA, T81.42XA, T81.43XA, T81.44XA or T81.49XA

0D164ZA Bypass Stomach to Jejunum, Percutaneous Endoscopic Approach
HAC When reported with principal diagnosis code E66.01 and secondary diagnosis code K68.11, K95.01, K95.81, T81.40XA, T81.41XA, T81.42XA, T81.43XA, T81.44XA or T81.49XA

0D164ZB Bypass Stomach to Ileum, Percutaneous Endoscopic Approach
HAC When reported with principal diagnosis code E66.01 and secondary diagnosis code K68.11, K95.01, K95.81, T81.40XA, T81.41XA, T81.42XA, T81.43XA, T81.44XA or T81.49XA

0D164ZL Bypass Stomach to Transverse Colon, Percutaneous Endoscopic Approach
HAC When reported with principal diagnosis E66.01 and secondary diagnosis code K68.11, K95.01, K95.81, T81.40XA, T81.41XA, T81.42XA, T81.43XA, T81.44XA or T81.49XA

0D16874 Bypass Stomach to Cutaneous with Autologous Tissue Substitute, Via Natural or Artificial Opening Endoscopic

0D16879 Bypass Stomach to Duodenum with Autologous Tissue Substitute, Via Natural or Artificial Opening Endoscopic
HAC When reported with principal diagnosis code E66.01 and secondary diagnosis code K68.11, K95.01, K95.81, T81.40XA, T81.41XA, T81.42XA, T81.43XA, T81.44XA or T81.49XA

0D1687A Bypass Stomach to Jejunum with Autologous Tissue Substitute, Via Natural or Artificial Opening Endoscopic
HAC When reported with principal diagnosis code E66.01 and secondary diagnosis code K68.11, K95.01, K95.81, T81.40XA, T81.41XA, T81.42XA, T81.43XA, T81.44XA or T81.49XA

0D1687B Bypass Stomach to Ileum with Autologous Tissue Substitute, Via Natural or Artificial Opening Endoscopic
HAC When reported with principal diagnosis code E66.01 and secondary diagnosis code K68.11, K95.01, K95.81, T81.40XA, T81.41XA, T81.42XA, T81.43XA, T81.44XA or T81.49XA

0D1687L Bypass Stomach to Transverse Colon with Autologous Tissue Substitute, Via Natural or Artificial Opening Endoscopic
HAC When reported with principal diagnosis code E66.01 and secondary diagnosis

♀ Female-only ♂ Male-only ▲ Limited Coverage ● Non-OR **HAC** HAC-associated procedure ▲ Non-covered procedures ✛ Cluster

code K68.11, K95.01, K95.81, T81.40XA, T81.41XA, T81.42XA, T81.43XA, T81.44XA or T81.49XA

0D168J4 Bypass Stomach to Cutaneous with Synthetic Substitute, Via Natural or Artificial Opening Endoscopic

0D168J9 Bypass Stomach to Duodenum with Synthetic Substitute, Via Natural or Artificial Opening Endoscopic

HAC When reported with principal diagnosis code E66.01 and secondary diagnosis code K68.11, K95.01, K95.81, T81.40XA, T81.41XA, T81.42XA, T81.43XA, T81.44XA or T81.49XA

0D168JA Bypass Stomach to Jejunum with Synthetic Substitute, Via Natural or Artificial Opening Endoscopic

HAC When reported with principal diagnosis code E66.01 and secondary diagnosis code K68.11, K95.01, K95.81, T81.40XA, T81.41XA, T81.42XA, T81.43XA, T81.44XA or T81.49XA

0D168JB Bypass Stomach to Ileum with Synthetic Substitute, Via Natural or Artificial Opening Endoscopic

HAC When reported with principal diagnosis code E66.01 and secondary diagnosis code K68.11, K95.01, K95.81, T81.40XA, T81.41XA, T81.42XA, T81.43XA, T81.44XA or T81.49XA

0D168JL Bypass Stomach to Transverse Colon with Synthetic Substitute, Via Natural or Artificial Opening Endoscopic

HAC When reported with principal diagnosis code E66.01 and secondary diagnosis code K68.11, K95.01, K95.81, T81.40XA, T81.41XA, T81.42XA, T81.43XA, T81.44XA or T81.49XA

0D168K4 Bypass Stomach to Cutaneous with Nonautologous Tissue Substitute, Via Natural or Artificial Opening Endoscopic

0D168K9 Bypass Stomach to Duodenum with Nonautologous Tissue Substitute, Via Natural or Artificial Opening Endoscopic

HAC When reported with principal diagnosis code E66.01 and secondary diagnosis code K68.11, K95.01, K95.81, T81.40XA, T81.41XA, T81.42XA, T81.43XA, T81.44XA or T81.49XA

0D168KA Bypass Stomach to Jejunum with Nonautologous Tissue Substitute, Via Natural or Artificial Opening Endoscopic

HAC When reported with principal diagnosis code E66.01 and secondary diagnosis code K68.11, K95.01, K95.81, T81.40XA, T81.41XA, T81.42XA, T81.43XA, T81.44XA or T81.49XA

0D168KB Bypass Stomach to Ileum with Nonautologous Tissue Substitute, Via Natural or Artificial Opening Endoscopic

HAC When reported with principal diagnosis E66.01 and secondary diagnosis code K68.11, K95.01, K95.81, T81.40XA, T81.41XA, T81.42XA, T81.43XA, T81.44XA or T81.49XA

0D168KL Bypass Stomach to Transverse Colon with Nonautologous Tissue Substitute, Via Natural or Artificial Opening Endoscopic

HAC When reported with principal diagnosis code E66.01 and secondary diagnosis code K68.11, K95.01, K95.81,

T81.40XA, T81.41XA, T81.42XA, T81.43XA, T81.44XA or T81.49XA

0D168Z4 Bypass Stomach to Cutaneous, Via Natural or Artificial Opening Endoscopic

0D168Z9 Bypass Stomach to Duodenum, Via Natural or Artificial Opening Endoscopic

HAC When reported with principal diagnosis code E66.01 and secondary diagnosis code K68.11, K95.01, K95.81, T81.40XA, T81.41XA, T81.42XA, T81.43XA, T81.44XA or T81.49XA

0D168ZA Bypass Stomach to Jejunum, Via Natural or Artificial Opening Endoscopic

HAC When reported with principal diagnosis code E66.01 and secondary diagnosis code K68.11, K95.01, K95.81, T81.40XA, T81.41XA, T81.42XA, T81.43XA, T81.44XA or T81.49XA

0D168ZB Bypass Stomach to Ileum, Via Natural or Artificial Opening Endoscopic

HAC When reported with principal diagnosis code E66.01 and secondary diagnosis code K68.11, K95.01, K95.81, T81.40XA, T81.41XA, T81.42XA, T81.43XA, T81.44XA or T81.49XA

0D168ZL Bypass Stomach to Transverse Colon, Via Natural or Artificial Opening Endoscopic

HAC When reported with principal diagnosis code E66.01 and secondary diagnosis code K68.11, K95.01, K95.81, T81.40XA, T81.41XA, T81.42XA, T81.43XA, T81.44XA or T81.49XA

0D18074 Bypass Small Intestine to Cutaneous with Autologous Tissue Substitute, Open Approach

0D18078 Bypass Small Intestine to Small Intestine with Autologous Tissue Substitute, Open Approach

0D1807H Bypass Small Intestine to Cecum with Autologous Tissue Substitute, Open Approach

0D1807K Bypass Small Intestine to Ascending Colon with Autologous Tissue Substitute, Open Approach

0D1807L Bypass Small Intestine to Transverse Colon with Autologous Tissue Substitute, Open Approach

0D1807M Bypass Small Intestine to Descending Colon with Autologous Tissue Substitute, Open Approach

0D1807N Bypass Small Intestine to Sigmoid Colon with Autologous Tissue Substitute, Open Approach

0D1807P Bypass Small Intestine to Rectum with Autologous Tissue Substitute, Open Approach

0D1807Q Bypass Small Intestine to Anus with Autologous Tissue Substitute, Open Approach

0D180J4 Bypass Small Intestine to Cutaneous with Synthetic Substitute, Open Approach

0D180J8 Bypass Small Intestine to Small Intestine with Synthetic Substitute, Open Approach

0D180JH Bypass Small Intestine to Cecum with Synthetic Substitute, Open Approach

0D180JK Bypass Small Intestine to Ascending Colon with Synthetic Substitute, Open Approach

0D180JL Bypass Small Intestine to Transverse Colon with Synthetic Substitute, Open Approach

0D180JM Bypass Small Intestine to Descending Colon with Synthetic Substitute, Open Approach

0D180JN Bypass Small Intestine to Sigmoid Colon with Synthetic Substitute, Open Approach

0D180JP Bypass Small Intestine to Rectum with Synthetic Substitute, Open Approach

0D180JQ Bypass Small Intestine to Anus with Synthetic Substitute, Open Approach

0D180K4 Bypass Small Intestine to Cutaneous with Nonautologous Tissue Substitute, Open Approach

0D180K8 Bypass Small Intestine to Small Intestine with Nonautologous Tissue Substitute, Open Approach

0D180KH Bypass Small Intestine to Cecum with Nonautologous Tissue Substitute, Open Approach

0D180KK Bypass Small Intestine to Ascending Colon with Nonautologous Tissue Substitute, Open Approach

0D180KL Bypass Small Intestine to Transverse Colon with Nonautologous Tissue Substitute, Open Approach

0D180KM Bypass Small Intestine to Descending Colon with Nonautologous Tissue Substitute, Open Approach

0D180KN Bypass Small Intestine to Sigmoid Colon with Nonautologous Tissue Substitute, Open Approach

0D180KP Bypass Small Intestine to Rectum with Nonautologous Tissue Substitute, Open Approach

0D180KQ Bypass Small Intestine to Anus with Nonautologous Tissue Substitute, Open Approach

0D180Z4 Bypass Small Intestine to Cutaneous, Open Approach

0D180Z8 Bypass Small Intestine to Small Intestine, Open Approach

0D180ZH Bypass Small Intestine to Cecum, Open Approach

0D180ZK Bypass Small Intestine to Ascending Colon, Open Approach

0D180ZL Bypass Small Intestine to Transverse Colon, Open Approach

0D180ZM Bypass Small Intestine to Descending Colon, Open Approach

0D180ZN Bypass Small Intestine to Sigmoid Colon, Open Approach

0D180ZP Bypass Small Intestine to Rectum, Open Approach

0D180ZQ Bypass Small Intestine to Anus, Open Approach

0D18474 Bypass Small Intestine to Cutaneous with Autologous Tissue Substitute, Percutaneous Endoscopic Approach

0D18478 Bypass Small Intestine to Small Intestine with Autologous Tissue Substitute, Percutaneous Endoscopic Approach

0D1847H Bypass Small Intestine to Cecum with Autologous Tissue Substitute, Percutaneous Endoscopic Approach

0D1847K Bypass Small Intestine to Ascending Colon with Autologous Tissue Substitute, Percutaneous Endoscopic Approach

0D1847L Bypass Small Intestine to Transverse Colon with Autologous Tissue Substitute, Percutaneous Endoscopic Approach

0D1847M Bypass Small Intestine to Descending Colon with Autologous Tissue Substitute, Percutaneous Endoscopic Approach

0D1847N Bypass Small Intestine to Sigmoid Colon with Autologous Tissue Substitute, Percutaneous Endoscopic Approach

0D1847P Bypass Small Intestine to Rectum with Autologous Tissue Substitute, Percutaneous Endoscopic Approach

0D1847Q Bypass Small Intestine to Anus with Autologous Tissue Substitute, Percutaneous Endoscopic Approach

0D184J4 Bypass Small Intestine to Cutaneous with Synthetic Substitute, Percutaneous Endoscopic Approach

0D184J8 Bypass Small Intestine to Small Intestine with Synthetic Substitute, Percutaneous Endoscopic Approach

0D184JH Bypass Small Intestine to Cecum with Synthetic Substitute, Percutaneous Endoscopic Approach

0D184JK Bypass Small Intestine to Ascending Colon with Synthetic Substitute, Percutaneous Endoscopic Approach

0D184JL Bypass Small Intestine to Transverse Colon with Synthetic Substitute, Percutaneous Endoscopic Approach

0D184JM Bypass Small Intestine to Descending Colon with Synthetic Substitute, Percutaneous Endoscopic Approach

0D184JN Bypass Small Intestine to Sigmoid Colon with Synthetic Substitute, Percutaneous Endoscopic Approach

0D184JP Bypass Small Intestine to Rectum with Synthetic Substitute, Percutaneous Endoscopic Approach

0D184JQ Bypass Small Intestine to Anus with Synthetic Substitute, Percutaneous Endoscopic Approach

0D184K4 Bypass Small Intestine to Cutaneous with Nonautologous Tissue Substitute, Percutaneous Endoscopic Approach

0D184K8 Bypass Small Intestine to Small Intestine with Nonautologous Tissue Substitute, Percutaneous Endoscopic Approach

0D184KH Bypass Small Intestine to Cecum with Nonautologous Tissue Substitute, Percutaneous Endoscopic Approach

0D184KK Bypass Small Intestine to Ascending Colon with Nonautologous Tissue Substitute, Percutaneous Endoscopic Approach

0D184KL Bypass Small Intestine to Transverse Colon with Nonautologous Tissue Substitute, Percutaneous Endoscopic Approach

0D184KM Bypass Small Intestine to Descending Colon with Nonautologous Tissue Substitute, Percutaneous Endoscopic Approach

0D184KN Bypass Small Intestine to Sigmoid Colon with Nonautologous Tissue Substitute, Percutaneous Endoscopic Approach

0D184KP Bypass Small Intestine to Rectum with Nonautologous Tissue Substitute, Percutaneous Endoscopic Approach

0D184KQ Bypass Small Intestine to Anus with Nonautologous Tissue Substitute, Percutaneous Endoscopic Approach

0D184Z4 Bypass Small Intestine to Cutaneous, Percutaneous Endoscopic Approach

0D184Z8 Bypass Small Intestine to Small Intestine, Percutaneous Endoscopic Approach

0D184ZH Bypass Small Intestine to Cecum, Percutaneous Endoscopic Approach

0D184ZK Bypass Small Intestine to Ascending Colon, Percutaneous Endoscopic Approach

0D184ZL Bypass Small Intestine to Transverse Colon, Percutaneous Endoscopic Approach

0D184ZM Bypass Small Intestine to Descending Colon, Percutaneous Endoscopic Approach

0D184ZN Bypass Small Intestine to Sigmoid Colon, Percutaneous Endoscopic Approach

0D184ZP Bypass Small Intestine to Rectum, Percutaneous Endoscopic Approach

0D184ZQ Bypass Small Intestine to Anus, Percutaneous Endoscopic Approach

0D18874 Bypass Small Intestine to Cutaneous with Autologous Tissue Substitute, Via Natural or Artificial Opening Endoscopic

0D18878 Bypass Small Intestine to Small Intestine with Autologous Tissue Substitute, Via Natural or Artificial Opening Endoscopic

0D1887H Bypass Small Intestine to Cecum with Autologous Tissue Substitute, Via Natural or Artificial Opening Endoscopic

0D1887K Bypass Small Intestine to Ascending Colon with Autologous Tissue Substitute, Via Natural or Artificial Opening Endoscopic

0D1887L Bypass Small Intestine to Transverse Colon with Autologous Tissue Substitute, Via Natural or Artificial Opening Endoscopic

0D1887M Bypass Small Intestine to Descending Colon with Autologous Tissue Substitute, Via Natural or Artificial Opening Endoscopic

0D1887N Bypass Small Intestine to Sigmoid Colon with Autologous Tissue Substitute, Via Natural or Artificial Opening Endoscopic

0D1887P Bypass Small Intestine to Rectum with Autologous Tissue Substitute, Via Natural or Artificial Opening Endoscopic

0D1887Q Bypass Small Intestine to Anus with Autologous Tissue Substitute, Via Natural or Artificial Opening Endoscopic

0D188J4 Bypass Small Intestine to Cutaneous with Synthetic Substitute, Via Natural or Artificial Opening Endoscopic

0D188J8 Bypass Small Intestine to Small Intestine with Synthetic Substitute, Via Natural or Artificial Opening Endoscopic

0D188JH Bypass Small Intestine to Cecum with Synthetic Substitute, Via Natural or Artificial Opening Endoscopic

0D188JK Bypass Small Intestine to Ascending Colon with Synthetic Substitute, Via Natural or Artificial Opening Endoscopic

0D188JL Bypass Small Intestine to Transverse Colon with Synthetic Substitute, Via Natural or Artificial Opening Endoscopic

0D188JM Bypass Small Intestine to Descending Colon with Synthetic Substitute, Via Natural or Artificial Opening Endoscopic

0D188JN Bypass Small Intestine to Sigmoid Colon with Synthetic Substitute, Via Natural or Artificial Opening Endoscopic

0D188JP Bypass Small Intestine to Rectum with Synthetic Substitute, Via Natural or Artificial Opening Endoscopic

0D188JQ Bypass Small Intestine to Anus with Synthetic Substitute, Via Natural or Artificial Opening Endoscopic

0D188K4 Bypass Small Intestine to Cutaneous with Nonautologous Tissue Substitute, Via Natural or Artificial Opening Endoscopic

0D188K8 Bypass Small Intestine to Small Intestine with Nonautologous Tissue Substitute, Via Natural or Artificial Opening Endoscopic

0D188KH Bypass Small Intestine to Cecum with Nonautologous Tissue Substitute, Via Natural or Artificial Opening Endoscopic

0D188KK Bypass Small Intestine to Ascending Colon with Nonautologous Tissue Substitute, Via Natural or Artificial Opening Endoscopic

0D188KL Bypass Small Intestine to Transverse Colon with Nonautologous Tissue Substitute, Via Natural or Artificial Opening Endoscopic

0D188KM Bypass Small Intestine to Descending Colon with Nonautologous Tissue Substitute, Via Natural or Artificial Opening Endoscopic

0D188KN Bypass Small Intestine to Sigmoid Colon with Nonautologous Tissue Substitute, Via Natural or Artificial Opening Endoscopic

0D188KP Bypass Small Intestine to Rectum with Nonautologous Tissue Substitute, Via Natural or Artificial Opening Endoscopic

0D188KQ Bypass Small Intestine to Anus with Nonautologous Tissue Substitute, Via Natural or Artificial Opening Endoscopic

0D188Z4 Bypass Small Intestine to Cutaneous, Via Natural or Artificial Opening Endoscopic

0D188Z8 Bypass Small Intestine to Small Intestine, Via Natural or Artificial Opening Endoscopic

0D188ZH Bypass Small Intestine to Cecum, Via Natural or Artificial Opening Endoscopic

0D188ZK Bypass Small Intestine to Ascending Colon, Via Natural or Artificial Opening Endoscopic

0D188ZL Bypass Small Intestine to Transverse Colon, Via Natural or Artificial Opening Endoscopic

0D188ZM Bypass Small Intestine to Descending Colon, Via Natural or Artificial Opening Endoscopic

0D188ZN Bypass Small Intestine to Sigmoid Colon, Via Natural or Artificial Opening Endoscopic

0D188ZP Bypass Small Intestine to Rectum, Via Natural or Artificial Opening Endoscopic

0D188ZQ Bypass Small Intestine to Anus, Via Natural or Artificial Opening Endoscopic

0D19074	Bypass Duodenum to Cutaneous with Autologous Tissue Substitute, Open Approach
0D19079	Bypass Duodenum to Duodenum with Autologous Tissue Substitute, Open Approach
0D1907A	Bypass Duodenum to Jejunum with Autologous Tissue Substitute, Open Approach
0D1907B	Bypass Duodenum to Ileum with Autologous Tissue Substitute, Open Approach
0D1907L	Bypass Duodenum to Transverse Colon with Autologous Tissue Substitute, Open Approach
0D190J4	Bypass Duodenum to Cutaneous with Synthetic Substitute, Open Approach
0D190J9	Bypass Duodenum to Duodenum with Synthetic Substitute, Open Approach
0D190JA	Bypass Duodenum to Jejunum with Synthetic Substitute, Open Approach
0D190JB	Bypass Duodenum to Ileum with Synthetic Substitute, Open Approach
0D190JL	Bypass Duodenum to Transverse Colon with Synthetic Substitute, Open Approach
0D190K4	Bypass Duodenum to Cutaneous with Nonautologous Tissue Substitute, Open Approach
0D190K9	Bypass Duodenum to Duodenum with Nonautologous Tissue Substitute, Open Approach
0D190KA	Bypass Duodenum to Jejunum with Nonautologous Tissue Substitute, Open Approach
0D190KB	Bypass Duodenum to Ileum with Nonautologous Tissue Substitute, Open Approach
0D190KL	Bypass Duodenum to Transverse Colon with Nonautologous Tissue Substitute, Open Approach
0D190Z4	Bypass Duodenum to Cutaneous, Open Approach
0D190Z9	Bypass Duodenum to Duodenum, Open Approach
0D190ZA	Bypass Duodenum to Jejunum, Open Approach
0D190ZB	Bypass Duodenum to Ileum, Open Approach
0D190ZL	Bypass Duodenum to Transverse Colon, Open Approach
0D193J4	Bypass Duodenum to Cutaneous with Synthetic Substitute, Percutaneous Approach
0D19474	Bypass Duodenum to Cutaneous with Autologous Tissue Substitute, Percutaneous Endoscopic Approach
0D19479	Bypass Duodenum to Duodenum with Autologous Tissue Substitute, Percutaneous Endoscopic Approach
0D1947A	Bypass Duodenum to Jejunum with Autologous Tissue Substitute, Percutaneous Endoscopic Approach
0D1947B	Bypass Duodenum to Ileum with Autologous Tissue Substitute, Percutaneous Endoscopic Approach
0D1947L	Bypass Duodenum to Transverse Colon with Autologous Tissue Substitute, Percutaneous Endoscopic Approach
0D194J4	Bypass Duodenum to Cutaneous with Synthetic Substitute, Percutaneous Endoscopic Approach
0D194J9	Bypass Duodenum to Duodenum with Synthetic Substitute, Percutaneous Endoscopic Approach

0D194JA	Bypass Duodenum to Jejunum with Synthetic Substitute, Percutaneous Endoscopic Approach
0D194JB	Bypass Duodenum to Ileum with Synthetic Substitute, Percutaneous Endoscopic Approach
0D194JL	Bypass Duodenum to Transverse Colon with Synthetic Substitute, Percutaneous Endoscopic Approach
0D194K4	Bypass Duodenum to Cutaneous with Nonautologous Tissue Substitute, Percutaneous Endoscopic Approach
0D194K9	Bypass Duodenum to Duodenum with Nonautologous Tissue Substitute, Percutaneous Endoscopic Approach
0D194KA	Bypass Duodenum to Jejunum with Nonautologous Tissue Substitute, Percutaneous Endoscopic Approach
0D194KB	Bypass Duodenum to Ileum with Nonautologous Tissue Substitute, Percutaneous Endoscopic Approach
0D194KL	Bypass Duodenum to Transverse Colon with Nonautologous Tissue Substitute, Percutaneous Endoscopic Approach
0D194Z4	Bypass Duodenum to Cutaneous, Percutaneous Endoscopic Approach
0D194Z9	Bypass Duodenum to Duodenum, Percutaneous Endoscopic Approach
0D194ZA	Bypass Duodenum to Jejunum, Percutaneous Endoscopic Approach
0D194ZB	Bypass Duodenum to Ileum, Percutaneous Endoscopic Approach
	AHA CC: 2Q, 2016, 31
0D194ZL	Bypass Duodenum to Transverse Colon, Percutaneous Endoscopic Approach
0D19874	Bypass Duodenum to Cutaneous with Autologous Tissue Substitute, Via Natural or Artificial Opening Endoscopic
0D19879	Bypass Duodenum to Duodenum with Autologous Tissue Substitute, Via Natural or Artificial Opening Endoscopic
0D1987A	Bypass Duodenum to Jejunum with Autologous Tissue Substitute, Via Natural or Artificial Opening Endoscopic
0D1987B	Bypass Duodenum to Ileum with Autologous Tissue Substitute, Via Natural or Artificial Opening Endoscopic
0D1987L	Bypass Duodenum to Transverse Colon with Autologous Tissue Substitute, Via Natural or Artificial Opening Endoscopic
0D198J4	Bypass Duodenum to Cutaneous with Synthetic Substitute, Via Natural or Artificial Opening Endoscopic
0D198J9	Bypass Duodenum to Duodenum with Synthetic Substitute, Via Natural or Artificial Opening Endoscopic
0D198JA	Bypass Duodenum to Jejunum with Synthetic Substitute, Via Natural or Artificial Opening Endoscopic
0D198JB	Bypass Duodenum to Ileum with Synthetic Substitute, Via Natural or Artificial Opening Endoscopic
0D198JL	Bypass Duodenum to Transverse Colon with Synthetic Substitute, Via Natural or Artificial Opening Endoscopic
0D198K4	Bypass Duodenum to Cutaneous with Nonautologous Tissue Substitute, Via Natural or Artificial Opening Endoscopic

0D198K9	Bypass Duodenum to Duodenum with Nonautologous Tissue Substitute, Via Natural or Artificial Opening Endoscopic
0D198KA	Bypass Duodenum to Jejunum with Nonautologous Tissue Substitute, Via Natural or Artificial Opening Endoscopic
0D198KB	Bypass Duodenum to Ileum with Nonautologous Tissue Substitute, Via Natural or Artificial Opening Endoscopic
0D198KL	Bypass Duodenum to Transverse Colon with Nonautologous Tissue Substitute, Via Natural or Artificial Opening Endoscopic
0D198Z4	Bypass Duodenum to Cutaneous, Via Natural or Artificial Opening Endoscopic
0D198Z9	Bypass Duodenum to Duodenum, Via Natural or Artificial Opening Endoscopic
0D198ZA	Bypass Duodenum to Jejunum, Via Natural or Artificial Opening Endoscopic
0D198ZB	Bypass Duodenum to Ileum, Via Natural or Artificial Opening Endoscopic
0D198ZL	Bypass Duodenum to Transverse Colon, Via Natural or Artificial Opening Endoscopic
0D1A074	Bypass Jejunum to Cutaneous with Autologous Tissue Substitute, Open Approach
0D1A07A	Bypass Jejunum to Jejunum with Autologous Tissue Substitute, Open Approach
0D1A07B	Bypass Jejunum to Ileum with Autologous Tissue Substitute, Open Approach
0D1A07H	Bypass Jejunum to Cecum with Autologous Tissue Substitute, Open Approach
0D1A07K	Bypass Jejunum to Ascending Colon with Autologous Tissue Substitute, Open Approach
0D1A07L	Bypass Jejunum to Transverse Colon with Autologous Tissue Substitute, Open Approach
0D1A07M	Bypass Jejunum to Descending Colon with Autologous Tissue Substitute, Open Approach
0D1A07N	Bypass Jejunum to Sigmoid Colon with Autologous Tissue Substitute, Open Approach
0D1A07P	Bypass Jejunum to Rectum with Autologous Tissue Substitute, Open Approach
0D1A07Q	Bypass Jejunum to Anus with Autologous Tissue Substitute, Open Approach
0D1A0J4	Bypass Jejunum to Cutaneous with Synthetic Substitute, Open Approach
0D1A0JA	Bypass Jejunum to Jejunum with Synthetic Substitute, Open Approach
0D1A0JB	Bypass Jejunum to Ileum with Synthetic Substitute, Open Approach
0D1A0JH	Bypass Jejunum to Cecum with Synthetic Substitute, Open Approach
0D1A0JK	Bypass Jejunum to Ascending Colon with Synthetic Substitute, Open Approach
0D1A0JL	Bypass Jejunum to Transverse Colon with Synthetic Substitute, Open Approach

0D1A0JM Bypass Jejunum to Descending Colon with Synthetic Substitute, Open Approach

0D1A0JN Bypass Jejunum to Sigmoid Colon with Synthetic Substitute, Open Approach

0D1A0JP Bypass Jejunum to Rectum with Synthetic Substitute, Open Approach

0D1A0JQ Bypass Jejunum to Anus with Synthetic Substitute, Open Approach

0D1A0K4 Bypass Jejunum to Cutaneous with Nonautologous Tissue Substitute, Open Approach

0D1A0KA Bypass Jejunum to Jejunum with Nonautologous Tissue Substitute, Open Approach

0D1A0KB Bypass Jejunum to Ileum with Nonautologous Tissue Substitute, Open Approach

0D1A0KH Bypass Jejunum to Cecum with Nonautologous Tissue Substitute, Open Approach

0D1A0KK Bypass Jejunum to Ascending Colon with Nonautologous Tissue Substitute, Open Approach

0D1A0KL Bypass Jejunum to Transverse Colon with Nonautologous Tissue Substitute, Open Approach

0D1A0KM Bypass Jejunum to Descending Colon with Nonautologous Tissue Substitute, Open Approach

0D1A0KN Bypass Jejunum to Sigmoid Colon with Nonautologous Tissue Substitute, Open Approach

0D1A0KP Bypass Jejunum to Rectum with Nonautologous Tissue Substitute, Open Approach

0D1A0KQ Bypass Jejunum to Anus with Nonautologous Tissue Substitute, Open Approach

0D1A0Z4 Bypass Jejunum to Cutaneous, Open Approach

0D1A0ZA Bypass Jejunum to Jejunum, Open Approach

0D1A0ZB Bypass Jejunum to Ileum, Open Approach

0D1A0ZH Bypass Jejunum to Cecum, Open Approach

0D1A0ZK Bypass Jejunum to Ascending Colon, Open Approach

0D1A0ZL Bypass Jejunum to Transverse Colon, Open Approach

0D1A0ZM Bypass Jejunum to Descending Colon, Open Approach

0D1A0ZN Bypass Jejunum to Sigmoid Colon, Open Approach

0D1A0ZP Bypass Jejunum to Rectum, Open Approach

0D1A0ZQ Bypass Jejunum to Anus, Open Approach

0D1A3J4 Bypass Jejunum to Cutaneous with Synthetic Substitute, Percutaneous Approach

0D1A474 Bypass Jejunum to Cutaneous with Autologous Tissue Substitute, Percutaneous Endoscopic Approach

0D1A47A Bypass Jejunum to Jejunum with Autologous Tissue Substitute, Percutaneous Endoscopic Approach

0D1A47B Bypass Jejunum to Ileum with Autologous Tissue Substitute, Percutaneous Endoscopic Approach

0D1A47H Bypass Jejunum to Cecum with Autologous Tissue Substitute, Percutaneous Endoscopic Approach

0D1A47K Bypass Jejunum to Ascending Colon with Autologous Tissue Substitute, Percutaneous Endoscopic Approach

0D1A47L Bypass Jejunum to Transverse Colon with Autologous Tissue Substitute, Percutaneous Endoscopic Approach

0D1A47M Bypass Jejunum to Descending Colon with Autologous Tissue Substitute, Percutaneous Endoscopic Approach

0D1A47N Bypass Jejunum to Sigmoid Colon with Autologous Tissue Substitute, Percutaneous Endoscopic Approach

0D1A47P Bypass Jejunum to Rectum with Autologous Tissue Substitute, Percutaneous Endoscopic Approach

0D1A47Q Bypass Jejunum to Anus with Autologous Tissue Substitute, Percutaneous Endoscopic Approach

0D1A4J4 Bypass Jejunum to Cutaneous with Synthetic Substitute, Percutaneous Endoscopic Approach

0D1A4JA Bypass Jejunum to Jejunum with Synthetic Substitute, Percutaneous Endoscopic Approach

0D1A4JB Bypass Jejunum to Ileum with Synthetic Substitute, Percutaneous Endoscopic Approach

0D1A4JH Bypass Jejunum to Cecum with Synthetic Substitute, Percutaneous Endoscopic Approach

0D1A4JK Bypass Jejunum to Ascending Colon with Synthetic Substitute, Percutaneous Endoscopic Approach

0D1A4JL Bypass Jejunum to Transverse Colon with Synthetic Substitute, Percutaneous Endoscopic Approach

0D1A4JM Bypass Jejunum to Descending Colon with Synthetic Substitute, Percutaneous Endoscopic Approach

0D1A4JN Bypass Jejunum to Sigmoid Colon with Synthetic Substitute, Percutaneous Endoscopic Approach

0D1A4JP Bypass Jejunum to Rectum with Synthetic Substitute, Percutaneous Endoscopic Approach

0D1A4JQ Bypass Jejunum to Anus with Synthetic Substitute, Percutaneous Endoscopic Approach

0D1A4K4 Bypass Jejunum to Cutaneous with Nonautologous Tissue Substitute, Percutaneous Endoscopic Approach

0D1A4KA Bypass Jejunum to Jejunum with Nonautologous Tissue Substitute, Percutaneous Endoscopic Approach

0D1A4KB Bypass Jejunum to Ileum with Nonautologous Tissue Substitute, Percutaneous Endoscopic Approach

0D1A4KH Bypass Jejunum to Cecum with Nonautologous Tissue Substitute, Percutaneous Endoscopic Approach

0D1A4KK Bypass Jejunum to Ascending Colon with Nonautologous Tissue Substitute, Percutaneous Endoscopic Approach

0D1A4KL Bypass Jejunum to Transverse Colon with Nonautologous Tissue Substitute, Percutaneous Endoscopic Approach

0D1A4KM Bypass Jejunum to Descending Colon with Nonautologous Tissue Substitute, Percutaneous Endoscopic Approach

0D1A4KN Bypass Jejunum to Sigmoid Colon with Nonautologous Tissue Substitute, Percutaneous Endoscopic Approach

0D1A4KP Bypass Jejunum to Rectum with Nonautologous Tissue Substitute, Percutaneous Endoscopic Approach

0D1A4KQ Bypass Jejunum to Anus with Nonautologous Tissue Substitute, Percutaneous Endoscopic Approach

0D1A4Z4 Bypass Jejunum to Cutaneous, Percutaneous Endoscopic Approach

0D1A4ZA Bypass Jejunum to Jejunum, Percutaneous Endoscopic Approach

0D1A4ZB Bypass Jejunum to Ileum, Percutaneous Endoscopic Approach

0D1A4ZH Bypass Jejunum to Cecum, Percutaneous Endoscopic Approach

0D1A4ZK Bypass Jejunum to Ascending Colon, Percutaneous Endoscopic Approach

0D1A4ZL Bypass Jejunum to Transverse Colon, Percutaneous Endoscopic Approach

0D1A4ZM Bypass Jejunum to Descending Colon, Percutaneous Endoscopic Approach

0D1A4ZN Bypass Jejunum to Sigmoid Colon, Percutaneous Endoscopic Approach

0D1A4ZP Bypass Jejunum to Rectum, Percutaneous Endoscopic Approach

0D1A4ZQ Bypass Jejunum to Anus, Percutaneous Endoscopic Approach

0D1A874 Bypass Jejunum to Cutaneous with Autologous Tissue Substitute, Via Natural or Artificial Opening Endoscopic

0D1A87A Bypass Jejunum to Jejunum with Autologous Tissue Substitute, Via Natural or Artificial Opening Endoscopic

0D1A87B Bypass Jejunum to Ileum with Autologous Tissue Substitute, Via Natural or Artificial Opening Endoscopic

0D1A87H Bypass Jejunum to Cecum with Autologous Tissue Substitute, Via Natural or Artificial Opening Endoscopic

0D1A87K Bypass Jejunum to Ascending Colon with Autologous Tissue Substitute, Via Natural or Artificial Opening Endoscopic

0D1A87L Bypass Jejunum to Transverse Colon with Autologous Tissue Substitute, Via Natural or Artificial Opening Endoscopic

0D1A87M Bypass Jejunum to Descending Colon with Autologous Tissue Substitute, Via Natural or Artificial Opening Endoscopic

0D1A87N Bypass Jejunum to Sigmoid Colon with Autologous Tissue Substitute, Via Natural or Artificial Opening Endoscopic

0D1A87P Bypass Jejunum to Rectum with Autologous Tissue Substitute, Via Natural or Artificial Opening Endoscopic

0D1A87Q Bypass Jejunum to Anus with Autologous Tissue Substitute, Via Natural or Artificial Opening Endoscopic

0D1A8J4 Bypass Jejunum to Cutaneous with Synthetic Substitute, Via Natural or Artificial Opening Endoscopic

0D1A8JA Bypass Jejunum to Jejunum with Synthetic Substitute, Via Natural or Artificial Opening Endoscopic

0D1A8JB Bypass Jejunum to Ileum with Synthetic Substitute, Via Natural or Artificial Opening Endoscopic

0D1A8JH Bypass Jejunum to Cecum with Synthetic Substitute, Via Natural or Artificial Opening Endoscopic

0D1A8JK Bypass Jejunum to Ascending Colon with Synthetic Substitute, Via Natural or Artificial Opening Endoscopic

0D1A8JL Bypass Jejunum to Transverse Colon with Synthetic Substitute, Via Natural or Artificial Opening Endoscopic

0D1A8JM Bypass Jejunum to Descending Colon with Synthetic Substitute, Via Natural or Artificial Opening Endoscopic

0D1A8JN Bypass Jejunum to Sigmoid Colon with Synthetic Substitute, Via Natural or Artificial Opening Endoscopic

0D1A8JP Bypass Jejunum to Rectum with Synthetic Substitute, Via Natural or Artificial Opening Endoscopic

0D1A8JQ Bypass Jejunum to Anus with Synthetic Substitute, Via Natural or Artificial Opening Endoscopic

0D1A8K4 Bypass Jejunum to Cutaneous with Nonautologous Tissue Substitute, Via Natural or Artificial Opening Endoscopic

0D1A8KA Bypass Jejunum to Jejunum with Nonautologous Tissue Substitute, Via Natural or Artificial Opening Endoscopic

0D1A8KB Bypass Jejunum to Ileum with Nonautologous Tissue Substitute, Via Natural or Artificial Opening Endoscopic

0D1A8KH Bypass Jejunum to Cecum with Nonautologous Tissue Substitute, Via Natural or Artificial Opening Endoscopic

0D1A8KK Bypass Jejunum to Ascending Colon with Nonautologous Tissue Substitute, Via Natural or Artificial Opening Endoscopic

0D1A8KL Bypass Jejunum to Transverse Colon with Nonautologous Tissue Substitute, Via Natural or Artificial Opening Endoscopic

0D1A8KM Bypass Jejunum to Descending Colon with Nonautologous Tissue Substitute, Via Natural or Artificial Opening Endoscopic

0D1A8KN Bypass Jejunum to Sigmoid Colon with Nonautologous Tissue Substitute, Via Natural or Artificial Opening Endoscopic

0D1A8KP Bypass Jejunum to Rectum with Nonautologous Tissue Substitute, Via Natural or Artificial Opening Endoscopic

0D1A8KQ Bypass Jejunum to Anus with Nonautologous Tissue Substitute, Via Natural or Artificial Opening Endoscopic

0D1A8Z4 Bypass Jejunum to Cutaneous, Via Natural or Artificial Opening Endoscopic

0D1A8ZA Bypass Jejunum to Jejunum, Via Natural or Artificial Opening Endoscopic

0D1A8ZB Bypass Jejunum to Ileum, Via Natural or Artificial Opening Endoscopic

0D1A8ZH Bypass Jejunum to Cecum, Via Natural or Artificial Opening Endoscopic

0D1A8ZK Bypass Jejunum to Ascending Colon, Via Natural or Artificial Opening Endoscopic

0D1A8ZL Bypass Jejunum to Transverse Colon, Via Natural or Artificial Opening Endoscopic

0D1A8ZM Bypass Jejunum to Descending Colon, Via Natural or Artificial Opening Endoscopic

0D1A8ZN Bypass Jejunum to Sigmoid Colon, Via Natural or Artificial Opening Endoscopic

0D1A8ZP Bypass Jejunum to Rectum, Via Natural or Artificial Opening Endoscopic

0D1A8ZQ Bypass Jejunum to Anus, Via Natural or Artificial Opening Endoscopic

0D1B074 Bypass Ileum to Cutaneous with Autologous Tissue Substitute, Open Approach

0D1B07B Bypass Ileum to Ileum with Autologous Tissue Substitute, Open Approach

0D1B07H Bypass Ileum to Cecum with Autologous Tissue Substitute, Open Approach

0D1B07K Bypass Ileum to Ascending Colon with Autologous Tissue Substitute, Open Approach

0D1B07L Bypass Ileum to Transverse Colon with Autologous Tissue Substitute, Open Approach

0D1B07M Bypass Ileum to Descending Colon with Autologous Tissue Substitute, Open Approach

0D1B07N Bypass Ileum to Sigmoid Colon with Autologous Tissue Substitute, Open Approach

0D1B07P Bypass Ileum to Rectum with Autologous Tissue Substitute, Open Approach

0D1B07Q Bypass Ileum to Anus with Autologous Tissue Substitute, Open Approach

0D1B0J4 Bypass Ileum to Cutaneous with Synthetic Substitute, Open Approach

0D1B0JB Bypass Ileum to Ileum with Synthetic Substitute, Open Approach

0D1B0JH Bypass Ileum to Cecum with Synthetic Substitute, Open Approach

0D1B0JK Bypass Ileum to Ascending Colon with Synthetic Substitute, Open Approach

0D1B0JL Bypass Ileum to Transverse Colon with Synthetic Substitute, Open Approach

0D1B0JM Bypass Ileum to Descending Colon with Synthetic Substitute, Open Approach

0D1B0JN Bypass Ileum to Sigmoid Colon with Synthetic Substitute, Open Approach

0D1B0JP Bypass Ileum to Rectum with Synthetic Substitute, Open Approach

0D1B0JQ Bypass Ileum to Anus with Synthetic Substitute, Open Approach

0D1B0K4 Bypass Ileum to Cutaneous with Nonautologous Tissue Substitute, Open Approach

0D1B0KB Bypass Ileum to Ileum with Nonautologous Tissue Substitute, Open Approach

0D1B0KH Bypass Ileum to Cecum with Nonautologous Tissue Substitute, Open Approach

0D1B0KK Bypass Ileum to Ascending Colon with Nonautologous Tissue Substitute, Open Approach

0D1B0KL Bypass Ileum to Transverse Colon with Nonautologous Tissue Substitute, Open Approach

0D1B0KM Bypass Ileum to Descending Colon with Nonautologous Tissue Substitute, Open Approach

0D1B0KN Bypass Ileum to Sigmoid Colon with Nonautologous Tissue Substitute, Open Approach

0D1B0KP Bypass Ileum to Rectum with Nonautologous Tissue Substitute, Open Approach

0D1B0KQ Bypass Ileum to Anus with Nonautologous Tissue Substitute, Open Approach

0D1B0Z4 Bypass Ileum to Cutaneous, Open Approach

0D1B0ZB Bypass Ileum to Ileum, Open Approach

0D1B0ZH Bypass Ileum to Cecum, Open Approach

0D1B0ZK Bypass Ileum to Ascending Colon, Open Approach

0D1B0ZL Bypass Ileum to Transverse Colon, Open Approach

0D1B0ZM Bypass Ileum to Descending Colon, Open Approach

0D1B0ZN Bypass Ileum to Sigmoid Colon, Open Approach

0D1B0ZP Bypass Ileum to Rectum, Open Approach

0D1B0ZQ Bypass Ileum to Anus, Open Approach

0D1B3J4 Bypass Ileum to Cutaneous with Synthetic Substitute, Percutaneous Approach

0D1B474 Bypass Ileum to Cutaneous with Autologous Tissue Substitute, Percutaneous Endoscopic Approach

0D1B47B Bypass Ileum to Ileum with Autologous Tissue Substitute, Percutaneous Endoscopic Approach

0D1B47H Bypass Ileum to Cecum with Autologous Tissue Substitute, Percutaneous Endoscopic Approach

0D1B47K Bypass Ileum to Ascending Colon with Autologous Tissue Substitute, Percutaneous Endoscopic Approach

0D1B47L Bypass Ileum to Transverse Colon with Autologous Tissue Substitute, Percutaneous Endoscopic Approach

0D1B47M Bypass Ileum to Descending Colon with Autologous Tissue Substitute, Percutaneous Endoscopic Approach

0D1B47N Bypass Ileum to Sigmoid Colon with Autologous Tissue Substitute, Percutaneous Endoscopic Approach

0D1B47P Bypass Ileum to Rectum with Autologous Tissue Substitute, Percutaneous Endoscopic Approach

0D1B47Q Bypass Ileum to Anus with Autologous Tissue Substitute, Percutaneous Endoscopic Approach

0D1B4J4 Bypass Ileum to Cutaneous with Synthetic Substitute, Percutaneous Endoscopic Approach

0D1B4JB Bypass Ileum to Ileum with Synthetic Substitute, Percutaneous Endoscopic Approach

0D1B4JH Bypass Ileum to Cecum with Synthetic Substitute, Percutaneous Endoscopic Approach

0D1B4JK Bypass Ileum to Ascending Colon with Synthetic Substitute, Percutaneous Endoscopic Approach

0D1B4JL Bypass Ileum to Transverse Colon with Synthetic Substitute, Percutaneous Endoscopic Approach

0D1B4JM Bypass Ileum to Descending Colon with Synthetic Substitute, Percutaneous Endoscopic Approach

0D1B4JN Bypass Ileum to Sigmoid Colon with Synthetic Substitute, Percutaneous Endoscopic Approach

0D1B4JP Bypass Ileum to Rectum with Synthetic Substitute, Percutaneous Endoscopic Approach

0D1B4JQ Bypass Ileum to Anus with Synthetic Substitute, Percutaneous Endoscopic Approach

0D1B4K4 Bypass Ileum to Cutaneous with Nonautologous Tissue Substitute, Percutaneous Endoscopic Approach

0D1B4KB Bypass Ileum to Ileum with Nonautologous Tissue Substitute, Percutaneous Endoscopic Approach

0D1B4KH Bypass Ileum to Cecum with Nonautologous Tissue Substitute, Percutaneous Endoscopic Approach

0D1B4KK Bypass Ileum to Ascending Colon with Nonautologous Tissue Substitute, Percutaneous Endoscopic Approach

0D1B4KL Bypass Ileum to Transverse Colon with Nonautologous Tissue Substitute, Percutaneous Endoscopic Approach

0D1B4KM Bypass Ileum to Descending Colon with Nonautologous Tissue Substitute, Percutaneous Endoscopic Approach

0D1B4KN Bypass Ileum to Sigmoid Colon with Nonautologous Tissue Substitute, Percutaneous Endoscopic Approach

0D1B4KP Bypass Ileum to Rectum with Nonautologous Tissue Substitute, Percutaneous Endoscopic Approach

0D1B4KQ Bypass Ileum to Anus with Nonautologous Tissue Substitute, Percutaneous Endoscopic Approach

0D1B4Z4 Bypass Ileum to Cutaneous, Percutaneous Endoscopic Approach

0D1B4ZB Bypass Ileum to Ileum, Percutaneous Endoscopic Approach

0D1B4ZH Bypass Ileum to Cecum, Percutaneous Endoscopic Approach

0D1B4ZK Bypass Ileum to Ascending Colon, Percutaneous Endoscopic Approach

0D1B4ZL Bypass Ileum to Transverse Colon, Percutaneous Endoscopic Approach

0D1B4ZM Bypass Ileum to Descending Colon, Percutaneous Endoscopic Approach

0D1B4ZN Bypass Ileum to Sigmoid Colon, Percutaneous Endoscopic Approach

0D1B4ZP Bypass Ileum to Rectum, Percutaneous Endoscopic Approach

0D1B4ZQ Bypass Ileum to Anus, Percutaneous Endoscopic Approach

0D1B874 Bypass Ileum to Cutaneous with Autologous Tissue Substitute, Via Natural or Artificial Opening Endoscopic

0D1B87B Bypass Ileum to Ileum with Autologous Tissue Substitute, Via Natural or Artificial Opening Endoscopic

0D1B87H Bypass Ileum to Cecum with Autologous Tissue Substitute, Via Natural or Artificial Opening Endoscopic

0D1B87K Bypass Ileum to Ascending Colon with Autologous Tissue Substitute, Via Natural or Artificial Opening Endoscopic

0D1B87L Bypass Ileum to Transverse Colon with Autologous Tissue Substitute, Via Natural or Artificial Opening Endoscopic

0D1B87M Bypass Ileum to Descending Colon with Autologous Tissue Substitute, Via Natural or Artificial Opening Endoscopic

0D1B87N Bypass Ileum to Sigmoid Colon with Autologous Tissue Substitute, Via Natural or Artificial Opening Endoscopic

0D1B87P Bypass Ileum to Rectum with Autologous Tissue Substitute, Via Natural or Artificial Opening Endoscopic

0D1B87Q Bypass Ileum to Anus with Autologous Tissue Substitute, Via Natural or Artificial Opening Endoscopic

0D1B8J4 Bypass Ileum to Cutaneous with Synthetic Substitute, Via Natural or Artificial Opening Endoscopic

0D1B8JB Bypass Ileum to Ileum with Synthetic Substitute, Via Natural or Artificial Opening Endoscopic

0D1B8JH Bypass Ileum to Cecum with Synthetic Substitute, Via Natural or Artificial Opening Endoscopic

0D1B8JK Bypass Ileum to Ascending Colon with Synthetic Substitute, Via Natural or Artificial Opening Endoscopic

0D1B8JL Bypass Ileum to Transverse Colon with Synthetic Substitute, Via Natural or Artificial Opening Endoscopic

0D1B8JM Bypass Ileum to Descending Colon with Synthetic Substitute, Via Natural or Artificial Opening Endoscopic

0D1B8JN Bypass Ileum to Sigmoid Colon with Synthetic Substitute, Via Natural or Artificial Opening Endoscopic

0D1B8JP Bypass Ileum to Rectum with Synthetic Substitute, Via Natural or Artificial Opening Endoscopic

0D1B8JQ Bypass Ileum to Anus with Synthetic Substitute, Via Natural or Artificial Opening Endoscopic

0D1B8K4 Bypass Ileum to Cutaneous with Nonautologous Tissue Substitute, Via Natural or Artificial Opening Endoscopic

0D1B8KB Bypass Ileum to Ileum with Nonautologous Tissue Substitute, Via Natural or Artificial Opening Endoscopic

0D1B8KH Bypass Ileum to Cecum with Nonautologous Tissue Substitute, Via Natural or Artificial Opening Endoscopic

0D1B8KK Bypass Ileum to Ascending Colon with Nonautologous Tissue Substitute, Via Natural or Artificial Opening Endoscopic

0D1B8KL Bypass Ileum to Transverse Colon with Nonautologous Tissue Substitute, Via Natural or Artificial Opening Endoscopic

0D1B8KM Bypass Ileum to Descending Colon with Nonautologous Tissue Substitute, Via Natural or Artificial Opening Endoscopic

0D1B8KN Bypass Ileum to Sigmoid Colon with Nonautologous Tissue Substitute, Via Natural or Artificial Opening Endoscopic

0D1B8KP Bypass Ileum to Rectum with Nonautologous Tissue Substitute, Via Natural or Artificial Opening Endoscopic

0D1B8KQ Bypass Ileum to Anus with Nonautologous Tissue Substitute, Via Natural or Artificial Opening Endoscopic

0D1B8Z4 Bypass Ileum to Cutaneous, Via Natural or Artificial Opening Endoscopic

0D1B8ZB Bypass Ileum to Ileum, Via Natural or Artificial Opening Endoscopic

0D1B8ZH Bypass Ileum to Cecum, Via Natural or Artificial Opening Endoscopic

0D1B8ZK Bypass Ileum to Ascending Colon, Via Natural or Artificial Opening Endoscopic

0D1B8ZL Bypass Ileum to Transverse Colon, Via Natural or Artificial Opening Endoscopic

0D1B8ZM Bypass Ileum to Descending Colon, Via Natural or Artificial Opening Endoscopic

0D1B8ZN Bypass Ileum to Sigmoid Colon, Via Natural or Artificial Opening Endoscopic

0D1B8ZP Bypass Ileum to Rectum, Via Natural or Artificial Opening Endoscopic

0D1B8ZQ Bypass Ileum to Anus, Via Natural or Artificial Opening Endoscopic

0D1E074 Bypass Large Intestine to Cutaneous with Autologous Tissue Substitute, Open Approach

0D1E07E Bypass Large Intestine to Large Intestine with Autologous Tissue Substitute, Open Approach

0D1E07P Bypass Large Intestine to Rectum with Autologous Tissue Substitute, Open Approach

0D1E0J4 Bypass Large Intestine to Cutaneous with Synthetic Substitute, Open Approach

0D1E0JE Bypass Large Intestine to Large Intestine with Synthetic Substitute, Open Approach

0D1E0JP Bypass Large Intestine to Rectum with Synthetic Substitute, Open Approach

0D1E0K4 Bypass Large Intestine to Cutaneous with Nonautologous Tissue Substitute, Open Approach

0D1E0KE Bypass Large Intestine to Large Intestine with Nonautologous Tissue Substitute, Open Approach

0D1E0KP Bypass Large Intestine to Rectum with Nonautologous Tissue Substitute, Open Approach

0D1E0Z4 Bypass Large Intestine to Cutaneous, Open Approach

0D1E0ZE Bypass Large Intestine to Large Intestine, Open Approach

0D1E0ZP Bypass Large Intestine to Rectum, Open Approach

0D1E474 Bypass Large Intestine to Cutaneous with Autologous Tissue Substitute, Percutaneous Endoscopic Approach

0D1E47E Bypass Large Intestine to Large Intestine with Autologous Tissue Substitute, Percutaneous Endoscopic Approach

0D1E47P Bypass Large Intestine to Rectum with Autologous Tissue Substitute, Percutaneous Endoscopic Approach

0D1E4J4 Bypass Large Intestine to Cutaneous with Synthetic Substitute, Percutaneous Endoscopic Approach

0D1E4JE Bypass Large Intestine to Large Intestine with Synthetic Substitute, Percutaneous Endoscopic Approach

0D1E4JP Bypass Large Intestine to Rectum with Synthetic Substitute, Percutaneous Endoscopic Approach

0D1E4K4 Bypass Large Intestine to Cutaneous with Nonautologous Tissue Substitute, Percutaneous Endoscopic Approach

♀ Female-only   ♂ Male-only   ▲ Limited Coverage   ● Non-OR   ▦ HAC-associated procedure   ▲ Non-covered procedures   ✛ Cluster

0D1E4KE Bypass Large Intestine to Large Intestine with Nonautologous Tissue Substitute, Percutaneous Endoscopic Approach

0D1E4KP Bypass Large Intestine to Rectum with Nonautologous Tissue Substitute, Percutaneous Endoscopic Approach

0D1E4Z4 Bypass Large Intestine to Cutaneous, Percutaneous Endoscopic Approach

0D1E4ZE Bypass Large Intestine to Large Intestine, Percutaneous Endoscopic Approach

0D1E4ZP Bypass Large Intestine to Rectum, Percutaneous Endoscopic Approach

0D1E874 Bypass Large Intestine to Cutaneous with Autologous Tissue Substitute, Via Natural or Artificial Opening Endoscopic

0D1E87E Bypass Large Intestine to Large Intestine with Autologous Tissue Substitute, Via Natural or Artificial Opening Endoscopic

0D1E87P Bypass Large Intestine to Rectum with Autologous Tissue Substitute, Via Natural or Artificial Opening Endoscopic

0D1E8J4 Bypass Large Intestine to Cutaneous with Synthetic Substitute, Via Natural or Artificial Opening Endoscopic

0D1E8JE Bypass Large Intestine to Large Intestine with Synthetic Substitute, Via Natural or Artificial Opening Endoscopic

0D1E8JP Bypass Large Intestine to Rectum with Synthetic Substitute, Via Natural or Artificial Opening Endoscopic

0D1E8K4 Bypass Large Intestine to Cutaneous with Nonautologous Tissue Substitute, Via Natural or Artificial Opening Endoscopic

0D1E8KE Bypass Large Intestine to Large Intestine with Nonautologous Tissue Substitute, Via Natural or Artificial Opening Endoscopic

0D1E8KP Bypass Large Intestine to Rectum with Nonautologous Tissue Substitute, Via Natural or Artificial Opening Endoscopic

0D1E8Z4 Bypass Large Intestine to Cutaneous, Via Natural or Artificial Opening Endoscopic

0D1E8ZE Bypass Large Intestine to Large Intestine, Via Natural or Artificial Opening Endoscopic

0D1E8ZP Bypass Large Intestine to Rectum, Via Natural or Artificial Opening Endoscopic

0D1H074 Bypass Cecum to Cutaneous with Autologous Tissue Substitute, Open Approach

0D1H07H Bypass Cecum to Cecum with Autologous Tissue Substitute, Open Approach

0D1H07K Bypass Cecum to Ascending Colon with Autologous Tissue Substitute, Open Approach

0D1H07L Bypass Cecum to Transverse Colon with Autologous Tissue Substitute, Open Approach

0D1H07M Bypass Cecum to Descending Colon with Autologous Tissue Substitute, Open Approach

0D1H07N Bypass Cecum to Sigmoid Colon with Autologous Tissue Substitute, Open Approach

0D1H07P Bypass Cecum to Rectum with Autologous Tissue Substitute, Open Approach

0D1H0J4 Bypass Cecum to Cutaneous with Synthetic Substitute, Open Approach

0D1H0JH Bypass Cecum to Cecum with Synthetic Substitute, Open Approach

0D1H0JK Bypass Cecum to Ascending Colon with Synthetic Substitute, Open Approach

0D1H0JL Bypass Cecum to Transverse Colon with Synthetic Substitute, Open Approach

0D1H0JM Bypass Cecum to Descending Colon with Synthetic Substitute, Open Approach

0D1H0JN Bypass Cecum to Sigmoid Colon with Synthetic Substitute, Open Approach

0D1H0JP Bypass Cecum to Rectum with Synthetic Substitute, Open Approach

0D1H0K4 Bypass Cecum to Cutaneous with Nonautologous Tissue Substitute, Open Approach

0D1H0KH Bypass Cecum to Cecum with Nonautologous Tissue Substitute, Open Approach

0D1H0KK Bypass Cecum to Ascending Colon with Nonautologous Tissue Substitute, Open Approach

0D1H0KL Bypass Cecum to Transverse Colon with Nonautologous Tissue Substitute, Open Approach

0D1H0KM Bypass Cecum to Descending Colon with Nonautologous Tissue Substitute, Open Approach

0D1H0KN Bypass Cecum to Sigmoid Colon with Nonautologous Tissue Substitute, Open Approach

0D1H0KP Bypass Cecum to Rectum with Nonautologous Tissue Substitute, Open Approach

0D1H0Z4 Bypass Cecum to Cutaneous, Open Approach

0D1H0ZH Bypass Cecum to Cecum, Open Approach

0D1H0ZK Bypass Cecum to Ascending Colon, Open Approach

0D1H0ZL Bypass Cecum to Transverse Colon, Open Approach

0D1H0ZM Bypass Cecum to Descending Colon, Open Approach

0D1H0ZN Bypass Cecum to Sigmoid Colon, Open Approach

0D1H0ZP Bypass Cecum to Rectum, Open Approach

0D1H3J4 Bypass Cecum to Cutaneous with Synthetic Substitute, Percutaneous Approach

0D1H474 Bypass Cecum to Cutaneous with Autologous Tissue Substitute, Percutaneous Endoscopic Approach

0D1H47H Bypass Cecum to Cecum with Autologous Tissue Substitute, Percutaneous Endoscopic Approach

0D1H47K Bypass Cecum to Ascending Colon with Autologous Tissue Substitute, Percutaneous Endoscopic Approach

0D1H47L Bypass Cecum to Transverse Colon with Autologous Tissue Substitute, Percutaneous Endoscopic Approach

0D1H47M Bypass Cecum to Descending Colon with Autologous Tissue Substitute, Percutaneous Endoscopic Approach

0D1H47N Bypass Cecum to Sigmoid Colon with Autologous Tissue Substitute, Percutaneous Endoscopic Approach

0D1H47P Bypass Cecum to Rectum with Autologous Tissue Substitute, Percutaneous Endoscopic Approach

0D1H4J4 Bypass Cecum to Cutaneous with Synthetic Substitute, Percutaneous Endoscopic Approach

0D1H4JH Bypass Cecum to Cecum with Synthetic Substitute, Percutaneous Endoscopic Approach

0D1H4JK Bypass Cecum to Ascending Colon with Synthetic Substitute, Percutaneous Endoscopic Approach

0D1H4JL Bypass Cecum to Transverse Colon with Synthetic Substitute, Percutaneous Endoscopic Approach

0D1H4JM Bypass Cecum to Descending Colon with Synthetic Substitute, Percutaneous Endoscopic Approach

0D1H4JN Bypass Cecum to Sigmoid Colon with Synthetic Substitute, Percutaneous Endoscopic Approach

0D1H4JP Bypass Cecum to Rectum with Synthetic Substitute, Percutaneous Endoscopic Approach

0D1H4K4 Bypass Cecum to Cutaneous with Nonautologous Tissue Substitute, Percutaneous Endoscopic Approach

0D1H4KH Bypass Cecum to Cecum with Nonautologous Tissue Substitute, Percutaneous Endoscopic Approach

0D1H4KK Bypass Cecum to Ascending Colon with Nonautologous Tissue Substitute, Percutaneous Endoscopic Approach

0D1H4KL Bypass Cecum to Transverse Colon with Nonautologous Tissue Substitute, Percutaneous Endoscopic Approach

0D1H4KM Bypass Cecum to Descending Colon with Nonautologous Tissue Substitute, Percutaneous Endoscopic Approach

0D1H4KN Bypass Cecum to Sigmoid Colon with Nonautologous Tissue Substitute, Percutaneous Endoscopic Approach

0D1H4KP Bypass Cecum to Rectum with Nonautologous Tissue Substitute, Percutaneous Endoscopic Approach

0D1H4Z4 Bypass Cecum to Cutaneous, Percutaneous Endoscopic Approach

0D1H4ZH Bypass Cecum to Cecum, Percutaneous Endoscopic Approach

0D1H4ZK Bypass Cecum to Ascending Colon, Percutaneous Endoscopic Approach

0D1H4ZL Bypass Cecum to Transverse Colon, Percutaneous Endoscopic Approach

0D1H4ZM Bypass Cecum to Descending Colon, Percutaneous Endoscopic Approach

0D1H4ZN Bypass Cecum to Sigmoid Colon, Percutaneous Endoscopic Approach

0D1H4ZP Bypass Cecum to Rectum, Percutaneous Endoscopic Approach

0D1H874 Bypass Cecum to Cutaneous with Autologous Tissue Substitute, Via Natural or Artificial Opening Endoscopic

0D1H87H Bypass Cecum to Cecum with Autologous Tissue Substitute, Via Natural or Artificial Opening Endoscopic

0D1H87K Bypass Cecum to Ascending Colon with Autologous Tissue Substitute, Via Natural or Artificial Opening Endoscopic

0D1H87L Bypass Cecum to Transverse Colon with Autologous Tissue Substitute, Via Natural or Artificial Opening Endoscopic

0D1H87M Bypass Cecum to Descending Colon with Autologous Tissue Substitute, Via Natural or Artificial Opening Endoscopic

0D1H87N Bypass Cecum to Sigmoid Colon with Autologous Tissue Substitute, Via Natural or Artificial Opening Endoscopic

0D1H87P Bypass Cecum to Rectum with Autologous Tissue Substitute, Via Natural or Artificial Opening Endoscopic

0D1H8J4 Bypass Cecum to Cutaneous with Synthetic Substitute, Via Natural or Artificial Opening Endoscopic

0D1H8JH Bypass Cecum to Cecum with Synthetic Substitute, Via Natural or Artificial Opening Endoscopic

0D1H8JK Bypass Cecum to Ascending Colon with Synthetic Substitute, Via Natural or Artificial Opening Endoscopic

0D1H8JL Bypass Cecum to Transverse Colon with Synthetic Substitute, Via Natural or Artificial Opening Endoscopic

0D1H8JM Bypass Cecum to Descending Colon with Synthetic Substitute, Via Natural or Artificial Opening Endoscopic

0D1H8JN Bypass Cecum to Sigmoid Colon with Synthetic Substitute, Via Natural or Artificial Opening Endoscopic

0D1H8JP Bypass Cecum to Rectum with Synthetic Substitute, Via Natural or Artificial Opening Endoscopic

0D1H8K4 Bypass Cecum to Cutaneous with Nonautologous Tissue Substitute, Via Natural or Artificial Opening Endoscopic

0D1H8KH Bypass Cecum to Cecum with Nonautologous Tissue Substitute, Via Natural or Artificial Opening Endoscopic

0D1H8KK Bypass Cecum to Ascending Colon with Nonautologous Tissue Substitute, Via Natural or Artificial Opening Endoscopic

0D1H8KL Bypass Cecum to Transverse Colon with Nonautologous Tissue Substitute, Via Natural or Artificial Opening Endoscopic

0D1H8KM Bypass Cecum to Descending Colon with Nonautologous Tissue Substitute, Via Natural or Artificial Opening Endoscopic

0D1H8KN Bypass Cecum to Sigmoid Colon with Nonautologous Tissue Substitute, Via Natural or Artificial Opening Endoscopic

0D1H8KP Bypass Cecum to Rectum with Nonautologous Tissue Substitute, Via Natural or Artificial Opening Endoscopic

0D1H8Z4 Bypass Cecum to Cutaneous, Via Natural or Artificial Opening Endoscopic

0D1H8ZH Bypass Cecum to Cecum, Via Natural or Artificial Opening Endoscopic

0D1H8ZK Bypass Cecum to Ascending Colon, Via Natural or Artificial Opening Endoscopic

0D1H8ZL Bypass Cecum to Transverse Colon, Via Natural or Artificial Opening Endoscopic

0D1H8ZM Bypass Cecum to Descending Colon, Via Natural or Artificial Opening Endoscopic

0D1H8ZN Bypass Cecum to Sigmoid Colon, Via Natural or Artificial Opening Endoscopic

0D1H8ZP Bypass Cecum to Rectum, Via Natural or Artificial Opening Endoscopic

0D1K074 Bypass Ascending Colon to Cutaneous with Autologous Tissue Substitute, Open Approach

0D1K07K Bypass Ascending Colon to Ascending Colon with Autologous Tissue Substitute, Open Approach

0D1K07L Bypass Ascending Colon to Transverse Colon with Autologous Tissue Substitute, Open Approach

0D1K07M Bypass Ascending Colon to Descending Colon with Autologous Tissue Substitute, Open Approach

0D1K07N Bypass Ascending Colon to Sigmoid Colon with Autologous Tissue Substitute, Open Approach

0D1K07P Bypass Ascending Colon to Rectum with Autologous Tissue Substitute, Open Approach

0D1K0J4 Bypass Ascending Colon to Cutaneous with Synthetic Substitute, Open Approach

0D1K0JK Bypass Ascending Colon to Ascending Colon with Synthetic Substitute, Open Approach

0D1K0JL Bypass Ascending Colon to Transverse Colon with Synthetic Substitute, Open Approach

0D1K0JM Bypass Ascending Colon to Descending Colon with Synthetic Substitute, Open Approach

0D1K0JN Bypass Ascending Colon to Sigmoid Colon with Synthetic Substitute, Open Approach

0D1K0JP Bypass Ascending Colon to Rectum with Synthetic Substitute, Open Approach

0D1K0K4 Bypass Ascending Colon to Cutaneous with Nonautologous Tissue Substitute, Open Approach

0D1K0KK Bypass Ascending Colon to Ascending Colon with Nonautologous Tissue Substitute, Open Approach

0D1K0KL Bypass Ascending Colon to Transverse Colon with Nonautologous Tissue Substitute, Open Approach

0D1K0KM Bypass Ascending Colon to Descending Colon with Nonautologous Tissue Substitute, Open Approach

0D1K0KN Bypass Ascending Colon to Sigmoid Colon with Nonautologous Tissue Substitute, Open Approach

0D1K0KP Bypass Ascending Colon to Rectum with Nonautologous Tissue Substitute, Open Approach

0D1K0Z4 Bypass Ascending Colon to Cutaneous, Open Approach

0D1K0ZK Bypass Ascending Colon to Ascending Colon, Open Approach

0D1K0ZL Bypass Ascending Colon to Transverse Colon, Open Approach

0D1K0ZM Bypass Ascending Colon to Descending Colon, Open Approach

0D1K0ZN Bypass Ascending Colon to Sigmoid Colon, Open Approach

0D1K0ZP Bypass Ascending Colon to Rectum, Open Approach

0D1K3J4 Bypass Ascending Colon to Cutaneous with Synthetic Substitute, Percutaneous Approach

0D1K474 Bypass Ascending Colon to Cutaneous with Autologous Tissue Substitute, Percutaneous Endoscopic Approach

0D1K47K Bypass Ascending Colon to Ascending Colon with Autologous Tissue Substitute, Percutaneous Endoscopic Approach

0D1K47L Bypass Ascending Colon to Transverse Colon with Autologous Tissue Substitute, Percutaneous Endoscopic Approach

0D1K47M Bypass Ascending Colon to Descending Colon with Autologous Tissue Substitute, Percutaneous Endoscopic Approach

0D1K47N Bypass Ascending Colon to Sigmoid Colon with Autologous Tissue Substitute, Percutaneous Endoscopic Approach

0D1K47P Bypass Ascending Colon to Rectum with Autologous Tissue Substitute, Percutaneous Endoscopic Approach

0D1K4J4 Bypass Ascending Colon to Cutaneous with Synthetic Substitute, Percutaneous Endoscopic Approach

0D1K4JK Bypass Ascending Colon to Ascending Colon with Synthetic Substitute, Percutaneous Endoscopic Approach

0D1K4JL Bypass Ascending Colon to Transverse Colon with Synthetic Substitute, Percutaneous Endoscopic Approach

0D1K4JM Bypass Ascending Colon to Descending Colon with Synthetic Substitute, Percutaneous Endoscopic Approach

0D1K4JN Bypass Ascending Colon to Sigmoid Colon with Synthetic Substitute, Percutaneous Endoscopic Approach

0D1K4JP Bypass Ascending Colon to Rectum with Synthetic Substitute, Percutaneous Endoscopic Approach

0D1K4K4 Bypass Ascending Colon to Cutaneous with Nonautologous Tissue Substitute, Percutaneous Endoscopic Approach

0D1K4KK Bypass Ascending Colon to Ascending Colon with Nonautologous Tissue Substitute, Percutaneous Endoscopic Approach

0D1K4KL Bypass Ascending Colon to Transverse Colon with Nonautologous Tissue Substitute, Percutaneous Endoscopic Approach

0D1K4KM Bypass Ascending Colon to Descending Colon with Nonautologous Tissue Substitute, Percutaneous Endoscopic Approach

0D1K4KN Bypass Ascending Colon to Sigmoid Colon with Nonautologous Tissue Substitute, Percutaneous Endoscopic Approach

0D1K4KP Bypass Ascending Colon to Rectum with Nonautologous Tissue Substitute, Percutaneous Endoscopic Approach

0D1K4Z4 Bypass Ascending Colon to Cutaneous, Percutaneous Endoscopic Approach

0D1K4ZK Bypass Ascending Colon to Ascending Colon, Percutaneous Endoscopic Approach

0D1K4ZL Bypass Ascending Colon to Transverse Colon, Percutaneous Endoscopic Approach

♀ Female-only   ♂ Male-only   ▲ Limited Coverage   ● Non-OR   HAC HAC-associated procedure   ▲ Non-covered procedures   ✚ Cluster

0D1K4ZM	Bypass Ascending Colon to Descending Colon, Percutaneous Endoscopic Approach
0D1K4ZN	Bypass Ascending Colon to Sigmoid Colon, Percutaneous Endoscopic Approach
0D1K4ZP	Bypass Ascending Colon to Rectum, Percutaneous Endoscopic Approach
0D1K874	Bypass Ascending Colon to Cutaneous with Autologous Tissue Substitute, Via Natural or Artificial Opening Endoscopic
0D1K87K	Bypass Ascending Colon to Ascending Colon with Autologous Tissue Substitute, Via Natural or Artificial Opening Endoscopic
0D1K87L	Bypass Ascending Colon to Transverse Colon with Autologous Tissue Substitute, Via Natural or Artificial Opening Endoscopic
0D1K87M	Bypass Ascending Colon to Descending Colon with Autologous Tissue Substitute, Via Natural or Artificial Opening Endoscopic
0D1K87N	Bypass Ascending Colon to Sigmoid Colon with Autologous Tissue Substitute, Via Natural or Artificial Opening Endoscopic
0D1K87P	Bypass Ascending Colon to Rectum with Autologous Tissue Substitute, Via Natural or Artificial Opening Endoscopic
0D1K8J4	Bypass Ascending Colon to Cutaneous with Synthetic Substitute, Via Natural or Artificial Opening Endoscopic
0D1K8JK	Bypass Ascending Colon to Ascending Colon with Synthetic Substitute, Via Natural or Artificial Opening Endoscopic
0D1K8JL	Bypass Ascending Colon to Transverse Colon with Synthetic Substitute, Via Natural or Artificial Opening Endoscopic
0D1K8JM	Bypass Ascending Colon to Descending Colon with Synthetic Substitute, Via Natural or Artificial Opening Endoscopic
0D1K8JN	Bypass Ascending Colon to Sigmoid Colon with Synthetic Substitute, Via Natural or Artificial Opening Endoscopic
0D1K8JP	Bypass Ascending Colon to Rectum with Synthetic Substitute, Via Natural or Artificial Opening Endoscopic
0D1K8K4	Bypass Ascending Colon to Cutaneous with Nonautologous Tissue Substitute, Via Natural or Artificial Opening Endoscopic
0D1K8KK	Bypass Ascending Colon to Ascending Colon with Nonautologous Tissue Substitute, Via Natural or Artificial Opening Endoscopic
0D1K8KL	Bypass Ascending Colon to Transverse Colon with Nonautologous Tissue Substitute, Via Natural or Artificial Opening Endoscopic
0D1K8KM	Bypass Ascending Colon to Descending Colon with Nonautologous Tissue Substitute, Via Natural or Artificial Opening Endoscopic
0D1K8KN	Bypass Ascending Colon to Sigmoid Colon with Nonautologous Tissue Substitute, Via Natural or Artificial Opening Endoscopic
0D1K8KP	Bypass Ascending Colon to Rectum with Nonautologous Tissue Substitute, Via Natural or Artificial Opening Endoscopic
0D1K8Z4	Bypass Ascending Colon to Cutaneous, Via Natural or Artificial Opening Endoscopic
0D1K8ZK	Bypass Ascending Colon to Ascending Colon, Via Natural or Artificial Opening Endoscopic
0D1K8ZL	Bypass Ascending Colon to Transverse Colon, Via Natural or Artificial Opening Endoscopic
0D1K8ZM	Bypass Ascending Colon to Descending Colon, Via Natural or Artificial Opening Endoscopic
0D1K8ZN	Bypass Ascending Colon to Sigmoid Colon, Via Natural or Artificial Opening Endoscopic
0D1K8ZP	Bypass Ascending Colon to Rectum, Via Natural or Artificial Opening Endoscopic
0D1L074	Bypass Transverse Colon to Cutaneous with Autologous Tissue Substitute, Open Approach
0D1L07L	Bypass Transverse Colon to Transverse Colon with Autologous Tissue Substitute, Open Approach
0D1L07M	Bypass Transverse Colon to Descending Colon with Autologous Tissue Substitute, Open Approach
0D1L07N	Bypass Transverse Colon to Sigmoid Colon with Autologous Tissue Substitute, Open Approach
0D1L07P	Bypass Transverse Colon to Rectum with Autologous Tissue Substitute, Open Approach
0D1L0J4	Bypass Transverse Colon to Cutaneous with Synthetic Substitute, Open Approach
0D1L0JL	Bypass Transverse Colon to Transverse Colon with Synthetic Substitute, Open Approach
0D1L0JM	Bypass Transverse Colon to Descending Colon with Synthetic Substitute, Open Approach
0D1L0JN	Bypass Transverse Colon to Sigmoid Colon with Synthetic Substitute, Open Approach
0D1L0JP	Bypass Transverse Colon to Rectum with Synthetic Substitute, Open Approach
0D1L0K4	Bypass Transverse Colon to Cutaneous with Nonautologous Tissue Substitute, Open Approach
0D1L0KL	Bypass Transverse Colon to Transverse Colon with Nonautologous Tissue Substitute, Open Approach
0D1L0KM	Bypass Transverse Colon to Descending Colon with Nonautologous Tissue Substitute, Open Approach
0D1L0KN	Bypass Transverse Colon to Sigmoid Colon with Nonautologous Tissue Substitute, Open Approach
0D1L0KP	Bypass Transverse Colon to Rectum with Nonautologous Tissue Substitute, Open Approach
0D1L0Z4	Bypass Transverse Colon to Cutaneous, Open Approach
0D1L0ZL	Bypass Transverse Colon to Transverse Colon, Open Approach
0D1L0ZM	Bypass Transverse Colon to Descending Colon, Open Approach
0D1L0ZN	Bypass Transverse Colon to Sigmoid Colon, Open Approach
0D1L0ZP	Bypass Transverse Colon to Rectum, Open Approach
0D1L3J4	Bypass Transverse Colon to Cutaneous with Synthetic Substitute, Percutaneous Approach
0D1L474	Bypass Transverse Colon to Cutaneous with Autologous Tissue Substitute, Percutaneous Endoscopic Approach
0D1L47L	Bypass Transverse Colon to Transverse Colon with Autologous Tissue Substitute, Percutaneous Endoscopic Approach
0D1L47M	Bypass Transverse Colon to Descending Colon with Autologous Tissue Substitute, Percutaneous Endoscopic Approach
0D1L47N	Bypass Transverse Colon to Sigmoid Colon with Autologous Tissue Substitute, Percutaneous Endoscopic Approach
0D1L47P	Bypass Transverse Colon to Rectum with Autologous Tissue Substitute, Percutaneous Endoscopic Approach
0D1L4J4	Bypass Transverse Colon to Cutaneous with Synthetic Substitute, Percutaneous Endoscopic Approach
0D1L4JL	Bypass Transverse Colon to Transverse Colon with Synthetic Substitute, Percutaneous Endoscopic Approach
0D1L4JM	Bypass Transverse Colon to Descending Colon with Synthetic Substitute, Percutaneous Endoscopic Approach
0D1L4JN	Bypass Transverse Colon to Sigmoid Colon with Synthetic Substitute, Percutaneous Endoscopic Approach
0D1L4JP	Bypass Transverse Colon to Rectum with Synthetic Substitute, Percutaneous Endoscopic Approach
0D1L4K4	Bypass Transverse Colon to Cutaneous with Nonautologous Tissue Substitute, Percutaneous Endoscopic Approach
0D1L4KL	Bypass Transverse Colon to Transverse Colon with Nonautologous Tissue Substitute, Percutaneous Endoscopic Approach
0D1L4KM	Bypass Transverse Colon to Descending Colon with Nonautologous Tissue Substitute, Percutaneous Endoscopic Approach
0D1L4KN	Bypass Transverse Colon to Sigmoid Colon with Nonautologous Tissue Substitute, Percutaneous Endoscopic Approach
0D1L4KP	Bypass Transverse Colon to Rectum with Nonautologous Tissue Substitute, Percutaneous Endoscopic Approach
0D1L4Z4	Bypass Transverse Colon to Cutaneous, Percutaneous Endoscopic Approach
0D1L4ZL	Bypass Transverse Colon to Transverse Colon, Percutaneous Endoscopic Approach
0D1L4ZM	Bypass Transverse Colon to Descending Colon, Percutaneous Endoscopic Approach
0D1L4ZN	Bypass Transverse Colon to Sigmoid Colon, Percutaneous Endoscopic Approach
0D1L4ZP	Bypass Transverse Colon to Rectum, Percutaneous Endoscopic Approach
0D1L874	Bypass Transverse Colon to Cutaneous with Autologous Tissue Substitute, Via Natural or Artificial Opening Endoscopic
0D1L87L	Bypass Transverse Colon to Transverse Colon with Autologous Tissue Substitute, Via Natural or Artificial Opening Endoscopic
0D1L87M	Bypass Transverse Colon to Descending Colon with Autologous Tissue Substitute, Via Natural or Artificial Opening Endoscopic

0D1L87N Bypass Transverse Colon to Sigmoid Colon with Autologous Tissue Substitute, Via Natural or Artificial Opening Endoscopic

0D1L87P Bypass Transverse Colon to Rectum with Autologous Tissue Substitute, Via Natural or Artificial Opening Endoscopic

0D1L8J4 Bypass Transverse Colon to Cutaneous with Synthetic Substitute, Via Natural or Artificial Opening Endoscopic

0D1L8JL Bypass Transverse Colon to Transverse Colon with Synthetic Substitute, Via Natural or Artificial Opening Endoscopic

0D1L8JM Bypass Transverse Colon to Descending Colon with Synthetic Substitute, Via Natural or Artificial Opening Endoscopic

0D1L8JN Bypass Transverse Colon to Sigmoid Colon with Synthetic Substitute, Via Natural or Artificial Opening Endoscopic

0D1L8JP Bypass Transverse Colon to Rectum with Synthetic Substitute, Via Natural or Artificial Opening Endoscopic

0D1L8K4 Bypass Transverse Colon to Cutaneous with Nonautologous Tissue Substitute, Via Natural or Artificial Opening Endoscopic

0D1L8KL Bypass Transverse Colon to Transverse Colon with Nonautologous Tissue Substitute, Via Natural or Artificial Opening Endoscopic

0D1L8KM Bypass Transverse Colon to Descending Colon with Nonautologous Tissue Substitute, Via Natural or Artificial Opening Endoscopic

0D1L8KN Bypass Transverse Colon to Sigmoid Colon with Nonautologous Tissue Substitute, Via Natural or Artificial Opening Endoscopic

0D1L8KP Bypass Transverse Colon to Rectum with Nonautologous Tissue Substitute, Via Natural or Artificial Opening Endoscopic

0D1L8Z4 Bypass Transverse Colon to Cutaneous, Via Natural or Artificial Opening Endoscopic

0D1L8ZL Bypass Transverse Colon to Transverse Colon, Via Natural or Artificial Opening Endoscopic

0D1L8ZM Bypass Transverse Colon to Descending Colon, Via Natural or Artificial Opening Endoscopic

0D1L8ZN Bypass Transverse Colon to Sigmoid Colon, Via Natural or Artificial Opening Endoscopic

0D1L8ZP Bypass Transverse Colon to Rectum, Via Natural or Artificial Opening Endoscopic

0D1M074 Bypass Descending Colon to Cutaneous with Autologous Tissue Substitute, Open Approach

0D1M07M Bypass Descending Colon to Descending Colon with Autologous Tissue Substitute, Open Approach

0D1M07N Bypass Descending Colon to Sigmoid Colon with Autologous Tissue Substitute, Open Approach

0D1M07P Bypass Descending Colon to Rectum with Autologous Tissue Substitute, Open Approach

0D1M0J4 Bypass Descending Colon to Cutaneous with Synthetic Substitute, Open Approach

0D1M0JM Bypass Descending Colon to Descending Colon with Synthetic Substitute, Open Approach

0D1M0JN Bypass Descending Colon to Sigmoid Colon with Synthetic Substitute, Open Approach

0D1M0JP Bypass Descending Colon to Rectum with Synthetic Substitute, Open Approach

0D1M0K4 Bypass Descending Colon to Cutaneous with Nonautologous Tissue Substitute, Open Approach

0D1M0KM Bypass Descending Colon to Descending Colon with Nonautologous Tissue Substitute, Open Approach

0D1M0KN Bypass Descending Colon to Sigmoid Colon with Nonautologous Tissue Substitute, Open Approach

0D1M0KP Bypass Descending Colon to Rectum with Nonautologous Tissue Substitute, Open Approach

0D1M0Z4 Bypass Descending Colon to Cutaneous, Open Approach

0D1M0ZM Bypass Descending Colon to Descending Colon, Open Approach

0D1M0ZN Bypass Descending Colon to Sigmoid Colon, Open Approach

0D1M0ZP Bypass Descending Colon to Rectum, Open Approach

0D1M3J4 Bypass Descending Colon to Cutaneous with Synthetic Substitute, Percutaneous Approach

0D1M474 Bypass Descending Colon to Cutaneous with Autologous Tissue Substitute, Percutaneous Endoscopic Approach

0D1M47M Bypass Descending Colon to Descending Colon with Autologous Tissue Substitute, Percutaneous Endoscopic Approach

0D1M47N Bypass Descending Colon to Sigmoid Colon with Autologous Tissue Substitute, Percutaneous Endoscopic Approach

0D1M47P Bypass Descending Colon to Rectum with Autologous Tissue Substitute, Percutaneous Endoscopic Approach

0D1M4J4 Bypass Descending Colon to Cutaneous with Synthetic Substitute, Percutaneous Endoscopic Approach

0D1M4JM Bypass Descending Colon to Descending Colon with Synthetic Substitute, Percutaneous Endoscopic Approach

0D1M4JN Bypass Descending Colon to Sigmoid Colon with Synthetic Substitute, Percutaneous Endoscopic Approach

0D1M4JP Bypass Descending Colon to Rectum with Synthetic Substitute, Percutaneous Endoscopic Approach

0D1M4K4 Bypass Descending Colon to Cutaneous with Nonautologous Tissue Substitute, Percutaneous Endoscopic Approach

0D1M4KM Bypass Descending Colon to Descending Colon with Nonautologous Tissue Substitute, Percutaneous Endoscopic Approach

0D1M4KN Bypass Descending Colon to Sigmoid Colon with Nonautologous Tissue Substitute, Percutaneous Endoscopic Approach

0D1M4KP Bypass Descending Colon to Rectum with Nonautologous Tissue Substitute, Percutaneous Endoscopic Approach

0D1M4Z4 Bypass Descending Colon to Cutaneous, Percutaneous Endoscopic Approach

0D1M4ZM Bypass Descending Colon to Descending Colon, Percutaneous Endoscopic Approach

0D1M4ZN Bypass Descending Colon to Sigmoid Colon, Percutaneous Endoscopic Approach

0D1M4ZP Bypass Descending Colon to Rectum, Percutaneous Endoscopic Approach

0D1M874 Bypass Descending Colon to Cutaneous with Autologous Tissue Substitute, Via Natural or Artificial Opening Endoscopic

0D1M87M Bypass Descending Colon to Descending Colon with Autologous Tissue Substitute, Via Natural or Artificial Opening Endoscopic

0D1M87N Bypass Descending Colon to Sigmoid Colon with Autologous Tissue Substitute, Via Natural or Artificial Opening Endoscopic

0D1M87P Bypass Descending Colon to Rectum with Autologous Tissue Substitute, Via Natural or Artificial Opening Endoscopic

0D1M8J4 Bypass Descending Colon to Cutaneous with Synthetic Substitute, Via Natural or Artificial Opening Endoscopic

0D1M8JM Bypass Descending Colon to Descending Colon with Synthetic Substitute, Via Natural or Artificial Opening Endoscopic

0D1M8JN Bypass Descending Colon to Sigmoid Colon with Synthetic Substitute, Via Natural or Artificial Opening Endoscopic

0D1M8JP Bypass Descending Colon to Rectum with Synthetic Substitute, Via Natural or Artificial Opening Endoscopic

0D1M8K4 Bypass Descending Colon to Cutaneous with Nonautologous Tissue Substitute, Via Natural or Artificial Opening Endoscopic

0D1M8KM Bypass Descending Colon to Descending Colon with Nonautologous Tissue Substitute, Via Natural or Artificial Opening Endoscopic

0D1M8KN Bypass Descending Colon to Sigmoid Colon with Nonautologous Tissue Substitute, Via Natural or Artificial Opening Endoscopic

0D1M8KP Bypass Descending Colon to Rectum with Nonautologous Tissue Substitute, Via Natural or Artificial Opening Endoscopic

0D1M8Z4 Bypass Descending Colon to Cutaneous, Via Natural or Artificial Opening Endoscopic

0D1M8ZM Bypass Descending Colon to Descending Colon, Via Natural or Artificial Opening Endoscopic

0D1M8ZN Bypass Descending Colon to Sigmoid Colon, Via Natural or Artificial Opening Endoscopic

0D1M8ZP Bypass Descending Colon to Rectum, Via Natural or Artificial Opening Endoscopic

0D1N074 Bypass Sigmoid Colon to Cutaneous with Autologous Tissue Substitute, Open Approach

0D1N07N Bypass Sigmoid Colon to Sigmoid Colon with Autologous Tissue Substitute, Open Approach

♀ Female-only   ♂ Male-only   ▲ Limited Coverage   ● Non-OR   🅷🅰🅲 HAC-associated procedure   ▲ Non-covered procedures   ✚ Cluster

0D1N07P Bypass Sigmoid Colon to Rectum with Autologous Tissue Substitute, Open Approach

0D1N0J4 Bypass Sigmoid Colon to Cutaneous with Synthetic Substitute, Open Approach

0D1N0JN Bypass Sigmoid Colon to Sigmoid Colon with Synthetic Substitute, Open Approach

0D1N0JP Bypass Sigmoid Colon to Rectum with Synthetic Substitute, Open Approach

0D1N0K4 Bypass Sigmoid Colon to Cutaneous with Nonautologous Tissue Substitute, Open Approach

0D1N0KN Bypass Sigmoid Colon to Sigmoid Colon with Nonautologous Tissue Substitute, Open Approach

0D1N0KP Bypass Sigmoid Colon to Rectum with Nonautologous Tissue Substitute, Open Approach

0D1N0Z4 Bypass Sigmoid Colon to Cutaneous, Open Approach
AHA CC: 4Q, 2014, 41-42

0D1N0ZN Bypass Sigmoid Colon to Sigmoid Colon, Open Approach

0D1N0ZP Bypass Sigmoid Colon to Rectum, Open Approach

0D1N3J4 Bypass Sigmoid Colon to Cutaneous with Synthetic Substitute, Percutaneous Approach

0D1N474 Bypass Sigmoid Colon to Cutaneous with Autologous Tissue Substitute, Percutaneous Endoscopic Approach

0D1N47N Bypass Sigmoid Colon to Sigmoid Colon with Autologous Tissue

Substitute, Percutaneous Endoscopic Approach

0D1N47P Bypass Sigmoid Colon to Rectum with Autologous Tissue Substitute, Percutaneous Endoscopic Approach

0D1N4J4 Bypass Sigmoid Colon to Cutaneous with Synthetic Substitute, Percutaneous Endoscopic Approach

0D1N4JN Bypass Sigmoid Colon to Sigmoid Colon with Synthetic Substitute, Percutaneous Endoscopic Approach

0D1N4JP Bypass Sigmoid Colon to Rectum with Synthetic Substitute, Percutaneous Endoscopic Approach

0D1N4K4 Bypass Sigmoid Colon to Cutaneous with Nonautologous Tissue Substitute, Percutaneous Endoscopic Approach

0D1N4KN Bypass Sigmoid Colon to Sigmoid Colon with Nonautologous Tissue Substitute, Percutaneous Endoscopic Approach

0D1N4KP Bypass Sigmoid Colon to Rectum with Nonautologous Tissue Substitute, Percutaneous Endoscopic Approach

0D1N4Z4 Bypass Sigmoid Colon to Cutaneous, Percutaneous Endoscopic Approach

0D1N4ZN Bypass Sigmoid Colon to Sigmoid Colon, Percutaneous Endoscopic Approach

0D1N4ZP Bypass Sigmoid Colon to Rectum, Percutaneous Endoscopic Approach

0D1N874 Bypass Sigmoid Colon to Cutaneous with Autologous Tissue Substitute, Via Natural or Artificial Opening Endoscopic

0D1N87N Bypass Sigmoid Colon to Sigmoid Colon with Autologous Tissue

Substitute, Via Natural or Artificial Opening Endoscopic

0D1N87P Bypass Sigmoid Colon to Rectum with Autologous Tissue Substitute, Via Natural or Artificial Opening Endoscopic

0D1N8J4 Bypass Sigmoid Colon to Cutaneous with Synthetic Substitute, Via Natural or Artificial Opening Endoscopic

0D1N8JN Bypass Sigmoid Colon to Sigmoid Colon with Synthetic Substitute, Via Natural or Artificial Opening Endoscopic

0D1N8JP Bypass Sigmoid Colon to Rectum with Synthetic Substitute, Via Natural or Artificial Opening Endoscopic

0D1N8K4 Bypass Sigmoid Colon to Cutaneous with Nonautologous Tissue Substitute, Via Natural or Artificial Opening Endoscopic

0D1N8KN Bypass Sigmoid Colon to Sigmoid Colon with Nonautologous Tissue Substitute, Via Natural or Artificial Opening Endoscopic

0D1N8KP Bypass Sigmoid Colon to Rectum with Nonautologous Tissue Substitute, Via Natural or Artificial Opening Endoscopic

0D1N8Z4 Bypass Sigmoid Colon to Cutaneous, Via Natural or Artificial Opening Endoscopic

0D1N8ZN Bypass Sigmoid Colon to Sigmoid Colon, Via Natural or Artificial Opening Endoscopic

0D1N8ZP Bypass Sigmoid Colon to Rectum, Via Natural or Artificial Opening Endoscopic

0D2 – Gastrointestinal System, Change

Review Coding Guideline B6.1c

0D20X0Z Change Drainage Device in Upper Intestinal Tract, External Approach

0D20XUZ Change Feeding Device in Upper Intestinal Tract, External Approach

0D20XYZ Change Other Device in Upper Intestinal Tract, External Approach

0D2DX0Z Change Drainage Device in Lower Intestinal Tract, External Approach

0D2DXUZ Change Feeding Device in Lower Intestinal Tract, External Approach
AHA CC: 1Q, 2019, 26-27

0D2DXYZ Change Other Device in Lower Intestinal Tract, External Approach

0D2UX0Z Change Drainage Device in Omentum, External Approach

0D2UXYZ Change Other Device in Omentum, External Approach

0D2VX0Z Change Drainage Device in Mesentery, External Approach

0D2VXYZ Change Other Device in Mesentery, External Approach

0D2WX0Z Change Drainage Device in Peritoneum, External Approach

0D2WXYZ Change Other Device in Peritoneum, External Approach

0D5 – Gastrointestinal System, Destruction

0D510ZZ Destruction of Upper Esophagus, Open Approach

0D513ZZ Destruction of Upper Esophagus, Percutaneous Approach

0D514ZZ Destruction of Upper Esophagus, Percutaneous Endoscopic Approach

0D517ZZ Destruction of Upper Esophagus, Via Natural or Artificial Opening

0D518ZZ Destruction of Upper Esophagus, Via Natural or Artificial Opening Endoscopic

0D520ZZ Destruction of Middle Esophagus, Open Approach

0D523ZZ Destruction of Middle Esophagus, Percutaneous Approach

0D524ZZ Destruction of Middle Esophagus, Percutaneous Endoscopic Approach

0D527ZZ Destruction of Middle Esophagus, Via Natural or Artificial Opening

0D528ZZ Destruction of Middle Esophagus, Via Natural or Artificial Opening Endoscopic

0D530ZZ Destruction of Lower Esophagus, Open Approach

0D533ZZ Destruction of Lower Esophagus, Percutaneous Approach

0D534ZZ Destruction of Lower Esophagus, Percutaneous Endoscopic Approach

0D537ZZ Destruction of Lower Esophagus, Via Natural or Artificial Opening

0D538ZZ Destruction of Lower Esophagus, Via Natural or Artificial Opening Endoscopic

0D540ZZ Destruction of Esophagogastric Junction, Open Approach

0D543ZZ Destruction of Esophagogastric Junction, Percutaneous Approach

0D544ZZ Destruction of Esophagogastric Junction, Percutaneous Endoscopic Approach

0D547ZZ Destruction of Esophagogastric Junction, Via Natural or Artificial Opening

0D548ZZ Destruction of Esophagogastric Junction, Via Natural or Artificial Opening Endoscopic

0D550ZZ Destruction of Esophagus, Open Approach

0D553ZZ Destruction of Esophagus, Percutaneous Approach

0D554ZZ Destruction of Esophagus, Percutaneous Endoscopic Approach

0D557ZZ Destruction of Esophagus, Via Natural or Artificial Opening

0D558ZZ Destruction of Esophagus, Via Natural or Artificial Opening Endoscopic

0D560ZZ Destruction of Stomach, Open Approach

0D563ZZ Destruction of Stomach, Percutaneous Approach

0D564ZZ	Destruction of Stomach, Percutaneous Endoscopic Approach
0D567ZZ	Destruction of Stomach, Via Natural or Artificial Opening
0D568ZZ	Destruction of Stomach, Via Natural or Artificial Opening Endoscopic
0D570ZZ	Destruction of Stomach, Pylorus, Open Approach
0D573ZZ	Destruction of Stomach, Pylorus, Percutaneous Approach
0D574ZZ	Destruction of Stomach, Pylorus, Percutaneous Endoscopic Approach
0D577ZZ	Destruction of Stomach, Pylorus, Via Natural or Artificial Opening
0D578ZZ	Destruction of Stomach, Pylorus, Via Natural or Artificial Opening Endoscopic
0D580ZZ	Destruction of Small Intestine, Open Approach
0D583ZZ	Destruction of Small Intestine, Percutaneous Approach
0D584ZZ	Destruction of Small Intestine, Percutaneous Endoscopic Approach
0D587ZZ	Destruction of Small Intestine, Via Natural or Artificial Opening
0D588ZZ	Destruction of Small Intestine, Via Natural or Artificial Opening Endoscopic
0D590ZZ	Destruction of Duodenum, Open Approach
0D593ZZ	Destruction of Duodenum, Percutaneous Approach
0D594ZZ	Destruction of Duodenum, Percutaneous Endoscopic Approach
0D597ZZ	Destruction of Duodenum, Via Natural or Artificial Opening
0D598ZZ	Destruction of Duodenum, Via Natural or Artificial Opening Endoscopic
0D5A0ZZ	Destruction of Jejunum, Open Approach
0D5A3ZZ	Destruction of Jejunum, Percutaneous Approach
0D5A4ZZ	Destruction of Jejunum, Percutaneous Endoscopic Approach
0D5A7ZZ	Destruction of Jejunum, Via Natural or Artificial Opening
0D5A8ZZ	Destruction of Jejunum, Via Natural or Artificial Opening Endoscopic
0D5B0ZZ	Destruction of Ileum, Open Approach
0D5B3ZZ	Destruction of Ileum, Percutaneous Approach
0D5B4ZZ	Destruction of Ileum, Percutaneous Endoscopic Approach
0D5B7ZZ	Destruction of Ileum, Via Natural or Artificial Opening
0D5B8ZZ	Destruction of Ileum, Via Natural or Artificial Opening Endoscopic
0D5C0ZZ	Destruction of Ileocecal Valve, Open Approach
0D5C3ZZ	Destruction of Ileocecal Valve, Percutaneous Approach
0D5C4ZZ	Destruction of Ileocecal Valve, Percutaneous Endoscopic Approach
0D5C7ZZ	Destruction of Ileocecal Valve, Via Natural or Artificial Opening
0D5C8ZZ	Destruction of Ileocecal Valve, Via Natural or Artificial Opening Endoscopic
0D5E0ZZ	Destruction of Large Intestine, Open Approach
0D5E3ZZ	Destruction of Large Intestine, Percutaneous Approach
0D5E4ZZ	Destruction of Large Intestine, Percutaneous Endoscopic Approach
0D5E7ZZ	Destruction of Large Intestine, Via Natural or Artificial Opening
0D5E8ZZ	Destruction of Large Intestine, Via Natural or Artificial Opening Endoscopic
0D5F0ZZ	Destruction of Right Large Intestine, Open Approach
0D5F3ZZ	Destruction of Right Large Intestine, Percutaneous Approach
0D5F4ZZ	Destruction of Right Large Intestine, Percutaneous Endoscopic Approach
0D5F7ZZ	Destruction of Right Large Intestine, Via Natural or Artificial Opening
0D5F8ZZ	Destruction of Right Large Intestine, Via Natural or Artificial Opening Endoscopic
0D5G0ZZ	Destruction of Left Large Intestine, Open Approach
0D5G3ZZ	Destruction of Left Large Intestine, Percutaneous Approach
0D5G4ZZ	Destruction of Left Large Intestine, Percutaneous Endoscopic Approach
0D5G7ZZ	Destruction of Left Large Intestine, Via Natural or Artificial Opening
0D5G8ZZ	Destruction of Left Large Intestine, Via Natural or Artificial Opening Endoscopic
0D5H0ZZ	Destruction of Cecum, Open Approach
0D5H3ZZ	Destruction of Cecum, Percutaneous Approach
0D5H4ZZ	Destruction of Cecum, Percutaneous Endoscopic Approach
0D5H7ZZ	Destruction of Cecum, Via Natural or Artificial Opening
0D5H8ZZ	Destruction of Cecum, Via Natural or Artificial Opening Endoscopic
0D5J0ZZ	Destruction of Appendix, Open Approach
0D5J3ZZ	Destruction of Appendix, Percutaneous Approach
0D5J4ZZ	Destruction of Appendix, Percutaneous Endoscopic Approach
0D5J7ZZ	Destruction of Appendix, Via Natural or Artificial Opening
0D5J8ZZ	Destruction of Appendix, Via Natural or Artificial Opening Endoscopic
0D5K0ZZ	Destruction of Ascending Colon, Open Approach
0D5K3ZZ	Destruction of Ascending Colon, Percutaneous Approach
0D5K4ZZ	Destruction of Ascending Colon, Percutaneous Endoscopic Approach
0D5K7ZZ	Destruction of Ascending Colon, Via Natural or Artificial Opening
0D5K8ZZ	Destruction of Ascending Colon, Via Natural or Artificial Opening Endoscopic
0D5L0ZZ	Destruction of Transverse Colon, Open Approach
0D5L3ZZ	Destruction of Transverse Colon, Percutaneous Approach
0D5L4ZZ	Destruction of Transverse Colon, Percutaneous Endoscopic Approach
0D5L7ZZ	Destruction of Transverse Colon, Via Natural or Artificial Opening
0D5L8ZZ	Destruction of Transverse Colon, Via Natural or Artificial Opening Endoscopic
0D5M0ZZ	Destruction of Descending Colon, Open Approach
0D5M3ZZ	Destruction of Descending Colon, Percutaneous Approach
0D5M4ZZ	Destruction of Descending Colon, Percutaneous Endoscopic Approach
0D5M7ZZ	Destruction of Descending Colon, Via Natural or Artificial Opening
0D5M8ZZ	Destruction of Descending Colon, Via Natural or Artificial Opening Endoscopic
0D5N0ZZ	Destruction of Sigmoid Colon, Open Approach
0D5N3ZZ	Destruction of Sigmoid Colon, Percutaneous Approach
0D5N4ZZ	Destruction of Sigmoid Colon, Percutaneous Endoscopic Approach
0D5N7ZZ	Destruction of Sigmoid Colon, Via Natural or Artificial Opening
0D5N8ZZ	Destruction of Sigmoid Colon, Via Natural or Artificial Opening Endoscopic
0D5P0ZZ	Destruction of Rectum, Open Approach
0D5P3ZZ	Destruction of Rectum, Percutaneous Approach
0D5P4ZZ	Destruction of Rectum, Percutaneous Endoscopic Approach
0D5P7ZZ	Destruction of Rectum, Via Natural or Artificial Opening
0D5P8ZZ	Destruction of Rectum, Via Natural or Artificial Opening Endoscopic
0D5Q0ZZ	Destruction of Anus, Open Approach
0D5Q3ZZ	Destruction of Anus, Percutaneous Approach
0D5Q4ZZ	Destruction of Anus, Percutaneous Endoscopic Approach
0D5Q7ZZ	Destruction of Anus, Via Natural or Artificial Opening
0D5Q8ZZ	Destruction of Anus, Via Natural or Artificial Opening Endoscopic
0D5QXZZ	Destruction of Anus, External Approach
0D5R0ZZ	Destruction of Anal Sphincter, Open Approach
0D5R3ZZ	Destruction of Anal Sphincter, Percutaneous Approach
0D5R4ZZ	Destruction of Anal Sphincter, Percutaneous Endoscopic Approach
0D5U0ZZ	Destruction of Omentum, Open Approach
0D5U3ZZ	Destruction of Omentum, Percutaneous Approach
0D5U4ZZ	Destruction of Omentum, Percutaneous Endoscopic Approach
0D5V0ZZ	Destruction of Mesentery, Open Approach
0D5V3ZZ	Destruction of Mesentery, Percutaneous Approach
0D5V4ZZ	Destruction of Mesentery, Percutaneous Endoscopic Approach
0D5W0ZZ	Destruction of Peritoneum, Open Approach
	AHA CC: 1Q, 2017, 34-35
0D5W3ZZ	Destruction of Peritoneum, Percutaneous Approach
0D5W4ZZ	Destruction of Peritoneum, Percutaneous Endoscopic Approach

0D7 – Gastrointestinal System, Dilation

0D710DZ	Dilation of Upper Esophagus with Intraluminal Device, Open Approach
0D710ZZ	Dilation of Upper Esophagus, Open Approach
0D713DZ	Dilation of Upper Esophagus with Intraluminal Device, Percutaneous Approach
0D713ZZ	Dilation of Upper Esophagus, Percutaneous Approach
0D714DZ	Dilation of Upper Esophagus with Intraluminal Device, Percutaneous Endoscopic Approach
0D714ZZ	Dilation of Upper Esophagus, Percutaneous Endoscopic Approach

0D717DZ Dilation of Upper Esophagus with Intraluminal Device, Via Natural or Artificial Opening

0D717ZZ Dilation of Upper Esophagus, Via Natural or Artificial Opening

0D718DZ Dilation of Upper Esophagus with Intraluminal Device, Via Natural or Artificial Opening Endoscopic

0D718ZZ Dilation of Upper Esophagus, Via Natural or Artificial Opening Endoscopic

0D720DZ Dilation of Middle Esophagus with Intraluminal Device, Open Approach

0D720ZZ Dilation of Middle Esophagus, Open Approach

0D723DZ Dilation of Middle Esophagus with Intraluminal Device, Percutaneous Approach

0D723ZZ Dilation of Middle Esophagus, Percutaneous Approach

0D724DZ Dilation of Middle Esophagus with Intraluminal Device, Percutaneous Endoscopic Approach

0D724ZZ Dilation of Middle Esophagus, Percutaneous Endoscopic Approach

0D727DZ Dilation of Middle Esophagus with Intraluminal Device, Via Natural or Artificial Opening

0D727ZZ Dilation of Middle Esophagus, Via Natural or Artificial Opening

0D728DZ Dilation of Middle Esophagus with Intraluminal Device, Via Natural or Artificial Opening Endoscopic

0D728ZZ Dilation of Middle Esophagus, Via Natural or Artificial Opening Endoscopic

0D730DZ Dilation of Lower Esophagus with Intraluminal Device, Open Approach

0D730ZZ Dilation of Lower Esophagus, Open Approach

0D733DZ Dilation of Lower Esophagus with Intraluminal Device, Percutaneous Approach

0D733ZZ Dilation of Lower Esophagus, Percutaneous Approach

0D734DZ Dilation of Lower Esophagus with Intraluminal Device, Percutaneous Endoscopic Approach

0D734ZZ Dilation of Lower Esophagus, Percutaneous Endoscopic Approach

0D737DZ Dilation of Lower Esophagus with Intraluminal Device, Via Natural or Artificial Opening

0D737ZZ Dilation of Lower Esophagus, Via Natural or Artificial Opening

0D738DZ Dilation of Lower Esophagus with Intraluminal Device, Via Natural or Artificial Opening Endoscopic

0D738ZZ Dilation of Lower Esophagus, Via Natural or Artificial Opening Endoscopic

0D740DZ Dilation of Esophagogastric Junction with Intraluminal Device, Open Approach

0D740ZZ Dilation of Esophagogastric Junction, Open Approach

0D743DZ Dilation of Esophagogastric Junction with Intraluminal Device, Percutaneous Approach

0D743ZZ Dilation of Esophagogastric Junction, Percutaneous Approach

0D744DZ Dilation of Esophagogastric Junction with Intraluminal Device, Percutaneous Endoscopic Approach

0D744ZZ Dilation of Esophagogastric Junction, Percutaneous Endoscopic Approach

0D747DZ Dilation of Esophagogastric Junction with Intraluminal Device, Via Natural or Artificial Opening

0D747ZZ Dilation of Esophagogastric Junction, Via Natural or Artificial Opening

0D748DZ Dilation of Esophagogastric Junction with Intraluminal Device, Via Natural or Artificial Opening Endoscopic

0D748ZZ Dilation of Esophagogastric Junction, Via Natural or Artificial Opening Endoscopic

0D750DZ Dilation of Esophagus with Intraluminal Device, Open Approach

0D750ZZ Dilation of Esophagus, Open Approach

0D753DZ Dilation of Esophagus with Intraluminal Device, Percutaneous Approach

0D753ZZ Dilation of Esophagus, Percutaneous Approach

0D754DZ Dilation of Esophagus with Intraluminal Device, Percutaneous Endoscopic Approach

0D754ZZ Dilation of Esophagus, Percutaneous Endoscopic Approach

0D757DZ Dilation of Esophagus with Intraluminal Device, Via Natural or Artificial Opening

0D757ZZ Dilation of Esophagus, Via Natural or Artificial Opening

0D758DZ Dilation of Esophagus with Intraluminal Device, Via Natural or Artificial Opening Endoscopic

0D758ZZ Dilation of Esophagus, Via Natural or Artificial Opening Endoscopic

0D760DZ Dilation of Stomach with Intraluminal Device, Open Approach

0D760ZZ Dilation of Stomach, Open Approach

0D763DZ Dilation of Stomach with Intraluminal Device, Percutaneous Approach

0D763ZZ Dilation of Stomach, Percutaneous Approach

0D764DZ Dilation of Stomach with Intraluminal Device, Percutaneous Endoscopic Approach

0D764ZZ Dilation of Stomach, Percutaneous Endoscopic Approach

0D767DZ Dilation of Stomach with Intraluminal Device, Via Natural or Artificial Opening

0D767ZZ Dilation of Stomach, Via Natural or Artificial Opening

0D768DZ Dilation of Stomach with Intraluminal Device, Via Natural or Artificial Opening Endoscopic

0D768ZZ Dilation of Stomach, Via Natural or Artificial Opening Endoscopic

AHA CC: 4Q, 2014, 40

0D770DZ Dilation of Stomach, Pylorus with Intraluminal Device, Open Approach

0D770ZZ Dilation of Stomach, Pylorus, Open Approach

0D773DZ Dilation of Stomach, Pylorus with Intraluminal Device, Percutaneous Approach

0D773ZZ Dilation of Stomach, Pylorus, Percutaneous Approach

0D774DZ Dilation of Stomach, Pylorus with Intraluminal Device, Percutaneous Endoscopic Approach

0D774ZZ Dilation of Stomach, Pylorus, Percutaneous Endoscopic Approach

0D777DZ Dilation of Stomach, Pylorus with Intraluminal Device, Via Natural or Artificial Opening

0D777ZZ Dilation of Stomach, Pylorus, Via Natural or Artificial Opening

0D778DZ Dilation of Stomach, Pylorus with Intraluminal Device, Via Natural or Artificial Opening Endoscopic

0D778ZZ Dilation of Stomach, Pylorus, Via Natural or Artificial Opening Endoscopic

0D780DZ Dilation of Small Intestine with Intraluminal Device, Open Approach

0D780ZZ Dilation of Small Intestine, Open Approach

0D783DZ Dilation of Small Intestine with Intraluminal Device, Percutaneous Approach

0D783ZZ Dilation of Small Intestine, Percutaneous Approach

0D784DZ Dilation of Small Intestine with Intraluminal Device, Percutaneous Endoscopic Approach

0D784ZZ Dilation of Small Intestine, Percutaneous Endoscopic Approach

0D787DZ Dilation of Small Intestine with Intraluminal Device, Via Natural or Artificial Opening

0D787ZZ Dilation of Small Intestine, Via Natural or Artificial Opening

0D788DZ Dilation of Small Intestine with Intraluminal Device, Via Natural or Artificial Opening Endoscopic

0D788ZZ Dilation of Small Intestine, Via Natural or Artificial Opening Endoscopic

0D790DZ Dilation of Duodenum with Intraluminal Device, Open Approach

0D790ZZ Dilation of Duodenum, Open Approach

0D793DZ Dilation of Duodenum with Intraluminal Device, Percutaneous Approach

0D793ZZ Dilation of Duodenum, Percutaneous Approach

0D794DZ Dilation of Duodenum with Intraluminal Device, Percutaneous Endoscopic Approach

0D794ZZ Dilation of Duodenum, Percutaneous Endoscopic Approach

0D797DZ Dilation of Duodenum with Intraluminal Device, Via Natural or Artificial Opening

0D797ZZ Dilation of Duodenum, Via Natural or Artificial Opening

0D798DZ Dilation of Duodenum with Intraluminal Device, Via Natural or Artificial Opening Endoscopic

0D798ZZ Dilation of Duodenum, Via Natural or Artificial Opening Endoscopic

0D7A0DZ Dilation of Jejunum with Intraluminal Device, Open Approach

0D7A0ZZ Dilation of Jejunum, Open Approach

0D7A3DZ Dilation of Jejunum with Intraluminal Device, Percutaneous Approach

0D7A3ZZ Dilation of Jejunum, Percutaneous Approach

0D7A4DZ Dilation of Jejunum with Intraluminal Device, Percutaneous Endoscopic Approach

0D7A4ZZ Dilation of Jejunum, Percutaneous Endoscopic Approach

0D7A7DZ Dilation of Jejunum with Intraluminal Device, Via Natural or Artificial Opening

0D7A7ZZ Dilation of Jejunum, Via Natural or Artificial Opening

0D7A8DZ Dilation of Jejunum with Intraluminal Device, Via Natural or Artificial Opening Endoscopic

0D7A8ZZ Dilation of Jejunum, Via Natural or Artificial Opening Endoscopic

AHA CC: 4Q, 2014, 40

0D7B0DZ Dilation of Ileum with Intraluminal Device, Open Approach

0D7B0ZZ Dilation of Ileum, Open Approach

0D7B3DZ Dilation of Ileum with Intraluminal Device, Percutaneous Approach

0D7B3ZZ Dilation of Ileum, Percutaneous Approach

0D7B4DZ Dilation of Ileum with Intraluminal Device, Percutaneous Endoscopic Approach

0D7B4ZZ Dilation of Ileum, Percutaneous Endoscopic Approach

0D7B7DZ Dilation of Ileum with Intraluminal Device, Via Natural or Artificial Opening

0D7B7ZZ Dilation of Ileum, Via Natural or Artificial Opening

0D7B8DZ Dilation of Ileum with Intraluminal Device, Via Natural or Artificial Opening Endoscopic

0D7B8ZZ Dilation of Ileum, Via Natural or Artificial Opening Endoscopic

0D7C0DZ Dilation of Ileocecal Valve with Intraluminal Device, Open Approach

0D7C0ZZ Dilation of Ileocecal Valve, Open Approach

0D7C3DZ Dilation of Ileocecal Valve with Intraluminal Device, Percutaneous Approach

0D7C3ZZ Dilation of Ileocecal Valve, Percutaneous Approach

0D7C4DZ Dilation of Ileocecal Valve with Intraluminal Device, Percutaneous Endoscopic Approach

0D7C4ZZ Dilation of Ileocecal Valve, Percutaneous Endoscopic Approach

0D7C7DZ Dilation of Ileocecal Valve with Intraluminal Device, Via Natural or Artificial Opening

0D7C7ZZ Dilation of Ileocecal Valve, Via Natural or Artificial Opening

0D7C8DZ Dilation of Ileocecal Valve with Intraluminal Device, Via Natural or Artificial Opening Endoscopic

0D7C8ZZ Dilation of Ileocecal Valve, Via Natural or Artificial Opening Endoscopic

0D7E0DZ Dilation of Large Intestine with Intraluminal Device, Open Approach

0D7E0ZZ Dilation of Large Intestine, Open Approach

0D7E3DZ Dilation of Large Intestine with Intraluminal Device, Percutaneous Approach

0D7E3ZZ Dilation of Large Intestine, Percutaneous Approach

0D7E4DZ Dilation of Large Intestine with Intraluminal Device, Percutaneous Endoscopic Approach

0D7E4ZZ Dilation of Large Intestine, Percutaneous Endoscopic Approach

0D7E7DZ Dilation of Large Intestine with Intraluminal Device, Via Natural or Artificial Opening

0D7E7ZZ Dilation of Large Intestine, Via Natural or Artificial Opening

0D7E8DZ Dilation of Large Intestine with Intraluminal Device, Via Natural or Artificial Opening Endoscopic

0D7E8ZZ Dilation of Large Intestine, Via Natural or Artificial Opening Endoscopic

0D7F0DZ Dilation of Right Large Intestine with Intraluminal Device, Open Approach

0D7F0ZZ Dilation of Right Large Intestine, Open Approach

0D7F3DZ Dilation of Right Large Intestine with Intraluminal Device, Percutaneous Approach

0D7F3ZZ Dilation of Right Large Intestine, Percutaneous Approach

0D7F4DZ Dilation of Right Large Intestine with Intraluminal Device, Percutaneous Endoscopic Approach

0D7F4ZZ Dilation of Right Large Intestine, Percutaneous Endoscopic Approach

0D7F7DZ Dilation of Right Large Intestine with Intraluminal Device, Via Natural or Artificial Opening

0D7F7ZZ Dilation of Right Large Intestine, Via Natural or Artificial Opening

0D7F8DZ Dilation of Right Large Intestine with Intraluminal Device, Via Natural or Artificial Opening Endoscopic

0D7F8ZZ Dilation of Right Large Intestine, Via Natural or Artificial Opening Endoscopic

0D7G0DZ Dilation of Left Large Intestine with Intraluminal Device, Open Approach

0D7G0ZZ Dilation of Left Large Intestine, Open Approach

0D7G3DZ Dilation of Left Large Intestine with Intraluminal Device, Percutaneous Approach

0D7G3ZZ Dilation of Left Large Intestine, Percutaneous Approach

0D7G4DZ Dilation of Left Large Intestine with Intraluminal Device, Percutaneous Endoscopic Approach

0D7G4ZZ Dilation of Left Large Intestine, Percutaneous Endoscopic Approach

0D7G7DZ Dilation of Left Large Intestine with Intraluminal Device, Via Natural or Artificial Opening

0D7G7ZZ Dilation of Left Large Intestine, Via Natural or Artificial Opening

0D7G8DZ Dilation of Left Large Intestine with Intraluminal Device, Via Natural or Artificial Opening Endoscopic

0D7G8ZZ Dilation of Left Large Intestine, Via Natural or Artificial Opening Endoscopic

0D7H0DZ Dilation of Cecum with Intraluminal Device, Open Approach

0D7H0ZZ Dilation of Cecum, Open Approach

0D7H3DZ Dilation of Cecum with Intraluminal Device, Percutaneous Approach

0D7H3ZZ Dilation of Cecum, Percutaneous Approach

0D7H4DZ Dilation of Cecum with Intraluminal Device, Percutaneous Endoscopic Approach

0D7H4ZZ Dilation of Cecum, Percutaneous Endoscopic Approach

0D7H7DZ Dilation of Cecum with Intraluminal Device, Via Natural or Artificial Opening

0D7H7ZZ Dilation of Cecum, Via Natural or Artificial Opening

0D7H8DZ Dilation of Cecum with Intraluminal Device, Via Natural or Artificial Opening Endoscopic

0D7H8ZZ Dilation of Cecum, Via Natural or Artificial Opening Endoscopic

0D7K0DZ Dilation of Ascending Colon with Intraluminal Device, Open Approach

0D7K0ZZ Dilation of Ascending Colon, Open Approach

0D7K3DZ Dilation of Ascending Colon with Intraluminal Device, Percutaneous Approach

0D7K3ZZ Dilation of Ascending Colon, Percutaneous Approach

0D7K4DZ Dilation of Ascending Colon with Intraluminal Device, Percutaneous Endoscopic Approach

0D7K4ZZ Dilation of Ascending Colon, Percutaneous Endoscopic Approach

0D7K7DZ Dilation of Ascending Colon with Intraluminal Device, Via Natural or Artificial Opening

0D7K7ZZ Dilation of Ascending Colon, Via Natural or Artificial Opening

0D7K8DZ Dilation of Ascending Colon with Intraluminal Device, Via Natural or Artificial Opening Endoscopic

0D7K8ZZ Dilation of Ascending Colon, Via Natural or Artificial Opening Endoscopic

0D7L0DZ Dilation of Transverse Colon with Intraluminal Device, Open Approach

0D7L0ZZ Dilation of Transverse Colon, Open Approach

0D7L3DZ Dilation of Transverse Colon with Intraluminal Device, Percutaneous Approach

0D7L3ZZ Dilation of Transverse Colon, Percutaneous Approach

0D7L4DZ Dilation of Transverse Colon with Intraluminal Device, Percutaneous Endoscopic Approach

0D7L4ZZ Dilation of Transverse Colon, Percutaneous Endoscopic Approach

0D7L7DZ Dilation of Transverse Colon with Intraluminal Device, Via Natural or Artificial Opening

0D7L7ZZ Dilation of Transverse Colon, Via Natural or Artificial Opening

0D7L8DZ Dilation of Transverse Colon with Intraluminal Device, Via Natural or Artificial Opening Endoscopic

0D7L8ZZ Dilation of Transverse Colon, Via Natural or Artificial Opening Endoscopic

0D7M0DZ Dilation of Descending Colon with Intraluminal Device, Open Approach

0D7M0ZZ Dilation of Descending Colon, Open Approach

0D7M3DZ Dilation of Descending Colon with Intraluminal Device, Percutaneous Approach

0D7M3ZZ Dilation of Descending Colon, Percutaneous Approach

0D7M4DZ Dilation of Descending Colon with Intraluminal Device, Percutaneous Endoscopic Approach

0D7M4ZZ Dilation of Descending Colon, Percutaneous Endoscopic Approach

0D7M7DZ Dilation of Descending Colon with Intraluminal Device, Via Natural or Artificial Opening

0D7M7ZZ Dilation of Descending Colon, Via Natural or Artificial Opening

0D7M8DZ Dilation of Descending Colon with Intraluminal Device, Via Natural or Artificial Opening Endoscopic

0D7M8ZZ Dilation of Descending Colon, Via Natural or Artificial Opening Endoscopic

0D7N0DZ Dilation of Sigmoid Colon with Intraluminal Device, Open Approach

0D7N0ZZ Dilation of Sigmoid Colon, Open Approach

0D7N3DZ Dilation of Sigmoid Colon with Intraluminal Device, Percutaneous Approach

0D7N3ZZ Dilation of Sigmoid Colon, Percutaneous Approach

♀ Female-only   ♂ Male-only   ▲ Limited Coverage   ● Non-OR   🅷🅰🅲 HAC-associated procedure   ▲ Non-covered procedures   ➕ Cluster

0D7N4DZ	Dilation of Sigmoid Colon with Intraluminal Device, Percutaneous Endoscopic Approach	
0D7N4ZZ	Dilation of Sigmoid Colon, Percutaneous Endoscopic Approach	
0D7N7DZ	Dilation of Sigmoid Colon with Intraluminal Device, Via Natural or Artificial Opening	
0D7N7ZZ	Dilation of Sigmoid Colon, Via Natural or Artificial Opening	
0D7N8DZ	Dilation of Sigmoid Colon with Intraluminal Device, Via Natural or Artificial Opening Endoscopic	
0D7N8ZZ	Dilation of Sigmoid Colon, Via Natural or Artificial Opening Endoscopic	
0D7P0DZ	Dilation of Rectum with Intraluminal Device, Open Approach	
0D7P0ZZ	Dilation of Rectum, Open Approach	
0D7P3DZ	Dilation of Rectum with Intraluminal Device, Percutaneous Approach	

0D7P3ZZ	Dilation of Rectum, Percutaneous Approach
0D7P4DZ	Dilation of Rectum with Intraluminal Device, Percutaneous Endoscopic Approach
0D7P4ZZ	Dilation of Rectum, Percutaneous Endoscopic Approach
0D7P7DZ	Dilation of Rectum with Intraluminal Device, Via Natural or Artificial Opening
0D7P7ZZ	Dilation of Rectum, Via Natural or Artificial Opening
0D7P8DZ	Dilation of Rectum with Intraluminal Device, Via Natural or Artificial Opening Endoscopic
0D7P8ZZ	Dilation of Rectum, Via Natural or Artificial Opening Endoscopic
0D7Q0DZ	Dilation of Anus with Intraluminal Device, Open Approach
0D7Q0ZZ	Dilation of Anus, Open Approach

0D7Q3DZ	Dilation of Anus with Intraluminal Device, Percutaneous Approach
0D7Q3ZZ	Dilation of Anus, Percutaneous Approach
0D7Q4DZ	Dilation of Anus with Intraluminal Device, Percutaneous Endoscopic Approach
0D7Q4ZZ	Dilation of Anus, Percutaneous Endoscopic Approach
0D7Q7DZ	Dilation of Anus with Intraluminal Device, Via Natural or Artificial Opening
0D7Q7ZZ	Dilation of Anus, Via Natural or Artificial Opening
0D7Q8DZ	Dilation of Anus with Intraluminal Device, Via Natural or Artificial Opening Endoscopic
0D7Q8ZZ	Dilation of Anus, Via Natural or Artificial Opening Endoscopic

0D8 – Gastrointestinal System, Division

Review Coding Guideline B3.14

0D840ZZ	Division of Esophagogastric Junction, Open Approach
0D843ZZ	Division of Esophagogastric Junction, Percutaneous Approach
0D844ZZ	Division of Esophagogastric Junction, Percutaneous Endoscopic Approach
	AHA CC: 3Q, 2017, 22-23
0D847ZZ	Division of Esophagogastric Junction, Via Natural or Artificial Opening

0D848ZZ	Division of Esophagogastric Junction, Via Natural or Artificial Opening Endoscopic
0D870ZZ	Division of Stomach, Pylorus, Open Approach
0D873ZZ	Division of Stomach, Pylorus, Percutaneous Approach
0D874ZZ	Division of Stomach, Pylorus, Percutaneous Endoscopic Approach
	AHA CC: 3Q, 2017, 23-24; 2Q, 2019, 15-16

0D877ZZ	Division of Stomach, Pylorus, Via Natural or Artificial Opening
0D878ZZ	Division of Stomach, Pylorus, Via Natural or Artificial Opening Endoscopic
0D8R0ZZ	Division of Anal Sphincter, Open Approach
0D8R3ZZ	Division of Anal Sphincter, Percutaneous Approach

0D9 – Gastrointestinal System, Drainage

Review Coding Guidelines B3.4a and B3.4b

Review Coding Guideline B6.2

0D9100Z	Drainage of Upper Esophagus with Drainage Device, Open Approach
0D910ZX	Drainage of Upper Esophagus, Open Approach, Diagnostic
0D910ZZ	Drainage of Upper Esophagus, Open Approach
0D9130Z	Drainage of Upper Esophagus with Drainage Device, Percutaneous Approach
0D913ZX	Drainage of Upper Esophagus, Percutaneous Approach, Diagnostic
0D913ZZ	Drainage of Upper Esophagus, Percutaneous Approach
0D9140Z	Drainage of Upper Esophagus with Drainage Device, Percutaneous Endoscopic Approach
0D914ZX	Drainage of Upper Esophagus, Percutaneous Endoscopic Approach, Diagnostic
0D914ZZ	Drainage of Upper Esophagus, Percutaneous Endoscopic Approach
0D9170Z	Drainage of Upper Esophagus with Drainage Device, Via Natural or Artificial Opening
0D917ZX	Drainage of Upper Esophagus, Via Natural or Artificial Opening, Diagnostic
0D917ZZ	Drainage of Upper Esophagus, Via Natural or Artificial Opening
0D9180Z	Drainage of Upper Esophagus with Drainage Device, Via Natural or Artificial Opening Endoscopic
0D918ZX	Drainage of Upper Esophagus, Via Natural or Artificial Opening Endoscopic, Diagnostic

0D918ZZ	Drainage of Upper Esophagus, Via Natural or Artificial Opening Endoscopic
0D9200Z	Drainage of Middle Esophagus with Drainage Device, Open Approach
0D920ZX	Drainage of Middle Esophagus, Open Approach, Diagnostic
0D920ZZ	Drainage of Middle Esophagus, Open Approach
0D9230Z	Drainage of Middle Esophagus with Drainage Device, Percutaneous Approach
0D923ZX	Drainage of Middle Esophagus, Percutaneous Approach, Diagnostic
0D923ZZ	Drainage of Middle Esophagus, Percutaneous Approach
0D9240Z	Drainage of Middle Esophagus with Drainage Device, Percutaneous Endoscopic Approach
0D924ZX	Drainage of Middle Esophagus, Percutaneous Endoscopic Approach, Diagnostic
0D924ZZ	Drainage of Middle Esophagus, Percutaneous Endoscopic Approach
0D9270Z	Drainage of Middle Esophagus with Drainage Device, Via Natural or Artificial Opening
0D927ZX	Drainage of Middle Esophagus, Via Natural or Artificial Opening, Diagnostic
0D927ZZ	Drainage of Middle Esophagus, Via Natural or Artificial Opening

0D9280Z	Drainage of Middle Esophagus with Drainage Device, Via Natural or Artificial Opening Endoscopic
0D928ZX	Drainage of Middle Esophagus, Via Natural or Artificial Opening Endoscopic, Diagnostic
0D928ZZ	Drainage of Middle Esophagus, Via Natural or Artificial Opening Endoscopic
0D9300Z	Drainage of Lower Esophagus with Drainage Device, Open Approach
0D930ZX	Drainage of Lower Esophagus, Open Approach, Diagnostic
0D930ZZ	Drainage of Lower Esophagus, Open Approach
0D9330Z	Drainage of Lower Esophagus with Drainage Device, Percutaneous Approach
0D933ZX	Drainage of Lower Esophagus, Percutaneous Approach, Diagnostic
0D933ZZ	Drainage of Lower Esophagus, Percutaneous Approach
0D9340Z	Drainage of Lower Esophagus with Drainage Device, Percutaneous Endoscopic Approach
0D934ZX	Drainage of Lower Esophagus, Percutaneous Endoscopic Approach, Diagnostic
0D934ZZ	Drainage of Lower Esophagus, Percutaneous Endoscopic Approach
0D9370Z	Drainage of Lower Esophagus with Drainage Device, Via Natural or Artificial Opening

♀ Female-only   ♂ Male-only   ▲ Limited Coverage   ● Non-OR   ▨ HAC-associated procedure   ▲ Non-covered procedures   ✛ Cluster

0D937ZX Drainage of Lower Esophagus, Via Natural or Artificial Opening, Diagnostic

0D937ZZ Drainage of Lower Esophagus, Via Natural or Artificial Opening

0D9380Z Drainage of Lower Esophagus with Drainage Device, Via Natural or Artificial Opening Endoscopic

0D938ZX Drainage of Lower Esophagus, Via Natural or Artificial Opening Endoscopic, Diagnostic

0D938ZZ Drainage of Lower Esophagus, Via Natural or Artificial Opening Endoscopic

0D9400Z Drainage of Esophagogastric Junction with Drainage Device, Open Approach

0D940ZX Drainage of Esophagogastric Junction, Open Approach, Diagnostic

0D940ZZ Drainage of Esophagogastric Junction, Open Approach

0D9430Z Drainage of Esophagogastric Junction with Drainage Device, Percutaneous Approach

0D943ZX Drainage of Esophagogastric Junction, Percutaneous Approach, Diagnostic

0D943ZZ Drainage of Esophagogastric Junction, Percutaneous Approach

0D9440Z Drainage of Esophagogastric Junction with Drainage Device, Percutaneous Endoscopic Approach

0D944ZX Drainage of Esophagogastric Junction, Percutaneous Endoscopic Approach, Diagnostic

0D944ZZ Drainage of Esophagogastric Junction, Percutaneous Endoscopic Approach

0D9470Z Drainage of Esophagogastric Junction with Drainage Device, Via Natural or Artificial Opening

0D947ZX Drainage of Esophagogastric Junction, Via Natural or Artificial Opening, Diagnostic

0D947ZZ Drainage of Esophagogastric Junction, Via Natural or Artificial Opening

0D9480Z Drainage of Esophagogastric Junction with Drainage Device, Via Natural or Artificial Opening Endoscopic

0D948ZX Drainage of Esophagogastric Junction, Via Natural or Artificial Opening Endoscopic, Diagnostic

0D948ZZ Drainage of Esophagogastric Junction, Via Natural or Artificial Opening Endoscopic

0D9500Z Drainage of Esophagus with Drainage Device, Open Approach

0D950ZX Drainage of Esophagus, Open Approach, Diagnostic

0D950ZZ Drainage of Esophagus, Open Approach

0D9530Z Drainage of Esophagus with Drainage Device, Percutaneous Approach

0D953ZX Drainage of Esophagus, Percutaneous Approach, Diagnostic

0D953ZZ Drainage of Esophagus, Percutaneous Approach

0D9540Z Drainage of Esophagus with Drainage Device, Percutaneous Endoscopic Approach

0D954ZX Drainage of Esophagus, Percutaneous Endoscopic Approach, Diagnostic

0D954ZZ Drainage of Esophagus, Percutaneous Endoscopic Approach

0D9570Z Drainage of Esophagus with Drainage Device, Via Natural or Artificial Opening

0D957ZX Drainage of Esophagus, Via Natural or Artificial Opening, Diagnostic

0D957ZZ Drainage of Esophagus, Via Natural or Artificial Opening

0D9580Z Drainage of Esophagus with Drainage Device, Via Natural or Artificial Opening Endoscopic

0D958ZX Drainage of Esophagus, Via Natural or Artificial Opening Endoscopic, Diagnostic

0D958ZZ Drainage of Esophagus, Via Natural or Artificial Opening Endoscopic

0D9600Z Drainage of Stomach with Drainage Device, Open Approach

0D960ZX Drainage of Stomach, Open Approach, Diagnostic

0D960ZZ Drainage of Stomach, Open Approach

0D9630Z Drainage of Stomach with Drainage Device, Percutaneous Approach

0D963ZX Drainage of Stomach, Percutaneous Approach, Diagnostic

0D963ZZ Drainage of Stomach, Percutaneous Approach

0D9640Z Drainage of Stomach with Drainage Device, Percutaneous Endoscopic Approach

0D964ZX Drainage of Stomach, Percutaneous Endoscopic Approach, Diagnostic

0D964ZZ Drainage of Stomach, Percutaneous Endoscopic Approach

0D9670Z Drainage of Stomach with Drainage Device, Via Natural or Artificial Opening

AHA CC: 2Q, 2015, 29

0D967ZX Drainage of Stomach, Via Natural or Artificial Opening, Diagnostic

0D967ZZ Drainage of Stomach, Via Natural or Artificial Opening

0D9680Z Drainage of Stomach with Drainage Device, Via Natural or Artificial Opening Endoscopic

0D968ZX Drainage of Stomach, Via Natural or Artificial Opening Endoscopic, Diagnostic

0D968ZZ Drainage of Stomach, Via Natural or Artificial Opening Endoscopic

0D9700Z Drainage of Stomach, Pylorus with Drainage Device, Open Approach

0D970ZX Drainage of Stomach, Pylorus, Open Approach, Diagnostic

0D970ZZ Drainage of Stomach, Pylorus, Open Approach

0D9730Z Drainage of Stomach, Pylorus with Drainage Device, Percutaneous Approach

0D973ZX Drainage of Stomach, Pylorus, Percutaneous Approach, Diagnostic

0D973ZZ Drainage of Stomach, Pylorus, Percutaneous Approach

0D9740Z Drainage of Stomach, Pylorus with Drainage Device, Percutaneous Endoscopic Approach

0D974ZX Drainage of Stomach, Pylorus, Percutaneous Endoscopic Approach, Diagnostic

0D974ZZ Drainage of Stomach, Pylorus, Percutaneous Endoscopic Approach

0D9770Z Drainage of Stomach, Pylorus with Drainage Device, Via Natural or Artificial Opening

0D977ZX Drainage of Stomach, Pylorus, Via Natural or Artificial Opening, Diagnostic

0D977ZZ Drainage of Stomach, Pylorus, Via Natural or Artificial Opening

0D9780Z Drainage of Stomach, Pylorus with Drainage Device, Via Natural or Artificial Opening Endoscopic

0D978ZX Drainage of Stomach, Pylorus, Via Natural or Artificial Opening Endoscopic, Diagnostic

0D978ZZ Drainage of Stomach, Pylorus, Via Natural or Artificial Opening Endoscopic

0D9800Z Drainage of Small Intestine with Drainage Device, Open Approach

0D980ZX Drainage of Small Intestine, Open Approach, Diagnostic

0D980ZZ Drainage of Small Intestine, Open Approach

0D9830Z Drainage of Small Intestine with Drainage Device, Percutaneous Approach

0D983ZX Drainage of Small Intestine, Percutaneous Approach, Diagnostic

0D983ZZ Drainage of Small Intestine, Percutaneous Approach

0D9840Z Drainage of Small Intestine with Drainage Device, Percutaneous Endoscopic Approach

0D984ZX Drainage of Small Intestine, Percutaneous Endoscopic Approach, Diagnostic

0D984ZZ Drainage of Small Intestine, Percutaneous Endoscopic Approach

0D9870Z Drainage of Small Intestine with Drainage Device, Via Natural or Artificial Opening

0D987ZX Drainage of Small Intestine, Via Natural or Artificial Opening, Diagnostic

0D987ZZ Drainage of Small Intestine, Via Natural or Artificial Opening

0D9880Z Drainage of Small Intestine with Drainage Device, Via Natural or Artificial Opening Endoscopic

0D988ZX Drainage of Small Intestine, Via Natural or Artificial Opening Endoscopic, Diagnostic

0D988ZZ Drainage of Small Intestine, Via Natural or Artificial Opening Endoscopic

0D9900Z Drainage of Duodenum with Drainage Device, Open Approach

0D990ZX Drainage of Duodenum, Open Approach, Diagnostic

0D990ZZ Drainage of Duodenum, Open Approach

0D9930Z Drainage of Duodenum with Drainage Device, Percutaneous Approach

0D993ZX Drainage of Duodenum, Percutaneous Approach, Diagnostic

0D993ZZ Drainage of Duodenum, Percutaneous Approach

0D9940Z Drainage of Duodenum with Drainage Device, Percutaneous Endoscopic Approach

0D994ZX Drainage of Duodenum, Percutaneous Endoscopic Approach, Diagnostic

0D994ZZ Drainage of Duodenum, Percutaneous Endoscopic Approach

0D9970Z Drainage of Duodenum with Drainage Device, Via Natural or Artificial Opening

0D997ZX Drainage of Duodenum, Via Natural or Artificial Opening, Diagnostic

0D997ZZ Drainage of Duodenum, Via Natural or Artificial Opening

0D9980Z Drainage of Duodenum with Drainage Device, Via Natural or Artificial Opening Endoscopic

♀ Female-only   ♂ Male-only   ▲ Limited Coverage   ● Non-OR   ᴴᴬᶜ HAC-associated procedure   ▲ Non-covered procedures   ✚ Cluster

0D998ZX Drainage of Duodenum, Via Natural or Artificial Opening Endoscopic, Diagnostic

0D998ZZ Drainage of Duodenum, Via Natural or Artificial Opening Endoscopic

0D9A00Z Drainage of Jejunum with Drainage Device, Open Approach

0D9A0ZX Drainage of Jejunum, Open Approach, Diagnostic

0D9A0ZZ Drainage of Jejunum, Open Approach

0D9A30Z Drainage of Jejunum with Drainage Device, Percutaneous Approach

0D9A3ZX Drainage of Jejunum, Percutaneous Approach, Diagnostic

0D9A3ZZ Drainage of Jejunum, Percutaneous Approach

0D9A40Z Drainage of Jejunum with Drainage Device, Percutaneous Endoscopic Approach

0D9A4ZX Drainage of Jejunum, Percutaneous Endoscopic Approach, Diagnostic

0D9A4ZZ Drainage of Jejunum, Percutaneous Endoscopic Approach

0D9A70Z Drainage of Jejunum with Drainage Device, Via Natural or Artificial Opening

0D9A7ZX Drainage of Jejunum, Via Natural or Artificial Opening, Diagnostic

0D9A7ZZ Drainage of Jejunum, Via Natural or Artificial Opening

0D9A80Z Drainage of Jejunum with Drainage Device, Via Natural or Artificial Opening Endoscopic

0D9A8ZX Drainage of Jejunum, Via Natural or Artificial Opening Endoscopic, Diagnostic

0D9A8ZZ Drainage of Jejunum, Via Natural or Artificial Opening Endoscopic

0D9B00Z Drainage of Ileum with Drainage Device, Open Approach

0D9B0ZX Drainage of Ileum, Open Approach, Diagnostic

0D9B0ZZ Drainage of Ileum, Open Approach

0D9B30Z Drainage of Ileum with Drainage Device, Percutaneous Approach

0D9B3ZX Drainage of Ileum, Percutaneous Approach, Diagnostic

0D9B3ZZ Drainage of Ileum, Percutaneous Approach

0D9B40Z Drainage of Ileum with Drainage Device, Percutaneous Endoscopic Approach

0D9B4ZX Drainage of Ileum, Percutaneous Endoscopic Approach, Diagnostic

0D9B4ZZ Drainage of Ileum, Percutaneous Endoscopic Approach

0D9B70Z Drainage of Ileum with Drainage Device, Via Natural or Artificial Opening

0D9B7ZX Drainage of Ileum, Via Natural or Artificial Opening, Diagnostic

0D9B7ZZ Drainage of Ileum, Via Natural or Artificial Opening

0D9B80Z Drainage of Ileum with Drainage Device, Via Natural or Artificial Opening Endoscopic

0D9B8ZX Drainage of Ileum, Via Natural or Artificial Opening Endoscopic, Diagnostic

0D9B8ZZ Drainage of Ileum, Via Natural or Artificial Opening Endoscopic

0D9C00Z Drainage of Ileocecal Valve with Drainage Device, Open Approach

0D9C0ZX Drainage of Ileocecal Valve, Open Approach, Diagnostic

0D9C0ZZ Drainage of Ileocecal Valve, Open Approach

0D9C30Z Drainage of Ileocecal Valve with Drainage Device, Percutaneous Approach

0D9C3ZX Drainage of Ileocecal Valve, Percutaneous Approach, Diagnostic

0D9C3ZZ Drainage of Ileocecal Valve, Percutaneous Approach

0D9C40Z Drainage of Ileocecal Valve with Drainage Device, Percutaneous Endoscopic Approach

0D9C4ZX Drainage of Ileocecal Valve, Percutaneous Endoscopic Approach, Diagnostic

0D9C4ZZ Drainage of Ileocecal Valve, Percutaneous Endoscopic Approach

0D9C70Z Drainage of Ileocecal Valve with Drainage Device, Via Natural or Artificial Opening

0D9C7ZX Drainage of Ileocecal Valve, Via Natural or Artificial Opening, Diagnostic

0D9C7ZZ Drainage of Ileocecal Valve, Via Natural or Artificial Opening

0D9C80Z Drainage of Ileocecal Valve with Drainage Device, Via Natural or Artificial Opening Endoscopic

0D9C8ZX Drainage of Ileocecal Valve, Via Natural or Artificial Opening Endoscopic, Diagnostic

0D9C8ZZ Drainage of Ileocecal Valve, Via Natural or Artificial Opening Endoscopic

0D9E00Z Drainage of Large Intestine with Drainage Device, Open Approach

0D9E0ZX Drainage of Large Intestine, Open Approach, Diagnostic

0D9E0ZZ Drainage of Large Intestine, Open Approach

0D9E30Z Drainage of Large Intestine with Drainage Device, Percutaneous Approach

0D9E3ZX Drainage of Large Intestine, Percutaneous Approach, Diagnostic

0D9E3ZZ Drainage of Large Intestine, Percutaneous Approach

0D9E40Z Drainage of Large Intestine with Drainage Device, Percutaneous Endoscopic Approach

0D9E4ZX Drainage of Large Intestine, Percutaneous Endoscopic Approach, Diagnostic

0D9E4ZZ Drainage of Large Intestine, Percutaneous Endoscopic Approach

0D9E70Z Drainage of Large Intestine with Drainage Device, Via Natural or Artificial Opening

0D9E7ZX Drainage of Large Intestine, Via Natural or Artificial Opening, Diagnostic

0D9E7ZZ Drainage of Large Intestine, Via Natural or Artificial Opening

0D9E80Z Drainage of Large Intestine with Drainage Device, Via Natural or Artificial Opening Endoscopic

0D9E8ZX Drainage of Large Intestine, Via Natural or Artificial Opening Endoscopic, Diagnostic

0D9E8ZZ Drainage of Large Intestine, Via Natural or Artificial Opening Endoscopic

0D9F00Z Drainage of Right Large Intestine with Drainage Device, Open Approach

0D9F0ZX Drainage of Right Large Intestine, Open Approach, Diagnostic

0D9F0ZZ Drainage of Right Large Intestine, Open Approach

0D9F30Z Drainage of Right Large Intestine with Drainage Device, Percutaneous Approach

0D9F3ZX Drainage of Right Large Intestine, Percutaneous Approach, Diagnostic

0D9F3ZZ Drainage of Right Large Intestine, Percutaneous Approach

0D9F40Z Drainage of Right Large Intestine with Drainage Device, Percutaneous Endoscopic Approach

0D9F4ZX Drainage of Right Large Intestine, Percutaneous Endoscopic Approach, Diagnostic

0D9F4ZZ Drainage of Right Large Intestine, Percutaneous Endoscopic Approach

0D9F70Z Drainage of Right Large Intestine with Drainage Device, Via Natural or Artificial Opening

0D9F7ZX Drainage of Right Large Intestine, Via Natural or Artificial Opening, Diagnostic

0D9F7ZZ Drainage of Right Large Intestine, Via Natural or Artificial Opening

0D9F80Z Drainage of Right Large Intestine with Drainage Device, Via Natural or Artificial Opening Endoscopic

0D9F8ZX Drainage of Right Large Intestine, Via Natural or Artificial Opening Endoscopic, Diagnostic

0D9F8ZZ Drainage of Right Large Intestine, Via Natural or Artificial Opening Endoscopic

0D9G00Z Drainage of Left Large Intestine with Drainage Device, Open Approach

0D9G0ZX Drainage of Left Large Intestine, Open Approach, Diagnostic

0D9G0ZZ Drainage of Left Large Intestine, Open Approach

0D9G30Z Drainage of Left Large Intestine with Drainage Device, Percutaneous Approach

0D9G3ZX Drainage of Left Large Intestine, Percutaneous Approach, Diagnostic

0D9G3ZZ Drainage of Left Large Intestine, Percutaneous Approach

0D9G40Z Drainage of Left Large Intestine with Drainage Device, Percutaneous Endoscopic Approach

0D9G4ZX Drainage of Left Large Intestine, Percutaneous Endoscopic Approach, Diagnostic

0D9G4ZZ Drainage of Left Large Intestine, Percutaneous Endoscopic Approach

0D9G70Z Drainage of Left Large Intestine with Drainage Device, Via Natural or Artificial Opening

0D9G7ZX Drainage of Left Large Intestine, Via Natural or Artificial Opening, Diagnostic

0D9G7ZZ Drainage of Left Large Intestine, Via Natural or Artificial Opening

0D9G80Z Drainage of Left Large Intestine with Drainage Device, Via Natural or Artificial Opening Endoscopic

0D9G8ZX Drainage of Left Large Intestine, Via Natural or Artificial Opening Endoscopic, Diagnostic

0D9G8ZZ Drainage of Left Large Intestine, Via Natural or Artificial Opening Endoscopic

0D9H00Z Drainage of Cecum with Drainage Device, Open Approach

0D9H0ZX Drainage of Cecum, Open Approach, Diagnostic

 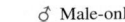

0D9H0ZZ Drainage of Cecum, Open Approach

0D9H30Z Drainage of Cecum with Drainage Device, Percutaneous Approach

0D9H3ZX Drainage of Cecum, Percutaneous Approach, Diagnostic

0D9H3ZZ Drainage of Cecum, Percutaneous Approach

0D9H40Z Drainage of Cecum with Drainage Device, Percutaneous Endoscopic Approach

0D9H4ZX Drainage of Cecum, Percutaneous Endoscopic Approach, Diagnostic

0D9H4ZZ Drainage of Cecum, Percutaneous Endoscopic Approach

0D9H70Z Drainage of Cecum with Drainage Device, Via Natural or Artificial Opening

0D9H7ZX Drainage of Cecum, Via Natural or Artificial Opening, Diagnostic

0D9H7ZZ Drainage of Cecum, Via Natural or Artificial Opening

0D9H80Z Drainage of Cecum with Drainage Device, Via Natural or Artificial Opening Endoscopic

0D9H8ZX Drainage of Cecum, Via Natural or Artificial Opening Endoscopic, Diagnostic

0D9H8ZZ Drainage of Cecum, Via Natural or Artificial Opening Endoscopic

0D9J00Z Drainage of Appendix with Drainage Device, Open Approach

0D9J0ZX Drainage of Appendix, Open Approach, Diagnostic

0D9J0ZZ Drainage of Appendix, Open Approach

0D9J30Z Drainage of Appendix with Drainage Device, Percutaneous Approach

0D9J3ZX Drainage of Appendix, Percutaneous Approach, Diagnostic

0D9J3ZZ Drainage of Appendix, Percutaneous Approach

0D9J40Z Drainage of Appendix with Drainage Device, Percutaneous Endoscopic Approach

0D9J4ZX Drainage of Appendix, Percutaneous Endoscopic Approach, Diagnostic

0D9J4ZZ Drainage of Appendix, Percutaneous Endoscopic Approach

0D9J70Z Drainage of Appendix with Drainage Device, Via Natural or Artificial Opening

0D9J7ZX Drainage of Appendix, Via Natural or Artificial Opening, Diagnostic

0D9J7ZZ Drainage of Appendix, Via Natural or Artificial Opening

0D9J80Z Drainage of Appendix with Drainage Device, Via Natural or Artificial Opening Endoscopic

0D9J8ZX Drainage of Appendix, Via Natural or Artificial Opening Endoscopic, Diagnostic

0D9J8ZZ Drainage of Appendix, Via Natural or Artificial Opening Endoscopic

0D9K00Z Drainage of Ascending Colon with Drainage Device, Open Approach

0D9K0ZX Drainage of Ascending Colon, Open Approach, Diagnostic

0D9K0ZZ Drainage of Ascending Colon, Open Approach

0D9K30Z Drainage of Ascending Colon with Drainage Device, Percutaneous Approach

0D9K3ZX Drainage of Ascending Colon, Percutaneous Approach, Diagnostic

0D9K3ZZ Drainage of Ascending Colon, Percutaneous Approach

0D9K40Z Drainage of Ascending Colon with Drainage Device, Percutaneous Endoscopic Approach

0D9K4ZX Drainage of Ascending Colon, Percutaneous Endoscopic Approach, Diagnostic

0D9K4ZZ Drainage of Ascending Colon, Percutaneous Endoscopic Approach

0D9K70Z Drainage of Ascending Colon with Drainage Device, Via Natural or Artificial Opening

0D9K7ZX Drainage of Ascending Colon, Via Natural or Artificial Opening, Diagnostic

0D9K7ZZ Drainage of Ascending Colon, Via Natural or Artificial Opening

0D9K80Z Drainage of Ascending Colon with Drainage Device, Via Natural or Artificial Opening Endoscopic

0D9K8ZX Drainage of Ascending Colon, Via Natural or Artificial Opening Endoscopic, Diagnostic

0D9K8ZZ Drainage of Ascending Colon, Via Natural or Artificial Opening Endoscopic

0D9L00Z Drainage of Transverse Colon with Drainage Device, Open Approach

0D9L0ZX Drainage of Transverse Colon, Open Approach, Diagnostic

0D9L0ZZ Drainage of Transverse Colon, Open Approach

0D9L30Z Drainage of Transverse Colon with Drainage Device, Percutaneous Approach

0D9L3ZX Drainage of Transverse Colon, Percutaneous Approach, Diagnostic

0D9L3ZZ Drainage of Transverse Colon, Percutaneous Approach

0D9L40Z Drainage of Transverse Colon with Drainage Device, Percutaneous Endoscopic Approach

0D9L4ZX Drainage of Transverse Colon, Percutaneous Endoscopic Approach, Diagnostic

0D9L4ZZ Drainage of Transverse Colon, Percutaneous Endoscopic Approach

0D9L70Z Drainage of Transverse Colon with Drainage Device, Via Natural or Artificial Opening

0D9L7ZX Drainage of Transverse Colon, Via Natural or Artificial Opening, Diagnostic

0D9L7ZZ Drainage of Transverse Colon, Via Natural or Artificial Opening

0D9L80Z Drainage of Transverse Colon with Drainage Device, Via Natural or Artificial Opening Endoscopic

0D9L8ZX Drainage of Transverse Colon, Via Natural or Artificial Opening Endoscopic, Diagnostic

0D9L8ZZ Drainage of Transverse Colon, Via Natural or Artificial Opening Endoscopic

0D9M00Z Drainage of Descending Colon with Drainage Device, Open Approach

0D9M0ZX Drainage of Descending Colon, Open Approach, Diagnostic

0D9M0ZZ Drainage of Descending Colon, Open Approach

0D9M30Z Drainage of Descending Colon with Drainage Device, Percutaneous Approach

0D9M3ZX Drainage of Descending Colon, Percutaneous Approach, Diagnostic

0D9M3ZZ Drainage of Descending Colon, Percutaneous Approach

0D9M40Z Drainage of Descending Colon with Drainage Device, Percutaneous Endoscopic Approach

0D9M4ZX Drainage of Descending Colon, Percutaneous Endoscopic Approach, Diagnostic

0D9M4ZZ Drainage of Descending Colon, Percutaneous Endoscopic Approach

0D9M70Z Drainage of Descending Colon with Drainage Device, Via Natural or Artificial Opening

0D9M7ZX Drainage of Descending Colon, Via Natural or Artificial Opening, Diagnostic

0D9M7ZZ Drainage of Descending Colon, Via Natural or Artificial Opening

0D9M80Z Drainage of Descending Colon with Drainage Device, Via Natural or Artificial Opening Endoscopic

0D9M8ZX Drainage of Descending Colon, Via Natural or Artificial Opening Endoscopic, Diagnostic

0D9M8ZZ Drainage of Descending Colon, Via Natural or Artificial Opening Endoscopic

0D9N00Z Drainage of Sigmoid Colon with Drainage Device, Open Approach

0D9N0ZX Drainage of Sigmoid Colon, Open Approach, Diagnostic

0D9N0ZZ Drainage of Sigmoid Colon, Open Approach

● **0D9N30Z** Drainage of Sigmoid Colon with Drainage Device, Percutaneous Approach

0D9N3ZX Drainage of Sigmoid Colon, Percutaneous Approach, Diagnostic

0D9N3ZZ Drainage of Sigmoid Colon, Percutaneous Approach

0D9N40Z Drainage of Sigmoid Colon with Drainage Device, Percutaneous Endoscopic Approach

0D9N4ZX Drainage of Sigmoid Colon, Percutaneous Endoscopic Approach, Diagnostic

0D9N4ZZ Drainage of Sigmoid Colon, Percutaneous Endoscopic Approach

0D9N70Z Drainage of Sigmoid Colon with Drainage Device, Via Natural or Artificial Opening

0D9N7ZX Drainage of Sigmoid Colon, Via Natural or Artificial Opening, Diagnostic

0D9N7ZZ Drainage of Sigmoid Colon, Via Natural or Artificial Opening

0D9N80Z Drainage of Sigmoid Colon with Drainage Device, Via Natural or Artificial Opening Endoscopic

0D9N8ZX Drainage of Sigmoid Colon, Via Natural or Artificial Opening Endoscopic, Diagnostic

0D9N8ZZ Drainage of Sigmoid Colon, Via Natural or Artificial Opening Endoscopic

0D9P00Z Drainage of Rectum with Drainage Device, Open Approach

0D9P0ZX Drainage of Rectum, Open Approach, Diagnostic

0D9P0ZZ Drainage of Rectum, Open Approach

0D9P30Z Drainage of Rectum with Drainage Device, Percutaneous Approach

0D9P3ZX Drainage of Rectum, Percutaneous Approach, Diagnostic

0D9P3ZZ Drainage of Rectum, Percutaneous Approach

0D9P40Z Drainage of Rectum with Drainage Device, Percutaneous Endoscopic Approach

♀ Female-only　　♂ Male-only　　▲ Limited Coverage　　● Non-OR　　**HAC** HAC-associated procedure　　▲ Non-covered procedures　　✚ Cluster

0D9P4ZX Drainage of Rectum, Percutaneous Endoscopic Approach, Diagnostic

0D9P4ZZ Drainage of Rectum, Percutaneous Endoscopic Approach

0D9P70Z Drainage of Rectum with Drainage Device, Via Natural or Artificial Opening

0D9P7ZX Drainage of Rectum, Via Natural or Artificial Opening, Diagnostic

0D9P7ZZ Drainage of Rectum, Via Natural or Artificial Opening

0D9P80Z Drainage of Rectum with Drainage Device, Via Natural or Artificial Opening Endoscopic

0D9P8ZX Drainage of Rectum, Via Natural or Artificial Opening Endoscopic, Diagnostic

0D9P8ZZ Drainage of Rectum, Via Natural or Artificial Opening Endoscopic

0D9Q00Z Drainage of Anus with Drainage Device, Open Approach

0D9Q0ZX Drainage of Anus, Open Approach, Diagnostic

0D9Q0ZZ Drainage of Anus, Open Approach

0D9Q30Z Drainage of Anus with Drainage Device, Percutaneous Approach

0D9Q3ZX Drainage of Anus, Percutaneous Approach, Diagnostic

0D9Q3ZZ Drainage of Anus, Percutaneous Approach

0D9Q40Z Drainage of Anus with Drainage Device, Percutaneous Endoscopic Approach

0D9Q4ZX Drainage of Anus, Percutaneous Endoscopic Approach, Diagnostic

0D9Q4ZZ Drainage of Anus, Percutaneous Endoscopic Approach

0D9Q70Z Drainage of Anus with Drainage Device, Via Natural or Artificial Opening

0D9Q7ZX Drainage of Anus, Via Natural or Artificial Opening, Diagnostic

0D9Q7ZZ Drainage of Anus, Via Natural or Artificial Opening

0D9Q80Z Drainage of Anus with Drainage Device, Via Natural or Artificial Opening Endoscopic

0D9Q8ZX Drainage of Anus, Via Natural or Artificial Opening Endoscopic, Diagnostic

0D9Q8ZZ Drainage of Anus, Via Natural or Artificial Opening Endoscopic

0D9QX0Z Drainage of Anus with Drainage Device, External Approach

0D9QXZX Drainage of Anus, External Approach, Diagnostic

0D9QXZZ Drainage of Anus, External Approach

0D9R00Z Drainage of Anal Sphincter with Drainage Device, Open Approach

0D9R0ZX Drainage of Anal Sphincter, Open Approach, Diagnostic

0D9R0ZZ Drainage of Anal Sphincter, Open Approach

0D9R30Z Drainage of Anal Sphincter with Drainage Device, Percutaneous Approach

0D9R3ZX Drainage of Anal Sphincter, Percutaneous Approach, Diagnostic

0D9R3ZZ Drainage of Anal Sphincter, Percutaneous Approach

0D9R40Z Drainage of Anal Sphincter with Drainage Device, Percutaneous Endoscopic Approach

0D9R4ZX Drainage of Anal Sphincter, Percutaneous Endoscopic Approach, Diagnostic

0D9R4ZZ Drainage of Anal Sphincter, Percutaneous Endoscopic Approach

0D9U00Z Drainage of Omentum with Drainage Device, Open Approach

0D9U0ZX Drainage of Omentum, Open Approach, Diagnostic

0D9U0ZZ Drainage of Omentum, Open Approach

0D9U30Z Drainage of Omentum with Drainage Device, Percutaneous Approach

0D9U3ZX Drainage of Omentum, Percutaneous Approach, Diagnostic

0D9U3ZZ Drainage of Omentum, Percutaneous Approach

0D9U40Z Drainage of Omentum with Drainage Device, Percutaneous Endoscopic Approach

0D9U4ZX Drainage of Omentum, Percutaneous Endoscopic Approach, Diagnostic

0D9U4ZZ Drainage of Omentum, Percutaneous Endoscopic Approach

0D9V00Z Drainage of Mesentery with Drainage Device, Open Approach

0D9V0ZX Drainage of Mesentery, Open Approach, Diagnostic

0D9V0ZZ Drainage of Mesentery, Open Approach

0D9V30Z Drainage of Mesentery with Drainage Device, Percutaneous Approach

0D9V3ZX Drainage of Mesentery, Percutaneous Approach, Diagnostic

0D9V3ZZ Drainage of Mesentery, Percutaneous Approach

0D9V40Z Drainage of Mesentery with Drainage Device, Percutaneous Endoscopic Approach

0D9V4ZX Drainage of Mesentery, Percutaneous Endoscopic Approach, Diagnostic

0D9V4ZZ Drainage of Mesentery, Percutaneous Endoscopic Approach

0D9W00Z Drainage of Peritoneum with Drainage Device, Open Approach

0D9W0ZX Drainage of Peritoneum, Open Approach, Diagnostic

0D9W0ZZ Drainage of Peritoneum, Open Approach

0D9W30Z Drainage of Peritoneum with Drainage Device, Percutaneous Approach

0D9W3ZX Drainage of Peritoneum, Percutaneous Approach, Diagnostic

0D9W3ZZ Drainage of Peritoneum, Percutaneous Approach

0D9W40Z Drainage of Peritoneum with Drainage Device, Percutaneous Endoscopic Approach

0D9W4ZX Drainage of Peritoneum, Percutaneous Endoscopic Approach, Diagnostic

0D9W4ZZ Drainage of Peritoneum, Percutaneous Endoscopic Approach

0DB – Gastrointestinal System, Excision

Review Coding Guidelines B3.4a and B3.4b

Review Coding Guideline B3.8

Review Coding Guideline B3.18

0DB10ZX Excision of Upper Esophagus, Open Approach, Diagnostic

0DB10ZZ Excision of Upper Esophagus, Open Approach

0DB13ZX Excision of Upper Esophagus, Percutaneous Approach, Diagnostic

0DB13ZZ Excision of Upper Esophagus, Percutaneous Approach

0DB14ZX Excision of Upper Esophagus, Percutaneous Endoscopic Approach, Diagnostic

0DB14ZZ Excision of Upper Esophagus, Percutaneous Endoscopic Approach

0DB17ZX Excision of Upper Esophagus, Via Natural or Artificial Opening, Diagnostic

0DB17ZZ Excision of Upper Esophagus, Via Natural or Artificial Opening

0DB18ZX Excision of Upper Esophagus, Via Natural or Artificial Opening Endoscopic, Diagnostic

0DB18ZZ Excision of Upper Esophagus, Via Natural or Artificial Opening Endoscopic

0DB20ZX Excision of Middle Esophagus, Open Approach, Diagnostic

0DB20ZZ Excision of Middle Esophagus, Open Approach

0DB23ZX Excision of Middle Esophagus, Percutaneous Approach, Diagnostic

0DB23ZZ Excision of Middle Esophagus, Percutaneous Approach

0DB24ZX Excision of Middle Esophagus, Percutaneous Endoscopic Approach, Diagnostic

0DB24ZZ Excision of Middle Esophagus, Percutaneous Endoscopic Approach

0DB27ZX Excision of Middle Esophagus, Via Natural or Artificial Opening, Diagnostic

0DB27ZZ Excision of Middle Esophagus, Via Natural or Artificial Opening

0DB28ZX Excision of Middle Esophagus, Via Natural or Artificial Opening Endoscopic, Diagnostic
AHA CC: 1Q, 2016, 24-25

0DB28ZZ Excision of Middle Esophagus, Via Natural or Artificial Opening Endoscopic

0DB30ZX Excision of Lower Esophagus, Open Approach, Diagnostic

0DB30ZZ Excision of Lower Esophagus, Open Approach

0DB33ZX Excision of Lower Esophagus, Percutaneous Approach, Diagnostic

0DB33ZZ Excision of Lower Esophagus, Percutaneous Approach

0DB34ZX Excision of Lower Esophagus, Percutaneous Endoscopic Approach, Diagnostic

0DB34ZZ Excision of Lower Esophagus, Percutaneous Endoscopic Approach

0DB37ZX Excision of Lower Esophagus, Via Natural or Artificial Opening, Diagnostic

0DB37ZZ Excision of Lower Esophagus, Via Natural or Artificial Opening

0DB38ZX Excision of Lower Esophagus, Via Natural or Artificial Opening Endoscopic, Diagnostic

0DB38ZZ Excision of Lower Esophagus, Via Natural or Artificial Opening Endoscopic

0DB40ZX Excision of Esophagogastric Junction, Open Approach, Diagnostic

0DB40ZZ Excision of Esophagogastric Junction, Open Approach

0DB43ZX Excision of Esophagogastric Junction, Percutaneous Approach, Diagnostic

0DB43ZZ Excision of Esophagogastric Junction, Percutaneous Approach

0DB44ZX Excision of Esophagogastric Junction, Percutaneous Endoscopic Approach, Diagnostic

0DB44ZZ Excision of Esophagogastric Junction, Percutaneous Endoscopic Approach

0DB47ZX Excision of Esophagogastric Junction, Via Natural or Artificial Opening, Diagnostic

0DB47ZZ Excision of Esophagogastric Junction, Via Natural or Artificial Opening

0DB48ZX Excision of Esophagogastric Junction, Via Natural or Artificial Opening Endoscopic, Diagnostic

0DB48ZZ Excision of Esophagogastric Junction, Via Natural or Artificial Opening Endoscopic

0DB50ZX Excision of Esophagus, Open Approach, Diagnostic

0DB50ZZ Excision of Esophagus, Open Approach

0DB53ZX Excision of Esophagus, Percutaneous Approach, Diagnostic

0DB53ZZ Excision of Esophagus, Percutaneous Approach

0DB54ZX Excision of Esophagus, Percutaneous Endoscopic Approach, Diagnostic

0DB54ZZ Excision of Esophagus, Percutaneous Endoscopic Approach

0DB57ZX Excision of Esophagus, Via Natural or Artificial Opening, Diagnostic

0DB57ZZ Excision of Esophagus, Via Natural or Artificial Opening

0DB58ZX Excision of Esophagus, Via Natural or Artificial Opening Endoscopic, Diagnostic

0DB58ZZ Excision of Esophagus, Via Natural or Artificial Opening Endoscopic

0DB60Z3 Excision of Stomach, Open Approach, Vertical

0DB60ZX Excision of Stomach, Open Approach, Diagnostic

0DB60ZZ Excision of Stomach, Open Approach
AHA CC: 2Q, 2017, 17-18; 1Q, 2019, 4-7

0DB63Z3 Excision of Stomach, Percutaneous Approach, Vertical

0DB63ZX Excision of Stomach, Percutaneous Approach, Diagnostic

0DB63ZZ Excision of Stomach, Percutaneous Approach

0DB64Z3 Excision of Stomach, Percutaneous Endoscopic Approach, Vertical
AHA CC: 2Q, 2016, 31

0DB64ZX Excision of Stomach, Percutaneous Endoscopic Approach, Diagnostic

0DB64ZZ Excision of Stomach, Percutaneous Endoscopic Approach

0DB67Z3 Excision of Stomach, Via Natural or Artificial Opening, Vertical

0DB67ZX Excision of Stomach, Via Natural or Artificial Opening, Diagnostic

0DB67ZZ Excision of Stomach, Via Natural or Artificial Opening

0DB68Z3 Excision of Stomach, Via Natural or Artificial Opening Endoscopic, Vertical

0DB68ZX Excision of Stomach, Via Natural or Artificial Opening Endoscopic, Diagnostic

0DB68ZZ Excision of Stomach, Via Natural or Artificial Opening Endoscopic

0DB70ZX Excision of Stomach, Pylorus, Open Approach, Diagnostic

0DB70ZZ Excision of Stomach, Pylorus, Open Approach

0DB73ZX Excision of Stomach, Pylorus, Percutaneous Approach, Diagnostic

0DB73ZZ Excision of Stomach, Pylorus, Percutaneous Approach

0DB74ZX Excision of Stomach, Pylorus, Percutaneous Endoscopic Approach, Diagnostic

0DB74ZZ Excision of Stomach, Pylorus, Percutaneous Endoscopic Approach

0DB77ZX Excision of Stomach, Pylorus, Via Natural or Artificial Opening, Diagnostic

0DB77ZZ Excision of Stomach, Pylorus, Via Natural or Artificial Opening

0DB78ZX Excision of Stomach, Pylorus, Via Natural or Artificial Opening Endoscopic, Diagnostic

0DB78ZZ Excision of Stomach, Pylorus, Via Natural or Artificial Opening Endoscopic

0DB80ZX Excision of Small Intestine, Open Approach, Diagnostic

0DB80ZZ Excision of Small Intestine, Open Approach
AHA CC: 2Q, 2021, 11-12

0DB83ZX Excision of Small Intestine, Percutaneous Approach, Diagnostic

0DB83ZZ Excision of Small Intestine, Percutaneous Approach

0DB84ZX Excision of Small Intestine, Percutaneous Endoscopic Approach, Diagnostic

0DB84ZZ Excision of Small Intestine, Percutaneous Endoscopic Approach

0DB87ZX Excision of Small Intestine, Via Natural or Artificial Opening, Diagnostic

0DB87ZZ Excision of Small Intestine, Via Natural or Artificial Opening

0DB88ZX Excision of Small Intestine, Via Natural or Artificial Opening Endoscopic, Diagnostic

0DB88ZZ Excision of Small Intestine, Via Natural or Artificial Opening Endoscopic

0DB90ZX Excision of Duodenum, Open Approach, Diagnostic

0DB90ZZ Excision of Duodenum, Open Approach
AHA CC: 3Q, 2014, 32-33; 1Q, 2019, 4-7

0DB93ZX Excision of Duodenum, Percutaneous Approach, Diagnostic

0DB93ZZ Excision of Duodenum, Percutaneous Approach

0DB94ZX Excision of Duodenum, Percutaneous Endoscopic Approach, Diagnostic

0DB94ZZ Excision of Duodenum, Percutaneous Endoscopic Approach

0DB97ZX Excision of Duodenum, Via Natural or Artificial Opening, Diagnostic

0DB97ZZ Excision of Duodenum, Via Natural or Artificial Opening

0DB98ZX Excision of Duodenum, Via Natural or Artificial Opening Endoscopic, Diagnostic

0DB98ZZ Excision of Duodenum, Via Natural or Artificial Opening Endoscopic

0DBA0ZX Excision of Jejunum, Open Approach, Diagnostic

0DBA0ZZ Excision of Jejunum, Open Approach
AHA CC: 1Q, 2019, 4-5

0DBA3ZX Excision of Jejunum, Percutaneous Approach, Diagnostic

0DBA3ZZ Excision of Jejunum, Percutaneous Approach

0DBA4ZX Excision of Jejunum, Percutaneous Endoscopic Approach, Diagnostic

0DBA4ZZ Excision of Jejunum, Percutaneous Endoscopic Approach
AHA CC: 2Q, 2019, 15-16

0DBA7ZX Excision of Jejunum, Via Natural or Artificial Opening, Diagnostic

0DBA7ZZ Excision of Jejunum, Via Natural or Artificial Opening

0DBA8ZX Excision of Jejunum, Via Natural or Artificial Opening Endoscopic, Diagnostic

0DBA8ZZ Excision of Jejunum, Via Natural or Artificial Opening Endoscopic

0DBB0ZX Excision of Ileum, Open Approach, Diagnostic

0DBB0ZZ Excision of Ileum, Open Approach
AHA CC: 3Q, 2014, 28-29; 3Q, 2016, 5-6

0DBB3ZX Excision of Ileum, Percutaneous Approach, Diagnostic

0DBB3ZZ Excision of Ileum, Percutaneous Approach

0DBB4ZX Excision of Ileum, Percutaneous Endoscopic Approach, Diagnostic

0DBB4ZZ Excision of Ileum, Percutaneous Endoscopic Approach

0DBB7ZX Excision of Ileum, Via Natural or Artificial Opening, Diagnostic

0DBB7ZZ Excision of Ileum, Via Natural or Artificial Opening

0DBB8ZX Excision of Ileum, Via Natural or Artificial Opening Endoscopic, Diagnostic

0DBB8ZZ Excision of Ileum, Via Natural or Artificial Opening Endoscopic

0DBC0ZX Excision of Ileocecal Valve, Open Approach, Diagnostic

0DBC0ZZ Excision of Ileocecal Valve, Open Approach

0DBC3ZX Excision of Ileocecal Valve, Percutaneous Approach, Diagnostic

0DBC3ZZ Excision of Ileocecal Valve, Percutaneous Approach

0DBC4ZX Excision of Ileocecal Valve, Percutaneous Endoscopic Approach, Diagnostic

0DBC4ZZ Excision of Ileocecal Valve, Percutaneous Endoscopic Approach

0DBC7ZX Excision of Ileocecal Valve, Via Natural or Artificial Opening, Diagnostic

0DBC7ZZ Excision of Ileocecal Valve, Via Natural or Artificial Opening

0DBC8ZX Excision of Ileocecal Valve, Via Natural or Artificial Opening Endoscopic, Diagnostic

0DBC8ZZ Excision of Ileocecal Valve, Via Natural or Artificial Opening Endoscopic

0DBE0ZX Excision of Large Intestine, Open Approach, Diagnostic

♀ Female-only   ♂ Male-only   ▲ Limited Coverage   ● Non-OR   ᴴᴬᶜ HAC-associated procedure   ▲ Non-covered procedures   ➕ Cluster

0DBE0ZZ Excision of Large Intestine, Open Approach

0DBE3ZX Excision of Large Intestine, Percutaneous Approach, Diagnostic

0DBE3ZZ Excision of Large Intestine, Percutaneous Approach

0DBE4ZX Excision of Large Intestine, Percutaneous Endoscopic Approach, Diagnostic

0DBE4ZZ Excision of Large Intestine, Percutaneous Endoscopic Approach

0DBE7ZX Excision of Large Intestine, Via Natural or Artificial Opening, Diagnostic

0DBE7ZZ Excision of Large Intestine, Via Natural or Artificial Opening

0DBE8ZX Excision of Large Intestine, Via Natural or Artificial Opening Endoscopic, Diagnostic

0DBE8ZZ Excision of Large Intestine, Via Natural or Artificial Opening Endoscopic

0DBF0ZX Excision of Right Large Intestine, Open Approach, Diagnostic

0DBF0ZZ Excision of Right Large Intestine, Open Approach

0DBF3ZX Excision of Right Large Intestine, Percutaneous Approach, Diagnostic

0DBF3ZZ Excision of Right Large Intestine, Percutaneous Approach

0DBF4ZX Excision of Right Large Intestine, Percutaneous Endoscopic Approach, Diagnostic

0DBF4ZZ Excision of Right Large Intestine, Percutaneous Endoscopic Approach

0DBF7ZX Excision of Right Large Intestine, Via Natural or Artificial Opening, Diagnostic

0DBF7ZZ Excision of Right Large Intestine, Via Natural or Artificial Opening

0DBF8ZX Excision of Right Large Intestine, Via Natural or Artificial Opening Endoscopic, Diagnostic

0DBF8ZZ Excision of Right Large Intestine, Via Natural or Artificial Opening Endoscopic

0DBG0ZX Excision of Left Large Intestine, Open Approach, Diagnostic

0DBG0ZZ Excision of Left Large Intestine, Open Approach

0DBG3ZX Excision of Left Large Intestine, Percutaneous Approach, Diagnostic

0DBG3ZZ Excision of Left Large Intestine, Percutaneous Approach

0DBG4ZX Excision of Left Large Intestine, Percutaneous Endoscopic Approach, Diagnostic

0DBG4ZZ Excision of Left Large Intestine, Percutaneous Endoscopic Approach

0DBG7ZX Excision of Left Large Intestine, Via Natural or Artificial Opening, Diagnostic

0DBG7ZZ Excision of Left Large Intestine, Via Natural or Artificial Opening

0DBG8ZX Excision of Left Large Intestine, Via Natural or Artificial Opening Endoscopic, Diagnostic

0DBG8ZZ Excision of Left Large Intestine, Via Natural or Artificial Opening Endoscopic

0DBGFZZ Excision of Left Large Intestine, Via Natural or Artificial Opening With Percutaneous Endoscopic Assistance

0DBH0ZX Excision of Cecum, Open Approach, Diagnostic

0DBH0ZZ Excision of Cecum, Open Approach

0DBH3ZX Excision of Cecum, Percutaneous Approach, Diagnostic

0DBH3ZZ Excision of Cecum, Percutaneous Approach

0DBH4ZX Excision of Cecum, Percutaneous Endoscopic Approach, Diagnostic

0DBH4ZZ Excision of Cecum, Percutaneous Endoscopic Approach

0DBH7ZX Excision of Cecum, Via Natural or Artificial Opening, Diagnostic

0DBH7ZZ Excision of Cecum, Via Natural or Artificial Opening

0DBH8ZX Excision of Cecum, Via Natural or Artificial Opening Endoscopic, Diagnostic

0DBH8ZZ Excision of Cecum, Via Natural or Artificial Opening Endoscopic

0DBJ0ZX Excision of Appendix, Open Approach, Diagnostic

0DBJ0ZZ Excision of Appendix, Open Approach

0DBJ3ZX Excision of Appendix, Percutaneous Approach, Diagnostic

0DBJ3ZZ Excision of Appendix, Percutaneous Approach

0DBJ4ZX Excision of Appendix, Percutaneous Endoscopic Approach, Diagnostic

0DBJ4ZZ Excision of Appendix, Percutaneous Endoscopic Approach

0DBJ7ZX Excision of Appendix, Via Natural or Artificial Opening, Diagnostic

0DBJ7ZZ Excision of Appendix, Via Natural or Artificial Opening

0DBJ8ZX Excision of Appendix, Via Natural or Artificial Opening Endoscopic, Diagnostic

0DBJ8ZZ Excision of Appendix, Via Natural or Artificial Opening Endoscopic

0DBK0ZX Excision of Ascending Colon, Open Approach, Diagnostic

0DBK0ZZ Excision of Ascending Colon, Open Approach

0DBK3ZX Excision of Ascending Colon, Percutaneous Approach, Diagnostic

0DBK3ZZ Excision of Ascending Colon, Percutaneous Approach

0DBK4ZX Excision of Ascending Colon, Percutaneous Endoscopic Approach, Diagnostic

0DBK4ZZ Excision of Ascending Colon, Percutaneous Endoscopic Approach

0DBK7ZX Excision of Ascending Colon, Via Natural or Artificial Opening, Diagnostic

0DBK7ZZ Excision of Ascending Colon, Via Natural or Artificial Opening

0DBK8ZX Excision of Ascending Colon, Via Natural or Artificial Opening Endoscopic, Diagnostic

0DBK8ZZ Excision of Ascending Colon, Via Natural or Artificial Opening Endoscopic
AHA CC: 1Q, 2017, 16

0DBL0ZX Excision of Transverse Colon, Open Approach, Diagnostic

0DBL0ZZ Excision of Transverse Colon, Open Approach

0DBL3ZX Excision of Transverse Colon, Percutaneous Approach, Diagnostic

0DBL3ZZ Excision of Transverse Colon, Percutaneous Approach

0DBL4ZX Excision of Transverse Colon, Percutaneous Endoscopic Approach, Diagnostic

0DBL4ZZ Excision of Transverse Colon, Percutaneous Endoscopic Approach

0DBL7ZX Excision of Transverse Colon, Via Natural or Artificial Opening, Diagnostic

0DBL7ZZ Excision of Transverse Colon, Via Natural or Artificial Opening

0DBL8ZX Excision of Transverse Colon, Via Natural or Artificial Opening Endoscopic, Diagnostic

0DBL8ZZ Excision of Transverse Colon, Via Natural or Artificial Opening Endoscopic

0DBLFZZ Excision of Transverse Colon, Via Natural or Artificial Opening With Percutaneous Endoscopic Assistance

0DBM0ZX Excision of Descending Colon, Open Approach, Diagnostic

0DBM0ZZ Excision of Descending Colon, Open Approach

0DBM3ZX Excision of Descending Colon, Percutaneous Approach, Diagnostic

0DBM3ZZ Excision of Descending Colon, Percutaneous Approach

0DBM4ZX Excision of Descending Colon, Percutaneous Endoscopic Approach, Diagnostic

0DBM4ZZ Excision of Descending Colon, Percutaneous Endoscopic Approach

0DBM7ZX Excision of Descending Colon, Via Natural or Artificial Opening, Diagnostic

0DBM7ZZ Excision of Descending Colon, Via Natural or Artificial Opening

0DBM8ZX Excision of Descending Colon, Via Natural or Artificial Opening Endoscopic, Diagnostic

0DBM8ZZ Excision of Descending Colon, Via Natural or Artificial Opening Endoscopic

0DBMFZZ Excision of Descending Colon, Via Natural or Artificial Opening With Percutaneous Endoscopic Assistance

0DBN0ZX Excision of Sigmoid Colon, Open Approach, Diagnostic

0DBN0ZZ Excision of Sigmoid Colon, Open Approach
AHA CC: 4Q, 2014, 40-41; 1Q, 2019, 27

0DBN3ZX Excision of Sigmoid Colon, Percutaneous Approach, Diagnostic

0DBN3ZZ Excision of Sigmoid Colon, Percutaneous Approach

0DBN4ZX Excision of Sigmoid Colon, Percutaneous Endoscopic Approach, Diagnostic

0DBN4ZZ Excision of Sigmoid Colon, Percutaneous Endoscopic Approach

0DBN7ZX Excision of Sigmoid Colon, Via Natural or Artificial Opening, Diagnostic

0DBN7ZZ Excision of Sigmoid Colon, Via Natural or Artificial Opening

0DBN8ZX Excision of Sigmoid Colon, Via Natural or Artificial Opening Endoscopic, Diagnostic

0DBN8ZZ Excision of Sigmoid Colon, Via Natural or Artificial Opening Endoscopic

0DBNFZZ Excision of Sigmoid Colon, Via Natural or Artificial Opening With Percutaneous Endoscopic Assistance

0DBP0ZX Excision of Rectum, Open Approach, Diagnostic

0DBP0ZZ Excision of Rectum, Open Approach
AHA CC: 1Q, 2019, 27

0DBP3ZX Excision of Rectum, Percutaneous Approach, Diagnostic

0DBP3ZZ Excision of Rectum, Percutaneous Approach	**0DBQ7ZZ** Excision of Anus, Via Natural or Artificial Opening	**0DBU3ZZ** Excision of Omentum, Percutaneous Approach
0DBP4ZX Excision of Rectum, Percutaneous Endoscopic Approach, Diagnostic	**0DBQ8ZX** Excision of Anus, Via Natural or Artificial Opening Endoscopic, Diagnostic	**0DBU4ZX** Excision of Omentum, Percutaneous Endoscopic Approach, Diagnostic
0DBP4ZZ Excision of Rectum, Percutaneous Endoscopic Approach	**0DBQ8ZZ** Excision of Anus, Via Natural or Artificial Opening Endoscopic	**0DBU4ZZ** Excision of Omentum, Percutaneous Endoscopic Approach
0DBP7ZX Excision of Rectum, Via Natural or Artificial Opening, Diagnostic	**0DBQXZX** Excision of Anus, External Approach, Diagnostic	**0DBV0ZX** Excision of Mesentery, Open Approach, Diagnostic
0DBP7ZZ Excision of Rectum, Via Natural or Artificial Opening	**0DBQXZZ** Excision of Anus, External Approach	**0DBV0ZZ** Excision of Mesentery, Open Approach
AHA CC: 1Q, 2016, 22	**0DBR0ZX** Excision of Anal Sphincter, Open Approach, Diagnostic	**0DBV3ZX** Excision of Mesentery, Percutaneous Approach, Diagnostic
0DBP8ZX Excision of Rectum, Via Natural or Artificial Opening Endoscopic, Diagnostic	**0DBR0ZZ** Excision of Anal Sphincter, Open Approach	**0DBV3ZZ** Excision of Mesentery, Percutaneous Approach
0DBP8ZZ Excision of Rectum, Via Natural or Artificial Opening Endoscopic	**0DBR3ZX** Excision of Anal Sphincter, Percutaneous Approach, Diagnostic	**0DBV4ZX** Excision of Mesentery, Percutaneous Endoscopic Approach, Diagnostic
0DBQ0ZX Excision of Anus, Open Approach, Diagnostic	**0DBR3ZZ** Excision of Anal Sphincter, Percutaneous Approach	**0DBV4ZZ** Excision of Mesentery, Percutaneous Endoscopic Approach
0DBQ0ZZ Excision of Anus, Open Approach	**0DBR4ZX** Excision of Anal Sphincter, Percutaneous Endoscopic Approach, Diagnostic	**0DBW0ZX** Excision of Peritoneum, Open Approach, Diagnostic
0DBQ3ZX Excision of Anus, Percutaneous Approach, Diagnostic		**0DBW0ZZ** Excision of Peritoneum, Open Approach
0DBQ3ZZ Excision of Anus, Percutaneous Approach	**0DBR4ZZ** Excision of Anal Sphincter, Percutaneous Endoscopic Approach	**0DBW3ZX** Excision of Peritoneum, Percutaneous Approach, Diagnostic
0DBQ4ZX Excision of Anus, Percutaneous Endoscopic Approach, Diagnostic	**0DBU0ZX** Excision of Omentum, Open Approach, Diagnostic	**0DBW3ZZ** Excision of Peritoneum, Percutaneous Approach
0DBQ4ZZ Excision of Anus, Percutaneous Endoscopic Approach	**0DBU0ZZ** Excision of Omentum, Open Approach	**0DBW4ZX** Excision of Peritoneum, Percutaneous Endoscopic Approach, Diagnostic
0DBQ7ZX Excision of Anus, Via Natural or Artificial Opening, Diagnostic	**0DBU3ZX** Excision of Omentum, Percutaneous Approach, Diagnostic	**0DBW4ZZ** Excision of Peritoneum, Percutaneous Endoscopic Approach

0DC – Gastrointestinal System, Extirpation

0DC10ZZ Extirpation of Matter from Upper Esophagus, Open Approach	**0DC43ZZ** Extirpation of Matter from Esophagogastric Junction, Percutaneous Approach	**0DC77ZZ** Extirpation of Matter from Stomach, Pylorus, Via Natural or Artificial Opening
0DC13ZZ Extirpation of Matter from Upper Esophagus, Percutaneous Approach	**0DC44ZZ** Extirpation of Matter from Esophagogastric Junction, Percutaneous Endoscopic Approach	**0DC78ZZ** Extirpation of Matter from Stomach, Pylorus, Via Natural or Artificial Opening Endoscopic
0DC14ZZ Extirpation of Matter from Upper Esophagus, Percutaneous Endoscopic Approach	**0DC47ZZ** Extirpation of Matter from Esophagogastric Junction, Via Natural or Artificial Opening	**0DC80ZZ** Extirpation of Matter from Small Intestine, Open Approach
0DC17ZZ Extirpation of Matter from Upper Esophagus, Via Natural or Artificial Opening	**0DC48ZZ** Extirpation of Matter from Esophagogastric Junction, Via Natural or Artificial Opening Endoscopic	**0DC83ZZ** Extirpation of Matter from Small Intestine, Percutaneous Approach
0DC18ZZ Extirpation of Matter from Upper Esophagus, Via Natural or Artificial Opening Endoscopic	**0DC50ZZ** Extirpation of Matter from Esophagus, Open Approach	**0DC84ZZ** Extirpation of Matter from Small Intestine, Percutaneous Endoscopic Approach
0DC20ZZ Extirpation of Matter from Middle Esophagus, Open Approach	**0DC53ZZ** Extirpation of Matter from Esophagus, Percutaneous Approach	**0DC87ZZ** Extirpation of Matter from Small Intestine, Via Natural or Artificial Opening
0DC23ZZ Extirpation of Matter from Middle Esophagus, Percutaneous Approach	**0DC54ZZ** Extirpation of Matter from Esophagus, Percutaneous Endoscopic Approach	**0DC88ZZ** Extirpation of Matter from Small Intestine, Via Natural or Artificial Opening Endoscopic
0DC24ZZ Extirpation of Matter from Middle Esophagus, Percutaneous Endoscopic Approach	**0DC57ZZ** Extirpation of Matter from Esophagus, Via Natural or Artificial Opening	**0DC90ZZ** Extirpation of Matter from Duodenum, Open Approach
0DC27ZZ Extirpation of Matter from Middle Esophagus, Via Natural or Artificial Opening	**0DC58ZZ** Extirpation of Matter from Esophagus, Via Natural or Artificial Opening Endoscopic	**0DC93ZZ** Extirpation of Matter from Duodenum, Percutaneous Approach
0DC28ZZ Extirpation of Matter from Middle Esophagus, Via Natural or Artificial Opening Endoscopic	**0DC60ZZ** Extirpation of Matter from Stomach, Open Approach	**0DC94ZZ** Extirpation of Matter from Duodenum, Percutaneous Endoscopic Approach
0DC30ZZ Extirpation of Matter from Lower Esophagus, Open Approach	**0DC63ZZ** Extirpation of Matter from Stomach, Percutaneous Approach	**0DC97ZZ** Extirpation of Matter from Duodenum, Via Natural or Artificial Opening
0DC33ZZ Extirpation of Matter from Lower Esophagus, Percutaneous Approach	**0DC64ZZ** Extirpation of Matter from Stomach, Percutaneous Endoscopic Approach	**0DC98ZZ** Extirpation of Matter from Duodenum, Via Natural or Artificial Opening Endoscopic
0DC34ZZ Extirpation of Matter from Lower Esophagus, Percutaneous Endoscopic Approach	**0DC67ZZ** Extirpation of Matter from Stomach, Via Natural or Artificial Opening	**0DCA0ZZ** Extirpation of Matter from Jejunum, Open Approach
0DC37ZZ Extirpation of Matter from Lower Esophagus, Via Natural or Artificial Opening	**0DC68ZZ** Extirpation of Matter from Stomach, Via Natural or Artificial Opening Endoscopic	**0DCA3ZZ** Extirpation of Matter from Jejunum, Percutaneous Approach
0DC38ZZ Extirpation of Matter from Lower Esophagus, Via Natural or Artificial Opening Endoscopic	**0DC70ZZ** Extirpation of Matter from Stomach, Pylorus, Open Approach	**0DCA4ZZ** Extirpation of Matter from Jejunum, Percutaneous Endoscopic Approach
0DC40ZZ Extirpation of Matter from Esophagogastric Junction, Open Approach	**0DC73ZZ** Extirpation of Matter from Stomach, Pylorus, Percutaneous Approach	**0DCA7ZZ** Extirpation of Matter from Jejunum, Via Natural or Artificial Opening
	0DC74ZZ Extirpation of Matter from Stomach, Pylorus, Percutaneous Endoscopic Approach	**0DCA8ZZ** Extirpation of Matter from Jejunum, Via Natural or Artificial Opening Endoscopic

♀ Female-only   ♂ Male-only   ▲ Limited Coverage   ● Non-OR   **HAC** HAC-associated procedure   ▲ Non-covered procedures   ✚ Cluster

0DCB0ZZ   Extirpation of Matter from Ileum, Open Approach

0DCB3ZZ   Extirpation of Matter from Ileum, Percutaneous Approach

0DCB4ZZ   Extirpation of Matter from Ileum, Percutaneous Endoscopic Approach

0DCB7ZZ   Extirpation of Matter from Ileum, Via Natural or Artificial Opening

0DCB8ZZ   Extirpation of Matter from Ileum, Via Natural or Artificial Opening Endoscopic

0DCC0ZZ   Extirpation of Matter from Ileocecal Valve, Open Approach

0DCC3ZZ   Extirpation of Matter from Ileocecal Valve, Percutaneous Approach

0DCC4ZZ   Extirpation of Matter from Ileocecal Valve, Percutaneous Endoscopic Approach

0DCC7ZZ   Extirpation of Matter from Ileocecal Valve, Via Natural or Artificial Opening

0DCC8ZZ   Extirpation of Matter from Ileocecal Valve, Via Natural or Artificial Opening Endoscopic

0DCE0ZZ   Extirpation of Matter from Large Intestine, Open Approach

0DCE3ZZ   Extirpation of Matter from Large Intestine, Percutaneous Approach

0DCE4ZZ   Extirpation of Matter from Large Intestine, Percutaneous Endoscopic Approach

0DCE7ZZ   Extirpation of Matter from Large Intestine, Via Natural or Artificial Opening

0DCE8ZZ   Extirpation of Matter from Large Intestine, Via Natural or Artificial Opening Endoscopic

0DCF0ZZ   Extirpation of Matter from Right Large Intestine, Open Approach

0DCF3ZZ   Extirpation of Matter from Right Large Intestine, Percutaneous Approach

0DCF4ZZ   Extirpation of Matter from Right Large Intestine, Percutaneous Endoscopic Approach

0DCF7ZZ   Extirpation of Matter from Right Large Intestine, Via Natural or Artificial Opening

0DCF8ZZ   Extirpation of Matter from Right Large Intestine, Via Natural or Artificial Opening Endoscopic

0DCG0ZZ   Extirpation of Matter from Left Large Intestine, Open Approach

0DCG3ZZ   Extirpation of Matter from Left Large Intestine, Percutaneous Approach

0DCG4ZZ   Extirpation of Matter from Left Large Intestine, Percutaneous Endoscopic Approach

0DCG7ZZ   Extirpation of Matter from Left Large Intestine, Via Natural or Artificial Opening

0DCG8ZZ   Extirpation of Matter from Left Large Intestine, Via Natural or Artificial Opening Endoscopic

0DCH0ZZ   Extirpation of Matter from Cecum, Open Approach

0DCH3ZZ   Extirpation of Matter from Cecum, Percutaneous Approach

0DCH4ZZ   Extirpation of Matter from Cecum, Percutaneous Endoscopic Approach

0DCH7ZZ   Extirpation of Matter from Cecum, Via Natural or Artificial Opening

0DCH8ZZ   Extirpation of Matter from Cecum, Via Natural or Artificial Opening Endoscopic

0DCJ0ZZ   Extirpation of Matter from Appendix, Open Approach

0DCJ3ZZ   Extirpation of Matter from Appendix, Percutaneous Approach

0DCJ4ZZ   Extirpation of Matter from Appendix, Percutaneous Endoscopic Approach

0DCJ7ZZ   Extirpation of Matter from Appendix, Via Natural or Artificial Opening

0DCJ8ZZ   Extirpation of Matter from Appendix, Via Natural or Artificial Opening Endoscopic

0DCK0ZZ   Extirpation of Matter from Ascending Colon, Open Approach

0DCK3ZZ   Extirpation of Matter from Ascending Colon, Percutaneous Approach

0DCK4ZZ   Extirpation of Matter from Ascending Colon, Percutaneous Endoscopic Approach

0DCK7ZZ   Extirpation of Matter from Ascending Colon, Via Natural or Artificial Opening

0DCK8ZZ   Extirpation of Matter from Ascending Colon, Via Natural or Artificial Opening Endoscopic

0DCL0ZZ   Extirpation of Matter from Transverse Colon, Open Approach

0DCL3ZZ   Extirpation of Matter from Transverse Colon, Percutaneous Approach

0DCL4ZZ   Extirpation of Matter from Transverse Colon, Percutaneous Endoscopic Approach

0DCL7ZZ   Extirpation of Matter from Transverse Colon, Via Natural or Artificial Opening

0DCL8ZZ   Extirpation of Matter from Transverse Colon, Via Natural or Artificial Opening Endoscopic

0DCM0ZZ   Extirpation of Matter from Descending Colon, Open Approach

0DCM3ZZ   Extirpation of Matter from Descending Colon, Percutaneous Approach

0DCM4ZZ   Extirpation of Matter from Descending Colon, Percutaneous Endoscopic Approach

0DCM7ZZ   Extirpation of Matter from Descending Colon, Via Natural or Artificial Opening

0DCM8ZZ   Extirpation of Matter from Descending Colon, Via Natural or Artificial Opening Endoscopic

0DCN0ZZ   Extirpation of Matter from Sigmoid Colon, Open Approach

0DCN3ZZ   Extirpation of Matter from Sigmoid Colon, Percutaneous Approach

0DCN4ZZ   Extirpation of Matter from Sigmoid Colon, Percutaneous Endoscopic Approach

0DCN7ZZ   Extirpation of Matter from Sigmoid Colon, Via Natural or Artificial Opening

0DCN8ZZ   Extirpation of Matter from Sigmoid Colon, Via Natural or Artificial Opening Endoscopic

0DCP0ZZ   Extirpation of Matter from Rectum, Open Approach

0DCP3ZZ   Extirpation of Matter from Rectum, Percutaneous Approach

0DCP4ZZ   Extirpation of Matter from Rectum, Percutaneous Endoscopic Approach

0DCP7ZZ   Extirpation of Matter from Rectum, Via Natural or Artificial Opening

0DCP8ZZ   Extirpation of Matter from Rectum, Via Natural or Artificial Opening Endoscopic

0DCQ0ZZ   Extirpation of Matter from Anus, Open Approach

0DCQ3ZZ   Extirpation of Matter from Anus, Percutaneous Approach

0DCQ4ZZ   Extirpation of Matter from Anus, Percutaneous Endoscopic Approach

0DCQ7ZZ   Extirpation of Matter from Anus, Via Natural or Artificial Opening

0DCQ8ZZ   Extirpation of Matter from Anus, Via Natural or Artificial Opening Endoscopic

0DCQXZZ   Extirpation of Matter from Anus, External Approach

0DCU0ZZ   Extirpation of Matter from Omentum, Open Approach

0DCU3ZZ   Extirpation of Matter from Omentum, Percutaneous Approach

0DCU4ZZ   Extirpation of Matter from Omentum, Percutaneous Endoscopic Approach

0DCV0ZZ   Extirpation of Matter from Mesentery, Open Approach

0DCV3ZZ   Extirpation of Matter from Mesentery, Percutaneous Approach

0DCV4ZZ   Extirpation of Matter from Mesentery, Percutaneous Endoscopic Approach

0DCW0ZZ   Extirpation of Matter from Peritoneum, Open Approach

0DCW3ZZ   Extirpation of Matter from Peritoneum, Percutaneous Approach

0DCW4ZZ   Extirpation of Matter from Peritoneum, Percutaneous Endoscopic Approach

0DD – Gastrointestinal System, Extraction

0DD13ZX   Extraction of Upper Esophagus, Percutaneous Approach, Diagnostic

0DD14ZX   Extraction of Upper Esophagus, Percutaneous Endoscopic Approach, Diagnostic

0DD18ZX   Extraction of Upper Esophagus, Via Natural or Artificial Opening Endoscopic, Diagnostic

0DD23ZX   Extraction of Middle Esophagus, Percutaneous Approach, Diagnostic

0DD24ZX   Extraction of Middle Esophagus, Percutaneous Endoscopic Approach, Diagnostic

0DD28ZX   Extraction of Middle Esophagus, Via Natural or Artificial Opening Endoscopic, Diagnostic

0DD33ZX   Extraction of Lower Esophagus, Percutaneous Approach, Diagnostic

0DD34ZX   Extraction of Lower Esophagus, Percutaneous Endoscopic Approach, Diagnostic

0DD38ZX   Extraction of Lower Esophagus, Via Natural or Artificial Opening Endoscopic, Diagnostic

0DD43ZX   Extraction of Esophagogastric Junction, Percutaneous Approach, Diagnostic

0DD44ZX   Extraction of Esophagogastric Junction, Percutaneous Endoscopic Approach, Diagnostic

0DD48ZX   Extraction of Esophagogastric Junction, Via Natural or Artificial Opening Endoscopic, Diagnostic

0DD53ZX	Extraction of Esophagus, Percutaneous Approach, Diagnostic	**0DDB8ZX**	Extraction of Ileum, Via Natural or Artificial Opening Endoscopic, Diagnostic	**0DDK3ZX**	Extraction of Ascending Colon, Percutaneous Approach, Diagnostic
0DD54ZX	Extraction of Esophagus, Percutaneous Endoscopic Approach, Diagnostic	**0DDC3ZX**	Extraction of Ileocecal Valve, Percutaneous Approach, Diagnostic	**0DDK4ZX**	Extraction of Ascending Colon, Percutaneous Endoscopic Approach, Diagnostic
0DD58ZX	Extraction of Esophagus, Via Natural or Artificial Opening Endoscopic, Diagnostic	**0DDC4ZX**	Extraction of Ileocecal Valve, Percutaneous Endoscopic Approach, Diagnostic	**0DDK8ZX**	Extraction of Ascending Colon, Via Natural or Artificial Opening Endoscopic, Diagnostic
0DD63ZX	Extraction of Stomach, Percutaneous Approach, Diagnostic	**0DDC8ZX**	Extraction of Ileocecal Valve, Via Natural or Artificial Opening Endoscopic, Diagnostic	**0DDL3ZX**	Extraction of Transverse Colon, Percutaneous Approach, Diagnostic
0DD64ZX	Extraction of Stomach, Percutaneous Endoscopic Approach, Diagnostic	**0DDE3ZX**	Extraction of Large Intestine, Percutaneous Approach, Diagnostic	**0DDL4ZX**	Extraction of Transverse Colon, Percutaneous Endoscopic Approach, Diagnostic
0DD68ZX	Extraction of Stomach, Via Natural or Artificial Opening Endoscopic, Diagnostic	**0DDE4ZX**	Extraction of Large Intestine, Percutaneous Endoscopic Approach, Diagnostic	**0DDL8ZX**	Extraction of Transverse Colon, Via Natural or Artificial Opening Endoscopic, Diagnostic
	AHA CC: 4Q, 2017, 42	**0DDE8ZX**	Extraction of Large Intestine, Via Natural or Artificial Opening Endoscopic, Diagnostic	**0DDM3ZX**	Extraction of Descending Colon, Percutaneous Approach, Diagnostic
0DD73ZX	Extraction of Stomach, Pylorus, Percutaneous Approach, Diagnostic	**0DDF3ZX**	Extraction of Right Large Intestine, Percutaneous Approach, Diagnostic	**0DDM4ZX**	Extraction of Descending Colon, Percutaneous Endoscopic Approach, Diagnostic
0DD74ZX	Extraction of Stomach, Pylorus, Percutaneous Endoscopic Approach, Diagnostic	**0DDF4ZX**	Extraction of Right Large Intestine, Percutaneous Endoscopic Approach, Diagnostic	**0DDM8ZX**	Extraction of Descending Colon, Via Natural or Artificial Opening Endoscopic, Diagnostic
0DD78ZX	Extraction of Stomach, Pylorus, Via Natural or Artificial Opening Endoscopic, Diagnostic	**0DDF8ZX**	Extraction of Right Large Intestine, Via Natural or Artificial Opening Endoscopic, Diagnostic	**0DDN3ZX**	Extraction of Sigmoid Colon, Percutaneous Approach, Diagnostic
0DD83ZX	Extraction of Small Intestine, Percutaneous Approach, Diagnostic	**0DDG3ZX**	Extraction of Left Large Intestine, Percutaneous Approach, Diagnostic	**0DDN4ZX**	Extraction of Sigmoid Colon, Percutaneous Endoscopic Approach, Diagnostic
0DD84ZX	Extraction of Small Intestine, Percutaneous Endoscopic Approach, Diagnostic	**0DDG4ZX**	Extraction of Left Large Intestine, Percutaneous Endoscopic Approach, Diagnostic	**0DDN8ZX**	Extraction of Sigmoid Colon, Via Natural or Artificial Opening Endoscopic, Diagnostic
0DD88ZX	Extraction of Small Intestine, Via Natural or Artificial Opening Endoscopic, Diagnostic	**0DDG8ZX**	Extraction of Left Large Intestine, Via Natural or Artificial Opening Endoscopic, Diagnostic	**0DDP3ZX**	Extraction of Rectum, Percutaneous Approach, Diagnostic
0DD93ZX	Extraction of Duodenum, Percutaneous Approach, Diagnostic	**0DDH3ZX**	Extraction of Cecum, Percutaneous Approach, Diagnostic	**0DDP4ZX**	Extraction of Rectum, Percutaneous Endoscopic Approach, Diagnostic
0DD94ZX	Extraction of Duodenum, Percutaneous Endoscopic Approach, Diagnostic	**0DDH4ZX**	Extraction of Cecum, Percutaneous Endoscopic Approach, Diagnostic	**0DDP8ZX**	Extraction of Rectum, Via Natural or Artificial Opening Endoscopic, Diagnostic
0DD98ZX	Extraction of Duodenum, Via Natural or Artificial Opening Endoscopic, Diagnostic	**0DDH8ZX**	Extraction of Cecum, Via Natural or Artificial Opening Endoscopic, Diagnostic		*AHA CC: 1Q, 2021, 20-21*
0DDA3ZX	Extraction of Jejunum, Percutaneous Approach, Diagnostic	**0DDJ3ZX**	Extraction of Appendix, Percutaneous Approach, Diagnostic	**0DDQ3ZX**	Extraction of Anus, Percutaneous Approach, Diagnostic
0DDA4ZX	Extraction of Jejunum, Percutaneous Endoscopic Approach, Diagnostic	**0DDJ4ZX**	Extraction of Appendix, Percutaneous Endoscopic Approach, Diagnostic	**0DDQ4ZX**	Extraction of Anus, Percutaneous Endoscopic Approach, Diagnostic
0DDA8ZX	Extraction of Jejunum, Via Natural or Artificial Opening Endoscopic, Diagnostic	**0DDJ8ZX**	Extraction of Appendix, Via Natural or Artificial Opening Endoscopic, Diagnostic	**0DDQ8ZX**	Extraction of Anus, Via Natural or Artificial Opening Endoscopic, Diagnostic
0DDB3ZX	Extraction of Ileum, Percutaneous Approach, Diagnostic			**0DDQXZX**	Extraction of Anus, External Approach, Diagnostic
0DDB4ZX	Extraction of Ileum, Percutaneous Endoscopic Approach, Diagnostic				

0DF – Gastrointestinal System, Fragmentation

0DF50ZZ	Fragmentation in Esophagus, Open Approach	**0DF68ZZ**	Fragmentation in Stomach, Via Natural or Artificial Opening Endoscopic	**0DF94ZZ**	Fragmentation in Duodenum, Percutaneous Endoscopic Approach
0DF53ZZ	Fragmentation in Esophagus, Percutaneous Approach	▲ **0DF6XZZ**	Fragmentation in Stomach, External Approach	**0DF97ZZ**	Fragmentation in Duodenum, Via Natural or Artificial Opening
0DF54ZZ	Fragmentation in Esophagus, Percutaneous Endoscopic Approach	**0DF80ZZ**	Fragmentation in Small Intestine, Open Approach	**0DF98ZZ**	Fragmentation in Duodenum, Via Natural or Artificial Opening Endoscopic
0DF57ZZ	Fragmentation in Esophagus, Via Natural or Artificial Opening	**0DF83ZZ**	Fragmentation in Small Intestine, Percutaneous Approach	▲ **0DF9XZZ**	Fragmentation in Duodenum, External Approach
0DF58ZZ	Fragmentation in Esophagus, Via Natural or Artificial Opening Endoscopic	**0DF84ZZ**	Fragmentation in Small Intestine, Percutaneous Endoscopic Approach	**0DFA0ZZ**	Fragmentation in Jejunum, Open Approach
▲ **0DF5XZZ**	Fragmentation in Esophagus, External Approach	**0DF87ZZ**	Fragmentation in Small Intestine, Via Natural or Artificial Opening	**0DFA3ZZ**	Fragmentation in Jejunum, Percutaneous Approach
0DF60ZZ	Fragmentation in Stomach, Open Approach	**0DF88ZZ**	Fragmentation in Small Intestine, Via Natural or Artificial Opening Endoscopic	**0DFA4ZZ**	Fragmentation in Jejunum, Percutaneous Endoscopic Approach
0DF63ZZ	Fragmentation in Stomach, Percutaneous Approach	▲ **0DF8XZZ**	Fragmentation in Small Intestine, External Approach	**0DFA7ZZ**	Fragmentation in Jejunum, Via Natural or Artificial Opening
0DF64ZZ	Fragmentation in Stomach, Percutaneous Endoscopic Approach	**0DF90ZZ**	Fragmentation in Duodenum, Open Approach	**0DFA8ZZ**	Fragmentation in Jejunum, Via Natural or Artificial Opening Endoscopic
0DF67ZZ	Fragmentation in Stomach, Via Natural or Artificial Opening	**0DF93ZZ**	Fragmentation in Duodenum, Percutaneous Approach	▲ **0DFAXZZ**	Fragmentation in Jejunum, External Approach

♀ Female-only   ♂ Male-only   ▲ Limited Coverage   ● Non-OR   ▨ HAC-associated procedure   ▲ Non-covered procedures   ✚ Cluster

0DFB0ZZ Fragmentation in Ileum, Open Approach

0DFB3ZZ Fragmentation in Ileum, Percutaneous Approach

0DFB4ZZ Fragmentation in Ileum, Percutaneous Endoscopic Approach

0DFB7ZZ Fragmentation in Ileum, Via Natural or Artificial Opening

0DFB8ZZ Fragmentation in Ileum, Via Natural or Artificial Opening Endoscopic

0DFBXZZ Fragmentation in Ileum, External Approach

0DFE0ZZ Fragmentation in Large Intestine, Open Approach

0DFE3ZZ Fragmentation in Large Intestine, Percutaneous Approach

0DFE4ZZ Fragmentation in Large Intestine, Percutaneous Endoscopic Approach

0DFE7ZZ Fragmentation in Large Intestine, Via Natural or Artificial Opening

0DFE8ZZ Fragmentation in Large Intestine, Via Natural or Artificial Opening Endoscopic

0DFEXZZ Fragmentation in Large Intestine, External Approach

0DFF0ZZ Fragmentation in Right Large Intestine, Open Approach

0DFF3ZZ Fragmentation in Right Large Intestine, Percutaneous Approach

0DFF4ZZ Fragmentation in Right Large Intestine, Percutaneous Endoscopic Approach

0DFF7ZZ Fragmentation in Right Large Intestine, Via Natural or Artificial Opening

0DFF8ZZ Fragmentation in Right Large Intestine, Via Natural or Artificial Opening Endoscopic

0DFFXZZ Fragmentation in Right Large Intestine, External Approach

0DFG0ZZ Fragmentation in Left Large Intestine, Open Approach

0DFG3ZZ Fragmentation in Left Large Intestine, Percutaneous Approach

0DFG4ZZ Fragmentation in Left Large Intestine, Percutaneous Endoscopic Approach

0DFG7ZZ Fragmentation in Left Large Intestine, Via Natural or Artificial Opening

0DFG8ZZ Fragmentation in Left Large Intestine, Via Natural or Artificial Opening Endoscopic

▲ 0DFGXZZ Fragmentation in Left Large Intestine, External Approach

0DFH0ZZ Fragmentation in Cecum, Open Approach

0DFH3ZZ Fragmentation in Cecum, Percutaneous Approach

0DFH4ZZ Fragmentation in Cecum, Percutaneous Endoscopic Approach

0DFH7ZZ Fragmentation in Cecum, Via Natural or Artificial Opening

0DFH8ZZ Fragmentation in Cecum, Via Natural or Artificial Opening Endoscopic

▲ 0DFHXZZ Fragmentation in Cecum, External Approach

0DFJ0ZZ Fragmentation in Appendix, Open Approach

0DFJ3ZZ Fragmentation in Appendix, Percutaneous Approach

0DFJ4ZZ Fragmentation in Appendix, Percutaneous Endoscopic Approach

0DFJ7ZZ Fragmentation in Appendix, Via Natural or Artificial Opening

0DFJ8ZZ Fragmentation in Appendix, Via Natural or Artificial Opening Endoscopic

▲ 0DFJXZZ Fragmentation in Appendix, External Approach

0DFK0ZZ Fragmentation in Ascending Colon, Open Approach

0DFK3ZZ Fragmentation in Ascending Colon, Percutaneous Approach

0DFK4ZZ Fragmentation in Ascending Colon, Percutaneous Endoscopic Approach

0DFK7ZZ Fragmentation in Ascending Colon, Via Natural or Artificial Opening

0DFK8ZZ Fragmentation in Ascending Colon, Via Natural or Artificial Opening Endoscopic

▲ 0DFKXZZ Fragmentation in Ascending Colon, External Approach

0DFL0ZZ Fragmentation in Transverse Colon, Open Approach

0DFL3ZZ Fragmentation in Transverse Colon, Percutaneous Approach

0DFL4ZZ Fragmentation in Transverse Colon, Percutaneous Endoscopic Approach

0DFL7ZZ Fragmentation in Transverse Colon, Via Natural or Artificial Opening

0DFL8ZZ Fragmentation in Transverse Colon, Via Natural or Artificial Opening Endoscopic

▲ 0DFLXZZ Fragmentation in Transverse Colon, External Approach

0DFM0ZZ Fragmentation in Descending Colon, Open Approach

0DFM3ZZ Fragmentation in Descending Colon, Percutaneous Approach

0DFM4ZZ Fragmentation in Descending Colon, Percutaneous Endoscopic Approach

0DFM7ZZ Fragmentation in Descending Colon, Via Natural or Artificial Opening

0DFM8ZZ Fragmentation in Descending Colon, Via Natural or Artificial Opening Endoscopic

▲ 0DFMXZZ Fragmentation in Descending Colon, External Approach

0DFN0ZZ Fragmentation in Sigmoid Colon, Open Approach

0DFN3ZZ Fragmentation in Sigmoid Colon, Percutaneous Approach

0DFN4ZZ Fragmentation in Sigmoid Colon, Percutaneous Endoscopic Approach

0DFN7ZZ Fragmentation in Sigmoid Colon, Via Natural or Artificial Opening

0DFN8ZZ Fragmentation in Sigmoid Colon, Via Natural or Artificial Opening Endoscopic

▲ 0DFNXZZ Fragmentation in Sigmoid Colon, External Approach

0DFP0ZZ Fragmentation in Rectum, Open Approach

0DFP3ZZ Fragmentation in Rectum, Percutaneous Approach

0DFP4ZZ Fragmentation in Rectum, Percutaneous Endoscopic Approach

0DFP7ZZ Fragmentation in Rectum, Via Natural or Artificial Opening

0DFP8ZZ Fragmentation in Rectum, Via Natural or Artificial Opening Endoscopic

▲ 0DFPXZZ Fragmentation in Rectum, External Approach

0DFQ0ZZ Fragmentation in Anus, Open Approach

0DFQ3ZZ Fragmentation in Anus, Percutaneous Approach

0DFQ4ZZ Fragmentation in Anus, Percutaneous Endoscopic Approach

0DFQ7ZZ Fragmentation in Anus, Via Natural or Artificial Opening

0DFQ8ZZ Fragmentation in Anus, Via Natural or Artificial Opening Endoscopic

▲ 0DFQXZZ Fragmentation in Anus, External Approach

0DH – Gastrointestinal System, Insertion

0DH00YZ Insertion of Other Device into Upper Intestinal Tract, Open Approach

0DH03YZ Insertion of Other Device into Upper Intestinal Tract, Percutaneous Approach

0DH04YZ Insertion of Other Device into Upper Intestinal Tract, Percutaneous Endoscopic Approach

0DH07YZ Insertion of Other Device into Upper Intestinal Tract, Via Natural or Artificial Opening

0DH08YZ Insertion of Other Device into Upper Intestinal Tract, Via Natural or Artificial Opening Endoscopic

0DH501Z Insertion of Radioactive Element into Esophagus, Open Approach

0DH502Z Insertion of Monitoring Device into Esophagus, Open Approach

0DH503Z Insertion of Infusion Device into Esophagus, Open Approach

0DH50DZ Insertion of Intraluminal Device into Esophagus, Open Approach

0DH50UZ Insertion of Feeding Device into Esophagus, Open Approach

0DH50YZ Insertion of Other Device into Esophagus, Open Approach

0DH531Z Insertion of Radioactive Element into Esophagus, Percutaneous Approach

0DH532Z Insertion of Monitoring Device into Esophagus, Percutaneous Approach

0DH533Z Insertion of Infusion Device into Esophagus, Percutaneous Approach

0DH53DZ Insertion of Intraluminal Device into Esophagus, Percutaneous Approach

0DH53UZ Insertion of Feeding Device into Esophagus, Percutaneous Approach

0DH53YZ Insertion of Other Device into Esophagus, Percutaneous Approach

0DH541Z Insertion of Radioactive Element into Esophagus, Percutaneous Endoscopic Approach

0DH542Z Insertion of Monitoring Device into Esophagus, Percutaneous Endoscopic Approach

0DH543Z Insertion of Infusion Device into Esophagus, Percutaneous Endoscopic Approach

0DH54DZ Insertion of Intraluminal Device into Esophagus, Percutaneous Endoscopic Approach

0DH54UZ Insertion of Feeding Device into Esophagus, Percutaneous Endoscopic Approach

0DH54YZ Insertion of Other Device into Esophagus, Percutaneous Endoscopic Approach

0DH571Z Insertion of Radioactive Element into Esophagus, Via Natural or Artificial Opening

0DH572Z Insertion of Monitoring Device into Esophagus, Via Natural or Artificial Opening

0DH573Z Insertion of Infusion Device into Esophagus, Via Natural or Artificial Opening

0DH57BZ Insertion of Airway into Esophagus, Via Natural or Artificial Opening

0DH57DZ Insertion of Intraluminal Device into Esophagus, Via Natural or Artificial Opening

0DH57UZ Insertion of Feeding Device into Esophagus, Via Natural or Artificial Opening

0DH57YZ Insertion of Other Device into Esophagus, Via Natural or Artificial Opening

0DH581Z Insertion of Radioactive Element into Esophagus, Via Natural or Artificial Opening Endoscopic

0DH582Z Insertion of Monitoring Device into Esophagus, Via Natural or Artificial Opening Endoscopic

0DH583Z Insertion of Infusion Device into Esophagus, Via Natural or Artificial Opening Endoscopic

0DH58BZ Insertion of Airway into Esophagus, Via Natural or Artificial Opening Endoscopic

0DH58DZ Insertion of Intraluminal Device into Esophagus, Via Natural or Artificial Opening Endoscopic

0DH58UZ Insertion of Feeding Device into Esophagus, Via Natural or Artificial Opening Endoscopic

0DH58YZ Insertion of Other Device into Esophagus, Via Natural or Artificial Opening Endoscopic

0DH601Z Insertion of Radioactive Element into Stomach, Open Approach

0DH602Z Insertion of Monitoring Device into Stomach, Open Approach

0DH603Z Insertion of Infusion Device into Stomach, Open Approach

0DH60DZ Insertion of Intraluminal Device into Stomach, Open Approach

0DH60MZ Insertion of Stimulator Lead into Stomach, Open Approach

0DH60UZ Insertion of Feeding Device into Stomach, Open Approach

0DH60YZ Insertion of Other Device into Stomach, Open Approach

0DH631Z Insertion of Radioactive Element into Stomach, Percutaneous Approach

0DH632Z Insertion of Monitoring Device into Stomach, Percutaneous Approach

0DH633Z Insertion of Infusion Device into Stomach, Percutaneous Approach

0DH63DZ Insertion of Intraluminal Device into Stomach, Percutaneous Approach

0DH63MZ Insertion of Stimulator Lead into Stomach, Percutaneous Approach

0DH63UZ Insertion of Feeding Device into Stomach, Percutaneous Approach
AHA CC: 4Q, 2013, 117

0DH63YZ Insertion of Other Device into Stomach, Percutaneous Approach

0DH641Z Insertion of Radioactive Element into Stomach, Percutaneous Endoscopic Approach

0DH642Z Insertion of Monitoring Device into Stomach, Percutaneous Endoscopic Approach

0DH643Z Insertion of Infusion Device into Stomach, Percutaneous Endoscopic Approach

0DH64DZ Insertion of Intraluminal Device into Stomach, Percutaneous Endoscopic Approach

0DH64MZ Insertion of Stimulator Lead into Stomach, Percutaneous Endoscopic Approach

0DH64UZ Insertion of Feeding Device into Stomach, Percutaneous Endoscopic Approach

0DH64YZ Insertion of Other Device into Stomach, Percutaneous Endoscopic Approach

0DH671Z Insertion of Radioactive Element into Stomach, Via Natural or Artificial Opening

0DH672Z Insertion of Monitoring Device into Stomach, Via Natural or Artificial Opening

0DH673Z Insertion of Infusion Device into Stomach, Via Natural or Artificial Opening

0DH67DZ Insertion of Intraluminal Device into Stomach, Via Natural or Artificial Opening

0DH67UZ Insertion of Feeding Device into Stomach, Via Natural or Artificial Opening
AHA CC: 3Q, 2016, 26-27

0DH67YZ Insertion of Other Device into Stomach, Via Natural or Artificial Opening

0DH681Z Insertion of Radioactive Element into Stomach, Via Natural or Artificial Opening Endoscopic

0DH682Z Insertion of Monitoring Device into Stomach, Via Natural or Artificial Opening Endoscopic

0DH683Z Insertion of Infusion Device into Stomach, Via Natural or Artificial Opening Endoscopic

0DH68DZ Insertion of Intraluminal Device into Stomach, Via Natural or Artificial Opening Endoscopic

0DH68UZ Insertion of Feeding Device into Stomach, Via Natural or Artificial Opening Endoscopic

0DH68YZ Insertion of Other Device into Stomach, Via Natural or Artificial Opening Endoscopic
AHA CC: 2Q, 2019, 18

0DH801Z Insertion of Radioactive Element into Small Intestine, Open Approach

0DH802Z Insertion of Monitoring Device into Small Intestine, Open Approach

0DH803Z Insertion of Infusion Device into Small Intestine, Open Approach

0DH80DZ Insertion of Intraluminal Device into Small Intestine, Open Approach

0DH80UZ Insertion of Feeding Device into Small Intestine, Open Approach

0DH831Z Insertion of Radioactive Element into Small Intestine, Percutaneous Approach

0DH832Z Insertion of Monitoring Device into Small Intestine, Percutaneous Approach

0DH833Z Insertion of Infusion Device into Small Intestine, Percutaneous Approach

0DH83DZ Insertion of Intraluminal Device into Small Intestine, Percutaneous Approach

0DH83UZ Insertion of Feeding Device into Small Intestine, Percutaneous Approach

0DH841Z Insertion of Radioactive Element into Small Intestine, Percutaneous Endoscopic Approach

0DH842Z Insertion of Monitoring Device into Small Intestine, Percutaneous Endoscopic Approach

0DH843Z Insertion of Infusion Device into Small Intestine, Percutaneous Endoscopic Approach

0DH84DZ Insertion of Intraluminal Device into Small Intestine, Percutaneous Endoscopic Approach

0DH84UZ Insertion of Feeding Device into Small Intestine, Percutaneous Endoscopic Approach

0DH871Z Insertion of Radioactive Element into Small Intestine, Via Natural or Artificial Opening

0DH872Z Insertion of Monitoring Device into Small Intestine, Via Natural or Artificial Opening

0DH873Z Insertion of Infusion Device into Small Intestine, Via Natural or Artificial Opening

0DH87DZ Insertion of Intraluminal Device into Small Intestine, Via Natural or Artificial Opening

0DH87UZ Insertion of Feeding Device into Small Intestine, Via Natural or Artificial Opening

0DH881Z Insertion of Radioactive Element into Small Intestine, Via Natural or Artificial Opening Endoscopic

0DH882Z Insertion of Monitoring Device into Small Intestine, Via Natural or Artificial Opening Endoscopic

0DH883Z Insertion of Infusion Device into Small Intestine, Via Natural or Artificial Opening Endoscopic

0DH88DZ Insertion of Intraluminal Device into Small Intestine, Via Natural or Artificial Opening Endoscopic

0DH88UZ Insertion of Feeding Device into Small Intestine, Via Natural or Artificial Opening Endoscopic

0DH901Z Insertion of Radioactive Element into Duodenum, Open Approach

0DH902Z Insertion of Monitoring Device into Duodenum, Open Approach

0DH903Z Insertion of Infusion Device into Duodenum, Open Approach

0DH90DZ Insertion of Intraluminal Device into Duodenum, Open Approach

0DH90UZ Insertion of Feeding Device into Duodenum, Open Approach

0DH931Z Insertion of Radioactive Element into Duodenum, Percutaneous Approach

0DH932Z Insertion of Monitoring Device into Duodenum, Percutaneous Approach

0DH933Z Insertion of Infusion Device into Duodenum, Percutaneous Approach

0DH93DZ Insertion of Intraluminal Device into Duodenum, Percutaneous Approach

0DH93UZ Insertion of Feeding Device into Duodenum, Percutaneous Approach

0DH941Z Insertion of Radioactive Element into Duodenum, Percutaneous Endoscopic Approach

0DH942Z Insertion of Monitoring Device into Duodenum, Percutaneous Endoscopic Approach

0DH943Z Insertion of Infusion Device into Duodenum, Percutaneous Endoscopic Approach

♀ Female-only   ♂ Male-only   ▲ Limited Coverage   ● Non-OR   🄷🄰🄲 HAC-associated procedure   ▲ Non-covered procedures   ✚ Cluster

0DH94DZ	Insertion of Intraluminal Device into Duodenum, Percutaneous Endoscopic Approach
0DH94UZ	Insertion of Feeding Device into Duodenum, Percutaneous Endoscopic Approach
0DH971Z	Insertion of Radioactive Element into Duodenum, Via Natural or Artificial Opening
0DH972Z	Insertion of Monitoring Device into Duodenum, Via Natural or Artificial Opening
0DH973Z	Insertion of Infusion Device into Duodenum, Via Natural or Artificial Opening
0DH97DZ	Insertion of Intraluminal Device into Duodenum, Via Natural or Artificial Opening
0DH97UZ	Insertion of Feeding Device into Duodenum, Via Natural or Artificial Opening
0DH981Z	Insertion of Radioactive Element into Duodenum, Via Natural or Artificial Opening Endoscopic
0DH982Z	Insertion of Monitoring Device into Duodenum, Via Natural or Artificial Opening Endoscopic
0DH983Z	Insertion of Infusion Device into Duodenum, Via Natural or Artificial Opening Endoscopic
0DH98DZ	Insertion of Intraluminal Device into Duodenum, Via Natural or Artificial Opening Endoscopic
0DH98UZ	Insertion of Feeding Device into Duodenum, Via Natural or Artificial Opening Endoscopic
0DHA01Z	Insertion of Radioactive Element into Jejunum, Open Approach
0DHA02Z	Insertion of Monitoring Device into Jejunum, Open Approach
0DHA03Z	Insertion of Infusion Device into Jejunum, Open Approach
0DHA0DZ	Insertion of Intraluminal Device into Jejunum, Open Approach
0DHA0UZ	Insertion of Feeding Device into Jejunum, Open Approach
0DHA31Z	Insertion of Radioactive Element into Jejunum, Percutaneous Approach
0DHA32Z	Insertion of Monitoring Device into Jejunum, Percutaneous Approach
0DHA33Z	Insertion of Infusion Device into Jejunum, Percutaneous Approach
0DHA3DZ	Insertion of Intraluminal Device into Jejunum, Percutaneous Approach
0DHA3UZ	Insertion of Feeding Device into Jejunum, Percutaneous Approach *AHA CC: 3Q, 2020, 43*
0DHA41Z	Insertion of Radioactive Element into Jejunum, Percutaneous Endoscopic Approach
0DHA42Z	Insertion of Monitoring Device into Jejunum, Percutaneous Endoscopic Approach
0DHA43Z	Insertion of Infusion Device into Jejunum, Percutaneous Endoscopic Approach
0DHA4DZ	Insertion of Intraluminal Device into Jejunum, Percutaneous Endoscopic Approach
0DHA4UZ	Insertion of Feeding Device into Jejunum, Percutaneous Endoscopic Approach
0DHA71Z	Insertion of Radioactive Element into Jejunum, Via Natural or Artificial Opening
0DHA72Z	Insertion of Monitoring Device into Jejunum, Via Natural or Artificial Opening
0DHA73Z	Insertion of Infusion Device into Jejunum, Via Natural or Artificial Opening
0DHA7DZ	Insertion of Intraluminal Device into Jejunum, Via Natural or Artificial Opening
0DHA7UZ	Insertion of Feeding Device into Jejunum, Via Natural or Artificial Opening
0DHA81Z	Insertion of Radioactive Element into Jejunum, Via Natural or Artificial Opening Endoscopic
0DHA82Z	Insertion of Monitoring Device into Jejunum, Via Natural or Artificial Opening Endoscopic
0DHA83Z	Insertion of Infusion Device into Jejunum, Via Natural or Artificial Opening Endoscopic
0DHA8DZ	Insertion of Intraluminal Device into Jejunum, Via Natural or Artificial Opening Endoscopic
0DHA8UZ	Insertion of Feeding Device into Jejunum, Via Natural or Artificial Opening Endoscopic
0DHB01Z	Insertion of Radioactive Element into Ileum, Open Approach
0DHB02Z	Insertion of Monitoring Device into Ileum, Open Approach
0DHB03Z	Insertion of Infusion Device into Ileum, Open Approach
0DHB0DZ	Insertion of Intraluminal Device into Ileum, Open Approach
0DHB0UZ	Insertion of Feeding Device into Ileum, Open Approach
0DHB31Z	Insertion of Radioactive Element into Ileum, Percutaneous Approach
0DHB32Z	Insertion of Monitoring Device into Ileum, Percutaneous Approach
0DHB33Z	Insertion of Infusion Device into Ileum, Percutaneous Approach
0DHB3DZ	Insertion of Intraluminal Device into Ileum, Percutaneous Approach
0DHB3UZ	Insertion of Feeding Device into Ileum, Percutaneous Approach
0DHB41Z	Insertion of Radioactive Element into Ileum, Percutaneous Endoscopic Approach
0DHB42Z	Insertion of Monitoring Device into Ileum, Percutaneous Endoscopic Approach
0DHB43Z	Insertion of Infusion Device into Ileum, Percutaneous Endoscopic Approach
0DHB4DZ	Insertion of Intraluminal Device into Ileum, Percutaneous Endoscopic Approach
0DHB4UZ	Insertion of Feeding Device into Ileum, Percutaneous Endoscopic Approach
0DHB71Z	Insertion of Radioactive Element into Ileum, Via Natural or Artificial Opening
0DHB72Z	Insertion of Monitoring Device into Ileum, Via Natural or Artificial Opening
0DHB73Z	Insertion of Infusion Device into Ileum, Via Natural or Artificial Opening
0DHB7DZ	Insertion of Intraluminal Device into Ileum, Via Natural or Artificial Opening
0DHB7UZ	Insertion of Feeding Device into Ileum, Via Natural or Artificial Opening
0DHB81Z	Insertion of Radioactive Element into Ileum, Via Natural or Artificial Opening Endoscopic
0DHB82Z	Insertion of Monitoring Device into Ileum, Via Natural or Artificial Opening Endoscopic
0DHB83Z	Insertion of Infusion Device into Ileum, Via Natural or Artificial Opening Endoscopic
0DHB8DZ	Insertion of Intraluminal Device into Ileum, Via Natural or Artificial Opening Endoscopic
0DHB8UZ	Insertion of Feeding Device into Ileum, Via Natural or Artificial Opening Endoscopic
0DHD0YZ	Insertion of Other Device into Lower Intestinal Tract, Open Approach
0DHD3YZ	Insertion of Other Device into Lower Intestinal Tract, Percutaneous Approach
0DHD4YZ	Insertion of Other Device into Lower Intestinal Tract, Percutaneous Endoscopic Approach
0DHD7YZ	Insertion of Other Device into Lower Intestinal Tract, Via Natural or Artificial Opening
0DHD8YZ	Insertion of Other Device into Lower Intestinal Tract, Via Natural or Artificial Opening Endoscopic
0DHE01Z	Insertion of Radioactive Element into Large Intestine, Open Approach
0DHE0DZ	Insertion of Intraluminal Device into Large Intestine, Open Approach
0DHE31Z	Insertion of Radioactive Element into Large Intestine, Percutaneous Approach
0DHE3DZ	Insertion of Intraluminal Device into Large Intestine, Percutaneous Approach
0DHE41Z	Insertion of Radioactive Element into Large Intestine, Percutaneous Endoscopic Approach
0DHE4DZ	Insertion of Intraluminal Device into Large Intestine, Percutaneous Endoscopic Approach
0DHE71Z	Insertion of Radioactive Element into Large Intestine, Via Natural or Artificial Opening
0DHE7DZ	Insertion of Intraluminal Device into Large Intestine, Via Natural or Artificial Opening
0DHE81Z	Insertion of Radioactive Element into Large Intestine, Via Natural or Artificial Opening Endoscopic
0DHE8DZ	Insertion of Intraluminal Device into Large Intestine, Via Natural or Artificial Opening Endoscopic
0DHP01Z	Insertion of Radioactive Element into Rectum, Open Approach
0DHP0DZ	Insertion of Intraluminal Device into Rectum, Open Approach
0DHP31Z	Insertion of Radioactive Element into Rectum, Percutaneous Approach
0DHP3DZ	Insertion of Intraluminal Device into Rectum, Percutaneous Approach
0DHP41Z	Insertion of Radioactive Element into Rectum, Percutaneous Endoscopic Approach
0DHP4DZ	Insertion of Intraluminal Device into Rectum, Percutaneous Endoscopic Approach
0DHP71Z	Insertion of Radioactive Element into Rectum, Via Natural or Artificial Opening
0DHP7DZ	Insertion of Intraluminal Device into Rectum, Via Natural or Artificial Opening

0DHP81Z Insertion of Radioactive Element into Rectum, Via Natural or Artificial Opening Endoscopic

0DHP8DZ Insertion of Intraluminal Device into Rectum, Via Natural or Artificial Opening Endoscopic

0DHQ0DZ Insertion of Intraluminal Device into Anus, Open Approach

0DHQ0LZ Insertion of Artificial Sphincter into Anus, Open Approach

0DHQ3DZ Insertion of Intraluminal Device into Anus, Percutaneous Approach

0DHQ3LZ Insertion of Artificial Sphincter into Anus, Percutaneous Approach

0DHQ4DZ Insertion of Intraluminal Device into Anus, Percutaneous Endoscopic Approach

0DHQ4LZ Insertion of Artificial Sphincter into Anus, Percutaneous Endoscopic Approach

0DHQ7DZ Insertion of Intraluminal Device into Anus, Via Natural or Artificial Opening

0DHQ8DZ Insertion of Intraluminal Device into Anus, Via Natural or Artificial Opening Endoscopic

0DHR0MZ Insertion of Stimulator Lead into Anal Sphincter, Open Approach

0DHR3MZ Insertion of Stimulator Lead into Anal Sphincter, Percutaneous Approach

0DHR4MZ Insertion of Stimulator Lead into Anal Sphincter, Percutaneous Endoscopic Approach

0DJ – Gastrointestinal System, Inspection

Review Coding Guidelines B3.11a, B3.11b and B3.11c

0DJ00ZZ Inspection of Upper Intestinal Tract, Open Approach

0DJ03ZZ Inspection of Upper Intestinal Tract, Percutaneous Approach

0DJ04ZZ Inspection of Upper Intestinal Tract, Percutaneous Endoscopic Approach

0DJ07ZZ Inspection of Upper Intestinal Tract, Via Natural or Artificial Opening
AHA CC: 2Q, 2016, 20-21

0DJ08ZZ Inspection of Upper Intestinal Tract, Via Natural or Artificial Opening Endoscopic
AHA CC: 3Q, 2015, 24-25

0DJ0XZZ Inspection of Upper Intestinal Tract, External Approach

0DJ60ZZ Inspection of Stomach, Open Approach

0DJ63ZZ Inspection of Stomach, Percutaneous Approach

0DJ64ZZ Inspection of Stomach, Percutaneous Endoscopic Approach

0DJ67ZZ Inspection of Stomach, Via Natural or Artificial Opening

0DJ68ZZ Inspection of Stomach, Via Natural or Artificial Opening Endoscopic

0DJ6XZZ Inspection of Stomach, External Approach

0DJD0ZZ Inspection of Lower Intestinal Tract, Open Approach
AHA CC: 1Q, 2019, 25-26

0DJD3ZZ Inspection of Lower Intestinal Tract, Percutaneous Approach

0DJD4ZZ Inspection of Lower Intestinal Tract, Percutaneous Endoscopic Approach

0DJD7ZZ Inspection of Lower Intestinal Tract, Via Natural or Artificial Opening

0DJD8ZZ Inspection of Lower Intestinal Tract, Via Natural or Artificial Opening Endoscopic
AHA CC: 2Q, 2017, 15-16

0DJDXZZ Inspection of Lower Intestinal Tract, External Approach

0DJU0ZZ Inspection of Omentum, Open Approach

0DJU3ZZ Inspection of Omentum, Percutaneous Approach

0DJU4ZZ Inspection of Omentum, Percutaneous Endoscopic Approach

0DJUXZZ Inspection of Omentum, External Approach

0DJV0ZZ Inspection of Mesentery, Open Approach

0DJV3ZZ Inspection of Mesentery, Percutaneous Approach

0DJV4ZZ Inspection of Mesentery, Percutaneous Endoscopic Approach

0DJVXZZ Inspection of Mesentery, External Approach

0DJW0ZZ Inspection of Peritoneum, Open Approach

0DJW3ZZ Inspection of Peritoneum, Percutaneous Approach

0DJW4ZZ Inspection of Peritoneum, Percutaneous Endoscopic Approach

0DJWXZZ Inspection of Peritoneum, External Approach

0DL – Gastrointestinal System, Occlusion

0DL10CZ Occlusion of Upper Esophagus with Extraluminal Device, Open Approach

0DL10DZ Occlusion of Upper Esophagus with Intraluminal Device, Open Approach

0DL10ZZ Occlusion of Upper Esophagus, Open Approach

0DL13CZ Occlusion of Upper Esophagus with Extraluminal Device, Percutaneous Approach

0DL13DZ Occlusion of Upper Esophagus with Intraluminal Device, Percutaneous Approach

0DL13ZZ Occlusion of Upper Esophagus, Percutaneous Approach

0DL14CZ Occlusion of Upper Esophagus with Extraluminal Device, Percutaneous Endoscopic Approach

0DL14DZ Occlusion of Upper Esophagus with Intraluminal Device, Percutaneous Endoscopic Approach

0DL14ZZ Occlusion of Upper Esophagus, Percutaneous Endoscopic Approach

0DL17DZ Occlusion of Upper Esophagus with Intraluminal Device, Via Natural or Artificial Opening

0DL17ZZ Occlusion of Upper Esophagus, Via Natural or Artificial Opening

0DL18DZ Occlusion of Upper Esophagus with Intraluminal Device, Via Natural or Artificial Opening Endoscopic

0DL18ZZ Occlusion of Upper Esophagus, Via Natural or Artificial Opening Endoscopic

0DL20CZ Occlusion of Middle Esophagus with Extraluminal Device, Open Approach

0DL20DZ Occlusion of Middle Esophagus with Intraluminal Device, Open Approach

0DL20ZZ Occlusion of Middle Esophagus, Open Approach

0DL23CZ Occlusion of Middle Esophagus with Extraluminal Device, Percutaneous Approach

0DL23DZ Occlusion of Middle Esophagus with Intraluminal Device, Percutaneous Approach

0DL23ZZ Occlusion of Middle Esophagus, Percutaneous Approach

0DL24CZ Occlusion of Middle Esophagus with Extraluminal Device, Percutaneous Endoscopic Approach

0DL24DZ Occlusion of Middle Esophagus with Intraluminal Device, Percutaneous Endoscopic Approach

0DL24ZZ Occlusion of Middle Esophagus, Percutaneous Endoscopic Approach

0DL27DZ Occlusion of Middle Esophagus with Intraluminal Device, Via Natural or Artificial Opening

0DL27ZZ Occlusion of Middle Esophagus, Via Natural or Artificial Opening

0DL28DZ Occlusion of Middle Esophagus with Intraluminal Device, Via Natural or Artificial Opening Endoscopic

0DL28ZZ Occlusion of Middle Esophagus, Via Natural or Artificial Opening Endoscopic

0DL30CZ Occlusion of Lower Esophagus with Extraluminal Device, Open Approach

0DL30DZ Occlusion of Lower Esophagus with Intraluminal Device, Open Approach

0DL30ZZ Occlusion of Lower Esophagus, Open Approach

0DL33CZ Occlusion of Lower Esophagus with Extraluminal Device, Percutaneous Approach

0DL33DZ Occlusion of Lower Esophagus with Intraluminal Device, Percutaneous Approach

0DL33ZZ Occlusion of Lower Esophagus, Percutaneous Approach

0DL34CZ Occlusion of Lower Esophagus with Extraluminal Device, Percutaneous Endoscopic Approach

0DL34DZ Occlusion of Lower Esophagus with Intraluminal Device, Percutaneous Endoscopic Approach

0DL34ZZ Occlusion of Lower Esophagus, Percutaneous Endoscopic Approach

0DL37DZ Occlusion of Lower Esophagus with Intraluminal Device, Via Natural or Artificial Opening

0DL37ZZ Occlusion of Lower Esophagus, Via Natural or Artificial Opening

0DL38DZ Occlusion of Lower Esophagus with Intraluminal Device, Via Natural or Artificial Opening Endoscopic

♀ Female-only   ♂ Male-only   ▲ Limited Coverage   ● Non-OR   HAC HAC-associated procedure   ▲ Non-covered procedures   Cluster

0DL38ZZ Occlusion of Lower Esophagus, Via Natural or Artificial Opening Endoscopic

0DL40CZ Occlusion of Esophagogastric Junction with Extraluminal Device, Open Approach

0DL40DZ Occlusion of Esophagogastric Junction with Intraluminal Device, Open Approach

0DL40ZZ Occlusion of Esophagogastric Junction, Open Approach

0DL43CZ Occlusion of Esophagogastric Junction with Extraluminal Device, Percutaneous Approach

0DL43DZ Occlusion of Esophagogastric Junction with Intraluminal Device, Percutaneous Approach

0DL43ZZ Occlusion of Esophagogastric Junction, Percutaneous Approach

0DL44CZ Occlusion of Esophagogastric Junction with Extraluminal Device, Percutaneous Endoscopic Approach

0DL44DZ Occlusion of Esophagogastric Junction with Intraluminal Device, Percutaneous Endoscopic Approach

0DL44ZZ Occlusion of Esophagogastric Junction, Percutaneous Endoscopic Approach

0DL47DZ Occlusion of Esophagogastric Junction with Intraluminal Device, Via Natural or Artificial Opening

0DL47ZZ Occlusion of Esophagogastric Junction, Via Natural or Artificial Opening

0DL48DZ Occlusion of Esophagogastric Junction with Intraluminal Device, Via Natural or Artificial Opening Endoscopic

0DL48ZZ Occlusion of Esophagogastric Junction, Via Natural or Artificial Opening Endoscopic

0DL50CZ Occlusion of Esophagus with Extraluminal Device, Open Approach

0DL50DZ Occlusion of Esophagus with Intraluminal Device, Open Approach

0DL50ZZ Occlusion of Esophagus, Open Approach

0DL53CZ Occlusion of Esophagus with Extraluminal Device, Percutaneous Approach

0DL53DZ Occlusion of Esophagus with Intraluminal Device, Percutaneous Approach

0DL53ZZ Occlusion of Esophagus, Percutaneous Approach

0DL54CZ Occlusion of Esophagus with Extraluminal Device, Percutaneous Endoscopic Approach

0DL54DZ Occlusion of Esophagus with Intraluminal Device, Percutaneous Endoscopic Approach

0DL54ZZ Occlusion of Esophagus, Percutaneous Endoscopic Approach

0DL57DZ Occlusion of Esophagus with Intraluminal Device, Via Natural or Artificial Opening

0DL57ZZ Occlusion of Esophagus, Via Natural or Artificial Opening

0DL58DZ Occlusion of Esophagus with Intraluminal Device, Via Natural or Artificial Opening Endoscopic

0DL58ZZ Occlusion of Esophagus, Via Natural or Artificial Opening Endoscopic

0DL60CZ Occlusion of Stomach with Extraluminal Device, Open Approach

0DL60DZ Occlusion of Stomach with Intraluminal Device, Open Approach

0DL60ZZ Occlusion of Stomach, Open Approach

0DL63CZ Occlusion of Stomach with Extraluminal Device, Percutaneous Approach

0DL63DZ Occlusion of Stomach with Intraluminal Device, Percutaneous Approach

0DL63ZZ Occlusion of Stomach, Percutaneous Approach

0DL64CZ Occlusion of Stomach with Extraluminal Device, Percutaneous Endoscopic Approach

0DL64DZ Occlusion of Stomach with Intraluminal Device, Percutaneous Endoscopic Approach

0DL64ZZ Occlusion of Stomach, Percutaneous Endoscopic Approach

0DL67DZ Occlusion of Stomach with Intraluminal Device, Via Natural or Artificial Opening

0DL67ZZ Occlusion of Stomach, Via Natural or Artificial Opening

0DL68DZ Occlusion of Stomach with Intraluminal Device, Via Natural or Artificial Opening Endoscopic

0DL68ZZ Occlusion of Stomach, Via Natural or Artificial Opening Endoscopic

0DL70CZ Occlusion of Stomach, Pylorus with Extraluminal Device, Open Approach

0DL70DZ Occlusion of Stomach, Pylorus with Intraluminal Device, Open Approach

0DL70ZZ Occlusion of Stomach, Pylorus, Open Approach

0DL73CZ Occlusion of Stomach, Pylorus with Extraluminal Device, Percutaneous Approach

0DL73DZ Occlusion of Stomach, Pylorus with Intraluminal Device, Percutaneous Approach

0DL73ZZ Occlusion of Stomach, Pylorus, Percutaneous Approach

0DL74CZ Occlusion of Stomach, Pylorus with Extraluminal Device, Percutaneous Endoscopic Approach

0DL74DZ Occlusion of Stomach, Pylorus with Intraluminal Device, Percutaneous Endoscopic Approach

0DL74ZZ Occlusion of Stomach, Pylorus, Percutaneous Endoscopic Approach

0DL77DZ Occlusion of Stomach, Pylorus with Intraluminal Device, Via Natural or Artificial Opening

0DL77ZZ Occlusion of Stomach, Pylorus, Via Natural or Artificial Opening

0DL78DZ Occlusion of Stomach, Pylorus with Intraluminal Device, Via Natural or Artificial Opening Endoscopic

0DL78ZZ Occlusion of Stomach, Pylorus, Via Natural or Artificial Opening Endoscopic

0DL80CZ Occlusion of Small Intestine with Extraluminal Device, Open Approach

0DL80DZ Occlusion of Small Intestine with Intraluminal Device, Open Approach

0DL80ZZ Occlusion of Small Intestine, Open Approach

0DL83CZ Occlusion of Small Intestine with Extraluminal Device, Percutaneous Approach

0DL83DZ Occlusion of Small Intestine with Intraluminal Device, Percutaneous Approach

0DL83ZZ Occlusion of Small Intestine, Percutaneous Approach

0DL84CZ Occlusion of Small Intestine with Extraluminal Device, Percutaneous Endoscopic Approach

0DL84DZ Occlusion of Small Intestine with Intraluminal Device, Percutaneous Endoscopic Approach

0DL84ZZ Occlusion of Small Intestine, Percutaneous Endoscopic Approach

0DL87DZ Occlusion of Small Intestine with Intraluminal Device, Via Natural or Artificial Opening

0DL87ZZ Occlusion of Small Intestine, Via Natural or Artificial Opening

0DL88DZ Occlusion of Small Intestine with Intraluminal Device, Via Natural or Artificial Opening Endoscopic

0DL88ZZ Occlusion of Small Intestine, Via Natural or Artificial Opening Endoscopic

0DL90CZ Occlusion of Duodenum with Extraluminal Device, Open Approach

0DL90DZ Occlusion of Duodenum with Intraluminal Device, Open Approach

0DL90ZZ Occlusion of Duodenum, Open Approach

0DL93CZ Occlusion of Duodenum with Extraluminal Device, Percutaneous Approach

0DL93DZ Occlusion of Duodenum with Intraluminal Device, Percutaneous Approach

0DL93ZZ Occlusion of Duodenum, Percutaneous Approach

0DL94CZ Occlusion of Duodenum with Extraluminal Device, Percutaneous Endoscopic Approach

0DL94DZ Occlusion of Duodenum with Intraluminal Device, Percutaneous Endoscopic Approach

0DL94ZZ Occlusion of Duodenum, Percutaneous Endoscopic Approach

0DL97DZ Occlusion of Duodenum with Intraluminal Device, Via Natural or Artificial Opening

0DL97ZZ Occlusion of Duodenum, Via Natural or Artificial Opening

0DL98DZ Occlusion of Duodenum with Intraluminal Device, Via Natural or Artificial Opening Endoscopic

0DL98ZZ Occlusion of Duodenum, Via Natural or Artificial Opening Endoscopic

0DLA0CZ Occlusion of Jejunum with Extraluminal Device, Open Approach

0DLA0DZ Occlusion of Jejunum with Intraluminal Device, Open Approach

0DLA0ZZ Occlusion of Jejunum, Open Approach

0DLA3CZ Occlusion of Jejunum with Extraluminal Device, Percutaneous Approach

0DLA3DZ Occlusion of Jejunum with Intraluminal Device, Percutaneous Approach

0DLA3ZZ Occlusion of Jejunum, Percutaneous Approach

0DLA4CZ Occlusion of Jejunum with Extraluminal Device, Percutaneous Endoscopic Approach

0DLA4DZ Occlusion of Jejunum with Intraluminal Device, Percutaneous Endoscopic Approach

0DLA4ZZ Occlusion of Jejunum, Percutaneous Endoscopic Approach

0DLA7DZ Occlusion of Jejunum with Intraluminal Device, Via Natural or Artificial Opening

0DLA7ZZ Occlusion of Jejunum, Via Natural or Artificial Opening

0DLA8DZ Occlusion of Jejunum with Intraluminal Device, Via Natural or Artificial Opening Endoscopic

0DLA8ZZ Occlusion of Jejunum, Via Natural or Artificial Opening Endoscopic

0DLB0CZ Occlusion of Ileum with Extraluminal Device, Open Approach

0DLB0DZ Occlusion of Ileum with Intraluminal Device, Open Approach

0DLB0ZZ Occlusion of Ileum, Open Approach

0DLB3CZ Occlusion of Ileum with Extraluminal Device, Percutaneous Approach

0DLB3DZ Occlusion of Ileum with Intraluminal Device, Percutaneous Approach

0DLB3ZZ Occlusion of Ileum, Percutaneous Approach

0DLB4CZ Occlusion of Ileum with Extraluminal Device, Percutaneous Endoscopic Approach

0DLB4DZ Occlusion of Ileum with Intraluminal Device, Percutaneous Endoscopic Approach

0DLB4ZZ Occlusion of Ileum, Percutaneous Endoscopic Approach

0DLB7DZ Occlusion of Ileum with Intraluminal Device, Via Natural or Artificial Opening

0DLB7ZZ Occlusion of Ileum, Via Natural or Artificial Opening

0DLB8DZ Occlusion of Ileum with Intraluminal Device, Via Natural or Artificial Opening Endoscopic

0DLB8ZZ Occlusion of Ileum, Via Natural or Artificial Opening Endoscopic

0DLC0CZ Occlusion of Ileocecal Valve with Extraluminal Device, Open Approach

0DLC0DZ Occlusion of Ileocecal Valve with Intraluminal Device, Open Approach

0DLC0ZZ Occlusion of Ileocecal Valve, Open Approach

0DLC3CZ Occlusion of Ileocecal Valve with Extraluminal Device, Percutaneous Approach

0DLC3DZ Occlusion of Ileocecal Valve with Intraluminal Device, Percutaneous Approach

0DLC3ZZ Occlusion of Ileocecal Valve, Percutaneous Approach

0DLC4CZ Occlusion of Ileocecal Valve with Extraluminal Device, Percutaneous Endoscopic Approach

0DLC4DZ Occlusion of Ileocecal Valve with Intraluminal Device, Percutaneous Endoscopic Approach

0DLC4ZZ Occlusion of Ileocecal Valve, Percutaneous Endoscopic Approach

0DLC7DZ Occlusion of Ileocecal Valve with Intraluminal Device, Via Natural or Artificial Opening

0DLC7ZZ Occlusion of Ileocecal Valve, Via Natural or Artificial Opening

0DLC8DZ Occlusion of Ileocecal Valve with Intraluminal Device, Via Natural or Artificial Opening Endoscopic

0DLC8ZZ Occlusion of Ileocecal Valve, Via Natural or Artificial Opening Endoscopic

0DLE0CZ Occlusion of Large Intestine with Extraluminal Device, Open Approach

0DLE0DZ Occlusion of Large Intestine with Intraluminal Device, Open Approach

0DLE0ZZ Occlusion of Large Intestine, Open Approach

0DLE3CZ Occlusion of Large Intestine with Extraluminal Device, Percutaneous Approach

0DLE3DZ Occlusion of Large Intestine with Intraluminal Device, Percutaneous Approach

0DLE3ZZ Occlusion of Large Intestine, Percutaneous Approach

0DLE4CZ Occlusion of Large Intestine with Extraluminal Device, Percutaneous Endoscopic Approach

0DLE4DZ Occlusion of Large Intestine with Intraluminal Device, Percutaneous Endoscopic Approach

0DLE4ZZ Occlusion of Large Intestine, Percutaneous Endoscopic Approach

0DLE7DZ Occlusion of Large Intestine with Intraluminal Device, Via Natural or Artificial Opening

0DLE7ZZ Occlusion of Large Intestine, Via Natural or Artificial Opening

0DLE8DZ Occlusion of Large Intestine with Intraluminal Device, Via Natural or Artificial Opening Endoscopic

0DLE8ZZ Occlusion of Large Intestine, Via Natural or Artificial Opening Endoscopic

0DLF0CZ Occlusion of Right Large Intestine with Extraluminal Device, Open Approach

0DLF0DZ Occlusion of Right Large Intestine with Intraluminal Device, Open Approach

0DLF0ZZ Occlusion of Right Large Intestine, Open Approach

0DLF3CZ Occlusion of Right Large Intestine with Extraluminal Device, Percutaneous Approach

0DLF3DZ Occlusion of Right Large Intestine with Intraluminal Device, Percutaneous Approach

0DLF3ZZ Occlusion of Right Large Intestine, Percutaneous Approach

0DLF4CZ Occlusion of Right Large Intestine with Extraluminal Device, Percutaneous Endoscopic Approach

0DLF4DZ Occlusion of Right Large Intestine with Intraluminal Device, Percutaneous Endoscopic Approach

0DLF4ZZ Occlusion of Right Large Intestine, Percutaneous Endoscopic Approach

0DLF7DZ Occlusion of Right Large Intestine with Intraluminal Device, Via Natural or Artificial Opening

0DLF7ZZ Occlusion of Right Large Intestine, Via Natural or Artificial Opening

0DLF8DZ Occlusion of Right Large Intestine with Intraluminal Device, Via Natural or Artificial Opening Endoscopic

0DLF8ZZ Occlusion of Right Large Intestine, Via Natural or Artificial Opening Endoscopic

0DLG0CZ Occlusion of Left Large Intestine with Extraluminal Device, Open Approach

0DLG0DZ Occlusion of Left Large Intestine with Intraluminal Device, Open Approach

0DLG0ZZ Occlusion of Left Large Intestine, Open Approach

0DLG3CZ Occlusion of Left Large Intestine with Extraluminal Device, Percutaneous Approach

0DLG3DZ Occlusion of Left Large Intestine with Intraluminal Device, Percutaneous Approach

0DLG3ZZ Occlusion of Left Large Intestine, Percutaneous Approach

0DLG4CZ Occlusion of Left Large Intestine with Extraluminal Device, Percutaneous Endoscopic Approach

0DLG4DZ Occlusion of Left Large Intestine with Intraluminal Device, Percutaneous Endoscopic Approach

0DLG4ZZ Occlusion of Left Large Intestine, Percutaneous Endoscopic Approach

0DLG7DZ Occlusion of Left Large Intestine with Intraluminal Device, Via Natural or Artificial Opening

0DLG7ZZ Occlusion of Left Large Intestine, Via Natural or Artificial Opening

0DLG8DZ Occlusion of Left Large Intestine with Intraluminal Device, Via Natural or Artificial Opening Endoscopic

0DLG8ZZ Occlusion of Left Large Intestine, Via Natural or Artificial Opening Endoscopic

0DLH0CZ Occlusion of Cecum with Extraluminal Device, Open Approach

0DLH0DZ Occlusion of Cecum with Intraluminal Device, Open Approach

0DLH0ZZ Occlusion of Cecum, Open Approach

0DLH3CZ Occlusion of Cecum with Extraluminal Device, Percutaneous Approach

0DLH3DZ Occlusion of Cecum with Intraluminal Device, Percutaneous Approach

0DLH3ZZ Occlusion of Cecum, Percutaneous Approach

0DLH4CZ Occlusion of Cecum with Extraluminal Device, Percutaneous Endoscopic Approach

0DLH4DZ Occlusion of Cecum with Intraluminal Device, Percutaneous Endoscopic Approach

0DLH4ZZ Occlusion of Cecum, Percutaneous Endoscopic Approach

0DLH7DZ Occlusion of Cecum with Intraluminal Device, Via Natural or Artificial Opening

0DLH7ZZ Occlusion of Cecum, Via Natural or Artificial Opening

0DLH8DZ Occlusion of Cecum with Intraluminal Device, Via Natural or Artificial Opening Endoscopic

0DLH8ZZ Occlusion of Cecum, Via Natural or Artificial Opening Endoscopic

0DLK0CZ Occlusion of Ascending Colon with Extraluminal Device, Open Approach

0DLK0DZ Occlusion of Ascending Colon with Intraluminal Device, Open Approach

0DLK0ZZ Occlusion of Ascending Colon, Open Approach

0DLK3CZ Occlusion of Ascending Colon with Extraluminal Device, Percutaneous Approach

0DLK3DZ Occlusion of Ascending Colon with Intraluminal Device, Percutaneous Approach

0DLK3ZZ Occlusion of Ascending Colon, Percutaneous Approach

0DLK4CZ Occlusion of Ascending Colon with Extraluminal Device, Percutaneous Endoscopic Approach

0DLK4DZ Occlusion of Ascending Colon with Intraluminal Device, Percutaneous Endoscopic Approach

0DLK4ZZ Occlusion of Ascending Colon, Percutaneous Endoscopic Approach

0DLK7DZ Occlusion of Ascending Colon with Intraluminal Device, Via Natural or Artificial Opening

♀ Female-only   ♂ Male-only   ▲ Limited Coverage   ● Non-OR   ▦ HAC-associated procedure   ▲ Non-covered procedures   ✛ Cluster

0DLK7ZZ	Occlusion of Ascending Colon, Via Natural or Artificial Opening
0DLK8DZ	Occlusion of Ascending Colon with Intraluminal Device, Via Natural or Artificial Opening Endoscopic
0DLK8ZZ	Occlusion of Ascending Colon, Via Natural or Artificial Opening Endoscopic
0DLL0CZ	Occlusion of Transverse Colon with Extraluminal Device, Open Approach
0DLL0DZ	Occlusion of Transverse Colon with Intraluminal Device, Open Approach
0DLL0ZZ	Occlusion of Transverse Colon, Open Approach
0DLL3CZ	Occlusion of Transverse Colon with Extraluminal Device, Percutaneous Approach
0DLL3DZ	Occlusion of Transverse Colon with Intraluminal Device, Percutaneous Approach
0DLL3ZZ	Occlusion of Transverse Colon, Percutaneous Approach
0DLL4CZ	Occlusion of Transverse Colon with Extraluminal Device, Percutaneous Endoscopic Approach
0DLL4DZ	Occlusion of Transverse Colon with Intraluminal Device, Percutaneous Endoscopic Approach
0DLL4ZZ	Occlusion of Transverse Colon, Percutaneous Endoscopic Approach
0DLL7DZ	Occlusion of Transverse Colon with Intraluminal Device, Via Natural or Artificial Opening
0DLL7ZZ	Occlusion of Transverse Colon, Via Natural or Artificial Opening
0DLL8DZ	Occlusion of Transverse Colon with Intraluminal Device, Via Natural or Artificial Opening Endoscopic
0DLL8ZZ	Occlusion of Transverse Colon, Via Natural or Artificial Opening Endoscopic
0DLM0CZ	Occlusion of Descending Colon with Extraluminal Device, Open Approach
0DLM0DZ	Occlusion of Descending Colon with Intraluminal Device, Open Approach
0DLM0ZZ	Occlusion of Descending Colon, Open Approach
0DLM3CZ	Occlusion of Descending Colon with Extraluminal Device, Percutaneous Approach
0DLM3DZ	Occlusion of Descending Colon with Intraluminal Device, Percutaneous Approach
0DLM3ZZ	Occlusion of Descending Colon, Percutaneous Approach
0DLM4CZ	Occlusion of Descending Colon with Extraluminal Device, Percutaneous Endoscopic Approach

0DLM4DZ	Occlusion of Descending Colon with Intraluminal Device, Percutaneous Endoscopic Approach
0DLM4ZZ	Occlusion of Descending Colon, Percutaneous Endoscopic Approach
0DLM7DZ	Occlusion of Descending Colon with Intraluminal Device, Via Natural or Artificial Opening
0DLM7ZZ	Occlusion of Descending Colon, Via Natural or Artificial Opening
0DLM8DZ	Occlusion of Descending Colon with Intraluminal Device, Via Natural or Artificial Opening Endoscopic
0DLM8ZZ	Occlusion of Descending Colon, Via Natural or Artificial Opening Endoscopic
0DLN0CZ	Occlusion of Sigmoid Colon with Extraluminal Device, Open Approach
0DLN0DZ	Occlusion of Sigmoid Colon with Intraluminal Device, Open Approach
0DLN0ZZ	Occlusion of Sigmoid Colon, Open Approach
0DLN3CZ	Occlusion of Sigmoid Colon with Extraluminal Device, Percutaneous Approach
0DLN3DZ	Occlusion of Sigmoid Colon with Intraluminal Device, Percutaneous Approach
0DLN3ZZ	Occlusion of Sigmoid Colon, Percutaneous Approach
0DLN4CZ	Occlusion of Sigmoid Colon with Extraluminal Device, Percutaneous Endoscopic Approach
0DLN4DZ	Occlusion of Sigmoid Colon with Intraluminal Device, Percutaneous Endoscopic Approach
0DLN4ZZ	Occlusion of Sigmoid Colon, Percutaneous Endoscopic Approach
0DLN7DZ	Occlusion of Sigmoid Colon with Intraluminal Device, Via Natural or Artificial Opening
0DLN7ZZ	Occlusion of Sigmoid Colon, Via Natural or Artificial Opening
0DLN8DZ	Occlusion of Sigmoid Colon with Intraluminal Device, Via Natural or Artificial Opening Endoscopic
0DLN8ZZ	Occlusion of Sigmoid Colon, Via Natural or Artificial Opening Endoscopic
0DLP0CZ	Occlusion of Rectum with Extraluminal Device, Open Approach
0DLP0DZ	Occlusion of Rectum with Intraluminal Device, Open Approach
0DLP0ZZ	Occlusion of Rectum, Open Approach
0DLP3CZ	Occlusion of Rectum with Extraluminal Device, Percutaneous Approach

0DLP3DZ	Occlusion of Rectum with Intraluminal Device, Percutaneous Approach
0DLP3ZZ	Occlusion of Rectum, Percutaneous Approach
0DLP4CZ	Occlusion of Rectum with Extraluminal Device, Percutaneous Endoscopic Approach
0DLP4DZ	Occlusion of Rectum with Intraluminal Device, Percutaneous Endoscopic Approach
0DLP4ZZ	Occlusion of Rectum, Percutaneous Endoscopic Approach
0DLP7DZ	Occlusion of Rectum with Intraluminal Device, Via Natural or Artificial Opening
0DLP7ZZ	Occlusion of Rectum, Via Natural or Artificial Opening
0DLP8DZ	Occlusion of Rectum with Intraluminal Device, Via Natural or Artificial Opening Endoscopic
0DLP8ZZ	Occlusion of Rectum, Via Natural or Artificial Opening Endoscopic
0DLQ0CZ	Occlusion of Anus with Extraluminal Device, Open Approach
0DLQ0DZ	Occlusion of Anus with Intraluminal Device, Open Approach
0DLQ0ZZ	Occlusion of Anus, Open Approach
0DLQ3CZ	Occlusion of Anus with Extraluminal Device, Percutaneous Approach
0DLQ3DZ	Occlusion of Anus with Intraluminal Device, Percutaneous Approach
0DLQ3ZZ	Occlusion of Anus, Percutaneous Approach
0DLQ4CZ	Occlusion of Anus with Extraluminal Device, Percutaneous Endoscopic Approach
0DLQ4DZ	Occlusion of Anus with Intraluminal Device, Percutaneous Endoscopic Approach
0DLQ4ZZ	Occlusion of Anus, Percutaneous Endoscopic Approach
0DLQ7DZ	Occlusion of Anus with Intraluminal Device, Via Natural or Artificial Opening
0DLQ7ZZ	Occlusion of Anus, Via Natural or Artificial Opening
0DLQ8DZ	Occlusion of Anus with Intraluminal Device, Via Natural or Artificial Opening Endoscopic
0DLQ8ZZ	Occlusion of Anus, Via Natural or Artificial Opening Endoscopic
0DLQXCZ	Occlusion of Anus with Extraluminal Device, External Approach
0DLQXDZ	Occlusion of Anus with Intraluminal Device, External Approach
0DLQXZZ	Occlusion of Anus, External Approach

0DM – Gastrointestinal System, Reattachment

0DM50ZZ	Reattachment of Esophagus, Open Approach
0DM54ZZ	Reattachment of Esophagus, Percutaneous Endoscopic Approach
0DM60ZZ	Reattachment of Stomach, Open Approach
0DM64ZZ	Reattachment of Stomach, Percutaneous Endoscopic Approach
0DM80ZZ	Reattachment of Small Intestine, Open Approach
0DM84ZZ	Reattachment of Small Intestine, Percutaneous Endoscopic Approach
0DM90ZZ	Reattachment of Duodenum, Open Approach

0DM94ZZ	Reattachment of Duodenum, Percutaneous Endoscopic Approach
0DMA0ZZ	Reattachment of Jejunum, Open Approach
0DMA4ZZ	Reattachment of Jejunum, Percutaneous Endoscopic Approach
0DMB0ZZ	Reattachment of Ileum, Open Approach
0DMB4ZZ	Reattachment of Ileum, Percutaneous Endoscopic Approach
0DME0ZZ	Reattachment of Large Intestine, Open Approach
0DME4ZZ	Reattachment of Large Intestine, Percutaneous Endoscopic Approach

0DMF0ZZ	Reattachment of Right Large Intestine, Open Approach
0DMF4ZZ	Reattachment of Right Large Intestine, Percutaneous Endoscopic Approach
0DMG0ZZ	Reattachment of Left Large Intestine, Open Approach
0DMG4ZZ	Reattachment of Left Large Intestine, Percutaneous Endoscopic Approach
0DMH0ZZ	Reattachment of Cecum, Open Approach
0DMH4ZZ	Reattachment of Cecum, Percutaneous Endoscopic Approach
0DMK0ZZ	Reattachment of Ascending Colon, Open Approach

0DMK4ZZ Reattachment of Ascending Colon, Percutaneous Endoscopic Approach
0DML0ZZ Reattachment of Transverse Colon, Open Approach
0DML4ZZ Reattachment of Transverse Colon, Percutaneous Endoscopic Approach

0DMM0ZZ Reattachment of Descending Colon, Open Approach
0DMM4ZZ Reattachment of Descending Colon, Percutaneous Endoscopic Approach
0DMN0ZZ Reattachment of Sigmoid Colon, Open Approach

0DMN4ZZ Reattachment of Sigmoid Colon, Percutaneous Endoscopic Approach
0DMP0ZZ Reattachment of Rectum, Open Approach
0DMP4ZZ Reattachment of Rectum, Percutaneous Endoscopic Approach

0DN – Gastrointestinal System, Release

Review Coding Guideline B3.13

Review Coding Guideline B3.14

0DN10ZZ Release Upper Esophagus, Open Approach
0DN13ZZ Release Upper Esophagus, Percutaneous Approach
0DN14ZZ Release Upper Esophagus, Percutaneous Endoscopic Approach
0DN17ZZ Release Upper Esophagus, Via Natural or Artificial Opening
0DN18ZZ Release Upper Esophagus, Via Natural or Artificial Opening Endoscopic
0DN20ZZ Release Middle Esophagus, Open Approach
0DN23ZZ Release Middle Esophagus, Percutaneous Approach
0DN24ZZ Release Middle Esophagus, Percutaneous Endoscopic Approach
0DN27ZZ Release Middle Esophagus, Via Natural or Artificial Opening
0DN28ZZ Release Middle Esophagus, Via Natural or Artificial Opening Endoscopic
0DN30ZZ Release Lower Esophagus, Open Approach
0DN33ZZ Release Lower Esophagus, Percutaneous Approach
0DN34ZZ Release Lower Esophagus, Percutaneous Endoscopic Approach
0DN37ZZ Release Lower Esophagus, Via Natural or Artificial Opening
0DN38ZZ Release Lower Esophagus, Via Natural or Artificial Opening Endoscopic
0DN40ZZ Release Esophagogastric Junction, Open Approach
0DN43ZZ Release Esophagogastric Junction, Percutaneous Approach
0DN44ZZ Release Esophagogastric Junction, Percutaneous Endoscopic Approach
0DN47ZZ Release Esophagogastric Junction, Via Natural or Artificial Opening
0DN48ZZ Release Esophagogastric Junction, Via Natural or Artificial Opening Endoscopic
0DN50ZZ Release Esophagus, Open Approach
AHA CC: 3Q, 2015, 15-16
0DN53ZZ Release Esophagus, Percutaneous Approach
0DN54ZZ Release Esophagus, Percutaneous Endoscopic Approach
0DN57ZZ Release Esophagus, Via Natural or Artificial Opening
0DN58ZZ Release Esophagus, Via Natural or Artificial Opening Endoscopic
0DN60ZZ Release Stomach, Open Approach
0DN63ZZ Release Stomach, Percutaneous Approach
0DN64ZZ Release Stomach, Percutaneous Endoscopic Approach
0DN67ZZ Release Stomach, Via Natural or Artificial Opening
0DN68ZZ Release Stomach, Via Natural or Artificial Opening Endoscopic
0DN70ZZ Release Stomach, Pylorus, Open Approach

0DN73ZZ Release Stomach, Pylorus, Percutaneous Approach
0DN74ZZ Release Stomach, Pylorus, Percutaneous Endoscopic Approach
0DN77ZZ Release Stomach, Pylorus, Via Natural or Artificial Opening
0DN78ZZ Release Stomach, Pylorus, Via Natural or Artificial Opening Endoscopic
0DN80ZZ Release Small Intestine, Open Approach
AHA CC: 4Q, 2017, 49-50
0DN83ZZ Release Small Intestine, Percutaneous Approach
0DN84ZZ Release Small Intestine, Percutaneous Endoscopic Approach
0DN87ZZ Release Small Intestine, Via Natural or Artificial Opening
0DN88ZZ Release Small Intestine, Via Natural or Artificial Opening Endoscopic
0DN90ZZ Release Duodenum, Open Approach
0DN93ZZ Release Duodenum, Percutaneous Approach
0DN94ZZ Release Duodenum, Percutaneous Endoscopic Approach
0DN97ZZ Release Duodenum, Via Natural or Artificial Opening
0DN98ZZ Release Duodenum, Via Natural or Artificial Opening Endoscopic
0DNA0ZZ Release Jejunum, Open Approach
0DNA3ZZ Release Jejunum, Percutaneous Approach
0DNA4ZZ Release Jejunum, Percutaneous Endoscopic Approach
0DNA7ZZ Release Jejunum, Via Natural or Artificial Opening
0DNA8ZZ Release Jejunum, Via Natural or Artificial Opening Endoscopic
0DNB0ZZ Release Ileum, Open Approach
0DNB3ZZ Release Ileum, Percutaneous Approach
0DNB4ZZ Release Ileum, Percutaneous Endoscopic Approach
0DNB7ZZ Release Ileum, Via Natural or Artificial Opening
0DNB8ZZ Release Ileum, Via Natural or Artificial Opening Endoscopic
0DNC0ZZ Release Ileocecal Valve, Open Approach
0DNC3ZZ Release Ileocecal Valve, Percutaneous Approach
0DNC4ZZ Release Ileocecal Valve, Percutaneous Endoscopic Approach
0DNC7ZZ Release Ileocecal Valve, Via Natural or Artificial Opening
0DNC8ZZ Release Ileocecal Valve, Via Natural or Artificial Opening Endoscopic
0DNE0ZZ Release Large Intestine, Open Approach
0DNE3ZZ Release Large Intestine, Percutaneous Approach
0DNE4ZZ Release Large Intestine, Percutaneous Endoscopic Approach
0DNE7ZZ Release Large Intestine, Via Natural or Artificial Opening

0DNE8ZZ Release Large Intestine, Via Natural or Artificial Opening Endoscopic
0DNF0ZZ Release Right Large Intestine, Open Approach
0DNF3ZZ Release Right Large Intestine, Percutaneous Approach
0DNF4ZZ Release Right Large Intestine, Percutaneous Endoscopic Approach
0DNF7ZZ Release Right Large Intestine, Via Natural or Artificial Opening
0DNF8ZZ Release Right Large Intestine, Via Natural or Artificial Opening Endoscopic
0DNG0ZZ Release Left Large Intestine, Open Approach
0DNG3ZZ Release Left Large Intestine, Percutaneous Approach
0DNG4ZZ Release Left Large Intestine, Percutaneous Endoscopic Approach
0DNG7ZZ Release Left Large Intestine, Via Natural or Artificial Opening
0DNG8ZZ Release Left Large Intestine, Via Natural or Artificial Opening Endoscopic
0DNH0ZZ Release Cecum, Open Approach
0DNH3ZZ Release Cecum, Percutaneous Approach
0DNH4ZZ Release Cecum, Percutaneous Endoscopic Approach
0DNH7ZZ Release Cecum, Via Natural or Artificial Opening
0DNH8ZZ Release Cecum, Via Natural or Artificial Opening Endoscopic
0DNJ0ZZ Release Appendix, Open Approach
0DNJ3ZZ Release Appendix, Percutaneous Approach
0DNJ4ZZ Release Appendix, Percutaneous Endoscopic Approach
0DNJ7ZZ Release Appendix, Via Natural or Artificial Opening
0DNJ8ZZ Release Appendix, Via Natural or Artificial Opening Endoscopic
0DNK0ZZ Release Ascending Colon, Open Approach
0DNK3ZZ Release Ascending Colon, Percutaneous Approach
0DNK4ZZ Release Ascending Colon, Percutaneous Endoscopic Approach
0DNK7ZZ Release Ascending Colon, Via Natural or Artificial Opening
0DNK8ZZ Release Ascending Colon, Via Natural or Artificial Opening Endoscopic
0DNL0ZZ Release Transverse Colon, Open Approach
0DNL3ZZ Release Transverse Colon, Percutaneous Approach
0DNL4ZZ Release Transverse Colon, Percutaneous Endoscopic Approach
0DNL7ZZ Release Transverse Colon, Via Natural or Artificial Opening
0DNL8ZZ Release Transverse Colon, Via Natural or Artificial Opening Endoscopic

♀ Female-only   ♂ Male-only   ▲ Limited Coverage   ● Non-OR   ▬ HAC-associated procedure   ▲ Non-covered procedures   ✚ Cluster

0DNM0ZZ	Release Descending Colon, Open Approach	
0DNM3ZZ	Release Descending Colon, Percutaneous Approach	
0DNM4ZZ	Release Descending Colon, Percutaneous Endoscopic Approach	
0DNM7ZZ	Release Descending Colon, Via Natural or Artificial Opening	
0DNM8ZZ	Release Descending Colon, Via Natural or Artificial Opening Endoscopic	
0DNN0ZZ	Release Sigmoid Colon, Open Approach	
0DNN3ZZ	Release Sigmoid Colon, Percutaneous Approach	
0DNN4ZZ	Release Sigmoid Colon, Percutaneous Endoscopic Approach	
0DNN7ZZ	Release Sigmoid Colon, Via Natural or Artificial Opening	
0DNN8ZZ	Release Sigmoid Colon, Via Natural or Artificial Opening Endoscopic	

0DNP0ZZ	Release Rectum, Open Approach
0DNP3ZZ	Release Rectum, Percutaneous Approach
0DNP4ZZ	Release Rectum, Percutaneous Endoscopic Approach
0DNP7ZZ	Release Rectum, Via Natural or Artificial Opening
0DNP8ZZ	Release Rectum, Via Natural or Artificial Opening Endoscopic
0DNQ0ZZ	Release Anus, Open Approach
0DNQ3ZZ	Release Anus, Percutaneous Approach
0DNQ4ZZ	Release Anus, Percutaneous Endoscopic Approach
0DNQ7ZZ	Release Anus, Via Natural or Artificial Opening
0DNQ8ZZ	Release Anus, Via Natural or Artificial Opening Endoscopic
0DNQXZZ	Release Anus, External Approach
0DNR0ZZ	Release Anal Sphincter, Open Approach

0DNR3ZZ	Release Anal Sphincter, Percutaneous Approach
0DNR4ZZ	Release Anal Sphincter, Percutaneous Endoscopic Approach
0DNU0ZZ	Release Omentum, Open Approach
0DNU3ZZ	Release Omentum, Percutaneous Approach
0DNU4ZZ	Release Omentum, Percutaneous Endoscopic Approach
0DNV0ZZ	Release Mesentery, Open Approach
0DNV3ZZ	Release Mesentery, Percutaneous Approach
0DNV4ZZ	Release Mesentery, Percutaneous Endoscopic Approach
0DNW0ZZ	Release Peritoneum, Open Approach
	AHA CC: 1Q, 2017, 35
0DNW3ZZ	Release Peritoneum, Percutaneous Approach
0DNW4ZZ	Release Peritoneum, Percutaneous Endoscopic Approach

0DP – Gastrointestinal System, Removal

Review Coding Guideline B6.1c

0DP000Z	Removal of Drainage Device from Upper Intestinal Tract, Open Approach
0DP002Z	Removal of Monitoring Device from Upper Intestinal Tract, Open Approach
0DP003Z	Removal of Infusion Device from Upper Intestinal Tract, Open Approach
0DP007Z	Removal of Autologous Tissue Substitute from Upper Intestinal Tract, Open Approach
0DP00CZ	Removal of Extraluminal Device from Upper Intestinal Tract, Open Approach
0DP00DZ	Removal of Intraluminal Device from Upper Intestinal Tract, Open Approach
0DP00JZ	Removal of Synthetic Substitute from Upper Intestinal Tract, Open Approach
0DP00KZ	Removal of Nonautologous Tissue Substitute from Upper Intestinal Tract, Open Approach
0DP00UZ	Removal of Feeding Device from Upper Intestinal Tract, Open Approach
0DP00YZ	Removal of Other Device from Upper Intestinal Tract, Open Approach
0DP030Z	Removal of Drainage Device from Upper Intestinal Tract, Percutaneous Approach
0DP032Z	Removal of Monitoring Device from Upper Intestinal Tract, Percutaneous Approach
0DP033Z	Removal of Infusion Device from Upper Intestinal Tract, Percutaneous Approach
0DP037Z	Removal of Autologous Tissue Substitute from Upper Intestinal Tract, Percutaneous Approach
0DP03CZ	Removal of Extraluminal Device from Upper Intestinal Tract, Percutaneous Approach
0DP03DZ	Removal of Intraluminal Device from Upper Intestinal Tract, Percutaneous Approach
0DP03JZ	Removal of Synthetic Substitute from Upper Intestinal Tract, Percutaneous Approach
0DP03KZ	Removal of Nonautologous Tissue Substitute from Upper Intestinal Tract, Percutaneous Approach
0DP03UZ	Removal of Feeding Device from Upper Intestinal Tract, Percutaneous Approach

0DP03YZ	Removal of Other Device from Upper Intestinal Tract, Percutaneous Approach
0DP040Z	Removal of Drainage Device from Upper Intestinal Tract, Percutaneous Endoscopic Approach
0DP042Z	Removal of Monitoring Device from Upper Intestinal Tract, Percutaneous Endoscopic Approach
0DP043Z	Removal of Infusion Device from Upper Intestinal Tract, Percutaneous Endoscopic Approach
0DP047Z	Removal of Autologous Tissue Substitute from Upper Intestinal Tract, Percutaneous Endoscopic Approach
0DP04CZ	Removal of Extraluminal Device from Upper Intestinal Tract, Percutaneous Endoscopic Approach
0DP04DZ	Removal of Intraluminal Device from Upper Intestinal Tract, Percutaneous Endoscopic Approach
0DP04JZ	Removal of Synthetic Substitute from Upper Intestinal Tract, Percutaneous Endoscopic Approach
0DP04KZ	Removal of Nonautologous Tissue Substitute from Upper Intestinal Tract, Percutaneous Endoscopic Approach
0DP04UZ	Removal of Feeding Device from Upper Intestinal Tract, Percutaneous Endoscopic Approach
0DP04YZ	Removal of Other Device from Upper Intestinal Tract, Percutaneous Endoscopic Approach
0DP070Z	Removal of Drainage Device from Upper Intestinal Tract, Via Natural or Artificial Opening
0DP072Z	Removal of Monitoring Device from Upper Intestinal Tract, Via Natural or Artificial Opening
0DP073Z	Removal of Infusion Device from Upper Intestinal Tract, Via Natural or Artificial Opening
0DP077Z	Removal of Autologous Tissue Substitute from Upper Intestinal Tract, Via Natural or Artificial Opening
0DP07CZ	Removal of Extraluminal Device from Upper Intestinal Tract, Via Natural or Artificial Opening

0DP07DZ	Removal of Intraluminal Device from Upper Intestinal Tract, Via Natural or Artificial Opening
0DP07JZ	Removal of Synthetic Substitute from Upper Intestinal Tract, Via Natural or Artificial Opening
0DP07KZ	Removal of Nonautologous Tissue Substitute from Upper Intestinal Tract, Via Natural or Artificial Opening
0DP07UZ	Removal of Feeding Device from Upper Intestinal Tract, Via Natural or Artificial Opening
0DP07YZ	Removal of Other Device from Upper Intestinal Tract, Via Natural or Artificial Opening
0DP080Z	Removal of Drainage Device from Upper Intestinal Tract, Via Natural or Artificial Opening Endoscopic
0DP082Z	Removal of Monitoring Device from Upper Intestinal Tract, Via Natural or Artificial Opening Endoscopic
0DP083Z	Removal of Infusion Device from Upper Intestinal Tract, Via Natural or Artificial Opening Endoscopic
0DP087Z	Removal of Autologous Tissue Substitute from Upper Intestinal Tract, Via Natural or Artificial Opening Endoscopic
0DP08CZ	Removal of Extraluminal Device from Upper Intestinal Tract, Via Natural or Artificial Opening Endoscopic
0DP08DZ	Removal of Intraluminal Device from Upper Intestinal Tract, Via Natural or Artificial Opening Endoscopic
0DP08JZ	Removal of Synthetic Substitute from Upper Intestinal Tract, Via Natural or Artificial Opening Endoscopic
0DP08KZ	Removal of Nonautologous Tissue Substitute from Upper Intestinal Tract, Via Natural or Artificial Opening Endoscopic
0DP08UZ	Removal of Feeding Device from Upper Intestinal Tract, Via Natural or Artificial Opening Endoscopic
0DP08YZ	Removal of Other Device from Upper Intestinal Tract, Via Natural or Artificial Opening Endoscopic
0DP0X0Z	Removal of Drainage Device from Upper Intestinal Tract, External Approach

0DP0X2Z Removal of Monitoring Device from Upper Intestinal Tract, External Approach

0DP0X3Z Removal of Infusion Device from Upper Intestinal Tract, External Approach

0DP0XDZ Removal of Intraluminal Device from Upper Intestinal Tract, External Approach

0DP0XUZ Removal of Feeding Device from Upper Intestinal Tract, External Approach

0DP501Z Removal of Radioactive Element from Esophagus, Open Approach

0DP502Z Removal of Monitoring Device from Esophagus, Open Approach

0DP503Z Removal of Infusion Device from Esophagus, Open Approach

0DP50UZ Removal of Feeding Device from Esophagus, Open Approach

0DP50YZ Removal of Other Device from Esophagus, Open Approach

0DP531Z Removal of Radioactive Element from Esophagus, Percutaneous Approach

0DP532Z Removal of Monitoring Device from Esophagus, Percutaneous Approach

0DP533Z Removal of Infusion Device from Esophagus, Percutaneous Approach

0DP53UZ Removal of Feeding Device from Esophagus, Percutaneous Approach

0DP53YZ Removal of Other Device from Esophagus, Percutaneous Approach

0DP541Z Removal of Radioactive Element from Esophagus, Percutaneous Endoscopic Approach

0DP542Z Removal of Monitoring Device from Esophagus, Percutaneous Endoscopic Approach

0DP543Z Removal of Infusion Device from Esophagus, Percutaneous Endoscopic Approach

0DP54UZ Removal of Feeding Device from Esophagus, Percutaneous Endoscopic Approach

0DP54YZ Removal of Other Device from Esophagus, Percutaneous Endoscopic Approach

0DP571Z Removal of Radioactive Element from Esophagus, Via Natural or Artificial Opening

0DP57DZ Removal of Intraluminal Device from Esophagus, Via Natural or Artificial Opening

0DP57YZ Removal of Other Device from Esophagus, Via Natural or Artificial Opening

0DP581Z Removal of Radioactive Element from Esophagus, Via Natural or Artificial Opening Endoscopic

0DP58DZ Removal of Intraluminal Device from Esophagus, Via Natural or Artificial Opening Endoscopic

0DP58YZ Removal of Other Device from Esophagus, Via Natural or Artificial Opening Endoscopic

0DP5X1Z Removal of Radioactive Element from Esophagus, External Approach

0DP5X2Z Removal of Monitoring Device from Esophagus, External Approach

0DP5X3Z Removal of Infusion Device from Esophagus, External Approach

0DP5XDZ Removal of Intraluminal Device from Esophagus, External Approach

0DP5XUZ Removal of Feeding Device from Esophagus, External Approach

0DP600Z Removal of Drainage Device from Stomach, Open Approach

0DP602Z Removal of Monitoring Device from Stomach, Open Approach

0DP603Z Removal of Infusion Device from Stomach, Open Approach

0DP607Z Removal of Autologous Tissue Substitute from Stomach, Open Approach

0DP60CZ Removal of Extraluminal Device from Stomach, Open Approach

0DP60DZ Removal of Intraluminal Device from Stomach, Open Approach

0DP60JZ Removal of Synthetic Substitute from Stomach, Open Approach

0DP60KZ Removal of Nonautologous Tissue Substitute from Stomach, Open Approach

0DP60MZ Removal of Stimulator Lead from Stomach, Open Approach

0DP60UZ Removal of Feeding Device from Stomach, Open Approach

0DP60YZ Removal of Other Device from Stomach, Open Approach

0DP630Z Removal of Drainage Device from Stomach, Percutaneous Approach

0DP632Z Removal of Monitoring Device from Stomach, Percutaneous Approach

0DP633Z Removal of Infusion Device from Stomach, Percutaneous Approach

0DP637Z Removal of Autologous Tissue Substitute from Stomach, Percutaneous Approach

0DP63CZ Removal of Extraluminal Device from Stomach, Percutaneous Approach

0DP63DZ Removal of Intraluminal Device from Stomach, Percutaneous Approach

0DP63JZ Removal of Synthetic Substitute from Stomach, Percutaneous Approach

0DP63KZ Removal of Nonautologous Tissue Substitute from Stomach, Percutaneous Approach

0DP63MZ Removal of Stimulator Lead from Stomach, Percutaneous Approach

0DP63UZ Removal of Feeding Device from Stomach, Percutaneous Approach

0DP63YZ Removal of Other Device from Stomach, Percutaneous Approach

0DP640Z Removal of Drainage Device from Stomach, Percutaneous Endoscopic Approach

0DP642Z Removal of Monitoring Device from Stomach, Percutaneous Endoscopic Approach

0DP643Z Removal of Infusion Device from Stomach, Percutaneous Endoscopic Approach

0DP647Z Removal of Autologous Tissue Substitute from Stomach, Percutaneous Endoscopic Approach

0DP64CZ Removal of Extraluminal Device from Stomach, Percutaneous Endoscopic Approach

0DP64DZ Removal of Intraluminal Device from Stomach, Percutaneous Endoscopic Approach

0DP64JZ Removal of Synthetic Substitute from Stomach, Percutaneous Endoscopic Approach

0DP64KZ Removal of Nonautologous Tissue Substitute from Stomach, Percutaneous Endoscopic Approach

0DP64MZ Removal of Stimulator Lead from Stomach, Percutaneous Endoscopic Approach

0DP64UZ Removal of Feeding Device from Stomach, Percutaneous Endoscopic Approach

0DP64YZ Removal of Other Device from Stomach, Percutaneous Endoscopic Approach

0DP670Z Removal of Drainage Device from Stomach, Via Natural or Artificial Opening

0DP672Z Removal of Monitoring Device from Stomach, Via Natural or Artificial Opening

0DP673Z Removal of Infusion Device from Stomach, Via Natural or Artificial Opening

0DP677Z Removal of Autologous Tissue Substitute from Stomach, Via Natural or Artificial Opening

0DP67CZ Removal of Extraluminal Device from Stomach, Via Natural or Artificial Opening

0DP67DZ Removal of Intraluminal Device from Stomach, Via Natural or Artificial Opening

0DP67JZ Removal of Synthetic Substitute from Stomach, Via Natural or Artificial Opening

0DP67KZ Removal of Nonautologous Tissue Substitute from Stomach, Via Natural or Artificial Opening

0DP67UZ Removal of Feeding Device from Stomach, Via Natural or Artificial Opening

0DP67YZ Removal of Other Device from Stomach, Via Natural or Artificial Opening

0DP680Z Removal of Drainage Device from Stomach, Via Natural or Artificial Opening Endoscopic

0DP682Z Removal of Monitoring Device from Stomach, Via Natural or Artificial Opening Endoscopic

0DP683Z Removal of Infusion Device from Stomach, Via Natural or Artificial Opening Endoscopic

0DP687Z Removal of Autologous Tissue Substitute from Stomach, Via Natural or Artificial Opening Endoscopic

0DP68CZ Removal of Extraluminal Device from Stomach, Via Natural or Artificial Opening Endoscopic

0DP68DZ Removal of Intraluminal Device from Stomach, Via Natural or Artificial Opening Endoscopic

0DP68JZ Removal of Synthetic Substitute from Stomach, Via Natural or Artificial Opening Endoscopic

0DP68KZ Removal of Nonautologous Tissue Substitute from Stomach, Via Natural or Artificial Opening Endoscopic

0DP68UZ Removal of Feeding Device from Stomach, Via Natural or Artificial Opening Endoscopic

0DP68YZ Removal of Other Device from Stomach, Via Natural or Artificial Opening Endoscopic

AHA CC: 2Q, 2019, 18-19

0DP6X0Z Removal of Drainage Device from Stomach, External Approach

0DP6X2Z Removal of Monitoring Device from Stomach, External Approach

0DP6X3Z Removal of Infusion Device from Stomach, External Approach

0DP6XDZ Removal of Intraluminal Device from Stomach, External Approach

♀ Female-only   ♂ Male-only   ▲ Limited Coverage   ● Non-OR   ▦ HAC-associated procedure   ▲ Non-covered procedures   ✚ Cluster

0DP6XUZ Removal of Feeding Device from Stomach, External Approach

0DPD00Z Removal of Drainage Device from Lower Intestinal Tract, Open Approach

0DPD02Z Removal of Monitoring Device from Lower Intestinal Tract, Open Approach

0DPD03Z Removal of Infusion Device from Lower Intestinal Tract, Open Approach

0DPD07Z Removal of Autologous Tissue Substitute from Lower Intestinal Tract, Open Approach

0DPD0CZ Removal of Extraluminal Device from Lower Intestinal Tract, Open Approach

0DPD0DZ Removal of Intraluminal Device from Lower Intestinal Tract, Open Approach

0DPD0JZ Removal of Synthetic Substitute from Lower Intestinal Tract, Open Approach

0DPD0KZ Removal of Nonautologous Tissue Substitute from Lower Intestinal Tract, Open Approach

0DPD0UZ Removal of Feeding Device from Lower Intestinal Tract, Open Approach

0DPD0YZ Removal of Other Device from Lower Intestinal Tract, Open Approach

0DPD30Z Removal of Drainage Device from Lower Intestinal Tract, Percutaneous Approach

0DPD32Z Removal of Monitoring Device from Lower Intestinal Tract, Percutaneous Approach

0DPD33Z Removal of Infusion Device from Lower Intestinal Tract, Percutaneous Approach

0DPD37Z Removal of Autologous Tissue Substitute from Lower Intestinal Tract, Percutaneous Approach

0DPD3CZ Removal of Extraluminal Device from Lower Intestinal Tract, Percutaneous Approach

0DPD3DZ Removal of Intraluminal Device from Lower Intestinal Tract, Percutaneous Approach

0DPD3JZ Removal of Synthetic Substitute from Lower Intestinal Tract, Percutaneous Approach

0DPD3KZ Removal of Nonautologous Tissue Substitute from Lower Intestinal Tract, Percutaneous Approach

0DPD3UZ Removal of Feeding Device from Lower Intestinal Tract, Percutaneous Approach

0DPD3YZ Removal of Other Device from Lower Intestinal Tract, Percutaneous Approach

0DPD40Z Removal of Drainage Device from Lower Intestinal Tract, Percutaneous Endoscopic Approach

0DPD42Z Removal of Monitoring Device from Lower Intestinal Tract, Percutaneous Endoscopic Approach

0DPD43Z Removal of Infusion Device from Lower Intestinal Tract, Percutaneous Endoscopic Approach

0DPD47Z Removal of Autologous Tissue Substitute from Lower Intestinal Tract, Percutaneous Endoscopic Approach

0DPD4CZ Removal of Extraluminal Device from Lower Intestinal Tract, Percutaneous Endoscopic Approach

0DPD4DZ Removal of Intraluminal Device from Lower Intestinal Tract, Percutaneous Endoscopic Approach

0DPD4JZ Removal of Synthetic Substitute from Lower Intestinal Tract, Percutaneous Endoscopic Approach

0DPD4KZ Removal of Nonautologous Tissue Substitute from Lower Intestinal Tract, Percutaneous Endoscopic Approach

0DPD4UZ Removal of Feeding Device from Lower Intestinal Tract, Percutaneous Endoscopic Approach

0DPD4YZ Removal of Other Device from Lower Intestinal Tract, Percutaneous Endoscopic Approach

0DPD70Z Removal of Drainage Device from Lower Intestinal Tract, Via Natural or Artificial Opening

0DPD72Z Removal of Monitoring Device from Lower Intestinal Tract, Via Natural or Artificial Opening

0DPD73Z Removal of Infusion Device from Lower Intestinal Tract, Via Natural or Artificial Opening

0DPD77Z Removal of Autologous Tissue Substitute from Lower Intestinal Tract, Via Natural or Artificial Opening

0DPD7CZ Removal of Extraluminal Device from Lower Intestinal Tract, Via Natural or Artificial Opening

0DPD7DZ Removal of Intraluminal Device from Lower Intestinal Tract, Via Natural or Artificial Opening

0DPD7JZ Removal of Synthetic Substitute from Lower Intestinal Tract, Via Natural or Artificial Opening

0DPD7KZ Removal of Nonautologous Tissue Substitute from Lower Intestinal Tract, Via Natural or Artificial Opening

0DPD7UZ Removal of Feeding Device from Lower Intestinal Tract, Via Natural or Artificial Opening

0DPD7YZ Removal of Other Device from Lower Intestinal Tract, Via Natural or Artificial Opening

0DPD80Z Removal of Drainage Device from Lower Intestinal Tract, Via Natural or Artificial Opening Endoscopic

0DPD82Z Removal of Monitoring Device from Lower Intestinal Tract, Via Natural or Artificial Opening Endoscopic

0DPD83Z Removal of Infusion Device from Lower Intestinal Tract, Via Natural or Artificial Opening Endoscopic

0DPD87Z Removal of Autologous Tissue Substitute from Lower Intestinal Tract, Via Natural or Artificial Opening Endoscopic

0DPD8CZ Removal of Extraluminal Device from Lower Intestinal Tract, Via Natural or Artificial Opening Endoscopic

0DPD8DZ Removal of Intraluminal Device from Lower Intestinal Tract, Via Natural or Artificial Opening Endoscopic

0DPD8JZ Removal of Synthetic Substitute from Lower Intestinal Tract, Via Natural or Artificial Opening Endoscopic

0DPD8KZ Removal of Nonautologous Tissue Substitute from Lower Intestinal Tract, Via Natural or Artificial Opening Endoscopic

0DPD8UZ Removal of Feeding Device from Lower Intestinal Tract, Via Natural or Artificial Opening Endoscopic

0DPD8YZ Removal of Other Device from Lower Intestinal Tract, Via Natural or Artificial Opening Endoscopic

0DPDX0Z Removal of Drainage Device from Lower Intestinal Tract, External Approach

0DPDX2Z Removal of Monitoring Device from Lower Intestinal Tract, External Approach

0DPDX3Z Removal of Infusion Device from Lower Intestinal Tract, External Approach

0DPDXDZ Removal of Intraluminal Device from Lower Intestinal Tract, External Approach

0DPDXUZ Removal of Feeding Device from Lower Intestinal Tract, External Approach

0DPP01Z Removal of Radioactive Element from Rectum, Open Approach

0DPP31Z Removal of Radioactive Element from Rectum, Percutaneous Approach

0DPP41Z Removal of Radioactive Element from Rectum, Percutaneous Endoscopic Approach

0DPP71Z Removal of Radioactive Element from Rectum, Via Natural or Artificial Opening

0DPP81Z Removal of Radioactive Element from Rectum, Via Natural or Artificial Opening Endoscopic

0DPPX1Z Removal of Radioactive Element from Rectum, External Approach

0DPQ0LZ Removal of Artificial Sphincter from Anus, Open Approach

0DPQ3LZ Removal of Artificial Sphincter from Anus, Percutaneous Approach

0DPQ4LZ Removal of Artificial Sphincter from Anus, Percutaneous Endoscopic Approach

0DPQ7LZ Removal of Artificial Sphincter from Anus, Via Natural or Artificial Opening

0DPQ8LZ Removal of Artificial Sphincter from Anus, Via Natural or Artificial Opening Endoscopic

0DPR0MZ Removal of Stimulator Lead from Anal Sphincter, Open Approach

0DPR3MZ Removal of Stimulator Lead from Anal Sphincter, Percutaneous Approach

0DPR4MZ Removal of Stimulator Lead from Anal Sphincter, Percutaneous Endoscopic Approach

0DPU00Z Removal of Drainage Device from Omentum, Open Approach

0DPU01Z Removal of Radioactive Element from Omentum, Open Approach

0DPU07Z Removal of Autologous Tissue Substitute from Omentum, Open Approach

0DPU0JZ Removal of Synthetic Substitute from Omentum, Open Approach

0DPU0KZ Removal of Nonautologous Tissue Substitute from Omentum, Open Approach

0DPU30Z Removal of Drainage Device from Omentum, Percutaneous Approach

0DPU31Z Removal of Radioactive Element from Omentum, Percutaneous Approach

0DPU37Z Removal of Autologous Tissue Substitute from Omentum, Percutaneous Approach

0DPU3JZ Removal of Synthetic Substitute from Omentum, Percutaneous Approach

0DPU3KZ Removal of Nonautologous Tissue Substitute from Omentum, Percutaneous Approach

0DPU40Z Removal of Drainage Device from Omentum, Percutaneous Endoscopic Approach

0DPU41Z Removal of Radioactive Element from Omentum, Percutaneous Endoscopic Approach

0DPU47Z Removal of Autologous Tissue Substitute from Omentum, Percutaneous Endoscopic Approach

0DPU4JZ Removal of Synthetic Substitute from Omentum, Percutaneous Endoscopic Approach

0DPU4KZ Removal of Nonautologous Tissue Substitute from Omentum, Percutaneous Endoscopic Approach

0DPV00Z Removal of Drainage Device from Mesentery, Open Approach

0DPV01Z Removal of Radioactive Element from Mesentery, Open Approach

0DPV07Z Removal of Autologous Tissue Substitute from Mesentery, Open Approach

0DPV0JZ Removal of Synthetic Substitute from Mesentery, Open Approach

0DPV0KZ Removal of Nonautologous Tissue Substitute from Mesentery, Open Approach

0DPV30Z Removal of Drainage Device from Mesentery, Percutaneous Approach

0DPV31Z Removal of Radioactive Element from Mesentery, Percutaneous Approach

0DPV37Z Removal of Autologous Tissue Substitute from Mesentery, Percutaneous Approach

0DPV3JZ Removal of Synthetic Substitute from Mesentery, Percutaneous Approach

0DPV3KZ Removal of Nonautologous Tissue Substitute from Mesentery, Percutaneous Approach

0DPV40Z Removal of Drainage Device from Mesentery, Percutaneous Endoscopic Approach

0DPV41Z Removal of Radioactive Element from Mesentery, Percutaneous Endoscopic Approach

0DPV47Z Removal of Autologous Tissue Substitute from Mesentery, Percutaneous Endoscopic Approach

0DPV4JZ Removal of Synthetic Substitute from Mesentery, Percutaneous Endoscopic Approach

0DPV4KZ Removal of Nonautologous Tissue Substitute from Mesentery, Percutaneous Endoscopic Approach

0DPW00Z Removal of Drainage Device from Peritoneum, Open Approach

0DPW01Z Removal of Radioactive Element from Peritoneum, Open Approach

0DPW07Z Removal of Autologous Tissue Substitute from Peritoneum, Open Approach

0DPW0JZ Removal of Synthetic Substitute from Peritoneum, Open Approach

0DPW0KZ Removal of Nonautologous Tissue Substitute from Peritoneum, Open Approach

0DPW30Z Removal of Drainage Device from Peritoneum, Percutaneous Approach

0DPW31Z Removal of Radioactive Element from Peritoneum, Percutaneous Approach

0DPW37Z Removal of Autologous Tissue Substitute from Peritoneum, Percutaneous Approach

0DPW3JZ Removal of Synthetic Substitute from Peritoneum, Percutaneous Approach

0DPW3KZ Removal of Nonautologous Tissue Substitute from Peritoneum, Percutaneous Approach

0DPW40Z Removal of Drainage Device from Peritoneum, Percutaneous Endoscopic Approach

0DPW41Z Removal of Radioactive Element from Peritoneum, Percutaneous Endoscopic Approach

0DPW47Z Removal of Autologous Tissue Substitute from Peritoneum, Percutaneous Endoscopic Approach

0DPW4JZ Removal of Synthetic Substitute from Peritoneum, Percutaneous Endoscopic Approach

0DPW4KZ Removal of Nonautologous Tissue Substitute from Peritoneum, Percutaneous Endoscopic Approach

0DQ – Gastrointestinal System, Repair

0DQ10ZZ Repair Upper Esophagus, Open Approach

0DQ13ZZ Repair Upper Esophagus, Percutaneous Approach

0DQ14ZZ Repair Upper Esophagus, Percutaneous Endoscopic Approach

0DQ17ZZ Repair Upper Esophagus, Via Natural or Artificial Opening

0DQ18ZZ Repair Upper Esophagus, Via Natural or Artificial Opening Endoscopic

0DQ20ZZ Repair Middle Esophagus, Open Approach

0DQ23ZZ Repair Middle Esophagus, Percutaneous Approach

0DQ24ZZ Repair Middle Esophagus, Percutaneous Endoscopic Approach

0DQ27ZZ Repair Middle Esophagus, Via Natural or Artificial Opening

0DQ28ZZ Repair Middle Esophagus, Via Natural or Artificial Opening Endoscopic

0DQ30ZZ Repair Lower Esophagus, Open Approach

0DQ33ZZ Repair Lower Esophagus, Percutaneous Approach

0DQ34ZZ Repair Lower Esophagus, Percutaneous Endoscopic Approach

0DQ37ZZ Repair Lower Esophagus, Via Natural or Artificial Opening

0DQ38ZZ Repair Lower Esophagus, Via Natural or Artificial Opening Endoscopic

0DQ40ZZ Repair Esophagogastric Junction, Open Approach

0DQ43ZZ Repair Esophagogastric Junction, Percutaneous Approach

0DQ44ZZ Repair Esophagogastric Junction, Percutaneous Endoscopic Approach

0DQ47ZZ Repair Esophagogastric Junction, Via Natural or Artificial Opening

0DQ48ZZ Repair Esophagogastric Junction, Via Natural or Artificial Opening Endoscopic

0DQ50ZZ Repair Esophagus, Open Approach

0DQ53ZZ Repair Esophagus, Percutaneous Approach

0DQ54ZZ Repair Esophagus, Percutaneous Endoscopic Approach

0DQ57ZZ Repair Esophagus, Via Natural or Artificial Opening

0DQ58ZZ Repair Esophagus, Via Natural or Artificial Opening Endoscopic

0DQ60ZZ Repair Stomach, Open Approach

0DQ63ZZ Repair Stomach, Percutaneous Approach

0DQ64ZZ Repair Stomach, Percutaneous Endoscopic Approach

AHA CC: 2Q, 2019, 15-16

0DQ67ZZ Repair Stomach, Via Natural or Artificial Opening

0DQ68ZZ Repair Stomach, Via Natural or Artificial Opening Endoscopic

0DQ70ZZ Repair Stomach, Pylorus, Open Approach

0DQ73ZZ Repair Stomach, Pylorus, Percutaneous Approach

0DQ74ZZ Repair Stomach, Pylorus, Percutaneous Endoscopic Approach

0DQ77ZZ Repair Stomach, Pylorus, Via Natural or Artificial Opening

0DQ78ZZ Repair Stomach, Pylorus, Via Natural or Artificial Opening Endoscopic

0DQ80ZZ Repair Small Intestine, Open Approach
➕ Ileostomy takedown when performed with code 0WQFXZ2, Repair of abdominal wall, stoma, external approach.

0DQ83ZZ Repair Small Intestine, Percutaneous Approach

0DQ84ZZ Repair Small Intestine, Percutaneous Endoscopic Approach

0DQ87ZZ Repair Small Intestine, Via Natural or Artificial Opening

0DQ88ZZ Repair Small Intestine, Via Natural or Artificial Opening Endoscopic

0DQ90ZZ Repair Duodenum, Open Approach
➕ Duodenostomy takedown when performed with code 0WQFXZ2, Repair of abdominal wall, stoma, external approach.

0DQ93ZZ Repair Duodenum, Percutaneous Approach

0DQ94ZZ Repair Duodenum, Percutaneous Endoscopic Approach

0DQ97ZZ Repair Duodenum, Via Natural or Artificial Opening

0DQ98ZZ Repair Duodenum, Via Natural or Artificial Opening Endoscopic

AHA CC: 4Q, 2014, 20

0DQA0ZZ Repair Jejunum, Open Approach
➕ Jejunostomy takedown when performed with code 0WQFXZ2, Repair of abdominal wall, stoma, external approach.

0DQA3ZZ Repair Jejunum, Percutaneous Approach

0DQA4ZZ Repair Jejunum, Percutaneous Endoscopic Approach

0DQA7ZZ Repair Jejunum, Via Natural or Artificial Opening

0DQA8ZZ Repair Jejunum, Via Natural or Artificial Opening Endoscopic

0DQB0ZZ Repair Ileum, Open Approach
➕ Ileostomy takedown when performed with code 0WQFXZ2, Repair of abdominal wall, stoma, external approach.

0DQB3ZZ Repair Ileum, Percutaneous Approach

0DQB4ZZ Repair Ileum, Percutaneous Endoscopic Approach

0DQB7ZZ Repair Ileum, Via Natural or Artificial Opening

0DQB8ZZ Repair Ileum, Via Natural or Artificial Opening Endoscopic

0DQC0ZZ Repair Ileocecal Valve, Open Approach

0DQC3ZZ Repair Ileocecal Valve, Percutaneous Approach

0DQC4ZZ Repair Ileocecal Valve, Percutaneous Endoscopic Approach

0DQC7ZZ Repair Ileocecal Valve, Via Natural or Artificial Opening

♀ Female-only   ♂ Male-only   ▲ Limited Coverage   ● Non-OR   HAC HAC-associated procedure   ▲ Non-covered procedures   ➕ Cluster

0DQC8ZZ	Repair Ileocecal Valve, Via Natural or Artificial Opening Endoscopic	
0DQE0ZZ	Repair Large Intestine, Open Approach	
⊞	Colostomy takedown when performed with code 0WQFXZ2, Repair of abdominal wall, stoma, external approach.	
0DQE3ZZ	Repair Large Intestine, Percutaneous Approach	
0DQE4ZZ	Repair Large Intestine, Percutaneous Endoscopic Approach	
0DQE7ZZ	Repair Large Intestine, Via Natural or Artificial Opening	
0DQE8ZZ	Repair Large Intestine, Via Natural or Artificial Opening Endoscopic	
0DQF0ZZ	Repair Right Large Intestine, Open Approach	
⊞	Colostomy takedown when performed with code 0WQFXZ2, Repair of abdominal wall, stoma, external approach.	
0DQF3ZZ	Repair Right Large Intestine, Percutaneous Approach	
0DQF4ZZ	Repair Right Large Intestine, Percutaneous Endoscopic Approach	
0DQF7ZZ	Repair Right Large Intestine, Via Natural or Artificial Opening	
0DQF8ZZ	Repair Right Large Intestine, Via Natural or Artificial Opening Endoscopic	
0DQG0ZZ	Repair Left Large Intestine, Open Approach	
⊞	Colostomy takedown when performed with code 0WQFXZ2, Repair of abdominal wall, stoma, external approach.	
0DQG3ZZ	Repair Left Large Intestine, Percutaneous Approach	
0DQG4ZZ	Repair Left Large Intestine, Percutaneous Endoscopic Approach	
0DQG7ZZ	Repair Left Large Intestine, Via Natural or Artificial Opening	
0DQG8ZZ	Repair Left Large Intestine, Via Natural or Artificial Opening Endoscopic	
0DQH0ZZ	Repair Cecum, Open Approach	
⊞	Cecostomy takedown when performed with code 0WQFXZ2, Repair of abdominal wall, stoma, external approach.	
0DQH3ZZ	Repair Cecum, Percutaneous Approach	
0DQH4ZZ	Repair Cecum, Percutaneous Endoscopic Approach	
0DQH7ZZ	Repair Cecum, Via Natural or Artificial Opening	

0DQH8ZZ	Repair Cecum, Via Natural or Artificial Opening Endoscopic
0DQJ0ZZ	Repair Appendix, Open Approach
0DQJ3ZZ	Repair Appendix, Percutaneous Approach
0DQJ4ZZ	Repair Appendix, Percutaneous Endoscopic Approach
0DQJ7ZZ	Repair Appendix, Via Natural or Artificial Opening
0DQJ8ZZ	Repair Appendix, Via Natural or Artificial Opening Endoscopic
0DQK0ZZ	Repair Ascending Colon, Open Approach
⊞	Colostomy takedown when performed with code 0WQFXZ2, Repair of abdominal wall, stoma, external approach.
0DQK3ZZ	Repair Ascending Colon, Percutaneous Approach
0DQK4ZZ	Repair Ascending Colon, Percutaneous Endoscopic Approach
0DQK7ZZ	Repair Ascending Colon, Via Natural or Artificial Opening
0DQK8ZZ	Repair Ascending Colon, Via Natural or Artificial Opening Endoscopic
0DQL0ZZ	Repair Transverse Colon, Open Approach
⊞	Colostomy takedown when performed with code 0WQFXZ2, Repair of abdominal wall, stoma, external approach.
0DQL3ZZ	Repair Transverse Colon, Percutaneous Approach
0DQL4ZZ	Repair Transverse Colon, Percutaneous Endoscopic Approach
0DQL7ZZ	Repair Transverse Colon, Via Natural or Artificial Opening
0DQL8ZZ	Repair Transverse Colon, Via Natural or Artificial Opening Endoscopic
0DQM0ZZ	Repair Descending Colon, Open Approach
⊞	Colostomy takedown when performed with code 0WQFXZ2, Repair of abdominal wall, stoma, external approach.
0DQM3ZZ	Repair Descending Colon, Percutaneous Approach
0DQM4ZZ	Repair Descending Colon, Percutaneous Endoscopic Approach
0DQM7ZZ	Repair Descending Colon, Via Natural or Artificial Opening
0DQM8ZZ	Repair Descending Colon, Via Natural or Artificial Opening Endoscopic
0DQN0ZZ	Repair Sigmoid Colon, Open Approach
⊞	Colostomy takedown when performed with code 0WQFXZ2, Repair of

	abdominal wall, stoma, external approach.
0DQN3ZZ	Repair Sigmoid Colon, Percutaneous Approach
0DQN4ZZ	Repair Sigmoid Colon, Percutaneous Endoscopic Approach
0DQN7ZZ	Repair Sigmoid Colon, Via Natural or Artificial Opening
0DQN8ZZ	Repair Sigmoid Colon, Via Natural or Artificial Opening Endoscopic
0DQP0ZZ	Repair Rectum, Open Approach
	AHA CC: 1Q, 2016, 7-8
0DQP3ZZ	Repair Rectum, Percutaneous Approach
0DQP4ZZ	Repair Rectum, Percutaneous Endoscopic Approach
0DQP7ZZ	Repair Rectum, Via Natural or Artificial Opening
0DQP8ZZ	Repair Rectum, Via Natural or Artificial Opening Endoscopic
0DQQ0ZZ	Repair Anus, Open Approach
0DQQ3ZZ	Repair Anus, Percutaneous Approach
0DQQ4ZZ	Repair Anus, Percutaneous Endoscopic Approach
0DQQ7ZZ	Repair Anus, Via Natural or Artificial Opening
0DQQ8ZZ	Repair Anus, Via Natural or Artificial Opening Endoscopic
0DQQXZZ	Repair Anus, External Approach
0DQR0ZZ	Repair Anal Sphincter, Open Approach
	AHA CC: 1Q, 2016, 7-8
0DQR3ZZ	Repair Anal Sphincter, Percutaneous Approach
0DQR4ZZ	Repair Anal Sphincter, Percutaneous Endoscopic Approach
0DQU0ZZ	Repair Omentum, Open Approach
0DQU3ZZ	Repair Omentum, Percutaneous Approach
0DQU4ZZ	Repair Omentum, Percutaneous Endoscopic Approach
0DQV0ZZ	Repair Mesentery, Open Approach
0DQV3ZZ	Repair Mesentery, Percutaneous Approach
0DQV4ZZ	Repair Mesentery, Percutaneous Endoscopic Approach
	AHA CC: 1Q, 2018, 11-12
0DQW0ZZ	Repair Peritoneum, Open Approach
0DQW3ZZ	Repair Peritoneum, Percutaneous Approach
0DQW4ZZ	Repair Peritoneum, Percutaneous Endoscopic Approach

0DR – Gastrointestinal System, Replacement

Review Coding Guideline B3.18

0DR507Z	Replacement of Esophagus with Autologous Tissue Substitute, Open Approach
0DR50JZ	Replacement of Esophagus with Synthetic Substitute, Open Approach
0DR50KZ	Replacement of Esophagus with Nonautologous Tissue Substitute, Open Approach
0DR547Z	Replacement of Esophagus with Autologous Tissue Substitute, Percutaneous Endoscopic Approach
0DR54JZ	Replacement of Esophagus with Synthetic Substitute, Percutaneous Endoscopic Approach

0DR54KZ	Replacement of Esophagus with Nonautologous Tissue Substitute, Percutaneous Endoscopic Approach
0DR577Z	Replacement of Esophagus with Autologous Tissue Substitute, Via Natural or Artificial Opening
0DR57JZ	Replacement of Esophagus with Synthetic Substitute, Via Natural or Artificial Opening
0DR57KZ	Replacement of Esophagus with Nonautologous Tissue Substitute, Via Natural or Artificial Opening
0DR587Z	Replacement of Esophagus with Autologous Tissue Substitute,

	Via Natural or Artificial Opening Endoscopic
0DR58JZ	Replacement of Esophagus with Synthetic Substitute, Via Natural or Artificial Opening Endoscopic
0DR58KZ	Replacement of Esophagus with Nonautologous Tissue Substitute, Via Natural or Artificial Opening Endoscopic
0DRR07Z	Replacement of Anal Sphincter with Autologous Tissue Substitute, Open Approach
0DRR0JZ	Replacement of Anal Sphincter with Synthetic Substitute, Open Approach

0DRR0KZ Replacement of Anal Sphincter with Nonautologous Tissue Substitute, Open Approach

0DRR47Z Replacement of Anal Sphincter with Autologous Tissue Substitute, Percutaneous Endoscopic Approach

0DRR4JZ Replacement of Anal Sphincter with Synthetic Substitute, Percutaneous Endoscopic Approach

0DRR4KZ Replacement of Anal Sphincter with Nonautologous Tissue Substitute, Percutaneous Endoscopic Approach

0DRU07Z Replacement of Omentum with Autologous Tissue Substitute, Open Approach

0DRU0JZ Replacement of Omentum with Synthetic Substitute, Open Approach

0DRU0KZ Replacement of Omentum with Nonautologous Tissue Substitute, Open Approach

0DRU47Z Replacement of Omentum with Autologous Tissue Substitute, Percutaneous Endoscopic Approach

0DRU4JZ Replacement of Omentum with Synthetic Substitute, Percutaneous Endoscopic Approach

0DRU4KZ Replacement of Omentum with Nonautologous Tissue Substitute, Percutaneous Endoscopic Approach

0DRV07Z Replacement of Mesentery with Autologous Tissue Substitute, Open Approach

0DRV0JZ Replacement of Mesentery with Synthetic Substitute, Open Approach

0DRV0KZ Replacement of Mesentery with Nonautologous Tissue Substitute, Open Approach

0DRV47Z Replacement of Mesentery with Autologous Tissue Substitute, Percutaneous Endoscopic Approach

0DRV4JZ Replacement of Mesentery with Synthetic Substitute, Percutaneous Endoscopic Approach

0DRV4KZ Replacement of Mesentery with Nonautologous Tissue Substitute, Percutaneous Endoscopic Approach

0DRW07Z Replacement of Peritoneum with Autologous Tissue Substitute, Open Approach

0DRW0JZ Replacement of Peritoneum with Synthetic Substitute, Open Approach

0DRW0KZ Replacement of Peritoneum with Nonautologous Tissue Substitute, Open Approach

0DRW47Z Replacement of Peritoneum with Autologous Tissue Substitute, Percutaneous Endoscopic Approach

0DRW4JZ Replacement of Peritoneum with Synthetic Substitute, Percutaneous Endoscopic Approach

0DRW4KZ Replacement of Peritoneum with Nonautologous Tissue Substitute, Percutaneous Endoscopic Approach

0DS – Gastrointestinal System, Reposition

0DS50ZZ Reposition Esophagus, Open Approach

0DS54ZZ Reposition Esophagus, Percutaneous Endoscopic Approach

0DS57ZZ Reposition Esophagus, Via Natural or Artificial Opening

0DS58ZZ Reposition Esophagus, Via Natural or Artificial Opening Endoscopic

0DS5XZZ Reposition Esophagus, External Approach

0DS60ZZ Reposition Stomach, Open Approach

0DS64ZZ Reposition Stomach, Percutaneous Endoscopic Approach

0DS67ZZ Reposition Stomach, Via Natural or Artificial Opening

0DS68ZZ Reposition Stomach, Via Natural or Artificial Opening Endoscopic

0DS6XZZ Reposition Stomach, External Approach

0DS80ZZ Reposition Small Intestine, Open Approach
AHA CC: 4Q, 2017, 49-50

0DS84ZZ Reposition Small Intestine, Percutaneous Endoscopic Approach

0DS87ZZ Reposition Small Intestine, Via Natural or Artificial Opening

0DS88ZZ Reposition Small Intestine, Via Natural or Artificial Opening Endoscopic

0DS90ZZ Reposition Duodenum, Open Approach

0DS94ZZ Reposition Duodenum, Percutaneous Endoscopic Approach

0DS97ZZ Reposition Duodenum, Via Natural or Artificial Opening

0DS98ZZ Reposition Duodenum, Via Natural or Artificial Opening Endoscopic

0DS9XZZ Reposition Duodenum, External Approach

0DSA0ZZ Reposition Jejunum, Open Approach

0DSA4ZZ Reposition Jejunum, Percutaneous Endoscopic Approach

0DSA7ZZ Reposition Jejunum, Via Natural or Artificial Opening

0DSA8ZZ Reposition Jejunum, Via Natural or Artificial Opening Endoscopic

0DSAXZZ Reposition Jejunum, External Approach

0DSB0ZZ Reposition Ileum, Open Approach

0DSB4ZZ Reposition Ileum, Percutaneous Endoscopic Approach

0DSB7ZZ Reposition Ileum, Via Natural or Artificial Opening
AHA CC: 3Q, 2017, 9-10

0DSB8ZZ Reposition Ileum, Via Natural or Artificial Opening Endoscopic

0DSBXZZ Reposition Ileum, External Approach

0DSE0ZZ Reposition Large Intestine, Open Approach
AHA CC: 4Q, 2017, 49-50

0DSE4ZZ Reposition Large Intestine, Percutaneous Endoscopic Approach

0DSE7ZZ Reposition Large Intestine, Via Natural or Artificial Opening

0DSE8ZZ Reposition Large Intestine, Via Natural or Artificial Opening Endoscopic

0DSH0ZZ Reposition Cecum, Open Approach

0DSH4ZZ Reposition Cecum, Percutaneous Endoscopic Approach

0DSH7ZZ Reposition Cecum, Via Natural or Artificial Opening

0DSH8ZZ Reposition Cecum, Via Natural or Artificial Opening Endoscopic

0DSHXZZ Reposition Cecum, External Approach

0DSK0ZZ Reposition Ascending Colon, Open Approach

0DSK4ZZ Reposition Ascending Colon, Percutaneous Endoscopic Approach

0DSK7ZZ Reposition Ascending Colon, Via Natural or Artificial Opening
AHA CC: 3Q, 2017, 9-10

0DSK8ZZ Reposition Ascending Colon, Via Natural or Artificial Opening Endoscopic

0DSKXZZ Reposition Ascending Colon, External Approach

0DSL0ZZ Reposition Transverse Colon, Open Approach

0DSL4ZZ Reposition Transverse Colon, Percutaneous Endoscopic Approach

0DSL7ZZ Reposition Transverse Colon, Via Natural or Artificial Opening

0DSL8ZZ Reposition Transverse Colon, Via Natural or Artificial Opening Endoscopic

0DSLXZZ Reposition Transverse Colon, External Approach

0DSM0ZZ Reposition Descending Colon, Open Approach

0DSM4ZZ Reposition Descending Colon, Percutaneous Endoscopic Approach
AHA CC: 3Q, 2016, 5-6

0DSM7ZZ Reposition Descending Colon, Via Natural or Artificial Opening

0DSM8ZZ Reposition Descending Colon, Via Natural or Artificial Opening Endoscopic

0DSMXZZ Reposition Descending Colon, External Approach

0DSN0ZZ Reposition Sigmoid Colon, Open Approach

0DSN4ZZ Reposition Sigmoid Colon, Percutaneous Endoscopic Approach

0DSN7ZZ Reposition Sigmoid Colon, Via Natural or Artificial Opening

0DSN8ZZ Reposition Sigmoid Colon, Via Natural or Artificial Opening Endoscopic

0DSNXZZ Reposition Sigmoid Colon, External Approach

0DSP0ZZ Reposition Rectum, Open Approach
AHA CC: 3Q, 2017, 17-18; 1Q, 2019, 30-31

0DSP4ZZ Reposition Rectum, Percutaneous Endoscopic Approach

0DSP7ZZ Reposition Rectum, Via Natural or Artificial Opening

0DSP8ZZ Reposition Rectum, Via Natural or Artificial Opening Endoscopic

0DSPXZZ Reposition Rectum, External Approach

0DSQ0ZZ Reposition Anus, Open Approach

0DSQ4ZZ Reposition Anus, Percutaneous Endoscopic Approach

0DSQ7ZZ Reposition Anus, Via Natural or Artificial Opening

0DSQ8ZZ Reposition Anus, Via Natural or Artificial Opening Endoscopic

0DSQXZZ Reposition Anus, External Approach

♀ Female-only   ♂ Male-only   ▲ Limited Coverage   ● Non-OR   ■ HAC-associated procedure   ▲ Non-covered procedures   ✚ Cluster

Review Coding Guideline B3.8

Review Coding Guideline B3.18

0DT10ZZ Resection of Upper Esophagus, Open Approach

0DT14ZZ Resection of Upper Esophagus, Percutaneous Endoscopic Approach

0DT17ZZ Resection of Upper Esophagus, Via Natural or Artificial Opening

0DT18ZZ Resection of Upper Esophagus, Via Natural or Artificial Opening Endoscopic

0DT20ZZ Resection of Middle Esophagus, Open Approach

0DT24ZZ Resection of Middle Esophagus, Percutaneous Endoscopic Approach

0DT27ZZ Resection of Middle Esophagus, Via Natural or Artificial Opening

0DT28ZZ Resection of Middle Esophagus, Via Natural or Artificial Opening Endoscopic

0DT30ZZ Resection of Lower Esophagus, Open Approach
    AHA CC: 1Q, 2019, 14-15

0DT34ZZ Resection of Lower Esophagus, Percutaneous Endoscopic Approach

0DT37ZZ Resection of Lower Esophagus, Via Natural or Artificial Opening

0DT38ZZ Resection of Lower Esophagus, Via Natural or Artificial Opening Endoscopic

0DT40ZZ Resection of Esophagogastric Junction, Open Approach

0DT44ZZ Resection of Esophagogastric Junction, Percutaneous Endoscopic Approach

0DT47ZZ Resection of Esophagogastric Junction, Via Natural or Artificial Opening

0DT48ZZ Resection of Esophagogastric Junction, Via Natural or Artificial Opening Endoscopic

0DT50ZZ Resection of Esophagus, Open Approach

0DT54ZZ Resection of Esophagus, Percutaneous Endoscopic Approach

0DT57ZZ Resection of Esophagus, Via Natural or Artificial Opening

0DT58ZZ Resection of Esophagus, Via Natural or Artificial Opening Endoscopic

0DT60ZZ Resection of Stomach, Open Approach

0DT64ZZ Resection of Stomach, Percutaneous Endoscopic Approach

0DT67ZZ Resection of Stomach, Via Natural or Artificial Opening

0DT68ZZ Resection of Stomach, Via Natural or Artificial Opening Endoscopic

0DT70ZZ Resection of Stomach, Pylorus, Open Approach

0DT74ZZ Resection of Stomach, Pylorus, Percutaneous Endoscopic Approach

0DT77ZZ Resection of Stomach, Pylorus, Via Natural or Artificial Opening

0DT78ZZ Resection of Stomach, Pylorus, Via Natural or Artificial Opening Endoscopic

0DT80ZZ Resection of Small Intestine, Open Approach

0DT84ZZ Resection of Small Intestine, Percutaneous Endoscopic Approach

0DT87ZZ Resection of Small Intestine, Via Natural or Artificial Opening

0DT88ZZ Resection of Small Intestine, Via Natural or Artificial Opening Endoscopic

0DT90ZZ Resection of Duodenum, Open Approach

  ✚ Pancreaticododenectomy when reported with Resection of the pancreas. *See table 0FT to construct the Resection code.*

0DT94ZZ Resection of Duodenum, Percutaneous Endoscopic Approach

0DT97ZZ Resection of Duodenum, Via Natural or Artificial Opening

0DT98ZZ Resection of Duodenum, Via Natural or Artificial Opening Endoscopic

0DTA0ZZ Resection of Jejunum, Open Approach

0DTA4ZZ Resection of Jejunum, Percutaneous Endoscopic Approach

0DTA7ZZ Resection of Jejunum, Via Natural or Artificial Opening

0DTA8ZZ Resection of Jejunum, Via Natural or Artificial Opening Endoscopic

0DTB0ZZ Resection of Ileum, Open Approach

0DTB4ZZ Resection of Ileum, Percutaneous Endoscopic Approach

0DTB7ZZ Resection of Ileum, Via Natural or Artificial Opening

0DTB8ZZ Resection of Ileum, Via Natural or Artificial Opening Endoscopic

0DTC0ZZ Resection of Ileocecal Valve, Open Approach

0DTC4ZZ Resection of Ileocecal Valve, Percutaneous Endoscopic Approach

0DTC7ZZ Resection of Ileocecal Valve, Via Natural or Artificial Opening

0DTC8ZZ Resection of Ileocecal Valve, Via Natural or Artificial Opening Endoscopic

0DTE0ZZ Resection of Large Intestine, Open Approach

0DTE4ZZ Resection of Large Intestine, Percutaneous Endoscopic Approach

0DTE7ZZ Resection of Large Intestine, Via Natural or Artificial Opening

0DTE8ZZ Resection of Large Intestine, Via Natural or Artificial Opening Endoscopic

0DTF0ZZ Resection of Right Large Intestine, Open Approach
    AHA CC: 3Q, 2014, 6-7; 4Q, 2014, 42-43

0DTF4ZZ Resection of Right Large Intestine, Percutaneous Endoscopic Approach

0DTF7ZZ Resection of Right Large Intestine, Via Natural or Artificial Opening

0DTF8ZZ Resection of Right Large Intestine, Via Natural or Artificial Opening Endoscopic

0DTG0ZZ Resection of Left Large Intestine, Open Approach

0DTG4ZZ Resection of Left Large Intestine, Percutaneous Endoscopic Approach

0DTG7ZZ Resection of Left Large Intestine, Via Natural or Artificial Opening

0DTG8ZZ Resection of Left Large Intestine, Via Natural or Artificial Opening Endoscopic

0DTGFZZ Resection of Left Large Intestine, Via Natural or Artificial Opening With Percutaneous Endoscopic Assistance

0DTH0ZZ Resection of Cecum, Open Approach
    AHA CC: 3Q, 2014, 6

0DTH4ZZ Resection of Cecum, Percutaneous Endoscopic Approach

0DTH7ZZ Resection of Cecum, Via Natural or Artificial Opening

0DTH8ZZ Resection of Cecum, Via Natural or Artificial Opening Endoscopic

0DTJ0ZZ Resection of Appendix, Open Approach
    AHA CC: 4Q, 2017, 49-50

0DTJ4ZZ Resection of Appendix, Percutaneous Endoscopic Approach

0DTJ7ZZ Resection of Appendix, Via Natural or Artificial Opening

0DTJ8ZZ Resection of Appendix, Via Natural or Artificial Opening Endoscopic

0DTK0ZZ Resection of Ascending Colon, Open Approach

0DTK4ZZ Resection of Ascending Colon, Percutaneous Endoscopic Approach

0DTK7ZZ Resection of Ascending Colon, Via Natural or Artificial Opening

0DTK8ZZ Resection of Ascending Colon, Via Natural or Artificial Opening Endoscopic

0DTL0ZZ Resection of Transverse Colon, Open Approach

0DTL4ZZ Resection of Transverse Colon, Percutaneous Endoscopic Approach

0DTL7ZZ Resection of Transverse Colon, Via Natural or Artificial Opening

0DTL8ZZ Resection of Transverse Colon, Via Natural or Artificial Opening Endoscopic

0DTLFZZ Resection of Transverse Colon, Via Natural or Artificial Opening With Percutaneous Endoscopic Assistance

0DTM0ZZ Resection of Descending Colon, Open Approach

0DTM4ZZ Resection of Descending Colon, Percutaneous Endoscopic Approach

0DTM7ZZ Resection of Descending Colon, Via Natural or Artificial Opening

0DTM8ZZ Resection of Descending Colon, Via Natural or Artificial Opening Endoscopic

0DTMFZZ Resection of Descending Colon, Via Natural or Artificial Opening With Percutaneous Endoscopic Assistance

0DTN0ZZ Resection of Sigmoid Colon, Open Approach

0DTN4ZZ Resection of Sigmoid Colon, Percutaneous Endoscopic Approach

0DTN7ZZ Resection of Sigmoid Colon, Via Natural or Artificial Opening

0DTN8ZZ Resection of Sigmoid Colon, Via Natural or Artificial Opening Endoscopic

0DTNFZZ Resection of Sigmoid Colon, Via Natural or Artificial Opening With Percutaneous Endoscopic Assistance

0DTP0ZZ Resection of Rectum, Open Approach
    AHA CC: 4Q, 2014, 40-41

0DTP4ZZ	Resection of Rectum, Percutaneous Endoscopic Approach	
0DTP7ZZ	Resection of Rectum, Via Natural or Artificial Opening	
0DTP8ZZ	Resection of Rectum, Via Natural or Artificial Opening Endoscopic	
0DTQ0ZZ	Resection of Anus, Open Approach	
	AHA CC: 4Q, 2014, 40-41	

0DTQ4ZZ Resection of Anus, Percutaneous Endoscopic Approach
0DTQ7ZZ Resection of Anus, Via Natural or Artificial Opening
0DTQ8ZZ Resection of Anus, Via Natural or Artificial Opening Endoscopic
0DTR0ZZ Resection of Anal Sphincter, Open Approach

0DTR4ZZ Resection of Anal Sphincter, Percutaneous Endoscopic Approach
0DTU0ZZ Resection of Omentum, Open Approach
0DTU4ZZ Resection of Omentum, Percutaneous Endoscopic Approach

0DU – Gastrointestinal System, Supplement

0DU107Z Supplement Upper Esophagus with Autologous Tissue Substitute, Open Approach
0DU10JZ Supplement Upper Esophagus with Synthetic Substitute, Open Approach
0DU10KZ Supplement Upper Esophagus with Nonautologous Tissue Substitute, Open Approach
0DU147Z Supplement Upper Esophagus with Autologous Tissue Substitute, Percutaneous Endoscopic Approach
0DU14JZ Supplement Upper Esophagus with Synthetic Substitute, Percutaneous Endoscopic Approach
0DU14KZ Supplement Upper Esophagus with Nonautologous Tissue Substitute, Percutaneous Endoscopic Approach
0DU177Z Supplement Upper Esophagus with Autologous Tissue Substitute, Via Natural or Artificial Opening
0DU17JZ Supplement Upper Esophagus with Synthetic Substitute, Via Natural or Artificial Opening
0DU17KZ Supplement Upper Esophagus with Nonautologous Tissue Substitute, Via Natural or Artificial Opening
0DU187Z Supplement Upper Esophagus with Autologous Tissue Substitute, Via Natural or Artificial Opening Endoscopic
0DU18JZ Supplement Upper Esophagus with Synthetic Substitute, Via Natural or Artificial Opening Endoscopic
0DU18KZ Supplement Upper Esophagus with Nonautologous Tissue Substitute, Via Natural or Artificial Opening Endoscopic
0DU207Z Supplement Middle Esophagus with Autologous Tissue Substitute, Open Approach
0DU20JZ Supplement Middle Esophagus with Synthetic Substitute, Open Approach
0DU20KZ Supplement Middle Esophagus with Nonautologous Tissue Substitute, Open Approach
0DU247Z Supplement Middle Esophagus with Autologous Tissue Substitute, Percutaneous Endoscopic Approach
0DU24JZ Supplement Middle Esophagus with Synthetic Substitute, Percutaneous Endoscopic Approach
0DU24KZ Supplement Middle Esophagus with Nonautologous Tissue Substitute, Percutaneous Endoscopic Approach
0DU277Z Supplement Middle Esophagus with Autologous Tissue Substitute, Via Natural or Artificial Opening
0DU27JZ Supplement Middle Esophagus with Synthetic Substitute, Via Natural or Artificial Opening

0DU27KZ Supplement Middle Esophagus with Nonautologous Tissue Substitute, Via Natural or Artificial Opening
0DU287Z Supplement Middle Esophagus with Autologous Tissue Substitute, Via Natural or Artificial Opening Endoscopic
0DU28JZ Supplement Middle Esophagus with Synthetic Substitute, Via Natural or Artificial Opening Endoscopic
0DU28KZ Supplement Middle Esophagus with Nonautologous Tissue Substitute, Via Natural or Artificial Opening Endoscopic
0DU307Z Supplement Lower Esophagus with Autologous Tissue Substitute, Open Approach
0DU30JZ Supplement Lower Esophagus with Synthetic Substitute, Open Approach
0DU30KZ Supplement Lower Esophagus with Nonautologous Tissue Substitute, Open Approach
0DU347Z Supplement Lower Esophagus with Autologous Tissue Substitute, Percutaneous Endoscopic Approach
0DU34JZ Supplement Lower Esophagus with Synthetic Substitute, Percutaneous Endoscopic Approach
0DU34KZ Supplement Lower Esophagus with Nonautologous Tissue Substitute, Percutaneous Endoscopic Approach
0DU377Z Supplement Lower Esophagus with Autologous Tissue Substitute, Via Natural or Artificial Opening
0DU37JZ Supplement Lower Esophagus with Synthetic Substitute, Via Natural or Artificial Opening
0DU37KZ Supplement Lower Esophagus with Nonautologous Tissue Substitute, Via Natural or Artificial Opening
0DU387Z Supplement Lower Esophagus with Autologous Tissue Substitute, Via Natural or Artificial Opening Endoscopic
0DU38JZ Supplement Lower Esophagus with Synthetic Substitute, Via Natural or Artificial Opening Endoscopic
0DU38KZ Supplement Lower Esophagus with Nonautologous Tissue Substitute, Via Natural or Artificial Opening Endoscopic
0DU407Z Supplement Esophagogastric Junction with Autologous Tissue Substitute, Open Approach
0DU40JZ Supplement Esophagogastric Junction with Synthetic Substitute, Open Approach
0DU40KZ Supplement Esophagogastric Junction with Nonautologous Tissue Substitute, Open Approach

0DU447Z Supplement Esophagogastric Junction with Autologous Tissue Substitute, Percutaneous Endoscopic Approach
0DU44JZ Supplement Esophagogastric Junction with Synthetic Substitute, Percutaneous Endoscopic Approach
0DU44KZ Supplement Esophagogastric Junction with Nonautologous Tissue Substitute, Percutaneous Endoscopic Approach
0DU477Z Supplement Esophagogastric Junction with Autologous Tissue Substitute, Via Natural or Artificial Opening
0DU47JZ Supplement Esophagogastric Junction with Synthetic Substitute, Via Natural or Artificial Opening
0DU47KZ Supplement Esophagogastric Junction with Nonautologous Tissue Substitute, Via Natural or Artificial Opening
0DU487Z Supplement Esophagogastric Junction with Autologous Tissue Substitute, Via Natural or Artificial Opening Endoscopic
0DU48JZ Supplement Esophagogastric Junction with Synthetic Substitute, Via Natural or Artificial Opening Endoscopic
0DU48KZ Supplement Esophagogastric Junction with Nonautologous Tissue Substitute, Via Natural or Artificial Opening Endoscopic
0DU507Z Supplement Esophagus with Autologous Tissue Substitute, Open Approach
0DU50JZ Supplement Esophagus with Synthetic Substitute, Open Approach
0DU50KZ Supplement Esophagus with Nonautologous Tissue Substitute, Open Approach
0DU547Z Supplement Esophagus with Autologous Tissue Substitute, Percutaneous Endoscopic Approach
0DU54JZ Supplement Esophagus with Synthetic Substitute, Percutaneous Endoscopic Approach
0DU54KZ Supplement Esophagus with Nonautologous Tissue Substitute, Percutaneous Endoscopic Approach
0DU577Z Supplement Esophagus with Autologous Tissue Substitute, Via Natural or Artificial Opening
0DU57JZ Supplement Esophagus with Synthetic Substitute, Via Natural or Artificial Opening
0DU57KZ Supplement Esophagus with Nonautologous Tissue Substitute, Via Natural or Artificial Opening
0DU587Z Supplement Esophagus with Autologous Tissue Substitute, Via Natural or Artificial Opening Endoscopic

♀ Female-only   ♂ Male-only   ▲ Limited Coverage   ● Non-OR   ⬛ HAC-associated procedure   ▲ Non-covered procedures   ✛ Cluster

0DU58JZ	Supplement Esophagus with Synthetic Substitute, Via Natural or Artificial Opening Endoscopic
0DU58KZ	Supplement Esophagus with Nonautologous Tissue Substitute, Via Natural or Artificial Opening Endoscopic
0DU607Z	Supplement Stomach with Autologous Tissue Substitute, Open Approach
0DU60JZ	Supplement Stomach with Synthetic Substitute, Open Approach
0DU60KZ	Supplement Stomach with Nonautologous Tissue Substitute, Open Approach
0DU647Z	Supplement Stomach with Autologous Tissue Substitute, Percutaneous Endoscopic Approach
0DU64JZ	Supplement Stomach with Synthetic Substitute, Percutaneous Endoscopic Approach
0DU64KZ	Supplement Stomach with Nonautologous Tissue Substitute, Percutaneous Endoscopic Approach
0DU677Z	Supplement Stomach with Autologous Tissue Substitute, Via Natural or Artificial Opening
0DU67JZ	Supplement Stomach with Synthetic Substitute, Via Natural or Artificial Opening
0DU67KZ	Supplement Stomach with Nonautologous Tissue Substitute, Via Natural or Artificial Opening
0DU687Z	Supplement Stomach with Autologous Tissue Substitute, Via Natural or Artificial Opening Endoscopic
0DU68JZ	Supplement Stomach with Synthetic Substitute, Via Natural or Artificial Opening Endoscopic
0DU68KZ	Supplement Stomach with Nonautologous Tissue Substitute, Via Natural or Artificial Opening Endoscopic
0DU707Z	Supplement Stomach, Pylorus with Autologous Tissue Substitute, Open Approach
0DU70JZ	Supplement Stomach, Pylorus with Synthetic Substitute, Open Approach
0DU70KZ	Supplement Stomach, Pylorus with Nonautologous Tissue Substitute, Open Approach
0DU747Z	Supplement Stomach, Pylorus with Autologous Tissue Substitute, Percutaneous Endoscopic Approach
0DU74JZ	Supplement Stomach, Pylorus with Synthetic Substitute, Percutaneous Endoscopic Approach
0DU74KZ	Supplement Stomach, Pylorus with Nonautologous Tissue Substitute, Percutaneous Endoscopic Approach
0DU777Z	Supplement Stomach, Pylorus with Autologous Tissue Substitute, Via Natural or Artificial Opening
0DU77JZ	Supplement Stomach, Pylorus with Synthetic Substitute, Via Natural or Artificial Opening
0DU77KZ	Supplement Stomach, Pylorus with Nonautologous Tissue Substitute, Via Natural or Artificial Opening
0DU787Z	Supplement Stomach, Pylorus with Autologous Tissue Substitute, Via Natural or Artificial Opening Endoscopic

0DU78JZ	Supplement Stomach, Pylorus with Synthetic Substitute, Via Natural or Artificial Opening Endoscopic
0DU78KZ	Supplement Stomach, Pylorus with Nonautologous Tissue Substitute, Via Natural or Artificial Opening Endoscopic
0DU807Z	Supplement Small Intestine with Autologous Tissue Substitute, Open Approach
0DU80JZ	Supplement Small Intestine with Synthetic Substitute, Open Approach
0DU80KZ	Supplement Small Intestine with Nonautologous Tissue Substitute, Open Approach
0DU847Z	Supplement Small Intestine with Autologous Tissue Substitute, Percutaneous Endoscopic Approach
0DU84JZ	Supplement Small Intestine with Synthetic Substitute, Percutaneous Endoscopic Approach
0DU84KZ	Supplement Small Intestine with Nonautologous Tissue Substitute, Percutaneous Endoscopic Approach
0DU877Z	Supplement Small Intestine with Autologous Tissue Substitute, Via Natural or Artificial Opening
0DU87JZ	Supplement Small Intestine with Synthetic Substitute, Via Natural or Artificial Opening
0DU87KZ	Supplement Small Intestine with Nonautologous Tissue Substitute, Via Natural or Artificial Opening
0DU887Z	Supplement Small Intestine with Autologous Tissue Substitute, Via Natural or Artificial Opening Endoscopic
0DU88JZ	Supplement Small Intestine with Synthetic Substitute, Via Natural or Artificial Opening Endoscopic
0DU88KZ	Supplement Small Intestine with Nonautologous Tissue Substitute, Via Natural or Artificial Opening Endoscopic
0DU907Z	Supplement Duodenum with Autologous Tissue Substitute, Open Approach
0DU90JZ	Supplement Duodenum with Synthetic Substitute, Open Approach
0DU90KZ	Supplement Duodenum with Nonautologous Tissue Substitute, Open Approach
0DU947Z	Supplement Duodenum with Autologous Tissue Substitute, Percutaneous Endoscopic Approach
0DU94JZ	Supplement Duodenum with Synthetic Substitute, Percutaneous Endoscopic Approach
0DU94KZ	Supplement Duodenum with Nonautologous Tissue Substitute, Percutaneous Endoscopic Approach
0DU977Z	Supplement Duodenum with Autologous Tissue Substitute, Via Natural or Artificial Opening
0DU97JZ	Supplement Duodenum with Synthetic Substitute, Via Natural or Artificial Opening
0DU97KZ	Supplement Duodenum with Nonautologous Tissue Substitute, Via Natural or Artificial Opening
0DU987Z	Supplement Duodenum with Autologous Tissue Substitute, Via Natural or Artificial Opening Endoscopic

0DU98JZ	Supplement Duodenum with Synthetic Substitute, Via Natural or Artificial Opening Endoscopic
0DU98KZ	Supplement Duodenum with Nonautologous Tissue Substitute, Via Natural or Artificial Opening Endoscopic
0DUA07Z	Supplement Jejunum with Autologous Tissue Substitute, Open Approach
0DUA0JZ	Supplement Jejunum with Synthetic Substitute, Open Approach
0DUA0KZ	Supplement Jejunum with Nonautologous Tissue Substitute, Open Approach
0DUA47Z	Supplement Jejunum with Autologous Tissue Substitute, Percutaneous Endoscopic Approach
0DUA4JZ	Supplement Jejunum with Synthetic Substitute, Percutaneous Endoscopic Approach
0DUA4KZ	Supplement Jejunum with Nonautologous Tissue Substitute, Percutaneous Endoscopic Approach
0DUA77Z	Supplement Jejunum with Autologous Tissue Substitute, Via Natural or Artificial Opening
0DUA7JZ	Supplement Jejunum with Synthetic Substitute, Via Natural or Artificial Opening
0DUA7KZ	Supplement Jejunum with Nonautologous Tissue Substitute, Via Natural or Artificial Opening
0DUA87Z	Supplement Jejunum with Autologous Tissue Substitute, Via Natural or Artificial Opening Endoscopic
0DUA8JZ	Supplement Jejunum with Synthetic Substitute, Via Natural or Artificial Opening Endoscopic
0DUA8KZ	Supplement Jejunum with Nonautologous Tissue Substitute, Via Natural or Artificial Opening Endoscopic
0DUB07Z	Supplement Ileum with Autologous Tissue Substitute, Open Approach
0DUB0JZ	Supplement Ileum with Synthetic Substitute, Open Approach
0DUB0KZ	Supplement Ileum with Nonautologous Tissue Substitute, Open Approach
0DUB47Z	Supplement Ileum with Autologous Tissue Substitute, Percutaneous Endoscopic Approach
0DUB4JZ	Supplement Ileum with Synthetic Substitute, Percutaneous Endoscopic Approach
0DUB4KZ	Supplement Ileum with Nonautologous Tissue Substitute, Percutaneous Endoscopic Approach
0DUB77Z	Supplement Ileum with Autologous Tissue Substitute, Via Natural or Artificial Opening
0DUB7JZ	Supplement Ileum with Synthetic Substitute, Via Natural or Artificial Opening
0DUB7KZ	Supplement Ileum with Nonautologous Tissue Substitute, Via Natural or Artificial Opening
0DUB87Z	Supplement Ileum with Autologous Tissue Substitute, Via Natural or Artificial Opening Endoscopic
0DUB8JZ	Supplement Ileum with Synthetic Substitute, Via Natural or Artificial Opening Endoscopic

♀ Female-only   ♂ Male-only   ▲ Limited Coverage   ● Non-OR   ᴴᴬᶜ HAC-associated procedure   ▲ Non-covered procedures   ✚ Cluster

0DUB8KZ Supplement Ileum with Nonautologous Tissue Substitute, Via Natural or Artificial Opening Endoscopic

0DUC07Z Supplement Ileocecal Valve with Autologous Tissue Substitute, Open Approach

0DUC0JZ Supplement Ileocecal Valve with Synthetic Substitute, Open Approach

0DUC0KZ Supplement Ileocecal Valve with Nonautologous Tissue Substitute, Open Approach

0DUC47Z Supplement Ileocecal Valve with Autologous Tissue Substitute, Percutaneous Endoscopic Approach

0DUC4JZ Supplement Ileocecal Valve with Synthetic Substitute, Percutaneous Endoscopic Approach

0DUC4KZ Supplement Ileocecal Valve with Nonautologous Tissue Substitute, Percutaneous Endoscopic Approach

0DUC77Z Supplement Ileocecal Valve with Autologous Tissue Substitute, Via Natural or Artificial Opening

0DUC7JZ Supplement Ileocecal Valve with Synthetic Substitute, Via Natural or Artificial Opening

0DUC7KZ Supplement Ileocecal Valve with Nonautologous Tissue Substitute, Via Natural or Artificial Opening

0DUC87Z Supplement Ileocecal Valve with Autologous Tissue Substitute, Via Natural or Artificial Opening Endoscopic

0DUC8JZ Supplement Ileocecal Valve with Synthetic Substitute, Via Natural or Artificial Opening Endoscopic

0DUC8KZ Supplement Ileocecal Valve with Nonautologous Tissue Substitute, Via Natural or Artificial Opening Endoscopic

0DUE07Z Supplement Large Intestine with Autologous Tissue Substitute, Open Approach
AHA CC: 2Q, 2021, 20-21

0DUE0JZ Supplement Large Intestine with Synthetic Substitute, Open Approach

0DUE0KZ Supplement Large Intestine with Nonautologous Tissue Substitute, Open Approach

0DUE47Z Supplement Large Intestine with Autologous Tissue Substitute, Percutaneous Endoscopic Approach

0DUE4JZ Supplement Large Intestine with Synthetic Substitute, Percutaneous Endoscopic Approach

0DUE4KZ Supplement Large Intestine with Nonautologous Tissue Substitute, Percutaneous Endoscopic Approach

0DUE77Z Supplement Large Intestine with Autologous Tissue Substitute, Via Natural or Artificial Opening

0DUE7JZ Supplement Large Intestine with Synthetic Substitute, Via Natural or Artificial Opening

0DUE7KZ Supplement Large Intestine with Nonautologous Tissue Substitute, Via Natural or Artificial Opening

0DUE87Z Supplement Large Intestine with Autologous Tissue Substitute, Via Natural or Artificial Opening Endoscopic

0DUE8JZ Supplement Large Intestine with Synthetic Substitute, Via Natural or Artificial Opening Endoscopic

0DUE8KZ Supplement Large Intestine with Nonautologous Tissue Substitute, Via Natural or Artificial Opening Endoscopic

0DUF07Z Supplement Right Large Intestine with Autologous Tissue Substitute, Open Approach

0DUF0JZ Supplement Right Large Intestine with Synthetic Substitute, Open Approach

0DUF0KZ Supplement Right Large Intestine with Nonautologous Tissue Substitute, Open Approach

0DUF47Z Supplement Right Large Intestine with Autologous Tissue Substitute, Percutaneous Endoscopic Approach

0DUF4JZ Supplement Right Large Intestine with Synthetic Substitute, Percutaneous Endoscopic Approach

0DUF4KZ Supplement Right Large Intestine with Nonautologous Tissue Substitute, Percutaneous Endoscopic Approach

0DUF77Z Supplement Right Large Intestine with Autologous Tissue Substitute, Via Natural or Artificial Opening

0DUF7JZ Supplement Right Large Intestine with Synthetic Substitute, Via Natural or Artificial Opening

0DUF7KZ Supplement Right Large Intestine with Nonautologous Tissue Substitute, Via Natural or Artificial Opening

0DUF87Z Supplement Right Large Intestine with Autologous Tissue Substitute, Via Natural or Artificial Opening Endoscopic

0DUF8JZ Supplement Right Large Intestine with Synthetic Substitute, Via Natural or Artificial Opening Endoscopic

0DUF8KZ Supplement Right Large Intestine with Nonautologous Tissue Substitute, Via Natural or Artificial Opening Endoscopic

0DUG07Z Supplement Left Large Intestine with Autologous Tissue Substitute, Open Approach

0DUG0JZ Supplement Left Large Intestine with Synthetic Substitute, Open Approach

0DUG0KZ Supplement Left Large Intestine with Nonautologous Tissue Substitute, Open Approach

0DUG47Z Supplement Left Large Intestine with Autologous Tissue Substitute, Percutaneous Endoscopic Approach

0DUG4JZ Supplement Left Large Intestine with Synthetic Substitute, Percutaneous Endoscopic Approach

0DUG4KZ Supplement Left Large Intestine with Nonautologous Tissue Substitute, Percutaneous Endoscopic Approach

0DUG77Z Supplement Left Large Intestine with Autologous Tissue Substitute, Via Natural or Artificial Opening

0DUG7JZ Supplement Left Large Intestine with Synthetic Substitute, Via Natural or Artificial Opening

0DUG7KZ Supplement Left Large Intestine with Nonautologous Tissue Substitute, Via Natural or Artificial Opening

0DUG87Z Supplement Left Large Intestine with Autologous Tissue Substitute, Via Natural or Artificial Opening Endoscopic

0DUG8JZ Supplement Left Large Intestine with Synthetic Substitute, Via Natural or Artificial Opening Endoscopic

0DUG8KZ Supplement Left Large Intestine with Nonautologous Tissue Substitute, Via Natural or Artificial Opening Endoscopic

0DUH07Z Supplement Cecum with Autologous Tissue Substitute, Open Approach

0DUH0JZ Supplement Cecum with Synthetic Substitute, Open Approach

0DUH0KZ Supplement Cecum with Nonautologous Tissue Substitute, Open Approach

0DUH47Z Supplement Cecum with Autologous Tissue Substitute, Percutaneous Endoscopic Approach

0DUH4JZ Supplement Cecum with Synthetic Substitute, Percutaneous Endoscopic Approach

0DUH4KZ Supplement Cecum with Nonautologous Tissue Substitute, Percutaneous Endoscopic Approach

0DUH77Z Supplement Cecum with Autologous Tissue Substitute, Via Natural or Artificial Opening

0DUH7JZ Supplement Cecum with Synthetic Substitute, Via Natural or Artificial Opening

0DUH7KZ Supplement Cecum with Nonautologous Tissue Substitute, Via Natural or Artificial Opening

0DUH87Z Supplement Cecum with Autologous Tissue Substitute, Via Natural or Artificial Opening Endoscopic

0DUH8JZ Supplement Cecum with Synthetic Substitute, Via Natural or Artificial Opening Endoscopic

0DUH8KZ Supplement Cecum with Nonautologous Tissue Substitute, Via Natural or Artificial Opening Endoscopic

0DUK07Z Supplement Ascending Colon with Autologous Tissue Substitute, Open Approach

0DUK0JZ Supplement Ascending Colon with Synthetic Substitute, Open Approach

0DUK0KZ Supplement Ascending Colon with Nonautologous Tissue Substitute, Open Approach

0DUK47Z Supplement Ascending Colon with Autologous Tissue Substitute, Percutaneous Endoscopic Approach

0DUK4JZ Supplement Ascending Colon with Synthetic Substitute, Percutaneous Endoscopic Approach

0DUK4KZ Supplement Ascending Colon with Nonautologous Tissue Substitute, Percutaneous Endoscopic Approach

0DUK77Z Supplement Ascending Colon with Autologous Tissue Substitute, Via Natural or Artificial Opening

0DUK7JZ Supplement Ascending Colon with Synthetic Substitute, Via Natural or Artificial Opening

0DUK7KZ Supplement Ascending Colon with Nonautologous Tissue Substitute, Via Natural or Artificial Opening

0DUK87Z Supplement Ascending Colon with Autologous Tissue Substitute, Via Natural or Artificial Opening Endoscopic

0DUK8JZ Supplement Ascending Colon with Synthetic Substitute, Via Natural or Artificial Opening Endoscopic

0DUK8KZ Supplement Ascending Colon with Nonautologous Tissue Substitute, Via Natural or Artificial Opening Endoscopic

0DUL07Z Supplement Transverse Colon with Autologous Tissue Substitute, Open Approach

0DUL0JZ Supplement Transverse Colon with Synthetic Substitute, Open Approach

0DUL0KZ Supplement Transverse Colon with Nonautologous Tissue Substitute, Open Approach

0DUL47Z Supplement Transverse Colon with Autologous Tissue Substitute, Percutaneous Endoscopic Approach

0DUL4JZ Supplement Transverse Colon with Synthetic Substitute, Percutaneous Endoscopic Approach

0DUL4KZ Supplement Transverse Colon with Nonautologous Tissue Substitute, Percutaneous Endoscopic Approach

0DUL77Z Supplement Transverse Colon with Autologous Tissue Substitute, Via Natural or Artificial Opening

0DUL7JZ Supplement Transverse Colon with Synthetic Substitute, Via Natural or Artificial Opening

0DUL7KZ Supplement Transverse Colon with Nonautologous Tissue Substitute, Via Natural or Artificial Opening

0DUL87Z Supplement Transverse Colon with Autologous Tissue Substitute, Via Natural or Artificial Opening Endoscopic

0DUL8JZ Supplement Transverse Colon with Synthetic Substitute, Via Natural or Artificial Opening Endoscopic

0DUL8KZ Supplement Transverse Colon with Nonautologous Tissue Substitute, Via Natural or Artificial Opening Endoscopic

0DUM07Z Supplement Descending Colon with Autologous Tissue Substitute, Open Approach

0DUM0JZ Supplement Descending Colon with Synthetic Substitute, Open Approach

0DUM0KZ Supplement Descending Colon with Nonautologous Tissue Substitute, Open Approach

0DUM47Z Supplement Descending Colon with Autologous Tissue Substitute, Percutaneous Endoscopic Approach

0DUM4JZ Supplement Descending Colon with Synthetic Substitute, Percutaneous Endoscopic Approach

0DUM4KZ Supplement Descending Colon with Nonautologous Tissue Substitute, Percutaneous Endoscopic Approach

0DUM77Z Supplement Descending Colon with Autologous Tissue Substitute, Via Natural or Artificial Opening

0DUM7JZ Supplement Descending Colon with Synthetic Substitute, Via Natural or Artificial Opening

0DUM7KZ Supplement Descending Colon with Nonautologous Tissue Substitute, Via Natural or Artificial Opening

0DUM87Z Supplement Descending Colon with Autologous Tissue Substitute, Via Natural or Artificial Opening Endoscopic

0DUM8JZ Supplement Descending Colon with Synthetic Substitute, Via Natural or Artificial Opening Endoscopic

0DUM8KZ Supplement Descending Colon with Nonautologous Tissue Substitute, Via Natural or Artificial Opening Endoscopic

0DUN07Z Supplement Sigmoid Colon with Autologous Tissue Substitute, Open Approach

0DUN0JZ Supplement Sigmoid Colon with Synthetic Substitute, Open Approach

0DUN0KZ Supplement Sigmoid Colon with Nonautologous Tissue Substitute, Open Approach

0DUN47Z Supplement Sigmoid Colon with Autologous Tissue Substitute, Percutaneous Endoscopic Approach

0DUN4JZ Supplement Sigmoid Colon with Synthetic Substitute, Percutaneous Endoscopic Approach

0DUN4KZ Supplement Sigmoid Colon with Nonautologous Tissue Substitute, Percutaneous Endoscopic Approach

0DUN77Z Supplement Sigmoid Colon with Autologous Tissue Substitute, Via Natural or Artificial Opening

0DUN7JZ Supplement Sigmoid Colon with Synthetic Substitute, Via Natural or Artificial Opening

0DUN7KZ Supplement Sigmoid Colon with Nonautologous Tissue Substitute, Via Natural or Artificial Opening

0DUN87Z Supplement Sigmoid Colon with Autologous Tissue Substitute, Via Natural or Artificial Opening Endoscopic

0DUN8JZ Supplement Sigmoid Colon with Synthetic Substitute, Via Natural or Artificial Opening Endoscopic

0DUN8KZ Supplement Sigmoid Colon with Nonautologous Tissue Substitute, Via Natural or Artificial Opening Endoscopic

0DUP07Z Supplement Rectum with Autologous Tissue Substitute, Open Approach

0DUP0JZ Supplement Rectum with Synthetic Substitute, Open Approach
AHA CC: 1Q, 2019, 30-31

0DUP0KZ Supplement Rectum with Nonautologous Tissue Substitute, Open Approach

0DUP47Z Supplement Rectum with Autologous Tissue Substitute, Percutaneous Endoscopic Approach
AHA CC: 1Q, 2021, 22-23

0DUP4JZ Supplement Rectum with Synthetic Substitute, Percutaneous Endoscopic Approach

0DUP4KZ Supplement Rectum with Nonautologous Tissue Substitute, Percutaneous Endoscopic Approach

0DUP77Z Supplement Rectum with Autologous Tissue Substitute, Via Natural or Artificial Opening

0DUP7JZ Supplement Rectum with Synthetic Substitute, Via Natural or Artificial Opening

0DUP7KZ Supplement Rectum with Nonautologous Tissue Substitute, Via Natural or Artificial Opening

0DUP87Z Supplement Rectum with Autologous Tissue Substitute, Via Natural or Artificial Opening Endoscopic

0DUP8JZ Supplement Rectum with Synthetic Substitute, Via Natural or Artificial Opening Endoscopic

0DUP8KZ Supplement Rectum with Nonautologous Tissue Substitute, Via Natural or Artificial Opening Endoscopic

0DUQ07Z Supplement Anus with Autologous Tissue Substitute, Open Approach

0DUQ0JZ Supplement Anus with Synthetic Substitute, Open Approach

0DUQ0KZ Supplement Anus with Nonautologous Tissue Substitute, Open Approach

0DUQ47Z Supplement Anus with Autologous Tissue Substitute, Percutaneous Endoscopic Approach

0DUQ4JZ Supplement Anus with Synthetic Substitute, Percutaneous Endoscopic Approach

0DUQ4KZ Supplement Anus with Nonautologous Tissue Substitute, Percutaneous Endoscopic Approach

0DUQ77Z Supplement Anus with Autologous Tissue Substitute, Via Natural or Artificial Opening

0DUQ7JZ Supplement Anus with Synthetic Substitute, Via Natural or Artificial Opening

0DUQ7KZ Supplement Anus with Nonautologous Tissue Substitute, Via Natural or Artificial Opening

0DUQ87Z Supplement Anus with Autologous Tissue Substitute, Via Natural or Artificial Opening Endoscopic

0DUQ8JZ Supplement Anus with Synthetic Substitute, Via Natural or Artificial Opening Endoscopic

0DUQ8KZ Supplement Anus with Nonautologous Tissue Substitute, Via Natural or Artificial Opening Endoscopic

0DUQX7Z Supplement Anus with Autologous Tissue Substitute, External Approach

0DUQXJZ Supplement Anus with Synthetic Substitute, External Approach

0DUQXKZ Supplement Anus with Nonautologous Tissue Substitute, External Approach

0DUR07Z Supplement Anal Sphincter with Autologous Tissue Substitute, Open Approach

0DUR0JZ Supplement Anal Sphincter with Synthetic Substitute, Open Approach

0DUR0KZ Supplement Anal Sphincter with Nonautologous Tissue Substitute, Open Approach

0DUR47Z Supplement Anal Sphincter with Autologous Tissue Substitute, Percutaneous Endoscopic Approach

0DUR4JZ Supplement Anal Sphincter with Synthetic Substitute, Percutaneous Endoscopic Approach

0DUR4KZ Supplement Anal Sphincter with Nonautologous Tissue Substitute, Percutaneous Endoscopic Approach

0DUU07Z Supplement Omentum with Autologous Tissue Substitute, Open Approach

0DUU0JZ Supplement Omentum with Synthetic Substitute, Open Approach

0DUU0KZ Supplement Omentum with Nonautologous Tissue Substitute, Open Approach

0DUU47Z Supplement Omentum with Autologous Tissue Substitute, Percutaneous Endoscopic Approach

0DUU4JZ Supplement Omentum with Synthetic Substitute, Percutaneous Endoscopic Approach

0DUU4KZ Supplement Omentum with Nonautologous Tissue Substitute, Percutaneous Endoscopic Approach

0DUV07Z Supplement Mesentery with Autologous Tissue Substitute, Open Approach

0DUV0JZ Supplement Mesentery with Synthetic Substitute, Open Approach

♀ Female-only ♂ Male-only ▲ Limited Coverage ● Non-OR 🅷🅰🅲 HAC-associated procedure ▲ Non-covered procedures ＋ Cluster 689

0DUL07Z–0DUV0JZ Medical and Surgical, Gastrointestinal System Code Listings

0DUV0KZ	Supplement Mesentery with Nonautologous Tissue Substitute, Open Approach
0DUV47Z	Supplement Mesentery with Autologous Tissue Substitute, Percutaneous Endoscopic Approach
0DUV4JZ	Supplement Mesentery with Synthetic Substitute, Percutaneous Endoscopic Approach
0DUV4KZ	Supplement Mesentery with Nonautologous Tissue Substitute, Percutaneous Endoscopic Approach
0DUW07Z	Supplement Peritoneum with Autologous Tissue Substitute, Open Approach
0DUW0JZ	Supplement Peritoneum with Synthetic Substitute, Open Approach
0DUW0KZ	Supplement Peritoneum with Nonautologous Tissue Substitute, Open Approach
0DUW47Z	Supplement Peritoneum with Autologous Tissue Substitute, Percutaneous Endoscopic Approach
0DUW4JZ	Supplement Peritoneum with Synthetic Substitute, Percutaneous Endoscopic Approach
0DUW4KZ	Supplement Peritoneum with Nonautologous Tissue Substitute, Percutaneous Endoscopic Approach

0DV – Gastrointestinal System, Restriction

0DV10CZ	Restriction of Upper Esophagus with Extraluminal Device, Open Approach
0DV10DZ	Restriction of Upper Esophagus with Intraluminal Device, Open Approach
0DV10ZZ	Restriction of Upper Esophagus, Open Approach
0DV13CZ	Restriction of Upper Esophagus with Extraluminal Device, Percutaneous Approach
0DV13DZ	Restriction of Upper Esophagus with Intraluminal Device, Percutaneous Approach
0DV13ZZ	Restriction of Upper Esophagus, Percutaneous Approach
0DV14CZ	Restriction of Upper Esophagus with Extraluminal Device, Percutaneous Endoscopic Approach
0DV14DZ	Restriction of Upper Esophagus with Intraluminal Device, Percutaneous Endoscopic Approach
0DV14ZZ	Restriction of Upper Esophagus, Percutaneous Endoscopic Approach
0DV17DZ	Restriction of Upper Esophagus with Intraluminal Device, Via Natural or Artificial Opening
0DV17ZZ	Restriction of Upper Esophagus, Via Natural or Artificial Opening
0DV18DZ	Restriction of Upper Esophagus with Intraluminal Device, Via Natural or Artificial Opening Endoscopic
0DV18ZZ	Restriction of Upper Esophagus, Via Natural or Artificial Opening Endoscopic
0DV20CZ	Restriction of Middle Esophagus with Extraluminal Device, Open Approach
0DV20DZ	Restriction of Middle Esophagus with Intraluminal Device, Open Approach
0DV20ZZ	Restriction of Middle Esophagus, Open Approach
0DV23CZ	Restriction of Middle Esophagus with Extraluminal Device, Percutaneous Approach
0DV23DZ	Restriction of Middle Esophagus with Intraluminal Device, Percutaneous Approach
0DV23ZZ	Restriction of Middle Esophagus, Percutaneous Approach
0DV24CZ	Restriction of Middle Esophagus with Extraluminal Device, Percutaneous Endoscopic Approach
0DV24DZ	Restriction of Middle Esophagus with Intraluminal Device, Percutaneous Endoscopic Approach
0DV24ZZ	Restriction of Middle Esophagus, Percutaneous Endoscopic Approach
0DV27DZ	Restriction of Middle Esophagus with Intraluminal Device, Via Natural or Artificial Opening
0DV27ZZ	Restriction of Middle Esophagus, Via Natural or Artificial Opening
0DV28DZ	Restriction of Middle Esophagus with Intraluminal Device, Via Natural or Artificial Opening Endoscopic
0DV28ZZ	Restriction of Middle Esophagus, Via Natural or Artificial Opening Endoscopic
0DV30CZ	Restriction of Lower Esophagus with Extraluminal Device, Open Approach
0DV30DZ	Restriction of Lower Esophagus with Intraluminal Device, Open Approach
0DV30ZZ	Restriction of Lower Esophagus, Open Approach
0DV33CZ	Restriction of Lower Esophagus with Extraluminal Device, Percutaneous Approach
0DV33DZ	Restriction of Lower Esophagus with Intraluminal Device, Percutaneous Approach
0DV33ZZ	Restriction of Lower Esophagus, Percutaneous Approach
0DV34CZ	Restriction of Lower Esophagus with Extraluminal Device, Percutaneous Endoscopic Approach
0DV34DZ	Restriction of Lower Esophagus with Intraluminal Device, Percutaneous Endoscopic Approach
0DV34ZZ	Restriction of Lower Esophagus, Percutaneous Endoscopic Approach
0DV37DZ	Restriction of Lower Esophagus with Intraluminal Device, Via Natural or Artificial Opening
0DV37ZZ	Restriction of Lower Esophagus, Via Natural or Artificial Opening
0DV38DZ	Restriction of Lower Esophagus with Intraluminal Device, Via Natural or Artificial Opening Endoscopic
0DV38ZZ	Restriction of Lower Esophagus, Via Natural or Artificial Opening Endoscopic
0DV40CZ	Restriction of Esophagogastric Junction with Extraluminal Device, Open Approach
0DV40DZ	Restriction of Esophagogastric Junction with Intraluminal Device, Open Approach
0DV40ZZ	Restriction of Esophagogastric Junction, Open Approach
	AHA CC: 2Q, 2016, 22-23
0DV43CZ	Restriction of Esophagogastric Junction with Extraluminal Device, Percutaneous Approach
0DV43DZ	Restriction of Esophagogastric Junction with Intraluminal Device, Percutaneous Approach
0DV43ZZ	Restriction of Esophagogastric Junction, Percutaneous Approach
0DV44CZ	Restriction of Esophagogastric Junction with Extraluminal Device, Percutaneous Endoscopic Approach
0DV44DZ	Restriction of Esophagogastric Junction with Intraluminal Device, Percutaneous Endoscopic Approach
0DV44ZZ	Restriction of Esophagogastric Junction, Percutaneous Endoscopic Approach
	AHA CC: 3Q, 2014, 28; 3Q, 2017, 22-23
0DV47DZ	Restriction of Esophagogastric Junction with Intraluminal Device, Via Natural or Artificial Opening
0DV47ZZ	Restriction of Esophagogastric Junction, Via Natural or Artificial Opening
0DV48DZ	Restriction of Esophagogastric Junction with Intraluminal Device, Via Natural or Artificial Opening Endoscopic
0DV48ZZ	Restriction of Esophagogastric Junction, Via Natural or Artificial Opening Endoscopic
0DV50CZ	Restriction of Esophagus with Extraluminal Device, Open Approach
0DV50DZ	Restriction of Esophagus with Intraluminal Device, Open Approach
0DV50ZZ	Restriction of Esophagus, Open Approach
0DV53CZ	Restriction of Esophagus with Extraluminal Device, Percutaneous Approach
0DV53DZ	Restriction of Esophagus with Intraluminal Device, Percutaneous Approach
0DV53ZZ	Restriction of Esophagus, Percutaneous Approach
0DV54CZ	Restriction of Esophagus with Extraluminal Device, Percutaneous Endoscopic Approach
0DV54DZ	Restriction of Esophagus with Intraluminal Device, Percutaneous Endoscopic Approach
0DV54ZZ	Restriction of Esophagus, Percutaneous Endoscopic Approach
0DV57DZ	Restriction of Esophagus with Intraluminal Device, Via Natural or Artificial Opening
0DV57ZZ	Restriction of Esophagus, Via Natural or Artificial Opening
0DV58DZ	Restriction of Esophagus with Intraluminal Device, Via Natural or Artificial Opening Endoscopic

♀ Female-only   ♂ Male-only   ▲ Limited Coverage   ● Non-OR   HAC HAC-associated procedure   ▲ Non-covered procedures   ✚ Cluster

0DV58ZZ Restriction of Esophagus, Via Natural or Artificial Opening Endoscopic

0DV60CZ Restriction of Stomach with Extraluminal Device, Open Approach

0DV60DZ Restriction of Stomach with Intraluminal Device, Open Approach

0DV60ZZ Restriction of Stomach, Open Approach

0DV63CZ Restriction of Stomach with Extraluminal Device, Percutaneous Approach

0DV63DZ Restriction of Stomach with Intraluminal Device, Percutaneous Approach

0DV63ZZ Restriction of Stomach, Percutaneous Approach

0DV64CZ Restriction of Stomach with Extraluminal Device, Percutaneous Endoscopic Approach

> [HAC] When reported with principal diagnosis code E66.01 and secondary diagnosis code K68.11, K95.01, K95.81, T81.40XA, T81.41XA, T81.42XA, T81.43XA, T81.44XA or T81.49XA

0DV64DZ Restriction of Stomach with Intraluminal Device, Percutaneous Endoscopic Approach

0DV64ZZ Restriction of Stomach, Percutaneous Endoscopic Approach

0DV67DZ Restriction of Stomach with Intraluminal Device, Via Natural or Artificial Opening

0DV67ZZ Restriction of Stomach, Via Natural or Artificial Opening

0DV68DZ Restriction of Stomach with Intraluminal Device, Via Natural or Artificial Opening Endoscopic

0DV68ZZ Restriction of Stomach, Via Natural or Artificial Opening Endoscopic

0DV70CZ Restriction of Stomach, Pylorus with Extraluminal Device, Open Approach

0DV70DZ Restriction of Stomach, Pylorus with Intraluminal Device, Open Approach

0DV70ZZ Restriction of Stomach, Pylorus, Open Approach

0DV73CZ Restriction of Stomach, Pylorus with Extraluminal Device, Percutaneous Approach

0DV73DZ Restriction of Stomach, Pylorus with Intraluminal Device, Percutaneous Approach

0DV73ZZ Restriction of Stomach, Pylorus, Percutaneous Approach

0DV74CZ Restriction of Stomach, Pylorus with Extraluminal Device, Percutaneous Endoscopic Approach

0DV74DZ Restriction of Stomach, Pylorus with Intraluminal Device, Percutaneous Endoscopic Approach

0DV74ZZ Restriction of Stomach, Pylorus, Percutaneous Endoscopic Approach

0DV77DZ Restriction of Stomach, Pylorus with Intraluminal Device, Via Natural or Artificial Opening

0DV77ZZ Restriction of Stomach, Pylorus, Via Natural or Artificial Opening

0DV78DZ Restriction of Stomach, Pylorus with Intraluminal Device, Via Natural or Artificial Opening Endoscopic

0DV78ZZ Restriction of Stomach, Pylorus, Via Natural or Artificial Opening Endoscopic

0DV80CZ Restriction of Small Intestine with Extraluminal Device, Open Approach

0DV80DZ Restriction of Small Intestine with Intraluminal Device, Open Approach

0DV80ZZ Restriction of Small Intestine, Open Approach

0DV83CZ Restriction of Small Intestine with Extraluminal Device, Percutaneous Approach

0DV83DZ Restriction of Small Intestine with Intraluminal Device, Percutaneous Approach

0DV83ZZ Restriction of Small Intestine, Percutaneous Approach

0DV84CZ Restriction of Small Intestine with Extraluminal Device, Percutaneous Endoscopic Approach

0DV84DZ Restriction of Small Intestine with Intraluminal Device, Percutaneous Endoscopic Approach

0DV84ZZ Restriction of Small Intestine, Percutaneous Endoscopic Approach

0DV87DZ Restriction of Small Intestine with Intraluminal Device, Via Natural or Artificial Opening

0DV87ZZ Restriction of Small Intestine, Via Natural or Artificial Opening

0DV88DZ Restriction of Small Intestine with Intraluminal Device, Via Natural or Artificial Opening Endoscopic

0DV88ZZ Restriction of Small Intestine, Via Natural or Artificial Opening Endoscopic

0DV90CZ Restriction of Duodenum with Extraluminal Device, Open Approach

0DV90DZ Restriction of Duodenum with Intraluminal Device, Open Approach

0DV90ZZ Restriction of Duodenum, Open Approach

0DV93CZ Restriction of Duodenum with Extraluminal Device, Percutaneous Approach

0DV93DZ Restriction of Duodenum with Intraluminal Device, Percutaneous Approach

0DV93ZZ Restriction of Duodenum, Percutaneous Approach

0DV94CZ Restriction of Duodenum with Extraluminal Device, Percutaneous Endoscopic Approach

0DV94DZ Restriction of Duodenum with Intraluminal Device, Percutaneous Endoscopic Approach

0DV94ZZ Restriction of Duodenum, Percutaneous Endoscopic Approach

0DV97DZ Restriction of Duodenum with Intraluminal Device, Via Natural or Artificial Opening

0DV97ZZ Restriction of Duodenum, Via Natural or Artificial Opening

0DV98DZ Restriction of Duodenum with Intraluminal Device, Via Natural or Artificial Opening Endoscopic

0DV98ZZ Restriction of Duodenum, Via Natural or Artificial Opening Endoscopic

0DVA0CZ Restriction of Jejunum with Extraluminal Device, Open Approach

0DVA0DZ Restriction of Jejunum with Intraluminal Device, Open Approach

0DVA0ZZ Restriction of Jejunum, Open Approach

0DVA3CZ Restriction of Jejunum with Extraluminal Device, Percutaneous Approach

0DVA3DZ Restriction of Jejunum with Intraluminal Device, Percutaneous Approach

0DVA3ZZ Restriction of Jejunum, Percutaneous Approach

0DVA4CZ Restriction of Jejunum with Extraluminal Device, Percutaneous Endoscopic Approach

0DVA4DZ Restriction of Jejunum with Intraluminal Device, Percutaneous Endoscopic Approach

0DVA4ZZ Restriction of Jejunum, Percutaneous Endoscopic Approach

0DVA7DZ Restriction of Jejunum with Intraluminal Device, Via Natural or Artificial Opening

0DVA7ZZ Restriction of Jejunum, Via Natural or Artificial Opening

0DVA8DZ Restriction of Jejunum with Intraluminal Device, Via Natural or Artificial Opening Endoscopic

0DVA8ZZ Restriction of Jejunum, Via Natural or Artificial Opening Endoscopic

0DVB0CZ Restriction of Ileum with Extraluminal Device, Open Approach

0DVB0DZ Restriction of Ileum with Intraluminal Device, Open Approach

0DVB0ZZ Restriction of Ileum, Open Approach

0DVB3CZ Restriction of Ileum with Extraluminal Device, Percutaneous Approach

0DVB3DZ Restriction of Ileum with Intraluminal Device, Percutaneous Approach

0DVB3ZZ Restriction of Ileum, Percutaneous Approach

0DVB4CZ Restriction of Ileum with Extraluminal Device, Percutaneous Endoscopic Approach

0DVB4DZ Restriction of Ileum with Intraluminal Device, Percutaneous Endoscopic Approach

0DVB4ZZ Restriction of Ileum, Percutaneous Endoscopic Approach

0DVB7DZ Restriction of Ileum with Intraluminal Device, Via Natural or Artificial Opening

0DVB7ZZ Restriction of Ileum, Via Natural or Artificial Opening

0DVB8DZ Restriction of Ileum with Intraluminal Device, Via Natural or Artificial Opening Endoscopic

0DVB8ZZ Restriction of Ileum, Via Natural or Artificial Opening Endoscopic

0DVC0CZ Restriction of Ileocecal Valve with Extraluminal Device, Open Approach

0DVC0DZ Restriction of Ileocecal Valve with Intraluminal Device, Open Approach

0DVC0ZZ Restriction of Ileocecal Valve, Open Approach

0DVC3CZ Restriction of Ileocecal Valve with Extraluminal Device, Percutaneous Approach

0DVC3DZ Restriction of Ileocecal Valve with Intraluminal Device, Percutaneous Approach

0DVC3ZZ Restriction of Ileocecal Valve, Percutaneous Approach

0DVC4CZ Restriction of Ileocecal Valve with Extraluminal Device, Percutaneous Endoscopic Approach

0DVC4DZ Restriction of Ileocecal Valve with Intraluminal Device, Percutaneous Endoscopic Approach

0DVC4ZZ	Restriction of Ileocecal Valve, Percutaneous Endoscopic Approach
0DVC7DZ	Restriction of Ileocecal Valve with Intraluminal Device, Via Natural or Artificial Opening
0DVC7ZZ	Restriction of Ileocecal Valve, Via Natural or Artificial Opening
0DVC8DZ	Restriction of Ileocecal Valve with Intraluminal Device, Via Natural or Artificial Opening Endoscopic
0DVC8ZZ	Restriction of Ileocecal Valve, Via Natural or Artificial Opening Endoscopic
0DVE0CZ	Restriction of Large Intestine with Extraluminal Device, Open Approach
0DVE0DZ	Restriction of Large Intestine with Intraluminal Device, Open Approach
0DVE0ZZ	Restriction of Large Intestine, Open Approach
0DVE3CZ	Restriction of Large Intestine with Extraluminal Device, Percutaneous Approach
0DVE3DZ	Restriction of Large Intestine with Intraluminal Device, Percutaneous Approach
0DVE3ZZ	Restriction of Large Intestine, Percutaneous Approach
0DVE4CZ	Restriction of Large Intestine with Extraluminal Device, Percutaneous Endoscopic Approach
0DVE4DZ	Restriction of Large Intestine with Intraluminal Device, Percutaneous Endoscopic Approach
0DVE4ZZ	Restriction of Large Intestine, Percutaneous Endoscopic Approach
0DVE7DZ	Restriction of Large Intestine with Intraluminal Device, Via Natural or Artificial Opening
0DVE7ZZ	Restriction of Large Intestine, Via Natural or Artificial Opening
0DVE8DZ	Restriction of Large Intestine with Intraluminal Device, Via Natural or Artificial Opening Endoscopic
0DVE8ZZ	Restriction of Large Intestine, Via Natural or Artificial Opening Endoscopic
0DVF0CZ	Restriction of Right Large Intestine with Extraluminal Device, Open Approach
0DVF0DZ	Restriction of Right Large Intestine with Intraluminal Device, Open Approach
0DVF0ZZ	Restriction of Right Large Intestine, Open Approach
0DVF3CZ	Restriction of Right Large Intestine with Extraluminal Device, Percutaneous Approach
0DVF3DZ	Restriction of Right Large Intestine with Intraluminal Device, Percutaneous Approach
0DVF3ZZ	Restriction of Right Large Intestine, Percutaneous Approach
0DVF4CZ	Restriction of Right Large Intestine with Extraluminal Device, Percutaneous Endoscopic Approach
0DVF4DZ	Restriction of Right Large Intestine with Intraluminal Device, Percutaneous Endoscopic Approach
0DVF4ZZ	Restriction of Right Large Intestine, Percutaneous Endoscopic Approach
0DVF7DZ	Restriction of Right Large Intestine with Intraluminal Device, Via Natural or Artificial Opening
0DVF7ZZ	Restriction of Right Large Intestine, Via Natural or Artificial Opening
0DVF8DZ	Restriction of Right Large Intestine with Intraluminal Device, Via Natural or Artificial Opening Endoscopic
0DVF8ZZ	Restriction of Right Large Intestine, Via Natural or Artificial Opening Endoscopic
0DVG0CZ	Restriction of Left Large Intestine with Extraluminal Device, Open Approach
0DVG0DZ	Restriction of Left Large Intestine with Intraluminal Device, Open Approach
0DVG0ZZ	Restriction of Left Large Intestine, Open Approach
0DVG3CZ	Restriction of Left Large Intestine with Extraluminal Device, Percutaneous Approach
0DVG3DZ	Restriction of Left Large Intestine with Intraluminal Device, Percutaneous Approach
0DVG3ZZ	Restriction of Left Large Intestine, Percutaneous Approach
0DVG4CZ	Restriction of Left Large Intestine with Extraluminal Device, Percutaneous Endoscopic Approach
0DVG4DZ	Restriction of Left Large Intestine with Intraluminal Device, Percutaneous Endoscopic Approach
0DVG4ZZ	Restriction of Left Large Intestine, Percutaneous Endoscopic Approach
0DVG7DZ	Restriction of Left Large Intestine with Intraluminal Device, Via Natural or Artificial Opening
0DVG7ZZ	Restriction of Left Large Intestine, Via Natural or Artificial Opening
0DVG8DZ	Restriction of Left Large Intestine with Intraluminal Device, Via Natural or Artificial Opening Endoscopic
0DVG8ZZ	Restriction of Left Large Intestine, Via Natural or Artificial Opening Endoscopic
0DVH0CZ	Restriction of Cecum with Extraluminal Device, Open Approach
0DVH0DZ	Restriction of Cecum with Intraluminal Device, Open Approach
0DVH0ZZ	Restriction of Cecum, Open Approach
0DVH3CZ	Restriction of Cecum with Extraluminal Device, Percutaneous Approach
0DVH3DZ	Restriction of Cecum with Intraluminal Device, Percutaneous Approach
0DVH3ZZ	Restriction of Cecum, Percutaneous Approach
0DVH4CZ	Restriction of Cecum with Extraluminal Device, Percutaneous Endoscopic Approach
0DVH4DZ	Restriction of Cecum with Intraluminal Device, Percutaneous Endoscopic Approach
0DVH4ZZ	Restriction of Cecum, Percutaneous Endoscopic Approach
0DVH7DZ	Restriction of Cecum with Intraluminal Device, Via Natural or Artificial Opening
0DVH7ZZ	Restriction of Cecum, Via Natural or Artificial Opening
0DVH8DZ	Restriction of Cecum with Intraluminal Device, Via Natural or Artificial Opening Endoscopic
0DVH8ZZ	Restriction of Cecum, Via Natural or Artificial Opening Endoscopic
0DVK0CZ	Restriction of Ascending Colon with Extraluminal Device, Open Approach
0DVK0DZ	Restriction of Ascending Colon with Intraluminal Device, Open Approach
0DVK0ZZ	Restriction of Ascending Colon, Open Approach
0DVK3CZ	Restriction of Ascending Colon with Extraluminal Device, Percutaneous Approach
0DVK3DZ	Restriction of Ascending Colon with Intraluminal Device, Percutaneous Approach
0DVK3ZZ	Restriction of Ascending Colon, Percutaneous Approach
0DVK4CZ	Restriction of Ascending Colon with Extraluminal Device, Percutaneous Endoscopic Approach
0DVK4DZ	Restriction of Ascending Colon with Intraluminal Device, Percutaneous Endoscopic Approach
0DVK4ZZ	Restriction of Ascending Colon, Percutaneous Endoscopic Approach
0DVK7DZ	Restriction of Ascending Colon with Intraluminal Device, Via Natural or Artificial Opening
0DVK7ZZ	Restriction of Ascending Colon, Via Natural or Artificial Opening
0DVK8DZ	Restriction of Ascending Colon with Intraluminal Device, Via Natural or Artificial Opening Endoscopic
0DVK8ZZ	Restriction of Ascending Colon, Via Natural or Artificial Opening Endoscopic
0DVL0CZ	Restriction of Transverse Colon with Extraluminal Device, Open Approach
0DVL0DZ	Restriction of Transverse Colon with Intraluminal Device, Open Approach
0DVL0ZZ	Restriction of Transverse Colon, Open Approach
0DVL3CZ	Restriction of Transverse Colon with Extraluminal Device, Percutaneous Approach
0DVL3DZ	Restriction of Transverse Colon with Intraluminal Device, Percutaneous Approach
0DVL3ZZ	Restriction of Transverse Colon, Percutaneous Approach
0DVL4CZ	Restriction of Transverse Colon with Extraluminal Device, Percutaneous Endoscopic Approach
0DVL4DZ	Restriction of Transverse Colon with Intraluminal Device, Percutaneous Endoscopic Approach
0DVL4ZZ	Restriction of Transverse Colon, Percutaneous Endoscopic Approach
0DVL7DZ	Restriction of Transverse Colon with Intraluminal Device, Via Natural or Artificial Opening
0DVL7ZZ	Restriction of Transverse Colon, Via Natural or Artificial Opening
0DVL8DZ	Restriction of Transverse Colon with Intraluminal Device, Via Natural or Artificial Opening Endoscopic
0DVL8ZZ	Restriction of Transverse Colon, Via Natural or Artificial Opening Endoscopic
0DVM0CZ	Restriction of Descending Colon with Extraluminal Device, Open Approach
0DVM0DZ	Restriction of Descending Colon with Intraluminal Device, Open Approach
0DVM0ZZ	Restriction of Descending Colon, Open Approach

♀ Female-only   ♂ Male-only   ▲ Limited Coverage   ● Non-OR   🅗🅐🅒 HAC-associated procedure   ▲ Non-covered procedures   ✚ Cluster

0DVM3CZ Restriction of Descending Colon with Extraluminal Device, Percutaneous Approach

0DVM3DZ Restriction of Descending Colon with Intraluminal Device, Percutaneous Approach

0DVM3ZZ Restriction of Descending Colon, Percutaneous Approach

0DVM4CZ Restriction of Descending Colon with Extraluminal Device, Percutaneous Endoscopic Approach

0DVM4DZ Restriction of Descending Colon with Intraluminal Device, Percutaneous Endoscopic Approach

0DVM4ZZ Restriction of Descending Colon, Percutaneous Endoscopic Approach

0DVM7DZ Restriction of Descending Colon with Intraluminal Device, Via Natural or Artificial Opening

0DVM7ZZ Restriction of Descending Colon, Via Natural or Artificial Opening

0DVM8DZ Restriction of Descending Colon with Intraluminal Device, Via Natural or Artificial Opening Endoscopic

0DVM8ZZ Restriction of Descending Colon, Via Natural or Artificial Opening Endoscopic

0DVN0CZ Restriction of Sigmoid Colon with Extraluminal Device, Open Approach

0DVN0DZ Restriction of Sigmoid Colon with Intraluminal Device, Open Approach

0DVN0ZZ Restriction of Sigmoid Colon, Open Approach

0DVN3CZ Restriction of Sigmoid Colon with Extraluminal Device, Percutaneous Approach

0DVN3DZ Restriction of Sigmoid Colon with Intraluminal Device, Percutaneous Approach

0DVN3ZZ Restriction of Sigmoid Colon, Percutaneous Approach

0DVN4CZ Restriction of Sigmoid Colon with Extraluminal Device, Percutaneous Endoscopic Approach

0DVN4DZ Restriction of Sigmoid Colon with Intraluminal Device, Percutaneous Endoscopic Approach

0DVN4ZZ Restriction of Sigmoid Colon, Percutaneous Endoscopic Approach

0DVN7DZ Restriction of Sigmoid Colon with Intraluminal Device, Via Natural or Artificial Opening

0DVN7ZZ Restriction of Sigmoid Colon, Via Natural or Artificial Opening

0DVN8DZ Restriction of Sigmoid Colon with Intraluminal Device, Via Natural or Artificial Opening Endoscopic

0DVN8ZZ Restriction of Sigmoid Colon, Via Natural or Artificial Opening Endoscopic

0DVP0CZ Restriction of Rectum with Extraluminal Device, Open Approach

0DVP0DZ Restriction of Rectum with Intraluminal Device, Open Approach

0DVP0ZZ Restriction of Rectum, Open Approach

0DVP3CZ Restriction of Rectum with Extraluminal Device, Percutaneous Approach

0DVP3DZ Restriction of Rectum with Intraluminal Device, Percutaneous Approach

0DVP3ZZ Restriction of Rectum, Percutaneous Approach

0DVP4CZ Restriction of Rectum with Extraluminal Device, Percutaneous Endoscopic Approach

0DVP4DZ Restriction of Rectum with Intraluminal Device, Percutaneous Endoscopic Approach

0DVP4ZZ Restriction of Rectum, Percutaneous Endoscopic Approach

0DVP7DZ Restriction of Rectum with Intraluminal Device, Via Natural or Artificial Opening

0DVP7ZZ Restriction of Rectum, Via Natural or Artificial Opening

0DVP8DZ Restriction of Rectum with Intraluminal Device, Via Natural or Artificial Opening Endoscopic

0DVP8ZZ Restriction of Rectum, Via Natural or Artificial Opening Endoscopic

0DVQ0CZ Restriction of Anus with Extraluminal Device, Open Approach

0DVQ0DZ Restriction of Anus with Intraluminal Device, Open Approach

0DVQ0ZZ Restriction of Anus, Open Approach

0DVQ3CZ Restriction of Anus with Extraluminal Device, Percutaneous Approach

0DVQ3DZ Restriction of Anus with Intraluminal Device, Percutaneous Approach

0DVQ3ZZ Restriction of Anus, Percutaneous Approach

0DVQ4CZ Restriction of Anus with Extraluminal Device, Percutaneous Endoscopic Approach

0DVQ4DZ Restriction of Anus with Intraluminal Device, Percutaneous Endoscopic Approach

0DVQ4ZZ Restriction of Anus, Percutaneous Endoscopic Approach

0DVQ7DZ Restriction of Anus with Intraluminal Device, Via Natural or Artificial Opening

0DVQ7ZZ Restriction of Anus, Via Natural or Artificial Opening

0DVQ8DZ Restriction of Anus with Intraluminal Device, Via Natural or Artificial Opening Endoscopic

0DVQ8ZZ Restriction of Anus, Via Natural or Artificial Opening Endoscopic

0DVQXCZ Restriction of Anus with Extraluminal Device, External Approach

0DVQXDZ Restriction of Anus with Intraluminal Device, External Approach

0DVQXZZ Restriction of Anus, External Approach

0DW – Gastrointestinal System, Revision

Review Coding Guideline B6.1c

0DW000Z Revision of Drainage Device in Upper Intestinal Tract, Open Approach

0DW002Z Revision of Monitoring Device in Upper Intestinal Tract, Open Approach

0DW003Z Revision of Infusion Device in Upper Intestinal Tract, Open Approach

0DW007Z Revision of Autologous Tissue Substitute in Upper Intestinal Tract, Open Approach

0DW00CZ Revision of Extraluminal Device in Upper Intestinal Tract, Open Approach

0DW00DZ Revision of Intraluminal Device in Upper Intestinal Tract, Open Approach

0DW00JZ Revision of Synthetic Substitute in Upper Intestinal Tract, Open Approach

0DW00KZ Revision of Nonautologous Tissue Substitute in Upper Intestinal Tract, Open Approach

0DW00UZ Revision of Feeding Device in Upper Intestinal Tract, Open Approach

0DW00YZ Revision of Other Device in Upper Intestinal Tract, Open Approach

0DW030Z Revision of Drainage Device in Upper Intestinal Tract, Percutaneous Approach

0DW032Z Revision of Monitoring Device in Upper Intestinal Tract, Percutaneous Approach

0DW033Z Revision of Infusion Device in Upper Intestinal Tract, Percutaneous Approach

0DW037Z Revision of Autologous Tissue Substitute in Upper Intestinal Tract, Percutaneous Approach

0DW03CZ Revision of Extraluminal Device in Upper Intestinal Tract, Percutaneous Approach

0DW03DZ Revision of Intraluminal Device in Upper Intestinal Tract, Percutaneous Approach

0DW03JZ Revision of Synthetic Substitute in Upper Intestinal Tract, Percutaneous Approach

0DW03KZ Revision of Nonautologous Tissue Substitute in Upper Intestinal Tract, Percutaneous Approach

0DW03UZ Revision of Feeding Device in Upper Intestinal Tract, Percutaneous Approach

0DW03YZ Revision of Other Device in Upper Intestinal Tract, Percutaneous Approach

0DW040Z Revision of Drainage Device in Upper Intestinal Tract, Percutaneous Endoscopic Approach

0DW042Z Revision of Monitoring Device in Upper Intestinal Tract, Percutaneous Endoscopic Approach

0DW043Z Revision of Infusion Device in Upper Intestinal Tract, Percutaneous Endoscopic Approach

0DW047Z Revision of Autologous Tissue Substitute in Upper Intestinal Tract, Percutaneous Endoscopic Approach

0DW04CZ Revision of Extraluminal Device in Upper Intestinal Tract, Percutaneous Endoscopic Approach

0DW04DZ Revision of Intraluminal Device in Upper Intestinal Tract, Percutaneous Endoscopic Approach

0DW04JZ Revision of Synthetic Substitute in Upper Intestinal Tract, Percutaneous Endoscopic Approach

0DW04KZ Revision of Nonautologous Tissue Substitute in Upper Intestinal Tract, Percutaneous Endoscopic Approach

0DW04UZ	Revision of Feeding Device in Upper Intestinal Tract, Percutaneous Endoscopic Approach
0DW04YZ	Revision of Other Device in Upper Intestinal Tract, Percutaneous Endoscopic Approach
0DW070Z	Revision of Drainage Device in Upper Intestinal Tract, Via Natural or Artificial Opening
0DW072Z	Revision of Monitoring Device in Upper Intestinal Tract, Via Natural or Artificial Opening
0DW073Z	Revision of Infusion Device in Upper Intestinal Tract, Via Natural or Artificial Opening
0DW077Z	Revision of Autologous Tissue Substitute in Upper Intestinal Tract, Via Natural or Artificial Opening
0DW07CZ	Revision of Extraluminal Device in Upper Intestinal Tract, Via Natural or Artificial Opening
0DW07DZ	Revision of Intraluminal Device in Upper Intestinal Tract, Via Natural or Artificial Opening
0DW07JZ	Revision of Synthetic Substitute in Upper Intestinal Tract, Via Natural or Artificial Opening
0DW07KZ	Revision of Nonautologous Tissue Substitute in Upper Intestinal Tract, Via Natural or Artificial Opening
0DW07UZ	Revision of Feeding Device in Upper Intestinal Tract, Via Natural or Artificial Opening
0DW07YZ	Revision of Other Device in Upper Intestinal Tract, Via Natural or Artificial Opening
0DW080Z	Revision of Drainage Device in Upper Intestinal Tract, Via Natural or Artificial Opening Endoscopic
0DW082Z	Revision of Monitoring Device in Upper Intestinal Tract, Via Natural or Artificial Opening Endoscopic
0DW083Z	Revision of Infusion Device in Upper Intestinal Tract, Via Natural or Artificial Opening Endoscopic
0DW087Z	Revision of Autologous Tissue Substitute in Upper Intestinal Tract, Via Natural or Artificial Opening Endoscopic
0DW08CZ	Revision of Extraluminal Device in Upper Intestinal Tract, Via Natural or Artificial Opening Endoscopic
0DW08DZ	Revision of Intraluminal Device in Upper Intestinal Tract, Via Natural or Artificial Opening Endoscopic
0DW08JZ	Revision of Synthetic Substitute in Upper Intestinal Tract, Via Natural or Artificial Opening Endoscopic
0DW08KZ	Revision of Nonautologous Tissue Substitute in Upper Intestinal Tract, Via Natural or Artificial Opening Endoscopic
0DW08UZ	Revision of Feeding Device in Upper Intestinal Tract, Via Natural or Artificial Opening Endoscopic
0DW08YZ	Revision of Other Device in Upper Intestinal Tract, Via Natural or Artificial Opening Endoscopic
0DW0X0Z	Revision of Drainage Device in Upper Intestinal Tract, External Approach
0DW0X2Z	Revision of Monitoring Device in Upper Intestinal Tract, External Approach
0DW0X3Z	Revision of Infusion Device in Upper Intestinal Tract, External Approach
0DW0X7Z	Revision of Autologous Tissue Substitute in Upper Intestinal Tract, External Approach
0DW0XCZ	Revision of Extraluminal Device in Upper Intestinal Tract, External Approach
0DW0XDZ	Revision of Intraluminal Device in Upper Intestinal Tract, External Approach
0DW0XJZ	Revision of Synthetic Substitute in Upper Intestinal Tract, External Approach
0DW0XKZ	Revision of Nonautologous Tissue Substitute in Upper Intestinal Tract, External Approach
0DW0XUZ	Revision of Feeding Device in Upper Intestinal Tract, External Approach
0DW50YZ	Revision of Other Device in Esophagus, Open Approach
0DW53YZ	Revision of Other Device in Esophagus, Percutaneous Approach
0DW54YZ	Revision of Other Device in Esophagus, Percutaneous Endoscopic Approach
0DW57DZ	Revision of Intraluminal Device in Esophagus, Via Natural or Artificial Opening
0DW57YZ	Revision of Other Device in Esophagus, Via Natural or Artificial Opening
0DW58DZ	Revision of Intraluminal Device in Esophagus, Via Natural or Artificial Opening Endoscopic
0DW58YZ	Revision of Other Device in Esophagus, Via Natural or Artificial Opening Endoscopic
0DW5XDZ	Revision of Intraluminal Device in Esophagus, External Approach
0DW600Z	Revision of Drainage Device in Stomach, Open Approach
0DW602Z	Revision of Monitoring Device in Stomach, Open Approach
0DW603Z	Revision of Infusion Device in Stomach, Open Approach
0DW607Z	Revision of Autologous Tissue Substitute in Stomach, Open Approach
0DW60CZ	Revision of Extraluminal Device in Stomach, Open Approach
0DW60DZ	Revision of Intraluminal Device in Stomach, Open Approach
0DW60JZ	Revision of Synthetic Substitute in Stomach, Open Approach
0DW60KZ	Revision of Nonautologous Tissue Substitute in Stomach, Open Approach
0DW60MZ	Revision of Stimulator Lead in Stomach, Open Approach
0DW60UZ	Revision of Feeding Device in Stomach, Open Approach
0DW60YZ	Revision of Other Device in Stomach, Open Approach
0DW630Z	Revision of Drainage Device in Stomach, Percutaneous Approach
0DW632Z	Revision of Monitoring Device in Stomach, Percutaneous Approach
0DW633Z	Revision of Infusion Device in Stomach, Percutaneous Approach
0DW637Z	Revision of Autologous Tissue Substitute in Stomach, Percutaneous Approach
0DW63CZ	Revision of Extraluminal Device in Stomach, Percutaneous Approach
	AHA CC: 1Q, 2018, 20
0DW63DZ	Revision of Intraluminal Device in Stomach, Percutaneous Approach
0DW63JZ	Revision of Synthetic Substitute in Stomach, Percutaneous Approach
0DW63KZ	Revision of Nonautologous Tissue Substitute in Stomach, Percutaneous Approach
0DW63MZ	Revision of Stimulator Lead in Stomach, Percutaneous Approach
0DW63UZ	Revision of Feeding Device in Stomach, Percutaneous Approach
0DW63YZ	Revision of Other Device in Stomach, Percutaneous Approach
0DW640Z	Revision of Drainage Device in Stomach, Percutaneous Endoscopic Approach
0DW642Z	Revision of Monitoring Device in Stomach, Percutaneous Endoscopic Approach
0DW643Z	Revision of Infusion Device in Stomach, Percutaneous Endoscopic Approach
0DW647Z	Revision of Autologous Tissue Substitute in Stomach, Percutaneous Endoscopic Approach
0DW64CZ	Revision of Extraluminal Device in Stomach, Percutaneous Endoscopic Approach
0DW64DZ	Revision of Intraluminal Device in Stomach, Percutaneous Endoscopic Approach
0DW64JZ	Revision of Synthetic Substitute in Stomach, Percutaneous Endoscopic Approach
0DW64KZ	Revision of Nonautologous Tissue Substitute in Stomach, Percutaneous Endoscopic Approach
0DW64MZ	Revision of Stimulator Lead in Stomach, Percutaneous Endoscopic Approach
0DW64UZ	Revision of Feeding Device in Stomach, Percutaneous Endoscopic Approach
0DW64YZ	Revision of Other Device in Stomach, Percutaneous Endoscopic Approach
0DW670Z	Revision of Drainage Device in Stomach, Via Natural or Artificial Opening
0DW672Z	Revision of Monitoring Device in Stomach, Via Natural or Artificial Opening
0DW673Z	Revision of Infusion Device in Stomach, Via Natural or Artificial Opening
0DW677Z	Revision of Autologous Tissue Substitute in Stomach, Via Natural or Artificial Opening
0DW67CZ	Revision of Extraluminal Device in Stomach, Via Natural or Artificial Opening
0DW67DZ	Revision of Intraluminal Device in Stomach, Via Natural or Artificial Opening
0DW67JZ	Revision of Synthetic Substitute in Stomach, Via Natural or Artificial Opening
0DW67KZ	Revision of Nonautologous Tissue Substitute in Stomach, Via Natural or Artificial Opening
0DW67UZ	Revision of Feeding Device in Stomach, Via Natural or Artificial Opening

♀ Female-only   ♂ Male-only   ▲ Limited Coverage   ● Non-OR   HAC HAC-associated procedure   ▲ Non-covered procedures   ✚ Cluster

0DW67YZ	Revision of Other Device in Stomach, Via Natural or Artificial Opening
0DW680Z	Revision of Drainage Device in Stomach, Via Natural or Artificial Opening Endoscopic
0DW682Z	Revision of Monitoring Device in Stomach, Via Natural or Artificial Opening Endoscopic
0DW683Z	Revision of Infusion Device in Stomach, Via Natural or Artificial Opening Endoscopic
0DW687Z	Revision of Autologous Tissue Substitute in Stomach, Via Natural or Artificial Opening Endoscopic
0DW68CZ	Revision of Extraluminal Device in Stomach, Via Natural or Artificial Opening Endoscopic
0DW68DZ	Revision of Intraluminal Device in Stomach, Via Natural or Artificial Opening Endoscopic
0DW68JZ	Revision of Synthetic Substitute in Stomach, Via Natural or Artificial Opening Endoscopic
0DW68KZ	Revision of Nonautologous Tissue Substitute in Stomach, Via Natural or Artificial Opening Endoscopic
0DW68UZ	Revision of Feeding Device in Stomach, Via Natural or Artificial Opening Endoscopic
0DW68YZ	Revision of Other Device in Stomach, Via Natural or Artificial Opening Endoscopic
0DW6X0Z	Revision of Drainage Device in Stomach, External Approach
0DW6X2Z	Revision of Monitoring Device in Stomach, External Approach
0DW6X3Z	Revision of Infusion Device in Stomach, External Approach
0DW6X7Z	Revision of Autologous Tissue Substitute in Stomach, External Approach
0DW6XCZ	Revision of Extraluminal Device in Stomach, External Approach
0DW6XDZ	Revision of Intraluminal Device in Stomach, External Approach
0DW6XJZ	Revision of Synthetic Substitute in Stomach, External Approach
0DW6XKZ	Revision of Nonautologous Tissue Substitute in Stomach, External Approach
0DW6XUZ	Revision of Feeding Device in Stomach, External Approach
0DW807Z	Revision of Autologous Tissue Substitute in Small Intestine, Open Approach

AHA CC: 1Q, 2021, 19-20

0DW80JZ	Revision of Synthetic Substitute in Small Intestine, Open Approach
0DW80KZ	Revision of Nonautologous Tissue Substitute in Small Intestine, Open Approach
0DW847Z	Revision of Autologous Tissue Substitute in Small Intestine, Percutaneous Endoscopic Approach
0DW84JZ	Revision of Synthetic Substitute in Small Intestine, Percutaneous Endoscopic Approach
0DW84KZ	Revision of Nonautologous Tissue Substitute in Small Intestine, Percutaneous Endoscopic Approach
0DW877Z	Revision of Autologous Tissue Substitute in Small Intestine, Via Natural or Artificial Opening

0DW87JZ	Revision of Synthetic Substitute in Small Intestine, Via Natural or Artificial Opening
0DW87KZ	Revision of Nonautologous Tissue Substitute in Small Intestine, Via Natural or Artificial Opening
0DW887Z	Revision of Autologous Tissue Substitute in Small Intestine, Via Natural or Artificial Opening Endoscopic
0DW88JZ	Revision of Synthetic Substitute in Small Intestine, Via Natural or Artificial Opening Endoscopic
0DW88KZ	Revision of Nonautologous Tissue Substitute in Small Intestine, Via Natural or Artificial Opening Endoscopic
0DWD00Z	Revision of Drainage Device in Lower Intestinal Tract, Open Approach
0DWD02Z	Revision of Monitoring Device in Lower Intestinal Tract, Open Approach
0DWD03Z	Revision of Infusion Device in Lower Intestinal Tract, Open Approach
0DWD07Z	Revision of Autologous Tissue Substitute in Lower Intestinal Tract, Open Approach
0DWD0CZ	Revision of Extraluminal Device in Lower Intestinal Tract, Open Approach
0DWD0DZ	Revision of Intraluminal Device in Lower Intestinal Tract, Open Approach
0DWD0JZ	Revision of Synthetic Substitute in Lower Intestinal Tract, Open Approach
0DWD0KZ	Revision of Nonautologous Tissue Substitute in Lower Intestinal Tract, Open Approach
0DWD0UZ	Revision of Feeding Device in Lower Intestinal Tract, Open Approach
0DWD0YZ	Revision of Other Device in Lower Intestinal Tract, Open Approach
0DWD30Z	Revision of Drainage Device in Lower Intestinal Tract, Percutaneous Approach
0DWD32Z	Revision of Monitoring Device in Lower Intestinal Tract, Percutaneous Approach
0DWD33Z	Revision of Infusion Device in Lower Intestinal Tract, Percutaneous Approach
0DWD37Z	Revision of Autologous Tissue Substitute in Lower Intestinal Tract, Percutaneous Approach
0DWD3CZ	Revision of Extraluminal Device in Lower Intestinal Tract, Percutaneous Approach
0DWD3DZ	Revision of Intraluminal Device in Lower Intestinal Tract, Percutaneous Approach
0DWD3JZ	Revision of Synthetic Substitute in Lower Intestinal Tract, Percutaneous Approach
0DWD3KZ	Revision of Nonautologous Tissue Substitute in Lower Intestinal Tract, Percutaneous Approach
0DWD3UZ	Revision of Feeding Device in Lower Intestinal Tract, Percutaneous Approach
0DWD3YZ	Revision of Other Device in Lower Intestinal Tract, Percutaneous Approach

0DWD40Z	Revision of Drainage Device in Lower Intestinal Tract, Percutaneous Endoscopic Approach
0DWD42Z	Revision of Monitoring Device in Lower Intestinal Tract, Percutaneous Endoscopic Approach
0DWD43Z	Revision of Infusion Device in Lower Intestinal Tract, Percutaneous Endoscopic Approach
0DWD47Z	Revision of Autologous Tissue Substitute in Lower Intestinal Tract, Percutaneous Endoscopic Approach
0DWD4CZ	Revision of Extraluminal Device in Lower Intestinal Tract, Percutaneous Endoscopic Approach
0DWD4DZ	Revision of Intraluminal Device in Lower Intestinal Tract, Percutaneous Endoscopic Approach
0DWD4JZ	Revision of Synthetic Substitute in Lower Intestinal Tract, Percutaneous Endoscopic Approach
0DWD4KZ	Revision of Nonautologous Tissue Substitute in Lower Intestinal Tract, Percutaneous Endoscopic Approach
0DWD4UZ	Revision of Feeding Device in Lower Intestinal Tract, Percutaneous Endoscopic Approach
0DWD4YZ	Revision of Other Device in Lower Intestinal Tract, Percutaneous Endoscopic Approach
0DWD70Z	Revision of Drainage Device in Lower Intestinal Tract, Via Natural or Artificial Opening
0DWD72Z	Revision of Monitoring Device in Lower Intestinal Tract, Via Natural or Artificial Opening
0DWD73Z	Revision of Infusion Device in Lower Intestinal Tract, Via Natural or Artificial Opening
0DWD77Z	Revision of Autologous Tissue Substitute in Lower Intestinal Tract, Via Natural or Artificial Opening
0DWD7CZ	Revision of Extraluminal Device in Lower Intestinal Tract, Via Natural or Artificial Opening
0DWD7DZ	Revision of Intraluminal Device in Lower Intestinal Tract, Via Natural or Artificial Opening
0DWD7JZ	Revision of Synthetic Substitute in Lower Intestinal Tract, Via Natural or Artificial Opening
0DWD7KZ	Revision of Nonautologous Tissue Substitute in Lower Intestinal Tract, Via Natural or Artificial Opening
0DWD7UZ	Revision of Feeding Device in Lower Intestinal Tract, Via Natural or Artificial Opening
0DWD7YZ	Revision of Other Device in Lower Intestinal Tract, Via Natural or Artificial Opening
0DWD80Z	Revision of Drainage Device in Lower Intestinal Tract, Via Natural or Artificial Opening Endoscopic
0DWD82Z	Revision of Monitoring Device in Lower Intestinal Tract, Via Natural or Artificial Opening Endoscopic
0DWD83Z	Revision of Infusion Device in Lower Intestinal Tract, Via Natural or Artificial Opening Endoscopic
0DWD87Z	Revision of Autologous Tissue Substitute in Lower Intestinal Tract, Via Natural or Artificial Opening Endoscopic

0DWD8CZ	Revision of Extraluminal Device in Lower Intestinal Tract, Via Natural or Artificial Opening Endoscopic
0DWD8DZ	Revision of Intraluminal Device in Lower Intestinal Tract, Via Natural or Artificial Opening Endoscopic
0DWD8JZ	Revision of Synthetic Substitute in Lower Intestinal Tract, Via Natural or Artificial Opening Endoscopic
0DWD8KZ	Revision of Nonautologous Tissue Substitute in Lower Intestinal Tract, Via Natural or Artificial Opening Endoscopic
0DWD8UZ	Revision of Feeding Device in Lower Intestinal Tract, Via Natural or Artificial Opening Endoscopic
0DWD8YZ	Revision of Other Device in Lower Intestinal Tract, Via Natural or Artificial Opening Endoscopic
0DWDX0Z	Revision of Drainage Device in Lower Intestinal Tract, External Approach
0DWDX2Z	Revision of Monitoring Device in Lower Intestinal Tract, External Approach
0DWDX3Z	Revision of Infusion Device in Lower Intestinal Tract, External Approach
0DWDX7Z	Revision of Autologous Tissue Substitute in Lower Intestinal Tract, External Approach
0DWDXCZ	Revision of Extraluminal Device in Lower Intestinal Tract, External Approach
0DWDXDZ	Revision of Intraluminal Device in Lower Intestinal Tract, External Approach
0DWDXJZ	Revision of Synthetic Substitute in Lower Intestinal Tract, External Approach
0DWDXKZ	Revision of Nonautologous Tissue Substitute in Lower Intestinal Tract, External Approach
0DWDXUZ	Revision of Feeding Device in Lower Intestinal Tract, External Approach
0DWE07Z	Revision of Autologous Tissue Substitute in Large Intestine, Open Approach
0DWE0JZ	Revision of Synthetic Substitute in Large Intestine, Open Approach
0DWE0KZ	Revision of Nonautologous Tissue Substitute in Large Intestine, Open Approach
0DWE47Z	Revision of Autologous Tissue Substitute in Large Intestine, Percutaneous Endoscopic Approach
0DWE4JZ	Revision of Synthetic Substitute in Large Intestine, Percutaneous Endoscopic Approach
0DWE4KZ	Revision of Nonautologous Tissue Substitute in Large Intestine, Percutaneous Endoscopic Approach
0DWE77Z	Revision of Autologous Tissue Substitute in Large Intestine, Via Natural or Artificial Opening

0DWE7JZ	Revision of Synthetic Substitute in Large Intestine, Via Natural or Artificial Opening
0DWE7KZ	Revision of Nonautologous Tissue Substitute in Large Intestine, Via Natural or Artificial Opening
0DWE87Z	Revision of Autologous Tissue Substitute in Large Intestine, Via Natural or Artificial Opening Endoscopic
0DWE8JZ	Revision of Synthetic Substitute in Large Intestine, Via Natural or Artificial Opening Endoscopic
0DWE8KZ	Revision of Nonautologous Tissue Substitute in Large Intestine, Via Natural or Artificial Opening Endoscopic
0DWQ0LZ	Revision of Artificial Sphincter in Anus, Open Approach
0DWQ3LZ	Revision of Artificial Sphincter in Anus, Percutaneous Approach
0DWQ4LZ	Revision of Artificial Sphincter in Anus, Percutaneous Endoscopic Approach
0DWQ7LZ	Revision of Artificial Sphincter in Anus, Via Natural or Artificial Opening
0DWQ8LZ	Revision of Artificial Sphincter in Anus, Via Natural or Artificial Opening Endoscopic
0DWR0MZ	Revision of Stimulator Lead in Anal Sphincter, Open Approach
0DWR3MZ	Revision of Stimulator Lead in Anal Sphincter, Percutaneous Approach
0DWR4MZ	Revision of Stimulator Lead in Anal Sphincter, Percutaneous Endoscopic Approach
0DWU00Z	Revision of Drainage Device in Omentum, Open Approach
0DWU07Z	Revision of Autologous Tissue Substitute in Omentum, Open Approach
0DWU0JZ	Revision of Synthetic Substitute in Omentum, Open Approach
0DWU0KZ	Revision of Nonautologous Tissue Substitute in Omentum, Open Approach
0DWU30Z	Revision of Drainage Device in Omentum, Percutaneous Approach
0DWU37Z	Revision of Autologous Tissue Substitute in Omentum, Percutaneous Approach
0DWU3JZ	Revision of Synthetic Substitute in Omentum, Percutaneous Approach
0DWU3KZ	Revision of Nonautologous Tissue Substitute in Omentum, Percutaneous Approach
0DWU40Z	Revision of Drainage Device in Omentum, Percutaneous Endoscopic Approach
0DWU47Z	Revision of Autologous Tissue Substitute in Omentum, Percutaneous Endoscopic Approach
0DWU4JZ	Revision of Synthetic Substitute in Omentum, Percutaneous Endoscopic Approach

0DWU4KZ	Revision of Nonautologous Tissue Substitute in Omentum, Percutaneous Endoscopic Approach
0DWV00Z	Revision of Drainage Device in Mesentery, Open Approach
0DWV07Z	Revision of Autologous Tissue Substitute in Mesentery, Open Approach
0DWV0JZ	Revision of Synthetic Substitute in Mesentery, Open Approach
0DWV0KZ	Revision of Nonautologous Tissue Substitute in Mesentery, Open Approach
0DWV30Z	Revision of Drainage Device in Mesentery, Percutaneous Approach
0DWV37Z	Revision of Autologous Tissue Substitute in Mesentery, Percutaneous Approach
0DWV3JZ	Revision of Synthetic Substitute in Mesentery, Percutaneous Approach
0DWV3KZ	Revision of Nonautologous Tissue Substitute in Mesentery, Percutaneous Approach
0DWV40Z	Revision of Drainage Device in Mesentery, Percutaneous Endoscopic Approach
0DWV47Z	Revision of Autologous Tissue Substitute in Mesentery, Percutaneous Endoscopic Approach
0DWV4JZ	Revision of Synthetic Substitute in Mesentery, Percutaneous Endoscopic Approach
0DWV4KZ	Revision of Nonautologous Tissue Substitute in Mesentery, Percutaneous Endoscopic Approach
0DWW00Z	Revision of Drainage Device in Peritoneum, Open Approach
0DWW07Z	Revision of Autologous Tissue Substitute in Peritoneum, Open Approach
0DWW0JZ	Revision of Synthetic Substitute in Peritoneum, Open Approach
0DWW0KZ	Revision of Nonautologous Tissue Substitute in Peritoneum, Open Approach
0DWW30Z	Revision of Drainage Device in Peritoneum, Percutaneous Approach
0DWW37Z	Revision of Autologous Tissue Substitute in Peritoneum, Percutaneous Approach
0DWW3JZ	Revision of Synthetic Substitute in Peritoneum, Percutaneous Approach
0DWW3KZ	Revision of Nonautologous Tissue Substitute in Peritoneum, Percutaneous Approach
0DWW40Z	Revision of Drainage Device in Peritoneum, Percutaneous Endoscopic Approach
0DWW47Z	Revision of Autologous Tissue Substitute in Peritoneum, Percutaneous Endoscopic Approach
0DWW4JZ	Revision of Synthetic Substitute in Peritoneum, Percutaneous Endoscopic Approach
0DWW4KZ	Revision of Nonautologous Tissue Substitute in Peritoneum, Percutaneous Endoscopic Approach

0DX – Gastrointestinal System, Transfer

0DX60Z5	Transfer Stomach to Esophagus, Open Approach
	AHA CC: 2Q, 2016, 22-23; 2Q, 2017, 18
0DX64Z5	Transfer Stomach to Esophagus, Percutaneous Endoscopic Approach
0DX80Z5	Transfer Small Intestine to Esophagus, Open Approach

0DX84Z5	Transfer Small Intestine to Esophagus, Percutaneous Endoscopic Approach
0DXE0Z5	Transfer Large Intestine to Esophagus, Open Approach
	AHA CC: 1Q, 2019, 14-15
♀ **0DXE0Z7**	Transfer Large Intestine to Vagina, Open Approach
	AHA CC: 4Q, 2019, 30

0DXE4Z5	Transfer Large Intestine to Esophagus, Percutaneous Endoscopic Approach
♀ **0DXE4Z7**	Transfer Large Intestine to Vagina, Percutaneous Endoscopic Approach

♀ Female-only   ♂ Male-only   ▲ Limited Coverage   ● Non-OR   ▦ HAC-associated procedure   ▲ Non-covered procedures   ✚ Cluster

Review Coding Guideline B3.16

0DY50Z0 Transplantation of Esophagus, Allogeneic, Open Approach

0DY50Z1 Transplantation of Esophagus, Syngeneic, Open Approach

0DY50Z2 Transplantation of Esophagus, Zooplastic, Open Approach

0DY60Z0 Transplantation of Stomach, Allogeneic, Open Approach

0DY60Z1 Transplantation of Stomach, Syngeneic, Open Approach

0DY60Z2 Transplantation of Stomach, Zooplastic, Open Approach

▲ **0DY80Z0** Transplantation of Small Intestine, Allogeneic, Open Approach

▲ **0DY80Z1** Transplantation of Small Intestine, Syngeneic, Open Approach

▲ **0DY80Z2** Transplantation of Small Intestine, Zooplastic, Open Approach

▲ **0DYE0Z0** Transplantation of Large Intestine, Allogeneic, Open Approach

▲ **0DYE0Z1** Transplantation of Large Intestine, Syngeneic, Open Approach`

▲ **0DYE0Z2** Transplantation of Large Intestine, Zooplastic, Open Approach

Surfaces and Bed of Liver

Diaphragm (*pulled up*)

Coronary ligament

Left triangular ligament

Right triangular ligament

Fibrous appendix of liver

Left lobe of liver

Right lobe of liver

Falciform ligament

Inferior border of liver

Inferior border of liver

Costal impressions

Round ligament (ligamentum teres) of liver (obliterated umbilical vein) forming free border of falciform ligament

Gallbladder (fundus)

Anterior view

Coronary ligament

Hepatic veins

Inferior vena cava

Bare area

Suprarenal impression

Hepatorenal portion of coronary ligament

Fibrous appendix of liver

Left triangular ligament

Right triangular ligament

Gastric impression

(Common) bile duct

Esophageal impression

Common hepatic duct

Cystic duct

Fissure for ligamentum venosum

Renal impression

Caudate lobe

Duodenal impression

Papillary process

Quadrate lobe

Caudate process

Gallbladder

Hepatic artery proper

Falciform ligament

Hepatic portal vein

Round ligament of liver

Fissure for ligamentum teres

Colic impression

Porta hepatis

Visceral surface

Falciform ligament

Coronary ligament

Left triangular ligament

Bare area

Inferior vena cava

Suprarenal gland

Right kidney

Left triangular ligament

Right triangular ligament

Fissure for ligamentum venosum

Superior recess of omental bursa

Groove for (inferior) vena cava

Duodenum

Transverse colon

Stomach

Posterior view

Bed of liver

Pancreas: Anatomy and Histology

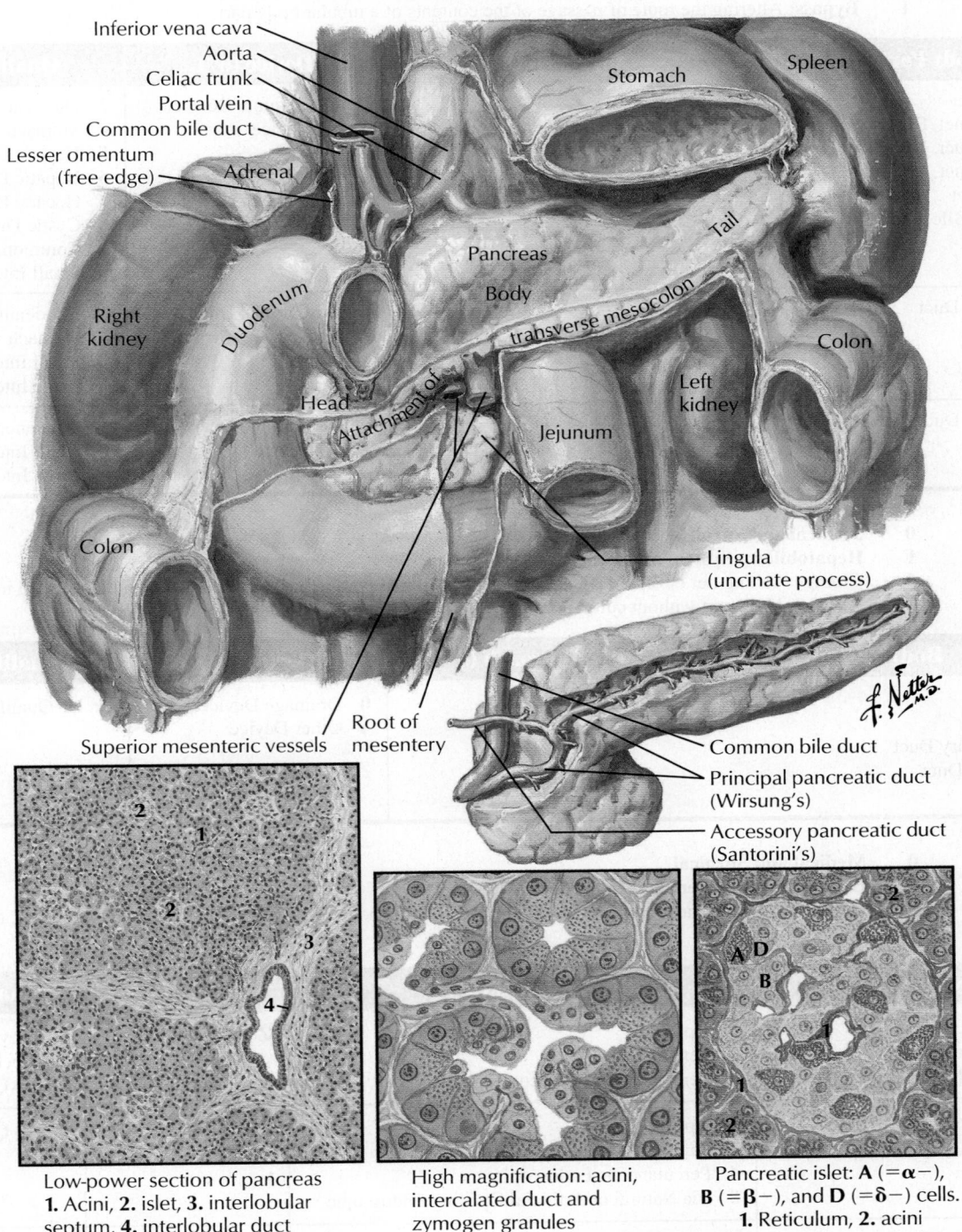

Inferior vena cava
Aorta
Celiac trunk
Portal vein
Common bile duct
Lesser omentum (free edge)
Adrenal
Stomach
Spleen
Pancreas
Body
Tail
transverse mesocolon
Right kidney
Duodenum
Colon
Left kidney
Head
Attachment of
Jejunum
Lingula (uncinate process)
Colon
Superior mesenteric vessels
Root of mesentery
Common bile duct
Principal pancreatic duct (Wirsung's)
Accessory pancreatic duct (Santorini's)

Low-power section of pancreas
1. Acini, **2.** islet, **3.** interlobular septum, **4.** interlobular duct

High magnification: acini, intercalated duct and zymogen granules

Pancreatic islet: **A** (=**α**−), **B** (=**β**−), and **D** (=**δ**−) cells.
1. Reticulum, **2.** acini

Hepatobiliary System and Pancreas Tables 0F1–0FY

Section	0	Medical and Surgical
Body System	F	Hepatobiliary System and Pancreas
Operation	1	**Bypass:** Altering the route of passage of the contents of a tubular body part

Body Part (4th)	Approach (5th)	Device (6th)	Qualifier (7th)
4 Gallbladder 5 Hepatic Duct, Right 6 Hepatic Duct, Left 7 Hepatic Duct, Common 8 Cystic Duct 9 Common Bile Duct	0 Open 4 Percutaneous Endoscopic	D Intraluminal Device Z No Device	3 Duodenum 4 Stomach 5 Hepatic Duct, Right 6 Hepatic Duct, Left 7 Hepatic Duct, Caudate 8 Cystic Duct 9 Common Bile Duct B Small Intestine
D Pancreatic Duct	0 Open 4 Percutaneous Endoscopic	D Intraluminal Device Z No Device	3 Duodenum 4 Stomach B Small Intestine C Large Intestine
F Pancreatic Duct, Accessory G Pancreas	0 Open 4 Percutaneous Endoscopic	D Intraluminal Device Z No Device	3 Duodenum B Small Intestine C Large Intestine

Section	0	Medical and Surgical
Body System	F	Hepatobiliary System and Pancreas
Operation	2	**Change:** Taking out or off a device from a body part and putting back an identical or similar device in or on the same body part without cutting or puncturing the skin or a mucous membrane

Body Part (4th)	Approach (5th)	Device (6th)	Qualifier (7th)
0 Liver 4 Gallbladder B Hepatobiliary Duct D Pancreatic Duct G Pancreas	X External	0 Drainage Device Y Other Device	Z No Qualifier

Section	0	Medical and Surgical
Body System	F	Hepatobiliary System and Pancreas
Operation	5	**Destruction:** Physical eradication of all or a portion of a body part by the direct use of energy, force, or a destructive agent

Body Part (4th)	Approach (5th)	Device (6th)	Qualifier (7th)
0 Liver 1 Liver, Right Lobe 2 Liver, Left Lobe	0 Open 3 Percutaneous 4 Percutaneous Endoscopic	Z No Device	F Irreversible Electroporation Z No Qualifier
4 Gallbladder	0 Open 3 Percutaneous 4 Percutaneous Endoscopic 8 Via Natural or Artificial Opening Endoscopic	Z No Device	Z No Qualifier
5 Hepatic Duct, Right 6 Hepatic Duct, Left 7 Hepatic Duct, Common 8 Cystic Duct 9 Common Bile Duct C Ampulla of Vater D Pancreatic Duct F Pancreatic Duct, Accessory	0 Open 3 Percutaneous 4 Percutaneous Endoscopic 7 Via Natural or Artificial Opening 8 Via Natural or Artificial Opening Endoscopic	Z No Device	Z No Qualifier
G Pancreas	0 Open 3 Percutaneous 4 Percutaneous Endoscopic	Z No Device	F Irreversible Electroporation Z No Qualifier
G Pancreas	8 Via Natural or Artificial Opening Endoscopic	Z No Device	Z No Qualifier

Section	0	Medical and Surgical
Body System	F	Hepatobiliary System and Pancreas
Operation	7	Dilation: Expanding an orifice or the lumen of a tubular body part

Body Part (4th)	Approach (5th)	Device (6th)	Qualifier (7th)
5 Hepatic Duct, Right 6 Hepatic Duct, Left 7 Hepatic Duct, Common 8 Cystic Duct 9 Common Bile Duct C Ampulla of Vater D Pancreatic Duct F Pancreatic Duct, Accessory	0 Open 3 Percutaneous 4 Percutaneous Endoscopic 7 Via Natural or Artificial Opening 8 Via Natural or Artificial Opening Endoscopic	D Intraluminal Device Z No Device	Z No Qualifier

Section	0	Medical and Surgical
Body System	F	Hepatobiliary System and Pancreas
Operation	8	Division: Cutting into a body part, without draining fluids and/or gases from the body part, in order to separate or transect a body part

Body Part (4th)	Approach (5th)	Device (6th)	Qualifier (7th)
0 Liver 1 Liver, Right Lobe 2 Liver, Left Lobe G Pancreas	0 Open 3 Percutaneous 4 Percutaneous Endoscopic	Z No Device	Z No Qualifier

Section	0	Medical and Surgical
Body System	F	Hepatobiliary System and Pancreas
Operation	9	Drainage: Taking or letting out fluids and/or gases from a body part

Body Part (4th)	Approach (5th)	Device (6th)	Qualifier (7th)
0 Liver 1 Liver, Right Lobe 2 Liver, Left Lobe	0 Open 3 Percutaneous 4 Percutaneous Endoscopic	0 Drainage Device	Z No Qualifier
0 Liver 1 Liver, Right Lobe 2 Liver, Left Lobe	0 Open 3 Percutaneous 4 Percutaneous Endoscopic	Z No Device	X Diagnostic Z No Qualifier
4 Gallbladder G Pancreas	0 Open 3 Percutaneous 4 Percutaneous Endoscopic 8 Via Natural or Artificial Opening Endoscopic	0 Drainage Device	Z No Qualifier
4 Gallbladder G Pancreas	0 Open 3 Percutaneous 4 Percutaneous Endoscopic 8 Via Natural or Artificial Opening Endoscopic	Z No Device	X Diagnostic Z No Qualifier
5 Hepatic Duct, Right 6 Hepatic Duct, Left 7 Hepatic Duct, Common 8 Cystic Duct 9 Common Bile Duct C Ampulla of Vater D Pancreatic Duct F Pancreatic Duct, Accessory	0 Open 3 Percutaneous 4 Percutaneous Endoscopic 7 Via Natural or Artificial Opening 8 Via Natural or Artificial Opening Endoscopic	0 Drainage Device	Z No Qualifier
5 Hepatic Duct, Right 6 Hepatic Duct, Left 7 Hepatic Duct, Common 8 Cystic Duct 9 Common Bile Duct C Ampulla of Vater D Pancreatic Duct F Pancreatic Duct, Accessory	0 Open 3 Percutaneous 4 Percutaneous Endoscopic 7 Via Natural or Artificial Opening 8 Via Natural or Artificial Opening Endoscopic	Z No Device	X Diagnostic Z No Qualifier

Section	0	Medical and Surgical
Body System	F	Hepatobiliary System and Pancreas
Operation	B	Excision: Cutting out or off, without replacement, a portion of a body part

Body Part (4th)	Approach (5th)	Device (6th)	Qualifier (7th)
0 Liver 1 Liver, Right Lobe 2 Liver, Left Lobe	0 Open 3 Percutaneous 4 Percutaneous Endoscopic	Z No Device	X Diagnostic Z No Qualifier
4 Gallbladder G Pancreas	0 Open 3 Percutaneous 4 Percutaneous Endoscopic 8 Via Natural or Artificial Opening Endoscopic	Z No Device	X Diagnostic Z No Qualifier
5 Hepatic Duct, Right 6 Hepatic Duct, Left 7 Hepatic Duct, Common 8 Cystic Duct 9 Common Bile Duct C Ampulla of Vater D Pancreatic Duct F Pancreatic Duct, Accessory	0 Open 3 Percutaneous 4 Percutaneous Endoscopic 7 Via Natural or Artificial Opening 8 Via Natural or Artificial Opening Endoscopic	Z No Device	X Diagnostic Z No Qualifier

Section	0	Medical and Surgical
Body System	F	Hepatobiliary System and Pancreas
Operation	C	Extirpation: Taking or cutting out solid matter from a body part

Body Part (4th)	Approach (5th)	Device (6th)	Qualifier (7th)
0 Liver 1 Liver, Right Lobe 2 Liver, Left Lobe	0 Open 3 Percutaneous 4 Percutaneous Endoscopic	Z No Device	Z No Qualifier
4 Gallbladder G Pancreas	0 Open 3 Percutaneous 4 Percutaneous Endoscopic 8 Via Natural or Artificial Opening Endoscopic	Z No Device	Z No Qualifier
5 Hepatic Duct, Right 6 Hepatic Duct, Left 7 Hepatic Duct, Common 8 Cystic Duct 9 Common Bile Duct C Ampulla of Vater D Pancreatic Duct F Pancreatic Duct, Accessory	0 Open 3 Percutaneous 4 Percutaneous Endoscopic 7 Via Natural or Artificial Opening 8 Via Natural or Artificial Opening Endoscopic	Z No Device	Z No Qualifier

Section	0	Medical and Surgical
Body System	F	Hepatobiliary System and Pancreas
Operation	D	Extraction: Pulling or stripping out or off all or a portion of a body part by the use of force

Body Part (4th)	Approach (5th)	Device (6th)	Qualifier (7th)
0 Liver 1 Liver, Right Lobe 2 Liver, Left Lobe	3 Percutaneous 4 Percutaneous Endoscopic	Z No Device	X Diagnostic
4 Gallbladder 5 Hepatic Duct, Right 6 Hepatic Duct, Left 7 Hepatic Duct, Common 8 Cystic Duct 9 Common Bile Duct C Ampulla of Vater D Pancreatic Duct F Pancreatic Duct, Accessory G Pancreas	3 Percutaneous 4 Percutaneous Endoscopic 8 Via Natural or Artificial Opening Endoscopic	Z No Device	X Diagnostic

Section	0	Medical and Surgical
Body System	F	Hepatobiliary System and Pancreas
Operation	F	Fragmentation: Breaking solid matter in a body part into pieces

Body Part (4th)	Approach (5th)	Device (6th)	Qualifier (7th)
4 Gallbladder 5 Hepatic Duct, Right 6 Hepatic Duct, Left 7 Hepatic Duct, Common 8 Cystic Duct 9 Common Bile Duct C Ampulla of Vater D Pancreatic Duct F Pancreatic Duct, Accessory	0 Open 3 Percutaneous 4 Percutaneous Endoscopic 7 Via Natural or Artificial Opening 8 Via Natural or Artificial Opening Endoscopic X External	Z No Device	Z No Qualifier

Section	0	Medical and Surgical
Body System	F	Hepatobiliary System and Pancreas
Operation	H	Insertion: Putting in a nonbiological appliance that monitors, assists, performs, or prevents a physiological function but does not physically take the place of a body part

Body Part (4th)	Approach (5th)	Device (6th)	Qualifier (7th)
0 Liver 4 Gallbladder G Pancreas	0 Open 3 Percutaneous 4 Percutaneous Endoscopic	1 Radioactive Element 2 Monitoring Device 3 Infusion Device Y Other Device	Z No Qualifier
1 Liver, Right Lobe 2 Liver, Left Lobe	0 Open 3 Percutaneous 4 Percutaneous Endoscopic	2 Monitoring Device 3 Infusion Device	Z No Qualifier
B Hepatobiliary Duct D Pancreatic Duct	0 Open 3 Percutaneous 4 Percutaneous Endoscopic 7 Via Natural or Artificial Opening 8 Via Natural or Artificial Opening Endoscopic	1 Radioactive Element 2 Monitoring Device 3 Infusion Device D Intraluminal Device Y Other Device	Z No Qualifier

Section	0	Medical and Surgical
Body System	F	Hepatobiliary System and Pancreas
Operation	J	Inspection: Visually and/or manually exploring a body part

Body Part (4th)	Approach (5th)	Device (6th)	Qualifier (7th)
0 Liver	0 Open 3 Percutaneous 4 Percutaneous Endoscopic X External	Z No Device	Z No Qualifier
4 Gallbladder G Pancreas	0 Open 3 Percutaneous 4 Percutaneous Endoscopic 8 Via Natural or Artificial Opening Endoscopic X External	Z No Device	Z No Qualifier
B Hepatobiliary Duct D Pancreatic Duct	0 Open 3 Percutaneous 4 Percutaneous Endoscopic 7 Via Natural or Artificial Opening 8 Via Natural or Artificial Opening Endoscopic	Z No Device	Z No Qualifier

Section	0	Medical and Surgical
Body System	F	Hepatobiliary System and Pancreas
Operation	L	**Occlusion:** Completely closing an orifice or the lumen of a tubular body part

Body Part (4th)	Approach (5th)	Device (6th)	Qualifier (7th)
5 Hepatic Duct, Right 6 Hepatic Duct, Left 7 Hepatic Duct, Common 8 Cystic Duct 9 Common Bile Duct C Ampulla of Vater D Pancreatic Duct F Pancreatic Duct, Accessory	0 Open 3 Percutaneous 4 Percutaneous Endoscopic	C Extraluminal Device D Intraluminal Device Z No Device	Z No Qualifier
5 Hepatic Duct, Right 6 Hepatic Duct, Left 7 Hepatic Duct, Common 8 Cystic Duct 9 Common Bile Duct C Ampulla of Vater D Pancreatic Duct F Pancreatic Duct, Accessory	7 Via Natural or Artificial Opening 8 Via Natural or Artificial Opening Endoscopic	D Intraluminal Device Z No Device	Z No Qualifier

Section	0	Medical and Surgical
Body System	F	Hepatobiliary System and Pancreas
Operation	M	**Reattachment:** Putting back in or on all or a portion of a separated body part to its normal location or other suitable location

Body Part (4th)	Approach (5th)	Device (6th)	Qualifier (7th)
0 Liver 1 Liver, Right Lobe 2 Liver, Left Lobe 4 Gallbladder 5 Hepatic Duct, Right 6 Hepatic Duct, Left 7 Hepatic Duct, Common 8 Cystic Duct 9 Common Bile Duct C Ampulla of Vater D Pancreatic Duct F Pancreatic Duct, Accessory G Pancreas	0 Open 4 Percutaneous Endoscopic	Z No Device	Z No Qualifier

Section	0	Medical and Surgical
Body System	F	Hepatobiliary System and Pancreas
Operation	N	**Release:** Freeing a body part from an abnormal physical constraint by cutting or by the use of force

Body Part (4th)	Approach (5th)	Device (6th)	Qualifier (7th)
0 Liver 1 Liver, Right Lobe 2 Liver, Left Lobe	0 Open 3 Percutaneous 4 Percutaneous Endoscopic	Z No Device	Z No Qualifier
4 Gallbladder G Pancreas	0 Open 3 Percutaneous 4 Percutaneous Endoscopic 8 Via Natural or Artificial Opening Endoscopic	Z No Device	Z No Qualifier
5 Hepatic Duct, Right 6 Hepatic Duct, Left 7 Hepatic Duct, Common 8 Cystic Duct 9 Common Bile Duct C Ampulla of Vater D Pancreatic Duct F Pancreatic Duct, Accessory	0 Open 3 Percutaneous 4 Percutaneous Endoscopic 7 Via Natural or Artificial Opening 8 Via Natural or Artificial Opening Endoscopic	Z No Device	Z No Qualifier

Section   0   **Medical and Surgical**
Body System   F   **Hepatobiliary System and Pancreas**
Operation   P   **Removal:** Taking out or off a device from a body part

Body Part (4th)	Approach (5th)	Device (6th)	Qualifier (7th)
0 Liver	**0** Open **3** Percutaneous **4** Percutaneous Endoscopic	**0** Drainage Device **2** Monitoring Device **3** Infusion Device **Y** Other Device	**Z** No Qualifier
0 Liver	**X** External	**0** Drainage Device **2** Monitoring Device **3** Infusion Device	**Z** No Qualifier
4 Gallbladder **G** Pancreas	**0** Open **3** Percutaneous **4** Percutaneous Endoscopic **X** External	**0** Drainage Device **2** Monitoring Device **3** Infusion Device **D** Intraluminal Device **Y** Other Device	**Z** No Qualifier
4 Gallbladder **G** Pancreas	**X** External	**0** Drainage Device **2** Monitoring Device **3** Infusion Device **D** Intraluminal Device	**Z** No Qualifier
B Hepatobiliary Duct **D** Pancreatic Duct	**0** Open **3** Percutaneous **4** Percutaneous Endoscopic **7** Via Natural or Artificial Opening **8** Via Natural or Artificial Opening Endoscopic	**0** Drainage Device **1** Radioactive Element **2** Monitoring Device **3** Infusion Device **7** Autologous Tissue Substitute **C** Extraluminal Device **D** Intraluminal Device **J** Synthetic Substitute **K** Nonautologous Tissue Substitute **Y** Other Device	**Z** No Qualifier
B Hepatobiliary Duct **D** Pancreatic Duct	**X** External	**0** Drainage Device **1** Radioactive Element **2** Monitoring Device **3** Infusion Device **D** Intraluminal Device	**Z** No Qualifier

Section   0   **Medical and Surgical**
Body System   F   **Hepatobiliary System and Pancreas**
Operation   Q   **Repair:** Restoring, to the extent possible, a body part to its normal anatomic structure and function

Body Part (4th)	Approach (5th)	Device (6th)	Qualifier (7th)
0 Liver **1** Liver, Right Lobe **2** Liver, Left Lobe	**0** Open **3** Percutaneous **4** Percutaneous Endoscopic	**Z** No Device	**Z** No Qualifier
4 Gallbladder **G** Pancreas	**0** Open **3** Percutaneous **4** Percutaneous Endoscopic **8** Via Natural or Artificial Opening Endoscopic	**Z** No Device	**Z** No Qualifier
5 Hepatic Duct, Right **6** Hepatic Duct, Left **7** Hepatic Duct, Common **8** Cystic Duct **9** Common Bile Duct **C** Ampulla of Vater **D** Pancreatic Duct **F** Pancreatic Duct, Accessory	**0** Open **3** Percutaneous **4** Percutaneous Endoscopic **7** Via Natural or Artificial Opening **8** Via Natural or Artificial Opening Endoscopic	**Z** No Device	**Z** No Qualifier

Section	0	Medical and Surgical
Body System	F	Hepatobiliary System and Pancreas
Operation	R	**Replacement:** Putting in or on biological or synthetic material that physically takes the place and/or function of all or a portion of a body part

Body Part (4th)	Approach (5th)	Device (6th)	Qualifier (7th)
5 Hepatic Duct, Right 6 Hepatic Duct, Left 7 Hepatic Duct, Common 8 Cystic Duct 9 Common Bile Duct C Ampulla of Vater D Pancreatic Duct F Pancreatic Duct, Accessory	0 Open 4 Percutaneous Endoscopic 8 Via Natural or Artificial Opening Endoscopic	7 Autologous Tissue Substitute J Synthetic Substitute K Nonautologous Tissue Substitute	Z No Qualifier

Section	0	Medical and Surgical
Body System	F	Hepatobiliary System and Pancreas
Operation	S	**Reposition:** Moving to its normal location, or other suitable location, all or a portion of a body part

Body Part (4th)	Approach (5th)	Device (6th)	Qualifier (7th)
0 Liver 4 Gallbladder 5 Hepatic Duct, Right 6 Hepatic Duct, Left 7 Hepatic Duct, Common 8 Cystic Duct 9 Common Bile Duct C Ampulla of Vater D Pancreatic Duct F Pancreatic Duct, Accessory G Pancreas	0 Open 4 Percutaneous Endoscopic	Z No Device	Z No Qualifier

Section	0	Medical and Surgical
Body System	F	Hepatobiliary System and Pancreas
Operation	T	**Resection:** Cutting out or off, without replacement, all of a body part

Body Part (4th)	Approach (5th)	Device (6th)	Qualifier (7th)
0 Liver 1 Liver, Right Lobe 2 Liver, Left Lobe 4 Gallbladder G Pancreas	0 Open 4 Percutaneous Endoscopic	Z No Device	Z No Qualifier
5 Hepatic Duct, Right 6 Hepatic Duct, Left 7 Hepatic Duct, Common 8 Cystic Duct 9 Common Bile Duct C Ampulla of Vater D Pancreatic Duct F Pancreatic Duct, Accessory	0 Open 4 Percutaneous Endoscopic 7 Via Natural or Artificial Opening 8 Via Natural or Artificial Opening Endoscopic	Z No Device	Z No Qualifier

Section	0	Medical and Surgical
Body System	F	Hepatobiliary System and Pancreas
Operation	U	**Supplement:** Putting in or on biological or synthetic material that physically reinforces and/or augments the function of a portion of a body part

Body Part (4th)	Approach (5th)	Device (6th)	Qualifier (7th)
5 Hepatic Duct, Right 6 Hepatic Duct, Left 7 Hepatic Duct, Common 8 Cystic Duct 9 Common Bile Duct C Ampulla of Vater D Pancreatic Duct F Pancreatic Duct, Accessory	0 Open 3 Percutaneous 4 Percutaneous Endoscopic 8 Via Natural or Artificial Opening Endoscopic	7 Autologous Tissue Substitute J Synthetic Substitute K Nonautologous Tissue Substitute	Z No Qualifier

Section	0	Medical and Surgical
Body System	F	Hepatobiliary System and Pancreas
Operation	V	Restriction: Partially closing an orifice or the lumen of a tubular body part

Body Part (4th)	Approach (5th)	Device (6th)	Qualifier (7th)
5 Hepatic Duct, Right 6 Hepatic Duct, Left 7 Hepatic Duct, Common 8 Cystic Duct 9 Common Bile Duct C Ampulla of Vater D Pancreatic Duct F Pancreatic Duct, Accessory	0 Open 3 Percutaneous 4 Percutaneous Endoscopic	C Extraluminal Device D Intraluminal Device Z No Device	Z No Qualifier
5 Hepatic Duct, Right 6 Hepatic Duct, Left 7 Hepatic Duct, Common 8 Cystic Duct 9 Common Bile Duct C Ampulla of Vater D Pancreatic Duct F Pancreatic Duct, Accessory	7 Via Natural or Artificial Opening 8 Via Natural or Artificial Opening Endoscopic	D Intraluminal Device Z No Device	Z No Qualifier

Section	0	Medical and Surgical
Body System	F	Hepatobiliary System and Pancreas
Operation	W	Revision: Correcting, to the extent possible, a portion of a malfunctioning device or the position of a displaced device

Body Part (4th)	Approach (5th)	Device (6th)	Qualifier (7th)
0 Liver	0 Open 3 Percutaneous 4 Percutaneous Endoscopic	0 Drainage Device 2 Monitoring Device 3 Infusion Device Y Other Device	Z No Qualifier
0 Liver	X External	0 Drainage Device 2 Monitoring Device 3 Infusion Device	Z No Qualifier
4 Gallbladder G Pancreas	0 Open 3 Percutaneous 4 Percutaneous Endoscopic	0 Drainage Device 2 Monitoring Device 3 Infusion Device D Intraluminal Device Y Other Device	Z No Qualifier
4 Gallbladder G Pancreas	X External	0 Drainage Device 2 Monitoring Device 3 Infusion Device D Intraluminal Device	Z No Qualifier
B Hepatobiliary Duct D Pancreatic Duct	0 Open 3 Percutaneous 4 Percutaneous Endoscopic 7 Via Natural or Artificial Opening 8 Via Natural or Artificial Opening Endoscopic	0 Drainage Device 2 Monitoring Device 3 Infusion Device 7 Autologous Tissue Substitute C Extraluminal Device D Intraluminal Device J Synthetic Substitute K Nonautologous Tissue Substitute Y Other Device	Z No Qualifier

Continued →

Section	0	Medical and Surgical
Body System	F	Hepatobiliary System and Pancreas
Operation	W	Revision: Correcting, to the extent possible, a portion of a malfunctioning device or the position of a displaced device

Body Part (4th)	Approach (5th)	Device (6th)	Qualifier (7th)
B Hepatobiliary Duct D Pancreatic Duct	X External	0 Drainage Device 2 Monitoring Device 3 Infusion Device 7 Autologous Tissue Substitute C Extraluminal Device D Intraluminal Device J Synthetic Substitute K Nonautologous Tissue Substitute	Z No Qualifier

Section	0	Medical and Surgical
Body System	F	Hepatobiliary System and Pancreas
Operation	Y	Transplantation: Putting in or on all or a portion of a living body part taken from another individual or animal to physically take the place and/or function of all or a portion of a similar body part

Body Part (4th)	Approach (5th)	Device (6th)	Qualifier (7th)
0 Liver G Pancreas	0 Open	Z No Device	0 Allogeneic 1 Syngeneic 2 Zooplastic

Hepatobiliary System and Pancreas Code Listing 0F1–0FY

0F1 – Hepatobiliary System and Pancreas, Bypass

Review Coding Guideline B3.6a

0F140D3 Bypass Gallbladder to Duodenum with Intraluminal Device, Open Approach
0F140D4 Bypass Gallbladder to Stomach with Intraluminal Device, Open Approach
0F140D5 Bypass Gallbladder to Right Hepatic Duct with Intraluminal Device, Open Approach
0F140D6 Bypass Gallbladder to Left Hepatic Duct with Intraluminal Device, Open Approach
0F140D7 Bypass Gallbladder to Caudate Hepatic Duct with Intraluminal Device, Open Approach
0F140D8 Bypass Gallbladder to Cystic Duct with Intraluminal Device, Open Approach
0F140D9 Bypass Gallbladder to Common Bile Duct with Intraluminal Device, Open Approach
0F140DB Bypass Gallbladder to Small Intestine with Intraluminal Device, Open Approach
0F140Z3 Bypass Gallbladder to Duodenum, Open Approach
0F140Z4 Bypass Gallbladder to Stomach, Open Approach
0F140Z5 Bypass Gallbladder to Right Hepatic Duct, Open Approach
0F140Z6 Bypass Gallbladder to Left Hepatic Duct, Open Approach
0F140Z7 Bypass Gallbladder to Caudate Hepatic Duct, Open Approach
0F140Z8 Bypass Gallbladder to Cystic Duct, Open Approach
0F140Z9 Bypass Gallbladder to Common Bile Duct, Open Approach
0F140ZB Bypass Gallbladder to Small Intestine, Open Approach
0F144D3 Bypass Gallbladder to Duodenum with Intraluminal Device, Percutaneous Endoscopic Approach
0F144D4 Bypass Gallbladder to Stomach with Intraluminal Device, Percutaneous Endoscopic Approach

0F144D5 Bypass Gallbladder to Right Hepatic Duct with Intraluminal Device, Percutaneous Endoscopic Approach
0F144D6 Bypass Gallbladder to Left Hepatic Duct with Intraluminal Device, Percutaneous Endoscopic Approach
0F144D7 Bypass Gallbladder to Caudate Hepatic Duct with Intraluminal Device, Percutaneous Endoscopic Approach
0F144D8 Bypass Gallbladder to Cystic Duct with Intraluminal Device, Percutaneous Endoscopic Approach
0F144D9 Bypass Gallbladder to Common Bile Duct with Intraluminal Device, Percutaneous Endoscopic Approach
0F144DB Bypass Gallbladder to Small Intestine with Intraluminal Device, Percutaneous Endoscopic Approach
0F144Z3 Bypass Gallbladder to Duodenum, Percutaneous Endoscopic Approach
0F144Z4 Bypass Gallbladder to Stomach, Percutaneous Endoscopic Approach
0F144Z5 Bypass Gallbladder to Right Hepatic Duct, Percutaneous Endoscopic Approach
0F144Z6 Bypass Gallbladder to Left Hepatic Duct, Percutaneous Endoscopic Approach
0F144Z7 Bypass Gallbladder to Caudate Hepatic Duct, Percutaneous Endoscopic Approach
0F144Z8 Bypass Gallbladder to Cystic Duct, Percutaneous Endoscopic Approach
0F144Z9 Bypass Gallbladder to Common Bile Duct, Percutaneous Endoscopic Approach
0F144ZB Bypass Gallbladder to Small Intestine, Percutaneous Endoscopic Approach
0F150D3 Bypass Right Hepatic Duct to Duodenum with Intraluminal Device, Open Approach
0F150D4 Bypass Right Hepatic Duct to Stomach with Intraluminal Device, Open Approach

0F150D5 Bypass Right Hepatic Duct to Right Hepatic Duct with Intraluminal Device, Open Approach
0F150D6 Bypass Right Hepatic Duct to Left Hepatic Duct with Intraluminal Device, Open Approach
0F150D7 Bypass Right Hepatic Duct to Caudate Hepatic Duct with Intraluminal Device, Open Approach
0F150D8 Bypass Right Hepatic Duct to Cystic Duct with Intraluminal Device, Open Approach
0F150D9 Bypass Right Hepatic Duct to Common Bile Duct with Intraluminal Device, Open Approach
0F150DB Bypass Right Hepatic Duct to Small Intestine with Intraluminal Device, Open Approach
0F150Z3 Bypass Right Hepatic Duct to Duodenum, Open Approach
0F150Z4 Bypass Right Hepatic Duct to Stomach, Open Approach
0F150Z5 Bypass Right Hepatic Duct to Right Hepatic Duct, Open Approach
0F150Z6 Bypass Right Hepatic Duct to Left Hepatic Duct, Open Approach
0F150Z7 Bypass Right Hepatic Duct to Caudate Hepatic Duct, Open Approach
0F150Z8 Bypass Right Hepatic Duct to Cystic Duct, Open Approach
0F150Z9 Bypass Right Hepatic Duct to Common Bile Duct, Open Approach
0F150ZB Bypass Right Hepatic Duct to Small Intestine, Open Approach
0F154D3 Bypass Right Hepatic Duct to Duodenum with Intraluminal Device, Percutaneous Endoscopic Approach
0F154D4 Bypass Right Hepatic Duct to Stomach with Intraluminal Device, Percutaneous Endoscopic Approach
0F154D5 Bypass Right Hepatic Duct to Right Hepatic Duct with Intraluminal Device, Percutaneous Endoscopic Approach

0F154D6 Bypass Right Hepatic Duct to Left Hepatic Duct with Intraluminal Device, Percutaneous Endoscopic Approach

0F154D7 Bypass Right Hepatic Duct to Caudate Hepatic Duct with Intraluminal Device, Percutaneous Endoscopic Approach

0F154D8 Bypass Right Hepatic Duct to Cystic Duct with Intraluminal Device, Percutaneous Endoscopic Approach

0F154D9 Bypass Right Hepatic Duct to Common Bile Duct with Intraluminal Device, Percutaneous Endoscopic Approach

0F154DB Bypass Right Hepatic Duct to Small Intestine with Intraluminal Device, Percutaneous Endoscopic Approach

0F154Z3 Bypass Right Hepatic Duct to Duodenum, Percutaneous Endoscopic Approach

0F154Z4 Bypass Right Hepatic Duct to Stomach, Percutaneous Endoscopic Approach

0F154Z5 Bypass Right Hepatic Duct to Right Hepatic Duct, Percutaneous Endoscopic Approach

0F154Z6 Bypass Right Hepatic Duct to Left Hepatic Duct, Percutaneous Endoscopic Approach

0F154Z7 Bypass Right Hepatic Duct to Caudate Hepatic Duct, Percutaneous Endoscopic Approach

0F154Z8 Bypass Right Hepatic Duct to Cystic Duct, Percutaneous Endoscopic Approach

0F154Z9 Bypass Right Hepatic Duct to Common Bile Duct, Percutaneous Endoscopic Approach

0F154ZB Bypass Right Hepatic Duct to Small Intestine, Percutaneous Endoscopic Approach

0F160D3 Bypass Left Hepatic Duct to Duodenum with Intraluminal Device, Open Approach

0F160D4 Bypass Left Hepatic Duct to Stomach with Intraluminal Device, Open Approach

0F160D5 Bypass Left Hepatic Duct to Right Hepatic Duct with Intraluminal Device, Open Approach

0F160D6 Bypass Left Hepatic Duct to Left Hepatic Duct with Intraluminal Device, Open Approach

0F160D7 Bypass Left Hepatic Duct to Caudate Hepatic Duct with Intraluminal Device, Open Approach

0F160D8 Bypass Left Hepatic Duct to Cystic Duct with Intraluminal Device, Open Approach

0F160D9 Bypass Left Hepatic Duct to Common Bile Duct with Intraluminal Device, Open Approach

0F160DB Bypass Left Hepatic Duct to Small Intestine with Intraluminal Device, Open Approach

0F160Z3 Bypass Left Hepatic Duct to Duodenum, Open Approach

0F160Z4 Bypass Left Hepatic Duct to Stomach, Open Approach

0F160Z5 Bypass Left Hepatic Duct to Right Hepatic Duct, Open Approach

0F160Z6 Bypass Left Hepatic Duct to Left Hepatic Duct, Open Approach

0F160Z7 Bypass Left Hepatic Duct to Caudate Hepatic Duct, Open Approach

0F160Z8 Bypass Left Hepatic Duct to Cystic Duct, Open Approach

0F160Z9 Bypass Left Hepatic Duct to Common Bile Duct, Open Approach

0F160ZB Bypass Left Hepatic Duct to Small Intestine, Open Approach

0F164D3 Bypass Left Hepatic Duct to Duodenum with Intraluminal Device, Percutaneous Endoscopic Approach

0F164D4 Bypass Left Hepatic Duct to Stomach with Intraluminal Device, Percutaneous Endoscopic Approach

0F164D5 Bypass Left Hepatic Duct to Right Hepatic Duct with Intraluminal Device, Percutaneous Endoscopic Approach

0F164D6 Bypass Left Hepatic Duct to Left Hepatic Duct with Intraluminal Device, Percutaneous Endoscopic Approach

0F164D7 Bypass Left Hepatic Duct to Caudate Hepatic Duct with Intraluminal Device, Percutaneous Endoscopic Approach

0F164D8 Bypass Left Hepatic Duct to Cystic Duct with Intraluminal Device, Percutaneous Endoscopic Approach

0F164D9 Bypass Left Hepatic Duct to Common Bile Duct with Intraluminal Device, Percutaneous Endoscopic Approach

0F164DB Bypass Left Hepatic Duct to Small Intestine with Intraluminal Device, Percutaneous Endoscopic Approach

0F164Z3 Bypass Left Hepatic Duct to Duodenum, Percutaneous Endoscopic Approach

0F164Z4 Bypass Left Hepatic Duct to Stomach, Percutaneous Endoscopic Approach

0F164Z5 Bypass Left Hepatic Duct to Right Hepatic Duct, Percutaneous Endoscopic Approach

0F164Z6 Bypass Left Hepatic Duct to Left Hepatic Duct, Percutaneous Endoscopic Approach

0F164Z7 Bypass Left Hepatic Duct to Caudate Hepatic Duct, Percutaneous Endoscopic Approach

0F164Z8 Bypass Left Hepatic Duct to Cystic Duct, Percutaneous Endoscopic Approach

0F164Z9 Bypass Left Hepatic Duct to Common Bile Duct, Percutaneous Endoscopic Approach

0F164ZB Bypass Left Hepatic Duct to Small Intestine, Percutaneous Endoscopic Approach

0F170D3 Bypass Common Hepatic Duct to Duodenum with Intraluminal Device, Open Approach

0F170D4 Bypass Common Hepatic Duct to Stomach with Intraluminal Device, Open Approach

0F170D5 Bypass Common Hepatic Duct to Right Hepatic Duct with Intraluminal Device, Open Approach

0F170D6 Bypass Common Hepatic Duct to Left Hepatic Duct with Intraluminal Device, Open Approach

0F170D7 Bypass Common Hepatic Duct to Caudate Hepatic Duct with Intraluminal Device, Open Approach

0F170D8 Bypass Common Hepatic Duct to Cystic Duct with Intraluminal Device, Open Approach

0F170D9 Bypass Common Hepatic Duct to Common Bile Duct with Intraluminal Device, Open Approach

0F170DB Bypass Common Hepatic Duct to Small Intestine with Intraluminal Device, Open Approach

0F170Z3 Bypass Common Hepatic Duct to Duodenum, Open Approach

0F170Z4 Bypass Common Hepatic Duct to Stomach, Open Approach

0F170Z5 Bypass Common Hepatic Duct to Right Hepatic Duct, Open Approach

0F170Z6 Bypass Common Hepatic Duct to Left Hepatic Duct, Open Approach

0F170Z7 Bypass Common Hepatic Duct to Caudate Hepatic Duct, Open Approach

0F170Z8 Bypass Common Hepatic Duct to Cystic Duct, Open Approach

0F170Z9 Bypass Common Hepatic Duct to Common Bile Duct, Open Approach

0F170ZB Bypass Common Hepatic Duct to Small Intestine, Open Approach

0F174D3 Bypass Common Hepatic Duct to Duodenum with Intraluminal Device, Percutaneous Endoscopic Approach

0F174D4 Bypass Common Hepatic Duct to Stomach with Intraluminal Device, Percutaneous Endoscopic Approach

0F174D5 Bypass Common Hepatic Duct to Right Hepatic Duct with Intraluminal Device, Percutaneous Endoscopic Approach

0F174D6 Bypass Common Hepatic Duct to Left Hepatic Duct with Intraluminal Device, Percutaneous Endoscopic Approach

0F174D7 Bypass Common Hepatic Duct to Caudate Hepatic Duct with Intraluminal Device, Percutaneous Endoscopic Approach

0F174D8 Bypass Common Hepatic Duct to Cystic Duct with Intraluminal Device, Percutaneous Endoscopic Approach

0F174D9 Bypass Common Hepatic Duct to Common Bile Duct with Intraluminal Device, Percutaneous Endoscopic Approach

0F174DB Bypass Common Hepatic Duct to Small Intestine with Intraluminal Device, Percutaneous Endoscopic Approach

0F174Z3 Bypass Common Hepatic Duct to Duodenum, Percutaneous Endoscopic Approach

0F174Z4 Bypass Common Hepatic Duct to Stomach, Percutaneous Endoscopic Approach

0F174Z5 Bypass Common Hepatic Duct to Right Hepatic Duct, Percutaneous Endoscopic Approach

0F174Z6 Bypass Common Hepatic Duct to Left Hepatic Duct, Percutaneous Endoscopic Approach

0F174Z7 Bypass Common Hepatic Duct to Caudate Hepatic Duct, Percutaneous Endoscopic Approach

0F174Z8 Bypass Common Hepatic Duct to Cystic Duct, Percutaneous Endoscopic Approach

0F174Z9 Bypass Common Hepatic Duct to Common Bile Duct, Percutaneous Endoscopic Approach

0F174ZB Bypass Common Hepatic Duct to Small Intestine, Percutaneous Endoscopic Approach

0F180D3 Bypass Cystic Duct to Duodenum with Intraluminal Device, Open Approach

0F180D4 Bypass Cystic Duct to Stomach with Intraluminal Device, Open Approach

0F180D5 Bypass Cystic Duct to Right Hepatic Duct with Intraluminal Device, Open Approach

0F180D6 Bypass Cystic Duct to Left Hepatic Duct with Intraluminal Device, Open Approach

0F180D7 Bypass Cystic Duct to Caudate Hepatic Duct with Intraluminal Device, Open Approach

0F180D8 Bypass Cystic Duct to Cystic Duct with Intraluminal Device, Open Approach

0F180D9 Bypass Cystic Duct to Common Bile Duct with Intraluminal Device, Open Approach

0F180DB Bypass Cystic Duct to Small Intestine with Intraluminal Device, Open Approach

0F180Z3 Bypass Cystic Duct to Duodenum, Open Approach

0F180Z4 Bypass Cystic Duct to Stomach, Open Approach

0F180Z5 Bypass Cystic Duct to Right Hepatic Duct, Open Approach

0F180Z6 Bypass Cystic Duct to Left Hepatic Duct, Open Approach

0F180Z7 Bypass Cystic Duct to Caudate Hepatic Duct, Open Approach

0F180Z8 Bypass Cystic Duct to Cystic Duct, Open Approach

0F180Z9 Bypass Cystic Duct to Common Bile Duct, Open Approach

0F180ZB Bypass Cystic Duct to Small Intestine, Open Approach

0F184D3 Bypass Cystic Duct to Duodenum with Intraluminal Device, Percutaneous Endoscopic Approach

0F184D4 Bypass Cystic Duct to Stomach with Intraluminal Device, Percutaneous Endoscopic Approach

0F184D5 Bypass Cystic Duct to Right Hepatic Duct with Intraluminal Device, Percutaneous Endoscopic Approach

0F184D6 Bypass Cystic Duct to Left Hepatic Duct with Intraluminal Device, Percutaneous Endoscopic Approach

0F184D7 Bypass Cystic Duct to Caudate Hepatic Duct with Intraluminal Device, Percutaneous Endoscopic Approach

0F184D8 Bypass Cystic Duct to Cystic Duct with Intraluminal Device, Percutaneous Endoscopic Approach

0F184D9 Bypass Cystic Duct to Common Bile Duct with Intraluminal Device, Percutaneous Endoscopic Approach

0F184DB Bypass Cystic Duct to Small Intestine with Intraluminal Device, Percutaneous Endoscopic Approach

0F184Z3 Bypass Cystic Duct to Duodenum, Percutaneous Endoscopic Approach

0F184Z4 Bypass Cystic Duct to Stomach, Percutaneous Endoscopic Approach

0F184Z5 Bypass Cystic Duct to Right Hepatic Duct, Percutaneous Endoscopic Approach

0F184Z6 Bypass Cystic Duct to Left Hepatic Duct, Percutaneous Endoscopic Approach

0F184Z7 Bypass Cystic Duct to Caudate Hepatic Duct, Percutaneous Endoscopic Approach

0F184Z8 Bypass Cystic Duct to Cystic Duct, Percutaneous Endoscopic Approach

0F184Z9 Bypass Cystic Duct to Common Bile Duct, Percutaneous Endoscopic Approach

0F184ZB Bypass Cystic Duct to Small Intestine, Percutaneous Endoscopic Approach

0F190D3 Bypass Common Bile Duct to Duodenum with Intraluminal Device, Open Approach

0F190D4 Bypass Common Bile Duct to Stomach with Intraluminal Device, Open Approach

0F190D5 Bypass Common Bile Duct to Right Hepatic Duct with Intraluminal Device, Open Approach

0F190D6 Bypass Common Bile Duct to Left Hepatic Duct with Intraluminal Device, Open Approach

0F190D7 Bypass Common Bile Duct to Caudate Hepatic Duct with Intraluminal Device, Open Approach

0F190D8 Bypass Common Bile Duct to Cystic Duct with Intraluminal Device, Open Approach

0F190D9 Bypass Common Bile Duct to Common Bile Duct with Intraluminal Device, Open Approach

0F190DB Bypass Common Bile Duct to Small Intestine with Intraluminal Device, Open Approach

0F190Z3 Bypass Common Bile Duct to Duodenum, Open Approach

0F190Z4 Bypass Common Bile Duct to Stomach, Open Approach

0F190Z5 Bypass Common Bile Duct to Right Hepatic Duct, Open Approach

0F190Z6 Bypass Common Bile Duct to Left Hepatic Duct, Open Approach

0F190Z7 Bypass Common Bile Duct to Caudate Hepatic Duct, Open Approach

0F190Z8 Bypass Common Bile Duct to Cystic Duct, Open Approach

0F190Z9 Bypass Common Bile Duct to Common Bile Duct, Open Approach

0F190ZB Bypass Common Bile Duct to Small Intestine, Open Approach

0F194D3 Bypass Common Bile Duct to Duodenum with Intraluminal Device, Percutaneous Endoscopic Approach

0F194D4 Bypass Common Bile Duct to Stomach with Intraluminal Device, Percutaneous Endoscopic Approach

0F194D5 Bypass Common Bile Duct to Right Hepatic Duct with Intraluminal Device, Percutaneous Endoscopic Approach

0F194D6 Bypass Common Bile Duct to Left Hepatic Duct with Intraluminal Device, Percutaneous Endoscopic Approach

0F194D7 Bypass Common Bile Duct to Caudate Hepatic Duct with Intraluminal Device, Percutaneous Endoscopic Approach

0F194D8 Bypass Common Bile Duct to Cystic Duct with Intraluminal Device, Percutaneous Endoscopic Approach

0F194D9 Bypass Common Bile Duct to Common Bile Duct with Intraluminal Device, Percutaneous Endoscopic Approach

0F194DB Bypass Common Bile Duct to Small Intestine with Intraluminal Device, Percutaneous Endoscopic Approach

0F194Z3 Bypass Common Bile Duct to Duodenum, Percutaneous Endoscopic Approach

0F194Z4 Bypass Common Bile Duct to Stomach, Percutaneous Endoscopic Approach

0F194Z5 Bypass Common Bile Duct to Right Hepatic Duct, Percutaneous Endoscopic Approach

0F194Z6 Bypass Common Bile Duct to Left Hepatic Duct, Percutaneous Endoscopic Approach

0F194Z7 Bypass Common Bile Duct to Caudate Hepatic Duct, Percutaneous Endoscopic Approach

0F194Z8 Bypass Common Bile Duct to Cystic Duct, Percutaneous Endoscopic Approach

0F194Z9 Bypass Common Bile Duct to Common Bile Duct, Percutaneous Endoscopic Approach

0F194ZB Bypass Common Bile Duct to Small Intestine, Percutaneous Endoscopic Approach

0F1D0D3 Bypass Pancreatic Duct to Duodenum with Intraluminal Device, Open Approach

0F1D0D4 Bypass Pancreatic Duct to Stomach with Intraluminal Device, Open Approach

0F1D0DB Bypass Pancreatic Duct to Small Intestine with Intraluminal Device, Open Approach

0F1D0DC Bypass Pancreatic Duct to Large Intestine with Intraluminal Device, Open Approach

0F1D0Z3 Bypass Pancreatic Duct to Duodenum, Open Approach

0F1D0Z4 Bypass Pancreatic Duct to Stomach, Open Approach

0F1D0ZB Bypass Pancreatic Duct to Small Intestine, Open Approach

0F1D0ZC Bypass Pancreatic Duct to Large Intestine, Open Approach

0F1D4D3 Bypass Pancreatic Duct to Duodenum with Intraluminal Device, Percutaneous Endoscopic Approach

0F1D4D4 Bypass Pancreatic Duct to Stomach with Intraluminal Device, Percutaneous Endoscopic Approach

0F1D4DB Bypass Pancreatic Duct to Small Intestine with Intraluminal Device, Percutaneous Endoscopic Approach

0F1D4DC Bypass Pancreatic Duct to Large Intestine with Intraluminal Device, Percutaneous Endoscopic Approach

0F1D4Z3 Bypass Pancreatic Duct to Duodenum, Percutaneous Endoscopic Approach

0F1D4Z4 Bypass Pancreatic Duct to Stomach, Percutaneous Endoscopic Approach

AHA CC: 4Q, 2020, 53-54

0F1D4ZB Bypass Pancreatic Duct to Small Intestine, Percutaneous Endoscopic Approach

0F1D4ZC Bypass Pancreatic Duct to Large Intestine, Percutaneous Endoscopic Approach

0F1F0D3 Bypass Accessory Pancreatic Duct to Duodenum with Intraluminal Device, Open Approach

0F1F0DB Bypass Accessory Pancreatic Duct to Small Intestine with Intraluminal Device, Open Approach

0F1F0DC Bypass Accessory Pancreatic Duct to Large Intestine with Intraluminal Device, Open Approach

0F1F0Z3 Bypass Accessory Pancreatic Duct to Duodenum, Open Approach

0F1F0ZB Bypass Accessory Pancreatic Duct to Small Intestine, Open Approach

0F1F0ZC Bypass Accessory Pancreatic Duct to Large Intestine, Open Approach

0F1F4D3 Bypass Accessory Pancreatic Duct to Duodenum with Intraluminal Device, Percutaneous Endoscopic Approach

0F1F4DB Bypass Accessory Pancreatic Duct to Small Intestine with Intraluminal Device, Percutaneous Endoscopic Approach

0F1F4DC Bypass Accessory Pancreatic Duct to Large Intestine with Intraluminal Device, Percutaneous Endoscopic Approach

0F1F4Z3 Bypass Accessory Pancreatic Duct to Duodenum, Percutaneous Endoscopic Approach

0F1F4ZB Bypass Accessory Pancreatic Duct to Small Intestine, Percutaneous Endoscopic Approach

♀ Female-only   ♂ Male-only   ▲ Limited Coverage   ● Non-OR   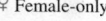 HAC-associated procedure   ▲ Non-covered procedures   ✚ Cluster

0F1F4ZC	Bypass Accessory Pancreatic Duct to Large Intestine, Percutaneous Endoscopic Approach	0F1G0ZB	Bypass Pancreas to Small Intestine, Open Approach	0F1G4DC	Bypass Pancreas to Large Intestine with Intraluminal Device, Percutaneous Endoscopic Approach
0F1G0D3	Bypass Pancreas to Duodenum with Intraluminal Device, Open Approach	0F1G0ZC	Bypass Pancreas to Large Intestine, Open Approach	0F1G4Z3	Bypass Pancreas to Duodenum, Percutaneous Endoscopic Approach
0F1G0DB	Bypass Pancreas to Small Intestine with Intraluminal Device, Open Approach	0F1G4D3	Bypass Pancreas to Duodenum with Intraluminal Device, Percutaneous Endoscopic Approach	0F1G4ZB	Bypass Pancreas to Small Intestine, Percutaneous Endoscopic Approach
0F1G0DC	Bypass Pancreas to Large Intestine with Intraluminal Device, Open Approach	0F1G4DB	Bypass Pancreas to Small Intestine with Intraluminal Device, Percutaneous Endoscopic Approach	0F1G4ZC	Bypass Pancreas to Large Intestine, Percutaneous Endoscopic Approach
0F1G0Z3	Bypass Pancreas to Duodenum, Open Approach				

0F2 – Hepatobiliary System and Pancreas, Change

Review Coding Guideline B6.1c

0F20X0Z	Change Drainage Device in Liver, External Approach	0F2BX0Z	Change Drainage Device in Hepatobiliary Duct, External Approach	0F2GX0Z	Change Drainage Device in Pancreas, External Approach
0F20XYZ	Change Other Device in Liver, External Approach	0F2BXYZ	Change Other Device in Hepatobiliary Duct, External Approach	0F2GXYZ	Change Other Device in Pancreas, External Approach
0F24X0Z	Change Drainage Device in Gallbladder, External Approach	0F2DX0Z	Change Drainage Device in Pancreatic Duct, External Approach		
0F24XYZ	Change Other Device in Gallbladder, External Approach	0F2DXYZ	Change Other Device in Pancreatic Duct, External Approach		

0F5 – Hepatobiliary System and Pancreas, Destruction

0F500ZF	Destruction of Liver using Irreversible Electroporation, Open Approach	0F548ZZ	Destruction of Gallbladder, Via Natural or Artificial Opening Endoscopic	0F590ZZ	Destruction of Common Bile Duct, Open Approach
0F500ZZ	Destruction of Liver, Open Approach	0F550ZZ	Destruction of Right Hepatic Duct, Open Approach	0F593ZZ	Destruction of Common Bile Duct, Percutaneous Approach
0F503ZF	Destruction of Liver using Irreversible Electroporation, Percutaneous Approach	0F553ZZ	Destruction of Right Hepatic Duct, Percutaneous Approach	0F594ZZ	Destruction of Common Bile Duct, Percutaneous Endoscopic Approach
0F503ZZ	Destruction of Liver, Percutaneous Approach	0F554ZZ	Destruction of Right Hepatic Duct, Percutaneous Endoscopic Approach	0F597ZZ	Destruction of Common Bile Duct, Via Natural or Artificial Opening
0F504ZF	Destruction of Liver using Irreversible Electroporation, Percutaneous Endoscopic Approach	0F557ZZ	Destruction of Right Hepatic Duct, Via Natural or Artificial Opening	0F598ZZ	Destruction of Common Bile Duct, Via Natural or Artificial Opening Endoscopic
0F504ZZ	Destruction of Liver, Percutaneous Endoscopic Approach	0F558ZZ	Destruction of Right Hepatic Duct, Via Natural or Artificial Opening Endoscopic	0F5C0ZZ	Destruction of Ampulla of Vater, Open Approach
0F510ZF	Destruction of Right Lobe Liver using Irreversible Electroporation, Open Approach	0F560ZZ	Destruction of Left Hepatic Duct, Open Approach	0F5C3ZZ	Destruction of Ampulla of Vater, Percutaneous Approach
0F510ZZ	Destruction of Right Lobe Liver, Open Approach	0F563ZZ	Destruction of Left Hepatic Duct, Percutaneous Approach	0F5C4ZZ	Destruction of Ampulla of Vater, Percutaneous Endoscopic Approach
0F513ZF	Destruction of Right Lobe Liver using Irreversible Electroporation, Percutaneous Approach	0F564ZZ	Destruction of Left Hepatic Duct, Percutaneous Endoscopic Approach	0F5C7ZZ	Destruction of Ampulla of Vater, Via Natural or Artificial Opening
0F513ZZ	Destruction of Right Lobe Liver, Percutaneous Approach	0F567ZZ	Destruction of Left Hepatic Duct, Via Natural or Artificial Opening	0F5C8ZZ	Destruction of Ampulla of Vater, Via Natural or Artificial Opening Endoscopic
0F514ZF	Destruction of Right Lobe Liver using Irreversible Electroporation, Percutaneous Endoscopic Approach	0F568ZZ	Destruction of Left Hepatic Duct, Via Natural or Artificial Opening Endoscopic	0F5D0ZZ	Destruction of Pancreatic Duct, Open Approach
0F514ZZ	Destruction of Right Lobe Liver, Percutaneous Endoscopic Approach	0F570ZZ	Destruction of Common Hepatic Duct, Open Approach	0F5D3ZZ	Destruction of Pancreatic Duct, Percutaneous Approach
0F520ZF	Destruction of Left Lobe Liver using Irreversible Electroporation, Open Approach	0F573ZZ	Destruction of Common Hepatic Duct, Percutaneous Approach	0F5D4ZZ	Destruction of Pancreatic Duct, Percutaneous Endoscopic Approach
0F520ZZ	Destruction of Left Lobe Liver, Open Approach	0F574ZZ	Destruction of Common Hepatic Duct, Percutaneous Endoscopic Approach	0F5D7ZZ	Destruction of Pancreatic Duct, Via Natural or Artificial Opening
0F523ZF	Destruction of Left Lobe Liver using Irreversible Electroporation, Percutaneous Approach	0F577ZZ	Destruction of Common Hepatic Duct, Via Natural or Artificial Opening	0F5D8ZZ	Destruction of Pancreatic Duct, Via Natural or Artificial Opening Endoscopic
0F523ZZ	Destruction of Left Lobe Liver, Percutaneous Approach	0F578ZZ	Destruction of Common Hepatic Duct, Via Natural or Artificial Opening Endoscopic	0F5F0ZZ	Destruction of Accessory Pancreatic Duct, Open Approach
0F524ZF	Destruction of Left Lobe Liver using Irreversible Electroporation, Percutaneous Endoscopic Approach	0F580ZZ	Destruction of Cystic Duct, Open Approach	0F5F3ZZ	Destruction of Accessory Pancreatic Duct, Percutaneous Approach
0F524ZZ	Destruction of Left Lobe Liver, Percutaneous Endoscopic Approach	0F583ZZ	Destruction of Cystic Duct, Percutaneous Approach	0F5F4ZZ	Destruction of Accessory Pancreatic Duct, Percutaneous Endoscopic Approach
0F540ZZ	Destruction of Gallbladder, Open Approach	0F584ZZ	Destruction of Cystic Duct, Percutaneous Endoscopic Approach	0F5F7ZZ	Destruction of Accessory Pancreatic Duct, Via Natural or Artificial Opening
0F543ZZ	Destruction of Gallbladder, Percutaneous Approach	0F587ZZ	Destruction of Cystic Duct, Via Natural or Artificial Opening	0F5F8ZZ	Destruction of Accessory Pancreatic Duct, Via Natural or Artificial Opening Endoscopic
0F544ZZ	Destruction of Gallbladder, Percutaneous Endoscopic Approach	0F588ZZ	Destruction of Cystic Duct, Via Natural or Artificial Opening Endoscopic	0F5G0ZF	Destruction of Pancreas using Irreversible Electroporation, Open Approach

| 0F5G0ZZ | Destruction of Pancreas, Open Approach |
| 0F5G3ZF | Destruction of Pancreas using Irreversible Electroporation, Percutaneous Approach |

| 0F5G3ZZ | Destruction of Pancreas, Percutaneous Approach |
| 0F5G4ZF | Destruction of Pancreas using Irreversible Electroporation, Percutaneous Endoscopic Approach |

AHA CC: 4Q, 2018, 39-40

| 0F5G4ZZ | Destruction of Pancreas, Percutaneous Endoscopic Approach |
| 0F5G8ZZ | Destruction of Pancreas, Via Natural or Artificial Opening Endoscopic |

0F7 – Hepatobiliary System and Pancreas, Dilation

0F750DZ	Dilation of Right Hepatic Duct with Intraluminal Device, Open Approach
0F750ZZ	Dilation of Right Hepatic Duct, Open Approach
0F753DZ	Dilation of Right Hepatic Duct with Intraluminal Device, Percutaneous Approach
0F753ZZ	Dilation of Right Hepatic Duct, Percutaneous Approach
0F754DZ	Dilation of Right Hepatic Duct with Intraluminal Device, Percutaneous Endoscopic Approach
0F754ZZ	Dilation of Right Hepatic Duct, Percutaneous Endoscopic Approach
0F757DZ	Dilation of Right Hepatic Duct with Intraluminal Device, Via Natural or Artificial Opening
0F757ZZ	Dilation of Right Hepatic Duct, Via Natural or Artificial Opening
0F758DZ	Dilation of Right Hepatic Duct with Intraluminal Device, Via Natural or Artificial Opening Endoscopic
0F758ZZ	Dilation of Right Hepatic Duct, Via Natural or Artificial Opening Endoscopic
0F760DZ	Dilation of Left Hepatic Duct with Intraluminal Device, Open Approach
0F760ZZ	Dilation of Left Hepatic Duct, Open Approach
0F763DZ	Dilation of Left Hepatic Duct with Intraluminal Device, Percutaneous Approach
0F763ZZ	Dilation of Left Hepatic Duct, Percutaneous Approach
0F764DZ	Dilation of Left Hepatic Duct with Intraluminal Device, Percutaneous Endoscopic Approach
0F764ZZ	Dilation of Left Hepatic Duct, Percutaneous Endoscopic Approach
0F767DZ	Dilation of Left Hepatic Duct with Intraluminal Device, Via Natural or Artificial Opening
0F767ZZ	Dilation of Left Hepatic Duct, Via Natural or Artificial Opening
0F768DZ	Dilation of Left Hepatic Duct with Intraluminal Device, Via Natural or Artificial Opening Endoscopic
0F768ZZ	Dilation of Left Hepatic Duct, Via Natural or Artificial Opening Endoscopic
0F770DZ	Dilation of Common Hepatic Duct with Intraluminal Device, Open Approach
0F770ZZ	Dilation of Common Hepatic Duct, Open Approach
0F773DZ	Dilation of Common Hepatic Duct with Intraluminal Device, Percutaneous Approach
0F773ZZ	Dilation of Common Hepatic Duct, Percutaneous Approach
0F774DZ	Dilation of Common Hepatic Duct with Intraluminal Device, Percutaneous Endoscopic Approach
0F774ZZ	Dilation of Common Hepatic Duct, Percutaneous Endoscopic Approach

0F777DZ	Dilation of Common Hepatic Duct with Intraluminal Device, Via Natural or Artificial Opening
0F777ZZ	Dilation of Common Hepatic Duct, Via Natural or Artificial Opening
0F778DZ	Dilation of Common Hepatic Duct with Intraluminal Device, Via Natural or Artificial Opening Endoscopic
0F778ZZ	Dilation of Common Hepatic Duct, Via Natural or Artificial Opening Endoscopic
0F780DZ	Dilation of Cystic Duct with Intraluminal Device, Open Approach
0F780ZZ	Dilation of Cystic Duct, Open Approach
0F783DZ	Dilation of Cystic Duct with Intraluminal Device, Percutaneous Approach
0F783ZZ	Dilation of Cystic Duct, Percutaneous Approach
0F784DZ	Dilation of Cystic Duct with Intraluminal Device, Percutaneous Endoscopic Approach
0F784ZZ	Dilation of Cystic Duct, Percutaneous Endoscopic Approach
0F787DZ	Dilation of Cystic Duct with Intraluminal Device, Via Natural or Artificial Opening
0F787ZZ	Dilation of Cystic Duct, Via Natural or Artificial Opening
0F788DZ	Dilation of Cystic Duct with Intraluminal Device, Via Natural or Artificial Opening Endoscopic
0F788ZZ	Dilation of Cystic Duct, Via Natural or Artificial Opening Endoscopic
0F790DZ	Dilation of Common Bile Duct with Intraluminal Device, Open Approach
0F790ZZ	Dilation of Common Bile Duct, Open Approach
0F793DZ	Dilation of Common Bile Duct with Intraluminal Device, Percutaneous Approach
0F793ZZ	Dilation of Common Bile Duct, Percutaneous Approach
0F794DZ	Dilation of Common Bile Duct with Intraluminal Device, Percutaneous Endoscopic Approach
0F794ZZ	Dilation of Common Bile Duct, Percutaneous Endoscopic Approach
0F797DZ	Dilation of Common Bile Duct with Intraluminal Device, Via Natural or Artificial Opening
0F797ZZ	Dilation of Common Bile Duct, Via Natural or Artificial Opening
0F798DZ	Dilation of Common Bile Duct with Intraluminal Device, Via Natural or Artificial Opening Endoscopic

AHA CC: 3Q, 2014, 15-16; 1Q, 2016, 25

0F798ZZ	Dilation of Common Bile Duct, Via Natural or Artificial Opening Endoscopic
0F7C0DZ	Dilation of Ampulla of Vater with Intraluminal Device, Open Approach
0F7C0ZZ	Dilation of Ampulla of Vater, Open Approach

0F7C3DZ	Dilation of Ampulla of Vater with Intraluminal Device, Percutaneous Approach
0F7C3ZZ	Dilation of Ampulla of Vater, Percutaneous Approach
0F7C4DZ	Dilation of Ampulla of Vater with Intraluminal Device, Percutaneous Endoscopic Approach
0F7C4ZZ	Dilation of Ampulla of Vater, Percutaneous Endoscopic Approach
0F7C7DZ	Dilation of Ampulla of Vater with Intraluminal Device, Via Natural or Artificial Opening
0F7C7ZZ	Dilation of Ampulla of Vater, Via Natural or Artificial Opening
0F7C8DZ	Dilation of Ampulla of Vater with Intraluminal Device, Via Natural or Artificial Opening Endoscopic
0F7C8ZZ	Dilation of Ampulla of Vater, Via Natural or Artificial Opening Endoscopic
0F7D0DZ	Dilation of Pancreatic Duct with Intraluminal Device, Open Approach
0F7D0ZZ	Dilation of Pancreatic Duct, Open Approach
0F7D3DZ	Dilation of Pancreatic Duct with Intraluminal Device, Percutaneous Approach
0F7D3ZZ	Dilation of Pancreatic Duct, Percutaneous Approach
0F7D4DZ	Dilation of Pancreatic Duct with Intraluminal Device, Percutaneous Endoscopic Approach
0F7D4ZZ	Dilation of Pancreatic Duct, Percutaneous Endoscopic Approach
0F7D7DZ	Dilation of Pancreatic Duct with Intraluminal Device, Via Natural or Artificial Opening
0F7D7ZZ	Dilation of Pancreatic Duct, Via Natural or Artificial Opening
0F7D8DZ	Dilation of Pancreatic Duct with Intraluminal Device, Via Natural or Artificial Opening Endoscopic

AHA CC: 1Q, 2016, 25; 3Q, 2016, 27-28

0F7D8ZZ	Dilation of Pancreatic Duct, Via Natural or Artificial Opening Endoscopic
0F7F0DZ	Dilation of Accessory Pancreatic Duct with Intraluminal Device, Open Approach
0F7F0ZZ	Dilation of Accessory Pancreatic Duct, Open Approach
0F7F3DZ	Dilation of Accessory Pancreatic Duct with Intraluminal Device, Percutaneous Approach
0F7F3ZZ	Dilation of Accessory Pancreatic Duct, Percutaneous Approach
0F7F4DZ	Dilation of Accessory Pancreatic Duct with Intraluminal Device, Percutaneous Endoscopic Approach
0F7F4ZZ	Dilation of Accessory Pancreatic Duct, Percutaneous Endoscopic Approach
0F7F7DZ	Dilation of Accessory Pancreatic Duct with Intraluminal Device, Via Natural or Artificial Opening

♀ Female-only   ♂ Male-only   ▲ Limited Coverage   ● Non-OR   HAC HAC-associated procedure   ▲ Non-covered procedures   ✚ Cluster

0F7F7ZZ	Dilation of Accessory Pancreatic Duct, Via Natural or Artificial Opening
0F7F8DZ	Dilation of Accessory Pancreatic Duct with Intraluminal Device, Via Natural or Artificial Opening Endoscopic
0F7F8ZZ	Dilation of Accessory Pancreatic Duct, Via Natural or Artificial Opening Endoscopic

0F8 – Hepatobiliary System and Pancreas, Division

Review Coding Guideline B3.14

0F800ZZ	Division of Liver, Open Approach
0F803ZZ	Division of Liver, Percutaneous Approach
0F804ZZ	Division of Liver, Percutaneous Endoscopic Approach
0F810ZZ	Division of Right Lobe Liver, Open Approach
0F813ZZ	Division of Right Lobe Liver, Percutaneous Approach
0F814ZZ	Division of Right Lobe Liver, Percutaneous Endoscopic Approach
0F820ZZ	Division of Left Lobe Liver, Open Approach
0F823ZZ	Division of Left Lobe Liver, Percutaneous Approach
0F824ZZ	Division of Left Lobe Liver, Percutaneous Endoscopic Approach
0F8G0ZZ	Division of Pancreas, Open Approach
0F8G3ZZ	Division of Pancreas, Percutaneous Approach
0F8G4ZZ	Division of Pancreas, Percutaneous Endoscopic Approach

0F9 – Hepatobiliary System and Pancreas, Drainage

Review Coding Guidelines B3.4a and B3.4b

Review Coding Guideline B6.2

0F9000Z	Drainage of Liver with Drainage Device, Open Approach
0F900ZX	Drainage of Liver, Open Approach, Diagnostic
0F900ZZ	Drainage of Liver, Open Approach
0F9030Z	Drainage of Liver with Drainage Device, Percutaneous Approach
0F903ZX	Drainage of Liver, Percutaneous Approach, Diagnostic
0F903ZZ	Drainage of Liver, Percutaneous Approach
0F9040Z	Drainage of Liver with Drainage Device, Percutaneous Endoscopic Approach
0F904ZX	Drainage of Liver, Percutaneous Endoscopic Approach, Diagnostic
0F904ZZ	Drainage of Liver, Percutaneous Endoscopic Approach
0F9100Z	Drainage of Right Lobe Liver with Drainage Device, Open Approach
0F910ZX	Drainage of Right Lobe Liver, Open Approach, Diagnostic
0F910ZZ	Drainage of Right Lobe Liver, Open Approach
0F9130Z	Drainage of Right Lobe Liver with Drainage Device, Percutaneous Approach
0F913ZX	Drainage of Right Lobe Liver, Percutaneous Approach, Diagnostic
0F913ZZ	Drainage of Right Lobe Liver, Percutaneous Approach
0F9140Z	Drainage of Right Lobe Liver with Drainage Device, Percutaneous Endoscopic Approach
0F914ZX	Drainage of Right Lobe Liver, Percutaneous Endoscopic Approach, Diagnostic
0F914ZZ	Drainage of Right Lobe Liver, Percutaneous Endoscopic Approach
0F9200Z	Drainage of Left Lobe Liver with Drainage Device, Open Approach
0F920ZX	Drainage of Left Lobe Liver, Open Approach, Diagnostic
0F920ZZ	Drainage of Left Lobe Liver, Open Approach
0F9230Z	Drainage of Left Lobe Liver with Drainage Device, Percutaneous Approach
0F923ZX	Drainage of Left Lobe Liver, Percutaneous Approach, Diagnostic
0F923ZZ	Drainage of Left Lobe Liver, Percutaneous Approach
0F9240Z	Drainage of Left Lobe Liver with Drainage Device, Percutaneous Endoscopic Approach
0F924ZX	Drainage of Left Lobe Liver, Percutaneous Endoscopic Approach, Diagnostic
0F924ZZ	Drainage of Left Lobe Liver, Percutaneous Endoscopic Approach
0F9400Z	Drainage of Gallbladder with Drainage Device, Open Approach
0F940ZX	Drainage of Gallbladder, Open Approach, Diagnostic
0F940ZZ	Drainage of Gallbladder, Open Approach
0F9430Z	Drainage of Gallbladder with Drainage Device, Percutaneous Approach
0F943ZX	Drainage of Gallbladder, Percutaneous Approach, Diagnostic
0F943ZZ	Drainage of Gallbladder, Percutaneous Approach
0F9440Z	Drainage of Gallbladder with Drainage Device, Percutaneous Endoscopic Approach
0F944ZX	Drainage of Gallbladder, Percutaneous Endoscopic Approach, Diagnostic
0F944ZZ	Drainage of Gallbladder, Percutaneous Endoscopic Approach
0F9480Z	Drainage of Gallbladder with Drainage Device, Via Natural or Artificial Opening Endoscopic
0F948ZX	Drainage of Gallbladder, Via Natural or Artificial Opening Endoscopic, Diagnostic
0F948ZZ	Drainage of Gallbladder, Via Natural or Artificial Opening Endoscopic
0F9500Z	Drainage of Right Hepatic Duct with Drainage Device, Open Approach
0F950ZX	Drainage of Right Hepatic Duct, Open Approach, Diagnostic
0F950ZZ	Drainage of Right Hepatic Duct, Open Approach
0F9530Z	Drainage of Right Hepatic Duct with Drainage Device, Percutaneous Approach
0F953ZX	Drainage of Right Hepatic Duct, Percutaneous Approach, Diagnostic
0F953ZZ	Drainage of Right Hepatic Duct, Percutaneous Approach
0F9540Z	Drainage of Right Hepatic Duct with Drainage Device, Percutaneous Endoscopic Approach
0F954ZX	Drainage of Right Hepatic Duct, Percutaneous Endoscopic Approach, Diagnostic
0F954ZZ	Drainage of Right Hepatic Duct, Percutaneous Endoscopic Approach
0F9570Z	Drainage of Right Hepatic Duct with Drainage Device, Via Natural or Artificial Opening
0F957ZX	Drainage of Right Hepatic Duct, Via Natural or Artificial Opening, Diagnostic
0F957ZZ	Drainage of Right Hepatic Duct, Via Natural or Artificial Opening
0F9580Z	Drainage of Right Hepatic Duct with Drainage Device, Via Natural or Artificial Opening Endoscopic
0F958ZX	Drainage of Right Hepatic Duct, Via Natural or Artificial Opening Endoscopic, Diagnostic
0F958ZZ	Drainage of Right Hepatic Duct, Via Natural or Artificial Opening Endoscopic
0F9600Z	Drainage of Left Hepatic Duct with Drainage Device, Open Approach
0F960ZX	Drainage of Left Hepatic Duct, Open Approach, Diagnostic
0F960ZZ	Drainage of Left Hepatic Duct, Open Approach
0F9630Z	Drainage of Left Hepatic Duct with Drainage Device, Percutaneous Approach *AHA CC: 1Q, 2015, 32*
0F963ZX	Drainage of Left Hepatic Duct, Percutaneous Approach, Diagnostic
0F963ZZ	Drainage of Left Hepatic Duct, Percutaneous Approach
0F9640Z	Drainage of Left Hepatic Duct with Drainage Device, Percutaneous Endoscopic Approach
0F964ZX	Drainage of Left Hepatic Duct, Percutaneous Endoscopic Approach, Diagnostic
0F964ZZ	Drainage of Left Hepatic Duct, Percutaneous Endoscopic Approach
0F9670Z	Drainage of Left Hepatic Duct with Drainage Device, Via Natural or Artificial Opening

0F967ZX Drainage of Left Hepatic Duct, Via Natural or Artificial Opening, Diagnostic

0F967ZZ Drainage of Left Hepatic Duct, Via Natural or Artificial Opening

0F9680Z Drainage of Left Hepatic Duct with Drainage Device, Via Natural or Artificial Opening Endoscopic

0F968ZX Drainage of Left Hepatic Duct, Via Natural or Artificial Opening Endoscopic, Diagnostic

0F968ZZ Drainage of Left Hepatic Duct, Via Natural or Artificial Opening Endoscopic

0F9700Z Drainage of Common Hepatic Duct with Drainage Device, Open Approach

0F970ZX Drainage of Common Hepatic Duct, Open Approach, Diagnostic

0F970ZZ Drainage of Common Hepatic Duct, Open Approach

0F9730Z Drainage of Common Hepatic Duct with Drainage Device, Percutaneous Approach

0F973ZX Drainage of Common Hepatic Duct, Percutaneous Approach, Diagnostic

0F973ZZ Drainage of Common Hepatic Duct, Percutaneous Approach

0F9740Z Drainage of Common Hepatic Duct with Drainage Device, Percutaneous Endoscopic Approach

0F974ZX Drainage of Common Hepatic Duct, Percutaneous Endoscopic Approach, Diagnostic

0F974ZZ Drainage of Common Hepatic Duct, Percutaneous Endoscopic Approach

0F9770Z Drainage of Common Hepatic Duct with Drainage Device, Via Natural or Artificial Opening

0F977ZX Drainage of Common Hepatic Duct, Via Natural or Artificial Opening, Diagnostic

0F977ZZ Drainage of Common Hepatic Duct, Via Natural or Artificial Opening

0F9780Z Drainage of Common Hepatic Duct with Drainage Device, Via Natural or Artificial Opening Endoscopic

0F978ZX Drainage of Common Hepatic Duct, Via Natural or Artificial Opening Endoscopic, Diagnostic

0F978ZZ Drainage of Common Hepatic Duct, Via Natural or Artificial Opening Endoscopic

0F9800Z Drainage of Cystic Duct with Drainage Device, Open Approach

0F980ZX Drainage of Cystic Duct, Open Approach, Diagnostic

0F980ZZ Drainage of Cystic Duct, Open Approach

0F9830Z Drainage of Cystic Duct with Drainage Device, Percutaneous Approach

0F983ZX Drainage of Cystic Duct, Percutaneous Approach, Diagnostic

0F983ZZ Drainage of Cystic Duct, Percutaneous Approach

0F9840Z Drainage of Cystic Duct with Drainage Device, Percutaneous Endoscopic Approach

0F984ZX Drainage of Cystic Duct, Percutaneous Endoscopic Approach, Diagnostic

0F984ZZ Drainage of Cystic Duct, Percutaneous Endoscopic Approach

0F9870Z Drainage of Cystic Duct with Drainage Device, Via Natural or Artificial Opening

0F987ZX Drainage of Cystic Duct, Via Natural or Artificial Opening, Diagnostic

0F987ZZ Drainage of Cystic Duct, Via Natural or Artificial Opening

0F9880Z Drainage of Cystic Duct with Drainage Device, Via Natural or Artificial Opening Endoscopic

0F988ZX Drainage of Cystic Duct, Via Natural or Artificial Opening Endoscopic, Diagnostic

0F988ZZ Drainage of Cystic Duct, Via Natural or Artificial Opening Endoscopic

0F9900Z Drainage of Common Bile Duct with Drainage Device, Open Approach

0F990ZX Drainage of Common Bile Duct, Open Approach, Diagnostic

0F990ZZ Drainage of Common Bile Duct, Open Approach

0F9930Z Drainage of Common Bile Duct with Drainage Device, Percutaneous Approach

0F993ZX Drainage of Common Bile Duct, Percutaneous Approach, Diagnostic

0F993ZZ Drainage of Common Bile Duct, Percutaneous Approach

0F9940Z Drainage of Common Bile Duct with Drainage Device, Percutaneous Endoscopic Approach

0F994ZX Drainage of Common Bile Duct, Percutaneous Endoscopic Approach, Diagnostic

0F994ZZ Drainage of Common Bile Duct, Percutaneous Endoscopic Approach

0F9970Z Drainage of Common Bile Duct with Drainage Device, Via Natural or Artificial Opening

0F997ZX Drainage of Common Bile Duct, Via Natural or Artificial Opening, Diagnostic

0F997ZZ Drainage of Common Bile Duct, Via Natural or Artificial Opening

0F9980Z Drainage of Common Bile Duct with Drainage Device, Via Natural or Artificial Opening Endoscopic

0F998ZX Drainage of Common Bile Duct, Via Natural or Artificial Opening Endoscopic, Diagnostic

0F998ZZ Drainage of Common Bile Duct, Via Natural or Artificial Opening Endoscopic

0F9C00Z Drainage of Ampulla of Vater with Drainage Device, Open Approach

0F9C0ZX Drainage of Ampulla of Vater, Open Approach, Diagnostic

0F9C0ZZ Drainage of Ampulla of Vater, Open Approach

0F9C30Z Drainage of Ampulla of Vater with Drainage Device, Percutaneous Approach

0F9C3ZX Drainage of Ampulla of Vater, Percutaneous Approach, Diagnostic

0F9C3ZZ Drainage of Ampulla of Vater, Percutaneous Approach

0F9C40Z Drainage of Ampulla of Vater with Drainage Device, Percutaneous Endoscopic Approach

0F9C4ZX Drainage of Ampulla of Vater, Percutaneous Endoscopic Approach, Diagnostic

0F9C4ZZ Drainage of Ampulla of Vater, Percutaneous Endoscopic Approach

0F9C70Z Drainage of Ampulla of Vater with Drainage Device, Via Natural or Artificial Opening

0F9C7ZX Drainage of Ampulla of Vater, Via Natural or Artificial Opening, Diagnostic

0F9C7ZZ Drainage of Ampulla of Vater, Via Natural or Artificial Opening

0F9C80Z Drainage of Ampulla of Vater with Drainage Device, Via Natural or Artificial Opening Endoscopic

0F9C8ZX Drainage of Ampulla of Vater, Via Natural or Artificial Opening Endoscopic, Diagnostic

0F9C8ZZ Drainage of Ampulla of Vater, Via Natural or Artificial Opening Endoscopic

0F9D00Z Drainage of Pancreatic Duct with Drainage Device, Open Approach

0F9D0ZX Drainage of Pancreatic Duct, Open Approach, Diagnostic

0F9D0ZZ Drainage of Pancreatic Duct, Open Approach

0F9D30Z Drainage of Pancreatic Duct with Drainage Device, Percutaneous Approach

0F9D3ZX Drainage of Pancreatic Duct, Percutaneous Approach, Diagnostic

0F9D3ZZ Drainage of Pancreatic Duct, Percutaneous Approach

0F9D40Z Drainage of Pancreatic Duct with Drainage Device, Percutaneous Endoscopic Approach

0F9D4ZX Drainage of Pancreatic Duct, Percutaneous Endoscopic Approach, Diagnostic

0F9D4ZZ Drainage of Pancreatic Duct, Percutaneous Endoscopic Approach

0F9D70Z Drainage of Pancreatic Duct with Drainage Device, Via Natural or Artificial Opening

0F9D7ZX Drainage of Pancreatic Duct, Via Natural or Artificial Opening, Diagnostic

0F9D7ZZ Drainage of Pancreatic Duct, Via Natural or Artificial Opening

0F9D80Z Drainage of Pancreatic Duct with Drainage Device, Via Natural or Artificial Opening Endoscopic

0F9D8ZX Drainage of Pancreatic Duct, Via Natural or Artificial Opening Endoscopic, Diagnostic

0F9D8ZZ Drainage of Pancreatic Duct, Via Natural or Artificial Opening Endoscopic

0F9F00Z Drainage of Accessory Pancreatic Duct with Drainage Device, Open Approach

0F9F0ZX Drainage of Accessory Pancreatic Duct, Open Approach, Diagnostic

0F9F0ZZ Drainage of Accessory Pancreatic Duct, Open Approach

0F9F30Z Drainage of Accessory Pancreatic Duct with Drainage Device, Percutaneous Approach

0F9F3ZX Drainage of Accessory Pancreatic Duct, Percutaneous Approach, Diagnostic

0F9F3ZZ Drainage of Accessory Pancreatic Duct, Percutaneous Approach

0F9F40Z Drainage of Accessory Pancreatic Duct with Drainage Device, Percutaneous Endoscopic Approach

0F9F4ZX Drainage of Accessory Pancreatic Duct, Percutaneous Endoscopic Approach, Diagnostic

0F9F4ZZ Drainage of Accessory Pancreatic Duct, Percutaneous Endoscopic Approach

0F9F70Z Drainage of Accessory Pancreatic Duct with Drainage Device, Via Natural or Artificial Opening

0F9F7ZX Drainage of Accessory Pancreatic Duct, Via Natural or Artificial Opening, Diagnostic

0F9F7ZZ Drainage of Accessory Pancreatic Duct, Via Natural or Artificial Opening

♀ Female-only   ♂ Male-only   ▲ Limited Coverage   ● Non-OR   ᴴᴬᶜ HAC-associated procedure   ▲ Non-covered procedures   ✚ Cluster

0F9F80Z Drainage of Accessory Pancreatic Duct with Drainage Device, Via Natural or Artificial Opening Endoscopic

0F9F8ZX Drainage of Accessory Pancreatic Duct, Via Natural or Artificial Opening Endoscopic, Diagnostic

0F9F8ZZ Drainage of Accessory Pancreatic Duct, Via Natural or Artificial Opening Endoscopic

0F9G00Z Drainage of Pancreas with Drainage Device, Open Approach

0F9G0ZX Drainage of Pancreas, Open Approach, Diagnostic

0F9G0ZZ Drainage of Pancreas, Open Approach

0F9G30Z Drainage of Pancreas with Drainage Device, Percutaneous Approach

0F9G3ZX Drainage of Pancreas, Percutaneous Approach, Diagnostic

0F9G3ZZ Drainage of Pancreas, Percutaneous Approach

0F9G40Z Drainage of Pancreas with Drainage Device, Percutaneous Endoscopic Approach

AHA CC: 3Q, 2014, 15-16

0F9G4ZX Drainage of Pancreas, Percutaneous Endoscopic Approach, Diagnostic

0F9G4ZZ Drainage of Pancreas, Percutaneous Endoscopic Approach

0F9G80Z Drainage of Pancreas with Drainage Device, Via Natural or Artificial Opening Endoscopic

AHA CC: 3Q, 2020, 34-35

0F9G8ZX Drainage of Pancreas, Via Natural or Artificial Opening Endoscopic, Diagnostic

0F9G8ZZ Drainage of Pancreas, Via Natural or Artificial Opening Endoscopic

0FB – Hepatobiliary System and Pancreas, Excision

Review Coding Guidelines B3.4a and B3.4b

Review Coding Guideline B3.8

Review Coding Guideline B3.18

0FB00ZX Excision of Liver, Open Approach, Diagnostic

AHA CC: 3Q, 2016, 41

0FB00ZZ Excision of Liver, Open Approach

0FB03ZX Excision of Liver, Percutaneous Approach, Diagnostic

0FB03ZZ Excision of Liver, Percutaneous Approach

0FB04ZX Excision of Liver, Percutaneous Endoscopic Approach, Diagnostic

0FB04ZZ Excision of Liver, Percutaneous Endoscopic Approach

0FB10ZX Excision of Right Lobe Liver, Open Approach, Diagnostic

0FB10ZZ Excision of Right Lobe Liver, Open Approach

0FB13ZX Excision of Right Lobe Liver, Percutaneous Approach, Diagnostic

0FB13ZZ Excision of Right Lobe Liver, Percutaneous Approach

0FB14ZX Excision of Right Lobe Liver, Percutaneous Endoscopic Approach, Diagnostic

0FB14ZZ Excision of Right Lobe Liver, Percutaneous Endoscopic Approach

0FB20ZX Excision of Left Lobe Liver, Open Approach, Diagnostic

0FB20ZZ Excision of Left Lobe Liver, Open Approach

0FB23ZX Excision of Left Lobe Liver, Percutaneous Approach, Diagnostic

0FB23ZZ Excision of Left Lobe Liver, Percutaneous Approach

0FB24ZX Excision of Left Lobe Liver, Percutaneous Endoscopic Approach, Diagnostic

0FB24ZZ Excision of Left Lobe Liver, Percutaneous Endoscopic Approach

0FB40ZX Excision of Gallbladder, Open Approach, Diagnostic

0FB40ZZ Excision of Gallbladder, Open Approach

0FB43ZX Excision of Gallbladder, Percutaneous Approach, Diagnostic

0FB43ZZ Excision of Gallbladder, Percutaneous Approach

0FB44ZX Excision of Gallbladder, Percutaneous Endoscopic Approach, Diagnostic

0FB44ZZ Excision of Gallbladder, Percutaneous Endoscopic Approach

0FB48ZX Excision of Gallbladder, Via Natural or Artificial Opening Endoscopic, Diagnostic

0FB48ZZ Excision of Gallbladder, Via Natural or Artificial Opening Endoscopic

0FB50ZX Excision of Right Hepatic Duct, Open Approach, Diagnostic

0FB50ZZ Excision of Right Hepatic Duct, Open Approach

0FB53ZX Excision of Right Hepatic Duct, Percutaneous Approach, Diagnostic

0FB53ZZ Excision of Right Hepatic Duct, Percutaneous Approach

0FB54ZX Excision of Right Hepatic Duct, Percutaneous Endoscopic Approach, Diagnostic

0FB54ZZ Excision of Right Hepatic Duct, Percutaneous Endoscopic Approach

0FB57ZX Excision of Right Hepatic Duct, Via Natural or Artificial Opening, Diagnostic

0FB57ZZ Excision of Right Hepatic Duct, Via Natural or Artificial Opening

0FB58ZX Excision of Right Hepatic Duct, Via Natural or Artificial Opening Endoscopic, Diagnostic

0FB58ZZ Excision of Right Hepatic Duct, Via Natural or Artificial Opening Endoscopic

0FB60ZX Excision of Left Hepatic Duct, Open Approach, Diagnostic

0FB60ZZ Excision of Left Hepatic Duct, Open Approach

0FB63ZX Excision of Left Hepatic Duct, Percutaneous Approach, Diagnostic

0FB63ZZ Excision of Left Hepatic Duct, Percutaneous Approach

0FB64ZX Excision of Left Hepatic Duct, Percutaneous Endoscopic Approach, Diagnostic

0FB64ZZ Excision of Left Hepatic Duct, Percutaneous Endoscopic Approach

0FB67ZX Excision of Left Hepatic Duct, Via Natural or Artificial Opening, Diagnostic

0FB67ZZ Excision of Left Hepatic Duct, Via Natural or Artificial Opening

0FB68ZX Excision of Left Hepatic Duct, Via Natural or Artificial Opening Endoscopic, Diagnostic

0FB68ZZ Excision of Left Hepatic Duct, Via Natural or Artificial Opening Endoscopic

0FB70ZX Excision of Common Hepatic Duct, Open Approach, Diagnostic

0FB70ZZ Excision of Common Hepatic Duct, Open Approach

0FB73ZX Excision of Common Hepatic Duct, Percutaneous Approach, Diagnostic

0FB73ZZ Excision of Common Hepatic Duct, Percutaneous Approach

0FB74ZX Excision of Common Hepatic Duct, Percutaneous Endoscopic Approach, Diagnostic

0FB74ZZ Excision of Common Hepatic Duct, Percutaneous Endoscopic Approach

0FB77ZX Excision of Common Hepatic Duct, Via Natural or Artificial Opening, Diagnostic

0FB77ZZ Excision of Common Hepatic Duct, Via Natural or Artificial Opening

0FB78ZX Excision of Common Hepatic Duct, Via Natural or Artificial Opening Endoscopic, Diagnostic

0FB78ZZ Excision of Common Hepatic Duct, Via Natural or Artificial Opening Endoscopic

0FB80ZX Excision of Cystic Duct, Open Approach, Diagnostic

0FB80ZZ Excision of Cystic Duct, Open Approach

0FB83ZX Excision of Cystic Duct, Percutaneous Approach, Diagnostic

0FB83ZZ Excision of Cystic Duct, Percutaneous Approach

0FB84ZX Excision of Cystic Duct, Percutaneous Endoscopic Approach, Diagnostic

0FB84ZZ Excision of Cystic Duct, Percutaneous Endoscopic Approach

0FB87ZX Excision of Cystic Duct, Via Natural or Artificial Opening, Diagnostic

0FB87ZZ Excision of Cystic Duct, Via Natural or Artificial Opening

0FB88ZX Excision of Cystic Duct, Via Natural or Artificial Opening Endoscopic, Diagnostic

0FB88ZZ Excision of Cystic Duct, Via Natural or Artificial Opening Endoscopic

0FB90ZX Excision of Common Bile Duct, Open Approach, Diagnostic

0FB90ZZ Excision of Common Bile Duct, Open Approach

AHA CC: 1Q, 2019, 4-7

0FB93ZX Excision of Common Bile Duct, Percutaneous Approach, Diagnostic

0FB93ZZ Excision of Common Bile Duct, Percutaneous Approach

0FB94ZX	Excision of Common Bile Duct, Percutaneous Endoscopic Approach, Diagnostic
0FB94ZZ	Excision of Common Bile Duct, Percutaneous Endoscopic Approach
0FB97ZX	Excision of Common Bile Duct, Via Natural or Artificial Opening, Diagnostic
0FB97ZZ	Excision of Common Bile Duct, Via Natural or Artificial Opening
0FB98ZX	Excision of Common Bile Duct, Via Natural or Artificial Opening Endoscopic, Diagnostic
	AHA CC: 1Q, 2016, 23-25
0FB98ZZ	Excision of Common Bile Duct, Via Natural or Artificial Opening Endoscopic
0FBC0ZX	Excision of Ampulla of Vater, Open Approach, Diagnostic
0FBC0ZZ	Excision of Ampulla of Vater, Open Approach
0FBC3ZX	Excision of Ampulla of Vater, Percutaneous Approach, Diagnostic
0FBC3ZZ	Excision of Ampulla of Vater, Percutaneous Approach
0FBC4ZX	Excision of Ampulla of Vater, Percutaneous Endoscopic Approach, Diagnostic
0FBC4ZZ	Excision of Ampulla of Vater, Percutaneous Endoscopic Approach
0FBC7ZX	Excision of Ampulla of Vater, Via Natural or Artificial Opening, Diagnostic
0FBC7ZZ	Excision of Ampulla of Vater, Via Natural or Artificial Opening

0FBC8ZX	Excision of Ampulla of Vater, Via Natural or Artificial Opening Endoscopic, Diagnostic
0FBC8ZZ	Excision of Ampulla of Vater, Via Natural or Artificial Opening Endoscopic
0FBD0ZX	Excision of Pancreatic Duct, Open Approach, Diagnostic
0FBD0ZZ	Excision of Pancreatic Duct, Open Approach
0FBD3ZX	Excision of Pancreatic Duct, Percutaneous Approach, Diagnostic
0FBD3ZZ	Excision of Pancreatic Duct, Percutaneous Approach
0FBD4ZX	Excision of Pancreatic Duct, Percutaneous Endoscopic Approach, Diagnostic
0FBD4ZZ	Excision of Pancreatic Duct, Percutaneous Endoscopic Approach
0FBD7ZX	Excision of Pancreatic Duct, Via Natural or Artificial Opening, Diagnostic
0FBD7ZZ	Excision of Pancreatic Duct, Via Natural or Artificial Opening
0FBD8ZX	Excision of Pancreatic Duct, Via Natural or Artificial Opening Endoscopic, Diagnostic
	AHA CC: 1Q, 2016, 25
0FBD8ZZ	Excision of Pancreatic Duct, Via Natural or Artificial Opening Endoscopic
0FBF0ZX	Excision of Accessory Pancreatic Duct, Open Approach, Diagnostic
0FBF0ZZ	Excision of Accessory Pancreatic Duct, Open Approach
0FBF3ZX	Excision of Accessory Pancreatic Duct, Percutaneous Approach, Diagnostic

0FBF3ZZ	Excision of Accessory Pancreatic Duct, Percutaneous Approach
0FBF4ZX	Excision of Accessory Pancreatic Duct, Percutaneous Endoscopic Approach, Diagnostic
0FBF4ZZ	Excision of Accessory Pancreatic Duct, Percutaneous Endoscopic Approach
0FBF7ZX	Excision of Accessory Pancreatic Duct, Via Natural or Artificial Opening, Diagnostic
0FBF7ZZ	Excision of Accessory Pancreatic Duct, Via Natural or Artificial Opening
0FBF8ZX	Excision of Accessory Pancreatic Duct, Via Natural or Artificial Opening Endoscopic, Diagnostic
0FBF8ZZ	Excision of Accessory Pancreatic Duct, Via Natural or Artificial Opening Endoscopic
0FBG0ZX	Excision of Pancreas, Open Approach, Diagnostic
0FBG0ZZ	Excision of Pancreas, Open Approach
	AHA CC: 3Q, 2014, 32-33; 1Q, 2019, 4-8
0FBG3ZX	Excision of Pancreas, Percutaneous Approach, Diagnostic
0FBG3ZZ	Excision of Pancreas, Percutaneous Approach
0FBG4ZX	Excision of Pancreas, Percutaneous Endoscopic Approach, Diagnostic
0FBG4ZZ	Excision of Pancreas, Percutaneous Endoscopic Approach
0FBG8ZX	Excision of Pancreas, Via Natural or Artificial Opening Endoscopic, Diagnostic
0FBG8ZZ	Excision of Pancreas, Via Natural or Artificial Opening Endoscopic

0FC – Hepatobiliary System and Pancreas, Extirpation

0FC00ZZ	Extirpation of Matter from Liver, Open Approach
0FC03ZZ	Extirpation of Matter from Liver, Percutaneous Approach
0FC04ZZ	Extirpation of Matter from Liver, Percutaneous Endoscopic Approach
0FC10ZZ	Extirpation of Matter from Right Lobe Liver, Open Approach
0FC13ZZ	Extirpation of Matter from Right Lobe Liver, Percutaneous Approach
0FC14ZZ	Extirpation of Matter from Right Lobe Liver, Percutaneous Endoscopic Approach
0FC20ZZ	Extirpation of Matter from Left Lobe Liver, Open Approach
0FC23ZZ	Extirpation of Matter from Left Lobe Liver, Percutaneous Approach
0FC24ZZ	Extirpation of Matter from Left Lobe Liver, Percutaneous Endoscopic Approach
0FC40ZZ	Extirpation of Matter from Gallbladder, Open Approach
0FC43ZZ	Extirpation of Matter from Gallbladder, Percutaneous Approach
0FC44ZZ	Extirpation of Matter from Gallbladder, Percutaneous Endoscopic Approach
0FC48ZZ	Extirpation of Matter from Gallbladder, Via Natural or Artificial Opening Endoscopic
0FC50ZZ	Extirpation of Matter from Right Hepatic Duct, Open Approach
0FC53ZZ	Extirpation of Matter from Right Hepatic Duct, Percutaneous Approach
0FC54ZZ	Extirpation of Matter from Right Hepatic Duct, Percutaneous Endoscopic Approach

0FC57ZZ	Extirpation of Matter from Right Hepatic Duct, Via Natural or Artificial Opening
0FC58ZZ	Extirpation of Matter from Right Hepatic Duct, Via Natural or Artificial Opening Endoscopic
0FC60ZZ	Extirpation of Matter from Left Hepatic Duct, Open Approach
0FC63ZZ	Extirpation of Matter from Left Hepatic Duct, Percutaneous Approach
0FC64ZZ	Extirpation of Matter from Left Hepatic Duct, Percutaneous Endoscopic Approach
0FC67ZZ	Extirpation of Matter from Left Hepatic Duct, Via Natural or Artificial Opening
0FC68ZZ	Extirpation of Matter from Left Hepatic Duct, Via Natural or Artificial Opening Endoscopic
0FC70ZZ	Extirpation of Matter from Common Hepatic Duct, Open Approach
0FC73ZZ	Extirpation of Matter from Common Hepatic Duct, Percutaneous Approach
0FC74ZZ	Extirpation of Matter from Common Hepatic Duct, Percutaneous Endoscopic Approach
0FC77ZZ	Extirpation of Matter from Common Hepatic Duct, Via Natural or Artificial Opening
0FC78ZZ	Extirpation of Matter from Common Hepatic Duct, Via Natural or Artificial Opening Endoscopic
0FC80ZZ	Extirpation of Matter from Cystic Duct, Open Approach
0FC83ZZ	Extirpation of Matter from Cystic Duct, Percutaneous Approach
0FC84ZZ	Extirpation of Matter from Cystic Duct, Percutaneous Endoscopic Approach

0FC87ZZ	Extirpation of Matter from Cystic Duct, Via Natural or Artificial Opening
0FC88ZZ	Extirpation of Matter from Cystic Duct, Via Natural or Artificial Opening Endoscopic
0FC90ZZ	Extirpation of Matter from Common Bile Duct, Open Approach
0FC93ZZ	Extirpation of Matter from Common Bile Duct, Percutaneous Approach
0FC94ZZ	Extirpation of Matter from Common Bile Duct, Percutaneous Endoscopic Approach
0FC97ZZ	Extirpation of Matter from Common Bile Duct, Via Natural or Artificial Opening
0FC98ZZ	Extirpation of Matter from Common Bile Duct, Via Natural or Artificial Opening Endoscopic
0FCC0ZZ	Extirpation of Matter from Ampulla of Vater, Open Approach
0FCC3ZZ	Extirpation of Matter from Ampulla of Vater, Percutaneous Approach
0FCC4ZZ	Extirpation of Matter from Ampulla of Vater, Percutaneous Endoscopic Approach
0FCC7ZZ	Extirpation of Matter from Ampulla of Vater, Via Natural or Artificial Opening
0FCC8ZZ	Extirpation of Matter from Ampulla of Vater, Via Natural or Artificial Opening Endoscopic
0FCD0ZZ	Extirpation of Matter from Pancreatic Duct, Open Approach
0FCD3ZZ	Extirpation of Matter from Pancreatic Duct, Percutaneous Approach
0FCD4ZZ	Extirpation of Matter from Pancreatic Duct, Percutaneous Endoscopic Approach

♀ Female-only ♂ Male-only ▲ Limited Coverage ● Non-OR ▦ HAC-associated procedure ▲ Non-covered procedures ✛ Cluster

0FCD7ZZ Extirpation of Matter from Pancreatic Duct, Via Natural or Artificial Opening
0FCD8ZZ Extirpation of Matter from Pancreatic Duct, Via Natural or Artificial Opening Endoscopic
0FCF0ZZ Extirpation of Matter from Accessory Pancreatic Duct, Open Approach
0FCF3ZZ Extirpation of Matter from Accessory Pancreatic Duct, Percutaneous Approach

0FCF4ZZ Extirpation of Matter from Accessory Pancreatic Duct, Percutaneous Endoscopic Approach
0FCF7ZZ Extirpation of Matter from Accessory Pancreatic Duct, Via Natural or Artificial Opening
0FCF8ZZ Extirpation of Matter from Accessory Pancreatic Duct, Via Natural or Artificial Opening Endoscopic

0FCG0ZZ Extirpation of Matter from Pancreas, Open Approach
0FCG3ZZ Extirpation of Matter from Pancreas, Percutaneous Approach
0FCG4ZZ Extirpation of Matter from Pancreas, Percutaneous Endoscopic Approach
0FCG8ZZ Extirpation of Matter from Pancreas, Via Natural or Artificial Opening Endoscopic

0FD – Hepatobiliary System and Pancreas, Extraction

Review Coding Guidelines B3.4a and B3.4b

0FD03ZX Extraction of Liver, Percutaneous Approach, Diagnostic
0FD04ZX Extraction of Liver, Percutaneous Endoscopic Approach, Diagnostic
0FD13ZX Extraction of Right Lobe Liver, Percutaneous Approach, Diagnostic
0FD14ZX Extraction of Right Lobe Liver, Percutaneous Endoscopic Approach, Diagnostic
0FD23ZX Extraction of Left Lobe Liver, Percutaneous Approach, Diagnostic
0FD24ZX Extraction of Left Lobe Liver, Percutaneous Endoscopic Approach, Diagnostic
0FD43ZX Extraction of Gallbladder, Percutaneous Approach, Diagnostic
0FD44ZX Extraction of Gallbladder, Percutaneous Endoscopic Approach, Diagnostic
0FD48ZX Extraction of Gallbladder, Via Natural or Artificial Opening Endoscopic, Diagnostic
0FD53ZX Extraction of Right Hepatic Duct, Percutaneous Approach, Diagnostic
0FD54ZX Extraction of Right Hepatic Duct, Percutaneous Endoscopic Approach, Diagnostic
0FD58ZX Extraction of Right Hepatic Duct, Via Natural or Artificial Opening Endoscopic, Diagnostic
0FD63ZX Extraction of Left Hepatic Duct, Percutaneous Approach, Diagnostic

0FD64ZX Extraction of Left Hepatic Duct, Percutaneous Endoscopic Approach, Diagnostic
0FD68ZX Extraction of Left Hepatic Duct, Via Natural or Artificial Opening Endoscopic, Diagnostic
0FD73ZX Extraction of Common Hepatic Duct, Percutaneous Approach, Diagnostic
0FD74ZX Extraction of Common Hepatic Duct, Percutaneous Endoscopic Approach, Diagnostic
0FD78ZX Extraction of Common Hepatic Duct, Via Natural or Artificial Opening Endoscopic, Diagnostic
0FD83ZX Extraction of Cystic Duct, Percutaneous Approach, Diagnostic
0FD84ZX Extraction of Cystic Duct, Percutaneous Endoscopic Approach, Diagnostic
0FD88ZX Extraction of Cystic Duct, Via Natural or Artificial Opening Endoscopic, Diagnostic
0FD93ZX Extraction of Common Bile Duct, Percutaneous Approach, Diagnostic
0FD94ZX Extraction of Common Bile Duct, Percutaneous Endoscopic Approach, Diagnostic
0FD98ZX Extraction of Common Bile Duct, Via Natural or Artificial Opening Endoscopic, Diagnostic
0FDC3ZX Extraction of Ampulla of Vater, Percutaneous Approach, Diagnostic

0FDC4ZX Extraction of Ampulla of Vater, Percutaneous Endoscopic Approach, Diagnostic
0FDC8ZX Extraction of Ampulla of Vater, Via Natural or Artificial Opening Endoscopic, Diagnostic
0FDD3ZX Extraction of Pancreatic Duct, Percutaneous Approach, Diagnostic
0FDD4ZX Extraction of Pancreatic Duct, Percutaneous Endoscopic Approach, Diagnostic
0FDD8ZX Extraction of Pancreatic Duct, Via Natural or Artificial Opening Endoscopic, Diagnostic
0FDF3ZX Extraction of Accessory Pancreatic Duct, Percutaneous Approach, Diagnostic
0FDF4ZX Extraction of Accessory Pancreatic Duct, Percutaneous Endoscopic Approach, Diagnostic
0FDF8ZX Extraction of Accessory Pancreatic Duct, Via Natural or Artificial Opening Endoscopic, Diagnostic
0FDG3ZX Extraction of Pancreas, Percutaneous Approach, Diagnostic
0FDG4ZX Extraction of Pancreas, Percutaneous Endoscopic Approach, Diagnostic
0FDG8ZX Extraction of Pancreas, Via Natural or Artificial Opening Endoscopic, Diagnostic

0FF – Hepatobiliary System and Pancreas, Fragmentation

0FF40ZZ Fragmentation in Gallbladder, Open Approach
0FF43ZZ Fragmentation in Gallbladder, Percutaneous Approach
0FF44ZZ Fragmentation in Gallbladder, Percutaneous Endoscopic Approach
0FF47ZZ Fragmentation in Gallbladder, Via Natural or Artificial Opening
0FF48ZZ Fragmentation in Gallbladder, Via Natural or Artificial Opening Endoscopic
▲ 0FF4XZZ Fragmentation in Gallbladder, External Approach
0FF50ZZ Fragmentation in Right Hepatic Duct, Open Approach
0FF53ZZ Fragmentation in Right Hepatic Duct, Percutaneous Approach
0FF54ZZ Fragmentation in Right Hepatic Duct, Percutaneous Endoscopic Approach
0FF57ZZ Fragmentation in Right Hepatic Duct, Via Natural or Artificial Opening
0FF58ZZ Fragmentation in Right Hepatic Duct, Via Natural or Artificial Opening Endoscopic
▲ 0FF5XZZ Fragmentation in Right Hepatic Duct, External Approach

0FF60ZZ Fragmentation in Left Hepatic Duct, Open Approach
0FF63ZZ Fragmentation in Left Hepatic Duct, Percutaneous Approach
0FF64ZZ Fragmentation in Left Hepatic Duct, Percutaneous Endoscopic Approach
0FF67ZZ Fragmentation in Left Hepatic Duct, Via Natural or Artificial Opening
0FF68ZZ Fragmentation in Left Hepatic Duct, Via Natural or Artificial Opening Endoscopic
▲ 0FF6XZZ Fragmentation in Left Hepatic Duct, External Approach
0FF70ZZ Fragmentation in Common Hepatic Duct, Open Approach
0FF73ZZ Fragmentation in Common Hepatic Duct, Percutaneous Approach
0FF74ZZ Fragmentation in Common Hepatic Duct, Percutaneous Endoscopic Approach
0FF77ZZ Fragmentation in Common Hepatic Duct, Via Natural or Artificial Opening
0FF78ZZ Fragmentation in Common Hepatic Duct, Via Natural or Artificial Opening Endoscopic
0FF7XZZ Fragmentation in Common Hepatic Duct, External Approach

0FF80ZZ Fragmentation in Cystic Duct, Open Approach
0FF83ZZ Fragmentation in Cystic Duct, Percutaneous Approach
0FF84ZZ Fragmentation in Cystic Duct, Percutaneous Endoscopic Approach
0FF87ZZ Fragmentation in Cystic Duct, Via Natural or Artificial Opening
0FF88ZZ Fragmentation in Cystic Duct, Via Natural or Artificial Opening Endoscopic
▲ 0FF8XZZ Fragmentation in Cystic Duct, External Approach
0FF90ZZ Fragmentation in Common Bile Duct, Open Approach
0FF93ZZ Fragmentation in Common Bile Duct, Percutaneous Approach
0FF94ZZ Fragmentation in Common Bile Duct, Percutaneous Endoscopic Approach
0FF97ZZ Fragmentation in Common Bile Duct, Via Natural or Artificial Opening
0FF98ZZ Fragmentation in Common Bile Duct, Via Natural or Artificial Opening Endoscopic
▲ 0FF9XZZ Fragmentation in Common Bile Duct, External Approach

0FFC0ZZ Fragmentation in Ampulla of Vater, Open Approach

0FFC3ZZ Fragmentation in Ampulla of Vater, Percutaneous Approach

0FFC4ZZ Fragmentation in Ampulla of Vater, Percutaneous Endoscopic Approach

0FFC7ZZ Fragmentation in Ampulla of Vater, Via Natural or Artificial Opening

0FFC8ZZ Fragmentation in Ampulla of Vater, Via Natural or Artificial Opening Endoscopic

▲ **0FFCXZZ** Fragmentation in Ampulla of Vater, External Approach

0FFD0ZZ Fragmentation in Pancreatic Duct, Open Approach

0FFD3ZZ Fragmentation in Pancreatic Duct, Percutaneous Approach

0FFD4ZZ Fragmentation in Pancreatic Duct, Percutaneous Endoscopic Approach

0FFD7ZZ Fragmentation in Pancreatic Duct, Via Natural or Artificial Opening

0FFD8ZZ Fragmentation in Pancreatic Duct, Via Natural or Artificial Opening Endoscopic

▲ **0FFDXZZ** Fragmentation in Pancreatic Duct, External Approach

0FFF0ZZ Fragmentation in Accessory Pancreatic Duct, Open Approach

0FFF3ZZ Fragmentation in Accessory Pancreatic Duct, Percutaneous Approach

0FFF4ZZ Fragmentation in Accessory Pancreatic Duct, Percutaneous Endoscopic Approach

0FFF7ZZ Fragmentation in Accessory Pancreatic Duct, Via Natural or Artificial Opening

● **0FFF8ZZ** Fragmentation in Accessory Pancreatic Duct, Via Natural or Artificial Opening Endoscopic

▲ **0FFFXZZ** Fragmentation in Accessory Pancreatic Duct, External Approach

0FH – Hepatobiliary System and Pancreas, Insertion

0FH001Z Insertion of Radioactive Element into Liver, Open Approach

0FH002Z Insertion of Monitoring Device into Liver, Open Approach

0FH003Z Insertion of Infusion Device into Liver, Open Approach

0FH00YZ Insertion of Other Device into Liver, Open Approach

0FH031Z Insertion of Radioactive Element into Liver, Percutaneous Approach

0FH032Z Insertion of Monitoring Device into Liver, Percutaneous Approach

0FH033Z Insertion of Infusion Device into Liver, Percutaneous Approach

0FH03YZ Insertion of Other Device into Liver, Percutaneous Approach

0FH041Z Insertion of Radioactive Element into Liver, Percutaneous Endoscopic Approach

0FH042Z Insertion of Monitoring Device into Liver, Percutaneous Endoscopic Approach

0FH043Z Insertion of Infusion Device into Liver, Percutaneous Endoscopic Approach

0FH04YZ Insertion of Other Device into Liver, Percutaneous Endoscopic Approach

0FH102Z Insertion of Monitoring Device into Right Lobe Liver, Open Approach

0FH103Z Insertion of Infusion Device into Right Lobe Liver, Open Approach

0FH132Z Insertion of Monitoring Device into Right Lobe Liver, Percutaneous Approach

0FH133Z Insertion of Infusion Device into Right Lobe Liver, Percutaneous Approach

0FH142Z Insertion of Monitoring Device into Right Lobe Liver, Percutaneous Endoscopic Approach

0FH143Z Insertion of Infusion Device into Right Lobe Liver, Percutaneous Endoscopic Approach

0FH202Z Insertion of Monitoring Device into Left Lobe Liver, Open Approach

0FH203Z Insertion of Infusion Device into Left Lobe Liver, Open Approach

0FH232Z Insertion of Monitoring Device into Left Lobe Liver, Percutaneous Approach

0FH233Z Insertion of Infusion Device into Left Lobe Liver, Percutaneous Approach

0FH242Z Insertion of Monitoring Device into Left Lobe Liver, Percutaneous Endoscopic Approach

0FH243Z Insertion of Infusion Device into Left Lobe Liver, Percutaneous Endoscopic Approach

0FH401Z Insertion of Radioactive Element into Gallbladder, Open Approach

0FH402Z Insertion of Monitoring Device into Gallbladder, Open Approach

0FH403Z Insertion of Infusion Device into Gallbladder, Open Approach

0FH40YZ Insertion of Other Device into Gallbladder, Open Approach

0FH431Z Insertion of Radioactive Element into Gallbladder, Percutaneous Approach

0FH432Z Insertion of Monitoring Device into Gallbladder, Percutaneous Approach

0FH433Z Insertion of Infusion Device into Gallbladder, Percutaneous Approach

0FH43YZ Insertion of Other Device into Gallbladder, Percutaneous Approach

0FH441Z Insertion of Radioactive Element into Gallbladder, Percutaneous Endoscopic Approach

0FH442Z Insertion of Monitoring Device into Gallbladder, Percutaneous Endoscopic Approach

0FH443Z Insertion of Infusion Device into Gallbladder, Percutaneous Endoscopic Approach

0FH44YZ Insertion of Other Device into Gallbladder, Percutaneous Endoscopic Approach

0FHB01Z Insertion of Radioactive Element into Hepatobiliary Duct, Open Approach

0FHB02Z Insertion of Monitoring Device into Hepatobiliary Duct, Open Approach

0FHB03Z Insertion of Infusion Device into Hepatobiliary Duct, Open Approach

0FHB0DZ Insertion of Intraluminal Device into Hepatobiliary Duct, Open Approach

0FHB0YZ Insertion of Other Device into Hepatobiliary Duct, Open Approach

0FHB31Z Insertion of Radioactive Element into Hepatobiliary Duct, Percutaneous Approach

0FHB32Z Insertion of Monitoring Device into Hepatobiliary Duct, Percutaneous Approach

0FHB33Z Insertion of Infusion Device into Hepatobiliary Duct, Percutaneous Approach

0FHB3DZ Insertion of Intraluminal Device into Hepatobiliary Duct, Percutaneous Approach

0FHB3YZ Insertion of Other Device into Hepatobiliary Duct, Percutaneous Approach

0FHB41Z Insertion of Radioactive Element into Hepatobiliary Duct, Percutaneous Endoscopic Approach

0FHB42Z Insertion of Monitoring Device into Hepatobiliary Duct, Percutaneous Endoscopic Approach

0FHB43Z Insertion of Infusion Device into Hepatobiliary Duct, Percutaneous Endoscopic Approach

0FHB4DZ Insertion of Intraluminal Device into Hepatobiliary Duct, Percutaneous Endoscopic Approach

0FHB4YZ Insertion of Other Device into Hepatobiliary Duct, Percutaneous Endoscopic Approach

0FHB71Z Insertion of Radioactive Element into Hepatobiliary Duct, Via Natural or Artificial Opening

0FHB72Z Insertion of Monitoring Device into Hepatobiliary Duct, Via Natural or Artificial Opening

0FHB73Z Insertion of Infusion Device into Hepatobiliary Duct, Via Natural or Artificial Opening

0FHB7DZ Insertion of Intraluminal Device into Hepatobiliary Duct, Via Natural or Artificial Opening

0FHB7YZ Insertion of Other Device into Hepatobiliary Duct, Via Natural or Artificial Opening

0FHB81Z Insertion of Radioactive Element into Hepatobiliary Duct, Via Natural or Artificial Opening Endoscopic

0FHB82Z Insertion of Monitoring Device into Hepatobiliary Duct, Via Natural or Artificial Opening Endoscopic

0FHB83Z Insertion of Infusion Device into Hepatobiliary Duct, Via Natural or Artificial Opening Endoscopic

0FHB8DZ Insertion of Intraluminal Device into Hepatobiliary Duct, Via Natural or Artificial Opening Endoscopic

0FHB8YZ Insertion of Other Device into Hepatobiliary Duct, Via Natural or Artificial Opening Endoscopic

0FHD01Z Insertion of Radioactive Element into Pancreatic Duct, Open Approach

0FHD02Z Insertion of Monitoring Device into Pancreatic Duct, Open Approach

0FHD03Z Insertion of Infusion Device into Pancreatic Duct, Open Approach

0FHD0DZ Insertion of Intraluminal Device into Pancreatic Duct, Open Approach

0FHD0YZ Insertion of Other Device into Pancreatic Duct, Open Approach

0FHD31Z Insertion of Radioactive Element into Pancreatic Duct, Percutaneous Approach

0FHD32Z Insertion of Monitoring Device into Pancreatic Duct, Percutaneous Approach

0FHD33Z Insertion of Infusion Device into Pancreatic Duct, Percutaneous Approach

♀ Female-only   ♂ Male-only   ▲ Limited Coverage   ● Non-OR   HAC HAC-associated procedure   ▲ Non-covered procedures   ✚ Cluster

0FHD3DZ Insertion of Intraluminal Device into Pancreatic Duct, Percutaneous Approach
0FHD3YZ Insertion of Other Device into Pancreatic Duct, Percutaneous Approach
0FHD41Z Insertion of Radioactive Element into Pancreatic Duct, Percutaneous Endoscopic Approach
0FHD42Z Insertion of Monitoring Device into Pancreatic Duct, Percutaneous Endoscopic Approach
0FHD43Z Insertion of Infusion Device into Pancreatic Duct, Percutaneous Endoscopic Approach
0FHD4DZ Insertion of Intraluminal Device into Pancreatic Duct, Percutaneous Endoscopic Approach
0FHD4YZ Insertion of Other Device into Pancreatic Duct, Percutaneous Endoscopic Approach
0FHD71Z Insertion of Radioactive Element into Pancreatic Duct, Via Natural or Artificial Opening
0FHD72Z Insertion of Monitoring Device into Pancreatic Duct, Via Natural or Artificial Opening

0FHD73Z Insertion of Infusion Device into Pancreatic Duct, Via Natural or Artificial Opening
0FHD7DZ Insertion of Intraluminal Device into Pancreatic Duct, Via Natural or Artificial Opening
0FHD7YZ Insertion of Other Device into Pancreatic Duct, Via Natural or Artificial Opening
0FHD81Z Insertion of Radioactive Element into Pancreatic Duct, Via Natural or Artificial Opening Endoscopic
0FHD82Z Insertion of Monitoring Device into Pancreatic Duct, Via Natural or Artificial Opening Endoscopic
0FHD83Z Insertion of Infusion Device into Pancreatic Duct, Via Natural or Artificial Opening Endoscopic
0FHD8DZ Insertion of Intraluminal Device into Pancreatic Duct, Via Natural or Artificial Opening Endoscopic
0FHD8YZ Insertion of Other Device into Pancreatic Duct, Via Natural or Artificial Opening Endoscopic
0FHG01Z Insertion of Radioactive Element into Pancreas, Open Approach

0FHG02Z Insertion of Monitoring Device into Pancreas, Open Approach
0FHG03Z Insertion of Infusion Device into Pancreas, Open Approach
0FHG0YZ Insertion of Other Device into Pancreas, Open Approach
0FHG31Z Insertion of Radioactive Element into Pancreas, Percutaneous Approach
0FHG32Z Insertion of Monitoring Device into Pancreas, Percutaneous Approach
0FHG33Z Insertion of Infusion Device into Pancreas, Percutaneous Approach
0FHG3YZ Insertion of Other Device into Pancreas, Percutaneous Approach
0FHG41Z Insertion of Radioactive Element into Pancreas, Percutaneous Endoscopic Approach
0FHG42Z Insertion of Monitoring Device into Pancreas, Percutaneous Endoscopic Approach
0FHG43Z Insertion of Infusion Device into Pancreas, Percutaneous Endoscopic Approach
0FHG4YZ Insertion of Other Device into Pancreas, Percutaneous Endoscopic Approach

0FJ – Hepatobiliary System and Pancreas, Inspection

Review Coding Guidelines B3.11a, B3.11b and B3.11c

0FJ00ZZ Inspection of Liver, Open Approach
0FJ03ZZ Inspection of Liver, Percutaneous Approach
0FJ04ZZ Inspection of Liver, Percutaneous Endoscopic Approach
0FJ0XZZ Inspection of Liver, External Approach
0FJ40ZZ Inspection of Gallbladder, Open Approach
0FJ43ZZ Inspection of Gallbladder, Percutaneous Approach
0FJ44ZZ Inspection of Gallbladder, Percutaneous Endoscopic Approach
0FJ48ZZ Inspection of Gallbladder, Via Natural or Artificial Opening Endoscopic
0FJ4XZZ Inspection of Gallbladder, External Approach

0FJB0ZZ Inspection of Hepatobiliary Duct, Open Approach
0FJB3ZZ Inspection of Hepatobiliary Duct, Percutaneous Approach
0FJB4ZZ Inspection of Hepatobiliary Duct, Percutaneous Endoscopic Approach
0FJB7ZZ Inspection of Hepatobiliary Duct, Via Natural or Artificial Opening
0FJB8ZZ Inspection of Hepatobiliary Duct, Via Natural or Artificial Opening Endoscopic
0FJD0ZZ Inspection of Pancreatic Duct, Open Approach
0FJD3ZZ Inspection of Pancreatic Duct, Percutaneous Approach

0FJD4ZZ Inspection of Pancreatic Duct, Percutaneous Endoscopic Approach
0FJD7ZZ Inspection of Pancreatic Duct, Via Natural or Artificial Opening
0FJD8ZZ Inspection of Pancreatic Duct, Via Natural or Artificial Opening Endoscopic
0FJG0ZZ Inspection of Pancreas, Open Approach
0FJG3ZZ Inspection of Pancreas, Percutaneous Approach
0FJG4ZZ Inspection of Pancreas, Percutaneous Endoscopic Approach
0FJG8ZZ Inspection of Pancreas, Via Natural or Artificial Opening Endoscopic
0FJGXZZ Inspection of Pancreas, External Approach

0FL – Hepatobiliary System and Pancreas, Occlusion

0FL50CZ Occlusion of Right Hepatic Duct with Extraluminal Device, Open Approach
0FL50DZ Occlusion of Right Hepatic Duct with Intraluminal Device, Open Approach
0FL50ZZ Occlusion of Right Hepatic Duct, Open Approach
0FL53CZ Occlusion of Right Hepatic Duct with Extraluminal Device, Percutaneous Approach
0FL53DZ Occlusion of Right Hepatic Duct with Intraluminal Device, Percutaneous Approach
0FL53ZZ Occlusion of Right Hepatic Duct, Percutaneous Approach
0FL54CZ Occlusion of Right Hepatic Duct with Extraluminal Device, Percutaneous Endoscopic Approach
0FL54DZ Occlusion of Right Hepatic Duct with Intraluminal Device, Percutaneous Endoscopic Approach
0FL54ZZ Occlusion of Right Hepatic Duct, Percutaneous Endoscopic Approach

0FL57DZ Occlusion of Right Hepatic Duct with Intraluminal Device, Via Natural or Artificial Opening
0FL57ZZ Occlusion of Right Hepatic Duct, Via Natural or Artificial Opening
0FL58DZ Occlusion of Right Hepatic Duct with Intraluminal Device, Via Natural or Artificial Opening Endoscopic
0FL58ZZ Occlusion of Right Hepatic Duct, Via Natural or Artificial Opening Endoscopic
0FL60CZ Occlusion of Left Hepatic Duct with Extraluminal Device, Open Approach
0FL60DZ Occlusion of Left Hepatic Duct with Intraluminal Device, Open Approach
0FL60ZZ Occlusion of Left Hepatic Duct, Open Approach
0FL63CZ Occlusion of Left Hepatic Duct with Extraluminal Device, Percutaneous Approach
0FL63DZ Occlusion of Left Hepatic Duct with Intraluminal Device, Percutaneous Approach

0FL63ZZ Occlusion of Left Hepatic Duct, Percutaneous Approach
0FL64CZ Occlusion of Left Hepatic Duct with Extraluminal Device, Percutaneous Endoscopic Approach
0FL64DZ Occlusion of Left Hepatic Duct with Intraluminal Device, Percutaneous Endoscopic Approach
0FL64ZZ Occlusion of Left Hepatic Duct, Percutaneous Endoscopic Approach
0FL67DZ Occlusion of Left Hepatic Duct with Intraluminal Device, Via Natural or Artificial Opening
0FL67ZZ Occlusion of Left Hepatic Duct, Via Natural or Artificial Opening
0FL68DZ Occlusion of Left Hepatic Duct with Intraluminal Device, Via Natural or Artificial Opening Endoscopic
0FL68ZZ Occlusion of Left Hepatic Duct, Via Natural or Artificial Opening Endoscopic
0FL70CZ Occlusion of Common Hepatic Duct with Extraluminal Device, Open Approach

0FL70DZ Occlusion of Common Hepatic Duct with Intraluminal Device, Open Approach

0FL70ZZ Occlusion of Common Hepatic Duct, Open Approach

0FL73CZ Occlusion of Common Hepatic Duct with Extraluminal Device, Percutaneous Approach

0FL73DZ Occlusion of Common Hepatic Duct with Intraluminal Device, Percutaneous Approach

0FL73ZZ Occlusion of Common Hepatic Duct, Percutaneous Approach

0FL74CZ Occlusion of Common Hepatic Duct with Extraluminal Device, Percutaneous Endoscopic Approach

0FL74DZ Occlusion of Common Hepatic Duct with Intraluminal Device, Percutaneous Endoscopic Approach

0FL74ZZ Occlusion of Common Hepatic Duct, Percutaneous Endoscopic Approach

0FL77DZ Occlusion of Common Hepatic Duct with Intraluminal Device, Via Natural or Artificial Opening

0FL77ZZ Occlusion of Common Hepatic Duct, Via Natural or Artificial Opening

0FL78DZ Occlusion of Common Hepatic Duct with Intraluminal Device, Via Natural or Artificial Opening Endoscopic

0FL78ZZ Occlusion of Common Hepatic Duct, Via Natural or Artificial Opening Endoscopic

0FL80CZ Occlusion of Cystic Duct with Extraluminal Device, Open Approach

0FL80DZ Occlusion of Cystic Duct with Intraluminal Device, Open Approach

0FL80ZZ Occlusion of Cystic Duct, Open Approach

0FL83CZ Occlusion of Cystic Duct with Extraluminal Device, Percutaneous Approach

0FL83DZ Occlusion of Cystic Duct with Intraluminal Device, Percutaneous Approach

0FL83ZZ Occlusion of Cystic Duct, Percutaneous Approach

0FL84CZ Occlusion of Cystic Duct with Extraluminal Device, Percutaneous Endoscopic Approach

0FL84DZ Occlusion of Cystic Duct with Intraluminal Device, Percutaneous Endoscopic Approach

0FL84ZZ Occlusion of Cystic Duct, Percutaneous Endoscopic Approach

0FL87DZ Occlusion of Cystic Duct with Intraluminal Device, Via Natural or Artificial Opening

0FL87ZZ Occlusion of Cystic Duct, Via Natural or Artificial Opening

0FL88DZ Occlusion of Cystic Duct with Intraluminal Device, Via Natural or Artificial Opening Endoscopic

0FL88ZZ Occlusion of Cystic Duct, Via Natural or Artificial Opening Endoscopic

0FL90CZ Occlusion of Common Bile Duct with Extraluminal Device, Open Approach

0FL90DZ Occlusion of Common Bile Duct with Intraluminal Device, Open Approach

0FL90ZZ Occlusion of Common Bile Duct, Open Approach

0FL93CZ Occlusion of Common Bile Duct with Extraluminal Device, Percutaneous Approach

0FL93DZ Occlusion of Common Bile Duct with Intraluminal Device, Percutaneous Approach

0FL93ZZ Occlusion of Common Bile Duct, Percutaneous Approach

0FL94CZ Occlusion of Common Bile Duct with Extraluminal Device, Percutaneous Endoscopic Approach

0FL94DZ Occlusion of Common Bile Duct with Intraluminal Device, Percutaneous Endoscopic Approach

0FL94ZZ Occlusion of Common Bile Duct, Percutaneous Endoscopic Approach

0FL97DZ Occlusion of Common Bile Duct with Intraluminal Device, Via Natural or Artificial Opening

0FL97ZZ Occlusion of Common Bile Duct, Via Natural or Artificial Opening

0FL98DZ Occlusion of Common Bile Duct with Intraluminal Device, Via Natural or Artificial Opening Endoscopic

0FL98ZZ Occlusion of Common Bile Duct, Via Natural or Artificial Opening Endoscopic

0FLC0CZ Occlusion of Ampulla of Vater with Extraluminal Device, Open Approach

0FLC0DZ Occlusion of Ampulla of Vater with Intraluminal Device, Open Approach

0FLC0ZZ Occlusion of Ampulla of Vater, Open Approach

0FLC3CZ Occlusion of Ampulla of Vater with Extraluminal Device, Percutaneous Approach

0FLC3DZ Occlusion of Ampulla of Vater with Intraluminal Device, Percutaneous Approach

0FLC3ZZ Occlusion of Ampulla of Vater, Percutaneous Approach

0FLC4CZ Occlusion of Ampulla of Vater with Extraluminal Device, Percutaneous Endoscopic Approach

0FLC4DZ Occlusion of Ampulla of Vater with Intraluminal Device, Percutaneous Endoscopic Approach

0FLC4ZZ Occlusion of Ampulla of Vater, Percutaneous Endoscopic Approach

0FLC7DZ Occlusion of Ampulla of Vater with Intraluminal Device, Via Natural or Artificial Opening

0FLC7ZZ Occlusion of Ampulla of Vater, Via Natural or Artificial Opening

0FLC8DZ Occlusion of Ampulla of Vater with Intraluminal Device, Via Natural or Artificial Opening Endoscopic

0FLC8ZZ Occlusion of Ampulla of Vater, Via Natural or Artificial Opening Endoscopic

0FLD0CZ Occlusion of Pancreatic Duct with Extraluminal Device, Open Approach

0FLD0DZ Occlusion of Pancreatic Duct with Intraluminal Device, Open Approach

0FLD0ZZ Occlusion of Pancreatic Duct, Open Approach

0FLD3CZ Occlusion of Pancreatic Duct with Extraluminal Device, Percutaneous Approach

0FLD3DZ Occlusion of Pancreatic Duct with Intraluminal Device, Percutaneous Approach

0FLD3ZZ Occlusion of Pancreatic Duct, Percutaneous Approach

0FLD4CZ Occlusion of Pancreatic Duct with Extraluminal Device, Percutaneous Endoscopic Approach

0FLD4DZ Occlusion of Pancreatic Duct with Intraluminal Device, Percutaneous Endoscopic Approach

0FLD4ZZ Occlusion of Pancreatic Duct, Percutaneous Endoscopic Approach

0FLD7DZ Occlusion of Pancreatic Duct with Intraluminal Device, Via Natural or Artificial Opening

0FLD7ZZ Occlusion of Pancreatic Duct, Via Natural or Artificial Opening

0FLD8DZ Occlusion of Pancreatic Duct with Intraluminal Device, Via Natural or Artificial Opening Endoscopic

0FLD8ZZ Occlusion of Pancreatic Duct, Via Natural or Artificial Opening Endoscopic

0FLF0CZ Occlusion of Accessory Pancreatic Duct with Extraluminal Device, Open Approach

0FLF0DZ Occlusion of Accessory Pancreatic Duct with Intraluminal Device, Open Approach

0FLF0ZZ Occlusion of Accessory Pancreatic Duct, Open Approach

0FLF3CZ Occlusion of Accessory Pancreatic Duct with Extraluminal Device, Percutaneous Approach

0FLF3DZ Occlusion of Accessory Pancreatic Duct with Intraluminal Device, Percutaneous Approach

0FLF3ZZ Occlusion of Accessory Pancreatic Duct, Percutaneous Approach

0FLF4CZ Occlusion of Accessory Pancreatic Duct with Extraluminal Device, Percutaneous Endoscopic Approach

0FLF4DZ Occlusion of Accessory Pancreatic Duct with Intraluminal Device, Percutaneous Endoscopic Approach

0FLF4ZZ Occlusion of Accessory Pancreatic Duct, Percutaneous Endoscopic Approach

0FLF7DZ Occlusion of Accessory Pancreatic Duct with Intraluminal Device, Via Natural or Artificial Opening

0FLF7ZZ Occlusion of Accessory Pancreatic Duct, Via Natural or Artificial Opening

0FLF8DZ Occlusion of Accessory Pancreatic Duct with Intraluminal Device, Via Natural or Artificial Opening Endoscopic

0FLF8ZZ Occlusion of Accessory Pancreatic Duct, Via Natural or Artificial Opening Endoscopic

0FM – Hepatobiliary System and Pancreas, Reattachment

0FM00ZZ Reattachment of Liver, Open Approach

0FM04ZZ Reattachment of Liver, Percutaneous Endoscopic Approach

0FM10ZZ Reattachment of Right Lobe Liver, Open Approach

0FM14ZZ Reattachment of Right Lobe Liver, Percutaneous Endoscopic Approach

0FM20ZZ Reattachment of Left Lobe Liver, Open Approach

0FM24ZZ Reattachment of Left Lobe Liver, Percutaneous Endoscopic Approach

♀ Female-only   ♂ Male-only   ▲ Limited Coverage   ● Non-OR   ▨ HAC-associated procedure   ▲ Non-covered procedures   ✚ Cluster

0FM40ZZ Reattachment of Gallbladder, Open Approach	**0FM74ZZ** Reattachment of Common Hepatic Duct, Percutaneous Endoscopic Approach	**0FMD0ZZ** Reattachment of Pancreatic Duct, Open Approach
0FM44ZZ Reattachment of Gallbladder, Percutaneous Endoscopic Approach	**0FM80ZZ** Reattachment of Cystic Duct, Open Approach	**0FMD4ZZ** Reattachment of Pancreatic Duct, Percutaneous Endoscopic Approach
0FM50ZZ Reattachment of Right Hepatic Duct, Open Approach	**0FM84ZZ** Reattachment of Cystic Duct, Percutaneous Endoscopic Approach	**0FMF0ZZ** Reattachment of Accessory Pancreatic Duct, Open Approach
0FM54ZZ Reattachment of Right Hepatic Duct, Percutaneous Endoscopic Approach	**0FM90ZZ** Reattachment of Common Bile Duct, Open Approach	**0FMF4ZZ** Reattachment of Accessory Pancreatic Duct, Percutaneous Endoscopic Approach
0FM60ZZ Reattachment of Left Hepatic Duct, Open Approach	**0FM94ZZ** Reattachment of Common Bile Duct, Percutaneous Endoscopic Approach	**0FMG0ZZ** Reattachment of Pancreas, Open Approach
0FM64ZZ Reattachment of Left Hepatic Duct, Percutaneous Endoscopic Approach	**0FMC0ZZ** Reattachment of Ampulla of Vater, Open Approach	**0FMG4ZZ** Reattachment of Pancreas, Percutaneous Endoscopic Approach
0FM70ZZ Reattachment of Common Hepatic Duct, Open Approach	**0FMC4ZZ** Reattachment of Ampulla of Vater, Percutaneous Endoscopic Approach	

0FN – Hepatobiliary System and Pancreas, Release

Review Coding Guideline B3.13

Review Coding Guideline B3.14

0FN00ZZ Release Liver, Open Approach	**0FN64ZZ** Release Left Hepatic Duct, Percutaneous Endoscopic Approach	**0FNC0ZZ** Release Ampulla of Vater, Open Approach
0FN03ZZ Release Liver, Percutaneous Approach	**0FN67ZZ** Release Left Hepatic Duct, Via Natural or Artificial Opening	**0FNC3ZZ** Release Ampulla of Vater, Percutaneous Approach
0FN04ZZ Release Liver, Percutaneous Endoscopic Approach	**0FN68ZZ** Release Left Hepatic Duct, Via Natural or Artificial Opening Endoscopic	**0FNC4ZZ** Release Ampulla of Vater, Percutaneous Endoscopic Approach
0FN10ZZ Release Right Lobe Liver, Open Approach	**0FN70ZZ** Release Common Hepatic Duct, Open Approach	**0FNC7ZZ** Release Ampulla of Vater, Via Natural or Artificial Opening
0FN13ZZ Release Right Lobe Liver, Percutaneous Approach	**0FN73ZZ** Release Common Hepatic Duct, Percutaneous Approach	**0FNC8ZZ** Release Ampulla of Vater, Via Natural or Artificial Opening Endoscopic
0FN14ZZ Release Right Lobe Liver, Percutaneous Endoscopic Approach	**0FN74ZZ** Release Common Hepatic Duct, Percutaneous Endoscopic Approach	**0FND0ZZ** Release Pancreatic Duct, Open Approach
0FN20ZZ Release Left Lobe Liver, Open Approach	**0FN77ZZ** Release Common Hepatic Duct, Via Natural or Artificial Opening	**0FND3ZZ** Release Pancreatic Duct, Percutaneous Approach
0FN23ZZ Release Left Lobe Liver, Percutaneous Approach	**0FN78ZZ** Release Common Hepatic Duct, Via Natural or Artificial Opening Endoscopic	**0FND4ZZ** Release Pancreatic Duct, Percutaneous Endoscopic Approach
0FN24ZZ Release Left Lobe Liver, Percutaneous Endoscopic Approach	**0FN80ZZ** Release Cystic Duct, Open Approach	**0FND7ZZ** Release Pancreatic Duct, Via Natural or Artificial Opening
0FN40ZZ Release Gallbladder, Open Approach	**0FN83ZZ** Release Cystic Duct, Percutaneous Approach	**0FND8ZZ** Release Pancreatic Duct, Via Natural or Artificial Opening Endoscopic
0FN43ZZ Release Gallbladder, Percutaneous Approach	**0FN84ZZ** Release Cystic Duct, Percutaneous Endoscopic Approach	**0FNF0ZZ** Release Accessory Pancreatic Duct, Open Approach
0FN44ZZ Release Gallbladder, Percutaneous Endoscopic Approach	**0FN87ZZ** Release Cystic Duct, Via Natural or Artificial Opening	**0FNF3ZZ** Release Accessory Pancreatic Duct, Percutaneous Approach
0FN48ZZ Release Gallbladder, Via Natural or Artificial Opening Endoscopic	**0FN88ZZ** Release Cystic Duct, Via Natural or Artificial Opening Endoscopic	**0FNF4ZZ** Release Accessory Pancreatic Duct, Percutaneous Endoscopic Approach
0FN50ZZ Release Right Hepatic Duct, Open Approach	**0FN90ZZ** Release Common Bile Duct, Open Approach	**0FNF7ZZ** Release Accessory Pancreatic Duct, Via Natural or Artificial Opening
0FN53ZZ Release Right Hepatic Duct, Percutaneous Approach	**0FN93ZZ** Release Common Bile Duct, Percutaneous Approach	**0FNF8ZZ** Release Accessory Pancreatic Duct, Via Natural or Artificial Opening Endoscopic
0FN54ZZ Release Right Hepatic Duct, Percutaneous Endoscopic Approach	**0FN94ZZ** Release Common Bile Duct, Percutaneous Endoscopic Approach	**0FNG0ZZ** Release Pancreas, Open Approach
0FN57ZZ Release Right Hepatic Duct, Via Natural or Artificial Opening	**0FN97ZZ** Release Common Bile Duct, Via Natural or Artificial Opening	**0FNG3ZZ** Release Pancreas, Percutaneous Approach
0FN58ZZ Release Right Hepatic Duct, Via Natural or Artificial Opening Endoscopic	**0FN98ZZ** Release Common Bile Duct, Via Natural or Artificial Opening Endoscopic	**0FNG4ZZ** Release Pancreas, Percutaneous Endoscopic Approach
0FN60ZZ Release Left Hepatic Duct, Open Approach		**0FNG8ZZ** Release Pancreas, Via Natural or Artificial Opening Endoscopic
0FN63ZZ Release Left Hepatic Duct, Percutaneous Approach		

0FP – Hepatobiliary System and Pancreas, Removal

Review Coding Guideline B6.1c

0FP000Z Removal of Drainage Device from Liver, Open Approach	**0FP032Z** Removal of Monitoring Device from Liver, Percutaneous Approach	**0FP042Z** Removal of Monitoring Device from Liver, Percutaneous Endoscopic Approach
0FP002Z Removal of Monitoring Device from Liver, Open Approach	**0FP033Z** Removal of Infusion Device from Liver, Percutaneous Approach	**0FP043Z** Removal of Infusion Device from Liver, Percutaneous Endoscopic Approach
0FP003Z Removal of Infusion Device from Liver, Open Approach	**0FP03YZ** Removal of Other Device from Liver, Percutaneous Approach	**0FP04YZ** Removal of Other Device from Liver, Percutaneous Endoscopic Approach
0FP00YZ Removal of Other Device from Liver, Open Approach	**0FP040Z** Removal of Drainage Device from Liver, Percutaneous Endoscopic Approach	**0FP0X0Z** Removal of Drainage Device from Liver, External Approach
0FP030Z Removal of Drainage Device from Liver, Percutaneous Approach		

0FP0X2Z Removal of Monitoring Device from Liver, External Approach

0FP0X3Z Removal of Infusion Device from Liver, External Approach

0FP400Z Removal of Drainage Device from Gallbladder, Open Approach

0FP402Z Removal of Monitoring Device from Gallbladder, Open Approach

0FP403Z Removal of Infusion Device from Gallbladder, Open Approach

0FP40DZ Removal of Intraluminal Device from Gallbladder, Open Approach

0FP40YZ Removal of Other Device from Gallbladder, Open Approach

0FP430Z Removal of Drainage Device from Gallbladder, Percutaneous Approach

0FP432Z Removal of Monitoring Device from Gallbladder, Percutaneous Approach

0FP433Z Removal of Infusion Device from Gallbladder, Percutaneous Approach

0FP43DZ Removal of Intraluminal Device from Gallbladder, Percutaneous Approach

0FP43YZ Removal of Other Device from Gallbladder, Percutaneous Approach

0FP440Z Removal of Drainage Device from Gallbladder, Percutaneous Endoscopic Approach

0FP442Z Removal of Monitoring Device from Gallbladder, Percutaneous Endoscopic Approach

0FP443Z Removal of Infusion Device from Gallbladder, Percutaneous Endoscopic Approach

0FP44DZ Removal of Intraluminal Device from Gallbladder, Percutaneous Endoscopic Approach

0FP44YZ Removal of Other Device from Gallbladder, Percutaneous Endoscopic Approach

0FP4X0Z Removal of Drainage Device from Gallbladder, External Approach

0FP4X2Z Removal of Monitoring Device from Gallbladder, External Approach

0FP4X3Z Removal of Infusion Device from Gallbladder, External Approach

0FP4XDZ Removal of Intraluminal Device from Gallbladder, External Approach

0FPB00Z Removal of Drainage Device from Hepatobiliary Duct, Open Approach

0FPB01Z Removal of Radioactive Element from Hepatobiliary Duct, Open Approach

0FPB02Z Removal of Monitoring Device from Hepatobiliary Duct, Open Approach

0FPB03Z Removal of Infusion Device from Hepatobiliary Duct, Open Approach

0FPB07Z Removal of Autologous Tissue Substitute from Hepatobiliary Duct, Open Approach

0FPB0CZ Removal of Extraluminal Device from Hepatobiliary Duct, Open Approach

0FPB0DZ Removal of Intraluminal Device from Hepatobiliary Duct, Open Approach

0FPB0JZ Removal of Synthetic Substitute from Hepatobiliary Duct, Open Approach

0FPB0KZ Removal of Nonautologous Tissue Substitute from Hepatobiliary Duct, Open Approach

0FPB0YZ Removal of Other Device from Hepatobiliary Duct, Open Approach

0FPB30Z Removal of Drainage Device from Hepatobiliary Duct, Percutaneous Approach

0FPB31Z Removal of Radioactive Element from Hepatobiliary Duct, Percutaneous Approach

0FPB32Z Removal of Monitoring Device from Hepatobiliary Duct, Percutaneous Approach

0FPB33Z Removal of Infusion Device from Hepatobiliary Duct, Percutaneous Approach

0FPB37Z Removal of Autologous Tissue Substitute from Hepatobiliary Duct, Percutaneous Approach

0FPB3CZ Removal of Extraluminal Device from Hepatobiliary Duct, Percutaneous Approach

0FPB3DZ Removal of Intraluminal Device from Hepatobiliary Duct, Percutaneous Approach

0FPB3JZ Removal of Synthetic Substitute from Hepatobiliary Duct, Percutaneous Approach

0FPB3KZ Removal of Nonautologous Tissue Substitute from Hepatobiliary Duct, Percutaneous Approach

0FPB3YZ Removal of Other Device from Hepatobiliary Duct, Percutaneous Approach

0FPB40Z Removal of Drainage Device from Hepatobiliary Duct, Percutaneous Endoscopic Approach

0FPB41Z Removal of Radioactive Element from Hepatobiliary Duct, Percutaneous Endoscopic Approach

0FPB42Z Removal of Monitoring Device from Hepatobiliary Duct, Percutaneous Endoscopic Approach

0FPB43Z Removal of Infusion Device from Hepatobiliary Duct, Percutaneous Endoscopic Approach

0FPB47Z Removal of Autologous Tissue Substitute from Hepatobiliary Duct, Percutaneous Endoscopic Approach

0FPB4CZ Removal of Extraluminal Device from Hepatobiliary Duct, Percutaneous Endoscopic Approach

0FPB4DZ Removal of Intraluminal Device from Hepatobiliary Duct, Percutaneous Endoscopic Approach

0FPB4JZ Removal of Synthetic Substitute from Hepatobiliary Duct, Percutaneous Endoscopic Approach

0FPB4KZ Removal of Nonautologous Tissue Substitute from Hepatobiliary Duct, Percutaneous Endoscopic Approach

0FPB4YZ Removal of Other Device from Hepatobiliary Duct, Percutaneous Endoscopic Approach

0FPB70Z Removal of Drainage Device from Hepatobiliary Duct, Via Natural or Artificial Opening

0FPB71Z Removal of Radioactive Element from Hepatobiliary Duct, Via Natural or Artificial Opening

0FPB72Z Removal of Monitoring Device from Hepatobiliary Duct, Via Natural or Artificial Opening

0FPB73Z Removal of Infusion Device from Hepatobiliary Duct, Via Natural or Artificial Opening

0FPB77Z Removal of Autologous Tissue Substitute from Hepatobiliary Duct, Via Natural or Artificial Opening

0FPB7CZ Removal of Extraluminal Device from Hepatobiliary Duct, Via Natural or Artificial Opening

0FPB7DZ Removal of Intraluminal Device from Hepatobiliary Duct, Via Natural or Artificial Opening

0FPB7JZ Removal of Synthetic Substitute from Hepatobiliary Duct, Via Natural or Artificial Opening

0FPB7KZ Removal of Nonautologous Tissue Substitute from Hepatobiliary Duct, Via Natural or Artificial Opening

0FPB7YZ Removal of Other Device from Hepatobiliary Duct, Via Natural or Artificial Opening

0FPB80Z Removal of Drainage Device from Hepatobiliary Duct, Via Natural or Artificial Opening Endoscopic

0FPB81Z Removal of Radioactive Element from Hepatobiliary Duct, Via Natural or Artificial Opening Endoscopic

0FPB82Z Removal of Monitoring Device from Hepatobiliary Duct, Via Natural or Artificial Opening Endoscopic

0FPB83Z Removal of Infusion Device from Hepatobiliary Duct, Via Natural or Artificial Opening Endoscopic

0FPB87Z Removal of Autologous Tissue Substitute from Hepatobiliary Duct, Via Natural or Artificial Opening Endoscopic

0FPB8CZ Removal of Extraluminal Device from Hepatobiliary Duct, Via Natural or Artificial Opening Endoscopic

0FPB8DZ Removal of Intraluminal Device from Hepatobiliary Duct, Via Natural or Artificial Opening Endoscopic

0FPB8JZ Removal of Synthetic Substitute from Hepatobiliary Duct, Via Natural or Artificial Opening Endoscopic

0FPB8KZ Removal of Nonautologous Tissue Substitute from Hepatobiliary Duct, Via Natural or Artificial Opening Endoscopic

0FPB8YZ Removal of Other Device from Hepatobiliary Duct, Via Natural or Artificial Opening Endoscopic

0FPBX0Z Removal of Drainage Device from Hepatobiliary Duct, External Approach

0FPBX1Z Removal of Radioactive Element from Hepatobiliary Duct, External Approach

0FPBX2Z Removal of Monitoring Device from Hepatobiliary Duct, External Approach

0FPBX3Z Removal of Infusion Device from Hepatobiliary Duct, External Approach

0FPBXDZ Removal of Intraluminal Device from Hepatobiliary Duct, External Approach

0FPD00Z Removal of Drainage Device from Pancreatic Duct, Open Approach

0FPD01Z Removal of Radioactive Element from Pancreatic Duct, Open Approach

0FPD02Z Removal of Monitoring Device from Pancreatic Duct, Open Approach

0FPD03Z Removal of Infusion Device from Pancreatic Duct, Open Approach

0FPD07Z Removal of Autologous Tissue Substitute from Pancreatic Duct, Open Approach

0FPD0CZ Removal of Extraluminal Device from Pancreatic Duct, Open Approach

0FPD0DZ Removal of Intraluminal Device from Pancreatic Duct, Open Approach

0FPD0JZ Removal of Synthetic Substitute from Pancreatic Duct, Open Approach

0FPD0KZ Removal of Nonautologous Tissue Substitute from Pancreatic Duct, Open Approach

0FPD0YZ Removal of Other Device from Pancreatic Duct, Open Approach

0FPD30Z Removal of Drainage Device from Pancreatic Duct, Percutaneous Approach

♀ Female-only   ♂ Male-only   ▲ Limited Coverage   ● Non-OR   HAC HAC-associated procedure   ▲ Non-covered procedures   ✚ Cluster

0FPD31Z Removal of Radioactive Element from Pancreatic Duct, Percutaneous Approach

0FPD32Z Removal of Monitoring Device from Pancreatic Duct, Percutaneous Approach

0FPD33Z Removal of Infusion Device from Pancreatic Duct, Percutaneous Approach

0FPD37Z Removal of Autologous Tissue Substitute from Pancreatic Duct, Percutaneous Approach

0FPD3CZ Removal of Extraluminal Device from Pancreatic Duct, Percutaneous Approach

0FPD3DZ Removal of Intraluminal Device from Pancreatic Duct, Percutaneous Approach

0FPD3JZ Removal of Synthetic Substitute from Pancreatic Duct, Percutaneous Approach

0FPD3KZ Removal of Nonautologous Tissue Substitute from Pancreatic Duct, Percutaneous Approach

0FPD3YZ Removal of Other Device from Pancreatic Duct, Percutaneous Approach

0FPD40Z Removal of Drainage Device from Pancreatic Duct, Percutaneous Endoscopic Approach

0FPD41Z Removal of Radioactive Element from Pancreatic Duct, Percutaneous Endoscopic Approach

0FPD42Z Removal of Monitoring Device from Pancreatic Duct, Percutaneous Endoscopic Approach

0FPD43Z Removal of Infusion Device from Pancreatic Duct, Percutaneous Endoscopic Approach

0FPD47Z Removal of Autologous Tissue Substitute from Pancreatic Duct, Percutaneous Endoscopic Approach

0FPD4CZ Removal of Extraluminal Device from Pancreatic Duct, Percutaneous Endoscopic Approach

0FPD4DZ Removal of Intraluminal Device from Pancreatic Duct, Percutaneous Endoscopic Approach

0FPD4JZ Removal of Synthetic Substitute from Pancreatic Duct, Percutaneous Endoscopic Approach

0FPD4KZ Removal of Nonautologous Tissue Substitute from Pancreatic Duct, Percutaneous Endoscopic Approach

0FPD4YZ Removal of Other Device from Pancreatic Duct, Percutaneous Endoscopic Approach

0FPD70Z Removal of Drainage Device from Pancreatic Duct, Via Natural or Artificial Opening

0FPD71Z Removal of Radioactive Element from Pancreatic Duct, Via Natural or Artificial Opening

0FPD72Z Removal of Monitoring Device from Pancreatic Duct, Via Natural or Artificial Opening

0FPD73Z Removal of Infusion Device from Pancreatic Duct, Via Natural or Artificial Opening

0FPD77Z Removal of Autologous Tissue Substitute from Pancreatic Duct, Via Natural or Artificial Opening

0FPD7CZ Removal of Extraluminal Device from Pancreatic Duct, Via Natural or Artificial Opening

0FPD7DZ Removal of Intraluminal Device from Pancreatic Duct, Via Natural or Artificial Opening

0FPD7JZ Removal of Synthetic Substitute from Pancreatic Duct, Via Natural or Artificial Opening

0FPD7KZ Removal of Nonautologous Tissue Substitute from Pancreatic Duct, Via Natural or Artificial Opening

0FPD7YZ Removal of Other Device from Pancreatic Duct, Via Natural or Artificial Opening

0FPD80Z Removal of Drainage Device from Pancreatic Duct, Via Natural or Artificial Opening Endoscopic

0FPD81Z Removal of Radioactive Element from Pancreatic Duct, Via Natural or Artificial Opening Endoscopic

0FPD82Z Removal of Monitoring Device from Pancreatic Duct, Via Natural or Artificial Opening Endoscopic

0FPD83Z Removal of Infusion Device from Pancreatic Duct, Via Natural or Artificial Opening Endoscopic

0FPD87Z Removal of Autologous Tissue Substitute from Pancreatic Duct, Via Natural or Artificial Opening Endoscopic

0FPD8CZ Removal of Extraluminal Device from Pancreatic Duct, Via Natural or Artificial Opening Endoscopic

0FPD8DZ Removal of Intraluminal Device from Pancreatic Duct, Via Natural or Artificial Opening Endoscopic

0FPD8JZ Removal of Synthetic Substitute from Pancreatic Duct, Via Natural or Artificial Opening Endoscopic

0FPD8KZ Removal of Nonautologous Tissue Substitute from Pancreatic Duct, Via Natural or Artificial Opening

0FPD8YZ Removal of Other Device from Pancreatic Duct, Via Natural or Artificial Opening Endoscopic

0FPDX0Z Removal of Drainage Device from Pancreatic Duct, External Approach

0FPDX1Z Removal of Radioactive Element from Pancreatic Duct, External Approach

0FPDX2Z Removal of Monitoring Device from Pancreatic Duct, External Approach

0FPDX3Z Removal of Infusion Device from Pancreatic Duct, External Approach

0FPDXDZ Removal of Intraluminal Device from Pancreatic Duct, External Approach

0FPG00Z Removal of Drainage Device from Pancreas, Open Approach

0FPG02Z Removal of Monitoring Device from Pancreas, Open Approach

0FPG03Z Removal of Infusion Device from Pancreas, Open Approach

0FPG0DZ Removal of Intraluminal Device from Pancreas, Open Approach

0FPG0YZ Removal of Other Device from Pancreas, Open Approach

0FPG30Z Removal of Drainage Device from Pancreas, Percutaneous Approach

0FPG32Z Removal of Monitoring Device from Pancreas, Percutaneous Approach

0FPG33Z Removal of Infusion Device from Pancreas, Percutaneous Approach

0FPG3DZ Removal of Intraluminal Device from Pancreas, Percutaneous Approach

0FPG3YZ Removal of Other Device from Pancreas, Percutaneous Approach

0FPG40Z Removal of Drainage Device from Pancreas, Percutaneous Endoscopic Approach

0FPG42Z Removal of Monitoring Device from Pancreas, Percutaneous Endoscopic Approach

0FPG43Z Removal of Infusion Device from Pancreas, Percutaneous Endoscopic Approach

0FPG4DZ Removal of Intraluminal Device from Pancreas, Percutaneous Endoscopic Approach

0FPG4YZ Removal of Other Device from Pancreas, Percutaneous Endoscopic Approach

0FPGX0Z Removal of Drainage Device from Pancreas, External Approach

0FPGX2Z Removal of Monitoring Device from Pancreas, External Approach

0FPGX3Z Removal of Infusion Device from Pancreas, External Approach

0FPGXDZ Removal of Intraluminal Device from Pancreas, External Approach

0FQ – Hepatobiliary System and Pancreas, Repair

0FQ00ZZ Repair Liver, Open Approach
AHA CC: 4Q, 2013, 109-111

0FQ03ZZ Repair Liver, Percutaneous Approach

0FQ04ZZ Repair Liver, Percutaneous Endoscopic Approach

0FQ10ZZ Repair Right Lobe Liver, Open Approach

0FQ13ZZ Repair Right Lobe Liver, Percutaneous Approach

0FQ14ZZ Repair Right Lobe Liver, Percutaneous Endoscopic Approach

0FQ20ZZ Repair Left Lobe Liver, Open Approach

0FQ23ZZ Repair Left Lobe Liver, Percutaneous Approach

0FQ24ZZ Repair Left Lobe Liver, Percutaneous Endoscopic Approach

0FQ40ZZ Repair Gallbladder, Open Approach

0FQ43ZZ Repair Gallbladder, Percutaneous Approach

0FQ44ZZ Repair Gallbladder, Percutaneous Endoscopic Approach

0FQ48ZZ Repair Gallbladder, Via Natural or Artificial Opening Endoscopic

0FQ50ZZ Repair Right Hepatic Duct, Open Approach

0FQ53ZZ Repair Right Hepatic Duct, Percutaneous Approach

0FQ54ZZ Repair Right Hepatic Duct, Percutaneous Endoscopic Approach

0FQ57ZZ Repair Right Hepatic Duct, Via Natural or Artificial Opening

0FQ58ZZ Repair Right Hepatic Duct, Via Natural or Artificial Opening Endoscopic

0FQ60ZZ Repair Left Hepatic Duct, Open Approach

0FQ63ZZ Repair Left Hepatic Duct, Percutaneous Approach

0FQ64ZZ Repair Left Hepatic Duct, Percutaneous Endoscopic Approach

0FQ67ZZ Repair Left Hepatic Duct, Via Natural or Artificial Opening

0FQ68ZZ Repair Left Hepatic Duct, Via Natural or Artificial Opening Endoscopic

0FQ70ZZ Repair Common Hepatic Duct, Open Approach

0FQ73ZZ Repair Common Hepatic Duct, Percutaneous Approach

0FQ74ZZ Repair Common Hepatic Duct, Percutaneous Endoscopic Approach

0FQ77ZZ Repair Common Hepatic Duct, Via Natural or Artificial Opening

0FQ78ZZ Repair Common Hepatic Duct, Via Natural or Artificial Opening Endoscopic

0FQ80ZZ Repair Cystic Duct, Open Approach

0FQ83ZZ Repair Cystic Duct, Percutaneous Approach

0FQ84ZZ Repair Cystic Duct, Percutaneous Endoscopic Approach

0FQ87ZZ Repair Cystic Duct, Via Natural or Artificial Opening

0FQ88ZZ Repair Cystic Duct, Via Natural or Artificial Opening Endoscopic

0FQ90ZZ Repair Common Bile Duct, Open Approach
AHA CC: 3Q, 2016, 27

0FQ93ZZ Repair Common Bile Duct, Percutaneous Approach

0FQ94ZZ Repair Common Bile Duct, Percutaneous Endoscopic Approach

0FQ97ZZ Repair Common Bile Duct, Via Natural or Artificial Opening

0FQ98ZZ Repair Common Bile Duct, Via Natural or Artificial Opening Endoscopic

0FQC0ZZ Repair Ampulla of Vater, Open Approach

0FQC3ZZ Repair Ampulla of Vater, Percutaneous Approach

0FQC4ZZ Repair Ampulla of Vater, Percutaneous Endoscopic Approach

0FQC7ZZ Repair Ampulla of Vater, Via Natural or Artificial Opening

0FQC8ZZ Repair Ampulla of Vater, Via Natural or Artificial Opening Endoscopic

0FQD0ZZ Repair Pancreatic Duct, Open Approach

0FQD3ZZ Repair Pancreatic Duct, Percutaneous Approach

0FQD4ZZ Repair Pancreatic Duct, Percutaneous Endoscopic Approach

0FQD7ZZ Repair Pancreatic Duct, Via Natural or Artificial Opening

0FQD8ZZ Repair Pancreatic Duct, Via Natural or Artificial Opening Endoscopic

0FQF0ZZ Repair Accessory Pancreatic Duct, Open Approach

0FQF3ZZ Repair Accessory Pancreatic Duct, Percutaneous Approach

0FQF4ZZ Repair Accessory Pancreatic Duct, Percutaneous Endoscopic Approach

0FQF7ZZ Repair Accessory Pancreatic Duct, Via Natural or Artificial Opening

0FQF8ZZ Repair Accessory Pancreatic Duct, Via Natural or Artificial Opening Endoscopic

0FQG0ZZ Repair Pancreas, Open Approach

0FQG3ZZ Repair Pancreas, Percutaneous Approach

0FQG4ZZ Repair Pancreas, Percutaneous Endoscopic Approach

0FQG8ZZ Repair Pancreas, Via Natural or Artificial Opening Endoscopic

0FR – Hepatobiliary System and Pancreas, Replacement

Review Coding Guideline B3.18

0FR507Z Replacement of Right Hepatic Duct with Autologous Tissue Substitute, Open Approach

0FR50JZ Replacement of Right Hepatic Duct with Synthetic Substitute, Open Approach

0FR50KZ Replacement of Right Hepatic Duct with Nonautologous Tissue Substitute, Open Approach

0FR547Z Replacement of Right Hepatic Duct with Autologous Tissue Substitute, Percutaneous Endoscopic Approach

0FR54JZ Replacement of Right Hepatic Duct with Synthetic Substitute, Percutaneous Endoscopic Approach

0FR54KZ Replacement of Right Hepatic Duct with Nonautologous Tissue Substitute, Percutaneous Endoscopic Approach

0FR587Z Replacement of Right Hepatic Duct with Autologous Tissue Substitute, Via Natural or Artificial Opening Endoscopic

0FR58JZ Replacement of Right Hepatic Duct with Synthetic Substitute, Via Natural or Artificial Opening Endoscopic

0FR58KZ Replacement of Right Hepatic Duct with Nonautologous Tissue Substitute, Via Natural or Artificial Opening Endoscopic

0FR607Z Replacement of Left Hepatic Duct with Autologous Tissue Substitute, Open Approach

0FR60JZ Replacement of Left Hepatic Duct with Synthetic Substitute, Open Approach

0FR60KZ Replacement of Left Hepatic Duct with Nonautologous Tissue Substitute, Open Approach

0FR647Z Replacement of Left Hepatic Duct with Autologous Tissue Substitute, Percutaneous Endoscopic Approach

0FR64JZ Replacement of Left Hepatic Duct with Synthetic Substitute, Percutaneous Endoscopic Approach

0FR64KZ Replacement of Left Hepatic Duct with Nonautologous Tissue Substitute, Percutaneous Endoscopic Approach

0FR687Z Replacement of Left Hepatic Duct with Autologous Tissue Substitute, Via Natural or Artificial Opening Endoscopic

0FR68JZ Replacement of Left Hepatic Duct with Synthetic Substitute, Via Natural or Artificial Opening Endoscopic

0FR68KZ Replacement of Left Hepatic Duct with Nonautologous Tissue Substitute, Via Natural or Artificial Opening Endoscopic

0FR707Z Replacement of Common Hepatic Duct with Autologous Tissue Substitute, Open Approach

0FR70JZ Replacement of Common Hepatic Duct with Synthetic Substitute, Open Approach

0FR70KZ Replacement of Common Hepatic Duct with Nonautologous Tissue Substitute, Open Approach

0FR747Z Replacement of Common Hepatic Duct with Autologous Tissue Substitute, Percutaneous Endoscopic Approach

0FR74JZ Replacement of Common Hepatic Duct with Synthetic Substitute, Percutaneous Endoscopic Approach

0FR74KZ Replacement of Common Hepatic Duct with Nonautologous Tissue Substitute, Percutaneous Endoscopic Approach

0FR787Z Replacement of Common Hepatic Duct with Autologous Tissue Substitute, Via Natural or Artificial Opening Endoscopic

0FR78JZ Replacement of Common Hepatic Duct with Synthetic Substitute, Via Natural or Artificial Opening Endoscopic

0FR78KZ Replacement of Common Hepatic Duct with Nonautologous Tissue Substitute, Via Natural or Artificial Opening Endoscopic

0FR807Z Replacement of Cystic Duct with Autologous Tissue Substitute, Open Approach

0FR80JZ Replacement of Cystic Duct with Synthetic Substitute, Open Approach

0FR80KZ Replacement of Cystic Duct with Nonautologous Tissue Substitute, Open Approach

0FR847Z Replacement of Cystic Duct with Autologous Tissue Substitute, Percutaneous Endoscopic Approach

0FR84JZ Replacement of Cystic Duct with Synthetic Substitute, Percutaneous Endoscopic Approach

0FR84KZ Replacement of Cystic Duct with Nonautologous Tissue Substitute, Percutaneous Endoscopic Approach

0FR887Z Replacement of Cystic Duct with Autologous Tissue Substitute, Via Natural or Artificial Opening Endoscopic

0FR88JZ Replacement of Cystic Duct with Synthetic Substitute, Via Natural or Artificial Opening Endoscopic

0FR88KZ Replacement of Cystic Duct with Nonautologous Tissue Substitute, Via Natural or Artificial Opening Endoscopic

0FR907Z Replacement of Common Bile Duct with Autologous Tissue Substitute, Open Approach

0FR90JZ Replacement of Common Bile Duct with Synthetic Substitute, Open Approach

0FR90KZ Replacement of Common Bile Duct with Nonautologous Tissue Substitute, Open Approach

0FR947Z Replacement of Common Bile Duct with Autologous Tissue Substitute, Percutaneous Endoscopic Approach

0FR94JZ Replacement of Common Bile Duct with Synthetic Substitute, Percutaneous Endoscopic Approach

0FR94KZ Replacement of Common Bile Duct with Nonautologous Tissue Substitute, Percutaneous Endoscopic Approach

0FR987Z Replacement of Common Bile Duct with Autologous Tissue Substitute, Via Natural or Artificial Opening Endoscopic

0FR98JZ Replacement of Common Bile Duct with Synthetic Substitute, Via Natural or Artificial Opening Endoscopic

0FR98KZ Replacement of Common Bile Duct with Nonautologous Tissue Substitute, Via Natural or Artificial Opening Endoscopic

♀ Female-only   ♂ Male-only   ▲ Limited Coverage   ● Non-OR   ⬛ HAC-associated procedure   ▲ Non-covered procedures   ✚ Cluster

0FRC07Z Replacement of Ampulla of Vater with Autologous Tissue Substitute, Open Approach

0FRC0JZ Replacement of Ampulla of Vater with Synthetic Substitute, Open Approach

0FRC0KZ Replacement of Ampulla of Vater with Nonautologous Tissue Substitute, Open Approach

0FRC47Z Replacement of Ampulla of Vater with Autologous Tissue Substitute, Percutaneous Endoscopic Approach

0FRC4JZ Replacement of Ampulla of Vater with Synthetic Substitute, Percutaneous Endoscopic Approach

0FRC4KZ Replacement of Ampulla of Vater with Nonautologous Tissue Substitute, Percutaneous Endoscopic Approach

0FRC87Z Replacement of Ampulla of Vater with Autologous Tissue Substitute, Via Natural or Artificial Opening Endoscopic

0FRC8JZ Replacement of Ampulla of Vater with Synthetic Substitute, Via Natural or Artificial Opening Endoscopic

0FRC8KZ Replacement of Ampulla of Vater with Nonautologous Tissue Substitute, Via Natural or Artificial Opening Endoscopic

0FRD07Z Replacement of Pancreatic Duct with Autologous Tissue Substitute, Open Approach

0FRD0JZ Replacement of Pancreatic Duct with Synthetic Substitute, Open Approach

0FRD0KZ Replacement of Pancreatic Duct with Nonautologous Tissue Substitute, Open Approach

0FRD47Z Replacement of Pancreatic Duct with Autologous Tissue Substitute, Percutaneous Endoscopic Approach

0FRD4JZ Replacement of Pancreatic Duct with Synthetic Substitute, Percutaneous Endoscopic Approach

0FRD4KZ Replacement of Pancreatic Duct with Nonautologous Tissue Substitute, Percutaneous Endoscopic Approach

0FRD87Z Replacement of Pancreatic Duct with Autologous Tissue Substitute, Via Natural or Artificial Opening Endoscopic

0FRD8JZ Replacement of Pancreatic Duct with Synthetic Substitute, Via Natural or Artificial Opening Endoscopic

0FRD8KZ Replacement of Pancreatic Duct with Nonautologous Tissue Substitute, Via Natural or Artificial Opening Endoscopic

0FRF07Z Replacement of Accessory Pancreatic Duct with Autologous Tissue Substitute, Open Approach

0FRF0JZ Replacement of Accessory Pancreatic Duct with Synthetic Substitute, Open Approach

0FRF0KZ Replacement of Accessory Pancreatic Duct with Nonautologous Tissue Substitute, Open Approach

0FRF47Z Replacement of Accessory Pancreatic Duct with Autologous Tissue Substitute, Percutaneous Endoscopic Approach

0FRF4JZ Replacement of Accessory Pancreatic Duct with Synthetic Substitute, Percutaneous Endoscopic Approach

0FRF4KZ Replacement of Accessory Pancreatic Duct with Nonautologous Tissue Substitute, Percutaneous Endoscopic Approach

0FRF87Z Replacement of Accessory Pancreatic Duct with Autologous Tissue Substitute, Via Natural or Artificial Opening Endoscopic

0FRF8JZ Replacement of Accessory Pancreatic Duct with Synthetic Substitute, Via Natural or Artificial Opening Endoscopic

0FRF8KZ Replacement of Accessory Pancreatic Duct with Nonautologous Tissue Substitute, Via Natural or Artificial Opening Endoscopic

0FS – Hepatobiliary System and Pancreas, Reposition

0FS00ZZ Reposition Liver, Open Approach

0FS04ZZ Reposition Liver, Percutaneous Endoscopic Approach

0FS40ZZ Reposition Gallbladder, Open Approach

0FS44ZZ Reposition Gallbladder, Percutaneous Endoscopic Approach

0FS50ZZ Reposition Right Hepatic Duct, Open Approach

0FS54ZZ Reposition Right Hepatic Duct, Percutaneous Endoscopic Approach

0FS60ZZ Reposition Left Hepatic Duct, Open Approach

0FS64ZZ Reposition Left Hepatic Duct, Percutaneous Endoscopic Approach

0FS70ZZ Reposition Common Hepatic Duct, Open Approach

0FS74ZZ Reposition Common Hepatic Duct, Percutaneous Endoscopic Approach

0FS80ZZ Reposition Cystic Duct, Open Approach

0FS84ZZ Reposition Cystic Duct, Percutaneous Endoscopic Approach

0FS90ZZ Reposition Common Bile Duct, Open Approach

0FS94ZZ Reposition Common Bile Duct, Percutaneous Endoscopic Approach

0FSC0ZZ Reposition Ampulla of Vater, Open Approach

0FSC4ZZ Reposition Ampulla of Vater, Percutaneous Endoscopic Approach

0FSD0ZZ Reposition Pancreatic Duct, Open Approach

0FSD4ZZ Reposition Pancreatic Duct, Percutaneous Endoscopic Approach

0FSF0ZZ Reposition Accessory Pancreatic Duct, Open Approach

0FSF4ZZ Reposition Accessory Pancreatic Duct, Percutaneous Endoscopic Approach

0FSG0ZZ Reposition Pancreas, Open Approach

0FSG4ZZ Reposition Pancreas, Percutaneous Endoscopic Approach

0FT – Hepatobiliary System and Pancreas, Resection

Review Coding Guideline B3.8

Review Coding Guideline B3.18

0FT00ZZ Resection of Liver, Open Approach
AHA CC: 4Q, 2012, 99-101

0FT04ZZ Resection of Liver, Percutaneous Endoscopic Approach

0FT10ZZ Resection of Right Lobe Liver, Open Approach

0FT14ZZ Resection of Right Lobe Liver, Percutaneous Endoscopic Approach

0FT20ZZ Resection of Left Lobe Liver, Open Approach

0FT24ZZ Resection of Left Lobe Liver, Percutaneous Endoscopic Approach

0FT40ZZ Resection of Gallbladder, Open Approach
AHA CC: 1Q, 2019, 4-5

0FT44ZZ Resection of Gallbladder, Percutaneous Endoscopic Approach

0FT50ZZ Resection of Right Hepatic Duct, Open Approach

0FT54ZZ Resection of Right Hepatic Duct, Percutaneous Endoscopic Approach

0FT57ZZ Resection of Right Hepatic Duct, Via Natural or Artificial Opening

0FT58ZZ Resection of Right Hepatic Duct, Via Natural or Artificial Opening Endoscopic

0FT60ZZ Resection of Left Hepatic Duct, Open Approach

0FT64ZZ Resection of Left Hepatic Duct, Percutaneous Endoscopic Approach

0FT67ZZ Resection of Left Hepatic Duct, Via Natural or Artificial Opening

0FT68ZZ Resection of Left Hepatic Duct, Via Natural or Artificial Opening Endoscopic

0FT70ZZ Resection of Common Hepatic Duct, Open Approach

0FT74ZZ Resection of Common Hepatic Duct, Percutaneous Endoscopic Approach

0FT77ZZ Resection of Common Hepatic Duct, Via Natural or Artificial Opening

0FT78ZZ Resection of Common Hepatic Duct, Via Natural or Artificial Opening Endoscopic

0FT80ZZ Resection of Cystic Duct, Open Approach

0FT84ZZ Resection of Cystic Duct, Percutaneous Endoscopic Approach

0FT87ZZ Resection of Cystic Duct, Via Natural or Artificial Opening

0FT88ZZ Resection of Cystic Duct, Via Natural or Artificial Opening Endoscopic

0FT90ZZ Resection of Common Bile Duct, Open Approach

0FT94ZZ Resection of Common Bile Duct, Percutaneous Endoscopic Approach

0FT97ZZ Resection of Common Bile Duct, Via Natural or Artificial Opening

0FT98ZZ Resection of Common Bile Duct, Via Natural or Artificial Opening Endoscopic

0FTC0ZZ Resection of Ampulla of Vater, Open Approach

0FTC4ZZ Resection of Ampulla of Vater, Percutaneous Endoscopic Approach

0FTC7ZZ Resection of Ampulla of Vater, Via Natural or Artificial Opening

0FTC8ZZ Resection of Ampulla of Vater, Via Natural or Artificial Opening Endoscopic

0FTD0ZZ Resection of Pancreatic Duct, Open Approach

0FTD4ZZ Resection of Pancreatic Duct, Percutaneous Endoscopic Approach

0FTD7ZZ Resection of Pancreatic Duct, Via Natural or Artificial Opening

0FTD8ZZ Resection of Pancreatic Duct, Via Natural or Artificial Opening Endoscopic

0FTF0ZZ Resection of Accessory Pancreatic Duct, Open Approach

0FTF4ZZ Resection of Accessory Pancreatic Duct, Percutaneous Endoscopic Approach

0FTF7ZZ Resection of Accessory Pancreatic Duct, Via Natural or Artificial Opening

0FTF8ZZ Resection of Accessory Pancreatic Duct, Via Natural or Artificial Opening Endoscopic

0FTG0ZZ Resection of Pancreas, Open Approach

0FTG4ZZ Resection of Pancreas, Percutaneous Endoscopic Approach

0FU – Hepatobiliary System and Pancreas, Supplement

0FU507Z Supplement Right Hepatic Duct with Autologous Tissue Substitute, Open Approach

0FU50JZ Supplement Right Hepatic Duct with Synthetic Substitute, Open Approach

0FU50KZ Supplement Right Hepatic Duct with Nonautologous Tissue Substitute, Open Approach

0FU537Z Supplement Right Hepatic Duct with Autologous Tissue Substitute, Percutaneous Approach

0FU53JZ Supplement Right Hepatic Duct with Synthetic Substitute, Percutaneous Approach

0FU53KZ Supplement Right Hepatic Duct with Nonautologous Tissue Substitute, Percutaneous Approach

0FU547Z Supplement Right Hepatic Duct with Autologous Tissue Substitute, Percutaneous Endoscopic Approach

0FU54JZ Supplement Right Hepatic Duct with Synthetic Substitute, Percutaneous Endoscopic Approach

0FU54KZ Supplement Right Hepatic Duct with Nonautologous Tissue Substitute, Percutaneous Endoscopic Approach

0FU587Z Supplement Right Hepatic Duct with Autologous Tissue Substitute, Via Natural or Artificial Opening Endoscopic

0FU58JZ Supplement Right Hepatic Duct with Synthetic Substitute, Via Natural or Artificial Opening Endoscopic

0FU58KZ Supplement Right Hepatic Duct with Nonautologous Tissue Substitute, Via Natural or Artificial Opening Endoscopic

0FU607Z Supplement Left Hepatic Duct with Autologous Tissue Substitute, Open Approach

0FU60JZ Supplement Left Hepatic Duct with Synthetic Substitute, Open Approach

0FU60KZ Supplement Left Hepatic Duct with Nonautologous Tissue Substitute, Open Approach

0FU637Z Supplement Left Hepatic Duct with Autologous Tissue Substitute, Percutaneous Approach

0FU63JZ Supplement Left Hepatic Duct with Synthetic Substitute, Percutaneous Approach

0FU63KZ Supplement Left Hepatic Duct with Nonautologous Tissue Substitute, Percutaneous Approach

0FU647Z Supplement Left Hepatic Duct with Autologous Tissue Substitute, Percutaneous Endoscopic Approach

0FU64JZ Supplement Left Hepatic Duct with Synthetic Substitute, Percutaneous Endoscopic Approach

0FU64KZ Supplement Left Hepatic Duct with Nonautologous Tissue Substitute, Percutaneous Endoscopic Approach

0FU687Z Supplement Left Hepatic Duct with Autologous Tissue Substitute, Via Natural or Artificial Opening Endoscopic

0FU68JZ Supplement Left Hepatic Duct with Synthetic Substitute, Via Natural or Artificial Opening Endoscopic

0FU68KZ Supplement Left Hepatic Duct with Nonautologous Tissue Substitute, Via Natural or Artificial Opening Endoscopic

0FU707Z Supplement Common Hepatic Duct with Autologous Tissue Substitute, Open Approach

0FU70JZ Supplement Common Hepatic Duct with Synthetic Substitute, Open Approach

0FU70KZ Supplement Common Hepatic Duct with Nonautologous Tissue Substitute, Open Approach

0FU737Z Supplement Common Hepatic Duct with Autologous Tissue Substitute, Percutaneous Approach

0FU73JZ Supplement Common Hepatic Duct with Synthetic Substitute, Percutaneous Approach

0FU73KZ Supplement Common Hepatic Duct with Nonautologous Tissue Substitute, Percutaneous Approach

0FU747Z Supplement Common Hepatic Duct with Autologous Tissue Substitute, Percutaneous Endoscopic Approach

0FU74JZ Supplement Common Hepatic Duct with Synthetic Substitute, Percutaneous Endoscopic Approach

0FU74KZ Supplement Common Hepatic Duct with Nonautologous Tissue Substitute, Percutaneous Endoscopic Approach

0FU787Z Supplement Common Hepatic Duct with Autologous Tissue Substitute, Via Natural or Artificial Opening Endoscopic

0FU78JZ Supplement Common Hepatic Duct with Synthetic Substitute, Via Natural or Artificial Opening Endoscopic

0FU78KZ Supplement Common Hepatic Duct with Nonautologous Tissue Substitute, Via Natural or Artificial Opening Endoscopic

0FU807Z Supplement Cystic Duct with Autologous Tissue Substitute, Open Approach

0FU80JZ Supplement Cystic Duct with Synthetic Substitute, Open Approach

0FU80KZ Supplement Cystic Duct with Nonautologous Tissue Substitute, Open Approach

0FU837Z Supplement Cystic Duct with Autologous Tissue Substitute, Percutaneous Approach

0FU83JZ Supplement Cystic Duct with Synthetic Substitute, Percutaneous Approach

0FU83KZ Supplement Cystic Duct with Nonautologous Tissue Substitute, Percutaneous Approach

0FU847Z Supplement Cystic Duct with Autologous Tissue Substitute, Percutaneous Endoscopic Approach

0FU84JZ Supplement Cystic Duct with Synthetic Substitute, Percutaneous Endoscopic Approach

0FU84KZ Supplement Cystic Duct with Nonautologous Tissue Substitute, Percutaneous Endoscopic Approach

0FU887Z Supplement Cystic Duct with Autologous Tissue Substitute, Via Natural or Artificial Opening Endoscopic

0FU88JZ Supplement Cystic Duct with Synthetic Substitute, Via Natural or Artificial Opening Endoscopic

0FU88KZ Supplement Cystic Duct with Nonautologous Tissue Substitute, Via Natural or Artificial Opening Endoscopic

0FU907Z Supplement Common Bile Duct with Autologous Tissue Substitute, Open Approach

0FU90JZ Supplement Common Bile Duct with Synthetic Substitute, Open Approach

0FU90KZ Supplement Common Bile Duct with Nonautologous Tissue Substitute, Open Approach

0FU937Z Supplement Common Bile Duct with Autologous Tissue Substitute, Percutaneous Approach

0FU93JZ Supplement Common Bile Duct with Synthetic Substitute, Percutaneous Approach

0FU93KZ Supplement Common Bile Duct with Nonautologous Tissue Substitute, Percutaneous Approach

0FU947Z Supplement Common Bile Duct with Autologous Tissue Substitute, Percutaneous Endoscopic Approach

0FU94JZ Supplement Common Bile Duct with Synthetic Substitute, Percutaneous Endoscopic Approach

♀ Female-only   ♂ Male-only   ▲ Limited Coverage   ● Non-OR   HAC HAC-associated procedure   ▲ Non-covered procedures   ✚ Cluster

0FU94KZ Supplement Common Bile Duct with Nonautologous Tissue Substitute, Percutaneous Endoscopic Approach

0FU987Z Supplement Common Bile Duct with Autologous Tissue Substitute, Via Natural or Artificial Opening Endoscopic

0FU98JZ Supplement Common Bile Duct with Synthetic Substitute, Via Natural or Artificial Opening Endoscopic

0FU98KZ Supplement Common Bile Duct with Nonautologous Tissue Substitute, Via Natural or Artificial Opening Endoscopic

0FUC07Z Supplement Ampulla of Vater with Autologous Tissue Substitute, Open Approach

0FUC0JZ Supplement Ampulla of Vater with Synthetic Substitute, Open Approach

0FUC0KZ Supplement Ampulla of Vater with Nonautologous Tissue Substitute, Open Approach

0FUC37Z Supplement Ampulla of Vater with Autologous Tissue Substitute, Percutaneous Approach

0FUC3JZ Supplement Ampulla of Vater with Synthetic Substitute, Percutaneous Approach

0FUC3KZ Supplement Ampulla of Vater with Nonautologous Tissue Substitute, Percutaneous Approach

0FUC47Z Supplement Ampulla of Vater with Autologous Tissue Substitute, Percutaneous Endoscopic Approach

0FUC4JZ Supplement Ampulla of Vater with Synthetic Substitute, Percutaneous Endoscopic Approach

0FUC4KZ Supplement Ampulla of Vater with Nonautologous Tissue Substitute, Percutaneous Endoscopic Approach

0FUC87Z Supplement Ampulla of Vater with Autologous Tissue Substitute, Via Natural or Artificial Opening Endoscopic

0FUC8JZ Supplement Ampulla of Vater with Synthetic Substitute, Via Natural or Artificial Opening Endoscopic

0FUC8KZ Supplement Ampulla of Vater with Nonautologous Tissue Substitute, Via Natural or Artificial Opening Endoscopic

0FUD07Z Supplement Pancreatic Duct with Autologous Tissue Substitute, Open Approach

0FUD0JZ Supplement Pancreatic Duct with Synthetic Substitute, Open Approach

0FUD0KZ Supplement Pancreatic Duct with Nonautologous Tissue Substitute, Open Approach

0FUD37Z Supplement Pancreatic Duct with Autologous Tissue Substitute, Percutaneous Approach

0FUD3JZ Supplement Pancreatic Duct with Synthetic Substitute, Percutaneous Approach

0FUD3KZ Supplement Pancreatic Duct with Nonautologous Tissue Substitute, Percutaneous Approach

0FUD47Z Supplement Pancreatic Duct with Autologous Tissue Substitute, Percutaneous Endoscopic Approach

0FUD4JZ Supplement Pancreatic Duct with Synthetic Substitute, Percutaneous Endoscopic Approach

0FUD4KZ Supplement Pancreatic Duct with Nonautologous Tissue Substitute, Percutaneous Endoscopic Approach

0FUD87Z Supplement Pancreatic Duct with Autologous Tissue Substitute, Via Natural or Artificial Opening Endoscopic

0FUD8JZ Supplement Pancreatic Duct with Synthetic Substitute, Via Natural or Artificial Opening Endoscopic

0FUD8KZ Supplement Pancreatic Duct with Nonautologous Tissue Substitute, Via Natural or Artificial Opening Endoscopic

0FUF07Z Supplement Accessory Pancreatic Duct with Autologous Tissue Substitute, Open Approach

0FUF0JZ Supplement Accessory Pancreatic Duct with Synthetic Substitute, Open Approach

0FUF0KZ Supplement Accessory Pancreatic Duct with Nonautologous Tissue Substitute, Open Approach

0FUF37Z Supplement Accessory Pancreatic Duct with Autologous Tissue Substitute, Percutaneous Approach

0FUF3JZ Supplement Accessory Pancreatic Duct with Synthetic Substitute, Percutaneous Approach

0FUF3KZ Supplement Accessory Pancreatic Duct with Nonautologous Tissue Substitute, Percutaneous Approach

0FUF47Z Supplement Accessory Pancreatic Duct with Autologous Tissue Substitute, Percutaneous Endoscopic Approach

0FUF4JZ Supplement Accessory Pancreatic Duct with Synthetic Substitute, Percutaneous Endoscopic Approach

0FUF4KZ Supplement Accessory Pancreatic Duct with Nonautologous Tissue Substitute, Percutaneous Endoscopic Approach

0FUF87Z Supplement Accessory Pancreatic Duct with Autologous Tissue Substitute, Via Natural or Artificial Opening Endoscopic

0FUF8JZ Supplement Accessory Pancreatic Duct with Synthetic Substitute, Via Natural or Artificial Opening Endoscopic

0FUF8KZ Supplement Accessory Pancreatic Duct with Nonautologous Tissue Substitute, Via Natural or Artificial Opening Endoscopic

0FV – Hepatobiliary System and Pancreas, Restriction

0FV50CZ Restriction of Right Hepatic Duct with Extraluminal Device, Open Approach

0FV50DZ Restriction of Right Hepatic Duct with Intraluminal Device, Open Approach

0FV50ZZ Restriction of Right Hepatic Duct, Open Approach

0FV53CZ Restriction of Right Hepatic Duct with Extraluminal Device, Percutaneous Approach

0FV53DZ Restriction of Right Hepatic Duct with Intraluminal Device, Percutaneous Approach

0FV53ZZ Restriction of Right Hepatic Duct, Percutaneous Approach

0FV54CZ Restriction of Right Hepatic Duct with Extraluminal Device, Percutaneous Endoscopic Approach

0FV54DZ Restriction of Right Hepatic Duct with Intraluminal Device, Percutaneous Endoscopic Approach

0FV54ZZ Restriction of Right Hepatic Duct, Percutaneous Endoscopic Approach

0FV57DZ Restriction of Right Hepatic Duct with Intraluminal Device, Via Natural or Artificial Opening

0FV57ZZ Restriction of Right Hepatic Duct, Via Natural or Artificial Opening

0FV58DZ Restriction of Right Hepatic Duct with Intraluminal Device, Via Natural or Artificial Opening Endoscopic

0FV58ZZ Restriction of Right Hepatic Duct, Via Natural or Artificial Opening Endoscopic

0FV60CZ Restriction of Left Hepatic Duct with Extraluminal Device, Open Approach

0FV60DZ Restriction of Left Hepatic Duct with Intraluminal Device, Open Approach

0FV60ZZ Restriction of Left Hepatic Duct, Open Approach

0FV63CZ Restriction of Left Hepatic Duct with Extraluminal Device, Percutaneous Approach

0FV63DZ Restriction of Left Hepatic Duct with Intraluminal Device, Percutaneous Approach

0FV63ZZ Restriction of Left Hepatic Duct, Percutaneous Approach

0FV64CZ Restriction of Left Hepatic Duct with Extraluminal Device, Percutaneous Endoscopic Approach

0FV64DZ Restriction of Left Hepatic Duct with Intraluminal Device, Percutaneous Endoscopic Approach

0FV64ZZ Restriction of Left Hepatic Duct, Percutaneous Endoscopic Approach

0FV67DZ Restriction of Left Hepatic Duct with Intraluminal Device, Via Natural or Artificial Opening

0FV67ZZ Restriction of Left Hepatic Duct, Via Natural or Artificial Opening

0FV68DZ Restriction of Left Hepatic Duct with Intraluminal Device, Via Natural or Artificial Opening Endoscopic

0FV68ZZ Restriction of Left Hepatic Duct, Via Natural or Artificial Opening Endoscopic

0FV70CZ Restriction of Common Hepatic Duct with Extraluminal Device, Open Approach

0FV70DZ Restriction of Common Hepatic Duct with Intraluminal Device, Open Approach

0FV70ZZ Restriction of Common Hepatic Duct, Open Approach

0FV73CZ Restriction of Common Hepatic Duct with Extraluminal Device, Percutaneous Approach

0FV73DZ Restriction of Common Hepatic Duct with Intraluminal Device, Percutaneous Approach

0FV73ZZ Restriction of Common Hepatic Duct, Percutaneous Approach

0FV74CZ Restriction of Common Hepatic Duct with Extraluminal Device, Percutaneous Endoscopic Approach

0FV74DZ Restriction of Common Hepatic Duct with Intraluminal Device, Percutaneous Endoscopic Approach

0FV74ZZ Restriction of Common Hepatic Duct, Percutaneous Endoscopic Approach

0FV77DZ Restriction of Common Hepatic Duct with Intraluminal Device, Via Natural or Artificial Opening

0FV77ZZ Restriction of Common Hepatic Duct, Via Natural or Artificial Opening

0FV78DZ Restriction of Common Hepatic Duct with Intraluminal Device, Via Natural or Artificial Opening Endoscopic

0FV78ZZ Restriction of Common Hepatic Duct, Via Natural or Artificial Opening Endoscopic

0FV80CZ Restriction of Cystic Duct with Extraluminal Device, Open Approach

0FV80DZ Restriction of Cystic Duct with Intraluminal Device, Open Approach

0FV80ZZ Restriction of Cystic Duct, Open Approach

0FV83CZ Restriction of Cystic Duct with Extraluminal Device, Percutaneous Approach

0FV83DZ Restriction of Cystic Duct with Intraluminal Device, Percutaneous Approach

0FV83ZZ Restriction of Cystic Duct, Percutaneous Approach

0FV84CZ Restriction of Cystic Duct with Extraluminal Device, Percutaneous Endoscopic Approach

0FV84DZ Restriction of Cystic Duct with Intraluminal Device, Percutaneous Endoscopic Approach

0FV84ZZ Restriction of Cystic Duct, Percutaneous Endoscopic Approach

0FV87DZ Restriction of Cystic Duct with Intraluminal Device, Via Natural or Artificial Opening

0FV87ZZ Restriction of Cystic Duct, Via Natural or Artificial Opening

0FV88DZ Restriction of Cystic Duct with Intraluminal Device, Via Natural or Artificial Opening Endoscopic

0FV88ZZ Restriction of Cystic Duct, Via Natural or Artificial Opening Endoscopic

0FV90CZ Restriction of Common Bile Duct with Extraluminal Device, Open Approach

0FV90DZ Restriction of Common Bile Duct with Intraluminal Device, Open Approach

0FV90ZZ Restriction of Common Bile Duct, Open Approach

0FV93CZ Restriction of Common Bile Duct with Extraluminal Device, Percutaneous Approach

0FV93DZ Restriction of Common Bile Duct with Intraluminal Device, Percutaneous Approach

0FV93ZZ Restriction of Common Bile Duct, Percutaneous Approach

0FV94CZ Restriction of Common Bile Duct with Extraluminal Device, Percutaneous Endoscopic Approach

0FV94DZ Restriction of Common Bile Duct with Intraluminal Device, Percutaneous Endoscopic Approach

0FV94ZZ Restriction of Common Bile Duct, Percutaneous Endoscopic Approach

0FV97DZ Restriction of Common Bile Duct with Intraluminal Device, Via Natural or Artificial Opening

0FV97ZZ Restriction of Common Bile Duct, Via Natural or Artificial Opening

0FV98DZ Restriction of Common Bile Duct with Intraluminal Device, Via Natural or Artificial Opening Endoscopic

0FV98ZZ Restriction of Common Bile Duct, Via Natural or Artificial Opening Endoscopic

0FVC0CZ Restriction of Ampulla of Vater with Extraluminal Device, Open Approach

0FVC0DZ Restriction of Ampulla of Vater with Intraluminal Device, Open Approach

0FVC0ZZ Restriction of Ampulla of Vater, Open Approach

0FVC3CZ Restriction of Ampulla of Vater with Extraluminal Device, Percutaneous Approach

0FVC3DZ Restriction of Ampulla of Vater with Intraluminal Device, Percutaneous Approach

0FVC3ZZ Restriction of Ampulla of Vater, Percutaneous Approach

0FVC4CZ Restriction of Ampulla of Vater with Extraluminal Device, Percutaneous Endoscopic Approach

0FVC4DZ Restriction of Ampulla of Vater with Intraluminal Device, Percutaneous Endoscopic Approach

0FVC4ZZ Restriction of Ampulla of Vater, Percutaneous Endoscopic Approach

0FVC7DZ Restriction of Ampulla of Vater with Intraluminal Device, Via Natural or Artificial Opening

0FVC7ZZ Restriction of Ampulla of Vater, Via Natural or Artificial Opening

0FVC8DZ Restriction of Ampulla of Vater with Intraluminal Device, Via Natural or Artificial Opening Endoscopic

0FVC8ZZ Restriction of Ampulla of Vater, Via Natural or Artificial Opening Endoscopic

0FVD0CZ Restriction of Pancreatic Duct with Extraluminal Device, Open Approach

0FVD0DZ Restriction of Pancreatic Duct with Intraluminal Device, Open Approach

0FVD0ZZ Restriction of Pancreatic Duct, Open Approach

0FVD3CZ Restriction of Pancreatic Duct with Extraluminal Device, Percutaneous Approach

0FVD3DZ Restriction of Pancreatic Duct with Intraluminal Device, Percutaneous Approach

0FVD3ZZ Restriction of Pancreatic Duct, Percutaneous Approach

0FVD4CZ Restriction of Pancreatic Duct with Extraluminal Device, Percutaneous Endoscopic Approach

0FVD4DZ Restriction of Pancreatic Duct with Intraluminal Device, Percutaneous Endoscopic Approach

0FVD4ZZ Restriction of Pancreatic Duct, Percutaneous Endoscopic Approach

0FVD7DZ Restriction of Pancreatic Duct with Intraluminal Device, Via Natural or Artificial Opening

0FVD7ZZ Restriction of Pancreatic Duct, Via Natural or Artificial Opening

0FVD8DZ Restriction of Pancreatic Duct with Intraluminal Device, Via Natural or Artificial Opening Endoscopic

0FVD8ZZ Restriction of Pancreatic Duct, Via Natural or Artificial Opening Endoscopic

0FVF0CZ Restriction of Accessory Pancreatic Duct with Extraluminal Device, Open Approach

0FVF0DZ Restriction of Accessory Pancreatic Duct with Intraluminal Device, Open Approach

0FVF0ZZ Restriction of Accessory Pancreatic Duct, Open Approach

0FVF3CZ Restriction of Accessory Pancreatic Duct with Extraluminal Device, Percutaneous Approach

0FVF3DZ Restriction of Accessory Pancreatic Duct with Intraluminal Device, Percutaneous Approach

0FVF3ZZ Restriction of Accessory Pancreatic Duct, Percutaneous Approach

0FVF4CZ Restriction of Accessory Pancreatic Duct with Extraluminal Device, Percutaneous Endoscopic Approach

0FVF4DZ Restriction of Accessory Pancreatic Duct with Intraluminal Device, Percutaneous Endoscopic Approach

0FVF4ZZ Restriction of Accessory Pancreatic Duct, Percutaneous Endoscopic Approach

0FVF7DZ Restriction of Accessory Pancreatic Duct with Intraluminal Device, Via Natural or Artificial Opening

0FVF7ZZ Restriction of Accessory Pancreatic Duct, Via Natural or Artificial Opening

0FVF8DZ Restriction of Accessory Pancreatic Duct with Intraluminal Device, Via Natural or Artificial Opening Endoscopic

0FVF8ZZ Restriction of Accessory Pancreatic Duct, Via Natural or Artificial Opening Endoscopic

0FW – Hepatobiliary System and Pancreas, Revision

Review Coding Guideline B6.1c

0FW000Z Revision of Drainage Device in Liver, Open Approach

0FW002Z Revision of Monitoring Device in Liver, Open Approach

0FW003Z Revision of Infusion Device in Liver, Open Approach

0FW00YZ Revision of Other Device in Liver, Open Approach

0FW030Z Revision of Drainage Device in Liver, Percutaneous Approach

0FW032Z Revision of Monitoring Device in Liver, Percutaneous Approach

♀ Female-only   ♂ Male-only   ▲ Limited Coverage   ● Non-OR   ▆ HAC-associated procedure   ▲ Non-covered procedures   ✚ Cluster

0FW033Z	Revision of Infusion Device in Liver, Percutaneous Approach
0FW03YZ	Revision of Other Device in Liver, Percutaneous Approach
0FW040Z	Revision of Drainage Device in Liver, Percutaneous Endoscopic Approach
0FW042Z	Revision of Monitoring Device in Liver, Percutaneous Endoscopic Approach
0FW043Z	Revision of Infusion Device in Liver, Percutaneous Endoscopic Approach
0FW04YZ	Revision of Other Device in Liver, Percutaneous Endoscopic Approach
0FW0X0Z	Revision of Drainage Device in Liver, External Approach
0FW0X2Z	Revision of Monitoring Device in Liver, External Approach
0FW0X3Z	Revision of Infusion Device in Liver, External Approach
0FW400Z	Revision of Drainage Device in Gallbladder, Open Approach
0FW402Z	Revision of Monitoring Device in Gallbladder, Open Approach
0FW403Z	Revision of Infusion Device in Gallbladder, Open Approach
0FW40DZ	Revision of Intraluminal Device in Gallbladder, Open Approach
0FW40YZ	Revision of Other Device in Gallbladder, Open Approach
0FW430Z	Revision of Drainage Device in Gallbladder, Percutaneous Approach
0FW432Z	Revision of Monitoring Device in Gallbladder, Percutaneous Approach
0FW433Z	Revision of Infusion Device in Gallbladder, Percutaneous Approach
0FW43DZ	Revision of Intraluminal Device in Gallbladder, Percutaneous Approach
0FW43YZ	Revision of Other Device in Gallbladder, Percutaneous Approach
0FW440Z	Revision of Drainage Device in Gallbladder, Percutaneous Endoscopic Approach
0FW442Z	Revision of Monitoring Device in Gallbladder, Percutaneous Endoscopic Approach
0FW443Z	Revision of Infusion Device in Gallbladder, Percutaneous Endoscopic Approach
0FW44DZ	Revision of Intraluminal Device in Gallbladder, Percutaneous Endoscopic Approach
0FW44YZ	Revision of Other Device in Gallbladder, Percutaneous Endoscopic Approach
0FW4X0Z	Revision of Drainage Device in Gallbladder, External Approach
0FW4X2Z	Revision of Monitoring Device in Gallbladder, External Approach
0FW4X3Z	Revision of Infusion Device in Gallbladder, External Approach
0FW4XDZ	Revision of Intraluminal Device in Gallbladder, External Approach
0FWB00Z	Revision of Drainage Device in Hepatobiliary Duct, Open Approach
0FWB02Z	Revision of Monitoring Device in Hepatobiliary Duct, Open Approach
0FWB03Z	Revision of Infusion Device in Hepatobiliary Duct, Open Approach
0FWB07Z	Revision of Autologous Tissue Substitute in Hepatobiliary Duct, Open Approach
0FWB0CZ	Revision of Extraluminal Device in Hepatobiliary Duct, Open Approach
0FWB0DZ	Revision of Intraluminal Device in Hepatobiliary Duct, Open Approach
0FWB0JZ	Revision of Synthetic Substitute in Hepatobiliary Duct, Open Approach
0FWB0KZ	Revision of Nonautologous Tissue Substitute in Hepatobiliary Duct, Open Approach
0FWB0YZ	Revision of Other Device in Hepatobiliary Duct, Open Approach
0FWB30Z	Revision of Drainage Device in Hepatobiliary Duct, Percutaneous Approach
0FWB32Z	Revision of Monitoring Device in Hepatobiliary Duct, Percutaneous Approach
0FWB33Z	Revision of Infusion Device in Hepatobiliary Duct, Percutaneous Approach
0FWB37Z	Revision of Autologous Tissue Substitute in Hepatobiliary Duct, Percutaneous Approach
0FWB3CZ	Revision of Extraluminal Device in Hepatobiliary Duct, Percutaneous Approach
0FWB3DZ	Revision of Intraluminal Device in Hepatobiliary Duct, Percutaneous Approach
0FWB3JZ	Revision of Synthetic Substitute in Hepatobiliary Duct, Percutaneous Approach
0FWB3KZ	Revision of Nonautologous Tissue Substitute in Hepatobiliary Duct, Percutaneous Approach
0FWB3YZ	Revision of Other Device in Hepatobiliary Duct, Percutaneous Approach
0FWB40Z	Revision of Drainage Device in Hepatobiliary Duct, Percutaneous Endoscopic Approach
0FWB42Z	Revision of Monitoring Device in Hepatobiliary Duct, Percutaneous Endoscopic Approach
0FWB43Z	Revision of Infusion Device in Hepatobiliary Duct, Percutaneous Endoscopic Approach
0FWB47Z	Revision of Autologous Tissue Substitute in Hepatobiliary Duct, Percutaneous Endoscopic Approach
0FWB4CZ	Revision of Extraluminal Device in Hepatobiliary Duct, Percutaneous Endoscopic Approach
0FWB4DZ	Revision of Intraluminal Device in Hepatobiliary Duct, Percutaneous Endoscopic Approach
0FWB4JZ	Revision of Synthetic Substitute in Hepatobiliary Duct, Percutaneous Endoscopic Approach
0FWB4KZ	Revision of Nonautologous Tissue Substitute in Hepatobiliary Duct, Percutaneous Endoscopic Approach
0FWB4YZ	Revision of Other Device in Hepatobiliary Duct, Percutaneous Endoscopic Approach
0FWB70Z	Revision of Drainage Device in Hepatobiliary Duct, Via Natural or Artificial Opening
0FWB72Z	Revision of Monitoring Device in Hepatobiliary Duct, Via Natural or Artificial Opening
0FWB73Z	Revision of Infusion Device in Hepatobiliary Duct, Via Natural or Artificial Opening
0FWB77Z	Revision of Autologous Tissue Substitute in Hepatobiliary Duct, Via Natural or Artificial Opening
0FWB7CZ	Revision of Extraluminal Device in Hepatobiliary Duct, Via Natural or Artificial Opening
0FWB7DZ	Revision of Intraluminal Device in Hepatobiliary Duct, Via Natural or Artificial Opening
0FWB7JZ	Revision of Synthetic Substitute in Hepatobiliary Duct, Via Natural or Artificial Opening
0FWB7KZ	Revision of Nonautologous Tissue Substitute in Hepatobiliary Duct, Via Natural or Artificial Opening
0FWB7YZ	Revision of Other Device in Hepatobiliary Duct, Via Natural or Artificial Opening
0FWB80Z	Revision of Drainage Device in Hepatobiliary Duct, Via Natural or Artificial Opening Endoscopic
0FWB82Z	Revision of Monitoring Device in Hepatobiliary Duct, Via Natural or Artificial Opening Endoscopic
0FWB83Z	Revision of Infusion Device in Hepatobiliary Duct, Via Natural or Artificial Opening Endoscopic
0FWB87Z	Revision of Autologous Tissue Substitute in Hepatobiliary Duct, Via Natural or Artificial Opening Endoscopic
0FWB8CZ	Revision of Extraluminal Device in Hepatobiliary Duct, Via Natural or Artificial Opening Endoscopic
0FWB8DZ	Revision of Intraluminal Device in Hepatobiliary Duct, Via Natural or Artificial Opening Endoscopic
0FWB8JZ	Revision of Synthetic Substitute in Hepatobiliary Duct, Via Natural or Artificial Opening Endoscopic
0FWB8KZ	Revision of Nonautologous Tissue Substitute in Hepatobiliary Duct, Via Natural or Artificial Opening Endoscopic
0FWB8YZ	Revision of Other Device in Hepatobiliary Duct, Via Natural or Artificial Opening Endoscopic
0FWBX0Z	Revision of Drainage Device in Hepatobiliary Duct, External Approach
0FWBX2Z	Revision of Monitoring Device in Hepatobiliary Duct, External Approach
0FWBX3Z	Revision of Infusion Device in Hepatobiliary Duct, External Approach
0FWBX7Z	Revision of Autologous Tissue Substitute in Hepatobiliary Duct, External Approach
0FWBXCZ	Revision of Extraluminal Device in Hepatobiliary Duct, External Approach
0FWBXDZ	Revision of Intraluminal Device in Hepatobiliary Duct, External Approach
0FWBXJZ	Revision of Synthetic Substitute in Hepatobiliary Duct, External Approach
0FWBXKZ	Revision of Nonautologous Tissue Substitute in Hepatobiliary Duct, External Approach

0FWD00Z Revision of Drainage Device in Pancreatic Duct, Open Approach

0FWD02Z Revision of Monitoring Device in Pancreatic Duct, Open Approach

0FWD03Z Revision of Infusion Device in Pancreatic Duct, Open Approach

0FWD07Z Revision of Autologous Tissue Substitute in Pancreatic Duct, Open Approach

0FWD0CZ Revision of Extraluminal Device in Pancreatic Duct, Open Approach

0FWD0DZ Revision of Intraluminal Device in Pancreatic Duct, Open Approach

0FWD0JZ Revision of Synthetic Substitute in Pancreatic Duct, Open Approach

0FWD0KZ Revision of Nonautologous Tissue Substitute in Pancreatic Duct, Open Approach

0FWD0YZ Revision of Other Device in Pancreatic Duct, Open Approach

0FWD30Z Revision of Drainage Device in Pancreatic Duct, Percutaneous Approach

0FWD32Z Revision of Monitoring Device in Pancreatic Duct, Percutaneous Approach

0FWD33Z Revision of Infusion Device in Pancreatic Duct, Percutaneous Approach

0FWD37Z Revision of Autologous Tissue Substitute in Pancreatic Duct, Percutaneous Approach

0FWD3CZ Revision of Extraluminal Device in Pancreatic Duct, Percutaneous Approach

0FWD3DZ Revision of Intraluminal Device in Pancreatic Duct, Percutaneous Approach

0FWD3JZ Revision of Synthetic Substitute in Pancreatic Duct, Percutaneous Approach

0FWD3KZ Revision of Nonautologous Tissue Substitute in Pancreatic Duct, Percutaneous Approach

0FWD3YZ Revision of Other Device in Pancreatic Duct, Percutaneous Approach

0FWD40Z Revision of Drainage Device in Pancreatic Duct, Percutaneous Endoscopic Approach

0FWD42Z Revision of Monitoring Device in Pancreatic Duct, Percutaneous Endoscopic Approach

0FWD43Z Revision of Infusion Device in Pancreatic Duct, Percutaneous Endoscopic Approach

0FWD47Z Revision of Autologous Tissue Substitute in Pancreatic Duct, Percutaneous Endoscopic Approach

0FWD4CZ Revision of Extraluminal Device in Pancreatic Duct, Percutaneous Endoscopic Approach

0FWD4DZ Revision of Intraluminal Device in Pancreatic Duct, Percutaneous Endoscopic Approach

0FWD4JZ Revision of Synthetic Substitute in Pancreatic Duct, Percutaneous Endoscopic Approach

0FWD4KZ Revision of Nonautologous Tissue Substitute in Pancreatic Duct, Percutaneous Endoscopic Approach

0FWD4YZ Revision of Other Device in Pancreatic Duct, Percutaneous Endoscopic Approach

0FWD70Z Revision of Drainage Device in Pancreatic Duct, Via Natural or Artificial Opening

0FWD72Z Revision of Monitoring Device in Pancreatic Duct, Via Natural or Artificial Opening

0FWD73Z Revision of Infusion Device in Pancreatic Duct, Via Natural or Artificial Opening

0FWD77Z Revision of Autologous Tissue Substitute in Pancreatic Duct, Via Natural or Artificial Opening

0FWD7CZ Revision of Extraluminal Device in Pancreatic Duct, Via Natural or Artificial Opening

0FWD7DZ Revision of Intraluminal Device in Pancreatic Duct, Via Natural or Artificial Opening

0FWD7JZ Revision of Synthetic Substitute in Pancreatic Duct, Via Natural or Artificial Opening

0FWD7KZ Revision of Nonautologous Tissue Substitute in Pancreatic Duct, Via Natural or Artificial Opening

0FWD7YZ Revision of Other Device in Pancreatic Duct, Via Natural or Artificial Opening

0FWD80Z Revision of Drainage Device in Pancreatic Duct, Via Natural or Artificial Opening Endoscopic

0FWD82Z Revision of Monitoring Device in Pancreatic Duct, Via Natural or Artificial Opening Endoscopic

0FWD83Z Revision of Infusion Device in Pancreatic Duct, Via Natural or Artificial Opening Endoscopic

0FWD87Z Revision of Autologous Tissue Substitute in Pancreatic Duct, Via Natural or Artificial Opening Endoscopic

0FWD8CZ Revision of Extraluminal Device in Pancreatic Duct, Via Natural or Artificial Opening Endoscopic

0FWD8DZ Revision of Intraluminal Device in Pancreatic Duct, Via Natural or Artificial Opening Endoscopic

0FWD8JZ Revision of Synthetic Substitute in Pancreatic Duct, Via Natural or Artificial Opening Endoscopic

0FWD8KZ Revision of Nonautologous Tissue Substitute in Pancreatic Duct, Via Natural or Artificial Opening Endoscopic

0FWD8YZ Revision of Other Device in Pancreatic Duct, Via Natural or Artificial Opening Endoscopic

0FWDX0Z Revision of Drainage Device in Pancreatic Duct, External Approach

0FWDX2Z Revision of Monitoring Device in Pancreatic Duct, External Approach

0FWDX3Z Revision of Infusion Device in Pancreatic Duct, External Approach

0FWDX7Z Revision of Autologous Tissue Substitute in Pancreatic Duct, External Approach

0FWDXCZ Revision of Extraluminal Device in Pancreatic Duct, External Approach

0FWDXDZ Revision of Intraluminal Device in Pancreatic Duct, External Approach

0FWDXJZ Revision of Synthetic Substitute in Pancreatic Duct, External Approach

0FWDXKZ Revision of Nonautologous Tissue Substitute in Pancreatic Duct, External Approach

0FWG00Z Revision of Drainage Device in Pancreas, Open Approach

0FWG02Z Revision of Monitoring Device in Pancreas, Open Approach

0FWG03Z Revision of Infusion Device in Pancreas, Open Approach

0FWG0DZ Revision of Intraluminal Device in Pancreas, Open Approach

0FWG0YZ Revision of Other Device in Pancreas, Open Approach

0FWG30Z Revision of Drainage Device in Pancreas, Percutaneous Approach

0FWG32Z Revision of Monitoring Device in Pancreas, Percutaneous Approach

0FWG33Z Revision of Infusion Device in Pancreas, Percutaneous Approach

0FWG3DZ Revision of Intraluminal Device in Pancreas, Percutaneous Approach

0FWG3YZ Revision of Other Device in Pancreas, Percutaneous Approach

0FWG40Z Revision of Drainage Device in Pancreas, Percutaneous Endoscopic Approach

0FWG42Z Revision of Monitoring Device in Pancreas, Percutaneous Endoscopic Approach

0FWG43Z Revision of Infusion Device in Pancreas, Percutaneous Endoscopic Approach

0FWG4DZ Revision of Intraluminal Device in Pancreas, Percutaneous Endoscopic Approach

0FWG4YZ Revision of Other Device in Pancreas, Percutaneous Endoscopic Approach

0FWGX0Z Revision of Drainage Device in Pancreas, External Approach

0FWGX2Z Revision of Monitoring Device in Pancreas, External Approach

0FWGX3Z Revision of Infusion Device in Pancreas, External Approach

0FWGXDZ Revision of Intraluminal Device in Pancreas, External Approach

0FY – Hepatobiliary System and Pancreas, Transplantation

Review Coding Guideline B3.16

▲ **0FY00Z0** Transplantation of Liver, Allogeneic, Open Approach

AHA CC: 4Q, 2012, 99-101; 3Q, 2014, 13-14

▲ **0FY00Z1** Transplantation of Liver, Syngeneic, Open Approach

▲ **0FY00Z2** Transplantation of Liver, Zooplastic, Open Approach

♀ Female-only   ♂ Male-only   ▲ Limited Coverage   ● Non-OR   HAC HAC-associated procedure   ▲ Non-covered procedures   ✚ Cluster

0FYG0Z0 Transplantation of Pancreas, Allogeneic, Open Approach

+ Pancreas/Kidney transplant when reported with Transplant of the Kidney. *See table 0TY to construct the Transplantation code.*

▲ *When reported without an associated kidney transplant code (0TY00Z0, 0TY00Z1, 0TY00Z2, 0TY10Z0, 0TY10Z1 or 0TY10Z2)*

▲ Procedure is covered when reported with one of the diagnosis codes in code range E10.10-E10.9, E89.1

▲ **0FYG0Z1** Transplantation of Pancreas, Syngeneic, Open Approah

+ Pancreas/Kidney transplant when reported with Transplant of the Kidney. *See table 0TY to construct the Transplantation code.*

▲ *When reported without an associated kidney transplant code (0TY00Z0, 0TY00Z1, 0TY00Z2, 0TY10Z0, 0TY10Z1 or 0TY10Z2)*

▲ Procedure is covered when reported with one of the diagnosis codes in code range E10.10-E10.9, E89.1

▲ **0FYG0Z2** Transplantation of Pancreas, Zooplastic, Open Approach

+ Pancreas/Kidney transplant when reported with Transplant of the Kidney. *See table 0TY to construct the Transplantation code.*

Endocrine System

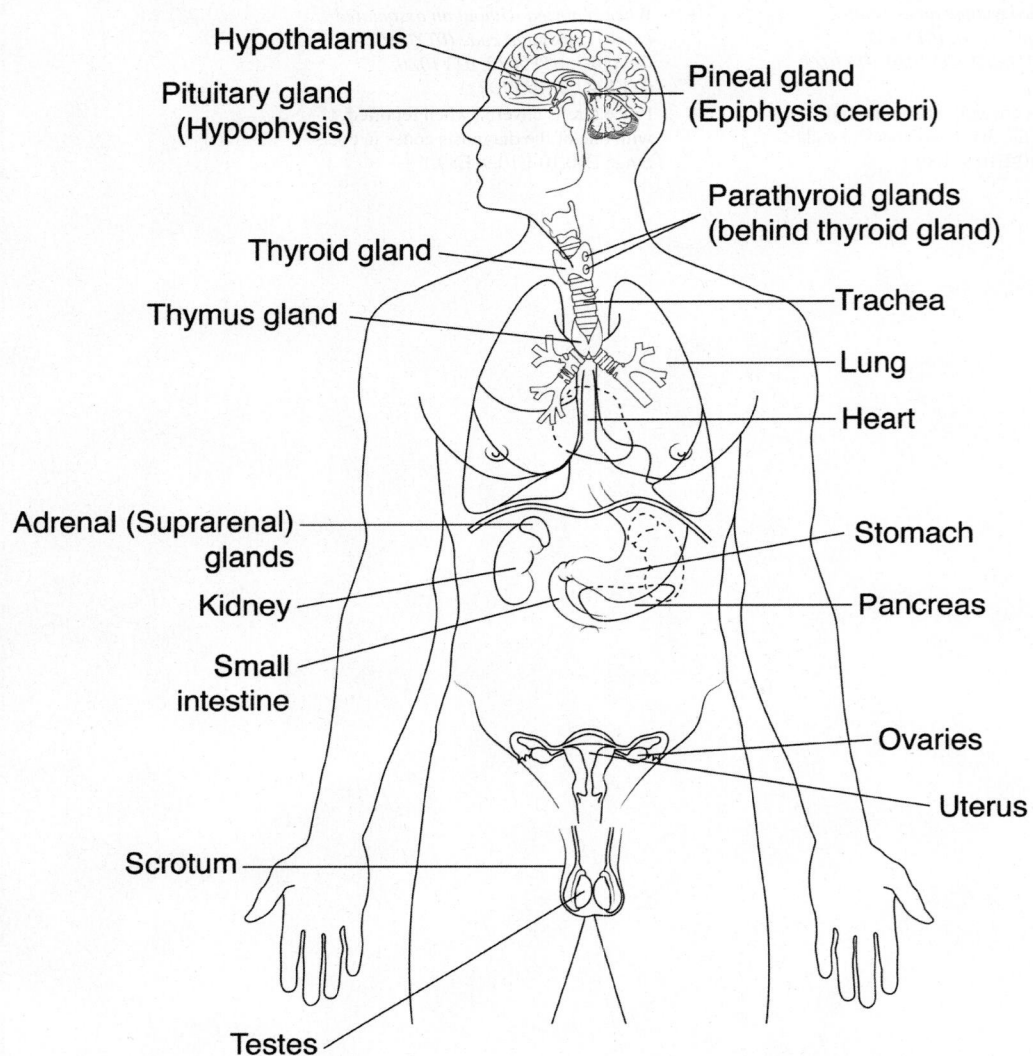

Hypothalamus

Pituitary gland
(Hypophysis)

Pineal gland
(Epiphysis cerebri)

Parathyroid glands
(behind thyroid gland)

Thyroid gland

Thymus gland

Trachea

Lung

Heart

Adrenal (Suprarenal)
glands

Stomach

Kidney

Pancreas

Small
intestine

Ovaries

Uterus

Scrotum

Testes

©AHIMA

Section	0	Medical and Surgical
Body System	G	Endocrine System
Operation	2	**Change:** Taking out or off a device from a body part and putting back an identical or similar device in or on the same body part without cutting or puncturing the skin or a mucous membrane

Body Part (4ᵗʰ)	Approach (5ᵗʰ)	Device (6ᵗʰ)	Qualifier (7ᵗʰ)
0 Pituitary Gland 1 Pineal Body 5 Adrenal Gland K Thyroid Gland R Parathyroid Gland S Endocrine Gland	X External	0 Drainage Device Y Other Device	Z No Qualifier

Section	0	Medical and Surgical
Body System	G	Endocrine System
Operation	5	**Destruction:** Physical eradication of all or a portion of a body part by the direct use of energy, force, or a destructive agent

Body Part (4ᵗʰ)	Approach (5ᵗʰ)	Device (6ᵗʰ)	Qualifier (7ᵗʰ)
0 Pituitary Gland 1 Pineal Body 2 Adrenal Gland, Left 3 Adrenal Gland, Right 4 Adrenal Glands, Bilateral 6 Carotid Body, Left 7 Carotid Body, Right 8 Carotid Bodies, Bilateral 9 Para-aortic Body B Coccygeal Glomus C Glomus Jugulare D Aortic Body F Paraganglion Extremity G Thyroid Gland Lobe, Left H Thyroid Gland Lobe, Right K Thyroid Gland L Superior Parathyroid Gland, Right M Superior Parathyroid Gland, Left N Inferior Parathyroid Gland, Right P Inferior Parathyroid Gland, Left Q Parathyroid Glands, Multiple R Parathyroid Gland	0 Open 3 Percutaneous 4 Percutaneous Endoscopic	Z No Device	Z No Qualifier

Section	0	Medical and Surgical
Body System	G	Endocrine System
Operation	8	**Division:** Cutting into a body part, without draining fluids and/or gases from the body part, in order to separate or transect a body part

Body Part (4ᵗʰ)	Approach (5ᵗʰ)	Device (6ᵗʰ)	Qualifier (7ᵗʰ)
0 Pituitary Gland J Thyroid Gland Isthmus	0 Open 3 Percutaneous 4 Percutaneous Endoscopic	Z No Device	Z No Qualifier

Section	0	Medical and Surgical
Body System	G	Endocrine System
Operation	9	Drainage: Taking or letting out fluids and/or gases from a body part

Body Part (4th)	Approach (5th)	Device (6th)	Qualifier (7th)
0 Pituitary Gland 1 Pineal Body 2 Adrenal Gland, Left 3 Adrenal Gland, Right 4 Adrenal Glands, Bilateral 6 Carotid Body, Left 7 Carotid Body, Right 8 Carotid Bodies, Bilateral 9 Para-aortic Body B Coccygeal Glomus C Glomus Jugulare D Aortic Body F Paraganglion Extremity G Thyroid Gland Lobe, Left H Thyroid Gland Lobe, Right K Thyroid Gland L Superior Parathyroid Gland, Right M Superior Parathyroid Gland, Left N Inferior Parathyroid Gland, Right P Inferior Parathyroid Gland, Left Q Parathyroid Glands, Multiple R Parathyroid Gland	0 Open 3 Percutaneous 4 Percutaneous Endoscopic	0 Drainage Device	Z No Qualifier
0 Pituitary Gland 1 Pineal Body 2 Adrenal Gland, Left 3 Adrenal Gland, Right 4 Adrenal Glands, Bilateral 6 Carotid Body, Left 7 Carotid Body, Right 8 Carotid Bodies, Bilateral 9 Para-aortic Body B Coccygeal Glomus C Glomus Jugulare D Aortic Body F Paraganglion Extremity G Thyroid Gland Lobe, Left H Thyroid Gland Lobe, Right K Thyroid Gland L Superior Parathyroid Gland, Right M Superior Parathyroid Gland, Left N Inferior Parathyroid Gland, Right P Inferior Parathyroid Gland, Left Q Parathyroid Glands, Multiple R Parathyroid Gland	0 Open 3 Percutaneous 4 Percutaneous Endoscopic	Z No Device	X Diagnostic Z No Qualifier

Section	0	Medical and Surgical
Body System	G	Endocrine System
Operation	B	Excision: Cutting out or off, without replacement, a portion of a body part

Body Part (4th)	Approach (5th)	Device (6th)	Qualifier (7th)
0 Pituitary Gland	0 Open	Z No Device	X Diagnostic
1 Pineal Body	3 Percutaneous		Z No Qualifier
2 Adrenal Gland, Left	4 Percutaneous Endoscopic		
3 Adrenal Gland, Right			
4 Adrenal Glands, Bilateral			
6 Carotid Body, Left			
7 Carotid Body, Right			
8 Carotid Bodies, Bilateral			
9 Para-aortic Body			
B Coccygeal Glomus			
C Glomus Jugulare			
D Aortic Body			
F Paraganglion Extremity			
G Thyroid Gland Lobe, Left			
H Thyroid Gland Lobe, Right			
J Thyroid Gland Isthmus			
L Superior Parathyroid Gland, Right			
M Superior Parathyroid Gland, Left			
N Inferior Parathyroid Gland, Right			
P Inferior Parathyroid Gland, Left			
Q Parathyroid Glands, Multiple			
R Parathyroid Gland			

Section	0	Medical and Surgical
Body System	G	Endocrine System
Operation	C	Extirpation: Taking or cutting out solid matter from a body part

Body Part (4th)	Approach (5th)	Device (6th)	Qualifier (7th)
0 Pituitary Gland	0 Open	Z No Device	Z No Qualifier
1 Pineal Body	3 Percutaneous		
2 Adrenal Gland, Left	4 Percutaneous Endoscopic		
3 Adrenal Gland, Right			
4 Adrenal Glands, Bilateral			
6 Carotid Body, Left			
7 Carotid Body, Right			
8 Carotid Bodies, Bilateral			
9 Para-aortic Body			
B Coccygeal Glomus			
C Glomus Jugulare			
D Aortic Body			
F Paraganglion Extremity			
G Thyroid Gland Lobe, Left			
H Thyroid Gland Lobe, Right			
K Thyroid Gland			
L Superior Parathyroid Gland, Right			
M Superior Parathyroid Gland, Left			
N Inferior Parathyroid Gland, Right			
P Inferior Parathyroid Gland, Left			
Q Parathyroid Glands, Multiple			
R Parathyroid Gland			

Section	0	Medical and Surgical
Body System	G	Endocrine System
Operation	H	Insertion: Putting in a nonbiological appliance that monitors, assists, performs, or prevents a physiological function but does not physically take the place of a body part

Body Part (4th)	Approach (5th)	Device (6th)	Qualifier (7th)
S Endocrine Gland	0 Open	1 Radioactive Element	Z No Qualifier
	3 Percutaneous	2 Monitoring Device	
	4 Percutaneous Endoscopic	3 Infusion Device	
		Y Other Device	

Section	0	Medical and Surgical
Body System	G	Endocrine System
Operation	J	**Inspection:** Visually and/or manually exploring a body part

Body Part (4th)	Approach (5th)	Device (6th)	Qualifier (7th)
0 Pituitary Gland 1 Pineal Body 5 Adrenal Gland K Thyroid Gland R Parathyroid Gland S Endocrine Gland	0 Open 3 Percutaneous 4 Percutaneous Endoscopic	Z No Device	Z No Qualifier

Section	0	Medical and Surgical
Body System	G	Endocrine System
Operation	M	**Reattachment:** Putting back in or on all or a portion of a separated body part to its normal location or other suitable location

Body Part (4th)	Approach (5th)	Device (6th)	Qualifier (7th)
2 Adrenal Gland, Left 3 Adrenal Gland, Right G Thyroid Gland Lobe, Left H Thyroid Gland Lobe, Right L Superior Parathyroid Gland, Right M Superior Parathyroid Gland, Left N Inferior Parathyroid Gland, Right P Inferior Parathyroid Gland, Left Q Parathyroid Glands, Multiple R Parathyroid Gland	0 Open 4 Percutaneous Endoscopic	Z No Device	Z No Qualifier

Section	0	Medical and Surgical
Body System	G	Endocrine System
Operation	N	**Release:** Freeing a body part from an abnormal physical constraint by cutting or by the use of force

Body Part (4th)	Approach (5th)	Device (6th)	Qualifier (7th)
0 Pituitary Gland 1 Pineal Body 2 Adrenal Gland, Left 3 Adrenal Gland, Right 4 Adrenal Glands, Bilateral 6 Carotid Body, Left 7 Carotid Body, Right 8 Carotid Bodies, Bilateral 9 Para-aortic Body B Coccygeal Glomus C Glomus Jugulare D Aortic Body F Paraganglion Extremity G Thyroid Gland Lobe, Left H Thyroid Gland Lobe, Right K Thyroid Gland L Superior Parathyroid Gland, Right M Superior Parathyroid Gland, Left N Inferior Parathyroid Gland, Right P Inferior Parathyroid Gland, Left Q Parathyroid Glands, Multiple R Parathyroid Gland	0 Open 3 Percutaneous 4 Percutaneous Endoscopic	Z No Device	Z No Qualifier

Section   0   **Medical and Surgical**
Body System   G   **Endocrine System**
Operation   P   **Removal:** Taking out or off a device from a body part

Body Part (4th)	Approach (5th)	Device (6th)	Qualifier (7th)
0 Pituitary Gland **1** Pineal Body **5** Adrenal Gland **K** Thyroid Gland **R** Parathyroid Gland	**0** Open **3** Percutaneous **4** Percutaneous Endoscopic **X** External	**0** Drainage Device	**Z** No Qualifier
S Endocrine Gland	**0** Open **3** Percutaneous **4** Percutaneous Endoscopic	**0** Drainage Device **2** Monitoring Device **3** Infusion Device **Y** Other Device	**Z** No Qualifier
S Endocrine Gland	**X** External	**0** Drainage Device **2** Monitoring Device **3** Infusion Device	**Z** No Qualifier

Section   0   **Medical and Surgical**
Body System   G   **Endocrine System**
Operation   Q   **Repair:** Restoring, to the extent possible, a body part to its normal anatomic structure and function

Body Part (4th)	Approach (5th)	Device (6th)	Qualifier (7th)
0 Pituitary Gland **1** Pineal Body **2** Adrenal Gland, Left **3** Adrenal Gland, Right **4** Adrenal Glands, Bilateral **6** Carotid Body, Left **7** Carotid Body, Right **8** Carotid Bodies, Bilateral **9** Para-aortic Body **B** Coccygeal Glomus **C** Glomus Jugulare **D** Aortic Body **F** Paraganglion Extremity **G** Thyroid Gland Lobe, Left **H** Thyroid Gland Lobe, Right **J** Thyroid Gland Isthmus **K** Thyroid Gland **L** Superior Parathyroid Gland, Right **M** Superior Parathyroid Gland, Left **N** Inferior Parathyroid Gland, Right **P** Inferior Parathyroid Gland, Left **Q** Parathyroid Glands, Multiple **R** Parathyroid Gland	**0** Open **3** Percutaneous **4** Percutaneous Endoscopic	**Z** No Device	**Z** No Qualifier

Section   0   **Medical and Surgical**
Body System   G   **Endocrine System**
Operation   S   **Reposition:** Moving to its normal location, or other suitable location, all or a portion of a body part

Body Part (4th)	Approach (5th)	Device (6th)	Qualifier (7th)
2 Adrenal Gland, Left **3** Adrenal Gland, Right **G** Thyroid Gland Lobe, Left **H** Thyroid Gland Lobe, Right **L** Superior Parathyroid Gland, Right **M** Superior Parathyroid Gland, Left **N** Inferior Parathyroid Gland, Right **P** Inferior Parathyroid Gland, Left **Q** Parathyroid Glands, Multiple **R** Parathyroid Gland	**0** Open **4** Percutaneous Endoscopic	**Z** No Device	**Z** No Qualifier

Section   0   **Medical and Surgical**
Body System   G   **Endocrine System**
Operation   T   **Resection:** Cutting out or off, without replacement, all of a body part

Body Part (4ᵗʰ)	Approach (5ᵗʰ)	Device (6ᵗʰ)	Qualifier (7ᵗʰ)
0 Pituitary Gland 1 Pineal Body 2 Adrenal Gland, Left 3 Adrenal Gland, Right 4 Adrenal Glands, Bilateral 6 Carotid Body, Left 7 Carotid Body, Right 8 Carotid Bodies, Bilateral 9 Para-aortic Body B Coccygeal Glomus C Glomus Jugulare D Aortic Body F Paraganglion Extremity G Thyroid Gland Lobe, Left H Thyroid Gland Lobe, Right J Thyroid Gland Isthmus K Thyroid Gland L Superior Parathyroid Gland, Right M Superior Parathyroid Gland, Left N Inferior Parathyroid Gland, Right P Inferior Parathyroid Gland, Left Q Parathyroid Glands, Multiple R Parathyroid Gland	0 Open 4 Percutaneous Endoscopic	Z No Device	Z No Qualifier

Section   0   **Medical and Surgical**
Body System   G   **Endocrine System**
Operation   W   **Revision:** Correcting, to the extent possible, a portion of a malfunctioning device or the position of a displaced device

Body Part (4ᵗʰ)	Approach (5ᵗʰ)	Device (6ᵗʰ)	Qualifier (7ᵗʰ)
0 Pituitary Gland 1 Pineal Body 5 Adrenal Gland K Thyroid Gland R Parathyroid Gland	0 Open 3 Percutaneous 4 Percutaneous Endoscopic X External	0 Drainage Device	Z No Qualifier
S Endocrine Gland	0 Open 3 Percutaneous 4 Percutaneous Endoscopic	0 Drainage Device 2 Monitoring Device 3 Infusion Device Y Other Device	Z No Qualifier
S Endocrine Gland	X External	0 Drainage Device 2 Monitoring Device 3 Infusion Device	Z No Qualifier

Endocrine System Code Listing 0G2–0GW

0G2 – Endocrine System, Change

Review Coding Guideline B6.1c

0G20X0Z Change Drainage Device in Pituitary Gland, External Approach
0G20XYZ Change Other Device in Pituitary Gland, External Approach
0G21X0Z Change Drainage Device in Pineal Body, External Approach
0G21XYZ Change Other Device in Pineal Body, External Approach

0G25X0Z Change Drainage Device in Adrenal Gland, External Approach
0G25XYZ Change Other Device in Adrenal Gland, External Approach
0G2KX0Z Change Drainage Device in Thyroid Gland, External Approach
0G2KXYZ Change Other Device in Thyroid Gland, External Approach

0G2RX0Z Change Drainage Device in Parathyroid Gland, External Approach
0G2RXYZ Change Other Device in Parathyroid Gland, External Approach
0G2SX0Z Change Drainage Device in Endocrine Gland, External Approach
0G2SXYZ Change Other Device in Endocrine Gland, External Approach

0G5 – Endocrine System, Destruction

0G500ZZ Destruction of Pituitary Gland, Open Approach

0G503ZZ Destruction of Pituitary Gland, Percutaneous Approach

0G504ZZ Destruction of Pituitary Gland, Percutaneous Endoscopic Approach

♀ Female-only   ♂ Male-only   ▲ Limited Coverage   ● Non-OR   HAC HAC-associated procedure   ▲ Non-covered procedures

0G510ZZ	Destruction of Pineal Body, Open Approach
0G513ZZ	Destruction of Pineal Body, Percutaneous Approach
0G514ZZ	Destruction of Pineal Body, Percutaneous Endoscopic Approach
0G520ZZ	Destruction of Left Adrenal Gland, Open Approach
0G523ZZ	Destruction of Left Adrenal Gland, Percutaneous Approach
0G524ZZ	Destruction of Left Adrenal Gland, Percutaneous Endoscopic Approach
0G530ZZ	Destruction of Right Adrenal Gland, Open Approach
0G533ZZ	Destruction of Right Adrenal Gland, Percutaneous Approach
0G534ZZ	Destruction of Right Adrenal Gland, Percutaneous Endoscopic Approach
0G540ZZ	Destruction of Bilateral Adrenal Glands, Open Approach
0G543ZZ	Destruction of Bilateral Adrenal Glands, Percutaneous Approach
0G544ZZ	Destruction of Bilateral Adrenal Glands, Percutaneous Endoscopic Approach
0G560ZZ	Destruction of Left Carotid Body, Open Approach
0G563ZZ	Destruction of Left Carotid Body, Percutaneous Approach
0G564ZZ	Destruction of Left Carotid Body, Percutaneous Endoscopic Approach
0G570ZZ	Destruction of Right Carotid Body, Open Approach
0G573ZZ	Destruction of Right Carotid Body, Percutaneous Approach
0G574ZZ	Destruction of Right Carotid Body, Percutaneous Endoscopic Approach
0G580ZZ	Destruction of Bilateral Carotid Bodies, Open Approach
0G583ZZ	Destruction of Bilateral Carotid Bodies, Percutaneous Approach
0G584ZZ	Destruction of Bilateral Carotid Bodies, Percutaneous Endoscopic Approach
0G590ZZ	Destruction of Para-aortic Body, Open Approach
0G593ZZ	Destruction of Para-aortic Body, Percutaneous Approach
0G594ZZ	Destruction of Para-aortic Body, Percutaneous Endoscopic Approach
0G5B0ZZ	Destruction of Coccygeal Glomus, Open Approach
0G5B3ZZ	Destruction of Coccygeal Glomus, Percutaneous Approach
0G5B4ZZ	Destruction of Coccygeal Glomus, Percutaneous Endoscopic Approach
0G5C0ZZ	Destruction of Glomus Jugulare, Open Approach
0G5C3ZZ	Destruction of Glomus Jugulare, Percutaneous Approach
0G5C4ZZ	Destruction of Glomus Jugulare, Percutaneous Endoscopic Approach
0G5D0ZZ	Destruction of Aortic Body, Open Approach
0G5D3ZZ	Destruction of Aortic Body, Percutaneous Approach
0G5D4ZZ	Destruction of Aortic Body, Percutaneous Endoscopic Approach
0G5F0ZZ	Destruction of Paraganglion Extremity, Open Approach
0G5F3ZZ	Destruction of Paraganglion Extremity, Percutaneous Approach
0G5F4ZZ	Destruction of Paraganglion Extremity, Percutaneous Endoscopic Approach
0G5G0ZZ	Destruction of Left Thyroid Gland Lobe, Open Approach
0G5G3ZZ	Destruction of Left Thyroid Gland Lobe, Percutaneous Approach
0G5G4ZZ	Destruction of Left Thyroid Gland Lobe, Percutaneous Endoscopic Approach
0G5H0ZZ	Destruction of Right Thyroid Gland Lobe, Open Approach
0G5H3ZZ	Destruction of Right Thyroid Gland Lobe, Percutaneous Approach
0G5H4ZZ	Destruction of Right Thyroid Gland Lobe, Percutaneous Endoscopic Approach
0G5K0ZZ	Destruction of Thyroid Gland, Open Approach
0G5K3ZZ	Destruction of Thyroid Gland, Percutaneous Approach
0G5K4ZZ	Destruction of Thyroid Gland, Percutaneous Endoscopic Approach
0G5L0ZZ	Destruction of Right Superior Parathyroid Gland, Open Approach
0G5L3ZZ	Destruction of Right Superior Parathyroid Gland, Percutaneous Approach
0G5L4ZZ	Destruction of Right Superior Parathyroid Gland, Percutaneous Endoscopic Approach
0G5M0ZZ	Destruction of Left Superior Parathyroid Gland, Open Approach
0G5M3ZZ	Destruction of Left Superior Parathyroid Gland, Percutaneous Approach
0G5M4ZZ	Destruction of Left Superior Parathyroid Gland, Percutaneous Endoscopic Approach
0G5N0ZZ	Destruction of Right Inferior Parathyroid Gland, Open Approach
0G5N3ZZ	Destruction of Right Inferior Parathyroid Gland, Percutaneous Approach
0G5N4ZZ	Destruction of Right Inferior Parathyroid Gland, Percutaneous Endoscopic Approach
0G5P0ZZ	Destruction of Left Inferior Parathyroid Gland, Open Approach
0G5P3ZZ	Destruction of Left Inferior Parathyroid Gland, Percutaneous Approach
0G5P4ZZ	Destruction of Left Inferior Parathyroid Gland, Percutaneous Endoscopic Approach
0G5Q0ZZ	Destruction of Multiple Parathyroid Glands, Open Approach
0G5Q3ZZ	Destruction of Multiple Parathyroid Glands, Percutaneous Approach
0G5Q4ZZ	Destruction of Multiple Parathyroid Glands, Percutaneous Endoscopic Approach
0G5R0ZZ	Destruction of Parathyroid Gland, Open Approach
0G5R3ZZ	Destruction of Parathyroid Gland, Percutaneous Approach
0G5R4ZZ	Destruction of Parathyroid Gland, Percutaneous Endoscopic Approach

0G8 – Endocrine System, Division

Review Coding Guideline B3.14

0G800ZZ	Division of Pituitary Gland, Open Approach
0G803ZZ	Division of Pituitary Gland, Percutaneous Approach
0G804ZZ	Division of Pituitary Gland, Percutaneous Endoscopic Approach
0G8J0ZZ	Division of Thyroid Gland Isthmus, Open Approach
0G8J3ZZ	Division of Thyroid Gland Isthmus, Percutaneous Approach
0G8J4ZZ	Division of Thyroid Gland Isthmus, Percutaneous Endoscopic Approach

0G9 – Endocrine System, Drainage

Review Coding Guidelines B3.4a and B3.4b

Review Coding Guideline B6.2

0G9000Z	Drainage of Pituitary Gland with Drainage Device, Open Approach
0G900ZX	Drainage of Pituitary Gland, Open Approach, Diagnostic
0G900ZZ	Drainage of Pituitary Gland, Open Approach
0G9030Z	Drainage of Pituitary Gland with Drainage Device, Percutaneous Approach
0G903ZX	Drainage of Pituitary Gland, Percutaneous Approach, Diagnostic
0G903ZZ	Drainage of Pituitary Gland, Percutaneous Approach
0G9040Z	Drainage of Pituitary Gland with Drainage Device, Percutaneous Endoscopic Approach
0G904ZX	Drainage of Pituitary Gland, Percutaneous Endoscopic Approach, Diagnostic
0G904ZZ	Drainage of Pituitary Gland, Percutaneous Endoscopic Approach
0G9100Z	Drainage of Pineal Body with Drainage Device, Open Approach
0G910ZX	Drainage of Pineal Body, Open Approach, Diagnostic
0G910ZZ	Drainage of Pineal Body, Open Approach
0G9130Z	Drainage of Pineal Body with Drainage Device, Percutaneous Approach
0G913ZX	Drainage of Pineal Body, Percutaneous Approach, Diagnostic
0G913ZZ	Drainage of Pineal Body, Percutaneous Approach
0G9140Z	Drainage of Pineal Body with Drainage Device, Percutaneous Endoscopic Approach
0G914ZX	Drainage of Pineal Body, Percutaneous Endoscopic Approach, Diagnostic
0G914ZZ	Drainage of Pineal Body, Percutaneous Endoscopic Approach
0G9200Z	Drainage of Left Adrenal Gland with Drainage Device, Open Approach

0G920ZX Drainage of Left Adrenal Gland, Open Approach, Diagnostic

0G920ZZ Drainage of Left Adrenal Gland, Open Approach

0G9230Z Drainage of Left Adrenal Gland with Drainage Device, Percutaneous Approach

0G923ZX Drainage of Left Adrenal Gland, Percutaneous Approach, Diagnostic

0G923ZZ Drainage of Left Adrenal Gland, Percutaneous Approach

0G9240Z Drainage of Left Adrenal Gland with Drainage Device, Percutaneous Endoscopic Approach

0G924ZX Drainage of Left Adrenal Gland, Percutaneous Endoscopic Approach, Diagnostic

0G924ZZ Drainage of Left Adrenal Gland, Percutaneous Endoscopic Approach

0G9300Z Drainage of Right Adrenal Gland with Drainage Device, Open Approach

0G930ZX Drainage of Right Adrenal Gland, Open Approach, Diagnostic

0G930ZZ Drainage of Right Adrenal Gland, Open Approach

0G9330Z Drainage of Right Adrenal Gland with Drainage Device, Percutaneous Approach

0G933ZX Drainage of Right Adrenal Gland, Percutaneous Approach, Diagnostic

0G933ZZ Drainage of Right Adrenal Gland, Percutaneous Approach

0G9340Z Drainage of Right Adrenal Gland with Drainage Device, Percutaneous Endoscopic Approach

0G934ZX Drainage of Right Adrenal Gland, Percutaneous Endoscopic Approach, Diagnostic

0G934ZZ Drainage of Right Adrenal Gland, Percutaneous Endoscopic Approach

0G9400Z Drainage of Bilateral Adrenal Glands with Drainage Device, Open Approach

0G940ZX Drainage of Bilateral Adrenal Glands, Open Approach, Diagnostic

0G940ZZ Drainage of Bilateral Adrenal Glands, Open Approach

0G9430Z Drainage of Bilateral Adrenal Glands with Drainage Device, Percutaneous Approach

0G943ZX Drainage of Bilateral Adrenal Glands, Percutaneous Approach, Diagnostic

0G943ZZ Drainage of Bilateral Adrenal Glands, Percutaneous Approach

0G9440Z Drainage of Bilateral Adrenal Glands with Drainage Device, Percutaneous Endoscopic Approach

0G944ZX Drainage of Bilateral Adrenal Glands, Percutaneous Endoscopic Approach, Diagnostic

0G944ZZ Drainage of Bilateral Adrenal Glands, Percutaneous Endoscopic Approach

0G9600Z Drainage of Left Carotid Body with Drainage Device, Open Approach

0G960ZX Drainage of Left Carotid Body, Open Approach, Diagnostic

0G960ZZ Drainage of Left Carotid Body, Open Approach

0G9630Z Drainage of Left Carotid Body with Drainage Device, Percutaneous Approach

0G963ZX Drainage of Left Carotid Body, Percutaneous Approach, Diagnostic

0G963ZZ Drainage of Left Carotid Body, Percutaneous Approach

0G9640Z Drainage of Left Carotid Body with Drainage Device, Percutaneous Endoscopic Approach

0G964ZX Drainage of Left Carotid Body, Percutaneous Endoscopic Approach, Diagnostic

0G964ZZ Drainage of Left Carotid Body, Percutaneous Endoscopic Approach

0G9700Z Drainage of Right Carotid Body with Drainage Device, Open Approach

0G970ZX Drainage of Right Carotid Body, Open Approach, Diagnostic

0G970ZZ Drainage of Right Carotid Body, Open Approach

0G9730Z Drainage of Right Carotid Body with Drainage Device, Percutaneous Approach

0G973ZX Drainage of Right Carotid Body, Percutaneous Approach, Diagnostic

0G973ZZ Drainage of Right Carotid Body, Percutaneous Approach

0G9740Z Drainage of Right Carotid Body with Drainage Device, Percutaneous Endoscopic Approach

0G974ZX Drainage of Right Carotid Body, Percutaneous Endoscopic Approach, Diagnostic

0G974ZZ Drainage of Right Carotid Body, Percutaneous Endoscopic Approach

0G9800Z Drainage of Bilateral Carotid Bodies with Drainage Device, Open Approach

0G980ZX Drainage of Bilateral Carotid Bodies, Open Approach, Diagnostic

0G980ZZ Drainage of Bilateral Carotid Bodies, Open Approach

0G9830Z Drainage of Bilateral Carotid Bodies with Drainage Device, Percutaneous Approach

0G983ZX Drainage of Bilateral Carotid Bodies, Percutaneous Approach, Diagnostic

0G983ZZ Drainage of Bilateral Carotid Bodies, Percutaneous Approach

0G9840Z Drainage of Bilateral Carotid Bodies with Drainage Device, Percutaneous Endoscopic Approach

0G984ZX Drainage of Bilateral Carotid Bodies, Percutaneous Endoscopic Approach, Diagnostic

0G984ZZ Drainage of Bilateral Carotid Bodies, Percutaneous Endoscopic Approach

0G9900Z Drainage of Para-aortic Body with Drainage Device, Open Approach

0G990ZX Drainage of Para-aortic Body, Open Approach, Diagnostic

0G990ZZ Drainage of Para-aortic Body, Open Approach

0G9930Z Drainage of Para-aortic Body with Drainage Device, Percutaneous Approach

0G993ZX Drainage of Para-aortic Body, Percutaneous Approach, Diagnostic

0G993ZZ Drainage of Para-aortic Body, Percutaneous Approach

0G9940Z Drainage of Para-aortic Body with Drainage Device, Percutaneous Endoscopic Approach

0G994ZX Drainage of Para-aortic Body, Percutaneous Endoscopic Approach, Diagnostic

0G994ZZ Drainage of Para-aortic Body, Percutaneous Endoscopic Approach

0G9B00Z Drainage of Coccygeal Glomus with Drainage Device, Open Approach

0G9B0ZX Drainage of Coccygeal Glomus, Open Approach, Diagnostic

0G9B0ZZ Drainage of Coccygeal Glomus, Open Approach

0G9B30Z Drainage of Coccygeal Glomus with Drainage Device, Percutaneous Approach

0G9B3ZX Drainage of Coccygeal Glomus, Percutaneous Approach, Diagnostic

0G9B3ZZ Drainage of Coccygeal Glomus, Percutaneous Approach

0G9B40Z Drainage of Coccygeal Glomus with Drainage Device, Percutaneous Endoscopic Approach

0G9B4ZX Drainage of Coccygeal Glomus, Percutaneous Endoscopic Approach, Diagnostic

0G9B4ZZ Drainage of Coccygeal Glomus, Percutaneous Endoscopic Approach

0G9C00Z Drainage of Glomus Jugulare with Drainage Device, Open Approach

0G9C0ZX Drainage of Glomus Jugulare, Open Approach, Diagnostic

0G9C0ZZ Drainage of Glomus Jugulare, Open Approach

0G9C30Z Drainage of Glomus Jugulare with Drainage Device, Percutaneous Approach

0G9C3ZX Drainage of Glomus Jugulare, Percutaneous Approach, Diagnostic

0G9C3ZZ Drainage of Glomus Jugulare, Percutaneous Approach

0G9C40Z Drainage of Glomus Jugulare with Drainage Device, Percutaneous Endoscopic Approach

0G9C4ZX Drainage of Glomus Jugulare, Percutaneous Endoscopic Approach, Diagnostic

0G9C4ZZ Drainage of Glomus Jugulare, Percutaneous Endoscopic Approach

0G9D00Z Drainage of Aortic Body with Drainage Device, Open Approach

0G9D0ZX Drainage of Aortic Body, Open Approach, Diagnostic

0G9D0ZZ Drainage of Aortic Body, Open Approach

0G9D30Z Drainage of Aortic Body with Drainage Device, Percutaneous Approach

0G9D3ZX Drainage of Aortic Body, Percutaneous Approach, Diagnostic

0G9D3ZZ Drainage of Aortic Body, Percutaneous Approach

0G9D40Z Drainage of Aortic Body with Drainage Device, Percutaneous Endoscopic Approach

0G9D4ZX Drainage of Aortic Body, Percutaneous Endoscopic Approach, Diagnostic

0G9D4ZZ Drainage of Aortic Body, Percutaneous Endoscopic Approach

0G9F00Z Drainage of Paraganglion Extremity with Drainage Device, Open Approach

0G9F0ZX Drainage of Paraganglion Extremity, Open Approach, Diagnostic

0G9F0ZZ Drainage of Paraganglion Extremity, Open Approach

0G9F30Z Drainage of Paraganglion Extremity with Drainage Device, Percutaneous Approach

0G9F3ZX Drainage of Paraganglion Extremity, Percutaneous Approach, Diagnostic

0G9F3ZZ Drainage of Paraganglion Extremity, Percutaneous Approach

0G9F40Z Drainage of Paraganglion Extremity with Drainage Device, Percutaneous Endoscopic Approach

0G9F4ZX Drainage of Paraganglion Extremity, Percutaneous Endoscopic Approach, Diagnostic

0G9F4ZZ Drainage of Paraganglion Extremity, Percutaneous Endoscopic Approach

0G9G00Z Drainage of Left Thyroid Gland Lobe with Drainage Device, Open Approach

0G9G0ZX Drainage of Left Thyroid Gland Lobe, Open Approach, Diagnostic

0G9G0ZZ Drainage of Left Thyroid Gland Lobe, Open Approach

0G9G30Z Drainage of Left Thyroid Gland Lobe with Drainage Device, Percutaneous Approach

♀ Female-only   ♂ Male-only   ▲ Limited Coverage   ● Non-OR   HAC HAC-associated procedure   ▲ Non-covered procedures   ✚ Cluste

0G9G3ZX Drainage of Left Thyroid Gland Lobe, Percutaneous Approach, Diagnostic

0G9G3ZZ Drainage of Left Thyroid Gland Lobe, Percutaneous Approach

0G9G40Z Drainage of Left Thyroid Gland Lobe with Drainage Device, Percutaneous Endoscopic Approach

0G9G4ZX Drainage of Left Thyroid Gland Lobe, Percutaneous Endoscopic Approach, Diagnostic

0G9G4ZZ Drainage of Left Thyroid Gland Lobe, Percutaneous Endoscopic Approach

0G9H00Z Drainage of Right Thyroid Gland Lobe with Drainage Device, Open Approach

0G9H0ZX Drainage of Right Thyroid Gland Lobe, Open Approach, Diagnostic

0G9H0ZZ Drainage of Right Thyroid Gland Lobe, Open Approach

0G9H30Z Drainage of Right Thyroid Gland Lobe with Drainage Device, Percutaneous Approach

0G9H3ZX Drainage of Right Thyroid Gland Lobe, Percutaneous Approach, Diagnostic

0G9H3ZZ Drainage of Right Thyroid Gland Lobe, Percutaneous Approach

0G9H40Z Drainage of Right Thyroid Gland Lobe with Drainage Device, Percutaneous Endoscopic Approach

0G9H4ZX Drainage of Right Thyroid Gland Lobe, Percutaneous Endoscopic Approach, Diagnostic

0G9H4ZZ Drainage of Right Thyroid Gland Lobe, Percutaneous Endoscopic Approach

0G9K00Z Drainage of Thyroid Gland with Drainage Device, Open Approach

0G9K0ZX Drainage of Thyroid Gland, Open Approach, Diagnostic

0G9K0ZZ Drainage of Thyroid Gland, Open Approach

0G9K30Z Drainage of Thyroid Gland with Drainage Device, Percutaneous Approach

0G9K3ZX Drainage of Thyroid Gland, Percutaneous Approach, Diagnostic

0G9K3ZZ Drainage of Thyroid Gland, Percutaneous Approach

0G9K40Z Drainage of Thyroid Gland with Drainage Device, Percutaneous Endoscopic Approach

0G9K4ZX Drainage of Thyroid Gland, Percutaneous Endoscopic Approach, Diagnostic

0G9K4ZZ Drainage of Thyroid Gland, Percutaneous Endoscopic Approach

0G9L00Z Drainage of Right Superior Parathyroid Gland with Drainage Device, Open Approach

0G9L0ZX Drainage of Right Superior Parathyroid Gland, Open Approach, Diagnostic

0G9L0ZZ Drainage of Right Superior Parathyroid Gland, Open Approach

0G9L30Z Drainage of Right Superior Parathyroid Gland with Drainage Device, Percutaneous Approach

0G9L3ZX Drainage of Right Superior Parathyroid Gland, Percutaneous Approach, Diagnostic

0G9L3ZZ Drainage of Right Superior Parathyroid Gland, Percutaneous Approach

0G9L40Z Drainage of Right Superior Parathyroid Gland with Drainage Device, Percutaneous Endoscopic Approach

0G9L4ZX Drainage of Right Superior Parathyroid Gland, Percutaneous Endoscopic Approach, Diagnostic

0G9L4ZZ Drainage of Right Superior Parathyroid Gland, Percutaneous Endoscopic Approach

0G9M00Z Drainage of Left Superior Parathyroid Gland with Drainage Device, Open Approach

0G9M0ZX Drainage of Left Superior Parathyroid Gland, Open Approach, Diagnostic

0G9M0ZZ Drainage of Left Superior Parathyroid Gland, Open Approach

0G9M30Z Drainage of Left Superior Parathyroid Gland with Drainage Device, Percutaneous Approach

0G9M3ZX Drainage of Left Superior Parathyroid Gland, Percutaneous Approach, Diagnostic

0G9M3ZZ Drainage of Left Superior Parathyroid Gland, Percutaneous Approach

0G9M40Z Drainage of Left Superior Parathyroid Gland with Drainage Device, Percutaneous Endoscopic Approach

0G9M4ZX Drainage of Left Superior Parathyroid Gland, Percutaneous Endoscopic Approach, Diagnostic

0G9M4ZZ Drainage of Left Superior Parathyroid Gland, Percutaneous Endoscopic Approach

0G9N00Z Drainage of Right Inferior Parathyroid Gland with Drainage Device, Open Approach

0G9N0ZX Drainage of Right Inferior Parathyroid Gland, Open Approach, Diagnostic

0G9N0ZZ Drainage of Right Inferior Parathyroid Gland, Open Approach

0G9N30Z Drainage of Right Inferior Parathyroid Gland with Drainage Device, Percutaneous Approach

0G9N3ZX Drainage of Right Inferior Parathyroid Gland, Percutaneous Approach, Diagnostic

0G9N3ZZ Drainage of Right Inferior Parathyroid Gland, Percutaneous Approach

0G9N40Z Drainage of Right Inferior Parathyroid Gland with Drainage Device, Percutaneous Endoscopic Approach

0G9N4ZX Drainage of Right Inferior Parathyroid Gland, Percutaneous Endoscopic Approach, Diagnostic

0G9N4ZZ Drainage of Right Inferior Parathyroid Gland, Percutaneous Endoscopic Approach

0G9P00Z Drainage of Left Inferior Parathyroid Gland with Drainage Device, Open Approach

0G9P0ZX Drainage of Left Inferior Parathyroid Gland, Open Approach, Diagnostic

0G9P0ZZ Drainage of Left Inferior Parathyroid Gland, Open Approach

0G9P30Z Drainage of Left Inferior Parathyroid Gland with Drainage Device, Percutaneous Approach

0G9P3ZX Drainage of Left Inferior Parathyroid Gland, Percutaneous Approach, Diagnostic

0G9P3ZZ Drainage of Left Inferior Parathyroid Gland, Percutaneous Approach

0G9P40Z Drainage of Left Inferior Parathyroid Gland with Drainage Device, Percutaneous Endoscopic Approach

0G9P4ZX Drainage of Left Inferior Parathyroid Gland, Percutaneous Endoscopic Approach, Diagnostic

0G9P4ZZ Drainage of Left Inferior Parathyroid Gland, Percutaneous Endoscopic Approach

0G9Q00Z Drainage of Multiple Parathyroid Glands with Drainage Device, Open Approach

0G9Q0ZX Drainage of Multiple Parathyroid Glands, Open Approach, Diagnostic

0G9Q0ZZ Drainage of Multiple Parathyroid Glands, Open Approach

0G9Q30Z Drainage of Multiple Parathyroid Glands with Drainage Device, Percutaneous Approach

0G9Q3ZX Drainage of Multiple Parathyroid Glands, Percutaneous Approach, Diagnostic

0G9Q3ZZ Drainage of Multiple Parathyroid Glands, Percutaneous Approach

0G9Q4ZX Drainage of Multiple Parathyroid Glands, Percutaneous Endoscopic Approach, Diagnostic

0G9Q4ZZ Drainage of Multiple Parathyroid Glands, Percutaneous Endoscopic Approach

0G9R00Z Drainage of Parathyroid Gland with Drainage Device, Open Approach

0G9R0ZX Drainage of Parathyroid Gland, Open Approach, Diagnostic

0G9R0ZZ Drainage of Parathyroid Gland, Open Approach

0G9R30Z Drainage of Parathyroid Gland with Drainage Device, Percutaneous Approach

0G9R3ZX Drainage of Parathyroid Gland, Percutaneous Approach, Diagnostic

0G9R3ZZ Drainage of Parathyroid Gland, Percutaneous Approach

0G9R40Z Drainage of Parathyroid Gland with Drainage Device, Percutaneous Endoscopic Approach

0G9R4ZX Drainage of Parathyroid Gland, Percutaneous Endoscopic Approach, Diagnostic

0G9R4ZZ Drainage of Parathyroid Gland, Percutaneous Endoscopic Approach

0GB – Endocrine System, Excision

Review Coding Guidelines B3.4a and B3.4b

Review Coding Guideline B3.8

Review Coding Guideline B3.18

0GB00ZX Excision of Pituitary Gland, Open Approach, Diagnostic

0GB00ZZ Excision of Pituitary Gland, Open Approach
AHA CC: 3Q, 2014, 22-23

0GB03ZX Excision of Pituitary Gland, Percutaneous Approach, Diagnostic

0GB03ZZ Excision of Pituitary Gland, Percutaneous Approach

0GB04ZX Excision of Pituitary Gland, Percutaneous Endoscopic Approach, Diagnostic

0GB04ZZ Excision of Pituitary Gland, Percutaneous Endoscopic Approach

0GB10ZX Excision of Pineal Body, Open Approach, Diagnostic
0GB10ZZ Excision of Pineal Body, Open Approach
0GB13ZX Excision of Pineal Body, Percutaneous Approach, Diagnostic
0GB13ZZ Excision of Pineal Body, Percutaneous Approach
0GB14ZX Excision of Pineal Body, Percutaneous Endoscopic Approach, Diagnostic
0GB14ZZ Excision of Pineal Body, Percutaneous Endoscopic Approach
0GB20ZX Excision of Left Adrenal Gland, Open Approach, Diagnostic
0GB20ZZ Excision of Left Adrenal Gland, Open Approach
0GB23ZX Excision of Left Adrenal Gland, Percutaneous Approach, Diagnostic
0GB23ZZ Excision of Left Adrenal Gland, Percutaneous Approach
0GB24ZX Excision of Left Adrenal Gland, Percutaneous Endoscopic Approach, Diagnostic
0GB24ZZ Excision of Left Adrenal Gland, Percutaneous Endoscopic Approach
0GB30ZX Excision of Right Adrenal Gland, Open Approach, Diagnostic
0GB30ZZ Excision of Right Adrenal Gland, Open Approach
0GB33ZX Excision of Right Adrenal Gland, Percutaneous Approach, Diagnostic
0GB33ZZ Excision of Right Adrenal Gland, Percutaneous Approach
0GB34ZX Excision of Right Adrenal Gland, Percutaneous Endoscopic Approach, Diagnostic
0GB34ZZ Excision of Right Adrenal Gland, Percutaneous Endoscopic Approach
0GB40ZX Excision of Bilateral Adrenal Glands, Open Approach, Diagnostic
0GB40ZZ Excision of Bilateral Adrenal Glands, Open Approach
0GB43ZX Excision of Bilateral Adrenal Glands, Percutaneous Approach, Diagnostic
0GB43ZZ Excision of Bilateral Adrenal Glands, Percutaneous Approach
0GB44ZX Excision of Bilateral Adrenal Glands, Percutaneous Endoscopic Approach, Diagnostic
0GB44ZZ Excision of Bilateral Adrenal Glands, Percutaneous Endoscopic Approach
0GB60ZX Excision of Left Carotid Body, Open Approach, Diagnostic
0GB60ZZ Excision of Left Carotid Body, Open Approach
0GB63ZX Excision of Left Carotid Body, Percutaneous Approach, Diagnostic
0GB63ZZ Excision of Left Carotid Body, Percutaneous Approach
0GB64ZX Excision of Left Carotid Body, Percutaneous Endoscopic Approach, Diagnostic
0GB64ZZ Excision of Left Carotid Body, Percutaneous Endoscopic Approach
0GB70ZX Excision of Right Carotid Body, Open Approach, Diagnostic
0GB70ZZ Excision of Right Carotid Body, Open Approach
0GB73ZX Excision of Right Carotid Body, Percutaneous Approach, Diagnostic
0GB73ZZ Excision of Right Carotid Body, Percutaneous Approach
0GB74ZX Excision of Right Carotid Body, Percutaneous Endoscopic Approach, Diagnostic

0GB74ZZ Excision of Right Carotid Body, Percutaneous Endoscopic Approach
0GB80ZX Excision of Bilateral Carotid Bodies, Open Approach, Diagnostic
0GB80ZZ Excision of Bilateral Carotid Bodies, Open Approach
0GB83ZX Excision of Bilateral Carotid Bodies, Percutaneous Approach, Diagnostic
0GB83ZZ Excision of Bilateral Carotid Bodies, Percutaneous Approach
0GB84ZX Excision of Bilateral Carotid Bodies, Percutaneous Endoscopic Approach, Diagnostic
0GB84ZZ Excision of Bilateral Carotid Bodies, Percutaneous Endoscopic Approach
0GB90ZX Excision of Para-aortic Body, Open Approach, Diagnostic
0GB90ZZ Excision of Para-aortic Body, Open Approach
AHA CC: 2Q, 2021, 7
0GB93ZX Excision of Para-aortic Body, Percutaneous Approach, Diagnostic
0GB93ZZ Excision of Para-aortic Body, Percutaneous Approach
0GB94ZX Excision of Para-aortic Body, Percutaneous Endoscopic Approach, Diagnostic
0GB94ZZ Excision of Para-aortic Body, Percutaneous Endoscopic Approach
0GBB0ZX Excision of Coccygeal Glomus, Open Approach, Diagnostic
0GBB0ZZ Excision of Coccygeal Glomus, Open Approach
0GBB3ZX Excision of Coccygeal Glomus, Percutaneous Approach, Diagnostic
0GBB3ZZ Excision of Coccygeal Glomus, Percutaneous Approach
0GBB4ZX Excision of Coccygeal Glomus, Percutaneous Endoscopic Approach, Diagnostic
0GBB4ZZ Excision of Coccygeal Glomus, Percutaneous Endoscopic Approach
0GBC0ZX Excision of Glomus Jugulare, Open Approach, Diagnostic
0GBC0ZZ Excision of Glomus Jugulare, Open Approach
0GBC3ZX Excision of Glomus Jugulare, Percutaneous Approach, Diagnostic
0GBC3ZZ Excision of Glomus Jugulare, Percutaneous Approach
0GBC4ZX Excision of Glomus Jugulare, Percutaneous Endoscopic Approach, Diagnostic
0GBC4ZZ Excision of Glomus Jugulare, Percutaneous Endoscopic Approach
0GBD0ZX Excision of Aortic Body, Open Approach, Diagnostic
0GBD0ZZ Excision of Aortic Body, Open Approach
0GBD3ZX Excision of Aortic Body, Percutaneous Approach, Diagnostic
0GBD3ZZ Excision of Aortic Body, Percutaneous Approach
0GBD4ZX Excision of Aortic Body, Percutaneous Endoscopic Approach, Diagnostic
0GBD4ZZ Excision of Aortic Body, Percutaneous Endoscopic Approach
0GBF0ZX Excision of Paraganglion Extremity, Open Approach, Diagnostic
0GBF0ZZ Excision of Paraganglion Extremity, Open Approach
0GBF3ZX Excision of Paraganglion Extremity, Percutaneous Approach, Diagnostic
0GBF3ZZ Excision of Paraganglion Extremity, Percutaneous Approach

0GBF4ZX Excision of Paraganglion Extremity, Percutaneous Endoscopic Approach, Diagnostic
0GBF4ZZ Excision of Paraganglion Extremity, Percutaneous Endoscopic Approach
0GBG0ZX Excision of Left Thyroid Gland Lobe, Open Approach, Diagnostic
0GBG0ZZ Excision of Left Thyroid Gland Lobe, Open Approach
AHA CC: 2Q, 2017, 20
0GBG3ZX Excision of Left Thyroid Gland Lobe, Percutaneous Approach, Diagnostic
0GBG3ZZ Excision of Left Thyroid Gland Lobe, Percutaneous Approach
0GBG4ZX Excision of Left Thyroid Gland Lobe, Percutaneous Endoscopic Approach, Diagnostic
0GBG4ZZ Excision of Left Thyroid Gland Lobe, Percutaneous Endoscopic Approach
0GBH0ZX Excision of Right Thyroid Gland Lobe, Open Approach, Diagnostic
0GBH0ZZ Excision of Right Thyroid Gland Lobe, Open Approach
AHA CC: 2Q, 2017, 20
0GBH3ZX Excision of Right Thyroid Gland Lobe, Percutaneous Approach, Diagnostic
0GBH3ZZ Excision of Right Thyroid Gland Lobe, Percutaneous Approach
0GBH4ZX Excision of Right Thyroid Gland Lobe, Percutaneous Endoscopic Approach, Diagnostic
0GBH4ZZ Excision of Right Thyroid Gland Lobe, Percutaneous Endoscopic Approach
0GBJ0ZX Excision of Thyroid Gland Isthmus, Open Approach, Diagnostic
0GBJ0ZZ Excision of Thyroid Gland Isthmus, Open Approach
0GBJ3ZX Excision of Thyroid Gland Isthmus, Percutaneous Approach, Diagnostic
0GBJ3ZZ Excision of Thyroid Gland Isthmus, Percutaneous Approach
0GBJ4ZX Excision of Thyroid Gland Isthmus, Percutaneous Endoscopic Approach, Diagnostic
0GBJ4ZZ Excision of Thyroid Gland Isthmus, Percutaneous Endoscopic Approach
0GBL0ZX Excision of Right Superior Parathyroid Gland, Open Approach, Diagnostic
0GBL0ZZ Excision of Right Superior Parathyroid Gland, Open Approach
0GBL3ZX Excision of Right Superior Parathyroid Gland, Percutaneous Approach, Diagnostic
0GBL3ZZ Excision of Right Superior Parathyroid Gland, Percutaneous Approach
0GBL4ZX Excision of Right Superior Parathyroid Gland, Percutaneous Endoscopic Approach, Diagnostic
0GBL4ZZ Excision of Right Superior Parathyroid Gland, Percutaneous Endoscopic Approach
0GBM0ZX Excision of Left Superior Parathyroid Gland, Open Approach, Diagnostic
0GBM0ZZ Excision of Left Superior Parathyroid Gland, Open Approach
0GBM3ZX Excision of Left Superior Parathyroid Gland, Percutaneous Approach, Diagnostic
0GBM3ZZ Excision of Left Superior Parathyroid Gland, Percutaneous Approach
0GBM4ZX Excision of Left Superior Parathyroid Gland, Percutaneous Endoscopic Approach, Diagnostic

♀ Female-only   ♂ Male-only   ▲ Limited Coverage   ● Non-OR   HAC HAC-associated procedure   ▲ Non-covered procedures   ✚ Cluster

0GBM4ZZ Excision of Left Superior Parathyroid Gland, Percutaneous Endoscopic Approach

0GBN0ZX Excision of Right Inferior Parathyroid Gland, Open Approach, Diagnostic

0GBN0ZZ Excision of Right Inferior Parathyroid Gland, Open Approach

0GBN3ZX Excision of Right Inferior Parathyroid Gland, Percutaneous Approach, Diagnostic

0GBN3ZZ Excision of Right Inferior Parathyroid Gland, Percutaneous Approach

0GBN4ZX Excision of Right Inferior Parathyroid Gland, Percutaneous Endoscopic Approach, Diagnostic

0GBN4ZZ Excision of Right Inferior Parathyroid Gland, Percutaneous Endoscopic Approach

0GBP0ZX Excision of Left Inferior Parathyroid Gland, Open Approach, Diagnostic

0GBP0ZZ Excision of Left Inferior Parathyroid Gland, Open Approach

0GBP3ZX Excision of Left Inferior Parathyroid Gland, Percutaneous Approach, Diagnostic

0GBP3ZZ Excision of Left Inferior Parathyroid Gland, Percutaneous Approach

0GBP4ZX Excision of Left Inferior Parathyroid Gland, Percutaneous Endoscopic Approach, Diagnostic

0GBP4ZZ Excision of Left Inferior Parathyroid Gland, Percutaneous Endoscopic Approach

0GBQ0ZX Excision of Multiple Parathyroid Glands, Open Approach, Diagnostic

0GBQ0ZZ Excision of Multiple Parathyroid Glands, Open Approach

0GBQ3ZX Excision of Multiple Parathyroid Glands, Percutaneous Approach, Diagnostic

0GBQ3ZZ Excision of Multiple Parathyroid Glands, Percutaneous Approach

0GBQ4ZX Excision of Multiple Parathyroid Glands, Percutaneous Endoscopic Approach, Diagnostic

0GBQ4ZZ Excision of Multiple Parathyroid Glands, Percutaneous Endoscopic Approach

0GBR0ZX Excision of Parathyroid Gland, Open Approach, Diagnostic

0GBR0ZZ Excision of Parathyroid Gland, Open Approach

0GBR3ZX Excision of Parathyroid Gland, Percutaneous Approach, Diagnostic

0GBR3ZZ Excision of Parathyroid Gland, Percutaneous Approach

0GBR4ZX Excision of Parathyroid Gland, Percutaneous Endoscopic Approach, Diagnostic

0GBR4ZZ Excision of Parathyroid Gland, Percutaneous Endoscopic Approach

0GC – Endocrine System, Extirpation

0GC00ZZ Extirpation of Matter from Pituitary Gland, Open Approach

0GC03ZZ Extirpation of Matter from Pituitary Gland, Percutaneous Approach

0GC04ZZ Extirpation of Matter from Pituitary Gland, Percutaneous Endoscopic Approach

0GC10ZZ Extirpation of Matter from Pineal Body, Open Approach

0GC13ZZ Extirpation of Matter from Pineal Body, Percutaneous Approach

0GC14ZZ Extirpation of Matter from Pineal Body, Percutaneous Endoscopic Approach

0GC20ZZ Extirpation of Matter from Left Adrenal Gland, Open Approach

0GC23ZZ Extirpation of Matter from Left Adrenal Gland, Percutaneous Approach

0GC24ZZ Extirpation of Matter from Left Adrenal Gland, Percutaneous Endoscopic Approach

0GC30ZZ Extirpation of Matter from Right Adrenal Gland, Open Approach

0GC33ZZ Extirpation of Matter from Right Adrenal Gland, Percutaneous Approach

0GC34ZZ Extirpation of Matter from Right Adrenal Gland, Percutaneous Endoscopic Approach

0GC40ZZ Extirpation of Matter from Bilateral Adrenal Glands, Open Approach

0GC43ZZ Extirpation of Matter from Bilateral Adrenal Glands, Percutaneous Approach

0GC44ZZ Extirpation of Matter from Bilateral Adrenal Glands, Percutaneous Endoscopic Approach

0GC60ZZ Extirpation of Matter from Left Carotid Body, Open Approach

0GC63ZZ Extirpation of Matter from Left Carotid Body, Percutaneous Approach

0GC64ZZ Extirpation of Matter from Left Carotid Body, Percutaneous Endoscopic Approach

0GC70ZZ Extirpation of Matter from Right Carotid Body, Open Approach

0GC73ZZ Extirpation of Matter from Right Carotid Body, Percutaneous Approach

0GC74ZZ Extirpation of Matter from Right Carotid Body, Percutaneous Endoscopic Approach

0GC80ZZ Extirpation of Matter from Bilateral Carotid Bodies, Open Approach

0GC83ZZ Extirpation of Matter from Bilateral Carotid Bodies, Percutaneous Approach

0GC84ZZ Extirpation of Matter from Bilateral Carotid Bodies, Percutaneous Endoscopic Approach

0GC90ZZ Extirpation of Matter from Para-aortic Body, Open Approach

0GC93ZZ Extirpation of Matter from Para-aortic Body, Percutaneous Approach

0GC94ZZ Extirpation of Matter from Para-aortic Body, Percutaneous Endoscopic Approach

0GCB0ZZ Extirpation of Matter from Coccygeal Glomus, Open Approach

0GCB3ZZ Extirpation of Matter from Coccygeal Glomus, Percutaneous Approach

0GCB4ZZ Extirpation of Matter from Coccygeal Glomus, Percutaneous Endoscopic Approach

0GCC0ZZ Extirpation of Matter from Glomus Jugulare, Open Approach

0GCC3ZZ Extirpation of Matter from Glomus Jugulare, Percutaneous Approach

0GCC4ZZ Extirpation of Matter from Glomus Jugulare, Percutaneous Endoscopic Approach

0GCD0ZZ Extirpation of Matter from Aortic Body, Open Approach

0GCD3ZZ Extirpation of Matter from Aortic Body, Percutaneous Approach

0GCD4ZZ Extirpation of Matter from Aortic Body, Percutaneous Endoscopic Approach

0GCF0ZZ Extirpation of Matter from Paraganglion Extremity, Open Approach

0GCF3ZZ Extirpation of Matter from Paraganglion Extremity, Percutaneous Approach

0GCF4ZZ Extirpation of Matter from Paraganglion Extremity, Percutaneous Endoscopic Approach

0GCG0ZZ Extirpation of Matter from Left Thyroid Gland Lobe, Open Approach

0GCG3ZZ Extirpation of Matter from Left Thyroid Gland Lobe, Percutaneous Approach

0GCG4ZZ Extirpation of Matter from Left Thyroid Gland Lobe, Percutaneous Endoscopic Approach

0GCH0ZZ Extirpation of Matter from Right Thyroid Gland Lobe, Open Approach

0GCH3ZZ Extirpation of Matter from Right Thyroid Gland Lobe, Percutaneous Approach

0GCH4ZZ Extirpation of Matter from Right Thyroid Gland Lobe, Percutaneous Endoscopic Approach

0GCK0ZZ Extirpation of Matter from Thyroid Gland, Open Approach

0GCK3ZZ Extirpation of Matter from Thyroid Gland, Percutaneous Approach

0GCK4ZZ Extirpation of Matter from Thyroid Gland, Percutaneous Endoscopic Approach

0GCL0ZZ Extirpation of Matter from Right Superior Parathyroid Gland, Open Approach

0GCL3ZZ Extirpation of Matter from Right Superior Parathyroid Gland, Percutaneous Approach

0GCL4ZZ Extirpation of Matter from Right Superior Parathyroid Gland, Percutaneous Endoscopic Approach

0GCM0ZZ Extirpation of Matter from Left Superior Parathyroid Gland, Open Approach

0GCM3ZZ Extirpation of Matter from Left Superior Parathyroid Gland, Percutaneous Approach

0GCM4ZZ Extirpation of Matter from Left Superior Parathyroid Gland, Percutaneous Endoscopic Approach

0GCN0ZZ Extirpation of Matter from Right Inferior Parathyroid Gland, Open Approach

0GCN3ZZ Extirpation of Matter from Right Inferior Parathyroid Gland, Percutaneous Approach

0GCN4ZZ Extirpation of Matter from Right Inferior Parathyroid Gland, Percutaneous Endoscopic Approach

0GCP0ZZ Extirpation of Matter from Left Inferior Parathyroid Gland, Open Approach

0GCP3ZZ Extirpation of Matter from Left Inferior Parathyroid Gland, Percutaneous Approach

0GCP4ZZ Extirpation of Matter from Left Inferior Parathyroid Gland, Percutaneous Endoscopic Approach

0GCQ0ZZ Extirpation of Matter from Multiple Parathyroid Glands, Open Approach

0GCQ3ZZ Extirpation of Matter from Multiple Parathyroid Glands, Percutaneous Approach

0GCQ4ZZ Extirpation of Matter from Multiple Parathyroid Glands, Percutaneous Endoscopic Approach

0GCR0ZZ Extirpation of Matter from Parathyroid Gland, Open Approach

0GCR3ZZ Extirpation of Matter from Parathyroid Gland, Percutaneous Approach

0GCR4ZZ Extirpation of Matter from Parathyroid Gland, Percutaneous Endoscopic Approach

0GH – Endocrine System, Insertion

0GHS01Z Insertion of Radioactive Element into Endocrine Gland, Open Approach

0GHS02Z Insertion of Monitoring Device into Endocrine Gland, Open Approach

0GHS03Z Insertion of Infusion Device into Endocrine Gland, Open Approach

0GHS0YZ Insertion of Other Device into Endocrine Gland, Open Approach

0GHS31Z Insertion of Radioactive Element into Endocrine Gland, Percutaneous Approach

0GHS32Z Insertion of Monitoring Device into Endocrine Gland, Percutaneous Approach

0GHS33Z Insertion of Infusion Device into Endocrine Gland, Percutaneous Approach

0GHS3YZ Insertion of Other Device into Endocrine Gland, Percutaneous Approach

0GHS41Z Insertion of Radioactive Element into Endocrine Gland, Percutaneous Endoscopic Approach

0GHS42Z Insertion of Monitoring Device into Endocrine Gland, Percutaneous Endoscopic Approach

0GHS43Z Insertion of Infusion Device into Endocrine Gland, Percutaneous Endoscopic Approach

0GHS4YZ Insertion of Other Device into Endocrine Gland, Percutaneous Endoscopic Approach

0GJ – Endocrine System, Inspection

Review Coding Guidelines B3.11a, B3.11b and B3.11c

0GJ00ZZ Inspection of Pituitary Gland, Open Approach

0GJ03ZZ Inspection of Pituitary Gland, Percutaneous Approach

0GJ04ZZ Inspection of Pituitary Gland, Percutaneous Endoscopic Approach

0GJ10ZZ Inspection of Pineal Body, Open Approach

0GJ13ZZ Inspection of Pineal Body, Percutaneous Approach

0GJ14ZZ Inspection Pineal Body, Percutaneous Endoscopic Approach

0GJ50ZZ Inspection of Adrenal Gland, Open Approach

0GJ53ZZ Inspection of Adrenal Gland, Percutaneous Approach

0GJ54ZZ Inspection of Adrenal Gland, Percutaneous Endoscopic Approach

0GJK0ZZ Inspection of Thyroid Gland, Open Approach

0GJK3ZZ Inspection of Thyroid Gland, Percutaneous Approach

0GJK4ZZ Inspection of Thyroid Gland, Percutaneous Endoscopic Approach

0GJR0ZZ Inspection of Parathyroid Gland, Open Approach

0GJR3ZZ Inspection of Parathyroid Gland, Percutaneous Approach

0GJR4ZZ Inspection of Parathyroid Gland, Percutaneous Endoscopic Approach

0GJS0ZZ Inspection of Endocrine Gland, Open Approach

0GJS3ZZ Inspection of Endocrine Gland, Percutaneous Approach

0GJS4ZZ Inspection of Endocrine Gland, Percutaneous Endoscopic Approach

0GM – Endocrine System, Reattachment

0GM20ZZ Reattachment of Left Adrenal Gland, Open Approach

0GM24ZZ Reattachment of Left Adrenal Gland, Percutaneous Endoscopic Approach

0GM30ZZ Reattachment of Right Adrenal Gland, Open Approach

0GM34ZZ Reattachment of Right Adrenal Gland, Percutaneous Endoscopic Approach

0GMG0ZZ Reattachment of Left Thyroid Gland Lobe, Open Approach

0GMG4ZZ Reattachment of Left Thyroid Gland Lobe, Percutaneous Endoscopic Approach

0GMH0ZZ Reattachment of Right Thyroid Gland Lobe, Open Approach

0GMH4ZZ Reattachment of Right Thyroid Gland Lobe, Percutaneous Endoscopic Approach

0GML0ZZ Reattachment of Right Superior Parathyroid Gland, Open Approach

0GML4ZZ Reattachment of Right Superior Parathyroid Gland, Percutaneous Endoscopic Approach

0GMM0ZZ Reattachment of Left Superior Parathyroid Gland, Open Approach

0GMM4ZZ Reattachment of Left Superior Parathyroid Gland, Percutaneous Endoscopic Approach

0GMN0ZZ Reattachment of Right Inferior Parathyroid Gland, Open Approach

0GMN4ZZ Reattachment of Right Inferior Parathyroid Gland, Percutaneous Endoscopic Approach

0GMP0ZZ Reattachment of Left Inferior Parathyroid Gland, Open Approach

0GMP4ZZ Reattachment of Left Inferior Parathyroid Gland, Percutaneous Endoscopic Approach

0GMQ0ZZ Reattachment of Multiple Parathyroid Glands, Open Approach

0GMQ4ZZ Reattachment of Multiple Parathyroid Glands, Percutaneous Endoscopic Approach

0GMR0ZZ Reattachment of Parathyroid Gland, Open Approach

0GMR4ZZ Reattachment of Parathyroid Gland, Percutaneous Endoscopic Approach

0GN – Endocrine System, Release

Review Coding Guideline B3.13

Review Coding Guideline B3.14

0GN00ZZ Release Pituitary Gland, Open Approach

0GN03ZZ Release Pituitary Gland, Percutaneous Approach

0GN04ZZ Release Pituitary Gland, Percutaneous Endoscopic Approach

0GN10ZZ Release Pineal Body, Open Approach

0GN13ZZ Release Pineal Body, Percutaneous Approach

0GN14ZZ Release Pineal Body, Percutaneous Endoscopic Approach

0GN20ZZ Release Left Adrenal Gland, Open Approach

0GN23ZZ Release Left Adrenal Gland, Percutaneous Approach

0GN24ZZ Release Left Adrenal Gland, Percutaneous Endoscopic Approach

0GN30ZZ Release Right Adrenal Gland, Open Approach

0GN33ZZ Release Right Adrenal Gland, Percutaneous Approach

0GN34ZZ Release Right Adrenal Gland, Percutaneous Endoscopic Approach

0GN40ZZ Release Bilateral Adrenal Glands, Open Approach

0GN43ZZ Release Bilateral Adrenal Glands, Percutaneous Approach

0GN44ZZ Release Bilateral Adrenal Glands, Percutaneous Endoscopic Approach

0GN60ZZ Release Left Carotid Body, Open Approach

0GN63ZZ Release Left Carotid Body, Percutaneous Approach

0GN64ZZ Release Left Carotid Body, Percutaneous Endoscopic Approach

0GN70ZZ Release Right Carotid Body, Open Approach

♀ Female-only   ♂ Male-only   ▲ Limited Coverage   ● Non-OR   HAC HAC-associated procedure   ▲ Non-covered procedures   ✚ Cluster

0GN73ZZ Release Right Carotid Body, Percutaneous Approach
0GN74ZZ Release Right Carotid Body, Percutaneous Endoscopic Approach
0GN80ZZ Release Bilateral Carotid Bodies, Open Approach
0GN83ZZ Release Bilateral Carotid Bodies, Percutaneous Approach
0GN84ZZ Release Bilateral Carotid Bodies, Percutaneous Endoscopic Approach
0GN90ZZ Release Para-aortic Body, Open Approach
0GN93ZZ Release Para-aortic Body, Percutaneous Approach
0GN94ZZ Release Para-aortic Body, Percutaneous Endoscopic Approach
0GNB0ZZ Release Coccygeal Glomus, Open Approach
0GNB3ZZ Release Coccygeal Glomus, Percutaneous Approach
0GNB4ZZ Release Coccygeal Glomus, Percutaneous Endoscopic Approach
0GNC0ZZ Release Glomus Jugulare, Open Approach
0GNC3ZZ Release Glomus Jugulare, Percutaneous Approach
0GNC4ZZ Release Glomus Jugulare, Percutaneous Endoscopic Approach
0GND0ZZ Release Aortic Body, Open Approach
0GND3ZZ Release Aortic Body, Percutaneous Approach
0GND4ZZ Release Aortic Body, Percutaneous Endoscopic Approach

0GNF0ZZ Release Paraganglion Extremity, Open Approach
0GNF3ZZ Release Paraganglion Extremity, Percutaneous Approach
0GNF4ZZ Release Paraganglion Extremity, Percutaneous Endoscopic Approach
0GNG0ZZ Release Left Thyroid Gland Lobe, Open Approach
0GNG3ZZ Release Left Thyroid Gland Lobe, Percutaneous Approach
0GNG4ZZ Release Left Thyroid Gland Lobe, Percutaneous Endoscopic Approach
0GNH0ZZ Release Right Thyroid Gland Lobe, Open Approach
0GNH3ZZ Release Right Thyroid Gland Lobe, Percutaneous Approach
0GNH4ZZ Release Right Thyroid Gland Lobe, Percutaneous Endoscopic Approach
0GNK0ZZ Release Thyroid Gland, Open Approach
0GNK3ZZ Release Thyroid Gland, Percutaneous Approach
0GNK4ZZ Release Thyroid Gland, Percutaneous Endoscopic Approach
0GNL0ZZ Release Right Superior Parathyroid Gland, Open Approach
0GNL3ZZ Release Right Superior Parathyroid Gland, Percutaneous Approach
0GNL4ZZ Release Right Superior Parathyroid Gland, Percutaneous Endoscopic Approach
0GNM0ZZ Release Left Superior Parathyroid Gland, Open Approach

0GNM3ZZ Release Left Superior Parathyroid Gland, Percutaneous Approach
0GNM4ZZ Release Left Superior Parathyroid Gland, Percutaneous Endoscopic Approach
0GNN0ZZ Release Right Inferior Parathyroid Gland, Open Approach
0GNN3ZZ Release Right Inferior Parathyroid Gland, Percutaneous Approach
0GNN4ZZ Release Right Inferior Parathyroid Gland, Percutaneous Endoscopic Approach
0GNP0ZZ Release Left Inferior Parathyroid Gland, Open Approach
0GNP3ZZ Release Left Inferior Parathyroid Gland, Percutaneous Approach
0GNP4ZZ Release Left Inferior Parathyroid Gland, Percutaneous Endoscopic Approach
0GNQ0ZZ Release Multiple Parathyroid Glands, Open Approach
0GNQ3ZZ Release Multiple Parathyroid Glands, Percutaneous Approach
0GNQ4ZZ Release Multiple Parathyroid Glands, Percutaneous Endoscopic Approach
0GNR0ZZ Release Parathyroid Gland, Open Approach
0GNR3ZZ Release Parathyroid Gland, Percutaneous Approach
0GNR4ZZ Release Parathyroid Gland, Percutaneous Endoscopic Approach

0GP – Endocrine System, Removal

Review Coding Guideline B6.1c

0GP000Z Removal of Drainage Device from Pituitary Gland, Open Approach
0GP030Z Removal of Drainage Device from Pituitary Gland, Percutaneous Approach
0GP040Z Removal of Drainage Device from Pituitary Gland, Percutaneous Endoscopic Approach
0GP0X0Z Removal of Drainage Device from Pituitary Gland, External Approach
0GP100Z Removal of Drainage Device from Pineal Body, Open Approach
0GP130Z Removal of Drainage Device from Pineal Body, Percutaneous Approach
0GP140Z Removal of Drainage Device from Pineal Body, Percutaneous Endoscopic Approach
0GP1X0Z Removal of Drainage Device from Pineal Body, External Approach
0GP500Z Removal of Drainage Device from Adrenal Gland, Open Approach
0GP530Z Removal of Drainage Device from Adrenal Gland, Percutaneous Approach
0GP540Z Removal of Drainage Device from Adrenal Gland, Percutaneous Endoscopic Approach
0GP5X0Z Removal of Drainage Device from Adrenal Gland, External Approach
0GPK00Z Removal of Drainage Device from Thyroid Gland, Open Approach

0GPK30Z Removal of Drainage Device from Thyroid Gland, Percutaneous Approach
0GPK40Z Removal of Drainage Device from Thyroid Gland, Percutaneous Endoscopic Approach
0GPKX0Z Removal of Drainage Device from Thyroid Gland, External Approach
0GPR00Z Removal of Drainage Device from Parathyroid Gland, Open Approach
0GPR30Z Removal of Drainage Device from Parathyroid Gland, Percutaneous Approach
0GPR40Z Removal of Drainage Device from Parathyroid Gland, Percutaneous Endoscopic Approach
0GPRX0Z Removal of Drainage Device from Parathyroid Gland, External Approach
0GPS00Z Removal of Drainage Device from Endocrine Gland, Open Approach
0GPS02Z Removal of Monitoring Device from Endocrine Gland, Open Approach
0GPS03Z Removal of Infusion Device from Endocrine Gland, Open Approach
0GPS0YZ Removal of Other Device from Endocrine Gland, Open Approach
0GPS30Z Removal of Drainage Device from Endocrine Gland, Percutaneous Approach

0GPS32Z Removal of Monitoring Device from Endocrine Gland, Percutaneous Approach
0GPS33Z Removal of Infusion Device from Endocrine Gland, Percutaneous Approach
0GPS3YZ Removal of Other Device from Endocrine Gland, Percutaneous Approach
0GPS40Z Removal of Drainage Device from Endocrine Gland, Percutaneous Endoscopic Approach
0GPS42Z Removal of Monitoring Device from Endocrine Gland, Percutaneous Endoscopic Approach
0GPS43Z Removal of Infusion Device from Endocrine Gland, Percutaneous Endoscopic Approach
0GPS4YZ Removal of Other Device from Endocrine Gland, Percutaneous Endoscopic Approach
0GPSX0Z Removal of Drainage Device from Endocrine Gland, External Approach
0GPSX2Z Removal of Monitoring Device from Endocrine Gland, External Approach
0GPSX3Z Removal of Infusion Device from Endocrine Gland, External Approach

0GQ – Endocrine System, Repair

0GQ00ZZ Repair Pituitary Gland, Open Approach
0GQ03ZZ Repair Pituitary Gland, Percutaneous Approach
0GQ04ZZ Repair Pituitary Gland, Percutaneous Endoscopic Approach
0GQ10ZZ Repair Pineal Body, Open Approach

0GQ13ZZ Repair Pineal Body, Percutaneous Approach
0GQ14ZZ Repair Pineal Body, Percutaneous Endoscopic Approach
0GQ20ZZ Repair Left Adrenal Gland, Open Approach

0GQ23ZZ Repair Left Adrenal Gland, Percutaneous Approach
0GQ24ZZ Repair Left Adrenal Gland, Percutaneous Endoscopic Approach
0GQ30ZZ Repair Right Adrenal Gland, Open Approach

0GQ33ZZ Repair Right Adrenal Gland, Percutaneous Approach	**0GQC0ZZ** Repair Glomus Jugulare, Open Approach	**0GQL0ZZ** Repair Right Superior Parathyroid Gland, Open Approach
0GQ34ZZ Repair Right Adrenal Gland, Percutaneous Endoscopic Approach	**0GQC3ZZ** Repair Glomus Jugulare, Percutaneous Approach	**0GQL3ZZ** Repair Right Superior Parathyroid Gland, Percutaneous Approach
0GQ40ZZ Repair Bilateral Adrenal Glands, Open Approach	**0GQC4ZZ** Repair Glomus Jugulare, Percutaneous Endoscopic Approach	**0GQL4ZZ** Repair Right Superior Parathyroid Gland, Percutaneous Endoscopic Approach
0GQ43ZZ Repair Bilateral Adrenal Glands, Percutaneous Approach	**0GQD0ZZ** Repair Aortic Body, Open Approach	**0GQM0ZZ** Repair Left Superior Parathyroid Gland, Open Approach
0GQ44ZZ Repair Bilateral Adrenal Glands, Percutaneous Endoscopic Approach	**0GQD3ZZ** Repair Aortic Body, Percutaneous Approach	**0GQM3ZZ** Repair Left Superior Parathyroid Gland, Percutaneous Approach
0GQ60ZZ Repair Left Carotid Body, Open Approach	**0GQD4ZZ** Repair Aortic Body, Percutaneous Endoscopic Approach	**0GQM4ZZ** Repair Left Superior Parathyroid Gland, Percutaneous Endoscopic Approach
0GQ63ZZ Repair Left Carotid Body, Percutaneous Approach	**0GQF0ZZ** Repair Paraganglion Extremity, Open Approach	**0GQN0ZZ** Repair Right Inferior Parathyroid Gland, Open Approach
0GQ64ZZ Repair Left Carotid Body, Percutaneous Endoscopic Approach	**0GQF3ZZ** Repair Paraganglion Extremity, Percutaneous Approach	**0GQN3ZZ** Repair Right Inferior Parathyroid Gland, Percutaneous Approach
0GQ70ZZ Repair Right Carotid Body, Open Approach	**0GQF4ZZ** Repair Paraganglion Extremity, Percutaneous Endoscopic Approach	**0GQN4ZZ** Repair Right Inferior Parathyroid Gland, Percutaneous Endoscopic Approach
0GQ73ZZ Repair Right Carotid Body, Percutaneous Approach	**0GQG0ZZ** Repair Left Thyroid Gland Lobe, Open Approach	**0GQP0ZZ** Repair Left Inferior Parathyroid Gland, Open Approach
0GQ74ZZ Repair Right Carotid Body, Percutaneous Endoscopic Approach	**0GQG3ZZ** Repair Left Thyroid Gland Lobe, Percutaneous Approach	**0GQP3ZZ** Repair Left Inferior Parathyroid Gland, Percutaneous Approach
0GQ80ZZ Repair Bilateral Carotid Bodies, Open Approach	**0GQG4ZZ** Repair Left Thyroid Gland Lobe, Percutaneous Endoscopic Approach	**0GQP4ZZ** Repair Left Inferior Parathyroid Gland, Percutaneous Endoscopic Approach
0GQ83ZZ Repair Bilateral Carotid Bodies, Percutaneous Approach	**0GQH0ZZ** Repair Right Thyroid Gland Lobe, Open Approach	**0GQQ0ZZ** Repair Multiple Parathyroid Glands, Open Approach
0GQ84ZZ Repair Bilateral Carotid Bodies, Percutaneous Endoscopic Approach	**0GQH3ZZ** Repair Right Thyroid Gland Lobe, Percutaneous Approach	**0GQQ3ZZ** Repair Multiple Parathyroid Glands, Percutaneous Approach
0GQ90ZZ Repair Para-aortic Body, Open Approach	**0GQH4ZZ** Repair Right Thyroid Gland Lobe, Percutaneous Endoscopic Approach	**0GQQ4ZZ** Repair Multiple Parathyroid Glands, Percutaneous Endoscopic Approach
0GQ93ZZ Repair Para-aortic Body, Percutaneous Approach	**0GQJ0ZZ** Repair Thyroid Gland Isthmus, Open Approach	**0GQR0ZZ** Repair Parathyroid Gland, Open Approach
0GQ94ZZ Repair Para-aortic Body, Percutaneous Endoscopic Approach	**0GQJ3ZZ** Repair Thyroid Gland Isthmus, Percutaneous Approach	**0GQR3ZZ** Repair Parathyroid Gland, Percutaneous Approach
0GQB0ZZ Repair Coccygeal Glomus, Open Approach	**0GQJ4ZZ** Repair Thyroid Gland Isthmus, Percutaneous Endoscopic Approach	**0GQR4ZZ** Repair Parathyroid Gland, Percutaneous Endoscopic Approach
0GQB3ZZ Repair Coccygeal Glomus, Percutaneous Approach	**0GQK0ZZ** Repair Thyroid Gland, Open Approach	
0GQB4ZZ Repair Coccygeal Glomus, Percutaneous Endoscopic Approach	**0GQK3ZZ** Repair Thyroid Gland, Percutaneous Approach	
	0GQK4ZZ Repair Thyroid Gland, Percutaneous Endoscopic Approach	

0GS – Endocrine System, Reposition

0GS20ZZ Reposition Left Adrenal Gland, Open Approach	**0GSL0ZZ** Reposition Right Superior Parathyroid Gland, Open Approach	**0GSP4ZZ** Reposition Left Inferior Parathyroid Gland, Percutaneous Endoscopic Approach
0GS24ZZ Reposition Left Adrenal Gland, Percutaneous Endoscopic Approach	**0GSL4ZZ** Reposition Right Superior Parathyroid Gland, Percutaneous Endoscopic Approach	**0GSQ0ZZ** Reposition Multiple Parathyroid Glands, Open Approach
0GS30ZZ Reposition Right Adrenal Gland, Open Approach	**0GSM0ZZ** Reposition Left Superior Parathyroid Gland, Open Approach	**0GSQ4ZZ** Reposition Multiple Parathyroid Glands, Percutaneous Endoscopic Approach
0GS34ZZ Reposition Right Adrenal Gland, Percutaneous Endoscopic Approach	**0GSM4ZZ** Reposition Left Superior Parathyroid Gland, Percutaneous Endoscopic Approach	**0GSR0ZZ** Reposition Parathyroid Gland, Open Approach
0GSG0ZZ Reposition Left Thyroid Gland Lobe, Open Approach	**0GSN0ZZ** Reposition Right Inferior Parathyroid Gland, Open Approach	**0GSR4ZZ** Reposition Parathyroid Gland, Percutaneous Endoscopic Approach
0GSG4ZZ Reposition Left Thyroid Gland Lobe, Percutaneous Endoscopic Approach	**0GSN4ZZ** Reposition Right Inferior Parathyroid Gland, Percutaneous Endoscopic Approach	
0GSH0ZZ Reposition Right Thyroid Gland Lobe, Open Approach	**0GSP0ZZ** Reposition Left Inferior Parathyroid Gland, Open Approach	
0GSH4ZZ Reposition Right Thyroid Gland Lobe, Percutaneous Endoscopic Approach		

0GT – Endocrine System, Resection

Review Coding Guideline B3.8

Review Coding Guideline B3.18

0GT00ZZ Resection of Pituitary Gland, Open Approach	**0GT20ZZ** Resection of Left Adrenal Gland, Open Approach	**0GT40ZZ** Resection of Bilateral Adrenal Glands, Open Approach
0GT04ZZ Resection of Pituitary Gland, Percutaneous Endoscopic Approach	**0GT24ZZ** Resection of Left Adrenal Gland, Percutaneous Endoscopic Approach	**0GT44ZZ** Resection of Bilateral Adrenal Glands, Percutaneous Endoscopic Approach
0GT10ZZ Resection of Pineal Body, Open Approach	**0GT30ZZ** Resection of Right Adrenal Gland, Open Approach	**0GT60ZZ** Resection of Left Carotid Body, Open Approach
0GT14ZZ Resection of Pineal Body, Percutaneous Endoscopic Approach	**0GT34ZZ** Resection of Right Adrenal Gland, Percutaneous Endoscopic Approach	**0GT64ZZ** Resection of Left Carotid Body, Percutaneous Endoscopic Approach

0GT70ZZ	Resection of Right Carotid Body, Open Approach
0GT74ZZ	Resection of Right Carotid Body, Percutaneous Endoscopic Approach
0GT80ZZ	Resection of Bilateral Carotid Bodies, Open Approach
0GT84ZZ	Resection of Bilateral Carotid Bodies, Percutaneous Endoscopic Approach
0GT90ZZ	Resection of Para-aortic Body, Open Approach
0GT94ZZ	Resection of Para-aortic Body, Percutaneous Endoscopic Approach
0GTB0ZZ	Resection of Coccygeal Glomus, Open Approach
0GTB4ZZ	Resection of Coccygeal Glomus, Percutaneous Endoscopic Approach
0GTC0ZZ	Resection of Glomus Jugulare, Open Approach
0GTC4ZZ	Resection of Glomus Jugulare, Percutaneous Endoscopic Approach
0GTD0ZZ	Resection of Aortic Body, Open Approach
0GTD4ZZ	Resection of Aortic Body, Percutaneous Endoscopic Approach
0GTF0ZZ	Resection of Paraganglion Extremity, Open Approach

0GTF4ZZ	Resection of Paraganglion Extremity, Percutaneous Endoscopic Approach
0GTG0ZZ	Resection of Left Thyroid Gland Lobe, Open Approach
0GTG4ZZ	Resection of Left Thyroid Gland Lobe, Percutaneous Endoscopic Approach
0GTH0ZZ	Resection of Right Thyroid Gland Lobe, Open Approach
0GTH4ZZ	Resection of Right Thyroid Gland Lobe, Percutaneous Endoscopic Approach
0GTJ0ZZ	Resection of Thyroid Gland Isthmus, Open Approach
0GTJ4ZZ	Resection of Thyroid Gland Isthmus, Percutaneous Endoscopic Approach
0GTK0ZZ	Resection of Thyroid Gland, Open Approach
0GTK4ZZ	Resection of Thyroid Gland, Percutaneous Endoscopic Approach
0GTL0ZZ	Resection of Right Superior Parathyroid Gland, Open Approach
0GTL4ZZ	Resection of Right Superior Parathyroid Gland, Percutaneous Endoscopic Approach

0GTM0ZZ	Resection of Left Superior Parathyroid Gland, Open Approach
0GTM4ZZ	Resection of Left Superior Parathyroid Gland, Percutaneous Endoscopic Approach
0GTN0ZZ	Resection of Right Inferior Parathyroid Gland, Open Approach
0GTN4ZZ	Resection of Right Inferior Parathyroid Gland, Percutaneous Endoscopic Approach
0GTP0ZZ	Resection of Left Inferior Parathyroid Gland, Open Approach
0GTP4ZZ	Resection of Left Inferior Parathyroid Gland, Percutaneous Endoscopic Approach
0GTQ0ZZ	Resection of Multiple Parathyroid Glands, Open Approach
0GTQ4ZZ	Resection of Multiple Parathyroid Glands, Percutaneous Endoscopic Approach
0GTR0ZZ	Resection of Parathyroid Gland, Open Approach
0GTR4ZZ	Resection of Parathyroid Gland, Percutaneous Endoscopic Approach

0GW – Endocrine System, Revision

Review Coding Guideline B6.1c

0GW000Z	Revision of Drainage Device in Pituitary Gland, Open Approach
0GW030Z	Revision of Drainage Device in Pituitary Gland, Percutaneous Approach
0GW040Z	Revision of Drainage Device in Pituitary Gland, Percutaneous Endoscopic Approach
0GW0X0Z	Revision of Drainage Device in Pituitary Gland, External Approach
0GW100Z	Revision of Drainage Device in Pineal Body, Open Approach
0GW130Z	Revision of Drainage Device in Pineal Body, Percutaneous Approach
0GW140Z	Revision of Drainage Device in Pineal Body, Percutaneous Endoscopic Approach
0GW1X0Z	Revision of Drainage Device in Pineal Body, External Approach
0GW500Z	Revision of Drainage Device in Adrenal Gland, Open Approach
0GW530Z	Revision of Drainage Device in Adrenal Gland, Percutaneous Approach
0GW540Z	Revision of Drainage Device in Adrenal Gland, Percutaneous Endoscopic Approach
0GW5X0Z	Revision of Drainage Device in Adrenal Gland, External Approach

0GWK00Z	Revision of Drainage Device in Thyroid Gland, Open Approach
0GWK30Z	Revision of Drainage Device in Thyroid Gland, Percutaneous Approach
0GWK40Z	Revision of Drainage Device in Thyroid Gland, Percutaneous Endoscopic Approach
0GWKX0Z	Revision of Drainage Device in Thyroid Gland, External Approach
0GWR00Z	Revision of Drainage Device in Parathyroid Gland, Open Approach
0GWR30Z	Revision of Drainage Device in Parathyroid Gland, Percutaneous Approach
0GWR40Z	Revision of Drainage Device in Parathyroid Gland, Percutaneous Endoscopic Approach
0GWRX0Z	Revision of Drainage Device in Parathyroid Gland, External Approach
0GWS00Z	Revision of Drainage Device in Endocrine Gland, Open Approach
0GWS02Z	Revision of Monitoring Device in Endocrine Gland, Open Approach
0GWS03Z	Revision of Infusion Device in Endocrine Gland, Open Approach
0GWS0YZ	Revision of Other Device in Endocrine Gland, Open Approach

0GWS30Z	Revision of Drainage Device in Endocrine Gland, Percutaneous Approach
0GWS32Z	Revision of Monitoring Device in Endocrine Gland, Percutaneous Approach
0GWS33Z	Revision of Infusion Device in Endocrine Gland, Percutaneous Approach
0GWS3YZ	Revision of Other Device in Endocrine Gland, Percutaneous Approach
0GWS40Z	Revision of Drainage Device in Endocrine Gland, Percutaneous Endoscopic Approach
0GWS42Z	Revision of Monitoring Device in Endocrine Gland, Percutaneous Endoscopic Approach
0GWS43Z	Revision of Infusion Device in Endocrine Gland, Percutaneous Endoscopic Approach
0GWS4YZ	Revision of Other Device in Endocrine Gland, Percutaneous Endoscopic Approach
0GWSX0Z	Revision of Drainage Device in Endocrine Gland, External Approach
0GWSX2Z	Revision of Monitoring Device in Endocrine Gland, External Approach
0GWSX3Z	Revision of Infusion Device in Endocrine Gland, External Approach

Cross-Section of the Skin Showing Layers and Types of Infections

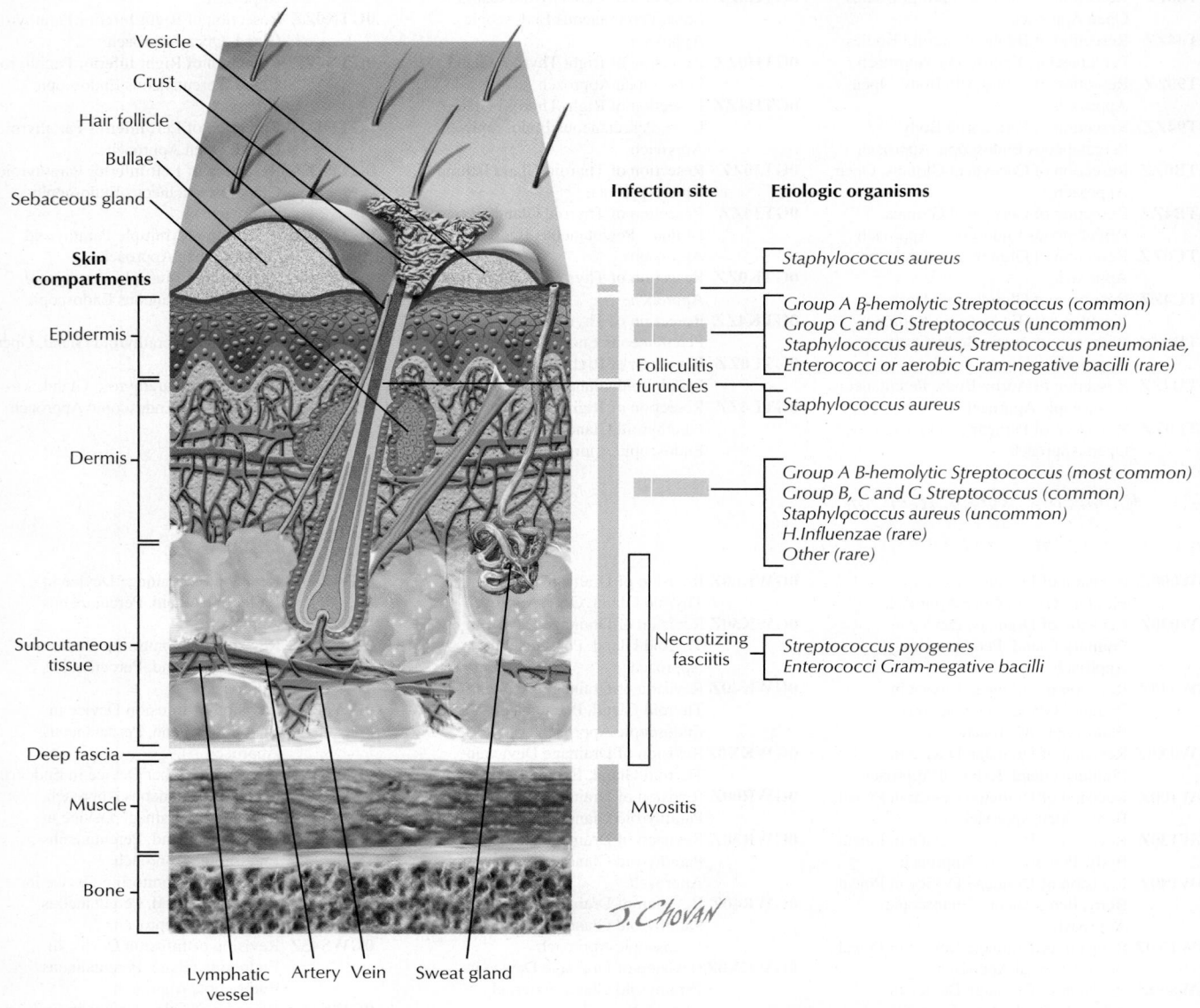

Vesicle
Crust
Hair follicle
Bullae
Sebaceous gland

Skin compartments

Epidermis

Dermis

Subcutaneous tissue

Deep fascia

Muscle

Bone

Lymphatic vessel   Artery Vein   Sweat gland

Infection site   **Etiologic organisms**

Staphylococcus aureus

Group A β-hemolytic Streptococcus (common)
Group C and G Streptococcus (uncommon)
Staphylococcus aureus, Streptococcus pneumoniae,
Enterococci or aerobic Gram-negative bacilli (rare)

Folliculitis
furuncles   *Staphylococcus aureus*

Group A B-hemolytic Streptococcus (most common)
Group B, C and G Streptococcus (common)
Staphylococcus aureus (uncommon)
H.Influenzae (rare)
Other (rare)

Necrotizing
fasciitis   *Streptococcus pyogenes*
Enterococci Gram-negative bacilli

Myositis

J. Chovan

Breast

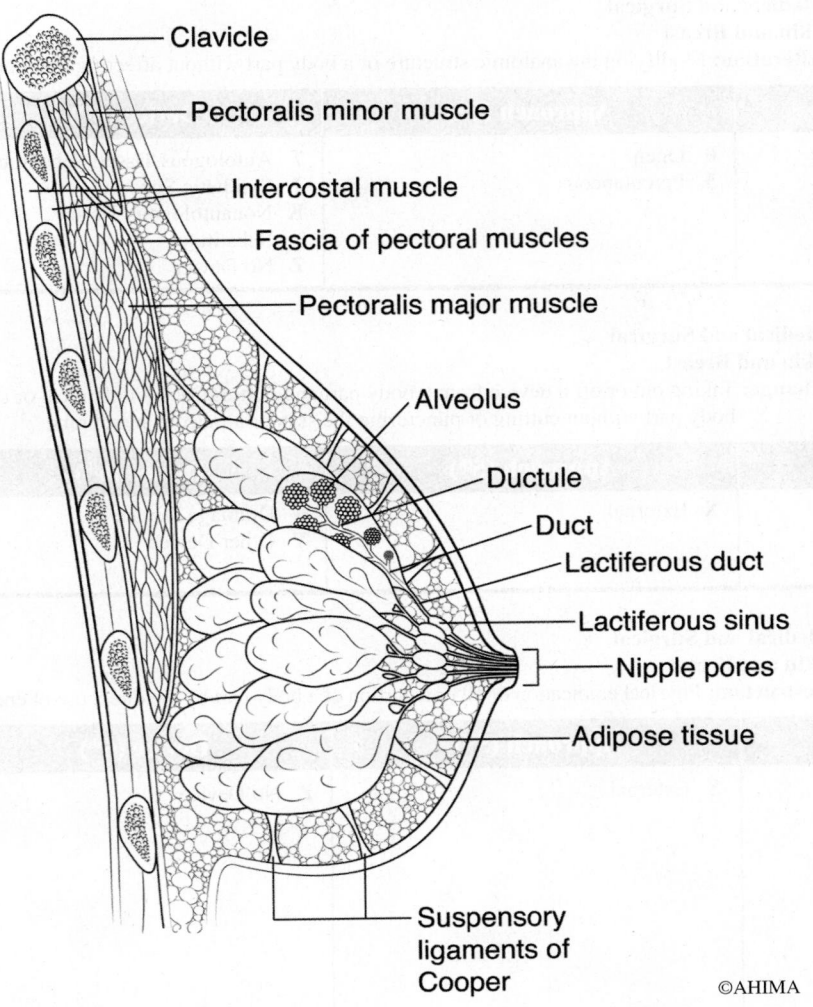

- Clavicle
- Pectoralis minor muscle
- Intercostal muscle
- Fascia of pectoral muscles
- Pectoralis major muscle
- Alveolus
- Ductule
- Duct
- Lactiferous duct
- Lactiferous sinus
- Nipple pores
- Adipose tissue
- Suspensory ligaments of Cooper

©AHIMA

Nail Bed

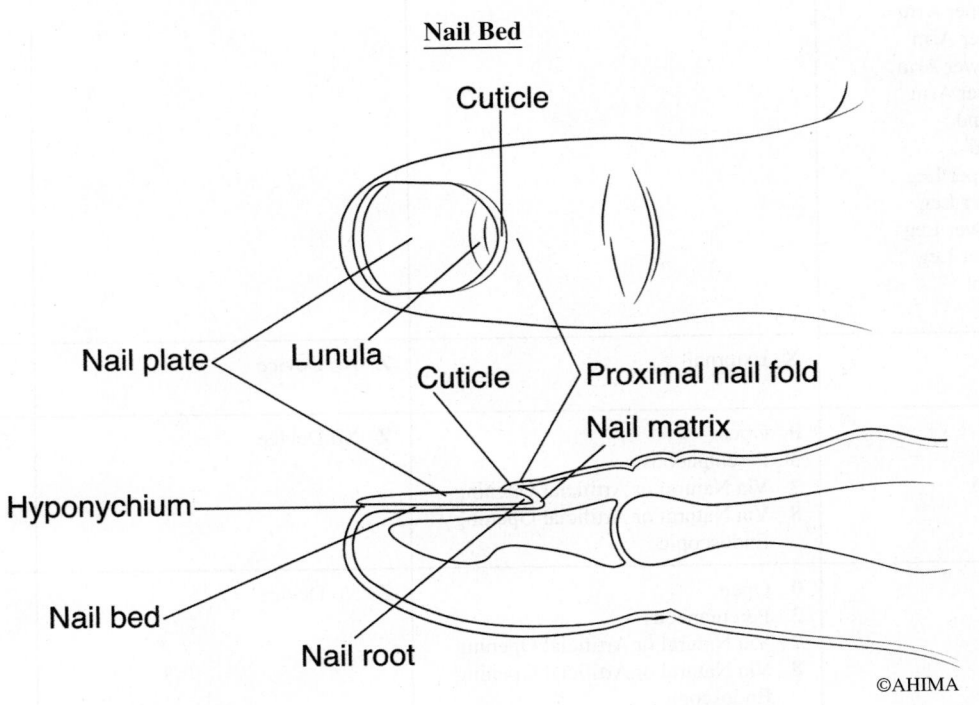

- Cuticle
- Nail plate
- Lunula
- Cuticle
- Proximal nail fold
- Nail matrix
- Hyponychium
- Nail bed
- Nail root

©AHIMA

Skin and Breast Tables 0H0–0HX

Section	0	Medical and Surgical
Body System	H	Skin and Breast
Operation	0	**Alteration:** Modifying the anatomic structure of a body part without affecting the function of the body part

Body Part (4th)	Approach (5th)	Device (6th)	Qualifier (7th)
T Breast, Right U Breast, Left V Breast, Bilateral	0 Open 3 Percutaneous	7 Autologous Tissue Substitute J Synthetic Substitute K Nonautologous Tissue Substitute Z No Device	Z No Qualifier

Section	0	Medical and Surgical
Body System	H	Skin and Breast
Operation	2	**Change:** Taking out or off a device from a body part and putting back an identical or similar device in or on the same body part without cutting or puncturing the skin or a mucous membrane

Body Part (4th)	Approach (5th)	Device (6th)	Qualifier (7th)
P Skin T Breast, Right U Breast, Left	X External	0 Drainage Device Y Other Device	Z No Qualifier

Section	0	Medical and Surgical
Body System	H	Skin and Breast
Operation	5	**Destruction:** Physical eradication of all or a portion of a body part by the direct use of energy, force, or a destructive agent

Body Part (4th)	Approach (5th)	Device (6th)	Qualifier (7th)
0 Skin, Scalp 1 Skin, Face 2 Skin, Right Ear 3 Skin, Left Ear 4 Skin, Neck 5 Skin, Chest 6 Skin, Back 7 Skin, Abdomen 8 Skin, Buttock 9 Skin, Perineum A Skin, Inguinal B Skin, Right Upper Arm C Skin, Left Upper Arm D Skin, Right Lower Arm E Skin, Left Lower Arm F Skin, Right Hand G Skin, Left Hand H Skin, Right Upper Leg J Skin, Left Upper Leg K Skin, Right Lower Leg L Skin, Left Lower Leg M Skin, Right Foot N Skin, Left Foot	X External	Z No Device	D Multiple Z No Qualifier
Q Finger Nail R Toe Nail	X External	Z No Device	Z No Qualifier
T Breast, Right U Breast, Left V Breast, Bilateral	0 Open 3 Percutaneous 7 Via Natural or Artificial Opening 8 Via Natural or Artificial Opening Endoscopic	Z No Device	Z No Qualifier
W Nipple, Right X Nipple, Left	0 Open 3 Percutaneous 7 Via Natural or Artificial Opening 8 Via Natural or Artificial Opening Endoscopic X External	Z No Device	Z No Qualifier

Section	0	Medical and Surgical
Body System	H	Skin and Breast
Operation	8	Division: Cutting into a body part, without draining fluids and/or gases from the body part, in order to separate or transect a body part

Body Part (4th)	Approach (5th)	Device (6th)	Qualifier (7th)
0 Skin, Scalp	X External	Z No Device	Z No Qualifier
1 Skin, Face			
2 Skin, Right Ear			
3 Skin, Left Ear			
4 Skin, Neck			
5 Skin, Chest			
6 Skin, Back			
7 Skin, Abdomen			
8 Skin, Buttock			
9 Skin, Perineum			
A Skin, Inguinal			
B Skin, Right Upper Arm			
C Skin, Left Upper Arm			
D Skin, Right Lower Arm			
E Skin, Left Lower Arm			
F Skin, Right Hand			
G Skin, Left Hand			
H Skin, Right Upper Leg			
J Skin, Left Upper Leg			
K Skin, Right Lower Leg			
L Skin, Left Lower Leg			
M Skin, Right Foot			
N Skin, Left Foot			

Section	0	Medical and Surgical
Body System	H	Skin and Breast
Operation	9	Drainage: Taking or letting out fluids and/or gases from a body part

Body Part (4th)	Approach (5th)	Device (6th)	Qualifier (7th)
0 Skin, Scalp	X External	0 Drainage Device	Z No Qualifier
1 Skin, Face			
2 Skin, Right Ear			
3 Skin, Left Ear			
4 Skin, Neck			
5 Skin, Chest			
6 Skin, Back			
7 Skin, Abdomen			
8 Skin, Buttock			
9 Skin, Perineum			
A Skin, Inguinal			
B Skin, Right Upper Arm			
C Skin, Left Upper Arm			
D Skin, Right Lower Arm			
E Skin, Left Lower Arm			
F Skin, Right Hand			
G Skin, Left Hand			
H Skin, Right Upper Leg			
J Skin, Left Upper Leg			
K Skin, Right Lower Leg			
L Skin, Left Lower Leg			
M Skin, Right Foot			
N Skin, Left Foot			
Q Finger Nail			
R Toe Nail			

Continued →

Section   0   **Medical and Surgical**
Body System   H   **Skin and Breast**
Operation   9   **Drainage:** Taking or letting out fluids and/or gases from a body part

Body Part (4th)	Approach (5th)	Device (6th)	Qualifier (7th)
0 Skin, Scalp 1 Skin, Face 2 Skin, Right Ear 3 Skin, Left Ear 4 Skin, Neck 5 Skin, Chest 6 Skin, Back 7 Skin, Abdomen 8 Skin, Buttock 9 Skin, Perineum A Skin, Inguinal B Skin, Right Upper Arm C Skin, Left Upper Arm D Skin, Right Lower Arm E Skin, Left Lower Arm F Skin, Right Hand G Skin, Left Hand H Skin, Right Upper Leg J Skin, Left Upper Leg K Skin, Right Lower Leg L Skin, Left Lower Leg M Skin, Right Foot N Skin, Left Foot Q Finger Nail R Toe Nail	X External	Z No Device	X Diagnostic Z No Qualifier
T Breast, Right U Breast, Left V Breast, Bilateral	0 Open 3 Percutaneous 7 Via Natural or Artificial Opening 8 Via Natural or Artificial Opening Endoscopic	0 Drainage Device	Z No Qualifier
T Breast, Right U Breast, Left V Breast, Bilateral	0 Open 3 Percutaneous 7 Via Natural or Artificial Opening 8 Via Natural or Artificial Opening Endoscopic	Z No Device	X Diagnostic Z No Qualifier
W Nipple, Right X Nipple, Left	0 Open 3 Percutaneous 7 Via Natural or Artificial Opening 8 Via Natural or Artificial Opening Endoscopic X External	0 Drainage Device	Z No Qualifier
W Nipple, Right X Nipple, Left	0 Open 3 Percutaneous 7 Via Natural or Artificial Opening 8 Via Natural or Artificial Opening Endoscopic X External	Z No Device	X Diagnostic Z No Qualifier

Section   **0**   **Medical and Surgical**
Body System   **H**   **Skin and Breast**
Operation   **B**   **Excision:** Cutting out or off, without replacement, a portion of a body part

Body Part (4th)	Approach (5th)	Device (6th)	Qualifier (7th)
0 Skin, Scalp **1** Skin, Face **2** Skin, Right Ear **3** Skin, Left Ear **4** Skin, Neck **5** Skin, Chest **6** Skin, Back **7** Skin, Abdomen **8** Skin, Buttock **9** Skin, Perineum **A** Skin, Inguinal **B** Skin, Right Upper Arm **C** Skin, Left Upper Arm **D** Skin, Right Lower Arm **E** Skin, Left Lower Arm **F** Skin, Right Hand **G** Skin, Left Hand **H** Skin, Right Upper Leg **J** Skin, Left Upper Leg **K** Skin, Right Lower Leg **L** Skin, Left Lower Leg **M** Skin, Right Foot **N** Skin, Left Foot **Q** Finger Nail **R** Toe Nail	**X** External	**Z** No Device	**X** Diagnostic **Z** No Qualifier
T Breast, Right **U** Breast, Left **V** Breast, Bilateral **Y** Supernumerary Breast	**0** Open **3** Percutaneous **7** Via Natural or Artificial Opening **8** Via Natural or Artificial Opening Endoscopic	**Z** No Device	**X** Diagnostic **Z** No Qualifier
W Nipple, Right **X** Nipple, Left	**0** Open **3** Percutaneous **7** Via Natural or Artificial Opening **8** Via Natural or Artificial Opening Endoscopic **X** External	**Z** No Device	**X** Diagnostic **Z** No Qualifier

Section   **0**   **Medical and Surgical**
Body System   **H**   **Skin and Breast**
Operation   **C**   **Extirpation:** Taking or cutting out solid matter from a body part

Body Part (4th)	Approach (5th)	Device (6th)	Qualifier (7th)
0 Skin, Scalp **1** Skin, Face **2** Skin, Right Ear **3** Skin, Left Ear **4** Skin, Neck **5** Skin, Chest **6** Skin, Back **7** Skin, Abdomen **8** Skin, Buttock **9** Skin, Perineum **A** Skin, Inguinal **B** Skin, Right Upper Arm **C** Skin, Left Upper Arm **D** Skin, Right Lower Arm **E** Skin, Left Lower Arm **F** Skin, Right Hand **G** Skin, Left Hand **H** Skin, Right Upper Leg **J** Skin, Left Upper Leg **K** Skin, Right Lower Leg **L** Skin, Left Lower Leg **M** Skin, Right Foot **N** Skin, Left Foot **Q** Finger Nail **R** Toe Nail	**X** External	**Z** No Device	**Z** No Qualifier
T Breast, Right **U** Breast, Left **V** Breast, Bilateral	**0** Open **3** Percutaneous **7** Via Natural or Artificial Opening **8** Via Natural or Artificial Opening Endoscopic	**Z** No Device	**Z** No Qualifier
W Nipple, Right **X** Nipple, Left	**0** Open **3** Percutaneous **7** Via Natural or Artificial Opening **8** Via Natural or Artificial Opening Endoscopic **X** External	**Z** No Device	**Z** No Qualifier

Section   **0**   **Medical and Surgical**
Body System   **H**   **Skin and Breast**
Operation   **D**   **Extraction:** Pulling or stripping out or off all or a portion of a body part by the use of force

Body Part (4th)	Approach (5th)	Device (6th)	Qualifier (7th)
0 Skin, Scalp **1** Skin, Face **2** Skin, Right Ear **3** Skin, Left Ear **4** Skin, Neck **5** Skin, Chest **6** Skin, Back **7** Skin, Abdomen **8** Skin, Buttock **9** Skin, Perineum **A** Skin, Inguinal **B** Skin, Right Upper Arm **C** Skin, Left Upper Arm **D** Skin, Right Lower Arm **E** Skin, Left Lower Arm **F** Skin, Right Hand **G** Skin, Left Hand **H** Skin, Right Upper Leg **J** Skin, Left Upper Leg **K** Skin, Right Lower Leg **L** Skin, Left Lower Leg **M** Skin, Right Foot **N** Skin, Left Foot **Q** Finger Nail **R** Toe Nail **S** Hair	**X** External	**Z** No Device	**Z** No Qualifier
T Breast, Right **U** Breast, Left **V** Breast, Bilateral **Y** Supernumerary Breast	**0** Open	**Z** No Device	**Z** No Qualifier

Section   **0**   **Medical and Surgical**
Body System   **H**   **Skin and Breast**
Operation   **H**   **Insertion:** Putting in a nonbiological appliance that monitors, assists, performs, or prevents a physiological function but does not physically take the place of a body part

Body Part (4th)	Approach (5th)	Device (6th)	Qualifier (7th)
P Skin	**X** External	**Y** Other Device	**Z** No Qualifier
T Breast, Right **U** Breast, Left	**0** Open **3** Percutaneous **7** Via Natural or Artificial Opening **8** Via Natural or Artificial Opening Endoscopic	**1** Radioactive Element **N** Tissue Expander **Y** Other Device	**Z** No Qualifier
V Breast, Bilateral	**0** Open **3** Percutaneous **7** Via Natural or Artificial Opening **8** Via Natural or Artificial Opening Endoscopic	**1** Radioactive Element **N** Tissue Expander	**Z** No Qualifier
W Nipple, Right **X** Nipple, Left	**0** Open **3** Percutaneous **7** Via Natural or Artificial Opening **8** Via Natural or Artificial Opening Endoscopic	**1** Radioactive Element **N** Tissue Expander	**Z** No Qualifier
W Nipple, Right **X** Nipple, Left	**X** External	**1** Radioactive Element	**Z** No Qualifier

Section	0	Medical and Surgical
Body System	H	Skin and Breast
Operation	J	Inspection: Visually and/or manually exploring a body part

Body Part (4th)	Approach (5th)	Device (6th)	Qualifier (7th)
P Skin Q Finger Nail R Toe Nail	X External	Z No Device	Z No Qualifier
T Breast, Right U Breast, Left	0 Open 3 Percutaneous 7 Via Natural or Artificial Opening 8 Via Natural or Artificial Opening Endoscopic	Z No Device	Z No Qualifier

Section	0	Medical and Surgical
Body System	H	Skin and Breast
Operation	M	Reattachment: Putting back in or on all or a portion of a separated body part to its normal location or other suitable location

Body Part (4th)	Approach (5th)	Device (6th)	Qualifier (7th)
0 Skin, Scalp 1 Skin, Face 2 Skin, Right Ear 3 Skin, Left Ear 4 Skin, Neck 5 Skin, Chest 6 Skin, Back 7 Skin, Abdomen 8 Skin, Buttock 9 Skin, Perineum A Skin, Inguinal B Skin, Right Upper Arm C Skin, Left Upper Arm D Skin, Right Lower Arm E Skin, Left Lower Arm F Skin, Right Hand G Skin, Left Hand H Skin, Right Upper Leg J Skin, Left Upper Leg K Skin, Right Lower Leg L Skin, Left Lower Leg M Skin, Right Foot N Skin, Left Foot T Breast, Right U Breast, Left V Breast, Bilateral W Nipple, Right X Nipple, Left	X External	Z No Device	Z No Qualifier

Section | 0 | Medical and Surgical
Body System | H | Skin and Breast
Operation | N | Release: Freeing a body part from an abnormal physical constraint by cutting or by the use of force

Body Part (4th)	Approach (5th)	Device (6th)	Qualifier (7th)
0 Skin, Scalp 1 Skin, Face 2 Skin, Right Ear 3 Skin, Left Ear 4 Skin, Neck 5 Skin, Chest 6 Skin, Back 7 Skin, Abdomen 8 Skin, Buttock 9 Skin, Perineum A Skin, Inguinal B Skin, Right Upper Arm C Skin, Left Upper Arm D Skin, Right Lower Arm E Skin, Left Lower Arm F Skin, Right Hand G Skin, Left Hand H Skin, Right Upper Leg J Skin, Left Upper Leg K Skin, Right Lower Leg L Skin, Left Lower Leg M Skin, Right Foot N Skin, Left Foot Q Finger Nail R Toe Nail	X External	Z No Device	Z No Qualifier
T Breast, Right U Breast, Left V Breast, Bilateral	0 Open 3 Percutaneous 7 Via Natural or Artificial Opening 8 Via Natural or Artificial Opening Endoscopic	Z No Device	Z No Qualifier
W Nipple, Right X Nipple, Left	0 Open 3 Percutaneous 7 Via Natural or Artificial Opening 8 Via Natural or Artificial Opening Endoscopic X External	Z No Device	Z No Qualifier

Section | 0 | Medical and Surgical
Body System | H | Skin and Breast
Operation | P | Removal: Taking out or off a device from a body part

Body Part (4th)	Approach (5th)	Device (6th)	Qualifier (7th)
P Skin	X External	0 Drainage Device 7 Autologous Tissue Substitute J Synthetic Substitute K Nonautologous Tissue Substitute Y Other Device	Z No Qualifier
Q Finger Nail R Toe Nail	X External	0 Drainage Device 7 Autologous Tissue Substitute J Synthetic Substitute K Nonautologous Tissue Substitute	Z No Qualifier
S Hair	X External	7 Autologous Tissue Substitute J Synthetic Substitute K Nonautologous Tissue Substitute	Z No Qualifier
T Breast, Right U Breast, Left	0 Open 3 Percutaneous 7 Via Natural or Artificial Opening 8 Via Natural or Artificial Opening Endoscopic	0 Drainage Device 1 Radioactive Element 7 Autologous Tissue Substitute J Synthetic Substitute K Nonautologous Tissue Substitute N Tissue Expander Y Other Device	Z No Qualifier

Section	0	Medical and Surgical
Body System	H	Skin and Breast
Operation	Q	**Repair:** Restoring, to the extent possible, a body part to its normal anatomic structure and function

Body Part (4th)	Approach (5th)	Device (6th)	Qualifier (7th)
0 Skin, Scalp 1 Skin, Face 2 Skin, Right Ear 3 Skin, Left Ear 4 Skin, Neck 5 Skin, Chest 6 Skin, Back 7 Skin, Abdomen 8 Skin, Buttock 9 Skin, Perineum A Skin, Inguinal B Skin, Right Upper Arm C Skin, Left Upper Arm D Skin, Right Lower Arm E Skin, Left Lower Arm F Skin, Right Hand G Skin, Left Hand H Skin, Right Upper Leg J Skin, Left Upper Leg K Skin, Right Lower Leg L Skin, Left Lower Leg M Skin, Right Foot N Skin, Left Foot Q Finger Nail R Toe Nail	X External	Z No Device	Z No Qualifier
T Breast, Right U Breast, Left V Breast, Bilateral Y Supernumerary Breast	0 Open 3 Percutaneous 7 Via Natural or Artificial Opening 8 Via Natural or Artificial Opening Endoscopic	Z No Device	Z No Qualifier
W Nipple, Right X Nipple, Left	0 Open 3 Percutaneous 7 Via Natural or Artificial Opening 8 Via Natural or Artificial Opening Endoscopic X External	Z No Device	Z No Qualifier

Section   **0**   **Medical and Surgical**
Body System   **H**   **Skin and Breast**
Operation   **R**   **Replacement:** Putting in or on biological or synthetic material that physically takes the place and/or function of all or a portion of a body part

Body Part (4th)	Approach (5th)	Device (6th)	Qualifier (7th)
0 Skin, Scalp **1** Skin, Face **2** Skin, Right Ear **3** Skin, Left Ear **4** Skin, Neck **5** Skin, Chest **6** Skin, Back **7** Skin, Abdomen **8** Skin, Buttock **9** Skin, Perineum **A** Skin, Inguinal **B** Skin, Right Upper Arm **C** Skin, Left Upper Arm **D** Skin, Right Lower Arm **E** Skin, Left Lower Arm **F** Skin, Right Hand **G** Skin, Left Hand **H** Skin, Right Upper Leg **J** Skin, Left Upper Leg **K** Skin, Right Lower Leg **L** Skin, Left Lower Leg **M** Skin, Right Foot **N** Skin, Left Foot	**X** External	**7** Autologous Tissue Substitute	**2** Cell Suspension Technique **3** Full Thickness **4** Partial Thickness
0 Skin, Scalp **1** Skin, Face **2** Skin, Right Ear **3** Skin, Left Ear **4** Skin, Neck **5** Skin, Chest **6** Skin, Back **7** Skin, Abdomen **8** Skin, Buttock **9** Skin, Perineum **A** Skin, Inguinal **B** Skin, Right Upper Arm **C** Skin, Left Upper Arm **D** Skin, Right Lower Arm **E** Skin, Left Lower Arm **F** Skin, Right Hand **G** Skin, Left Hand **H** Skin, Right Upper Leg **J** Skin, Left Upper Leg **K** Skin, Right Lower Leg **L** Skin, Left Lower Leg **M** Skin, Right Foot **N** Skin, Left Foot	**X** External	**J** Synthetic Substitute	**3** Full Thickness **4** Partial Thickness **Z** No Qualifier

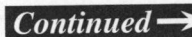

Continued →

Section	0	Medical and Surgical	
Body System	H	Skin and Breast	
Operation	R	Replacement: Putting in or on biological or synthetic material that physically takes the place and/or function of all or a portion of a body part	

Body Part (4th)	Approach (5th)	Device (6th)	Qualifier (7th)
0 Skin, Scalp 1 Skin, Face 2 Skin, Right Ear 3 Skin, Left Ear 4 Skin, Neck 5 Skin, Chest 6 Skin, Back 7 Skin, Abdomen 8 Skin, Buttock 9 Skin, Perineum A Skin, Inguinal B Skin, Right Upper Arm C Skin, Left Upper Arm D Skin, Right Lower Arm E Skin, Left Lower Arm F Skin, Right Hand G Skin, Left Hand H Skin, Right Upper Leg J Skin, Left Upper Leg K Skin, Right Lower Leg L Skin, Left Lower Leg M Skin, Right Foot N Skin, Left Foot	X External	K Nonautologous Tissue Substitute	3 Full Thickness 4 Partial Thickness
Q Finger Nail R Toe Nail S Hair	X External	7 Autologous Tissue Substitute J Synthetic Substitute K Nonautologous Tissue Substitute	Z No Qualifier
T Breast, Right U Breast, Left V Breast, Bilateral	0 Open	7 Autologous Tissue Substitute	5 Latissimus Dorsi Myocutaneous Flap 6 Transverse Rectus Abdominis Myocutaneous Flap 7 Deep Inferior Epigastric Artery Perforator Flap 8 Superficial Inferior Epigastric Artery Flap 9 Gluteal Artery Perforator Flap Z No Qualifier
T Breast, Right U Breast, Left V Breast, Bilateral	0 Open	J Synthetic Substitute K Nonautologous Tissue Substitute	Z No Qualifier
T Breast, Right U Breast, Left V Breast, Bilateral	3 Percutaneous	7 Autologous Tissue Substitute J Synthetic Substitute K Nonautologous Tissue Substitute	Z No Qualifier
W Nipple, Right X Nipple, Left	0 Open 3 Percutaneous X External	7 Autologous Tissue Substitute J Synthetic Substitute K Nonautologous Tissue Substitute	Z No Qualifier

Section	0	Medical and Surgical	
Body System	H	Skin and Breast	
Operation	S	Reposition: Moving to its normal location, or other suitable location, all or a portion of a body part	

Body Part (4th)	Approach (5th)	Device (6th)	Qualifier (7th)
S Hair W Nipple, Right X Nipple, Left	X External	Z No Device	Z No Qualifier
T Breast, Right U Breast, Left V Breast, Bilateral	0 Open	Z No Device	Z No Qualifier

Section 0 Medical and Surgical
Body System H Skin and Breast
Operation T Resection: Cutting out or off, without replacement, all of a body part

Body Part (4th)	Approach (5th)	Device (6th)	Qualifier (7th)
Q Finger Nail R Toe Nail W Nipple, Right X Nipple, Left	X External	Z No Device	Z No Qualifier
T Breast, Right U Breast, Left V Breast, Bilateral Y Supernumerary Breast	0 Open	Z No Device	Z No Qualifier

Section 0 Medical and Surgical
Body System H Skin and Breast
Operation U Supplement: Putting in or on biological or synthetic material that physically reinforces and/or augments the function of a portion of a body part

Body Part (4th)	Approach (5th)	Device (6th)	Qualifier (7th)
T Breast, Right U Breast, Left V Breast, Bilateral	0 Open 3 Percutaneous 7 Via Natural or Artificial Opening 8 Via Natural or Artificial Opening Endoscopic	7 Autologous Tissue Substitute J Synthetic Substitute K Nonautologous Tissue Substitute	Z No Qualifier
W Nipple, Right X Nipple, Left	0 Open 3 Percutaneous 7 Via Natural or Artificial Opening 8 Via Natural or Artificial Opening Endoscopic X External	7 Autologous Tissue Substitute J Synthetic Substitute K Nonautologous Tissue Substitute	Z No Qualifier

Section 0 Medical and Surgical
Body System H Skin and Breast
Operation W Revision: Correcting, to the extent possible, a portion of a malfunctioning device or the position of a displaced device

Body Part (4th)	Approach (5th)	Device (6th)	Qualifier (7th)
P Skin	X External	0 Drainage Device 7 Autologous Tissue Substitute J Synthetic Substitute K Nonautologous Tissue Substitute Y Other Device	Z No Qualifier
Q Finger Nail R Toe Nail	X External	0 Drainage Device 7 Autologous Tissue Substitute J Synthetic Substitute K Nonautologous Tissue Substitute	Z No Qualifier
S Hair	X External	7 Autologous Tissue Substitute J Synthetic Substitute K Nonautologous Tissue Substitute	Z No Qualifier
T Breast, Right U Breast, Left	0 Open 3 Percutaneous 7 Via Natural or Artificial Opening 8 Via Natural or Artificial Opening Endoscopic	0 Drainage Device 7 Autologous Tissue Substitute J Synthetic Substitute K Nonautologous Tissue Substitute N Tissue Expander Y Other Device	Z No Qualifier

Section	0	Medical and Surgical
Body System	H	Skin and Breast
Operation	X	**Transfer:** Moving, without taking out, all or a portion of a body part to another location to take over the function of all or a portion of a body part

Body Part (4th)	Approach (5th)	Device (6th)	Qualifier (7th)
0 Skin, Scalp **1** Skin, Face **2** Skin, Right Ear **3** Skin, Left Ear **4** Skin, Neck **5** Skin, Chest **6** Skin, Back **7** Skin, Abdomen **8** Skin, Buttock **9** Skin, Perineum **A** Skin, Inguinal **B** Skin, Right Upper Arm **C** Skin, Left Upper Arm **D** Skin, Right Lower Arm **E** Skin, Left Lower Arm **F** Skin, Right Hand **G** Skin, Left Hand **H** Skin, Right Upper Leg **J** Skin, Left Upper Leg **K** Skin, Right Lower Leg **L** Skin, Left Lower Leg **M** Skin, Right Foot **N** Skin, Left Foot	**X** External	**Z** No Device	**Z** No Qualifier

Skin and Breast Code Listing 0H0–0HX

0H0 – Skin and Breast, Alteration

0H0T07Z Alteration of Right Breast with Autologous Tissue Substitute, Open Approach

0H0T0JZ Alteration of Right Breast with Synthetic Substitute, Open Approach

0H0T0KZ Alteration of Right Breast with Nonautologous Tissue Substitute, Open Approach

0H0T0ZZ Alteration of Right Breast, Open Approach

0H0T37Z Alteration of Right Breast with Autologous Tissue Substitute, Percutaneous Approach

0H0T3JZ Alteration of Right Breast with Synthetic Substitute, Percutaneous Approach

0H0T3KZ Alteration of Right Breast with Nonautologous Tissue Substitute, Percutaneous Approach

0H0T3ZZ Alteration of Right Breast, Percutaneous Approach

0H0U07Z Alteration of Left Breast with Autologous Tissue Substitute, Open Approach

0H0U0JZ Alteration of Left Breast with Synthetic Substitute, Open Approach

0H0U0KZ Alteration of Left Breast with Nonautologous Tissue Substitute, Open Approach

0H0U0ZZ Alteration of Left Breast, Open Approach

0H0U37Z Alteration of Left Breast with Autologous Tissue Substitute, Percutaneous Approach

0H0U3JZ Alteration of Left Breast with Synthetic Substitute, Percutaneous Approach

0H0U3KZ Alteration of Left Breast with Nonautologous Tissue Substitute, Percutaneous Approach

0H0U3ZZ Alteration of Left Breast, Percutaneous Approach

0H0V07Z Alteration of Bilateral Breast with Autologous Tissue Substitute, Open Approach

0H0V0JZ Alteration of Bilateral Breast with Synthetic Substitute, Open Approach

0H0V0KZ Alteration of Bilateral Breast with Nonautologous Tissue Substitute, Open Approach

0H0V0ZZ Alteration of Bilateral Breast, Open Approach

0H0V37Z Alteration of Bilateral Breast with Autologous Tissue Substitute, Percutaneous Approach

0H0V3JZ Alteration of Bilateral Breast with Synthetic Substitute, Percutaneous Approach

0H0V3KZ Alteration of Bilateral Breast with Nonautologous Tissue Substitute, Percutaneous Approach

0H0V3ZZ Alteration of Bilateral Breast, Percutaneous Approach

0H2 – Skin and Breast, Change

Review Coding Guideline B6.1c

0H2PX0Z Change Drainage Device in Skin, External Approach

0H2PXYZ Change Other Device in Skin, External Approach

0H2TX0Z Change Drainage Device in Right Breast, External Approach

0H2TXYZ Change Other Device in Right Breast, External Approach

0H2UX0Z Change Drainage Device in Left Breast, External Approach

0H2UXYZ Change Other Device in Left Breast, External Approach

0H5 – Skin and Breast, Destruction

● **0H50XZD** Destruction of Scalp Skin, Multiple, External Approach

● **0H50XZZ** Destruction of Scalp Skin, External Approach

● **0H51XZD** Destruction of Face Skin, Multiple, External Approach

● **0H51XZZ** Destruction of Face Skin, External Approach

0H52XZD Destruction of Right Ear Skin, Multiple, External Approach

0H52XZZ Destruction of Right Ear Skin, External Approach

0H53XZD Destruction of Left Ear Skin, Multiple, External Approach

0H53XZZ Destruction of Left Ear Skin, External Approach

● **0H54XZD** Destruction of Neck Skin, Multiple, External Approach

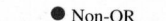

♀ Female-only   ♂ Male-only   ▲ Limited Coverage   ● Non-OR   HAC HAC-associated procedure   ▲ Non-covered procedures   ✛ Cluster

0H54XZZ   Destruction of Neck Skin, External Approach

0H55XZD   Destruction of Chest Skin, Multiple, External Approach

0H55XZZ   Destruction of Chest Skin, External Approach

0H56XZD   Destruction of Back Skin, Multiple, External Approach

0H56XZZ   Destruction of Back Skin, External Approach

0H57XZD   Destruction of Abdomen Skin, Multiple, External Approach

0H57XZZ   Destruction of Abdomen Skin, External Approach

0H58XZD   Destruction of Buttock Skin, Multiple, External Approach

0H58XZZ   Destruction of Buttock Skin, External Approach

0H59XZD   Destruction of Perineum Skin, Multiple, External Approach

0H59XZZ   Destruction of Perineum Skin, External Approach

0H5AXZD   Destruction of Inguinal Skin, Multiple, External Approach

0H5AXZZ   Destruction of Inguinal Skin, External Approach

0H5BXZD   Destruction of Right Upper Arm Skin, Multiple, External Approach

0H5BXZZ   Destruction of Right Upper Arm Skin, External Approach

0H5CXZD   Destruction of Left Upper Arm Skin, Multiple, External Approach

0H5CXZZ   Destruction of Left Upper Arm Skin, External Approach

0H5DXZD   Destruction of Right Lower Arm Skin, Multiple, External Approach

0H5DXZZ   Destruction of Right Lower Arm Skin, External Approach

0H5EXZD   Destruction of Left Lower Arm Skin, Multiple, External Approach

0H5EXZZ   Destruction of Left Lower Arm Skin, External Approach

0H5FXZD   Destruction of Right Hand Skin, Multiple, External Approach

● 0H5FXZZ   Destruction of Right Hand Skin, External Approach

● 0H5GXZD   Destruction of Left Hand Skin, Multiple, External Approach

● 0H5GXZZ   Destruction of Left Hand Skin, External Approach

● 0H5HXZD   Destruction of Right Upper Leg Skin, Multiple, External Approach

● 0H5HXZZ   Destruction of Right Upper Leg Skin, External Approach

● 0H5JXZD   Destruction of Left Upper Leg Skin, Multiple, External Approach

● 0H5JXZZ   Destruction of Left Upper Leg Skin, External Approach

● 0H5KXZD   Destruction of Right Lower Leg Skin, Multiple, External Approach

● 0H5KXZZ   Destruction of Right Lower Leg Skin, External Approach

● 0H5LXZD   Destruction of Left Lower Leg Skin, Multiple, External Approach

● 0H5LXZZ   Destruction of Left Lower Leg Skin, External Approach

● 0H5MXZD   Destruction of Right Foot Skin, Multiple, External Approach

● 0H5MXZZ   Destruction of Right Foot Skin, External Approach

● 0H5NXZD   Destruction of Left Foot Skin, Multiple, External Approach

● 0H5NXZZ   Destruction of Left Foot Skin, External Approach

● 0H5QXZZ   Destruction of Finger Nail, External Approach

● 0H5RXZZ   Destruction of Toe Nail, External Approach

0H5T0ZZ   Destruction of Right Breast, Open Approach

0H5T3ZZ   Destruction of Right Breast, Percutaneous Approach

0H5T7ZZ   Destruction of Right Breast, Via Natural or Artificial Opening

0H5T8ZZ   Destruction of Right Breast, Via Natural or Artificial Opening Endoscopic

0H5TXZZ   Destruction of Right Breast, External Approach

0H5U0ZZ   Destruction of Left Breast, Open Approach

0H5U3ZZ   Destruction of Left Breast, Percutaneous Approach

0H5U7ZZ   Destruction of Left Breast, Via Natural or Artificial Opening

0H5U8ZZ   Destruction of Left Breast, Via Natural or Artificial Opening Endoscopic

0H5UXZZ   Destruction of Left Breast, External Approach

0H5V0ZZ   Destruction of Bilateral Breast, Open Approach

0H5V3ZZ   Destruction of Bilateral Breast, Percutaneous Approach

0H5V7ZZ   Destruction of Bilateral Breast, Via Natural or Artificial Opening

0H5V8ZZ   Destruction of Bilateral Breast, Via Natural or Artificial Opening Endoscopic

0H5VXZZ   Destruction of Bilateral Breast, External Approach

0H5W0ZZ   Destruction of Right Nipple, Open Approach

0H5W3ZZ   Destruction of Right Nipple, Percutaneous Approach

0H5W7ZZ   Destruction of Right Nipple, Via Natural or Artificial Opening

0H5W8ZZ   Destruction of Right Nipple, Via Natural or Artificial Opening Endoscopic

0H5WXZZ   Destruction of Right Nipple, External Approach

0H5X0ZZ   Destruction of Left Nipple, Open Approach

0H5X3ZZ   Destruction of Left Nipple, Percutaneous Approach

0H5X7ZZ   Destruction of Left Nipple, Via Natural or Artificial Opening

0H5X8ZZ   Destruction of Left Nipple, Via Natural or Artificial Opening Endoscopic

0H5XXZZ   Destruction of Left Nipple, External Approach

0H8 – Skin and Breast, Division

Review Coding Guideline B3.14

0H80XZZ   Division of Scalp Skin, External Approach

0H81XZZ   Division of Face Skin, External Approach

0H82XZZ   Division of Right Ear Skin, External Approach

0H83XZZ   Division of Left Ear Skin, External Approach

0H84XZZ   Division of Neck Skin, External Approach

0H85XZZ   Division of Chest Skin, External Approach

0H86XZZ   Division of Back Skin, External Approach

0H87XZZ   Division of Abdomen Skin, External Approach

0H88XZZ   Division of Buttock Skin, External Approach

0H89XZZ   Division of Perineum Skin, External Approach

0H8AXZZ   Division of Inguinal Skin, External Approach

0H8BXZZ   Division of Right Upper Arm Skin, External Approach

0H8CXZZ   Division of Left Upper Arm Skin, External Approach

0H8DXZZ   Division of Right Lower Arm Skin, External Approach

0H8EXZZ   Division of Left Lower Arm Skin, External Approach

0H8FXZZ   Division of Right Hand Skin, External Approach

0H8GXZZ   Division of Left Hand Skin, External Approach

0H8HXZZ   Division of Right Upper Leg Skin, External Approach

0H8JXZZ   Division of Left Upper Leg Skin, External Approach

0H8KXZZ   Division of Right Lower Leg Skin, External Approach

0H8LXZZ   Division of Left Lower Leg Skin, External Approach

0H8MXZZ   Division of Right Foot Skin, External Approach

0H8NXZZ   Division of Left Foot Skin, External Approach

0H9 – Skin and Breast, Drainage

Review Coding Guidelines B3.4a and B3.4b

Review Coding Guideline B6.2

0H90X0Z   Drainage of Scalp Skin with Drainage Device, External Approach

0H90XZX   Drainage of Scalp Skin, External Approach, Diagnostic

0H90XZZ   Drainage of Scalp Skin, External Approach

0H91X0Z   Drainage of Face Skin with Drainage Device, External Approach

0H91XZX   Drainage of Face Skin, External Approach, Diagnostic

0H91XZZ   Drainage of Face Skin, External Approach

0H92X0Z   Drainage of Right Ear Skin with Drainage Device, External Approach

0H92XZX   Drainage of Right Ear Skin, External Approach, Diagnostic

0H92XZZ   Drainage of Right Ear Skin, External Approach

♀ Female-only   ♂ Male-only   ▲ Limited Coverage   ● Non-OR   HAC HAC-associated procedure   ▲ Non-covered procedures   ✛ Cluster

0H93X0Z	Drainage of Left Ear Skin with Drainage Device, External Approach
0H93XZX	Drainage of Left Ear Skin, External Approach, Diagnostic
0H93XZZ	Drainage of Left Ear Skin, External Approach
0H94X0Z	Drainage of Neck Skin with Drainage Device, External Approach
0H94XZX	Drainage of Neck Skin, External Approach, Diagnostic
0H94XZZ	Drainage of Neck Skin, External Approach
0H95X0Z	Drainage of Chest Skin with Drainage Device, External Approach
0H95XZX	Drainage of Chest Skin, External Approach, Diagnostic
0H95XZZ	Drainage of Chest Skin, External Approach
0H96X0Z	Drainage of Back Skin with Drainage Device, External Approach
0H96XZX	Drainage of Back Skin, External Approach, Diagnostic
0H96XZZ	Drainage of Back Skin, External Approach
0H97X0Z	Drainage of Abdomen Skin with Drainage Device, External Approach
0H97XZX	Drainage of Abdomen Skin, External Approach, Diagnostic
0H97XZZ	Drainage of Abdomen Skin, External Approach
0H98X0Z	Drainage of Buttock Skin with Drainage Device, External Approach
0H98XZX	Drainage of Buttock Skin, External Approach, Diagnostic
0H98XZZ	Drainage of Buttock Skin, External Approach
0H99X0Z	Drainage of Perineum Skin with Drainage Device, External Approach
0H99XZX	Drainage of Perineum Skin, External Approach, Diagnostic
0H99XZZ	Drainage of Perineum Skin, External Approach
0H9AX0Z	Drainage of Inguinal Skin with Drainage Device, External Approach
0H9AXZX	Drainage of Inguinal Skin, External Approach, Diagnostic
0H9AXZZ	Drainage of Inguinal Skin, External Approach
0H9BX0Z	Drainage of Right Upper Arm Skin with Drainage Device, External Approach
0H9BXZX	Drainage of Right Upper Arm Skin, External Approach, Diagnostic
0H9BXZZ	Drainage of Right Upper Arm Skin, External Approach
0H9CX0Z	Drainage of Left Upper Arm Skin with Drainage Device, External Approach
0H9CXZX	Drainage of Left Upper Arm Skin, External Approach, Diagnostic
0H9CXZZ	Drainage of Left Upper Arm Skin, External Approach
0H9DX0Z	Drainage of Right Lower Arm Skin with Drainage Device, External Approach
0H9DXZX	Drainage of Right Lower Arm Skin, External Approach, Diagnostic
0H9DXZZ	Drainage of Right Lower Arm Skin, External Approach
0H9EX0Z	Drainage of Left Lower Arm Skin with Drainage Device, External Approach
0H9EXZX	Drainage of Left Lower Arm Skin, External Approach, Diagnostic
0H9EXZZ	Drainage of Left Lower Arm Skin, External Approach
0H9FX0Z	Drainage of Right Hand Skin with Drainage Device, External Approach
0H9FXZX	Drainage of Right Hand Skin, External Approach, Diagnostic
0H9FXZZ	Drainage of Right Hand Skin, External Approach
0H9GX0Z	Drainage of Left Hand Skin with Drainage Device, External Approach
0H9GXZX	Drainage of Left Hand Skin, External Approach, Diagnostic
0H9GXZZ	Drainage of Left Hand Skin, External Approach
0H9HX0Z	Drainage of Right Upper Leg Skin with Drainage Device, External Approach
0H9HXZX	Drainage of Right Upper Leg Skin, External Approach, Diagnostic
0H9HXZZ	Drainage of Right Upper Leg Skin, External Approach
0H9JX0Z	Drainage of Left Upper Leg Skin with Drainage Device, External Approach
0H9JXZX	Drainage of Left Upper Leg Skin, External Approach, Diagnostic
0H9JXZZ	Drainage of Left Upper Leg Skin, External Approach
0H9KX0Z	Drainage of Right Lower Leg Skin with Drainage Device, External Approach
0H9KXZX	Drainage of Right Lower Leg Skin, External Approach, Diagnostic
0H9KXZZ	Drainage of Right Lower Leg Skin, External Approach
0H9LX0Z	Drainage of Left Lower Leg Skin with Drainage Device, External Approach
0H9LXZX	Drainage of Left Lower Leg Skin, External Approach, Diagnostic
0H9LXZZ	Drainage of Left Lower Leg Skin, External Approach
0H9MX0Z	Drainage of Right Foot Skin with Drainage Device, External Approach
0H9MXZX	Drainage of Right Foot Skin, External Approach, Diagnostic
0H9MXZZ	Drainage of Right Foot Skin, External Approach
0H9NX0Z	Drainage of Left Foot Skin with Drainage Device, External Approach
0H9NXZX	Drainage of Left Foot Skin, External Approach, Diagnostic
0H9NXZZ	Drainage of Left Foot Skin, External Approach
0H9QX0Z	Drainage of Finger Nail with Drainage Device, External Approach
0H9QXZX	Drainage of Finger Nail, External Approach, Diagnostic
0H9QXZZ	Drainage of Finger Nail, External Approach
0H9RX0Z	Drainage of Toe Nail with Drainage Device, External Approach
0H9RXZX	Drainage of Toe Nail, External Approach, Diagnostic
0H9RXZZ	Drainage of Toe Nail, External Approach
0H9T00Z	Drainage of Right Breast with Drainage Device, Open Approach
0H9T0ZX	Drainage of Right Breast, Open Approach, Diagnostic
0H9T0ZZ	Drainage of Right Breast, Open Approach
0H9T30Z	Drainage of Right Breast with Drainage Device, Percutaneous Approach
0H9T3ZX	Drainage of Right Breast, Percutaneous Approach, Diagnostic
0H9T3ZZ	Drainage of Right Breast, Percutaneous Approach
0H9T70Z	Drainage of Right Breast with Drainage Device, Via Natural or Artificial Opening
0H9T7ZX	Drainage of Right Breast, Via Natural or Artificial Opening, Diagnostic
0H9T7ZZ	Drainage of Right Breast, Via Natural or Artificial Opening
0H9T80Z	Drainage of Right Breast with Drainage Device, Via Natural or Artificial Opening Endoscopic
0H9T8ZX	Drainage of Right Breast, Via Natural or Artificial Opening Endoscopic, Diagnostic
0H9T8ZZ	Drainage of Right Breast, Via Natural or Artificial Opening Endoscopic
0H9U00Z	Drainage of Left Breast with Drainage Device, Open Approach
0H9U0ZX	Drainage of Left Breast, Open Approach, Diagnostic
0H9U0ZZ	Drainage of Left Breast, Open Approach
0H9U30Z	Drainage of Left Breast with Drainage Device, Percutaneous Approach
0H9U3ZX	Drainage of Left Breast, Percutaneous Approach, Diagnostic
0H9U3ZZ	Drainage of Left Breast, Percutaneous Approach
0H9U70Z	Drainage of Left Breast with Drainage Device, Via Natural or Artificial Opening
0H9U7ZX	Drainage of Left Breast, Via Natural or Artificial Opening, Diagnostic
0H9U7ZZ	Drainage of Left Breast, Via Natural or Artificial Opening
0H9U80Z	Drainage of Left Breast with Drainage Device, Via Natural or Artificial Opening Endoscopic
0H9U8ZX	Drainage of Left Breast, Via Natural or Artificial Opening Endoscopic, Diagnostic
0H9U8ZZ	Drainage of Left Breast, Via Natural or Artificial Opening Endoscopic
0H9V00Z	Drainage of Bilateral Breast with Drainage Device, Open Approach
0H9V0ZX	Drainage of Bilateral Breast, Open Approach, Diagnostic
0H9V0ZZ	Drainage of Bilateral Breast, Open Approach
0H9V30Z	Drainage of Bilateral Breast with Drainage Device, Percutaneous Approach
0H9V3ZX	Drainage of Bilateral Breast, Percutaneous Approach, Diagnostic
0H9V3ZZ	Drainage of Bilateral Breast, Percutaneous Approach
0H9V70Z	Drainage of Bilateral Breast with Drainage Device, Via Natural or Artificial Opening
0H9V7ZX	Drainage of Bilateral Breast, Via Natural or Artificial Opening, Diagnostic
0H9V7ZZ	Drainage of Bilateral Breast, Via Natural or Artificial Opening
0H9V80Z	Drainage of Bilateral Breast with Drainage Device, Via Natural or Artificial Opening Endoscopic
0H9V8ZX	Drainage of Bilateral Breast, Via Natural or Artificial Opening Endoscopic, Diagnostic
0H9V8ZZ	Drainage of Bilateral Breast, Via Natural or Artificial Opening Endoscopic
0H9W00Z	Drainage of Right Nipple with Drainage Device, Open Approach
0H9W0ZX	Drainage of Right Nipple, Open Approach, Diagnostic
0H9W0ZZ	Drainage of Right Nipple, Open Approach
0H9W30Z	Drainage of Right Nipple with Drainage Device, Percutaneous Approach
0H9W3ZX	Drainage of Right Nipple, Percutaneous Approach, Diagnostic
0H9W3ZZ	Drainage of Right Nipple, Percutaneous Approach
0H9W70Z	Drainage of Right Nipple with Drainage Device, Via Natural or Artificial Opening
0H9W7ZX	Drainage of Right Nipple, Via Natural or Artificial Opening, Diagnostic
0H9W7ZZ	Drainage of Right Nipple, Via Natural or Artificial Opening

♀ Female-only   ♂ Male-only   ▲ Limited Coverage   ● Non-OR   HAC HAC-associated procedure   ▲ Non-covered procedures   ✚ Cluster

0H9W80Z	Drainage of Right Nipple with Drainage Device, Via Natural or Artificial Opening Endoscopic
0H9W8ZX	Drainage of Right Nipple, Via Natural or Artificial Opening Endoscopic, Diagnostic
0H9W8ZZ	Drainage of Right Nipple, Via Natural or Artificial Opening Endoscopic
0H9WX0Z	Drainage of Right Nipple with Drainage Device, External Approach
0H9WXZX	Drainage of Right Nipple, External Approach, Diagnostic
0H9WXZZ	Drainage of Right Nipple, External Approach
0H9X00Z	Drainage of Left Nipple with Drainage Device, Open Approach

0H9X0ZX	Drainage of Left Nipple, Open Approach, Diagnostic
0H9X0ZZ	Drainage of Left Nipple, Open Approach
0H9X30Z	Drainage of Left Nipple with Drainage Device, Percutaneous Approach
0H9X3ZX	Drainage of Left Nipple, Percutaneous Approach, Diagnostic
0H9X3ZZ	Drainage of Left Nipple, Percutaneous Approach
0H9X70Z	Drainage of Left Nipple with Drainage Device, Via Natural or Artificial Opening
0H9X7ZX	Drainage of Left Nipple, Via Natural or Artificial Opening, Diagnostic
0H9X7ZZ	Drainage of Left Nipple, Via Natural or Artificial Opening

0H9X80Z	Drainage of Left Nipple with Drainage Device, Via Natural or Artificial Opening Endoscopic
0H9X8ZX	Drainage of Left Nipple, Via Natural or Artificial Opening Endoscopic, Diagnostic
0H9X8ZZ	Drainage of Left Nipple, Via Natural or Artificial Opening Endoscopic
0H9XX0Z	Drainage of Left Nipple with Drainage Device, External Approach
0H9XXZX	Drainage of Left Nipple, External Approach, Diagnostic
0H9XXZZ	Drainage of Left Nipple, External Approach

0HB – Skin and Breast, Excision

Review Coding Guidelines 3B.4a and 3B.4b

Review Coding Guideline B3.5

Review Coding Guideline B3.8

Review Coding Guideline B3.18

0HB0XZX	Excision of Scalp Skin, External Approach, Diagnostic
0HB0XZZ	Excision of Scalp Skin, External Approach
0HB1XZX	Excision of Face Skin, External Approach, Diagnostic
0HB1XZZ	Excision of Face Skin, External Approach
0HB2XZX	Excision of Right Ear Skin, External Approach, Diagnostic
0HB2XZZ	Excision of Right Ear Skin, External Approach
0HB3XZX	Excision of Left Ear Skin, External Approach, Diagnostic
0HB3XZZ	Excision of Left Ear Skin, External Approach
0HB4XZX	Excision of Neck Skin, External Approach, Diagnostic
0HB4XZZ	Excision of Neck Skin, External Approach
0HB5XZX	Excision of Chest Skin, External Approach, Diagnostic
0HB5XZZ	Excision of Chest Skin, External Approach
0HB6XZX	Excision of Back Skin, External Approach, Diagnostic
0HB6XZZ	Excision of Back Skin, External Approach
0HB7XZX	Excision of Abdomen Skin, External Approach, Diagnostic
0HB7XZZ	Excision of Abdomen Skin, External Approach
0HB8XZX	Excision of Buttock Skin, External Approach, Diagnostic
0HB8XZZ	Excision of Buttock Skin, External Approach

AHA CC: 3Q, 2015, 3

0HB9XZX	Excision of Perineum Skin, External Approach, Diagnostic
● 0HB9XZZ	Excision of Perineum Skin, External Approach
0HBAXZX	Excision of Inguinal Skin, External Approach, Diagnostic
0HBAXZZ	Excision of Inguinal Skin, External Approach
0HBBXZX	Excision of Right Upper Arm Skin, External Approach, Diagnostic
0HBBXZZ	Excision of Right Upper Arm Skin, External Approach

0HBCXZX	Excision of Left Upper Arm Skin, External Approach, Diagnostic
0HBCXZZ	Excision of Left Upper Arm Skin, External Approach
0HBDXZX	Excision of Right Lower Arm Skin, External Approach, Diagnostic
0HBDXZZ	Excision of Right Lower Arm Skin, External Approach
0HBEXZX	Excision of Left Lower Arm Skin, External Approach, Diagnostic
0HBEXZZ	Excision of Left Lower Arm Skin, External Approach
0HBFXZX	Excision of Right Hand Skin, External Approach, Diagnostic
0HBFXZZ	Excision of Right Hand Skin, External Approach
0HBGXZX	Excision of Left Hand Skin, External Approach, Diagnostic
● 0HBGXZZ	Excision of Left Hand Skin, External Approach
0HBHXZX	Excision of Right Upper Leg Skin, External Approach, Diagnostic
0HBHXZZ	Excision of Right Upper Leg Skin, External Approach

AHA CC: 1Q, 2020, 31-32

0HBJXZX	Excision of Left Upper Leg Skin, External Approach, Diagnostic
0HBJXZZ	Excision of Left Upper Leg Skin, External Approach

AHA CC: 3Q, 2016, 29-30

0HBKXZX	Excision of Right Lower Leg Skin, External Approach, Diagnostic
0HBKXZZ	Excision of Right Lower Leg Skin, External Approach
0HBLXZX	Excision of Left Lower Leg Skin, External Approach, Diagnostic
0HBLXZZ	Excision of Left Lower Leg Skin, External Approach
0HBMXZX	Excision of Right Foot Skin, External Approach, Diagnostic
0HBMXZZ	Excision of Right Foot Skin, External Approach
0HBNXZX	Excision of Left Foot Skin, External Approach, Diagnostic
0HBNXZZ	Excision of Left Foot Skin, External Approach
0HBQXZX	Excision of Finger Nail, External Approach, Diagnostic

0HBQXZZ	Excision of Finger Nail, External Approach
0HBRXZX	Excision of Toe Nail, External Approach, Diagnostic
0HBRXZZ	Excision of Toe Nail, External Approach
0HBT0ZX	Excision of Right Breast, Open Approach, Diagnostic
0HBT0ZZ	Excision of Right Breast, Open Approach

AHA CC: 1Q, 2018, 14-15

0HBT3ZX	Excision of Right Breast, Percutaneous Approach, Diagnostic
0HBT3ZZ	Excision of Right Breast, Percutaneous Approach
0HBT7ZX	Excision of Right Breast, Via Natural or Artificial Opening, Diagnostic
0HBT7ZZ	Excision of Right Breast, Via Natural or Artificial Opening
0HBT8ZX	Excision of Right Breast, Via Natural or Artificial Opening Endoscopic, Diagnostic
0HBT8ZZ	Excision of Right Breast, Via Natural or Artificial Opening Endoscopic
0HBU0ZX	Excision of Left Breast, Open Approach, Diagnostic
0HBU0ZZ	Excision of Left Breast, Open Approach
0HBU3ZX	Excision of Left Breast, Percutaneous Approach, Diagnostic
0HBU3ZZ	Excision of Left Breast, Percutaneous Approach
0HBU7ZX	Excision of Left Breast, Via Natural or Artificial Opening, Diagnostic
0HBU7ZZ	Excision of Left Breast, Via Natural or Artificial Opening
0HBU8ZX	Excision of Left Breast, Via Natural or Artificial Opening Endoscopic, Diagnostic
0HBU8ZZ	Excision of Left Breast, Via Natural or Artificial Opening Endoscopic
0HBV0ZX	Excision of Bilateral Breast, Open Approach, Diagnostic
0HBV0ZZ	Excision of Bilateral Breast, Open Approach
0HBV3ZX	Excision of Bilateral Breast, Percutaneous Approach, Diagnostic
0HBV3ZZ	Excision of Bilateral Breast, Percutaneous Approach
0HBV7ZX	Excision of Bilateral Breast, Via Natural or Artificial Opening, Diagnostic

0HBV7ZZ Excision of Bilateral Breast, Via Natural or Artificial Opening

0HBV8ZX Excision of Bilateral Breast, Via Natural or Artificial Opening Endoscopic, Diagnostic

0HBV8ZZ Excision of Bilateral Breast, Via Natural or Artificial Opening Endoscopic

0HBW0ZX Excision of Right Nipple, Open Approach, Diagnostic

0HBW0ZZ Excision of Right Nipple, Open Approach

0HBW3ZX Excision of Right Nipple, Percutaneous Approach, Diagnostic

0HBW3ZZ Excision of Right Nipple, Percutaneous Approach

0HBW7ZX Excision of Right Nipple, Via Natural or Artificial Opening, Diagnostic

0HBW7ZZ Excision of Right Nipple, Via Natural or Artificial Opening

0HBW8ZX Excision of Right Nipple, Via Natural or Artificial Opening Endoscopic, Diagnostic

0HBW8ZZ Excision of Right Nipple, Via Natural or Artificial Opening Endoscopic

0HBWXZX Excision of Right Nipple, External Approach, Diagnostic

0HBWXZZ Excision of Right Nipple, External Approach

0HBX0ZX Excision of Left Nipple, Open Approach, Diagnostic

0HBX0ZZ Excision of Left Nipple, Open Approach

0HBX3ZX Excision of Left Nipple, Percutaneous Approach, Diagnostic

0HBX3ZZ Excision of Left Nipple, Percutaneous Approach

0HBX7ZX Excision of Left Nipple, Via Natural or Artificial Opening, Diagnostic

0HBX7ZZ Excision of Left Nipple, Via Natural or Artificial Opening

0HBX8ZX Excision of Left Nipple, Via Natural or Artificial Opening Endoscopic, Diagnostic

0HBX8ZZ Excision of Left Nipple, Via Natural or Artificial Opening Endoscopic

0HBXXZX Excision of Left Nipple, External Approach, Diagnostic

0HBXXZZ Excision of Left Nipple, External Approach

0HBY0ZX Excision of Supernumerary Breast, Open Approach, Diagnostic

0HBY0ZZ Excision of Supernumerary Breast, Open Approach

0HBY3ZX Excision of Supernumerary Breast, Percutaneous Approach, Diagnostic

0HBY3ZZ Excision of Supernumerary Breast, Percutaneous Approach

0HBY7ZX Excision of Supernumerary Breast, Via Natural or Artificial Opening, Diagnostic

0HBY7ZZ Excision of Supernumerary Breast, Via Natural or Artificial Opening

0HBY8ZX Excision of Supernumerary Breast, Via Natural or Artificial Opening Endoscopic, Diagnostic

0HBY8ZZ Excision of Supernumerary Breast, Via Natural or Artificial Opening Endoscopic

0HC – Skin and Breast, Extirpation

0HC0XZZ Extirpation of Matter from Scalp Skin, External Approach

0HC1XZZ Extirpation of Matter from Face Skin, External Approach

0HC2XZZ Extirpation of Matter from Right Ear Skin, External Approach

0HC3XZZ Extirpation of Matter from Left Ear Skin, External Approach

0HC4XZZ Extirpation of Matter from Neck Skin, External Approach

0HC5XZZ Extirpation of Matter from Chest Skin, External Approach

0HC6XZZ Extirpation of Matter from Back Skin, External Approach

0HC7XZZ Extirpation of Matter from Abdomen Skin, External Approach

0HC8XZZ Extirpation of Matter from Buttock Skin, External Approach

0HC9XZZ Extirpation of Matter from Perineum Skin, External Approach

0HCAXZZ Extirpation of Matter from Inguinal Skin, External Approach

0HCBXZZ Extirpation of Matter from Right Upper Arm Skin, External Approach

0HCCXZZ Extirpation of Matter from Left Upper Arm Skin, External Approach

0HCDXZZ Extirpation of Matter from Right Lower Arm Skin, External Approach

0HCEXZZ Extirpation of Matter from Left Lower Arm Skin, External Approach

0HCFXZZ Extirpation of Matter from Right Hand Skin, External Approach

0HCGXZZ Extirpation of Matter from Left Hand Skin, External Approach

0HCHXZZ Extirpation of Matter from Right Upper Leg Skin, External Approach

0HCJXZZ Extirpation of Matter from Left Upper Leg Skin, External Approach

0HCKXZZ Extirpation of Matter from Right Lower Leg Skin, External Approach

0HCLXZZ Extirpation of Matter from Left Lower Leg Skin, External Approach

0HCMXZZ Extirpation of Matter from Right Foot Skin, External Approach

0HCNXZZ Extirpation of Matter from Left Foot Skin, External Approach

0HCQXZZ Extirpation of Matter from Finger Nail, External Approach

0HCRXZZ Extirpation of Matter from Toe Nail, External Approach

0HCT0ZZ Extirpation of Matter from Right Breast, Open Approach

0HCT3ZZ Extirpation of Matter from Right Breast, Percutaneous Approach

0HCT7ZZ Extirpation of Matter from Right Breast, Via Natural or Artificial Opening

0HCT8ZZ Extirpation of Matter from Right Breast, Via Natural or Artificial Opening Endoscopic

0HCU0ZZ Extirpation of Matter from Left Breast, Open Approach

0HCU3ZZ Extirpation of Matter from Left Breast, Percutaneous Approach

0HCU7ZZ Extirpation of Matter from Left Breast, Via Natural or Artificial Opening

0HCU8ZZ Extirpation of Matter from Left Breast, Via Natural or Artificial Opening Endoscopic

0HCV0ZZ Extirpation of Matter from Bilateral Breast, Open Approach

0HCV3ZZ Extirpation of Matter from Bilateral Breast, Percutaneous Approach

0HCV7ZZ Extirpation of Matter from Bilateral Breast, Via Natural or Artificial Opening

0HCV8ZZ Extirpation of Matter from Bilateral Breast, Via Natural or Artificial Opening Endoscopic

0HCW0ZZ Extirpation of Matter from Right Nipple, Open Approach

0HCW3ZZ Extirpation of Matter from Right Nipple, Percutaneous Approach

0HCW7ZZ Extirpation of Matter from Right Nipple, Via Natural or Artificial Opening

0HCW8ZZ Extirpation of Matter from Right Nipple, Via Natural or Artificial Opening Endoscopic

0HCWXZZ Extirpation of Matter from Right Nipple, External Approach

0HCX0ZZ Extirpation of Matter from Left Nipple, Open Approach

0HCX3ZZ Extirpation of Matter from Left Nipple, Percutaneous Approach

0HCX7ZZ Extirpation of Matter from Left Nipple, Via Natural or Artificial Opening

0HCX8ZZ Extirpation of Matter from Left Nipple, Via Natural or Artificial Opening Endoscopic

0HCXXZZ Extirpation of Matter from Left Nipple, External Approach

0HD – Skin and Breast, Extraction

0HD0XZZ Extraction of Scalp Skin, External Approach

0HD1XZZ Extraction of Face Skin, External Approach

0HD2XZZ Extraction of Right Ear Skin, External Approach

0HD3XZZ Extraction of Left Ear Skin, External Approach

0HD4XZZ Extraction of Neck Skin, External Approach

0HD5XZZ Extraction of Chest Skin, External Approach

0HD6XZZ Extraction of Back Skin, External Approach

AHA CC: 3Q, 2015, 5-6

0HD7XZZ Extraction of Abdomen Skin, External Approach

0HD8XZZ Extraction of Buttock Skin, External Approach

0HD9XZZ Extraction of Perineum Skin, External Approach

0HDAXZZ Extraction of Inguinal Skin, External Approach

0HDBXZZ Extraction of Right Upper Arm Skin, External Approach

0HDCXZZ Extraction of Left Upper Arm Skin, External Approach

0HDDXZZ Extraction of Right Lower Arm Skin, External Approach

0HDEXZZ Extraction of Left Lower Arm Skin, External Approach

0HDFXZZ Extraction of Right Hand Skin, External Approach

0HDGXZZ Extraction of Left Hand Skin, External Approach

0HDHXZZ Extraction of Right Upper Leg Skin, External Approach

AHA CC: 3Q, 2015, 5

0HDJXZZ Extraction of Left Upper Leg Skin, External Approach

0HDKXZZ Extraction of Right Lower Leg Skin, External Approach

0HDLXZZ Extraction of Left Lower Leg Skin, External Approach

♀ Female-only   ♂ Male-only   ▲ Limited Coverage   ● Non-OR   HAC HAC-associated procedure   ▲ Non-covered procedures   ✛ Cluster

0HDMXZZ Extraction of Right Foot Skin, External Approach
0HDNXZZ Extraction of Left Foot Skin, External Approach
0HDQXZZ Extraction of Finger Nail, External Approach

0HDRXZZ Extraction of Toe Nail, External Approach
0HDSXZZ Extraction of Hair, External Approach
0HDT0ZZ Extraction of Right Breast, Open Approach

0HDU0ZZ Extraction of Left Breast, Open Approach
0HDV0ZZ Extraction of Bilateral Breast, Open Approach
0HDY0ZZ Extraction of Supernumerary Breast, Open Approach

0HH – Skin and Breast, Insertion

0HHPXYZ Insertion of Other Device into Skin, External Approach
0HHT01Z Insertion of Radioactive Element into Right Breast, Open Approach
0HHT0NZ Insertion of Tissue Expander into Right Breast, Open Approach
AHA CC: 4Q, 2017, 67
0HHT0YZ Insertion of Other Device into Right Breast, Open Approach
0HHT31Z Insertion of Radioactive Element into Right Breast, Percutaneous Approach
0HHT3NZ Insertion of Tissue Expander into Right Breast, Percutaneous Approach
0HHT3YZ Insertion of Other Device into Right Breast, Percutaneous Approach
0HHT71Z Insertion of Radioactive Element into Right Breast, Via Natural or Artificial Opening
0HHT7NZ Insertion of Tissue Expander into Right Breast, Via Natural or Artificial Opening
0HHT7YZ Insertion of Other Device into Right Breast, Via Natural or Artificial Opening
0HHT81Z Insertion of Radioactive Element into Right Breast, Via Natural or Artificial Opening Endoscopic
0HHT8NZ Insertion of Tissue Expander into Right Breast, Via Natural or Artificial Opening Endoscopic
0HHT8YZ Insertion of Other Device into Right Breast, Via Natural or Artificial Opening Endoscopic
0HHU01Z Insertion of Radioactive Element into Left Breast, Open Approach
0HHU0NZ Insertion of Tissue Expander into Left Breast, Open Approach
0HHU0YZ Insertion of Other Device into Left Breast, Open Approach
AHA CC: 4Q, 2013, 107
0HHU31Z Insertion of Radioactive Element into Left Breast, Percutaneous Approach
0HHU3NZ Insertion of Tissue Expander into Left Breast, Percutaneous Approach

0HHU3YZ Insertion of Other Device into Left Breast, Percutaneous Approach
0HHU71Z Insertion of Radioactive Element into Left Breast, Via Natural or Artificial Opening
0HHU7NZ Insertion of Tissue Expander into Left Breast, Via Natural or Artificial Opening
0HHU7YZ Insertion of Other Device into Left Breast, Via Natural or Artificial Opening
0HHU81Z Insertion of Radioactive Element into Left Breast, Via Natural or Artificial Opening Endoscopic
0HHU8NZ Insertion of Tissue Expander into Left Breast, Via Natural or Artificial Opening Endoscopic
0HHU8YZ Insertion of Other Device into Left Breast, Via Natural or Artificial Opening Endoscopic
0HHV01Z Insertion of Radioactive Element into Bilateral Breast, Open Approach
0HHV0NZ Insertion of Tissue Expander into Bilateral Breast, Open Approach
AHA CC: 2Q, 2014, 12
0HHV31Z Insertion of Radioactive Element into Bilateral Breast, Percutaneous Approach
0HHV3NZ Insertion of Tissue Expander into Bilateral Breast, Percutaneous Approach
0HHV71Z Insertion of Radioactive Element into Bilateral Breast, Via Natural or Artificial Opening
0HHV7NZ Insertion of Tissue Expander into Bilateral Breast, Via Natural or Artificial Opening
0HHV81Z Insertion of Radioactive Element into Bilateral Breast, Via Natural or Artificial Opening Endoscopic
0HHV8NZ Insertion of Tissue Expander into Bilateral Breast, Via Natural or Artificial Opening Endoscopic
0HHW01Z Insertion of Radioactive Element into Right Nipple, Open Approach

0HHW0NZ Insertion of Tissue Expander into Right Nipple, Open Approach
0HHW31Z Insertion of Radioactive Element into Right Nipple, Percutaneous Approach
0HHW3NZ Insertion of Tissue Expander into Right Nipple, Percutaneous Approach
0HHW71Z Insertion of Radioactive Element into Right Nipple, Via Natural or Artificial Opening
0HHW7NZ Insertion of Tissue Expander into Right Nipple, Via Natural or Artificial Opening
0HHW81Z Insertion of Radioactive Element into Right Nipple, Via Natural or Artificial Opening Endoscopic
0HHW8NZ Insertion of Tissue Expander into Right Nipple, Via Natural or Artificial Opening Endoscopic
0HHWX1Z Insertion of Radioactive Element into Right Nipple, External Approach
0HHX01Z Insertion of Radioactive Element into Left Nipple, Open Approach
0HHX0NZ Insertion of Tissue Expander into Left Nipple, Open Approach
0HHX31Z Insertion of Radioactive Element into Left Nipple, Percutaneous Approach
0HHX3NZ Insertion of Tissue Expander into Left Nipple, Percutaneous Approach
0HHX71Z Insertion of Radioactive Element into Left Nipple, Via Natural or Artificial Opening
0HHX7NZ Insertion of Tissue Expander into Left Nipple, Via Natural or Artificial Opening
0HHX81Z Insertion of Radioactive Element into Left Nipple, Via Natural or Artificial Opening Endoscopic
0HHX8NZ Insertion of Tissue Expander into Left Nipple, Via Natural or Artificial Opening Endoscopic
0HHXX1Z Insertion of Radioactive Element into Left Nipple, External Approach

0HJ – Skin and Breast, Inspection

Review Coding Guideline B3.5

Review Coding Guidelines B3.11a, B3.11b and B3.11c

0HJPXZZ Inspection of Skin, External Approach
0HJQXZZ Inspection of Finger Nail, External Approach
0HJRXZZ Inspection of Toe Nail, External Approach
0HJT0ZZ Inspection of Right Breast, Open Approach

0HJT3ZZ Inspection of Right Breast, Percutaneous Approach
0HJT7ZZ Inspection of Right Breast, Via Natural or Artificial Opening
0HJT8ZZ Inspection of Right Breast, Via Natural or Artificial Opening Endoscopic
0HJU0ZZ Inspection of Left Breast, Open Approach

0HJU3ZZ Inspection of Left Breast, Percutaneous Approach
0HJU7ZZ Inspection of Left Breast, Via Natural or Artificial Opening
0HJU8ZZ Inspection of Left Breast, Via Natural or Artificial Opening Endoscopic

0HM – Skin and Breast, Reattachment

0HM0XZZ Reattachment of Scalp Skin, External Approach
0HM1XZZ Reattachment of Face Skin, External Approach

0HM2XZZ Reattachment of Right Ear Skin, External Approach
0HM3XZZ Reattachment of Left Ear Skin, External Approach

0HM4XZZ Reattachment of Neck Skin, External Approach
0HM5XZZ Reattachment of Chest Skin, External Approach

♀ Female-only   ♂ Male-only   ▲ Limited Coverage   ● Non-OR   HAC HAC-associated procedure   ▲ Non-covered procedures   ✚ Cluster

0HM6XZZ	Reattachment of Back Skin, External Approach
0HM7XZZ	Reattachment of Abdomen Skin, External Approach
0HM8XZZ	Reattachment of Buttock Skin, External Approach
0HM9XZZ	Reattachment of Perineum Skin, External Approach
0HMAXZZ	Reattachment of Inguinal Skin, External Approach
0HMBXZZ	Reattachment of Right Upper Arm Skin, External Approach
0HMCXZZ	Reattachment of Left Upper Arm Skin, External Approach
0HMDXZZ	Reattachment of Right Lower Arm Skin, External Approach

0HMEXZZ	Reattachment of Left Lower Arm Skin, External Approach
0HMFXZZ	Reattachment of Right Hand Skin, External Approach
0HMGXZZ	Reattachment of Left Hand Skin, External Approach
0HMHXZZ	Reattachment of Right Upper Leg Skin, External Approach
0HMJXZZ	Reattachment of Left Upper Leg Skin, External Approach
0HMKXZZ	Reattachment of Right Lower Leg Skin, External Approach
0HMLXZZ	Reattachment of Left Lower Leg Skin, External Approach
0HMMXZZ	Reattachment of Right Foot Skin, External Approach

0HMNXZZ	Reattachment of Left Foot Skin, External Approach
0HMTXZZ	Reattachment of Right Breast, External Approach
0HMUXZZ	Reattachment of Left Breast, External Approach
0HMVXZZ	Reattachment of Bilateral Breast, External Approach
0HMWXZZ	Reattachment of Right Nipple, External Approach
0HMXXZZ	Reattachment of Left Nipple, External Approach

0HN – Skin and Breast, Release

Review Coding Guideline B3.13

Review Coding Guideline B3.14

0HN0XZZ	Release Scalp Skin, External Approach
0HN1XZZ	Release Face Skin, External Approach
0HN2XZZ	Release Right Ear Skin, External Approach
0HN3XZZ	Release Left Ear Skin, External Approach
0HN4XZZ	Release Neck Skin, External Approach
0HN5XZZ	Release Chest Skin, External Approach
0HN6XZZ	Release Back Skin, External Approach
0HN7XZZ	Release Abdomen Skin, External Approach
0HN8XZZ	Release Buttock Skin, External Approach
0HN9XZZ	Release Perineum Skin, External Approach
0HNAXZZ	Release Inguinal Skin, External Approach
0HNBXZZ	Release Right Upper Arm Skin, External Approach
0HNCXZZ	Release Left Upper Arm Skin, External Approach
0HNDXZZ	Release Right Lower Arm Skin, External Approach
0HNEXZZ	Release Left Lower Arm Skin, External Approach
0HNFXZZ	Release Right Hand Skin, External Approach

0HNGXZZ	Release Left Hand Skin, External Approach
0HNHXZZ	Release Right Upper Leg Skin, External Approach
0HNJXZZ	Release Left Upper Leg Skin, External Approach
0HNKXZZ	Release Right Lower Leg Skin, External Approach
0HNLXZZ	Release Left Lower Leg Skin, External Approach
0HNMXZZ	Release Right Foot Skin, External Approach
0HNNXZZ	Release Left Foot Skin, External Approach
0HNQXZZ	Release Finger Nail, External Approach
0HNRXZZ	Release Toe Nail, External Approach
0HNT0ZZ	Release Right Breast, Open Approach
0HNT3ZZ	Release Right Breast, Percutaneous Approach
0HNT7ZZ	Release Right Breast, Via Natural or Artificial Opening
0HNT8ZZ	Release Right Breast, Via Natural or Artificial Opening Endoscopic
0HNU0ZZ	Release Left Breast, Open Approach
0HNU3ZZ	Release Left Breast, Percutaneous Approach
0HNU7ZZ	Release Left Breast, Via Natural or Artificial Opening
0HNU8ZZ	Release Left Breast, Via Natural or Artificial Opening Endoscopic

0HNV0ZZ	Release Bilateral Breast, Open Approach
0HNV3ZZ	Release Bilateral Breast, Percutaneous Approach
0HNV7ZZ	Release Bilateral Breast, Via Natural or Artificial Opening
0HNV8ZZ	Release Bilateral Breast, Via Natural or Artificial Opening Endoscopic
0HNW0ZZ	Release Right Nipple, Open Approach
0HNW3ZZ	Release Right Nipple, Percutaneous Approach
0HNW7ZZ	Release Right Nipple, Via Natural or Artificial Opening
0HNW8ZZ	Release Right Nipple, Via Natural or Artificial Opening Endoscopic
0HNWXZZ	Release Right Nipple, External Approach
0HNX0ZZ	Release Left Nipple, Open Approach
0HNX3ZZ	Release Left Nipple, Percutaneous Approach
0HNX7ZZ	Release Left Nipple, Via Natural or Artificial Opening
0HNX8ZZ	Release Left Nipple, Via Natural or Artificial Opening Endoscopic
0HNXXZZ	Release Left Nipple, External Approach

0HP – Skin and Breast, Removal

Review Coding Guideline B6.1c

0HPPX0Z	Removal of Drainage Device from Skin, External Approach
0HPPX7Z	Removal of Autologous Tissue Substitute from Skin, External Approach
0HPPXJZ	Removal of Synthetic Substitute from Skin, External Approach
0HPPXKZ	Removal of Nonautologous Tissue Substitute from Skin, External Approach
0HPPXYZ	Removal of Other Device from Skin, External Approach
0HPQX0Z	Removal of Drainage Device from Finger Nail, External Approach
0HPQX7Z	Removal of Autologous Tissue Substitute from Finger Nail, External Approach

0HPQXJZ	Removal of Synthetic Substitute from Finger Nail, External Approach
0HPQXKZ	Removal of Nonautologous Tissue Substitute from Finger Nail, External Approach
0HPRX0Z	Removal of Drainage Device from Toe Nail, External Approach
0HPRX7Z	Removal of Autologous Tissue Substitute from Toe Nail, External Approach
0HPRXJZ	Removal of Synthetic Substitute from Toe Nail, External Approach
0HPRXKZ	Removal of Nonautologous Tissue Substitute from Toe Nail, External Approach
0HPSX7Z	Removal of Autologous Tissue Substitute from Hair, External Approach

0HPSXJZ	Removal of Synthetic Substitute from Hair, External Approach
0HPSXKZ	Removal of Nonautologous Tissue Substitute from Hair, External Approach
0HPT00Z	Removal of Drainage Device from Right Breast, Open Approach
0HPT01Z	Removal of Radioactive Element from Right Breast, Open Approach
0HPT07Z	Removal of Autologous Tissue Substitute from Right Breast, Open Approach
	AHA CC: 2Q, 2016, 27
0HPT0JZ	Removal of Synthetic Substitute from Right Breast, Open Approach
0HPT0KZ	Removal of Nonautologous Tissue Substitute from Right Breast, Open Approach

♀ Female-only   ♂ Male-only   ▲ Limited Coverage   ● Non-OR   HAC HAC-associated procedure   ▲ Non-covered procedures   ✚ Cluster

0HPT0NZ Removal of Tissue Expander from Right Breast, Open Approach
AHA CC: 3Q, 2018, 13-14
0HPT0YZ Removal of Other Device from Right Breast, Open Approach
0HPT30Z Removal of Drainage Device from Right Breast, Percutaneous Approach
0HPT31Z Removal of Radioactive Element from Right Breast, Percutaneous Approach
0HPT37Z Removal of Autologous Tissue Substitute from Right Breast, Percutaneous Approach
0HPT3JZ Removal of Synthetic Substitute from Right Breast, Percutaneous Approach
0HPT3KZ Removal of Nonautologous Tissue Substitute from Right Breast, Percutaneous Approach
0HPT3NZ Removal of Tissue Expander from Right Breast, Percutaneous Approach
0HPT3YZ Removal of Other Device from Right Breast, Percutaneous Approach
0HPT70Z Removal of Drainage Device from Right Breast, Via Natural or Artificial Opening
0HPT71Z Removal of Radioactive Element from Right Breast, Via Natural or Artificial Opening
0HPT77Z Removal of Autologous Tissue Substitute from Right Breast, Via Natural or Artificial Opening
0HPT7JZ Removal of Synthetic Substitute from Right Breast, Via Natural or Artificial Opening
0HPT7KZ Removal of Nonautologous Tissue Substitute from Right Breast, Via Natural or Artificial Opening
0HPT7NZ Removal of Tissue Expander from Right Breast, Via Natural or Artificial Opening
0HPT7YZ Removal of Other Device from Right Breast, Via Natural or Artificial Opening
0HPT80Z Removal of Drainage Device from Right Breast, Via Natural or Artificial Opening Endoscopic
0HPT81Z Removal of Radioactive Element from Right Breast, Via Natural or Artificial Opening Endoscopic

0HPT87Z Removal of Autologous Tissue Substitute from Right Breast, Via Natural or Artificial Opening Endoscopic
0HPT8JZ Removal of Synthetic Substitute from Right Breast, Via Natural or Artificial Opening Endoscopic
0HPT8KZ Removal of Nonautologous Tissue Substitute from Right Breast, Via Natural or Artificial Opening Endoscopic
0HPT8NZ Removal of Tissue Expander from Right Breast, Via Natural or Artificial Opening Endoscopic
0HPT8YZ Removal of Other Device from Right Breast, Via Natural or Artificial Opening Endoscopic
0HPU00Z Removal of Drainage Device from Left Breast, Open Approach
0HPU01Z Removal of Radioactive Element from Left Breast, Open Approach
0HPU07Z Removal of Autologous Tissue Substitute from Left Breast, Open Approach
AHA CC: 2Q, 2016, 27
0HPU0JZ Removal of Synthetic Substitute from Left Breast, Open Approach
0HPU0KZ Removal of Nonautologous Tissue Substitute from Left Breast, Open Approach
0HPU0NZ Removal of Tissue Expander from Left Breast, Open Approach
0HPU0YZ Removal of Other Device from Left Breast, Open Approach
0HPU30Z Removal of Drainage Device from Left Breast, Percutaneous Approach
0HPU31Z Removal of Radioactive Element from Left Breast, Percutaneous Approach
0HPU37Z Removal of Autologous Tissue Substitute from Left Breast, Percutaneous Approach
0HPU3JZ Removal of Synthetic Substitute from Left Breast, Percutaneous Approach
0HPU3KZ Removal of Nonautologous Tissue Substitute from Left Breast, Percutaneous Approach
0HPU3NZ Removal of Tissue Expander from Left Breast, Percutaneous Approach

0HPU3YZ Removal of Other Device from Left Breast, Percutaneous Approach
0HPU70Z Removal of Drainage Device from Left Breast, Via Natural or Artificial Opening
0HPU71Z Removal of Radioactive Element from Left Breast, Via Natural or Artificial Opening
0HPU77Z Removal of Autologous Tissue Substitute from Left Breast, Via Natural or Artificial Opening
0HPU7JZ Removal of Synthetic Substitute from Left Breast, Via Natural or Artificial Opening
0HPU7KZ Removal of Nonautologous Tissue Substitute from Left Breast, Via Natural or Artificial Opening
0HPU7NZ Removal of Tissue Expander from Left Breast, Via Natural or Artificial Opening
0HPU7YZ Removal of Other Device from Left Breast, Via Natural or Artificial Opening
0HPU80Z Removal of Drainage Device from Left Breast, Via Natural or Artificial Opening Endoscopic
0HPU81Z Removal of Radioactive Element from Left Breast, Via Natural or Artificial Opening Endoscopic
0HPU87Z Removal of Autologous Tissue Substitute from Left Breast, Via Natural or Artificial Opening Endoscopic
0HPU8JZ Removal of Synthetic Substitute from Left Breast, Via Natural or Artificial Opening Endoscopic
0HPU8KZ Removal of Nonautologous Tissue Substitute from Left Breast, Via Natural or Artificial Opening Endoscopic
0HPU8NZ Removal of Tissue Expander from Left Breast, Via Natural or Artificial Opening Endoscopic
0HPU8YZ Removal of Other Device from Left Breast, Via Natural or Artificial Opening Endoscopic

0HQ – Skin and Breast, Repair

Review Coding Guideline B3.5

0HQ0XZZ Repair Scalp Skin, External Approach
0HQ1XZZ Repair Face Skin, External Approach
0HQ2XZZ Repair Right Ear Skin, External Approach
0HQ3XZZ Repair Left Ear Skin, External Approach
0HQ4XZZ Repair Neck Skin, External Approach
0HQ5XZZ Repair Chest Skin, External Approach
0HQ6XZZ Repair Back Skin, External Approach
0HQ7XZZ Repair Abdomen Skin, External Approach
0HQ8XZZ Repair Buttock Skin, External Approach
● 0HQ9XZZ Repair Perineum Skin, External Approach
AHA CC: 1Q, 2016, 7
0HQAXZZ Repair Inguinal Skin, External Approach
0HQBXZZ Repair Right Upper Arm Skin, External Approach
0HQCXZZ Repair Left Upper Arm Skin, External Approach

0HQDXZZ Repair Right Lower Arm Skin, External Approach
0HQEXZZ Repair Left Lower Arm Skin, External Approach
AHA CC: 4Q, 2014, 31-32
0HQFXZZ Repair Right Hand Skin, External Approach
0HQGXZZ Repair Left Hand Skin, External Approach
0HQHXZZ Repair Right Upper Leg Skin, External Approach
0HQJXZZ Repair Left Upper Leg Skin, External Approach
0HQKXZZ Repair Right Lower Leg Skin, External Approach
0HQLXZZ Repair Left Lower Leg Skin, External Approach
0HQMXZZ Repair Right Foot Skin, External Approach
0HQNXZZ Repair Left Foot Skin, External Approach
0HQQXZZ Repair Finger Nail, External Approach

0HQRXZZ Repair Toe Nail, External Approach
0HQT0ZZ Repair Right Breast, Open Approach
0HQT3ZZ Repair Right Breast, Percutaneous Approach
0HQT7ZZ Repair Right Breast, Via Natural or Artificial Opening
0HQT8ZZ Repair Right Breast, Via Natural or Artificial Opening Endoscopic
0HQU0ZZ Repair Left Breast, Open Approach
0HQU3ZZ Repair Left Breast, Percutaneous Approach
0HQU7ZZ Repair Left Breast, Via Natural or Artificial Opening
0HQU8ZZ Repair Left Breast, Via Natural or Artificial Opening Endoscopic
0HQV0ZZ Repair Bilateral Breast, Open Approach
0HQV3ZZ Repair Bilateral Breast, Percutaneous Approach
0HQV7ZZ Repair Bilateral Breast, Via Natural or Artificial Opening
0HQV8ZZ Repair Bilateral Breast, Via Natural or Artificial Opening Endoscopic

♀ Female-only ♂ Male-only ▲ Limited Coverage ● Non-OR HAC HAC-associated procedure ▲ Non-covered procedures ✛ Cluster

0HQW0ZZ Repair Right Nipple, Open Approach

0HQW3ZZ Repair Right Nipple, Percutaneous Approach

0HQW7ZZ Repair Right Nipple, Via Natural or Artificial Opening

0HQW8ZZ Repair Right Nipple, Via Natural or Artificial Opening Endoscopic

0HQWXZZ Repair Right Nipple, External Approach

0HQX0ZZ Repair Left Nipple, Open Approach

0HQX3ZZ Repair Left Nipple, Percutaneous Approach

0HQX7ZZ Repair Left Nipple, Via Natural or Artificial Opening

0HQX8ZZ Repair Left Nipple, Via Natural or Artificial Opening Endoscopic

0HQXXZZ Repair Left Nipple, External Approach

0HQY0ZZ Repair Supernumerary Breast, Open Approach

0HQY3ZZ Repair Supernumerary Breast, Percutaneous Approach

0HQY7ZZ Repair Supernumerary Breast, Via Natural or Artificial Opening

0HQY8ZZ Repair Supernumerary Breast, Via Natural or Artificial Opening Endoscopic

0HR – Skin and Breast, Replacement

Review Coding Guideline B3.18

0HR0X72 Replacement of Scalp Skin with Autologous Tissue Substitute, Cell Suspension Technique, External Approach

0HR0X73 Replacement of Scalp Skin with Autologous Tissue Substitute, Full Thickness, External Approach

0HR0X74 Replacement of Scalp Skin with Autologous Tissue Substitute, Partial Thickness, External Approach

0HR0XJ3 Replacement of Scalp Skin with Synthetic Substitute, Full Thickness, External Approach

0HR0XJ4 Replacement of Scalp Skin with Synthetic Substitute, Partial Thickness, External Approach

0HR0XJZ Replacement of Scalp Skin with Synthetic Substitute, External Approach

0HR0XK3 Replacement of Scalp Skin with Nonautologous Tissue Substitute, Full Thickness, External Approach

0HR0XK4 Replacement of Scalp Skin with Nonautologous Tissue Substitute, Partial Thickness, External Approach

0HR1X72 Replacement of Face Skin with Autologous Tissue Substitute, Cell Suspension Technique, External Approach

0HR1X73 Replacement of Face Skin with Autologous Tissue Substitute, Full Thickness, External Approach

0HR1X74 Replacement of Face Skin with Autologous Tissue Substitute, Partial Thickness, External Approach

0HR1XJ3 Replacement of Face Skin with Synthetic Substitute, Full Thickness, External Approach

0HR1XJ4 Replacement of Face Skin with Synthetic Substitute, Partial Thickness, External Approach

0HR1XJZ Replacement of Face Skin with Synthetic Substitute, External Approach

0HR1XK3 Replacement of Face Skin with Nonautologous Tissue Substitute, Full Thickness, External Approach

0HR1XK4 Replacement of Face Skin with Nonautologous Tissue Substitute, Partial Thickness, External Approach

0HR2X72 Replacement of Right Ear Skin with Autologous Tissue Substitute, Cell Suspension Technique, External Approach

0HR2X73 Replacement of Right Ear Skin with Autologous Tissue Substitute, Full Thickness, External Approach

0HR2X74 Replacement of Right Ear Skin with Autologous Tissue Substitute, Partial Thickness, External Approach

0HR2XJ3 Replacement of Right Ear Skin with Synthetic Substitute, Full Thickness, External Approach

0HR2XJ4 Replacement of Right Ear Skin with Synthetic Substitute, Partial Thickness, External Approach

0HR2XJZ Replacement of Right Ear Skin with Synthetic Substitute, External Approach

0HR2XK3 Replacement of Right Ear Skin with Nonautologous Tissue Substitute, Full Thickness, External Approach

0HR2XK4 Replacement of Right Ear Skin with Nonautologous Tissue Substitute, Partial Thickness, External Approach

0HR3X72 Replacement of Left Ear Skin with Autologous Tissue Substitute, Cell Suspension Technique, External Approach

0HR3X73 Replacement of Left Ear Skin with Autologous Tissue Substitute, Full Thickness, External Approach

0HR3X74 Replacement of Left Ear Skin with Autologous Tissue Substitute, Partial Thickness, External Approach

0HR3XJ3 Replacement of Left Ear Skin with Synthetic Substitute, Full Thickness, External Approach

0HR3XJ4 Replacement of Left Ear Skin with Synthetic Substitute, Partial Thickness, External Approach

0HR3XJZ Replacement of Left Ear Skin with Synthetic Substitute, External Approach

0HR3XK3 Replacement of Left Ear Skin with Nonautologous Tissue Substitute, Full Thickness, External Approach

0HR3XK4 Replacement of Left Ear Skin with Nonautologous Tissue Substitute, Partial Thickness, External Approach

0HR4X72 Replacement of Neck Skin with Autologous Tissue Substitute, Cell Suspension Technique, External Approach

0HR4X72 Replacement of Neck Skin with Autologous Tissue Substitute, Cell Suspension Technique, External Approach

0HR4X73 Replacement of Neck Skin with Autologous Tissue Substitute, Full Thickness, External Approach

0HR4X74 Replacement of Neck Skin with Autologous Tissue Substitute, Partial Thickness, External Approach

0HR4XJ3 Replacement of Neck Skin with Synthetic Substitute, Full Thickness, External Approach

0HR4XJ4 Replacement of Neck Skin with Synthetic Substitute, Partial Thickness, External Approach

0HR4XJZ Replacement of Neck Skin with Synthetic Substitute, External Approach

0HR4XK3 Replacement of Neck Skin with Nonautologous Tissue Substitute, Full Thickness, External Approach

0HR4XK4 Replacement of Neck Skin with Nonautologous Tissue Substitute, Partial Thickness, External Approach

0HR5X72 Replacement of Chest Skin with Autologous Tissue Substitute, Cell Suspension Technique, External Approach

0HR5X73 Replacement of Chest Skin with Autologous Tissue Substitute, Full Thickness, External Approach

0HR5X74 Replacement of Chest Skin with Autologous Tissue Substitute, Partial Thickness, External Approach

0HR5XJ3 Replacement of Chest Skin with Synthetic Substitute, Full Thickness, External Approach

0HR5XJ4 Replacement of Chest Skin with Synthetic Substitute, Partial Thickness, External Approach

0HR5XJZ Replacement of Chest Skin with Synthetic Substitute, External Approach

0HR5XK3 Replacement of Chest Skin with Nonautologous Tissue Substitute, Full Thickness, External Approach

0HR5XK4 Replacement of Chest Skin with Nonautologous Tissue Substitute, Partial Thickness, External Approach

0HR6X72 Replacement of Back Skin with Autologous Tissue Substitute, Cell Suspension Technique, External Approach

0HR6X73 Replacement of Back Skin with Autologous Tissue Substitute, Full Thickness, External Approach

0HR6X74 Replacement of Back Skin with Autologous Tissue Substitute, Partial Thickness, External Approach

0HR6XJ3 Replacement of Back Skin with Synthetic Substitute, Full Thickness, External Approach

0HR6XJ4 Replacement of Back Skin with Synthetic Substitute, Partial Thickness, External Approach

0HR6XJZ Replacement of Back Skin with Synthetic Substitute, External Approach

0HR6XK3 Replacement of Back Skin with Nonautologous Tissue Substitute, Full Thickness, External Approach

0HR6XK4 Replacement of Back Skin with Nonautologous Tissue Substitute, Partial Thickness, External Approach

0HR7X72 Replacement of Abdomen Skin with Autologous Tissue Substitute, Cell Suspension Technique, External Approach

0HR7X73 Replacement of Abdomen Skin with Autologous Tissue Substitute, Full Thickness, External Approach

0HR7X74 Replacement of Abdomen Skin with Autologous Tissue Substitute, Partial Thickness, External Approach

♀ Female-only   ♂ Male-only   ▲ Limited Coverage   ● Non-OR   ▦ HAC-associated procedure   ▲ Non-covered procedures   ✚ Cluster

0HR7XJ3 Replacement of Abdomen Skin with Synthetic Substitute, Full Thickness, External Approach

0HR7XJ4 Replacement of Abdomen Skin with Synthetic Substitute, Partial Thickness, External Approach

0HR7XJZ Replacement of Abdomen Skin with Synthetic Substitute, External Approach

0HR7XK3 Replacement of Abdomen Skin with Nonautologous Tissue Substitute, Full Thickness, External Approach

0HR7XK4 Replacement of Abdomen Skin with Nonautologous Tissue Substitute, Partial Thickness, External Approach

0HR8X72 Replacement of Buttock Skin with Autologous Tissue Substitute, Cell Suspension Technique, External Approach

0HR8X73 Replacement of Buttock Skin with Autologous Tissue Substitute, Full Thickness, External Approach

0HR8X74 Replacement of Buttock Skin with Autologous Tissue Substitute, Partial Thickness, External Approach

0HR8XJ3 Replacement of Buttock Skin with Synthetic Substitute, Full Thickness, External Approach

0HR8XJ4 Replacement of Buttock Skin with Synthetic Substitute, Partial Thickness, External Approach

0HR8XJZ Replacement of Buttock Skin with Synthetic Substitute, External Approach

0HR8XK3 Replacement of Buttock Skin with Nonautologous Tissue Substitute, Full Thickness, External Approach

0HR8XK4 Replacement of Buttock Skin with Nonautologous Tissue Substitute, Partial Thickness, External Approach

0HR9X72 Replacement of Perineum Skin with Autologous Tissue Substitute, Cell Suspension Technique, External Approach

0HR9X73 Replacement of Perineum Skin with Autologous Tissue Substitute, Full Thickness, External Approach

0HR9X74 Replacement of Perineum Skin with Autologous Tissue Substitute, Partial Thickness, External Approach

0HR9XJ3 Replacement of Perineum Skin with Synthetic Substitute, Full Thickness, External Approach

0HR9XJ4 Replacement of Perineum Skin with Synthetic Substitute, Partial Thickness, External Approach

0HR9XJZ Replacement of Perineum Skin with Synthetic Substitute, External Approach

0HR9XK3 Replacement of Perineum Skin with Nonautologous Tissue Substitute, Full Thickness, External Approach

0HR9XK4 Replacement of Perineum Skin with Nonautologous Tissue Substitute, Partial Thickness, External Approach

0HRAX72 Replacement of Inguinal Skin with Autologous Tissue Substitute, Cell Suspension Technique, External Approach

0HRAX73 Replacement of Inguinal Skin with Autologous Tissue Substitute, Full Thickness, External Approach

0HRAX74 Replacement of Inguinal Skin with Autologous Tissue Substitute, Partial Thickness, External Approach

0HRAXJ3 Replacement of Inguinal Skin with Synthetic Substitute, Full Thickness, External Approach

0HRAXJ4 Replacement of Inguinal Skin with Synthetic Substitute, Partial Thickness, External Approach

0HRAXJZ Replacement of Inguinal Skin with Synthetic Substitute, External Approach

0HRAXK3 Replacement of Inguinal Skin with Nonautologous Tissue Substitute, Full Thickness, External Approach

0HRAXK4 Replacement of Inguinal Skin with Nonautologous Tissue Substitute, Partial Thickness, External Approach

0HRBX72 Replacement of Right Upper Arm Skin with Autologous Tissue Substitute, Cell Suspension Technique, External Approach

0HRBX73 Replacement of Right Upper Arm Skin with Autologous Tissue Substitute, Full Thickness, External Approach

0HRBX74 Replacement of Right Upper Arm Skin with Autologous Tissue Substitute, Partial Thickness, External Approach

0HRBXJ3 Replacement of Right Upper Arm Skin with Synthetic Substitute, Full Thickness, External Approach

0HRBXJ4 Replacement of Right Upper Arm Skin with Synthetic Substitute, Partial Thickness, External Approach

0HRBXJZ Replacement of Right Upper Arm Skin with Synthetic Substitute, External Approach

0HRBXK3 Replacement of Right Upper Arm Skin with Nonautologous Tissue Substitute, Full Thickness, External Approach

0HRBXK4 Replacement of Right Upper Arm Skin with Nonautologous Tissue Substitute, Partial Thickness, External Approach

0HRCX72 Replacement of Left Upper Arm Skin with Autologous Tissue Substitute, Cell Suspension Technique, External Approach

0HRCX73 Replacement of Left Upper Arm Skin with Autologous Tissue Substitute, Full Thickness, External Approach

0HRCX74 Replacement of Left Upper Arm Skin with Autologous Tissue Substitute, Partial Thickness, External Approach

0HRCXJ3 Replacement of Left Upper Arm Skin with Synthetic Substitute, Full Thickness, External Approach

0HRCXJ4 Replacement of Left Upper Arm Skin with Synthetic Substitute, Partial Thickness, External Approach

0HRCXJZ Replacement of Left Upper Arm Skin with Synthetic Substitute, External Approach

0HRCXK3 Replacement of Left Upper Arm Skin with Nonautologous Tissue Substitute, Full Thickness, External Approach

0HRCXK4 Replacement of Left Upper Arm Skin with Nonautologous Tissue Substitute, Partial Thickness, External Approach

0HRDX72 Replacement of Right Lower Arm Skin with Autologous Tissue Substitute, Cell Suspension Technique, External Approach

0HRDX73 Replacement of Right Lower Arm Skin with Autologous Tissue Substitute, Full Thickness, External Approach

0HRDX74 Replacement of Right Lower Arm Skin with Autologous Tissue Substitute, Partial Thickness, External Approach

0HRDXJ3 Replacement of Right Lower Arm Skin with Synthetic Substitute, Full Thickness, External Approach

0HRDXJ4 Replacement of Right Lower Arm Skin with Synthetic Substitute, Partial Thickness, External Approach

0HRDXJZ Replacement of Right Lower Arm Skin with Synthetic Substitute, External Approach

0HRDXK3 Replacement of Right Lower Arm Skin with Nonautologous Tissue Substitute, Full Thickness, External Approach

0HRDXK4 Replacement of Right Lower Arm Skin with Nonautologous Tissue Substitute, Partial Thickness, External Approach

0HREX72 Replacement of Left Lower Arm Skin with Autologous Tissue Substitute, Cell Suspension Technique, External Approach

0HREX73 Replacement of Left Lower Arm Skin with Autologous Tissue Substitute, Full Thickness, External Approach

0HREX74 Replacement of Left Lower Arm Skin with Autologous Tissue Substitute, Partial Thickness, External Approach

0HREXJ3 Replacement of Left Lower Arm Skin with Synthetic Substitute, Full Thickness, External Approach

0HREXJ4 Replacement of Left Lower Arm Skin with Synthetic Substitute, Partial Thickness, External Approach

0HREXJZ Replacement of Left Lower Arm Skin with Synthetic Substitute, External Approach

0HREXK3 Replacement of Left Lower Arm Skin with Nonautologous Tissue Substitute, Full Thickness, External Approach

0HREXK4 Replacement of Left Lower Arm Skin with Nonautologous Tissue Substitute, Partial Thickness, External Approach

0HRFX72 Replacement of Right Hand Skin with Autologous Tissue Substitute, Cell Suspension Technique, External Approach

0HRFX73 Replacement of Right Hand Skin with Autologous Tissue Substitute, Full Thickness, External Approach

0HRFX74 Replacement of Right Hand Skin with Autologous Tissue Substitute, Partial Thickness, External Approach

0HRFXJ3 Replacement of Right Hand Skin with Synthetic Substitute, Full Thickness, External Approach

0HRFXJ4 Replacement of Right Hand Skin with Synthetic Substitute, Partial Thickness, External Approach

0HRFXJZ Replacement of Right Hand Skin with Synthetic Substitute, External Approach

0HRFXK3 Replacement of Right Hand Skin with Nonautologous Tissue Substitute, Full Thickness, External Approach

0HRFXK4 Replacement of Right Hand Skin with Nonautologous Tissue Substitute, Partial Thickness, External Approach

0HRGX72 Replacement of Left Hand Skin with Autologous Tissue Substitute, Cell Suspension Technique, External Approach

0HRGX73 Replacement of Left Hand Skin with Autologous Tissue Substitute, Full Thickness, External Approach

0HRGX74 Replacement of Left Hand Skin with Autologous Tissue Substitute, Partial Thickness, External Approach

0HRGXJ3 Replacement of Left Hand Skin with Synthetic Substitute, Full Thickness, External Approach

0HRGXJ4	Replacement of Left Hand Skin with Synthetic Substitute, Partial Thickness, External Approach
0HRGXJZ	Replacement of Left Hand Skin with Synthetic Substitute, External Approach
0HRGXK3	Replacement of Left Hand Skin with Nonautologous Tissue Substitute, Full Thickness, External Approach
0HRGXK4	Replacement of Left Hand Skin with Nonautologous Tissue Substitute, Partial Thickness, External Approach
0HRHX72	Replacement of Right Upper Leg Skin with Autologous Tissue Substitute, Cell Suspension Technique, External Approach
0HRHX73	Replacement of Right Upper Leg Skin with Autologous Tissue Substitute, Full Thickness, External Approach
0HRHX74	Replacement of Right Upper Leg Skin with Autologous Tissue Substitute, Partial Thickness, External Approach
0HRHXJ3	Replacement of Right Upper Leg Skin with Synthetic Substitute, Full Thickness, External Approach
0HRHXJ4	Replacement of Right Upper Leg Skin with Synthetic Substitute, Partial Thickness, External Approach
0HRHXJZ	Replacement of Right Upper Leg Skin with Synthetic Substitute, External Approach
0HRHXK3	Replacement of Right Upper Leg Skin with Nonautologous Tissue Substitute, Full Thickness, External Approach
0HRHXK4	Replacement of Right Upper Leg Skin with Nonautologous Tissue Substitute, Partial Thickness, External Approach
0HRJX72	Replacement of Left Upper Leg Skin with Autologous Tissue Substitute, Cell Suspension Technique, External Approach
0HRJX73	Replacement of Left Upper Leg Skin with Autologous Tissue Substitute, Full Thickness, External Approach
0HRJX74	Replacement of Left Upper Leg Skin with Autologous Tissue Substitute, Partial Thickness, External Approach
0HRJXJ3	Replacement of Left Upper Leg Skin with Synthetic Substitute, Full Thickness, External Approach
0HRJXJ4	Replacement of Left Upper Leg Skin with Synthetic Substitute, Partial Thickness, External Approach
0HRJXJZ	Replacement of Left Upper Leg Skin with Synthetic Substitute, External Approach
0HRJXK3	Replacement of Left Upper Leg Skin with Nonautologous Tissue Substitute, Full Thickness, External Approach
0HRJXK4	Replacement of Left Upper Leg Skin with Nonautologous Tissue Substitute, Partial Thickness, External Approach
0HRKX72	Replacement of Right Lower Leg Skin with Autologous Tissue Substitute, Cell Suspension Technique, External Approach
0HRKX73	Replacement of Right Lower Leg Skin with Autologous Tissue Substitute, Full Thickness, External Approach
0HRKX74	Replacement of Right Lower Leg Skin with Autologous Tissue Substitute, Partial Thickness, External Approach
0HRKXJ3	Replacement of Right Lower Leg Skin with Synthetic Substitute, Full Thickness, External Approach
0HRKXJ4	Replacement of Right Lower Leg Skin with Synthetic Substitute, Partial Thickness, External Approach
0HRKXJZ	Replacement of Right Lower Leg Skin with Synthetic Substitute, External Approach
0HRKXK3	Replacement of Right Lower Leg Skin with Nonautologous Tissue Substitute, Full Thickness, External Approach
0HRKXK4	Replacement of Right Lower Leg Skin with Nonautologous Tissue Substitute, Partial Thickness, External Approach
0HRLX72	Replacement of Left Lower Leg Skin with Autologous Tissue Substitute, Cell Suspension Technique, External Approach
0HRLX73	Replacement of Left Lower Leg Skin with Autologous Tissue Substitute, Full Thickness, External Approach
0HRLX74	Replacement of Left Lower Leg Skin with Autologous Tissue Substitute, Partial Thickness, External Approach
0HRLXJ3	Replacement of Left Lower Leg Skin with Synthetic Substitute, Full Thickness, External Approach
0HRLXJ4	Replacement of Left Lower Leg Skin with Synthetic Substitute, Partial Thickness, External Approach
0HRLXJZ	Replacement of Left Lower Leg Skin with Synthetic Substitute, External Approach
0HRLXK3	Replacement of Left Lower Leg Skin with Nonautologous Tissue Substitute, Full Thickness, External Approach
0HRLXK4	Replacement of Left Lower Leg Skin with Nonautologous Tissue Substitute, Partial Thickness, External Approach
0HRMX72	Replacement of Right Foot Skin with Autologous Tissue Substitute, Cell Suspension Technique, External Approach
0HRMX73	Replacement of Right Foot Skin with Autologous Tissue Substitute, Full Thickness, External Approach
0HRMX74	Replacement of Right Foot Skin with Autologous Tissue Substitute, Partial Thickness, External Approach
0HRMXJ3	Replacement of Right Foot Skin with Synthetic Substitute, Full Thickness, External Approach
0HRMXJ4	Replacement of Right Foot Skin with Synthetic Substitute, Partial Thickness, External Approach
0HRMXJZ	Replacement of Right Foot Skin with Synthetic Substitute, External Approach
0HRMXK3	Replacement of Right Foot Skin with Nonautologous Tissue Substitute, Full Thickness, External Approach

AHA CC: 1Q, 2017, 35-36

0HRMXK4	Replacement of Right Foot Skin with Nonautologous Tissue Substitute, Partial Thickness, External Approach
0HRNX72	Replacement of Left Foot Skin with Autologous Tissue Substitute, Cell Suspension Technique, External Approach
0HRNX73	Replacement of Left Foot Skin with Autologous Tissue Substitute, Full Thickness, External Approach
0HRNX74	Replacement of Left Foot Skin with Autologous Tissue Substitute, Partial Thickness, External Approach
0HRNXJ3	Replacement of Left Foot Skin with Synthetic Substitute, Full Thickness, External Approach
0HRNXJ4	Replacement of Left Foot Skin with Synthetic Substitute, Partial Thickness, External Approach
0HRNXJZ	Replacement of Left Foot Skin with Synthetic Substitute, External Approach
0HRNXK3	Replacement of Left Foot Skin with Nonautologous Tissue Substitute, Full Thickness, External Approach

AHA CC: 3Q, 2014, 14-15

0HRNXK4	Replacement of Left Foot Skin with Nonautologous Tissue Substitute, Partial Thickness, External Approach
0HRQX7Z	Replacement of Finger Nail with Autologous Tissue Substitute, External Approach
0HRQXJZ	Replacement of Finger Nail with Synthetic Substitute, External Approach
0HRQXKZ	Replacement of Finger Nail with Nonautologous Tissue Substitute, External Approach
0HRRX7Z	Replacement of Toe Nail with Autologous Tissue Substitute, External Approach
0HRRXJZ	Replacement of Toe Nail with Synthetic Substitute, External Approach
0HRRXKZ	Replacement of Toe Nail with Nonautologous Tissue Substitute, External Approach
0HRSX7Z	Replacement of Hair with Autologous Tissue Substitute, External Approach
0HRSXJZ	Replacement of Hair with Synthetic Substitute, External Approach
0HRSXKZ	Replacement of Hair with Nonautologous Tissue Substitute, External Approach
0HRT075	Replacement of Right Breast using Latissimus Dorsi Myocutaneous Flap, Open Approach
0HRT076	Replacement of Right Breast using Transverse Rectus Abdominis Myocutaneous Flap, Open Approach
0HRT077	Replacement of Right Breast using Deep Inferior Epigastric Artery Perforator Flap, Open Approach
0HRT078	Replacement of Right Breast using Superficial Inferior Epigastric Artery Flap, Open Approach
0HRT079	Replacement of Right Breast using Gluteal Artery Perforator Flap, Open Approach
0HRT07Z	Replacement of Right Breast with Autologous Tissue Substitute, Open Approach
0HRT0JZ	Replacement of Right Breast with Synthetic Substitute, Open Approach
0HRT0KZ	Replacement of Right Breast with Nonautologous Tissue Substitute, Open Approach
0HRT37Z	Replacement of Right Breast with Autologous Tissue Substitute, Percutaneous Approach
⊞	Breast replacement when reported with Extraction of subcutaneous tissue and fascia (4th characters 6,7,8,9,L or M). *See table 0JD to construct the Extraction code.*
0HRT3JZ	Replacement of Right Breast with Synthetic Substitute, Percutaneous Approach
0HRT3KZ	Replacement of Right Breast with Nonautologous Tissue Substitute, Percutaneous Approach
0HRU075	Replacement of Left Breast using Latissimus Dorsi Myocutaneous Flap, Open Approach

♀ Female-only   ♂ Male-only   ▲ Limited Coverage   ● Non-OR   ▪ HAC-associated procedure   ▲ Non-covered procedures   ⊞ Cluster

0HRU076 Replacement of Left Breast using Transverse Rectus Abdominis Myocutaneous Flap, Open Approach

0HRU077 Replacement of Left Breast using Deep Inferior Epigastric Artery Perforator Flap, Open Approach

0HRU078 Replacement of Left Breast using Superficial Inferior Epigastric Artery Flap, Open Approach

0HRU079 Replacement of Left Breast using Gluteal Artery Perforator Flap, Open Approach

0HRU07Z Replacement of Left Breast with Autologous Tissue Substitute, Open Approach
AHA CC: 1Q, 2020, 27-28

0HRU0JZ Replacement of Left Breast with Synthetic Substitute, Open Approach

0HRU0KZ Replacement of Left Breast with Nonautologous Tissue Substitute, Open Approach

0HRU37Z Replacement of Left Breast with Autologous Tissue Substitute, Percutaneous Approach

➕ Breast replacement when reported with Extraction of subcutaneous tissue and fascia (4th characters 6,7,8,9,L or M). *See table 0JD to construct the Extraction code.*

0HRU3JZ Replacement of Left Breast with Synthetic Substitute, Percutaneous Approach

0HRU3KZ Replacement of Left Breast with Nonautologous Tissue Substitute, Percutaneous Approach

0HRV075 Replacement of Bilateral Breast using Latissimus Dorsi Myocutaneous Flap, Open Approach

0HRV076 Replacement of Bilateral Breast using Transverse Rectus Abdominis Myocutaneous Flap, Open Approach

0HRV077 Replacement of Bilateral Breast using Deep Inferior Epigastric Artery Perforator Flap, Open Approach
AHA CC: 3Q, 2018, 13-14

0HRV078 Replacement of Bilateral Breast using Superficial Inferior Epigastric Artery Flap, Open Approach

0HRV079 Replacement of Bilateral Breast using Gluteal Artery Perforator Flap, Open Approach

0HRV07Z Replacement of Bilateral Breast with Autologous Tissue Substitute, Open Approach

0HRV0JZ Replacement of Bilateral Breast with Synthetic Substitute, Open Approach

0HRV0KZ Replacement of Bilateral Breast with Nonautologous Tissue Substitute, Open Approach

0HRV37Z Replacement of Bilateral Breast with Autologous Tissue Substitute, Percutaneous Approach

➕ Breast replacement when reported with Extraction of subcutaneous tissue and fascia (4th characters 6,7,8,9,L or M). *See table 0JD to construct the Extraction code.*

0HRV3JZ Replacement of Bilateral Breast with Synthetic Substitute, Percutaneous Approach

0HRV3KZ Replacement of Bilateral Breast with Nonautologous Tissue Substitute, Percutaneous Approach

0HRW07Z Replacement of Right Nipple with Autologous Tissue Substitute, Open Approach

0HRW0JZ Replacement of Right Nipple with Synthetic Substitute, Open Approach

0HRW0KZ Replacement of Right Nipple with Nonautologous Tissue Substitute, Open Approach

0HRW37Z Replacement of Right Nipple with Autologous Tissue Substitute, Percutaneous Approach

0HRW3JZ Replacement of Right Nipple with Synthetic Substitute, Percutaneous Approach

0HRW3KZ Replacement of Right Nipple with Nonautologous Tissue Substitute, Percutaneous Approach

0HRWX7Z Replacement of Right Nipple with Autologous Tissue Substitute, External Approach

0HRWXJZ Replacement of Right Nipple with Synthetic Substitute, External Approach

0HRWXKZ Replacement of Right Nipple with Nonautologous Tissue Substitute, External Approach

0HRX07Z Replacement of Left Nipple with Autologous Tissue Substitute, Open Approach

0HRX0JZ Replacement of Left Nipple with Synthetic Substitute, Open Approach

0HRX0KZ Replacement of Left Nipple with Nonautologous Tissue Substitute, Open Approach

0HRX37Z Replacement of Left Nipple with Autologous Tissue Substitute, Percutaneous Approach

0HRX3JZ Replacement of Left Nipple with Synthetic Substitute, Percutaneous Approach

0HRX3KZ Replacement of Left Nipple with Nonautologous Tissue Substitute, Percutaneous Approach

0HRXX7Z Replacement of Left Nipple with Autologous Tissue Substitute, External Approach

0HRXXJZ Replacement of Left Nipple with Synthetic Substitute, External Approach

0HRXXKZ Replacement of Left Nipple with Nonautologous Tissue Substitute, External Approach

0HS – Skin and Breast, Reposition

0HSSXZZ Reposition Hair, External Approach

0HST0ZZ Reposition Right Breast, Open Approach

0HSU0ZZ Reposition Left Breast, Open Approach

0HSV0ZZ Reposition Bilateral Breast, Open Approach

0HSWXZZ Reposition Right Nipple, External Approach

0HSXXZZ Reposition Left Nipple, External Approach

0HT – Skin and Breast, Resection

Review Coding Guideline B3.8

Review Coding Guideline B3.18

0HTQXZZ Resection of Finger Nail, External Approach

0HTRXZZ Resection of Toe Nail, External Approach

0HTT0ZZ Resection of Right Breast, Open Approach
AHA CC: 4Q, 2014, 34

0HTU0ZZ Resection of Left Breast, Open Approach
AHA CC: 3Q, 2018, 13-14

0HTV0ZZ Resection of Bilateral Breast, Open Approach
AHA CC: 2Q, 2021, 16-17

0HTWXZZ Resection of Right Nipple, External Approach

0HTXXZZ Resection of Left Nipple, External Approach

0HTY0ZZ Resection of Supernumerary Breast, Open Approach

0HU – Skin and Breast, Supplement

0HUT07Z Supplement Right Breast with Autologous Tissue Substitute, Open Approach

0HUT0JZ Supplement Right Breast with Synthetic Substitute, Open Approach

0HUT0KZ Supplement Right Breast with Nonautologous Tissue Substitute, Open Approach

0HUT37Z Supplement Right Breast with Autologous Tissue Substitute, Percutaneous Approach

0HUT3JZ Supplement Right Breast with Synthetic Substitute, Percutaneous Approach

0HUT3KZ Supplement Right Breast with Nonautologous Tissue Substitute, Percutaneous Approach

0HUT77Z Supplement Right Breast with Autologous Tissue Substitute, Via Natural or Artificial Opening

0HUT7JZ Supplement Right Breast with Synthetic Substitute, Via Natural or Artificial Opening

0HUT7KZ Supplement Right Breast with Nonautologous Tissue Substitute, Via Natural or Artificial Opening

---

♀ Female-only ♂ Male-only ▲ Limited Coverage ● Non-OR ⬛ HAC-associated procedure ▲ Non-covered procedures ➕ Cluster

0HUT87Z	Supplement Right Breast with Autologous Tissue Substitute, Via Natural or Artificial Opening Endoscopic	
0HUT8JZ	Supplement Right Breast with Synthetic Substitute, Via Natural or Artificial Opening Endoscopic	
0HUT8KZ	Supplement Right Breast with Nonautologous Tissue Substitute, Via Natural or Artificial Opening Endoscopic	
0HUU07Z	Supplement Left Breast with Autologous Tissue Substitute, Open Approach	
0HUU0JZ	Supplement Left Breast with Synthetic Substitute, Open Approach	
0HUU0KZ	Supplement Left Breast with Nonautologous Tissue Substitute, Open Approach	
0HUU37Z	Supplement Left Breast with Autologous Tissue Substitute, Percutaneous Approach	
0HUU3JZ	Supplement Left Breast with Synthetic Substitute, Percutaneous Approach	
0HUU3KZ	Supplement Left Breast with Nonautologous Tissue Substitute, Percutaneous Approach	
0HUU77Z	Supplement Left Breast with Autologous Tissue Substitute, Via Natural or Artificial Opening	
0HUU7JZ	Supplement Left Breast with Synthetic Substitute, Via Natural or Artificial Opening	
0HUU7KZ	Supplement Left Breast with Nonautologous Tissue Substitute, Via Natural or Artificial Opening	
0HUU87Z	Supplement Left Breast with Autologous Tissue Substitute, Via Natural or Artificial Opening Endoscopic	
0HUU8JZ	Supplement Left Breast with Synthetic Substitute, Via Natural or Artificial Opening Endoscopic	
0HUU8KZ	Supplement Left Breast with Nonautologous Tissue Substitute, Via Natural or Artificial Opening Endoscopic	
0HUV07Z	Supplement Bilateral Breast with Autologous Tissue Substitute, Open Approach	
0HUV0JZ	Supplement Bilateral Breast with Synthetic Substitute, Open Approach	
0HUV0KZ	Supplement Bilateral Breast with Nonautologous Tissue Substitute, Open Approach	
0HUV37Z	Supplement Bilateral Breast with Autologous Tissue Substitute, Percutaneous Approach	

0HUV3JZ	Supplement Bilateral Breast with Synthetic Substitute, Percutaneous Approach
0HUV3KZ	Supplement Bilateral Breast with Nonautologous Tissue Substitute, Percutaneous Approach
0HUV77Z	Supplement Bilateral Breast with Autologous Tissue Substitute, Via Natural or Artificial Opening
0HUV7JZ	Supplement Bilateral Breast with Synthetic Substitute, Via Natural or Artificial Opening
0HUV7KZ	Supplement Bilateral Breast with Nonautologous Tissue Substitute, Via Natural or Artificial Opening
0HUV87Z	Supplement Bilateral Breast with Autologous Tissue Substitute, Via Natural or Artificial Opening Endoscopic
0HUV8JZ	Supplement Bilateral Breast with Synthetic Substitute, Via Natural or Artificial Opening Endoscopic
0HUV8KZ	Supplement Bilateral Breast with Nonautologous Tissue Substitute, Via Natural or Artificial Opening Endoscopic
0HUW07Z	Supplement Right Nipple with Autologous Tissue Substitute, Open Approach
0HUW0JZ	Supplement Right Nipple with Synthetic Substitute, Open Approach
0HUW0KZ	Supplement Right Nipple with Nonautologous Tissue Substitute, Open Approach
0HUW37Z	Supplement Right Nipple with Autologous Tissue Substitute, Percutaneous Approach
0HUW3JZ	Supplement Right Nipple with Synthetic Substitute, Percutaneous Approach
0HUW3KZ	Supplement Right Nipple with Nonautologous Tissue Substitute, Percutaneous Approach
0HUW77Z	Supplement Right Nipple with Autologous Tissue Substitute, Via Natural or Artificial Opening
0HUW7JZ	Supplement Right Nipple with Synthetic Substitute, Via Natural or Artificial Opening
0HUW7KZ	Supplement Right Nipple with Nonautologous Tissue Substitute, Via Natural or Artificial Opening
0HUW87Z	Supplement Right Nipple with Autologous Tissue Substitute, Via Natural or Artificial Opening Endoscopic
0HUW8JZ	Supplement Right Nipple with Synthetic Substitute, Via Natural or Artificial Opening Endoscopic

0HUW8KZ	Supplement Right Nipple with Nonautologous Tissue Substitute, Via Natural or Artificial Opening Endoscopic
0HUWX7Z	Supplement Right Nipple with Autologous Tissue Substitute, External Approach
0HUWXJZ	Supplement Right Nipple with Synthetic Substitute, External Approach
0HUWXKZ	Supplement Right Nipple with Nonautologous Tissue Substitute, External Approach
0HUX07Z	Supplement Left Nipple with Autologous Tissue Substitute, Open Approach
0HUX0JZ	Supplement Left Nipple with Synthetic Substitute, Open Approach
0HUX0KZ	Supplement Left Nipple with Nonautologous Tissue Substitute, Open Approach
0HUX37Z	Supplement Left Nipple with Autologous Tissue Substitute, Percutaneous Approach
0HUX3JZ	Supplement Left Nipple with Synthetic Substitute, Percutaneous Approach
0HUX3KZ	Supplement Left Nipple with Nonautologous Tissue Substitute, Percutaneous Approach
0HUX77Z	Supplement Left Nipple with Autologous Tissue Substitute, Via Natural or Artificial Opening
0HUX7JZ	Supplement Left Nipple with Synthetic Substitute, Via Natural or Artificial Opening
0HUX7KZ	Supplement Left Nipple with Nonautologous Tissue Substitute, Via Natural or Artificial Opening
0HUX87Z	Supplement Left Nipple with Autologous Tissue Substitute, Via Natural or Artificial Opening Endoscopic
0HUX8JZ	Supplement Left Nipple with Synthetic Substitute, Via Natural or Artificial Opening Endoscopic
0HUX8KZ	Supplement Left Nipple with Nonautologous Tissue Substitute, Via Natural or Artificial Opening Endoscopic
0HUXX7Z	Supplement Left Nipple with Autologous Tissue Substitute, External Approach
0HUXXJZ	Supplement Left Nipple with Synthetic Substitute, External Approach
0HUXXKZ	Supplement Left Nipple with Nonautologous Tissue Substitute, External Approach

0HW – Skin and Breast, Revision

Review Coding Guideline B6.1c

0HWPX0Z	Revision of Drainage Device in Skin, External Approach	
0HWPX7Z	Revision of Autologous Tissue Substitute in Skin, External Approach	
0HWPXJZ	Revision of Synthetic Substitute in Skin, External Approach	
0HWPXKZ	Revision of Nonautologous Tissue Substitute in Skin, External Approach	
0HWPXYZ	Revision of Other Device in Skin, External Approach	

0HWQX0Z	Revision of Drainage Device in Finger Nail, External Approach
0HWQX7Z	Revision of Autologous Tissue Substitute in Finger Nail, External Approach
0HWQXJZ	Revision of Synthetic Substitute in Finger Nail, External Approach
0HWQXKZ	Revision of Nonautologous Tissue Substitute in Finger Nail, External Approach

0HWRX0Z	Revision of Drainage Device in Toe Nail, External Approach
0HWRX7Z	Revision of Autologous Tissue Substitute in Toe Nail, External Approach
0HWRXJZ	Revision of Synthetic Substitute in Toe Nail, External Approach
0HWRXKZ	Revision of Nonautologous Tissue Substitute in Toe Nail, External Approach

♀ Female-only ♂ Male-only ▲ Limited Coverage ● Non-OR HAC HAC-associated procedure ▲ Non-covered procedures ✚ Cluster

0HWSX7Z	Revision of Autologous Tissue Substitute in Hair, External Approach
0HWSXJZ	Revision of Synthetic Substitute in Hair, External Approach
0HWSXKZ	Revision of Nonautologous Tissue Substitute in Hair, External Approach
0HWT00Z	Revision of Drainage Device in Right Breast, Open Approach
0HWT07Z	Revision of Autologous Tissue Substitute in Right Breast, Open Approach
0HWT0JZ	Revision of Synthetic Substitute in Right Breast, Open Approach
0HWT0KZ	Revision of Nonautologous Tissue Substitute in Right Breast, Open Approach
0HWT0NZ	Revision of Tissue Expander in Right Breast, Open Approach
0HWT0YZ	Revision of Other Device in Right Breast, Open Approach
0HWT30Z	Revision of Drainage Device in Right Breast, Percutaneous Approach
0HWT37Z	Revision of Autologous Tissue Substitute in Right Breast, Percutaneous Approach
0HWT3JZ	Revision of Synthetic Substitute in Right Breast, Percutaneous Approach
0HWT3KZ	Revision of Nonautologous Tissue Substitute in Right Breast, Percutaneous Approach
0HWT3NZ	Revision of Tissue Expander in Right Breast, Percutaneous Approach
0HWT3YZ	Revision of Other Device in Right Breast, Percutaneous Approach
0HWT70Z	Revision of Drainage Device in Right Breast, Via Natural or Artificial Opening
0HWT77Z	Revision of Autologous Tissue Substitute in Right Breast, Via Natural or Artificial Opening
0HWT7JZ	Revision of Synthetic Substitute in Right Breast, Via Natural or Artificial Opening

0HWT7KZ	Revision of Nonautologous Tissue Substitute in Right Breast, Via Natural or Artificial Opening
0HWT7NZ	Revision of Tissue Expander in Right Breast, Via Natural or Artificial Opening
0HWT7YZ	Revision of Other Device in Right Breast, Via Natural or Artificial Opening
0HWT80Z	Revision of Drainage Device in Right Breast, Via Natural or Artificial Opening Endoscopic
0HWT87Z	Revision of Autologous Tissue Substitute in Right Breast, Via Natural or Artificial Opening Endoscopic
0HWT8JZ	Revision of Synthetic Substitute in Right Breast, Via Natural or Artificial Opening Endoscopic
0HWT8KZ	Revision of Nonautologous Tissue Substitute in Right Breast, Via Natural or Artificial Opening Endoscopic
0HWT8NZ	Revision of Tissue Expander in Right Breast, Via Natural or Artificial Opening Endoscopic
0HWT8YZ	Revision of Other Device in Right Breast, Via Natural or Artificial Opening Endoscopic
0HWU00Z	Revision of Drainage Device in Left Breast, Open Approach
0HWU07Z	Revision of Autologous Tissue Substitute in Left Breast, Open Approach
0HWU0JZ	Revision of Synthetic Substitute in Left Breast, Open Approach
0HWU0KZ	Revision of Nonautologous Tissue Substitute in Left Breast, Open Approach
0HWU0NZ	Revision of Tissue Expander in Left Breast, Open Approach
0HWU0YZ	Revision of Other Device in Left Breast, Open Approach
0HWU30Z	Revision of Drainage Device in Left Breast, Percutaneous Approach
0HWU37Z	Revision of Autologous Tissue Substitute in Left Breast, Percutaneous Approach
0HWU3JZ	Revision of Synthetic Substitute in Left Breast, Percutaneous Approach

0HWU3KZ	Revision of Nonautologous Tissue Substitute in Left Breast, Percutaneous Approach
0HWU3NZ	Revision of Tissue Expander in Left Breast, Percutaneous Approach
0HWU3YZ	Revision of Other Device in Left Breast, Percutaneous Approach
0HWU70Z	Revision of Drainage Device in Left Breast, Via Natural or Artificial Opening
0HWU77Z	Revision of Autologous Tissue Substitute in Left Breast, Via Natural or Artificial Opening
0HWU7JZ	Revision of Synthetic Substitute in Left Breast, Via Natural or Artificial Opening
0HWU7KZ	Revision of Nonautologous Tissue Substitute in Left Breast, Via Natural or Artificial Opening
0HWU7NZ	Revision of Tissue Expander in Left Breast, Via Natural or Artificial Opening
0HWU7YZ	Revision of Other Device in Left Breast, Via Natural or Artificial Opening
0HWU80Z	Revision of Drainage Device in Left Breast, Via Natural or Artificial Opening Endoscopic
0HWU87Z	Revision of Autologous Tissue Substitute in Left Breast, Via Natural or Artificial Opening Endoscopic
0HWU8JZ	Revision of Synthetic Substitute in Left Breast, Via Natural or Artificial Opening Endoscopic
0HWU8KZ	Revision of Nonautologous Tissue Substitute in Left Breast, Via Natural or Artificial Opening Endoscopic
0HWU8NZ	Revision of Tissue Expander in Left Breast, Via Natural or Artificial Opening Endoscopic
0HWU8YZ	Revision of Other Device in Left Breast, Via Natural or Artificial Opening Endoscopic

0HX – Skin and Breast, Transfer

Review Coding Guideline B3.17

0HX0XZZ	Transfer Scalp Skin, External Approach
0HX1XZZ	Transfer Face Skin, External Approach
0HX2XZZ	Transfer Right Ear Skin, External Approach
0HX3XZZ	Transfer Left Ear Skin, External Approach
0HX4XZZ	Transfer Neck Skin, External Approach
0HX5XZZ	Transfer Chest Skin, External Approach
0HX6XZZ	Transfer Back Skin, External Approach
0HX7XZZ	Transfer Abdomen Skin, External Approach
0HX8XZZ	Transfer Buttock Skin, External Approach

0HX9XZZ	Transfer Perineum Skin, External Approach
0HXAXZZ	Transfer Inguinal Skin, External Approach
0HXBXZZ	Transfer Right Upper Arm Skin, External Approach
0HXCXZZ	Transfer Left Upper Arm Skin, External Approach
0HXDXZZ	Transfer Right Lower Arm Skin, External Approach
0HXEXZZ	Transfer Left Lower Arm Skin, External Approach
0HXFXZZ	Transfer Right Hand Skin, External Approach
0HXGXZZ	Transfer Left Hand Skin, External Approach

0HXHXZZ	Transfer Right Upper Leg Skin, External Approach
0HXJXZZ	Transfer Left Upper Leg Skin, External Approach
0HXKXZZ	Transfer Right Lower Leg Skin, External Approach
0HXLXZZ	Transfer Left Lower Leg Skin, External Approach
0HXMXZZ	Transfer Right Foot Skin, External Approach
0HXNXZZ	Transfer Left Foot Skin, External Approach

Cross-Section of the Skin Showing Layer and Types of Infections

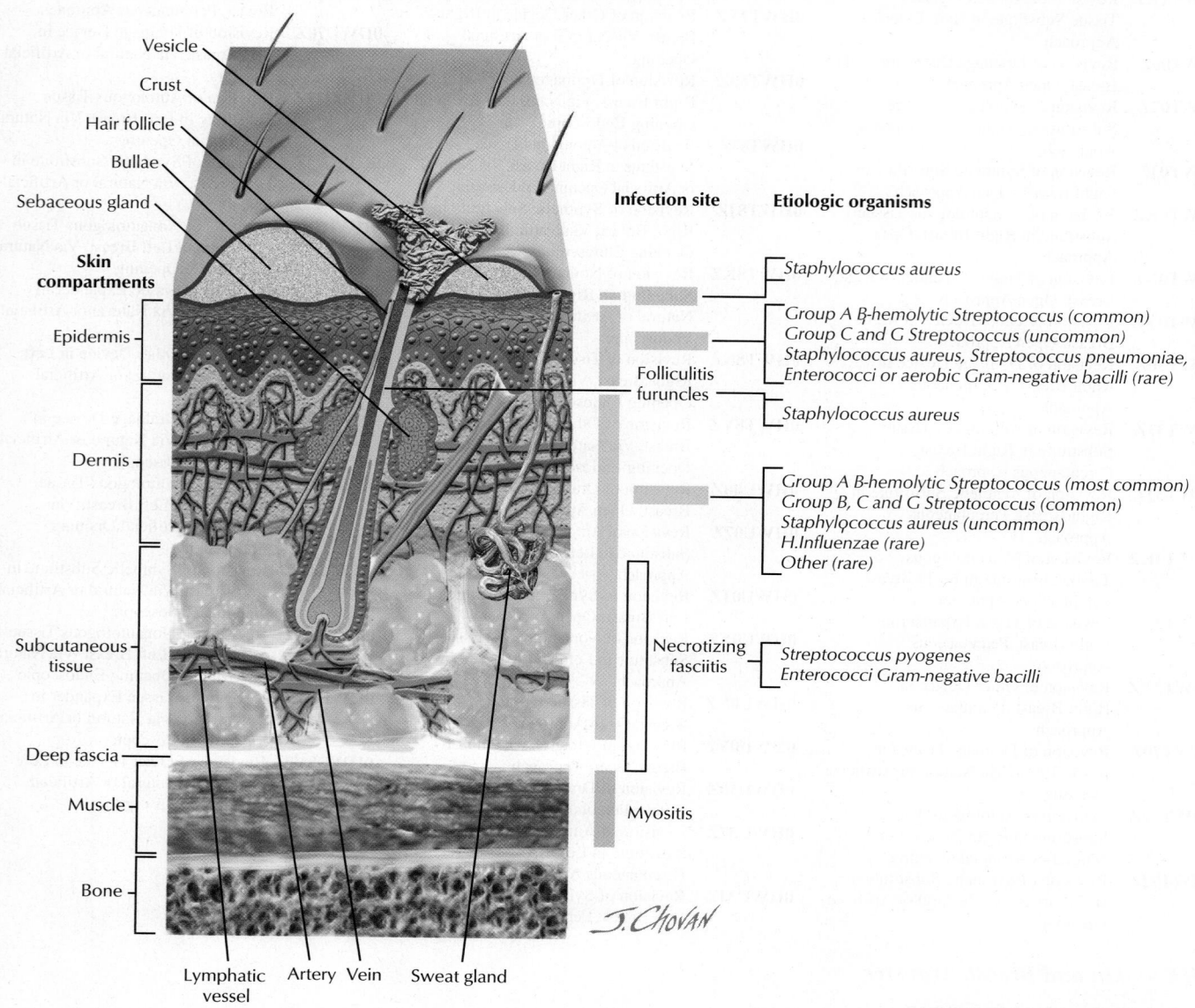

Vesicle
Crust
Hair follicle
Bullae
Sebaceous gland

Skin compartments

Epidermis

Dermis

Subcutaneous tissue

Deep fascia

Muscle

Bone

Lymphatic vessel   Artery   Vein   Sweat gland

Infection site   **Etiologic organisms**

Staphylococcus aureus

Folliculitis furuncles

Group A B-hemolytic Streptococcus (common)
Group C and G Streptococcus (uncommon)
Staphylococcus aureus, Streptococcus pneumoniae,
Enterococci or aerobic Gram-negative bacilli (rare)

Staphylococcus aureus

Group A B-hemolytic Streptococcus (most common)
Group B, C and G Streptococcus (common)
Staphylococcus aureus (uncommon)
H.Influenzae (rare)
Other (rare)

Necrotizing fasciitis

Streptococcus pyogenes
Enterococci Gram-negative bacilli

Myositis

J. Chovan

Subcutaneous Tissue and Fascia Tables 0J0–0JX

Section	0	Medical and Surgical
Body System	J	Subcutaneous Tissue and Fascia
Operation	0	**Alteration:** Modifying the anatomic structure of a body part without affecting the function of the body part

Body Part (4th)	Approach (5th)	Device (6th)	Qualifier (7th)
1 Subcutaneous Tissue and Fascia, Face 4 Subcutaneous Tissue and Fascia, Right Neck 5 Subcutaneous Tissue and Fascia, Left Neck 6 Subcutaneous Tissue and Fascia, Chest 7 Subcutaneous Tissue and Fascia, Back 8 Subcutaneous Tissue and Fascia, Abdomen 9 Subcutaneous Tissue and Fascia, Buttock D Subcutaneous Tissue and Fascia, Right Upper Arm F Subcutaneous Tissue and Fascia, Left Upper Arm G Subcutaneous Tissue and Fascia, Right Lower Arm H Subcutaneous Tissue and Fascia, Left Lower Arm L Subcutaneous Tissue and Fascia, Right Upper Leg M Subcutaneous Tissue and Fascia, Left Upper Leg N Subcutaneous Tissue and Fascia, Right Lower Leg P Subcutaneous Tissue and Fascia, Left Lower Leg	0 Open 3 Percutaneous	Z No Device	Z No Qualifier

Section	0	Medical and Surgical
Body System	J	Subcutaneous Tissue and Fascia
Operation	2	**Change:** Taking out or off a device from a body part and putting back an identical or similar device in or on the same body part without cutting or puncturing the skin or a mucous membrane

Body Part (4th)	Approach (5th)	Device (6th)	Qualifier (7th)
S Subcutaneous Tissue and Fascia, Head and Neck T Subcutaneous Tissue and Fascia, Trunk V Subcutaneous Tissue and Fascia, Upper Extremity W Subcutaneous Tissue and Fascia, Lower Extremity	X External	0 Drainage Device Y Other Device	Z No Qualifier

Section	0	Medical and Surgical
Body System	J	Subcutaneous Tissue and Fascia
Operation	5	**Destruction:** Physical eradication of all or a portion of a body part by the direct use of energy, force, or a destructive agent

Body Part (4th)	Approach (5th)	Device (6th)	Qualifier (7th)
0 Subcutaneous Tissue and Fascia, Scalp 1 Subcutaneous Tissue and Fascia, Face 4 Subcutaneous Tissue and Fascia, Right Neck 5 Subcutaneous Tissue and Fascia, Left Neck 6 Subcutaneous Tissue and Fascia, Chest 7 Subcutaneous Tissue and Fascia, Back 8 Subcutaneous Tissue and Fascia, Abdomen 9 Subcutaneous Tissue and Fascia, Buttock B Subcutaneous Tissue and Fascia, Perineum C Subcutaneous Tissue and Fascia, Pelvic Region D Subcutaneous Tissue and Fascia, Right Upper Arm F Subcutaneous Tissue and Fascia, Left Upper Arm G Subcutaneous Tissue and Fascia, Right Lower Arm H Subcutaneous Tissue and Fascia, Left Lower Arm J Subcutaneous Tissue and Fascia, Right Hand K Subcutaneous Tissue and Fascia, Left Hand L Subcutaneous Tissue and Fascia, Right Upper Leg M Subcutaneous Tissue and Fascia, Left Upper Leg N Subcutaneous Tissue and Fascia, Right Lower Leg P Subcutaneous Tissue and Fascia, Left Lower Leg Q Subcutaneous Tissue and Fascia, Right Foot R Subcutaneous Tissue and Fascia, Left Foot	0 Open 3 Percutaneous	Z No Device	Z No Qualifier

Section 0 **Medical and Surgical**
Body System J **Subcutaneous Tissue and Fascia**
Operation 8 **Division:** Cutting into a body part, without draining fluids and/or gases from the body part, in order to separate or transect a body part

Body Part (4th)	Approach (5th)	Device (6th)	Qualifier (7th)
0 Subcutaneous Tissue and Fascia, Scalp	0 Open	Z No Device	Z No Qualifier
1 Subcutaneous Tissue and Fascia, Face	3 Percutaneous		
4 Subcutaneous Tissue and Fascia, Right Neck			
5 Subcutaneous Tissue and Fascia, Left Neck			
6 Subcutaneous Tissue and Fascia, Chest			
7 Subcutaneous Tissue and Fascia, Back			
8 Subcutaneous Tissue and Fascia, Abdomen			
9 Subcutaneous Tissue and Fascia, Buttock			
B Subcutaneous Tissue and Fascia, Perineum			
C Subcutaneous Tissue and Fascia, Pelvic Region			
D Subcutaneous Tissue and Fascia, Right Upper Arm			
F Subcutaneous Tissue and Fascia, Left Upper Arm			
G Subcutaneous Tissue and Fascia, Right Lower Arm			
H Subcutaneous Tissue and Fascia, Left Lower Arm			
J Subcutaneous Tissue and Fascia, Right Hand			
K Subcutaneous Tissue and Fascia, Left Hand			
L Subcutaneous Tissue and Fascia, Right Upper Leg			
M Subcutaneous Tissue and Fascia, Left Upper Leg			
N Subcutaneous Tissue and Fascia, Right Lower Leg			
P Subcutaneous Tissue and Fascia, Left Lower Leg			
Q Subcutaneous Tissue and Fascia, Right Foot			
R Subcutaneous Tissue and Fascia, Left Foot			
S Subcutaneous Tissue and Fascia, Head and Neck			
T Subcutaneous Tissue and Fascia, Trunk			
V Subcutaneous Tissue and Fascia, Upper Extremity			
W Subcutaneous Tissue and Fascia, Lower Extremity			

Section 0 **Medical and Surgical**
Body System J **Subcutaneous Tissue and Fascia**
Operation 9 **Drainage:** Taking or letting out fluids and/or gases from a body part

Body Part (4th)	Approach (5th)	Device (6th)	Qualifier (7th)
0 Subcutaneous Tissue and Fascia, Scalp	0 Open	0 Drainage Device	Z No Qualifier
1 Subcutaneous Tissue and Fascia, Face	3 Percutaneous		
4 Subcutaneous Tissue and Fascia, Right Neck			
5 Subcutaneous Tissue and Fascia, Left Neck			
6 Subcutaneous Tissue and Fascia, Chest			
7 Subcutaneous Tissue and Fascia, Back			
8 Subcutaneous Tissue and Fascia, Abdomen			
9 Subcutaneous Tissue and Fascia, Buttock			
B Subcutaneous Tissue and Fascia, Perineum			
C Subcutaneous Tissue and Fascia, Pelvic Region			
D Subcutaneous Tissue and Fascia, Right Upper Arm			
F Subcutaneous Tissue and Fascia, Left Upper Arm			
G Subcutaneous Tissue and Fascia, Right Lower Arm			
H Subcutaneous Tissue and Fascia, Left Lower Arm			
J Subcutaneous Tissue and Fascia, Right Hand			
K Subcutaneous Tissue and Fascia, Left Hand			
L Subcutaneous Tissue and Fascia, Right Upper Leg			
M Subcutaneous Tissue and Fascia, Left Upper Leg			
N Subcutaneous Tissue and Fascia, Right Lower Leg			
P Subcutaneous Tissue and Fascia, Left Lower Leg			
Q Subcutaneous Tissue and Fascia, Right Foot			
R Subcutaneous Tissue and Fascia, Left Foot			

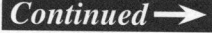

Continued →

Section	0	Medical and Surgical
Body System	J	Subcutaneous Tissue and Fascia
Operation	9	Drainage: Taking or letting out fluids and/or gases from a body part

Body Part (4th)	Approach (5th)	Device (6th)	Qualifier (7th)
0 Subcutaneous Tissue and Fascia, Scalp 1 Subcutaneous Tissue and Fascia, Face 4 Subcutaneous Tissue and Fascia, Right Neck 5 Subcutaneous Tissue and Fascia, Left Neck 6 Subcutaneous Tissue and Fascia, Chest 7 Subcutaneous Tissue and Fascia, Back 8 Subcutaneous Tissue and Fascia, Abdomen 9 Subcutaneous Tissue and Fascia, Buttock B Subcutaneous Tissue and Fascia, Perineum C Subcutaneous Tissue and Fascia, Pelvic Region D Subcutaneous Tissue and Fascia, Right Upper Arm F Subcutaneous Tissue and Fascia, Left Upper Arm G Subcutaneous Tissue and Fascia, Right Lower Arm H Subcutaneous Tissue and Fascia, Left Lower Arm J Subcutaneous Tissue and Fascia, Right Hand K Subcutaneous Tissue and Fascia, Left Hand L Subcutaneous Tissue and Fascia, Right Upper Leg M Subcutaneous Tissue and Fascia, Left Upper Leg N Subcutaneous Tissue and Fascia, Right Lower Leg P Subcutaneous Tissue and Fascia, Left Lower Leg Q Subcutaneous Tissue and Fascia, Right Foot R Subcutaneous Tissue and Fascia, Left Foot	0 Open 3 Percutaneous	Z No Device	X Diagnostic Z No Qualifier

Section	0	Medical and Surgical
Body System	J	Subcutaneous Tissue and Fascia
Operation	B	Excision: Cutting out or off, without replacement, a portion of a body part

Body Part (4th)	Approach (5th)	Device (6th)	Qualifier (7th)
0 Subcutaneous Tissue and Fascia, Scalp 1 Subcutaneous Tissue and Fascia, Face 4 Subcutaneous Tissue and Fascia, Right Neck 5 Subcutaneous Tissue and Fascia, Left Neck 6 Subcutaneous Tissue and Fascia, Chest 7 Subcutaneous Tissue and Fascia, Back 8 Subcutaneous Tissue and Fascia, Abdomen 9 Subcutaneous Tissue and Fascia, Buttock B Subcutaneous Tissue and Fascia, Perineum C Subcutaneous Tissue and Fascia, Pelvic Region D Subcutaneous Tissue and Fascia, Right Upper Arm F Subcutaneous Tissue and Fascia, Left Upper Arm G Subcutaneous Tissue and Fascia, Right Lower Arm H Subcutaneous Tissue and Fascia, Left Lower Arm J Subcutaneous Tissue and Fascia, Right Hand K Subcutaneous Tissue and Fascia, Left Hand L Subcutaneous Tissue and Fascia, Right Upper Leg M Subcutaneous Tissue and Fascia, Left Upper Leg N Subcutaneous Tissue and Fascia, Right Lower Leg P Subcutaneous Tissue and Fascia, Left Lower Leg Q Subcutaneous Tissue and Fascia, Right Foot R Subcutaneous Tissue and Fascia, Left Foot	0 Open 3 Percutaneous	Z No Device	X Diagnostic Z No Qualifier

Section	0	Medical and Surgical
Body System	J	Subcutaneous Tissue and Fascia
Operation	C	Extirpation: Taking or cutting out solid matter from a body part

Body Part (4th)	Approach (5th)	Device (6th)	Qualifier (7th)
0 Subcutaneous Tissue and Fascia, Scalp 1 Subcutaneous Tissue and Fascia, Face 4 Subcutaneous Tissue and Fascia, Right Neck 5 Subcutaneous Tissue and Fascia, Left Neck 6 Subcutaneous Tissue and Fascia, Chest 7 Subcutaneous Tissue and Fascia, Back 8 Subcutaneous Tissue and Fascia, Abdomen 9 Subcutaneous Tissue and Fascia, Buttock B Subcutaneous Tissue and Fascia, Perineum C Subcutaneous Tissue and Fascia, Pelvic Region D Subcutaneous Tissue and Fascia, Right Upper Arm F Subcutaneous Tissue and Fascia, Left Upper Arm G Subcutaneous Tissue and Fascia, Right Lower Arm H Subcutaneous Tissue and Fascia, Left Lower Arm J Subcutaneous Tissue and Fascia, Right Hand K Subcutaneous Tissue and Fascia, Left Hand L Subcutaneous Tissue and Fascia, Right Upper Leg M Subcutaneous Tissue and Fascia, Left Upper Leg N Subcutaneous Tissue and Fascia, Right Lower Leg P Subcutaneous Tissue and Fascia, Left Lower Leg Q Subcutaneous Tissue and Fascia, Right Foot R Subcutaneous Tissue and Fascia, Left Foot	0 Open 3 Percutaneous	Z No Device	Z No Qualifier

Section	0	Medical and Surgical
Body System	J	Subcutaneous Tissue and Fascia
Operation	D	Extraction: Pulling or stripping out or off all or a portion of a body part by the use of force

Body Part (4th)	Approach (5th)	Device (6th)	Qualifier (7th)
0 Subcutaneous Tissue and Fascia, Scalp 1 Subcutaneous Tissue and Fascia, Face 4 Subcutaneous Tissue and Fascia, Right Neck 5 Subcutaneous Tissue and Fascia, Left Neck 6 Subcutaneous Tissue and Fascia, Chest 7 Subcutaneous Tissue and Fascia, Back 8 Subcutaneous Tissue and Fascia, Abdomen 9 Subcutaneous Tissue and Fascia, Buttock B Subcutaneous Tissue and Fascia, Perineum C Subcutaneous Tissue and Fascia, Pelvic Region D Subcutaneous Tissue and Fascia, Right Upper Arm F Subcutaneous Tissue and Fascia, Left Upper Arm G Subcutaneous Tissue and Fascia, Right Lower Arm H Subcutaneous Tissue and Fascia, Left Lower Arm J Subcutaneous Tissue and Fascia, Right Hand K Subcutaneous Tissue and Fascia, Left Hand L Subcutaneous Tissue and Fascia, Right Upper Leg M Subcutaneous Tissue and Fascia, Left Upper Leg N Subcutaneous Tissue and Fascia, Right Lower Leg P Subcutaneous Tissue and Fascia, Left Lower Leg Q Subcutaneous Tissue and Fascia, Right Foot R Subcutaneous Tissue and Fascia, Left Foot	0 Open 3 Percutaneous	Z No Device	Z No Qualifier

Section	0	Medical and Surgical
Body System	J	Subcutaneous Tissue and Fascia
Operation	H	**Insertion:** Putting in a nonbiological appliance that monitors, assists, performs, or prevents a physiological function but does not physically take the place of a body part

Body Part (4th)	Approach (5th)	Device (6th)	Qualifier (7th)
0 Subcutaneous Tissue and Fascia, Scalp 1 Subcutaneous Tissue and Fascia, Face 4 Subcutaneous Tissue and Fascia, Right Neck 5 Subcutaneous Tissue and Fascia, Left Neck 9 Subcutaneous Tissue and Fascia, Buttock B Subcutaneous Tissue and Fascia, Perineum C Subcutaneous Tissue and Fascia, Pelvic Region J Subcutaneous Tissue and Fascia, Right Hand K Subcutaneous Tissue and Fascia, Left Hand Q Subcutaneous Tissue and Fascia, Right Foot R Subcutaneous Tissue and Fascia, Left Foot	0 Open 3 Percutaneous	N Tissue Expander	Z No Qualifier
6 Subcutaneous Tissue and Fascia, Chest	0 Open 3 Percutaneous	0 Monitoring Device, Hemodynamic 2 Monitoring Device 4 Pacemaker, Single Chamber 5 Pacemaker, Single Chamber Rate Responsive 6 Pacemaker, Dual Chamber 7 Cardiac Resynchronization Pacemaker Pulse Generator 8 Defibrillator Generator 9 Cardiac Resynchronization Defibrillator Pulse Generator A Contractility Modulation Device B Stimulator Generator, Single Array C Stimulator Generator, Single Array Rechargeable D Stimulator Generator, Multiple Array E Stimulator Generator, Multiple Array Rechargeable F Subcutaneous Defibrillator Lead H Contraceptive Device M Stimulator Generator N Tissue Expander P Cardiac Rhythm Related Device V Infusion Device, Pump W Vascular Access Device, Totally Implantable X Vascular Access Device, Tunneled Y Other Device	Z No Qualifier
7 Subcutaneous Tissue and Fascia, Back	0 Open 3 Percutaneous	B Stimulator Generator, Single Array C Stimulator Generator, Single Array Rechargeable D Stimulator Generator, Multiple Array E Stimulator Generator, Multiple Array Rechargeable M Stimulator Generator N Tissue Expander V Infusion Device, Pump Y Other Device	Z No Qualifier

Continued →

Section	0	**Medical and Surgical**
Body System	J	**Subcutaneous Tissue and Fascia**
Operation	H	**Insertion:** Putting in a nonbiological appliance that monitors, assists, performs, or prevents a physiological function but does not physically take the place of a body part

Body Part (4th)	Approach (5th)	Device (6th)	Qualifier (7th)
8 Subcutaneous Tissue and Fascia, Abdomen	0 Open 3 Percutaneous	0 Monitoring Device, Hemodynamic 2 Monitoring Device 4 Pacemaker, Single Chamber 5 Pacemaker, Single Chamber Rate Responsive 6 Pacemaker, Dual Chamber 7 Cardiac Resynchronization Pacemaker Pulse Generator 8 Defibrillator Generator 9 Cardiac Resynchronization Defibrillator Pulse Generator A Contractility Modulation Device B Stimulator Generator, Single Array C Stimulator Generator, Single Array Rechargeable D Stimulator Generator, Multiple Array E Stimulator Generator, Multiple Array Rechargeable H Contraceptive Device M Stimulator Generator N Tissue Expander P Cardiac Rhythm Related Device V Infusion Device, Pump W Vascular Access Device Totally Implantable X Vascular Access Device, Tunneled Y Other Device	Z No Qualifier
D Subcutaneous Tissue and Fascia, Right Upper Arm F Subcutaneous Tissue and Fascia, Left Upper Arm G Subcutaneous Tissue and Fascia, Right Lower Arm H Subcutaneous Tissue and Fascia, Left Lower Arm L Subcutaneous Tissue and Fascia, Right Upper Leg M Subcutaneous Tissue and Fascia, Left Upper Leg N Subcutaneous Tissue and Fascia, Right Lower Leg P Subcutaneous Tissue and Fascia, Left Lower Leg	0 Open 3 Percutaneous	H Contraceptive Device N Tissue Expander V Infusion Device, Pump W Vascular Access Device, Totally Implantable X Vascular Access Device, Tunneled	Z No Qualifier
S Subcutaneous Tissue and Fascia, Head and Neck V Subcutaneous Tissue and Fascia, Upper Extremity W Subcutaneous Tissue and Fascia, Lower Extremity	0 Open 3 Percutaneous	1 Radioactive Element 3 Infusion Device Y Other Device	Z No Qualifier
T Subcutaneous Tissue and Fascia, Trunk	0 Open 3 Percutaneous	1 Radioactive Element 3 Infusion Device V Infusion Device, Pump Y Other Device	Z No Qualifier

Section	0	**Medical and Surgical**
Body System	J	**Subcutaneous Tissue and Fascia**
Operation	J	**Inspection:** Visually and/or manually exploring a body part

Body Part (4th)	Approach (5th)	Device (6th)	Qualifier (7th)
S Subcutaneous Tissue and Fascia, Head and Neck T Subcutaneous Tissue and Fascia, Trunk V Subcutaneous Tissue and Fascia, Upper Extremity W Subcutaneous Tissue and Fascia, Lower Extremity	0 Open 3 Percutaneous X External	Z No Device	Z No Qualifier

Section 0 Medical and Surgical
Body System J Subcutaneous Tissue and Fascia
Operation N **Release:** Freeing a body part from an abnormal physical constraint by cutting or by the use of force

Body Part (4ᵗʰ)	Approach (5ᵗʰ)	Device (6ᵗʰ)	Qualifier (7ᵗʰ)
0 Subcutaneous Tissue and Fascia, Scalp 1 Subcutaneous Tissue and Fascia, Face 4 Subcutaneous Tissue and Fascia, Right Neck 5 Subcutaneous Tissue and Fascia, Left Neck 6 Subcutaneous Tissue and Fascia, Chest 7 Subcutaneous Tissue and Fascia, Back 8 Subcutaneous Tissue and Fascia, Abdomen 9 Subcutaneous Tissue and Fascia, Buttock B Subcutaneous Tissue and Fascia, Perineum C Subcutaneous Tissue and Fascia, Pelvic Region D Subcutaneous Tissue and Fascia, Right Upper Arm F Subcutaneous Tissue and Fascia, Left Upper Arm G Subcutaneous Tissue and Fascia, Right Lower Arm H Subcutaneous Tissue and Fascia, Left Lower Arm J Subcutaneous Tissue and Fascia, Right Hand K Subcutaneous Tissue and Fascia, Left Hand L Subcutaneous Tissue and Fascia, Right Upper Leg M Subcutaneous Tissue and Fascia, Left Upper Leg N Subcutaneous Tissue and Fascia, Right Lower Leg P Subcutaneous Tissue and Fascia, Left Lower Leg Q Subcutaneous Tissue and Fascia, Right Foot R Subcutaneous Tissue and Fascia, Left Foot	0 Open 3 Percutaneous X External	Z No Device	Z No Qualifier

Section 0 Medical and Surgical
Body System J Subcutaneous Tissue and Fascia
Operation P **Removal:** Taking out or off a device from a body part

Body Part (4ᵗʰ)	Approach (5ᵗʰ)	Device (6ᵗʰ)	Qualifier (7ᵗʰ)
S Subcutaneous Tissue and Fascia, Head and Neck	0 Open 3 Percutaneous	0 Drainage Device 1 Radioactive Element 3 Infusion Device 7 Autologous Tissue Substitute J Synthetic Substitute K Nonautologous Tissue Substitute N Tissue Expander Y Other Device	Z No Qualifier
S Subcutaneous Tissue and Fascia, Head and Neck	X External	0 Drainage Device 1 Radioactive Element 3 Infusion Device	Z No Qualifier
T Subcutaneous Tissue and Fascia, Trunk	0 Open 3 Percutaneous	0 Drainage Device 1 Radioactive Element 2 Monitoring Device 3 Infusion Device 7 Autologous Tissue Substitute F Subcutaneous Defibrillator Lead H Contraceptive Device J Synthetic Substitute K Nonautologous Tissue Substitute M Stimulator Generator N Tissue Expander P Cardiac Rhythm Related Device V Infusion Device, Pump W Vascular Access Device, Totally Implantable X Vascular Access Device, Tunneled Y Other Device	Z No Qualifier

Continued →

Section	0	Medical and Surgical
Body System	J	Subcutaneous Tissue and Fascia
Operation	P	**Removal:** Taking out or off a device from a body part

Body Part (4th)	Approach (5th)	Device (6th)	Qualifier (7th)
T Subcutaneous Tissue and Fascia, Trunk	X External	0 Drainage Device 1 Radioactive Element 2 Monitoring Device 3 Infusion Device H Contraceptive Device V Infusion Device, Pump X Vascular Access Device, Tunneled	Z No Qualifier
V Subcutaneous Tissue and Fascia, Upper Extremity W Subcutaneous Tissue and Fascia, Lower Extremity	0 Open 3 Percutaneous	0 Drainage Device 1 Radioactive Element 3 Infusion Device 7 Autologous Tissue Substitute H Contraceptive Device J Synthetic Substitute K Nonautologous Tissue Substitute N Tissue Expander V Infusion Device, Pump W Vascular Access Device, Totally Implantable X Vascular Access Device, Tunneled Y Other Device	Z No Qualifier
V Subcutaneous Tissue and Fascia, Upper Extremity W Subcutaneous Tissue and Fascia, Lower Extremity	X External	0 Drainage Device 1 Radioactive Element 3 Infusion Device H Contraceptive Device V Infusion Device, Pump X Vascular Access Device, Tunneled	Z No Qualifier

Section	0	Medical and Surgical
Body System	J	Subcutaneous Tissue and Fascia
Operation	Q	**Repair:** Restoring, to the extent possible, a body part to its normal anatomic structure and function

Body Part (4th)	Approach (5th)	Device (6th)	Qualifier (7th)
0 Subcutaneous Tissue and Fascia, Scalp 1 Subcutaneous Tissue and Fascia, Face 4 Subcutaneous Tissue and Fascia, Right Neck 5 Subcutaneous Tissue and Fascia, Left Neck 6 Subcutaneous Tissue and Fascia, Chest 7 Subcutaneous Tissue and Fascia, Back 8 Subcutaneous Tissue and Fascia, Abdomen 9 Subcutaneous Tissue and Fascia, Buttock B Subcutaneous Tissue and Fascia, Perineum C Subcutaneous Tissue and Fascia, Pelvic Region D Subcutaneous Tissue and Fascia, Right Upper Arm F Subcutaneous Tissue and Fascia, Left Upper Arm G Subcutaneous Tissue and Fascia, Right Lower Arm H Subcutaneous Tissue and Fascia, Left Lower Arm J Subcutaneous Tissue and Fascia, Right Hand K Subcutaneous Tissue and Fascia, Left Hand L Subcutaneous Tissue and Fascia, Right Upper Leg M Subcutaneous Tissue and Fascia, Left Upper Leg N Subcutaneous Tissue and Fascia, Right Lower Leg P Subcutaneous Tissue and Fascia, Left Lower Leg Q Subcutaneous Tissue and Fascia, Right Foot R Subcutaneous Tissue and Fascia, Left Foot	0 Open 3 Percutaneous	Z No Device	Z No Qualifier

Section   **0**   **Medical and Surgical**
Body System   **J**   **Subcutaneous Tissue and Fascia**
Operation   **R**   **Replacement:** Putting in or on biological or synthetic material that physically takes the place and/or function of all or a portion of a body part

Body Part (4th)	Approach (5th)	Device (6th)	Qualifier (7th)
0 Subcutaneous Tissue and Fascia, Scalp	**0** Open	**7** Autologous Tissue Substitute	**Z** No Qualifier
1 Subcutaneous Tissue and Fascia, Face	**3** Percutaneous	**J** Synthetic Substitute	
4 Subcutaneous Tissue and Fascia, Right Neck		**K** Nonautologous Tissue	
5 Subcutaneous Tissue and Fascia, Left Neck		Substitute	
6 Subcutaneous Tissue and Fascia, Chest			
7 Subcutaneous Tissue and Fascia, Back			
8 Subcutaneous Tissue and Fascia, Abdomen			
9 Subcutaneous Tissue and Fascia, Buttock			
B Subcutaneous Tissue and Fascia, Perineum			
C Subcutaneous Tissue and Fascia, Pelvic Region			
D Subcutaneous Tissue and Fascia, Right Upper Arm			
F Subcutaneous Tissue and Fascia, Left Upper Arm			
G Subcutaneous Tissue and Fascia, Right Lower Arm			
H Subcutaneous Tissue and Fascia, Left Lower Arm			
J Subcutaneous Tissue and Fascia, Right Hand			
K Subcutaneous Tissue and Fascia, Left Hand			
L Subcutaneous Tissue and Fascia, Right Upper Leg			
M Subcutaneous Tissue and Fascia, Left Upper Leg			
N Subcutaneous Tissue and Fascia, Right Lower Leg			
P Subcutaneous Tissue and Fascia, Left Lower Leg			
Q Subcutaneous Tissue and Fascia, Right Foot			
R Subcutaneous Tissue and Fascia, Left Foot			

Section   **0**   **Medical and Surgical**
Body System   **J**   **Subcutaneous Tissue and Fascia**
Operation   **U**   **Supplement:** Putting in or on biological or synthetic material that physically reinforces and/or augments the function of a portion of a body part

Body Part (4th)	Approach (5th)	Device (6th)	Qualifier (7th)
0 Subcutaneous Tissue and Fascia, Scalp	**0** Open	**7** Autologous Tissue Substitute	**Z** No Qualifier
1 Subcutaneous Tissue and Fascia, Face	**3** Percutaneous	**J** Synthetic Substitute	
4 Subcutaneous Tissue and Fascia, Right Neck		**K** Nonautologous Tissue Substitute	
5 Subcutaneous Tissue and Fascia, Left Neck			
6 Subcutaneous Tissue and Fascia, Chest			
7 Subcutaneous Tissue and Fascia, Back			
8 Subcutaneous Tissue and Fascia, Abdomen			
9 Subcutaneous Tissue and Fascia, Buttock			
B Subcutaneous Tissue and Fascia, Perineum			
C Subcutaneous Tissue and Fascia, Pelvic Region			
D Subcutaneous Tissue and Fascia, Right Upper Arm			
F Subcutaneous Tissue and Fascia, Left Upper Arm			
G Subcutaneous Tissue and Fascia, Right Lower Arm			
H Subcutaneous Tissue and Fascia, Left Lower Arm			
J Subcutaneous Tissue and Fascia, Right Hand			
K Subcutaneous Tissue and Fascia, Left Hand			
L Subcutaneous Tissue and Fascia, Right Upper Leg			
M Subcutaneous Tissue and Fascia, Left Upper Leg			
N Subcutaneous Tissue and Fascia, Right Lower Leg			
P Subcutaneous Tissue and Fascia, Left Lower Leg			
Q Subcutaneous Tissue and Fascia, Right Foot			
R Subcutaneous Tissue and Fascia, Left Foot			

Section   **0**   **Medical and Surgical**
Body System   **J**   **Subcutaneous Tissue and Fascia**
Operation   **W**   **Revision:** Correcting, to the extent possible, a portion of a malfunctioning device or the position of a displaced device

Body Part (4th)	Approach (5th)	Device (6th)	Qualifier (7th)
S Subcutaneous Tissue and Fascia, Head and Neck	**0** Open **3** Percutaneous	**0** Drainage Device **3** Infusion Device **7** Autologous Tissue Substitute **J** Synthetic Substitute **K** Nonautologous Tissue Substitute **N** Tissue Expander **Y** Other Device	**Z** No Qualifier
S Subcutaneous Tissue and Fascia, Head and Neck	**X** External	**0** Drainage Device **3** Infusion Device **7** Autologous Tissue Substitute **J** Synthetic Substitute **K** Nonautologous Tissue Substitute **N** Tissue Expander	**Z** No Qualifier
T Subcutaneous Tissue and Fascia, Trunk	**0** Open **3** Percutaneous	**0** Drainage Device **2** Monitoring Device **3** Infusion Device **7** Autologous Tissue Substitute **F** Subcutaneous Defibrillator Lead **H** Contraceptive Device **J** Synthetic Substitute **K** Nonautologous Tissue Substitute **M** Stimulator Generator **N** Tissue Expander **P** Cardiac Rhythm Related Device **V** Infusion Device, Pump **W** Vascular Access Device, Totally Implantable **X** Vascular Access Device, Tunneled **Y** Other Device	**Z** No Qualifier
T Subcutaneous Tissue and Fascia, Trunk	**X** External	**0** Drainage Device **2** Monitoring Device **3** Infusion Device **7** Autologous Tissue Substitute **F** Subcutaneous Defibrillator Lead **H** Contraceptive Device **J** Synthetic Substitute **K** Nonautologous Tissue Substitute **M** Stimulator Generator **N** Tissue Expander **P** Cardiac Rhythm Related Device **V** Infusion Device, Pump **W** Vascular Access Device, Totally Implantable **X** Vascular Access Device, Tunneled	**Z** No Qualifier
V Subcutaneous Tissue and Fascia, Upper Extremity **W** Subcutaneous Tissue and Fascia, Lower Extremity	**0** Open **3** Percutaneous	**0** Drainage Device **3** Infusion Device **7** Autologous Tissue Substitute **H** Contraceptive Device **J** Synthetic Substitute **K** Nonautologous Tissue Substitute **N** Tissue Expander **V** Infusion Device, Pump **W** Vascular Access Device, Totally Implantable **X** Vascular Access Device, Tunneled **Y** Other Device	**Z** No Qualifier

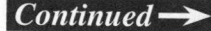

Continued →

Section	0	Medical and Surgical
Body System	J	Subcutaneous Tissue and Fascia
Operation	W	Revision: Correcting, to the extent possible, a portion of a malfunctioning device or the position of a displaced device

Body Part (4th)	Approach (5th)	Device (6th)	Qualifier (7th)
V Subcutaneous Tissue and Fascia, Upper Extremity W Subcutaneous Tissue and Fascia, Lower Extremity	X External	0 Drainage Device 3 Infusion Device 7 Autologous Tissue Substitute H Contraceptive Device J Synthetic Substitute K Nonautologous Tissue Substitute N Tissue Expander V Infusion Device, Pump W Vascular Access Device, Totally Implantable X Vascular Access Device, Tunneled	Z No Qualifier

Section	0	Medical and Surgical
Body System	J	Subcutaneous Tissue and Fascia
Operation	X	Transfer: Moving, without taking out, all or a portion of a body part to another location to take over the function of all or a portion of a body part

Body Part (4th)	Approach (5th)	Device (6th)	Qualifier (7th)
0 Subcutaneous Tissue and Fascia, Scalp 1 Subcutaneous Tissue and Fascia, Face 4 Subcutaneous Tissue and Fascia, Right Neck 5 Subcutaneous Tissue and Fascia, Left Neck 6 Subcutaneous Tissue and Fascia, Chest 7 Subcutaneous Tissue and Fascia, Back 8 Subcutaneous Tissue and Fascia, Abdomen 9 Subcutaneous Tissue and Fascia, Buttock B Subcutaneous Tissue and Fascia, Perineum C Subcutaneous Tissue and Fascia, Pelvic Region D Subcutaneous Tissue and Fascia, Right Upper Arm F Subcutaneous Tissue and Fascia, Left Upper Arm G Subcutaneous Tissue and Fascia, Right Lower Arm H Subcutaneous Tissue and Fascia, Left Lower Arm J Subcutaneous Tissue and Fascia, Right Hand K Subcutaneous Tissue and Fascia, Left Hand L Subcutaneous Tissue and Fascia, Right Upper Leg M Subcutaneous Tissue and Fascia, Left Upper Leg N Subcutaneous Tissue and Fascia, Right Lower Leg P Subcutaneous Tissue and Fascia, Left Lower Leg Q Subcutaneous Tissue and Fascia, Right Foot R Subcutaneous Tissue and Fascia, Left Foot	0 Open 3 Percutaneous	Z No Device	B Skin and Subcutaneous Tissue C Skin, Subcutaneous Tissue and Fascia Z No Qualifier

Subcutaneous Tissue and Fascia Code Listing 0J0–0JX

Review Coding Guideline B4.5

Review Coding Guideline B4.6

0J0 – Subcutaneous Tissue and Fascia, Alteration

0J010ZZ Alteration of Face Subcutaneous Tissue and Fascia, Open Approach

0J013ZZ Alteration of Face Subcutaneous Tissue and Fascia, Percutaneous Approach

0J040ZZ Alteration of Right Neck Subcutaneous Tissue and Fascia, Open Approach

0J043ZZ Alteration of Right Neck Subcutaneous Tissue and Fascia, Percutaneous Approach

0J050ZZ Alteration of Left Neck Subcutaneous Tissue and Fascia, Open Approach

0J053ZZ Alteration of Left Neck Subcutaneous Tissue and Fascia, Percutaneous Approach

0J060ZZ Alteration of Chest Subcutaneous Tissue and Fascia, Open Approach

0J063ZZ Alteration of Chest Subcutaneous Tissue and Fascia, Percutaneous Approach

0J070ZZ Alteration of Back Subcutaneous Tissue and Fascia, Open Approach

0J073ZZ Alteration of Back Subcutaneous Tissue and Fascia, Percutaneous Approach

0J080ZZ Alteration of Abdomen Subcutaneous Tissue and Fascia, Open Approach

0J083ZZ Alteration of Abdomen Subcutaneous Tissue and Fascia, Percutaneous Approach

0J090ZZ Alteration of Buttock Subcutaneous Tissue and Fascia, Open Approach

0J093ZZ Alteration of Buttock Subcutaneous Tissue and Fascia, Percutaneous Approach

0J0D0ZZ Alteration of Right Upper Arm Subcutaneous Tissue and Fascia, Open Approach

0J0D3ZZ Alteration of Right Upper Arm Subcutaneous Tissue and Fascia, Percutaneous Approach

0J0F0ZZ Alteration of Left Upper Arm Subcutaneous Tissue and Fascia, Open Approach

0J0F3ZZ Alteration of Left Upper Arm Subcutaneous Tissue and Fascia, Percutaneous Approach

0J0G0ZZ Alteration of Right Lower Arm Subcutaneous Tissue and Fascia, Open Approach

0J0G3ZZ Alteration of Right Lower Arm Subcutaneous Tissue and Fascia, Percutaneous Approach

0J0H0ZZ Alteration of Left Lower Arm Subcutaneous Tissue and Fascia, Open Approach

♀ Female-only   ♂ Male-only   ▲ Limited Coverage   ● Non-OR   HAC HAC-associated procedure   ▲ Non-covered procedures   ✚ Cluster

0J0H3ZZ	Alteration of Left Lower Arm Subcutaneous Tissue and Fascia, Percutaneous Approach	
0J0L0ZZ	Alteration of Right Upper Leg Subcutaneous Tissue and Fascia, Open Approach	
0J0L3ZZ	Alteration of Right Upper Leg Subcutaneous Tissue and Fascia, Percutaneous Approach	

0J0M0ZZ Alteration of Left Upper Leg Subcutaneous Tissue and Fascia, Open Approach

0J0M3ZZ Alteration of Left Upper Leg Subcutaneous Tissue and Fascia, Percutaneous Approach

0J0N0ZZ Alteration of Right Lower Leg Subcutaneous Tissue and Fascia, Open Approach

0J0N3ZZ Alteration of Right Lower Leg Subcutaneous Tissue and Fascia, Percutaneous Approach

0J0P0ZZ Alteration of Left Lower Leg Subcutaneous Tissue and Fascia, Open Approach

0J0P3ZZ Alteration of Left Lower Leg Subcutaneous Tissue and Fascia, Percutaneous Approach

0J2 – Subcutaneous Tissue and Fascia, Change

Review Coding Guideline B6.1c

0J2SX0Z Change Drainage Device in Head and Neck Subcutaneous Tissue and Fascia, External Approach

0J2SXYZ Change Other Device in Head and Neck Subcutaneous Tissue and Fascia, External Approach

0J2TX0Z Change Drainage Device in Trunk Subcutaneous Tissue and Fascia, External Approach

0J2TXYZ Change Other Device in Trunk Subcutaneous Tissue and Fascia, External Approach
AHA CC: 2Q, 2017, 26; 3Q, 2018, 10

0J2VX0Z Change Drainage Device in Upper Extremity Subcutaneous Tissue and Fascia, External Approach

0J2VXYZ Change Other Device in Upper Extremity Subcutaneous Tissue and Fascia, External Approach

0J2WX0Z Change Drainage Device in Lower Extremity Subcutaneous Tissue and Fascia, External Approach

0J2WXYZ Change Other Device in Lower Extremity Subcutaneous Tissue and Fascia, External Approach

0J5 – Subcutaneous Tissue and Fascia, Destruction

● **0J500ZZ** Destruction of Scalp Subcutaneous Tissue and Fascia, Open Approach

● **0J503ZZ** Destruction of Scalp Subcutaneous Tissue and Fascia, Percutaneous Approach

● **0J510ZZ** Destruction of Face Subcutaneous Tissue and Fascia, Open Approach

● **0J513ZZ** Destruction of Face Subcutaneous Tissue and Fascia, Percutaneous Approach

● **0J540ZZ** Destruction of Right Neck Subcutaneous Tissue and Fascia, Open Approach

● **0J543ZZ** Destruction of Right Neck Subcutaneous Tissue and Fascia, Percutaneous Approach

● **0J550ZZ** Destruction of Left Neck Subcutaneous Tissue and Fascia, Open Approach

● **0J553ZZ** Destruction of Left Neck Subcutaneous Tissue and Fascia, Percutaneous Approach

● **0J560ZZ** Destruction of Chest Subcutaneous Tissue and Fascia, Open Approach

● **0J563ZZ** Destruction of Chest Subcutaneous Tissue and Fascia, Percutaneous Approach

● **0J570ZZ** Destruction of Back Subcutaneous Tissue and Fascia, Open Approach

● **0J573ZZ** Destruction of Back Subcutaneous Tissue and Fascia, Percutaneous Approach

● **0J580ZZ** Destruction of Abdomen Subcutaneous Tissue and Fascia, Open Approach

● **0J583ZZ** Destruction of Abdomen Subcutaneous Tissue and Fascia, Percutaneous Approach

● **0J590ZZ** Destruction of Buttock Subcutaneous Tissue and Fascia, Open Approach

● **0J593ZZ** Destruction of Buttock Subcutaneous Tissue and Fascia, Percutaneous Approach

● **0J5B0ZZ** Destruction of Perineum Subcutaneous Tissue and Fascia, Open Approach

● **0J5B3ZZ** Destruction of Perineum Subcutaneous Tissue and Fascia, Percutaneous Approach

● **0J5C0ZZ** Destruction of Pelvic Region Subcutaneous Tissue and Fascia, Open Approach

● **0J5C3ZZ** Destruction of Pelvic Region Subcutaneous Tissue and Fascia, Percutaneous Approach

● **0J5D0ZZ** Destruction of Right Upper Arm Subcutaneous Tissue and Fascia, Open Approach

● **0J5D3ZZ** Destruction of Right Upper Arm Subcutaneous Tissue and Fascia, Percutaneous Approach

● **0J5F0ZZ** Destruction of Left Upper Arm Subcutaneous Tissue and Fascia, Open Approach

● **0J5F3ZZ** Destruction of Left Upper Arm Subcutaneous Tissue and Fascia, Percutaneous Approach

● **0J5G0ZZ** Destruction of Right Lower Arm Subcutaneous Tissue and Fascia, Open Approach

● **0J5G3ZZ** Destruction of Right Lower Arm Subcutaneous Tissue and Fascia, Percutaneous Approach

● **0J5H0ZZ** Destruction of Left Lower Arm Subcutaneous Tissue and Fascia, Open Approach

● **0J5H3ZZ** Destruction of Left Lower Arm Subcutaneous Tissue and Fascia, Percutaneous Approach

● **0J5J0ZZ** Destruction of Right Hand Subcutaneous Tissue and Fascia, Open Approach

● **0J5J3ZZ** Destruction of Right Hand Subcutaneous Tissue and Fascia, Percutaneous Approach

● **0J5K0ZZ** Destruction of Left Hand Subcutaneous Tissue and Fascia, Open Approach

● **0J5K3ZZ** Destruction of Left Hand Subcutaneous Tissue and Fascia, Percutaneous Approach

● **0J5L0ZZ** Destruction of Right Upper Leg Subcutaneous Tissue and Fascia, Open Approach

● **0J5L3ZZ** Destruction of Right Upper Leg Subcutaneous Tissue and Fascia, Percutaneous Approach

● **0J5M0ZZ** Destruction of Left Upper Leg Subcutaneous Tissue and Fascia, Open Approach

● **0J5M3ZZ** Destruction of Left Upper Leg Subcutaneous Tissue and Fascia, Percutaneous Approach

● **0J5N0ZZ** Destruction of Right Lower Leg Subcutaneous Tissue and Fascia, Open Approach

● **0J5N3ZZ** Destruction of Right Lower Leg Subcutaneous Tissue and Fascia, Percutaneous Approach

● **0J5P0ZZ** Destruction of Left Lower Leg Subcutaneous Tissue and Fascia, Open Approach

● **0J5P3ZZ** Destruction of Left Lower Leg Subcutaneous Tissue and Fascia, Percutaneous Approach

● **0J5Q0ZZ** Destruction of Right Foot Subcutaneous Tissue and Fascia, Open Approach

● **0J5Q3ZZ** Destruction of Right Foot Subcutaneous Tissue and Fascia, Percutaneous Approach

● **0J5R0ZZ** Destruction of Left Foot Subcutaneous Tissue and Fascia, Open Approach

● **0J5R3ZZ** Destruction of Left Foot Subcutaneous Tissue and Fascia, Percutaneous Approach

0J8 – Subcutaneous Tissue and Fascia, Division

Review Coding Guideline B3.14

0J800ZZ Division of Scalp Subcutaneous Tissue and Fascia, Open Approach

0J803ZZ Division of Scalp Subcutaneous Tissue and Fascia, Percutaneous Approach

0J810ZZ Division of Face Subcutaneous Tissue and Fascia, Open Approach

---

788 ♀ Female-only   ♂ Male-only   ▲ Limited Coverage   ● Non-OR   **HAC** HAC-associated procedure   ▲ Non-covered procedures   ✛ Cluster

0J813ZZ Division of Face Subcutaneous Tissue and Fascia, Percutaneous Approach

0J840ZZ Division of Right Neck Subcutaneous Tissue and Fascia, Open Approach

0J843ZZ Division of Right Neck Subcutaneous Tissue and Fascia, Percutaneous Approach

0J850ZZ Division of Left Neck Subcutaneous Tissue and Fascia, Open Approach

0J853ZZ Division of Left Neck Subcutaneous Tissue and Fascia, Percutaneous Approach

0J860ZZ Division of Chest Subcutaneous Tissue and Fascia, Open Approach

0J863ZZ Division of Chest Subcutaneous Tissue and Fascia, Percutaneous Approach

0J870ZZ Division of Back Subcutaneous Tissue and Fascia, Open Approach

0J873ZZ Division of Back Subcutaneous Tissue and Fascia, Percutaneous Approach

0J880ZZ Division of Abdomen Subcutaneous Tissue and Fascia, Open Approach

0J883ZZ Division of Abdomen Subcutaneous Tissue and Fascia, Percutaneous Approach

0J890ZZ Division of Buttock Subcutaneous Tissue and Fascia, Open Approach

0J893ZZ Division of Buttock Subcutaneous Tissue and Fascia, Percutaneous Approach

0J8B0ZZ Division of Perineum Subcutaneous Tissue and Fascia, Open Approach

0J8B3ZZ Division of Perineum Subcutaneous Tissue and Fascia, Percutaneous Approach

0J8C0ZZ Division of Pelvic Region Subcutaneous Tissue and Fascia, Open Approach

0J8C3ZZ Division of Pelvic Region Subcutaneous Tissue and Fascia, Percutaneous Approach

0J8D0ZZ Division of Right Upper Arm Subcutaneous Tissue and Fascia, Open Approach

0J8D3ZZ Division of Right Upper Arm Subcutaneous Tissue and Fascia, Percutaneous Approach

0J8F0ZZ Division of Left Upper Arm Subcutaneous Tissue and Fascia, Open Approach

0J8F3ZZ Division of Left Upper Arm Subcutaneous Tissue and Fascia, Percutaneous Approach

0J8G0ZZ Division of Right Lower Arm Subcutaneous Tissue and Fascia, Open Approach

0J8G3ZZ Division of Right Lower Arm Subcutaneous Tissue and Fascia, Percutaneous Approach

0J8H0ZZ Division of Left Lower Arm Subcutaneous Tissue and Fascia, Open Approach

0J8H3ZZ Division of Left Lower Arm Subcutaneous Tissue and Fascia, Percutaneous Approach

0J8J0ZZ Division of Right Hand Subcutaneous Tissue and Fascia, Open Approach

0J8J3ZZ Division of Right Hand Subcutaneous Tissue and Fascia, Percutaneous Approach

0J8K0ZZ Division of Left Hand Subcutaneous Tissue and Fascia, Open Approach

0J8K3ZZ Division of Left Hand Subcutaneous Tissue and Fascia, Percutaneous Approach

0J8L0ZZ Division of Right Upper Leg Subcutaneous Tissue and Fascia, Open Approach

0J8L3ZZ Division of Right Upper Leg Subcutaneous Tissue and Fascia, Percutaneous Approach

0J8M0ZZ Division of Left Upper Leg Subcutaneous Tissue and Fascia, Open Approach

0J8M3ZZ Division of Left Upper Leg Subcutaneous Tissue and Fascia, Percutaneous Approach

0J8N0ZZ Division of Right Lower Leg Subcutaneous Tissue and Fascia, Open Approach

0J8N3ZZ Division of Right Lower Leg Subcutaneous Tissue and Fascia, Percutaneous Approach

0J8P0ZZ Division of Left Lower Leg Subcutaneous Tissue and Fascia, Open Approach

0J8P3ZZ Division of Left Lower Leg Subcutaneous Tissue and Fascia, Percutaneous Approach

0J8Q0ZZ Division of Right Foot Subcutaneous Tissue and Fascia, Open Approach

0J8Q3ZZ Division of Right Foot Subcutaneous Tissue and Fascia, Percutaneous Approach

0J8R0ZZ Division of Left Foot Subcutaneous Tissue and Fascia, Open Approach

0J8R3ZZ Division of Left Foot Subcutaneous Tissue and Fascia, Percutaneous Approach

0J8S0ZZ Division of Head and Neck Subcutaneous Tissue and Fascia, Open Approach

0J8S3ZZ Division of Head and Neck Subcutaneous Tissue and Fascia, Percutaneous Approach

0J8T0ZZ Division of Trunk Subcutaneous Tissue and Fascia, Open Approach

0J8T3ZZ Division of Trunk Subcutaneous Tissue and Fascia, Percutaneous Approach

0J8V0ZZ Division of Upper Extremity Subcutaneous Tissue and Fascia, Open Approach

0J8V3ZZ Division of Upper Extremity Subcutaneous Tissue and Fascia, Percutaneous Approach

0J8W0ZZ Division of Lower Extremity Subcutaneous Tissue and Fascia, Open Approach

0J8W3ZZ Division of Lower Extremity Subcutaneous Tissue and Fascia, Percutaneous Approach

0J9 – Subcutaneous Tissue and Fascia, Drainage

Review Coding Guidelines B3.4a and B3.4b

Review Coding Guideline B6.2

0J9000Z Drainage of Scalp Subcutaneous Tissue and Fascia with Drainage Device, Open Approach

0J900ZX Drainage of Scalp Subcutaneous Tissue and Fascia, Open Approach, Diagnostic

0J900ZZ Drainage of Scalp Subcutaneous Tissue and Fascia, Open Approach

0J9030Z Drainage of Scalp Subcutaneous Tissue and Fascia with Drainage Device, Percutaneous Approach

0J903ZX Drainage of Scalp Subcutaneous Tissue and Fascia, Percutaneous Approach, Diagnostic

0J903ZZ Drainage of Scalp Subcutaneous Tissue and Fascia, Percutaneous Approach

0J9100Z Drainage of Face Subcutaneous Tissue and Fascia with Drainage Device, Open Approach

0J910ZX Drainage of Face Subcutaneous Tissue and Fascia, Open Approach, Diagnostic

0J910ZZ Drainage of Face Subcutaneous Tissue and Fascia, Open Approach
AHA CC: 3Q, 2018, 16

0J9130Z Drainage of Face Subcutaneous Tissue and Fascia with Drainage Device, Percutaneous Approach

0J913ZX Drainage of Face Subcutaneous Tissue and Fascia, Percutaneous Approach, Diagnostic

0J913ZZ Drainage of Face Subcutaneous Tissue and Fascia, Percutaneous Approach

0J9400Z Drainage of Right Neck Subcutaneous Tissue and Fascia with Drainage Device, Open Approach

0J940ZX Drainage of Right Neck Subcutaneous Tissue and Fascia, Open Approach, Diagnostic

0J940ZZ Drainage of Right Neck Subcutaneous Tissue and Fascia, Open Approach
AHA CC: 3Q, 2018, 16-17

0J9430Z Drainage of Right Neck Subcutaneous Tissue and Fascia with Drainage Device, Percutaneous Approach

0J943ZX Drainage of Right Neck Subcutaneous Tissue and Fascia, Percutaneous Approach, Diagnostic

0J943ZZ Drainage of Right Neck Subcutaneous Tissue and Fascia, Percutaneous Approach

0J9500Z Drainage of Left Neck Subcutaneous Tissue and Fascia with Drainage Device, Open Approach

0J950ZX Drainage of Left Neck Subcutaneous Tissue and Fascia, Open Approach, Diagnostic

0J950ZZ Drainage of Left Neck Subcutaneous Tissue and Fascia, Open Approach

0J9530Z Drainage of Left Neck Subcutaneous Tissue and Fascia with Drainage Device, Percutaneous Approach

0J953ZX Drainage of Left Neck Subcutaneous Tissue and Fascia, Percutaneous Approach, Diagnostic

0J953ZZ Drainage of Left Neck Subcutaneous Tissue and Fascia, Percutaneous Approach

0J9600Z Drainage of Chest Subcutaneous Tissue and Fascia with Drainage Device, Open Approach

---

♀ Female-only   ♂ Male-only   ▲ Limited Coverage   ● Non-OR   ▨ HAC-associated procedure   ▲ Non-covered procedures   ➕ Cluster

0J960ZX Drainage of Chest Subcutaneous Tissue and Fascia, Open Approach, Diagnostic

0J960ZZ Drainage of Chest Subcutaneous Tissue and Fascia, Open Approach
AHA CC: 3Q, 2015, 23-24

0J9630Z Drainage of Chest Subcutaneous Tissue and Fascia with Drainage Device, Percutaneous Approach

0J963ZX Drainage of Chest Subcutaneous Tissue and Fascia, Percutaneous Approach, Diagnostic

0J963ZZ Drainage of Chest Subcutaneous Tissue and Fascia, Percutaneous Approach

0J9700Z Drainage of Back Subcutaneous Tissue and Fascia with Drainage Device, Open Approach

0J970ZX Drainage of Back Subcutaneous Tissue and Fascia, Open Approach, Diagnostic

0J970ZZ Drainage of Back Subcutaneous Tissue and Fascia, Open Approach

0J9730Z Drainage of Back Subcutaneous Tissue and Fascia with Drainage Device, Percutaneous Approach

0J973ZX Drainage of Back Subcutaneous Tissue and Fascia, Percutaneous Approach, Diagnostic

0J973ZZ Drainage of Back Subcutaneous Tissue and Fascia, Percutaneous Approach

0J9800Z Drainage of Abdomen Subcutaneous Tissue and Fascia with Drainage Device, Open Approach

0J980ZX Drainage of Abdomen Subcutaneous Tissue and Fascia, Open Approach, Diagnostic

0J980ZZ Drainage of Abdomen Subcutaneous Tissue and Fascia, Open Approach

0J9830Z Drainage of Abdomen Subcutaneous Tissue and Fascia with Drainage Device, Percutaneous Approach

0J983ZX Drainage of Abdomen Subcutaneous Tissue and Fascia, Percutaneous Approach, Diagnostic

0J983ZZ Drainage of Abdomen Subcutaneous Tissue and Fascia, Percutaneous Approach

0J9900Z Drainage of Buttock Subcutaneous Tissue and Fascia with Drainage Device, Open Approach

0J990ZX Drainage of Buttock Subcutaneous Tissue and Fascia, Open Approach, Diagnostic

0J990ZZ Drainage of Buttock Subcutaneous Tissue and Fascia, Open Approach

0J9930Z Drainage of Buttock Subcutaneous Tissue and Fascia with Drainage Device, Percutaneous Approach

0J993ZX Drainage of Buttock Subcutaneous Tissue and Fascia, Percutaneous Approach, Diagnostic

0J993ZZ Drainage of Buttock Subcutaneous Tissue and Fascia, Percutaneous Approach

0J9B00Z Drainage of Perineum Subcutaneous Tissue and Fascia with Drainage Device, Open Approach

0J9B0ZX Drainage of Perineum Subcutaneous Tissue and Fascia, Open Approach, Diagnostic

0J9B0ZZ Drainage of Perineum Subcutaneous Tissue and Fascia, Open Approach

0J9B30Z Drainage of Perineum Subcutaneous Tissue and Fascia with Drainage Device, Percutaneous Approach

0J9B3ZX Drainage of Perineum Subcutaneous Tissue and Fascia, Percutaneous Approach, Diagnostic

0J9B3ZZ Drainage of Perineum Subcutaneous Tissue and Fascia, Percutaneous Approach

0J9C00Z Drainage of Pelvic Region Subcutaneous Tissue and Fascia with Drainage Device, Open Approach

0J9C0ZX Drainage of Pelvic Region Subcutaneous Tissue and Fascia, Open Approach, Diagnostic

0J9C0ZZ Drainage of Pelvic Region Subcutaneous Tissue and Fascia, Open Approach
AHA CC: 3Q, 2015, 23-24

0J9C30Z Drainage of Pelvic Region Subcutaneous Tissue and Fascia with Drainage Device, Percutaneous Approach

0J9C3ZX Drainage of Pelvic Region Subcutaneous Tissue and Fascia, Percutaneous Approach, Diagnostic

0J9C3ZZ Drainage of Pelvic Region Subcutaneous Tissue and Fascia, Percutaneous Approach

0J9D00Z Drainage of Right Upper Arm Subcutaneous Tissue and Fascia with Drainage Device, Open Approach

0J9D0ZX Drainage of Right Upper Arm Subcutaneous Tissue and Fascia, Open Approach, Diagnostic

0J9D0ZZ Drainage of Right Upper Arm Subcutaneous Tissue and Fascia, Open Approach
AHA CC: 3Q, 2015, 23-24

0J9D30Z Drainage of Right Upper Arm Subcutaneous Tissue and Fascia with Drainage Device, Percutaneous Approach

0J9D3ZX Drainage of Right Upper Arm Subcutaneous Tissue and Fascia, Percutaneous Approach, Diagnostic

0J9D3ZZ Drainage of Right Upper Arm Subcutaneous Tissue and Fascia, Percutaneous Approach

0J9F00Z Drainage of Left Upper Arm Subcutaneous Tissue and Fascia with Drainage Device, Open Approach

0J9F0ZX Drainage of Left Upper Arm Subcutaneous Tissue and Fascia, Open Approach, Diagnostic

0J9F0ZZ Drainage of Left Upper Arm Subcutaneous Tissue and Fascia, Open Approach
AHA CC: 3Q, 2015, 23-24

0J9F30Z Drainage of Left Upper Arm Subcutaneous Tissue and Fascia with Drainage Device, Percutaneous Approach

0J9F3ZX Drainage of Left Upper Arm Subcutaneous Tissue and Fascia, Percutaneous Approach, Diagnostic

0J9F3ZZ Drainage of Left Upper Arm Subcutaneous Tissue and Fascia, Percutaneous Approach

0J9G00Z Drainage of Right Lower Arm Subcutaneous Tissue and Fascia with Drainage Device, Open Approach

0J9G0ZX Drainage of Right Lower Arm Subcutaneous Tissue and Fascia, Open Approach, Diagnostic

0J9G0ZZ Drainage of Right Lower Arm Subcutaneous Tissue and Fascia, Open Approach

0J9G30Z Drainage of Right Lower Arm Subcutaneous Tissue and Fascia with Drainage Device, Percutaneous Approach

0J9G3ZX Drainage of Right Lower Arm Subcutaneous Tissue and Fascia, Percutaneous Approach, Diagnostic

0J9G3ZZ Drainage of Right Lower Arm Subcutaneous Tissue and Fascia, Percutaneous Approach

0J9H00Z Drainage of Left Lower Arm Subcutaneous Tissue and Fascia with Drainage Device, Open Approach

0J9H0ZX Drainage of Left Lower Arm Subcutaneous Tissue and Fascia, Open Approach, Diagnostic

0J9H0ZZ Drainage of Left Lower Arm Subcutaneous Tissue and Fascia, Open Approach

0J9H30Z Drainage of Left Lower Arm Subcutaneous Tissue and Fascia with Drainage Device, Percutaneous Approach

0J9H3ZX Drainage of Left Lower Arm Subcutaneous Tissue and Fascia, Percutaneous Approach, Diagnostic

0J9H3ZZ Drainage of Left Lower Arm Subcutaneous Tissue and Fascia, Percutaneous Approach

0J9J00Z Drainage of Right Hand Subcutaneous Tissue and Fascia with Drainage Device, Open Approach

0J9J0ZX Drainage of Right Hand Subcutaneous Tissue and Fascia, Open Approach, Diagnostic

0J9J0ZZ Drainage of Right Hand Subcutaneous Tissue and Fascia, Open Approach

0J9J30Z Drainage of Right Hand Subcutaneous Tissue and Fascia with Drainage Device, Percutaneous Approach

0J9J3ZX Drainage of Right Hand Subcutaneous Tissue and Fascia, Percutaneous Approach, Diagnostic

0J9J3ZZ Drainage of Right Hand Subcutaneous Tissue and Fascia, Percutaneous Approach

0J9K00Z Drainage of Left Hand Subcutaneous Tissue and Fascia with Drainage Device, Open Approach

0J9K0ZX Drainage of Left Hand Subcutaneous Tissue and Fascia, Open Approach, Diagnostic

0J9K0ZZ Drainage of Left Hand Subcutaneous Tissue and Fascia, Open Approach

0J9K30Z Drainage of Left Hand Subcutaneous Tissue and Fascia with Drainage Device, Percutaneous Approach

0J9K3ZX Drainage of Left Hand Subcutaneous Tissue and Fascia, Percutaneous Approach, Diagnostic

0J9K3ZZ Drainage of Left Hand Subcutaneous Tissue and Fascia, Percutaneous Approach

0J9L00Z Drainage of Right Upper Leg Subcutaneous Tissue and Fascia with Drainage Device, Open Approach

0J9L0ZX Drainage of Right Upper Leg Subcutaneous Tissue and Fascia, Open Approach, Diagnostic

0J9L0ZZ Drainage of Right Upper Leg Subcutaneous Tissue and Fascia, Open Approach
AHA CC: 3Q, 2015, 23-24

0J9L30Z Drainage of Right Upper Leg Subcutaneous Tissue and Fascia with Drainage Device, Percutaneous Approach

0J9L3ZX Drainage of Right Upper Leg Subcutaneous Tissue and Fascia, Percutaneous Approach, Diagnostic

♀ Female-only   ♂ Male-only   ▲ Limited Coverage   ● Non-OR   ⬛ HAC-associated procedure   ▲ Non-covered procedures   ✚ Cluster

0J9L3ZZ	Drainage of Right Upper Leg Subcutaneous Tissue and Fascia, Percutaneous Approach
0J9M00Z	Drainage of Left Upper Leg Subcutaneous Tissue and Fascia with Drainage Device, Open Approach
0J9M0ZX	Drainage of Left Upper Leg Subcutaneous Tissue and Fascia, Open Approach, Diagnostic
0J9M0ZZ	Drainage of Left Upper Leg Subcutaneous Tissue and Fascia, Open Approach
	AHA CC: 3Q, 2015, 23-24
0J9M30Z	Drainage of Left Upper Leg Subcutaneous Tissue and Fascia with Drainage Device, Percutaneous Approach
0J9M3ZX	Drainage of Left Upper Leg Subcutaneous Tissue and Fascia, Percutaneous Approach, Diagnostic
0J9M3ZZ	Drainage of Left Upper Leg Subcutaneous Tissue and Fascia, Percutaneous Approach
0J9N00Z	Drainage of Right Lower Leg Subcutaneous Tissue and Fascia with Drainage Device, Open Approach
0J9N0ZX	Drainage of Right Lower Leg Subcutaneous Tissue and Fascia, Open Approach, Diagnostic
0J9N0ZZ	Drainage of Right Lower Leg Subcutaneous Tissue and Fascia, Open Approach
0J9N30Z	Drainage of Right Lower Leg Subcutaneous Tissue and Fascia with Drainage Device, Percutaneous Approach
0J9N3ZX	Drainage of Right Lower Leg Subcutaneous Tissue and Fascia, Percutaneous Approach, Diagnostic
0J9N3ZZ	Drainage of Right Lower Leg Subcutaneous Tissue and Fascia, Percutaneous Approach
0J9P00Z	Drainage of Left Lower Leg Subcutaneous Tissue and Fascia with Drainage Device, Open Approach
0J9P0ZX	Drainage of Left Lower Leg Subcutaneous Tissue and Fascia, Open Approach, Diagnostic
0J9P0ZZ	Drainage of Left Lower Leg Subcutaneous Tissue and Fascia, Open Approach
0J9P30Z	Drainage of Left Lower Leg Subcutaneous Tissue and Fascia with Drainage Device, Percutaneous Approach
0J9P3ZX	Drainage of Left Lower Leg Subcutaneous Tissue and Fascia, Percutaneous Approach, Diagnostic
0J9P3ZZ	Drainage of Left Lower Leg Subcutaneous Tissue and Fascia, Percutaneous Approach
0J9Q00Z	Drainage of Right Foot Subcutaneous Tissue and Fascia with Drainage Device, Open Approach
0J9Q0ZX	Drainage of Right Foot Subcutaneous Tissue and Fascia, Open Approach, Diagnostic
0J9Q0ZZ	Drainage of Right Foot Subcutaneous Tissue and Fascia, Open Approach
0J9Q30Z	Drainage of Right Foot Subcutaneous Tissue and Fascia with Drainage Device, Percutaneous Approach
0J9Q3ZX	Drainage of Right Foot Subcutaneous Tissue and Fascia, Percutaneous Approach, Diagnostic
0J9Q3ZZ	Drainage of Right Foot Subcutaneous Tissue and Fascia, Percutaneous Approach
0J9R00Z	Drainage of Left Foot Subcutaneous Tissue and Fascia with Drainage Device, Open Approach
0J9R0ZX	Drainage of Left Foot Subcutaneous Tissue and Fascia, Open Approach, Diagnostic
0J9R0ZZ	Drainage of Left Foot Subcutaneous Tissue and Fascia, Open Approach
0J9R30Z	Drainage of Left Foot Subcutaneous Tissue and Fascia with Drainage Device, Percutaneous Approach
0J9R3ZX	Drainage of Left Foot Subcutaneous Tissue and Fascia, Percutaneous Approach, Diagnostic
0J9R3ZZ	Drainage of Left Foot Subcutaneous Tissue and Fascia, Percutaneous Approach

0JB – Subcutaneous Tissue and Fascia, Excision

Review Coding Guidelines B3.4a and B3.4b

Review Coding Guideline B3.5

Review Coding Guideline B3.8

Review Coding Guideline B3.18

0JB00ZX	Excision of Scalp Subcutaneous Tissue and Fascia, Open Approach, Diagnostic
0JB00ZZ	Excision of Scalp Subcutaneous Tissue and Fascia, Open Approach
0JB03ZX	Excision of Scalp Subcutaneous Tissue and Fascia, Percutaneous Approach, Diagnostic
● **0JB03ZZ**	Excision of Scalp Subcutaneous Tissue and Fascia, Percutaneous Approach
0JB10ZX	Excision of Face Subcutaneous Tissue and Fascia, Open Approach, Diagnostic
0JB10ZZ	Excision of Face Subcutaneous Tissue and Fascia, Open Approach
0JB13ZX	Excision of Face Subcutaneous Tissue and Fascia, Percutaneous Approach, Diagnostic
0JB13ZZ	Excision of Face Subcutaneous Tissue and Fascia, Percutaneous Approach
0JB40ZX	Excision of Right Neck Subcutaneous Tissue and Fascia, Open Approach, Diagnostic
0JB40ZZ	Excision of Right Neck Subcutaneous Tissue and Fascia, Open Approach
0JB43ZX	Excision of Right Neck Subcutaneous Tissue and Fascia, Percutaneous Approach, Diagnostic
● **0JB43ZZ**	Excision of Right Neck Subcutaneous Tissue and Fascia, Percutaneous Approach
0JB50ZX	Excision of Left Neck Subcutaneous Tissue and Fascia, Open Approach, Diagnostic
0JB50ZZ	Excision of Left Neck Subcutaneous Tissue and Fascia, Open Approach
0JB53ZX	Excision of Left Neck Subcutaneous Tissue and Fascia, Percutaneous Approach, Diagnostic
● **0JB53ZZ**	Excision of Left Neck Subcutaneous Tissue and Fascia, Percutaneous Approach
0JB60ZX	Excision of Chest Subcutaneous Tissue and Fascia, Open Approach, Diagnostic
0JB60ZZ	Excision of Chest Subcutaneous Tissue and Fascia, Open Approach
0JB63ZX	Excision of Chest Subcutaneous Tissue and Fascia, Percutaneous Approach, Diagnostic
● **0JB63ZZ**	Excision of Chest Subcutaneous Tissue and Fascia, Percutaneous Approach
0JB70ZX	Excision of Back Subcutaneous Tissue and Fascia, Open Approach, Diagnostic
0JB70ZZ	Excision of Back Subcutaneous Tissue and Fascia, Open Approach
	AHA CC: 1Q, 2018, 7-8
0JB73ZX	Excision of Back Subcutaneous Tissue and Fascia, Percutaneous Approach, Diagnostic
● **0JB73ZZ**	Excision of Back Subcutaneous Tissue and Fascia, Percutaneous Approach
0JB80ZX	Excision of Abdomen Subcutaneous Tissue and Fascia, Open Approach, Diagnostic
0JB80ZZ	Excision of Abdomen Subcutaneous Tissue and Fascia, Open Approach
	AHA CC: 3Q, 2014, 22-23; 4Q, 2014, 39-40; 1Q, 2020, 31-32
0JB83ZX	Excision of Abdomen Subcutaneous Tissue and Fascia, Percutaneous Approach, Diagnostic
● **0JB83ZZ**	Excision of Abdomen Subcutaneous Tissue and Fascia, Percutaneous Approach
0JB90ZX	Excision of Buttock Subcutaneous Tissue and Fascia, Open Approach, Diagnostic
0JB90ZZ	Excision of Buttock Subcutaneous Tissue and Fascia, Open Approach
	AHA CC: 3Q, 2015, 6-7
0JB93ZX	Excision of Buttock Subcutaneous Tissue and Fascia, Percutaneous Approach, Diagnostic
● **0JB93ZZ**	Excision of Buttock Subcutaneous Tissue and Fascia, Percutaneous Approach
	AHA CC: 3Q, 2019, 25
0JBB0ZX	Excision of Perineum Subcutaneous Tissue and Fascia, Open Approach, Diagnostic
0JBB0ZZ	Excision of Perineum Subcutaneous Tissue and Fascia, Open Approach
	AHA CC: 1Q, 2015, 29-30
0JBB3ZX	Excision of Perineum Subcutaneous Tissue and Fascia, Percutaneous Approach, Diagnostic
● **0JBB3ZZ**	Excision of Perineum Subcutaneous Tissue and Fascia, Percutaneous Approach
0JBC0ZX	Excision of Pelvic Region Subcutaneous Tissue and Fascia, Open Approach, Diagnostic

0JBC0ZZ Excision of Pelvic Region Subcutaneous Tissue and Fascia, Open Approach

0JBC3ZX Excision of Pelvic Region Subcutaneous Tissue and Fascia, Percutaneous Approach, Diagnostic

● **0JBC3ZZ** Excision of Pelvic Region Subcutaneous Tissue and Fascia, Percutaneous Approach

0JBD0ZX Excision of Right Upper Arm Subcutaneous Tissue and Fascia, Open Approach, Diagnostic

0JBD0ZZ Excision of Right Upper Arm Subcutaneous Tissue and Fascia, Open Approach

0JBD3ZX Excision of Right Upper Arm Subcutaneous Tissue and Fascia, Percutaneous Approach, Diagnostic

● **0JBD3ZZ** Excision of Right Upper Arm Subcutaneous Tissue and Fascia, Percutaneous Approach

0JBF0ZX Excision of Left Upper Arm Subcutaneous Tissue and Fascia, Open Approach, Diagnostic

0JBF0ZZ Excision of Left Upper Arm Subcutaneous Tissue and Fascia, Open Approach

0JBF3ZX Excision of Left Upper Arm Subcutaneous Tissue and Fascia, Percutaneous Approach, Diagnostic

● **0JBF3ZZ** Excision of Left Upper Arm Subcutaneous Tissue and Fascia, Percutaneous Approach

0JBG0ZX Excision of Right Lower Arm Subcutaneous Tissue and Fascia, Open Approach, Diagnostic

0JBG0ZZ Excision of Right Lower Arm Subcutaneous Tissue and Fascia, Open Approach

0JBG3ZX Excision of Right Lower Arm Subcutaneous Tissue and Fascia, Percutaneous Approach, Diagnostic

● **0JBG3ZZ** Excision of Right Lower Arm Subcutaneous Tissue and Fascia, Percutaneous Approach

0JBH0ZX Excision of Left Lower Arm Subcutaneous Tissue and Fascia, Open Approach, Diagnostic

0JBH0ZZ Excision of Left Lower Arm Subcutaneous Tissue and Fascia, Open Approach
AHA CC: 2Q, 2015, 13

0JBH3ZX Excision of Left Lower Arm Subcutaneous Tissue and Fascia, Percutaneous Approach, Diagnostic

● **0JBH3ZZ** Excision of Left Lower Arm Subcutaneous Tissue and Fascia, Percutaneous Approach

0JBJ0ZX Excision of Right Hand Subcutaneous Tissue and Fascia, Open Approach, Diagnostic

0JBJ0ZZ Excision of Right Hand Subcutaneous Tissue and Fascia, Open Approach

0JBJ3ZX Excision of Right Hand Subcutaneous Tissue and Fascia, Percutaneous Approach, Diagnostic

0JBJ3ZZ Excision of Right Hand Subcutaneous Tissue and Fascia, Percutaneous Approach

0JBK0ZX Excision of Left Hand Subcutaneous Tissue and Fascia, Open Approach, Diagnostic

0JBK0ZZ Excision of Left Hand Subcutaneous Tissue and Fascia, Open Approach

0JBK3ZX Excision of Left Hand Subcutaneous Tissue and Fascia, Percutaneous Approach, Diagnostic

0JBK3ZZ Excision of Left Hand Subcutaneous Tissue and Fascia, Percutaneous Approach

0JBL0ZX Excision of Right Upper Leg Subcutaneous Tissue and Fascia, Open Approach, Diagnostic

0JBL0ZZ Excision of Right Upper Leg Subcutaneous Tissue and Fascia, Open Approach

0JBL3ZX Excision of Right Upper Leg Subcutaneous Tissue and Fascia, Percutaneous Approach, Diagnostic

● **0JBL3ZZ** Excision of Right Upper Leg Subcutaneous Tissue and Fascia, Percutaneous Approach

0JBM0ZX Excision of Left Upper Leg Subcutaneous Tissue and Fascia, Open Approach, Diagnostic

0JBM0ZZ Excision of Left Upper Leg Subcutaneous Tissue and Fascia, Open Approach

0JBM3ZX Excision of Left Upper Leg Subcutaneous Tissue and Fascia, Percutaneous Approach, Diagnostic

● **0JBM3ZZ** Excision of Left Upper Leg Subcutaneous Tissue and Fascia, Percutaneous Approach

0JBN0ZX Excision of Right Lower Leg Subcutaneous Tissue and Fascia, Open Approach, Diagnostic

0JBN0ZZ Excision of Right Lower Leg Subcutaneous Tissue and Fascia, Open Approach

0JBN3ZX Excision of Right Lower Leg Subcutaneous Tissue and Fascia, Percutaneous Approach, Diagnostic

● **0JBN3ZZ** Excision of Right Lower Leg Subcutaneous Tissue and Fascia, Percutaneous Approach

0JBP0ZX Excision of Left Lower Leg Subcutaneous Tissue and Fascia, Open Approach, Diagnostic

0JBP0ZZ Excision of Left Lower Leg Subcutaneous Tissue and Fascia, Open Approach

0JBP3ZX Excision of Left Lower Leg Subcutaneous Tissue and Fascia, Percutaneous Approach, Diagnostic

● **0JBP3ZZ** Excision of Left Lower Leg Subcutaneous Tissue and Fascia, Percutaneous Approach

0JBQ0ZX Excision of Right Foot Subcutaneous Tissue and Fascia, Open Approach, Diagnostic

0JBQ0ZZ Excision of Right Foot Subcutaneous Tissue and Fascia, Open Approach

0JBQ3ZX Excision of Right Foot Subcutaneous Tissue and Fascia, Percutaneous Approach, Diagnostic

● **0JBQ3ZZ** Excision of Right Foot Subcutaneous Tissue and Fascia, Percutaneous Approach

0JBR0ZX Excision of Left Foot Subcutaneous Tissue and Fascia, Open Approach, Diagnostic

0JBR0ZZ Excision of Left Foot Subcutaneous Tissue and Fascia, Open Approach

0JBR3ZX Excision of Left Foot Subcutaneous Tissue and Fascia, Percutaneous Approach, Diagnostic

● **0JBR3ZZ** Excision of Left Foot Subcutaneous Tissue and Fascia, Percutaneous Approach

0JC – Subcutaneous Tissue and Fascia, Extirpation

0JC00ZZ Extirpation of Matter from Scalp Subcutaneous Tissue and Fascia, Open Approach

0JC03ZZ Extirpation of Matter from Scalp Subcutaneous Tissue and Fascia, Percutaneous Approach

0JC10ZZ Extirpation of Matter from Face Subcutaneous Tissue and Fascia, Open Approach

0JC13ZZ Extirpation of Matter from Face Subcutaneous Tissue and Fascia, Percutaneous Approach

0JC40ZZ Extirpation of Matter from Right Neck Subcutaneous Tissue and Fascia, Open Approach

0JC43ZZ Extirpation of Matter from Right Neck Subcutaneous Tissue and Fascia, Percutaneous Approach

0JC50ZZ Extirpation of Matter from Left Neck Subcutaneous Tissue and Fascia, Open Approach

0JC53ZZ Extirpation of Matter from Left Neck Subcutaneous Tissue and Fascia, Percutaneous Approach

0JC60ZZ Extirpation of Matter from Chest Subcutaneous Tissue and Fascia, Open Approach

0JC63ZZ Extirpation of Matter from Chest Subcutaneous Tissue and Fascia, Percutaneous Approach

0JC70ZZ Extirpation of Matter from Back Subcutaneous Tissue and Fascia, Open Approach

0JC73ZZ Extirpation of Matter from Back Subcutaneous Tissue and Fascia, Percutaneous Approach

0JC80ZZ Extirpation of Matter from Abdomen Subcutaneous Tissue and Fascia, Open Approach
AHA CC: 3Q, 2017, 22

0JC83ZZ Extirpation of Matter from Abdomen Subcutaneous Tissue and Fascia, Percutaneous Approach

0JC90ZZ Extirpation of Matter from Buttock Subcutaneous Tissue and Fascia, Open Approach

0JC93ZZ Extirpation of Matter from Buttock Subcutaneous Tissue and Fascia, Percutaneous Approach

0JCB0ZZ Extirpation of Matter from Perineum Subcutaneous Tissue and Fascia, Open Approach

0JCB3ZZ Extirpation of Matter from Perineum Subcutaneous Tissue and Fascia, Percutaneous Approach

0JCC0ZZ Extirpation of Matter from Pelvic Region Subcutaneous Tissue and Fascia, Open Approach

0JCC3ZZ Extirpation of Matter from Pelvic Region Subcutaneous Tissue and Fascia, Percutaneous Approach

0JCD0ZZ Extirpation of Matter from Right Upper Arm Subcutaneous Tissue and Fascia, Open Approach

0JCD3ZZ Extirpation of Matter from Right Upper Arm Subcutaneous Tissue and Fascia, Percutaneous Approach

0JCF0ZZ Extirpation of Matter from Left Upper Arm Subcutaneous Tissue and Fascia, Open Approach

0JCF3ZZ Extirpation of Matter from Left Upper Arm Subcutaneous Tissue and Fascia, Percutaneous Approach

0JCG0ZZ Extirpation of Matter from Right Lower Arm Subcutaneous Tissue and Fascia, Open Approach

0JCG3ZZ Extirpation of Matter from Right Lower Arm Subcutaneous Tissue and Fascia, Percutaneous Approach

0JCH0ZZ Extirpation of Matter from Left Lower Arm Subcutaneous Tissue and Fascia, Open Approach

0JCH3ZZ Extirpation of Matter from Left Lower Arm Subcutaneous Tissue and Fasciva, Percutaneous Approach

0JCJ0ZZ Extirpation of Matter from Right Hand Subcutaneous Tissue and Fascia, Open Approach

0JCJ3ZZ Extirpation of Matter from Right Hand Subcutaneous Tissue and Fascia, Percutaneous Approach

0JCK0ZZ Extirpation of Matter from Left Hand Subcutaneous Tissue and Fascia, Open Approach

0JCK3ZZ Extirpation of Matter from Left Hand Subcutaneous Tissue and Fascia, Percutaneous Approach

0JCL0ZZ Extirpation of Matter from Right Upper Leg Subcutaneous Tissue and Fascia, Open Approach

0JCL3ZZ Extirpation of Matter from Right Upper Leg Subcutaneous Tissue and Fascia, Percutaneous Approach

0JCM0ZZ Extirpation of Matter from Left Upper Leg Subcutaneous Tissue and Fascia, Open Approach

0JCM3ZZ Extirpation of Matter from Left Upper Leg Subcutaneous Tissue and Fascia, Percutaneous Approach

0JCN0ZZ Extirpation of Matter from Right Lower Leg Subcutaneous Tissue and Fascia, Open Approach

0JCN3ZZ Extirpation of Matter from Right Lower Leg Subcutaneous Tissue and Fascia, Percutaneous Approach

0JCP0ZZ Extirpation of Matter from Left Lower Leg Subcutaneous Tissue and Fascia, Open Approach

0JCP3ZZ Extirpation of Matter from Left Lower Leg Subcutaneous Tissue and Fascia, Percutaneous Approach

0JCQ0ZZ Extirpation of Matter from Right Foot Subcutaneous Tissue and Fascia, Open Approach

0JCQ3ZZ Extirpation of Matter from Right Foot Subcutaneous Tissue and Fascia, Percutaneous Approach

0JCR0ZZ Extirpation of Matter from Left Foot Subcutaneous Tissue and Fascia, Open Approach

0JCR3ZZ Extirpation of Matter from Left Foot Subcutaneous Tissue and Fascia, Percutaneous Approach

0JD – Subcutaneous Tissue and Fascia, Extraction

0JD00ZZ Extraction of Scalp Subcutaneous Tissue and Fascia, Open Approach

0JD03ZZ Extraction of Scalp Subcutaneous Tissue and Fascia, Percutaneous Approach

0JD10ZZ Extraction of Face Subcutaneous Tissue and Fascia, Open Approach

0JD13ZZ Extraction of Face Subcutaneous Tissue and Fascia, Percutaneous Approach

0JD40ZZ Extraction of Right Neck Subcutaneous Tissue and Fascia, Open Approach

0JD43ZZ Extraction of Right Neck Subcutaneous Tissue and Fascia, Percutaneous Approach

0JD50ZZ Extraction of Left Neck Subcutaneous Tissue and Fascia, Open Approach

0JD53ZZ Extraction of Left Neck Subcutaneous Tissue and Fascia, Percutaneous Approach

0JD60ZZ Extraction of Chest Subcutaneous Tissue and Fascia, Open Approach

● **0JD63ZZ** Extraction of Chest Subcutaneous Tissue and Fascia, Percutaneous Approach

0JD70ZZ Extraction of Back Subcutaneous Tissue and Fascia, Open Approach
AHA CC: 3Q, 2016, 21

● **0JD73ZZ** Extraction of Back Subcutaneous Tissue and Fascia, Percutaneous Approach

0JD80ZZ Extraction of Abdomen Subcutaneous Tissue and Fascia, Open Approach

● **0JD83ZZ** Extraction of Abdomen Subcutaneous Tissue and Fascia, Percutaneous Approach

0JD90ZZ Extraction of Buttock Subcutaneous Tissue and Fascia, Open Approach

● **0JD93ZZ** Extraction of Buttock Subcutaneous Tissue and Fascia, Percutaneous Approach

0JDB0ZZ Extraction of Perineum Subcutaneous Tissue and Fascia, Open Approach

0JDB3ZZ Extraction of Perineum Subcutaneous Tissue and Fascia, Percutaneous Approach

0JDC0ZZ Extraction of Pelvic Region Subcutaneous Tissue and Fascia, Open Approach
AHA CC: 1Q, 2015, 23

0JDC3ZZ Extraction of Pelvic Region Subcutaneous Tissue and Fascia, Percutaneous Approach

0JDD0ZZ Extraction of Right Upper Arm Subcutaneous Tissue and Fascia, Open Approach

0JDD3ZZ Extraction of Right Upper Arm Subcutaneous Tissue and Fascia, Percutaneous Approach

0JDF0ZZ Extraction of Left Upper Arm Subcutaneous Tissue and Fascia, Open Approach

0JDF3ZZ Extraction of Left Upper Arm Subcutaneous Tissue and Fascia, Percutaneous Approach

0JDG0ZZ Extraction of Right Lower Arm Subcutaneous Tissue and Fascia, Open Approach

0JDG3ZZ Extraction of Right Lower Arm Subcutaneous Tissue and Fascia, Percutaneous Approach

0JDH0ZZ Extraction of Left Lower Arm Subcutaneous Tissue and Fascia, Open Approach

0JDH3ZZ Extraction of Left Lower Arm Subcutaneous Tissue and Fascia, Percutaneous Approach

0JDJ0ZZ Extraction of Right Hand Subcutaneous Tissue and Fascia, Open Approach

0JDJ3ZZ Extraction of Right Hand Subcutaneous Tissue and Fascia, Percutaneous Approach

0JDK0ZZ Extraction of Left Hand Subcutaneous Tissue and Fascia, Open Approach

0JDK3ZZ Extraction of Left Hand Subcutaneous Tissue and Fascia, Percutaneous Approach

0JDL0ZZ Extraction of Right Upper Leg Subcutaneous Tissue and Fascia, Open Approach
AHA CC: 1Q, 2016, 40

● **0JDL3ZZ** Extraction of Right Upper Leg Subcutaneous Tissue and Fascia, Percutaneous Approach

0JDM0ZZ Extraction of Left Upper Leg Subcutaneous Tissue and Fascia, Open Approach

● **0JDM3ZZ** Extraction of Left Upper Leg Subcutaneous Tissue and Fascia, Percutaneous Approach

0JDN0ZZ Extraction of Right Lower Leg Subcutaneous Tissue and Fascia, Open Approach
AHA CC: 3Q, 2016, 20-21

0JDN3ZZ Extraction of Right Lower Leg Subcutaneous Tissue and Fascia, Percutaneous Approach

0JDP0ZZ Extraction of Left Lower Leg Subcutaneous Tissue and Fascia, Open Approach

0JDP3ZZ Extraction of Left Lower Leg Subcutaneous Tissue and Fascia, Percutaneous Approach

0JDQ0ZZ Extraction of Right Foot Subcutaneous Tissue and Fascia, Open Approach

0JDQ3ZZ Extraction of Right Foot Subcutaneous Tissue and Fascia, Percutaneous Approach

0JDR0ZZ Extraction of Left Foot Subcutaneous Tissue and Fascia, Open Approach
AHA CC: 3Q, 2016, 22

0JDR3ZZ Extraction of Left Foot Subcutaneous Tissue and Fascia, Percutaneous Approach

0JH – Subcutaneous Tissue and Fascia, Insertion

0JH00NZ Insertion of Tissue Expander into Scalp Subcutaneous Tissue and Fascia, Open Approach

0JH03NZ Insertion of Tissue Expander into Scalp Subcutaneous Tissue and Fascia, Percutaneous Approach

0JH10NZ Insertion of Tissue Expander into Face Subcutaneous Tissue and Fascia, Open Approach

0JH13NZ Insertion of Tissue Expander into Face Subcutaneous Tissue and Fascia, Percutaneous Approach

0JH40NZ Insertion of Tissue Expander into Right Neck Subcutaneous Tissue and Fascia, Open Approach

0JH43NZ Insertion of Tissue Expander into Right Neck Subcutaneous Tissue and Fascia, Percutaneous Approach

0JH50NZ Insertion of Tissue Expander into Left Neck Subcutaneous Tissue and Fascia, Open Approach

0JH53NZ Insertion of Tissue Expander into Left Neck Subcutaneous Tissue and Fascia, Percutaneous Approach

0JH600Z Insertion of Hemodynamic Monitoring Device into Chest Subcutaneous Tissue and Fascia, Open Approach

0JH602Z Insertion of Monitoring Device into Chest Subcutaneous Tissue and Fascia, Open Approach

● **0JH604Z** Insertion of Pacemaker, Single Chamber into Chest Subcutaneous Tissue and Fascia, Open Approach

   HAC With a secondary diagnosis code of K68.11, T81.40XA, T81.41XA, T81.42XA, T81.43XA, T81.44XA, T82.6XXA, T82.7XXA

   + Insertion of pacemaker is part of the pacemaker cluster for MS-DRG assignment when reported with pacemaker lead code. *See table 02H to construct pacemaker lead Insertion code.*

● **0JH605Z** Insertion of Pacemaker, Single Chamber Rate Responsive into Chest Subcutaneous Tissue and Fascia, Open Approach

   HAC With a secondary diagnosis code of K68.11, T81.40XA, T81.41XA, T81.42XA, T81.43XA, T81.44XA, T82.6XXA, T82.7XXA

   + Insertion of pacemaker is part of the pacemaker cluster for MS-DRG assignment when reported with pacemaker lead code. *See table 02H to construct pacemaker lead Insertion code.*

● **0JH606Z** Insertion of Pacemaker, Dual Chamber into Chest Subcutaneous Tissue and Fascia, Open Approach

   HAC With a secondary diagnosis code of K68.11, T81.40XA, T81.41XA, T81.42XA, T81.43XA, T81.44XA, T82.6XXA, T82.7XXA

   + Insertion of pacemaker is part of the pacemaker cluster for MS-DRG assignment when reported with pacemaker lead code. *See table 02H to construct pacemaker lead Insertion code.*

● **0JH607Z** Insertion of Cardiac Resynchronization Pacemaker Pulse Generator into Chest Subcutaneous Tissue and Fascia, Open Approach

   HAC With a secondary diagnosis code of K68.11, T81.40XA, T81.41XA, T81.42XA, T81.43XA, T81.44XA, T82.6XXA, T82.7XXA

   + Insertion of pacemaker is part of the pacemaker cluster for MS-DRG assignment when reported with pacemaker lead code. *See table 02H to construct pacemaker lead Insertion code.*

0JH608Z Insertion of Defibrillator Generator into Chest Subcutaneous Tissue and Fascia, Open Approach

   AHA CC: 4Q, 2012, 104-106

   HAC With a secondary diagnosis code of K68.11, T81.40XA, T81.41XA, T81.42XA, T81.43XA, T81.44XA, T82.6XXA, T82.7XXA

   + Cardioverter-Defibrillator lead(s)/generator when reported with Insertion of a defibrillator cardiac lead (6th character K) into the coronary vein, atrium, or ventricle. Also applicable with Insertion of pacemaker cardiac lead, defibrillator cardiac lead or cardiac lead (6th characters J, K, M) into the pericardium. *See table 02H to construct the Insertion code.*

0JH609Z Insertion of Cardiac Resynchronization Defibrillator Pulse Generator into Chest Subcutaneous Tissue and Fascia, Open Approach

   HAC With a secondary diagnosis code of K68.11, T81.40XA, T81.41XA, T81.42XA, T81.43XA, T81.44XA, T82.6XXA, T82.7XXA

   + Cardioverter-Defibrillator lead(s)/generator when reported with Insertion of a defibrillator cardiac lead (6th character K) into the atrium, or ventricle. Also applicable with Insertion of pacemaker cardiac lead, defibrillator cardiac lead or cardiac lead (6th characters J, K, M) into the coronary vein or pericardium. *See table 02H to construct the Insertion code.*

0JH60AZ Insertion of Contractility Modulation Device into Chest Subcutaneous Tissue and Fascia, Open Approach

   + Cardioverter-Defibrillator lead(s)/generator when reported with Insertion of a cardiac lead (6th character M) into the left ventricle. *See table 02H to construct the Insertion code.*

0JH60BZ Insertion of Single Array Stimulator Generator into Chest Subcutaneous Tissue and Fascia, Open Approach

   + Neurotransmitter/Neurostimulator when reported with an Insertion of a neurostimulator lead (6th character M) into the cranial nerve, spinal canal or spinal cord. *See table 00H to construct the Insertion code.* Also applicable when reported with Insertion of neurostimulator lead (6th character M) into the peripheral nerve. *See table 01H to construct the Insertion code.* Also applicable when reported with Insertion of neurostimulator lead (6th character M) into upper vein. *See table 05H to construct the Insertion code.* Also applicable when reported with Insertion of a stimulator lead (6th character M) into the stomach. *See table 0DH to construct the Insertion code.*

0JH60CZ Insertion of Single Array Rechargeable Stimulator Generator into Chest Subcutaneous Tissue and Fascia, Open Approach

   + Neurotransmitter/Neurostimulator when reported with an Insertion of a neurostimulator lead (6th character M) into the cranial nerve, spinal canal or spinal cord. *See table 00H to construct the Insertion code.* Also applicable when reported with Insertion of neurostimulator lead (6th character M) into the peripheral nerve. *See table 01H to construct the Insertion code.* Also applicable when reported with Insertion of neurostimulator lead (6th character M) into upper vein. *See table 05H to construct the Insertion code.* Also applicable when reported with Insertion of a stimulator lead (6th character M) into the stomach. *See table 0DH to construct the Insertion code.*

0JH60DZ Insertion of Multiple Array Stimulator Generator into Chest Subcutaneous Tissue and Fascia, Open Approach

   + Major brain device implant when reported with an Insertion of a neurostimulator lead (6th character M) into the brain or cerebral ventricle. *See table 00H to construct the Insertion code.*

   + Neurotransmitter/Neurostimulator when reported with an Insertion of a neurostimulator lead (6th character M) into the cranial nerve, spinal canal or spinal cord. *See table 00H to construct the Insertion code.* Also applicable when reported with Insertion of neurostimulator lead (6th character M) into the peripheral nerve. *See table 01H to construct the Insertion code.* Also applicable when reported with Insertion of neurostimulator lead (6th character M) into upper vein. *See table 05H to construct the Insertion code.* Also applicable when reported with Insertion of a stimulator lead (6th character M) into the stomach. *See table 0DH to construct the Insertion code.*

0JH60EZ Insertion of Multiple Array Rechargeable Stimulator Generator into Chest Subcutaneous Tissue and Fascia, Open Approach

   + Major brain device implant when reported with an Insertion of a neurostimulator lead (6th character M) into the brain or cerebral ventricle. *See table 00H to construct the Insertion code.*

   + Neurotransmitter/Neurostimulator when reported with an Insertion of a neurostimulator lead (6th character M) into the cranial nerve, spinal canal or spinal cord. *See table 00H to construct the Insertion code.* Also applicable when reported with Insertion of neurostimulator lead (6th character M) into the peripheral nerve. *See table 01H to construct the Insertion code.* Also applicable when reported with Insertion of neurostimulator lead (6th character M) into upper vein. *See table 05H to construct the Insertion code.* Also applicable when reported with Insertion of a stimulator lead (6th character M) into the stomach. *See table 0DH to construct the Insertion code.*

0JH60FZ Insertion of Subcutaneous Defibrillator Lead into Chest Subcutaneous Tissue and Fascia, Open Approach

● **0JH60HZ** Insertion of Contraceptive Device into Chest Subcutaneous Tissue and Fascia, Open Approach

0JH60MZ Insertion of Stimulator Generator into Chest Subcutaneous Tissue and Fascia, Open Approach

AHA CC: 4Q, 2016, 98-99

0JH60NZ Insertion of Tissue Expander into Chest Subcutaneous Tissue and Fascia, Open Approach

0JH60PZ Insertion of Cardiac Rhythm Related Device into Chest Subcutaneous Tissue and Fascia, Open Approach

AHA CC: 4Q, 2012, 104-106

HAC With a secondary diagnosis code of K68.11, T81.40XA, T81.41XA, T81.42XA, T81.43XA, T81.44XA, T82.6XXA, T82.7XXA

+ Insertion of pacemaker is part of the pacemaker cluster for MS-DRG assignment when reported with pacemaker lead code. See table 02H to construct pacemaker lead Insertion code.

0JH60VZ Insertion of Infusion Pump into Chest Subcutaneous Tissue and Fascia, Open Approach

0JH60WZ Insertion of Totally Implantable Vascular Access Device into Chest Subcutaneous Tissue and Fascia, Open Approach

AHA CC: 4Q, 2017, 63-64

0JH60XZ Insertion of Tunneled Vascular Access Device into Chest Subcutaneous Tissue and Fascia, Open Approach

AHA CC: 2Q, 2015, 33-34

0JH60YZ Insertion of Other Device into Chest Subcutaneous Tissue and Fascia, Open Approach

0JH630Z Insertion of Hemodynamic Monitoring Device into Chest Subcutaneous Tissue and Fascia, Percutaneous Approach

0JH632Z Insertion of Monitoring Device into Chest Subcutaneous Tissue and Fascia, Percutaneous Approach

● **0JH634Z** Insertion of Pacemaker, Single Chamber into Chest Subcutaneous Tissue and Fascia, Percutaneous Approach

HAC With a secondary diagnosis code of K68.11, T81.40XA, T81.41XA, T81.42XA, T81.43XA, T81.44XA, T82.6XXA, T82.7XXA

+ Insertion of pacemaker is part of the pacemaker cluster for MS-DRG assignment when reported with pacemaker lead code. *See table 02H to construct pacemaker lead Insertion code.*

● **0JH635Z** Insertion of Pacemaker, Single Chamber Rate Responsive into Chest Subcutaneous Tissue and Fascia, Percutaneous Approach

HAC With a secondary diagnosis code of K68.11, T81.40XA, T81.41XA, T81.42XA, T81.43XA, T81.44XA, T82.6XXA, T82.7XXA

+ Insertion of pacemaker is part of the pacemaker cluster for MS-DRG assignment when reported with pacemaker lead code. *See table 02H to construct pacemaker lead Insertion code.*

● **0JH636Z** Insertion of Pacemaker, Dual Chamber into Chest Subcutaneous Tissue and Fascia, Percutaneous Approach

HAC With a secondary diagnosis code of K68.11, T81.40XA, T81.41XA,

T81.42XA, T81.43XA, T81.44XA, T82.6XXA, T82.7XXA

+ Insertion of pacemaker is part of the pacemaker cluster for MS-DRG assignment when reported with pacemaker lead code. *See table 02H to construct pacemaker lead Insertion code.*

● **0JH637Z** Insertion of Cardiac Resynchronization Pacemaker Pulse Generator into Chest Subcutaneous Tissue and Fascia, Percutaneous Approach

HAC With a secondary diagnosis code of K68.11, T81.40XA, T81.41XA, T81.42XA, T81.43XA, T81.44XA, T82.6XXA, T82.7XXA

+ Insertion of pacemaker is part of the pacemaker cluster for MS-DRG assignment when reported with pacemaker lead code. *See table 02H to construct pacemaker lead Insertion code.*

0JH638Z Insertion of Defibrillator Generator into Chest Subcutaneous Tissue and Fascia, Percutaneous Approach

HAC With a secondary diagnosis code of K68.11, T81.40XA, T81.41XA, T81.42XA, T81.43XA, T81.44XA, T82.6XXA, T82.7XXA

+ Cardioverter-Defibrillator lead(s)/ generator when reported with Insertion of a defibrillator cardiac lead (6th character K) into the coronary vein, atrium, or ventricle. Also applicable with Insertion of pacemaker cardiac lead, defibrillator cardiac lead or cardiac lead (6th characters J, K, M) into the pericardium. *See table 02H to construct the Insertion code.*

0JH639Z Insertion of Cardiac Resynchronization Defibrillator Pulse Generator into Chest Subcutaneous Tissue and Fascia, Percutaneous Approach

HAC With a secondary diagnosis code of K68.11, T81.40XA, T81.41XA, T81.42XA, T81.43XA, T81.44XA, T82.6XXA, T82.7XXA

+ Cardioverter-Defibrillator lead(s)/ generator when reported with Insertion of a defibrillator cardiac lead (6th character K) into the atrium, or ventricle. Also applicable with Insertion of pacemaker cardiac lead, defibrillator cardiac lead or cardiac lead (6th characters J, K, M) into the coronary vein or pericardium. *See table 02H to construct the Insertion code.*

0JH63AZ Insertion of Contractility Modulation Device into Chest Subcutaneous Tissue and Fascia, Percutaneous Approach

+ Cardioverter-Defibrillator lead(s)/ generator when reported with Insertion of a cardiac lead (6th character M) into the left ventricle. *See table 02H to construct the Insertion code.*

0JH63BZ Insertion of Single Array Stimulator Generator into Chest Subcutaneous Tissue and Fascia, Percutaneous Approach

+ Neurotransmitter/Neurostimulator when reported with an Insertion of a neurostimulator lead (6th character M) into the cranial nerve, spinal canal or spinal cord. *See table 00H to construct the Insertion code.* Also applicable when reported with Insertion of

neurostimulator lead (6th character M) into the peripheral nerve. *See table 01H to construct the Insertion code.* Also applicable when reported with Insertion of neurostimulator lead (6th character M) into upper vein. *See table 05H to construct the Insertion code.* Also applicable when reported with Insertion of a stimulator lead (6th character M) into the stomach. *See table 0DH to construct the Insertion code.*

0JH63CZ Insertion of Single Array Rechargeable Stimulator Generator into Chest Subcutaneous Tissue and Fascia, Percutaneous Approach

+ Neurotransmitter/Neurostimulator when reported with an Insertion of a neurostimulator lead (6th character M) into the cranial nerve, spinal canal or spinal cord. *See table 00H to construct the Insertion code.* Also applicable when reported with Insertion of neurostimulator lead (6th character M) into the peripheral nerve. *See table 01H to construct the Insertion code.* Also applicable when reported with Insertion of neurostimulator lead (6th character M) into upper vein. *See table 05H to construct the Insertion code.* Also applicable when reported with Insertion of a stimulator lead (6th character M) into the stomach. *See table 0DH to construct the Insertion code.*

0JH63DZ Insertion of Multiple Array Stimulator Generator into Chest Subcutaneous Tissue and Fascia, Percutaneous Approach

+ Major brain device implant when reported with an Insertion of a neurostimulator lead (6th character M) into the brain or cerebral ventricle. *See table 00H to construct the Insertion code.*

+ Neurotransmitter/Neurostimulator when reported with an Insertion of a neurostimulator lead (6th character M) into the cranial nerve, spinal canal or spinal cord. *See table 00H to construct the Insertion code.* Also applicable when reported with Insertion of neurostimulator lead (6th character M) into the peripheral nerve. *See table 01H to construct the Insertion code.* Also applicable when reported with Insertion of neurostimulator lead (6th character M) into upper vein. *See table 05H to construct the Insertion code.* Also applicable when reported with Insertion of a stimulator lead (6th character M) into the stomach. *See table 0DH to construct the Insertion code.*

0JH63EZ Insertion of Multiple Array Rechargeable Stimulator Generator into Chest Subcutaneous Tissue and Fascia, Percutaneous Approach

+ Major brain device implant when reported with an Insertion of a neurostimulator lead (6th character M) into the brain or cerebral ventricle. *See table 00H to construct the Insertion code.*

+ Neurotransmitter/Neurostimulator when reported with an Insertion of a neurostimulator lead (6th character M) into the cranial nerve, spinal canal or spinal cord. *See table 00H to construct*

the Insertion code. Also applicable when reported with Insertion of neurostimulator lead (6th character M) into the peripheral nerve. See table 01H to construct the Insertion code. Also applicable when reported with Insertion of neurostimulator lead (6th character M) into upper vein. See table 05H to construct the Insertion code. Also applicable when reported with Insertion of a stimulator lead (6th character M) into the stomach. See table 0DH to construct the Insertion code.

0JH63FZ Insertion of Subcutaneous Defibrillator Lead into Chest Subcutaneous Tissue and Fascia, Percutaneous Approach

● **0JH63HZ** Insertion of Contraceptive Device into Chest Subcutaneous Tissue and Fascia, Percutaneous Approach

0JH63MZ Insertion of Stimulator Generator into Chest Subcutaneous Tissue and Fascia, Percutaneous Approach

0JH63NZ Insertion of Tissue Expander into Chest Subcutaneous Tissue and Fascia, Percutaneous Approach

● **0JH63PZ** Insertion of Cardiac Rhythm Related Device into Chest Subcutaneous Tissue and Fascia, Percutaneous Approach

HAC With a secondary diagnosis code of K68.11, T81.40XA, T81.41XA, T81.42XA, T81.43XA, T81.44XA, T82.6XXA, T82.7XXA

+ Insertion of pacemaker is part of the pacemaker cluster for MS-DRG assignment when reported with pacemaker lead code. *See table 02H to construct pacemaker lead Insertion code.*

0JH63VZ Insertion of Infusion Pump into Chest Subcutaneous Tissue and Fascia, Percutaneous Approach

AHA CC: 4Q, 2015, 14-15

● **0JH63WZ** Insertion of Totally Implantable Vascular Access Device into Chest Subcutaneous Tissue and Fascia, Percutaneous Approach

● **0JH63XZ** Insertion of Tunneled Vascular Access Device into Chest Subcutaneous Tissue and Fascia, Percutaneous Approach

AHA CC: 4Q, 2015, 30-32; 2Q, 2016, 15-16; 2Q, 2017, 24-26

HAC With secondary diagnosis code J95.811

0JH63YZ Insertion of Other Device into Chest Subcutaneous Tissue and Fascia, Percutaneous Approach

0JH70BZ Insertion of Single Array Stimulator Generator into Back Subcutaneous Tissue and Fascia, Open Approach

+ Neurotransmitter/Neurostimulator when reported with an Insertion of a neurostimulator lead (6th character M) into the cranial nerve, spinal canal or spinal cord. *See table 00H to construct the Insertion code. Also applicable when reported with Insertion of neurostimulator lead (6th character M) into the peripheral nerve. See table 01H to construct the Insertion code. Also applicable when reported with Insertion of neurostimulator lead (6th character M) into upper vein. See table 05H to construct the Insertion code. Also applicable when reported with Insertion of a stimulator lead (6th character M) into the stomach. See table 0DH to construct the Insertion code.*

0JH70CZ Insertion of Single Array Rechargeable Stimulator Generator into Back Subcutaneous Tissue and Fascia, Open Approach

+ Neurotransmitter/Neurostimulator when reported with an Insertion of a neurostimulator lead (6th character M) into the cranial nerve, spinal canal or spinal cord. *See table 00H to construct the Insertion code. Also applicable when reported with Insertion of neurostimulator lead (6th character M) into the peripheral nerve. See table 01H to construct the Insertion code. Also applicable when reported with Insertion of neurostimulator lead (6th character M) into upper vein. See table 05H to construct the Insertion code. Also applicable when reported with Insertion of a stimulator lead (6th character M) into the stomach. See table 0DH to construct the Insertion code.*

0JH70DZ Insertion of Multiple Array Stimulator Generator into Back Subcutaneous Tissue and Fascia, Open Approach

+ Major brain device implant when reported with an Insertion of a neurostimulator lead (6th character M) into the brain or cerebral ventricle. *See table 00H to construct the Insertion code.*

+ Neurotransmitter/Neurostimulator when reported with an Insertion of a neurostimulator lead (6th character M) into the cranial nerve, spinal canal or spinal cord. *See table 00H to construct the Insertion code. Also applicable when reported with Insertion of neurostimulator lead (6th character M) into the peripheral nerve. See table 01H to construct the Insertion code. Also applicable when reported with Insertion of neurostimulator lead (6th character M) into upper vein. See table 05H to construct the Insertion code. Also applicable when reported with Insertion of a stimulator lead (6th character M) into the stomach. See table 0DH to construct the Insertion code.*

0JH70EZ Insertion of Multiple Array Rechargeable Stimulator Generator into Back Subcutaneous Tissue and Fascia, Open Approach

+ Major brain device implant when reported with an Insertion of a neurostimulator lead (6th character M) into the brain or cerebral ventricle. *See table 00H to construct the Insertion code.*

+ Neurotransmitter/Neurostimulator when reported with an Insertion of a neurostimulator lead (6th character M) into the cranial nerve, spinal canal or spinal cord. *See table 00H to construct the Insertion code. Also applicable when reported with Insertion of neurostimulator lead (6th character M) into the peripheral nerve. See table 01H to construct the Insertion code. Also applicable when reported with Insertion of neurostimulator lead (6th character M) into upper vein. See table 05H to construct the Insertion code. Also applicable when reported with Insertion of a stimulator lead (6th character M) into the stomach. See table 0DH to construct the Insertion code.*

▲ **0JH70MZ** Insertion of Stimulator Generator into Back Subcutaneous Tissue and Fascia, Open Approach

0JH70NZ Insertion of Tissue Expander into Back Subcutaneous Tissue and Fascia, Open Approach

0JH70VZ Insertion of Infusion Pump into Back Subcutaneous Tissue and Fascia, Open Approach

0JH70YZ Insertion of Other Device into Back Subcutaneous Tissue and Fascia, Open Approach

0JH73BZ Insertion of Single Array Stimulator Generator into Back Subcutaneous Tissue and Fascia, Percutaneous Approach

+ Neurotransmitter/Neurostimulator when reported with an Insertion of a neurostimulator lead (6th character M) into the cranial nerve, spinal canal or spinal cord. *See table 00H to construct the Insertion code. Also applicable when reported with Insertion of neurostimulator lead (6th character M) into the peripheral nerve. See table 01H to construct the Insertion code. Also applicable when reported with Insertion of neurostimulator lead (6th character M) into upper vein. See table 05H to construct the Insertion code. Also applicable when reported with Insertion of a stimulator lead (6th character M) into the stomach. See table 0DH to construct the Insertion code.*

0JH73CZ Insertion of Single Array Rechargeable Stimulator Generator into Back Subcutaneous Tissue and Fascia, Percutaneous Approach

+ Neurotransmitter/Neurostimulator when reported with an Insertion of a neurostimulator lead (6th character M) into the cranial nerve, spinal canal or spinal cord. *See table 00H to construct the Insertion code. Also applicable when reported with Insertion of neurostimulator lead (6th character M) into the peripheral nerve. See table 01H to construct the Insertion code. Also applicable when reported with Insertion of neurostimulator lead (6th character M) into upper vein. See table 05H to construct the Insertion code. Also applicable when reported with Insertion of a stimulator lead (6th character M) into the stomach. See table 0DH to construct the Insertion code.*

0JH73DZ Insertion of Multiple Array Stimulator Generator into Back Subcutaneous Tissue and Fascia, Percutaneous Approach

+ Major brain device implant when reported with an Insertion of a neurostimulator lead (6th character M) into the brain or cerebral ventricle. *See table 00H to construct the Insertion code.*

+ Neurotransmitter/Neurostimulator when reported with an Insertion of a neurostimulator lead (6th character M) into the cranial nerve, spinal canal or spinal cord. *See table 00H to construct the Insertion code. Also applicable when reported with Insertion of neurostimulator lead (6th character M) into the peripheral nerve. See table 01H to construct the Insertion code. Also applicable when reported with Insertion*

of neurostimulator lead (6th character M) into upper vein. *See table 05H to construct the Insertion code.* Also applicable when reported with Insertion of a stimulator lead (6th character M) into the stomach. *See table 0DH to construct the Insertion code.*

0JH73EZ Insertion of Multiple Array Rechargeable Stimulator Generator into Back Subcutaneous Tissue and Fascia, Percutaneous Approach

+ Major brain device implant when reported with an Insertion of a neurostimulator lead (6th character M) into the brain or cerebral ventricle. *See table 00H to construct the Insertion code.*

+ Neurotransmitter/Neurostimulator when reported with an Insertion of a neurostimulator lead (6th character M) into the cranial nerve, spinal canal or spinal cord. *See table 00H to construct the Insertion code.* Also applicable when reported with Insertion of neurostimulator lead (6th character M) into the peripheral nerve. *See table 01H to construct the Insertion code.* Also applicable when reported with Insertion of neurostimulator lead (6th character M) into upper vein. *See table 05H to construct the Insertion code.* Also applicable when reported with Insertion of a stimulator lead (6th character M) into the stomach. *See table 0DH to construct the Insertion code.*

0JH73MZ Insertion of Stimulator Generator into Back Subcutaneous Tissue and Fascia, Percutaneous Approach

0JH73NZ Insertion of Tissue Expander into Back Subcutaneous Tissue and Fascia, Percutaneous Approach

0JH73VZ Insertion of Infusion Pump into Back Subcutaneous Tissue and Fascia, Percutaneous Approach

0JH73YZ Insertion of Other Device into Back Subcutaneous Tissue and Fascia, Percutaneous Approach

0JH800Z Insertion of Hemodynamic Monitoring Device into Abdomen Subcutaneous Tissue and Fascia, Open Approach

● **0JH802Z** Insertion of Monitoring Device into Abdomen Subcutaneous Tissue and Fascia, Open Approach

● **0JH804Z** Insertion of Pacemaker, Single Chamber into Abdomen Subcutaneous Tissue and Fascia, Open Approach

HAC With a secondary diagnosis code of K68.11, T81.40XA, T81.41XA, T81.42XA, T81.43XA, T81.44XA, T82.6XXA, T82.7XXA

+ Insertion of pacemaker is part of the pacemaker cluster for MS-DRG assignment when reported with pacemaker lead code. *See table 02H to construct pacemaker lead Insertion code.*

● **0JH805Z** Insertion of Pacemaker, Single Chamber Rate Responsive into Abdomen Subcutaneous Tissue and Fascia, Open Approach

HAC With a secondary diagnosis code of K68.11, T81.40XA, T81.41XA, T81.42XA, T81.43XA, T81.44XA, T82.6XXA, T82.7XXA

+ Insertion of pacemaker is part of the pacemaker cluster for MS-DRG

assignment when reported with pacemaker lead code. *See table 02H to construct pacemaker lead Insertion code.*

● **0JH806Z** Insertion of Pacemaker, Dual Chamber into Abdomen Subcutaneous Tissue and Fascia, Open Approach

HAC With a secondary diagnosis code of K68.11, T81.40XA, T81.41XA, T81.42XA, T81.43XA, T81.44XA, T82.6XXA, T82.7XXA

+ Insertion of pacemaker is part of the pacemaker cluster for MS-DRG assignment when reported with pacemaker lead code. *See table 02H to construct pacemaker lead Insertion code.*

● **0JH807Z** Insertion of Cardiac Resynchronization Pacemaker Pulse Generator into Abdomen Subcutaneous Tissue and Fascia, Open Approach

HAC With a secondary diagnosis code of K68.11, T81.40XA, T81.41XA, T81.42XA, T81.43XA, T81.44XA, T82.6XXA, T82.7XXA

+ Insertion of pacemaker is part of the pacemaker cluster for MS-DRG assignment when reported with pacemaker lead code. *See table 02H to construct pacemaker lead Insertion code.*

0JH808Z Insertion of Defibrillator Generator into Abdomen Subcutaneous Tissue and Fascia, Open Approach

HAC With a secondary diagnosis code of K68.11, T81.40XA, T81.41XA, T81.42XA, T81.43XA, T81.44XA, T82.6XXA, T82.7XXA

+ Cardioverter-Defibrillator lead(s)/generator when reported with Insertion of a defibrillator cardiac lead (6th character K) into the coronary vein, atrium, or ventricle. Also applicable with Insertion of pacemaker cardiac lead, defibrillator cardiac lead or cardiac lead (6th characters J, K, M) into the pericardium. *See table 02H to construct the Insertion code.*

0JH809Z Insertion of Cardiac Resynchronization Defibrillator Pulse Generator into Abdomen Subcutaneous Tissue and Fascia, Open Approach

HAC With a secondary diagnosis code of K68.11, T81.40XA, T81.41XA, T81.42XA, T81.43XA, T81.44XA, T82.6XXA, T82.7XXA

+ Cardioverter-Defibrillator lead(s)/generator when reported with Insertion of a defibrillator cardiac lead (6th character K) into the atrium, or ventricle. Also applicable with Insertion of pacemaker cardiac lead, defibrillator cardiac lead or cardiac lead (6th characters J, K, M) into the coronary vein or pericardium. *See table 02H to construct the Insertion code.*

0JH80AZ Insertion of Contractility Modulation Device into Abdomen Subcutaneous Tissue and Fascia, Open Approach

+ Cardioverter-Defibrillator lead(s)/generator when reported with Insertion of a cardiac lead (6th character M) into the left ventricle. *See table 02H to construct the Insertion code.*

0JH80BZ Insertion of Single Array Stimulator Generator into Abdomen Subcutaneous Tissue and Fascia, Open Approach

+ Neurotransmitter/Neurostimulator when reported with an Insertion of a neurostimulator lead (6th character M) into the cranial nerve, spinal canal or spinal cord. *See table 00H to construct the Insertion code.* Also applicable when reported with Insertion of neurostimulator lead (6th character M) into the peripheral nerve. *See table 01H to construct the Insertion code.* Also applicable when reported with Insertion of neurostimulator lead (6th character M) into upper vein. *See table 05H to construct the Insertion code.* Also applicable when reported with Insertion of a stimulator lead (6th character M) into the stomach. *See table 0DH to construct the Insertion code.*

0JH80CZ Insertion of Single Array Rechargeable Stimulator Generator into Abdomen Subcutaneous Tissue and Fascia, Open Approach

+ Neurotransmitter/Neurostimulator when reported with an Insertion of a neurostimulator lead (6th character M) into the cranial nerve, spinal canal or spinal cord. *See table 00H to construct the Insertion code.* Also applicable when reported with Insertion of neurostimulator lead (6th character M) into the peripheral nerve. *See table 01H to construct the Insertion code.* Also applicable when reported with Insertion of neurostimulator lead (6th character M) into upper vein. *See table 05H to construct the Insertion code.* Also applicable when reported with Insertion of a stimulator lead (6th character M) into the stomach. *See table 0DH to construct the Insertion code.*

0JH80DZ Insertion of Multiple Array Stimulator Generator into Abdomen Subcutaneous Tissue and Fascia, Open Approach

+ Major brain device implant when reported with an Insertion of a neurostimulator lead (6th character M) into the brain or cerebral ventricle. *See table 00H to construct the Insertion code.*

+ Neurotransmitter/Neurostimulator when reported with an Insertion of a neurostimulator lead (6th character M) into the cranial nerve, spinal canal or spinal cord. *See table 00H to construct the Insertion code.* Also applicable when reported with Insertion of neurostimulator lead (6th character M) into the peripheral nerve. *See table 01H to construct the Insertion code.* Also applicable when reported with Insertion of neurostimulator lead (6th character M) into upper vein. *See table 05H to construct the Insertion code.* Also applicable when reported with Insertion of a stimulator lead (6th character M) into the stomach. *See table 0DH to construct the Insertion code.*

0JH80EZ Insertion of Multiple Array Rechargeable Stimulator Generator into Abdomen Subcutaneous Tissue and Fascia, Open Approach

+ Major brain device implant when reported with an Insertion of a neurostimulator lead (6th character M)

into the brain or cerebral ventricle. *See table 00H to construct the Insertion code.*

+ Neurotransmitter/Neurostimulator when reported with an Insertion of a neurostimulator lead (6th character M) into the cranial nerve, spinal canal or spinal cord. *See table 00H to construct the Insertion code. Also applicable when reported with Insertion of neurostimulator lead (6th character M) into the peripheral nerve. See table 01H to construct the Insertion code. Also applicable when reported with Insertion of neurostimulator lead (6th character M) into upper vein. See table 05H to construct the Insertion code. Also applicable when reported with Insertion of a stimulator lead (6th character M) into the stomach. See table 0DH to construct the Insertion code.*

● **0JH80HZ** Insertion of Contraceptive Device into Abdomen Subcutaneous Tissue and Fascia, Open Approach

▲ **0JH80MZ** Insertion of Stimulator Generator into Abdomen Subcutaneous Tissue and Fascia, Open Approach

0JH80NZ Insertion of Tissue Expander into Abdomen Subcutaneous Tissue and Fascia, Open Approach

● **0JH80PZ** Insertion of Cardiac Rhythm Related Device into Abdomen Subcutaneous Tissue and Fascia, Open Approach

HAC With a secondary diagnosis code of K68.11, T81.40XA, T81.41XA, T81.42XA, T81.43XA, T81.44XA, T82.6XXA, T82.7XXA

+ Insertion of pacemaker is part of the pacemaker cluster for MS-DRG assignment when reported with pacemaker lead code. *See table 02H to construct pacemaker lead Insertion code.*

0JH80VZ Insertion of Infusion Pump into Abdomen Subcutaneous Tissue and Fascia, Open Approach
AHA CC: 3Q, 2014, 19-20

0JH80WZ Insertion of Totally Implantable Vascular Access Device into Abdomen Subcutaneous Tissue and Fascia, Open Approach
AHA CC: 2Q, 2016, 14

● **0JH80XZ** Insertion of Tunneled Vascular Access Device into Abdomen Subcutaneous Tissue and Fascia, Open Approach

0JH80YZ Insertion of Other Device into Abdomen Subcutaneous Tissue and Fascia, Open Approach
AHA CC: 4Q, 2020, 55

0JH830Z Insertion of Hemodynamic Monitoring Device into Abdomen Subcutaneous Tissue and Fascia, Percutaneous Approach

● **0JH832Z** Insertion of Monitoring Device into Abdomen Subcutaneous Tissue and Fascia, Percutaneous Approach

● **0JH834Z** Insertion of Pacemaker, Single Chamber into Abdomen Subcutaneous Tissue and Fascia, Percutaneous Approach

HAC With a secondary diagnosis code of K68.11, T81.40XA, T81.41XA, T81.42XA, T81.43XA, T81.44XA, T82.6XXA, T82.7XXA

+ Insertion of pacemaker is part of the pacemaker cluster for MS-DRG

assignment when reported with pacemaker lead code. *See table 02H to construct pacemaker lead Insertion code.*

● **0JH835Z** Insertion of Pacemaker, Single Chamber Rate Responsive into Abdomen Subcutaneous Tissue and Fascia, Percutaneous Approach

HAC With a secondary diagnosis code of K68.11, T81.40XA, T81.41XA, T81.42XA, T81.43XA, T81.44XA, T82.6XXA, T82.7XXA

+ Insertion of pacemaker is part of the pacemaker cluster for MS-DRG assignment when reported with pacemaker lead code. *See table 02H to construct pacemaker lead Insertion code.*

● **0JH836Z** Insertion of Pacemaker, Dual Chamber into Abdomen Subcutaneous Tissue and Fascia, Percutaneous Approach

HAC With a secondary diagnosis code of K68.11, T81.40XA, T81.41XA, T81.42XA, T81.43XA, T81.44XA, T82.6XXA, T82.7XXA

+ Insertion of pacemaker is part of the pacemaker cluster for MS-DRG assignment when reported with pacemaker lead code. *See table 02H to construct pacemaker lead Insertion code.*

● **0JH837Z** Insertion of Cardiac Resynchronization Pacemaker Pulse Generator into Abdomen Subcutaneous Tissue and Fascia, Percutaneous Approach

HAC With a secondary diagnosis code of K68.11, T81.40XA, T81.41XA, T81.42XA, T81.43XA, T81.44XA, T82.6XXA, T82.7XXA

+ Insertion of pacemaker is part of the pacemaker cluster for MS-DRG assignment when reported with pacemaker lead code. *See table 02H to construct pacemaker lead Insertion code.*

0JH838Z Insertion of Defibrillator Generator into Abdomen Subcutaneous Tissue and Fascia, Percutaneous Approach

HAC With a secondary diagnosis code of K68.11, T81.40XA, T81.41XA, T81.42XA, T81.43XA, T81.44XA, T82.6XXA, T82.7XXA

+ Cardioverter-Defibrillator lead(s)/ generator when reported with Insertion of a defibrillator cardiac lead (6th character K) into the coronary vein, atrium, or ventricle. Also applicable with Insertion of pacemaker cardiac lead, defibrillator cardiac lead or cardiac lead (6th characters J, K, M) into the pericardium. *See table 02H to construct the Insertion code.*

0JH839Z Insertion of Cardiac Resynchronization Defibrillator Pulse Generator into Abdomen Subcutaneous Tissue and Fascia, Percutaneous Approach

HAC With a secondary diagnosis code of K68.11, T81.40XA, T81.41XA, T81.42XA, T81.43XA, T81.44XA, T82.6XXA, T82.7XXA

+ Cardioverter-Defibrillator lead(s)/ generator when reported with Insertion of a defibrillator cardiac lead (6th character K) into the atrium, or ventricle. Also applicable with Insertion of pacemaker cardiac lead, defibrillator

cardiac lead or cardiac lead (6th characters J, K, M) into the coronary vein or pericardium. *See table 02H to construct the Insertion code.*

0JH83AZ Insertion of Contractility Modulation Device into Abdomen Subcutaneous Tissue and Fascia, Percutaneous Approach

+ Cardioverter-Defibrillator lead(s)/ generator when reported with Insertion of a cardiac lead (6th character M) into the left ventricle. *See table 02H to construct the Insertion code.*

0JH83BZ Insertion of Single Array Stimulator Generator into Abdomen Subcutaneous Tissue and Fascia, Percutaneous Approach

+ Neurotransmitter/Neurostimulator when reported with an Insertion of a neurostimulator lead (6th character M) into the cranial nerve, spinal canal or spinal cord. *See table 00H to construct the Insertion code. Also applicable when reported with Insertion of neurostimulator lead (6th character M) into the peripheral nerve. See table 01H to construct the Insertion code. Also applicable when reported with Insertion of neurostimulator lead (6th character M) into upper vein. See table 05H to construct the Insertion code. Also applicable when reported with Insertion of a stimulator lead (6th character M) into the stomach. See table 0DH to construct the Insertion code.*

0JH83CZ Insertion of Single Array Rechargeable Stimulator Generator into Abdomen Subcutaneous Tissue and Fascia, Percutaneous Approach

+ Neurotransmitter/Neurostimulator when reported with an Insertion of a neurostimulator lead (6th character M) into the cranial nerve, spinal canal or spinal cord. *See table 00H to construct the Insertion code. Also applicable when reported with Insertion of neurostimulator lead (6th character M) into the peripheral nerve. See table 01H to construct the Insertion code. Also applicable when reported with Insertion of neurostimulator lead (6th character M) into upper vein. See table 05H to construct the Insertion code. Also applicable when reported with Insertion of a stimulator lead (6th character M) into the stomach. See table 0DH to construct the Insertion code.*

0JH83DZ Insertion of Multiple Array Stimulator Generator into Abdomen Subcutaneous Tissue and Fascia, Percutaneous Approach

+ Major brain device implant when reported with an Insertion of a neurostimulator lead (6th character M) into the brain or cerebral ventricle. *See table 00H to construct the Insertion code.*

+ Neurotransmitter/Neurostimulator when reported with an Insertion of a neurostimulator lead (6th character M) into the cranial nerve, spinal canal or spinal cord. *See table 00H to construct the Insertion code. Also applicable when reported with Insertion of neurostimulator lead (6th character M) into the peripheral nerve. See table 01H to construct the Insertion code. Also*

applicable when reported with Insertion of neurostimulator lead (6th character M) into upper vein. *See table 05H to construct the Insertion code.* Also applicable when reported with Insertion of a stimulator lead (6th character M) into the stomach. *See table 0DH to construct the Insertion code.*

0JH83EZ Insertion of Multiple Array Rechargeable Stimulator Generator into Abdomen Subcutaneous Tissue and Fascia, Percutaneous Approach

＋ Major brain device implant when reported with an Insertion of a neurostimulator lead (6th character M) into the brain or cerebral ventricle. *See table 00H to construct the Insertion code.*

＋ Neurotransmitter/Neurostimulator when reported with an Insertion of a neurostimulator lead (6th character M) into the cranial nerve, spinal canal or spinal cord. *See table 00H to construct the Insertion code.* Also applicable when reported with Insertion of neurostimulator lead (6th character M) into the peripheral nerve. *See table 01H to construct the Insertion code.* Also applicable when reported with Insertion of neurostimulator lead (6th character M) into upper vein. *See table 05H to construct the Insertion code.* Also applicable when reported with Insertion of a stimulator lead (6th character M) into the stomach. *See table 0DH to construct the Insertion code.*

● **0JH83HZ** Insertion of Contraceptive Device into Abdomen Subcutaneous Tissue and Fascia, Percutaneous Approach

▲ **0JH83MZ** Insertion of Stimulator Generator into Abdomen Subcutaneous Tissue and Fascia, Percutaneous Approach

0JH83NZ Insertion of Tissue Expander into Abdomen Subcutaneous Tissue and Fascia, Percutaneous Approach

● **0JH83PZ** Insertion of Cardiac Rhythm Related Device into Abdomen Subcutaneous Tissue and Fascia, Percutaneous Approach

HAC With a secondary diagnosis code of K68.11, T81.40XA, T81.41XA, T81.42XA, T81.43XA, T81.44XA, T82.6XXA, T82.7XXA

＋ Insertion of pacemaker is part of the pacemaker cluster for MS-DRG assignment when reported with pacemaker lead code. *See table 02H to construct pacemaker lead Insertion code.*

0JH83VZ Insertion of Infusion Pump into Abdomen Subcutaneous Tissue and Fascia, Percutaneous Approach

● **0JH83WZ** Insertion of Totally Implantable Vascular Access Device into Abdomen Subcutaneous Tissue and Fascia, Percutaneous Approach

● **0JH83XZ** Insertion of Tunneled Vascular Access Device into Abdomen Subcutaneous Tissue and Fascia, Percutaneous Approach

0JH83YZ Insertion of Other Device into Abdomen Subcutaneous Tissue and Fascia, Percutaneous Approach

0JH90NZ Insertion of Tissue Expander into Buttock Subcutaneous Tissue and Fascia, Open Approach

0JH93NZ Insertion of Tissue Expander into Buttock Subcutaneous Tissue and Fascia, Percutaneous Approach

0JHB0NZ Insertion of Tissue Expander into Perineum Subcutaneous Tissue and Fascia, Open Approach

0JHB3NZ Insertion of Tissue Expander into Perineum Subcutaneous Tissue and Fascia, Percutaneous Approach

0JHC0NZ Insertion of Tissue Expander into Pelvic Region Subcutaneous Tissue and Fascia, Open Approach

0JHC3NZ Insertion of Tissue Expander into Pelvic Region Subcutaneous Tissue and Fascia, Percutaneous Approach

0JHD0HZ Insertion of Contraceptive Device into Right Upper Arm Subcutaneous Tissue and Fascia, Open Approach

0JHD0NZ Insertion of Tissue Expander into Right Upper Arm Subcutaneous Tissue and Fascia, Open Approach

0JHD0VZ Insertion of Infusion Pump into Right Upper Arm Subcutaneous Tissue and Fascia, Open Approach

0JHD0WZ Insertion of Totally Implantable Vascular Access Device into Right Upper Arm Subcutaneous Tissue and Fascia, Open Approach

● **0JHD0XZ** Insertion of Tunneled Vascular Access Device into Right Upper Arm Subcutaneous Tissue and Fascia, Open Approach

0JHD3HZ Insertion of Contraceptive Device into Right Upper Arm Subcutaneous Tissue and Fascia, Percutaneous Approach

0JHD3NZ Insertion of Tissue Expander into Right Upper Arm Subcutaneous Tissue and Fascia, Percutaneous Approach

0JHD3VZ Insertion of Infusion Pump into Right Upper Arm Subcutaneous Tissue and Fascia, Percutaneous Approach

● **0JHD3WZ** Insertion of Totally Implantable Vascular Access Device into Right Upper Arm Subcutaneous Tissue and Fascia, Percutaneous Approach

● **0JHD3XZ** Insertion of Tunneled Vascular Access Device into Right Upper Arm Subcutaneous Tissue and Fascia, Percutaneous Approach

0JHF0HZ Insertion of Contraceptive Device into Left Upper Arm Subcutaneous Tissue and Fascia, Open Approach

0JHF0NZ Insertion of Tissue Expander into Left Upper Arm Subcutaneous Tissue and Fascia, Open Approach

0JHF0VZ Insertion of Infusion Pump into Left Upper Arm Subcutaneous Tissue and Fascia, Open Approach

0JHF0WZ Insertion of Totally Implantable Vascular Access Device into Left Upper Arm Subcutaneous Tissue and Fascia, Open Approach

● **0JHF0XZ** Insertion of Tunneled Vascular Access Device into Left Upper Arm Subcutaneous Tissue and Fascia, Open Approach

0JHF3HZ Insertion of Contraceptive Device into Left Upper Arm Subcutaneous Tissue and Fascia, Percutaneous Approach

0JHF3NZ Insertion of Tissue Expander into Left Upper Arm Subcutaneous Tissue and Fascia, Percutaneous Approach

0JHF3VZ Insertion of Infusion Pump into Left Upper Arm Subcutaneous Tissue and Fascia, Percutaneous Approach

● **0JHF3WZ** Insertion of Totally Implantable Vascular Access Device into Left Upper Arm Subcutaneous Tissue and Fascia, Percutaneous Approach

● **0JHF3XZ** Insertion of Tunneled Vascular Access Device into Left Upper Arm Subcutaneous Tissue and Fascia, Percutaneous Approach

0JHG0HZ Insertion of Contraceptive Device into Right Lower Arm Subcutaneous Tissue and Fascia, Open Approach

0JHG0NZ Insertion of Tissue Expander into Right Lower Arm Subcutaneous Tissue and Fascia, Open Approach

0JHG0VZ Insertion of Infusion Pump into Right Lower Arm Subcutaneous Tissue and Fascia, Open Approach

0JHG0WZ Insertion of Totally Implantable Vascular Access Device into Right Lower Arm Subcutaneous Tissue and Fascia, Open Approach

● **0JHG0XZ** Insertion of Tunneled Vascular Access Device into Right Lower Arm Subcutaneous Tissue and Fascia, Open Approach

0JHG3HZ Insertion of Contraceptive Device into Right Lower Arm Subcutaneous Tissue and Fascia, Percutaneous Approach

0JHG3NZ Insertion of Tissue Expander into Right Lower Arm Subcutaneous Tissue and Fascia, Percutaneous Approach

0JHG3VZ Insertion of Infusion Pump into Right Lower Arm Subcutaneous Tissue and Fascia, Percutaneous Approach

● **0JHG3WZ** Insertion of Totally Implantable Vascular Access Device into Right Lower Arm Subcutaneous Tissue and Fascia, Percutaneous Approach

● **0JHG3XZ** Insertion of Tunneled Vascular Access Device into Right Lower Arm Subcutaneous Tissue and Fascia, Percutaneous Approach

0JHH0HZ Insertion of Contraceptive Device into Left Lower Arm Subcutaneous Tissue and Fascia, Open Approach

0JHH0NZ Insertion of Tissue Expander into Left Lower Arm Subcutaneous Tissue and Fascia, Open Approach

0JHH0VZ Insertion of Infusion Pump into Left Lower Arm Subcutaneous Tissue and Fascia, Open Approach

0JHH0WZ Insertion of Totally Implantable Vascular Access Device into Left Lower Arm Subcutaneous Tissue and Fascia, Open Approach

● **0JHH0XZ** Insertion of Tunneled Vascular Access Device into Left Lower Arm Subcutaneous Tissue and Fascia, Open Approach

0JHH3HZ Insertion of Contraceptive Device into Left Lower Arm Subcutaneous Tissue and Fascia, Percutaneous Approach

0JHH3NZ Insertion of Tissue Expander into Left Lower Arm Subcutaneous Tissue and Fascia, Percutaneous Approach

0JHH3VZ Insertion of Infusion Pump into Left Lower Arm Subcutaneous Tissue and Fascia, Percutaneous Approach

● **0JHH3WZ** Insertion of Totally Implantable Vascular Access Device into Left Lower Arm Subcutaneous Tissue and Fascia, Percutaneous Approach

● **0JHH3XZ** Insertion of Tunneled Vascular Access Device into Left Lower Arm Subcutaneous Tissue and Fascia, Percutaneous Approach

♀ Female-only ♂ Male-only ▲ Limited Coverage ● Non-OR HAC HAC-associated procedure ▲ Non-covered procedures ＋ Cluster

0JHJ0NZ Insertion of Tissue Expander into Right Hand Subcutaneous Tissue and Fascia, Open Approach

0JHJ3NZ Insertion of Tissue Expander into Right Hand Subcutaneous Tissue and Fascia, Percutaneous Approach

0JHK0NZ Insertion of Tissue Expander into Left Hand Subcutaneous Tissue and Fascia, Open Approach

0JHK3NZ Insertion of Tissue Expander into Left Hand Subcutaneous Tissue and Fascia, Percutaneous Approach

0JHL0HZ Insertion of Contraceptive Device into Right Upper Leg Subcutaneous Tissue and Fascia, Open Approach

0JHL0NZ Insertion of Tissue Expander into Right Upper Leg Subcutaneous Tissue and Fascia, Open Approach

0JHL0VZ Insertion of Infusion Pump into Right Upper Leg Subcutaneous Tissue and Fascia, Open Approach

0JHL0WZ Insertion of Totally Implantable Vascular Access Device into Right Upper Leg Subcutaneous Tissue and Fascia, Open Approach

● 0JHL0XZ Insertion of Tunneled Vascular Access Device into Right Upper Leg Subcutaneous Tissue and Fascia, Open Approach

0JHL3HZ Insertion of Contraceptive Device into Right Upper Leg Subcutaneous Tissue and Fascia, Percutaneous Approach

0JHL3NZ Insertion of Tissue Expander into Right Upper Leg Subcutaneous Tissue and Fascia, Percutaneous Approach

0JHL3VZ Insertion of Infusion Pump into Right Upper Leg Subcutaneous Tissue and Fascia, Percutaneous Approach

● 0JHL3WZ Insertion of Totally Implantable Vascular Access Device into Right Upper Leg Subcutaneous Tissue and Fascia, Percutaneous Approach

● 0JHL3XZ Insertion of Tunneled Vascular Access Device into Right Upper Leg Subcutaneous Tissue and Fascia, Percutaneous Approach

0JHM0HZ Insertion of Contraceptive Device into Left Upper Leg Subcutaneous Tissue and Fascia, Open Approach

0JHM0NZ Insertion of Tissue Expander into Left Upper Leg Subcutaneous Tissue and Fascia, Open Approach

0JHM0VZ Insertion of Infusion Pump into Left Upper Leg Subcutaneous Tissue and Fascia, Open Approach

0JHM0WZ Insertion of Totally Implantable Vascular Access Device into Left Upper Leg Subcutaneous Tissue and Fascia, Open Approach

● 0JHM0XZ Insertion of Tunneled Vascular Access Device into Left Upper Leg Subcutaneous Tissue and Fascia, Open Approach

0JHM3HZ Insertion of Contraceptive Device into Left Upper Leg Subcutaneous Tissue and Fascia, Percutaneous Approach

0JHM3NZ Insertion of Tissue Expander into Left Upper Leg Subcutaneous Tissue and Fascia, Percutaneous Approach

0JHM3VZ Insertion of Infusion Pump into Left Upper Leg Subcutaneous Tissue and Fascia, Percutaneous Approach

● 0JHM3WZ Insertion of Totally Implantable Vascular Access Device into Left Upper Leg Subcutaneous Tissue and Fascia, Percutaneous Approach

● 0JHM3XZ Insertion of Tunneled Vascular Access Device into Left Upper Leg Subcutaneous Tissue and Fascia, Percutaneous Approach

0JHN0HZ Insertion of Contraceptive Device into Right Lower Leg Subcutaneous Tissue and Fascia, Open Approach

0JHN0NZ Insertion of Tissue Expander into Right Lower Leg Subcutaneous Tissue and Fascia, Open Approach

0JHN0VZ Insertion of Infusion Pump into Right Lower Leg Subcutaneous Tissue and Fascia, Open Approach

0JHN0WZ Insertion of Totally Implantable Vascular Access Device into Right Lower Leg Subcutaneous Tissue and Fascia, Open Approach

● 0JHN0XZ Insertion of Tunneled Vascular Access Device into Right Lower Leg Subcutaneous Tissue and Fascia, Open Approach

● 0JHN3HZ Insertion of Contraceptive Device into Right Lower Leg Subcutaneous Tissue and Fascia, Percutaneous Approach

0JHN3NZ Insertion of Tissue Expander into Right Lower Leg Subcutaneous Tissue and Fascia, Percutaneous Approach

0JHN3VZ Insertion of Infusion Pump into Right Lower Leg Subcutaneous Tissue and Fascia, Percutaneous Approach

● 0JHN3WZ Insertion of Totally Implantable Vascular Access Device into Right Lower Leg Subcutaneous Tissue and Fascia, Percutaneous Approach

● 0JHN3XZ Insertion of Tunneled Vascular Access Device into Right Lower Leg Subcutaneous Tissue and Fascia, Percutaneous Approach

● 0JHP0HZ Insertion of Contraceptive Device into Left Lower Leg Subcutaneous Tissue and Fascia, Open Approach

0JHP0NZ Insertion of Tissue Expander into Left Lower Leg Subcutaneous Tissue and Fascia, Open Approach

0JHP0VZ Insertion of Infusion Pump into Left Lower Leg Subcutaneous Tissue and Fascia, Open Approach

0JHP0WZ Insertion of Totally Implantable Vascular Access Device into Left Lower Leg Subcutaneous Tissue and Fascia, Open Approach

● 0JHP0XZ Insertion of Tunneled Vascular Access Device into Left Lower Leg Subcutaneous Tissue and Fascia, Open Approach

● 0JHP3HZ Insertion of Contraceptive Device into Left Lower Leg Subcutaneous Tissue and Fascia, Percutaneous Approach

0JHP3NZ Insertion of Tissue Expander into Left Lower Leg Subcutaneous Tissue and Fascia, Percutaneous Approach

0JHP3VZ Insertion of Infusion Pump into Left Lower Leg Subcutaneous Tissue and Fascia, Percutaneous Approach

● 0JHP3WZ Insertion of Totally Implantable Vascular Access Device into Left Lower Leg Subcutaneous Tissue and Fascia, Percutaneous Approach

● 0JHP3XZ Insertion of Tunneled Vascular Access Device into Left Lower Leg Subcutaneous Tissue and Fascia, Percutaneous Approach

0JHQ0NZ Insertion of Tissue Expander into Right Foot Subcutaneous Tissue and Fascia, Open Approach

0JHQ3NZ Insertion of Tissue Expander into Right Foot Subcutaneous Tissue and Fascia, Percutaneous Approach

0JHR0NZ Insertion of Tissue Expander into Left Foot Subcutaneous Tissue and Fascia, Open Approach

0JHR3NZ Insertion of Tissue Expander into Left Foot Subcutaneous Tissue and Fascia, Percutaneous Approach

0JHS01Z Insertion of Radioactive Element into Head and Neck Subcutaneous Tissue and Fascia, Open Approach

0JHS03Z Insertion of Infusion Device into Head and Neck Subcutaneous Tissue and Fascia, Open Approach

0JHS0YZ Insertion of Other Device into Head and Neck Subcutaneous Tissue and Fascia, Open Approach

0JHS31Z Insertion of Radioactive Element into Head and Neck Subcutaneous Tissue and Fascia, Percutaneous Approach

0JHS33Z Insertion of Infusion Device into Head and Neck Subcutaneous Tissue and Fascia, Percutaneous Approach
AHA CC: 2Q, 2020, 15-16

0JHS3YZ Insertion of Other Device into Head and Neck Subcutaneous Tissue and Fascia, Percutaneous Approach

0JHT01Z Insertion of Radioactive Element into Trunk Subcutaneous Tissue and Fascia, Open Approach

0JHT03Z Insertion of Infusion Device into Trunk Subcutaneous Tissue and Fascia, Open Approach
AHA CC: 2Q, 2020, 16-17

0JHT0VZ Insertion of Infusion Pump into Trunk Subcutaneous Tissue and Fascia, Open Approach

0JHT0YZ Insertion of Other Device into Trunk Subcutaneous Tissue and Fascia, Open Approach
AHA CC: 4Q, 2018, 4-43

0JHT31Z Insertion of Radioactive Element into Trunk Subcutaneous Tissue and Fascia, Percutaneous Approach

0JHT33Z Insertion of Infusion Device into Trunk Subcutaneous Tissue and Fascia, Percutaneous Approach

0JHT3VZ Insertion of Infusion Pump into Trunk Subcutaneous Tissue and Fascia, Percutaneous Approach

0JHT3YZ Insertion of Other Device into Trunk Subcutaneous Tissue and Fascia, Percutaneous Approach

0JHV01Z Insertion of Radioactive Element into Upper Extremity Subcutaneous Tissue and Fascia, Open Approach

0JHV03Z Insertion of Infusion Device into Upper Extremity Subcutaneous Tissue and Fascia, Open Approach

0JHV0YZ Insertion of Other Device into Upper Extremity Subcutaneous Tissue and Fascia, Open Approach

0JHV31Z Insertion of Radioactive Element into Upper Extremity Subcutaneous Tissue and Fascia, Percutaneous Approach

0JHV33Z Insertion of Infusion Device into Upper Extremity Subcutaneous Tissue and Fascia, Percutaneous Approach

0JHV3YZ Insertion of Other Device into Upper Extremity Subcutaneous Tissue and Fascia, Percutaneous Approach

♀ Female-only   ♂ Male-only   ▲ Limited Coverage   ● Non-OR   ᴴᴬᶜ HAC-associated procedure   ▲ Non-covered procedures   ✚ Cluster

0JHW01Z	Insertion of Radioactive Element into Lower Extremity Subcutaneous Tissue and Fascia, Open Approach	0JHW0YZ	Insertion of Other Device into Lower Extremity Subcutaneous Tissue and Fascia, Open Approach	0JHW33Z	Insertion of Infusion Device into Lower Extremity Subcutaneous Tissue and Fascia, Percutaneous Approach
0JHW03Z	Insertion of Infusion Device into Lower Extremity Subcutaneous Tissue and Fascia, Open Approach	0JHW31Z	Insertion of Radioactive Element into Lower Extremity Subcutaneous Tissue and Fascia, Percutaneous Approach	0JHW3YZ	Insertion of Other Device into Lower Extremity Subcutaneous Tissue and Fascia, Percutaneous Approach

0JJ – Subcutaneous Tissue and Fascia, Inspection

Review Coding Guideline B3.5

Review Coding Guidelines B3.11a, B3.11b and B3.11c

0JJS0ZZ	Inspection of Head and Neck Subcutaneous Tissue and Fascia, Open Approach	0JJT3ZZ	Inspection of Trunk Subcutaneous Tissue and Fascia, Percutaneous Approach	0JJVXZZ	Inspection of Upper Extremity Subcutaneous Tissue and Fascia, External Approach
0JJS3ZZ	Inspection of Head and Neck Subcutaneous Tissue and Fascia, Percutaneous Approach	0JJTXZZ	Inspection of Trunk Subcutaneous Tissue and Fascia, External Approach	0JJW0ZZ	Inspection of Lower Extremity Subcutaneous Tissue and Fascia, Open Approach
0JJSXZZ	Inspection of Head and Neck Subcutaneous Tissue and Fascia, External Approach	0JJV0ZZ	Inspection of Upper Extremity Subcutaneous Tissue and Fascia, Open Approach	0JJW3ZZ	Inspection of Lower Extremity Subcutaneous Tissue and Fascia, Percutaneous Approach
0JJT0ZZ	Inspection of Trunk Subcutaneous Tissue and Fascia, Open Approach	0JJV3ZZ	Inspection of Upper Extremity Subcutaneous Tissue and Fascia, Percutaneous Approach	0JJWXZZ	Inspection of Lower Extremity Subcutaneous Tissue and Fascia, External Approach

0JN – Subcutaneous Tissue and Fascia, Release

Review Coding Guideline B3.13

Review Coding Guideline B3.14

0JN00ZZ	Release Scalp Subcutaneous Tissue and Fascia, Open Approach	0JN8XZZ	Release Abdomen Subcutaneous Tissue and Fascia, External Approach	0JNGXZZ	Release Right Lower Arm Subcutaneous Tissue and Fascia, External Approach
0JN03ZZ	Release Scalp Subcutaneous Tissue and Fascia, Percutaneous Approach	0JN90ZZ	Release Buttock Subcutaneous Tissue and Fascia, Open Approach	0JNH0ZZ	Release Left Lower Arm Subcutaneous Tissue and Fascia, Open Approach
0JN0XZZ	Release Scalp Subcutaneous Tissue and Fascia, External Approach	0JN93ZZ	Release Buttock Subcutaneous Tissue and Fascia, Percutaneous Approach	0JNH3ZZ	Release Left Lower Arm Subcutaneous Tissue and Fascia, Percutaneous Approach
0JN10ZZ	Release Face Subcutaneous Tissue and Fascia, Open Approach	0JN9XZZ	Release Buttock Subcutaneous Tissue and Fascia, External Approach	0JNHXZZ	Release Left Lower Arm Subcutaneous Tissue and Fascia, External Approach
0JN13ZZ	Release Face Subcutaneous Tissue and Fascia, Percutaneous Approach	0JNB0ZZ	Release Perineum Subcutaneous Tissue and Fascia, Open Approach	0JNJ0ZZ	Release Right Hand Subcutaneous Tissue and Fascia, Open Approach
0JN1XZZ	Release Face Subcutaneous Tissue and Fascia, External Approach	0JNB3ZZ	Release Perineum Subcutaneous Tissue and Fascia, Percutaneous Approach	0JNJ3ZZ	Release Right Hand Subcutaneous Tissue and Fascia, Percutaneous Approach
0JN40ZZ	Release Right Neck Subcutaneous Tissue and Fascia, Open Approach	0JNBXZZ	Release Perineum Subcutaneous Tissue and Fascia, External Approach	0JNJXZZ	Release Right Hand Subcutaneous Tissue and Fascia, External Approach
0JN43ZZ	Release Right Neck Subcutaneous Tissue and Fascia, Percutaneous Approach	0JNC0ZZ	Release Pelvic Region Subcutaneous Tissue and Fascia, Open Approach	0JNK0ZZ	Release Left Hand Subcutaneous Tissue and Fascia, Open Approach
0JN4XZZ	Release Right Neck Subcutaneous Tissue and Fascia, External Approach	0JNC3ZZ	Release Pelvic Region Subcutaneous Tissue and Fascia, Percutaneous Approach	0JNK3ZZ	Release Left Hand Subcutaneous Tissue and Fascia, Percutaneous Approach
0JN50ZZ	Release Left Neck Subcutaneous Tissue and Fascia, Open Approach	0JNCXZZ	Release Pelvic Region Subcutaneous Tissue and Fascia, External Approach	0JNKXZZ	Release Left Hand Subcutaneous Tissue and Fascia, External Approach
0JN53ZZ	Release Left Neck Subcutaneous Tissue and Fascia, Percutaneous Approach	0JND0ZZ	Release Right Upper Arm Subcutaneous Tissue and Fascia, Open Approach	0JNL0ZZ	Release Right Upper Leg Subcutaneous Tissue and Fascia, Open Approach
0JN5XZZ	Release Left Neck Subcutaneous Tissue and Fascia, External Approach	0JND3ZZ	Release Right Upper Arm Subcutaneous Tissue and Fascia, Percutaneous Approach		*AHA CC: 3Q, 2017, 11-12*
0JN60ZZ	Release Chest Subcutaneous Tissue and Fascia, Open Approach	0JNDXZZ	Release Right Upper Arm Subcutaneous Tissue and Fascia, External Approach	0JNL3ZZ	Release Right Upper Leg Subcutaneous Tissue and Fascia, Percutaneous Approach
0JN63ZZ	Release Chest Subcutaneous Tissue and Fascia, Percutaneous Approach	0JNF0ZZ	Release Left Upper Arm Subcutaneous Tissue and Fascia, Open Approach	0JNLXZZ	Release Right Upper Leg Subcutaneous Tissue and Fascia, External Approach
0JN6XZZ	Release Chest Subcutaneous Tissue and Fascia, External Approach	0JNF3ZZ	Release Left Upper Arm Subcutaneous Tissue and Fascia, Percutaneous Approach	0JNM0ZZ	Release Left Upper Leg Subcutaneous Tissue and Fascia, Open Approach
0JN70ZZ	Release Back Subcutaneous Tissue and Fascia, Open Approach	0JNFXZZ	Release Left Upper Arm Subcutaneous Tissue and Fascia, External Approach		*AHA CC: 3Q, 2017, 11-12*
0JN73ZZ	Release Back Subcutaneous Tissue and Fascia, Percutaneous Approach	0JNG0ZZ	Release Right Lower Arm Subcutaneous Tissue and Fascia, Open Approach	0JNM3ZZ	Release Left Upper Leg Subcutaneous Tissue and Fascia, Percutaneous Approach
0JN7XZZ	Release Back Subcutaneous Tissue and Fascia, External Approach	0JNG3ZZ	Release Right Lower Arm Subcutaneous Tissue and Fascia, Percutaneous Approach	0JNMXZZ	Release Left Upper Leg Subcutaneous Tissue and Fascia, External Approach
0JN80ZZ	Release Abdomen Subcutaneous Tissue and Fascia, Open Approach			0JNN0ZZ	Release Right Lower Leg Subcutaneous Tissue and Fascia, Open Approach
0JN83ZZ	Release Abdomen Subcutaneous Tissue and Fascia, Percutaneous Approach				*AHA CC: 3Q, 2017, 11-12*

0JNN3ZZ Release Right Lower Leg Subcutaneous Tissue and Fascia, Percutaneous Approach

0JNNXZZ Release Right Lower Leg Subcutaneous Tissue and Fascia, External Approach

0JNP0ZZ Release Left Lower Leg Subcutaneous Tissue and Fascia, Open Approach
AHA CC: 3Q, 2017, 11-12

0JNP3ZZ Release Left Lower Leg Subcutaneous Tissue and Fascia, Percutaneous Approach

0JNPXZZ Release Left Lower Leg Subcutaneous Tissue and Fascia, External Approach

0JNQ0ZZ Release Right Foot Subcutaneous Tissue and Fascia, Open Approach
AHA CC: 3Q, 2017, 11-12

0JNQ3ZZ Release Right Foot Subcutaneous Tissue and Fascia, Percutaneous Approach

0JNQXZZ Release Right Foot Subcutaneous Tissue and Fascia, External Approach

0JNR0ZZ Release Left Foot Subcutaneous Tissue and Fascia, Open Approach
AHA CC: 3Q, 2017, 11-12

0JNR3ZZ Release Left Foot Subcutaneous Tissue and Fascia, Percutaneous Approach

0JNRXZZ Release Left Foot Subcutaneous Tissue and Fascia, External Approach

0JP – Subcutaneous Tissue and Fascia, Removal

Review Coding Guideline B6.1c

0JPS00Z Removal of Drainage Device from Head and Neck Subcutaneous Tissue and Fascia, Open Approach

0JPS01Z Removal of Radioactive Element from Head and Neck Subcutaneous Tissue and Fascia, Open Approach

0JPS03Z Removal of Infusion Device from Head and Neck Subcutaneous Tissue and Fascia, Open Approach

0JPS07Z Removal of Autologous Tissue Substitute from Head and Neck Subcutaneous Tissue and Fascia, Open Approach

0JPS0JZ Removal of Synthetic Substitute from Head and Neck Subcutaneous Tissue and Fascia, Open Approach

0JPS0KZ Removal of Nonautologous Tissue Substitute from Head and Neck Subcutaneous Tissue and Fascia, Open Approach

0JPS0NZ Removal of Tissue Expander from Head and Neck Subcutaneous Tissue and Fascia, Open Approach

0JPS0YZ Removal of Other Device from Head and Neck Subcutaneous Tissue and Fascia, Open Approach

0JPS30Z Removal of Drainage Device from Head and Neck Subcutaneous Tissue and Fascia, Percutaneous Approach

0JPS31Z Removal of Radioactive Element from Head and Neck Subcutaneous Tissue and Fascia, Percutaneous Approach

0JPS33Z Removal of Infusion Device from Head and Neck Subcutaneous Tissue and Fascia, Percutaneous Approach

0JPS37Z Removal of Autologous Tissue Substitute from Head and Neck Subcutaneous Tissue and Fascia, Percutaneous Approach

0JPS3JZ Removal of Synthetic Substitute from Head and Neck Subcutaneous Tissue and Fascia, Percutaneous Approach

0JPS3KZ Removal of Nonautologous Tissue Substitute from Head and Neck Subcutaneous Tissue and Fascia, Percutaneous Approach

0JPS3NZ Removal of Tissue Expander from Head and Neck Subcutaneous Tissue and Fascia, Percutaneous Approach

0JPS3YZ Removal of Other Device from Head and Neck Subcutaneous Tissue and Fascia, Percutaneous Approach

0JPSX0Z Removal of Drainage Device from Head and Neck Subcutaneous Tissue and Fascia, External Approach

0JPSX1Z Removal of Radioactive Element from Head and Neck Subcutaneous Tissue and Fascia, External Approach

0JPSX3Z Removal of Infusion Device from Head and Neck Subcutaneous Tissue and Fascia, External Approach

0JPT00Z Removal of Drainage Device from Trunk Subcutaneous Tissue and Fascia, Open Approach

0JPT01Z Removal of Radioactive Element from Trunk Subcutaneous Tissue and Fascia, Open Approach

0JPT02Z Removal of Monitoring Device from Trunk Subcutaneous Tissue and Fascia, Open Approach

0JPT03Z Removal of Infusion Device from Trunk Subcutaneous Tissue and Fascia, Open Approach

0JPT07Z Removal of Autologous Tissue Substitute from Trunk Subcutaneous Tissue and Fascia, Open Approach

0JPT0FZ Removal of Subcutaneous Defibrillator Lead from Trunk Subcutaneous Tissue and Fascia, Open Approach
HAC With a secondary diagnosis code of K68.11, T81.40XA, T81.41XA, T81.42XA, T81.43XA, T81.44XA, T81.49XA, T82.6XXA, T82.7XXA

0JPT0HZ Removal of Contraceptive Device from Trunk Subcutaneous Tissue and Fascia, Open Approach

0JPT0JZ Removal of Synthetic Substitute from Trunk Subcutaneous Tissue and Fascia, Open Approach

0JPT0KZ Removal of Nonautologous Tissue Substitute from Trunk Subcutaneous Tissue and Fascia, Open Approach

0JPT0MZ Removal of Stimulator Generator from Trunk Subcutaneous Tissue and Fascia, Open Approach

0JPT0NZ Removal of Tissue Expander from Trunk Subcutaneous Tissue and Fascia, Open Approach
AHA CC: 4Q, 2013, 109-111

0JPT0PZ Removal of Cardiac Rhythm Related Device from Trunk Subcutaneous Tissue and Fascia, Open Approach
AHA CC: 4Q, 2012, 104-106
HAC With a secondary diagnosis code of K68.11, T81.40XA, T81.41XA, T81.42XA, T81.43XA, T81.44XA, T82.6XXA, T82.7XXA

0JPT0VZ Removal of Infusion Pump from Trunk Subcutaneous Tissue and Fascia, Open Approach
AHA CC: 3Q, 2014, 19-20

0JPT0WZ Removal of Totally Implantable Vascular Access Device from Trunk Subcutaneous Tissue and Fascia, Open Approach

0JPT0XZ Removal of Tunneled Vascular Access Device from Trunk Subcutaneous Tissue and Fascia, Open Approach

AHA CC: 4Q, 2015, 31-32; 2Q, 2016, 15-16

0JPT0YZ Removal of Other Device from Trunk Subcutaneous Tissue and Fascia, Open Approach

0JPT30Z Removal of Drainage Device from Trunk Subcutaneous Tissue and Fascia, Percutaneous Approach

0JPT31Z Removal of Radioactive Element from Trunk Subcutaneous Tissue and Fascia, Percutaneous Approach

0JPT32Z Removal of Monitoring Device from Trunk Subcutaneous Tissue and Fascia, Percutaneous Approach

0JPT33Z Removal of Infusion Device from Trunk Subcutaneous Tissue and Fascia, Percutaneous Approach

0JPT37Z Removal of Autologous Tissue Substitute from Trunk Subcutaneous Tissue and Fascia, Percutaneous Approach

0JPT3FZ Removal of Subcutaneous Defibrillator Lead from Trunk Subcutaneous Tissue and Fascia, Percutaneous Approach
HAC With a secondary diagnosis code of K68.11, T81.40XA, T81.41XA, T81.42XA, T81.43XA, T81.44XA, T81.49XA, T82.6XXA, T82.7XXA

0JPT3HZ Removal of Contraceptive Device from Trunk Subcutaneous Tissue and Fascia, Percutaneous Approach

0JPT3JZ Removal of Synthetic Substitute from Trunk Subcutaneous Tissue and Fascia, Percutaneous Approach
AHA CC: 4Q, 2018, 86

0JPT3KZ Removal of Nonautologous Tissue Substitute from Trunk Subcutaneous Tissue and Fascia, Percutaneous Approach

0JPT3MZ Removal of Stimulator Generator from Trunk Subcutaneous Tissue and Fascia, Percutaneous Approach

0JPT3NZ Removal of Tissue Expander from Trunk Subcutaneous Tissue and Fascia, Percutaneous Approach

0JPT3PZ Removal of Cardiac Rhythm Related Device from Trunk Subcutaneous Tissue and Fascia, Percutaneous Approach
HAC With a secondary diagnosis code of K68.11, T81.40XA, T81.41XA, T81.42XA, T81.43XA, T81.44XA, T82.6XXA, T82.7XXA

0JPT3VZ Removal of Infusion Pump from Trunk Subcutaneous Tissue and Fascia, Percutaneous Approach

0JPT3WZ Removal of Totally Implantable Vascular Access Device from Trunk Subcutaneous Tissue and Fascia, Percutaneous Approach

♀ Female-only　　♂ Male-only　　▲ Limited Coverage　　● Non-OR　　HAC HAC-associated procedure　　▲ Non-covered procedures　　✚ Cluster

0JPT3XZ Removal of Tunneled Vascular Access Device from Trunk Subcutaneous Tissue and Fascia, Percutaneous Approach

0JPT3YZ Removal of Other Device from Trunk Subcutaneous Tissue and Fascia, Percutaneous Approach
AHA CC: 3Q, 2018, 29

0JPTX0Z Removal of Drainage Device from Trunk Subcutaneous Tissue and Fascia, External Approach

0JPTX1Z Removal of Radioactive Element from Trunk Subcutaneous Tissue and Fascia, External Approach

0JPTX2Z Removal of Monitoring Device from Trunk Subcutaneous Tissue and Fascia, External Approach

0JPTX3Z Removal of Infusion Device from Trunk Subcutaneous Tissue and Fascia, External Approach

0JPTXHZ Removal of Contraceptive Device from Trunk Subcutaneous Tissue and Fascia, External Approach

0JPTXVZ Removal of Infusion Pump from Trunk Subcutaneous Tissue and Fascia, External Approach

0JPTXXZ Removal of Tunneled Vascular Access Device from Trunk Subcutaneous Tissue and Fascia, External Approach

0JPV00Z Removal of Drainage Device from Upper Extremity Subcutaneous Tissue and Fascia, Open Approach

0JPV01Z Removal of Radioactive Element from Upper Extremity Subcutaneous Tissue and Fascia, Open Approach

0JPV03Z Removal of Infusion Device from Upper Extremity Subcutaneous Tissue and Fascia, Open Approach

0JPV07Z Removal of Autologous Tissue Substitute from Upper Extremity Subcutaneous Tissue and Fascia, Open Approach

0JPV0HZ Removal of Contraceptive Device from Upper Extremity Subcutaneous Tissue and Fascia, Open Approach

0JPV0JZ Removal of Synthetic Substitute from Upper Extremity Subcutaneous Tissue and Fascia, Open Approach

0JPV0KZ Removal of Nonautologous Tissue Substitute from Upper Extremity Subcutaneous Tissue and Fascia, Open Approach

0JPV0NZ Removal of Tissue Expander from Upper Extremity Subcutaneous Tissue and Fascia, Open Approach

0JPV0VZ Removal of Infusion Pump from Upper Extremity Subcutaneous Tissue and Fascia, Open Approach

0JPV0WZ Removal of Totally Implantable Vascular Access Device from Upper Extremity Subcutaneous Tissue and Fascia, Open Approach

0JPV0XZ Removal of Tunneled Vascular Access Device from Upper Extremity Subcutaneous Tissue and Fascia, Open Approach

0JPV0YZ Removal of Other Device from Upper Extremity Subcutaneous Tissue and Fascia, Open Approach

0JPV30Z Removal of Drainage Device from Upper Extremity Subcutaneous Tissue and Fascia, Percutaneous Approach

0JPV31Z Removal of Radioactive Element from Upper Extremity Subcutaneous Tissue and Fascia, Percutaneous Approach

0JPV33Z Removal of Infusion Device from Upper Extremity Subcutaneous Tissue and Fascia, Percutaneous Approach

0JPV37Z Removal of Autologous Tissue Substitute from Upper Extremity Subcutaneous Tissue and Fascia, Percutaneous Approach

0JPV3HZ Removal of Contraceptive Device from Upper Extremity Subcutaneous Tissue and Fascia, Percutaneous Approach

0JPV3JZ Removal of Synthetic Substitute from Upper Extremity Subcutaneous Tissue and Fascia, Percutaneous Approach

0JPV3KZ Removal of Nonautologous Tissue Substitute from Upper Extremity Subcutaneous Tissue and Fascia, Percutaneous Approach

0JPV3NZ Removal of Tissue Expander from Upper Extremity Subcutaneous Tissue and Fascia, Percutaneous Approach

0JPV3VZ Removal of Infusion Pump from Upper Extremity Subcutaneous Tissue and Fascia, Percutaneous Approach

0JPV3WZ Removal of Totally Implantable Vascular Access Device from Upper Extremity Subcutaneous Tissue and Fascia, Percutaneous Approach

0JPV3XZ Removal of Tunneled Vascular Access Device from Upper Extremity Subcutaneous Tissue and Fascia, Percutaneous Approach

0JPV3YZ Removal of Other Device from Upper Extremity Subcutaneous Tissue and Fascia, Percutaneous Approach

0JPVX0Z Removal of Drainage Device from Upper Extremity Subcutaneous Tissue and Fascia, External Approach

0JPVX1Z Removal of Radioactive Element from Upper Extremity Subcutaneous Tissue and Fascia, External Approach

0JPVX3Z Removal of Infusion Device from Upper Extremity Subcutaneous Tissue and Fascia, External Approach

0JPVXHZ Removal of Contraceptive Device from Upper Extremity Subcutaneous Tissue and Fascia, External Approach

0JPVXVZ Removal of Infusion Pump from Upper Extremity Subcutaneous Tissue and Fascia, External Approach

0JPVXXZ Removal of Tunneled Vascular Access Device from Upper Extremity Subcutaneous Tissue and Fascia, External Approach

0JPW00Z Removal of Drainage Device from Lower Extremity Subcutaneous Tissue and Fascia, Open Approach

0JPW01Z Removal of Radioactive Element from Lower Extremity Subcutaneous Tissue and Fascia, Open Approach

0JPW03Z Removal of Infusion Device from Lower Extremity Subcutaneous Tissue and Fascia, Open Approach

0JPW07Z Removal of Autologous Tissue Substitute from Lower Extremity Subcutaneous Tissue and Fascia, Open Approach

0JPW0HZ Removal of Contraceptive Device from Lower Extremity Subcutaneous Tissue and Fascia, Open Approach

0JPW0JZ Removal of Synthetic Substitute from Lower Extremity Subcutaneous Tissue and Fascia, Open Approach

0JPW0KZ Removal of Nonautologous Tissue Substitute from Lower Extremity Subcutaneous Tissue and Fascia, Open Approach

0JPW0NZ Removal of Tissue Expander from Lower Extremity Subcutaneous Tissue and Fascia, Open Approach

0JPW0VZ Removal of Infusion Pump from Lower Extremity Subcutaneous Tissue and Fascia, Open Approach

0JPW0WZ Removal of Totally Implantable Vascular Access Device from Lower Extremity Subcutaneous Tissue and Fascia, Open Approach

0JPW0XZ Removal of Tunneled Vascular Access Device from Lower Extremity Subcutaneous Tissue and Fascia, Open Approach

0JPW0YZ Removal of Other Device from Lower Extremity Subcutaneous Tissue and Fascia, Open Approach

0JPW30Z Removal of Drainage Device from Lower Extremity Subcutaneous Tissue and Fascia, Percutaneous Approach

0JPW31Z Removal of Radioactive Element from Lower Extremity Subcutaneous Tissue and Fascia, Percutaneous Approach

0JPW33Z Removal of Infusion Device from Lower Extremity Subcutaneous Tissue and Fascia, Percutaneous Approach

0JPW37Z Removal of Autologous Tissue Substitute from Lower Extremity Subcutaneous Tissue and Fascia, Percutaneous Approach

0JPW3HZ Removal of Contraceptive Device from Lower Extremity Subcutaneous Tissue and Fascia, Percutaneous Approach

0JPW3JZ Removal of Synthetic Substitute from Lower Extremity Subcutaneous Tissue and Fascia, Percutaneous Approach

0JPW3KZ Removal of Nonautologous Tissue Substitute from Lower Extremity Subcutaneous Tissue and Fascia, Percutaneous Approach

0JPW3NZ Removal of Tissue Expander from Lower Extremity Subcutaneous Tissue and Fascia, Percutaneous Approach

0JPW3VZ Removal of Infusion Pump from Lower Extremity Subcutaneous Tissue and Fascia, Percutaneous Approach

0JPW3WZ Removal of Totally Implantable Vascular Access Device from Lower Extremity Subcutaneous Tissue and Fascia, Percutaneous Approach

0JPW3XZ Removal of Tunneled Vascular Access Device from Lower Extremity Subcutaneous Tissue and Fascia, Percutaneous Approach

0JPW3YZ Removal of Other Device from Lower Extremity Subcutaneous Tissue and Fascia, Percutaneous Approach

0JPWX0Z Removal of Drainage Device from Lower Extremity Subcutaneous Tissue and Fascia, External Approach

0JPWX1Z Removal of Radioactive Element from Lower Extremity Subcutaneous Tissue and Fascia, External Approach

0JPWX3Z Removal of Infusion Device from Lower Extremity Subcutaneous Tissue and Fascia, External Approach

0JPWXHZ Removal of Contraceptive Device from Lower Extremity Subcutaneous Tissue and Fascia, External Approach

0JPWXVZ   Removal of Infusion Pump from Lower Extremity Subcutaneous Tissue and Fascia, External Approach

0JPWXXZ   Removal of Tunneled Vascular Access Device from Lower Extremity Subcutaneous Tissue and Fascia, External Approach

0JQ – Subcutaneous Tissue and Fascia, Repair

Review Coding Guideline B3.5

0JQ00ZZ   Repair Scalp Subcutaneous Tissue and Fascia, Open Approach
0JQ03ZZ   Repair Scalp Subcutaneous Tissue and Fascia, Percutaneous Approach
0JQ10ZZ   Repair Face Subcutaneous Tissue and Fascia, Open Approach
0JQ13ZZ   Repair Face Subcutaneous Tissue and Fascia, Percutaneous Approach
0JQ40ZZ   Repair Right Neck Subcutaneous Tissue and Fascia, Open Approach
0JQ43ZZ   Repair Right Neck Subcutaneous Tissue and Fascia, Percutaneous Approach
0JQ50ZZ   Repair Left Neck Subcutaneous Tissue and Fascia, Open Approach
0JQ53ZZ   Repair Left Neck Subcutaneous Tissue and Fascia, Percutaneous Approach
0JQ60ZZ   Repair Chest Subcutaneous Tissue and Fascia, Open Approach
0JQ63ZZ   Repair Chest Subcutaneous Tissue and Fascia, Percutaneous Approach
0JQ70ZZ   Repair Back Subcutaneous Tissue and Fascia, Open Approach
0JQ73ZZ   Repair Back Subcutaneous Tissue and Fascia, Percutaneous Approach
0JQ80ZZ   Repair Abdomen Subcutaneous Tissue and Fascia, Open Approach
0JQ83ZZ   Repair Abdomen Subcutaneous Tissue and Fascia, Percutaneous Approach
0JQ90ZZ   Repair Buttock Subcutaneous Tissue and Fascia, Open Approach
0JQ93ZZ   Repair Buttock Subcutaneous Tissue and Fascia, Percutaneous Approach
0JQB0ZZ   Repair Perineum Subcutaneous Tissue and Fascia, Open Approach

0JQB3ZZ   Repair Perineum Subcutaneous Tissue and Fascia, Percutaneous Approach
0JQC0ZZ   Repair Pelvic Region Subcutaneous Tissue and Fascia, Open Approach
            AHA CC: 4Q, 2014, 44-45; 3Q, 2017, 19
0JQC3ZZ   Repair Pelvic Region Subcutaneous Tissue and Fascia, Percutaneous Approach
0JQD0ZZ   Repair Right Upper Arm Subcutaneous Tissue and Fascia, Open Approach
0JQD3ZZ   Repair Right Upper Arm Subcutaneous Tissue and Fascia, Percutaneous Approach
0JQF0ZZ   Repair Left Upper Arm Subcutaneous Tissue and Fascia, Open Approach
0JQF3ZZ   Repair Left Upper Arm Subcutaneous Tissue and Fascia, Percutaneous Approach
0JQG0ZZ   Repair Right Lower Arm Subcutaneous Tissue and Fascia, Open Approach
0JQG3ZZ   Repair Right Lower Arm Subcutaneous Tissue and Fascia, Percutaneous Approach
0JQH0ZZ   Repair Left Lower Arm Subcutaneous Tissue and Fascia, Open Approach
0JQH3ZZ   Repair Left Lower Arm Subcutaneous Tissue and Fascia, Percutaneous Approach
0JQJ0ZZ   Repair Right Hand Subcutaneous Tissue and Fascia, Open Approach
0JQJ3ZZ   Repair Right Hand Subcutaneous Tissue and Fascia, Percutaneous Approach
0JQK0ZZ   Repair Left Hand Subcutaneous Tissue and Fascia, Open Approach

0JQK3ZZ   Repair Left Hand Subcutaneous Tissue and Fascia, Percutaneous Approach
0JQL0ZZ   Repair Right Upper Leg Subcutaneous Tissue and Fascia, Open Approach
0JQL3ZZ   Repair Right Upper Leg Subcutaneous Tissue and Fascia, Percutaneous Approach
0JQM0ZZ   Repair Left Upper Leg Subcutaneous Tissue and Fascia, Open Approach
0JQM3ZZ   Repair Left Upper Leg Subcutaneous Tissue and Fascia, Percutaneous Approach
0JQN0ZZ   Repair Right Lower Leg Subcutaneous Tissue and Fascia, Open Approach
0JQN3ZZ   Repair Right Lower Leg Subcutaneous Tissue and Fascia, Percutaneous Approach
0JQP0ZZ   Repair Left Lower Leg Subcutaneous Tissue and Fascia, Open Approach
0JQP3ZZ   Repair Left Lower Leg Subcutaneous Tissue and Fascia, Percutaneous Approach
0JQQ0ZZ   Repair Right Foot Subcutaneous Tissue and Fascia, Open Approach
0JQQ3ZZ   Repair Right Foot Subcutaneous Tissue and Fascia, Percutaneous Approach
0JQR0ZZ   Repair Left Foot Subcutaneous Tissue and Fascia, Open Approach
0JQR3ZZ   Repair Left Foot Subcutaneous Tissue and Fascia, Percutaneous Approach

0JR – Subcutaneous Tissue and Fascia, Replacement

Review Coding Guideline B3.18

0JR007Z   Replacement of Scalp Subcutaneous Tissue and Fascia with Autologous Tissue Substitute, Open Approach
0JR00JZ   Replacement of Scalp Subcutaneous Tissue and Fascia with Synthetic Substitute, Open Approach
0JR00KZ   Replacement of Scalp Subcutaneous Tissue and Fascia with Nonautologous Tissue Substitute, Open Approach
0JR037Z   Replacement of Scalp Subcutaneous Tissue and Fascia with Autologous Tissue Substitute, Percutaneous Approach
0JR03JZ   Replacement of Scalp Subcutaneous Tissue and Fascia with Synthetic Substitute, Percutaneous Approach
0JR03KZ   Replacement of Scalp Subcutaneous Tissue and Fascia with Nonautologous Tissue Substitute, Percutaneous Approach
0JR107Z   Replacement of Face Subcutaneous Tissue and Fascia with Autologous Tissue Substitute, Open Approach
            AHA CC: 2Q, 2015, 13
0JR10JZ   Replacement of Face Subcutaneous Tissue and Fascia with Synthetic Substitute, Open Approach

0JR10KZ   Replacement of Face Subcutaneous Tissue and Fascia with Nonautologous Tissue Substitute, Open Approach
0JR137Z   Replacement of Face Subcutaneous Tissue and Fascia with Autologous Tissue Substitute, Percutaneous Approach
0JR13JZ   Replacement of Face Subcutaneous Tissue and Fascia with Synthetic Substitute, Percutaneous Approach
0JR13KZ   Replacement of Face Subcutaneous Tissue and Fascia with Nonautologous Tissue Substitute, Percutaneous Approach
0JR407Z   Replacement of Right Neck Subcutaneous Tissue and Fascia with Autologous Tissue Substitute, Open Approach
0JR40JZ   Replacement of Right Neck Subcutaneous Tissue and Fascia with Synthetic Substitute, Open Approach
0JR40KZ   Replacement of Right Neck Subcutaneous Tissue and Fascia with Nonautologous Tissue Substitute, Open Approach
0JR437Z   Replacement of Right Neck Subcutaneous Tissue and Fascia with Autologous Tissue Substitute, Percutaneous Approach

0JR43JZ   Replacement of Right Neck Subcutaneous Tissue and Fascia with Synthetic Substitute, Percutaneous Approach
0JR43KZ   Replacement of Right Neck Subcutaneous Tissue and Fascia with Nonautologous Tissue Substitute, Percutaneous Approach
0JR507Z   Replacement of Left Neck Subcutaneous Tissue and Fascia with Autologous Tissue Substitute, Open Approach
0JR50JZ   Replacement of Left Neck Subcutaneous Tissue and Fascia with Synthetic Substitute, Open Approach
0JR50KZ   Replacement of Left Neck Subcutaneous Tissue and Fascia with Nonautologous Tissue Substitute, Open Approach
0JR537Z   Replacement of Left Neck Subcutaneous Tissue and Fascia with Autologous Tissue Substitute, Percutaneous Approach
0JR53JZ   Replacement of Left Neck Subcutaneous Tissue and Fascia with Synthetic Substitute, Percutaneous Approach

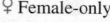 ♀ Female-only   ♂ Male-only   ▲ Limited Coverage   ● Non-OR   HAC HAC-associated procedure   ▲ Non-covered procedures   ✚ Cluster

0JR53KZ Replacement of Left Neck Subcutaneous Tissue and Fascia with Nonautologous Tissue Substitute, Percutaneous Approach

0JR607Z Replacement of Chest Subcutaneous Tissue and Fascia with Autologous Tissue Substitute, Open Approach

0JR60JZ Replacement of Chest Subcutaneous Tissue and Fascia with Synthetic Substitute, Open Approach

0JR60KZ Replacement of Chest Subcutaneous Tissue and Fascia with Nonautologous Tissue Substitute, Open Approach

0JR637Z Replacement of Chest Subcutaneous Tissue and Fascia with Autologous Tissue Substitute, Percutaneous Approach

0JR63JZ Replacement of Chest Subcutaneous Tissue and Fascia with Synthetic Substitute, Percutaneous Approach

0JR63KZ Replacement of Chest Subcutaneous Tissue and Fascia with Nonautologous Tissue Substitute, Percutaneous Approach

0JR707Z Replacement of Back Subcutaneous Tissue and Fascia with Autologous Tissue Substitute, Open Approach

0JR70JZ Replacement of Back Subcutaneous Tissue and Fascia with Synthetic Substitute, Open Approach

0JR70KZ Replacement of Back Subcutaneous Tissue and Fascia with Nonautologous Tissue Substitute, Open Approach

0JR737Z Replacement of Back Subcutaneous Tissue and Fascia with Autologous Tissue Substitute, Percutaneous Approach

0JR73JZ Replacement of Back Subcutaneous Tissue and Fascia with Synthetic Substitute, Percutaneous Approach

0JR73KZ Replacement of Back Subcutaneous Tissue and Fascia with Nonautologous Tissue Substitute, Percutaneous Approach

0JR807Z Replacement of Abdomen Subcutaneous Tissue and Fascia with Autologous Tissue Substitute, Open Approach

0JR80JZ Replacement of Abdomen Subcutaneous Tissue and Fascia with Synthetic Substitute, Open Approach

0JR80KZ Replacement of Abdomen Subcutaneous Tissue and Fascia with Nonautologous Tissue Substitute, Open Approach

0JR837Z Replacement of Abdomen Subcutaneous Tissue and Fascia with Autologous Tissue Substitute, Percutaneous Approach

0JR83JZ Replacement of Abdomen Subcutaneous Tissue and Fascia with Synthetic Substitute, Percutaneous Approach

0JR83KZ Replacement of Abdomen Subcutaneous Tissue and Fascia with Nonautologous Tissue Substitute, Percutaneous Approach

0JR907Z Replacement of Buttock Subcutaneous Tissue and Fascia with Autologous Tissue Substitute, Open Approach

0JR90JZ Replacement of Buttock Subcutaneous Tissue and Fascia with Synthetic Substitute, Open Approach

0JR90KZ Replacement of Buttock Subcutaneous Tissue and Fascia with Nonautologous Tissue Substitute, Open Approach

0JR937Z Replacement of Buttock Subcutaneous Tissue and Fascia with Autologous Tissue Substitute, Percutaneous Approach

0JR93JZ Replacement of Buttock Subcutaneous Tissue and Fascia with Synthetic Substitute, Percutaneous Approach

0JR93KZ Replacement of Buttock Subcutaneous Tissue and Fascia with Nonautologous Tissue Substitute, Percutaneous Approach

0JRB07Z Replacement of Perineum Subcutaneous Tissue and Fascia with Autologous Tissue Substitute, Open Approach

0JRB0JZ Replacement of Perineum Subcutaneous Tissue and Fascia with Synthetic Substitute, Open Approach

0JRB0KZ Replacement of Perineum Subcutaneous Tissue and Fascia with Nonautologous Tissue Substitute, Open Approach

0JRB37Z Replacement of Perineum Subcutaneous Tissue and Fascia with Autologous Tissue Substitute, Percutaneous Approach

0JRB3JZ Replacement of Perineum Subcutaneous Tissue and Fascia with Synthetic Substitute, Percutaneous Approach

0JRB3KZ Replacement of Perineum Subcutaneous Tissue and Fascia with Nonautologous Tissue Substitute, Percutaneous Approach

0JRC07Z Replacement of Pelvic Region Subcutaneous Tissue and Fascia with Autologous Tissue Substitute, Open Approach

0JRC0JZ Replacement of Pelvic Region Subcutaneous Tissue and Fascia with Synthetic Substitute, Open Approach

0JRC0KZ Replacement of Pelvic Region Subcutaneous Tissue and Fascia with Nonautologous Tissue Substitute, Open Approach

0JRC37Z Replacement of Pelvic Region Subcutaneous Tissue and Fascia with Autologous Tissue Substitute, Percutaneous Approach

0JRC3JZ Replacement of Pelvic Region Subcutaneous Tissue and Fascia with Synthetic Substitute, Percutaneous Approach

0JRC3KZ Replacement of Pelvic Region Subcutaneous Tissue and Fascia with Nonautologous Tissue Substitute, Percutaneous Approach

0JRD07Z Replacement of Right Upper Arm Subcutaneous Tissue and Fascia with Autologous Tissue Substitute, Open Approach

0JRD0JZ Replacement of Right Upper Arm Subcutaneous Tissue and Fascia with Synthetic Substitute, Open Approach

0JRD0KZ Replacement of Right Upper Arm Subcutaneous Tissue and Fascia with Nonautologous Tissue Substitute, Open Approach

0JRD37Z Replacement of Right Upper Arm Subcutaneous Tissue and Fascia with Autologous Tissue Substitute, Percutaneous Approach

0JRD3JZ Replacement of Right Upper Arm Subcutaneous Tissue and Fascia with Synthetic Substitute, Percutaneous Approach

0JRD3KZ Replacement of Right Upper Arm Subcutaneous Tissue and Fascia with Nonautologous Tissue Substitute, Percutaneous Approach

0JRF07Z Replacement of Left Upper Arm Subcutaneous Tissue and Fascia with Autologous Tissue Substitute, Open Approach

0JRF0JZ Replacement of Left Upper Arm Subcutaneous Tissue and Fascia with Synthetic Substitute, Open Approach

0JRF0KZ Replacement of Left Upper Arm Subcutaneous Tissue and Fascia with Nonautologous Tissue Substitute, Open Approach

0JRF37Z Replacement of Left Upper Arm Subcutaneous Tissue and Fascia with Autologous Tissue Substitute, Percutaneous Approach

0JRF3JZ Replacement of Left Upper Arm Subcutaneous Tissue and Fascia with Synthetic Substitute, Percutaneous Approach

0JRF3KZ Replacement of Left Upper Arm Subcutaneous Tissue and Fascia with Nonautologous Tissue Substitute, Percutaneous Approach

0JRG07Z Replacement of Right Lower Arm Subcutaneous Tissue and Fascia with Autologous Tissue Substitute, Open Approach

0JRG0JZ Replacement of Right Lower Arm Subcutaneous Tissue and Fascia with Synthetic Substitute, Open Approach

0JRG0KZ Replacement of Right Lower Arm Subcutaneous Tissue and Fascia with Nonautologous Tissue Substitute, Open Approach

0JRG37Z Replacement of Right Lower Arm Subcutaneous Tissue and Fascia with Autologous Tissue Substitute, Percutaneous Approach

0JRG3JZ Replacement of Right Lower Arm Subcutaneous Tissue and Fascia with Synthetic Substitute, Percutaneous Approach

0JRG3KZ Replacement of Right Lower Arm Subcutaneous Tissue and Fascia with Nonautologous Tissue Substitute, Percutaneous Approach

0JRH07Z Replacement of Left Lower Arm Subcutaneous Tissue and Fascia with Autologous Tissue Substitute, Open Approach

0JRH0JZ Replacement of Left Lower Arm Subcutaneous Tissue and Fascia with Synthetic Substitute, Open Approach

0JRH0KZ Replacement of Left Lower Arm Subcutaneous Tissue and Fascia with Nonautologous Tissue Substitute, Open Approach

0JRH37Z Replacement of Left Lower Arm Subcutaneous Tissue and Fascia with Autologous Tissue Substitute, Percutaneous Approach

0JRH3JZ Replacement of Left Lower Arm Subcutaneous Tissue and Fascia with Synthetic Substitute, Percutaneous Approach

0JRH3KZ Replacement of Left Lower Arm Subcutaneous Tissue and Fascia with Nonautologous Tissue Substitute, Percutaneous Approach

0JRJ07Z Replacement of Right Hand Subcutaneous Tissue and Fascia with Autologous Tissue Substitute, Open Approach

0JRJ0JZ Replacement of Right Hand Subcutaneous Tissue and Fascia with Synthetic Substitute, Open Approach

0JRJ0KZ Replacement of Right Hand Subcutaneous Tissue and Fascia with Nonautologous Tissue Substitute, Open Approach

0JRJ37Z Replacement of Right Hand Subcutaneous Tissue and Fascia with Autologous Tissue Substitute, Percutaneous Approach

0JRJ3JZ Replacement of Right Hand Subcutaneous Tissue and Fascia with Synthetic Substitute, Percutaneous Approach

0JRJ3KZ Replacement of Right Hand Subcutaneous Tissue and Fascia with Nonautologous Tissue Substitute, Percutaneous Approach

0JRK07Z Replacement of Left Hand Subcutaneous Tissue and Fascia with Autologous Tissue Substitute, Open Approach

0JRK0JZ Replacement of Left Hand Subcutaneous Tissue and Fascia with Synthetic Substitute, Open Approach

0JRK0KZ Replacement of Left Hand Subcutaneous Tissue and Fascia with Nonautologous Tissue Substitute, Open Approach

0JRK37Z Replacement of Left Hand Subcutaneous Tissue and Fascia with Autologous Tissue Substitute, Percutaneous Approach

0JRK3JZ Replacement of Left Hand Subcutaneous Tissue and Fascia with Synthetic Substitute, Percutaneous Approach

0JRK3KZ Replacement of Left Hand Subcutaneous Tissue and Fascia with Nonautologous Tissue Substitute, Percutaneous Approach

0JRL07Z Replacement of Right Upper Leg Subcutaneous Tissue and Fascia with Autologous Tissue Substitute, Open Approach

0JRL0JZ Replacement of Right Upper Leg Subcutaneous Tissue and Fascia with Synthetic Substitute, Open Approach

0JRL0KZ Replacement of Right Upper Leg Subcutaneous Tissue and Fascia with Nonautologous Tissue Substitute, Open Approach

0JRL37Z Replacement of Right Upper Leg Subcutaneous Tissue and Fascia with Autologous Tissue Substitute, Percutaneous Approach

0JRL3JZ Replacement of Right Upper Leg Subcutaneous Tissue and Fascia with Synthetic Substitute, Percutaneous Approach

0JRL3KZ Replacement of Right Upper Leg Subcutaneous Tissue and Fascia with Nonautologous Tissue Substitute, Percutaneous Approach

0JRM07Z Replacement of Left Upper Leg Subcutaneous Tissue and Fascia with Autologous Tissue Substitute, Open Approach

0JRM0JZ Replacement of Left Upper Leg Subcutaneous Tissue and Fascia with Synthetic Substitute, Open Approach

0JRM0KZ Replacement of Left Upper Leg Subcutaneous Tissue and Fascia with Nonautologous Tissue Substitute, Open Approach

0JRM37Z Replacement of Left Upper Leg Subcutaneous Tissue and Fascia with Autologous Tissue Substitute, Percutaneous Approach

0JRM3JZ Replacement of Left Upper Leg Subcutaneous Tissue and Fascia with Synthetic Substitute, Percutaneous Approach

0JRM3KZ Replacement of Left Upper Leg Subcutaneous Tissue and Fascia with Nonautologous Tissue Substitute, Percutaneous Approach

0JRN07Z Replacement of Right Lower Leg Subcutaneous Tissue and Fascia with Autologous Tissue Substitute, Open Approach

0JRN0JZ Replacement of Right Lower Leg Subcutaneous Tissue and Fascia with Synthetic Substitute, Open Approach

0JRN0KZ Replacement of Right Lower Leg Subcutaneous Tissue and Fascia with Nonautologous Tissue Substitute, Open Approach

0JRN37Z Replacement of Right Lower Leg Subcutaneous Tissue and Fascia with Autologous Tissue Substitute, Percutaneous Approach

0JRN3JZ Replacement of Right Lower Leg Subcutaneous Tissue and Fascia with Synthetic Substitute, Percutaneous Approach

0JRN3KZ Replacement of Right Lower Leg Subcutaneous Tissue and Fascia with Nonautologous Tissue Substitute, Percutaneous Approach

0JRP07Z Replacement of Left Lower Leg Subcutaneous Tissue and Fascia with Autologous Tissue Substitute, Open Approach

0JRP0JZ Replacement of Left Lower Leg Subcutaneous Tissue and Fascia with Synthetic Substitute, Open Approach

0JRP0KZ Replacement of Left Lower Leg Subcutaneous Tissue and Fascia with Nonautologous Tissue Substitute, Open Approach

0JRP37Z Replacement of Left Lower Leg Subcutaneous Tissue and Fascia with Autologous Tissue Substitute, Percutaneous Approach

0JRP3JZ Replacement of Left Lower Leg Subcutaneous Tissue and Fascia with Synthetic Substitute, Percutaneous Approach

0JRP3KZ Replacement of Left Lower Leg Subcutaneous Tissue and Fascia with Nonautologous Tissue Substitute, Percutaneous Approach

0JRQ07Z Replacement of Right Foot Subcutaneous Tissue and Fascia with Autologous Tissue Substitute, Open Approach

0JRQ0JZ Replacement of Right Foot Subcutaneous Tissue and Fascia with Synthetic Substitute, Open Approach

0JRQ0KZ Replacement of Right Foot Subcutaneous Tissue and Fascia with Nonautologous Tissue Substitute, Open Approach

0JRQ37Z Replacement of Right Foot Subcutaneous Tissue and Fascia with Autologous Tissue Substitute, Percutaneous Approach

0JRQ3JZ Replacement of Right Foot Subcutaneous Tissue and Fascia with Synthetic Substitute, Percutaneous Approach

0JRQ3KZ Replacement of Right Foot Subcutaneous Tissue and Fascia with Nonautologous Tissue Substitute, Percutaneous Approach

0JRR07Z Replacement of Left Foot Subcutaneous Tissue and Fascia with Autologous Tissue Substitute, Open Approach

0JRR0JZ Replacement of Left Foot Subcutaneous Tissue and Fascia with Synthetic Substitute, Open Approach

0JRR0KZ Replacement of Left Foot Subcutaneous Tissue and Fascia with Nonautologous Tissue Substitute, Open Approach

0JRR37Z Replacement of Left Foot Subcutaneous Tissue and Fascia with Autologous Tissue Substitute, Percutaneous Approach

0JRR3JZ Replacement of Left Foot Subcutaneous Tissue and Fascia with Synthetic Substitute, Percutaneous Approach

0JRR3KZ Replacement of Left Foot Subcutaneous Tissue and Fascia with Nonautologous Tissue Substitute, Percutaneous Approach

0JU – Subcutaneous Tissue and Fascia, Supplement

0JU007Z Supplement of Scalp Subcutaneous Tissue and Fascia with Autologous Tissue Substitute, Open Approach

0JU00JZ Supplement of Scalp Subcutaneous Tissue and Fascia with Synthetic Substitute, Open Approach

0JU00KZ Supplement of Scalp Subcutaneous Tissue and Fascia with Nonautologous Tissue Substitute, Open Approach

0JU037Z Supplement of Scalp Subcutaneous Tissue and Fascia with Autologous Tissue Substitute, Percutaneous Approach

0JU03JZ Supplement of Scalp Subcutaneous Tissue and Fascia with Synthetic Substitute, Percutaneous Approach

0JU03KZ Supplement of Scalp Subcutaneous Tissue and Fascia with Nonautologous Tissue Substitute, Percutaneous Approach

0JU107Z Supplement of Face Subcutaneous Tissue and Fascia with Autologous Tissue Substitute, Open Approach

0JU10JZ Supplement of Face Subcutaneous Tissue and Fascia with Synthetic Substitute, Open Approach

0JU10KZ Supplement of Face Subcutaneous Tissue and Fascia with Nonautologous Tissue Substitute, Open Approach

0JU137Z Supplement of Face Subcutaneous Tissue and Fascia with Autologous Tissue Substitute, Percutaneous Approach

0JU13JZ Supplement of Face Subcutaneous Tissue and Fascia with Synthetic Substitute, Percutaneous Approach

0JU13KZ Supplement of Face Subcutaneous Tissue and Fascia with Nonautologous Tissue Substitute, Percutaneous Approach

♀ Female-only ♂ Male-only ▲ Limited Coverage ● Non-OR ᴴᴬᶜ HAC-associated procedure ▲ Non-covered procedures ✚ Cluster

0JU407Z Supplement of Right Neck Subcutaneous Tissue and Fascia with Autologous Tissue Substitute, Open Approach

0JU40JZ Supplement of Right Neck Subcutaneous Tissue and Fascia with Synthetic Substitute, Open Approach

0JU40KZ Supplement of Right Neck Subcutaneous Tissue and Fascia with Nonautologous Tissue Substitute, Open Approach

0JU437Z Supplement of Right Neck Subcutaneous Tissue and Fascia with Autologous Tissue Substitute, Percutaneous Approach

0JU43JZ Supplement of Right Neck Subcutaneous Tissue and Fascia with Synthetic Substitute, Percutaneous Approach

0JU43KZ Supplement of Right Neck Subcutaneous Tissue and Fascia with Nonautologous Tissue Substitute, Percutaneous Approach

0JU507Z Supplement of Left Neck Subcutaneous Tissue and Fascia with Autologous Tissue Substitute, Open Approach

0JU50JZ Supplement of Left Neck Subcutaneous Tissue and Fascia with Synthetic Substitute, Open Approach

0JU50KZ Supplement of Left Neck Subcutaneous Tissue and Fascia with Nonautologous Tissue Substitute, Open Approach

0JU537Z Supplement of Left Neck Subcutaneous Tissue and Fascia with Autologous Tissue Substitute, Percutaneous Approach

0JU53JZ Supplement of Left Neck Subcutaneous Tissue and Fascia with Synthetic Substitute, Percutaneous Approach

0JU53KZ Supplement of Left Neck Subcutaneous Tissue and Fascia with Nonautologous Tissue Substitute, Percutaneous Approach

0JU607Z Supplement of Chest Subcutaneous Tissue and Fascia with Autologous Tissue Substitute, Open Approach

0JU60JZ Supplement of Chest Subcutaneous Tissue and Fascia with Synthetic Substitute, Open Approach

0JU60KZ Supplement of Chest Subcutaneous Tissue and Fascia with Nonautologous Tissue Substitute, Open Approach

0JU637Z Supplement of Chest Subcutaneous Tissue and Fascia with Autologous Tissue Substitute, Percutaneous Approach

0JU63JZ Supplement of Chest Subcutaneous Tissue and Fascia with Synthetic Substitute, Percutaneous Approach

0JU63KZ Supplement of Chest Subcutaneous Tissue and Fascia with Nonautologous Tissue Substitute, Percutaneous Approach

0JU707Z Supplement of Back Subcutaneous Tissue and Fascia with Autologous Tissue Substitute, Open Approach
AHA CC: 1Q, 2018, 7-8

0JU70JZ Supplement of Back Subcutaneous Tissue and Fascia with Synthetic Substitute, Open Approach

0JU70KZ Supplement of Back Subcutaneous Tissue and Fascia with Nonautologous Tissue Substitute, Open Approach

0JU737Z Supplement of Back Subcutaneous Tissue and Fascia with Autologous Tissue Substitute, Percutaneous Approach

0JU73JZ Supplement of Back Subcutaneous Tissue and Fascia with Synthetic Substitute, Percutaneous Approach

0JU73KZ Supplement of Back Subcutaneous Tissue and Fascia with Nonautologous Tissue Substitute, Percutaneous Approach

0JU807Z Supplement of Abdomen Subcutaneous Tissue and Fascia with Autologous Tissue Substitute, Open Approach

0JU80JZ Supplement of Abdomen Subcutaneous Tissue and Fascia with Synthetic Substitute, Open Approach

0JU80KZ Supplement of Abdomen Subcutaneous Tissue and Fascia with Nonautologous Tissue Substitute, Open Approach

0JU837Z Supplement of Abdomen Subcutaneous Tissue and Fascia with Autologous Tissue Substitute, Percutaneous Approach

0JU83JZ Supplement of Abdomen Subcutaneous Tissue and Fascia with Synthetic Substitute, Percutaneous Approach

0JU83KZ Supplement of Abdomen Subcutaneous Tissue and Fascia with Nonautologous Tissue Substitute, Percutaneous Approach

0JU907Z Supplement of Buttock Subcutaneous Tissue and Fascia with Autologous Tissue Substitute, Open Approach

0JU90JZ Supplement of Buttock Subcutaneous Tissue and Fascia with Synthetic Substitute, Open Approach

0JU90KZ Supplement of Buttock Subcutaneous Tissue and Fascia with Nonautologous Tissue Substitute, Open Approach

0JU937Z Supplement of Buttock Subcutaneous Tissue and Fascia with Autologous Tissue Substitute, Percutaneous Approach

0JU93JZ Supplement of Buttock Subcutaneous Tissue and Fascia with Synthetic Substitute, Percutaneous Approach

0JU93KZ Supplement of Buttock Subcutaneous Tissue and Fascia with Nonautologous Tissue Substitute, Percutaneous Approach

0JUB07Z Supplement of Perineum Subcutaneous Tissue and Fascia with Autologous Tissue Substitute, Open Approach

0JUB0JZ Supplement of Perineum Subcutaneous Tissue and Fascia with Synthetic Substitute, Open Approach

0JUB0KZ Supplement of Perineum Subcutaneous Tissue and Fascia with Nonautologous Tissue Substitute, Open Approach

0JUB37Z Supplement of Perineum Subcutaneous Tissue and Fascia with Autologous Tissue Substitute, Percutaneous Approach

0JUB3JZ Supplement of Perineum Subcutaneous Tissue and Fascia with Synthetic Substitute, Percutaneous Approach

0JUB3KZ Supplement of Perineum Subcutaneous Tissue and Fascia with Nonautologous Tissue Substitute, Percutaneous Approach

0JUC07Z Supplement of Pelvic Region Subcutaneous Tissue and Fascia with Autologous Tissue Substitute, Open Approach

0JUC0JZ Supplement of Pelvic Region Subcutaneous Tissue and Fascia with Synthetic Substitute, Open Approach

0JUC0KZ Supplement of Pelvic Region Subcutaneous Tissue and Fascia with Nonautologous Tissue Substitute, Open Approach

0JUC37Z Supplement of Pelvic Region Subcutaneous Tissue and Fascia with Autologous Tissue Substitute, Percutaneous Approach

0JUC3JZ Supplement of Pelvic Region Subcutaneous Tissue and Fascia with Synthetic Substitute, Percutaneous Approach

0JUC3KZ Supplement of Pelvic Region Subcutaneous Tissue and Fascia with Nonautologous Tissue Substitute, Percutaneous Approach

0JUD07Z Supplement of Right Upper Arm Subcutaneous Tissue and Fascia with Autologous Tissue Substitute, Open Approach

0JUD0JZ Supplement of Right Upper Arm Subcutaneous Tissue and Fascia with Synthetic Substitute, Open Approach

0JUD0KZ Supplement of Right Upper Arm Subcutaneous Tissue and Fascia with Nonautologous Tissue Substitute, Open Approach

0JUD37Z Supplement of Right Upper Arm Subcutaneous Tissue and Fascia with Autologous Tissue Substitute, Percutaneous Approach

0JUD3JZ Supplement of Right Upper Arm Subcutaneous Tissue and Fascia with Synthetic Substitute, Percutaneous Approach

0JUD3KZ Supplement of Right Upper Arm Subcutaneous Tissue and Fascia with Nonautologous Tissue Substitute, Percutaneous Approach

0JUF07Z Supplement of Left Upper Arm Subcutaneous Tissue and Fascia with Autologous Tissue Substitute, Open Approach

0JUF0JZ Supplement of Left Upper Arm Subcutaneous Tissue and Fascia with Synthetic Substitute, Open Approach

0JUF0KZ Supplement of Left Upper Arm Subcutaneous Tissue and Fascia with Nonautologous Tissue Substitute, Open Approach

0JUF37Z Supplement of Left Upper Arm Subcutaneous Tissue and Fascia with Autologous Tissue Substitute, Percutaneous Approach

0JUF3JZ Supplement of Left Upper Arm Subcutaneous Tissue and Fascia with Synthetic Substitute, Percutaneous Approach

0JUF3KZ Supplement of Left Upper Arm Subcutaneous Tissue and Fascia with Nonautologous Tissue Substitute, Percutaneous Approach

0JUG07Z Supplement of Right Lower Arm Subcutaneous Tissue and Fascia with Autologous Tissue Substitute, Open Approach

0JUG0JZ Supplement of Right Lower Arm Subcutaneous Tissue and Fascia with Synthetic Substitute, Open Approach

0JUG0KZ Supplement of Right Lower Arm Subcutaneous Tissue and Fascia with Nonautologous Tissue Substitute, Open Approach

0JUG37Z Supplement of Right Lower Arm Subcutaneous Tissue and Fascia with Autologous Tissue Substitute, Percutaneous Approach

0JUG3JZ Supplement of Right Lower Arm Subcutaneous Tissue and Fascia with Synthetic Substitute, Percutaneous Approach

0JUG3KZ Supplement of Right Lower Arm Subcutaneous Tissue and Fascia with Nonautologous Tissue Substitute, Percutaneous Approach

0JUH07Z Supplement of Left Lower Arm Subcutaneous Tissue and Fascia with Autologous Tissue Substitute, Open Approach

0JUH0JZ Supplement of Left Lower Arm Subcutaneous Tissue and Fascia with Synthetic Substitute, Open Approach

0JUH0KZ Supplement of Left Lower Arm Subcutaneous Tissue and Fascia with Nonautologous Tissue Substitute, Open Approach
AHA CC: 2Q, 2018, 20

0JUH37Z Supplement of Left Lower Arm Subcutaneous Tissue and Fascia with Autologous Tissue Substitute, Percutaneous Approach

0JUH3JZ Supplement of Left Lower Arm Subcutaneous Tissue and Fascia with Synthetic Substitute, Percutaneous Approach

0JUH3KZ Supplement of Left Lower Arm Subcutaneous Tissue and Fascia with Nonautologous Tissue Substitute, Percutaneous Approach

0JUJ07Z Supplement of Right Hand Subcutaneous Tissue and Fascia with Autologous Tissue Substitute, Open Approach

0JUJ0JZ Supplement of Right Hand Subcutaneous Tissue and Fascia with Synthetic Substitute, Open Approach

0JUJ0KZ Supplement of Right Hand Subcutaneous Tissue and Fascia with Nonautologous Tissue Substitute, Open Approach

0JUJ37Z Supplement of Right Hand Subcutaneous Tissue and Fascia with Autologous Tissue Substitute, Percutaneous Approach

0JUJ3JZ Supplement of Right Hand Subcutaneous Tissue and Fascia with Synthetic Substitute, Percutaneous Approach

0JUJ3KZ Supplement of Right Hand Subcutaneous Tissue and Fascia with Nonautologous Tissue Substitute, Percutaneous Approach

0JUK07Z Supplement of Left Hand Subcutaneous Tissue and Fascia with Autologous Tissue Substitute, Open Approach

0JUK0JZ Supplement of Left Hand Subcutaneous Tissue and Fascia with Synthetic Substitute, Open Approach

0JUK0KZ Supplement of Left Hand Subcutaneous Tissue and Fascia with Nonautologous Tissue Substitute, Open Approach

0JUK37Z Supplement of Left Hand Subcutaneous Tissue and Fascia with Autologous Tissue Substitute, Percutaneous Approach

0JUK3JZ Supplement of Left Hand Subcutaneous Tissue and Fascia with Synthetic Substitute, Percutaneous Approach

0JUK3KZ Supplement of Left Hand Subcutaneous Tissue and Fascia with Nonautologous Tissue Substitute, Percutaneous Approach

0JUL07Z Supplement of Right Upper Leg Subcutaneous Tissue and Fascia with Autologous Tissue Substitute, Open Approach

0JUL0JZ Supplement of Right Upper Leg Subcutaneous Tissue and Fascia with Synthetic Substitute, Open Approach

0JUL0KZ Supplement of Right Upper Leg Subcutaneous Tissue and Fascia with Nonautologous Tissue Substitute, Open Approach

0JUL37Z Supplement of Right Upper Leg Subcutaneous Tissue and Fascia with Autologous Tissue Substitute, Percutaneous Approach

0JUL3JZ Supplement of Right Upper Leg Subcutaneous Tissue and Fascia with Synthetic Substitute, Percutaneous Approach

0JUL3KZ Supplement of Right Upper Leg Subcutaneous Tissue and Fascia with Nonautologous Tissue Substitute, Percutaneous Approach

0JUM07Z Supplement of Left Upper Leg Subcutaneous Tissue and Fascia with Autologous Tissue Substitute, Open Approach

0JUM0JZ Supplement of Left Upper Leg Subcutaneous Tissue and Fascia with Synthetic Substitute, Open Approach

0JUM0KZ Supplement of Left Upper Leg Subcutaneous Tissue and Fascia with Nonautologous Tissue Substitute, Open Approach

0JUM37Z Supplement of Left Upper Leg Subcutaneous Tissue and Fascia with Autologous Tissue Substitute, Percutaneous Approach

0JUM3JZ Supplement of Left Upper Leg Subcutaneous Tissue and Fascia with Synthetic Substitute, Percutaneous Approach

0JUM3KZ Supplement of Left Upper Leg Subcutaneous Tissue and Fascia with Nonautologous Tissue Substitute, Percutaneous Approach

0JUN07Z Supplement of Right Lower Leg Subcutaneous Tissue and Fascia with Autologous Tissue Substitute, Open Approach

0JUN0JZ Supplement of Right Lower Leg Subcutaneous Tissue and Fascia with Synthetic Substitute, Open Approach

0JUN0KZ Supplement of Right Lower Leg Subcutaneous Tissue and Fascia with Nonautologous Tissue Substitute, Open Approach

0JUN37Z Supplement of Right Lower Leg Subcutaneous Tissue and Fascia with Autologous Tissue Substitute, Percutaneous Approach

0JUN3JZ Supplement of Right Lower Leg Subcutaneous Tissue and Fascia with Synthetic Substitute, Percutaneous Approach

0JUN3KZ Supplement of Right Lower Leg Subcutaneous Tissue and Fascia with Nonautologous Tissue Substitute, Percutaneous Approach

0JUP07Z Supplement of Left Lower Leg Subcutaneous Tissue and Fascia with Autologous Tissue Substitute, Open Approach

0JUP0JZ Supplement of Left Lower Leg Subcutaneous Tissue and Fascia with Synthetic Substitute, Open Approach

0JUP0KZ Supplement of Left Lower Leg Subcutaneous Tissue and Fascia with Nonautologous Tissue Substitute, Open Approach

0JUP37Z Supplement of Left Lower Leg Subcutaneous Tissue and Fascia with Autologous Tissue Substitute, Percutaneous Approach

0JUP3JZ Supplement of Left Lower Leg Subcutaneous Tissue and Fascia with Synthetic Substitute, Percutaneous Approach

0JUP3KZ Supplement of Left Lower Leg Subcutaneous Tissue and Fascia with Nonautologous Tissue Substitute, Percutaneous Approach

0JUQ07Z Supplement of Right Foot Subcutaneous Tissue and Fascia with Autologous Tissue Substitute, Open Approach

0JUQ0JZ Supplement of Right Foot Subcutaneous Tissue and Fascia with Synthetic Substitute, Open Approach

0JUQ0KZ Supplement of Right Foot Subcutaneous Tissue and Fascia with Nonautologous Tissue Substitute, Open Approach

0JUQ37Z Supplement of Right Foot Subcutaneous Tissue and Fascia with Autologous Tissue Substitute, Percutaneous Approach

0JUQ3JZ Supplement of Right Foot Subcutaneous Tissue and Fascia with Synthetic Substitute, Percutaneous Approach

0JUQ3KZ Supplement of Right Foot Subcutaneous Tissue and Fascia with Nonautologous Tissue Substitute, Percutaneous Approach

0JUR07Z Supplement of Left Foot Subcutaneous Tissue and Fascia with Autologous Tissue Substitute, Open Approach

0JUR0JZ Supplement of Left Foot Subcutaneous Tissue and Fascia with Synthetic Substitute, Open Approach

0JUR0KZ Supplement of Left Foot Subcutaneous Tissue and Fascia with Nonautologous Tissue Substitute, Open Approach

0JUR37Z Supplement of Left Foot Subcutaneous Tissue and Fascia with Autologous Tissue Substitute, Percutaneous Approach

0JUR3JZ Supplement of Left Foot Subcutaneous Tissue and Fascia with Synthetic Substitute, Percutaneous Approach

0JUR3KZ Supplement of Left Foot Subcutaneous Tissue and Fascia with Nonautologous Tissue Substitute, Percutaneous Approach

Review Coding Guideline B6.1c

0JWS00Z	Revision of Drainage Device in Head and Neck Subcutaneous Tissue and Fascia, Open Approach	
0JWS03Z	Revision of Infusion Device in Head and Neck Subcutaneous Tissue and Fascia, Open Approach	
0JWS07Z	Revision of Autologous Tissue Substitute in Head and Neck Subcutaneous Tissue and Fascia, Open Approach	
0JWS0JZ	Revision of Synthetic Substitute in Head and Neck Subcutaneous Tissue and Fascia, Open Approach	

AHA CC: 2Q, 2015, 9-10

0JWS0KZ	Revision of Nonautologous Tissue Substitute in Head and Neck Subcutaneous Tissue and Fascia, Open Approach
0JWS0NZ	Revision of Tissue Expander in Head and Neck Subcutaneous Tissue and Fascia, Open Approach
0JWS0YZ	Revision of Other Device in Head and Neck Subcutaneous Tissue and Fascia, Open Approach
0JWS30Z	Revision of Drainage Device in Head and Neck Subcutaneous Tissue and Fascia, Percutaneous Approach
0JWS33Z	Revision of Infusion Device in Head and Neck Subcutaneous Tissue and Fascia, Percutaneous Approach
0JWS37Z	Revision of Autologous Tissue Substitute in Head and Neck Subcutaneous Tissue and Fascia, Percutaneous Approach
● **0JWS3JZ**	Revision of Synthetic Substitute in Head and Neck Subcutaneous Tissue and Fascia, Percutaneous Approach
● **0JWS3KZ**	Revision of Nonautologous Tissue Substitute in Head and Neck Subcutaneous Tissue and Fascia, Percutaneous Approach
● **0JWS3NZ**	Revision of Tissue Expander in Head and Neck Subcutaneous Tissue and Fascia, Percutaneous Approach
● **0JWS3YZ**	Revision of Other Device in Head and Neck Subcutaneous Tissue and Fascia, Percutaneous Approach
0JWSX0Z	Revision of Drainage Device in Head and Neck Subcutaneous Tissue and Fascia, External Approach
0JWSX3Z	Revision of Infusion Device in Head and Neck Subcutaneous Tissue and Fascia, External Approach
0JWSX7Z	Revision of Autologous Tissue Substitute in Head and Neck Subcutaneous Tissue and Fascia, External Approach
0JWSXJZ	Revision of Synthetic Substitute in Head and Neck Subcutaneous Tissue and Fascia, External Approach
0JWSXKZ	Revision of Nonautologous Tissue Substitute in Head and Neck Subcutaneous Tissue and Fascia, External Approach

0JWSXNZ	Revision of Tissue Expander in Head and Neck Subcutaneous Tissue and Fascia, External Approach
● **0JWT00Z**	Revision of Drainage Device in Trunk Subcutaneous Tissue and Fascia, Open Approach
0JWT02Z	Revision of Monitoring Device in Trunk Subcutaneous Tissue and Fascia, Open Approach
● **0JWT03Z**	Revision of Infusion Device in Trunk Subcutaneous Tissue and Fascia, Open Approach
● **0JWT07Z**	Revision of Autologous Tissue Substitute in Trunk Subcutaneous Tissue and Fascia, Open Approach
0JWT0FZ	Revision of Subcutaneous Defibrillator Lead in Trunk Subcutaneous Tissue and Fascia, Open Approach

HAC With a secondary diagnosis code of K68.11, T81.40XA, T81.41XA, T81.42XA, T81.43XA, T81.44XA, T81.49XA, T82.6XXA, T82.7XXA

● **0JWT0HZ**	Revision of Contraceptive Device in Trunk Subcutaneous Tissue and Fascia, Open Approach
● **0JWT0JZ**	Revision of Synthetic Substitute in Trunk Subcutaneous Tissue and Fascia, Open Approach

AHA CC: 1Q, 2018, 8-9

● **0JWT0KZ**	Revision of Nonautologous Tissue Substitute in Trunk Subcutaneous Tissue and Fascia, Open Approach
● **0JWT0MZ**	Revision of Stimulator Generator in Trunk Subcutaneous Tissue and Fascia, Open Approach
● **0JWT0NZ**	Revision of Tissue Expander in Trunk Subcutaneous Tissue and Fascia, Open Approach
0JWT0PZ	Revision of Cardiac Rhythm Related Device in Trunk Subcutaneous Tissue and Fascia, Open Approach

AHA CC: 4Q, 2012, 104-106

HAC With a secondary diagnosis code of K68.11, T81.40XA, T81.41XA, T81.42XA, T81.43XA, T81.44XA, T82.6XXA, T82.7XXA

● **0JWT0VZ**	Revision of Infusion Pump in Trunk Subcutaneous Tissue and Fascia, Open Approach
● **0JWT0WZ**	Revision of Totally Implantable Vascular Access Device in Trunk Subcutaneous Tissue and Fascia, Open Approach
● **0JWT0XZ**	Revision of Tunneled Vascular Access Device in Trunk Subcutaneous Tissue and Fascia, Open Approach
0JWT0YZ	Revision of Other Device in Trunk Subcutaneous Tissue and Fascia, Open Approach
● **0JWT30Z**	Revision of Drainage Device in Trunk Subcutaneous Tissue and Fascia, Percutaneous Approach
0JWT32Z	Revision of Monitoring Device in Trunk Subcutaneous Tissue and Fascia, Percutaneous Approach

● **0JWT33Z**	Revision of Infusion Device in Trunk Subcutaneous Tissue and Fascia, Percutaneous Approach

AHA CC: 4Q, 2015, 33

● **0JWT37Z**	Revision of Autologous Tissue Substitute in Trunk Subcutaneous Tissue and Fascia, Percutaneous Approach
0JWT3FZ	Revision of Subcutaneous Defibrillator Lead in Trunk Subcutaneous Tissue and Fascia, Percutaneous Approach

HAC With a secondary diagnosis code of K68.11, T81.40XA, T81.41XA, T81.42XA, T81.43XA, T81.44XA, T81.49XA, T82.6XXA, T82.7XXA

● **0JWT3HZ**	Revision of Contraceptive Device in Trunk Subcutaneous Tissue and Fascia, Percutaneous Approach
● **0JWT3JZ**	Revision of Synthetic Substitute in Trunk Subcutaneous Tissue and Fascia, Percutaneous Approach
● **0JWT3KZ**	Revision of Nonautologous Tissue Substitute in Trunk Subcutaneous Tissue and Fascia, Percutaneous Approach
● **0JWT3MZ**	Revision of Stimulator Generator in Trunk Subcutaneous Tissue and Fascia, Percutaneous Approach
● **0JWT3NZ**	Revision of Tissue Expander in Trunk Subcutaneous Tissue and Fascia, Percutaneous Approach
0JWT3PZ	Revision of Cardiac Rhythm Related Device in Trunk Subcutaneous Tissue and Fascia, Percutaneous Approach

HAC With a secondary diagnosis code of K68.11, T81.40XA, T81.41XA, T81.42XA, T81.43XA, T81.44XA T82.6XXA, T82.7XXA

● **0JWT3VZ**	Revision of Infusion Pump in Trunk Subcutaneous Tissue and Fascia, Percutaneous Approach
● **0JWT3WZ**	Revision of Totally Implantable Vascular Access Device in Trunk Subcutaneous Tissue and Fascia, Percutaneous Approach
● **0JWT3XZ**	Revision of Tunneled Vascular Access Device in Trunk Subcutaneous Tissue and Fascia, Percutaneous Approach
0JWT3YZ	Revision of Other Device in Trunk Subcutaneous Tissue and Fascia, Percutaneous Approach
0JWTX0Z	Revision of Drainage Device in Trunk Subcutaneous Tissue and Fascia, External Approach
0JWTX2Z	Revision of Monitoring Device in Trunk Subcutaneous Tissue and Fascia, External Approach
0JWTX3Z	Revision of Infusion Device in Trunk Subcutaneous Tissue and Fascia, External Approach
0JWTX7Z	Revision of Autologous Tissue Substitute in Trunk Subcutaneous Tissue and Fascia, External Approach
0JWTXFZ	Revision of Subcutaneous Defibrillator Lead in Trunk Subcutaneous Tissue and Fascia, External Approach

♀ Female-only	♂ Male-only	▲ Limited Coverage	● Non-OR	HAC HAC-associated procedure	▲ Non-covered procedures	+ Cluster

0JWTXHZ Revision of Contraceptive Device in Trunk Subcutaneous Tissue and Fascia, External Approach

0JWTXJZ Revision of Synthetic Substitute in Trunk Subcutaneous Tissue and Fascia, External Approach

0JWTXKZ Revision of Nonautologous Tissue Substitute in Trunk Subcutaneous Tissue and Fascia, External Approach

● **0JWTXMZ** Revision of Stimulator Generator in Trunk Subcutaneous Tissue and Fascia, External Approach

0JWTXNZ Revision of Tissue Expander in Trunk Subcutaneous Tissue and Fascia, External Approach

0JWTXPZ Revision of Cardiac Rhythm Related Device in Trunk Subcutaneous Tissue and Fascia, External Approach

0JWTXVZ Revision of Infusion Pump in Trunk Subcutaneous Tissue and Fascia, External Approach

0JWTXWZ Revision of Totally Implantable Vascular Access Device in Trunk Subcutaneous Tissue and Fascia, External Approach

0JWTXXZ Revision of Tunneled Vascular Access Device in Trunk Subcutaneous Tissue and Fascia, External Approach

● **0JWV00Z** Revision of Drainage Device in Upper Extremity Subcutaneous Tissue and Fascia, Open Approach

● **0JWV03Z** Revision of Infusion Device in Upper Extremity Subcutaneous Tissue and Fascia, Open Approach

● **0JWV07Z** Revision of Autologous Tissue Substitute in Upper Extremity Subcutaneous Tissue and Fascia, Open Approach

● **0JWV0HZ** Revision of Contraceptive Device in Upper Extremity Subcutaneous Tissue and Fascia, Open Approach

● **0JWV0JZ** Revision of Synthetic Substitute in Upper Extremity Subcutaneous Tissue and Fascia, Open Approach

● **0JWV0KZ** Revision of Nonautologous Tissue Substitute in Upper Extremity Subcutaneous Tissue and Fascia, Open Approach

● **0JWV0NZ** Revision of Tissue Expander in Upper Extremity Subcutaneous Tissue and Fascia, Open Approach

● **0JWV0VZ** Revision of Infusion Pump in Upper Extremity Subcutaneous Tissue and Fascia, Open Approach

● **0JWV0WZ** Revision of Totally Implantable Vascular Access Device in Upper Extremity Subcutaneous Tissue and Fascia, Open Approach

● **0JWV0XZ** Revision of Tunneled Vascular Access Device in Upper Extremity Subcutaneous Tissue and Fascia, Open Approach

● **0JWV0YZ** Revision of Other Device in Upper Extremity Subcutaneous Tissue and Fascia, Open Approach

● **0JWV30Z** Revision of Drainage Device in Upper Extremity Subcutaneous Tissue and Fascia, Percutaneous Approach

● **0JWV33Z** Revision of Infusion Device in Upper Extremity Subcutaneous Tissue and Fascia, Percutaneous Approach

● **0JWV37Z** Revision of Autologous Tissue Substitute in Upper Extremity Subcutaneous Tissue and Fascia, Percutaneous Approach

● **0JWV3HZ** Revision of Contraceptive Device in Upper Extremity Subcutaneous Tissue and Fascia, Percutaneous Approach

● **0JWV3JZ** Revision of Synthetic Substitute in Upper Extremity Subcutaneous Tissue and Fascia, Percutaneous Approach

● **0JWV3KZ** Revision of Nonautologous Tissue Substitute in Upper Extremity Subcutaneous Tissue and Fascia, Percutaneous Approach

● **0JWV3NZ** Revision of Tissue Expander in Upper Extremity Subcutaneous Tissue and Fascia, Percutaneous Approach

● **0JWV3VZ** Revision of Infusion Pump in Upper Extremity Subcutaneous Tissue and Fascia, Percutaneous Approach

● **0JWV3WZ** Revision of Totally Implantable Vascular Access Device in Upper Extremity Subcutaneous Tissue and Fascia, Percutaneous Approach

● **0JWV3XZ** Revision of Tunneled Vascular Access Device in Upper Extremity Subcutaneous Tissue and Fascia, Percutaneous Approach

● **0JWV3YZ** Revision of Other Device in Upper Extremity Subcutaneous Tissue and Fascia, Percutaneous Approach

0JWVX0Z Revision of Drainage Device in Upper Extremity Subcutaneous Tissue and Fascia, External Approach

0JWVX3Z Revision of Infusion Device in Upper Extremity Subcutaneous Tissue and Fascia, External Approach

0JWVX7Z Revision of Autologous Tissue Substitute in Upper Extremity Subcutaneous Tissue and Fascia, External Approach

0JWVXHZ Revision of Contraceptive Device in Upper Extremity Subcutaneous Tissue and Fascia, External Approach

0JWVXJZ Revision of Synthetic Substitute in Upper Extremity Subcutaneous Tissue and Fascia, External Approach

0JWVXKZ Revision of Nonautologous Tissue Substitute in Upper Extremity Subcutaneous Tissue and Fascia, External Approach

0JWVXNZ Revision of Tissue Expander in Upper Extremity Subcutaneous Tissue and Fascia, External Approach

0JWVXVZ Revision of Infusion Pump in Upper Extremity Subcutaneous Tissue and Fascia, External Approach

0JWVXWZ Revision of Totally Implantable Vascular Access Device in Upper Extremity Subcutaneous Tissue and Fascia, External Approach

0JWVXXZ Revision of Tunneled Vascular Access Device in Upper Extremity Subcutaneous Tissue and Fascia, External Approach

● **0JWW00Z** Revision of Drainage Device in Lower Extremity Subcutaneous Tissue and Fascia, Open Approach

● **0JWW03Z** Revision of Infusion Device in Lower Extremity Subcutaneous Tissue and Fascia, Open Approach

● **0JWW07Z** Revision of Autologous Tissue Substitute in Lower Extremity Subcutaneous Tissue and Fascia, Open Approach

● **0JWW0HZ** Revision of Contraceptive Device in Lower Extremity Subcutaneous Tissue and Fascia, Open Approach

● **0JWW0JZ** Revision of Synthetic Substitute in Lower Extremity Subcutaneous Tissue and Fascia, Open Approach

● **0JWW0KZ** Revision of Nonautologous Tissue Substitute in Lower Extremity Subcutaneous Tissue and Fascia, Open Approach

● **0JWW0NZ** Revision of Tissue Expander in Lower Extremity Subcutaneous Tissue and Fascia, Open Approach

● **0JWW0VZ** Revision of Infusion Pump in Lower Extremity Subcutaneous Tissue and Fascia, Open Approach

● **0JWW0WZ** Revision of Totally Implantable Vascular Access Device in Lower Extremity Subcutaneous Tissue and Fascia, Open Approach

● **0JWW0XZ** Revision of Tunneled Vascular Access Device in Lower Extremity Subcutaneous Tissue and Fascia, Open Approach

● **0JWW0YZ** Revision of Other Device in Lower Extremity Subcutaneous Tissue and Fascia, Open Approach

● **0JWW30Z** Revision of Drainage Device in Lower Extremity Subcutaneous Tissue and Fascia, Percutaneous Approach

● **0JWW33Z** Revision of Infusion Device in Lower Extremity Subcutaneous Tissue and Fascia, Percutaneous Approach

● **0JWW37Z** Revision of Autologous Tissue Substitute in Lower Extremity Subcutaneous Tissue and Fascia, Percutaneous Approach

● **0JWW3HZ** Revision of Contraceptive Device in Lower Extremity Subcutaneous Tissue and Fascia, Percutaneous Approach

● **0JWW3JZ** Revision of Synthetic Substitute in Lower Extremity Subcutaneous Tissue and Fascia, Percutaneous Approach

● **0JWW3KZ** Revision of Nonautologous Tissue Substitute in Lower Extremity Subcutaneous Tissue and Fascia, Percutaneous Approach

● **0JWW3NZ** Revision of Tissue Expander in Lower Extremity Subcutaneous Tissue and Fascia, Percutaneous Approach

● **0JWW3VZ** Revision of Infusion Pump in Lower Extremity Subcutaneous Tissue and Fascia, Percutaneous Approach

● **0JWW3WZ** Revision of Totally Implantable Vascular Access Device in Lower Extremity Subcutaneous Tissue and Fascia, Percutaneous Approach

● **0JWW3XZ** Revision of Tunneled Vascular Access Device in Lower Extremity Subcutaneous Tissue and Fascia, Percutaneous Approach

● **0JWW3YZ** Revision of Other Device in Lower Extremity Subcutaneous Tissue and Fascia, Percutaneous Approach

0JWWX0Z Revision of Drainage Device in Lower Extremity Subcutaneous Tissue and Fascia, External Approach

0JWWX3Z Revision of Infusion Device in Lower Extremity Subcutaneous Tissue and Fascia, External Approach

0JWWX7Z Revision of Autologous Tissue Substitute in Lower Extremity Subcutaneous Tissue and Fascia, External Approach

0JWWXHZ Revision of Contraceptive Device in Lower Extremity Subcutaneous Tissue and Fascia, External Approach

♀ Female-only ♂ Male-only ▲ Limited Coverage ● Non-OR ■ᴴᴬᶜ HAC-associated procedure ▲ Non-covered procedures ✚ Cluster

0JWWXJZ Revision of Synthetic Substitute in Lower Extremity Subcutaneous Tissue and Fascia, External Approach

0JWWXKZ Revision of Nonautologous Tissue Substitute in Lower Extremity Subcutaneous Tissue and Fascia, External Approach

0JWWXNZ Revision of Tissue Expander in Lower Extremity Subcutaneous Tissue and Fascia, External Approach

0JWWXVZ Revision of Infusion Pump in Lower Extremity Subcutaneous Tissue and Fascia, External Approach

0JWWXWZ Revision of Totally Implantable Vascular Access Device in Lower Extremity Subcutaneous Tissue and Fascia, External Approach

0JWWXXZ Revision of Tunneled Vascular Access Device in Lower Extremity Subcutaneous Tissue and Fascia, External Approach

0JX – Subcutaneous Tissue and Fascia, Transfer

Review Coding Guideline B3.17

0JX00ZB Transfer Scalp Subcutaneous Tissue and Fascia with Skin and Subcutaneous Tissue, Open Approach

0JX00ZC Transfer Scalp Subcutaneous Tissue and Fascia with Skin, Subcutaneous Tissue and Fascia, Open Approach
AHA CC: 1Q, 2018, 10

0JX00ZZ Transfer Scalp Subcutaneous Tissue and Fascia, Open Approach

0JX03ZB Transfer Scalp Subcutaneous Tissue and Fascia with Skin and Subcutaneous Tissue, Percutaneous Approach

0JX03ZC Transfer Scalp Subcutaneous Tissue and Fascia with Skin, Subcutaneous Tissue and Fascia, Percutaneous Approach

0JX03ZZ Transfer Scalp Subcutaneous Tissue and Fascia, Percutaneous Approach

0JX10ZB Transfer Face Subcutaneous Tissue and Fascia with Skin and Subcutaneous Tissue, Open Approach

0JX10ZC Transfer Face Subcutaneous Tissue and Fascia with Skin, Subcutaneous Tissue and Fascia, Open Approach

0JX10ZZ Transfer Face Subcutaneous Tissue and Fascia, Open Approach

0JX13ZB Transfer Face Subcutaneous Tissue and Fascia with Skin and Subcutaneous Tissue, Percutaneous Approach

0JX13ZC Transfer Face Subcutaneous Tissue and Fascia with Skin, Subcutaneous Tissue and Fascia, Percutaneous Approach

0JX13ZZ Transfer Face Subcutaneous Tissue and Fascia, Percutaneous Approach

0JX40ZB Transfer Right Neck Subcutaneous Tissue and Fascia with Skin and Subcutaneous Tissue, Open Approach

0JX40ZC Transfer Right Neck Subcutaneous Tissue and Fascia with Skin, Subcutaneous Tissue and Fascia, Open Approach

0JX40ZZ Transfer Right Neck Subcutaneous Tissue and Fascia, Open Approach

0JX43ZB Transfer Right Neck Subcutaneous Tissue and Fascia with Skin and Subcutaneous Tissue, Percutaneous Approach

0JX43ZC Transfer Right Neck Subcutaneous Tissue and Fascia with Skin, Subcutaneous Tissue and Fascia, Percutaneous Approach

0JX43ZZ Transfer Right Neck Subcutaneous Tissue and Fascia, Percutaneous Approach

0JX50ZB Transfer Left Neck Subcutaneous Tissue and Fascia with Skin and Subcutaneous Tissue, Open Approach

0JX50ZC Transfer Left Neck Subcutaneous Tissue and Fascia with Skin, Subcutaneous Tissue and Fascia, Open Approach

0JX50ZZ Transfer Left Neck Subcutaneous Tissue and Fascia, Open Approach

0JX53ZB Transfer Left Neck Subcutaneous Tissue and Fascia with Skin and Subcutaneous Tissue, Percutaneous Approach

0JX53ZC Transfer Left Neck Subcutaneous Tissue and Fascia with Skin, Subcutaneous Tissue and Fascia, Percutaneous Approach

0JX53ZZ Transfer Left Neck Subcutaneous Tissue and Fascia, Percutaneous Approach

0JX60ZB Transfer Chest Subcutaneous Tissue and Fascia with Skin and Subcutaneous Tissue, Open Approach
AHA CC: 4Q, 2013, 109-111; 2Q, 2021, 16-17

0JX60ZC Transfer Chest Subcutaneous Tissue and Fascia with Skin, Subcutaneous Tissue and Fascia, Open Approach

0JX60ZZ Transfer Chest Subcutaneous Tissue and Fascia, Open Approach

0JX63ZB Transfer Chest Subcutaneous Tissue and Fascia with Skin and Subcutaneous Tissue, Percutaneous Approach

0JX63ZC Transfer Chest Subcutaneous Tissue and Fascia with Skin, Subcutaneous Tissue and Fascia, Percutaneous Approach

0JX63ZZ Transfer Chest Subcutaneous Tissue and Fascia, Percutaneous Approach

0JX70ZB Transfer Back Subcutaneous Tissue and Fascia with Skin and Subcutaneous Tissue, Open Approach

0JX70ZC Transfer Back Subcutaneous Tissue and Fascia with Skin, Subcutaneous Tissue and Fascia, Open Approach

0JX70ZZ Transfer Back Subcutaneous Tissue and Fascia, Open Approach

0JX73ZB Transfer Back Subcutaneous Tissue and Fascia with Skin and Subcutaneous Tissue, Percutaneous Approach

0JX73ZC Transfer Back Subcutaneous Tissue and Fascia with Skin, Subcutaneous Tissue and Fascia, Percutaneous Approach

0JX73ZZ Transfer Back Subcutaneous Tissue and Fascia, Percutaneous Approach

0JX80ZB Transfer Abdomen Subcutaneous Tissue and Fascia with Skin and Subcutaneous Tissue, Open Approach
AHA CC: 4Q, 2013, 109-111

0JX80ZC Transfer Abdomen Subcutaneous Tissue and Fascia with Skin, Subcutaneous Tissue and Fascia, Open Approach

0JX80ZZ Transfer Abdomen Subcutaneous Tissue and Fascia, Open Approach

0JX83ZB Transfer Abdomen Subcutaneous Tissue and Fascia with Skin and Subcutaneous Tissue, Percutaneous Approach

0JX83ZC Transfer Abdomen Subcutaneous Tissue and Fascia with Skin, Subcutaneous Tissue and Fascia, Percutaneous Approach

0JX83ZZ Transfer Abdomen Subcutaneous Tissue and Fascia, Percutaneous Approach

0JX90ZB Transfer Buttock Subcutaneous Tissue and Fascia with Skin and Subcutaneous Tissue, Open Approach

0JX90ZC Transfer Buttock Subcutaneous Tissue and Fascia with Skin, Subcutaneous Tissue and Fascia, Open Approach

0JX90ZZ Transfer Buttock Subcutaneous Tissue and Fascia, Open Approach

0JX93ZB Transfer Buttock Subcutaneous Tissue and Fascia with Skin and Subcutaneous Tissue, Percutaneous Approach

0JX93ZC Transfer Buttock Subcutaneous Tissue and Fascia with Skin, Subcutaneous Tissue and Fascia, Percutaneous Approach

0JX93ZZ Transfer Buttock Subcutaneous Tissue and Fascia, Percutaneous Approach

0JXB0ZB Transfer Perineum Subcutaneous Tissue and Fascia with Skin and Subcutaneous Tissue, Open Approach

0JXB0ZC Transfer Perineum Subcutaneous Tissue and Fascia with Skin, Subcutaneous Tissue and Fascia, Open Approach

0JXB0ZZ Transfer Perineum Subcutaneous Tissue and Fascia, Open Approach

0JXB3ZB Transfer Perineum Subcutaneous Tissue and Fascia with Skin and Subcutaneous Tissue, Percutaneous Approach

0JXB3ZC Transfer Perineum Subcutaneous Tissue and Fascia with Skin, Subcutaneous Tissue and Fascia, Percutaneous Approach

0JXB3ZZ Transfer Perineum Subcutaneous Tissue and Fascia, Percutaneous Approach

0JXC0ZB Transfer Pelvic Region Subcutaneous Tissue and Fascia with Skin and Subcutaneous Tissue, Open Approach

0JXC0ZC Transfer Pelvic Region Subcutaneous Tissue and Fascia with Skin, Subcutaneous Tissue and Fascia, Open Approach

0JXC0ZZ Transfer Pelvic Region Subcutaneous Tissue and Fascia, Open Approach

0JXC3ZB Transfer Pelvic Region Subcutaneous Tissue and Fascia with Skin and Subcutaneous Tissue, Percutaneous Approach

0JXC3ZC Transfer Pelvic Region Subcutaneous Tissue and Fascia with Skin, Subcutaneous Tissue and Fascia, Percutaneous Approach

---

♀ Female-only   ♂ Male-only   ▲ Limited Coverage   ● Non-OR   HAC HAC-associated procedure   ▲ Non-covered procedures   ✚ Cluster

0JXC3ZZ Transfer Pelvic Region Subcutaneous Tissue and Fascia, Percutaneous Approach

0JXD0ZB Transfer Right Upper Arm Subcutaneous Tissue and Fascia with Skin and Subcutaneous Tissue, Open Approach

0JXD0ZC Transfer Right Upper Arm Subcutaneous Tissue and Fascia with Skin, Subcutaneous Tissue and Fascia, Open Approach

0JXD0ZZ Transfer Right Upper Arm Subcutaneous Tissue and Fascia, Open Approach

0JXD3ZB Transfer Right Upper Arm Subcutaneous Tissue and Fascia with Skin and Subcutaneous Tissue, Percutaneous Approach

0JXD3ZC Transfer Right Upper Arm Subcutaneous Tissue and Fascia with Skin, Subcutaneous Tissue and Fascia, Percutaneous Approach

0JXD3ZZ Transfer Right Upper Arm Subcutaneous Tissue and Fascia, Percutaneous Approach

0JXF0ZB Transfer Left Upper Arm Subcutaneous Tissue and Fascia with Skin and Subcutaneous Tissue, Open Approach

0JXF0ZC Transfer Left Upper Arm Subcutaneous Tissue and Fascia with Skin, Subcutaneous Tissue and Fascia, Open Approach

0JXF0ZZ Transfer Left Upper Arm Subcutaneous Tissue and Fascia, Open Approach

0JXF3ZB Transfer Left Upper Arm Subcutaneous Tissue and Fascia with Skin and Subcutaneous Tissue, Percutaneous Approach

0JXF3ZC Transfer Left Upper Arm Subcutaneous Tissue and Fascia with Skin, Subcutaneous Tissue and Fascia, Percutaneous Approach

0JXF3ZZ Transfer Left Upper Arm Subcutaneous Tissue and Fascia, Percutaneous Approach

0JXG0ZB Transfer Right Lower Arm Subcutaneous Tissue and Fascia with Skin and Subcutaneous Tissue, Open Approach

0JXG0ZC Transfer Right Lower Arm Subcutaneous Tissue and Fascia with Skin, Subcutaneous Tissue and Fascia, Open Approach

0JXG0ZZ Transfer Right Lower Arm Subcutaneous Tissue and Fascia, Open Approach

0JXG3ZB Transfer Right Lower Arm Subcutaneous Tissue and Fascia with Skin and Subcutaneous Tissue, Percutaneous Approach

0JXG3ZC Transfer Right Lower Arm Subcutaneous Tissue and Fascia with Skin, Subcutaneous Tissue and Fascia, Percutaneous Approach

0JXG3ZZ Transfer Right Lower Arm Subcutaneous Tissue and Fascia, Percutaneous Approach

0JXH0ZB Transfer Left Lower Arm Subcutaneous Tissue and Fascia with Skin and Subcutaneous Tissue, Open Approach

0JXH0ZC Transfer Left Lower Arm Subcutaneous Tissue and Fascia with Skin, Subcutaneous Tissue and Fascia, Open Approach

0JXH0ZZ Transfer Left Lower Arm Subcutaneous Tissue and Fascia, Open Approach

0JXH3ZB Transfer Left Lower Arm Subcutaneous Tissue and Fascia with Skin and Subcutaneous Tissue, Percutaneous Approach

0JXH3ZC Transfer Left Lower Arm Subcutaneous Tissue and Fascia with Skin, Subcutaneous Tissue and Fascia, Percutaneous Approach

0JXH3ZZ Transfer Left Lower Arm Subcutaneous Tissue and Fascia, Percutaneous Approach

0JXJ0ZB Transfer Right Hand Subcutaneous Tissue and Fascia with Skin and Subcutaneous Tissue, Open Approach

0JXJ0ZC Transfer Right Hand Subcutaneous Tissue and Fascia with Skin, Subcutaneous Tissue and Fascia, Open Approach

0JXJ0ZZ Transfer Right Hand Subcutaneous Tissue and Fascia, Open Approach

0JXJ3ZB Transfer Right Hand Subcutaneous Tissue and Fascia with Skin and Subcutaneous Tissue, Percutaneous Approach

0JXJ3ZC Transfer Right Hand Subcutaneous Tissue and Fascia with Skin, Subcutaneous Tissue and Fascia, Percutaneous Approach

0JXJ3ZZ Transfer Right Hand Subcutaneous Tissue and Fascia, Percutaneous Approach

0JXK0ZB Transfer Left Hand Subcutaneous Tissue and Fascia with Skin and Subcutaneous Tissue, Open Approach

0JXK0ZC Transfer Left Hand Subcutaneous Tissue and Fascia with Skin, Subcutaneous Tissue and Fascia, Open Approach

0JXK0ZZ Transfer Left Hand Subcutaneous Tissue and Fascia, Open Approach

0JXK3ZB Transfer Left Hand Subcutaneous Tissue and Fascia with Skin and Subcutaneous Tissue, Percutaneous Approach

0JXK3ZC Transfer Left Hand Subcutaneous Tissue and Fascia with Skin, Subcutaneous Tissue and Fascia, Percutaneous Approach

0JXK3ZZ Transfer Left Hand Subcutaneous Tissue and Fascia, Percutaneous Approach

0JXL0ZB Transfer Right Upper Leg Subcutaneous Tissue and Fascia with Skin and Subcutaneous Tissue, Open Approach

0JXL0ZC Transfer Right Upper Leg Subcutaneous Tissue and Fascia with Skin, Subcutaneous Tissue and Fascia, Open Approach

0JXL0ZZ Transfer Right Upper Leg Subcutaneous Tissue and Fascia, Open Approach

0JXL3ZB Transfer Right Upper Leg Subcutaneous Tissue and Fascia with Skin and Subcutaneous Tissue, Percutaneous Approach

0JXL3ZC Transfer Right Upper Leg Subcutaneous Tissue and Fascia with Skin, Subcutaneous Tissue and Fascia, Percutaneous Approach

0JXL3ZZ Transfer Right Upper Leg Subcutaneous Tissue and Fascia, Percutaneous Approach

0JXM0ZB Transfer Left Upper Leg Subcutaneous Tissue and Fascia with Skin and Subcutaneous Tissue, Open Approach

0JXM0ZC Transfer Left Upper Leg Subcutaneous Tissue and Fascia with Skin, Subcutaneous Tissue and Fascia, Open Approach

0JXM0ZZ Transfer Left Upper Leg Subcutaneous Tissue and Fascia, Open Approach

0JXM3ZB Transfer Left Upper Leg Subcutaneous Tissue and Fascia with Skin and Subcutaneous Tissue, Percutaneous Approach

0JXM3ZC Transfer Left Upper Leg Subcutaneous Tissue and Fascia with Skin, Subcutaneous Tissue and Fascia, Percutaneous Approach

0JXM3ZZ Transfer Left Upper Leg Subcutaneous Tissue and Fascia, Percutaneous Approach

0JXN0ZB Transfer Right Lower Leg Subcutaneous Tissue and Fascia with Skin and Subcutaneous Tissue, Open Approach

0JXN0ZC Transfer Right Lower Leg Subcutaneous Tissue and Fascia with Skin, Subcutaneous Tissue and Fascia, Open Approach

AHA CC: 3Q, 2014, 18-19

0JXN0ZZ Transfer Right Lower Leg Subcutaneous Tissue and Fascia, Open Approach

0JXN3ZB Transfer Right Lower Leg Subcutaneous Tissue and Fascia with Skin and Subcutaneous Tissue, Percutaneous Approach

0JXN3ZC Transfer Right Lower Leg Subcutaneous Tissue and Fascia with Skin, Subcutaneous Tissue and Fascia, Percutaneous Approach

0JXN3ZZ Transfer Right Lower Leg Subcutaneous Tissue and Fascia, Percutaneous Approach

0JXP0ZB Transfer Left Lower Leg Subcutaneous Tissue and Fascia with Skin and Subcutaneous Tissue, Open Approach

0JXP0ZC Transfer Left Lower Leg Subcutaneous Tissue and Fascia with Skin, Subcutaneous Tissue and Fascia, Open Approach

0JXP0ZZ Transfer Left Lower Leg Subcutaneous Tissue and Fascia, Open Approach

0JXP3ZB Transfer Left Lower Leg Subcutaneous Tissue and Fascia with Skin and Subcutaneous Tissue, Percutaneous Approach

0JXP3ZC Transfer Left Lower Leg Subcutaneous Tissue and Fascia with Skin, Subcutaneous Tissue and Fascia, Percutaneous Approach

0JXP3ZZ Transfer Left Lower Leg Subcutaneous Tissue and Fascia, Percutaneous Approach

0JXQ0ZB Transfer Right Foot Subcutaneous Tissue and Fascia with Skin and Subcutaneous Tissue, Open Approach

0JXQ0ZC Transfer Right Foot Subcutaneous Tissue and Fascia with Skin, Subcutaneous Tissue and Fascia, Open Approach

0JXQ0ZZ Transfer Right Foot Subcutaneous Tissue and Fascia, Open Approach

0JXQ3ZB Transfer Right Foot Subcutaneous Tissue and Fascia with Skin and Subcutaneous Tissue, Percutaneous Approach

♀ Female-only   ♂ Male-only   ▲ Limited Coverage   ● Non-OR   🅷🅰🅲 HAC-associated procedure   ▲ Non-covered procedures   ➕ Cluster

0JXQ3ZC Transfer Right Foot Subcutaneous Tissue and Fascia with Skin, Subcutaneous Tissue and Fascia, Percutaneous Approach

0JXQ3ZZ Transfer Right Foot Subcutaneous Tissue and Fascia, Percutaneous Approach

0JXR0ZB Transfer Left Foot Subcutaneous Tissue and Fascia with Skin and Subcutaneous Tissue, Open Approach

0JXR0ZC Transfer Left Foot Subcutaneous Tissue and Fascia with Skin, Subcutaneous Tissue and Fascia, Open Approach

0JXR0ZZ Transfer Left Foot Subcutaneous Tissue and Fascia, Open Approach

0JXR3ZB Transfer Left Foot Subcutaneous Tissue and Fascia with Skin and Subcutaneous Tissue, Percutaneous Approach

0JXR3ZC Transfer Left Foot Subcutaneous Tissue and Fascia with Skin, Subcutaneous Tissue and Fascia, Percutaneous Approach

0JXR3ZZ Transfer Left Foot Subcutaneous Tissue and Fascia, Percutaneous Approach

Muscles

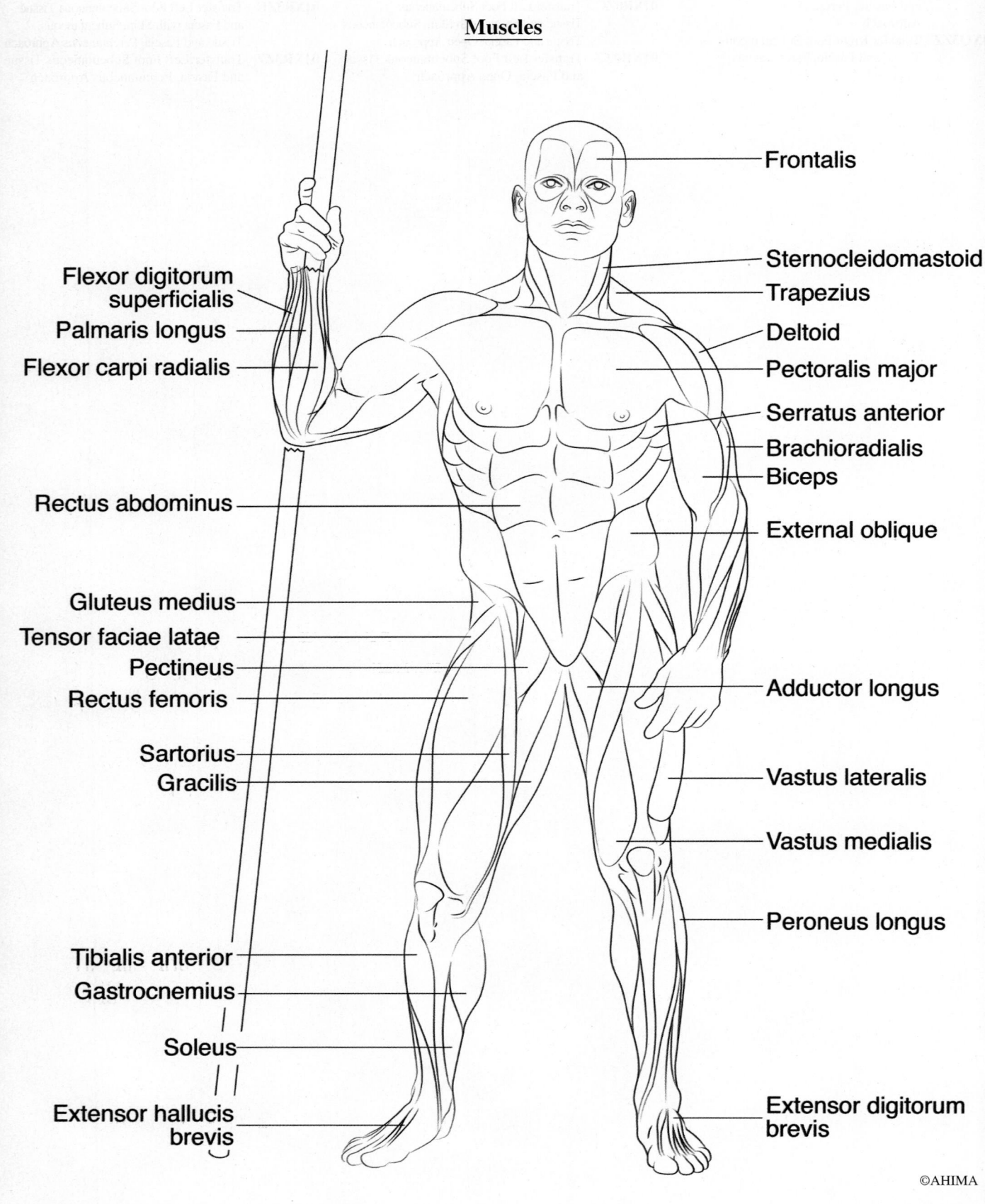

Frontalis

Sternocleidomastoid

Trapezius

Deltoid

Pectoralis major

Serratus anterior

Brachioradialis

Biceps

External oblique

Adductor longus

Vastus lateralis

Vastus medialis

Peroneus longus

Extensor digitorum brevis

Flexor digitorum superficialis

Palmaris longus

Flexor carpi radialis

Rectus abdominus

Gluteus medius

Tensor faciae latae

Pectineus

Rectus femoris

Sartorius

Gracilis

Tibialis anterior

Gastrocnemius

Soleus

Extensor hallucis brevis

©AHIMA

Muscles of the Hand

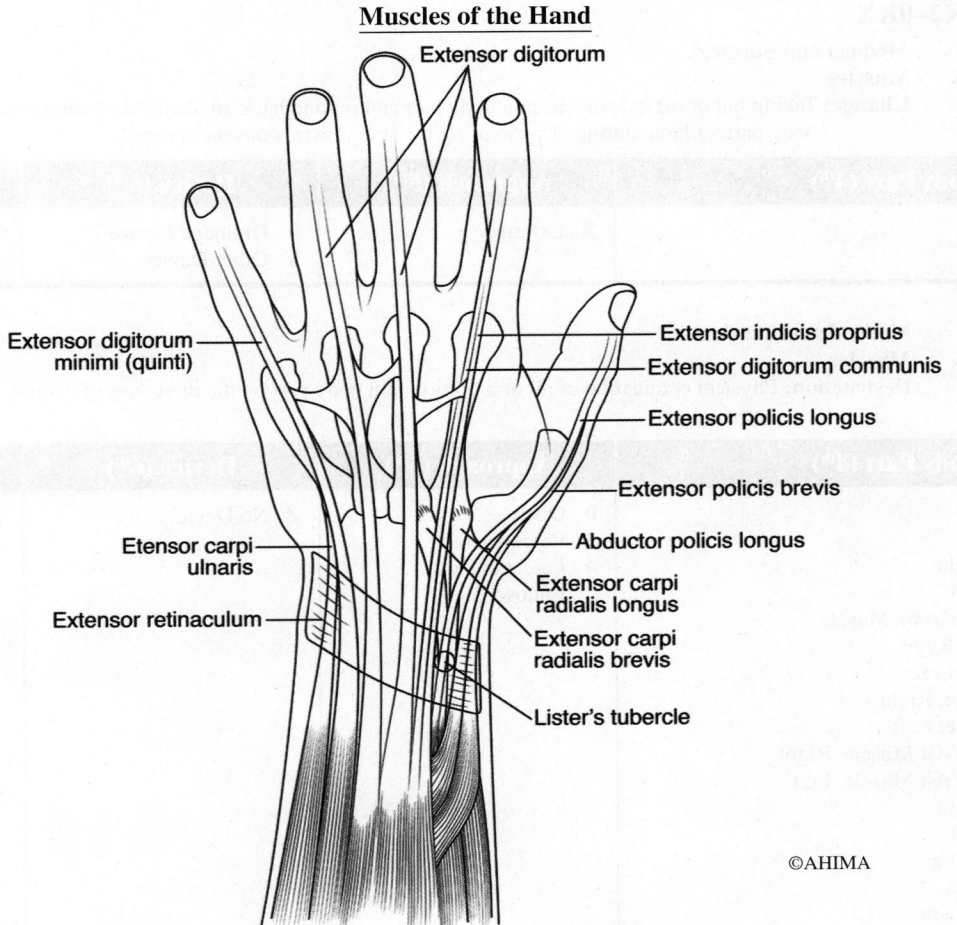

Extensor digitorum

Extensor digitorum minimi (quinti)

Etensor carpi ulnaris

Extensor retinaculum

Extensor indicis proprius

Extensor digitorum communis

Extensor policis longus

Extensor policis brevis

Abductor policis longus

Extensor carpi radialis longus

Extensor carpi radialis brevis

Lister's tubercle

©AHIMA

Muscles of the Foot

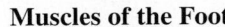

Lateral View

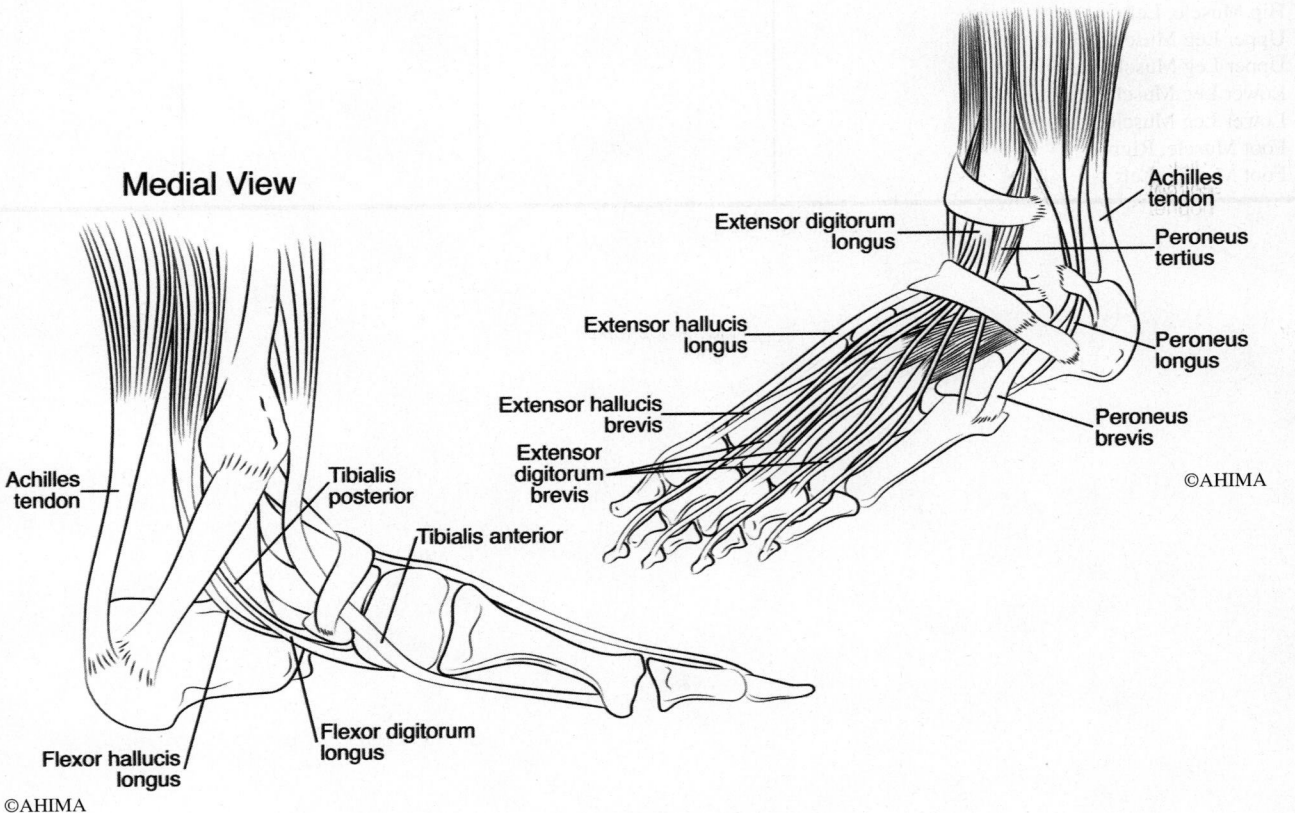

Extensor digitorum longus

Extensor hallucis longus

Extensor hallucis brevis

Extensor digitorum brevis

Achilles tendon

Peroneus tertius

Peroneus longus

Peroneus brevis

©AHIMA

Medial View

Achilles tendon

Tibialis posterior

Tibialis anterior

Flexor hallucis longus

Flexor digitorum longus

©AHIMA

Muscles Tables 0K2–0KX

Section	0	Medical and Surgical
Body System	K	Muscles
Operation	2	**Change:** Taking out or off a device from a body part and putting back an identical or similar device in or on the same body part without cutting or puncturing the skin or a mucous membrane

Body Part (4th)	Approach (5th)	Device (6th)	Qualifier (7th)
X Upper Muscle **Y** Lower Muscle	**X** External	**0** Drainage Device **Y** Other Device	**Z** No Qualifier

Section	0	Medical and Surgical
Body System	K	Muscles
Operation	5	**Destruction:** Physical eradication of all or a portion of a body part by the direct use of energy, force, or a destructive agent

Body Part (4th)	Approach (5th)	Device (6th)	Qualifier (7th)
0 Head Muscle **1** Facial Muscle **2** Neck Muscle, Right **3** Neck Muscle, Left **4** Tongue, Palate, Pharynx Muscle **5** Shoulder Muscle, Right **6** Shoulder Muscle, Left **7** Upper Arm Muscle, Right **8** Upper Arm Muscle, Left **9** Lower Arm and Wrist Muscle, Right **B** Lower Arm and Wrist Muscle, Left **C** Hand Muscle, Right **D** Hand Muscle, Left **F** Trunk Muscle, Right **G** Trunk Muscle, Left **H** Thorax Muscle, Right **J** Thorax Muscle, Left **K** Abdomen Muscle, Right **L** Abdomen Muscle, Left **M** Perineum Muscle **N** Hip Muscle, Right **P** Hip Muscle, Left **Q** Upper Leg Muscle, Right **R** Upper Leg Muscle, Left **S** Lower Leg Muscle, Right **T** Lower Leg Muscle, Left **V** Foot Muscle, Right **W** Foot Muscle, Left	**0** Open **3** Percutaneous **4** Percutaneous Endoscopic	**Z** No Device	**Z** No Qualifier

Section	0	Medical and Surgical
Body System	K	Muscles
Operation	8	**Division:** Cutting into a body part, without draining fluids and/or gases from the body part, in order to separate or transect a body part

Body Part (4th)	Approach (5th)	Device (6th)	Qualifier (7th)
0 Head Muscle **1** Facial Muscle **2** Neck Muscle, Right **3** Neck Muscle, Left **5** Shoulder Muscle, Right **6** Shoulder Muscle, Left **7** Upper Arm Muscle, Right **8** Upper Arm Muscle, Left **9** Lower Arm and Wrist Muscle, Right **B** Lower Arm and Wrist Muscle, Left **C** Hand Muscle, Right **D** Hand Muscle, Left **F** Trunk Muscle, Right **G** Trunk Muscle, Left **H** Thorax Muscle, Right **J** Thorax Muscle, Left **K** Abdomen Muscle, Right **L** Abdomen Muscle, Left **M** Perineum Muscle **N** Hip Muscle, Right **P** Hip Muscle, Left **Q** Upper Leg Muscle, Right **R** Upper Leg Muscle, Left **S** Lower Leg Muscle, Right **T** Lower Leg Muscle, Left **V** Foot Muscle, Right **W** Foot Muscle, Left	**0** Open **3** Percutaneous **4** Percutaneous Endoscopic	**Z** No Device	**Z** No Qualifier
4 Tongue, Palate, Pharynx Muscle	**0** Open **3** Percutaneous **4** Percutaneous Endoscopic **7** Via Natural or Artificial Opening **8** Via Natural or Artificial Opening Endoscopic	**Z** No Device	**Z** No Qualifier

Body Part (4ᵗʰ)	Approach (5ᵗʰ)	Device (6ᵗʰ)	Qualifier (7ᵗʰ)
0 Head Muscle 1 Facial Muscle 2 Neck Muscle, Right 3 Neck Muscle, Left 4 Tongue, Palate, Pharynx Muscle 5 Shoulder Muscle, Right 6 Shoulder Muscle, Left 7 Upper Arm Muscle, Right 8 Upper Arm Muscle, Left 9 Lower Arm and Wrist Muscle, Right B Lower Arm and Wrist Muscle, Left C Hand Muscle, Right D Hand Muscle, Left F Trunk Muscle, Right G Trunk Muscle, Left H Thorax Muscle, Right J Thorax Muscle, Left K Abdomen Muscle, Right L Abdomen Muscle, Left M Perineum Muscle N Hip Muscle, Right P Hip Muscle, Left Q Upper Leg Muscle, Right R Upper Leg Muscle, Left S Lower Leg Muscle, Right T Lower Leg Muscle, Left V Foot Muscle, Right W Foot Muscle, Left	0 Open 3 Percutaneous 4 Percutaneous Endoscopic	0 Drainage Device	Z No Qualifier
0 Head Muscle 1 Facial Muscle 2 Neck Muscle, Right 3 Neck Muscle, Left 4 Tongue, Palate, Pharynx Muscle 5 Shoulder Muscle, Right 6 Shoulder Muscle, Left 7 Upper Arm Muscle, Right 8 Upper Arm Muscle, Left 9 Lower Arm and Wrist Muscle, Right B Lower Arm and Wrist Muscle, Left C Hand Muscle, Right D Hand Muscle, Left F Trunk Muscle, Right G Trunk Muscle, Left H Thorax Muscle, Right J Thorax Muscle, Left K Abdomen Muscle, Right L Abdomen Muscle, Left M Perineum Muscle N Hip Muscle, Right P Hip Muscle, Left Q Upper Leg Muscle, Right R Upper Leg Muscle, Left S Lower Leg Muscle, Right T Lower Leg Muscle, Left V Foot Muscle, Right W Foot Muscle, Left	0 Open 3 Percutaneous 4 Percutaneous Endoscopic	Z No Device	X Diagnostic Z No Qualifier

Section	0	Medical and Surgical
Body System	K	Muscles
Operation	B	**Excision:** Cutting out or off, without replacement, a portion of a body part

Body Part (4th)	Approach (5th)	Device (6th)	Qualifier (7th)
0 Head Muscle 1 Facial Muscle 2 Neck Muscle, Right 3 Neck Muscle, Left 4 Tongue, Palate, Pharynx Muscle 5 Shoulder Muscle, Right 6 Shoulder Muscle, Left 7 Upper Arm Muscle, Right 8 Upper Arm Muscle, Left 9 Lower Arm and Wrist Muscle, Right B Lower Arm and Wrist Muscle, Left C Hand Muscle, Right D Hand Muscle, Left F Trunk Muscle, Right G Trunk Muscle, Left H Thorax Muscle, Right J Thorax Muscle, Left K Abdomen Muscle, Right L Abdomen Muscle, Left M Perineum Muscle N Hip Muscle, Right P Hip Muscle, Left Q Upper Leg Muscle, Right R Upper Leg Muscle, Left S Lower Leg Muscle, Right T Lower Leg Muscle, Left V Foot Muscle, Right W Foot Muscle, Left	0 Open 3 Percutaneous 4 Percutaneous Endoscopic	Z No Device	X Diagnostic Z No Qualifier

Section	0	Medical and Surgical
Body System	K	Muscles
Operation	C	**Extirpation:** Taking or cutting out solid matter from a body part

Body Part (4th)	Approach (5th)	Device (6th)	Qualifier (7th)
0 Head Muscle 1 Facial Muscle 2 Neck Muscle, Right 3 Neck Muscle, Left 4 Tongue, Palate, Pharynx Muscle 5 Shoulder Muscle, Right 6 Shoulder Muscle, Left 7 Upper Arm Muscle, Right 8 Upper Arm Muscle, Left 9 Lower Arm and Wrist Muscle, Right B Lower Arm and Wrist Muscle, Left C Hand Muscle, Right D Hand Muscle, Left F Trunk Muscle, Right G Trunk Muscle, Left H Thorax Muscle, Right J Thorax Muscle, Left K Abdomen Muscle, Right L Abdomen Muscle, Left M Perineum Muscle N Hip Muscle, Right P Hip Muscle, Left Q Upper Leg Muscle, Right R Upper Leg Muscle, Left S Lower Leg Muscle, Right T Lower Leg Muscle, Left V Foot Muscle, Right W Foot Muscle, Left	0 Open 3 Percutaneous 4 Percutaneous Endoscopic	Z No Device	Z No Qualifier

Section	0	Medical and Surgical
Body System	K	Muscles
Operation	D	**Extraction:** Pulling or stripping out or off all or a portion of a body part by the use of force

Body Part (4th)	Approach (5th)	Device (6th)	Qualifier (7th)
0 Head Muscle	0 Open	Z No Device	Z No Qualifier
1 Facial Muscle			
2 Neck Muscle, Right			
3 Neck Muscle, Left			
4 Tongue, Palate, Pharynx Muscle			
5 Shoulder Muscle, Right			
6 Shoulder Muscle, Left			
7 Upper Arm Muscle, Right			
8 Upper Arm Muscle, Left			
9 Lower Arm and Wrist Muscle, Right			
B Lower Arm and Wrist Muscle, Left			
C Hand Muscle, Right			
D Hand Muscle, Left			
F Trunk Muscle, Right			
G Trunk Muscle, Left			
H Thorax Muscle, Right			
J Thorax Muscle, Left			
K Abdomen Muscle, Right			
L Abdomen Muscle, Left			
M Perineum			
N Hip Muscle, Right			
P Hip Muscle, Left			
Q Upper Leg Muscle, Right			
R Upper Leg Muscle, Left			
S Lower Leg Muscle, Right			
T Lower Leg Muscle, Left			
V Foot Muscle, Right			
W Foot Muscle, Left			

Section	0	Medical and Surgical
Body System	K	Muscles
Operation	H	**Insertion:** Putting in a nonbiological appliance that monitors, assists, performs, or prevents a physiological function but does not physically take the place of a body part

Body Part (4th)	Approach (5th)	Device (6th)	Qualifier (7th)
X Upper Muscle	0 Open	M Stimulator Lead	Z No Qualifier
Y Lower Muscle	3 Percutaneous	Y Other Device	
	4 Percutaneous Endoscopic		

Section	0	Medical and Surgical
Body System	K	Muscles
Operation	J	**Inspection:** Visually and/or manually exploring a body part

Body Part (4th)	Approach (5th)	Device (6th)	Qualifier (7th)
X Upper Muscle	0 Open	Z No Device	Z No Qualifier
Y Lower Muscle	3 Percutaneous		
	4 Percutaneous Endoscopic		
	X External		

Section	0	Medical and Surgical
Body System	K	Muscles
Operation	M	**Reattachment:** Putting back in or on all or a portion of a separated body part to its normal location or other suitable location

Body Part (4th)	Approach (5th)	Device (6th)	Qualifier (7th)
0 Head Muscle 1 Facial Muscle 2 Neck Muscle, Right 3 Neck Muscle, Left 4 Tongue, Palate, Pharynx Muscle 5 Shoulder Muscle, Right 6 Shoulder Muscle, Left 7 Upper Arm Muscle, Right 8 Upper Arm Muscle, Left 9 Lower Arm and Wrist Muscle, Right B Lower Arm and Wrist Muscle, Left C Hand Muscle, Right D Hand Muscle, Left F Trunk Muscle, Right G Trunk Muscle, Left H Thorax Muscle, Right J Thorax Muscle, Left K Abdomen Muscle, Right L Abdomen Muscle, Left M Perineum Muscle N Hip Muscle, Right P Hip Muscle, Left Q Upper Leg Muscle, Right R Upper Leg Muscle, Left S Lower Leg Muscle, Right T Lower Leg Muscle, Left V Foot Muscle, Right W Foot Muscle, Left	0 Open 4 Percutaneous Endoscopic	Z No Device	Z No Qualifier

Section	0	Medical and Surgical
Body System	K	Muscles
Operation	N	**Release:** Freeing a body part from an abnormal physical constraint by cutting or by the use of force

Body Part (4th)	Approach (5th)	Device (6th)	Qualifier (7th)
0 Head Muscle 1 Facial Muscle 2 Neck Muscle, Right 3 Neck Muscle, Left 4 Tongue, Palate, Pharynx Muscle 5 Shoulder Muscle, Right 6 Shoulder Muscle, Left 7 Upper Arm Muscle, Right 8 Upper Arm Muscle, Left 9 Lower Arm and Wrist Muscle, Right B Lower Arm and Wrist Muscle, Left C Hand Muscle, Right D Hand Muscle, Left F Trunk Muscle, Right G Trunk Muscle, Left H Thorax Muscle, Right J Thorax Muscle, Left K Abdomen Muscle, Right L Abdomen Muscle, Left M Perineum Muscle N Hip Muscle, Right P Hip Muscle, Left Q Upper Leg Muscle, Right R Upper Leg Muscle, Left S Lower Leg Muscle, Right T Lower Leg Muscle, Left V Foot Muscle, Right W Foot Muscle, Left	0 Open 3 Percutaneous 4 Percutaneous Endoscopic X External	Z No Device	Z No Qualifier

Section	0	Medical and Surgical
Body System	K	Muscles
Operation	P	**Removal:** Taking out or off a device from a body part

Body Part (4th)	Approach (5th)	Device (6th)	Qualifier (7th)
X Upper Muscle Y Lower Muscle	0 Open 3 Percutaneous 4 Percutaneous Endoscopic	0 Drainage Device 7 Autologous Tissue Substitute J Synthetic Substitute K Nonautologous Tissue Substitute M Stimulator Lead Y Other Device	Z No Qualifier
X Upper Muscle Y Lower Muscle	X External	0 Drainage Device M Stimulator Lead	Z No Qualifier

Section	0	Medical and Surgical
Body System	K	Muscles
Operation	Q	**Repair:** Restoring, to the extent possible, a body part to its normal anatomic structure and function

Body Part (4th)	Approach (5th)	Device (6th)	Qualifier (7th)
0 Head Muscle 1 Facial Muscle 2 Neck Muscle, Right 3 Neck Muscle, Left 4 Tongue, Palate, Pharynx Muscle 5 Shoulder Muscle, Right 6 Shoulder Muscle, Left 7 Upper Arm Muscle, Right 8 Upper Arm Muscle, Left 9 Lower Arm and Wrist Muscle, Right B Lower Arm and Wrist Muscle, Left C Hand Muscle, Right D Hand Muscle, Left F Trunk Muscle, Right G Trunk Muscle, Left H Thorax Muscle, Right J Thorax Muscle, Left K Abdomen Muscle, Right L Abdomen Muscle, Left M Perineum Muscle N Hip Muscle, Right P Hip Muscle, Left Q Upper Leg Muscle, Right R Upper Leg Muscle, Left S Lower Leg Muscle, Right T Lower Leg Muscle, Left V Foot Muscle, Right W Foot Muscle, Left	0 Open 3 Percutaneous 4 Percutaneous Endoscopic	Z No Device	Z No Qualifier

Section   0   **Medical and Surgical**
Body System   K   **Muscles**
Operation   R   **Replacement:** Putting in or on biological or synthetic material that physically takes the place and/or function of all or a portion of a body part

Body Part (4ᵗʰ)	Approach (5ᵗʰ)	Device (6ᵗʰ)	Qualifier (7ᵗʰ)
0 Head Muscle	0 Open	7 Autologous Tissue	Z No Qualifier
1 Facial Muscle	4 Percutaneous Endoscopic	Substitute	
2 Neck Muscle, Right		J Synthetic Substitute	
3 Neck Muscle, Left		K Nonautologous Tissue	
4 Tongue, Palate, Pharynx Muscle		Substitute	
5 Shoulder Muscle, Right			
6 Shoulder Muscle, Left			
7 Upper Arm Muscle, Right			
8 Upper Arm Muscle, Left			
9 Lower Arm and Wrist Muscle, Right			
B Lower Arm and Wrist Muscle, Left			
C Hand Muscle, Right			
D Hand Muscle, Left			
F Trunk Muscle, Right			
G Trunk Muscle, Left			
H Thorax Muscle, Right			
J Thorax Muscle, Left			
K Abdomen Muscle, Right			
L Abdomen Muscle, Left			
M Perineum			
N Hip Muscle, Right			
P Hip Muscle, Left			
Q Upper Leg Muscle, Right			
R Upper Leg Muscle, Left			
S Lower Leg Muscle, Right			
T Lower Leg Muscle, Left			
V Foot Muscle, Right			
W Foot Muscle, Left			

Section   0   **Medical and Surgical**
Body System   K   **Muscles**
Operation   S   **Reposition:** Moving to its normal location, or other suitable location, all or a portion of a body part

Body Part (4ᵗʰ)	Approach (5ᵗʰ)	Device (6ᵗʰ)	Qualifier (7ᵗʰ)
0 Head Muscle	0 Open	Z No Device	Z No Qualifier
1 Facial Muscle	4 Percutaneous Endoscopic		
2 Neck Muscle, Right			
3 Neck Muscle, Left			
4 Tongue, Palate, Pharynx Muscle			
5 Shoulder Muscle, Right			
6 Shoulder Muscle, Left			
7 Upper Arm Muscle, Right			
8 Upper Arm Muscle, Left			
9 Lower Arm and Wrist Muscle, Right			
B Lower Arm and Wrist Muscle, Left			
C Hand Muscle, Right			
D Hand Muscle, Left			
F Trunk Muscle, Right			
G Trunk Muscle, Left			
H Thorax Muscle, Right			
J Thorax Muscle, Left			
K Abdomen Muscle, Right			
L Abdomen Muscle, Left			
M Perineum Muscle			
N Hip Muscle, Right			
P Hip Muscle, Left			
Q Upper Leg Muscle, Right			
R Upper Leg Muscle, Left			
S Lower Leg Muscle, Right			
T Lower Leg Muscle, Left			
V Foot Muscle, Right			
W Foot Muscle, Left			

Section	0	Medical and Surgical
Body System	K	Muscles
Operation	T	**Resection:** Cutting out or off, without replacement, all of a body part

Body Part (4th)	Approach (5th)	Device (6th)	Qualifier (7th)
0 Head Muscle 1 Facial Muscle 2 Neck Muscle, Right 3 Neck Muscle, Left 4 Tongue, Palate, Pharynx Muscle 5 Shoulder Muscle, Right 6 Shoulder Muscle, Left 7 Upper Arm Muscle, Right 8 Upper Arm Muscle, Left 9 Lower Arm and Wrist Muscle, Right B Lower Arm and Wrist Muscle, Left C Hand Muscle, Right D Hand Muscle, Left F Trunk Muscle, Right G Trunk Muscle, Left H Thorax Muscle, Right J Thorax Muscle, Left K Abdomen Muscle, Right L Abdomen Muscle, Left M Perineum Muscle N Hip Muscle, Right P Hip Muscle, Left Q Upper Leg Muscle, Right R Upper Leg Muscle, Left S Lower Leg Muscle, Right T Lower Leg Muscle, Left V Foot Muscle, Right W Foot Muscle, Left	0 Open 4 Percutaneous Endoscopic	Z No Device	Z No Qualifier

Section	0	Medical and Surgical
Body System	K	Muscles
Operation	U	**Supplement:** Putting in or on biological or synthetic material that physically reinforces and/or augments the function of a portion of a body part

Body Part (4th)	Approach (5th)	Device (6th)	Qualifier (7th)
0 Head Muscle 1 Facial Muscle 2 Neck Muscle, Right 3 Neck Muscle, Left 4 Tongue, Palate, Pharynx Muscle 5 Shoulder Muscle, Right 6 Shoulder Muscle, Left 7 Upper Arm Muscle, Right 8 Upper Arm Muscle, Left 9 Lower Arm and Wrist Muscle, Right B Lower Arm and Wrist Muscle, Left C Hand Muscle, Right D Hand Muscle, Left F Trunk Muscle, Right G Trunk Muscle, Left H Thorax Muscle, Right J Thorax Muscle, Left K Abdomen Muscle, Right L Abdomen Muscle, Left M Perineum Muscle N Hip Muscle, Right P Hip Muscle, Left Q Upper Leg Muscle, Right R Upper Leg Muscle, Left S Lower Leg Muscle, Right T Lower Leg Muscle, Left V Foot Muscle, Right W Foot Muscle, Left	0 Open 4 Percutaneous Endoscopic	7 Autologous Tissue Substitute J Synthetic Substitute K Nonautologous Tissue Substitute	Z No Qualifier

Section	0	Medical and Surgical
Body System	K	Muscles
Operation	W	**Revision:** Correcting, to the extent possible, a portion of a malfunctioning device or the position of a displaced device

Body Part (4th)	Approach (5th)	Device (6th)	Qualifier (7th)
X Upper Muscle Y Lower Muscle	0 Open 3 Percutaneous 4 Percutaneous Endoscopic	0 Drainage Device 7 Autologous Tissue Substitute J Synthetic Substitute K Nonautologous Tissue Substitute M Stimulator Lead Y Other Device	Z No Qualifier
X Upper Muscle Y Lower Muscle	X External	0 Drainage Device 7 Autologous Tissue Substitute J Synthetic Substitute K Nonautologous Tissue Substitute M Stimulator Lead	Z No Qualifier

Section	0	Medical and Surgical
Body System	K	Muscles
Operation	X	**Transfer:** Moving, without taking out, all or a portion of a body part to another location to take over the function of all or a portion of a body part

Body Part (4th)	Approach (5th)	Device (6th)	Qualifier (7th)
0 Head Muscle 1 Facial Muscle 2 Neck Muscle, Right 3 Neck Muscle, Left 4 Tongue, Palate, Pharynx Muscle 5 Shoulder Muscle, Right 6 Shoulder Muscle, Left 7 Upper Arm Muscle, Right 8 Upper Arm Muscle, Left 9 Lower Arm and Wrist Muscle, Right B Lower Arm and Wrist Muscle, Left C Hand Muscle, Right D Hand Muscle, Left H Thorax Muscle, Right J Thorax Muscle, Left M Perineum Muscle N Hip Muscle, Right P Hip Muscle, Left Q Upper Leg Muscle, Right R Upper Leg Muscle, Left S Lower Leg Muscle, Right T Lower Leg Muscle, Left V Foot Muscle, Right W Foot Muscle, Left	0 Open 4 Percutaneous Endoscopic	Z No Device	0 Skin 1 Subcutaneous Tissue 2 Skin and Subcutaneous Tissue Z No Qualifier
F Trunk Muscle, Right G Trunk Muscle, Left	0 Open 4 Percutaneous Endoscopic	Z No Device	0 Skin 1 Subcutaneous Tissue 2 Skin and Subcutaneous Tissue 5 Latissimus Dorsi Myocutaneous Flap 7 Deep Inferior Epigastric Artery Perforator Flap 8 Superficial Inferior Epigastric Artery Flap 9 Gluteal Artery Perforator Flap Z No Qualifier
K Abdomen Muscle, Right L Abdomen Muscle, Left	0 Open 4 Percutaneous Endoscopic	Z No Device	0 Skin 1 Subcutaneous Tissue 2 Skin and Subcutaneous Tissue 6 Transverse Rectus Abdominis Myocutaneous Flap Z No Qualifier

Muscles Code Listing 0K2–0KX

0K2 – Muscles, Change

Review Coding Guideline B6.1c

0K2XX0Z Change Drainage Device in Upper Muscle, External Approach

0K2XXYZ Change Other Device in Upper Muscle, External Approach

0K2YX0Z Change Drainage Device in Lower Muscle, External Approach

0K2YXYZ Change Other Device in Lower Muscle, External Approach

0K5 – Muscles, Destruction

0K500ZZ Destruction of Head Muscle, Open Approach

0K503ZZ Destruction of Head Muscle, Percutaneous Approach

0K504ZZ Destruction of Head Muscle, Percutaneous Endoscopic Approach

0K510ZZ Destruction of Facial Muscle, Open Approach

0K513ZZ Destruction of Facial Muscle, Percutaneous Approach

0K514ZZ Destruction of Facial Muscle, Percutaneous Endoscopic Approach

0K520ZZ Destruction of Right Neck Muscle, Open Approach

0K523ZZ Destruction of Right Neck Muscle, Percutaneous Approach

0K524ZZ Destruction of Right Neck Muscle, Percutaneous Endoscopic Approach

0K530ZZ Destruction of Left Neck Muscle, Open Approach

0K533ZZ Destruction of Left Neck Muscle, Percutaneous Approach

0K534ZZ Destruction of Left Neck Muscle, Percutaneous Endoscopic Approach

0K540ZZ Destruction of Tongue, Palate, Pharynx Muscle, Open Approach

0K543ZZ Destruction of Tongue, Palate, Pharynx Muscle, Percutaneous Approach

0K544ZZ Destruction of Tongue, Palate, Pharynx Muscle, Percutaneous Endoscopic Approach

0K550ZZ Destruction of Right Shoulder Muscle, Open Approach

0K553ZZ Destruction of Right Shoulder Muscle, Percutaneous Approach

0K554ZZ Destruction of Right Shoulder Muscle, Percutaneous Endoscopic Approach

0K560ZZ Destruction of Left Shoulder Muscle, Open Approach

0K563ZZ Destruction of Left Shoulder Muscle, Percutaneous Approach

0K564ZZ Destruction of Left Shoulder Muscle, Percutaneous Endoscopic Approach

0K570ZZ Destruction of Right Upper Arm Muscle, Open Approach

0K573ZZ Destruction of Right Upper Arm Muscle, Percutaneous Approach

0K574ZZ Destruction of Right Upper Arm Muscle, Percutaneous Endoscopic Approach

0K580ZZ Destruction of Left Upper Arm Muscle, Open Approach

0K583ZZ Destruction of Left Upper Arm Muscle, Percutaneous Approach

0K584ZZ Destruction of Left Upper Arm Muscle, Percutaneous Endoscopic Approach

0K590ZZ Destruction of Right Lower Arm and Wrist Muscle, Open Approach

0K593ZZ Destruction of Right Lower Arm and Wrist Muscle, Percutaneous Approach

0K594ZZ Destruction of Right Lower Arm and Wrist Muscle, Percutaneous Endoscopic Approach

0K5B0ZZ Destruction of Left Lower Arm and Wrist Muscle, Open Approach

0K5B3ZZ Destruction of Left Lower Arm and Wrist Muscle, Percutaneous Approach

0K5B4ZZ Destruction of Left Lower Arm and Wrist Muscle, Percutaneous Endoscopic Approach

0K5C0ZZ Destruction of Right Hand Muscle, Open Approach

0K5C3ZZ Destruction of Right Hand Muscle, Percutaneous Approach

0K5C4ZZ Destruction of Right Hand Muscle, Percutaneous Endoscopic Approach

0K5D0ZZ Destruction of Left Hand Muscle, Open Approach

0K5D3ZZ Destruction of Left Hand Muscle, Percutaneous Approach

0K5D4ZZ Destruction of Left Hand Muscle, Percutaneous Endoscopic Approach

0K5F0ZZ Destruction of Right Trunk Muscle, Open Approach

0K5F3ZZ Destruction of Right Trunk Muscle, Percutaneous Approach

0K5F4ZZ Destruction of Right Trunk Muscle, Percutaneous Endoscopic Approach

0K5G0ZZ Destruction of Left Trunk Muscle, Open Approach

0K5G3ZZ Destruction of Left Trunk Muscle, Percutaneous Approach

0K5G4ZZ Destruction of Left Trunk Muscle, Percutaneous Endoscopic Approach

0K5H0ZZ Destruction of Right Thorax Muscle, Open Approach

0K5H3ZZ Destruction of Right Thorax Muscle, Percutaneous Approach

0K5H4ZZ Destruction of Right Thorax Muscle, Percutaneous Endoscopic Approach

0K5J0ZZ Destruction of Left Thorax Muscle, Open Approach

0K5J3ZZ Destruction of Left Thorax Muscle, Percutaneous Approach

0K5J4ZZ Destruction of Left Thorax Muscle, Percutaneous Endoscopic Approach

0K5K0ZZ Destruction of Right Abdomen Muscle, Open Approach

0K5K3ZZ Destruction of Right Abdomen Muscle, Percutaneous Approach

0K5K4ZZ Destruction of Right Abdomen Muscle, Percutaneous Endoscopic Approach

0K5L0ZZ Destruction of Left Abdomen Muscle, Open Approach

0K5L3ZZ Destruction of Left Abdomen Muscle, Percutaneous Approach

0K5L4ZZ Destruction of Left Abdomen Muscle, Percutaneous Endoscopic Approach

0K5M0ZZ Destruction of Perineum Muscle, Open Approach

0K5M3ZZ Destruction of Perineum Muscle, Percutaneous Approach

0K5M4ZZ Destruction of Perineum Muscle, Percutaneous Endoscopic Approach

0K5N0ZZ Destruction of Right Hip Muscle, Open Approach

0K5N3ZZ Destruction of Right Hip Muscle, Percutaneous Approach

0K5N4ZZ Destruction of Right Hip Muscle, Percutaneous Endoscopic Approach

0K5P0ZZ Destruction of Left Hip Muscle, Open Approach

0K5P3ZZ Destruction of Left Hip Muscle, Percutaneous Approach

0K5P4ZZ Destruction of Left Hip Muscle, Percutaneous Endoscopic Approach

0K5Q0ZZ Destruction of Right Upper Leg Muscle, Open Approach

0K5Q3ZZ Destruction of Right Upper Leg Muscle, Percutaneous Approach

0K5Q4ZZ Destruction of Right Upper Leg Muscle, Percutaneous Endoscopic Approach

0K5R0ZZ Destruction of Left Upper Leg Muscle, Open Approach

0K5R3ZZ Destruction of Left Upper Leg Muscle, Percutaneous Approach

0K5R4ZZ Destruction of Left Upper Leg Muscle, Percutaneous Endoscopic Approach

0K5S0ZZ Destruction of Right Lower Leg Muscle, Open Approach

0K5S3ZZ Destruction of Right Lower Leg Muscle, Percutaneous Approach

0K5S4ZZ Destruction of Right Lower Leg Muscle, Percutaneous Endoscopic Approach

0K5T0ZZ Destruction of Left Lower Leg Muscle, Open Approach

0K5T3ZZ Destruction of Left Lower Leg Muscle, Percutaneous Approach

0K5T4ZZ Destruction of Left Lower Leg Muscle, Percutaneous Endoscopic Approach

0K5V0ZZ Destruction of Right Foot Muscle, Open Approach

0K5V3ZZ Destruction of Right Foot Muscle, Percutaneous Approach

0K5V4ZZ Destruction of Right Foot Muscle, Percutaneous Endoscopic Approach

0K5W0ZZ Destruction of Left Foot Muscle, Open Approach

0K5W3ZZ Destruction of Left Foot Muscle, Percutaneous Approach

0K5W4ZZ Destruction of Left Foot Muscle, Percutaneous Endoscopic Approach

0K8 – Muscles, Division

Review Coding Guideline B3.14

0K800ZZ Division of Head Muscle, Open Approach

0K803ZZ Division of Head Muscle, Percutaneous Approach

0K804ZZ Division of Head Muscle, Percutaneous Endoscopic Approach

♀ Female-only   ♂ Male-only   ▲ Limited Coverage   ● Non-OR   ▨ HAC-associated procedure   ▲ Non-covered procedures   ✚ Cluster

0K810ZZ Division of Facial Muscle, Open Approach

0K813ZZ Division of Facial Muscle, Percutaneous Approach

0K814ZZ Division of Facial Muscle, Percutaneous Endoscopic Approach

0K820ZZ Division of Right Neck Muscle, Open Approach

0K823ZZ Division of Right Neck Muscle, Percutaneous Approach

0K824ZZ Division of Right Neck Muscle, Percutaneous Endoscopic Approach

0K830ZZ Division of Left Neck Muscle, Open Approach

0K833ZZ Division of Left Neck Muscle, Percutaneous Approach

0K834ZZ Division of Left Neck Muscle, Percutaneous Endoscopic Approach

0K840ZZ Division of Tongue, Palate, Pharynx Muscle, Open Approach

0K843ZZ Division of Tongue, Palate, Pharynx Muscle, Percutaneous Approach

0K844ZZ Division of Tongue, Palate, Pharynx Muscle, Percutaneous Endoscopic Approach

AHA CC: 2Q, 2020, 25

0K847ZZ Division of Tongue, Palate, Pharynx Muscle, Via Natural or Artificial Opening

0K848ZZ Division of Tongue, Palate, Pharynx Muscle, Via Natural or Artificial Opening Endoscopic

0K850ZZ Division of Right Shoulder Muscle, Open Approach

0K853ZZ Division of Right Shoulder Muscle, Percutaneous Approach

0K854ZZ Division of Right Shoulder Muscle, Percutaneous Endoscopic Approach

0K860ZZ Division of Left Shoulder Muscle, Open Approach

0K863ZZ Division of Left Shoulder Muscle, Percutaneous Approach

0K864ZZ Division of Left Shoulder Muscle, Percutaneous Endoscopic Approach

0K870ZZ Division of Right Upper Arm Muscle, Open Approach

0K873ZZ Division of Right Upper Arm Muscle, Percutaneous Approach

0K874ZZ Division of Right Upper Arm Muscle, Percutaneous Endoscopic Approach

0K880ZZ Division of Left Upper Arm Muscle, Open Approach

0K883ZZ Division of Left Upper Arm Muscle, Percutaneous Approach

0K884ZZ Division of Left Upper Arm Muscle, Percutaneous Endoscopic Approach

0K890ZZ Division of Right Lower Arm and Wrist Muscle, Open Approach

0K893ZZ Division of Right Lower Arm and Wrist Muscle, Percutaneous Approach

0K894ZZ Division of Right Lower Arm and Wrist Muscle, Percutaneous Endoscopic Approach

0K8B0ZZ Division of Left Lower Arm and Wrist Muscle, Open Approach

0K8B3ZZ Division of Left Lower Arm and Wrist Muscle, Percutaneous Approach

0K8B4ZZ Division of Left Lower Arm and Wrist Muscle, Percutaneous Endoscopic Approach

0K8C0ZZ Division of Right Hand Muscle, Open Approach

0K8C3ZZ Division of Right Hand Muscle, Percutaneous Approach

0K8C4ZZ Division of Right Hand Muscle, Percutaneous Endoscopic Approach

0K8D0ZZ Division of Left Hand Muscle, Open Approach

0K8D3ZZ Division of Left Hand Muscle, Percutaneous Approach

0K8D4ZZ Division of Left Hand Muscle, Percutaneous Endoscopic Approach

0K8F0ZZ Division of Right Trunk Muscle, Open Approach

0K8F3ZZ Division of Right Trunk Muscle, Percutaneous Approach

0K8F4ZZ Division of Right Trunk Muscle, Percutaneous Endoscopic Approach

0K8G0ZZ Division of Left Trunk Muscle, Open Approach

0K8G3ZZ Division of Left Trunk Muscle, Percutaneous Approach

0K8G4ZZ Division of Left Trunk Muscle, Percutaneous Endoscopic Approach

0K8H0ZZ Division of Right Thorax Muscle, Open Approach

0K8H3ZZ Division of Right Thorax Muscle, Percutaneous Approach

0K8H4ZZ Division of Right Thorax Muscle, Percutaneous Endoscopic Approach

0K8J0ZZ Division of Left Thorax Muscle, Open Approach

0K8J3ZZ Division of Left Thorax Muscle, Percutaneous Approach

0K8J4ZZ Division of Left Thorax Muscle, Percutaneous Endoscopic Approach

0K8K0ZZ Division of Right Abdomen Muscle, Open Approach

0K8K3ZZ Division of Right Abdomen Muscle, Percutaneous Approach

0K8K4ZZ Division of Right Abdomen Muscle, Percutaneous Endoscopic Approach

0K8L0ZZ Division of Left Abdomen Muscle, Open Approach

0K8L3ZZ Division of Left Abdomen Muscle, Percutaneous Approach

0K8L4ZZ Division of Left Abdomen Muscle, Percutaneous Endoscopic Approach

0K8M0ZZ Division of Perineum Muscle, Open Approach

0K8M3ZZ Division of Perineum Muscle, Percutaneous Approach

0K8M4ZZ Division of Perineum Muscle, Percutaneous Endoscopic Approach

0K8N0ZZ Division of Right Hip Muscle, Open Approach

0K8N3ZZ Division of Right Hip Muscle, Percutaneous Approach

0K8N4ZZ Division of Right Hip Muscle, Percutaneous Endoscopic Approach

0K8P0ZZ Division of Left Hip Muscle, Open Approach

0K8P3ZZ Division of Left Hip Muscle, Percutaneous Approach

0K8P4ZZ Division of Left Hip Muscle, Percutaneous Endoscopic Approach

0K8Q0ZZ Division of Right Upper Leg Muscle, Open Approach

0K8Q3ZZ Division of Right Upper Leg Muscle, Percutaneous Approach

0K8Q4ZZ Division of Right Upper Leg Muscle, Percutaneous Endoscopic Approach

0K8R0ZZ Division of Left Upper Leg Muscle, Open Approach

0K8R3ZZ Division of Left Upper Leg Muscle, Percutaneous Approach

0K8R4ZZ Division of Left Upper Leg Muscle, Percutaneous Endoscopic Approach

0K8S0ZZ Division of Right Lower Leg Muscle, Open Approach

0K8S3ZZ Division of Right Lower Leg Muscle, Percutaneous Approach

0K8S4ZZ Division of Right Lower Leg Muscle, Percutaneous Endoscopic Approach

0K8T0ZZ Division of Left Lower Leg Muscle, Open Approach

0K8T3ZZ Division of Left Lower Leg Muscle, Percutaneous Approach

0K8T4ZZ Division of Left Lower Leg Muscle, Percutaneous Endoscopic Approach

0K8V0ZZ Division of Right Foot Muscle, Open Approach

0K8V3ZZ Division of Right Foot Muscle, Percutaneous Approach

0K8V4ZZ Division of Right Foot Muscle, Percutaneous Endoscopic Approach

0K8W0ZZ Division of Left Foot Muscle, Open Approach

0K8W3ZZ Division of Left Foot Muscle, Percutaneous Approach

0K8W4ZZ Division of Left Foot Muscle, Percutaneous Endoscopic Approach

0K9 – Muscles, Drainage

Review Coding Guidelines B3.4a and B3.4b

Review Coding Guideline B6.2

0K9000Z Drainage of Head Muscle with Drainage Device, Open Approach

0K900ZX Drainage of Head Muscle, Open Approach, Diagnostic

0K900ZZ Drainage of Head Muscle, Open Approach

0K9030Z Drainage of Head Muscle with Drainage Device, Percutaneous Approach

0K903ZX Drainage of Head Muscle, Percutaneous Approach, Diagnostic

0K903ZZ Drainage of Head Muscle, Percutaneous Approach

0K9040Z Drainage of Head Muscle with Drainage Device, Percutaneous Endoscopic Approach

0K904ZX Drainage of Head Muscle, Percutaneous Endoscopic Approach, Diagnostic

0K904ZZ Drainage of Head Muscle, Percutaneous Endoscopic Approach

0K9100Z Drainage of Facial Muscle with Drainage Device, Open Approach

0K910ZX Drainage of Facial Muscle, Open Approach, Diagnostic

0K910ZZ Drainage of Facial Muscle, Open Approach

0K9130Z Drainage of Facial Muscle with Drainage Device, Percutaneous Approach

0K913ZX Drainage of Facial Muscle, Percutaneous Approach, Diagnostic

0K913ZZ Drainage of Facial Muscle, Percutaneous Approach

0K9140Z Drainage of Facial Muscle with Drainage Device, Percutaneous Endoscopic Approach

0K914ZX Drainage of Facial Muscle, Percutaneous Endoscopic Approach, Diagnostic

0K914ZZ Drainage of Facial Muscle, Percutaneous Endoscopic Approach

0K9200Z Drainage of Right Neck Muscle with Drainage Device, Open Approach

0K920ZX Drainage of Right Neck Muscle, Open Approach, Diagnostic

0K920ZZ Drainage of Right Neck Muscle, Open Approach

0K9230Z Drainage of Right Neck Muscle with Drainage Device, Percutaneous Approach

0K923ZX Drainage of Right Neck Muscle, Percutaneous Approach, Diagnostic

0K923ZZ Drainage of Right Neck Muscle, Percutaneous Approach

0K9240Z Drainage of Right Neck Muscle with Drainage Device, Percutaneous Endoscopic Approach

0K924ZX Drainage of Right Neck Muscle, Percutaneous Endoscopic Approach, Diagnostic

0K924ZZ Drainage of Right Neck Muscle, Percutaneous Endoscopic Approach

0K9300Z Drainage of Left Neck Muscle with Drainage Device, Open Approach

0K930ZX Drainage of Left Neck Muscle, Open Approach, Diagnostic

0K930ZZ Drainage of Left Neck Muscle, Open Approach

0K9330Z Drainage of Left Neck Muscle with Drainage Device, Percutaneous Approach

0K933ZX Drainage of Left Neck Muscle, Percutaneous Approach, Diagnostic

0K933ZZ Drainage of Left Neck Muscle, Percutaneous Approach

0K9340Z Drainage of Left Neck Muscle with Drainage Device, Percutaneous Endoscopic Approach

0K934ZX Drainage of Left Neck Muscle, Percutaneous Endoscopic Approach, Diagnostic

0K934ZZ Drainage of Left Neck Muscle, Percutaneous Endoscopic Approach

0K9400Z Drainage of Tongue, Palate, Pharynx Muscle with Drainage Device, Open Approach

0K940ZX Drainage of Tongue, Palate, Pharynx Muscle, Open Approach, Diagnostic

0K940ZZ Drainage of Tongue, Palate, Pharynx Muscle, Open Approach

0K9430Z Drainage of Tongue, Palate, Pharynx Muscle with Drainage Device, Percutaneous Approach

0K943ZX Drainage of Tongue, Palate, Pharynx Muscle, Percutaneous Approach, Diagnostic

0K943ZZ Drainage of Tongue, Palate, Pharynx Muscle, Percutaneous Approach

0K9440Z Drainage of Tongue, Palate, Pharynx Muscle with Drainage Device, Percutaneous Endoscopic Approach

0K944ZX Drainage of Tongue, Palate, Pharynx Muscle, Percutaneous Endoscopic Approach, Diagnostic

0K944ZZ Drainage of Tongue, Palate, Pharynx Muscle, Percutaneous Endoscopic Approach

0K9500Z Drainage of Right Shoulder Muscle with Drainage Device, Open Approach

0K950ZX Drainage of Right Shoulder Muscle, Open Approach, Diagnostic

0K950ZZ Drainage of Right Shoulder Muscle, Open Approach

0K9530Z Drainage of Right Shoulder Muscle with Drainage Device, Percutaneous Approach

0K953ZX Drainage of Right Shoulder Muscle, Percutaneous Approach, Diagnostic

0K953ZZ Drainage of Right Shoulder Muscle, Percutaneous Approach

0K9540Z Drainage of Right Shoulder Muscle with Drainage Device, Percutaneous Endoscopic Approach

0K954ZX Drainage of Right Shoulder Muscle, Percutaneous Endoscopic Approach, Diagnostic

0K954ZZ Drainage of Right Shoulder Muscle, Percutaneous Endoscopic Approach

0K9600Z Drainage of Left Shoulder Muscle with Drainage Device, Open Approach

0K960ZX Drainage of Left Shoulder Muscle, Open Approach, Diagnostic

0K960ZZ Drainage of Left Shoulder Muscle, Open Approach

0K9630Z Drainage of Left Shoulder Muscle with Drainage Device, Percutaneous Approach

0K963ZX Drainage of Left Shoulder Muscle, Percutaneous Approach, Diagnostic

0K963ZZ Drainage of Left Shoulder Muscle, Percutaneous Approach

0K9640Z Drainage of Left Shoulder Muscle with Drainage Device, Percutaneous Endoscopic Approach

0K964ZX Drainage of Left Shoulder Muscle, Percutaneous Endoscopic Approach, Diagnostic

0K964ZZ Drainage of Left Shoulder Muscle, Percutaneous Endoscopic Approach

0K9700Z Drainage of Right Upper Arm Muscle with Drainage Device, Open Approach

0K970ZX Drainage of Right Upper Arm Muscle, Open Approach, Diagnostic

0K970ZZ Drainage of Right Upper Arm Muscle, Open Approach

0K9730Z Drainage of Right Upper Arm Muscle with Drainage Device, Percutaneous Approach

0K973ZX Drainage of Right Upper Arm Muscle, Percutaneous Approach, Diagnostic

0K973ZZ Drainage of Right Upper Arm Muscle, Percutaneous Approach

0K9740Z Drainage of Right Upper Arm Muscle with Drainage Device, Percutaneous Endoscopic Approach

0K974ZX Drainage of Right Upper Arm Muscle, Percutaneous Endoscopic Approach, Diagnostic

0K974ZZ Drainage of Right Upper Arm Muscle, Percutaneous Endoscopic Approach

0K9800Z Drainage of Left Upper Arm Muscle with Drainage Device, Open Approach

0K980ZX Drainage of Left Upper Arm Muscle, Open Approach, Diagnostic

0K980ZZ Drainage of Left Upper Arm Muscle, Open Approach

0K9830Z Drainage of Left Upper Arm Muscle with Drainage Device, Percutaneous Approach

0K983ZX Drainage of Left Upper Arm Muscle, Percutaneous Approach, Diagnostic

0K983ZZ Drainage of Left Upper Arm Muscle, Percutaneous Approach

0K9840Z Drainage of Left Upper Arm Muscle with Drainage Device, Percutaneous Endoscopic Approach

0K984ZX Drainage of Left Upper Arm Muscle, Percutaneous Endoscopic Approach, Diagnostic

0K984ZZ Drainage of Left Upper Arm Muscle, Percutaneous Endoscopic Approach

0K9900Z Drainage of Right Lower Arm and Wrist Muscle with Drainage Device, Open Approach

0K990ZX Drainage of Right Lower Arm and Wrist Muscle, Open Approach, Diagnostic

0K990ZZ Drainage of Right Lower Arm and Wrist Muscle, Open Approach

0K9930Z Drainage of Right Lower Arm and Wrist Muscle with Drainage Device, Percutaneous Approach

0K993ZX Drainage of Right Lower Arm and Wrist Muscle, Percutaneous Approach, Diagnostic

0K993ZZ Drainage of Right Lower Arm and Wrist Muscle, Percutaneous Approach

0K9940Z Drainage of Right Lower Arm and Wrist Muscle with Drainage Device, Percutaneous Endoscopic Approach

0K994ZX Drainage of Right Lower Arm and Wrist Muscle, Percutaneous Endoscopic Approach, Diagnostic

0K994ZZ Drainage of Right Lower Arm and Wrist Muscle, Percutaneous Endoscopic Approach

0K9B00Z Drainage of Left Lower Arm and Wrist Muscle with Drainage Device, Open Approach

0K9B0ZX Drainage of Left Lower Arm and Wrist Muscle, Open Approach, Diagnostic

0K9B0ZZ Drainage of Left Lower Arm and Wrist Muscle, Open Approach

0K9B30Z Drainage of Left Lower Arm and Wrist Muscle with Drainage Device, Percutaneous Approach

0K9B3ZX Drainage of Left Lower Arm and Wrist Muscle, Percutaneous Approach, Diagnostic

0K9B3ZZ Drainage of Left Lower Arm and Wrist Muscle, Percutaneous Approach

0K9B40Z Drainage of Left Lower Arm and Wrist Muscle with Drainage Device, Percutaneous Endoscopic Approach

0K9B4ZX Drainage of Left Lower Arm and Wrist Muscle, Percutaneous Endoscopic Approach, Diagnostic

0K9B4ZZ Drainage of Left Lower Arm and Wrist Muscle, Percutaneous Endoscopic Approach

0K9C00Z Drainage of Right Hand Muscle with Drainage Device, Open Approach

0K9C0ZX Drainage of Right Hand Muscle, Open Approach, Diagnostic

0K9C0ZZ Drainage of Right Hand Muscle, Open Approach

0K9C30Z Drainage of Right Hand Muscle with Drainage Device, Percutaneous Approach

0K9C3ZX Drainage of Right Hand Muscle, Percutaneous Approach, Diagnostic

0K9C3ZZ Drainage of Right Hand Muscle, Percutaneous Approach

0K9C40Z Drainage of Right Hand Muscle with Drainage Device, Percutaneous Endoscopic Approach

0K9C4ZX Drainage of Right Hand Muscle, Percutaneous Endoscopic Approach, Diagnostic

0K9C4ZZ Drainage of Right Hand Muscle, Percutaneous Endoscopic Approach

0K9D00Z Drainage of Left Hand Muscle with Drainage Device, Open Approach

♀ Female-only   ♂ Male-only   ▲ Limited Coverage   ● Non-OR   [HAC] HAC-associated procedure   ▲ Non-covered procedures   ✚ Cluster

0K9D0ZX Drainage of Left Hand Muscle, Open Approach, Diagnostic

0K9D0ZZ Drainage of Left Hand Muscle, Open Approach

0K9D30Z Drainage of Left Hand Muscle with Drainage Device, Percutaneous Approach

0K9D3ZX Drainage of Left Hand Muscle, Percutaneous Approach, Diagnostic

0K9D3ZZ Drainage of Left Hand Muscle, Percutaneous Approach

0K9D40Z Drainage of Left Hand Muscle with Drainage Device, Percutaneous Endoscopic Approach

0K9D4ZX Drainage of Left Hand Muscle, Percutaneous Endoscopic Approach, Diagnostic

0K9D4ZZ Drainage of Left Hand Muscle, Percutaneous Endoscopic Approach

0K9F00Z Drainage of Right Trunk Muscle with Drainage Device, Open Approach

0K9F0ZX Drainage of Right Trunk Muscle, Open Approach, Diagnostic

0K9F0ZZ Drainage of Right Trunk Muscle, Open Approach

0K9F30Z Drainage of Right Trunk Muscle with Drainage Device, Percutaneous Approach

0K9F3ZX Drainage of Right Trunk Muscle, Percutaneous Approach, Diagnostic

0K9F3ZZ Drainage of Right Trunk Muscle, Percutaneous Approach

0K9F40Z Drainage of Right Trunk Muscle with Drainage Device, Percutaneous Endoscopic Approach

0K9F4ZX Drainage of Right Trunk Muscle, Percutaneous Endoscopic Approach, Diagnostic

0K9F4ZZ Drainage of Right Trunk Muscle, Percutaneous Endoscopic Approach

0K9G00Z Drainage of Left Trunk Muscle with Drainage Device, Open Approach

0K9G0ZX Drainage of Left Trunk Muscle, Open Approach, Diagnostic

0K9G0ZZ Drainage of Left Trunk Muscle, Open Approach

0K9G30Z Drainage of Left Trunk Muscle with Drainage Device, Percutaneous Approach

0K9G3ZX Drainage of Left Trunk Muscle, Percutaneous Approach, Diagnostic

0K9G3ZZ Drainage of Left Trunk Muscle, Percutaneous Approach

0K9G40Z Drainage of Left Trunk Muscle with Drainage Device, Percutaneous Endoscopic Approach

0K9G4ZX Drainage of Left Trunk Muscle, Percutaneous Endoscopic Approach, Diagnostic

0K9G4ZZ Drainage of Left Trunk Muscle, Percutaneous Endoscopic Approach

0K9H00Z Drainage of Right Thorax Muscle with Drainage Device, Open Approach

0K9H0ZX Drainage of Right Thorax Muscle, Open Approach, Diagnostic

0K9H0ZZ Drainage of Right Thorax Muscle, Open Approach

0K9H30Z Drainage of Right Thorax Muscle with Drainage Device, Percutaneous Approach

0K9H3ZX Drainage of Right Thorax Muscle, Percutaneous Approach, Diagnostic

0K9H3ZZ Drainage of Right Thorax Muscle, Percutaneous Approach

0K9H40Z Drainage of Right Thorax Muscle with Drainage Device, Percutaneous Endoscopic Approach

0K9H4ZX Drainage of Right Thorax Muscle, Percutaneous Endoscopic Approach, Diagnostic

0K9H4ZZ Drainage of Right Thorax Muscle, Percutaneous Endoscopic Approach

0K9J00Z Drainage of Left Thorax Muscle with Drainage Device, Open Approach

0K9J0ZX Drainage of Left Thorax Muscle, Open Approach, Diagnostic

0K9J0ZZ Drainage of Left Thorax Muscle, Open Approach

0K9J30Z Drainage of Left Thorax Muscle with Drainage Device, Percutaneous Approach

0K9J3ZX Drainage of Left Thorax Muscle, Percutaneous Approach, Diagnostic

0K9J3ZZ Drainage of Left Thorax Muscle, Percutaneous Approach

0K9J40Z Drainage of Left Thorax Muscle with Drainage Device, Percutaneous Endoscopic Approach

0K9J4ZX Drainage of Left Thorax Muscle, Percutaneous Endoscopic Approach, Diagnostic

0K9J4ZZ Drainage of Left Thorax Muscle, Percutaneous Endoscopic Approach

0K9K00Z Drainage of Right Abdomen Muscle with Drainage Device, Open Approach

0K9K0ZX Drainage of Right Abdomen Muscle, Open Approach, Diagnostic

0K9K0ZZ Drainage of Right Abdomen Muscle, Open Approach

0K9K30Z Drainage of Right Abdomen Muscle with Drainage Device, Percutaneous Approach

0K9K3ZX Drainage of Right Abdomen Muscle, Percutaneous Approach, Diagnostic

0K9K3ZZ Drainage of Right Abdomen Muscle, Percutaneous Approach

0K9K40Z Drainage of Right Abdomen Muscle with Drainage Device, Percutaneous Endoscopic Approach

0K9K4ZX Drainage of Right Abdomen Muscle, Percutaneous Endoscopic Approach, Diagnostic

0K9K4ZZ Drainage of Right Abdomen Muscle, Percutaneous Endoscopic Approach

0K9L00Z Drainage of Left Abdomen Muscle with Drainage Device, Open Approach

0K9L0ZX Drainage of Left Abdomen Muscle, Open Approach, Diagnostic

0K9L0ZZ Drainage of Left Abdomen Muscle, Open Approach

0K9L30Z Drainage of Left Abdomen Muscle with Drainage Device, Percutaneous Approach

0K9L3ZX Drainage of Left Abdomen Muscle, Percutaneous Approach, Diagnostic

0K9L3ZZ Drainage of Left Abdomen Muscle, Percutaneous Approach

0K9L40Z Drainage of Left Abdomen Muscle with Drainage Device, Percutaneous Endoscopic Approach

0K9L4ZX Drainage of Left Abdomen Muscle, Percutaneous Endoscopic Approach, Diagnostic

0K9L4ZZ Drainage of Left Abdomen Muscle, Percutaneous Endoscopic Approach

0K9M00Z Drainage of Perineum Muscle with Drainage Device, Open Approach

0K9M0ZX Drainage of Perineum Muscle, Open Approach, Diagnostic

0K9M0ZZ Drainage of Perineum Muscle, Open Approach

0K9M30Z Drainage of Perineum Muscle with Drainage Device, Percutaneous Approach

0K9M3ZX Drainage of Perineum Muscle, Percutaneous Approach, Diagnostic

0K9M3ZZ Drainage of Perineum Muscle, Percutaneous Approach

0K9M40Z Drainage of Perineum Muscle with Drainage Device, Percutaneous Endoscopic Approach

0K9M4ZX Drainage of Perineum Muscle, Percutaneous Endoscopic Approach, Diagnostic

0K9M4ZZ Drainage of Perineum Muscle, Percutaneous Endoscopic Approach

0K9N00Z Drainage of Right Hip Muscle with Drainage Device, Open Approach

0K9N0ZX Drainage of Right Hip Muscle, Open Approach, Diagnostic

0K9N0ZZ Drainage of Right Hip Muscle, Open Approach

0K9N30Z Drainage of Right Hip Muscle with Drainage Device, Percutaneous Approach

0K9N3ZX Drainage of Right Hip Muscle, Percutaneous Approach, Diagnostic

0K9N3ZZ Drainage of Right Hip Muscle, Percutaneous Approach

0K9N40Z Drainage of Right Hip Muscle with Drainage Device, Percutaneous Endoscopic Approach

0K9N4ZX Drainage of Right Hip Muscle, Percutaneous Endoscopic Approach, Diagnostic

0K9N4ZZ Drainage of Right Hip Muscle, Percutaneous Endoscopic Approach

0K9P00Z Drainage of Left Hip Muscle with Drainage Device, Open Approach

0K9P0ZX Drainage of Left Hip Muscle, Open Approach, Diagnostic

0K9P0ZZ Drainage of Left Hip Muscle, Open Approach

0K9P30Z Drainage of Left Hip Muscle with Drainage Device, Percutaneous Approach

0K9P3ZX Drainage of Left Hip Muscle, Percutaneous Approach, Diagnostic

0K9P3ZZ Drainage of Left Hip Muscle, Percutaneous Approach

0K9P40Z Drainage of Left Hip Muscle with Drainage Device, Percutaneous Endoscopic Approach

0K9P4ZX Drainage of Left Hip Muscle, Percutaneous Endoscopic Approach, Diagnostic

0K9P4ZZ Drainage of Left Hip Muscle, Percutaneous Endoscopic Approach

0K9Q00Z Drainage of Right Upper Leg Muscle with Drainage Device, Open Approach

0K9Q0ZX Drainage of Right Upper Leg Muscle, Open Approach, Diagnostic

0K9Q0ZZ Drainage of Right Upper Leg Muscle, Open Approach

0K9Q30Z Drainage of Right Upper Leg Muscle with Drainage Device, Percutaneous Approach

0K9Q3ZX Drainage of Right Upper Leg Muscle, Percutaneous Approach, Diagnostic

0K9Q3ZZ Drainage of Right Upper Leg Muscle, Percutaneous Approach

0K9Q40Z Drainage of Right Upper Leg Muscle with Drainage Device, Percutaneous Endoscopic Approach

0K9Q4ZX Drainage of Right Upper Leg Muscle, Percutaneous Endoscopic Approach, Diagnostic

0K9Q4ZZ Drainage of Right Upper Leg Muscle, Percutaneous Endoscopic Approach

♀ Female-only   ♂ Male-only   ▲ Limited Coverage   ● Non-OR   HAC HAC-associated procedure   ▲ Non-covered procedures   + Cluster

0K9R00Z	Drainage of Left Upper Leg Muscle with Drainage Device, Open Approach	
0K9R0ZX	Drainage of Left Upper Leg Muscle, Open Approach, Diagnostic	
0K9R0ZZ	Drainage of Left Upper Leg Muscle, Open Approach	
0K9R30Z	Drainage of Left Upper Leg Muscle with Drainage Device, Percutaneous Approach	
0K9R3ZX	Drainage of Left Upper Leg Muscle, Percutaneous Approach, Diagnostic	
0K9R3ZZ	Drainage of Left Upper Leg Muscle, Percutaneous Approach	
0K9R40Z	Drainage of Left Upper Leg Muscle with Drainage Device, Percutaneous Endoscopic Approach	
0K9R4ZX	Drainage of Left Upper Leg Muscle, Percutaneous Endoscopic Approach, Diagnostic	
0K9R4ZZ	Drainage of Left Upper Leg Muscle, Percutaneous Endoscopic Approach	
0K9S00Z	Drainage of Right Lower Leg Muscle with Drainage Device, Open Approach	
0K9S0ZX	Drainage of Right Lower Leg Muscle, Open Approach, Diagnostic	
0K9S0ZZ	Drainage of Right Lower Leg Muscle, Open Approach	
0K9S30Z	Drainage of Right Lower Leg Muscle with Drainage Device, Percutaneous Approach	
0K9S3ZX	Drainage of Right Lower Leg Muscle, Percutaneous Approach, Diagnostic	
0K9S3ZZ	Drainage of Right Lower Leg Muscle, Percutaneous Approach	
0K9S40Z	Drainage of Right Lower Leg Muscle with Drainage Device, Percutaneous Endoscopic Approach	
0K9S4ZX	Drainage of Right Lower Leg Muscle, Percutaneous Endoscopic Approach, Diagnostic	
0K9S4ZZ	Drainage of Right Lower Leg Muscle, Percutaneous Endoscopic Approach	
0K9T00Z	Drainage of Left Lower Leg Muscle with Drainage Device, Open Approach	
0K9T0ZX	Drainage of Left Lower Leg Muscle, Open Approach, Diagnostic	
0K9T0ZZ	Drainage of Left Lower Leg Muscle, Open Approach	
0K9T30Z	Drainage of Left Lower Leg Muscle with Drainage Device, Percutaneous Approach	
0K9T3ZX	Drainage of Left Lower Leg Muscle, Percutaneous Approach, Diagnostic	
0K9T3ZZ	Drainage of Left Lower Leg Muscle, Percutaneous Approach	
0K9T40Z	Drainage of Left Lower Leg Muscle with Drainage Device, Percutaneous Endoscopic Approach	
0K9T4ZX	Drainage of Left Lower Leg Muscle, Percutaneous Endoscopic Approach, Diagnostic	
0K9T4ZZ	Drainage of Left Lower Leg Muscle, Percutaneous Endoscopic Approach	
0K9V00Z	Drainage of Right Foot Muscle with Drainage Device, Open Approach	
0K9V0ZX	Drainage of Right Foot Muscle, Open Approach, Diagnostic	
0K9V0ZZ	Drainage of Right Foot Muscle, Open Approach	
0K9V30Z	Drainage of Right Foot Muscle with Drainage Device, Percutaneous Approach	
0K9V3ZX	Drainage of Right Foot Muscle, Percutaneous Approach, Diagnostic	
0K9V3ZZ	Drainage of Right Foot Muscle, Percutaneous Approach	
0K9V40Z	Drainage of Right Foot Muscle with Drainage Device, Percutaneous Endoscopic Approach	
0K9V4ZX	Drainage of Right Foot Muscle, Percutaneous Endoscopic Approach, Diagnostic	
0K9V4ZZ	Drainage of Right Foot Muscle, Percutaneous Endoscopic Approach	
0K9W00Z	Drainage of Left Foot Muscle with Drainage Device, Open Approach	
0K9W0ZX	Drainage of Left Foot Muscle, Open Approach, Diagnostic	
0K9W0ZZ	Drainage of Left Foot Muscle, Open Approach	
0K9W30Z	Drainage of Left Foot Muscle with Drainage Device, Percutaneous Approach	
0K9W3ZX	Drainage of Left Foot Muscle, Percutaneous Approach, Diagnostic	
0K9W3ZZ	Drainage of Left Foot Muscle, Percutaneous Approach	
0K9W40Z	Drainage of Left Foot Muscle with Drainage Device, Percutaneous Endoscopic Approach	
0K9W4ZX	Drainage of Left Foot Muscle, Percutaneous Endoscopic Approach, Diagnostic	
0K9W4ZZ	Drainage of Left Foot Muscle, Percutaneous Endoscopic Approach	

0KB – Muscles, Excision

Review Coding Guidelines B3.4a and B3.4b

Review Coding Guideline B3.5

Review Coding Guideline B3.8

Review Coding Guideline B3.18

0KB00ZX	Excision of Head Muscle, Open Approach, Diagnostic
0KB00ZZ	Excision of Head Muscle, Open Approach
0KB03ZX	Excision of Head Muscle, Percutaneous Approach, Diagnostic
0KB03ZZ	Excision of Head Muscle, Percutaneous Approach
0KB04ZX	Excision of Head Muscle, Percutaneous Endoscopic Approach, Diagnostic
0KB04ZZ	Excision of Head Muscle, Percutaneous Endoscopic Approach
0KB10ZX	Excision of Facial Muscle, Open Approach, Diagnostic
0KB10ZZ	Excision of Facial Muscle, Open Approach
0KB13ZX	Excision of Facial Muscle, Percutaneous Approach, Diagnostic
0KB13ZZ	Excision of Facial Muscle, Percutaneous Approach
0KB14ZX	Excision of Facial Muscle, Percutaneous Endoscopic Approach, Diagnostic
0KB14ZZ	Excision of Facial Muscle, Percutaneous Endoscopic Approach
0KB20ZX	Excision of Right Neck Muscle, Open Approach, Diagnostic
0KB20ZZ	Excision of Right Neck Muscle, Open Approach
0KB23ZX	Excision of Right Neck Muscle, Percutaneous Approach, Diagnostic
0KB23ZZ	Excision of Right Neck Muscle, Percutaneous Approach
0KB24ZX	Excision of Right Neck Muscle, Percutaneous Endoscopic Approach, Diagnostic
0KB24ZZ	Excision of Right Neck Muscle, Percutaneous Endoscopic Approach
0KB30ZX	Excision of Left Neck Muscle, Open Approach, Diagnostic
0KB30ZZ	Excision of Left Neck Muscle, Open Approach
0KB33ZX	Excision of Left Neck Muscle, Percutaneous Approach, Diagnostic
0KB33ZZ	Excision of Left Neck Muscle, Percutaneous Approach
0KB34ZX	Excision of Left Neck Muscle, Percutaneous Endoscopic Approach, Diagnostic
0KB34ZZ	Excision of Left Neck Muscle, Percutaneous Endoscopic Approach
0KB40ZX	Excision of Tongue, Palate, Pharynx Muscle, Open Approach, Diagnostic
0KB40ZZ	Excision of Tongue, Palate, Pharynx Muscle, Open Approach
0KB43ZX	Excision of Tongue, Palate, Pharynx Muscle, Percutaneous Approach, Diagnostic
0KB43ZZ	Excision of Tongue, Palate, Pharynx Muscle, Percutaneous Approach
0KB44ZX	Excision of Tongue, Palate, Pharynx Muscle, Percutaneous Endoscopic Approach, Diagnostic
0KB44ZZ	Excision of Tongue, Palate, Pharynx Muscle, Percutaneous Endoscopic Approach
0KB50ZX	Excision of Right Shoulder Muscle, Open Approach, Diagnostic
0KB50ZZ	Excision of Right Shoulder Muscle, Open Approach
0KB53ZX	Excision of Right Shoulder Muscle, Percutaneous Approach, Diagnostic
0KB53ZZ	Excision of Right Shoulder Muscle, Percutaneous Approach
0KB54ZX	Excision of Right Shoulder Muscle, Percutaneous Endoscopic Approach, Diagnostic
0KB54ZZ	Excision of Right Shoulder Muscle, Percutaneous Endoscopic Approach
0KB60ZX	Excision of Left Shoulder Muscle, Open Approach, Diagnostic
0KB60ZZ	Excision of Left Shoulder Muscle, Open Approach
0KB63ZX	Excision of Left Shoulder Muscle, Percutaneous Approach, Diagnostic
0KB63ZZ	Excision of Left Shoulder Muscle, Percutaneous Approach

♀ Female-only   ♂ Male-only   ▲ Limited Coverage   ● Non-OR   HAC HAC-associated procedure   ▲ Non-covered procedures   ✚ Cluster

0KB64ZX Excision of Left Shoulder Muscle, Percutaneous Endoscopic Approach, Diagnostic

0KB64ZZ Excision of Left Shoulder Muscle, Percutaneous Endoscopic Approach

0KB70ZX Excision of Right Upper Arm Muscle, Open Approach, Diagnostic

0KB70ZZ Excision of Right Upper Arm Muscle, Open Approach

0KB73ZX Excision of Right Upper Arm Muscle, Percutaneous Approach, Diagnostic

0KB73ZZ Excision of Right Upper Arm Muscle, Percutaneous Approach

0KB74ZX Excision of Right Upper Arm Muscle, Percutaneous Endoscopic Approach, Diagnostic

0KB74ZZ Excision of Right Upper Arm Muscle, Percutaneous Endoscopic Approach

0KB80ZX Excision of Left Upper Arm Muscle, Open Approach, Diagnostic

0KB80ZZ Excision of Left Upper Arm Muscle, Open Approach

0KB83ZX Excision of Left Upper Arm Muscle, Percutaneous Approach, Diagnostic

0KB83ZZ Excision of Left Upper Arm Muscle, Percutaneous Approach

0KB84ZX Excision of Left Upper Arm Muscle, Percutaneous Endoscopic Approach, Diagnostic

0KB84ZZ Excision of Left Upper Arm Muscle, Percutaneous Endoscopic Approach

0KB90ZX Excision of Right Lower Arm and Wrist Muscle, Open Approach, Diagnostic

0KB90ZZ Excision of Right Lower Arm and Wrist Muscle, Open Approach

0KB93ZX Excision of Right Lower Arm and Wrist Muscle, Percutaneous Approach, Diagnostic

0KB93ZZ Excision of Right Lower Arm and Wrist Muscle, Percutaneous Approach

0KB94ZX Excision of Right Lower Arm and Wrist Muscle, Percutaneous Endoscopic Approach, Diagnostic

0KB94ZZ Excision of Right Lower Arm and Wrist Muscle, Percutaneous Endoscopic Approach

0KBB0ZX Excision of Left Lower Arm and Wrist Muscle, Open Approach, Diagnostic

0KBB0ZZ Excision of Left Lower Arm and Wrist Muscle, Open Approach

0KBB3ZX Excision of Left Lower Arm and Wrist Muscle, Percutaneous Approach, Diagnostic

0KBB3ZZ Excision of Left Lower Arm and Wrist Muscle, Percutaneous Approach

0KBB4ZX Excision of Left Lower Arm and Wrist Muscle, Percutaneous Endoscopic Approach, Diagnostic

0KBB4ZZ Excision of Left Lower Arm and Wrist Muscle, Percutaneous Endoscopic Approach

0KBC0ZX Excision of Right Hand Muscle, Open Approach, Diagnostic

0KBC0ZZ Excision of Right Hand Muscle, Open Approach

0KBC3ZX Excision of Right Hand Muscle, Percutaneous Approach, Diagnostic

0KBC3ZZ Excision of Right Hand Muscle, Percutaneous Approach

0KBC4ZX Excision of Right Hand Muscle, Percutaneous Endoscopic Approach, Diagnostic

0KBC4ZZ Excision of Right Hand Muscle, Percutaneous Endoscopic Approach

0KBD0ZX Excision of Left Hand Muscle, Open Approach, Diagnostic

0KBD0ZZ Excision of Left Hand Muscle, Open Approach

0KBD3ZX Excision of Left Hand Muscle, Percutaneous Approach, Diagnostic

0KBD3ZZ Excision of Left Hand Muscle, Percutaneous Approach

0KBD4ZX Excision of Left Hand Muscle, Percutaneous Endoscopic Approach, Diagnostic

0KBD4ZZ Excision of Left Hand Muscle, Percutaneous Endoscopic Approach

0KBF0ZX Excision of Right Trunk Muscle, Open Approach, Diagnostic

0KBF0ZZ Excision of Right Trunk Muscle, Open Approach

0KBF3ZX Excision of Right Trunk Muscle, Percutaneous Approach, Diagnostic

0KBF3ZZ Excision of Right Trunk Muscle, Percutaneous Approach

0KBF4ZX Excision of Right Trunk Muscle, Percutaneous Endoscopic Approach, Diagnostic

0KBF4ZZ Excision of Right Trunk Muscle, Percutaneous Endoscopic Approach

0KBG0ZX Excision of Left Trunk Muscle, Open Approach, Diagnostic

0KBG0ZZ Excision of Left Trunk Muscle, Open Approach

0KBG3ZX Excision of Left Trunk Muscle, Percutaneous Approach, Diagnostic

0KBG3ZZ Excision of Left Trunk Muscle, Percutaneous Approach

0KBG4ZX Excision of Left Trunk Muscle, Percutaneous Endoscopic Approach, Diagnostic

0KBG4ZZ Excision of Left Trunk Muscle, Percutaneous Endoscopic Approach

0KBH0ZX Excision of Right Thorax Muscle, Open Approach, Diagnostic

0KBH0ZZ Excision of Right Thorax Muscle, Open Approach

0KBH3ZX Excision of Right Thorax Muscle, Percutaneous Approach, Diagnostic

0KBH3ZZ Excision of Right Thorax Muscle, Percutaneous Approach

0KBH4ZX Excision of Right Thorax Muscle, Percutaneous Endoscopic Approach, Diagnostic

0KBH4ZZ Excision of Right Thorax Muscle, Percutaneous Endoscopic Approach

0KBJ0ZX Excision of Left Thorax Muscle, Open Approach, Diagnostic

0KBJ0ZZ Excision of Left Thorax Muscle, Open Approach

0KBJ3ZX Excision of Left Thorax Muscle, Percutaneous Approach, Diagnostic

0KBJ3ZZ Excision of Left Thorax Muscle, Percutaneous Approach

0KBJ4ZX Excision of Left Thorax Muscle, Percutaneous Endoscopic Approach, Diagnostic

0KBJ4ZZ Excision of Left Thorax Muscle, Percutaneous Endoscopic Approach

0KBK0ZX Excision of Right Abdomen Muscle, Open Approach, Diagnostic

0KBK0ZZ Excision of Right Abdomen Muscle, Open Approach

0KBK3ZX Excision of Right Abdomen Muscle, Percutaneous Approach, Diagnostic

0KBK3ZZ Excision of Right Abdomen Muscle, Percutaneous Approach

0KBK4ZX Excision of Right Abdomen Muscle, Percutaneous Endoscopic Approach, Diagnostic

0KBK4ZZ Excision of Right Abdomen Muscle, Percutaneous Endoscopic Approach

0KBL0ZX Excision of Left Abdomen Muscle, Open Approach, Diagnostic

0KBL0ZZ Excision of Left Abdomen Muscle, Open Approach

0KBL3ZX Excision of Left Abdomen Muscle, Percutaneous Approach, Diagnostic

0KBL3ZZ Excision of Left Abdomen Muscle, Percutaneous Approach

0KBL4ZX Excision of Left Abdomen Muscle, Percutaneous Endoscopic Approach, Diagnostic

0KBL4ZZ Excision of Left Abdomen Muscle, Percutaneous Endoscopic Approach

0KBM0ZX Excision of Perineum Muscle, Open Approach, Diagnostic

0KBM0ZZ Excision of Perineum Muscle, Open Approach

0KBM3ZX Excision of Perineum Muscle, Percutaneous Approach, Diagnostic

0KBM3ZZ Excision of Perineum Muscle, Percutaneous Approach

0KBM4ZX Excision of Perineum Muscle, Percutaneous Endoscopic Approach, Diagnostic

0KBM4ZZ Excision of Perineum Muscle, Percutaneous Endoscopic Approach

0KBN0ZX Excision of Right Hip Muscle, Open Approach, Diagnostic

0KBN0ZZ Excision of Right Hip Muscle, Open Approach
AHA CC: 3Q, 2016, 20

0KBN3ZX Excision of Right Hip Muscle, Percutaneous Approach, Diagnostic

0KBN3ZZ Excision of Right Hip Muscle, Percutaneous Approach

0KBN4ZX Excision of Right Hip Muscle, Percutaneous Endoscopic Approach, Diagnostic

0KBN4ZZ Excision of Right Hip Muscle, Percutaneous Endoscopic Approach

0KBP0ZX Excision of Left Hip Muscle, Open Approach, Diagnostic

0KBP0ZZ Excision of Left Hip Muscle, Open Approach
AHA CC: 3Q, 2016, 20; 4Q, 2019, 43-44

0KBP3ZX Excision of Left Hip Muscle, Percutaneous Approach, Diagnostic

0KBP3ZZ Excision of Left Hip Muscle, Percutaneous Approach

0KBP4ZX Excision of Left Hip Muscle, Percutaneous Endoscopic Approach, Diagnostic

0KBP4ZZ Excision of Left Hip Muscle, Percutaneous Endoscopic Approach

0KBQ0ZX Excision of Right Upper Leg Muscle, Open Approach, Diagnostic

0KBQ0ZZ Excision of Right Upper Leg Muscle, Open Approach

0KBQ3ZX Excision of Right Upper Leg Muscle, Percutaneous Approach, Diagnostic

0KBQ3ZZ Excision of Right Upper Leg Muscle, Percutaneous Approach

0KBQ4ZX Excision of Right Upper Leg Muscle, Percutaneous Endoscopic Approach, Diagnostic

0KBQ4ZZ Excision of Right Upper Leg Muscle, Percutaneous Endoscopic Approach

0KBR0ZX Excision of Left Upper Leg Muscle, Open Approach, Diagnostic

0KBR0ZZ Excision of Left Upper Leg Muscle, Open Approach
AHA CC: 1Q, 2020, 27-28

0KBR3ZX Excision of Left Upper Leg Muscle, Percutaneous Approach, Diagnostic

0KBR3ZZ	Excision of Left Upper Leg Muscle, Percutaneous Approach	**0KBT0ZX**	Excision of Left Lower Leg Muscle, Open Approach, Diagnostic
0KBR4ZX	Excision of Left Upper Leg Muscle, Percutaneous Endoscopic Approach, Diagnostic	**0KBT0ZZ**	Excision of Left Lower Leg Muscle, Open Approach
0KBR4ZZ	Excision of Left Upper Leg Muscle, Percutaneous Endoscopic Approach	**0KBT3ZX**	Excision of Left Lower Leg Muscle, Percutaneous Approach, Diagnostic
0KBS0ZX	Excision of Right Lower Leg Muscle, Open Approach, Diagnostic	**0KBT3ZZ**	Excision of Left Lower Leg Muscle, Percutaneous Approach
0KBS0ZZ	Excision of Right Lower Leg Muscle, Open Approach	**0KBT4ZX**	Excision of Left Lower Leg Muscle, Percutaneous Endoscopic Approach, Diagnostic
0KBS3ZX	Excision of Right Lower Leg Muscle, Percutaneous Approach, Diagnostic	**0KBT4ZZ**	Excision of Left Lower Leg Muscle, Percutaneous Endoscopic Approach
0KBS3ZZ	Excision of Right Lower Leg Muscle, Percutaneous Approach	**0KBV0ZX**	Excision of Right Foot Muscle, Open Approach, Diagnostic
0KBS4ZX	Excision of Right Lower Leg Muscle, Percutaneous Endoscopic Approach, Diagnostic	**0KBV0ZZ**	Excision of Right Foot Muscle, Open Approach
0KBS4ZZ	Excision of Right Lower Leg Muscle, Percutaneous Endoscopic Approach	**0KBV3ZX**	Excision of Right Foot Muscle, Percutaneous Approach, Diagnostic
		0KBV3ZZ	Excision of Right Foot Muscle, Percutaneous Approach

0KBV4ZX	Excision of Right Foot Muscle, Percutaneous Endoscopic Approach, Diagnostic
0KBV4ZZ	Excision of Right Foot Muscle, Percutaneous Endoscopic Approach
0KBW0ZX	Excision of Left Foot Muscle, Open Approach, Diagnostic
0KBW0ZZ	Excision of Left Foot Muscle, Open Approach
0KBW3ZX	Excision of Left Foot Muscle, Percutaneous Approach, Diagnostic
0KBW3ZZ	Excision of Left Foot Muscle, Percutaneous Approach
0KBW4ZX	Excision of Left Foot Muscle, Percutaneous Endoscopic Approach, Diagnostic
0KBW4ZZ	Excision of Left Foot Muscle, Percutaneous Endoscopic Approach

0KC – Muscles, Extirpation

0KC00ZZ	Extirpation of Matter from Head Muscle, Open Approach	**0KC70ZZ**	Extirpation of Matter from Right Upper Arm Muscle, Open Approach
0KC03ZZ	Extirpation of Matter from Head Muscle, Percutaneous Approach	**0KC73ZZ**	Extirpation of Matter from Right Upper Arm Muscle, Percutaneous Approach
0KC04ZZ	Extirpation of Matter from Head Muscle, Percutaneous Endoscopic Approach	**0KC74ZZ**	Extirpation of Matter from Right Upper Arm Muscle, Percutaneous Endoscopic Approach
0KC10ZZ	Extirpation of Matter from Facial Muscle, Open Approach	**0KC80ZZ**	Extirpation of Matter from Left Upper Arm Muscle, Open Approach
0KC13ZZ	Extirpation of Matter from Facial Muscle, Percutaneous Approach	**0KC83ZZ**	Extirpation of Matter from Left Upper Arm Muscle, Percutaneous Approach
0KC14ZZ	Extirpation of Matter from Facial Muscle, Percutaneous Endoscopic Approach	**0KC84ZZ**	Extirpation of Matter from Left Upper Arm Muscle, Percutaneous Endoscopic Approach
0KC20ZZ	Extirpation of Matter from Right Neck Muscle, Open Approach	**0KC90ZZ**	Extirpation of Matter from Right Lower Arm and Wrist Muscle, Open Approach
0KC23ZZ	Extirpation of Matter from Right Neck Muscle, Percutaneous Approach	**0KC93ZZ**	Extirpation of Matter from Right Lower Arm and Wrist Muscle, Percutaneous Approach
0KC24ZZ	Extirpation of Matter from Right Neck Muscle, Percutaneous Endoscopic Approach	**0KC94ZZ**	Extirpation of Matter from Right Lower Arm and Wrist Muscle, Percutaneous Endoscopic Approach
0KC30ZZ	Extirpation of Matter from Left Neck Muscle, Open Approach	**0KCB0ZZ**	Extirpation of Matter from Left Lower Arm and Wrist Muscle, Open Approach
0KC33ZZ	Extirpation of Matter from Left Neck Muscle, Percutaneous Approach	**0KCB3ZZ**	Extirpation of Matter from Left Lower Arm and Wrist Muscle, Percutaneous Approach
0KC34ZZ	Extirpation of Matter from Left Neck Muscle, Percutaneous Endoscopic Approach	**0KCB4ZZ**	Extirpation of Matter from Left Lower Arm and Wrist Muscle, Percutaneous Endoscopic Approach
0KC40ZZ	Extirpation of Matter from Tongue, Palate, Pharynx Muscle, Open Approach	**0KCC0ZZ**	Extirpation of Matter from Right Hand Muscle, Open Approach
0KC43ZZ	Extirpation of Matter from Tongue, Palate, Pharynx Muscle, Percutaneous Approach	**0KCC3ZZ**	Extirpation of Matter from Right Hand Muscle, Percutaneous Approach
0KC44ZZ	Extirpation of Matter from Tongue, Palate, Pharynx Muscle, Percutaneous Endoscopic Approach	**0KCC4ZZ**	Extirpation of Matter from Right Hand Muscle, Percutaneous Endoscopic Approach
0KC50ZZ	Extirpation of Matter from Right Shoulder Muscle, Open Approach	**0KCD0ZZ**	Extirpation of Matter from Left Hand Muscle, Open Approach
0KC53ZZ	Extirpation of Matter from Right Shoulder Muscle, Percutaneous Approach	**0KCD3ZZ**	Extirpation of Matter from Left Hand Muscle, Percutaneous Approach
0KC54ZZ	Extirpation of Matter from Right Shoulder Muscle, Percutaneous Endoscopic Approach	**0KCD4ZZ**	Extirpation of Matter from Left Hand Muscle, Percutaneous Endoscopic Approach
0KC60ZZ	Extirpation of Matter from Left Shoulder Muscle, Open Approach	**0KCF0ZZ**	Extirpation of Matter from Right Trunk Muscle, Open Approach
0KC63ZZ	Extirpation of Matter from Left Shoulder Muscle, Percutaneous Approach	**0KCF3ZZ**	Extirpation of Matter from Right Trunk Muscle, Percutaneous Approach
0KC64ZZ	Extirpation of Matter from Left Shoulder Muscle, Percutaneous Endoscopic Approach	**0KCF4ZZ**	Extirpation of Matter from Right Trunk Muscle, Percutaneous Endoscopic Approach

0KCG0ZZ	Extirpation of Matter from Left Trunk Muscle, Open Approach
0KCG3ZZ	Extirpation of Matter from Left Trunk Muscle, Percutaneous Approach
0KCG4ZZ	Extirpation of Matter from Left Trunk Muscle, Percutaneous Endoscopic Approach
0KCH0ZZ	Extirpation of Matter from Right Thorax Muscle, Open Approach
0KCH3ZZ	Extirpation of Matter from Right Thorax Muscle, Percutaneous Approach
0KCH4ZZ	Extirpation of Matter from Right Thorax Muscle, Percutaneous Endoscopic Approach
0KCJ0ZZ	Extirpation of Matter from Left Thorax Muscle, Open Approach
0KCJ3ZZ	Extirpation of Matter from Left Thorax Muscle, Percutaneous Approach
0KCJ4ZZ	Extirpation of Matter from Left Thorax Muscle, Percutaneous Endoscopic Approach
0KCK0ZZ	Extirpation of Matter from Right Abdomen Muscle, Open Approach
0KCK3ZZ	Extirpation of Matter from Right Abdomen Muscle, Percutaneous Approach
0KCK4ZZ	Extirpation of Matter from Right Abdomen Muscle, Percutaneous Endoscopic Approach
0KCL0ZZ	Extirpation of Matter from Left Abdomen Muscle, Open Approach
0KCL3ZZ	Extirpation of Matter from Left Abdomen Muscle, Percutaneous Approach
0KCL4ZZ	Extirpation of Matter from Left Abdomen Muscle, Percutaneous Endoscopic Approach
0KCM0ZZ	Extirpation of Matter from Perineum Muscle, Open Approach
0KCM3ZZ	Extirpation of Matter from Perineum Muscle, Percutaneous Approach
0KCM4ZZ	Extirpation of Matter from Perineum Muscle, Percutaneous Endoscopic Approach
0KCN0ZZ	Extirpation of Matter from Right Hip Muscle, Open Approach
0KCN3ZZ	Extirpation of Matter from Right Hip Muscle, Percutaneous Approach
0KCN4ZZ	Extirpation of Matter from Right Hip Muscle, Percutaneous Endoscopic Approach

♀ Female-only ♂ Male-only ▲ Limited Coverage ● Non-OR 🄷🄰🄲 HAC-associated procedure ▲ Non-covered procedures ✚ Cluster

0KCP0ZZ Extirpation of Matter from Left Hip Muscle, Open Approach

0KCP3ZZ Extirpation of Matter from Left Hip Muscle, Percutaneous Approach

0KCP4ZZ Extirpation of Matter from Left Hip Muscle, Percutaneous Endoscopic Approach

0KCQ0ZZ Extirpation of Matter from Right Upper Leg Muscle, Open Approach

0KCQ3ZZ Extirpation of Matter from Right Upper Leg Muscle, Percutaneous Approach

0KCQ4ZZ Extirpation of Matter from Right Upper Leg Muscle, Percutaneous Endoscopic Approach

0KCR0ZZ Extirpation of Matter from Left Upper Leg Muscle, Open Approach

0KCR3ZZ Extirpation of Matter from Left Upper Leg Muscle, Percutaneous Approach

0KCR4ZZ Extirpation of Matter from Left Upper Leg Muscle, Percutaneous Endoscopic Approach

0KCS0ZZ Extirpation of Matter from Right Lower Leg Muscle, Open Approach

0KCS3ZZ Extirpation of Matter from Right Lower Leg Muscle, Percutaneous Approach

0KCS4ZZ Extirpation of Matter from Right Lower Leg Muscle, Percutaneous Endoscopic Approach

0KCT0ZZ Extirpation of Matter from Left Lower Leg Muscle, Open Approach

0KCT3ZZ Extirpation of Matter from Left Lower Leg Muscle, Percutaneous Approach

0KCT4ZZ Extirpation of Matter from Left Lower Leg Muscle, Percutaneous Endoscopic Approach

0KCV0ZZ Extirpation of Matter from Right Foot Muscle, Open Approach

0KCV3ZZ Extirpation of Matter from Right Foot Muscle, Percutaneous Approach

0KCV4ZZ Extirpation of Matter from Right Foot Muscle, Percutaneous Endoscopic Approach

0KCW0ZZ Extirpation of Matter from Left Foot Muscle, Open Approach

0KCW3ZZ Extirpation of Matter from Left Foot Muscle, Percutaneous Approach

0KCW4ZZ Extirpation of Matter from Left Foot Muscle, Percutaneous Endoscopic Approach

0KD – Muscles, Extraction

0KD00ZZ Extraction of Head Muscle, Open Approach

0KD10ZZ Extraction of Facial Muscle, Open Approach

0KD20ZZ Extraction of Right Neck Muscle, Open Approach

0KD30ZZ Extraction of Left Neck Muscle, Open Approach

0KD40ZZ Extraction of Tongue, Palate, Pharynx Muscle, Open Approach

0KD50ZZ Extraction of Right Shoulder Muscle, Open Approach

0KD60ZZ Extraction of Left Shoulder Muscle, Open Approach

0KD70ZZ Extraction of Right Upper Arm Muscle, Open Approach

0KD80ZZ Extraction of Left Upper Arm Muscle, Open Approach

0KD90ZZ Extraction of Right Lower Arm and Wrist Muscle, Open Approach

0KDB0ZZ Extraction of Left Lower Arm and Wrist Muscle, Open Approach

0KDC0ZZ Extraction of Right Hand Muscle, Open Approach

0KDD0ZZ Extraction of Left Hand Muscle, Open Approach

0KDF0ZZ Extraction of Right Trunk Muscle, Open Approach

0KDG0ZZ Extraction of Left Trunk Muscle, Open Approach

0KDH0ZZ Extraction of Right Thorax Muscle, Open Approach

0KDJ0ZZ Extraction of Left Thorax Muscle, Open Approach

0KDK0ZZ Extraction of Right Abdomen Muscle, Open Approach

0KDL0ZZ Extraction of Left Abdomen Muscle, Open Approach

0KDM0ZZ Extraction of Perineum Muscle, Open Approach

0KDN0ZZ Extraction of Right Hip Muscle, Open Approach

0KDP0ZZ Extraction of Left Hip Muscle, Open Approach

0KDQ0ZZ Extraction of Right Upper Leg Muscle, Open Approach

0KDR0ZZ Extraction of Left Upper Leg Muscle, Open Approach

0KDS0ZZ Extraction of Right Lower Leg Muscle, Open Approach

AHA CC: 4Q, 2017, 42

0KDT0ZZ Extraction of Left Lower Leg Muscle, Open Approach

0KDV0ZZ Extraction of Right Foot Muscle, Open Approach

0KDW0ZZ Extraction of Left Foot Muscle, Open Approach

0KH – Muscles, Insertion

0KHX0MZ Insertion of Stimulator Lead into Upper Muscle, Open Approach

0KHX0YZ Insertion of Other Device into Upper Muscle, Open Approach

0KHX3MZ Insertion of Stimulator Lead into Upper Muscle, Percutaneous Approach

0KHX3YZ Insertion of Other Device into Upper Muscle, Percutaneous Approach

0KHX4MZ Insertion of Stimulator Lead into Upper Muscle, Percutaneous Endoscopic Approach

0KHX4YZ Insertion of Other Device into Upper Muscle, Percutaneous Endoscopic Approach

0KHY0MZ Insertion of Stimulator Lead into Lower Muscle, Open Approach

0KHY0YZ Insertion of Other Device into Lower Muscle, Open Approach

0KHY3MZ Insertion of Stimulator Lead into Lower Muscle, Percutaneous Approach

0KHY3YZ Insertion of Other Device into Lower Muscle, Percutaneous Approach

AHA CC: 4Q, 2020, 63-64

0KHY4MZ Insertion of Stimulator Lead into Lower Muscle, Percutaneous Endoscopic Approach

0KHY4YZ Insertion of Other Device into Lower Muscle, Percutaneous Endoscopic Approach

0KJ – Muscles, Inspection

Review Coding Guideline B3.5

Review Coding Guidelines B3.11a, B3.11b and B3.11c

0KJX0ZZ Inspection of Upper Muscle, Open Approach

0KJX3ZZ Inspection of Upper Muscle, Percutaneous Approach

0KJX4ZZ Inspection of Upper Muscle, Percutaneous Endoscopic Approach

0KJXXZZ Inspection of Upper Muscle, External Approach

0KJY0ZZ Inspection of Lower Muscle, Open Approach

0KJY3ZZ Inspection of Lower Muscle, Percutaneous Approach

0KJY4ZZ Inspection of Lower Muscle, Percutaneous Endoscopic Approach

0KJYXZZ Inspection of Lower Muscle, External Approach

0KM – Muscles, Reattachment

0KM00ZZ Reattachment of Head Muscle, Open Approach

0KM04ZZ Reattachment of Head Muscle, Percutaneous Endoscopic Approach

0KM10ZZ Reattachment of Facial Muscle, Open Approach

0KM14ZZ Reattachment of Facial Muscle, Percutaneous Endoscopic Approach

0KM20ZZ Reattachment of Right Neck Muscle, Open Approach

0KM24ZZ Reattachment of Right Neck Muscle, Percutaneous Endoscopic Approach

0KM30ZZ	Reattachment of Left Neck Muscle, Open Approach
0KM34ZZ	Reattachment of Left Neck Muscle, Percutaneous Endoscopic Approach
0KM40ZZ	Reattachment of Tongue, Palate, Pharynx Muscle, Open Approach
0KM44ZZ	Reattachment of Tongue, Palate, Pharynx Muscle, Percutaneous Endoscopic Approach
0KM50ZZ	Reattachment of Right Shoulder Muscle, Open Approach
0KM54ZZ	Reattachment of Right Shoulder Muscle, Percutaneous Endoscopic Approach
0KM60ZZ	Reattachment of Left Shoulder Muscle, Open Approach
0KM64ZZ	Reattachment of Left Shoulder Muscle, Percutaneous Endoscopic Approach
0KM70ZZ	Reattachment of Right Upper Arm Muscle, Open Approach
0KM74ZZ	Reattachment of Right Upper Arm Muscle, Percutaneous Endoscopic Approach
0KM80ZZ	Reattachment of Left Upper Arm Muscle, Open Approach
0KM84ZZ	Reattachment of Left Upper Arm Muscle, Percutaneous Endoscopic Approach
0KM90ZZ	Reattachment of Right Lower Arm and Wrist Muscle, Open Approach
0KM94ZZ	Reattachment of Right Lower Arm and Wrist Muscle, Percutaneous Endoscopic Approach
0KMB0ZZ	Reattachment of Left Lower Arm and Wrist Muscle, Open Approach
0KMB4ZZ	Reattachment of Left Lower Arm and Wrist Muscle, Percutaneous Endoscopic Approach
0KMC0ZZ	Reattachment of Right Hand Muscle, Open Approach
0KMC4ZZ	Reattachment of Right Hand Muscle, Percutaneous Endoscopic Approach
0KMD0ZZ	Reattachment of Left Hand Muscle, Open Approach
0KMD4ZZ	Reattachment of Left Hand Muscle, Percutaneous Endoscopic Approach
0KMF0ZZ	Reattachment of Right Trunk Muscle, Open Approach
0KMF4ZZ	Reattachment of Right Trunk Muscle, Percutaneous Endoscopic Approach
0KMG0ZZ	Reattachment of Left Trunk Muscle, Open Approach
0KMG4ZZ	Reattachment of Left Trunk Muscle, Percutaneous Endoscopic Approach
0KMH0ZZ	Reattachment of Right Thorax Muscle, Open Approach
0KMH4ZZ	Reattachment of Right Thorax Muscle, Percutaneous Endoscopic Approach
0KMJ0ZZ	Reattachment of Left Thorax Muscle, Open Approach
0KMJ4ZZ	Reattachment of Left Thorax Muscle, Percutaneous Endoscopic Approach
0KMK0ZZ	Reattachment of Right Abdomen Muscle, Open Approach
0KMK4ZZ	Reattachment of Right Abdomen Muscle, Percutaneous Endoscopic Approach
0KML0ZZ	Reattachment of Left Abdomen Muscle, Open Approach
0KML4ZZ	Reattachment of Left Abdomen Muscle, Percutaneous Endoscopic Approach
0KMM0ZZ	Reattachment of Perineum Muscle, Open Approach
0KMM4ZZ	Reattachment of Perineum Muscle, Percutaneous Endoscopic Approach
0KMN0ZZ	Reattachment of Right Hip Muscle, Open Approach
0KMN4ZZ	Reattachment of Right Hip Muscle, Percutaneous Endoscopic Approach
0KMP0ZZ	Reattachment of Left Hip Muscle, Open Approach
0KMP4ZZ	Reattachment of Left Hip Muscle, Percutaneous Endoscopic Approach
0KMQ0ZZ	Reattachment of Right Upper Leg Muscle, Open Approach
0KMQ4ZZ	Reattachment of Right Upper Leg Muscle, Percutaneous Endoscopic Approach
0KMR0ZZ	Reattachment of Left Upper Leg Muscle, Open Approach
0KMR4ZZ	Reattachment of Left Upper Leg Muscle, Percutaneous Endoscopic Approach
0KMS0ZZ	Reattachment of Right Lower Leg Muscle, Open Approach
0KMS4ZZ	Reattachment of Right Lower Leg Muscle, Percutaneous Endoscopic Approach
0KMT0ZZ	Reattachment of Left Lower Leg Muscle, Open Approach
0KMT4ZZ	Reattachment of Left Lower Leg Muscle, Percutaneous Endoscopic Approach
0KMV0ZZ	Reattachment of Right Foot Muscle, Open Approach
0KMV4ZZ	Reattachment of Right Foot Muscle, Percutaneous Endoscopic Approach
0KMW0ZZ	Reattachment of Left Foot Muscle, Open Approach
0KMW4ZZ	Reattachment of Left Foot Muscle, Percutaneous Endoscopic Approach

0KN – Muscles, Release

Review Coding Guideline B3.13

Review Coding Guideline B3.14

0KN00ZZ	Release Head Muscle, Open Approach
0KN03ZZ	Release Head Muscle, Percutaneous Approach
0KN04ZZ	Release Head Muscle, Percutaneous Endoscopic Approach
0KN0XZZ	Release Head Muscle, External Approach
0KN10ZZ	Release Facial Muscle, Open Approach
0KN13ZZ	Release Facial Muscle, Percutaneous Approach
0KN14ZZ	Release Facial Muscle, Percutaneous Endoscopic Approach
0KN1XZZ	Release Facial Muscle, External Approach
0KN20ZZ	Release Right Neck Muscle, Open Approach
0KN23ZZ	Release Right Neck Muscle, Percutaneous Approach
0KN24ZZ	Release Right Neck Muscle, Percutaneous Endoscopic Approach
0KN2XZZ	Release Right Neck Muscle, External Approach
0KN30ZZ	Release Left Neck Muscle, Open Approach
0KN33ZZ	Release Left Neck Muscle, Percutaneous Approach
0KN34ZZ	Release Left Neck Muscle, Percutaneous Endoscopic Approach
0KN3XZZ	Release Left Neck Muscle, External Approach
0KN40ZZ	Release Tongue, Palate, Pharynx Muscle, Open Approach
0KN43ZZ	Release Tongue, Palate, Pharynx Muscle, Percutaneous Approach
0KN44ZZ	Release Tongue, Palate, Pharynx Muscle, Percutaneous Endoscopic Approach
0KN4XZZ	Release Tongue, Palate, Pharynx Muscle, External Approach
0KN50ZZ	Release Right Shoulder Muscle, Open Approach
0KN53ZZ	Release Right Shoulder Muscle, Percutaneous Approach
0KN54ZZ	Release Right Shoulder Muscle, Percutaneous Endoscopic Approach
0KN5XZZ	Release Right Shoulder Muscle, External Approach
0KN60ZZ	Release Left Shoulder Muscle, Open Approach
0KN63ZZ	Release Left Shoulder Muscle, Percutaneous Approach
0KN64ZZ	Release Left Shoulder Muscle, Percutaneous Endoscopic Approach
0KN6XZZ	Release Left Shoulder Muscle, External Approach
0KN70ZZ	Release Right Upper Arm Muscle, Open Approach
0KN73ZZ	Release Right Upper Arm Muscle, Percutaneous Approach
0KN74ZZ	Release Right Upper Arm Muscle, Percutaneous Endoscopic Approach
0KN7XZZ	Release Right Upper Arm Muscle, External Approach
0KN80ZZ	Release Left Upper Arm Muscle, Open Approach
0KN83ZZ	Release Left Upper Arm Muscle, Percutaneous Approach
0KN84ZZ	Release Left Upper Arm Muscle, Percutaneous Endoscopic Approach
	AHA CC: 2Q, 2015, 22-23
0KN8XZZ	Release Left Upper Arm Muscle, External Approach
0KN90ZZ	Release Right Lower Arm and Wrist Muscle, Open Approach
0KN93ZZ	Release Right Lower Arm and Wrist Muscle, Percutaneous Approach
0KN94ZZ	Release Right Lower Arm and Wrist Muscle, Percutaneous Endoscopic Approach
0KN9XZZ	Release Right Lower Arm and Wrist Muscle, External Approach
0KNB0ZZ	Release Left Lower Arm and Wrist Muscle, Open Approach
0KNB3ZZ	Release Left Lower Arm and Wrist Muscle, Percutaneous Approach
0KNB4ZZ	Release Left Lower Arm and Wrist Muscle, Percutaneous Endoscopic Approach
0KNBXZZ	Release Left Lower Arm and Wrist Muscle, External Approach
0KNC0ZZ	Release Right Hand Muscle, Open Approach

0KNC3ZZ Release Right Hand Muscle, Percutaneous Approach

0KNC4ZZ Release Right Hand Muscle, Percutaneous Endoscopic Approach

0KNCXZZ Release Right Hand Muscle, External Approach

0KND0ZZ Release Left Hand Muscle, Open Approach

0KND3ZZ Release Left Hand Muscle, Percutaneous Approach

0KND4ZZ Release Left Hand Muscle, Percutaneous Endoscopic Approach

0KNDXZZ Release Left Hand Muscle, External Approach

0KNF0ZZ Release Right Trunk Muscle, Open Approach

0KNF3ZZ Release Right Trunk Muscle, Percutaneous Approach

0KNF4ZZ Release Right Trunk Muscle, Percutaneous Endoscopic Approach

0KNFXZZ Release Right Trunk Muscle, External Approach

0KNG0ZZ Release Left Trunk Muscle, Open Approach

0KNG3ZZ Release Left Trunk Muscle, Percutaneous Approach

0KNG4ZZ Release Left Trunk Muscle, Percutaneous Endoscopic Approach

0KNGXZZ Release Left Trunk Muscle, External Approach

0KNH0ZZ Release Right Thorax Muscle, Open Approach

0KNH3ZZ Release Right Thorax Muscle, Percutaneous Approach

0KNH4ZZ Release Right Thorax Muscle, Percutaneous Endoscopic Approach

0KNHXZZ Release Right Thorax Muscle, External Approach

0KNJ0ZZ Release Left Thorax Muscle, Open Approach

0KNJ3ZZ Release Left Thorax Muscle, Percutaneous Approach

0KNJ4ZZ Release Left Thorax Muscle, Percutaneous Endoscopic Approach

0KNJXZZ Release Left Thorax Muscle, External Approach

0KNK0ZZ Release Right Abdomen Muscle, Open Approach
AHA CC: 4Q, 2014, 39-40

0KNK3ZZ Release Right Abdomen Muscle, Percutaneous Approach

0KNK4ZZ Release Right Abdomen Muscle, Percutaneous Endoscopic Approach

0KNKXZZ Release Right Abdomen Muscle, External Approach

0KNL0ZZ Release Left Abdomen Muscle, Open Approach
AHA CC: 4Q, 2014, 39-40

0KNL3ZZ Release Left Abdomen Muscle, Percutaneous Approach

0KNL4ZZ Release Left Abdomen Muscle, Percutaneous Endoscopic Approach

0KNLXZZ Release Left Abdomen Muscle, External Approach

0KNM0ZZ Release Perineum Muscle, Open Approach

0KNM3ZZ Release Perineum Muscle, Percutaneous Approach

0KNM4ZZ Release Perineum Muscle, Percutaneous Endoscopic Approach

0KNMXZZ Release Perineum Muscle, External Approach

0KNN0ZZ Release Right Hip Muscle, Open Approach

0KNN3ZZ Release Right Hip Muscle, Percutaneous Approach

0KNN4ZZ Release Right Hip Muscle, Percutaneous Endoscopic Approach

0KNNXZZ Release Right Hip Muscle, External Approach

0KNP0ZZ Release Left Hip Muscle, Open Approach

0KNP3ZZ Release Left Hip Muscle, Percutaneous Approach

0KNP4ZZ Release Left Hip Muscle, Percutaneous Endoscopic Approach

0KNPXZZ Release Left Hip Muscle, External Approach

0KNQ0ZZ Release Right Upper Leg Muscle, Open Approach

0KNQ3ZZ Release Right Upper Leg Muscle, Percutaneous Approach

0KNQ4ZZ Release Right Upper Leg Muscle, Percutaneous Endoscopic Approach

0KNQXZZ Release Right Upper Leg Muscle, External Approach

0KNR0ZZ Release Left Upper Leg Muscle, Open Approach

0KNR3ZZ Release Left Upper Leg Muscle, Percutaneous Approach

0KNR4ZZ Release Left Upper Leg Muscle, Percutaneous Endoscopic Approach

0KNRXZZ Release Left Upper Leg Muscle, External Approach

0KNS0ZZ Release Right Lower Leg Muscle, Open Approach

0KNS3ZZ Release Right Lower Leg Muscle, Percutaneous Approach

0KNS4ZZ Release Right Lower Leg Muscle, Percutaneous Endoscopic Approach

0KNSXZZ Release Right Lower Leg Muscle, External Approach

0KNT0ZZ Release Left Lower Leg Muscle, Open Approach
AHA CC: 2Q, 2017, 12-14

0KNT3ZZ Release Left Lower Leg Muscle, Percutaneous Approach

0KNT4ZZ Release Left Lower Leg Muscle, Percutaneous Endoscopic Approach

0KNTXZZ Release Left Lower Leg Muscle, External Approach

0KNV0ZZ Release Right Foot Muscle, Open Approach
AHA CC: 2Q, 2017, 12-14

0KNV3ZZ Release Right Foot Muscle, Percutaneous Approach

0KNV4ZZ Release Right Foot Muscle, Percutaneous Endoscopic Approach

0KNVXZZ Release Right Foot Muscle, External Approach

0KNW0ZZ Release Left Foot Muscle, Open Approach

0KNW3ZZ Release Left Foot Muscle, Percutaneous Approach

0KNW4ZZ Release Left Foot Muscle, Percutaneous Endoscopic Approach

0KNWXZZ Release Left Foot Muscle, External Approach

0KP – Muscles, Removal

Review Coding Guideline B6.1c

0KPX00Z Removal of Drainage Device from Upper Muscle, Open Approach

0KPX07Z Removal of Autologous Tissue Substitute from Upper Muscle, Open Approach

0KPX0JZ Removal of Synthetic Substitute from Upper Muscle, Open Approach

0KPX0KZ Removal of Nonautologous Tissue Substitute from Upper Muscle, Open Approach

0KPX0MZ Removal of Stimulator Lead from Upper Muscle, Open Approach

0KPX0YZ Removal of Other Device from Upper Muscle, Open Approach

0KPX30Z Removal of Drainage Device from Upper Muscle, Percutaneous Approach

0KPX37Z Removal of Autologous Tissue Substitute from Upper Muscle, Percutaneous Approach

0KPX3JZ Removal of Synthetic Substitute from Upper Muscle, Percutaneous Approach

0KPX3KZ Removal of Nonautologous Tissue Substitute from Upper Muscle, Percutaneous Approach

0KPX3MZ Removal of Stimulator Lead from Upper Muscle, Percutaneous Approach

0KPX3YZ Removal of Other Device from Upper Muscle, Percutaneous Approach

0KPX40Z Removal of Drainage Device from Upper Muscle, Percutaneous Endoscopic Approach

0KPX47Z Removal of Autologous Tissue Substitute from Upper Muscle, Percutaneous Endoscopic Approach

0KPX4JZ Removal of Synthetic Substitute from Upper Muscle, Percutaneous Endoscopic Approach

0KPX4KZ Removal of Nonautologous Tissue Substitute from Upper Muscle, Percutaneous Endoscopic Approach

0KPX4MZ Removal of Stimulator Lead from Upper Muscle, Percutaneous Endoscopic Approach

0KPX4YZ Removal of Other Device from Upper Muscle, Percutaneous Endoscopic Approach

0KPXX0Z Removal of Drainage Device from Upper Muscle, External Approach

0KPXXMZ Removal of Stimulator Lead from Upper Muscle, External Approach

0KPY00Z Removal of Drainage Device from Lower Muscle, Open Approach

0KPY07Z Removal of Autologous Tissue Substitute from Lower Muscle, Open Approach

0KPY0JZ Removal of Synthetic Substitute from Lower Muscle, Open Approach

0KPY0KZ Removal of Nonautologous Tissue Substitute from Lower Muscle, Open Approach

0KPY0MZ Removal of Stimulator Lead from Lower Muscle, Open Approach

0KPY0YZ Removal of Other Device from Lower Muscle, Open Approach

0KPY30Z Removal of Drainage Device from Lower Muscle, Percutaneous Approach

0KPY37Z Removal of Autologous Tissue Substitute from Lower Muscle, Percutaneous Approach

0KPY3JZ Removal of Synthetic Substitute from Lower Muscle, Percutaneous Approach

0KPY3KZ Removal of Nonautologous Tissue Substitute from Lower Muscle, Percutaneous Approach	**0KPY47Z** Removal of Autologous Tissue Substitute from Lower Muscle, Percutaneous Endoscopic Approach	**0KPY4YZ** Removal of Other Device from Lower Muscle, Percutaneous Endoscopic Approach
0KPY3MZ Removal of Stimulator Lead from Lower Muscle, Percutaneous Approach	**0KPY4JZ** Removal of Synthetic Substitute from Lower Muscle, Percutaneous Endoscopic Approach	**0KPYX0Z** Removal of Drainage Device from Lower Muscle, External Approach
0KPY3YZ Removal of Other Device from Lower Muscle, Percutaneous Approach	**0KPY4KZ** Removal of Nonautologous Tissue Substitute from Lower Muscle, Percutaneous Endoscopic Approach	**0KPYXMZ** Removal of Stimulator Lead from Lower Muscle, External Approach
0KPY40Z Removal of Drainage Device from Lower Muscle, Percutaneous Endoscopic Approach	**0KPY4MZ** Removal of Stimulator Lead from Lower Muscle, Percutaneous Endoscopic Approach	

0KQ – Muscles, Repair

Review Coding Guideline B3.5

0KQ00ZZ Repair Head Muscle, Open Approach	**0KQ94ZZ** Repair Right Lower Arm and Wrist Muscle, Percutaneous Endoscopic Approach	**0KQM0ZZ** Repair Perineum Muscle, Open Approach
0KQ03ZZ Repair Head Muscle, Percutaneous Approach	**0KQB0ZZ** Repair Left Lower Arm and Wrist Muscle, Open Approach	*AHA CC: 4Q, 2013, 120; 1Q, 2016, 7; 2Q, 2016, 34-35*
0KQ04ZZ Repair Head Muscle, Percutaneous Endoscopic Approach	**0KQB3ZZ** Repair Left Lower Arm and Wrist Muscle, Percutaneous Approach	**0KQM3ZZ** Repair Perineum Muscle, Percutaneous Approach
0KQ10ZZ Repair Facial Muscle, Open Approach	**0KQB4ZZ** Repair Left Lower Arm and Wrist Muscle, Percutaneous Endoscopic Approach	**0KQM4ZZ** Repair Perineum Muscle, Percutaneous Endoscopic Approach
0KQ13ZZ Repair Facial Muscle, Percutaneous Approach	**0KQC0ZZ** Repair Right Hand Muscle, Open Approach	**0KQN0ZZ** Repair Right Hip Muscle, Open Approach
0KQ14ZZ Repair Facial Muscle, Percutaneous Endoscopic Approach	**0KQC3ZZ** Repair Right Hand Muscle, Percutaneous Approach	**0KQN3ZZ** Repair Right Hip Muscle, Percutaneous Approach
0KQ20ZZ Repair Right Neck Muscle, Open Approach	**0KQC4ZZ** Repair Right Hand Muscle, Percutaneous Endoscopic Approach	**0KQN4ZZ** Repair Right Hip Muscle, Percutaneous Endoscopic Approach
0KQ23ZZ Repair Right Neck Muscle, Percutaneous Approach	**0KQD0ZZ** Repair Left Hand Muscle, Open Approach	**0KQP0ZZ** Repair Left Hip Muscle, Open Approach
0KQ24ZZ Repair Right Neck Muscle, Percutaneous Endoscopic Approach	**0KQD3ZZ** Repair Left Hand Muscle, Percutaneous Approach	**0KQP3ZZ** Repair Left Hip Muscle, Percutaneous Approach
0KQ30ZZ Repair Left Neck Muscle, Open Approach	**0KQD4ZZ** Repair Left Hand Muscle, Percutaneous Endoscopic Approach	**0KQP4ZZ** Repair Left Hip Muscle, Percutaneous Endoscopic Approach
0KQ33ZZ Repair Left Neck Muscle, Percutaneous Approach	**0KQF0ZZ** Repair Right Trunk Muscle, Open Approach	**0KQQ0ZZ** Repair Right Upper Leg Muscle, Open Approach
0KQ34ZZ Repair Left Neck Muscle, Percutaneous Endoscopic Approach	**0KQF3ZZ** Repair Right Trunk Muscle, Percutaneous Approach	**0KQQ3ZZ** Repair Right Upper Leg Muscle, Percutaneous Approach
0KQ40ZZ Repair Tongue, Palate, Pharynx Muscle, Open Approach	**0KQF4ZZ** Repair Right Trunk Muscle, Percutaneous Endoscopic Approach	**0KQQ4ZZ** Repair Right Upper Leg Muscle, Percutaneous Endoscopic Approach
0KQ43ZZ Repair Tongue, Palate, Pharynx Muscle, Percutaneous Approach	**0KQG0ZZ** Repair Left Trunk Muscle, Open Approach	**0KQR0ZZ** Repair Left Upper Leg Muscle, Open Approach
0KQ44ZZ Repair Tongue, Palate, Pharynx Muscle, Percutaneous Endoscopic Approach	**0KQG3ZZ** Repair Left Trunk Muscle, Percutaneous Approach	**0KQR3ZZ** Repair Left Upper Leg Muscle, Percutaneous Approach
0KQ50ZZ Repair Right Shoulder Muscle, Open Approach	**0KQG4ZZ** Repair Left Trunk Muscle, Percutaneous Endoscopic Approach	**0KQR4ZZ** Repair Left Upper Leg Muscle, Percutaneous Endoscopic Approach
0KQ53ZZ Repair Right Shoulder Muscle, Percutaneous Approach	**0KQH0ZZ** Repair Right Thorax Muscle, Open Approach	**0KQS0ZZ** Repair Right Lower Leg Muscle, Open Approach
0KQ54ZZ Repair Right Shoulder Muscle, Percutaneous Endoscopic Approach	**0KQH3ZZ** Repair Right Thorax Muscle, Percutaneous Approach	**0KQS3ZZ** Repair Right Lower Leg Muscle, Percutaneous Approach
0KQ60ZZ Repair Left Shoulder Muscle, Open Approach	**0KQH4ZZ** Repair Right Thorax Muscle, Percutaneous Endoscopic Approach	**0KQS4ZZ** Repair Right Lower Leg Muscle, Percutaneous Endoscopic Approach
0KQ63ZZ Repair Left Shoulder Muscle, Percutaneous Approach	**0KQJ0ZZ** Repair Left Thorax Muscle, Open Approach	**0KQT0ZZ** Repair Left Lower Leg Muscle, Open Approach
0KQ64ZZ Repair Left Shoulder Muscle, Percutaneous Endoscopic Approach	**0KQJ3ZZ** Repair Left Thorax Muscle, Percutaneous Approach	**0KQT3ZZ** Repair Left Lower Leg Muscle, Percutaneous Approach
0KQ70ZZ Repair Right Upper Arm Muscle, Open Approach	**0KQJ4ZZ** Repair Left Thorax Muscle, Percutaneous Endoscopic Approach	**0KQT4ZZ** Repair Left Lower Leg Muscle, Percutaneous Endoscopic Approach
0KQ73ZZ Repair Right Upper Arm Muscle, Percutaneous Approach	**0KQK0ZZ** Repair Right Abdomen Muscle, Open Approach	**0KQV0ZZ** Repair Right Foot Muscle, Open Approach
0KQ74ZZ Repair Right Upper Arm Muscle, Percutaneous Endoscopic Approach	**0KQK3ZZ** Repair Right Abdomen Muscle, Percutaneous Approach	**0KQV3ZZ** Repair Right Foot Muscle, Percutaneous Approach
0KQ80ZZ Repair Left Upper Arm Muscle, Open Approach	**0KQK4ZZ** Repair Right Abdomen Muscle, Percutaneous Endoscopic Approach	**0KQV4ZZ** Repair Right Foot Muscle, Percutaneous Endoscopic Approach
0KQ83ZZ Repair Left Upper Arm Muscle, Percutaneous Approach	**0KQL0ZZ** Repair Left Abdomen Muscle, Open Approach	**0KQW0ZZ** Repair Left Foot Muscle, Open Approach
0KQ84ZZ Repair Left Upper Arm Muscle, Percutaneous Endoscopic Approach	**0KQL3ZZ** Repair Left Abdomen Muscle, Percutaneous Approach	**0KQW3ZZ** Repair Left Foot Muscle, Percutaneous Approach
0KQ90ZZ Repair Right Lower Arm and Wrist Muscle, Open Approach	**0KQL4ZZ** Repair Left Abdomen Muscle, Percutaneous Endoscopic Approach	**0KQW4ZZ** Repair Left Foot Muscle, Percutaneous Endoscopic Approach
0KQ93ZZ Repair Right Lower Arm and Wrist Muscle, Percutaneous Approach		

Review Coding Guideline B3.18

0KR007Z Replacement of Head Muscle with Autologous Tissue Substitute, Open Approach

0KR00JZ Replacement of Head Muscle with Synthetic Substitute, Open Approach

0KR00KZ Replacement of Head Muscle with Nonautologous Tissue Substitute, Open Approach

0KR047Z Replacement of Head Muscle with Autologous Tissue Substitute, Percutaneous Endoscopic Approach

0KR04JZ Replacement of Head Muscle with Synthetic Substitute, Percutaneous Endoscopic Approach

0KR04KZ Replacement of Head Muscle with Nonautologous Tissue Substitute, Percutaneous Endoscopic Approach

0KR107Z Replacement of Facial Muscle with Autologous Tissue Substitute, Open Approach

0KR10JZ Replacement of Facial Muscle with Synthetic Substitute, Open Approach

0KR10KZ Replacement of Facial Muscle with Nonautologous Tissue Substitute, Open Approach

0KR147Z Replacement of Facial Muscle with Autologous Tissue Substitute, Percutaneous Endoscopic Approach

0KR14JZ Replacement of Facial Muscle with Synthetic Substitute, Percutaneous Endoscopic Approach

0KR14KZ Replacement of Facial Muscle with Nonautologous Tissue Substitute, Percutaneous Endoscopic Approach

0KR207Z Replacement of Right Neck Muscle with Autologous Tissue Substitute, Open Approach

0KR20JZ Replacement of Right Neck Muscle with Synthetic Substitute, Open Approach

0KR20KZ Replacement of Right Neck Muscle with Nonautologous Tissue Substitute, Open Approach

0KR247Z Replacement of Right Neck Muscle with Autologous Tissue Substitute, Percutaneous Endoscopic Approach

0KR24JZ Replacement of Right Neck Muscle with Synthetic Substitute, Percutaneous Endoscopic Approach

0KR24KZ Replacement of Right Neck Muscle with Nonautologous Tissue Substitute, Percutaneous Endoscopic Approach

0KR307Z Replacement of Left Neck Muscle with Autologous Tissue Substitute, Open Approach

0KR30JZ Replacement of Left Neck Muscle with Synthetic Substitute, Open Approach

0KR30KZ Replacement of Left Neck Muscle with Nonautologous Tissue Substitute, Open Approach

0KR347Z Replacement of Left Neck Muscle with Autologous Tissue Substitute, Percutaneous Endoscopic Approach

0KR34JZ Replacement of Left Neck Muscle with Synthetic Substitute, Percutaneous Endoscopic Approach

0KR34KZ Replacement of Left Neck Muscle with Nonautologous Tissue Substitute, Percutaneous Endoscopic Approach

0KR407Z Replacement of Tongue, Palate, Pharynx Muscle with Autologous Tissue Substitute, Open Approach

0KR40JZ Replacement of Tongue, Palate, Pharynx Muscle with Synthetic Substitute, Open Approach

0KR40KZ Replacement of Tongue, Palate, Pharynx Muscle with Nonautologous Tissue Substitute, Open Approach

0KR447Z Replacement of Tongue, Palate, Pharynx Muscle with Autologous Tissue Substitute, Percutaneous Endoscopic Approach

0KR44JZ Replacement of Tongue, Palate, Pharynx Muscle with Synthetic Substitute, Percutaneous Endoscopic Approach

0KR44KZ Replacement of Tongue, Palate, Pharynx Muscle with Nonautologous Tissue Substitute, Percutaneous Endoscopic Approach

0KR507Z Replacement of Right Shoulder Muscle with Autologous Tissue Substitute, Open Approach

0KR50JZ Replacement of Right Shoulder Muscle with Synthetic Substitute, Open Approach

0KR50KZ Replacement of Right Shoulder Muscle with Nonautologous Tissue Substitute, Open Approach

0KR547Z Replacement of Right Shoulder Muscle with Autologous Tissue Substitute, Percutaneous Endoscopic Approach

0KR54JZ Replacement of Right Shoulder Muscle with Synthetic Substitute, Percutaneous Endoscopic Approach

0KR54KZ Replacement of Right Shoulder Muscle with Nonautologous Tissue Substitute, Percutaneous Endoscopic Approach

0KR607Z Replacement of Left Shoulder Muscle with Autologous Tissue Substitute, Open Approach

0KR60JZ Replacement of Left Shoulder Muscle with Synthetic Substitute, Open Approach

0KR60KZ Replacement of Left Shoulder Muscle with Nonautologous Tissue Substitute, Open Approach

0KR647Z Replacement of Left Shoulder Muscle with Autologous Tissue Substitute, Percutaneous Endoscopic Approach

0KR64JZ Replacement of Left Shoulder Muscle with Synthetic Substitute, Percutaneous Endoscopic Approach

0KR64KZ Replacement of Left Shoulder Muscle with Nonautologous Tissue Substitute, Percutaneous Endoscopic Approach

0KR707Z Replacement of Right Upper Arm Muscle with Autologous Tissue Substitute, Open Approach

0KR70JZ Replacement of Right Upper Arm Muscle with Synthetic Substitute, Open Approach

0KR70KZ Replacement of Right Upper Arm Muscle with Nonautologous Tissue Substitute, Open Approach

0KR747Z Replacement of Right Upper Arm Muscle with Autologous Tissue Substitute, Percutaneous Endoscopic Approach

0KR74JZ Replacement of Right Upper Arm Muscle with Synthetic Substitute, Percutaneous Endoscopic Approach

0KR74KZ Replacement of Right Upper Arm Muscle with Nonautologous Tissue Substitute, Percutaneous Endoscopic Approach

0KR807Z Replacement of Left Upper Arm Muscle with Autologous Tissue Substitute, Open Approach

0KR80JZ Replacement of Left Upper Arm Muscle with Synthetic Substitute, Open Approach

0KR80KZ Replacement of Left Upper Arm Muscle with Nonautologous Tissue Substitute, Open Approach

0KR847Z Replacement of Left Upper Arm Muscle with Autologous Tissue Substitute, Percutaneous Endoscopic Approach

0KR84JZ Replacement of Left Upper Arm Muscle with Synthetic Substitute, Percutaneous Endoscopic Approach

0KR84KZ Replacement of Left Upper Arm Muscle with Nonautologous Tissue Substitute, Percutaneous Endoscopic Approach

0KR907Z Replacement of Right Lower Arm and Wrist Muscle with Autologous Tissue Substitute, Open Approach

0KR90JZ Replacement of Right Lower Arm and Wrist Muscle with Synthetic Substitute, Open Approach

0KR90KZ Replacement of Right Lower Arm and Wrist Muscle with Nonautologous Tissue Substitute, Open Approach

0KR947Z Replacement of Right Lower Arm and Wrist Muscle with Autologous Tissue Substitute, Percutaneous Endoscopic Approach

0KR94JZ Replacement of Right Lower Arm and Wrist Muscle with Synthetic Substitute, Percutaneous Endoscopic Approach

0KR94KZ Replacement of Right Lower Arm and Wrist Muscle with Nonautologous Tissue Substitute, Percutaneous Endoscopic Approach

0KRB07Z Replacement of Left Lower Arm and Wrist Muscle with Autologous Tissue Substitute, Open Approach

0KRB0JZ Replacement of Left Lower Arm and Wrist Muscle with Synthetic Substitute, Open Approach

0KRB0KZ Replacement of Left Lower Arm and Wrist Muscle with Nonautologous Tissue Substitute, Open Approach

0KRB47Z Replacement of Left Lower Arm and Wrist Muscle with Autologous Tissue Substitute, Percutaneous Endoscopic Approach

0KRB4JZ Replacement of Left Lower Arm and Wrist Muscle with Synthetic Substitute, Percutaneous Endoscopic Approach

0KRB4KZ Replacement of Left Lower Arm and Wrist Muscle with Nonautologous Tissue Substitute, Percutaneous Endoscopic Approach

0KRC07Z Replacement of Right Hand Muscle with Autologous Tissue Substitute, Open Approach

0KRC0JZ Replacement of Right Hand Muscle with Synthetic Substitute, Open Approach

0KRC0KZ Replacement of Right Hand Muscle with Nonautologous Tissue Substitute, Open Approach

0KRC47Z Replacement of Right Hand Muscle with Autologous Tissue Substitute, Percutaneous Endoscopic Approach

0KRC4JZ Replacement of Right Hand Muscle with Synthetic Substitute, Percutaneous Endoscopic Approach

0KRC4KZ Replacement of Right Hand Muscle with Nonautologous Tissue Substitute, Percutaneous Endoscopic Approach

0KRD07Z Replacement of Left Hand Muscle with Autologous Tissue Substitute, Open Approach

0KRD0JZ Replacement of Left Hand Muscle with Synthetic Substitute, Open Approach

0KRD0KZ Replacement of Left Hand Muscle with Nonautologous Tissue Substitute, Open Approach

0KRD47Z Replacement of Left Hand Muscle with Autologous Tissue Substitute, Percutaneous Endoscopic Approach

0KRD4JZ Replacement of Left Hand Muscle with Synthetic Substitute, Percutaneous Endoscopic Approach

0KRD4KZ Replacement of Left Hand Muscle with Nonautologous Tissue Substitute, Percutaneous Endoscopic Approach

0KRF07Z Replacement of Right Trunk Muscle with Autologous Tissue Substitute, Open Approach

0KRF0JZ Replacement of Right Trunk Muscle with Synthetic Substitute, Open Approach

0KRF0KZ Replacement of Right Trunk Muscle with Nonautologous Tissue Substitute, Open Approach

0KRF47Z Replacement of Right Trunk Muscle with Autologous Tissue Substitute, Percutaneous Endoscopic Approach

0KRF4JZ Replacement of Right Trunk Muscle with Synthetic Substitute, Percutaneous Endoscopic Approach

0KRF4KZ Replacement of Right Trunk Muscle with Nonautologous Tissue Substitute, Percutaneous Endoscopic Approach

0KRG07Z Replacement of Left Trunk Muscle with Autologous Tissue Substitute, Open Approach

0KRG0JZ Replacement of Left Trunk Muscle with Synthetic Substitute, Open Approach

0KRG0KZ Replacement of Left Trunk Muscle with Nonautologous Tissue Substitute, Open Approach

0KRG47Z Replacement of Left Trunk Muscle with Autologous Tissue Substitute, Percutaneous Endoscopic Approach

0KRG4JZ Replacement of Left Trunk Muscle with Synthetic Substitute, Percutaneous Endoscopic Approach

0KRG4KZ Replacement of Left Trunk Muscle with Nonautologous Tissue Substitute, Percutaneous Endoscopic Approach

0KRH07Z Replacement of Right Thorax Muscle with Autologous Tissue Substitute, Open Approach

0KRH0JZ Replacement of Right Thorax Muscle with Synthetic Substitute, Open Approach

0KRH0KZ Replacement of Right Thorax Muscle with Nonautologous Tissue Substitute, Open Approach

0KRH47Z Replacement of Right Thorax Muscle with Autologous Tissue Substitute, Percutaneous Endoscopic Approach

0KRH4JZ Replacement of Right Thorax Muscle with Synthetic Substitute, Percutaneous Endoscopic Approach

0KRH4KZ Replacement of Right Thorax Muscle with Nonautologous Tissue Substitute, Percutaneous Endoscopic Approach

0KRJ07Z Replacement of Left Thorax Muscle with Autologous Tissue Substitute, Open Approach

0KRJ0JZ Replacement of Left Thorax Muscle with Synthetic Substitute, Open Approach

0KRJ0KZ Replacement of Left Thorax Muscle with Nonautologous Tissue Substitute, Open Approach

0KRJ47Z Replacement of Left Thorax Muscle with Autologous Tissue Substitute, Percutaneous Endoscopic Approach

0KRJ4JZ Replacement of Left Thorax Muscle with Synthetic Substitute, Percutaneous Endoscopic Approach

0KRJ4KZ Replacement of Left Thorax Muscle with Nonautologous Tissue Substitute, Percutaneous Endoscopic Approach

0KRK07Z Replacement of Right Abdomen Muscle with Autologous Tissue Substitute, Open Approach

0KRK0JZ Replacement of Right Abdomen Muscle with Synthetic Substitute, Open Approach

0KRK0KZ Replacement of Right Abdomen Muscle with Nonautologous Tissue Substitute, Open Approach

0KRK47Z Replacement of Right Abdomen Muscle with Autologous Tissue Substitute, Percutaneous Endoscopic Approach

0KRK4JZ Replacement of Right Abdomen Muscle with Synthetic Substitute, Percutaneous Endoscopic Approach

0KRK4KZ Replacement of Right Abdomen Muscle with Nonautologous Tissue Substitute, Percutaneous Endoscopic Approach

0KRL07Z Replacement of Left Abdomen Muscle with Autologous Tissue Substitute, Open Approach

0KRL0JZ Replacement of Left Abdomen Muscle with Synthetic Substitute, Open Approach

0KRL0KZ Replacement of Left Abdomen Muscle with Nonautologous Tissue Substitute, Open Approach

0KRL47Z Replacement of Left Abdomen Muscle with Autologous Tissue Substitute, Percutaneous Endoscopic Approach

0KRL4JZ Replacement of Left Abdomen Muscle with Synthetic Substitute, Percutaneous Endoscopic Approach

0KRL4KZ Replacement of Left Abdomen Muscle with Nonautologous Tissue Substitute, Percutaneous Endoscopic Approach

0KRM07Z Replacement of Perineum Muscle with Autologous Tissue Substitute, Open Approach

0KRM0JZ Replacement of Perineum Muscle with Synthetic Substitute, Open Approach

0KRM0KZ Replacement of Perineum Muscle with Nonautologous Tissue Substitute, Open Approach

0KRM47Z Replacement of Perineum Muscle with Autologous Tissue Substitute, Percutaneous Endoscopic Approach

0KRM4JZ Replacement of Perineum Muscle with Synthetic Substitute, Percutaneous Endoscopic Approach

0KRM4KZ Replacement of Perineum Muscle with Nonautologous Tissue Substitute, Percutaneous Endoscopic Approach

0KRN07Z Replacement of Right Hip Muscle with Autologous Tissue Substitute, Open Approach

0KRN0JZ Replacement of Right Hip Muscle with Synthetic Substitute, Open Approach

0KRN0KZ Replacement of Right Hip Muscle with Nonautologous Tissue Substitute, Open Approach

0KRN47Z Replacement of Right Hip Muscle with Autologous Tissue Substitute, Percutaneous Endoscopic Approach

0KRN4JZ Replacement of Right Hip Muscle with Synthetic Substitute, Percutaneous Endoscopic Approach

0KRN4KZ Replacement of Right Hip Muscle with Nonautologous Tissue Substitute, Percutaneous Endoscopic Approach

0KRP07Z Replacement of Left Hip Muscle with Autologous Tissue Substitute, Open Approach

0KRP0JZ Replacement of Left Hip Muscle with Synthetic Substitute, Open Approach

0KRP0KZ Replacement of Left Hip Muscle with Nonautologous Tissue Substitute, Open Approach

0KRP47Z Replacement of Left Hip Muscle with Autologous Tissue Substitute, Percutaneous Endoscopic Approach

0KRP4JZ Replacement of Left Hip Muscle with Synthetic Substitute, Percutaneous Endoscopic Approach

0KRP4KZ Replacement of Left Hip Muscle with Nonautologous Tissue Substitute, Percutaneous Endoscopic Approach

0KRQ07Z Replacement of Right Upper Leg Muscle with Autologous Tissue Substitute, Open Approach

0KRQ0JZ Replacement of Right Upper Leg Muscle with Synthetic Substitute, Open Approach

0KRQ0KZ Replacement of Right Upper Leg Muscle with Nonautologous Tissue Substitute, Open Approach

0KRQ47Z Replacement of Right Upper Leg Muscle with Autologous Tissue Substitute, Percutaneous Endoscopic Approach

0KRQ4JZ Replacement of Right Upper Leg Muscle with Synthetic Substitute, Percutaneous Endoscopic Approach

0KRQ4KZ Replacement of Right Upper Leg Muscle with Nonautologous Tissue Substitute, Percutaneous Endoscopic Approach

0KRR07Z Replacement of Left Upper Leg Muscle with Autologous Tissue Substitute, Open Approach

0KRR0JZ Replacement of Left Upper Leg Muscle with Synthetic Substitute, Open Approach

0KRR0KZ Replacement of Left Upper Leg Muscle with Nonautologous Tissue Substitute, Open Approach

0KRR47Z Replacement of Left Upper Leg Muscle with Autologous Tissue Substitute, Percutaneous Endoscopic Approach

0KRR4JZ Replacement of Left Upper Leg Muscle with Synthetic Substitute, Percutaneous Endoscopic Approach

0KRR4KZ Replacement of Left Upper Leg Muscle with Nonautologous Tissue Substitute, Percutaneous Endoscopic Approach

0KRS07Z Replacement of Right Lower Leg Muscle with Autologous Tissue Substitute, Open Approach

0KRS0JZ Replacement of Right Lower Leg Muscle with Synthetic Substitute, Open Approach

♀ Female-only   ♂ Male-only   ▲ Limited Coverage   ● Non-OR   HAC HAC-associated procedure   ▲ Non-covered procedures   ✚ Cluster

0KRS0KZ	Replacement of Right Lower Leg Muscle with Nonautologous Tissue Substitute, Open Approach
0KRS47Z	Replacement of Right Lower Leg Muscle with Autologous Tissue Substitute, Percutaneous Endoscopic Approach
0KRS4JZ	Replacement of Right Lower Leg Muscle with Synthetic Substitute, Percutaneous Endoscopic Approach
0KRS4KZ	Replacement of Right Lower Leg Muscle with Nonautologous Tissue Substitute, Percutaneous Endoscopic Approach
0KRT07Z	Replacement of Left Lower Leg Muscle with Autologous Tissue Substitute, Open Approach
0KRT0JZ	Replacement of Left Lower Leg Muscle with Synthetic Substitute, Open Approach
0KRT0KZ	Replacement of Left Lower Leg Muscle with Nonautologous Tissue Substitute, Open Approach
0KRT47Z	Replacement of Left Lower Leg Muscle with Autologous Tissue Substitute, Percutaneous Endoscopic Approach
0KRT4JZ	Replacement of Left Lower Leg Muscle with Synthetic Substitute, Percutaneous Endoscopic Approach
0KRT4KZ	Replacement of Left Lower Leg Muscle with Nonautologous Tissue Substitute, Percutaneous Endoscopic Approach
0KRV07Z	Replacement of Right Foot Muscle with Autologous Tissue Substitute, Open Approach
0KRV0JZ	Replacement of Right Foot Muscle with Synthetic Substitute, Open Approach
0KRV0KZ	Replacement of Right Foot Muscle with Nonautologous Tissue Substitute, Open Approach
0KRV47Z	Replacement of Right Foot Muscle with Autologous Tissue Substitute, Percutaneous Endoscopic Approach
0KRV4JZ	Replacement of Right Foot Muscle with Synthetic Substitute, Percutaneous Endoscopic Approach
0KRV4KZ	Replacement of Right Foot Muscle with Nonautologous Tissue Substitute, Percutaneous Endoscopic Approach
0KRW07Z	Replacement of Left Foot Muscle with Autologous Tissue Substitute, Open Approach
0KRW0JZ	Replacement of Left Foot Muscle with Synthetic Substitute, Open Approach
0KRW0KZ	Replacement of Left Foot Muscle with Nonautologous Tissue Substitute, Open Approach
0KRW47Z	Replacement of Left Foot Muscle with Autologous Tissue Substitute, Percutaneous Endoscopic Approach
0KRW4JZ	Replacement of Left Foot Muscle with Synthetic Substitute, Percutaneous Endoscopic Approach
0KRW4KZ	Replacement of Left Foot Muscle with Nonautologous Tissue Substitute, Percutaneous Endoscopic Approach

0KS – Muscles, Reposition

0KS00ZZ	Reposition Head Muscle, Open Approach
0KS04ZZ	Reposition Head Muscle, Percutaneous Endoscopic Approach
0KS10ZZ	Reposition Facial Muscle, Open Approach
0KS14ZZ	Reposition Facial Muscle, Percutaneous Endoscopic Approach
0KS20ZZ	Reposition Right Neck Muscle, Open Approach
0KS24ZZ	Reposition Right Neck Muscle, Percutaneous Endoscopic Approach
0KS30ZZ	Reposition Left Neck Muscle, Open Approach
0KS34ZZ	Reposition Left Neck Muscle, Percutaneous Endoscopic Approach
0KS40ZZ	Reposition Tongue, Palate, Pharynx Muscle, Open Approach
0KS44ZZ	Reposition Tongue, Palate, Pharynx Muscle, Percutaneous Endoscopic Approach
0KS50ZZ	Reposition Right Shoulder Muscle, Open Approach
0KS54ZZ	Reposition Right Shoulder Muscle, Percutaneous Endoscopic Approach
0KS60ZZ	Reposition Left Shoulder Muscle, Open Approach
0KS64ZZ	Reposition Left Shoulder Muscle, Percutaneous Endoscopic Approach
0KS70ZZ	Reposition Right Upper Arm Muscle, Open Approach
0KS74ZZ	Reposition Right Upper Arm Muscle, Percutaneous Endoscopic Approach
0KS80ZZ	Reposition Left Upper Arm Muscle, Open Approach
0KS84ZZ	Reposition Left Upper Arm Muscle, Percutaneous Endoscopic Approach
0KS90ZZ	Reposition Right Lower Arm and Wrist Muscle, Open Approach
0KS94ZZ	Reposition Right Lower Arm and Wrist Muscle, Percutaneous Endoscopic Approach
0KSB0ZZ	Reposition Left Lower Arm and Wrist Muscle, Open Approach
0KSB4ZZ	Reposition Left Lower Arm and Wrist Muscle, Percutaneous Endoscopic Approach
0KSC0ZZ	Reposition Right Hand Muscle, Open Approach
0KSC4ZZ	Reposition Right Hand Muscle, Percutaneous Endoscopic Approach
0KSD0ZZ	Reposition Left Hand Muscle, Open Approach
0KSD4ZZ	Reposition Left Hand Muscle, Percutaneous Endoscopic Approach
0KSF0ZZ	Reposition Right Trunk Muscle, Open Approach
0KSF4ZZ	Reposition Right Trunk Muscle, Percutaneous Endoscopic Approach
0KSG0ZZ	Reposition Left Trunk Muscle, Open Approach
0KSG4ZZ	Reposition Left Trunk Muscle, Percutaneous Endoscopic Approach
0KSH0ZZ	Reposition Right Thorax Muscle, Open Approach
0KSH4ZZ	Reposition Right Thorax Muscle, Percutaneous Endoscopic Approach
0KSJ0ZZ	Reposition Left Thorax Muscle, Open Approach
0KSJ4ZZ	Reposition Left Thorax Muscle, Percutaneous Endoscopic Approach
0KSK0ZZ	Reposition Right Abdomen Muscle, Open Approach
0KSK4ZZ	Reposition Right Abdomen Muscle, Percutaneous Endoscopic Approach
0KSL0ZZ	Reposition Left Abdomen Muscle, Open Approach
0KSL4ZZ	Reposition Left Abdomen Muscle, Percutaneous Endoscopic Approach
0KSM0ZZ	Reposition Perineum Muscle, Open Approach
0KSM4ZZ	Reposition Perineum Muscle, Percutaneous Endoscopic Approach
0KSN0ZZ	Reposition Right Hip Muscle, Open Approach
0KSN4ZZ	Reposition Right Hip Muscle, Percutaneous Endoscopic Approach
0KSP0ZZ	Reposition Left Hip Muscle, Open Approach
0KSP4ZZ	Reposition Left Hip Muscle, Percutaneous Endoscopic Approach
0KSQ0ZZ	Reposition Right Upper Leg Muscle, Open Approach
0KSQ4ZZ	Reposition Right Upper Leg Muscle, Percutaneous Endoscopic Approach
0KSR0ZZ	Reposition Left Upper Leg Muscle, Open Approach
0KSR4ZZ	Reposition Left Upper Leg Muscle, Percutaneous Endoscopic Approach
0KSS0ZZ	Reposition Right Lower Leg Muscle, Open Approach
0KSS4ZZ	Reposition Right Lower Leg Muscle, Percutaneous Endoscopic Approach
0KST0ZZ	Reposition Left Lower Leg Muscle, Open Approach
0KST4ZZ	Reposition Left Lower Leg Muscle, Percutaneous Endoscopic Approach
0KSV0ZZ	Reposition Right Foot Muscle, Open Approach
0KSV4ZZ	Reposition Right Foot Muscle, Percutaneous Endoscopic Approach
0KSW0ZZ	Reposition Left Foot Muscle, Open Approach
0KSW4ZZ	Reposition Left Foot Muscle, Percutaneous Endoscopic Approach

0KT – Muscles, Resection

Review Coding Guideline B3.8

Review Coding Guideline B3.18

0KT00ZZ	Resection of Head Muscle, Open Approach
0KT04ZZ	Resection of Head Muscle, Percutaneous Endoscopic Approach
0KT10ZZ	Resection of Facial Muscle, Open Approach
0KT14ZZ	Resection of Facial Muscle, Percutaneous Endoscopic Approach
0KT20ZZ	Resection of Right Neck Muscle, Open Approach
0KT24ZZ	Resection of Right Neck Muscle, Percutaneous Endoscopic Approach

0KT30ZZ Resection of Left Neck Muscle, Open Approach
AHA CC: 2Q, 2016, 12-14

0KT34ZZ Resection of Left Neck Muscle, Percutaneous Endoscopic Approach

0KT40ZZ Resection of Tongue, Palate, Pharynx Muscle, Open Approach

0KT44ZZ Resection of Tongue, Palate, Pharynx Muscle, Percutaneous Endoscopic Approach

0KT50ZZ Resection of Right Shoulder Muscle, Open Approach

0KT54ZZ Resection of Right Shoulder Muscle, Percutaneous Endoscopic Approach

0KT60ZZ Resection of Left Shoulder Muscle, Open Approach

0KT64ZZ Resection of Left Shoulder Muscle, Percutaneous Endoscopic Approach

0KT70ZZ Resection of Right Upper Arm Muscle, Open Approach

0KT74ZZ Resection of Right Upper Arm Muscle, Percutaneous Endoscopic Approach

0KT80ZZ Resection of Left Upper Arm Muscle, Open Approach

0KT84ZZ Resection of Left Upper Arm Muscle, Percutaneous Endoscopic Approach

0KT90ZZ Resection of Right Lower Arm and Wrist Muscle, Open Approach

0KT94ZZ Resection of Right Lower Arm and Wrist Muscle, Percutaneous Endoscopic Approach

0KTB0ZZ Resection of Left Lower Arm and Wrist Muscle, Open Approach

0KTB4ZZ Resection of Left Lower Arm and Wrist Muscle, Percutaneous Endoscopic Approach

0KTC0ZZ Resection of Right Hand Muscle, Open Approach

0KTC4ZZ Resection of Right Hand Muscle, Percutaneous Endoscopic Approach

0KTD0ZZ Resection of Left Hand Muscle, Open Approach

0KTD4ZZ Resection of Left Hand Muscle, Percutaneous Endoscopic Approach

0KTF0ZZ Resection of Right Trunk Muscle, Open Approach

0KTF4ZZ Resection of Right Trunk Muscle, Percutaneous Endoscopic Approach

0KTG0ZZ Resection of Left Trunk Muscle, Open Approach

0KTG4ZZ Resection of Left Trunk Muscle, Percutaneous Endoscopic Approach

0KTH0ZZ Resection of Right Thorax Muscle, Open Approach

0KTH4ZZ Resection of Right Thorax Muscle, Percutaneous Endoscopic Approach

0KTJ0ZZ Resection of Left Thorax Muscle, Open Approach

0KTJ4ZZ Resection of Left Thorax Muscle, Percutaneous Endoscopic Approach

0KTK0ZZ Resection of Right Abdomen Muscle, Open Approach

0KTK4ZZ Resection of Right Abdomen Muscle, Percutaneous Endoscopic Approach

0KTL0ZZ Resection of Left Abdomen Muscle, Open Approach

0KTL4ZZ Resection of Left Abdomen Muscle, Percutaneous Endoscopic Approach

0KTM0ZZ Resection of Perineum Muscle, Open Approach
AHA CC: 4Q, 2014, 40-41; 1Q, 2015, 38

0KTM4ZZ Resection of Perineum Muscle, Percutaneous Endoscopic Approach

0KTN0ZZ Resection of Right Hip Muscle, Open Approach

0KTN4ZZ Resection of Right Hip Muscle, Percutaneous Endoscopic Approach

0KTP0ZZ Resection of Left Hip Muscle, Open Approach

0KTP4ZZ Resection of Left Hip Muscle, Percutaneous Endoscopic Approach

0KTQ0ZZ Resection of Right Upper Leg Muscle, Open Approach

0KTQ4ZZ Resection of Right Upper Leg Muscle, Percutaneous Endoscopic Approach

0KTR0ZZ Resection of Left Upper Leg Muscle, Open Approach

0KTR4ZZ Resection of Left Upper Leg Muscle, Percutaneous Endoscopic Approach

0KTS0ZZ Resection of Right Lower Leg Muscle, Open Approach

0KTS4ZZ Resection of Right Lower Leg Muscle, Percutaneous Endoscopic Approach

0KTT0ZZ Resection of Left Lower Leg Muscle, Open Approach

0KTT4ZZ Resection of Left Lower Leg Muscle, Percutaneous Endoscopic Approach

0KTV0ZZ Resection of Right Foot Muscle, Open Approach

0KTV4ZZ Resection of Right Foot Muscle, Percutaneous Endoscopic Approach

0KTW0ZZ Resection of Left Foot Muscle, Open Approach

0KTW4ZZ Resection of Left Foot Muscle, Percutaneous Endoscopic Approach

0KU – Muscles, Supplement

0KU007Z Supplement Head Muscle with Autologous Tissue Substitute, Open Approach

0KU00JZ Supplement Head Muscle with Synthetic Substitute, Open Approach

0KU00KZ Supplement Head Muscle with Nonautologous Tissue Substitute, Open Approach

0KU047Z Supplement Head Muscle with Autologous Tissue Substitute, Percutaneous Endoscopic Approach

0KU04JZ Supplement Head Muscle with Synthetic Substitute, Percutaneous Endoscopic Approach

0KU04KZ Supplement Head Muscle with Nonautologous Tissue Substitute, Percutaneous Endoscopic Approach

0KU107Z Supplement Facial Muscle with Autologous Tissue Substitute, Open Approach

0KU10JZ Supplement Facial Muscle with Synthetic Substitute, Open Approach

0KU10KZ Supplement Facial Muscle with Nonautologous Tissue Substitute, Open Approach

0KU147Z Supplement Facial Muscle with Autologous Tissue Substitute, Percutaneous Endoscopic Approach

0KU14JZ Supplement Facial Muscle with Synthetic Substitute, Percutaneous Endoscopic Approach

0KU14KZ Supplement Facial Muscle with Nonautologous Tissue Substitute, Percutaneous Endoscopic Approach

0KU207Z Supplement Right Neck Muscle with Autologous Tissue Substitute, Open Approach

0KU20JZ Supplement Right Neck Muscle with Synthetic Substitute, Open Approach

0KU20KZ Supplement Right Neck Muscle with Nonautologous Tissue Substitute, Open Approach

0KU247Z Supplement Right Neck Muscle with Autologous Tissue Substitute, Percutaneous Endoscopic Approach

0KU24JZ Supplement Right Neck Muscle with Synthetic Substitute, Percutaneous Endoscopic Approach

0KU24KZ Supplement Right Neck Muscle with Nonautologous Tissue Substitute, Percutaneous Endoscopic Approach

0KU307Z Supplement Left Neck Muscle with Autologous Tissue Substitute, Open Approach

0KU30JZ Supplement Left Neck Muscle with Synthetic Substitute, Open Approach

0KU30KZ Supplement Left Neck Muscle with Nonautologous Tissue Substitute, Open Approach

0KU347Z Supplement Left Neck Muscle with Autologous Tissue Substitute, Percutaneous Endoscopic Approach

0KU34JZ Supplement Left Neck Muscle with Synthetic Substitute, Percutaneous Endoscopic Approach

0KU34KZ Supplement Left Neck Muscle with Nonautologous Tissue Substitute, Percutaneous Endoscopic Approach

0KU407Z Supplement Tongue, Palate, Pharynx Muscle with Autologous Tissue Substitute, Open Approach

0KU40JZ Supplement Tongue, Palate, Pharynx Muscle with Synthetic Substitute, Open Approach

0KU40KZ Supplement Tongue, Palate, Pharynx Muscle with Nonautologous Tissue Substitute, Open Approach

0KU447Z Supplement Tongue, Palate, Pharynx Muscle with Autologous Tissue Substitute, Percutaneous Endoscopic Approach

0KU44JZ Supplement Tongue, Palate, Pharynx Muscle with Synthetic Substitute, Percutaneous Endoscopic Approach

0KU44KZ Supplement Tongue, Palate, Pharynx Muscle with Nonautologous Tissue Substitute, Percutaneous Endoscopic Approach

0KU507Z Supplement Right Shoulder Muscle with Autologous Tissue Substitute, Open Approach

0KU50JZ Supplement Right Shoulder Muscle with Synthetic Substitute, Open Approach

0KU50KZ Supplement Right Shoulder Muscle with Nonautologous Tissue Substitute, Open Approach

0KU547Z Supplement Right Shoulder Muscle with Autologous Tissue Substitute, Percutaneous Endoscopic Approach

0KU54JZ Supplement Right Shoulder Muscle with Synthetic Substitute, Percutaneous Endoscopic Approach

0KU54KZ Supplement Right Shoulder Muscle with Nonautologous Tissue Substitute, Percutaneous Endoscopic Approach

♀ Female-only   ♂ Male-only   ▲ Limited Coverage   ● Non-OR   HAC HAC-associated procedure   ▲ Non-covered procedures   ✛ Cluster

0KU607Z   Supplement Left Shoulder Muscle with Autologous Tissue Substitute, Open Approach

0KU60JZ   Supplement Left Shoulder Muscle with Synthetic Substitute, Open Approach

0KU60KZ   Supplement Left Shoulder Muscle with Nonautologous Tissue Substitute, Open Approach

0KU647Z   Supplement Left Shoulder Muscle with Autologous Tissue Substitute, Percutaneous Endoscopic Approach

0KU64JZ   Supplement Left Shoulder Muscle with Synthetic Substitute, Percutaneous Endoscopic Approach

0KU64KZ   Supplement Left Shoulder Muscle with Nonautologous Tissue Substitute, Percutaneous Endoscopic Approach

0KU707Z   Supplement Right Upper Arm Muscle with Autologous Tissue Substitute, Open Approach

0KU70JZ   Supplement Right Upper Arm Muscle with Synthetic Substitute, Open Approach

0KU70KZ   Supplement Right Upper Arm Muscle with Nonautologous Tissue Substitute, Open Approach

0KU747Z   Supplement Right Upper Arm Muscle with Autologous Tissue Substitute, Percutaneous Endoscopic Approach

0KU74JZ   Supplement Right Upper Arm Muscle with Synthetic Substitute, Percutaneous Endoscopic Approach

0KU74KZ   Supplement Right Upper Arm Muscle with Nonautologous Tissue Substitute, Percutaneous Endoscopic Approach

0KU807Z   Supplement Left Upper Arm Muscle with Autologous Tissue Substitute, Open Approach

0KU80JZ   Supplement Left Upper Arm Muscle with Synthetic Substitute, Open Approach

0KU80KZ   Supplement Left Upper Arm Muscle with Nonautologous Tissue Substitute, Open Approach

0KU847Z   Supplement Left Upper Arm Muscle with Autologous Tissue Substitute, Percutaneous Endoscopic Approach

0KU84JZ   Supplement Left Upper Arm Muscle with Synthetic Substitute, Percutaneous Endoscopic Approach

0KU84KZ   Supplement Left Upper Arm Muscle with Nonautologous Tissue Substitute, Percutaneous Endoscopic Approach

0KU907Z   Supplement Right Lower Arm and Wrist Muscle with Autologous Tissue Substitute, Open Approach

0KU90JZ   Supplement Right Lower Arm and Wrist Muscle with Synthetic Substitute, Open Approach

0KU90KZ   Supplement Right Lower Arm and Wrist Muscle with Nonautologous Tissue Substitute, Open Approach

0KU947Z   Supplement Right Lower Arm and Wrist Muscle with Autologous Tissue Substitute, Percutaneous Endoscopic Approach

0KU94JZ   Supplement Right Lower Arm and Wrist Muscle with Synthetic Substitute, Percutaneous Endoscopic Approach

0KU94KZ   Supplement Right Lower Arm and Wrist Muscle with Nonautologous Tissue Substitute, Percutaneous Endoscopic Approach

0KUB07Z   Supplement Left Lower Arm and Wrist Muscle with Autologous Tissue Substitute, Open Approach

0KUB0JZ   Supplement Left Lower Arm and Wrist Muscle with Synthetic Substitute, Open Approach

0KUB0KZ   Supplement Left Lower Arm and Wrist Muscle with Nonautologous Tissue Substitute, Open Approach

0KUB47Z   Supplement Left Lower Arm and Wrist Muscle with Autologous Tissue Substitute, Percutaneous Endoscopic Approach

0KUB4JZ   Supplement Left Lower Arm and Wrist Muscle with Synthetic Substitute, Percutaneous Endoscopic Approach

0KUB4KZ   Supplement Left Lower Arm and Wrist Muscle with Nonautologous Tissue Substitute, Percutaneous Endoscopic Approach

0KUC07Z   Supplement Right Hand Muscle with Autologous Tissue Substitute, Open Approach

0KUC0JZ   Supplement Right Hand Muscle with Synthetic Substitute, Open Approach

0KUC0KZ   Supplement Right Hand Muscle with Nonautologous Tissue Substitute, Open Approach

0KUC47Z   Supplement Right Hand Muscle with Autologous Tissue Substitute, Percutaneous Endoscopic Approach

0KUC4JZ   Supplement Right Hand Muscle with Synthetic Substitute, Percutaneous Endoscopic Approach

0KUC4KZ   Supplement Right Hand Muscle with Nonautologous Tissue Substitute, Percutaneous Endoscopic Approach

0KUD07Z   Supplement Left Hand Muscle with Autologous Tissue Substitute, Open Approach

0KUD0JZ   Supplement Left Hand Muscle with Synthetic Substitute, Open Approach

0KUD0KZ   Supplement Left Hand Muscle with Nonautologous Tissue Substitute, Open Approach

0KUD47Z   Supplement Left Hand Muscle with Autologous Tissue Substitute, Percutaneous Endoscopic Approach

0KUD4JZ   Supplement Left Hand Muscle with Synthetic Substitute, Percutaneous Endoscopic Approach

0KUD4KZ   Supplement Left Hand Muscle with Nonautologous Tissue Substitute, Percutaneous Endoscopic Approach

0KUF07Z   Supplement Right Trunk Muscle with Autologous Tissue Substitute, Open Approach

0KUF0JZ   Supplement Right Trunk Muscle with Synthetic Substitute, Open Approach

0KUF0KZ   Supplement Right Trunk Muscle with Nonautologous Tissue Substitute, Open Approach

0KUF47Z   Supplement Right Trunk Muscle with Autologous Tissue Substitute, Percutaneous Endoscopic Approach

0KUF4JZ   Supplement Right Trunk Muscle with Synthetic Substitute, Percutaneous Endoscopic Approach

0KUF4KZ   Supplement Right Trunk Muscle with Nonautologous Tissue Substitute, Percutaneous Endoscopic Approach

0KUG07Z   Supplement Left Trunk Muscle with Autologous Tissue Substitute, Open Approach

0KUG0JZ   Supplement Left Trunk Muscle with Synthetic Substitute, Open Approach

0KUG0KZ   Supplement Left Trunk Muscle with Nonautologous Tissue Substitute, Open Approach

0KUG47Z   Supplement Left Trunk Muscle with Autologous Tissue Substitute, Percutaneous Endoscopic Approach

0KUG4JZ   Supplement Left Trunk Muscle with Synthetic Substitute, Percutaneous Endoscopic Approach

0KUG4KZ   Supplement Left Trunk Muscle with Nonautologous Tissue Substitute, Percutaneous Endoscopic Approach

0KUH07Z   Supplement Right Thorax Muscle with Autologous Tissue Substitute, Open Approach

0KUH0JZ   Supplement Right Thorax Muscle with Synthetic Substitute, Open Approach

0KUH0KZ   Supplement Right Thorax Muscle with Nonautologous Tissue Substitute, Open Approach

0KUH47Z   Supplement Right Thorax Muscle with Autologous Tissue Substitute, Percutaneous Endoscopic Approach

0KUH4JZ   Supplement Right Thorax Muscle with Synthetic Substitute, Percutaneous Endoscopic Approach

0KUH4KZ   Supplement Right Thorax Muscle with Nonautologous Tissue Substitute, Percutaneous Endoscopic Approach

0KUJ07Z   Supplement Left Thorax Muscle with Autologous Tissue Substitute, Open Approach

0KUJ0JZ   Supplement Left Thorax Muscle with Synthetic Substitute, Open Approach

0KUJ0KZ   Supplement Left Thorax Muscle with Nonautologous Tissue Substitute, Open Approach

0KUJ47Z   Supplement Left Thorax Muscle with Autologous Tissue Substitute, Percutaneous Endoscopic Approach

0KUJ4JZ   Supplement Left Thorax Muscle with Synthetic Substitute, Percutaneous Endoscopic Approach

0KUJ4KZ   Supplement Left Thorax Muscle with Nonautologous Tissue Substitute, Percutaneous Endoscopic Approach

0KUK07Z   Supplement Right Abdomen Muscle with Autologous Tissue Substitute, Open Approach

0KUK0JZ   Supplement Right Abdomen Muscle with Synthetic Substitute, Open Approach

0KUK0KZ   Supplement Right Abdomen Muscle with Nonautologous Tissue Substitute, Open Approach

0KUK47Z   Supplement Right Abdomen Muscle with Autologous Tissue Substitute, Percutaneous Endoscopic Approach

0KUK4JZ   Supplement Right Abdomen Muscle with Synthetic Substitute, Percutaneous Endoscopic Approach

0KUK4KZ   Supplement Right Abdomen Muscle with Nonautologous Tissue Substitute, Percutaneous Endoscopic Approach

0KUL07Z   Supplement Left Abdomen Muscle with Autologous Tissue Substitute, Open Approach

0KUL0JZ   Supplement Left Abdomen Muscle with Synthetic Substitute, Open Approach

0KUL0KZ   Supplement Left Abdomen Muscle with Nonautologous Tissue Substitute, Open Approach

0KUL47Z   Supplement Left Abdomen Muscle with Autologous Tissue Substitute, Percutaneous Endoscopic Approach

0KUL4JZ   Supplement Left Abdomen Muscle with Synthetic Substitute, Percutaneous Endoscopic Approach

0KUL4KZ   Supplement Left Abdomen Muscle with Nonautologous Tissue Substitute, Percutaneous Endoscopic Approach

0KUM07Z   Supplement Perineum Muscle with Autologous Tissue Substitute, Open Approach

0KUM0JZ   Supplement Perineum Muscle with Synthetic Substitute, Open Approach

0KUM0KZ   Supplement Perineum Muscle with Nonautologous Tissue Substitute, Open Approach

0KUM47Z   Supplement Perineum Muscle with Autologous Tissue Substitute, Percutaneous Endoscopic Approach

0KUM4JZ   Supplement Perineum Muscle with Synthetic Substitute, Percutaneous Endoscopic Approach

0KUM4KZ   Supplement Perineum Muscle with Nonautologous Tissue Substitute, Percutaneous Endoscopic Approach

0KUN07Z   Supplement Right Hip Muscle with Autologous Tissue Substitute, Open Approach

0KUN0JZ   Supplement Right Hip Muscle with Synthetic Substitute, Open Approach

0KUN0KZ   Supplement Right Hip Muscle with Nonautologous Tissue Substitute, Open Approach

0KUN47Z   Supplement Right Hip Muscle with Autologous Tissue Substitute, Percutaneous Endoscopic Approach

0KUN4JZ   Supplement Right Hip Muscle with Synthetic Substitute, Percutaneous Endoscopic Approach

0KUN4KZ   Supplement Right Hip Muscle with Nonautologous Tissue Substitute, Percutaneous Endoscopic Approach

0KUP07Z   Supplement Left Hip Muscle with Autologous Tissue Substitute, Open Approach

0KUP0JZ   Supplement Left Hip Muscle with Synthetic Substitute, Open Approach

0KUP0KZ   Supplement Left Hip Muscle with Nonautologous Tissue Substitute, Open Approach

0KUP47Z   Supplement Left Hip Muscle with Autologous Tissue Substitute, Percutaneous Endoscopic Approach

0KUP4JZ   Supplement Left Hip Muscle with Synthetic Substitute, Percutaneous Endoscopic Approach

0KUP4KZ   Supplement Left Hip Muscle with Nonautologous Tissue Substitute, Percutaneous Endoscopic Approach

0KUQ07Z   Supplement Right Upper Leg Muscle with Autologous Tissue Substitute, Open Approach

0KUQ0JZ   Supplement Right Upper Leg Muscle with Synthetic Substitute, Open Approach

0KUQ0KZ   Supplement Right Upper Leg Muscle with Nonautologous Tissue Substitute, Open Approach

0KUQ47Z   Supplement Right Upper Leg Muscle with Autologous Tissue Substitute, Percutaneous Endoscopic Approach

0KUQ4JZ   Supplement Right Upper Leg Muscle with Synthetic Substitute, Percutaneous Endoscopic Approach

0KUQ4KZ   Supplement Right Upper Leg Muscle with Nonautologous Tissue Substitute, Percutaneous Endoscopic Approach

0KUR07Z   Supplement Left Upper Leg Muscle with Autologous Tissue Substitute, Open Approach

0KUR0JZ   Supplement Left Upper Leg Muscle with Synthetic Substitute, Open Approach

0KUR0KZ   Supplement Left Upper Leg Muscle with Nonautologous Tissue Substitute, Open Approach

0KUR47Z   Supplement Left Upper Leg Muscle with Autologous Tissue Substitute, Percutaneous Endoscopic Approach

0KUR4JZ   Supplement Left Upper Leg Muscle with Synthetic Substitute, Percutaneous Endoscopic Approach

0KUR4KZ   Supplement Left Upper Leg Muscle with Nonautologous Tissue Substitute, Percutaneous Endoscopic Approach

0KUS07Z   Supplement Right Lower Leg Muscle with Autologous Tissue Substitute, Open Approach

0KUS0JZ   Supplement Right Lower Leg Muscle with Synthetic Substitute, Open Approach

0KUS0KZ   Supplement Right Lower Leg Muscle with Nonautologous Tissue Substitute, Open Approach

0KUS47Z   Supplement Right Lower Leg Muscle with Autologous Tissue Substitute, Percutaneous Endoscopic Approach

0KUS4JZ   Supplement Right Lower Leg Muscle with Synthetic Substitute, Percutaneous Endoscopic Approach

0KUS4KZ   Supplement Right Lower Leg Muscle with Nonautologous Tissue Substitute, Percutaneous Endoscopic Approach

0KUT07Z   Supplement Left Lower Leg Muscle with Autologous Tissue Substitute, Open Approach

0KUT0JZ   Supplement Left Lower Leg Muscle with Synthetic Substitute, Open Approach

0KUT0KZ   Supplement Left Lower Leg Muscle with Nonautologous Tissue Substitute, Open Approach

0KUT47Z   Supplement Left Lower Leg Muscle with Autologous Tissue Substitute, Percutaneous Endoscopic Approach

0KUT4JZ   Supplement Left Lower Leg Muscle with Synthetic Substitute, Percutaneous Endoscopic Approach

0KUT4KZ   Supplement Left Lower Leg Muscle with Nonautologous Tissue Substitute, Percutaneous Endoscopic Approach

0KUV07Z   Supplement Right Foot Muscle with Autologous Tissue Substitute, Open Approach

0KUV0JZ   Supplement Right Foot Muscle with Synthetic Substitute, Open Approach

0KUV0KZ   Supplement Right Foot Muscle with Nonautologous Tissue Substitute, Open Approach

0KUV47Z   Supplement Right Foot Muscle with Autologous Tissue Substitute, Percutaneous Endoscopic Approach

0KUV4JZ   Supplement Right Foot Muscle with Synthetic Substitute, Percutaneous Endoscopic Approach

0KUV4KZ   Supplement Right Foot Muscle with Nonautologous Tissue Substitute, Percutaneous Endoscopic Approach

0KUW07Z   Supplement Left Foot Muscle with Autologous Tissue Substitute, Open Approach

0KUW0JZ   Supplement Left Foot Muscle with Synthetic Substitute, Open Approach

0KUW0KZ   Supplement Left Foot Muscle with Nonautologous Tissue Substitute, Open Approach

0KUW47Z   Supplement Left Foot Muscle with Autologous Tissue Substitute, Percutaneous Endoscopic Approach

0KUW4JZ   Supplement Left Foot Muscle with Synthetic Substitute, Percutaneous Endoscopic Approach

0KUW4KZ   Supplement Left Foot Muscle with Nonautologous Tissue Substitute, Percutaneous Endoscopic Approach

0KW – Muscles, Revision

Review Coding Guideline B6.1c

0KWX00Z   Revision of Drainage Device in Upper Muscle, Open Approach

0KWX07Z   Revision of Autologous Tissue Substitute in Upper Muscle, Open Approach

0KWX0JZ   Revision of Synthetic Substitute in Upper Muscle, Open Approach

0KWX0KZ   Revision of Nonautologous Tissue Substitute in Upper Muscle, Open Approach

0KWX0MZ   Revision of Stimulator Lead in Upper Muscle, Open Approach

0KWX0YZ   Revision of Other Device in Upper Muscle, Open Approach

0KWX30Z   Revision of Drainage Device in Upper Muscle, Percutaneous Approach

0KWX37Z   Revision of Autologous Tissue Substitute in Upper Muscle, Percutaneous Approach

0KWX3JZ   Revision of Synthetic Substitute in Upper Muscle, Percutaneous Approach

0KWX3KZ   Revision of Nonautologous Tissue Substitute in Upper Muscle, Percutaneous Approach

0KWX3MZ   Revision of Stimulator Lead in Upper Muscle, Percutaneous Approach

0KWX3YZ   Revision of Other Device in Upper Muscle, Percutaneous Approach

0KWX40Z   Revision of Drainage Device in Upper Muscle, Percutaneous Endoscopic Approach

0KWX47Z   Revision of Autologous Tissue Substitute in Upper Muscle, Percutaneous Endoscopic Approach

0KWX4JZ   Revision of Synthetic Substitute in Upper Muscle, Percutaneous Endoscopic Approach

0KWX4KZ   Revision of Nonautologous Tissue Substitute in Upper Muscle, Percutaneous Endoscopic Approach

0KWX4MZ   Revision of Stimulator Lead in Upper Muscle, Percutaneous Endoscopic Approach

0KWX4YZ   Revision of Other Device in Upper Muscle, Percutaneous Endoscopic Approach

0KWXX0Z   Revision of Drainage Device in Upper Muscle, External Approach

0KWXX7Z Revision of Autologous Tissue Substitute in Upper Muscle, External Approach

0KWXXJZ Revision of Synthetic Substitute in Upper Muscle, External Approach

0KWXXKZ Revision of Nonautologous Tissue Substitute in Upper Muscle, External Approach

0KWXXMZ Revision of Stimulator Lead in Upper Muscle, External Approach

0KWY00Z Revision of Drainage Device in Lower Muscle, Open Approach

0KWY07Z Revision of Autologous Tissue Substitute in Lower Muscle, Open Approach

0KWY0JZ Revision of Synthetic Substitute in Lower Muscle, Open Approach

0KWY0KZ Revision of Nonautologous Tissue Substitute in Lower Muscle, Open Approach

0KWY0MZ Revision of Stimulator Lead in Lower Muscle, Open Approach

0KWY0YZ Revision of Other Device in Lower Muscle, Open Approach

0KWY30Z Revision of Drainage Device in Lower Muscle, Percutaneous Approach

0KWY37Z Revision of Autologous Tissue Substitute in Lower Muscle, Percutaneous Approach

0KWY3JZ Revision of Synthetic Substitute in Lower Muscle, Percutaneous Approach

0KWY3KZ Revision of Nonautologous Tissue Substitute in Lower Muscle, Percutaneous Approach

0KWY3MZ Revision of Stimulator Lead in Lower Muscle, Percutaneous Approach

0KWY3YZ Revision of Other Device in Lower Muscle, Percutaneous Approach

0KWY40Z Revision of Drainage Device in Lower Muscle, Percutaneous Endoscopic Approach

0KWY47Z Revision of Autologous Tissue Substitute in Lower Muscle, Percutaneous Endoscopic Approach

0KWY4JZ Revision of Synthetic Substitute in Lower Muscle, Percutaneous Endoscopic Approach

0KWY4KZ Revision of Nonautologous Tissue Substitute in Lower Muscle, Percutaneous Endoscopic Approach

0KWY4MZ Revision of Stimulator Lead in Lower Muscle, Percutaneous Endoscopic Approach

0KWY4YZ Revision of Other Device in Lower Muscle, Percutaneous Endoscopic Approach

0KWYX0Z Revision of Drainage Device in Lower Muscle, External Approach

0KWYX7Z Revision of Autologous Tissue Substitute in Lower Muscle, External Approach

0KWYXJZ Revision of Synthetic Substitute in Lower Muscle, External Approach

0KWYXKZ Revision of Nonautologous Tissue Substitute in Lower Muscle, External Approach

0KWYXMZ Revision of Stimulator Lead in Lower Muscle, External Approach

0KX – Muscles, Transfer

Review Coding Guideline B3.17

0KX00Z0 Transfer Head Muscle with Skin, Open Approach

0KX00Z1 Transfer Head Muscle with Subcutaneous Tissue, Open Approach

0KX00Z2 Transfer Head Muscle with Skin and Subcutaneous Tissue, Open Approach

0KX00ZZ Transfer Head Muscle, Open Approach

0KX04Z0 Transfer Head Muscle with Skin, Percutaneous Endoscopic Approach

0KX04Z1 Transfer Head Muscle with Subcutaneous Tissue, Percutaneous Endoscopic Approach

0KX04Z2 Transfer Head Muscle with Skin and Subcutaneous Tissue, Percutaneous Endoscopic Approach

0KX04ZZ Transfer Head Muscle, Percutaneous Endoscopic Approach

0KX10Z0 Transfer Facial Muscle with Skin, Open Approach

0KX10Z1 Transfer Facial Muscle with Subcutaneous Tissue, Open Approach

0KX10Z2 Transfer Facial Muscle with Skin and Subcutaneous Tissue, Open Approach

AHA CC: 3Q, 2015, 33

0KX10ZZ Transfer Facial Muscle, Open Approach

0KX14Z0 Transfer Facial Muscle with Skin, Percutaneous Endoscopic Approach

0KX14Z1 Transfer Facial Muscle with Subcutaneous Tissue, Percutaneous Endoscopic Approach

0KX14Z2 Transfer Facial Muscle with Skin and Subcutaneous Tissue, Percutaneous Endoscopic Approach

0KX14ZZ Transfer Facial Muscle, Percutaneous Endoscopic Approach

0KX20Z0 Transfer Right Neck Muscle with Skin, Open Approach

0KX20Z1 Transfer Right Neck Muscle with Subcutaneous Tissue, Open Approach

0KX20Z2 Transfer Right Neck Muscle with Skin and Subcutaneous Tissue, Open Approach

0KX20ZZ Transfer Right Neck Muscle, Open Approach

0KX24Z0 Transfer Right Neck Muscle with Skin, Percutaneous Endoscopic Approach

0KX24Z1 Transfer Right Neck Muscle with Subcutaneous Tissue, Percutaneous Endoscopic Approach

0KX24Z2 Transfer Right Neck Muscle with Skin and Subcutaneous Tissue, Percutaneous Endoscopic Approach

0KX24ZZ Transfer Right Neck Muscle, Percutaneous Endoscopic Approach

0KX30Z0 Transfer Left Neck Muscle with Skin, Open Approach

0KX30Z1 Transfer Left Neck Muscle with Subcutaneous Tissue, Open Approach

0KX30Z2 Transfer Left Neck Muscle with Skin and Subcutaneous Tissue, Open Approach

0KX30ZZ Transfer Left Neck Muscle, Open Approach

0KX34Z0 Transfer Left Neck Muscle with Skin, Percutaneous Endoscopic Approach

0KX34Z1 Transfer Left Neck Muscle with Subcutaneous Tissue, Percutaneous Endoscopic Approach

0KX34Z2 Transfer Left Neck Muscle with Skin and Subcutaneous Tissue, Percutaneous Endoscopic Approach

0KX34ZZ Transfer Left Neck Muscle, Percutaneous Endoscopic Approach

0KX40Z0 Transfer Tongue, Palate, Pharynx Muscle with Skin, Open Approach

0KX40Z1 Transfer Tongue, Palate, Pharynx Muscle with Subcutaneous Tissue, Open Approach

0KX40Z2 Transfer Tongue, Palate, Pharynx Muscle with Skin and Subcutaneous Tissue, Open Approach

AHA CC: 2Q, 2015, 26

0KX40ZZ Transfer Tongue, Palate, Pharynx Muscle, Open Approach

0KX44Z0 Transfer Tongue, Palate, Pharynx Muscle with Skin, Percutaneous Endoscopic Approach

0KX44Z1 Transfer Tongue, Palate, Pharynx Muscle with Subcutaneous Tissue, Percutaneous Endoscopic Approach

0KX44Z2 Transfer Tongue, Palate, Pharynx Muscle with Skin and Subcutaneous Tissue, Percutaneous Endoscopic Approach

0KX44ZZ Transfer Tongue, Palate, Pharynx Muscle, Percutaneous Endoscopic Approach

0KX50Z0 Transfer Right Shoulder Muscle with Skin, Open Approach

0KX50Z1 Transfer Right Shoulder Muscle with Subcutaneous Tissue, Open Approach

0KX50Z2 Transfer Right Shoulder Muscle with Skin and Subcutaneous Tissue, Open Approach

0KX50ZZ Transfer Right Shoulder Muscle, Open Approach

0KX54Z0 Transfer Right Shoulder Muscle with Skin, Percutaneous Endoscopic Approach

0KX54Z1 Transfer Right Shoulder Muscle with Subcutaneous Tissue, Percutaneous Endoscopic Approach

0KX54Z2 Transfer Right Shoulder Muscle with Skin and Subcutaneous Tissue, Percutaneous Endoscopic Approach

0KX54ZZ Transfer Right Shoulder Muscle, Percutaneous Endoscopic Approach

0KX60Z0 Transfer Left Shoulder Muscle with Skin, Open Approach

0KX60Z1 Transfer Left Shoulder Muscle with Subcutaneous Tissue, Open Approach

0KX60Z2 Transfer Left Shoulder Muscle with Skin and Subcutaneous Tissue, Open Approach

0KX60ZZ Transfer Left Shoulder Muscle, Open Approach

0KX64Z0 Transfer Left Shoulder Muscle with Skin, Percutaneous Endoscopic Approach

0KX64Z1 Transfer Left Shoulder Muscle with Subcutaneous Tissue, Percutaneous Endoscopic Approach

0KX64Z2 Transfer Left Shoulder Muscle with Skin and Subcutaneous Tissue, Percutaneous Endoscopic Approach

0KX64ZZ Transfer Left Shoulder Muscle, Percutaneous Endoscopic Approach

0KX70Z0 Transfer Right Upper Arm Muscle with Skin, Open Approach

0KX70Z1 Transfer Right Upper Arm Muscle with Subcutaneous Tissue, Open Approach

0KX70Z2 Transfer Right Upper Arm Muscle with Skin and Subcutaneous Tissue, Open Approach

0KX70ZZ Transfer Right Upper Arm Muscle, Open Approach

0KX74Z0 Transfer Right Upper Arm Muscle with Skin, Percutaneous Endoscopic Approach

0KX74Z1 Transfer Right Upper Arm Muscle with Subcutaneous Tissue, Percutaneous Endoscopic Approach

0KX74Z2 Transfer Right Upper Arm Muscle with Skin and Subcutaneous Tissue, Percutaneous Endoscopic Approach

0KX74ZZ Transfer Right Upper Arm Muscle, Percutaneous Endoscopic Approach

0KX80Z0 Transfer Left Upper Arm Muscle with Skin, Open Approach

0KX80Z1 Transfer Left Upper Arm Muscle with Subcutaneous Tissue, Open Approach

0KX80Z2 Transfer Left Upper Arm Muscle with Skin and Subcutaneous Tissue, Open Approach

0KX80ZZ Transfer Left Upper Arm Muscle, Open Approach

0KX84Z0 Transfer Left Upper Arm Muscle with Skin, Percutaneous Endoscopic Approach

0KX84Z1 Transfer Left Upper Arm Muscle with Subcutaneous Tissue, Percutaneous Endoscopic Approach

0KX84Z2 Transfer Left Upper Arm Muscle with Skin and Subcutaneous Tissue, Percutaneous Endoscopic Approach

0KX84ZZ Transfer Left Upper Arm Muscle, Percutaneous Endoscopic Approach

0KX90Z0 Transfer Right Lower Arm and Wrist Muscle with Skin, Open Approach

0KX90Z1 Transfer Right Lower Arm and Wrist Muscle with Subcutaneous Tissue, Open Approach

0KX90Z2 Transfer Right Lower Arm and Wrist Muscle with Skin and Subcutaneous Tissue, Open Approach

0KX90ZZ Transfer Right Lower Arm and Wrist Muscle, Open Approach

0KX94Z0 Transfer Right Lower Arm and Wrist Muscle with Skin, Percutaneous Endoscopic Approach

0KX94Z1 Transfer Right Lower Arm and Wrist Muscle with Subcutaneous Tissue, Percutaneous Endoscopic Approach

0KX94Z2 Transfer Right Lower Arm and Wrist Muscle with Skin and Subcutaneous Tissue, Percutaneous Endoscopic Approach

0KX94ZZ Transfer Right Lower Arm and Wrist Muscle, Percutaneous Endoscopic Approach

0KXB0Z0 Transfer Left Lower Arm and Wrist Muscle with Skin, Open Approach

0KXB0Z1 Transfer Left Lower Arm and Wrist Muscle with Subcutaneous Tissue, Open Approach

0KXB0Z2 Transfer Left Lower Arm and Wrist Muscle with Skin and Subcutaneous Tissue, Open Approach

0KXB0ZZ Transfer Left Lower Arm and Wrist Muscle, Open Approach

0KXB4Z0 Transfer Left Lower Arm and Wrist Muscle with Skin, Percutaneous Endoscopic Approach

0KXB4Z1 Transfer Left Lower Arm and Wrist Muscle with Subcutaneous Tissue, Percutaneous Endoscopic Approach

0KXB4Z2 Transfer Left Lower Arm and Wrist Muscle with Skin and Subcutaneous Tissue, Percutaneous Endoscopic Approach

0KXB4ZZ Transfer Left Lower Arm and Wrist Muscle, Percutaneous Endoscopic Approach

0KXC0Z0 Transfer Right Hand Muscle with Skin, Open Approach

0KXC0Z1 Transfer Right Hand Muscle with Subcutaneous Tissue, Open Approach

0KXC0Z2 Transfer Right Hand Muscle with Skin and Subcutaneous Tissue, Open Approach

0KXC0ZZ Transfer Right Hand Muscle, Open Approach

0KXC4Z0 Transfer Right Hand Muscle with Skin, Percutaneous Endoscopic Approach

0KXC4Z1 Transfer Right Hand Muscle with Subcutaneous Tissue, Percutaneous Endoscopic Approach

0KXC4Z2 Transfer Right Hand Muscle with Skin and Subcutaneous Tissue, Percutaneous Endoscopic Approach

0KXC4ZZ Transfer Right Hand Muscle, Percutaneous Endoscopic Approach

0KXD0Z0 Transfer Left Hand Muscle with Skin, Open Approach

0KXD0Z1 Transfer Left Hand Muscle with Subcutaneous Tissue, Open Approach

0KXD0Z2 Transfer Left Hand Muscle with Skin and Subcutaneous Tissue, Open Approach

0KXD0ZZ Transfer Left Hand Muscle, Open Approach

0KXD4Z0 Transfer Left Hand Muscle with Skin, Percutaneous Endoscopic Approach

0KXD4Z1 Transfer Left Hand Muscle with Subcutaneous Tissue, Percutaneous Endoscopic Approach

0KXD4Z2 Transfer Left Hand Muscle with Skin and Subcutaneous Tissue, Percutaneous Endoscopic Approach

0KXD4ZZ Transfer Left Hand Muscle, Percutaneous Endoscopic Approach

0KXF0Z0 Transfer Right Trunk Muscle with Skin, Open Approach

0KXF0Z1 Transfer Right Trunk Muscle with Subcutaneous Tissue, Open Approach

0KXF0Z2 Transfer Right Trunk Muscle with Skin and Subcutaneous Tissue, Open Approach

AHA CC: 2Q, 2014, 12

0KXF0Z5 Transfer Right Trunk Muscle, Latissimus Dorsi Myocutaneous Flap, Open Approach

AHA CC: 4Q, 2017, 67

0KXF0Z7 Transfer Right Trunk Muscle, Deep Inferior Epigastric Artery Perforator Flap, Open Approach

0KXF0Z8 Transfer Right Trunk Muscle, Superficial Inferior Epigastric Artery Flap, Open Approach

0KXF0Z9 Transfer Right Trunk Muscle, Gluteal Artery Perforator Flap, Open Approach

0KXF0ZZ Transfer Right Trunk Muscle, Open Approach

0KXF4Z0 Transfer Right Trunk Muscle with Skin, Percutaneous Endoscopic Approach

0KXF4Z1 Transfer Right Trunk Muscle with Subcutaneous Tissue, Percutaneous Endoscopic Approach

0KXF4Z2 Transfer Right Trunk Muscle with Skin and Subcutaneous Tissue, Percutaneous Endoscopic Approach

0KXF4Z5 Transfer Right Trunk Muscle, Latissimus Dorsi Myocutaneous Flap, Percutaneous Endoscopic Approach

0KXF4Z7 Transfer Right Trunk Muscle, Deep Inferior Epigastric Artery Perforator Flap, Percutaneous Endoscopic Approach

0KXF4Z8 Transfer Right Trunk Muscle, Superficial Inferior Epigastric Artery Flap, Percutaneous Endoscopic Approach

0KXF4Z9 Transfer Right Trunk Muscle, Gluteal Artery Perforator Flap, Percutaneous Endoscopic Approach

0KXF4ZZ Transfer Right Trunk Muscle, Percutaneous Endoscopic Approach

0KXG0Z0 Transfer Left Trunk Muscle with Skin, Open Approach

0KXG0Z1 Transfer Left Trunk Muscle with Subcutaneous Tissue, Open Approach

0KXG0Z2 Transfer Left Trunk Muscle with Skin and Subcutaneous Tissue, Open Approach

0KXG0Z5 Transfer Left Trunk Muscle, Latissimus Dorsi Myocutaneous Flap, Open Approach

0KXG0Z7 Transfer Left Trunk Muscle, Deep Inferior Epigastric Artery Perforator Flap, Open Approach

0KXG0Z8 Transfer Left Trunk Muscle, Superficial Inferior Epigastric Artery Flap, Open Approach

0KXG0Z9 Transfer Left Trunk Muscle, Gluteal Artery Perforator Flap, Open Approach

0KXG0ZZ Transfer Left Trunk Muscle, Open Approach

0KXG4Z0 Transfer Left Trunk Muscle with Skin, Percutaneous Endoscopic Approach

0KXG4Z1 Transfer Left Trunk Muscle with Subcutaneous Tissue, Percutaneous Endoscopic Approach

0KXG4Z2 Transfer Left Trunk Muscle with Skin and Subcutaneous Tissue, Percutaneous Endoscopic Approach

0KXG4Z5 Transfer Left Trunk Muscle, Latissimus Dorsi Myocutaneous Flap, Percutaneous Endoscopic Approach

0KXG4Z7 Transfer Left Trunk Muscle, Deep Inferior Epigastric Artery Perforator Flap, Percutaneous Endoscopic Approach

0KXG4Z8 Transfer Left Trunk Muscle, Superficial Inferior Epigastric Artery Flap, Percutaneous Endoscopic Approach

0KXG4Z9 Transfer Left Trunk Muscle, Gluteal Artery Perforator Flap, Percutaneous Endoscopic Approach

0KXG4ZZ Transfer Left Trunk Muscle, Percutaneous Endoscopic Approach

0KXH0Z0 Transfer Right Thorax Muscle with Skin, Open Approach

0KXH0Z1 Transfer Right Thorax Muscle with Subcutaneous Tissue, Open Approach

♀ Female-only   ♂ Male-only   ▲ Limited Coverage   ● Non-OR   ▦ HAC-associated procedure   ▲ Non-covered procedures   ✚ Cluster

0KXH0Z2 Transfer Right Thorax Muscle with Skin and Subcutaneous Tissue, Open Approach
0KXH0ZZ Transfer Right Thorax Muscle, Open Approach
0KXH4Z0 Transfer Right Thorax Muscle with Skin, Percutaneous Endoscopic Approach
0KXH4Z1 Transfer Right Thorax Muscle with Subcutaneous Tissue, Percutaneous Endoscopic Approach
0KXH4Z2 Transfer Right Thorax Muscle with Skin and Subcutaneous Tissue, Percutaneous Endoscopic Approach
0KXH4ZZ Transfer Right Thorax Muscle, Percutaneous Endoscopic Approach
0KXJ0Z0 Transfer Left Thorax Muscle with Skin, Open Approach
0KXJ0Z1 Transfer Left Thorax Muscle with Subcutaneous Tissue, Open Approach
0KXJ0Z2 Transfer Left Thorax Muscle with Skin and Subcutaneous Tissue, Open Approach
0KXJ0ZZ Transfer Left Thorax Muscle, Open Approach
0KXJ4Z0 Transfer Left Thorax Muscle with Skin, Percutaneous Endoscopic Approach
0KXJ4Z1 Transfer Left Thorax Muscle with Subcutaneous Tissue, Percutaneous Endoscopic Approach
0KXJ4Z2 Transfer Left Thorax Muscle with Skin and Subcutaneous Tissue, Percutaneous Endoscopic Approach
0KXJ4ZZ Transfer Left Thorax Muscle, Percutaneous Endoscopic Approach
0KXK0Z0 Transfer Right Abdomen Muscle with Skin, Open Approach
0KXK0Z1 Transfer Right Abdomen Muscle with Subcutaneous Tissue, Open Approach
0KXK0Z2 Transfer Right Abdomen Muscle with Skin and Subcutaneous Tissue, Open Approach
0KXK0Z6 Transfer Right Abdomen Muscle, Transverse Rectus Abdominis Myocutaneous Flap, Open Approach
AHA CC: 4Q, 2014, 41
0KXK0ZZ Transfer Right Abdomen Muscle, Open Approach
0KXK4Z0 Transfer Right Abdomen Muscle with Skin, Percutaneous Endoscopic Approach
0KXK4Z1 Transfer Right Abdomen Muscle with Subcutaneous Tissue, Percutaneous Endoscopic Approach
0KXK4Z2 Transfer Right Abdomen Muscle with Skin and Subcutaneous Tissue, Percutaneous Endoscopic Approach
0KXK4Z6 Transfer Right Abdomen Muscle, Transverse Rectus Abdominis Myocutaneous Flap, Percutaneous Endoscopic Approach
0KXK4ZZ Transfer Right Abdomen Muscle, Percutaneous Endoscopic Approach
0KXL0Z0 Transfer Left Abdomen Muscle with Skin, Open Approach
0KXL0Z1 Transfer Left Abdomen Muscle with Subcutaneous Tissue, Open Approach
0KXL0Z2 Transfer Left Abdomen Muscle with Skin and Subcutaneous Tissue, Open Approach
0KXL0Z6 Transfer Left Abdomen Muscle, Transverse Rectus Abdominis Myocutaneous Flap, Open Approach
AHA CC: 2Q, 2014, 10-11
0KXL0ZZ Transfer Left Abdomen Muscle, Open Approach
0KXL4Z0 Transfer Left Abdomen Muscle with Skin, Percutaneous Endoscopic Approach
0KXL4Z1 Transfer Left Abdomen Muscle with Subcutaneous Tissue, Percutaneous Endoscopic Approach
0KXL4Z2 Transfer Left Abdomen Muscle with Skin and Subcutaneous Tissue, Percutaneous Endoscopic Approach
0KXL4Z6 Transfer Left Abdomen Muscle, Transverse Rectus Abdominis Myocutaneous Flap, Percutaneous Endoscopic Approach
0KXL4ZZ Transfer Left Abdomen Muscle, Percutaneous Endoscopic Approach
0KXM0Z0 Transfer Perineum Muscle with Skin, Open Approach
0KXM0Z1 Transfer Perineum Muscle with Subcutaneous Tissue, Open Approach
0KXM0Z2 Transfer Perineum Muscle with Skin and Subcutaneous Tissue, Open Approach
0KXM0ZZ Transfer Perineum Muscle, Open Approach
0KXM4Z0 Transfer Perineum Muscle with Skin, Percutaneous Endoscopic Approach
0KXM4Z1 Transfer Perineum Muscle with Subcutaneous Tissue, Percutaneous Endoscopic Approach
0KXM4Z2 Transfer Perineum Muscle with Skin and Subcutaneous Tissue, Percutaneous Endoscopic Approach
0KXM4ZZ Transfer Perineum Muscle, Percutaneous Endoscopic Approach
0KXN0Z0 Transfer Right Hip Muscle with Skin, Open Approach
0KXN0Z1 Transfer Right Hip Muscle with Subcutaneous Tissue, Open Approach
0KXN0Z2 Transfer Right Hip Muscle with Skin and Subcutaneous Tissue, Open Approach
0KXN0ZZ Transfer Right Hip Muscle, Open Approach
0KXN4Z0 Transfer Right Hip Muscle with Skin, Percutaneous Endoscopic Approach
0KXN4Z1 Transfer Right Hip Muscle with Subcutaneous Tissue, Percutaneous Endoscopic Approach
0KXN4Z2 Transfer Right Hip Muscle with Skin and Subcutaneous Tissue, Percutaneous Endoscopic Approach
0KXN4ZZ Transfer Right Hip Muscle, Percutaneous Endoscopic Approach
0KXP0Z0 Transfer Left Hip Muscle with Skin, Open Approach
0KXP0Z1 Transfer Left Hip Muscle with Subcutaneous Tissue, Open Approach
0KXP0Z2 Transfer Left Hip Muscle with Skin and Subcutaneous Tissue, Open Approach
0KXP0ZZ Transfer Left Hip Muscle, Open Approach
0KXP4Z0 Transfer Left Hip Muscle with Skin, Percutaneous Endoscopic Approach
0KXP4Z1 Transfer Left Hip Muscle with Subcutaneous Tissue, Percutaneous Endoscopic Approach
0KXP4Z2 Transfer Left Hip Muscle with Skin and Subcutaneous Tissue, Percutaneous Endoscopic Approach
0KXP4ZZ Transfer Left Hip Muscle, Percutaneous Endoscopic Approach
0KXQ0Z0 Transfer Right Upper Leg Muscle with Skin, Open Approach
0KXQ0Z1 Transfer Right Upper Leg Muscle with Subcutaneous Tissue, Open Approach
0KXQ0Z2 Transfer Right Upper Leg Muscle with Skin and Subcutaneous Tissue, Open Approach
0KXQ0ZZ Transfer Right Upper Leg Muscle, Open Approach
AHA CC: 3Q, 2016, 30-31
0KXQ4Z0 Transfer Right Upper Leg Muscle with Skin, Percutaneous Endoscopic Approach
0KXQ4Z1 Transfer Right Upper Leg Muscle with Subcutaneous Tissue, Percutaneous Endoscopic Approach
0KXQ4Z2 Transfer Right Upper Leg Muscle with Skin and Subcutaneous Tissue, Percutaneous Endoscopic Approach
0KXQ4ZZ Transfer Right Upper Leg Muscle, Percutaneous Endoscopic Approach
0KXR0Z0 Transfer Left Upper Leg Muscle with Skin, Open Approach
0KXR0Z1 Transfer Left Upper Leg Muscle with Subcutaneous Tissue, Open Approach
0KXR0Z2 Transfer Left Upper Leg Muscle with Skin and Subcutaneous Tissue, Open Approach
0KXR0ZZ Transfer Left Upper Leg Muscle, Open Approach
AHA CC: 3Q, 2016, 30-31
0KXR4Z0 Transfer Left Upper Leg Muscle with Skin, Percutaneous Endoscopic Approach
0KXR4Z1 Transfer Left Upper Leg Muscle with Subcutaneous Tissue, Percutaneous Endoscopic Approach
0KXR4Z2 Transfer Left Upper Leg Muscle with Skin and Subcutaneous Tissue, Percutaneous Endoscopic Approach
0KXR4ZZ Transfer Left Upper Leg Muscle, Percutaneous Endoscopic Approach
0KXS0Z0 Transfer Right Lower Leg Muscle with Skin, Open Approach
0KXS0Z1 Transfer Right Lower Leg Muscle with Subcutaneous Tissue, Open Approach
0KXS0Z2 Transfer Right Lower Leg Muscle with Skin and Subcutaneous Tissue, Open Approach
0KXS0ZZ Transfer Right Lower Leg Muscle, Open Approach
0KXS4Z0 Transfer Right Lower Leg Muscle with Skin, Percutaneous Endoscopic Approach
0KXS4Z1 Transfer Right Lower Leg Muscle with Subcutaneous Tissue, Percutaneous Endoscopic Approach
0KXS4Z2 Transfer Right Lower Leg Muscle with Skin and Subcutaneous Tissue, Percutaneous Endoscopic Approach
0KXS4ZZ Transfer Right Lower Leg Muscle, Percutaneous Endoscopic Approach
0KXT0Z0 Transfer Left Lower Leg Muscle with Skin, Open Approach
0KXT0Z1 Transfer Left Lower Leg Muscle with Subcutaneous Tissue, Open Approach
0KXT0Z2 Transfer Left Lower Leg Muscle with Skin and Subcutaneous Tissue, Open Approach
0KXT0ZZ Transfer Left Lower Leg Muscle, Open Approach
0KXT4Z0 Transfer Left Lower Leg Muscle with Skin, Percutaneous Endoscopic Approach
0KXT4Z1 Transfer Left Lower Leg Muscle with Subcutaneous Tissue, Percutaneous Endoscopic Approach

0KXT4Z2 Transfer Left Lower Leg Muscle with Skin and Subcutaneous Tissue, Percutaneous Endoscopic Approach

0KXT4ZZ Transfer Left Lower Leg Muscle, Percutaneous Endoscopic Approach

0KXV0Z0 Transfer Right Foot Muscle with Skin, Open Approach

0KXV0Z1 Transfer Right Foot Muscle with Subcutaneous Tissue, Open Approach

0KXV0Z2 Transfer Right Foot Muscle with Skin and Subcutaneous Tissue, Open Approach

0KXV0ZZ Transfer Right Foot Muscle, Open Approach

0KXV4Z0 Transfer Right Foot Muscle with Skin, Percutaneous Endoscopic Approach

0KXV4Z1 Transfer Right Foot Muscle with Subcutaneous Tissue, Percutaneous Endoscopic Approach

0KXV4Z2 Transfer Right Foot Muscle with Skin and Subcutaneous Tissue, Percutaneous Endoscopic Approach

0KXV4ZZ Transfer Right Foot Muscle, Percutaneous Endoscopic Approach

0KXW0Z0 Transfer Left Foot Muscle with Skin, Open Approach

0KXW0Z1 Transfer Left Foot Muscle with Subcutaneous Tissue, Open Approach

0KXW0Z2 Transfer Left Foot Muscle with Skin and Subcutaneous Tissue, Open Approach

0KXW0ZZ Transfer Left Foot Muscle, Open Approach

0KXW4Z0 Transfer Left Foot Muscle with Skin, Percutaneous Endoscopic Approach

0KXW4Z1 Transfer Left Foot Muscle with Subcutaneous Tissue, Percutaneous Endoscopic Approach

0KXW4Z2 Transfer Left Foot Muscle with Skin and Subcutaneous Tissue, Percutaneous Endoscopic Approach

0KXW4ZZ Transfer Left Foot Muscle, Percutaneous Endoscopic Approach

Shoulder Tendons and Ligaments

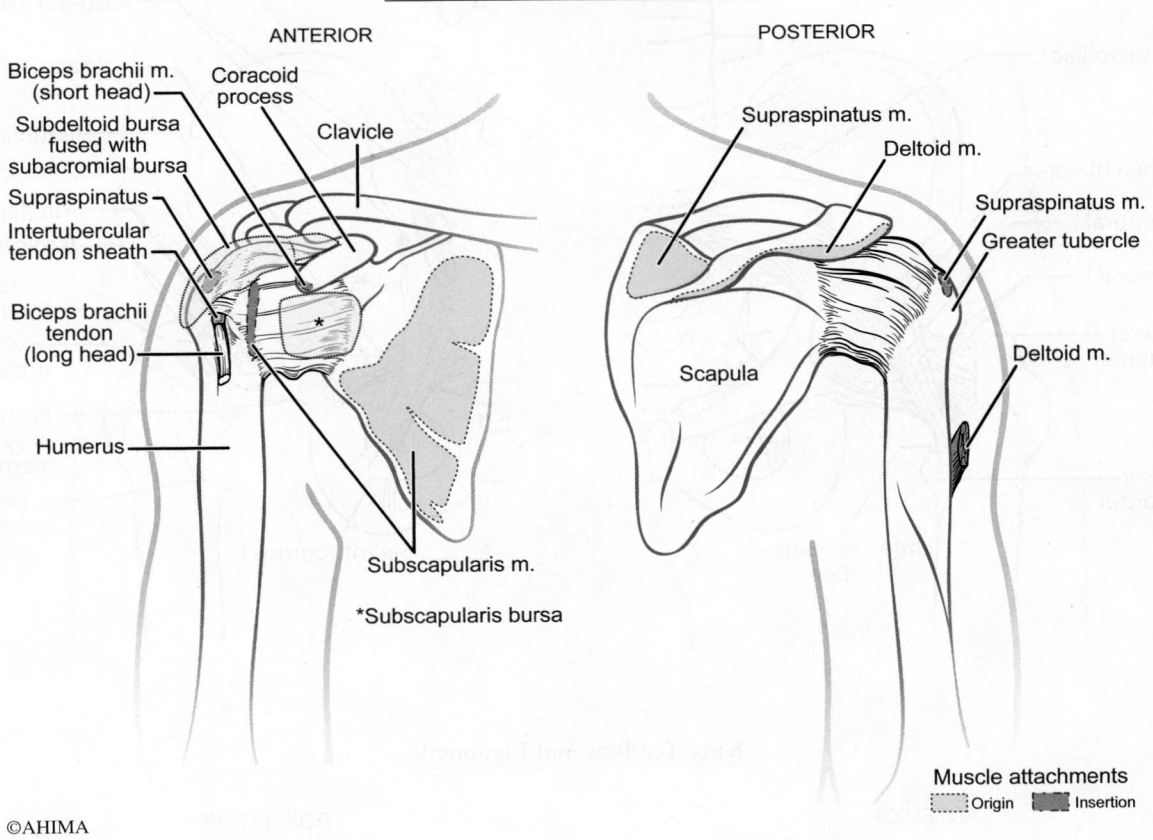

ANTERIOR

- Biceps brachii m. (short head)
- Coracoid process
- Clavicle
- Subdeltoid bursa fused with subacromial bursa
- Supraspinatus
- Intertubercular tendon sheath
- Biceps brachii tendon (long head)
- Humerus
- Subscapularis m.

*Subscapularis bursa

POSTERIOR

- Supraspinatus m.
- Deltoid m.
- Supraspinatus m.
- Greater tubercle
- Deltoid m.
- Scapula

Muscle attachments
[ ] Origin   [■] Insertion

©AHIMA

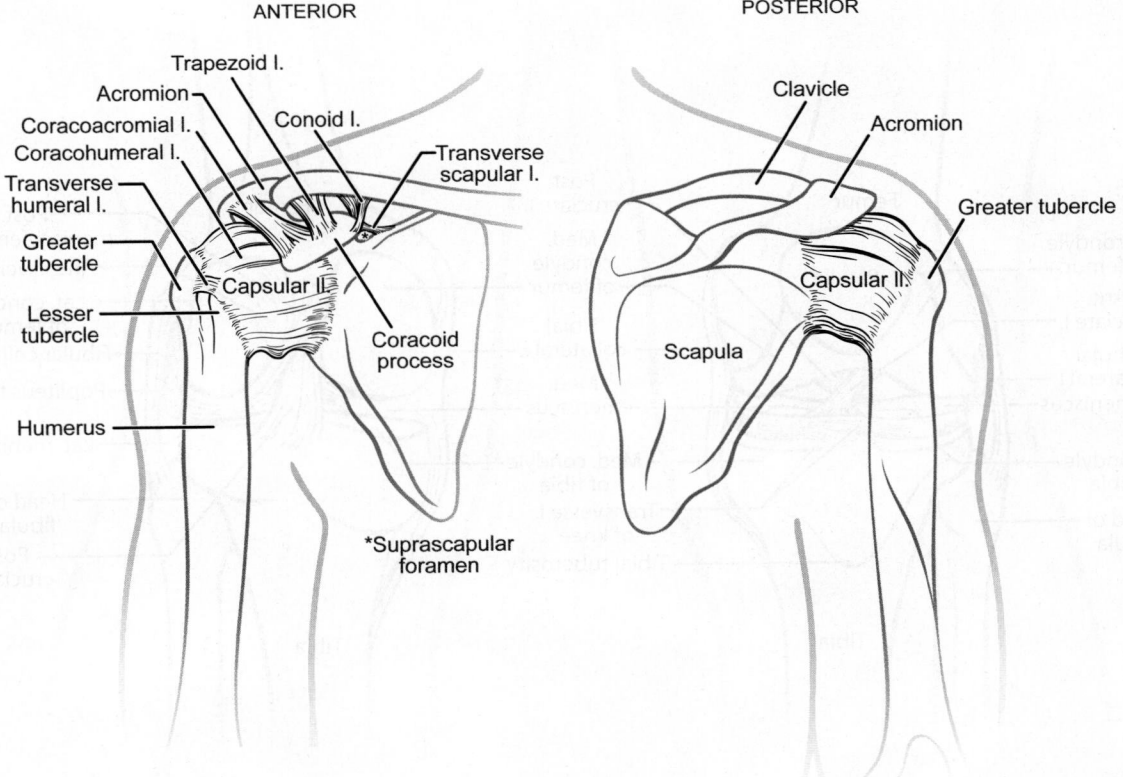

ANTERIOR

- Trapezoid l.
- Acromion
- Coracoacromial l.
- Coracohumeral l.
- Conoid l.
- Transverse humeral l.
- Transverse scapular l.
- Greater tubercle
- Capsular ll
- Lesser tubercle
- Coracoid process
- Humerus

*Suprascapular foramen

POSTERIOR

- Clavicle
- Acromion
- Greater tubercle
- Capsular ll
- Scapula

©AHIMA

Hip Tendons and Ligaments

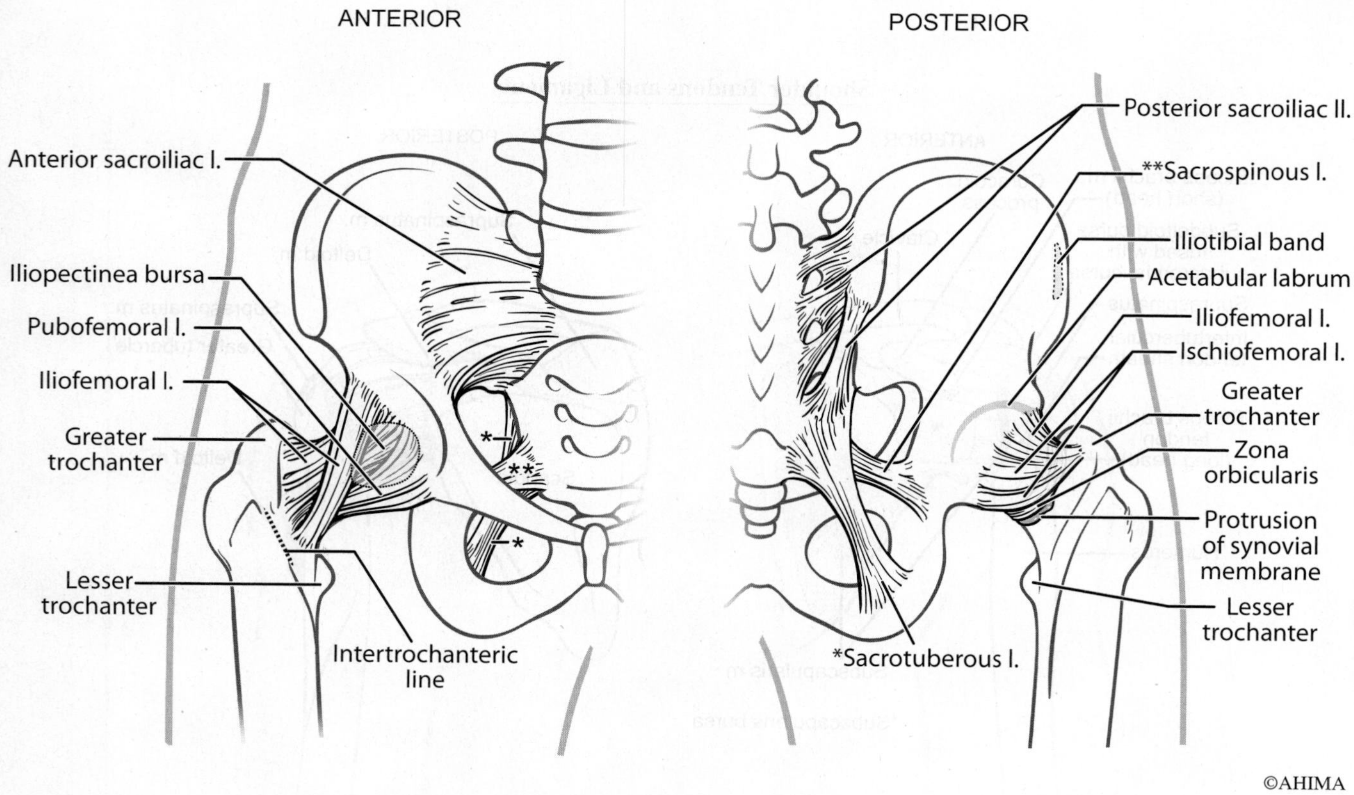

ANTERIOR

POSTERIOR

Anterior sacroiliac l.

Iliopectinea bursa

Pubofemoral l.

Iliofemoral l.

Greater trochanter

Lesser trochanter

*

**

*

Intertrochanteric line

Posterior sacroiliac ll.

**Sacrospinous l.

Iliotibial band

Acetabular labrum

Iliofemoral l.

Ischiofemoral l.

Greater trochanter

Zona orbicularis

Protrusion of synovial membrane

Lesser trochanter

*Sacrotuberous l.

©AHIMA

Knee Tendons and Ligaments

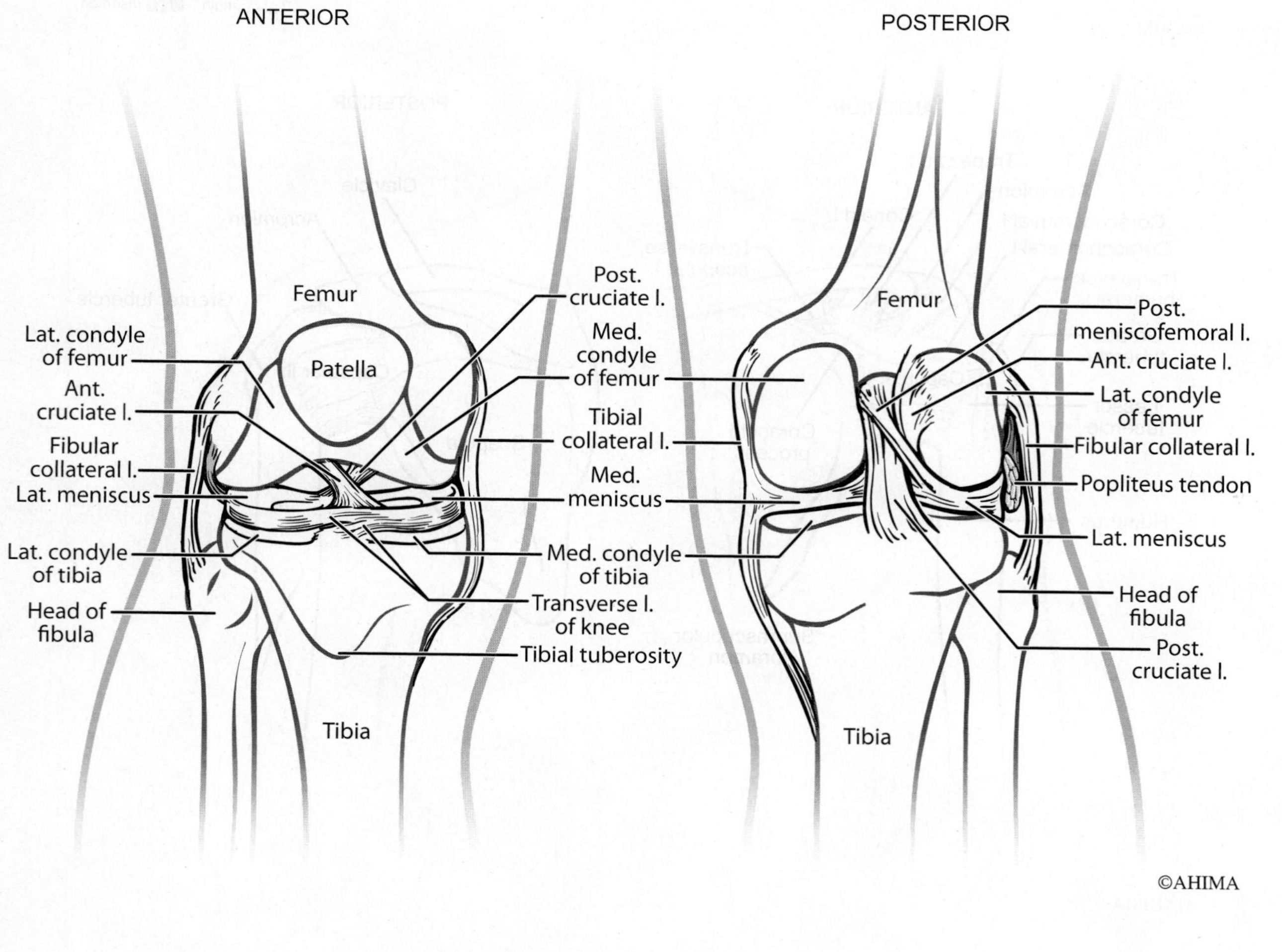

ANTERIOR

POSTERIOR

Femur

Lat. condyle of femur

Ant. cruciate l.

Fibular collateral l.

Lat. meniscus

Lat. condyle of tibia

Head of fibula

Patella

Tibia

Post. cruciate l.

Med. condyle of femur

Tibial collateral l.

Med. meniscus

Med. condyle of tibia

Transverse l. of knee

Tibial tuberosity

Femur

Post. meniscofemoral l.

Ant. cruciate l.

Lat. condyle of femur

Fibular collateral l.

Popliteus tendon

Lat. meniscus

Head of fibula

Post. cruciate l.

Tibia

©AHIMA

Tendons Tables 0L2–0LX

Section	0	Medical and Surgical
Body System	L	Tendons
Operation	2	Change: Taking out or off a device from a body part and putting back an identical or similar device in or on the same body part without cutting or puncturing the skin or a mucous membrane

Body Part (4th)	Approach (5th)	Device (6th)	Qualifier (7th)
X Upper Tendon Y Lower Tendon	X External	0 Drainage Device Y Other Device	Z No Qualifier

Section	0	Medical and Surgical
Body System	L	Tendons
Operation	5	Destruction: Physical eradication of all or a portion of a body part by the direct use of energy, force, or a destructive agent

Body Part (4th)	Approach (5th)	Device (6th)	Qualifier (7th)
0 Head and Neck Tendon 1 Shoulder Tendon, Right 2 Shoulder Tendon, Left 3 Upper Arm Tendon, Right 4 Upper Arm Tendon, Left 5 Lower Arm and Wrist Tendon, Right 6 Lower Arm and Wrist Tendon, Left 7 Hand Tendon, Right 8 Hand Tendon, Left 9 Trunk Tendon, Right B Trunk Tendon, Left C Thorax Tendon, Right D Thorax Tendon, Left F Abdomen Tendon, Right G Abdomen Tendon, Left H Perineum Tendon J Hip Tendon, Right K Hip Tendon, Left L Upper Leg Tendon, Right M Upper Leg Tendon, Left N Lower Leg Tendon, Right P Lower Leg Tendon, Left Q Knee Tendon, Right R Knee Tendon, Left S Ankle Tendon, Right T Ankle Tendon, Left V Foot Tendon, Right W Foot Tendon, Left	0 Open 3 Percutaneous 4 Percutaneous Endoscopic	Z No Device	Z No Qualifier

Section	0	Medical and Surgical
Body System	L	Tendons
Operation	8	**Division:** Cutting into a body part, without draining fluids and/or gases from the body part, in order to separate or transect a body part

Body Part (4th)	Approach (5th)	Device (6th)	Qualifier (7th)
0 Head and Neck Tendon 1 Shoulder Tendon, Right 2 Shoulder Tendon, Left 3 Upper Arm Tendon, Right 4 Upper Arm Tendon, Left 5 Lower Arm and Wrist Tendon, Right 6 Lower Arm and Wrist Tendon, Left 7 Hand Tendon, Right 8 Hand Tendon, Left 9 Trunk Tendon, Right B Trunk Tendon, Left C Thorax Tendon, Right D Thorax Tendon, Left F Abdomen Tendon, Right G Abdomen Tendon, Left H Perineum Tendon J Hip Tendon, Right K Hip Tendon, Left L Upper Leg Tendon, Right M Upper Leg Tendon, Left N Lower Leg Tendon, Right P Lower Leg Tendon, Left Q Knee Tendon, Right R Knee Tendon, Left S Ankle Tendon, Right T Ankle Tendon, Left V Foot Tendon, Right W Foot Tendon, Left	0 Open 3 Percutaneous 4 Percutaneous Endoscopic	Z No Device	Z No Qualifier

Section	0	Medical and Surgical
Body System	L	Tendons
Operation	9	**Drainage:** Taking or letting out fluids and/or gases from a body part

Body Part (4th)	Approach (5th)	Device (6th)	Qualifier (7th)
0 Head and Neck Tendon 1 Shoulder Tendon, Right 2 Shoulder Tendon, Left 3 Upper Arm Tendon, Right 4 Upper Arm Tendon, Left 5 Lower Arm and Wrist Tendon, Right 6 Lower Arm and Wrist Tendon, Left 7 Hand Tendon, Right 8 Hand Tendon, Left 9 Trunk Tendon, Right B Trunk Tendon, Left C Thorax Tendon, Right D Thorax Tendon, Left F Abdomen Tendon, Right G Abdomen Tendon, Left H Perineum Tendon J Hip Tendon, Right K Hip Tendon, Left L Upper Leg Tendon, Right M Upper Leg Tendon, Left N Lower Leg Tendon, Right P Lower Leg Tendon, Left Q Knee Tendon, Right R Knee Tendon, Left S Ankle Tendon, Right T Ankle Tendon, Left V Foot Tendon, Right W Foot Tendon, Left	0 Open 3 Percutaneous 4 Percutaneous Endoscopic	0 Drainage Device	Z No Qualifier

Continued →

Section   **0**   **Medical and Surgical**
Body System   **L**   **Tendons**
Operation   **9**   **Drainage:** Taking or letting out fluids and/or gases from a body part

Body Part (4ᵗʰ)	Approach (5ᵗʰ)	Device (6ᵗʰ)	Qualifier (7ᵗʰ)
0 Head and Neck Tendon	0 Open	Z No Device	X Diagnostic
1 Shoulder Tendon, Right	3 Percutaneous		Z No Qualifier
2 Shoulder Tendon, Left	4 Percutaneous Endoscopic		
3 Upper Arm Tendon, Right			
4 Upper Arm Tendon, Left			
5 Lower Arm and Wrist Tendon, Right			
6 Lower Arm and Wrist Tendon, Left			
7 Hand Tendon, Right			
8 Hand Tendon, Left			
9 Trunk Tendon, Right			
B Trunk Tendon, Left			
C Thorax Tendon, Right			
D Thorax Tendon, Left			
F Abdomen Tendon, Right			
G Abdomen Tendon, Left			
H Perineum Tendon			
J Hip Tendon, Right			
K Hip Tendon, Left			
L Upper Leg Tendon, Right			
M Upper Leg Tendon, Left			
N Lower Leg Tendon, Right			
P Lower Leg Tendon, Left			
Q Knee Tendon, Right			
R Knee Tendon, Left			
S Ankle Tendon, Right			
T Ankle Tendon, Left			
V Foot Tendon, Right			
W Foot Tendon, Left			

Section   **0**   **Medical and Surgical**
Body System   **L**   **Tendons**
Operation   **B**   **Excision:** Cutting out or off, without replacement, a portion of a body part

Body Part (4ᵗʰ)	Approach (5ᵗʰ)	Device (6ᵗʰ)	Qualifier (7ᵗʰ)
0 Head and Neck Tendon	0 Open	Z No Device	X Diagnostic
1 Shoulder Tendon, Right	3 Percutaneous		Z No Qualifier
2 Shoulder Tendon, Left	4 Percutaneous Endoscopic		
3 Upper Arm Tendon, Right			
4 Upper Arm Tendon, Left			
5 Lower Arm and Wrist Tendon, Right			
6 Lower Arm and Wrist Tendon, Left			
7 Hand Tendon, Right			
8 Hand Tendon, Left			
9 Trunk Tendon, Right			
B Trunk Tendon, Left			
C Thorax Tendon, Right			
D Thorax Tendon, Left			
F Abdomen Tendon, Right			
G Abdomen Tendon, Left			
H Perineum Tendon			
J Hip Tendon, Right			
K Hip Tendon, Left			
L Upper Leg Tendon, Right			
M Upper Leg Tendon, Left			
N Lower Leg Tendon, Right			
P Lower Leg Tendon, Left			
Q Knee Tendon, Right			
R Knee Tendon, Left			
S Ankle Tendon, Right			
T Ankle Tendon, Left			
V Foot Tendon, Right			
W Foot Tendon, Left			

Section	0	Medical and Surgical
Body System	L	Tendons
Operation	C	Extirpation: Taking or cutting out solid matter from a body part

Body Part (4th)	Approach (5th)	Device (6th)	Qualifier (7th)
0 Head and Neck Tendon 1 Shoulder Tendon, Right 2 Shoulder Tendon, Left 3 Upper Arm Tendon, Right 4 Upper Arm Tendon, Left 5 Lower Arm and Wrist Tendon, Right 6 Lower Arm and Wrist Tendon, Left 7 Hand Tendon, Right 8 Hand Tendon, Left 9 Trunk Tendon, Right B Trunk Tendon, Left C Thorax Tendon, Right D Thorax Tendon, Left F Abdomen Tendon, Right G Abdomen Tendon, Left H Perineum Tendon J Hip Tendon, Right K Hip Tendon, Left L Upper Leg Tendon, Right M Upper Leg Tendon, Left N Lower Leg Tendon, Right P Lower Leg Tendon, Left Q Knee Tendon, Right R Knee Tendon, Left S Ankle Tendon, Right T Ankle Tendon, Left V Foot Tendon, Right W Foot Tendon, Left	0 Open 3 Percutaneous 4 Percutaneous Endoscopic	Z No Device	Z No Qualifier

Section	0	Medical and Surgical
Body System	L	Tendons
Operation	D	Extraction: Pulling or stripping out or off all or a portion of a body part by the use of force

Body Part (4th)	Approach (5th)	Device (6th)	Qualifier (7th)
0 Head and Neck Tendon 1 Shoulder Tendon, Right 2 Shoulder Tendon, Left 3 Upper Arm Tendon, Right 4 Upper Arm Tendon, Left 5 Lower Arm and Wrist Tendon, Right 6 Lower Arm and Wrist Tendon, Left 7 Hand Tendon, Right 8 Hand Tendon, Left 9 Trunk Tendon, Right B Trunk Tendon, Left C Thorax Tendon, Right D Thorax Tendon, Left F Abdomen Tendon, Right G Abdomen Tendon, Left H Perineum Tendon J Hip Tendon, Right K Hip Tendon, Left L Upper Leg Tendon, Right M Upper Leg Tendon, Left N Lower Leg Tendon, Right P Lower Leg Tendon, Left Q Knee Tendon, Right R Knee Tendon, Left S Ankle Tendon, Right T Ankle Tendon, Left V Foot Tendon, Right W Foot Tendon, Left	0 Open	Z No Device	Z No Qualifier

Section   **0**   **Medical and Surgical**
Body System   **L**   **Tendons**
Operation   **H**   **Inspection:** Putting in a nonbiological appliance that monitors, assists, performs, or prevents a physiological function but does not physically take the place of a body part

Body Part (4th)	Approach (5th)	Device (6th)	Qualifier (7th)
X Upper Tendon **Y** Lower Tendon	**0** Open **3** Percutaneous **4** Percutaneous Endoscopic	**Y** Other Device	**Z** No Qualifier

Section   **0**   **Medical and Surgical**
Body System   **L**   **Tendons**
Operation   **J**   **Inspection:** Visually and/or manually exploring a body part

Body Part (4th)	Approach (5th)	Device (6th)	Qualifier (7th)
X Upper Tendon **Y** Lower Tendon	**0** Open **3** Percutaneous **4** Percutaneous Endoscopic **X** External	**Z** No Device	**Z** No Qualifier

Section   **0**   **Medical and Surgical**
Body System   **L**   **Tendons**
Operation   **M**   **Reattachment:** Putting back in or on all or a portion of a separated body part to its normal location or other suitable location

Body Part (4th)	Approach (5th)	Device (6th)	Qualifier (7th)
0 Head and Neck Tendon **1** Shoulder Tendon, Right **2** Shoulder Tendon, Left **3** Upper Arm Tendon, Right **4** Upper Arm Tendon, Left **5** Lower Arm and Wrist Tendon, Right **6** Lower Arm and Wrist Tendon, Left **7** Hand Tendon, Right **8** Hand Tendon, Left **9** Trunk Tendon, Right **B** Trunk Tendon, Left **C** Thorax Tendon, Right **D** Thorax Tendon, Left **F** Abdomen Tendon, Right **G** Abdomen Tendon, Left **H** Perineum Tendon **J** Hip Tendon, Right **K** Hip Tendon, Left **L** Upper Leg Tendon, Right **M** Upper Leg Tendon, Left **N** Lower Leg Tendon, Right **P** Lower Leg Tendon, Left **Q** Knee Tendon, Right **R** Knee Tendon, Left **S** Ankle Tendon, Right **T** Ankle Tendon, Left **V** Foot Tendon, Right **W** Foot Tendon, Left	**0** Open **4** Percutaneous Endoscopic	**Z** No Device	**Z** No Qualifier

Section   **0**   **Medical and Surgical**
Body System   **L**   **Tendons**
Operation   **N**   **Release:** Freeing a body part from an abnormal physical constraint by cutting or by the use of force

Body Part (4ᵗʰ)	Approach (5ᵗʰ)	Device (6ᵗʰ)	Qualifier (7ᵗʰ)
0 Head and Neck Tendon	0 Open	Z No Device	Z No Qualifier
1 Shoulder Tendon, Right	3 Percutaneous		
2 Shoulder Tendon, Left	4 Percutaneous Endoscopic		
3 Upper Arm Tendon, Right	X External		
4 Upper Arm Tendon, Left			
5 Lower Arm and Wrist Tendon, Right			
6 Lower Arm and Wrist Tendon, Left			
7 Hand Tendon, Right			
8 Hand Tendon, Left			
9 Trunk Tendon, Right			
B Trunk Tendon, Left			
C Thorax Tendon, Right			
D Thorax Tendon, Left			
F Abdomen Tendon, Right			
G Abdomen Tendon, Left			
H Perineum Tendon			
J Hip Tendon, Right			
K Hip Tendon, Left			
L Upper Leg Tendon, Right			
M Upper Leg Tendon, Left			
N Lower Leg Tendon, Right			
P Lower Leg Tendon, Left			
Q Knee Tendon, Right			
R Knee Tendon, Left			
S Ankle Tendon, Right			
T Ankle Tendon, Left			
V Foot Tendon, Right			
W Foot Tendon, Left			

Section   **0**   **Medical and Surgical**
Body System   **L**   **Tendons**
Operation   **P**   **Removal:** Taking out or off a device from a body part

Body Part (4ᵗʰ)	Approach (5ᵗʰ)	Device (6ᵗʰ)	Qualifier (7ᵗʰ)
X Upper Tendon	0 Open	0 Drainage Device	Z No Qualifier
Y Lower Tendon	3 Percutaneous	7 Autologous Tissue Substitute	
	4 Percutaneous Endoscopic	J Synthetic Substitute	
		K Nonautologous Tissue Substitute	
		Y Other Device	
X Upper Tendon	X External	0 Drainage Device	Z No Qualifier
Y Lower Tendon			

Section	0	Medical and Surgical
Body System	L	Tendons
Operation	Q	Repair: Restoring, to the extent possible, a body part to its normal anatomic structure and function

Body Part (4th)	Approach (5th)	Device (6th)	Qualifier (7th)
0 Head and Neck Tendon	0 Open	Z No Device	Z No Qualifier
1 Shoulder Tendon, Right	3 Percutaneous		
2 Shoulder Tendon, Left	4 Percutaneous Endoscopic		
3 Upper Arm Tendon, Right			
4 Upper Arm Tendon, Left			
5 Lower Arm and Wrist Tendon, Right			
6 Lower Arm and Wrist Tendon, Left			
7 Hand Tendon, Right			
8 Hand Tendon, Left			
9 Trunk Tendon, Right			
B Trunk Tendon, Left			
C Thorax Tendon, Right			
D Thorax Tendon, Left			
F Abdomen Tendon, Right			
G Abdomen Tendon, Left			
H Perineum Tendon			
J Hip Tendon, Right			
K Hip Tendon, Left			
L Upper Leg Tendon, Right			
M Upper Leg Tendon, Left			
N Lower Leg Tendon, Right			
P Lower Leg Tendon, Left			
Q Knee Tendon, Right			
R Knee Tendon, Left			
S Ankle Tendon, Right			
T Ankle Tendon, Left			
V Foot Tendon, Right			
W Foot Tendon, Left			

Section	0	Medical and Surgical
Body System	L	Tendons
Operation	R	Replacement: Putting in or on biological or synthetic material that physically takes the place and/or function of all or a portion of a body part

Body Part (4th)	Approach (5th)	Device (6th)	Qualifier (7th)
0 Head and Neck Tendon	0 Open	7 Autologous Tissue Substitute	Z No Qualifier
1 Shoulder Tendon, Right	4 Percutaneous Endoscopic	J Synthetic Substitute	
2 Shoulder Tendon, Left		K Nonautologous Tissue Substitute	
3 Upper Arm Tendon, Right			
4 Upper Arm Tendon, Left			
5 Lower Arm and Wrist Tendon, Right			
6 Lower Arm and Wrist Tendon, Left			
7 Hand Tendon, Right			
8 Hand Tendon, Left			
9 Trunk Tendon, Right			
B Trunk Tendon, Left			
C Thorax Tendon, Right			
D Thorax Tendon, Left			
F Abdomen Tendon, Right			
G Abdomen Tendon, Left			
H Perineum Tendon			
J Hip Tendon, Right			
K Hip Tendon, Left			
L Upper Leg Tendon, Right			
M Upper Leg Tendon, Left			
N Lower Leg Tendon, Right			
P Lower Leg Tendon, Left			
Q Knee Tendon, Right			
R Knee Tendon, Left			
S Ankle Tendon, Right			
T Ankle Tendon, Left			
V Foot Tendon, Right			
W Foot Tendon, Left			

Section	0	Medical and Surgical
Body System	L	Tendons
Operation	S	Reposition: Moving to its normal location, or other suitable location, all or a portion of a body part

Body Part (4th)	Approach (5th)	Device (6th)	Qualifier (7th)
0 Head and Neck Tendon 1 Shoulder Tendon, Right 2 Shoulder Tendon, Left 3 Upper Arm Tendon, Right 4 Upper Arm Tendon, Left 5 Lower Arm and Wrist Tendon, Right 6 Lower Arm and Wrist Tendon, Left 7 Hand Tendon, Right 8 Hand Tendon, Left 9 Trunk Tendon, Right B Trunk Tendon, Left C Thorax Tendon, Right D Thorax Tendon, Left F Abdomen Tendon, Right G Abdomen Tendon, Left H Perineum Tendon J Hip Tendon, Right K Hip Tendon, Left L Upper Leg Tendon, Right M Upper Leg Tendon, Left N Lower Leg Tendon, Right P Lower Leg Tendon, Left Q Knee Tendon, Right R Knee Tendon, Left S Ankle Tendon, Right T Ankle Tendon, Left V Foot Tendon, Right W Foot Tendon, Left	0 Open 4 Percutaneous Endoscopic	Z No Device	Z No Qualifier

Section	0	Medical and Surgical
Body System	L	Tendons
Operation	T	Resection: Cutting out or off, without replacement, all of a body part

Body Part (4th)	Approach (5th)	Device (6th)	Qualifier (7th)
0 Head and Neck Tendon 1 Shoulder Tendon, Right 2 Shoulder Tendon, Left 3 Upper Arm Tendon, Right 4 Upper Arm Tendon, Left 5 Lower Arm and Wrist Tendon, Right 6 Lower Arm and Wrist Tendon, Left 7 Hand Tendon, Right 8 Hand Tendon, Left 9 Trunk Tendon, Right B Trunk Tendon, Left C Thorax Tendon, Right D Thorax Tendon, Left F Abdomen Tendon, Right G Abdomen Tendon, Left H Perineum Tendon J Hip Tendon, Right K Hip Tendon, Left L Upper Leg Tendon, Right M Upper Leg Tendon, Left N Lower Leg Tendon, Right P Lower Leg Tendon, Left Q Knee Tendon, Right R Knee Tendon, Left S Ankle Tendon, Right T Ankle Tendon, Left V Foot Tendon, Right W Foot Tendon, Left	0 Open 4 Percutaneous Endoscopic	Z No Device	Z No Qualifier

Section   0   **Medical and Surgical**
Body System   L   **Tendons**
Operation   U   **Supplement:** Putting in or on biological or synthetic material that physically reinforces and/or augments the function of a portion of a body part

Body Part (4th)	Approach (5th)	Device (6th)	Qualifier (7th)
0 Head and Neck Tendon	0 Open	7 Autologous Tissue Substitute	Z No Qualifier
1 Shoulder Tendon, Right	4 Percutaneous Endoscopic	J Synthetic Substitute	
2 Shoulder Tendon, Left		K Nonautologous Tissue Substitute	
3 Upper Arm Tendon, Right			
4 Upper Arm Tendon, Left			
5 Lower Arm and Wrist Tendon, Right			
6 Lower Arm and Wrist Tendon, Left			
7 Hand Tendon, Right			
8 Hand Tendon, Left			
9 Trunk Tendon, Right			
B Trunk Tendon, Left			
C Thorax Tendon, Right			
D Thorax Tendon, Left			
F Abdomen Tendon, Right			
G Abdomen Tendon, Left			
H Perineum Tendon			
J Hip Tendon, Right			
K Hip Tendon, Left			
L Upper Leg Tendon, Right			
M Upper Leg Tendon, Left			
N Lower Leg Tendon, Right			
P Lower Leg Tendon, Left			
Q Knee Tendon, Right			
R Knee Tendon, Left			
S Ankle Tendon, Right			
T Ankle Tendon, Left			
V Foot Tendon, Right			
W Foot Tendon, Left			

Section   0   **Medical and Surgical**
Body System   L   **Tendons**
Operation   W   **Revision:** Correcting, to the extent possible, a portion of a malfunctioning device or the position of a displaced device

Body Part (4th)	Approach (5th)	Device (6th)	Qualifier (7th)
X Upper Tendon Y Lower Tendon	0 Open 3 Percutaneous 4 Percutaneous Endoscopic	0 Drainage Device 7 Autologous Tissue Substitute J Synthetic Substitute K Nonautologous Tissue Substitute Y Other Device	Z No Qualifier
X Upper Tendon Y Lower Tendon	X External	0 Drainage Device 7 Autologous Tissue Substitute J Synthetic Substitute K Nonautologous Tissue Substitute	Z No Qualifier

Section	0	Medical and Surgical
Body System	L	Tendons
Operation	X	**Transfer:** Moving, without taking out, all or a portion of a body part to another location to take over the function of all or a portion of a body part

Body Part (4th)	Approach (5th)	Device (6th)	Qualifier (7th)
0 Head and Neck Tendon 1 Shoulder Tendon, Right 2 Shoulder Tendon, Left 3 Upper Arm Tendon, Right 4 Upper Arm Tendon, Left 5 Lower Arm and Wrist Tendon, Right 6 Lower Arm and Wrist Tendon, Left 7 Hand Tendon, Right 8 Hand Tendon, Left 9 Trunk Tendon, Right B Trunk Tendon, Left C Thorax Tendon, Right D Thorax Tendon, Left F Abdomen Tendon, Right G Abdomen Tendon, Left H Perineum Tendon J Hip Tendon, Right K Hip Tendon, Left L Upper Leg Tendon, Right M Upper Leg Tendon, Left N Lower Leg Tendon, Right P Lower Leg Tendon, Left Q Knee Tendon, Right R Knee Tendon, Left S Ankle Tendon, Right T Ankle Tendon, Left V Foot Tendon, Right W Foot Tendon, Left	0 Open 4 Percutaneous Endoscopic	Z No Device	Z No Qualifier

Tendons Code Listing 0L2–0LX

Review Coding Guideline B4.5

0L2 – Tendons, Change

Review Coding Guideline B6.1c

0L2XX0Z Change Drainage Device in Upper Tendon, External Approach
0L2XXYZ Change Other Device in Upper Tendon, External Approach

0L2YX0Z Change Drainage Device in Lower Tendon, External Approach

0L2YXYZ Change Other Device in Lower Tendon, External Approach

0L5 – Tendons, Destruction

0L500ZZ Destruction of Head and Neck Tendon, Open Approach
0L503ZZ Destruction of Head and Neck Tendon, Percutaneous Approach
0L504ZZ Destruction of Head and Neck Tendon, Percutaneous Endoscopic Approach
0L510ZZ Destruction of Right Shoulder Tendon, Open Approach
0L513ZZ Destruction of Right Shoulder Tendon, Percutaneous Approach
0L514ZZ Destruction of Right Shoulder Tendon, Percutaneous Endoscopic Approach
0L520ZZ Destruction of Left Shoulder Tendon, Open Approach
0L523ZZ Destruction of Left Shoulder Tendon, Percutaneous Approach
0L524ZZ Destruction of Left Shoulder Tendon, Percutaneous Endoscopic Approach
0L530ZZ Destruction of Right Upper Arm Tendon, Open Approach

0L533ZZ Destruction of Right Upper Arm Tendon, Percutaneous Approach
0L534ZZ Destruction of Right Upper Arm Tendon, Percutaneous Endoscopic Approach
0L540ZZ Destruction of Left Upper Arm Tendon, Open Approach
0L543ZZ Destruction of Left Upper Arm Tendon, Percutaneous Approach
0L544ZZ Destruction of Left Upper Arm Tendon, Percutaneous Endoscopic Approach
0L550ZZ Destruction of Right Lower Arm and Wrist Tendon, Open Approach
0L553ZZ Destruction of Right Lower Arm and Wrist Tendon, Percutaneous Approach
0L554ZZ Destruction of Right Lower Arm and Wrist Tendon, Percutaneous Endoscopic Approach
0L560ZZ Destruction of Left Lower Arm and Wrist Tendon, Open Approach
0L563ZZ Destruction of Left Lower Arm and Wrist Tendon, Percutaneous Approach

0L564ZZ Destruction of Left Lower Arm and Wrist Tendon, Percutaneous Endoscopic Approach
0L570ZZ Destruction of Right Hand Tendon, Open Approach
0L573ZZ Destruction of Right Hand Tendon, Percutaneous Approach
0L574ZZ Destruction of Right Hand Tendon, Percutaneous Endoscopic Approach
0L580ZZ Destruction of Left Hand Tendon, Open Approach
0L583ZZ Destruction of Left Hand Tendon, Percutaneous Approach
0L584ZZ Destruction of Left Hand Tendon, Percutaneous Endoscopic Approach
0L590ZZ Destruction of Right Trunk Tendon, Open Approach
0L593ZZ Destruction of Right Trunk Tendon, Percutaneous Approach
0L594ZZ Destruction of Right Trunk Tendon, Percutaneous Endoscopic Approach

♀ Female-only   ♂ Male-only   ▲ Limited Coverage   ● Non-OR   HAC HAC-associated procedure   ▲ Non-covered procedures   ✚ Cluster

0L5B0ZZ Destruction of Left Trunk Tendon, Open Approach

0L5B3ZZ Destruction of Left Trunk Tendon, Percutaneous Approach

0L5B4ZZ Destruction of Left Trunk Tendon, Percutaneous Endoscopic Approach

0L5C0ZZ Destruction of Right Thorax Tendon, Open Approach

0L5C3ZZ Destruction of Right Thorax Tendon, Percutaneous Approach

0L5C4ZZ Destruction of Right Thorax Tendon, Percutaneous Endoscopic Approach

0L5D0ZZ Destruction of Left Thorax Tendon, Open Approach

0L5D3ZZ Destruction of Left Thorax Tendon, Percutaneous Approach

0L5D4ZZ Destruction of Left Thorax Tendon, Percutaneous Endoscopic Approach

0L5F0ZZ Destruction of Right Abdomen Tendon, Open Approach

0L5F3ZZ Destruction of Right Abdomen Tendon, Percutaneous Approach

0L5F4ZZ Destruction of Right Abdomen Tendon, Percutaneous Endoscopic Approach

0L5G0ZZ Destruction of Left Abdomen Tendon, Open Approach

0L5G3ZZ Destruction of Left Abdomen Tendon, Percutaneous Approach

0L5G4ZZ Destruction of Left Abdomen Tendon, Percutaneous Endoscopic Approach

0L5H0ZZ Destruction of Perineum Tendon, Open Approach

0L5H3ZZ Destruction of Perineum Tendon, Percutaneous Approach

0L5H4ZZ Destruction of Perineum Tendon, Percutaneous Endoscopic Approach

0L5J0ZZ Destruction of Right Hip Tendon, Open Approach

0L5J3ZZ Destruction of Right Hip Tendon, Percutaneous Approach

0L5J4ZZ Destruction of Right Hip Tendon, Percutaneous Endoscopic Approach

0L5K0ZZ Destruction of Left Hip Tendon, Open Approach

0L5K3ZZ Destruction of Left Hip Tendon, Percutaneous Approach

0L5K4ZZ Destruction of Left Hip Tendon, Percutaneous Endoscopic Approach

0L5L0ZZ Destruction of Right Upper Leg Tendon, Open Approach

0L5L3ZZ Destruction of Right Upper Leg Tendon, Percutaneous Approach

0L5L4ZZ Destruction of Right Upper Leg Tendon, Percutaneous Endoscopic Approach

0L5M0ZZ Destruction of Left Upper Leg Tendon, Open Approach

0L5M3ZZ Destruction of Left Upper Leg Tendon, Percutaneous Approach

0L5M4ZZ Destruction of Left Upper Leg Tendon, Percutaneous Endoscopic Approach

0L5N0ZZ Destruction of Right Lower Leg Tendon, Open Approach

0L5N3ZZ Destruction of Right Lower Leg Tendon, Percutaneous Approach

0L5N4ZZ Destruction of Right Lower Leg Tendon, Percutaneous Endoscopic Approach

0L5P0ZZ Destruction of Left Lower Leg Tendon, Open Approach

0L5P3ZZ Destruction of Left Lower Leg Tendon, Percutaneous Approach

0L5P4ZZ Destruction of Left Lower Leg Tendon, Percutaneous Endoscopic Approach

0L5Q0ZZ Destruction of Right Knee Tendon, Open Approach

0L5Q3ZZ Destruction of Right Knee Tendon, Percutaneous Approach

0L5Q4ZZ Destruction of Right Knee Tendon, Percutaneous Endoscopic Approach

0L5R0ZZ Destruction of Left Knee Tendon, Open Approach

0L5R3ZZ Destruction of Left Knee Tendon, Percutaneous Approach

0L5R4ZZ Destruction of Left Knee Tendon, Percutaneous Endoscopic Approach

0L5S0ZZ Destruction of Right Ankle Tendon, Open Approach

0L5S3ZZ Destruction of Right Ankle Tendon, Percutaneous Approach

0L5S4ZZ Destruction of Right Ankle Tendon, Percutaneous Endoscopic Approach

0L5T0ZZ Destruction of Left Ankle Tendon, Open Approach

0L5T3ZZ Destruction of Left Ankle Tendon, Percutaneous Approach

0L5T4ZZ Destruction of Left Ankle Tendon, Percutaneous Endoscopic Approach

0L5V0ZZ Destruction of Right Foot Tendon, Open Approach

0L5V3ZZ Destruction of Right Foot Tendon, Percutaneous Approach

0L5V4ZZ Destruction of Right Foot Tendon, Percutaneous Endoscopic Approach

0L5W0ZZ Destruction of Left Foot Tendon, Open Approach

0L5W3ZZ Destruction of Left Foot Tendon, Percutaneous Approach

0L5W4ZZ Destruction of Left Foot Tendon, Percutaneous Endoscopic Approach

0L8 – Tendons, Division

Review Coding Guideline B3.14

0L800ZZ Division of Head and Neck Tendon, Open Approach

0L803ZZ Division of Head and Neck Tendon, Percutaneous Approach

0L804ZZ Division of Head and Neck Tendon, Percutaneous Endoscopic Approach

0L810ZZ Division of Right Shoulder Tendon, Open Approach

0L813ZZ Division of Right Shoulder Tendon, Percutaneous Approach

0L814ZZ Division of Right Shoulder Tendon, Percutaneous Endoscopic Approach

0L820ZZ Division of Left Shoulder Tendon, Open Approach

0L823ZZ Division of Left Shoulder Tendon, Percutaneous Approach

0L824ZZ Division of Left Shoulder Tendon, Percutaneous Endoscopic Approach

0L830ZZ Division of Right Upper Arm Tendon, Open Approach

0L833ZZ Division of Right Upper Arm Tendon, Percutaneous Approach

0L834ZZ Division of Right Upper Arm Tendon, Percutaneous Endoscopic Approach

0L840ZZ Division of Left Upper Arm Tendon, Open Approach

0L843ZZ Division of Left Upper Arm Tendon, Percutaneous Approach

0L844ZZ Division of Left Upper Arm Tendon, Percutaneous Endoscopic Approach

0L850ZZ Division of Right Lower Arm and Wrist Tendon, Open Approach

0L853ZZ Division of Right Lower Arm and Wrist Tendon, Percutaneous Approach

0L854ZZ Division of Right Lower Arm and Wrist Tendon, Percutaneous Endoscopic Approach

0L860ZZ Division of Left Lower Arm and Wrist Tendon, Open Approach

0L863ZZ Division of Left Lower Arm and Wrist Tendon, Percutaneous Approach

0L864ZZ Division of Left Lower Arm and Wrist Tendon, Percutaneous Endoscopic Approach

0L870ZZ Division of Right Hand Tendon, Open Approach

0L873ZZ Division of Right Hand Tendon, Percutaneous Approach

0L874ZZ Division of Right Hand Tendon, Percutaneous Endoscopic Approach

0L880ZZ Division of Left Hand Tendon, Open Approach

0L883ZZ Division of Left Hand Tendon, Percutaneous Approach

0L884ZZ Division of Left Hand Tendon, Percutaneous Endoscopic Approach

0L890ZZ Division of Right Trunk Tendon, Open Approach

0L893ZZ Division of Right Trunk Tendon, Percutaneous Approach

0L894ZZ Division of Right Trunk Tendon, Percutaneous Endoscopic Approach

0L8B0ZZ Division of Left Trunk Tendon, Open Approach

0L8B3ZZ Division of Left Trunk Tendon, Percutaneous Approach

0L8B4ZZ Division of Left Trunk Tendon, Percutaneous Endoscopic Approach

0L8C0ZZ Division of Right Thorax Tendon, Open Approach

0L8C3ZZ Division of Right Thorax Tendon, Percutaneous Approach

0L8C4ZZ Division of Right Thorax Tendon, Percutaneous Endoscopic Approach

0L8D0ZZ Division of Left Thorax Tendon, Open Approach

0L8D3ZZ Division of Left Thorax Tendon, Percutaneous Approach

0L8D4ZZ Division of Left Thorax Tendon, Percutaneous Endoscopic Approach

0L8F0ZZ Division of Right Abdomen Tendon, Open Approach

0L8F3ZZ Division of Right Abdomen Tendon, Percutaneous Approach

0L8F4ZZ Division of Right Abdomen Tendon, Percutaneous Endoscopic Approach

0L8G0ZZ Division of Left Abdomen Tendon, Open Approach

0L8G3ZZ Division of Left Abdomen Tendon, Percutaneous Approach

0L8G4ZZ Division of Left Abdomen Tendon, Percutaneous Endoscopic Approach

0L8H0ZZ Division of Perineum Tendon, Open Approach

0L8H3ZZ Division of Perineum Tendon, Percutaneous Approach

♀ Female-only   ♂ Male-only   ▲ Limited Coverage   ● Non-OR   ᴴᴬᶜ HAC-associated procedure   ▲ Non-covered procedures   ✚ Cluster

0L8H4ZZ	Division of Perineum Tendon, Percutaneous Endoscopic Approach
0L8J0ZZ	Division of Right Hip Tendon, Open Approach
	AHA CC: 3Q, 2016, 30-31
0L8J3ZZ	Division of Right Hip Tendon, Percutaneous Approach
0L8J4ZZ	Division of Right Hip Tendon, Percutaneous Endoscopic Approach
0L8K0ZZ	Division of Left Hip Tendon, Open Approach
0L8K3ZZ	Division of Left Hip Tendon, Percutaneous Approach
0L8K4ZZ	Division of Left Hip Tendon, Percutaneous Endoscopic Approach
0L8L0ZZ	Division of Right Upper Leg Tendon, Open Approach
0L8L3ZZ	Division of Right Upper Leg Tendon, Percutaneous Approach
0L8L4ZZ	Division of Right Upper Leg Tendon, Percutaneous Endoscopic Approach
0L8M0ZZ	Division of Left Upper Leg Tendon, Open Approach
0L8M3ZZ	Division of Left Upper Leg Tendon, Percutaneous Approach

0L8M4ZZ	Division of Left Upper Leg Tendon, Percutaneous Endoscopic Approach
0L8N0ZZ	Division of Right Lower Leg Tendon, Open Approach
0L8N3ZZ	Division of Right Lower Leg Tendon, Percutaneous Approach
0L8N4ZZ	Division of Right Lower Leg Tendon, Percutaneous Endoscopic Approach
0L8P0ZZ	Division of Left Lower Leg Tendon, Open Approach
0L8P3ZZ	Division of Left Lower Leg Tendon, Percutaneous Approach
0L8P4ZZ	Division of Left Lower Leg Tendon, Percutaneous Endoscopic Approach
0L8Q0ZZ	Division of Right Knee Tendon, Open Approach
0L8Q3ZZ	Division of Right Knee Tendon, Percutaneous Approach
0L8Q4ZZ	Division of Right Knee Tendon, Percutaneous Endoscopic Approach
0L8R0ZZ	Division of Left Knee Tendon, Open Approach
0L8R3ZZ	Division of Left Knee Tendon, Percutaneous Approach
0L8R4ZZ	Division of Left Knee Tendon, Percutaneous Endoscopic Approach

0L8S0ZZ	Division of Right Ankle Tendon, Open Approach
0L8S3ZZ	Division of Right Ankle Tendon, Percutaneous Approach
0L8S4ZZ	Division of Right Ankle Tendon, Percutaneous Endoscopic Approach
0L8T0ZZ	Division of Left Ankle Tendon, Open Approach
0L8T3ZZ	Division of Left Ankle Tendon, Percutaneous Approach
0L8T4ZZ	Division of Left Ankle Tendon, Percutaneous Endoscopic Approach
0L8V0ZZ	Division of Right Foot Tendon, Open Approach
0L8V3ZZ	Division of Right Foot Tendon, Percutaneous Approach
0L8V4ZZ	Division of Right Foot Tendon, Percutaneous Endoscopic Approach
0L8W0ZZ	Division of Left Foot Tendon, Open Approach
0L8W3ZZ	Division of Left Foot Tendon, Percutaneous Approach
0L8W4ZZ	Division of Left Foot Tendon, Percutaneous Endoscopic Approach

0L9 – Tendons, Drainage

Review Coding Guidelines B3.4a and B3.4b

Review Coding Guideline B6.2

0L9000Z	Drainage of Head and Neck Tendon with Drainage Device, Open Approach
0L900ZX	Drainage of Head and Neck Tendon, Open Approach, Diagnostic
0L900ZZ	Drainage of Head and Neck Tendon, Open Approach
0L9030Z	Drainage of Head and Neck Tendon with Drainage Device, Percutaneous Approach
0L903ZX	Drainage of Head and Neck Tendon, Percutaneous Approach, Diagnostic
0L903ZZ	Drainage of Head and Neck Tendon, Percutaneous Approach
0L9040Z	Drainage of Head and Neck Tendon with Drainage Device, Percutaneous Endoscopic Approach
0L904ZX	Drainage of Head and Neck Tendon, Percutaneous Endoscopic Approach, Diagnostic
0L904ZZ	Drainage of Head and Neck Tendon, Percutaneous Endoscopic Approach
0L9100Z	Drainage of Right Shoulder Tendon with Drainage Device, Open Approach
0L910ZX	Drainage of Right Shoulder Tendon, Open Approach, Diagnostic
0L910ZZ	Drainage of Right Shoulder Tendon, Open Approach
0L9130Z	Drainage of Right Shoulder Tendon with Drainage Device, Percutaneous Approach
0L913ZX	Drainage of Right Shoulder Tendon, Percutaneous Approach, Diagnostic
0L913ZZ	Drainage of Right Shoulder Tendon, Percutaneous Approach
0L9140Z	Drainage of Right Shoulder Tendon with Drainage Device, Percutaneous Endoscopic Approach
0L914ZX	Drainage of Right Shoulder Tendon, Percutaneous Endoscopic Approach, Diagnostic
0L914ZZ	Drainage of Right Shoulder Tendon, Percutaneous Endoscopic Approach
0L9200Z	Drainage of Left Shoulder Tendon with Drainage Device, Open Approach

0L920ZX	Drainage of Left Shoulder Tendon, Open Approach, Diagnostic
0L920ZZ	Drainage of Left Shoulder Tendon, Open Approach
0L9230Z	Drainage of Left Shoulder Tendon with Drainage Device, Percutaneous Approach
0L923ZX	Drainage of Left Shoulder Tendon, Percutaneous Approach, Diagnostic
0L923ZZ	Drainage of Left Shoulder Tendon, Percutaneous Approach
0L9240Z	Drainage of Left Shoulder Tendon with Drainage Device, Percutaneous Endoscopic Approach
0L924ZX	Drainage of Left Shoulder Tendon, Percutaneous Endoscopic Approach, Diagnostic
0L924ZZ	Drainage of Left Shoulder Tendon, Percutaneous Endoscopic Approach
0L9300Z	Drainage of Right Upper Arm Tendon with Drainage Device, Open Approach
0L930ZX	Drainage of Right Upper Arm Tendon, Open Approach, Diagnostic
0L930ZZ	Drainage of Right Upper Arm Tendon, Open Approach
0L9330Z	Drainage of Right Upper Arm Tendon with Drainage Device, Percutaneous Approach
0L933ZX	Drainage of Right Upper Arm Tendon, Percutaneous Approach, Diagnostic
0L933ZZ	Drainage of Right Upper Arm Tendon, Percutaneous Approach
0L9340Z	Drainage of Right Upper Arm Tendon with Drainage Device, Percutaneous Endoscopic Approach
0L934ZX	Drainage of Right Upper Arm Tendon, Percutaneous Endoscopic Approach, Diagnostic
0L934ZZ	Drainage of Right Upper Arm Tendon, Percutaneous Endoscopic Approach
0L9400Z	Drainage of Left Upper Arm Tendon with Drainage Device, Open Approach

0L940ZX	Drainage of Left Upper Arm Tendon, Open Approach, Diagnostic
0L940ZZ	Drainage of Left Upper Arm Tendon, Open Approach
0L9430Z	Drainage of Left Upper Arm Tendon with Drainage Device, Percutaneous Approach
0L943ZX	Drainage of Left Upper Arm Tendon, Percutaneous Approach, Diagnostic
0L943ZZ	Drainage of Left Upper Arm Tendon, Percutaneous Approach
0L9440Z	Drainage of Left Upper Arm Tendon with Drainage Device, Percutaneous Endoscopic Approach
0L944ZX	Drainage of Left Upper Arm Tendon, Percutaneous Endoscopic Approach, Diagnostic
0L944ZZ	Drainage of Left Upper Arm Tendon, Percutaneous Endoscopic Approach
0L9500Z	Drainage of Right Lower Arm and Wrist Tendon with Drainage Device, Open Approach
0L950ZX	Drainage of Right Lower Arm and Wrist Tendon, Open Approach, Diagnostic
0L950ZZ	Drainage of Right Lower Arm and Wrist Tendon, Open Approach
0L9530Z	Drainage of Right Lower Arm and Wrist Tendon with Drainage Device, Percutaneous Approach
0L953ZX	Drainage of Right Lower Arm and Wrist Tendon, Percutaneous Approach, Diagnostic
0L953ZZ	Drainage of Right Lower Arm and Wrist Tendon, Percutaneous Approach
0L9540Z	Drainage of Right Lower Arm and Wrist Tendon with Drainage Device, Percutaneous Endoscopic Approach
0L954ZX	Drainage of Right Lower Arm and Wrist Tendon, Percutaneous Endoscopic Approach, Diagnostic
0L954ZZ	Drainage of Right Lower Arm and Wrist Tendon, Percutaneous Endoscopic Approach

♀ Female-only   ♂ Male-only   ▲ Limited Coverage   ● Non-OR   **HAC** HAC-associated procedure   ▲ Non-covered procedures   ✚ Cluster

0L9600Z Drainage of Left Lower Arm and Wrist Tendon with Drainage Device, Open Approach

0L960ZX Drainage of Left Lower Arm and Wrist Tendon, Open Approach, Diagnostic

0L960ZZ Drainage of Left Lower Arm and Wrist Tendon, Open Approach

0L9630Z Drainage of Left Lower Arm and Wrist Tendon with Drainage Device, Percutaneous Approach

0L963ZX Drainage of Left Lower Arm and Wrist Tendon, Percutaneous Approach, Diagnostic

0L963ZZ Drainage of Left Lower Arm and Wrist Tendon, Percutaneous Approach

0L9640Z Drainage of Left Lower Arm and Wrist Tendon with Drainage Device, Percutaneous Endoscopic Approach

0L964ZX Drainage of Left Lower Arm and Wrist Tendon, Percutaneous Endoscopic Approach, Diagnostic

0L964ZZ Drainage of Left Lower Arm and Wrist Tendon, Percutaneous Endoscopic Approach

0L9700Z Drainage of Right Hand Tendon with Drainage Device, Open Approach

0L970ZX Drainage of Right Hand Tendon, Open Approach, Diagnostic

0L970ZZ Drainage of Right Hand Tendon, Open Approach

0L9730Z Drainage of Right Hand Tendon with Drainage Device, Percutaneous Approach

0L973ZX Drainage of Right Hand Tendon, Percutaneous Approach, Diagnostic

0L973ZZ Drainage of Right Hand Tendon, Percutaneous Approach

0L9740Z Drainage of Right Hand Tendon with Drainage Device, Percutaneous Endoscopic Approach

0L974ZX Drainage of Right Hand Tendon, Percutaneous Endoscopic Approach, Diagnostic

0L974ZZ Drainage of Right Hand Tendon, Percutaneous Endoscopic Approach

0L9800Z Drainage of Left Hand Tendon with Drainage Device, Open Approach

0L980ZX Drainage of Left Hand Tendon, Open Approach, Diagnostic

0L980ZZ Drainage of Left Hand Tendon, Open Approach

0L9830Z Drainage of Left Hand Tendon with Drainage Device, Percutaneous Approach

0L983ZX Drainage of Left Hand Tendon, Percutaneous Approach, Diagnostic

0L983ZZ Drainage of Left Hand Tendon, Percutaneous Approach

0L9840Z Drainage of Left Hand Tendon with Drainage Device, Percutaneous Endoscopic Approach

0L984ZX Drainage of Left Hand Tendon, Percutaneous Endoscopic Approach, Diagnostic

0L984ZZ Drainage of Left Hand Tendon, Percutaneous Endoscopic Approach

0L9900Z Drainage of Right Trunk Tendon with Drainage Device, Open Approach

0L990ZX Drainage of Right Trunk Tendon, Open Approach, Diagnostic

0L990ZZ Drainage of Right Trunk Tendon, Open Approach

0L9930Z Drainage of Right Trunk Tendon with Drainage Device, Percutaneous Approach

0L993ZX Drainage of Right Trunk Tendon, Percutaneous Approach, Diagnostic

0L993ZZ Drainage of Right Trunk Tendon, Percutaneous Approach

0L9940Z Drainage of Right Trunk Tendon with Drainage Device, Percutaneous Endoscopic Approach

0L994ZX Drainage of Right Trunk Tendon, Percutaneous Endoscopic Approach, Diagnostic

0L994ZZ Drainage of Right Trunk Tendon, Percutaneous Endoscopic Approach

0L9B00Z Drainage of Left Trunk Tendon with Drainage Device, Open Approach

0L9B0ZX Drainage of Left Trunk Tendon, Open Approach, Diagnostic

0L9B0ZZ Drainage of Left Trunk Tendon, Open Approach

0L9B30Z Drainage of Left Trunk Tendon with Drainage Device, Percutaneous Approach

0L9B3ZX Drainage of Left Trunk Tendon, Percutaneous Approach, Diagnostic

0L9B3ZZ Drainage of Left Trunk Tendon, Percutaneous Approach

0L9B40Z Drainage of Left Trunk Tendon with Drainage Device, Percutaneous Endoscopic Approach

0L9B4ZX Drainage of Left Trunk Tendon, Percutaneous Endoscopic Approach, Diagnostic

0L9B4ZZ Drainage of Left Trunk Tendon, Percutaneous Endoscopic Approach

0L9C00Z Drainage of Right Thorax Tendon with Drainage Device, Open Approach

0L9C0ZX Drainage of Right Thorax Tendon, Open Approach, Diagnostic

0L9C0ZZ Drainage of Right Thorax Tendon, Open Approach

0L9C30Z Drainage of Right Thorax Tendon with Drainage Device, Percutaneous Approach

0L9C3ZX Drainage of Right Thorax Tendon, Percutaneous Approach, Diagnostic

0L9C3ZZ Drainage of Right Thorax Tendon, Percutaneous Approach

0L9C40Z Drainage of Right Thorax Tendon with Drainage Device, Percutaneous Endoscopic Approach

0L9C4ZX Drainage of Right Thorax Tendon, Percutaneous Endoscopic Approach, Diagnostic

0L9C4ZZ Drainage of Right Thorax Tendon, Percutaneous Endoscopic Approach

0L9D00Z Drainage of Left Thorax Tendon with Drainage Device, Open Approach

0L9D0ZX Drainage of Left Thorax Tendon, Open Approach, Diagnostic

0L9D0ZZ Drainage of Left Thorax Tendon, Open Approach

0L9D30Z Drainage of Left Thorax Tendon with Drainage Device, Percutaneous Approach

0L9D3ZX Drainage of Left Thorax Tendon, Percutaneous Approach, Diagnostic

0L9D3ZZ Drainage of Left Thorax Tendon, Percutaneous Approach

0L9D40Z Drainage of Left Thorax Tendon with Drainage Device, Percutaneous Endoscopic Approach

0L9D4ZX Drainage of Left Thorax Tendon, Percutaneous Endoscopic Approach, Diagnostic

0L9D4ZZ Drainage of Left Thorax Tendon, Percutaneous Endoscopic Approach

0L9F00Z Drainage of Right Abdomen Tendon with Drainage Device, Open Approach

0L9F0ZX Drainage of Right Abdomen Tendon, Open Approach, Diagnostic

0L9F0ZZ Drainage of Right Abdomen Tendon, Open Approach

0L9F30Z Drainage of Right Abdomen Tendon with Drainage Device, Percutaneous Approach

0L9F3ZX Drainage of Right Abdomen Tendon, Percutaneous Approach, Diagnostic

0L9F3ZZ Drainage of Right Abdomen Tendon, Percutaneous Approach

0L9F40Z Drainage of Right Abdomen Tendon with Drainage Device, Percutaneous Endoscopic Approach

0L9F4ZX Drainage of Right Abdomen Tendon, Percutaneous Endoscopic Approach, Diagnostic

0L9F4ZZ Drainage of Right Abdomen Tendon, Percutaneous Endoscopic Approach

0L9G00Z Drainage of Left Abdomen Tendon with Drainage Device, Open Approach

0L9G0ZX Drainage of Left Abdomen Tendon, Open Approach, Diagnostic

0L9G0ZZ Drainage of Left Abdomen Tendon, Open Approach

0L9G30Z Drainage of Left Abdomen Tendon with Drainage Device, Percutaneous Approach

0L9G3ZX Drainage of Left Abdomen Tendon, Percutaneous Approach, Diagnostic

0L9G3ZZ Drainage of Left Abdomen Tendon, Percutaneous Approach

0L9G40Z Drainage of Left Abdomen Tendon with Drainage Device, Percutaneous Endoscopic Approach

0L9G4ZX Drainage of Left Abdomen Tendon, Percutaneous Endoscopic Approach, Diagnostic

0L9G4ZZ Drainage of Left Abdomen Tendon, Percutaneous Endoscopic Approach

0L9H00Z Drainage of Perineum Tendon with Drainage Device, Open Approach

0L9H0ZX Drainage of Perineum Tendon, Open Approach, Diagnostic

0L9H0ZZ Drainage of Perineum Tendon, Open Approach

0L9H30Z Drainage of Perineum Tendon with Drainage Device, Percutaneous Approach

0L9H3ZX Drainage of Perineum Tendon, Percutaneous Approach, Diagnostic

0L9H3ZZ Drainage of Perineum Tendon, Percutaneous Approach

0L9H40Z Drainage of Perineum Tendon with Drainage Device, Percutaneous Endoscopic Approach

0L9H4ZX Drainage of Perineum Tendon, Percutaneous Endoscopic Approach, Diagnostic

0L9H4ZZ Drainage of Perineum Tendon, Percutaneous Endoscopic Approach

0L9J00Z Drainage of Right Hip Tendon with Drainage Device, Open Approach

0L9J0ZX Drainage of Right Hip Tendon, Open Approach, Diagnostic

0L9J0ZZ Drainage of Right Hip Tendon, Open Approach

0L9J30Z Drainage of Right Hip Tendon with Drainage Device, Percutaneous Approach

0L9J3ZX Drainage of Right Hip Tendon, Percutaneous Approach, Diagnostic

0L9J3ZZ Drainage of Right Hip Tendon, Percutaneous Approach

0L9J40Z Drainage of Right Hip Tendon with Drainage Device, Percutaneous Endoscopic Approach

0L9J4ZX Drainage of Right Hip Tendon, Percutaneous Endoscopic Approach, Diagnostic

0L9J4ZZ Drainage of Right Hip Tendon, Percutaneous Endoscopic Approach

0L9K00Z Drainage of Left Hip Tendon with Drainage Device, Open Approach

0L9K0ZX Drainage of Left Hip Tendon, Open Approach, Diagnostic

0L9K0ZZ Drainage of Left Hip Tendon, Open Approach

0L9K30Z Drainage of Left Hip Tendon with Drainage Device, Percutaneous Approach

0L9K3ZX Drainage of Left Hip Tendon, Percutaneous Approach, Diagnostic

0L9K3ZZ Drainage of Left Hip Tendon, Percutaneous Approach

0L9K40Z Drainage of Left Hip Tendon with Drainage Device, Percutaneous Endoscopic Approach

0L9K4ZX Drainage of Left Hip Tendon, Percutaneous Endoscopic Approach, Diagnostic

0L9K4ZZ Drainage of Left Hip Tendon, Percutaneous Endoscopic Approach

0L9L00Z Drainage of Right Upper Leg Tendon with Drainage Device, Open Approach

0L9L0ZX Drainage of Right Upper Leg Tendon, Open Approach, Diagnostic

0L9L0ZZ Drainage of Right Upper Leg Tendon, Open Approach

0L9L30Z Drainage of Right Upper Leg Tendon with Drainage Device, Percutaneous Approach

0L9L3ZX Drainage of Right Upper Leg Tendon, Percutaneous Approach, Diagnostic

0L9L3ZZ Drainage of Right Upper Leg Tendon, Percutaneous Approach

0L9L40Z Drainage of Right Upper Leg Tendon with Drainage Device, Percutaneous Endoscopic Approach

0L9L4ZX Drainage of Right Upper Leg Tendon, Percutaneous Endoscopic Approach, Diagnostic

0L9L4ZZ Drainage of Right Upper Leg Tendon, Percutaneous Endoscopic Approach

0L9M00Z Drainage of Left Upper Leg Tendon with Drainage Device, Open Approach

0L9M0ZX Drainage of Left Upper Leg Tendon, Open Approach, Diagnostic

0L9M0ZZ Drainage of Left Upper Leg Tendon, Open Approach

0L9M30Z Drainage of Left Upper Leg Tendon with Drainage Device, Percutaneous Approach

0L9M3ZX Drainage of Left Upper Leg Tendon, Percutaneous Approach, Diagnostic

0L9M3ZZ Drainage of Left Upper Leg Tendon, Percutaneous Approach

0L9M40Z Drainage of Left Upper Leg Tendon with Drainage Device, Percutaneous Endoscopic Approach

0L9M4ZX Drainage of Left Upper Leg Tendon, Percutaneous Endoscopic Approach, Diagnostic

0L9M4ZZ Drainage of Left Upper Leg Tendon, Percutaneous Endoscopic Approach

0L9N00Z Drainage of Right Lower Leg Tendon with Drainage Device, Open Approach

0L9N0ZX Drainage of Right Lower Leg Tendon, Open Approach, Diagnostic

0L9N0ZZ Drainage of Right Lower Leg Tendon, Open Approach

0L9N30Z Drainage of Right Lower Leg Tendon with Drainage Device, Percutaneous Approach

0L9N3ZX Drainage of Right Lower Leg Tendon, Percutaneous Approach, Diagnostic

0L9N3ZZ Drainage of Right Lower Leg Tendon, Percutaneous Approach

0L9N40Z Drainage of Right Lower Leg Tendon with Drainage Device, Percutaneous Endoscopic Approach

0L9N4ZX Drainage of Right Lower Leg Tendon, Percutaneous Endoscopic Approach, Diagnostic

0L9N4ZZ Drainage of Right Lower Leg Tendon, Percutaneous Endoscopic Approach

0L9P00Z Drainage of Left Lower Leg Tendon with Drainage Device, Open Approach

0L9P0ZX Drainage of Left Lower Leg Tendon, Open Approach, Diagnostic

0L9P0ZZ Drainage of Left Lower Leg Tendon, Open Approach

0L9P30Z Drainage of Left Lower Leg Tendon with Drainage Device, Percutaneous Approach

0L9P3ZX Drainage of Left Lower Leg Tendon, Percutaneous Approach, Diagnostic

0L9P3ZZ Drainage of Left Lower Leg Tendon, Percutaneous Approach

0L9P40Z Drainage of Left Lower Leg Tendon with Drainage Device, Percutaneous Endoscopic Approach

0L9P4ZX Drainage of Left Lower Leg Tendon, Percutaneous Endoscopic Approach, Diagnostic

0L9P4ZZ Drainage of Left Lower Leg Tendon, Percutaneous Endoscopic Approach

0L9Q00Z Drainage of Right Knee Tendon with Drainage Device, Open Approach

0L9Q0ZX Drainage of Right Knee Tendon, Open Approach, Diagnostic

0L9Q0ZZ Drainage of Right Knee Tendon, Open Approach

0L9Q30Z Drainage of Right Knee Tendon with Drainage Device, Percutaneous Approach

0L9Q3ZX Drainage of Right Knee Tendon, Percutaneous Approach, Diagnostic

0L9Q3ZZ Drainage of Right Knee Tendon, Percutaneous Approach

0L9Q40Z Drainage of Right Knee Tendon with Drainage Device, Percutaneous Endoscopic Approach

0L9Q4ZX Drainage of Right Knee Tendon, Percutaneous Endoscopic Approach, Diagnostic

0L9Q4ZZ Drainage of Right Knee Tendon, Percutaneous Endoscopic Approach

0L9R00Z Drainage of Left Knee Tendon with Drainage Device, Open Approach

0L9R0ZX Drainage of Left Knee Tendon, Open Approach, Diagnostic

0L9R0ZZ Drainage of Left Knee Tendon, Open Approach

0L9R30Z Drainage of Left Knee Tendon with Drainage Device, Percutaneous Approach

0L9R3ZX Drainage of Left Knee Tendon, Percutaneous Approach, Diagnostic

0L9R3ZZ Drainage of Left Knee Tendon, Percutaneous Approach

0L9R40Z Drainage of Left Knee Tendon with Drainage Device, Percutaneous Endoscopic Approach

0L9R4ZX Drainage of Left Knee Tendon, Percutaneous Endoscopic Approach, Diagnostic

0L9R4ZZ Drainage of Left Knee Tendon, Percutaneous Endoscopic Approach

0L9S00Z Drainage of Right Ankle Tendon with Drainage Device, Open Approach

0L9S0ZX Drainage of Right Ankle Tendon, Open Approach, Diagnostic

0L9S0ZZ Drainage of Right Ankle Tendon, Open Approach

0L9S30Z Drainage of Right Ankle Tendon with Drainage Device, Percutaneous Approach

0L9S3ZX Drainage of Right Ankle Tendon, Percutaneous Approach, Diagnostic

0L9S3ZZ Drainage of Right Ankle Tendon, Percutaneous Approach

0L9S40Z Drainage of Right Ankle Tendon with Drainage Device, Percutaneous Endoscopic Approach

0L9S4ZX Drainage of Right Ankle Tendon, Percutaneous Endoscopic Approach, Diagnostic

0L9S4ZZ Drainage of Right Ankle Tendon, Percutaneous Endoscopic Approach

0L9T00Z Drainage of Left Ankle Tendon with Drainage Device, Open Approach

0L9T0ZX Drainage of Left Ankle Tendon, Open Approach, Diagnostic

0L9T0ZZ Drainage of Left Ankle Tendon, Open Approach

0L9T30Z Drainage of Left Ankle Tendon with Drainage Device, Percutaneous Approach

0L9T3ZX Drainage of Left Ankle Tendon, Percutaneous Approach, Diagnostic

0L9T3ZZ Drainage of Left Ankle Tendon, Percutaneous Approach

0L9T40Z Drainage of Left Ankle Tendon with Drainage Device, Percutaneous Endoscopic Approach

0L9T4ZX Drainage of Left Ankle Tendon, Percutaneous Endoscopic Approach, Diagnostic

0L9T4ZZ Drainage of Left Ankle Tendon, Percutaneous Endoscopic Approach

0L9V00Z Drainage of Right Foot Tendon with Drainage Device, Open Approach

0L9V0ZX Drainage of Right Foot Tendon, Open Approach, Diagnostic

0L9V0ZZ Drainage of Right Foot Tendon, Open Approach

0L9V30Z Drainage of Right Foot Tendon with Drainage Device, Percutaneous Approach

0L9V3ZX Drainage of Right Foot Tendon, Percutaneous Approach, Diagnostic

0L9V3ZZ Drainage of Right Foot Tendon, Percutaneous Approach

0L9V40Z Drainage of Right Foot Tendon with Drainage Device, Percutaneous Endoscopic Approach

0L9V4ZX Drainage of Right Foot Tendon, Percutaneous Endoscopic Approach, Diagnostic

0L9V4ZZ Drainage of Right Foot Tendon, Percutaneous Endoscopic Approach

0L9W00Z Drainage of Left Foot Tendon with Drainage Device, Open Approach

0L9W0ZX Drainage of Left Foot Tendon, Open Approach, Diagnostic

0L9W0ZZ Drainage of Left Foot Tendon, Open Approach

♀ Female-only   ♂ Male-only   ▲ Limited Coverage   ● Non-OR   🅗🅐🅒 HAC-associated procedure   ▲ Non-covered procedures   ➕ Cluster

0L9W30Z Drainage of Left Foot Tendon with Drainage Device, Percutaneous Approach
0L9W3ZX Drainage of Left Foot Tendon, Percutaneous Approach, Diagnostic

0L9W3ZZ Drainage of Left Foot Tendon, Percutaneous Approach
0L9W40Z Drainage of Left Foot Tendon with Drainage Device, Percutaneous Endoscopic Approach

0L9W4ZX Drainage of Left Foot Tendon, Percutaneous Endoscopic Approach, Diagnostic
0L9W4ZZ Drainage of Left Foot Tendon, Percutaneous Endoscopic Approach

0LB – Tendons, Excision

Review Coding Guidelines B3.4a and B3.4b

Review Coding Guideline B3.5

Review Coding Guideline B3.8

Review Coding Guideline B3.18

0LB00ZX Excision of Head and Neck Tendon, Open Approach, Diagnostic
0LB00ZZ Excision of Head and Neck Tendon, Open Approach
0LB03ZX Excision of Head and Neck Tendon, Percutaneous Approach, Diagnostic
0LB03ZZ Excision of Head and Neck Tendon, Percutaneous Approach
0LB04ZX Excision of Head and Neck Tendon, Percutaneous Endoscopic Approach, Diagnostic
0LB04ZZ Excision of Head and Neck Tendon, Percutaneous Endoscopic Approach
0LB10ZX Excision of Right Shoulder Tendon, Open Approach, Diagnostic
0LB10ZZ Excision of Right Shoulder Tendon, Open Approach
0LB13ZX Excision of Right Shoulder Tendon, Percutaneous Approach, Diagnostic
0LB13ZZ Excision of Right Shoulder Tendon, Percutaneous Approach
0LB14ZX Excision of Right Shoulder Tendon, Percutaneous Endoscopic Approach, Diagnostic
0LB14ZZ Excision of Right Shoulder Tendon, Percutaneous Endoscopic Approach
0LB20ZX Excision of Left Shoulder Tendon, Open Approach, Diagnostic
0LB20ZZ Excision of Left Shoulder Tendon, Open Approach
0LB23ZX Excision of Left Shoulder Tendon, Percutaneous Approach, Diagnostic
0LB23ZZ Excision of Left Shoulder Tendon, Percutaneous Approach
0LB24ZX Excision of Left Shoulder Tendon, Percutaneous Endoscopic Approach, Diagnostic
0LB24ZZ Excision of Left Shoulder Tendon, Percutaneous Endoscopic Approach
0LB30ZX Excision of Right Upper Arm Tendon, Open Approach, Diagnostic
0LB30ZZ Excision of Right Upper Arm Tendon, Open Approach
0LB33ZX Excision of Right Upper Arm Tendon, Percutaneous Approach, Diagnostic
0LB33ZZ Excision of Right Upper Arm Tendon, Percutaneous Approach
0LB34ZX Excision of Right Upper Arm Tendon, Percutaneous Endoscopic Approach, Diagnostic
0LB34ZZ Excision of Right Upper Arm Tendon, Percutaneous Endoscopic Approach
0LB40ZX Excision of Left Upper Arm Tendon, Open Approach, Diagnostic
0LB40ZZ Excision of Left Upper Arm Tendon, Open Approach
0LB43ZX Excision of Left Upper Arm Tendon, Percutaneous Approach, Diagnostic
0LB43ZZ Excision of Left Upper Arm Tendon, Percutaneous Approach

0LB44ZX Excision of Left Upper Arm Tendon, Percutaneous Endoscopic Approach, Diagnostic
0LB44ZZ Excision of Left Upper Arm Tendon, Percutaneous Endoscopic Approach
0LB50ZX Excision of Right Lower Arm and Wrist Tendon, Open Approach, Diagnostic
0LB50ZZ Excision of Right Lower Arm and Wrist Tendon, Open Approach
0LB53ZX Excision of Right Lower Arm and Wrist Tendon, Percutaneous Approach, Diagnostic
0LB53ZZ Excision of Right Lower Arm and Wrist Tendon, Percutaneous Approach
0LB54ZX Excision of Right Lower Arm and Wrist Tendon, Percutaneous Endoscopic Approach, Diagnostic
0LB54ZZ Excision of Right Lower Arm and Wrist Tendon, Percutaneous Endoscopic Approach
0LB60ZX Excision of Left Lower Arm and Wrist Tendon, Open Approach, Diagnostic
0LB60ZZ Excision of Left Lower Arm and Wrist Tendon, Open Approach
AHA CC: 3Q, 2015, 26-27
0LB63ZX Excision of Left Lower Arm and Wrist Tendon, Percutaneous Approach, Diagnostic
0LB63ZZ Excision of Left Lower Arm and Wrist Tendon, Percutaneous Approach
0LB64ZX Excision of Left Lower Arm and Wrist Tendon, Percutaneous Endoscopic Approach, Diagnostic
0LB64ZZ Excision of Left Lower Arm and Wrist Tendon, Percutaneous Endoscopic Approach
0LB70ZX Excision of Right Hand Tendon, Open Approach, Diagnostic
0LB70ZZ Excision of Right Hand Tendon, Open Approach
0LB73ZX Excision of Right Hand Tendon, Percutaneous Approach, Diagnostic
0LB73ZZ Excision of Right Hand Tendon, Percutaneous Approach
0LB74ZX Excision of Right Hand Tendon, Percutaneous Endoscopic Approach, Diagnostic
0LB74ZZ Excision of Right Hand Tendon, Percutaneous Endoscopic Approach
0LB80ZX Excision of Left Hand Tendon, Open Approach, Diagnostic
0LB80ZZ Excision of Left Hand Tendon, Open Approach
0LB83ZX Excision of Left Hand Tendon, Percutaneous Approach, Diagnostic
0LB83ZZ Excision of Left Hand Tendon, Percutaneous Approach
0LB84ZX Excision of Left Hand Tendon, Percutaneous Endoscopic Approach, Diagnostic

0LB84ZZ Excision of Left Hand Tendon, Percutaneous Endoscopic Approach
0LB90ZX Excision of Right Trunk Tendon, Open Approach, Diagnostic
0LB90ZZ Excision of Right Trunk Tendon, Open Approach
0LB93ZX Excision of Right Trunk Tendon, Percutaneous Approach, Diagnostic
0LB93ZZ Excision of Right Trunk Tendon, Percutaneous Approach
0LB94ZX Excision of Right Trunk Tendon, Percutaneous Endoscopic Approach, Diagnostic
0LB94ZZ Excision of Right Trunk Tendon, Percutaneous Endoscopic Approach
0LBB0ZX Excision of Left Trunk Tendon, Open Approach, Diagnostic
0LBB0ZZ Excision of Left Trunk Tendon, Open Approach
0LBB3ZX Excision of Left Trunk Tendon, Percutaneous Approach, Diagnostic
0LBB3ZZ Excision of Left Trunk Tendon, Percutaneous Approach
0LBB4ZX Excision of Left Trunk Tendon, Percutaneous Endoscopic Approach, Diagnostic
0LBB4ZZ Excision of Left Trunk Tendon, Percutaneous Endoscopic Approach
0LBC0ZX Excision of Right Thorax Tendon, Open Approach, Diagnostic
0LBC0ZZ Excision of Right Thorax Tendon, Open Approach
0LBC3ZX Excision of Right Thorax Tendon, Percutaneous Approach, Diagnostic
0LBC3ZZ Excision of Right Thorax Tendon, Percutaneous Approach
0LBC4ZX Excision of Right Thorax Tendon, Percutaneous Endoscopic Approach, Diagnostic
0LBC4ZZ Excision of Right Thorax Tendon, Percutaneous Endoscopic Approach
0LBD0ZX Excision of Left Thorax Tendon, Open Approach, Diagnostic
0LBD0ZZ Excision of Left Thorax Tendon, Open Approach
0LBD3ZX Excision of Left Thorax Tendon, Percutaneous Approach, Diagnostic
0LBD3ZZ Excision of Left Thorax Tendon, Percutaneous Approach
0LBD4ZX Excision of Left Thorax Tendon, Percutaneous Endoscopic Approach, Diagnostic
0LBD4ZZ Excision of Left Thorax Tendon, Percutaneous Endoscopic Approach
0LBF0ZX Excision of Right Abdomen Tendon, Open Approach, Diagnostic
0LBF0ZZ Excision of Right Abdomen Tendon, Open Approach
0LBF3ZX Excision of Right Abdomen Tendon, Percutaneous Approach, Diagnostic

♀ Female-only   ♂ Male-only   ▲ Limited Coverage   ● Non-OR   [HAC] HAC-associated procedure   ▲ Non-covered procedures   ✚ Cluster

0LBF3ZZ Excision of Right Abdomen Tendon, Percutaneous Approach
0LBF4ZX Excision of Right Abdomen Tendon, Percutaneous Endoscopic Approach, Diagnostic
0LBF4ZZ Excision of Right Abdomen Tendon, Percutaneous Endoscopic Approach
0LBG0ZX Excision of Left Abdomen Tendon, Open Approach, Diagnostic
0LBG0ZZ Excision of Left Abdomen Tendon, Open Approach
0LBG3ZX Excision of Left Abdomen Tendon, Percutaneous Approach, Diagnostic
0LBG3ZZ Excision of Left Abdomen Tendon, Percutaneous Approach
0LBG4ZX Excision of Left Abdomen Tendon, Percutaneous Endoscopic Approach, Diagnostic
0LBG4ZZ Excision of Left Abdomen Tendon, Percutaneous Endoscopic Approach
0LBH0ZX Excision of Perineum Tendon, Open Approach, Diagnostic
0LBH0ZZ Excision of Perineum Tendon, Open Approach
0LBH3ZX Excision of Perineum Tendon, Percutaneous Approach, Diagnostic
0LBH3ZZ Excision of Perineum Tendon, Percutaneous Approach
0LBH4ZX Excision of Perineum Tendon, Percutaneous Endoscopic Approach, Diagnostic
0LBH4ZZ Excision of Perineum Tendon, Percutaneous Endoscopic Approach
0LBJ0ZX Excision of Right Hip Tendon, Open Approach, Diagnostic
0LBJ0ZZ Excision of Right Hip Tendon, Open Approach
0LBJ3ZX Excision of Right Hip Tendon, Percutaneous Approach, Diagnostic
0LBJ3ZZ Excision of Right Hip Tendon, Percutaneous Approach
0LBJ4ZX Excision of Right Hip Tendon, Percutaneous Endoscopic Approach, Diagnostic
0LBJ4ZZ Excision of Right Hip Tendon, Percutaneous Endoscopic Approach
0LBK0ZX Excision of Left Hip Tendon, Open Approach, Diagnostic
0LBK0ZZ Excision of Left Hip Tendon, Open Approach
0LBK3ZX Excision of Left Hip Tendon, Percutaneous Approach, Diagnostic
0LBK3ZZ Excision of Left Hip Tendon, Percutaneous Approach
0LBK4ZX Excision of Left Hip Tendon, Percutaneous Endoscopic Approach, Diagnostic
0LBK4ZZ Excision of Left Hip Tendon, Percutaneous Endoscopic Approach
0LBL0ZX Excision of Right Upper Leg Tendon, Open Approach, Diagnostic
0LBL0ZZ Excision of Right Upper Leg Tendon, Open Approach
AHA CC: 2Q, 2017, 21-22

0LBL3ZX Excision of Right Upper Leg Tendon, Percutaneous Approach, Diagnostic
0LBL3ZZ Excision of Right Upper Leg Tendon, Percutaneous Approach
0LBL4ZX Excision of Right Upper Leg Tendon, Percutaneous Endoscopic Approach, Diagnostic
0LBL4ZZ Excision of Right Upper Leg Tendon, Percutaneous Endoscopic Approach
0LBM0ZX Excision of Left Upper Leg Tendon, Open Approach, Diagnostic
0LBM0ZZ Excision of Left Upper Leg Tendon, Open Approach
0LBM3ZX Excision of Left Upper Leg Tendon, Percutaneous Approach, Diagnostic
0LBM3ZZ Excision of Left Upper Leg Tendon, Percutaneous Approach
0LBM4ZX Excision of Left Upper Leg Tendon, Percutaneous Endoscopic Approach, Diagnostic
0LBM4ZZ Excision of Left Upper Leg Tendon, Percutaneous Endoscopic Approach
0LBN0ZX Excision of Right Lower Leg Tendon, Open Approach, Diagnostic
0LBN0ZZ Excision of Right Lower Leg Tendon, Open Approach
0LBN3ZX Excision of Right Lower Leg Tendon, Percutaneous Approach, Diagnostic
0LBN3ZZ Excision of Right Lower Leg Tendon, Percutaneous Approach
0LBN4ZX Excision of Right Lower Leg Tendon, Percutaneous Endoscopic Approach, Diagnostic
0LBN4ZZ Excision of Right Lower Leg Tendon, Percutaneous Endoscopic Approach
0LBP0ZX Excision of Left Lower Leg Tendon, Open Approach, Diagnostic
0LBP0ZZ Excision of Left Lower Leg Tendon, Open Approach
AHA CC: 3Q, 2014, 18-19

0LBP3ZX Excision of Left Lower Leg Tendon, Percutaneous Approach, Diagnostic
0LBP3ZZ Excision of Left Lower Leg Tendon, Percutaneous Approach
0LBP4ZX Excision of Left Lower Leg Tendon, Percutaneous Endoscopic Approach, Diagnostic
0LBP4ZZ Excision of Left Lower Leg Tendon, Percutaneous Endoscopic Approach
0LBQ0ZX Excision of Right Knee Tendon, Open Approach, Diagnostic
0LBQ0ZZ Excision of Right Knee Tendon, Open Approach
0LBQ3ZX Excision of Right Knee Tendon, Percutaneous Approach, Diagnostic
0LBQ3ZZ Excision of Right Knee Tendon, Percutaneous Approach
0LBQ4ZX Excision of Right Knee Tendon, Percutaneous Endoscopic Approach, Diagnostic
0LBQ4ZZ Excision of Right Knee Tendon, Percutaneous Endoscopic Approach
0LBR0ZX Excision of Left Knee Tendon, Open Approach, Diagnostic

0LBR0ZZ Excision of Left Knee Tendon, Open Approach
0LBR3ZX Excision of Left Knee Tendon, Percutaneous Approach, Diagnostic
0LBR3ZZ Excision of Left Knee Tendon, Percutaneous Approach
0LBR4ZX Excision of Left Knee Tendon, Percutaneous Endoscopic Approach, Diagnostic
0LBR4ZZ Excision of Left Knee Tendon, Percutaneous Endoscopic Approach
0LBS0ZX Excision of Right Ankle Tendon, Open Approach, Diagnostic
0LBS0ZZ Excision of Right Ankle Tendon, Open Approach
0LBS3ZX Excision of Right Ankle Tendon, Percutaneous Approach, Diagnostic
0LBS3ZZ Excision of Right Ankle Tendon, Percutaneous Approach
0LBS4ZX Excision of Right Ankle Tendon, Percutaneous Endoscopic Approach, Diagnostic
0LBS4ZZ Excision of Right Ankle Tendon, Percutaneous Endoscopic Approach
0LBT0ZX Excision of Left Ankle Tendon, Open Approach, Diagnostic
0LBT0ZZ Excision of Left Ankle Tendon, Open Approach
AHA CC: 3Q, 2014, 14-15

0LBT3ZX Excision of Left Ankle Tendon, Percutaneous Approach, Diagnostic
0LBT3ZZ Excision of Left Ankle Tendon, Percutaneous Approach
0LBT4ZX Excision of Left Ankle Tendon, Percutaneous Endoscopic Approach, Diagnostic
0LBT4ZZ Excision of Left Ankle Tendon, Percutaneous Endoscopic Approach
0LBV0ZX Excision of Right Foot Tendon, Open Approach, Diagnostic
0LBV0ZZ Excision of Right Foot Tendon, Open Approach
0LBV3ZX Excision of Right Foot Tendon, Percutaneous Approach, Diagnostic
0LBV3ZZ Excision of Right Foot Tendon, Percutaneous Approach
0LBV4ZX Excision of Right Foot Tendon, Percutaneous Endoscopic Approach, Diagnostic
0LBV4ZZ Excision of Right Foot Tendon, Percutaneous Endoscopic Approach
0LBW0ZX Excision of Left Foot Tendon, Open Approach, Diagnostic
0LBW0ZZ Excision of Left Foot Tendon, Open Approach
0LBW3ZX Excision of Left Foot Tendon, Percutaneous Approach, Diagnostic
0LBW3ZZ Excision of Left Foot Tendon, Percutaneous Approach
0LBW4ZX Excision of Left Foot Tendon, Percutaneous Endoscopic Approach, Diagnostic
0LBW4ZZ Excision of Left Foot Tendon, Percutaneous Endoscopic Approach

0LC – Tendons, Extirpation

0LC00ZZ Extirpation of Matter from Head and Neck Tendon, Open Approach
0LC03ZZ Extirpation of Matter from Head and Neck Tendon, Percutaneous Approach
0LC04ZZ Extirpation of Matter from Head and Neck Tendon, Percutaneous Endoscopic Approach
0LC10ZZ Extirpation of Matter from Right Shoulder Tendon, Open Approach

0LC13ZZ Extirpation of Matter from Right Shoulder Tendon, Percutaneous Approach
0LC14ZZ Extirpation of Matter from Right Shoulder Tendon, Percutaneous Endoscopic Approach
0LC20ZZ Extirpation of Matter from Left Shoulder Tendon, Open Approach

0LC23ZZ Extirpation of Matter from Left Shoulder Tendon, Percutaneous Approach
0LC24ZZ Extirpation of Matter from Left Shoulder Tendon, Percutaneous Endoscopic Approach
0LC30ZZ Extirpation of Matter from Right Upper Arm Tendon, Open Approach

♀ Female-only   ♂ Male-only   ▲ Limited Coverage   ● Non-OR   ⬛ HAC-associated procedure   ▲ Non-covered procedures   ✚ Cluster

0LC33ZZ	Extirpation of Matter from Right Upper Arm Tendon, Percutaneous Approach	**0LCC3ZZ**	Extirpation of Matter from Right Thorax Tendon, Percutaneous Approach	**0LCM4ZZ**	Extirpation of Matter from Left Upper Leg Tendon, Percutaneous Endoscopic Approach
0LC34ZZ	Extirpation of Matter from Right Upper Arm Tendon, Percutaneous Endoscopic Approach	**0LCC4ZZ**	Extirpation of Matter from Right Thorax Tendon, Percutaneous Endoscopic Approach	**0LCN0ZZ**	Extirpation of Matter from Right Lower Leg Tendon, Open Approach
0LC40ZZ	Extirpation of Matter from Left Upper Arm Tendon, Open Approach	**0LCD0ZZ**	Extirpation of Matter from Left Thorax Tendon, Open Approach	**0LCN3ZZ**	Extirpation of Matter from Right Lower Leg Tendon, Percutaneous Approach
0LC43ZZ	Extirpation of Matter from Left Upper Arm Tendon, Percutaneous Approach	**0LCD3ZZ**	Extirpation of Matter from Left Thorax Tendon, Percutaneous Approach	**0LCN4ZZ**	Extirpation of Matter from Right Lower Leg Tendon, Percutaneous Endoscopic Approach
0LC44ZZ	Extirpation of Matter from Left Upper Arm Tendon, Percutaneous Endoscopic Approach	**0LCD4ZZ**	Extirpation of Matter from Left Thorax Tendon, Percutaneous Endoscopic Approach	**0LCP0ZZ**	Extirpation of Matter from Left Lower Leg Tendon, Open Approach
0LC50ZZ	Extirpation of Matter from Right Lower Arm and Wrist Tendon, Open Approach	**0LCF0ZZ**	Extirpation of Matter from Right Abdomen Tendon, Open Approach	**0LCP3ZZ**	Extirpation of Matter from Left Lower Leg Tendon, Percutaneous Approach
0LC53ZZ	Extirpation of Matter from Right Lower Arm and Wrist Tendon, Percutaneous Approach	**0LCF3ZZ**	Extirpation of Matter from Right Abdomen Tendon, Percutaneous Approach	**0LCP4ZZ**	Extirpation of Matter from Left Lower Leg Tendon, Percutaneous Endoscopic Approach
0LC54ZZ	Extirpation of Matter from Right Lower Arm and Wrist Tendon, Percutaneous Endoscopic Approach	**0LCF4ZZ**	Extirpation of Matter from Right Abdomen Tendon, Percutaneous Endoscopic Approach	**0LCQ0ZZ**	Extirpation of Matter from Right Knee Tendon, Open Approach
0LC60ZZ	Extirpation of Matter from Left Lower Arm and Wrist Tendon, Open Approach	**0LCG0ZZ**	Extirpation of Matter from Left Abdomen Tendon, Open Approach	**0LCQ3ZZ**	Extirpation of Matter from Right Knee Tendon, Percutaneous Approach
0LC63ZZ	Extirpation of Matter from Left Lower Arm and Wrist Tendon, Percutaneous Approach	**0LCG3ZZ**	Extirpation of Matter from Left Abdomen Tendon, Percutaneous Approach	**0LCQ4ZZ**	Extirpation of Matter from Right Knee Tendon, Percutaneous Endoscopic Approach
0LC64ZZ	Extirpation of Matter from Left Lower Arm and Wrist Tendon, Percutaneous Endoscopic Approach	**0LCG4ZZ**	Extirpation of Matter from Left Abdomen Tendon, Percutaneous Endoscopic Approach	**0LCR0ZZ**	Extirpation of Matter from Left Knee Tendon, Open Approach
0LC70ZZ	Extirpation of Matter from Right Hand Tendon, Open Approach	**0LCH0ZZ**	Extirpation of Matter from Perineum Tendon, Open Approach	**0LCR3ZZ**	Extirpation of Matter from Left Knee Tendon, Percutaneous Approach
0LC73ZZ	Extirpation of Matter from Right Hand Tendon, Percutaneous Approach	**0LCH3ZZ**	Extirpation of Matter from Perineum Tendon, Percutaneous Approach	**0LCR4ZZ**	Extirpation of Matter from Left Knee Tendon, Percutaneous Endoscopic Approach
0LC74ZZ	Extirpation of Matter from Right Hand Tendon, Percutaneous Endoscopic Approach	**0LCH4ZZ**	Extirpation of Matter from Perineum Tendon, Percutaneous Endoscopic Approach	**0LCS0ZZ**	Extirpation of Matter from Right Ankle Tendon, Open Approach
0LC80ZZ	Extirpation of Matter from Left Hand Tendon, Open Approach	**0LCJ0ZZ**	Extirpation of Matter from Right Hip Tendon, Open Approach	**0LCS3ZZ**	Extirpation of Matter from Right Ankle Tendon, Percutaneous Approach
0LC83ZZ	Extirpation of Matter from Left Hand Tendon, Percutaneous Approach	**0LCJ3ZZ**	Extirpation of Matter from Right Hip Tendon, Percutaneous Approach	**0LCS4ZZ**	Extirpation of Matter from Right Ankle Tendon, Percutaneous Endoscopic Approach
0LC84ZZ	Extirpation of Matter from Left Hand Tendon, Percutaneous Endoscopic Approach	**0LCJ4ZZ**	Extirpation of Matter from Right Hip Tendon, Percutaneous Endoscopic Approach	**0LCT0ZZ**	Extirpation of Matter from Left Ankle Tendon, Open Approach
0LC90ZZ	Extirpation of Matter from Right Trunk Tendon, Open Approach	**0LCK0ZZ**	Extirpation of Matter from Left Hip Tendon, Open Approach	**0LCT3ZZ**	Extirpation of Matter from Left Ankle Tendon, Percutaneous Approach
0LC93ZZ	Extirpation of Matter from Right Trunk Tendon, Percutaneous Approach	**0LCK3ZZ**	Extirpation of Matter from Left Hip Tendon, Percutaneous Approach	**0LCT4ZZ**	Extirpation of Matter from Left Ankle Tendon, Percutaneous Endoscopic Approach
0LC94ZZ	Extirpation of Matter from Right Trunk Tendon, Percutaneous Endoscopic Approach	**0LCK4ZZ**	Extirpation of Matter from Left Hip Tendon, Percutaneous Endoscopic Approach	**0LCV0ZZ**	Extirpation of Matter from Right Foot Tendon, Open Approach
0LCB0ZZ	Extirpation of Matter from Left Trunk Tendon, Open Approach	**0LCL0ZZ**	Extirpation of Matter from Right Upper Leg Tendon, Open Approach	**0LCV3ZZ**	Extirpation of Matter from Right Foot Tendon, Percutaneous Approach
0LCB3ZZ	Extirpation of Matter from Left Trunk Tendon, Percutaneous Approach	**0LCL3ZZ**	Extirpation of Matter from Right Upper Leg Tendon, Percutaneous Approach	**0LCV4ZZ**	Extirpation of Matter from Right Foot Tendon, Percutaneous Endoscopic Approach
0LCB4ZZ	Extirpation of Matter from Left Trunk Tendon, Percutaneous Endoscopic Approach	**0LCL4ZZ**	Extirpation of Matter from Right Upper Leg Tendon, Percutaneous Endoscopic Approach	**0LCW0ZZ**	Extirpation of Matter from Left Foot Tendon, Open Approach
0LCC0ZZ	Extirpation of Matter from Right Thorax Tendon, Open Approach	**0LCM0ZZ**	Extirpation of Matter from Left Upper Leg Tendon, Open Approach	**0LCW3ZZ**	Extirpation of Matter from Left Foot Tendon, Percutaneous Approach
		0LCM3ZZ	Extirpation of Matter from Left Upper Leg Tendon, Percutaneous Approach	**0LCW4ZZ**	Extirpation of Matter from Left Foot Tendon, Percutaneous Endoscopic Approach

0LD – Tendons, Extraction

0LD00ZZ	Extraction of Head and Neck Tendon, Open Approach	**0LD60ZZ**	Extraction of Left Lower Arm and Wrist Tendon, Open Approach	**0LDD0ZZ**	Extraction of Left Thorax Tendon, Open Approach
0LD10ZZ	Extraction of Right Shoulder Tendon, Open Approach	**0LD70ZZ**	Extraction of Right Hand Tendon, Open Approach	**0LDF0ZZ**	Extraction of Right Abdomen Tendon, Open Approach
0LD20ZZ	Extraction of Left Shoulder Tendon, Open Approach	**0LD80ZZ**	Extraction of Left Hand Tendon, Open Approach	**0LDG0ZZ**	Extraction of Left Abdomen Tendon, Open Approach
0LD30ZZ	Extraction of Right Upper Arm Tendon, Open Approach	**0LD90ZZ**	Extraction of Right Trunk Tendon, Open Approach	**0LDH0ZZ**	Extraction of Perineum Tendon, Open Approach
0LD40ZZ	Extraction of Left Upper Arm Tendon, Open Approach	**0LDB0ZZ**	Extraction of Left Trunk Tendon, Open Approach	**0LDJ0ZZ**	Extraction of Right Hip Tendon, Open Approach
0LD50ZZ	Extraction of Right Lower Arm and Wrist Tendon, Open Approach	**0LDC0ZZ**	Extraction of Right Thorax Tendon, Open Approach	**0LDK0ZZ**	Extraction of Left Hip Tendon, Open Approach

0LDL0ZZ	Extraction of Right Upper Leg Tendon, Open Approach
0LDM0ZZ	Extraction of Left Upper Leg Tendon, Open Approach
0LDN0ZZ	Extraction of Right Lower Leg Tendon, Open Approach
0LDP0ZZ	Extraction of Left Lower Leg Tendon, Open Approach
0LDQ0ZZ	Extraction of Right Knee Tendon, Open Approach
0LDR0ZZ	Extraction of Left Knee Tendon, Open Approach
0LDS0ZZ	Extraction of Right Ankle Tendon, Open Approach
0LDT0ZZ	Extraction of Left Ankle Tendon, Open Approach
0LDV0ZZ	Extraction of Right Foot Tendon, Open Approach
0LDW0ZZ	Extraction of Left Foot Tendon, Open Approach

0LH – Tendons, Insertion

0LHX0YZ	Insertion of Other Device into Upper Tendon, Open Approach
0LHX3YZ	Insertion of Other Device into Upper Tendon, Percutaneous Approach
0LHX4YZ	Insertion of Other Device into Upper Tendon, Percutaneous Endoscopic Approach
0LHY0YZ	Insertion of Other Device into Lower Tendon, Open Approach
0LHY3YZ	Insertion of Other Device into Lower Tendon, Percutaneous Approach
0LHY4YZ	Insertion of Other Device into Lower Tendon, Percutaneous Endoscopic Approach

0LJ – Tendons, Inspection

Review Coding Guidelines B3.5

Review Coding Guidelines B3.11a, B3.11b and B3.11c

0LJX0ZZ	Inspection of Upper Tendon, Open Approach
0LJX3ZZ	Inspection of Upper Tendon, Percutaneous Approach
0LJX4ZZ	Inspection of Upper Tendon, Percutaneous Endoscopic Approach
0LJXXZZ	Inspection of Upper Tendon, External Approach
0LJY0ZZ	Inspection of Lower Tendon, Open Approach
0LJY3ZZ	Inspection of Lower Tendon, Percutaneous Approach
0LJY4ZZ	Inspection of Lower Tendon, Percutaneous Endoscopic Approach
0LJYXZZ	Inspection of Lower Tendon, External Approach

0LM – Tendons, Reattachment

0LM00ZZ	Reattachment of Head and Neck Tendon, Open Approach
0LM04ZZ	Reattachment of Head and Neck Tendon, Percutaneous Endoscopic Approach
0LM10ZZ	Reattachment of Right Shoulder Tendon, Open Approach
0LM14ZZ	Reattachment of Right Shoulder Tendon, Percutaneous Endoscopic Approach
0LM20ZZ	Reattachment of Left Shoulder Tendon, Open Approach
0LM24ZZ	Reattachment of Left Shoulder Tendon, Percutaneous Endoscopic Approach
0LM30ZZ	Reattachment of Right Upper Arm Tendon, Open Approach
0LM34ZZ	Reattachment of Right Upper Arm Tendon, Percutaneous Endoscopic Approach
0LM40ZZ	Reattachment of Left Upper Arm Tendon, Open Approach
0LM44ZZ	Reattachment of Left Upper Arm Tendon, Percutaneous Endoscopic Approach
0LM50ZZ	Reattachment of Right Lower Arm and Wrist Tendon, Open Approach
0LM54ZZ	Reattachment of Right Lower Arm and Wrist Tendon, Percutaneous Endoscopic Approach
0LM60ZZ	Reattachment of Left Lower Arm and Wrist Tendon, Open Approach
0LM64ZZ	Reattachment of Left Lower Arm and Wrist Tendon, Percutaneous Endoscopic Approach
0LM70ZZ	Reattachment of Right Hand Tendon, Open Approach
0LM74ZZ	Reattachment of Right Hand Tendon, Percutaneous Endoscopic Approach
0LM80ZZ	Reattachment of Left Hand Tendon, Open Approach
0LM84ZZ	Reattachment of Left Hand Tendon, Percutaneous Endoscopic Approach
0LM90ZZ	Reattachment of Right Trunk Tendon, Open Approach
0LM94ZZ	Reattachment of Right Trunk Tendon, Percutaneous Endoscopic Approach
0LMB0ZZ	Reattachment of Left Trunk Tendon, Open Approach
0LMB4ZZ	Reattachment of Left Trunk Tendon, Percutaneous Endoscopic Approach
0LMC0ZZ	Reattachment of Right Thorax Tendon, Open Approach
0LMC4ZZ	Reattachment of Right Thorax Tendon, Percutaneous Endoscopic Approach
0LMD0ZZ	Reattachment of Left Thorax Tendon, Open Approach
0LMD4ZZ	Reattachment of Left Thorax Tendon, Percutaneous Endoscopic Approach
0LMF0ZZ	Reattachment of Right Abdomen Tendon, Open Approach
0LMF4ZZ	Reattachment of Right Abdomen Tendon, Percutaneous Endoscopic Approach
0LMG0ZZ	Reattachment of Left Abdomen Tendon, Open Approach
0LMG4ZZ	Reattachment of Left Abdomen Tendon, Percutaneous Endoscopic Approach
0LMH0ZZ	Reattachment of Perineum Tendon, Open Approach
0LMH4ZZ	Reattachment of Perineum Tendon, Percutaneous Endoscopic Approach
0LMJ0ZZ	Reattachment of Right Hip Tendon, Open Approach
0LMJ4ZZ	Reattachment of Right Hip Tendon, Percutaneous Endoscopic Approach
0LMK0ZZ	Reattachment of Left Hip Tendon, Open Approach
0LMK4ZZ	Reattachment of Left Hip Tendon, Percutaneous Endoscopic Approach
0LML0ZZ	Reattachment of Right Upper Leg Tendon, Open Approach
0LML4ZZ	Reattachment of Right Upper Leg Tendon, Percutaneous Endoscopic Approach
0LMM0ZZ	Reattachment of Left Upper Leg Tendon, Open Approach
0LMM4ZZ	Reattachment of Left Upper Leg Tendon, Percutaneous Endoscopic Approach
0LMN0ZZ	Reattachment of Right Lower Leg Tendon, Open Approach
0LMN4ZZ	Reattachment of Right Lower Leg Tendon, Percutaneous Endoscopic Approach
0LMP0ZZ	Reattachment of Left Lower Leg Tendon, Open Approach
0LMP4ZZ	Reattachment of Left Lower Leg Tendon, Percutaneous Endoscopic Approach
0LMQ0ZZ	Reattachment of Right Knee Tendon, Open Approach
0LMQ4ZZ	Reattachment of Right Knee Tendon, Percutaneous Endoscopic Approach
0LMR0ZZ	Reattachment of Left Knee Tendon, Open Approach
0LMR4ZZ	Reattachment of Left Knee Tendon, Percutaneous Endoscopic Approach
0LMS0ZZ	Reattachment of Right Ankle Tendon, Open Approach
0LMS4ZZ	Reattachment of Right Ankle Tendon, Percutaneous Endoscopic Approach
0LMT0ZZ	Reattachment of Left Ankle Tendon, Open Approach
0LMT4ZZ	Reattachment of Left Ankle Tendon, Percutaneous Endoscopic Approach
0LMV0ZZ	Reattachment of Right Foot Tendon, Open Approach
0LMV4ZZ	Reattachment of Right Foot Tendon, Percutaneous Endoscopic Approach
0LMW0ZZ	Reattachment of Left Foot Tendon, Open Approach
0LMW4ZZ	Reattachment of Left Foot Tendon, Percutaneous Endoscopic Approach

Review Coding Guideline B3.13

Review Coding Guideline B3.14

0LN00ZZ	Release Head and Neck Tendon, Open Approach
0LN03ZZ	Release Head and Neck Tendon, Percutaneous Approach
0LN04ZZ	Release Head and Neck Tendon, Percutaneous Endoscopic Approach
0LN0XZZ	Release Head and Neck Tendon, External Approach
0LN10ZZ	Release Right Shoulder Tendon, Open Approach
0LN13ZZ	Release Right Shoulder Tendon, Percutaneous Approach
0LN14ZZ	Release Right Shoulder Tendon, Percutaneous Endoscopic Approach
0LN1XZZ	Release Right Shoulder Tendon, External Approach
0LN20ZZ	Release Left Shoulder Tendon, Open Approach
0LN23ZZ	Release Left Shoulder Tendon, Percutaneous Approach
0LN24ZZ	Release Left Shoulder Tendon, Percutaneous Endoscopic Approach
0LN2XZZ	Release Left Shoulder Tendon, External Approach
0LN30ZZ	Release Right Upper Arm Tendon, Open Approach
0LN33ZZ	Release Right Upper Arm Tendon, Percutaneous Approach
0LN34ZZ	Release Right Upper Arm Tendon, Percutaneous Endoscopic Approach
0LN3XZZ	Release Right Upper Arm Tendon, External Approach
0LN40ZZ	Release Left Upper Arm Tendon, Open Approach
0LN43ZZ	Release Left Upper Arm Tendon, Percutaneous Approach
0LN44ZZ	Release Left Upper Arm Tendon, Percutaneous Endoscopic Approach
0LN4XZZ	Release Left Upper Arm Tendon, External Approach
0LN50ZZ	Release Right Lower Arm and Wrist Tendon, Open Approach
0LN53ZZ	Release Right Lower Arm and Wrist Tendon, Percutaneous Approach
0LN54ZZ	Release Right Lower Arm and Wrist Tendon, Percutaneous Endoscopic Approach
0LN5XZZ	Release Right Lower Arm and Wrist Tendon, External Approach
0LN60ZZ	Release Left Lower Arm and Wrist Tendon, Open Approach
0LN63ZZ	Release Left Lower Arm and Wrist Tendon, Percutaneous Approach
0LN64ZZ	Release Left Lower Arm and Wrist Tendon, Percutaneous Endoscopic Approach
0LN6XZZ	Release Left Lower Arm and Wrist Tendon, External Approach
0LN70ZZ	Release Right Hand Tendon, Open Approach
0LN73ZZ	Release Right Hand Tendon, Percutaneous Approach
0LN74ZZ	Release Right Hand Tendon, Percutaneous Endoscopic Approach
0LN7XZZ	Release Right Hand Tendon, External Approach
0LN80ZZ	Release Left Hand Tendon, Open Approach
0LN83ZZ	Release Left Hand Tendon, Percutaneous Approach
0LN84ZZ	Release Left Hand Tendon, Percutaneous Endoscopic Approach
0LN8XZZ	Release Left Hand Tendon, External Approach
0LN90ZZ	Release Right Trunk Tendon, Open Approach
0LN93ZZ	Release Right Trunk Tendon, Percutaneous Approach
0LN94ZZ	Release Right Trunk Tendon, Percutaneous Endoscopic Approach
0LN9XZZ	Release Right Trunk Tendon, External Approach
0LNB0ZZ	Release Left Trunk Tendon, Open Approach
0LNB3ZZ	Release Left Trunk Tendon, Percutaneous Approach
0LNB4ZZ	Release Left Trunk Tendon, Percutaneous Endoscopic Approach
0LNBXZZ	Release Left Trunk Tendon, External Approach
0LNC0ZZ	Release Right Thorax Tendon, Open Approach
0LNC3ZZ	Release Right Thorax Tendon, Percutaneous Approach
0LNC4ZZ	Release Right Thorax Tendon, Percutaneous Endoscopic Approach
0LNCXZZ	Release Right Thorax Tendon, External Approach
0LND0ZZ	Release Left Thorax Tendon, Open Approach
0LND3ZZ	Release Left Thorax Tendon, Percutaneous Approach
0LND4ZZ	Release Left Thorax Tendon, Percutaneous Endoscopic Approach
0LNDXZZ	Release Left Thorax Tendon, External Approach
0LNF0ZZ	Release Right Abdomen Tendon, Open Approach
0LNF3ZZ	Release Right Abdomen Tendon, Percutaneous Approach
0LNF4ZZ	Release Right Abdomen Tendon, Percutaneous Endoscopic Approach
0LNFXZZ	Release Right Abdomen Tendon, External Approach
0LNG0ZZ	Release Left Abdomen Tendon, Open Approach
0LNG3ZZ	Release Left Abdomen Tendon, Percutaneous Approach
0LNG4ZZ	Release Left Abdomen Tendon, Percutaneous Endoscopic Approach
0LNGXZZ	Release Left Abdomen Tendon, External Approach
0LNH0ZZ	Release Perineum Tendon, Open Approach
0LNH3ZZ	Release Perineum Tendon, Percutaneous Approach
0LNH4ZZ	Release Perineum Tendon, Percutaneous Endoscopic Approach
0LNHXZZ	Release Perineum Tendon, External Approach
0LNJ0ZZ	Release Right Hip Tendon, Open Approach
0LNJ3ZZ	Release Right Hip Tendon, Percutaneous Approach
0LNJ4ZZ	Release Right Hip Tendon, Percutaneous Endoscopic Approach
0LNJXZZ	Release Right Hip Tendon, External Approach
0LNK0ZZ	Release Left Hip Tendon, Open Approach
0LNK3ZZ	Release Left Hip Tendon, Percutaneous Approach
0LNK4ZZ	Release Left Hip Tendon, Percutaneous Endoscopic Approach
0LNKXZZ	Release Left Hip Tendon, External Approach
0LNL0ZZ	Release Right Upper Leg Tendon, Open Approach
0LNL3ZZ	Release Right Upper Leg Tendon, Percutaneous Approach
0LNL4ZZ	Release Right Upper Leg Tendon, Percutaneous Endoscopic Approach
0LNLXZZ	Release Right Upper Leg Tendon, External Approach
0LNM0ZZ	Release Left Upper Leg Tendon, Open Approach
0LNM3ZZ	Release Left Upper Leg Tendon, Percutaneous Approach
0LNM4ZZ	Release Left Upper Leg Tendon, Percutaneous Endoscopic Approach
0LNMXZZ	Release Left Upper Leg Tendon, External Approach
0LNN0ZZ	Release Right Lower Leg Tendon, Open Approach
0LNN3ZZ	Release Right Lower Leg Tendon, Percutaneous Approach
0LNN4ZZ	Release Right Lower Leg Tendon, Percutaneous Endoscopic Approach
0LNNXZZ	Release Right Lower Leg Tendon, External Approach
0LNP0ZZ	Release Left Lower Leg Tendon, Open Approach
0LNP3ZZ	Release Left Lower Leg Tendon, Percutaneous Approach
0LNP4ZZ	Release Left Lower Leg Tendon, Percutaneous Endoscopic Approach
0LNPXZZ	Release Left Lower Leg Tendon, External Approach
0LNQ0ZZ	Release Right Knee Tendon, Open Approach
0LNQ3ZZ	Release Right Knee Tendon, Percutaneous Approach
0LNQ4ZZ	Release Right Knee Tendon, Percutaneous Endoscopic Approach
0LNQXZZ	Release Right Knee Tendon, External Approach
0LNR0ZZ	Release Left Knee Tendon, Open Approach
0LNR3ZZ	Release Left Knee Tendon, Percutaneous Approach
0LNR4ZZ	Release Left Knee Tendon, Percutaneous Endoscopic Approach
0LNRXZZ	Release Left Knee Tendon, External Approach
0LNS0ZZ	Release Right Ankle Tendon, Open Approach
0LNS3ZZ	Release Right Ankle Tendon, Percutaneous Approach
0LNS4ZZ	Release Right Ankle Tendon, Percutaneous Endoscopic Approach
0LNSXZZ	Release Right Ankle Tendon, External Approach
0LNT0ZZ	Release Left Ankle Tendon, Open Approach
0LNT3ZZ	Release Left Ankle Tendon, Percutaneous Approach
0LNT4ZZ	Release Left Ankle Tendon, Percutaneous Endoscopic Approach
0LNTXZZ	Release Left Ankle Tendon, External Approach

♀ Female-only   ♂ Male-only   ▲ Limited Coverage   ● Non-OR   ⬛ HAC-associated procedure   ▲ Non-covered procedures   ➕ Cluster

0LNV0ZZ Release Right Foot Tendon, Open Approach	**0LNVXZZ** Release Right Foot Tendon, External Approach	**0LNW4ZZ** Release Left Foot Tendon, Percutaneous Endoscopic Approach
0LNV3ZZ Release Right Foot Tendon, Percutaneous Approach	**0LNW0ZZ** Release Left Foot Tendon, Open Approach	**0LNWXZZ** Release Left Foot Tendon, External Approach
0LNV4ZZ Release Right Foot Tendon, Percutaneous Endoscopic Approach	**0LNW3ZZ** Release Left Foot Tendon, Percutaneous Approach	

0LP – Tendons, Removal

Review Coding Guideline B6.1c

0LPX00Z Removal of Drainage Device from Upper Tendon, Open Approach	**0LPX47Z** Removal of Autologous Tissue Substitute from Upper Tendon, Percutaneous Endoscopic Approach	**0LPY37Z** Removal of Autologous Tissue Substitute from Lower Tendon, Percutaneous Approach
0LPX07Z Removal of Autologous Tissue Substitute from Upper Tendon, Open Approach	**0LPX4JZ** Removal of Synthetic Substitute from Upper Tendon, Percutaneous Endoscopic Approach	**0LPY3JZ** Removal of Synthetic Substitute from Lower Tendon, Percutaneous Approach
0LPX0JZ Removal of Synthetic Substitute from Upper Tendon, Open Approach	**0LPX4KZ** Removal of Nonautologous Tissue Substitute from Upper Tendon, Percutaneous Endoscopic Approach	**0LPY3KZ** Removal of Nonautologous Tissue Substitute from Lower Tendon, Percutaneous Approach
0LPX0KZ Removal of Nonautologous Tissue Substitute from Upper Tendon, Open Approach	**0LPX4YZ** Removal of Other Device from Upper Tendon, Percutaneous Endoscopic Approach	**0LPY3YZ** Removal of Other Device from Lower Tendon, Percutaneous Approach
0LPX0YZ Removal of Other Device from Upper Tendon, Open Approach	**0LPXX0Z** Removal of Drainage Device from Upper Tendon, External Approach	**0LPY40Z** Removal of Drainage Device from Lower Tendon, Percutaneous Endoscopic Approach
0LPX30Z Removal of Drainage Device from Upper Tendon, Percutaneous Approach	**0LPY00Z** Removal of Drainage Device from Lower Tendon, Open Approach	**0LPY47Z** Removal of Autologous Tissue Substitute from Lower Tendon, Percutaneous Endoscopic Approach
0LPX37Z Removal of Autologous Tissue Substitute from Upper Tendon, Percutaneous Approach	**0LPY07Z** Removal of Autologous Tissue Substitute from Lower Tendon, Open Approach	**0LPY4JZ** Removal of Synthetic Substitute from Lower Tendon, Percutaneous Endoscopic Approach
0LPX3JZ Removal of Synthetic Substitute from Upper Tendon, Percutaneous Approach	**0LPY0JZ** Removal of Synthetic Substitute from Lower Tendon, Open Approach	**0LPY4KZ** Removal of Nonautologous Tissue Substitute from Lower Tendon, Percutaneous Endoscopic Approach
0LPX3KZ Removal of Nonautologous Tissue Substitute from Upper Tendon, Percutaneous Approach	**0LPY0KZ** Removal of Nonautologous Tissue Substitute from Lower Tendon, Open Approach	**0LPY4YZ** Removal of Other Device from Lower Tendon, Percutaneous Endoscopic Approach
0LPX3YZ Removal of Other Device from Upper Tendon, Percutaneous Approach	**0LPY0YZ** Removal of Other Device from Lower Tendon, Open Approach	**0LPYX0Z** Removal of Drainage Device from Lower Tendon, External Approach
0LPX40Z Removal of Drainage Device from Upper Tendon, Percutaneous Endoscopic Approach	**0LPY30Z** Removal of Drainage Device from Lower Tendon, Percutaneous Approach	

0LQ – Tendons, Repair

Review Coding Guideline B3.5

0LQ00ZZ Repair Head and Neck Tendon, Open Approach	**0LQ50ZZ** Repair Right Lower Arm and Wrist Tendon, Open Approach	**0LQB0ZZ** Repair Left Trunk Tendon, Open Approach
0LQ03ZZ Repair Head and Neck Tendon, Percutaneous Approach	**0LQ53ZZ** Repair Right Lower Arm and Wrist Tendon, Percutaneous Approach	**0LQB3ZZ** Repair Left Trunk Tendon, Percutaneous Approach
0LQ04ZZ Repair Head and Neck Tendon, Percutaneous Endoscopic Approach	**0LQ54ZZ** Repair Right Lower Arm and Wrist Tendon, Percutaneous Endoscopic Approach	**0LQB4ZZ** Repair Left Trunk Tendon, Percutaneous Endoscopic Approach
0LQ10ZZ Repair Right Shoulder Tendon, Open Approach	**0LQ60ZZ** Repair Left Lower Arm and Wrist Tendon, Open Approach	**0LQC0ZZ** Repair Right Thorax Tendon, Open Approach
0LQ13ZZ Repair Right Shoulder Tendon, Percutaneous Approach	**0LQ63ZZ** Repair Left Lower Arm and Wrist Tendon, Percutaneous Approach	**0LQC3ZZ** Repair Right Thorax Tendon, Percutaneous Approach
0LQ14ZZ Repair Right Shoulder Tendon, Percutaneous Endoscopic Approach	**0LQ64ZZ** Repair Left Lower Arm and Wrist Tendon, Percutaneous Endoscopic Approach	**0LQC4ZZ** Repair Right Thorax Tendon, Percutaneous Endoscopic Approach
AHA CC: 3Q, 2013, 20-22; 3Q, 2016, 32-33	**0LQ70ZZ** Repair Right Hand Tendon, Open Approach	**0LQD0ZZ** Repair Left Thorax Tendon, Open Approach
0LQ20ZZ Repair Left Shoulder Tendon, Open Approach	**0LQ73ZZ** Repair Right Hand Tendon, Percutaneous Approach	**0LQD3ZZ** Repair Left Thorax Tendon, Percutaneous Approach
0LQ23ZZ Repair Left Shoulder Tendon, Percutaneous Approach	**0LQ74ZZ** Repair Right Hand Tendon, Percutaneous Endoscopic Approach	**0LQD4ZZ** Repair Left Thorax Tendon, Percutaneous Endoscopic Approach
0LQ24ZZ Repair Left Shoulder Tendon, Percutaneous Endoscopic Approach	**0LQ80ZZ** Repair Left Hand Tendon, Open Approach	**0LQF0ZZ** Repair Right Abdomen Tendon, Open Approach
0LQ30ZZ Repair Right Upper Arm Tendon, Open Approach	**0LQ83ZZ** Repair Left Hand Tendon, Percutaneous Approach	**0LQF3ZZ** Repair Right Abdomen Tendon, Percutaneous Approach
0LQ33ZZ Repair Right Upper Arm Tendon, Percutaneous Approach	**0LQ84ZZ** Repair Left Hand Tendon, Percutaneous Endoscopic Approach	**0LQF4ZZ** Repair Right Abdomen Tendon, Percutaneous Endoscopic Approach
0LQ34ZZ Repair Right Upper Arm Tendon, Percutaneous Endoscopic Approach	**0LQ90ZZ** Repair Right Trunk Tendon, Open Approach	**0LQG0ZZ** Repair Left Abdomen Tendon, Open Approach
0LQ40ZZ Repair Left Upper Arm Tendon, Open Approach	**0LQ93ZZ** Repair Right Trunk Tendon, Percutaneous Approach	**0LQG3ZZ** Repair Left Abdomen Tendon, Percutaneous Approach
0LQ43ZZ Repair Left Upper Arm Tendon, Percutaneous Approach	**0LQ94ZZ** Repair Right Trunk Tendon, Percutaneous Endoscopic Approach	**0LQG4ZZ** Repair Left Abdomen Tendon, Percutaneous Endoscopic Approach
0LQ44ZZ Repair Left Upper Arm Tendon, Percutaneous Endoscopic Approach		**0LQH0ZZ** Repair Perineum Tendon, Open Approach

♀ Female-only   ♂ Male-only   ▲ Limited Coverage   ● Non-OR   ▦ HAC-associated procedure   ▲ Non-covered procedures   ✚ Cluster

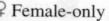

0LQH3ZZ Repair Perineum Tendon, Percutaneous Approach

0LQH4ZZ Repair Perineum Tendon, Percutaneous Endoscopic Approach

0LQJ0ZZ Repair Right Hip Tendon, Open Approach

0LQJ3ZZ Repair Right Hip Tendon, Percutaneous Approach

0LQJ4ZZ Repair Right Hip Tendon, Percutaneous Endoscopic Approach

0LQK0ZZ Repair Left Hip Tendon, Open Approach

0LQK3ZZ Repair Left Hip Tendon, Percutaneous Approach

0LQK4ZZ Repair Left Hip Tendon, Percutaneous Endoscopic Approach

0LQL0ZZ Repair Right Upper Leg Tendon, Open Approach

0LQL3ZZ Repair Right Upper Leg Tendon, Percutaneous Approach

0LQL4ZZ Repair Right Upper Leg Tendon, Percutaneous Endoscopic Approach

0LQM0ZZ Repair Left Upper Leg Tendon, Open Approach

0LQM3ZZ Repair Left Upper Leg Tendon, Percutaneous Approach

0LQM4ZZ Repair Left Upper Leg Tendon, Percutaneous Endoscopic Approach

0LQN0ZZ Repair Right Lower Leg Tendon, Open Approach

0LQN3ZZ Repair Right Lower Leg Tendon, Percutaneous Approach

0LQN4ZZ Repair Right Lower Leg Tendon, Percutaneous Endoscopic Approach

0LQP0ZZ Repair Left Lower Leg Tendon, Open Approach

0LQP3ZZ Repair Left Lower Leg Tendon, Percutaneous Approach

0LQP4ZZ Repair Left Lower Leg Tendon, Percutaneous Endoscopic Approach

0LQQ0ZZ Repair Right Knee Tendon, Open Approach

0LQQ3ZZ Repair Right Knee Tendon, Percutaneous Approach

0LQQ4ZZ Repair Right Knee Tendon, Percutaneous Endoscopic Approach

0LQR0ZZ Repair Left Knee Tendon, Open Approach

0LQR3ZZ Repair Left Knee Tendon, Percutaneous Approach

0LQR4ZZ Repair Left Knee Tendon, Percutaneous Endoscopic Approach

0LQS0ZZ Repair Right Ankle Tendon, Open Approach

0LQS3ZZ Repair Right Ankle Tendon, Percutaneous Approach

0LQS4ZZ Repair Right Ankle Tendon, Percutaneous Endoscopic Approach

0LQT0ZZ Repair Left Ankle Tendon, Open Approach

0LQT3ZZ Repair Left Ankle Tendon, Percutaneous Approach

0LQT4ZZ Repair Left Ankle Tendon, Percutaneous Endoscopic Approach

0LQV0ZZ Repair Right Foot Tendon, Open Approach

0LQV3ZZ Repair Right Foot Tendon, Percutaneous Approach

0LQV4ZZ Repair Right Foot Tendon, Percutaneous Endoscopic Approach

0LQW0ZZ Repair Left Foot Tendon, Open Approach

0LQW3ZZ Repair Left Foot Tendon, Percutaneous Approach

0LQW4ZZ Repair Left Foot Tendon, Percutaneous Endoscopic Approach

0LR – Tendons, Replacement

Review Coding Guideline B3.18

0LR007Z Replacement of Head and Neck Tendon with Autologous Tissue Substitute, Open Approach

0LR00JZ Replacement of Head and Neck Tendon with Synthetic Substitute, Open Approach

0LR00KZ Replacement of Head and Neck Tendon with Nonautologous Tissue Substitute, Open Approach

0LR047Z Replacement of Head and Neck Tendon with Autologous Tissue Substitute, Percutaneous Endoscopic Approach

0LR04JZ Replacement of Head and Neck Tendon with Synthetic Substitute, Percutaneous Endoscopic Approach

0LR04KZ Replacement of Head and Neck Tendon with Nonautologous Tissue Substitute, Percutaneous Endoscopic Approach

0LR107Z Replacement of Right Shoulder Tendon with Autologous Tissue Substitute, Open Approach

0LR10JZ Replacement of Right Shoulder Tendon with Synthetic Substitute, Open Approach

0LR10KZ Replacement of Right Shoulder Tendon with Nonautologous Tissue Substitute, Open Approach

0LR147Z Replacement of Right Shoulder Tendon with Autologous Tissue Substitute, Percutaneous Endoscopic Approach

0LR14JZ Replacement of Right Shoulder Tendon with Synthetic Substitute, Percutaneous Endoscopic Approach

0LR14KZ Replacement of Right Shoulder Tendon with Nonautologous Tissue Substitute, Percutaneous Endoscopic Approach

0LR207Z Replacement of Left Shoulder Tendon with Autologous Tissue Substitute, Open Approach

0LR20JZ Replacement of Left Shoulder Tendon with Synthetic Substitute, Open Approach

0LR20KZ Replacement of Left Shoulder Tendon with Nonautologous Tissue Substitute, Open Approach

0LR247Z Replacement of Left Shoulder Tendon with Autologous Tissue Substitute, Percutaneous Endoscopic Approach

0LR24JZ Replacement of Left Shoulder Tendon with Synthetic Substitute, Percutaneous Endoscopic Approach

0LR24KZ Replacement of Left Shoulder Tendon with Nonautologous Tissue Substitute, Percutaneous Endoscopic Approach

0LR307Z Replacement of Right Upper Arm Tendon with Autologous Tissue Substitute, Open Approach

0LR30JZ Replacement of Right Upper Arm Tendon with Synthetic Substitute, Open Approach

0LR30KZ Replacement of Right Upper Arm Tendon with Nonautologous Tissue Substitute, Open Approach

0LR347Z Replacement of Right Upper Arm Tendon with Autologous Tissue Substitute, Percutaneous Endoscopic Approach

0LR34JZ Replacement of Right Upper Arm Tendon with Synthetic Substitute, Percutaneous Endoscopic Approach

0LR34KZ Replacement of Right Upper Arm Tendon with Nonautologous Tissue Substitute, Percutaneous Endoscopic Approach

0LR407Z Replacement of Left Upper Arm Tendon with Autologous Tissue Substitute, Open Approach

0LR40JZ Replacement of Left Upper Arm Tendon with Synthetic Substitute, Open Approach

0LR40KZ Replacement of Left Upper Arm Tendon with Nonautologous Tissue Substitute, Open Approach

0LR447Z Replacement of Left Upper Arm Tendon with Autologous Tissue Substitute, Percutaneous Endoscopic Approach

0LR44JZ Replacement of Left Upper Arm Tendon with Synthetic Substitute, Percutaneous Endoscopic Approach

0LR44KZ Replacement of Left Upper Arm Tendon with Nonautologous Tissue Substitute, Percutaneous Endoscopic Approach

0LR507Z Replacement of Right Lower Arm and Wrist Tendon with Autologous Tissue Substitute, Open Approach

0LR50JZ Replacement of Right Lower Arm and Wrist Tendon with Synthetic Substitute, Open Approach

0LR50KZ Replacement of Right Lower Arm and Wrist Tendon with Nonautologous Tissue Substitute, Open Approach

0LR547Z Replacement of Right Lower Arm and Wrist Tendon with Autologous Tissue Substitute, Percutaneous Endoscopic Approach

0LR54JZ Replacement of Right Lower Arm and Wrist Tendon with Synthetic Substitute, Percutaneous Endoscopic Approach

0LR54KZ Replacement of Right Lower Arm and Wrist Tendon with Nonautologous Tissue Substitute, Percutaneous Endoscopic Approach

0LR607Z Replacement of Left Lower Arm and Wrist Tendon with Autologous Tissue Substitute, Open Approach

0LR60JZ Replacement of Left Lower Arm and Wrist Tendon with Synthetic Substitute, Open Approach

0LR60KZ Replacement of Left Lower Arm and Wrist Tendon with Nonautologous Tissue Substitute, Open Approach

0LR647Z Replacement of Left Lower Arm and Wrist Tendon with Autologous Tissue Substitute, Percutaneous Endoscopic Approach

0LR64JZ Replacement of Left Lower Arm and Wrist Tendon with Synthetic Substitute, Percutaneous Endoscopic Approach

0LR64KZ Replacement of Left Lower Arm and Wrist Tendon with Nonautologous Tissue Substitute, Percutaneous Endoscopic Approach

0LR707Z Replacement of Right Hand Tendon with Autologous Tissue Substitute, Open Approach

0LR70JZ Replacement of Right Hand Tendon with Synthetic Substitute, Open Approach

0LR70KZ Replacement of Right Hand Tendon with Nonautologous Tissue Substitute, Open Approach

0LR747Z Replacement of Right Hand Tendon with Autologous Tissue Substitute, Percutaneous Endoscopic Approach

0LR74JZ Replacement of Right Hand Tendon with Synthetic Substitute, Percutaneous Endoscopic Approach

0LR74KZ Replacement of Right Hand Tendon with Nonautologous Tissue Substitute, Percutaneous Endoscopic Approach

0LR807Z Replacement of Left Hand Tendon with Autologous Tissue Substitute, Open Approach

0LR80JZ Replacement of Left Hand Tendon with Synthetic Substitute, Open Approach

0LR80KZ Replacement of Left Hand Tendon with Nonautologous Tissue Substitute, Open Approach

0LR847Z Replacement of Left Hand Tendon with Autologous Tissue Substitute, Percutaneous Endoscopic Approach

0LR84JZ Replacement of Left Hand Tendon with Synthetic Substitute, Percutaneous Endoscopic Approach

0LR84KZ Replacement of Left Hand Tendon with Nonautologous Tissue Substitute, Percutaneous Endoscopic Approach

0LR907Z Replacement of Right Trunk Tendon with Autologous Tissue Substitute, Open Approach

0LR90JZ Replacement of Right Trunk Tendon with Synthetic Substitute, Open Approach

0LR90KZ Replacement of Right Trunk Tendon with Nonautologous Tissue Substitute, Open Approach

0LR947Z Replacement of Right Trunk Tendon with Autologous Tissue Substitute, Percutaneous Endoscopic Approach

0LR94JZ Replacement of Right Trunk Tendon with Synthetic Substitute, Percutaneous Endoscopic Approach

0LR94KZ Replacement of Right Trunk Tendon with Nonautologous Tissue Substitute, Percutaneous Endoscopic Approach

0LRB07Z Replacement of Left Trunk Tendon with Autologous Tissue Substitute, Open Approach

0LRB0JZ Replacement of Left Trunk Tendon with Synthetic Substitute, Open Approach

0LRB0KZ Replacement of Left Trunk Tendon with Nonautologous Tissue Substitute, Open Approach

0LRB47Z Replacement of Left Trunk Tendon with Autologous Tissue Substitute, Percutaneous Endoscopic Approach

0LRB4JZ Replacement of Left Trunk Tendon with Synthetic Substitute, Percutaneous Endoscopic Approach

0LRB4KZ Replacement of Left Trunk Tendon with Nonautologous Tissue Substitute, Percutaneous Endoscopic Approach

0LRC07Z Replacement of Right Thorax Tendon with Autologous Tissue Substitute, Open Approach

0LRC0JZ Replacement of Right Thorax Tendon with Synthetic Substitute, Open Approach

0LRC0KZ Replacement of Right Thorax Tendon with Nonautologous Tissue Substitute, Open Approach

0LRC47Z Replacement of Right Thorax Tendon with Autologous Tissue Substitute, Percutaneous Endoscopic Approach

0LRC4JZ Replacement of Right Thorax Tendon with Synthetic Substitute, Percutaneous Endoscopic Approach

0LRC4KZ Replacement of Right Thorax Tendon with Nonautologous Tissue Substitute, Percutaneous Endoscopic Approach

0LRD07Z Replacement of Left Thorax Tendon with Autologous Tissue Substitute, Open Approach

0LRD0JZ Replacement of Left Thorax Tendon with Synthetic Substitute, Open Approach

0LRD0KZ Replacement of Left Thorax Tendon with Nonautologous Tissue Substitute, Open Approach

0LRD47Z Replacement of Left Thorax Tendon with Autologous Tissue Substitute, Percutaneous Endoscopic Approach

0LRD4JZ Replacement of Left Thorax Tendon with Synthetic Substitute, Percutaneous Endoscopic Approach

0LRD4KZ Replacement of Left Thorax Tendon with Nonautologous Tissue Substitute, Percutaneous Endoscopic Approach

0LRF07Z Replacement of Right Abdomen Tendon with Autologous Tissue Substitute, Open Approach

0LRF0JZ Replacement of Right Abdomen Tendon with Synthetic Substitute, Open Approach

0LRF0KZ Replacement of Right Abdomen Tendon with Nonautologous Tissue Substitute, Open Approach

0LRF47Z Replacement of Right Abdomen Tendon with Autologous Tissue Substitute, Percutaneous Endoscopic Approach

0LRF4JZ Replacement of Right Abdomen Tendon with Synthetic Substitute, Percutaneous Endoscopic Approach

0LRF4KZ Replacement of Right Abdomen Tendon with Nonautologous Tissue Substitute, Percutaneous Endoscopic Approach

0LRG07Z Replacement of Left Abdomen Tendon with Autologous Tissue Substitute, Open Approach

0LRG0JZ Replacement of Left Abdomen Tendon with Synthetic Substitute, Open Approach

0LRG0KZ Replacement of Left Abdomen Tendon with Nonautologous Tissue Substitute, Open Approach

0LRG47Z Replacement of Left Abdomen Tendon with Autologous Tissue Substitute, Percutaneous Endoscopic Approach

0LRG4JZ Replacement of Left Abdomen Tendon with Synthetic Substitute, Percutaneous Endoscopic Approach

0LRG4KZ Replacement of Left Abdomen Tendon with Nonautologous Tissue Substitute, Percutaneous Endoscopic Approach

0LRH07Z Replacement of Perineum Tendon with Autologous Tissue Substitute, Open Approach

0LRH0JZ Replacement of Perineum Tendon with Synthetic Substitute, Open Approach

0LRH0KZ Replacement of Perineum Tendon with Nonautologous Tissue Substitute, Open Approach

0LRH47Z Replacement of Perineum Tendon with Autologous Tissue Substitute, Percutaneous Endoscopic Approach

0LRH4JZ Replacement of Perineum Tendon with Synthetic Substitute, Percutaneous Endoscopic Approach

0LRH4KZ Replacement of Perineum Tendon with Nonautologous Tissue Substitute, Percutaneous Endoscopic Approach

0LRJ07Z Replacement of Right Hip Tendon with Autologous Tissue Substitute, Open Approach

0LRJ0JZ Replacement of Right Hip Tendon with Synthetic Substitute, Open Approach

0LRJ0KZ Replacement of Right Hip Tendon with Nonautologous Tissue Substitute, Open Approach

0LRJ47Z Replacement of Right Hip Tendon with Autologous Tissue Substitute, Percutaneous Endoscopic Approach

0LRJ4JZ Replacement of Right Hip Tendon with Synthetic Substitute, Percutaneous Endoscopic Approach

0LRJ4KZ Replacement of Right Hip Tendon with Nonautologous Tissue Substitute, Percutaneous Endoscopic Approach

0LRK07Z Replacement of Left Hip Tendon with Autologous Tissue Substitute, Open Approach

0LRK0JZ Replacement of Left Hip Tendon with Synthetic Substitute, Open Approach

0LRK0KZ Replacement of Left Hip Tendon with Nonautologous Tissue Substitute, Open Approach

0LRK47Z Replacement of Left Hip Tendon with Autologous Tissue Substitute, Percutaneous Endoscopic Approach

0LRK4JZ Replacement of Left Hip Tendon with Synthetic Substitute, Percutaneous Endoscopic Approach

0LRK4KZ Replacement of Left Hip Tendon with Nonautologous Tissue Substitute, Percutaneous Endoscopic Approach

0LRL07Z Replacement of Right Upper Leg Tendon with Autologous Tissue Substitute, Open Approach

0LRL0JZ Replacement of Right Upper Leg Tendon with Synthetic Substitute, Open Approach

0LRL0KZ Replacement of Right Upper Leg Tendon with Nonautologous Tissue Substitute, Open Approach

0LRL47Z Replacement of Right Upper Leg Tendon with Autologous Tissue Substitute, Percutaneous Endoscopic Approach

0LRL4JZ Replacement of Right Upper Leg Tendon with Synthetic Substitute, Percutaneous Endoscopic Approach

0LRL4KZ Replacement of Right Upper Leg Tendon with Nonautologous Tissue Substitute, Percutaneous Endoscopic Approach

0LRM07Z Replacement of Left Upper Leg Tendon with Autologous Tissue Substitute, Open Approach

0LRM0JZ Replacement of Left Upper Leg Tendon with Synthetic Substitute, Open Approach

0LRM0KZ Replacement of Left Upper Leg Tendon with Nonautologous Tissue Substitute, Open Approach

♀ Female-only   ♂ Male-only   ▲ Limited Coverage   ● Non-OR   ▦ HAC-associated procedure   ▲ Non-covered procedures   ✛ Cluster

0LRM47Z	Replacement of Left Upper Leg Tendon with Autologous Tissue Substitute, Percutaneous Endoscopic Approach	**0LRQ0JZ**	Replacement of Right Knee Tendon with Synthetic Substitute, Open Approach	**0LRT0JZ**	Replacement of Left Ankle Tendon with Synthetic Substitute, Open Approach
0LRM4JZ	Replacement of Left Upper Leg Tendon with Synthetic Substitute, Percutaneous Endoscopic Approach	**0LRQ0KZ**	Replacement of Right Knee Tendon with Nonautologous Tissue Substitute, Open Approach	**0LRT0KZ**	Replacement of Left Ankle Tendon with Nonautologous Tissue Substitute, Open Approach
0LRM4KZ	Replacement of Left Upper Leg Tendon with Nonautologous Tissue Substitute, Percutaneous Endoscopic Approach	**0LRQ47Z**	Replacement of Right Knee Tendon with Autologous Tissue Substitute, Percutaneous Endoscopic Approach	**0LRT47Z**	Replacement of Left Ankle Tendon with Autologous Tissue Substitute, Percutaneous Endoscopic Approach
0LRN07Z	Replacement of Right Lower Leg Tendon with Autologous Tissue Substitute, Open Approach	**0LRQ4JZ**	Replacement of Right Knee Tendon with Synthetic Substitute, Percutaneous Endoscopic Approach	**0LRT4JZ**	Replacement of Left Ankle Tendon with Synthetic Substitute, Percutaneous Endoscopic Approach
0LRN0JZ	Replacement of Right Lower Leg Tendon with Synthetic Substitute, Open Approach	**0LRQ4KZ**	Replacement of Right Knee Tendon with Nonautologous Tissue Substitute, Percutaneous Endoscopic Approach	**0LRT4KZ**	Replacement of Left Ankle Tendon with Nonautologous Tissue Substitute, Percutaneous Endoscopic Approach
0LRN0KZ	Replacement of Right Lower Leg Tendon with Nonautologous Tissue Substitute, Open Approach	**0LRR07Z**	Replacement of Left Knee Tendon with Autologous Tissue Substitute, Open Approach	**0LRV07Z**	Replacement of Right Foot Tendon with Autologous Tissue Substitute, Open Approach
0LRN47Z	Replacement of Right Lower Leg Tendon with Autologous Tissue Substitute, Percutaneous Endoscopic Approach	**0LRR0JZ**	Replacement of Left Knee Tendon with Synthetic Substitute, Open Approach	**0LRV0JZ**	Replacement of Right Foot Tendon with Synthetic Substitute, Open Approach
0LRN4JZ	Replacement of Right Lower Leg Tendon with Synthetic Substitute, Percutaneous Endoscopic Approach	**0LRR0KZ**	Replacement of Left Knee Tendon with Nonautologous Tissue Substitute, Open Approach	**0LRV0KZ**	Replacement of Right Foot Tendon with Nonautologous Tissue Substitute, Open Approach
0LRN4KZ	Replacement of Right Lower Leg Tendon with Nonautologous Tissue Substitute, Percutaneous Endoscopic Approach	**0LRR47Z**	Replacement of Left Knee Tendon with Autologous Tissue Substitute, Percutaneous Endoscopic Approach	**0LRV47Z**	Replacement of Right Foot Tendon with Autologous Tissue Substitute, Percutaneous Endoscopic Approach
0LRP07Z	Replacement of Left Lower Leg Tendon with Autologous Tissue Substitute, Open Approach	**0LRR4JZ**	Replacement of Left Knee Tendon with Synthetic Substitute, Percutaneous Endoscopic Approach	**0LRV4JZ**	Replacement of Right Foot Tendon with Synthetic Substitute, Percutaneous Endoscopic Approach
0LRP0JZ	Replacement of Left Lower Leg Tendon with Synthetic Substitute, Open Approach	**0LRR4KZ**	Replacement of Left Knee Tendon with Nonautologous Tissue Substitute, Percutaneous Endoscopic Approach	**0LRV4KZ**	Replacement of Right Foot Tendon with Nonautologous Tissue Substitute, Percutaneous Endoscopic Approach
0LRP0KZ	Replacement of Left Lower Leg Tendon with Nonautologous Tissue Substitute, Open Approach	**0LRS07Z**	Replacement of Right Ankle Tendon with Autologous Tissue Substitute, Open Approach	**0LRW07Z**	Replacement of Left Foot Tendon with Autologous Tissue Substitute, Open Approach
0LRP47Z	Replacement of Left Lower Leg Tendon with Autologous Tissue Substitute, Percutaneous Endoscopic Approach	**0LRS0JZ**	Replacement of Right Ankle Tendon with Synthetic Substitute, Open Approach	**0LRW0JZ**	Replacement of Left Foot Tendon with Synthetic Substitute, Open Approach
0LRP4JZ	Replacement of Left Lower Leg Tendon with Synthetic Substitute, Percutaneous Endoscopic Approach	**0LRS0KZ**	Replacement of Right Ankle Tendon with Nonautologous Tissue Substitute, Open Approach	**0LRW0KZ**	Replacement of Left Foot Tendon with Nonautologous Tissue Substitute, Open Approach
0LRP4KZ	Replacement of Left Lower Leg Tendon with Nonautologous Tissue Substitute, Percutaneous Endoscopic Approach	**0LRS47Z**	Replacement of Right Ankle Tendon with Autologous Tissue Substitute, Percutaneous Endoscopic Approach	**0LRW47Z**	Replacement of Left Foot Tendon with Autologous Tissue Substitute, Percutaneous Endoscopic Approach
0LRQ07Z	Replacement of Right Knee Tendon with Autologous Tissue Substitute, Open Approach	**0LRS4JZ**	Replacement of Right Ankle Tendon with Synthetic Substitute, Percutaneous Endoscopic Approach	**0LRW4JZ**	Replacement of Left Foot Tendon with Synthetic Substitute, Percutaneous Endoscopic Approach
		0LRS4KZ	Replacement of Right Ankle Tendon with Nonautologous Tissue Substitute, Percutaneous Endoscopic Approach	**0LRW4KZ**	Replacement of Left Foot Tendon with Nonautologous Tissue Substitute, Percutaneous Endoscopic Approach
		0LRT07Z	Replacement of Left Ankle Tendon with Autologous Tissue Substitute, Open Approach		

0LS – Tendons, Reposition

0LS00ZZ	Reposition Head and Neck Tendon, Open Approach	**0LS40ZZ**	Reposition Left Upper Arm Tendon, Open Approach	**0LS80ZZ**	Reposition Left Hand Tendon, Open Approach
0LS04ZZ	Reposition Head and Neck Tendon, Percutaneous Endoscopic Approach		*AHA CC: 3Q, 2015, 14-15*	**0LS84ZZ**	Reposition Left Hand Tendon, Percutaneous Endoscopic Approach
0LS10ZZ	Reposition Right Shoulder Tendon, Open Approach	**0LS44ZZ**	Reposition Left Upper Arm Tendon, Percutaneous Endoscopic Approach	**0LS90ZZ**	Reposition Right Trunk Tendon, Open Approach
0LS14ZZ	Reposition Right Shoulder Tendon, Percutaneous Endoscopic Approach	**0LS50ZZ**	Reposition Right Lower Arm and Wrist Tendon, Open Approach	**0LS94ZZ**	Reposition Right Trunk Tendon, Percutaneous Endoscopic Approach
0LS20ZZ	Reposition Left Shoulder Tendon, Open Approach	**0LS54ZZ**	Reposition Right Lower Arm and Wrist Tendon, Percutaneous Endoscopic Approach	**0LSB0ZZ**	Reposition Left Trunk Tendon, Open Approach
0LS24ZZ	Reposition Left Shoulder Tendon, Percutaneous Endoscopic Approach	**0LS60ZZ**	Reposition Left Lower Arm and Wrist Tendon, Open Approach	**0LSB4ZZ**	Reposition Left Trunk Tendon, Percutaneous Endoscopic Approach
0LS30ZZ	Reposition Right Upper Arm Tendon, Open Approach	**0LS64ZZ**	Reposition Left Lower Arm and Wrist Tendon, Percutaneous Endoscopic Approach	**0LSC0ZZ**	Reposition Right Thorax Tendon, Open Approach
	AHA CC: 3Q, 2016, 32-33	**0LS70ZZ**	Reposition Right Hand Tendon, Open Approach	**0LSC4ZZ**	Reposition Right Thorax Tendon, Percutaneous Endoscopic Approach
0LS34ZZ	Reposition Right Upper Arm Tendon, Percutaneous Endoscopic Approach	**0LS74ZZ**	Reposition Right Hand Tendon, Percutaneous Endoscopic Approach	**0LSD0ZZ**	Reposition Left Thorax Tendon, Open Approach

0LSD4ZZ	Reposition Left Thorax Tendon, Percutaneous Endoscopic Approach	
0LSF0ZZ	Reposition Right Abdomen Tendon, Open Approach	
0LSF4ZZ	Reposition Right Abdomen Tendon, Percutaneous Endoscopic Approach	
0LSG0ZZ	Reposition Left Abdomen Tendon, Open Approach	
0LSG4ZZ	Reposition Left Abdomen Tendon, Percutaneous Endoscopic Approach	
0LSH0ZZ	Reposition Perineum Tendon, Open Approach	
0LSH4ZZ	Reposition Perineum Tendon, Percutaneous Endoscopic Approach	
0LSJ0ZZ	Reposition Right Hip Tendon, Open Approach	
0LSJ4ZZ	Reposition Right Hip Tendon, Percutaneous Endoscopic Approach	
0LSK0ZZ	Reposition Left Hip Tendon, Open Approach	
0LSK4ZZ	Reposition Left Hip Tendon, Percutaneous Endoscopic Approach	

0LSL0ZZ	Reposition Right Upper Leg Tendon, Open Approach
0LSL4ZZ	Reposition Right Upper Leg Tendon, Percutaneous Endoscopic Approach
0LSM0ZZ	Reposition Left Upper Leg Tendon, Open Approach
0LSM4ZZ	Reposition Left Upper Leg Tendon, Percutaneous Endoscopic Approach
0LSN0ZZ	Reposition Right Lower Leg Tendon, Open Approach
0LSN4ZZ	Reposition Right Lower Leg Tendon, Percutaneous Endoscopic Approach
0LSP0ZZ	Reposition Left Lower Leg Tendon, Open Approach
0LSP4ZZ	Reposition Left Lower Leg Tendon, Percutaneous Endoscopic Approach
0LSQ0ZZ	Reposition Right Knee Tendon, Open Approach
0LSQ4ZZ	Reposition Right Knee Tendon, Percutaneous Endoscopic Approach

0LSR0ZZ	Reposition Left Knee Tendon, Open Approach
0LSR4ZZ	Reposition Left Knee Tendon, Percutaneous Endoscopic Approach
0LSS0ZZ	Reposition Right Ankle Tendon, Open Approach
0LSS4ZZ	Reposition Right Ankle Tendon, Percutaneous Endoscopic Approach
0LST0ZZ	Reposition Left Ankle Tendon, Open Approach
0LST4ZZ	Reposition Left Ankle Tendon, Percutaneous Endoscopic Approach
0LSV0ZZ	Reposition Right Foot Tendon, Open Approach
0LSV4ZZ	Reposition Right Foot Tendon, Percutaneous Endoscopic Approach
0LSW0ZZ	Reposition Left Foot Tendon, Open Approach
0LSW4ZZ	Reposition Left Foot Tendon, Percutaneous Endoscopic Approach

0LT – Tendons, Resection

Review Coding Guideline B3.8

Review Coding Guideline B3.18

0LT00ZZ	Resection of Head and Neck Tendon, Open Approach
0LT04ZZ	Resection of Head and Neck Tendon, Percutaneous Endoscopic Approach
0LT10ZZ	Resection of Right Shoulder Tendon, Open Approach
0LT14ZZ	Resection of Right Shoulder Tendon, Percutaneous Endoscopic Approach
0LT20ZZ	Resection of Left Shoulder Tendon, Open Approach
0LT24ZZ	Resection of Left Shoulder Tendon, Percutaneous Endoscopic Approach
0LT30ZZ	Resection of Right Upper Arm Tendon, Open Approach
0LT34ZZ	Resection of Right Upper Arm Tendon, Percutaneous Endoscopic Approach
0LT40ZZ	Resection of Left Upper Arm Tendon, Open Approach
0LT44ZZ	Resection of Left Upper Arm Tendon, Percutaneous Endoscopic Approach
0LT50ZZ	Resection of Right Lower Arm and Wrist Tendon, Open Approach
0LT54ZZ	Resection of Right Lower Arm and Wrist Tendon, Percutaneous Endoscopic Approach
0LT60ZZ	Resection of Left Lower Arm and Wrist Tendon, Open Approach
0LT64ZZ	Resection of Left Lower Arm and Wrist Tendon, Percutaneous Endoscopic Approach
0LT70ZZ	Resection of Right Hand Tendon, Open Approach
0LT74ZZ	Resection of Right Hand Tendon, Percutaneous Endoscopic Approach
0LT80ZZ	Resection of Left Hand Tendon, Open Approach
0LT84ZZ	Resection of Left Hand Tendon, Percutaneous Endoscopic Approach

0LT90ZZ	Resection of Right Trunk Tendon, Open Approach
0LT94ZZ	Resection of Right Trunk Tendon, Percutaneous Endoscopic Approach
0LTB0ZZ	Resection of Left Trunk Tendon, Open Approach
0LTB4ZZ	Resection of Left Trunk Tendon, Percutaneous Endoscopic Approach
0LTC0ZZ	Resection of Right Thorax Tendon, Open Approach
0LTC4ZZ	Resection of Right Thorax Tendon, Percutaneous Endoscopic Approach
0LTD0ZZ	Resection of Left Thorax Tendon, Open Approach
0LTD4ZZ	Resection of Left Thorax Tendon, Percutaneous Endoscopic Approach
0LTF0ZZ	Resection of Right Abdomen Tendon, Open Approach
0LTF4ZZ	Resection of Right Abdomen Tendon, Percutaneous Endoscopic Approach
0LTG0ZZ	Resection of Left Abdomen Tendon, Open Approach
0LTG4ZZ	Resection of Left Abdomen Tendon, Percutaneous Endoscopic Approach
0LTH0ZZ	Resection of Perineum Tendon, Open Approach
0LTH4ZZ	Resection of Perineum Tendon, Percutaneous Endoscopic Approach
0LTJ0ZZ	Resection of Right Hip Tendon, Open Approach
0LTJ4ZZ	Resection of Right Hip Tendon, Percutaneous Endoscopic Approach
0LTK0ZZ	Resection of Left Hip Tendon, Open Approach
0LTK4ZZ	Resection of Left Hip Tendon, Percutaneous Endoscopic Approach
0LTL0ZZ	Resection of Right Upper Leg Tendon, Open Approach

0LTL4ZZ	Resection of Right Upper Leg Tendon, Percutaneous Endoscopic Approach
0LTM0ZZ	Resection of Left Upper Leg Tendon, Open Approach
0LTM4ZZ	Resection of Left Upper Leg Tendon, Percutaneous Endoscopic Approach
0LTN0ZZ	Resection of Right Lower Leg Tendon, Open Approach
0LTN4ZZ	Resection of Right Lower Leg Tendon, Percutaneous Endoscopic Approach
0LTP0ZZ	Resection of Left Lower Leg Tendon, Open Approach
0LTP4ZZ	Resection of Left Lower Leg Tendon, Percutaneous Endoscopic Approach
0LTQ0ZZ	Resection of Right Knee Tendon, Open Approach
0LTQ4ZZ	Resection of Right Knee Tendon, Percutaneous Endoscopic Approach
0LTR0ZZ	Resection of Left Knee Tendon, Open Approach
0LTR4ZZ	Resection of Left Knee Tendon, Percutaneous Endoscopic Approach
0LTS0ZZ	Resection of Right Ankle Tendon, Open Approach
0LTS4ZZ	Resection of Right Ankle Tendon, Percutaneous Endoscopic Approach
0LTT0ZZ	Resection of Left Ankle Tendon, Open Approach
0LTT4ZZ	Resection of Left Ankle Tendon, Percutaneous Endoscopic Approach
0LTV0ZZ	Resection of Right Foot Tendon, Open Approach
0LTV4ZZ	Resection of Right Foot Tendon, Percutaneous Endoscopic Approach
0LTW0ZZ	Resection of Left Foot Tendon, Open Approach
0LTW4ZZ	Resection of Left Foot Tendon, Percutaneous Endoscopic Approach

0LU – Tendons, Supplement

0LU007Z	Supplement Head and Neck Tendon with Autologous Tissue Substitute, Open Approach
0LU00JZ	Supplement Head and Neck Tendon with Synthetic Substitute, Open Approach

0LU00KZ	Supplement Head and Neck Tendon with Nonautologous Tissue Substitute, Open Approach
0LU047Z	Supplement Head and Neck Tendon with Autologous Tissue Substitute, Percutaneous Endoscopic Approach

0LU04JZ	Supplement Head and Neck Tendon with Synthetic Substitute, Percutaneous Endoscopic Approach
0LU04KZ	Supplement Head and Neck Tendon with Nonautologous Tissue Substitute, Percutaneous Endoscopic Approach

♀ Female-only   ♂ Male-only   ▲ Limited Coverage   ● Non-OR   ▨ HAC-associated procedure   ▲ Non-covered procedures   ✚ Cluster

0LU107Z Supplement Right Shoulder Tendon with Autologous Tissue Substitute, Open Approach

0LU10JZ Supplement Right Shoulder Tendon with Synthetic Substitute, Open Approach

0LU10KZ Supplement Right Shoulder Tendon with Nonautologous Tissue Substitute, Open Approach

0LU147Z Supplement Right Shoulder Tendon with Autologous Tissue Substitute, Percutaneous Endoscopic Approach

0LU14JZ Supplement Right Shoulder Tendon with Synthetic Substitute, Percutaneous Endoscopic Approach

0LU14KZ Supplement Right Shoulder Tendon with Nonautologous Tissue Substitute, Percutaneous Endoscopic Approach

0LU207Z Supplement Left Shoulder Tendon with Autologous Tissue Substitute, Open Approach

0LU20JZ Supplement Left Shoulder Tendon with Synthetic Substitute, Open Approach

0LU20KZ Supplement Left Shoulder Tendon with Nonautologous Tissue Substitute, Open Approach

0LU247Z Supplement Left Shoulder Tendon with Autologous Tissue Substitute, Percutaneous Endoscopic Approach

0LU24JZ Supplement Left Shoulder Tendon with Synthetic Substitute, Percutaneous Endoscopic Approach

0LU24KZ Supplement Left Shoulder Tendon with Nonautologous Tissue Substitute, Percutaneous Endoscopic Approach

0LU307Z Supplement Right Upper Arm Tendon with Autologous Tissue Substitute, Open Approach

0LU30JZ Supplement Right Upper Arm Tendon with Synthetic Substitute, Open Approach

0LU30KZ Supplement Right Upper Arm Tendon with Nonautologous Tissue Substitute, Open Approach

0LU347Z Supplement Right Upper Arm Tendon with Autologous Tissue Substitute, Percutaneous Endoscopic Approach

0LU34JZ Supplement Right Upper Arm Tendon with Synthetic Substitute, Percutaneous Endoscopic Approach

0LU34KZ Supplement Right Upper Arm Tendon with Nonautologous Tissue Substitute, Percutaneous Endoscopic Approach

0LU407Z Supplement Left Upper Arm Tendon with Autologous Tissue Substitute, Open Approach

0LU40JZ Supplement Left Upper Arm Tendon with Synthetic Substitute, Open Approach

0LU40KZ Supplement Left Upper Arm Tendon with Nonautologous Tissue Substitute, Open Approach

0LU447Z Supplement Left Upper Arm Tendon with Autologous Tissue Substitute, Percutaneous Endoscopic Approach

0LU44JZ Supplement Left Upper Arm Tendon with Synthetic Substitute, Percutaneous Endoscopic Approach

0LU44KZ Supplement Left Upper Arm Tendon with Nonautologous Tissue Substitute, Percutaneous Endoscopic Approach

0LU507Z Supplement Right Lower Arm and Wrist Tendon with Autologous Tissue Substitute, Open Approach

0LU50JZ Supplement Right Lower Arm and Wrist Tendon with Synthetic Substitute, Open Approach

0LU50KZ Supplement Right Lower Arm and Wrist Tendon with Nonautologous Tissue Substitute, Open Approach

0LU547Z Supplement Right Lower Arm and Wrist Tendon with Autologous Tissue Substitute, Percutaneous Endoscopic Approach

0LU54JZ Supplement Right Lower Arm and Wrist Tendon with Synthetic Substitute, Percutaneous Endoscopic Approach

0LU54KZ Supplement Right Lower Arm and Wrist Tendon with Nonautologous Tissue Substitute, Percutaneous Endoscopic Approach

0LU607Z Supplement Left Lower Arm and Wrist Tendon with Autologous Tissue Substitute, Open Approach

0LU60JZ Supplement Left Lower Arm and Wrist Tendon with Synthetic Substitute, Open Approach

0LU60KZ Supplement Left Lower Arm and Wrist Tendon with Nonautologous Tissue Substitute, Open Approach

0LU647Z Supplement Left Lower Arm and Wrist Tendon with Autologous Tissue Substitute, Percutaneous Endoscopic Approach

0LU64JZ Supplement Left Lower Arm and Wrist Tendon with Synthetic Substitute, Percutaneous Endoscopic Approach

0LU64KZ Supplement Left Lower Arm and Wrist Tendon with Nonautologous Tissue Substitute, Percutaneous Endoscopic Approach

0LU707Z Supplement Right Hand Tendon with Autologous Tissue Substitute, Open Approach

0LU70JZ Supplement Right Hand Tendon with Synthetic Substitute, Open Approach

0LU70KZ Supplement Right Hand Tendon with Nonautologous Tissue Substitute, Open Approach

0LU747Z Supplement Right Hand Tendon with Autologous Tissue Substitute, Percutaneous Endoscopic Approach

0LU74JZ Supplement Right Hand Tendon with Synthetic Substitute, Percutaneous Endoscopic Approach

0LU74KZ Supplement Right Hand Tendon with Nonautologous Tissue Substitute, Percutaneous Endoscopic Approach

0LU807Z Supplement Left Hand Tendon with Autologous Tissue Substitute, Open Approach

0LU80JZ Supplement Left Hand Tendon with Synthetic Substitute, Open Approach

0LU80KZ Supplement Left Hand Tendon with Nonautologous Tissue Substitute, Open Approach

0LU847Z Supplement Left Hand Tendon with Autologous Tissue Substitute, Percutaneous Endoscopic Approach

0LU84JZ Supplement Left Hand Tendon with Synthetic Substitute, Percutaneous Endoscopic Approach

0LU84KZ Supplement Left Hand Tendon with Nonautologous Tissue Substitute, Percutaneous Endoscopic Approach

0LU907Z Supplement Right Trunk Tendon with Autologous Tissue Substitute, Open Approach

0LU90JZ Supplement Right Trunk Tendon with Synthetic Substitute, Open Approach

0LU90KZ Supplement Right Trunk Tendon with Nonautologous Tissue Substitute, Open Approach

0LU947Z Supplement Right Trunk Tendon with Autologous Tissue Substitute, Percutaneous Endoscopic Approach

0LU94JZ Supplement Right Trunk Tendon with Synthetic Substitute, Percutaneous Endoscopic Approach

0LU94KZ Supplement Right Trunk Tendon with Nonautologous Tissue Substitute, Percutaneous Endoscopic Approach

0LUB07Z Supplement Left Trunk Tendon with Autologous Tissue Substitute, Open Approach

0LUB0JZ Supplement Left Trunk Tendon with Synthetic Substitute, Open Approach

0LUB0KZ Supplement Left Trunk Tendon with Nonautologous Tissue Substitute, Open Approach

0LUB47Z Supplement Left Trunk Tendon with Autologous Tissue Substitute, Percutaneous Endoscopic Approach

0LUB4JZ Supplement Left Trunk Tendon with Synthetic Substitute, Percutaneous Endoscopic Approach

0LUB4KZ Supplement Left Trunk Tendon with Nonautologous Tissue Substitute, Percutaneous Endoscopic Approach

0LUC07Z Supplement Right Thorax Tendon with Autologous Tissue Substitute, Open Approach

0LUC0JZ Supplement Right Thorax Tendon with Synthetic Substitute, Open Approach

0LUC0KZ Supplement Right Thorax Tendon with Nonautologous Tissue Substitute, Open Approach

0LUC47Z Supplement Right Thorax Tendon with Autologous Tissue Substitute, Percutaneous Endoscopic Approach

0LUC4JZ Supplement Right Thorax Tendon with Synthetic Substitute, Percutaneous Endoscopic Approach

0LUC4KZ Supplement Right Thorax Tendon with Nonautologous Tissue Substitute, Percutaneous Endoscopic Approach

0LUD07Z Supplement Left Thorax Tendon with Autologous Tissue Substitute, Open Approach

0LUD0JZ Supplement Left Thorax Tendon with Synthetic Substitute, Open Approach

0LUD0KZ Supplement Left Thorax Tendon with Nonautologous Tissue Substitute, Open Approach

0LUD47Z Supplement Left Thorax Tendon with Autologous Tissue Substitute, Percutaneous Endoscopic Approach

0LUD4JZ Supplement Left Thorax Tendon with Synthetic Substitute, Percutaneous Endoscopic Approach

0LUD4KZ Supplement Left Thorax Tendon with Nonautologous Tissue Substitute, Percutaneous Endoscopic Approach

0LUF07Z Supplement Right Abdomen Tendon with Autologous Tissue Substitute, Open Approach

0LUF0JZ Supplement Right Abdomen Tendon with Synthetic Substitute, Open Approach

0LUF0KZ Supplement Right Abdomen Tendon with Nonautologous Tissue Substitute, Open Approach

0LUF47Z Supplement Right Abdomen Tendon with Autologous Tissue Substitute, Percutaneous Endoscopic Approach

0LUF4JZ Supplement Right Abdomen Tendon with Synthetic Substitute, Percutaneous Endoscopic Approach

0LUF4KZ Supplement Right Abdomen Tendon with Nonautologous Tissue Substitute, Percutaneous Endoscopic Approach

0LUG07Z Supplement Left Abdomen Tendon with Autologous Tissue Substitute, Open Approach

0LUG0JZ Supplement Left Abdomen Tendon with Synthetic Substitute, Open Approach

0LUG0KZ Supplement Left Abdomen Tendon with Nonautologous Tissue Substitute, Open Approach

0LUG47Z Supplement Left Abdomen Tendon with Autologous Tissue Substitute, Percutaneous Endoscopic Approach

0LUG4JZ Supplement Left Abdomen Tendon with Synthetic Substitute, Percutaneous Endoscopic Approach

0LUG4KZ Supplement Left Abdomen Tendon with Nonautologous Tissue Substitute, Percutaneous Endoscopic Approach

0LUH07Z Supplement Perineum Tendon with Autologous Tissue Substitute, Open Approach

0LUH0JZ Supplement Perineum Tendon with Synthetic Substitute, Open Approach

0LUH0KZ Supplement Perineum Tendon with Nonautologous Tissue Substitute, Open Approach

0LUH47Z Supplement Perineum Tendon with Autologous Tissue Substitute, Percutaneous Endoscopic Approach

0LUH4JZ Supplement Perineum Tendon with Synthetic Substitute, Percutaneous Endoscopic Approach

0LUH4KZ Supplement Perineum Tendon with Nonautologous Tissue Substitute, Percutaneous Endoscopic Approach

0LUJ07Z Supplement Right Hip Tendon with Autologous Tissue Substitute, Open Approach

0LUJ0JZ Supplement Right Hip Tendon with Synthetic Substitute, Open Approach

0LUJ0KZ Supplement Right Hip Tendon with Nonautologous Tissue Substitute, Open Approach

0LUJ47Z Supplement Right Hip Tendon with Autologous Tissue Substitute, Percutaneous Endoscopic Approach

0LUJ4JZ Supplement Right Hip Tendon with Synthetic Substitute, Percutaneous Endoscopic Approach

0LUJ4KZ Supplement Right Hip Tendon with Nonautologous Tissue Substitute, Percutaneous Endoscopic Approach

0LUK07Z Supplement Left Hip Tendon with Autologous Tissue Substitute, Open Approach

0LUK0JZ Supplement Left Hip Tendon with Synthetic Substitute, Open Approach

0LUK0KZ Supplement Left Hip Tendon with Nonautologous Tissue Substitute, Open Approach

0LUK47Z Supplement Left Hip Tendon with Autologous Tissue Substitute, Percutaneous Endoscopic Approach

0LUK4JZ Supplement Left Hip Tendon with Synthetic Substitute, Percutaneous Endoscopic Approach

0LUK4KZ Supplement Left Hip Tendon with Nonautologous Tissue Substitute, Percutaneous Endoscopic Approach

0LUL07Z Supplement Right Upper Leg Tendon with Autologous Tissue Substitute, Open Approach

0LUL0JZ Supplement Right Upper Leg Tendon with Synthetic Substitute, Open Approach

0LUL0KZ Supplement Right Upper Leg Tendon with Nonautologous Tissue Substitute, Open Approach

0LUL47Z Supplement Right Upper Leg Tendon with Autologous Tissue Substitute, Percutaneous Endoscopic Approach

0LUL4JZ Supplement Right Upper Leg Tendon with Synthetic Substitute, Percutaneous Endoscopic Approach

0LUL4KZ Supplement Right Upper Leg Tendon with Nonautologous Tissue Substitute, Percutaneous Endoscopic Approach

0LUM07Z Supplement Left Upper Leg Tendon with Autologous Tissue Substitute, Open Approach

0LUM0JZ Supplement Left Upper Leg Tendon with Synthetic Substitute, Open Approach

0LUM0KZ Supplement Left Upper Leg Tendon with Nonautologous Tissue Substitute, Open Approach
AHA CC: 2Q, 2015, 11

0LUM47Z Supplement Left Upper Leg Tendon with Autologous Tissue Substitute, Percutaneous Endoscopic Approach

0LUM4JZ Supplement Left Upper Leg Tendon with Synthetic Substitute, Percutaneous Endoscopic Approach

0LUM4KZ Supplement Left Upper Leg Tendon with Nonautologous Tissue Substitute, Percutaneous Endoscopic Approach

0LUN07Z Supplement Right Lower Leg Tendon with Autologous Tissue Substitute, Open Approach

0LUN0JZ Supplement Right Lower Leg Tendon with Synthetic Substitute, Open Approach

0LUN0KZ Supplement Right Lower Leg Tendon with Nonautologous Tissue Substitute, Open Approach

0LUN47Z Supplement Right Lower Leg Tendon with Autologous Tissue Substitute, Percutaneous Endoscopic Approach

0LUN4JZ Supplement Right Lower Leg Tendon with Synthetic Substitute, Percutaneous Endoscopic Approach

0LUN4KZ Supplement Right Lower Leg Tendon with Nonautologous Tissue Substitute, Percutaneous Endoscopic Approach

0LUP07Z Supplement Left Lower Leg Tendon with Autologous Tissue Substitute, Open Approach

0LUP0JZ Supplement Left Lower Leg Tendon with Synthetic Substitute, Open Approach

0LUP0KZ Supplement Left Lower Leg Tendon with Nonautologous Tissue Substitute, Open Approach

0LUP47Z Supplement Left Lower Leg Tendon with Autologous Tissue Substitute, Percutaneous Endoscopic Approach

0LUP4JZ Supplement Left Lower Leg Tendon with Synthetic Substitute, Percutaneous Endoscopic Approach

0LUP4KZ Supplement Left Lower Leg Tendon with Nonautologous Tissue Substitute, Percutaneous Endoscopic Approach

0LUQ07Z Supplement Right Knee Tendon with Autologous Tissue Substitute, Open Approach

0LUQ0JZ Supplement Right Knee Tendon with Synthetic Substitute, Open Approach

0LUQ0KZ Supplement Right Knee Tendon with Nonautologous Tissue Substitute, Open Approach
AHA CC: 2Q, 2015, 11

0LUQ47Z Supplement Right Knee Tendon with Autologous Tissue Substitute, Percutaneous Endoscopic Approach

0LUQ4JZ Supplement Right Knee Tendon with Synthetic Substitute, Percutaneous Endoscopic Approach

0LUQ4KZ Supplement Right Knee Tendon with Nonautologous Tissue Substitute, Percutaneous Endoscopic Approach

0LUR07Z Supplement Left Knee Tendon with Autologous Tissue Substitute, Open Approach

0LUR0JZ Supplement Left Knee Tendon with Synthetic Substitute, Open Approach

0LUR0KZ Supplement Left Knee Tendon with Nonautologous Tissue Substitute, Open Approach

0LUR47Z Supplement Left Knee Tendon with Autologous Tissue Substitute, Percutaneous Endoscopic Approach

0LUR4JZ Supplement Left Knee Tendon with Synthetic Substitute, Percutaneous Endoscopic Approach

0LUR4KZ Supplement Left Knee Tendon with Nonautologous Tissue Substitute, Percutaneous Endoscopic Approach

0LUS07Z Supplement Right Ankle Tendon with Autologous Tissue Substitute, Open Approach

0LUS0JZ Supplement Right Ankle Tendon with Synthetic Substitute, Open Approach

0LUS0KZ Supplement Right Ankle Tendon with Nonautologous Tissue Substitute, Open Approach

0LUS47Z Supplement Right Ankle Tendon with Autologous Tissue Substitute, Percutaneous Endoscopic Approach

0LUS4JZ Supplement Right Ankle Tendon with Synthetic Substitute, Percutaneous Endoscopic Approach

0LUS4KZ Supplement Right Ankle Tendon with Nonautologous Tissue Substitute, Percutaneous Endoscopic Approach

0LUT07Z Supplement Left Ankle Tendon with Autologous Tissue Substitute, Open Approach

0LUT0JZ Supplement Left Ankle Tendon with Synthetic Substitute, Open Approach

0LUT0KZ Supplement Left Ankle Tendon with Nonautologous Tissue Substitute, Open Approach

0LUT47Z Supplement Left Ankle Tendon with Autologous Tissue Substitute, Percutaneous Endoscopic Approach

0LUT4JZ Supplement Left Ankle Tendon with Synthetic Substitute, Percutaneous Endoscopic Approach

0LUT4KZ Supplement Left Ankle Tendon with Nonautologous Tissue Substitute, Percutaneous Endoscopic Approach

0LUV07Z Supplement Right Foot Tendon with Autologous Tissue Substitute, Open Approach

0LUV0JZ Supplement Right Foot Tendon with Synthetic Substitute, Open Approach

♀ Female-only ♂ Male-only ▲ Limited Coverage ● Non-OR **HAC** HAC-associated procedure ▲ Non-covered procedures ✚ Cluster

0LUV0KZ Supplement Right Foot Tendon with Nonautologous Tissue Substitute, Open Approach

0LUV47Z Supplement Right Foot Tendon with Autologous Tissue Substitute, Percutaneous Endoscopic Approach

0LUV4JZ Supplement Right Foot Tendon with Synthetic Substitute, Percutaneous Endoscopic Approach

0LUV4KZ Supplement Right Foot Tendon with Nonautologous Tissue

Substitute, Percutaneous Endoscopic Approach

0LUW07Z Supplement Left Foot Tendon with Autologous Tissue Substitute, Open Approach

0LUW0JZ Supplement Left Foot Tendon with Synthetic Substitute, Open Approach

0LUW0KZ Supplement Left Foot Tendon with Nonautologous Tissue Substitute, Open Approach

0LUW47Z Supplement Left Foot Tendon with Autologous Tissue Substitute, Percutaneous Endoscopic Approach

0LUW4JZ Supplement Left Foot Tendon with Synthetic Substitute, Percutaneous Endoscopic Approach

0LUW4KZ Supplement Left Foot Tendon with Nonautologous Tissue Substitute, Percutaneous Endoscopic Approach

0LW – Tendons, Revision

Review Coding Guideline B6.1c

0LWX00Z Revision of Drainage Device in Upper Tendon, Open Approach

0LWX07Z Revision of Autologous Tissue Substitute in Upper Tendon, Open Approach

0LWX0JZ Revision of Synthetic Substitute in Upper Tendon, Open Approach

0LWX0KZ Revision of Nonautologous Tissue Substitute in Upper Tendon, Open Approach

0LWX0YZ Revision of Other Device in Upper Tendon, Open Approach

0LWX30Z Revision of Drainage Device in Upper Tendon, Percutaneous Approach

0LWX37Z Revision of Autologous Tissue Substitute in Upper Tendon, Percutaneous Approach

0LWX3JZ Revision of Synthetic Substitute in Upper Tendon, Percutaneous Approach

0LWX3KZ Revision of Nonautologous Tissue Substitute in Upper Tendon, Percutaneous Approach

0LWX3YZ Revision of Other Device in Upper Tendon, Percutaneous Approach

0LWX40Z Revision of Drainage Device in Upper Tendon, Percutaneous Endoscopic Approach

0LWX47Z Revision of Autologous Tissue Substitute in Upper Tendon, Percutaneous Endoscopic Approach

0LWX4JZ Revision of Synthetic Substitute in Upper Tendon, Percutaneous Endoscopic Approach

0LWX4KZ Revision of Nonautologous Tissue Substitute in Upper Tendon, Percutaneous Endoscopic Approach

0LWX4YZ Revision of Other Device in Upper Tendon, Percutaneous Endoscopic Approach

0LWXX0Z Revision of Drainage Device in Upper Tendon, External Approach

0LWXX7Z Revision of Autologous Tissue Substitute in Upper Tendon, External Approach

0LWXXJZ Revision of Synthetic Substitute in Upper Tendon, External Approach

0LWXXKZ Revision of Nonautologous Tissue Substitute in Upper Tendon, External Approach

0LWY00Z Revision of Drainage Device in Lower Tendon, Open Approach

0LWY07Z Revision of Autologous Tissue Substitute in Lower Tendon, Open Approach

0LWY0JZ Revision of Synthetic Substitute in Lower Tendon, Open Approach

0LWY0KZ Revision of Nonautologous Tissue Substitute in Lower Tendon, Open Approach

0LWY0YZ Revision of Other Device in Lower Tendon, Open Approach

0LWY30Z Revision of Drainage Device in Lower Tendon, Percutaneous Approach

0LWY37Z Revision of Autologous Tissue Substitute in Lower Tendon, Percutaneous Approach

0LWY3JZ Revision of Synthetic Substitute in Lower Tendon, Percutaneous Approach

0LWY3KZ Revision of Nonautologous Tissue Substitute in Lower Tendon, Percutaneous Approach

0LWY3YZ Revision of Other Device in Lower Tendon, Percutaneous Approach

0LWY40Z Revision of Drainage Device in Lower Tendon, Percutaneous Endoscopic Approach

0LWY47Z Revision of Autologous Tissue Substitute in Lower Tendon, Percutaneous Endoscopic Approach

0LWY4JZ Revision of Synthetic Substitute in Lower Tendon, Percutaneous Endoscopic Approach

0LWY4KZ Revision of Nonautologous Tissue Substitute in Lower Tendon, Percutaneous Endoscopic Approach

0LWY4YZ Revision of Other Device in Lower Tendon, Percutaneous Endoscopic Approach

0LWYX0Z Revision of Drainage Device in Lower Tendon, External Approach

0LWYX7Z Revision of Autologous Tissue Substitute in Lower Tendon, External Approach

0LWYXJZ Revision of Synthetic Substitute in Lower Tendon, External Approach

0LWYXKZ Revision of Nonautologous Tissue Substitute in Lower Tendon, External Approach

0LX – Tendons, Transfer

0LX00ZZ Transfer Head and Neck Tendon, Open Approach

0LX04ZZ Transfer Head and Neck Tendon, Percutaneous Endoscopic Approach

0LX10ZZ Transfer Right Shoulder Tendon, Open Approach

0LX14ZZ Transfer Right Shoulder Tendon, Percutaneous Endoscopic Approach

0LX20ZZ Transfer Left Shoulder Tendon, Open Approach

0LX24ZZ Transfer Left Shoulder Tendon, Percutaneous Endoscopic Approach

0LX30ZZ Transfer Right Upper Arm Tendon, Open Approach

0LX34ZZ Transfer Right Upper Arm Tendon, Percutaneous Endoscopic Approach

0LX40ZZ Transfer Left Upper Arm Tendon, Open Approach

0LX44ZZ Transfer Left Upper Arm Tendon, Percutaneous Endoscopic Approach

0LX50ZZ Transfer Right Lower Arm and Wrist Tendon, Open Approach

0LX54ZZ Transfer Right Lower Arm and Wrist Tendon, Percutaneous Endoscopic Approach

0LX60ZZ Transfer Left Lower Arm and Wrist Tendon, Open Approach

0LX64ZZ Transfer Left Lower Arm and Wrist Tendon, Percutaneous Endoscopic Approach

0LX70ZZ Transfer Right Hand Tendon, Open Approach

0LX74ZZ Transfer Right Hand Tendon, Percutaneous Endoscopic Approach

0LX80ZZ Transfer Left Hand Tendon, Open Approach

0LX84ZZ Transfer Left Hand Tendon, Percutaneous Endoscopic Approach

0LX90ZZ Transfer Right Trunk Tendon, Open Approach

0LX94ZZ Transfer Right Trunk Tendon, Percutaneous Endoscopic Approach

0LXB0ZZ Transfer Left Trunk Tendon, Open Approach

0LXB4ZZ Transfer Left Trunk Tendon, Percutaneous Endoscopic Approach

0LXC0ZZ Transfer Right Thorax Tendon, Open Approach

0LXC4ZZ Transfer Right Thorax Tendon, Percutaneous Endoscopic Approach

0LXD0ZZ Transfer Left Thorax Tendon, Open Approach

0LXD4ZZ Transfer Left Thorax Tendon, Percutaneous Endoscopic Approach

0LXF0ZZ Transfer Right Abdomen Tendon, Open Approach

0LXF4ZZ Transfer Right Abdomen Tendon, Percutaneous Endoscopic Approach

0LXG0ZZ Transfer Left Abdomen Tendon, Open Approach

0LXG4ZZ Transfer Left Abdomen Tendon, Percutaneous Endoscopic Approach

0LXH0ZZ Transfer Perineum Tendon, Open Approach

0LXH4ZZ Transfer Perineum Tendon, Percutaneous Endoscopic Approach

0LXJ0ZZ	Transfer Right Hip Tendon, Open Approach
0LXJ4ZZ	Transfer Right Hip Tendon, Percutaneous Endoscopic Approach
0LXK0ZZ	Transfer Left Hip Tendon, Open Approach
0LXK4ZZ	Transfer Left Hip Tendon, Percutaneous Endoscopic Approach
0LXL0ZZ	Transfer Right Upper Leg Tendon, Open Approach
0LXL4ZZ	Transfer Right Upper Leg Tendon, Percutaneous Endoscopic Approach
0LXM0ZZ	Transfer Left Upper Leg Tendon, Open Approach
0LXM4ZZ	Transfer Left Upper Leg Tendon, Percutaneous Endoscopic Approach

0LXN0ZZ	Transfer Right Lower Leg Tendon, Open Approach
0LXN4ZZ	Transfer Right Lower Leg Tendon, Percutaneous Endoscopic Approach
0LXP0ZZ	Transfer Left Lower Leg Tendon, Open Approach
0LXP4ZZ	Transfer Left Lower Leg Tendon, Percutaneous Endoscopic Approach
0LXQ0ZZ	Transfer Right Knee Tendon, Open Approach
0LXQ4ZZ	Transfer Right Knee Tendon, Percutaneous Endoscopic Approach
0LXR0ZZ	Transfer Left Knee Tendon, Open Approach
0LXR4ZZ	Transfer Left Knee Tendon, Percutaneous Endoscopic Approach

0LXS0ZZ	Transfer Right Ankle Tendon, Open Approach
0LXS4ZZ	Transfer Right Ankle Tendon, Percutaneous Endoscopic Approach
0LXT0ZZ	Transfer Left Ankle Tendon, Open Approach
0LXT4ZZ	Transfer Left Ankle Tendon, Percutaneous Endoscopic Approach
0LXV0ZZ	Transfer Right Foot Tendon, Open Approach
0LXV4ZZ	Transfer Right Foot Tendon, Percutaneous Endoscopic Approach
0LXW0ZZ	Transfer Left Foot Tendon, Open Approach
0LXW4ZZ	Transfer Left Foot Tendon, Percutaneous Endoscopic Approach

Bursa of the Knee

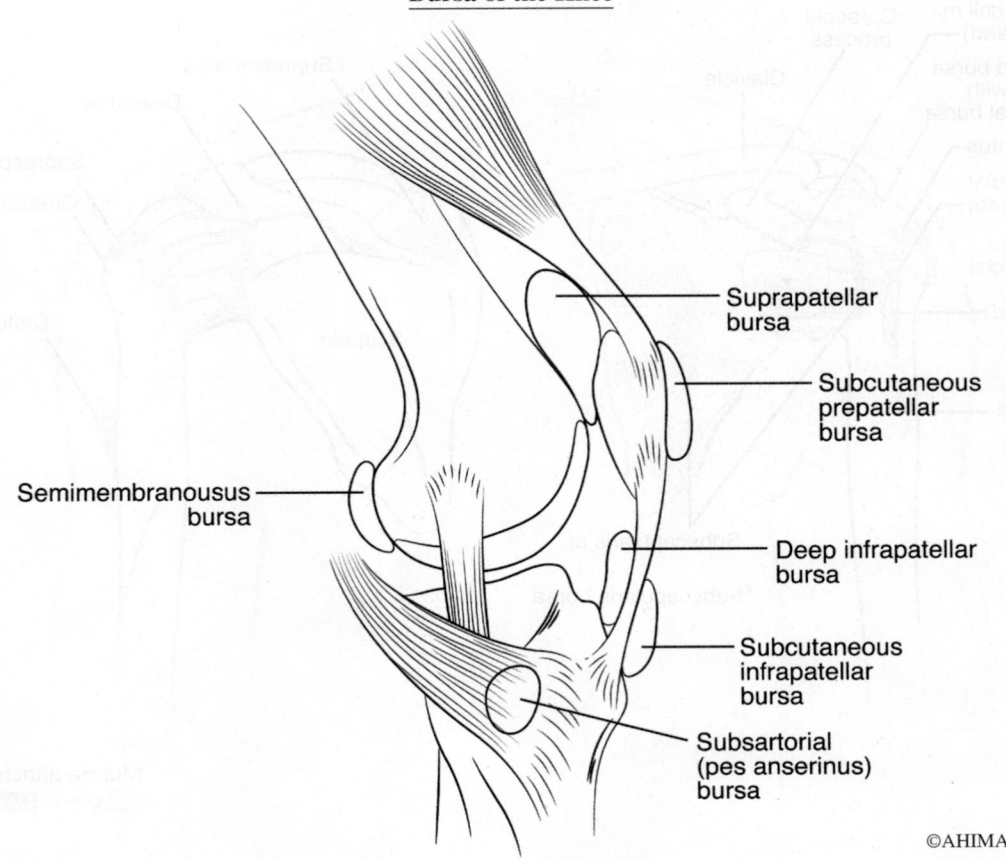

Suprapatellar bursa

Subcutaneous prepatellar bursa

Semimembranousus bursa

Deep infrapatellar bursa

Subcutaneous infrapatellar bursa

Subsartorial (pes anserinus) bursa

©AHIMA

Ligaments of the Knee

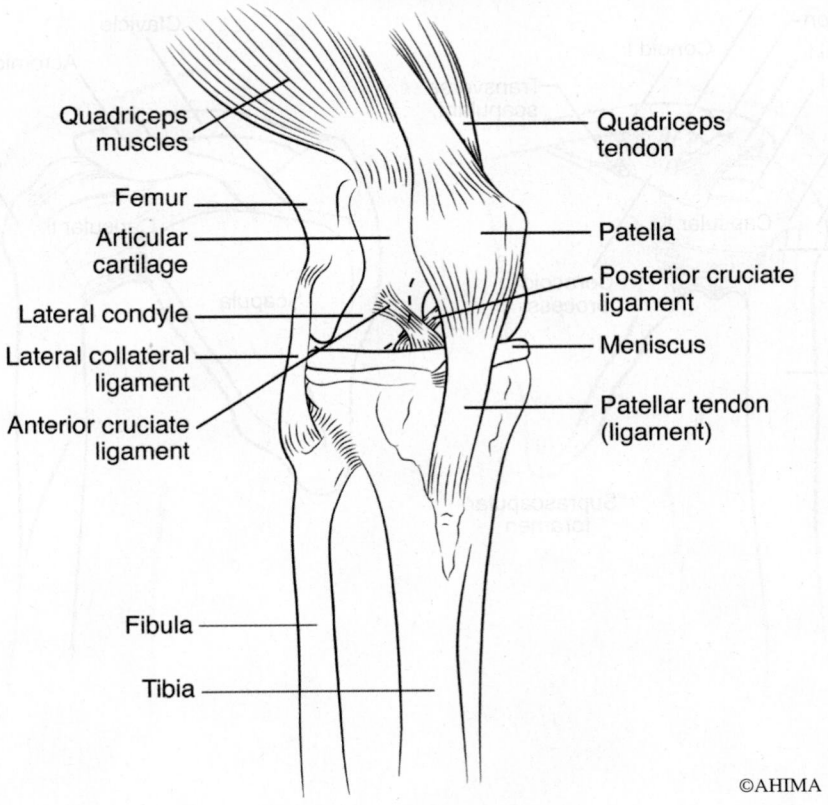

Quadriceps muscles

Femur

Articular cartilage

Lateral condyle

Lateral collateral ligament

Anterior cruciate ligament

Fibula

Tibia

Quadriceps tendon

Patella

Posterior cruciate ligament

Meniscus

Patellar tendon (ligament)

©AHIMA

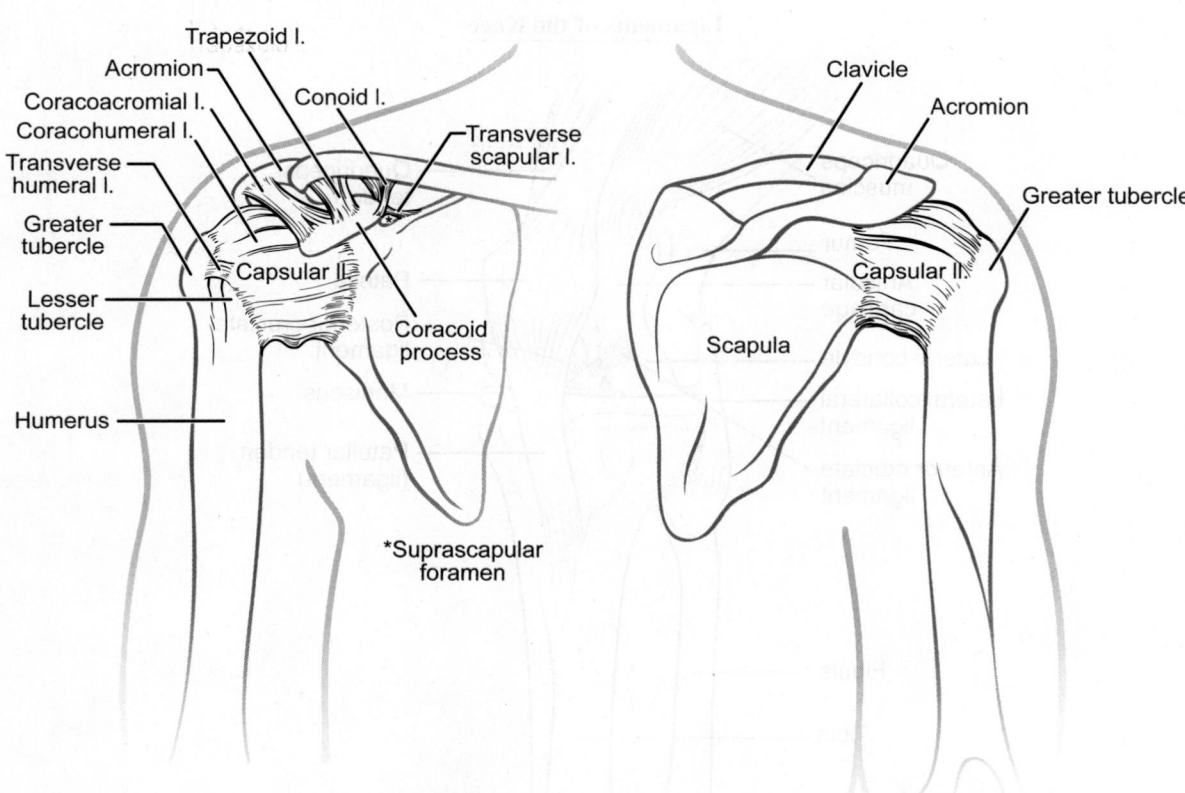

ANTERIOR

Biceps brachii m.
(short head)
Coracoid process
Clavicle

Subdeltoid bursa
fused with
subacromial bursa

Supraspinatus

Intertubercular
tendon sheath

Biceps brachii
tendon
(long head)

Humerus

Subscapularis m.

*Subscapularis bursa

POSTERIOR

Supraspinatus m.
Deltoid m.
Supraspinatus m.
Greater tubercle
Deltoid m.
Scapula

Muscle attachments
Origin   Insertion

©AHIMA

ANTERIOR

Trapezoid l.
Acromion
Coracoacromial l.
Coracohumeral l.
Transverse
humeral l.
Greater
tubercle
Lesser
tubercle
Humerus

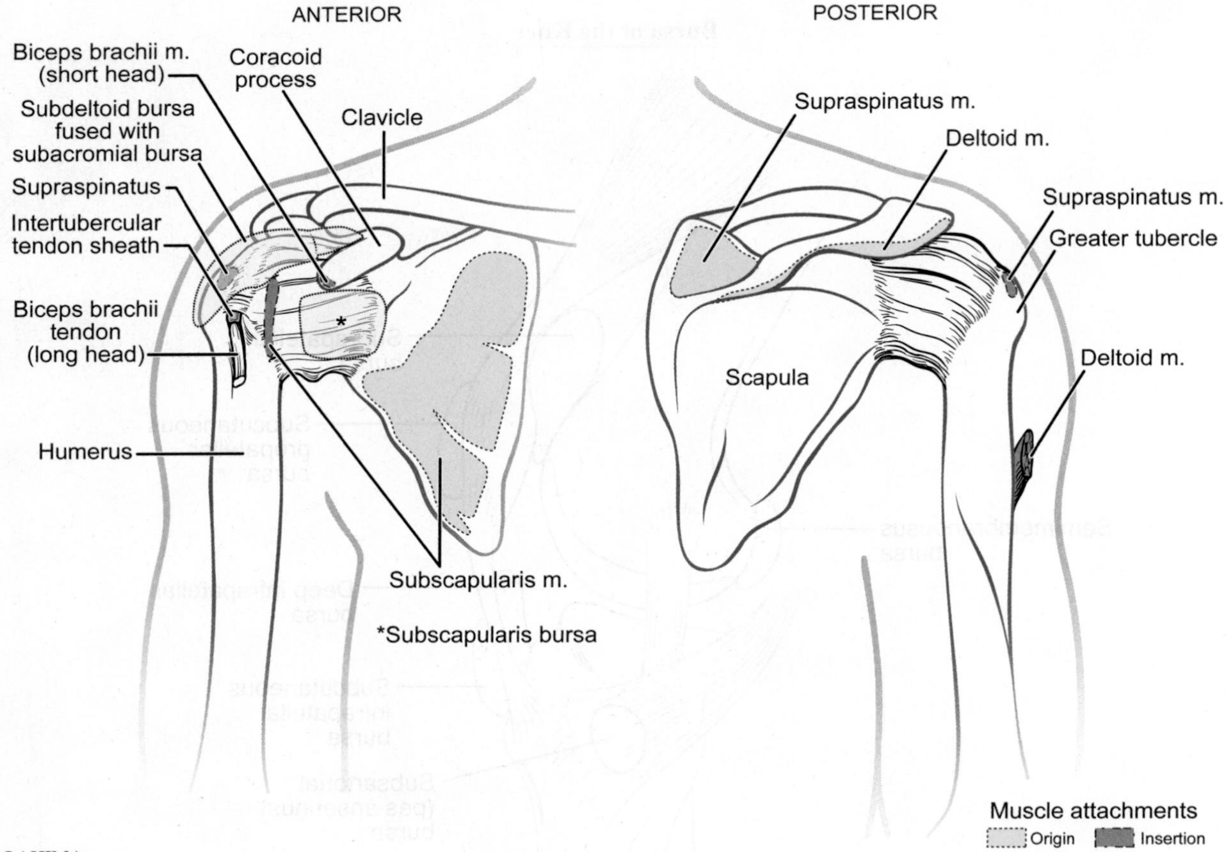

Conoid l.
Transverse
scapular l.
Capsular l.
Coracoid
process

*Suprascapular
foramen

POSTERIOR

Clavicle
Acromion
Greater tubercle
Capsular l.
Scapula

©AHIMA

Knee Tendons and Ligaments

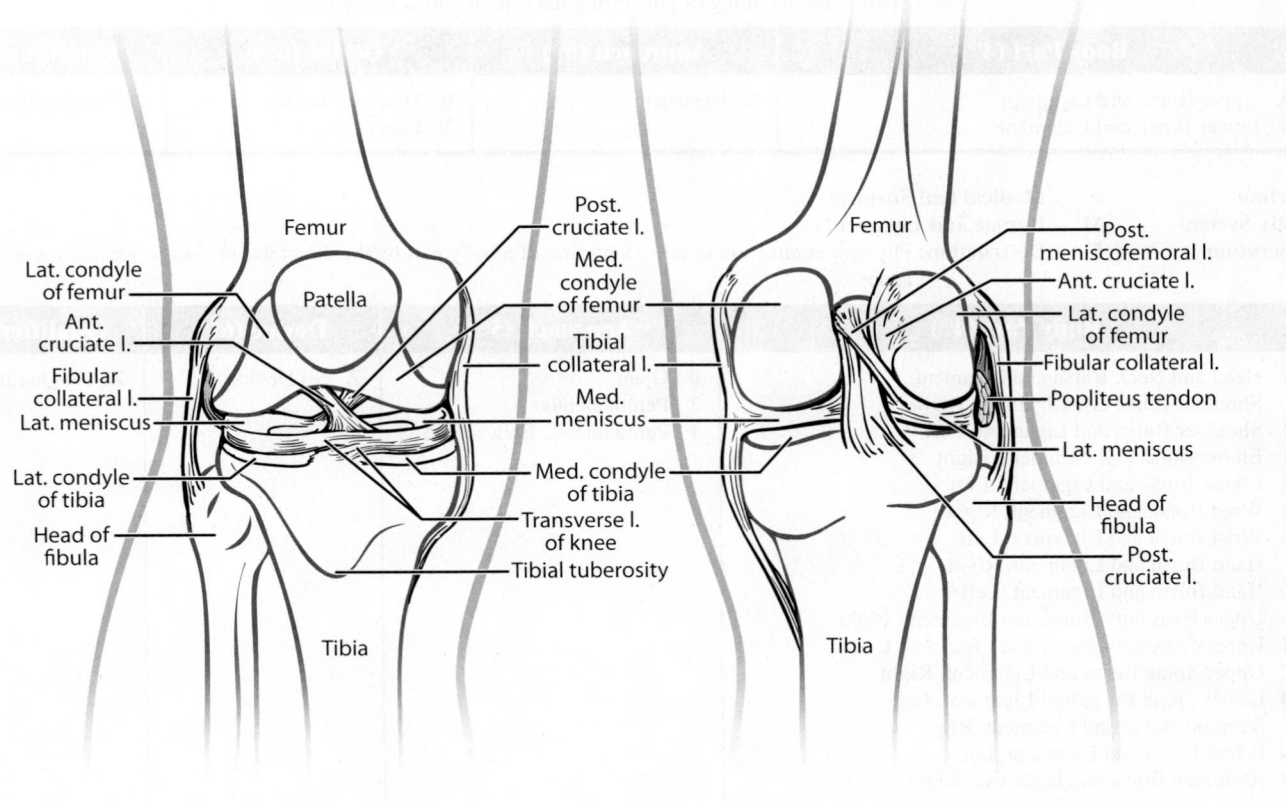

ANTERIOR

POSTERIOR

Femur

Patella

Lat. condyle of femur

Ant. cruciate l.

Fibular collateral l.

Lat. meniscus

Lat. condyle of tibia

Head of fibula

Tibia

Post. cruciate l.

Med. condyle of femur

Tibial collateral l.

Med. meniscus

Med. condyle of tibia

Transverse l. of knee

Tibial tuberosity

Femur

Post. meniscofemoral l.

Ant. cruciate l.

Lat. condyle of femur

Fibular collateral l.

Popliteus tendon

Lat. meniscus

Head of fibula

Post. cruciate l.

Tibia

©AHIMA

Hip Tendons and Ligaments

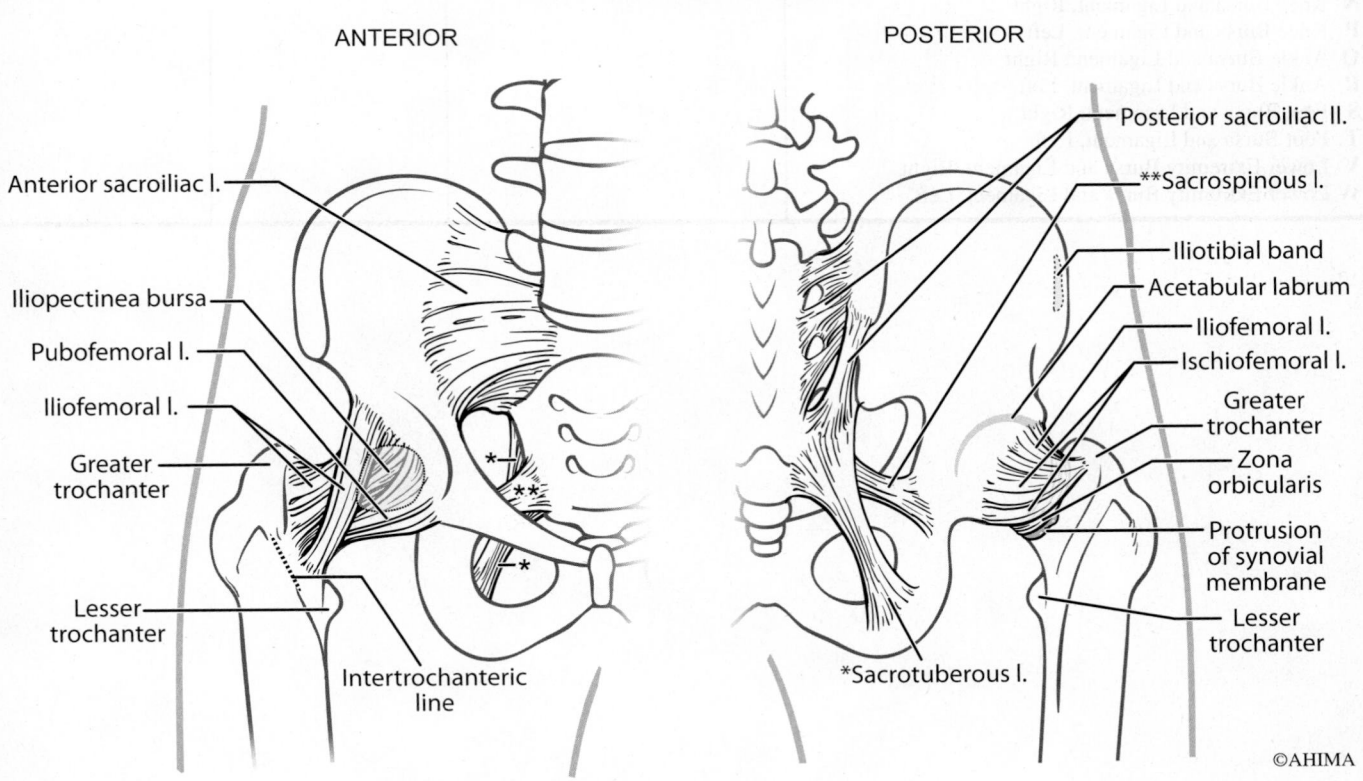

ANTERIOR

POSTERIOR

Anterior sacroiliac l.

Iliopectinea bursa

Pubofemoral l.

Iliofemoral l.

Greater trochanter

Lesser trochanter

Intertrochanteric line

*
**
*

Posterior sacroiliac ll.

**Sacrospinous l.

Iliotibial band

Acetabular labrum

Iliofemoral l.

Ischiofemoral l.

Greater trochanter

Zona orbicularis

Protrusion of synovial membrane

Lesser trochanter

*Sacrotuberous l.

©AHIMA

Bursae and Ligaments Tables 0M2–0MX

Section	0	Medical and Surgical
Body System	M	Bursae and Ligaments
Operation	2	**Change:** Taking out or off a device from a body part and putting back an identical or similar device in or on the same body part without cutting or puncturing the skin or a mucous membrane

Body Part (4th)	Approach (5th)	Device (6th)	Qualifier (7th)
X Upper Bursa and Ligament Y Lower Bursa and Ligament	X External	0 Drainage Device Y Other Device	Z No Qualifier

Section	0	Medical and Surgical
Body System	M	Bursae and Ligaments
Operation	5	**Destruction:** Physical eradication of all or a portion of a body part by the direct use of energy, force, or a destructive agent

Body Part (4th)	Approach (5th)	Device (6th)	Qualifier (7th)
0 Head and Neck Bursa and Ligament 1 Shoulder Bursa and Ligament, Right 2 Shoulder Bursa and Ligament, Left 3 Elbow Bursa and Ligament, Right 4 Elbow Bursa and Ligament, Left 5 Wrist Bursa and Ligament, Right 6 Wrist Bursa and Ligament, Left 7 Hand Bursa and Ligament, Right 8 Hand Bursa and Ligament, Left 9 Upper Extremity Bursa and Ligament, Right B Upper Extremity Bursa and Ligament, Left C Upper Spine Bursa and Ligament, Right D Lower Spine Bursa and Ligament, Left F Sternum Bursa and Ligament, Right G Rib(s) Bursa and Ligament, Left H Abdomen Bursa and Ligament, Right J Abdomen Bursa and Ligament, Left K Perineum Bursa and Ligament L Hip Bursa and Ligament, Right M Hip Bursa and Ligament, Left N Knee Bursa and Ligament, Right P Knee Bursa and Ligament, Left Q Ankle Bursa and Ligament, Right R Ankle Bursa and Ligament, Left S Foot Bursa and Ligament, Right T Foot Bursa and Ligament, Left V Lower Extremity Bursa and Ligament, Right W Lower Extremity Bursa and Ligament, Left	0 Open 3 Percutaneous 4 Percutaneous Endoscopic	Z No Device	Z No Qualifier

Section	0	Medical and Surgical
Body System	M	Bursae and Ligaments
Operation	8	**Division:** Cutting into a body part, without draining fluids and/or gases from the body part, in order to separate or transect a body part

Body Part (4th)	Approach (5th)	Device (6th)	Qualifier (7th)
0 Head and Neck Bursa and Ligament 1 Shoulder Bursa and Ligament, Right 2 Shoulder Bursa and Ligament, Left 3 Elbow Bursa and Ligament, Right 4 Elbow Bursa and Ligament, Left 5 Wrist Bursa and Ligament, Right 6 Wrist Bursa and Ligament, Left 7 Hand Bursa and Ligament, Right 8 Hand Bursa and Ligament, Left 9 Upper Extremity Bursa and Ligament, Right B Upper Extremity Bursa and Ligament, Left C Upper Spine Bursa and Ligament, Right D Lower Spine Bursa and Ligament, Left F Sternum Bursa and Ligament, Right G Rib(s) Bursa and Ligament, Left H Abdomen Bursa and Ligament, Right J Abdomen Bursa and Ligament, Left K Perineum Bursa and Ligament L Hip Bursa and Ligament, Right M Hip Bursa and Ligament, Left N Knee Bursa and Ligament, Right P Knee Bursa and Ligament, Left Q Ankle Bursa and Ligament, Right R Ankle Bursa and Ligament, Left S Foot Bursa and Ligament, Right T Foot Bursa and Ligament, Left V Lower Extremity Bursa and Ligament, Right W Lower Extremity Bursa and Ligament, Left	0 Open 3 Percutaneous 4 Percutaneous Endoscopic	Z No Device	Z No Qualifier

Section	0	Medical and Surgical
Body System	M	Bursae and Ligaments
Operation	9	**Drainage:** Taking or letting out fluids and/or gases from a body part

Body Part (4th)	Approach (5th)	Device (6th)	Qualifier (7th)
0 Head and Neck Bursa and Ligament 1 Shoulder Bursa and Ligament, Right 2 Shoulder Bursa and Ligament, Left 3 Elbow Bursa and Ligament, Right 4 Elbow Bursa and Ligament, Left 5 Wrist Bursa and Ligament, Right 6 Wrist Bursa and Ligament, Left 7 Hand Bursa and Ligament, Right 8 Hand Bursa and Ligament, Left 9 Upper Extremity Bursa and Ligament, Right B Upper Extremity Bursa and Ligament, Left C Upper Spine Bursa and Ligament, Right D Lower Spine Bursa and Ligament, Left F Sternum Bursa and Ligament, Right G Rib(s) Bursa and Ligament, Left H Abdomen Bursa and Ligament, Right J Abdomen Bursa and Ligament, Left K Perineum Bursa and Ligament L Hip Bursa and Ligament, Right M Hip Bursa and Ligament, Left N Knee Bursa and Ligament, Right P Knee Bursa and Ligament, Left Q Ankle Bursa and Ligament, Right R Ankle Bursa and Ligament, Left S Foot Bursa and Ligament, Right T Foot Bursa and Ligament, Left V Lower Extremity Bursa and Ligament, Right W Lower Extremity Bursa and Ligament, Left	0 Open 3 Percutaneous 4 Percutaneous Endoscopic	0 Drainage Device	Z No Qualifier

Continued →

Section	0	Medical and Surgical
Body System	M	Bursae and Ligaments
Operation	9	Drainage: Taking or letting out fluids and/or gases from a body part

Body Part (4th)	Approach (5th)	Device (6th)	Qualifier (7th)
0 Head and Neck Bursa and Ligament	0 Open	Z No Device	X Diagnostic
1 Shoulder Bursa and Ligament, Right	3 Percutaneous		Z No Qualifier
2 Shoulder Bursa and Ligament, Left	4 Percutaneous Endoscopic		
3 Elbow Bursa and Ligament, Right			
4 Elbow Bursa and Ligament, Left			
5 Wrist Bursa and Ligament, Right			
6 Wrist Bursa and Ligament, Left			
7 Hand Bursa and Ligament, Right			
8 Hand Bursa and Ligament, Left			
9 Upper Extremity Bursa and Ligament, Right			
B Upper Extremity Bursa and Ligament, Left			
C Upper Spine Bursa and Ligament, Right			
D Lower Spine Bursa and Ligament, Left			
F Sternum Bursa and Ligament, Right			
G Rib(s) Bursa and Ligament, Left			
H Abdomen Bursa and Ligament, Right			
J Abdomen Bursa and Ligament, Left			
K Perineum Bursa and Ligament			
L Hip Bursa and Ligament, Right			
M Hip Bursa and Ligament, Left			
N Knee Bursa and Ligament, Right			
P Knee Bursa and Ligament, Left			
Q Ankle Bursa and Ligament, Right			
R Ankle Bursa and Ligament, Left			
S Foot Bursa and Ligament, Right			
T Foot Bursa and Ligament, Left			
V Lower Extremity Bursa and Ligament, Right			
W Lower Extremity Bursa and Ligament, Left			

Section	0	Medical and Surgical
Body System	M	Bursae and Ligaments
Operation	B	Excision: Cutting out or off, without replacement, a portion of a body part

Body Part (4th)	Approach (5th)	Device (6th)	Qualifier (7th)
0 Head and Neck Bursa and Ligament	0 Open	Z No Device	X Diagnostic
1 Shoulder Bursa and Ligament, Right	3 Percutaneous		Z No Qualifier
2 Shoulder Bursa and Ligament, Left	4 Percutaneous Endoscopic		
3 Elbow Bursa and Ligament, Right			
4 Elbow Bursa and Ligament, Left			
5 Wrist Bursa and Ligament, Right			
6 Wrist Bursa and Ligament, Left			
7 Hand Bursa and Ligament, Right			
8 Hand Bursa and Ligament, Left			
9 Upper Extremity Bursa and Ligament, Right			
B Upper Extremity Bursa and Ligament, Left			
C Upper Spine Bursa and Ligament, Right			
D Lower Spine Bursa and Ligament, Left			
F Sternum Bursa and Ligament, Right			
G Rib(s) Bursa and Ligament, Left			
H Abdomen Bursa and Ligament, Right			
J Abdomen Bursa and Ligament, Left			
K Perineum Bursa and Ligament			
L Hip Bursa and Ligament, Right			
M Hip Bursa and Ligament, Left			
N Knee Bursa and Ligament, Right			
P Knee Bursa and Ligament, Left			
Q Ankle Bursa and Ligament, Right			
R Ankle Bursa and Ligament, Left			
S Foot Bursa and Ligament, Right			
T Foot Bursa and Ligament, Left			
V Lower Extremity Bursa and Ligament, Right			
W Lower Extremity Bursa and Ligament, Left			

Section | 0 | Medical and Surgical
Body System | M | Bursae and Ligaments
Operation | C | **Extirpation:** Taking or cutting out solid matter from a body part

Body Part (4th)	Approach (5th)	Device (6th)	Qualifier (7th)
0 Head and Neck Bursa and Ligament	0 Open	Z No Device	Z No Qualifier
1 Shoulder Bursa and Ligament, Right	3 Percutaneous		
2 Shoulder Bursa and Ligament, Left	4 Percutaneous Endoscopic		
3 Elbow Bursa and Ligament, Right			
4 Elbow Bursa and Ligament, Left			
5 Wrist Bursa and Ligament, Right			
6 Wrist Bursa and Ligament, Left			
7 Hand Bursa and Ligament, Right			
8 Hand Bursa and Ligament, Left			
9 Upper Extremity Bursa and Ligament, Right			
B Upper Extremity Bursa and Ligament, Left			
C Upper Spine Bursa and Ligament, Right			
D Trunk Bursa and Ligament, Left			
F Sternum Bursa and Ligament, Right			
G Rib(s) Bursa and Ligament, Left			
H Abdomen Bursa and Ligament, Right			
J Abdomen Bursa and Ligament, Left			
K Perineum Bursa and Ligament			
L Hip Bursa and Ligament, Right			
M Hip Bursa and Ligament, Left			
N Knee Bursa and Ligament, Right			
P Knee Bursa and Ligament, Left			
Q Ankle Bursa and Ligament, Right			
R Ankle Bursa and Ligament, Left			
S Foot Bursa and Ligament, Right			
T Foot Bursa and Ligament, Left			
V Lower Extremity Bursa and Ligament, Right			
W Lower Extremity Bursa and Ligament, Left			

Section | 0 | Medical and Surgical
Body System | M | Bursae and Ligaments
Operation | D | **Extraction:** Pulling or stripping out or off all or a portion of a body part by the use of force

Body Part (4th)	Approach (5th)	Device (6th)	Qualifier (7th)
0 Head and Neck Bursa and Ligament	0 Open	Z No Device	Z No Qualifier
1 Shoulder Bursa and Ligament, Right	3 Percutaneous		
2 Shoulder Bursa and Ligament, Left	4 Percutaneous Endoscopic		
3 Elbow Bursa and Ligament, Right			
4 Elbow Bursa and Ligament, Left			
5 Wrist Bursa and Ligament, Right			
6 Wrist Bursa and Ligament, Left			
7 Hand Bursa and Ligament, Right			
8 Hand Bursa and Ligament, Left			
9 Upper Extremity Bursa and Ligament, Right			
B Upper Extremity Bursa and Ligament, Left			
C Upper Spine Bursa and Ligament, Right			
D Lower Spine Bursa and Ligament, Left			
F Sternum Bursa and Ligament, Right			
G Rib(s) Bursa and Ligament, Left			
H Abdomen Bursa and Ligament, Right			
J Abdomen Bursa and Ligament, Left			
K Perineum Bursa and Ligament			
L Hip Bursa and Ligament, Right			
M Hip Bursa and Ligament, Left			
N Knee Bursa and Ligament, Right			
P Knee Bursa and Ligament, Left			
Q Ankle Bursa and Ligament, Right			
R Ankle Bursa and Ligament, Left			
S Foot Bursa and Ligament, Right			
T Foot Bursa and Ligament, Left			
V Lower Extremity Bursa and Ligament, Right			
W Lower Extremity Bursa and Ligament, Left			

Section	0	Medical and Surgical
Body System	M	Bursae and Ligaments
Operation	H	Insertion: Putting in a nonbiological appliance that monitors, assists, performs, or prevents a physiological function but does not physically take the place of a body part

Body Part (4th)	Approach (5th)	Device (6th)	Qualifier (7th)
X Upper Bursa and Ligament Y Lower Bursa and Ligament	0 Open 3 Percutaneous 4 Percutaneous Endoscopic	Y Other Device	Z No Qualifier

Section	0	Medical and Surgical
Body System	M	Bursae and Ligaments
Operation	J	Inspection: Visually and/or manually exploring a body part

Body Part (4th)	Approach (5th)	Device (6th)	Qualifier (7th)
X Upper Bursa and Ligament Y Lower Bursa and Ligament	0 Open 3 Percutaneous 4 Percutaneous Endoscopic X External	Z No Device	Z No Qualifier

Section	0	Medical and Surgical
Body System	M	Bursae and Ligaments
Operation	M	Reattachment: Putting back in or on all or a portion of a separated body part to its normal location or other suitable location

Body Part (4th)	Approach (5th)	Device (6th)	Qualifier (7th)
0 Head and Neck Bursa and Ligament 1 Shoulder Bursa and Ligament, Right 2 Shoulder Bursa and Ligament, Left 3 Elbow Bursa and Ligament, Right 4 Elbow Bursa and Ligament, Left 5 Wrist Bursa and Ligament, Right 6 Wrist Bursa and Ligament, Left 7 Hand Bursa and Ligament, Right 8 Hand Bursa and Ligament, Left 9 Upper Extremity Bursa and Ligament, Right B Upper Extremity Bursa and Ligament, Left C Upper Spine Bursa and Ligament, Right D Lower Spine Bursa and Ligament, Left F Sternum Bursa and Ligament, Right G Rib(s) Bursa and Ligament, Left H Abdomen Bursa and Ligament, Right J Abdomen Bursa and Ligament, Left K Perineum Bursa and Ligament L Hip Bursa and Ligament, Right M Hip Bursa and Ligament, Left N Knee Bursa and Ligament, Right P Knee Bursa and Ligament, Left Q Ankle Bursa and Ligament, Right R Ankle Bursa and Ligament, Left S Foot Bursa and Ligament, Right T Foot Bursa and Ligament, Left V Lower Extremity Bursa and Ligament, Right W Lower Extremity Bursa and Ligament, Left	0 Open 4 Percutaneous Endoscopic	Z No Device	Z No Qualifier

Section   **0**   **Medical and Surgical**
Body System   **M**   **Bursae and Ligaments**
Operation   **N**   **Release:** Freeing a body part from an abnormal physical constraint by cutting or by the use of force

Body Part (4th)	Approach (5th)	Device (6th)	Qualifier (7th)
0 Head and Neck Bursa and Ligament	0 Open	Z No Device	Z No Qualifier
1 Shoulder Bursa and Ligament, Right	3 Percutaneous		
2 Shoulder Bursa and Ligament, Left	4 Percutaneous Endoscopic		
3 Elbow Bursa and Ligament, Right	X External		
4 Elbow Bursa and Ligament, Left			
5 Wrist Bursa and Ligament, Right			
6 Wrist Bursa and Ligament, Left			
7 Hand Bursa and Ligament, Right			
8 Hand Bursa and Ligament, Left			
9 Upper Extremity Bursa and Ligament, Right			
B Upper Extremity Bursa and Ligament, Left			
C Upper Spine Bursa and Ligament, Right			
D Lower Spine Bursa and Ligament, Left			
F Sternum Bursa and Ligament, Right			
G Rib(s) Bursa and Ligament, Left			
H Abdomen Bursa and Ligament, Right			
J Abdomen Bursa and Ligament, Left			
K Perineum Bursa and Ligament			
L Hip Bursa and Ligament, Right			
M Hip Bursa and Ligament, Left			
N Knee Bursa and Ligament, Right			
P Knee Bursa and Ligament, Left			
Q Ankle Bursa and Ligament, Right			
R Ankle Bursa and Ligament, Left			
S Foot Bursa and Ligament, Right			
T Foot Bursa and Ligament, Left			
V Lower Extremity Bursa and Ligament, Right			
W Lower Extremity Bursa and Ligament, Left			

Section   **0**   **Medical and Surgical**
Body System   **M**   **Bursae and Ligaments**
Operation   **P**   **Removal:** Taking out or off a device from a body part

Body Part (4th)	Approach (5th)	Device (6th)	Qualifier (7th)
X Upper Bursa and Ligament	0 Open	0 Drainage Device	Z No Qualifier
Y Lower Bursa and Ligament	3 Percutaneous	7 Autologous Tissue Substitute	
	4 Percutaneous Endoscopic	J Synthetic Substitute	
		K Nonautologous Tissue Substitute	
		Y Other Device	
X Upper Bursa and Ligament	X External	0 Drainage Device	Z No Qualifier
Y Lower Bursa and Ligament			

Section	0	Medical and Surgical
Body System	M	Bursae and Ligaments
Operation	Q	**Repair:** Restoring, to the extent possible, a body part to its normal anatomic structure and function

Body Part (4ᵗʰ)	Approach (5ᵗʰ)	Device (6ᵗʰ)	Qualifier (7ᵗʰ)
0 Head and Neck Bursa and Ligament 1 Shoulder Bursa and Ligament, Right 2 Shoulder Bursa and Ligament, Left 3 Elbow Bursa and Ligament, Right 4 Elbow Bursa and Ligament, Left 5 Wrist Bursa and Ligament, Right 6 Wrist Bursa and Ligament, Left 7 Hand Bursa and Ligament, Right 8 Hand Bursa and Ligament, Left 9 Upper Extremity Bursa and Ligament, Right B Upper Extremity Bursa and Ligament, Left C Upper Spine Bursa and Ligament, Right D Lower Spine Bursa and Ligament, Left F Sternum Bursa and Ligament, Right G Rib(s) Bursa and Ligament, Left H Abdomen Bursa and Ligament, Right J Abdomen Bursa and Ligament, Left K Perineum Bursa and Ligament L Hip Bursa and Ligament, Right M Hip Bursa and Ligament, Left N Knee Bursa and Ligament, Right P Knee Bursa and Ligament, Left Q Ankle Bursa and Ligament, Right R Ankle Bursa and Ligament, Left S Foot Bursa and Ligament, Right T Foot Bursa and Ligament, Left V Lower Extremity Bursa and Ligament, Right W Lower Extremity Bursa and Ligament, Left	0 Open 3 Percutaneous 4 Percutaneous Endoscopic	Z No Device	Z No Qualifier

Section	0	Medical and Surgical
Body System	M	Bursae and Ligaments
Operation	R	**Replacement:** Putting in or on biological or synthetic material that physically takes the place and/or function of all or a portion of a body part

Body Part (4ᵗʰ)	Approach (5ᵗʰ)	Device (6ᵗʰ)	Qualifier (7ᵗʰ)
0 Head and Neck Bursa and Ligament 1 Shoulder Bursa and Ligament, Right 2 Shoulder Bursa and Ligament, Left 3 Elbow Bursa and Ligament, Right 4 Elbow Bursa and Ligament, Left 5 Wrist Bursa and Ligament, Right 6 Wrist Bursa and Ligament, Left 7 Hand Bursa and Ligament, Right 8 Hand Bursa and Ligament, Left 9 Upper Extremity Bursa and Ligament, Right B Upper Extremity Bursa and Ligament, Left C Upper Spine Bursa and Ligament D Lower Spine Bursa and Ligament F Sternum Bursa and Ligament G Rib(s) Bursa and Ligament H Abdomen Bursa and Ligament, Right J Abdomen Bursa and Ligament, Left K Perineum Bursa and Ligament L Hip Bursa and Ligament, Right M Hip Bursa and Ligament, Left N Knee Bursa and Ligament, Right P Knee Bursa and Ligament, Left Q Ankle Bursa and Ligament, Right R Ankle Bursa and Ligament, Left S Foot Bursa and Ligament, Right T Foot Bursa and Ligament, Left V Lower Extremity Bursa and Ligament, Right W Lower Extremity Bursa and Ligament, Left	0 Open 4 Percutaneous Endoscopic	7 Autologous Tissue Substitute J Synthetic Substitute K Nonautologous Tissue Substitute	Z No Qualifier

Section   **0**   **Medical and Surgical**
Body System   **M**   **Bursae and Ligaments**
Operation   **S**   **Reposition:** Moving to its normal location, or other suitable location, all or a portion of a body part

Body Part (4ᵗʰ)	Approach (5ᵗʰ)	Device (6ᵗʰ)	Qualifier (7ᵗʰ)
0 Head and Neck Bursa and Ligament	0 Open	Z No Device	Z No Qualifier
1 Shoulder Bursa and Ligament, Right	4 Percutaneous Endoscopic		
2 Shoulder Bursa and Ligament, Left			
3 Elbow Bursa and Ligament, Right			
4 Elbow Bursa and Ligament, Left			
5 Wrist Bursa and Ligament, Right			
6 Wrist Bursa and Ligament, Left			
7 Hand Bursa and Ligament, Right			
8 Hand Bursa and Ligament, Left			
9 Upper Extremity Bursa and Ligament, Right			
B Upper Extremity Bursa and Ligament, Left			
C Upper Spine Bursa and Ligament, Right			
D Lower Spine Bursa and Ligament, Left			
F Sternum Bursa and Ligament, Right			
G Rib(s) Bursa and Ligament, Left			
H Abdomen Bursa and Ligament, Right			
J Abdomen Bursa and Ligament, Left			
K Perineum Bursa and Ligament			
L Hip Bursa and Ligament, Right			
M Hip Bursa and Ligament, Left			
N Knee Bursa and Ligament, Right			
P Knee Bursa and Ligament, Left			
Q Ankle Bursa and Ligament, Right			
R Ankle Bursa and Ligament, Left			
S Foot Bursa and Ligament, Right			
T Foot Bursa and Ligament, Left			
V Lower Extremity Bursa and Ligament, Right			
W Lower Extremity Bursa and Ligament, Left			

Section   **0**   **Medical and Surgical**
Body System   **M**   **Bursae and Ligaments**
Operation   **T**   **Resection:** Cutting out or off, without replacement, all of a body part

Body Part (4ᵗʰ)	Approach (5ᵗʰ)	Device (6ᵗʰ)	Qualifier (7ᵗʰ)
0 Head and Neck Bursa and Ligament	0 Open	Z No Device	Z No Qualifier
1 Shoulder Bursa and Ligament, Right	4 Percutaneous Endoscopic		
2 Shoulder Bursa and Ligament, Left			
3 Elbow Bursa and Ligament, Right			
4 Elbow Bursa and Ligament, Left			
5 Wrist Bursa and Ligament, Right			
6 Wrist Bursa and Ligament, Left			
7 Hand Bursa and Ligament, Right			
8 Hand Bursa and Ligament, Left			
9 Upper Extremity Bursa and Ligament, Right			
B Upper Extremity Bursa and Ligament, Left			
C Upper Spine Bursa and Ligament, Right			
D Lower Spine Bursa and Ligament, Left			
F Sternum Bursa and Ligament, Right			
G Rib(s) Bursa and Ligament, Left			
H Abdomen Bursa and Ligament, Right			
J Abdomen Bursa and Ligament, Left			
K Perineum Bursa and Ligament			
L Hip Bursa and Ligament, Right			
M Hip Bursa and Ligament, Left			
N Knee Bursa and Ligament, Right			
P Knee Bursa and Ligament, Left			
Q Ankle Bursa and Ligament, Right			
R Ankle Bursa and Ligament, Left			
S Foot Bursa and Ligament, Right			
T Foot Bursa and Ligament, Left			
V Lower Extremity Bursa and Ligament, Right			
W Lower Extremity Bursa and Ligament, Left			

Section	0	Medical and Surgical
Body System	M	Bursae and Ligaments
Operation	U	Supplement: Putting in or on biological or synthetic material that physically reinforces and/or augments the function of a portion of a body part

Body Part (4th)	Approach (5th)	Device (6th)	Qualifier (7th)
0 Head and Neck Bursa and Ligament 1 Shoulder Bursa and Ligament, Right 2 Shoulder Bursa and Ligament, Left 3 Elbow Bursa and Ligament, Right 4 Elbow Bursa and Ligament, Left 5 Wrist Bursa and Ligament, Right 6 Wrist Bursa and Ligament, Left 7 Hand Bursa and Ligament, Right 8 Hand Bursa and Ligament, Left 9 Upper Extremity Bursa and Ligament, Right B Upper Extremity Bursa and Ligament, Left C Upper Spine Bursa and Ligament, Right D Lower Spine Bursa and Ligament, Left F Sternum Bursa and Ligament, Right G Rib(s) Bursa and Ligament, Left H Abdomen Bursa and Ligament, Right J Abdomen Bursa and Ligament, Left K Perineum Bursa and Ligament L Hip Bursa and Ligament, Right M Hip Bursa and Ligament, Left N Knee Bursa and Ligament, Right P Knee Bursa and Ligament, Left Q Ankle Bursa and Ligament, Right R Ankle Bursa and Ligament, Left S Foot Bursa and Ligament, Right T Foot Bursa and Ligament, Left V Lower Extremity Bursa and Ligament, Right W Lower Extremity Bursa and Ligament, Left	0 Open 4 Percutaneous Endoscopic	7 Autologous Tissue Substitute J Synthetic Substitute K Nonautologous Tissue Substitute	Z No Qualifier

Section	0	Medical and Surgical
Body System	M	Bursae and Ligaments
Operation	W	Revision: Correcting, to the extent possible, a portion of a malfunctioning device or the position of a displaced device

Body Part (4th)	Approach (5th)	Device (6th)	Qualifier (7th)
X Upper Bursa and Ligament Y Lower Bursa and Ligament	0 Open 3 Percutaneous 4 Percutaneous Endoscopic	0 Drainage Device 7 Autologous Tissue Substitute J Synthetic Substitute K Nonautologous Tissue Substitute Y Other Device	Z No Qualifier
X Upper Bursa and Ligament Y Lower Bursa and Ligament	X External	0 Drainage Device 7 Autologous Tissue Substitute J Synthetic Substitute K Nonautologous Tissue Substitute	Z No Qualifier

Section	0	Medical and Surgical
Body System	M	Bursae and Ligaments
Operation	X	**Transfer:** Moving, without taking out, all or a portion of a body part to another location to take over the function of all or a portion of a body part

Body Part (4th)	Approach (5th)	Device (6th)	Qualifier (7th)
0 Head and Neck Bursa and Ligament 1 Shoulder Bursa and Ligament, Right 2 Shoulder Bursa and Ligament, Left 3 Elbow Bursa and Ligament, Right 4 Elbow Bursa and Ligament, Left 5 Wrist Bursa and Ligament, Right 6 Wrist Bursa and Ligament, Left 7 Hand Bursa and Ligament, Right 8 Hand Bursa and Ligament, Left 9 Upper Extremity Bursa and Ligament, Right B Upper Extremity Bursa and Ligament, Left C Upper Spine Bursa and Ligament, Right D Lower Spine Bursa and Ligament, Left F Sternum Bursa and Ligament, Right G Rib(s) Bursa and Ligament, Left H Abdomen Bursa and Ligament, Right J Abdomen Bursa and Ligament, Left K Perineum Bursa and Ligament L Hip Bursa and Ligament, Right M Hip Bursa and Ligament, Left N Knee Bursa and Ligament, Right P Knee Bursa and Ligament, Left Q Ankle Bursa and Ligament, Right R Ankle Bursa and Ligament, Left S Foot Bursa and Ligament, Right T Foot Bursa and Ligament, Left V Lower Extremity Bursa and Ligament, Right W Lower Extremity Bursa and Ligament, Left	0 Open 4 Percutaneous Endoscopic	Z No Device	Z No Qualifier

Bursae and Ligaments Code Listing 0M2–0MX

Review Coding Guideline B4.5

0M2 – Bursae and Ligaments, Change

0M2XX0Z Change Drainage Device in Upper Bursa and Ligament, External Approach

0M2XXYZ Change Other Device in Upper Bursa and Ligament, External Approach

0M2YX0Z Change Drainage Device in Lower Bursa and Ligament, External Approach

0M2YXYZ Change Other Device in Lower Bursa and Ligament, External Approach

0M5 – Bursae and Ligaments, Destruction

Review Coding Guideline B6.1c

0M500ZZ Destruction of Head and Neck Bursa and Ligament, Open Approach

0M503ZZ Destruction of Head and Neck Bursa and Ligament, Percutaneous Approach

0M504ZZ Destruction of Head and Neck Bursa and Ligament, Percutaneous Endoscopic Approach

0M510ZZ Destruction of Right Shoulder Bursa and Ligament, Open Approach

0M513ZZ Destruction of Right Shoulder Bursa and Ligament, Percutaneous Approach

0M514ZZ Destruction of Right Shoulder Bursa and Ligament, Percutaneous Endoscopic Approach

0M520ZZ Destruction of Left Shoulder Bursa and Ligament, Open Approach

0M523ZZ Destruction of Left Shoulder Bursa and Ligament, Percutaneous Approach

0M524ZZ Destruction of Left Shoulder Bursa and Ligament, Percutaneous Endoscopic Approach

0M530ZZ Destruction of Right Elbow Bursa and Ligament, Open Approach

0M533ZZ Destruction of Right Elbow Bursa and Ligament, Percutaneous Approach

0M534ZZ Destruction of Right Elbow Bursa and Ligament, Percutaneous Endoscopic Approach

0M540ZZ Destruction of Left Elbow Bursa and Ligament, Open Approach

0M543ZZ Destruction of Left Elbow Bursa and Ligament, Percutaneous Approach

0M544ZZ Destruction of Left Elbow Bursa and Ligament, Percutaneous Endoscopic Approach

0M550ZZ Destruction of Right Wrist Bursa and Ligament, Open Approach

0M553ZZ Destruction of Right Wrist Bursa and Ligament, Percutaneous Approach

0M554ZZ Destruction of Right Wrist Bursa and Ligament, Percutaneous Endoscopic Approach

0M560ZZ Destruction of Left Wrist Bursa and Ligament, Open Approach

0M563ZZ Destruction of Left Wrist Bursa and Ligament, Percutaneous Approach

0M564ZZ Destruction of Left Wrist Bursa and Ligament, Percutaneous Endoscopic Approach

0M570ZZ Destruction of Right Hand Bursa and Ligament, Open Approach

0M573ZZ Destruction of Right Hand Bursa and Ligament, Percutaneous Approach

0M574ZZ Destruction of Right Hand Bursa and Ligament, Percutaneous Endoscopic Approach

♀ Female-only   ♂ Male-only   ▲ Limited Coverage   ● Non-OR   HAC HAC-associated procedure   ▲ Non-covered procedures   ✚ Cluster

0M580ZZ	Destruction of Left Hand Bursa and Ligament, Open Approach	**0M5G4ZZ**	Destruction of Rib(s) Bursa and Ligament, Percutaneous Endoscopic Approach	**0M5P4ZZ**	Destruction of Left Knee Bursa and Ligament, Percutaneous Endoscopic Approach
0M583ZZ	Destruction of Left Hand Bursa and Ligament, Percutaneous Approach	**0M5H0ZZ**	Destruction of Right Abdomen Bursa and Ligament, Open Approach	**0M5Q0ZZ**	Destruction of Right Ankle Bursa and Ligament, Open Approach
0M584ZZ	Destruction of Left Hand Bursa and Ligament, Percutaneous Endoscopic Approach	**0M5H3ZZ**	Destruction of Right Abdomen Bursa and Ligament, Percutaneous Approach	**0M5Q3ZZ**	Destruction of Right Ankle Bursa and Ligament, Percutaneous Approach
0M590ZZ	Destruction of Right Upper Extremity Bursa and Ligament, Open Approach	**0M5H4ZZ**	Destruction of Right Abdomen Bursa and Ligament, Percutaneous Endoscopic Approach	**0M5Q4ZZ**	Destruction of Right Ankle Bursa and Ligament, Percutaneous Endoscopic Approach
0M593ZZ	Destruction of Right Upper Extremity Bursa and Ligament, Percutaneous Approach	**0M5J0ZZ**	Destruction of Left Abdomen Bursa and Ligament, Open Approach	**0M5R0ZZ**	Destruction of Left Ankle Bursa and Ligament, Open Approach
0M594ZZ	Destruction of Right Upper Extremity Bursa and Ligament, Percutaneous Endoscopic Approach	**0M5J3ZZ**	Destruction of Left Abdomen Bursa and Ligament, Percutaneous Approach	**0M5R3ZZ**	Destruction of Left Ankle Bursa and Ligament, Percutaneous Approach
0M5B0ZZ	Destruction of Left Upper Extremity Bursa and Ligament, Open Approach	**0M5J4ZZ**	Destruction of Left Abdomen Bursa and Ligament, Percutaneous Endoscopic Approach	**0M5R4ZZ**	Destruction of Left Ankle Bursa and Ligament, Percutaneous Endoscopic Approach
0M5B3ZZ	Destruction of Left Upper Extremity Bursa and Ligament, Percutaneous Approach	**0M5K0ZZ**	Destruction of Perineum Bursa and Ligament, Open Approach	**0M5S0ZZ**	Destruction of Right Foot Bursa and Ligament, Open Approach
0M5B4ZZ	Destruction of Left Upper Extremity Bursa and Ligament, Percutaneous Endoscopic Approach	**0M5K3ZZ**	Destruction of Perineum Bursa and Ligament, Percutaneous Approach	**0M5S3ZZ**	Destruction of Right Foot Bursa and Ligament, Percutaneous Approach
0M5C0ZZ	Destruction of Upper Spine Bursa and Ligament, Open Approach	**0M5K4ZZ**	Destruction of Perineum Bursa and Ligament, Percutaneous Endoscopic Approach	**0M5S4ZZ**	Destruction of Right Foot Bursa and Ligament, Percutaneous Endoscopic Approach
0M5C3ZZ	Destruction of Upper Spine Bursa and Ligament, Percutaneous Approach	**0M5L0ZZ**	Destruction of Right Hip Bursa and Ligament, Open Approach	**0M5T0ZZ**	Destruction of Left Foot Bursa and Ligament, Open Approach
0M5C4ZZ	Destruction of Upper Spine Bursa and Ligament, Percutaneous Endoscopic Approach	**0M5L3ZZ**	Destruction of Right Hip Bursa and Ligament, Percutaneous Approach	**0M5T3ZZ**	Destruction of Left Foot Bursa and Ligament, Percutaneous Approach
0M5D0ZZ	Destruction of Lower Spine Bursa and Ligament, Open Approach	**0M5L4ZZ**	Destruction of Right Hip Bursa and Ligament, Percutaneous Endoscopic Approach	**0M5T4ZZ**	Destruction of Left Foot Bursa and Ligament, Percutaneous Endoscopic Approach
0M5D3ZZ	Destruction of Lower Spine Bursa and Ligament, Percutaneous Approach	**0M5M0ZZ**	Destruction of Left Hip Bursa and Ligament, Open Approach	**0M5V0ZZ**	Destruction of Right Lower Extremity Bursa and Ligament, Open Approach
0M5D4ZZ	Destruction of Lower Spine Bursa and Ligament, Percutaneous Endoscopic Approach	**0M5M3ZZ**	Destruction of Left Hip Bursa and Ligament, Percutaneous Approach	**0M5V3ZZ**	Destruction of Right Lower Extremity Bursa and Ligament, Percutaneous Approach
0M5F0ZZ	Destruction of Sternum Bursa and Ligament, Open Approach	**0M5M4ZZ**	Destruction of Left Hip Bursa and Ligament, Percutaneous Endoscopic Approach	**0M5V4ZZ**	Destruction of Right Lower Extremity Bursa and Ligament, Percutaneous Endoscopic Approach
0M5F3ZZ	Destruction of Sternum Bursa and Ligament, Percutaneous Approach	**0M5N0ZZ**	Destruction of Right Knee Bursa and Ligament, Open Approach	**0M5W0ZZ**	Destruction of Left Lower Extremity Bursa and Ligament, Open Approach
0M5F4ZZ	Destruction of Sternum Bursa and Ligament, Percutaneous Endoscopic Approach	**0M5N3ZZ**	Destruction of Right Knee Bursa and Ligament, Percutaneous Approach	**0M5W3ZZ**	Destruction of Left Lower Extremity Bursa and Ligament, Percutaneous Approach
0M5G0ZZ	Destruction of Rib(s) Bursa and Ligament, Open Approach	**0M5N4ZZ**	Destruction of Right Knee Bursa and Ligament, Percutaneous Endoscopic Approach	**0M5W4ZZ**	Destruction of Left Lower Extremity Bursa and Ligament, Percutaneous Endoscopic Approach
0M5G3ZZ	Destruction of Rib(s) Bursa and Ligament, Percutaneous Approach	**0M5P0ZZ**	Destruction of Left Knee Bursa and Ligament, Open Approach		
		0M5P3ZZ	Destruction of Left Knee Bursa and Ligament, Percutaneous Approach		

0M8 – Bursae and Ligaments, Division

Review Coding Guideline B3.14

0M800ZZ	Division of Head and Neck Bursa and Ligament, Open Approach	**0M830ZZ**	Division of Right Elbow Bursa and Ligament, Open Approach	**0M860ZZ**	Division of Left Wrist Bursa and Ligament, Open Approach
0M803ZZ	Division of Head and Neck Bursa and Ligament, Percutaneous Approach	**0M833ZZ**	Division of Right Elbow Bursa and Ligament, Percutaneous Approach	**0M863ZZ**	Division of Left Wrist Bursa and Ligament, Percutaneous Approach
0M804ZZ	Division of Head and Neck Bursa and Ligament, Percutaneous Endoscopic Approach	**0M834ZZ**	Division of Right Elbow Bursa and Ligament, Percutaneous Endoscopic Approach	**0M864ZZ**	Division of Left Wrist Bursa and Ligament, Percutaneous Endoscopic Approach
0M810ZZ	Division of Right Shoulder Bursa and Ligament, Open Approach	**0M840ZZ**	Division of Left Elbow Bursa and Ligament, Open Approach	**0M870ZZ**	Division of Right Hand Bursa and Ligament, Open Approach
0M813ZZ	Division of Right Shoulder Bursa and Ligament, Percutaneous Approach	**0M843ZZ**	Division of Left Elbow Bursa and Ligament, Percutaneous Approach	**0M873ZZ**	Division of Right Hand Bursa and Ligament, Percutaneous Approach
0M814ZZ	Division of Right Shoulder Bursa and Ligament, Percutaneous Endoscopic Approach	**0M844ZZ**	Division of Left Elbow Bursa and Ligament, Percutaneous Endoscopic Approach	**0M874ZZ**	Division of Right Hand Bursa and Ligament, Percutaneous Endoscopic Approach
0M820ZZ	Division of Left Shoulder Bursa and Ligament, Open Approach	**0M850ZZ**	Division of Right Wrist Bursa and Ligament, Open Approach	**0M880ZZ**	Division of Left Hand Bursa and Ligament, Open Approach
0M823ZZ	Division of Left Shoulder Bursa and Ligament, Percutaneous Approach	**0M853ZZ**	Division of Right Wrist Bursa and Ligament, Percutaneous Approach	**0M883ZZ**	Division of Left Hand Bursa and Ligament, Percutaneous Approach
0M824ZZ	Division of Left Shoulder Bursa and Ligament, Percutaneous Endoscopic Approach	**0M854ZZ**	Division of Right Wrist Bursa and Ligament, Percutaneous Endoscopic Approach	**0M884ZZ**	Division of Left Hand Bursa and Ligament, Percutaneous Endoscopic Approach

♀ Female-only   ♂ Male-only   ▲ Limited Coverage   ● Non-OR   **HAC** HAC-associated procedure   ▲ Non-covered procedures   ✚ Cluster

0M890ZZ	Division of Right Upper Extremity Bursa and Ligament, Open Approach
0M893ZZ	Division of Right Upper Extremity Bursa and Ligament, Percutaneous Approach
0M894ZZ	Division of Right Upper Extremity Bursa and Ligament, Percutaneous Endoscopic Approach
0M8B0ZZ	Division of Left Upper Extremity Bursa and Ligament, Open Approach
0M8B3ZZ	Division of Left Upper Extremity Bursa and Ligament, Percutaneous Approach
0M8B4ZZ	Division of Left Upper Extremity Bursa and Ligament, Percutaneous Endoscopic Approach
0M8C0ZZ	Division of Upper Spine Bursa and Ligament, Open Approach
0M8C3ZZ	Division of Upper Spine Bursa and Ligament, Percutaneous Approach
0M8C4ZZ	Division of Upper Spine Bursa and Ligament, Percutaneous Endoscopic Approach
0M8D0ZZ	Division of Lower Spine Bursa and Ligament, Open Approach
0M8D3ZZ	Division of Lower Spine Bursa and Ligament, Percutaneous Approach
0M8D4ZZ	Division of Lower Spine Bursa and Ligament, Percutaneous Endoscopic Approach
0M8F0ZZ	Division of Sternum Bursa and Ligament, Open Approach
0M8F3ZZ	Division of Sternum Bursa and Ligament, Percutaneous Approach
0M8F4ZZ	Division of Sternum Bursa and Ligament, Percutaneous Endoscopic Approach
0M8G0ZZ	Division of Rib(s) Bursa and Ligament, Open Approach
0M8G3ZZ	Division of Rib(s) Bursa and Ligament, Percutaneous Approach
0M8G4ZZ	Division of Rib(s) Bursa and Ligament, Percutaneous Endoscopic Approach
0M8H0ZZ	Division of Right Abdomen Bursa and Ligament, Open Approach
0M8H3ZZ	Division of Right Abdomen Bursa and Ligament, Percutaneous Approach
0M8H4ZZ	Division of Right Abdomen Bursa and Ligament, Percutaneous Endoscopic Approach
0M8J0ZZ	Division of Left Abdomen Bursa and Ligament, Open Approach
0M8J3ZZ	Division of Left Abdomen Bursa and Ligament, Percutaneous Approach
0M8J4ZZ	Division of Left Abdomen Bursa and Ligament, Percutaneous Endoscopic Approach
0M8K0ZZ	Division of Perineum Bursa and Ligament, Open Approach
0M8K3ZZ	Division of Perineum Bursa and Ligament, Percutaneous Approach
0M8K4ZZ	Division of Perineum Bursa and Ligament, Percutaneous Endoscopic Approach
0M8L0ZZ	Division of Right Hip Bursa and Ligament, Open Approach
0M8L3ZZ	Division of Right Hip Bursa and Ligament, Percutaneous Approach
0M8L4ZZ	Division of Right Hip Bursa and Ligament, Percutaneous Endoscopic Approach
0M8M0ZZ	Division of Left Hip Bursa and Ligament, Open Approach
0M8M3ZZ	Division of Left Hip Bursa and Ligament, Percutaneous Approach
0M8M4ZZ	Division of Left Hip Bursa and Ligament, Percutaneous Endoscopic Approach
0M8N0ZZ	Division of Right Knee Bursa and Ligament, Open Approach
0M8N3ZZ	Division of Right Knee Bursa and Ligament, Percutaneous Approach
0M8N4ZZ	Division of Right Knee Bursa and Ligament, Percutaneous Endoscopic Approach
0M8P0ZZ	Division of Left Knee Bursa and Ligament, Open Approach
0M8P3ZZ	Division of Left Knee Bursa and Ligament, Percutaneous Approach
0M8P4ZZ	Division of Left Knee Bursa and Ligament, Percutaneous Endoscopic Approach
0M8Q0ZZ	Division of Right Ankle Bursa and Ligament, Open Approach
0M8Q3ZZ	Division of Right Ankle Bursa and Ligament, Percutaneous Approach
0M8Q4ZZ	Division of Right Ankle Bursa and Ligament, Percutaneous Endoscopic Approach
0M8R0ZZ	Division of Left Ankle Bursa and Ligament, Open Approach
0M8R3ZZ	Division of Left Ankle Bursa and Ligament, Percutaneous Approach
0M8R4ZZ	Division of Left Ankle Bursa and Ligament, Percutaneous Endoscopic Approach
0M8S0ZZ	Division of Right Foot Bursa and Ligament, Open Approach
0M8S3ZZ	Division of Right Foot Bursa and Ligament, Percutaneous Approach
0M8S4ZZ	Division of Right Foot Bursa and Ligament, Percutaneous Endoscopic Approach
0M8T0ZZ	Division of Left Foot Bursa and Ligament, Open Approach
0M8T3ZZ	Division of Left Foot Bursa and Ligament, Percutaneous Approach
0M8T4ZZ	Division of Left Foot Bursa and Ligament, Percutaneous Endoscopic Approach
0M8V0ZZ	Division of Right Lower Extremity Bursa and Ligament, Open Approach
0M8V3ZZ	Division of Right Lower Extremity Bursa and Ligament, Percutaneous Approach
0M8V4ZZ	Division of Right Lower Extremity Bursa and Ligament, Percutaneous Endoscopic Approach
0M8W0ZZ	Division of Left Lower Extremity Bursa and Ligament, Open Approach
0M8W3ZZ	Division of Left Lower Extremity Bursa and Ligament, Percutaneous Approach
0M8W4ZZ	Division of Left Lower Extremity Bursa and Ligament, Percutaneous Endoscopic Approach

0M9 – Bursae and Ligaments, Drainage

Review Coding Guidelines B3.4a and B3.4b

Review Coding Guideline B6.2

0M9000Z	Drainage of Head and Neck Bursa and Ligament with Drainage Device, Open Approach
0M900ZX	Drainage of Head and Neck Bursa and Ligament, Open Approach, Diagnostic
0M900ZZ	Drainage of Head and Neck Bursa and Ligament, Open Approach
0M9030Z	Drainage of Head and Neck Bursa and Ligament with Drainage Device, Percutaneous Approach
0M903ZX	Drainage of Head and Neck Bursa and Ligament, Percutaneous Approach, Diagnostic
0M903ZZ	Drainage of Head and Neck Bursa and Ligament, Percutaneous Approach
0M9040Z	Drainage of Head and Neck Bursa and Ligament with Drainage Device, Percutaneous Endoscopic Approach
0M904ZX	Drainage of Head and Neck Bursa and Ligament, Percutaneous Endoscopic Approach, Diagnostic
0M904ZZ	Drainage of Head and Neck Bursa and Ligament, Percutaneous Endoscopic Approach
0M9100Z	Drainage of Right Shoulder Bursa and Ligament with Drainage Device, Open Approach
0M910ZX	Drainage of Right Shoulder Bursa and Ligament, Open Approach, Diagnostic
0M910ZZ	Drainage of Right Shoulder Bursa and Ligament, Open Approach
0M9130Z	Drainage of Right Shoulder Bursa and Ligament with Drainage Device, Percutaneous Approach
0M913ZX	Drainage of Right Shoulder Bursa and Ligament, Percutaneous Approach, Diagnostic
0M913ZZ	Drainage of Right Shoulder Bursa and Ligament, Percutaneous Approach
0M9140Z	Drainage of Right Shoulder Bursa and Ligament with Drainage Device, Percutaneous Endoscopic Approach
0M914ZX	Drainage of Right Shoulder Bursa and Ligament, Percutaneous Endoscopic Approach, Diagnostic
0M914ZZ	Drainage of Right Shoulder Bursa and Ligament, Percutaneous Endoscopic Approach
0M9200Z	Drainage of Left Shoulder Bursa and Ligament with Drainage Device, Open Approach
0M920ZX	Drainage of Left Shoulder Bursa and Ligament, Open Approach, Diagnostic
0M920ZZ	Drainage of Left Shoulder Bursa and Ligament, Open Approach
0M9230Z	Drainage of Left Shoulder Bursa and Ligament with Drainage Device, Percutaneous Approach
0M923ZX	Drainage of Left Shoulder Bursa and Ligament, Percutaneous Approach, Diagnostic
0M923ZZ	Drainage of Left Shoulder Bursa and Ligament, Percutaneous Approach

0M9240Z Drainage of Left Shoulder Bursa and Ligament with Drainage Device, Percutaneous Endoscopic Approach

0M924ZX Drainage of Left Shoulder Bursa and Ligament, Percutaneous Endoscopic Approach, Diagnostic

0M924ZZ Drainage of Left Shoulder Bursa and Ligament, Percutaneous Endoscopic Approach

0M9300Z Drainage of Right Elbow Bursa and Ligament with Drainage Device, Open Approach

0M930ZX Drainage of Right Elbow Bursa and Ligament, Open Approach, Diagnostic

0M930ZZ Drainage of Right Elbow Bursa and Ligament, Open Approach

0M9330Z Drainage of Right Elbow Bursa and Ligament with Drainage Device, Percutaneous Approach

0M933ZX Drainage of Right Elbow Bursa and Ligament, Percutaneous Approach, Diagnostic

0M933ZZ Drainage of Right Elbow Bursa and Ligament, Percutaneous Approach

0M9340Z Drainage of Right Elbow Bursa and Ligament with Drainage Device, Percutaneous Endoscopic Approach

0M934ZX Drainage of Right Elbow Bursa and Ligament, Percutaneous Endoscopic Approach, Diagnostic

0M934ZZ Drainage of Right Elbow Bursa and Ligament, Percutaneous Endoscopic Approach

0M9400Z Drainage of Left Elbow Bursa and Ligament with Drainage Device, Open Approach

0M940ZX Drainage of Left Elbow Bursa and Ligament, Open Approach, Diagnostic

0M940ZZ Drainage of Left Elbow Bursa and Ligament, Open Approach

0M9430Z Drainage of Left Elbow Bursa and Ligament with Drainage Device, Percutaneous Approach

0M943ZX Drainage of Left Elbow Bursa and Ligament, Percutaneous Approach, Diagnostic

0M943ZZ Drainage of Left Elbow Bursa and Ligament, Percutaneous Approach

0M9440Z Drainage of Left Elbow Bursa and Ligament with Drainage Device, Percutaneous Endoscopic Approach

0M944ZX Drainage of Left Elbow Bursa and Ligament, Percutaneous Endoscopic Approach, Diagnostic

0M944ZZ Drainage of Left Elbow Bursa and Ligament, Percutaneous Endoscopic Approach

0M9500Z Drainage of Right Wrist Bursa and Ligament with Drainage Device, Open Approach

0M950ZX Drainage of Right Wrist Bursa and Ligament, Open Approach, Diagnostic

0M950ZZ Drainage of Right Wrist Bursa and Ligament, Open Approach

0M9530Z Drainage of Right Wrist Bursa and Ligament with Drainage Device, Percutaneous Approach

0M953ZX Drainage of Right Wrist Bursa and Ligament, Percutaneous Approach, Diagnostic

0M953ZZ Drainage of Right Wrist Bursa and Ligament, Percutaneous Approach

0M9540Z Drainage of Right Wrist Bursa and Ligament with Drainage Device, Percutaneous Endoscopic Approach

0M954ZX Drainage of Right Wrist Bursa and Ligament, Percutaneous Endoscopic Approach, Diagnostic

0M954ZZ Drainage of Right Wrist Bursa and Ligament, Percutaneous Endoscopic Approach

0M9600Z Drainage of Left Wrist Bursa and Ligament with Drainage Device, Open Approach

0M960ZX Drainage of Left Wrist Bursa and Ligament, Open Approach, Diagnostic

0M960ZZ Drainage of Left Wrist Bursa and Ligament, Open Approach

0M9630Z Drainage of Left Wrist Bursa and Ligament with Drainage Device, Percutaneous Approach

0M963ZX Drainage of Left Wrist Bursa and Ligament, Percutaneous Approach, Diagnostic

0M963ZZ Drainage of Left Wrist Bursa and Ligament, Percutaneous Approach

0M9640Z Drainage of Left Wrist Bursa and Ligament with Drainage Device, Percutaneous Endoscopic Approach

0M964ZX Drainage of Left Wrist Bursa and Ligament, Percutaneous Endoscopic Approach, Diagnostic

0M964ZZ Drainage of Left Wrist Bursa and Ligament, Percutaneous Endoscopic Approach

0M9700Z Drainage of Right Hand Bursa and Ligament with Drainage Device, Open Approach

0M970ZX Drainage of Right Hand Bursa and Ligament, Open Approach, Diagnostic

0M970ZZ Drainage of Right Hand Bursa and Ligament, Open Approach

0M9730Z Drainage of Right Hand Bursa and Ligament with Drainage Device, Percutaneous Approach

0M973ZX Drainage of Right Hand Bursa and Ligament, Percutaneous Approach, Diagnostic

0M973ZZ Drainage of Right Hand Bursa and Ligament, Percutaneous Approach

0M9740Z Drainage of Right Hand Bursa and Ligament with Drainage Device, Percutaneous Endoscopic Approach

0M974ZX Drainage of Right Hand Bursa and Ligament, Percutaneous Endoscopic Approach, Diagnostic

0M974ZZ Drainage of Right Hand Bursa and Ligament, Percutaneous Endoscopic Approach

0M9800Z Drainage of Left Hand Bursa and Ligament with Drainage Device, Open Approach

0M980ZX Drainage of Left Hand Bursa and Ligament, Open Approach, Diagnostic

0M980ZZ Drainage of Left Hand Bursa and Ligament, Open Approach

0M9830Z Drainage of Left Hand Bursa and Ligament with Drainage Device, Percutaneous Approach

0M983ZX Drainage of Left Hand Bursa and Ligament, Percutaneous Approach, Diagnostic

0M983ZZ Drainage of Left Hand Bursa and Ligament, Percutaneous Approach

0M9840Z Drainage of Left Hand Bursa and Ligament with Drainage Device, Percutaneous Endoscopic Approach

0M984ZX Drainage of Left Hand Bursa and Ligament, Percutaneous Endoscopic Approach, Diagnostic

0M984ZZ Drainage of Left Hand Bursa and Ligament, Percutaneous Endoscopic Approach

0M9900Z Drainage of Right Upper Extremity Bursa and Ligament with Drainage Device, Open Approach

0M990ZX Drainage of Right Upper Extremity Bursa and Ligament, Open Approach, Diagnostic

0M990ZZ Drainage of Right Upper Extremity Bursa and Ligament, Open Approach

0M9930Z Drainage of Right Upper Extremity Bursa and Ligament with Drainage Device, Percutaneous Approach

0M993ZX Drainage of Right Upper Extremity Bursa and Ligament, Percutaneous Approach, Diagnostic

0M993ZZ Drainage of Right Upper Extremity Bursa and Ligament, Percutaneous Approach

0M9940Z Drainage of Right Upper Extremity Bursa and Ligament with Drainage Device, Percutaneous Endoscopic Approach

0M994ZX Drainage of Right Upper Extremity Bursa and Ligament, Percutaneous Endoscopic Approach, Diagnostic

0M994ZZ Drainage of Right Upper Extremity Bursa and Ligament, Percutaneous Endoscopic Approach

0M9B00Z Drainage of Left Upper Extremity Bursa and Ligament with Drainage Device, Open Approach

0M9B0ZX Drainage of Left Upper Extremity Bursa and Ligament, Open Approach, Diagnostic

0M9B0ZZ Drainage of Left Upper Extremity Bursa and Ligament, Open Approach

0M9B30Z Drainage of Left Upper Extremity Bursa and Ligament with Drainage Device, Percutaneous Approach

0M9B3ZX Drainage of Left Upper Extremity Bursa and Ligament, Percutaneous Approach, Diagnostic

0M9B3ZZ Drainage of Left Upper Extremity Bursa and Ligament, Percutaneous Approach

0M9B40Z Drainage of Left Upper Extremity Bursa and Ligament with Drainage Device, Percutaneous Endoscopic Approach

0M9B4ZX Drainage of Left Upper Extremity Bursa and Ligament, Percutaneous Endoscopic Approach, Diagnostic

0M9B4ZZ Drainage of Left Upper Extremity Bursa and Ligament, Percutaneous Endoscopic Approach

0M9C00Z Drainage of Upper Spine Bursa and Ligament with Drainage Device, Open Approach

0M9C0ZX Drainage of Upper Spine Bursa and Ligament, Open Approach, Diagnostic

0M9C0ZZ Drainage of Upper Spine Bursa and Ligament, Open Approach

0M9C30Z Drainage of Upper Spine Bursa and Ligament with Drainage Device, Percutaneous Approach

0M9C3ZX Drainage of Upper Spine Bursa and Ligament, Percutaneous Approach, Diagnostic

0M9C3ZZ Drainage of Upper Spine Bursa and Ligament, Percutaneous Approach

0M9C40Z Drainage of Upper Spine Bursa and Ligament with Drainage Device, Percutaneous Endoscopic Approach

♀ Female-only   ♂ Male-only   ▲ Limited Coverage   ● Non-OR   **HAC** HAC-associated procedure   ▲ Non-covered procedures   ✚ Cluster

0M9C4ZX Drainage of Upper Spine Bursa and Ligament, Percutaneous Endoscopic Approach, Diagnostic

0M9C4ZZ Drainage of Upper Spine Bursa and Ligament, Percutaneous Endoscopic Approach

0M9D00Z Drainage of Lower Spine Bursa and Ligament with Drainage Device, Open Approach

0M9D0ZX Drainage of Lower Spine Bursa and Ligament, Open Approach, Diagnostic

0M9D0ZZ Drainage of Lower Spine Bursa and Ligament, Open Approach

0M9D30Z Drainage of Lower Spine Bursa and Ligament with Drainage Device, Percutaneous Approach

0M9D3ZX Drainage of Lower Spine Bursa and Ligament, Percutaneous Approach, Diagnostic

0M9D3ZZ Drainage of Lower Spine Bursa and Ligament, Percutaneous Approach

0M9D40Z Drainage of Lower Spine Bursa and Ligament with Drainage Device, Percutaneous Endoscopic Approach

0M9D4ZX Drainage of Lower Spine Bursa and Ligament, Percutaneous Endoscopic Approach, Diagnostic

0M9D4ZZ Drainage of Lower Spine Bursa and Ligament, Percutaneous Endoscopic Approach

0M9F00Z Drainage of Sternum Bursa and Ligament with Drainage Device, Open Approach

0M9F0ZX Drainage of Sternum Bursa and Ligament, Open Approach, Diagnostic

0M9F0ZZ Drainage of Sternum Bursa and Ligament, Open Approach

0M9F30Z Drainage of Sternum Bursa and Ligament with Drainage Device, Percutaneous Approach

0M9F3ZX Drainage of Sternum Bursa and Ligament, Percutaneous Approach, Diagnostic

0M9F3ZZ Drainage of Sternum Bursa and Ligament, Percutaneous Approach

0M9F40Z Drainage of Sternum Bursa and Ligament with Drainage Device, Percutaneous Endoscopic Approach

0M9F4ZX Drainage of Sternum Bursa and Ligament, Percutaneous Endoscopic Approach, Diagnostic

0M9F4ZZ Drainage of Sternum Bursa and Ligament, Percutaneous Endoscopic Approach

0M9G00Z Drainage of Rib(s) Bursa and Ligament with Drainage Device, Open Approach

0M9G0ZX Drainage of Rib(s) Bursa and Ligament, Open Approach, Diagnostic

0M9G0ZZ Drainage of Rib(s) Bursa and Ligament, Open Approach

0M9G30Z Drainage of Rib(s) Bursa and Ligament with Drainage Device, Percutaneous Approach

0M9G3ZX Drainage of Rib(s) Bursa and Ligament, Percutaneous Approach, Diagnostic

0M9G3ZZ Drainage of Rib(s) Bursa and Ligament, Percutaneous Approach

0M9G40Z Drainage of Rib(s) Bursa and Ligament with Drainage Device, Percutaneous Endoscopic Approach

0M9G4ZX Drainage of Rib(s) Bursa and Ligament, Percutaneous Endoscopic Approach, Diagnostic

0M9G4ZZ Drainage of Rib(s) Bursa and Ligament, Percutaneous Endoscopic Approach

0M9H00Z Drainage of Right Abdomen Bursa and Ligament with Drainage Device, Open Approach

0M9H0ZX Drainage of Right Abdomen Bursa and Ligament, Open Approach, Diagnostic

0M9H0ZZ Drainage of Right Abdomen Bursa and Ligament, Open Approach

0M9H30Z Drainage of Right Abdomen Bursa and Ligament with Drainage Device, Percutaneous Approach

0M9H3ZX Drainage of Right Abdomen Bursa and Ligament, Percutaneous Approach, Diagnostic

0M9H3ZZ Drainage of Right Abdomen Bursa and Ligament, Percutaneous Approach

0M9H40Z Drainage of Right Abdomen Bursa and Ligament with Drainage Device, Percutaneous Endoscopic Approach

0M9H4ZX Drainage of Right Abdomen Bursa and Ligament, Percutaneous Endoscopic Approach, Diagnostic

0M9H4ZZ Drainage of Right Abdomen Bursa and Ligament, Percutaneous Endoscopic Approach

0M9J00Z Drainage of Left Abdomen Bursa and Ligament with Drainage Device, Open Approach

0M9J0ZX Drainage of Left Abdomen Bursa and Ligament, Open Approach, Diagnostic

0M9J0ZZ Drainage of Left Abdomen Bursa and Ligament, Open Approach

0M9J30Z Drainage of Left Abdomen Bursa and Ligament with Drainage Device, Percutaneous Approach

0M9J3ZX Drainage of Left Abdomen Bursa and Ligament, Percutaneous Approach, Diagnostic

0M9J3ZZ Drainage of Left Abdomen Bursa and Ligament, Percutaneous Approach

0M9J40Z Drainage of Left Abdomen Bursa and Ligament with Drainage Device, Percutaneous Endoscopic Approach

0M9J4ZX Drainage of Left Abdomen Bursa and Ligament, Percutaneous Endoscopic Approach, Diagnostic

0M9J4ZZ Drainage of Left Abdomen Bursa and Ligament, Percutaneous Endoscopic Approach

0M9K00Z Drainage of Perineum Bursa and Ligament with Drainage Device, Open Approach

0M9K0ZX Drainage of Perineum Bursa and Ligament, Open Approach, Diagnostic

0M9K0ZZ Drainage of Perineum Bursa and Ligament, Open Approach

0M9K30Z Drainage of Perineum Bursa and Ligament with Drainage Device, Percutaneous Approach

0M9K3ZX Drainage of Perineum Bursa and Ligament, Percutaneous Approach, Diagnostic

0M9K3ZZ Drainage of Perineum Bursa and Ligament, Percutaneous Approach

0M9K40Z Drainage of Perineum Bursa and Ligament with Drainage Device, Percutaneous Endoscopic Approach

0M9K4ZX Drainage of Perineum Bursa and Ligament, Percutaneous Endoscopic Approach, Diagnostic

0M9K4ZZ Drainage of Perineum Bursa and Ligament, Percutaneous Endoscopic Approach

0M9L00Z Drainage of Right Hip Bursa and Ligament with Drainage Device, Open Approach

0M9L0ZX Drainage of Right Hip Bursa and Ligament, Open Approach, Diagnostic

0M9L0ZZ Drainage of Right Hip Bursa and Ligament, Open Approach

0M9L30Z Drainage of Right Hip Bursa and Ligament with Drainage Device, Percutaneous Approach

0M9L3ZX Drainage of Right Hip Bursa and Ligament, Percutaneous Approach, Diagnostic

0M9L3ZZ Drainage of Right Hip Bursa and Ligament, Percutaneous Approach

0M9L40Z Drainage of Right Hip Bursa and Ligament with Drainage Device, Percutaneous Endoscopic Approach

0M9L4ZX Drainage of Right Hip Bursa and Ligament, Percutaneous Endoscopic Approach, Diagnostic

0M9L4ZZ Drainage of Right Hip Bursa and Ligament, Percutaneous Endoscopic Approach

0M9M00Z Drainage of Left Hip Bursa and Ligament with Drainage Device, Open Approach

0M9M0ZX Drainage of Left Hip Bursa and Ligament, Open Approach, Diagnostic

0M9M0ZZ Drainage of Left Hip Bursa and Ligament, Open Approach

0M9M30Z Drainage of Left Hip Bursa and Ligament with Drainage Device, Percutaneous Approach

0M9M3ZX Drainage of Left Hip Bursa and Ligament, Percutaneous Approach, Diagnostic

0M9M3ZZ Drainage of Left Hip Bursa and Ligament, Percutaneous Approach

0M9M40Z Drainage of Left Hip Bursa and Ligament with Drainage Device, Percutaneous Endoscopic Approach

0M9M4ZX Drainage of Left Hip Bursa and Ligament, Percutaneous Endoscopic Approach, Diagnostic

0M9M4ZZ Drainage of Left Hip Bursa and Ligament, Percutaneous Endoscopic Approach

0M9N00Z Drainage of Right Knee Bursa and Ligament with Drainage Device, Open Approach

0M9N0ZX Drainage of Right Knee Bursa and Ligament, Open Approach, Diagnostic

0M9N0ZZ Drainage of Right Knee Bursa and Ligament, Open Approach

0M9N30Z Drainage of Right Knee Bursa and Ligament with Drainage Device, Percutaneous Approach

0M9N3ZX Drainage of Right Knee Bursa and Ligament, Percutaneous Approach, Diagnostic

0M9N3ZZ Drainage of Right Knee Bursa and Ligament, Percutaneous Approach

0M9N40Z Drainage of Right Knee Bursa and Ligament with Drainage Device, Percutaneous Endoscopic Approach

0M9N4ZX Drainage of Right Knee Bursa and Ligament, Percutaneous Endoscopic Approach, Diagnostic

0M9N4ZZ Drainage of Right Knee Bursa and Ligament, Percutaneous Endoscopic Approach

Code	Description	Code	Description	Code	Description
0M9P00Z	Drainage of Left Knee Bursa and Ligament with Drainage Device, Open Approach	0M9R3ZX	Drainage of Left Ankle Bursa and Ligament, Percutaneous Approach, Diagnostic	0M9T4ZZ	Drainage of Left Foot Bursa and Ligament, Percutaneous Endoscopic Approach
0M9P0ZX	Drainage of Left Knee Bursa and Ligament, Open Approach, Diagnostic	0M9R3ZZ	Drainage of Left Ankle Bursa and Ligament, Percutaneous Approach	0M9V00Z	Drainage of Right Lower Extremity Bursa and Ligament with Drainage Device, Open Approach
0M9P0ZZ	Drainage of Left Knee Bursa and Ligament, Open Approach	0M9R40Z	Drainage of Left Ankle Bursa and Ligament with Drainage Device, Percutaneous Endoscopic Approach	0M9V0ZX	Drainage of Right Lower Extremity Bursa and Ligament, Open Approach, Diagnostic
0M9P30Z	Drainage of Left Knee Bursa and Ligament with Drainage Device, Percutaneous Approach	0M9R4ZX	Drainage of Left Ankle Bursa and Ligament, Percutaneous Endoscopic Approach, Diagnostic	0M9V0ZZ	Drainage of Right Lower Extremity Bursa and Ligament, Open Approach
0M9P3ZX	Drainage of Left Knee Bursa and Ligament, Percutaneous Approach, Diagnostic	0M9R4ZZ	Drainage of Left Ankle Bursa and Ligament, Percutaneous Endoscopic Approach	0M9V30Z	Drainage of Right Lower Extremity Bursa and Ligament with Drainage Device, Percutaneous Approach
0M9P3ZZ	Drainage of Left Knee Bursa and Ligament, Percutaneous Approach	0M9S00Z	Drainage of Right Foot Bursa and Ligament with Drainage Device, Open Approach	0M9V3ZX	Drainage of Right Lower Extremity Bursa and Ligament, Percutaneous Approach, Diagnostic
0M9P40Z	Drainage of Left Knee Bursa and Ligament with Drainage Device, Percutaneous Endoscopic Approach	0M9S0ZX	Drainage of Right Foot Bursa and Ligament, Open Approach, Diagnostic	0M9V3ZZ	Drainage of Right Lower Extremity Bursa and Ligament, Percutaneous Approach
0M9P4ZX	Drainage of Left Knee Bursa and Ligament, Percutaneous Endoscopic Approach, Diagnostic	0M9S0ZZ	Drainage of Right Foot Bursa and Ligament, Open Approach	0M9V40Z	Drainage of Right Lower Extremity Bursa and Ligament with Drainage Device, Percutaneous Endoscopic Approach
0M9P4ZZ	Drainage of Left Knee Bursa and Ligament, Percutaneous Endoscopic Approach	0M9S30Z	Drainage of Right Foot Bursa and Ligament with Drainage Device, Percutaneous Approach	0M9V4ZX	Drainage of Right Lower Extremity Bursa and Ligament, Percutaneous Endoscopic Approach, Diagnostic
0M9Q00Z	Drainage of Right Ankle Bursa and Ligament with Drainage Device, Open Approach	0M9S3ZX	Drainage of Right Foot Bursa and Ligament, Percutaneous Approach, Diagnostic	0M9V4ZZ	Drainage of Right Lower Extremity Bursa and Ligament, Percutaneous Endoscopic Approach
0M9Q0ZX	Drainage of Right Ankle Bursa and Ligament, Open Approach, Diagnostic	0M9S3ZZ	Drainage of Right Foot Bursa and Ligament, Percutaneous Approach	0M9W00Z	Drainage of Left Lower Extremity Bursa and Ligament with Drainage Device, Open Approach
0M9Q0ZZ	Drainage of Right Ankle Bursa and Ligament, Open Approach	0M9S40Z	Drainage of Right Foot Bursa and Ligament with Drainage Device, Percutaneous Endoscopic Approach	0M9W0ZX	Drainage of Left Lower Extremity Bursa and Ligament, Open Approach, Diagnostic
0M9Q30Z	Drainage of Right Ankle Bursa and Ligament with Drainage Device, Percutaneous Approach	0M9S4ZX	Drainage of Right Foot Bursa and Ligament, Percutaneous Endoscopic Approach, Diagnostic	0M9W0ZZ	Drainage of Left Lower Extremity Bursa and Ligament, Open Approach
0M9Q3ZX	Drainage of Right Ankle Bursa and Ligament, Percutaneous Approach, Diagnostic	0M9S4ZZ	Drainage of Right Foot Bursa and Ligament, Percutaneous Endoscopic Approach	0M9W30Z	Drainage of Left Lower Extremity Bursa and Ligament with Drainage Device, Percutaneous Approach
0M9Q3ZZ	Drainage of Right Ankle Bursa and Ligament, Percutaneous Approach	0M9T00Z	Drainage of Left Foot Bursa and Ligament with Drainage Device, Open Approach	0M9W3ZX	Drainage of Left Lower Extremity Bursa and Ligament, Percutaneous Approach, Diagnostic
0M9Q40Z	Drainage of Right Ankle Bursa and Ligament with Drainage Device, Percutaneous Endoscopic Approach	0M9T0ZX	Drainage of Left Foot Bursa and Ligament, Open Approach, Diagnostic	0M9W3ZZ	Drainage of Left Lower Extremity Bursa and Ligament, Percutaneous Approach
0M9Q4ZX	Drainage of Right Ankle Bursa and Ligament, Percutaneous Endoscopic Approach, Diagnostic	0M9T0ZZ	Drainage of Left Foot Bursa and Ligament, Open Approach	0M9W40Z	Drainage of Left Lower Extremity Bursa and Ligament with Drainage Device, Percutaneous Endoscopic Approach
0M9Q4ZZ	Drainage of Right Ankle Bursa and Ligament, Percutaneous Endoscopic Approach	0M9T30Z	Drainage of Left Foot Bursa and Ligament with Drainage Device, Percutaneous Approach	0M9W4ZX	Drainage of Left Lower Extremity Bursa and Ligament, Percutaneous Endoscopic Approach, Diagnostic
0M9R00Z	Drainage of Left Ankle Bursa and Ligament with Drainage Device, Open Approach	0M9T3ZX	Drainage of Left Foot Bursa and Ligament, Percutaneous Approach, Diagnostic	0M9W4ZZ	Drainage of Left Lower Extremity Bursa and Ligament, Percutaneous Endoscopic Approach
0M9R0ZX	Drainage of Left Ankle Bursa and Ligament, Open Approach, Diagnostic	0M9T3ZZ	Drainage of Left Foot Bursa and Ligament, Percutaneous Approach		
0M9R0ZZ	Drainage of Left Ankle Bursa and Ligament, Open Approach	0M9T40Z	Drainage of Left Foot Bursa and Ligament with Drainage Device, Percutaneous Endoscopic Approach		
0M9R30Z	Drainage of Left Ankle Bursa and Ligament with Drainage Device, Percutaneous Approach	0M9T4ZX	Drainage of Left Foot Bursa and Ligament, Percutaneous Endoscopic Approach, Diagnostic		

0MB – Bursae and Ligaments, Excision

Review Coding Guidelines B3.4a and B3.4b

Review Coding Guideline B3.5

Review Coding Guideline B3.8

Review Coding Guideline B3.18

Code	Description	Code	Description	Code	Description
0MB00ZX	Excision of Head and Neck Bursa and Ligament, Open Approach, Diagnostic	0MB03ZX	Excision of Head and Neck Bursa and Ligament, Percutaneous Approach, Diagnostic	0MB04ZX	Excision of Head and Neck Bursa and Ligament, Percutaneous Endoscopic Approach, Diagnostic
0MB00ZZ	Excision of Head and Neck Bursa and Ligament, Open Approach	0MB03ZZ	Excision of Head and Neck Bursa and Ligament, Percutaneous Approach	0MB04ZZ	Excision of Head and Neck Bursa and Ligament, Percutaneous Endoscopic Approach

♀ Female-only   ♂ Male-only   ▲ Limited Coverage   ● Non-OR   HAC HAC-associated procedure   ▲ Non-covered procedures   ✚ Cluster

0MB10ZX Excision of Right Shoulder Bursa and Ligament, Open Approach, Diagnostic

0MB10ZZ Excision of Right Shoulder Bursa and Ligament, Open Approach

0MB13ZX Excision of Right Shoulder Bursa and Ligament, Percutaneous Approach, Diagnostic

0MB13ZZ Excision of Right Shoulder Bursa and Ligament, Percutaneous Approach

0MB14ZX Excision of Right Shoulder Bursa and Ligament, Percutaneous Endoscopic Approach, Diagnostic

0MB14ZZ Excision of Right Shoulder Bursa and Ligament, Percutaneous Endoscopic Approach

0MB20ZX Excision of Left Shoulder Bursa and Ligament, Open Approach, Diagnostic

0MB20ZZ Excision of Left Shoulder Bursa and Ligament, Open Approach

0MB23ZX Excision of Left Shoulder Bursa and Ligament, Percutaneous Approach, Diagnostic

0MB23ZZ Excision of Left Shoulder Bursa and Ligament, Percutaneous Approach

0MB24ZX Excision of Left Shoulder Bursa and Ligament, Percutaneous Endoscopic Approach, Diagnostic

0MB24ZZ Excision of Left Shoulder Bursa and Ligament, Percutaneous Endoscopic Approach

0MB30ZX Excision of Right Elbow Bursa and Ligament, Open Approach, Diagnostic

0MB30ZZ Excision of Right Elbow Bursa and Ligament, Open Approach

0MB33ZX Excision of Right Elbow Bursa and Ligament, Percutaneous Approach, Diagnostic

0MB33ZZ Excision of Right Elbow Bursa and Ligament, Percutaneous Approach

0MB34ZX Excision of Right Elbow Bursa and Ligament, Percutaneous Endoscopic Approach, Diagnostic

0MB34ZZ Excision of Right Elbow Bursa and Ligament, Percutaneous Endoscopic Approach

0MB40ZX Excision of Left Elbow Bursa and Ligament, Open Approach, Diagnostic

0MB40ZZ Excision of Left Elbow Bursa and Ligament, Open Approach

0MB43ZX Excision of Left Elbow Bursa and Ligament, Percutaneous Approach, Diagnostic

0MB43ZZ Excision of Left Elbow Bursa and Ligament, Percutaneous Approach

0MB44ZX Excision of Left Elbow Bursa and Ligament, Percutaneous Endoscopic Approach, Diagnostic

0MB44ZZ Excision of Left Elbow Bursa and Ligament, Percutaneous Endoscopic Approach

0MB50ZX Excision of Right Wrist Bursa and Ligament, Open Approach, Diagnostic

0MB50ZZ Excision of Right Wrist Bursa and Ligament, Open Approach

0MB53ZX Excision of Right Wrist Bursa and Ligament, Percutaneous Approach, Diagnostic

0MB53ZZ Excision of Right Wrist Bursa and Ligament, Percutaneous Approach

0MB54ZX Excision of Right Wrist Bursa and Ligament, Percutaneous Endoscopic Approach, Diagnostic

0MB54ZZ Excision of Right Wrist Bursa and Ligament, Percutaneous Endoscopic Approach

0MB60ZX Excision of Left Wrist Bursa and Ligament, Open Approach, Diagnostic

0MB60ZZ Excision of Left Wrist Bursa and Ligament, Open Approach

0MB63ZX Excision of Left Wrist Bursa and Ligament, Percutaneous Approach, Diagnostic

0MB63ZZ Excision of Left Wrist Bursa and Ligament, Percutaneous Approach

0MB64ZX Excision of Left Wrist Bursa and Ligament, Percutaneous Endoscopic Approach, Diagnostic

0MB64ZZ Excision of Left Wrist Bursa and Ligament, Percutaneous Endoscopic Approach

0MB70ZX Excision of Right Hand Bursa and Ligament, Open Approach, Diagnostic

0MB70ZZ Excision of Right Hand Bursa and Ligament, Open Approach

0MB73ZX Excision of Right Hand Bursa and Ligament, Percutaneous Approach, Diagnostic

0MB73ZZ Excision of Right Hand Bursa and Ligament, Percutaneous Approach

0MB74ZX Excision of Right Hand Bursa and Ligament, Percutaneous Endoscopic Approach, Diagnostic

0MB74ZZ Excision of Right Hand Bursa and Ligament, Percutaneous Endoscopic Approach

0MB80ZX Excision of Left Hand Bursa and Ligament, Open Approach, Diagnostic

0MB80ZZ Excision of Left Hand Bursa and Ligament, Open Approach

0MB83ZX Excision of Left Hand Bursa and Ligament, Percutaneous Approach, Diagnostic

0MB83ZZ Excision of Left Hand Bursa and Ligament, Percutaneous Approach

0MB84ZX Excision of Left Hand Bursa and Ligament, Percutaneous Endoscopic Approach, Diagnostic

0MB84ZZ Excision of Left Hand Bursa and Ligament, Percutaneous Endoscopic Approach

0MB90ZX Excision of Right Upper Extremity Bursa and Ligament, Open Approach, Diagnostic

0MB90ZZ Excision of Right Upper Extremity Bursa and Ligament, Open Approach

0MB93ZX Excision of Right Upper Extremity Bursa and Ligament, Percutaneous Approach, Diagnostic

0MB93ZZ Excision of Right Upper Extremity Bursa and Ligament, Percutaneous Approach

0MB94ZX Excision of Right Upper Extremity Bursa and Ligament, Percutaneous Endoscopic Approach, Diagnostic

0MB94ZZ Excision of Right Upper Extremity Bursa and Ligament, Percutaneous Endoscopic Approach

0MBB0ZX Excision of Left Upper Extremity Bursa and Ligament, Open Approach, Diagnostic

0MBB0ZZ Excision of Left Upper Extremity Bursa and Ligament, Open Approach

0MBB3ZX Excision of Left Upper Extremity Bursa and Ligament, Percutaneous Approach, Diagnostic

0MBB3ZZ Excision of Left Upper Extremity Bursa and Ligament, Percutaneous Approach

0MBB4ZX Excision of Left Upper Extremity Bursa and Ligament, Percutaneous Endoscopic Approach, Diagnostic

0MBB4ZZ Excision of Left Upper Extremity Bursa and Ligament, Percutaneous Endoscopic Approach

0MBC0ZX Excision of Upper Spine Bursa and Ligament, Open Approach, Diagnostic

0MBC0ZZ Excision of Upper Spine Bursa and Ligament, Open Approach

0MBC3ZX Excision of Upper Spine Bursa and Ligament, Percutaneous Approach, Diagnostic

0MBC3ZZ Excision of Upper Spine Bursa and Ligament, Percutaneous Approach

0MBC4ZX Excision of Upper Spine Bursa and Ligament, Percutaneous Endoscopic Approach, Diagnostic

0MBC4ZZ Excision of Upper Spine Bursa and Ligament, Percutaneous Endoscopic Approach

0MBD0ZX Excision of Lower Spine Bursa and Ligament, Open Approach, Diagnostic

0MBD0ZZ Excision of Lower Spine Bursa and Ligament, Open Approach

0MBD3ZX Excision of Lower Spine Bursa and Ligament, Percutaneous Approach, Diagnostic

0MBD3ZZ Excision of Lower Spine Bursa and Ligament, Percutaneous Approach

0MBD4ZX Excision of Lower Spine Bursa and Ligament, Percutaneous Endoscopic Approach, Diagnostic

0MBD4ZZ Excision of Lower Spine Bursa and Ligament, Percutaneous Endoscopic Approach

0MBF0ZX Excision of Sternum Bursa and Ligament, Open Approach, Diagnostic

0MBF0ZZ Excision of Sternum Bursa and Ligament, Open Approach

0MBF3ZX Excision of Sternum Bursa and Ligament, Percutaneous Approach, Diagnostic

0MBF3ZZ Excision of Sternum Bursa and Ligament, Percutaneous Approach

0MBF4ZX Excision of Sternum Bursa and Ligament, Percutaneous Endoscopic Approach, Diagnostic

0MBF4ZZ Excision of Sternum Bursa and Ligament, Percutaneous Endoscopic Approach

0MBG0ZX Excision of Rib(s) Bursa and Ligament, Open Approach, Diagnostic

0MBG0ZZ Excision of Rib(s) Bursa and Ligament, Open Approach

0MBG3ZX Excision of Rib(s) Bursa and Ligament, Percutaneous Approach, Diagnostic

0MBG3ZZ Excision of Rib(s) Bursa and Ligament, Percutaneous Approach

0MBG4ZX Excision of Rib(s) Bursa and Ligament, Percutaneous Endoscopic Approach, Diagnostic

0MBG4ZZ Excision of Rib(s) Bursa and Ligament, Percutaneous Endoscopic Approach

0MBH0ZX Excision of Right Abdomen Bursa and Ligament, Open Approach, Diagnostic

0MBH0ZZ Excision of Right Abdomen Bursa and Ligament, Open Approach

0MBH3ZX Excision of Right Abdomen Bursa and Ligament, Percutaneous Approach, Diagnostic

0MBH3ZZ Excision of Right Abdomen Bursa and Ligament, Percutaneous Approach

0MBH4ZX Excision of Right Abdomen Bursa and Ligament, Percutaneous Endoscopic Approach, Diagnostic

0MBH4ZZ Excision of Right Abdomen Bursa and Ligament, Percutaneous Endoscopic Approach

0MBJ0ZX Excision of Left Abdomen Bursa and Ligament, Open Approach, Diagnostic

0MBJ0ZZ	Excision of Left Abdomen Bursa and Ligament, Open Approach	**0MBN3ZX**	Excision of Right Knee Bursa and Ligament, Percutaneous Approach, Diagnostic	**0MBS3ZX**	Excision of Right Foot Bursa and Ligament, Percutaneous Approach, Diagnostic
0MBJ3ZX	Excision of Left Abdomen Bursa and Ligament, Percutaneous Approach, Diagnostic	**0MBN3ZZ**	Excision of Right Knee Bursa and Ligament, Percutaneous Approach	**0MBS3ZZ**	Excision of Right Foot Bursa and Ligament, Percutaneous Approach
0MBJ3ZZ	Excision of Left Abdomen Bursa and Ligament, Percutaneous Approach	**0MBN4ZX**	Excision of Right Knee Bursa and Ligament, Percutaneous Endoscopic Approach, Diagnostic	**0MBS4ZX**	Excision of Right Foot Bursa and Ligament, Percutaneous Endoscopic Approach, Diagnostic
0MBJ4ZX	Excision of Left Abdomen Bursa and Ligament, Percutaneous Endoscopic Approach, Diagnostic	**0MBN4ZZ**	Excision of Right Knee Bursa and Ligament, Percutaneous Endoscopic Approach	**0MBS4ZZ**	Excision of Right Foot Bursa and Ligament, Percutaneous Endoscopic Approach
0MBJ4ZZ	Excision of Left Abdomen Bursa and Ligament, Percutaneous Endoscopic Approach	**0MBP0ZX**	Excision of Left Knee Bursa and Ligament, Open Approach, Diagnostic	**0MBT0ZZ**	Excision of Left Foot Bursa and Ligament, Open Approach, Diagnostic
0MBK0ZX	Excision of Perineum Bursa and Ligament, Open Approach, Diagnostic	**0MBP0ZZ**	Excision of Left Knee Bursa and Ligament, Open Approach	**0MBT0ZZ**	Excision of Left Foot Bursa and Ligament, Open Approach
0MBK0ZZ	Excision of Perineum Bursa and Ligament, Open Approach	**0MBP3ZX**	Excision of Left Knee Bursa and Ligament, Percutaneous Approach, Diagnostic	**0MBT3ZX**	Excision of Left Foot Bursa and Ligament, Percutaneous Approach, Diagnostic
0MBK3ZX	Excision of Perineum Bursa and Ligament, Percutaneous Approach, Diagnostic	**0MBP3ZZ**	Excision of Left Knee Bursa and Ligament, Percutaneous Approach	**0MBT3ZZ**	Excision of Left Foot Bursa and Ligament, Percutaneous Approach
0MBK3ZZ	Excision of Perineum Bursa and Ligament, Percutaneous Approach	**0MBP4ZX**	Excision of Left Knee Bursa and Ligament, Percutaneous Endoscopic Approach, Diagnostic	**0MBT4ZX**	Excision of Left Foot Bursa and Ligament, Percutaneous Endoscopic Approach, Diagnostic
0MBK4ZX	Excision of Perineum Bursa and Ligament, Percutaneous Endoscopic Approach, Diagnostic	**0MBP4ZZ**	Excision of Left Knee Bursa and Ligament, Percutaneous Endoscopic Approach	**0MBT4ZZ**	Excision of Left Foot Bursa and Ligament, Percutaneous Endoscopic Approach
0MBK4ZZ	Excision of Perineum Bursa and Ligament, Percutaneous Endoscopic Approach	**0MBQ0ZX**	Excision of Right Ankle Bursa and Ligament, Open Approach, Diagnostic	**0MBV0ZX**	Excision of Right Lower Extremity Bursa and Ligament, Open Approach, Diagnostic
0MBL0ZX	Excision of Right Hip Bursa and Ligament, Open Approach, Diagnostic	**0MBQ0ZZ**	Excision of Right Ankle Bursa and Ligament, Open Approach	**0MBV0ZZ**	Excision of Right Lower Extremity Bursa and Ligament, Open Approach
0MBL0ZZ	Excision of Right Hip Bursa and Ligament, Open Approach	**0MBQ3ZX**	Excision of Right Ankle Bursa and Ligament, Percutaneous Approach, Diagnostic	**0MBV3ZX**	Excision of Right Lower Extremity Bursa and Ligament, Percutaneous Approach, Diagnostic
0MBL3ZX	Excision of Right Hip Bursa and Ligament, Percutaneous Approach, Diagnostic	**0MBQ3ZZ**	Excision of Right Ankle Bursa and Ligament, Percutaneous Approach	**0MBV3ZZ**	Excision of Right Lower Extremity Bursa and Ligament, Percutaneous Approach
0MBL3ZZ	Excision of Right Hip Bursa and Ligament, Percutaneous Approach	**0MBQ4ZX**	Excision of Right Ankle Bursa and Ligament, Percutaneous Endoscopic Approach, Diagnostic	**0MBV4ZX**	Excision of Right Lower Extremity Bursa and Ligament, Percutaneous Endoscopic Approach, Diagnostic
0MBL4ZX	Excision of Right Hip Bursa and Ligament, Percutaneous Endoscopic Approach, Diagnostic	**0MBQ4ZZ**	Excision of Right Ankle Bursa and Ligament, Percutaneous Endoscopic Approach	**0MBV4ZZ**	Excision of Right Lower Extremity Bursa and Ligament, Percutaneous Endoscopic Approach
0MBL4ZZ	Excision of Right Hip Bursa and Ligament, Percutaneous Endoscopic Approach	**0MBR0ZX**	Excision of Left Ankle Bursa and Ligament, Open Approach, Diagnostic	**0MBW0ZX**	Excision of Left Lower Extremity Bursa and Ligament, Open Approach, Diagnostic
0MBM0ZX	Excision of Left Hip Bursa and Ligament, Open Approach, Diagnostic	**0MBR0ZZ**	Excision of Left Ankle Bursa and Ligament, Open Approach	**0MBW0ZZ**	Excision of Left Lower Extremity Bursa and Ligament, Open Approach
0MBM0ZZ	Excision of Left Hip Bursa and Ligament, Open Approach	**0MBR3ZX**	Excision of Left Ankle Bursa and Ligament, Percutaneous Approach, Diagnostic	**0MBW3ZX**	Excision of Left Lower Extremity Bursa and Ligament, Percutaneous Approach, Diagnostic
0MBM3ZX	Excision of Left Hip Bursa and Ligament, Percutaneous Approach, Diagnostic	**0MBR3ZZ**	Excision of Left Ankle Bursa and Ligament, Percutaneous Approach	**0MBW3ZZ**	Excision of Left Lower Extremity Bursa and Ligament, Percutaneous Approach
0MBM3ZZ	Excision of Left Hip Bursa and Ligament, Percutaneous Approach	**0MBR4ZX**	Excision of Left Ankle Bursa and Ligament, Percutaneous Endoscopic Approach, Diagnostic	**0MBW4ZX**	Excision of Left Lower Extremity Bursa and Ligament, Percutaneous Endoscopic Approach, Diagnostic
0MBM4ZX	Excision of Left Hip Bursa and Ligament, Percutaneous Endoscopic Approach, Diagnostic	**0MBR4ZZ**	Excision of Left Ankle Bursa and Ligament, Percutaneous Endoscopic Approach	**0MBW4ZZ**	Excision of Left Lower Extremity Bursa and Ligament, Percutaneous Endoscopic Approach
0MBM4ZZ	Excision of Left Hip Bursa and Ligament, Percutaneous Endoscopic Approach	**0MBS0ZX**	Excision of Right Foot Bursa and Ligament, Open Approach, Diagnostic		
0MBN0ZX	Excision of Right Knee Bursa and Ligament, Open Approach, Diagnostic	**0MBS0ZZ**	Excision of Right Foot Bursa and Ligament, Open Approach		
0MBN0ZZ	Excision of Right Knee Bursa and Ligament, Open Approach				

0MC – Bursae and Ligaments, Extirpation

0MC00ZZ	Extirpation of Matter from Head and Neck Bursa and Ligament, Open Approach	**0MC13ZZ**	Extirpation of Matter from Right Shoulder Bursa and Ligament, Percutaneous Approach	**0MC24ZZ**	Extirpation of Matter from Left Shoulder Bursa and Ligament, Percutaneous Endoscopic Approach
0MC03ZZ	Extirpation of Matter from Head and Neck Bursa and Ligament, Percutaneous Approach	**0MC14ZZ**	Extirpation of Matter from Right Shoulder Bursa and Ligament, Percutaneous Endoscopic Approach	**0MC30ZZ**	Extirpation of Matter from Right Elbow Bursa and Ligament, Open Approach
0MC04ZZ	Extirpation of Matter from Head and Neck Bursa and Ligament, Percutaneous Endoscopic Approach	**0MC20ZZ**	Extirpation of Matter from Left Shoulder Bursa and Ligament, Open Approach	**0MC33ZZ**	Extirpation of Matter from Right Elbow Bursa and Ligament, Percutaneous Approach
0MC10ZZ	Extirpation of Matter from Right Shoulder Bursa and Ligament, Open Approach	**0MC23ZZ**	Extirpation of Matter from Left Shoulder Bursa and Ligament, Percutaneous Approach	**0MC34ZZ**	Extirpation of Matter from Right Elbow Bursa and Ligament, Percutaneous Endoscopic Approach

♀ Female-only   ♂ Male-only   ▲ Limited Coverage   ● Non-OR   🄷🄰🄲 HAC-associated procedure   ▲ Non-covered procedures   ✚ Cluster

0MC40ZZ Extirpation of Matter from Left Elbow Bursa and Ligament, Open Approach

0MC43ZZ Extirpation of Matter from Left Elbow Bursa and Ligament, Percutaneous Approach

0MC44ZZ Extirpation of Matter from Left Elbow Bursa and Ligament, Percutaneous Endoscopic Approach

0MC50ZZ Extirpation of Matter from Right Wrist Bursa and Ligament, Open Approach

0MC53ZZ Extirpation of Matter from Right Wrist Bursa and Ligament, Percutaneous Approach

0MC54ZZ Extirpation of Matter from Right Wrist Bursa and Ligament, Percutaneous Endoscopic Approach

0MC60ZZ Extirpation of Matter from Left Wrist Bursa and Ligament, Open Approach

0MC63ZZ Extirpation of Matter from Left Wrist Bursa and Ligament, Percutaneous Approach

0MC64ZZ Extirpation of Matter from Left Wrist Bursa and Ligament, Percutaneous Endoscopic Approach

0MC70ZZ Extirpation of Matter from Right Hand Bursa and Ligament, Open Approach

0MC73ZZ Extirpation of Matter from Right Hand Bursa and Ligament, Percutaneous Approach

0MC74ZZ Extirpation of Matter from Right Hand Bursa and Ligament, Percutaneous Endoscopic Approach

0MC80ZZ Extirpation of Matter from Left Hand Bursa and Ligament, Open Approach

0MC83ZZ Extirpation of Matter from Left Hand Bursa and Ligament, Percutaneous Approach

0MC84ZZ Extirpation of Matter from Left Hand Bursa and Ligament, Percutaneous Endoscopic Approach

0MC90ZZ Extirpation of Matter from Right Upper Extremity Bursa and Ligament, Open Approach

0MC93ZZ Extirpation of Matter from Right Upper Extremity Bursa and Ligament, Percutaneous Approach

0MC94ZZ Extirpation of Matter from Right Upper Extremity Bursa and Ligament, Percutaneous Endoscopic Approach

0MCB0ZZ Extirpation of Matter from Left Upper Extremity Bursa and Ligament, Open Approach

0MCB3ZZ Extirpation of Matter from Left Upper Extremity Bursa and Ligament, Percutaneous Approach

0MCB4ZZ Extirpation of Matter from Left Upper Extremity Bursa and Ligament, Percutaneous Endoscopic Approach

0MCC0ZZ Extirpation of Matter from Upper Spine Bursa and Ligament, Open Approach

0MCC3ZZ Extirpation of Matter from Upper Spine Bursa and Ligament, Percutaneous Approach

0MCC4ZZ Extirpation of Matter from Upper Spine Bursa and Ligament, Percutaneous Endoscopic Approach

0MCD0ZZ Extirpation of Matter from Lower Spine Bursa and Ligament, Open Approach

0MCD3ZZ Extirpation of Matter from Lower Spine Bursa and Ligament, Percutaneous Approach

0MCD4ZZ Extirpation of Matter from Lower Spine Bursa and Ligament, Percutaneous Endoscopic Approach

0MCF0ZZ Extirpation of Matter from Sternum Bursa and Ligament, Open Approach

0MCF3ZZ Extirpation of Matter from Sternum Bursa and Ligament, Percutaneous Approach

0MCF4ZZ Extirpation of Matter from Sternum Bursa and Ligament, Percutaneous Endoscopic Approach

0MCG0ZZ Extirpation of Matter from Rib(s) Bursa and Ligament, Open Approach

0MCG3ZZ Extirpation of Matter from Rib(s) Bursa and Ligament, Percutaneous Approach

0MCG4ZZ Extirpation of Matter from Rib(s) Bursa and Ligament, Percutaneous Endoscopic Approach

0MCH0ZZ Extirpation of Matter from Right Abdomen Bursa and Ligament, Open Approach

0MCH3ZZ Extirpation of Matter from Right Abdomen Bursa and Ligament, Percutaneous Approach

0MCH4ZZ Extirpation of Matter from Right Abdomen Bursa and Ligament, Percutaneous Endoscopic Approach

0MCJ0ZZ Extirpation of Matter from Left Abdomen Bursa and Ligament, Open Approach

0MCJ3ZZ Extirpation of Matter from Left Abdomen Bursa and Ligament, Percutaneous Approach

0MCJ4ZZ Extirpation of Matter from Left Abdomen Bursa and Ligament, Percutaneous Endoscopic Approach

0MCK0ZZ Extirpation of Matter from Perineum Bursa and Ligament, Open Approach

0MCK3ZZ Extirpation of Matter from Perineum Bursa and Ligament, Percutaneous Approach

0MCK4ZZ Extirpation of Matter from Perineum Bursa and Ligament, Percutaneous Endoscopic Approach

0MCL0ZZ Extirpation of Matter from Right Hip Bursa and Ligament, Open Approach

0MCL3ZZ Extirpation of Matter from Right Hip Bursa and Ligament, Percutaneous Approach

0MCL4ZZ Extirpation of Matter from Right Hip Bursa and Ligament, Percutaneous Endoscopic Approach

0MCM0ZZ Extirpation of Matter from Left Hip Bursa and Ligament, Open Approach

0MCM3ZZ Extirpation of Matter from Left Hip Bursa and Ligament, Percutaneous Approach

0MCM4ZZ Extirpation of Matter from Left Hip Bursa and Ligament, Percutaneous Endoscopic Approach

0MCN0ZZ Extirpation of Matter from Right Knee Bursa and Ligament, Open Approach

0MCN3ZZ Extirpation of Matter from Right Knee Bursa and Ligament, Percutaneous Approach

0MCN4ZZ Extirpation of Matter from Right Knee Bursa and Ligament, Percutaneous Endoscopic Approach

0MCP0ZZ Extirpation of Matter from Left Knee Bursa and Ligament, Open Approach

0MCP3ZZ Extirpation of Matter from Left Knee Bursa and Ligament, Percutaneous Approach

0MCP4ZZ Extirpation of Matter from Left Knee Bursa and Ligament, Percutaneous Endoscopic Approach

0MCQ0ZZ Extirpation of Matter from Right Ankle Bursa and Ligament, Open Approach

0MCQ3ZZ Extirpation of Matter from Right Ankle Bursa and Ligament, Percutaneous Approach

0MCQ4ZZ Extirpation of Matter from Right Ankle Bursa and Ligament, Percutaneous Endoscopic Approach

0MCR0ZZ Extirpation of Matter from Left Ankle Bursa and Ligament, Open Approach

0MCR3ZZ Extirpation of Matter from Left Ankle Bursa and Ligament, Percutaneous Approach

0MCR4ZZ Extirpation of Matter from Left Ankle Bursa and Ligament, Percutaneous Endoscopic Approach

0MCS0ZZ Extirpation of Matter from Right Foot Bursa and Ligament, Open Approach

0MCS3ZZ Extirpation of Matter from Right Foot Bursa and Ligament, Percutaneous Approach

0MCS4ZZ Extirpation of Matter from Right Foot Bursa and Ligament, Percutaneous Endoscopic Approach

0MCT0ZZ Extirpation of Matter from Left Foot Bursa and Ligament, Open Approach

0MCT3ZZ Extirpation of Matter from Left Foot Bursa and Ligament, Percutaneous Approach

0MCT4ZZ Extirpation of Matter from Left Foot Bursa and Ligament, Percutaneous Endoscopic Approach

0MCV0ZZ Extirpation of Matter from Right Lower Extremity Bursa and Ligament, Open Approach

0MCV3ZZ Extirpation of Matter from Right Lower Extremity Bursa and Ligament, Percutaneous Approach

0MCV4ZZ Extirpation of Matter from Right Lower Extremity Bursa and Ligament, Percutaneous Endoscopic Approach

0MCW0ZZ Extirpation of Matter from Left Lower Extremity Bursa and Ligament, Open Approach

0MCW3ZZ Extirpation of Matter from Left Lower Extremity Bursa and Ligament, Percutaneous Approach

0MCW4ZZ Extirpation of Matter from Left Lower Extremity Bursa and Ligament, Percutaneous Endoscopic Approach

0MD – Bursae and Ligaments, Extraction

0MD00ZZ Extraction of Head and Neck Bursa and Ligament, Open Approach

0MD03ZZ Extraction of Head and Neck Bursa and Ligament, Percutaneous Approach

0MD04ZZ Extraction of Head and Neck Bursa and Ligament, Percutaneous Endoscopic Approach

0MD10ZZ Extraction of Right Shoulder Bursa and Ligament, Open Approach

0MD13ZZ Extraction of Right Shoulder Bursa and Ligament, Percutaneous Approach

0MD14ZZ Extraction of Right Shoulder Bursa and Ligament, Percutaneous Endoscopic Approach

0MD20ZZ Extraction of Left Shoulder Bursa and Ligament, Open Approach

0MD23ZZ Extraction of Left Shoulder Bursa and Ligament, Percutaneous Approach

0MD24ZZ Extraction of Left Shoulder Bursa and Ligament, Percutaneous Endoscopic Approach

0MD30ZZ Extraction of Right Elbow Bursa and Ligament, Open Approach

0MD33ZZ Extraction of Right Elbow Bursa and Ligament, Percutaneous Approach

0MD34ZZ Extraction of Right Elbow Bursa and Ligament, Percutaneous Endoscopic Approach

0MD40ZZ Extraction of Left Elbow Bursa and Ligament, Open Approach

0MD43ZZ Extraction of Left Elbow Bursa and Ligament, Percutaneous Approach

0MD44ZZ Extraction of Left Elbow Bursa and Ligament, Percutaneous Endoscopic Approach

0MD50ZZ Extraction of Right Wrist Bursa and Ligament, Open Approach

0MD53ZZ Extraction of Right Wrist Bursa and Ligament, Percutaneous Approach

0MD54ZZ Extraction of Right Wrist Bursa and Ligament, Percutaneous Endoscopic Approach

0MD60ZZ Extraction of Left Wrist Bursa and Ligament, Open Approach

0MD63ZZ Extraction of Left Wrist Bursa and Ligament, Percutaneous Approach

0MD64ZZ Extraction of Left Wrist Bursa and Ligament, Percutaneous Endoscopic Approach

0MD70ZZ Extraction of Right Hand Bursa and Ligament, Open Approach

0MD73ZZ Extraction of Right Hand Bursa and Ligament, Percutaneous Approach

0MD74ZZ Extraction of Right Hand Bursa and Ligament, Percutaneous Endoscopic Approach

0MD80ZZ Extraction of Left Hand Bursa and Ligament, Open Approach

0MD83ZZ Extraction of Left Hand Bursa and Ligament, Percutaneous Approach

0MD84ZZ Extraction of Left Hand Bursa and Ligament, Percutaneous Endoscopic Approach

0MD90ZZ Extraction of Right Upper Extremity Bursa and Ligament, Open Approach

0MD93ZZ Extraction of Right Upper Extremity Bursa and Ligament, Percutaneous Approach

0MD94ZZ Extraction of Right Upper Extremity Bursa and Ligament, Percutaneous Endoscopic Approach

0MDB0ZZ Extraction of Left Upper Extremity Bursa and Ligament, Open Approach

0MDB3ZZ Extraction of Left Upper Extremity Bursa and Ligament, Percutaneous Approach

0MDB4ZZ Extraction of Left Upper Extremity Bursa and Ligament, Percutaneous Endoscopic Approach

0MDC0ZZ Extraction of Upper Spine Bursa and Ligament, Open Approach

0MDC3ZZ Extraction of Upper Spine Bursa and Ligament, Percutaneous Approach

0MDC4ZZ Extraction of Upper Spine Bursa and Ligament, Percutaneous Endoscopic Approach

0MDD0ZZ Extraction of Lower Spine Bursa and Ligament, Open Approach

0MDD3ZZ Extraction of Lower Spine Bursa and Ligament, Percutaneous Approach

0MDD4ZZ Extraction of Lower Spine Bursa and Ligament, Percutaneous Endoscopic Approach

0MDF0ZZ Extraction of Sternum Bursa and Ligament, Open Approach

0MDF3ZZ Extraction of Sternum Bursa and Ligament, Percutaneous Approach

0MDF4ZZ Extraction of Sternum Bursa and Ligament, Percutaneous Endoscopic Approach

0MDG0ZZ Extraction of Rib(s) Bursa and Ligament, Open Approach

0MDG3ZZ Extraction of Rib(s) Bursa and Ligament, Percutaneous Approach

0MDG4ZZ Extraction of Rib(s) Bursa and Ligament, Percutaneous Endoscopic Approach

0MDH0ZZ Extraction of Right Abdomen Bursa and Ligament, Open Approach

0MDH3ZZ Extraction of Right Abdomen Bursa and Ligament, Percutaneous Approach

0MDH4ZZ Extraction of Right Abdomen Bursa and Ligament, Percutaneous Endoscopic Approach

0MDJ0ZZ Extraction of Left Abdomen Bursa and Ligament, Open Approach

0MDJ3ZZ Extraction of Left Abdomen Bursa and Ligament, Percutaneous Approach

0MDJ4ZZ Extraction of Left Abdomen Bursa and Ligament, Percutaneous Endoscopic Approach

0MDK0ZZ Extraction of Perineum Bursa and Ligament, Open Approach

0MDK3ZZ Extraction of Perineum Bursa and Ligament, Percutaneous Approach

0MDK4ZZ Extraction of Perineum Bursa and Ligament, Percutaneous Endoscopic Approach

0MDL0ZZ Extraction of Right Hip Bursa and Ligament, Open Approach

0MDL3ZZ Extraction of Right Hip Bursa and Ligament, Percutaneous Approach

0MDL4ZZ Extraction of Right Hip Bursa and Ligament, Percutaneous Endoscopic Approach

0MDM0ZZ Extraction of Left Hip Bursa and Ligament, Open Approach

0MDM3ZZ Extraction of Left Hip Bursa and Ligament, Percutaneous Approach

0MDM4ZZ Extraction of Left Hip Bursa and Ligament, Percutaneous Endoscopic Approach

0MDN0ZZ Extraction of Right Knee Bursa and Ligament, Open Approach

0MDN3ZZ Extraction of Right Knee Bursa and Ligament, Percutaneous Approach

0MDN4ZZ Extraction of Right Knee Bursa and Ligament, Percutaneous Endoscopic Approach

0MDP0ZZ Extraction of Left Knee Bursa and Ligament, Open Approach

0MDP3ZZ Extraction of Left Knee Bursa and Ligament, Percutaneous Approach

0MDP4ZZ Extraction of Left Knee Bursa and Ligament, Percutaneous Endoscopic Approach

0MDQ0ZZ Extraction of Right Ankle Bursa and Ligament, Open Approach

0MDQ3ZZ Extraction of Right Ankle Bursa and Ligament, Percutaneous Approach

0MDQ4ZZ Extraction of Right Ankle Bursa and Ligament, Percutaneous Endoscopic Approach

0MDR0ZZ Extraction of Left Ankle Bursa and Ligament, Open Approach

0MDR3ZZ Extraction of Left Ankle Bursa and Ligament, Percutaneous Approach

0MDR4ZZ Extraction of Left Ankle Bursa and Ligament, Percutaneous Endoscopic Approach

0MDS0ZZ Extraction of Right Foot Bursa and Ligament, Open Approach

0MDS3ZZ Extraction of Right Foot Bursa and Ligament, Percutaneous Approach

0MDS4ZZ Extraction of Right Foot Bursa and Ligament, Percutaneous Endoscopic Approach

0MDT0ZZ Extraction of Left Foot Bursa and Ligament, Open Approach

0MDT3ZZ Extraction of Left Foot Bursa and Ligament, Percutaneous Approach

0MDT4ZZ Extraction of Left Foot Bursa and Ligament, Percutaneous Endoscopic Approach

0MDV0ZZ Extraction of Right Lower Extremity Bursa and Ligament, Open Approach

0MDV3ZZ Extraction of Right Lower Extremity Bursa and Ligament, Percutaneous Approach

0MDV4ZZ Extraction of Right Lower Extremity Bursa and Ligament, Percutaneous Endoscopic Approach

0MDW0ZZ Extraction of Left Lower Extremity Bursa and Ligament, Open Approach

0MDW3ZZ Extraction of Left Lower Extremity Bursa and Ligament, Percutaneous Approach

0MDW4ZZ Extraction of Left Lower Extremity Bursa and Ligament, Percutaneous Endoscopic Approach

0MH – Bursae and Ligaments, Insertion

0MHX0YZ Insertion of Other Device into Upper Bursa and Ligament, Open Approach

0MHX3YZ Insertion of Other Device into Upper Bursa and Ligament, Percutaneous Approach

0MHX4YZ Insertion of Other Device into Upper Bursa and Ligament, Percutaneous Endoscopic Approach

0MHY0YZ Insertion of Other Device into Lower Bursa and Ligament, Open Approach

0MHY3YZ Insertion of Other Device into Lower Bursa and Ligament, Percutaneous Approach

0MHY4YZ Insertion of Other Device into Lower Bursa and Ligament, Percutaneous Endoscopic Approach

♀ Female-only　　♂ Male-only　　▲ Limited Coverage　　● Non-OR　　HAC HAC-associated procedure　　▲ Non-covered procedures　　➕ Cluster

0MJ – Bursae and Ligaments, Inspection

Review Coding Guideline B3.5

Review Coding Guidelines B3.11a, B3.11b and B3.11c

0MJX0ZZ Inspection of Upper Bursa and Ligament, Open Approach

0MJX3ZZ Inspection of Upper Bursa and Ligament, Percutaneous Approach

0MJX4ZZ Inspection of Upper Bursa and Ligament, Percutaneous Endoscopic Approach

0MJXXZZ Inspection of Upper Bursa and Ligament, External Approach

0MJY0ZZ Inspection of Lower Bursa and Ligament, Open Approach

0MJY3ZZ Inspection of Lower Bursa and Ligament, Percutaneous Approach

0MJY4ZZ Inspection of Lower Bursa and Ligament, Percutaneous Endoscopic Approach

0MJYXZZ Inspection of Lower Bursa and Ligament, External Approach

0MM – Bursae and Ligaments, Reattachment

0MM00ZZ Reattachment of Head and Neck Bursa and Ligament, Open Approach

0MM04ZZ Reattachment of Head and Neck Bursa and Ligament, Percutaneous Endoscopic Approach

0MM10ZZ Reattachment of Right Shoulder Bursa and Ligament, Open Approach

0MM14ZZ Reattachment of Right Shoulder Bursa and Ligament, Percutaneous Endoscopic Approach
AHA CC: 3Q, 2013, 20-22

0MM20ZZ Reattachment of Left Shoulder Bursa and Ligament, Open Approach

0MM24ZZ Reattachment of Left Shoulder Bursa and Ligament, Percutaneous Endoscopic Approach

0MM30ZZ Reattachment of Right Elbow Bursa and Ligament, Open Approach

0MM34ZZ Reattachment of Right Elbow Bursa and Ligament, Percutaneous Endoscopic Approach

0MM40ZZ Reattachment of Left Elbow Bursa and Ligament, Open Approach

0MM44ZZ Reattachment of Left Elbow Bursa and Ligament, Percutaneous Endoscopic Approach

0MM50ZZ Reattachment of Right Wrist Bursa and Ligament, Open Approach

0MM54ZZ Reattachment of Right Wrist Bursa and Ligament, Percutaneous Endoscopic Approach

0MM60ZZ Reattachment of Left Wrist Bursa and Ligament, Open Approach

0MM64ZZ Reattachment of Left Wrist Bursa and Ligament, Percutaneous Endoscopic Approach

0MM70ZZ Reattachment of Right Hand Bursa and Ligament, Open Approach

0MM74ZZ Reattachment of Right Hand Bursa and Ligament, Percutaneous Endoscopic Approach

0MM80ZZ Reattachment of Left Hand Bursa and Ligament, Open Approach

0MM84ZZ Reattachment of Left Hand Bursa and Ligament, Percutaneous Endoscopic Approach

0MM90ZZ Reattachment of Right Upper Extremity Bursa and Ligament, Open Approach

0MM94ZZ Reattachment of Right Upper Extremity Bursa and Ligament, Percutaneous Endoscopic Approach

0MMB0ZZ Reattachment of Left Upper Extremity Bursa and Ligament, Open Approach

0MMB4ZZ Reattachment of Left Upper Extremity Bursa and Ligament, Percutaneous Endoscopic Approach

0MMC0ZZ Reattachment of Upper Spine Bursa and Ligament, Open Approach

0MMC4ZZ Reattachment of Upper Spine Bursa and Ligament, Percutaneous Endoscopic Approach

0MMD0ZZ Reattachment of Lower Spine Bursa and Ligament, Open Approach

0MMD4ZZ Reattachment of Lower Spine Bursa and Ligament, Percutaneous Endoscopic Approach

0MMF0ZZ Reattachment of Sternum Bursa and Ligament, Open Approach

0MMF4ZZ Reattachment of Sternum Bursa and Ligament, Percutaneous Endoscopic Approach

0MMG0ZZ Reattachment of Rib(s) Bursa and Ligament, Open Approach

0MMG4ZZ Reattachment of Rib(s) Bursa and Ligament, Percutaneous Endoscopic Approach

0MMH0ZZ Reattachment of Right Abdomen Bursa and Ligament, Open Approach

0MMH4ZZ Reattachment of Right Abdomen Bursa and Ligament, Percutaneous Endoscopic Approach

0MMJ0ZZ Reattachment of Left Abdomen Bursa and Ligament, Open Approach

0MMJ4ZZ Reattachment of Left Abdomen Bursa and Ligament, Percutaneous Endoscopic Approach

0MMK0ZZ Reattachment of Perineum Bursa and Ligament, Open Approach

0MMK4ZZ Reattachment of Perineum Bursa and Ligament, Percutaneous Endoscopic Approach

0MML0ZZ Reattachment of Right Hip Bursa and Ligament, Open Approach

0MML4ZZ Reattachment of Right Hip Bursa and Ligament, Percutaneous Endoscopic Approach

0MMM0ZZ Reattachment of Left Hip Bursa and Ligament, Open Approach

0MMM4ZZ Reattachment of Left Hip Bursa and Ligament, Percutaneous Endoscopic Approach

0MMN0ZZ Reattachment of Right Knee Bursa and Ligament, Open Approach

0MMN4ZZ Reattachment of Right Knee Bursa and Ligament, Percutaneous Endoscopic Approach

0MMP0ZZ Reattachment of Left Knee Bursa and Ligament, Open Approach

0MMP4ZZ Reattachment of Left Knee Bursa and Ligament, Percutaneous Endoscopic Approach

0MMQ0ZZ Reattachment of Right Ankle Bursa and Ligament, Open Approach

0MMQ4ZZ Reattachment of Right Ankle Bursa and Ligament, Percutaneous Endoscopic Approach

0MMR0ZZ Reattachment of Left Ankle Bursa and Ligament, Open Approach

0MMR4ZZ Reattachment of Left Ankle Bursa and Ligament, Percutaneous Endoscopic Approach

0MMS0ZZ Reattachment of Right Foot Bursa and Ligament, Open Approach

0MMS4ZZ Reattachment of Right Foot Bursa and Ligament, Percutaneous Endoscopic Approach

0MMT0ZZ Reattachment of Left Foot Bursa and Ligament, Open Approach

0MMT4ZZ Reattachment of Left Foot Bursa and Ligament, Percutaneous Endoscopic Approach

0MMV0ZZ Reattachment of Right Lower Extremity Bursa and Ligament, Open Approach

0MMV4ZZ Reattachment of Right Lower Extremity Bursa and Ligament, Percutaneous Endoscopic Approach

0MMW0ZZ Reattachment of Left Lower Extremity Bursa and Ligament, Open Approach

0MMW4ZZ Reattachment of Left Lower Extremity Bursa and Ligament, Percutaneous Endoscopic Approach

0MN – Bursae and Ligaments, Release

Review Coding Guideline B3.13

Review Coding Guideline B3.14

0MN00ZZ Release Head and Neck Bursa and Ligament, Open Approach

0MN03ZZ Release Head and Neck Bursa and Ligament, Percutaneous Approach

0MN04ZZ Release Head and Neck Bursa and Ligament, Percutaneous Endoscopic Approach

0MN0XZZ	Release Head and Neck Bursa and Ligament, External Approach
0MN10ZZ	Release Right Shoulder Bursa and Ligament, Open Approach
0MN13ZZ	Release Right Shoulder Bursa and Ligament, Percutaneous Approach
0MN14ZZ	Release Right Shoulder Bursa and Ligament, Percutaneous Endoscopic Approach
0MN1XZZ	Release Right Shoulder Bursa and Ligament, External Approach
0MN20ZZ	Release Left Shoulder Bursa and Ligament, Open Approach
0MN23ZZ	Release Left Shoulder Bursa and Ligament, Percutaneous Approach
0MN24ZZ	Release Left Shoulder Bursa and Ligament, Percutaneous Endoscopic Approach
0MN2XZZ	Release Left Shoulder Bursa and Ligament, External Approach
0MN30ZZ	Release Right Elbow Bursa and Ligament, Open Approach
0MN33ZZ	Release Right Elbow Bursa and Ligament, Percutaneous Approach
0MN34ZZ	Release Right Elbow Bursa and Ligament, Percutaneous Endoscopic Approach
0MN3XZZ	Release Right Elbow Bursa and Ligament, External Approach
0MN40ZZ	Release Left Elbow Bursa and Ligament, Open Approach
0MN43ZZ	Release Left Elbow Bursa and Ligament, Percutaneous Approach
0MN44ZZ	Release Left Elbow Bursa and Ligament, Percutaneous Endoscopic Approach
0MN4XZZ	Release Left Elbow Bursa and Ligament, External Approach
0MN50ZZ	Release Right Wrist Bursa and Ligament, Open Approach
0MN53ZZ	Release Right Wrist Bursa and Ligament, Percutaneous Approach
0MN54ZZ	Release Right Wrist Bursa and Ligament, Percutaneous Endoscopic Approach
0MN5XZZ	Release Right Wrist Bursa and Ligament, External Approach
0MN60ZZ	Release Left Wrist Bursa and Ligament, Open Approach
0MN63ZZ	Release Left Wrist Bursa and Ligament, Percutaneous Approach
0MN64ZZ	Release Left Wrist Bursa and Ligament, Percutaneous Endoscopic Approach
0MN6XZZ	Release Left Wrist Bursa and Ligament, External Approach
0MN70ZZ	Release Right Hand Bursa and Ligament, Open Approach
0MN73ZZ	Release Right Hand Bursa and Ligament, Percutaneous Approach
0MN74ZZ	Release Right Hand Bursa and Ligament, Percutaneous Endoscopic Approach
0MN7XZZ	Release Right Hand Bursa and Ligament, External Approach
0MN80ZZ	Release Left Hand Bursa and Ligament, Open Approach
0MN83ZZ	Release Left Hand Bursa and Ligament, Percutaneous Approach
0MN84ZZ	Release Left Hand Bursa and Ligament, Percutaneous Endoscopic Approach
0MN8XZZ	Release Left Hand Bursa and Ligament, External Approach
0MN90ZZ	Release Right Upper Extremity Bursa and Ligament, Open Approach
0MN93ZZ	Release Right Upper Extremity Bursa and Ligament, Percutaneous Approach
0MN94ZZ	Release Right Upper Extremity Bursa and Ligament, Percutaneous Endoscopic Approach
0MN9XZZ	Release Right Upper Extremity Bursa and Ligament, External Approach
0MNB0ZZ	Release Left Upper Extremity Bursa and Ligament, Open Approach
0MNB3ZZ	Release Left Upper Extremity Bursa and Ligament, Percutaneous Approach
0MNB4ZZ	Release Left Upper Extremity Bursa and Ligament, Percutaneous Endoscopic Approach
0MNBXZZ	Release Left Upper Extremity Bursa and Ligament, External Approach
0MNC0ZZ	Release Upper Spine Bursa and Ligament, Open Approach
0MNC3ZZ	Release Upper Spine Bursa and Ligament, Percutaneous Approach
0MNC4ZZ	Release Upper Spine Bursa and Ligament, Percutaneous Endoscopic Approach
0MNCXZZ	Release Upper Spine Bursa and Ligament, External Approach
0MND0ZZ	Release Lower Spine Bursa and Ligament, Open Approach
0MND3ZZ	Release Lower Spine Bursa and Ligament, Percutaneous Approach
0MND4ZZ	Release Lower Spine Bursa and Ligament, Percutaneous Endoscopic Approach
0MNDXZZ	Release Lower Spine Bursa and Ligament, External Approach
0MNF0ZZ	Release Sternum Bursa and Ligament, Open Approach
0MNF3ZZ	Release Sternum Bursa and Ligament, Percutaneous Approach
0MNF4ZZ	Release Sternum Bursa and Ligament, Percutaneous Endoscopic Approach
0MNFXZZ	Release Sternum Bursa and Ligament, External Approach
0MNG0ZZ	Release Rib(s) Bursa and Ligament, Open Approach
0MNG3ZZ	Release Rib(s) Bursa and Ligament, Percutaneous Approach
0MNG4ZZ	Release Rib(s) Bursa and Ligament, Percutaneous Endoscopic Approach
0MNGXZZ	Release Rib(s) Bursa and Ligament, External Approach
0MNH0ZZ	Release Right Abdomen Bursa and Ligament, Open Approach
0MNH3ZZ	Release Right Abdomen Bursa and Ligament, Percutaneous Approach
0MNH4ZZ	Release Right Abdomen Bursa and Ligament, Percutaneous Endoscopic Approach
0MNHXZZ	Release Right Abdomen Bursa and Ligament, External Approach
0MNJ0ZZ	Release Left Abdomen Bursa and Ligament, Open Approach
0MNJ3ZZ	Release Left Abdomen Bursa and Ligament, Percutaneous Approach
0MNJ4ZZ	Release Left Abdomen Bursa and Ligament, Percutaneous Endoscopic Approach
0MNJXZZ	Release Left Abdomen Bursa and Ligament, External Approach
0MNK0ZZ	Release Perineum Bursa and Ligament, Open Approach
0MNK3ZZ	Release Perineum Bursa and Ligament, Percutaneous Approach
0MNK4ZZ	Release Perineum Bursa and Ligament, Percutaneous Endoscopic Approach
0MNKXZZ	Release Perineum Bursa and Ligament, External Approach
0MNL0ZZ	Release Right Hip Bursa and Ligament, Open Approach
0MNL3ZZ	Release Right Hip Bursa and Ligament, Percutaneous Approach
0MNL4ZZ	Release Right Hip Bursa and Ligament, Percutaneous Endoscopic Approach
0MNLXZZ	Release Right Hip Bursa and Ligament, External Approach
0MNM0ZZ	Release Left Hip Bursa and Ligament, Open Approach
0MNM3ZZ	Release Left Hip Bursa and Ligament, Percutaneous Approach
0MNM4ZZ	Release Left Hip Bursa and Ligament, Percutaneous Endoscopic Approach
0MNMXZZ	Release Left Hip Bursa and Ligament, External Approach
0MNN0ZZ	Release Right Knee Bursa and Ligament, Open Approach
0MNN3ZZ	Release Right Knee Bursa and Ligament, Percutaneous Approach
0MNN4ZZ	Release Right Knee Bursa and Ligament, Percutaneous Endoscopic Approach
0MNNXZZ	Release Right Knee Bursa and Ligament, External Approach
0MNP0ZZ	Release Left Knee Bursa and Ligament, Open Approach
0MNP3ZZ	Release Left Knee Bursa and Ligament, Percutaneous Approach
0MNP4ZZ	Release Left Knee Bursa and Ligament, Percutaneous Endoscopic Approach
0MNPXZZ	Release Left Knee Bursa and Ligament, External Approach
0MNQ0ZZ	Release Right Ankle Bursa and Ligament, Open Approach
0MNQ3ZZ	Release Right Ankle Bursa and Ligament, Percutaneous Approach
0MNQ4ZZ	Release Right Ankle Bursa and Ligament, Percutaneous Endoscopic Approach
0MNQXZZ	Release Right Ankle Bursa and Ligament, External Approach
0MNR0ZZ	Release Left Ankle Bursa and Ligament, Open Approach
0MNR3ZZ	Release Left Ankle Bursa and Ligament, Percutaneous Approach
0MNR4ZZ	Release Left Ankle Bursa and Ligament, Percutaneous Endoscopic Approach
0MNRXZZ	Release Left Ankle Bursa and Ligament, External Approach
0MNS0ZZ	Release Right Foot Bursa and Ligament, Open Approach
0MNS3ZZ	Release Right Foot Bursa and Ligament, Percutaneous Approach
0MNS4ZZ	Release Right Foot Bursa and Ligament, Percutaneous Endoscopic Approach
0MNSXZZ	Release Right Foot Bursa and Ligament, External Approach
0MNT0ZZ	Release Left Foot Bursa and Ligament, Open Approach
0MNT3ZZ	Release Left Foot Bursa and Ligament, Percutaneous Approach
0MNT4ZZ	Release Left Foot Bursa and Ligament, Percutaneous Endoscopic Approach
0MNTXZZ	Release Left Foot Bursa and Ligament, External Approach
0MNV0ZZ	Release Right Lower Extremity Bursa and Ligament, Open Approach
0MNV3ZZ	Release Right Lower Extremity Bursa and Ligament, Percutaneous Approach

♀ Female-only   ♂ Male-only   ▲ Limited Coverage   ● Non-OR   HAC HAC-associated procedure   ▲ Non-covered procedures   ✚ Cluster

0MNV4ZZ Release Right Lower Extremity Bursa and Ligament, Percutaneous Endoscopic Approach
0MNVXZZ Release Right Lower Extremity Bursa and Ligament, External Approach

0MNW0ZZ Release Left Lower Extremity Bursa and Ligament, Open Approach
0MNW3ZZ Release Left Lower Extremity Bursa and Ligament, Percutaneous Approach

0MNW4ZZ Release Left Lower Extremity Bursa and Ligament, Percutaneous Endoscopic Approach
0MNWXZZ Release Left Lower Extremity Bursa and Ligament, External Approach

0MP – Bursae and Ligaments, Removal

Review Coding Guideline B6.1c

0MPX00Z Removal of Drainage Device from Upper Bursa and Ligament, Open Approach
0MPX07Z Removal of Autologous Tissue Substitute from Upper Bursa and Ligament, Open Approach
0MPX0JZ Removal of Synthetic Substitute from Upper Bursa and Ligament, Open Approach
0MPX0KZ Removal of Nonautologous Tissue Substitute from Upper Bursa and Ligament, Open Approach
0MPX0YZ Removal of Other Device from Upper Bursa and Ligament, Open Approach
0MPX30Z Removal of Drainage Device from Upper Bursa and Ligament, Percutaneous Approach
0MPX37Z Removal of Autologous Tissue Substitute from Upper Bursa and Ligament, Percutaneous Approach
0MPX3JZ Removal of Synthetic Substitute from Upper Bursa and Ligament, Percutaneous Approach
0MPX3KZ Removal of Nonautologous Tissue Substitute from Upper Bursa and Ligament, Percutaneous Approach
0MPX3YZ Removal of Other Device from Upper Bursa and Ligament, Percutaneous Approach
0MPX40Z Removal of Drainage Device from Upper Bursa and Ligament, Percutaneous Endoscopic Approach
0MPX47Z Removal of Autologous Tissue Substitute from Upper Bursa and

Ligament, Percutaneous Endoscopic Approach
0MPX4JZ Removal of Synthetic Substitute from Upper Bursa and Ligament, Percutaneous Endoscopic Approach
0MPX4KZ Removal of Nonautologous Tissue Substitute from Upper Bursa and Ligament, Percutaneous Endoscopic Approach
0MPX4YZ Removal of Other Device from Upper Bursa and Ligament, Percutaneous Endoscopic Approach
0MPXX0Z Removal of Drainage Device from Upper Bursa and Ligament, External Approach
0MPY00Z Removal of Drainage Device from Lower Bursa and Ligament, Open Approach
0MPY07Z Removal of Autologous Tissue Substitute from Lower Bursa and Ligament, Open Approach
0MPY0JZ Removal of Synthetic Substitute from Lower Bursa and Ligament, Open Approach
0MPY0KZ Removal of Nonautologous Tissue Substitute from Lower Bursa and Ligament, Open Approach
0MPY0YZ Removal of Other Device from Lower Bursa and Ligament, Open Approach
0MPY30Z Removal of Drainage Device from Lower Bursa and Ligament, Percutaneous Approach

0MPY37Z Removal of Autologous Tissue Substitute from Lower Bursa and Ligament, Percutaneous Approach
0MPY3JZ Removal of Synthetic Substitute from Lower Bursa and Ligament, Percutaneous Approach
0MPY3KZ Removal of Nonautologous Tissue Substitute from Lower Bursa and Ligament, Percutaneous Approach
0MPY3YZ Removal of Other Device from Lower Bursa and Ligament, Percutaneous Approach
0MPY40Z Removal of Drainage Device from Lower Bursa and Ligament, Percutaneous Endoscopic Approach
0MPY47Z Removal of Autologous Tissue Substitute from Lower Bursa and Ligament, Percutaneous Endoscopic Approach
0MPY4JZ Removal of Synthetic Substitute from Lower Bursa and Ligament, Percutaneous Endoscopic Approach
0MPY4KZ Removal of Nonautologous Tissue Substitute from Lower Bursa and Ligament, Percutaneous Endoscopic Approach
0MPY4YZ Removal of Other Device from Lower Bursa and Ligament, Percutaneous Endoscopic Approach
0MPYX0Z Removal of Drainage Device from Lower Bursa and Ligament, External Approach

0MQ – Bursae and Ligaments, Repair

Review Coding Guideline B3.5

0MQ00ZZ Repair Head and Neck Bursa and Ligament, Open Approach
AHA CC: 3Q, 2014, 9
0MQ03ZZ Repair Head and Neck Bursa and Ligament, Percutaneous Approach
0MQ04ZZ Repair Head and Neck Bursa and Ligament, Percutaneous Endoscopic Approach
0MQ10ZZ Repair Right Shoulder Bursa and Ligament, Open Approach
0MQ13ZZ Repair Right Shoulder Bursa and Ligament, Percutaneous Approach
0MQ14ZZ Repair Right Shoulder Bursa and Ligament, Percutaneous Endoscopic Approach
0MQ20ZZ Repair Left Shoulder Bursa and Ligament, Open Approach
0MQ23ZZ Repair Left Shoulder Bursa and Ligament, Percutaneous Approach
0MQ24ZZ Repair Left Shoulder Bursa and Ligament, Percutaneous Endoscopic Approach
0MQ30ZZ Repair Right Elbow Bursa and Ligament, Open Approach

0MQ33ZZ Repair Right Elbow Bursa and Ligament, Percutaneous Approach
0MQ34ZZ Repair Right Elbow Bursa and Ligament, Percutaneous Endoscopic Approach
0MQ40ZZ Repair Left Elbow Bursa and Ligament, Open Approach
0MQ43ZZ Repair Left Elbow Bursa and Ligament, Percutaneous Approach
0MQ44ZZ Repair Left Elbow Bursa and Ligament, Percutaneous Endoscopic Approach
0MQ50ZZ Repair Right Wrist Bursa and Ligament, Open Approach
0MQ53ZZ Repair Right Wrist Bursa and Ligament, Percutaneous Approach
0MQ54ZZ Repair Right Wrist Bursa and Ligament, Percutaneous Endoscopic Approach
0MQ60ZZ Repair Left Wrist Bursa and Ligament, Open Approach
0MQ63ZZ Repair Left Wrist Bursa and Ligament, Percutaneous Approach

0MQ64ZZ Repair Left Wrist Bursa and Ligament, Percutaneous Endoscopic Approach
0MQ70ZZ Repair Right Hand Bursa and Ligament, Open Approach
0MQ73ZZ Repair Right Hand Bursa and Ligament, Percutaneous Approach
0MQ74ZZ Repair Right Hand Bursa and Ligament, Percutaneous Endoscopic Approach
0MQ80ZZ Repair Left Hand Bursa and Ligament, Open Approach
0MQ83ZZ Repair Left Hand Bursa and Ligament, Percutaneous Approach
0MQ84ZZ Repair Left Hand Bursa and Ligament, Percutaneous Endoscopic Approach
0MQ90ZZ Repair Right Upper Extremity Bursa and Ligament, Open Approach
0MQ93ZZ Repair Right Upper Extremity Bursa and Ligament, Percutaneous Approach
0MQ94ZZ Repair Right Upper Extremity Bursa and Ligament, Percutaneous Endoscopic Approach

♀ Female-only ♂ Male-only ▲ Limited Coverage ● Non-OR HAC HAC-associated procedure ▲ Non-covered procedures ✚ Cluster **901**

0MQB0ZZ Repair Left Upper Extremity Bursa and Ligament, Open Approach

0MQB3ZZ Repair Left Upper Extremity Bursa and Ligament, Percutaneous Approach

0MQB4ZZ Repair Left Upper Extremity Bursa and Ligament, Percutaneous Endoscopic Approach

0MQC0ZZ Repair Upper Spine Bursa and Ligament, Open Approach

0MQC3ZZ Repair Upper Spine Bursa and Ligament, Percutaneous Approach

0MQC4ZZ Repair Upper Spine Bursa and Ligament, Percutaneous Endoscopic Approach

0MQD0ZZ Repair Lower Spine Bursa and Ligament, Open Approach

0MQD3ZZ Repair Lower Spine Bursa and Ligament, Percutaneous Approach

0MQD4ZZ Repair Lower Spine and Ligament, Percutaneous Endoscopic Approach

0MQF0ZZ Repair Sternum Bursa and Ligament, Open Approach

0MQF3ZZ Repair Sternum Bursa and Ligament, Percutaneous Approach

0MQF4ZZ Repair Sternum Bursa and Ligament, Percutaneous Endoscopic Approach

0MQG0ZZ Repair Rib(s) Bursa and Ligament, Open Approach

0MQG3ZZ Repair Rib(s) Bursa and Ligament, Percutaneous Approach

0MQG4ZZ Repair Rib(s) Bursa and Ligament, Percutaneous Endoscopic Approach

0MQH0ZZ Repair Right Abdomen Bursa and Ligament, Open Approach

0MQH3ZZ Repair Right Abdomen Bursa and Ligament, Percutaneous Approach

0MQH4ZZ Repair Right Abdomen Bursa and Ligament, Percutaneous Endoscopic Approach

0MQJ0ZZ Repair Left Abdomen Bursa and Ligament, Open Approach

0MQJ3ZZ Repair Left Abdomen Bursa and Ligament, Percutaneous Approach

0MQJ4ZZ Repair Left Abdomen Bursa and Ligament, Percutaneous Endoscopic Approach

0MQK0ZZ Repair Perineum Bursa and Ligament, Open Approach

0MQK3ZZ Repair Perineum Bursa and Ligament, Percutaneous Approach

0MQK4ZZ Repair Perineum Bursa and Ligament, Percutaneous Endoscopic Approach

0MQL0ZZ Repair Right Hip Bursa and Ligament, Open Approach

0MQL3ZZ Repair Right Hip Bursa and Ligament, Percutaneous Approach

0MQL4ZZ Repair Right Hip Bursa and Ligament, Percutaneous Endoscopic Approach

0MQM0ZZ Repair Left Hip Bursa and Ligament, Open Approach

0MQM3ZZ Repair Left Hip Bursa and Ligament, Percutaneous Approach

0MQM4ZZ Repair Left Hip Bursa and Ligament, Percutaneous Endoscopic Approach

0MQN0ZZ Repair Right Knee Bursa and Ligament, Open Approach

0MQN3ZZ Repair Right Knee Bursa and Ligament, Percutaneous Approach

0MQN4ZZ Repair Right Knee Bursa and Ligament, Percutaneous Endoscopic Approach

0MQP0ZZ Repair Left Knee Bursa and Ligament, Open Approach

0MQP3ZZ Repair Left Knee Bursa and Ligament, Percutaneous Approach

0MQP4ZZ Repair Left Knee Bursa and Ligament, Percutaneous Endoscopic Approach

0MQQ0ZZ Repair Right Ankle Bursa and Ligament, Open Approach

0MQQ3ZZ Repair Right Ankle Bursa and Ligament, Percutaneous Approach

0MQQ4ZZ Repair Right Ankle Bursa and Ligament, Percutaneous Endoscopic Approach

0MQR0ZZ Repair Left Ankle Bursa and Ligament, Open Approach

0MQR3ZZ Repair Left Ankle Bursa and Ligament, Percutaneous Approach

0MQR4ZZ Repair Left Ankle Bursa and Ligament, Percutaneous Endoscopic Approach

0MQS0ZZ Repair Right Foot Bursa and Ligament, Open Approach

0MQS3ZZ Repair Right Foot Bursa and Ligament, Percutaneous Approach

0MQS4ZZ Repair Right Foot Bursa and Ligament, Percutaneous Endoscopic Approach

0MQT0ZZ Repair Left Foot Bursa and Ligament, Open Approach

0MQT3ZZ Repair Left Foot Bursa and Ligament, Percutaneous Approach

0MQT4ZZ Repair Left Foot Bursa and Ligament, Percutaneous Endoscopic Approach

0MQV0ZZ Repair Right Lower Extremity Bursa and Ligament, Open Approach

0MQV3ZZ Repair Right Lower Extremity Bursa and Ligament, Percutaneous Approach

0MQV4ZZ Repair Right Lower Extremity Bursa and Ligament, Percutaneous Endoscopic Approach

0MQW0ZZ Repair Left Lower Extremity Bursa and Ligament, Open Approach

0MQW3ZZ Repair Left Lower Extremity Bursa and Ligament, Percutaneous Approach

0MQW4ZZ Repair Left Lower Extremity Bursa and Ligament, Percutaneous Endoscopic Approach

0MR – Bursae and Ligaments, Replacement

Review Coding Guideline B3.18

0MR007Z Replacement of Head and Neck Bursa and Ligament with Autologous Tissue Substitute, Open Approach

0MR00JZ Replacement of Head and Neck Bursa and Ligament with Synthetic Substitute, Open Approach

0MR00KZ Replacement of Head and Neck Bursa and Ligament with Nonautologous Tissue Substitute, Open Approach

0MR047Z Replacement of Head and Neck Bursa and Ligament with Autologous Tissue Substitute, Percutaneous Endoscopic Approach

0MR04JZ Replacement of Head and Neck Bursa and Ligament with Synthetic Substitute, Percutaneous Endoscopic Approach

0MR04KZ Replacement of Head and Neck Bursa and Ligament with Nonautologous Tissue Substitute, Percutaneous Endoscopic Approach

0MR107Z Replacement of Right Shoulder Bursa and Ligament with Autologous Tissue Substitute, Open Approach

0MR10JZ Replacement of Right Shoulder Bursa and Ligament with Synthetic Substitute, Open Approach

0MR10KZ Replacement of Right Shoulder Bursa and Ligament with Nonautologous Tissue Substitute, Open Approach

0MR147Z Replacement of Right Shoulder Bursa and Ligament with Autologous Tissue Substitute, Percutaneous Endoscopic Approach

0MR14JZ Replacement of Right Shoulder Bursa and Ligament with Synthetic Substitute, Percutaneous Endoscopic Approach

0MR14KZ Replacement of Right Shoulder Bursa and Ligament with Nonautologous Tissue Substitute, Percutaneous Endoscopic Approach

0MR207Z Replacement of Left Shoulder Bursa and Ligament with Autologous Tissue Substitute, Open Approach

0MR20JZ Replacement of Left Shoulder Bursa and Ligament with Synthetic Substitute, Open Approach

0MR20KZ Replacement of Left Shoulder Bursa and Ligament with Nonautologous Tissue Substitute, Open Approach

0MR247Z Replacement of Left Shoulder Bursa and Ligament with Autologous Tissue Substitute, Percutaneous Endoscopic Approach

0MR24JZ Replacement of Left Shoulder Bursa and Ligament with Synthetic Substitute, Percutaneous Endoscopic Approach

0MR24KZ Replacement of Left Shoulder Bursa and Ligament with Nonautologous Tissue Substitute, Percutaneous Endoscopic Approach

0MR307Z Replacement of Right Elbow Bursa and Ligament with Autologous Tissue Substitute, Open Approach

0MR30JZ Replacement of Right Elbow Bursa and Ligament with Synthetic Substitute, Open Approach

0MR30KZ Replacement of Right Elbow Bursa and Ligament with Nonautologous Tissue Substitute, Open Approach

0MR347Z Replacement of Right Elbow Bursa and Ligament with Autologous Tissue Substitute, Percutaneous Endoscopic Approach

0MR34JZ Replacement of Right Elbow Bursa and Ligament with Synthetic Substitute, Percutaneous Endoscopic Approach

0MR34KZ Replacement of Right Elbow Bursa and Ligament with Nonautologous Tissue Substitute, Percutaneous Endoscopic Approach

0MR407Z Replacement of Left Elbow Bursa and Ligament with Autologous Tissue Substitute, Open Approach

0MR40JZ Replacement of Left Elbow Bursa and Ligament with Synthetic Substitute, Open Approach

♀ Female-only　　♂ Male-only　　▲ Limited Coverage　　● Non-OR　　HAC HAC-associated procedure　　▲ Non-covered procedures　　✚ Cluster

0MR40KZ Replacement of Left Elbow Bursa and Ligament with Nonautologous Tissue Substitute, Open Approach

0MR447Z Replacement of Left Elbow Bursa and Ligament with Autologous Tissue Substitute, Percutaneous Endoscopic Approach

0MR44JZ Replacement of Left Elbow Bursa and Ligament with Synthetic Substitute, Percutaneous Endoscopic Approach

0MR44KZ Replacement of Left Elbow Bursa and Ligament with Nonautologous Tissue Substitute, Percutaneous Endoscopic Approach

0MR507Z Replacement of Right Wrist Bursa and Ligament with Autologous Tissue Substitute, Open Approach

0MR50JZ Replacement of Right Wrist Bursa and Ligament with Synthetic Substitute, Open Approach

0MR50KZ Replacement of Right Wrist Bursa and Ligament with Nonautologous Tissue Substitute, Open Approach

0MR547Z Replacement of Right Wrist Bursa and Ligament with Autologous Tissue Substitute, Percutaneous Endoscopic Approach

0MR54JZ Replacement of Right Wrist Bursa and Ligament with Synthetic Substitute, Percutaneous Endoscopic Approach

0MR54KZ Replacement of Right Wrist Bursa and Ligament with Nonautologous Tissue Substitute, Percutaneous Endoscopic Approach

0MR607Z Replacement of Left Wrist Bursa and Ligament with Autologous Tissue Substitute, Open Approach

0MR60JZ Replacement of Left Wrist Bursa and Ligament with Synthetic Substitute, Open Approach

0MR60KZ Replacement of Left Wrist Bursa and Ligament with Nonautologous Tissue Substitute, Open Approach

0MR647Z Replacement of Left Wrist Bursa and Ligament with Autologous Tissue Substitute, Percutaneous Endoscopic Approach

0MR64JZ Replacement of Left Wrist Bursa and Ligament with Synthetic Substitute, Percutaneous Endoscopic Approach

0MR64KZ Replacement of Left Wrist Bursa and Ligament with Nonautologous Tissue Substitute, Percutaneous Endoscopic Approach

0MR707Z Replacement of Right Hand Bursa and Ligament with Autologous Tissue Substitute, Open Approach

0MR70JZ Replacement of Right Hand Bursa and Ligament with Synthetic Substitute, Open Approach

0MR70KZ Replacement of Right Hand Bursa and Ligament with Nonautologous Tissue Substitute, Open Approach

0MR747Z Replacement of Right Hand Bursa and Ligament with Autologous Tissue Substitute, Percutaneous Endoscopic Approach

0MR74JZ Replacement of Right Hand Bursa and Ligament with Synthetic Substitute, Percutaneous Endoscopic Approach

0MR74KZ Replacement of Right Hand Bursa and Ligament with Nonautologous Tissue Substitute, Percutaneous Endoscopic Approach

0MR807Z Replacement of Left Hand Bursa and Ligament with Autologous Tissue Substitute, Open Approach

0MR80JZ Replacement of Left Hand Bursa and Ligament with Synthetic Substitute, Open Approach

0MR80KZ Replacement of Left Hand Bursa and Ligament with Nonautologous Tissue Substitute, Open Approach

0MR847Z Replacement of Left Hand Bursa and Ligament with Autologous Tissue Substitute, Percutaneous Endoscopic Approach

0MR84JZ Replacement of Left Hand Bursa and Ligament with Synthetic Substitute, Percutaneous Endoscopic Approach

0MR84KZ Replacement of Left Hand Bursa and Ligament with Nonautologous Tissue Substitute, Percutaneous Endoscopic Approach

0MR907Z Replacement of Right Upper Extremity Bursa and Ligament with Autologous Tissue Substitute, Open Approach

0MR90JZ Replacement of Right Upper Extremity Bursa and Ligament with Synthetic Substitute, Open Approach

0MR90KZ Replacement of Right Upper Extremity Bursa and Ligament with Nonautologous Tissue Substitute, Open Approach

0MR947Z Replacement of Right Upper Extremity Bursa and Ligament with Autologous Tissue Substitute, Percutaneous Endoscopic Approach

0MR94JZ Replacement of Right Upper Extremity Bursa and Ligament with Synthetic Substitute, Percutaneous Endoscopic Approach

0MR94KZ Replacement of Right Upper Extremity Bursa and Ligament with Nonautologous Tissue Substitute, Percutaneous Endoscopic Approach

0MRB07Z Replacement of Left Upper Extremity Bursa and Ligament with Autologous Tissue Substitute, Open Approach

0MRB0JZ Replacement of Left Upper Extremity Bursa and Ligament with Synthetic Substitute, Open Approach

0MRB0KZ Replacement of Left Upper Extremity Bursa and Ligament with Nonautologous Tissue Substitute, Open Approach

0MRB47Z Replacement of Left Upper Extremity Bursa and Ligament with Autologous Tissue Substitute, Percutaneous Endoscopic Approach

0MRB4JZ Replacement of Left Upper Extremity Bursa and Ligament with Synthetic Substitute, Percutaneous Endoscopic Approach

0MRB4KZ Replacement of Left Upper Extremity Bursa and Ligament with Nonautologous Tissue Substitute, Percutaneous Endoscopic Approach

0MRC07Z Replacement of Upper Spine Bursa and Ligament with Autologous Tissue Substitute, Open Approach

0MRC0JZ Replacement of Upper Spine Bursa and Ligament with Synthetic Substitute, Open Approach

0MRC0KZ Replacement of Upper Spine Bursa and Ligament with Nonautologous Tissue Substitute, Open Approach

0MRC47Z Replacement of Upper Spine Bursa and Ligament with Autologous Tissue Substitute, Percutaneous Endoscopic Approach

0MRC4JZ Replacement of Upper Spine Bursa and Ligament with Synthetic Substitute, Percutaneous Endoscopic Approach

0MRC4KZ Replacement of Upper Spine Bursa and Ligament with Nonautologous Tissue Substitute, Percutaneous Endoscopic Approach

0MRD07Z Replacement of Lower Spine Bursa and Ligament with Autologous Tissue Substitute, Open Approach

0MRD0JZ Replacement of Lower Spine Bursa and Ligament with Synthetic Substitute, Open Approach

0MRD0KZ Replacement of Lower Spine Bursa and Ligament with Nonautologous Tissue Substitute, Open Approach

0MRD47Z Replacement of Lower Spine Bursa and Ligament with Autologous Tissue Substitute, Percutaneous Endoscopic Approach

0MRD4JZ Replacement of Lower Spine Bursa and Ligament with Synthetic Substitute, Percutaneous Endoscopic Approach

0MRD4KZ Replacement of Lower Spine Bursa and Ligament with Nonautologous Tissue Substitute, Percutaneous Endoscopic Approach

0MRF07Z Replacement of Sternum Bursa and Ligament with Autologous Tissue Substitute, Open Approach

0MRF0JZ Replacement of Sternum Bursa and Ligament with Synthetic Substitute, Open Approach

0MRF0KZ Replacement of Sternum Bursa and Ligament with Nonautologous Tissue Substitute, Open Approach

0MRF47Z Replacement of Sternum Bursa and Ligament with Autologous Tissue Substitute, Percutaneous Endoscopic Approach

0MRF4JZ Replacement of Sternum Bursa and Ligament with Synthetic Substitute, Percutaneous Endoscopic Approach

0MRF4KZ Replacement of Sternum Bursa and Ligament with Nonautologous Tissue Substitute, Percutaneous Endoscopic Approach

0MRG07Z Replacement of Rib(s) Bursa and Ligament with Autologous Tissue Substitute, Open Approach

0MRG0JZ Replacement of Rib(s) Bursa and Ligament with Synthetic Substitute, Open Approach

0MRG0KZ Replacement of Rib(s) Bursa and Ligament with Nonautologous Tissue Substitute, Open Approach

0MRG47Z Replacement of Rib(s) Bursa and Ligament with Autologous Tissue Substitute, Percutaneous Endoscopic Approach

0MRG4JZ Replacement of Rib(s) Bursa and Ligament with Synthetic Substitute, Percutaneous Endoscopic Approach

0MRG4KZ Replacement of Rib(s) Bursa and Ligament with Nonautologous Tissue Substitute, Percutaneous Endoscopic Approach

0MRH07Z Replacement of Right Abdomen Bursa and Ligament with Autologous Tissue Substitute, Open Approach

0MRH0JZ Replacement of Right Abdomen Bursa and Ligament with Synthetic Substitute, Open Approach

0MRH0KZ Replacement of Right Abdomen Bursa and Ligament with Nonautologous Tissue Substitute, Open Approach

0MRH47Z Replacement of Right Abdomen Bursa and Ligament with Autologous Tissue Substitute, Percutaneous Endoscopic Approach

0MRH4JZ Replacement of Right Abdomen Bursa and Ligament with Synthetic Substitute, Percutaneous Endoscopic Approach

0MRH4KZ Replacement of Right Abdomen Bursa and Ligament with Nonautologous Tissue Substitute, Percutaneous Endoscopic Approach

0MRJ07Z Replacement of Left Abdomen Bursa and Ligament with Autologous Tissue Substitute, Open Approach

0MRJ0JZ Replacement of Left Abdomen Bursa and Ligament with Synthetic Substitute, Open Approach

0MRJ0KZ Replacement of Left Abdomen Bursa and Ligament with Nonautologous Tissue Substitute, Open Approach

0MRJ47Z Replacement of Left Abdomen Bursa and Ligament with Autologous Tissue Substitute, Percutaneous Endoscopic Approach

0MRJ4JZ Replacement of Left Abdomen Bursa and Ligament with Synthetic Substitute, Percutaneous Endoscopic Approach

0MRJ4KZ Replacement of Left Abdomen Bursa and Ligament with Nonautologous Tissue Substitute, Percutaneous Endoscopic Approach

0MRK07Z Replacement of Perineum Bursa and Ligament with Autologous Tissue Substitute, Open Approach

0MRK0JZ Replacement of Perineum Bursa and Ligament with Synthetic Substitute, Open Approach

0MRK0KZ Replacement of Perineum Bursa and Ligament with Nonautologous Tissue Substitute, Open Approach

0MRK47Z Replacement of Perineum Bursa and Ligament with Autologous Tissue Substitute, Percutaneous Endoscopic Approach

0MRK4JZ Replacement of Perineum Bursa and Ligament with Synthetic Substitute, Percutaneous Endoscopic Approach

0MRK4KZ Replacement of Perineum Bursa and Ligament with Nonautologous Tissue Substitute, Percutaneous Endoscopic Approach

0MRL07Z Replacement of Right Hip Bursa and Ligament with Autologous Tissue Substitute, Open Approach

0MRL0JZ Replacement of Right Hip Bursa and Ligament with Synthetic Substitute, Open Approach

0MRL0KZ Replacement of Right Hip Bursa and Ligament with Nonautologous Tissue Substitute, Open Approach

0MRL47Z Replacement of Right Hip Bursa and Ligament with Autologous Tissue Substitute, Percutaneous Endoscopic Approach

0MRL4JZ Replacement of Right Hip Bursa and Ligament with Synthetic Substitute, Percutaneous Endoscopic Approach

0MRL4KZ Replacement of Right Hip Bursa and Ligament with Nonautologous Tissue Substitute, Percutaneous Endoscopic Approach

0MRM07Z Replacement of Left Hip Bursa and Ligament with Autologous Tissue Substitute, Open Approach

0MRM0JZ Replacement of Left Hip Bursa and Ligament with Synthetic Substitute, Open Approach

0MRM0KZ Replacement of Left Hip Bursa and Ligament with Nonautologous Tissue Substitute, Open Approach

0MRM47Z Replacement of Left Hip Bursa and Ligament with Autologous Tissue Substitute, Percutaneous Endoscopic Approach

0MRM4JZ Replacement of Left Hip Bursa and Ligament with Synthetic Substitute, Percutaneous Endoscopic Approach

0MRM4KZ Replacement of Left Hip Bursa and Ligament with Nonautologous Tissue Substitute, Percutaneous Endoscopic Approach

0MRN07Z Replacement of Right Knee Bursa and Ligament with Autologous Tissue Substitute, Open Approach

0MRN0JZ Replacement of Right Knee Bursa and Ligament with Synthetic Substitute, Open Approach

0MRN0KZ Replacement of Right Knee Bursa and Ligament with Nonautologous Tissue Substitute, Open Approach

0MRN47Z Replacement of Right Knee Bursa and Ligament with Autologous Tissue Substitute, Percutaneous Endoscopic Approach

0MRN4JZ Replacement of Right Knee Bursa and Ligament with Synthetic Substitute, Percutaneous Endoscopic Approach

0MRN4KZ Replacement of Right Knee Bursa and Ligament with Nonautologous Tissue Substitute, Percutaneous Endoscopic Approach

0MRP07Z Replacement of Left Knee Bursa and Ligament with Autologous Tissue Substitute, Open Approach

0MRP0JZ Replacement of Left Knee Bursa and Ligament with Synthetic Substitute, Open Approach

0MRP0KZ Replacement of Left Knee Bursa and Ligament with Nonautologous Tissue Substitute, Open Approach

0MRP47Z Replacement of Left Knee Bursa and Ligament with Autologous Tissue Substitute, Percutaneous Endoscopic Approach

0MRP4JZ Replacement of Left Knee Bursa and Ligament with Synthetic Substitute, Percutaneous Endoscopic Approach

0MRP4KZ Replacement of Left Knee Bursa and Ligament with Nonautologous Tissue Substitute, Percutaneous Endoscopic Approach

0MRQ07Z Replacement of Right Ankle Bursa and Ligament with Autologous Tissue Substitute, Open Approach

0MRQ0JZ Replacement of Right Ankle Bursa and Ligament with Synthetic Substitute, Open Approach

0MRQ0KZ Replacement of Right Ankle Bursa and Ligament with Nonautologous Tissue Substitute, Open Approach

0MRQ47Z Replacement of Right Ankle Bursa and Ligament with Autologous Tissue Substitute, Percutaneous Endoscopic Approach

0MRQ4JZ Replacement of Right Ankle Bursa and Ligament with Synthetic Substitute, Percutaneous Endoscopic Approach

0MRQ4KZ Replacement of Right Ankle Bursa and Ligament with Nonautologous Tissue Substitute, Percutaneous Endoscopic Approach

0MRR07Z Replacement of Left Ankle Bursa and Ligament with Autologous Tissue Substitute, Open Approach

0MRR0JZ Replacement of Left Ankle Bursa and Ligament with Synthetic Substitute, Open Approach

0MRR0KZ Replacement of Left Ankle Bursa and Ligament with Nonautologous Tissue Substitute, Open Approach

0MRR47Z Replacement of Left Ankle Bursa and Ligament with Autologous Tissue Substitute, Percutaneous Endoscopic Approach

0MRR4JZ Replacement of Left Ankle Bursa and Ligament with Synthetic Substitute, Percutaneous Endoscopic Approach

0MRR4KZ Replacement of Left Ankle Bursa and Ligament with Nonautologous Tissue Substitute, Percutaneous Endoscopic Approach

0MRS07Z Replacement of Right Foot Bursa and Ligament with Autologous Tissue Substitute, Open Approach

0MRS0JZ Replacement of Right Foot Bursa and Ligament with Synthetic Substitute, Open Approach

0MRS0KZ Replacement of Right Foot Bursa and Ligament with Nonautologous Tissue Substitute, Open Approach

0MRS47Z Replacement of Right Foot Bursa and Ligament with Autologous Tissue Substitute, Percutaneous Endoscopic Approach

0MRS4JZ Replacement of Right Foot Bursa and Ligament with Synthetic Substitute, Percutaneous Endoscopic Approach

0MRS4KZ Replacement of Right Foot Bursa and Ligament with Nonautologous Tissue Substitute, Percutaneous Endoscopic Approach

0MRT07Z Replacement of Left Foot Bursa and Ligament with Autologous Tissue Substitute, Open Approach

0MRT0JZ Replacement of Left Foot Bursa and Ligament with Synthetic Substitute, Open Approach

0MRT0KZ Replacement of Left Foot Bursa and Ligament with Nonautologous Tissue Substitute, Open Approach

0MRT47Z Replacement of Left Foot Bursa and Ligament with Autologous Tissue Substitute, Percutaneous Endoscopic Approach

0MRT4JZ Replacement of Left Foot Bursa and Ligament with Synthetic Substitute, Percutaneous Endoscopic Approach

0MRT4KZ Replacement of Left Foot Bursa and Ligament with Nonautologous Tissue Substitute, Percutaneous Endoscopic Approach

0MRV07Z Replacement of Right Lower Extremity Bursa and Ligament with Autologous Tissue Substitute, Open Approach

0MRV0JZ Replacement of Right Lower Extremity Bursa and Ligament with Synthetic Substitute, Open Approach

0MRV0KZ Replacement of Right Lower Extremity Bursa and Ligament with Nonautologous Tissue Substitute, Open Approach

♀ Female-only   ♂ Male-only   ▲ Limited Coverage   ● Non-OR   HAC HAC-associated procedure   ▲ Non-covered procedures   ✚ Cluster

0MRV47Z	Replacement of Right Lower Extremity Bursa and Ligament with Autologous Tissue Substitute, Percutaneous Endoscopic Approach
0MRV4JZ	Replacement of Right Lower Extremity Bursa and Ligament with Synthetic Substitute, Percutaneous Endoscopic Approach
0MRV4KZ	Replacement of Right Lower Extremity Bursa and Ligament with Nonautologous Tissue Substitute, Percutaneous Endoscopic Approach

0MRW07Z	Replacement of Left Lower Extremity Bursa and Ligament with Autologous Tissue Substitute, Open Approach
0MRW0JZ	Replacement of Left Lower Extremity Bursa and Ligament with Synthetic Substitute, Open Approach
0MRW0KZ	Replacement of Left Lower Extremity Bursa and Ligament with Nonautologous Tissue Substitute, Open Approach
0MRW47Z	Replacement of Left Lower Extremity Bursa and Ligament with Autologous Tissue Substitute, Percutaneous Endoscopic Approach
0MRW4JZ	Replacement of Left Lower Extremity Bursa and Ligament with Synthetic Substitute, Percutaneous Endoscopic Approach
0MRW4KZ	Replacement of Left Lower Extremity Bursa and Ligament with Nonautologous Tissue Substitute, Percutaneous Endoscopic Approach

0MS – Bursae and Ligaments, Reposition

0MS00ZZ	Reposition Head and Neck Bursa and Ligament, Open Approach
0MS04ZZ	Reposition Head and Neck Bursa and Ligament, Percutaneous Endoscopic Approach
0MS10ZZ	Reposition Right Shoulder Bursa and Ligament, Open Approach
0MS14ZZ	Reposition Right Shoulder Bursa and Ligament, Percutaneous Endoscopic Approach
0MS20ZZ	Reposition Left Shoulder Bursa and Ligament, Open Approach
0MS24ZZ	Reposition Left Shoulder Bursa and Ligament, Percutaneous Endoscopic Approach
0MS30ZZ	Reposition Right Elbow Bursa and Ligament, Open Approach
0MS34ZZ	Reposition Right Elbow Bursa and Ligament, Percutaneous Endoscopic Approach
0MS40ZZ	Reposition Left Elbow Bursa and Ligament, Open Approach
0MS44ZZ	Reposition Left Elbow Bursa and Ligament, Percutaneous Endoscopic Approach
0MS50ZZ	Reposition Right Wrist Bursa and Ligament, Open Approach
0MS54ZZ	Reposition Right Wrist Bursa and Ligament, Percutaneous Endoscopic Approach
0MS60ZZ	Reposition Left Wrist Bursa and Ligament, Open Approach
0MS64ZZ	Reposition Left Wrist Bursa and Ligament, Percutaneous Endoscopic Approach
0MS70ZZ	Reposition Right Hand Bursa and Ligament, Open Approach
0MS74ZZ	Reposition Right Hand Bursa and Ligament, Percutaneous Endoscopic Approach
0MS80ZZ	Reposition Left Hand Bursa and Ligament, Open Approach
0MS84ZZ	Reposition Left Hand Bursa and Ligament, Percutaneous Endoscopic Approach
0MS90ZZ	Reposition Right Upper Extremity Bursa and Ligament, Open Approach

0MS94ZZ	Reposition Right Upper Extremity Bursa and Ligament, Percutaneous Endoscopic Approach
0MSB0ZZ	Reposition Left Upper Extremity Bursa and Ligament, Open Approach
0MSB4ZZ	Reposition Left Upper Extremity Bursa and Ligament, Percutaneous Endoscopic Approach
0MSC0ZZ	Reposition Upper Spine Bursa and Ligament, Open Approach
0MSC4ZZ	Reposition Upper Spine Bursa and Ligament, Percutaneous Endoscopic Approach
0MSD0ZZ	Reposition Lower Spine Bursa and Ligament, Open Approach
0MSD4ZZ	Reposition Lower Spine Bursa and Ligament, Percutaneous Endoscopic Approach
0MSF0ZZ	Reposition Sternum Bursa and Ligament, Open Approach
0MSF4ZZ	Reposition Sternum Bursa and Ligament, Percutaneous Endoscopic Approach
0MSG0ZZ	Reposition Rib(s) Bursa and Ligament, Open Approach
0MSG4ZZ	Reposition Rib(s) Bursa and Ligament, Percutaneous Endoscopic Approach
0MSH0ZZ	Reposition Right Abdomen Bursa and Ligament, Open Approach
0MSH4ZZ	Reposition Right Abdomen Bursa and Ligament, Percutaneous Endoscopic Approach
0MSJ0ZZ	Reposition Left Abdomen Bursa and Ligament, Open Approach
0MSJ4ZZ	Reposition Left Abdomen Bursa and Ligament, Percutaneous Endoscopic Approach
0MSK0ZZ	Reposition Perineum Bursa and Ligament, Open Approach
0MSK4ZZ	Reposition Perineum Bursa and Ligament, Percutaneous Endoscopic Approach
0MSL0ZZ	Reposition Right Hip Bursa and Ligament, Open Approach
0MSL4ZZ	Reposition Right Hip Bursa and Ligament, Percutaneous Endoscopic Approach

0MSM0ZZ	Reposition Left Hip Bursa and Ligament, Open Approach
0MSM4ZZ	Reposition Left Hip Bursa and Ligament, Percutaneous Endoscopic Approach
0MSN0ZZ	Reposition Right Knee Bursa and Ligament, Open Approach
0MSN4ZZ	Reposition Right Knee Bursa and Ligament, Percutaneous Endoscopic Approach
0MSP0ZZ	Reposition Left Knee Bursa and Ligament, Open Approach
0MSP4ZZ	Reposition Left Knee Bursa and Ligament, Percutaneous Endoscopic Approach
0MSQ0ZZ	Reposition Right Ankle Bursa and Ligament, Open Approach
0MSQ4ZZ	Reposition Right Ankle Bursa and Ligament, Percutaneous Endoscopic Approach
0MSR0ZZ	Reposition Left Ankle Bursa and Ligament, Open Approach
0MSR4ZZ	Reposition Left Ankle Bursa and Ligament, Percutaneous Endoscopic Approach
0MSS0ZZ	Reposition Right Foot Bursa and Ligament, Open Approach
0MSS4ZZ	Reposition Right Foot Bursa and Ligament, Percutaneous Endoscopic Approach
0MST0ZZ	Reposition Left Foot Bursa and Ligament, Open Approach
0MST4ZZ	Reposition Left Foot Bursa and Ligament, Percutaneous Endoscopic Approach
0MSV0ZZ	Reposition Right Lower Extremity Bursa and Ligament, Open Approach
0MSV4ZZ	Reposition Right Lower Extremity Bursa and Ligament, Percutaneous Endoscopic Approach
0MSW0ZZ	Reposition Left Lower Extremity Bursa and Ligament, Open Approach
0MSW4ZZ	Reposition Left Lower Extremity Bursa and Ligament, Percutaneous Endoscopic Approach

0MT – Bursae and Ligaments, Resection

Review Coding Guideline B3.8

Review Coding Guideline B3.18

| 0MT00ZZ | Resection of Head and Neck Bursa and Ligament, Open Approach |
| 0MT04ZZ | Resection of Head and Neck Bursa and Ligament, Percutaneous Endoscopic Approach |

| 0MT10ZZ | Resection of Right Shoulder Bursa and Ligament, Open Approach |
| 0MT14ZZ | Resection of Right Shoulder Bursa and Ligament, Percutaneous Endoscopic Approach |

| 0MT20ZZ | Resection of Left Shoulder Bursa and Ligament, Open Approach |
| 0MT24ZZ | Resection of Left Shoulder Bursa and Ligament, Percutaneous Endoscopic Approach |

0MT30ZZ	Resection of Right Elbow Bursa and Ligament, Open Approach
0MT34ZZ	Resection of Right Elbow Bursa and Ligament, Percutaneous Endoscopic Approach
0MT40ZZ	Resection of Left Elbow Bursa and Ligament, Open Approach
0MT44ZZ	Resection of Left Elbow Bursa and Ligament, Percutaneous Endoscopic Approach
0MT50ZZ	Resection of Right Wrist Bursa and Ligament, Open Approach
0MT54ZZ	Resection of Right Wrist Bursa and Ligament, Percutaneous Endoscopic Approach
0MT60ZZ	Resection of Left Wrist Bursa and Ligament, Open Approach
0MT64ZZ	Resection of Left Wrist Bursa and Ligament, Percutaneous Endoscopic Approach
0MT70ZZ	Resection of Right Hand Bursa and Ligament, Open Approach
0MT74ZZ	Resection of Right Hand Bursa and Ligament, Percutaneous Endoscopic Approach
0MT80ZZ	Resection of Left Hand Bursa and Ligament, Open Approach
0MT84ZZ	Resection of Left Hand Bursa and Ligament, Percutaneous Endoscopic Approach
0MT90ZZ	Resection of Right Upper Extremity Bursa and Ligament, Open Approach
0MT94ZZ	Resection of Right Upper Extremity Bursa and Ligament, Percutaneous Endoscopic Approach
0MTB0ZZ	Resection of Left Upper Extremity Bursa and Ligament, Open Approach
0MTB4ZZ	Resection of Left Upper Extremity Bursa and Ligament, Percutaneous Endoscopic Approach
0MTC0ZZ	Resection of Upper Spine Bursa and Ligament, Open Approach

0MTC4ZZ	Resection of Upper Spine Bursa and Ligament, Percutaneous Endoscopic Approach
0MTD0ZZ	Resection of Lower Spine Bursa and Ligament, Open Approach
0MTD4ZZ	Resection of Lower Spine Bursa and Ligament, Percutaneous Endoscopic Approach
0MTF0ZZ	Resection of Sternum Bursa and Ligament, Open Approach
0MTF4ZZ	Resection of Sternum Bursa and Ligament, Percutaneous Endoscopic Approach
0MTG0ZZ	Resection of Rib(s) Bursa and Ligament, Open Approach
0MTG4ZZ	Resection of Rib(s) Bursa and Ligament, Percutaneous Endoscopic Approach
0MTH0ZZ	Resection of Right Abdomen Bursa and Ligament, Open Approach
0MTH4ZZ	Resection of Right Abdomen Bursa and Ligament, Percutaneous Endoscopic Approach
0MTJ0ZZ	Resection of Left Abdomen Bursa and Ligament, Open Approach
0MTJ4ZZ	Resection of Left Abdomen Bursa and Ligament, Percutaneous Endoscopic Approach
0MTK0ZZ	Resection of Perineum Bursa and Ligament, Open Approach
0MTK4ZZ	Resection of Perineum Bursa and Ligament, Percutaneous Endoscopic Approach
0MTL0ZZ	Resection of Right Hip Bursa and Ligament, Open Approach
0MTL4ZZ	Resection of Right Hip Bursa and Ligament, Percutaneous Endoscopic Approach
0MTM0ZZ	Resection of Left Hip Bursa and Ligament, Open Approach
0MTM4ZZ	Resection of Left Hip Bursa and Ligament, Percutaneous Endoscopic Approach

0MTN0ZZ	Resection of Right Knee Bursa and Ligament, Open Approach
0MTN4ZZ	Resection of Right Knee Bursa and Ligament, Percutaneous Endoscopic Approach
0MTP0ZZ	Resection of Left Knee Bursa and Ligament, Open Approach
0MTP4ZZ	Resection of Left Knee Bursa and Ligament, Percutaneous Endoscopic Approach
0MTQ0ZZ	Resection of Right Ankle Bursa and Ligament, Open Approach
0MTQ4ZZ	Resection of Right Ankle Bursa and Ligament, Percutaneous Endoscopic Approach
0MTR0ZZ	Resection of Left Ankle Bursa and Ligament, Open Approach
0MTR4ZZ	Resection of Left Ankle Bursa and Ligament, Percutaneous Endoscopic Approach
0MTS0ZZ	Resection of Right Foot Bursa and Ligament, Open Approach
0MTS4ZZ	Resection of Right Foot Bursa and Ligament, Percutaneous Endoscopic Approach
0MTT0ZZ	Resection of Left Foot Bursa and Ligament, Open Approach
0MTT4ZZ	Resection of Left Foot Bursa and Ligament, Percutaneous Endoscopic Approach
0MTV0ZZ	Resection of Right Lower Extremity Bursa and Ligament, Open Approach
0MTV4ZZ	Resection of Right Lower Extremity Bursa and Ligament, Percutaneous Endoscopic Approach
0MTW0ZZ	Resection of Left Lower Extremity Bursa and Ligament, Open Approach
0MTW4ZZ	Resection of Left Lower Extremity Bursa and Ligament, Percutaneous Endoscopic Approach

0MU – Bursae and Ligaments, Supplement

0MU007Z	Supplement Head and Neck Bursa and Ligament with Autologous Tissue Substitute, Open Approach
0MU00JZ	Supplement Head and Neck Bursa and Ligament with Synthetic Substitute, Open Approach
0MU00KZ	Supplement Head and Neck Bursa and Ligament with Nonautologous Tissue Substitute, Open Approach
0MU047Z	Supplement Head and Neck Bursa and Ligament with Autologous Tissue Substitute, Percutaneous Endoscopic Approach
0MU04JZ	Supplement Head and Neck Bursa and Ligament with Synthetic Substitute, Percutaneous Endoscopic Approach
0MU04KZ	Supplement Head and Neck Bursa and Ligament with Nonautologous Tissue Substitute, Percutaneous Endoscopic Approach
0MU107Z	Supplement Right Shoulder Bursa and Ligament with Autologous Tissue Substitute, Open Approach
0MU10JZ	Supplement Right Shoulder Bursa and Ligament with Synthetic Substitute, Open Approach
0MU10KZ	Supplement Right Shoulder Bursa and Ligament with Nonautologous Tissue Substitute, Open Approach

0MU147Z	Supplement Right Shoulder Bursa and Ligament with Autologous Tissue Substitute, Percutaneous Endoscopic Approach
0MU14JZ	Supplement Right Shoulder Bursa and Ligament with Synthetic Substitute, Percutaneous Endoscopic Approach
0MU14KZ	Supplement Right Shoulder Bursa and Ligament with Nonautologous Tissue Substitute, Percutaneous Endoscopic Approach
0MU207Z	Supplement Left Shoulder Bursa and Ligament with Autologous Tissue Substitute, Open Approach
0MU20JZ	Supplement Left Shoulder Bursa and Ligament with Synthetic Substitute, Open Approach
0MU20KZ	Supplement Left Shoulder Bursa and Ligament with Nonautologous Tissue Substitute, Open Approach
0MU247Z	Supplement Left Shoulder Bursa and Ligament with Autologous Tissue Substitute, Percutaneous Endoscopic Approach
0MU24JZ	Supplement Left Shoulder Bursa and Ligament with Synthetic Substitute, Percutaneous Endoscopic Approach

0MU24KZ	Supplement Left Shoulder Bursa and Ligament with Nonautologous Tissue Substitute, Percutaneous Endoscopic Approach
0MU307Z	Supplement Right Elbow Bursa and Ligament with Autologous Tissue Substitute, Open Approach
0MU30JZ	Supplement Right Elbow Bursa and Ligament with Synthetic Substitute, Open Approach
0MU30KZ	Supplement Right Elbow Bursa and Ligament with Nonautologous Tissue Substitute, Open Approach
0MU347Z	Supplement Right Elbow Bursa and Ligament with Autologous Tissue Substitute, Percutaneous Endoscopic Approach
0MU34JZ	Supplement Right Elbow Bursa and Ligament with Synthetic Substitute, Percutaneous Endoscopic Approach
0MU34KZ	Supplement Right Elbow Bursa and Ligament with Nonautologous Tissue Substitute, Percutaneous Endoscopic Approach
0MU407Z	Supplement Left Elbow Bursa and Ligament with Autologous Tissue Substitute, Open Approach
0MU40JZ	Supplement Left Elbow Bursa and Ligament with Synthetic Substitute, Open Approach

♀ Female-only   ♂ Male-only   ▲ Limited Coverage   ● Non-OR   HAC HAC-associated procedure   ▲ Non-covered procedures   ✚ Cluster

0MU40KZ	Supplement Left Elbow Bursa and Ligament with Nonautologous Tissue Substitute, Open Approach
0MU447Z	Supplement Left Elbow Bursa and Ligament with Autologous Tissue Substitute, Percutaneous Endoscopic Approach
0MU44JZ	Supplement Left Elbow Bursa and Ligament with Synthetic Substitute, Percutaneous Endoscopic Approach
0MU44KZ	Supplement Left Elbow Bursa and Ligament with Nonautologous Tissue Substitute, Percutaneous Endoscopic Approach
0MU507Z	Supplement Right Wrist Bursa and Ligament with Autologous Tissue Substitute, Open Approach
0MU50JZ	Supplement Right Wrist Bursa and Ligament with Synthetic Substitute, Open Approach
0MU50KZ	Supplement Right Wrist Bursa and Ligament with Nonautologous Tissue Substitute, Open Approach
0MU547Z	Supplement Right Wrist Bursa and Ligament with Autologous Tissue Substitute, Percutaneous Endoscopic Approach
0MU54JZ	Supplement Right Wrist Bursa and Ligament with Synthetic Substitute, Percutaneous Endoscopic Approach
0MU54KZ	Supplement Right Wrist Bursa and Ligament with Nonautologous Tissue Substitute, Percutaneous Endoscopic Approach
0MU607Z	Supplement Left Wrist Bursa and Ligament with Autologous Tissue Substitute, Open Approach
0MU60JZ	Supplement Left Wrist Bursa and Ligament with Synthetic Substitute, Open Approach
0MU60KZ	Supplement Left Wrist Bursa and Ligament with Nonautologous Tissue Substitute, Open Approach
0MU647Z	Supplement Left Wrist Bursa and Ligament with Autologous Tissue Substitute, Percutaneous Endoscopic Approach
0MU64JZ	Supplement Left Wrist Bursa and Ligament with Synthetic Substitute, Percutaneous Endoscopic Approach
0MU64KZ	Supplement Left Wrist Bursa and Ligament with Nonautologous Tissue Substitute, Percutaneous Endoscopic Approach
0MU707Z	Supplement Right Hand Bursa and Ligament with Autologous Tissue Substitute, Open Approach
0MU70JZ	Supplement Right Hand Bursa and Ligament with Synthetic Substitute, Open Approach
0MU70KZ	Supplement Right Hand Bursa and Ligament with Nonautologous Tissue Substitute, Open Approach
0MU747Z	Supplement Right Hand Bursa and Ligament with Autologous Tissue Substitute, Percutaneous Endoscopic Approach
0MU74JZ	Supplement Right Hand Bursa and Ligament with Synthetic Substitute, Percutaneous Endoscopic Approach
0MU74KZ	Supplement Right Hand Bursa and Ligament with Nonautologous Tissue Substitute, Percutaneous Endoscopic Approach

0MU807Z	Supplement Left Hand Bursa and Ligament with Autologous Tissue Substitute, Open Approach
0MU80JZ	Supplement Left Hand Bursa and Ligament with Synthetic Substitute, Open Approach
0MU80KZ	Supplement Left Hand Bursa and Ligament with Nonautologous Tissue Substitute, Open Approach
0MU847Z	Supplement Left Hand Bursa and Ligament with Autologous Tissue Substitute, Percutaneous Endoscopic Approach
0MU84JZ	Supplement Left Hand Bursa and Ligament with Synthetic Substitute, Percutaneous Endoscopic Approach
0MU84KZ	Supplement Left Hand Bursa and Ligament with Nonautologous Tissue Substitute, Percutaneous Endoscopic Approach
0MU907Z	Supplement Right Upper Extremity Bursa and Ligament with Autologous Tissue Substitute, Open Approach
0MU90JZ	Supplement Right Upper Extremity Bursa and Ligament with Synthetic Substitute, Open Approach
0MU90KZ	Supplement Right Upper Extremity Bursa and Ligament with Nonautologous Tissue Substitute, Open Approach
0MU947Z	Supplement Right Upper Extremity Bursa and Ligament with Autologous Tissue Substitute, Percutaneous Endoscopic Approach
0MU94JZ	Supplement Right Upper Extremity Bursa and Ligament with Synthetic Substitute, Percutaneous Endoscopic Approach
0MU94KZ	Supplement Right Upper Extremity Bursa and Ligament with Nonautologous Tissue Substitute, Percutaneous Endoscopic Approach
0MUB07Z	Supplement Left Upper Extremity Bursa and Ligament with Autologous Tissue Substitute, Open Approach
0MUB0JZ	Supplement Left Upper Extremity Bursa and Ligament with Synthetic Substitute, Open Approach
0MUB0KZ	Supplement Left Upper Extremity Bursa and Ligament with Nonautologous Tissue Substitute, Open Approach
0MUB47Z	Supplement Left Upper Extremity Bursa and Ligament with Autologous Tissue Substitute, Percutaneous Endoscopic Approach
0MUB4JZ	Supplement Left Upper Extremity Bursa and Ligament with Synthetic Substitute, Percutaneous Endoscopic Approach
0MUB4KZ	Supplement Left Upper Extremity Bursa and Ligament with Nonautologous Tissue Substitute, Percutaneous Endoscopic Approach
0MUC07Z	Supplement Upper Spine Bursa and Ligament with Autologous Tissue Substitute, Open Approach
0MUC0JZ	Supplement Upper Spine Bursa and Ligament with Synthetic Substitute, Open Approach
0MUC0KZ	Supplement Upper Spine Bursa and Ligament with Nonautologous Tissue Substitute, Open Approach
0MUC47Z	Supplement Upper Spine Bursa and Ligament with Autologous Tissue Substitute, Percutaneous Endoscopic Approach

0MUC4JZ	Supplement Upper Spine Bursa and Ligament with Synthetic Substitute, Percutaneous Endoscopic Approach
0MUC4KZ	Supplement Upper Spine Bursa and Ligament with Nonautologous Tissue Substitute, Percutaneous Endoscopic Approach
0MUD07Z	Supplement Lower Spine Bursa and Ligament with Autologous Tissue Substitute, Open Approach
0MUD0JZ	Supplement Lower Spine Bursa and Ligament with Synthetic Substitute, Open Approach
0MUD0KZ	Supplement Lower Spine Bursa and Ligament with Nonautologous Tissue Substitute, Open Approach
0MUD47Z	Supplement Lower Spine Bursa and Ligament with Autologous Tissue Substitute, Percutaneous Endoscopic Approach
0MUD4JZ	Supplement Lower Spine Bursa and Ligament with Synthetic Substitute, Percutaneous Endoscopic Approach
0MUD4KZ	Supplement Lower Spine Bursa and Ligament with Nonautologous Tissue Substitute, Percutaneous Endoscopic Approach
0MUF07Z	Supplement Sternum Bursa and Ligament with Autologous Tissue Substitute, Open Approach
0MUF0JZ	Supplement Sternum Bursa and Ligament with Synthetic Substitute, Open Approach
0MUF0KZ	Supplement Sternum Bursa and Ligament with Nonautologous Tissue Substitute, Open Approach
0MUF47Z	Supplement Sternum Bursa and Ligament with Autologous Tissue Substitute, Percutaneous Endoscopic Approach
0MUF4JZ	Supplement Sternum Bursa and Ligament with Synthetic Substitute, Percutaneous Endoscopic Approach
0MUF4KZ	Supplement Sternum Bursa and Ligament with Nonautologous Tissue Substitute, Percutaneous Endoscopic Approach
0MUG07Z	Supplement Rib(s) Bursa and Ligament with Autologous Tissue Substitute, Open Approach
0MUG0JZ	Supplement Rib(s) Bursa and Ligament with Synthetic Substitute, Open Approach
0MUG0KZ	Supplement Rib(s) Bursa and Ligament with Nonautologous Tissue Substitute, Open Approach
0MUG47Z	Supplement Rib(s) Bursa and Ligament with Autologous Tissue Substitute, Percutaneous Endoscopic Approach
0MUG4JZ	Supplement Rib(s) Bursa and Ligament with Synthetic Substitute, Percutaneous Endoscopic Approach
0MUG4KZ	Supplement Rib(s) Bursa and Ligament with Nonautologous Tissue Substitute, Percutaneous Endoscopic Approach
0MUH07Z	Supplement Right Abdomen Bursa and Ligament with Autologous Tissue Substitute, Open Approach
0MUH0JZ	Supplement Right Abdomen Bursa and Ligament with Synthetic Substitute, Open Approach
0MUH0KZ	Supplement Right Abdomen Bursa and Ligament with Nonautologous Tissue Substitute, Open Approach

♀ Female-only	♂ Male-only	▲ Limited Coverage	● Non-OR	☒ HAC-associated procedure	▲ Non-covered procedures	➕ Cluster

0MUH47Z Supplement Right Abdomen Bursa and Ligament with Autologous Tissue Substitute, Percutaneous Endoscopic Approach

0MUH4JZ Supplement Right Abdomen Bursa and Ligament with Synthetic Substitute, Percutaneous Endoscopic Approach

0MUH4KZ Supplement Right Abdomen Bursa and Ligament with Nonautologous Tissue Substitute, Percutaneous Endoscopic Approach

0MUJ07Z Supplement Left Abdomen Bursa and Ligament with Autologous Tissue Substitute, Open Approach

0MUJ0JZ Supplement Left Abdomen Bursa and Ligament with Synthetic Substitute, Open Approach

0MUJ0KZ Supplement Left Abdomen Bursa and Ligament with Nonautologous Tissue Substitute, Open Approach

0MUJ47Z Supplement Left Abdomen Bursa and Ligament with Autologous Tissue Substitute, Percutaneous Endoscopic Approach

0MUJ4JZ Supplement Left Abdomen Bursa and Ligament with Synthetic Substitute, Percutaneous Endoscopic Approach

0MUJ4KZ Supplement Left Abdomen Bursa and Ligament with Nonautologous Tissue Substitute, Percutaneous Endoscopic Approach

0MUK07Z Supplement Perineum Bursa and Ligament with Autologous Tissue Substitute, Open Approach

0MUK0JZ Supplement Perineum Bursa and Ligament with Synthetic Substitute, Open Approach

0MUK0KZ Supplement Perineum Bursa and Ligament with Nonautologous Tissue Substitute, Open Approach

0MUK47Z Supplement Perineum Bursa and Ligament with Autologous Tissue Substitute, Percutaneous Endoscopic Approach

0MUK4JZ Supplement Perineum Bursa and Ligament with Synthetic Substitute, Percutaneous Endoscopic Approach

0MUK4KZ Supplement Perineum Bursa and Ligament with Nonautologous Tissue Substitute, Percutaneous Endoscopic Approach

0MUL07Z Supplement Right Hip Bursa and Ligament with Autologous Tissue Substitute, Open Approach

0MUL0JZ Supplement Right Hip Bursa and Ligament with Synthetic Substitute, Open Approach

0MUL0KZ Supplement Right Hip Bursa and Ligament with Nonautologous Tissue Substitute, Open Approach

0MUL47Z Supplement Right Hip Bursa and Ligament with Autologous Tissue Substitute, Percutaneous Endoscopic Approach

0MUL4JZ Supplement Right Hip Bursa and Ligament with Synthetic Substitute, Percutaneous Endoscopic Approach

0MUL4KZ Supplement Right Hip Bursa and Ligament with Nonautologous Tissue Substitute, Percutaneous Endoscopic Approach

0MUM07Z Supplement Left Hip Bursa and Ligament with Autologous Tissue Substitute, Open Approach

0MUM0JZ Supplement Left Hip Bursa and Ligament with Synthetic Substitute, Open Approach

0MUM0KZ Supplement Left Hip Bursa and Ligament with Nonautologous Tissue Substitute, Open Approach

0MUM47Z Supplement Left Hip Bursa and Ligament with Autologous Tissue Substitute, Percutaneous Endoscopic Approach

0MUM4JZ Supplement Left Hip Bursa and Ligament with Synthetic Substitute, Percutaneous Endoscopic Approach

0MUM4KZ Supplement Left Hip Bursa and Ligament with Nonautologous Tissue Substitute, Percutaneous Endoscopic Approach

0MUN07Z Supplement Right Knee Bursa and Ligament with Autologous Tissue Substitute, Open Approach

0MUN0JZ Supplement Right Knee Bursa and Ligament with Synthetic Substitute, Open Approach

0MUN0KZ Supplement Right Knee Bursa and Ligament with Nonautologous Tissue Substitute, Open Approach

0MUN47Z Supplement Right Knee Bursa and Ligament with Autologous Tissue Substitute, Percutaneous Endoscopic Approach

AHA CC: 2Q, 2017, 21-22

0MUN4JZ Supplement Right Knee Bursa and Ligament with Synthetic Substitute, Percutaneous Endoscopic Approach

0MUN4KZ Supplement Right Knee Bursa and Ligament with Nonautologous Tissue Substitute, Percutaneous Endoscopic Approach

0MUP07Z Supplement Left Knee Bursa and Ligament with Autologous Tissue Substitute, Open Approach

0MUP0JZ Supplement Left Knee Bursa and Ligament with Synthetic Substitute, Open Approach

0MUP0KZ Supplement Left Knee Bursa and Ligament with Nonautologous Tissue Substitute, Open Approach

0MUP47Z Supplement Left Knee Bursa and Ligament with Autologous Tissue Substitute, Percutaneous Endoscopic Approach

0MUP4JZ Supplement Left Knee Bursa and Ligament with Synthetic Substitute, Percutaneous Endoscopic Approach

0MUP4KZ Supplement Left Knee Bursa and Ligament with Nonautologous Tissue Substitute, Percutaneous Endoscopic Approach

0MUQ07Z Supplement Right Ankle Bursa and Ligament with Autologous Tissue Substitute, Open Approach

0MUQ0JZ Supplement Right Ankle Bursa and Ligament with Synthetic Substitute, Open Approach

0MUQ0KZ Supplement Right Ankle Bursa and Ligament with Nonautologous Tissue Substitute, Open Approach

0MUQ47Z Supplement Right Ankle Bursa and Ligament with Autologous Tissue Substitute, Percutaneous Endoscopic Approach

0MUQ4JZ Supplement Right Ankle Bursa and Ligament with Synthetic Substitute, Percutaneous Endoscopic Approach

0MUQ4KZ Supplement Right Ankle Bursa and Ligament with Nonautologous Tissue Substitute, Percutaneous Endoscopic Approach

0MUR07Z Supplement Left Ankle Bursa and Ligament with Autologous Tissue Substitute, Open Approach

0MUR0JZ Supplement Left Ankle Bursa and Ligament with Synthetic Substitute, Open Approach

0MUR0KZ Supplement Left Ankle Bursa and Ligament with Nonautologous Tissue Substitute, Open Approach

0MUR47Z Supplement Left Ankle Bursa and Ligament with Autologous Tissue Substitute, Percutaneous Endoscopic Approach

0MUR4JZ Supplement Left Ankle Bursa and Ligament with Synthetic Substitute, Percutaneous Endoscopic Approach

0MUR4KZ Supplement Left Ankle Bursa and Ligament with Nonautologous Tissue Substitute, Percutaneous Endoscopic Approach

0MUS07Z Supplement Right Foot Bursa and Ligament with Autologous Tissue Substitute, Open Approach

0MUS0JZ Supplement Right Foot Bursa and Ligament with Synthetic Substitute, Open Approach

0MUS0KZ Supplement Right Foot Bursa and Ligament with Nonautologous Tissue Substitute, Open Approach

0MUS47Z Supplement Right Foot Bursa and Ligament with Autologous Tissue Substitute, Percutaneous Endoscopic Approach

0MUS4JZ Supplement Right Foot Bursa and Ligament with Synthetic Substitute, Percutaneous Endoscopic Approach

0MUS4KZ Supplement Right Foot Bursa and Ligament with Nonautologous Tissue Substitute, Percutaneous Endoscopic Approach

0MUT07Z Supplement Left Foot Bursa and Ligament with Autologous Tissue Substitute, Open Approach

0MUT0JZ Supplement Left Foot Bursa and Ligament with Synthetic Substitute, Open Approach

0MUT0KZ Supplement Left Foot Bursa and Ligament with Nonautologous Tissue Substitute, Open Approach

0MUT47Z Supplement Left Foot Bursa and Ligament with Autologous Tissue Substitute, Percutaneous Endoscopic Approach

0MUT4JZ Supplement Left Foot Bursa and Ligament with Synthetic Substitute, Percutaneous Endoscopic Approach

0MUT4KZ Supplement Left Foot Bursa and Ligament with Nonautologous Tissue Substitute, Percutaneous Endoscopic Approach

0MUV07Z Supplement Right Lower Extremity Bursa and Ligament with Autologous Tissue Substitute, Open Approach

0MUV0JZ Supplement Right Lower Extremity Bursa and Ligament with Synthetic Substitute, Open Approach

0MUV0KZ Supplement Right Lower Extremity Bursa and Ligament with Nonautologous Tissue Substitute, Open Approach

♀ Female-only   ♂ Male-only   ▲ Limited Coverage   ● Non-OR   ⬛ HAC-associated procedure   ▲ Non-covered procedures   ✚ Cluster

0MUV47Z   Supplement Right Lower Extremity Bursa and Ligament with Autologous Tissue Substitute, Percutaneous Endoscopic Approach
0MUV4JZ   Supplement Right Lower Extremity Bursa and Ligament with Synthetic Substitute, Percutaneous Endoscopic Approach
0MUV4KZ   Supplement Right Lower Extremity Bursa and Ligament with Nonautologous Tissue Substitute, Percutaneous Endoscopic Approach

0MUW07Z   Supplement Left Lower Extremity Bursa and Ligament with Autologous Tissue Substitute, Open Approach
0MUW0JZ   Supplement Left Lower Extremity Bursa and Ligament with Synthetic Substitute, Open Approach
0MUW0KZ   Supplement Left Lower Extremity Bursa and Ligament with Nonautologous Tissue Substitute, Open Approach
0MUW47Z   Supplement Left Lower Extremity Bursa and Ligament with Autologous

Tissue Substitute, Percutaneous Endoscopic Approach
0MUW4JZ   Supplement Left Lower Extremity Bursa and Ligament with Synthetic Substitute, Percutaneous Endoscopic Approach
0MUW4KZ   Supplement Left Lower Extremity Bursa and Ligament with Nonautologous Tissue Substitute, Percutaneous Endoscopic Approach

0MW – Bursae and Ligaments, Revision

Review Coding Guideline B6.1c

0MWX00Z   Revision of Drainage Device in Upper Bursa and Ligament, Open Approach
0MWX07Z   Revision of Autologous Tissue Substitute in Upper Bursa and Ligament, Open Approach
0MWX0JZ   Revision of Synthetic Substitute in Upper Bursa and Ligament, Open Approach
0MWX0KZ   Revision of Nonautologous Tissue Substitute in Upper Bursa and Ligament, Open Approach
0MWX0YZ   Revision of Other Device in Upper Bursa and Ligament, Open Approach
0MWX30Z   Revision of Drainage Device in Upper Bursa and Ligament, Percutaneous Approach
0MWX37Z   Revision of Autologous Tissue Substitute in Upper Bursa and Ligament, Percutaneous Approach
0MWX3JZ   Revision of Synthetic Substitute in Upper Bursa and Ligament, Percutaneous Approach
0MWX3KZ   Revision of Nonautologous Tissue Substitute in Upper Bursa and Ligament, Percutaneous Approach
0MWX3YZ   Revision of Other Device in Upper Bursa and Ligament, Percutaneous Approach
0MWX40Z   Revision of Drainage Device in Upper Bursa and Ligament, Percutaneous Endoscopic Approach
0MWX47Z   Revision of Autologous Tissue Substitute in Upper Bursa and Ligament, Percutaneous Endoscopic Approach
0MWX4JZ   Revision of Synthetic Substitute in Upper Bursa and Ligament, Percutaneous Endoscopic Approach

0MWX4KZ   Revision of Nonautologous Tissue Substitute in Upper Bursa and Ligament, Percutaneous Endoscopic Approach
0MWX4YZ   Revision of Other Device in Upper Bursa and Ligament, Percutaneous Endoscopic Approach
0MWXX0Z   Revision of Drainage Device in Upper Bursa and Ligament, External Approach
0MWXX7Z   Revision of Autologous Tissue Substitute in Upper Bursa and Ligament, External Approach
0MWXXJZ   Revision of Synthetic Substitute in Upper Bursa and Ligament, External Approach
0MWXXKZ   Revision of Nonautologous Tissue Substitute in Upper Bursa and Ligament, External Approach
0MWY00Z   Revision of Drainage Device in Lower Bursa and Ligament, Open Approach
0MWY07Z   Revision of Autologous Tissue Substitute in Lower Bursa and Ligament, Open Approach
0MWY0JZ   Revision of Synthetic Substitute in Lower Bursa and Ligament, Open Approach
0MWY0KZ   Revision of Nonautologous Tissue Substitute in Lower Bursa and Ligament, Open Approach
0MWY0YZ   Revision of Other Device in Lower Bursa and Ligament, Open Approach
0MWY30Z   Revision of Drainage Device in Lower Bursa and Ligament, Percutaneous Approach
0MWY37Z   Revision of Autologous Tissue Substitute in Lower Bursa and Ligament, Percutaneous Approach

0MWY3JZ   Revision of Synthetic Substitute in Lower Bursa and Ligament, Percutaneous Approach
0MWY3KZ   Revision of Nonautologous Tissue Substitute in Lower Bursa and Ligament, Percutaneous Approach
0MWY3YZ   Revision of Other Device in Lower Bursa and Ligament, Percutaneous Approach
0MWY40Z   Revision of Drainage Device in Lower Bursa and Ligament, Percutaneous Endoscopic Approach
0MWY47Z   Revision of Autologous Tissue Substitute in Lower Bursa and Ligament, Percutaneous Endoscopic Approach
0MWY4JZ   Revision of Synthetic Substitute in Lower Bursa and Ligament, Percutaneous Endoscopic Approach
0MWY4KZ   Revision of Nonautologous Tissue Substitute in Lower Bursa and Ligament, Percutaneous Endoscopic Approach
0MWY4YZ   Revision of Other Device in Lower Bursa and Ligament, Percutaneous Endoscopic Approach
0MWYX0Z   Revision of Drainage Device in Lower Bursa and Ligament, External Approach
0MWYX7Z   Revision of Autologous Tissue Substitute in Lower Bursa and Ligament, External Approach
0MWYXJZ   Revision of Synthetic Substitute in Lower Bursa and Ligament, External Approach
0MWYXKZ   Revision of Nonautologous Tissue Substitute in Lower Bursa and Ligament, External Approach

0MX – Bursae and Ligaments, Transfer

0MX00ZZ   Transfer Head and Neck Bursa and Ligament, Open Approach
0MX04ZZ   Transfer Head and Neck Bursa and Ligament, Percutaneous Endoscopic Approach
0MX10ZZ   Transfer Right Shoulder Bursa and Ligament, Open Approach
0MX14ZZ   Transfer Right Shoulder Bursa and Ligament, Percutaneous Endoscopic Approach
0MX20ZZ   Transfer Left Shoulder Bursa and Ligament, Open Approach
0MX24ZZ   Transfer Left Shoulder Bursa and Ligament, Percutaneous Endoscopic Approach

0MX30ZZ   Transfer Right Elbow Bursa and Ligament, Open Approach
0MX34ZZ   Transfer Right Elbow Bursa and Ligament, Percutaneous Endoscopic Approach
0MX40ZZ   Transfer Left Elbow Bursa and Ligament, Open Approach
0MX44ZZ   Transfer Left Elbow Bursa and Ligament, Percutaneous Endoscopic Approach
0MX50ZZ   Transfer Right Wrist Bursa and Ligament, Open Approach
0MX54ZZ   Transfer Right Wrist Bursa and Ligament, Percutaneous Endoscopic Approach

0MX60ZZ   Transfer Left Wrist Bursa and Ligament, Open Approach
0MX64ZZ   Transfer Left Wrist Bursa and Ligament, Percutaneous Endoscopic Approach
0MX70ZZ   Transfer Right Hand Bursa and Ligament, Open Approach
0MX74ZZ   Transfer Right Hand Bursa and Ligament, Percutaneous Endoscopic Approach
0MX80ZZ   Transfer Left Hand Bursa and Ligament, Open Approach
0MX84ZZ   Transfer Left Hand Bursa and Ligament, Percutaneous Endoscopic Approach

0MX90ZZ	Transfer Right Upper Extremity Bursa and Ligament, Open Approach
0MX94ZZ	Transfer Right Upper Extremity Bursa and Ligament, Percutaneous Endoscopic Approach
0MXB0ZZ	Transfer Left Upper Extremity Bursa and Ligament, Open Approach
0MXB4ZZ	Transfer Left Upper Extremity Bursa and Ligament, Percutaneous Endoscopic Approach
0MXC0ZZ	Transfer Upper Spine Bursa and Ligament, Open Approach
0MXC4ZZ	Transfer Upper Spine Bursa and Ligament, Percutaneous Endoscopic Approach
0MXD0ZZ	Transfer Lower Spine Bursa and Ligament, Open Approach
0MXD4ZZ	Transfer Lower Spine Bursa and Ligament, Percutaneous Endoscopic Approach
0MXF0ZZ	Transfer Sternum Bursa and Ligament, Open Approach
0MXF4ZZ	Transfer Sternum Bursa and Ligament, Percutaneous Endoscopic Approach
0MXG0ZZ	Transfer Rib(s) Bursa and Ligament, Open Approach
0MXG4ZZ	Transfer Rib(s) Bursa and Ligament, Percutaneous Endoscopic Approach
0MXH0ZZ	Transfer Right Abdomen Bursa and Ligament, Open Approach

0MXH4ZZ	Transfer Right Abdomen Bursa and Ligament, Percutaneous Endoscopic Approach
0MXJ0ZZ	Transfer Left Abdomen Bursa and Ligament, Open Approach
0MXJ4ZZ	Transfer Left Abdomen Bursa and Ligament, Percutaneous Endoscopic Approach
0MXK0ZZ	Transfer Perineum Bursa and Ligament, Open Approach
0MXK4ZZ	Transfer Perineum Bursa and Ligament, Percutaneous Endoscopic Approach
0MXL0ZZ	Transfer Right Hip Bursa and Ligament, Open Approach
0MXL4ZZ	Transfer Right Hip Bursa and Ligament, Percutaneous Endoscopic Approach
0MXM0ZZ	Transfer Left Hip Bursa and Ligament, Open Approach
0MXM4ZZ	Transfer Left Hip Bursa and Ligament, Percutaneous Endoscopic Approach
0MXN0ZZ	Transfer Right Knee Bursa and Ligament, Open Approach
0MXN4ZZ	Transfer Right Knee Bursa and Ligament, Percutaneous Endoscopic Approach
0MXP0ZZ	Transfer Left Knee Bursa and Ligament, Open Approach
0MXP4ZZ	Transfer Left Knee Bursa and Ligament, Percutaneous Endoscopic Approach

0MXQ0ZZ	Transfer Right Ankle Bursa and Ligament, Open Approach
0MXQ4ZZ	Transfer Right Ankle Bursa and Ligament, Percutaneous Endoscopic Approach
0MXR0ZZ	Transfer Left Ankle Bursa and Ligament, Open Approach
0MXR4ZZ	Transfer Left Ankle Bursa and Ligament, Percutaneous Endoscopic Approach
0MXS0ZZ	Transfer Right Foot Bursa and Ligament, Open Approach
0MXS4ZZ	Transfer Right Foot Bursa and Ligament, Percutaneous Endoscopic Approach
0MXT0ZZ	Transfer Left Foot Bursa and Ligament, Open Approach
0MXT4ZZ	Transfer Left Foot Bursa and Ligament, Percutaneous Endoscopic Approach
0MXV0ZZ	Transfer Right Lower Extremity Bursa and Ligament, Open Approach
0MXV4ZZ	Transfer Right Lower Extremity Bursa and Ligament, Percutaneous Endoscopic Approach
0MXW0ZZ	Transfer Left Lower Extremity Bursa and Ligament, Open Approach
0MXW4ZZ	Transfer Left Lower Extremity Bursa and Ligament, Percutaneous Endoscopic Approach

Head and Facial Bones

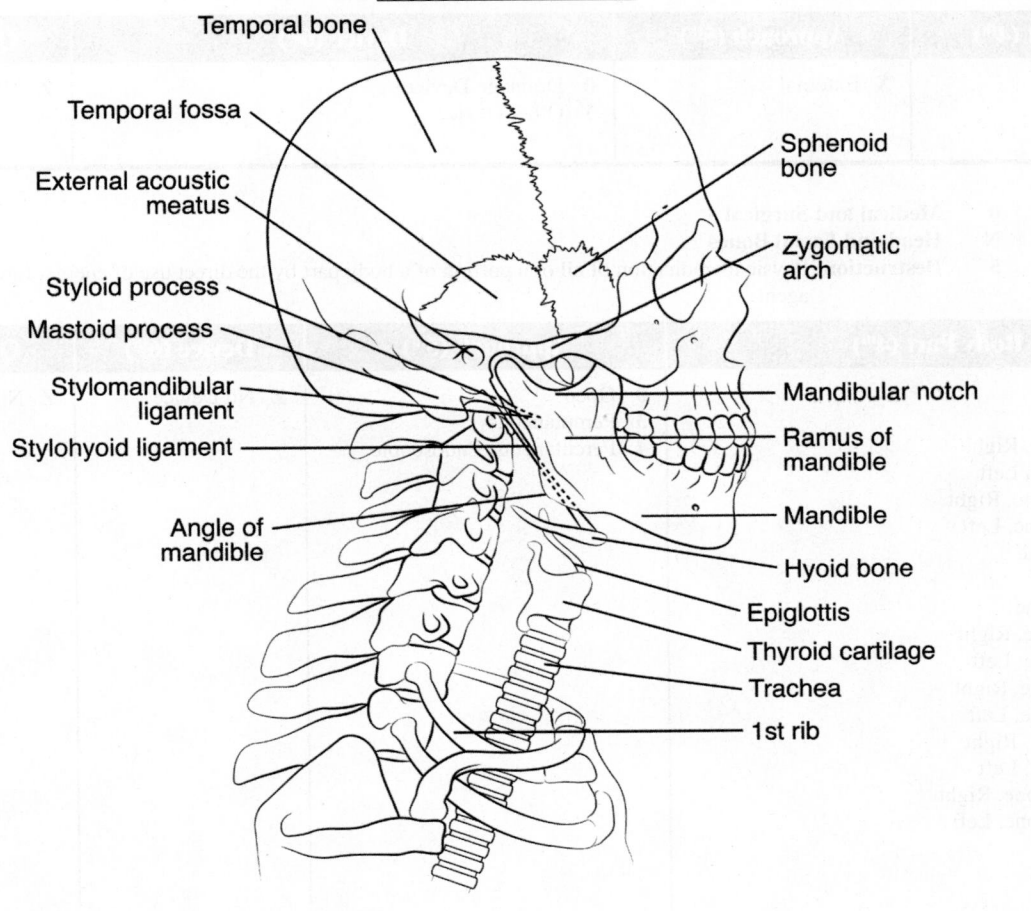

Temporal bone

Temporal fossa

External acoustic meatus

Styloid process

Mastoid process

Stylomandibular ligament

Stylohyoid ligament

Angle of mandible

Sphenoid bone

Zygomatic arch

Mandibular notch

Ramus of mandible

Mandible

Hyoid bone

Epiglottis

Thyroid cartilage

Trachea

1st rib

©AHIMA

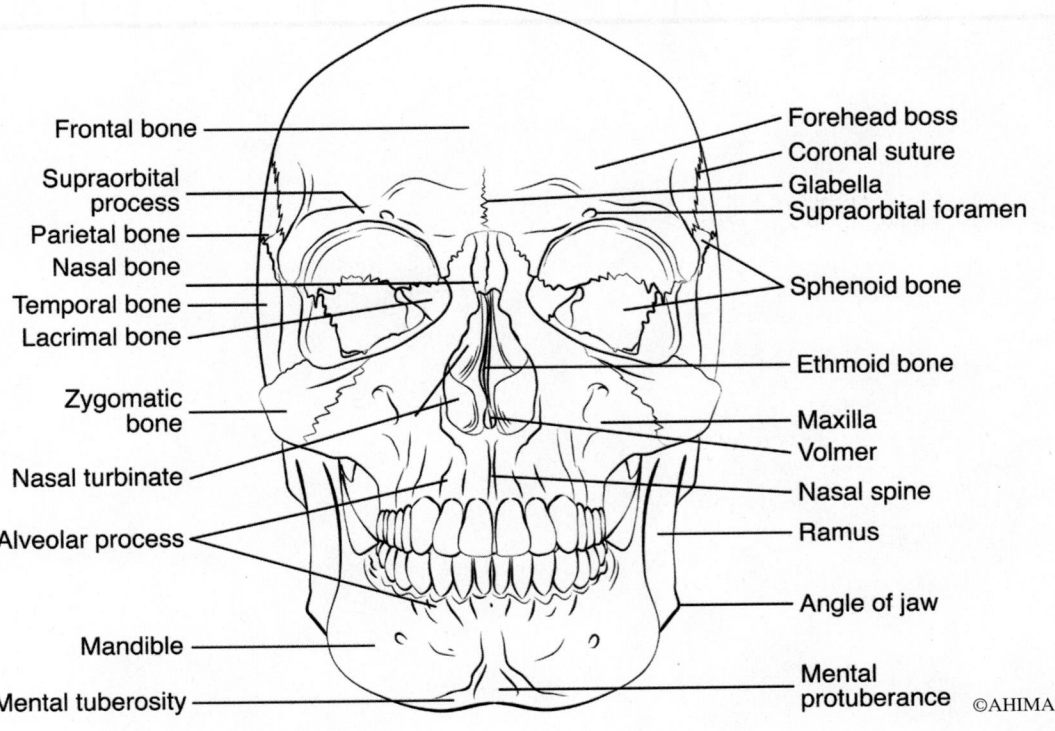

Frontal bone

Supraorbital process

Parietal bone

Nasal bone

Temporal bone

Lacrimal bone

Zygomatic bone

Nasal turbinate

Alveolar process

Mandible

Mental tuberosity

Forehead boss

Coronal suture

Glabella

Supraorbital foramen

Sphenoid bone

Ethmoid bone

Maxilla

Volmer

Nasal spine

Ramus

Angle of jaw

Mental protuberance

©AHIMA

Section	0	Medical and Surgical
Body System	N	Head and Facial Bones
Operation	2	Change: Taking out or off a device from a body part and putting back an identical or similar device in or on the same body part without cutting or puncturing the skin or a mucous membrane

Body Part (4th)	Approach (5th)	Device (6th)	Qualifier (7th)
0 Skull B Nasal Bone W Facial Bone	X External	0 Drainage Device Y Other Device	Z No Qualifier

Section	0	Medical and Surgical
Body System	N	Head and Facial Bones
Operation	5	Destruction: Physical eradication of all or a portion of a body part by the direct use of energy, force, or a destructive agent

Body Part (4th)	Approach (5th)	Device (6th)	Qualifier (7th)
0 Skull 1 Frontal Bone 3 Parietal Bone, Right 4 Parietal Bone, Left 5 Temporal Bone, Right 6 Temporal Bone, Left 7 Occipital Bone B Nasal Bone C Sphenoid Bone F Ethmoid Bone, Right G Ethmoid Bone, Left H Lacrimal Bone, Right J Lacrimal Bone, Left K Palatine Bone, Right L Palatine Bone, Left M Zygomatic Bone, Right N Zygomatic Bone, Left P Orbit, Right Q Orbit, Left R Maxilla T Mandible, Right V Mandible, Left X Hyoid Bone	0 Open 3 Percutaneous 4 Percutaneous Endoscopic	Z No Device	Z No Qualifier

Section   0   **Medical and Surgical**
Body System   N   **Head and Facial Bones**
Operation   8   **Division:** Cutting into a body part, without draining fluids and/or gases from the body part, in order to separate or transect a body part

Body Part (4ᵗʰ)	Approach (5ᵗʰ)	Device (6ᵗʰ)	Qualifier (7ᵗʰ)
0 Skull	0 Open	**Z** No Device	**Z** No Qualifier
1 Frontal Bone	3 Percutaneous		
3 Parietal Bone, Right	4 Percutaneous Endoscopic		
4 Parietal Bone, Left			
5 Temporal Bone, Right			
6 Temporal Bone, Left			
7 Occipital Bone			
B Nasal Bone			
C Sphenoid Bone			
F Ethmoid Bone, Right			
G Ethmoid Bone, Left			
H Lacrimal Bone, Right			
J Lacrimal Bone, Left			
K Palatine Bone, Right			
L Palatine Bone, Left			
M Zygomatic Bone, Right			
N Zygomatic Bone, Left			
P Orbit, Right			
Q Orbit, Left			
R Maxilla			
T Mandible, Right			
V Mandible, Left			
X Hyoid Bone			

Section   0   **Medical and Surgical**
Body System   N   **Head and Facial Bones**
Operation   9   **Drainage:** Taking or letting out fluids and/or gases from a body part

Body Part (4ᵗʰ)	Approach (5ᵗʰ)	Device (6ᵗʰ)	Qualifier (7ᵗʰ)
0 Skull	0 Open	0 Drainage Device	**Z** No Qualifier
1 Frontal Bone	3 Percutaneous		
3 Parietal Bone, Right	4 Percutaneous Endoscopic		
4 Parietal Bone, Left			
5 Temporal Bone, Right			
6 Temporal Bone, Left			
7 Occipital Bone			
B Nasal Bone			
C Sphenoid Bone			
F Ethmoid Bone, Right			
G Ethmoid Bone, Left			
H Lacrimal Bone, Right			
J Lacrimal Bone, Left			
K Palatine Bone, Right			
L Palatine Bone, Left			
M Zygomatic Bone, Right			
N Zygomatic Bone, Left			
P Orbit, Right			
Q Orbit, Left			
R Maxilla			
T Mandible, Right			
V Mandible, Left			
X Hyoid Bone			

Continued →

Section	0	Medical and Surgical
Body System	N	Head and Facial Bones
Operation	9	Drainage: Taking or letting out fluids and/or gases from a body part

Body Part (4th)	Approach (5th)	Device (6th)	Qualifier (7th)
0 Skull 1 Frontal Bone 3 Parietal Bone, Right 4 Parietal Bone, Left 5 Temporal Bone, Right 6 Temporal Bone, Left 7 Occipital Bone B Nasal Bone C Sphenoid Bone F Ethmoid Bone, Right G Ethmoid Bone, Left H Lacrimal Bone, Right J Lacrimal Bone, Left K Palatine Bone, Right L Palatine Bone, Left M Zygomatic Bone, Right N Zygomatic Bone, Left P Orbit, Right Q Orbit, Left R Maxilla T Mandible, Right V Mandible, Left X Hyoid Bone	0 Open 3 Percutaneous 4 Percutaneous Endoscopic	Z No Device	X Diagnostic Z No Qualifier

Section	0	Medical and Surgical
Body System	N	Head and Facial Bones
Operation	B	Excision: Cutting out or off, without replacement, a portion of a body part

Body Part (4th)	Approach (5th)	Device (6th)	Qualifier (7th)
0 Skull 1 Frontal Bone 3 Parietal Bone, Right 4 Parietal Bone, Left 5 Temporal Bone, Right 6 Temporal Bone, Left 7 Occipital Bone B Nasal Bone C Sphenoid Bone F Ethmoid Bone, Right G Ethmoid Bone, Left H Lacrimal Bone, Right J Lacrimal Bone, Left K Palatine Bone, Right L Palatine Bone, Left M Zygomatic Bone, Right N Zygomatic Bone, Left P Orbit, Right Q Orbit, Left R Maxilla T Mandible, Right V Mandible, Left X Hyoid Bone	0 Open 3 Percutaneous 4 Percutaneous Endoscopic	Z No Device	X Diagnostic Z No Qualifier

Section	0	Medical and Surgical
Body System	N	Head and Facial Bones
Operation	C	Extirpation: Taking or cutting out solid matter from a body part

Body Part (4th)	Approach (5th)	Device (6th)	Qualifier (7th)
1 Frontal Bone	0 Open	Z No Device	Z No Qualifier
3 Parietal Bone, Right	3 Percutaneous		
4 Parietal Bone, Left	4 Percutaneous Endoscopic		
5 Temporal Bone, Right			
6 Temporal Bone, Left			
7 Occipital Bone			
B Nasal Bone			
C Sphenoid Bone			
F Ethmoid Bone, Right			
G Ethmoid Bone, Left			
H Lacrimal Bone, Right			
J Lacrimal Bone, Left			
K Palatine Bone, Right			
L Palatine Bone, Left			
M Zygomatic Bone, Right			
N Zygomatic Bone, Left			
P Orbit, Right			
Q Orbit, Left			
R Maxilla			
T Mandible, Right			
V Mandible, Left			
X Hyoid Bone			

Section	0	Medical and Surgical
Body System	N	Head and Facial Bones
Operation	D	Extraction: Pulling or stripping out or off all or a portion of a body part by the use of force

Body Part (4th)	Approach (5th)	Device (6th)	Qualifier (7th)
0 Skull	0 Open	Z No Device	Z No Qualifier
1 Frontal Bone			
3 Parietal Bone, Right			
4 Parietal Bone, Left			
5 Temporal Bone, Right			
6 Temporal Bone, Left			
7 Occipital Bone			
B Nasal Bone			
C Sphenoid Bone			
F Ethmoid Bone, Right			
G Ethmoid Bone, Left			
H Lacrimal Bone, Right			
J Lacrimal Bone, Left			
K Palatine Bone, Right			
L Palatine Bone, Left			
M Zygomatic Bone, Right			
N Zygomatic Bone, Left			
P Orbit, Right			
Q Orbit, Left			
R Maxilla			
T Mandible, Right			
V Mandible, Left			
X Hyoid Bone			

Section	0	**Medical and Surgical**
Body System	N	**Head and Facial Bones**
Operation	H	**Insertion:** Putting in a nonbiological appliance that monitors, assists, performs, or prevents a physiological function but does not physically take the place of a body part

Body Part (4th)	Approach (5th)	Device (6th)	Qualifier (7th)
0 Skull	**0** Open	**3** Infusion Device **4** Internal Fixation Device **5** External Fixation Device **M** Bone Growth Stimulator **N** Neurostimulator Generator	**Z** No Qualifier
0 Skull	**3** Percutaneous **4** Percutaneous Endoscopic	**3** Infusion Device **4** Internal Fixation Device **5** External Fixation Device **M** Bone Growth Stimulator	**Z** No Qualifier
1 Frontal Bone **3** Parietal Bone, Right **4** Parietal Bone, Left **7** Occipital Bone **C** Sphenoid Bone **F** Ethmoid Bone, Right **G** Ethmoid Bone, Left **H** Lacrimal Bone, Right **J** Lacrimal Bone, Left **K** Palatine Bone, Right **L** Palatine Bone, Left **M** Zygomatic Bone, Right **N** Zygomatic Bone, Left **P** Orbit, Right **Q** Orbit, Left **X** Hyoid Bone	**0** Open **3** Percutaneous **4** Percutaneous Endoscopic	**4** Internal Fixation Device	**Z** No Qualifier
5 Temporal Bone, Right **6** Temporal Bone, Left	**0** Open **3** Percutaneous **4** Percutaneous Endoscopic	**4** Internal Fixation Device **S** Hearing Device	**Z** No Qualifier
B Nasal Bone	**0** Open **3** Percutaneous **4** Percutaneous Endoscopic	**4** Internal Fixation Device **M** Bone Growth Stimulator	**Z** No Qualifier
R Maxilla **T** Mandible, Right **V** Mandible, Left	**0** Open **3** Percutaneous **4** Percutaneous Endoscopic	**4** Internal Fixation Device **5** External Fixation Device	**Z** No Qualifier
W Facial Bone	**0** Open **3** Percutaneous **4** Percutaneous Endoscopic	**M** Bone Growth Stimulator	**Z** No Qualifier

Section   0   **Medical and Surgical**
Body System   N   **Head and Facial Bones**
Operation   J   **Inspection:** Visually and/or manually exploring a body part

Body Part (4ᵗʰ)	Approach (5ᵗʰ)	Device (6ᵗʰ)	Qualifier (7ᵗʰ)
0 Skull B Nasal Bone W Facial Bone	0 Open 3 Percutaneous 4 Percutaneous Endoscopic X External	Z No Device	Z No Qualifier

Section   0   **Medical and Surgical**
Body System   N   **Head and Facial Bones**
Operation   N   **Release:** Freeing a body part from an abnormal physical constraint by cutting or by the use of force

Body Part (4ᵗʰ)	Approach (5ᵗʰ)	Device (6ᵗʰ)	Qualifier (7ᵗʰ)
1 Frontal Bone 3 Parietal Bone, Right 4 Parietal Bone, Left 5 Temporal Bone, Right 6 Temporal Bone, Left 7 Occipital Bone B Nasal Bone C Sphenoid Bone F Ethmoid Bone, Right G Ethmoid Bone, Left H Lacrimal Bone, Right J Lacrimal Bone, Left K Palatine Bone, Right L Palatine Bone, Left M Zygomatic Bone, Right N Zygomatic Bone, Left P Orbit, Right Q Orbit, Left R Maxilla T Mandible, Right V Mandible, Left X Hyoid Bone	0 Open 3 Percutaneous 4 Percutaneous Endoscopic	Z No Device	Z No Qualifier

Section	0	Medical and Surgical
Body System	N	Head and Facial Bones
Operation	P	Removal: Taking out or off a device from a body part

Body Part (4th)	Approach (5th)	Device (6th)	Qualifier (7th)
0 Skull	0 Open	0 Drainage Device 4 Internal Fixation Device 5 External Fixation Device 7 Autologous Tissue Substitute J Synthetic Substitute K Nonautologous Tissue Substitute M Bone Growth Stimulator N Neurostimulator Generator S Hearing Device	Z No Qualifier
0 Skull	3 Percutaneous 4 Percutaneous Endoscopic	0 Drainage Device 4 Internal Fixation Device 5 External Fixation Device 7 Autologous Tissue Substitute J Synthetic Substitute K Nonautologous Tissue Substitute M Bone Growth Stimulator S Hearing Device	Z No Qualifier
0 Skull	X External	0 Drainage Device 4 Internal Fixation Device 5 External Fixation Device M Bone Growth Stimulator S Hearing Device	Z No Qualifier
B Nasal Bone W Facial Bone	0 Open 3 Percutaneous 4 Percutaneous Endoscopic	0 Drainage Device 4 Internal Fixation Device 7 Autologous Tissue Substitute J Synthetic Substitute K Nonautologous Tissue Substitute M Bone Growth Stimulator	Z No Qualifier
B Nasal Bone W Facial Bone	X External	0 Drainage Device 4 Internal Fixation Device M Bone Growth Stimulator	Z No Qualifier

Section   **0**   **Medical and Surgical**
Body System   **N**   **Head and Facial Bones**
Operation   **Q**   **Repair:** Restoring, to the extent possible, a body part to its normal anatomic structure and function

Body Part (4ᵗʰ)	Approach (5ᵗʰ)	Device (6ᵗʰ)	Qualifier (7ᵗʰ)
0 Skull **1** Frontal Bone **3** Parietal Bone, Right **4** Parietal Bone, Left **5** Temporal Bone, Right **6** Temporal Bone, Left **7** Occipital Bone **B** Nasal Bone **C** Sphenoid Bone **F** Ethmoid Bone, Right **G** Ethmoid Bone, Left **H** Lacrimal Bone, Right **J** Lacrimal Bone, Left **K** Palatine Bone, Right **L** Palatine Bone, Left **M** Zygomatic Bone, Right **N** Zygomatic Bone, Left **P** Orbit, Right **Q** Orbit, Left **R** Maxilla **T** Mandible, Right **V** Mandible, Left **X** Hyoid Bone	**0** Open **3** Percutaneous **4** Percutaneous Endoscopic **X** External	**Z** No Device	**Z** No Qualifier

Section   **0**   **Medical and Surgical**
Body System   **N**   **Head and Facial Bones**
Operation   **R**   **Replacement:** Putting in or on biological or synthetic material that physically takes the place and/or function of all or a portion of a body part

Body Part (4ᵗʰ)	Approach (5ᵗʰ)	Device (6ᵗʰ)	Qualifier (7ᵗʰ)
0 Skull **1** Frontal Bone **3** Parietal Bone, Right **4** Parietal Bone, Left **5** Temporal Bone, Right **6** Temporal Bone, Left **7** Occipital Bone **B** Nasal Bone **C** Sphenoid Bone **F** Ethmoid Bone, Right **G** Ethmoid Bone, Left **H** Lacrimal Bone, Right **J** Lacrimal Bone, Left **K** Palatine Bone, Right **L** Palatine Bone, Left **M** Zygomatic Bone, Right **N** Zygomatic Bone, Left **P** Orbit, Right **Q** Orbit, Left **R** Maxilla **T** Mandible, Right **V** Mandible, Left **X** Hyoid Bone	**0** Open **3** Percutaneous **4** Percutaneous Endoscopic	**7** Autologous Tissue Substitute **J** Synthetic Substitute **K** Nonautologous Tissue Substitute	**Z** No Qualifier

Section	0	Medical and Surgical
Body System	N	Head and Facial Bones
Operation	S	**Reposition:** Moving to its normal location, or other suitable location, all or a portion of a body part

Body Part (4th)	Approach (5th)	Device (6th)	Qualifier (7th)
0 Skull **R** Maxilla **T** Mandible, Right **V** Mandible, Left	**0** Open **3** Percutaneous **4** Percutaneous Endoscopic	**4** Internal Fixation Device **5** External Fixation Device **Z** No Device	**Z** No Qualifier
0 Skull **R** Maxilla **T** Mandible, Right **V** Mandible, Left	**X** External	**Z** No Device	**Z** No Qualifier
1 Frontal Bone **3** Parietal Bone, Right **4** Parietal Bone, Left **5** Temporal Bone, Right **6** Temporal Bone, Left **7** Occipital Bone **B** Nasal Bone **C** Sphenoid Bone **F** Ethmoid Bone, Right **G** Ethmoid Bone, Left **H** Lacrimal Bone, Right **J** Lacrimal Bone, Left **K** Palatine Bone, Right **L** Palatine Bone, Left **M** Zygomatic Bone, Right **N** Zygomatic Bone, Left **P** Orbit, Right **Q** Orbit, Left **X** Hyoid Bone	**0** Open **3** Percutaneous **4** Percutaneous Endoscopic	**4** Internal Fixation Device **Z** No Device	**Z** No Qualifier
1 Frontal Bone **3** Parietal Bone, Right **4** Parietal Bone, Left **5** Temporal Bone, Right **6** Temporal Bone, Left **7** Occipital Bone **B** Nasal Bone **C** Sphenoid Bone **F** Ethmoid Bone, Right **G** Ethmoid Bone, Left **H** Lacrimal Bone, Right **J** Lacrimal Bone, Left **K** Palatine Bone, Right **L** Palatine Bone, Left **M** Zygomatic Bone, Right **N** Zygomatic Bone, Left **P** Orbit, Right **Q** Orbit, Left **X** Hyoid Bone	**X** External	**Z** No Device	**Z** No Qualifier

Section 0 **Medical and Surgical**
Body System N **Head and Facial Bones**
Operation T **Resection:** Cutting out or off, without replacement, all of a body part

Body Part (4th)	Approach (5th)	Device (6th)	Qualifier (7th)
1 Frontal Bone	0 Open	Z No Device	Z No Qualifier
3 Parietal Bone, Right			
4 Parietal Bone, Left			
5 Temporal Bone, Right			
6 Temporal Bone, Left			
7 Occipital Bone			
B Nasal Bone			
C Sphenoid Bone			
F Ethmoid Bone, Right			
G Ethmoid Bone, Left			
H Lacrimal Bone, Right			
J Lacrimal Bone, Left			
K Palatine Bone, Right			
L Palatine Bone, Left			
M Zygomatic Bone, Right			
N Zygomatic Bone, Left			
P Orbit, Right			
Q Orbit, Left			
R Maxilla			
T Mandible, Right			
V Mandible, Left			
X Hyoid Bone			

Section 0 **Medical and Surgical**
Body System N **Head and Facial Bones**
Operation U **Supplement:** Putting in or on biological or synthetic material that physically reinforces and/or augments the function of a portion of a body part

Body Part (4th)	Approach (5th)	Device (6th)	Qualifier (7th)
0 Skull	0 Open	7 Autologous Tissue Substitute	Z No Qualifier
1 Frontal Bone	3 Percutaneous	J Synthetic Substitute	
3 Parietal Bone, Right	4 Percutaneous Endoscopic	K Nonautologous Tissue Substitute	
4 Parietal Bone, Left			
5 Temporal Bone, Right			
6 Temporal Bone, Left			
7 Occipital Bone			
B Nasal Bone			
C Sphenoid Bone			
F Ethmoid Bone, Right			
G Ethmoid Bone, Left			
H Lacrimal Bone, Right			
J Lacrimal Bone, Left			
K Palatine Bone, Right			
L Palatine Bone, Left			
M Zygomatic Bone, Right			
N Zygomatic Bone, Left			
P Orbit, Right			
Q Orbit, Left			
R Maxilla			
T Mandible, Right			
V Mandible, Left			
X Hyoid Bone			

Section	0	Medical and Surgical
Body System	N	Head and Facial Bones
Operation	W	Revision: Correcting, to the extent possible, a portion of a malfunctioning device or the position of a displaced device

Body Part (4th)	Approach (5th)	Device (6th)	Qualifier (7th)
0 Skull	0 Open	0 Drainage Device 4 Internal Fixation Device 5 External Fixation Device 7 Autologous Tissue Substitute J Synthetic Substitute K Nonautologous Tissue Substitute M Bone Growth Stimulator N Neurostimulator Generator S Hearing Device	Z No Qualifier
0 Skull	3 Percutaneous 4 Percutaneous Endoscopic X External	0 Drainage Device 4 Internal Fixation Device 5 External Fixation Device 7 Autologous Tissue Substitute J Synthetic Substitute K Nonautologous Tissue Substitute M Bone Growth Stimulator S Hearing Device	Z No Qualifier
B Nasal Bone W Facial Bone	0 Open 3 Percutaneous 4 Percutaneous Endoscopic X External	0 Drainage Device 4 Internal Fixation Device 7 Autologous Tissue Substitute J Synthetic Substitute K Nonautologous Tissue Substitute M Bone Growth Stimulator	Z No Qualifier

Head and Facial Bones Code Listing 0N2–0NW

0N2 – Head and Facial Bones, Change

Review Coding Guideline B6.1c

0N20X0Z Change Drainage Device in Skull, External Approach
0N20XYZ Change Other Device in Skull, External Approach

0N2BX0Z Change Drainage Device in Nasal Bone, External Approach
0N2BXYZ Change Other Device in Nasal Bone, External Approach

0N2WX0Z Change Drainage Device in Facial Bone, External Approach
0N2WXYZ Change Other Device in Facial Bone, External Approach

0N5 – Head and Facial Bones, Destruction

0N500ZZ Destruction of Skull, Open Approach
0N503ZZ Destruction of Skull, Percutaneous Approach
0N504ZZ Destruction of Skull, Percutaneous Endoscopic Approach
0N510ZZ Destruction of Frontal Bone, Open Approach
0N513ZZ Destruction of Frontal Bone, Percutaneous Approach
0N514ZZ Destruction of Frontal Bone, Percutaneous Endoscopic Approach
0N530ZZ Destruction of Right Parietal Bone, Open Approach
0N533ZZ Destruction of Right Parietal Bone, Percutaneous Approach
0N534ZZ Destruction of Right Parietal Bone, Percutaneous Endoscopic Approach
0N540ZZ Destruction of Left Parietal Bone, Open Approach
0N543ZZ Destruction of Left Parietal Bone, Percutaneous Approach
0N544ZZ Destruction of Left Parietal Bone, Percutaneous Endoscopic Approach
0N550ZZ Destruction of Right Temporal Bone, Open Approach

0N553ZZ Destruction of Right Temporal Bone, Percutaneous Approach
0N554ZZ Destruction of Right Temporal Bone, Percutaneous Endoscopic Approach
0N560ZZ Destruction of Left Temporal Bone, Open Approach
0N563ZZ Destruction of Left Temporal Bone, Percutaneous Approach
0N564ZZ Destruction of Left Temporal Bone, Percutaneous Endoscopic Approach
0N570ZZ Destruction of Occipital Bone, Open Approach
0N573ZZ Destruction of Occipital Bone, Percutaneous Approach
0N574ZZ Destruction of Occipital Bone, Percutaneous Endoscopic Approach
0N5B0ZZ Destruction of Nasal Bone, Open Approach
0N5B3ZZ Destruction of Nasal Bone, Percutaneous Approach
0N5B4ZZ Destruction of Nasal Bone, Percutaneous Endoscopic Approach
0N5C0ZZ Destruction of Sphenoid Bone, Open Approach
0N5C3ZZ Destruction of Sphenoid Bone, Percutaneous Approach

0N5C4ZZ Destruction of Sphenoid Bone, Percutaneous Endoscopic Approach
0N5F0ZZ Destruction of Right Ethmoid Bone, Open Approach
0N5F3ZZ Destruction of Right Ethmoid Bone, Percutaneous Approach
0N5F4ZZ Destruction of Right Ethmoid Bone, Percutaneous Endoscopic Approach
0N5G0ZZ Destruction of Left Ethmoid Bone, Open Approach
0N5G3ZZ Destruction of Left Ethmoid Bone, Percutaneous Approach
0N5G4ZZ Destruction of Left Ethmoid Bone, Percutaneous Endoscopic Approach
0N5H0ZZ Destruction of Right Lacrimal Bone, Open Approach
0N5H3ZZ Destruction of Right Lacrimal Bone, Percutaneous Approach
0N5H4ZZ Destruction of Right Lacrimal Bone, Percutaneous Endoscopic Approach
0N5J0ZZ Destruction of Left Lacrimal Bone, Open Approach
0N5J3ZZ Destruction of Left Lacrimal Bone, Percutaneous Approach
0N5J4ZZ Destruction of Left Lacrimal Bone, Percutaneous Endoscopic Approach

♀ Female-only   ♂ Male-only   ▲ Limited Coverage   ● Non-OR   HAC HAC-associated procedure   ▲ Non-covered procedures   ✛ Cluster

0N5K0ZZ	Destruction of Right Palatine Bone, Open Approach
0N5K3ZZ	Destruction of Right Palatine Bone, Percutaneous Approach
0N5K4ZZ	Destruction of Right Palatine Bone, Percutaneous Endoscopic Approach
0N5L0ZZ	Destruction of Left Palatine Bone, Open Approach
0N5L3ZZ	Destruction of Left Palatine Bone, Percutaneous Approach
0N5L4ZZ	Destruction of Left Palatine Bone, Percutaneous Endoscopic Approach
0N5M0ZZ	Destruction of Right Zygomatic Bone, Open Approach
0N5M3ZZ	Destruction of Right Zygomatic Bone, Percutaneous Approach
0N5M4ZZ	Destruction of Right Zygomatic Bone, Percutaneous Endoscopic Approach
0N5N0ZZ	Destruction of Left Zygomatic Bone, Open Approach
0N5N3ZZ	Destruction of Left Zygomatic Bone, Percutaneous Approach
0N5N4ZZ	Destruction of Left Zygomatic Bone, Percutaneous Endoscopic Approach
0N5P0ZZ	Destruction of Right Orbit, Open Approach
0N5P3ZZ	Destruction of Right Orbit, Percutaneous Approach
0N5P4ZZ	Destruction of Right Orbit, Percutaneous Endoscopic Approach
0N5Q0ZZ	Destruction of Left Orbit, Open Approach
0N5Q3ZZ	Destruction of Left Orbit, Percutaneous Approach
0N5Q4ZZ	Destruction of Left Orbit, Percutaneous Endoscopic Approach
0N5R0ZZ	Destruction of Maxilla, Open Approach
0N5R3ZZ	Destruction of Maxilla, Percutaneous Approach
0N5R4ZZ	Destruction of Maxilla, Percutaneous Endoscopic Approach
0N5T0ZZ	Destruction of Right Mandible, Open Approach
0N5T3ZZ	Destruction of Right Mandible, Percutaneous Approach
0N5T4ZZ	Destruction of Right Mandible, Percutaneous Endoscopic Approach
0N5V0ZZ	Destruction of Left Mandible, Open Approach
0N5V3ZZ	Destruction of Left Mandible, Percutaneous Approach
0N5V4ZZ	Destruction of Left Mandible, Percutaneous Endoscopic Approach
0N5X0ZZ	Destruction of Hyoid Bone, Open Approach
0N5X3ZZ	Destruction of Hyoid Bone, Percutaneous Approach
0N5X4ZZ	Destruction of Hyoid Bone, Percutaneous Endoscopic Approach

0N8 – Head and Facial Bones, Division

Review Coding Guideline B3.14

0N800ZZ	Division of Skull, Open Approach
0N803ZZ	Division of Skull, Percutaneous Approach
0N804ZZ	Division of Skull, Percutaneous Endoscopic Approach
0N810ZZ	Division of Frontal Bone, Open Approach
0N813ZZ	Division of Frontal Bone, Percutaneous Approach
0N814ZZ	Division of Frontal Bone, Percutaneous Endoscopic Approach
0N830ZZ	Division of Right Parietal Bone, Open Approach
0N833ZZ	Division of Right Parietal Bone, Percutaneous Approach
0N834ZZ	Division of Right Parietal Bone, Percutaneous Endoscopic Approach
0N840ZZ	Division of Left Parietal Bone, Open Approach
0N843ZZ	Division of Left Parietal Bone, Percutaneous Approach
0N844ZZ	Division of Left Parietal Bone, Percutaneous Endoscopic Approach
0N850ZZ	Division of Right Temporal Bone, Open Approach
0N853ZZ	Division of Right Temporal Bone, Percutaneous Approach
0N854ZZ	Division of Right Temporal Bone, Percutaneous Endoscopic Approach
0N860ZZ	Division of Left Temporal Bone, Open Approach
0N863ZZ	Division of Left Temporal Bone, Percutaneous Approach
0N864ZZ	Division of Left Temporal Bone, Percutaneous Endoscopic Approach
0N870ZZ	Division of Occipital Bone, Open Approach
0N873ZZ	Division of Occipital Bone, Percutaneous Approach
0N874ZZ	Division of Occipital Bone, Percutaneous Endoscopic Approach
0N8B0ZZ	Division of Nasal Bone, Open Approach
0N8B3ZZ	Division of Nasal Bone, Percutaneous Approach
0N8B4ZZ	Division of Nasal Bone, Percutaneous Endoscopic Approach
0N8C0ZZ	Division of Sphenoid Bone, Open Approach
0N8C3ZZ	Division of Sphenoid Bone, Percutaneous Approach
0N8C4ZZ	Division of Sphenoid Bone, Percutaneous Endoscopic Approach
0N8F0ZZ	Division of Right Ethmoid Bone, Open Approach
0N8F3ZZ	Division of Right Ethmoid Bone, Percutaneous Approach
0N8F4ZZ	Division of Right Ethmoid Bone, Percutaneous Endoscopic Approach
0N8G0ZZ	Division of Left Ethmoid Bone, Open Approach
0N8G3ZZ	Division of Left Ethmoid Bone, Percutaneous Approach
0N8G4ZZ	Division of Left Ethmoid Bone, Percutaneous Endoscopic Approach
0N8H0ZZ	Division of Right Lacrimal Bone, Open Approach
0N8H3ZZ	Division of Right Lacrimal Bone, Percutaneous Approach
0N8H4ZZ	Division of Right Lacrimal Bone, Percutaneous Endoscopic Approach
0N8J0ZZ	Division of Left Lacrimal Bone, Open Approach
0N8J3ZZ	Division of Left Lacrimal Bone, Percutaneous Approach
0N8J4ZZ	Division of Left Lacrimal Bone, Percutaneous Endoscopic Approach
0N8K0ZZ	Division of Right Palatine Bone, Open Approach
0N8K3ZZ	Division of Right Palatine Bone, Percutaneous Approach
0N8K4ZZ	Division of Right Palatine Bone, Percutaneous Endoscopic Approach
0N8L0ZZ	Division of Left Palatine Bone, Open Approach
0N8L3ZZ	Division of Left Palatine Bone, Percutaneous Approach
0N8L4ZZ	Division of Left Palatine Bone, Percutaneous Endoscopic Approach
0N8M0ZZ	Division of Right Zygomatic Bone, Open Approach
0N8M3ZZ	Division of Right Zygomatic Bone, Percutaneous Approach
0N8M4ZZ	Division of Right Zygomatic Bone, Percutaneous Endoscopic Approach
0N8N0ZZ	Division of Left Zygomatic Bone, Open Approach
0N8N3ZZ	Division of Left Zygomatic Bone, Percutaneous Approach
0N8N4ZZ	Division of Left Zygomatic Bone, Percutaneous Endoscopic Approach
0N8P0ZZ	Division of Right Orbit, Open Approach
0N8P3ZZ	Division of Right Orbit, Percutaneous Approach
0N8P4ZZ	Division of Right Orbit, Percutaneous Endoscopic Approach
0N8Q0ZZ	Division of Left Orbit, Open Approach
0N8Q3ZZ	Division of Left Orbit, Percutaneous Approach
0N8Q4ZZ	Division of Left Orbit, Percutaneous Endoscopic Approach
0N8R0ZZ	Division of Maxilla, Open Approach
0N8R3ZZ	Division of Maxilla, Percutaneous Approach
0N8R4ZZ	Division of Maxilla, Percutaneous Endoscopic Approach
0N8T0ZZ	Division of Right Mandible, Open Approach
0N8T3ZZ	Division of Right Mandible, Percutaneous Approach
0N8T4ZZ	Division of Right Mandible, Percutaneous Endoscopic Approach
0N8V0ZZ	Division of Left Mandible, Open Approach
0N8V3ZZ	Division of Left Mandible, Percutaneous Approach
0N8V4ZZ	Division of Left Mandible, Percutaneous Endoscopic Approach
0N8X0ZZ	Division of Hyoid Bone, Open Approach
0N8X3ZZ	Division of Hyoid Bone, Percutaneous Approach
0N8X4ZZ	Division of Hyoid Bone, Percutaneous Endoscopic Approach

0N9 – Head and Facial Bones, Drainage

Review Coding Guidelines B3.4a and B3.4b

Review Coding Guideline B6.2

0N9000Z Drainage of Skull with Drainage Device, Open Approach

0N900ZX Drainage of Skull, Open Approach, Diagnostic

0N900ZZ Drainage of Skull, Open Approach

0N9030Z Drainage of Skull with Drainage Device, Percutaneous Approach

0N903ZX Drainage of Skull, Percutaneous Approach, Diagnostic

0N903ZZ Drainage of Skull, Percutaneous Approach

0N9040Z Drainage of Skull with Drainage Device, Percutaneous Endoscopic Approach

0N904ZX Drainage of Skull, Percutaneous Endoscopic Approach, Diagnostic

0N904ZZ Drainage of Skull, Percutaneous Endoscopic Approach

0N9100Z Drainage of Frontal Bone with Drainage Device, Open Approach

0N910ZX Drainage of Frontal Bone, Open Approach, Diagnostic

0N910ZZ Drainage of Frontal Bone, Open Approach

0N9130Z Drainage of Frontal Bone with Drainage Device, Percutaneous Approach

0N913ZX Drainage of Frontal Bone, Percutaneous Approach, Diagnostic

0N913ZZ Drainage of Frontal Bone, Percutaneous Approach

0N9140Z Drainage of Frontal Bone with Drainage Device, Percutaneous Endoscopic Approach

0N914ZX Drainage of Frontal Bone, Percutaneous Endoscopic Approach, Diagnostic

0N914ZZ Drainage of Frontal Bone, Percutaneous Endoscopic Approach

0N9300Z Drainage of Right Parietal Bone with Drainage Device, Open Approach

0N930ZX Drainage of Right Parietal Bone, Open Approach, Diagnostic

0N930ZZ Drainage of Right Parietal Bone, Open Approach

0N9330Z Drainage of Right Parietal Bone with Drainage Device, Percutaneous Approach

0N933ZX Drainage of Right Parietal Bone, Percutaneous Approach, Diagnostic

0N933ZZ Drainage of Right Parietal Bone, Percutaneous Approach

0N9340Z Drainage of Right Parietal Bone with Drainage Device, Percutaneous Endoscopic Approach

0N934ZX Drainage of Right Parietal Bone, Percutaneous Endoscopic Approach, Diagnostic

0N934ZZ Drainage of Right Parietal Bone, Percutaneous Endoscopic Approach

0N9400Z Drainage of Left Parietal Bone with Drainage Device, Open Approach

0N940ZX Drainage of Left Parietal Bone, Open Approach, Diagnostic

0N940ZZ Drainage of Left Parietal Bone, Open Approach

0N9430Z Drainage of Left Parietal Bone with Drainage Device, Percutaneous Approach

0N943ZX Drainage of Left Parietal Bone, Percutaneous Approach, Diagnostic

0N943ZZ Drainage of Left Parietal Bone, Percutaneous Approach

0N9440Z Drainage of Left Parietal Bone with Drainage Device, Percutaneous Endoscopic Approach

0N944ZX Drainage of Left Parietal Bone, Percutaneous Endoscopic Approach, Diagnostic

0N944ZZ Drainage of Left Parietal Bone, Percutaneous Endoscopic Approach

0N9500Z Drainage of Right Temporal Bone with Drainage Device, Open Approach

0N950ZX Drainage of Right Temporal Bone, Open Approach, Diagnostic

0N950ZZ Drainage of Right Temporal Bone, Open Approach

0N9530Z Drainage of Right Temporal Bone with Drainage Device, Percutaneous Approach

0N953ZX Drainage of Right Temporal Bone, Percutaneous Approach, Diagnostic

0N953ZZ Drainage of Right Temporal Bone, Percutaneous Approach

0N9540Z Drainage of Right Temporal Bone with Drainage Device, Percutaneous Endoscopic Approach

0N954ZX Drainage of Right Temporal Bone, Percutaneous Endoscopic Approach, Diagnostic

0N954ZZ Drainage of Right Temporal Bone, Percutaneous Endoscopic Approach

0N9600Z Drainage of Left Temporal Bone with Drainage Device, Open Approach

0N960ZX Drainage of Left Temporal Bone, Open Approach, Diagnostic

0N960ZZ Drainage of Left Temporal Bone, Open Approach

0N9630Z Drainage of Left Temporal Bone with Drainage Device, Percutaneous Approach

0N963ZX Drainage of Left Temporal Bone, Percutaneous Approach, Diagnostic

0N963ZZ Drainage of Left Temporal Bone, Percutaneous Approach

0N9640Z Drainage of Left Temporal Bone with Drainage Device, Percutaneous Endoscopic Approach

0N964ZX Drainage of Left Temporal Bone, Percutaneous Endoscopic Approach, Diagnostic

0N964ZZ Drainage of Left Temporal Bone, Percutaneous Endoscopic Approach

0N9700Z Drainage of Occipital Bone with Drainage Device, Open Approach

0N970ZX Drainage of Occipital Bone, Open Approach, Diagnostic

0N970ZZ Drainage of Occipital Bone, Open Approach

0N9730Z Drainage of Occipital Bone with Drainage Device, Percutaneous Approach

0N973ZX Drainage of Occipital Bone, Percutaneous Approach, Diagnostic

0N973ZZ Drainage of Occipital Bone, Percutaneous Approach

0N9740Z Drainage of Occipital Bone with Drainage Device, Percutaneous Endoscopic Approach

0N974ZX Drainage of Occipital Bone, Percutaneous Endoscopic Approach, Diagnostic

0N974ZZ Drainage of Occipital Bone, Percutaneous Endoscopic Approach

0N9B00Z Drainage of Nasal Bone with Drainage Device, Open Approach

0N9B0ZX Drainage of Nasal Bone, Open Approach, Diagnostic

0N9B0ZZ Drainage of Nasal Bone, Open Approach

0N9B30Z Drainage of Nasal Bone with Drainage Device, Percutaneous Approach

0N9B3ZX Drainage of Nasal Bone, Percutaneous Approach, Diagnostic

0N9B3ZZ Drainage of Nasal Bone, Percutaneous Approach

0N9B40Z Drainage of Nasal Bone with Drainage Device, Percutaneous Endoscopic Approach

0N9B4ZX Drainage of Nasal Bone, Percutaneous Endoscopic Approach, Diagnostic

0N9B4ZZ Drainage of Nasal Bone, Percutaneous Endoscopic Approach

0N9C00Z Drainage of Sphenoid Bone with Drainage Device, Open Approach

0N9C0ZX Drainage of Sphenoid Bone, Open Approach, Diagnostic

0N9C0ZZ Drainage of Sphenoid Bone, Open Approach

0N9C30Z Drainage of Sphenoid Bone with Drainage Device, Percutaneous Approach

0N9C3ZX Drainage of Sphenoid Bone, Percutaneous Approach, Diagnostic

0N9C3ZZ Drainage of Sphenoid Bone, Percutaneous Approach

0N9C40Z Drainage of Sphenoid Bone with Drainage Device, Percutaneous Endoscopic Approach

0N9C4ZX Drainage of Sphenoid Bone, Percutaneous Endoscopic Approach, Diagnostic

0N9C4ZZ Drainage of Sphenoid Bone, Percutaneous Endoscopic Approach

0N9F00Z Drainage of Right Ethmoid Bone with Drainage Device, Open Approach

0N9F0ZX Drainage of Right Ethmoid Bone, Open Approach, Diagnostic

0N9F0ZZ Drainage of Right Ethmoid Bone, Open Approach

0N9F30Z Drainage of Right Ethmoid Bone with Drainage Device, Percutaneous Approach

0N9F3ZX Drainage of Right Ethmoid Bone, Percutaneous Approach, Diagnostic

0N9F3ZZ Drainage of Right Ethmoid Bone, Percutaneous Approach

0N9F40Z Drainage of Right Ethmoid Bone with Drainage Device, Percutaneous Endoscopic Approach

0N9F4ZX Drainage of Right Ethmoid Bone, Percutaneous Endoscopic Approach, Diagnostic

0N9F4ZZ Drainage of Right Ethmoid Bone, Percutaneous Endoscopic Approach

0N9G00Z Drainage of Left Ethmoid Bone with Drainage Device, Open Approach

0N9G0ZX Drainage of Left Ethmoid Bone, Open Approach, Diagnostic

0N9G0ZZ Drainage of Left Ethmoid Bone, Open Approach

0N9G30Z Drainage of Left Ethmoid Bone with Drainage Device, Percutaneous Approach

0N9G3ZX Drainage of Left Ethmoid Bone, Percutaneous Approach, Diagnostic

0N9G3ZZ Drainage of Left Ethmoid Bone, Percutaneous Approach

0N9G40Z Drainage of Left Ethmoid Bone with Drainage Device, Percutaneous Endoscopic Approach

0N9G4ZX Drainage of Left Ethmoid Bone, Percutaneous Endoscopic Approach, Diagnostic

0N9G4ZZ Drainage of Left Ethmoid Bone, Percutaneous Endoscopic Approach

0N9H00Z Drainage of Right Lacrimal Bone with Drainage Device, Open Approach

0N9H0ZX Drainage of Right Lacrimal Bone, Open Approach, Diagnostic

0N9H0ZZ Drainage of Right Lacrimal Bone, Open Approach

0N9H30Z Drainage of Right Lacrimal Bone with Drainage Device, Percutaneous Approach

0N9H3ZX Drainage of Right Lacrimal Bone, Percutaneous Approach, Diagnostic

0N9H3ZZ Drainage of Right Lacrimal Bone, Percutaneous Approach

0N9H40Z Drainage of Right Lacrimal Bone with Drainage Device, Percutaneous Endoscopic Approach

0N9H4ZX Drainage of Right Lacrimal Bone, Percutaneous Endoscopic Approach, Diagnostic

0N9H4ZZ Drainage of Right Lacrimal Bone, Percutaneous Endoscopic Approach

0N9J00Z Drainage of Left Lacrimal Bone with Drainage Device, Open Approach

0N9J0ZX Drainage of Left Lacrimal Bone, Open Approach, Diagnostic

0N9J0ZZ Drainage of Left Lacrimal Bone, Open Approach

0N9J30Z Drainage of Left Lacrimal Bone with Drainage Device, Percutaneous Approach

0N9J3ZX Drainage of Left Lacrimal Bone, Percutaneous Approach, Diagnostic

0N9J3ZZ Drainage of Left Lacrimal Bone, Percutaneous Approach

0N9J40Z Drainage of Left Lacrimal Bone with Drainage Device, Percutaneous Endoscopic Approach

0N9J4ZX Drainage of Left Lacrimal Bone, Percutaneous Endoscopic Approach, Diagnostic

0N9J4ZZ Drainage of Left Lacrimal Bone, Percutaneous Endoscopic Approach

0N9K00Z Drainage of Right Palatine Bone with Drainage Device, Open Approach

0N9K0ZX Drainage of Right Palatine Bone, Open Approach, Diagnostic

0N9K0ZZ Drainage of Right Palatine Bone, Open Approach

0N9K30Z Drainage of Right Palatine Bone with Drainage Device, Percutaneous Approach

0N9K3ZX Drainage of Right Palatine Bone, Percutaneous Approach, Diagnostic

0N9K3ZZ Drainage of Right Palatine Bone, Percutaneous Approach

0N9K40Z Drainage of Right Palatine Bone with Drainage Device, Percutaneous Endoscopic Approach

0N9K4ZX Drainage of Right Palatine Bone, Percutaneous Endoscopic Approach, Diagnostic

0N9K4ZZ Drainage of Right Palatine Bone, Percutaneous Endoscopic Approach

0N9L00Z Drainage of Left Palatine Bone with Drainage Device, Open Approach

0N9L0ZX Drainage of Left Palatine Bone, Open Approach, Diagnostic

0N9L0ZZ Drainage of Left Palatine Bone, Open Approach

0N9L30Z Drainage of Left Palatine Bone with Drainage Device, Percutaneous Approach

0N9L3ZX Drainage of Left Palatine Bone, Percutaneous Approach, Diagnostic

0N9L3ZZ Drainage of Left Palatine Bone, Percutaneous Approach

0N9L40Z Drainage of Left Palatine Bone with Drainage Device, Percutaneous Endoscopic Approach

0N9L4ZX Drainage of Left Palatine Bone, Percutaneous Endoscopic Approach, Diagnostic

0N9L4ZZ Drainage of Left Palatine Bone, Percutaneous Endoscopic Approach

0N9M00Z Drainage of Right Zygomatic Bone with Drainage Device, Open Approach

0N9M0ZX Drainage of Right Zygomatic Bone, Open Approach, Diagnostic

0N9M0ZZ Drainage of Right Zygomatic Bone, Open Approach

0N9M30Z Drainage of Right Zygomatic Bone with Drainage Device, Percutaneous Approach

0N9M3ZX Drainage of Right Zygomatic Bone, Percutaneous Approach, Diagnostic

0N9M3ZZ Drainage of Right Zygomatic Bone, Percutaneous Approach

0N9M40Z Drainage of Right Zygomatic Bone with Drainage Device, Percutaneous Endoscopic Approach

0N9M4ZX Drainage of Right Zygomatic Bone, Percutaneous Endoscopic Approach, Diagnostic

0N9M4ZZ Drainage of Right Zygomatic Bone, Percutaneous Endoscopic Approach

0N9N00Z Drainage of Left Zygomatic Bone with Drainage Device, Open Approach

0N9N0ZX Drainage of Left Zygomatic Bone, Open Approach, Diagnostic

0N9N0ZZ Drainage of Left Zygomatic Bone, Open Approach

0N9N30Z Drainage of Left Zygomatic Bone with Drainage Device, Percutaneous Approach

0N9N3ZX Drainage of Left Zygomatic Bone, Percutaneous Approach, Diagnostic

0N9N3ZZ Drainage of Left Zygomatic Bone, Percutaneous Approach

0N9N40Z Drainage of Left Zygomatic Bone with Drainage Device, Percutaneous Endoscopic Approach

0N9N4ZX Drainage of Left Zygomatic Bone, Percutaneous Endoscopic Approach, Diagnostic

0N9N4ZZ Drainage of Left Zygomatic Bone, Percutaneous Endoscopic Approach

0N9P00Z Drainage of Right Orbit with Drainage Device, Open Approach

0N9P0ZX Drainage of Right Orbit, Open Approach, Diagnostic

0N9P0ZZ Drainage of Right Orbit, Open Approach

0N9P30Z Drainage of Right Orbit with Drainage Device, Percutaneous Approach

0N9P3ZX Drainage of Right Orbit, Percutaneous Approach, Diagnostic

0N9P3ZZ Drainage of Right Orbit, Percutaneous Approach

0N9P40Z Drainage of Right Orbit with Drainage Device, Percutaneous Endoscopic Approach

0N9P4ZX Drainage of Right Orbit, Percutaneous Endoscopic Approach, Diagnostic

0N9P4ZZ Drainage of Right Orbit, Percutaneous Endoscopic Approach

0N9Q00Z Drainage of Left Orbit with Drainage Device, Open Approach

0N9Q0ZX Drainage of Left Orbit, Open Approach, Diagnostic

0N9Q0ZZ Drainage of Left Orbit, Open Approach

0N9Q30Z Drainage of Left Orbit with Drainage Device, Percutaneous Approach

0N9Q3ZX Drainage of Left Orbit, Percutaneous Approach, Diagnostic

0N9Q3ZZ Drainage of Left Orbit, Percutaneous Approach

0N9Q40Z Drainage of Left Orbit with Drainage Device, Percutaneous Endoscopic Approach

0N9Q4ZX Drainage of Left Orbit, Percutaneous Endoscopic Approach, Diagnostic

0N9Q4ZZ Drainage of Left Orbit, Percutaneous Endoscopic Approach

0N9R00Z Drainage of Maxilla with Drainage Device, Open Approach

0N9R0ZX Drainage of Maxilla, Open Approach, Diagnostic

0N9R0ZZ Drainage of Maxilla, Open Approach

0N9R30Z Drainage of Maxilla with Drainage Device, Percutaneous Approach

0N9R3ZX Drainage of Maxilla, Percutaneous Approach, Diagnostic

0N9R3ZZ Drainage of Maxilla, Percutaneous Approach

0N9R40Z Drainage of Maxilla with Drainage Device, Percutaneous Endoscopic Approach

0N9R4ZX Drainage of Maxilla, Percutaneous Endoscopic Approach, Diagnostic

0N9R4ZZ Drainage of Maxilla, Percutaneous Endoscopic Approach

0N9T00Z Drainage of Right Mandible with Drainage Device, Open Approach

0N9T0ZX Drainage of Right Mandible, Open Approach, Diagnostic

0N9T0ZZ Drainage of Right Mandible, Open Approach

0N9T30Z Drainage of Right Mandible with Drainage Device, Percutaneous Approach

0N9T3ZX Drainage of Right Mandible, Percutaneous Approach, Diagnostic

0N9T3ZZ Drainage of Right Mandible, Percutaneous Approach

0N9T40Z Drainage of Right Mandible with Drainage Device, Percutaneous Endoscopic Approach

0N9T4ZX Drainage of Right Mandible, Percutaneous Endoscopic Approach, Diagnostic

0N9T4ZZ Drainage of Right Mandible, Percutaneous Endoscopic Approach

0N9V00Z Drainage of Left Mandible with Drainage Device, Open Approach

0N9V0ZX Drainage of Left Mandible, Open Approach, Diagnostic

0N9V0ZZ Drainage of Left Mandible, Open Approach

0N9V30Z Drainage of Left Mandible with Drainage Device, Percutaneous Approach

0N9V3ZX Drainage of Left Mandible, Percutaneous Approach, Diagnostic

0N9V3ZZ Drainage of Left Mandible, Percutaneous Approach

0N9V40Z Drainage of Left Mandible with Drainage Device, Percutaneous Endoscopic Approach

0N9V4ZX Drainage of Left Mandible, Percutaneous Endoscopic Approach, Diagnostic

0N9V4ZZ Drainage of Left Mandible, Percutaneous Endoscopic Approach

0N9X00Z Drainage of Hyoid Bone with Drainage Device, Open Approach

0N9X0ZX Drainage of Hyoid Bone, Open Approach, Diagnostic

0N9X0ZZ Drainage of Hyoid Bone, Open Approach

0N9X30Z Drainage of Hyoid Bone with Drainage Device, Percutaneous Approach

0N9X3ZX Drainage of Hyoid Bone, Percutaneous Approach, Diagnostic

0N9X3ZZ Drainage of Hyoid Bone, Percutaneous Approach

0N9X40Z Drainage of Hyoid Bone with Drainage Device, Percutaneous Endoscopic Approach

0N9X4ZX Drainage of Hyoid Bone, Percutaneous Endoscopic Approach, Diagnostic

0N9X4ZZ Drainage of Hyoid Bone, Percutaneous Endoscopic Approach

0NB – Head and Facial Bones, Excision

Review Coding Guidelines B3.4a and B3.4b

Review Coding Guideline B3.5

Review Coding Guideline B3.8

Review Coding Guideline B3.18

0NB00ZX Excision of Skull, Open Approach, Diagnostic

0NB00ZZ Excision of Skull, Open Approach

0NB03ZX Excision of Skull, Percutaneous Approach, Diagnostic

0NB03ZZ Excision of Skull, Percutaneous Approach

0NB04ZX Excision of Skull, Percutaneous Endoscopic Approach, Diagnostic

0NB04ZZ Excision of Skull, Percutaneous Endoscopic Approach

0NB10ZX Excision of Frontal Bone, Open Approach, Diagnostic

0NB10ZZ Excision of Frontal Bone, Open Approach

0NB13ZX Excision of Frontal Bone, Percutaneous Approach, Diagnostic

0NB13ZZ Excision of Frontal Bone, Percutaneous Approach

0NB14ZX Excision of Frontal Bone, Percutaneous Endoscopic Approach, Diagnostic

0NB14ZZ Excision of Frontal Bone, Percutaneous Endoscopic Approach

0NB30ZX Excision of Right Parietal Bone, Open Approach, Diagnostic

0NB30ZZ Excision of Right Parietal Bone, Open Approach

0NB33ZX Excision of Right Parietal Bone, Percutaneous Approach, Diagnostic

0NB33ZZ Excision of Right Parietal Bone, Percutaneous Approach

0NB34ZX Excision of Right Parietal Bone, Percutaneous Endoscopic Approach, Diagnostic

0NB34ZZ Excision of Right Parietal Bone, Percutaneous Endoscopic Approach

0NB40ZX Excision of Left Parietal Bone, Open Approach, Diagnostic

0NB40ZZ Excision of Left Parietal Bone, Open Approach

0NB43ZX Excision of Left Parietal Bone, Percutaneous Approach, Diagnostic

0NB43ZZ Excision of Left Parietal Bone, Percutaneous Approach

0NB44ZX Excision of Left Parietal Bone, Percutaneous Endoscopic Approach, Diagnostic

0NB44ZZ Excision of Left Parietal Bone, Percutaneous Endoscopic Approach

0NB50ZX Excision of Right Temporal Bone, Open Approach, Diagnostic

0NB50ZZ Excision of Right Temporal Bone, Open Approach

0NB53ZX Excision of Right Temporal Bone, Percutaneous Approach, Diagnostic

0NB53ZZ Excision of Right Temporal Bone, Percutaneous Approach

0NB54ZX Excision of Right Temporal Bone, Percutaneous Endoscopic Approach, Diagnostic

0NB54ZZ Excision of Right Temporal Bone, Percutaneous Endoscopic Approach

0NB60ZX Excision of Left Temporal Bone, Open Approach, Diagnostic

0NB60ZZ Excision of Left Temporal Bone, Open Approach

0NB63ZX Excision of Left Temporal Bone, Percutaneous Approach, Diagnostic

0NB63ZZ Excision of Left Temporal Bone, Percutaneous Approach

0NB64ZX Excision of Left Temporal Bone, Percutaneous Endoscopic Approach, Diagnostic

0NB64ZZ Excision of Left Temporal Bone, Percutaneous Endoscopic Approach

0NB70ZX Excision of Occipital Bone, Open Approach, Diagnostic

0NB70ZZ Excision of Occipital Bone, Open Approach

0NB73ZX Excision of Occipital Bone, Percutaneous Approach, Diagnostic

0NB73ZZ Excision of Occipital Bone, Percutaneous Approach

0NB74ZX Excision of Occipital Bone, Percutaneous Endoscopic Approach, Diagnostic

0NB74ZZ Excision of Occipital Bone, Percutaneous Endoscopic Approach

0NBB0ZX Excision of Nasal Bone, Open Approach, Diagnostic

0NBB0ZZ Excision of Nasal Bone, Open Approach
AHA CC: 1Q, 2017, 20-21

0NBB3ZX Excision of Nasal Bone, Percutaneous Approach, Diagnostic

0NBB3ZZ Excision of Nasal Bone, Percutaneous Approach

0NBB4ZX Excision of Nasal Bone, Percutaneous Endoscopic Approach, Diagnostic

0NBB4ZZ Excision of Nasal Bone, Percutaneous Endoscopic Approach

0NBC0ZX Excision of Sphenoid Bone, Open Approach, Diagnostic

0NBC0ZZ Excision of Sphenoid Bone, Open Approach

0NBC3ZX Excision of Sphenoid Bone, Percutaneous Approach, Diagnostic

0NBC3ZZ Excision of Sphenoid Bone, Percutaneous Approach

0NBC4ZX Excision of Sphenoid Bone, Percutaneous Endoscopic Approach, Diagnostic

0NBC4ZZ Excision of Sphenoid Bone, Percutaneous Endoscopic Approach

0NBF0ZX Excision of Right Ethmoid Bone, Open Approach, Diagnostic

0NBF0ZZ Excision of Right Ethmoid Bone, Open Approach

0NBF3ZX Excision of Right Ethmoid Bone, Percutaneous Approach, Diagnostic

0NBF3ZZ Excision of Right Ethmoid Bone, Percutaneous Approach

0NBF4ZX Excision of Right Ethmoid Bone, Percutaneous Endoscopic Approach, Diagnostic

0NBF4ZZ Excision of Right Ethmoid Bone, Percutaneous Endoscopic Approach

0NBG0ZX Excision of Left Ethmoid Bone, Open Approach, Diagnostic

0NBG0ZZ Excision of Left Ethmoid Bone, Open Approach

0NBG3ZX Excision of Left Ethmoid Bone, Percutaneous Approach, Diagnostic

0NBG3ZZ Excision of Left Ethmoid Bone, Percutaneous Approach

0NBG4ZX Excision of Left Ethmoid Bone, Percutaneous Endoscopic Approach, Diagnostic

0NBG4ZZ Excision of Left Ethmoid Bone, Percutaneous Endoscopic Approach

0NBH0ZX Excision of Right Lacrimal Bone, Open Approach, Diagnostic

0NBH0ZZ Excision of Right Lacrimal Bone, Open Approach

0NBH3ZX Excision of Right Lacrimal Bone, Percutaneous Approach, Diagnostic

0NBH3ZZ Excision of Right Lacrimal Bone, Percutaneous Approach

0NBH4ZX Excision of Right Lacrimal Bone, Percutaneous Endoscopic Approach, Diagnostic

0NBH4ZZ Excision of Right Lacrimal Bone, Percutaneous Endoscopic Approach

0NBJ0ZX Excision of Left Lacrimal Bone, Open Approach, Diagnostic

0NBJ0ZZ Excision of Left Lacrimal Bone, Open Approach

0NBJ3ZX Excision of Left Lacrimal Bone, Percutaneous Approach, Diagnostic

0NBJ3ZZ Excision of Left Lacrimal Bone, Percutaneous Approach

0NBJ4ZX Excision of Left Lacrimal Bone, Percutaneous Endoscopic Approach, Diagnostic

0NBJ4ZZ Excision of Left Lacrimal Bone, Percutaneous Endoscopic Approach

0NBK0ZX Excision of Right Palatine Bone, Open Approach, Diagnostic

0NBK0ZZ Excision of Right Palatine Bone, Open Approach

0NBK3ZX Excision of Right Palatine Bone, Percutaneous Approach, Diagnostic

0NBK3ZZ Excision of Right Palatine Bone, Percutaneous Approach

♀ Female-only   ♂ Male-only   ▲ Limited Coverage   ● Non-OR   🅗🅐🅒 HAC-associated procedure   ▲ Non-covered procedures   ✚ Cluster

0NBK4ZX Excision of Right Palatine Bone, Percutaneous Endoscopic Approach, Diagnostic

0NBK4ZZ Excision of Right Palatine Bone, Percutaneous Endoscopic Approach

0NBL0ZX Excision of Left Palatine Bone, Open Approach, Diagnostic

0NBL0ZZ Excision of Left Palatine Bone, Open Approach

0NBL3ZX Excision of Left Palatine Bone, Percutaneous Approach, Diagnostic

0NBL3ZZ Excision of Left Palatine Bone, Percutaneous Approach

0NBL4ZX Excision of Left Palatine Bone, Percutaneous Endoscopic Approach, Diagnostic

0NBL4ZZ Excision of Left Palatine Bone, Percutaneous Endoscopic Approach

0NBM0ZX Excision of Right Zygomatic Bone, Open Approach, Diagnostic

0NBM0ZZ Excision of Right Zygomatic Bone, Open Approach

0NBM3ZX Excision of Right Zygomatic Bone, Percutaneous Approach, Diagnostic

0NBM3ZZ Excision of Right Zygomatic Bone, Percutaneous Approach

0NBM4ZX Excision of Right Zygomatic Bone, Percutaneous Endoscopic Approach, Diagnostic

0NBM4ZZ Excision of Right Zygomatic Bone, Percutaneous Endoscopic Approach

0NBN0ZX Excision of Left Zygomatic Bone, Open Approach, Diagnostic

0NBN0ZZ Excision of Left Zygomatic Bone, Open Approach

0NBN3ZX Excision of Left Zygomatic Bone, Percutaneous Approach, Diagnostic

0NBN3ZZ Excision of Left Zygomatic Bone, Percutaneous Approach

0NBN4ZX Excision of Left Zygomatic Bone, Percutaneous Endoscopic Approach, Diagnostic

0NBN4ZZ Excision of Left Zygomatic Bone, Percutaneous Endoscopic Approach

0NBP0ZX Excision of Right Orbit, Open Approach, Diagnostic

0NBP0ZZ Excision of Right Orbit, Open Approach

0NBP3ZX Excision of Right Orbit, Percutaneous Approach, Diagnostic

0NBP3ZZ Excision of Right Orbit, Percutaneous Approach

0NBP4ZX Excision of Right Orbit, Percutaneous Endoscopic Approach, Diagnostic

0NBP4ZZ Excision of Right Orbit, Percutaneous Endoscopic Approach

0NBQ0ZX Excision of Left Orbit, Open Approach, Diagnostic

0NBQ0ZZ Excision of Left Orbit, Open Approach
AHA CC: 2Q, 2015, 12-13

0NBQ3ZX Excision of Left Orbit, Percutaneous Approach, Diagnostic

0NBQ3ZZ Excision of Left Orbit, Percutaneous Approach

0NBQ4ZX Excision of Left Orbit, Percutaneous Endoscopic Approach, Diagnostic

0NBQ4ZZ Excision of Left Orbit, Percutaneous Endoscopic Approach

0NBR0ZX Excision of Maxilla, Open Approach, Diagnostic

0NBR0ZZ Excision of Maxilla, Open Approach
AHA CC: 1Q, 2021, 21-22

0NBR3ZX Excision of Maxilla, Percutaneous Approach, Diagnostic

0NBR3ZZ Excision of Maxilla, Percutaneous Approach

0NBR4ZX Excision of Maxilla, Percutaneous Endoscopic Approach, Diagnostic

0NBR4ZZ Excision of Maxilla, Percutaneous Endoscopic Approach

0NBT0ZX Excision of Right Mandible, Open Approach, Diagnostic

0NBT0ZZ Excision of Right Mandible, Open Approach

0NBT3ZX Excision of Right Mandible, Percutaneous Approach, Diagnostic

0NBT3ZZ Excision of Right Mandible, Percutaneous Approach

0NBT4ZX Excision of Right Mandible, Percutaneous Endoscopic Approach, Diagnostic

0NBT4ZZ Excision of Right Mandible, Percutaneous Endoscopic Approach

0NBV0ZX Excision of Left Mandible, Open Approach, Diagnostic

0NBV0ZZ Excision of Left Mandible, Open Approach

0NBV3ZX Excision of Left Mandible, Percutaneous Approach, Diagnostic

0NBV3ZZ Excision of Left Mandible, Percutaneous Approach

0NBV4ZX Excision of Left Mandible, Percutaneous Endoscopic Approach, Diagnostic

0NBV4ZZ Excision of Left Mandible, Percutaneous Endoscopic Approach

0NBX0ZX Excision of Hyoid Bone, Open Approach, Diagnostic

0NBX0ZZ Excision of Hyoid Bone, Open Approach

0NBX3ZX Excision of Hyoid Bone, Percutaneous Approach, Diagnostic

0NBX3ZZ Excision of Hyoid Bone, Percutaneous Approach

0NBX4ZX Excision of Hyoid Bone, Percutaneous Endoscopic Approach, Diagnostic

0NBX4ZZ Excision of Hyoid Bone, Percutaneous Endoscopic Approach

0NC – Head and Facial Bones, Extirpation

0NC10ZZ Extirpation of Matter from Frontal Bone, Open Approach

0NC13ZZ Extirpation of Matter from Frontal Bone, Percutaneous Approach

0NC14ZZ Extirpation of Matter from Frontal Bone, Percutaneous Endoscopic Approach

0NC30ZZ Extirpation of Matter from Right Parietal Bone, Open Approach

0NC33ZZ Extirpation of Matter from Right Parietal Bone, Percutaneous Approach

0NC34ZZ Extirpation of Matter from Right Parietal Bone, Percutaneous Endoscopic Approach

0NC40ZZ Extirpation of Matter from Left Parietal Bone, Open Approach

0NC43ZZ Extirpation of Matter from Left Parietal Bone, Percutaneous Approach

0NC44ZZ Extirpation of Matter from Left Parietal Bone, Percutaneous Endoscopic Approach

0NC50ZZ Extirpation of Matter from Right Temporal Bone, Open Approach

0NC53ZZ Extirpation of Matter from Right Temporal Bone, Percutaneous Approach

0NC54ZZ Extirpation of Matter from Right Temporal Bone, Percutaneous Endoscopic Approach

0NC60ZZ Extirpation of Matter from Left Temporal Bone, Open Approach

0NC63ZZ Extirpation of Matter from Left Temporal Bone, Percutaneous Approach

0NC64ZZ Extirpation of Matter from Left Temporal Bone, Percutaneous Endoscopic Approach

0NC70ZZ Extirpation of Matter from Occipital Bone, Open Approach

0NC73ZZ Extirpation of Matter from Occipital Bone, Percutaneous Approach

0NC74ZZ Extirpation of Matter from Occipital Bone, Percutaneous Endoscopic Approach

0NCB0ZZ Extirpation of Matter from Nasal Bone, Open Approach

0NCB3ZZ Extirpation of Matter from Nasal Bone, Percutaneous Approach

0NCB4ZZ Extirpation of Matter from Nasal Bone, Percutaneous Endoscopic Approach

0NCC0ZZ Extirpation of Matter from Sphenoid Bone, Open Approach

0NCC3ZZ Extirpation of Matter from Sphenoid Bone, Percutaneous Approach

0NCC4ZZ Extirpation of Matter from Sphenoid Bone, Percutaneous Endoscopic Approach

0NCF0ZZ Extirpation of Matter from Right Ethmoid Bone, Open Approach

0NCF3ZZ Extirpation of Matter from Right Ethmoid Bone, Percutaneous Approach

0NCF4ZZ Extirpation of Matter from Right Ethmoid Bone, Percutaneous Endoscopic Approach

0NCG0ZZ Extirpation of Matter from Left Ethmoid Bone, Open Approach

0NCG3ZZ Extirpation of Matter from Left Ethmoid Bone, Percutaneous Approach

0NCG4ZZ Extirpation of Matter from Left Ethmoid Bone, Percutaneous Endoscopic Approach

0NCH0ZZ Extirpation of Matter from Right Lacrimal Bone, Open Approach

0NCH3ZZ Extirpation of Matter from Right Lacrimal Bone, Percutaneous Approach

0NCH4ZZ Extirpation of Matter from Right Lacrimal Bone, Percutaneous Endoscopic Approach

0NCJ0ZZ Extirpation of Matter from Left Lacrimal Bone, Open Approach

0NCJ3ZZ Extirpation of Matter from Left Lacrimal Bone, Percutaneous Approach

0NCJ4ZZ Extirpation of Matter from Left Lacrimal Bone, Percutaneous Endoscopic Approach

0NCK0ZZ Extirpation of Matter from Right Palatine Bone, Open Approach

0NCK3ZZ Extirpation of Matter from Right Palatine Bone, Percutaneous Approach

0NCK4ZZ Extirpation of Matter from Right Palatine Bone, Percutaneous Endoscopic Approach

0NCL0ZZ Extirpation of Matter from Left Palatine Bone, Open Approach

0NCL3ZZ Extirpation of Matter from Left Palatine Bone, Percutaneous Approach
0NCL4ZZ Extirpation of Matter from Left Palatine Bone, Percutaneous Endoscopic Approach
0NCM0ZZ Extirpation of Matter from Right Zygomatic Bone, Open Approach
0NCM3ZZ Extirpation of Matter from Right Zygomatic Bone, Percutaneous Approach
0NCM4ZZ Extirpation of Matter from Right Zygomatic Bone, Percutaneous Endoscopic Approach
0NCN0ZZ Extirpation of Matter from Left Zygomatic Bone, Open Approach
0NCN3ZZ Extirpation of Matter from Left Zygomatic Bone, Percutaneous Approach
0NCN4ZZ Extirpation of Matter from Left Zygomatic Bone, Percutaneous Endoscopic Approach

0NCP0ZZ Extirpation of Matter from Right Orbit, Open Approach
0NCP3ZZ Extirpation of Matter from Right Orbit, Percutaneous Approach
0NCP4ZZ Extirpation of Matter from Right Orbit, Percutaneous Endoscopic Approach
0NCQ0ZZ Extirpation of Matter from Left Orbit, Open Approach
0NCQ3ZZ Extirpation of Matter from Left Orbit, Percutaneous Approach
0NCQ4ZZ Extirpation of Matter from Left Orbit, Percutaneous Endoscopic Approach
0NCR0ZZ Extirpation of Matter from Maxilla, Open Approach
0NCR3ZZ Extirpation of Matter from Maxilla, Percutaneous Approach
0NCR4ZZ Extirpation of Matter from Maxilla, Percutaneous Endoscopic Approach
0NCT0ZZ Extirpation of Matter from Right Mandible, Open Approach

0NCT3ZZ Extirpation of Matter from Right Mandible, Percutaneous Approach
0NCT4ZZ Extirpation of Matter from Right Mandible, Percutaneous Endoscopic Approach
0NCV0ZZ Extirpation of Matter from Left Mandible, Open Approach
0NCV3ZZ Extirpation of Matter from Left Mandible, Percutaneous Approach
0NCV4ZZ Extirpation of Matter from Left Mandible, Percutaneous Endoscopic Approach
0NCX0ZZ Extirpation of Matter from Hyoid Bone, Open Approach
0NCX3ZZ Extirpation of Matter from Hyoid Bone, Percutaneous Approach
0NCX4ZZ Extirpation of Matter from Hyoid Bone, Percutaneous Endoscopic Approach

0ND – Head and Facial Bones, Extraction

0ND00ZZ Extraction of Skull, Open Approach
0ND10ZZ Extraction of Frontal Bone, Open Approach
0ND30ZZ Extraction of Right Parietal Bone, Open Approach
0ND40ZZ Extraction of Left Parietal Bone, Open Approach
0ND50ZZ Extraction of Right Temporal Bone, Open Approach
0ND60ZZ Extraction of Left Temporal Bone, Open Approach
0ND70ZZ Extraction of Occipital Bone, Open Approach
0NDB0ZZ Extraction of Nasal Bone, Open Approach

0NDC0ZZ Extraction of Sphenoid Bone, Open Approach
0NDF0ZZ Extraction of Right Ethmoid Bone, Open Approach
0NDG0ZZ Extraction of Left Ethmoid Bone, Open Approach
0NDH0ZZ Extraction of Right Lacrimal Bone, Open Approach
0NDJ0ZZ Extraction of Left Lacrimal Bone, Open Approach
0NDK0ZZ Extraction of Right Palatine Bone, Open Approach
0NDL0ZZ Extraction of Left Palatine Bone, Open Approach

0NDM0ZZ Extraction of Right Zygomatic Bone, Open Approach
0NDN0ZZ Extraction of Left Zygomatic Bone, Open Approach
0NDP0ZZ Extraction of Right Orbit, Open Approach
0NDQ0ZZ Extraction of Left Orbit, Open Approach
0NDR0ZZ Extraction of Maxilla, Open Approach
0NDT0ZZ Extraction of Right Mandible, Open Approach
0NDV0ZZ Extraction of Left Mandible, Open Approach
0NDX0ZZ Extraction of Hyoid Bone, Open Approach

0NH – Head and Facial Bones, Insertion

0NH003Z Insertion of Infusion Device into Skull, Open Approach
0NH004Z Insertion of Internal Fixation Device into Skull, Open Approach
AHA CC: 3Q, 2015, 13-14
0NH005Z Insertion of External Fixation Device into Skull, Open Approach
0NH00MZ Insertion of Bone Growth Stimulator into Skull, Open Approach
0NH00NZ Insertion of Neurostimulator Generator into Skull, Open Approach
+ Major brain device implant when reported with an Insertion of a neurostimulator lead (6th character M) into the brain or cerebral ventricle. See table 00H to construct the Insertion code.
0NH033Z Insertion of Infusion Device into Skull, Percutaneous Approach
0NH034Z Insertion of Internal Fixation Device into Skull, Percutaneous Approach
0NH035Z Insertion of External Fixation Device into Skull, Percutaneous Approach
0NH03MZ Insertion of Bone Growth Stimulator into Skull, Percutaneous Approach
0NH043Z Insertion of Infusion Device into Skull, Percutaneous Endoscopic Approach
0NH044Z Insertion of Internal Fixation Device into Skull, Percutaneous Endoscopic Approach
0NH045Z Insertion of External Fixation Device into Skull, Percutaneous Endoscopic Approach

0NH04MZ Insertion of Bone Growth Stimulator into Skull, Percutaneous Endoscopic Approach
0NH104Z Insertion of Internal Fixation Device into Frontal Bone, Open Approach
0NH134Z Insertion of Internal Fixation Device into Frontal Bone, Percutaneous Approach
0NH144Z Insertion of Internal Fixation Device into Frontal Bone, Percutaneous Endoscopic Approach
0NH304Z Insertion of Internal Fixation Device into Right Parietal Bone, Open Approach
0NH334Z Insertion of Internal Fixation Device into Right Parietal Bone, Percutaneous Approach
0NH344Z Insertion of Internal Fixation Device into Right Parietal Bone, Percutaneous Endoscopic Approach
0NH404Z Insertion of Internal Fixation Device into Left Parietal Bone, Open Approach
0NH434Z Insertion of Internal Fixation Device into Left Parietal Bone, Percutaneous Approach
0NH444Z Insertion of Internal Fixation Device into Left Parietal Bone, Percutaneous Endoscopic Approach
0NH504Z Insertion of Internal Fixation Device into Right Temporal Bone, Open Approach
0NH50SZ Insertion of Hearing Device into Right Temporal Bone, Open Approach

0NH534Z Insertion of Internal Fixation Device into Right Temporal Bone, Percutaneous Approach
0NH53SZ Insertion of Hearing Device into Right Temporal Bone, Percutaneous Approach
0NH544Z Insertion of Internal Fixation Device into Right Temporal Bone, Percutaneous Endoscopic Approach
0NH54SZ Insertion of Hearing Device into Right Temporal Bone, Percutaneous Endoscopic Approach
0NH604Z Insertion of Internal Fixation Device into Left Temporal Bone, Open Approach
0NH60SZ Insertion of Hearing Device into Left Temporal Bone, Open Approach
0NH634Z Insertion of Internal Fixation Device into Left Temporal Bone, Percutaneous Approach
0NH63SZ Insertion of Hearing Device into Left Temporal Bone, Percutaneous Approach
0NH644Z Insertion of Internal Fixation Device into Left Temporal Bone, Percutaneous Endoscopic Approach
0NH64SZ Insertion of Hearing Device into Left Temporal Bone, Percutaneous Endoscopic Approach
0NH704Z Insertion of Internal Fixation Device into Occipital Bone, Open Approach
0NH734Z Insertion of Internal Fixation Device into Occipital Bone, Percutaneous Approach

♀ Female-only   ♂ Male-only   ▲ Limited Coverage   ● Non-OR   ▥ HAC-associated procedure   ▲ Non-covered procedures   + Cluster

0NH744Z Insertion of Internal Fixation Device into Occipital Bone, Percutaneous Endoscopic Approach

0NHB04Z Insertion of Internal Fixation Device into Nasal Bone, Open Approach

0NHB0MZ Insertion of Bone Growth Stimulator into Nasal Bone, Open Approach

0NHB34Z Insertion of Internal Fixation Device into Nasal Bone, Percutaneous Approach

0NHB3MZ Insertion of Bone Growth Stimulator into Nasal Bone, Percutaneous Approach

0NHB44Z Insertion of Internal Fixation Device into Nasal Bone, Percutaneous Endoscopic Approach

0NHB4MZ Insertion of Bone Growth Stimulator into Nasal Bone, Percutaneous Endoscopic Approach

0NHC04Z Insertion of Internal Fixation Device into Sphenoid Bone, Open Approach

0NHC34Z Insertion of Internal Fixation Device into Sphenoid Bone, Percutaneous Approach

0NHC44Z Insertion of Internal Fixation Device into Sphenoid Bone, Percutaneous Endoscopic Approach

0NHF04Z Insertion of Internal Fixation Device into Right Ethmoid Bone, Open Approach

0NHF34Z Insertion of Internal Fixation Device into Right Ethmoid Bone, Percutaneous Approach

0NHF44Z Insertion of Internal Fixation Device into Right Ethmoid Bone, Percutaneous Endoscopic Approach

0NHG04Z Insertion of Internal Fixation Device into Left Ethmoid Bone, Open Approach

0NHG34Z Insertion of Internal Fixation Device into Left Ethmoid Bone, Percutaneous Approach

0NHG44Z Insertion of Internal Fixation Device into Left Ethmoid Bone, Percutaneous Endoscopic Approach

0NHH04Z Insertion of Internal Fixation Device into Right Lacrimal Bone, Open Approach

0NHH34Z Insertion of Internal Fixation Device into Right Lacrimal Bone, Percutaneous Approach

0NHH44Z Insertion of Internal Fixation Device into Right Lacrimal Bone, Percutaneous Endoscopic Approach

0NHJ04Z Insertion of Internal Fixation Device into Left Lacrimal Bone, Open Approach

0NHJ34Z Insertion of Internal Fixation Device into Left Lacrimal Bone, Percutaneous Approach

0NHJ44Z Insertion of Internal Fixation Device into Left Lacrimal Bone, Percutaneous Endoscopic Approach

0NHK04Z Insertion of Internal Fixation Device into Right Palatine Bone, Open Approach

0NHK34Z Insertion of Internal Fixation Device into Right Palatine Bone, Percutaneous Approach

0NHK44Z Insertion of Internal Fixation Device into Right Palatine Bone, Percutaneous Endoscopic Approach

0NHL04Z Insertion of Internal Fixation Device into Left Palatine Bone, Open Approach

0NHL34Z Insertion of Internal Fixation Device into Left Palatine Bone, Percutaneous Approach

0NHL44Z Insertion of Internal Fixation Device into Left Palatine Bone, Percutaneous Endoscopic Approach

0NHM04Z Insertion of Internal Fixation Device into Right Zygomatic Bone, Open Approach

0NHM34Z Insertion of Internal Fixation Device into Right Zygomatic Bone, Percutaneous Approach

0NHM44Z Insertion of Internal Fixation Device into Right Zygomatic Bone, Percutaneous Endoscopic Approach

0NHN04Z Insertion of Internal Fixation Device into Left Zygomatic Bone, Open Approach

0NHN34Z Insertion of Internal Fixation Device into Left Zygomatic Bone, Percutaneous Approach

0NHN44Z Insertion of Internal Fixation Device into Left Zygomatic Bone, Percutaneous Endoscopic Approach

0NHP04Z Insertion of Internal Fixation Device into Right Orbit, Open Approach

0NHP34Z Insertion of Internal Fixation Device into Right Orbit, Percutaneous Approach

0NHP44Z Insertion of Internal Fixation Device into Right Orbit, Percutaneous Endoscopic Approach

0NHQ04Z Insertion of Internal Fixation Device into Left Orbit, Open Approach

0NHQ34Z Insertion of Internal Fixation Device into Left Orbit, Percutaneous Approach

0NHQ44Z Insertion of Internal Fixation Device into Left Orbit, Percutaneous Endoscopic Approach

0NHR04Z Insertion of Internal Fixation Device into Maxilla, Open Approach

0NHR05Z Insertion of External Fixation Device into Maxilla, Open Approach

0NHR34Z Insertion of Internal Fixation Device into Maxilla, Percutaneous Approach

0NHR35Z Insertion of External Fixation Device into Maxilla, Percutaneous Approach

0NHR44Z Insertion of Internal Fixation Device into Maxilla, Percutaneous Endoscopic Approach

0NHR45Z Insertion of External Fixation Device into Maxilla, Percutaneous Endoscopic Approach

0NHT04Z Insertion of Internal Fixation Device into Right Mandible, Open Approach

0NHT05Z Insertion of External Fixation Device into Right Mandible, Open Approach

0NHT34Z Insertion of Internal Fixation Device into Right Mandible, Percutaneous Approach

0NHT35Z Insertion of External Fixation Device into Right Mandible, Percutaneous Approach

0NHT44Z Insertion of Internal Fixation Device into Right Mandible, Percutaneous Endoscopic Approach

0NHT45Z Insertion of External Fixation Device into Right Mandible, Percutaneous Endoscopic Approach

0NHV04Z Insertion of Internal Fixation Device into Left Mandible, Open Approach

0NHV05Z Insertion of External Fixation Device into Left Mandible, Open Approach

0NHV34Z Insertion of Internal Fixation Device into Left Mandible, Percutaneous Approach

0NHV35Z Insertion of External Fixation Device into Left Mandible, Percutaneous Approach

0NHV44Z Insertion of Internal Fixation Device into Left Mandible, Percutaneous Endoscopic Approach

0NHV45Z Insertion of External Fixation Device into Left Mandible, Percutaneous Endoscopic Approach

0NHW0MZ Insertion of Bone Growth Stimulator into Facial Bone, Open Approach

0NHW3MZ Insertion of Bone Growth Stimulator into Facial Bone, Percutaneous Approach

0NHW4MZ Insertion of Bone Growth Stimulator into Facial Bone, Percutaneous Endoscopic Approach

0NHX04Z Insertion of Internal Fixation Device into Hyoid Bone, Open Approach

0NHX34Z Insertion of Internal Fixation Device into Hyoid Bone, Percutaneous Approach

0NHX44Z Insertion of Internal Fixation Device into Hyoid Bone, Percutaneous Endoscopic Approach

0NJ – Head and Facial Bones, Inspection

Review Coding Guideline B3.5

Review Coding Guidelines B3.11a, B3.11b and B3.11c

0NJ00ZZ Inspection of Skull, Open Approach

0NJ03ZZ Inspection of Skull, Percutaneous Approach

0NJ04ZZ Inspection of Skull, Percutaneous Endoscopic Approach

0NJ0XZZ Inspection of Skull, External Approach

0NJB0ZZ Inspection of Nasal Bone, Open Approach

0NJB3ZZ Inspection of Nasal Bone, Percutaneous Approach

0NJB4ZZ Inspection of Nasal Bone, Percutaneous Endoscopic Approach

0NJBXZZ Inspection of Nasal Bone, External Approach

0NJW0ZZ Inspection of Facial Bone, Open Approach

0NJW3ZZ Inspection of Facial Bone, Percutaneous Approach

0NJW4ZZ Inspection of Facial Bone, Percutaneous Endoscopic Approach

0NJWXZZ Inspection of Facial Bone, External Approach

0NN – Head and Facial Bones, Release

Review Coding Guideline B3.13

Review Coding Guideline B3.14

0NN10ZZ	Release Frontal Bone, Open Approach
0NN13ZZ	Release Frontal Bone, Percutaneous Approach
0NN14ZZ	Release Frontal Bone, Percutaneous Endoscopic Approach
0NN30ZZ	Release Right Parietal Bone, Open Approach
0NN33ZZ	Release Right Parietal Bone, Percutaneous Approach
0NN34ZZ	Release Right Parietal Bone, Percutaneous Endoscopic Approach
0NN40ZZ	Release Left Parietal Bone, Open Approach
0NN43ZZ	Release Left Parietal Bone, Percutaneous Approach
0NN44ZZ	Release Left Parietal Bone, Percutaneous Endoscopic Approach
0NN50ZZ	Release Right Temporal Bone, Open Approach
0NN53ZZ	Release Right Temporal Bone, Percutaneous Approach
0NN54ZZ	Release Right Temporal Bone, Percutaneous Endoscopic Approach
0NN60ZZ	Release Left Temporal Bone, Open Approach
0NN63ZZ	Release Left Temporal Bone, Percutaneous Approach
0NN64ZZ	Release Left Temporal Bone, Percutaneous Endoscopic Approach
0NN70ZZ	Release Occipital Bone, Open Approach
0NN73ZZ	Release Occipital Bone, Percutaneous Approach
0NN74ZZ	Release Occipital Bone, Percutaneous Endoscopic Approach
0NNB0ZZ	Release Nasal Bone, Open Approach
0NNB3ZZ	Release Nasal Bone, Percutaneous Approach
0NNB4ZZ	Release Nasal Bone, Percutaneous Endoscopic Approach
0NNC0ZZ	Release Sphenoid Bone, Open Approach
0NNC3ZZ	Release Sphenoid Bone, Percutaneous Approach
0NNC4ZZ	Release Sphenoid Bone, Percutaneous Endoscopic Approach
0NNF0ZZ	Release Right Ethmoid Bone, Open Approach
0NNF3ZZ	Release Right Ethmoid Bone, Percutaneous Approach
0NNF4ZZ	Release Right Ethmoid Bone, Percutaneous Endoscopic Approach
0NNG0ZZ	Release Left Ethmoid Bone, Open Approach
0NNG3ZZ	Release Left Ethmoid Bone, Percutaneous Approach
0NNG4ZZ	Release Left Ethmoid Bone, Percutaneous Endoscopic Approach
0NNH0ZZ	Release Right Lacrimal Bone, Open Approach
0NNH3ZZ	Release Right Lacrimal Bone, Percutaneous Approach
0NNH4ZZ	Release Right Lacrimal Bone, Percutaneous Endoscopic Approach
0NNJ0ZZ	Release Left Lacrimal Bone, Open Approach
0NNJ3ZZ	Release Left Lacrimal Bone, Percutaneous Approach
0NNJ4ZZ	Release Left Lacrimal Bone, Percutaneous Endoscopic Approach
0NNK0ZZ	Release Right Palatine Bone, Open Approach
0NNK3ZZ	Release Right Palatine Bone, Percutaneous Approach
0NNK4ZZ	Release Right Palatine Bone, Percutaneous Endoscopic Approach
0NNL0ZZ	Release Left Palatine Bone, Open Approach
0NNL3ZZ	Release Left Palatine Bone, Percutaneous Approach
0NNL4ZZ	Release Left Palatine Bone, Percutaneous Endoscopic Approach
0NNM0ZZ	Release Right Zygomatic Bone, Open Approach
0NNM3ZZ	Release Right Zygomatic Bone, Percutaneous Approach
0NNM4ZZ	Release Right Zygomatic Bone, Percutaneous Endoscopic Approach
0NNN0ZZ	Release Left Zygomatic Bone, Open Approach
0NNN3ZZ	Release Left Zygomatic Bone, Percutaneous Approach
0NNN4ZZ	Release Left Zygomatic Bone, Percutaneous Endoscopic Approach
0NNP0ZZ	Release Right Orbit, Open Approach
0NNP3ZZ	Release Right Orbit, Percutaneous Approach
0NNP4ZZ	Release Right Orbit, Percutaneous Endoscopic Approach
0NNQ0ZZ	Release Left Orbit, Open Approach
0NNQ3ZZ	Release Left Orbit, Percutaneous Approach
0NNQ4ZZ	Release Left Orbit, Percutaneous Endoscopic Approach
0NNR0ZZ	Release Maxilla, Open Approach
0NNR3ZZ	Release Maxilla, Percutaneous Approach
0NNR4ZZ	Release Maxilla, Percutaneous Endoscopic Approach
0NNT0ZZ	Release Right Mandible, Open Approach
0NNT3ZZ	Release Right Mandible, Percutaneous Approach
0NNT4ZZ	Release Right Mandible, Percutaneous Endoscopic Approach
0NNV0ZZ	Release Left Mandible, Open Approach
0NNV3ZZ	Release Left Mandible, Percutaneous Approach
0NNV4ZZ	Release Left Mandible, Percutaneous Endoscopic Approach
0NNX0ZZ	Release Hyoid Bone, Open Approach
0NNX3ZZ	Release Hyoid Bone, Percutaneous Approach
0NNX4ZZ	Release Hyoid Bone, Percutaneous Endoscopic Approach

0NP – Head and Facial Bones, Removal

Review Coding Guideline B6.1c

0NP000Z	Removal of Drainage Device from Skull, Open Approach
0NP004Z	Removal of Internal Fixation Device from Skull, Open Approach
	AHA CC: 3Q, 2015, 13-14
0NP005Z	Removal of External Fixation Device from Skull, Open Approach
0NP007Z	Removal of Autologous Tissue Substitute from Skull, Open Approach
0NP00JZ	Removal of Synthetic Substitute from Skull, Open Approach
0NP00KZ	Removal of Nonautologous Tissue Substitute from Skull, Open Approach
0NP00MZ	Removal of Bone Growth Stimulator from Skull, Open Approach
0NP00NZ	Removal of Neurostimulator Generator from Skull, Open Approach
0NP00SZ	Removal of Hearing Device from Skull, Open Approach
0NP030Z	Removal of Drainage Device from Skull, Percutaneous Approach
0NP034Z	Removal of Internal Fixation Device from Skull, Percutaneous Approach
0NP035Z	Removal of External Fixation Device from Skull, Percutaneous Approach
0NP037Z	Removal of Autologous Tissue Substitute from Skull, Percutaneous Approach
0NP03JZ	Removal of Synthetic Substitute from Skull, Percutaneous Approach
0NP03KZ	Removal of Nonautologous Tissue Substitute from Skull, Percutaneous Approach
0NP03MZ	Removal of Bone Growth Stimulator from Skull, Percutaneous Approach
0NP03SZ	Removal of Hearing Device from Skull, Percutaneous Approach
0NP040Z	Removal of Drainage Device from Skull, Percutaneous Endoscopic Approach
0NP044Z	Removal of Internal Fixation Device from Skull, Percutaneous Endoscopic Approach
0NP045Z	Removal of External Fixation Device from Skull, Percutaneous Endoscopic Approach
0NP047Z	Removal of Autologous Tissue Substitute from Skull, Percutaneous Endoscopic Approach
0NP04JZ	Removal of Synthetic Substitute from Skull, Percutaneous Endoscopic Approach
0NP04KZ	Removal of Nonautologous Tissue Substitute from Skull, Percutaneous Endoscopic Approach
0NP04MZ	Removal of Bone Growth Stimulator from Skull, Percutaneous Endoscopic Approach
0NP04SZ	Removal of Hearing Device from Skull, Percutaneous Endoscopic Approach
0NP0X0Z	Removal of Drainage Device from Skull, External Approach
0NP0X4Z	Removal of Internal Fixation Device from Skull, External Approach
0NP0X5Z	Removal of External Fixation Device from Skull, External Approach
0NP0XMZ	Removal of Bone Growth Stimulator from Skull, External Approach

♀ Female-only   ♂ Male-only   ▲ Limited Coverage   ● Non-OR   HAC HAC-associated procedure   ▲ Non-covered procedures   ✚ Cluster

0NP0XSZ Removal of Hearing Device from Skull, External Approach
0NPB00Z Removal of Drainage Device from Nasal Bone, Open Approach
0NPB04Z Removal of Internal Fixation Device from Nasal Bone, Open Approach
0NPB07Z Removal of Autologous Tissue Substitute from Nasal Bone, Open Approach
0NPB0JZ Removal of Synthetic Substitute from Nasal Bone, Open Approach
0NPB0KZ Removal of Nonautologous Tissue Substitute from Nasal Bone, Open Approach
0NPB0MZ Removal of Bone Growth Stimulator from Nasal Bone, Open Approach
0NPB30Z Removal of Drainage Device from Nasal Bone, Percutaneous Approach
0NPB34Z Removal of Internal Fixation Device from Nasal Bone, Percutaneous Approach
0NPB37Z Removal of Autologous Tissue Substitute from Nasal Bone, Percutaneous Approach
0NPB3JZ Removal of Synthetic Substitute from Nasal Bone, Percutaneous Approach
0NPB3KZ Removal of Nonautologous Tissue Substitute from Nasal Bone, Percutaneous Approach
0NPB3MZ Removal of Bone Growth Stimulator from Nasal Bone, Percutaneous Approach
0NPB40Z Removal of Drainage Device from Nasal Bone, Percutaneous Endoscopic Approach
0NPB44Z Removal of Internal Fixation Device from Nasal Bone, Percutaneous Endoscopic Approach

0NPB47Z Removal of Autologous Tissue Substitute from Nasal Bone, Percutaneous Endoscopic Approach
0NPB4JZ Removal of Synthetic Substitute from Nasal Bone, Percutaneous Endoscopic Approach
0NPB4KZ Removal of Nonautologous Tissue Substitute from Nasal Bone, Percutaneous Endoscopic Approach
0NPB4MZ Removal of Bone Growth Stimulator from Nasal Bone, Percutaneous Endoscopic Approach
0NPBX0Z Removal of Drainage Device from Nasal Bone, External Approach
0NPBX4Z Removal of Internal Fixation Device from Nasal Bone, External Approach
0NPBXMZ Removal of Bone Growth Stimulator from Nasal Bone, External Approach
0NPW00Z Removal of Drainage Device from Facial Bone, Open Approach
0NPW04Z Removal of Internal Fixation Device from Facial Bone, Open Approach
0NPW07Z Removal of Autologous Tissue Substitute from Facial Bone, Open Approach
0NPW0JZ Removal of Synthetic Substitute from Facial Bone, Open Approach
0NPW0KZ Removal of Nonautologous Tissue Substitute from Facial Bone, Open Approach
0NPW0MZ Removal of Bone Growth Stimulator from Facial Bone, Open Approach
0NPW30Z Removal of Drainage Device from Facial Bone, Percutaneous Approach
0NPW34Z Removal of Internal Fixation Device from Facial Bone, Percutaneous Approach

0NPW37Z Removal of Autologous Tissue Substitute from Facial Bone, Percutaneous Approach
0NPW3JZ Removal of Synthetic Substitute from Facial Bone, Percutaneous Approach
0NPW3KZ Removal of Nonautologous Tissue Substitute from Facial Bone, Percutaneous Approach
0NPW3MZ Removal of Bone Growth Stimulator from Facial Bone, Percutaneous Approach
0NPW40Z Removal of Drainage Device from Facial Bone, Percutaneous Endoscopic Approach
0NPW44Z Removal of Internal Fixation Device from Facial Bone, Percutaneous Endoscopic Approach
0NPW47Z Removal of Autologous Tissue Substitute from Facial Bone, Percutaneous Endoscopic Approach
0NPW4JZ Removal of Synthetic Substitute from Facial Bone, Percutaneous Endoscopic Approach
0NPW4KZ Removal of Nonautologous Tissue Substitute from Facial Bone, Percutaneous Endoscopic Approach
0NPW4MZ Removal of Bone Growth Stimulator from Facial Bone, Percutaneous Endoscopic Approach
0NPWX0Z Removal of Drainage Device from Facial Bone, External Approach
0NPWX4Z Removal of Internal Fixation Device from Facial Bone, External Approach
0NPWXMZ Removal of Bone Growth Stimulator from Facial Bone, External Approach

0NQ – Head and Facial Bones, Repair

Review Coding Guideline B3.5

0NQ00ZZ Repair Skull, Open Approach
0NQ03ZZ Repair Skull, Percutaneous Approach
0NQ04ZZ Repair Skull, Percutaneous Endoscopic Approach
0NQ0XZZ Repair Skull, External Approach
0NQ10ZZ Repair Frontal Bone, Open Approach
0NQ13ZZ Repair Frontal Bone, Percutaneous Approach
0NQ14ZZ Repair Frontal Bone, Percutaneous Endoscopic Approach
0NQ1XZZ Repair Frontal Bone, External Approach
0NQ30ZZ Repair Right Parietal Bone, Open Approach
0NQ33ZZ Repair Right Parietal Bone, Percutaneous Approach
0NQ34ZZ Repair Right Parietal Bone, Percutaneous Endoscopic Approach
0NQ3XZZ Repair Right Parietal Bone, External Approach
0NQ40ZZ Repair Left Parietal Bone, Open Approach
0NQ43ZZ Repair Left Parietal Bone, Percutaneous Approach
0NQ44ZZ Repair Left Parietal Bone, Percutaneous Endoscopic Approach
0NQ4XZZ Repair Left Parietal Bone, External Approach
0NQ50ZZ Repair Right Temporal Bone, Open Approach
0NQ53ZZ Repair Right Temporal Bone, Percutaneous Approach
0NQ54ZZ Repair Right Temporal Bone, Percutaneous Endoscopic Approach

0NQ5XZZ Repair Right Temporal Bone, External Approach
0NQ60ZZ Repair Left Temporal Bone, Open Approach
0NQ63ZZ Repair Left Temporal Bone, Percutaneous Approach
0NQ64ZZ Repair Left Temporal Bone, Percutaneous Endoscopic Approach
0NQ6XZZ Repair Left Temporal Bone, External Approach
0NQ70ZZ Repair Occipital Bone, Open Approach
0NQ73ZZ Repair Occipital Bone, Percutaneous Approach
0NQ74ZZ Repair Occipital Bone, Percutaneous Endoscopic Approach
0NQ7XZZ Repair Occipital Bone, External Approach
0NQB0ZZ Repair Nasal Bone, Open Approach
0NQB3ZZ Repair Nasal Bone, Percutaneous Approach
0NQB4ZZ Repair Nasal Bone, Percutaneous Endoscopic Approach
0NQBXZZ Repair Nasal Bone, External Approach
0NQC0ZZ Repair Sphenoid Bone, Open Approach
0NQC3ZZ Repair Sphenoid Bone, Percutaneous Approach
0NQC4ZZ Repair Sphenoid Bone, Percutaneous Endoscopic Approach
0NQCXZZ Repair Sphenoid Bone, External Approach
0NQF0ZZ Repair Right Ethmoid Bone, Open Approach

0NQF3ZZ Repair Right Ethmoid Bone, Percutaneous Approach
0NQF4ZZ Repair Right Ethmoid Bone, Percutaneous Endoscopic Approach
0NQFXZZ Repair Right Ethmoid Bone, External Approach
0NQG0ZZ Repair Left Ethmoid Bone, Open Approach
0NQG3ZZ Repair Left Ethmoid Bone, Percutaneous Approach
0NQG4ZZ Repair Left Ethmoid Bone, Percutaneous Endoscopic Approach
0NQGXZZ Repair Left Ethmoid Bone, External Approach
0NQH0ZZ Repair Right Lacrimal Bone, Open Approach
0NQH3ZZ Repair Right Lacrimal Bone, Percutaneous Approach
0NQH4ZZ Repair Right Lacrimal Bone, Percutaneous Endoscopic Approach
0NQHXZZ Repair Right Lacrimal Bone, External Approach
0NQJ0ZZ Repair Left Lacrimal Bone, Open Approach
0NQJ3ZZ Repair Left Lacrimal Bone, Percutaneous Approach
0NQJ4ZZ Repair Left Lacrimal Bone, Percutaneous Endoscopic Approach
0NQJXZZ Repair Left Lacrimal Bone, External Approach
0NQK0ZZ Repair Right Palatine Bone, Open Approach

0NQK3ZZ Repair Right Palatine Bone, Percutaneous Approach

0NQK4ZZ Repair Right Palatine Bone, Percutaneous Endoscopic Approach

0NQKXZZ Repair Right Palatine Bone, External Approach

0NQL0ZZ Repair Left Palatine Bone, Open Approach

0NQL3ZZ Repair Left Palatine Bone, Percutaneous Approach

0NQL4ZZ Repair Left Palatine Bone, Percutaneous Endoscopic Approach

0NQLXZZ Repair Left Palatine Bone, External Approach

0NQM0ZZ Repair Right Zygomatic Bone, Open Approach

0NQM3ZZ Repair Right Zygomatic Bone, Percutaneous Approach

0NQM4ZZ Repair Right Zygomatic Bone, Percutaneous Endoscopic Approach

0NQMXZZ Repair Right Zygomatic Bone, External Approach

0NQN0ZZ Repair Left Zygomatic Bone, Open Approach

0NQN3ZZ Repair Left Zygomatic Bone, Percutaneous Approach

0NQN4ZZ Repair Left Zygomatic Bone, Percutaneous Endoscopic Approach

0NQNXZZ Repair Left Zygomatic Bone, External Approach

0NQP0ZZ Repair Right Orbit, Open Approach

0NQP3ZZ Repair Right Orbit, Percutaneous Approach

0NQP4ZZ Repair Right Orbit, Percutaneous Endoscopic Approach

0NQPXZZ Repair Right Orbit, External Approach

0NQQ0ZZ Repair Left Orbit, Open Approach

0NQQ3ZZ Repair Left Orbit, Percutaneous Approach

0NQQ4ZZ Repair Left Orbit, Percutaneous Endoscopic Approach

0NQQXZZ Repair Left Orbit, External Approach

0NQR0ZZ Repair Maxilla, Open Approach

0NQR3ZZ Repair Maxilla, Percutaneous Approach

0NQR4ZZ Repair Maxilla, Percutaneous Endoscopic Approach

0NQRXZZ Repair Maxilla, External Approach

0NQT0ZZ Repair Right Mandible, Open Approach

0NQT3ZZ Repair Right Mandible, Percutaneous Approach

0NQT4ZZ Repair Right Mandible, Percutaneous Endoscopic Approach

0NQTXZZ Repair Right Mandible, External Approach

0NQV0ZZ Repair Left Mandible, Open Approach

0NQV3ZZ Repair Left Mandible, Percutaneous Approach

0NQV4ZZ Repair Left Mandible, Percutaneous Endoscopic Approach

0NQVXZZ Repair Left Mandible, External Approach

0NQX0ZZ Repair Hyoid Bone, Open Approach

0NQX3ZZ Repair Hyoid Bone, Percutaneous Approach

0NQX4ZZ Repair Hyoid Bone, Percutaneous Endoscopic Approach

0NQXXZZ Repair Hyoid Bone, External Approach

0NR – Head and Facial Bones, Replacement

Review Coding Guideline B3.18

0NR007Z Replacement of Skull with Autologous Tissue Substitute, Open Approach

0NR00JZ Replacement of Skull with Synthetic Substitute, Open Approach
AHA CC: 3Q, 2014, 7-8

0NR00KZ Replacement of Skull with Nonautologous Tissue Substitute, Open Approach

0NR037Z Replacement of Skull with Autologous Tissue Substitute, Percutaneous Approach

0NR03JZ Replacement of Skull with Synthetic Substitute, Percutaneous Approach

0NR03KZ Replacement of Skull with Nonautologous Tissue Substitute, Percutaneous Approach

0NR047Z Replacement of Skull with Autologous Tissue Substitute, Percutaneous Endoscopic Approach

0NR04JZ Replacement of Skull with Synthetic Substitute, Percutaneous Endoscopic Approach

0NR04KZ Replacement of Skull with Nonautologous Tissue Substitute, Percutaneous Endoscopic Approach

0NR107Z Replacement of Frontal Bone with Autologous Tissue Substitute, Open Approach

0NR10JZ Replacement of Frontal Bone with Synthetic Substitute, Open Approach

0NR10KZ Replacement of Frontal Bone with Nonautologous Tissue Substitute, Open Approach

0NR137Z Replacement of Frontal Bone with Autologous Tissue Substitute, Percutaneous Approach

0NR13JZ Replacement of Frontal Bone with Synthetic Substitute, Percutaneous Approach

0NR13KZ Replacement of Frontal Bone with Nonautologous Tissue Substitute, Percutaneous Approach

0NR147Z Replacement of Frontal Bone with Autologous Tissue Substitute, Percutaneous Endoscopic Approach

0NR14JZ Replacement of Frontal Bone with Synthetic Substitute, Percutaneous Endoscopic Approach

0NR14KZ Replacement of Frontal Bone with Nonautologous Tissue Substitute, Percutaneous Endoscopic Approach

0NR307Z Replacement of Right Parietal Bone with Autologous Tissue Substitute, Open Approach

0NR30JZ Replacement of Right Parietal Bone with Synthetic Substitute, Open Approach

0NR30KZ Replacement of Right Parietal Bone with Nonautologous Tissue Substitute, Open Approach

0NR337Z Replacement of Right Parietal Bone with Autologous Tissue Substitute, Percutaneous Approach

0NR33JZ Replacement of Right Parietal Bone with Synthetic Substitute, Percutaneous Approach

0NR33KZ Replacement of Right Parietal Bone with Nonautologous Tissue Substitute, Percutaneous Approach

0NR347Z Replacement of Right Parietal Bone with Autologous Tissue Substitute, Percutaneous Endoscopic Approach

0NR34JZ Replacement of Right Parietal Bone with Synthetic Substitute, Percutaneous Endoscopic Approach

0NR34KZ Replacement of Right Parietal Bone with Nonautologous Tissue Substitute, Percutaneous Endoscopic Approach

0NR407Z Replacement of Left Parietal Bone with Autologous Tissue Substitute, Open Approach

0NR40JZ Replacement of Left Parietal Bone with Synthetic Substitute, Open Approach

0NR40KZ Replacement of Left Parietal Bone with Nonautologous Tissue Substitute, Open Approach

0NR437Z Replacement of Left Parietal Bone with Autologous Tissue Substitute, Percutaneous Approach

0NR43JZ Replacement of Left Parietal Bone with Synthetic Substitute, Percutaneous Approach

0NR43KZ Replacement of Left Parietal Bone with Nonautologous Tissue Substitute, Percutaneous Approach

0NR447Z Replacement of Left Parietal Bone with Autologous Tissue Substitute, Percutaneous Endoscopic Approach

0NR44JZ Replacement of Left Parietal Bone with Synthetic Substitute, Percutaneous Endoscopic Approach

0NR44KZ Replacement of Left Parietal Bone with Nonautologous Tissue Substitute, Percutaneous Endoscopic Approach

0NR507Z Replacement of Right Temporal Bone with Autologous Tissue Substitute, Open Approach

0NR50JZ Replacement of Right Temporal Bone with Synthetic Substitute, Open Approach

0NR50KZ Replacement of Right Temporal Bone with Nonautologous Tissue Substitute, Open Approach

0NR537Z Replacement of Right Temporal Bone with Autologous Tissue Substitute, Percutaneous Approach

0NR53JZ Replacement of Right Temporal Bone with Synthetic Substitute, Percutaneous Approach

0NR53KZ Replacement of Right Temporal Bone with Nonautologous Tissue Substitute, Percutaneous Approach

0NR547Z Replacement of Right Temporal Bone with Autologous Tissue Substitute, Percutaneous Endoscopic Approach

0NR54JZ Replacement of Right Temporal Bone with Synthetic Substitute, Percutaneous Endoscopic Approach

0NR54KZ Replacement of Right Temporal Bone with Nonautologous Tissue Substitute, Percutaneous Endoscopic Approach

0NR607Z Replacement of Left Temporal Bone with Autologous Tissue Substitute, Open Approach

0NR60JZ Replacement of Left Temporal Bone with Synthetic Substitute, Open Approach

0NR60KZ Replacement of Left Temporal Bone with Nonautologous Tissue Substitute, Open Approach

0NR637Z Replacement of Left Temporal Bone with Autologous Tissue Substitute, Percutaneous Approach

♀ Female-only   ♂ Male-only   ▲ Limited Coverage   ● Non-OR   HAC HAC-associated procedure   ▲ Non-covered procedures   ✚ Cluster

0NR63JZ Replacement of Left Temporal Bone with Synthetic Substitute, Percutaneous Approach

0NR63KZ Replacement of Left Temporal Bone with Nonautologous Tissue Substitute, Percutaneous Approach

0NR647Z Replacement of Left Temporal Bone with Autologous Tissue Substitute, Percutaneous Endoscopic Approach

0NR64JZ Replacement of Left Temporal Bone with Synthetic Substitute, Percutaneous Endoscopic Approach

0NR64KZ Replacement of Left Temporal Bone with Nonautologous Tissue Substitute, Percutaneous Endoscopic Approach

0NR707Z Replacement of Occipital Bone with Autologous Tissue Substitute, Open Approach

0NR70JZ Replacement of Occipital Bone with Synthetic Substitute, Open Approach
AHA CC: 3Q, 2017, 17

0NR70KZ Replacement of Occipital Bone with Nonautologous Tissue Substitute, Open Approach

0NR737Z Replacement of Occipital Bone with Autologous Tissue Substitute, Percutaneous Approach

0NR73JZ Replacement of Occipital Bone with Synthetic Substitute, Percutaneous Approach

0NR73KZ Replacement of Occipital Bone with Nonautologous Tissue Substitute, Percutaneous Approach

0NR747Z Replacement of Occipital Bone with Autologous Tissue Substitute, Percutaneous Endoscopic Approach

0NR74JZ Replacement of Occipital Bone with Synthetic Substitute, Percutaneous Endoscopic Approach

0NR74KZ Replacement of Occipital Bone with Nonautologous Tissue Substitute, Percutaneous Endoscopic Approach

0NRB07Z Replacement of Nasal Bone with Autologous Tissue Substitute, Open Approach

0NRB0JZ Replacement of Nasal Bone with Synthetic Substitute, Open Approach

0NRB0KZ Replacement of Nasal Bone with Nonautologous Tissue Substitute, Open Approach

0NRB37Z Replacement of Nasal Bone with Autologous Tissue Substitute, Percutaneous Approach

0NRB3JZ Replacement of Nasal Bone with Synthetic Substitute, Percutaneous Approach

0NRB3KZ Replacement of Nasal Bone with Nonautologous Tissue Substitute, Percutaneous Approach

0NRB47Z Replacement of Nasal Bone with Autologous Tissue Substitute, Percutaneous Endoscopic Approach

0NRB4JZ Replacement of Nasal Bone with Synthetic Substitute, Percutaneous Endoscopic Approach

0NRB4KZ Replacement of Nasal Bone with Nonautologous Tissue Substitute, Percutaneous Endoscopic Approach

0NRC07Z Replacement of Sphenoid Bone with Autologous Tissue Substitute, Open Approach

0NRC0JZ Replacement of Sphenoid Bone with Synthetic Substitute, Open Approach

0NRC0KZ Replacement of Sphenoid Bone with Nonautologous Tissue Substitute, Open Approach

0NRC37Z Replacement of Sphenoid Bone with Autologous Tissue Substitute, Percutaneous Approach

0NRC3JZ Replacement of Sphenoid Bone with Synthetic Substitute, Percutaneous Approach

0NRC3KZ Replacement of Sphenoid Bone with Nonautologous Tissue Substitute, Percutaneous Approach

0NRC47Z Replacement of Sphenoid Bone with Autologous Tissue Substitute, Percutaneous Endoscopic Approach

0NRC4JZ Replacement of Sphenoid Bone with Synthetic Substitute, Percutaneous Endoscopic Approach

0NRC4KZ Replacement of Sphenoid Bone with Nonautologous Tissue Substitute, Percutaneous Endoscopic Approach

0NRF07Z Replacement of Right Ethmoid Bone with Autologous Tissue Substitute, Open Approach

0NRF0JZ Replacement of Right Ethmoid Bone with Synthetic Substitute, Open Approach

0NRF0KZ Replacement of Right Ethmoid Bone with Nonautologous Tissue Substitute, Open Approach

0NRF37Z Replacement of Right Ethmoid Bone with Autologous Tissue Substitute, Percutaneous Approach

0NRF3JZ Replacement of Right Ethmoid Bone with Synthetic Substitute, Percutaneous Approach

0NRF3KZ Replacement of Right Ethmoid Bone with Nonautologous Tissue Substitute, Percutaneous Approach

0NRF47Z Replacement of Right Ethmoid Bone with Autologous Tissue Substitute, Percutaneous Endoscopic Approach

0NRF4JZ Replacement of Right Ethmoid Bone with Synthetic Substitute, Percutaneous Endoscopic Approach

0NRF4KZ Replacement of Right Ethmoid Bone with Nonautologous Tissue Substitute, Percutaneous Endoscopic Approach

0NRG07Z Replacement of Left Ethmoid Bone with Autologous Tissue Substitute, Open Approach

0NRG0JZ Replacement of Left Ethmoid Bone with Synthetic Substitute, Open Approach

0NRG0KZ Replacement of Left Ethmoid Bone with Nonautologous Tissue Substitute, Open Approach

0NRG37Z Replacement of Left Ethmoid Bone with Autologous Tissue Substitute, Percutaneous Approach

0NRG3JZ Replacement of Left Ethmoid Bone with Synthetic Substitute, Percutaneous Approach

0NRG3KZ Replacement of Left Ethmoid Bone with Nonautologous Tissue Substitute, Percutaneous Approach

0NRG47Z Replacement of Left Ethmoid Bone with Autologous Tissue Substitute, Percutaneous Endoscopic Approach

0NRG4JZ Replacement of Left Ethmoid Bone with Synthetic Substitute, Percutaneous Endoscopic Approach

0NRG4KZ Replacement of Left Ethmoid Bone with Nonautologous Tissue Substitute, Percutaneous Endoscopic Approach

0NRH07Z Replacement of Right Lacrimal Bone with Autologous Tissue Substitute, Open Approach

0NRH0JZ Replacement of Right Lacrimal Bone with Synthetic Substitute, Open Approach

0NRH0KZ Replacement of Right Lacrimal Bone with Nonautologous Tissue Substitute, Open Approach

0NRH37Z Replacement of Right Lacrimal Bone with Autologous Tissue Substitute, Percutaneous Approach

0NRH3JZ Replacement of Right Lacrimal Bone with Synthetic Substitute, Percutaneous Approach

0NRH3KZ Replacement of Right Lacrimal Bone with Nonautologous Tissue Substitute, Percutaneous Approach

0NRH47Z Replacement of Right Lacrimal Bone with Autologous Tissue Substitute, Percutaneous Endoscopic Approach

0NRH4JZ Replacement of Right Lacrimal Bone with Synthetic Substitute, Percutaneous Endoscopic Approach

0NRH4KZ Replacement of Right Lacrimal Bone with Nonautologous Tissue Substitute, Percutaneous Endoscopic Approach

0NRJ07Z Replacement of Left Lacrimal Bone with Autologous Tissue Substitute, Open Approach

0NRJ0JZ Replacement of Left Lacrimal Bone with Synthetic Substitute, Open Approach

0NRJ0KZ Replacement of Left Lacrimal Bone with Nonautologous Tissue Substitute, Open Approach

0NRJ37Z Replacement of Left Lacrimal Bone with Autologous Tissue Substitute, Percutaneous Approach

0NRJ3JZ Replacement of Left Lacrimal Bone with Synthetic Substitute, Percutaneous Approach

0NRJ3KZ Replacement of Left Lacrimal Bone with Nonautologous Tissue Substitute, Percutaneous Approach

0NRJ47Z Replacement of Left Lacrimal Bone with Autologous Tissue Substitute, Percutaneous Endoscopic Approach

0NRJ4JZ Replacement of Left Lacrimal Bone with Synthetic Substitute, Percutaneous Endoscopic Approach

0NRJ4KZ Replacement of Left Lacrimal Bone with Nonautologous Tissue Substitute, Percutaneous Endoscopic Approach

0NRK07Z Replacement of Right Palatine Bone with Autologous Tissue Substitute, Open Approach

0NRK0JZ Replacement of Right Palatine Bone with Synthetic Substitute, Open Approach

0NRK0KZ Replacement of Right Palatine Bone with Nonautologous Tissue Substitute, Open Approach

0NRK37Z Replacement of Right Palatine Bone with Autologous Tissue Substitute, Percutaneous Approach

0NRK3JZ Replacement of Right Palatine Bone with Synthetic Substitute, Percutaneous Approach

0NRK3KZ Replacement of Right Palatine Bone with Nonautologous Tissue Substitute, Percutaneous Approach

0NRK47Z Replacement of Right Palatine Bone with Autologous Tissue Substitute, Percutaneous Endoscopic Approach

0NRK4JZ Replacement of Right Palatine Bone with Synthetic Substitute, Percutaneous Endoscopic Approach

0NRK4KZ Replacement of Right Palatine Bone with Nonautologous Tissue Substitute, Percutaneous Endoscopic Approach

0NRL07Z Replacement of Left Palatine Bone with Autologous Tissue Substitute, Open Approach

0NRL0JZ Replacement of Left Palatine Bone with Synthetic Substitute, Open Approach

0NRL0KZ Replacement of Left Palatine Bone with Nonautologous Tissue Substitute, Open Approach

0NRL37Z Replacement of Left Palatine Bone with Autologous Tissue Substitute, Percutaneous Approach

0NRL3JZ Replacement of Left Palatine Bone with Synthetic Substitute, Percutaneous Approach

0NRL3KZ Replacement of Left Palatine Bone with Nonautologous Tissue Substitute, Percutaneous Approach

0NRL47Z Replacement of Left Palatine Bone with Autologous Tissue Substitute, Percutaneous Endoscopic Approach

0NRL4JZ Replacement of Left Palatine Bone with Synthetic Substitute, Percutaneous Endoscopic Approach

0NRL4KZ Replacement of Left Palatine Bone with Nonautologous Tissue Substitute, Percutaneous Endoscopic Approach

0NRM07Z Replacement of Right Zygomatic Bone with Autologous Tissue Substitute, Open Approach

0NRM0JZ Replacement of Right Zygomatic Bone with Synthetic Substitute, Open Approach

0NRM0KZ Replacement of Right Zygomatic Bone with Nonautologous Tissue Substitute, Open Approach

0NRM37Z Replacement of Right Zygomatic Bone with Autologous Tissue Substitute, Percutaneous Approach

0NRM3JZ Replacement of Right Zygomatic Bone with Synthetic Substitute, Percutaneous Approach

0NRM3KZ Replacement of Right Zygomatic Bone with Nonautologous Tissue Substitute, Percutaneous Approach

0NRM47Z Replacement of Right Zygomatic Bone with Autologous Tissue Substitute, Percutaneous Endoscopic Approach

0NRM4JZ Replacement of Right Zygomatic Bone with Synthetic Substitute, Percutaneous Endoscopic Approach

0NRM4KZ Replacement of Right Zygomatic Bone with Nonautologous Tissue Substitute, Percutaneous Endoscopic Approach

0NRN07Z Replacement of Left Zygomatic Bone with Autologous Tissue Substitute, Open Approach

0NRN0JZ Replacement of Left Zygomatic Bone with Synthetic Substitute, Open Approach

0NRN0KZ Replacement of Left Zygomatic Bone with Nonautologous Tissue Substitute, Open Approach

0NRN37Z Replacement of Left Zygomatic Bone with Autologous Tissue Substitute, Percutaneous Approach

0NRN3JZ Replacement of Left Zygomatic Bone with Synthetic Substitute, Percutaneous Approach

0NRN3KZ Replacement of Left Zygomatic Bone with Nonautologous Tissue Substitute, Percutaneous Approach

0NRN47Z Replacement of Left Zygomatic Bone with Autologous Tissue Substitute, Percutaneous Endoscopic Approach

0NRN4JZ Replacement of Left Zygomatic Bone with Synthetic Substitute, Percutaneous Endoscopic Approach

0NRN4KZ Replacement of Left Zygomatic Bone with Nonautologous Tissue Substitute, Percutaneous Endoscopic Approach

0NRP07Z Replacement of Right Orbit with Autologous Tissue Substitute, Open Approach

0NRP0JZ Replacement of Right Orbit with Synthetic Substitute, Open Approach

0NRP0KZ Replacement of Right Orbit with Nonautologous Tissue Substitute, Open Approach

0NRP37Z Replacement of Right Orbit with Autologous Tissue Substitute, Percutaneous Approach

0NRP3JZ Replacement of Right Orbit with Synthetic Substitute, Percutaneous Approach

0NRP3KZ Replacement of Right Orbit with Nonautologous Tissue Substitute, Percutaneous Approach

0NRP47Z Replacement of Right Orbit with Autologous Tissue Substitute, Percutaneous Endoscopic Approach

0NRP4JZ Replacement of Right Orbit with Synthetic Substitute, Percutaneous Endoscopic Approach

0NRP4KZ Replacement of Right Orbit with Nonautologous Tissue Substitute, Percutaneous Endoscopic Approach

0NRQ07Z Replacement of Left Orbit with Autologous Tissue Substitute, Open Approach

0NRQ0JZ Replacement of Left Orbit with Synthetic Substitute, Open Approach

0NRQ0KZ Replacement of Left Orbit with Nonautologous Tissue Substitute, Open Approach

0NRQ37Z Replacement of Left Orbit with Autologous Tissue Substitute, Percutaneous Approach

0NRQ3JZ Replacement of Left Orbit with Synthetic Substitute, Percutaneous Approach

0NRQ3KZ Replacement of Left Orbit with Nonautologous Tissue Substitute, Percutaneous Approach

0NRQ47Z Replacement of Left Orbit with Autologous Tissue Substitute, Percutaneous Endoscopic Approach

0NRQ4JZ Replacement of Left Orbit with Synthetic Substitute, Percutaneous Endoscopic Approach

0NRQ4KZ Replacement of Left Orbit with Nonautologous Tissue Substitute, Percutaneous Endoscopic Approach

0NRR07Z Replacement of Maxilla with Autologous Tissue Substitute, Open Approach

0NRR0JZ Replacement of Maxilla with Synthetic Substitute, Open Approach
AHA CC: 1Q, 2021, 21-22

0NRR0KZ Replacement of Maxilla with Nonautologous Tissue Substitute, Open Approach

0NRR37Z Replacement of Maxilla with Autologous Tissue Substitute, Percutaneous Approach

0NRR3JZ Replacement of Maxilla with Synthetic Substitute, Percutaneous Approach

0NRR3KZ Replacement of Maxilla with Nonautologous Tissue Substitute, Percutaneous Approach

0NRR47Z Replacement of Maxilla with Autologous Tissue Substitute, Percutaneous Endoscopic Approach

0NRR4JZ Replacement of Right Maxilla with Synthetic Substitute, Percutaneous Endoscopic Approach

0NRR4KZ Replacement of Maxilla with Nonautologous Tissue Substitute, Percutaneous Endoscopic Approach

0NRT07Z Replacement of Right Mandible with Autologous Tissue Substitute, Open Approach

0NRT0JZ Replacement of Right Mandible with Synthetic Substitute, Open Approach

0NRT0KZ Replacement of Right Mandible with Nonautologous Tissue Substitute, Open Approach

0NRT37Z Replacement of Right Mandible with Autologous Tissue Substitute, Percutaneous Approach

0NRT3JZ Replacement of Right Mandible with Synthetic Substitute, Percutaneous Approach

0NRT3KZ Replacement of Right Mandible with Nonautologous Tissue Substitute, Percutaneous Approach

0NRT47Z Replacement of Right Mandible with Autologous Tissue Substitute, Percutaneous Endoscopic Approach

0NRT4JZ Replacement of Right Mandible with Synthetic Substitute, Percutaneous Endoscopic Approach

0NRT4KZ Replacement of Right Mandible with Nonautologous Tissue Substitute, Percutaneous Endoscopic Approach

0NRV07Z Replacement of Left Mandible with Autologous Tissue Substitute, Open Approach
AHA CC: 1Q, 2017, 23-24

0NRV0JZ Replacement of Left Mandible with Synthetic Substitute, Open Approach
AHA CC: 1Q, 2017, 23-24

0NRV0KZ Replacement of Left Mandible with Nonautologous Tissue Substitute, Open Approach

0NRV37Z Replacement of Left Mandible with Autologous Tissue Substitute, Percutaneous Approach

0NRV3JZ Replacement of Left Mandible with Synthetic Substitute, Percutaneous Approach

0NRV3KZ Replacement of Left Mandible with Nonautologous Tissue Substitute, Percutaneous Approach

0NRV47Z Replacement of Left Mandible with Autologous Tissue Substitute, Percutaneous Endoscopic Approach

0NRV4JZ Replacement of Left Mandible with Synthetic Substitute, Percutaneous Endoscopic Approach

0NRV4KZ Replacement of Left Mandible with Nonautologous Tissue Substitute, Percutaneous Endoscopic Approach

0NRX07Z Replacement of Hyoid Bone with Autologous Tissue Substitute, Open Approach

0NRX0JZ Replacement of Hyoid Bone with Synthetic Substitute, Open Approach

0NRX0KZ Replacement of Hyoid Bone with Nonautologous Tissue Substitute, Open Approach

0NRX37Z Replacement of Hyoid Bone with Autologous Tissue Substitute, Percutaneous Approach

♀ Female-only   ♂ Male-only   ▲ Limited Coverage   ● Non-OR   HAC HAC-associated procedure   ▲ Non-covered procedures   ✚ Cluster

0NRX3JZ	Replacement of Hyoid Bone with Synthetic Substitute, Percutaneous Approach
0NRX3KZ	Replacement of Hyoid Bone with Nonautologous Tissue Substitute, Percutaneous Approach
0NRX47Z	Replacement of Hyoid Bone with Autologous Tissue Substitute, Percutaneous Endoscopic Approach
0NRX4JZ	Replacement of Hyoid Bone with Synthetic Substitute, Percutaneous Endoscopic Approach
0NRX4KZ	Replacement of Hyoid Bone with Nonautologous Tissue Substitute, Percutaneous Endoscopic Approach

0NS – Head and Facial Bones, Reposition

Review Coding Guideline B3.15

0NS004Z Reposition Skull with Internal Fixation Device, Open Approach
AHA CC: 3Q, 2017, 22

0NS005Z Reposition Skull with External Fixation Device, Open Approach
AHA CC: 3Q, 2013, 24-25

0NS00ZZ Reposition Skull, Open Approach
AHA CC: 3Q, 2015, 17-18; 2Q, 2016, 30

0NS034Z Reposition Skull with Internal Fixation Device, Percutaneous Approach

0NS035Z Reposition Skull with External Fixation Device, Percutaneous Approach

0NS03ZZ Reposition Skull, Percutaneous Approach

0NS044Z Reposition Skull with Internal Fixation Device, Percutaneous Endoscopic Approach

0NS045Z Reposition Skull with External Fixation Device, Percutaneous Endoscopic Approach

0NS04ZZ Reposition Skull, Percutaneous Endoscopic Approach

0NS0XZZ Reposition Skull, External Approach

0NS104Z Reposition Frontal Bone with Internal Fixation Device, Open Approach
AHA CC: 3Q, 2013, 25

0NS10ZZ Reposition Frontal Bone, Open Approach

0NS134Z Reposition Frontal Bone with Internal Fixation Device, Percutaneous Approach

0NS13ZZ Reposition Frontal Bone, Percutaneous Approach

0NS144Z Reposition Frontal Bone with Internal Fixation Device, Percutaneous Endoscopic Approach

0NS14ZZ Reposition Frontal Bone, Percutaneous Endoscopic Approach

0NS1XZZ Reposition Frontal Bone, External Approach

0NS304Z Reposition Right Parietal Bone with Internal Fixation Device, Open Approach

0NS30ZZ Reposition Right Parietal Bone, Open Approach

0NS334Z Reposition Right Parietal Bone with Internal Fixation Device, Percutaneous Approach

0NS33ZZ Reposition Right Parietal Bone, Percutaneous Approach

0NS344Z Reposition Right Parietal Bone with Internal Fixation Device, Percutaneous Endoscopic Approach

0NS34ZZ Reposition Right Parietal Bone, Percutaneous Endoscopic Approach

0NS3XZZ Reposition Right Parietal Bone, External Approach

0NS404Z Reposition Left Parietal Bone with Internal Fixation Device, Open Approach

0NS40ZZ Reposition Left Parietal Bone, Open Approach

0NS434Z Reposition Left Parietal Bone with Internal Fixation Device, Percutaneous Approach

0NS43ZZ Reposition Left Parietal Bone, Percutaneous Approach

0NS444Z Reposition Left Parietal Bone with Internal Fixation Device, Percutaneous Endoscopic Approach

0NS44ZZ Reposition Left Parietal Bone, Percutaneous Endoscopic Approach

0NS4XZZ Reposition Left Parietal Bone, External Approach

0NS504Z Reposition Right Temporal Bone with Internal Fixation Device, Open Approach
AHA CC: 3Q, 2015, 27-28

0NS50ZZ Reposition Right Temporal Bone, Open Approach

0NS534Z Reposition Right Temporal Bone with Internal Fixation Device, Percutaneous Approach

0NS53ZZ Reposition Right Temporal Bone, Percutaneous Approach

0NS544Z Reposition Right Temporal Bone with Internal Fixation Device, Percutaneous Endoscopic Approach

0NS54ZZ Reposition Right Temporal Bone, Percutaneous Endoscopic Approach

0NS5XZZ Reposition Right Temporal Bone, External Approach

0NS604Z Reposition Left Temporal Bone with Internal Fixation Device, Open Approach

0NS60ZZ Reposition Left Temporal Bone, Open Approach

0NS634Z Reposition Left Temporal Bone with Internal Fixation Device, Percutaneous Approach

0NS63ZZ Reposition Left Temporal Bone, Percutaneous Approach

0NS644Z Reposition Left Temporal Bone with Internal Fixation Device, Percutaneous Endoscopic Approach

0NS64ZZ Reposition Left Temporal Bone, Percutaneous Endoscopic Approach

0NS6XZZ Reposition Left Temporal Bone, External Approach

0NS704Z Reposition Occipital Bone with Internal Fixation Device, Open Approach

0NS70ZZ Reposition Occipital Bone, Open Approach

0NS734Z Reposition Occipital Bone with Internal Fixation Device, Percutaneous Approach

0NS73ZZ Reposition Occipital Bone, Percutaneous Approach

0NS744Z Reposition Occipital Bone with Internal Fixation Device, Percutaneous Endoscopic Approach

0NS74ZZ Reposition Occipital Bone, Percutaneous Endoscopic Approach

0NS7XZZ Reposition Occipital Bone, External Approach

0NSB04Z Reposition Nasal Bone with Internal Fixation Device, Open Approach

0NSB0ZZ Reposition Nasal Bone, Open Approach

0NSB34Z Reposition Nasal Bone with Internal Fixation Device, Percutaneous Approach

0NSB3ZZ Reposition Nasal Bone, Percutaneous Approach

0NSB44Z Reposition Nasal Bone with Internal Fixation Device, Percutaneous Endoscopic Approach

0NSB4ZZ Reposition Nasal Bone, Percutaneous Endoscopic Approach

0NSBXZZ Reposition Nasal Bone, External Approach

0NSC04Z Reposition Sphenoid Bone with Internal Fixation Device, Open Approach

0NSC0ZZ Reposition Sphenoid Bone, Open Approach

0NSC34Z Reposition Sphenoid Bone with Internal Fixation Device, Percutaneous Approach

0NSC3ZZ Reposition Sphenoid Bone, Percutaneous Approach

0NSC44Z Reposition Sphenoid Bone with Internal Fixation Device, Percutaneous Endoscopic Approach

0NSC4ZZ Reposition Sphenoid Bone, Percutaneous Endoscopic Approach

0NSCXZZ Reposition Sphenoid Bone, External Approach

0NSF04Z Reposition Right Ethmoid Bone with Internal Fixation Device, Open Approach

0NSF0ZZ Reposition Right Ethmoid Bone, Open Approach

0NSF34Z Reposition Right Ethmoid Bone with Internal Fixation Device, Percutaneous Approach

0NSF3ZZ Reposition Right Ethmoid Bone, Percutaneous Approach

0NSF44Z Reposition Right Ethmoid Bone with Internal Fixation Device, Percutaneous Endoscopic Approach

0NSF4ZZ Reposition Right Ethmoid Bone, Percutaneous Endoscopic Approach

0NSFXZZ Reposition Right Ethmoid Bone, External Approach

0NSG04Z Reposition Left Ethmoid Bone with Internal Fixation Device, Open Approach

0NSG0ZZ Reposition Left Ethmoid Bone, Open Approach

0NSG34Z Reposition Left Ethmoid Bone with Internal Fixation Device, Percutaneous Approach

0NSG3ZZ Reposition Left Ethmoid Bone, Percutaneous Approach

0NSG44Z Reposition Left Ethmoid Bone with Internal Fixation Device, Percutaneous Endoscopic Approach

0NSG4ZZ Reposition Left Ethmoid Bone, Percutaneous Endoscopic Approach

0NSGXZZ Reposition Left Ethmoid Bone, External Approach

0NSH04Z Reposition Right Lacrimal Bone with Internal Fixation Device, Open Approach

0NSH0ZZ Reposition Right Lacrimal Bone, Open Approach

0NSH34Z Reposition Right Lacrimal Bone with Internal Fixation Device, Percutaneous Approach

0NSH3ZZ	Reposition Right Lacrimal Bone, Percutaneous Approach
0NSH44Z	Reposition Right Lacrimal Bone with Internal Fixation Device, Percutaneous Endoscopic Approach
0NSH4ZZ	Reposition Right Lacrimal Bone, Percutaneous Endoscopic Approach
0NSHXZZ	Reposition Right Lacrimal Bone, External Approach
0NSJ04Z	Reposition Left Lacrimal Bone with Internal Fixation Device, Open Approach
0NSJ0ZZ	Reposition Left Lacrimal Bone, Open Approach
0NSJ34Z	Reposition Left Lacrimal Bone with Internal Fixation Device, Percutaneous Approach
0NSJ3ZZ	Reposition Left Lacrimal Bone, Percutaneous Approach
0NSJ44Z	Reposition Left Lacrimal Bone with Internal Fixation Device, Percutaneous Endoscopic Approach
0NSJ4ZZ	Reposition Left Lacrimal Bone, Percutaneous Endoscopic Approach
0NSJXZZ	Reposition Left Lacrimal Bone, External Approach
0NSK04Z	Reposition Right Palatine Bone with Internal Fixation Device, Open Approach
0NSK0ZZ	Reposition Right Palatine Bone, Open Approach
0NSK34Z	Reposition Right Palatine Bone with Internal Fixation Device, Percutaneous Approach
0NSK3ZZ	Reposition Right Palatine Bone, Percutaneous Approach
0NSK44Z	Reposition Right Palatine Bone with Internal Fixation Device, Percutaneous Endoscopic Approach
0NSK4ZZ	Reposition Right Palatine Bone, Percutaneous Endoscopic Approach
0NSKXZZ	Reposition Right Palatine Bone, External Approach
0NSL04Z	Reposition Left Palatine Bone with Internal Fixation Device, Open Approach
0NSL0ZZ	Reposition Left Palatine Bone, Open Approach
0NSL34Z	Reposition Left Palatine Bone with Internal Fixation Device, Percutaneous Approach
0NSL3ZZ	Reposition Left Palatine Bone, Percutaneous Approach
0NSL44Z	Reposition Left Palatine Bone with Internal Fixation Device, Percutaneous Endoscopic Approach
0NSL4ZZ	Reposition Left Palatine Bone, Percutaneous Endoscopic Approach
0NSLXZZ	Reposition Left Palatine Bone, External Approach
0NSM04Z	Reposition Right Zygomatic Bone with Internal Fixation Device, Open Approach
0NSM0ZZ	Reposition Right Zygomatic Bone, Open Approach
0NSM34Z	Reposition Right Zygomatic Bone with Internal Fixation Device, Percutaneous Approach
0NSM3ZZ	Reposition Right Zygomatic Bone, Percutaneous Approach
0NSM44Z	Reposition Right Zygomatic Bone with Internal Fixation Device, Percutaneous Endoscopic Approach
0NSM4ZZ	Reposition Right Zygomatic Bone, Percutaneous Endoscopic Approach
0NSMXZZ	Reposition Right Zygomatic Bone, External Approach
0NSN04Z	Reposition Left Zygomatic Bone with Internal Fixation Device, Open Approach
0NSN0ZZ	Reposition Left Zygomatic Bone, Open Approach
0NSN34Z	Reposition Left Zygomatic Bone with Internal Fixation Device, Percutaneous Approach
0NSN3ZZ	Reposition Left Zygomatic Bone, Percutaneous Approach
0NSN44Z	Reposition Left Zygomatic Bone with Internal Fixation Device, Percutaneous Endoscopic Approach
0NSN4ZZ	Reposition Left Zygomatic Bone, Percutaneous Endoscopic Approach
0NSNXZZ	Reposition Left Zygomatic Bone, External Approach
0NSP04Z	Reposition Right Orbit with Internal Fixation Device, Open Approach
0NSP0ZZ	Reposition Right Orbit, Open Approach
0NSP34Z	Reposition Right Orbit with Internal Fixation Device, Percutaneous Approach
0NSP3ZZ	Reposition Right Orbit, Percutaneous Approach
0NSP44Z	Reposition Right Orbit with Internal Fixation Device, Percutaneous Endoscopic Approach
0NSP4ZZ	Reposition Right Orbit, Percutaneous Endoscopic Approach
0NSPXZZ	Reposition Right Orbit, External Approach
0NSQ04Z	Reposition Left Orbit with Internal Fixation Device, Open Approach
0NSQ0ZZ	Reposition Left Orbit, Open Approach
0NSQ34Z	Reposition Left Orbit with Internal Fixation Device, Percutaneous Approach
0NSQ3ZZ	Reposition Left Orbit, Percutaneous Approach
0NSQ44Z	Reposition Left Orbit with Internal Fixation Device, Percutaneous Endoscopic Approach
0NSQ4ZZ	Reposition Left Orbit, Percutaneous Endoscopic Approach
0NSQXZZ	Reposition Left Orbit, External Approach
0NSR04Z	Reposition Maxilla with Internal Fixation Device, Open Approach *AHA CC: 3Q, 2014, 23-24*
0NSR05Z	Reposition Maxilla with External Fixation Device, Open Approach
0NSR0ZZ	Reposition Maxilla, Open Approach *AHA CC: 1Q, 2017, 20-21*
0NSR34Z	Reposition Maxilla with Internal Fixation Device, Percutaneous Approach
0NSR35Z	Reposition Maxilla with External Fixation Device, Percutaneous Approach
0NSR3ZZ	Reposition Maxilla, Percutaneous Approach
0NSR44Z	Reposition Maxilla with Internal Fixation Device, Percutaneous Endoscopic Approach
0NSR45Z	Reposition Maxilla with External Fixation Device, Percutaneous Endoscopic Approach
0NSR4ZZ	Reposition Maxilla, Percutaneous Endoscopic Approach
0NSRXZZ	Reposition Maxilla, External Approach
0NST04Z	Reposition Right Mandible with Internal Fixation Device, Open Approach
0NST05Z	Reposition Right Mandible with External Fixation Device, Open Approach
0NST0ZZ	Reposition Right Mandible, Open Approach
0NST34Z	Reposition Right Mandible with Internal Fixation Device, Percutaneous Approach
0NST35Z	Reposition Right Mandible with External Fixation Device, Percutaneous Approach
0NST3ZZ	Reposition Right Mandible, Percutaneous Approach
0NST44Z	Reposition Right Mandible with Internal Fixation Device, Percutaneous Endoscopic Approach
0NST45Z	Reposition Right Mandible with External Fixation Device, Percutaneous Endoscopic Approach
0NST4ZZ	Reposition Right Mandible, Percutaneous Endoscopic Approach
0NSTXZZ	Reposition Right Mandible, External Approach
0NSV04Z	Reposition Left Mandible with Internal Fixation Device, Open Approach
0NSV05Z	Reposition Left Mandible with External Fixation Device, Open Approach
0NSV0ZZ	Reposition Left Mandible, Open Approach
0NSV34Z	Reposition Left Mandible with Internal Fixation Device, Percutaneous Approach
0NSV35Z	Reposition Left Mandible with External Fixation Device, Percutaneous Approach
0NSV3ZZ	Reposition Left Mandible, Percutaneous Approach
0NSV44Z	Reposition Left Mandible with Internal Fixation Device, Percutaneous Endoscopic Approach
0NSV45Z	Reposition Left Mandible with External Fixation Device, Percutaneous Endoscopic Approach
0NSV4ZZ	Reposition Left Mandible, Percutaneous Endoscopic Approach
0NSVXZZ	Reposition Left Mandible, External Approach
0NSX04Z	Reposition Hyoid Bone with Internal Fixation Device, Open Approach
0NSX0ZZ	Reposition Hyoid Bone, Open Approach
0NSX34Z	Reposition Hyoid Bone with Internal Fixation Device, Percutaneous Approach
0NSX3ZZ	Reposition Hyoid Bone, Percutaneous Approach
0NSX44Z	Reposition Hyoid Bone with Internal Fixation Device, Percutaneous Endoscopic Approach
0NSX4ZZ	Reposition Hyoid Bone, Percutaneous Endoscopic Approach
0NSXXZZ	Reposition Hyoid Bone, External Approach

♀ Female-only   ♂ Male-only   ▲ Limited Coverage   ● Non-OR   ▇ HAC-associated procedure   ▲ Non-covered procedures   ✛ Cluster

0NT – Head and Facial Bones, Resection

Review Coding Guideline B3.8

Review Coding Guideline B3.18

0NT10ZZ Resection of Frontal Bone, Open Approach
0NT30ZZ Resection of Right Parietal Bone, Open Approach
0NT40ZZ Resection of Left Parietal Bone, Open Approach
0NT50ZZ Resection of Right Temporal Bone, Open Approach
0NT60ZZ Resection of Left Temporal Bone, Open Approach
0NT70ZZ Resection of Occipital Bone, Open Approach
0NTB0ZZ Resection of Nasal Bone, Open Approach

0NTC0ZZ Resection of Sphenoid Bone, Open Approach
0NTF0ZZ Resection of Right Ethmoid Bone, Open Approach
0NTG0ZZ Resection of Left Ethmoid Bone, Open Approach
0NTH0ZZ Resection of Right Lacrimal Bone, Open Approach
0NTJ0ZZ Resection of Left Lacrimal Bone, Open Approach
0NTK0ZZ Resection of Right Palatine Bone, Open Approach
0NTL0ZZ Resection of Left Palatine Bone, Open Approach

0NTM0ZZ Resection of Right Zygomatic Bone, Open Approach
0NTN0ZZ Resection of Left Zygomatic Bone, Open Approach
0NTP0ZZ Resection of Right Orbit, Open Approach
0NTQ0ZZ Resection of Left Orbit, Open Approach
0NTR0ZZ Resection of Maxilla, Open Approach
0NTT0ZZ Resection of Right Mandible, Open Approach
0NTV0ZZ Resection of Left Mandible, Open Approach
0NTX0ZZ Resection of Hyoid Bone, Open Approach

0NU – Head and Facial Bones, Supplement

0NU007Z Supplement Skull with Autologous Tissue Substitute, Open Approach
0NU00JZ Supplement Skull with Synthetic Substitute, Open Approach
AHA CC: 3Q, 2013, 24-25
0NU00KZ Supplement Skull with Nonautologous Tissue Substitute, Open Approach
0NU037Z Supplement Skull with Autologous Tissue Substitute, Percutaneous Approach
0NU03JZ Supplement Skull with Synthetic Substitute, Percutaneous Approach
0NU03KZ Supplement Skull with Nonautologous Tissue Substitute, Percutaneous Approach
0NU047Z Supplement Skull with Autologous Tissue Substitute, Percutaneous Endoscopic Approach
0NU04JZ Supplement Skull with Synthetic Substitute, Percutaneous Endoscopic Approach
0NU04KZ Supplement Skull with Nonautologous Tissue Substitute, Percutaneous Endoscopic Approach
0NU107Z Supplement Frontal Bone with Autologous Tissue Substitute, Open Approach
0NU10JZ Supplement Frontal Bone with Synthetic Substitute, Open Approach
0NU10KZ Supplement Frontal Bone with Nonautologous Tissue Substitute, Open Approach
0NU137Z Supplement Frontal Bone with Autologous Tissue Substitute, Percutaneous Approach
0NU13JZ Supplement Frontal Bone with Synthetic Substitute, Percutaneous Approach
0NU13KZ Supplement Frontal Bone with Nonautologous Tissue Substitute, Percutaneous Approach
0NU147Z Supplement Frontal Bone with Autologous Tissue Substitute, Percutaneous Endoscopic Approach
0NU14JZ Supplement Frontal Bone with Synthetic Substitute, Percutaneous Endoscopic Approach
0NU14KZ Supplement Frontal Bone with Nonautologous Tissue Substitute, Percutaneous Endoscopic Approach
0NU307Z Supplement Right Parietal Bone with Autologous Tissue Substitute, Open Approach

0NU30JZ Supplement Right Parietal Bone with Synthetic Substitute, Open Approach
0NU30KZ Supplement Right Parietal Bone with Nonautologous Tissue Substitute, Open Approach
0NU337Z Supplement Right Parietal Bone with Autologous Tissue Substitute, Percutaneous Approach
0NU33JZ Supplement Right Parietal Bone with Synthetic Substitute, Percutaneous Approach
0NU33KZ Supplement Right Parietal Bone with Nonautologous Tissue Substitute, Percutaneous Approach
0NU347Z Supplement Right Parietal Bone with Autologous Tissue Substitute, Percutaneous Endoscopic Approach
0NU34JZ Supplement Right Parietal Bone with Synthetic Substitute, Percutaneous Endoscopic Approach
0NU34KZ Supplement Right Parietal Bone with Nonautologous Tissue Substitute, Percutaneous Endoscopic Approach
0NU407Z Supplement Left Parietal Bone with Autologous Tissue Substitute, Open Approach
0NU40JZ Supplement Left Parietal Bone with Synthetic Substitute, Open Approach
0NU40KZ Supplement Left Parietal Bone with Nonautologous Tissue Substitute, Open Approach
0NU437Z Supplement Left Parietal Bone with Autologous Tissue Substitute, Percutaneous Approach
0NU43JZ Supplement Left Parietal Bone with Synthetic Substitute, Percutaneous Approach
0NU43KZ Supplement Left Parietal Bone with Nonautologous Tissue Substitute, Percutaneous Approach
0NU447Z Supplement Left Parietal Bone with Autologous Tissue Substitute, Percutaneous Endoscopic Approach
0NU44JZ Supplement Left Parietal Bone with Synthetic Substitute, Percutaneous Endoscopic Approach
0NU44KZ Supplement Left Parietal Bone with Nonautologous Tissue Substitute, Percutaneous Endoscopic Approach
0NU507Z Supplement Right Temporal Bone with Autologous Tissue Substitute, Open Approach

0NU50JZ Supplement Right Temporal Bone with Synthetic Substitute, Open Approach
0NU50KZ Supplement Right Temporal Bone with Nonautologous Tissue Substitute, Open Approach
0NU537Z Supplement Right Temporal Bone with Autologous Tissue Substitute, Percutaneous Approach
0NU53JZ Supplement Right Temporal Bone with Synthetic Substitute, Percutaneous Approach
0NU53KZ Supplement Right Temporal Bone with Nonautologous Tissue Substitute, Percutaneous Approach
0NU547Z Supplement Right Temporal Bone with Autologous Tissue Substitute, Percutaneous Endoscopic Approach
0NU54JZ Supplement Right Temporal Bone with Synthetic Substitute, Percutaneous Endoscopic Approach
0NU54KZ Supplement Right Temporal Bone with Nonautologous Tissue Substitute, Percutaneous Endoscopic Approach
0NU607Z Supplement Left Temporal Bone with Autologous Tissue Substitute, Open Approach
0NU60JZ Supplement Left Temporal Bone with Synthetic Substitute, Open Approach
0NU60KZ Supplement Left Temporal Bone with Nonautologous Tissue Substitute, Open Approach
0NU637Z Supplement Left Temporal Bone with Autologous Tissue Substitute, Percutaneous Approach
0NU63JZ Supplement Left Temporal Bone with Synthetic Substitute, Percutaneous Approach
0NU63KZ Supplement Left Temporal Bone with Nonautologous Tissue Substitute, Percutaneous Approach
0NU647Z Supplement Left Temporal Bone with Autologous Tissue Substitute, Percutaneous Endoscopic Approach
0NU64JZ Supplement Left Temporal Bone with Synthetic Substitute, Percutaneous Endoscopic Approach
0NU64KZ Supplement Left Temporal Bone with Nonautologous Tissue Substitute, Percutaneous Endoscopic Approach
0NU707Z Supplement Occipital Bone with Autologous Tissue Substitute, Open Approach

0NU70JZ Supplement Occipital Bone with Synthetic Substitute, Open Approach

0NU70KZ Supplement Occipital Bone with Nonautologous Tissue Substitute, Open Approach

0NU737Z Supplement Occipital Bone with Autologous Tissue Substitute, Percutaneous Approach

0NU73JZ Supplement Occipital Bone with Synthetic Substitute, Percutaneous Approach

0NU73KZ Supplement Occipital Bone with Nonautologous Tissue Substitute, Percutaneous Approach

0NU747Z Supplement Occipital Bone with Autologous Tissue Substitute, Percutaneous Endoscopic Approach

0NU74JZ Supplement Occipital Bone with Synthetic Substitute, Percutaneous Endoscopic Approach

0NU74KZ Supplement Occipital Bone with Nonautologous Tissue Substitute, Percutaneous Endoscopic Approach

0NUB07Z Supplement Nasal Bone with Autologous Tissue Substitute, Open Approach

0NUB0JZ Supplement Nasal Bone with Synthetic Substitute, Open Approach

0NUB0KZ Supplement Nasal Bone with Nonautologous Tissue Substitute, Open Approach

0NUB37Z Supplement Nasal Bone with Autologous Tissue Substitute, Percutaneous Approach

0NUB3JZ Supplement Nasal Bone with Synthetic Substitute, Percutaneous Approach

0NUB3KZ Supplement Nasal Bone with Nonautologous Tissue Substitute, Percutaneous Approach

0NUB47Z Supplement Nasal Bone with Autologous Tissue Substitute, Percutaneous Endoscopic Approach

0NUB4JZ Supplement Nasal Bone with Synthetic Substitute, Percutaneous Endoscopic Approach

0NUB4KZ Supplement Nasal Bone with Nonautologous Tissue Substitute, Percutaneous Endoscopic Approach

0NUC07Z Supplement Sphenoid Bone with Autologous Tissue Substitute, Open Approach

0NUC0JZ Supplement Sphenoid Bone with Synthetic Substitute, Open Approach

0NUC0KZ Supplement Sphenoid Bone with Nonautologous Tissue Substitute, Open Approach

0NUC37Z Supplement Sphenoid Bone with Autologous Tissue Substitute, Percutaneous Approach

0NUC3JZ Supplement Sphenoid Bone with Synthetic Substitute, Percutaneous Approach

0NUC3KZ Supplement Sphenoid Bone with Nonautologous Tissue Substitute, Percutaneous Approach

0NUC47Z Supplement Sphenoid Bone with Autologous Tissue Substitute, Percutaneous Endoscopic Approach

0NUC4JZ Supplement Sphenoid Bone with Synthetic Substitute, Percutaneous Endoscopic Approach

0NUC4KZ Supplement Sphenoid Bone with Nonautologous Tissue Substitute, Percutaneous Endoscopic Approach

0NUF07Z Supplement Right Ethmoid Bone with Autologous Tissue Substitute, Open Approach

0NUF0JZ Supplement Right Ethmoid Bone with Synthetic Substitute, Open Approach

0NUF0KZ Supplement Right Ethmoid Bone with Nonautologous Tissue Substitute, Open Approach

0NUF37Z Supplement Right Ethmoid Bone with Autologous Tissue Substitute, Percutaneous Approach

0NUF3JZ Supplement Right Ethmoid Bone with Synthetic Substitute, Percutaneous Approach

0NUF3KZ Supplement Right Ethmoid Bone with Nonautologous Tissue Substitute, Percutaneous Approach

0NUF47Z Supplement Right Ethmoid Bone with Autologous Tissue Substitute, Percutaneous Endoscopic Approach

0NUF4JZ Supplement Right Ethmoid Bone with Synthetic Substitute, Percutaneous Endoscopic Approach

0NUF4KZ Supplement Right Ethmoid Bone with Nonautologous Tissue Substitute, Percutaneous Endoscopic Approach

0NUG07Z Supplement Left Ethmoid Bone with Autologous Tissue Substitute, Open Approach

0NUG0JZ Supplement Left Ethmoid Bone with Synthetic Substitute, Open Approach

0NUG0KZ Supplement Left Ethmoid Bone with Nonautologous Tissue Substitute, Open Approach

0NUG37Z Supplement Left Ethmoid Bone with Autologous Tissue Substitute, Percutaneous Approach

0NUG3JZ Supplement Left Ethmoid Bone with Synthetic Substitute, Percutaneous Approach

0NUG3KZ Supplement Left Ethmoid Bone with Nonautologous Tissue Substitute, Percutaneous Approach

0NUG47Z Supplement Left Ethmoid Bone with Autologous Tissue Substitute, Percutaneous Endoscopic Approach

0NUG4JZ Supplement Left Ethmoid Bone with Synthetic Substitute, Percutaneous Endoscopic Approach

0NUG4KZ Supplement Left Ethmoid Bone with Nonautologous Tissue Substitute, Percutaneous Endoscopic Approach

0NUH07Z Supplement Right Lacrimal Bone with Autologous Tissue Substitute, Open Approach

0NUH0JZ Supplement Right Lacrimal Bone with Synthetic Substitute, Open Approach

0NUH0KZ Supplement Right Lacrimal Bone with Nonautologous Tissue Substitute, Open Approach

0NUH37Z Supplement Right Lacrimal Bone with Autologous Tissue Substitute, Percutaneous Approach

0NUH3JZ Supplement Right Lacrimal Bone with Synthetic Substitute, Percutaneous Approach

0NUH3KZ Supplement Right Lacrimal Bone with Nonautologous Tissue Substitute, Percutaneous Approach

0NUH47Z Supplement Right Lacrimal Bone with Autologous Tissue Substitute, Percutaneous Endoscopic Approach

0NUH4JZ Supplement Right Lacrimal Bone with Synthetic Substitute, Percutaneous Endoscopic Approach

0NUH4KZ Supplement Right Lacrimal Bone with Nonautologous Tissue Substitute, Percutaneous Endoscopic Approach

0NUJ07Z Supplement Left Lacrimal Bone with Autologous Tissue Substitute, Open Approach

0NUJ0JZ Supplement Left Lacrimal Bone with Synthetic Substitute, Open Approach

0NUJ0KZ Supplement Left Lacrimal Bone with Nonautologous Tissue Substitute, Open Approach

0NUJ37Z Supplement Left Lacrimal Bone with Autologous Tissue Substitute, Percutaneous Approach

0NUJ3JZ Supplement Left Lacrimal Bone with Synthetic Substitute, Percutaneous Approach

0NUJ3KZ Supplement Left Lacrimal Bone with Nonautologous Tissue Substitute, Percutaneous Approach

0NUJ47Z Supplement Left Lacrimal Bone with Autologous Tissue Substitute, Percutaneous Endoscopic Approach

0NUJ4JZ Supplement Left Lacrimal Bone with Synthetic Substitute, Percutaneous Endoscopic Approach

0NUJ4KZ Supplement Left Lacrimal Bone with Nonautologous Tissue Substitute, Percutaneous Endoscopic Approach

0NUK07Z Supplement Right Palatine Bone with Autologous Tissue Substitute, Open Approach

0NUK0JZ Supplement Right Palatine Bone with Synthetic Substitute, Open Approach

0NUK0KZ Supplement Right Palatine Bone with Nonautologous Tissue Substitute, Open Approach

0NUK37Z Supplement Right Palatine Bone with Autologous Tissue Substitute, Percutaneous Approach

0NUK3JZ Supplement Right Palatine Bone with Synthetic Substitute, Percutaneous Approach

0NUK3KZ Supplement Right Palatine Bone with Nonautologous Tissue Substitute, Percutaneous Approach

0NUK47Z Supplement Right Palatine Bone with Autologous Tissue Substitute, Percutaneous Endoscopic Approach

0NUK4JZ Supplement Right Palatine Bone with Synthetic Substitute, Percutaneous Endoscopic Approach

0NUK4KZ Supplement Right Palatine Bone with Nonautologous Tissue Substitute, Percutaneous Endoscopic Approach

0NUL07Z Supplement Left Palatine Bone with Autologous Tissue Substitute, Open Approach

0NUL0JZ Supplement Left Palatine Bone with Synthetic Substitute, Open Approach

0NUL0KZ Supplement Left Palatine Bone with Nonautologous Tissue Substitute, Open Approach

0NUL37Z Supplement Left Palatine Bone with Autologous Tissue Substitute, Percutaneous Approach

0NUL3JZ Supplement Left Palatine Bone with Synthetic Substitute, Percutaneous Approach

0NUL3KZ Supplement Left Palatine Bone with Nonautologous Tissue Substitute, Percutaneous Approach

0NUL47Z Supplement Left Palatine Bone with Autologous Tissue Substitute, Percutaneous Endoscopic Approach

0NUL4JZ Supplement Left Palatine Bone with Synthetic Substitute, Percutaneous Endoscopic Approach

0NUL4KZ   Supplement Left Palatine Bone with Nonautologous Tissue Substitute, Percutaneous Endoscopic Approach

0NUM07Z   Supplement Right Zygomatic Bone with Autologous Tissue Substitute, Open Approach

0NUM0JZ   Supplement Right Zygomatic Bone with Synthetic Substitute, Open Approach

0NUM0KZ   Supplement Right Zygomatic Bone with Nonautologous Tissue Substitute, Open Approach

0NUM37Z   Supplement Right Zygomatic Bone with Autologous Tissue Substitute, Percutaneous Approach

0NUM3JZ   Supplement Right Zygomatic Bone with Synthetic Substitute, Percutaneous Approach

0NUM3KZ   Supplement Right Zygomatic Bone with Nonautologous Tissue Substitute, Percutaneous Approach

0NUM47Z   Supplement Right Zygomatic Bone with Autologous Tissue Substitute, Percutaneous Endoscopic Approach

0NUM4JZ   Supplement Right Zygomatic Bone with Synthetic Substitute, Percutaneous Endoscopic Approach

0NUM4KZ   Supplement Right Zygomatic Bone with Nonautologous Tissue Substitute, Percutaneous Endoscopic Approach

0NUN07Z   Supplement Left Zygomatic Bone with Autologous Tissue Substitute, Open Approach

0NUN0JZ   Supplement Left Zygomatic Bone with Synthetic Substitute, Open Approach

0NUN0KZ   Supplement Left Zygomatic Bone with Nonautologous Tissue Substitute, Open Approach

0NUN37Z   Supplement Left Zygomatic Bone with Autologous Tissue Substitute, Percutaneous Approach

0NUN3JZ   Supplement Left Zygomatic Bone with Synthetic Substitute, Percutaneous Approach

0NUN3KZ   Supplement Left Zygomatic Bone with Nonautologous Tissue Substitute, Percutaneous Approach

0NUN47Z   Supplement Left Zygomatic Bone with Autologous Tissue Substitute, Percutaneous Endoscopic Approach

0NUN4JZ   Supplement Left Zygomatic Bone with Synthetic Substitute, Percutaneous Endoscopic Approach

0NUN4KZ   Supplement Left Zygomatic Bone with Nonautologous Tissue Substitute, Percutaneous Endoscopic Approach

0NUP07Z   Supplement Right Orbit with Autologous Tissue Substitute, Open Approach

0NUP0JZ   Supplement Right Orbit with Synthetic Substitute, Open Approach

0NUP0KZ   Supplement Right Orbit with Nonautologous Tissue Substitute, Open Approach

0NUP37Z   Supplement Right Orbit with Autologous Tissue Substitute, Percutaneous Approach

0NUP3JZ   Supplement Right Orbit with Synthetic Substitute, Percutaneous Approach

0NUP3KZ   Supplement Right Orbit with Nonautologous Tissue Substitute, Percutaneous Approach

0NUP47Z   Supplement Right Orbit with Autologous Tissue Substitute, Percutaneous Endoscopic Approach

0NUP4JZ   Supplement Right Orbit with Synthetic Substitute, Percutaneous Endoscopic Approach

0NUP4KZ   Supplement Right Orbit with Nonautologous Tissue Substitute, Percutaneous Endoscopic Approach

0NUQ07Z   Supplement Left Orbit with Autologous Tissue Substitute, Open Approach

0NUQ0JZ   Supplement Left Orbit with Synthetic Substitute, Open Approach

0NUQ0KZ   Supplement Left Orbit with Nonautologous Tissue Substitute, Open Approach

0NUQ37Z   Supplement Left Orbit with Autologous Tissue Substitute, Percutaneous Approach

0NUQ3JZ   Supplement Left Orbit with Synthetic Substitute, Percutaneous Approach

0NUQ3KZ   Supplement Left Orbit with Nonautologous Tissue Substitute, Percutaneous Approach

0NUQ47Z   Supplement Left Orbit with Autologous Tissue Substitute, Percutaneous Endoscopic Approach

0NUQ4JZ   Supplement Left Orbit with Synthetic Substitute, Percutaneous Endoscopic Approach

0NUQ4KZ   Supplement Left Orbit with Nonautologous Tissue Substitute, Percutaneous Endoscopic Approach

0NUR07Z   Supplement Maxilla with Autologous Tissue Substitute, Open Approach

AHA CC: 3Q, 2016, 29-30

0NUR0JZ   Supplement Maxilla with Synthetic Substitute, Open Approach

0NUR0KZ   Supplement Maxilla with Nonautologous Tissue Substitute, Open Approach

0NUR37Z   Supplement Maxilla with Autologous Tissue Substitute, Percutaneous Approach

0NUR3JZ   Supplement Maxilla with Synthetic Substitute, Percutaneous Approach

0NUR3KZ   Supplement Maxilla with Nonautologous Tissue Substitute, Percutaneous Approach

0NUR47Z   Supplement Maxilla with Autologous Tissue Substitute, Percutaneous Endoscopic Approach

0NUR4JZ   Supplement Maxilla with Synthetic Substitute, Percutaneous Endoscopic Approach

0NUR4KZ   Supplement Maxilla with Nonautologous Tissue Substitute, Percutaneous Endoscopic Approach

0NUT07Z   Supplement Right Mandible with Autologous Tissue Substitute, Open Approach

0NUT0JZ   Supplement Right Mandible with Synthetic Substitute, Open Approach

0NUT0KZ   Supplement Right Mandible with Nonautologous Tissue Substitute, Open Approach

0NUT37Z   Supplement Right Mandible with Autologous Tissue Substitute, Percutaneous Approach

0NUT3JZ   Supplement Right Mandible with Synthetic Substitute, Percutaneous Approach

0NUT3KZ   Supplement Right Mandible with Nonautologous Tissue Substitute, Percutaneous Approach

0NUT47Z   Supplement Right Mandible with Autologous Tissue Substitute, Percutaneous Endoscopic Approach

0NUT4JZ   Supplement Right Mandible with Synthetic Substitute, Percutaneous Endoscopic Approach

0NUT4KZ   Supplement Right Mandible with Nonautologous Tissue Substitute, Percutaneous Endoscopic Approach

0NUV07Z   Supplement Left Mandible with Autologous Tissue Substitute, Open Approach

0NUV0JZ   Supplement Left Mandible with Synthetic Substitute, Open Approach

0NUV0KZ   Supplement Left Mandible with Nonautologous Tissue Substitute, Open Approach

0NUV37Z   Supplement Left Mandible with Autologous Tissue Substitute, Percutaneous Approach

0NUV3JZ   Supplement Left Mandible with Synthetic Substitute, Percutaneous Approach

0NUV3KZ   Supplement Left Mandible with Nonautologous Tissue Substitute, Percutaneous Approach

0NUV47Z   Supplement Left Mandible with Autologous Tissue Substitute, Percutaneous Endoscopic Approach

0NUV4JZ   Supplement Left Mandible with Synthetic Substitute, Percutaneous Endoscopic Approach

0NUV4KZ   Supplement Left Mandible with Nonautologous Tissue Substitute, Percutaneous Endoscopic Approach

0NUX07Z   Supplement Hyoid Bone with Autologous Tissue Substitute, Open Approach

0NUX0JZ   Supplement Hyoid Bone with Synthetic Substitute, Open Approach

0NUX0KZ   Supplement Hyoid Bone with Nonautologous Tissue Substitute, Open Approach

0NUX37Z   Supplement Hyoid Bone with Autologous Tissue Substitute, Percutaneous Approach

0NUX3JZ   Supplement Hyoid Bone with Synthetic Substitute, Percutaneous Approach

0NUX3KZ   Supplement Hyoid Bone with Nonautologous Tissue Substitute, Percutaneous Approach

0NUX47Z   Supplement Hyoid Bone with Autologous Tissue Substitute, Percutaneous Endoscopic Approach

0NUX4JZ   Supplement Hyoid Bone with Synthetic Substitute, Percutaneous Endoscopic Approach

0NUX4KZ   Supplement Hyoid Bone with Nonautologous Tissue Substitute, Percutaneous Endoscopic Approach

0NW – Head and Facial Bones, Revision

Review Coding Guideline B6.1c

0NW000Z   Revision of Drainage Device in Skull, Open Approach

0NW004Z   Revision of Internal Fixation Device in Skull, Open Approach

0NW005Z   Revision of External Fixation Device in Skull, Open Approach

0NW007Z   Revision of Autologous Tissue Substitute in Skull, Open Approach

0NW00JZ   Revision of Synthetic Substitute in Skull, Open Approach

0NW00KZ   Revision of Nonautologous Tissue Substitute in Skull, Open Approach

0NW00MZ	Revision of Bone Growth Stimulator in Skull, Open Approach	**0NWB00Z**	Revision of Drainage Device in Nasal Bone, Open Approach	**0NWW00Z**	Revision of Drainage Device in Facial Bone, Open Approach
0NW00NZ	Revision of Neurostimulator Generator in Skull, Open Approach	**0NWB04Z**	Revision of Internal Fixation Device in Nasal Bone, Open Approach	**0NWW04Z**	Revision of Internal Fixation Device in Facial Bone, Open Approach
0NW00SZ	Revision of Hearing Device in Skull, Open Approach	**0NWB07Z**	Revision of Autologous Tissue Substitute in Nasal Bone, Open Approach	**0NWW07Z**	Revision of Autologous Tissue Substitute in Facial Bone, Open Approach
0NW030Z	Revision of Drainage Device in Skull, Percutaneous Approach	**0NWB0JZ**	Revision of Synthetic Substitute in Nasal Bone, Open Approach	**0NWW0JZ**	Revision of Synthetic Substitute in Facial Bone, Open Approach
0NW034Z	Revision of Internal Fixation Device in Skull, Percutaneous Approach	**0NWB0KZ**	Revision of Nonautologous Tissue Substitute in Nasal Bone, Open Approach	**0NWW0KZ**	Revision of Nonautologous Tissue Substitute in Facial Bone, Open Approach
0NW035Z	Revision of External Fixation Device in Skull, Percutaneous Approach	**0NWB0MZ**	Revision of Bone Growth Stimulator in Nasal Bone, Open Approach	**0NWW0MZ**	Revision of Bone Growth Stimulator in Facial Bone, Open Approach
0NW037Z	Revision of Autologous Tissue Substitute in Skull, Percutaneous Approach	**0NWB30Z**	Revision of Drainage Device in Nasal Bone, Percutaneous Approach	**0NWW30Z**	Revision of Drainage Device in Facial Bone, Percutaneous Approach
0NW03JZ	Revision of Synthetic Substitute in Skull, Percutaneous Approach	**0NWB34Z**	Revision of Internal Fixation Device in Nasal Bone, Percutaneous Approach	**0NWW34Z**	Revision of Internal Fixation Device in Facial Bone, Percutaneous Approach
0NW03KZ	Revision of Nonautologous Tissue Substitute in Skull, Percutaneous Approach	**0NWB37Z**	Revision of Autologous Tissue Substitute in Nasal Bone, Percutaneous Approach	**0NWW37Z**	Revision of Autologous Tissue Substitute in Facial Bone, Percutaneous Approach
0NW03MZ	Revision of Bone Growth Stimulator in Skull, Percutaneous Approach	**0NWB3JZ**	Revision of Synthetic Substitute in Nasal Bone, Percutaneous Approach	**0NWW3JZ**	Revision of Synthetic Substitute in Facial Bone, Percutaneous Approach
0NW03SZ	Revision of Hearing Device in Skull, Percutaneous Approach	**0NWB3KZ**	Revision of Nonautologous Tissue Substitute in Nasal Bone, Percutaneous Approach	**0NWW3KZ**	Revision of Nonautologous Tissue Substitute in Facial Bone, Percutaneous Approach
0NW040Z	Revision of Drainage Device in Skull, Percutaneous Endoscopic Approach	**0NWB3MZ**	Revision of Bone Growth Stimulator in Nasal Bone, Percutaneous Approach	**0NWW3MZ**	Revision of Bone Growth Stimulator in Facial Bone, Percutaneous Approach
0NW044Z	Revision of Internal Fixation Device in Skull, Percutaneous Endoscopic Approach	**0NWB40Z**	Revision of Drainage Device in Nasal Bone, Percutaneous Endoscopic Approach	**0NWW40Z**	Revision of Drainage Device in Facial Bone, Percutaneous Endoscopic Approach
0NW045Z	Revision of External Fixation Device in Skull, Percutaneous Endoscopic Approach	**0NWB44Z**	Revision of Internal Fixation Device in Nasal Bone, Percutaneous Endoscopic Approach	**0NWW44Z**	Revision of Internal Fixation Device in Facial Bone, Percutaneous Endoscopic Approach
0NW047Z	Revision of Autologous Tissue Substitute in Skull, Percutaneous Endoscopic Approach	**0NWB47Z**	Revision of Autologous Tissue Substitute in Nasal Bone, Percutaneous Endoscopic Approach	**0NWW47Z**	Revision of Autologous Tissue Substitute in Facial Bone, Percutaneous Endoscopic Approach
0NW04JZ	Revision of Synthetic Substitute in Skull, Percutaneous Endoscopic Approach	**0NWB4JZ**	Revision of Synthetic Substitute in Nasal Bone, Percutaneous Endoscopic Approach	**0NWW4JZ**	Revision of Synthetic Substitute in Facial Bone, Percutaneous Endoscopic Approach
0NW04KZ	Revision of Nonautologous Tissue Substitute in Skull, Percutaneous Endoscopic Approach	**0NWB4KZ**	Revision of Nonautologous Tissue Substitute in Nasal Bone, Percutaneous Endoscopic Approach	**0NWW4KZ**	Revision of Nonautologous Tissue Substitute in Facial Bone, Percutaneous Endoscopic Approach
0NW04MZ	Revision of Bone Growth Stimulator in Skull, Percutaneous Endoscopic Approach	**0NWB4MZ**	Revision of Bone Growth Stimulator in Nasal Bone, Percutaneous Endoscopic Approach	**0NWW4MZ**	Revision of Bone Growth Stimulator in Facial Bone, Percutaneous Endoscopic Approach
0NW04SZ	Revision of Hearing Device in Skull, Percutaneous Endoscopic Approach	**0NWBX0Z**	Revision of Drainage Device in Nasal Bone, External Approach	**0NWWX0Z**	Revision of Drainage Device in Facial Bone, External Approach
0NW0X0Z	Revision of Drainage Device in Skull, External Approach	**0NWBX4Z**	Revision of Internal Fixation Device in Nasal Bone, External Approach	**0NWWX4Z**	Revision of Internal Fixation Device in Facial Bone, External Approach
0NW0X4Z	Revision of Internal Fixation Device in Skull, External Approach	**0NWBX7Z**	Revision of Autologous Tissue Substitute in Nasal Bone, External Approach	**0NWWX7Z**	Revision of Autologous Tissue Substitute in Facial Bone, External Approach
0NW0X5Z	Revision of External Fixation Device in Skull, External Approach	**0NWBXJZ**	Revision of Synthetic Substitute in Nasal Bone, External Approach	**0NWWXJZ**	Revision of Synthetic Substitute in Facial Bone, External Approach
0NW0X7Z	Revision of Autologous Tissue Substitute in Skull, External Approach	**0NWBXKZ**	Revision of Nonautologous Tissue Substitute in Nasal Bone, External Approach	**0NWWXKZ**	Revision of Nonautologous Tissue Substitute in Facial Bone, External Approach
0NW0XJZ	Revision of Synthetic Substitute in Skull, External Approach	**0NWBXMZ**	Revision of Bone Growth Stimulator in Nasal Bone, External Approach	**0NWWXMZ**	Revision of Bone Growth Stimulator in Facial Bone, External Approach
0NW0XKZ	Revision of Nonautologous Tissue Substitute in Skull, External Approach				
0NW0XMZ	Revision of Bone Growth Stimulator in Skull, External Approach				
0NW0XSZ	Revision of Hearing Device in Skull, External Approach				

Bones - Front and Back Views

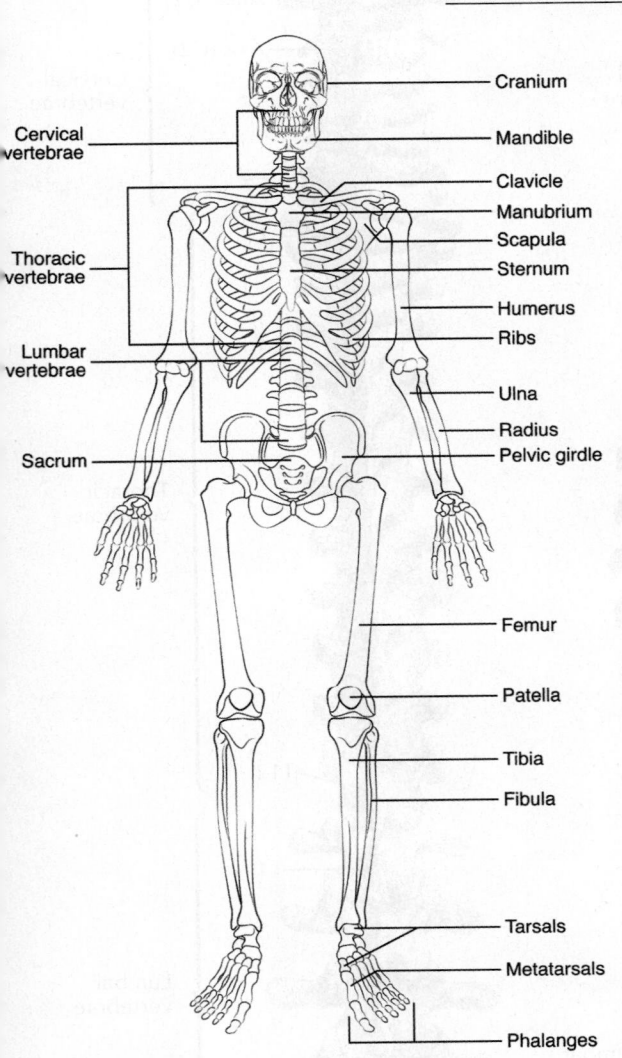

Cranium
Mandible
Clavicle
Manubrium
Scapula
Sternum
Humerus
Ribs
Ulna
Radius
Pelvic girdle

Cervical vertebrae
Thoracic vertebrae
Lumbar vertebrae
Sacrum

Femur
Patella
Tibia
Fibula

Tarsals
Metatarsals
Phalanges

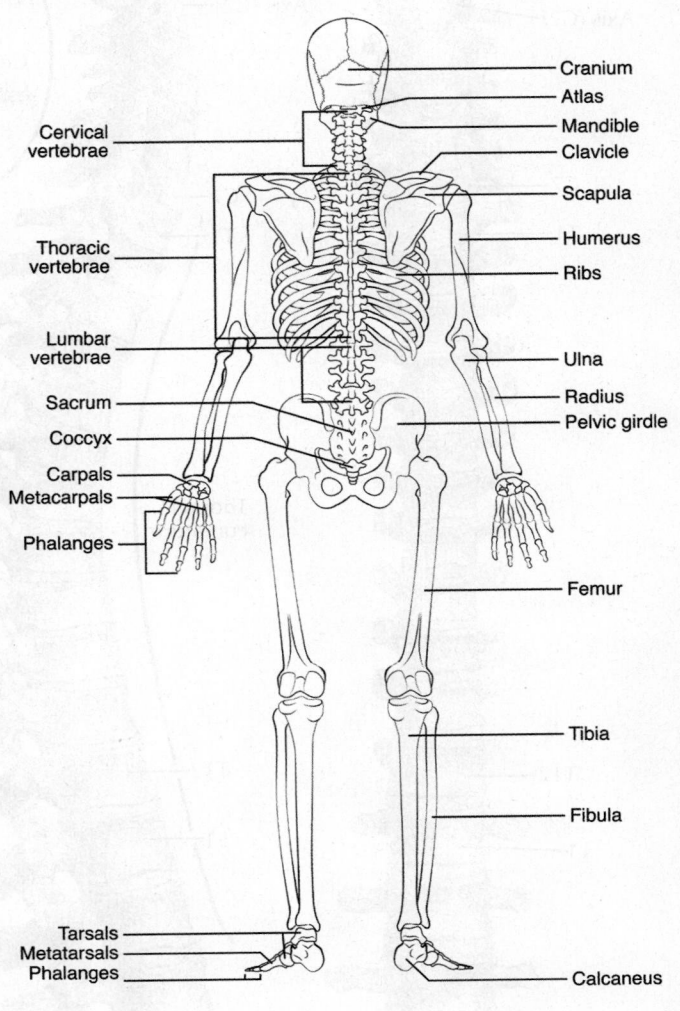

Cervical vertebrae
Thoracic vertebrae
Lumbar vertebrae
Sacrum
Coccyx
Carpals
Metacarpals
Phalanges

Cranium
Atlas
Mandible
Clavicle
Scapula
Humerus
Ribs
Ulna
Radius
Pelvic girdle

Femur

Tibia

Fibula

Tarsals
Metatarsals
Phalanges
Calcaneus

©AHIMA

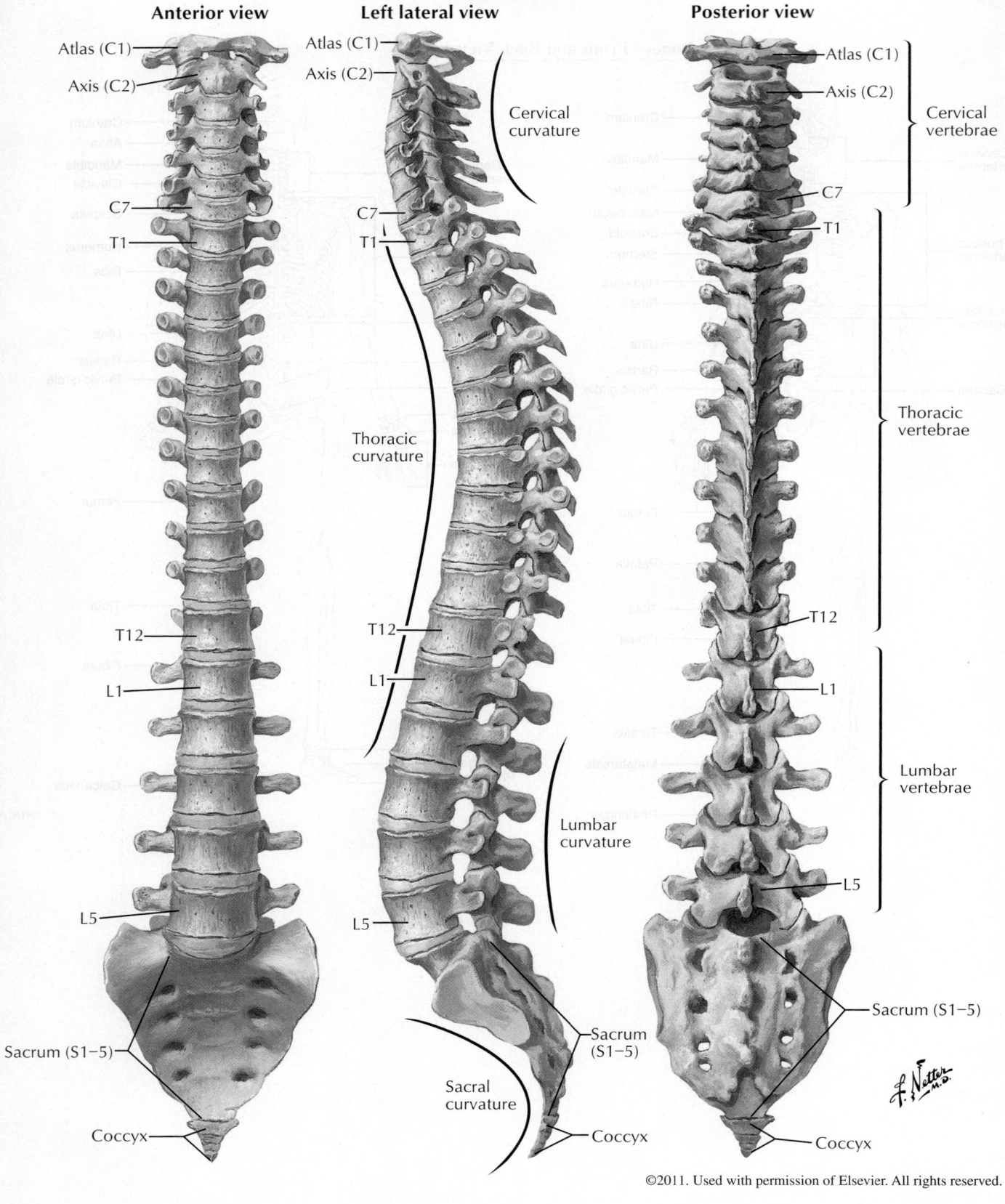

Anterior view

Atlas (C1)
Axis (C2)
C7
T1
T12
L1
L5
Sacrum (S1–5)
Coccyx

Left lateral view

Atlas (C1)
Axis (C2)
Cervical curvature
C7
T1
Thoracic curvature
T12
L1
Lumbar curvature
L5
Sacrum (S1–5)
Sacral curvature
Coccyx

Posterior view

Atlas (C1)
Axis (C2)
Cervical vertebrae
C7
T1
Thoracic vertebrae
T12
L1
Lumbar vertebrae
L5
Sacrum (S1–5)
Coccyx

Medical and Surgical, Upper Bones

Cross-section Spine

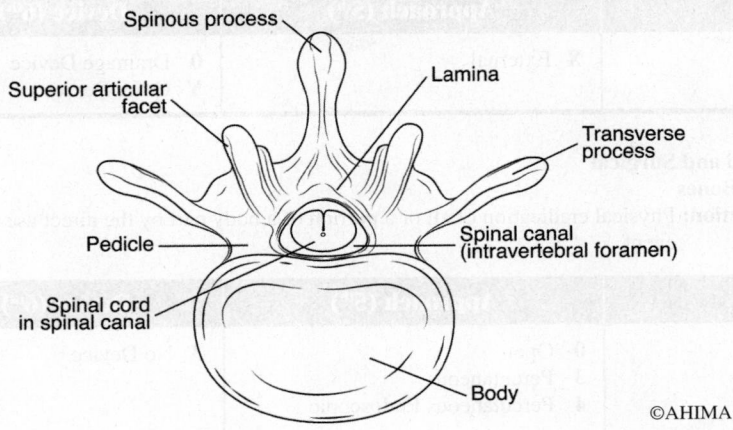

Spinous process

Lamina

Superior articular facet

Transverse process

Pedicle

Spinal canal (intravertebral foramen)

Spinal cord in spinal canal

Body

©AHIMA

Hand Bones

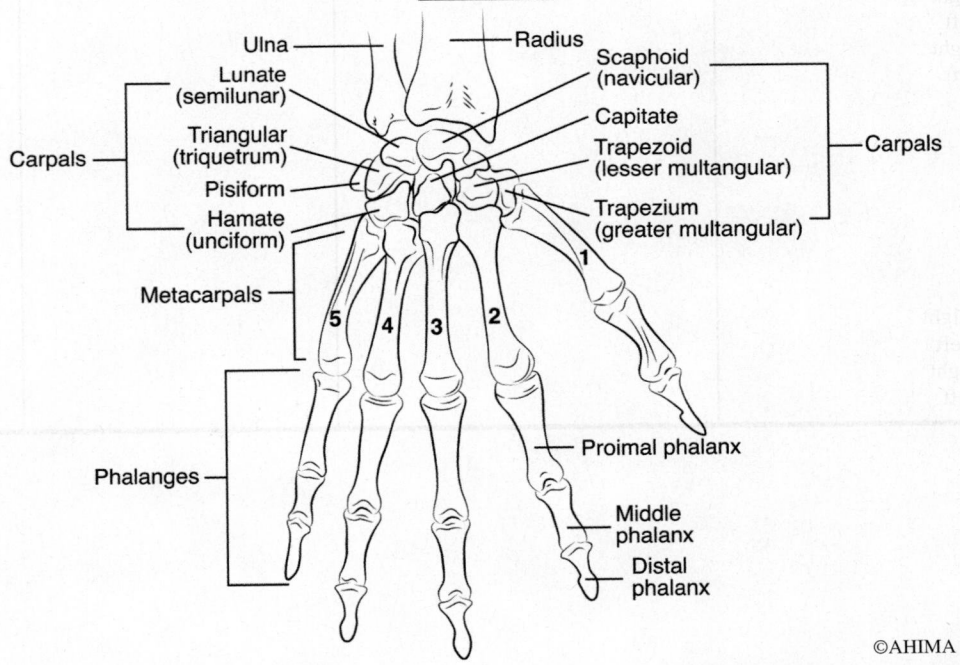

Ulna

Radius

Lunate (semilunar)

Scaphoid (navicular)

Triangular (triquetrum)

Capitate

Carpals

Trapezoid (lesser multangular)

Pisiform

Hamate (unciform)

Trapezium (greater multangular)

Carpals

Metacarpals

Phalanges

Proimal phalanx

Middle phalanx

Distal phalanx

©AHIMA

Upper Bones Tables 0P2–0PW

Section	0	Medical and Surgical
Body System	P	Upper Bones
Operation	2	**Change:** Taking out or off a device from a body part and putting back an identical or similar device in or on the same body part without cutting or puncturing the skin or a mucous membrane

Body Part (4th)	Approach (5th)	Device (6th)	Qualifier (7th)
Y Upper Bone	X External	0 Drainage Device Y Other Device	Z No Qualifier

Section	0	Medical and Surgical
Body System	P	Upper Bones
Operation	5	**Destruction:** Physical eradication of all or a portion of a body part by the direct use of energy, force, or a destructive agent

Body Part (4th)	Approach (5th)	Device (6th)	Qualifier (7th)
0 Sternum 1 Ribs, 1 to 2 2 Ribs, 3 or More 3 Cervical Vertebra 4 Thoracic Vertebra 5 Scapula, Right 6 Scapula, Left 7 Glenoid Cavity, Right 8 Glenoid Cavity, Left 9 Clavicle, Right B Clavicle, Left C Humeral Head, Right D Humeral Head, Left F Humeral Shaft, Right G Humeral Shaft, Left H Radius, Right J Radius, Left K Ulna, Right L Ulna, Left M Carpal, Right N Carpal, Left P Metacarpal, Right Q Metacarpal, Left R Thumb Phalanx, Right S Thumb Phalanx, Left T Finger Phalanx, Right V Finger Phalanx, Left	0 Open 3 Percutaneous 4 Percutaneous Endoscopic	Z No Device	Z No Qualifier

Section	0	Medical and Surgical
Body System	P	Upper Bones
Operation	8	**Division:** Cutting into a body part, without draining fluids and/or gases from the body part, in order to separate or transect a body part

Body Part (4th)	Approach (5th)	Device (6th)	Qualifier (7th)
0 Sternum 1 Ribs, 1 to 2 2 Ribs, 3 or More 3 Cervical Vertebra 4 Thoracic Vertebra 5 Scapula, Right 6 Scapula, Left 7 Glenoid Cavity, Right 8 Glenoid Cavity, Left 9 Clavicle, Right B Clavicle, Left C Humeral Head, Right D Humeral Head, Left F Humeral Shaft, Right G Humeral Shaft, Left H Radius, Right J Radius, Left K Ulna, Right L Ulna, Left M Carpal, Right N Carpal, Left P Metacarpal, Right Q Metacarpal, Left R Thumb Phalanx, Right S Thumb Phalanx, Left T Finger Phalanx, Right V Finger Phalanx, Left	0 Open 3 Percutaneous 4 Percutaneous Endoscopic	Z No Device	Z No Qualifier

Section	0	Medical and Surgical
Body System	P	Upper Bones
Operation	9	**Drainage:** Taking or letting out fluids and/or gases from a body part

Body Part (4th)	Approach (5th)	Device (6th)	Qualifier (7th)
0 Sternum 1 Ribs, 1 to 2 2 Ribs, 3 or More 3 Cervical Vertebra 4 Thoracic Vertebra 5 Scapula, Right 6 Scapula, Left 7 Glenoid Cavity, Right 8 Glenoid Cavity, Left 9 Clavicle, Right B Clavicle, Left C Humeral Head, Right D Humeral Head, Left F Humeral Shaft, Right G Humeral Shaft, Left H Radius, Right J Radius, Left K Ulna, Right L Ulna, Left M Carpal, Right N Carpal, Left P Metacarpal, Right Q Metacarpal, Left R Thumb Phalanx, Right S Thumb Phalanx, Left T Finger Phalanx, Right V Finger Phalanx, Left	0 Open 3 Percutaneous 4 Percutaneous Endoscopic	0 Drainage Device	Z No Qualifier

Continued →

Section   **0**   **Medical and Surgical**
Body System   **P**   **Upper Bones**
Operation   **9**   **Drainage:** Taking or letting out fluids and/or gases from a body part

Body Part (4ᵗʰ)	Approach (5ᵗʰ)	Device (6ᵗʰ)	Qualifier (7ᵗʰ)
0 Sternum	**0** Open	**Z** No Device	**X** Diagnostic
1 Ribs, 1 to 2	**3** Percutaneous		**Z** No Qualifier
2 Ribs, 3 or More	**4** Percutaneous Endoscopic		
3 Cervical Vertebra			
4 Thoracic Vertebra			
5 Scapula, Right			
6 Scapula, Left			
7 Glenoid Cavity, Right			
8 Glenoid Cavity, Left			
9 Clavicle, Right			
B Clavicle, Left			
C Humeral Head, Right			
D Humeral Head, Left			
F Humeral Shaft, Right			
G Humeral Shaft, Left			
H Radius, Right			
J Radius, Left			
K Ulna, Right			
L Ulna, Left			
M Carpal, Right			
N Carpal, Left			
P Metacarpal, Right			
Q Metacarpal, Left			
R Thumb Phalanx, Right			
S Thumb Phalanx, Left			
T Finger Phalanx, Right			
V Finger Phalanx, Left			

Section   **0**   **Medical and Surgical**
Body System   **P**   **Upper Bones**
Operation   **B**   **Excision:** Cutting out or off, without replacement, a portion of a body part

Body Part (4ᵗʰ)	Approach (5ᵗʰ)	Device (6ᵗʰ)	Qualifier (7ᵗʰ)
0 Sternum	**0** Open	**Z** No Device	**X** Diagnostic
1 Ribs, 1 to 2	**3** Percutaneous		**Z** No Qualifier
2 Ribs, 3 or More	**4** Percutaneous Endoscopic		
3 Cervical Vertebra			
4 Thoracic Vertebra			
5 Scapula, Right			
6 Scapula, Left			
7 Glenoid Cavity, Right			
8 Glenoid Cavity, Left			
9 Clavicle, Right			
B Clavicle, Left			
C Humeral Head, Right			
D Humeral Head, Left			
F Humeral Shaft, Right			
G Humeral Shaft, Left			
H Radius, Right			
J Radius, Left			
K Ulna, Right			
L Ulna, Left			
M Carpal, Right			
N Carpal, Left			
P Metacarpal, Right			
Q Metacarpal, Left			
R Thumb Phalanx, Right			
S Thumb Phalanx, Left			
T Finger Phalanx, Right			
V Finger Phalanx, Left			

Section   **0**   **Medical and Surgical**
Body System   **P**   **Upper Bones**
Operation   **C**   **Extirpation:** Taking or cutting out solid matter from a body part

Body Part (4th)	Approach (5th)	Device (6th)	Qualifier (7th)
0 Sternum	**0** Open	**Z** No Device	**Z** No Qualifier
1 Ribs, 1 to 2	**3** Percutaneous		
2 Ribs, 3 or More	**4** Percutaneous Endoscopic		
3 Cervical Vertebra			
4 Thoracic Vertebra			
5 Scapula, Right			
6 Scapula, Left			
7 Glenoid Cavity, Right			
8 Glenoid Cavity, Left			
9 Clavicle, Right			
B Clavicle, Left			
C Humeral Head, Right			
D Humeral Head, Left			
F Humeral Shaft, Right			
G Humeral Shaft, Left			
H Radius, Right			
J Radius, Left			
K Ulna, Right			
L Ulna, Left			
M Carpal, Right			
N Carpal, Left			
P Metacarpal, Right			
Q Metacarpal, Left			
R Thumb Phalanx, Right			
S Thumb Phalanx, Left			
T Finger Phalanx, Right			
V Finger Phalanx, Left			

Section   **0**   **Medical and Surgical**
Body System   **P**   **Upper Bones**
Operation   **D**   **Extraction:** Pulling or stripping out or off all or a portion of a body part by the use of force

Body Part (4th)	Approach (5th)	Device (6th)	Qualifier (7th)
0 Sternum	**0** Open	**Z** No Device	**Z** No Qualifier
1 Ribs, 1 to 2			
2 Ribs, 3 or More			
3 Cervical Vertebra			
4 Thoracic Vertebra			
5 Scapula, Right			
6 Scapula, Left			
7 Glenoid Cavity, Right			
8 Glenoid Cavity, Left			
9 Clavical, Right			
B Clavical, Left			
C Humeral Head, Right			
D Humeral Head, Left			
F Humeral Shaft, Right			
G Humeral Shaft, Left			
H Radius, Right			
J Radius, Left			
K Ulna, Right			
L Ulna, Left			
M Carpal, Right			
N Carpal, Left			
P Metacarpal, Right			
Q Metacarpal, Left			
R Thumb Phalanx, Right			
S Thumb Phalanx, Left			
T Finger Phalanx, Right			
V Finger Phalanx, Left			

Section 0 **Medical and Surgical**
Body System P **Upper Bones**
Operation H **Insertion:** Putting in a nonbiological appliance that monitors, assists, performs, or prevents a physiological function but does not physically take the place of a body part

Body Part (4th)	Approach (5th)	Device (6th)	Qualifier (7th)
0 Sternum	0 Open 3 Percutaneous 4 Percutaneous Endoscopic	0 Internal Fixation Device, Rigid Plate 4 Internal Fixation Device	Z No Qualifier
1 Ribs, 1 to 2 2 Ribs, 3 or More 3 Cervical Vertebra 4 Thoracic Vertebra 5 Scapula, Right 6 Scapula, Left 7 Glenoid Cavity, Right 8 Glenoid Cavity, Left 9 Clavicle, Right B Clavicle, Left	0 Open 3 Percutaneous 4 Percutaneous Endoscopic	4 Internal Fixation Device	Z No Qualifier
C Humeral Head, Right D Humeral Head, Left H Radius, Right J Radius, Left K Ulna, Right L Ulna, Left	0 Open 3 Percutaneous 4 Percutaneous Endoscopic	4 Internal Fixation Device 5 External Fixation Device 6 Internal Fixation Device, Intramedullary 8 External Fixation Device, Limb Lengthening B External Fixation Device, Monoplanar C External Fixation Device, Ring D External Fixation Device, Hybrid	Z No Qualifier
F Humeral Shaft, Right G Humeral Shaft, Left	0 Open 3 Percutaneous 4 Percutaneous Endoscopic	4 Internal Fixation Device 5 External Fixation Device 6 Internal Fixation Device, Intramedullary 7 Internal Fixation Device, Intramedullary Limb Lengthening 8 External Fixation Device, Limb Lengthening B External Fixation Device, Monoplanar C External Fixation Device, Ring D External Fixation Device, Hybrid	Z No Qualifier
M Carpal, Right N Carpal, Left P Metacarpal, Right Q Metacarpal, Left R Thumb Phalanx, Right S Thumb Phalanx, Left T Finger Phalanx, Right V Finger Phalanx, Left	0 Open 3 Percutaneous 4 Percutaneous Endoscopic	4 Internal Fixation Device 5 External Fixation Device	Z No Qualifier
Y Upper Bone	0 Open 3 Percutaneous 4 Percutaneous Endoscopic	M Bone Growth Stimulator	Z No Qualifier

Section 0 **Medical and Surgical**
Body System P **Upper Bones**
Operation J **Inspection:** Visually and/or manually exploring a body part

Body Part (4th)	Approach (5th)	Device (6th)	Qualifier (7th)
Y Upper Bone	0 Open 3 Percutaneous 4 Percutaneous Endoscopic X External	Z No Device	Z No Qualifier

Section	0	Medical and Surgical
Body System	P	Upper Bones
Operation	N	Release: Freeing a body part from an abnormal physical constraint by cutting or by the use of force

Body Part (4th)	Approach (5th)	Device (6th)	Qualifier (7th)
0 Sternum 1 Ribs, 1 to 2 2 Ribs, 3 or More 3 Cervical Vertebra 4 Thoracic Vertebra 5 Scapula, Right 6 Scapula, Left 7 Glenoid Cavity, Right 8 Glenoid Cavity, Left 9 Clavicle, Right B Clavicle, Left C Humeral Head, Right D Humeral Head, Left F Humeral Shaft, Right G Humeral Shaft, Left H Radius, Right J Radius, Left K Ulna, Right L Ulna, Left M Carpal, Right N Carpal, Left P Metacarpal, Right Q Metacarpal, Left R Thumb Phalanx, Right S Thumb Phalanx, Left T Finger Phalanx, Right V Finger Phalanx, Left	0 Open 3 Percutaneous 4 Percutaneous Endoscopic	Z No Device	Z No Qualifier

Section	0	Medical and Surgical
Body System	P	Upper Bones
Operation	P	Removal: Taking out or off a device from a body part

Body Part (4th)	Approach (5th)	Device (6th)	Qualifier (7th)
0 Sternum 1 Ribs, 1 to 2 2 Ribs, 3 or More 3 Cervical Vertebra 4 Thoracic Vertebra 5 Scapula, Right 6 Scapula, Left 7 Glenoid Cavity, Right 8 Glenoid Cavity, Left 9 Clavicle, Right B Clavicle, Left	0 Open 3 Percutaneous 4 Percutaneous Endoscopic	4 Internal Fixation Device 7 Autologous Tissue Substitute J Synthetic Substitute K Nonautologous Tissue Substitute	Z No Qualifier
0 Sternum 1 Ribs, 1 to 2 2 Ribs, 3 or More 3 Cervical Vertebra 4 Thoracic Vertebra 5 Scapula, Right 6 Scapula, Left 7 Glenoid Cavity, Right 8 Glenoid Cavity, Left 9 Clavicle, Right B Clavicle, Left	X External	4 Internal Fixation Device	Z No Qualifier

Continued →

Section	0	Medical and Surgical
Body System	P	Upper Bones
Operation	P	**Removal:** Taking out or off a device from a body part

Body Part (4ᵗʰ)	Approach (5ᵗʰ)	Device (6ᵗʰ)	Qualifier (7ᵗʰ)
C Humeral Head, Right D Humeral Head, Left F Humeral Shaft, Right G Humeral Shaft, Left H Radius, Right J Radius, Left K Ulna, Right L Ulna, Left M Carpal, Right N Carpal, Left P Metacarpal, Right Q Metacarpal, Left R Thumb Phalanx, Right S Thumb Phalanx, Left T Finger Phalanx, Right V Finger Phalanx, Left	0 Open 3 Percutaneous 4 Percutaneous Endoscopic	4 Internal Fixation Device 5 External Fixation Device 7 Autologous Tissue Substitute J Synthetic Substitute K Nonautologous Tissue Substitute	Z No Qualifier
C Humeral Head, Right D Humeral Head, Left F Humeral Shaft, Right G Humeral Shaft, Left H Radius, Right J Radius, Left K Ulna, Right L Ulna, Left M Carpal, Right N Carpal, Left P Metacarpal, Right Q Metacarpal, Left R Thumb Phalanx, Right S Thumb Phalanx, Left T Finger Phalanx, Right V Finger Phalanx, Left	X External	4 Internal Fixation Device 5 External Fixation Device	Z No Qualifier
Y Upper Bone	0 Open 3 Percutaneous 4 Percutaneous Endoscopic X External	0 Drainage Device M Bone Growth Stimulator	Z No Qualifier

Section	0	Medical and Surgical
Body System	P	Upper Bones
Operation	Q	Repair: Restoring, to the extent possible, a body part to its normal anatomic structure and function

Body Part (4th)	Approach (5th)	Device (6th)	Qualifier (7th)
0 Sternum	0 Open	Z No Device	Z No Qualifier
1 Ribs, 1 to 2	3 Percutaneous		
2 Ribs, 3 or More	4 Percutaneous Endoscopic		
3 Cervical Vertebra	X External		
4 Thoracic Vertebra			
5 Scapula, Right			
6 Scapula, Left			
7 Glenoid Cavity, Right			
8 Glenoid Cavity, Left			
9 Clavicle, Right			
B Clavicle, Left			
C Humeral Head, Right			
D Humeral Head, Left			
F Humeral Shaft, Right			
G Humeral Shaft, Left			
H Radius, Right			
J Radius, Left			
K Ulna, Right			
L Ulna, Left			
M Carpal, Right			
N Carpal, Left			
P Metacarpal, Right			
Q Metacarpal, Left			
R Thumb Phalanx, Right			
S Thumb Phalanx, Left			
T Finger Phalanx, Right			
V Finger Phalanx, Left			

Section	0	Medical and Surgical
Body System	P	Upper Bones
Operation	R	Replacement: Putting in or on biological or synthetic material that physically takes the place and/or function of all or a portion of a body part

Body Part (4th)	Approach (5th)	Device (6th)	Qualifier (7th)
0 Sternum	0 Open	7 Autologous Tissue Substitute	Z No Qualifier
1 Ribs, 1 to 2	3 Percutaneous	J Synthetic Substitute	
2 Ribs, 3 or More	4 Percutaneous Endoscopic	K Nonautologous Tissue Substitute	
3 Cervical Vertebra			
4 Thoracic Vertebra			
5 Scapula, Right			
6 Scapula, Left			
7 Glenoid Cavity, Right			
8 Glenoid Cavity, Left			
9 Clavicle, Right			
B Clavicle, Left			
C Humeral Head, Right			
D Humeral Head, Left			
F Humeral Shaft, Right			
G Humeral Shaft, Left			
H Radius, Right			
J Radius, Left			
K Ulna, Right			
L Ulna, Left			
M Carpal, Right			
N Carpal, Left			
P Metacarpal, Right			
Q Metacarpal, Left			
R Thumb Phalanx, Right			
S Thumb Phalanx, Left			
T Finger Phalanx, Right			
V Finger Phalanx, Left			

Section	0	Medical and Surgical
Body System	P	Upper Bones
Operation	S	**Reposition:** Moving to its normal location, or other suitable location, all or a portion of a body part

Body Part (4ᵗʰ)	Approach (5ᵗʰ)	Device (6ᵗʰ)	Qualifier (7ᵗʰ)
0 Sternum	**0** Open **3** Percutaneous **4** Percutaneous Endoscopic	**0** Internal Fixation Device, Rigid Plate **4** Internal Fixation Device **Z** No Device	**Z** No Qualifier
0 Sternum	**X** External	**Z** No Device	**Z** No Qualifier
1 Ribs, 1 to 2 **2** Ribs, 3 or More **3** Cervical Vertebra **5** Scapula, Right **6** Scapula, Left **7** Glenoid Cavity, Right **8** Glenoid Cavity, Left **9** Clavicle, Right **B** Clavicle, Left	**0** Open **3** Percutaneous **4** Percutaneous Endoscopic	**4** Internal Fixation Device **Z** No Device	**Z** No Qualifier
1 Ribs, 1 to 2 **2** Ribs, 3 or More **3** Cervical Vertebra **5** Scapula, Right **6** Scapula, Left **7** Glenoid Cavity, Right **8** Glenoid Cavity, Left **9** Clavicle, Right **B** Clavicle, Left	**X** External	**Z** No Device	**Z** No Qualifier
4 Thoracic Vertebra	**0** Open **4** Percutaneous Endoscopic	**3** Spinal Stabilization Device, Vertebral Body Tether **4** Internal Fixation Device **Z** No Device	**Z** No Qualifier
4 Thoracic Vertebra	**3** Percutaneous	**4** Internal Fixation Device **Z** No Device	**Z** No Qualifier
4 Thoracic Vertebra	**X** External	**Z** No Device	**Z** No Qualifier
C Humeral Head, Right **D** Humeral Head, Left **F** Humeral Shaft, Right **G** Humeral Shaft, Left **H** Radius, Right **J** Radius, Left **K** Ulna, Right **L** Ulna, Left	**0** Open **3** Percutaneous **4** Percutaneous Endoscopic	**4** Internal Fixation Device **5** External Fixation Device **6** Internal Fixation Device, Intramedullary **B** External Fixation Device, Monoplanar **C** External Fixation Device, Ring **D** External Fixation Device, Hybrid **Z** No Device	**Z** No Qualifier
C Humeral Head, Right **D** Humeral Head, Left **F** Humeral Shaft, Right **G** Humeral Shaft, Left **H** Radius, Right **J** Radius, Left **K** Ulna, Right **L** Ulna, Left	**X** External	**Z** No Device	**Z** No Qualifier
M Carpal, Right **N** Carpal, Left **P** Metacarpal, Right **Q** Metacarpal, Left **R** Thumb Phalanx, Right **S** Thumb Phalanx, Left **T** Finger Phalanx, Right **V** Finger Phalanx, Left	**0** Open **3** Percutaneous **4** Percutaneous Endoscopic	**4** Internal Fixation Device **5** External Fixation Device **Z** No Device	**Z** No Qualifier
M Carpal, Right **N** Carpal, Left **P** Metacarpal, Right **Q** Metacarpal, Left **R** Thumb Phalanx, Right **S** Thumb Phalanx, Left **T** Finger Phalanx, Right **V** Finger Phalanx, Left	**X** External	**Z** No Device	**Z** No Qualifier

Section   **0**   **Medical and Surgical**
Body System   **P**   **Upper Bones**
Operation   **T**   **Resection:** Cutting out or off, without replacement, all of a body part

Body Part (4ᵗʰ)	Approach (5ᵗʰ)	Device (6ᵗʰ)	Qualifier (7ᵗʰ)
0 Sternum	**0** Open	**Z** No Device	**Z** No Qualifier
1 Ribs, 1 to 2			
2 Ribs, 3 or More			
5 Scapula, Right			
6 Scapula, Left			
7 Glenoid Cavity, Right			
8 Glenoid Cavity, Left			
9 Clavicle, Right			
B Clavicle, Left			
C Humeral Head, Right			
D Humeral Head, Left			
F Humeral Shaft, Right			
G Humeral Shaft, Left			
H Radius, Right			
J Radius, Left			
K Ulna, Right			
L Ulna, Left			
M Carpal, Right			
N Carpal, Left			
P Metacarpal, Right			
Q Metacarpal, Left			
R Thumb Phalanx, Right			
S Thumb Phalanx, Left			
T Finger Phalanx, Right			
V Finger Phalanx, Left			

Section   **0**   **Medical and Surgical**
Body System   **P**   **Upper Bones**
Operation   **U**   **Supplement:** Putting in or on biological or synthetic material that physically reinforces and/or augments the function of a portion of a body part

Body Part (4ᵗʰ)	Approach (5ᵗʰ)	Device (6ᵗʰ)	Qualifier (7ᵗʰ)
0 Sternum	**0** Open	**7** Autologous Tissue Substitute	**Z** No Qualifier
1 Ribs, 1 to 2	**3** Percutaneous	**J** Synthetic Substitute	
2 Ribs, 3 or More	**4** Percutaneous Endoscopic	**K** Nonautologous Tissue Substitute	
3 Cervical Vertebra			
4 Thoracic Vertebra			
5 Scapula, Right			
6 Scapula, Left			
7 Glenoid Cavity, Right			
8 Glenoid Cavity, Left			
9 Clavicle, Right			
B Clavicle, Left			
C Humeral Head, Right			
D Humeral Head, Left			
F Humeral Shaft, Right			
G Humeral Shaft, Left			
H Radius, Right			
J Radius, Left			
K Ulna, Right			
L Ulna, Left			
M Carpal, Right			
N Carpal, Left			
P Metacarpal, Right			
Q Metacarpal, Left			
R Thumb Phalanx, Right			
S Thumb Phalanx, Left			
T Finger Phalanx, Right			
V Finger Phalanx, Left			

Section **0** **Medical and Surgical**
Body System **P** **Upper Bones**
Operation **W** **Revision:** Correcting, to the extent possible, a portion of a malfunctioning device or the position of a displaced device

Body Part (4th)	Approach (5th)	Device (6th)	Qualifier (7th)
0 Sternum **1** Ribs, 1 to 2 **2** Ribs, 3 or More **3** Cervical Vertebra **4** Thoracic Vertebra **5** Scapula, Right **6** Scapula, Left **7** Glenoid Cavity, Right **8** Glenoid Cavity, Left **9** Clavicle, Right **B** Clavicle, Left	**0** Open **3** Percutaneous **4** Percutaneous Endoscopic **X** External	**4** Internal Fixation Device **7** Autologous Tissue Substitute **J** Synthetic Substitute **K** Nonautologous Tissue Substitute	**Z** No Qualifier
C Humeral Head, Right **D** Humeral Head, Left **F** Humeral Shaft, Right **G** Humeral Shaft, Left **H** Radius, Right **J** Radius, Left **K** Ulna, Right **L** Ulna, Left **M** Carpal, Right **N** Carpal, Left **P** Metacarpal, Right **Q** Metacarpal, Left **R** Thumb Phalanx, Right **S** Thumb Phalanx, Left **T** Finger Phalanx, Right **V** Finger Phalanx, Left	**0** Open **3** Percutaneous **4** Percutaneous Endoscopic **X** External	**4** Internal Fixation Device **5** External Fixation Device **7** Autologous Tissue Substitute **J** Synthetic Substitute **K** Nonautologous Tissue Substitute	**Z** No Qualifier
Y Upper Bone	**0** Open **3** Percutaneous **4** Percutaneous Endoscopic **X** External	**0** Drainage Device **M** Bone Growth Stimulator	**Z** No Qualifier

Upper Bones Code Listing 0P2–0PW

0P2 – Upper Bones, Change

Review Coding Guideline B6.1c

0P2YX0Z Change Drainage Device in Upper Bone, External Approach

0P2YXYZ Change Other Device in Upper Bone, External Approach

0P5 – Upper Bones, Destruction

0P500ZZ Destruction of Sternum, Open Approach

0P503ZZ Destruction of Sternum, Percutaneous Approach

0P504ZZ Destruction of Sternum, Percutaneous Endoscopic Approach

0P510ZZ Destruction of I to 2 Ribs, Open Approach

0P513ZZ Destruction of I to 2 Ribs, Percutaneous Approach

0P514ZZ Destruction of I to 2 Ribs, Percutaneous Endoscopic Approach

0P520ZZ Destruction of 3 or More Ribs, Open Approach

0P523ZZ Destruction of 3 or More Ribs, Percutaneous Approach

0P524ZZ Destruction of 3 or More Ribs, Percutaneous Endoscopic Approach

0P530ZZ Destruction of Cervical Vertebra, Open Approach

0P533ZZ Destruction of Cervical Vertebra, Percutaneous Approach

0P534ZZ Destruction of Cervical Vertebra, Percutaneous Endoscopic Approach

0P540ZZ Destruction of Thoracic Vertebra, Open Approach

0P543ZZ Destruction of Thoracic Vertebra, Percutaneous Approach

0P544ZZ Destruction of Thoracic Vertebra, Percutaneous Endoscopic Approach

0P550ZZ Destruction of Right Scapula, Open Approach

0P553ZZ Destruction of Right Scapula, Percutaneous Approach

0P554ZZ Destruction of Right Scapula, Percutaneous Endoscopic Approach

0P560ZZ Destruction of Left Scapula, Open Approach

0P563ZZ Destruction of Left Scapula, Percutaneous Approach

0P564ZZ Destruction of Left Scapula, Percutaneous Endoscopic Approach

0P570ZZ Destruction of Right Glenoid Cavity, Open Approach

0P573ZZ Destruction of Right Glenoid Cavity, Percutaneous Approach

0P574ZZ Destruction of Right Glenoid Cavity, Percutaneous Endoscopic Approach

0P580ZZ Destruction of Left Glenoid Cavity, Open Approach

0P583ZZ Destruction of Left Glenoid Cavity, Percutaneous Approach

0P584ZZ Destruction of Left Glenoid Cavity, Percutaneous Endoscopic Approach

0P590ZZ Destruction of Right Clavicle, Open Approach

0P593ZZ Destruction of Right Clavicle, Percutaneous Approach

0P594ZZ Destruction of Right Clavicle, Percutaneous Endoscopic Approach

♀ Female-only   ♂ Male-only   ▲ Limited Coverage   ● Non-OR   HAC HAC-associated procedure   ▲ Non-covered procedures   ✚ Cluster

0P5B0ZZ	Destruction of Left Clavicle, Open Approach
0P5B3ZZ	Destruction of Left Clavicle, Percutaneous Approach
0P5B4ZZ	Destruction of Left Clavicle, Percutaneous Endoscopic Approach
0P5C0ZZ	Destruction of Right Humeral Head, Open Approach
0P5C3ZZ	Destruction of Right Humeral Head, Percutaneous Approach
0P5C4ZZ	Destruction of Right Humeral Head, Percutaneous Endoscopic Approach
0P5D0ZZ	Destruction of Left Humeral Head, Open Approach
0P5D3ZZ	Destruction of Left Humeral Head, Percutaneous Approach
0P5D4ZZ	Destruction of Left Humeral Head, Percutaneous Endoscopic Approach
0P5F0ZZ	Destruction of Right Humeral Shaft, Open Approach
0P5F3ZZ	Destruction of Right Humeral Shaft, Percutaneous Approach
0P5F4ZZ	Destruction of Right Humeral Shaft, Percutaneous Endoscopic Approach
0P5G0ZZ	Destruction of Left Humeral Shaft, Open Approach
0P5G3ZZ	Destruction of Left Humeral Shaft, Percutaneous Approach
0P5G4ZZ	Destruction of Left Humeral Shaft, Percutaneous Endoscopic Approach
0P5H0ZZ	Destruction of Right Radius, Open Approach
0P5H3ZZ	Destruction of Right Radius, Percutaneous Approach

0P5H4ZZ	Destruction of Right Radius, Percutaneous Endoscopic Approach
0P5J0ZZ	Destruction of Left Radius, Open Approach
0P5J3ZZ	Destruction of Left Radius, Percutaneous Approach
0P5J4ZZ	Destruction of Left Radius, Percutaneous Endoscopic Approach
0P5K0ZZ	Destruction of Right Ulna, Open Approach
0P5K3ZZ	Destruction of Right Ulna, Percutaneous Approach
0P5K4ZZ	Destruction of Right Ulna, Percutaneous Endoscopic Approach
0P5L0ZZ	Destruction of Left Ulna, Open Approach
0P5L3ZZ	Destruction of Left Ulna, Percutaneous Approach
0P5L4ZZ	Destruction of Left Ulna, Percutaneous Endoscopic Approach
0P5M0ZZ	Destruction of Right Carpal, Open Approach
0P5M3ZZ	Destruction of Right Carpal, Percutaneous Approach
0P5M4ZZ	Destruction of Right Carpal, Percutaneous Endoscopic Approach
0P5N0ZZ	Destruction of Left Carpal, Open Approach
0P5N3ZZ	Destruction of Left Carpal, Percutaneous Approach
0P5N4ZZ	Destruction of Left Carpal, Percutaneous Endoscopic Approach
0P5P0ZZ	Destruction of Right Metacarpal, Open Approach

0P5P3ZZ	Destruction of Right Metacarpal, Percutaneous Approach
0P5P4ZZ	Destruction of Right Metacarpal, Percutaneous Endoscopic Approach
0P5Q0ZZ	Destruction of Left Metacarpal, Open Approach
0P5Q3ZZ	Destruction of Left Metacarpal, Percutaneous Approach
0P5Q4ZZ	Destruction of Left Metacarpal, Percutaneous Endoscopic Approach
0P5R0ZZ	Destruction of Right Thumb Phalanx, Open Approach
0P5R3ZZ	Destruction of Right Thumb Phalanx, Percutaneous Approach
0P5R4ZZ	Destruction of Right Thumb Phalanx, Percutaneous Endoscopic Approach
0P5S0ZZ	Destruction of Left Thumb Phalanx, Open Approach
0P5S3ZZ	Destruction of Left Thumb Phalanx, Percutaneous Approach
0P5S4ZZ	Destruction of Left Thumb Phalanx, Percutaneous Endoscopic Approach
0P5T0ZZ	Destruction of Right Finger Phalanx, Open Approach
0P5T3ZZ	Destruction of Right Finger Phalanx, Percutaneous Approach
0P5T4ZZ	Destruction of Right Finger Phalanx, Percutaneous Endoscopic Approach
0P5V0ZZ	Destruction of Left Finger Phalanx, Open Approach
0P5V3ZZ	Destruction of Left Finger Phalanx, Percutaneous Approach
0P5V4ZZ	Destruction of Left Finger Phalanx, Percutaneous Endoscopic Approach

0P8 – Upper Bones, Division

Review Coding Guideline B3.14

0P800ZZ	Division of Sternum, Open Approach
0P803ZZ	Division of Sternum, Percutaneous Approach
0P804ZZ	Division of Sternum, Percutaneous Endoscopic Approach
0P810ZZ	Division of I to 2 Ribs, Open Approach
0P813ZZ	Division of I to 2 Ribs, Percutaneous Approach
0P814ZZ	Division of I to 2 Ribs, Percutaneous Endoscopic Approach
0P820ZZ	Division of 3 or More Ribs, Open Approach
0P823ZZ	Division of 3 or More Ribs, Percutaneous Approach
0P824ZZ	Division of 3 or More Ribs, Percutaneous Endoscopic Approach
0P830ZZ	Division of Cervical Vertebra, Open Approach
0P833ZZ	Division of Cervical Vertebra, Percutaneous Approach
0P834ZZ	Division of Cervical Vertebra, Percutaneous Endoscopic Approach
0P840ZZ	Division of Thoracic Vertebra, Open Approach
0P843ZZ	Division of Thoracic Vertebra, Percutaneous Approach
0P844ZZ	Division of Thoracic Vertebra, Percutaneous Endoscopic Approach
0P850ZZ	Division of Right Scapula, Open Approach
0P853ZZ	Division of Right Scapula, Percutaneous Approach
0P854ZZ	Division of Right Scapula, Percutaneous Endoscopic Approach
0P860ZZ	Division of Left Scapula, Open Approach
0P863ZZ	Division of Left Scapula, Percutaneous Approach

0P864ZZ	Division of Left Scapula, Percutaneous Endoscopic Approach
0P870ZZ	Division of Right Glenoid Cavity, Open Approach
0P873ZZ	Division of Right Glenoid Cavity, Percutaneous Approach
0P874ZZ	Division of Right Glenoid Cavity, Percutaneous Endoscopic Approach
0P880ZZ	Division of Left Glenoid Cavity, Open Approach
0P883ZZ	Division of Left Glenoid Cavity, Percutaneous Approach
0P884ZZ	Division of Left Glenoid Cavity, Percutaneous Endoscopic Approach
0P890ZZ	Division of Right Clavicle, Open Approach
0P893ZZ	Division of Right Clavicle, Percutaneous Approach
0P894ZZ	Division of Right Clavicle, Percutaneous Endoscopic Approach
0P8B0ZZ	Division of Left Clavicle, Open Approach
0P8B3ZZ	Division of Left Clavicle, Percutaneous Approach
0P8B4ZZ	Division of Left Clavicle, Percutaneous Endoscopic Approach
0P8C0ZZ	Division of Right Humeral Head, Open Approach
0P8C3ZZ	Division of Right Humeral Head, Percutaneous Approach
0P8C4ZZ	Division of Right Humeral Head, Percutaneous Endoscopic Approach
0P8D0ZZ	Division of Left Humeral Head, Open Approach
0P8D3ZZ	Division of Left Humeral Head, Percutaneous Approach
0P8D4ZZ	Division of Left Humeral Head, Percutaneous Endoscopic Approach

0P8F0ZZ	Division of Right Humeral Shaft, Open Approach
0P8F3ZZ	Division of Right Humeral Shaft, Percutaneous Approach
0P8F4ZZ	Division of Right Humeral Shaft, Percutaneous Endoscopic Approach
0P8G0ZZ	Division of Left Humeral Shaft, Open Approach
0P8G3ZZ	Division of Left Humeral Shaft, Percutaneous Approach
0P8G4ZZ	Division of Left Humeral Shaft, Percutaneous Endoscopic Approach
0P8H0ZZ	Division of Right Radius, Open Approach
0P8H3ZZ	Division of Right Radius, Percutaneous Approach
0P8H4ZZ	Division of Right Radius, Percutaneous Endoscopic Approach
0P8J0ZZ	Division of Left Radius, Open Approach
0P8J3ZZ	Division of Left Radius, Percutaneous Approach
0P8J4ZZ	Division of Left Radius, Percutaneous Endoscopic Approach
0P8K0ZZ	Division of Right Ulna, Open Approach
0P8K3ZZ	Division of Right Ulna, Percutaneous Approach
0P8K4ZZ	Division of Right Ulna, Percutaneous Endoscopic Approach
0P8L0ZZ	Division of Left Ulna, Open Approach
0P8L3ZZ	Division of Left Ulna, Percutaneous Approach
0P8L4ZZ	Division of Left Ulna, Percutaneous Endoscopic Approach
0P8M0ZZ	Division of Right Carpal, Open Approach
0P8M3ZZ	Division of Right Carpal, Percutaneous Approach
0P8M4ZZ	Division of Right Carpal, Percutaneous Endoscopic Approach

♀ Female-only   ♂ Male-only   ▲ Limited Coverage   ● Non-OR   ▦ HAC-associated procedure   ▲ Non-covered procedures   ✚ Cluster

0P8N0ZZ	Division of Left Carpal, Open Approach
0P8N3ZZ	Division of Left Carpal, Percutaneous Approach
0P8N4ZZ	Division of Left Carpal, Percutaneous Endoscopic Approach
0P8P0ZZ	Division of Right Metacarpal, Open Approach
0P8P3ZZ	Division of Right Metacarpal, Percutaneous Approach
0P8P4ZZ	Division of Right Metacarpal, Percutaneous Endoscopic Approach
0P8Q0ZZ	Division of Left Metacarpal, Open Approach

0P8Q3ZZ	Division of Left Metacarpal, Percutaneous Approach
0P8Q4ZZ	Division of Left Metacarpal, Percutaneous Endoscopic Approach
0P8R0ZZ	Division of Right Thumb Phalanx, Open Approach
0P8R3ZZ	Division of Right Thumb Phalanx, Percutaneous Approach
0P8R4ZZ	Division of Right Thumb Phalanx, Percutaneous Endoscopic Approach
0P8S0ZZ	Division of Left Thumb Phalanx, Open Approach
0P8S3ZZ	Division of Left Thumb Phalanx, Percutaneous Approach

0P8S4ZZ	Division of Left Thumb Phalanx, Percutaneous Endoscopic Approach
0P8T0ZZ	Division of Right Finger Phalanx, Open Approach
0P8T3ZZ	Division of Right Finger Phalanx, Percutaneous Approach
0P8T4ZZ	Division of Right Finger Phalanx, Percutaneous Endoscopic Approach
0P8V0ZZ	Division of Left Finger Phalanx, Open Approach
0P8V3ZZ	Division of Left Finger Phalanx, Percutaneous Approach
0P8V4ZZ	Division of Left Finger Phalanx, Percutaneous Endoscopic Approach

0P9 – Upper Bones, Drainage

Review Coding Guidelines B3.4a and B3.4b

Review Coding Guideline B6.2

0P9000Z	Drainage of Sternum with Drainage Device, Open Approach
0P900ZX	Drainage of Sternum, Open Approach, Diagnostic
0P900ZZ	Drainage of Sternum, Open Approach
0P9030Z	Drainage of Sternum with Drainage Device, Percutaneous Approach
0P903ZX	Drainage of Sternum, Percutaneous Approach, Diagnostic
0P903ZZ	Drainage of Sternum, Percutaneous Approach
0P9040Z	Drainage of Sternum with Drainage Device, Percutaneous Endoscopic Approach
0P904ZX	Drainage of Sternum, Percutaneous Endoscopic Approach, Diagnostic
0P904ZZ	Drainage of Sternum, Percutaneous Endoscopic Approach
0P9100Z	Drainage of I to 2 Ribs with Drainage Device, Open Approach
0P910ZX	Drainage of I to 2 Ribs, Open Approach, Diagnostic
0P910ZZ	Drainage of I to 2 Ribs, Open Approach
0P9130Z	Drainage of I to 2 Ribs with Drainage Device, Percutaneous Approach
0P913ZX	Drainage of I to 2 Ribs, Percutaneous Approach, Diagnostic
0P913ZZ	Drainage of I to 2 Ribs, Percutaneous Approach
0P9140Z	Drainage of I to 2 Ribs with Drainage Device, Percutaneous Endoscopic Approach
0P914ZX	Drainage of I to 2 Ribs, Percutaneous Endoscopic Approach, Diagnostic
0P914ZZ	Drainage of I to 2 Ribs, Percutaneous Endoscopic Approach
0P9200Z	Drainage of 3 or More Ribs with Drainage Device, Open Approach
0P920ZX	Drainage of 3 or More Ribs, Open Approach, Diagnostic
0P920ZZ	Drainage of 3 or More Ribs, Open Approach
0P9230Z	Drainage of 3 or More Ribs with Drainage Device, Percutaneous Approach
0P923ZX	Drainage of 3 or More Ribs, Percutaneous Approach, Diagnostic
0P923ZZ	Drainage of 3 or More Ribs, Percutaneous Approach
0P9240Z	Drainage of 3 or More Ribs with Drainage Device, Percutaneous Endoscopic Approach
0P924ZX	Drainage of 3 or More Ribs, Percutaneous Endoscopic Approach, Diagnostic

0P924ZZ	Drainage of 3 or More Ribs, Percutaneous Endoscopic Approach
0P9300Z	Drainage of Cervical Vertebra with Drainage Device, Open Approach
0P930ZX	Drainage of Cervical Vertebra, Open Approach, Diagnostic
0P930ZZ	Drainage of Cervical Vertebra, Open Approach
0P9330Z	Drainage of Cervical Vertebra with Drainage Device, Percutaneous Approach
0P933ZX	Drainage of Cervical Vertebra, Percutaneous Approach, Diagnostic
0P933ZZ	Drainage of Cervical Vertebra, Percutaneous Approach
0P9340Z	Drainage of Cervical Vertebra with Drainage Device, Percutaneous Endoscopic Approach
0P934ZX	Drainage of Cervical Vertebra, Percutaneous Endoscopic Approach, Diagnostic
0P934ZZ	Drainage of Cervical Vertebra, Percutaneous Endoscopic Approach
0P9400Z	Drainage of Thoracic Vertebra with Drainage Device, Open Approach
0P940ZX	Drainage of Thoracic Vertebra, Open Approach, Diagnostic
0P940ZZ	Drainage of Thoracic Vertebra, Open Approach
0P9430Z	Drainage of Thoracic Vertebra with Drainage Device, Percutaneous Approach
0P943ZX	Drainage of Thoracic Vertebra, Percutaneous Approach, Diagnostic
0P943ZZ	Drainage of Thoracic Vertebra, Percutaneous Approach
0P9440Z	Drainage of Thoracic Vertebra with Drainage Device, Percutaneous Endoscopic Approach
0P944ZX	Drainage of Thoracic Vertebra, Percutaneous Endoscopic Approach, Diagnostic
0P944ZZ	Drainage of Thoracic Vertebra, Percutaneous Endoscopic Approach
0P9500Z	Drainage of Right Scapula with Drainage Device, Open Approach
0P950ZX	Drainage of Right Scapula, Open Approach, Diagnostic
0P950ZZ	Drainage of Right Scapula, Open Approach
0P9530Z	Drainage of Right Scapula with Drainage Device, Percutaneous Approach
0P953ZX	Drainage of Right Scapula, Percutaneous Approach, Diagnostic
0P953ZZ	Drainage of Right Scapula, Percutaneous Approach

0P9540Z	Drainage of Right Scapula with Drainage Device, Percutaneous Endoscopic Approach
0P954ZX	Drainage of Right Scapula, Percutaneous Endoscopic Approach, Diagnostic
0P954ZZ	Drainage of Right Scapula, Percutaneous Endoscopic Approach
0P9600Z	Drainage of Left Scapula with Drainage Device, Open Approach
0P960ZX	Drainage of Left Scapula, Open Approach, Diagnostic
0P960ZZ	Drainage of Left Scapula, Open Approach
0P9630Z	Drainage of Left Scapula with Drainage Device, Percutaneous Approach
0P963ZX	Drainage of Left Scapula, Percutaneous Approach, Diagnostic
0P963ZZ	Drainage of Left Scapula, Percutaneous Approach
0P9640Z	Drainage of Left Scapula with Drainage Device, Percutaneous Endoscopic Approach
0P964ZX	Drainage of Left Scapula, Percutaneous Endoscopic Approach, Diagnostic
0P964ZZ	Drainage of Left Scapula, Percutaneous Endoscopic Approach
0P9700Z	Drainage of Right Glenoid Cavity with Drainage Device, Open Approach
0P970ZX	Drainage of Right Glenoid Cavity, Open Approach, Diagnostic
0P970ZZ	Drainage of Right Glenoid Cavity, Open Approach
0P9730Z	Drainage of Right Glenoid Cavity with Drainage Device, Percutaneous Approach
0P973ZX	Drainage of Right Glenoid Cavity, Percutaneous Approach, Diagnostic
0P973ZZ	Drainage of Right Glenoid Cavity, Percutaneous Approach
0P9740Z	Drainage of Right Glenoid Cavity with Drainage Device, Percutaneous Endoscopic Approach
0P974ZX	Drainage of Right Glenoid Cavity, Percutaneous Endoscopic Approach, Diagnostic
0P974ZZ	Drainage of Right Glenoid Cavity, Percutaneous Endoscopic Approach
0P9800Z	Drainage of Left Glenoid Cavity with Drainage Device, Open Approach
0P980ZX	Drainage of Left Glenoid Cavity, Open Approach, Diagnostic
0P980ZZ	Drainage of Left Glenoid Cavity, Open Approach
0P9830Z	Drainage of Left Glenoid Cavity with Drainage Device, Percutaneous Approach

♀ Female-only   ♂ Male-only   ▲ Limited Coverage   ● Non-OR   HAC HAC-associated procedure   ▲ Non-covered procedures   ✚ Cluster

0P983ZX Drainage of Left Glenoid Cavity, Percutaneous Approach, Diagnostic

0P983ZZ Drainage of Left Glenoid Cavity, Percutaneous Approach

0P9840Z Drainage of Left Glenoid Cavity with Drainage Device, Percutaneous Endoscopic Approach

0P984ZX Drainage of Left Glenoid Cavity, Percutaneous Endoscopic Approach, Diagnostic

0P984ZZ Drainage of Left Glenoid Cavity, Percutaneous Endoscopic Approach

0P9900Z Drainage of Right Clavicle with Drainage Device, Open Approach

0P990ZX Drainage of Right Clavicle, Open Approach, Diagnostic

0P990ZZ Drainage of Right Clavicle, Open Approach

0P9930Z Drainage of Right Clavicle with Drainage Device, Percutaneous Approach

0P993ZX Drainage of Right Clavicle, Percutaneous Approach, Diagnostic

0P993ZZ Drainage of Right Clavicle, Percutaneous Approach

0P9940Z Drainage of Right Clavicle with Drainage Device, Percutaneous Endoscopic Approach

0P994ZX Drainage of Right Clavicle, Percutaneous Endoscopic Approach, Diagnostic

0P994ZZ Drainage of Right Clavicle, Percutaneous Endoscopic Approach

0P9B00Z Drainage of Left Clavicle with Drainage Device, Open Approach

0P9B0ZX Drainage of Left Clavicle, Open Approach, Diagnostic

0P9B0ZZ Drainage of Left Clavicle, Open Approach

0P9B30Z Drainage of Left Clavicle with Drainage Device, Percutaneous Approach

0P9B3ZX Drainage of Left Clavicle, Percutaneous Approach, Diagnostic

0P9B3ZZ Drainage of Left Clavicle, Percutaneous Approach

0P9B40Z Drainage of Left Clavicle with Drainage Device, Percutaneous Endoscopic Approach

0P9B4ZX Drainage of Left Clavicle, Percutaneous Endoscopic Approach, Diagnostic

0P9B4ZZ Drainage of Left Clavicle, Percutaneous Endoscopic Approach

0P9C00Z Drainage of Right Humeral Head with Drainage Device, Open Approach

0P9C0ZX Drainage of Right Humeral Head, Open Approach, Diagnostic

0P9C0ZZ Drainage of Right Humeral Head, Open Approach

0P9C30Z Drainage of Right Humeral Head with Drainage Device, Percutaneous Approach

0P9C3ZX Drainage of Right Humeral Head, Percutaneous Approach, Diagnostic

0P9C3ZZ Drainage of Right Humeral Head, Percutaneous Approach

0P9C40Z Drainage of Right Humeral Head with Drainage Device, Percutaneous Endoscopic Approach

0P9C4ZX Drainage of Right Humeral Head, Percutaneous Endoscopic Approach, Diagnostic

0P9C4ZZ Drainage of Right Humeral Head, Percutaneous Endoscopic Approach

0P9D00Z Drainage of Left Humeral Head with Drainage Device, Open Approach

0P9D0ZX Drainage of Left Humeral Head, Open Approach, Diagnostic

0P9D0ZZ Drainage of Left Humeral Head, Open Approach

0P9D30Z Drainage of Left Humeral Head with Drainage Device, Percutaneous Approach

0P9D3ZX Drainage of Left Humeral Head, Percutaneous Approach, Diagnostic

0P9D3ZZ Drainage of Left Humeral Head, Percutaneous Approach

0P9D40Z Drainage of Left Humeral Head with Drainage Device, Percutaneous Endoscopic Approach

0P9D4ZX Drainage of Left Humeral Head, Percutaneous Endoscopic Approach, Diagnostic

0P9D4ZZ Drainage of Left Humeral Head, Percutaneous Endoscopic Approach

0P9F00Z Drainage of Right Humeral Shaft with Drainage Device, Open Approach

0P9F0ZX Drainage of Right Humeral Shaft, Open Approach, Diagnostic

0P9F0ZZ Drainage of Right Humeral Shaft, Open Approach

0P9F30Z Drainage of Right Humeral Shaft with Drainage Device, Percutaneous Approach

0P9F3ZX Drainage of Right Humeral Shaft, Percutaneous Approach, Diagnostic

0P9F3ZZ Drainage of Right Humeral Shaft, Percutaneous Approach

0P9F40Z Drainage of Right Humeral Shaft with Drainage Device, Percutaneous Endoscopic Approach

0P9F4ZX Drainage of Right Humeral Shaft, Percutaneous Endoscopic Approach, Diagnostic

0P9F4ZZ Drainage of Right Humeral Shaft, Percutaneous Endoscopic Approach

0P9G00Z Drainage of Left Humeral Shaft with Drainage Device, Open Approach

0P9G0ZX Drainage of Left Humeral Shaft, Open Approach, Diagnostic

0P9G0ZZ Drainage of Left Humeral Shaft, Open Approach

0P9G30Z Drainage of Left Humeral Shaft with Drainage Device, Percutaneous Approach

0P9G3ZX Drainage of Left Humeral Shaft, Percutaneous Approach, Diagnostic

0P9G3ZZ Drainage of Left Humeral Shaft, Percutaneous Approach

0P9G40Z Drainage of Left Humeral Shaft with Drainage Device, Percutaneous Endoscopic Approach

0P9G4ZX Drainage of Left Humeral Shaft, Percutaneous Endoscopic Approach, Diagnostic

0P9G4ZZ Drainage of Left Humeral Shaft, Percutaneous Endoscopic Approach

0P9H00Z Drainage of Right Radius with Drainage Device, Open Approach

0P9H0ZX Drainage of Right Radius, Open Approach, Diagnostic

0P9H0ZZ Drainage of Right Radius, Open Approach

0P9H30Z Drainage of Right Radius with Drainage Device, Percutaneous Approach

0P9H3ZX Drainage of Right Radius, Percutaneous Approach, Diagnostic

0P9H3ZZ Drainage of Right Radius, Percutaneous Approach

0P9H40Z Drainage of Right Radius with Drainage Device, Percutaneous Endoscopic Approach

0P9H4ZX Drainage of Right Radius, Percutaneous Endoscopic Approach, Diagnostic

0P9H4ZZ Drainage of Right Radius, Percutaneous Endoscopic Approach

0P9J00Z Drainage of Left Radius with Drainage Device, Open Approach

0P9J0ZX Drainage of Left Radius, Open Approach, Diagnostic

0P9J0ZZ Drainage of Left Radius, Open Approach

0P9J30Z Drainage of Left Radius with Drainage Device, Percutaneous Approach

0P9J3ZX Drainage of Left Radius, Percutaneous Approach, Diagnostic

0P9J3ZZ Drainage of Left Radius, Percutaneous Approach

0P9J40Z Drainage of Left Radius with Drainage Device, Percutaneous Endoscopic Approach

0P9J4ZX Drainage of Left Radius, Percutaneous Endoscopic Approach, Diagnostic

0P9J4ZZ Drainage of Left Radius, Percutaneous Endoscopic Approach

0P9K00Z Drainage of Right Ulna with Drainage Device, Open Approach

0P9K0ZX Drainage of Right Ulna, Open Approach, Diagnostic

0P9K0ZZ Drainage of Right Ulna, Open Approach

0P9K30Z Drainage of Right Ulna with Drainage Device, Percutaneous Approach

0P9K3ZX Drainage of Right Ulna, Percutaneous Approach, Diagnostic

0P9K3ZZ Drainage of Right Ulna, Percutaneous Approach

0P9K40Z Drainage of Right Ulna with Drainage Device, Percutaneous Endoscopic Approach

0P9K4ZX Drainage of Right Ulna, Percutaneous Endoscopic Approach, Diagnostic

0P9K4ZZ Drainage of Right Ulna, Percutaneous Endoscopic Approach

0P9L00Z Drainage of Left Ulna with Drainage Device, Open Approach

0P9L0ZX Drainage of Left Ulna, Open Approach, Diagnostic

0P9L0ZZ Drainage of Left Ulna, Open Approach

0P9L30Z Drainage of Left Ulna with Drainage Device, Percutaneous Approach

0P9L3ZX Drainage of Left Ulna, Percutaneous Approach, Diagnostic

0P9L3ZZ Drainage of Left Ulna, Percutaneous Approach

0P9L40Z Drainage of Left Ulna with Drainage Device, Percutaneous Endoscopic Approach

0P9L4ZX Drainage of Left Ulna, Percutaneous Endoscopic Approach, Diagnostic

0P9L4ZZ Drainage of Left Ulna, Percutaneous Endoscopic Approach

0P9M00Z Drainage of Right Carpal with Drainage Device, Open Approach

0P9M0ZX Drainage of Right Carpal, Open Approach, Diagnostic

0P9M0ZZ Drainage of Right Carpal, Open Approach

0P9M30Z Drainage of Right Carpal with Drainage Device, Percutaneous Approach

0P9M3ZX Drainage of Right Carpal, Percutaneous Approach, Diagnostic

0P9M3ZZ Drainage of Right Carpal, Percutaneous Approach

0P9M40Z Drainage of Right Carpal with Drainage Device, Percutaneous Endoscopic Approach

0P9M4ZX Drainage of Right Carpal, Percutaneous Endoscopic Approach, Diagnostic

0P9M4ZZ Drainage of Right Carpal, Percutaneous Endoscopic Approach

0P9N00Z	Drainage of Left Carpal with Drainage Device, Open Approach
0P9N0ZX	Drainage of Left Carpal, Open Approach, Diagnostic
0P9N0ZZ	Drainage of Left Carpal, Open Approach
0P9N30Z	Drainage of Left Carpal with Drainage Device, Percutaneous Approach
0P9N3ZX	Drainage of Left Carpal, Percutaneous Approach, Diagnostic
0P9N3ZZ	Drainage of Left Carpal, Percutaneous Approach
0P9N40Z	Drainage of Left Carpal with Drainage Device, Percutaneous Endoscopic Approach
0P9N4ZX	Drainage of Left Carpal, Percutaneous Endoscopic Approach, Diagnostic
0P9N4ZZ	Drainage of Left Carpal, Percutaneous Endoscopic Approach
0P9P00Z	Drainage of Right Metacarpal with Drainage Device, Open Approach
0P9P0ZX	Drainage of Right Metacarpal, Open Approach, Diagnostic
0P9P0ZZ	Drainage of Right Metacarpal, Open Approach
0P9P30Z	Drainage of Right Metacarpal with Drainage Device, Percutaneous Approach
0P9P3ZX	Drainage of Right Metacarpal, Percutaneous Approach, Diagnostic
0P9P3ZZ	Drainage of Right Metacarpal, Percutaneous Approach
0P9P40Z	Drainage of Right Metacarpal with Drainage Device, Percutaneous Endoscopic Approach
0P9P4ZX	Drainage of Right Metacarpal, Percutaneous Endoscopic Approach, Diagnostic
0P9P4ZZ	Drainage of Right Metacarpal, Percutaneous Endoscopic Approach
0P9Q00Z	Drainage of Left Metacarpal with Drainage Device, Open Approach
0P9Q0ZX	Drainage of Left Metacarpal, Open Approach, Diagnostic
0P9Q0ZZ	Drainage of Left Metacarpal, Open Approach
0P9Q30Z	Drainage of Left Metacarpal with Drainage Device, Percutaneous Approach
0P9Q3ZX	Drainage of Left Metacarpal, Percutaneous Approach, Diagnostic
0P9Q3ZZ	Drainage of Left Metacarpal, Percutaneous Approach
0P9Q40Z	Drainage of Left Metacarpal with Drainage Device, Percutaneous Endoscopic Approach
0P9Q4ZX	Drainage of Left Metacarpal, Percutaneous Endoscopic Approach, Diagnostic
0P9Q4ZZ	Drainage of Left Metacarpal, Percutaneous Endoscopic Approach
0P9R00Z	Drainage of Right Thumb Phalanx with Drainage Device, Open Approach
0P9R0ZX	Drainage of Right Thumb Phalanx, Open Approach, Diagnostic
0P9R0ZZ	Drainage of Right Thumb Phalanx, Open Approach
0P9R30Z	Drainage of Right Thumb Phalanx with Drainage Device, Percutaneous Approach
0P9R3ZX	Drainage of Right Thumb Phalanx, Percutaneous Approach, Diagnostic
0P9R3ZZ	Drainage of Right Thumb Phalanx, Percutaneous Approach
0P9R40Z	Drainage of Right Thumb Phalanx with Drainage Device, Percutaneous Endoscopic Approach
0P9R4ZX	Drainage of Right Thumb Phalanx, Percutaneous Endoscopic Approach, Diagnostic
0P9R4ZZ	Drainage of Right Thumb Phalanx, Percutaneous Endoscopic Approach
0P9S00Z	Drainage of Left Thumb Phalanx with Drainage Device, Open Approach
0P9S0ZX	Drainage of Left Thumb Phalanx, Open Approach, Diagnostic
0P9S0ZZ	Drainage of Left Thumb Phalanx, Open Approach
0P9S30Z	Drainage of Left Thumb Phalanx with Drainage Device, Percutaneous Approach
0P9S3ZX	Drainage of Left Thumb Phalanx, Percutaneous Approach, Diagnostic
0P9S3ZZ	Drainage of Left Thumb Phalanx, Percutaneous Approach
0P9S40Z	Drainage of Left Thumb Phalanx with Drainage Device, Percutaneous Endoscopic Approach
0P9S4ZX	Drainage of Left Thumb Phalanx, Percutaneous Endoscopic Approach, Diagnostic
0P9S4ZZ	Drainage of Left Thumb Phalanx, Percutaneous Endoscopic Approach
0P9T00Z	Drainage of Right Finger Phalanx with Drainage Device, Open Approach
0P9T0ZX	Drainage of Right Finger Phalanx, Open Approach, Diagnostic
0P9T0ZZ	Drainage of Right Finger Phalanx, Open Approach
0P9T30Z	Drainage of Right Finger Phalanx with Drainage Device, Percutaneous Approach
0P9T3ZX	Drainage of Right Finger Phalanx, Percutaneous Approach, Diagnostic
0P9T3ZZ	Drainage of Right Finger Phalanx, Percutaneous Approach
0P9T40Z	Drainage of Right Finger Phalanx with Drainage Device, Percutaneous Endoscopic Approach
0P9T4ZX	Drainage of Right Finger Phalanx, Percutaneous Endoscopic Approach, Diagnostic
0P9T4ZZ	Drainage of Right Finger Phalanx, Percutaneous Endoscopic Approach
0P9V00Z	Drainage of Left Finger Phalanx with Drainage Device, Open Approach
0P9V0ZX	Drainage of Left Finger Phalanx, Open Approach, Diagnostic
0P9V0ZZ	Drainage of Left Finger Phalanx, Open Approach
0P9V30Z	Drainage of Left Finger Phalanx with Drainage Device, Percutaneous Approach
0P9V3ZX	Drainage of Left Finger Phalanx, Percutaneous Approach, Diagnostic
0P9V3ZZ	Drainage of Left Finger Phalanx, Percutaneous Approach
0P9V40Z	Drainage of Left Finger Phalanx with Drainage Device, Percutaneous Endoscopic Approach
0P9V4ZX	Drainage of Left Finger Phalanx, Percutaneous Endoscopic Approach, Diagnostic
0P9V4ZZ	Drainage of Left Finger Phalanx, Percutaneous Endoscopic Approach

0PB – Upper Bones, Excision

Review Coding Guideline B3.5

Review Coding Guidelines B3.4a and B3.4b

Review Coding Guideline B3.8

Review Coding Guideline B3.18

0PB00ZX	Excision of Sternum, Open Approach, Diagnostic
0PB00ZZ	Excision of Sternum, Open Approach
0PB03ZX	Excision of Sternum, Percutaneous Approach, Diagnostic
0PB03ZZ	Excision of Sternum, Percutaneous Approach
0PB04ZX	Excision of Sternum, Percutaneous Endoscopic Approach, Diagnostic
0PB04ZZ	Excision of Sternum, Percutaneous Endoscopic Approach
0PB10ZX	Excision of I to 2 Ribs, Open Approach, Diagnostic
0PB10ZZ	Excision of I to 2 Ribs, Open Approach
	AHA CC: 4Q, 2012, 101-102; 4Q, 2013, 109-111
0PB13ZX	Excision of I to 2 Ribs, Percutaneous Approach, Diagnostic
0PB13ZZ	Excision of I to 2 Ribs, Percutaneous Approach
0PB14ZX	Excision of I to 2 Ribs, Percutaneous Endoscopic Approach, Diagnostic
0PB14ZZ	Excision of I to 2 Ribs, Percutaneous Endoscopic Approach
0PB20ZX	Excision of 3 or More Ribs, Open Approach, Diagnostic
0PB20ZZ	Excision of 3 or More Ribs, Open Approach
	AHA CC: 4Q, 2013, 109-111
0PB23ZX	Excision of 3 or More Ribs, Percutaneous Approach, Diagnostic
0PB23ZZ	Excision of 3 or More Ribs, Percutaneous Approach
0PB24ZX	Excision of 3 or More Ribs, Percutaneous Endoscopic Approach, Diagnostic
0PB24ZZ	Excision of 3 or More Ribs, Percutaneous Endoscopic Approach
0PB30ZX	Excision of Cervical Vertebra, Open Approach, Diagnostic
0PB30ZZ	Excision of Cervical Vertebra, Open Approach
0PB33ZX	Excision of Cervical Vertebra, Percutaneous Approach, Diagnostic
0PB33ZZ	Excision of Cervical Vertebra, Percutaneous Approach
0PB34ZX	Excision of Cervical Vertebra, Percutaneous Endoscopic Approach, Diagnostic
0PB34ZZ	Excision of Cervical Vertebra, Percutaneous Endoscopic Approach
0PB40ZX	Excision of Thoracic Vertebra, Open Approach, Diagnostic
0PB40ZZ	Excision of Thoracic Vertebra, Open Approach
0PB43ZX	Excision of Thoracic Vertebra, Percutaneous Approach, Diagnostic

♀ Female-only   ♂ Male-only   ▲ Limited Coverage   ● Non-OR   ▦ HAC-associated procedure   ▲ Non-covered procedures   ✚ Cluster

0PB43ZZ Excision of Thoracic Vertebra, Percutaneous Approach

0PB44ZX Excision of Thoracic Vertebra, Percutaneous Endoscopic Approach, Diagnostic

0PB44ZZ Excision of Thoracic Vertebra, Percutaneous Endoscopic Approach

0PB50ZX Excision of Right Scapula, Open Approach, Diagnostic

0PB50ZZ Excision of Right Scapula, Open Approach

0PB53ZX Excision of Right Scapula, Percutaneous Approach, Diagnostic

0PB53ZZ Excision of Right Scapula, Percutaneous Approach

0PB54ZX Excision of Right Scapula, Percutaneous Endoscopic Approach, Diagnostic

0PB54ZZ Excision of Right Scapula, Percutaneous Endoscopic Approach
AHA CC: 3Q, 2013, 20-22

0PB60ZX Excision of Left Scapula, Open Approach, Diagnostic

0PB60ZZ Excision of Left Scapula, Open Approach

0PB63ZX Excision of Left Scapula, Percutaneous Approach, Diagnostic

0PB63ZZ Excision of Left Scapula, Percutaneous Approach

0PB64ZX Excision of Left Scapula, Percutaneous Endoscopic Approach, Diagnostic

0PB64ZZ Excision of Left Scapula, Percutaneous Endoscopic Approach

0PB70ZX Excision of Right Glenoid Cavity, Open Approach, Diagnostic

0PB70ZZ Excision of Right Glenoid Cavity, Open Approach

0PB73ZX Excision of Right Glenoid Cavity, Percutaneous Approach, Diagnostic

0PB73ZZ Excision of Right Glenoid Cavity, Percutaneous Approach

0PB74ZX Excision of Right Glenoid Cavity, Percutaneous Endoscopic Approach, Diagnostic

0PB74ZZ Excision of Right Glenoid Cavity, Percutaneous Endoscopic Approach

0PB80ZX Excision of Left Glenoid Cavity, Open Approach, Diagnostic

0PB80ZZ Excision of Left Glenoid Cavity, Open Approach

0PB83ZX Excision of Left Glenoid Cavity, Percutaneous Approach, Diagnostic

0PB83ZZ Excision of Left Glenoid Cavity, Percutaneous Approach

0PB84ZX Excision of Left Glenoid Cavity, Percutaneous Endoscopic Approach, Diagnostic

0PB84ZZ Excision of Left Glenoid Cavity, Percutaneous Endoscopic Approach

0PB90ZX Excision of Right Clavicle, Open Approach, Diagnostic

0PB90ZZ Excision of Right Clavicle, Open Approach

0PB93ZX Excision of Right Clavicle, Percutaneous Approach, Diagnostic

0PB93ZZ Excision of Right Clavicle, Percutaneous Approach

0PB94ZX Excision of Right Clavicle, Percutaneous Endoscopic Approach, Diagnostic

0PB94ZZ Excision of Right Clavicle, Percutaneous Endoscopic Approach

0PBB0ZX Excision of Left Clavicle, Open Approach, Diagnostic

0PBB0ZZ Excision of Left Clavicle, Open Approach

0PBB3ZX Excision of Left Clavicle, Percutaneous Approach, Diagnostic

0PBB3ZZ Excision of Left Clavicle, Percutaneous Approach

0PBB4ZX Excision of Left Clavicle, Percutaneous Endoscopic Approach, Diagnostic

0PBB4ZZ Excision of Left Clavicle, Percutaneous Endoscopic Approach

0PBC0ZX Excision of Right Humeral Head, Open Approach, Diagnostic

0PBC0ZZ Excision of Right Humeral Head, Open Approach

0PBC3ZX Excision of Right Humeral Head, Percutaneous Approach, Diagnostic

0PBC3ZZ Excision of Right Humeral Head, Percutaneous Approach

0PBC4ZX Excision of Right Humeral Head, Percutaneous Endoscopic Approach, Diagnostic

0PBC4ZZ Excision of Right Humeral Head, Percutaneous Endoscopic Approach

0PBD0ZX Excision of Left Humeral Head, Open Approach, Diagnostic

0PBD0ZZ Excision of Left Humeral Head, Open Approach

0PBD3ZX Excision of Left Humeral Head, Percutaneous Approach, Diagnostic

0PBD3ZZ Excision of Left Humeral Head, Percutaneous Approach

0PBD4ZX Excision of Left Humeral Head, Percutaneous Endoscopic Approach, Diagnostic

0PBD4ZZ Excision of Left Humeral Head, Percutaneous Endoscopic Approach

0PBF0ZX Excision of Right Humeral Shaft, Open Approach, Diagnostic

0PBF0ZZ Excision of Right Humeral Shaft, Open Approach

0PBF3ZX Excision of Right Humeral Shaft, Percutaneous Approach, Diagnostic

0PBF3ZZ Excision of Right Humeral Shaft, Percutaneous Approach

0PBF4ZX Excision of Right Humeral Shaft, Percutaneous Endoscopic Approach, Diagnostic

0PBF4ZZ Excision of Right Humeral Shaft, Percutaneous Endoscopic Approach

0PBG0ZX Excision of Left Humeral Shaft, Open Approach, Diagnostic

0PBG0ZZ Excision of Left Humeral Shaft, Open Approach

0PBG3ZX Excision of Left Humeral Shaft, Percutaneous Approach, Diagnostic

0PBG3ZZ Excision of Left Humeral Shaft, Percutaneous Approach

0PBG4ZX Excision of Left Humeral Shaft, Percutaneous Endoscopic Approach, Diagnostic

0PBG4ZZ Excision of Left Humeral Shaft, Percutaneous Endoscopic Approach

0PBH0ZX Excision of Right Radius, Open Approach, Diagnostic

0PBH0ZZ Excision of Right Radius, Open Approach

0PBH3ZX Excision of Right Radius, Percutaneous Approach, Diagnostic

0PBH3ZZ Excision of Right Radius, Percutaneous Approach

0PBH4ZX Excision of Right Radius, Percutaneous Endoscopic Approach, Diagnostic

0PBH4ZZ Excision of Right Radius, Percutaneous Endoscopic Approach

0PBJ0ZX Excision of Left Radius, Open Approach, Diagnostic

0PBJ0ZZ Excision of Left Radius, Open Approach

0PBJ3ZX Excision of Left Radius, Percutaneous Approach, Diagnostic

0PBJ3ZZ Excision of Left Radius, Percutaneous Approach

0PBJ4ZX Excision of Left Radius, Percutaneous Endoscopic Approach, Diagnostic

0PBJ4ZZ Excision of Left Radius, Percutaneous Endoscopic Approach

0PBK0ZX Excision of Right Ulna, Open Approach, Diagnostic

0PBK0ZZ Excision of Right Ulna, Open Approach

0PBK3ZX Excision of Right Ulna, Percutaneous Approach, Diagnostic

0PBK3ZZ Excision of Right Ulna, Percutaneous Approach

0PBK4ZX Excision of Right Ulna, Percutaneous Endoscopic Approach, Diagnostic

0PBK4ZZ Excision of Right Ulna, Percutaneous Endoscopic Approach

0PBL0ZX Excision of Left Ulna, Open Approach, Diagnostic

0PBL0ZZ Excision of Left Ulna, Open Approach

0PBL3ZX Excision of Left Ulna, Percutaneous Approach, Diagnostic

0PBL3ZZ Excision of Left Ulna, Percutaneous Approach

0PBL4ZX Excision of Left Ulna, Percutaneous Endoscopic Approach, Diagnostic

0PBL4ZZ Excision of Left Ulna, Percutaneous Endoscopic Approach

0PBM0ZX Excision of Right Carpal, Open Approach, Diagnostic

0PBM0ZZ Excision of Right Carpal, Open Approach

0PBM3ZX Excision of Right Carpal, Percutaneous Approach, Diagnostic

0PBM3ZZ Excision of Right Carpal, Percutaneous Approach

0PBM4ZX Excision of Right Carpal, Percutaneous Endoscopic Approach, Diagnostic

0PBM4ZZ Excision of Right Carpal, Percutaneous Endoscopic Approach

0PBN0ZX Excision of Left Carpal, Open Approach, Diagnostic

0PBN0ZZ Excision of Left Carpal, Open Approach

0PBN3ZX Excision of Left Carpal, Percutaneous Approach, Diagnostic

0PBN3ZZ Excision of Left Carpal, Percutaneous Approach

0PBN4ZX Excision of Left Carpal, Percutaneous Endoscopic Approach, Diagnostic

0PBN4ZZ Excision of Left Carpal, Percutaneous Endoscopic Approach

0PBP0ZX Excision of Right Metacarpal, Open Approach, Diagnostic

0PBP0ZZ Excision of Right Metacarpal, Open Approach

0PBP3ZX Excision of Right Metacarpal, Percutaneous Approach, Diagnostic

0PBP3ZZ Excision of Right Metacarpal, Percutaneous Approach

0PBP4ZX Excision of Right Metacarpal, Percutaneous Endoscopic Approach, Diagnostic

0PBP4ZZ Excision of Right Metacarpal, Percutaneous Endoscopic Approach

0PBQ0ZX Excision of Left Metacarpal, Open Approach, Diagnostic

0PBQ0ZZ Excision of Left Metacarpal, Open Approach

0PBQ3ZX Excision of Left Metacarpal, Percutaneous Approach, Diagnostic

0PBQ3ZZ Excision of Left Metacarpal, Percutaneous Approach

0PBQ4ZX Excision of Left Metacarpal, Percutaneous Endoscopic Approach, Diagnostic

0PBQ4ZZ Excision of Left Metacarpal, Percutaneous Endoscopic Approach

0PBR0ZX Excision of Right Thumb Phalanx, Open Approach, Diagnostic

0PBR0ZZ Excision of Right Thumb Phalanx, Open Approach

0PBR3ZX Excision of Right Thumb Phalanx, Percutaneous Approach, Diagnostic

0PBR3ZZ Excision of Right Thumb Phalanx, Percutaneous Approach

0PBR4ZX Excision of Right Thumb Phalanx, Percutaneous Endoscopic Approach, Diagnostic

0PBR4ZZ Excision of Right Thumb Phalanx, Percutaneous Endoscopic Approach

0PBS0ZX Excision of Left Thumb Phalanx, Open Approach, Diagnostic

0PBS0ZZ Excision of Left Thumb Phalanx, Open Approach

0PBS3ZX Excision of Left Thumb Phalanx, Percutaneous Approach, Diagnostic

0PBS3ZZ Excision of Left Thumb Phalanx, Percutaneous Approach

0PBS4ZX Excision of Left Thumb Phalanx, Percutaneous Endoscopic Approach, Diagnostic

0PBS4ZZ Excision of Left Thumb Phalanx, Percutaneous Endoscopic Approach

0PBT0ZX Excision of Right Finger Phalanx, Open Approach, Diagnostic

0PBT0ZZ Excision of Right Finger Phalanx, Open Approach

0PBT3ZX Excision of Right Finger Phalanx, Percutaneous Approach, Diagnostic

0PBT3ZZ Excision of Right Finger Phalanx, Percutaneous Approach

0PBT4ZX Excision of Right Finger Phalanx, Percutaneous Endoscopic Approach, Diagnostic

0PBT4ZZ Excision of Right Finger Phalanx, Percutaneous Endoscopic Approach

0PBV0ZX Excision of Left Finger Phalanx, Open Approach, Diagnostic

0PBV0ZZ Excision of Left Finger Phalanx, Open Approach

0PBV3ZX Excision of Left Finger Phalanx, Percutaneous Approach, Diagnostic

0PBV3ZZ Excision of Left Finger Phalanx, Percutaneous Approach

0PBV4ZX Excision of Left Finger Phalanx, Percutaneous Endoscopic Approach, Diagnostic

0PBV4ZZ Excision of Left Finger Phalanx, Percutaneous Endoscopic Approach

0PC – Upper Bones, Extirpation

0PC00ZZ Extirpation of Matter from Sternum, Open Approach
AHA CC: 3Q, 2019, 19

0PC03ZZ Extirpation of Matter from Sternum, Percutaneous Approach

0PC04ZZ Extirpation of Matter from Sternum, Percutaneous Endoscopic Approach

0PC10ZZ Extirpation of Matter from I to 2 Ribs, Open Approach

0PC13ZZ Extirpation of Matter from I to 2 Ribs, Percutaneous Approach

0PC14ZZ Extirpation of Matter from I to 2 Ribs, Percutaneous Endoscopic Approach

0PC20ZZ Extirpation of Matter from 3 or More Ribs, Open Approach

0PC23ZZ Extirpation of Matter from 3 or More Ribs, Percutaneous Approach

0PC24ZZ Extirpation of Matter from 3 or More Ribs, Percutaneous Endoscopic Approach

0PC30ZZ Extirpation of Matter from Cervical Vertebra, Open Approach

0PC33ZZ Extirpation of Matter from Cervical Vertebra, Percutaneous Approach

0PC34ZZ Extirpation of Matter from Cervical Vertebra, Percutaneous Endoscopic Approach

0PC40ZZ Extirpation of Matter from Thoracic Vertebra, Open Approach

0PC43ZZ Extirpation of Matter from Thoracic Vertebra, Percutaneous Approach

0PC44ZZ Extirpation of Matter from Thoracic Vertebra, Percutaneous Endoscopic Approach

0PC50ZZ Extirpation of Matter from Right Scapula, Open Approach

0PC53ZZ Extirpation of Matter from Right Scapula, Percutaneous Approach

0PC54ZZ Extirpation of Matter from Right Scapula, Percutaneous Endoscopic Approach

0PC60ZZ Extirpation of Matter from Left Scapula, Open Approach

0PC63ZZ Extirpation of Matter from Left Scapula, Percutaneous Approach

0PC64ZZ Extirpation of Matter from Left Scapula, Percutaneous Endoscopic Approach

0PC70ZZ Extirpation of Matter from Right Glenoid Cavity, Open Approach

0PC73ZZ Extirpation of Matter from Right Glenoid Cavity, Percutaneous Approach

0PC74ZZ Extirpation of Matter from Right Glenoid Cavity, Percutaneous Endoscopic Approach

0PC80ZZ Extirpation of Matter from Left Glenoid Cavity, Open Approach

0PC83ZZ Extirpation of Matter from Left Glenoid Cavity, Percutaneous Approach

0PC84ZZ Extirpation of Matter from Left Glenoid Cavity, Percutaneous Endoscopic Approach

0PC90ZZ Extirpation of Matter from Right Clavicle, Open Approach

0PC93ZZ Extirpation of Matter from Right Clavicle, Percutaneous Approach

0PC94ZZ Extirpation of Matter from Right Clavicle, Percutaneous Endoscopic Approach

0PCB0ZZ Extirpation of Matter from Left Clavicle, Open Approach

0PCB3ZZ Extirpation of Matter from Left Clavicle, Percutaneous Approach

0PCB4ZZ Extirpation of Matter from Left Clavicle, Percutaneous Endoscopic Approach

0PCC0ZZ Extirpation of Matter from Right Humeral Head, Open Approach

0PCC3ZZ Extirpation of Matter from Right Humeral Head, Percutaneous Approach

0PCC4ZZ Extirpation of Matter from Right Humeral Head, Percutaneous Endoscopic Approach

0PCD0ZZ Extirpation of Matter from Left Humeral Head, Open Approach

0PCD3ZZ Extirpation of Matter from Left Humeral Head, Percutaneous Approach

0PCD4ZZ Extirpation of Matter from Left Humeral Head, Percutaneous Endoscopic Approach

0PCF0ZZ Extirpation of Matter from Right Humeral Shaft, Open Approach

0PCF3ZZ Extirpation of Matter from Right Humeral Shaft, Percutaneous Approach

0PCF4ZZ Extirpation of Matter from Right Humeral Shaft, Percutaneous Endoscopic Approach

0PCG0ZZ Extirpation of Matter from Left Humeral Shaft, Open Approach

0PCG3ZZ Extirpation of Matter from Left Humeral Shaft, Percutaneous Approach

0PCG4ZZ Extirpation of Matter from Left Humeral Shaft, Percutaneous Endoscopic Approach

0PCH0ZZ Extirpation of Matter from Right Radius, Open Approach

0PCH3ZZ Extirpation of Matter from Right Radius, Percutaneous Approach

0PCH4ZZ Extirpation of Matter from Right Radius, Percutaneous Endoscopic Approach

0PCJ0ZZ Extirpation of Matter from Left Radius, Open Approach

0PCJ3ZZ Extirpation of Matter from Left Radius, Percutaneous Approach

0PCJ4ZZ Extirpation of Matter from Left Radius, Percutaneous Endoscopic Approach

0PCK0ZZ Extirpation of Matter from Right Ulna, Open Approach

0PCK3ZZ Extirpation of Matter from Right Ulna, Percutaneous Approach

0PCK4ZZ Extirpation of Matter from Right Ulna, Percutaneous Endoscopic Approach

0PCL0ZZ Extirpation of Matter from Left Ulna, Open Approach

0PCL3ZZ Extirpation of Matter from Left Ulna, Percutaneous Approach

0PCL4ZZ Extirpation of Matter from Left Ulna, Percutaneous Endoscopic Approach

0PCM0ZZ Extirpation of Matter from Right Carpal, Open Approach

0PCM3ZZ Extirpation of Matter from Right Carpal, Percutaneous Approach

0PCM4ZZ Extirpation of Matter from Right Carpal, Percutaneous Endoscopic Approach

0PCN0ZZ Extirpation of Matter from Left Carpal, Open Approach

0PCN3ZZ Extirpation of Matter from Left Carpal, Percutaneous Approach

0PCN4ZZ Extirpation of Matter from Left Carpal, Percutaneous Endoscopic Approach

0PCP0ZZ Extirpation of Matter from Right Metacarpal, Open Approach

0PCP3ZZ Extirpation of Matter from Right Metacarpal, Percutaneous Approach

0PCP4ZZ Extirpation of Matter from Right Metacarpal, Percutaneous Endoscopic Approach

0PCQ0ZZ Extirpation of Matter from Left Metacarpal, Open Approach

0PCQ3ZZ Extirpation of Matter from Left Metacarpal, Percutaneous Approach

0PCQ4ZZ Extirpation of Matter from Left Metacarpal, Percutaneous Endoscopic Approach

0PCR0ZZ Extirpation of Matter from Right Thumb Phalanx, Open Approach

0PCR3ZZ Extirpation of Matter from Right Thumb Phalanx, Percutaneous Approach

0PCR4ZZ Extirpation of Matter from Right Thumb Phalanx, Percutaneous Endoscopic Approach

0PCS0ZZ Extirpation of Matter from Left Thumb Phalanx, Open Approach

0PCS3ZZ Extirpation of Matter from Left Thumb Phalanx, Percutaneous Approach
0PCS4ZZ Extirpation of Matter from Left Thumb Phalanx, Percutaneous Endoscopic Approach
0PCT0ZZ Extirpation of Matter from Right Finger Phalanx, Open Approach

0PCT3ZZ Extirpation of Matter from Right Finger Phalanx, Percutaneous Approach
0PCT4ZZ Extirpation of Matter from Right Finger Phalanx, Percutaneous Endoscopic Approach
0PCV0ZZ Extirpation of Matter from Left Finger Phalanx, Open Approach

0PCV3ZZ Extirpation of Matter from Left Finger Phalanx, Percutaneous Approach
0PCV4ZZ Extirpation of Matter from Left Finger Phalanx, Percutaneous Endoscopic Approach

0PD – Upper Bones, Extraction

0PD00ZZ Extraction of Sternum, Open Approach
0PD10ZZ Extraction of 1 to 2 Ribs, Open Approach
0PD20ZZ Extraction of 3 or More Ribs, Open Approach
0PD30ZZ Extraction of Cervical Vertebra, Open Approach
0PD40ZZ Extraction of Thoracic Vertebra, Open Approach
0PD50ZZ Extraction of Right Scapula, Open Approach
0PD60ZZ Extraction of Left Scapula, Open Approach
0PD70ZZ Extraction of Right Glenoid Cavity, Open Approach
0PD80ZZ Extraction of Left Glenoid Cavity, Open Approach

0PD90ZZ Extraction of Right Clavicle, Open Approach
0PDB0ZZ Extraction of Left Clavicle, Open Approach
0PDC0ZZ Extraction of Right Humeral Head, Open Approach
0PDD0ZZ Extraction of Left Humeral Head, Open Approach
0PDF0ZZ Extraction of Right Humeral Shaft, Open Approach
0PDG0ZZ Extraction of Left Humeral Shaft, Open Approach
0PDH0ZZ Extraction of Right Radius, Open Approach
0PDJ0ZZ Extraction of Left Radius, Open Approach
0PDK0ZZ Extraction of Right Ulna, Open Approach

0PDL0ZZ Extraction of Left Ulna, Open Approach
0PDM0ZZ Extraction of Right Carpal, Open Approach
0PDN0ZZ Extraction of Left Carpal, Open Approach
0PDP0ZZ Extraction of Right Metacarpal, Open Approach
0PDQ0ZZ Extraction of Left Metacarpal, Open Approach
0PDR0ZZ Extraction of Right Thumb Phalanx, Open Approach
0PDS0ZZ Extraction of Left Thumb Phalanx, Open Approach
0PDT0ZZ Extraction of Right Finger Phalanx, Open Approach
0PDV0ZZ Extraction of Left Finger Phalanx, Open Approach

0PH – Upper Bones, Insertion

0PH000Z Insertion of Rigid Plate Internal Fixation Device into Sternum, Open Approach
AHA CC: 1Q, 2020, 29-30
0PH004Z Insertion of Internal Fixation Device into Sternum, Open Approach
0PH030Z Insertion of Rigid Plate Internal Fixation Device into Sternum, Percutaneous Approach
0PH034Z Insertion of Internal Fixation Device into Sternum, Percutaneous Approach
AHA CC: 2Q, 2017, 23-24; 2Q, 2019, 40
0PH040Z Insertion of Rigid Plate Internal Fixation Device into Sternum, Percutaneous Endoscopic Approach
0PH044Z Insertion of Internal Fixation Device into Sternum, Percutaneous Endoscopic Approach
0PH104Z Insertion of Internal Fixation Device into I to 2 Ribs, Open Approach
0PH134Z Insertion of Internal Fixation Device into I to 2 Ribs, Percutaneous Approach
0PH144Z Insertion of Internal Fixation Device into I to 2 Ribs, Percutaneous Endoscopic Approach
0PH204Z Insertion of Internal Fixation Device into 3 or More Ribs, Open Approach
0PH234Z Insertion of Internal Fixation Device into 3 or More Ribs, Percutaneous Approach
0PH244Z Insertion of Internal Fixation Device into 3 or More Ribs, Percutaneous Endoscopic Approach
0PH304Z Insertion of Internal Fixation Device into Cervical Vertebra, Open Approach
0PH334Z Insertion of Internal Fixation Device into Cervical Vertebra, Percutaneous Approach
0PH344Z Insertion of Internal Fixation Device into Cervical Vertebra, Percutaneous Endoscopic Approach
0PH404Z Insertion of Internal Fixation Device into Thoracic Vertebra, Open Approach
AHA CC: 4Q, 2014, 28-29
0PH434Z Insertion of Internal Fixation Device into Thoracic Vertebra, Percutaneous Approach

0PH444Z Insertion of Internal Fixation Device into Thoracic Vertebra, Percutaneous Endoscopic Approach
0PH504Z Insertion of Internal Fixation Device into Right Scapula, Open Approach
AHA CC: 4Q, 2018, 12-13
0PH534Z Insertion of Internal Fixation Device into Right Scapula, Percutaneous Approach
0PH544Z Insertion of Internal Fixation Device into Right Scapula, Percutaneous Endoscopic Approach
0PH604Z Insertion of Internal Fixation Device into Left Scapula, Open Approach
0PH634Z Insertion of Internal Fixation Device into Left Scapula, Percutaneous Approach
0PH644Z Insertion of Internal Fixation Device into Left Scapula, Percutaneous Endoscopic Approach
0PH704Z Insertion of Internal Fixation Device into Right Glenoid Cavity, Open Approach
0PH734Z Insertion of Internal Fixation Device into Right Glenoid Cavity, Percutaneous Approach
0PH744Z Insertion of Internal Fixation Device into Right Glenoid Cavity, Percutaneous Endoscopic Approach
0PH804Z Insertion of Internal Fixation Device into Left Glenoid Cavity, Open Approach
0PH834Z Insertion of Internal Fixation Device into Left Glenoid Cavity, Percutaneous Approach
0PH844Z Insertion of Internal Fixation Device into Left Glenoid Cavity, Percutaneous Endoscopic Approach
0PH904Z Insertion of Internal Fixation Device into Right Clavicle, Open Approach
0PH934Z Insertion of Internal Fixation Device into Right Clavicle, Percutaneous Approach
0PH944Z Insertion of Internal Fixation Device into Right Clavicle, Percutaneous Endoscopic Approach

0PHB04Z Insertion of Internal Fixation Device into Left Clavicle, Open Approach
0PHB34Z Insertion of Internal Fixation Device into Left Clavicle, Percutaneous Approach
0PHB44Z Insertion of Internal Fixation Device into Left Clavicle, Percutaneous Endoscopic Approach
0PHC04Z Insertion of Internal Fixation Device into Right Humeral Head, Open Approach
0PHC05Z Insertion of External Fixation Device into Right Humeral Head, Open Approach
0PHC06Z Insertion of Intramedullary Internal Fixation Device into Right Humeral Head, Open Approach
0PHC08Z Insertion of Limb Lengthening External Fixation Device into Right Humeral Head, Open Approach
0PHC0BZ Insertion of Monoplanar External Fixation Device into Right Humeral Head, Open Approach
0PHC0CZ Insertion of Ring External Fixation Device into Right Humeral Head, Open Approach
0PHC0DZ Insertion of Hybrid External Fixation Device into Right Humeral Head, Open Approach
0PHC34Z Insertion of Internal Fixation Device into Right Humeral Head, Percutaneous Approach
0PHC35Z Insertion of External Fixation Device into Right Humeral Head, Percutaneous Approach
0PHC36Z Insertion of Intramedullary Internal Fixation Device into Right Humeral Head, Percutaneous Approach
0PHC38Z Insertion of Limb Lengthening External Fixation Device into Right Humeral Head, Percutaneous Approach
0PHC3BZ Insertion of Monoplanar External Fixation Device into Right Humeral Head, Percutaneous Approach
0PHC3CZ Insertion of Ring External Fixation Device into Right Humeral Head, Percutaneous Approach

0PHC3DZ Insertion of Hybrid External Fixation Device into Right Humeral Head, Percutaneous Approach

0PHC44Z Insertion of Internal Fixation Device into Right Humeral Head, Percutaneous Endoscopic Approach

0PHC45Z Insertion of External Fixation Device into Right Humeral Head, Percutaneous Endoscopic Approach

0PHC46Z Insertion of Intramedullary Internal Fixation Device into Right Humeral Head, Percutaneous Endoscopic Approach

0PHC48Z Insertion of Limb Lengthening External Fixation Device into Right Humeral Head, Percutaneous Endoscopic Approach

0PHC4BZ Insertion of Monoplanar External Fixation Device into Right Humeral Head, Percutaneous Endoscopic Approach

0PHC4CZ Insertion of Ring External Fixation Device into Right Humeral Head, Percutaneous Endoscopic Approach

0PHC4DZ Insertion of Hybrid External Fixation Device into Right Humeral Head, Percutaneous Endoscopic Approach

0PHD04Z Insertion of Internal Fixation Device into Left Humeral Head, Open Approach

0PHD05Z Insertion of External Fixation Device into Left Humeral Head, Open Approach

0PHD06Z Insertion of Intramedullary Internal Fixation Device into Left Humeral Head, Open Approach

0PHD08Z Insertion of Limb Lengthening External Fixation Device into Left Humeral Head, Open Approach

0PHD0BZ Insertion of Monoplanar External Fixation Device into Left Humeral Head, Open Approach

0PHD0CZ Insertion of Ring External Fixation Device into Left Humeral Head, Open Approach

0PHD0DZ Insertion of Hybrid External Fixation Device into Left Humeral Head, Open Approach

0PHD34Z Insertion of Internal Fixation Device into Left Humeral Head, Percutaneous Approach

0PHD35Z Insertion of External Fixation Device into Left Humeral Head, Percutaneous Approach

0PHD36Z Insertion of Intramedullary Internal Fixation Device into Left Humeral Head, Percutaneous Approach

0PHD38Z Insertion of Limb Lengthening External Fixation Device into Left Humeral Head, Percutaneous Approach

0PHD3BZ Insertion of Monoplanar External Fixation Device into Left Humeral Head, Percutaneous Approach

0PHD3CZ Insertion of Ring External Fixation Device into Left Humeral Head, Percutaneous Approach

0PHD3DZ Insertion of Hybrid External Fixation Device into Left Humeral Head, Percutaneous Approach

0PHD44Z Insertion of Internal Fixation Device into Left Humeral Head, Percutaneous Endoscopic Approach

0PHD45Z Insertion of External Fixation Device into Left Humeral Head, Percutaneous Endoscopic Approach

0PHD46Z Insertion of Intramedullary Internal Fixation Device into Left Humeral Head, Percutaneous Endoscopic Approach

0PHD48Z Insertion of Limb Lengthening External Fixation Device into Left Humeral Head, Percutaneous Endoscopic Approach

0PHD4BZ Insertion of Monoplanar External Fixation Device into Left Humeral Head, Percutaneous Endoscopic Approach

0PHD4CZ Insertion of Ring External Fixation Device into Left Humeral Head, Percutaneous Endoscopic Approach

0PHD4DZ Insertion of Hybrid External Fixation Device into Left Humeral Head, Percutaneous Endoscopic Approach

0PHF04Z Insertion of Internal Fixation Device into Right Humeral Shaft, Open Approach

0PHF05Z Insertion of External Fixation Device into Right Humeral Shaft, Open Approach

0PHF06Z Insertion of Intramedullary Internal Fixation Device into Right Humeral Shaft, Open Approach

0PHF07Z Insertion of Intramedullary Limb Lengthening Internal Fixation Device into Right Humeral Shaft, Open Approach

0PHF08Z Insertion of Limb Lengthening External Fixation Device into Right Humeral Shaft, Open Approach

0PHF0BZ Insertion of Monoplanar External Fixation Device into Right Humeral Shaft, Open Approach

0PHF0CZ Insertion of Ring External Fixation Device into Right Humeral Shaft, Open Approach

0PHF0DZ Insertion of Hybrid External Fixation Device into Right Humeral Shaft, Open Approach

0PHF34Z Insertion of Internal Fixation Device into Right Humeral Shaft, Percutaneous Approach

0PHF35Z Insertion of External Fixation Device into Right Humeral Shaft, Percutaneous Approach

0PHF36Z Insertion of Intramedullary Internal Fixation Device into Right Humeral Shaft, Percutaneous Approach

0PHF37Z Insertion of Intramedullary Limb Lengthening Internal Fixation Device into Right Humeral Shaft, Percutaneous Approach

0PHF38Z Insertion of Limb Lengthening External Fixation Device into Right Humeral Shaft, Percutaneous Approach

0PHF3BZ Insertion of Monoplanar External Fixation Device into Right Humeral Shaft, Percutaneous Approach

0PHF3CZ Insertion of Ring External Fixation Device into Right Humeral Shaft, Percutaneous Approach

0PHF3DZ Insertion of Hybrid External Fixation Device into Right Humeral Shaft, Percutaneous Approach

0PHF44Z Insertion of Internal Fixation Device into Right Humeral Shaft, Percutaneous Endoscopic Approach

0PHF45Z Insertion of External Fixation Device into Right Humeral Shaft, Percutaneous Endoscopic Approach

0PHF46Z Insertion of Intramedullary Internal Fixation Device into Right Humeral Shaft, Percutaneous Endoscopic Approach

0PHF47Z Insertion of Intramedullary Limb Lengthening Internal Fixation Device into Right Humeral Shaft, Percutaneous Endoscopic Approach

0PHF48Z Insertion of Limb Lengthening External Fixation Device into Right Humeral Shaft, Percutaneous Endoscopic Approach

0PHF4BZ Insertion of Monoplanar External Fixation Device into Right Humeral Shaft, Percutaneous Endoscopic Approach

0PHF4CZ Insertion of Ring External Fixation Device into Right Humeral Shaft, Percutaneous Endoscopic Approach

0PHF4DZ Insertion of Hybrid External Fixation Device into Right Humeral Shaft, Percutaneous Endoscopic Approach

0PHG04Z Insertion of Internal Fixation Device into Left Humeral Shaft, Open Approach

0PHG05Z Insertion of External Fixation Device into Left Humeral Shaft, Open Approach

0PHG06Z Insertion of Intramedullary Internal Fixation Device into Left Humeral Shaft, Open Approach

0PHG07Z Insertion of Intramedullary Limb Lengthening Internal Fixation Device into Left Humeral Shaft, Open Approach

0PHG08Z Insertion of Limb Lengthening External Fixation Device into Left Humeral Shaft, Open Approach

0PHG0BZ Insertion of Monoplanar External Fixation Device into Left Humeral Shaft, Open Approach

0PHG0CZ Insertion of Ring External Fixation Device into Left Humeral Shaft, Open Approach

0PHG0DZ Insertion of Hybrid External Fixation Device into Left Humeral Shaft, Open Approach

0PHG34Z Insertion of Internal Fixation Device into Left Humeral Shaft, Percutaneous Approach

0PHG35Z Insertion of External Fixation Device into Left Humeral Shaft, Percutaneous Approach

0PHG36Z Insertion of Intramedullary Internal Fixation Device into Left Humeral Shaft, Percutaneous Approach

0PHG37Z Insertion of Intramedullary Limb Lengthening Internal Fixation Device into Left Humeral Shaft, Percutaneous Approach

0PHG38Z Insertion of Limb Lengthening External Fixation Device into Left Humeral Shaft, Percutaneous Approach

0PHG3BZ Insertion of Monoplanar External Fixation Device into Left Humeral Shaft, Percutaneous Approach

0PHG3CZ Insertion of Ring External Fixation Device into Left Humeral Shaft, Percutaneous Approach

0PHG3DZ Insertion of Hybrid External Fixation Device into Left Humeral Shaft, Percutaneous Approach

0PHG44Z Insertion of Internal Fixation Device into Left Humeral Shaft, Percutaneous Endoscopic Approach

0PHG45Z Insertion of External Fixation Device into Left Humeral Shaft, Percutaneous Endoscopic Approach

0PHG46Z Insertion of Intramedullary Internal Fixation Device into Left Humeral Shaft, Percutaneous Endoscopic Approach

0PHG47Z Insertion of Intramedullary Limb Lengthening Internal Fixation Device into Left Humeral Shaft, Percutaneous Endoscopic Approach

0PHG48Z Insertion of Limb Lengthening External Fixation Device into Left Humeral Shaft, Percutaneous Endoscopic Approach

0PHG4BZ Insertion of Monoplanar External Fixation Device into Left Humeral Shaft, Percutaneous Endoscopic Approach

0PHG4CZ Insertion of Ring External Fixation Device into Left Humeral Shaft, Percutaneous Endoscopic Approach

0PHG4DZ Insertion of Hybrid External Fixation Device into Left Humeral Shaft, Percutaneous Endoscopic Approach

0PHH04Z Insertion of Internal Fixation Device into Right Radius, Open Approach

0PHH05Z Insertion of External Fixation Device into Right Radius, Open Approach

0PHH06Z Insertion of Intramedullary Internal Fixation Device into Right Radius, Open Approach

0PHH08Z Insertion of Limb Lengthening External Fixation Device into Right Radius, Open Approach

0PHH0BZ Insertion of Monoplanar External Fixation Device into Right Radius, Open Approach

0PHH0CZ Insertion of Ring External Fixation Device into Right Radius, Open Approach

0PHH0DZ Insertion of Hybrid External Fixation Device into Right Radius, Open Approach

0PHH34Z Insertion of Internal Fixation Device into Right Radius, Percutaneous Approach

0PHH35Z Insertion of External Fixation Device into Right Radius, Percutaneous Approach

0PHH36Z Insertion of Intramedullary Internal Fixation Device into Right Radius, Percutaneous Approach

0PHH38Z Insertion of Limb Lengthening External Fixation Device into Right Radius, Percutaneous Approach

0PHH3BZ Insertion of Monoplanar External Fixation Device into Right Radius, Percutaneous Approach

0PHH3CZ Insertion of Ring External Fixation Device into Right Radius, Percutaneous Approach

0PHH3DZ Insertion of Hybrid External Fixation Device into Right Radius, Percutaneous Approach

0PHH44Z Insertion of Internal Fixation Device into Right Radius, Percutaneous Endoscopic Approach

0PHH45Z Insertion of External Fixation Device into Right Radius, Percutaneous Endoscopic Approach

0PHH46Z Insertion of Intramedullary Internal Fixation Device into Right Radius, Percutaneous Endoscopic Approach

0PHH48Z Insertion of Limb Lengthening External Fixation Device into Right Radius, Percutaneous Endoscopic Approach

0PHH4BZ Insertion of Monoplanar External Fixation Device into Right Radius, Percutaneous Endoscopic Approach

0PHH4CZ Insertion of Ring External Fixation Device into Right Radius, Percutaneous Endoscopic Approach

0PHH4DZ Insertion of Hybrid External Fixation Device into Right Radius, Percutaneous Endoscopic Approach

0PHJ04Z Insertion of Internal Fixation Device into Left Radius, Open Approach

0PHJ05Z Insertion of External Fixation Device into Left Radius, Open Approach

0PHJ06Z Insertion of Intramedullary Internal Fixation Device into Left Radius, Open Approach

0PHJ08Z Insertion of Limb Lengthening External Fixation Device into Left Radius, Open Approach

0PHJ0BZ Insertion of Monoplanar External Fixation Device into Left Radius, Open Approach

0PHJ0CZ Insertion of Ring External Fixation Device into Left Radius, Open Approach

0PHJ0DZ Insertion of Hybrid External Fixation Device into Left Radius, Open Approach

0PHJ34Z Insertion of Internal Fixation Device into Left Radius, Percutaneous Approach

0PHJ35Z Insertion of External Fixation Device into Left Radius, Percutaneous Approach

0PHJ36Z Insertion of Intramedullary Internal Fixation Device into Left Radius, Percutaneous Approach

0PHJ38Z Insertion of Limb Lengthening External Fixation Device into Left Radius, Percutaneous Approach

0PHJ3BZ Insertion of Monoplanar External Fixation Device into Left Radius, Percutaneous Approach

0PHJ3CZ Insertion of Ring External Fixation Device into Left Radius, Percutaneous Approach

0PHJ3DZ Insertion of Hybrid External Fixation Device into Left Radius, Percutaneous Approach

0PHJ44Z Insertion of Internal Fixation Device into Left Radius, Percutaneous Endoscopic Approach

0PHJ45Z Insertion of External Fixation Device into Left Radius, Percutaneous Endoscopic Approach

0PHJ46Z Insertion of Intramedullary Internal Fixation Device into Left Radius, Percutaneous Endoscopic Approach

0PHJ48Z Insertion of Limb Lengthening External Fixation Device into Left Radius, Percutaneous Endoscopic Approach

0PHJ4BZ Insertion of Monoplanar External Fixation Device into Left Radius, Percutaneous Endoscopic Approach

0PHJ4CZ Insertion of Ring External Fixation Device into Left Radius, Percutaneous Endoscopic Approach

0PHJ4DZ Insertion of Hybrid External Fixation Device into Left Radius, Percutaneous Endoscopic Approach

0PHK04Z Insertion of Internal Fixation Device into Right Ulna, Open Approach

0PHK05Z Insertion of External Fixation Device into Right Ulna, Open Approach

0PHK06Z Insertion of Intramedullary Internal Fixation Device into Right Ulna, Open Approach

0PHK08Z Insertion of Limb Lengthening External Fixation Device into Right Ulna, Open Approach

0PHK0BZ Insertion of Monoplanar External Fixation Device into Right Ulna, Open Approach

0PHK0CZ Insertion of Ring External Fixation Device into Right Ulna, Open Approach

0PHK0DZ Insertion of Hybrid External Fixation Device into Right Ulna, Open Approach

0PHK34Z Insertion of Internal Fixation Device into Right Ulna, Percutaneous Approach

0PHK35Z Insertion of External Fixation Device into Right Ulna, Percutaneous Approach

0PHK36Z Insertion of Intramedullary Internal Fixation Device into Right Ulna, Percutaneous Approach

0PHK38Z Insertion of Limb Lengthening External Fixation Device into Right Ulna, Percutaneous Approach

0PHK3BZ Insertion of Monoplanar External Fixation Device into Right Ulna, Percutaneous Approach

0PHK3CZ Insertion of Ring External Fixation Device into Right Ulna, Percutaneous Approach

0PHK3DZ Insertion of Hybrid External Fixation Device into Right Ulna, Percutaneous Approach

0PHK44Z Insertion of Internal Fixation Device into Right Ulna, Percutaneous Endoscopic Approach

0PHK45Z Insertion of External Fixation Device into Right Ulna, Percutaneous Endoscopic Approach

0PHK46Z Insertion of Intramedullary Internal Fixation Device into Right Ulna, Percutaneous Endoscopic Approach

0PHK48Z Insertion of Limb Lengthening External Fixation Device into Right Ulna, Percutaneous Endoscopic Approach

0PHK4BZ Insertion of Monoplanar External Fixation Device into Right Ulna, Percutaneous Endoscopic Approach

0PHK4CZ Insertion of Ring External Fixation Device into Right Ulna, Percutaneous Endoscopic Approach

0PHK4DZ Insertion of Hybrid External Fixation Device into Right Ulna, Percutaneous Endoscopic Approach

0PHL04Z Insertion of Internal Fixation Device into Left Ulna, Open Approach

0PHL05Z Insertion of External Fixation Device into Left Ulna, Open Approach

0PHL06Z Insertion of Intramedullary Internal Fixation Device into Left Ulna, Open Approach

0PHL08Z Insertion of Limb Lengthening External Fixation Device into Left Ulna, Open Approach

0PHL0BZ Insertion of Monoplanar External Fixation Device into Left Ulna, Open Approach

0PHL0CZ Insertion of Ring External Fixation Device into Left Ulna, Open Approach

0PHL0DZ Insertion of Hybrid External Fixation Device into Left Ulna, Open Approach

0PHL34Z Insertion of Internal Fixation Device into Left Ulna, Percutaneous Approach

0PHL35Z Insertion of External Fixation Device into Left Ulna, Percutaneous Approach

0PHL36Z Insertion of Intramedullary Internal Fixation Device into Left Ulna, Percutaneous Approach

0PHL38Z Insertion of Limb Lengthening External Fixation Device into Left Ulna, Percutaneous Approach

0PHL3BZ Insertion of Monoplanar External Fixation Device into Left Ulna, Percutaneous Approach

0PHL3CZ Insertion of Ring External Fixation Device into Left Ulna, Percutaneous Approach

0PHL3DZ Insertion of Hybrid External Fixation Device into Left Ulna, Percutaneous Approach

0PHL44Z	Insertion of Internal Fixation Device into Left Ulna, Percutaneous Endoscopic Approach
0PHL45Z	Insertion of External Fixation Device into Left Ulna, Percutaneous Endoscopic Approach
0PHL46Z	Insertion of Intramedullary Internal Fixation Device into Left Ulna, Percutaneous Endoscopic Approach
0PHL48Z	Insertion of Limb Lengthening External Fixation Device into Left Ulna, Percutaneous Endoscopic Approach
0PHL4BZ	Insertion of Monoplanar External Fixation Device into Left Ulna, Percutaneous Endoscopic Approach
0PHL4CZ	Insertion of Ring External Fixation Device into Left Ulna, Percutaneous Endoscopic Approach
0PHL4DZ	Insertion of Hybrid External Fixation Device into Left Ulna, Percutaneous Endoscopic Approach
0PHM04Z	Insertion of Internal Fixation Device into Right Carpal, Open Approach
0PHM05Z	Insertion of External Fixation Device into Right Carpal, Open Approach
0PHM34Z	Insertion of Internal Fixation Device into Right Carpal, Percutaneous Approach
0PHM35Z	Insertion of External Fixation Device into Right Carpal, Percutaneous Approach
0PHM44Z	Insertion of Internal Fixation Device into Right Carpal, Percutaneous Endoscopic Approach
0PHM45Z	Insertion of External Fixation Device into Right Carpal, Percutaneous Endoscopic Approach
0PHN04Z	Insertion of Internal Fixation Device into Left Carpal, Open Approach
0PHN05Z	Insertion of External Fixation Device into Left Carpal, Open Approach
0PHN34Z	Insertion of Internal Fixation Device into Left Carpal, Percutaneous Approach
0PHN35Z	Insertion of External Fixation Device into Left Carpal, Percutaneous Approach
0PHN44Z	Insertion of Internal Fixation Device into Left Carpal, Percutaneous Endoscopic Approach
0PHN45Z	Insertion of External Fixation Device into Left Carpal, Percutaneous Endoscopic Approach
0PHP04Z	Insertion of Internal Fixation Device into Right Metacarpal, Open Approach
0PHP05Z	Insertion of External Fixation Device into Right Metacarpal, Open Approach
0PHP34Z	Insertion of Internal Fixation Device into Right Metacarpal, Percutaneous Approach
0PHP35Z	Insertion of External Fixation Device into Right Metacarpal, Percutaneous Approach
0PHP44Z	Insertion of Internal Fixation Device into Right Metacarpal, Percutaneous Endoscopic Approach
0PHP45Z	Insertion of External Fixation Device into Right Metacarpal, Percutaneous Endoscopic Approach
0PHQ04Z	Insertion of Internal Fixation Device into Left Metacarpal, Open Approach
0PHQ05Z	Insertion of External Fixation Device into Left Metacarpal, Open Approach
0PHQ34Z	Insertion of Internal Fixation Device into Left Metacarpal, Percutaneous Approach
0PHQ35Z	Insertion of External Fixation Device into Left Metacarpal, Percutaneous Approach
0PHQ44Z	Insertion of Internal Fixation Device into Left Metacarpal, Percutaneous Endoscopic Approach
0PHQ45Z	Insertion of External Fixation Device into Left Metacarpal, Percutaneous Endoscopic Approach
0PHR04Z	Insertion of Internal Fixation Device into Right Thumb Phalanx, Open Approach
0PHR05Z	Insertion of External Fixation Device into Right Thumb Phalanx, Open Approach
0PHR34Z	Insertion of Internal Fixation Device into Right Thumb Phalanx, Percutaneous Approach
0PHR35Z	Insertion of External Fixation Device into Right Thumb Phalanx, Percutaneous Approach
0PHR44Z	Insertion of Internal Fixation Device into Right Thumb Phalanx, Percutaneous Endoscopic Approach
0PHR45Z	Insertion of External Fixation Device into Right Thumb Phalanx, Percutaneous Endoscopic Approach
0PHS04Z	Insertion of Internal Fixation Device into Left Thumb Phalanx, Open Approach
0PHS05Z	Insertion of External Fixation Device into Left Thumb Phalanx, Open Approach
0PHS34Z	Insertion of Internal Fixation Device into Left Thumb Phalanx, Percutaneous Approach
0PHS35Z	Insertion of External Fixation Device into Left Thumb Phalanx, Percutaneous Approach
0PHS44Z	Insertion of Internal Fixation Device into Left Thumb Phalanx, Percutaneous Endoscopic Approach
0PHS45Z	Insertion of External Fixation Device into Left Thumb Phalanx, Percutaneous Endoscopic Approach
0PHT04Z	Insertion of Internal Fixation Device into Right Finger Phalanx, Open Approach
0PHT05Z	Insertion of External Fixation Device into Right Finger Phalanx, Open Approach
0PHT34Z	Insertion of Internal Fixation Device into Right Finger Phalanx, Percutaneous Approach
0PHT35Z	Insertion of External Fixation Device into Right Finger Phalanx, Percutaneous Approach
0PHT44Z	Insertion of Internal Fixation Device into Right Finger Phalanx, Percutaneous Endoscopic Approach
0PHT45Z	Insertion of External Fixation Device into Right Finger Phalanx, Percutaneous Endoscopic Approach
0PHV04Z	Insertion of Internal Fixation Device into Left Finger Phalanx, Open Approach
0PHV05Z	Insertion of External Fixation Device into Left Finger Phalanx, Open Approach
0PHV34Z	Insertion of Internal Fixation Device into Left Finger Phalanx, Percutaneous Approach
0PHV35Z	Insertion of External Fixation Device into Left Finger Phalanx, Percutaneous Approach
0PHV44Z	Insertion of Internal Fixation Device into Left Finger Phalanx, Percutaneous Endoscopic Approach
0PHV45Z	Insertion of External Fixation Device into Left Finger Phalanx, Percutaneous Endoscopic Approach
0PHY0MZ	Insertion of Bone Growth Stimulator into Upper Bone, Open Approach
0PHY3MZ	Insertion of Bone Growth Stimulator into Upper Bone, Percutaneous Approach
0PHY4MZ	Insertion of Bone Growth Stimulator into Upper Bone, Percutaneous Endoscopic Approach

0PJ – Upper Bones, Inspection

Review Coding Guideline B3.5

Review Coding Guidelines B3.11a, B3.11b and B3.11c

0PJY0ZZ	Inspection of Upper Bone, Open Approach
0PJY3ZZ	Inspection of Upper Bone, Percutaneous Approach
0PJY4ZZ	Inspection of Upper Bone, Percutaneous Endoscopic Approach
0PJYXZZ	Inspection of Upper Bone, External Approach

0PN – Upper Bones, Release

Review Coding Guideline B3.13

Review Coding Guideline B3.14

0PN00ZZ	Release Sternum, Open Approach
0PN03ZZ	Release Sternum, Percutaneous Approach
0PN04ZZ	Release Sternum, Percutaneous Endoscopic Approach
0PN10ZZ	Release I to 2 Ribs, Open Approach
0PN13ZZ	Release I to 2 Ribs, Percutaneous Approach
0PN14ZZ	Release I to 2 Ribs, Percutaneous Endoscopic Approach
0PN20ZZ	Release 3 or More Ribs, Open Approach
0PN23ZZ	Release 3 or More Ribs, Percutaneous Approach
0PN24ZZ	Release 3 or More Ribs, Percutaneous Endoscopic Approach

0PN30ZZ	Release Cervical Vertebra, Open Approach
0PN33ZZ	Release Cervical Vertebra, Percutaneous Approach
0PN34ZZ	Release Cervical Vertebra, Percutaneous Endoscopic Approach
0PN40ZZ	Release Thoracic Vertebra, Open Approach
0PN43ZZ	Release Thoracic Vertebra, Percutaneous Approach
0PN44ZZ	Release Thoracic Vertebra, Percutaneous Endoscopic Approach
0PN50ZZ	Release Right Scapula, Open Approach
0PN53ZZ	Release Right Scapula, Percutaneous Approach
0PN54ZZ	Release Right Scapula, Percutaneous Endoscopic Approach
0PN60ZZ	Release Left Scapula, Open Approach
0PN63ZZ	Release Left Scapula, Percutaneous Approach
0PN64ZZ	Release Left Scapula, Percutaneous Endoscopic Approach
0PN70ZZ	Release Right Glenoid Cavity, Open Approach
0PN73ZZ	Release Right Glenoid Cavity, Percutaneous Approach
0PN74ZZ	Release Right Glenoid Cavity, Percutaneous Endoscopic Approach
0PN80ZZ	Release Left Glenoid Cavity, Open Approach
0PN83ZZ	Release Left Glenoid Cavity, Percutaneous Approach
0PN84ZZ	Release Left Glenoid Cavity, Percutaneous Endoscopic Approach
0PN90ZZ	Release Right Clavicle, Open Approach
0PN93ZZ	Release Right Clavicle, Percutaneous Approach
0PN94ZZ	Release Right Clavicle, Percutaneous Endoscopic Approach
0PNB0ZZ	Release Left Clavicle, Open Approach
0PNB3ZZ	Release Left Clavicle, Percutaneous Approach
0PNB4ZZ	Release Left Clavicle, Percutaneous Endoscopic Approach

0PNC0ZZ	Release Right Humeral Head, Open Approach
0PNC3ZZ	Release Right Humeral Head, Percutaneous Approach
0PNC4ZZ	Release Right Humeral Head, Percutaneous Endoscopic Approach
0PND0ZZ	Release Left Humeral Head, Open Approach
0PND3ZZ	Release Left Humeral Head, Percutaneous Approach
0PND4ZZ	Release Left Humeral Head, Percutaneous Endoscopic Approach
0PNF0ZZ	Release Right Humeral Shaft, Open Approach
0PNF3ZZ	Release Right Humeral Shaft, Percutaneous Approach
0PNF4ZZ	Release Right Humeral Shaft, Percutaneous Endoscopic Approach
0PNG0ZZ	Release Left Humeral Shaft, Open Approach
0PNG3ZZ	Release Left Humeral Shaft, Percutaneous Approach
0PNG4ZZ	Release Left Humeral Shaft, Percutaneous Endoscopic Approach
0PNH0ZZ	Release Right Radius, Open Approach
0PNH3ZZ	Release Right Radius, Percutaneous Approach
0PNH4ZZ	Release Right Radius, Percutaneous Endoscopic Approach
0PNJ0ZZ	Release Left Radius, Open Approach
0PNJ3ZZ	Release Left Radius, Percutaneous Approach
0PNJ4ZZ	Release Left Radius, Percutaneous Endoscopic Approach
0PNK0ZZ	Release Right Ulna, Open Approach
0PNK3ZZ	Release Right Ulna, Percutaneous Approach
0PNK4ZZ	Release Right Ulna, Percutaneous Endoscopic Approach
0PNL0ZZ	Release Left Ulna, Open Approach
0PNL3ZZ	Release Left Ulna, Percutaneous Approach
0PNL4ZZ	Release Left Ulna, Percutaneous Endoscopic Approach
0PNM0ZZ	Release Right Carpal, Open Approach

0PNM3ZZ	Release Right Carpal, Percutaneous Approach
0PNM4ZZ	Release Right Carpal, Percutaneous Endoscopic Approach
0PNN0ZZ	Release Left Carpal, Open Approach
0PNN3ZZ	Release Left Carpal, Percutaneous Approach
0PNN4ZZ	Release Left Carpal, Percutaneous Endoscopic Approach
0PNP0ZZ	Release Right Metacarpal, Open Approach
0PNP3ZZ	Release Right Metacarpal, Percutaneous Approach
0PNP4ZZ	Release Right Metacarpal, Percutaneous Endoscopic Approach
0PNQ0ZZ	Release Left Metacarpal, Open Approach
0PNQ3ZZ	Release Left Metacarpal, Percutaneous Approach
0PNQ4ZZ	Release Left Metacarpal, Percutaneous Endoscopic Approach
0PNR0ZZ	Release Right Thumb Phalanx, Open Approach
0PNR3ZZ	Release Right Thumb Phalanx, Percutaneous Approach
0PNR4ZZ	Release Right Thumb Phalanx, Percutaneous Endoscopic Approach
0PNS0ZZ	Release Left Thumb Phalanx, Open Approach
0PNS3ZZ	Release Left Thumb Phalanx, Percutaneous Approach
0PNS4ZZ	Release Left Thumb Phalanx, Percutaneous Endoscopic Approach
0PNT0ZZ	Release Right Finger Phalanx, Open Approach
0PNT3ZZ	Release Right Finger Phalanx, Percutaneous Approach
0PNT4ZZ	Release Right Finger Phalanx, Percutaneous Endoscopic Approach
0PNV0ZZ	Release Left Finger Phalanx, Open Approach
0PNV3ZZ	Release Left Finger Phalanx, Percutaneous Approach
0PNV4ZZ	Release Left Finger Phalanx, Percutaneous Endoscopic Approach

0PP – Upper Bones, Removal

Review Coding Guideline B6.1c

0PP004Z	Removal of Internal Fixation Device from Sternum, Open Approach
0PP007Z	Removal of Autologous Tissue Substitute from Sternum, Open Approach
0PP00JZ	Removal of Synthetic Substitute from Sternum, Open Approach
0PP00KZ	Removal of Nonautologous Tissue Substitute from Sternum, Open Approach
0PP034Z	Removal of Internal Fixation Device from Sternum, Percutaneous Approach
0PP037Z	Removal of Autologous Tissue Substitute from Sternum, Percutaneous Approach
0PP03JZ	Removal of Synthetic Substitute from Sternum, Percutaneous Approach
0PP03KZ	Removal of Nonautologous Tissue Substitute from Sternum, Percutaneous Approach
0PP044Z	Removal of Internal Fixation Device from Sternum, Percutaneous Endoscopic Approach
0PP047Z	Removal of Autologous Tissue Substitute from Sternum, Percutaneous

	Endoscopic Approach
0PP04JZ	Removal of Synthetic Substitute from Sternum, Percutaneous Endoscopic Approach
0PP04KZ	Removal of Nonautologous Tissue Substitute from Sternum, Percutaneous Endoscopic Approach
0PP0X4Z	Removal of Internal Fixation Device from Sternum, External Approach
0PP104Z	Removal of Internal Fixation Device from I to 2 Ribs, Open Approach
0PP107Z	Removal of Autologous Tissue Substitute from I to 2 Ribs, Open Approach
0PP10JZ	Removal of Synthetic Substitute from I to 2 Ribs, Open Approach
0PP10KZ	Removal of Nonautologous Tissue Substitute from I to 2 Ribs, Open Approach
0PP134Z	Removal of Internal Fixation Device from I to 2 Ribs, Percutaneous Approach
0PP137Z	Removal of Autologous Tissue Substitute from I to 2 Ribs, Percutaneous Approach

0PP13JZ	Removal of Synthetic Substitute from I to 2 Ribs, Percutaneous Approach
0PP13KZ	Removal of Nonautologous Tissue Substitute from I to 2 Ribs, Percutaneous Approach
0PP144Z	Removal of Internal Fixation Device from I to 2 Ribs, Percutaneous Endoscopic Approach
0PP147Z	Removal of Autologous Tissue Substitute from I to 2 Ribs, Percutaneous Endoscopic Approach
0PP14JZ	Removal of Synthetic Substitute from I to 2 Ribs, Percutaneous Endoscopic Approach
0PP14KZ	Removal of Nonautologous Tissue Substitute from I to 2 Ribs, Percutaneous Endoscopic Approach
0PP1X4Z	Removal of Internal Fixation Device from I to 2 Ribs, External Approach
0PP204Z	Removal of Internal Fixation Device from 3 or More Ribs, Open Approach
0PP207Z	Removal of Autologous Tissue Substitute from 3 or More Ribs, Open Approach
0PP20JZ	Removal of Synthetic Substitute from 3 or More Ribs, Open Approach

♀ Female-only   ♂ Male-only   ▲ Limited Coverage   ● Non-OR   ⬛ HAC-associated procedure   ▲ Non-covered procedures   ✛ Cluster

0PP20KZ Removal of Nonautologous Tissue Substitute from 3 or More Ribs, Open Approach

0PP234Z Removal of Internal Fixation Device from 3 or More Ribs, Percutaneous Approach

0PP237Z Removal of Autologous Tissue Substitute from 3 or More Ribs, Percutaneous Approach

0PP23JZ Removal of Synthetic Substitute from 3 or More Ribs, Percutaneous Approach

0PP23KZ Removal of Nonautologous Tissue Substitute from 3 or More Ribs, Percutaneous Approach

0PP244Z Removal of Internal Fixation Device from 3 or More Ribs, Percutaneous Endoscopic Approach

0PP247Z Removal of Autologous Tissue Substitute from 3 or More Ribs, Percutaneous Endoscopic Approach

0PP24JZ Removal of Synthetic Substitute from 3 or More Ribs, Percutaneous Endoscopic Approach

0PP24KZ Removal of Nonautologous Tissue Substitute from 3 or More Ribs, Percutaneous Endoscopic Approach

0PP2X4Z Removal of Internal Fixation Device from 3 or More Ribs, External Approach

0PP304Z Removal of Internal Fixation Device from Cervical Vertebra, Open Approach

0PP307Z Removal of Autologous Tissue Substitute from Cervical Vertebra, Open Approach

0PP30JZ Removal of Synthetic Substitute from Cervical Vertebra, Open Approach

0PP30KZ Removal of Nonautologous Tissue Substitute from Cervical Vertebra, Open Approach

0PP334Z Removal of Internal Fixation Device from Cervical Vertebra, Percutaneous Approach

0PP337Z Removal of Autologous Tissue Substitute from Cervical Vertebra, Percutaneous Approach

0PP33JZ Removal of Synthetic Substitute from Cervical Vertebra, Percutaneous Approach

0PP33KZ Removal of Nonautologous Tissue Substitute from Cervical Vertebra, Percutaneous Approach

0PP344Z Removal of Internal Fixation Device from Cervical Vertebra, Percutaneous Endoscopic Approach

0PP347Z Removal of Autologous Tissue Substitute from Cervical Vertebra, Percutaneous Endoscopic Approach

0PP34JZ Removal of Synthetic Substitute from Cervical Vertebra, Percutaneous Endoscopic Approach

0PP34KZ Removal of Nonautologous Tissue Substitute from Cervical Vertebra, Percutaneous Endoscopic Approach

0PP3X4Z Removal of Internal Fixation Device from Cervical Vertebra, External Approach

0PP404Z Removal of Internal Fixation Device from Thoracic Vertebra, Open Approach

AHA CC: 4Q, 2014, 28-29

0PP407Z Removal of Autologous Tissue Substitute from Thoracic Vertebra, Open Approach

0PP40JZ Removal of Synthetic Substitute from Thoracic Vertebra, Open Approach

0PP40KZ Removal of Nonautologous Tissue Substitute from Thoracic Vertebra, Open Approach

0PP434Z Removal of Internal Fixation Device from Thoracic Vertebra, Percutaneous Approach

0PP437Z Removal of Autologous Tissue Substitute from Thoracic Vertebra, Percutaneous Approach

0PP43JZ Removal of Synthetic Substitute from Thoracic Vertebra, Percutaneous Approach

0PP43KZ Removal of Nonautologous Tissue Substitute from Thoracic Vertebra, Percutaneous Approach

0PP444Z Removal of Internal Fixation Device from Thoracic Vertebra, Percutaneous Endoscopic Approach

0PP447Z Removal of Autologous Tissue Substitute from Thoracic Vertebra, Percutaneous Endoscopic Approach

0PP44JZ Removal of Synthetic Substitute from Thoracic Vertebra, Percutaneous Endoscopic Approach

0PP44KZ Removal of Nonautologous Tissue Substitute from Thoracic Vertebra, Percutaneous Endoscopic Approach

0PP4X4Z Removal of Internal Fixation Device from Thoracic Vertebra, External Approach

0PP504Z Removal of Internal Fixation Device from Right Scapula, Open Approach

0PP507Z Removal of Autologous Tissue Substitute from Right Scapula, Open Approach

0PP50JZ Removal of Synthetic Substitute from Right Scapula, Open Approach

0PP50KZ Removal of Nonautologous Tissue Substitute from Right Scapula, Open Approach

0PP534Z Removal of Internal Fixation Device from Right Scapula, Percutaneous Approach

0PP537Z Removal of Autologous Tissue Substitute from Right Scapula, Percutaneous Approach

0PP53JZ Removal of Synthetic Substitute from Right Scapula, Percutaneous Approach

0PP53KZ Removal of Nonautologous Tissue Substitute from Right Scapula, Percutaneous Approach

0PP544Z Removal of Internal Fixation Device from Right Scapula, Percutaneous Endoscopic Approach

0PP547Z Removal of Autologous Tissue Substitute from Right Scapula, Percutaneous Endoscopic Approach

0PP54JZ Removal of Synthetic Substitute from Right Scapula, Percutaneous Endoscopic Approach

0PP54KZ Removal of Nonautologous Tissue Substitute from Right Scapula, Percutaneous Endoscopic Approach

0PP5X4Z Removal of Internal Fixation Device from Right Scapula, External Approach

0PP604Z Removal of Internal Fixation Device from Left Scapula, Open Approach

0PP607Z Removal of Autologous Tissue Substitute from Left Scapula, Open Approach

0PP60JZ Removal of Synthetic Substitute from Left Scapula, Open Approach

0PP60KZ Removal of Nonautologous Tissue Substitute from Left Scapula, Open Approach

0PP634Z Removal of Internal Fixation Device from Left Scapula, Percutaneous Approach

0PP637Z Removal of Autologous Tissue Substitute from Left Scapula, Percutaneous Approach

0PP63JZ Removal of Synthetic Substitute from Left Scapula, Percutaneous Approach

0PP63KZ Removal of Nonautologous Tissue Substitute from Left Scapula, Percutaneous Approach

0PP644Z Removal of Internal Fixation Device from Left Scapula, Percutaneous Endoscopic Approach

0PP647Z Removal of Autologous Tissue Substitute from Left Scapula, Percutaneous Endoscopic Approach

0PP64JZ Removal of Synthetic Substitute from Left Scapula, Percutaneous Endoscopic Approach

0PP64KZ Removal of Nonautologous Tissue Substitute from Left Scapula, Percutaneous Endoscopic Approach

0PP6X4Z Removal of Internal Fixation Device from Left Scapula, External Approach

0PP704Z Removal of Internal Fixation Device from Right Glenoid Cavity, Open Approach

0PP707Z Removal of Autologous Tissue Substitute from Right Glenoid Cavity, Open Approach

0PP70JZ Removal of Synthetic Substitute from Right Glenoid Cavity, Open Approach

0PP70KZ Removal of Nonautologous Tissue Substitute from Right Glenoid Cavity, Open Approach

0PP734Z Removal of Internal Fixation Device from Right Glenoid Cavity, Percutaneous Approach

0PP737Z Removal of Autologous Tissue Substitute from Right Glenoid Cavity, Percutaneous Approach

0PP73JZ Removal of Synthetic Substitute from Right Glenoid Cavity, Percutaneous Approach

0PP73KZ Removal of Nonautologous Tissue Substitute from Right Glenoid Cavity, Percutaneous Approach

0PP744Z Removal of Internal Fixation Device from Right Glenoid Cavity, Percutaneous Endoscopic Approach

0PP747Z Removal of Autologous Tissue Substitute from Right Glenoid Cavity, Percutaneous Endoscopic Approach

0PP74JZ Removal of Synthetic Substitute from Right Glenoid Cavity, Percutaneous Endoscopic Approach

0PP74KZ Removal of Nonautologous Tissue Substitute from Right Glenoid Cavity, Percutaneous Endoscopic Approach

0PP7X4Z Removal of Internal Fixation Device from Right Glenoid Cavity, External Approach

0PP804Z Removal of Internal Fixation Device from Left Glenoid Cavity, Open Approach

0PP807Z Removal of Autologous Tissue Substitute from Left Glenoid Cavity, Open Approach

0PP80JZ Removal of Synthetic Substitute from Left Glenoid Cavity, Open Approach

0PP80KZ Removal of Nonautologous Tissue Substitute from Left Glenoid Cavity, Open Approach

0PP834Z Removal of Internal Fixation Device from Left Glenoid Cavity, Percutaneous Approach

0PP837Z Removal of Autologous Tissue Substitute from Left Glenoid Cavity, Percutaneous Approach

0PP83JZ Removal of Synthetic Substitute from Left Glenoid Cavity, Percutaneous Approach

0PP83KZ Removal of Nonautologous Tissue Substitute from Left Glenoid Cavity, Percutaneous Approach

0PP844Z Removal of Internal Fixation Device from Left Glenoid Cavity, Percutaneous Endoscopic Approach

0PP847Z Removal of Autologous Tissue Substitute from Left Glenoid Cavity, Percutaneous Endoscopic Approach

0PP84JZ Removal of Synthetic Substitute from Left Glenoid Cavity, Percutaneous Endoscopic Approach

0PP84KZ Removal of Nonautologous Tissue Substitute from Left Glenoid Cavity, Percutaneous Endoscopic Approach

0PP8X4Z Removal of Internal Fixation Device from Left Glenoid Cavity, External Approach

0PP904Z Removal of Internal Fixation Device from Right Clavicle, Open Approach

0PP907Z Removal of Autologous Tissue Substitute from Right Clavicle, Open Approach

0PP90JZ Removal of Synthetic Substitute from Right Clavicle, Open Approach

0PP90KZ Removal of Nonautologous Tissue Substitute from Right Clavicle, Open Approach

0PP934Z Removal of Internal Fixation Device from Right Clavicle, Percutaneous Approach

0PP937Z Removal of Autologous Tissue Substitute from Right Clavicle, Percutaneous Approach

0PP93JZ Removal of Synthetic Substitute from Right Clavicle, Percutaneous Approach

0PP93KZ Removal of Nonautologous Tissue Substitute from Right Clavicle, Percutaneous Approach

0PP944Z Removal of Internal Fixation Device from Right Clavicle, Percutaneous Endoscopic Approach

0PP947Z Removal of Autologous Tissue Substitute from Right Clavicle, Percutaneous Endoscopic Approach

0PP94JZ Removal of Synthetic Substitute from Right Clavicle, Percutaneous Endoscopic Approach

0PP94KZ Removal of Nonautologous Tissue Substitute from Right Clavicle, Percutaneous Endoscopic Approach

0PP9X4Z Removal of Internal Fixation Device from Right Clavicle, External Approach

0PPB04Z Removal of Internal Fixation Device from Left Clavicle, Open Approach

0PPB07Z Removal of Autologous Tissue Substitute from Left Clavicle, Open Approach

0PPB0JZ Removal of Synthetic Substitute from Left Clavicle, Open Approach

0PPB0KZ Removal of Nonautologous Tissue Substitute from Left Clavicle, Open Approach

0PPB34Z Removal of Internal Fixation Device from Left Clavicle, Percutaneous Approach

0PPB37Z Removal of Autologous Tissue Substitute from Left Clavicle, Percutaneous Approach

0PPB3JZ Removal of Synthetic Substitute from Left Clavicle, Percutaneous Approach

0PPB3KZ Removal of Nonautologous Tissue Substitute from Left Clavicle, Percutaneous Approach

0PPB44Z Removal of Internal Fixation Device from Left Clavicle, Percutaneous Endoscopic Approach

0PPB47Z Removal of Autologous Tissue Substitute from Left Clavicle, Percutaneous Endoscopic Approach

0PPB4JZ Removal of Synthetic Substitute from Left Clavicle, Percutaneous Endoscopic Approach

0PPB4KZ Removal of Nonautologous Tissue Substitute from Left Clavicle, Percutaneous Endoscopic Approach

0PPBX4Z Removal of Internal Fixation Device from Left Clavicle, External Approach

0PPC04Z Removal of Internal Fixation Device from Right Humeral Head, Open Approach

0PPC05Z Removal of External Fixation Device from Right Humeral Head, Open Approach

0PPC07Z Removal of Autologous Tissue Substitute from Right Humeral Head, Open Approach

0PPC0JZ Removal of Synthetic Substitute from Right Humeral Head, Open Approach

0PPC0KZ Removal of Nonautologous Tissue Substitute from Right Humeral Head, Open Approach

0PPC34Z Removal of Internal Fixation Device from Right Humeral Head, Percutaneous Approach

0PPC35Z Removal of External Fixation Device from Right Humeral Head, Percutaneous Approach

0PPC37Z Removal of Autologous Tissue Substitute from Right Humeral Head, Percutaneous Approach

0PPC3JZ Removal of Synthetic Substitute from Right Humeral Head, Percutaneous Approach

0PPC3KZ Removal of Nonautologous Tissue Substitute from Right Humeral Head, Percutaneous Approach

0PPC44Z Removal of Internal Fixation Device from Right Humeral Head, Percutaneous Endoscopic Approach

0PPC45Z Removal of External Fixation Device from Right Humeral Head, Percutaneous Endoscopic Approach

0PPC47Z Removal of Autologous Tissue Substitute from Right Humeral Head, Percutaneous Endoscopic Approach

0PPC4JZ Removal of Synthetic Substitute from Right Humeral Head, Percutaneous Endoscopic Approach

0PPC4KZ Removal of Nonautologous Tissue Substitute from Right Humeral Head, Percutaneous Endoscopic Approach

0PPCX4Z Removal of Internal Fixation Device from Right Humeral Head, External Approach

0PPCX5Z Removal of External Fixation Device from Right Humeral Head, External Approach

0PPD04Z Removal of Internal Fixation Device from Left Humeral Head, Open Approach

0PPD05Z Removal of External Fixation Device from Left Humeral Head, Open Approach

0PPD07Z Removal of Autologous Tissue Substitute from Left Humeral Head, Open Approach

0PPD0JZ Removal of Synthetic Substitute from Left Humeral Head, Open Approach

0PPD0KZ Removal of Nonautologous Tissue Substitute from Left Humeral Head, Open Approach

0PPD34Z Removal of Internal Fixation Device from Left Humeral Head, Percutaneous Approach

0PPD35Z Removal of External Fixation Device from Left Humeral Head, Percutaneous Approach

0PPD37Z Removal of Autologous Tissue Substitute from Left Humeral Head, Percutaneous Approach

0PPD3JZ Removal of Synthetic Substitute from Left Humeral Head, Percutaneous Approach

0PPD3KZ Removal of Nonautologous Tissue Substitute from Left Humeral Head, Percutaneous Approach

0PPD44Z Removal of Internal Fixation Device from Left Humeral Head, Percutaneous Endoscopic Approach

0PPD45Z Removal of External Fixation Device from Left Humeral Head, Percutaneous Endoscopic Approach

0PPD47Z Removal of Autologous Tissue Substitute from Left Humeral Head, Percutaneous Endoscopic Approach

0PPD4JZ Removal of Synthetic Substitute from Left Humeral Head, Percutaneous Endoscopic Approach

0PPD4KZ Removal of Nonautologous Tissue Substitute from Left Humeral Head, Percutaneous Endoscopic Approach

0PPDX4Z Removal of Internal Fixation Device from Left Humeral Head, External Approach

0PPDX5Z Removal of External Fixation Device from Left Humeral Head, External Approach

0PPF04Z Removal of Internal Fixation Device from Right Humeral Shaft, Open Approach

0PPF05Z Removal of External Fixation Device from Right Humeral Shaft, Open Approach

0PPF07Z Removal of Autologous Tissue Substitute from Right Humeral Shaft, Open Approach

0PPF0JZ Removal of Synthetic Substitute from Right Humeral Shaft, Open Approach

0PPF0KZ Removal of Nonautologous Tissue Substitute from Right Humeral Shaft, Open Approach

0PPF34Z Removal of Internal Fixation Device from Right Humeral Shaft, Percutaneous Approach

0PPF35Z Removal of External Fixation Device from Right Humeral Shaft, Percutaneous Approach

0PPF37Z Removal of Autologous Tissue Substitute from Right Humeral Shaft, Percutaneous Approach

0PPF3JZ Removal of Synthetic Substitute from Right Humeral Shaft, Percutaneous Approach

0PPF3KZ Removal of Nonautologous Tissue Substitute from Right Humeral Shaft, Percutaneous Approach

0PPF44Z Removal of Internal Fixation Device from Right Humeral Shaft, Percutaneous Endoscopic Approach

0PPF45Z Removal of External Fixation Device from Right Humeral Shaft, Percutaneous Endoscopic Approach

0PPF47Z Removal of Autologous Tissue Substitute from Right Humeral Shaft, Percutaneous Endoscopic Approach

0PPF4JZ Removal of Synthetic Substitute from Right Humeral Shaft, Percutaneous Endoscopic Approach

0PPF4KZ Removal of Nonautologous Tissue Substitute from Right Humeral Shaft, Percutaneous Endoscopic Approach

0PPFX4Z Removal of Internal Fixation Device from Right Humeral Shaft, External Approach

0PPFX5Z Removal of External Fixation Device from Right Humeral Shaft, External Approach

0PPG04Z Removal of Internal Fixation Device from Left Humeral Shaft, Open Approach

0PPG05Z Removal of External Fixation Device from Left Humeral Shaft, Open Approach

0PPG07Z Removal of Autologous Tissue Substitute from Left Humeral Shaft, Open Approach

0PPG0JZ Removal of Synthetic Substitute from Left Humeral Shaft, Open Approach

0PPG0KZ Removal of Nonautologous Tissue Substitute from Left Humeral Shaft, Open Approach

0PPG34Z Removal of Internal Fixation Device from Left Humeral Shaft, Percutaneous Approach

0PPG35Z Removal of External Fixation Device from Left Humeral Shaft, Percutaneous Approach

0PPG37Z Removal of Autologous Tissue Substitute from Left Humeral Shaft, Percutaneous Approach

0PPG3JZ Removal of Synthetic Substitute from Left Humeral Shaft, Percutaneous Approach

0PPG3KZ Removal of Nonautologous Tissue Substitute from Left Humeral Shaft, Percutaneous Approach

0PPG44Z Removal of Internal Fixation Device from Left Humeral Shaft, Percutaneous Endoscopic Approach

0PPG45Z Removal of External Fixation Device from Left Humeral Shaft, Percutaneous Endoscopic Approach

0PPG47Z Removal of Autologous Tissue Substitute from Left Humeral Shaft, Percutaneous Endoscopic Approach

0PPG4JZ Removal of Synthetic Substitute from Left Humeral Shaft, Percutaneous Endoscopic Approach

0PPG4KZ Removal of Nonautologous Tissue Substitute from Left Humeral Shaft, Percutaneous Endoscopic Approach

0PPGX4Z Removal of Internal Fixation Device from Left Humeral Shaft, External Approach

0PPGX5Z Removal of External Fixation Device from Left Humeral Shaft, External Approach

0PPH04Z Removal of Internal Fixation Device from Right Radius, Open Approach

0PPH05Z Removal of External Fixation Device from Right Radius, Open Approach

0PPH07Z Removal of Autologous Tissue Substitute from Right Radius, Open Approach

0PPH0JZ Removal of Synthetic Substitute from Right Radius, Open Approach

0PPH0KZ Removal of Nonautologous Tissue Substitute from Right Radius, Open Approach

0PPH34Z Removal of Internal Fixation Device from Right Radius, Percutaneous Approach

0PPH35Z Removal of External Fixation Device from Right Radius, Percutaneous Approach

0PPH37Z Removal of Autologous Tissue Substitute from Right Radius, Percutaneous Approach

0PPH3JZ Removal of Synthetic Substitute from Right Radius, Percutaneous Approach

0PPH3KZ Removal of Nonautologous Tissue Substitute from Right Radius, Percutaneous Approach

0PPH44Z Removal of Internal Fixation Device from Right Radius, Percutaneous Endoscopic Approach

0PPH45Z Removal of External Fixation Device from Right Radius, Percutaneous Endoscopic Approach

0PPH47Z Removal of Autologous Tissue Substitute from Right Radius, Percutaneous Endoscopic Approach

0PPH4JZ Removal of Synthetic Substitute from Right Radius, Percutaneous Endoscopic Approach

0PPH4KZ Removal of Nonautologous Tissue Substitute from Right Radius, Percutaneous Endoscopic Approach

0PPHX4Z Removal of Internal Fixation Device from Right Radius, External Approach

0PPHX5Z Removal of External Fixation Device from Right Radius, External Approach

0PPJ04Z Removal of Internal Fixation Device from Left Radius, Open Approach

0PPJ05Z Removal of External Fixation Device from Left Radius, Open Approach

0PPJ07Z Removal of Autologous Tissue Substitute from Left Radius, Open Approach

0PPJ0JZ Removal of Synthetic Substitute from Left Radius, Open Approach

0PPJ0KZ Removal of Nonautologous Tissue Substitute from Left Radius, Open Approach

0PPJ34Z Removal of Internal Fixation Device from Left Radius, Percutaneous Approach

0PPJ35Z Removal of External Fixation Device from Left Radius, Percutaneous Approach

0PPJ37Z Removal of Autologous Tissue Substitute from Left Radius, Percutaneous Approach

0PPJ3JZ Removal of Synthetic Substitute from Left Radius, Percutaneous Approach

0PPJ3KZ Removal of Nonautologous Tissue Substitute from Left Radius, Percutaneous Approach

0PPJ44Z Removal of Internal Fixation Device from Left Radius, Percutaneous Endoscopic Approach

0PPJ45Z Removal of External Fixation Device from Left Radius, Percutaneous Endoscopic Approach

0PPJ47Z Removal of Autologous Tissue Substitute from Left Radius, Percutaneous Endoscopic Approach

0PPJ4JZ Removal of Synthetic Substitute from Left Radius, Percutaneous Endoscopic Approach

0PPJ4KZ Removal of Nonautologous Tissue Substitute from Left Radius, Percutaneous Endoscopic Approach

0PPJX4Z Removal of Internal Fixation Device from Left Radius, External Approach

0PPJX5Z Removal of External Fixation Device from Left Radius, External Approach

0PPK04Z Removal of Internal Fixation Device from Right Ulna, Open Approach

0PPK05Z Removal of External Fixation Device from Right Ulna, Open Approach

0PPK07Z Removal of Autologous Tissue Substitute from Right Ulna, Open Approach

0PPK0JZ Removal of Synthetic Substitute from Right Ulna, Open Approach

0PPK0KZ Removal of Nonautologous Tissue Substitute from Right Ulna, Open Approach

0PPK34Z Removal of Internal Fixation Device from Right Ulna, Percutaneous Approach

0PPK35Z Removal of External Fixation Device from Right Ulna, Percutaneous Approach

0PPK37Z Removal of Autologous Tissue Substitute from Right Ulna, Percutaneous Approach

0PPK3JZ Removal of Synthetic Substitute from Right Ulna, Percutaneous Approach

0PPK3KZ Removal of Nonautologous Tissue Substitute from Right Ulna, Percutaneous Approach

0PPK44Z Removal of Internal Fixation Device from Right Ulna, Percutaneous Endoscopic Approach

0PPK45Z Removal of External Fixation Device from Right Ulna, Percutaneous Endoscopic Approach

0PPK47Z Removal of Autologous Tissue Substitute from Right Ulna, Percutaneous Endoscopic Approach

0PPK4JZ Removal of Synthetic Substitute from Right Ulna, Percutaneous Endoscopic Approach

0PPK4KZ Removal of Nonautologous Tissue Substitute from Right Ulna, Percutaneous Endoscopic Approach

0PPKX4Z Removal of Internal Fixation Device from Right Ulna, External Approach

0PPKX5Z Removal of External Fixation Device from Right Ulna, External Approach

0PPL04Z Removal of Internal Fixation Device from Left Ulna, Open Approach

0PPL05Z Removal of External Fixation Device from Left Ulna, Open Approach

0PPL07Z Removal of Autologous Tissue Substitute from Left Ulna, Open Approach

0PPL0JZ Removal of Synthetic Substitute from Left Ulna, Open Approach

0PPL0KZ Removal of Nonautologous Tissue Substitute from Left Ulna, Open Approach

0PPL34Z Removal of Internal Fixation Device from Left Ulna, Percutaneous Approach

0PPL35Z Removal of External Fixation Device from Left Ulna, Percutaneous Approach

0PPL37Z Removal of Autologous Tissue Substitute from Left Ulna, Percutaneous Approach

0PPL3JZ Removal of Synthetic Substitute from Left Ulna, Percutaneous Approach

0PPL3KZ Removal of Nonautologous Tissue Substitute from Left Ulna, Percutaneous Approach

0PPL44Z Removal of Internal Fixation Device from Left Ulna, Percutaneous Endoscopic Approach

0PPL45Z Removal of External Fixation Device from Left Ulna, Percutaneous Endoscopic Approach

0PPL47Z Removal of Autologous Tissue Substitute from Left Ulna, Percutaneous Endoscopic Approach

0PPL4JZ Removal of Synthetic Substitute from Left Ulna, Percutaneous Endoscopic Approach

0PPL4KZ Removal of Nonautologous Tissue Substitute from Left Ulna, Percutaneous Endoscopic Approach

0PPLX4Z Removal of Internal Fixation Device from Left Ulna, External Approach

0PPLX5Z Removal of External Fixation Device from Left Ulna, External Approach

0PPM04Z Removal of Internal Fixation Device from Right Carpal, Open Approach

0PPM05Z Removal of External Fixation Device from Right Carpal, Open Approach

0PPM07Z Removal of Autologous Tissue Substitute from Right Carpal, Open Approach

0PPM0JZ Removal of Synthetic Substitute from Right Carpal, Open Approach

0PPM0KZ Removal of Nonautologous Tissue Substitute from Right Carpal, Open Approach

0PPM34Z Removal of Internal Fixation Device from Right Carpal, Percutaneous Approach

0PPM35Z Removal of External Fixation Device from Right Carpal, Percutaneous Approach

0PPM37Z Removal of Autologous Tissue Substitute from Right Carpal, Percutaneous Approach

0PPM3JZ Removal of Synthetic Substitute from Right Carpal, Percutaneous Approach

0PPM3KZ Removal of Nonautologous Tissue Substitute from Right Carpal, Percutaneous Approach

0PPM44Z Removal of Internal Fixation Device from Right Carpal, Percutaneous Endoscopic Approach

0PPM45Z Removal of External Fixation Device from Right Carpal, Percutaneous Endoscopic Approach

0PPM47Z Removal of Autologous Tissue Substitute from Right Carpal, Percutaneous Endoscopic Approach

0PPM4JZ Removal of Synthetic Substitute from Right Carpal, Percutaneous Endoscopic Approach

0PPM4KZ Removal of Nonautologous Tissue Substitute from Right Carpal, Percutaneous Endoscopic Approach

0PPMX4Z Removal of Internal Fixation Device from Right Carpal, External Approach

0PPMX5Z Removal of External Fixation Device from Right Carpal, External Approach

0PPN04Z Removal of Internal Fixation Device from Left Carpal, Open Approach

0PPN05Z Removal of External Fixation Device from Left Carpal, Open Approach

0PPN07Z Removal of Autologous Tissue Substitute from Left Carpal, Open Approach

0PPN0JZ Removal of Synthetic Substitute from Left Carpal, Open Approach

0PPN0KZ Removal of Nonautologous Tissue Substitute from Left Carpal, Open Approach

0PPN34Z Removal of Internal Fixation Device from Left Carpal, Percutaneous Approach

0PPN35Z Removal of External Fixation Device from Left Carpal, Percutaneous Approach

0PPN37Z Removal of Autologous Tissue Substitute from Left Carpal, Percutaneous Approach

0PPN3JZ Removal of Synthetic Substitute from Left Carpal, Percutaneous Approach

0PPN3KZ Removal of Nonautologous Tissue Substitute from Left Carpal, Percutaneous Approach

0PPN44Z Removal of Internal Fixation Device from Left Carpal, Percutaneous Endoscopic Approach

0PPN45Z Removal of External Fixation Device from Left Carpal, Percutaneous Endoscopic Approach

0PPN47Z Removal of Autologous Tissue Substitute from Left Carpal, Percutaneous Endoscopic Approach

0PPN4JZ Removal of Synthetic Substitute from Left Carpal, Percutaneous Endoscopic Approach

0PPN4KZ Removal of Nonautologous Tissue Substitute from Left Carpal, Percutaneous Endoscopic Approach

0PPNX4Z Removal of Internal Fixation Device from Left Carpal, External Approach

0PPNX5Z Removal of External Fixation Device from Left Carpal, External Approach

0PPP04Z Removal of Internal Fixation Device from Right Metacarpal, Open Approach

0PPP05Z Removal of External Fixation Device from Right Metacarpal, Open Approach

0PPP07Z Removal of Autologous Tissue Substitute from Right Metacarpal, Open Approach

0PPP0JZ Removal of Synthetic Substitute from Right Metacarpal, Open Approach

0PPP0KZ Removal of Nonautologous Tissue Substitute from Right Metacarpal, Open Approach

0PPP34Z Removal of Internal Fixation Device from Right Metacarpal, Percutaneous Approach

0PPP35Z Removal of External Fixation Device from Right Metacarpal, Percutaneous Approach

0PPP37Z Removal of Autologous Tissue Substitute from Right Metacarpal, Percutaneous Approach

0PPP3JZ Removal of Synthetic Substitute from Right Metacarpal, Percutaneous Approach

0PPP3KZ Removal of Nonautologous Tissue Substitute from Right Metacarpal, Percutaneous Approach

0PPP44Z Removal of Internal Fixation Device from Right Metacarpal, Percutaneous Endoscopic Approach

0PPP45Z Removal of External Fixation Device from Right Metacarpal, Percutaneous Endoscopic Approach

0PPP47Z Removal of Autologous Tissue Substitute from Right Metacarpal, Percutaneous Endoscopic Approach

0PPP4JZ Removal of Synthetic Substitute from Right Metacarpal, Percutaneous Endoscopic Approach

0PPP4KZ Removal of Nonautologous Tissue Substitute from Right Metacarpal, Percutaneous Endoscopic Approach

0PPPX4Z Removal of Internal Fixation Device from Right Metacarpal, External Approach

0PPPX5Z Removal of External Fixation Device from Right Metacarpal, External Approach

0PPQ04Z Removal of Internal Fixation Device from Left Metacarpal, Open Approach

0PPQ05Z Removal of External Fixation Device from Left Metacarpal, Open Approach

0PPQ07Z Removal of Autologous Tissue Substitute from Left Metacarpal, Open Approach

0PPQ0JZ Removal of Synthetic Substitute from Left Metacarpal, Open Approach

0PPQ0KZ Removal of Nonautologous Tissue Substitute from Left Metacarpal, Open Approach

0PPQ34Z Removal of Internal Fixation Device from Left Metacarpal, Percutaneous Approach

0PPQ35Z Removal of External Fixation Device from Left Metacarpal, Percutaneous Approach

0PPQ37Z Removal of Autologous Tissue Substitute from Left Metacarpal, Percutaneous Approach

0PPQ3JZ Removal of Synthetic Substitute from Left Metacarpal, Percutaneous Approach

0PPQ3KZ Removal of Nonautologous Tissue Substitute from Left Metacarpal, Percutaneous Approach

0PPQ44Z Removal of Internal Fixation Device from Left Metacarpal, Percutaneous Endoscopic Approach

0PPQ45Z Removal of External Fixation Device from Left Metacarpal, Percutaneous Endoscopic Approach

0PPQ47Z Removal of Autologous Tissue Substitute from Left Metacarpal, Percutaneous Endoscopic Approach

0PPQ4JZ Removal of Synthetic Substitute from Left Metacarpal, Percutaneous Endoscopic Approach

0PPQ4KZ Removal of Nonautologous Tissue Substitute from Left Metacarpal, Percutaneous Endoscopic Approach

0PPQX4Z Removal of Internal Fixation Device from Left Metacarpal, External Approach

0PPQX5Z Removal of External Fixation Device from Left Metacarpal, External Approach

0PPR04Z Removal of Internal Fixation Device from Right Thumb Phalanx, Open Approach

0PPR05Z Removal of External Fixation Device from Right Thumb Phalanx, Open Approach

0PPR07Z Removal of Autologous Tissue Substitute from Right Thumb Phalanx, Open Approach

0PPR0JZ Removal of Synthetic Substitute from Right Thumb Phalanx, Open Approach

0PPR0KZ Removal of Nonautologous Tissue Substitute from Right Thumb Phalanx, Open Approach

0PPR34Z Removal of Internal Fixation Device from Right Thumb Phalanx, Percutaneous Approach

0PPR35Z Removal of External Fixation Device from Right Thumb Phalanx, Percutaneous Approach

0PPR37Z Removal of Autologous Tissue Substitute from Right Thumb Phalanx, Percutaneous Approach

0PPR3JZ Removal of Synthetic Substitute from Right Thumb Phalanx, Percutaneous Approach

0PPR3KZ Removal of Nonautologous Tissue Substitute from Right Thumb Phalanx, Percutaneous Approach

0PPR44Z Removal of Internal Fixation Device from Right Thumb Phalanx, Percutaneous Endoscopic Approach

0PPR45Z Removal of External Fixation Device from Right Thumb Phalanx, Percutaneous Endoscopic Approach

0PPR47Z Removal of Autologous Tissue Substitute from Right Thumb Phalanx, Percutaneous Endoscopic Approach

0PPR4JZ Removal of Synthetic Substitute from Right Thumb Phalanx, Percutaneous Endoscopic Approach

0PPR4KZ Removal of Nonautologous Tissue Substitute from Right Thumb Phalanx, Percutaneous Endoscopic Approach

0PPRX4Z Removal of Internal Fixation Device from Right Thumb Phalanx, External Approach

0PPRX5Z Removal of External Fixation Device from Right Thumb Phalanx, External Approach

0PPS04Z Removal of Internal Fixation Device from Left Thumb Phalanx, Open Approach

0PPS05Z Removal of External Fixation Device from Left Thumb Phalanx, Open Approach

0PPS07Z Removal of Autologous Tissue Substitute from Left Thumb Phalanx, Open Approach

0PPS0JZ Removal of Synthetic Substitute from Left Thumb Phalanx, Open Approach

0PPS0KZ Removal of Nonautologous Tissue Substitute from Left Thumb Phalanx, Open Approach

0PPS34Z Removal of Internal Fixation Device from Left Thumb Phalanx, Percutaneous Approach

0PPS35Z Removal of External Fixation Device from Left Thumb Phalanx, Percutaneous Approach

0PPS37Z Removal of Autologous Tissue Substitute from Left Thumb Phalanx, Percutaneous Approach

0PPS3JZ Removal of Synthetic Substitute from Left Thumb Phalanx, Percutaneous Approach

0PPS3KZ Removal of Nonautologous Tissue Substitute from Left Thumb Phalanx, Percutaneous Approach

0PPS44Z Removal of Internal Fixation Device from Left Thumb Phalanx, Percutaneous Endoscopic Approach

0PPS45Z Removal of External Fixation Device from Left Thumb Phalanx, Percutaneous Endoscopic Approach

0PPS47Z Removal of Autologous Tissue Substitute from Left Thumb Phalanx, Percutaneous Endoscopic Approach

0PPS4JZ Removal of Synthetic Substitute from Left Thumb Phalanx, Percutaneous Endoscopic Approach

0PPS4KZ Removal of Nonautologous Tissue Substitute from Left Thumb Phalanx, Percutaneous Endoscopic Approach

0PPSX4Z Removal of Internal Fixation Device from Left Thumb Phalanx, External Approach

0PPSX5Z Removal of External Fixation Device from Left Thumb Phalanx, External Approach

0PPT04Z Removal of Internal Fixation Device from Right Finger Phalanx, Open Approach

0PPT05Z Removal of External Fixation Device from Right Finger Phalanx, Open Approach

0PPT07Z Removal of Autologous Tissue Substitute from Right Finger Phalanx, Open Approach

0PPT0JZ Removal of Synthetic Substitute from Right Finger Phalanx, Open Approach

0PPT0KZ Removal of Nonautologous Tissue Substitute from Right Finger Phalanx, Open Approach

0PPT34Z Removal of Internal Fixation Device from Right Finger Phalanx, Percutaneous Approach

0PPT35Z Removal of External Fixation Device from Right Finger Phalanx, Percutaneous Approach

0PPT37Z Removal of Autologous Tissue Substitute from Right Finger Phalanx, Percutaneous Approach

0PPT3JZ Removal of Synthetic Substitute from Right Finger Phalanx, Percutaneous Approach

0PPT3KZ Removal of Nonautologous Tissue Substitute from Right Finger Phalanx, Percutaneous Approach

0PPT44Z Removal of Internal Fixation Device from Right Finger Phalanx, Percutaneous Endoscopic Approach

0PPT45Z Removal of External Fixation Device from Right Finger Phalanx, Percutaneous Endoscopic Approach

0PPT47Z Removal of Autologous Tissue Substitute from Right Finger Phalanx, Percutaneous Endoscopic Approach

0PPT4JZ Removal of Synthetic Substitute from Right Finger Phalanx, Percutaneous Endoscopic Approach

0PPT4KZ Removal of Nonautologous Tissue Substitute from Right Finger Phalanx, Percutaneous Endoscopic Approach

0PPTX4Z Removal of Internal Fixation Device from Right Finger Phalanx, External Approach

0PPTX5Z Removal of External Fixation Device from Right Finger Phalanx, External Approach

0PPV04Z Removal of Internal Fixation Device from Left Finger Phalanx, Open Approach

0PPV05Z Removal of External Fixation Device from Left Finger Phalanx, Open Approach

0PPV07Z Removal of Autologous Tissue Substitute from Left Finger Phalanx, Open Approach

0PPV0JZ Removal of Synthetic Substitute from Left Finger Phalanx, Open Approach

0PPV0KZ Removal of Nonautologous Tissue Substitute from Left Finger Phalanx, Open Approach

0PPV34Z Removal of Internal Fixation Device from Left Finger Phalanx, Percutaneous Approach

0PPV35Z Removal of External Fixation Device from Left Finger Phalanx, Percutaneous Approach

0PPV37Z Removal of Autologous Tissue Substitute from Left Finger Phalanx, Percutaneous Approach

0PPV3JZ Removal of Synthetic Substitute from Left Finger Phalanx, Percutaneous Approach

0PPV3KZ Removal of Nonautologous Tissue Substitute from Left Finger Phalanx, Percutaneous Approach

0PPV44Z Removal of Internal Fixation Device from Left Finger Phalanx, Percutaneous Endoscopic Approach

0PPV45Z Removal of External Fixation Device from Left Finger Phalanx, Percutaneous Endoscopic Approach

0PPV47Z Removal of Autologous Tissue Substitute from Left Finger Phalanx, Percutaneous Endoscopic Approach

0PPV4JZ Removal of Synthetic Substitute from Left Finger Phalanx, Percutaneous Endoscopic Approach

0PPV4KZ Removal of Nonautologous Tissue Substitute from Left Finger Phalanx, Percutaneous Endoscopic Approach

0PPVX4Z Removal of Internal Fixation Device from Left Finger Phalanx, External Approach

0PPVX5Z Removal of External Fixation Device from Left Finger Phalanx, External Approach

0PPY00Z Removal of Drainage Device from Upper Bone, Open Approach

0PPY0MZ Removal of Bone Growth Stimulator from Upper Bone, Open Approach

0PPY30Z Removal of Drainage Device from Upper Bone, Percutaneous Approach

0PPY3MZ Removal of Bone Growth Stimulator from Upper Bone, Percutaneous Approach

0PPY40Z Removal of Drainage Device from Upper Bone, Percutaneous Endoscopic Approach

0PPY4MZ Removal of Bone Growth Stimulator from Upper Bone, Percutaneous Endoscopic Approach

0PPYX0Z Removal of Drainage Device from Upper Bone, External Approach

0PPYXMZ Removal of Bone Growth Stimulator from Upper Bone, External Approach

0PQ – Upper Bones, Repair

Review Coding Guideline B3.5

0PQ00ZZ Repair Sternum, Open Approach

0PQ03ZZ Repair Sternum, Percutaneous Approach

0PQ04ZZ Repair Sternum, Percutaneous Endoscopic Approach

0PQ0XZZ Repair Sternum, External Approach

0PQ10ZZ Repair I to 2 Ribs, Open Approach

0PQ13ZZ Repair I to 2 Ribs, Percutaneous Approach

0PQ14ZZ Repair I to 2 Ribs, Percutaneous Endoscopic Approach

0PQ1XZZ Repair I to 2 Ribs, External Approach

0PQ20ZZ Repair 3 or More Ribs, Open Approach

♀ Female-only   ♂ Male-only   ▲ Limited Coverage   ● Non-OR   HAC HAC-associated procedure   ▲ Non-covered procedures   ✚ Cluster

0PQ23ZZ	Repair 3 or More Ribs, Percutaneous Approach	
0PQ24ZZ	Repair 3 or More Ribs, Percutaneous Endoscopic Approach	
0PQ2XZZ	Repair 3 or More Ribs, External Approach	
0PQ30ZZ	Repair Cervical Vertebra, Open Approach	
0PQ33ZZ	Repair Cervical Vertebra, Percutaneous Approach	
0PQ34ZZ	Repair Cervical Vertebra, Percutaneous Endoscopic Approach	
0PQ3XZZ	Repair Cervical Vertebra, External Approach	
0PQ40ZZ	Repair Thoracic Vertebra, Open Approach	
0PQ43ZZ	Repair Thoracic Vertebra, Percutaneous Approach	
0PQ44ZZ	Repair Thoracic Vertebra, Percutaneous Endoscopic Approach	
0PQ4XZZ	Repair Thoracic Vertebra, External Approach	
0PQ50ZZ	Repair Right Scapula, Open Approach	
0PQ53ZZ	Repair Right Scapula, Percutaneous Approach	
0PQ54ZZ	Repair Right Scapula, Percutaneous Endoscopic Approach	
0PQ5XZZ	Repair Right Scapula, External Approach	
0PQ60ZZ	Repair Left Scapula, Open Approach	
0PQ63ZZ	Repair Left Scapula, Percutaneous Approach	
0PQ64ZZ	Repair Left Scapula, Percutaneous Endoscopic Approach	
0PQ6XZZ	Repair Left Scapula, External Approach	
0PQ70ZZ	Repair Right Glenoid Cavity, Open Approach	
0PQ73ZZ	Repair Right Glenoid Cavity, Percutaneous Approach	
0PQ74ZZ	Repair Right Glenoid Cavity, Percutaneous Endoscopic Approach	
0PQ7XZZ	Repair Right Glenoid Cavity, External Approach	
0PQ80ZZ	Repair Left Glenoid Cavity, Open Approach	
0PQ83ZZ	Repair Left Glenoid Cavity, Percutaneous Approach	
0PQ84ZZ	Repair Left Glenoid Cavity, Percutaneous Endoscopic Approach	
0PQ8XZZ	Repair Left Glenoid Cavity, External Approach	
0PQ90ZZ	Repair Right Clavicle, Open Approach	
0PQ93ZZ	Repair Right Clavicle, Percutaneous Approach	
0PQ94ZZ	Repair Right Clavicle, Percutaneous Endoscopic Approach	
0PQ9XZZ	Repair Right Clavicle, External Approach	
0PQB0ZZ	Repair Left Clavicle, Open Approach	
0PQB3ZZ	Repair Left Clavicle, Percutaneous Approach	

0PQB4ZZ	Repair Left Clavicle, Percutaneous Endoscopic Approach
0PQBXZZ	Repair Left Clavicle, External Approach
0PQC0ZZ	Repair Right Humeral Head, Open Approach
0PQC3ZZ	Repair Right Humeral Head, Percutaneous Approach
0PQC4ZZ	Repair Right Humeral Head, Percutaneous Endoscopic Approach
0PQCXZZ	Repair Right Humeral Head, External Approach
0PQD0ZZ	Repair Left Humeral Head, Open Approach
0PQD3ZZ	Repair Left Humeral Head, Percutaneous Approach
0PQD4ZZ	Repair Left Humeral Head, Percutaneous Endoscopic Approach
0PQDXZZ	Repair Left Humeral Head, External Approach
0PQF0ZZ	Repair Right Humeral Shaft, Open Approach
0PQF3ZZ	Repair Right Humeral Shaft, Percutaneous Approach
0PQF4ZZ	Repair Right Humeral Shaft, Percutaneous Endoscopic Approach
0PQFXZZ	Repair Right Humeral Shaft, External Approach
0PQG0ZZ	Repair Left Humeral Shaft, Open Approach
0PQG3ZZ	Repair Left Humeral Shaft, Percutaneous Approach
0PQG4ZZ	Repair Left Humeral Shaft, Percutaneous Endoscopic Approach
0PQGXZZ	Repair Left Humeral Shaft, External Approach
0PQH0ZZ	Repair Right Radius, Open Approach
0PQH3ZZ	Repair Right Radius, Percutaneous Approach
0PQH4ZZ	Repair Right Radius, Percutaneous Endoscopic Approach
0PQHXZZ	Repair Right Radius, External Approach
0PQJ0ZZ	Repair Left Radius, Open Approach
0PQJ3ZZ	Repair Left Radius, Percutaneous Approach
0PQJ4ZZ	Repair Left Radius, Percutaneous Endoscopic Approach
0PQJXZZ	Repair Left Radius, External Approach
0PQK0ZZ	Repair Right Ulna, Open Approach
0PQK3ZZ	Repair Right Ulna, Percutaneous Approach
0PQK4ZZ	Repair Right Ulna, Percutaneous Endoscopic Approach
0PQKXZZ	Repair Right Ulna, External Approach
0PQL0ZZ	Repair Left Ulna, Open Approach
0PQL3ZZ	Repair Left Ulna, Percutaneous Approach
0PQL4ZZ	Repair Left Ulna, Percutaneous Endoscopic Approach
0PQLXZZ	Repair Left Ulna, External Approach
0PQM0ZZ	Repair Right Carpal, Open Approach

0PQM3ZZ	Repair Right Carpal, Percutaneous Approach
0PQM4ZZ	Repair Right Carpal, Percutaneous Endoscopic Approach
0PQMXZZ	Repair Right Carpal, External Approach
0PQN0ZZ	Repair Left Carpal, Open Approach
0PQN3ZZ	Repair Left Carpal, Percutaneous Approach
0PQN4ZZ	Repair Left Carpal, Percutaneous Endoscopic Approach
0PQNXZZ	Repair Left Carpal, External Approach
0PQP0ZZ	Repair Right Metacarpal, Open Approach
0PQP3ZZ	Repair Right Metacarpal, Percutaneous Approach
0PQP4ZZ	Repair Right Metacarpal, Percutaneous Endoscopic Approach
0PQPXZZ	Repair Right Metacarpal, External Approach
0PQQ0ZZ	Repair Left Metacarpal, Open Approach
0PQQ3ZZ	Repair Left Metacarpal, Percutaneous Approach
0PQQ4ZZ	Repair Left Metacarpal, Percutaneous Endoscopic Approach
0PQQXZZ	Repair Left Metacarpal, External Approach
0PQR0ZZ	Repair Right Thumb Phalanx, Open Approach
0PQR3ZZ	Repair Right Thumb Phalanx, Percutaneous Approach
0PQR4ZZ	Repair Right Thumb Phalanx, Percutaneous Endoscopic Approach
0PQRXZZ	Repair Right Thumb Phalanx, External Approach
0PQS0ZZ	Repair Left Thumb Phalanx, Open Approach
0PQS3ZZ	Repair Left Thumb Phalanx, Percutaneous Approach
0PQS4ZZ	Repair Left Thumb Phalanx, Percutaneous Endoscopic Approach
0PQSXZZ	Repair Left Thumb Phalanx, External Approach
0PQT0ZZ	Repair Right Finger Phalanx, Open Approach
0PQT3ZZ	Repair Right Finger Phalanx, Percutaneous Approach
0PQT4ZZ	Repair Right Finger Phalanx, Percutaneous Endoscopic Approach
0PQTXZZ	Repair Right Finger Phalanx, External Approach
0PQV0ZZ	Repair Left Finger Phalanx, Open Approach
0PQV3ZZ	Repair Left Finger Phalanx, Percutaneous Approach
0PQV4ZZ	Repair Left Finger Phalanx, Percutaneous Endoscopic Approach
0PQVXZZ	Repair Left Finger Phalanx, External Approach

0PR – Upper Bones, Replacement

Review Coding Guideline B3.18

0PR007Z	Replacement of Sternum with Autologous Tissue Substitute, Open Approach
0PR00JZ	Replacement of Sternum with Synthetic Substitute, Open Approach
0PR00KZ	Replacement of Sternum with Nonautologous Tissue Substitute, Open Approach
0PR037Z	Replacement of Sternum with Autologous Tissue Substitute, Percutaneous Approach
0PR03JZ	Replacement of Sternum with Synthetic Substitute, Percutaneous Approach
0PR03KZ	Replacement of Sternum with Nonautologous Tissue Substitute, Percutaneous Approach
0PR047Z	Replacement of Sternum with Autologous Tissue Substitute, Percutaneous Endoscopic Approach
0PR04JZ	Replacement of Sternum with Synthetic Substitute, Percutaneous Endoscopic Approach
0PR04KZ	Replacement of Sternum with Nonautologous Tissue Substitute, Percutaneous Endoscopic Approach
0PR107Z	Replacement of I to 2 Ribs with Autologous Tissue Substitute, Open Approach

0PR10JZ Replacement of I to 2 Ribs with Synthetic Substitute, Open Approach

0PR10KZ Replacement of I to 2 Ribs with Nonautologous Tissue Substitute, Open Approach

0PR137Z Replacement of I to 2 Ribs with Autologous Tissue Substitute, Percutaneous Approach

0PR13JZ Replacement of I to 2 Ribs with Synthetic Substitute, Percutaneous Approach

0PR13KZ Replacement of I to 2 Ribs with Nonautologous Tissue Substitute, Percutaneous Approach

0PR147Z Replacement of I to 2 Ribs with Autologous Tissue Substitute, Percutaneous Endoscopic Approach

0PR14JZ Replacement of I to 2 Ribs with Synthetic Substitute, Percutaneous Endoscopic Approach

0PR14KZ Replacement of I to 2 Ribs with Nonautologous Tissue Substitute, Percutaneous Endoscopic Approach

0PR207Z Replacement of 3 or More Ribs with Autologous Tissue Substitute, Open Approach

0PR20JZ Replacement of 3 or More Ribs with Synthetic Substitute, Open Approach

0PR20KZ Replacement of 3 or More Ribs with Nonautologous Tissue Substitute, Open Approach

0PR237Z Replacement of 3 or More Ribs with Autologous Tissue Substitute, Percutaneous Approach

0PR23JZ Replacement of 3 or More Ribs with Synthetic Substitute, Percutaneous Approach

0PR23KZ Replacement of 3 or More Ribs with Nonautologous Tissue Substitute, Percutaneous Approach

0PR247Z Replacement of 3 or More Ribs with Autologous Tissue Substitute, Percutaneous Endoscopic Approach

0PR24JZ Replacement of 3 or More Ribs with Synthetic Substitute, Percutaneous Endoscopic Approach

0PR24KZ Replacement of 3 or More Ribs with Nonautologous Tissue Substitute, Percutaneous Endoscopic Approach

0PR307Z Replacement of Cervical Vertebra with Autologous Tissue Substitute, Open Approach

0PR30JZ Replacement of Cervical Vertebra with Synthetic Substitute, Open Approach

0PR30KZ Replacement of Cervical Vertebra with Nonautologous Tissue Substitute, Open Approach

0PR337Z Replacement of Cervical Vertebra with Autologous Tissue Substitute, Percutaneous Approach

0PR33JZ Replacement of Cervical Vertebra with Synthetic Substitute, Percutaneous Approach

0PR33KZ Replacement of Cervical Vertebra with Nonautologous Tissue Substitute, Percutaneous Approach

0PR347Z Replacement of Cervical Vertebra with Autologous Tissue Substitute, Percutaneous Endoscopic Approach

0PR34JZ Replacement of Cervical Vertebra with Synthetic Substitute, Percutaneous Endoscopic Approach

0PR34KZ Replacement of Cervical Vertebra with Nonautologous Tissue Substitute, Percutaneous Endoscopic Approach

0PR407Z Replacement of Thoracic Vertebra with Autologous Tissue Substitute, Open Approach

0PR40JZ Replacement of Thoracic Vertebra with Synthetic Substitute, Open Approach

0PR40KZ Replacement of Thoracic Vertebra with Nonautologous Tissue Substitute, Open Approach

0PR437Z Replacement of Thoracic Vertebra with Autologous Tissue Substitute, Percutaneous Approach

0PR43JZ Replacement of Thoracic Vertebra with Synthetic Substitute, Percutaneous Approach

0PR43KZ Replacement of Thoracic Vertebra with Nonautologous Tissue Substitute, Percutaneous Approach

0PR447Z Replacement of Thoracic Vertebra with Autologous Tissue Substitute, Percutaneous Endoscopic Approach

0PR44JZ Replacement of Thoracic Vertebra with Synthetic Substitute, Percutaneous Endoscopic Approach

0PR44KZ Replacement of Thoracic Vertebra with Nonautologous Tissue Substitute, Percutaneous Endoscopic Approach

0PR507Z Replacement of Right Scapula with Autologous Tissue Substitute, Open Approach

0PR50JZ Replacement of Right Scapula with Synthetic Substitute, Open Approach

0PR50KZ Replacement of Right Scapula with Nonautologous Tissue Substitute, Open Approach

0PR537Z Replacement of Right Scapula with Autologous Tissue Substitute, Percutaneous Approach

0PR53JZ Replacement of Right Scapula with Synthetic Substitute, Percutaneous Approach

0PR53KZ Replacement of Right Scapula with Nonautologous Tissue Substitute, Percutaneous Approach

0PR547Z Replacement of Right Scapula with Autologous Tissue Substitute, Percutaneous Endoscopic Approach

0PR54JZ Replacement of Right Scapula with Synthetic Substitute, Percutaneous Endoscopic Approach

0PR54KZ Replacement of Right Scapula with Nonautologous Tissue Substitute, Percutaneous Endoscopic Approach

0PR607Z Replacement of Left Scapula with Autologous Tissue Substitute, Open Approach

0PR60JZ Replacement of Left Scapula with Synthetic Substitute, Open Approach

0PR60KZ Replacement of Left Scapula with Nonautologous Tissue Substitute, Open Approach

0PR637Z Replacement of Left Scapula with Autologous Tissue Substitute, Percutaneous Approach

0PR63JZ Replacement of Left Scapula with Synthetic Substitute, Percutaneous Approach

0PR63KZ Replacement of Left Scapula with Nonautologous Tissue Substitute, Percutaneous Approach

0PR647Z Replacement of Left Scapula with Autologous Tissue Substitute, Percutaneous Endoscopic Approach

0PR64JZ Replacement of Left Scapula with Synthetic Substitute, Percutaneous Endoscopic Approach

0PR64KZ Replacement of Left Scapula with Nonautologous Tissue Substitute, Percutaneous Endoscopic Approach

0PR707Z Replacement of Right Glenoid Cavity with Autologous Tissue Substitute, Open Approach

0PR70JZ Replacement of Right Glenoid Cavity with Synthetic Substitute, Open Approach

0PR70KZ Replacement of Right Glenoid Cavity with Nonautologous Tissue Substitute, Open Approach

0PR737Z Replacement of Right Glenoid Cavity with Autologous Tissue Substitute, Percutaneous Approach

0PR73JZ Replacement of Right Glenoid Cavity with Synthetic Substitute, Percutaneous Approach

0PR73KZ Replacement of Right Glenoid Cavity with Nonautologous Tissue Substitute, Percutaneous Approach

0PR747Z Replacement of Right Glenoid Cavity with Autologous Tissue Substitute, Percutaneous Endoscopic Approach

0PR74JZ Replacement of Right Glenoid Cavity with Synthetic Substitute, Percutaneous Endoscopic Approach

0PR74KZ Replacement of Right Glenoid Cavity with Nonautologous Tissue Substitute, Percutaneous Endoscopic Approach

0PR807Z Replacement of Left Glenoid Cavity with Autologous Tissue Substitute, Open Approach

0PR80JZ Replacement of Left Glenoid Cavity with Synthetic Substitute, Open Approach

0PR80KZ Replacement of Left Glenoid Cavity with Nonautologous Tissue Substitute, Open Approach

0PR837Z Replacement of Left Glenoid Cavity with Autologous Tissue Substitute, Percutaneous Approach

0PR83JZ Replacement of Left Glenoid Cavity with Synthetic Substitute, Percutaneous Approach

0PR83KZ Replacement of Left Glenoid Cavity with Nonautologous Tissue Substitute, Percutaneous Approach

0PR847Z Replacement of Left Glenoid Cavity with Autologous Tissue Substitute, Percutaneous Endoscopic Approach

0PR84JZ Replacement of Left Glenoid Cavity with Synthetic Substitute, Percutaneous Endoscopic Approach

0PR84KZ Replacement of Left Glenoid Cavity with Nonautologous Tissue Substitute, Percutaneous Endoscopic Approach

0PR907Z Replacement of Right Clavicle with Autologous Tissue Substitute, Open Approach

0PR90JZ Replacement of Right Clavicle with Synthetic Substitute, Open Approach

0PR90KZ Replacement of Right Clavicle with Nonautologous Tissue Substitute, Open Approach

0PR937Z Replacement of Right Clavicle with Autologous Tissue Substitute, Percutaneous Approach

0PR93JZ Replacement of Right Clavicle with Synthetic Substitute, Percutaneous Approach

0PR93KZ Replacement of Right Clavicle with Nonautologous Tissue Substitute, Percutaneous Approach

0PR947Z Replacement of Right Clavicle with Autologous Tissue Substitute, Percutaneous Endoscopic Approach

♀ Female-only   ♂ Male-only   ▲ Limited Coverage   ● Non-OR   ▦ HAC-associated procedure   ▲ Non-covered procedures   ✚ Cluster

0PR94JZ	Replacement of Right Clavicle with Synthetic Substitute, Percutaneous Endoscopic Approach
0PR94KZ	Replacement of Right Clavicle with Nonautologous Tissue Substitute, Percutaneous Endoscopic Approach
0PRB07Z	Replacement of Left Clavicle with Autologous Tissue Substitute, Open Approach
0PRB0JZ	Replacement of Left Clavicle with Synthetic Substitute, Open Approach
0PRB0KZ	Replacement of Left Clavicle with Nonautologous Tissue Substitute, Open Approach
0PRB37Z	Replacement of Left Clavicle with Autologous Tissue Substitute, Percutaneous Approach
0PRB3JZ	Replacement of Left Clavicle with Synthetic Substitute, Percutaneous Approach
0PRB3KZ	Replacement of Left Clavicle with Nonautologous Tissue Substitute, Percutaneous Approach
0PRB47Z	Replacement of Left Clavicle with Autologous Tissue Substitute, Percutaneous Endoscopic Approach
0PRB4JZ	Replacement of Left Clavicle with Synthetic Substitute, Percutaneous Endoscopic Approach
0PRB4KZ	Replacement of Left Clavicle with Nonautologous Tissue Substitute, Percutaneous Endoscopic Approach
0PRC07Z	Replacement of Right Humeral Head with Autologous Tissue Substitute, Open Approach
0PRC0JZ	Replacement of Right Humeral Head with Synthetic Substitute, Open Approach
0PRC0KZ	Replacement of Right Humeral Head with Nonautologous Tissue Substitute, Open Approach
0PRC37Z	Replacement of Right Humeral Head with Autologous Tissue Substitute, Percutaneous Approach
0PRC3JZ	Replacement of Right Humeral Head with Synthetic Substitute, Percutaneous Approach
0PRC3KZ	Replacement of Right Humeral Head with Nonautologous Tissue Substitute, Percutaneous Approach
0PRC47Z	Replacement of Right Humeral Head with Autologous Tissue Substitute, Percutaneous Endoscopic Approach
0PRC4JZ	Replacement of Right Humeral Head with Synthetic Substitute, Percutaneous Endoscopic Approach
0PRC4KZ	Replacement of Right Humeral Head with Nonautologous Tissue Substitute, Percutaneous Endoscopic Approach
0PRD07Z	Replacement of Left Humeral Head with Autologous Tissue Substitute, Open Approach
0PRD0JZ	Replacement of Left Humeral Head with Synthetic Substitute, Open Approach
0PRD0KZ	Replacement of Left Humeral Head with Nonautologous Tissue Substitute, Open Approach
0PRD37Z	Replacement of Left Humeral Head with Autologous Tissue Substitute, Percutaneous Approach
0PRD3JZ	Replacement of Left Humeral Head with Synthetic Substitute, Percutaneous Approach
0PRD3KZ	Replacement of Left Humeral Head with Nonautologous Tissue Substitute, Percutaneous Approach

0PRD47Z	Replacement of Left Humeral Head with Autologous Tissue Substitute, Percutaneous Endoscopic Approach
0PRD4JZ	Replacement of Left Humeral Head with Synthetic Substitute, Percutaneous Endoscopic Approach
0PRD4KZ	Replacement of Left Humeral Head with Nonautologous Tissue Substitute, Percutaneous Endoscopic Approach
0PRF07Z	Replacement of Right Humeral Shaft with Autologous Tissue Substitute, Open Approach
0PRF0JZ	Replacement of Right Humeral Shaft with Synthetic Substitute, Open Approach
0PRF0KZ	Replacement of Right Humeral Shaft with Nonautologous Tissue Substitute, Open Approach
0PRF37Z	Replacement of Right Humeral Shaft with Autologous Tissue Substitute, Percutaneous Approach
0PRF3JZ	Replacement of Right Humeral Shaft with Synthetic Substitute, Percutaneous Approach
0PRF3KZ	Replacement of Right Humeral Shaft with Nonautologous Tissue Substitute, Percutaneous Approach
0PRF47Z	Replacement of Right Humeral Shaft with Autologous Tissue Substitute, Percutaneous Endoscopic Approach
0PRF4JZ	Replacement of Right Humeral Shaft with Synthetic Substitute, Percutaneous Endoscopic Approach
0PRF4KZ	Replacement of Right Humeral Shaft with Nonautologous Tissue Substitute, Percutaneous Endoscopic Approach
0PRG07Z	Replacement of Left Humeral Shaft with Autologous Tissue Substitute, Open Approach
0PRG0JZ	Replacement of Left Humeral Shaft with Synthetic Substitute, Open Approach
0PRG0KZ	Replacement of Left Humeral Shaft with Nonautologous Tissue Substitute, Open Approach
0PRG37Z	Replacement of Left Humeral Shaft with Autologous Tissue Substitute, Percutaneous Approach
0PRG3JZ	Replacement of Left Humeral Shaft with Synthetic Substitute, Percutaneous Approach
0PRG3KZ	Replacement of Left Humeral Shaft with Nonautologous Tissue Substitute, Percutaneous Approach
0PRG47Z	Replacement of Left Humeral Shaft with Autologous Tissue Substitute, Percutaneous Endoscopic Approach
0PRG4JZ	Replacement of Left Humeral Shaft with Synthetic Substitute, Percutaneous Endoscopic Approach
0PRG4KZ	Replacement of Left Humeral Shaft with Nonautologous Tissue Substitute, Percutaneous Endoscopic Approach
0PRH07Z	Replacement of Right Radius with Autologous Tissue Substitute, Open Approach
0PRH0JZ	Replacement of Right Radius with Synthetic Substitute, Open Approach
	AHA CC: 4Q, 2018, 92-93
0PRH0KZ	Replacement of Right Radius with Nonautologous Tissue Substitute, Open Approach
0PRH37Z	Replacement of Right Radius with Autologous Tissue Substitute, Percutaneous Approach

0PRH3JZ	Replacement of Right Radius with Synthetic Substitute, Percutaneous Approach
0PRH3KZ	Replacement of Right Radius with Nonautologous Tissue Substitute, Percutaneous Approach
0PRH47Z	Replacement of Right Radius with Autologous Tissue Substitute, Percutaneous Endoscopic Approach
0PRH4JZ	Replacement of Right Radius with Synthetic Substitute, Percutaneous Endoscopic Approach
0PRH4KZ	Replacement of Right Radius with Nonautologous Tissue Substitute, Percutaneous Endoscopic Approach
0PRJ07Z	Replacement of Left Radius with Autologous Tissue Substitute, Open Approach
0PRJ0JZ	Replacement of Left Radius with Synthetic Substitute, Open Approach
0PRJ0KZ	Replacement of Left Radius with Nonautologous Tissue Substitute, Open Approach
0PRJ37Z	Replacement of Left Radius with Autologous Tissue Substitute, Percutaneous Approach
0PRJ3JZ	Replacement of Left Radius with Synthetic Substitute, Percutaneous Approach
0PRJ3KZ	Replacement of Left Radius with Nonautologous Tissue Substitute, Percutaneous Approach
0PRJ47Z	Replacement of Left Radius with Autologous Tissue Substitute, Percutaneous Endoscopic Approach
0PRJ4JZ	Replacement of Left Radius with Synthetic Substitute, Percutaneous Endoscopic Approach
0PRJ4KZ	Replacement of Left Radius with Nonautologous Tissue Substitute, Percutaneous Endoscopic Approach
0PRK07Z	Replacement of Right Ulna with Autologous Tissue Substitute, Open Approach
0PRK0JZ	Replacement of Right Ulna with Synthetic Substitute, Open Approach
0PRK0KZ	Replacement of Right Ulna with Nonautologous Tissue Substitute, Open Approach
0PRK37Z	Replacement of Right Ulna with Autologous Tissue Substitute, Percutaneous Approach
0PRK3JZ	Replacement of Right Ulna with Synthetic Substitute, Percutaneous Approach
0PRK3KZ	Replacement of Right Ulna with Nonautologous Tissue Substitute, Percutaneous Approach
0PRK47Z	Replacement of Right Ulna with Autologous Tissue Substitute, Percutaneous Endoscopic Approach
0PRK4JZ	Replacement of Right Ulna with Synthetic Substitute, Percutaneous Endoscopic Approach
0PRK4KZ	Replacement of Right Ulna with Nonautologous Tissue Substitute, Percutaneous Endoscopic Approach
0PRL07Z	Replacement of Left Ulna with Autologous Tissue Substitute, Open Approach
0PRL0JZ	Replacement of Left Ulna with Synthetic Substitute, Open Approach
0PRL0KZ	Replacement of Left Ulna with Nonautologous Tissue Substitute, Open Approach

♀ Female-only   ♂ Male-only   ▲ Limited Coverage   ● Non-OR   ▰▰ HAC-associated procedure   ▲ Non-covered procedures   ✚ Cluster

0PRL37Z Replacement of Left Ulna with Autologous Tissue Substitute, Percutaneous Approach

0PRL3JZ Replacement of Left Ulna with Synthetic Substitute, Percutaneous Approach

0PRL3KZ Replacement of Left Ulna with Nonautologous Tissue Substitute, Percutaneous Approach

0PRL47Z Replacement of Left Ulna with Autologous Tissue Substitute, Percutaneous Endoscopic Approach

0PRL4JZ Replacement of Left Ulna with Synthetic Substitute, Percutaneous Endoscopic Approach

0PRL4KZ Replacement of Left Ulna with Nonautologous Tissue Substitute, Percutaneous Endoscopic Approach

0PRM07Z Replacement of Right Carpal with Autologous Tissue Substitute, Open Approach

0PRM0JZ Replacement of Right Carpal with Synthetic Substitute, Open Approach

0PRM0KZ Replacement of Right Carpal with Nonautologous Tissue Substitute, Open Approach

0PRM37Z Replacement of Right Carpal with Autologous Tissue Substitute, Percutaneous Approach

0PRM3JZ Replacement of Right Carpal with Synthetic Substitute, Percutaneous Approach

0PRM3KZ Replacement of Right Carpal with Nonautologous Tissue Substitute, Percutaneous Approach

0PRM47Z Replacement of Right Carpal with Autologous Tissue Substitute, Percutaneous Endoscopic Approach

0PRM4JZ Replacement of Right Carpal with Synthetic Substitute, Percutaneous Endoscopic Approach

0PRM4KZ Replacement of Right Carpal with Nonautologous Tissue Substitute, Percutaneous Endoscopic Approach

0PRN07Z Replacement of Left Carpal with Autologous Tissue Substitute, Open Approach

0PRN0JZ Replacement of Left Carpal with Synthetic Substitute, Open Approach

0PRN0KZ Replacement of Left Carpal with Nonautologous Tissue Substitute, Open Approach

0PRN37Z Replacement of Left Carpal with Autologous Tissue Substitute, Percutaneous Approach

0PRN3JZ Replacement of Left Carpal with Synthetic Substitute, Percutaneous Approach

0PRN3KZ Replacement of Left Carpal with Nonautologous Tissue Substitute, Percutaneous Approach

0PRN47Z Replacement of Left Carpal with Autologous Tissue Substitute, Percutaneous Endoscopic Approach

0PRN4JZ Replacement of Left Carpal with Synthetic Substitute, Percutaneous Endoscopic Approach

0PRN4KZ Replacement of Left Carpal with Nonautologous Tissue Substitute, Percutaneous Endoscopic Approach

0PRP07Z Replacement of Right Metacarpal with Autologous Tissue Substitute, Open Approach

0PRP0JZ Replacement of Right Metacarpal with Synthetic Substitute, Open Approach

0PRP0KZ Replacement of Right Metacarpal with Nonautologous Tissue Substitute, Open Approach

0PRP37Z Replacement of Right Metacarpal with Autologous Tissue Substitute, Percutaneous Approach

0PRP3JZ Replacement of Right Metacarpal with Synthetic Substitute, Percutaneous Approach

0PRP3KZ Replacement of Right Metacarpal with Nonautologous Tissue Substitute, Percutaneous Approach

0PRP47Z Replacement of Right Metacarpal with Autologous Tissue Substitute, Percutaneous Endoscopic Approach

0PRP4JZ Replacement of Right Metacarpal with Synthetic Substitute, Percutaneous Endoscopic Approach

0PRP4KZ Replacement of Right Metacarpal with Nonautologous Tissue Substitute, Percutaneous Endoscopic Approach

0PRQ07Z Replacement of Left Metacarpal with Autologous Tissue Substitute, Open Approach

0PRQ0JZ Replacement of Left Metacarpal with Synthetic Substitute, Open Approach

0PRQ0KZ Replacement of Left Metacarpal with Nonautologous Tissue Substitute, Open Approach

0PRQ37Z Replacement of Left Metacarpal with Autologous Tissue Substitute, Percutaneous Approach

0PRQ3JZ Replacement of Left Metacarpal with Synthetic Substitute, Percutaneous Approach

0PRQ3KZ Replacement of Left Metacarpal with Nonautologous Tissue Substitute, Percutaneous Approach

0PRQ47Z Replacement of Left Metacarpal with Autologous Tissue Substitute, Percutaneous Endoscopic Approach

0PRQ4JZ Replacement of Left Metacarpal with Synthetic Substitute, Percutaneous Endoscopic Approach

0PRQ4KZ Replacement of Left Metacarpal with Nonautologous Tissue Substitute, Percutaneous Endoscopic Approach

0PRR07Z Replacement of Right Thumb Phalanx with Autologous Tissue Substitute, Open Approach

0PRR0JZ Replacement of Right Thumb Phalanx with Synthetic Substitute, Open Approach

0PRR0KZ Replacement of Right Thumb Phalanx with Nonautologous Tissue Substitute, Open Approach

0PRR37Z Replacement of Right Thumb Phalanx with Autologous Tissue Substitute, Percutaneous Approach

0PRR3JZ Replacement of Right Thumb Phalanx with Synthetic Substitute, Percutaneous Approach

0PRR3KZ Replacement of Right Thumb Phalanx with Nonautologous Tissue Substitute, Percutaneous Approach

0PRR47Z Replacement of Right Thumb Phalanx with Autologous Tissue Substitute, Percutaneous Endoscopic Approach

0PRR4JZ Replacement of Right Thumb Phalanx with Synthetic Substitute, Percutaneous Endoscopic Approach

0PRR4KZ Replacement of Right Thumb Phalanx with Nonautologous Tissue Substitute, Percutaneous Endoscopic Approach

0PRS07Z Replacement of Left Thumb Phalanx with Autologous Tissue Substitute, Open Approach

0PRS0JZ Replacement of Left Thumb Phalanx with Synthetic Substitute, Open Approach

0PRS0KZ Replacement of Left Thumb Phalanx with Nonautologous Tissue Substitute, Open Approach

0PRS37Z Replacement of Left Thumb Phalanx with Autologous Tissue Substitute, Percutaneous Approach

0PRS3JZ Replacement of Left Thumb Phalanx with Synthetic Substitute, Percutaneous Approach

0PRS3KZ Replacement of Left Thumb Phalanx with Nonautologous Tissue Substitute, Percutaneous Approach

0PRS47Z Replacement of Left Thumb Phalanx with Autologous Tissue Substitute, Percutaneous Endoscopic Approach

0PRS4JZ Replacement of Left Thumb Phalanx with Synthetic Substitute, Percutaneous Endoscopic Approach

0PRS4KZ Replacement of Left Thumb Phalanx with Nonautologous Tissue Substitute, Percutaneous Endoscopic Approach

0PRT07Z Replacement of Right Finger Phalanx with Autologous Tissue Substitute, Open Approach

0PRT0JZ Replacement of Right Finger Phalanx with Synthetic Substitute, Open Approach

0PRT0KZ Replacement of Right Finger Phalanx with Nonautologous Tissue Substitute, Open Approach

0PRT37Z Replacement of Right Finger Phalanx with Autologous Tissue Substitute, Percutaneous Approach

0PRT3JZ Replacement of Right Finger Phalanx with Synthetic Substitute, Percutaneous Approach

0PRT3KZ Replacement of Right Finger Phalanx with Nonautologous Tissue Substitute, Percutaneous Approach

0PRT47Z Replacement of Right Finger Phalanx with Autologous Tissue Substitute, Percutaneous Endoscopic Approach

0PRT4JZ Replacement of Right Finger Phalanx with Synthetic Substitute, Percutaneous Endoscopic Approach

0PRT4KZ Replacement of Right Finger Phalanx with Nonautologous Tissue Substitute, Percutaneous Endoscopic Approach

0PRV07Z Replacement of Left Finger Phalanx with Autologous Tissue Substitute, Open Approach

0PRV0JZ Replacement of Left Finger Phalanx with Synthetic Substitute, Open Approach

0PRV0KZ Replacement of Left Finger Phalanx with Nonautologous Tissue Substitute, Open Approach

0PRV37Z Replacement of Left Finger Phalanx with Autologous Tissue Substitute, Percutaneous Approach

0PRV3JZ Replacement of Left Finger Phalanx with Synthetic Substitute, Percutaneous Approach

0PRV3KZ Replacement of Left Finger Phalanx with Nonautologous Tissue Substitute, Percutaneous Approach

♀ Female-only   ♂ Male-only   ▲ Limited Coverage   ● Non-OR   🅷🅰🅲 HAC-associated procedure   ▲ Non-covered procedures   ➕ Cluster

0PRV47Z Replacement of Left Finger Phalanx with Autologous Tissue Substitute, Percutaneous Endoscopic Approach

0PRV4JZ Replacement of Left Finger Phalanx with Synthetic Substitute, Percutaneous Endoscopic Approach

0PRV4KZ Replacement of Left Finger Phalanx with Nonautologous Tissue Substitute, Percutaneous Endoscopic Approach

0PS – Upper Bones, Reposition

Review Coding Guideline B3.15

0PS000Z Reposition Sternum with Rigid Plate Internal Fixation Device, Open Approach

0PS004Z Reposition Sternum with Internal Fixation Device, Open Approach

0PS00ZZ Reposition Sternum, Open Approach
AHA CC: 4Q, 2015, 34

0PS030Z Reposition Sternum with Rigid Plate Internal Fixation Device, Percutaneous Approach

0PS034Z Reposition Sternum with Internal Fixation Device, Percutaneous Approach

0PS03ZZ Reposition Sternum, Percutaneous Approach

0PS040Z Reposition Sternum with Rigid Plate Internal Fixation Device, Percutaneous Endoscopic Approach

0PS044Z Reposition Sternum with Internal Fixation Device, Percutaneous Endoscopic Approach

0PS04ZZ Reposition Sternum, Percutaneous Endoscopic Approach

0PS0XZZ Reposition Sternum, External Approach

0PS104Z Reposition I to 2 Ribs with Internal Fixation Device, Open Approach

0PS10ZZ Reposition I to 2 Ribs, Open Approach

0PS134Z Reposition I to 2 Ribs with Internal Fixation Device, Percutaneous Approach

0PS13ZZ Reposition I to 2 Ribs, Percutaneous Approach

0PS144Z Reposition I to 2 Ribs with Internal Fixation Device, Percutaneous Endoscopic Approach

0PS14ZZ Reposition I to 2 Ribs, Percutaneous Endoscopic Approach

0PS1XZZ Reposition I to 2 Ribs, External Approach

0PS204Z Reposition 3 or More Ribs with Internal Fixation Device, Open Approach
AHA CC: 4Q, 2014, 26; 4Q, 2017, 53

0PS20ZZ Reposition 3 or More Ribs, Open Approach

0PS234Z Reposition 3 or More Ribs with Internal Fixation Device, Percutaneous Approach

0PS23ZZ Reposition 3 or More Ribs, Percutaneous Approach

0PS244Z Reposition 3 or More Ribs with Internal Fixation Device, Percutaneous Endoscopic Approach

0PS24ZZ Reposition 3 or More Ribs, Percutaneous Endoscopic Approach

0PS2XZZ Reposition 3 or More Ribs, External Approach

0PS304Z Reposition Cervical Vertebra with Internal Fixation Device, Open Approach

0PS30ZZ Reposition Cervical Vertebra, Open Approach

0PS334Z Reposition Cervical Vertebra with Internal Fixation Device, Percutaneous Approach

0PS33ZZ Reposition Cervical Vertebra, Percutaneous Approach

➕ *See table 0PU to construct a code for Supplement with synthetic substitute.*

0PS344Z Reposition Cervical Vertebra with Internal Fixation Device, Percutaneous Endoscopic Approach

0PS34ZZ Reposition Cervical Vertebra, Percutaneous Endoscopic Approach

0PS3XZZ Reposition Cervical Vertebra, External Approach
AHA CC: 2Q, 2015, 35

0PS403Z Reposition Thoracic Vertebra with Spinal Stabilization Device, Vertebral Body Tether, Open Approach

0PS404Z Reposition Thoracic Vertebra with Internal Fixation Device, Open Approach
AHA CC: 1Q, 2020, 33-34

0PS40ZZ Reposition Thoracic Vertebra, Open Approach

0PS434Z Reposition Thoracic Vertebra with Internal Fixation Device, Percutaneous Approach

0PS43ZZ Reposition Thoracic Vertebra, Percutaneous Approach

➕ *See table 0PU to construct a code for Supplement with synthetic substitute.*

0PS443Z Reposition Thoracic Vertebra with Spinal Stabilization Device, Vertebral Body Tether, Percutaneous Endoscopic Approach

0PS444Z Reposition Thoracic Vertebra with Internal Fixation Device, Percutaneous Endoscopic Approach
AHA CC: 3Q, 2018, 26-27

0PS44ZZ Reposition Thoracic Vertebra, Percutaneous Endoscopic Approach

0PS4XZZ Reposition Thoracic Vertebra, External Approach
AHA CC: 1Q, 2016, 21

0PS504Z Reposition Right Scapula with Internal Fixation Device, Open Approach

0PS50ZZ Reposition Right Scapula, Open Approach

0PS534Z Reposition Right Scapula with Internal Fixation Device, Percutaneous Approach

0PS53ZZ Reposition Right Scapula, Percutaneous Approach

0PS544Z Reposition Right Scapula with Internal Fixation Device, Percutaneous Endoscopic Approach

0PS54ZZ Reposition Right Scapula, Percutaneous Endoscopic Approach

0PS5XZZ Reposition Right Scapula, External Approach

0PS604Z Reposition Left Scapula with Internal Fixation Device, Open Approach

0PS60ZZ Reposition Left Scapula, Open Approach

0PS634Z Reposition Left Scapula with Internal Fixation Device, Percutaneous Approach

0PS63ZZ Reposition Left Scapula, Percutaneous Approach

0PS644Z Reposition Left Scapula with Internal Fixation Device, Percutaneous Endoscopic Approach

0PS64ZZ Reposition Left Scapula, Percutaneous Endoscopic Approach

0PS6XZZ Reposition Left Scapula, External Approach

0PS704Z Reposition Right Glenoid Cavity with Internal Fixation Device, Open Approach

0PS70ZZ Reposition Right Glenoid Cavity, Open Approach

0PS734Z Reposition Right Glenoid Cavity with Internal Fixation Device, Percutaneous Approach

0PS73ZZ Reposition Right Glenoid Cavity, Percutaneous Approach

0PS744Z Reposition Right Glenoid Cavity with Internal Fixation Device, Percutaneous Endoscopic Approach

0PS74ZZ Reposition Right Glenoid Cavity, Percutaneous Endoscopic Approach

0PS7XZZ Reposition Right Glenoid Cavity, External Approach

0PS804Z Reposition Left Glenoid Cavity with Internal Fixation Device, Open Approach

0PS80ZZ Reposition Left Glenoid Cavity, Open Approach

0PS834Z Reposition Left Glenoid Cavity with Internal Fixation Device, Percutaneous Approach

0PS83ZZ Reposition Left Glenoid Cavity, Percutaneous Approach

0PS844Z Reposition Left Glenoid Cavity with Internal Fixation Device, Percutaneous Endoscopic Approach

0PS84ZZ Reposition Left Glenoid Cavity, Percutaneous Endoscopic Approach

0PS8XZZ Reposition Left Glenoid Cavity, External Approach

0PS904Z Reposition Right Clavicle with Internal Fixation Device, Open Approach

0PS90ZZ Reposition Right Clavicle, Open Approach

0PS934Z Reposition Right Clavicle with Internal Fixation Device, Percutaneous Approach

0PS93ZZ Reposition Right Clavicle, Percutaneous Approach

0PS944Z Reposition Right Clavicle with Internal Fixation Device, Percutaneous Endoscopic Approach

0PS94ZZ Reposition Right Clavicle, Percutaneous Endoscopic Approach

0PS9XZZ Reposition Right Clavicle, External Approach

0PSB04Z Reposition Left Clavicle with Internal Fixation Device, Open Approach

0PSB0ZZ Reposition Left Clavicle, Open Approach

0PSB34Z Reposition Left Clavicle with Internal Fixation Device, Percutaneous Approach

0PSB3ZZ Reposition Left Clavicle, Percutaneous Approach

0PSB44Z Reposition Left Clavicle with Internal Fixation Device, Percutaneous Endoscopic Approach

0PSB4ZZ Reposition Left Clavicle, Percutaneous Endoscopic Approach

0PSBXZZ Reposition Left Clavicle, External Approach

0PSC04Z Reposition Right Humeral Head with Internal Fixation Device, Open Approach

0PSC05Z Reposition Right Humeral Head with External Fixation Device, Open Approach

0PSC06Z Reposition Right Humeral Head with Intramedullary Internal Fixation Device, Open Approach

0PSC0BZ Reposition Right Humeral Head with Monoplanar External Fixation Device, Open Approach

0PSC0CZ Reposition Right Humeral Head with Ring External Fixation Device, Open Approach

0PSC0DZ Reposition Right Humeral Head with Hybrid External Fixation Device, Open Approach

0PSC0ZZ Reposition Right Humeral Head, Open Approach

0PSC34Z Reposition Right Humeral Head with Internal Fixation Device, Percutaneous Approach

0PSC35Z Reposition Right Humeral Head with External Fixation Device, Percutaneous Approach

0PSC36Z Reposition Right Humeral Head with Intramedullary Internal Fixation Device, Percutaneous Approach

0PSC3BZ Reposition Right Humeral Head with Monoplanar External Fixation Device, Percutaneous Approach

0PSC3CZ Reposition Right Humeral Head with Ring External Fixation Device, Percutaneous Approach

0PSC3DZ Reposition Right Humeral Head with Hybrid External Fixation Device, Percutaneous Approach

0PSC3ZZ Reposition Right Humeral Head, Percutaneous Approach

0PSC44Z Reposition Right Humeral Head with Internal Fixation Device, Percutaneous Endoscopic Approach

0PSC45Z Reposition Right Humeral Head with External Fixation Device, Percutaneous Endoscopic Approach

0PSC46Z Reposition Right Humeral Head with Intramedullary Internal Fixation Device, Percutaneous Endoscopic Approach

0PSC4BZ Reposition Right Humeral Head with Monoplanar External Fixation Device, Percutaneous Endoscopic Approach

0PSC4CZ Reposition Right Humeral Head with Ring External Fixation Device, Percutaneous Endoscopic Approach

0PSC4DZ Reposition Right Humeral Head with Hybrid External Fixation Device, Percutaneous Endoscopic Approach

0PSC4ZZ Reposition Right Humeral Head, Percutaneous Endoscopic Approach

0PSCXZZ Reposition Right Humeral Head, External Approach

0PSD04Z Reposition Left Humeral Head with Internal Fixation Device, Open Approach

0PSD05Z Reposition Left Humeral Head with External Fixation Device, Open Approach

0PSD06Z Reposition Left Humeral Head with Intramedullary Internal Fixation Device, Open Approach

0PSD0BZ Reposition Left Humeral Head with Monoplanar External Fixation Device, Open Approach

0PSD0CZ Reposition Left Humeral Head with Ring External Fixation Device, Open Approach

0PSD0DZ Reposition Left Humeral Head with Hybrid External Fixation Device, Open Approach

0PSD0ZZ Reposition Left Humeral Head, Open Approach

0PSD34Z Reposition Left Humeral Head with Internal Fixation Device, Percutaneous Approach

0PSD35Z Reposition Left Humeral Head with External Fixation Device, Percutaneous Approach

0PSD36Z Reposition Left Humeral Head with Intramedullary Internal Fixation Device, Percutaneous Approach

0PSD3BZ Reposition Left Humeral Head with Monoplanar External Fixation Device, Percutaneous Approach

0PSD3CZ Reposition Left Humeral Head with Ring External Fixation Device, Percutaneous Approach

0PSD3DZ Reposition Left Humeral Head with Hybrid External Fixation Device, Percutaneous Approach

0PSD3ZZ Reposition Left Humeral Head, Percutaneous Approach

0PSD44Z Reposition Left Humeral Head with Internal Fixation Device, Percutaneous Endoscopic Approach

0PSD45Z Reposition Left Humeral Head with External Fixation Device, Percutaneous Endoscopic Approach

0PSD46Z Reposition Left Humeral Head with Intramedullary Internal Fixation Device, Percutaneous Endoscopic Approach

0PSD4BZ Reposition Left Humeral Head with Monoplanar External Fixation Device, Percutaneous Endoscopic Approach

0PSD4CZ Reposition Left Humeral Head with Ring External Fixation Device, Percutaneous Endoscopic Approach

0PSD4DZ Reposition Left Humeral Head with Hybrid External Fixation Device, Percutaneous Endoscopic Approach

0PSD4ZZ Reposition Left Humeral Head, Percutaneous Endoscopic Approach

0PSDXZZ Reposition Left Humeral Head, External Approach

0PSF04Z Reposition Right Humeral Shaft with Internal Fixation Device, Open Approach

0PSF05Z Reposition Right Humeral Shaft with External Fixation Device, Open Approach

0PSF06Z Reposition Right Humeral Shaft with Intramedullary Internal Fixation Device, Open Approach

0PSF0BZ Reposition Right Humeral Shaft with Monoplanar External Fixation Device, Open Approach

0PSF0CZ Reposition Right Humeral Shaft with Ring External Fixation Device, Open Approach

0PSF0DZ Reposition Right Humeral Shaft with Hybrid External Fixation Device, Open Approach

0PSF0ZZ Reposition Right Humeral Shaft, Open Approach

0PSF34Z Reposition Right Humeral Shaft with Internal Fixation Device, Percutaneous Approach

0PSF35Z Reposition Right Humeral Shaft with External Fixation Device, Percutaneous Approach

0PSF36Z Reposition Right Humeral Shaft with Intramedullary Internal Fixation Device, Percutaneous Approach

0PSF3BZ Reposition Right Humeral Shaft with Monoplanar External Fixation Device, Percutaneous Approach

0PSF3CZ Reposition Right Humeral Shaft with Ring External Fixation Device, Percutaneous Approach

0PSF3DZ Reposition Right Humeral Shaft with Hybrid External Fixation Device, Percutaneous Approach

0PSF3ZZ Reposition Right Humeral Shaft, Percutaneous Approach

0PSF44Z Reposition Right Humeral Shaft with Internal Fixation Device, Percutaneous Endoscopic Approach

0PSF45Z Reposition Right Humeral Shaft with External Fixation Device, Percutaneous Endoscopic Approach

0PSF46Z Reposition Right Humeral Shaft with Intramedullary Internal Fixation Device, Percutaneous Endoscopic Approach

0PSF4BZ Reposition Right Humeral Shaft with Monoplanar External Fixation Device, Percutaneous Endoscopic Approach

0PSF4CZ Reposition Right Humeral Shaft with Ring External Fixation Device, Percutaneous Endoscopic Approach

0PSF4DZ Reposition Right Humeral Shaft with Hybrid External Fixation Device, Percutaneous Endoscopic Approach

0PSF4ZZ Reposition Right Humeral Shaft, Percutaneous Endoscopic Approach

0PSFXZZ Reposition Right Humeral Shaft, External Approach

0PSG04Z Reposition Left Humeral Shaft with Internal Fixation Device, Open Approach

0PSG05Z Reposition Left Humeral Shaft with External Fixation Device, Open Approach

0PSG06Z Reposition Left Humeral Shaft with Intramedullary Internal Fixation Device, Open Approach

0PSG0BZ Reposition Left Humeral Shaft with Monoplanar External Fixation Device, Open Approach

0PSG0CZ Reposition Left Humeral Shaft with Ring External Fixation Device, Open Approach

0PSG0DZ Reposition Left Humeral Shaft with Hybrid External Fixation Device, Open Approach

0PSG0ZZ Reposition Left Humeral Shaft, Open Approach

0PSG34Z Reposition Left Humeral Shaft with Internal Fixation Device, Percutaneous Approach

0PSG35Z Reposition Left Humeral Shaft with External Fixation Device, Percutaneous Approach

0PSG36Z Reposition Left Humeral Shaft with Intramedullary Internal Fixation Device, Percutaneous Approach

0PSG3BZ Reposition Left Humeral Shaft with Monoplanar External Fixation Device, Percutaneous Approach

0PSG3CZ Reposition Left Humeral Shaft with Ring External Fixation Device, Percutaneous Approach

0PSG3DZ Reposition Left Humeral Shaft with Hybrid External Fixation Device, Percutaneous Approach

0PSG3ZZ Reposition Left Humeral Shaft, Percutaneous Approach

0PSG44Z Reposition Left Humeral Shaft with Internal Fixation Device, Percutaneous Endoscopic Approach

0PSG45Z Reposition Left Humeral Shaft with External Fixation Device, Percutaneous Endoscopic Approach

0PSG46Z Reposition Left Humeral Shaft with Intramedullary Internal Fixation Device, Percutaneous Endoscopic Approach

0PSG4BZ Reposition Left Humeral Shaft with Monoplanar External Fixation Device, Percutaneous Endoscopic Approach

0PSG4CZ Reposition Left Humeral Shaft with Ring External Fixation Device, Percutaneous Endoscopic Approach

0PSG4DZ Reposition Left Humeral Shaft with Hybrid External Fixation Device, Percutaneous Endoscopic Approach

0PSG4ZZ Reposition Left Humeral Shaft, Percutaneous Endoscopic Approach

0PSGXZZ Reposition Left Humeral Shaft, External Approach

0PSH04Z Reposition Right Radius with Internal Fixation Device, Open Approach

0PSH05Z Reposition Right Radius with External Fixation Device, Open Approach

0PSH06Z Reposition Right Radius with Intramedullary Internal Fixation Device, Open Approach

0PSH0BZ Reposition Right Radius with Monoplanar External Fixation Device, Open Approach

0PSH0CZ Reposition Right Radius with Ring External Fixation Device, Open Approach

0PSH0DZ Reposition Right Radius with Hybrid External Fixation Device, Open Approach

0PSH0ZZ Reposition Right Radius, Open Approach

0PSH34Z Reposition Right Radius with Internal Fixation Device, Percutaneous Approach

0PSH35Z Reposition Right Radius with External Fixation Device, Percutaneous Approach

0PSH36Z Reposition Right Radius with Intramedullary Internal Fixation Device, Percutaneous Approach

0PSH3BZ Reposition Right Radius with Monoplanar External Fixation Device, Percutaneous Approach

0PSH3CZ Reposition Right Radius with Ring External Fixation Device, Percutaneous Approach

0PSH3DZ Reposition Right Radius with Hybrid External Fixation Device, Percutaneous Approach

0PSH3ZZ Reposition Right Radius, Percutaneous Approach

0PSH44Z Reposition Right Radius with Internal Fixation Device, Percutaneous Endoscopic Approach

0PSH45Z Reposition Right Radius with External Fixation Device, Percutaneous Endoscopic Approach

0PSH46Z Reposition Right Radius with Intramedullary Internal Fixation Device, Percutaneous Endoscopic Approach

0PSH4BZ Reposition Right Radius with Monoplanar External Fixation Device, Percutaneous Endoscopic Approach

0PSH4CZ Reposition Right Radius with Ring External Fixation Device, Percutaneous Endoscopic Approach

0PSH4DZ Reposition Right Radius with Hybrid External Fixation Device, Percutaneous Endoscopic Approach

0PSH4ZZ Reposition Right Radius, Percutaneous Endoscopic Approach

0PSHXZZ Reposition Right Radius, External Approach

0PSJ04Z Reposition Left Radius with Internal Fixation Device, Open Approach
AHA CC: 3Q, 2014, 33-34; 4Q, 2014, 32-33

0PSJ05Z Reposition Left Radius with External Fixation Device, Open Approach

0PSJ06Z Reposition Left Radius with Intramedullary Internal Fixation Device, Open Approach

0PSJ0BZ Reposition Left Radius with Monoplanar External Fixation Device, Open Approach

0PSJ0CZ Reposition Left Radius with Ring External Fixation Device, Open Approach

0PSJ0DZ Reposition Left Radius with Hybrid External Fixation Device, Open Approach

0PSJ0ZZ Reposition Left Radius, Open Approach

0PSJ34Z Reposition Left Radius with Internal Fixation Device, Percutaneous Approach

0PSJ35Z Reposition Left Radius with External Fixation Device, Percutaneous Approach

0PSJ36Z Reposition Left Radius with Intramedullary Internal Fixation Device, Percutaneous Approach

0PSJ3BZ Reposition Left Radius with Monoplanar External Fixation Device, Percutaneous Approach

0PSJ3CZ Reposition Left Radius with Ring External Fixation Device, Percutaneous Approach

0PSJ3DZ Reposition Left Radius with Hybrid External Fixation Device, Percutaneous Approach

0PSJ3ZZ Reposition Left Radius, Percutaneous Approach

0PSJ44Z Reposition Left Radius with Internal Fixation Device, Percutaneous Endoscopic Approach

0PSJ45Z Reposition Left Radius with External Fixation Device, Percutaneous Endoscopic Approach

0PSJ46Z Reposition Left Radius with Intramedullary Internal Fixation Device, Percutaneous Endoscopic Approach

0PSJ4BZ Reposition Left Radius with Monoplanar External Fixation Device, Percutaneous Endoscopic Approach

0PSJ4CZ Reposition Left Radius with Ring External Fixation Device, Percutaneous Endoscopic Approach

0PSJ4DZ Reposition Left Radius with Hybrid External Fixation Device, Percutaneous Endoscopic Approach

0PSJ4ZZ Reposition Left Radius, Percutaneous Endoscopic Approach

0PSJXZZ Reposition Left Radius, External Approach

0PSK04Z Reposition Right Ulna with Internal Fixation Device, Open Approach

0PSK05Z Reposition Right Ulna with External Fixation Device, Open Approach

0PSK06Z Reposition Right Ulna with Intramedullary Internal Fixation Device, Open Approach

0PSK0BZ Reposition Right Ulna with Monoplanar External Fixation Device, Open Approach

0PSK0CZ Reposition Right Ulna with Ring External Fixation Device, Open Approach

0PSK0DZ Reposition Right Ulna with Hybrid External Fixation Device, Open Approach

0PSK0ZZ Reposition Right Ulna, Open Approach

0PSK34Z Reposition Right Ulna with Internal Fixation Device, Percutaneous Approach

0PSK35Z Reposition Right Ulna with External Fixation Device, Percutaneous Approach

0PSK36Z Reposition Right Ulna with Intramedullary Internal Fixation Device, Percutaneous Approach

0PSK3BZ Reposition Right Ulna with Monoplanar External Fixation Device, Percutaneous Approach

0PSK3CZ Reposition Right Ulna with Ring External Fixation Device, Percutaneous Approach

0PSK3DZ Reposition Right Ulna with Hybrid External Fixation Device, Percutaneous Approach

0PSK3ZZ Reposition Right Ulna, Percutaneous Approach

0PSK44Z Reposition Right Ulna with Internal Fixation Device, Percutaneous Endoscopic Approach

0PSK45Z Reposition Right Ulna with External Fixation Device, Percutaneous Endoscopic Approach

0PSK46Z Reposition Right Ulna with Intramedullary Internal Fixation Device, Percutaneous Endoscopic Approach

0PSK4BZ Reposition Right Ulna with Monoplanar External Fixation Device, Percutaneous Endoscopic Approach

0PSK4CZ Reposition Right Ulna with Ring External Fixation Device, Percutaneous Endoscopic Approach

0PSK4DZ Reposition Right Ulna with Hybrid External Fixation Device, Percutaneous Endoscopic Approach

0PSK4ZZ Reposition Right Ulna, Percutaneous Endoscopic Approach

0PSKXZZ Reposition Right Ulna, External Approach

0PSL04Z Reposition Left Ulna with Internal Fixation Device, Open Approach
AHA CC: 4Q, 2014, 32-33

0PSL05Z Reposition Left Ulna with External Fixation Device, Open Approach

0PSL06Z Reposition Left Ulna with Intramedullary Internal Fixation Device, Open Approach

0PSL0BZ Reposition Left Ulna with Monoplanar External Fixation Device, Open Approach

0PSL0CZ Reposition Left Ulna with Ring External Fixation Device, Open Approach

0PSL0DZ Reposition Left Ulna with Hybrid External Fixation Device, Open Approach

0PSL0ZZ Reposition Left Ulna, Open Approach

0PSL34Z Reposition Left Ulna with Internal Fixation Device, Percutaneous Approach

0PSL35Z Reposition Left Ulna with External Fixation Device, Percutaneous Approach

0PSL36Z   Reposition Left Ulna with Intramedullary Internal Fixation Device, Percutaneous Approach

0PSL3BZ   Reposition Left Ulna with Monoplanar External Fixation Device, Percutaneous Approach

0PSL3CZ   Reposition Left Ulna with Ring External Fixation Device, Percutaneous Approach

0PSL3DZ   Reposition Left Ulna with Hybrid External Fixation Device, Percutaneous Approach

0PSL3ZZ   Reposition Left Ulna, Percutaneous Approach

0PSL44Z   Reposition Left Ulna with Internal Fixation Device, Percutaneous Endoscopic Approach

0PSL45Z   Reposition Left Ulna with External Fixation Device, Percutaneous Endoscopic Approach

0PSL46Z   Reposition Left Ulna with Intramedullary Internal Fixation Device, Percutaneous Endoscopic Approach

0PSL4BZ   Reposition Left Ulna with Monoplanar External Fixation Device, Percutaneous Endoscopic Approach

0PSL4CZ   Reposition Left Ulna with Ring External Fixation Device, Percutaneous Endoscopic Approach

0PSL4DZ   Reposition Left Ulna with Hybrid External Fixation Device, Percutaneous Endoscopic Approach

0PSL4ZZ   Reposition Left Ulna, Percutaneous Endoscopic Approach

0PSLXZZ   Reposition Left Ulna, External Approach

0PSM04Z   Reposition Right Carpal with Internal Fixation Device, Open Approach

0PSM05Z   Reposition Right Carpal with External Fixation Device, Open Approach

0PSM0ZZ   Reposition Right Carpal, Open Approach

0PSM34Z   Reposition Right Carpal with Internal Fixation Device, Percutaneous Approach

0PSM35Z   Reposition Right Carpal with External Fixation Device, Percutaneous Approach

0PSM3ZZ   Reposition Right Carpal, Percutaneous Approach

0PSM44Z   Reposition Right Carpal with Internal Fixation Device, Percutaneous Endoscopic Approach

0PSM45Z   Reposition Right Carpal with External Fixation Device, Percutaneous Endoscopic Approach

0PSM4ZZ   Reposition Right Carpal, Percutaneous Endoscopic Approach

0PSMXZZ   Reposition Right Carpal, External Approach

0PSN04Z   Reposition Left Carpal with Internal Fixation Device, Open Approach

0PSN05Z   Reposition Left Carpal with External Fixation Device, Open Approach

0PSN0ZZ   Reposition Left Carpal, Open Approach

0PSN34Z   Reposition Left Carpal with Internal Fixation Device, Percutaneous Approach

0PSN35Z   Reposition Left Carpal with External Fixation Device, Percutaneous Approach

0PSN3ZZ   Reposition Left Carpal, Percutaneous Approach

0PSN44Z   Reposition Left Carpal with Internal Fixation Device, Percutaneous Endoscopic Approach

0PSN45Z   Reposition Left Carpal with External Fixation Device, Percutaneous Endoscopic Approach

0PSN4ZZ   Reposition Left Carpal, Percutaneous Endoscopic Approach

0PSNXZZ   Reposition Left Carpal, External Approach

0PSP04Z   Reposition Right Metacarpal with Internal Fixation Device, Open Approach

0PSP05Z   Reposition Right Metacarpal with External Fixation Device, Open Approach

0PSP0ZZ   Reposition Right Metacarpal, Open Approach

0PSP34Z   Reposition Right Metacarpal with Internal Fixation Device, Percutaneous Approach

0PSP35Z   Reposition Right Metacarpal with External Fixation Device, Percutaneous Approach

0PSP3ZZ   Reposition Right Metacarpal, Percutaneous Approach

0PSP44Z   Reposition Right Metacarpal with Internal Fixation Device, Percutaneous Endoscopic Approach

0PSP45Z   Reposition Right Metacarpal with External Fixation Device, Percutaneous Endoscopic Approach

0PSP4ZZ   Reposition Right Metacarpal, Percutaneous Endoscopic Approach

0PSPXZZ   Reposition Right Metacarpal, External Approach

0PSQ04Z   Reposition Left Metacarpal with Internal Fixation Device, Open Approach

0PSQ05Z   Reposition Left Metacarpal with External Fixation Device, Open Approach

0PSQ0ZZ   Reposition Left Metacarpal, Open Approach

0PSQ34Z   Reposition Left Metacarpal with Internal Fixation Device, Percutaneous Approach

0PSQ35Z   Reposition Left Metacarpal with External Fixation Device, Percutaneous Approach

0PSQ3ZZ   Reposition Left Metacarpal, Percutaneous Approach

0PSQ44Z   Reposition Left Metacarpal with Internal Fixation Device, Percutaneous Endoscopic Approach

0PSQ45Z   Reposition Left Metacarpal with External Fixation Device, Percutaneous Endoscopic Approach

0PSQ4ZZ   Reposition Left Metacarpal, Percutaneous Endoscopic Approach

0PSQXZZ   Reposition Left Metacarpal, External Approach

0PSR04Z   Reposition Right Thumb Phalanx with Internal Fixation Device, Open Approach

0PSR05Z   Reposition Right Thumb Phalanx with External Fixation Device, Open Approach

0PSR0ZZ   Reposition Right Thumb Phalanx, Open Approach

0PSR34Z   Reposition Right Thumb Phalanx with Internal Fixation Device, Percutaneous Approach

0PSR35Z   Reposition Right Thumb Phalanx with External Fixation Device, Percutaneous Approach

0PSR3ZZ   Reposition Right Thumb Phalanx, Percutaneous Approach

0PSR44Z   Reposition Right Thumb Phalanx with Internal Fixation Device, Percutaneous Endoscopic Approach

0PSR45Z   Reposition Right Thumb Phalanx with External Fixation Device, Percutaneous Endoscopic Approach

0PSR4ZZ   Reposition Right Thumb Phalanx, Percutaneous Endoscopic Approach

0PSRXZZ   Reposition Right Thumb Phalanx, External Approach

0PSS04Z   Reposition Left Thumb Phalanx with Internal Fixation Device, Open Approach

0PSS05Z   Reposition Left Thumb Phalanx with External Fixation Device, Open Approach

0PSS0ZZ   Reposition Left Thumb Phalanx, Open Approach

0PSS34Z   Reposition Left Thumb Phalanx with Internal Fixation Device, Percutaneous Approach

0PSS35Z   Reposition Left Thumb Phalanx with External Fixation Device, Percutaneous Approach

0PSS3ZZ   Reposition Left Thumb Phalanx, Percutaneous Approach

0PSS44Z   Reposition Left Thumb Phalanx with Internal Fixation Device, Percutaneous Endoscopic Approach

0PSS45Z   Reposition Left Thumb Phalanx with External Fixation Device, Percutaneous Endoscopic Approach

0PSS4ZZ   Reposition Left Thumb Phalanx, Percutaneous Endoscopic Approach

0PSSXZZ   Reposition Left Thumb Phalanx, External Approach

0PST04Z   Reposition Right Finger Phalanx with Internal Fixation Device, Open Approach

0PST05Z   Reposition Right Finger Phalanx with External Fixation Device, Open Approach

0PST0ZZ   Reposition Right Finger Phalanx, Open Approach

0PST34Z   Reposition Right Finger Phalanx with Internal Fixation Device, Percutaneous Approach

0PST35Z   Reposition Right Finger Phalanx with External Fixation Device, Percutaneous Approach

0PST3ZZ   Reposition Right Finger Phalanx, Percutaneous Approach

0PST44Z   Reposition Right Finger Phalanx with Internal Fixation Device, Percutaneous Endoscopic Approach

0PST45Z   Reposition Right Finger Phalanx with External Fixation Device, Percutaneous Endoscopic Approach

0PST4ZZ   Reposition Right Finger Phalanx, Percutaneous Endoscopic Approach

0PSTXZZ   Reposition Right Finger Phalanx, External Approach

0PSV04Z   Reposition Left Finger Phalanx with Internal Fixation Device, Open Approach

0PSV05Z   Reposition Left Finger Phalanx with External Fixation Device, Open Approach

0PSV0ZZ   Reposition Left Finger Phalanx, Open Approach

0PSV34Z   Reposition Left Finger Phalanx with Internal Fixation Device, Percutaneous Approach

♀ Female-only   ♂ Male-only   ▲ Limited Coverage   ● Non-OR   ⬛ HAC-associated procedure   ▲ Non-covered procedures   ✚ Cluster

0PSV35Z Reposition Left Finger Phalanx with External Fixation Device, Percutaneous Approach

0PSV3ZZ Reposition Left Finger Phalanx, Percutaneous Approach

0PSV44Z Reposition Left Finger Phalanx with Internal Fixation Device, Percutaneous Endoscopic Approach

0PSV45Z Reposition Left Finger Phalanx with External Fixation Device, Percutaneous Endoscopic Approach

0PSV4ZZ Reposition Left Finger Phalanx, Percutaneous Endoscopic Approach

0PSVXZZ Reposition Left Finger Phalanx, External Approach

0PT – Upper Bones, Resection

Review Coding Guideline B3.8

Review Coding Guideline B3.18

0PT00ZZ Resection of Sternum, Open Approach
0PT10ZZ Resection of I to 2 Ribs, Open Approach
0PT20ZZ Resection of 3 or More Ribs, Open Approach
0PT50ZZ Resection of Right Scapula, Open Approach
0PT60ZZ Resection of Left Scapula, Open Approach
0PT70ZZ Resection of Right Glenoid Cavity, Open Approach
0PT80ZZ Resection of Left Glenoid Cavity, Open Approach
0PT90ZZ Resection of Right Clavicle, Open Approach
0PTB0ZZ Resection of Left Clavicle, Open Approach

0PTC0ZZ Resection of Right Humeral Head, Open Approach
0PTD0ZZ Resection of Left Humeral Head, Open Approach
0PTF0ZZ Resection of Right Humeral Shaft, Open Approach
0PTG0ZZ Resection of Left Humeral Shaft, Open Approach
0PTH0ZZ Resection of Right Radius, Open Approach
0PTJ0ZZ Resection of Left Radius, Open Approach
0PTK0ZZ Resection of Right Ulna, Open Approach
0PTL0ZZ Resection of Left Ulna, Open Approach
0PTM0ZZ Resection of Right Carpal, Open Approach

0PTN0ZZ Resection of Left Carpal, Open Approach
    AHA CC: 3Q, 2015, 26-27
0PTP0ZZ Resection of Right Metacarpal, Open Approach
0PTQ0ZZ Resection of Left Metacarpal, Open Approach
0PTR0ZZ Resection of Right Thumb Phalanx, Open Approach
0PTS0ZZ Resection of Left Thumb Phalanx, Open Approach
0PTT0ZZ Resection of Right Finger Phalanx, Open Approach
0PTV0ZZ Resection of Left Finger Phalanx, Open Approach

0PU – Upper Bones, Supplement

0PU007Z Supplement Sternum with Autologous Tissue Substitute, Open Approach
0PU00JZ Supplement Sternum with Synthetic Substitute, Open Approach
    AHA CC: 4Q, 2013, 109-111
0PU00KZ Supplement Sternum with Nonautologous Tissue Substitute, Open Approach
0PU037Z Supplement Sternum with Autologous Tissue Substitute, Percutaneous Approach
0PU03JZ Supplement Sternum with Synthetic Substitute, Percutaneous Approach
0PU03KZ Supplement Sternum with Nonautologous Tissue Substitute, Percutaneous Approach
0PU047Z Supplement Sternum with Autologous Tissue Substitute, Percutaneous Endoscopic Approach
0PU04JZ Supplement Sternum with Synthetic Substitute, Percutaneous Endoscopic Approach
0PU04KZ Supplement Sternum with Nonautologous Tissue Substitute, Percutaneous Endoscopic Approach
0PU107Z Supplement I to 2 Ribs with Autologous Tissue Substitute, Open Approach
0PU10JZ Supplement I to 2 Ribs with Synthetic Substitute, Open Approach
0PU10KZ Supplement I to 2 Ribs with Nonautologous Tissue Substitute, Open Approach
0PU137Z Supplement I to 2 Ribs with Autologous Tissue Substitute, Percutaneous Approach
0PU13JZ Supplement I to 2 Ribs with Synthetic Substitute, Percutaneous Approach
0PU13KZ Supplement I to 2 Ribs with Nonautologous Tissue Substitute, Percutaneous Approach

0PU147Z Supplement I to 2 Ribs with Autologous Tissue Substitute, Percutaneous Endoscopic Approach
0PU14JZ Supplement I to 2 Ribs with Synthetic Substitute, Percutaneous Endoscopic Approach
0PU14KZ Supplement I to 2 Ribs with Nonautologous Tissue Substitute, Percutaneous Endoscopic Approach
0PU207Z Supplement 3 or More Ribs with Autologous Tissue Substitute, Open Approach
0PU20JZ Supplement 3 or More Ribs with Synthetic Substitute, Open Approach
0PU20KZ Supplement 3 or More Ribs with Nonautologous Tissue Substitute, Open Approach
0PU237Z Supplement 3 or More Ribs with Autologous Tissue Substitute, Percutaneous Approach
0PU23JZ Supplement 3 or More Ribs with Synthetic Substitute, Percutaneous Approach
0PU23KZ Supplement 3 or More Ribs with Nonautologous Tissue Substitute, Percutaneous Approach
0PU247Z Supplement 3 or More Ribs with Autologous Tissue Substitute, Percutaneous Endoscopic Approach
0PU24JZ Supplement 3 or More Ribs with Synthetic Substitute, Percutaneous Endoscopic Approach
0PU24KZ Supplement 3 or More Ribs with Nonautologous Tissue Substitute, Percutaneous Endoscopic Approach
0PU307Z Supplement Cervical Vertebra with Autologous Tissue Substitute, Open Approach
0PU30JZ Supplement Cervical Vertebra with Synthetic Substitute, Open Approach

0PU30KZ Supplement Cervical Vertebra with Nonautologous Tissue Substitute, Open Approach
    AHA CC: 2Q, 2015, 20-21
0PU337Z Supplement Cervical Vertebra with Autologous Tissue Substitute, Percutaneous Approach
0PU33JZ Supplement Cervical Vertebra with Synthetic Substitute, Percutaneous Approach
0PU33KZ Supplement Cervical Vertebra with Nonautologous Tissue Substitute, Percutaneous Approach
0PU347Z Supplement Cervical Vertebra with Autologous Tissue Substitute, Percutaneous Endoscopic Approach
0PU34JZ Supplement Cervical Vertebra with Synthetic Substitute, Percutaneous Endoscopic Approach
0PU34KZ Supplement Cervical Vertebra with Nonautologous Tissue Substitute, Percutaneous Endoscopic Approach
0PU407Z Supplement Thoracic Vertebra with Autologous Tissue Substitute, Open Approach
0PU40JZ Supplement Thoracic Vertebra with Synthetic Substitute, Open Approach
0PU40KZ Supplement Thoracic Vertebra with Nonautologous Tissue Substitute, Open Approach
0PU437Z Supplement Thoracic Vertebra with Autologous Tissue Substitute, Percutaneous Approach
0PU43JZ Supplement Thoracic Vertebra with Synthetic Substitute, Percutaneous Approach
0PU43KZ Supplement Thoracic Vertebra with Nonautologous Tissue Substitute, Percutaneous Approach
0PU447Z Supplement Thoracic Vertebra with Autologous Tissue Substitute, Percutaneous Endoscopic Approach

0PU44JZ Supplement Thoracic Vertebra with Synthetic Substitute, Percutaneous Endoscopic Approach

0PU44KZ Supplement Thoracic Vertebra with Nonautologous Tissue Substitute, Percutaneous Endoscopic Approach

0PU507Z Supplement Right Scapula with Autologous Tissue Substitute, Open Approach
AHA CC: 4Q, 2018, 12-13

0PU50JZ Supplement Right Scapula with Synthetic Substitute, Open Approach

0PU50KZ Supplement Right Scapula with Nonautologous Tissue Substitute, Open Approach
AHA CC: 4Q, 2018, 12-13

0PU537Z Supplement Right Scapula with Autologous Tissue Substitute, Percutaneous Approach

0PU53JZ Supplement Right Scapula with Synthetic Substitute, Percutaneous Approach

0PU53KZ Supplement Right Scapula with Nonautologous Tissue Substitute, Percutaneous Approach

0PU547Z Supplement Right Scapula with Autologous Tissue Substitute, Percutaneous Endoscopic Approach

0PU54JZ Supplement Right Scapula with Synthetic Substitute, Percutaneous Endoscopic Approach

0PU54KZ Supplement Right Scapula with Nonautologous Tissue Substitute, Percutaneous Endoscopic Approach

0PU607Z Supplement Left Scapula with Autologous Tissue Substitute, Open Approach

0PU60JZ Supplement Left Scapula with Synthetic Substitute, Open Approach

0PU60KZ Supplement Left Scapula with Nonautologous Tissue Substitute, Open Approach

0PU637Z Supplement Left Scapula with Autologous Tissue Substitute, Percutaneous Approach

0PU63JZ Supplement Left Scapula with Synthetic Substitute, Percutaneous Approach

0PU63KZ Supplement Left Scapula with Nonautologous Tissue Substitute, Percutaneous Approach

0PU647Z Supplement Left Scapula with Autologous Tissue Substitute, Percutaneous Endoscopic Approach

0PU64JZ Supplement Left Scapula with Synthetic Substitute, Percutaneous Endoscopic Approach

0PU64KZ Supplement Left Scapula with Nonautologous Tissue Substitute, Percutaneous Endoscopic Approach

0PU707Z Supplement Right Glenoid Cavity with Autologous Tissue Substitute, Open Approach

0PU70JZ Supplement Right Glenoid Cavity with Synthetic Substitute, Open Approach

0PU70KZ Supplement Right Glenoid Cavity with Nonautologous Tissue Substitute, Open Approach

0PU737Z Supplement Right Glenoid Cavity with Autologous Tissue Substitute, Percutaneous Approach

0PU73JZ Supplement Right Glenoid Cavity with Synthetic Substitute, Percutaneous Approach

0PU73KZ Supplement Right Glenoid Cavity with Nonautologous Tissue Substitute, Percutaneous Approach

0PU747Z Supplement Right Glenoid Cavity with Autologous Tissue Substitute, Percutaneous Endoscopic Approach

0PU74JZ Supplement Right Glenoid Cavity with Synthetic Substitute, Percutaneous Endoscopic Approach

0PU74KZ Supplement Right Glenoid Cavity with Nonautologous Tissue Substitute, Percutaneous Endoscopic Approach

0PU807Z Supplement Left Glenoid Cavity with Autologous Tissue Substitute, Open Approach

0PU80JZ Supplement Left Glenoid Cavity with Synthetic Substitute, Open Approach

0PU80KZ Supplement Left Glenoid Cavity with Nonautologous Tissue Substitute, Open Approach

0PU837Z Supplement Left Glenoid Cavity with Autologous Tissue Substitute, Percutaneous Approach

0PU83JZ Supplement Left Glenoid Cavity with Synthetic Substitute, Percutaneous Approach

0PU83KZ Supplement Left Glenoid Cavity with Nonautologous Tissue Substitute, Percutaneous Approach

0PU847Z Supplement Left Glenoid Cavity with Autologous Tissue Substitute, Percutaneous Endoscopic Approach

0PU84JZ Supplement Left Glenoid Cavity with Synthetic Substitute, Percutaneous Endoscopic Approach

0PU84KZ Supplement Left Glenoid Cavity with Nonautologous Tissue Substitute, Percutaneous Endoscopic Approach

0PU907Z Supplement Right Clavicle with Autologous Tissue Substitute, Open Approach

0PU90JZ Supplement Right Clavicle with Synthetic Substitute, Open Approach

0PU90KZ Supplement Right Clavicle with Nonautologous Tissue Substitute, Open Approach

0PU937Z Supplement Right Clavicle with Autologous Tissue Substitute, Percutaneous Approach

0PU93JZ Supplement Right Clavicle with Synthetic Substitute, Percutaneous Approach

0PU93KZ Supplement Right Clavicle with Nonautologous Tissue Substitute, Percutaneous Approach

0PU947Z Supplement Right Clavicle with Autologous Tissue Substitute, Percutaneous Endoscopic Approach

0PU94JZ Supplement Right Clavicle with Synthetic Substitute, Percutaneous Endoscopic Approach

0PU94KZ Supplement Right Clavicle with Nonautologous Tissue Substitute, Percutaneous Endoscopic Approach

0PUB07Z Supplement Left Clavicle with Autologous Tissue Substitute, Open Approach

0PUB0JZ Supplement Left Clavicle with Synthetic Substitute, Open Approach

0PUB0KZ Supplement Left Clavicle with Nonautologous Tissue Substitute, Open Approach

0PUB37Z Supplement Left Clavicle with Autologous Tissue Substitute, Percutaneous Approach

0PUB3JZ Supplement Left Clavicle with Synthetic Substitute, Percutaneous Approach

0PUB3KZ Supplement Left Clavicle with Nonautologous Tissue Substitute, Percutaneous Approach

0PUB47Z Supplement Left Clavicle with Autologous Tissue Substitute, Percutaneous Endoscopic Approach

0PUB4JZ Supplement Left Clavicle with Synthetic Substitute, Percutaneous Endoscopic Approach

0PUB4KZ Supplement Left Clavicle with Nonautologous Tissue Substitute, Percutaneous Endoscopic Approach

0PUC07Z Supplement Right Humeral Head with Autologous Tissue Substitute, Open Approach

0PUC0JZ Supplement Right Humeral Head with Synthetic Substitute, Open Approach

0PUC0KZ Supplement Right Humeral Head with Nonautologous Tissue Substitute, Open Approach

0PUC37Z Supplement Right Humeral Head with Autologous Tissue Substitute, Percutaneous Approach

0PUC3JZ Supplement Right Humeral Head with Synthetic Substitute, Percutaneous Approach

0PUC3KZ Supplement Right Humeral Head with Nonautologous Tissue Substitute, Percutaneous Approach

0PUC47Z Supplement Right Humeral Head with Autologous Tissue Substitute, Percutaneous Endoscopic Approach

0PUC4JZ Supplement Right Humeral Head with Synthetic Substitute, Percutaneous Endoscopic Approach

0PUC4KZ Supplement Right Humeral Head with Nonautologous Tissue Substitute, Percutaneous Endoscopic Approach

0PUD07Z Supplement Left Humeral Head with Autologous Tissue Substitute, Open Approach

0PUD0JZ Supplement Left Humeral Head with Synthetic Substitute, Open Approach

0PUD0KZ Supplement Left Humeral Head with Nonautologous Tissue Substitute, Open Approach

0PUD37Z Supplement Left Humeral Head with Autologous Tissue Substitute, Percutaneous Approach

0PUD3JZ Supplement Left Humeral Head with Synthetic Substitute, Percutaneous Approach

0PUD3KZ Supplement Left Humeral Head with Nonautologous Tissue Substitute, Percutaneous Approach

0PUD47Z Supplement Left Humeral Head with Autologous Tissue Substitute, Percutaneous Endoscopic Approach

0PUD4JZ Supplement Left Humeral Head with Synthetic Substitute, Percutaneous Endoscopic Approach

0PUD4KZ Supplement Left Humeral Head with Nonautologous Tissue Substitute, Percutaneous Endoscopic Approach

0PUF07Z Supplement Right Humeral Shaft with Autologous Tissue Substitute, Open Approach

0PUF0JZ Supplement Right Humeral Shaft with Synthetic Substitute, Open Approach

0PUF0KZ Supplement Right Humeral Shaft with Nonautologous Tissue Substitute, Open Approach

0PUF37Z Supplement Right Humeral Shaft with Autologous Tissue Substitute, Percutaneous Approach

♀ Female-only ♂ Male-only ▲ Limited Coverage ● Non-OR ▨ HAC-associated procedure ▲ Non-covered procedures ✚ Cluster

0PUF3JZ	Supplement Right Humeral Shaft with Synthetic Substitute, Percutaneous Approach
0PUF3KZ	Supplement Right Humeral Shaft with Nonautologous Tissue Substitute, Percutaneous Approach
0PUF47Z	Supplement Right Humeral Shaft with Autologous Tissue Substitute, Percutaneous Endoscopic Approach
0PUF4JZ	Supplement Right Humeral Shaft with Synthetic Substitute, Percutaneous Endoscopic Approach
0PUF4KZ	Supplement Right Humeral Shaft with Nonautologous Tissue Substitute, Percutaneous Endoscopic Approach
0PUG07Z	Supplement Left Humeral Shaft with Autologous Tissue Substitute, Open Approach
0PUG0JZ	Supplement Left Humeral Shaft with Synthetic Substitute, Open Approach
0PUG0KZ	Supplement Left Humeral Shaft with Nonautologous Tissue Substitute, Open Approach
0PUG37Z	Supplement Left Humeral Shaft with Autologous Tissue Substitute, Percutaneous Approach
0PUG3JZ	Supplement Left Humeral Shaft with Synthetic Substitute, Percutaneous Approach
0PUG3KZ	Supplement Left Humeral Shaft with Nonautologous Tissue Substitute, Percutaneous Approach
0PUG47Z	Supplement Left Humeral Shaft with Autologous Tissue Substitute, Percutaneous Endoscopic Approach
0PUG4JZ	Supplement Left Humeral Shaft with Synthetic Substitute, Percutaneous Endoscopic Approach
0PUG4KZ	Supplement Left Humeral Shaft with Nonautologous Tissue Substitute, Percutaneous Endoscopic Approach
0PUH07Z	Supplement Right Radius with Autologous Tissue Substitute, Open Approach
0PUH0JZ	Supplement Right Radius with Synthetic Substitute, Open Approach
0PUH0KZ	Supplement Right Radius with Nonautologous Tissue Substitute, Open Approach
0PUH37Z	Supplement Right Radius with Autologous Tissue Substitute, Percutaneous Approach
0PUH3JZ	Supplement Right Radius with Synthetic Substitute, Percutaneous Approach
0PUH3KZ	Supplement Right Radius with Nonautologous Tissue Substitute, Percutaneous Approach
0PUH47Z	Supplement Right Radius with Autologous Tissue Substitute, Percutaneous Endoscopic Approach
0PUH4JZ	Supplement Right Radius with Synthetic Substitute, Percutaneous Endoscopic Approach
0PUH4KZ	Supplement Right Radius with Nonautologous Tissue Substitute, Percutaneous Endoscopic Approach
0PUJ07Z	Supplement Left Radius with Autologous Tissue Substitute, Open Approach
0PUJ0JZ	Supplement Left Radius with Synthetic Substitute, Open Approach
0PUJ0KZ	Supplement Left Radius with Nonautologous Tissue Substitute, Open Approach

0PUJ37Z	Supplement Left Radius with Autologous Tissue Substitute, Percutaneous Approach
0PUJ3JZ	Supplement Left Radius with Synthetic Substitute, Percutaneous Approach
0PUJ3KZ	Supplement Left Radius with Nonautologous Tissue Substitute, Percutaneous Approach
0PUJ47Z	Supplement Left Radius with Autologous Tissue Substitute, Percutaneous Endoscopic Approach
0PUJ4JZ	Supplement Left Radius with Synthetic Substitute, Percutaneous Endoscopic Approach
0PUJ4KZ	Supplement Left Radius with Nonautologous Tissue Substitute, Percutaneous Endoscopic Approach
0PUK07Z	Supplement Right Ulna with Autologous Tissue Substitute, Open Approach
0PUK0JZ	Supplement Right Ulna with Synthetic Substitute, Open Approach
0PUK0KZ	Supplement Right Ulna with Nonautologous Tissue Substitute, Open Approach
0PUK37Z	Supplement Right Ulna with Autologous Tissue Substitute, Percutaneous Approach
0PUK3JZ	Supplement Right Ulna with Synthetic Substitute, Percutaneous Approach
0PUK3KZ	Supplement Right Ulna with Nonautologous Tissue Substitute, Percutaneous Approach
0PUK47Z	Supplement Right Ulna with Autologous Tissue Substitute, Percutaneous Endoscopic Approach
0PUK4JZ	Supplement Right Ulna with Synthetic Substitute, Percutaneous Endoscopic Approach
0PUK4KZ	Supplement Right Ulna with Nonautologous Tissue Substitute, Percutaneous Endoscopic Approach
0PUL07Z	Supplement Left Ulna with Autologous Tissue Substitute, Open Approach
0PUL0JZ	Supplement Left Ulna with Synthetic Substitute, Open Approach
0PUL0KZ	Supplement Left Ulna with Nonautologous Tissue Substitute, Open Approach
0PUL37Z	Supplement Left Ulna with Autologous Tissue Substitute, Percutaneous Approach
0PUL3JZ	Supplement Left Ulna with Synthetic Substitute, Percutaneous Approach
0PUL3KZ	Supplement Left Ulna with Nonautologous Tissue Substitute, Percutaneous Approach
0PUL47Z	Supplement Left Ulna with Autologous Tissue Substitute, Percutaneous Endoscopic Approach
0PUL4JZ	Supplement Left Ulna with Synthetic Substitute, Percutaneous Endoscopic Approach
0PUL4KZ	Supplement Left Ulna with Nonautologous Tissue Substitute, Percutaneous Endoscopic Approach
0PUM07Z	Supplement Right Carpal with Autologous Tissue Substitute, Open Approach
0PUM0JZ	Supplement Right Carpal with Synthetic Substitute, Open Approach
0PUM0KZ	Supplement Right Carpal with Nonautologous Tissue Substitute, Open Approach

0PUM37Z	Supplement Right Carpal with Autologous Tissue Substitute, Percutaneous Approach
0PUM3JZ	Supplement Right Carpal with Synthetic Substitute, Percutaneous Approach
0PUM3KZ	Supplement Right Carpal with Nonautologous Tissue Substitute, Percutaneous Approach
0PUM47Z	Supplement Right Carpal with Autologous Tissue Substitute, Percutaneous Endoscopic Approach
0PUM4JZ	Supplement Right Carpal with Synthetic Substitute, Percutaneous Endoscopic Approach
0PUM4KZ	Supplement Right Carpal with Nonautologous Tissue Substitute, Percutaneous Endoscopic Approach
0PUN07Z	Supplement Left Carpal with Autologous Tissue Substitute, Open Approach
0PUN0JZ	Supplement Left Carpal with Synthetic Substitute, Open Approach
0PUN0KZ	Supplement Left Carpal with Nonautologous Tissue Substitute, Open Approach
0PUN37Z	Supplement Left Carpal with Autologous Tissue Substitute, Percutaneous Approach
0PUN3JZ	Supplement Left Carpal with Synthetic Substitute, Percutaneous Approach
0PUN3KZ	Supplement Left Carpal with Nonautologous Tissue Substitute, Percutaneous Approach
0PUN47Z	Supplement Left Carpal with Autologous Tissue Substitute, Percutaneous Endoscopic Approach
0PUN4JZ	Supplement Left Carpal with Synthetic Substitute, Percutaneous Endoscopic Approach
0PUN4KZ	Supplement Left Carpal with Nonautologous Tissue Substitute, Percutaneous Endoscopic Approach
0PUP07Z	Supplement Right Metacarpal with Autologous Tissue Substitute, Open Approach
0PUP0JZ	Supplement Right Metacarpal with Synthetic Substitute, Open Approach
0PUP0KZ	Supplement Right Metacarpal with Nonautologous Tissue Substitute, Open Approach
0PUP37Z	Supplement Right Metacarpal with Autologous Tissue Substitute, Percutaneous Approach
0PUP3JZ	Supplement Right Metacarpal with Synthetic Substitute, Percutaneous Approach
0PUP3KZ	Supplement Right Metacarpal with Nonautologous Tissue Substitute, Percutaneous Approach
0PUP47Z	Supplement Right Metacarpal with Autologous Tissue Substitute, Percutaneous Endoscopic Approach
0PUP4JZ	Supplement Right Metacarpal with Synthetic Substitute, Percutaneous Endoscopic Approach
0PUP4KZ	Supplement Right Metacarpal with Nonautologous Tissue Substitute, Percutaneous Endoscopic Approach
0PUQ07Z	Supplement Left Metacarpal with Autologous Tissue Substitute, Open Approach
0PUQ0JZ	Supplement Left Metacarpal with Synthetic Substitute, Open Approach
0PUQ0KZ	Supplement Left Metacarpal with Nonautologous Tissue Substitute, Open Approach

---

♀ Female-only   ♂ Male-only   ▲ Limited Coverage   ● Non-OR   **HAC** HAC-associated procedure   ▲ Non-covered procedures   ✚ Cluster

0PUQ37Z   Supplement Left Metacarpal with Autologous Tissue Substitute, Percutaneous Approach

0PUQ3JZ   Supplement Left Metacarpal with Synthetic Substitute, Percutaneous Approach

0PUQ3KZ   Supplement Left Metacarpal with Nonautologous Tissue Substitute, Percutaneous Approach

0PUQ47Z   Supplement Left Metacarpal with Autologous Tissue Substitute, Percutaneous Endoscopic Approach

0PUQ4JZ   Supplement Left Metacarpal with Synthetic Substitute, Percutaneous Endoscopic Approach

0PUQ4KZ   Supplement Left Metacarpal with Nonautologous Tissue Substitute, Percutaneous Endoscopic Approach

0PUR07Z   Supplement Right Thumb Phalanx with Autologous Tissue Substitute, Open Approach

0PUR0JZ   Supplement Right Thumb Phalanx with Synthetic Substitute, Open Approach

0PUR0KZ   Supplement Right Thumb Phalanx with Nonautologous Tissue Substitute, Open Approach

0PUR37Z   Supplement Right Thumb Phalanx with Autologous Tissue Substitute, Percutaneous Approach

0PUR3JZ   Supplement Right Thumb Phalanx with Synthetic Substitute, Percutaneous Approach

0PUR3KZ   Supplement Right Thumb Phalanx with Nonautologous Tissue Substitute, Percutaneous Approach

0PUR47Z   Supplement Right Thumb Phalanx with Autologous Tissue Substitute, Percutaneous Endoscopic Approach

0PUR4JZ   Supplement Right Thumb Phalanx with Synthetic Substitute, Percutaneous Endoscopic Approach

0PUR4KZ   Supplement Right Thumb Phalanx with Nonautologous Tissue Substitute, Percutaneous Endoscopic Approach

0PUS07Z   Supplement Left Thumb Phalanx with Autologous Tissue Substitute, Open Approach

0PUS0JZ   Supplement Left Thumb Phalanx with Synthetic Substitute, Open Approach

0PUS0KZ   Supplement Left Thumb Phalanx with Nonautologous Tissue Substitute, Open Approach

0PUS37Z   Supplement Left Thumb Phalanx with Autologous Tissue Substitute, Percutaneous Approach

0PUS3JZ   Supplement Left Thumb Phalanx with Synthetic Substitute, Percutaneous Approach

0PUS3KZ   Supplement Left Thumb Phalanx with Nonautologous Tissue Substitute, Percutaneous Approach

0PUS47Z   Supplement Left Thumb Phalanx with Autologous Tissue Substitute, Percutaneous Endoscopic Approach

0PUS4JZ   Supplement Left Thumb Phalanx with Synthetic Substitute, Percutaneous Endoscopic Approach

0PUS4KZ   Supplement Left Thumb Phalanx with Nonautologous Tissue Substitute, Percutaneous Endoscopic Approach

0PUT07Z   Supplement Right Finger Phalanx with Autologous Tissue Substitute, Open Approach

0PUT0JZ   Supplement Right Finger Phalanx with Synthetic Substitute, Open Approach

0PUT0KZ   Supplement Right Finger Phalanx with Nonautologous Tissue Substitute, Open Approach

0PUT37Z   Supplement Right Finger Phalanx with Autologous Tissue Substitute, Percutaneous Approach

0PUT3JZ   Supplement Right Finger Phalanx with Synthetic Substitute, Percutaneous Approach

0PUT3KZ   Supplement Right Finger Phalanx with Nonautologous Tissue Substitute, Percutaneous Approach

0PUT47Z   Supplement Right Finger Phalanx with Autologous Tissue Substitute, Percutaneous Endoscopic Approach

0PUT4JZ   Supplement Right Finger Phalanx with Synthetic Substitute, Percutaneous Endoscopic Approach

0PUT4KZ   Supplement Right Finger Phalanx with Nonautologous Tissue Substitute, Percutaneous Endoscopic Approach

0PUV07Z   Supplement Left Finger Phalanx with Autologous Tissue Substitute, Open Approach

0PUV0JZ   Supplement Left Finger Phalanx with Synthetic Substitute, Open Approach

0PUV0KZ   Supplement Left Finger Phalanx with Nonautologous Tissue Substitute, Open Approach

0PUV37Z   Supplement Left Finger Phalanx with Autologous Tissue Substitute, Percutaneous Approach

0PUV3JZ   Supplement Left Finger Phalanx with Synthetic Substitute, Percutaneous Approach

0PUV3KZ   Supplement Left Finger Phalanx with Nonautologous Tissue Substitute, Percutaneous Approach

0PUV47Z   Supplement Left Finger Phalanx with Autologous Tissue Substitute, Percutaneous Endoscopic Approach

0PUV4JZ   Supplement Left Finger Phalanx with Synthetic Substitute, Percutaneous Endoscopic Approach

0PUV4KZ   Supplement Left Finger Phalanx with Nonautologous Tissue Substitute, Percutaneous Endoscopic Approach

0PW – Upper Bones, Revision

Review Coding Guideline B6.1c

0PW004Z   Revision of Internal Fixation Device in Sternum, Open Approach

0PW007Z   Revision of Autologous Tissue Substitute in Sternum, Open Approach

0PW00JZ   Revision of Synthetic Substitute in Sternum, Open Approach

0PW00KZ   Revision of Nonautologous Tissue Substitute in Sternum, Open Approach

0PW034Z   Revision of Internal Fixation Device in Sternum, Percutaneous Approach

0PW037Z   Revision of Autologous Tissue Substitute in Sternum, Percutaneous Approach

0PW03JZ   Revision of Synthetic Substitute in Sternum, Percutaneous Approach

0PW03KZ   Revision of Nonautologous Tissue Substitute in Sternum, Percutaneous Approach

0PW044Z   Revision of Internal Fixation Device in Sternum, Percutaneous Endoscopic Approach

0PW047Z   Revision of Autologous Tissue Substitute in Sternum, Percutaneous Endoscopic Approach

0PW04JZ   Revision of Synthetic Substitute in Sternum, Percutaneous Endoscopic Approach

0PW04KZ   Revision of Nonautologous Tissue Substitute in Sternum, Percutaneous Endoscopic Approach

0PW0X4Z   Revision of Internal Fixation Device in Sternum, External Approach

0PW0X7Z   Revision of Autologous Tissue Substitute in Sternum, External Approach

0PW0XJZ   Revision of Synthetic Substitute in Sternum, External Approach

0PW0XKZ   Revision of Nonautologous Tissue Substitute in Sternum, External Approach

0PW104Z   Revision of Internal Fixation Device in I to 2 Ribs, Open Approach
AHA CC: 4Q, 2014, 26-27

0PW107Z   Revision of Autologous Tissue Substitute in I to 2 Ribs, Open Approach

0PW10JZ   Revision of Synthetic Substitute in I to 2 Ribs, Open Approach

0PW10KZ   Revision of Nonautologous Tissue Substitute in I to 2 Ribs, Open Approach

0PW134Z   Revision of Internal Fixation Device in I to 2 Ribs, Percutaneous Approach

0PW137Z   Revision of Autologous Tissue Substitute in I to 2 Ribs, Percutaneous Approach

0PW13JZ   Revision of Synthetic Substitute in I to 2 Ribs, Percutaneous Approach

0PW13KZ   Revision of Nonautologous Tissue Substitute in I to 2 Ribs, Percutaneous Approach

0PW144Z   Revision of Internal Fixation Device in I to 2 Ribs, Percutaneous Endoscopic Approach

0PW147Z   Revision of Autologous Tissue Substitute in I to 2 Ribs, Percutaneous Endoscopic Approach

0PW14JZ   Revision of Synthetic Substitute in I to 2 Ribs, Percutaneous Endoscopic Approach

0PW14KZ   Revision of Nonautologous Tissue Substitute in I to 2 Ribs, Percutaneous Endoscopic Approach

0PW1X4Z   Revision of Internal Fixation Device in I to 2 Ribs, External Approach

0PW1X7Z   Revision of Autologous Tissue Substitute in I to 2 Ribs, External Approach

0PW1XJZ   Revision of Synthetic Substitute in I to 2 Ribs, External Approach

0PW1XKZ   Revision of Nonautologous Tissue Substitute in I to 2 Ribs, External Approach

0PW204Z   Revision of Internal Fixation Device in 3 or More Ribs, Open Approach
AHA CC: 4Q, 2014, 26-27

♀ Female-only   ♂ Male-only   ▲ Limited Coverage   ● Non-OR   **HAC** HAC-associated procedure   ▲ Non-covered procedures   ✚ Cluster

0PW207Z	Revision of Autologous Tissue Substitute in 3 or More Ribs, Open Approach
0PW20JZ	Revision of Synthetic Substitute in 3 or 3 or More Ribs, Open Approach
0PW20KZ	Revision of Nonautologous Tissue Substitute in 3 or More Ribs, Open Approach
0PW234Z	Revision of Internal Fixation Device in 3 or More Ribs, Percutaneous Approach
0PW237Z	Revision of Autologous Tissue Substitute in 3 or More Ribs, Percutaneous Approach
0PW23JZ	Revision of Synthetic Substitute in 3 or More Ribs, Percutaneous Approach
0PW23KZ	Revision of Nonautologous Tissue Substitute in 3 or More Ribs, Percutaneous Approach
0PW244Z	Revision of Internal Fixation Device in 3 or More Ribs, Percutaneous Endoscopic Approach
0PW247Z	Revision of Autologous Tissue Substitute in 3 or More Ribs, Percutaneous Endoscopic Approach
0PW24JZ	Revision of Synthetic Substitute in 3 or More Ribs, Percutaneous Endoscopic Approach
0PW24KZ	Revision of Nonautologous Tissue Substitute in 3 or More Ribs, Percutaneous Endoscopic Approach
0PW2X4Z	Revision of Internal Fixation Device in 3 or More Ribs, External Approach
0PW2X7Z	Revision of Autologous Tissue Substitute in 3 or More Ribs, External Approach
0PW2XJZ	Revision of Synthetic Substitute in 3 or More Ribs, External Approach
0PW2XKZ	Revision of Nonautologous Tissue Substitute in 3 or More Ribs, External Approach
0PW304Z	Revision of Internal Fixation Device in Cervical Vertebra, Open Approach
0PW307Z	Revision of Autologous Tissue Substitute in Cervical Vertebra, Open Approach
0PW30JZ	Revision of Synthetic Substitute in Cervical Vertebra, Open Approach
0PW30KZ	Revision of Nonautologous Tissue Substitute in Cervical Vertebra, Open Approach
0PW334Z	Revision of Internal Fixation Device in Cervical Vertebra, Percutaneous Approach
0PW337Z	Revision of Autologous Tissue Substitute in Cervical Vertebra, Percutaneous Approach
0PW33JZ	Revision of Synthetic Substitute in Cervical Vertebra, Percutaneous Approach
0PW33KZ	Revision of Nonautologous Tissue Substitute in Cervical Vertebra, Percutaneous Approach
0PW344Z	Revision of Internal Fixation Device in Cervical Vertebra, Percutaneous Endoscopic Approach
0PW347Z	Revision of Autologous Tissue Substitute in Cervical Vertebra, Percutaneous Endoscopic Approach
0PW34JZ	Revision of Synthetic Substitute in Cervical Vertebra, Percutaneous Endoscopic Approach

0PW34KZ	Revision of Nonautologous Tissue Substitute in Cervical Vertebra, Percutaneous Endoscopic Approach
0PW3X4Z	Revision of Internal Fixation Device in Cervical Vertebra, External Approach
0PW3X7Z	Revision of Autologous Tissue Substitute in Cervical Vertebra, External Approach
0PW3XJZ	Revision of Synthetic Substitute in Cervical Vertebra, External Approach
0PW3XKZ	Revision of Nonautologous Tissue Substitute in Cervical Vertebra, External Approach
0PW404Z	Revision of Internal Fixation Device in Thoracic Vertebra, Open Approach
	AHA CC: 4Q, 2014, 27-28
0PW407Z	Revision of Autologous Tissue Substitute in Thoracic Vertebra, Open Approach
0PW40JZ	Revision of Synthetic Substitute in Thoracic Vertebra, Open Approach
0PW40KZ	Revision of Nonautologous Tissue Substitute in Thoracic Vertebra, Open Approach
0PW434Z	Revision of Internal Fixation Device in Thoracic Vertebra, Percutaneous Approach
0PW437Z	Revision of Autologous Tissue Substitute in Thoracic Vertebra, Percutaneous Approach
0PW43JZ	Revision of Synthetic Substitute in Thoracic Vertebra, Percutaneous Approach
0PW43KZ	Revision of Nonautologous Tissue Substitute in Thoracic Vertebra, Percutaneous Approach
0PW444Z	Revision of Internal Fixation Device in Thoracic Vertebra, Percutaneous Endoscopic Approach
0PW447Z	Revision of Autologous Tissue Substitute in Thoracic Vertebra, Percutaneous Endoscopic Approach
0PW44JZ	Revision of Synthetic Substitute in Thoracic Vertebra, Percutaneous Endoscopic Approach
0PW44KZ	Revision of Nonautologous Tissue Substitute in Thoracic Vertebra, Percutaneous Endoscopic Approach
0PW4X4Z	Revision of Internal Fixation Device in Thoracic Vertebra, External Approach
0PW4X7Z	Revision of Autologous Tissue Substitute in Thoracic Vertebra, External Approach
0PW4XJZ	Revision of Synthetic Substitute in Thoracic Vertebra, External Approach
0PW4XKZ	Revision of Nonautologous Tissue Substitute in Thoracic Vertebra, External Approach
0PW504Z	Revision of Internal Fixation Device in Right Scapula, Open Approach
0PW507Z	Revision of Autologous Tissue Substitute in Right Scapula, Open Approach
0PW50JZ	Revision of Synthetic Substitute in Right Scapula, Open Approach
0PW50KZ	Revision of Nonautologous Tissue Substitute in Right Scapula, Open Approach
0PW534Z	Revision of Internal Fixation Device in Right Scapula, Percutaneous Approach
0PW537Z	Revision of Autologous Tissue Substitute in Right Scapula, Percutaneous Approach

0PW53JZ	Revision of Synthetic Substitute in Right Scapula, Percutaneous Approach
0PW53KZ	Revision of Nonautologous Tissue Substitute in Right Scapula, Percutaneous Approach
0PW544Z	Revision of Internal Fixation Device in Right Scapula, Percutaneous Endoscopic Approach
0PW547Z	Revision of Autologous Tissue Substitute in Right Scapula, Percutaneous Endoscopic Approach
0PW54JZ	Revision of Synthetic Substitute in Right Scapula, Percutaneous Endoscopic Approach
0PW54KZ	Revision of Nonautologous Tissue Substitute in Right Scapula, Percutaneous Endoscopic Approach
0PW5X4Z	Revision of Internal Fixation Device in Right Scapula, External Approach
0PW5X7Z	Revision of Autologous Tissue Substitute in Right Scapula, External Approach
0PW5XJZ	Revision of Synthetic Substitute in Right Scapula, External Approach
0PW5XKZ	Revision of Nonautologous Tissue Substitute in Right Scapula, External Approach
0PW604Z	Revision of Internal Fixation Device in Left Scapula, Open Approach
0PW607Z	Revision of Autologous Tissue Substitute in Left Scapula, Open Approach
0PW60JZ	Revision of Synthetic Substitute in Left Scapula, Open Approach
0PW60KZ	Revision of Nonautologous Tissue Substitute in Left Scapula, Open Approach
0PW634Z	Revision of Internal Fixation Device in Left Scapula, Percutaneous Approach
0PW637Z	Revision of Autologous Tissue Substitute in Left Scapula, Percutaneous Approach
0PW63JZ	Revision of Synthetic Substitute in Left Scapula, Percutaneous Approach
0PW63KZ	Revision of Nonautologous Tissue Substitute in Left Scapula, Percutaneous Approach
0PW644Z	Revision of Internal Fixation Device in Left Scapula, Percutaneous Endoscopic Approach
0PW647Z	Revision of Autologous Tissue Substitute in Left Scapula, Percutaneous Endoscopic Approach
0PW64JZ	Revision of Synthetic Substitute in Left Scapula, Percutaneous Endoscopic Approach
0PW64KZ	Revision of Nonautologous Tissue Substitute in Left Scapula, Percutaneous Endoscopic Approach
0PW6X4Z	Revision of Internal Fixation Device in Left Scapula, External Approach
0PW6X7Z	Revision of Autologous Tissue Substitute in Left Scapula, External Approach
0PW6XJZ	Revision of Synthetic Substitute in Left Scapula, External Approach
0PW6XKZ	Revision of Nonautologous Tissue Substitute in Left Scapula, External Approach
0PW704Z	Revision of Internal Fixation Device in Right Glenoid Cavity, Open Approach
0PW707Z	Revision of Autologous Tissue Substitute in Right Glenoid Cavity, Open Approach

0PW70JZ Revision of Synthetic Substitute in Right Glenoid Cavity, Open Approach

0PW70KZ Revision of Nonautologous Tissue Substitute in Right Glenoid Cavity, Open Approach

0PW734Z Revision of Internal Fixation Device in Right Glenoid Cavity, Percutaneous Approach

0PW737Z Revision of Autologous Tissue Substitute in Right Glenoid Cavity, Percutaneous Approach

0PW73JZ Revision of Synthetic Substitute in Right Glenoid Cavity, Percutaneous Approach

0PW73KZ Revision of Nonautologous Tissue Substitute in Right Glenoid Cavity, Percutaneous Approach

0PW744Z Revision of Internal Fixation Device in Right Glenoid Cavity, Percutaneous Endoscopic Approach

0PW747Z Revision of Autologous Tissue Substitute in Right Glenoid Cavity, Percutaneous Endoscopic Approach

0PW74JZ Revision of Synthetic Substitute in Right Glenoid Cavity, Percutaneous Endoscopic Approach

0PW74KZ Revision of Nonautologous Tissue Substitute in Right Glenoid Cavity, Percutaneous Endoscopic Approach

0PW7X4Z Revision of Internal Fixation Device in Right Glenoid Cavity, External Approach

0PW7X7Z Revision of Autologous Tissue Substitute in Right Glenoid Cavity, External Approach

0PW7XJZ Revision of Synthetic Substitute in Right Glenoid Cavity, External Approach

0PW7XKZ Revision of Nonautologous Tissue Substitute in Right Glenoid Cavity, External Approach

0PW804Z Revision of Internal Fixation Device in Left Glenoid Cavity, Open Approach

0PW807Z Revision of Autologous Tissue Substitute in Left Glenoid Cavity, Open Approach

0PW80JZ Revision of Synthetic Substitute in Left Glenoid Cavity, Open Approach

0PW80KZ Revision of Nonautologous Tissue Substitute in Left Glenoid Cavity, Open Approach

0PW834Z Revision of Internal Fixation Device in Left Glenoid Cavity, Percutaneous Approach

0PW837Z Revision of Autologous Tissue Substitute in Left Glenoid Cavity, Percutaneous Approach

0PW83JZ Revision of Synthetic Substitute in Left Glenoid Cavity, Percutaneous Approach

0PW83KZ Revision of Nonautologous Tissue Substitute in Left Glenoid Cavity, Percutaneous Approach

0PW844Z Revision of Internal Fixation Device in Left Glenoid Cavity, Percutaneous Endoscopic Approach

0PW847Z Revision of Autologous Tissue Substitute in Left Glenoid Cavity, Percutaneous Endoscopic Approach

0PW84JZ Revision of Synthetic Substitute in Left Glenoid Cavity, Percutaneous Endoscopic Approach

0PW84KZ Revision of Nonautologous Tissue Substitute in Left Glenoid Cavity, Percutaneous Endoscopic Approach

0PW8X4Z Revision of Internal Fixation Device in Left Glenoid Cavity, External Approach

0PW8X7Z Revision of Autologous Tissue Substitute in Left Glenoid Cavity, External Approach

0PW8XJZ Revision of Synthetic Substitute in Left Glenoid Cavity, External Approach

0PW8XKZ Revision of Nonautologous Tissue Substitute in Left Glenoid Cavity, External Approach

0PW904Z Revision of Internal Fixation Device in Right Clavicle, Open Approach

0PW907Z Revision of Autologous Tissue Substitute in Right Clavicle, Open Approach

0PW90JZ Revision of Synthetic Substitute in Right Clavicle, Open Approach

0PW90KZ Revision of Nonautologous Tissue Substitute in Right Clavicle, Open Approach

0PW934Z Revision of Internal Fixation Device in Right Clavicle, Percutaneous Approach

0PW937Z Revision of Autologous Tissue Substitute in Right Clavicle, Percutaneous Approach

0PW93JZ Revision of Synthetic Substitute in Right Clavicle, Percutaneous Approach

0PW93KZ Revision of Nonautologous Tissue Substitute in Right Clavicle, Percutaneous Approach

0PW944Z Revision of Internal Fixation Device in Right Clavicle, Percutaneous Endoscopic Approach

0PW947Z Revision of Autologous Tissue Substitute in Right Clavicle, Percutaneous Endoscopic Approach

0PW94JZ Revision of Synthetic Substitute in Right Clavicle, Percutaneous Endoscopic Approach

0PW94KZ Revision of Nonautologous Tissue Substitute in Right Clavicle, Percutaneous Endoscopic Approach

0PW9X4Z Revision of Internal Fixation Device in Right Clavicle, External Approach

0PW9X7Z Revision of Autologous Tissue Substitute in Right Clavicle, External Approach

0PW9XJZ Revision of Synthetic Substitute in Right Clavicle, External Approach

0PW9XKZ Revision of Nonautologous Tissue Substitute in Right Clavicle, External Approach

0PWB04Z Revision of Internal Fixation Device in Left Clavicle, Open Approach

0PWB07Z Revision of Autologous Tissue Substitute in Left Clavicle, Open Approach

0PWB0JZ Revision of Synthetic Substitute in Left Clavicle, Open Approach

0PWB0KZ Revision of Nonautologous Tissue Substitute in Left Clavicle, Open Approach

0PWB34Z Revision of Internal Fixation Device in Left Clavicle, Percutaneous Approach

0PWB37Z Revision of Autologous Tissue Substitute in Left Clavicle, Percutaneous Approach

0PWB3JZ Revision of Synthetic Substitute in Left Clavicle, Percutaneous Approach

0PWB3KZ Revision of Nonautologous Tissue Substitute in Left Clavicle, Percutaneous Approach

0PWB44Z Revision of Internal Fixation Device in Left Clavicle, Percutaneous Endoscopic Approach

0PWB47Z Revision of Autologous Tissue Substitute in Left Clavicle, Percutaneous Endoscopic Approach

0PWB4JZ Revision of Synthetic Substitute in Left Clavicle, Percutaneous Endoscopic Approach

0PWB4KZ Revision of Nonautologous Tissue Substitute in Left Clavicle, Percutaneous Endoscopic Approach

0PWBX4Z Revision of Internal Fixation Device in Left Clavicle, External Approach

0PWBX7Z Revision of Autologous Tissue Substitute in Left Clavicle, External Approach

0PWBXJZ Revision of Synthetic Substitute in Left Clavicle, External Approach

0PWBXKZ Revision of Nonautologous Tissue Substitute in Left Clavicle, External Approach

0PWC04Z Revision of Internal Fixation Device in Right Humeral Head, Open Approach

0PWC05Z Revision of External Fixation Device in Right Humeral Head, Open Approach

0PWC07Z Revision of Autologous Tissue Substitute in Right Humeral Head, Open Approach

0PWC0JZ Revision of Synthetic Substitute in Right Humeral Head, Open Approach

0PWC0KZ Revision of Nonautologous Tissue Substitute in Right Humeral Head, Open Approach

0PWC34Z Revision of Internal Fixation Device in Right Humeral Head, Percutaneous Approach

0PWC35Z Revision of External Fixation Device in Right Humeral Head, Percutaneous Approach

0PWC37Z Revision of Autologous Tissue Substitute in Right Humeral Head, Percutaneous Approach

0PWC3JZ Revision of Synthetic Substitute in Right Humeral Head, Percutaneous Approach

0PWC3KZ Revision of Nonautologous Tissue Substitute in Right Humeral Head, Percutaneous Approach

0PWC44Z Revision of Internal Fixation Device in Right Humeral Head, Percutaneous Endoscopic Approach

0PWC45Z Revision of External Fixation Device in Right Humeral Head, Percutaneous Endoscopic Approach

0PWC47Z Revision of Autologous Tissue Substitute in Right Humeral Head, Percutaneous Endoscopic Approach

0PWC4JZ Revision of Synthetic Substitute in Right Humeral Head, Percutaneous Endoscopic Approach

0PWC4KZ Revision of Nonautologous Tissue Substitute in Right Humeral Head, Percutaneous Endoscopic Approach

0PWCX4Z Revision of Internal Fixation Device in Right Humeral Head, External Approach

0PWCX5Z Revision of External Fixation Device in Right Humeral Head, External Approach

0PWCX7Z Revision of Autologous Tissue Substitute in Right Humeral Head, External Approach

0PWCXJZ Revision of Synthetic Substitute in Right Humeral Head, External Approach

0PWCXKZ Revision of Nonautologous Tissue Substitute in Right Humeral Head, External Approach

0PWD04Z Revision of Internal Fixation Device in Left Humeral Head, Open Approach

0PWD05Z Revision of External Fixation Device in Left Humeral Head, Open Approach

0PWD07Z Revision of Autologous Tissue Substitute in Left Humeral Head, Open Approach

0PWD0JZ Revision of Synthetic Substitute in Left Humeral Head, Open Approach

0PWD0KZ Revision of Nonautologous Tissue Substitute in Left Humeral Head, Open Approach

0PWD34Z Revision of Internal Fixation Device in Left Humeral Head, Percutaneous Approach

0PWD35Z Revision of External Fixation Device in Left Humeral Head, Percutaneous Approach

0PWD37Z Revision of Autologous Tissue Substitute in Left Humeral Head, Percutaneous Approach

0PWD3JZ Revision of Synthetic Substitute in Left Humeral Head, Percutaneous Approach

0PWD3KZ Revision of Nonautologous Tissue Substitute in Left Humeral Head, Percutaneous Approach

0PWD44Z Revision of Internal Fixation Device in Left Humeral Head, Percutaneous Endoscopic Approach

0PWD45Z Revision of External Fixation Device in Left Humeral Head, Percutaneous Endoscopic Approach

0PWD47Z Revision of Autologous Tissue Substitute in Left Humeral Head, Percutaneous Endoscopic Approach

0PWD4JZ Revision of Synthetic Substitute in Left Humeral Head, Percutaneous Endoscopic Approach

0PWD4KZ Revision of Nonautologous Tissue Substitute in Left Humeral Head, Percutaneous Endoscopic Approach

0PWDX4Z Revision of Internal Fixation Device in Left Humeral Head, External Approach

0PWDX5Z Revision of External Fixation Device in Left Humeral Head, External Approach

0PWDX7Z Revision of Autologous Tissue Substitute in Left Humeral Head, External Approach

0PWDXJZ Revision of Synthetic Substitute in Left Humeral Head, External Approach

0PWDXKZ Revision of Nonautologous Tissue Substitute in Left Humeral Head, External Approach

0PWF04Z Revision of Internal Fixation Device in Right Humeral Shaft, Open Approach

0PWF05Z Revision of External Fixation Device in Right Humeral Shaft, Open Approach

0PWF07Z Revision of Autologous Tissue Substitute in Right Humeral Shaft, Open Approach

0PWF0JZ Revision of Synthetic Substitute in Right Humeral Shaft, Open Approach

0PWF0KZ Revision of Nonautologous Tissue Substitute in Right Humeral Shaft, Open Approach

0PWF34Z Revision of Internal Fixation Device in Right Humeral Shaft, Percutaneous Approach

0PWF35Z Revision of External Fixation Device in Right Humeral Shaft, Percutaneous Approach

0PWF37Z Revision of Autologous Tissue Substitute in Right Humeral Shaft, Percutaneous Approach

0PWF3JZ Revision of Synthetic Substitute in Right Humeral Shaft, Percutaneous Approach

0PWF3KZ Revision of Nonautologous Tissue Substitute in Right Humeral Shaft, Percutaneous Approach

0PWF44Z Revision of Internal Fixation Device in Right Humeral Shaft, Percutaneous Endoscopic Approach

0PWF45Z Revision of External Fixation Device in Right Humeral Shaft, Percutaneous Endoscopic Approach

0PWF47Z Revision of Autologous Tissue Substitute in Right Humeral Shaft, Percutaneous Endoscopic Approach

0PWF4JZ Revision of Synthetic Substitute in Right Humeral Shaft, Percutaneous Endoscopic Approach

0PWF4KZ Revision of Nonautologous Tissue Substitute in Right Humeral Shaft, Percutaneous Endoscopic Approach

0PWFX4Z Revision of Internal Fixation Device in Right Humeral Shaft, External Approach

0PWFX5Z Revision of External Fixation Device in Right Humeral Shaft, External Approach

0PWFX7Z Revision of Autologous Tissue Substitute in Right Humeral Shaft, External Approach

0PWFXJZ Revision of Synthetic Substitute in Right Humeral Shaft, External Approach

0PWFXKZ Revision of Nonautologous Tissue Substitute in Right Humeral Shaft, External Approach

0PWG04Z Revision of Internal Fixation Device in Left Humeral Shaft, Open Approach

0PWG05Z Revision of External Fixation Device in Left Humeral Shaft, Open Approach

0PWG07Z Revision of Autologous Tissue Substitute in Left Humeral Shaft, Open Approach

0PWG0JZ Revision of Synthetic Substitute in Left Humeral Shaft, Open Approach

0PWG0KZ Revision of Nonautologous Tissue Substitute in Left Humeral Shaft, Open Approach

0PWG34Z Revision of Internal Fixation Device in Left Humeral Shaft, Percutaneous Approach

0PWG35Z Revision of External Fixation Device in Left Humeral Shaft, Percutaneous Approach

0PWG37Z Revision of Autologous Tissue Substitute in Left Humeral Shaft, Percutaneous Approach

0PWG3JZ Revision of Synthetic Substitute in Left Humeral Shaft, Percutaneous Approach

0PWG3KZ Revision of Nonautologous Tissue Substitute in Left Humeral Shaft, Percutaneous Approach

0PWG44Z Revision of Internal Fixation Device in Left Humeral Shaft, Percutaneous Endoscopic Approach

0PWG45Z Revision of External Fixation Device in Left Humeral Shaft, Percutaneous Endoscopic Approach

0PWG47Z Revision of Autologous Tissue Substitute in Left Humeral Shaft, Percutaneous Endoscopic Approach

0PWG4JZ Revision of Synthetic Substitute in Left Humeral Shaft, Percutaneous Endoscopic Approach

0PWG4KZ Revision of Nonautologous Tissue Substitute in Left Humeral Shaft, Percutaneous Endoscopic Approach

0PWGX4Z Revision of Internal Fixation Device in Left Humeral Shaft, External Approach

0PWGX5Z Revision of External Fixation Device in Left Humeral Shaft, External Approach

0PWGX7Z Revision of Autologous Tissue Substitute in Left Humeral Shaft, External Approach

0PWGXJZ Revision of Synthetic Substitute in Left Humeral Shaft, External Approach

0PWGXKZ Revision of Nonautologous Tissue Substitute in Left Humeral Shaft, External Approach

0PWH04Z Revision of Internal Fixation Device in Right Radius, Open Approach

0PWH05Z Revision of External Fixation Device in Right Radius, Open Approach

0PWH07Z Revision of Autologous Tissue Substitute in Right Radius, Open Approach

0PWH0JZ Revision of Synthetic Substitute in Right Radius, Open Approach

0PWH0KZ Revision of Nonautologous Tissue Substitute in Right Radius, Open Approach

0PWH34Z Revision of Internal Fixation Device in Right Radius, Percutaneous Approach

0PWH35Z Revision of External Fixation Device in Right Radius, Percutaneous Approach

0PWH37Z Revision of Autologous Tissue Substitute in Right Radius, Percutaneous Approach

0PWH3JZ Revision of Synthetic Substitute in Right Radius, Percutaneous Approach

0PWH3KZ Revision of Nonautologous Tissue Substitute in Right Radius, Percutaneous Approach

0PWH44Z	Revision of Internal Fixation Device in Right Radius, Percutaneous Endoscopic Approach
0PWH45Z	Revision of External Fixation Device in Right Radius, Percutaneous Endoscopic Approach
0PWH47Z	Revision of Autologous Tissue Substitute in Right Radius, Percutaneous Endoscopic Approach
0PWH4JZ	Revision of Synthetic Substitute in Right Radius, Percutaneous Endoscopic Approach
0PWH4KZ	Revision of Nonautologous Tissue Substitute in Right Radius, Percutaneous Endoscopic Approach
0PWHX4Z	Revision of Internal Fixation Device in Right Radius, External Approach
0PWHX5Z	Revision of External Fixation Device in Right Radius, External Approach
0PWHX7Z	Revision of Autologous Tissue Substitute in Right Radius, External Approach
0PWHXJZ	Revision of Synthetic Substitute in Right Radius, External Approach
0PWHXKZ	Revision of Nonautologous Tissue Substitute in Right Radius, External Approach
0PWJ04Z	Revision of Internal Fixation Device in Left Radius, Open Approach
0PWJ05Z	Revision of External Fixation Device in Left Radius, Open Approach
0PWJ07Z	Revision of Autologous Tissue Substitute in Left Radius, Open Approach
0PWJ0JZ	Revision of Synthetic Substitute in Left Radius, Open Approach
0PWJ0KZ	Revision of Nonautologous Tissue Substitute in Left Radius, Open Approach
0PWJ34Z	Revision of Internal Fixation Device in Left Radius, Percutaneous Approach
0PWJ35Z	Revision of External Fixation Device in Left Radius, Percutaneous Approach
0PWJ37Z	Revision of Autologous Tissue Substitute in Left Radius, Percutaneous Approach
0PWJ3JZ	Revision of Synthetic Substitute in Left Radius, Percutaneous Approach
0PWJ3KZ	Revision of Nonautologous Tissue Substitute in Left Radius, Percutaneous Approach
0PWJ44Z	Revision of Internal Fixation Device in Left Radius, Percutaneous Endoscopic Approach
0PWJ45Z	Revision of External Fixation Device in Left Radius, Percutaneous Endoscopic Approach
0PWJ47Z	Revision of Autologous Tissue Substitute in Left Radius, Percutaneous Endoscopic Approach
0PWJ4JZ	Revision of Synthetic Substitute in Left Radius, Percutaneous Endoscopic Approach
0PWJ4KZ	Revision of Nonautologous Tissue Substitute in Left Radius, Percutaneous Endoscopic Approach
0PWJX4Z	Revision of Internal Fixation Device in Left Radius, External Approach
0PWJX5Z	Revision of External Fixation Device in Left Radius, External Approach
0PWJX7Z	Revision of Autologous Tissue Substitute in Left Radius, External Approach
0PWJXJZ	Revision of Synthetic Substitute in Left Radius, External Approach
0PWJXKZ	Revision of Nonautologous Tissue Substitute in Left Radius, External Approach
0PWK04Z	Revision of Internal Fixation Device in Right Ulna, Open Approach
0PWK05Z	Revision of External Fixation Device in Right Ulna, Open Approach
0PWK07Z	Revision of Autologous Tissue Substitute in Right Ulna, Open Approach
0PWK0JZ	Revision of Synthetic Substitute in Right Ulna, Open Approach
0PWK0KZ	Revision of Nonautologous Tissue Substitute in Right Ulna, Open Approach
0PWK34Z	Revision of Internal Fixation Device in Right Ulna, Percutaneous Approach
0PWK35Z	Revision of External Fixation Device in Right Ulna, Percutaneous Approach
0PWK37Z	Revision of Autologous Tissue Substitute in Right Ulna, Percutaneous Approach
0PWK3JZ	Revision of Synthetic Substitute in Right Ulna, Percutaneous Approach
0PWK3KZ	Revision of Nonautologous Tissue Substitute in Right Ulna, Percutaneous Approach
0PWK44Z	Revision of Internal Fixation Device in Right Ulna, Percutaneous Endoscopic Approach
0PWK45Z	Revision of External Fixation Device in Right Ulna, Percutaneous Endoscopic Approach
0PWK47Z	Revision of Autologous Tissue Substitute in Right Ulna, Percutaneous Endoscopic Approach
0PWK4JZ	Revision of Synthetic Substitute in Right Ulna, Percutaneous Endoscopic Approach
0PWK4KZ	Revision of Nonautologous Tissue Substitute in Right Ulna, Percutaneous Endoscopic Approach
0PWKX4Z	Revision of Internal Fixation Device in Right Ulna, External Approach
0PWKX5Z	Revision of External Fixation Device in Right Ulna, External Approach
0PWKX7Z	Revision of Autologous Tissue Substitute in Right Ulna, External Approach
0PWKXJZ	Revision of Synthetic Substitute in Right Ulna, External Approach
0PWKXKZ	Revision of Nonautologous Tissue Substitute in Right Ulna, External Approach
0PWL04Z	Revision of Internal Fixation Device in Left Ulna, Open Approach
0PWL05Z	Revision of External Fixation Device in Left Ulna, Open Approach
0PWL07Z	Revision of Autologous Tissue Substitute in Left Ulna, Open Approach
0PWL0JZ	Revision of Synthetic Substitute in Left Ulna, Open Approach
0PWL0KZ	Revision of Nonautologous Tissue Substitute in Left Ulna, Open Approach
0PWL34Z	Revision of Internal Fixation Device in Left Ulna, Percutaneous Approach
0PWL35Z	Revision of External Fixation Device in Left Ulna, Percutaneous Approach
0PWL37Z	Revision of Autologous Tissue Substitute in Left Ulna, Percutaneous Approach
0PWL3JZ	Revision of Synthetic Substitute in Left Ulna, Percutaneous Approach
0PWL3KZ	Revision of Nonautologous Tissue Substitute in Left Ulna, Percutaneous Approach
0PWL44Z	Revision of Internal Fixation Device in Left Ulna, Percutaneous Endoscopic Approach
0PWL45Z	Revision of External Fixation Device in Left Ulna, Percutaneous Endoscopic Approach
0PWL47Z	Revision of Autologous Tissue Substitute in Left Ulna, Percutaneous Endoscopic Approach
0PWL4JZ	Revision of Synthetic Substitute in Left Ulna, Percutaneous Endoscopic Approach
0PWL4KZ	Revision of Nonautologous Tissue Substitute in Left Ulna, Percutaneous Endoscopic Approach
0PWLX4Z	Revision of Internal Fixation Device in Left Ulna, External Approach
0PWLX5Z	Revision of External Fixation Device in Left Ulna, External Approach
0PWLX7Z	Revision of Autologous Tissue Substitute in Left Ulna, External Approach
0PWLXJZ	Revision of Synthetic Substitute in Left Ulna, External Approach
0PWLXKZ	Revision of Nonautologous Tissue Substitute in Left Ulna, External Approach
0PWM04Z	Revision of Internal Fixation Device in Right Carpal, Open Approach
0PWM05Z	Revision of External Fixation Device in Right Carpal, Open Approach
0PWM07Z	Revision of Autologous Tissue Substitute in Right Carpal, Open Approach
0PWM0JZ	Revision of Synthetic Substitute in Right Carpal, Open Approach
0PWM0KZ	Revision of Nonautologous Tissue Substitute in Right Carpal, Open Approach
0PWM34Z	Revision of Internal Fixation Device in Right Carpal, Percutaneous Approach
0PWM35Z	Revision of External Fixation Device in Right Carpal, Percutaneous Approach
0PWM37Z	Revision of Autologous Tissue Substitute in Right Carpal, Percutaneous Approach
0PWM3JZ	Revision of Synthetic Substitute in Right Carpal, Percutaneous Approach
0PWM3KZ	Revision of Nonautologous Tissue Substitute in Right Carpal, Percutaneous Approach
0PWM44Z	Revision of Internal Fixation Device in Right Carpal, Percutaneous Endoscopic Approach

♀ Female-only ♂ Male-only ▲ Limited Coverage ● Non-OR ᴴᴬᶜ HAC-associated procedure ▲ Non-covered procedures ✚ Cluster

0PWM45Z Revision of External Fixation Device in Right Carpal, Percutaneous Endoscopic Approach

0PWM47Z Revision of Autologous Tissue Substitute in Right Carpal, Percutaneous Endoscopic Approach

0PWM4JZ Revision of Synthetic Substitute in Right Carpal, Percutaneous Endoscopic Approach

0PWM4KZ Revision of Nonautologous Tissue Substitute in Right Carpal, Percutaneous Endoscopic Approach

0PWMX4Z Revision of Internal Fixation Device in Right Carpal, External Approach

0PWMX5Z Revision of External Fixation Device in Right Carpal, External Approach

0PWMX7Z Revision of Autologous Tissue Substitute in Right Carpal, External Approach

0PWMXJZ Revision of Synthetic Substitute in Right Carpal, External Approach

0PWMXKZ Revision of Nonautologous Tissue Substitute in Right Carpal, External Approach

0PWN04Z Revision of Internal Fixation Device in Left Carpal, Open Approach

0PWN05Z Revision of External Fixation Device in Left Carpal, Open Approach

0PWN07Z Revision of Autologous Tissue Substitute in Left Carpal, Open Approach

0PWN0JZ Revision of Synthetic Substitute in Left Carpal, Open Approach

0PWN0KZ Revision of Nonautologous Tissue Substitute in Left Carpal, Open Approach

0PWN34Z Revision of Internal Fixation Device in Left Carpal, Percutaneous Approach

0PWN35Z Revision of External Fixation Device in Left Carpal, Percutaneous Approach

0PWN37Z Revision of Autologous Tissue Substitute in Left Carpal, Percutaneous Approach

0PWN3JZ Revision of Synthetic Substitute in Left Carpal, Percutaneous Approach

0PWN3KZ Revision of Nonautologous Tissue Substitute in Left Carpal, Percutaneous Approach

0PWN44Z Revision of Internal Fixation Device in Left Carpal, Percutaneous Endoscopic Approach

0PWN45Z Revision of External Fixation Device in Left Carpal, Percutaneous Endoscopic Approach

0PWN47Z Revision of Autologous Tissue Substitute in Left Carpal, Percutaneous Endoscopic Approach

0PWN4JZ Revision of Synthetic Substitute in Left Carpal, Percutaneous Endoscopic Approach

0PWN4KZ Revision of Nonautologous Tissue Substitute in Left Carpal, Percutaneous Endoscopic Approach

0PWNX4Z Revision of Internal Fixation Device in Left Carpal, External Approach

0PWNX5Z Revision of External Fixation Device in Left Carpal, External Approach

0PWNX7Z Revision of Autologous Tissue Substitute in Left Carpal, External Approach

0PWNXJZ Revision of Synthetic Substitute in Left Carpal, External Approach

0PWNXKZ Revision of Nonautologous Tissue Substitute in Left Carpal, External Approach

0PWP04Z Revision of Internal Fixation Device in Right Metacarpal, Open Approach

0PWP05Z Revision of External Fixation Device in Right Metacarpal, Open Approach

0PWP07Z Revision of Autologous Tissue Substitute in Right Metacarpal, Open Approach

0PWP0JZ Revision of Synthetic Substitute in Right Metacarpal, Open Approach

0PWP0KZ Revision of Nonautologous Tissue Substitute in Right Metacarpal, Open Approach

0PWP34Z Revision of Internal Fixation Device in Right Metacarpal, Percutaneous Approach

0PWP35Z Revision of External Fixation Device in Right Metacarpal, Percutaneous Approach

0PWP37Z Revision of Autologous Tissue Substitute in Right Metacarpal, Percutaneous Approach

0PWP3JZ Revision of Synthetic Substitute in Right Metacarpal, Percutaneous Approach

0PWP3KZ Revision of Nonautologous Tissue Substitute in Right Metacarpal, Percutaneous Approach

0PWP44Z Revision of Internal Fixation Device in Right Metacarpal, Percutaneous Endoscopic Approach

0PWP45Z Revision of External Fixation Device in Right Metacarpal, Percutaneous Endoscopic Approach

0PWP47Z Revision of Autologous Tissue Substitute in Right Metacarpal, Percutaneous Endoscopic Approach

0PWP4JZ Revision of Synthetic Substitute in Right Metacarpal, Percutaneous Endoscopic Approach

0PWP4KZ Revision of Nonautologous Tissue Substitute in Right Metacarpal, Percutaneous Endoscopic Approach

0PWPX4Z Revision of Internal Fixation Device in Right Metacarpal, External Approach

0PWPX5Z Revision of External Fixation Device in Right Metacarpal, External Approach

0PWPX7Z Revision of Autologous Tissue Substitute in Right Metacarpal, External Approach

0PWPXJZ Revision of Synthetic Substitute in Right Metacarpal, External Approach

0PWPXKZ Revision of Nonautologous Tissue Substitute in Right Metacarpal, External Approach

0PWQ04Z Revision of Internal Fixation Device in Left Metacarpal, Open Approach

0PWQ05Z Revision of External Fixation Device in Left Metacarpal, Open Approach

0PWQ07Z Revision of Autologous Tissue Substitute in Left Metacarpal, Open Approach

0PWQ0JZ Revision of Synthetic Substitute in Left Metacarpal, Open Approach

0PWQ0KZ Revision of Nonautologous Tissue Substitute in Left Metacarpal, Open Approach

0PWQ34Z Revision of Internal Fixation Device in Left Metacarpal, Percutaneous Approach

0PWQ35Z Revision of External Fixation Device in Left Metacarpal, Percutaneous Approach

0PWQ37Z Revision of Autologous Tissue Substitute in Left Metacarpal, Percutaneous Approach

0PWQ3JZ Revision of Synthetic Substitute in Left Metacarpal, Percutaneous Approach

0PWQ3KZ Revision of Nonautologous Tissue Substitute in Left Metacarpal, Percutaneous Approach

0PWQ44Z Revision of Internal Fixation Device in Left Metacarpal, Percutaneous Endoscopic Approach

0PWQ45Z Revision of External Fixation Device in Left Metacarpal, Percutaneous Endoscopic Approach

0PWQ47Z Revision of Autologous Tissue Substitute in Left Metacarpal, Percutaneous Endoscopic Approach

0PWQ4JZ Revision of Synthetic Substitute in Left Metacarpal, Percutaneous Endoscopic Approach

0PWQ4KZ Revision of Nonautologous Tissue Substitute in Left Metacarpal, Percutaneous Endoscopic Approach

0PWQX4Z Revision of Internal Fixation Device in Left Metacarpal, External Approach

0PWQX5Z Revision of External Fixation Device in Left Metacarpal, External Approach

0PWQX7Z Revision of Autologous Tissue Substitute in Left Metacarpal, External Approach

0PWQXJZ Revision of Synthetic Substitute in Left Metacarpal, External Approach

0PWQXKZ Revision of Nonautologous Tissue Substitute in Left Metacarpal, External Approach

0PWR04Z Revision of Internal Fixation Device in Right Thumb Phalanx, Open Approach

0PWR05Z Revision of External Fixation Device in Right Thumb Phalanx, Open Approach

0PWR07Z Revision of Autologous Tissue Substitute in Right Thumb Phalanx, Open Approach

0PWR0JZ Revision of Synthetic Substitute in Right Thumb Phalanx, Open Approach

0PWR0KZ Revision of Nonautologous Tissue Substitute in Right Thumb Phalanx, Open Approach

0PWR34Z Revision of Internal Fixation Device in Right Thumb Phalanx, Percutaneous Approach

0PWR35Z Revision of External Fixation Device in Right Thumb Phalanx, Percutaneous Approach

0PWR37Z Revision of Autologous Tissue Substitute in Right Thumb Phalanx, Percutaneous Approach

0PWR3JZ Revision of Synthetic Substitute in Right Thumb Phalanx, Percutaneous Approach

0PWR3KZ Revision of Nonautologous Tissue Substitute in Right Thumb Phalanx, Percutaneous Approach

0PWR44Z Revision of Internal Fixation Device in Right Thumb Phalanx, Percutaneous Endoscopic Approach

0PWR45Z Revision of External Fixation Device in Right Thumb Phalanx, Percutaneous Endoscopic Approach

0PWR47Z Revision of Autologous Tissue Substitute in Right Thumb Phalanx, Percutaneous Endoscopic Approach

0PWR4JZ Revision of Synthetic Substitute in Right Thumb Phalanx, Percutaneous Endoscopic Approach

0PWR4KZ Revision of Nonautologous Tissue Substitute in Right Thumb Phalanx, Percutaneous Endoscopic Approach

0PWRX4Z Revision of Internal Fixation Device in Right Thumb Phalanx, External Approach

0PWRX5Z Revision of External Fixation Device in Right Thumb Phalanx, External Approach

0PWRX7Z Revision of Autologous Tissue Substitute in Right Thumb Phalanx, External Approach

0PWRXJZ Revision of Synthetic Substitute in Right Thumb Phalanx, External Approach

0PWRXKZ Revision of Nonautologous Tissue Substitute in Right Thumb Phalanx, External Approach

0PWS04Z Revision of Internal Fixation Device in Left Thumb Phalanx, Open Approach

0PWS05Z Revision of External Fixation Device in Left Thumb Phalanx, Open Approach

0PWS07Z Revision of Autologous Tissue Substitute in Left Thumb Phalanx, Open Approach

0PWS0JZ Revision of Synthetic Substitute in Left Thumb Phalanx, Open Approach

0PWS0KZ Revision of Nonautologous Tissue Substitute in Left Thumb Phalanx, Open Approach

0PWS34Z Revision of Internal Fixation Device in Left Thumb Phalanx, Percutaneous Approach

0PWS35Z Revision of External Fixation Device in Left Thumb Phalanx, Percutaneous Approach

0PWS37Z Revision of Autologous Tissue Substitute in Left Thumb Phalanx, Percutaneous Approach

0PWS3JZ Revision of Synthetic Substitute in Left Thumb Phalanx, Percutaneous Approach

0PWS3KZ Revision of Nonautologous Tissue Substitute in Left Thumb Phalanx, Percutaneous Approach

0PWS44Z Revision of Internal Fixation Device in Left Thumb Phalanx, Percutaneous Endoscopic Approach

0PWS45Z Revision of External Fixation Device in Left Thumb Phalanx, Percutaneous Endoscopic Approach

0PWS47Z Revision of Autologous Tissue Substitute in Left Thumb Phalanx, Percutaneous Endoscopic Approach

0PWS4JZ Revision of Synthetic Substitute in Left Thumb Phalanx, Percutaneous Endoscopic Approach

0PWS4KZ Revision of Nonautologous Tissue Substitute in Left Thumb Phalanx, Percutaneous Endoscopic Approach

0PWSX4Z Revision of Internal Fixation Device in Left Thumb Phalanx, External Approach

0PWSX5Z Revision of External Fixation Device in Left Thumb Phalanx, External Approach

0PWSX7Z Revision of Autologous Tissue Substitute in Left Thumb Phalanx, External Approach

0PWSXJZ Revision of Synthetic Substitute in Left Thumb Phalanx, External Approach

0PWSXKZ Revision of Nonautologous Tissue Substitute in Left Thumb Phalanx, External Approach

0PWT04Z Revision of Internal Fixation Device in Right Finger Phalanx, Open Approach

0PWT05Z Revision of External Fixation Device in Right Finger Phalanx, Open Approach

0PWT07Z Revision of Autologous Tissue Substitute in Right Finger Phalanx, Open Approach

0PWT0JZ Revision of Synthetic Substitute in Right Finger Phalanx, Open Approach

0PWT0KZ Revision of Nonautologous Tissue Substitute in Right Finger Phalanx, Open Approach

0PWT34Z Revision of Internal Fixation Device in Right Finger Phalanx, Percutaneous Approach

0PWT35Z Revision of External Fixation Device in Right Finger Phalanx, Percutaneous Approach

0PWT37Z Revision of Autologous Tissue Substitute in Right Finger Phalanx, Percutaneous Approach

0PWT3JZ Revision of Synthetic Substitute in Right Finger Phalanx, Percutaneous Approach

0PWT3KZ Revision of Nonautologous Tissue Substitute in Right Finger Phalanx, Percutaneous Approach

0PWT44Z Revision of Internal Fixation Device in Right Finger Phalanx, Percutaneous Endoscopic Approach

0PWT45Z Revision of External Fixation Device in Right Finger Phalanx, Percutaneous Endoscopic Approach

0PWT47Z Revision of Autologous Tissue Substitute in Right Finger Phalanx, Percutaneous Endoscopic Approach

0PWT4JZ Revision of Synthetic Substitute in Right Finger Phalanx, Percutaneous Endoscopic Approach

0PWT4KZ Revision of Nonautologous Tissue Substitute in Right Finger Phalanx, Percutaneous Endoscopic Approach

0PWTX4Z Revision of Internal Fixation Device in Right Finger Phalanx, External Approach

0PWTX5Z Revision of External Fixation Device in Right Finger Phalanx, External Approach

0PWTX7Z Revision of Autologous Tissue Substitute in Right Finger Phalanx, External Approach

0PWTXJZ Revision of Synthetic Substitute in Right Finger Phalanx, External Approach

0PWTXKZ Revision of Nonautologous Tissue Substitute in Right Finger Phalanx, External Approach

0PWV04Z Revision of Internal Fixation Device in Left Finger Phalanx, Open Approach

0PWV05Z Revision of External Fixation Device in Left Finger Phalanx, Open Approach

0PWV07Z Revision of Autologous Tissue Substitute in Left Finger Phalanx, Open Approach

0PWV0JZ Revision of Synthetic Substitute in Left Finger Phalanx, Open Approach

0PWV0KZ Revision of Nonautologous Tissue Substitute in Left Finger Phalanx, Open Approach

0PWV34Z Revision of Internal Fixation Device in Left Finger Phalanx, Percutaneous Approach

0PWV35Z Revision of External Fixation Device in Left Finger Phalanx, Percutaneous Approach

0PWV37Z Revision of Autologous Tissue Substitute in Left Finger Phalanx, Percutaneous Approach

0PWV3JZ Revision of Synthetic Substitute in Left Finger Phalanx, Percutaneous Approach

0PWV3KZ Revision of Nonautologous Tissue Substitute in Left Finger Phalanx, Percutaneous Approach

0PWV44Z Revision of Internal Fixation Device in Left Finger Phalanx, Percutaneous Endoscopic Approach

0PWV45Z Revision of External Fixation Device in Left Finger Phalanx, Percutaneous Endoscopic Approach

0PWV47Z Revision of Autologous Tissue Substitute in Left Finger Phalanx, Percutaneous Endoscopic Approach

0PWV4JZ Revision of Synthetic Substitute in Left Finger Phalanx, Percutaneous Endoscopic Approach

0PWV4KZ Revision of Nonautologous Tissue Substitute in Left Finger Phalanx, Percutaneous Endoscopic Approach

0PWVX4Z Revision of Internal Fixation Device in Left Finger Phalanx, External Approach

0PWVX5Z Revision of External Fixation Device in Left Finger Phalanx, External Approach

0PWVX7Z Revision of Autologous Tissue Substitute in Left Finger Phalanx, External Approach

0PWVXJZ Revision of Synthetic Substitute in Left Finger Phalanx, External Approach

0PWVXKZ Revision of Nonautologous Tissue Substitute in Left Finger Phalanx, External Approach

0PWY00Z Revision of Drainage Device in Upper Bone, Open Approach

0PWY0MZ Revision of Bone Growth Stimulator in Upper Bone, Open Approach

0PWY30Z Revision of Drainage Device in Upper Bone, Percutaneous Approach

0PWY3MZ Revision of Bone Growth Stimulator in Upper Bone, Percutaneous Approach

0PWY40Z Revision of Drainage Device in Upper Bone, Percutaneous Endoscopic Approach

0PWY4MZ Revision of Bone Growth Stimulator in Upper Bone, Percutaneous Endoscopic Approach

0PWYX0Z Revision of Drainage Device in Upper Bone, External Approach

0PWYXMZ Revision of Bone Growth Stimulator in Upper Bone, External Approach

Bones - Front and Back Views

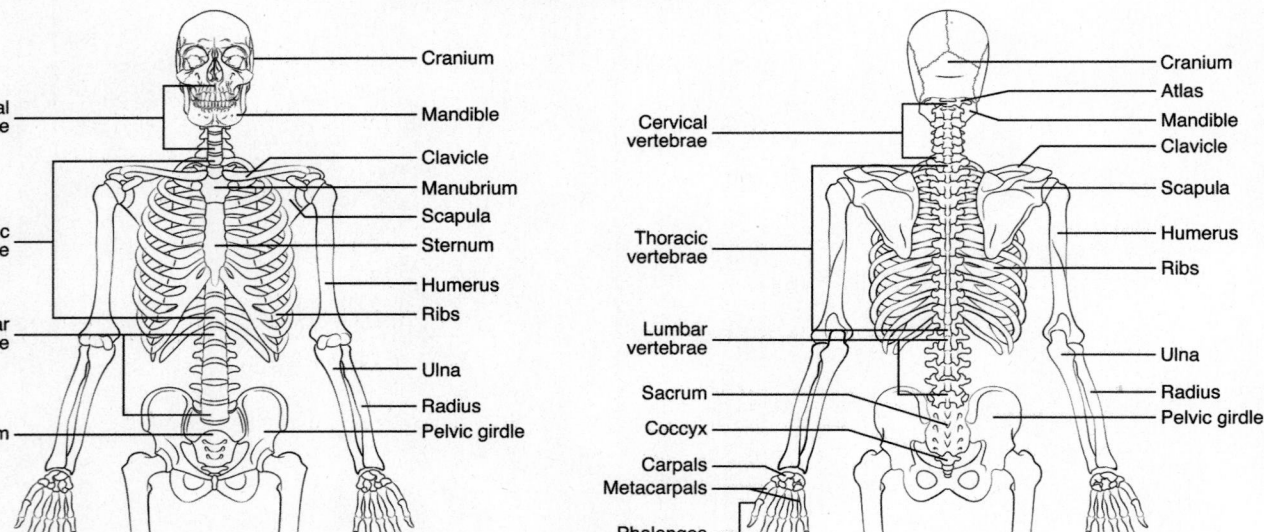

Front View labels:
- Cranium
- Cervical vertebrae
- Mandible
- Clavicle
- Manubrium
- Thoracic vertebrae
- Scapula
- Sternum
- Humerus
- Ribs
- Lumbar vertebrae
- Ulna
- Radius
- Sacrum
- Pelvic girdle
- Femur
- Patella
- Tibia
- Fibula
- Tarsals
- Metatarsals
- Phalanges

Back View labels:
- Cranium
- Atlas
- Cervical vertebrae
- Mandible
- Clavicle
- Scapula
- Thoracic vertebrae
- Humerus
- Ribs
- Lumbar vertebrae
- Sacrum
- Ulna
- Coccyx
- Radius
- Carpals
- Pelvic girdle
- Metacarpals
- Phalanges
- Femur
- Tibia
- Fibula
- Tarsals
- Metatarsals
- Phalanges
- Calcaneus

©AHIMA

Vertebral Column

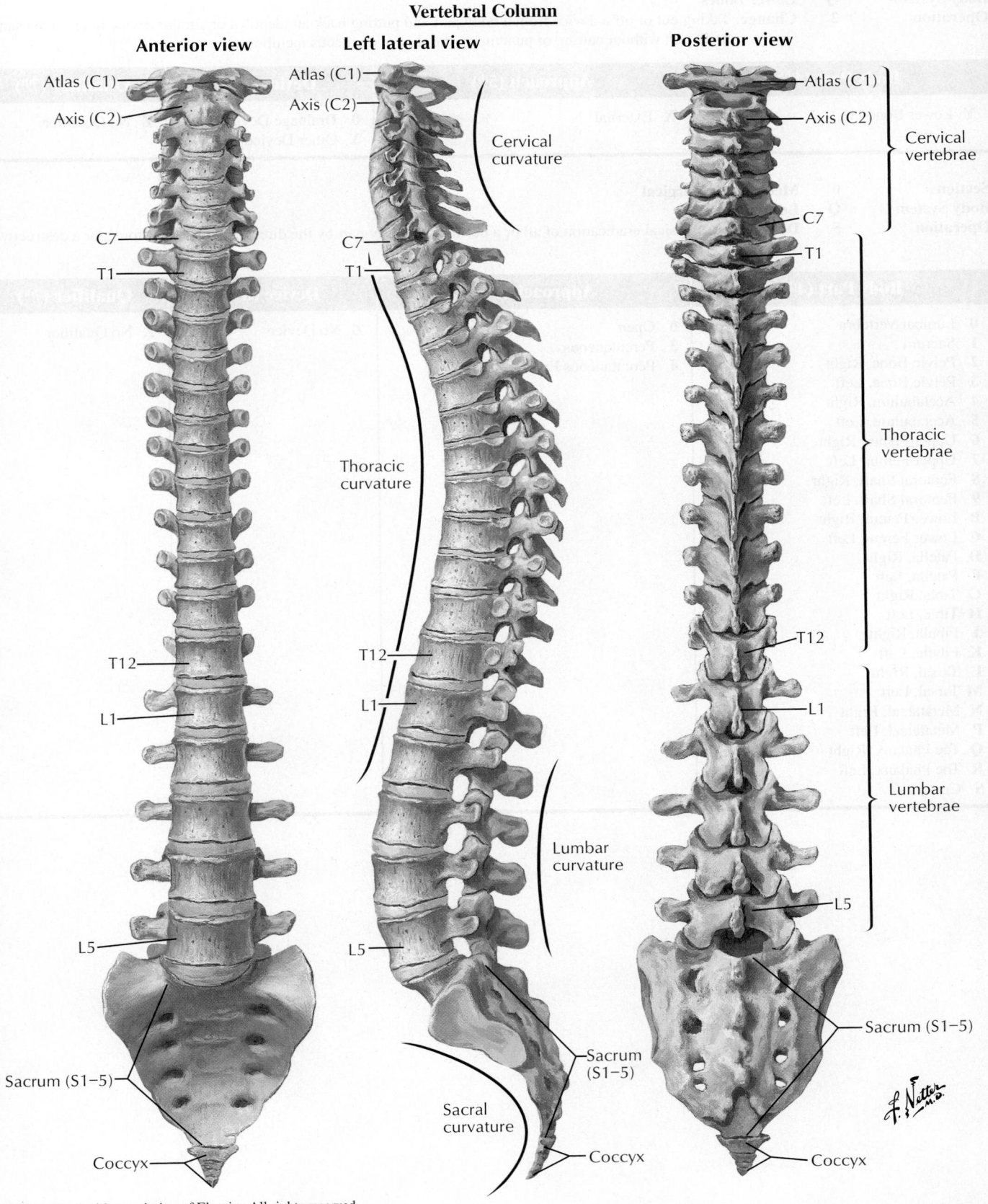

Anterior view

Atlas (C1)
Axis (C2)

C7
T1

T12

L1

L5

Sacrum (S1–5)

Coccyx

Left lateral view

Atlas (C1)
Axis (C2)

Cervical
curvature

C7
T1

Thoracic
curvature

T12
L1

Lumbar
curvature

L5

Sacrum
(S1–5)

Sacral
curvature

Coccyx

Posterior view

Atlas (C1)
Axis (C2)

Cervical
vertebrae

C7
T1

Thoracic
vertebrae

T12

L1

Lumbar
vertebrae

L5

Sacrum (S1–5)

Coccyx

F. Netter
M.S.

Medical and Surgical, Lower Bones

Lower Bones Tables 0Q2–0QW

Section	0	Medical and Surgical
Body System	Q	Lower Bones
Operation	2	Change: Taking out or off a device from a body part and putting back an identical or similar device in or on the same body part without cutting or puncturing the skin or a mucous membrane

Body Part (4th)	Approach (5th)	Device (6th)	Qualifier (7th)
Y Lower Bone	X External	0 Drainage Device Y Other Device	Z No Qualifier

Section	0	Medical and Surgical
Body System	Q	Lower Bones
Operation	5	Destruction: Physical eradication of all or a portion of a body part by the direct use of energy, force, or a destructive agent

Body Part (4th)	Approach (5th)	Device (6th)	Qualifier (7th)
0 Lumbar Vertebra 1 Sacrum 2 Pelvic Bone, Right 3 Pelvic Bone, Left 4 Acetabulum, Right 5 Acetabulum, Left 6 Upper Femur, Right 7 Upper Femur, Left 8 Femoral Shaft, Right 9 Femoral Shaft, Left B Lower Femur, Right C Lower Femur, Left D Patella, Right F Patella, Left G Tibia, Right H Tibia, Left J Fibula, Right K Fibula, Left L Tarsal, Right M Tarsal, Left N Metatarsal, Right P Metatarsal, Left Q Toe Phalanx, Right R Toe Phalanx, Left S Coccyx	0 Open 3 Percutaneous 4 Percutaneous Endoscopic	Z No Device	Z No Qualifier

Medical and Surgical, Lower Bones Tables

Section	0	Medical and Surgical
Body System	Q	Lower Bones
Operation	8	**Division:** Cutting into a body part, without draining fluids and/or gases from the body part, in order to separate or transect a body part

Body Part (4ᵗʰ)	Approach (5ᵗʰ)	Device (6ᵗʰ)	Qualifier (7ᵗʰ)
0 Lumbar Vertebra 1 Sacrum 2 Pelvic Bone, Right 3 Pelvic Bone, Left 4 Acetabulum, Right 5 Acetabulum, Left 6 Upper Femur, Right 7 Upper Femur, Left 8 Femoral Shaft, Right 9 Femoral Shaft, Left B Lower Femur, Right C Lower Femur, Left D Patella, Right F Patella, Left G Tibia, Right H Tibia, Left J Fibula, Right K Fibula, Left L Tarsal, Right M Tarsal, Left N Metatarsal, Right P Metatarsal, Left Q Toe Phalanx, Right R Toe Phalanx, Left S Coccyx	0 Open 3 Percutaneous 4 Percutaneous Endoscopic	Z No Device	Z No Qualifier

Section	0	Medical and Surgical
Body System	Q	Lower Bones
Operation	9	**Drainage:** Taking or letting out fluids and/or gases from a body part

Body Part (4ᵗʰ)	Approach (5ᵗʰ)	Device (6ᵗʰ)	Qualifier (7ᵗʰ)
0 Lumbar Vertebra 1 Sacrum 2 Pelvic Bone, Right 3 Pelvic Bone, Left 4 Acetabulum, Right 5 Acetabulum, Left 6 Upper Femur, Right 7 Upper Femur, Left 8 Femoral Shaft, Right 9 Femoral Shaft, Left B Lower Femur, Right C Lower Femur, Left D Patella, Right F Patella, Left G Tibia, Right H Tibia, Left J Fibula, Right K Fibula, Left L Tarsal, Right M Tarsal, Left N Metatarsal, Right P Metatarsal, Left Q Toe Phalanx, Right R Toe Phalanx, Left S Coccyx	0 Open 3 Percutaneous 4 Percutaneous Endoscopic	0 Drainage Device	Z No Qualifier

Continued →

Section	0	Medical and Surgical
Body System	Q	Lower Bones
Operation	9	Drainage: Taking or letting out fluids and/or gases from a body part

Body Part (4th)	Approach (5th)	Device (6th)	Qualifier (7th)
0 Lumbar Vertebra	0 Open	Z No Device	X Diagnostic
1 Sacrum	3 Percutaneous		Z No Qualifier
2 Pelvic Bone, Right	4 Percutaneous Endoscopic		
3 Pelvic Bone, Left			
4 Acetabulum, Right			
5 Acetabulum, Left			
6 Upper Femur, Right			
7 Upper Femur, Left			
8 Femoral Shaft, Right			
9 Femoral Shaft, Left			
B Lower Femur, Right			
C Lower Femur, Left			
D Patella, Right			
F Patella, Left			
G Tibia, Right			
H Tibia, Left			
J Fibula, Right			
K Fibula, Left			
L Tarsal, Right			
M Tarsal, Left			
N Metatarsal, Right			
P Metatarsal, Left			
Q Toe Phalanx, Right			
R Toe Phalanx, Left			
S Coccyx			

Section	0	Medical and Surgical
Body System	Q	Lower Bones
Operation	B	Excision: Cutting out or off, without replacement, a portion of a body part

Body Part (4th)	Approach (5th)	Device (6th)	Qualifier (7th)
0 Lumbar Vertebra	0 Open	Z No Device	X Diagnostic
1 Sacrum	3 Percutaneous		Z No Qualifier
2 Pelvic Bone, Right	4 Percutaneous Endoscopic		
3 Pelvic Bone, Left			
4 Acetabulum, Right			
5 Acetabulum, Left			
6 Upper Femur, Right			
7 Upper Femur, Left			
8 Femoral Shaft, Right			
9 Femoral Shaft, Left			
B Lower Femur, Right			
C Lower Femur, Left			
D Patella, Right			
F Patella, Left			
G Tibia, Right			
H Tibia, Left			
J Fibula, Right			
K Fibula, Left			
L Tarsal, Right			
M Tarsal, Left			
Q Toe Phalanx, Right			
R Toe Phalanx, Left			
S Coccyx			
N Metatarsal, Right	0 Open	Z No Device	2 Sesamoid Bone(s) 1st Toe
P Metatarsal, Left	3 Percutaneous		X Diagnostic
	4 Percutaneous Endoscopic		Z No Qualifier

Section   **0**   **Medical and Surgical**
Body System   **Q**   **Lower Bones**
Operation   **C**   **Extirpation:** Taking or cutting out solid matter from a body part

Body Part (4ᵗʰ)	Approach (5ᵗʰ)	Device (6ᵗʰ)	Qualifier (7ᵗʰ)
0 Lumbar Vertebra	0 Open	Z No Device	Z No Qualifier
1 Sacrum	3 Percutaneous		
2 Pelvic Bone, Right	4 Percutaneous Endoscopic		
3 Pelvic Bone, Left			
4 Acetabulum, Right			
5 Acetabulum, Left			
6 Upper Femur, Right			
7 Upper Femur, Left			
8 Femoral Shaft, Right			
9 Femoral Shaft, Left			
B Lower Femur, Right			
C Lower Femur, Left			
D Patella, Right			
F Patella, Left			
G Tibia, Right			
H Tibia, Left			
J Fibula, Right			
K Fibula, Left			
L Tarsal, Right			
M Tarsal, Left			
N Metatarsal, Right			
P Metatarsal, Left			
Q Toe Phalanx, Right			
R Toe Phalanx, Left			
S Coccyx			

Section   **0**   **Medical and Surgical**
Body System   **Q**   **Lower Bones**
Operation   **D**   **Extraction:** Pulling or stripping out or off all or a portion of a body part by the use of force

Body Part (4ᵗʰ)	Approach (5ᵗʰ)	Device (6ᵗʰ)	Qualifier (7ᵗʰ)
0 Lumbar Vertebra	0 Open	Z No Device	Z No Qualifier
1 Sacrum			
2 Pelvic Bone, Right			
3 Pelvic Bone, Left			
4 Acetabulum, Right			
5 Acetabulum, Left			
6 Upper Femur, Right			
7 Upper Femur, Left			
8 Femoral Shaft, Right			
9 Femoral Shaft, Left			
B Lower Femur, Right			
C Lower Femur, Left			
D Patella, Right			
F Patella, Left			
G Tibia, Right			
H Tibia, Left			
J Fibula, Right			
K Fibula, Left			
L Tarsal, Right			
M Tarsal, Left			
N Metatarsal, Right			
P Metatarsal, Left			
Q Toe Phalanx, Right			
R Toe Phalanx, Left			
S Coccyx			

Section	0	Medical and Surgical
Body System	Q	Lower Bones
Operation	H	Insertion: Putting in a nonbiological appliance that monitors, assists, performs, or prevents a physiological function but does not physically take the place of a body part

Body Part (4th)	Approach (5th)	Device (6th)	Qualifier (7th)
0 Lumbar Vertebra 1 Sacrum 2 Pelvic Bone, Right 3 Pelvic Bone, Left 4 Acetabulum, Right 5 Acetabulum, Left D Patella, Right F Patella, Left L Tarsal, Right M Tarsal, Left N Metatarsal, Right P Metatarsal, Left Q Toe Phalanx, Right R Toe Phalanx, Left S Coccyx	0 Open 3 Percutaneous 4 Percutaneous Endoscopic	4 Internal Fixation Device 5 External Fixation Device	Z No Qualifier
6 Upper Femur, Right 7 Upper Femur, Left B Lower Femur, Right C Lower Femur, Left J Fibula, Right K Fibula, Left	0 Open 3 Percutaneous 4 Percutaneous Endoscopic	4 Internal Fixation Device 5 External Fixation Device 6 Internal Fixation Device, Intramedullary 8 External Fixation Device, Limb Lengthening B External Fixation Device, Monoplanar C External Fixation Device, Ring D External Fixation Device, Hybrid	Z No Qualifier
8 Femoral Shaft, Right 9 Femoral Shaft, Left G Tibia, Right H Tibia, Left	0 Open 3 Percutaneous 4 Percutaneous Endoscopic	4 Internal Fixation Device 5 External Fixation Device 6 Internal Fixation Device, Intramedullary 7 Internal Fixation Device, Intramedullary Limb Lengthening 8 External Fixation Device, Limb Lengthening B External Fixation Device, Monoplanar C External Fixation Device, Ring D External Fixation Device, Hybrid	Z No Qualifier
Y Lower Bone	0 Open 3 Percutaneous 4 Percutaneous Endoscopic	M Bone Growth Stimulator	Z No Qualifier

Section	0	Medical and Surgical
Body System	Q	Lower Bones
Operation	J	Inspection: Visually and/or manually exploring a body part

Body Part (4th)	Approach (5th)	Device (6th)	Qualifier (7th)
Y Lower Bone	0 Open 3 Percutaneous 4 Percutaneous Endoscopic X External	Z No Device	Z No Qualifier

Section   0   **Medical and Surgical**
Body System   Q   **Lower Bones**
Operation   N   **Release:** Freeing a body part from an abnormal physical constraint by cutting or by the use of force

Body Part (4th)	Approach (5th)	Device (6th)	Qualifier (7th)
0 Lumbar Vertebra	0 Open	Z No Device	Z No Qualifier
1 Sacrum	3 Percutaneous		
2 Pelvic Bone, Right	4 Percutaneous Endoscopic		
3 Pelvic Bone, Left			
4 Acetabulum, Right			
5 Acetabulum, Left			
6 Upper Femur, Right			
7 Upper Femur, Left			
8 Femoral Shaft, Right			
9 Femoral Shaft, Left			
B Lower Femur, Right			
C Lower Femur, Left			
D Patella, Right			
F Patella, Left			
G Tibia, Right			
H Tibia, Left			
J Fibula, Right			
K Fibula, Left			
L Tarsal, Right			
M Tarsal, Left			
N Metatarsal, Right			
P Metatarsal, Left			
Q Toe Phalanx, Right			
R Toe Phalanx, Left			
S Coccyx			

Section   0   **Medical and Surgical**
Body System   Q   **Lower Bones**
Operation   P   **Removal:** Taking out or off a device from a body part

Body Part (4th)	Approach (5th)	Device (6th)	Qualifier (7th)
0 Lumbar Vertebra	0 Open	4 Internal Fixation Device	Z No Qualifier
1 Sacrum	3 Percutaneous	5 External Fixation Device	
2 Pelvic Bone, Right	4 Percutaneous Endoscopic	7 Autologous Tissue Substitute	
3 Pelvic Bone, Left		J Synthetic Substitute	
4 Acetabulum, Right		K Nonautologous Tissue Substitute	
5 Acetabulum, Left			
6 Upper Femur, Right			
7 Upper Femur, Left			
8 Femoral Shaft, Right			
9 Femoral Shaft, Left			
B Lower Femur, Right			
C Lower Femur, Left			
D Patella, Right			
F Patella, Left			
G Tibia, Right			
H Tibia, Left			
J Fibula, Right			
K Fibula, Left			
L Tarsal, Right			
M Tarsal, Left			
N Metatarsal, Right			
P Metatarsal, Left			
Q Toe Phalanx, Right			
R Toe Phalanx, Left			
S Coccyx			

Continued →

Section	0	Medical and Surgical
Body System	Q	Lower Bones
Operation	P	**Removal:** Taking out or off a device from a body part

Body Part (4ᵗʰ)	Approach (5ᵗʰ)	Device (6ᵗʰ)	Qualifier (7ᵗʰ)
0 Lumbar Vertebra 1 Sacrum 2 Pelvic Bone, Right 3 Pelvic Bone, Left 4 Acetabulum, Right 5 Acetabulum, Left 6 Upper Femur, Right 7 Upper Femur, Left 8 Femoral Shaft, Right 9 Femoral Shaft, Left B Lower Femur, Right C Lower Femur, Left D Patella, Right F Patella, Left G Tibia, Right H Tibia, Left J Fibula, Right K Fibula, Left L Tarsal, Right M Tarsal, Left N Metatarsal, Right P Metatarsal, Left Q Toe Phalanx, Right R Toe Phalanx, Left S Coccyx	X External	4 Internal Fixation Device 5 External Fixation Device	Z No Qualifier
Y Lower Bone	0 Open 3 Percutaneous 4 Percutaneous Endoscopic X External	0 Drainage Device M Bone Growth Stimulator	Z No Qualifier

Section	0	Medical and Surgical
Body System	Q	Lower Bones
Operation	Q	**Repair:** Restoring, to the extent possible, a body part to its normal anatomic structure and function

Body Part (4th)	Approach (5th)	Device (6th)	Qualifier (7th)
0 Lumbar Vertebra 1 Sacrum 2 Pelvic Bone, Right 3 Pelvic Bone, Left 4 Acetabulum, Right 5 Acetabulum, Left 6 Upper Femur, Right 7 Upper Femur, Left 8 Femoral Shaft, Right 9 Femoral Shaft, Left B Lower Femur, Right C Lower Femur, Left D Patella, Right F Patella, Left G Tibia, Right H Tibia, Left J Fibula, Right K Fibula, Left L Tarsal, Right M Tarsal, Left N Metatarsal, Right P Metatarsal, Left Q Toe Phalanx, Right R Toe Phalanx, Left S Coccyx	0 Open 3 Percutaneous 4 Percutaneous Endoscopic X External	Z No Device	Z No Qualifier

Section	0	Medical and Surgical
Body System	Q	Lower Bones
Operation	R	**Replacement:** Putting in or on biological or synthetic material that physically takes the place and/or function of all or a portion of a body part

Body Part (4th)	Approach (5th)	Device (6th)	Qualifier (7th)
0 Lumbar Vertebra 1 Sacrum 2 Pelvic Bone, Right 3 Pelvic Bone, Left 4 Acetabulum, Right 5 Acetabulum, Left 6 Upper Femur, Right 7 Upper Femur, Left 8 Femoral Shaft, Right 9 Femoral Shaft, Left B Lower Femur, Right C Lower Femur, Left D Patella, Right F Patella, Left G Tibia, Right H Tibia, Left J Fibula, Right K Fibula, Left L Tarsal, Right M Tarsal, Left N Metatarsal, Right P Metatarsal, Left Q Toe Phalanx, Right R Toe Phalanx, Left S Coccyx	0 Open 3 Percutaneous 4 Percutaneous Endoscopic	7 Autologous Tissue Substitute J Synthetic Substitute K Nonautologous Tissue Substitute	Z No Qualifier

Section   0   **Medical and Surgical**
Body System   Q   **Lower Bones**
Operation   S   **Reposition:** Moving to its normal location, or other suitable location, all or a portion of a body part

Body Part (4ᵗʰ)	Approach (5ᵗʰ)	Device (6ᵗʰ)	Qualifier (7ᵗʰ)
0 Lumbar Vertebra	**0** Open **4** Percutaneous Endoscopic	**3** Spinal Stabilization Device, Vertebral Body Tether **4** Internal Fixation Device **Z** No Device	**Z** No Qualifier
0 Lumbar Vertebra	**3** Percutaneous	**4** Internal Fixation Device **Z** No Device	**Z** No Qualifier
0 Lumbar Vertebra	**X** External	**Z** No Device	**Z** No Qualifier
1 Sacrum **4** Acetabulum, Right **5** Acetabulum, Left **S** Coccyx	**0** Open **3** Percutaneous **4** Percutaneous Endoscopic	**4** Internal Fixation Device **Z** No Device	**Z** No Qualifier
1 Sacrum **4** Acetabulum, Right **5** Acetabulum, Left **S** Coccyx	**X** External	**Z** No Device	**Z** No Qualifier
2 Pelvic Bone, Right **3** Pelvic Bone, Left **D** Patella, Right **F** Patella, Left **L** Tarsal, Right **M** Tarsal, Left **Q** Toe Phalanx, Right **R** Toe Phalanx, Left	**0** Open **3** Percutaneous **4** Percutaneous Endoscopic	**4** Internal Fixation Device **5** External Fixation Device **Z** No Device	**Z** No Qualifier
2 Pelvic Bone, Right **3** Pelvic Bone, Left **D** Patella, Right **F** Patella, Left **L** Tarsal, Right **M** Tarsal, Left **Q** Toe Phalanx, Right **R** Toe Phalanx, Left	**X** External	**Z** No Device	**Z** No Qualifier
6 Upper Femur, Right **7** Upper Femur, Left **8** Femoral Shaft, Right **9** Femoral Shaft, Left **B** Lower Femur, Right **C** Lower Femur, Left **G** Tibia, Right **H** Tibia, Left **J** Fibula, Right **K** Fibula, Left	**0** Open **3** Percutaneous **4** Percutaneous Endoscopic	**4** Internal Fixation Device **5** External Fixation Device **6** Internal Fixation Device, Intramedullary **B** External Fixation Device, Monoplanar **C** External Fixation Device, Ring **D** External Fixation Device, Hybrid **Z** No Device	**Z** No Qualifier
6 Upper Femur, Right **7** Upper Femur, Left **8** Femoral Shaft, Right **9** Femoral Shaft, Left **B** Lower Femur, Right **C** Lower Femur, Left **G** Tibia, Right **H** Tibia, Left **J** Fibula, Right **K** Fibula, Left	**X** External	**Z** No Device	**Z** No Qualifier
N Metatarsal, Right **P** Metatarsal, Left	**0** Open **3** Percutaneous **4** Percutaneous Endoscopic	**4** Internal Fixation Device **5** External Fixation Device **Z** No Device	**2** Sesamoid Bone(s) 1st Toe **Z** No Qualifier
N Metatarsal, Right **P** Metatarsal, Left	**X** External	**Z** No Device	**2** Sesamoid Bone(s) 1st Toe **Z** No Qualifier

Section 0 **Medical and Surgical**
Body System Q **Lower Bones**
Operation T **Resection:** Cutting out or off, without replacement, all of a body part

Body Part (4th)	Approach (5th)	Device (6th)	Qualifier (7th)
2 Pelvic Bone, Right	0 Open	Z No Device	Z No Qualifier
3 Pelvic Bone, Left			
4 Acetabulum, Right			
5 Acetabulum, Left			
6 Upper Femur, Right			
7 Upper Femur, Left			
8 Femoral Shaft, Right			
9 Femoral Shaft, Left			
B Lower Femur, Right			
C Lower Femur, Left			
D Patella, Right			
F Patella, Left			
G Tibia, Right			
H Tibia, Left			
J Fibula, Right			
K Fibula, Left			
L Tarsal, Right			
M Tarsal, Left			
N Metatarsal, Right			
P Metatarsal, Left			
Q Toe Phalanx, Right			
R Toe Phalanx, Left			
S Coccyx			

Section 0 **Medical and Surgical**
Body System Q **Lower Bones**
Operation U **Supplement:** Putting in or on biological or synthetic material that physically reinforces and/or augments the function of a portion of a body part

Body Part (4th)	Approach (5th)	Device (6th)	Qualifier (7th)
0 Lumbar Vertebra	0 Open	7 Autologous Tissue Substitute	Z No Qualifier
1 Sacrum	3 Percutaneous	J Synthetic Substitute	
2 Pelvic Bone, Right	4 Percutaneous Endoscopic	K Nonautologous Tissue Substitute	
3 Pelvic Bone, Left			
4 Acetabulum, Right			
5 Acetabulum, Left			
6 Upper Femur, Right			
7 Upper Femur, Left			
8 Femoral Shaft, Right			
9 Femoral Shaft, Left			
B Lower Femur, Right			
C Lower Femur, Left			
D Patella, Right			
F Patella, Left			
G Tibia, Right			
H Tibia, Left			
J Fibula, Right			
K Fibula, Left			
L Tarsal, Right			
M Tarsal, Left			
N Metatarsal, Right			
P Metatarsal, Left			
Q Toe Phalanx, Right			
R Toe Phalanx, Left			
S Coccyx			

Section 0 **Medical and Surgical**
Body System Q **Lower Bones**
Operation W **Revision:** Correcting, to the extent possible, a portion of a malfunctioning device or the position of a displaced device

Body Part (4ᵗʰ)	Approach (5ᵗʰ)	Device (6ᵗʰ)	Qualifier (7ᵗʰ)
0 Lumbar Vertebra **1** Sacrum **4** Acetabulum, Right **5** Acetabulum, Left **S** Coccyx	**0** Open **3** Percutaneous **4** Percutaneous Endoscopic **X** External	**4** Internal Fixation Device **7** Autologous Tissue Substitute **J** Synthetic Substitute **K** Nonautologous Tissue Substitute	**Z** No Qualifier
2 Pelvic Bone, Right **3** Pelvic Bone, Left **6** Upper Femur, Right **7** Upper Femur, Left **8** Femoral Shaft, Right **9** Femoral Shaft, Left **B** Lower Femur, Right **C** Lower Femur, Left **D** Patella, Right **F** Patella, Left **G** Tibia, Right **H** Tibia, Left **J** Fibula, Right **K** Fibula, Left **L** Tarsal, Right **M** Tarsal, Left **N** Metatarsal, Right **P** Metatarsal, Left **Q** Toe Phalanx, Right **R** Toe Phalanx, Left	**0** Open **3** Percutaneous **4** Percutaneous Endoscopic **X** External	**4** Internal Fixation Device **5** External Fixation Device **7** Autologous Tissue Substitute **J** Synthetic Substitute **K** Nonautologous Tissue Substitute	**Z** No Qualifier
Y Lower Bone	**0** Open **3** Percutaneous **4** Percutaneous Endoscopic **X** External	**0** Drainage Device **M** Bone Growth Stimulator	**Z** No Qualifier

Lower Bones Code Listing 0Q2–0QW

0Q2 – Lower Bones, Change

Review Coding Guideline B6.1c

0Q2YX0Z Change Drainage Device in Lower Bone, External Approach

0Q2YXYZ Change Other Device in Lower Bone, External Approach

0Q5 – Lower Bones, Destruction

0Q500ZZ Destruction of Lumbar Vertebra, Open Approach
0Q503ZZ Destruction of Lumbar Vertebra, Percutaneous Approach
0Q504ZZ Destruction of Lumbar Vertebra, Percutaneous Endoscopic Approach
0Q510ZZ Destruction of Sacrum, Open Approach
0Q513ZZ Destruction of Sacrum, Percutaneous Approach
0Q514ZZ Destruction of Sacrum, Percutaneous Endoscopic Approach
0Q520ZZ Destruction of Right Pelvic Bone, Open Approach
0Q523ZZ Destruction of Right Pelvic Bone, Percutaneous Approach
0Q524ZZ Destruction of Right Pelvic Bone, Percutaneous Endoscopic Approach
0Q530ZZ Destruction of Left Pelvic Bone, Open Approach
0Q533ZZ Destruction of Left Pelvic Bone, Percutaneous Approach
0Q534ZZ Destruction of Left Pelvic Bone, Percutaneous Endoscopic Approach

0Q540ZZ Destruction of Right Acetabulum, Open Approach
0Q543ZZ Destruction of Right Acetabulum, Percutaneous Approach
0Q544ZZ Destruction of Right Acetabulum, Percutaneous Endoscopic Approach
0Q550ZZ Destruction of Left Acetabulum, Open Approach
0Q553ZZ Destruction of Left Acetabulum, Percutaneous Approach
0Q554ZZ Destruction of Left Acetabulum, Percutaneous Endoscopic Approach
0Q560ZZ Destruction of Right Upper Femur, Open Approach
0Q563ZZ Destruction of Right Upper Femur, Percutaneous Approach
0Q564ZZ Destruction of Right Upper Femur, Percutaneous Endoscopic Approach
0Q570ZZ Destruction of Left Upper Femur, Open Approach
0Q573ZZ Destruction of Left Upper Femur, Percutaneous Approach

0Q574ZZ Destruction of Left Upper Femur, Percutaneous Endoscopic Approach
0Q580ZZ Destruction of Right Femoral Shaft, Open Approach
0Q583ZZ Destruction of Right Femoral Shaft, Percutaneous Approach
0Q584ZZ Destruction of Right Femoral Shaft, Percutaneous Endoscopic Approach
0Q590ZZ Destruction of Left Femoral Shaft, Open Approach
0Q593ZZ Destruction of Left Femoral Shaft, Percutaneous Approach
0Q594ZZ Destruction of Left Femoral Shaft, Percutaneous Endoscopic Approach
0Q5B0ZZ Destruction of Right Lower Femur, Open Approach
0Q5B3ZZ Destruction of Right Lower Femur, Percutaneous Approach
0Q5B4ZZ Destruction of Right Lower Femur, Percutaneous Endoscopic Approach
0Q5C0ZZ Destruction of Left Lower Femur, Open Approach

♀ Female-only   ♂ Male-only   ▲ Limited Coverage   ● Non-OR   ▩ HAC-associated procedure   ▲ Non-covered procedures   ✚ Cluster

0Q5C3ZZ	Destruction of Left Lower Femur, Percutaneous Approach
0Q5C4ZZ	Destruction of Left Lower Femur, Percutaneous Endoscopic Approach
0Q5D0ZZ	Destruction of Right Patella, Open Approach
0Q5D3ZZ	Destruction of Right Patella, Percutaneous Approach
0Q5D4ZZ	Destruction of Right Patella, Percutaneous Endoscopic Approach
0Q5F0ZZ	Destruction of Left Patella, Open Approach
0Q5F3ZZ	Destruction of Left Patella, Percutaneous Approach
0Q5F4ZZ	Destruction of Left Patella, Percutaneous Endoscopic Approach
0Q5G0ZZ	Destruction of Right Tibia, Open Approach
0Q5G3ZZ	Destruction of Right Tibia, Percutaneous Approach
0Q5G4ZZ	Destruction of Right Tibia, Percutaneous Endoscopic Approach
0Q5H0ZZ	Destruction of Left Tibia, Open Approach
0Q5H3ZZ	Destruction of Left Tibia, Percutaneous Approach
0Q5H4ZZ	Destruction of Left Tibia, Percutaneous Endoscopic Approach

0Q5J0ZZ	Destruction of Right Fibula, Open Approach
0Q5J3ZZ	Destruction of Right Fibula, Percutaneous Approach
0Q5J4ZZ	Destruction of Right Fibula, Percutaneous Endoscopic Approach
0Q5K0ZZ	Destruction of Left Fibula, Open Approach
0Q5K3ZZ	Destruction of Left Fibula, Percutaneous Approach
0Q5K4ZZ	Destruction of Left Fibula, Percutaneous Endoscopic Approach
0Q5L0ZZ	Destruction of Right Tarsal, Open Approach
0Q5L3ZZ	Destruction of Right Tarsal, Percutaneous Approach
0Q5L4ZZ	Destruction of Right Tarsal, Percutaneous Endoscopic Approach
0Q5M0ZZ	Destruction of Left Tarsal, Open Approach
0Q5M3ZZ	Destruction of Left Tarsal, Percutaneous Approach
0Q5M4ZZ	Destruction of Left Tarsal, Percutaneous Endoscopic Approach
0Q5N0ZZ	Destruction of Right Metatarsal, Open Approach

0Q5N3ZZ	Destruction of Right Metatarsal, Percutaneous Approach
0Q5N4ZZ	Destruction of Right Metatarsal, Percutaneous Endoscopic Approach
0Q5P0ZZ	Destruction of Left Metatarsal, Open Approach
0Q5P3ZZ	Destruction of Left Metatarsal, Percutaneous Approach
0Q5P4ZZ	Destruction of Left Metatarsal, Percutaneous Endoscopic Approach
0Q5Q0ZZ	Destruction of Right Toe Phalanx, Open Approach
0Q5Q3ZZ	Destruction of Right Toe Phalanx, Percutaneous Approach
0Q5Q4ZZ	Destruction of Right Toe Phalanx, Percutaneous Endoscopic Approach
0Q5R0ZZ	Destruction of Left Toe Phalanx, Open Approach
0Q5R3ZZ	Destruction of Left Toe Phalanx, Percutaneous Approach
0Q5R4ZZ	Destruction of Left Toe Phalanx, Percutaneous Endoscopic Approach
0Q5S0ZZ	Destruction of Coccyx, Open Approach
0Q5S3ZZ	Destruction of Coccyx, Percutaneous Approach
0Q5S4ZZ	Destruction of Coccyx, Percutaneous Endoscopic Approach

0Q8 – Lower Bones, Division

Review Coding Guideline B3.14

0Q800ZZ	Division of Lumbar Vertebra, Open Approach
0Q803ZZ	Division of Lumbar Vertebra, Percutaneous Approach
0Q804ZZ	Division of Lumbar Vertebra, Percutaneous Endoscopic Approach
0Q810ZZ	Division of Sacrum, Open Approach
0Q813ZZ	Division of Sacrum, Percutaneous Approach
0Q814ZZ	Division of Sacrum, Percutaneous Endoscopic Approach
0Q820ZZ	Division of Right Pelvic Bone, Open Approach
0Q823ZZ	Division of Right Pelvic Bone, Percutaneous Approach
0Q824ZZ	Division of Right Pelvic Bone, Percutaneous Endoscopic Approach
0Q830ZZ	Division of Left Pelvic Bone, Open Approach
0Q833ZZ	Division of Left Pelvic Bone, Percutaneous Approach
0Q834ZZ	Division of Left Pelvic Bone, Percutaneous Endoscopic Approach
0Q840ZZ	Division of Right Acetabulum, Open Approach
0Q843ZZ	Division of Right Acetabulum, Percutaneous Approach
0Q844ZZ	Division of Right Acetabulum, Percutaneous Endoscopic Approach
0Q850ZZ	Division of Left Acetabulum, Open Approach
0Q853ZZ	Division of Left Acetabulum, Percutaneous Approach
0Q854ZZ	Division of Left Acetabulum, Percutaneous Endoscopic Approach
0Q860ZZ	Division of Right Upper Femur, Open Approach
0Q863ZZ	Division of Right Upper Femur, Percutaneous Approach
0Q864ZZ	Division of Right Upper Femur, Percutaneous Endoscopic Approach
0Q870ZZ	Division of Left Upper Femur, Open Approach

0Q873ZZ	Division of Left Upper Femur, Percutaneous Approach
0Q874ZZ	Division of Left Upper Femur, Percutaneous Endoscopic Approach
0Q880ZZ	Division of Right Femoral Shaft, Open Approach
0Q883ZZ	Division of Right Femoral Shaft, Percutaneous Approach
0Q884ZZ	Division of Right Femoral Shaft, Percutaneous Endoscopic Approach
0Q890ZZ	Division of Left Femoral Shaft, Open Approach
0Q893ZZ	Division of Left Femoral Shaft, Percutaneous Approach
0Q894ZZ	Division of Left Femoral Shaft, Percutaneous Endoscopic Approach
0Q8B0ZZ	Division of Right Lower Femur, Open Approach
0Q8B3ZZ	Division of Right Lower Femur, Percutaneous Approach
0Q8B4ZZ	Division of Right Lower Femur, Percutaneous Endoscopic Approach
0Q8C0ZZ	Division of Left Lower Femur, Open Approach
0Q8C3ZZ	Division of Left Lower Femur, Percutaneous Approach
0Q8C4ZZ	Division of Left Lower Femur, Percutaneous Endoscopic Approach
0Q8D0ZZ	Division of Right Patella, Open Approach
0Q8D3ZZ	Division of Right Patella, Percutaneous Approach
0Q8D4ZZ	Division of Right Patella, Percutaneous Endoscopic Approach
0Q8F0ZZ	Division of Left Patella, Open Approach
0Q8F3ZZ	Division of Left Patella, Percutaneous Approach
0Q8F4ZZ	Division of Left Patella, Percutaneous Endoscopic Approach
0Q8G0ZZ	Division of Right Tibia, Open Approach
0Q8G3ZZ	Division of Right Tibia, Percutaneous Approach

0Q8G4ZZ	Division of Right Tibia, Percutaneous Endoscopic Approach
0Q8H0ZZ	Division of Left Tibia, Open Approach
0Q8H3ZZ	Division of Left Tibia, Percutaneous Approach
0Q8H4ZZ	Division of Left Tibia, Percutaneous Endoscopic Approach
0Q8J0ZZ	Division of Right Fibula, Open Approach
0Q8J3ZZ	Division of Right Fibula, Percutaneous Approach
0Q8J4ZZ	Division of Right Fibula, Percutaneous Endoscopic Approach
0Q8K0ZZ	Division of Left Fibula, Open Approach
0Q8K3ZZ	Division of Left Fibula, Percutaneous Approach
0Q8K4ZZ	Division of Left Fibula, Percutaneous Endoscopic Approach
0Q8L0ZZ	Division of Right Tarsal, Open Approach
0Q8L3ZZ	Division of Right Tarsal, Percutaneous Approach
0Q8L4ZZ	Division of Right Tarsal, Percutaneous Endoscopic Approach
0Q8M0ZZ	Division of Left Tarsal, Open Approach
0Q8M3ZZ	Division of Left Tarsal, Percutaneous Approach
0Q8M4ZZ	Division of Left Tarsal, Percutaneous Endoscopic Approach
0Q8N0ZZ	Division of Right Metatarsal, Open Approach
0Q8N3ZZ	Division of Right Metatarsal, Percutaneous Approach
0Q8N4ZZ	Division of Right Metatarsal, Percutaneous Endoscopic Approach
0Q8P0ZZ	Division of Left Metatarsal, Open Approach
0Q8P3ZZ	Division of Left Metatarsal, Percutaneous Approach
0Q8P4ZZ	Division of Left Metatarsal, Percutaneous Endoscopic Approach
0Q8Q0ZZ	Division of Right Toe Phalanx, Open Approach
0Q8Q3ZZ	Division of Right Toe Phalanx, Percutaneous Approach

0Q8Q4ZZ Division of Right Toe Phalanx, Percutaneous Endoscopic Approach
0Q8R0ZZ Division of Left Toe Phalanx, Open Approach
0Q8R3ZZ Division of Left Toe Phalanx, Percutaneous Approach

0Q8R4ZZ Division of Left Toe Phalanx, Percutaneous Endoscopic Approach
0Q8S0ZZ Division of Coccyx, Open Approach
0Q8S3ZZ Division of Coccyx, Percutaneous Approach

0Q8S4ZZ Division of Coccyx, Percutaneous Endoscopic Approach

0Q9 – Lower Bones, Drainage

Review Coding Guidelines B3.4a and B3.4b

Review Coding Guideline B6.2

0Q9000Z Drainage of Lumbar Vertebra with Drainage Device, Open Approach
0Q900ZX Drainage of Lumbar Vertebra, Open Approach, Diagnostic
0Q900ZZ Drainage of Lumbar Vertebra, Open Approach
0Q9030Z Drainage of Lumbar Vertebra with Drainage Device, Percutaneous Approach
0Q903ZX Drainage of Lumbar Vertebra, Percutaneous Approach, Diagnostic
0Q903ZZ Drainage of Lumbar Vertebra, Percutaneous Approach
0Q9040Z Drainage of Lumbar Vertebra with Drainage Device, Percutaneous Endoscopic Approach
0Q904ZX Drainage of Lumbar Vertebra, Percutaneous Endoscopic Approach, Diagnostic
0Q904ZZ Drainage of Lumbar Vertebra, Percutaneous Endoscopic Approach
0Q9100Z Drainage of Sacrum with Drainage Device, Open Approach
0Q910ZX Drainage of Sacrum, Open Approach, Diagnostic
0Q910ZZ Drainage of Sacrum, Open Approach
0Q9130Z Drainage of Sacrum with Drainage Device, Percutaneous Approach
0Q913ZX Drainage of Sacrum, Percutaneous Approach, Diagnostic
0Q913ZZ Drainage of Sacrum, Percutaneous Approach
0Q9140Z Drainage of Sacrum with Drainage Device, Percutaneous Endoscopic Approach
0Q914ZX Drainage of Sacrum, Percutaneous Endoscopic Approach, Diagnostic
0Q914ZZ Drainage of Sacrum, Percutaneous Endoscopic Approach
0Q9200Z Drainage of Right Pelvic Bone with Drainage Device, Open Approach
0Q920ZX Drainage of Right Pelvic Bone, Open Approach, Diagnostic
0Q920ZZ Drainage of Right Pelvic Bone, Open Approach
0Q9230Z Drainage of Right Pelvic Bone with Drainage Device, Percutaneous Approach
0Q923ZX Drainage of Right Pelvic Bone, Percutaneous Approach, Diagnostic
0Q923ZZ Drainage of Right Pelvic Bone, Percutaneous Approach
0Q9240Z Drainage of Right Pelvic Bone with Drainage Device, Percutaneous Endoscopic Approach
0Q924ZX Drainage of Right Pelvic Bone, Percutaneous Endoscopic Approach, Diagnostic
0Q924ZZ Drainage of Right Pelvic Bone, Percutaneous Endoscopic Approach
0Q9300Z Drainage of Left Pelvic Bone with Drainage Device, Open Approach
0Q930ZX Drainage of Left Pelvic Bone, Open Approach, Diagnostic

0Q930ZZ Drainage of Left Pelvic Bone, Open Approach
0Q9330Z Drainage of Left Pelvic Bone with Drainage Device, Percutaneous Approach
0Q933ZX Drainage of Left Pelvic Bone, Percutaneous Approach, Diagnostic
0Q933ZZ Drainage of Left Pelvic Bone, Percutaneous Approach
0Q9340Z Drainage of Left Pelvic Bone with Drainage Device, Percutaneous Endoscopic Approach
0Q934ZX Drainage of Left Pelvic Bone, Percutaneous Endoscopic Approach, Diagnostic
0Q934ZZ Drainage of Left Pelvic Bone, Percutaneous Endoscopic Approach
0Q9400Z Drainage of Right Acetabulum with Drainage Device, Open Approach
0Q940ZX Drainage of Right Acetabulum, Open Approach, Diagnostic
0Q940ZZ Drainage of Right Acetabulum, Open Approach
0Q9430Z Drainage of Right Acetabulum with Drainage Device, Percutaneous Approach
0Q943ZX Drainage of Right Acetabulum, Percutaneous Approach, Diagnostic
0Q943ZZ Drainage of Right Acetabulum, Percutaneous Approach
0Q9440Z Drainage of Right Acetabulum with Drainage Device, Percutaneous Endoscopic Approach
0Q944ZX Drainage of Right Acetabulum, Percutaneous Endoscopic Approach, Diagnostic
0Q944ZZ Drainage of Right Acetabulum, Percutaneous Endoscopic Approach
0Q9500Z Drainage of Left Acetabulum with Drainage Device, Open Approach
0Q950ZX Drainage of Left Acetabulum, Open Approach, Diagnostic
0Q950ZZ Drainage of Left Acetabulum, Open Approach
0Q9530Z Drainage of Left Acetabulum with Drainage Device, Percutaneous Approach
0Q953ZX Drainage of Left Acetabulum, Percutaneous Approach, Diagnostic
0Q953ZZ Drainage of Left Acetabulum, Percutaneous Approach
0Q9540Z Drainage of Left Acetabulum with Drainage Device, Percutaneous Endoscopic Approach
0Q954ZX Drainage of Left Acetabulum, Percutaneous Endoscopic Approach, Diagnostic
0Q954ZZ Drainage of Left Acetabulum, Percutaneous Endoscopic Approach
0Q9600Z Drainage of Right Upper Femur with Drainage Device, Open Approach
0Q960ZX Drainage of Right Upper Femur, Open Approach, Diagnostic
0Q960ZZ Drainage of Right Upper Femur, Open Approach

0Q9630Z Drainage of Right Upper Femur with Drainage Device, Percutaneous Approach
0Q963ZX Drainage of Right Upper Femur, Percutaneous Approach, Diagnostic
0Q963ZZ Drainage of Right Upper Femur, Percutaneous Approach
0Q9640Z Drainage of Right Upper Femur with Drainage Device, Percutaneous Endoscopic Approach
0Q964ZX Drainage of Right Upper Femur, Percutaneous Endoscopic Approach, Diagnostic
0Q964ZZ Drainage of Right Upper Femur, Percutaneous Endoscopic Approach
0Q9700Z Drainage of Left Upper Femur with Drainage Device, Open Approach
0Q970ZX Drainage of Left Upper Femur, Open Approach, Diagnostic
0Q970ZZ Drainage of Left Upper Femur, Open Approach
0Q9730Z Drainage of Left Upper Femur with Drainage Device, Percutaneous Approach
0Q973ZX Drainage of Left Upper Femur, Percutaneous Approach, Diagnostic
0Q973ZZ Drainage of Left Upper Femur, Percutaneous Approach
0Q9740Z Drainage of Left Upper Femur with Drainage Device, Percutaneous Endoscopic Approach
0Q974ZX Drainage of Left Upper Femur, Percutaneous Endoscopic Approach, Diagnostic
0Q974ZZ Drainage of Left Upper Femur, Percutaneous Endoscopic Approach
0Q9800Z Drainage of Right Femoral Shaft with Drainage Device, Open Approach
0Q980ZX Drainage of Right Femoral Shaft, Open Approach, Diagnostic
0Q980ZZ Drainage of Right Femoral Shaft, Open Approach
0Q9830Z Drainage of Right Femoral Shaft with Drainage Device, Percutaneous Approach
0Q983ZX Drainage of Right Femoral Shaft, Percutaneous Approach, Diagnostic
0Q983ZZ Drainage of Right Femoral Shaft, Percutaneous Approach
0Q9840Z Drainage of Right Femoral Shaft with Drainage Device, Percutaneous Endoscopic Approach
0Q984ZX Drainage of Right Femoral Shaft, Percutaneous Endoscopic Approach, Diagnostic
0Q984ZZ Drainage of Right Femoral Shaft, Percutaneous Endoscopic Approach
0Q9900Z Drainage of Left Femoral Shaft with Drainage Device, Open Approach
0Q990ZX Drainage of Left Femoral Shaft, Open Approach, Diagnostic
0Q990ZZ Drainage of Left Femoral Shaft, Open Approach
0Q9930Z Drainage of Left Femoral Shaft with Drainage Device, Percutaneous Approach

0Q993ZX Drainage of Left Femoral Shaft, Percutaneous Approach, Diagnostic

0Q993ZZ Drainage of Left Femoral Shaft, Percutaneous Approach

0Q9940Z Drainage of Left Femoral Shaft with Drainage Device, Percutaneous Endoscopic Approach

0Q994ZX Drainage of Left Femoral Shaft, Percutaneous Endoscopic Approach, Diagnostic

0Q994ZZ Drainage of Left Femoral Shaft, Percutaneous Endoscopic Approach

0Q9B00Z Drainage of Right Lower Femur with Drainage Device, Open Approach

0Q9B0ZX Drainage of Right Lower Femur, Open Approach, Diagnostic

0Q9B0ZZ Drainage of Right Lower Femur, Open Approach

0Q9B30Z Drainage of Right Lower Femur with Drainage Device, Percutaneous Approach

0Q9B3ZX Drainage of Right Lower Femur, Percutaneous Approach, Diagnostic

0Q9B3ZZ Drainage of Right Lower Femur, Percutaneous Approach

0Q9B40Z Drainage of Right Lower Femur with Drainage Device, Percutaneous Endoscopic Approach

0Q9B4ZX Drainage of Right Lower Femur, Percutaneous Endoscopic Approach, Diagnostic

0Q9B4ZZ Drainage of Right Lower Femur, Percutaneous Endoscopic Approach

0Q9C00Z Drainage of Left Lower Femur with Drainage Device, Open Approach

0Q9C0ZX Drainage of Left Lower Femur, Open Approach, Diagnostic

0Q9C0ZZ Drainage of Left Lower Femur, Open Approach

0Q9C30Z Drainage of Left Lower Femur with Drainage Device, Percutaneous Approach

0Q9C3ZX Drainage of Left Lower Femur, Percutaneous Approach, Diagnostic

0Q9C3ZZ Drainage of Left Lower Femur, Percutaneous Approach

0Q9C40Z Drainage of Left Lower Femur with Drainage Device, Percutaneous Endoscopic Approach

0Q9C4ZX Drainage of Left Lower Femur, Percutaneous Endoscopic Approach, Diagnostic

0Q9C4ZZ Drainage of Left Lower Femur, Percutaneous Endoscopic Approach

0Q9D00Z Drainage of Right Patella with Drainage Device, Open Approach

0Q9D0ZX Drainage of Right Patella, Open Approach, Diagnostic

0Q9D0ZZ Drainage of Right Patella, Open Approach

0Q9D30Z Drainage of Right Patella with Drainage Device, Percutaneous Approach

0Q9D3ZX Drainage of Right Patella, Percutaneous Approach, Diagnostic

0Q9D3ZZ Drainage of Right Patella, Percutaneous Approach

0Q9D40Z Drainage of Right Patella with Drainage Device, Percutaneous Endoscopic Approach

0Q9D4ZX Drainage of Right Patella, Percutaneous Endoscopic Approach, Diagnostic

0Q9D4ZZ Drainage of Right Patella, Percutaneous Endoscopic Approach

0Q9F00Z Drainage of Left Patella with Drainage Device, Open Approach

0Q9F0ZX Drainage of Left Patella, Open Approach, Diagnostic

0Q9F0ZZ Drainage of Left Patella, Open Approach

0Q9F30Z Drainage of Left Patella with Drainage Device, Percutaneous Approach

0Q9F3ZX Drainage of Left Patella, Percutaneous Approach, Diagnostic

0Q9F3ZZ Drainage of Left Patella, Percutaneous Approach

0Q9F40Z Drainage of Left Patella with Drainage Device, Percutaneous Endoscopic Approach

0Q9F4ZX Drainage of Left Patella, Percutaneous Endoscopic Approach, Diagnostic

0Q9F4ZZ Drainage of Left Patella, Percutaneous Endoscopic Approach

0Q9G00Z Drainage of Right Tibia with Drainage Device, Open Approach

0Q9G0ZX Drainage of Right Tibia, Open Approach, Diagnostic

0Q9G0ZZ Drainage of Right Tibia, Open Approach

0Q9G30Z Drainage of Right Tibia with Drainage Device, Percutaneous Approach

0Q9G3ZX Drainage of Right Tibia, Percutaneous Approach, Diagnostic

0Q9G3ZZ Drainage of Right Tibia, Percutaneous Approach

0Q9G40Z Drainage of Right Tibia with Drainage Device, Percutaneous Endoscopic Approach

0Q9G4ZX Drainage of Right Tibia, Percutaneous Endoscopic Approach, Diagnostic

0Q9G4ZZ Drainage of Right Tibia, Percutaneous Endoscopic Approach

0Q9H00Z Drainage of Left Tibia with Drainage Device, Open Approach

0Q9H0ZX Drainage of Left Tibia, Open Approach, Diagnostic

0Q9H0ZZ Drainage of Left Tibia, Open Approach

0Q9H30Z Drainage of Left Tibia with Drainage Device, Percutaneous Approach

0Q9H3ZX Drainage of Left Tibia, Percutaneous Approach, Diagnostic

0Q9H3ZZ Drainage of Left Tibia, Percutaneous Approach

0Q9H40Z Drainage of Left Tibia with Drainage Device, Percutaneous Endoscopic Approach

0Q9H4ZX Drainage of Left Tibia, Percutaneous Endoscopic Approach, Diagnostic

0Q9H4ZZ Drainage of Left Tibia, Percutaneous Endoscopic Approach

0Q9J00Z Drainage of Right Fibula with Drainage Device, Open Approach

0Q9J0ZX Drainage of Right Fibula, Open Approach, Diagnostic

0Q9J0ZZ Drainage of Right Fibula, Open Approach

0Q9J30Z Drainage of Right Fibula with Drainage Device, Percutaneous Approach

0Q9J3ZX Drainage of Right Fibula, Percutaneous Approach, Diagnostic

0Q9J3ZZ Drainage of Right Fibula, Percutaneous Approach

0Q9J40Z Drainage of Right Fibula with Drainage Device, Percutaneous Endoscopic Approach

0Q9J4ZX Drainage of Right Fibula, Percutaneous Endoscopic Approach, Diagnostic

0Q9J4ZZ Drainage of Right Fibula, Percutaneous Endoscopic Approach

0Q9K00Z Drainage of Left Fibula with Drainage Device, Open Approach

0Q9K0ZX Drainage of Left Fibula, Open Approach, Diagnostic

0Q9K0ZZ Drainage of Left Fibula, Open Approach

0Q9K30Z Drainage of Left Fibula with Drainage Device, Percutaneous Approach

0Q9K3ZX Drainage of Left Fibula, Percutaneous Approach, Diagnostic

0Q9K3ZZ Drainage of Left Fibula, Percutaneous Approach

0Q9K40Z Drainage of Left Fibula with Drainage Device, Percutaneous Endoscopic Approach

0Q9K4ZX Drainage of Left Fibula, Percutaneous Endoscopic Approach, Diagnostic

0Q9K4ZZ Drainage of Left Fibula, Percutaneous Endoscopic Approach

0Q9L00Z Drainage of Right Tarsal with Drainage Device, Open Approach

0Q9L0ZX Drainage of Right Tarsal, Open Approach, Diagnostic

0Q9L0ZZ Drainage of Right Tarsal, Open Approach

0Q9L30Z Drainage of Right Tarsal with Drainage Device, Percutaneous Approach

0Q9L3ZX Drainage of Right Tarsal, Percutaneous Approach, Diagnostic

0Q9L3ZZ Drainage of Right Tarsal, Percutaneous Approach

0Q9L40Z Drainage of Right Tarsal with Drainage Device, Percutaneous Endoscopic Approach

0Q9L4ZX Drainage of Right Tarsal, Percutaneous Endoscopic Approach, Diagnostic

0Q9L4ZZ Drainage of Right Tarsal, Percutaneous Endoscopic Approach

0Q9M00Z Drainage of Left Tarsal with Drainage Device, Open Approach

0Q9M0ZX Drainage of Left Tarsal, Open Approach, Diagnostic

0Q9M0ZZ Drainage of Left Tarsal, Open Approach

0Q9M30Z Drainage of Left Tarsal with Drainage Device, Percutaneous Approach

0Q9M3ZX Drainage of Left Tarsal, Percutaneous Approach, Diagnostic

0Q9M3ZZ Drainage of Left Tarsal, Percutaneous Approach

0Q9M40Z Drainage of Left Tarsal with Drainage Device, Percutaneous Endoscopic Approach

0Q9M4ZX Drainage of Left Tarsal, Percutaneous Endoscopic Approach, Diagnostic

0Q9M4ZZ Drainage of Left Tarsal, Percutaneous Endoscopic Approach

0Q9N00Z Drainage of Right Metatarsal with Drainage Device, Open Approach

0Q9N0ZX Drainage of Right Metatarsal, Open Approach, Diagnostic

0Q9N0ZZ Drainage of Right Metatarsal, Open Approach

0Q9N30Z Drainage of Right Metatarsal with Drainage Device, Percutaneous Approach

0Q9N3ZX Drainage of Right Metatarsal, Percutaneous Approach, Diagnostic

0Q9N3ZZ Drainage of Right Metatarsal, Percutaneous Approach

0Q9N40Z Drainage of Right Metatarsal with Drainage Device, Percutaneous Endoscopic Approach

0Q9N4ZX Drainage of Right Metatarsal, Percutaneous Endoscopic Approach, Diagnostic

0Q9N4ZZ Drainage of Right Metatarsal, Percutaneous Endoscopic Approach

0Q9P00Z Drainage of Left Metatarsal with Drainage Device, Open Approach

0Q9P0ZX Drainage of Left Metatarsal, Open Approach, Diagnostic

0Q9P0ZZ Drainage of Left Metatarsal, Open Approach

♀ Female-only   ♂ Male-only   ▲ Limited Coverage   ● Non-OR   🅷🅰🅲 HAC-associated procedure   ▲ Non-covered procedures   ✚ Cluster

0Q9P30Z Drainage of Left Metatarsal with Drainage Device, Percutaneous Approach

0Q9P3ZX Drainage of Left Metatarsal, Percutaneous Approach, Diagnostic

0Q9P3ZZ Drainage of Left Metatarsal, Percutaneous Approach

0Q9P40Z Drainage of Left Metatarsal with Drainage Device, Percutaneous Endoscopic Approach

0Q9P4ZX Drainage of Left Metatarsal, Percutaneous Endoscopic Approach, Diagnostic

0Q9P4ZZ Drainage of Left Metatarsal, Percutaneous Endoscopic Approach

0Q9Q00Z Drainage of Right Toe Phalanx with Drainage Device, Open Approach

0Q9Q0ZX Drainage of Right Toe Phalanx, Open Approach, Diagnostic

0Q9Q0ZZ Drainage of Right Toe Phalanx, Open Approach

0Q9Q30Z Drainage of Right Toe Phalanx with Drainage Device, Percutaneous Approach

0Q9Q3ZX Drainage of Right Toe Phalanx, Percutaneous Approach, Diagnostic

0Q9Q3ZZ Drainage of Right Toe Phalanx, Percutaneous Approach

0Q9Q40Z Drainage of Right Toe Phalanx with Drainage Device, Percutaneous Endoscopic Approach

0Q9Q4ZX Drainage of Right Toe Phalanx, Percutaneous Endoscopic Approach, Diagnostic

0Q9Q4ZZ Drainage of Right Toe Phalanx, Percutaneous Endoscopic Approach

0Q9R00Z Drainage of Left Toe Phalanx with Drainage Device, Open Approach

0Q9R0ZX Drainage of Left Toe Phalanx, Open Approach, Diagnostic

0Q9R0ZZ Drainage of Left Toe Phalanx, Open Approach

0Q9R30Z Drainage of Left Toe Phalanx with Drainage Device, Percutaneous Approach

0Q9R3ZX Drainage of Left Toe Phalanx, Percutaneous Approach, Diagnostic

0Q9R3ZZ Drainage of Left Toe Phalanx, Percutaneous Approach

0Q9R40Z Drainage of Left Toe Phalanx with Drainage Device, Percutaneous Endoscopic Approach

0Q9R4ZX Drainage of Left Toe Phalanx, Percutaneous Endoscopic Approach, Diagnostic

0Q9R4ZZ Drainage of Left Toe Phalanx, Percutaneous Endoscopic Approach

0Q9S00Z Drainage of Coccyx with Drainage Device, Open Approach

0Q9S0ZX Drainage of Coccyx, Open Approach, Diagnostic

0Q9S0ZZ Drainage of Coccyx, Open Approach

0Q9S30Z Drainage of Coccyx with Drainage Device, Percutaneous Approach

0Q9S3ZX Drainage of Coccyx, Percutaneous Approach, Diagnostic

0Q9S3ZZ Drainage of Coccyx, Percutaneous Approach

0Q9S40Z Drainage of Coccyx with Drainage Device, Percutaneous Endoscopic Approach

0Q9S4ZX Drainage of Coccyx, Percutaneous Endoscopic Approach, Diagnostic

0Q9S4ZZ Drainage of Coccyx, Percutaneous Endoscopic Approach

0QB – Lower Bones, Excision

Review Coding Guidelines B3.4a and B3.4b

Review Coding Guideline B3.5

Review Coding Guideline B3.8

Review Coding Guideline B3.18

0QB00ZX Excision of Lumbar Vertebra, Open Approach, Diagnostic

0QB00ZZ Excision of Lumbar Vertebra, Open Approach

0QB03ZX Excision of Lumbar Vertebra, Percutaneous Approach, Diagnostic

0QB03ZZ Excision of Lumbar Vertebra, Percutaneous Approach

0QB04ZX Excision of Lumbar Vertebra, Percutaneous Endoscopic Approach, Diagnostic

0QB04ZZ Excision of Lumbar Vertebra, Percutaneous Endoscopic Approach

0QB10ZX Excision of Sacrum, Open Approach, Diagnostic

0QB10ZZ Excision of Sacrum, Open Approach
AHA CC: 2Q, 2020, 26

0QB13ZX Excision of Sacrum, Percutaneous Approach, Diagnostic

0QB13ZZ Excision of Sacrum, Percutaneous Approach

0QB14ZX Excision of Sacrum, Percutaneous Endoscopic Approach, Diagnostic

0QB14ZZ Excision of Sacrum, Percutaneous Endoscopic Approach

0QB20ZX Excision of Right Pelvic Bone, Open Approach, Diagnostic

0QB20ZZ Excision of Right Pelvic Bone, Open Approach
AHA CC: 2Q, 2014, 6-7; 4Q, 2018, 12-13

0QB23ZX Excision of Right Pelvic Bone, Percutaneous Approach, Diagnostic

0QB23ZZ Excision of Right Pelvic Bone, Percutaneous Approach

0QB24ZX Excision of Right Pelvic Bone, Percutaneous Endoscopic Approach, Diagnostic

0QB24ZZ Excision of Right Pelvic Bone, Percutaneous Endoscopic Approach

0QB30ZX Excision of Left Pelvic Bone, Open Approach, Diagnostic

0QB30ZZ Excision of Left Pelvic Bone, Open Approach
AHA CC: 2Q, 2019, 19-20

0QB33ZX Excision of Left Pelvic Bone, Percutaneous Approach, Diagnostic

0QB33ZZ Excision of Left Pelvic Bone, Percutaneous Approach

0QB34ZX Excision of Left Pelvic Bone, Percutaneous Endoscopic Approach, Diagnostic

0QB34ZZ Excision of Left Pelvic Bone, Percutaneous Endoscopic Approach

0QB40ZX Excision of Right Acetabulum, Open Approach, Diagnostic

0QB40ZZ Excision of Right Acetabulum, Open Approach

0QB43ZX Excision of Right Acetabulum, Percutaneous Approach, Diagnostic

0QB43ZZ Excision of Right Acetabulum, Percutaneous Approach

0QB44ZX Excision of Right Acetabulum, Percutaneous Endoscopic Approach, Diagnostic

0QB44ZZ Excision of Right Acetabulum, Percutaneous Endoscopic Approach

0QB50ZX Excision of Left Acetabulum, Open Approach, Diagnostic

0QB50ZZ Excision of Left Acetabulum, Open Approach

0QB53ZX Excision of Left Acetabulum, Percutaneous Approach, Diagnostic

0QB53ZZ Excision of Left Acetabulum, Percutaneous Approach

0QB54ZX Excision of Left Acetabulum, Percutaneous Endoscopic Approach, Diagnostic

0QB54ZZ Excision of Left Acetabulum, Percutaneous Endoscopic Approach

0QB60ZX Excision of Right Upper Femur, Open Approach, Diagnostic

0QB60ZZ Excision of Right Upper Femur, Open Approach

0QB63ZX Excision of Right Upper Femur, Percutaneous Approach, Diagnostic

0QB63ZZ Excision of Right Upper Femur, Percutaneous Approach

0QB64ZX Excision of Right Upper Femur, Percutaneous Endoscopic Approach, Diagnostic

0QB64ZZ Excision of Right Upper Femur, Percutaneous Endoscopic Approach

0QB70ZX Excision of Left Upper Femur, Open Approach, Diagnostic

0QB70ZZ Excision of Left Upper Femur, Open Approach

0QB73ZX Excision of Left Upper Femur, Percutaneous Approach, Diagnostic

0QB73ZZ Excision of Left Upper Femur, Percutaneous Approach

0QB74ZX Excision of Left Upper Femur, Percutaneous Endoscopic Approach, Diagnostic

0QB74ZZ Excision of Left Upper Femur, Percutaneous Endoscopic Approach
AHA CC: 4Q, 2014, 25-26

0QB80ZX Excision of Right Femoral Shaft, Open Approach, Diagnostic

0QB80ZZ Excision of Right Femoral Shaft, Open Approach

0QB83ZX Excision of Right Femoral Shaft, Percutaneous Approach, Diagnostic

0QB83ZZ Excision of Right Femoral Shaft, Percutaneous Approach

0QB84ZX Excision of Right Femoral Shaft, Percutaneous Endoscopic Approach, Diagnostic

0QB84ZZ Excision of Right Femoral Shaft, Percutaneous Endoscopic Approach

0QB90ZX Excision of Left Femoral Shaft, Open Approach, Diagnostic

♀ Female-only   ♂ Male-only   ▲ Limited Coverage   ● Non-OR   HAC HAC-associated procedure   ▲ Non-covered procedures   ✚ Cluster

0QB90ZZ	Excision of Left Femoral Shaft, Open Approach
0QB93ZX	Excision of Left Femoral Shaft, Percutaneous Approach, Diagnostic
0QB93ZZ	Excision of Left Femoral Shaft, Percutaneous Approach
0QB94ZX	Excision of Left Femoral Shaft, Percutaneous Endoscopic Approach, Diagnostic
0QB94ZZ	Excision of Left Femoral Shaft, Percutaneous Endoscopic Approach
0QBB0ZX	Excision of Right Lower Femur, Open Approach, Diagnostic
0QBB0ZZ	Excision of Right Lower Femur, Open Approach
0QBB3ZX	Excision of Right Lower Femur, Percutaneous Approach, Diagnostic
0QBB3ZZ	Excision of Right Lower Femur, Percutaneous Approach
0QBB4ZX	Excision of Right Lower Femur, Percutaneous Endoscopic Approach, Diagnostic
0QBB4ZZ	Excision of Right Lower Femur, Percutaneous Endoscopic Approach
0QBC0ZX	Excision of Left Lower Femur, Open Approach, Diagnostic
0QBC0ZZ	Excision of Left Lower Femur, Open Approach
0QBC3ZX	Excision of Left Lower Femur, Percutaneous Approach, Diagnostic
0QBC3ZZ	Excision of Left Lower Femur, Percutaneous Approach
0QBC4ZX	Excision of Left Lower Femur, Percutaneous Endoscopic Approach, Diagnostic
0QBC4ZZ	Excision of Left Lower Femur, Percutaneous Endoscopic Approach
0QBD0ZX	Excision of Right Patella, Open Approach, Diagnostic
0QBD0ZZ	Excision of Right Patella, Open Approach
0QBD3ZX	Excision of Right Patella, Percutaneous Approach, Diagnostic
0QBD3ZZ	Excision of Right Patella, Percutaneous Approach
0QBD4ZX	Excision of Right Patella, Percutaneous Endoscopic Approach, Diagnostic
0QBD4ZZ	Excision of Right Patella, Percutaneous Endoscopic Approach
0QBF0ZX	Excision of Left Patella, Open Approach, Diagnostic
0QBF0ZZ	Excision of Left Patella, Open Approach
0QBF3ZX	Excision of Left Patella, Percutaneous Approach, Diagnostic
0QBF3ZZ	Excision of Left Patella, Percutaneous Approach
0QBF4ZX	Excision of Left Patella, Percutaneous Endoscopic Approach, Diagnostic
0QBF4ZZ	Excision of Left Patella, Percutaneous Endoscopic Approach
0QBG0ZX	Excision of Right Tibia, Open Approach, Diagnostic
0QBG0ZZ	Excision of Right Tibia, Open Approach
0QBG3ZX	Excision of Right Tibia, Percutaneous Approach, Diagnostic
0QBG3ZZ	Excision of Right Tibia, Percutaneous Approach
0QBG4ZX	Excision of Right Tibia, Percutaneous Endoscopic Approach, Diagnostic
0QBG4ZZ	Excision of Right Tibia, Percutaneous Endoscopic Approach

0QBH0ZX	Excision of Left Tibia, Open Approach, Diagnostic
0QBH0ZZ	Excision of Left Tibia, Open Approach
0QBH3ZX	Excision of Left Tibia, Percutaneous Approach, Diagnostic
0QBH3ZZ	Excision of Left Tibia, Percutaneous Approach
0QBH4ZX	Excision of Left Tibia, Percutaneous Endoscopic Approach, Diagnostic
0QBH4ZZ	Excision of Left Tibia, Percutaneous Endoscopic Approach
0QBJ0ZX	Excision of Right Fibula, Open Approach, Diagnostic
0QBJ0ZZ	Excision of Right Fibula, Open Approach
	AHA CC: 1Q, 2017, 23-24
0QBJ3ZX	Excision of Right Fibula, Percutaneous Approach, Diagnostic
0QBJ3ZZ	Excision of Right Fibula, Percutaneous Approach
0QBJ4ZX	Excision of Right Fibula, Percutaneous Endoscopic Approach, Diagnostic
0QBJ4ZZ	Excision of Right Fibula, Percutaneous Endoscopic Approach
0QBK0ZX	Excision of Left Fibula, Open Approach, Diagnostic
0QBK0ZZ	Excision of Left Fibula, Open Approach
	AHA CC: 2Q, 2013, 39-40
0QBK3ZX	Excision of Left Fibula, Percutaneous Approach, Diagnostic
0QBK3ZZ	Excision of Left Fibula, Percutaneous Approach
0QBK4ZX	Excision of Left Fibula, Percutaneous Endoscopic Approach, Diagnostic
0QBK4ZZ	Excision of Left Fibula, Percutaneous Endoscopic Approach
0QBL0ZX	Excision of Right Tarsal, Open Approach, Diagnostic
0QBL0ZZ	Excision of Right Tarsal, Open Approach
	AHA CC: 3Q, 2018, 17-18
0QBL3ZX	Excision of Right Tarsal, Percutaneous Approach, Diagnostic
0QBL3ZZ	Excision of Right Tarsal, Percutaneous Approach
0QBL4ZX	Excision of Right Tarsal, Percutaneous Endoscopic Approach, Diagnostic
0QBL4ZZ	Excision of Right Tarsal, Percutaneous Endoscopic Approach
0QBM0ZX	Excision of Left Tarsal, Open Approach, Diagnostic
0QBM0ZZ	Excision of Left Tarsal, Open Approach
0QBM3ZX	Excision of Left Tarsal, Percutaneous Approach, Diagnostic
0QBM3ZZ	Excision of Left Tarsal, Percutaneous Approach
0QBM4ZX	Excision of Left Tarsal, Percutaneous Endoscopic Approach, Diagnostic
0QBM4ZZ	Excision of Left Tarsal, Percutaneous Endoscopic Approach
0QBN0Z2	Excision of Right Metatarsal, Sesamoid Bone(s) 1st Toe, Open Approach
0QBN0ZX	Excision of Right Metatarsal, Open Approach, Diagnostic
0QBN0ZZ	Excision of Right Metatarsal, Open Approach
	AHA CC: 2Q, 2021, 18-19
0QBN3Z2	Excision of Right Metatarsal, Sesamoid Bone(s) 1st Toe, Percutaneous Approach

0QBN3ZX	Excision of Right Metatarsal, Percutaneous Approach, Diagnostic
0QBN3ZZ	Excision of Right Metatarsal, Percutaneous Approach
0QBN4Z2	Excision of Right Metatarsal, Sesamoid Bone(s) 1st Toe, Percutaneous Endoscopic Approach
0QBN4ZX	Excision of Right Metatarsal, Percutaneous Endoscopic Approach, Diagnostic
0QBN4ZZ	Excision of Right Metatarsal, Percutaneous Endoscopic Approach
0QBP0Z2	Excision of Left Metatarsal, Sesamoid Bone(s) 1st Toe, Open Approach
0QBP0ZX	Excision of Left Metatarsal, Open Approach, Diagnostic
0QBP0ZZ	Excision of Left Metatarsal, Open Approach
0QBP3Z2	Excision of Left Metatarsal, Sesamoid Bone(s) 1st Toe, Percutaneous Approach
0QBP3ZX	Excision of Left Metatarsal, Percutaneous Approach, Diagnostic
0QBP3ZZ	Excision of Left Metatarsal, Percutaneous Approach
0QBP4Z2	Excision of Left Metatarsal, Sesamoid Bone(s) 1st Toe, Percutaneous Endoscopic Approach
0QBP4ZX	Excision of Left Metatarsal, Percutaneous Endoscopic Approach, Diagnostic
0QBP4ZZ	Excision of Left Metatarsal, Percutaneous Endoscopic Approach
0QBQ0ZX	Excision of Right Toe Phalanx, Open Approach, Diagnostic
0QBQ0ZZ	Excision of Right Toe Phalanx, Open Approach
0QBQ3ZX	Excision of Right Toe Phalanx, Percutaneous Approach, Diagnostic
0QBQ3ZZ	Excision of Right Toe Phalanx, Percutaneous Approach
0QBQ4ZX	Excision of Right Toe Phalanx, Percutaneous Endoscopic Approach, Diagnostic
0QBQ4ZZ	Excision of Right Toe Phalanx, Percutaneous Endoscopic Approach
0QBR0ZX	Excision of Left Toe Phalanx, Open Approach, Diagnostic
0QBR0ZZ	Excision of Left Toe Phalanx, Open Approach
0QBR3ZX	Excision of Left Toe Phalanx, Percutaneous Approach, Diagnostic
0QBR3ZZ	Excision of Left Toe Phalanx, Percutaneous Approach
0QBR4ZX	Excision of Left Toe Phalanx, Percutaneous Endoscopic Approach, Diagnostic
0QBR4ZZ	Excision of Left Toe Phalanx, Percutaneous Endoscopic Approach
0QBS0ZX	Excision of Coccyx, Open Approach, Diagnostic
0QBS0ZZ	Excision of Coccyx, Open Approach
	AHA CC: 3Q, 2015, 3-4
0QBS3ZX	Excision of Coccyx, Percutaneous Approach, Diagnostic
0QBS3ZZ	Excision of Coccyx, Percutaneous Approach
0QBS4ZX	Excision of Coccyx, Percutaneous Endoscopic Approach, Diagnostic
0QBS4ZZ	Excision of Coccyx, Percutaneous Endoscopic Approach

♀ Female-only   ♂ Male-only   ▲ Limited Coverage   ● Non-OR   ▨ HAC-associated procedure   ▲ Non-covered procedures   ✚ Cluster

0QC – Lower Bones, Extirpation

0QC00ZZ Extirpation of Matter from Lumbar Vertebra, Open Approach

0QC03ZZ Extirpation of Matter from Lumbar Vertebra, Percutaneous Approach

0QC04ZZ Extirpation of Matter from Lumbar Vertebra, Percutaneous Endoscopic Approach

0QC10ZZ Extirpation of Matter from Sacrum, Open Approach

0QC13ZZ Extirpation of Matter from Sacrum, Percutaneous Approach

0QC14ZZ Extirpation of Matter from Sacrum, Percutaneous Endoscopic Approach

0QC20ZZ Extirpation of Matter from Right Pelvic Bone, Open Approach

0QC23ZZ Extirpation of Matter from Right Pelvic Bone, Percutaneous Approach

0QC24ZZ Extirpation of Matter from Right Pelvic Bone, Percutaneous Endoscopic Approach

0QC30ZZ Extirpation of Matter from Left Pelvic Bone, Open Approach

0QC33ZZ Extirpation of Matter from Left Pelvic Bone, Percutaneous Approach

0QC34ZZ Extirpation of Matter from Left Pelvic Bone, Percutaneous Endoscopic Approach

0QC40ZZ Extirpation of Matter from Right Acetabulum, Open Approach

0QC43ZZ Extirpation of Matter from Right Acetabulum, Percutaneous Approach

0QC44ZZ Extirpation of Matter from Right Acetabulum, Percutaneous Endoscopic Approach

0QC50ZZ Extirpation of Matter from Left Acetabulum, Open Approach

0QC53ZZ Extirpation of Matter from Left Acetabulum, Percutaneous Approach

0QC54ZZ Extirpation of Matter from Left Acetabulum, Percutaneous Endoscopic Approach

0QC60ZZ Extirpation of Matter from Right Upper Femur, Open Approach

0QC63ZZ Extirpation of Matter from Right Upper Femur, Percutaneous Approach

0QC64ZZ Extirpation of Matter from Right Upper Femur, Percutaneous Endoscopic Approach

0QC70ZZ Extirpation of Matter from Left Upper Femur, Open Approach

0QC73ZZ Extirpation of Matter from Left Upper Femur, Percutaneous Approach

0QC74ZZ Extirpation of Matter from Left Upper Femur, Percutaneous Endoscopic Approach

0QC80ZZ Extirpation of Matter from Right Femoral Shaft, Open Approach

0QC83ZZ Extirpation of Matter from Right Femoral Shaft, Percutaneous Approach

0QC84ZZ Extirpation of Matter from Right Femoral Shaft, Percutaneous Endoscopic Approach

0QC90ZZ Extirpation of Matter from Left Femoral Shaft, Open Approach

0QC93ZZ Extirpation of Matter from Left Femoral Shaft, Percutaneous Approach

0QC94ZZ Extirpation of Matter from Left Femoral Shaft, Percutaneous Endoscopic Approach

0QCB0ZZ Extirpation of Matter from Right Lower Femur, Open Approach

0QCB3ZZ Extirpation of Matter from Right Lower Femur, Percutaneous Approach

0QCB4ZZ Extirpation of Matter from Right Lower Femur, Percutaneous Endoscopic Approach

0QCC0ZZ Extirpation of Matter from Left Lower Femur, Open Approach

0QCC3ZZ Extirpation of Matter from Left Lower Femur, Percutaneous Approach

0QCC4ZZ Extirpation of Matter from Left Lower Femur, Percutaneous Endoscopic Approach

0QCD0ZZ Extirpation of Matter from Right Patella, Open Approach

0QCD3ZZ Extirpation of Matter from Right Patella, Percutaneous Approach

0QCD4ZZ Extirpation of Matter from Right Patella, Percutaneous Endoscopic Approach

0QCF0ZZ Extirpation of Matter from Left Patella, Open Approach

0QCF3ZZ Extirpation of Matter from Left Patella, Percutaneous Approach

0QCF4ZZ Extirpation of Matter from Left Patella, Percutaneous Endoscopic Approach

0QCG0ZZ Extirpation of Matter from Right Tibia, Open Approach

0QCG3ZZ Extirpation of Matter from Right Tibia, Percutaneous Approach

0QCG4ZZ Extirpation of Matter from Right Tibia, Percutaneous Endoscopic Approach

0QCH0ZZ Extirpation of Matter from Left Tibia, Open Approach

0QCH3ZZ Extirpation of Matter from Left Tibia, Percutaneous Approach

0QCH4ZZ Extirpation of Matter from Left Tibia, Percutaneous Endoscopic Approach

0QCJ0ZZ Extirpation of Matter from Right Fibula, Open Approach

0QCJ3ZZ Extirpation of Matter from Right Fibula, Percutaneous Approach

0QCJ4ZZ Extirpation of Matter from Right Fibula, Percutaneous Endoscopic Approach

0QCK0ZZ Extirpation of Matter from Left Fibula, Open Approach

0QCK3ZZ Extirpation of Matter from Left Fibula, Percutaneous Approach

0QCK4ZZ Extirpation of Matter from Left Fibula, Percutaneous Endoscopic Approach

0QCL0ZZ Extirpation of Matter from Right Tarsal, Open Approach

0QCL3ZZ Extirpation of Matter from Right Tarsal, Percutaneous Approach

0QCL4ZZ Extirpation of Matter from Right Tarsal, Percutaneous Endoscopic Approach

0QCM0ZZ Extirpation of Matter from Left Tarsal, Open Approach

0QCM3ZZ Extirpation of Matter from Left Tarsal, Percutaneous Approach

0QCM4ZZ Extirpation of Matter from Left Tarsal, Percutaneous Endoscopic Approach

0QCN0ZZ Extirpation of Matter from Right Metatarsal, Open Approach

0QCN3ZZ Extirpation of Matter from Right Metatarsal, Percutaneous Approach

0QCN4ZZ Extirpation of Matter from Right Metatarsal, Percutaneous Endoscopic Approach

0QCP0ZZ Extirpation of Matter from Left Metatarsal, Open Approach

0QCP3ZZ Extirpation of Matter from Left Metatarsal, Percutaneous Approach

0QCP4ZZ Extirpation of Matter from Left Metatarsal, Percutaneous Endoscopic Approach

0QCQ0ZZ Extirpation of Matter from Right Toe Phalanx, Open Approach

0QCQ3ZZ Extirpation of Matter from Right Toe Phalanx, Percutaneous Approach

0QCQ4ZZ Extirpation of Matter from Right Toe Phalanx, Percutaneous Endoscopic Approach

0QCR0ZZ Extirpation of Matter from Left Toe Phalanx, Open Approach

0QCR3ZZ Extirpation of Matter from Left Toe Phalanx, Percutaneous Approach

0QCR4ZZ Extirpation of Matter from Left Toe Phalanx, Percutaneous Endoscopic Approach

0QCS0ZZ Extirpation of Matter from Coccyx, Open Approach

0QCS3ZZ Extirpation of Matter from Coccyx, Percutaneous Approach

0QCS4ZZ Extirpation of Matter from Coccyx, Percutaneous Endoscopic Approach

0QD – Lower Bones, Extraction

0QD00ZZ Extraction of Lumbar Vertebra, Open Approach

0QD10ZZ Extraction of Sacrum, Open Approach

0QD20ZZ Extraction of Right Pelvic Bone, Open Approach

0QD30ZZ Extraction of Left Pelvic Bone, Open Approach

0QD40ZZ Extraction of Right Acetabulum, Open Approach

0QD50ZZ Extraction of Left Acetabulum, Open Approach

0QD60ZZ Extraction of Right Upper Femur, Open Approach

0QD70ZZ Extraction of Left Upper Femur, Open Approach

0QD80ZZ Extraction of Right Femoral Shaft, Open Approach

0QD90ZZ Extraction of Left Femoral Shaft, Open Approach

0QDB0ZZ Extraction of Right Lower Femur, Open Approach

0QDC0ZZ Extraction of Left Lower Femur, Open Approach

0QDD0ZZ Extraction of Right Patella, Open Approach

0QDF0ZZ Extraction of Left Patella, Open Approach

0QDG0ZZ Extraction of Right Tibia, Open Approach

0QDH0ZZ Extraction of Left Tibia, Open Approach

0QDJ0ZZ Extraction of Right Fibula, Open Approach

0QDK0ZZ Extraction of Left Fibula, Open Approach

0QDL0ZZ Extraction of Right Tarsal, Open Approach

0QDM0ZZ Extraction of Left Tarsal, Open Approach

0QDN0ZZ Extraction of Right Metatarsal, Open Approach

0QDP0ZZ Extraction of Left Metatarsal, Open Approach

♀ Female-only   ♂ Male-only   ▲ Limited Coverage   ● Non-OR   HAC HAC-associated procedure   ▲ Non-covered procedures   ✚ Cluster

| 0QDQ0ZZ | Extraction of Right Toe Phalanx, Open Approach | 0QDR0ZZ | Extraction of Left Toe Phalanx, Open Approach | 0QDS0ZZ | Extraction of Coccyx, Open Approach |

0QH – Lower Bones, Insertion

0QH004Z Insertion of Internal Fixation Device into Lumbar Vertebra, Open Approach

0QH005Z Insertion of External Fixation Device into Lumbar Vertebra, Open Approach

0QH034Z Insertion of Internal Fixation Device into Lumbar Vertebra, Percutaneous Approach

0QH035Z Insertion of External Fixation Device into Lumbar Vertebra, Percutaneous Approach

0QH044Z Insertion of Internal Fixation Device into Lumbar Vertebra, Percutaneous Endoscopic Approach

0QH045Z Insertion of External Fixation Device into Lumbar Vertebra, Percutaneous Endoscopic Approach

0QH104Z Insertion of Internal Fixation Device into Sacrum, Open Approach

0QH105Z Insertion of External Fixation Device into Sacrum, Open Approach

0QH134Z Insertion of Internal Fixation Device into Sacrum, Percutaneous Approach

0QH135Z Insertion of External Fixation Device into Sacrum, Percutaneous Approach

0QH144Z Insertion of Internal Fixation Device into Sacrum, Percutaneous Endoscopic Approach

0QH145Z Insertion of External Fixation Device into Sacrum, Percutaneous Endoscopic Approach

0QH204Z Insertion of Internal Fixation Device into Right Pelvic Bone, Open Approach
AHA CC: 1Q, 2017, 21-22

0QH205Z Insertion of External Fixation Device into Right Pelvic Bone, Open Approach

0QH234Z Insertion of Internal Fixation Device into Right Pelvic Bone, Percutaneous Approach

0QH235Z Insertion of External Fixation Device into Right Pelvic Bone, Percutaneous Approach

0QH244Z Insertion of Internal Fixation Device into Right Pelvic Bone, Percutaneous Endoscopic Approach

0QH245Z Insertion of External Fixation Device into Right Pelvic Bone, Percutaneous Endoscopic Approach

0QH304Z Insertion of Internal Fixation Device into Left Pelvic Bone, Open Approach
AHA CC: 1Q, 2017, 21-22

0QH305Z Insertion of External Fixation Device into Left Pelvic Bone, Open Approach

0QH334Z Insertion of Internal Fixation Device into Left Pelvic Bone, Percutaneous Approach

0QH335Z Insertion of External Fixation Device into Left Pelvic Bone, Percutaneous Approach

0QH344Z Insertion of Internal Fixation Device into Left Pelvic Bone, Percutaneous Endoscopic Approach

0QH345Z Insertion of External Fixation Device into Left Pelvic Bone, Percutaneous Endoscopic Approach

0QH404Z Insertion of Internal Fixation Device into Right Acetabulum, Open Approach

0QH405Z Insertion of External Fixation Device into Right Acetabulum, Open Approach

0QH434Z Insertion of Internal Fixation Device into Right Acetabulum, Percutaneous Approach

0QH435Z Insertion of External Fixation Device into Right Acetabulum, Percutaneous Approach

0QH444Z Insertion of Internal Fixation Device into Right Acetabulum, Percutaneous Endoscopic Approach

0QH445Z Insertion of External Fixation Device into Right Acetabulum, Percutaneous Endoscopic Approach

0QH504Z Insertion of Internal Fixation Device into Left Acetabulum, Open Approach

0QH505Z Insertion of External Fixation Device into Left Acetabulum, Open Approach

0QH534Z Insertion of Internal Fixation Device into Left Acetabulum, Percutaneous Approach

0QH535Z Insertion of External Fixation Device into Left Acetabulum, Percutaneous Approach

0QH544Z Insertion of Internal Fixation Device into Left Acetabulum, Percutaneous Endoscopic Approach

0QH545Z Insertion of External Fixation Device into Left Acetabulum, Percutaneous Endoscopic Approach

0QH604Z Insertion of Internal Fixation Device into Right Upper Femur, Open Approach

0QH605Z Insertion of External Fixation Device into Right Upper Femur, Open Approach

0QH606Z Insertion of Intramedullary Internal Fixation Device into Right Upper Femur, Open Approach

0QH608Z Insertion of Limb Lengthening External Fixation Device into Right Upper Femur, Open Approach

0QH60BZ Insertion of Monoplanar External Fixation Device into Right Upper Femur, Open Approach

0QH60CZ Insertion of Ring External Fixation Device into Right Upper Femur, Open Approach

0QH60DZ Insertion of Hybrid External Fixation Device into Right Upper Femur, Open Approach

0QH634Z Insertion of Internal Fixation Device into Right Upper Femur, Percutaneous Approach

0QH635Z Insertion of External Fixation Device into Right Upper Femur, Percutaneous Approach

0QH636Z Insertion of Intramedullary Internal Fixation Device into Right Upper Femur, Percutaneous Approach

0QH638Z Insertion of Limb Lengthening External Fixation Device into Right Upper Femur, Percutaneous Approach

0QH63BZ Insertion of Monoplanar External Fixation Device into Right Upper Femur, Percutaneous Approach

0QH63CZ Insertion of Ring External Fixation Device into Right Upper Femur, Percutaneous Approach

0QH63DZ Insertion of Hybrid External Fixation Device into Right Upper Femur, Percutaneous Approach

0QH644Z Insertion of Internal Fixation Device into Right Upper Femur, Percutaneous Endoscopic Approach

0QH645Z Insertion of External Fixation Device into Right Upper Femur, Percutaneous Endoscopic Approach

0QH646Z Insertion of Intramedullary Internal Fixation Device into Right Upper Femur, Percutaneous Endoscopic Approach

0QH648Z Insertion of Limb Lengthening External Fixation Device into Right Upper Femur, Percutaneous Endoscopic Approach

0QH64BZ Insertion of Monoplanar External Fixation Device into Right Upper Femur, Percutaneous Endoscopic Approach

0QH64CZ Insertion of Ring External Fixation Device into Right Upper Femur, Percutaneous Endoscopic Approach

0QH64DZ Insertion of Hybrid External Fixation Device into Right Upper Femur, Percutaneous Endoscopic Approach

0QH704Z Insertion of Internal Fixation Device into Left Upper Femur, Open Approach

0QH705Z Insertion of External Fixation Device into Left Upper Femur, Open Approach

0QH706Z Insertion of Intramedullary Internal Fixation Device into Left Upper Femur, Open Approach

0QH708Z Insertion of Limb Lengthening External Fixation Device into Left Upper Femur, Open Approach

0QH70BZ Insertion of Monoplanar External Fixation Device into Left Upper Femur, Open Approach

0QH70CZ Insertion of Ring External Fixation Device into Left Upper Femur, Open Approach

0QH70DZ Insertion of Hybrid External Fixation Device into Left Upper Femur, Open Approach

0QH734Z Insertion of Internal Fixation Device into Left Upper Femur, Percutaneous Approach

0QH735Z Insertion of External Fixation Device into Left Upper Femur, Percutaneous Approach

0QH736Z Insertion of Intramedullary Internal Fixation Device into Left Upper Femur, Percutaneous Approach

0QH738Z Insertion of Limb Lengthening External Fixation Device into Left Upper Femur, Percutaneous Approach

0QH73BZ Insertion of Monoplanar External Fixation Device into Left Upper Femur, Percutaneous Approach

0QH73CZ Insertion of Ring External Fixation Device into Left Upper Femur, Percutaneous Approach

0QH73DZ Insertion of Hybrid External Fixation Device into Left Upper Femur, Percutaneous Approach

0QH744Z Insertion of Internal Fixation Device into Left Upper Femur, Percutaneous Endoscopic Approach

0QH745Z Insertion of External Fixation Device into Left Upper Femur, Percutaneous Endoscopic Approach

0QH746Z Insertion of Intramedullary Internal Fixation Device into Left Upper Femur, Percutaneous Endoscopic Approach

0QH748Z Insertion of Limb Lengthening External Fixation Device into Left Upper Femur, Percutaneous Endoscopic Approach

0QH74BZ Insertion of Monoplanar External Fixation Device into Left Upper Femur, Percutaneous Endoscopic Approach

0QH74CZ Insertion of Ring External Fixation Device into Left Upper Femur, Percutaneous Endoscopic Approach

0QH74DZ Insertion of Hybrid External Fixation Device into Left Upper Femur, Percutaneous Endoscopic Approach

0QH804Z Insertion of Internal Fixation Device into Right Femoral Shaft, Open Approach

0QH805Z Insertion of External Fixation Device into Right Femoral Shaft, Open Approach

0QH806Z Insertion of Intramedullary Internal Fixation Device into Right Femoral Shaft, Open Approach

0QH807Z Insertion of Intramedullary Limb Lengthening Internal Fixation Device into Right Femoral Shaft, Open Approach

0QH808Z Insertion of Limb Lengthening External Fixation Device into Right Femoral Shaft, Open Approach

0QH80BZ Insertion of Monoplanar External Fixation Device into Right Femoral Shaft, Open Approach

0QH80CZ Insertion of Ring External Fixation Device into Right Femoral Shaft, Open Approach

0QH80DZ Insertion of Hybrid External Fixation Device into Right Femoral Shaft, Open Approach

0QH834Z Insertion of Internal Fixation Device into Right Femoral Shaft, Percutaneous Approach

0QH835Z Insertion of External Fixation Device into Right Femoral Shaft, Percutaneous Approach

0QH836Z Insertion of Intramedullary Internal Fixation Device into Right Femoral Shaft, Percutaneous Approach

0QH837Z Insertion of Intramedullary Limb Lengthening Internal Fixation Device into Right Femoral Shaft, Percutaneous Approach

0QH838Z Insertion of Limb Lengthening External Fixation Device into Right Femoral Shaft, Percutaneous Approach

0QH83BZ Insertion of Monoplanar External Fixation Device into Right Femoral Shaft, Percutaneous Approach

0QH83CZ Insertion of Ring External Fixation Device into Right Femoral Shaft, Percutaneous Approach

0QH83DZ Insertion of Hybrid External Fixation Device into Right Femoral Shaft, Percutaneous Approach

0QH844Z Insertion of Internal Fixation Device into Right Femoral Shaft, Percutaneous Endoscopic Approach

0QH845Z Insertion of External Fixation Device into Right Femoral Shaft, Percutaneous Endoscopic Approach

0QH846Z Insertion of Intramedullary Internal Fixation Device into Right Femoral Shaft, Percutaneous Endoscopic Approach

0QH847Z Insertion of Intramedullary Limb Lengthening Internal Fixation Device into Right Femoral Shaft, Percutaneous Endoscopic Approach

0QH848Z Insertion of Limb Lengthening External Fixation Device into Right Femoral Shaft, Percutaneous Endoscopic Approach

0QH84BZ Insertion of Monoplanar External Fixation Device into Right Femoral Shaft, Percutaneous Endoscopic Approach

0QH84CZ Insertion of Ring External Fixation Device into Right Femoral Shaft, Percutaneous Endoscopic Approach

0QH84DZ Insertion of Hybrid External Fixation Device into Right Femoral Shaft, Percutaneous Endoscopic Approach

0QH904Z Insertion of Internal Fixation Device into Left Femoral Shaft, Open Approach

0QH905Z Insertion of External Fixation Device into Left Femoral Shaft, Open Approach

0QH906Z Insertion of Intramedullary Internal Fixation Device into Left Femoral Shaft, Open Approach

0QH907Z Insertion of Intramedullary Limb Lengthening Internal Fixation Device into Left Femoral Shaft, Open Approach

0QH908Z Insertion of Limb Lengthening External Fixation Device into Left Femoral Shaft, Open Approach

0QH90BZ Insertion of Monoplanar External Fixation Device into Left Femoral Shaft, Open Approach

0QH90CZ Insertion of Ring External Fixation Device into Left Femoral Shaft, Open Approach

0QH90DZ Insertion of Hybrid External Fixation Device into Left Femoral Shaft, Open Approach

0QH934Z Insertion of Internal Fixation Device into Left Femoral Shaft, Percutaneous Approach

0QH935Z Insertion of External Fixation Device into Left Femoral Shaft, Percutaneous Approach

0QH936Z Insertion of Intramedullary Internal Fixation Device into Left Femoral Shaft, Percutaneous Approach

0QH937Z Insertion of Intramedullary Limb Lengthening Internal Fixation Device into Left Femoral Shaft, Percutaneous Approach

0QH938Z Insertion of Limb Lengthening External Fixation Device into Left Femoral Shaft, Percutaneous Approach

0QH93BZ Insertion of Monoplanar External Fixation Device into Left Femoral Shaft, Percutaneous Approach

0QH93CZ Insertion of Ring External Fixation Device into Left Femoral Shaft, Percutaneous Approach

0QH93DZ Insertion of Hybrid External Fixation Device into Left Femoral Shaft, Percutaneous Approach

0QH944Z Insertion of Internal Fixation Device into Left Femoral Shaft, Percutaneous Endoscopic Approach

0QH945Z Insertion of External Fixation Device into Left Femoral Shaft, Percutaneous Endoscopic Approach

0QH946Z Insertion of Intramedullary Internal Fixation Device into Left Femoral Shaft, Percutaneous Endoscopic Approach

0QH947Z Insertion of Intramedullary Limb Lengthening Internal Fixation Device into Left Femoral Shaft, Percutaneous Endoscopic Approach

0QH948Z Insertion of Limb Lengthening External Fixation Device into Left Femoral Shaft, Percutaneous Endoscopic Approach

0QH94BZ Insertion of Monoplanar External Fixation Device into Left Femoral Shaft, Percutaneous Endoscopic Approach

0QH94CZ Insertion of Ring External Fixation Device into Left Femoral Shaft, Percutaneous Endoscopic Approach

0QH94DZ Insertion of Hybrid External Fixation Device into Left Femoral Shaft, Percutaneous Endoscopic Approach

0QHB04Z Insertion of Internal Fixation Device into Right Lower Femur, Open Approach

0QHB05Z Insertion of External Fixation Device into Right Lower Femur, Open Approach

0QHB06Z Insertion of Intramedullary Internal Fixation Device into Right Lower Femur, Open Approach

0QHB08Z Insertion of Limb Lengthening External Fixation Device into Right Lower Femur, Open Approach

0QHB0BZ Insertion of Monoplanar External Fixation Device into Right Lower Femur, Open Approach

0QHB0CZ Insertion of Ring External Fixation Device into Right Lower Femur, Open Approach

0QHB0DZ Insertion of Hybrid External Fixation Device into Right Lower Femur, Open Approach

0QHB34Z Insertion of Internal Fixation Device into Right Lower Femur, Percutaneous Approach

0QHB35Z Insertion of External Fixation Device into Right Lower Femur, Percutaneous Approach

0QHB36Z Insertion of Intramedullary Internal Fixation Device into Right Lower Femur, Percutaneous Approach

0QHB38Z Insertion of Limb Lengthening External Fixation Device into Right Lower Femur, Percutaneous Approach

0QHB3BZ Insertion of Monoplanar External Fixation Device into Right Lower Femur, Percutaneous Approach

0QHB3CZ Insertion of Ring External Fixation Device into Right Lower Femur, Percutaneous Approach

0QHB3DZ Insertion of Hybrid External Fixation Device into Right Lower Femur, Percutaneous Approach

0QHB44Z Insertion of Internal Fixation Device into Right Lower Femur, Percutaneous Endoscopic Approach

0QHB45Z Insertion of External Fixation Device into Right Lower Femur, Percutaneous Endoscopic Approach

0QHB46Z Insertion of Intramedullary Internal Fixation Device into Right Lower Femur, Percutaneous Endoscopic Approach

0QHB48Z Insertion of Limb Lengthening External Fixation Device into Right Lower Femur, Percutaneous Endoscopic Approach

0QHB4BZ Insertion of Monoplanar External Fixation Device into Right Lower Femur, Percutaneous Endoscopic Approach

0QHB4CZ Insertion of Ring External Fixation Device into Right Lower Femur, Percutaneous Endoscopic Approach

0QHB4DZ Insertion of Hybrid External Fixation Device into Right Lower Femur, Percutaneous Endoscopic Approach

0QHC04Z Insertion of Internal Fixation Device into Left Lower Femur, Open Approach

0QHC05Z Insertion of External Fixation Device into Left Lower Femur, Open Approach

♀ Female-only   ♂ Male-only   ▲ Limited Coverage   ● Non-OR   ▉ HAC-associated procedure   ▲ Non-covered procedures   ✚ Cluster

0QHC06Z Insertion of Intramedullary Internal Fixation Device into Left Lower Femur, Open Approach

0QHC08Z Insertion of Limb Lengthening External Fixation Device into Left Lower Femur, Open Approach

0QHC0BZ Insertion of Monoplanar External Fixation Device into Left Lower Femur, Open Approach

0QHC0CZ Insertion of Ring External Fixation Device into Left Lower Femur, Open Approach

0QHC0DZ Insertion of Hybrid External Fixation Device into Left Lower Femur, Open Approach

0QHC34Z Insertion of Internal Fixation Device into Left Lower Femur, Percutaneous Approach

0QHC35Z Insertion of External Fixation Device into Left Lower Femur, Percutaneous Approach

0QHC36Z Insertion of Intramedullary Internal Fixation Device into Left Lower Femur, Percutaneous Approach

0QHC38Z Insertion of Limb Lengthening External Fixation Device into Left Lower Femur, Percutaneous Approach

0QHC3BZ Insertion of Monoplanar External Fixation Device into Left Lower Femur, Percutaneous Approach

0QHC3CZ Insertion of Ring External Fixation Device into Left Lower Femur, Percutaneous Approach

0QHC3DZ Insertion of Hybrid External Fixation Device into Left Lower Femur, Percutaneous Approach

0QHC44Z Insertion of Internal Fixation Device into Left Lower Femur, Percutaneous Endoscopic Approach

0QHC45Z Insertion of External Fixation Device into Left Lower Femur, Percutaneous Endoscopic Approach

0QHC46Z Insertion of Intramedullary Internal Fixation Device into Left Lower Femur, Percutaneous Endoscopic Approach

0QHC48Z Insertion of Limb Lengthening External Fixation Device into Left Lower Femur, Percutaneous Endoscopic Approach

0QHC4BZ Insertion of Monoplanar External Fixation Device into Left Lower Femur, Percutaneous Endoscopic Approach

0QHC4CZ Insertion of Ring External Fixation Device into Left Lower Femur, Percutaneous Endoscopic Approach

0QHC4DZ Insertion of Hybrid External Fixation Device into Left Lower Femur, Percutaneous Endoscopic Approach

0QHD04Z Insertion of Internal Fixation Device into Right Patella, Open Approach

0QHD05Z Insertion of External Fixation Device into Right Patella, Open Approach

0QHD34Z Insertion of Internal Fixation Device into Right Patella, Percutaneous Approach

0QHD35Z Insertion of External Fixation Device into Right Patella, Percutaneous Approach

0QHD44Z Insertion of Internal Fixation Device into Right Patella, Percutaneous Endoscopic Approach

0QHD45Z Insertion of External Fixation Device into Right Patella, Percutaneous Endoscopic Approach

0QHF04Z Insertion of Internal Fixation Device into Left Patella, Open Approach

0QHF05Z Insertion of External Fixation Device into Left Patella, Open Approach

0QHF34Z Insertion of Internal Fixation Device into Left Patella, Percutaneous Approach

0QHF35Z Insertion of External Fixation Device into Left Patella, Percutaneous Approach

0QHF44Z Insertion of Internal Fixation Device into Left Patella, Percutaneous Endoscopic Approach

0QHF45Z Insertion of External Fixation Device into Left Patella, Percutaneous Endoscopic Approach

0QHG04Z Insertion of Internal Fixation Device into Right Tibia, Open Approach

AHA CC: 3Q, 2016, 34-35

0QHG05Z Insertion of External Fixation Device into Right Tibia, Open Approach

0QHG06Z Insertion of Intramedullary Internal Fixation Device into Right Tibia, Open Approach

0QHG07Z Insertion of Intramedullary Limb Lengthening Internal Fixation Device into Right Tibia, Open Approach

0QHG08Z Insertion of Limb Lengthening External Fixation Device into Right Tibia, Open Approach

0QHG0BZ Insertion of Monoplanar External Fixation Device into Right Tibia, Open Approach

0QHG0CZ Insertion of Ring External Fixation Device into Right Tibia, Open Approach

0QHG0DZ Insertion of Hybrid External Fixation Device into Right Tibia, Open Approach

0QHG34Z Insertion of Internal Fixation Device into Right Tibia, Percutaneous Approach

0QHG35Z Insertion of External Fixation Device into Right Tibia, Percutaneous Approach

0QHG36Z Insertion of Intramedullary Internal Fixation Device into Right Tibia, Percutaneous Approach

0QHG37Z Insertion of Intramedullary Limb Lengthening Internal Fixation Device into Right Tibia, Percutaneous Approach

0QHG38Z Insertion of Limb Lengthening External Fixation Device into Right Tibia, Percutaneous Approach

0QHG3BZ Insertion of Monoplanar External Fixation Device into Right Tibia, Percutaneous Approach

0QHG3CZ Insertion of Ring External Fixation Device into Right Tibia, Percutaneous Approach

0QHG3DZ Insertion of Hybrid External Fixation Device into Right Tibia, Percutaneous Approach

0QHG44Z Insertion of Internal Fixation Device into Right Tibia, Percutaneous Endoscopic Approach

0QHG45Z Insertion of External Fixation Device into Right Tibia, Percutaneous Endoscopic Approach

0QHG46Z Insertion of Intramedullary Internal Fixation Device into Right Tibia, Percutaneous Endoscopic Approach

0QHG47Z Insertion of Intramedullary Limb Lengthening Internal Fixation Device into Right Tibia, Percutaneous Endoscopic Approach

0QHG48Z Insertion of Limb Lengthening External Fixation Device into Right Tibia, Percutaneous Endoscopic Approach

0QHG4BZ Insertion of Monoplanar External Fixation Device into Right Tibia, Percutaneous Endoscopic Approach

0QHG4CZ Insertion of Ring External Fixation Device into Right Tibia, Percutaneous Endoscopic Approach

0QHG4DZ Insertion of Hybrid External Fixation Device into Right Tibia, Percutaneous Endoscopic Approach

0QHH04Z Insertion of Internal Fixation Device into Left Tibia, Open Approach

0QHH05Z Insertion of External Fixation Device into Left Tibia, Open Approach

0QHH06Z Insertion of Intramedullary Internal Fixation Device into Left Tibia, Open Approach

0QHH07Z Insertion of Intramedullary Limb Lengthening Internal Fixation Device into Left Tibia, Open Approach

0QHH08Z Insertion of Limb Lengthening External Fixation Device into Left Tibia, Open Approach

0QHH0BZ Insertion of Monoplanar External Fixation Device into Left Tibia, Open Approach

0QHH0CZ Insertion of Ring External Fixation Device into Left Tibia, Open Approach

0QHH0DZ Insertion of Hybrid External Fixation Device into Left Tibia, Open Approach

0QHH34Z Insertion of Internal Fixation Device into Left Tibia, Percutaneous Approach

0QHH35Z Insertion of External Fixation Device into Left Tibia, Percutaneous Approach

0QHH36Z Insertion of Intramedullary Internal Fixation Device into Left Tibia, Percutaneous Approach

0QHH37Z Insertion of Intramedullary Limb Lengthening Internal Fixation Device into Left Tibia, Percutaneous Approach

0QHH38Z Insertion of Limb Lengthening External Fixation Device into Left Tibia, Percutaneous Approach

0QHH3BZ Insertion of Monoplanar External Fixation Device into Left Tibia, Percutaneous Approach

0QHH3CZ Insertion of Ring External Fixation Device into Left Tibia, Percutaneous Approach

0QHH3DZ Insertion of Hybrid External Fixation Device into Left Tibia, Percutaneous Approach

0QHH44Z Insertion of Internal Fixation Device into Left Tibia, Percutaneous Endoscopic Approach

0QHH45Z Insertion of External Fixation Device into Left Tibia, Percutaneous Endoscopic Approach

0QHH46Z Insertion of Intramedullary Internal Fixation Device into Left Tibia, Percutaneous Endoscopic Approach

0QHH47Z Insertion of Intramedullary Limb Lengthening Internal Fixation Device into Left Tibia, Percutaneous Endoscopic Approach

0QHH48Z Insertion of Limb Lengthening External Fixation Device into Left Tibia, Percutaneous Endoscopic Approach

0QHH4BZ Insertion of Monoplanar External Fixation Device into Left Tibia, Percutaneous Endoscopic Approach

0QHH4CZ Insertion of Ring External Fixation Device into Left Tibia, Percutaneous Endoscopic Approach

0QHH4DZ Insertion of Hybrid External Fixation Device into Left Tibia, Percutaneous Endoscopic Approach

0QHJ04Z Insertion of Internal Fixation Device into Right Fibula, Open Approach
AHA CC: 3Q, 2016, 34-35

0QHJ05Z Insertion of External Fixation Device into Right Fibula, Open Approach

0QHJ06Z Insertion of Intramedullary Internal Fixation Device into Right Fibula, Open Approach

0QHJ08Z Insertion of Limb Lengthening External Fixation Device into Right Fibula, Open Approach

0QHJ0BZ Insertion of Monoplanar External Fixation Device into Right Fibula, Open Approach

0QHJ0CZ Insertion of Ring External Fixation Device into Right Fibula, Open Approach

0QHJ0DZ Insertion of Hybrid External Fixation Device into Right Fibula, Open Approach

0QHJ34Z Insertion of Internal Fixation Device into Right Fibula, Percutaneous Approach

0QHJ35Z Insertion of External Fixation Device into Right Fibula, Percutaneous Approach

0QHJ36Z Insertion of Intramedullary Internal Fixation Device into Right Fibula, Percutaneous Approach

0QHJ38Z Insertion of Limb Lengthening External Fixation Device into Right Fibula, Percutaneous Approach

0QHJ3BZ Insertion of Monoplanar External Fixation Device into Right Fibula, Percutaneous Approach

0QHJ3CZ Insertion of Ring External Fixation Device into Right Fibula, Percutaneous Approach

0QHJ3DZ Insertion of Hybrid External Fixation Device into Right Fibula, Percutaneous Approach

0QHJ44Z Insertion of Internal Fixation Device into Right Fibula, Percutaneous Endoscopic Approach

0QHJ45Z Insertion of External Fixation Device into Right Fibula, Percutaneous Endoscopic Approach

0QHJ46Z Insertion of Intramedullary Internal Fixation Device into Right Fibula, Percutaneous Endoscopic Approach

0QHJ48Z Insertion of Limb Lengthening External Fixation Device into Right Fibula, Percutaneous Endoscopic Approach

0QHJ4BZ Insertion of Monoplanar External Fixation Device into Right Fibula, Percutaneous Endoscopic Approach

0QHJ4CZ Insertion of Ring External Fixation Device into Right Fibula, Percutaneous Endoscopic Approach

0QHJ4DZ Insertion of Hybrid External Fixation Device into Right Fibula, Percutaneous Endoscopic Approach

0QHK04Z Insertion of Internal Fixation Device into Left Fibula, Open Approach

0QHK05Z Insertion of External Fixation Device into Left Fibula, Open Approach

0QHK06Z Insertion of Intramedullary Internal Fixation Device into Left Fibula, Open Approach

0QHK08Z Insertion of Limb Lengthening External Fixation Device into Left Fibula, Open Approach

0QHK0BZ Insertion of Monoplanar External Fixation Device into Left Fibula, Open Approach

0QHK0CZ Insertion of Ring External Fixation Device into Left Fibula, Open Approach

0QHK0DZ Insertion of Hybrid External Fixation Device into Left Fibula, Open Approach

0QHK34Z Insertion of Internal Fixation Device into Left Fibula, Percutaneous Approach

0QHK35Z Insertion of External Fixation Device into Left Fibula, Percutaneous Approach

0QHK36Z Insertion of Intramedullary Internal Fixation Device into Left Fibula, Percutaneous Approach

0QHK38Z Insertion of Limb Lengthening External Fixation Device into Left Fibula, Percutaneous Approach

0QHK3BZ Insertion of Monoplanar External Fixation Device into Left Fibula, Percutaneous Approach

0QHK3CZ Insertion of Ring External Fixation Device into Left Fibula, Percutaneous Approach

0QHK3DZ Insertion of Hybrid External Fixation Device into Left Fibula, Percutaneous Approach

0QHK44Z Insertion of Internal Fixation Device into Left Fibula, Percutaneous Endoscopic Approach

0QHK45Z Insertion of External Fixation Device into Left Fibula, Percutaneous Endoscopic Approach

0QHK46Z Insertion of Intramedullary Internal Fixation Device into Left Fibula, Percutaneous Endoscopic Approach

0QHK48Z Insertion of Limb Lengthening External Fixation Device into Left Fibula, Percutaneous Endoscopic Approach

0QHK4BZ Insertion of Monoplanar External Fixation Device into Left Fibula, Percutaneous Endoscopic Approach

0QHK4CZ Insertion of Ring External Fixation Device into Left Fibula, Percutaneous Endoscopic Approach

0QHK4DZ Insertion of Hybrid External Fixation Device into Left Fibula, Percutaneous Endoscopic Approach

0QHL04Z Insertion of Internal Fixation Device into Right Tarsal, Open Approach

0QHL05Z Insertion of External Fixation Device into Right Tarsal, Open Approach

0QHL34Z Insertion of Internal Fixation Device into Right Tarsal, Percutaneous Approach

0QHL35Z Insertion of External Fixation Device into Right Tarsal, Percutaneous Approach

0QHL44Z Insertion of Internal Fixation Device into Right Tarsal, Percutaneous Endoscopic Approach

0QHL45Z Insertion of External Fixation Device into Right Tarsal, Percutaneous Endoscopic Approach

0QHM04Z Insertion of Internal Fixation Device into Left Tarsal, Open Approach

0QHM05Z Insertion of External Fixation Device into Left Tarsal, Open Approach

0QHM34Z Insertion of Internal Fixation Device into Left Tarsal, Percutaneous Approach

0QHM35Z Insertion of External Fixation Device into Left Tarsal, Percutaneous Approach

0QHM44Z Insertion of Internal Fixation Device into Left Tarsal, Percutaneous Endoscopic Approach

0QHM45Z Insertion of External Fixation Device into Left Tarsal, Percutaneous Endoscopic Approach

0QHN04Z Insertion of Internal Fixation Device into Right Metatarsal, Open Approach

0QHN05Z Insertion of External Fixation Device into Right Metatarsal, Open Approach

0QHN34Z Insertion of Internal Fixation Device into Right Metatarsal, Percutaneous Approach

0QHN35Z Insertion of External Fixation Device into Right Metatarsal, Percutaneous Approach

0QHN44Z Insertion of Internal Fixation Device into Right Metatarsal, Percutaneous Endoscopic Approach

0QHN45Z Insertion of External Fixation Device into Right Metatarsal, Percutaneous Endoscopic Approach

0QHP04Z Insertion of Internal Fixation Device into Left Metatarsal, Open Approach

0QHP05Z Insertion of External Fixation Device into Left Metatarsal, Open Approach

0QHP34Z Insertion of Internal Fixation Device into Left Metatarsal, Percutaneous Approach

0QHP35Z Insertion of External Fixation Device into Left Metatarsal, Percutaneous Approach

0QHP44Z Insertion of Internal Fixation Device into Left Metatarsal, Percutaneous Endoscopic Approach

0QHP45Z Insertion of External Fixation Device into Left Metatarsal, Percutaneous Endoscopic Approach

0QHQ04Z Insertion of Internal Fixation Device into Right Toe Phalanx, Open Approach

0QHQ05Z Insertion of External Fixation Device into Right Toe Phalanx, Open Approach

0QHQ34Z Insertion of Internal Fixation Device into Right Toe Phalanx, Percutaneous Approach

0QHQ35Z Insertion of External Fixation Device into Right Toe Phalanx, Percutaneous Approach

0QHQ44Z Insertion of Internal Fixation Device into Right Toe Phalanx, Percutaneous Endoscopic Approach

0QHQ45Z Insertion of External Fixation Device into Right Toe Phalanx, Percutaneous Endoscopic Approach

0QHR04Z Insertion of Internal Fixation Device into Left Toe Phalanx, Open Approach

0QHR05Z Insertion of External Fixation Device into Left Toe Phalanx, Open Approach

0QHR34Z Insertion of Internal Fixation Device into Left Toe Phalanx, Percutaneous Approach

0QHR35Z Insertion of External Fixation Device into Left Toe Phalanx, Percutaneous Approach

0QHR44Z Insertion of Internal Fixation Device into Left Toe Phalanx, Percutaneous Endoscopic Approach

♀ Female-only   ♂ Male-only   ▲ Limited Coverage   ● Non-OR   ▥ HAC-associated procedure   ▲ Non-covered procedures   ✛ Cluster

0QHR45Z	Insertion of External Fixation Device into Left Toe Phalanx, Percutaneous Endoscopic Approach
0QHS04Z	Insertion of Internal Fixation Device into Coccyx, Open Approach
0QHS05Z	Insertion of External Fixation Device into Coccyx, Open Approach
0QHS34Z	Insertion of Internal Fixation Device into Coccyx, Percutaneous Approach

0QHS35Z	Insertion of External Fixation Device into Coccyx, Percutaneous Approach
0QHS44Z	Insertion of Internal Fixation Device into Coccyx, Percutaneous Endoscopic Approach
0QHS45Z	Insertion of External Fixation Device into Coccyx, Percutaneous Endoscopic Approach

0QHY0MZ	Insertion of Bone Growth Stimulator into Lower Bone, Open Approach
0QHY3MZ	Insertion of Bone Growth Stimulator into Lower Bone, Percutaneous Approach
0QHY4MZ	Insertion of Bone Growth Stimulator into Lower Bone, Percutaneous Endoscopic Approach

0QJ – Lower Bones, Inspection

Review Coding Guideline B3.5

Review Coding Guidelines B3.11a, B3.11b and B3.11c

0QJY0ZZ	Inspection of Lower Bone, Open Approach
0QJY3ZZ	Inspection of Lower Bone, Percutaneous Approach

0QJY4ZZ	Inspection of Lower Bone, Percutaneous Endoscopic Approach
0QJYXZZ	Inspection of Lower Bone, External Approach

0QN – Lower Bones, Release

Review Coding Guideline B3.13

Review Coding Guideline B3.14

0QN00ZZ	Release Lumbar Vertebra, Open Approach
0QN03ZZ	Release Lumbar Vertebra, Percutaneous Approach
0QN04ZZ	Release Lumbar Vertebra, Percutaneous Endoscopic Approach
0QN10ZZ	Release Sacrum, Open Approach
0QN13ZZ	Release Sacrum, Percutaneous Approach
0QN14ZZ	Release Sacrum, Percutaneous Endoscopic Approach
0QN20ZZ	Release Right Pelvic Bone, Open Approach
0QN23ZZ	Release Right Pelvic Bone, Percutaneous Approach
0QN24ZZ	Release Right Pelvic Bone, Percutaneous Endoscopic Approach
0QN30ZZ	Release Left Pelvic Bone, Open Approach
0QN33ZZ	Release Left Pelvic Bone, Percutaneous Approach
0QN34ZZ	Release Left Pelvic Bone, Percutaneous Endoscopic Approach
0QN40ZZ	Release Right Acetabulum, Open Approach
0QN43ZZ	Release Right Acetabulum, Percutaneous Approach
0QN44ZZ	Release Right Acetabulum, Percutaneous Endoscopic Approach
0QN50ZZ	Release Left Acetabulum, Open Approach
0QN53ZZ	Release Left Acetabulum, Percutaneous Approach
0QN54ZZ	Release Left Acetabulum, Percutaneous Endoscopic Approach
0QN60ZZ	Release Right Upper Femur, Open Approach
0QN63ZZ	Release Right Upper Femur, Percutaneous Approach
0QN64ZZ	Release Right Upper Femur, Percutaneous Endoscopic Approach
0QN70ZZ	Release Left Upper Femur, Open Approach
0QN73ZZ	Release Left Upper Femur, Percutaneous Approach
0QN74ZZ	Release Left Upper Femur, Percutaneous Endoscopic Approach

0QN80ZZ	Release Right Femoral Shaft, Open Approach
0QN83ZZ	Release Right Femoral Shaft, Percutaneous Approach
0QN84ZZ	Release Right Femoral Shaft, Percutaneous Endoscopic Approach
0QN90ZZ	Release Left Femoral Shaft, Open Approach
0QN93ZZ	Release Left Femoral Shaft, Percutaneous Approach
0QN94ZZ	Release Left Femoral Shaft, Percutaneous Endoscopic Approach
0QNB0ZZ	Release Right Lower Femur, Open Approach
0QNB3ZZ	Release Right Lower Femur, Percutaneous Approach
0QNB4ZZ	Release Right Lower Femur, Percutaneous Endoscopic Approach
0QNC0ZZ	Release Left Lower Femur, Open Approach
0QNC3ZZ	Release Left Lower Femur, Percutaneous Approach
0QNC4ZZ	Release Left Lower Femur, Percutaneous Endoscopic Approach
0QND0ZZ	Release Right Patella, Open Approach
0QND3ZZ	Release Right Patella, Percutaneous Approach
0QND4ZZ	Release Right Patella, Percutaneous Endoscopic Approach
0QNF0ZZ	Release Left Patella, Open Approach
0QNF3ZZ	Release Left Patella, Percutaneous Approach
0QNF4ZZ	Release Left Patella, Percutaneous Endoscopic Approach
0QNG0ZZ	Release Right Tibia, Open Approach
0QNG3ZZ	Release Right Tibia, Percutaneous Approach
0QNG4ZZ	Release Right Tibia, Percutaneous Endoscopic Approach
0QNH0ZZ	Release Left Tibia, Open Approach
0QNH3ZZ	Release Left Tibia, Percutaneous Approach
0QNH4ZZ	Release Left Tibia, Percutaneous Endoscopic Approach
0QNJ0ZZ	Release Right Fibula, Open Approach
0QNJ3ZZ	Release Right Fibula, Percutaneous Approach

0QNJ4ZZ	Release Right Fibula, Percutaneous Endoscopic Approach
0QNK0ZZ	Release Left Fibula, Open Approach
0QNK3ZZ	Release Left Fibula, Percutaneous Approach
0QNK4ZZ	Release Left Fibula, Percutaneous Endoscopic Approach
0QNL0ZZ	Release Right Tarsal, Open Approach
0QNL3ZZ	Release Right Tarsal, Percutaneous Approach
0QNL4ZZ	Release Right Tarsal, Percutaneous Endoscopic Approach
0QNM0ZZ	Release Left Tarsal, Open Approach
0QNM3ZZ	Release Left Tarsal, Percutaneous Approach
0QNM4ZZ	Release Left Tarsal, Percutaneous Endoscopic Approach
0QNN0ZZ	Release Right Metatarsal, Open Approach
0QNN3ZZ	Release Right Metatarsal, Percutaneous Approach
0QNN4ZZ	Release Right Metatarsal, Percutaneous Endoscopic Approach
0QNP0ZZ	Release Left Metatarsal, Open Approach
0QNP3ZZ	Release Left Metatarsal, Percutaneous Approach
0QNP4ZZ	Release Left Metatarsal, Percutaneous Endoscopic Approach
0QNQ0ZZ	Release Right Toe Phalanx, Open Approach
0QNQ3ZZ	Release Right Toe Phalanx, Percutaneous Approach
0QNQ4ZZ	Release Right Toe Phalanx, Percutaneous Endoscopic Approach
0QNR0ZZ	Release Left Toe Phalanx, Open Approach
0QNR3ZZ	Release Left Toe Phalanx, Percutaneous Approach
0QNR4ZZ	Release Left Toe Phalanx, Percutaneous Endoscopic Approach
0QNS0ZZ	Release Coccyx, Open Approach
0QNS3ZZ	Release Coccyx, Percutaneous Approach
0QNS4ZZ	Release Coccyx, Percutaneous Endoscopic Approach

Review Coding Guideline B6.1c

0QP004Z Removal of Internal Fixation Device from Lumbar Vertebra, Open Approach
AHA CC: 4Q, 2017, 75

0QP005Z Removal of External Fixation Device from Lumbar Vertebra, Open Approach

0QP007Z Removal of Autologous Tissue Substitute from Lumbar Vertebra, Open Approach

0QP00JZ Removal of Synthetic Substitute from Lumbar Vertebra, Open Approach

0QP00KZ Removal of Nonautologous Tissue Substitute from Lumbar Vertebra, Open Approach

0QP034Z Removal of Internal Fixation Device from Lumbar Vertebra, Percutaneous Approach

0QP035Z Removal of External Fixation Device from Lumbar Vertebra, Percutaneous Approach

0QP037Z Removal of Autologous Tissue Substitute from Lumbar Vertebra, Percutaneous Approach

0QP03JZ Removal of Synthetic Substitute from Lumbar Vertebra, Percutaneous Approach

0QP03KZ Removal of Nonautologous Tissue Substitute from Lumbar Vertebra, Percutaneous Approach

0QP044Z Removal of Internal Fixation Device from Lumbar Vertebra, Percutaneous Endoscopic Approach

0QP045Z Removal of External Fixation Device from Lumbar Vertebra, Percutaneous Endoscopic Approach

0QP047Z Removal of Autologous Tissue Substitute from Lumbar Vertebra, Percutaneous Endoscopic Approach

0QP04JZ Removal of Synthetic Substitute from Lumbar Vertebra, Percutaneous Endoscopic Approach

0QP04KZ Removal of Nonautologous Tissue Substitute from Lumbar Vertebra, Percutaneous Endoscopic Approach

0QP0X4Z Removal of Internal Fixation Device from Lumbar Vertebra, External Approach

0QP0X5Z Removal of External Fixation Device from Lumbar Vertebra, External Approach

0QP104Z Removal of Internal Fixation Device from Sacrum, Open Approach

0QP105Z Removal of External Fixation Device from Sacrum, Open Approach

0QP107Z Removal of Autologous Tissue Substitute from Sacrum, Open Approach

0QP10JZ Removal of Synthetic Substitute from Sacrum, Open Approach

0QP10KZ Removal of Nonautologous Tissue Substitute from Sacrum, Open Approach

0QP134Z Removal of Internal Fixation Device from Sacrum, Percutaneous Approach

0QP135Z Removal of External Fixation Device from Sacrum, Percutaneous Approach

0QP137Z Removal of Autologous Tissue Substitute from Sacrum, Percutaneous Approach

0QP13JZ Removal of Synthetic Substitute from Sacrum, Percutaneous Approach

0QP13KZ Removal of Nonautologous Tissue Substitute from Sacrum, Percutaneous Approach

0QP144Z Removal of Internal Fixation Device from Sacrum, Percutaneous Endoscopic Approach

0QP145Z Removal of External Fixation Device from Sacrum, Percutaneous Endoscopic Approach

0QP147Z Removal of Autologous Tissue Substitute from Sacrum, Percutaneous Endoscopic Approach

0QP14JZ Removal of Synthetic Substitute from Sacrum, Percutaneous Endoscopic Approach

0QP14KZ Removal of Nonautologous Tissue Substitute from Sacrum, Percutaneous Endoscopic Approach

0QP1X4Z Removal of Internal Fixation Device from Sacrum, External Approach

0QP1X5Z Removal of External Fixation Device from Sacrum, External Approach

0QP204Z Removal of Internal Fixation Device from Right Pelvic Bone, Open Approach

0QP205Z Removal of External Fixation Device from Right Pelvic Bone, Open Approach

0QP207Z Removal of Autologous Tissue Substitute from Right Pelvic Bone, Open Approach

0QP20JZ Removal of Synthetic Substitute from Right Pelvic Bone, Open Approach

0QP20KZ Removal of Nonautologous Tissue Substitute from Right Pelvic Bone, Open Approach

0QP234Z Removal of Internal Fixation Device from Right Pelvic Bone, Percutaneous Approach

0QP235Z Removal of External Fixation Device from Right Pelvic Bone, Percutaneous Approach

0QP237Z Removal of Autologous Tissue Substitute from Right Pelvic Bone, Percutaneous Approach

0QP23JZ Removal of Synthetic Substitute from Right Pelvic Bone, Percutaneous Approach

0QP23KZ Removal of Nonautologous Tissue Substitute from Right Pelvic Bone, Percutaneous Approach

0QP244Z Removal of Internal Fixation Device from Right Pelvic Bone, Percutaneous Endoscopic Approach

0QP245Z Removal of External Fixation Device from Right Pelvic Bone, Percutaneous Endoscopic Approach

0QP247Z Removal of Autologous Tissue Substitute from Right Pelvic Bone, Percutaneous Endoscopic Approach

0QP24JZ Removal of Synthetic Substitute from Right Pelvic Bone, Percutaneous Endoscopic Approach

0QP24KZ Removal of Nonautologous Tissue Substitute from Right Pelvic Bone, Percutaneous Endoscopic Approach

0QP2X4Z Removal of Internal Fixation Device from Right Pelvic Bone, External Approach

0QP2X5Z Removal of External Fixation Device from Right Pelvic Bone, External Approach

0QP304Z Removal of Internal Fixation Device from Left Pelvic Bone, Open Approach

0QP305Z Removal of External Fixation Device from Left Pelvic Bone, Open Approach

0QP307Z Removal of Autologous Tissue Substitute from Left Pelvic Bone, Open Approach

0QP30JZ Removal of Synthetic Substitute from Left Pelvic Bone, Open Approach

0QP30KZ Removal of Nonautologous Tissue Substitute from Left Pelvic Bone, Open Approach

0QP334Z Removal of Internal Fixation Device from Left Pelvic Bone, Percutaneous Approach

0QP335Z Removal of External Fixation Device from Left Pelvic Bone, Percutaneous Approach

0QP337Z Removal of Autologous Tissue Substitute from Left Pelvic Bone, Percutaneous Approach

0QP33JZ Removal of Synthetic Substitute from Left Pelvic Bone, Percutaneous Approach

0QP33KZ Removal of Nonautologous Tissue Substitute from Left Pelvic Bone, Percutaneous Approach

0QP344Z Removal of Internal Fixation Device from Left Pelvic Bone, Percutaneous Endoscopic Approach

0QP345Z Removal of External Fixation Device from Left Pelvic Bone, Percutaneous Endoscopic Approach

0QP347Z Removal of Autologous Tissue Substitute from Left Pelvic Bone, Percutaneous Endoscopic Approach

0QP34JZ Removal of Synthetic Substitute from Left Pelvic Bone, Percutaneous Endoscopic Approach

0QP34KZ Removal of Nonautologous Tissue Substitute from Left Pelvic Bone, Percutaneous Endoscopic Approach

0QP3X4Z Removal of Internal Fixation Device from Left Pelvic Bone, External Approach

0QP3X5Z Removal of External Fixation Device from Left Pelvic Bone, External Approach

0QP404Z Removal of Internal Fixation Device from Right Acetabulum, Open Approach

0QP405Z Removal of External Fixation Device from Right Acetabulum, Open Approach

0QP407Z Removal of Autologous Tissue Substitute from Right Acetabulum, Open Approach

0QP40JZ Removal of Synthetic Substitute from Right Acetabulum, Open Approach

0QP40KZ Removal of Nonautologous Tissue Substitute from Right Acetabulum, Open Approach

0QP434Z Removal of Internal Fixation Device from Right Acetabulum, Percutaneous Approach

0QP435Z Removal of External Fixation Device from Right Acetabulum, Percutaneous Approach

0QP437Z Removal of Autologous Tissue Substitute from Right Acetabulum, Percutaneous Approach

0QP43JZ Removal of Synthetic Substitute from Right Acetabulum, Percutaneous Approach

0QP43KZ Removal of Nonautologous Tissue Substitute from Right Acetabulum, Percutaneous Approach

♀ Female-only   ♂ Male-only   ▲ Limited Coverage   ● Non-OR   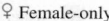 HAC-associated procedure   ▲ Non-covered procedures   ✛ Cluster

0QP444Z Removal of Internal Fixation Device from Right Acetabulum, Percutaneous Endoscopic Approach

0QP445Z Removal of External Fixation Device from Right Acetabulum, Percutaneous Endoscopic Approach

0QP447Z Removal of Autologous Tissue Substitute from Right Acetabulum, Percutaneous Endoscopic Approach

0QP44JZ Removal of Synthetic Substitute from Right Acetabulum, Percutaneous Endoscopic Approach

0QP44KZ Removal of Nonautologous Tissue Substitute from Right Acetabulum, Percutaneous Endoscopic Approach

0QP4X4Z Removal of Internal Fixation Device from Right Acetabulum, External Approach

0QP4X5Z Removal of External Fixation Device from Right Acetabulum, External Approach

0QP504Z Removal of Internal Fixation Device from Left Acetabulum, Open Approach

0QP505Z Removal of External Fixation Device from Left Acetabulum, Open Approach

0QP507Z Removal of Autologous Tissue Substitute from Left Acetabulum, Open Approach

0QP50JZ Removal of Synthetic Substitute from Left Acetabulum, Open Approach

0QP50KZ Removal of Nonautologous Tissue Substitute from Left Acetabulum, Open Approach

0QP534Z Removal of Internal Fixation Device from Left Acetabulum, Percutaneous Approach

0QP535Z Removal of External Fixation Device from Left Acetabulum, Percutaneous Approach

0QP537Z Removal of Autologous Tissue Substitute from Left Acetabulum, Percutaneous Approach

0QP53JZ Removal of Synthetic Substitute from Left Acetabulum, Percutaneous Approach

0QP53KZ Removal of Nonautologous Tissue Substitute from Left Acetabulum, Percutaneous Approach

0QP544Z Removal of Internal Fixation Device from Left Acetabulum, Percutaneous Endoscopic Approach

0QP545Z Removal of External Fixation Device from Left Acetabulum, Percutaneous Endoscopic Approach

0QP547Z Removal of Autologous Tissue Substitute from Left Acetabulum, Percutaneous Endoscopic Approach

0QP54JZ Removal of Synthetic Substitute from Left Acetabulum, Percutaneous Endoscopic Approach

0QP54KZ Removal of Nonautologous Tissue Substitute from Left Acetabulum, Percutaneous Endoscopic Approach

0QP5X4Z Removal of Internal Fixation Device from Left Acetabulum, External Approach

0QP5X5Z Removal of External Fixation Device from Left Acetabulum, External Approach

0QP604Z Removal of Internal Fixation Device from Right Upper Femur, Open Approach

0QP605Z Removal of External Fixation Device from Right Upper Femur, Open Approach

0QP607Z Removal of Autologous Tissue Substitute from Right Upper Femur, Open Approach

0QP60JZ Removal of Synthetic Substitute from Right Upper Femur, Open Approach

0QP60KZ Removal of Nonautologous Tissue Substitute from Right Upper Femur, Open Approach

0QP634Z Removal of Internal Fixation Device from Right Upper Femur, Percutaneous Approach

0QP635Z Removal of External Fixation Device from Right Upper Femur, Percutaneous Approach

0QP637Z Removal of Autologous Tissue Substitute from Right Upper Femur, Percutaneous Approach

0QP63JZ Removal of Synthetic Substitute from Right Upper Femur, Percutaneous Approach

0QP63KZ Removal of Nonautologous Tissue Substitute from Right Upper Femur, Percutaneous Approach

0QP644Z Removal of Internal Fixation Device from Right Upper Femur, Percutaneous Endoscopic Approach

0QP645Z Removal of External Fixation Device from Right Upper Femur, Percutaneous Endoscopic Approach

0QP647Z Removal of Autologous Tissue Substitute from Right Upper Femur, Percutaneous Endoscopic Approach

0QP64JZ Removal of Synthetic Substitute from Right Upper Femur, Percutaneous Endoscopic Approach

0QP64KZ Removal of Nonautologous Tissue Substitute from Right Upper Femur, Percutaneous Endoscopic Approach

0QP6X4Z Removal of Internal Fixation Device from Right Upper Femur, External Approach

0QP6X5Z Removal of External Fixation Device from Right Upper Femur, External Approach

0QP704Z Removal of Internal Fixation Device from Left Upper Femur, Open Approach

0QP705Z Removal of External Fixation Device from Left Upper Femur, Open Approach

0QP707Z Removal of Autologous Tissue Substitute from Left Upper Femur, Open Approach

0QP70JZ Removal of Synthetic Substitute from Left Upper Femur, Open Approach

0QP70KZ Removal of Nonautologous Tissue Substitute from Left Upper Femur, Open Approach

0QP734Z Removal of Internal Fixation Device from Left Upper Femur, Percutaneous Approach

0QP735Z Removal of External Fixation Device from Left Upper Femur, Percutaneous Approach

0QP737Z Removal of Autologous Tissue Substitute from Left Upper Femur, Percutaneous Approach

0QP73JZ Removal of Synthetic Substitute from Left Upper Femur, Percutaneous Approach

0QP73KZ Removal of Nonautologous Tissue Substitute from Left Upper Femur, Percutaneous Approach

0QP744Z Removal of Internal Fixation Device from Left Upper Femur, Percutaneous Endoscopic Approach

0QP745Z Removal of External Fixation Device from Left Upper Femur, Percutaneous Endoscopic Approach

0QP747Z Removal of Autologous Tissue Substitute from Left Upper Femur, Percutaneous Endoscopic Approach

0QP74JZ Removal of Synthetic Substitute from Left Upper Femur, Percutaneous Endoscopic Approach

0QP74KZ Removal of Nonautologous Tissue Substitute from Left Upper Femur, Percutaneous Endoscopic Approach

0QP7X4Z Removal of Internal Fixation Device from Left Upper Femur, External Approach

0QP7X5Z Removal of External Fixation Device from Left Upper Femur, External Approach

0QP804Z Removal of Internal Fixation Device from Right Femoral Shaft, Open Approach

0QP805Z Removal of External Fixation Device from Right Femoral Shaft, Open Approach

0QP807Z Removal of Autologous Tissue Substitute from Right Femoral Shaft, Open Approach

0QP80JZ Removal of Synthetic Substitute from Right Femoral Shaft, Open Approach

0QP80KZ Removal of Nonautologous Tissue Substitute from Right Femoral Shaft, Open Approach

0QP834Z Removal of Internal Fixation Device from Right Femoral Shaft, Percutaneous Approach

0QP835Z Removal of External Fixation Device from Right Femoral Shaft, Percutaneous Approach

0QP837Z Removal of Autologous Tissue Substitute from Right Femoral Shaft, Percutaneous Approach

0QP83JZ Removal of Synthetic Substitute from Right Femoral Shaft, Percutaneous Approach

0QP83KZ Removal of Nonautologous Tissue Substitute from Right Femoral Shaft, Percutaneous Approach

0QP844Z Removal of Internal Fixation Device from Right Femoral Shaft, Percutaneous Endoscopic Approach

0QP845Z Removal of External Fixation Device from Right Femoral Shaft, Percutaneous Endoscopic Approach

0QP847Z Removal of Autologous Tissue Substitute from Right Femoral Shaft, Percutaneous Endoscopic Approach

0QP84JZ Removal of Synthetic Substitute from Right Femoral Shaft, Percutaneous Endoscopic Approach

0QP84KZ Removal of Nonautologous Tissue Substitute from Right Femoral Shaft, Percutaneous Endoscopic Approach

0QP8X4Z Removal of Internal Fixation Device from Right Femoral Shaft, External Approach

0QP8X5Z Removal of External Fixation Device from Right Femoral Shaft, External Approach

0QP904Z Removal of Internal Fixation Device from Left Femoral Shaft, Open Approach

0QP905Z Removal of External Fixation Device from Left Femoral Shaft, Open Approach

0QP907Z Removal of Autologous Tissue Substitute from Left Femoral Shaft, Open Approach

0QP90JZ Removal of Synthetic Substitute from Left Femoral Shaft, Open Approach

0QP90KZ Removal of Nonautologous Tissue Substitute from Left Femoral Shaft, Open Approach

0QP934Z Removal of Internal Fixation Device from Left Femoral Shaft, Percutaneous Approach

0QP935Z Removal of External Fixation Device from Left Femoral Shaft, Percutaneous Approach

0QP937Z Removal of Autologous Tissue Substitute from Left Femoral Shaft, Percutaneous Approach

0QP93JZ Removal of Synthetic Substitute from Left Femoral Shaft, Percutaneous Approach

0QP93KZ Removal of Nonautologous Tissue Substitute from Left Femoral Shaft, Percutaneous Approach

0QP944Z Removal of Internal Fixation Device from Left Femoral Shaft, Percutaneous Endoscopic Approach

0QP945Z Removal of External Fixation Device from Left Femoral Shaft, Percutaneous Endoscopic Approach

0QP947Z Removal of Autologous Tissue Substitute from Left Femoral Shaft, Percutaneous Endoscopic Approach

0QP94JZ Removal of Synthetic Substitute from Left Femoral Shaft, Percutaneous Endoscopic Approach

0QP94KZ Removal of Nonautologous Tissue Substitute from Left Femoral Shaft, Percutaneous Endoscopic Approach

0QP9X4Z Removal of Internal Fixation Device from Left Femoral Shaft, External Approach

0QP9X5Z Removal of External Fixation Device from Left Femoral Shaft, External Approach

0QPB04Z Removal of Internal Fixation Device from Right Lower Femur, Open Approach

0QPB05Z Removal of External Fixation Device from Right Lower Femur, Open Approach

0QPB07Z Removal of Autologous Tissue Substitute from Right Lower Femur, Open Approach

0QPB0JZ Removal of Synthetic Substitute from Right Lower Femur, Open Approach

0QPB0KZ Removal of Nonautologous Tissue Substitute from Right Lower Femur, Open Approach

0QPB34Z Removal of Internal Fixation Device from Right Lower Femur, Percutaneous Approach

0QPB35Z Removal of External Fixation Device from Right Lower Femur, Percutaneous Approach

0QPB37Z Removal of Autologous Tissue Substitute from Right Lower Femur, Percutaneous Approach

0QPB3JZ Removal of Synthetic Substitute from Right Lower Femur, Percutaneous Approach

0QPB3KZ Removal of Nonautologous Tissue Substitute from Right Lower Femur, Percutaneous Approach

0QPB44Z Removal of Internal Fixation Device from Right Lower Femur, Percutaneous Endoscopic Approach

0QPB45Z Removal of External Fixation Device from Right Lower Femur, Percutaneous Endoscopic Approach

0QPB47Z Removal of Autologous Tissue Substitute from Right Lower Femur, Percutaneous Endoscopic Approach

0QPB4JZ Removal of Synthetic Substitute from Right Lower Femur, Percutaneous Endoscopic Approach

0QPB4KZ Removal of Nonautologous Tissue Substitute from Right Lower Femur, Percutaneous Endoscopic Approach

0QPBX4Z Removal of Internal Fixation Device from Right Lower Femur, External Approach

0QPBX5Z Removal of External Fixation Device from Right Lower Femur, External Approach

0QPC04Z Removal of Internal Fixation Device from Left Lower Femur, Open Approach

0QPC05Z Removal of External Fixation Device from Left Lower Femur, Open Approach

0QPC07Z Removal of Autologous Tissue Substitute from Left Lower Femur, Open Approach

0QPC0JZ Removal of Synthetic Substitute from Left Lower Femur, Open Approach

0QPC0KZ Removal of Nonautologous Tissue Substitute from Left Lower Femur, Open Approach

0QPC34Z Removal of Internal Fixation Device from Left Lower Femur, Percutaneous Approach

0QPC35Z Removal of External Fixation Device from Left Lower Femur, Percutaneous Approach

0QPC37Z Removal of Autologous Tissue Substitute from Left Lower Femur, Percutaneous Approach

0QPC3JZ Removal of Synthetic Substitute from Left Lower Femur, Percutaneous Approach

0QPC3KZ Removal of Nonautologous Tissue Substitute from Left Lower Femur, Percutaneous Approach

0QPC44Z Removal of Internal Fixation Device from Left Lower Femur, Percutaneous Endoscopic Approach

0QPC45Z Removal of External Fixation Device from Left Lower Femur, Percutaneous Endoscopic Approach

0QPC47Z Removal of Autologous Tissue Substitute from Left Lower Femur, Percutaneous Endoscopic Approach

0QPC4JZ Removal of Synthetic Substitute from Left Lower Femur, Percutaneous Endoscopic Approach

0QPC4KZ Removal of Nonautologous Tissue Substitute from Left Lower Femur, Percutaneous Endoscopic Approach

0QPCX4Z Removal of Internal Fixation Device from Left Lower Femur, External Approach

0QPCX5Z Removal of External Fixation Device from Left Lower Femur, External Approach

0QPD04Z Removal of Internal Fixation Device from Right Patella, Open Approach

0QPD05Z Removal of External Fixation Device from Right Patella, Open Approach

0QPD07Z Removal of Autologous Tissue Substitute from Right Patella, Open Approach

0QPD0JZ Removal of Synthetic Substitute from Right Patella, Open Approach

0QPD0KZ Removal of Nonautologous Tissue Substitute from Right Patella, Open Approach

0QPD34Z Removal of Internal Fixation Device from Right Patella, Percutaneous Approach

0QPD35Z Removal of External Fixation Device from Right Patella, Percutaneous Approach

0QPD37Z Removal of Autologous Tissue Substitute from Right Patella, Percutaneous Approach

0QPD3JZ Removal of Synthetic Substitute from Right Patella, Percutaneous Approach

0QPD3KZ Removal of Nonautologous Tissue Substitute from Right Patella, Percutaneous Approach

0QPD44Z Removal of Internal Fixation Device from Right Patella, Percutaneous Endoscopic Approach

0QPD45Z Removal of External Fixation Device from Right Patella, Percutaneous Endoscopic Approach

0QPD47Z Removal of Autologous Tissue Substitute from Right Patella, Percutaneous Endoscopic Approach

0QPD4JZ Removal of Synthetic Substitute from Right Patella, Percutaneous Endoscopic Approach

0QPD4KZ Removal of Nonautologous Tissue Substitute from Right Patella, Percutaneous Endoscopic Approach

0QPDX4Z Removal of Internal Fixation Device from Right Patella, External Approach

0QPDX5Z Removal of External Fixation Device from Right Patella, External Approach

0QPF04Z Removal of Internal Fixation Device from Left Patella, Open Approach

0QPF05Z Removal of External Fixation Device from Left Patella, Open Approach

0QPF07Z Removal of Autologous Tissue Substitute from Left Patella, Open Approach

0QPF0JZ Removal of Synthetic Substitute from Left Patella, Open Approach

0QPF0KZ Removal of Nonautologous Tissue Substitute from Left Patella, Open Approach

0QPF34Z Removal of Internal Fixation Device from Left Patella, Percutaneous Approach

0QPF35Z Removal of External Fixation Device from Left Patella, Percutaneous Approach

0QPF37Z Removal of Autologous Tissue Substitute from Left Patella, Percutaneous Approach

0QPF3JZ Removal of Synthetic Substitute from Left Patella, Percutaneous Approach

0QPF3KZ Removal of Nonautologous Tissue Substitute from Left Patella, Percutaneous Approach

0QPF44Z Removal of Internal Fixation Device from Left Patella, Percutaneous Endoscopic Approach

0QPF45Z Removal of External Fixation Device from Left Patella, Percutaneous Endoscopic Approach

0QPF47Z Removal of Autologous Tissue Substitute from Left Patella, Percutaneous Endoscopic Approach

0QPF4JZ Removal of Synthetic Substitute from Left Patella, Percutaneous Endoscopic Approach

0QPF4KZ Removal of Nonautologous Tissue Substitute from Left Patella, Percutaneous Endoscopic Approach

0QPFX4Z Removal of Internal Fixation Device from Left Patella, External Approach

0QPFX5Z   Removal of External Fixation Device from Left Patella, External Approach

0QPG04Z   Removal of Internal Fixation Device from Right Tibia, Open Approach
AHA CC: 2Q, 2015, 6-7

0QPG05Z   Removal of External Fixation Device from Right Tibia, Open Approach

0QPG07Z   Removal of Autologous Tissue Substitute from Right Tibia, Open Approach

0QPG0JZ   Removal of Synthetic Substitute from Right Tibia, Open Approach

0QPG0KZ   Removal of Nonautologous Tissue Substitute from Right Tibia, Open Approach

0QPG34Z   Removal of Internal Fixation Device from Right Tibia, Percutaneous Approach

0QPG35Z   Removal of External Fixation Device from Right Tibia, Percutaneous Approach

0QPG37Z   Removal of Autologous Tissue Substitute from Right Tibia, Percutaneous Approach

0QPG3JZ   Removal of Synthetic Substitute from Right Tibia, Percutaneous Approach

0QPG3KZ   Removal of Nonautologous Tissue Substitute from Right Tibia, Percutaneous Approach

0QPG44Z   Removal of Internal Fixation Device from Right Tibia, Percutaneous Endoscopic Approach

0QPG45Z   Removal of External Fixation Device from Right Tibia, Percutaneous Endoscopic Approach

0QPG47Z   Removal of Autologous Tissue Substitute from Right Tibia, Percutaneous Endoscopic Approach

0QPG4JZ   Removal of Synthetic Substitute from Right Tibia, Percutaneous Endoscopic Approach

0QPG4KZ   Removal of Nonautologous Tissue Substitute from Right Tibia, Percutaneous Endoscopic Approach

0QPGX4Z   Removal of Internal Fixation Device from Right Tibia, External Approach

0QPGX5Z   Removal of External Fixation Device from Right Tibia, External Approach

0QPH04Z   Removal of Internal Fixation Device from Left Tibia, Open Approach

0QPH05Z   Removal of External Fixation Device from Left Tibia, Open Approach

0QPH07Z   Removal of Autologous Tissue Substitute from Left Tibia, Open Approach

0QPH0JZ   Removal of Synthetic Substitute from Left Tibia, Open Approach

0QPH0KZ   Removal of Nonautologous Tissue Substitute from Left Tibia, Open Approach

0QPH34Z   Removal of Internal Fixation Device from Left Tibia, Percutaneous Approach

0QPH35Z   Removal of External Fixation Device from Left Tibia, Percutaneous Approach

0QPH37Z   Removal of Autologous Tissue Substitute from Left Tibia, Percutaneous Approach

0QPH3JZ   Removal of Synthetic Substitute from Left Tibia, Percutaneous Approach

0QPH3KZ   Removal of Nonautologous Tissue Substitute from Left Tibia, Percutaneous Approach

0QPH44Z   Removal of Internal Fixation Device from Left Tibia, Percutaneous Endoscopic Approach

0QPH45Z   Removal of External Fixation Device from Left Tibia, Percutaneous Endoscopic Approach

0QPH47Z   Removal of Autologous Tissue Substitute from Left Tibia, Percutaneous Endoscopic Approach

0QPH4JZ   Removal of Synthetic Substitute from Left Tibia, Percutaneous Endoscopic Approach

0QPH4KZ   Removal of Nonautologous Tissue Substitute from Left Tibia, Percutaneous Endoscopic Approach

0QPHX4Z   Removal of Internal Fixation Device from Left Tibia, External Approach

0QPHX5Z   Removal of External Fixation Device from Left Tibia, External Approach

0QPJ04Z   Removal of Internal Fixation Device from Right Fibula, Open Approach

0QPJ05Z   Removal of External Fixation Device from Right Fibula, Open Approach

0QPJ07Z   Removal of Autologous Tissue Substitute from Right Fibula, Open Approach

0QPJ0JZ   Removal of Synthetic Substitute from Right Fibula, Open Approach

0QPJ0KZ   Removal of Nonautologous Tissue Substitute from Right Fibula, Open Approach

0QPJ34Z   Removal of Internal Fixation Device from Right Fibula, Percutaneous Approach

0QPJ35Z   Removal of External Fixation Device from Right Fibula, Percutaneous Approach

0QPJ37Z   Removal of Autologous Tissue Substitute from Right Fibula, Percutaneous Approach

0QPJ3JZ   Removal of Synthetic Substitute from Right Fibula, Percutaneous Approach

0QPJ3KZ   Removal of Nonautologous Tissue Substitute from Right Fibula, Percutaneous Approach

0QPJ44Z   Removal of Internal Fixation Device from Right Fibula, Percutaneous Endoscopic Approach

0QPJ45Z   Removal of External Fixation Device from Right Fibula, Percutaneous Endoscopic Approach

0QPJ47Z   Removal of Autologous Tissue Substitute from Right Fibula, Percutaneous Endoscopic Approach

0QPJ4JZ   Removal of Synthetic Substitute from Right Fibula, Percutaneous Endoscopic Approach

0QPJ4KZ   Removal of Nonautologous Tissue Substitute from Right Fibula, Percutaneous Endoscopic Approach

0QPJX4Z   Removal of Internal Fixation Device from Right Fibula, External Approach

0QPJX5Z   Removal of External Fixation Device from Right Fibula, External Approach

0QPK04Z   Removal of Internal Fixation Device from Left Fibula, Open Approach

0QPK05Z   Removal of External Fixation Device from Left Fibula, Open Approach

0QPK07Z   Removal of Autologous Tissue Substitute from Left Fibula, Open Approach

0QPK0JZ   Removal of Synthetic Substitute from Left Fibula, Open Approach

0QPK0KZ   Removal of Nonautologous Tissue Substitute from Left Fibula, Open Approach

0QPK34Z   Removal of Internal Fixation Device from Left Fibula, Percutaneous Approach

0QPK35Z   Removal of External Fixation Device from Left Fibula, Percutaneous Approach

0QPK37Z   Removal of Autologous Tissue Substitute from Left Fibula, Percutaneous Approach

0QPK3JZ   Removal of Synthetic Substitute from Left Fibula, Percutaneous Approach

0QPK3KZ   Removal of Nonautologous Tissue Substitute from Left Fibula, Percutaneous Approach

0QPK44Z   Removal of Internal Fixation Device from Left Fibula, Percutaneous Endoscopic Approach

0QPK45Z   Removal of External Fixation Device from Left Fibula, Percutaneous Endoscopic Approach

0QPK47Z   Removal of Autologous Tissue Substitute from Left Fibula, Percutaneous Endoscopic Approach

0QPK4JZ   Removal of Synthetic Substitute from Left Fibula, Percutaneous Endoscopic Approach

0QPK4KZ   Removal of Nonautologous Tissue Substitute from Left Fibula, Percutaneous Endoscopic Approach

0QPKX4Z   Removal of Internal Fixation Device from Left Fibula, External Approach

0QPKX5Z   Removal of External Fixation Device from Left Fibula, External Approach

0QPL04Z   Removal of Internal Fixation Device from Right Tarsal, Open Approach

0QPL05Z   Removal of External Fixation Device from Right Tarsal, Open Approach

0QPL07Z   Removal of Autologous Tissue Substitute from Right Tarsal, Open Approach

0QPL0JZ   Removal of Synthetic Substitute from Right Tarsal, Open Approach

0QPL0KZ   Removal of Nonautologous Tissue Substitute from Right Tarsal, Open Approach

0QPL34Z   Removal of Internal Fixation Device from Right Tarsal, Percutaneous Approach

0QPL35Z   Removal of External Fixation Device from Right Tarsal, Percutaneous Approach

0QPL37Z   Removal of Autologous Tissue Substitute from Right Tarsal, Percutaneous Approach

0QPL3JZ   Removal of Synthetic Substitute from Right Tarsal, Percutaneous Approach

0QPL3KZ   Removal of Nonautologous Tissue Substitute from Right Tarsal, Percutaneous Approach

0QPL44Z   Removal of Internal Fixation Device from Right Tarsal, Percutaneous Endoscopic Approach

0QPL45Z   Removal of External Fixation Device from Right Tarsal, Percutaneous Endoscopic Approach

0QPL47Z   Removal of Autologous Tissue Substitute from Right Tarsal, Percutaneous Endoscopic Approach

0QPL4JZ   Removal of Synthetic Substitute from Right Tarsal, Percutaneous Endoscopic Approach

0QPL4KZ   Removal of Nonautologous Tissue Substitute from Right Tarsal, Percutaneous Endoscopic Approach

0QPLX4Z   Removal of Internal Fixation Device from Right Tarsal, External Approach

0QPLX5Z Removal of External Fixation Device from Right Tarsal, External Approach

0QPM04Z Removal of Internal Fixation Device from Left Tarsal, Open Approach

0QPM05Z Removal of External Fixation Device from Left Tarsal, Open Approach

0QPM07Z Removal of Autologous Tissue Substitute from Left Tarsal, Open Approach

0QPM0JZ Removal of Synthetic Substitute from Left Tarsal, Open Approach

0QPM0KZ Removal of Nonautologous Tissue Substitute from Left Tarsal, Open Approach

0QPM34Z Removal of Internal Fixation Device from Left Tarsal, Percutaneous Approach

0QPM35Z Removal of External Fixation Device from Left Tarsal, Percutaneous Approach

0QPM37Z Removal of Autologous Tissue Substitute from Left Tarsal, Percutaneous Approach

0QPM3JZ Removal of Synthetic Substitute from Left Tarsal, Percutaneous Approach

0QPM3KZ Removal of Nonautologous Tissue Substitute from Left Tarsal, Percutaneous Approach

0QPM44Z Removal of Internal Fixation Device from Left Tarsal, Percutaneous Endoscopic Approach

0QPM45Z Removal of External Fixation Device from Left Tarsal, Percutaneous Endoscopic Approach

0QPM47Z Removal of Autologous Tissue Substitute from Left Tarsal, Percutaneous Endoscopic Approach

0QPM4JZ Removal of Synthetic Substitute from Left Tarsal, Percutaneous Endoscopic Approach

0QPM4KZ Removal of Nonautologous Tissue Substitute from Left Tarsal, Percutaneous Endoscopic Approach

0QPMX4Z Removal of Internal Fixation Device from Left Tarsal, External Approach

0QPMX5Z Removal of External Fixation Device from Left Tarsal, External Approach

0QPN04Z Removal of Internal Fixation Device from Right Metatarsal, Open Approach

0QPN05Z Removal of External Fixation Device from Right Metatarsal, Open Approach

0QPN07Z Removal of Autologous Tissue Substitute from Right Metatarsal, Open Approach

0QPN0JZ Removal of Synthetic Substitute from Right Metatarsal, Open Approach

0QPN0KZ Removal of Nonautologous Tissue Substitute from Right Metatarsal, Open Approach

0QPN34Z Removal of Internal Fixation Device from Right Metatarsal, Percutaneous Approach

0QPN35Z Removal of External Fixation Device from Right Metatarsal, Percutaneous Approach

0QPN37Z Removal of Autologous Tissue Substitute from Right Metatarsal, Percutaneous Approach

0QPN3JZ Removal of Synthetic Substitute from Right Metatarsal, Percutaneous Approach

0QPN3KZ Removal of Nonautologous Tissue Substitute from Right Metatarsal, Percutaneous Approach

0QPN44Z Removal of Internal Fixation Device from Right Metatarsal, Percutaneous Endoscopic Approach

0QPN45Z Removal of External Fixation Device from Right Metatarsal, Percutaneous Endoscopic Approach

0QPN47Z Removal of Autologous Tissue Substitute from Right Metatarsal, Percutaneous Endoscopic Approach

0QPN4JZ Removal of Synthetic Substitute from Right Metatarsal, Percutaneous Endoscopic Approach

0QPN4KZ Removal of Nonautologous Tissue Substitute from Right Metatarsal, Percutaneous Endoscopic Approach

0QPNX4Z Removal of Internal Fixation Device from Right Metatarsal, External Approach

0QPNX5Z Removal of External Fixation Device from Right Metatarsal, External Approach

0QPP04Z Removal of Internal Fixation Device from Left Metatarsal, Open Approach

0QPP05Z Removal of External Fixation Device from Left Metatarsal, Open Approach

0QPP07Z Removal of Autologous Tissue Substitute from Left Metatarsal, Open Approach

0QPP0JZ Removal of Synthetic Substitute from Left Metatarsal, Open Approach

0QPP0KZ Removal of Nonautologous Tissue Substitute from Left Metatarsal, Open Approach

0QPP34Z Removal of Internal Fixation Device from Left Metatarsal, Percutaneous Approach

0QPP35Z Removal of External Fixation Device from Left Metatarsal, Percutaneous Approach

0QPP37Z Removal of Autologous Tissue Substitute from Left Metatarsal, Percutaneous Approach

0QPP3JZ Removal of Synthetic Substitute from Left Metatarsal, Percutaneous Approach

0QPP3KZ Removal of Nonautologous Tissue Substitute from Left Metatarsal, Percutaneous Approach

0QPP44Z Removal of Internal Fixation Device from Left Metatarsal, Percutaneous Endoscopic Approach

0QPP45Z Removal of External Fixation Device from Left Metatarsal, Percutaneous Endoscopic Approach

0QPP47Z Removal of Autologous Tissue Substitute from Left Metatarsal, Percutaneous Endoscopic Approach

0QPP4JZ Removal of Synthetic Substitute from Left Metatarsal, Percutaneous Endoscopic Approach

0QPP4KZ Removal of Nonautologous Tissue Substitute from Left Metatarsal, Percutaneous Endoscopic Approach

0QPPX4Z Removal of Internal Fixation Device from Left Metatarsal, External Approach

0QPPX5Z Removal of External Fixation Device from Left Metatarsal, External Approach

0QPQ04Z Removal of Internal Fixation Device from Right Toe Phalanx, Open Approach

0QPQ05Z Removal of External Fixation Device from Right Toe Phalanx, Open Approach

0QPQ07Z Removal of Autologous Tissue Substitute from Right Toe Phalanx, Open Approach

0QPQ0JZ Removal of Synthetic Substitute from Right Toe Phalanx, Open Approach

0QPQ0KZ Removal of Nonautologous Tissue Substitute from Right Toe Phalanx, Open Approach

0QPQ34Z Removal of Internal Fixation Device from Right Toe Phalanx, Percutaneous Approach

0QPQ35Z Removal of External Fixation Device from Right Toe Phalanx, Percutaneous Approach

0QPQ37Z Removal of Autologous Tissue Substitute from Right Toe Phalanx, Percutaneous Approach

0QPQ3JZ Removal of Synthetic Substitute from Right Toe Phalanx, Percutaneous Approach

0QPQ3KZ Removal of Nonautologous Tissue Substitute from Right Toe Phalanx, Percutaneous Approach

0QPQ44Z Removal of Internal Fixation Device from Right Toe Phalanx, Percutaneous Endoscopic Approach

0QPQ45Z Removal of External Fixation Device from Right Toe Phalanx, Percutaneous Endoscopic Approach

0QPQ47Z Removal of Autologous Tissue Substitute from Right Toe Phalanx, Percutaneous Endoscopic Approach

0QPQ4JZ Removal of Synthetic Substitute from Right Toe Phalanx, Percutaneous Endoscopic Approach

0QPQ4KZ Removal of Nonautologous Tissue Substitute from Right Toe Phalanx, Percutaneous Endoscopic Approach

0QPQX4Z Removal of Internal Fixation Device from Right Toe Phalanx, External Approach

0QPQX5Z Removal of External Fixation Device from Right Toe Phalanx, External Approach

0QPR04Z Removal of Internal Fixation Device from Left Toe Phalanx, Open Approach

0QPR05Z Removal of External Fixation Device from Left Toe Phalanx, Open Approach

0QPR07Z Removal of Autologous Tissue Substitute from Left Toe Phalanx, Open Approach

0QPR0JZ Removal of Synthetic Substitute from Left Toe Phalanx, Open Approach

0QPR0KZ Removal of Nonautologous Tissue Substitute from Left Toe Phalanx, Open Approach

0QPR34Z Removal of Internal Fixation Device from Left Toe Phalanx, Percutaneous Approach

0QPR35Z Removal of External Fixation Device from Left Toe Phalanx, Percutaneous Approach

0QPR37Z Removal of Autologous Tissue Substitute from Left Toe Phalanx, Percutaneous Approach

0QPR3JZ Removal of Synthetic Substitute from Left Toe Phalanx, Percutaneous Approach

0QPR3KZ Removal of Nonautologous Tissue Substitute from Left Toe Phalanx, Percutaneous Approach

0QPR44Z Removal of Internal Fixation Device from Left Toe Phalanx, Percutaneous Endoscopic Approach

0QPR45Z Removal of External Fixation Device from Left Toe Phalanx, Percutaneous Endoscopic Approach

♀ Female-only　　♂ Male-only　　▲ Limited Coverage　　● Non-OR　　HAC HAC-associated procedure　　▲ Non-covered procedures　　✚ Cluster

0QPR47Z Removal of Autologous Tissue Substitute from Left Toe Phalanx, Percutaneous Endoscopic Approach	**0QPS34Z** Removal of Internal Fixation Device from Coccyx, Percutaneous Approach	**0QPSX4Z** Removal of Internal Fixation Device from Coccyx, External Approach
0QPR4JZ Removal of Synthetic Substitute from Left Toe Phalanx, Percutaneous Endoscopic Approach	**0QPS35Z** Removal of External Fixation Device from Coccyx, Percutaneous Approach	**0QPSX5Z** Removal of External Fixation Device from Coccyx, External Approach
0QPR4KZ Removal of Nonautologous Tissue Substitute from Left Toe Phalanx, Percutaneous Endoscopic Approach	**0QPS37Z** Removal of Autologous Tissue Substitute from Coccyx, Percutaneous Approach	**0QPY00Z** Removal of Drainage Device from Lower Bone, Open Approach
0QPRX4Z Removal of Internal Fixation Device from Left Toe Phalanx, External Approach	**0QPS3JZ** Removal of Synthetic Substitute from Coccyx, Percutaneous Approach	**0QPY0MZ** Removal of Bone Growth Stimulator from Lower Bone, Open Approach
0QPRX5Z Removal of External Fixation Device from Left Toe Phalanx, External Approach	**0QPS3KZ** Removal of Nonautologous Tissue Substitute from Coccyx, Percutaneous Approach	**0QPY30Z** Removal of Drainage Device from Lower Bone, Percutaneous Approach
0QPS04Z Removal of Internal Fixation Device from Coccyx, Open Approach	**0QPS44Z** Removal of Internal Fixation Device from Coccyx, Percutaneous Endoscopic Approach	**0QPY3MZ** Removal of Bone Growth Stimulator from Lower Bone, Percutaneous Approach
0QPS05Z Removal of External Fixation Device from Coccyx, Open Approach	**0QPS45Z** Removal of External Fixation Device from Coccyx, Percutaneous Endoscopic Approach	**0QPY40Z** Removal of Drainage Device from Lower Bone, Percutaneous Endoscopic Approach
0QPS07Z Removal of Autologous Tissue Substitute from Coccyx, Open Approach	**0QPS47Z** Removal of Autologous Tissue Substitute from Coccyx, Percutaneous Endoscopic Approach	**0QPY4MZ** Removal of Bone Growth Stimulator from Lower Bone, Percutaneous Endoscopic Approach
0QPS0JZ Removal of Synthetic Substitute from Coccyx, Open Approach	**0QPS4JZ** Removal of Synthetic Substitute from Coccyx, Percutaneous Endoscopic Approach	**0QPYX0Z** Removal of Drainage Device from Lower Bone, External Approach
0QPS0KZ Removal of Nonautologous Tissue Substitute from Coccyx, Open Approach	**0QPS4KZ** Removal of Nonautologous Tissue Substitute from Coccyx, Percutaneous Endoscopic Approach	**0QPYXMZ** Removal of Bone Growth Stimulator from Lower Bone, External Approach

0QQ – Lower Bones, Repair

Review Coding Guideline B3.5

0QQ00ZZ Repair Lumbar Vertebra, Open Approach	**0QQ53ZZ** Repair Left Acetabulum, Percutaneous Approach	**0QQBXZZ** Repair Right Lower Femur, External Approach
0QQ03ZZ Repair Lumbar Vertebra, Percutaneous Approach	**0QQ54ZZ** Repair Left Acetabulum, Percutaneous Endoscopic Approach	**0QQC0ZZ** Repair Left Lower Femur, Open Approach
0QQ04ZZ Repair Lumbar Vertebra, Percutaneous Endoscopic Approach	**0QQ5XZZ** Repair Left Acetabulum, External Approach	**0QQC3ZZ** Repair Left Lower Femur, Percutaneous Approach
0QQ0XZZ Repair Lumbar Vertebra, External Approach	**0QQ60ZZ** Repair Right Upper Femur, Open Approach	**0QQC4ZZ** Repair Left Lower Femur, Percutaneous Endoscopic Approach
0QQ10ZZ Repair Sacrum, Open Approach	**0QQ63ZZ** Repair Right Upper Femur, Percutaneous Approach	**0QQCXZZ** Repair Left Lower Femur, External Approach
AHA CC: 3Q, 2014, 24	**0QQ64ZZ** Repair Right Upper Femur, Percutaneous Endoscopic Approach	**0QQD0ZZ** Repair Right Patella, Open Approach
0QQ13ZZ Repair Sacrum, Percutaneous Approach	**0QQ6XZZ** Repair Right Upper Femur, External Approach	**0QQD3ZZ** Repair Right Patella, Percutaneous Approach
0QQ14ZZ Repair Sacrum, Percutaneous Endoscopic Approach	**0QQ70ZZ** Repair Left Upper Femur, Open Approach	**0QQD4ZZ** Repair Right Patella, Percutaneous Endoscopic Approach
0QQ1XZZ Repair Sacrum, External Approach	**0QQ73ZZ** Repair Left Upper Femur, Percutaneous Approach	**0QQDXZZ** Repair Right Patella, External Approach
0QQ20ZZ Repair Right Pelvic Bone, Open Approach	**0QQ74ZZ** Repair Left Upper Femur, Percutaneous Endoscopic Approach	**0QQF0ZZ** Repair Left Patella, Open Approach
AHA CC: 1Q, 2018, 15	**0QQ7XZZ** Repair Left Upper Femur, External Approach	**0QQF3ZZ** Repair Left Patella, Percutaneous Approach
0QQ23ZZ Repair Right Pelvic Bone, Percutaneous Approach	**0QQ80ZZ** Repair Right Femoral Shaft, Open Approach	**0QQF4ZZ** Repair Left Patella, Percutaneous Endoscopic Approach
0QQ24ZZ Repair Right Pelvic Bone, Percutaneous Endoscopic Approach	**0QQ83ZZ** Repair Right Femoral Shaft, Percutaneous Approach	**0QQFXZZ** Repair Left Patella, External Approach
0QQ2XZZ Repair Right Pelvic Bone, External Approach	**0QQ84ZZ** Repair Right Femoral Shaft, Percutaneous Endoscopic Approach	**0QQG0ZZ** Repair Right Tibia, Open Approach
0QQ30ZZ Repair Left Pelvic Bone, Open Approach	**0QQ8XZZ** Repair Right Femoral Shaft, External Approach	**0QQG3ZZ** Repair Right Tibia, Percutaneous Approach
AHA CC: 1Q, 2018, 15	**0QQ90ZZ** Repair Left Femoral Shaft, Open Approach	**0QQG4ZZ** Repair Right Tibia, Percutaneous Endoscopic Approach
0QQ33ZZ Repair Left Pelvic Bone, Percutaneous Approach	**0QQ93ZZ** Repair Left Femoral Shaft, Percutaneous Approach	**0QQGXZZ** Repair Right Tibia, External Approach
0QQ34ZZ Repair Left Pelvic Bone, Percutaneous Endoscopic Approach	**0QQ94ZZ** Repair Left Femoral Shaft, Percutaneous Endoscopic Approach	**0QQH0ZZ** Repair Left Tibia, Open Approach
0QQ3XZZ Repair Left Pelvic Bone, External Approach	**0QQ9XZZ** Repair Left Femoral Shaft, External Approach	**0QQH3ZZ** Repair Left Tibia, Percutaneous Approach
0QQ40ZZ Repair Right Acetabulum, Open Approach	**0QQB0ZZ** Repair Right Lower Femur, Open Approach	**0QQH4ZZ** Repair Left Tibia, Percutaneous Endoscopic Approach
0QQ43ZZ Repair Right Acetabulum, Percutaneous Approach	**0QQB3ZZ** Repair Right Lower Femur, Percutaneous Approach	**0QQHXZZ** Repair Left Tibia, External Approach
0QQ44ZZ Repair Right Acetabulum, Percutaneous Endoscopic Approach	**0QQB4ZZ** Repair Right Lower Femur, Percutaneous Endoscopic Approach	**0QQJ0ZZ** Repair Right Fibula, Open Approach
0QQ4XZZ Repair Right Acetabulum, External Approach		**0QQJ3ZZ** Repair Right Fibula, Percutaneous Approach
0QQ50ZZ Repair Left Acetabulum, Open Approach		**0QQJ4ZZ** Repair Right Fibula, Percutaneous Endoscopic Approach
		0QQJXZZ Repair Right Fibula, External Approach

0QQK0ZZ	Repair Left Fibula, Open Approach	0QQN0ZZ	Repair Right Metatarsal, Open Approach	0QQQ4ZZ	Repair Right Toe Phalanx, Percutaneous Endoscopic Approach
0QQK3ZZ	Repair Left Fibula, Percutaneous Approach	0QQN3ZZ	Repair Right Metatarsal, Percutaneous Approach	0QQQXZZ	Repair Right Toe Phalanx, External Approach
0QQK4ZZ	Repair Left Fibula, Percutaneous Endoscopic Approach	0QQN4ZZ	Repair Right Metatarsal, Percutaneous Endoscopic Approach	0QQR0ZZ	Repair Left Toe Phalanx, Open Approach
0QQKXZZ	Repair Left Fibula, External Approach	0QQNXZZ	Repair Right Metatarsal, External Approach	0QQR3ZZ	Repair Left Toe Phalanx, Percutaneous Approach
0QQL0ZZ	Repair Right Tarsal, Open Approach	0QQP0ZZ	Repair Left Metatarsal, Open Approach	0QQR4ZZ	Repair Left Toe Phalanx, Percutaneous Endoscopic Approach
0QQL3ZZ	Repair Right Tarsal, Percutaneous Approach	0QQP3ZZ	Repair Left Metatarsal, Percutaneous Approach	0QQRXZZ	Repair Left Toe Phalanx, External Approach
0QQL4ZZ	Repair Right Tarsal, Percutaneous Endoscopic Approach	0QQP4ZZ	Repair Left Metatarsal, Percutaneous Endoscopic Approach	0QQS0ZZ	Repair Coccyx, Open Approach
0QQLXZZ	Repair Right Tarsal, External Approach	0QQPXZZ	Repair Left Metatarsal, External Approach	0QQS3ZZ	Repair Coccyx, Percutaneous Approach
0QQM0ZZ	Repair Left Tarsal, Open Approach	0QQQ0ZZ	Repair Right Toe Phalanx, Open Approach	0QQS4ZZ	Repair Coccyx, Percutaneous Endoscopic Approach
0QQM3ZZ	Repair Left Tarsal, Percutaneous Approach	0QQQ3ZZ	Repair Right Toe Phalanx, Percutaneous Approach	0QQSXZZ	Repair Coccyx, External Approach
0QQM4ZZ	Repair Left Tarsal, Percutaneous Endoscopic Approach				
0QQMXZZ	Repair Left Tarsal, External Approach				

0QR – Lower Bones, Replacement

Review Coding Guideline B3.18

0QR007Z	Replacement of Lumbar Vertebra with Autologous Tissue Substitute, Open Approach	0QR207Z	Replacement of Right Pelvic Bone with Autologous Tissue Substitute, Open Approach	0QR34KZ	Replacement of Left Pelvic Bone with Nonautologous Tissue Substitute, Percutaneous Endoscopic Approach
0QR00JZ	Replacement of Lumbar Vertebra with Synthetic Substitute, Open Approach	0QR20JZ	Replacement of Right Pelvic Bone with Synthetic Substitute, Open Approach	0QR407Z	Replacement of Right Acetabulum with Autologous Tissue Substitute, Open Approach
0QR00KZ	Replacement of Lumbar Vertebra with Nonautologous Tissue Substitute, Open Approach	0QR20KZ	Replacement of Right Pelvic Bone with Nonautologous Tissue Substitute, Open Approach	0QR40JZ	Replacement of Right Acetabulum with Synthetic Substitute, Open Approach
0QR037Z	Replacement of Lumbar Vertebra with Autologous Tissue Substitute, Percutaneous Approach	0QR237Z	Replacement of Right Pelvic Bone with Autologous Tissue Substitute, Percutaneous Approach	0QR40KZ	Replacement of Right Acetabulum with Nonautologous Tissue Substitute, Open Approach
0QR03JZ	Replacement of Lumbar Vertebra with Synthetic Substitute, Percutaneous Approach	0QR23JZ	Replacement of Right Pelvic Bone with Synthetic Substitute, Percutaneous Approach	0QR437Z	Replacement of Right Acetabulum with Autologous Tissue Substitute, Percutaneous Approach
0QR03KZ	Replacement of Lumbar Vertebra with Nonautologous Tissue Substitute, Percutaneous Approach	0QR23KZ	Replacement of Right Pelvic Bone with Nonautologous Tissue Substitute, Percutaneous Approach	0QR43JZ	Replacement of Right Acetabulum with Synthetic Substitute, Percutaneous Approach
0QR047Z	Replacement of Lumbar Vertebra with Autologous Tissue Substitute, Percutaneous Endoscopic Approach	0QR247Z	Replacement of Right Pelvic Bone with Autologous Tissue Substitute, Percutaneous Endoscopic Approach	0QR43KZ	Replacement of Right Acetabulum with Nonautologous Tissue Substitute, Percutaneous Approach
0QR04JZ	Replacement of Lumbar Vertebra with Synthetic Substitute, Percutaneous Endoscopic Approach	0QR24JZ	Replacement of Right Pelvic Bone with Synthetic Substitute, Percutaneous Endoscopic Approach	0QR447Z	Replacement of Right Acetabulum with Autologous Tissue Substitute, Percutaneous Endoscopic Approach
0QR04KZ	Replacement of Lumbar Vertebra with Nonautologous Tissue Substitute, Percutaneous Endoscopic Approach	0QR24KZ	Replacement of Right Pelvic Bone with Nonautologous Tissue Substitute, Percutaneous Endoscopic Approach	0QR44JZ	Replacement of Right Acetabulum with Synthetic Substitute, Percutaneous Endoscopic Approach
0QR107Z	Replacement of Sacrum with Autologous Tissue Substitute, Open Approach	0QR307Z	Replacement of Left Pelvic Bone with Autologous Tissue Substitute, Open Approach	0QR44KZ	Replacement of Right Acetabulum with Nonautologous Tissue Substitute, Percutaneous Endoscopic Approach
0QR10JZ	Replacement of Sacrum with Synthetic Substitute, Open Approach	0QR30JZ	Replacement of Left Pelvic Bone with Synthetic Substitute, Open Approach	0QR507Z	Replacement of Left Acetabulum with Autologous Tissue Substitute, Open Approach
0QR10KZ	Replacement of Sacrum with Nonautologous Tissue Substitute, Open Approach	0QR30KZ	Replacement of Left Pelvic Bone with Nonautologous Tissue Substitute, Open Approach	0QR50JZ	Replacement of Left Acetabulum with Synthetic Substitute, Open Approach
0QR137Z	Replacement of Sacrum with Autologous Tissue Substitute, Percutaneous Approach	0QR337Z	Replacement of Left Pelvic Bone with Autologous Tissue Substitute, Percutaneous Approach	0QR50KZ	Replacement of Left Acetabulum with Nonautologous Tissue Substitute, Open Approach
0QR13JZ	Replacement of Sacrum with Synthetic Substitute, Percutaneous Approach	0QR33JZ	Replacement of Left Pelvic Bone with Synthetic Substitute, Percutaneous Approach	0QR537Z	Replacement of Left Acetabulum with Autologous Tissue Substitute, Percutaneous Approach
0QR13KZ	Replacement of Sacrum with Nonautologous Tissue Substitute, Percutaneous Approach	0QR33KZ	Replacement of Left Pelvic Bone with Nonautologous Tissue Substitute, Percutaneous Approach	0QR53JZ	Replacement of Left Acetabulum with Synthetic Substitute, Percutaneous Approach
0QR147Z	Replacement of Sacrum with Autologous Tissue Substitute, Percutaneous Endoscopic Approach	0QR347Z	Replacement of Left Pelvic Bone with Autologous Tissue Substitute, Percutaneous Endoscopic Approach	0QR53KZ	Replacement of Left Acetabulum with Nonautologous Tissue Substitute, Percutaneous Approach
0QR14JZ	Replacement of Sacrum with Synthetic Substitute, Percutaneous Endoscopic Approach	0QR34JZ	Replacement of Left Pelvic Bone with Synthetic Substitute, Percutaneous Endoscopic Approach	0QR547Z	Replacement of Left Acetabulum with Autologous Tissue Substitute, Percutaneous Endoscopic Approach
0QR14KZ	Replacement of Sacrum with Nonautologous Tissue Substitute, Percutaneous Endoscopic Approach				

♀ Female-only   ♂ Male-only   ▲ Limited Coverage   ● Non-OR   ⬛ HAC-associated procedure   ▲ Non-covered procedures   ✚ Cluster

0QR54JZ	Replacement of Left Acetabulum with Synthetic Substitute, Percutaneous Endoscopic Approach
0QR54KZ	Replacement of Left Acetabulum with Nonautologous Tissue Substitute, Percutaneous Endoscopic Approach
0QR607Z	Replacement of Right Upper Femur with Autologous Tissue Substitute, Open Approach
0QR60JZ	Replacement of Right Upper Femur with Synthetic Substitute, Open Approach
0QR60KZ	Replacement of Right Upper Femur with Nonautologous Tissue Substitute, Open Approach
0QR637Z	Replacement of Right Upper Femur with Autologous Tissue Substitute, Percutaneous Approach
0QR63JZ	Replacement of Right Upper Femur with Synthetic Substitute, Percutaneous Approach
0QR63KZ	Replacement of Right Upper Femur with Nonautologous Tissue Substitute, Percutaneous Approach
0QR647Z	Replacement of Right Upper Femur with Autologous Tissue Substitute, Percutaneous Endoscopic Approach
0QR64JZ	Replacement of Right Upper Femur with Synthetic Substitute, Percutaneous Endoscopic Approach
0QR64KZ	Replacement of Right Upper Femur with Nonautologous Tissue Substitute, Percutaneous Endoscopic Approach
0QR707Z	Replacement of Left Upper Femur with Autologous Tissue Substitute, Open Approach
0QR70JZ	Replacement of Left Upper Femur with Synthetic Substitute, Open Approach
0QR70KZ	Replacement of Left Upper Femur with Nonautologous Tissue Substitute, Open Approach
0QR737Z	Replacement of Left Upper Femur with Autologous Tissue Substitute, Percutaneous Approach
0QR73JZ	Replacement of Left Upper Femur with Synthetic Substitute, Percutaneous Approach
0QR73KZ	Replacement of Left Upper Femur with Nonautologous Tissue Substitute, Percutaneous Approach
0QR747Z	Replacement of Left Upper Femur with Autologous Tissue Substitute, Percutaneous Endoscopic Approach
0QR74JZ	Replacement of Left Upper Femur with Synthetic Substitute, Percutaneous Endoscopic Approach
0QR74KZ	Replacement of Left Upper Femur with Nonautologous Tissue Substitute, Percutaneous Endoscopic Approach
0QR807Z	Replacement of Right Femoral Shaft with Autologous Tissue Substitute, Open Approach
0QR80JZ	Replacement of Right Femoral Shaft with Synthetic Substitute, Open Approach
0QR80KZ	Replacement of Right Femoral Shaft with Nonautologous Tissue Substitute, Open Approach
0QR837Z	Replacement of Right Femoral Shaft with Autologous Tissue Substitute, Percutaneous Approach
0QR83JZ	Replacement of Right Femoral Shaft with Synthetic Substitute, Percutaneous Approach
0QR83KZ	Replacement of Right Femoral Shaft with Nonautologous Tissue Substitute, Percutaneous Approach

0QR847Z	Replacement of Right Femoral Shaft with Autologous Tissue Substitute, Percutaneous Endoscopic Approach
0QR84JZ	Replacement of Right Femoral Shaft with Synthetic Substitute, Percutaneous Endoscopic Approach
0QR84KZ	Replacement of Right Femoral Shaft with Nonautologous Tissue Substitute, Percutaneous Endoscopic Approach
0QR907Z	Replacement of Left Femoral Shaft with Autologous Tissue Substitute, Open Approach
0QR90JZ	Replacement of Left Femoral Shaft with Synthetic Substitute, Open Approach
0QR90KZ	Replacement of Left Femoral Shaft with Nonautologous Tissue Substitute, Open Approach
0QR937Z	Replacement of Left Femoral Shaft with Autologous Tissue Substitute, Percutaneous Approach
0QR93JZ	Replacement of Left Femoral Shaft with Synthetic Substitute, Percutaneous Approach
0QR93KZ	Replacement of Left Femoral Shaft with Nonautologous Tissue Substitute, Percutaneous Approach
0QR947Z	Replacement of Left Femoral Shaft with Autologous Tissue Substitute, Percutaneous Endoscopic Approach
0QR94JZ	Replacement of Left Femoral Shaft with Synthetic Substitute, Percutaneous Endoscopic Approach
0QR94KZ	Replacement of Left Femoral Shaft with Nonautologous Tissue Substitute, Percutaneous Endoscopic Approach
0QRB07Z	Replacement of Right Lower Femur with Autologous Tissue Substitute, Open Approach
0QRB0JZ	Replacement of Right Lower Femur with Synthetic Substitute, Open Approach
0QRB0KZ	Replacement of Right Lower Femur with Nonautologous Tissue Substitute, Open Approach
0QRB37Z	Replacement of Right Lower Femur with Autologous Tissue Substitute, Percutaneous Approach
0QRB3JZ	Replacement of Right Lower Femur with Synthetic Substitute, Percutaneous Approach
0QRB3KZ	Replacement of Right Lower Femur with Nonautologous Tissue Substitute, Percutaneous Approach
0QRB47Z	Replacement of Right Lower Femur with Autologous Tissue Substitute, Percutaneous Endoscopic Approach
0QRB4JZ	Replacement of Right Lower Femur with Synthetic Substitute, Percutaneous Endoscopic Approach
0QRB4KZ	Replacement of Right Lower Femur with Nonautologous Tissue Substitute, Percutaneous Endoscopic Approach
0QRC07Z	Replacement of Left Lower Femur with Autologous Tissue Substitute, Open Approach
0QRC0JZ	Replacement of Left Lower Femur with Synthetic Substitute, Open Approach
0QRC0KZ	Replacement of Left Lower Femur with Nonautologous Tissue Substitute, Open Approach
0QRC37Z	Replacement of Left Lower Femur with Autologous Tissue Substitute, Percutaneous Approach
0QRC3JZ	Replacement of Left Lower Femur with Synthetic Substitute, Percutaneous Approach

0QRC3KZ	Replacement of Left Lower Femur with Nonautologous Tissue Substitute, Percutaneous Approach
0QRC47Z	Replacement of Left Lower Femur with Autologous Tissue Substitute, Percutaneous Endoscopic Approach
0QRC4JZ	Replacement of Left Lower Femur with Synthetic Substitute, Percutaneous Endoscopic Approach
0QRC4KZ	Replacement of Left Lower Femur with Nonautologous Tissue Substitute, Percutaneous Endoscopic Approach
0QRD07Z	Replacement of Right Patella with Autologous Tissue Substitute, Open Approach
0QRD0JZ	Replacement of Right Patella with Synthetic Substitute, Open Approach
0QRD0KZ	Replacement of Right Patella with Nonautologous Tissue Substitute, Open Approach
0QRD37Z	Replacement of Right Patella with Autologous Tissue Substitute, Percutaneous Approach
0QRD3JZ	Replacement of Right Patella with Synthetic Substitute, Percutaneous Approach
0QRD3KZ	Replacement of Right Patella with Nonautologous Tissue Substitute, Percutaneous Approach
0QRD47Z	Replacement of Right Patella with Autologous Tissue Substitute, Percutaneous Endoscopic Approach
0QRD4JZ	Replacement of Right Patella with Synthetic Substitute, Percutaneous Endoscopic Approach
0QRD4KZ	Replacement of Right Patella with Nonautologous Tissue Substitute, Percutaneous Endoscopic Approach
0QRF07Z	Replacement of Left Patella with Autologous Tissue Substitute, Open Approach
0QRF0JZ	Replacement of Left Patella with Synthetic Substitute, Open Approach
0QRF0KZ	Replacement of Left Patella with Nonautologous Tissue Substitute, Open Approach
0QRF37Z	Replacement of Left Patella with Autologous Tissue Substitute, Percutaneous Approach
0QRF3JZ	Replacement of Left Patella with Synthetic Substitute, Percutaneous Approach
0QRF3KZ	Replacement of Left Patella with Nonautologous Tissue Substitute, Percutaneous Approach
0QRF47Z	Replacement of Left Patella with Autologous Tissue Substitute, Percutaneous Endoscopic Approach
0QRF4JZ	Replacement of Left Patella with Synthetic Substitute, Percutaneous Endoscopic Approach
0QRF4KZ	Replacement of Left Patella with Nonautologous Tissue Substitute, Percutaneous Endoscopic Approach
0QRG07Z	Replacement of Right Tibia with Autologous Tissue Substitute, Open Approach
0QRG0JZ	Replacement of Right Tibia with Synthetic Substitute, Open Approach
0QRG0KZ	Replacement of Right Tibia with Nonautologous Tissue Substitute, Open Approach
0QRG37Z	Replacement of Right Tibia with Autologous Tissue Substitute, Percutaneous Approach

♀ Female-only   ♂ Male-only   ▲ Limited Coverage   ● Non-OR   🔠 HAC-associated procedure   ▲ Non-covered procedures   ✚ Cluster

0QRG3JZ	Replacement of Right Tibia with Synthetic Substitute, Percutaneous Approach
0QRG3KZ	Replacement of Right Tibia with Nonautologous Tissue Substitute, Percutaneous Approach
0QRG47Z	Replacement of Right Tibia with Autologous Tissue Substitute, Percutaneous Endoscopic Approach
0QRG4JZ	Replacement of Right Tibia with Synthetic Substitute, Percutaneous Endoscopic Approach
0QRG4KZ	Replacement of Right Tibia with Nonautologous Tissue Substitute, Percutaneous Endoscopic Approach
0QRH07Z	Replacement of Left Tibia with Autologous Tissue Substitute, Open Approach
0QRH0JZ	Replacement of Left Tibia with Synthetic Substitute, Open Approach
0QRH0KZ	Replacement of Left Tibia with Nonautologous Tissue Substitute, Open Approach
0QRH37Z	Replacement of Left Tibia with Autologous Tissue Substitute, Percutaneous Approach
0QRH3JZ	Replacement of Left Tibia with Synthetic Substitute, Percutaneous Approach
0QRH3KZ	Replacement of Left Tibia with Nonautologous Tissue Substitute, Percutaneous Approach
0QRH47Z	Replacement of Left Tibia with Autologous Tissue Substitute, Percutaneous Endoscopic Approach
0QRH4JZ	Replacement of Left Tibia with Synthetic Substitute, Percutaneous Endoscopic Approach
0QRH4KZ	Replacement of Left Tibia with Nonautologous Tissue Substitute, Percutaneous Endoscopic Approach
0QRJ07Z	Replacement of Right Fibula with Autologous Tissue Substitute, Open Approach
0QRJ0JZ	Replacement of Right Fibula with Synthetic Substitute, Open Approach
0QRJ0KZ	Replacement of Right Fibula with Nonautologous Tissue Substitute, Open Approach
0QRJ37Z	Replacement of Right Fibula with Autologous Tissue Substitute, Percutaneous Approach
0QRJ3JZ	Replacement of Right Fibula with Synthetic Substitute, Percutaneous Approach
0QRJ3KZ	Replacement of Right Fibula with Nonautologous Tissue Substitute, Percutaneous Approach
0QRJ47Z	Replacement of Right Fibula with Autologous Tissue Substitute, Percutaneous Endoscopic Approach
0QRJ4JZ	Replacement of Right Fibula with Synthetic Substitute, Percutaneous Endoscopic Approach
0QRJ4KZ	Replacement of Right Fibula with Nonautologous Tissue Substitute, Percutaneous Endoscopic Approach
0QRK07Z	Replacement of Left Fibula with Autologous Tissue Substitute, Open Approach
0QRK0JZ	Replacement of Left Fibula with Synthetic Substitute, Open Approach
0QRK0KZ	Replacement of Left Fibula with Nonautologous Tissue Substitute, Open Approach
0QRK37Z	Replacement of Left Fibula with Autologous Tissue Substitute, Percutaneous Approach
0QRK3JZ	Replacement of Left Fibula with Synthetic Substitute, Percutaneous Approach
0QRK3KZ	Replacement of Left Fibula with Nonautologous Tissue Substitute, Percutaneous Approach
0QRK47Z	Replacement of Left Fibula with Autologous Tissue Substitute, Percutaneous Endoscopic Approach
0QRK4JZ	Replacement of Left Fibula with Synthetic Substitute, Percutaneous Endoscopic Approach
0QRK4KZ	Replacement of Left Fibula with Nonautologous Tissue Substitute, Percutaneous Endoscopic Approach
0QRL07Z	Replacement of Right Tarsal with Autologous Tissue Substitute, Open Approach
0QRL0JZ	Replacement of Right Tarsal with Synthetic Substitute, Open Approach
0QRL0KZ	Replacement of Right Tarsal with Nonautologous Tissue Substitute, Open Approach
0QRL37Z	Replacement of Right Tarsal with Autologous Tissue Substitute, Percutaneous Approach
0QRL3JZ	Replacement of Right Tarsal with Synthetic Substitute, Percutaneous Approach
0QRL3KZ	Replacement of Right Tarsal with Nonautologous Tissue Substitute, Percutaneous Approach
0QRL47Z	Replacement of Right Tarsal with Autologous Tissue Substitute, Percutaneous Endoscopic Approach
0QRL4JZ	Replacement of Right Tarsal with Synthetic Substitute, Percutaneous Endoscopic Approach
0QRL4KZ	Replacement of Right Tarsal with Nonautologous Tissue Substitute, Percutaneous Endoscopic Approach
0QRM07Z	Replacement of Left Tarsal with Autologous Tissue Substitute, Open Approach
0QRM0JZ	Replacement of Left Tarsal with Synthetic Substitute, Open Approach
0QRM0KZ	Replacement of Left Tarsal with Nonautologous Tissue Substitute, Open Approach
0QRM37Z	Replacement of Left Tarsal with Autologous Tissue Substitute, Percutaneous Approach
0QRM3JZ	Replacement of Left Tarsal with Synthetic Substitute, Percutaneous Approach
0QRM3KZ	Replacement of Left Tarsal with Nonautologous Tissue Substitute, Percutaneous Approach
0QRM47Z	Replacement of Left Tarsal with Autologous Tissue Substitute, Percutaneous Endoscopic Approach
0QRM4JZ	Replacement of Left Tarsal with Synthetic Substitute, Percutaneous Endoscopic Approach
0QRM4KZ	Replacement of Left Tarsal with Nonautologous Tissue Substitute, Percutaneous Endoscopic Approach
0QRN07Z	Replacement of Right Metatarsal with Autologous Tissue Substitute, Open Approach
0QRN0JZ	Replacement of Right Metatarsal with Synthetic Substitute, Open Approach
0QRN0KZ	Replacement of Right Metatarsal with Nonautologous Tissue Substitute, Open Approach
0QRN37Z	Replacement of Right Metatarsal with Autologous Tissue Substitute, Percutaneous Approach
0QRN3JZ	Replacement of Right Metatarsal with Synthetic Substitute, Percutaneous Approach
0QRN3KZ	Replacement of Right Metatarsal with Nonautologous Tissue Substitute, Percutaneous Approach
0QRN47Z	Replacement of Right Metatarsal with Autologous Tissue Substitute, Percutaneous Endoscopic Approach
0QRN4JZ	Replacement of Right Metatarsal with Synthetic Substitute, Percutaneous Endoscopic Approach
0QRN4KZ	Replacement of Right Metatarsal with Nonautologous Tissue Substitute, Percutaneous Endoscopic Approach
0QRP07Z	Replacement of Left Metatarsal with Autologous Tissue Substitute, Open Approach
0QRP0JZ	Replacement of Left Metatarsal with Synthetic Substitute, Open Approach
0QRP0KZ	Replacement of Left Metatarsal with Nonautologous Tissue Substitute, Open Approach
0QRP37Z	Replacement of Left Metatarsal with Autologous Tissue Substitute, Percutaneous Approach
0QRP3JZ	Replacement of Left Metatarsal with Synthetic Substitute, Percutaneous Approach
0QRP3KZ	Replacement of Left Metatarsal with Nonautologous Tissue Substitute, Percutaneous Approach
0QRP47Z	Replacement of Left Metatarsal with Autologous Tissue Substitute, Percutaneous Endoscopic Approach
0QRP4JZ	Replacement of Left Metatarsal with Synthetic Substitute, Percutaneous Endoscopic Approach
0QRP4KZ	Replacement of Left Metatarsal with Nonautologous Tissue Substitute, Percutaneous Endoscopic Approach
0QRQ07Z	Replacement of Right Toe Phalanx with Autologous Tissue Substitute, Open Approach
0QRQ0JZ	Replacement of Right Toe Phalanx with Synthetic Substitute, Open Approach
0QRQ0KZ	Replacement of Right Toe Phalanx with Nonautologous Tissue Substitute, Open Approach
0QRQ37Z	Replacement of Right Toe Phalanx with Autologous Tissue Substitute, Percutaneous Approach
0QRQ3JZ	Replacement of Right Toe Phalanx with Synthetic Substitute, Percutaneous Approach
0QRQ3KZ	Replacement of Right Toe Phalanx with Nonautologous Tissue Substitute, Percutaneous Approach
0QRQ47Z	Replacement of Right Toe Phalanx with Autologous Tissue Substitute, Percutaneous Endoscopic Approach
0QRQ4JZ	Replacement of Right Toe Phalanx with Synthetic Substitute, Percutaneous Endoscopic Approach
0QRQ4KZ	Replacement of Right Toe Phalanx with Nonautologous Tissue Substitute, Percutaneous Endoscopic Approach
0QRR07Z	Replacement of Left Toe Phalanx with Autologous Tissue Substitute, Open Approach

♀ Female-only　　♂ Male-only　　▲ Limited Coverage　　● Non-OR　　HAC HAC-associated procedure　　▲ Non-covered procedures　　✚ Cluster

0QRR0JZ Replacement of Left Toe Phalanx with Synthetic Substitute, Open Approach

0QRR0KZ Replacement of Left Toe Phalanx with Nonautologous Tissue Substitute, Open Approach

0QRR37Z Replacement of Left Toe Phalanx with Autologous Tissue Substitute, Percutaneous Approach

0QRR3JZ Replacement of Left Toe Phalanx with Synthetic Substitute, Percutaneous Approach

0QRR3KZ Replacement of Left Toe Phalanx with Nonautologous Tissue Substitute, Percutaneous Approach

0QRR47Z Replacement of Left Toe Phalanx with Autologous Tissue Substitute, Percutaneous Endoscopic Approach

0QRR4JZ Replacement of Left Toe Phalanx with Synthetic Substitute, Percutaneous Endoscopic Approach

0QRR4KZ Replacement of Left Toe Phalanx with Nonautologous Tissue Substitute, Percutaneous Endoscopic Approach

0QRS07Z Replacement of Coccyx with Autologous Tissue Substitute, Open Approach

0QRS0JZ Replacement of Coccyx with Synthetic Substitute, Open Approach

0QRS0KZ Replacement of Coccyx with Nonautologous Tissue Substitute, Open Approach

0QRS37Z Replacement of Coccyx with Autologous Tissue Substitute, Percutaneous Approach

0QRS3JZ Replacement of Coccyx with Synthetic Substitute, Percutaneous Approach

0QRS3KZ Replacement of Coccyx with Nonautologous Tissue Substitute, Percutaneous Approach

0QRS47Z Replacement of Coccyx with Autologous Tissue Substitute, Percutaneous Endoscopic Approach

0QRS4JZ Replacement of Coccyx with Synthetic Substitute, Percutaneous Endoscopic Approach

0QRS4KZ Replacement of Coccyx with Nonautologous Tissue Substitute, Percutaneous Endoscopic Approach

0QS – Lower Bones, Reposition

Review Coding Guideline B3.15

0QS003Z Reposition Lumbar Vertebra with Spinal Stabilization Device, Vertebral Body Tether, Open Approach

0QS004Z Reposition Lumbar Vertebra with Internal Fixation Device, Open Approach
AHA CC: 1Q, 2020, 33-34

0QS00ZZ Reposition Lumbar Vertebra, Open Approach

0QS034Z Reposition Lumbar Vertebra with Internal Fixation Device, Percutaneous Approach

0QS03ZZ Reposition Lumbar Vertebra, Percutaneous Approach

➕ *See table 0QU to construct a code for Supplement of with synthetic substitute.*

0QS043Z Reposition Lumbar Vertebra with Spinal Stabilization Device, Vertebral Body Tether, Percutaneous Endoscopic Approach

0QS044Z Reposition Lumbar Vertebra with Internal Fixation Device, Percutaneous Endoscopic Approach

0QS04ZZ Reposition Lumbar Vertebra, Percutaneous Endoscopic Approach

0QS0XZZ Reposition Lumbar Vertebra, External Approach

0QS104Z Reposition Sacrum with Internal Fixation Device, Open Approach

0QS10ZZ Reposition Sacrum, Open Approach

0QS134Z Reposition Sacrum with Internal Fixation Device, Percutaneous Approach

0QS13ZZ Reposition Sacrum, Percutaneous Approach

➕ *See table 0QU to construct a code for Supplement of with synthetic substitute.*

0QS144Z Reposition Sacrum with Internal Fixation Device, Percutaneous Endoscopic Approach

0QS14ZZ Reposition Sacrum, Percutaneous Endoscopic Approach

0QS1XZZ Reposition Sacrum, External Approach

0QS204Z Reposition Right Pelvic Bone with Internal Fixation Device, Open Approach

0QS205Z Reposition Right Pelvic Bone with External Fixation Device, Open Approach

0QS20ZZ Reposition Right Pelvic Bone, Open Approach

0QS234Z Reposition Right Pelvic Bone with Internal Fixation Device, Percutaneous Approach

0QS235Z Reposition Right Pelvic Bone with External Fixation Device, Percutaneous Approach

0QS23ZZ Reposition Right Pelvic Bone, Percutaneous Approach

0QS244Z Reposition Right Pelvic Bone with Internal Fixation Device, Percutaneous Endoscopic Approach

0QS245Z Reposition Right Pelvic Bone with External Fixation Device, Percutaneous Endoscopic Approach

0QS24ZZ Reposition Right Pelvic Bone, Percutaneous Endoscopic Approach

0QS2XZZ Reposition Right Pelvic Bone, External Approach

0QS304Z Reposition Left Pelvic Bone with Internal Fixation Device, Open Approach

0QS305Z Reposition Left Pelvic Bone with External Fixation Device, Open Approach

0QS30ZZ Reposition Left Pelvic Bone, Open Approach

0QS334Z Reposition Left Pelvic Bone with Internal Fixation Device, Percutaneous Approach

0QS335Z Reposition Left Pelvic Bone with External Fixation Device, Percutaneous Approach

0QS33ZZ Reposition Left Pelvic Bone, Percutaneous Approach

0QS344Z Reposition Left Pelvic Bone with Internal Fixation Device, Percutaneous Endoscopic Approach

0QS345Z Reposition Left Pelvic Bone with External Fixation Device, Percutaneous Endoscopic Approach

0QS34ZZ Reposition Left Pelvic Bone, Percutaneous Endoscopic Approach

0QS3XZZ Reposition Left Pelvic Bone, External Approach

0QS404Z Reposition Right Acetabulum with Internal Fixation Device, Open Approach

0QS40ZZ Reposition Right Acetabulum, Open Approach

0QS434Z Reposition Right Acetabulum with Internal Fixation Device, Percutaneous Approach

0QS43ZZ Reposition Right Acetabulum, Percutaneous Approach

0QS444Z Reposition Right Acetabulum with Internal Fixation Device, Percutaneous Endoscopic Approach

0QS44ZZ Reposition Right Acetabulum, Percutaneous Endoscopic Approach

0QS4XZZ Reposition Right Acetabulum, External Approach

0QS504Z Reposition Left Acetabulum with Internal Fixation Device, Open Approach
AHA CC: 2Q, 2016, 32; 1Q, 2018, 25

0QS50ZZ Reposition Left Acetabulum, Open Approach

0QS534Z Reposition Left Acetabulum with Internal Fixation Device, Percutaneous Approach

0QS53ZZ Reposition Left Acetabulum, Percutaneous Approach

0QS544Z Reposition Left Acetabulum with Internal Fixation Device, Percutaneous Endoscopic Approach

0QS54ZZ Reposition Left Acetabulum, Percutaneous Endoscopic Approach

0QS5XZZ Reposition Left Acetabulum, External Approach

0QS604Z Reposition Right Upper Femur with Internal Fixation Device, Open Approach

0QS605Z Reposition Right Upper Femur with External Fixation Device, Open Approach

0QS606Z Reposition Right Upper Femur with Intramedullary Internal Fixation Device, Open Approach

0QS60BZ Reposition Right Upper Femur with Monoplanar External Fixation Device, Open Approach

0QS60CZ Reposition Right Upper Femur with Ring External Fixation Device, Open Approach

0QS60DZ Reposition Right Upper Femur with Hybrid External Fixation Device, Open Approach

0QS60ZZ Reposition Right Upper Femur, Open Approach

0QS634Z Reposition Right Upper Femur with Internal Fixation Device, Percutaneous Approach

0QS635Z Reposition Right Upper Femur with External Fixation Device, Percutaneous Approach

0QS636Z Reposition Right Upper Femur with Intramedullary Internal Fixation Device, Percutaneous Approach

0QS63BZ Reposition Right Upper Femur with Monoplanar External Fixation Device, Percutaneous Approach

0QS63CZ Reposition Right Upper Femur with Ring External Fixation Device, Percutaneous Approach

0QS63DZ Reposition Right Upper Femur with Hybrid External Fixation Device, Percutaneous Approach

0QS63ZZ Reposition Right Upper Femur, Percutaneous Approach

0QS644Z Reposition Right Upper Femur with Internal Fixation Device, Percutaneous Endoscopic Approach

0QS645Z Reposition Right Upper Femur with External Fixation Device, Percutaneous Endoscopic Approach

0QS646Z Reposition Right Upper Femur with Intramedullary Internal Fixation Device, Percutaneous Endoscopic Approach

0QS64BZ Reposition Right Upper Femur with Monoplanar External Fixation Device, Percutaneous Endoscopic Approach

0QS64CZ Reposition Right Upper Femur with Ring External Fixation Device, Percutaneous Endoscopic Approach

0QS64DZ Reposition Right Upper Femur with Hybrid External Fixation Device, Percutaneous Endoscopic Approach

0QS64ZZ Reposition Right Upper Femur, Percutaneous Endoscopic Approach

0QS6XZZ Reposition Right Upper Femur, External Approach

0QS704Z Reposition Left Upper Femur with Internal Fixation Device, Open Approach

0QS705Z Reposition Left Upper Femur with External Fixation Device, Open Approach

0QS706Z Reposition Left Upper Femur with Intramedullary Internal Fixation Device, Open Approach

0QS70BZ Reposition Left Upper Femur with Monoplanar External Fixation Device, Open Approach

0QS70CZ Reposition Left Upper Femur with Ring External Fixation Device, Open Approach

0QS70DZ Reposition Left Upper Femur with Hybrid External Fixation Device, Open Approach

0QS70ZZ Reposition Left Upper Femur, Open Approach

0QS734Z Reposition Left Upper Femur with Internal Fixation Device, Percutaneous Approach

0QS735Z Reposition Left Upper Femur with External Fixation Device, Percutaneous Approach

0QS736Z Reposition Left Upper Femur with Intramedullary Internal Fixation Device, Percutaneous Approach

0QS73BZ Reposition Left Upper Femur with Monoplanar External Fixation Device, Percutaneous Approach

0QS73CZ Reposition Left Upper Femur with Ring External Fixation Device, Percutaneous Approach

0QS73DZ Reposition Left Upper Femur with Hybrid External Fixation Device, Percutaneous Approach

0QS73ZZ Reposition Left Upper Femur, Percutaneous Approach

0QS744Z Reposition Left Upper Femur with Internal Fixation Device, Percutaneous Endoscopic Approach

0QS745Z Reposition Left Upper Femur with External Fixation Device, Percutaneous Endoscopic Approach

0QS746Z Reposition Left Upper Femur with Intramedullary Internal Fixation Device, Percutaneous Endoscopic Approach

0QS74BZ Reposition Left Upper Femur with Monoplanar External Fixation Device, Percutaneous Endoscopic Approach

0QS74CZ Reposition Left Upper Femur with Ring External Fixation Device, Percutaneous Endoscopic Approach

0QS74DZ Reposition Left Upper Femur with Hybrid External Fixation Device, Percutaneous Endoscopic Approach

0QS74ZZ Reposition Left Upper Femur, Percutaneous Endoscopic Approach

0QS7XZZ Reposition Left Upper Femur, External Approach

0QS804Z Reposition Right Femoral Shaft with Internal Fixation Device, Open Approach

0QS805Z Reposition Right Femoral Shaft with External Fixation Device, Open Approach

0QS806Z Reposition Right Femoral Shaft with Intramedullary Internal Fixation Device, Open Approach

0QS80BZ Reposition Right Femoral Shaft with Monoplanar External Fixation Device, Open Approach

0QS80CZ Reposition Right Femoral Shaft with Ring External Fixation Device, Open Approach

0QS80DZ Reposition Right Femoral Shaft with Hybrid External Fixation Device, Open Approach

0QS80ZZ Reposition Right Femoral Shaft, Open Approach

0QS834Z Reposition Right Femoral Shaft with Internal Fixation Device, Percutaneous Approach

0QS835Z Reposition Right Femoral Shaft with External Fixation Device, Percutaneous Approach

0QS836Z Reposition Right Femoral Shaft with Intramedullary Internal Fixation Device, Percutaneous Approach

0QS83BZ Reposition Right Femoral Shaft with Monoplanar External Fixation Device, Percutaneous Approach

0QS83CZ Reposition Right Femoral Shaft with Ring External Fixation Device, Percutaneous Approach

0QS83DZ Reposition Right Femoral Shaft with Hybrid External Fixation Device, Percutaneous Approach

0QS83ZZ Reposition Right Femoral Shaft, Percutaneous Approach

0QS844Z Reposition Right Femoral Shaft with Internal Fixation Device, Percutaneous Endoscopic Approach

0QS845Z Reposition Right Femoral Shaft with External Fixation Device, Percutaneous Endoscopic Approach

0QS846Z Reposition Right Femoral Shaft with Intramedullary Internal Fixation Device, Percutaneous Endoscopic Approach

0QS84BZ Reposition Right Femoral Shaft with Monoplanar External Fixation Device, Percutaneous Endoscopic Approach

0QS84CZ Reposition Right Femoral Shaft with Ring External Fixation Device, Percutaneous Endoscopic Approach

0QS84DZ Reposition Right Femoral Shaft with Hybrid External Fixation Device, Percutaneous Endoscopic Approach

0QS84ZZ Reposition Right Femoral Shaft, Percutaneous Endoscopic Approach

0QS8XZZ Reposition Right Femoral Shaft, External Approach

0QS904Z Reposition Left Femoral Shaft with Internal Fixation Device, Open Approach

AHA CC: 3Q, 2019, 26

0QS905Z Reposition Left Femoral Shaft with External Fixation Device, Open Approach

0QS906Z Reposition Left Femoral Shaft with Intramedullary Internal Fixation Device, Open Approach

0QS90BZ Reposition Left Femoral Shaft with Monoplanar External Fixation Device, Open Approach

0QS90CZ Reposition Left Femoral Shaft with Ring External Fixation Device, Open Approach

0QS90DZ Reposition Left Femoral Shaft with Hybrid External Fixation Device, Open Approach

0QS90ZZ Reposition Left Femoral Shaft, Open Approach

0QS934Z Reposition Left Femoral Shaft with Internal Fixation Device, Percutaneous Approach

0QS935Z Reposition Left Femoral Shaft with External Fixation Device, Percutaneous Approach

0QS936Z Reposition Left Femoral Shaft with Intramedullary Internal Fixation Device, Percutaneous Approach

0QS93BZ Reposition Left Femoral Shaft with Monoplanar External Fixation Device, Percutaneous Approach

0QS93CZ Reposition Left Femoral Shaft with Ring External Fixation Device, Percutaneous Approach

0QS93DZ Reposition Left Femoral Shaft with Hybrid External Fixation Device, Percutaneous Approach

0QS93ZZ Reposition Left Femoral Shaft, Percutaneous Approach

0QS944Z Reposition Left Femoral Shaft with Internal Fixation Device, Percutaneous Endoscopic Approach

0QS945Z Reposition Left Femoral Shaft with External Fixation Device, Percutaneous Endoscopic Approach

0QS946Z Reposition Left Femoral Shaft with Intramedullary Internal Fixation Device, Percutaneous Endoscopic Approach

0QS94BZ Reposition Left Femoral Shaft with Monoplanar External Fixation Device, Percutaneous Endoscopic Approach

0QS94CZ Reposition Left Femoral Shaft with Ring External Fixation Device, Percutaneous Endoscopic Approach

0QS94DZ Reposition Left Femoral Shaft with Hybrid External Fixation Device, Percutaneous Endoscopic Approach

0QS94ZZ Reposition Left Femoral Shaft, Percutaneous Endoscopic Approach

0QS9XZZ Reposition Left Femoral Shaft, External Approach

0QSB04Z Reposition Right Lower Femur with Internal Fixation Device, Open Approach

0QSB05Z Reposition Right Lower Femur with External Fixation Device, Open Approach

0QSB06Z Reposition Right Lower Femur with Intramedullary Internal Fixation Device, Open Approach

♀ Female-only   ♂ Male-only   ▲ Limited Coverage   ● Non-OR   **HAC** HAC-associated procedure   ▲ Non-covered procedures   ✚ Cluster

0QSB0BZ Reposition Right Lower Femur with Monoplanar External Fixation Device, Open Approach

0QSB0CZ Reposition Right Lower Femur with Ring External Fixation Device, Open Approach

0QSB0DZ Reposition Right Lower Femur with Hybrid External Fixation Device, Open Approach

0QSB0ZZ Reposition Right Lower Femur, Open Approach

0QSB34Z Reposition Right Lower Femur with Internal Fixation Device, Percutaneous Approach

0QSB35Z Reposition Right Lower Femur with External Fixation Device, Percutaneous Approach

0QSB36Z Reposition Right Lower Femur with Intramedullary Internal Fixation Device, Percutaneous Approach

0QSB3BZ Reposition Right Lower Femur with Monoplanar External Fixation Device, Percutaneous Approach

0QSB3CZ Reposition Right Lower Femur with Ring External Fixation Device, Percutaneous Approach

0QSB3DZ Reposition Right Lower Femur with Hybrid External Fixation Device, Percutaneous Approach

0QSB3ZZ Reposition Right Lower Femur, Percutaneous Approach

0QSB44Z Reposition Right Lower Femur with Internal Fixation Device, Percutaneous Endoscopic Approach

0QSB45Z Reposition Right Lower Femur with External Fixation Device, Percutaneous Endoscopic Approach

0QSB46Z Reposition Right Lower Femur with Intramedullary Internal Fixation Device, Percutaneous Endoscopic Approach

0QSB4BZ Reposition Right Lower Femur with Monoplanar External Fixation Device, Percutaneous Endoscopic Approach

0QSB4CZ Reposition Right Lower Femur with Ring External Fixation Device, Percutaneous Endoscopic Approach

0QSB4DZ Reposition Right Lower Femur with Hybrid External Fixation Device, Percutaneous Endoscopic Approach

0QSB4ZZ Reposition Right Lower Femur, Percutaneous Endoscopic Approach

0QSBXZZ Reposition Right Lower Femur, External Approach

0QSC04Z Reposition Left Lower Femur with Internal Fixation Device, Open Approach
AHA CC: 4Q, 2014, 31

0QSC05Z Reposition Left Lower Femur with External Fixation Device, Open Approach

0QSC06Z Reposition Left Lower Femur with Intramedullary Internal Fixation Device, Open Approach

0QSC0BZ Reposition Left Lower Femur with Monoplanar External Fixation Device, Open Approach

0QSC0CZ Reposition Left Lower Femur with Ring External Fixation Device, Open Approach

0QSC0DZ Reposition Left Lower Femur with Hybrid External Fixation Device, Open Approach

0QSC0ZZ Reposition Left Lower Femur, Open Approach

0QSC34Z Reposition Left Lower Femur with Internal Fixation Device, Percutaneous Approach

0QSC35Z Reposition Left Lower Femur with External Fixation Device, Percutaneous Approach

0QSC36Z Reposition Left Lower Femur with Intramedullary Internal Fixation Device, Percutaneous Approach

0QSC3BZ Reposition Left Lower Femur with Monoplanar External Fixation Device, Percutaneous Approach

0QSC3CZ Reposition Left Lower Femur with Ring External Fixation Device, Percutaneous Approach

0QSC3DZ Reposition Left Lower Femur with Hybrid External Fixation Device, Percutaneous Approach

0QSC3ZZ Reposition Left Lower Femur, Percutaneous Approach

0QSC44Z Reposition Left Lower Femur with Internal Fixation Device, Percutaneous Endoscopic Approach

0QSC45Z Reposition Left Lower Femur with External Fixation Device, Percutaneous Endoscopic Approach

0QSC46Z Reposition Left Lower Femur with Intramedullary Internal Fixation Device, Percutaneous Endoscopic Approach

0QSC4BZ Reposition Left Lower Femur with Monoplanar External Fixation Device, Percutaneous Endoscopic Approach

0QSC4CZ Reposition Left Lower Femur with Ring External Fixation Device, Percutaneous Endoscopic Approach

0QSC4DZ Reposition Left Lower Femur with Hybrid External Fixation Device, Percutaneous Endoscopic Approach

0QSC4ZZ Reposition Left Lower Femur, Percutaneous Endoscopic Approach

0QSCXZZ Reposition Left Lower Femur, External Approach

0QSD04Z Reposition Right Patella with Internal Fixation Device, Open Approach

0QSD05Z Reposition Right Patella with External Fixation Device, Open Approach

0QSD0ZZ Reposition Right Patella, Open Approach

0QSD34Z Reposition Right Patella with Internal Fixation Device, Percutaneous Approach

0QSD35Z Reposition Right Patella with External Fixation Device, Percutaneous Approach

0QSD3ZZ Reposition Right Patella, Percutaneous Approach

0QSD44Z Reposition Right Patella with Internal Fixation Device, Percutaneous Endoscopic Approach

0QSD45Z Reposition Right Patella with External Fixation Device, Percutaneous Endoscopic Approach

0QSD4ZZ Reposition Right Patella, Percutaneous Endoscopic Approach

0QSDXZZ Reposition Right Patella, External Approach

0QSF04Z Reposition Left Patella with Internal Fixation Device, Open Approach
AHA CC: 3Q, 2016, 34-35

0QSF05Z Reposition Left Patella with External Fixation Device, Open Approach

0QSF0ZZ Reposition Left Patella, Open Approach

0QSF34Z Reposition Left Patella with Internal Fixation Device, Percutaneous Approach

0QSF35Z Reposition Left Patella with External Fixation Device, Percutaneous Approach

0QSF3ZZ Reposition Left Patella, Percutaneous Approach

0QSF44Z Reposition Left Patella with Internal Fixation Device, Percutaneous Endoscopic Approach

0QSF45Z Reposition Left Patella with External Fixation Device, Percutaneous Endoscopic Approach

0QSF4ZZ Reposition Left Patella, Percutaneous Endoscopic Approach

0QSFXZZ Reposition Left Patella, External Approach

0QSG04Z Reposition Right Tibia with Internal Fixation Device, Open Approach

0QSG05Z Reposition Right Tibia with External Fixation Device, Open Approach

0QSG06Z Reposition Right Tibia with Intramedullary Internal Fixation Device, Open Approach

0QSG0BZ Reposition Right Tibia with Monoplanar External Fixation Device, Open Approach

0QSG0CZ Reposition Right Tibia with Ring External Fixation Device, Open Approach

0QSG0DZ Reposition Right Tibia with Hybrid External Fixation Device, Open Approach

0QSG0ZZ Reposition Right Tibia, Open Approach

0QSG34Z Reposition Right Tibia with Internal Fixation Device, Percutaneous Approach

0QSG35Z Reposition Right Tibia with External Fixation Device, Percutaneous Approach

0QSG36Z Reposition Right Tibia with Intramedullary Internal Fixation Device, Percutaneous Approach

0QSG3BZ Reposition Right Tibia with Monoplanar External Fixation Device, Percutaneous Approach

0QSG3CZ Reposition Right Tibia with Ring External Fixation Device, Percutaneous Approach

0QSG3DZ Reposition Right Tibia with Hybrid External Fixation Device, Percutaneous Approach

0QSG3ZZ Reposition Right Tibia, Percutaneous Approach

0QSG44Z Reposition Right Tibia with Internal Fixation Device, Percutaneous Endoscopic Approach

0QSG45Z Reposition Right Tibia with External Fixation Device, Percutaneous Endoscopic Approach

0QSG46Z Reposition Right Tibia with Intramedullary Internal Fixation Device, Percutaneous Endoscopic Approach

0QSG4BZ Reposition Right Tibia with Monoplanar External Fixation Device, Percutaneous Endoscopic Approach

0QSG4CZ Reposition Right Tibia with Ring External Fixation Device, Percutaneous Endoscopic Approach

0QSG4DZ Reposition Right Tibia with Hybrid External Fixation Device, Percutaneous Endoscopic Approach

0QSG4ZZ Reposition Right Tibia, Percutaneous Endoscopic Approach

0QSGXZZ Reposition Right Tibia, External Approach

0QSH04Z Reposition Left Tibia with Internal Fixation Device, Open Approach
AHA CC: 4Q, 2014, 30-31; 3Q, 2016, 34-35

0QSH05Z Reposition Left Tibia with External Fixation Device, Open Approach

0QSH06Z Reposition Left Tibia with Intramedullary Internal Fixation Device, Open Approach

0QSH0BZ Reposition Left Tibia with Monoplanar External Fixation Device, Open Approach

0QSH0CZ Reposition Left Tibia with Ring External Fixation Device, Open Approach

0QSH0DZ Reposition Left Tibia with Hybrid External Fixation Device, Open Approach

0QSH0ZZ Reposition Left Tibia, Open Approach

0QSH34Z Reposition Left Tibia with Internal Fixation Device, Percutaneous Approach

0QSH35Z Reposition Left Tibia with External Fixation Device, Percutaneous Approach

0QSH36Z Reposition Left Tibia with Intramedullary Internal Fixation Device, Percutaneous Approach

0QSH3BZ Reposition Left Tibia with Monoplanar External Fixation Device, Percutaneous Approach

0QSH3CZ Reposition Left Tibia with Ring External Fixation Device, Percutaneous Approach

0QSH3DZ Reposition Left Tibia with Hybrid External Fixation Device, Percutaneous Approach

0QSH3ZZ Reposition Left Tibia, Percutaneous Approach

0QSH44Z Reposition Left Tibia with Internal Fixation Device, Percutaneous Endoscopic Approach

0QSH45Z Reposition Left Tibia with External Fixation Device, Percutaneous Endoscopic Approach

0QSH46Z Reposition Left Tibia with Intramedullary Internal Fixation Device, Percutaneous Endoscopic Approach

0QSH4BZ Reposition Left Tibia with Monoplanar External Fixation Device, Percutaneous Endoscopic Approach

0QSH4CZ Reposition Left Tibia with Ring External Fixation Device, Percutaneous Endoscopic Approach

0QSH4DZ Reposition Left Tibia with Hybrid External Fixation Device, Percutaneous Endoscopic Approach

0QSH4ZZ Reposition Left Tibia, Percutaneous Endoscopic Approach

0QSHXZZ Reposition Left Tibia, External Approach

0QSJ04Z Reposition Right Fibula with Internal Fixation Device, Open Approach

0QSJ05Z Reposition Right Fibula with External Fixation Device, Open Approach

0QSJ06Z Reposition Right Fibula with Intramedullary Internal Fixation Device, Open Approach

0QSJ0BZ Reposition Right Fibula with Monoplanar External Fixation Device, Open Approach

0QSJ0CZ Reposition Right Fibula with Ring External Fixation Device, Open Approach

0QSJ0DZ Reposition Right Fibula with Hybrid External Fixation Device, Open Approach

0QSJ0ZZ Reposition Right Fibula, Open Approach

0QSJ34Z Reposition Right Fibula with Internal Fixation Device, Percutaneous Approach

0QSJ35Z Reposition Right Fibula with External Fixation Device, Percutaneous Approach

0QSJ36Z Reposition Right Fibula with Intramedullary Internal Fixation Device, Percutaneous Approach

0QSJ3BZ Reposition Right Fibula with Monoplanar External Fixation Device, Percutaneous Approach

0QSJ3CZ Reposition Right Fibula with Ring External Fixation Device, Percutaneous Approach

0QSJ3DZ Reposition Right Fibula with Hybrid External Fixation Device, Percutaneous Approach

0QSJ3ZZ Reposition Right Fibula, Percutaneous Approach

0QSJ44Z Reposition Right Fibula with Internal Fixation Device, Percutaneous Endoscopic Approach

0QSJ45Z Reposition Right Fibula with External Fixation Device, Percutaneous Endoscopic Approach

0QSJ46Z Reposition Right Fibula with Intramedullary Internal Fixation Device, Percutaneous Endoscopic Approach

0QSJ4BZ Reposition Right Fibula with Monoplanar External Fixation Device, Percutaneous Endoscopic Approach

0QSJ4CZ Reposition Right Fibula with Ring External Fixation Device, Percutaneous Endoscopic Approach

0QSJ4DZ Reposition Right Fibula with Hybrid External Fixation Device, Percutaneous Endoscopic Approach

0QSJ4ZZ Reposition Right Fibula, Percutaneous Endoscopic Approach

0QSJXZZ Reposition Right Fibula, External Approach

0QSK04Z Reposition Left Fibula with Internal Fixation Device, Open Approach

0QSK05Z Reposition Left Fibula with External Fixation Device, Open Approach

0QSK06Z Reposition Left Fibula with Intramedullary Internal Fixation Device, Open Approach

0QSK0BZ Reposition Left Fibula with Monoplanar External Fixation Device, Open Approach

0QSK0CZ Reposition Left Fibula with Ring External Fixation Device, Open Approach

0QSK0DZ Reposition Left Fibula with Hybrid External Fixation Device, Open Approach

0QSK0ZZ Reposition Left Fibula, Open Approach
AHA CC: 3Q, 2016, 34-35

0QSK34Z Reposition Left Fibula with Internal Fixation Device, Percutaneous Approach

0QSK35Z Reposition Left Fibula with External Fixation Device, Percutaneous Approach

0QSK36Z Reposition Left Fibula with Intramedullary Internal Fixation Device, Percutaneous Approach

0QSK3BZ Reposition Left Fibula with Monoplanar External Fixation Device, Percutaneous Approach

0QSK3CZ Reposition Left Fibula with Ring External Fixation Device, Percutaneous Approach

0QSK3DZ Reposition Left Fibula with Hybrid External Fixation Device, Percutaneous Approach

0QSK3ZZ Reposition Left Fibula, Percutaneous Approach

0QSK44Z Reposition Left Fibula with Internal Fixation Device, Percutaneous Endoscopic Approach

0QSK45Z Reposition Left Fibula with External Fixation Device, Percutaneous Endoscopic Approach

0QSK46Z Reposition Left Fibula with Intramedullary Internal Fixation Device, Percutaneous Endoscopic Approach

0QSK4BZ Reposition Left Fibula with Monoplanar External Fixation Device, Percutaneous Endoscopic Approach

0QSK4CZ Reposition Left Fibula with Ring External Fixation Device, Percutaneous Endoscopic Approach

0QSK4DZ Reposition Left Fibula with Hybrid External Fixation Device, Percutaneous Endoscopic Approach

0QSK4ZZ Reposition Left Fibula, Percutaneous Endoscopic Approach

0QSKXZZ Reposition Left Fibula, External Approach

0QSL04Z Reposition Right Tarsal with Internal Fixation Device, Open Approach
AHA CC: 1Q, 2018, 13

0QSL05Z Reposition Right Tarsal with External Fixation Device, Open Approach

0QSL0ZZ Reposition Right Tarsal, Open Approach

0QSL34Z Reposition Right Tarsal with Internal Fixation Device, Percutaneous Approach

0QSL35Z Reposition Right Tarsal with External Fixation Device, Percutaneous Approach

0QSL3ZZ Reposition Right Tarsal, Percutaneous Approach

0QSL44Z Reposition Right Tarsal with Internal Fixation Device, Percutaneous Endoscopic Approach

0QSL45Z Reposition Right Tarsal with External Fixation Device, Percutaneous Endoscopic Approach

0QSL4ZZ Reposition Right Tarsal, Percutaneous Endoscopic Approach

0QSLXZZ Reposition Right Tarsal, External Approach

0QSM04Z Reposition Left Tarsal with Internal Fixation Device, Open Approach
AHA CC: 1Q, 2018, 13

0QSM05Z Reposition Left Tarsal with External Fixation Device, Open Approach

0QSM0ZZ Reposition Left Tarsal, Open Approach

0QSM34Z Reposition Left Tarsal with Internal Fixation Device, Percutaneous Approach

0QSM35Z Reposition Left Tarsal with External Fixation Device, Percutaneous Approach

0QSM3ZZ Reposition Left Tarsal, Percutaneous Approach

0QSM44Z Reposition Left Tarsal with Internal Fixation Device, Percutaneous Endoscopic Approach

0QSM45Z Reposition Left Tarsal with External Fixation Device, Percutaneous Endoscopic Approach

♀ Female-only   ♂ Male-only   ▲ Limited Coverage   ● Non-OR   HAC HAC-associated procedure   ▲ Non-covered procedures   ✚ Cluster

0QSM4ZZ	Reposition Left Tarsal, Percutaneous Endoscopic Approach
0QSMXZZ	Reposition Left Tarsal, External Approach
0QSN042	Reposition Right Metatarsal, Sesamoid Bone(s) 1st Toe, with Internal Fixation Device, Open Approach
0QSN04Z	Reposition Right Metatarsal with Internal Fixation Device, Open Approach
0QSN052	Reposition Right Metatarsal, Sesamoid Bone(s) 1st Toe, with External Fixation Device, Open Approach
0QSN05Z	Reposition Right Metatarsal with External Fixation Device, Open Approach
0QSN0Z2	Reposition Right Metatarsal, Sesamoid Bone(s) 1st Toe, Open Approach
0QSN0ZZ	Reposition Right Metatarsal, Open Approach
0QSN342	Reposition Right Metatarsal, Sesamoid Bone(s) 1st Toe, with Internal Fixation Device, Percutaneous Approach
0QSN34Z	Reposition Right Metatarsal with Internal Fixation Device, Percutaneous Approach
0QSN352	Reposition Right Metatarsal, Sesamoid Bone(s) 1st Toe, with External Fixation Device, Percutaneous Approach
0QSN35Z	Reposition Right Metatarsal with External Fixation Device, Percutaneous Approach
0QSN3Z2	Reposition Right Metatarsal, Sesamoid Bone(s) 1st Toe, Percutaneous Approach
0QSN3ZZ	Reposition Right Metatarsal, Percutaneous Approach
0QSN442	Reposition Right Metatarsal, Sesamoid Bone(s) 1st Toe, with Internal Fixation Device, Percutaneous Endoscopic Approach
0QSN44Z	Reposition Right Metatarsal with Internal Fixation Device, Percutaneous Endoscopic Approach
0QSN452	Reposition Right Metatarsal, Sesamoid Bone(s) 1st Toe, with External Fixation Device, Percutaneous Endoscopic Approach
0QSN45Z	Reposition Right Metatarsal with External Fixation Device, Percutaneous Endoscopic Approach
0QSN4Z2	Reposition Right Metatarsal, Sesamoid Bone(s) 1st Toe, Percutaneous Endoscopic Approach
0QSN4ZZ	Reposition Right Metatarsal, Percutaneous Endoscopic Approach
0QSNXZ2	Reposition Right Metatarsal, Sesamoid Bone(s) 1st Toe, External Approach
0QSNXZZ	Reposition Right Metatarsal, External Approach
0QSP042	Reposition Left Metatarsal, Sesamoid Bone(s) 1st Toe, with Internal Fixation Device, Open Approach

0QSP04Z	Reposition Left Metatarsal with Internal Fixation Device, Open Approach
0QSP052	Reposition Left Metatarsal, Sesamoid Bone(s) 1st Toe, with External Fixation Device, Open Approach
0QSP05Z	Reposition Left Metatarsal with External Fixation Device, Open Approach
0QSP0Z2	Reposition Left Metatarsal, Sesamoid Bone(s) 1st Toe, Open Approach
0QSP0ZZ	Reposition Left Metatarsal, Open Approach
0QSP342	Reposition Left Metatarsal, Sesamoid Bone(s) 1st Toe, with Internal Fixation Device, Percutaneous Approach
0QSP34Z	Reposition Left Metatarsal with Internal Fixation Device, Percutaneous Approach
0QSP352	Reposition Left Metatarsal, Sesamoid Bone(s) 1st Toe, with External Fixation Device, Percutaneous Approach
0QSP35Z	Reposition Left Metatarsal with External Fixation Device, Percutaneous Approach
0QSP3Z2	Reposition Left Metatarsal, Sesamoid Bone(s) 1st Toe, Percutaneous Approach
0QSP3ZZ	Reposition Left Metatarsal, Percutaneous Approach
0QSP442	Reposition Left Metatarsal, Sesamoid Bone(s) 1st Toe, with Internal Fixation Device, Percutaneous Endoscopic Approach
0QSP44Z	Reposition Left Metatarsal with Internal Fixation Device, Percutaneous Endoscopic Approach
0QSP452	Reposition Left Metatarsal, Sesamoid Bone(s) 1st Toe, with External Fixation Device, Percutaneous Endoscopic Approach
0QSP45Z	Reposition Left Metatarsal with External Fixation Device, Percutaneous Endoscopic Approach
0QSP4Z2	Reposition Left Metatarsal, Sesamoid Bone(s) 1st Toe, Percutaneous Endoscopic Approach
0QSP4ZZ	Reposition Left Metatarsal, Percutaneous Endoscopic Approach
0QSPXZ2	Reposition Left Metatarsal, Sesamoid Bone(s) 1st Toe, External Approach
0QSPXZZ	Reposition Left Metatarsal, External Approach
0QSQ04Z	Reposition Right Toe Phalanx with Internal Fixation Device, Open Approach
0QSQ05Z	Reposition Right Toe Phalanx with External Fixation Device, Open Approach
0QSQ0ZZ	Reposition Right Toe Phalanx, Open Approach

0QSQ34Z	Reposition Right Toe Phalanx with Internal Fixation Device, Percutaneous Approach
0QSQ35Z	Reposition Right Toe Phalanx with External Fixation Device, Percutaneous Approach
0QSQ3ZZ	Reposition Right Toe Phalanx, Percutaneous Approach
0QSQ44Z	Reposition Right Toe Phalanx with Internal Fixation Device, Percutaneous Endoscopic Approach
0QSQ45Z	Reposition Right Toe Phalanx with External Fixation Device, Percutaneous Endoscopic Approach
0QSQ4ZZ	Reposition Right Toe Phalanx, Percutaneous Endoscopic Approach
0QSQXZZ	Reposition Right Toe Phalanx, External Approach
0QSR04Z	Reposition Left Toe Phalanx with Internal Fixation Device, Open Approach
0QSR05Z	Reposition Left Toe Phalanx with External Fixation Device, Open Approach
0QSR0ZZ	Reposition Left Toe Phalanx, Open Approach
0QSR34Z	Reposition Left Toe Phalanx with Internal Fixation Device, Percutaneous Approach
0QSR35Z	Reposition Left Toe Phalanx with External Fixation Device, Percutaneous Approach
0QSR3ZZ	Reposition Left Toe Phalanx, Percutaneous Approach
0QSR44Z	Reposition Left Toe Phalanx with Internal Fixation Device, Percutaneous Endoscopic Approach
0QSR45Z	Reposition Left Toe Phalanx with External Fixation Device, Percutaneous Endoscopic Approach
0QSR4ZZ	Reposition Left Toe Phalanx, Percutaneous Endoscopic Approach
0QSRXZZ	Reposition Left Toe Phalanx, External Approach
0QSS04Z	Reposition Coccyx with Internal Fixation Device, Open Approach
0QSS0ZZ	Reposition Coccyx, Open Approach
0QSS34Z	Reposition Coccyx with Internal Fixation Device, Percutaneous Approach
0QSS3ZZ	Reposition Coccyx, Percutaneous Approach
✚	*See table 0QU to construct a code for Supplement of with synthetic substitute.*
0QSS44Z	Reposition Coccyx with Internal Fixation Device, Percutaneous Endoscopic Approach
0QSS4ZZ	Reposition Coccyx, Percutaneous Endoscopic Approach
0QSSXZZ	Reposition Coccyx, External Approach

0QT – Lower Bones, Resection

Review Coding Guideline B3.8

Review Coding Guideline B3.18

0QT20ZZ	Resection of Right Pelvic Bone, Open Approach
0QT30ZZ	Resection of Left Pelvic Bone, Open Approach
0QT40ZZ	Resection of Right Acetabulum, Open Approach

0QT50ZZ	Resection of Left Acetabulum, Open Approach
0QT60ZZ	Resection of Right Upper Femur, Open Approach
	AHA CC: 3Q, 2016, 30-31

0QT70ZZ	Resection of Left Upper Femur, Open Approach
	AHA CC: 3Q, 2015, 26; 3Q, 2016, 30-31
0QT80ZZ	Resection of Right Femoral Shaft, Open Approach

♀ Female-only	♂ Male-only	▲ Limited Coverage	● Non-OR	▨ HAC-associated procedure	▲ Non-covered procedures	✚ Cluster

0QT90ZZ Resection of Left Femoral Shaft, Open Approach

0QTB0ZZ Resection of Right Lower Femur, Open Approach

0QTC0ZZ Resection of Left Lower Femur, Open Approach
AHA CC: 4Q, 2014, 30-31

0QTD0ZZ Resection of Right Patella, Open Approach

0QTF0ZZ Resection of Left Patella, Open Approach

0QTG0ZZ Resection of Right Tibia, Open Approach

0QTH0ZZ Resection of Left Tibia, Open Approach

0QTJ0ZZ Resection of Right Fibula, Open Approach

0QTK0ZZ Resection of Left Fibula, Open Approach

0QTL0ZZ Resection of Right Tarsal, Open Approach

0QTM0ZZ Resection of Left Tarsal, Open Approach

0QTN0ZZ Resection of Right Metatarsal, Open Approach

0QTP0ZZ Resection of Left Metatarsal, Open Approach

0QTQ0ZZ Resection of Right Toe Phalanx, Open Approach

0QTR0ZZ Resection of Left Toe Phalanx, Open Approach

0QTS0ZZ Resection of Coccyx, Open Approach

0QU – Lower Bones, Supplement

0QU007Z Supplement Lumbar Vertebra with Autologous Tissue Substitute, Open Approach

0QU00JZ Supplement Lumbar Vertebra with Synthetic Substitute, Open Approach

0QU00KZ Supplement Lumbar Vertebra with Nonautologous Tissue Substitute, Open Approach

0QU037Z Supplement Lumbar Vertebra with Autologous Tissue Substitute, Percutaneous Approach

0QU03JZ Supplement Lumbar Vertebra with Synthetic Substitute, Percutaneous Approach
AHA CC: 2Q, 2014, 12-13; 2Q, 2019, 35

0QU03KZ Supplement Lumbar Vertebra with Nonautologous Tissue Substitute, Percutaneous Approach

0QU047Z Supplement Lumbar Vertebra with Autologous Tissue Substitute, Percutaneous Endoscopic Approach

0QU04JZ Supplement Lumbar Vertebra with Synthetic Substitute, Percutaneous Endoscopic Approach

0QU04KZ Supplement Lumbar Vertebra with Nonautologous Tissue Substitute, Percutaneous Endoscopic Approach

0QU107Z Supplement Sacrum with Autologous Tissue Substitute, Open Approach

0QU10JZ Supplement Sacrum with Synthetic Substitute, Open Approach

0QU10KZ Supplement Sacrum with Nonautologous Tissue Substitute, Open Approach

0QU137Z Supplement Sacrum with Autologous Tissue Substitute, Percutaneous Approach

0QU13JZ Supplement Sacrum with Synthetic Substitute, Percutaneous Approach

0QU13KZ Supplement Sacrum with Nonautologous Tissue Substitute, Percutaneous Approach

0QU147Z Supplement Sacrum with Autologous Tissue Substitute, Percutaneous Endoscopic Approach

0QU14JZ Supplement Sacrum with Synthetic Substitute, Percutaneous Endoscopic Approach

0QU14KZ Supplement Sacrum with Nonautologous Tissue Substitute, Percutaneous Endoscopic Approach

0QU207Z Supplement Right Pelvic Bone with Autologous Tissue Substitute, Open Approach

0QU20JZ Supplement Right Pelvic Bone with Synthetic Substitute, Open Approach
AHA CC: 2Q, 2013, 35-36

0QU20KZ Supplement Right Pelvic Bone with Nonautologous Tissue Substitute, Open Approach

0QU237Z Supplement Right Pelvic Bone with Autologous Tissue Substitute, Percutaneous Approach

0QU23JZ Supplement Right Pelvic Bone with Synthetic Substitute, Percutaneous Approach

0QU23KZ Supplement Right Pelvic Bone with Nonautologous Tissue Substitute, Percutaneous Approach

0QU247Z Supplement Right Pelvic Bone with Autologous Tissue Substitute, Percutaneous Endoscopic Approach

0QU24JZ Supplement Right Pelvic Bone with Synthetic Substitute, Percutaneous Endoscopic Approach

0QU24KZ Supplement Right Pelvic Bone with Nonautologous Tissue Substitute, Percutaneous Endoscopic Approach

0QU307Z Supplement Left Pelvic Bone with Autologous Tissue Substitute, Open Approach

0QU30JZ Supplement Left Pelvic Bone with Synthetic Substitute, Open Approach

0QU30KZ Supplement Left Pelvic Bone with Nonautologous Tissue Substitute, Open Approach

0QU337Z Supplement Left Pelvic Bone with Autologous Tissue Substitute, Percutaneous Approach

0QU33JZ Supplement Left Pelvic Bone with Synthetic Substitute, Percutaneous Approach

0QU33KZ Supplement Left Pelvic Bone with Nonautologous Tissue Substitute, Percutaneous Approach

0QU347Z Supplement Left Pelvic Bone with Autologous Tissue Substitute, Percutaneous Endoscopic Approach

0QU34JZ Supplement Left Pelvic Bone with Synthetic Substitute, Percutaneous Endoscopic Approach

0QU34KZ Supplement Left Pelvic Bone with Nonautologous Tissue Substitute, Percutaneous Endoscopic Approach

0QU407Z Supplement Right Acetabulum with Autologous Tissue Substitute, Open Approach

0QU40JZ Supplement Right Acetabulum with Synthetic Substitute, Open Approach

0QU40KZ Supplement Right Acetabulum with Nonautologous Tissue Substitute, Open Approach

0QU437Z Supplement Right Acetabulum with Autologous Tissue Substitute, Percutaneous Approach

0QU43JZ Supplement Right Acetabulum with Synthetic Substitute, Percutaneous Approach

0QU43KZ Supplement Right Acetabulum with Nonautologous Tissue Substitute, Percutaneous Approach

0QU447Z Supplement Right Acetabulum with Autologous Tissue Substitute, Percutaneous Endoscopic Approach

0QU44JZ Supplement Right Acetabulum with Synthetic Substitute, Percutaneous Endoscopic Approach

0QU44KZ Supplement Right Acetabulum with Nonautologous Tissue Substitute, Percutaneous Endoscopic Approach

0QU507Z Supplement Left Acetabulum with Autologous Tissue Substitute, Open Approach

0QU50JZ Supplement Left Acetabulum with Synthetic Substitute, Open Approach
AHA CC: 3Q, 2015, 18-19

0QU50KZ Supplement Left Acetabulum with Nonautologous Tissue Substitute, Open Approach

0QU537Z Supplement Left Acetabulum with Autologous Tissue Substitute, Percutaneous Approach

0QU53JZ Supplement Left Acetabulum with Synthetic Substitute, Percutaneous Approach

0QU53KZ Supplement Left Acetabulum with Nonautologous Tissue Substitute, Percutaneous Approach

0QU547Z Supplement Left Acetabulum with Autologous Tissue Substitute, Percutaneous Endoscopic Approach

0QU54JZ Supplement Left Acetabulum with Synthetic Substitute, Percutaneous Endoscopic Approach

0QU54KZ Supplement Left Acetabulum with Nonautologous Tissue Substitute, Percutaneous Endoscopic Approach

0QU607Z Supplement Right Upper Femur with Autologous Tissue Substitute, Open Approach

0QU60JZ Supplement Right Upper Femur with Synthetic Substitute, Open Approach

0QU60KZ Supplement Right Upper Femur with Nonautologous Tissue Substitute, Open Approach

0QU637Z Supplement Right Upper Femur with Autologous Tissue Substitute, Percutaneous Approach

0QU63JZ Supplement Right Upper Femur with Synthetic Substitute, Percutaneous Approach

0QU63KZ Supplement Right Upper Femur with Nonautologous Tissue Substitute, Percutaneous Approach

0QU647Z Supplement Right Upper Femur with Autologous Tissue Substitute, Percutaneous Endoscopic Approach

0QU64JZ Supplement Right Upper Femur with Synthetic Substitute, Percutaneous Endoscopic Approach

0QU64KZ Supplement Right Upper Femur with Nonautologous Tissue Substitute, Percutaneous Endoscopic Approach

0QU707Z Supplement Left Upper Femur with Autologous Tissue Substitute, Open Approach

♀ Female-only ♂ Male-only ▲ Limited Coverage ● Non-OR ▦ HAC-associated procedure ▲ Non-covered procedures ✚ Cluster

0QU70JZ Supplement Left Upper Femur with Synthetic Substitute, Open Approach

0QU70KZ Supplement Left Upper Femur with Nonautologous Tissue Substitute, Open Approach

0QU737Z Supplement Left Upper Femur with Autologous Tissue Substitute, Percutaneous Approach

0QU73JZ Supplement Left Upper Femur with Synthetic Substitute, Percutaneous Approach

0QU73KZ Supplement Left Upper Femur with Nonautologous Tissue Substitute, Percutaneous Approach

0QU747Z Supplement Left Upper Femur with Autologous Tissue Substitute, Percutaneous Endoscopic Approach

0QU74JZ Supplement Left Upper Femur with Synthetic Substitute, Percutaneous Endoscopic Approach

0QU74KZ Supplement Left Upper Femur with Nonautologous Tissue Substitute, Percutaneous Endoscopic Approach

0QU807Z Supplement Right Femoral Shaft with Autologous Tissue Substitute, Open Approach

0QU80JZ Supplement Right Femoral Shaft with Synthetic Substitute, Open Approach

0QU80KZ Supplement Right Femoral Shaft with Nonautologous Tissue Substitute, Open Approach

0QU837Z Supplement Right Femoral Shaft with Autologous Tissue Substitute, Percutaneous Approach

0QU83JZ Supplement Right Femoral Shaft with Synthetic Substitute, Percutaneous Approach

0QU83KZ Supplement Right Femoral Shaft with Nonautologous Tissue Substitute, Percutaneous Approach

0QU847Z Supplement Right Femoral Shaft with Autologous Tissue Substitute, Percutaneous Endoscopic Approach

0QU84JZ Supplement Right Femoral Shaft with Synthetic Substitute, Percutaneous Endoscopic Approach

0QU84KZ Supplement Right Femoral Shaft with Nonautologous Tissue Substitute, Percutaneous Endoscopic Approach

0QU907Z Supplement Left Femoral Shaft with Autologous Tissue Substitute, Open Approach

0QU90JZ Supplement Left Femoral Shaft with Synthetic Substitute, Open Approach

0QU90KZ Supplement Left Femoral Shaft with Nonautologous Tissue Substitute, Open Approach

AHA CC: 3Q, 2019, 26

0QU937Z Supplement Left Femoral Shaft with Autologous Tissue Substitute, Percutaneous Approach

0QU93JZ Supplement Left Femoral Shaft with Synthetic Substitute, Percutaneous Approach

0QU93KZ Supplement Left Femoral Shaft with Nonautologous Tissue Substitute, Percutaneous Approach

0QU947Z Supplement Left Femoral Shaft with Autologous Tissue Substitute, Percutaneous Endoscopic Approach

0QU94JZ Supplement Left Femoral Shaft with Synthetic Substitute, Percutaneous Endoscopic Approach

0QU94KZ Supplement Left Femoral Shaft with Nonautologous Tissue Substitute, Percutaneous Endoscopic Approach

0QUB07Z Supplement Right Lower Femur with Autologous Tissue Substitute, Open Approach

0QUB0JZ Supplement Right Lower Femur with Synthetic Substitute, Open Approach

0QUB0KZ Supplement Right Lower Femur with Nonautologous Tissue Substitute, Open Approach

0QUB37Z Supplement Right Lower Femur with Autologous Tissue Substitute, Percutaneous Approach

0QUB3JZ Supplement Right Lower Femur with Synthetic Substitute, Percutaneous Approach

0QUB3KZ Supplement Right Lower Femur with Nonautologous Tissue Substitute, Percutaneous Approach

0QUB47Z Supplement Right Lower Femur with Autologous Tissue Substitute, Percutaneous Endoscopic Approach

0QUB4JZ Supplement Right Lower Femur with Synthetic Substitute, Percutaneous Endoscopic Approach

0QUB4KZ Supplement Right Lower Femur with Nonautologous Tissue Substitute, Percutaneous Endoscopic Approach

0QUC07Z Supplement Left Lower Femur with Autologous Tissue Substitute, Open Approach

0QUC0JZ Supplement Left Lower Femur with Synthetic Substitute, Open Approach

0QUC0KZ Supplement Left Lower Femur with Nonautologous Tissue Substitute, Open Approach

AHA CC: 4Q, 2014, 31

0QUC37Z Supplement Left Lower Femur with Autologous Tissue Substitute, Percutaneous Approach

0QUC3JZ Supplement Left Lower Femur with Synthetic Substitute, Percutaneous Approach

0QUC3KZ Supplement Left Lower Femur with Nonautologous Tissue Substitute, Percutaneous Approach

0QUC47Z Supplement Left Lower Femur with Autologous Tissue Substitute, Percutaneous Endoscopic Approach

0QUC4JZ Supplement Left Lower Femur with Synthetic Substitute, Percutaneous Endoscopic Approach

0QUC4KZ Supplement Left Lower Femur with Nonautologous Tissue Substitute, Percutaneous Endoscopic Approach

0QUD07Z Supplement Right Patella with Autologous Tissue Substitute, Open Approach

0QUD0JZ Supplement Right Patella with Synthetic Substitute, Open Approach

0QUD0KZ Supplement Right Patella with Nonautologous Tissue Substitute, Open Approach

0QUD37Z Supplement Right Patella with Autologous Tissue Substitute, Percutaneous Approach

0QUD3JZ Supplement Right Patella with Synthetic Substitute, Percutaneous Approach

0QUD3KZ Supplement Right Patella with Nonautologous Tissue Substitute, Percutaneous Approach

0QUD47Z Supplement Right Patella with Autologous Tissue Substitute, Percutaneous Endoscopic Approach

0QUD4JZ Supplement Right Patella with Synthetic Substitute, Percutaneous Endoscopic Approach

0QUD4KZ Supplement Right Patella with Nonautologous Tissue Substitute, Percutaneous Endoscopic Approach

0QUF07Z Supplement Left Patella with Autologous Tissue Substitute, Open Approach

0QUF0JZ Supplement Left Patella with Synthetic Substitute, Open Approach

0QUF0KZ Supplement Left Patella with Nonautologous Tissue Substitute, Open Approach

0QUF37Z Supplement Left Patella with Autologous Tissue Substitute, Percutaneous Approach

0QUF3JZ Supplement Left Patella with Synthetic Substitute, Percutaneous Approach

0QUF3KZ Supplement Left Patella with Nonautologous Tissue Substitute, Percutaneous Approach

0QUF47Z Supplement Left Patella with Autologous Tissue Substitute, Percutaneous Endoscopic Approach

0QUF4JZ Supplement Left Patella with Synthetic Substitute, Percutaneous Endoscopic Approach

0QUF4KZ Supplement Left Patella with Nonautologous Tissue Substitute, Percutaneous Endoscopic Approach

0QUG07Z Supplement Right Tibia with Autologous Tissue Substitute, Open Approach

0QUG0JZ Supplement Right Tibia with Synthetic Substitute, Open Approach

0QUG0KZ Supplement Right Tibia with Nonautologous Tissue Substitute, Open Approach

0QUG37Z Supplement Right Tibia with Autologous Tissue Substitute, Percutaneous Approach

0QUG3JZ Supplement Right Tibia with Synthetic Substitute, Percutaneous Approach

0QUG3KZ Supplement Right Tibia with Nonautologous Tissue Substitute, Percutaneous Approach

0QUG47Z Supplement Right Tibia with Autologous Tissue Substitute, Percutaneous Endoscopic Approach

0QUG4JZ Supplement Right Tibia with Synthetic Substitute, Percutaneous Endoscopic Approach

0QUG4KZ Supplement Right Tibia with Nonautologous Tissue Substitute, Percutaneous Endoscopic Approach

0QUH07Z Supplement Left Tibia with Autologous Tissue Substitute, Open Approach

0QUH0JZ Supplement Left Tibia with Synthetic Substitute, Open Approach

0QUH0KZ Supplement Left Tibia with Nonautologous Tissue Substitute, Open Approach

0QUH37Z Supplement Left Tibia with Autologous Tissue Substitute, Percutaneous Approach

0QUH3JZ Supplement Left Tibia with Synthetic Substitute, Percutaneous Approach

0QUH3KZ Supplement Left Tibia with Nonautologous Tissue Substitute, Percutaneous Approach

0QUH47Z Supplement Left Tibia with Autologous Tissue Substitute, Percutaneous Endoscopic Approach

0QUH4JZ Supplement Left Tibia with Synthetic Substitute, Percutaneous Endoscopic Approach

0QUH4KZ Supplement Left Tibia with Nonautologous Tissue Substitute, Percutaneous Endoscopic Approach

0QUJ07Z Supplement Right Fibula with Autologous Tissue Substitute, Open Approach

0QUJ0JZ Supplement Right Fibula with Synthetic Substitute, Open Approach

0QUJ0KZ Supplement Right Fibula with Nonautologous Tissue Substitute, Open Approach

0QUJ37Z Supplement Right Fibula with Autologous Tissue Substitute, Percutaneous Approach

0QUJ3JZ Supplement Right Fibula with Synthetic Substitute, Percutaneous Approach

0QUJ3KZ Supplement Right Fibula with Nonautologous Tissue Substitute, Percutaneous Approach

0QUJ47Z Supplement Right Fibula with Autologous Tissue Substitute, Percutaneous Endoscopic Approach

0QUJ4JZ Supplement Right Fibula with Synthetic Substitute, Percutaneous Endoscopic Approach

0QUJ4KZ Supplement Right Fibula with Nonautologous Tissue Substitute, Percutaneous Endoscopic Approach

0QUK07Z Supplement Left Fibula with Autologous Tissue Substitute, Open Approach

0QUK0JZ Supplement Left Fibula with Synthetic Substitute, Open Approach

0QUK0KZ Supplement Left Fibula with Nonautologous Tissue Substitute, Open Approach

0QUK37Z Supplement Left Fibula with Autologous Tissue Substitute, Percutaneous Approach

0QUK3JZ Supplement Left Fibula with Synthetic Substitute, Percutaneous Approach

0QUK3KZ Supplement Left Fibula with Nonautologous Tissue Substitute, Percutaneous Approach

0QUK47Z Supplement Left Fibula with Autologous Tissue Substitute, Percutaneous Endoscopic Approach

0QUK4JZ Supplement Left Fibula with Synthetic Substitute, Percutaneous Endoscopic Approach

0QUK4KZ Supplement Left Fibula with Nonautologous Tissue Substitute, Percutaneous Endoscopic Approach

0QUL07Z Supplement Right Tarsal with Autologous Tissue Substitute, Open Approach

0QUL0JZ Supplement Right Tarsal with Synthetic Substitute, Open Approach

0QUL0KZ Supplement Right Tarsal with Nonautologous Tissue Substitute, Open Approach

0QUL37Z Supplement Right Tarsal with Autologous Tissue Substitute, Percutaneous Approach

0QUL3JZ Supplement Right Tarsal with Synthetic Substitute, Percutaneous Approach

0QUL3KZ Supplement Right Tarsal with Nonautologous Tissue Substitute, Percutaneous Approach

0QUL47Z Supplement Right Tarsal with Autologous Tissue Substitute, Percutaneous Endoscopic Approach

0QUL4JZ Supplement Right Tarsal with Synthetic Substitute, Percutaneous Endoscopic Approach

0QUL4KZ Supplement Right Tarsal with Nonautologous Tissue Substitute, Percutaneous Endoscopic Approach

0QUM07Z Supplement Left Tarsal with Autologous Tissue Substitute, Open Approach

0QUM0JZ Supplement Left Tarsal with Synthetic Substitute, Open Approach

0QUM0KZ Supplement Left Tarsal with Nonautologous Tissue Substitute, Open Approach

0QUM37Z Supplement Left Tarsal with Autologous Tissue Substitute, Percutaneous Approach

0QUM3JZ Supplement Left Tarsal with Synthetic Substitute, Percutaneous Approach

0QUM3KZ Supplement Left Tarsal with Nonautologous Tissue Substitute, Percutaneous Approach

0QUM47Z Supplement Left Tarsal with Autologous Tissue Substitute, Percutaneous Endoscopic Approach

0QUM4JZ Supplement Left Tarsal with Synthetic Substitute, Percutaneous Endoscopic Approach

0QUM4KZ Supplement Left Tarsal with Nonautologous Tissue Substitute, Percutaneous Endoscopic Approach

0QUN07Z Supplement Right Metatarsal with Autologous Tissue Substitute, Open Approach

0QUN0JZ Supplement Right Metatarsal with Synthetic Substitute, Open Approach

0QUN0KZ Supplement Right Metatarsal with Nonautologous Tissue Substitute, Open Approach

0QUN37Z Supplement Right Metatarsal with Autologous Tissue Substitute, Percutaneous Approach

0QUN3JZ Supplement Right Metatarsal with Synthetic Substitute, Percutaneous Approach

0QUN3KZ Supplement Right Metatarsal with Nonautologous Tissue Substitute, Percutaneous Approach

0QUN47Z Supplement Right Metatarsal with Autologous Tissue Substitute, Percutaneous Endoscopic Approach

0QUN4JZ Supplement Right Metatarsal with Synthetic Substitute, Percutaneous Endoscopic Approach

0QUN4KZ Supplement Right Metatarsal with Nonautologous Tissue Substitute, Percutaneous Endoscopic Approach

0QUP07Z Supplement Left Metatarsal with Autologous Tissue Substitute, Open Approach

0QUP0JZ Supplement Left Metatarsal with Synthetic Substitute, Open Approach

0QUP0KZ Supplement Left Metatarsal with Nonautologous Tissue Substitute, Open Approach

0QUP37Z Supplement Left Metatarsal with Autologous Tissue Substitute, Percutaneous Approach

0QUP3JZ Supplement Left Metatarsal with Synthetic Substitute, Percutaneous Approach

0QUP3KZ Supplement Left Metatarsal with Nonautologous Tissue Substitute, Percutaneous Approach

0QUP47Z Supplement Left Metatarsal with Autologous Tissue Substitute, Percutaneous Endoscopic Approach

0QUP4JZ Supplement Left Metatarsal with Synthetic Substitute, Percutaneous Endoscopic Approach

0QUP4KZ Supplement Left Metatarsal with Nonautologous Tissue Substitute, Percutaneous Endoscopic Approach

0QUQ07Z Supplement Right Toe Phalanx with Autologous Tissue Substitute, Open Approach

0QUQ0JZ Supplement Right Toe Phalanx with Synthetic Substitute, Open Approach

0QUQ0KZ Supplement Right Toe Phalanx with Nonautologous Tissue Substitute, Open Approach

0QUQ37Z Supplement Right Toe Phalanx with Autologous Tissue Substitute, Percutaneous Approach

0QUQ3JZ Supplement Right Toe Phalanx with Synthetic Substitute, Percutaneous Approach

0QUQ3KZ Supplement Right Toe Phalanx with Nonautologous Tissue Substitute, Percutaneous Approach

0QUQ47Z Supplement Right Toe Phalanx with Autologous Tissue Substitute, Percutaneous Endoscopic Approach

0QUQ4JZ Supplement Right Toe Phalanx with Synthetic Substitute, Percutaneous Endoscopic Approach

0QUQ4KZ Supplement Right Toe Phalanx with Nonautologous Tissue Substitute, Percutaneous Endoscopic Approach

0QUR07Z Supplement Left Toe Phalanx with Autologous Tissue Substitute, Open Approach

0QUR0JZ Supplement Left Toe Phalanx with Synthetic Substitute, Open Approach

0QUR0KZ Supplement Left Toe Phalanx with Nonautologous Tissue Substitute, Open Approach

0QUR37Z Supplement Left Toe Phalanx with Autologous Tissue Substitute, Percutaneous Approach

0QUR3JZ Supplement Left Toe Phalanx with Synthetic Substitute, Percutaneous Approach

0QUR3KZ Supplement Left Toe Phalanx with Nonautologous Tissue Substitute, Percutaneous Approach

0QUR47Z Supplement Left Toe Phalanx with Autologous Tissue Substitute, Percutaneous Endoscopic Approach

0QUR4JZ Supplement Left Toe Phalanx with Synthetic Substitute, Percutaneous Endoscopic Approach

0QUR4KZ Supplement Left Toe Phalanx with Nonautologous Tissue Substitute, Percutaneous Endoscopic Approach

0QUS07Z Supplement Coccyx with Autologous Tissue Substitute, Open Approach

0QUS0JZ Supplement Coccyx with Synthetic Substitute, Open Approach

0QUS0KZ Supplement Coccyx with Nonautologous Tissue Substitute, Open Approach

0QUS37Z Supplement Coccyx with Autologous Tissue Substitute, Percutaneous Approach

0QUS3JZ Supplement Coccyx with Synthetic Substitute, Percutaneous Approach

0QUS3KZ Supplement Coccyx with Nonautologous Tissue Substitute, Percutaneous Approach

♀ Female-only   ♂ Male-only   ▲ Limited Coverage   ● Non-OR   HAC HAC-associated procedure   ▲ Non-covered procedures   ➕ Cluster

0QUS47Z Supplement Coccyx with Autologous Tissue Substitute, Percutaneous Endoscopic Approach

0QUS4JZ Supplement Coccyx with Synthetic Substitute, Percutaneous Endoscopic Approach

0QUS4KZ Supplement Coccyx with Nonautologous Tissue Substitute, Percutaneous Endoscopic Approach

0QW – Lower Bones, Revision

Review Coding Guideline B6.1c

0QW004Z Revision of Internal Fixation Device in Lumbar Vertebra, Open Approach

0QW007Z Revision of Autologous Tissue Substitute in Lumbar Vertebra, Open Approach

0QW00JZ Revision of Synthetic Substitute in Lumbar Vertebra, Open Approach

0QW00KZ Revision of Nonautologous Tissue Substitute in Lumbar Vertebra, Open Approach

0QW034Z Revision of Internal Fixation Device in Lumbar Vertebra, Percutaneous Approach
AHA CC: 4Q, 2017, 75

0QW037Z Revision of Autologous Tissue Substitute in Lumbar Vertebra, Percutaneous Approach

0QW03JZ Revision of Synthetic Substitute in Lumbar Vertebra, Percutaneous Approach

0QW03KZ Revision of Nonautologous Tissue Substitute in Lumbar Vertebra, Percutaneous Approach

0QW044Z Revision of Internal Fixation Device in Lumbar Vertebra, Percutaneous Endoscopic Approach

0QW047Z Revision of Autologous Tissue Substitute in Lumbar Vertebra, Percutaneous Endoscopic Approach

0QW04JZ Revision of Synthetic Substitute in Lumbar Vertebra, Percutaneous Endoscopic Approach

0QW04KZ Revision of Nonautologous Tissue Substitute in Lumbar Vertebra, Percutaneous Endoscopic Approach

0QW0X4Z Revision of Internal Fixation Device in Lumbar Vertebra, External Approach

0QW0X7Z Revision of Autologous Tissue Substitute in Lumbar Vertebra, External Approach

0QW0XJZ Revision of Synthetic Substitute in Lumbar Vertebra, External Approach

0QW0XKZ Revision of Nonautologous Tissue Substitute in Lumbar Vertebra, External Approach

0QW104Z Revision of Internal Fixation Device in Sacrum, Open Approach

0QW107Z Revision of Autologous Tissue Substitute in Sacrum, Open Approach

0QW10JZ Revision of Synthetic Substitute in Sacrum, Open Approach

0QW10KZ Revision of Nonautologous Tissue Substitute in Sacrum, Open Approach

0QW134Z Revision of Internal Fixation Device in Sacrum, Percutaneous Approach

0QW137Z Revision of Autologous Tissue Substitute in Sacrum, Percutaneous Approach

0QW13JZ Revision of Synthetic Substitute in Sacrum, Percutaneous Approach

0QW13KZ Revision of Nonautologous Tissue Substitute in Sacrum, Percutaneous Approach

0QW144Z Revision of Internal Fixation Device in Sacrum, Percutaneous Endoscopic Approach

0QW147Z Revision of Autologous Tissue Substitute in Sacrum, Percutaneous Endoscopic Approach

0QW14JZ Revision of Synthetic Substitute in Sacrum, Percutaneous Endoscopic Approach

0QW14KZ Revision of Nonautologous Tissue Substitute in Sacrum, Percutaneous Endoscopic Approach

0QW1X4Z Revision of Internal Fixation Device in Sacrum, External Approach

0QW1X7Z Revision of Autologous Tissue Substitute in Sacrum, External Approach

0QW1XJZ Revision of Synthetic Substitute in Sacrum, External Approach

0QW1XKZ Revision of Nonautologous Tissue Substitute in Sacrum, External Approach

0QW204Z Revision of Internal Fixation Device in Right Pelvic Bone, Open Approach

0QW205Z Revision of External Fixation Device in Right Pelvic Bone, Open Approach

0QW207Z Revision of Autologous Tissue Substitute in Right Pelvic Bone, Open Approach

0QW20JZ Revision of Synthetic Substitute in Right Pelvic Bone, Open Approach

0QW20KZ Revision of Nonautologous Tissue Substitute in Right Pelvic Bone, Open Approach

0QW234Z Revision of Internal Fixation Device in Right Pelvic Bone, Percutaneous Approach

0QW235Z Revision of External Fixation Device in Right Pelvic Bone, Percutaneous Approach

0QW237Z Revision of Autologous Tissue Substitute in Right Pelvic Bone, Percutaneous Approach

0QW23JZ Revision of Synthetic Substitute in Right Pelvic Bone, Percutaneous Approach

0QW23KZ Revision of Nonautologous Tissue Substitute in Right Pelvic Bone, Percutaneous Approach

0QW244Z Revision of Internal Fixation Device in Right Pelvic Bone, Percutaneous Endoscopic Approach

0QW245Z Revision of External Fixation Device in Right Pelvic Bone, Percutaneous Endoscopic Approach

0QW247Z Revision of Autologous Tissue Substitute in Right Pelvic Bone, Percutaneous Endoscopic Approach

0QW24JZ Revision of Synthetic Substitute in Right Pelvic Bone, Percutaneous Endoscopic Approach

0QW24KZ Revision of Nonautologous Tissue Substitute in Right Pelvic Bone, Percutaneous Endoscopic Approach

0QW2X4Z Revision of Internal Fixation Device in Right Pelvic Bone, External Approach

0QW2X5Z Revision of External Fixation Device in Right Pelvic Bone, External Approach

0QW2X7Z Revision of Autologous Tissue Substitute in Right Pelvic Bone, External Approach

0QW2XJZ Revision of Synthetic Substitute in Right Pelvic Bone, External Approach

0QW2XKZ Revision of Nonautologous Tissue Substitute in Right Pelvic Bone, External Approach

0QW304Z Revision of Internal Fixation Device in Left Pelvic Bone, Open Approach

0QW305Z Revision of External Fixation Device in Left Pelvic Bone, Open Approach

0QW307Z Revision of Autologous Tissue Substitute in Left Pelvic Bone, Open Approach

0QW30JZ Revision of Synthetic Substitute in Left Pelvic Bone, Open Approach

0QW30KZ Revision of Nonautologous Tissue Substitute in Left Pelvic Bone, Open Approach

0QW334Z Revision of Internal Fixation Device in Left Pelvic Bone, Percutaneous Approach

0QW335Z Revision of External Fixation Device in Left Pelvic Bone, Percutaneous Approach

0QW337Z Revision of Autologous Tissue Substitute in Left Pelvic Bone, Percutaneous Approach

0QW33JZ Revision of Synthetic Substitute in Left Pelvic Bone, Percutaneous Approach

0QW33KZ Revision of Nonautologous Tissue Substitute in Left Pelvic Bone, Percutaneous Approach

0QW344Z Revision of Internal Fixation Device in Left Pelvic Bone, Percutaneous Endoscopic Approach

0QW345Z Revision of External Fixation Device in Left Pelvic Bone, Percutaneous Endoscopic Approach

0QW347Z Revision of Autologous Tissue Substitute in Left Pelvic Bone, Percutaneous Endoscopic Approach

0QW34JZ Revision of Synthetic Substitute in Left Pelvic Bone, Percutaneous Endoscopic Approach

0QW34KZ Revision of Nonautologous Tissue Substitute in Left Pelvic Bone, Percutaneous Endoscopic Approach

0QW3X4Z Revision of Internal Fixation Device in Left Pelvic Bone, External Approach

0QW3X5Z Revision of External Fixation Device in Left Pelvic Bone, External Approach

0QW3X7Z Revision of Autologous Tissue Substitute in Left Pelvic Bone, External Approach

0QW3XJZ Revision of Synthetic Substitute in Left Pelvic Bone, External Approach

0QW3XKZ Revision of Nonautologous Tissue Substitute in Left Pelvic Bone, External Approach

0QW404Z Revision of Internal Fixation Device in Right Acetabulum, Open Approach

0QW407Z Revision of Autologous Tissue Substitute in Right Acetabulum, Open Approach

0QW40JZ Revision of Synthetic Substitute in Right Acetabulum, Open Approach

0QW40KZ Revision of Nonautologous Tissue Substitute in Right Acetabulum, Open Approach

0QW434Z Revision of Internal Fixation Device in Right Acetabulum, Percutaneous Approach

0QW437Z Revision of Autologous Tissue Substitute in Right Acetabulum, Percutaneous Approach

0QW43JZ Revision of Synthetic Substitute in Right Acetabulum, Percutaneous Approach

0QW43KZ Revision of Nonautologous Tissue Substitute in Right Acetabulum, Percutaneous Approach

0QW444Z Revision of Internal Fixation Device in Right Acetabulum, Percutaneous Endoscopic Approach

0QW447Z Revision of Autologous Tissue Substitute in Right Acetabulum, Percutaneous Endoscopic Approach

0QW44JZ Revision of Synthetic Substitute in Right Acetabulum, Percutaneous Endoscopic Approach

0QW44KZ Revision of Nonautologous Tissue Substitute in Right Acetabulum, Percutaneous Endoscopic Approach

0QW4X4Z Revision of Internal Fixation Device in Right Acetabulum, External Approach

0QW4X7Z Revision of Autologous Tissue Substitute in Right Acetabulum, External Approach

0QW4XJZ Revision of Synthetic Substitute in Right Acetabulum, External Approach

0QW4XKZ Revision of Nonautologous Tissue Substitute in Right Acetabulum, External Approach

0QW504Z Revision of Internal Fixation Device in Left Acetabulum, Open Approach

0QW507Z Revision of Autologous Tissue Substitute in Left Acetabulum, Open Approach

0QW50JZ Revision of Synthetic Substitute in Left Acetabulum, Open Approach

0QW50KZ Revision of Nonautologous Tissue Substitute in Left Acetabulum, Open Approach

0QW534Z Revision of Internal Fixation Device in Left Acetabulum, Percutaneous Approach

0QW537Z Revision of Autologous Tissue Substitute in Left Acetabulum, Percutaneous Approach

0QW53JZ Revision of Synthetic Substitute in Left Acetabulum, Percutaneous Approach

0QW53KZ Revision of Nonautologous Tissue Substitute in Left Acetabulum, Percutaneous Approach

0QW544Z Revision of Internal Fixation Device in Left Acetabulum, Percutaneous Endoscopic Approach

0QW547Z Revision of Autologous Tissue Substitute in Left Acetabulum, Percutaneous Endoscopic Approach

0QW54JZ Revision of Synthetic Substitute in Left Acetabulum, Percutaneous Endoscopic Approach

0QW54KZ Revision of Nonautologous Tissue Substitute in Left Acetabulum, Percutaneous Endoscopic Approach

0QW5X4Z Revision of Internal Fixation Device in Left Acetabulum, External Approach

0QW5X7Z Revision of Autologous Tissue Substitute in Left Acetabulum, External Approach

0QW5XJZ Revision of Synthetic Substitute in Left Acetabulum, External Approach

0QW5XKZ Revision of Nonautologous Tissue Substitute in Left Acetabulum, External Approach

0QW604Z Revision of Internal Fixation Device in Right Upper Femur, Open Approach

0QW605Z Revision of External Fixation Device in Right Upper Femur, Open Approach

0QW607Z Revision of Autologous Tissue Substitute in Right Upper Femur, Open Approach

0QW60JZ Revision of Synthetic Substitute in Right Upper Femur, Open Approach

0QW60KZ Revision of Nonautologous Tissue Substitute in Right Upper Femur, Open Approach

0QW634Z Revision of Internal Fixation Device in Right Upper Femur, Percutaneous Approach

0QW635Z Revision of External Fixation Device in Right Upper Femur, Percutaneous Approach

0QW637Z Revision of Autologous Tissue Substitute in Right Upper Femur, Percutaneous Approach

0QW63JZ Revision of Synthetic Substitute in Right Upper Femur, Percutaneous Approach

0QW63KZ Revision of Nonautologous Tissue Substitute in Right Upper Femur, Percutaneous Approach

0QW644Z Revision of Internal Fixation Device in Right Upper Femur, Percutaneous Endoscopic Approach

0QW645Z Revision of External Fixation Device in Right Upper Femur, Percutaneous Endoscopic Approach

0QW647Z Revision of Autologous Tissue Substitute in Right Upper Femur, Percutaneous Endoscopic Approach

0QW64JZ Revision of Synthetic Substitute in Right Upper Femur, Percutaneous Endoscopic Approach

0QW64KZ Revision of Nonautologous Tissue Substitute in Right Upper Femur, Percutaneous Endoscopic Approach

0QW6X4Z Revision of Internal Fixation Device in Right Upper Femur, External Approach

0QW6X5Z Revision of External Fixation Device in Right Upper Femur, External Approach

0QW6X7Z Revision of Autologous Tissue Substitute in Right Upper Femur, External Approach

0QW6XJZ Revision of Synthetic Substitute in Right Upper Femur, External Approach

0QW6XKZ Revision of Nonautologous Tissue Substitute in Right Upper Femur, External Approach

0QW704Z Revision of Internal Fixation Device in Left Upper Femur, Open Approach

0QW705Z Revision of External Fixation Device in Left Upper Femur, Open Approach

0QW707Z Revision of Autologous Tissue Substitute in Left Upper Femur, Open Approach

0QW70JZ Revision of Synthetic Substitute in Left Upper Femur, Open Approach

0QW70KZ Revision of Nonautologous Tissue Substitute in Left Upper Femur, Open Approach

0QW734Z Revision of Internal Fixation Device in Left Upper Femur, Percutaneous Approach

0QW735Z Revision of External Fixation Device in Left Upper Femur, Percutaneous Approach

0QW737Z Revision of Autologous Tissue Substitute in Left Upper Femur, Percutaneous Approach

0QW73JZ Revision of Synthetic Substitute in Left Upper Femur, Percutaneous Approach

0QW73KZ Revision of Nonautologous Tissue Substitute in Left Upper Femur, Percutaneous Approach

0QW744Z Revision of Internal Fixation Device in Left Upper Femur, Percutaneous Endoscopic Approach

0QW745Z Revision of External Fixation Device in Left Upper Femur, Percutaneous Endoscopic Approach

0QW747Z Revision of Autologous Tissue Substitute in Left Upper Femur, Percutaneous Endoscopic Approach

0QW74JZ Revision of Synthetic Substitute in Left Upper Femur, Percutaneous Endoscopic Approach

0QW74KZ Revision of Nonautologous Tissue Substitute in Left Upper Femur, Percutaneous Endoscopic Approach

0QW7X4Z Revision of Internal Fixation Device in Left Upper Femur, External Approach

0QW7X5Z Revision of External Fixation Device in Left Upper Femur, External Approach

0QW7X7Z Revision of Autologous Tissue Substitute in Left Upper Femur, External Approach

0QW7XJZ Revision of Synthetic Substitute in Left Upper Femur, External Approach

0QW7XKZ Revision of Nonautologous Tissue Substitute in Left Upper Femur, External Approach

0QW804Z Revision of Internal Fixation Device in Right Femoral Shaft, Open Approach

0QW805Z Revision of External Fixation Device in Right Femoral Shaft, Open Approach

0QW807Z Revision of Autologous Tissue Substitute in Right Femoral Shaft, Open Approach

0QW80JZ Revision of Synthetic Substitute in Right Femoral Shaft, Open Approach

0QW80KZ Revision of Nonautologous Tissue Substitute in Right Femoral Shaft, Open Approach

0QW834Z Revision of Internal Fixation Device in Right Femoral Shaft, Percutaneous Approach

0QW835Z Revision of External Fixation Device in Right Femoral Shaft, Percutaneous Approach

0QW837Z Revision of Autologous Tissue Substitute in Right Femoral Shaft, Percutaneous Approach

0QW83JZ Revision of Synthetic Substitute in Right Femoral Shaft, Percutaneous Approach

0QW83KZ Revision of Nonautologous Tissue Substitute in Right Femoral Shaft, Percutaneous Approach

♀ Female-only ♂ Male-only ▲ Limited Coverage ● Non-OR ▨ HAC-associated procedure ▲ Non-covered procedures ✚ Cluster

0QW844Z	Revision of Internal Fixation Device in Right Femoral Shaft, Percutaneous Endoscopic Approach
0QW845Z	Revision of External Fixation Device in Right Femoral Shaft, Percutaneous Endoscopic Approach
0QW847Z	Revision of Autologous Tissue Substitute in Right Femoral Shaft, Percutaneous Endoscopic Approach
0QW84JZ	Revision of Synthetic Substitute in Right Femoral Shaft, Percutaneous Endoscopic Approach
0QW84KZ	Revision of Nonautologous Tissue Substitute in Right Femoral Shaft, Percutaneous Endoscopic Approach
0QW8X4Z	Revision of Internal Fixation Device in Right Femoral Shaft, External Approach
0QW8X5Z	Revision of External Fixation Device in Right Femoral Shaft, External Approach
0QW8X7Z	Revision of Autologous Tissue Substitute in Right Femoral Shaft, External Approach
0QW8XJZ	Revision of Synthetic Substitute in Right Femoral Shaft, External Approach
0QW8XKZ	Revision of Nonautologous Tissue Substitute in Right Femoral Shaft, External Approach
0QW904Z	Revision of Internal Fixation Device in Left Femoral Shaft, Open Approach
0QW905Z	Revision of External Fixation Device in Left Femoral Shaft, Open Approach
0QW907Z	Revision of Autologous Tissue Substitute in Left Femoral Shaft, Open Approach
0QW90JZ	Revision of Synthetic Substitute in Left Femoral Shaft, Open Approach
0QW90KZ	Revision of Nonautologous Tissue Substitute in Left Femoral Shaft, Open Approach
0QW934Z	Revision of Internal Fixation Device in Left Femoral Shaft, Percutaneous Approach
0QW935Z	Revision of External Fixation Device in Left Femoral Shaft, Percutaneous Approach
0QW937Z	Revision of Autologous Tissue Substitute in Left Femoral Shaft, Percutaneous Approach
0QW93JZ	Revision of Synthetic Substitute in Left Femoral Shaft, Percutaneous Approach
0QW93KZ	Revision of Nonautologous Tissue Substitute in Left Femoral Shaft, Percutaneous Approach
0QW944Z	Revision of Internal Fixation Device in Left Femoral Shaft, Percutaneous Endoscopic Approach
0QW945Z	Revision of External Fixation Device in Left Femoral Shaft, Percutaneous Endoscopic Approach
0QW947Z	Revision of Autologous Tissue Substitute in Left Femoral Shaft, Percutaneous Endoscopic Approach
0QW94JZ	Revision of Synthetic Substitute in Left Femoral Shaft, Percutaneous Endoscopic Approach
0QW94KZ	Revision of Nonautologous Tissue Substitute in Left Femoral Shaft, Percutaneous Endoscopic Approach
0QW9X4Z	Revision of Internal Fixation Device in Left Femoral Shaft, External Approach
0QW9X5Z	Revision of External Fixation Device in Left Femoral Shaft, External Approach
0QW9X7Z	Revision of Autologous Tissue Substitute in Left Femoral Shaft, External Approach
0QW9XJZ	Revision of Synthetic Substitute in Left Femoral Shaft, External Approach
0QW9XKZ	Revision of Nonautologous Tissue Substitute in Left Femoral Shaft, External Approach
0QWB04Z	Revision of Internal Fixation Device in Right Lower Femur, Open Approach
0QWB05Z	Revision of External Fixation Device in Right Lower Femur, Open Approach
0QWB07Z	Revision of Autologous Tissue Substitute in Right Lower Femur, Open Approach
0QWB0JZ	Revision of Synthetic Substitute in Right Lower Femur, Open Approach
0QWB0KZ	Revision of Nonautologous Tissue Substitute in Right Lower Femur, Open Approach
0QWB34Z	Revision of Internal Fixation Device in Right Lower Femur, Percutaneous Approach
0QWB35Z	Revision of External Fixation Device in Right Lower Femur, Percutaneous Approach
0QWB37Z	Revision of Autologous Tissue Substitute in Right Lower Femur, Percutaneous Approach
0QWB3JZ	Revision of Synthetic Substitute in Right Lower Femur, Percutaneous Approach
0QWB3KZ	Revision of Nonautologous Tissue Substitute in Right Lower Femur, Percutaneous Approach
0QWB44Z	Revision of Internal Fixation Device in Right Lower Femur, Percutaneous Endoscopic Approach
0QWB45Z	Revision of External Fixation Device in Right Lower Femur, Percutaneous Endoscopic Approach
0QWB47Z	Revision of Autologous Tissue Substitute in Right Lower Femur, Percutaneous Endoscopic Approach
0QWB4JZ	Revision of Synthetic Substitute in Right Lower Femur, Percutaneous Endoscopic Approach
0QWB4KZ	Revision of Nonautologous Tissue Substitute in Right Lower Femur, Percutaneous Endoscopic Approach
0QWBX4Z	Revision of Internal Fixation Device in Right Lower Femur, External Approach
0QWBX5Z	Revision of External Fixation Device in Right Lower Femur, External Approach
0QWBX7Z	Revision of Autologous Tissue Substitute in Right Lower Femur, External Approach
0QWBXJZ	Revision of Synthetic Substitute in Right Lower Femur, External Approach
0QWBXKZ	Revision of Nonautologous Tissue Substitute in Right Lower Femur, External Approach
0QWC04Z	Revision of Internal Fixation Device in Left Lower Femur, Open Approach
0QWC05Z	Revision of External Fixation Device in Left Lower Femur, Open Approach
0QWC07Z	Revision of Autologous Tissue Substitute in Left Lower Femur, Open Approach
0QWC0JZ	Revision of Synthetic Substitute in Left Lower Femur, Open Approach
0QWC0KZ	Revision of Nonautologous Tissue Substitute in Left Lower Femur, Open Approach
0QWC34Z	Revision of Internal Fixation Device in Left Lower Femur, Percutaneous Approach
0QWC35Z	Revision of External Fixation Device in Left Lower Femur, Percutaneous Approach
0QWC37Z	Revision of Autologous Tissue Substitute in Left Lower Femur, Percutaneous Approach
0QWC3JZ	Revision of Synthetic Substitute in Left Lower Femur, Percutaneous Approach
0QWC3KZ	Revision of Nonautologous Tissue Substitute in Left Lower Femur, Percutaneous Approach
0QWC44Z	Revision of Internal Fixation Device in Left Lower Femur, Percutaneous Endoscopic Approach
0QWC45Z	Revision of External Fixation Device in Left Lower Femur, Percutaneous Endoscopic Approach
0QWC47Z	Revision of Autologous Tissue Substitute in Left Lower Femur, Percutaneous Endoscopic Approach
0QWC4JZ	Revision of Synthetic Substitute in Left Lower Femur, Percutaneous Endoscopic Approach
0QWC4KZ	Revision of Nonautologous Tissue Substitute in Left Lower Femur, Percutaneous Endoscopic Approach
0QWCX4Z	Revision of Internal Fixation Device in Left Lower Femur, External Approach
0QWCX5Z	Revision of External Fixation Device in Left Lower Femur, External Approach
0QWCX7Z	Revision of Autologous Tissue Substitute in Left Lower Femur, External Approach
0QWCXJZ	Revision of Synthetic Substitute in Left Lower Femur, External Approach
0QWCXKZ	Revision of Nonautologous Tissue Substitute in Left Lower Femur, External Approach
0QWD04Z	Revision of Internal Fixation Device in Right Patella, Open Approach
0QWD05Z	Revision of External Fixation Device in Right Patella, Open Approach
0QWD07Z	Revision of Autologous Tissue Substitute in Right Patella, Open Approach
0QWD0JZ	Revision of Synthetic Substitute in Right Patella, Open Approach
0QWD0KZ	Revision of Nonautologous Tissue Substitute in Right Patella, Open Approach
0QWD34Z	Revision of Internal Fixation Device in Right Patella, Percutaneous Approach
0QWD35Z	Revision of External Fixation Device in Right Patella, Percutaneous Approach
0QWD37Z	Revision of Autologous Tissue Substitute in Right Patella, Percutaneous Approach
0QWD3JZ	Revision of Synthetic Substitute in Right Patella, Percutaneous Approach

0QWD3KZ Revision of Nonautologous Tissue Substitute in Right Patella, Percutaneous Approach

0QWD44Z Revision of Internal Fixation Device in Right Patella, Percutaneous Endoscopic Approach

0QWD45Z Revision of External Fixation Device in Right Patella, Percutaneous Endoscopic Approach

0QWD47Z Revision of Autologous Tissue Substitute in Right Patella, Percutaneous Endoscopic Approach

0QWD4JZ Revision of Synthetic Substitute in Right Patella, Percutaneous Endoscopic Approach

0QWD4KZ Revision of Nonautologous Tissue Substitute in Right Patella, Percutaneous Endoscopic Approach

0QWDX4Z Revision of Internal Fixation Device in Right Patella, External Approach

0QWDX5Z Revision of External Fixation Device in Right Patella, External Approach

0QWDX7Z Revision of Autologous Tissue Substitute in Right Patella, External Approach

0QWDXJZ Revision of Synthetic Substitute in Right Patella, External Approach

0QWDXKZ Revision of Nonautologous Tissue Substitute in Right Patella, External Approach

0QWF04Z Revision of Internal Fixation Device in Left Patella, Open Approach

0QWF05Z Revision of External Fixation Device in Left Patella, Open Approach

0QWF07Z Revision of Autologous Tissue Substitute in Left Patella, Open Approach

0QWF0JZ Revision of Synthetic Substitute in Left Patella, Open Approach

0QWF0KZ Revision of Nonautologous Tissue Substitute in Left Patella, Open Approach

0QWF34Z Revision of Internal Fixation Device in Left Patella, Percutaneous Approach

0QWF35Z Revision of External Fixation Device in Left Patella, Percutaneous Approach

0QWF37Z Revision of Autologous Tissue Substitute in Left Patella, Percutaneous Approach

0QWF3JZ Revision of Synthetic Substitute in Left Patella, Percutaneous Approach

0QWF3KZ Revision of Nonautologous Tissue Substitute in Left Patella, Percutaneous Approach

0QWF44Z Revision of Internal Fixation Device in Left Patella, Percutaneous Endoscopic Approach

0QWF45Z Revision of External Fixation Device in Left Patella, Percutaneous Endoscopic Approach

0QWF47Z Revision of Autologous Tissue Substitute in Left Patella, Percutaneous Endoscopic Approach

0QWF4JZ Revision of Synthetic Substitute in Left Patella, Percutaneous Endoscopic Approach

0QWF4KZ Revision of Nonautologous Tissue Substitute in Left Patella, Percutaneous Endoscopic Approach

0QWFX4Z Revision of Internal Fixation Device in Left Patella, External Approach

0QWFX5Z Revision of External Fixation Device in Left Patella, External Approach

0QWFX7Z Revision of Autologous Tissue Substitute in Left Patella, External Approach

0QWFXJZ Revision of Synthetic Substitute in Left Patella, External Approach

0QWFXKZ Revision of Nonautologous Tissue Substitute in Left Patella, External Approach

0QWG04Z Revision of Internal Fixation Device in Right Tibia, Open Approach

0QWG05Z Revision of External Fixation Device in Right Tibia, Open Approach

0QWG07Z Revision of Autologous Tissue Substitute in Right Tibia, Open Approach

0QWG0JZ Revision of Synthetic Substitute in Right Tibia, Open Approach

0QWG0KZ Revision of Nonautologous Tissue Substitute in Right Tibia, Open Approach

0QWG34Z Revision of Internal Fixation Device in Right Tibia, Percutaneous Approach

0QWG35Z Revision of External Fixation Device in Right Tibia, Percutaneous Approach

0QWG37Z Revision of Autologous Tissue Substitute in Right Tibia, Percutaneous Approach

0QWG3JZ Revision of Synthetic Substitute in Right Tibia, Percutaneous Approach

0QWG3KZ Revision of Nonautologous Tissue Substitute in Right Tibia, Percutaneous Approach

0QWG44Z Revision of Internal Fixation Device in Right Tibia, Percutaneous Endoscopic Approach

0QWG45Z Revision of External Fixation Device in Right Tibia, Percutaneous Endoscopic Approach

0QWG47Z Revision of Autologous Tissue Substitute in Right Tibia, Percutaneous Endoscopic Approach

0QWG4JZ Revision of Synthetic Substitute in Right Tibia, Percutaneous Endoscopic Approach

0QWG4KZ Revision of Nonautologous Tissue Substitute in Right Tibia, Percutaneous Endoscopic Approach

0QWGX4Z Revision of Internal Fixation Device in Right Tibia, External Approach

0QWGX5Z Revision of External Fixation Device in Right Tibia, External Approach

0QWGX7Z Revision of Autologous Tissue Substitute in Right Tibia, External Approach

0QWGXJZ Revision of Synthetic Substitute in Right Tibia, External Approach

0QWGXKZ Revision of Nonautologous Tissue Substitute in Right Tibia, External Approach

0QWH04Z Revision of Internal Fixation Device in Left Tibia, Open Approach

0QWH05Z Revision of External Fixation Device in Left Tibia, Open Approach

0QWH07Z Revision of Autologous Tissue Substitute in Left Tibia, Open Approach

0QWH0JZ Revision of Synthetic Substitute in Left Tibia, Open Approach

0QWH0KZ Revision of Nonautologous Tissue Substitute in Left Tibia, Open Approach

0QWH34Z Revision of Internal Fixation Device in Left Tibia, Percutaneous Approach

0QWH35Z Revision of External Fixation Device in Left Tibia, Percutaneous Approach

0QWH37Z Revision of Autologous Tissue Substitute in Left Tibia, Percutaneous Approach

0QWH3JZ Revision of Synthetic Substitute in Left Tibia, Percutaneous Approach

0QWH3KZ Revision of Nonautologous Tissue Substitute in Left Tibia, Percutaneous Approach

0QWH44Z Revision of Internal Fixation Device in Left Tibia, Percutaneous Endoscopic Approach

0QWH45Z Revision of External Fixation Device in Left Tibia, Percutaneous Endoscopic Approach

0QWH47Z Revision of Autologous Tissue Substitute in Left Tibia, Percutaneous Endoscopic Approach

0QWH4JZ Revision of Synthetic Substitute in Left Tibia, Percutaneous Endoscopic Approach

0QWH4KZ Revision of Nonautologous Tissue Substitute in Left Tibia, Percutaneous Endoscopic Approach

0QWHX4Z Revision of Internal Fixation Device in Left Tibia, External Approach

0QWHX5Z Revision of External Fixation Device in Left Tibia, External Approach

0QWHX7Z Revision of Autologous Tissue Substitute in Left Tibia, External Approach

0QWHXJZ Revision of Synthetic Substitute in Left Tibia, External Approach

0QWHXKZ Revision of Nonautologous Tissue Substitute in Left Tibia, External Approach

0QWJ04Z Revision of Internal Fixation Device in Right Fibula, Open Approach

0QWJ05Z Revision of External Fixation Device in Right Fibula, Open Approach

0QWJ07Z Revision of Autologous Tissue Substitute in Right Fibula, Open Approach

0QWJ0JZ Revision of Synthetic Substitute in Right Fibula, Open Approach

0QWJ0KZ Revision of Nonautologous Tissue Substitute in Right Fibula, Open Approach

0QWJ34Z Revision of Internal Fixation Device in Right Fibula, Percutaneous Approach

0QWJ35Z Revision of External Fixation Device in Right Fibula, Percutaneous Approach

0QWJ37Z Revision of Autologous Tissue Substitute in Right Fibula, Percutaneous Approach

0QWJ3JZ Revision of Synthetic Substitute in Right Fibula, Percutaneous Approach

0QWJ3KZ Revision of Nonautologous Tissue Substitute in Right Fibula, Percutaneous Approach

0QWJ44Z Revision of Internal Fixation Device in Right Fibula, Percutaneous Endoscopic Approach

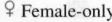

0QWJ45Z	Revision of External Fixation Device in Right Fibula, Percutaneous Endoscopic Approach
0QWJ47Z	Revision of Autologous Tissue Substitute in Right Fibula, Percutaneous Endoscopic Approach
0QWJ4JZ	Revision of Synthetic Substitute in Right Fibula, Percutaneous Endoscopic Approach
0QWJ4KZ	Revision of Nonautologous Tissue Substitute in Right Fibula, Percutaneous Endoscopic Approach
0QWJX4Z	Revision of Internal Fixation Device in Right Fibula, External Approach
0QWJX5Z	Revision of External Fixation Device in Right Fibula, External Approach
0QWJX7Z	Revision of Autologous Tissue Substitute in Right Fibula, External Approach
0QWJXJZ	Revision of Synthetic Substitute in Right Fibula, External Approach
0QWJXKZ	Revision of Nonautologous Tissue Substitute in Right Fibula, External Approach
0QWK04Z	Revision of Internal Fixation Device in Left Fibula, Open Approach
0QWK05Z	Revision of External Fixation Device in Left Fibula, Open Approach
0QWK07Z	Revision of Autologous Tissue Substitute in Left Fibula, Open Approach
0QWK0JZ	Revision of Synthetic Substitute in Left Fibula, Open Approach
0QWK0KZ	Revision of Nonautologous Tissue Substitute in Left Fibula, Open Approach
0QWK34Z	Revision of Internal Fixation Device in Left Fibula, Percutaneous Approach
0QWK35Z	Revision of External Fixation Device in Left Fibula, Percutaneous Approach
0QWK37Z	Revision of Autologous Tissue Substitute in Left Fibula, Percutaneous Approach
0QWK3JZ	Revision of Synthetic Substitute in Left Fibula, Percutaneous Approach
0QWK3KZ	Revision of Nonautologous Tissue Substitute in Left Fibula, Percutaneous Approach
0QWK44Z	Revision of Internal Fixation Device in Left Fibula, Percutaneous Endoscopic Approach
0QWK45Z	Revision of External Fixation Device in Left Fibula, Percutaneous Endoscopic Approach
0QWK47Z	Revision of Autologous Tissue Substitute in Left Fibula, Percutaneous Endoscopic Approach
0QWK4JZ	Revision of Synthetic Substitute in Left Fibula, Percutaneous Endoscopic Approach
0QWK4KZ	Revision of Nonautologous Tissue Substitute in Left Fibula, Percutaneous Endoscopic Approach
0QWKX4Z	Revision of Internal Fixation Device in Left Fibula, External Approach
0QWKX5Z	Revision of External Fixation Device in Left Fibula, External Approach
0QWKX7Z	Revision of Autologous Tissue Substitute in Left Fibula, External Approach
0QWKXJZ	Revision of Synthetic Substitute in Left Fibula, External Approach

0QWKXKZ	Revision of Nonautologous Tissue Substitute in Left Fibula, External Approach
0QWL04Z	Revision of Internal Fixation Device in Right Tarsal, Open Approach
0QWL05Z	Revision of External Fixation Device in Right Tarsal, Open Approach
0QWL07Z	Revision of Autologous Tissue Substitute in Right Tarsal, Open Approach
0QWL0JZ	Revision of Synthetic Substitute in Right Tarsal, Open Approach
0QWL0KZ	Revision of Nonautologous Tissue Substitute in Right Tarsal, Open Approach
0QWL34Z	Revision of Internal Fixation Device in Right Tarsal, Percutaneous Approach
0QWL35Z	Revision of External Fixation Device in Right Tarsal, Percutaneous Approach
0QWL37Z	Revision of Autologous Tissue Substitute in Right Tarsal, Percutaneous Approach
0QWL3JZ	Revision of Synthetic Substitute in Right Tarsal, Percutaneous Approach
0QWL3KZ	Revision of Nonautologous Tissue Substitute in Right Tarsal, Percutaneous Approach
0QWL44Z	Revision of Internal Fixation Device in Right Tarsal, Percutaneous Endoscopic Approach
0QWL45Z	Revision of External Fixation Device in Right Tarsal, Percutaneous Endoscopic Approach
0QWL47Z	Revision of Autologous Tissue Substitute in Right Tarsal, Percutaneous Endoscopic Approach
0QWL4JZ	Revision of Synthetic Substitute in Right Tarsal, Percutaneous Endoscopic Approach
0QWL4KZ	Revision of Nonautologous Tissue Substitute in Right Tarsal, Percutaneous Endoscopic Approach
0QWLX4Z	Revision of Internal Fixation Device in Right Tarsal, External Approach
0QWLX5Z	Revision of External Fixation Device in Right Tarsal, External Approach
0QWLX7Z	Revision of Autologous Tissue Substitute in Right Tarsal, External Approach
0QWLXJZ	Revision of Synthetic Substitute in Right Tarsal, External Approach
0QWLXKZ	Revision of Nonautologous Tissue Substitute in Right Tarsal, External Approach
0QWM04Z	Revision of Internal Fixation Device in Left Tarsal, Open Approach
0QWM05Z	Revision of External Fixation Device in Left Tarsal, Open Approach
0QWM07Z	Revision of Autologous Tissue Substitute in Left Tarsal, Open Approach
0QWM0JZ	Revision of Synthetic Substitute in Left Tarsal, Open Approach
0QWM0KZ	Revision of Nonautologous Tissue Substitute in Left Tarsal, Open Approach
0QWM34Z	Revision of Internal Fixation Device in Left Tarsal, Percutaneous Approach
0QWM35Z	Revision of External Fixation Device in Left Tarsal, Percutaneous Approach

0QWM37Z	Revision of Autologous Tissue Substitute in Left Tarsal, Percutaneous Approach
0QWM3JZ	Revision of Synthetic Substitute in Left Tarsal, Percutaneous Approach
0QWM3KZ	Revision of Nonautologous Tissue Substitute in Left Tarsal, Percutaneous Approach
0QWM44Z	Revision of Internal Fixation Device in Left Tarsal, Percutaneous Endoscopic Approach
0QWM45Z	Revision of External Fixation Device in Left Tarsal, Percutaneous Endoscopic Approach
0QWM47Z	Revision of Autologous Tissue Substitute in Left Tarsal, Percutaneous Endoscopic Approach
0QWM4JZ	Revision of Synthetic Substitute in Left Tarsal, Percutaneous Endoscopic Approach
0QWM4KZ	Revision of Nonautologous Tissue Substitute in Left Tarsal, Percutaneous Endoscopic Approach
0QWMX4Z	Revision of Internal Fixation Device in Left Tarsal, External Approach
0QWMX5Z	Revision of External Fixation Device in Left Tarsal, External Approach
0QWMX7Z	Revision of Autologous Tissue Substitute in Left Tarsal, External Approach
0QWMXJZ	Revision of Synthetic Substitute in Left Tarsal, External Approach
0QWMXKZ	Revision of Nonautologous Tissue Substitute in Left Tarsal, External Approach
0QWN04Z	Revision of Internal Fixation Device in Right Metatarsal, Open Approach
0QWN05Z	Revision of External Fixation Device in Right Metatarsal, Open Approach
0QWN07Z	Revision of Autologous Tissue Substitute in Right Metatarsal, Open Approach
0QWN0JZ	Revision of Synthetic Substitute in Right Metatarsal, Open Approach
0QWN0KZ	Revision of Nonautologous Tissue Substitute in Right Metatarsal, Open Approach
0QWN34Z	Revision of Internal Fixation Device in Right Metatarsal, Percutaneous Approach
0QWN35Z	Revision of External Fixation Device in Right Metatarsal, Percutaneous Approach
0QWN37Z	Revision of Autologous Tissue Substitute in Right Metatarsal, Percutaneous Approach
0QWN3JZ	Revision of Synthetic Substitute in Right Metatarsal, Percutaneous Approach
0QWN3KZ	Revision of Nonautologous Tissue Substitute in Right Metatarsal, Percutaneous Approach
0QWN44Z	Revision of Internal Fixation Device in Right Metatarsal, Percutaneous Endoscopic Approach
0QWN45Z	Revision of External Fixation Device in Right Metatarsal, Percutaneous Endoscopic Approach
0QWN47Z	Revision of Autologous Tissue Substitute in Right Metatarsal, Percutaneous Endoscopic Approach
0QWN4JZ	Revision of Synthetic Substitute in Right Metatarsal, Percutaneous Endoscopic Approach

0QWN4KZ Revision of Nonautologous Tissue Substitute in Right Metatarsal, Percutaneous Endoscopic Approach

0QWNX4Z Revision of Internal Fixation Device in Right Metatarsal, External Approach

0QWNX5Z Revision of External Fixation Device in Right Metatarsal, External Approach

0QWNX7Z Revision of Autologous Tissue Substitute in Right Metatarsal, External Approach

0QWNXJZ Revision of Synthetic Substitute in Right Metatarsal, External Approach

0QWNXKZ Revision of Nonautologous Tissue Substitute in Right Metatarsal, External Approach

0QWP04Z Revision of Internal Fixation Device in Left Metatarsal, Open Approach

0QWP05Z Revision of External Fixation Device in Left Metatarsal, Open Approach

0QWP07Z Revision of Autologous Tissue Substitute in Left Metatarsal, Open Approach

0QWP0JZ Revision of Synthetic Substitute in Left Metatarsal, Open Approach

0QWP0KZ Revision of Nonautologous Tissue Substitute in Left Metatarsal, Open Approach

0QWP34Z Revision of Internal Fixation Device in Left Metatarsal, Percutaneous Approach

0QWP35Z Revision of External Fixation Device in Left Metatarsal, Percutaneous Approach

0QWP37Z Revision of Autologous Tissue Substitute in Left Metatarsal, Percutaneous Approach

0QWP3JZ Revision of Synthetic Substitute in Left Metatarsal, Percutaneous Approach

0QWP3KZ Revision of Nonautologous Tissue Substitute in Left Metatarsal, Percutaneous Approach

0QWP44Z Revision of Internal Fixation Device in Left Metatarsal, Percutaneous Endoscopic Approach

0QWP45Z Revision of External Fixation Device in Left Metatarsal, Percutaneous Endoscopic Approach

0QWP47Z Revision of Autologous Tissue Substitute in Left Metatarsal, Percutaneous Endoscopic Approach

0QWP4JZ Revision of Synthetic Substitute in Left Metatarsal, Percutaneous Endoscopic Approach

0QWP4KZ Revision of Nonautologous Tissue Substitute in Left Metatarsal, Percutaneous Endoscopic Approach

0QWPX4Z Revision of Internal Fixation Device in Left Metatarsal, External Approach

0QWPX5Z Revision of External Fixation Device in Left Metatarsal, External Approach

0QWPX7Z Revision of Autologous Tissue Substitute in Left Metatarsal, External Approach

0QWPXJZ Revision of Synthetic Substitute in Left Metatarsal, External Approach

0QWPXKZ Revision of Nonautologous Tissue Substitute in Left Metatarsal, External Approach

0QWQ04Z Revision of Internal Fixation Device in Right Toe Phalanx, Open Approach

0QWQ05Z Revision of External Fixation Device in Right Toe Phalanx, Open Approach

0QWQ07Z Revision of Autologous Tissue Substitute in Right Toe Phalanx, Open Approach

0QWQ0JZ Revision of Synthetic Substitute in Right Toe Phalanx, Open Approach

0QWQ0KZ Revision of Nonautologous Tissue Substitute in Right Toe Phalanx, Open Approach

0QWQ34Z Revision of Internal Fixation Device in Right Toe Phalanx, Percutaneous Approach

0QWQ35Z Revision of External Fixation Device in Right Toe Phalanx, Percutaneous Approach

0QWQ37Z Revision of Autologous Tissue Substitute in Right Toe Phalanx, Percutaneous Approach

0QWQ3JZ Revision of Synthetic Substitute in Right Toe Phalanx, Percutaneous Approach

0QWQ3KZ Revision of Nonautologous Tissue Substitute in Right Toe Phalanx, Percutaneous Approach

0QWQ44Z Revision of Internal Fixation Device in Right Toe Phalanx, Percutaneous Endoscopic Approach

0QWQ45Z Revision of External Fixation Device in Right Toe Phalanx, Percutaneous Endoscopic Approach

0QWQ47Z Revision of Autologous Tissue Substitute in Right Toe Phalanx, Percutaneous Endoscopic Approach

0QWQ4JZ Revision of Synthetic Substitute in Right Toe Phalanx, Percutaneous Endoscopic Approach

0QWQ4KZ Revision of Nonautologous Tissue Substitute in Right Toe Phalanx, Percutaneous Endoscopic Approach

0QWQX4Z Revision of Internal Fixation Device in Right Toe Phalanx, External Approach

0QWQX5Z Revision of External Fixation Device in Right Toe Phalanx, External Approach

0QWQX7Z Revision of Autologous Tissue Substitute in Right Toe Phalanx, External Approach

0QWQXJZ Revision of Synthetic Substitute in Right Toe Phalanx, External Approach

0QWQXKZ Revision of Nonautologous Tissue Substitute in Right Toe Phalanx, External Approach

0QWR04Z Revision of Internal Fixation Device in Left Toe Phalanx, Open Approach

0QWR05Z Revision of External Fixation Device in Left Toe Phalanx, Open Approach

0QWR07Z Revision of Autologous Tissue Substitute in Left Toe Phalanx, Open Approach

0QWR0JZ Revision of Synthetic Substitute in Left Toe Phalanx, Open Approach

0QWR0KZ Revision of Nonautologous Tissue Substitute in Left Toe Phalanx, Open Approach

0QWR34Z Revision of Internal Fixation Device in Left Toe Phalanx, Percutaneous Approach

0QWR35Z Revision of External Fixation Device in Left Toe Phalanx, Percutaneous Approach

0QWR37Z Revision of Autologous Tissue Substitute in Left Toe Phalanx, Percutaneous Approach

0QWR3JZ Revision of Synthetic Substitute in Left Toe Phalanx, Percutaneous Approach

0QWR3KZ Revision of Nonautologous Tissue Substitute in Left Toe Phalanx, Percutaneous Approach

0QWR44Z Revision of Internal Fixation Device in Left Toe Phalanx, Percutaneous Endoscopic Approach

0QWR45Z Revision of External Fixation Device in Left Toe Phalanx, Percutaneous Endoscopic Approach

0QWR47Z Revision of Autologous Tissue Substitute in Left Toe Phalanx, Percutaneous Endoscopic Approach

0QWR4JZ Revision of Synthetic Substitute in Left Toe Phalanx, Percutaneous Endoscopic Approach

0QWR4KZ Revision of Nonautologous Tissue Substitute in Left Toe Phalanx, Percutaneous Endoscopic Approach

0QWRX4Z Revision of Internal Fixation Device in Left Toe Phalanx, External Approach

0QWRX5Z Revision of External Fixation Device in Left Toe Phalanx, External Approach

0QWRX7Z Revision of Autologous Tissue Substitute in Left Toe Phalanx, External Approach

0QWRXJZ Revision of Synthetic Substitute in Left Toe Phalanx, External Approach

0QWRXKZ Revision of Nonautologous Tissue Substitute in Left Toe Phalanx, External Approach

0QWS04Z Revision of Internal Fixation Device in Coccyx, Open Approach

0QWS07Z Revision of Autologous Tissue Substitute in Coccyx, Open Approach

0QWS0JZ Revision of Synthetic Substitute in Coccyx, Open Approach

0QWS0KZ Revision of Nonautologous Tissue Substitute in Coccyx, Open Approach

0QWS34Z Revision of Internal Fixation Device in Coccyx, Percutaneous Approach

0QWS37Z Revision of Autologous Tissue Substitute in Coccyx, Percutaneous Approach

0QWS3JZ Revision of Synthetic Substitute in Coccyx, Percutaneous Approach

0QWS3KZ Revision of Nonautologous Tissue Substitute in Coccyx, Percutaneous Approach

0QWS44Z Revision of Internal Fixation Device in Coccyx, Percutaneous Endoscopic Approach

0QWS47Z Revision of Autologous Tissue Substitute in Coccyx, Percutaneous Endoscopic Approach

0QWS4JZ Revision of Synthetic Substitute in Coccyx, Percutaneous Endoscopic Approach

0QWS4KZ Revision of Nonautologous Tissue Substitute in Coccyx, Percutaneous Endoscopic Approach

0QWSX4Z Revision of Internal Fixation Device in Coccyx, External Approach

0QWSX7Z Revision of Autologous Tissue Substitute in Coccyx, External Approach

0QWSXJZ Revision of Synthetic Substitute in Coccyx, External Approach

♀ Female-only ♂ Male-only ▲ Limited Coverage ● Non-OR █ HAC-associated procedure ▲ Non-covered procedures ✚ Cluster

0QWSXKZ Revision of Nonautologous Tissue Substitute in Coccyx, External Approach

0QWY00Z Revision of Drainage Device in Lower Bone, Open Approach

0QWY0MZ Revision of Bone Growth Stimulator in Lower Bone, Open Approach

0QWY30Z Revision of Drainage Device in Lower Bone, Percutaneous Approach

0QWY3MZ Revision of Bone Growth Stimulator in Lower Bone, Percutaneous Approach

0QWY40Z Revision of Drainage Device in Lower Bone, Percutaneous Endoscopic Approach

0QWY4MZ Revision of Bone Growth Stimulator in Lower Bone, Percutaneous Endoscopic Approach

0QWYX0Z Revision of Drainage Device in Lower Bone, External Approach

0QWYXMZ Revision of Bone Growth Stimulator in Lower Bone, External Approach

Intervertebral Joint

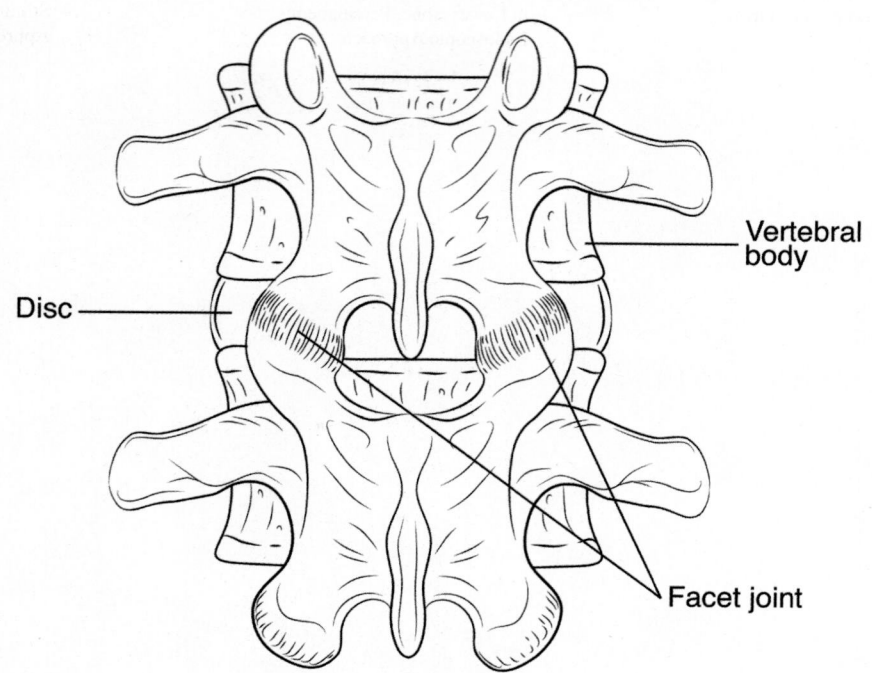

Vertebral
body

Disc

Facet joint

©AHIMA

Shoulder

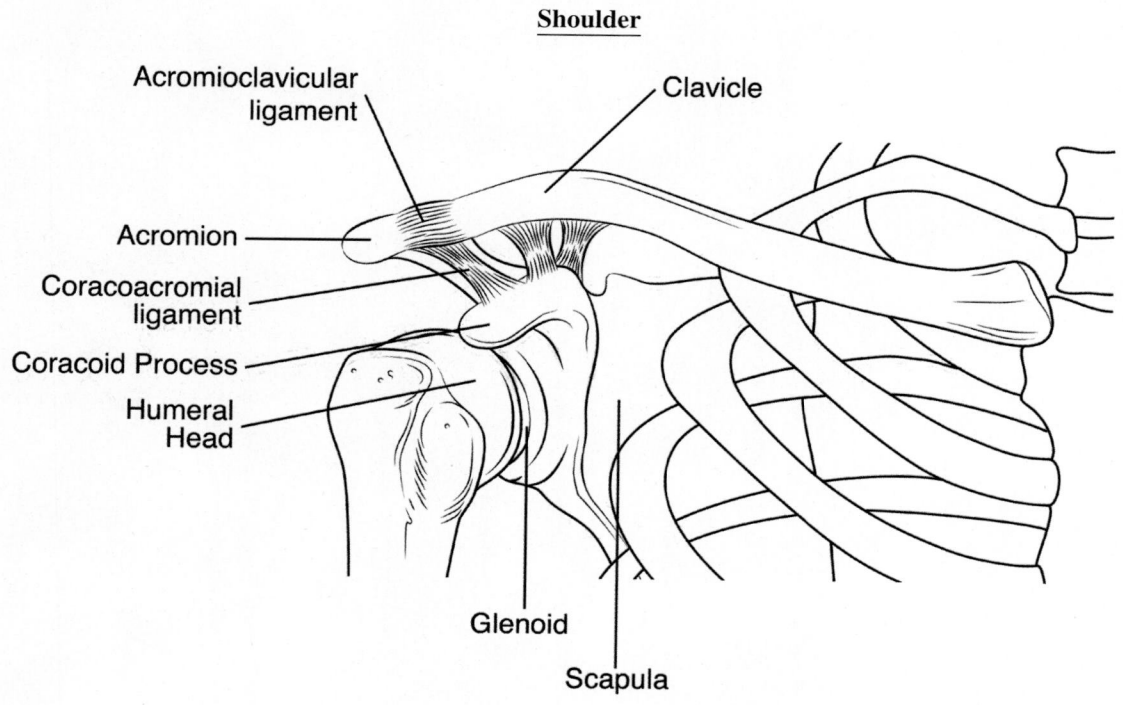

Acromioclavicular
ligament

Clavicle

Acromion

Coracoacromial
ligament

Coracoid Process

Humeral
Head

Glenoid

Scapula

©AHIMA

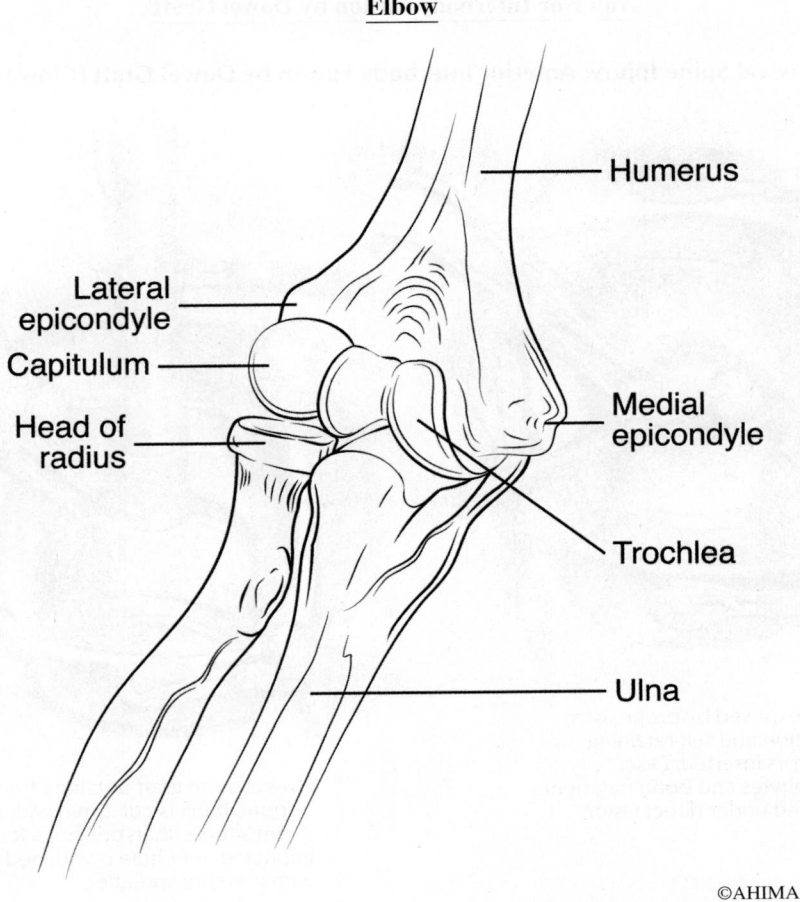

Humerus

Lateral
epicondyle

Capitulum

Head of
radius

Medial
epicondyle

Trochlea

Ulna

©AHIMA

Wrist

Capitate

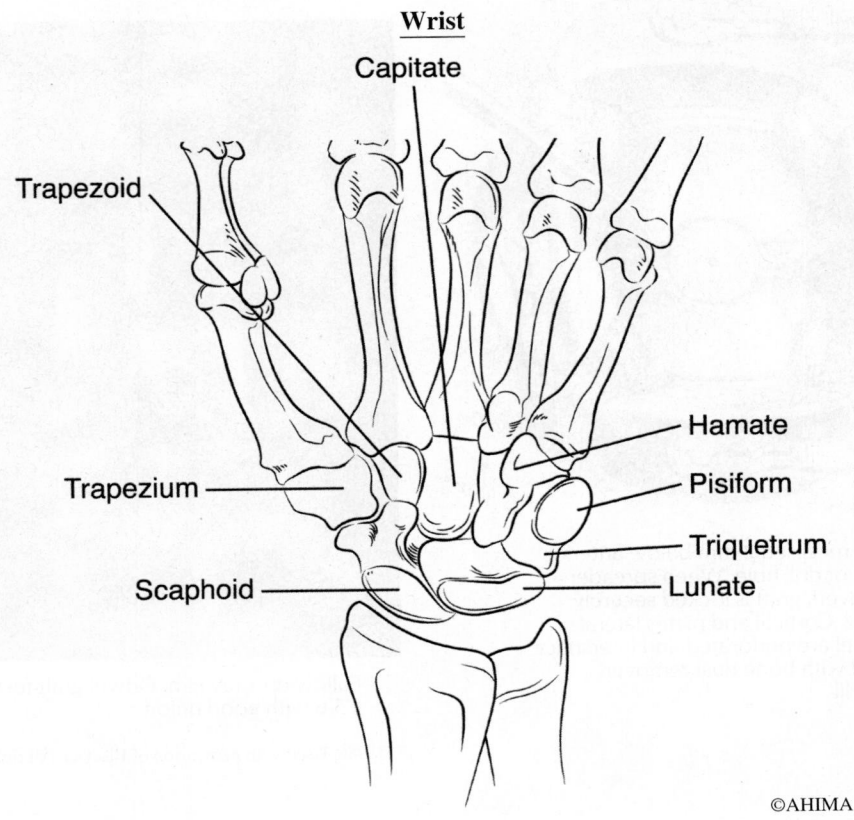

Trapezoid

Trapezium

Scaphoid

Hamate

Pisiform

Triquetrum

Lunate

©AHIMA

Cervical Spine Injury: Anterior Interbody Fusion by Dowel Graft (Cloward)

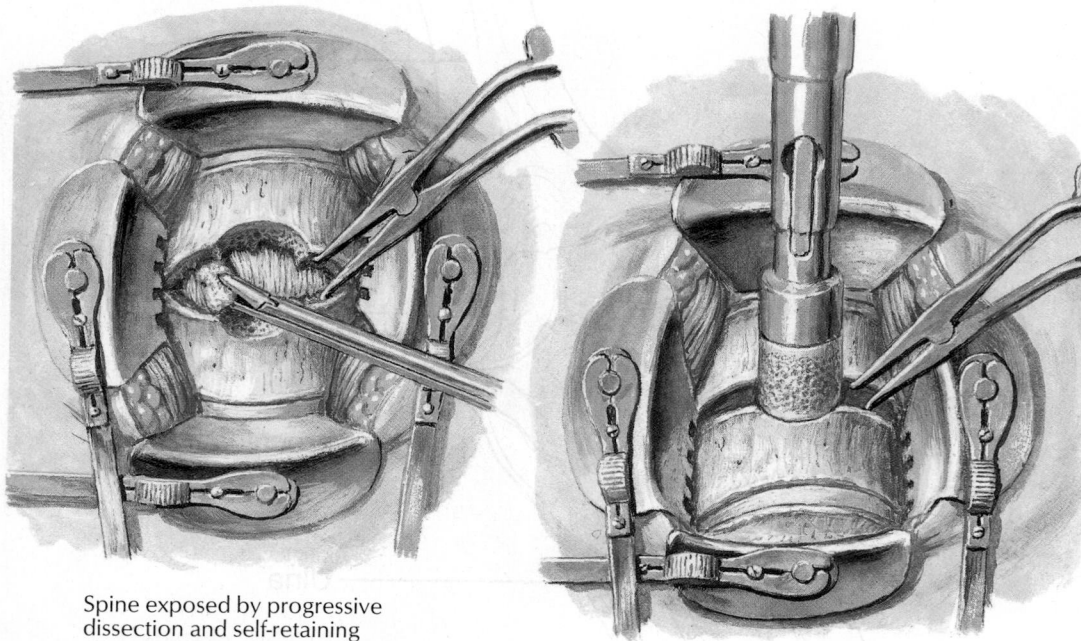

Spine exposed by progressive dissection and self-retaining retractors inserted. Disc, osteophytes and bone fragments removed under direct vision

Dowel bone graft obtained from ilium or bone bank is cut 2 mm wider and 2 mm shorter than drill hole. It is impacted after hole is widened with vertebra spreader

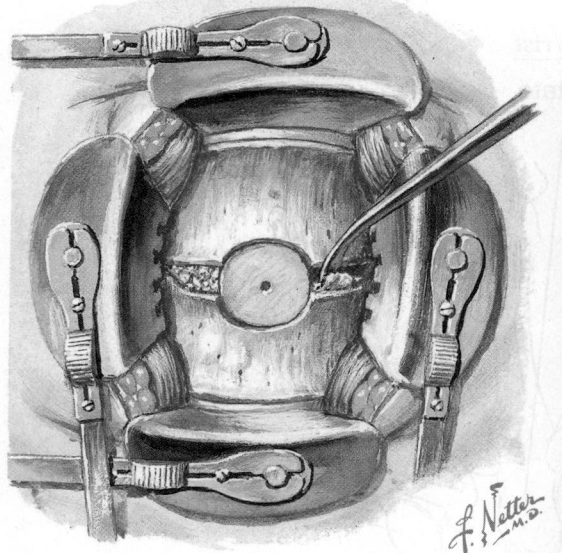

Dowel recessed 2 mm below anterior margin of drill hole. When spreader is removed, graft is locked securely in place. Cortical end plates lateral to dowel are perforated and interspace packed with bone dust removed from drill

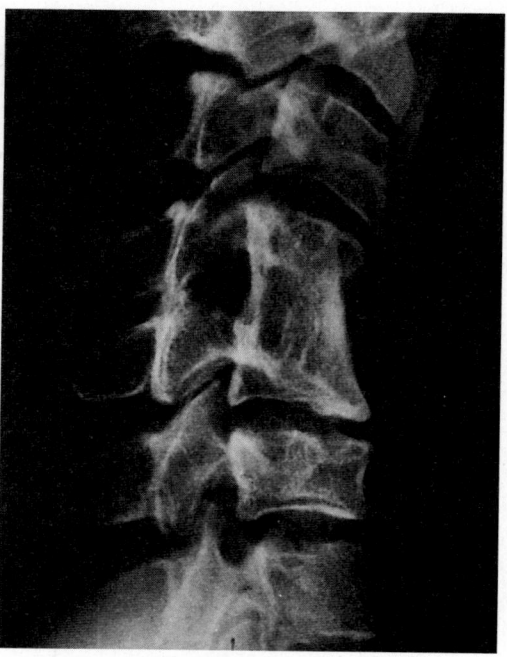

Follow-up x-ray film. Dowel graft fusion of C5-6 with good union

Section	0	Medical and Surgical
Body System	R	Upper Joints
Operation	2	**Change:** Taking out or off a device from a body part and putting back an identical or similar device in or on the same body part without cutting or puncturing the skin or a mucous membrane

Body Part (4th)	Approach (5th)	Device (6th)	Qualifier (7th)
Y Upper Joint	**X** External	**0** Drainage Device **Y** Other Device	**Z** No Qualifier

Section	0	Medical and Surgical
Body System	R	Upper Joints
Operation	5	**Destruction:** Physical eradication of all or a portion of a body part by the direct use of energy, force, or a destructive agent

Body Part (4th)	Approach (5th)	Device (6th)	Qualifier (7th)
0 Occipital-cervical Joint **1** Cervical Vertebral Joint **3** Cervical Vertebral Disc **4** Cervicothoracic Vertebral Joint **5** Cervicothoracic Vertebral Disc **6** Thoracic Vertebral Joint **9** Thoracic Vertebral Disc **A** Thoracolumbar Vertebral Joint **B** Thoracolumbar Vertebral Disc **C** Temporomandibular Joint, Right **D** Temporomandibular Joint, Left **E** Sternoclavicular Joint, Right **F** Sternoclavicular Joint, Left **G** Acromioclavicular Joint, Right **H** Acromioclavicular Joint, Left **J** Shoulder Joint, Right **K** Shoulder Joint, Left **L** Elbow Joint, Right **M** Elbow Joint, Left **N** Wrist Joint, Right **P** Wrist Joint, Left **Q** Carpal Joint, Right **R** Carpal Joint, Left **S** Carpometacarpal Joint, Right **T** Carpometacarpal Joint, Left **U** Metacarpophalangeal Joint, Right **V** Metacarpophalangeal Joint, Left **W** Finger Phalangeal Joint, Right **X** Finger Phalangeal Joint, Left	**0** Open **3** Percutaneous **4** Percutaneous Endoscopic	**Z** No Device	**Z** No Qualifier

Section	0	Medical and Surgical
Body System	R	Upper Joints
Operation	9	Drainage: Taking or letting out fluids and/or gases from a body part

Body Part (4th)	Approach (5th)	Device (6th)	Qualifier (7th)
0 Occipital-cervical Joint 1 Cervical Vertebral Joint 3 Cervical Vertebral Disc 4 Cervicothoracic Vertebral Joint 5 Cervicothoracic Vertebral Disc 6 Thoracic Vertebral Joint 9 Thoracic Vertebral Disc A Thoracolumbar Vertebral Joint B Thoracolumbar Vertebral Disc C Temporomandibular Joint, Right D Temporomandibular Joint, Left E Sternoclavicular Joint, Right F Sternoclavicular Joint, Left G Acromioclavicular Joint, Right H Acromioclavicular Joint, Left J Shoulder Joint, Right K Shoulder Joint, Left L Elbow Joint, Right M Elbow Joint, Left N Wrist Joint, Right P Wrist Joint, Left Q Carpal Joint, Right R Carpal Joint, Left S Carpometacarpal Joint, Right T Carpometacarpal Joint, Left U Metacarpophalangeal Joint, Right V Metacarpophalangeal Joint, Left W Finger Phalangeal Joint, Right X Finger Phalangeal Joint, Left	0 Open 3 Percutaneous 4 Percutaneous Endoscopic	0 Drainage Device	Z No Qualifier
0 Occipital-cervical Joint 1 Cervical Vertebral Joint 3 Cervical Vertebral Disc 4 Cervicothoracic Vertebral Joint 5 Cervicothoracic Vertebral Disc 6 Thoracic Vertebral Joint 9 Thoracic Vertebral Disc A Thoracolumbar Vertebral Joint B Thoracolumbar Vertebral Disc C Temporomandibular Joint, Right D Temporomandibular Joint, Left E Sternoclavicular Joint, Right F Sternoclavicular Joint, Left G Acromioclavicular Joint, Right H Acromioclavicular Joint, Left J Shoulder Joint, Right K Shoulder Joint, Left L Elbow Joint, Right M Elbow Joint, Left N Wrist Joint, Right P Wrist Joint, Left Q Carpal Joint, Right R Carpal Joint, Left S Carpometacarpal Joint, Right T Carpometacarpal Joint, Left U Metacarpophalangeal Joint, Right V Metacarpophalangeal Joint, Left W Finger Phalangeal Joint, Right X Finger Phalangeal Joint, Left	0 Open 3 Percutaneous 4 Percutaneous Endoscopic	Z No Device	X Diagnostic Z No Qualifier

Section	0	Medical and Surgical
Body System	R	Upper Joints
Operation	B	Excision: Cutting out or off, without replacement, a portion of a body part

Body Part (4th)	Approach (5th)	Device (6th)	Qualifier (7th)
0 Occipital-cervical Joint 1 Cervical Vertebral Joint 3 Cervical Vertebral Disc 4 Cervicothoracic Vertebral Joint 5 Cervicothoracic Vertebral Disc 6 Thoracic Vertebral Joint 9 Thoracic Vertebral Disc A Thoracolumbar Vertebral Joint B Thoracolumbar Vertebral Disc C Temporomandibular Joint, Right D Temporomandibular Joint, Left E Sternoclavicular Joint, Right F Sternoclavicular Joint, Left G Acromioclavicular Joint, Right H Acromioclavicular Joint, Left J Shoulder Joint, Right K Shoulder Joint, Left L Elbow Joint, Right M Elbow Joint, Left N Wrist Joint, Right P Wrist Joint, Left Q Carpal Joint, Right R Carpal Joint, Left S Carpometacarpal Joint, Right T Carpometacarpal Joint, Left U Metacarpophalangeal Joint, Right V Metacarpophalangeal Joint, Left W Finger Phalangeal Joint, Right X Finger Phalangeal Joint, Left	0 Open 3 Percutaneous 4 Percutaneous Endoscopic	Z No Device	X Diagnostic Z No Qualifier

Section	0	Medical and Surgical
Body System	R	Upper Joints
Operation	C	Extirpation: Taking or cutting out solid matter from a body part

Body Part (4th)	Approach (5th)	Device (6th)	Qualifier (7th)
0 Occipital-cervical Joint	0 Open	Z No Device	Z No Qualifier
1 Cervical Vertebral Joint	3 Percutaneous		
3 Cervical Vertebral Disc	4 Percutaneous Endoscopic		
4 Cervicothoracic Vertebral Joint			
5 Cervicothoracic Vertebral Disc			
6 Thoracic Vertebral Joint			
9 Thoracic Vertebral Disc			
A Thoracolumbar Vertebral Joint			
B Thoracolumbar Vertebral Disc			
C Temporomandibular Joint, Right			
D Temporomandibular Joint, Left			
E Sternoclavicular Joint, Right			
F Sternoclavicular Joint, Left			
G Acromioclavicular Joint, Right			
H Acromioclavicular Joint, Left			
J Shoulder Joint, Right			
K Shoulder Joint, Left			
L Elbow Joint, Right			
M Elbow Joint, Left			
N Wrist Joint, Right			
P Wrist Joint, Left			
Q Carpal Joint, Right			
R Carpal Joint, Left			
S Carpometacarpal Joint, Right			
T Carpometacarpal Joint, Left			
U Metacarpophalangeal Joint, Right			
V Metacarpophalangeal Joint, Left			
W Finger Phalangeal Joint, Right			
X Finger Phalangeal Joint, Left			

Section	0	Medical and Surgical
Body System	R	Upper Joints
Operation	G	Fusion: Joining together portions of an articular body part rendering the articular body part immobile

Body Part (4th)	Approach (5th)	Device (6th)	Qualifier (7th)
0 Occipital-cervical Joint 1 Cervical Vertebral Joint 2 Cervical Vertebral Joints, 2 or more 4 Cervicothoracic Vertebral Joint 6 Thoracic Vertebral Joint 7 Thoracic Vertebral Joints, 2 to 7 8 Thoracic Vertebral Joints, 8 or more A Thoracolumbar Vertebral Joint	0 Open 3 Percutaneous 4 Percutaneous Endoscopic	7 Autologous Tissue Substitute J Synthetic Substitute K Nonautologous Tissue Substitute	0 Anterior Approach, Anterior Column 1 Posterior Approach, Posterior Column J Posterior Approach, Anterior Column
0 Occipital-cervical Joint 1 Cervical Vertebral Joint 2 Cervical Vertebral Joints, 2 or more 4 Cervicothoracic Vertebral Joint 6 Thoracic Vertebral Joint 7 Thoracic Vertebral Joints, 2 to 7 8 Thoracic Vertebral Joints, 8 or more A Thoracolumbar Vertebral Joint	0 Open 3 Percutaneous 4 Percutaneous Endoscopic	A Interbody Fusion Device	0 Anterior Approach, Anterior Column J Posterior Approach, Anterior Column
C Temporomandibular Joint, Right D Temporomandibular Joint, Left E Sternoclavicular Joint, Right F Sternoclavicular Joint, Left G Acromioclavicular Joint, Right H Acromioclavicular Joint, Left J Shoulder Joint, Right K Shoulder Joint, Left	0 Open 3 Percutaneous 4 Percutaneous Endoscopic	4 Internal Fixation Device 7 Autologous Tissue Substitute J Synthetic Substitute K Nonautologous Tissue Substitute	Z No Qualifier

Continued →

Section	0	Medical and Surgical
Body System	R	Upper Joints
Operation	G	**Fusion:** Joining together portions of an articular body part rendering the articular body part immobile

Body Part (4th)	Approach (5th)	Device (6th)	Qualifier (7th)
L Elbow Joint, Right M Elbow Joint, Left N Wrist Joint, Right P Wrist Joint, Left Q Carpal Joint, Right R Carpal Joint, Left S Carpometacarpal Joint, Right T Carpometacarpal Joint, Left U Metacarpophalangeal Joint, Right V Metacarpophalangeal Joint, Left W Finger Phalangeal Joint, Right X Finger Phalangeal Joint, Left	0 Open 3 Percutaneous 4 Percutaneous Endoscopic	3 Internal Fixation Device, Sustained Compression 4 Internal Fixation Device 5 External Fixation Device 7 Autologous Tissue Substitute J Synthetic Substitute K Nonautologous Tissue Substitute	Z No Qualifier

Section	0	Medical and Surgical
Body System	R	Upper Joints
Operation	H	**Insertion:** Putting in a nonbiological appliance that monitors, assists, performs, or prevents a physiological function but does not physically take the place of a body part

Body Part (4th)	Approach (5th)	Device (6th)	Qualifier (7th)
0 Occipital-cervical Joint 1 Cervical Vertebral Joint 4 Cervicothoracic Vertebral Joint 6 Thoracic Vertebral Joint A Thoracolumbar Vertebral Joint	0 Open 3 Percutaneous 4 Percutaneous Endoscopic	3 Infusion Device 4 Internal Fixation Device 8 Spacer B Spinal Stabilization Device, Interspinous Process C Spinal Stabilization Device, Pedicle-Based D Spinal Stabilization Device, Facet Replacement	Z No Qualifier
3 Cervical Vertebral Disc 5 Cervicothoracic Vertebral Disc 9 Thoracic Vertebral Disc B Thoracolumbar Vertebral Disc	0 Open 3 Percutaneous 4 Percutaneous Endoscopic	3 Infusion Device	Z No Qualifier
C Temporomandibular Joint, Right D Temporomandibular Joint, Left E Sternoclavicular Joint, Right F Sternoclavicular Joint, Left G Acromioclavicular Joint, Right H Acromioclavicular Joint, Left J Shoulder Joint, Right K Shoulder Joint, Left	0 Open 3 Percutaneous 4 Percutaneous Endoscopic	3 Infusion Device 4 Internal Fixation Device 8 Spacer	Z No Qualifier
L Elbow Joint, Right M Elbow Joint, Left N Wrist Joint, Right P Wrist Joint, Left Q Carpal Joint, Right R Carpal Joint, Left S Carpometacarpal Joint, Right T Carpometacarpal Joint, Left U Metacarpophalangeal Joint, Right V Metacarpophalangeal Joint, Left W Finger Phalangeal Joint, Right X Finger Phalangeal Joint, Left	0 Open 3 Percutaneous 4 Percutaneous Endoscopic	3 Infusion Device 4 Internal Fixation Device 5 External Fixation Device 8 Spacer	Z No Qualifier

Section	0	Medical and Surgical
Body System	R	Upper Joints
Operation	J	Inspection: Visually and/or manually exploring a body part

Body Part (4th)	Approach (5th)	Device (6th)	Qualifier (7th)
0 Occipital-cervical Joint	0 Open	Z No Device	Z No Qualifier
1 Cervical Vertebral Joint	3 Percutaneous		
3 Cervical Vertebral Disc	4 Percutaneous Endoscopic		
4 Cervicothoracic Vertebral Joint	X External		
5 Cervicothoracic Vertebral Disc			
6 Thoracic Vertebral Joint			
9 Thoracic Vertebral Disc			
A Thoracolumbar Vertebral Joint			
B Thoracolumbar Vertebral Disc			
C Temporomandibular Joint, Right			
D Temporomandibular Joint, Left			
E Sternoclavicular Joint, Right			
F Sternoclavicular Joint, Left			
G Acromioclavicular Joint, Right			
H Acromioclavicular Joint, Left			
J Shoulder Joint, Right			
K Shoulder Joint, Left			
L Elbow Joint, Right			
M Elbow Joint, Left			
N Wrist Joint, Right			
P Wrist Joint, Left			
Q Carpal Joint, Right			
R Carpal Joint, Left			
S Carpometacarpal Joint, Right			
T Carpometacarpal Joint, Left			
U Metacarpophalangeal Joint, Right			
V Metacarpophalangeal Joint, Left			
W Finger Phalangeal Joint, Right			
X Finger Phalangeal Joint, Left			

Section	0	Medical and Surgical
Body System	R	Upper Joints
Operation	N	Release: Freeing a body part from an abnormal physical constraint by cutting or by the use of force

Body Part (4th)	Approach (5th)	Device (6th)	Qualifier (7th)
0 Occipital-cervical Joint	0 Open	Z No Device	Z No Qualifier
1 Cervical Vertebral Joint	3 Percutaneous		
3 Cervical Vertebral Disc	4 Percutaneous Endoscopic		
4 Cervicothoracic Vertebral Joint	X External		
5 Cervicothoracic Vertebral Disc			
6 Thoracic Vertebral Joint			
9 Thoracic Vertebral Disc			
A Thoracolumbar Vertebral Joint			
B Thoracolumbar Vertebral Disc			
C Temporomandibular Joint, Right			
D Temporomandibular Joint, Left			
E Sternoclavicular Joint, Right			
F Sternoclavicular Joint, Left			
G Acromioclavicular Joint, Right			
H Acromioclavicular Joint, Left			
J Shoulder Joint, Right			
K Shoulder Joint, Left			
L Elbow Joint, Right			
M Elbow Joint, Left			
N Wrist Joint, Right			
P Wrist Joint, Left			
Q Carpal Joint, Right			
R Carpal Joint, Left			
S Carpometacarpal Joint, Right			
T Carpometacarpal Joint, Left			
U Metacarpophalangeal Joint, Right			
V Metacarpophalangeal Joint, Left			
W Finger Phalangeal Joint, Right			
X Finger Phalangeal Joint, Left			

Section	0	Medical and Surgical
Body System	R	Upper Joints
Operation	P	Removal: Taking out or off a device from a body part

Body Part (4th)	Approach (5th)	Device (6th)	Qualifier (7th)
0 Occipital-cervical Joint 1 Cervical Vertebral Joint 4 Cervicothoracic Vertebral Joint 6 Thoracic Vertebral Joint A Thoracolumbar Vertebral Joint	0 Open 3 Percutaneous 4 Percutaneous Endoscopic	0 Drainage Device 3 Infusion Device 4 Internal Fixation Device 7 Autologous Tissue Substitute 8 Spacer A Interbody Fusion Device J Synthetic Substitute K Nonautologous Tissue Substitute	Z No Qualifier
0 Occipital-cervical Joint 1 Cervical Vertebral Joint 4 Cervicothoracic Vertebral Joint 6 Thoracic Vertebral Joint A Thoracolumbar Vertebral Joint	X External	0 Drainage Device 3 Infusion Device 4 Internal Fixation Device	Z No Qualifier
3 Cervical Vertebral Disc 5 Cervicothoracic Vertebral Disc 9 Thoracic Vertebral Disc B Thoracolumbar Vertebral Disc	0 Open 3 Percutaneous 4 Percutaneous Endoscopic	0 Drainage Device 3 Infusion Device 7 Autologous Tissue Substitute J Synthetic Substitute K Nonautologous Tissue Substitute	Z No Qualifier
3 Cervical Vertebral Disc 5 Cervicothoracic Vertebral Disc 9 Thoracic Vertebral Disc B Thoracolumbar Vertebral Disc	X External	0 Drainage Device 3 Infusion Device	Z No Qualifier
C Temporomandibular Joint, Right D Temporomandibular Joint, Left E Sternoclavicular Joint, Right F Sternoclavicular Joint, Left G Acromioclavicular Joint, Right H Acromioclavicular Joint, Left	0 Open 3 Percutaneous 4 Percutaneous Endoscopic	0 Drainage Device 3 Infusion Device 4 Internal Fixation Device 7 Autologous Tissue Substitute 8 Spacer J Synthetic Substitute K Nonautologous Tissue Substitute	Z No Qualifier
C Temporomandibular Joint, Right D Temporomandibular Joint, Left E Sternoclavicular Joint, Right F Sternoclavicular Joint, Left G Acromioclavicular Joint, Right H Acromioclavicular Joint, Left	X External	0 Drainage Device 3 Infusion Device 4 Internal Fixation Device	Z No Qualifier
J Shoulder Joint, Right K Shoulder Joint, Left	0 Open 3 Percutaneous 4 Percutaneous Endoscopic	0 Drainage Device 3 Infusion Device 4 Internal Fixation Device 7 Autologous Tissue Substitute 8 Spacer K Nonautologous Tissue Substitute	Z No Qualifier
J Shoulder Joint, Right K Shoulder Joint, Left	0 Open 3 Percutaneous 4 Percutaneous Endoscopic	J Synthetic Substitute	6 Humeral Surface 7 Glenoid Surface Z No Device
J Shoulder Joint, Right K Shoulder Joint, Left	X External	0 Drainage Device 3 Infusion Device 4 Internal Fixation Device	Z No Qualifier

Continued →

Section	0	Medical and Surgical
Body System	R	Upper Joints
Operation	P	Removal: Taking out or off a device from a body part

Body Part (4th)	Approach (5th)	Device (6th)	Qualifier (7th)
L Elbow Joint, Right M Elbow Joint, Left N Wrist Joint, Right P Wrist Joint, Left Q Carpal Joint, Right R Carpal Joint, Left S Carpometacarpal Joint, Right T Carpometacarpal Joint, Left U Metacarpophalangeal Joint, Right V Metacarpophalangeal Joint, Left W Finger Phalangeal Joint, Right X Finger Phalangeal Joint, Left	0 Open 3 Percutaneous 4 Percutaneous Endoscopic	0 Drainage Device 3 Infusion Device 4 Internal Fixation Device 5 External Fixation Device 7 Autologous Tissue Substitute 8 Spacer J Synthetic Substitute K Nonautologous Tissue Substitute	Z No Qualifier
L Elbow Joint, Right M Elbow Joint, Left N Wrist Joint, Right P Wrist Joint, Left Q Carpal Joint, Right R Carpal Joint, Left S Carpometacarpal Joint, Right T Carpometacarpal Joint, Left U Metacarpophalangeal Joint, Right V Metacarpophalangeal Joint, Left W Finger Phalangeal Joint, Right X Finger Phalangeal Joint, Left	X External	0 Drainage Device 3 Infusion Device 4 Internal Fixation Device 5 External Fixation Device	Z No Qualifier

Section	0	Medical and Surgical
Body System	R	Upper Joints
Operation	Q	Repair: Restoring, to the extent possible, a body part to its normal anatomic structure and function

Body Part (4th)	Approach (5th)	Device (6th)	Qualifier (7th)
0 Occipital-cervical Joint 1 Cervical Vertebral Joint 3 Cervical Vertebral Disc 4 Cervicothoracic Vertebral Joint 5 Cervicothoracic Vertebral Disc 6 Thoracic Vertebral Joint 9 Thoracic Vertebral Disc A Thoracolumbar Vertebral Joint B Thoracolumbar Vertebral Disc C Temporomandibular Joint, Right D Temporomandibular Joint, Left E Sternoclavicular Joint, Right F Sternoclavicular Joint, Left G Acromioclavicular Joint, Right H Acromioclavicular Joint, Left J Shoulder Joint, Right K Shoulder Joint, Left L Elbow Joint, Right M Elbow Joint, Left N Wrist Joint, Right P Wrist Joint, Left Q Carpal Joint, Right R Carpal Joint, Left S Carpometacarpal Joint, Right T Carpometacarpal Joint, Left U Metacarpophalangeal Joint, Right V Metacarpophalangeal Joint, Left W Finger Phalangeal Joint, Right X Finger Phalangeal Joint, Left	0 Open 3 Percutaneous 4 Percutaneous Endoscopic X External	Z No Device	Z No Qualifier

Section   **0**   **Medical and Surgical**
Body System   **R**   **Upper Joints**
Operation   **R**   **Replacement:** Putting in or on biological or synthetic material that physically takes the place and/or function of all or a portion of a body part

Body Part (4ᵗʰ)	Approach (5ᵗʰ)	Device (6ᵗʰ)	Qualifier (7ᵗʰ)
0 Occipital-cervical Joint **1** Cervical Vertebral Joint **3** Cervical Vertebral Disc **4** Cervicothoracic Vertebral Joint **5** Cervicothoracic Vertebral Disc **6** Thoracic Vertebral Joint **9** Thoracic Vertebral Disc **A** Thoracolumbar Vertebral Joint **B** Thoracolumbar Vertebral Disc **C** Temporomandibular Joint, Right **D** Temporomandibular Joint, Left **E** Sternoclavicular Joint, Right **F** Sternoclavicular Joint, Left **G** Acromioclavicular Joint, Right **H** Acromioclavicular Joint, Left **L** Elbow Joint, Right **M** Elbow Joint, Left **N** Wrist Joint, Right **P** Wrist Joint, Left **Q** Carpal Joint, Right **R** Carpal Joint, Left **S** Carpometacarpal Joint, Right **T** Carpometacarpal Joint, Left **U** Metacarpophalangeal Joint, Right **V** Metacarpophalangeal Joint, Left **W** Finger Phalangeal Joint, Right **X** Finger Phalangeal Joint, Left	**0** Open	**7** Autologous Tissue Substitute **J** Synthetic Substitute **K** Nonautologous Tissue Substitute	**Z** No Qualifier
J Shoulder Joint, Right **K** Shoulder Joint, Left	**0** Open	**0** Synthetic Substitute, Reverse Ball and Socket **7** Autologous Tissue Substitute **K** Nonautologous Tissue Substitute	**Z** No Qualifier
J Shoulder Joint, Right **K** Shoulder Joint, Left	**0** Open	**J** Synthetic Substitute	**6** Humeral Surface **7** Glenoid Surface **Z** No Qualifier

Section   **0**   **Medical and Surgical**
Body System   **R**   **Upper Joints**
Operation   **S**   **Reposition:** Moving to its normal location, or other suitable location, all or a portion of a body part

Body Part (4ᵗʰ)	Approach (5ᵗʰ)	Device (6ᵗʰ)	Qualifier (7ᵗʰ)
0 Occipital-cervical Joint **1** Cervical Vertebral Joint **4** Cervicothoracic Vertebral Joint **6** Thoracic Vertebral Joint **A** Thoracolumbar Vertebral Joint **C** Temporomandibular Joint, Right **D** Temporomandibular Joint, Left **E** Sternoclavicular Joint, Right **F** Sternoclavicular Joint, Left **G** Acromioclavicular Joint, Right **H** Acromioclavicular Joint, Left **J** Shoulder Joint, Right **K** Shoulder Joint, Left	**0** Open **3** Percutaneous **4** Percutaneous Endoscopic **X** External	**4** Internal Fixation Device **Z** No Device	**Z** No Qualifier

Continued →

Section	0	Medical and Surgical
Body System	R	Upper Joints
Operation	S	Reposition: Moving to its normal location, or other suitable location, all or a portion of a body part

Body Part (4th)	Approach (5th)	Device (6th)	Qualifier (7th)
L Elbow Joint, Right M Elbow Joint, Left N Wrist Joint, Right P Wrist Joint, Left Q Carpal Joint, Right R Carpal Joint, Left S Carpometacarpal Joint, Right T Carpometacarpal Joint, Left U Metacarpophalangeal Joint, Right V Metacarpophalangeal Joint, Left W Finger Phalangeal Joint, Right X Finger Phalangeal Joint, Left	0 Open 3 Percutaneous 4 Percutaneous Endoscopic X External	4 Internal Fixation Device 5 External Fixation Device Z No Device	Z No Qualifier

Section	0	Medical and Surgical
Body System	R	Upper Joints
Operation	T	Resection: Cutting out or off, without replacement, all of a body part

Body Part (4th)	Approach (5th)	Device (6th)	Qualifier (7th)
3 Cervical Vertebral Disc 4 Cervicothoracic Vertebral Joint 5 Cervicothoracic Vertebral Disc 9 Thoracic Vertebral Disc B Thoracolumbar Vertebral Disc C Temporomandibular Joint, Right D Temporomandibular Joint, Left E Sternoclavicular Joint, Right F Sternoclavicular Joint, Left G Acromioclavicular Joint, Right H Acromioclavicular Joint, Left J Shoulder Joint, Right K Shoulder Joint, Left L Elbow Joint, Right M Elbow Joint, Left N Wrist Joint, Right P Wrist Joint, Left Q Carpal Joint, Right R Carpal Joint, Left S Carpometacarpal Joint, Right T Carpometacarpal Joint, Left U Metacarpophalangeal Joint, Right V Metacarpophalangeal Joint, Left W Finger Phalangeal Joint, Right X Finger Phalangeal Joint, Left	0 Open	Z No Device	Z No Qualifier

Section 0 Medical and Surgical
Body System R Upper Joints
Operation U Supplement: Putting in or on biological or synthetic material that physically reinforces and/or augments the function of a portion of a body part

Body Part (4th)	Approach (5th)	Device (6th)	Qualifier (7th)
0 Occipital-cervical Joint 1 Cervical Vertebral Joint 3 Cervical Vertebral Disc 4 Cervicothoracic Vertebral Joint 5 Cervicothoracic Vertebral Disc 6 Thoracic Vertebral Joint 9 Thoracic Vertebral Disc A Thoracolumbar Vertebral Joint B Thoracolumbar Vertebral Disc C Temporomandibular Joint, Right D Temporomandibular Joint, Left E Sternoclavicular Joint, Right F Sternoclavicular Joint, Left G Acromioclavicular Joint, Right H Acromioclavicular Joint, Left J Shoulder Joint, Right K Shoulder Joint, Left L Elbow Joint, Right M Elbow Joint, Left N Wrist Joint, Right P Wrist Joint, Left Q Carpal Joint, Right R Carpal Joint, Left S Carpometacarpal Joint, Right T Carpometacarpal Joint, Left U Metacarpophalangeal Joint, Right V Metacarpophalangeal Joint, Left W Finger Phalangeal Joint, Right X Finger Phalangeal Joint, Left	0 Open 3 Percutaneous 4 Percutaneous Endoscopic	7 Autologous Tissue Substitute J Synthetic Substitute K Nonautologous Tissue Substitute	Z No Qualifier

Section 0 Medical and Surgical
Body System R Upper Joints
Operation W Revision: Correcting, to the extent possible, a portion of a malfunctioning device or the position of a displaced device

Body Part (4th)	Approach (5th)	Device (6th)	Qualifier (7th)
0 Occipital-cervical Joint 1 Cervical Vertebral Joint 4 Cervicothoracic Vertebral Joint 6 Thoracic Vertebral Joint A Thoracolumbar Vertebral Joint	0 Open 3 Percutaneous 4 Percutaneous Endoscopic X External	0 Drainage Device 3 Infusion Device 4 Internal Fixation Device 7 Autologous Tissue Substitute 8 Spacer A Interbody Fusion Device J Synthetic Substitute K Nonautologous Tissue Substitute	Z No Qualifier
3 Cervical Vertebral Disc 5 Cervicothoracic Vertebral Disc 9 Thoracic Vertebral Disc B Thoracolumbar Vertebral Disc	0 Open 3 Percutaneous 4 Percutaneous Endoscopic X External	0 Drainage Device 3 Infusion Device 7 Autologous Tissue Substitute J Synthetic Substitute K Nonautologous Tissue Substitute	Z No Qualifier
C Temporomandibular Joint, Right D Temporomandibular Joint, Left E Sternoclavicular Joint, Right F Sternoclavicular Joint, Left G Acromioclavicular Joint, Right H Acromioclavicular Joint, Left	0 Open 3 Percutaneous 4 Percutaneous Endoscopic X External	0 Drainage Device 3 Infusion Device 4 Internal Fixation Device 7 Autologous Tissue Substitute 8 Spacer J Synthetic Substitute K Nonautologous Tissue Substitute	Z No Qualifier

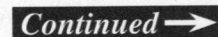

Continued ➡

Section	**0**	**Medical and Surgical**	
Body System	**R**	**Upper Joints**	
Operation	**W**	**Revision:** Correcting, to the extent possible, a portion of a malfunctioning device or the position of a displaced device	

Body Part (4th)	Approach (5th)	Device (6th)	Qualifier (7th)
J Shoulder Joint, Right **K** Shoulder Joint, Left	**0** Open **3** Percutaneous **4** Percutaneous Endoscopic **X** External	**0** Drainage Device **3** Infusion Device **4** Internal Fixation Device **7** Autologous Tissue Substitute **8** Spacer **K** Nonautologous Tissue Substitute	**Z** No Qualifier
J Shoulder Joint, Right **K** Shoulder Joint, Left	**0** Open **3** Percutaneous **4** Percutaneous Endoscopic **X** External	**J** Synthetic Substitute	**6** Humeral Surface **7** Glenoid Surface **Z** No Device
L Elbow Joint, Right **M** Elbow Joint, Left **N** Wrist Joint, Right **P** Wrist Joint, Left **Q** Carpal Joint, Right **R** Carpal Joint, Left **S** Carpometacarpal Joint, Right **T** Carpometacarpal Joint, Left **U** Metacarpophalangeal Joint, Right **V** Metacarpophalangeal Joint, Left **W** Finger Phalangeal Joint, Right **X** Finger Phalangeal Joint, Left	**0** Open **3** Percutaneous **4** Percutaneous Endoscopic **X** External	**0** Drainage Device **3** Infusion Device **4** Internal Fixation Device **5** External Fixation Device **7** Autologous Tissue Substitute **8** Spacer **J** Synthetic Substitute **K** Nonautologous Tissue Substitute	**Z** No Qualifier

Upper Joints Code Listing 0R2–0RW

Review Coding Guideline B4.5

0R2 – Upper Joints, Change

Review Coding Guideline B6.1c

0R2YX0Z Change Drainage Device in Upper Joint, External Approach

0R2YXYZ Change Other Device in Upper Joint, External Approach

0R5 – Upper Joints, Destruction

0R500ZZ Destruction of Occipital-cervical Joint, Open Approach

0R503ZZ Destruction of Occipital-cervical Joint, Percutaneous Approach

0R504ZZ Destruction of Occipital-cervical Joint, Percutaneous Endoscopic Approach

0R510ZZ Destruction of Cervical Vertebral Joint, Open Approach

0R513ZZ Destruction of Cervical Vertebral Joint, Percutaneous Approach

0R514ZZ Destruction of Cervical Vertebral Joint, Percutaneous Endoscopic Approach

0R530ZZ Destruction of Cervical Vertebral Disc, Open Approach

0R533ZZ Destruction of Cervical Vertebral Disc, Percutaneous Approach

0R534ZZ Destruction of Cervical Vertebral Disc, Percutaneous Endoscopic Approach

0R540ZZ Destruction of Cervicothoracic Vertebral Joint, Open Approach

0R543ZZ Destruction of Cervicothoracic Vertebral Joint, Percutaneous Approach

0R544ZZ Destruction of Cervicothoracic Vertebral Joint, Percutaneous Endoscopic Approach

0R550ZZ Destruction of Cervicothoracic Vertebral Disc, Open Approach

0R553ZZ Destruction of Cervicothoracic Vertebral Disc, Percutaneous Approach

0R554ZZ Destruction of Cervicothoracic Vertebral Disc, Percutaneous Endoscopic Approach

0R560ZZ Destruction of Thoracic Vertebral Joint, Open Approach

0R563ZZ Destruction of Thoracic Vertebral Joint, Percutaneous Approach

0R564ZZ Destruction of Thoracic Vertebral Joint, Percutaneous Endoscopic Approach

0R590ZZ Destruction of Thoracic Vertebral Disc, Open Approach

0R593ZZ Destruction of Thoracic Vertebral Disc, Percutaneous Approach

0R594ZZ Destruction of Thoracic Vertebral Disc, Percutaneous Endoscopic Approach

0R5A0ZZ Destruction of Thoracolumbar Vertebral Joint, Open Approach

0R5A3ZZ Destruction of Thoracolumbar Vertebral Joint, Percutaneous Approach

0R5A4ZZ Destruction of Thoracolumbar Vertebral Joint, Percutaneous Endoscopic Approach

0R5B0ZZ Destruction of Thoracolumbar Vertebral Disc, Open Approach

0R5B3ZZ Destruction of Thoracolumbar Vertebral Disc, Percutaneous Approach

0R5B4ZZ Destruction of Thoracolumbar Vertebral Disc, Percutaneous Endoscopic Approach

0R5C0ZZ Destruction of Right Temporomandibular Joint, Open Approach

0R5C3ZZ Destruction of Right Temporomandibular Joint, Percutaneous Approach

0R5C4ZZ Destruction of Right Temporomandibular Joint, Percutaneous Endoscopic Approach

0R5D0ZZ Destruction of Left Temporomandibular Joint, Open Approach

0R5D3ZZ Destruction of Left Temporomandibular Joint, Percutaneous Approach

0R5D4ZZ Destruction of Left Temporomandibular Joint, Percutaneous Endoscopic Approach

0R5E0ZZ Destruction of Right Sternoclavicular Joint, Open Approach

0R5E3ZZ Destruction of Right Sternoclavicular Joint, Percutaneous Approach

0R5E4ZZ Destruction of Right Sternoclavicular Joint, Percutaneous Endoscopic Approach

♀ Female-only   ♂ Male-only   ▲ Limited Coverage   ● Non-OR   HAC HAC-associated procedure   ▲ Non-covered procedures   ✚ Cluster

0R5F0ZZ Destruction of Left Sternoclavicular Joint, Open Approach
0R5F3ZZ Destruction of Left Sternoclavicular Joint, Percutaneous Approach
0R5F4ZZ Destruction of Left Sternoclavicular Joint, Percutaneous Endoscopic Approach
0R5G0ZZ Destruction of Right Acromioclavicular Joint, Open Approach
0R5G3ZZ Destruction of Right Acromioclavicular Joint, Percutaneous Approach
0R5G4ZZ Destruction of Right Acromioclavicular Joint, Percutaneous Endoscopic Approach
0R5H0ZZ Destruction of Left Acromioclavicular Joint, Open Approach
0R5H3ZZ Destruction of Left Acromioclavicular Joint, Percutaneous Approach
0R5H4ZZ Destruction of Left Acromioclavicular Joint, Percutaneous Endoscopic Approach
0R5J0ZZ Destruction of Right Shoulder Joint, Open Approach
0R5J3ZZ Destruction of Right Shoulder Joint, Percutaneous Approach
0R5J4ZZ Destruction of Right Shoulder Joint, Percutaneous Endoscopic Approach
0R5K0ZZ Destruction of Left Shoulder Joint, Open Approach
0R5K3ZZ Destruction of Left Shoulder Joint, Percutaneous Approach
0R5K4ZZ Destruction of Left Shoulder Joint, Percutaneous Endoscopic Approach
0R5L0ZZ Destruction of Right Elbow Joint, Open Approach
0R5L3ZZ Destruction of Right Elbow Joint, Percutaneous Approach
0R5L4ZZ Destruction of Right Elbow Joint, Percutaneous Endoscopic Approach

0R5M0ZZ Destruction of Left Elbow Joint, Open Approach
0R5M3ZZ Destruction of Left Elbow Joint, Percutaneous Approach
0R5M4ZZ Destruction of Left Elbow Joint, Percutaneous Endoscopic Approach
0R5N0ZZ Destruction of Right Wrist Joint, Open Approach
0R5N3ZZ Destruction of Right Wrist Joint, Percutaneous Approach
0R5N4ZZ Destruction of Right Wrist Joint, Percutaneous Endoscopic Approach
0R5P0ZZ Destruction of Left Wrist Joint, Open Approach
0R5P3ZZ Destruction of Left Wrist Joint, Percutaneous Approach
0R5P4ZZ Destruction of Left Wrist Joint, Percutaneous Endoscopic Approach
0R5Q0ZZ Destruction of Right Carpal Joint, Open Approach
0R5Q3ZZ Destruction of Right Carpal Joint, Percutaneous Approach
0R5Q4ZZ Destruction of Right Carpal Joint, Percutaneous Endoscopic Approach
0R5R0ZZ Destruction of Left Carpal Joint, Open Approach
0R5R3ZZ Destruction of Left Carpal Joint, Percutaneous Approach
0R5R4ZZ Destruction of Left Carpal Joint, Percutaneous Endoscopic Approach
0R5S0ZZ Destruction of Right Carpometacarpal Joint, Open Approach
0R5S3ZZ Destruction of Right Carpometacarpal Joint, Percutaneous Approach
0R5S4ZZ Destruction of Right Carpometacarpal Joint, Percutaneous Endoscopic Approach
0R5T0ZZ Destruction of Left Carpometacarpal Joint, Open Approach

0R5T3ZZ Destruction of Left Carpometacarpal Joint, Percutaneous Approach
0R5T4ZZ Destruction of Left Carpometacarpal Joint, Percutaneous Endoscopic Approach
0R5U0ZZ Destruction of Right Metacarpophalangeal Joint, Open Approach
0R5U3ZZ Destruction of Right Metacarpophalangeal Joint, Percutaneous Approach
0R5U4ZZ Destruction of Right Metacarpophalangeal Joint, Percutaneous Endoscopic Approach
0R5V0ZZ Destruction of Left Metacarpophalangeal Joint, Open Approach
0R5V3ZZ Destruction of Left Metacarpophalangeal Joint, Percutaneous Approach
0R5V4ZZ Destruction of Left Metacarpophalangeal Joint, Percutaneous Endoscopic Approach
0R5W0ZZ Destruction of Right Finger Phalangeal Joint, Open Approach
0R5W3ZZ Destruction of Right Finger Phalangeal Joint, Percutaneous Approach
0R5W4ZZ Destruction of Right Finger Phalangeal Joint, Percutaneous Endoscopic Approach
0R5X0ZZ Destruction of Left Finger Phalangeal Joint, Open Approach
0R5X3ZZ Destruction of Left Finger Phalangeal Joint, Percutaneous Approach
0R5X4ZZ Destruction of Left Finger Phalangeal Joint, Percutaneous Endoscopic Approach

0R9 – Upper Joints, Drainage

Review Coding Guidelines B3.4a and B3.4b

Review Coding Guideline B6.2

0R9000Z Drainage of Occipital-cervical Joint with Drainage Device, Open Approach
0R900ZX Drainage of Occipital-cervical Joint, Open Approach, Diagnostic
0R900ZZ Drainage of Occipital-cervical Joint, Open Approach
0R9030Z Drainage of Occipital-cervical Joint with Drainage Device, Percutaneous Approach
0R903ZX Drainage of Occipital-cervical Joint, Percutaneous Approach, Diagnostic
0R903ZZ Drainage of Occipital-cervical Joint, Percutaneous Approach
0R9040Z Drainage of Occipital-cervical Joint with Drainage Device, Percutaneous Endoscopic Approach
0R904ZX Drainage of Occipital-cervical Joint, Percutaneous Endoscopic Approach, Diagnostic
0R904ZZ Drainage of Occipital-cervical Joint, Percutaneous Endoscopic Approach
0R9100Z Drainage of Cervical Vertebral Joint with Drainage Device, Open Approach
0R910ZX Drainage of Cervical Vertebral Joint, Open Approach, Diagnostic
0R910ZZ Drainage of Cervical Vertebral Joint, Open Approach
0R9130Z Drainage of Cervical Vertebral Joint with Drainage Device, Percutaneous Approach

0R913ZX Drainage of Cervical Vertebral Joint, Percutaneous Approach, Diagnostic
0R913ZZ Drainage of Cervical Vertebral Joint, Percutaneous Approach
0R9140Z Drainage of Cervical Vertebral Joint with Drainage Device, Percutaneous Endoscopic Approach
0R914ZX Drainage of Cervical Vertebral Joint, Percutaneous Endoscopic Approach, Diagnostic
0R914ZZ Drainage of Cervical Vertebral Joint, Percutaneous Endoscopic Approach
0R9300Z Drainage of Cervical Vertebral Disc with Drainage Device, Open Approach
0R930ZX Drainage of Cervical Vertebral Disc, Open Approach, Diagnostic
0R930ZZ Drainage of Cervical Vertebral Disc, Open Approach
0R9330Z Drainage of Cervical Vertebral Disc with Drainage Device, Percutaneous Approach
0R933ZX Drainage of Cervical Vertebral Disc, Percutaneous Approach, Diagnostic
0R933ZZ Drainage of Cervical Vertebral Disc, Percutaneous Approach
0R9340Z Drainage of Cervical Vertebral Disc with Drainage Device, Percutaneous Endoscopic Approach

0R934ZX Drainage of Cervical Vertebral Disc, Percutaneous Endoscopic Approach, Diagnostic
0R934ZZ Drainage of Cervical Vertebral Disc, Percutaneous Endoscopic Approach
0R9400Z Drainage of Cervicothoracic Vertebral Joint with Drainage Device, Open Approach
0R940ZX Drainage of Cervicothoracic Vertebral Joint, Open Approach, Diagnostic
0R940ZZ Drainage of Cervicothoracic Vertebral Joint, Open Approach
0R9430Z Drainage of Cervicothoracic Vertebral Joint with Drainage Device, Percutaneous Approach
0R943ZX Drainage of Cervicothoracic Vertebral Joint, Percutaneous Approach, Diagnostic
0R943ZZ Drainage of Cervicothoracic Vertebral Joint, Percutaneous Approach
0R9440Z Drainage of Cervicothoracic Vertebral Joint with Drainage Device, Percutaneous Endoscopic Approach
0R944ZX Drainage of Cervicothoracic Vertebral Joint, Percutaneous Endoscopic Approach, Diagnostic
0R944ZZ Drainage of Cervicothoracic Vertebral Joint, Percutaneous Endoscopic Approach

0R9500Z Drainage of Cervicothoracic Vertebral Disc with Drainage Device, Open Approach

0R950ZX Drainage of Cervicothoracic Vertebral Disc, Open Approach, Diagnostic

0R950ZZ Drainage of Cervicothoracic Vertebral Disc, Open Approach

0R9530Z Drainage of Cervicothoracic Vertebral Disc with Drainage Device, Percutaneous Approach

0R953ZX Drainage of Cervicothoracic Vertebral Disc, Percutaneous Approach, Diagnostic

0R953ZZ Drainage of Cervicothoracic Vertebral Disc, Percutaneous Approach

0R9540Z Drainage of Cervicothoracic Vertebral Disc with Drainage Device, Percutaneous Endoscopic Approach

0R954ZX Drainage of Cervicothoracic Vertebral Disc, Percutaneous Endoscopic Approach, Diagnostic

0R954ZZ Drainage of Cervicothoracic Vertebral Disc, Percutaneous Endoscopic Approach

0R9600Z Drainage of Thoracic Vertebral Joint with Drainage Device, Open Approach

0R960ZX Drainage of Thoracic Vertebral Joint, Open Approach, Diagnostic

0R960ZZ Drainage of Thoracic Vertebral Joint, Open Approach

0R9630Z Drainage of Thoracic Vertebral Joint with Drainage Device, Percutaneous Approach

0R963ZX Drainage of Thoracic Vertebral Joint, Percutaneous Approach, Diagnostic

0R963ZZ Drainage of Thoracic Vertebral Joint, Percutaneous Approach

0R9640Z Drainage of Thoracic Vertebral Joint with Drainage Device, Percutaneous Endoscopic Approach

0R964ZX Drainage of Thoracic Vertebral Joint, Percutaneous Endoscopic Approach, Diagnostic

0R964ZZ Drainage of Thoracic Vertebral Joint, Percutaneous Endoscopic Approach

0R9900Z Drainage of Thoracic Vertebral Disc with Drainage Device, Open Approach

0R990ZX Drainage of Thoracic Vertebral Disc, Open Approach, Diagnostic

0R990ZZ Drainage of Thoracic Vertebral Disc, Open Approach

0R9930Z Drainage of Thoracic Vertebral Disc with Drainage Device, Percutaneous Approach

0R993ZX Drainage of Thoracic Vertebral Disc, Percutaneous Approach, Diagnostic

0R993ZZ Drainage of Thoracic Vertebral Disc, Percutaneous Approach

0R9940Z Drainage of Thoracic Vertebral Disc with Drainage Device, Percutaneous Endoscopic Approach

0R994ZX Drainage of Thoracic Vertebral Disc, Percutaneous Endoscopic Approach, Diagnostic

0R994ZZ Drainage of Thoracic Vertebral Disc, Percutaneous Endoscopic Approach

0R9A00Z Drainage of Thoracolumbar Vertebral Joint with Drainage Device, Open Approach

0R9A0ZX Drainage of Thoracolumbar Vertebral Joint, Open Approach, Diagnostic

0R9A0ZZ Drainage of Thoracolumbar Vertebral Joint, Open Approach

0R9A30Z Drainage of Thoracolumbar Vertebral Joint with Drainage Device, Percutaneous Approach

0R9A3ZX Drainage of Thoracolumbar Vertebral Joint, Percutaneous Approach, Diagnostic

0R9A3ZZ Drainage of Thoracolumbar Vertebral Joint, Percutaneous Approach

0R9A40Z Drainage of Thoracolumbar Vertebral Joint with Drainage Device, Percutaneous Endoscopic Approach

0R9A4ZX Drainage of Thoracolumbar Vertebral Joint, Percutaneous Endoscopic Approach, Diagnostic

0R9A4ZZ Drainage of Thoracolumbar Vertebral Joint, Percutaneous Endoscopic Approach

0R9B00Z Drainage of Thoracolumbar Vertebral Disc with Drainage Device, Open Approach

0R9B0ZX Drainage of Thoracolumbar Vertebral Disc, Open Approach, Diagnostic

0R9B0ZZ Drainage of Thoracolumbar Vertebral Disc, Open Approach

0R9B30Z Drainage of Thoracolumbar Vertebral Disc with Drainage Device, Percutaneous Approach

0R9B3ZX Drainage of Thoracolumbar Vertebral Disc, Percutaneous Approach, Diagnostic

0R9B3ZZ Drainage of Thoracolumbar Vertebral Disc, Percutaneous Approach

0R9B40Z Drainage of Thoracolumbar Vertebral Disc with Drainage Device, Percutaneous Endoscopic Approach

0R9B4ZX Drainage of Thoracolumbar Vertebral Disc, Percutaneous Endoscopic Approach, Diagnostic

0R9B4ZZ Drainage of Thoracolumbar Vertebral Disc, Percutaneous Endoscopic Approach

0R9C00Z Drainage of Right Temporomandibular Joint with Drainage Device, Open Approach

0R9C0ZX Drainage of Right Temporomandibular Joint, Open Approach, Diagnostic

0R9C0ZZ Drainage of Right Temporomandibular Joint, Open Approach

0R9C30Z Drainage of Right Temporomandibular Joint with Drainage Device, Percutaneous Approach

0R9C3ZX Drainage of Right Temporomandibular Joint, Percutaneous Approach, Diagnostic

0R9C3ZZ Drainage of Right Temporomandibular Joint, Percutaneous Approach

0R9C40Z Drainage of Right Temporomandibular Joint with Drainage Device, Percutaneous Endoscopic Approach

0R9C4ZX Drainage of Right Temporomandibular Joint, Percutaneous Endoscopic Approach, Diagnostic

0R9C4ZZ Drainage of Right Temporomandibular Joint, Percutaneous Endoscopic Approach

0R9D00Z Drainage of Left Temporomandibular Joint with Drainage Device, Open Approach

0R9D0ZX Drainage of Left Temporomandibular Joint, Open Approach, Diagnostic

0R9D0ZZ Drainage of Left Temporomandibular Joint, Open Approach

0R9D30Z Drainage of Left Temporomandibular Joint with Drainage Device, Percutaneous Approach

0R9D3ZX Drainage of Left Temporomandibular Joint, Percutaneous Approach, Diagnostic

0R9D3ZZ Drainage of Left Temporomandibular Joint, Percutaneous Approach

0R9D40Z Drainage of Left Temporomandibular Joint with Drainage Device, Percutaneous Endoscopic Approach

0R9D4ZX Drainage of Left Temporomandibular Joint, Percutaneous Endoscopic Approach, Diagnostic

0R9D4ZZ Drainage of Left Temporomandibular Joint, Percutaneous Endoscopic Approach

0R9E00Z Drainage of Right Sternoclavicular Joint with Drainage Device, Open Approach

0R9E0ZX Drainage of Right Sternoclavicular Joint, Open Approach, Diagnostic

0R9E0ZZ Drainage of Right Sternoclavicular Joint, Open Approach

0R9E30Z Drainage of Right Sternoclavicular Joint with Drainage Device, Percutaneous Approach

0R9E3ZX Drainage of Right Sternoclavicular Joint, Percutaneous Approach, Diagnostic

0R9E3ZZ Drainage of Right Sternoclavicular Joint, Percutaneous Approach

0R9E40Z Drainage of Right Sternoclavicular Joint with Drainage Device, Percutaneous Endoscopic Approach

0R9E4ZX Drainage of Right Sternoclavicular Joint, Percutaneous Endoscopic Approach, Diagnostic

0R9E4ZZ Drainage of Right Sternoclavicular Joint, Percutaneous Endoscopic Approach

0R9F00Z Drainage of Left Sternoclavicular Joint with Drainage Device, Open Approach

0R9F0ZX Drainage of Left Sternoclavicular Joint, Open Approach, Diagnostic

0R9F0ZZ Drainage of Left Sternoclavicular Joint, Open Approach

0R9F30Z Drainage of Left Sternoclavicular Joint with Drainage Device, Percutaneous Approach

0R9F3ZX Drainage of Left Sternoclavicular Joint, Percutaneous Approach, Diagnostic

0R9F3ZZ Drainage of Left Sternoclavicular Joint, Percutaneous Approach

0R9F40Z Drainage of Left Sternoclavicular Joint with Drainage Device, Percutaneous Endoscopic Approach

0R9F4ZX Drainage of Left Sternoclavicular Joint, Percutaneous Endoscopic Approach, Diagnostic

0R9F4ZZ Drainage of Left Sternoclavicular Joint, Percutaneous Endoscopic Approach

0R9G00Z Drainage of Right Acromioclavicular Joint with Drainage Device, Open Approach

0R9G0ZX Drainage of Right Acromioclavicular Joint, Open Approach, Diagnostic

0R9G0ZZ Drainage of Right Acromioclavicular Joint, Open Approach

0R9G30Z Drainage of Right Acromioclavicular Joint with Drainage Device, Percutaneous Approach

0R9G3ZX Drainage of Right Acromioclavicular Joint, Percutaneous Approach, Diagnostic

0R9G3ZZ Drainage of Right Acromioclavicular Joint, Percutaneous Approach

0R9G40Z Drainage of Right Acromioclavicular Joint with Drainage Device, Percutaneous Endoscopic Approach

0R9G4ZX Drainage of Right Acromioclavicular Joint, Percutaneous Endoscopic Approach, Diagnostic

♀ Female-only   ♂ Male-only   ▲ Limited Coverage   ● Non-OR   ᴴᴬᶜ HAC-associated procedure   ▲ Non-covered procedures   ✚ Cluster

0R9G4ZZ	Drainage of Right Acromioclavicular Joint, Percutaneous Endoscopic Approach
0R9H00Z	Drainage of Left Acromioclavicular Joint with Drainage Device, Open Approach
0R9H0ZX	Drainage of Left Acromioclavicular Joint, Open Approach, Diagnostic
0R9H0ZZ	Drainage of Left Acromioclavicular Joint, Open Approach
0R9H30Z	Drainage of Left Acromioclavicular Joint with Drainage Device, Percutaneous Approach
0R9H3ZX	Drainage of Left Acromioclavicular Joint, Percutaneous Approach, Diagnostic
0R9H3ZZ	Drainage of Left Acromioclavicular Joint, Percutaneous Approach
0R9H40Z	Drainage of Left Acromioclavicular Joint with Drainage Device, Percutaneous Endoscopic Approach
0R9H4ZX	Drainage of Left Acromioclavicular Joint, Percutaneous Endoscopic Approach, Diagnostic
0R9H4ZZ	Drainage of Left Acromioclavicular Joint, Percutaneous Endoscopic Approach
0R9J00Z	Drainage of Right Shoulder Joint with Drainage Device, Open Approach
0R9J0ZX	Drainage of Right Shoulder Joint, Open Approach, Diagnostic
0R9J0ZZ	Drainage of Right Shoulder Joint, Open Approach
0R9J30Z	Drainage of Right Shoulder Joint with Drainage Device, Percutaneous Approach
0R9J3ZX	Drainage of Right Shoulder Joint, Percutaneous Approach, Diagnostic
0R9J3ZZ	Drainage of Right Shoulder Joint, Percutaneous Approach
0R9J40Z	Drainage of Right Shoulder Joint with Drainage Device, Percutaneous Endoscopic Approach
0R9J4ZX	Drainage of Right Shoulder Joint, Percutaneous Endoscopic Approach, Diagnostic
0R9J4ZZ	Drainage of Right Shoulder Joint, Percutaneous Endoscopic Approach
0R9K00Z	Drainage of Left Shoulder Joint with Drainage Device, Open Approach
0R9K0ZX	Drainage of Left Shoulder Joint, Open Approach, Diagnostic
0R9K0ZZ	Drainage of Left Shoulder Joint, Open Approach
0R9K30Z	Drainage of Left Shoulder Joint with Drainage Device, Percutaneous Approach
0R9K3ZX	Drainage of Left Shoulder Joint, Percutaneous Approach, Diagnostic
0R9K3ZZ	Drainage of Left Shoulder Joint, Percutaneous Approach
0R9K40Z	Drainage of Left Shoulder Joint with Drainage Device, Percutaneous Endoscopic Approach
0R9K4ZX	Drainage of Left Shoulder Joint, Percutaneous Endoscopic Approach, Diagnostic
0R9K4ZZ	Drainage of Left Shoulder Joint, Percutaneous Endoscopic Approach
0R9L00Z	Drainage of Right Elbow Joint with Drainage Device, Open Approach
0R9L0ZX	Drainage of Right Elbow Joint, Open Approach, Diagnostic
0R9L0ZZ	Drainage of Right Elbow Joint, Open Approach

0R9L30Z	Drainage of Right Elbow Joint with Drainage Device, Percutaneous Approach
0R9L3ZX	Drainage of Right Elbow Joint, Percutaneous Approach, Diagnostic
0R9L3ZZ	Drainage of Right Elbow Joint, Percutaneous Approach
0R9L40Z	Drainage of Right Elbow Joint with Drainage Device, Percutaneous Endoscopic Approach
0R9L4ZX	Drainage of Right Elbow Joint, Percutaneous Endoscopic Approach, Diagnostic
0R9L4ZZ	Drainage of Right Elbow Joint, Percutaneous Endoscopic Approach
0R9M00Z	Drainage of Left Elbow Joint with Drainage Device, Open Approach
0R9M0ZX	Drainage of Left Elbow Joint, Open Approach, Diagnostic
0R9M0ZZ	Drainage of Left Elbow Joint, Open Approach
0R9M30Z	Drainage of Left Elbow Joint with Drainage Device, Percutaneous Approach
0R9M3ZX	Drainage of Left Elbow Joint, Percutaneous Approach, Diagnostic
0R9M3ZZ	Drainage of Left Elbow Joint, Percutaneous Approach
0R9M40Z	Drainage of Left Elbow Joint with Drainage Device, Percutaneous Endoscopic Approach
0R9M4ZX	Drainage of Left Elbow Joint, Percutaneous Endoscopic Approach, Diagnostic
0R9M4ZZ	Drainage of Left Elbow Joint, Percutaneous Endoscopic Approach
0R9N00Z	Drainage of Right Wrist Joint with Drainage Device, Open Approach
0R9N0ZX	Drainage of Right Wrist Joint, Open Approach, Diagnostic
0R9N0ZZ	Drainage of Right Wrist Joint, Open Approach
0R9N30Z	Drainage of Right Wrist Joint with Drainage Device, Percutaneous Approach
0R9N3ZX	Drainage of Right Wrist Joint, Percutaneous Approach, Diagnostic
0R9N3ZZ	Drainage of Right Wrist Joint, Percutaneous Approach
0R9N40Z	Drainage of Right Wrist Joint with Drainage Device, Percutaneous Endoscopic Approach
0R9N4ZX	Drainage of Right Wrist Joint, Percutaneous Endoscopic Approach, Diagnostic
0R9N4ZZ	Drainage of Right Wrist Joint, Percutaneous Endoscopic Approach
0R9P00Z	Drainage of Left Wrist Joint with Drainage Device, Open Approach
0R9P0ZX	Drainage of Left Wrist Joint, Open Approach, Diagnostic
0R9P0ZZ	Drainage of Left Wrist Joint, Open Approach
0R9P30Z	Drainage of Left Wrist Joint with Drainage Device, Percutaneous Approach
0R9P3ZX	Drainage of Left Wrist Joint, Percutaneous Approach, Diagnostic
0R9P3ZZ	Drainage of Left Wrist Joint, Percutaneous Approach
0R9P40Z	Drainage of Left Wrist Joint with Drainage Device, Percutaneous Endoscopic Approach
0R9P4ZX	Drainage of Left Wrist Joint, Percutaneous Endoscopic Approach, Diagnostic

0R9P4ZZ	Drainage of Left Wrist Joint, Percutaneous Endoscopic Approach
0R9Q00Z	Drainage of Right Carpal Joint with Drainage Device, Open Approach
0R9Q0ZX	Drainage of Right Carpal Joint, Open Approach, Diagnostic
0R9Q0ZZ	Drainage of Right Carpal Joint, Open Approach
0R9Q30Z	Drainage of Right Carpal Joint with Drainage Device, Percutaneous Approach
0R9Q3ZX	Drainage of Right Carpal Joint, Percutaneous Approach, Diagnostic
0R9Q3ZZ	Drainage of Right Carpal Joint, Percutaneous Approach
0R9Q40Z	Drainage of Right Carpal Joint with Drainage Device, Percutaneous Endoscopic Approach
0R9Q4ZX	Drainage of Right Carpal Joint, Percutaneous Endoscopic Approach, Diagnostic
0R9Q4ZZ	Drainage of Right Carpal Joint, Percutaneous Endoscopic Approach
0R9R00Z	Drainage of Left Carpal Joint with Drainage Device, Open Approach
0R9R0ZX	Drainage of Left Carpal Joint, Open Approach, Diagnostic
0R9R0ZZ	Drainage of Left Carpal Joint, Open Approach
0R9R30Z	Drainage of Left Carpal Joint with Drainage Device, Percutaneous Approach
0R9R3ZX	Drainage of Left Carpal Joint, Percutaneous Approach, Diagnostic
0R9R3ZZ	Drainage of Left Carpal Joint, Percutaneous Approach
0R9R40Z	Drainage of Left Carpal Joint with Drainage Device, Percutaneous Endoscopic Approach
0R9R4ZX	Drainage of Left Carpal Joint, Percutaneous Endoscopic Approach, Diagnostic
0R9R4ZZ	Drainage of Left Carpal Joint, Percutaneous Endoscopic Approach
0R9S00Z	Drainage of Right Carpometacarpal Joint with Drainage Device, Open Approach
0R9S0ZX	Drainage of Right Carpometacarpal Joint, Open Approach, Diagnostic
0R9S0ZZ	Drainage of Right Carpometacarpal Joint, Open Approach
0R9S30Z	Drainage of Right Carpometacarpal Joint with Drainage Device, Percutaneous Approach
0R9S3ZX	Drainage of Right Carpometacarpal Joint, Percutaneous Approach, Diagnostic
0R9S3ZZ	Drainage of Right Carpometacarpal Joint, Percutaneous Approach
0R9S40Z	Drainage of Right Carpometacarpal Joint with Drainage Device, Percutaneous Endoscopic Approach
0R9S4ZX	Drainage of Right Carpometacarpal Joint, Percutaneous Endoscopic Approach, Diagnostic
0R9S4ZZ	Drainage of Right Carpometacarpal Joint, Percutaneous Endoscopic Approach
0R9T00Z	Drainage of Left Carpometacarpal Joint with Drainage Device, Open Approach
0R9T0ZX	Drainage of Left Carpometacarpal Joint, Open Approach, Diagnostic
0R9T0ZZ	Drainage of Left Carpometacarpal Joint, Open Approach

♀ Female-only   ♂ Male-only   ▲ Limited Coverage   ● Non-OR   ᴴᴬᶜ HAC-associated procedure   ▲ Non-covered procedures   ➕ Cluster

0R9T30Z	Drainage of Left Carpometacarpal Joint with Drainage Device, Percutaneous Approach	**0R9U4ZX**	Drainage of Right Metacarpophalangeal Joint, Percutaneous Endoscopic Approach, Diagnostic	**0R9W3ZX**	Drainage of Right Finger Phalangeal Joint, Percutaneous Approach, Diagnostic
0R9T3ZX	Drainage of Left Carpometacarpal Joint, Percutaneous Approach, Diagnostic	**0R9U4ZZ**	Drainage of Right Metacarpophalangeal Joint, Percutaneous Endoscopic Approach	**0R9W3ZZ**	Drainage of Right Finger Phalangeal Joint, Percutaneous Approach
0R9T3ZZ	Drainage of Left Carpometacarpal Joint, Percutaneous Approach	**0R9V00Z**	Drainage of Left Metacarpophalangeal Joint with Drainage Device, Open Approach	**0R9W40Z**	Drainage of Right Finger Phalangeal Joint with Drainage Device, Percutaneous Endoscopic Approach
0R9T40Z	Drainage of Left Carpometacarpal Joint with Drainage Device, Percutaneous Endoscopic Approach	**0R9V0ZX**	Drainage of Left Metacarpophalangeal Joint, Open Approach, Diagnostic	**0R9W4ZX**	Drainage of Right Finger Phalangeal Joint, Percutaneous Endoscopic Approach, Diagnostic
0R9T4ZX	Drainage of Left Carpometacarpal Joint, Percutaneous Endoscopic Approach, Diagnostic	**0R9V0ZZ**	Drainage of Left Metacarpophalangeal Joint, Open Approach	**0R9W4ZZ**	Drainage of Right Finger Phalangeal Joint, Percutaneous Endoscopic Approach
0R9T4ZZ	Drainage of Left Carpometacarpal Joint, Percutaneous Endoscopic Approach	**0R9V30Z**	Drainage of Left Metacarpophalangeal Joint with Drainage Device, Percutaneous Approach	**0R9X00Z**	Drainage of Left Finger Phalangeal Joint with Drainage Device, Open Approach
0R9U00Z	Drainage of Right Metacarpophalangeal Joint with Drainage Device, Open Approach	**0R9V3ZX**	Drainage of Left Metacarpophalangeal Joint, Percutaneous Approach, Diagnostic	**0R9X0ZX**	Drainage of Left Finger Phalangeal Joint, Open Approach, Diagnostic
0R9U0ZX	Drainage of Right Metacarpophalangeal Joint, Open Approach, Diagnostic	**0R9V3ZZ**	Drainage of Left Metacarpophalangeal Joint, Percutaneous Approach	**0R9X0ZZ**	Drainage of Left Finger Phalangeal Joint, Open Approach
0R9U0ZZ	Drainage of Right Metacarpophalangeal Joint, Open Approach	**0R9V40Z**	Drainage of Left Metacarpophalangeal Joint with Drainage Device, Percutaneous Endoscopic Approach	**0R9X30Z**	Drainage of Left Finger Phalangeal Joint with Drainage Device, Percutaneous Approach
0R9U30Z	Drainage of Right Metacarpophalangeal Joint with Drainage Device, Percutaneous Approach	**0R9V4ZX**	Drainage of Left Metacarpophalangeal Joint, Percutaneous Endoscopic Approach, Diagnostic	**0R9X3ZX**	Drainage of Left Finger Phalangeal Joint, Percutaneous Approach, Diagnostic
0R9U3ZX	Drainage of Right Metacarpophalangeal Joint, Percutaneous Approach, Diagnostic	**0R9V4ZZ**	Drainage of Left Metacarpophalangeal Joint, Percutaneous Endoscopic Approach	**0R9X3ZZ**	Drainage of Left Finger Phalangeal Joint, Percutaneous Approach
0R9U3ZZ	Drainage of Right Metacarpophalangeal Joint, Percutaneous Approach	**0R9W00Z**	Drainage of Right Finger Phalangeal Joint with Drainage Device, Open Approach	**0R9X40Z**	Drainage of Left Finger Phalangeal Joint with Drainage Device, Percutaneous Endoscopic Approach
0R9U40Z	Drainage of Right Metacarpophalangeal Joint with Drainage Device, Percutaneous Endoscopic Approach	**0R9W0ZX**	Drainage of Right Finger Phalangeal Joint, Open Approach, Diagnostic	**0R9X4ZX**	Drainage of Left Finger Phalangeal Joint, Percutaneous Endoscopic Approach, Diagnostic
		0R9W0ZZ	Drainage of Right Finger Phalangeal Joint, Open Approach	**0R9X4ZZ**	Drainage of Left Finger Phalangeal Joint, Percutaneous Endoscopic Approach
		0R9W30Z	Drainage of Right Finger Phalangeal Joint with Drainage Device, Percutaneous Approach		

0RB – Upper Joints, Excision

Review Coding Guidelines B3.4a and B3.4b

Review Coding Guideline B3.5

Review Coding Guideline B3.8

Review Coding Guideline B3.18

0RB00ZX	Excision of Occipital-cervical Joint, Open Approach, Diagnostic	**0RB30ZX**	Excision of Cervical Vertebral Disc, Open Approach, Diagnostic	**0RB44ZZ**	Excision of Cervicothoracic Vertebral Joint, Percutaneous Endoscopic Approach
0RB00ZZ	Excision of Occipital-cervical Joint, Open Approach	**0RB30ZZ**	Excision of Cervical Vertebral Disc, Open Approach	**0RB50ZX**	Excision of Cervicothoracic Vertebral Disc, Open Approach, Diagnostic
0RB03ZX	Excision of Occipital-cervical Joint, Percutaneous Approach, Diagnostic	**0RB33ZX**	Excision of Cervical Vertebral Disc, Percutaneous Approach, Diagnostic	**0RB50ZZ**	Excision of Cervicothoracic Vertebral Disc, Open Approach
0RB03ZZ	Excision of Occipital-cervical Joint, Percutaneous Approach	**0RB33ZZ**	Excision of Cervical Vertebral Disc, Percutaneous Approach	**0RB53ZX**	Excision of Cervicothoracic Vertebral Disc, Percutaneous Approach, Diagnostic
0RB04ZX	Excision of Occipital-cervical Joint, Percutaneous Endoscopic Approach, Diagnostic	**0RB34ZX**	Excision of Cervical Vertebral Disc, Percutaneous Endoscopic Approach, Diagnostic	**0RB53ZZ**	Excision of Cervicothoracic Vertebral Disc, Percutaneous Approach
0RB04ZZ	Excision of Occipital-cervical Joint, Percutaneous Endoscopic Approach	**0RB34ZZ**	Excision of Cervical Vertebral Disc, Percutaneous Endoscopic Approach	**0RB54ZX**	Excision of Cervicothoracic Vertebral Disc, Percutaneous Endoscopic Approach, Diagnostic
0RB10ZX	Excision of Cervical Vertebral Joint, Open Approach, Diagnostic	**0RB40ZX**	Excision of Cervicothoracic Vertebral Joint, Open Approach, Diagnostic	**0RB54ZZ**	Excision of Cervicothoracic Vertebral Disc, Percutaneous Endoscopic Approach
0RB10ZZ	Excision of Cervical Vertebral Joint, Open Approach	**0RB40ZZ**	Excision of Cervicothoracic Vertebral Joint, Open Approach	**0RB60ZX**	Excision of Thoracic Vertebral Joint, Open Approach, Diagnostic
0RB13ZX	Excision of Cervical Vertebral Joint, Percutaneous Approach, Diagnostic	**0RB43ZX**	Excision of Cervicothoracic Vertebral Joint, Percutaneous Approach, Diagnostic	**0RB60ZZ**	Excision of Thoracic Vertebral Joint, Open Approach
0RB13ZZ	Excision of Cervical Vertebral Joint, Percutaneous Approach	**0RB43ZZ**	Excision of Cervicothoracic Vertebral Joint, Percutaneous Approach	**0RB63ZX**	Excision of Thoracic Vertebral Joint, Percutaneous Approach, Diagnostic
0RB14ZX	Excision of Cervical Vertebral Joint, Percutaneous Endoscopic Approach, Diagnostic	**0RB44ZX**	Excision of Cervicothoracic Vertebral Joint, Percutaneous Endoscopic Approach, Diagnostic	**0RB63ZZ**	Excision of Thoracic Vertebral Joint, Percutaneous Approach
0RB14ZZ	Excision of Cervical Vertebral Joint, Percutaneous Endoscopic Approach				

♀ Female-only   ♂ Male-only   ▲ Limited Coverage   ● Non-OR   **HAC** HAC-associated procedure   ▲ Non-covered procedures   ✚ Cluster

0RB64ZX	Excision of Thoracic Vertebral Joint, Percutaneous Endoscopic Approach, Diagnostic
0RB64ZZ	Excision of Thoracic Vertebral Joint, Percutaneous Endoscopic Approach
0RB90ZX	Excision of Thoracic Vertebral Disc, Open Approach, Diagnostic
0RB90ZZ	Excision of Thoracic Vertebral Disc, Open Approach
0RB93ZX	Excision of Thoracic Vertebral Disc, Percutaneous Approach, Diagnostic
0RB93ZZ	Excision of Thoracic Vertebral Disc, Percutaneous Approach
0RB94ZX	Excision of Thoracic Vertebral Disc, Percutaneous Endoscopic Approach, Diagnostic
0RB94ZZ	Excision of Thoracic Vertebral Disc, Percutaneous Endoscopic Approach
0RBA0ZX	Excision of Thoracolumbar Vertebral Joint, Open Approach, Diagnostic
0RBA0ZZ	Excision of Thoracolumbar Vertebral Joint, Open Approach
0RBA3ZX	Excision of Thoracolumbar Vertebral Joint, Percutaneous Approach, Diagnostic
0RBA3ZZ	Excision of Thoracolumbar Vertebral Joint, Percutaneous Approach
0RBA4ZX	Excision of Thoracolumbar Vertebral Joint, Percutaneous Endoscopic Approach, Diagnostic
0RBA4ZZ	Excision of Thoracolumbar Vertebral Joint, Percutaneous Endoscopic Approach
0RBB0ZX	Excision of Thoracolumbar Vertebral Disc, Open Approach, Diagnostic
0RBB0ZZ	Excision of Thoracolumbar Vertebral Disc, Open Approach
0RBB3ZX	Excision of Thoracolumbar Vertebral Disc, Percutaneous Approach, Diagnostic
0RBB3ZZ	Excision of Thoracolumbar Vertebral Disc, Percutaneous Approach
0RBB4ZX	Excision of Thoracolumbar Vertebral Disc, Percutaneous Endoscopic Approach, Diagnostic
0RBB4ZZ	Excision of Thoracolumbar Vertebral Disc, Percutaneous Endoscopic Approach
0RBC0ZX	Excision of Right Temporomandibular Joint, Open Approach, Diagnostic
0RBC0ZZ	Excision of Right Temporomandibular Joint, Open Approach
0RBC3ZX	Excision of Right Temporomandibular Joint, Percutaneous Approach, Diagnostic
0RBC3ZZ	Excision of Right Temporomandibular Joint, Percutaneous Approach
0RBC4ZX	Excision of Right Temporomandibular Joint, Percutaneous Endoscopic Approach, Diagnostic
0RBC4ZZ	Excision of Right Temporomandibular Joint, Percutaneous Endoscopic Approach
0RBD0ZX	Excision of Left Temporomandibular Joint, Open Approach, Diagnostic
0RBD0ZZ	Excision of Left Temporomandibular Joint, Open Approach
0RBD3ZX	Excision of Left Temporomandibular Joint, Percutaneous Approach, Diagnostic
0RBD3ZZ	Excision of Left Temporomandibular Joint, Percutaneous Approach
0RBD4ZX	Excision of Left Temporomandibular Joint, Percutaneous Endoscopic Approach, Diagnostic
0RBD4ZZ	Excision of Left Temporomandibular Joint, Percutaneous Endoscopic Approach
0RBE0ZX	Excision of Right Sternoclavicular Joint, Open Approach, Diagnostic
0RBE0ZZ	Excision of Right Sternoclavicular Joint, Open Approach
0RBE3ZX	Excision of Right Sternoclavicular Joint, Percutaneous Approach, Diagnostic
0RBE3ZZ	Excision of Right Sternoclavicular Joint, Percutaneous Approach
0RBE4ZX	Excision of Right Sternoclavicular Joint, Percutaneous Endoscopic Approach, Diagnostic
0RBE4ZZ	Excision of Right Sternoclavicular Joint, Percutaneous Endoscopic Approach
0RBF0ZX	Excision of Left Sternoclavicular Joint, Open Approach, Diagnostic
0RBF0ZZ	Excision of Left Sternoclavicular Joint, Open Approach
0RBF3ZX	Excision of Left Sternoclavicular Joint, Percutaneous Approach, Diagnostic
0RBF3ZZ	Excision of Left Sternoclavicular Joint, Percutaneous Approach
0RBF4ZX	Excision of Left Sternoclavicular Joint, Percutaneous Endoscopic Approach, Diagnostic
0RBF4ZZ	Excision of Left Sternoclavicular Joint, Percutaneous Endoscopic Approach
0RBG0ZX	Excision of Right Acromioclavicular Joint, Open Approach, Diagnostic
0RBG0ZZ	Excision of Right Acromioclavicular Joint, Open Approach
0RBG3ZX	Excision of Right Acromioclavicular Joint, Percutaneous Approach, Diagnostic
0RBG3ZZ	Excision of Right Acromioclavicular Joint, Percutaneous Approach
0RBG4ZX	Excision of Right Acromioclavicular Joint, Percutaneous Endoscopic Approach, Diagnostic
0RBG4ZZ	Excision of Right Acromioclavicular Joint, Percutaneous Endoscopic Approach
0RBH0ZX	Excision of Left Acromioclavicular Joint, Open Approach, Diagnostic
0RBH0ZZ	Excision of Left Acromioclavicular Joint, Open Approach
0RBH3ZX	Excision of Left Acromioclavicular Joint, Percutaneous Approach, Diagnostic
0RBH3ZZ	Excision of Left Acromioclavicular Joint, Percutaneous Approach
0RBH4ZX	Excision of Left Acromioclavicular Joint, Percutaneous Endoscopic Approach, Diagnostic
0RBH4ZZ	Excision of Left Acromioclavicular Joint, Percutaneous Endoscopic Approach
0RBJ0ZX	Excision of Right Shoulder Joint, Open Approach, Diagnostic
0RBJ0ZZ	Excision of Right Shoulder Joint, Open Approach
0RBJ3ZX	Excision of Right Shoulder Joint, Percutaneous Approach, Diagnostic
0RBJ3ZZ	Excision of Right Shoulder Joint, Percutaneous Approach
0RBJ4ZX	Excision of Right Shoulder Joint, Percutaneous Endoscopic Approach, Diagnostic
0RBJ4ZZ	Excision of Right Shoulder Joint, Percutaneous Endoscopic Approach
0RBK0ZX	Excision of Left Shoulder Joint, Open Approach, Diagnostic
0RBK0ZZ	Excision of Left Shoulder Joint, Open Approach
0RBK3ZX	Excision of Left Shoulder Joint, Percutaneous Approach, Diagnostic
0RBK3ZZ	Excision of Left Shoulder Joint, Percutaneous Approach
0RBK4ZX	Excision of Left Shoulder Joint, Percutaneous Endoscopic Approach, Diagnostic
0RBK4ZZ	Excision of Left Shoulder Joint, Percutaneous Endoscopic Approach
0RBL0ZX	Excision of Right Elbow Joint, Open Approach, Diagnostic
0RBL0ZZ	Excision of Right Elbow Joint, Open Approach
0RBL3ZX	Excision of Right Elbow Joint, Percutaneous Approach, Diagnostic
0RBL3ZZ	Excision of Right Elbow Joint, Percutaneous Approach
0RBL4ZX	Excision of Right Elbow Joint, Percutaneous Endoscopic Approach, Diagnostic
0RBL4ZZ	Excision of Right Elbow Joint, Percutaneous Endoscopic Approach
0RBM0ZX	Excision of Left Elbow Joint, Open Approach, Diagnostic
0RBM0ZZ	Excision of Left Elbow Joint, Open Approach
0RBM3ZX	Excision of Left Elbow Joint, Percutaneous Approach, Diagnostic
0RBM3ZZ	Excision of Left Elbow Joint, Percutaneous Approach
0RBM4ZX	Excision of Left Elbow Joint, Percutaneous Endoscopic Approach, Diagnostic
0RBM4ZZ	Excision of Left Elbow Joint, Percutaneous Endoscopic Approach
0RBN0ZX	Excision of Right Wrist Joint, Open Approach, Diagnostic
0RBN0ZZ	Excision of Right Wrist Joint, Open Approach
0RBN3ZX	Excision of Right Wrist Joint, Percutaneous Approach, Diagnostic
0RBN3ZZ	Excision of Right Wrist Joint, Percutaneous Approach
0RBN4ZX	Excision of Right Wrist Joint, Percutaneous Endoscopic Approach, Diagnostic
0RBN4ZZ	Excision of Right Wrist Joint, Percutaneous Endoscopic Approach
0RBP0ZX	Excision of Left Wrist Joint, Open Approach, Diagnostic
0RBP0ZZ	Excision of Left Wrist Joint, Open Approach
0RBP3ZX	Excision of Left Wrist Joint, Percutaneous Approach, Diagnostic
0RBP3ZZ	Excision of Left Wrist Joint, Percutaneous Approach
0RBP4ZX	Excision of Left Wrist Joint, Percutaneous Endoscopic Approach, Diagnostic
0RBP4ZZ	Excision of Left Wrist Joint, Percutaneous Endoscopic Approach
0RBQ0ZX	Excision of Right Carpal Joint, Open Approach, Diagnostic
0RBQ0ZZ	Excision of Right Carpal Joint, Open Approach
0RBQ3ZX	Excision of Right Carpal Joint, Percutaneous Approach, Diagnostic
0RBQ3ZZ	Excision of Right Carpal Joint, Percutaneous Approach
0RBQ4ZX	Excision of Right Carpal Joint, Percutaneous Endoscopic Approach, Diagnostic
0RBQ4ZZ	Excision of Right Carpal Joint, Percutaneous Endoscopic Approach

0RBR0ZX Excision of Left Carpal Joint, Open Approach, Diagnostic

0RBR0ZZ Excision of Left Carpal Joint, Open Approach

0RBR3ZX Excision of Left Carpal Joint, Percutaneous Approach, Diagnostic

0RBR3ZZ Excision of Left Carpal Joint, Percutaneous Approach

0RBR4ZX Excision of Left Carpal Joint, Percutaneous Endoscopic Approach, Diagnostic

0RBR4ZZ Excision of Left Carpal Joint, Percutaneous Endoscopic Approach

0RBS0ZX Excision of Right Carpometacarpal Joint, Open Approach, Diagnostic

0RBS0ZZ Excision of Right Carpometacarpal Joint, Open Approach

0RBS3ZX Excision of Right Carpometacarpal Joint, Percutaneous Approach, Diagnostic

0RBS3ZZ Excision of Right Carpometacarpal Joint, Percutaneous Approach

0RBS4ZX Excision of Right Carpometacarpal Joint, Percutaneous Endoscopic Approach, Diagnostic

0RBS4ZZ Excision of Right Carpometacarpal Joint, Percutaneous Endoscopic Approach

0RBT0ZX Excision of Left Carpometacarpal Joint, Open Approach, Diagnostic

0RBT0ZZ Excision of Left Carpometacarpal Joint, Open Approach

0RBT3ZX Excision of Left Carpometacarpal Joint, Percutaneous Approach, Diagnostic

0RBT3ZZ Excision of Left Carpometacarpal Joint, Percutaneous Approach

0RBT4ZX Excision of Left Carpometacarpal Joint, Percutaneous Endoscopic Approach, Diagnostic

0RBT4ZZ Excision of Left Carpometacarpal Joint, Percutaneous Endoscopic Approach

0RBU0ZX Excision of Right Metacarpophalangeal Joint, Open Approach, Diagnostic

0RBU0ZZ Excision of Right Metacarpophalangeal Joint, Open Approach

0RBU3ZX Excision of Right Metacarpophalangeal Joint, Percutaneous Approach, Diagnostic

0RBU3ZZ Excision of Right Metacarpophalangeal Joint, Percutaneous Approach

0RBU4ZX Excision of Right Metacarpophalangeal Joint, Percutaneous Endoscopic Approach, Diagnostic

0RBU4ZZ Excision of Right Metacarpophalangeal Joint, Percutaneous Endoscopic Approach

0RBV0ZX Excision of Left Metacarpophalangeal Joint, Open Approach, Diagnostic

0RBV0ZZ Excision of Left Metacarpophalangeal Joint, Open Approach

0RBV3ZX Excision of Left Metacarpophalangeal Joint, Percutaneous Approach, Diagnostic

0RBV3ZZ Excision of Left Metacarpophalangeal Joint, Percutaneous Approach

0RBV4ZX Excision of Left Metacarpophalangeal Joint, Percutaneous Endoscopic Approach, Diagnostic

0RBV4ZZ Excision of Left Metacarpophalangeal Joint, Percutaneous Endoscopic Approach

0RBW0ZX Excision of Right Finger Phalangeal Joint, Open Approach, Diagnostic

0RBW0ZZ Excision of Right Finger Phalangeal Joint, Open Approach

0RBW3ZX Excision of Right Finger Phalangeal Joint, Percutaneous Approach, Diagnostic

0RBW3ZZ Excision of Right Finger Phalangeal Joint, Percutaneous Approach

0RBW4ZX Excision of Right Finger Phalangeal Joint, Percutaneous Endoscopic Approach, Diagnostic

0RBW4ZZ Excision of Right Finger Phalangeal Joint, Percutaneous Endoscopic Approach

0RBX0ZX Excision of Left Finger Phalangeal Joint, Open Approach, Diagnostic

0RBX0ZZ Excision of Left Finger Phalangeal Joint, Open Approach

0RBX3ZX Excision of Left Finger Phalangeal Joint, Percutaneous Approach, Diagnostic

0RBX3ZZ Excision of Left Finger Phalangeal Joint, Percutaneous Approach

0RBX4ZX Excision of Left Finger Phalangeal Joint, Percutaneous Endoscopic Approach, Diagnostic

0RBX4ZZ Excision of Left Finger Phalangeal Joint, Percutaneous Endoscopic Approach

0RC – Upper Joints, Extirpation

0RC00ZZ Extirpation of Matter from Occipital-cervical Joint, Open Approach

0RC03ZZ Extirpation of Matter from Occipital-cervical Joint, Percutaneous Approach

0RC04ZZ Extirpation of Matter from Occipital-cervical Joint, Percutaneous Endoscopic Approach

0RC10ZZ Extirpation of Matter from Cervical Vertebral Joint, Open Approach

0RC13ZZ Extirpation of Matter from Cervical Vertebral Joint, Percutaneous Approach

0RC14ZZ Extirpation of Matter from Cervical Vertebral Joint, Percutaneous Endoscopic Approach

0RC30ZZ Extirpation of Matter from Cervical Vertebral Disc, Open Approach

0RC33ZZ Extirpation of Matter from Cervical Vertebral Disc, Percutaneous Approach

0RC34ZZ Extirpation of Matter from Cervical Vertebral Disc, Percutaneous Endoscopic Approach

0RC40ZZ Extirpation of Matter from Cervicothoracic Vertebral Joint, Open Approach

0RC43ZZ Extirpation of Matter from Cervicothoracic Vertebral Joint, Percutaneous Approach

0RC44ZZ Extirpation of Matter from Cervicothoracic Vertebral Joint, Percutaneous Endoscopic Approach

0RC50ZZ Extirpation of Matter from Cervicothoracic Vertebral Disc, Open Approach

0RC53ZZ Extirpation of Matter from Cervicothoracic Vertebral Disc, Percutaneous Approach

0RC54ZZ Extirpation of Matter from Cervicothoracic Vertebral Disc, Percutaneous Endoscopic Approach

0RC60ZZ Extirpation of Matter from Thoracic Vertebral Joint, Open Approach

0RC63ZZ Extirpation of Matter from Thoracic Vertebral Joint, Percutaneous Approach

0RC64ZZ Extirpation of Matter from Thoracic Vertebral Joint, Percutaneous Endoscopic Approach

0RC90ZZ Extirpation of Matter from Thoracic Vertebral Disc, Open Approach

0RC93ZZ Extirpation of Matter from Thoracic Vertebral Disc, Percutaneous Approach

0RC94ZZ Extirpation of Matter from Thoracic Vertebral Disc, Percutaneous Endoscopic Approach

0RCA0ZZ Extirpation of Matter from Thoracolumbar Vertebral Joint, Open Approach

0RCA3ZZ Extirpation of Matter from Thoracolumbar Vertebral Joint, Percutaneous Approach

0RCA4ZZ Extirpation of Matter from Thoracolumbar Vertebral Joint, Percutaneous Endoscopic Approach

0RCB0ZZ Extirpation of Matter from Thoracolumbar Vertebral Disc, Open Approach

0RCB3ZZ Extirpation of Matter from Thoracolumbar Vertebral Disc, Percutaneous Approach

0RCB4ZZ Extirpation of Matter from Thoracolumbar Vertebral Disc, Percutaneous Endoscopic Approach

0RCC0ZZ Extirpation of Matter from Right Temporomandibular Joint, Open Approach

0RCC3ZZ Extirpation of Matter from Right Temporomandibular Joint, Percutaneous Approach

0RCC4ZZ Extirpation of Matter from Right Temporomandibular Joint, Percutaneous Endoscopic Approach

0RCD0ZZ Extirpation of Matter from Left Temporomandibular Joint, Open Approach

0RCD3ZZ Extirpation of Matter from Left Temporomandibular Joint, Percutaneous Approach

0RCD4ZZ Extirpation of Matter from Left Temporomandibular Joint, Percutaneous Endoscopic Approach

0RCE0ZZ Extirpation of Matter from Right Sternoclavicular Joint, Open Approach

0RCE3ZZ Extirpation of Matter from Right Sternoclavicular Joint, Percutaneous Approach

0RCE4ZZ Extirpation of Matter from Right Sternoclavicular Joint, Percutaneous Endoscopic Approach

0RCF0ZZ Extirpation of Matter from Left Sternoclavicular Joint, Open Approach

0RCF3ZZ Extirpation of Matter from Left Sternoclavicular Joint, Percutaneous Approach

0RCF4ZZ Extirpation of Matter from Left Sternoclavicular Joint, Percutaneous Endoscopic Approach

0RCG0ZZ Extirpation of Matter from Right Acromioclavicular Joint, Open Approach

♀ Female-only   ♂ Male-only   ▲ Limited Coverage   ● Non-OR   HAC HAC-associated procedure   ▲ Non-covered procedures   ✚ Cluster

0RCG3ZZ	Extirpation of Matter from Right Acromioclavicular Joint, Percutaneous Approach
0RCG4ZZ	Extirpation of Matter from Right Acromioclavicular Joint, Percutaneous Endoscopic Approach
0RCH0ZZ	Extirpation of Matter from Left Acromioclavicular Joint, Open Approach
0RCH3ZZ	Extirpation of Matter from Left Acromioclavicular Joint, Percutaneous Approach
0RCH4ZZ	Extirpation of Matter from Left Acromioclavicular Joint, Percutaneous Endoscopic Approach
0RCJ0ZZ	Extirpation of Matter from Right Shoulder Joint, Open Approach
0RCJ3ZZ	Extirpation of Matter from Right Shoulder Joint, Percutaneous Approach
0RCJ4ZZ	Extirpation of Matter from Right Shoulder Joint, Percutaneous Endoscopic Approach
0RCK0ZZ	Extirpation of Matter from Left Shoulder Joint, Open Approach
0RCK3ZZ	Extirpation of Matter from Left Shoulder Joint, Percutaneous Approach
0RCK4ZZ	Extirpation of Matter from Left Shoulder Joint, Percutaneous Endoscopic Approach
0RCL0ZZ	Extirpation of Matter from Right Elbow Joint, Open Approach
0RCL3ZZ	Extirpation of Matter from Right Elbow Joint, Percutaneous Approach
0RCL4ZZ	Extirpation of Matter from Right Elbow Joint, Percutaneous Endoscopic Approach
0RCM0ZZ	Extirpation of Matter from Left Elbow Joint, Open Approach
0RCM3ZZ	Extirpation of Matter from Left Elbow Joint, Percutaneous Approach
0RCM4ZZ	Extirpation of Matter from Left Elbow Joint, Percutaneous Endoscopic Approach
0RCN0ZZ	Extirpation of Matter from Right Wrist Joint, Open Approach
0RCN3ZZ	Extirpation of Matter from Right Wrist Joint, Percutaneous Approach
0RCN4ZZ	Extirpation of Matter from Right Wrist Joint, Percutaneous Endoscopic Approach
0RCP0ZZ	Extirpation of Matter from Left Wrist Joint, Open Approach
0RCP3ZZ	Extirpation of Matter from Left Wrist Joint, Percutaneous Approach
0RCP4ZZ	Extirpation of Matter from Left Wrist Joint, Percutaneous Endoscopic Approach
0RCQ0ZZ	Extirpation of Matter from Right Carpal Joint, Open Approach
0RCQ3ZZ	Extirpation of Matter from Right Carpal Joint, Percutaneous Approach
0RCQ4ZZ	Extirpation of Matter from Right Carpal Joint, Percutaneous Endoscopic Approach
0RCR0ZZ	Extirpation of Matter from Left Carpal Joint, Open Approach
0RCR3ZZ	Extirpation of Matter from Left Carpal Joint, Percutaneous Approach
0RCR4ZZ	Extirpation of Matter from Left Carpal Joint, Percutaneous Endoscopic Approach
0RCS0ZZ	Extirpation of Matter from Right Carpometacarpal Joint, Open Approach
0RCS3ZZ	Extirpation of Matter from Right Carpometacarpal Joint, Percutaneous Approach
0RCS4ZZ	Extirpation of Matter from Right Carpometacarpal Joint, Percutaneous Endoscopic Approach
0RCT0ZZ	Extirpation of Matter from Left Carpometacarpal Joint, Open Approach
0RCT3ZZ	Extirpation of Matter from Left Carpometacarpal Joint, Percutaneous Approach
0RCT4ZZ	Extirpation of Matter from Left Carpometacarpal Joint, Percutaneous Endoscopic Approach
0RCU0ZZ	Extirpation of Matter from Right Metacarpophalangeal Joint, Open Approach
0RCU3ZZ	Extirpation of Matter from Right Metacarpophalangeal Joint, Percutaneous Approach
0RCU4ZZ	Extirpation of Matter from Right Metacarpophalangeal Joint, Percutaneous Endoscopic Approach
0RCV0ZZ	Extirpation of Matter from Left Metacarpophalangeal Joint, Open Approach
0RCV3ZZ	Extirpation of Matter from Left Metacarpophalangeal Joint, Percutaneous Approach
0RCV4ZZ	Extirpation of Matter from Left Metacarpophalangeal Joint, Percutaneous Endoscopic Approach
0RCW0ZZ	Extirpation of Matter from Right Finger Phalangeal Joint, Open Approach
0RCW3ZZ	Extirpation of Matter from Right Finger Phalangeal Joint, Percutaneous Approach
0RCW4ZZ	Extirpation of Matter from Right Finger Phalangeal Joint, Percutaneous Endoscopic Approach
0RCX0ZZ	Extirpation of Matter from Left Finger Phalangeal Joint, Open Approach
0RCX3ZZ	Extirpation of Matter from Left Finger Phalangeal Joint, Percutaneous Approach
0RCX4ZZ	Extirpation of Matter from Left Finger Phalangeal Joint, Percutaneous Endoscopic Approach

0RG – Upper Joints, Fusion

For Fusion procedures involving the vertebral joints

Review Coding Guidelines B3.10a, B3.10b and B3.10c

0RG0070 Fusion of Occipital-cervical Joint with Autologous Tissue Substitute, Anterior Approach, Anterior Column, Open Approach

HAC When reported with secondary diagnosis code K68.11, T81.40XA, T81.41XA, T81.42XA, T81.43XA, T81.44XA or T81.49XA, T84.60XA, T84.610A, T84.611A, T84.612A, T84.613A, T84.614A, T84.615A, T84.619A, T84.63XA, T84.69XA, T84.7XXA

0RG0071 Fusion of Occipital-cervical Joint with Autologous Tissue Substitute, Posterior Approach, Posterior Column, Open Approach

HAC When reported with secondary diagnosis code K68.11, T81.40XA, T81.41XA, T81.42XA, T81.43XA, T81.44XA or T81.49XA, T84.60XA, T84.610A, T84.611A, T84.612A, T84.613A, T84.614A, T84.615A, T84.619A, T84.63XA, T84.69XA, T84.7XXA

0RG007J Fusion of Occipital-cervical Joint with Autologous Tissue Substitute, Posterior Approach, Anterior Column, Open Approach

HAC When reported with secondary diagnosis code K68.11, T81.40XA, T81.41XA, T81.42XA, T81.43XA, T81.44XA or T81.49XA, T84.60XA, T84.610A, T84.611A, T84.612A, T84.613A, T84.614A, T84.615A, T84.619A, T84.63XA, T84.69XA, T84.7XXA

0RG00A0 Fusion of Occipital-cervical Joint with Interbody Fusion Device, Anterior Approach, Anterior Column, Open Approach

HAC When reported with secondary diagnosis code K68.11, T81.40XA, T81.41XA, T81.42XA, T81.43XA, T81.44XA or T81.49XA, T84.60XA, T84.610A, T84.611A, T84.612A, T84.613A, T84.614A, T84.615A, T84.619A, T84.63XA, T84.69XA, T84.7XXA

0RG00AJ Fusion of Occipital-cervical Joint with Interbody Fusion Device, Posterior Approach, Anterior Column, Open Approach

HAC When reported with secondary diagnosis code K68.11, T81.40XA, T81.41XA, T81.42XA, T81.43XA, T81.44XA or T81.49XA, T84.60XA, T84.610A, T84.611A, T84.612A, T84.613A, T84.614A, T84.615A, T84.619A, T84.63XA, T84.69XA, T84.7XXA

0RG00J0 Fusion of Occipital-cervical Joint with Synthetic Substitute, Anterior Approach, Anterior Column, Open Approach

HAC When reported with secondary diagnosis code K68.11, T81.40XA, T81.41XA, T81.42XA, T81.43XA, T81.44XA or T81.49XA, T84.60XA, T84.610A, T84.611A, T84.612A, T84.613A, T84.614A, T84.615A, T84.619A, T84.63XA, T84.69XA, T84.7XXA

0RG00J1 Fusion of Occipital-cervical Joint with Synthetic Substitute, Posterior Approach, Posterior Column, Open Approach

HAC When reported with secondary diagnosis code K68.11, T81.40XA,

T81.41XA, T81.42XA, T81.43XA,
T81.44XA or T81.49XA, T84.60XA,
T84.610A, T84.611A, T84.612A,
T84.613A, T84.614A, T84.615A,
T84.619A, T84.63XA, T84.69XA,
T84.7XXA

0RG00JJ Fusion of Occipital-cervical Joint
with Synthetic Substitute, Posterior
Approach, Anterior Column, Open
Approach

HAC When reported with secondary
diagnosis code K68.11, T81.40XA,
T81.41XA, T81.42XA, T81.43XA,
T81.44XA or T81.49XA, T84.60XA,
T84.610A, T84.611A, T84.612A,
T84.613A, T84.614A, T84.615A,
T84.619A, T84.63XA, T84.69XA,
T84.7XXA

0RG00K0 Fusion of Occipital-cervical Joint with
Nonautologous Tissue Substitute,
Anterior Approach, Anterior Column,
Open Approach

HAC When reported with secondary
diagnosis code K68.11, T81.40XA,
T81.41XA, T81.42XA, T81.43XA,
T81.44XA or T81.49XA, T84.60XA,
T84.610A, T84.611A, T84.612A,
T84.613A, T84.614A, T84.615A,
T84.619A, T84.63XA, T84.69XA,
T84.7XXA

0RG00K1 Fusion of Occipital-cervical Joint with
Nonautologous Tissue Substitute,
Posterior Approach, Posterior Column,
Open Approach

HAC When reported with secondary
diagnosis code K68.11, T81.40XA,
T81.41XA, T81.42XA, T81.43XA,
T81.44XA or T81.49XA, T84.60XA,
T84.610A, T84.611A, T84.612A,
T84.613A, T84.614A, T84.615A,
T84.619A, T84.63XA, T84.69XA,
T84.7XXA

0RG00KJ Fusion of Occipital-cervical Joint with
Nonautologous Tissue Substitute,
Posterior Approach, Anterior Column,
Open Approach

HAC When reported with secondary
diagnosis code K68.11, T81.40XA,
T81.41XA, T81.42XA, T81.43XA,
T81.44XA or T81.49XA, T84.60XA,
T84.610A, T84.611A, T84.612A,
T84.613A, T84.614A, T84.615A,
T84.619A, T84.63XA, T84.69XA,
T84.7XXA

0RG0370 Fusion of Occipital-cervical Joint
with Autologous Tissue Substitute,
Anterior Approach, Anterior Column,
Percutaneous Approach

HAC When reported with secondary
diagnosis code K68.11, T81.40XA,
T81.41XA, T81.42XA, T81.43XA,
T81.44XA or T81.49XA, T84.60XA,
T84.610A, T84.611A, T84.612A,
T84.613A, T84.614A, T84.615A,
T84.619A, T84.63XA, T84.69XA,
T84.7XXA

0RG0371 Fusion of Occipital-cervical Joint
with Autologous Tissue Substitute,
Posterior Approach, Posterior Column,
Percutaneous Approach

HAC When reported with secondary
diagnosis code K68.11, T81.40XA,
T81.41XA, T81.42XA, T81.43XA,
T81.44XA or T81.49XA, T84.60XA,
T84.610A, T84.611A, T84.612A,
T84.613A, T84.614A, T84.615A,

T84.619A, T84.63XA, T84.69XA,
T84.7XXA

0RG037J Fusion of Occipital-cervical Joint
with Autologous Tissue Substitute,
Posterior Approach, Anterior Column,
Percutaneous Approach

HAC When reported with secondary
diagnosis code K68.11, T81.40XA,
T81.41XA, T81.42XA, T81.43XA,
T81.44XA or T81.49XA, T84.60XA,
T84.610A, T84.611A, T84.612A,
T84.613A, T84.614A, T84.615A,
T84.619A, T84.63XA, T84.69XA,
T84.7XXA

0RG03A0 Fusion of Occipital-cervical Joint
with Interbody Fusion Device,
Anterior Approach, Anterior Column,
Percutaneous Approach

HAC When reported with secondary
diagnosis code K68.11, T81.40XA,
T81.41XA, T81.42XA, T81.43XA,
T81.44XA or T81.49XA, T84.60XA,
T84.610A, T84.611A, T84.612A,
T84.613A, T84.614A, T84.615A,
T84.619A, T84.63XA, T84.69XA,
T84.7XXA

0RG03AJ Fusion of Occipital-cervical Joint
with Interbody Fusion Device,
Posterior Approach, Anterior Column,
Percutaneous Approach

HAC When reported with secondary
diagnosis code K68.11, T81.40XA,
T81.41XA, T81.42XA, T81.43XA,
T81.44XA or T81.49XA, T84.60XA,
T84.610A, T84.611A, T84.612A,
T84.613A, T84.614A, T84.615A,
T84.619A, T84.63XA, T84.69XA,
T84.7XXA

0RG03J0 Fusion of Occipital-cervical Joint
with Synthetic Substitute, Anterior
Approach, Anterior Column,
Percutaneous Approach

HAC When reported with secondary
diagnosis code K68.11, T81.40XA,
T81.41XA, T81.42XA, T81.43XA,
T81.44XA or T81.49XA, T84.60XA,
T84.610A, T84.611A, T84.612A,
T84.613A, T84.614A, T84.615A,
T84.619A, T84.63XA, T84.69XA,
T84.7XXA

0RG03J1 Fusion of Occipital-cervical Joint
with Synthetic Substitute, Posterior
Approach, Posterior Column,
Percutaneous Approach

HAC When reported with secondary
diagnosis code K68.11, T81.40XA,
T81.41XA, T81.42XA, T81.43XA,
T81.44XA or T81.49XA, T84.60XA,
T84.610A, T84.611A, T84.612A,
T84.613A, T84.614A, T84.615A,
T84.619A, T84.63XA, T84.69XA,
T84.7XXA

0RG03JJ Fusion of Occipital-cervical Joint
with Synthetic Substitute, Posterior
Approach, Anterior Column,
Percutaneous Approach

HAC When reported with secondary
diagnosis code K68.11, T81.40XA,
T81.41XA, T81.42XA, T81.43XA,
T81.44XA or T81.49XA, T84.60XA,
T84.610A, T84.611A, T84.612A,
T84.613A, T84.614A, T84.615A,
T84.619A, T84.63XA, T84.69XA,
T84.7XXA

0RG03K0 Fusion of Occipital-cervical Joint with
Nonautologous Tissue Substitute,

Anterior Approach, Anterior Column,
Percutaneous Approach

HAC When reported with secondary
diagnosis code K68.11, T81.40XA,
T81.41XA, T81.42XA, T81.43XA,
T81.44XA or T81.49XA, T84.60XA,
T84.610A, T84.611A, T84.612A,
T84.613A, T84.614A, T84.615A,
T84.619A, T84.63XA, T84.69XA,
T84.7XXA

0RG03K1 Fusion of Occipital-cervical Joint with
Nonautologous Tissue Substitute,
Posterior Approach, Posterior Column,
Percutaneous Approach

HAC When reported with secondary
diagnosis code K68.11, T81.40XA,
T81.41XA, T81.42XA, T81.43XA,
T81.44XA or T81.49XA, T84.60XA,
T84.610A, T84.611A, T84.612A,
T84.613A, T84.614A, T84.615A,
T84.619A, T84.63XA, T84.69XA,
T84.7XXA

0RG03KJ Fusion of Occipital-cervical Joint with
Nonautologous Tissue Substitute,
Posterior Approach, Anterior Column,
Percutaneous Approach

HAC When reported with secondary
diagnosis code K68.11, T81.40XA,
T81.41XA, T81.42XA, T81.43XA,
T81.44XA or T81.49XA, T84.60XA,
T84.610A, T84.611A, T84.612A,
T84.613A, T84.614A, T84.615A,
T84.619A, T84.63XA, T84.69XA,
T84.7XXA

0RG0470 Fusion of Occipital-cervical Joint
with Autologous Tissue Substitute,
Anterior Approach, Anterior Column,
Percutaneous Endoscopic Approach

HAC When reported with secondary
diagnosis code K68.11, T81.40XA,
T81.41XA, T81.42XA, T81.43XA,
T81.44XA or T81.49XA, T84.60XA,
T84.610A, T84.611A, T84.612A,
T84.613A, T84.614A, T84.615A,
T84.619A, T84.63XA, T84.69XA,
T84.7XXA

0RG0471 Fusion of Occipital-cervical Joint
with Autologous Tissue Substitute,
Posterior Approach, Posterior Column,
Percutaneous Endoscopic Approach

HAC When reported with secondary
diagnosis code K68.11, T81.40XA,
T81.41XA, T81.42XA, T81.43XA,
T81.44XA or T81.49XA, T84.60XA,
T84.610A, T84.611A, T84.612A,
T84.613A, T84.614A, T84.615A,
T84.619A, T84.63XA, T84.69XA,
T84.7XXA

0RG047J Fusion of Occipital-cervical Joint
with Autologous Tissue Substitute,
Posterior Approach, Anterior Column,
Percutaneous Endoscopic Approach

HAC When reported with secondary
diagnosis code K68.11, T81.40XA,
T81.41XA, T81.42XA, T81.43XA,
T81.44XA or T81.49XA, T84.60XA,
T84.610A, T84.611A, T84.612A,
T84.613A, T84.614A, T84.615A,
T84.619A, T84.63XA, T84.69XA,
T84.7XXA

0RG04A0 Fusion of Occipital-cervical Joint
with Interbody Fusion Device,
Anterior Approach, Anterior Column,
Percutaneous Endoscopic Approach

HAC When reported with secondary
diagnosis code K68.11, T81.40XA,

♀ Female-only   ♂ Male-only   ▲ Limited Coverage   ● Non-OR   HAC HAC-associated procedure   ▲ Non-covered procedures   ✚ Cluster

T81.41XA, T81.42XA, T81.43XA,
T81.44XA or T81.49XA, T84.60XA,
T84.610A, T84.611A, T84.612A,
T84.613A, T84.614A, T84.615A,
T84.619A, T84.63XA, T84.69XA,
T84.7XXA

0RG04AJ Fusion of Occipital-cervical Joint
with Interbody Fusion Device,
Posterior Approach, Anterior
Column, Percutaneous Endoscopic
Approach

HAC When reported with secondary
diagnosis code K68.11, T81.40XA,
T81.41XA, T81.42XA, T81.43XA,
T81.44XA or T81.49XA, T84.60XA,
T84.610A, T84.611A, T84.612A,
T84.613A, T84.614A, T84.615A,
T84.619A, T84.63XA, T84.69XA,
T84.7XXA

0RG04J0 Fusion of Occipital-cervical
Joint with Synthetic Substitute,
Anterior Approach, Anterior
Column, Percutaneous Endoscopic
Approach

HAC When reported with secondary
diagnosis code K68.11, T81.40XA,
T81.41XA, T81.42XA, T81.43XA,
T81.44XA or T81.49XA, T84.60XA,
T84.610A, T84.611A, T84.612A,
T84.613A, T84.614A, T84.615A,
T84.619A, T84.63XA, T84.69XA,
T84.7XXA

0RG04J1 Fusion of Occipital-cervical Joint
with Synthetic Substitute, Posterior
Approach, Posterior Column,
Percutaneous Endoscopic Approach

HAC When reported with secondary
diagnosis code K68.11, T81.40XA,
T81.41XA, T81.42XA, T81.43XA,
T81.44XA or T81.49XA, T84.60XA,
T84.610A, T84.611A, T84.612A,
T84.613A, T84.614A, T84.615A,
T84.619A, T84.63XA, T84.69XA,
T84.7XXA

0RG04JJ Fusion of Occipital-cervical
Joint with Synthetic Substitute,
Posterior Approach, Anterior
Column, Percutaneous Endoscopic
Approach

HAC When reported with secondary
diagnosis code K68.11, T81.40XA,
T81.41XA, T81.42XA, T81.43XA,
T81.44XA or T81.49XA, T84.60XA,
T84.610A, T84.611A, T84.612A,
T84.613A, T84.614A, T84.615A,
T84.619A, T84.63XA, T84.69XA,
T84.7XXA

0RG04K0 Fusion of Occipital-cervical Joint
with Nonautologous Tissue Substitute,
Anterior Approach, Anterior Column,
Percutaneous Endoscopic Approach

HAC When reported with secondary
diagnosis code K68.11, T81.40XA,
T81.41XA, T81.42XA, T81.43XA,
T81.44XA or T81.49XA, T84.60XA,
T84.610A, T84.611A, T84.612A,
T84.613A, T84.614A, T84.615A,
T84.619A, T84.63XA, T84.69XA,
T84.7XXA

0RG04K1 Fusion of Occipital-cervical Joint
with Nonautologous Tissue Substitute,
Posterior Approach, Posterior
Column, Percutaneous Endoscopic
Approach

HAC When reported with secondary
diagnosis code K68.11, T81.40XA,

T81.41XA, T81.42XA, T81.43XA,
T81.44XA or T81.49XA, T84.60XA,
T84.610A, T84.611A, T84.612A,
T84.613A, T84.614A, T84.615A,
T84.619A, T84.63XA, T84.69XA,
T84.7XXA

0RG04KJ Fusion of Occipital-cervical
Joint with Nonautologous
Tissue Substitute, Posterior
Approach, Anterior Column,
Percutaneous Endoscopic
Approach

HAC When reported with secondary
diagnosis code K68.11, T81.40XA,
T81.41XA, T81.42XA, T81.43XA,
T81.44XA or T81.49XA, T84.60XA,
T84.610A, T84.611A, T84.612A,
T84.613A, T84.614A, T84.615A,
T84.619A, T84.63XA, T84.69XA,
T84.7XXA

0RG1070 Fusion of Cervical Vertebral Joint with
Autologous Tissue Substitute, Anterior
Approach, Anterior Column, Open
Approach

HAC When reported with secondary
diagnosis code K68.11, T81.40XA,
T81.41XA, T81.42XA, T81.43XA,
T81.44XA or T81.49XA, T84.60XA,
T84.610A, T84.611A, T84.612A,
T84.613A, T84.614A, T84.615A,
T84.619A, T84.63XA, T84.69XA,
T84.7XXA

0RG1071 Fusion of Cervical Vertebral Joint with
Autologous Tissue Substitute, Posterior
Approach, Posterior Column, Open
Approach

HAC When reported with secondary
diagnosis code K68.11, T81.40XA,
T81.41XA, T81.42XA, T81.43XA,
T81.44XA or T81.49XA, T84.60XA,
T84.610A, T84.611A, T84.612A,
T84.613A, T84.614A, T84.615A,
T84.619A, T84.63XA, T84.69XA,
T84.7XXA

0RG107J Fusion of Cervical Vertebral Joint with
Autologous Tissue Substitute, Posterior
Approach, Anterior Column, Open
Approach

HAC When reported with secondary
diagnosis code K68.11, T81.40XA,
T81.41XA, T81.42XA, T81.43XA,
T81.44XA or T81.49XA, T84.60XA,
T84.610A, T84.611A, T84.612A,
T84.613A, T84.614A, T84.615A,
T84.619A, T84.63XA, T84.69XA,
T84.7XXA

0RG10A0 Fusion of Cervical Vertebral Joint with
Interbody Fusion Device, Anterior
Approach, Anterior Column, Open
Approach

HAC When reported with secondary
diagnosis code K68.11, T81.40XA,
T81.41XA, T81.42XA, T81.43XA,
T81.44XA or T81.49XA, T84.60XA,
T84.610A, T84.611A, T84.612A,
T84.613A, T84.614A, T84.615A,
T84.619A, T84.63XA, T84.69XA,
T84.7XXA

0RG10AJ Fusion of Cervical Vertebral Joint with
Interbody Fusion Device, Posterior
Approach, Anterior Column, Open
Approach

HAC When reported with secondary
diagnosis code K68.11, T81.40XA,
T81.41XA, T81.42XA, T81.43XA,
T81.44XA or T81.49XA, T84.60XA,

T84.610A, T84.611A, T84.612A,
T84.613A, T84.614A, T84.615A,
T84.619A, T84.63XA, T84.69XA,
T84.7XXA

0RG10J0 Fusion of Cervical Vertebral Joint
with Synthetic Substitute, Anterior
Approach, Anterior Column, Open
Approach

HAC When reported with secondary
diagnosis code K68.11, T81.40XA,
T81.41XA, T81.42XA, T81.43XA,
T81.44XA or T81.49XA, T84.60XA,
T84.610A, T84.611A, T84.612A,
T84.613A, T84.614A, T84.615A,
T84.619A, T84.63XA, T84.69XA,
T84.7XXA

0RG10J1 Fusion of Cervical Vertebral Joint
with Synthetic Substitute, Posterior
Approach, Posterior Column, Open
Approach

HAC When reported with secondary
diagnosis code K68.11, T81.40XA,
T81.41XA, T81.42XA, T81.43XA,
T81.44XA or T81.49XA, T84.60XA,
T84.610A, T84.611A, T84.612A,
T84.613A, T84.614A, T84.615A,
T84.619A, T84.63XA, T84.69XA,
T84.7XXA

0RG10JJ Fusion of Cervical Vertebral Joint
with Synthetic Substitute, Posterior
Approach, Anterior Column, Open
Approach

HAC When reported with secondary
diagnosis code K68.11, T81.40XA,
T81.41XA, T81.42XA, T81.43XA,
T81.44XA or T81.49XA, T84.60XA,
T84.610A, T84.611A, T84.612A,
T84.613A, T84.614A, T84.615A,
T84.619A, T84.63XA, T84.69XA,
T84.7XXA

0RG10K0 Fusion of Cervical Vertebral Joint
with Nonautologous Tissue Substitute,
Anterior Approach, Anterior Column,
Open Approach

HAC When reported with secondary
diagnosis code K68.11, T81.40XA,
T81.41XA, T81.42XA, T81.43XA,
T81.44XA or T81.49XA, T84.60XA,
T84.610A, T84.611A, T84.612A,
T84.613A, T84.614A, T84.615A,
T84.619A, T84.63XA, T84.69XA,
T84.7XXA

0RG10K1 Fusion of Cervical Vertebral Joint
with Nonautologous Tissue Substitute,
Posterior Approach, Posterior Column,
Open Approach

HAC When reported with secondary
diagnosis code K68.11, T81.40XA,
T81.41XA, T81.42XA, T81.43XA,
T81.44XA or T81.49XA, T84.60XA,
T84.610A, T84.611A, T84.612A,
T84.613A, T84.614A, T84.615A,
T84.619A, T84.63XA, T84.69XA,
T84.7XXA

0RG10KJ Fusion of Cervical Vertebral Joint
with Nonautologous Tissue Substitute,
Posterior Approach, Anterior Column,
Open Approach

HAC When reported with secondary
diagnosis code K68.11, T81.40XA,
T81.41XA, T81.42XA, T81.43XA,
T81.44XA or T81.49XA, T84.60XA,
T84.610A, T84.611A, T84.612A,
T84.613A, T84.614A, T84.615A,
T84.619A, T84.63XA, T84.69XA,
T84.7XXA

0RG1370 Fusion of Cervical Vertebral Joint with Autologous Tissue Substitute, Anterior Approach, Anterior Column, Percutaneous Approach

HAC When reported with secondary diagnosis code K68.11, T81.40XA, T81.41XA, T81.42XA, T81.43XA, T81.44XA or T81.49XA, T84.60XA, T84.610A, T84.611A, T84.612A, T84.613A, T84.614A, T84.615A, T84.619A, T84.63XA, T84.69XA, T84.7XXA

0RG1371 Fusion of Cervical Vertebral Joint with Autologous Tissue Substitute, Posterior Approach, Posterior Column, Percutaneous Approach

HAC When reported with secondary diagnosis code K68.11, T81.40XA, T81.41XA, T81.42XA, T81.43XA, T81.44XA or T81.49XA, T84.60XA, T84.610A, T84.611A, T84.612A, T84.613A, T84.614A, T84.615A, T84.619A, T84.63XA, T84.69XA, T84.7XXA

0RG137J Fusion of Cervical Vertebral Joint with Autologous Tissue Substitute, Posterior Approach, Anterior Column, Percutaneous Approach

HAC When reported with secondary diagnosis code K68.11, T81.40XA, T81.41XA, T81.42XA, T81.43XA, T81.44XA or T81.49XA, T84.60XA, T84.610A, T84.611A, T84.612A, T84.613A, T84.614A, T84.615A, T84.619A, T84.63XA, T84.69XA, T84.7XXA

0RG13A0 Fusion of Cervical Vertebral Joint with Interbody Fusion Device, Anterior Approach, Anterior Column, Percutaneous Approach

HAC When reported with secondary diagnosis code K68.11, T81.40XA, T81.41XA, T81.42XA, T81.43XA, T81.44XA or T81.49XA, T84.60XA, T84.610A, T84.611A, T84.612A, T84.613A, T84.614A, T84.615A, T84.619A, T84.63XA, T84.69XA, T84.7XXA

0RG13AJ Fusion of Cervical Vertebral Joint with Interbody Fusion Device, Posterior Approach, Anterior Column, Percutaneous Approach

HAC When reported with secondary diagnosis code K68.11, T81.40XA, T81.41XA, T81.42XA, T81.43XA, T81.44XA or T81.49XA, T84.60XA, T84.610A, T84.611A, T84.612A, T84.613A, T84.614A, T84.615A, T84.619A, T84.63XA, T84.69XA, T84.7XXA

0RG13J0 Fusion of Cervical Vertebral Joint with Synthetic Substitute, Anterior Approach, Anterior Column, Percutaneous Approach

HAC When reported with secondary diagnosis code K68.11, T81.40XA, T81.41XA, T81.42XA, T81.43XA, T81.44XA or T81.49XA, T84.60XA, T84.610A, T84.611A, T84.612A, T84.613A, T84.614A, T84.615A, T84.619A, T84.63XA, T84.69XA, T84.7XXA

0RG13J1 Fusion of Cervical Vertebral Joint with Synthetic Substitute, Posterior Approach, Posterior Column, Percutaneous Approach

HAC When reported with secondary diagnosis code K68.11, T81.40XA, T81.41XA, T81.42XA, T81.43XA, T81.44XA or T81.49XA, T84.60XA, T84.610A, T84.611A, T84.612A, T84.613A, T84.614A, T84.615A, T84.619A, T84.63XA, T84.69XA, T84.7XXA

0RG13JJ Fusion of Cervical Vertebral Joint with Synthetic Substitute, Posterior Approach, Anterior Column, Percutaneous Approach

HAC When reported with secondary diagnosis code K68.11, T81.40XA, T81.41XA, T81.42XA, T81.43XA, T81.44XA or T81.49XA, T84.60XA, T84.610A, T84.611A, T84.612A, T84.613A, T84.614A, T84.615A, T84.619A, T84.63XA, T84.69XA, T84.7XXA

0RG13K0 Fusion of Cervical Vertebral Joint with Nonautologous Tissue Substitute, Anterior Approach, Anterior Column, Percutaneous Approach

HAC When reported with secondary diagnosis code K68.11, T81.40XA, T81.41XA, T81.42XA, T81.43XA, T81.44XA or T81.49XA, T84.60XA, T84.610A, T84.611A, T84.612A, T84.613A, T84.614A, T84.615A, T84.619A, T84.63XA, T84.69XA, T84.7XXA

0RG13K1 Fusion of Cervical Vertebral Joint with Nonautologous Tissue Substitute, Posterior Approach, Posterior Column, Percutaneous Approach

HAC When reported with secondary diagnosis code K68.11, T81.40XA, T81.41XA, T81.42XA, T81.43XA, T81.44XA or T81.49XA, T84.60XA, T84.610A, T84.611A, T84.612A, T84.613A, T84.614A, T84.615A, T84.619A, T84.63XA, T84.69XA, T84.7XXA

0RG13KJ Fusion of Cervical Vertebral Joint with Nonautologous Tissue Substitute, Posterior Approach, Anterior Column, Percutaneous Approach

HAC When reported with secondary diagnosis code K68.11, T81.40XA, T81.41XA, T81.42XA, T81.43XA, T81.44XA or T81.49XA, T84.60XA, T84.610A, T84.611A, T84.612A, T84.613A, T84.614A, T84.615A, T84.619A, T84.63XA, T84.69XA, T84.7XXA

0RG1470 Fusion of Cervical Vertebral Joint with Autologous Tissue Substitute, Anterior Approach, Anterior Column, Percutaneous Endoscopic Approach

HAC When reported with secondary diagnosis code K68.11, T81.40XA, T81.41XA, T81.42XA, T81.43XA, T81.44XA or T81.49XA, T84.60XA, T84.610A, T84.611A, T84.612A, T84.613A, T84.614A, T84.615A, T84.619A, T84.63XA, T84.69XA, T84.7XXA

0RG1471 Fusion of Cervical Vertebral Joint with Autologous Tissue Substitute, Posterior Approach, Posterior Column, Percutaneous Endoscopic Approach

HAC When reported with secondary diagnosis code K68.11, T81.40XA, T81.41XA, T81.42XA, T81.43XA, T81.44XA or T81.49XA, T84.60XA, T84.610A, T84.611A, T84.612A, T84.613A, T84.614A, T84.615A, T84.619A, T84.63XA, T84.69XA, T84.7XXA

0RG147J Fusion of Cervical Vertebral Joint with Autologous Tissue Substitute, Posterior Approach, Anterior Column, Percutaneous Endoscopic Approach

HAC When reported with secondary diagnosis code K68.11, T81.40XA, T81.41XA, T81.42XA, T81.43XA, T81.44XA or T81.49XA, T84.60XA, T84.610A, T84.611A, T84.612A, T84.613A, T84.614A, T84.615A, T84.619A, T84.63XA, T84.69XA, T84.7XXA

0RG14A0 Fusion of Cervical Vertebral Joint with Interbody Fusion Device, Anterior Approach, Anterior Column, Percutaneous Endoscopic Approach

HAC When reported with secondary diagnosis code K68.11, T81.40XA, T81.41XA, T81.42XA, T81.43XA, T81.44XA or T81.49XA, T84.60XA, T84.610A, T84.611A, T84.612A, T84.613A, T84.614A, T84.615A, T84.619A, T84.63XA, T84.69XA, T84.7XXA

0RG14AJ Fusion of Cervical Vertebral Joint with Interbody Fusion Device, Posterior Approach, Anterior Column, Percutaneous Endoscopic Approach

HAC When reported with secondary diagnosis code K68.11, T81.40XA, T81.41XA, T81.42XA, T81.43XA, T81.44XA or T81.49XA, T84.60XA, T84.610A, T84.611A, T84.612A, T84.613A, T84.614A, T84.615A, T84.619A, T84.63XA, T84.69XA, T84.7XXA

0RG14J0 Fusion of Cervical Vertebral Joint with Synthetic Substitute, Anterior Approach, Anterior Column, Percutaneous Endoscopic Approach

HAC When reported with secondary diagnosis code K68.11, T81.40XA, T81.41XA, T81.42XA, T81.43XA, T81.44XA or T81.49XA, T84.60XA, T84.610A, T84.611A, T84.612A, T84.613A, T84.614A, T84.615A, T84.619A, T84.63XA, T84.69XA, T84.7XXA

0RG14J1 Fusion of Cervical Vertebral Joint with Synthetic Substitute, Posterior Approach, Posterior Column, Percutaneous Endoscopic Approach

HAC When reported with secondary diagnosis code K68.11, T81.40XA, T81.41XA, T81.42XA, T81.43XA, T81.44XA or T81.49XA, T84.60XA, T84.610A, T84.611A, T84.612A, T84.613A, T84.614A, T84.615A, T84.619A, T84.63XA, T84.69XA, T84.7XXA

0RG14JJ Fusion of Cervical Vertebral Joint with Synthetic Substitute, Posterior Approach, Anterior Column, Percutaneous Endoscopic Approach

HAC When reported with secondary diagnosis code K68.11, T81.40XA, T81.41XA, T81.42XA, T81.43XA, T81.44XA or T81.49XA, T84.60XA, T84.610A, T84.611A, T84.612A, T84.613A, T84.614A, T84.615A, T84.619A, T84.63XA, T84.69XA, T84.7XXA

♀ Female-only ♂ Male-only ▲ Limited Coverage ● Non-OR HAC HAC-associated procedure ▲ Non-covered procedures ✚ Cluster

0RG14K0 Fusion of Cervical Vertebral Joint with Nonautologous Tissue Substitute, Anterior Approach, Anterior Column, Percutaneous Endoscopic Approach

HAC When reported with secondary diagnosis code K68.11, T81.40XA, T81.41XA, T81.42XA, T81.43XA, T81.44XA or T81.49XA, T84.60XA, T84.610A, T84.611A, T84.612A, T84.613A, T84.614A, T84.615A, T84.619A, T84.63XA, T84.69XA, T84.7XXA

0RG14K1 Fusion of Cervical Vertebral Joint with Nonautologous Tissue Substitute, Posterior Approach, Posterior Column, Percutaneous Endoscopic Approach

HAC When reported with secondary diagnosis code K68.11, T81.40XA, T81.41XA, T81.42XA, T81.43XA, T81.44XA or T81.49XA, T84.60XA, T84.610A, T84.611A, T84.612A, T84.613A, T84.614A, T84.615A, T84.619A, T84.63XA, T84.69XA, T84.7XXA

0RG14KJ Fusion of Cervical Vertebral Joint with Nonautologous Tissue Substitute, Posterior Approach, Anterior Column, Percutaneous Endoscopic Approach

HAC When reported with secondary diagnosis code K68.11, T81.40XA, T81.41XA, T81.42XA, T81.43XA, T81.44XA or T81.49XA, T84.60XA, T84.610A, T84.611A, T84.612A, T84.613A, T84.614A, T84.615A, T84.619A, T84.63XA, T84.69XA, T84.7XXA

0RG2070 Fusion of 2 or more Cervical Vertebral Joints with Autologous Tissue Substitute, Anterior Approach, Anterior Column, Open Approach

HAC When reported with secondary diagnosis code K68.11, T81.40XA, T81.41XA, T81.42XA, T81.43XA, T81.44XA or T81.49XA, T84.60XA, T84.610A, T84.611A, T84.612A, T84.613A, T84.614A, T84.615A, T84.619A, T84.63XA, T84.69XA, T84.7XXA

0RG2071 Fusion of 2 or more Cervical Vertebral Joints with Autologous Tissue Substitute, Posterior Approach, Posterior Column, Open Approach

HAC When reported with secondary diagnosis code K68.11, T81.40XA, T81.41XA, T81.42XA, T81.43XA, T81.44XA or T81.49XA, T84.60XA, T84.610A, T84.611A, T84.612A, T84.613A, T84.614A, T84.615A, T84.619A, T84.63XA, T84.69XA, T84.7XXA

0RG207J Fusion of 2 or more Cervical Vertebral Joints with Autologous Tissue Substitute, Posterior Approach, Anterior Column, Open Approach

HAC When reported with secondary diagnosis code K68.11, T81.40XA, T81.41XA, T81.42XA, T81.43XA, T81.44XA or T81.49XA, T84.60XA, T84.610A, T84.611A, T84.612A, T84.613A, T84.614A, T84.615A, T84.619A, T84.63XA, T84.69XA, T84.7XXA

0RG20A0 Fusion of 2 or more Cervical Vertebral Joints with Interbody Fusion Device, Anterior Approach, Anterior Column, Open Approach

AHA CC: 3Q, 2019, 28

HAC When reported with secondary diagnosis code K68.11, T81.40XA, T81.41XA, T81.42XA, T81.43XA, T81.44XA or T81.49XA, T84.60XA, T84.610A, T84.611A, T84.612A, T84.613A, T84.614A, T84.615A, T84.619A, T84.63XA, T84.69XA, T84.7XXA

0RG20AJ Fusion of 2 or more Cervical Vertebral Joints with Interbody Fusion Device, Posterior Approach, Anterior Column, Open Approach

HAC When reported with secondary diagnosis code K68.11, T81.40XA, T81.41XA, T81.42XA, T81.43XA, T81.44XA or T81.49XA, T84.60XA, T84.610A, T84.611A, T84.612A, T84.613A, T84.614A, T84.615A, T84.619A, T84.63XA, T84.69XA, T84.7XXA

0RG20J0 Fusion of 2 or more Cervical Vertebral Joints with Synthetic Substitute, Anterior Approach, Anterior Column, Open Approach

HAC When reported with secondary diagnosis code K68.11, T81.40XA, T81.41XA, T81.42XA, T81.43XA, T81.44XA or T81.49XA, T84.60XA, T84.610A, T84.611A, T84.612A, T84.613A, T84.614A, T84.615A, T84.619A, T84.63XA, T84.69XA, T84.7XXA

0RG20J1 Fusion of 2 or more Cervical Vertebral Joints with Synthetic Substitute, Posterior Approach, Posterior Column, Open Approach

HAC When reported with secondary diagnosis code K68.11, T81.40XA, T81.41XA, T81.42XA, T81.43XA, T81.44XA or T81.49XA, T84.60XA, T84.610A, T84.611A, T84.612A, T84.613A, T84.614A, T84.615A, T84.619A, T84.63XA, T84.69XA, T84.7XXA

0RG20JJ Fusion of 2 or more Cervical Vertebral Joints with Synthetic Substitute, Posterior Approach, Anterior Column, Open Approach

HAC When reported with secondary diagnosis code K68.11, T81.40XA, T81.41XA, T81.42XA, T81.43XA, T81.44XA or T81.49XA, T84.60XA, T84.610A, T84.611A, T84.612A, T84.613A, T84.614A, T84.615A, T84.619A, T84.63XA, T84.69XA, T84.7XXA

0RG20K0 Fusion of 2 or more Cervical Vertebral Joints with Nonautologous Tissue Substitute, Anterior Approach, Anterior Column, Open Approach

HAC When reported with secondary diagnosis code K68.11, T81.40XA, T81.41XA, T81.42XA, T81.43XA, T81.44XA or T81.49XA, T84.60XA, T84.610A, T84.611A, T84.612A, T84.613A, T84.614A, T84.615A, T84.619A, T84.63XA, T84.69XA, T84.7XXA

0RG20K1 Fusion of 2 or more Cervical Vertebral Joints with Nonautologous Tissue Substitute, Posterior Approach, Posterior Column, Open Approach

HAC When reported with secondary diagnosis code K68.11, T81.40XA, T81.41XA, T81.42XA, T81.43XA, T81.44XA or T81.49XA, T84.60XA, T84.610A, T84.611A, T84.612A, T84.613A, T84.614A, T84.615A, T84.619A, T84.63XA, T84.69XA, T84.7XXA

0RG20KJ Fusion of 2 or more Cervical Vertebral Joints with Nonautologous Tissue Substitute, Posterior Approach, Anterior Column, Open Approach

HAC When reported with secondary diagnosis code K68.11, T81.40XA, T81.41XA, T81.42XA, T81.43XA, T81.44XA or T81.49XA, T84.60XA, T84.610A, T84.611A, T84.612A, T84.613A, T84.614A, T84.615A, T84.619A, T84.63XA, T84.69XA, T84.7XXA

0RG2370 Fusion of 2 or more Cervical Vertebral Joints with Autologous Tissue Substitute, Anterior Approach, Anterior Column, Percutaneous Approach

HAC When reported with secondary diagnosis code K68.11, T81.40XA, T81.41XA, T81.42XA, T81.43XA, T81.44XA or T81.49XA, T84.60XA, T84.610A, T84.611A, T84.612A, T84.613A, T84.614A, T84.615A, T84.619A, T84.63XA, T84.69XA, T84.7XXA

0RG2371 Fusion of 2 or more Cervical Vertebral Joints with Autologous Tissue Substitute, Posterior Approach, Posterior Column, Percutaneous Approach

AHA CC: 2Q, 2019, 19-20

HAC When reported with secondary diagnosis code K68.11, T81.40XA, T81.41XA, T81.42XA, T81.43XA, T81.44XA or T81.49XA, T84.60XA, T84.610A, T84.611A, T84.612A, T84.613A, T84.614A, T84.615A, T84.619A, T84.63XA, T84.69XA, T84.7XXA

0RG237J Fusion of 2 or more Cervical Vertebral Joints with Autologous Tissue Substitute, Posterior Approach, Anterior Column, Percutaneous Approach

HAC When reported with secondary diagnosis code K68.11, T81.40XA, T81.41XA, T81.42XA, T81.43XA, T81.44XA or T81.49XA, T84.60XA, T84.610A, T84.611A, T84.612A, T84.613A, T84.614A, T84.615A, T84.619A, T84.63XA, T84.69XA, T84.7XXA

0RG23A0 Fusion of 2 or more Cervical Vertebral Joints with Interbody Fusion Device, Anterior Approach, Anterior Column, Percutaneous Approach

When reported with secondary diagnosis code K68.11, T81.40XA, T81.41XA, T81.42XA, T81.43XA, T81.44XA or T81.49XA, T84.60XA, T84.610A, T84.611A, T84.612A, T84.613A, T84.614A, T84.615A, T84.619A, T84.63XA, T84.69XA, T84.7XXA

0RG23AJ Fusion of 2 or more Cervical Vertebral Joints with Interbody Fusion Device, Posterior Approach, Anterior Column, Percutaneous Approach

When reported with secondary diagnosis code K68.11, T81.40XA, T81.41XA, T81.42XA, T81.43XA, T81.44XA or T81.49XA, T84.60XA, T84.610A, T84.611A, T84.612A, T84.613A, T84.614A, T84.615A, T84.619A, T84.63XA, T84.69XA, T84.7XXA

0RG23J0 Fusion of 2 or more Cervical Vertebral Joints with Synthetic Substitute, Anterior Approach, Anterior Column, Percutaneous Approach

HAC When reported with secondary diagnosis code K68.11, T81.40XA, T81.41XA, T81.42XA, T81.43XA, T81.44XA or T81.49XA, T84.60XA, T84.610A, T84.611A, T84.612A, T84.613A, T84.614A, T84.615A, T84.619A, T84.63XA, T84.69XA, T84.7XXA

0RG23J1 Fusion of 2 or more Cervical Vertebral Joints with Synthetic Substitute, Posterior Approach, Posterior Column, Percutaneous Approach

HAC When reported with secondary diagnosis code K68.11, T81.40XA, T81.41XA, T81.42XA, T81.43XA, T81.44XA or T81.49XA, T84.60XA, T84.610A, T84.611A, T84.612A, T84.613A, T84.614A, T84.615A, T84.619A, T84.63XA, T84.69XA, T84.7XXA

0RG23JJ Fusion of 2 or more Cervical Vertebral Joints with Synthetic Substitute, Posterior Approach, Anterior Column, Percutaneous Approach

HAC When reported with secondary diagnosis code K68.11, T81.40XA, T81.41XA, T81.42XA, T81.43XA, T81.44XA or T81.49XA, T84.60XA, T84.610A, T84.611A, T84.612A, T84.613A, T84.614A, T84.615A, T84.619A, T84.63XA, T84.69XA, T84.7XXA

0RG23K0 Fusion of 2 or more Cervical Vertebral Joints with Nonautologous Tissue Substitute, Anterior Approach, Anterior Column, Percutaneous Approach

HAC When reported with secondary diagnosis code K68.11, T81.40XA, T81.41XA, T81.42XA, T81.43XA, T81.44XA or T81.49XA, T84.60XA, T84.610A, T84.611A, T84.612A, T84.613A, T84.614A, T84.615A, T84.619A, T84.63XA, T84.69XA, T84.7XXA

0RG23K1 Fusion of 2 or more Cervical Vertebral Joints with Nonautologous Tissue Substitute, Posterior Approach, Posterior Column, Percutaneous Approach

HAC When reported with secondary diagnosis code K68.11, T81.40XA, T81.41XA, T81.42XA, T81.43XA, T81.44XA or T81.49XA, T84.60XA, T84.610A, T84.611A, T84.612A, T84.613A, T84.614A, T84.615A, T84.619A, T84.63XA, T84.69XA, T84.7XXA

0RG23KJ Fusion of 2 or more Cervical Vertebral Joints with Nonautologous Tissue Substitute, Posterior Approach, Anterior Column, Percutaneous Approach

HAC When reported with secondary diagnosis code K68.11, T81.40XA,

T81.41XA, T81.42XA, T81.43XA, T81.44XA or T81.49XA, T84.60XA, T84.610A, T84.611A, T84.612A, T84.613A, T84.614A, T84.615A, T84.619A, T84.63XA, T84.69XA, T84.7XXA

0RG2470 Fusion of 2 or more Cervical Vertebral Joints with Autologous Tissue Substitute, Anterior Approach, Anterior Column, Percutaneous Endoscopic Approach

HAC When reported with secondary diagnosis code K68.11, T81.40XA, T81.41XA, T81.42XA, T81.43XA, T81.44XA or T81.49XA, T84.60XA, T84.610A, T84.611A, T84.612A, T84.613A, T84.614A, T84.615A, T84.619A, T84.63XA, T84.69XA, T84.7XXA

0RG2471 Fusion of 2 or more Cervical Vertebral Joints with Autologous Tissue Substitute, Posterior Approach, Posterior Column, Percutaneous Endoscopic Approach

HAC When reported with secondary diagnosis code K68.11, T81.40XA, T81.41XA, T81.42XA, T81.43XA, T81.44XA or T81.49XA, T84.60XA, T84.610A, T84.611A, T84.612A, T84.613A, T84.614A, T84.615A, T84.619A, T84.63XA, T84.69XA, T84.7XXA

0RG247J Fusion of 2 or more Cervical Vertebral Joints with Autologous Tissue Substitute, Posterior Approach, Anterior Column, Percutaneous Endoscopic Approach

HAC When reported with secondary diagnosis code K68.11, T81.40XA, T81.41XA, T81.42XA, T81.43XA, T81.44XA or T81.49XA, T84.60XA, T84.610A, T84.611A, T84.612A, T84.613A, T84.614A, T84.615A, T84.619A, T84.63XA, T84.69XA, T84.7XXA

0RG24A0 Fusion of 2 or more Cervical Vertebral Joints with Interbody Fusion Device, Anterior Approach, Anterior Column, Percutaneous Endoscopic Approach

HAC When reported with secondary diagnosis code K68.11, T81.40XA, T81.41XA, T81.42XA, T81.43XA, T81.44XA or T81.49XA, T84.60XA, T84.610A, T84.611A, T84.612A, T84.613A, T84.614A, T84.615A, T84.619A, T84.63XA, T84.69XA, T84.7XXA

0RG24AJ Fusion of 2 or more Cervical Vertebral Joints with Interbody Fusion Device, Posterior Approach, Anterior Column, Percutaneous Endoscopic Approach

HAC When reported with secondary diagnosis code K68.11, T81.40XA, T81.41XA, T81.42XA, T81.43XA, T81.44XA or T81.49XA, T84.60XA, T84.610A, T84.611A, T84.612A, T84.613A, T84.614A, T84.615A, T84.619A, T84.63XA, T84.69XA, T84.7XXA

0RG24J0 Fusion of 2 or more Cervical Vertebral Joints with Synthetic Substitute, Anterior Approach, Anterior Column, Percutaneous Endoscopic Approach

HAC When reported with secondary diagnosis code K68.11, T81.40XA, T81.41XA, T81.42XA, T81.43XA,

T81.44XA or T81.49XA, T84.60XA, T84.610A, T84.611A, T84.612A, T84.613A, T84.614A, T84.615A, T84.619A, T84.63XA, T84.69XA, T84.7XXA

0RG24J1 Fusion of 2 or more Cervical Vertebral Joints with Synthetic Substitute, Posterior Approach, Posterior Column, Percutaneous Endoscopic Approach

HAC When reported with secondary diagnosis code K68.11, T81.40XA, T81.41XA, T81.42XA, T81.43XA, T81.44XA or T81.49XA, T84.60XA, T84.610A, T84.611A, T84.612A, T84.613A, T84.614A, T84.615A, T84.619A, T84.63XA, T84.69XA, T84.7XXA

0RG24JJ Fusion of 2 or more Cervical Vertebral Joints with Synthetic Substitute, Posterior Approach, Anterior Column, Percutaneous Endoscopic Approach

HAC When reported with secondary diagnosis code K68.11, T81.40XA, T81.41XA, T81.42XA, T81.43XA, T81.44XA or T81.49XA, T84.60XA, T84.610A, T84.611A, T84.612A, T84.613A, T84.614A, T84.615A, T84.619A, T84.63XA, T84.69XA, T84.7XXA

0RG24K0 Fusion of 2 or more Cervical Vertebral Joints with Nonautologous Tissue Substitute, Anterior Approach, Anterior Column, Percutaneous Endoscopic Approach

HAC When reported with secondary diagnosis code K68.11, T81.40XA, T81.41XA, T81.42XA, T81.43XA, T81.44XA or T81.49XA, T84.60XA, T84.610A, T84.611A, T84.612A, T84.613A, T84.614A, T84.615A, T84.619A, T84.63XA, T84.69XA, T84.7XXA

0RG24K1 Fusion of 2 or more Cervical Vertebral Joints with Nonautologous Tissue Substitute, Posterior Approach, Posterior Column, Percutaneous Endoscopic Approach

HAC When reported with secondary diagnosis code K68.11, T81.40XA, T81.41XA, T81.42XA, T81.43XA, T81.44XA or T81.49XA, T84.60XA, T84.610A, T84.611A, T84.612A, T84.613A, T84.614A, T84.615A, T84.619A, T84.63XA, T84.69XA, T84.7XXA

0RG24KJ Fusion of 2 or more Cervical Vertebral Joints with Nonautologous Tissue Substitute, Posterior Approach, Anterior Column, Percutaneous Endoscopic Approach

HAC When reported with secondary diagnosis code K68.11, T81.40XA, T81.41XA, T81.42XA, T81.43XA, T81.44XA or T81.49XA, T84.60XA, T84.610A, T84.611A, T84.612A, T84.613A, T84.614A, T84.615A, T84.619A, T84.63XA, T84.69XA, T84.7XXA

0RG4070 Fusion of Cervicothoracic Vertebral Joint with Autologous Tissue Substitute, Anterior Approach, Anterior Column, Open Approach

HAC When reported with secondary diagnosis code K68.11, T81.40XA, T81.41XA, T81.42XA, T81.43XA, T81.44XA or T81.49XA, T84.60XA,

♀ Female-only   ♂ Male-only   ▲ Limited Coverage   ● Non-OR   HAC HAC-associated procedure   ▲ Non-covered procedures   ✚ Cluster

T84.610A, T84.611A, T84.612A,
T84.613A, T84.614A, T84.615A,
T84.619A, T84.63XA, T84.69XA,
T84.7XXA

0RG4071 Fusion of Cervicothoracic Vertebral
Joint with Autologous Tissue
Substitute, Posterior Approach,
Posterior Column, Open Approach

[HAC] When reported with secondary
diagnosis code K68.11, T81.40XA,
T81.41XA, T81.42XA, T81.43XA,
T81.44XA or T81.49XA, T84.60XA,
T84.610A, T84.611A, T84.612A,
T84.613A, T84.614A, T84.615A,
T84.619A, T84.63XA, T84.69XA,
T84.7XXA

0RG407J Fusion of Cervicothoracic Vertebral
Joint with Autologous Tissue
Substitute, Posterior Approach,
Anterior Column, Open
Approach

[HAC] When reported with secondary
diagnosis code K68.11, T81.40XA,
T81.41XA, T81.42XA, T81.43XA,
T81.44XA or T81.49XA, T84.60XA,
T84.610A, T84.611A, T84.612A,
T84.613A, T84.614A, T84.615A,
T84.619A, T84.63XA, T84.69XA,
T84.7XXA

0RG40A0 Fusion of Cervicothoracic Vertebral
Joint with Interbody Fusion Device,
Anterior Approach, Anterior Column,
Open Approach

AHA CC: 1Q, 2013, 29-30; 2Q, 2014, 7-8

[HAC] When reported with secondary
diagnosis code K68.11, T81.40XA,
T81.41XA, T81.42XA, T81.43XA,
T81.44XA or T81.49XA, T84.60XA,
T84.610A, T84.611A, T84.612A,
T84.613A, T84.614A, T84.615A,
T84.619A, T84.63XA, T84.69XA,
T84.7XXA

0RG40AJ Fusion of Cervicothoracic Vertebral
Joint with Interbody Fusion Device,
Posterior Approach, Anterior Column,
Open Approach

[HAC] When reported with secondary
diagnosis code K68.11, T81.40XA,
T81.41XA, T81.42XA, T81.43XA,
T81.44XA or T81.49XA, T84.60XA,
T84.610A, T84.611A, T84.612A,
T84.613A, T84.614A, T84.615A,
T84.619A, T84.63XA, T84.69XA,
T84.7XXA

0RG40J0 Fusion of Cervicothoracic Vertebral
Joint with Synthetic Substitute,
Anterior Approach, Anterior Column,
Open Approach

[HAC] When reported with secondary
diagnosis code K68.11, T81.40XA,
T81.41XA, T81.42XA, T81.43XA,
T81.44XA or T81.49XA, T84.60XA,
T84.610A, T84.611A, T84.612A,
T84.613A, T84.614A, T84.615A,
T84.619A, T84.63XA, T84.69XA,
T84.7XXA

0RG40J1 Fusion of Cervicothoracic Vertebral
Joint with Synthetic Substitute,
Posterior Approach, Posterior Column,
Open Approach

[HAC] When reported with secondary
diagnosis code K68.11, T81.40XA,
T81.41XA, T81.42XA, T81.43XA,
T81.44XA or T81.49XA, T84.60XA,
T84.610A, T84.611A, T84.612A,
T84.613A, T84.614A, T84.615A,

T84.619A, T84.63XA, T84.69XA,
T84.7XXA

0RG40JJ Fusion of Cervicothoracic Vertebral
Joint with Synthetic Substitute,
Posterior Approach, Anterior Column,
Open Approach

[HAC] When reported with secondary
diagnosis code K68.11, T81.40XA,
T81.41XA, T81.42XA, T81.43XA,
T81.44XA or T81.49XA, T84.60XA,
T84.610A, T84.611A, T84.612A,
T84.613A, T84.614A, T84.615A,
T84.619A, T84.63XA, T84.69XA,
T84.7XXA

0RG40K0 Fusion of Cervicothoracic Vertebral
Joint with Nonautologous Tissue
Substitute, Anterior Approach, Anterior
Column, Open Approach

[HAC] When reported with secondary
diagnosis code K68.11, T81.40XA,
T81.41XA, T81.42XA, T81.43XA,
T81.44XA or T81.49XA, T84.60XA,
T84.610A, T84.611A, T84.612A,
T84.613A, T84.614A, T84.615A,
T84.619A, T84.63XA, T84.69XA,
T84.7XXA

0RG40K1 Fusion of Cervicothoracic Vertebral
Joint with Nonautologous Tissue
Substitute, Posterior Approach,
Posterior Column, Open Approach

[HAC] When reported with secondary
diagnosis code K68.11, T81.40XA,
T81.41XA, T81.42XA, T81.43XA,
T81.44XA or T81.49XA, T84.60XA,
T84.610A, T84.611A, T84.612A,
T84.613A, T84.614A, T84.615A,
T84.619A, T84.63XA, T84.69XA,
T84.7XXA

0RG40KJ Fusion of Cervicothoracic Vertebral
Joint with Nonautologous Tissue
Substitute, Posterior Approach,
Anterior Column, Open Approach

[HAC] When reported with secondary
diagnosis code K68.11, T81.40XA,
T81.41XA, T81.42XA, T81.43XA,
T81.44XA or T81.49XA, T84.60XA,
T84.610A, T84.611A, T84.612A,
T84.613A, T84.614A, T84.615A,
T84.619A, T84.63XA, T84.69XA,
T84.7XXA

0RG4370 Fusion of Cervicothoracic Vertebral
Joint with Autologous Tissue
Substitute, Anterior Approach,
Anterior Column, Percutaneous
Approach

[HAC] When reported with secondary
diagnosis code K68.11, T81.40XA,
T81.41XA, T81.42XA, T81.43XA,
T81.44XA or T81.49XA, T84.60XA,
T84.610A, T84.611A, T84.612A,
T84.613A, T84.614A, T84.615A,
T84.619A, T84.63XA, T84.69XA,
T84.7XXA

0RG4371 Fusion of Cervicothoracic Vertebral
Joint with Autologous Tissue
Substitute, Posterior Approach,
Posterior Column, Percutaneous
Approach

[HAC] When reported with secondary
diagnosis code K68.11, T81.40XA,
T81.41XA, T81.42XA, T81.43XA,
T81.44XA or T81.49XA, T84.60XA,
T84.610A, T84.611A, T84.612A,
T84.613A, T84.614A, T84.615A,
T84.619A, T84.63XA, T84.69XA,
T84.7XXA

0RG437J Fusion of Cervicothoracic Vertebral
Joint with Autologous Tissue
Substitute, Posterior Approach,
Anterior Column, Percutaneous
Approach

[HAC] When reported with secondary
diagnosis code K68.11, T81.40XA,
T81.41XA, T81.42XA, T81.43XA,
T81.44XA or T81.49XA, T84.60XA,
T84.610A, T84.611A, T84.612A,
T84.613A, T84.614A, T84.615A,
T84.619A, T84.63XA, T84.69XA,
T84.7XXA

0RG43A0 Fusion of Cervicothoracic
Vertebral Joint with Interbody
Fusion Device, Anterior Approach,
Anterior Column, Percutaneous
Approach

[HAC] When reported with secondary
diagnosis code K68.11, T81.40XA,
T81.41XA, T81.42XA, T81.43XA,
T81.44XA or T81.49XA, T84.60XA,
T84.610A, T84.611A, T84.612A,
T84.613A, T84.614A, T84.615A,
T84.619A, T84.63XA, T84.69XA,
T84.7XXA

0RG43AJ Fusion of Cervicothoracic
Vertebral Joint with Interbody
Fusion Device, Posterior Approach,
Anterior Column, Percutaneous
Approach

[HAC] When reported with secondary
diagnosis code K68.11, T81.40XA,
T81.41XA, T81.42XA, T81.43XA,
T81.44XA or T81.49XA, T84.60XA,
T84.610A, T84.611A, T84.612A,
T84.613A, T84.614A, T84.615A,
T84.619A, T84.63XA, T84.69XA,
T84.7XXA

0RG43J0 Fusion of Cervicothoracic
Vertebral Joint with Synthetic
Substitute, Anterior Approach,
Anterior Column, Percutaneous
Approach

[HAC] When reported with secondary
diagnosis code K68.11, T81.40XA,
T81.41XA, T81.42XA, T81.43XA,
T81.44XA or T81.49XA, T84.60XA,
T84.610A, T84.611A, T84.612A,
T84.613A, T84.614A, T84.615A,
T84.619A, T84.63XA, T84.69XA,
T84.7XXA

0RG43J1 Fusion of Cervicothoracic Vertebral
Joint with Synthetic Substitute,
Posterior Approach, Posterior Column,
Percutaneous Approach

[HAC] When reported with secondary
diagnosis code K68.11, T81.40XA,
T81.41XA, T81.42XA, T81.43XA,
T81.44XA or T81.49XA, T84.60XA,
T84.610A, T84.611A, T84.612A,
T84.613A, T84.614A, T84.615A,
T84.619A, T84.63XA, T84.69XA,
T84.7XXA

0RG43JJ Fusion of Cervicothoracic Vertebral
Joint with Synthetic Substitute,
Posterior Approach, Anterior Column,
Percutaneous Approach

[HAC] When reported with secondary
diagnosis code K68.11, T81.40XA,
T81.41XA, T81.42XA, T81.43XA,
T81.44XA or T81.49XA, T84.60XA,
T84.610A, T84.611A, T84.612A,
T84.613A, T84.614A, T84.615A,
T84.619A, T84.63XA, T84.69XA,
T84.7XXA

0RG43K0 Fusion of Cervicothoracic Vertebral Joint with Nonautologous Tissue Substitute, Anterior Approach, Anterior Column, Percutaneous Approach

HAC When reported with secondary diagnosis code K68.11, T81.40XA, T81.41XA, T81.42XA, T81.43XA, T81.44XA or T81.49XA, T84.60XA, T84.610A, T84.611A, T84.612A, T84.613A, T84.614A, T84.615A, T84.619A, T84.63XA, T84.69XA, T84.7XXA

0RG43K1 Fusion of Cervicothoracic Vertebral Joint with Nonautologous Tissue Substitute, Posterior Approach, Posterior Column, Percutaneous Approach

HAC When reported with secondary diagnosis code K68.11, T81.40XA, T81.41XA, T81.42XA, T81.43XA, T81.44XA or T81.49XA, T84.60XA, T84.610A, T84.611A, T84.612A, T84.613A, T84.614A, T84.615A, T84.619A, T84.63XA, T84.69XA, T84.7XXA

0RG43KJ Fusion of Cervicothoracic Vertebral Joint with Nonautologous Tissue Substitute, Posterior Approach, Anterior Column, Percutaneous Approach

HAC When reported with secondary diagnosis code K68.11, T81.40XA, T81.41XA, T81.42XA, T81.43XA, T81.44XA or T81.49XA, T84.60XA, T84.610A, T84.611A, T84.612A, T84.613A, T84.614A, T84.615A, T84.619A, T84.63XA, T84.69XA, T84.7XXA

0RG4470 Fusion of Cervicothoracic Vertebral Joint with Autologous Tissue Substitute, Anterior Approach, Anterior Column, Percutaneous Endoscopic Approach

HAC When reported with secondary diagnosis code K68.11, T81.40XA, T81.41XA, T81.42XA, T81.43XA, T81.44XA or T81.49XA, T84.60XA, T84.610A, T84.611A, T84.612A, T84.613A, T84.614A, T84.615A, T84.619A, T84.63XA, T84.69XA, T84.7XXA

0RG4471 Fusion of Cervicothoracic Vertebral Joint with Autologous Tissue Substitute, Posterior Approach, Posterior Column, Percutaneous Endoscopic Approach

HAC When reported with secondary diagnosis code K68.11, T81.40XA, T81.41XA, T81.42XA, T81.43XA, T81.44XA or T81.49XA, T84.60XA, T84.610A, T84.611A, T84.612A, T84.613A, T84.614A, T84.615A, T84.619A, T84.63XA, T84.69XA, T84.7XXA

0RG447J Fusion of Cervicothoracic Vertebral Joint with Autologous Tissue Substitute, Posterior Approach, Anterior Column, Percutaneous Endoscopic Approach

HAC When reported with secondary diagnosis code K68.11, T81.40XA, T81.41XA, T81.42XA, T81.43XA, T81.44XA or T81.49XA, T84.60XA, T84.610A, T84.611A, T84.612A, T84.613A, T84.614A, T84.615A, T84.619A, T84.63XA, T84.69XA, T84.7XXA

0RG44A0 Fusion of Cervicothoracic Vertebral Joint with Interbody Fusion Device, Anterior Approach, Anterior Column, Percutaneous Endoscopic Approach

HAC When reported with secondary diagnosis code K68.11, T81.40XA, T81.41XA, T81.42XA, T81.43XA, T81.44XA or T81.49XA, T84.60XA, T84.610A, T84.611A, T84.612A, T84.613A, T84.614A, T84.615A, T84.619A, T84.63XA, T84.69XA, T84.7XXA

0RG44AJ Fusion of Cervicothoracic Vertebral Joint with Interbody Fusion Device, Posterior Approach, Anterior Column, Percutaneous Endoscopic Approach

HAC When reported with secondary diagnosis code K68.11, T81.40XA, T81.41XA, T81.42XA, T81.43XA, T81.44XA or T81.49XA, T84.60XA, T84.610A, T84.611A, T84.612A, T84.613A, T84.614A, T84.615A, T84.619A, T84.63XA, T84.69XA, T84.7XXA

0RG44J0 Fusion of Cervicothoracic Vertebral Joint with Synthetic Substitute, Anterior Approach, Anterior Column, Percutaneous Endoscopic Approach

HAC When reported with secondary diagnosis code K68.11, T81.40XA, T81.41XA, T81.42XA, T81.43XA, T81.44XA or T81.49XA, T84.60XA, T84.610A, T84.611A, T84.612A, T84.613A, T84.614A, T84.615A, T84.619A, T84.63XA, T84.69XA, T84.7XXA

0RG44J1 Fusion of Cervicothoracic Vertebral Joint with Synthetic Substitute, Posterior Approach, Posterior Column, Percutaneous Endoscopic Approach

HAC When reported with secondary diagnosis code K68.11, T81.40XA, T81.41XA, T81.42XA, T81.43XA, T81.44XA or T81.49XA, T84.60XA, T84.610A, T84.611A, T84.612A, T84.613A, T84.614A, T84.615A, T84.619A, T84.63XA, T84.69XA, T84.7XXA

0RG44JJ Fusion of Cervicothoracic Vertebral Joint with Synthetic Substitute, Posterior Approach, Anterior Column, Percutaneous Endoscopic Approach

HAC When reported with secondary diagnosis code K68.11, T81.40XA, T81.41XA, T81.42XA, T81.43XA, T81.44XA or T81.49XA, T84.60XA, T84.610A, T84.611A, T84.612A, T84.613A, T84.614A, T84.615A, T84.619A, T84.63XA, T84.69XA, T84.7XXA

0RG44K0 Fusion of Cervicothoracic Vertebral Joint with Nonautologous Tissue Substitute, Anterior Approach, Anterior Column, Percutaneous Endoscopic Approach

HAC When reported with secondary diagnosis code K68.11, T81.40XA, T81.41XA, T81.42XA, T81.43XA, T81.44XA or T81.49XA, T84.60XA, T84.610A, T84.611A, T84.612A, T84.613A, T84.614A, T84.615A, T84.619A, T84.63XA, T84.69XA, T84.7XXA

0RG44K1 Fusion of Cervicothoracic Vertebral Joint with Nonautologous Tissue Substitute, Posterior Approach, Posterior Column, Percutaneous Endoscopic Approach

HAC When reported with secondary diagnosis code K68.11, T81.40XA, T81.41XA, T81.42XA, T81.43XA, T81.44XA or T81.49XA, T84.60XA, T84.610A, T84.611A, T84.612A, T84.613A, T84.614A, T84.615A, T84.619A, T84.63XA, T84.69XA, T84.7XXA

0RG44KJ Fusion of Cervicothoracic Vertebral Joint with Nonautologous Tissue Substitute, Posterior Approach, Anterior Column, Percutaneous Endoscopic Approach

HAC When reported with secondary diagnosis code K68.11, T81.40XA, T81.41XA, T81.42XA, T81.43XA, T81.44XA or T81.49XA, T84.60XA, T84.610A, T84.611A, T84.612A, T84.613A, T84.614A, T84.615A, T84.619A, T84.63XA, T84.69XA, T84.7XXA

0RG6070 Fusion of Thoracic Vertebral Joint with Autologous Tissue Substitute, Anterior Approach, Anterior Column, Open Approach

HAC When reported with secondary diagnosis code K68.11, T81.40XA, T81.41XA, T81.42XA, T81.43XA, T81.44XA or T81.49XA, T84.60XA, T84.610A, T84.611A, T84.612A, T84.613A, T84.614A, T84.615A, T84.619A, T84.63XA, T84.69XA, T84.7XXA

0RG6071 Fusion of Thoracic Vertebral Joint with Autologous Tissue Substitute, Posterior Approach, Posterior Column, Open Approach

HAC When reported with secondary diagnosis code K68.11, T81.40XA, T81.41XA, T81.42XA, T81.43XA, T81.44XA or T81.49XA, T84.60XA, T84.610A, T84.611A, T84.612A, T84.613A, T84.614A, T84.615A, T84.619A, T84.63XA, T84.69XA, T84.7XXA

0RG607J Fusion of Thoracic Vertebral Joint with Autologous Tissue Substitute, Posterior Approach, Anterior Column, Open Approach

HAC When reported with secondary diagnosis code K68.11, T81.40XA, T81.41XA, T81.42XA, T81.43XA, T81.44XA or T81.49XA, T84.60XA, T84.610A, T84.611A, T84.612A, T84.613A, T84.614A, T84.615A, T84.619A, T84.63XA, T84.69XA, T84.7XXA

0RG60A0 Fusion of Thoracic Vertebral Joint with Interbody Fusion Device, Anterior Approach, Anterior Column, Open Approach

HAC When reported with secondary diagnosis code K68.11, T81.40XA, T81.41XA, T81.42XA, T81.43XA, T81.44XA or T81.49XA, T84.60XA, T84.610A, T84.611A, T84.612A, T84.613A, T84.614A, T84.615A, T84.619A, T84.63XA, T84.69XA, T84.7XXA

0RG60AJ Fusion of Thoracic Vertebral Joint with Interbody Fusion Device, Posterior Approach, Anterior Column, Open Approach

HAC When reported with secondary diagnosis code K68.11, T81.40XA,

T81.41XA, T81.42XA, T81.43XA,
T81.44XA or T81.49XA, T84.60XA,
T84.610A, T84.611A, T84.612A,
T84.613A, T84.614A, T84.615A,
T84.619A, T84.63XA, T84.69XA,
T84.7XXA

0RG60J0 Fusion of Thoracic Vertebral Joint
with Synthetic Substitute, Anterior
Approach, Anterior Column, Open
Approach

HAC When reported with secondary
diagnosis code K68.11, T81.40XA,
T81.41XA, T81.42XA, T81.43XA,
T81.44XA or T81.49XA, T84.60XA,
T84.610A, T84.611A, T84.612A,
T84.613A, T84.614A, T84.615A,
T84.619A, T84.63XA, T84.69XA,
T84.7XXA

0RG60J1 Fusion of Thoracic Vertebral Joint
with Synthetic Substitute, Posterior
Approach, Posterior Column, Open
Approach

HAC When reported with secondary
diagnosis code K68.11, T81.40XA,
T81.41XA, T81.42XA, T81.43XA,
T81.44XA or T81.49XA, T84.60XA,
T84.610A, T84.611A, T84.612A,
T84.613A, T84.614A, T84.615A,
T84.619A, T84.63XA, T84.69XA,
T84.7XXA

0RG60JJ Fusion of Thoracic Vertebral Joint with
Synthetic Substitute, Posterior Approach,
Anterior Column, Open Approach

HAC When reported with secondary
diagnosis code K68.11, T81.40XA,
T81.41XA, T81.42XA, T81.43XA,
T81.44XA or T81.49XA, T84.60XA,
T84.610A, T84.611A, T84.612A,
T84.613A, T84.614A, T84.615A,
T84.619A, T84.63XA, T84.69XA,
T84.7XXA

0RG60K0 Fusion of Thoracic Vertebral Joint
with Nonautologous Tissue Substitute,
Anterior Approach, Anterior Column,
Open Approach

HAC When reported with secondary
diagnosis code K68.11, T81.40XA,
T81.41XA, T81.42XA, T81.43XA,
T81.44XA or T81.49XA, T84.60XA,
T84.610A, T84.611A, T84.612A,
T84.613A, T84.614A, T84.615A,
T84.619A, T84.63XA, T84.69XA,
T84.7XXA

0RG60K1 Fusion of Thoracic Vertebral Joint
with Nonautologous Tissue Substitute,
Posterior Approach, Posterior Column,
Open Approach

HAC When reported with secondary
diagnosis code K68.11, T81.40XA,
T81.41XA, T81.42XA, T81.43XA,
T81.44XA or T81.49XA, T84.60XA,
T84.610A, T84.611A, T84.612A,
T84.613A, T84.614A, T84.615A,
T84.619A, T84.63XA, T84.69XA,
T84.7XXA

0RG60KJ Fusion of Thoracic Vertebral Joint
with Nonautologous Tissue Substitute,
Posterior Approach, Anterior Column,
Open Approach

HAC When reported with secondary
diagnosis code K68.11, T81.40XA,
T81.41XA, T81.42XA, T81.43XA,
T81.44XA or T81.49XA, T84.60XA,
T84.610A, T84.611A, T84.612A,
T84.613A, T84.614A, T84.615A,
T84.619A, T84.63XA, T84.69XA,
T84.7XXA

0RG6370 Fusion of Thoracic Vertebral Joint
with Autologous Tissue Substitute,
Anterior Approach, Anterior Column,
Percutaneous Approach

HAC When reported with secondary
diagnosis code K68.11, T81.40XA,
T81.41XA, T81.42XA, T81.43XA,
T81.44XA or T81.49XA, T84.60XA,
T84.610A, T84.611A, T84.612A,
T84.613A, T84.614A, T84.615A,
T84.619A, T84.63XA, T84.69XA,
T84.7XXA

0RG6371 Fusion of Thoracic Vertebral Joint
with Autologous Tissue Substitute,
Posterior Approach, Posterior Column,
Percutaneous Approach

HAC When reported with secondary
diagnosis code K68.11, T81.40XA,
T81.41XA, T81.42XA, T81.43XA,
T81.44XA or T81.49XA, T84.60XA,
T84.610A, T84.611A, T84.612A,
T84.613A, T84.614A, T84.615A,
T84.619A, T84.63XA, T84.69XA,
T84.7XXA

0RG637J Fusion of Thoracic Vertebral
Joint with Autologous Tissue
Substitute, Posterior Approach,
Anterior Column, Percutaneous
Approach

HAC When reported with secondary
diagnosis code K68.11, T81.40XA,
T81.41XA, T81.42XA, T81.43XA,
T81.44XA or T81.49XA, T84.60XA,
T84.610A, T84.611A, T84.612A,
T84.613A, T84.614A, T84.615A,
T84.619A, T84.63XA, T84.69XA,
T84.7XXA

0RG63A0 Fusion of Thoracic Vertebral Joint
with Interbody Fusion Device,
Anterior Approach, Anterior Column,
Percutaneous Approach

HAC When reported with secondary
diagnosis code K68.11, T81.40XA,
T81.41XA, T81.42XA, T81.43XA,
T81.44XA or T81.49XA, T84.60XA,
T84.610A, T84.611A, T84.612A,
T84.613A, T84.614A, T84.615A,
T84.619A, T84.63XA, T84.69XA,
T84.7XXA

0RG63AJ Fusion of Thoracic Vertebral Joint
with Interbody Fusion Device,
Posterior Approach, Anterior Column,
Percutaneous Approach

HAC When reported with secondary
diagnosis code K68.11, T81.40XA,
T81.41XA, T81.42XA, T81.43XA,
T81.44XA or T81.49XA, T84.60XA,
T84.610A, T84.611A, T84.612A,
T84.613A, T84.614A, T84.615A,
T84.619A, T84.63XA, T84.69XA,
T84.7XXA

0RG63J0 Fusion of Thoracic Vertebral Joint
with Synthetic Substitute, Anterior
Approach, Anterior Column,
Percutaneous Approach

HAC When reported with secondary
diagnosis code K68.11, T81.40XA,
T81.41XA, T81.42XA, T81.43XA,
T81.44XA or T81.49XA, T84.60XA,
T84.610A, T84.611A, T84.612A,
T84.613A, T84.614A, T84.615A,
T84.619A, T84.63XA, T84.69XA,
T84.7XXA

0RG63J1 Fusion of Thoracic Vertebral Joint
with Synthetic Substitute, Posterior
Approach, Posterior Column,
Percutaneous Approach

When reported with secondary
diagnosis code K68.11, T81.40XA,
T81.41XA, T81.42XA, T81.43XA,
T81.44XA or T81.49XA, T84.60XA,
T84.610A, T84.611A, T84.612A,
T84.613A, T84.614A, T84.615A,
T84.619A, T84.63XA, T84.69XA,
T84.7XXA

0RG63JJ Fusion of Thoracic Vertebral Joint
with Synthetic Substitute, Posterior
Approach, Anterior Column,
Percutaneous Approach

HAC When reported with secondary
diagnosis code K68.11, T81.40XA,
T81.41XA, T81.42XA, T81.43XA,
T81.44XA or T81.49XA, T84.60XA,
T84.610A, T84.611A, T84.612A,
T84.613A, T84.614A, T84.615A,
T84.619A, T84.63XA, T84.69XA,
T84.7XXA

0RG63K0 Fusion of Thoracic Vertebral Joint
with Nonautologous Tissue Substitute,
Anterior Approach, Anterior Column,
Percutaneous Approach

HAC When reported with secondary
diagnosis code K68.11, T81.40XA,
T81.41XA, T81.42XA, T81.43XA,
T81.44XA or T81.49XA, T84.60XA,
T84.610A, T84.611A, T84.612A,
T84.613A, T84.614A, T84.615A,
T84.619A, T84.63XA, T84.69XA,
T84.7XXA

0RG63K1 Fusion of Thoracic Vertebral Joint
with Nonautologous Tissue Substitute,
Posterior Approach, Posterior Column,
Percutaneous Approach

HAC When reported with secondary
diagnosis code K68.11, T81.40XA,
T81.41XA, T81.42XA, T81.43XA,
T81.44XA or T81.49XA, T84.60XA,
T84.610A, T84.611A, T84.612A,
T84.613A, T84.614A, T84.615A,
T84.619A, T84.63XA, T84.69XA,
T84.7XXA

0RG63KJ Fusion of Thoracic Vertebral Joint
with Nonautologous Tissue Substitute,
Posterior Approach, Anterior Column,
Percutaneous Approach

HAC When reported with secondary
diagnosis code K68.11, T81.40XA,
T81.41XA, T81.42XA, T81.43XA,
T81.44XA or T81.49XA, T84.60XA,
T84.610A, T84.611A, T84.612A,
T84.613A, T84.614A, T84.615A,
T84.619A, T84.63XA, T84.69XA,
T84.7XXA

0RG6470 Fusion of Thoracic Vertebral Joint
with Autologous Tissue Substitute,
Anterior Approach, Anterior
Column, Percutaneous Endoscopic
Approach

HAC When reported with secondary
diagnosis code K68.11, T81.40XA,
T81.41XA, T81.42XA, T81.43XA,
T81.44XA or T81.49XA, T84.60XA,
T84.610A, T84.611A, T84.612A,
T84.613A, T84.614A, T84.615A,
T84.619A, T84.63XA, T84.69XA,
T84.7XXA

0RG6471 Fusion of Thoracic Vertebral Joint
with Autologous Tissue Substitute,
Posterior Approach, Posterior
Column, Percutaneous Endoscopic
Approach

HAC When reported with secondary
diagnosis code K68.11, T81.40XA,
T81.41XA, T81.42XA, T81.43XA,

T81.44XA or T81.49XA, T84.60XA, T84.610A, T84.611A, T84.612A, T84.613A, T84.614A, T84.615A, T84.619A, T84.63XA, T84.69XA, T84.7XXA

0RG647J Fusion of Thoracic Vertebral Joint with Autologous Tissue Substitute, Posterior Approach, Anterior Column, Percutaneous Endoscopic Approach

HAC When reported with secondary diagnosis code K68.11, T81.4XXA, T84.60XA, T84.610A, T84.611A, T84.612A, T84.613A, T84.614A, T84.615A, T84.619A, T84.63XA, T84.69XA, T84.7XXA

0RG64A0 Fusion of Thoracic Vertebral Joint with Interbody Fusion Device, Anterior Approach, Anterior Column, Percutaneous Endoscopic Approach

HAC When reported with secondary diagnosis code K68.11, T81.4XXA, T84.60XA, T84.610A, T84.611A, T84.612A, T84.613A, T84.614A, T84.615A, T84.619A, T84.63XA, T84.69XA, T84.7XXA

0RG64AJ Fusion of Thoracic Vertebral Joint with Interbody Fusion Device, Posterior Approach, Anterior Column, Percutaneous Endoscopic Approach

HAC When reported with secondary diagnosis code K68.11, T81.40XA, T81.41XA, T81.42XA, T81.43XA, T81.44XA or T81.49XA, T84.60XA, T84.610A, T84.611A, T84.612A, T84.613A, T84.614A, T84.615A, T84.619A, T84.63XA, T84.69XA, T84.7XXA

0RG64J0 Fusion of Thoracic Vertebral Joint with Synthetic Substitute, Anterior Approach, Anterior Column, Percutaneous Endoscopic Approach

HAC When reported with secondary diagnosis code K68.11, T81.40XA, T81.41XA, T81.42XA, T81.43XA, T81.44XA or T81.49XA, T84.60XA, T84.610A, T84.611A, T84.612A, T84.613A, T84.614A, T84.615A, T84.619A, T84.63XA, T84.69XA, T84.7XXA

0RG64J1 Fusion of Thoracic Vertebral Joint with Synthetic Substitute, Posterior Approach, Posterior Column, Percutaneous Endoscopic Approach

HAC When reported with secondary diagnosis code K68.11, T81.40XA, T81.41XA, T81.42XA, T81.43XA, T81.44XA or T81.49XA, T84.60XA, T84.610A, T84.611A, T84.612A, T84.613A, T84.614A, T84.615A, T84.619A, T84.63XA, T84.69XA, T84.7XXA

0RG64JJ Fusion of Thoracic Vertebral Joint with Synthetic Substitute, Posterior Approach, Anterior Column, Percutaneous Endoscopic Approach

HAC When reported with secondary diagnosis code K68.11, T81.40XA, T81.41XA, T81.42XA, T81.43XA, T81.44XA or T81.49XA, T84.60XA, T84.610A, T84.611A, T84.612A, T84.613A, T84.614A, T84.615A, T84.619A, T84.63XA, T84.69XA, T84.7XXA

0RG64K0 Fusion of Thoracic Vertebral Joint with Nonautologous Tissue Substitute, Anterior Approach, Anterior Column, Percutaneous Endoscopic Approach

HAC When reported with secondary diagnosis code K68.11, T81.40XA, T81.41XA, T81.42XA, T81.43XA, T81.44XA or T81.49XA, T84.60XA, T84.610A, T84.611A, T84.612A, T84.613A, T84.614A, T84.615A, T84.619A, T84.63XA, T84.69XA, T84.7XXA

0RG64K1 Fusion of Thoracic Vertebral Joint with Nonautologous Tissue Substitute, Posterior Approach, Posterior Column, Percutaneous Endoscopic Approach

HAC When reported with secondary diagnosis code K68.11, T81.40XA, T81.41XA, T81.42XA, T81.43XA, T81.44XA or T81.49XA, T84.60XA, T84.610A, T84.611A, T84.612A, T84.613A, T84.614A, T84.615A, T84.619A, T84.63XA, T84.69XA, T84.7XXA

0RG64KJ Fusion of Thoracic Vertebral Joint with Nonautologous Tissue Substitute, Posterior Approach, Anterior Column, Percutaneous Endoscopic Approach

HAC When reported with secondary diagnosis code K68.11, T81.40XA, T81.41XA, T81.42XA, T81.43XA, T81.44XA or T81.49XA, T84.60XA, T84.610A, T84.611A, T84.612A, T84.613A, T84.614A, T84.615A, T84.619A, T84.63XA, T84.69XA, T84.7XXA

0RG7070 Fusion of 2 to 7 Thoracic Vertebral Joints with Autologous Tissue Substitute, Anterior Approach, Anterior Column, Open Approach

HAC When reported with secondary diagnosis code K68.11, T81.40XA, T81.41XA, T81.42XA, T81.43XA, T81.44XA or T81.49XA, T84.60XA, T84.610A, T84.611A, T84.612A, T84.613A, T84.614A, T84.615A, T84.619A, T84.63XA, T84.69XA, T84.7XXA

➕ Fusion of nine or more joints when reported with Fusion of two or more lumbar vertebral joints. *See code XRGC0F3 or table 0SG to construct Fusion code.*

0RG7071 Fusion of 2 to 7 Thoracic Vertebral Joints with Autologous Tissue Substitute, Posterior Approach, Posterior Column, Open Approach

AHA CC: 1Q, 2013, 21-23

HAC When reported with secondary diagnosis code K68.11, T81.40XA, T81.41XA, T81.42XA, T81.43XA, T81.44XA or T81.49XA, T84.60XA, T84.610A, T84.611A, T84.612A, T84.613A, T84.614A, T84.615A, T84.619A, T84.63XA, T84.69XA, T84.7XXA

➕ Fusion of nine or more joints when reported with Fusion of two or more lumbar vertebral joints. *See code XRGC0F3 or table 0SG to construct Fusion code.*

0RG707J Fusion of 2 to 7 Thoracic Vertebral Joints with Autologous Tissue Substitute, Posterior Approach, Anterior Column, Open Approach

HAC When reported with secondary diagnosis code K68.11, T81.40XA, T81.41XA, T81.42XA, T81.43XA, T81.44XA or T81.49XA, T84.60XA,

T84.610A, T84.611A, T84.612A, T84.613A, T84.614A, T84.615A, T84.619A, T84.63XA, T84.69XA, T84.7XXA

➕ Fusion of nine or more joints when reported with Fusion of two or more lumbar vertebral joints. *See code XRGC0F3 or table 0SG to construct Fusion code.*

0RG70A0 Fusion of 2 to 7 Thoracic Vertebral Joints with Interbody Fusion Device, Anterior Approach, Anterior Column, Open Approach

HAC When reported with secondary diagnosis code K68.11, T81.40XA, T81.41XA, T81.42XA, T81.43XA, T81.44XA or T81.49XA, T84.60XA, T84.610A, T84.611A, T84.612A, T84.613A, T84.614A, T84.615A, T84.619A, T84.63XA, T84.69XA, T84.7XXA

➕ Fusion of nine or more joints when reported with Fusion of two or more lumbar vertebral joints. *See code XRGC0F3 or table 0SG to construct Fusion code.*

0RG70AJ Fusion of 2 to 7 Thoracic Vertebral Joints with Interbody Fusion Device, Posterior Approach, Anterior Column, Open Approach

HAC When reported with secondary diagnosis code K68.11, T81.40XA, T81.41XA, T81.42XA, T81.43XA, T81.44XA or T81.49XA, T84.60XA, T84.610A, T84.611A, T84.612A, T84.613A, T84.614A, T84.615A, T84.619A, T84.63XA, T84.69XA, T84.7XXA

➕ Fusion of nine or more joints when reported with Fusion of two or more lumbar vertebral joints. *See code XRGC0F3 or table 0SG to construct Fusion code.*

0RG70J0 Fusion of 2 to 7 Thoracic Vertebral Joints with Synthetic Substitute, Anterior Approach, Anterior Column, Open Approach

HAC When reported with secondary diagnosis code K68.11, T81.40XA, T81.41XA, T81.42XA, T81.43XA, T81.44XA or T81.49XA, T84.60XA, T84.610A, T84.611A, T84.612A, T84.613A, T84.614A, T84.615A, T84.619A, T84.63XA, T84.69XA, T84.7XXA

➕ Fusion of nine or more joints when reported with Fusion of two or more lumbar vertebral joints. *See code XRGC0F3 or table 0SG to construct Fusion code.*

0RG70J1 Fusion of 2 to 7 Thoracic Vertebral Joints with Synthetic Substitute, Posterior Approach, Posterior Column, Open Approach

HAC When reported with secondary diagnosis code K68.11, T81.40XA, T81.41XA, T81.42XA, T81.43XA, T81.44XA or T81.49XA, T84.60XA, T84.610A, T84.611A, T84.612A, T84.613A, T84.614A, T84.615A, T84.619A, T84.63XA, T84.69XA, T84.7XXA

➕ Fusion of nine or more joints when reported with Fusion of two or more lumbar vertebral joints. *See code XRGC0F3 or table 0SG to construct Fusion code.*

0RG70JJ Fusion of 2 to 7 Thoracic Vertebral Joints with Synthetic Substitute, Posterior Approach, Anterior Column, Open Approach

HAC When reported with secondary diagnosis code K68.11, T81.40XA, T81.41XA, T81.42XA, T81.43XA, T81.44XA or T81.49XA, T84.60XA, T84.610A, T84.611A, T84.612A, T84.613A, T84.614A, T84.615A, T84.619A, T84.63XA, T84.69XA, T84.7XXA

+ Fusion of nine or more joints when reported with Fusion of two or more lumbar vertebral joints. *See code XRGC0F3 or table 0SG to construct Fusion code.*

0RG70K0 Fusion of 2 to 7 Thoracic Vertebral Joints with Nonautologous Tissue Substitute, Anterior Approach, Anterior Column, Open Approach

HAC When reported with secondary diagnosis code K68.11, T81.40XA, T81.41XA, T81.42XA, T81.43XA, T81.44XA or T81.49XA, T84.60XA, T84.610A, T84.611A, T84.612A, T84.613A, T84.614A, T84.615A, T84.619A, T84.63XA, T84.69XA, T84.7XXA

+ Fusion of nine or more joints when reported with Fusion of two or more lumbar vertebral joints. *See code XRGC0F3 or table 0SG to construct Fusion code.*

0RG70K1 Fusion of 2 to 7 Thoracic Vertebral Joints with Nonautologous Tissue Substitute, Posterior Approach, Posterior Column, Open Approach

HAC When reported with secondary diagnosis code K68.11, T81.40XA, T81.41XA, T81.42XA, T81.43XA, T81.44XA or T81.49XA, T84.60XA, T84.610A, T84.611A, T84.612A, T84.613A, T84.614A, T84.615A, T84.619A, T84.63XA, T84.69XA, T84.7XXA

+ Fusion of nine or more joints when reported with Fusion of two or more lumbar vertebral joints. *See code XRGC0F3 or table 0SG to construct Fusion code.*

0RG70KJ Fusion of 2 to 7 Thoracic Vertebral Joints with Nonautologous Tissue Substitute, Posterior Approach, Anterior Column, Open Approach

HAC When reported with secondary diagnosis code K68.11, T81.40XA, T81.41XA, T81.42XA, T81.43XA, T81.44XA or T81.49XA, T84.60XA, T84.610A, T84.611A, T84.612A, T84.613A, T84.614A, T84.615A, T84.619A, T84.63XA, T84.69XA, T84.7XXA

+ Fusion of nine or more joints when reported with Fusion of two or more lumbar vertebral joints. *See code XRGC0F3 or table 0SG to construct Fusion code.*

0RG7370 Fusion of 2 to 7 Thoracic Vertebral Joints with Autologous Tissue Substitute, Anterior Approach, Anterior Column, Percutaneous Approach

HAC When reported with secondary diagnosis code K68.11, T81.40XA, T81.41XA, T81.42XA, T81.43XA, T81.44XA or T81.49XA, T84.60XA, T84.610A, T84.611A, T84.612A, T84.613A, T84.614A, T84.615A,

T84.619A, T84.63XA, T84.69XA, T84.7XXA

+ Fusion of nine or more joints when reported with Fusion of two or more lumbar vertebral joints. *See code XRGC0F3 or table 0SG to construct Fusion code.*

0RG7371 Fusion of 2 to 7 Thoracic Vertebral Joints with Autologous Tissue Substitute, Posterior Approach, Posterior Column, Percutaneous Approach

HAC When reported with secondary diagnosis code K68.11, T81.40XA, T81.41XA, T81.42XA, T81.43XA, T81.44XA or T81.49XA, T84.60XA, T84.610A, T84.611A, T84.612A, T84.613A, T84.614A, T84.615A, T84.619A, T84.63XA, T84.69XA, T84.7XXA

+ Fusion of nine or more joints when reported with Fusion of two or more lumbar vertebral joints. *See code XRGC0F3 or table 0SG to construct Fusion code.*

0RG737J Fusion of 2 to 7 Thoracic Vertebral Joints with Autologous Tissue Substitute, Posterior Approach, Anterior Column, Percutaneous Approach

HAC When reported with secondary diagnosis code K68.11, T81.40XA, T81.41XA, T81.42XA, T81.43XA, T81.44XA or T81.49XA, T84.60XA, T84.610A, T84.611A, T84.612A, T84.613A, T84.614A, T84.615A, T84.619A, T84.63XA, T84.69XA, T84.7XXA

+ Fusion of nine or more joints when reported with Fusion of two or more lumbar vertebral joints. *See code XRGC0F3 or table 0SG to construct Fusion code.*

0RG73A0 Fusion of 2 to 7 Thoracic Vertebral Joints with Interbody Fusion Device, Anterior Approach, Anterior Column, Percutaneous Approach

HAC When reported with secondary diagnosis code K68.11, T81.40XA, T81.41XA, T81.42XA, T81.43XA, T81.44XA or T81.49XA, T84.60XA, T84.610A, T84.611A, T84.612A, T84.613A, T84.614A, T84.615A, T84.619A, T84.63XA, T84.69XA, T84.7XXA

+ Fusion of nine or more joints when reported with Fusion of two or more lumbar vertebral joints. *See code XRGC0F3 or table 0SG to construct Fusion code.*

0RG73AJ Fusion of 2 to 7 Thoracic Vertebral Joints with Interbody Fusion Device, Posterior Approach, Anterior Column, Percutaneous Approach

HAC When reported with secondary diagnosis code K68.11, T81.40XA, T81.41XA, T81.42XA, T81.43XA, T81.44XA or T81.49XA, T84.60XA, T84.610A, T84.611A, T84.612A, T84.613A, T84.614A, T84.615A, T84.619A, T84.63XA, T84.69XA, T84.7XXA

+ Fusion of nine or more joints when reported with Fusion of two or more lumbar vertebral joints. *See code XRGC0F3 or table 0SG to construct Fusion code.*

0RG73J0 Fusion of 2 to 7 Thoracic Vertebral Joints with Synthetic Substitute, Anterior Approach, Anterior Column, Percutaneous Approach

HAC When reported with secondary diagnosis code K68.11, T81.40XA, T81.41XA, T81.42XA, T81.43XA, T81.44XA or T81.49XA, T84.60XA, T84.610A, T84.611A, T84.612A, T84.613A, T84.614A, T84.615A, T84.619A, T84.63XA, T84.69XA, T84.7XXA

+ Fusion of nine or more joints when reported with Fusion of two or more lumbar vertebral joints. *See code XRGC0F3 or table 0SG to construct Fusion code.*

0RG73J1 Fusion of 2 to 7 Thoracic Vertebral Joints with Synthetic Substitute, Posterior Approach, Posterior Column, Percutaneous Approach

HAC When reported with secondary diagnosis code K68.11, T81.40XA, T81.41XA, T81.42XA, T81.43XA, T81.44XA or T81.49XA, T84.60XA, T84.610A, T84.611A, T84.612A, T84.613A, T84.614A, T84.615A, T84.619A, T84.63XA, T84.69XA, T84.7XXA

+ Fusion of nine or more joints when reported with Fusion of two or more lumbar vertebral joints. *See code XRGC0F3 or table 0SG to construct Fusion code.*

0RG73JJ Fusion of 2 to 7 Thoracic Vertebral Joints with Synthetic Substitute, Posterior Approach, Anterior Column, Percutaneous Approach

HAC When reported with secondary diagnosis code K68.11, T81.40XA, T81.41XA, T81.42XA, T81.43XA, T81.44XA or T81.49XA, T84.60XA, T84.610A, T84.611A, T84.612A, T84.613A, T84.614A, T84.615A, T84.619A, T84.63XA, T84.69XA, T84.7XXA

+ Fusion of nine or more joints when reported with Fusion of two or more lumbar vertebral joints. *See code XRGC0F3 or table 0SG to construct Fusion code.*

0RG73K0 Fusion of 2 to 7 Thoracic Vertebral Joints with Nonautologous Tissue Substitute, Anterior Approach, Anterior Column, Percutaneous Approach

HAC When reported with secondary diagnosis code K68.11, T81.40XA, T81.41XA, T81.42XA, T81.43XA, T81.44XA or T81.49XA, T84.60XA, T84.610A, T84.611A, T84.612A, T84.613A, T84.614A, T84.615A, T84.619A, T84.63XA, T84.69XA, T84.7XXA

+ Fusion of nine or more joints when reported with Fusion of two or more lumbar vertebral joints. *See code XRGC0F3 or table 0SG to construct Fusion code.*

0RG73K1 Fusion of 2 to 7 Thoracic Vertebral Joints with Nonautologous Tissue Substitute, Posterior Approach, Posterior Column, Percutaneous Approach

HAC When reported with secondary diagnosis code K68.11, T81.40XA, T81.41XA, T81.42XA, T81.43XA,

T81.44XA or T81.49XA, T84.60XA,
T84.610A, T84.611A, T84.612A,
T84.613A, T84.614A, T84.615A,
T84.619A, T84.63XA, T84.69XA,
T84.7XXA

+ Fusion of nine or more joints when
reported with Fusion of two or more
lumbar vertebral joints. *See code
XRGC0F3 or table 0SG to construct
Fusion code.*

0RG73KJ Fusion of 2 to 7 Thoracic Vertebral
Joints
with Nonautologous Tissue Substitute,
Posterior Approach, Anterior Column,
Percutaneous Approach

HAC When reported with secondary
diagnosis code K68.11, T81.40XA,
T81.41XA, T81.42XA, T81.43XA,
T81.44XA or T81.49XA, T84.60XA,
T84.610A, T84.611A, T84.612A,
T84.613A, T84.614A, T84.615A,
T84.619A, T84.63XA, T84.69XA,
T84.7XXA

+ Fusion of nine or more joints when
reported with Fusion of two or more
lumbar vertebral joints. *See code
XRGC0F3 or table 0SG to construct
Fusion code.*

0RG7470 Fusion of 2 to 7 Thoracic Vertebral
Joints with Autologous Tissue
Substitute, Anterior Approach, Anterior
Column, Percutaneous Endoscopic
Approach

HAC When reported with secondary
diagnosis code K68.11, T81.40XA,
T81.41XA, T81.42XA, T81.43XA,
T81.44XA or T81.49XA, T84.60XA,
T84.610A, T84.611A, T84.612A,
T84.613A, T84.614A, T84.615A,
T84.619A, T84.63XA, T84.69XA,
T84.7XXA

+ Fusion of nine or more joints when
reported with Fusion of two or more
lumbar vertebral joints. *See code
XRGC0F3 or table 0SG to construct
Fusion code.*

0RG7471 Fusion of 2 to 7 Thoracic Vertebral
Joints with Autologous Tissue
Substitute, Posterior Approach,
Posterior Column, Percutaneous
Endoscopic Approach

HAC When reported with secondary
diagnosis code K68.11, T81.40XA,
T81.41XA, T81.42XA, T81.43XA,
T81.44XA or T81.49XA, T84.60XA,
T84.610A, T84.611A, T84.612A,
T84.613A, T84.614A, T84.615A,
T84.619A, T84.63XA, T84.69XA,
T84.7XXA

+ Fusion of nine or more joints when
reported with Fusion of two or more
lumbar vertebral joints. *See code
XRGC0F3 or table 0SG to construct
Fusion code.*

0RG747J Fusion of 2 to 7 Thoracic Vertebral
Joints with Autologous Tissue
Substitute, Posterior Approach,
Anterior Column, Percutaneous
Endoscopic Approach

HAC When reported with secondary
diagnosis code K68.11, T81.40XA,
T81.41XA, T81.42XA, T81.43XA,
T81.44XA or T81.49XA, T84.60XA,
T84.610A, T84.611A, T84.612A,
T84.613A, T84.614A, T84.615A,
T84.619A, T84.63XA, T84.69XA,
T84.7XXA

+ Fusion of nine or more joints when
reported with Fusion of two or more
lumbar vertebral joints. *See code
XRGC0F3 or table 0SG to construct
Fusion code.*

0RG74A0 Fusion of 2 to 7 Thoracic Vertebral
Joints with Interbody Fusion Device,
Anterior Approach, Anterior Column,
Percutaneous Endoscopic Approach

HAC When reported with secondary
diagnosis code K68.11, T81.40XA,
T81.41XA, T81.42XA, T81.43XA,
T81.44XA or T81.49XA, T84.60XA,
T84.610A, T84.611A, T84.612A,
T84.613A, T84.614A, T84.615A,
T84.619A, T84.63XA, T84.69XA,
T84.7XXA

+ Fusion of nine or more joints when
reported with Fusion of two or more
lumbar vertebral joints. *See code
XRGC0F3 or table 0SG to construct
Fusion code.*

0RG74AJ Fusion of 2 to 7 Thoracic Vertebral
Joints with Interbody Fusion Device,
Posterior Approach, Anterior Column,
Percutaneous Endoscopic Approach

HAC When reported with secondary
diagnosis code K68.11, T81.40XA,
T81.41XA, T81.42XA, T81.43XA,
T81.44XA or T81.49XA, T84.60XA,
T84.610A, T84.611A, T84.612A,
T84.613A, T84.614A, T84.615A,
T84.619A, T84.63XA, T84.69XA,
T84.7XXA

+ Fusion of nine or more joints when
reported with Fusion of two or more
lumbar vertebral joints. *See code
XRGC0F3 or table 0SG to construct
Fusion code.*

0RG74J0 Fusion of 2 to 7 Thoracic Vertebral
Joints with Synthetic Substitute,
Anterior Approach, Anterior Column,
Percutaneous Endoscopic Approach

HAC When reported with secondary
diagnosis code K68.11, T81.40XA,
T81.41XA, T81.42XA, T81.43XA,
T81.44XA or T81.49XA, T84.60XA,
T84.610A, T84.611A, T84.612A,
T84.613A, T84.614A, T84.615A,
T84.619A, T84.63XA, T84.69XA,
T84.7XXA

+ Fusion of nine or more joints when
reported with Fusion of two or more
lumbar vertebral joints. *See code
XRGC0F3 or table 0SG to construct
Fusion code.*

0RG74J1 Fusion of 2 to 7 Thoracic Vertebral
Joints with Synthetic Substitute,
Posterior Approach, Posterior Column,
Percutaneous Endoscopic Approach

HAC When reported with secondary
diagnosis code K68.11, T81.40XA,
T81.41XA, T81.42XA, T81.43XA,
T81.44XA or T81.49XA, T84.60XA,
T84.610A, T84.611A, T84.612A,
T84.613A, T84.614A, T84.615A,
T84.619A, T84.63XA, T84.69XA,
T84.7XXA

+ Fusion of nine or more joints when
reported with Fusion of two or more
lumbar vertebral joints. *See code
XRGC0F3 or table 0SG to construct
Fusion code.*

0RG74JJ Fusion of 2 to 7 Thoracic Vertebral
Joints with Synthetic Substitute,
Posterior Approach, Anterior Column,
Percutaneous Endoscopic Approach

HAC When reported with secondary
diagnosis code K68.11, T81.40XA,
T81.41XA, T81.42XA, T81.43XA,
T81.44XA or T81.49XA, T84.60XA,
T84.610A, T84.611A, T84.612A,
T84.613A, T84.614A, T84.615A,
T84.619A, T84.63XA, T84.69XA,
T84.7XXA

+ Fusion of nine or more joints when
reported with Fusion of two or more
lumbar vertebral joints. *See code
XRGC0F3 or table 0SG to construct
Fusion code.*

0RG74K0 Fusion of 2 to 7 Thoracic Vertebral
Joints with Nonautologous Tissue
Substitute, Anterior Approach, Anterior
Column, Percutaneous Endoscopic
Approach

HAC When reported with secondary
diagnosis code K68.11, T81.40XA,
T81.41XA, T81.42XA, T81.43XA,
T81.44XA or T81.49XA, T84.60XA,
T84.610A, T84.611A, T84.612A,
T84.613A, T84.614A, T84.615A,
T84.619A, T84.63XA, T84.69XA,
T84.7XXA

+ Fusion of nine or more joints when
reported with Fusion of two or more
lumbar vertebral joints. *See code
XRGC0F3 or table 0SG to construct
Fusion code.*

0RG74K1 Fusion of 2 to 7 Thoracic Vertebral
Joints
with Nonautologous Tissue Substitute,
Posterior Approach, Posterior Column,
Percutaneous Endoscopic Approach

HAC When reported with secondary
diagnosis code K68.11, T81.40XA,
T81.41XA, T81.42XA, T81.43XA,
T81.44XA or T81.49XA, T84.60XA,
T84.610A, T84.611A, T84.612A,
T84.613A, T84.614A, T84.615A,
T84.619A, T84.63XA, T84.69XA,
T84.7XXA

+ Fusion of nine or more joints when
reported with Fusion of two or more
lumbar vertebral joints. *See code
XRGC0F3 or table 0SG to construct
Fusion code.*

0RG74KJ Fusion of 2 to 7 Thoracic Vertebral
Joints
with Nonautologous Tissue Substitute,
Posterior Approach, Anterior Column,
Percutaneous Endoscopic Approach

HAC When reported with secondary
diagnosis code K68.11, T81.40XA,
T81.41XA, T81.42XA, T81.43XA,
T81.44XA or T81.49XA, T84.60XA,
T84.610A, T84.611A, T84.612A,
T84.613A, T84.614A, T84.615A,
T84.619A, T84.63XA, T84.69XA,
T84.7XXA

+ Fusion of nine or more joints when
reported with Fusion of two or more
lumbar vertebral joints. *See code
XRGC0F3 or table 0SG to construct
Fusion code.*

0RG8070 Fusion of 8 or more Thoracic Vertebral
Joints with Autologous Tissue
Substitute, Anterior Approach, Anterior
Column, Open Approach

HAC When reported with secondary
diagnosis code K68.11, T81.40XA,
T81.41XA, T81.42XA, T81.43XA,
T81.44XA or T81.49XA, T84.60XA,
T84.610A, T84.611A, T84.612A,
T84.613A, T84.614A, T84.615A,

1070   ♀ Female-only   ♂ Male-only   ▲ Limited Coverage   ● Non-OR   HAC HAC-associated procedure   ▲ Non-covered procedures   + Cluster

T84.619A, T84.63XA, T84.69XA,
T84.7XXA

0RG8071 Fusion of 8 or more Thoracic
Vertebral Joints with Autologous
Tissue Substitute, Posterior Approach,
Posterior Column, Open Approach
- *HAC* When reported with secondary
diagnosis code K68.11, T81.40XA,
T81.41XA, T81.42XA, T81.43XA,
T81.44XA or T81.49XA, T84.60XA,
T84.610A, T84.611A, T84.612A,
T84.613A, T84.614A, T84.615A,
T84.619A, T84.63XA, T84.69XA,
T84.7XXA

0RG807J Fusion of 8 or more Thoracic Vertebral
Joints with Autologous
Tissue Substitute, Posterior
Approach, Anterior Column, Open
Approach
- *HAC* When reported with secondary
diagnosis code K68.11, T81.40XA,
T81.41XA, T81.42XA, T81.43XA,
T81.44XA or T81.49XA, T84.60XA,
T84.610A, T84.611A, T84.612A,
T84.613A, T84.614A, T84.615A,
T84.619A, T84.63XA, T84.69XA,
T84.7XXA

0RG80A0 Fusion of 8 or more Thoracic
Vertebral Joints with Interbody
Fusion Device, Anterior
Approach, Anterior Column, Open
Approach
- *HAC* When reported with secondary
diagnosis code K68.11, T81.40XA,
T81.41XA, T81.42XA, T81.43XA,
T81.44XA or T81.49XA, T84.60XA,
T84.610A, T84.611A, T84.612A,
T84.613A, T84.614A, T84.615A,
T84.619A, T84.63XA, T84.69XA,
T84.7XXA

0RG80AJ Fusion of 8 or more Thoracic
Vertebral Joints with Interbody
Fusion Device, Posterior
Approach, Anterior Column, Open
Approach
- *HAC* When reported with secondary
diagnosis code K68.11, T81.40XA,
T81.41XA, T81.42XA, T81.43XA,
T81.44XA or T81.49XA, T84.60XA,
T84.610A, T84.611A, T84.612A,
T84.613A, T84.614A, T84.615A,
T84.619A, T84.63XA, T84.69XA,
T84.7XXA

0RG80J0 Fusion of 8 or more Thoracic Vertebral
Joints with Synthetic Substitute,
Anterior Approach, Anterior Column,
Open Approach
- *HAC* When reported with secondary
diagnosis code K68.11, T81.40XA,
T81.41XA, T81.42XA, T81.43XA,
T81.44XA or T81.49XA, T84.60XA,
T84.610A, T84.611A, T84.612A,
T84.613A, T84.614A, T84.615A,
T84.619A, T84.63XA, T84.69XA,
T84.7XXA

0RG80J1 Fusion of 8 or more Thoracic Vertebral
Joints with Synthetic Substitute,
Posterior Approach, Posterior Column,
Open Approach
- *HAC* When reported with secondary
diagnosis code K68.11, T81.40XA,
T81.41XA, T81.42XA, T81.43XA,
T81.44XA or T81.49XA, T84.60XA,
T84.610A, T84.611A, T84.612A,
T84.613A, T84.614A, T84.615A,
T84.619A, T84.63XA, T84.69XA,
T84.7XXA

0RG80JJ Fusion of 8 or more Thoracic Vertebral
Joints with Synthetic Substitute,
Posterior Approach, Anterior Column,
Open Approach
- *HAC* When reported with secondary
diagnosis code K68.11, T81.40XA,
T81.41XA, T81.42XA, T81.43XA,
T81.44XA or T81.49XA, T84.60XA,
T84.610A, T84.611A, T84.612A,
T84.613A, T84.614A, T84.615A,
T84.619A, T84.63XA, T84.69XA,
T84.7XXA

0RG80K0 Fusion of 8 or more Thoracic Vertebral
Joints with Nonautologous Tissue
Substitute, Anterior Approach, Anterior
Column, Open Approach
- *HAC* When reported with secondary
diagnosis code K68.11, T81.40XA,
T81.41XA, T81.42XA, T81.43XA,
T81.44XA or T81.49XA, T84.60XA,
T84.610A, T84.611A, T84.612A,
T84.613A, T84.614A, T84.615A,
T84.619A, T84.63XA, T84.69XA,
T84.7XXA

0RG80K1 Fusion of 8 or more Thoracic Vertebral
Joints with Nonautologous Tissue
Substitute, Posterior Approach,
Posterior Column, Open Approach
- *HAC* When reported with secondary
diagnosis code K68.11, T81.40XA,
T81.41XA, T81.42XA, T81.43XA,
T81.44XA or T81.49XA, T84.60XA,
T84.610A, T84.611A, T84.612A,
T84.613A, T84.614A, T84.615A,
T84.619A, T84.63XA, T84.69XA,
T84.7XXA

0RG80KJ Fusion of 8 or more Thoracic Vertebral
Joints with Nonautologous Tissue
Substitute, Posterior Approach,
Anterior Column, Open Approach
- *HAC* When reported with secondary
diagnosis code K68.11, T81.40XA,
T81.41XA, T81.42XA, T81.43XA,
T81.44XA or T81.49XA, T84.60XA,
T84.610A, T84.611A, T84.612A,
T84.613A, T84.614A, T84.615A,
T84.619A, T84.63XA, T84.69XA,
T84.7XXA

0RG8370 Fusion of 8 or more Thoracic
Vertebral Joints with Autologous
Tissue Substitute, Anterior Approach,
Anterior Column, Percutaneous
Approach
- *HAC* When reported with secondary
diagnosis code K68.11, T81.40XA,
T81.41XA, T81.42XA, T81.43XA,
T81.44XA or T81.49XA, T84.60XA,
T84.610A, T84.611A, T84.612A,
T84.613A, T84.614A, T84.615A,
T84.619A, T84.63XA, T84.69XA,
T84.7XXA

0RG8371 Fusion of 8 or more Thoracic
Vertebral Joints with Autologous
Tissue Substitute, Posterior Approach,
Posterior Column, Percutaneous
Approach
- *HAC* When reported with secondary
diagnosis code K68.11, T81.40XA,
T81.41XA, T81.42XA, T81.43XA,
T81.44XA or T81.49XA, T84.60XA,
T84.610A, T84.611A, T84.612A,
T84.613A, T84.614A, T84.615A,
T84.619A, T84.63XA, T84.69XA,
T84.7XXA

0RG837J Fusion of 8 or more Thoracic
Vertebral Joints with Autologous
Tissue Substitute, Posterior Approach,

Anterior Column, Percutaneous
Approach
- *HAC* When reported with secondary
diagnosis code K68.11, T81.40XA,
T81.41XA, T81.42XA, T81.43XA,
T81.44XA or T81.49XA, T84.60XA,
T84.610A, T84.611A, T84.612A,
T84.613A, T84.614A, T84.615A,
T84.619A, T84.63XA, T84.69XA,
T84.7XXA

0RG83A0 Fusion of 8 or more Thoracic Vertebral
Joints with Interbody Fusion Device,
Anterior Approach, Anterior Column,
Percutaneous Approach
- *HAC* When reported with secondary
diagnosis code K68.11, T81.40XA,
T81.41XA, T81.42XA, T81.43XA,
T81.44XA or T81.49XA, T84.60XA,
T84.610A, T84.611A, T84.612A,
T84.613A, T84.614A, T84.615A,
T84.619A, T84.63XA, T84.69XA,
T84.7XXA

0RG83AJ Fusion of 8 or more Thoracic Vertebral
Joints with Interbody Fusion Device,
Posterior Approach, Anterior Column,
Percutaneous Approach
- *HAC* When reported with secondary
diagnosis code K68.11, T81.40XA,
T81.41XA, T81.42XA, T81.43XA,
T81.44XA or T81.49XA, T84.60XA,
T84.610A, T84.611A, T84.612A,
T84.613A, T84.614A, T84.615A,
T84.619A, T84.63XA, T84.69XA,
T84.7XXA

0RG83J0 Fusion of 8 or more Thoracic Vertebral
Joints with Synthetic Substitute,
Anterior Approach, Anterior Column,
Percutaneous Approach
- *HAC* When reported with secondary
diagnosis code K68.11, T81.40XA,
T81.41XA, T81.42XA, T81.43XA,
T81.44XA or T81.49XA, T84.60XA,
T84.610A, T84.611A, T84.612A,
T84.613A, T84.614A, T84.615A,
T84.619A, T84.63XA, T84.69XA,
T84.7XXA

0RG83J1 Fusion of 8 or more Thoracic
Vertebral Joints with Synthetic
Substitute, Posterior Approach,
Posterior Column, Percutaneous
Approach
- *HAC* When reported with secondary
diagnosis code K68.11, T81.40XA,
T81.41XA, T81.42XA, T81.43XA,
T81.44XA or T81.49XA, T84.60XA,
T84.610A, T84.611A, T84.612A,
T84.613A, T84.614A, T84.615A,
T84.619A, T84.63XA, T84.69XA,
T84.7XXA

0RG83JJ Fusion of 8 or more Thoracic
Vertebral Joints with Synthetic
Substitute, Posterior Approach,
Anterior Column, Percutaneous
Approach
- *HAC* When reported with secondary
diagnosis code K68.11, T81.40XA,
T81.41XA, T81.42XA, T81.43XA,
T81.44XA or T81.49XA, T84.60XA,
T84.610A, T84.611A, T84.612A,
T84.613A, T84.614A, T84.615A,
T84.619A, T84.63XA, T84.69XA,
T84.7XXA

0RG83K0 Fusion of 8 or more Thoracic
Vertebral Joints with Nonautologous
Tissue Substitute, Anterior Approach,
Anterior Column, Percutaneous
Approach

When reported with secondary diagnosis code K68.11, T81.40XA, T81.41XA, T81.42XA, T81.43XA, T81.44XA or T81.49XA, T84.60XA, T84.610A, T84.611A, T84.612A, T84.613A, T84.614A, T84.615A, T84.619A, T84.63XA, T84.69XA, T84.7XXA

0RG83K1 Fusion of 8 or more Thoracic Vertebral Joints with Nonautologous Tissue Substitute, Posterior Approach, Posterior Column, Percutaneous Approach

When reported with secondary diagnosis code K68.11, T81.40XA, T81.41XA, T81.42XA, T81.43XA, T81.44XA or T81.49XA, T84.60XA, T84.610A, T84.611A, T84.612A, T84.613A, T84.614A, T84.615A, T84.619A, T84.63XA, T84.69XA, T84.7XXA

0RG83KJ Fusion of 8 or more Thoracic Vertebral Joints with Nonautologous Tissue Substitute, Posterior Approach, Anterior Column, Percutaneous Approach

When reported with secondary diagnosis code K68.11, T81.40XA, T81.41XA, T81.42XA, T81.43XA, T81.44XA or T81.49XA, T84.60XA, T84.610A, T84.611A, T84.612A, T84.613A, T84.614A, T84.615A, T84.619A, T84.63XA, T84.69XA, T84.7XXA

0RG8470 Fusion of 8 or more Thoracic Vertebral Joints with Autologous Tissue Substitute, Anterior Approach, Anterior Column, Percutaneous Endoscopic Approach

When reported with secondary diagnosis code K68.11, T81.40XA, T81.41XA, T81.42XA, T81.43XA, T81.44XA or T81.49XA, T84.60XA, T84.610A, T84.611A, T84.612A, T84.613A, T84.614A, T84.615A, T84.619A, T84.63XA, T84.69XA, T84.7XXA

0RG8471 Fusion of 8 or more Thoracic Vertebral Joints with Autologous Tissue Substitute, Posterior Approach, Posterior Column, Percutaneous Endoscopic Approach

When reported with secondary diagnosis code K68.11, T81.40XA, T81.41XA, T81.42XA, T81.43XA, T81.44XA or T81.49XA, T84.60XA, T84.610A, T84.611A, T84.612A, T84.613A, T84.614A, T84.615A, T84.619A, T84.63XA, T84.69XA, T84.7XXA

0RG847J Fusion of 8 or more Thoracic Vertebral Joints with Autologous Tissue Substitute, Posterior Approach, Anterior Column, Percutaneous Endoscopic Approach

When reported with secondary diagnosis code K68.11, T81.40XA, T81.41XA, T81.42XA, T81.43XA, T81.44XA or T81.49XA, T84.60XA, T84.610A, T84.611A, T84.612A, T84.613A, T84.614A, T84.615A, T84.619A, T84.63XA, T84.69XA, T84.7XXA

0RG84A0 Fusion of 8 or more Thoracic Vertebral Joints with Interbody Fusion Device,

Anterior Approach, Anterior Column, Percutaneous Endoscopic Approach

When reported with secondary diagnosis code K68.11, T81.40XA, T81.41XA, T81.42XA, T81.43XA, T81.44XA or T81.49XA, T84.60XA, T84.610A, T84.611A, T84.612A, T84.613A, T84.614A, T84.615A, T84.619A, T84.63XA, T84.69XA, T84.7XXA

0RG84AJ Fusion of 8 or more Thoracic Vertebral Joints with Interbody Fusion Device, Posterior Approach, Anterior Column, Percutaneous Endoscopic Approach

When reported with secondary diagnosis code K68.11, T81.40XA, T81.41XA, T81.42XA, T81.43XA, T81.44XA or T81.49XA, T84.60XA, T84.610A, T84.611A, T84.612A, T84.613A, T84.614A, T84.615A, T84.619A, T84.63XA, T84.69XA, T84.7XXA

0RG84J0 Fusion of 8 or more Thoracic Vertebral Joints with Synthetic Substitute, Anterior Approach, Anterior Column, Percutaneous Endoscopic Approach

When reported with secondary diagnosis code K68.11, T81.40XA, T81.41XA, T81.42XA, T81.43XA, T81.44XA or T81.49XA, T84.60XA, T84.610A, T84.611A, T84.612A, T84.613A, T84.614A, T84.615A, T84.619A, T84.63XA, T84.69XA, T84.7XXA

0RG84J1 Fusion of 8 or more Thoracic Vertebral Joints with Synthetic Substitute, Posterior Approach, Posterior Column, Percutaneous Endoscopic Approach

When reported with secondary diagnosis code K68.11, T81.40XA, T81.41XA, T81.42XA, T81.43XA, T81.44XA or T81.49XA, T84.60XA, T84.610A, T84.611A, T84.612A, T84.613A, T84.614A, T84.615A, T84.619A, T84.63XA, T84.69XA, T84.7XXA

0RG84JJ Fusion of 8 or more Thoracic Vertebral Joints with Synthetic Substitute, Posterior Approach, Anterior Column, Percutaneous Endoscopic Approach

When reported with secondary diagnosis code K68.11, T81.40XA, T81.41XA, T81.42XA, T81.43XA, T81.44XA or T81.49XA, T84.60XA, T84.610A, T84.611A, T84.612A, T84.613A, T84.614A, T84.615A, T84.619A, T84.63XA, T84.69XA, T84.7XXA

0RG84K0 Fusion of 8 or more Thoracic Vertebral Joints with Nonautologous Tissue Substitute, Anterior Approach, Anterior Column, Percutaneous Endoscopic Approach

When reported with secondary diagnosis code K68.11, T81.40XA, T81.41XA, T81.42XA, T81.43XA, T81.44XA or T81.49XA, T84.60XA, T84.610A, T84.611A, T84.612A, T84.613A, T84.614A, T84.615A, T84.619A, T84.63XA, T84.69XA, T84.7XXA

0RG84K1 Fusion of 8 or more Thoracic Vertebral Joints with Nonautologous Tissue Substitute, Posterior Approach, Posterior Column, Percutaneous Endoscopic Approach

When reported with secondary diagnosis code K68.11, T81.40XA, T81.41XA, T81.42XA, T81.43XA, T81.44XA or T81.49XA, T84.60XA, T84.610A, T84.611A, T84.612A, T84.613A, T84.614A, T84.615A, T84.619A, T84.63XA, T84.69XA, T84.7XXA

0RG84KJ Fusion of 8 or more Thoracic Vertebral Joints with Nonautologous Tissue Substitute, Posterior Approach, Anterior Column, Percutaneous Endoscopic Approach

When reported with secondary diagnosis code K68.11, T81.40XA, T81.41XA, T81.42XA, T81.43XA, T81.44XA or T81.49XA, T84.60XA, T84.610A, T84.611A, T84.612A, T84.613A, T84.614A, T84.615A, T84.619A, T84.63XA, T84.69XA, T84.7XXA

0RGA070 Fusion of Thoracolumbar Vertebral Joint with Autologous Tissue Substitute, Anterior Approach, Anterior Column, Open Approach

When reported with secondary diagnosis code K68.11, T81.40XA, T81.41XA, T81.42XA, T81.43XA, T81.44XA or T81.49XA, T84.60XA, T84.610A, T84.611A, T84.612A, T84.613A, T84.614A, T84.615A, T84.619A, T84.63XA, T84.69XA, T84.7XXA

0RGA071 Fusion of Thoracolumbar Vertebral Joint with Autologous Tissue Substitute, Posterior Approach, Posterior Column, Open Approach

AHA CC: 1Q, 2013, 21-23

When reported with secondary diagnosis code K68.11, T81.40XA, T81.41XA, T81.42XA, T81.43XA, T81.44XA or T81.49XA, T84.60XA, T84.610A, T84.611A, T84.612A, T84.613A, T84.614A, T84.615A, T84.619A, T84.63XA, T84.69XA, T84.7XXA

0RGA07J Fusion of Thoracolumbar Vertebral Joint with Autologous Tissue Substitute, Posterior Approach, Anterior Column, Open Approach

When reported with secondary diagnosis code K68.11, T81.40XA, T81.41XA, T81.42XA, T81.43XA, T81.44XA or T81.49XA, T84.60XA, T84.610A, T84.611A, T84.612A, T84.613A, T84.614A, T84.615A, T84.619A, T84.63XA, T84.69XA, T84.7XXA

0RGA0A0 Fusion of Thoracolumbar Vertebral Joint with Interbody Fusion Device, Anterior Approach, Anterior Column, Open Approach

When reported with secondary diagnosis code K68.11, T81.40XA, T81.41XA, T81.42XA, T81.43XA, T81.44XA or T81.49XA, T84.60XA, T84.610A, T84.611A, T84.612A, T84.613A, T84.614A, T84.615A, T84.619A, T84.63XA, T84.69XA, T84.7XXA

0RGA0AJ Fusion of Thoracolumbar Vertebral Joint with Interbody Fusion Device, Posterior Approach, Anterior Column, Open Approach

When reported with secondary diagnosis code K68.11, T81.40XA, T81.41XA, T81.42XA, T81.43XA,

♀ Female-only   ♂ Male-only   ▲ Limited Coverage   ● Non-OR   ᴴᴬᶜ HAC-associated procedure   ▲ Non-covered procedures   ✚ Cluster

T81.44XA or T81.49XA, T84.60XA,
T84.610A, T84.611A, T84.612A,
T84.613A, T84.614A, T84.615A,
T84.619A, T84.63XA, T84.69XA,
T84.7XXA

0RGA0J0 Fusion of Thoracolumbar Vertebral
Joint with Synthetic Substitute,
Anterior Approach, Anterior Column,
Open Approach

HAC   When reported with secondary
diagnosis code K68.11, T81.40XA,
T81.41XA, T81.42XA, T81.43XA,
T81.44XA or T81.49XA, T84.60XA,
T84.610A, T84.611A, T84.612A,
T84.613A, T84.614A, T84.615A,
T84.619A, T84.63XA, T84.69XA,
T84.7XXA

0RGA0J1 Fusion of Thoracolumbar Vertebral
Joint with Synthetic Substitute,
Posterior Approach, Posterior Column,
Open Approach

HAC   When reported with secondary
diagnosis code K68.11, T81.40XA,
T81.41XA, T81.42XA, T81.43XA,
T81.44XA or T81.49XA, T84.60XA,
T84.610A, T84.611A, T84.612A,
T84.613A, T84.614A, T84.615A,
T84.619A, T84.63XA, T84.69XA,
T84.7XXA

0RGA0JJ Fusion of Thoracolumbar Vertebral
Joint with Synthetic Substitute,
Posterior Approach, Anterior Column,
Open Approach

HAC   When reported with secondary
diagnosis code K68.11, T81.40XA,
T81.41XA, T81.42XA, T81.43XA,
T81.44XA or T81.49XA, T84.60XA,
T84.610A, T84.611A, T84.612A,
T84.613A, T84.614A, T84.615A,
T84.619A, T84.63XA, T84.69XA,
T84.7XXA

0RGA0K0 Fusion of Thoracolumbar Vertebral
Joint with Nonautologous Tissue
Substitute, Anterior Approach, Anterior
Column, Open Approach

HAC   When reported with secondary
diagnosis code K68.11, T81.40XA,
T81.41XA, T81.42XA, T81.43XA,
T81.44XA or T81.49XA, T84.60XA,
T84.610A, T84.611A, T84.612A,
T84.613A, T84.614A, T84.615A,
T84.619A, T84.63XA, T84.69XA,
T84.7XXA

0RGA0K1 Fusion of Thoracolumbar Vertebral
Joint with Nonautologous Tissue
Substitute, Posterior Approach,
Posterior Column, Open Approach

HAC   When reported with secondary
diagnosis code K68.11, T81.40XA,
T81.41XA, T81.42XA, T81.43XA,
T81.44XA or T81.49XA, T84.60XA,
T84.610A, T84.611A, T84.612A,
T84.613A, T84.614A, T84.615A,
T84.619A, T84.63XA, T84.69XA,
T84.7XXA

0RGA0KJ Fusion of Thoracolumbar Vertebral
Joint with Nonautologous Tissue
Substitute, Posterior Approach,
Anterior Column, Open Approach

HAC   When reported with secondary
diagnosis code K68.11, T81.40XA,
T81.41XA, T81.42XA, T81.43XA,
T81.44XA or T81.49XA, T84.60XA,
T84.610A, T84.611A, T84.612A,
T84.613A, T84.614A, T84.615A,
T84.619A, T84.63XA, T84.69XA,
T84.7XXA

0RGA370 Fusion of Thoracolumbar Vertebral
Joint with Autologous Tissue
Substitute, Anterior Approach, Anterior
Column, Percutaneous Approach

HAC   When reported with secondary
diagnosis code K68.11, T81.40XA,
T81.41XA, T81.42XA, T81.43XA,
T81.44XA or T81.49XA, T84.60XA,
T84.610A, T84.611A, T84.612A,
T84.613A, T84.614A, T84.615A,
T84.619A, T84.63XA, T84.69XA,
T84.7XXA

0RGA371 Fusion of Thoracolumbar
Vertebral Joint with Autologous
Tissue Substitute, Posterior
Approach, Posterior Column,
Percutaneous Approach

HAC   When reported with secondary
diagnosis code K68.11, T81.40XA,
T81.41XA, T81.42XA, T81.43XA,
T81.44XA or T81.49XA, T84.60XA,
T84.610A, T84.611A, T84.612A,
T84.613A, T84.614A, T84.615A,
T84.619A, T84.63XA, T84.69XA,
T84.7XXA

0RGA37J Fusion of Thoracolumbar Vertebral
Joint with Autologous Tissue
Substitute, Posterior Approach,
Anterior Column, Percutaneous
Approach

HAC   When reported with secondary
diagnosis code K68.11, T81.40XA,
T81.41XA, T81.42XA, T81.43XA,
T81.44XA or T81.49XA, T84.60XA,
T84.610A, T84.611A, T84.612A,
T84.613A, T84.614A, T84.615A,
T84.619A, T84.63XA, T84.69XA,
T84.7XXA

0RGA3A0 Fusion of Thoracolumbar Vertebral
Joint with Interbody Fusion Device,
Anterior Approach, Anterior Column,
Percutaneous Approach

HAC   When reported with secondary
diagnosis code K68.11, T81.40XA,
T81.41XA, T81.42XA, T81.43XA,
T81.44XA or T81.49XA, T84.60XA,
T84.610A, T84.611A, T84.612A,
T84.613A, T84.614A, T84.615A,
T84.619A, T84.63XA, T84.69XA,
T84.7XXA

0RGA3AJ Fusion of Thoracolumbar Vertebral
Joint with Interbody Fusion Device,
Posterior Approach, Anterior Column,
Percutaneous Approach

HAC   When reported with secondary
diagnosis code K68.11, T81.40XA,
T81.41XA, T81.42XA, T81.43XA,
T81.44XA or T81.49XA, T84.60XA,
T84.610A, T84.611A, T84.612A,
T84.613A, T84.614A, T84.615A,
T84.619A, T84.63XA, T84.69XA,
T84.7XXA

0RGA3J0 Fusion of Thoracolumbar Vertebral
Joint with Synthetic Substitute,
Anterior Approach, Anterior Column,
Percutaneous Approach

HAC   When reported with secondary
diagnosis code K68.11, T81.40XA,
T81.41XA, T81.42XA, T81.43XA,
T81.44XA or T81.49XA, T84.60XA,
T84.610A, T84.611A, T84.612A,
T84.613A, T84.614A, T84.615A,
T84.619A, T84.63XA, T84.69XA,
T84.7XXA

0RGA3J1 Fusion of Thoracolumbar
Vertebral Joint with Synthetic
Substitute, Posterior Approach,

Posterior Column, Percutaneous
Approach

HAC   When reported with secondary
diagnosis code K68.11, T81.40XA,
T81.41XA, T81.42XA, T81.43XA,
T81.44XA or T81.49XA, T84.60XA,
T84.610A, T84.611A, T84.612A,
T84.613A, T84.614A, T84.615A,
T84.619A, T84.63XA, T84.69XA,
T84.7XXA

0RGA3JJ Fusion of Thoracolumbar Vertebral
Joint with Synthetic Substitute,
Posterior Approach, Anterior Column,
Percutaneous Approach

HAC   When reported with secondary
diagnosis code K68.11, T81.40XA,
T81.41XA, T81.42XA, T81.43XA,
T81.44XA or T81.49XA, T84.60XA,
T84.610A, T84.611A, T84.612A,
T84.613A, T84.614A, T84.615A,
T84.619A, T84.63XA, T84.69XA,
T84.7XXA

0RGA3K0 Fusion of Thoracolumbar Vertebral
Joint with Nonautologous Tissue
Substitute, Anterior Approach,
Anterior Column, Percutaneous
Approach

HAC   When reported with secondary
diagnosis code K68.11, T81.40XA,
T81.41XA, T81.42XA, T81.43XA,
T81.44XA or T81.49XA, T84.60XA,
T84.610A, T84.611A, T84.612A,
T84.613A, T84.614A, T84.615A,
T84.619A, T84.63XA, T84.69XA,
T84.7XXA

0RGA3K1 Fusion of Thoracolumbar Vertebral
Joint with Nonautologous Tissue
Substitute, Posterior Approach,
Posterior Column, Percutaneous
Approach

HAC   When reported with secondary
diagnosis code K68.11, T81.40XA,
T81.41XA, T81.42XA, T81.43XA,
T81.44XA or T81.49XA, T84.60XA,
T84.610A, T84.611A, T84.612A,
T84.613A, T84.614A, T84.615A,
T84.619A, T84.63XA, T84.69XA,
T84.7XXA

0RGA3KJ Fusion of Thoracolumbar Vertebral
Joint with Nonautologous Tissue
Substitute, Posterior Approach, Anterior
Column, Percutaneous Approach

HAC   When reported with secondary
diagnosis code K68.11, T81.40XA,
T81.41XA, T81.42XA, T81.43XA,
T81.44XA or T81.49XA, T84.60XA,
T84.610A, T84.611A, T84.612A,
T84.613A, T84.614A, T84.615A,
T84.619A, T84.63XA, T84.69XA,
T84.7XXA

0RGA470 Fusion of Thoracolumbar Vertebral
Joint with Autologous Tissue Substitute,
Anterior Approach, Anterior Column,
Percutaneous Endoscopic Approach

HAC   When reported with secondary
diagnosis code K68.11, T81.40XA,
T81.41XA, T81.42XA, T81.43XA,
T81.44XA or T81.49XA, T84.60XA,
T84.610A, T84.611A, T84.612A,
T84.613A, T84.614A, T84.615A,
T84.619A, T84.63XA, T84.69XA,
T84.7XXA

0RGA471 Fusion of Thoracolumbar Vertebral
Joint with Autologous Tissue
Substitute, Posterior Approach,
Posterior Column, Percutaneous
Endoscopic Approach

When reported with secondary diagnosis code K68.11, T81.40XA, T81.41XA, T81.42XA, T81.43XA, T81.44XA or T81.49XA, T84.60XA, T84.610A, T84.611A, T84.612A, T84.613A, T84.614A, T84.615A, T84.619A, T84.63XA, T84.69XA, T84.7XXA

0RGA47J Fusion of Thoracolumbar Vertebral Joint with Autologous Tissue Substitute, Posterior Approach, Anterior Column, Percutaneous Endoscopic Approach

HAC When reported with secondary diagnosis code K68.11, T81.40XA, T81.41XA, T81.42XA, T81.43XA, T81.44XA or T81.49XA, T84.60XA, T84.610A, T84.611A, T84.612A, T84.613A, T84.614A, T84.615A, T84.619A, T84.63XA, T84.69XA, T84.7XXA

0RGA4A0 Fusion of Thoracolumbar Vertebral Joint with Interbody Fusion Device, Anterior Approach, Anterior Column, Percutaneous Endoscopic Approach

HAC When reported with secondary diagnosis code K68.11, T81.40XA, T81.41XA, T81.42XA, T81.43XA, T81.44XA or T81.49XA, T84.60XA, T84.610A, T84.611A, T84.612A, T84.613A, T84.614A, T84.615A, T84.619A, T84.63XA, T84.69XA, T84.7XXA

0RGA4AJ Fusion of Thoracolumbar Vertebral Joint with Interbody Fusion Device, Posterior Approach, Anterior Column, Percutaneous Endoscopic Approach

HAC When reported with secondary diagnosis code K68.11, T81.40XA, T81.41XA, T81.42XA, T81.43XA, T81.44XA or T81.49XA, T84.60XA, T84.610A, T84.611A, T84.612A, T84.613A, T84.614A, T84.615A, T84.619A, T84.63XA, T84.69XA, T84.7XXA

0RGA4J0 Fusion of Thoracolumbar Vertebral Joint with Synthetic Substitute, Anterior Approach, Anterior Column, Percutaneous Endoscopic Approach

HAC When reported with secondary diagnosis code K68.11, T81.40XA, T81.41XA, T81.42XA, T81.43XA, T81.44XA or T81.49XA, T84.60XA, T84.610A, T84.611A, T84.612A, T84.613A, T84.614A, T84.615A, T84.619A, T84.63XA, T84.69XA, T84.7XXA

0RGA4J1 Fusion of Thoracolumbar Vertebral Joint with Synthetic Substitute, Posterior Approach, Posterior Column, Percutaneous Endoscopic Approach

HAC When reported with secondary diagnosis code K68.11, T81.40XA, T81.41XA, T81.42XA, T81.43XA, T81.44XA or T81.49XA, T84.60XA, T84.610A, T84.611A, T84.612A, T84.613A, T84.614A, T84.615A, T84.619A, T84.63XA, T84.69XA, T84.7XXA

0RGA4JJ Fusion of Thoracolumbar Vertebral Joint with Synthetic Substitute, Posterior Approach, Anterior Column, Percutaneous Endoscopic Approach

HAC When reported with secondary diagnosis code K68.11, T81.40XA,

T81.41XA, T81.42XA, T81.43XA, T81.44XA or T81.49XA, T84.60XA, T84.610A, T84.611A, T84.612A, T84.613A, T84.614A, T84.615A, T84.619A, T84.63XA, T84.69XA, T84.7XXA

0RGA4K0 Fusion of Thoracolumbar Vertebral Joint with Nonautologous Tissue Substitute, Anterior Approach, Anterior Column, Percutaneous Endoscopic Approach

HAC When reported with secondary diagnosis code K68.11, T81.40XA, T81.41XA, T81.42XA, T81.43XA, T81.44XA or T81.49XA, T84.60XA, T84.610A, T84.611A, T84.612A, T84.613A, T84.614A, T84.615A, T84.619A, T84.63XA, T84.69XA, T84.7XXA

0RGA4K1 Fusion of Thoracolumbar Vertebral Joint with Nonautologous Tissue Substitute, Posterior Approach, Posterior Column, Percutaneous Endoscopic Approach

HAC When reported with secondary diagnosis code K68.11, T81.40XA, T81.41XA, T81.42XA, T81.43XA, T81.44XA or T81.49XA, T84.60XA, T84.610A, T84.611A, T84.612A, T84.613A, T84.614A, T84.615A, T84.619A, T84.63XA, T84.69XA, T84.7XXA

0RGA4KJ Fusion of Thoracolumbar Vertebral Joint with Nonautologous Tissue Substitute, Posterior Approach, Anterior Column, Percutaneous Endoscopic Approach

HAC When reported with secondary diagnosis code K68.11, T81.40XA, T81.41XA, T81.42XA, T81.43XA, T81.44XA or T81.49XA, T84.60XA, T84.610A, T84.611A, T84.612A, T84.613A, T84.614A, T84.615A, T84.619A, T84.63XA, T84.69XA, T84.7XXA

0RGC04Z Fusion of Right Temporomandibular Joint with Internal Fixation Device, Open Approach

0RGC07Z Fusion of Right Temporomandibular Joint with Autologous Tissue Substitute, Open Approach

0RGC0JZ Fusion of Right Temporomandibular Joint with Synthetic Substitute, Open Approach

0RGC0KZ Fusion of Right Temporomandibular Joint with Nonautologous Tissue Substitute, Open Approach

0RGC34Z Fusion of Right Temporomandibular Joint with Internal Fixation Device, Percutaneous Approach

0RGC37Z Fusion of Right Temporomandibular Joint with Autologous Tissue Substitute, Percutaneous Approach

0RGC3JZ Fusion of Right Temporomandibular Joint with Synthetic Substitute, Percutaneous Approach

0RGC3KZ Fusion of Right Temporomandibular Joint with Nonautologous Tissue Substitute, Percutaneous Approach

0RGC44Z Fusion of Right Temporomandibular Joint with Internal Fixation Device, Percutaneous Endoscopic Approach

0RGC47Z Fusion of Right Temporomandibular Joint with Autologous Tissue Substitute, Percutaneous Endoscopic Approach

0RGC4JZ Fusion of Right Temporomandibular Joint with Synthetic Substitute, Percutaneous Endoscopic Approach

0RGC4KZ Fusion of Right Temporomandibular Joint with Nonautologous Tissue Substitute, Percutaneous Endoscopic Approach

0RGD04Z Fusion of Left Temporomandibular Joint with Internal Fixation Device, Open Approach

0RGD07Z Fusion of Left Temporomandibular Joint with Autologous Tissue Substitute, Open Approach

0RGD0JZ Fusion of Left Temporomandibular Joint with Synthetic Substitute, Open Approach

0RGD0KZ Fusion of Left Temporomandibular Joint with Nonautologous Tissue Substitute, Open Approach

0RGD34Z Fusion of Left Temporomandibular Joint with Internal Fixation Device, Percutaneous Approach

0RGD37Z Fusion of Left Temporomandibular Joint with Autologous Tissue Substitute, Percutaneous Approach

0RGD3JZ Fusion of Left Temporomandibular Joint with Synthetic Substitute, Percutaneous Approach

0RGD3KZ Fusion of Left Temporomandibular Joint with Nonautologous Tissue Substitute, Percutaneous Approach

0RGD44Z Fusion of Left Temporomandibular Joint with Internal Fixation Device, Percutaneous Endoscopic Approach

0RGD47Z Fusion of Left Temporomandibular Joint with Autologous Tissue Substitute, Percutaneous Endoscopic Approach

0RGD4JZ Fusion of Left Temporomandibular Joint with Synthetic Substitute, Percutaneous Endoscopic Approach

0RGD4KZ Fusion of Left Temporomandibular Joint with Nonautologous Tissue Substitute, Percutaneous Endoscopic Approach

0RGE04Z Fusion of Right Sternoclavicular Joint with Internal Fixation Device, Open Approach

HAC When reported with secondary diagnosis code K68.11, T81.40XA, T81.41XA, T81.42XA, T81.43XA, T81.44XA or T81.49XA, T84.60XA, T84.610A, T84.611A, T84.612A, T84.613A, T84.614A, T84.615A, T84.619A, T84.63XA, T84.69XA, T84.7XXA

0RGE07Z Fusion of Right Sternoclavicular Joint with Autologous Tissue Substitute, Open Approach

HAC When reported with secondary diagnosis code K68.11, T81.40XA, T81.41XA, T81.42XA, T81.43XA, T81.44XA or T81.49XA, T84.60XA, T84.610A, T84.611A, T84.612A, T84.613A, T84.614A, T84.615A, T84.619A, T84.63XA, T84.69XA, T84.7XXA

0RGE0JZ Fusion of Right Sternoclavicular Joint with Synthetic Substitute, Open Approach

HAC When reported with secondary diagnosis code K68.11, T81.40XA, T81.41XA, T81.42XA, T81.43XA, T81.44XA or T81.49XA, T84.60XA, T84.610A, T84.611A, T84.612A, T84.613A, T84.614A, T84.615A,

♀ Female-only   ♂ Male-only   ▲ Limited Coverage   ● Non-OR   HAC HAC-associated procedure   ▲ Non-covered procedures   ✚ Cluster

T84.619A, T84.63XA, T84.69XA, T84.7XXA

0RGE0KZ Fusion of Right Sternoclavicular Joint with Nonautologous Tissue Substitute, Open Approach

> HAC When reported with secondary diagnosis code K68.11, T81.40XA, T81.41XA, T81.42XA, T81.43XA, T81.44XA or T81.49XA, T84.60XA, T84.610A, T84.611A, T84.612A, T84.613A, T84.614A, T84.615A, T84.619A, T84.63XA, T84.69XA, T84.7XXA

0RGE34Z Fusion of Right Sternoclavicular Joint with Internal Fixation Device, Percutaneous Approach

> HAC When reported with secondary diagnosis code K68.11, T81.40XA, T81.41XA, T81.42XA, T81.43XA, T81.44XA or T81.49XA, T84.60XA, T84.610A, T84.611A, T84.612A, T84.613A, T84.614A, T84.615A, T84.619A, T84.63XA, T84.69XA, T84.7XXA

0RGE37Z Fusion of Right Sternoclavicular Joint with Autologous Tissue Substitute, Percutaneous Approach

> HAC When reported with secondary diagnosis code K68.11, T81.40XA, T81.41XA, T81.42XA, T81.43XA, T81.44XA or T81.49XA, T84.60XA, T84.610A, T84.611A, T84.612A, T84.613A, T84.614A, T84.615A, T84.619A, T84.63XA, T84.69XA, T84.7XXA

0RGE3JZ Fusion of Right Sternoclavicular Joint with Synthetic Substitute, Percutaneous Approach

> HAC When reported with secondary diagnosis code K68.11, T81.40XA, T81.41XA, T81.42XA, T81.43XA, T81.44XA or T81.49XA, T84.60XA, T84.610A, T84.611A, T84.612A, T84.613A, T84.614A, T84.615A, T84.619A, T84.63XA, T84.69XA, T84.7XXA

0RGE3KZ Fusion of Right Sternoclavicular Joint with Nonautologous Tissue Substitute, Percutaneous Approach

> HAC When reported with secondary diagnosis code K68.11, T81.40XA, T81.41XA, T81.42XA, T81.43XA, T81.44XA or T81.49XA, T84.60XA, T84.610A, T84.611A, T84.612A, T84.613A, T84.614A, T84.615A, T84.619A, T84.63XA, T84.69XA, T84.7XXA

0RGE44Z Fusion of Right Sternoclavicular Joint with Internal Fixation Device, Percutaneous Endoscopic Approach

> HAC When reported with secondary diagnosis code K68.11, T81.40XA, T81.41XA, T81.42XA, T81.43XA, T81.44XA or T81.49XA, T84.60XA, T84.610A, T84.611A, T84.612A, T84.613A, T84.614A, T84.615A, T84.619A, T84.63XA, T84.69XA, T84.7XXA

0RGE47Z Fusion of Right Sternoclavicular Joint with Autologous Tissue Substitute, Percutaneous Endoscopic Approach

> HAC When reported with secondary diagnosis code K68.11, T81.40XA, T81.41XA, T81.42XA, T81.43XA, T81.44XA or T81.49XA, T84.60XA, T84.610A, T84.611A, T84.612A, T84.613A, T84.614A, T84.615A,

T84.619A, T84.63XA, T84.69XA, T84.7XXA

0RGE4JZ Fusion of Right Sternoclavicular Joint with Synthetic Substitute, Percutaneous Endoscopic Approach

> HAC When reported with secondary diagnosis code K68.11, T81.40XA, T81.41XA, T81.42XA, T81.43XA, T81.44XA or T81.49XA, T84.60XA, T84.610A, T84.611A, T84.612A, T84.613A, T84.614A, T84.615A, T84.619A, T84.63XA, T84.69XA, T84.7XXA

0RGE4KZ Fusion of Right Sternoclavicular Joint with Nonautologous Tissue Substitute, Percutaneous Endoscopic Approach

> HAC When reported with secondary diagnosis code K68.11, T81.40XA, T81.41XA, T81.42XA, T81.43XA, T81.44XA or T81.49XA, T84.60XA, T84.610A, T84.611A, T84.612A, T84.613A, T84.614A, T84.615A, T84.619A, T84.63XA, T84.69XA, T84.7XXA

0RGF04Z Fusion of Left Sternoclavicular Joint with Internal Fixation Device, Open Approach

> HAC When reported with secondary diagnosis code K68.11, T81.40XA, T81.41XA, T81.42XA, T81.43XA, T81.44XA or T81.49XA, T84.60XA, T84.610A, T84.611A, T84.612A, T84.613A, T84.614A, T84.615A, T84.619A, T84.63XA, T84.69XA, T84.7XXA

0RGF07Z Fusion of Left Sternoclavicular Joint with Autologous Tissue Substitute, Open Approach

> HAC When reported with secondary diagnosis code K68.11, T81.40XA, T81.41XA, T81.42XA, T81.43XA, T81.44XA or T81.49XA, T84.60XA, T84.610A, T84.611A, T84.612A, T84.613A, T84.614A, T84.615A, T84.619A, T84.63XA, T84.69XA, T84.7XXA

0RGF0JZ Fusion of Left Sternoclavicular Joint with Synthetic Substitute, Open Approach

> HAC When reported with secondary diagnosis code K68.11, T81.40XA, T81.41XA, T81.42XA, T81.43XA, T81.44XA or T81.49XA, T84.60XA, T84.610A, T84.611A, T84.612A, T84.613A, T84.614A, T84.615A, T84.619A, T84.63XA, T84.69XA, T84.7XXA

0RGF0KZ Fusion of Left Sternoclavicular Joint with Nonautologous Tissue Substitute, Open Approach

> HAC When reported with secondary diagnosis code K68.11, T81.40XA, T81.41XA, T81.42XA, T81.43XA, T81.44XA or T81.49XA, T84.60XA, T84.610A, T84.611A, T84.612A, T84.613A, T84.614A, T84.615A, T84.619A, T84.63XA, T84.69XA, T84.7XXA

0RGF34Z Fusion of Left Sternoclavicular Joint with Internal Fixation Device, Percutaneous Approach

> HAC When reported with secondary diagnosis code K68.11, T81.40XA, T81.41XA, T81.42XA, T81.43XA, T81.44XA or T81.49XA, T84.60XA, T84.610A, T84.611A, T84.612A, T84.613A, T84.614A, T84.615A,

T84.619A, T84.63XA, T84.69XA, T84.7XXA

0RGF37Z Fusion of Left Sternoclavicular Joint with Autologous Tissue Substitute, Percutaneous Approach

> HAC When reported with secondary diagnosis code K68.11, T81.40XA, T81.41XA, T81.42XA, T81.43XA, T81.44XA or T81.49XA, T84.60XA, T84.610A, T84.611A, T84.612A, T84.613A, T84.614A, T84.615A, T84.619A, T84.63XA, T84.69XA, T84.7XXA

0RGF3JZ Fusion of Left Sternoclavicular Joint with Synthetic Substitute, Percutaneous Approach

> HAC When reported with secondary diagnosis code K68.11, T81.40XA, T81.41XA, T81.42XA, T81.43XA, T81.44XA or T81.49XA, T84.60XA, T84.610A, T84.611A, T84.612A, T84.613A, T84.614A, T84.615A, T84.619A, T84.63XA, T84.69XA, T84.7XXA

0RGF3KZ Fusion of Left Sternoclavicular Joint with Nonautologous Tissue Substitute, Percutaneous Approach

> HAC When reported with secondary diagnosis code K68.11, T81.40XA, T81.41XA, T81.42XA, T81.43XA, T81.44XA or T81.49XA, T84.60XA, T84.610A, T84.611A, T84.612A, T84.613A, T84.614A, T84.615A, T84.619A, T84.63XA, T84.69XA, T84.7XXA

0RGF44Z Fusion of Left Sternoclavicular Joint with Internal Fixation Device, Percutaneous Endoscopic Approach

> HAC When reported with secondary diagnosis code K68.11, T81.40XA, T81.41XA, T81.42XA, T81.43XA, T81.44XA or T81.49XA, T84.60XA, T84.610A, T84.611A, T84.612A, T84.613A, T84.614A, T84.615A, T84.619A, T84.63XA, T84.69XA, T84.7XXA

0RGF47Z Fusion of Left Sternoclavicular Joint with Autologous Tissue Substitute, Percutaneous Endoscopic Approach

> HAC When reported with secondary diagnosis code K68.11, T81.40XA, T81.41XA, T81.42XA, T81.43XA, T81.44XA or T81.49XA, T84.60XA, T84.610A, T84.611A, T84.612A, T84.613A, T84.614A, T84.615A, T84.619A, T84.63XA, T84.69XA, T84.7XXA

0RGF4JZ Fusion of Left Sternoclavicular Joint with Synthetic Substitute, Percutaneous Endoscopic Approach

> HAC When reported with secondary diagnosis code K68.11, T81.40XA, T81.41XA, T81.42XA, T81.43XA, T81.44XA or T81.49XA, T84.60XA, T84.610A, T84.611A, T84.612A, T84.613A, T84.614A, T84.615A, T84.619A, T84.63XA, T84.69XA, T84.7XXA

0RGF4KZ Fusion of Left Sternoclavicular Joint with Nonautologous Tissue Substitute, Percutaneous Endoscopic Approach

> HAC When reported with secondary diagnosis code K68.11, T81.40XA, T81.41XA, T81.42XA, T81.43XA, T81.44XA or T81.49XA, T84.60XA, T84.610A, T84.611A, T84.612A,

T84.613A, T84.614A, T84.615A,
T84.619A, T84.63XA, T84.69XA,
T84.7XXA

0RGG04Z Fusion of Right Acromioclavicular
Joint with Internal Fixation Device,
Open Approach

HAC When reported with secondary
diagnosis code K68.11, T81.40XA,
T81.41XA, T81.42XA, T81.43XA,
T81.44XA or T81.49XA, T84.60XA,
T84.610A, T84.611A, T84.612A,
T84.613A, T84.614A, T84.615A,
T84.619A, T84.63XA, T84.69XA,
T84.7XXA

0RGG07Z Fusion of Right Acromioclavicular
Joint with Autologous Tissue
Substitute, Open Approach

HAC When reported with secondary
diagnosis code K68.11, T81.40XA,
T81.41XA, T81.42XA, T81.43XA,
T81.44XA or T81.49XA, T84.60XA,
T84.610A, T84.611A, T84.612A,
T84.613A, T84.614A, T84.615A,
T84.619A, T84.63XA, T84.69XA,
T84.7XXA

0RGG0JZ Fusion of Right Acromioclavicular
Joint
with Synthetic Substitute, Open
Approach

HAC When reported with secondary
diagnosis code K68.11, T81.40XA,
T81.41XA, T81.42XA, T81.43XA,
T81.44XA or T81.49XA, T84.60XA,
T84.610A, T84.611A, T84.612A,
T84.613A, T84.614A, T84.615A,
T84.619A, T84.63XA, T84.69XA,
T84.7XXA

0RGG0KZ Fusion of Right Acromioclavicular
Joint with Nonautologous Tissue
Substitute, Open Approach

HAC When reported with secondary
diagnosis code K68.11, T81.40XA,
T81.41XA, T81.42XA, T81.43XA,
T81.44XA or T81.49XA, T84.60XA,
T84.610A, T84.611A, T84.612A,
T84.613A, T84.614A, T84.615A,
T84.619A, T84.63XA, T84.69XA,
T84.7XXA

0RGG34Z Fusion of Right Acromioclavicular
Joint with Internal Fixation Device,
Percutaneous Approach

HAC When reported with secondary
diagnosis code K68.11, T81.40XA,
T81.41XA, T81.42XA, T81.43XA,
T81.44XA or T81.49XA, T84.60XA,
T84.610A, T84.611A, T84.612A,
T84.613A, T84.614A, T84.615A,
T84.619A, T84.63XA, T84.69XA,
T84.7XXA

0RGG37Z Fusion of Right Acromioclavicular
Joint with Autologous Tissue
Substitute, Percutaneous Approach

HAC When reported with secondary
diagnosis code K68.11, T81.40XA,
T81.41XA, T81.42XA, T81.43XA,
T81.44XA or T81.49XA, T84.60XA,
T84.610A, T84.611A, T84.612A,
T84.613A, T84.614A, T84.615A,
T84.619A, T84.63XA, T84.69XA,
T84.7XXA

0RGG3JZ Fusion of Right Acromioclavicular
Joint with Synthetic Substitute,
Percutaneous Approach

HAC When reported with secondary
diagnosis code K68.11, T81.40XA,
T81.41XA, T81.42XA, T81.43XA,
T81.44XA or T81.49XA, T84.60XA,

T84.610A, T84.611A, T84.612A,
T84.613A, T84.614A, T84.615A,
T84.619A, T84.63XA, T84.69XA,
T84.7XXA

0RGG3KZ Fusion of Right Acromioclavicular
Joint with Nonautologous Tissue
Substitute, Percutaneous Approach

HAC When reported with secondary
diagnosis code K68.11, T81.40XA,
T81.41XA, T81.42XA, T81.43XA,
T81.44XA or T81.49XA, T84.60XA,
T84.610A, T84.611A, T84.612A,
T84.613A, T84.614A, T84.615A,
T84.619A, T84.63XA, T84.69XA,
T84.7XXA

0RGG44Z Fusion of Right Acromioclavicular
Joint with Internal Fixation Device,
Percutaneous Endoscopic Approach

HAC When reported with secondary
diagnosis code K68.11, T81.40XA,
T81.41XA, T81.42XA, T81.43XA,
T81.44XA or T81.49XA, T84.60XA,
T84.610A, T84.611A, T84.612A,
T84.613A, T84.614A, T84.615A,
T84.619A, T84.63XA, T84.69XA,
T84.7XXA

0RGG47Z Fusion of Right Acromioclavicular
Joint with Autologous Tissue
Substitute, Percutaneous Endoscopic
Approach

HAC When reported with secondary
diagnosis code K68.11, T81.40XA,
T81.41XA, T81.42XA, T81.43XA,
T81.44XA or T81.49XA, T84.60XA,
T84.610A, T84.611A, T84.612A,
T84.613A, T84.614A, T84.615A,
T84.619A, T84.63XA, T84.69XA,
T84.7XXA

0RGG4JZ Fusion of Right Acromioclavicular
Joint with Synthetic Substitute,
Percutaneous Endoscopic Approach

HAC When reported with secondary
diagnosis code K68.11, T81.40XA,
T81.41XA, T81.42XA, T81.43XA,
T81.44XA or T81.49XA, T84.60XA,
T84.610A, T84.611A, T84.612A,
T84.613A, T84.614A, T84.615A,
T84.619A, T84.63XA, T84.69XA,
T84.7XXA

0RGG4KZ Fusion of Right Acromioclavicular
Joint
with Nonautologous Tissue Substitute,
Percutaneous Endoscopic Approach

HAC When reported with secondary
diagnosis code K68.11, T81.40XA,
T81.41XA, T81.42XA, T81.43XA,
T81.44XA or T81.49XA, T84.60XA,
T84.610A, T84.611A, T84.612A,
T84.613A, T84.614A, T84.615A,
T84.619A, T84.63XA, T84.69XA,
T84.7XXA

0RGH04Z Fusion of Left Acromioclavicular Joint
with Internal Fixation Device, Open
Approach

HAC When reported with secondary
diagnosis code K68.11, T81.40XA,
T81.41XA, T81.42XA, T81.43XA,
T81.44XA or T81.49XA, T84.60XA,
T84.610A, T84.611A, T84.612A,
T84.613A, T84.614A, T84.615A,
T84.619A, T84.63XA, T84.69XA,
T84.7XXA

0RGH07Z Fusion of Left Acromioclavicular Joint
with Autologous Tissue Substitute,
Open Approach

HAC When reported with secondary
diagnosis code K68.11, T81.40XA,

T81.41XA, T81.42XA, T81.43XA,
T81.44XA or T81.49XA, T84.60XA,
T84.610A, T84.611A, T84.612A,
T84.613A, T84.614A, T84.615A,
T84.619A, T84.63XA, T84.69XA,
T84.7XXA

0RGH0JZ Fusion of Left Acromioclavicular Joint
with Synthetic Substitute, Open
Approach

HAC When reported with secondary
diagnosis code K68.11, T81.40XA,
T81.41XA, T81.42XA, T81.43XA,
T81.44XA or T81.49XA, T84.60XA,
T84.610A, T84.611A, T84.612A,
T84.613A, T84.614A, T84.615A,
T84.619A, T84.63XA, T84.69XA,
T84.7XXA

0RGH0KZ Fusion of Left Acromioclavicular Joint
with Nonautologous Tissue Substitute,
Open Approach

HAC When reported with secondary
diagnosis code K68.11, T81.40XA,
T81.41XA, T81.42XA, T81.43XA,
T81.44XA or T81.49XA, T84.60XA,
T84.610A, T84.611A, T84.612A,
T84.613A, T84.614A, T84.615A,
T84.619A, T84.63XA, T84.69XA,
T84.7XXA

0RGH34Z Fusion of Left Acromioclavicular
Joint with Internal Fixation Device,
Percutaneous Approach

HAC When reported with secondary
diagnosis code K68.11, T81.40XA,
T81.41XA, T81.42XA, T81.43XA,
T81.44XA or T81.49XA, T84.60XA,
T84.610A, T84.611A, T84.612A,
T84.613A, T84.614A, T84.615A,
T84.619A, T84.63XA, T84.69XA,
T84.7XXA

0RGH37Z Fusion of Left Acromioclavicular Joint
with Autologous Tissue Substitute,
Percutaneous Approach

HAC When reported with secondary
diagnosis code K68.11, T81.40XA,
T81.41XA, T81.42XA, T81.43XA,
T81.44XA or T81.49XA, T84.60XA,
T84.610A, T84.611A, T84.612A,
T84.613A, T84.614A, T84.615A,
T84.619A, T84.63XA, T84.69XA,
T84.7XXA

0RGH3JZ Fusion of Left Acromioclavicular Joint
with Synthetic Substitute, Percutaneous
Approach

HAC When reported with secondary
diagnosis code K68.11, T81.40XA,
T81.41XA, T81.42XA, T81.43XA,
T81.44XA or T81.49XA, T84.60XA,
T84.610A, T84.611A, T84.612A,
T84.613A, T84.614A, T84.615A,
T84.619A, T84.63XA, T84.69XA,
T84.7XXA

0RGH3KZ Fusion of Left Acromioclavicular Joint
with Nonautologous Tissue Substitute,
Percutaneous Approach

HAC When reported with secondary
diagnosis code K68.11, T81.40XA,
T81.41XA, T81.42XA, T81.43XA,
T81.44XA or T81.49XA, T84.60XA,
T84.610A, T84.611A, T84.612A,
T84.613A, T84.614A, T84.615A,
T84.619A, T84.63XA, T84.69XA,
T84.7XXA

0RGH44Z Fusion of Left Acromioclavicular
Joint with Internal Fixation Device,
Percutaneous Endoscopic Approach

HAC When reported with secondary
diagnosis code K68.11, T81.40XA,

T81.41XA, T81.42XA, T81.43XA,
T81.44XA or T81.49XA, T84.60XA,
T84.610A, T84.611A, T84.612A,
T84.613A, T84.614A, T84.615A,
T84.619A, T84.63XA, T84.69XA,
T84.7XXA

0RGH47Z Fusion of Left Acromioclavicular Joint with Autologous Tissue Substitute, Percutaneous Endoscopic Approach

HAC   When reported with secondary diagnosis code K68.11, T81.40XA, T81.41XA, T81.42XA, T81.43XA, T81.44XA or T81.49XA, T84.60XA, T84.610A, T84.611A, T84.612A, T84.613A, T84.614A, T84.615A, T84.619A, T84.63XA, T84.69XA, T84.7XXA

0RGH4JZ Fusion of Left Acromioclavicular Joint with Synthetic Substitute, Percutaneous Endoscopic Approach

HAC   When reported with secondary diagnosis code K68.11, T81.40XA, T81.41XA, T81.42XA, T81.43XA, T81.44XA or T81.49XA, T84.60XA, T84.610A, T84.611A, T84.612A, T84.613A, T84.614A, T84.615A, T84.619A, T84.63XA, T84.69XA, T84.7XXA

0RGH4KZ Fusion of Left Acromioclavicular Joint with Nonautologous Tissue Substitute, Percutaneous Endoscopic Approach

HAC   When reported with secondary diagnosis code K68.11, T81.40XA, T81.41XA, T81.42XA, T81.43XA, T81.44XA or T81.49XA, T84.60XA, T84.610A, T84.611A, T84.612A, T84.613A, T84.614A, T84.615A, T84.619A, T84.63XA, T84.69XA, T84.7XXA

0RGJ04Z Fusion of Right Shoulder Joint with Internal Fixation Device, Open Approach

HAC   When reported with secondary diagnosis code K68.11, T81.40XA, T81.41XA, T81.42XA, T81.43XA, T81.44XA or T81.49XA, T84.60XA, T84.610A, T84.611A, T84.612A, T84.613A, T84.614A, T84.615A, T84.619A, T84.63XA, T84.69XA, T84.7XXA

0RGJ07Z Fusion of Right Shoulder Joint with Autologous Tissue Substitute, Open Approach

HAC   When reported with secondary diagnosis code K68.11, T81.40XA, T81.41XA, T81.42XA, T81.43XA, T81.44XA or T81.49XA, T84.60XA, T84.610A, T84.611A, T84.612A, T84.613A, T84.614A, T84.615A, T84.619A, T84.63XA, T84.69XA, T84.7XXA

0RGJ0JZ Fusion of Right Shoulder Joint with Synthetic Substitute, Open Approach

HAC   When reported with secondary diagnosis code K68.11, T81.40XA, T81.41XA, T81.42XA, T81.43XA, T81.44XA or T81.49XA, T84.60XA, T84.610A, T84.611A, T84.612A, T84.613A, T84.614A, T84.615A, T84.619A, T84.63XA, T84.69XA, T84.7XXA

0RGJ0KZ Fusion of Right Shoulder Joint with Nonautologous Tissue Substitute, Open Approach

HAC   When reported with secondary diagnosis code K68.11, T81.40XA,

---

T81.41XA, T81.42XA, T81.43XA,
T81.44XA or T81.49XA, T84.60XA,
T84.610A, T84.611A, T84.612A,
T84.613A, T84.614A, T84.615A,
T84.619A, T84.63XA, T84.69XA,
T84.7XXA

0RGJ34Z Fusion of Right Shoulder Joint with Internal Fixation Device, Percutaneous Approach

HAC   When reported with secondary diagnosis code K68.11, T81.40XA, T81.41XA, T81.42XA, T81.43XA, T81.44XA or T81.49XA, T84.60XA, T84.610A, T84.611A, T84.612A, T84.613A, T84.614A, T84.615A, T84.619A, T84.63XA, T84.69XA, T84.7XXA

0RGJ37Z Fusion of Right Shoulder Joint with Autologous Tissue Substitute, Percutaneous Approach

HAC   When reported with secondary diagnosis code K68.11, T81.40XA, T81.41XA, T81.42XA, T81.43XA, T81.44XA or T81.49XA, T84.60XA, T84.610A, T84.611A, T84.612A, T84.613A, T84.614A, T84.615A, T84.619A, T84.63XA, T84.69XA, T84.7XXA

0RGJ3JZ Fusion of Right Shoulder Joint with Synthetic Substitute, Percutaneous Approach

HAC   When reported with secondary diagnosis code K68.11, T81.40XA, T81.41XA, T81.42XA, T81.43XA, T81.44XA or T81.49XA, T84.60XA, T84.610A, T84.611A, T84.612A, T84.613A, T84.614A, T84.615A, T84.619A, T84.63XA, T84.69XA, T84.7XXA

0RGJ3KZ Fusion of Right Shoulder Joint with Nonautologous Tissue Substitute, Percutaneous Approach

HAC   When reported with secondary diagnosis code K68.11, T81.40XA, T81.41XA, T81.42XA, T81.43XA, T81.44XA or T81.49XA, T84.60XA, T84.610A, T84.611A, T84.612A, T84.613A, T84.614A, T84.615A, T84.619A, T84.63XA, T84.69XA, T84.7XXA

0RGJ44Z Fusion of Right Shoulder Joint with Internal Fixation Device, Percutaneous Endoscopic Approach

HAC   When reported with secondary diagnosis code K68.11, T81.40XA, T81.41XA, T81.42XA, T81.43XA, T81.44XA or T81.49XA, T84.60XA, T84.610A, T84.611A, T84.612A, T84.613A, T84.614A, T84.615A, T84.619A, T84.63XA, T84.69XA, T84.7XXA

0RGJ47Z Fusion of Right Shoulder Joint with Autologous Tissue Substitute, Percutaneous Endoscopic Approach

HAC   When reported with secondary diagnosis code K68.11, T81.40XA, T81.41XA, T81.42XA, T81.43XA, T81.44XA or T81.49XA, T84.60XA, T84.610A, T84.611A, T84.612A, T84.613A, T84.614A, T84.615A, T84.619A, T84.63XA, T84.69XA, T84.7XXA

0RGJ4JZ Fusion of Right Shoulder Joint with Synthetic Substitute, Percutaneous Endoscopic Approach

HAC   When reported with secondary diagnosis code K68.11, T81.40XA,

---

T81.41XA, T81.42XA, T81.43XA,
T81.44XA or T81.49XA, T84.60XA,
T84.610A, T84.611A, T84.612A,
T84.613A, T84.614A, T84.615A,
T84.619A, T84.63XA, T84.69XA,
T84.7XXA

0RGJ4KZ Fusion of Right Shoulder Joint with Nonautologous Tissue Substitute, Percutaneous Endoscopic Approach

HAC   When reported with secondary diagnosis code K68.11, T81.40XA, T81.41XA, T81.42XA, T81.43XA, T81.44XA or T81.49XA, T84.60XA, T84.610A, T84.611A, T84.612A, T84.613A, T84.614A, T84.615A, T84.619A, T84.63XA, T84.69XA, T84.7XXA

0RGK04Z Fusion of Left Shoulder Joint with Internal Fixation Device, Open Approach

HAC   When reported with secondary diagnosis code K68.11, T81.40XA, T81.41XA, T81.42XA, T81.43XA, T81.44XA or T81.49XA, T84.60XA, T84.610A, T84.611A, T84.612A, T84.613A, T84.614A, T84.615A, T84.619A, T84.63XA, T84.69XA, T84.7XXA

0RGK07Z Fusion of Left Shoulder Joint with Autologous Tissue Substitute, Open Approach

HAC   When reported with secondary diagnosis code K68.11, T81.40XA, T81.41XA, T81.42XA, T81.43XA, T81.44XA or T81.49XA, T84.60XA, T84.610A, T84.611A, T84.612A, T84.613A, T84.614A, T84.615A, T84.619A, T84.63XA, T84.69XA, T84.7XXA

0RGK0JZ Fusion of Left Shoulder Joint with Synthetic Substitute, Open Approach

HAC   When reported with secondary diagnosis code K68.11, T81.40XA, T81.41XA, T81.42XA, T81.43XA, T81.44XA or T81.49XA, T84.60XA, T84.610A, T84.611A, T84.612A, T84.613A, T84.614A, T84.615A, T84.619A, T84.63XA, T84.69XA, T84.7XXA

0RGK0KZ Fusion of Left Shoulder Joint with Nonautologous Tissue Substitute, Open Approach

HAC   When reported with secondary diagnosis code K68.11, T81.40XA, T81.41XA, T81.42XA, T81.43XA, T81.44XA or T81.49XA, T84.60XA, T84.610A, T84.611A, T84.612A, T84.613A, T84.614A, T84.615A, T84.619A, T84.63XA, T84.69XA, T84.7XXA

0RGK34Z Fusion of Left Shoulder Joint with Internal Fixation Device, Percutaneous Approach

HAC   When reported with secondary diagnosis code K68.11, T81.40XA, T81.41XA, T81.42XA, T81.43XA, T81.44XA or T81.49XA, T84.60XA, T84.610A, T84.611A, T84.612A, T84.613A, T84.614A, T84.615A, T84.619A, T84.63XA, T84.69XA, T84.7XXA

0RGK37Z Fusion of Left Shoulder Joint with Autologous Tissue Substitute, Percutaneous Approach

HAC   When reported with secondary diagnosis code K68.11, T81.40XA, T81.41XA, T81.42XA, T81.43XA,

---

♀ Female-only   ♂ Male-only   ▲ Limited Coverage   ● Non-OR   HAC HAC-associated procedure   ▲ Non-covered procedures   ✛ Cluster

T81.44XA or T81.49XA, T84.60XA,
T84.610A, T84.611A, T84.612A,
T84.613A, T84.614A, T84.615A,
T84.619A, T84.63XA, T84.69XA,
T84.7XXA

0RGK3JZ Fusion of Left Shoulder Joint with
Synthetic Substitute, Percutaneous
Approach

HAC When reported with secondary
diagnosis code K68.11, T81.40XA,
T81.41XA, T81.42XA, T81.43XA,
T81.44XA or T81.49XA, T84.60XA,
T84.610A, T84.611A, T84.612A,
T84.613A, T84.614A, T84.615A,
T84.619A, T84.63XA, T84.69XA,
T84.7XXA

0RGK3KZ Fusion of Left Shoulder Joint with
Nonautologous Tissue Substitute,
Percutaneous Approach

HAC When reported with secondary
diagnosis code K68.11, T81.40XA,
T81.41XA, T81.42XA, T81.43XA,
T81.44XA or T81.49XA, T84.60XA,
T84.610A, T84.611A, T84.612A,
T84.613A, T84.614A, T84.615A,
T84.619A, T84.63XA, T84.69XA,
T84.7XXA

0RGK44Z Fusion of Left Shoulder Joint with
Internal Fixation Device, Percutaneous
Endoscopic Approach

HAC When reported with secondary
diagnosis code K68.11, T81.40XA,
T81.41XA, T81.42XA, T81.43XA,
T81.44XA or T81.49XA, T84.60XA,
T84.610A, T84.611A, T84.612A,
T84.613A, T84.614A, T84.615A,
T84.619A, T84.63XA, T84.69XA,
T84.7XXA

0RGK47Z Fusion of Left Shoulder Joint with
Autologous Tissue Substitute,
Percutaneous Endoscopic Approach

HAC When reported with secondary
diagnosis code K68.11, T81.40XA,
T81.41XA, T81.42XA, T81.43XA,
T81.44XA or T81.49XA, T84.60XA,
T84.610A, T84.611A, T84.612A,
T84.613A, T84.614A, T84.615A,
T84.619A, T84.63XA, T84.69XA,
T84.7XXA

0RGK4JZ Fusion of Left Shoulder Joint with
Synthetic Substitute, Percutaneous
Endoscopic Approach

HAC When reported with secondary
diagnosis code K68.11, T81.40XA,
T81.41XA, T81.42XA, T81.43XA,
T81.44XA or T81.49XA, T84.60XA,
T84.610A, T84.611A, T84.612A,
T84.613A, T84.614A, T84.615A,
T84.619A, T84.63XA, T84.69XA,
T84.7XXA

0RGK4KZ Fusion of Left Shoulder Joint with
Nonautologous Tissue Substitute,
Percutaneous Endoscopic Approach

HAC When reported with secondary
diagnosis code K68.11, T81.40XA,
T81.41XA, T81.42XA, T81.43XA,
T81.44XA or T81.49XA, T84.60XA,
T84.610A, T84.611A, T84.612A,
T84.613A, T84.614A, T84.615A,
T84.619A, T84.63XA, T84.69XA,
T84.7XXA

0RGL03Z Fusion of Right Elbow Joint with
Sustained Compression Internal
Fixation Device, Open Approach

0RGL04Z Fusion of Right Elbow Joint with
Internal Fixation Device, Open
Approach

HAC When reported with secondary
diagnosis code K68.11, T81.40XA,
T81.41XA, T81.42XA, T81.43XA,
T81.44XA or T81.49XA, T84.60XA,
T84.610A, T84.611A, T84.612A,
T84.613A, T84.614A, T84.615A,
T84.619A, T84.63XA, T84.69XA,
T84.7XXA

0RGL05Z Fusion of Right Elbow Joint with
External Fixation Device, Open
Approach

HAC When reported with secondary
diagnosis code K68.11, T81.40XA,
T81.41XA, T81.42XA, T81.43XA,
T81.44XA or T81.49XA, T84.60XA,
T84.610A, T84.611A, T84.612A,
T84.613A, T84.614A, T84.615A,
T84.619A, T84.63XA, T84.69XA,
T84.7XXA

0RGL07Z Fusion of Right Elbow Joint with
Autologous Tissue Substitute, Open
Approach

HAC When reported with secondary
diagnosis code K68.11, T81.40XA,
T81.41XA, T81.42XA, T81.43XA,
T81.44XA or T81.49XA, T84.60XA,
T84.610A, T84.611A, T84.612A,
T84.613A, T84.614A, T84.615A,
T84.619A, T84.63XA, T84.69XA,
T84.7XXA

0RGL0JZ Fusion of Right Elbow Joint with
Synthetic Substitute, Open Approach

HAC When reported with secondary
diagnosis code K68.11, T81.40XA,
T81.41XA, T81.42XA, T81.43XA,
T81.44XA or T81.49XA, T84.60XA,
T84.610A, T84.611A, T84.612A,
T84.613A, T84.614A, T84.615A,
T84.619A, T84.63XA, T84.69XA,
T84.7XXA

0RGL0KZ Fusion of Right Elbow Joint with
Nonautologous Tissue Substitute, Open
Approach

HAC When reported with secondary
diagnosis code K68.11, T81.40XA,
T81.41XA, T81.42XA, T81.43XA,
T81.44XA or T81.49XA, T84.60XA,
T84.610A, T84.611A, T84.612A,
T84.613A, T84.614A, T84.615A,
T84.619A, T84.63XA, T84.69XA,
T84.7XXA

0RGL33Z Fusion of Right Elbow Joint with
Sustained Compression Internal
Fixation Device, Percutaneous
Approach

0RGL34Z Fusion of Right Elbow Joint with
Internal Fixation Device, Percutaneous
Approach

HAC When reported with secondary
diagnosis code K68.11, T81.40XA,
T81.41XA, T81.42XA, T81.43XA,
T81.44XA or T81.49XA, T84.60XA,
T84.610A, T84.611A, T84.612A,
T84.613A, T84.614A, T84.615A,
T84.619A, T84.63XA, T84.69XA,
T84.7XXA

0RGL35Z Fusion of Right Elbow Joint with
External Fixation Device, Percutaneous
Approach

HAC When reported with secondary
diagnosis code K68.11, T81.40XA,
T81.41XA, T81.42XA, T81.43XA,
T81.44XA or T81.49XA, T84.60XA,
T84.610A, T84.611A, T84.612A,
T84.613A, T84.614A, T84.615A,
T84.619A, T84.63XA, T84.69XA,
T84.7XXA

0RGL37Z Fusion of Right Elbow Joint with
Autologous Tissue Substitute,
Percutaneous Approach

HAC When reported with secondary
diagnosis code K68.11, T81.40XA,
T81.41XA, T81.42XA, T81.43XA,
T81.44XA or T81.49XA, T84.60XA,
T84.610A, T84.611A, T84.612A,
T84.613A, T84.614A, T84.615A,
T84.619A, T84.63XA, T84.69XA,
T84.7XXA

0RGL3JZ Fusion of Right Elbow Joint with
Synthetic Substitute, Percutaneous
Approach

HAC When reported with secondary diagnosis
code K68.11, T81.40XA, T81.41XA,
T81.42XA, T81.43XA, T81.44XA or
T81.49XA, T84.60XA, T84.610A,
T84.611A, T84.612A, T84.613A,
T84.614A, T84.615A, T84.619A,
T84.63XA, T84.69XA, T84.7XXA

0RGL3KZ Fusion of Right Elbow Joint with
Nonautologous Tissue Substitute,
Percutaneous Approach

HAC When reported with secondary
diagnosis code K68.11, T81.40XA,
T81.41XA, T81.42XA, T81.43XA,
T81.44XA or T81.49XA, T84.60XA,
T84.610A, T84.611A, T84.612A,
T84.613A, T84.614A, T84.615A,
T84.619A, T84.63XA, T84.69XA,
T84.7XXA

0RGL43Z Fusion of Right Elbow Joint with
Sustained Compression Internal
Fixation Device, Percutaneous
Endoscopic Approach

0RGL44Z Fusion of Right Elbow Joint with
Internal Fixation Device, Percutaneous
Endoscopic Approach

HAC When reported with secondary
diagnosis code K68.11, T81.40XA,
T81.41XA, T81.42XA, T81.43XA,
T81.44XA or T81.49XA, T84.60XA,
T84.610A, T84.611A, T84.612A,
T84.613A, T84.614A, T84.615A,
T84.619A, T84.63XA, T84.69XA,
T84.7XXA

0RGL45Z Fusion of Right Elbow Joint with
External Fixation Device, Percutaneous
Endoscopic Approach

HAC When reported with secondary
diagnosis code K68.11, T81.40XA,
T81.41XA, T81.42XA, T81.43XA,
T81.44XA or T81.49XA, T84.60XA,
T84.610A, T84.611A, T84.612A,
T84.613A, T84.614A, T84.615A,
T84.619A, T84.63XA, T84.69XA,
T84.7XXA

0RGL47Z Fusion of Right Elbow Joint with
Autologous Tissue Substitute,
Percutaneous Endoscopic Approach

HAC When reported with secondary
diagnosis code K68.11, T81.40XA,
T81.41XA, T81.42XA, T81.43XA,
T81.44XA or T81.49XA, T84.60XA,
T84.610A, T84.611A, T84.612A,
T84.613A, T84.614A, T84.615A,
T84.619A, T84.63XA, T84.69XA,
T84.7XXA

0RGL4JZ Fusion of Right Elbow Joint with
Synthetic Substitute, Percutaneous
Endoscopic Approach

HAC When reported with secondary
diagnosis code K68.11, T81.40XA,
T81.41XA, T81.42XA, T81.43XA,
T81.44XA or T81.49XA, T84.60XA,
T84.610A, T84.611A, T84.612A,

♀ Female-only   ♂ Male-only   ▲ Limited Coverage   ● Non-OR   HAC HAC-associated procedure   ▲ Non-covered procedures   ✛ Cluster

T84.613A, T84.614A, T84.615A,
T84.619A, T84.63XA, T84.69XA,
T84.7XXA

0RGL4KZ Fusion of Right Elbow Joint with Nonautologous Tissue Substitute, Percutaneous Endoscopic Approach

HAC When reported with secondary diagnosis code K68.11, T81.40XA, T81.41XA, T81.42XA, T81.43XA, T81.44XA or T81.49XA, T84.60XA, T84.610A, T84.611A, T84.612A, T84.613A, T84.614A, T84.615A, T84.619A, T84.63XA, T84.69XA, T84.7XXA

0RGM03Z Fusion of Left Elbow Joint with Sustained Compression Internal Fixation Device, Open Approach

0RGM04Z Fusion of Left Elbow Joint with Internal Fixation Device, Open Approach

HAC When reported with secondary diagnosis code K68.11, T81.40XA, T81.41XA, T81.42XA, T81.43XA, T81.44XA or T81.49XA, T84.60XA, T84.610A, T84.611A, T84.612A, T84.613A, T84.614A, T84.615A, T84.619A, T84.63XA, T84.69XA, T84.7XXA

0RGM05Z Fusion of Left Elbow Joint with External Fixation Device, Open Approach

HAC When reported with secondary diagnosis code K68.11, T81.40XA, T81.41XA, T81.42XA, T81.43XA, T81.44XA or T81.49XA, T84.60XA, T84.610A, T84.611A, T84.612A, T84.613A, T84.614A, T84.615A, T84.619A, T84.63XA, T84.69XA, T84.7XXA

0RGM07Z Fusion of Left Elbow Joint with Autologous Tissue Substitute, Open Approach

HAC When reported with secondary diagnosis code K68.11, T81.40XA, T81.41XA, T81.42XA, T81.43XA, T81.44XA or T81.49XA, T84.60XA, T84.610A, T84.611A, T84.612A, T84.613A, T84.614A, T84.615A, T84.619A, T84.63XA, T84.69XA, T84.7XXA

0RGM0JZ Fusion of Left Elbow Joint with Synthetic Substitute, Open Approach

HAC When reported with secondary diagnosis code K68.11, T81.40XA, T81.41XA, T81.42XA, T81.43XA, T81.44XA or T81.49XA, T84.60XA, T84.610A, T84.611A, T84.612A, T84.613A, T84.614A, T84.615A, T84.619A, T84.63XA, T84.69XA, T84.7XXA

0RGM0KZ Fusion of Left Elbow Joint with Nonautologous Tissue Substitute, Open Approach

HAC When reported with secondary diagnosis code K68.11, T81.40XA, T81.41XA, T81.42XA, T81.43XA, T81.44XA or T81.49XA, T84.60XA, T84.610A, T84.611A, T84.612A, T84.613A, T84.614A, T84.615A, T84.619A, T84.63XA, T84.69XA, T84.7XXA

0RGM33Z Fusion of Left Elbow Joint with Sustained Compression Internal Fixation Device, Percutaneous Approach

0RGM34Z Fusion of Left Elbow Joint with Internal Fixation Device, Percutaneous Approach

HAC When reported with secondary diagnosis code K68.11, T81.40XA, T81.41XA, T81.42XA, T81.43XA, T81.44XA or T81.49XA, T84.60XA, T84.610A, T84.611A, T84.612A, T84.613A, T84.614A, T84.615A, T84.619A, T84.63XA, T84.69XA, T84.7XXA

0RGM35Z Fusion of Left Elbow Joint with External Fixation Device, Percutaneous Approach

HAC When reported with secondary diagnosis code K68.11, T81.40XA, T81.41XA, T81.42XA, T81.43XA, T81.44XA or T81.49XA, T84.60XA, T84.610A, T84.611A, T84.612A, T84.613A, T84.614A, T84.615A, T84.619A, T84.63XA, T84.69XA, T84.7XXA

0RGM37Z Fusion of Left Elbow Joint with Autologous Tissue Substitute, Percutaneous Approach

HAC When reported with secondary diagnosis code K68.11, T81.40XA, T81.41XA, T81.42XA, T81.43XA, T81.44XA or T81.49XA, T84.60XA, T84.610A, T84.611A, T84.612A, T84.613A, T84.614A, T84.615A, T84.619A, T84.63XA, T84.69XA, T84.7XXA

0RGM3JZ Fusion of Left Elbow Joint with Synthetic Substitute, Percutaneous Approach

HAC When reported with secondary diagnosis code K68.11, T81.40XA, T81.41XA, T81.42XA, T81.43XA, T81.44XA or T81.49XA, T84.60XA, T84.610A, T84.611A, T84.612A, T84.613A, T84.614A, T84.615A, T84.619A, T84.63XA, T84.69XA, T84.7XXA

0RGM3KZ Fusion of Left Elbow Joint with Nonautologous Tissue Substitute, Percutaneous Approach

HAC When reported with secondary diagnosis code K68.11, T81.40XA, T81.41XA, T81.42XA, T81.43XA, T81.44XA or T81.49XA, T84.60XA, T84.610A, T84.611A, T84.612A, T84.613A, T84.614A, T84.615A, T84.619A, T84.63XA, T84.69XA, T84.7XXA

0RGM43Z Fusion of Left Elbow Joint with Sustained Compression Internal Fixation Device, Percutaneous Endoscopic Approach

0RGM44Z Fusion of Left Elbow Joint with Internal Fixation Device, Percutaneous Endoscopic Approach

HAC When reported with secondary diagnosis code K68.11, T81.40XA, T81.41XA, T81.42XA, T81.43XA, T81.44XA or T81.49XA, T84.60XA, T84.610A, T84.611A, T84.612A, T84.613A, T84.614A, T84.615A, T84.619A, T84.63XA, T84.69XA, T84.7XXA

0RGM45Z Fusion of Left Elbow Joint with External Fixation Device, Percutaneous Endoscopic Approach

HAC When reported with secondary diagnosis code K68.11, T81.40XA, T81.41XA, T81.42XA, T81.43XA, T81.44XA or T81.49XA, T84.60XA, T84.610A, T84.611A, T84.612A, T84.613A, T84.614A, T84.615A,

T84.619A, T84.63XA, T84.69XA, T84.7XXA

0RGM47Z Fusion of Left Elbow Joint with Autologous Tissue Substitute, Percutaneous Endoscopic Approach

HAC When reported with secondary diagnosis code K68.11, T81.40XA, T81.41XA, T81.42XA, T81.43XA, T81.44XA or T81.49XA, T84.60XA, T84.610A, T84.611A, T84.612A, T84.613A, T84.614A, T84.615A, T84.619A, T84.63XA, T84.69XA, T84.7XXA

0RGM4JZ Fusion of Left Elbow Joint with Synthetic Substitute, Percutaneous Endoscopic Approach

HAC When reported with secondary diagnosis code K68.11, T81.40XA, T81.41XA, T81.42XA, T81.43XA, T81.44XA or T81.49XA, T84.60XA, T84.610A, T84.611A, T84.612A, T84.613A, T84.614A, T84.615A, T84.619A, T84.63XA, T84.69XA, T84.7XXA

0RGM4KZ Fusion of Left Elbow Joint with Nonautologous Tissue Substitute, Percutaneous Endoscopic Approach

HAC When reported with secondary diagnosis code K68.11, T81.40XA, T81.41XA, T81.42XA, T81.43XA, T81.44XA or T81.49XA, T84.60XA, T84.610A, T84.611A, T84.612A, T84.613A, T84.614A, T84.615A, T84.619A, T84.63XA, T84.69XA, T84.7XXA

0RGN03Z Fusion of Right Wrist Joint with Sustained Compression Internal Fixation Device, Open Approach

0RGN04Z Fusion of Right Wrist Joint with Internal Fixation Device, Open Approach

0RGN05Z Fusion of Right Wrist Joint with External Fixation Device, Open Approach

0RGN07Z Fusion of Right Wrist Joint with Autologous Tissue Substitute, Open Approach

0RGN0JZ Fusion of Right Wrist Joint with Synthetic Substitute, Open Approach

0RGN0KZ Fusion of Right Wrist Joint with Nonautologous Tissue Substitute, Open Approach

0RGN33Z Fusion of Right Wrist Joint with Sustained Compression Internal Fixation Device, Percutaneous Approach

0RGN34Z Fusion of Right Wrist Joint with Internal Fixation Device, Percutaneous Approach

0RGN35Z Fusion of Right Wrist Joint with External Fixation Device, Percutaneous Approach

0RGN37Z Fusion of Right Wrist Joint with Autologous Tissue Substitute, Percutaneous Approach

0RGN3JZ Fusion of Right Wrist Joint with Synthetic Substitute, Percutaneous Approach

0RGN3KZ Fusion of Right Wrist Joint with Nonautologous Tissue Substitute, Percutaneous Approach

0RGN43Z Fusion of Right Wrist Joint with Sustained Compression Internal Fixation Device, Percutaneous Endoscopic Approach

0RGN44Z Fusion of Right Wrist Joint with Internal Fixation Device, Percutaneous Endoscopic Approach

0RGN45Z Fusion of Right Wrist Joint with External Fixation Device, Percutaneous Endoscopic Approach

0RGN47Z Fusion of Right Wrist Joint with Autologous Tissue Substitute, Percutaneous Endoscopic Approach

0RGN4JZ Fusion of Right Wrist Joint with Synthetic Substitute, Percutaneous Endoscopic Approach

0RGN4KZ Fusion of Right Wrist Joint with Nonautologous Tissue Substitute, Percutaneous Endoscopic Approach

0RGP03Z Fusion of Left Wrist Joint with Sustained Compression Internal Fixation Device, Open Approach

0RGP04Z Fusion of Left Wrist Joint with Internal Fixation Device, Open Approach

0RGP05Z Fusion of Left Wrist Joint with External Fixation Device, Open Approach

0RGP07Z Fusion of Left Wrist Joint with Autologous Tissue Substitute, Open Approach

0RGP0JZ Fusion of Left Wrist Joint with Synthetic Substitute, Open Approach

0RGP0KZ Fusion of Left Wrist Joint with Nonautologous Tissue Substitute, Open Approach

0RGP33Z Fusion of Left Wrist Joint with Sustained Compression Internal Fixation Device, Percutaneous Approach

0RGP34Z Fusion of Left Wrist Joint with Internal Fixation Device, Percutaneous Approach

0RGP35Z Fusion of Left Wrist Joint with External Fixation Device, Percutaneous Approach

0RGP37Z Fusion of Left Wrist Joint with Autologous Tissue Substitute, Percutaneous Approach

0RGP3JZ Fusion of Left Wrist Joint with Synthetic Substitute, Percutaneous Approach

0RGP3KZ Fusion of Left Wrist Joint with Nonautologous Tissue Substitute, Percutaneous Approach

0RGP43Z Fusion of Left Wrist Joint with Sustained Compression Internal Fixation Device, Percutaneous Endoscopic Approach

0RGP44Z Fusion of Left Wrist Joint with Internal Fixation Device, Percutaneous Endoscopic Approach

0RGP45Z Fusion of Left Wrist Joint with External Fixation Device, Percutaneous Endoscopic Approach

0RGP47Z Fusion of Left Wrist Joint with Autologous Tissue Substitute, Percutaneous Endoscopic Approach

0RGP4JZ Fusion of Left Wrist Joint with Synthetic Substitute, Percutaneous Endoscopic Approach

0RGP4KZ Fusion of Left Wrist Joint with Nonautologous Tissue Substitute, Percutaneous Endoscopic Approach

0RGQ03Z Fusion of Right Carpal Joint with Sustained Compression Internal Fixation Device, Open Approach

0RGQ04Z Fusion of Right Carpal Joint with Internal Fixation Device, Open Approach

0RGQ05Z Fusion of Right Carpal Joint with External Fixation Device, Open Approach

0RGQ07Z Fusion of Right Carpal Joint with Autologous Tissue Substitute, Open Approach

0RGQ0JZ Fusion of Right Carpal Joint with Synthetic Substitute, Open Approach

0RGQ0KZ Fusion of Right Carpal Joint with Nonautologous Tissue Substitute, Open Approach

0RGQ33Z Fusion of Right Carpal Joint with Sustained Compression Internal Fixation Device, Percutaneous Approach

0RGQ34Z Fusion of Right Carpal Joint with Internal Fixation Device, Percutaneous Approach

0RGQ35Z Fusion of Right Carpal Joint with External Fixation Device, Percutaneous Approach

0RGQ37Z Fusion of Right Carpal Joint with Autologous Tissue Substitute, Percutaneous Approach

0RGQ3JZ Fusion of Right Carpal Joint with Synthetic Substitute, Percutaneous Approach

0RGQ3KZ Fusion of Right Carpal Joint with Nonautologous Tissue Substitute, Percutaneous Approach

0RGQ44Z Fusion of Right Carpal Joint with Internal Fixation Device, Percutaneous Endoscopic Approach

0RGQ43Z Fusion of Right Carpal Joint with Sustained Compression Internal Fixation Device, Percutaneous Endoscopic Approach

0RGQ45Z Fusion of Right Carpal Joint with External Fixation Device, Percutaneous Endoscopic Approach

0RGQ47Z Fusion of Right Carpal Joint with Autologous Tissue Substitute, Percutaneous Endoscopic Approach

0RGQ4JZ Fusion of Right Carpal Joint with Synthetic Substitute, Percutaneous Endoscopic Approach

0RGQ4KZ Fusion of Right Carpal Joint with Nonautologous Tissue Substitute, Percutaneous Endoscopic Approach

0RGR03Z Fusion of Left Carpal Joint with Sustained Compression Internal Fixation Device, Open Approach

0RGR04Z Fusion of Left Carpal Joint with Internal Fixation Device, Open Approach

0RGR05Z Fusion of Left Carpal Joint with External Fixation Device, Open Approach

0RGR07Z Fusion of Left Carpal Joint with Autologous Tissue Substitute, Open Approach

0RGR0JZ Fusion of Left Carpal Joint with Synthetic Substitute, Open Approach

0RGR0KZ Fusion of Left Carpal Joint with Nonautologous Tissue Substitute, Open Approach

0RGR33Z Fusion of Left Carpal Joint with Sustained Compression Internal Fixation Device, Percutaneous Approach

0RGR34Z Fusion of Left Carpal Joint with Internal Fixation Device, Percutaneous Approach

0RGR35Z Fusion of Left Carpal Joint with External Fixation Device, Percutaneous Approach

0RGR37Z Fusion of Left Carpal Joint with Autologous Tissue Substitute, Percutaneous Approach

0RGR3JZ Fusion of Left Carpal Joint with Synthetic Substitute, Percutaneous Approach

0RGR3KZ Fusion of Left Carpal Joint with Nonautologous Tissue Substitute, Percutaneous Approach

0RGR43Z Fusion of Left Carpal Joint with Sustained Compression Internal Fixation Device, Percutaneous Endoscopic Approach

0RGR44Z Fusion of Left Carpal Joint with Internal Fixation Device, Percutaneous Endoscopic Approach

0RGR45Z Fusion of Left Carpal Joint with External Fixation Device, Percutaneous Endoscopic Approach

0RGR47Z Fusion of Left Carpal Joint with Autologous Tissue Substitute, Percutaneous Endoscopic Approach

0RGR4JZ Fusion of Left Carpal Joint with Synthetic Substitute, Percutaneous Endoscopic Approach

0RGR4KZ Fusion of Left Carpal Joint with Nonautologous Tissue Substitute, Percutaneous Endoscopic Approach

0RGS03Z Fusion of Right Carpometacarpal Joint with Sustained Compression Internal Fixation Device, Open Approach

0RGS04Z Fusion of Right Carpometacarpal Joint with Internal Fixation Device, Open Approach

0RGS05Z Fusion of Right Carpometacarpal Joint with External Fixation Device, Open Approach

0RGS07Z Fusion of Right Carpometacarpal Joint with Autologous Tissue Substitute, Open Approach

0RGS0JZ Fusion of Right Carpometacarpal Joint with Synthetic Substitute, Open Approach

0RGS0KZ Fusion of Right Carpometacarpal Joint with Nonautologous Tissue Substitute, Open Approach

0RGS33Z Fusion of Right Carpometacarpal Joint with Sustained Compression Internal Fixation Device, Percutaneous Approach

0RGS34Z Fusion of Right Carpometacarpal Joint with Internal Fixation Device, Percutaneous Approach

0RGS35Z Fusion of Right Carpometacarpal Joint with External Fixation Device, Percutaneous Approach

0RGS37Z Fusion of Right Carpometacarpal Joint with Autologous Tissue Substitute, Percutaneous Approach

0RGS3JZ Fusion of Right Carpometacarpal Joint with Synthetic Substitute, Percutaneous Approach

0RGS3KZ Fusion of Right Carpometacarpal Joint with Nonautologous Tissue Substitute, Percutaneous Approach

0RGS43Z Fusion of Right Carpometacarpal Joint with Sustained Compression Internal Fixation Device, Percutaneous Endoscopic Approach

0RGS44Z Fusion of Right Carpometacarpal Joint with Internal Fixation Device, Percutaneous Endoscopic Approach

♀ Female-only   ♂ Male-only   ▲ Limited Coverage   ● Non-OR   ▥ HAC-associated procedure   ▲ Non-covered procedures   ✚ Cluster

0RGS45Z Fusion of Right Carpometacarpal Joint with External Fixation Device, Percutaneous Endoscopic Approach

0RGS47Z Fusion of Right Carpometacarpal Joint with Autologous Tissue Substitute, Percutaneous Endoscopic Approach

0RGS4JZ Fusion of Right Carpometacarpal Joint with Synthetic Substitute, Percutaneous Endoscopic Approach

0RGS4KZ Fusion of Right Carpometacarpal Joint with Nonautologous Tissue Substitute, Percutaneous Endoscopic Approach

0RGT03Z Fusion of Left Carpometacarpal Joint with Sustained Compression Internal Fixation Device, Open Approach

0RGT04Z Fusion of Left Carpometacarpal Joint with Internal Fixation Device, Open Approach

0RGT05Z Fusion of Left Carpometacarpal Joint with External Fixation Device, Open Approach

0RGT07Z Fusion of Left Carpometacarpal Joint with Autologous Tissue Substitute, Open Approach

0RGT0JZ Fusion of Left Carpometacarpal Joint with Synthetic Substitute, Open Approach

0RGT0KZ Fusion of Left Carpometacarpal Joint with Nonautologous Tissue Substitute, Open Approach

0RGT33Z Fusion of Left Carpometacarpal Joint with Sustained Compression Internal Fixation Device, Percutaneous Approach

0RGT34Z Fusion of Left Carpometacarpal Joint with Internal Fixation Device, Percutaneous Approach

0RGT35Z Fusion of Left Carpometacarpal Joint with External Fixation Device, Percutaneous Approach

0RGT37Z Fusion of Left Carpometacarpal Joint with Autologous Tissue Substitute, Percutaneous Approach

0RGT3JZ Fusion of Left Carpometacarpal Joint with Synthetic Substitute, Percutaneous Approach

0RGT3KZ Fusion of Left Carpometacarpal Joint with Nonautologous Tissue Substitute, Percutaneous Approach

0RGT43Z Fusion of Left Carpometacarpal Joint with Sustained Compression Internal Fixation Device, Percutaneous Endoscopic Approach

0RGT44Z Fusion of Left Carpometacarpal Joint with Internal Fixation Device, Percutaneous Endoscopic Approach

0RGT45Z Fusion of Left Carpometacarpal Joint with External Fixation Device, Percutaneous Endoscopic Approach

0RGT47Z Fusion of Left Carpometacarpal Joint with Autologous Tissue Substitute, Percutaneous Endoscopic Approach

0RGT4JZ Fusion of Left Carpometacarpal Joint with Synthetic Substitute, Percutaneous Endoscopic Approach

0RGT4KZ Fusion of Left Carpometacarpal Joint with Nonautologous Tissue Substitute, Percutaneous Endoscopic Approach

0RGU03Z Fusion of Right Metacarpophalangeal Joint with Sustained Compression Internal Fixation Device, Open Approach

0RGU04Z Fusion of Right Metacarpophalangeal Joint with Internal Fixation Device, Open Approach

0RGU05Z Fusion of Right Metacarpophalangeal Joint with External Fixation Device, Open Approach

0RGU07Z Fusion of Right Metacarpophalangeal Joint with Autologous Tissue Substitute, Open Approach

0RGU0JZ Fusion of Right Metacarpophalangeal Joint with Synthetic Substitute, Open Approach

0RGU0KZ Fusion of Right Metacarpophalangeal Joint with Nonautologous Tissue Substitute, Open Approach

0RGU33Z Fusion of Right Metacarpophalangeal Joint with Sustained Compression Internal Fixation Device, Percutaneous Approach

0RGU34Z Fusion of Right Metacarpophalangeal Joint with Internal Fixation Device, Percutaneous Approach

0RGU35Z Fusion of Right Metacarpophalangeal Joint with External Fixation Device, Percutaneous Approach

0RGU37Z Fusion of Right Metacarpophalangeal Joint with Autologous Tissue Substitute, Percutaneous Approach

0RGU3JZ Fusion of Right Metacarpophalangeal Joint with Synthetic Substitute, Percutaneous Approach

0RGU3KZ Fusion of Right Metacarpophalangeal Joint with Nonautologous Tissue Substitute, Percutaneous Approach

0RGU43Z Fusion of Right Metacarpophalangeal Joint with Sustained Compression Internal Fixation Device, Percutaneous Endoscopic Approach

0RGU44Z Fusion of Right Metacarpophalangeal Joint with Internal Fixation Device, Percutaneous Endoscopic Approach

0RGU45Z Fusion of Right Metacarpophalangeal Joint with External Fixation Device, Percutaneous Endoscopic Approach

0RGU47Z Fusion of Right Metacarpophalangeal Joint with Autologous Tissue Substitute, Percutaneous Endoscopic Approach

0RGU4JZ Fusion of Right Metacarpophalangeal Joint with Synthetic Substitute, Percutaneous Endoscopic Approach

0RGU4KZ Fusion of Right Metacarpophalangeal Joint with Nonautologous Tissue Substitute, Percutaneous Endoscopic Approach

0RGV03Z Fusion of Left Metacarpophalangeal Joint with Sustained Compression Internal Fixation Device, Open Approach

0RGV04Z Fusion of Left Metacarpophalangeal Joint with Internal Fixation Device, Open Approach

0RGV05Z Fusion of Left Metacarpophalangeal Joint with External Fixation Device, Open Approach

0RGV07Z Fusion of Left Metacarpophalangeal Joint with Autologous Tissue Substitute, Open Approach

0RGV0JZ Fusion of Left Metacarpophalangeal Joint with Synthetic Substitute, Open Approach

0RGV0KZ Fusion of Left Metacarpophalangeal Joint with Nonautologous Tissue Substitute, Open Approach

0RGV33Z Fusion of Left Metacarpophalangeal Joint with Sustained Compression Internal Fixation Device, Percutaneous Approach

0RGV34Z Fusion of Left Metacarpophalangeal Joint with Internal Fixation Device, Percutaneous Approach

0RGV35Z Fusion of Left Metacarpophalangeal Joint with External Fixation Device, Percutaneous Approach

0RGV37Z Fusion of Left Metacarpophalangeal Joint with Autologous Tissue Substitute, Percutaneous Approach

0RGV3JZ Fusion of Left Metacarpophalangeal Joint with Synthetic Substitute, Percutaneous Approach

0RGV3KZ Fusion of Left Metacarpophalangeal Joint with Nonautologous Tissue Substitute, Percutaneous Approach

0RGV43Z Fusion of Left Metacarpophalangeal Joint with Sustained Compression Internal Fixation Device, Percutaneous Endoscopic Approach

0RGV44Z Fusion of Left Metacarpophalangeal Joint with Internal Fixation Device, Percutaneous Endoscopic Approach

0RGV45Z Fusion of Left Metacarpophalangeal Joint with External Fixation Device, Percutaneous Endoscopic Approach

0RGV47Z Fusion of Left Metacarpophalangeal Joint with Autologous Tissue Substitute, Percutaneous Endoscopic Approach

0RGV4JZ Fusion of Left Metacarpophalangeal Joint with Synthetic Substitute, Percutaneous Endoscopic Approach

0RGV4KZ Fusion of Left Metacarpophalangeal Joint with Nonautologous Tissue Substitute, Percutaneous Endoscopic Approach

0RGW03Z Fusion of Right Finger Phalangeal Joint with Sustained Compression Internal Fixation Device, Open Approach

0RGW04Z Fusion of Right Finger Phalangeal Joint with Internal Fixation Device, Open Approach

AHA CC: 4Q, 2017, 62

0RGW05Z Fusion of Right Finger Phalangeal Joint with External Fixation Device, Open Approach

0RGW07Z Fusion of Right Finger Phalangeal Joint with Autologous Tissue Substitute, Open Approach

0RGW0JZ Fusion of Right Finger Phalangeal Joint with Synthetic Substitute, Open Approach

0RGW0KZ Fusion of Right Finger Phalangeal Joint with Nonautologous Tissue Substitute, Open Approach

0RGW33Z Fusion of Right Finger Phalangeal Joint with Sustained Compression Internal Fixation Device, Percutaneous Approach

0RGW34Z Fusion of Right Finger Phalangeal Joint with Internal Fixation Device, Percutaneous Approach

0RGW35Z Fusion of Right Finger Phalangeal Joint with External Fixation Device, Percutaneous Approach

0RGW37Z Fusion of Right Finger Phalangeal Joint with Autologous Tissue Substitute, Percutaneous Approach

0RGW3JZ Fusion of Right Finger Phalangeal Joint with Synthetic Substitute, Percutaneous Approach

0RGW3KZ Fusion of Right Finger Phalangeal Joint with Nonautologous Tissue Substitute, Percutaneous Approach

0RGW43Z Fusion of Right Finger Phalangeal Joint with Sustained Compression Internal Fixation Device, Percutaneous Endoscopic Approach

0RGW44Z Fusion of Right Finger Phalangeal Joint with Internal Fixation Device, Percutaneous Endoscopic Approach

0RGW45Z Fusion of Right Finger Phalangeal Joint with External Fixation Device, Percutaneous Endoscopic Approach

0RGW47Z Fusion of Right Finger Phalangeal Joint with Autologous Tissue Substitute, Percutaneous Endoscopic Approach

0RGW4JZ Fusion of Right Finger Phalangeal Joint with Synthetic Substitute, Percutaneous Endoscopic Approach

0RGW4KZ Fusion of Right Finger Phalangeal Joint with Nonautologous Tissue Substitute, Percutaneous Endoscopic Approach

0RGX03Z Fusion of Left Finger Phalangeal Joint with Sustained Compression Internal Fixation Device, Open Approach

0RGX04Z Fusion of Left Finger Phalangeal Joint with Internal Fixation Device, Open Approach

0RGX05Z Fusion of Left Finger Phalangeal Joint with External Fixation Device, Open Approach

0RGX07Z Fusion of Left Finger Phalangeal Joint with Autologous Tissue Substitute, Open Approach

0RGX0JZ Fusion of Left Finger Phalangeal Joint with Synthetic Substitute, Open Approach

0RGX0KZ Fusion of Left Finger Phalangeal Joint with Nonautologous Tissue Substitute, Open Approach

0RGX33Z Fusion of Left Finger Phalangeal Joint with Sustained Compression Internal Fixation Device, Percutaneous Approach

0RGX34Z Fusion of Left Finger Phalangeal Joint with Internal Fixation Device, Percutaneous Approach

0RGX35Z Fusion of Left Finger Phalangeal Joint with External Fixation Device, Percutaneous Approach

0RGX37Z Fusion of Left Finger Phalangeal Joint with Autologous Tissue Substitute, Percutaneous Approach

0RGX3JZ Fusion of Left Finger Phalangeal Joint with Synthetic Substitute, Percutaneous Approach

0RGX3KZ Fusion of Left Finger Phalangeal Joint with Nonautologous Tissue Substitute, Percutaneous Approach

0RGX43Z Fusion of Left Finger Phalangeal Joint with Sustained Compression Internal Fixation Device, Percutaneous Endoscopic Approach

0RGX44Z Fusion of Left Finger Phalangeal Joint with Internal Fixation Device, Percutaneous Endoscopic Approach

0RGX45Z Fusion of Left Finger Phalangeal Joint with External Fixation Device, Percutaneous Endoscopic Approach

0RGX47Z Fusion of Left Finger Phalangeal Joint with Autologous Tissue Substitute, Percutaneous Endoscopic Approach

0RGX4JZ Fusion of Left Finger Phalangeal Joint with Synthetic Substitute, Percutaneous Endoscopic Approach

0RGX4KZ Fusion of Left Finger Phalangeal Joint with Nonautologous Tissue Substitute, Percutaneous Endoscopic Approach

0RH – Upper Joints, Insertion

0RH003Z Insertion of Infusion Device into Occipital-cervical Joint, Open Approach

0RH004Z Insertion of Internal Fixation Device into Occipital-cervical Joint, Open Approach

0RH008Z Insertion of Spacer into Occipital-cervical Joint, Open Approach

0RH00BZ Insertion of Interspinous Process Spinal Stabilization Device into Occipital-cervical Joint, Open Approach

0RH00CZ Insertion of Pedicle-Based Spinal Stabilization Device into Occipital-cervical Joint, Open Approach

0RH00DZ Insertion of Facet Replacement Spinal Stabilization Device into Occipital-cervical Joint, Open Approach

0RH033Z Insertion of Infusion Device into Occipital-cervical Joint, Percutaneous Approach

0RH034Z Insertion of Internal Fixation Device into Occipital-cervical Joint, Percutaneous Approach

0RH038Z Insertion of Spacer into Occipital-cervical Joint, Percutaneous Approach

0RH03BZ Insertion of Interspinous Process Spinal Stabilization Device into Occipital-cervical Joint, Percutaneous Approach

0RH03CZ Insertion of Pedicle-Based Spinal Stabilization Device into Occipital-cervical Joint, Percutaneous Approach

0RH03DZ Insertion of Facet Replacement Spinal Stabilization Device into Occipital-cervical Joint, Percutaneous Approach

0RH043Z Insertion of Infusion Device into Occipital-cervical Joint, Percutaneous Endoscopic Approach

0RH044Z Insertion of Internal Fixation Device into Occipital-cervical Joint, Percutaneous Endoscopic Approach

0RH048Z Insertion of Spacer into Occipital-cervical Joint, Percutaneous Endoscopic Approach

0RH04BZ Insertion of Interspinous Process Spinal Stabilization Device into Occipital-cervical Joint, Percutaneous Endoscopic Approach

0RH04CZ Insertion of Pedicle-Based Spinal Stabilization Device into Occipital-cervical Joint, Percutaneous Endoscopic Approach

0RH04DZ Insertion of Facet Replacement Spinal Stabilization Device into Occipital-cervical Joint, Percutaneous Endoscopic Approach

0RH103Z Insertion of Infusion Device into Cervical Vertebral Joint, Open Approach

0RH104Z Insertion of Internal Fixation Device into Cervical Vertebral Joint, Open Approach

0RH108Z Insertion of Spacer into Cervical Vertebral Joint, Open Approach

0RH10BZ Insertion of Interspinous Process Spinal Stabilization Device into Cervical Vertebral Joint, Open Approach

0RH10CZ Insertion of Pedicle-Based Spinal Stabilization Device into Cervical Vertebral Joint, Open Approach

0RH10DZ Insertion of Facet Replacement Spinal Stabilization Device into Cervical Vertebral Joint, Open Approach

0RH133Z Insertion of Infusion Device into Cervical Vertebral Joint, Percutaneous Approach

0RH134Z Insertion of Internal Fixation Device into Cervical Vertebral Joint, Percutaneous Approach

0RH138Z Insertion of Spacer into Cervical Vertebral Joint, Percutaneous Approach

0RH13BZ Insertion of Interspinous Process Spinal Stabilization Device into Cervical Vertebral Joint, Percutaneous Approach

0RH13CZ Insertion of Pedicle-Based Spinal Stabilization Device into Cervical Vertebral Joint, Percutaneous Approach

0RH13DZ Insertion of Facet Replacement Spinal Stabilization Device into Cervical Vertebral Joint, Percutaneous Approach

0RH143Z Insertion of Infusion Device into Cervical Vertebral Joint, Percutaneous Endoscopic Approach

0RH144Z Insertion of Internal Fixation Device into Cervical Vertebral Joint, Percutaneous Endoscopic Approach

0RH148Z Insertion of Spacer into Cervical Vertebral Joint, Percutaneous Endoscopic Approach

0RH14BZ Insertion of Interspinous Process Spinal Stabilization Device into Cervical Vertebral Joint, Percutaneous Endoscopic Approach

0RH14CZ Insertion of Pedicle-Based Spinal Stabilization Device into Cervical Vertebral Joint, Percutaneous Endoscopic Approach

0RH14DZ Insertion of Facet Replacement Spinal Stabilization Device into Cervical Vertebral Joint, Percutaneous Endoscopic Approach

0RH303Z Insertion of Infusion Device into Cervical Vertebral Disc, Open Approach

0RH333Z Insertion of Infusion Device into Cervical Vertebral Disc, Percutaneous Approach

0RH343Z Insertion of Infusion Device into Cervical Vertebral Disc, Percutaneous Endoscopic Approach

0RH403Z Insertion of Infusion Device into Cervicothoracic Vertebral Joint, Open Approach

♀ Female-only ♂ Male-only ▲ Limited Coverage ● Non-OR ᴴᴬᶜ HAC-associated procedure ▲ Non-covered procedures ✚ Cluster

0RH404Z Insertion of Internal Fixation Device into Cervicothoracic Vertebral Joint, Open Approach

0RH408Z Insertion of Spacer into Cervicothoracic Vertebral Joint, Open Approach

0RH40BZ Insertion of Interspinous Process Spinal Stabilization Device into Cervicothoracic Vertebral Joint, Open Approach

0RH40CZ Insertion of Pedicle-Based Spinal Stabilization Device into Cervicothoracic Vertebral Joint, Open Approach

0RH40DZ Insertion of Facet Replacement Spinal Stabilization Device into Cervicothoracic Vertebral Joint, Open Approach

0RH433Z Insertion of Infusion Device into Cervicothoracic Vertebral Joint, Percutaneous Approach

0RH434Z Insertion of Internal Fixation Device into Cervicothoracic Vertebral Joint, Percutaneous Approach

0RH438Z Insertion of Spacer into Cervicothoracic Vertebral Joint, Percutaneous Approach

0RH43BZ Insertion of Interspinous Process Spinal Stabilization Device into Cervicothoracic Vertebral Joint, Percutaneous Approach

0RH43CZ Insertion of Pedicle-Based Spinal Stabilization Device into Cervicothoracic Vertebral Joint, Percutaneous Approach

0RH43DZ Insertion of Facet Replacement Spinal Stabilization Device into Cervicothoracic Vertebral Joint, Percutaneous Approach

0RH443Z Insertion of Infusion Device into Cervicothoracic Vertebral Joint, Percutaneous Endoscopic Approach

0RH444Z Insertion of Internal Fixation Device into Cervicothoracic Vertebral Joint, Percutaneous Endoscopic Approach

0RH448Z Insertion of Spacer into Cervicothoracic Vertebral Joint, Percutaneous Endoscopic Approach

0RH44BZ Insertion of Interspinous Process Spinal Stabilization Device into Cervicothoracic Vertebral Joint, Percutaneous Endoscopic Approach

0RH44CZ Insertion of Pedicle-Based Spinal Stabilization Device into Cervicothoracic Vertebral Joint, Percutaneous Endoscopic Approach

0RH44DZ Insertion of Facet Replacement Spinal Stabilization Device into Cervicothoracic Vertebral Joint, Percutaneous Endoscopic Approach

0RH503Z Insertion of Infusion Device into Cervicothoracic Vertebral Disc, Open Approach

0RH533Z Insertion of Infusion Device into Cervicothoracic Vertebral Disc, Percutaneous Approach

0RH543Z Insertion of Infusion Device into Cervicothoracic Vertebral Disc, Percutaneous Endoscopic Approach

0RH603Z Insertion of Infusion Device into Thoracic Vertebral Joint, Open Approach

0RH604Z Insertion of Internal Fixation Device into Thoracic Vertebral Joint, Open Approach

0RH608Z Insertion of Spacer into Thoracic Vertebral Joint, Open Approach

0RH60BZ Insertion of Interspinous Process Spinal Stabilization Device into Thoracic Vertebral Joint, Open Approach

0RH60CZ Insertion of Pedicle-Based Spinal Stabilization Device into Thoracic Vertebral Joint, Open Approach

0RH60DZ Insertion of Facet Replacement Spinal Stabilization Device into Thoracic Vertebral Joint, Open Approach

0RH633Z Insertion of Infusion Device into Thoracic Vertebral Joint, Percutaneous Approach

0RH634Z Insertion of Internal Fixation Device into Thoracic Vertebral Joint, Percutaneous Approach

0RH638Z Insertion of Spacer into Thoracic Vertebral Joint, Percutaneous Approach

0RH63BZ Insertion of Interspinous Process Spinal Stabilization Device into Thoracic Vertebral Joint, Percutaneous Approach

0RH63CZ Insertion of Pedicle-Based Spinal Stabilization Device into Thoracic Vertebral Joint, Percutaneous Approach

0RH63DZ Insertion of Facet Replacement Spinal Stabilization Device into Thoracic Vertebral Joint, Percutaneous Approach

0RH643Z Insertion of Infusion Device into Thoracic Vertebral Joint, Percutaneous Endoscopic Approach

0RH644Z Insertion of Internal Fixation Device into Thoracic Vertebral Joint, Percutaneous Endoscopic Approach

0RH648Z Insertion of Spacer into Thoracic Vertebral Joint, Percutaneous Endoscopic Approach

0RH64BZ Insertion of Interspinous Process Spinal Stabilization Device into Thoracic Vertebral Joint, Percutaneous Endoscopic Approach

0RH64CZ Insertion of Pedicle-Based Spinal Stabilization Device into Thoracic Vertebral Joint, Percutaneous Endoscopic Approach

0RH64DZ Insertion of Facet Replacement Spinal Stabilization Device into Thoracic Vertebral Joint, Percutaneous Endoscopic Approach

0RH903Z Insertion of Infusion Device into Thoracic Vertebral Disc, Open Approach

0RH933Z Insertion of Infusion Device into Thoracic Vertebral Disc, Percutaneous Approach

0RH943Z Insertion of Infusion Device into Thoracic Vertebral Disc, Percutaneous Endoscopic Approach

0RHA03Z Insertion of Infusion Device into Thoracolumbar Vertebral Joint, Open Approach

0RHA04Z Insertion of Internal Fixation Device into Thoracolumbar Vertebral Joint, Open Approach

0RHA08Z Insertion of Spacer into Thoracolumbar Vertebral Joint, Open Approach

0RHA0BZ Insertion of Interspinous Process Spinal Stabilization Device into Thoracolumbar Vertebral Joint, Open Approach

0RHA0CZ Insertion of Pedicle-Based Spinal Stabilization Device into Thoracolumbar Vertebral Joint, Open Approach

0RHA0DZ Insertion of Facet Replacement Spinal Stabilization Device into Thoracolumbar Vertebral Joint, Open Approach

0RHA33Z Insertion of Infusion Device into Thoracolumbar Vertebral Joint, Percutaneous Approach

0RHA34Z Insertion of Internal Fixation Device into Thoracolumbar Vertebral Joint, Percutaneous Approach

0RHA38Z Insertion of Spacer into Thoracolumbar Vertebral Joint, Percutaneous Approach

0RHA3BZ Insertion of Interspinous Process Spinal Stabilization Device into Thoracolumbar Vertebral Joint, Percutaneous Approach

0RHA3CZ Insertion of Pedicle-Based Spinal Stabilization Device into Thoracolumbar Vertebral Joint, Percutaneous Approach

0RHA3DZ Insertion of Facet Replacement Spinal Stabilization Device into Thoracolumbar Vertebral Joint, Percutaneous Approach

0RHA43Z Insertion of Infusion Device into Thoracolumbar Vertebral Joint, Percutaneous Endoscopic Approach

0RHA44Z Insertion of Internal Fixation Device into Thoracolumbar Vertebral Joint, Percutaneous Endoscopic Approach

0RHA48Z Insertion of Spacer into Thoracolumbar Vertebral Joint, Percutaneous Endoscopic Approach

0RHA4BZ Insertion of Interspinous Process Spinal Stabilization Device into Thoracolumbar Vertebral Joint, Percutaneous Endoscopic Approach

0RHA4CZ Insertion of Pedicle-Based Spinal Stabilization Device into Thoracolumbar Vertebral Joint, Percutaneous Endoscopic Approach

0RHA4DZ Insertion of Facet Replacement Spinal Stabilization Device into Thoracolumbar Vertebral Joint, Percutaneous Endoscopic Approach

0RHB03Z Insertion of Infusion Device into Thoracolumbar Vertebral Disc, Open Approach

0RHB33Z Insertion of Infusion Device into Thoracolumbar Vertebral Disc, Percutaneous Approach

0RHB43Z Insertion of Infusion Device into Thoracolumbar Vertebral Disc, Percutaneous Endoscopic Approach

0RHC03Z Insertion of Infusion Device into Right Temporomandibular Joint, Open Approach

0RHC04Z Insertion of Internal Fixation Device into Right Temporomandibular Joint, Open Approach

0RHC08Z Insertion of Spacer into Right Temporomandibular Joint, Open Approach

0RHC33Z Insertion of Infusion Device into Right Temporomandibular Joint, Percutaneous Approach

0RHC34Z Insertion of Internal Fixation Device into Right Temporomandibular Joint, Percutaneous Approach

---

♀ Female-only   ♂ Male-only   ▲ Limited Coverage   ● Non-OR   ▦ HAC-associated procedure   ▲ Non-covered procedures   ✚ Cluster   **1083**

0RHC38Z	Insertion of Spacer into Right Temporomandibular Joint, Percutaneous Approach
0RHC43Z	Insertion of Infusion Device into Right Temporomandibular Joint, Percutaneous Endoscopic Approach
0RHC44Z	Insertion of Internal Fixation Device into Right Temporomandibular Joint, Percutaneous Endoscopic Approach
0RHC48Z	Insertion of Spacer into Right Temporomandibular Joint, Percutaneous Endoscopic Approach
0RHD03Z	Insertion of Infusion Device into Left Temporomandibular Joint, Open Approach
0RHD04Z	Insertion of Internal Fixation Device into Left Temporomandibular Joint, Open Approach
0RHD08Z	Insertion of Spacer into Left Temporomandibular Joint, Open Approach
0RHD33Z	Insertion of Infusion Device into Left Temporomandibular Joint, Percutaneous Approach
0RHD34Z	Insertion of Internal Fixation Device into Left Temporomandibular Joint, Percutaneous Approach
0RHD38Z	Insertion of Spacer into Left Temporomandibular Joint, Percutaneous Approach
0RHD43Z	Insertion of Infusion Device into Left Temporomandibular Joint, Percutaneous Endoscopic Approach
0RHD44Z	Insertion of Internal Fixation Device into Left Temporomandibular Joint, Percutaneous Endoscopic Approach
0RHD48Z	Insertion of Spacer into Left Temporomandibular Joint, Percutaneous Endoscopic Approach
0RHE03Z	Insertion of Infusion Device into Right Sternoclavicular Joint, Open Approach
0RHE04Z	Insertion of Internal Fixation Device into Right Sternoclavicular Joint, Open Approach
0RHE08Z	Insertion of Spacer into Right Sternoclavicular Joint, Open Approach
0RHE33Z	Insertion of Infusion Device into Right Sternoclavicular Joint, Percutaneous Approach
0RHE34Z	Insertion of Internal Fixation Device into Right Sternoclavicular Joint, Percutaneous Approach
0RHE38Z	Insertion of Spacer into Right Sternoclavicular Joint, Percutaneous Approach
0RHE43Z	Insertion of Infusion Device into Right Sternoclavicular Joint, Percutaneous Endoscopic Approach
0RHE44Z	Insertion of Internal Fixation Device into Right Sternoclavicular Joint, Percutaneous Endoscopic Approach
0RHE48Z	Insertion of Spacer into Right Sternoclavicular Joint, Percutaneous Endoscopic Approach
0RHF03Z	Insertion of Infusion Device into Left Sternoclavicular Joint, Open Approach
0RHF04Z	Insertion of Internal Fixation Device into Left Sternoclavicular Joint, Open Approach
0RHF08Z	Insertion of Spacer into Left Sternoclavicular Joint, Open Approach
0RHF33Z	Insertion of Infusion Device into Left Sternoclavicular Joint, Percutaneous Approach
0RHF34Z	Insertion of Internal Fixation Device into Left Sternoclavicular Joint, Percutaneous Approach
0RHF38Z	Insertion of Spacer into Left Sternoclavicular Joint, Percutaneous Approach
0RHF43Z	Insertion of Infusion Device into Left Sternoclavicular Joint, Percutaneous Endoscopic Approach
0RHF44Z	Insertion of Internal Fixation Device into Left Sternoclavicular Joint, Percutaneous Endoscopic Approach
0RHF48Z	Insertion of Spacer into Left Sternoclavicular Joint, Percutaneous Endoscopic Approach
0RHG03Z	Insertion of Infusion Device into Right Acromioclavicular Joint, Open Approach
0RHG04Z	Insertion of Internal Fixation Device into Right Acromioclavicular Joint, Open Approach
0RHG08Z	Insertion of Spacer into Right Acromioclavicular Joint, Open Approach
0RHG33Z	Insertion of Infusion Device into Right Acromioclavicular Joint, Percutaneous Approach
0RHG34Z	Insertion of Internal Fixation Device into Right Acromioclavicular Joint, Percutaneous Approach
0RHG38Z	Insertion of Spacer into Right Acromioclavicular Joint, Percutaneous Approach
0RHG43Z	Insertion of Infusion Device into Right Acromioclavicular Joint, Percutaneous Endoscopic Approach
0RHG44Z	Insertion of Internal Fixation Device into Right Acromioclavicular Joint, Percutaneous Endoscopic Approach
0RHG48Z	Insertion of Spacer into Right Acromioclavicular Joint, Percutaneous Endoscopic Approach
0RHH03Z	Insertion of Infusion Device into Left Acromioclavicular Joint, Open Approach
0RHH04Z	Insertion of Internal Fixation Device into Left Acromioclavicular Joint, Open Approach
0RHH08Z	Insertion of Spacer into Left Acromioclavicular Joint, Open Approach
0RHH33Z	Insertion of Infusion Device into Left Acromioclavicular Joint, Percutaneous Approach
0RHH34Z	Insertion of Internal Fixation Device into Left Acromioclavicular Joint, Percutaneous Approach
0RHH38Z	Insertion of Spacer into Left Acromioclavicular Joint, Percutaneous Approach
0RHH43Z	Insertion of Infusion Device into Left Acromioclavicular Joint, Percutaneous Endoscopic Approach
0RHH44Z	Insertion of Internal Fixation Device into Left Acromioclavicular Joint, Percutaneous Endoscopic Approach
0RHH48Z	Insertion of Spacer into Left Acromioclavicular Joint, Percutaneous Endoscopic Approach
0RHJ03Z	Insertion of Infusion Device into Right Shoulder Joint, Open Approach
0RHJ04Z	Insertion of Internal Fixation Device into Right Shoulder Joint, Open Approach
	AHA CC: 3Q, 2016, 32-33
0RHJ08Z	Insertion of Spacer into Right Shoulder Joint, Open Approach
0RHJ33Z	Insertion of Infusion Device into Right Shoulder Joint, Percutaneous Approach
0RHJ34Z	Insertion of Internal Fixation Device into Right Shoulder Joint, Percutaneous Approach
0RHJ38Z	Insertion of Spacer into Right Shoulder Joint, Percutaneous Approach
0RHJ43Z	Insertion of Infusion Device into Right Shoulder Joint, Percutaneous Endoscopic Approach
0RHJ44Z	Insertion of Internal Fixation Device into Right Shoulder Joint, Percutaneous Endoscopic Approach
0RHJ48Z	Insertion of Spacer into Right Shoulder Joint, Percutaneous Endoscopic Approach
0RHK03Z	Insertion of Infusion Device into Left Shoulder Joint, Open Approach
0RHK04Z	Insertion of Internal Fixation Device into Left Shoulder Joint, Open Approach
0RHK08Z	Insertion of Spacer into Left Shoulder Joint, Open Approach
0RHK33Z	Insertion of Infusion Device into Left Shoulder Joint, Percutaneous Approach
0RHK34Z	Insertion of Internal Fixation Device into Left Shoulder Joint, Percutaneous Approach
0RHK38Z	Insertion of Spacer into Left Shoulder Joint, Percutaneous Approach
0RHK43Z	Insertion of Infusion Device into Left Shoulder Joint, Percutaneous Endoscopic Approach
0RHK44Z	Insertion of Internal Fixation Device into Left Shoulder Joint, Percutaneous Endoscopic Approach
0RHK48Z	Insertion of Spacer into Left Shoulder Joint, Percutaneous Endoscopic Approach
0RHL03Z	Insertion of Infusion Device into Right Elbow Joint, Open Approach
0RHL04Z	Insertion of Internal Fixation Device into Right Elbow Joint, Open Approach
0RHL05Z	Insertion of External Fixation Device into Right Elbow Joint, Open Approach
0RHL08Z	Insertion of Spacer into Right Elbow Joint, Open Approach
0RHL33Z	Insertion of Infusion Device into Right Elbow Joint, Percutaneous Approach
0RHL34Z	Insertion of Internal Fixation Device into Right Elbow Joint, Percutaneous Approach
0RHL35Z	Insertion of External Fixation Device into Right Elbow Joint, Percutaneous Approach
0RHL38Z	Insertion of Spacer into Right Elbow Joint, Percutaneous Approach
0RHL43Z	Insertion of Infusion Device into Right Elbow Joint, Percutaneous Endoscopic Approach
0RHL44Z	Insertion of Internal Fixation Device into Right Elbow Joint, Percutaneous Endoscopic Approach
0RHL45Z	Insertion of External Fixation Device into Right Elbow Joint, Percutaneous Endoscopic Approach
0RHL48Z	Insertion of Spacer into Right Elbow Joint, Percutaneous Endoscopic Approach
0RHM03Z	Insertion of Infusion Device into Left Elbow Joint, Open Approach
0RHM04Z	Insertion of Internal Fixation Device into Left Elbow Joint, Open Approach

♀ Female-only   ♂ Male-only   ▲ Limited Coverage   ● Non-OR   ▥ HAC-associated procedure   ▲ Non-covered procedures   ✚ Cluster

0RHM05Z Insertion of External Fixation Device into Left Elbow Joint, Open Approach

0RHM08Z Insertion of Spacer into Left Elbow Joint, Open Approach

0RHM33Z Insertion of Infusion Device into Left Elbow Joint, Percutaneous Approach

0RHM34Z Insertion of Internal Fixation Device into Left Elbow Joint, Percutaneous Approach

0RHM35Z Insertion of External Fixation Device into Left Elbow Joint, Percutaneous Approach

0RHM38Z Insertion of Spacer into Left Elbow Joint, Percutaneous Approach

0RHM43Z Insertion of Infusion Device into Left Elbow Joint, Percutaneous Endoscopic Approach

0RHM44Z Insertion of Internal Fixation Device into Left Elbow Joint, Percutaneous Endoscopic Approach

0RHM45Z Insertion of External Fixation Device into Left Elbow Joint, Percutaneous Endoscopic Approach

0RHM48Z Insertion of Spacer into Left Elbow Joint, Percutaneous Endoscopic Approach

0RHN03Z Insertion of Infusion Device into Right Wrist Joint, Open Approach

0RHN04Z Insertion of Internal Fixation Device into Right Wrist Joint, Open Approach

0RHN05Z Insertion of External Fixation Device into Right Wrist Joint, Open Approach

0RHN08Z Insertion of Spacer into Right Wrist Joint, Open Approach

0RHN33Z Insertion of Infusion Device into Right Wrist Joint, Percutaneous Approach

0RHN34Z Insertion of Internal Fixation Device into Right Wrist Joint, Percutaneous Approach

0RHN35Z Insertion of External Fixation Device into Right Wrist Joint, Percutaneous Approach

0RHN38Z Insertion of Spacer into Right Wrist Joint, Percutaneous Approach

0RHN43Z Insertion of Infusion Device into Right Wrist Joint, Percutaneous Endoscopic Approach

0RHN44Z Insertion of Internal Fixation Device into Right Wrist Joint, Percutaneous Endoscopic Approach

0RHN45Z Insertion of External Fixation Device into Right Wrist Joint, Percutaneous Endoscopic Approach

0RHN48Z Insertion of Spacer into Right Wrist Joint, Percutaneous Endoscopic Approach

0RHP03Z Insertion of Infusion Device into Left Wrist Joint, Open Approach

0RHP04Z Insertion of Internal Fixation Device into Left Wrist Joint, Open Approach

0RHP05Z Insertion of External Fixation Device into Left Wrist Joint, Open Approach

0RHP08Z Insertion of Spacer into Left Wrist Joint, Open Approach

0RHP33Z Insertion of Infusion Device into Left Wrist Joint, Percutaneous Approach

0RHP34Z Insertion of Internal Fixation Device into Left Wrist Joint, Percutaneous Approach

0RHP35Z Insertion of External Fixation Device into Left Wrist Joint, Percutaneous Approach

0RHP38Z Insertion of Spacer into Left Wrist Joint, Percutaneous Approach

0RHP43Z Insertion of Infusion Device into Left Wrist Joint, Percutaneous Endoscopic Approach

0RHP44Z Insertion of Internal Fixation Device into Left Wrist Joint, Percutaneous Endoscopic Approach

0RHP45Z Insertion of External Fixation Device into Left Wrist Joint, Percutaneous Endoscopic Approach

0RHP48Z Insertion of Spacer into Left Wrist Joint, Percutaneous Endoscopic Approach

0RHQ03Z Insertion of Infusion Device into Right Carpal Joint, Open Approach

0RHQ04Z Insertion of Internal Fixation Device into Right Carpal Joint, Open Approach

0RHQ05Z Insertion of External Fixation Device into Right Carpal Joint, Open Approach

0RHQ08Z Insertion of Spacer into Right Carpal Joint, Open Approach

0RHQ33Z Insertion of Infusion Device into Right Carpal Joint, Percutaneous Approach

0RHQ34Z Insertion of Internal Fixation Device into Right Carpal Joint, Percutaneous Approach

0RHQ35Z Insertion of External Fixation Device into Right Carpal Joint, Percutaneous Approach

0RHQ38Z Insertion of Spacer into Right Carpal Joint, Percutaneous Approach

0RHQ43Z Insertion of Infusion Device into Right Carpal Joint, Percutaneous Endoscopic Approach

0RHQ44Z Insertion of Internal Fixation Device into Right Carpal Joint, Percutaneous Endoscopic Approach

0RHQ45Z Insertion of External Fixation Device into Right Carpal Joint, Percutaneous Endoscopic Approach

0RHQ48Z Insertion of Spacer into Right Carpal Joint, Percutaneous Endoscopic Approach

0RHR03Z Insertion of Infusion Device into Left Carpal Joint, Open Approach

0RHR04Z Insertion of Internal Fixation Device into Left Carpal Joint, Open Approach

0RHR05Z Insertion of External Fixation Device into Left Carpal Joint, Open Approach

0RHR08Z Insertion of Spacer into Left Carpal Joint, Open Approach

0RHR33Z Insertion of Infusion Device into Left Carpal Joint, Percutaneous Approach

0RHR34Z Insertion of Internal Fixation Device into Left Carpal Joint, Percutaneous Approach

0RHR35Z Insertion of External Fixation Device into Left Carpal Joint, Percutaneous Approach

0RHR38Z Insertion of Spacer into Left Carpal Joint, Percutaneous Approach

0RHR43Z Insertion of Infusion Device into Left Carpal Joint, Percutaneous Endoscopic Approach

0RHR44Z Insertion of Internal Fixation Device into Left Carpal Joint, Percutaneous Endoscopic Approach

0RHR45Z Insertion of External Fixation Device into Left Carpal Joint, Percutaneous Endoscopic Approach

0RHR48Z Insertion of Spacer into Left Carpal Joint, Percutaneous Endoscopic Approach

0RHS03Z Insertion of Infusion Device into Right Carpometacarpal Joint, Open Approach

0RHS04Z Insertion of Internal Fixation Device into Right Carpometacarpal Joint, Open Approach

0RHS05Z Insertion of External Fixation Device into Right Carpometacarpal Joint, Open Approach

0RHS08Z Insertion of Spacer into Right Carpometacarpal Joint, Open Approach

0RHS33Z Insertion of Infusion Device into Right Carpometacarpal Joint, Percutaneous Approach

0RHS34Z Insertion of Internal Fixation Device into Right Carpometacarpal Joint, Percutaneous Approach

0RHS35Z Insertion of External Fixation Device into Right Carpometacarpal Joint, Percutaneous Approach

0RHS38Z Insertion of Spacer into Right Carpometacarpal Joint, Percutaneous Approach

0RHS43Z Insertion of Infusion Device into Right Carpometacarpal Joint, Percutaneous Endoscopic Approach

0RHS44Z Insertion of Internal Fixation Device into Right Carpometacarpal Joint, Percutaneous Endoscopic Approach

0RHS45Z Insertion of External Fixation Device into Right Carpometacarpal Joint, Percutaneous Endoscopic Approach

0RHS48Z Insertion of Spacer into Right Carpometacarpal Joint, Percutaneous Endoscopic Approach

0RHT03Z Insertion of Infusion Device into Left Carpometacarpal Joint, Open Approach

0RHT04Z Insertion of Internal Fixation Device into Left Carpometacarpal Joint, Open Approach

0RHT05Z Insertion of External Fixation Device into Left Carpometacarpal Joint, Open Approach

0RHT08Z Insertion of Spacer into Left Carpometacarpal Joint, Open Approach

0RHT33Z Insertion of Infusion Device into Left Carpometacarpal Joint, Percutaneous Approach

0RHT34Z Insertion of Internal Fixation Device into Left Carpometacarpal Joint, Percutaneous Approach

0RHT35Z Insertion of External Fixation Device into Left Carpometacarpal Joint, Percutaneous Approach

0RHT38Z Insertion of Spacer into Left Carpometacarpal Joint, Percutaneous Approach

0RHT43Z Insertion of Infusion Device into Left Carpometacarpal Joint, Percutaneous Endoscopic Approach

0RHT44Z Insertion of Internal Fixation Device into Left Carpometacarpal Joint, Percutaneous Endoscopic Approach

0RHT45Z Insertion of External Fixation Device into Left Carpometacarpal Joint, Percutaneous Endoscopic Approach

0RHT48Z Insertion of Spacer into Left Carpometacarpal Joint, Percutaneous Endoscopic Approach

0RHU03Z Insertion of Infusion Device into Right Metacarpophalangeal Joint, Open Approach

0RHU04Z Insertion of Internal Fixation Device into Right Metacarpophalangeal Joint, Open Approach

0RHU05Z Insertion of External Fixation Device into Right Metacarpophalangeal Joint, Open Approach

0RHU08Z Insertion of Spacer into Right Metacarpophalangeal Joint, Open Approach

0RHU33Z Insertion of Infusion Device into Right Metacarpophalangeal Joint, Percutaneous Approach

0RHU34Z Insertion of Internal Fixation Device into Right Metacarpophalangeal Joint, Percutaneous Approach

0RHU35Z Insertion of External Fixation Device into Right Metacarpophalangeal Joint, Percutaneous Approach

0RHU38Z Insertion of Spacer into Right Metacarpophalangeal Joint, Percutaneous Approach

0RHU43Z Insertion of Infusion Device into Right Metacarpophalangeal Joint, Percutaneous Endoscopic Approach

0RHU44Z Insertion of Internal Fixation Device into Right Metacarpophalangeal Joint, Percutaneous Endoscopic Approach

0RHU45Z Insertion of External Fixation Device into Right Metacarpophalangeal Joint, Percutaneous Endoscopic Approach

0RHU48Z Insertion of Spacer into Right Metacarpophalangeal Joint, Percutaneous Endoscopic Approach

0RHV03Z Insertion of Infusion Device into Left Metacarpophalangeal Joint, Open Approach

0RHV04Z Insertion of Internal Fixation Device into Left Metacarpophalangeal Joint, Open Approach

0RHV05Z Insertion of External Fixation Device into Left Metacarpophalangeal Joint, Open Approach

0RHV08Z Insertion of Spacer into Left Metacarpophalangeal Joint, Open Approach

0RHV33Z Insertion of Infusion Device into Left Metacarpophalangeal Joint, Percutaneous Approach

0RHV34Z Insertion of Internal Fixation Device into Left Metacarpophalangeal Joint, Percutaneous Approach

0RHV35Z Insertion of External Fixation Device into Left Metacarpophalangeal Joint, Percutaneous Approach

0RHV38Z Insertion of Spacer into Left Metacarpophalangeal Joint, Percutaneous Approach

0RHV43Z Insertion of Infusion Device into Left Metacarpophalangeal Joint, Percutaneous Endoscopic Approach

0RHV44Z Insertion of Internal Fixation Device into Left Metacarpophalangeal Joint, Percutaneous Endoscopic Approach

0RHV45Z Insertion of External Fixation Device into Left Metacarpophalangeal Joint, Percutaneous Endoscopic Approach

0RHV48Z Insertion of Spacer into Left Metacarpophalangeal Joint, Percutaneous Endoscopic Approach

0RHW03Z Insertion of Infusion Device into Right Finger Phalangeal Joint, Open Approach

0RHW04Z Insertion of Internal Fixation Device into Right Finger Phalangeal Joint, Open Approach

0RHW05Z Insertion of External Fixation Device into Right Finger Phalangeal Joint, Open Approach

0RHW08Z Insertion of Spacer into Right Finger Phalangeal Joint, Open Approach

0RHW33Z Insertion of Infusion Device into Right Finger Phalangeal Joint, Percutaneous Approach

0RHW34Z Insertion of Internal Fixation Device into Right Finger Phalangeal Joint, Percutaneous Approach

0RHW35Z Insertion of External Fixation Device into Right Finger Phalangeal Joint, Percutaneous Approach

0RHW38Z Insertion of Spacer into Right Finger Phalangeal Joint, Percutaneous Approach

0RHW43Z Insertion of Infusion Device into Right Finger Phalangeal Joint, Percutaneous Endoscopic Approach

0RHW44Z Insertion of Internal Fixation Device into Right Finger Phalangeal Joint, Percutaneous Endoscopic Approach

0RHW45Z Insertion of External Fixation Device into Right Finger Phalangeal Joint, Percutaneous Endoscopic Approach

0RHW48Z Insertion of Spacer into Right Finger Phalangeal Joint, Percutaneous Endoscopic Approach

0RHX03Z Insertion of Infusion Device into Left Finger Phalangeal Joint, Open Approach

0RHX04Z Insertion of Internal Fixation Device into Left Finger Phalangeal Joint, Open Approach

0RHX05Z Insertion of External Fixation Device into Left Finger Phalangeal Joint, Open Approach

0RHX08Z Insertion of Spacer into Left Finger Phalangeal Joint, Open Approach

0RHX33Z Insertion of Infusion Device into Left Finger Phalangeal Joint, Percutaneous Approach

0RHX34Z Insertion of Internal Fixation Device into Left Finger Phalangeal Joint, Percutaneous Approach

0RHX35Z Insertion of External Fixation Device into Left Finger Phalangeal Joint, Percutaneous Approach

0RHX38Z Insertion of Spacer into Left Finger Phalangeal Joint, Percutaneous Approach

0RHX43Z Insertion of Infusion Device into Left Finger Phalangeal Joint, Percutaneous Endoscopic Approach

0RHX44Z Insertion of Internal Fixation Device into Left Finger Phalangeal Joint, Percutaneous Endoscopic Approach

0RHX45Z Insertion of External Fixation Device into Left Finger Phalangeal Joint, Percutaneous Endoscopic Approach

0RHX48Z Insertion of Spacer into Left Finger Phalangeal Joint, Percutaneous Endoscopic Approach

0RJ – Upper Joints, Inspection

Review Coding Guideline B3.5

Review Coding Guidelines B3.11a, B3.11b and B3.11c

0RJ00ZZ Inspection of Occipital-cervical Joint, Open Approach

0RJ03ZZ Inspection of Occipital-cervical Joint, Percutaneous Approach

0RJ04ZZ Inspection of Occipital-cervical Joint, Percutaneous Endoscopic Approach

0RJ0XZZ Inspection of Occipital-cervical Joint, External Approach

0RJ10ZZ Inspection of Cervical Vertebral Joint, Open Approach

0RJ13ZZ Inspection of Cervical Vertebral Joint, Percutaneous Approach

0RJ14ZZ Inspection of Cervical Vertebral Joint, Percutaneous Endoscopic Approach

0RJ1XZZ Inspection of Cervical Vertebral Joint, External Approach

0RJ30ZZ Inspection of Cervical Vertebral Disc, Open Approach

0RJ33ZZ Inspection of Cervical Vertebral Disc, Percutaneous Approach

0RJ34ZZ Inspection of Cervical Vertebral Disc, Percutaneous Endoscopic Approach

0RJ3XZZ Inspection of Cervical Vertebral Disc, External Approach

0RJ40ZZ Inspection of Cervicothoracic Vertebral Joint, Open Approach

0RJ43ZZ Inspection of Cervicothoracic Vertebral Joint, Percutaneous Approach

0RJ44ZZ Inspection of Cervicothoracic Vertebral Joint, Percutaneous Endoscopic Approach

0RJ4XZZ Inspection of Cervicothoracic Vertebral Joint, External Approach

0RJ50ZZ Inspection of Cervicothoracic Vertebral Disc, Open Approach

0RJ53ZZ Inspection of Cervicothoracic Vertebral Disc, Percutaneous Approach

0RJ54ZZ Inspection of Cervicothoracic Vertebral Disc, Percutaneous Endoscopic Approach

0RJ5XZZ Inspection of Cervicothoracic Vertebral Disc, External Approach

0RJ60ZZ Inspection of Thoracic Vertebral Joint, Open Approach

0RJ63ZZ Inspection of Thoracic Vertebral Joint, Percutaneous Approach

0RJ64ZZ Inspection of Thoracic Vertebral Joint, Percutaneous Endoscopic Approach

0RJ6XZZ Inspection of Thoracic Vertebral Joint, External Approach

0RJ90ZZ Inspection of Thoracic Vertebral Disc, Open Approach

0RJ93ZZ Inspection of Thoracic Vertebral Disc, Percutaneous Approach

0RJ94ZZ Inspection of Thoracic Vertebral Disc, Percutaneous Endoscopic Approach

0RJ9XZZ Inspection of Thoracic Vertebral Disc, External Approach

0RJA0ZZ Inspection of Thoracolumbar Vertebral Joint, Open Approach

0RJA3ZZ Inspection of Thoracolumbar Vertebral Joint, Percutaneous Approach

0RJA4ZZ Inspection of Thoracolumbar Vertebral Joint, Percutaneous Endoscopic Approach

0RJAXZZ Inspection of Thoracolumbar Vertebral Joint, External Approach

♀ Female-only   ♂ Male-only   ▲ Limited Coverage   ● Non-OR   ▦ HAC-associated procedure   ▲ Non-covered procedures   ✚ Cluster

0RJB0ZZ Inspection of Thoracolumbar Vertebral Disc, Open Approach

0RJB3ZZ Inspection of Thoracolumbar Vertebral Disc, Percutaneous Approach

0RJB4ZZ Inspection of Thoracolumbar Vertebral Disc, Percutaneous Endoscopic Approach

0RJBXZZ Inspection of Thoracolumbar Vertebral Disc, External Approach

0RJC0ZZ Inspection of Right Temporomandibular Joint, Open Approach

0RJC3ZZ Inspection of Right Temporomandibular Joint, Percutaneous Approach

0RJC4ZZ Inspection of Right Temporomandibular Joint, Percutaneous Endoscopic Approach

0RJCXZZ Inspection of Right Temporomandibular Joint, External Approach

0RJD0ZZ Inspection of Left Temporomandibular Joint, Open Approach

0RJD3ZZ Inspection of Left Temporomandibular Joint, Percutaneous Approach

0RJD4ZZ Inspection of Left Temporomandibular Joint, Percutaneous Endoscopic Approach

0RJDXZZ Inspection of Left Temporomandibular Joint, External Approach

0RJE0ZZ Inspection of Right Sternoclavicular Joint, Open Approach

0RJE3ZZ Inspection of Right Sternoclavicular Joint, Percutaneous Approach

0RJE4ZZ Inspection of Right Sternoclavicular Joint, Percutaneous Endoscopic Approach

0RJEXZZ Inspection of Right Sternoclavicular Joint, External Approach

0RJF0ZZ Inspection of Left Sternoclavicular Joint, Open Approach

0RJF3ZZ Inspection of Left Sternoclavicular Joint, Percutaneous Approach

0RJF4ZZ Inspection of Left Sternoclavicular Joint, Percutaneous Endoscopic Approach

0RJFXZZ Inspection of Left Sternoclavicular Joint, External Approach

0RJG0ZZ Inspection of Right Acromioclavicular Joint, Open Approach

0RJG3ZZ Inspection of Right Acromioclavicular Joint, Percutaneous Approach

0RJG4ZZ Inspection of Right Acromioclavicular Joint, Percutaneous Endoscopic Approach

0RJGXZZ Inspection of Right Acromioclavicular Joint, External Approach

0RJH0ZZ Inspection of Left Acromioclavicular Joint, Open Approach

0RJH3ZZ Inspection of Left Acromioclavicular Joint, Percutaneous Approach

0RJH4ZZ Inspection of Left Acromioclavicular Joint, Percutaneous Endoscopic Approach

0RJHXZZ Inspection of Left Acromioclavicular Joint, External Approach

0RJJ0ZZ Inspection of Right Shoulder Joint, Open Approach

0RJJ3ZZ Inspection of Right Shoulder Joint, Percutaneous Approach

0RJJ4ZZ Inspection of Right Shoulder Joint, Percutaneous Endoscopic Approach

0RJJXZZ Inspection of Right Shoulder Joint, External Approach

0RJK0ZZ Inspection of Left Shoulder Joint, Open Approach

0RJK3ZZ Inspection of Left Shoulder Joint, Percutaneous Approach

0RJK4ZZ Inspection of Left Shoulder Joint, Percutaneous Endoscopic Approach

0RJKXZZ Inspection of Left Shoulder Joint, External Approach

0RJL0ZZ Inspection of Right Elbow Joint, Open Approach

0RJL3ZZ Inspection of Right Elbow Joint, Percutaneous Approach

0RJL4ZZ Inspection of Right Elbow Joint, Percutaneous Endoscopic Approach

0RJLXZZ Inspection of Right Elbow Joint, External Approach

0RJM0ZZ Inspection of Left Elbow Joint, Open Approach

0RJM3ZZ Inspection of Left Elbow Joint, Percutaneous Approach

0RJM4ZZ Inspection of Left Elbow Joint, Percutaneous Endoscopic Approach

0RJMXZZ Inspection of Left Elbow Joint, External Approach

0RJN0ZZ Inspection of Right Wrist Joint, Open Approach

0RJN3ZZ Inspection of Right Wrist Joint, Percutaneous Approach

0RJN4ZZ Inspection of Right Wrist Joint, Percutaneous Endoscopic Approach

0RJNXZZ Inspection of Right Wrist Joint, External Approach

0RJP0ZZ Inspection of Left Wrist Joint, Open Approach

0RJP3ZZ Inspection of Left Wrist Joint, Percutaneous Approach

0RJP4ZZ Inspection of Left Wrist Joint, Percutaneous Endoscopic Approach

0RJPXZZ Inspection of Left Wrist Joint, External Approach

0RJQ0ZZ Inspection of Right Carpal Joint, Open Approach

0RJQ3ZZ Inspection of Right Carpal Joint, Percutaneous Approach

0RJQ4ZZ Inspection of Right Carpal Joint, Percutaneous Endoscopic Approach

0RJQXZZ Inspection of Right Carpal Joint, External Approach

0RJR0ZZ Inspection of Left Carpal Joint, Open Approach

0RJR3ZZ Inspection of Left Carpal Joint, Percutaneous Approach

0RJR4ZZ Inspection of Left Carpal Joint, Percutaneous Endoscopic Approach

0RJRXZZ Inspection of Left Carpal Joint, External Approach

0RJS0ZZ Inspection of Right Carpometacarpal Joint, Open Approach

0RJS3ZZ Inspection of Right Carpometacarpal Joint, Percutaneous Approach

0RJS4ZZ Inspection of Right Carpometacarpal Joint, Percutaneous Endoscopic Approach

0RJSXZZ Inspection of Right Carpometacarpal Joint, External Approach

0RJT0ZZ Inspection of Left Carpometacarpal Joint, Open Approach

0RJT3ZZ Inspection of Left Carpometacarpal Joint, Percutaneous Approach

0RJT4ZZ Inspection of Left Carpometacarpal Joint, Percutaneous Endoscopic Approach

0RJTXZZ Inspection of Left Carpometacarpal Joint, External Approach

0RJU0ZZ Inspection of Right Metacarpophalangeal Joint, Open Approach

0RJU3ZZ Inspection of Right Metacarpophalangeal Joint, Percutaneous Approach

0RJU4ZZ Inspection of Right Metacarpophalangeal Joint, Percutaneous Endoscopic Approach

0RJUXZZ Inspection of Right Metacarpophalangeal Joint, External Approach

0RJV0ZZ Inspection of Left Metacarpophalangeal Joint, Open Approach

0RJV3ZZ Inspection of Left Metacarpophalangeal Joint, Percutaneous Approach

0RJV4ZZ Inspection of Left Metacarpophalangeal Joint, Percutaneous Endoscopic Approach

0RJVXZZ Inspection of Left Metacarpophalangeal Joint, External Approach

0RJW0ZZ Inspection of Right Finger Phalangeal Joint, Open Approach

0RJW3ZZ Inspection of Right Finger Phalangeal Joint, Percutaneous Approach

0RJW4ZZ Inspection of Right Finger Phalangeal Joint, Percutaneous Endoscopic Approach

0RJWXZZ Inspection of Right Finger Phalangeal Joint, External Approach

0RJX0ZZ Inspection of Left Finger Phalangeal Joint, Open Approach

0RJX3ZZ Inspection of Left Finger Phalangeal Joint, Percutaneous Approach

0RJX4ZZ Inspection of Left Finger Phalangeal Joint, Percutaneous Endoscopic Approach

0RJXXZZ Inspection of Left Finger Phalangeal Joint, External Approach

0RN – Upper Joints, Release

Review Coding Guideline B3.13

0RN00ZZ Release Occipital-cervical Joint, Open Approach

0RN03ZZ Release Occipital-cervical Joint, Percutaneous Approach

0RN04ZZ Release Occipital-cervical Joint, Percutaneous Endoscopic Approach

0RN0XZZ Release Occipital-cervical Joint, External Approach

0RN10ZZ Release Cervical Vertebral Joint, Open Approach

0RN13ZZ Release Cervical Vertebral Joint, Percutaneous Approach

0RN14ZZ Release Cervical Vertebral Joint, Percutaneous Endoscopic Approach

0RN1XZZ Release Cervical Vertebral Joint, External Approach

0RN30ZZ Release Cervical Vertebral Disc, Open Approach

0RN33ZZ Release Cervical Vertebral Disc, Percutaneous Approach

0RN34ZZ Release Cervical Vertebral Disc, Percutaneous Endoscopic Approach

0RN3XZZ Release Cervical Vertebral Disc, External Approach

♀ Female-only   ♂ Male-only   ▲ Limited Coverage   ● Non-OR   ▥ HAC-associated procedure   ▲ Non-covered procedures   ✚ Cluster

0RN40ZZ	Release Cervicothoracic Vertebral Joint, Open Approach
0RN43ZZ	Release Cervicothoracic Vertebral Joint, Percutaneous Approach
0RN44ZZ	Release Cervicothoracic Vertebral Joint, Percutaneous Endoscopic Approach
0RN4XZZ	Release Cervicothoracic Vertebral Joint, External Approach
0RN50ZZ	Release Cervicothoracic Vertebral Disc, Open Approach
0RN53ZZ	Release Cervicothoracic Vertebral Disc, Percutaneous Approach
0RN54ZZ	Release Cervicothoracic Vertebral Disc, Percutaneous Endoscopic Approach
0RN5XZZ	Release Cervicothoracic Vertebral Disc, External Approach
0RN60ZZ	Release Thoracic Vertebral Joint, Open Approach
0RN63ZZ	Release Thoracic Vertebral Joint, Percutaneous Approach
0RN64ZZ	Release Thoracic Vertebral Joint, Percutaneous Endoscopic Approach
0RN6XZZ	Release Thoracic Vertebral Joint, External Approach
0RN90ZZ	Release Thoracic Vertebral Disc, Open Approach
0RN93ZZ	Release Thoracic Vertebral Disc, Percutaneous Approach
0RN94ZZ	Release Thoracic Vertebral Disc, Percutaneous Endoscopic Approach
0RN9XZZ	Release Thoracic Vertebral Disc, External Approach
0RNA0ZZ	Release Thoracolumbar Vertebral Joint, Open Approach
0RNA3ZZ	Release Thoracolumbar Vertebral Joint, Percutaneous Approach
0RNA4ZZ	Release Thoracolumbar Vertebral Joint, Percutaneous Endoscopic Approach
0RNAXZZ	Release Thoracolumbar Vertebral Joint, External Approach
0RNB0ZZ	Release Thoracolumbar Vertebral Disc, Open Approach
0RNB3ZZ	Release Thoracolumbar Vertebral Disc, Percutaneous Approach
0RNB4ZZ	Release Thoracolumbar Vertebral Disc, Percutaneous Endoscopic Approach
0RNBXZZ	Release Thoracolumbar Vertebral Disc, External Approach
0RNC0ZZ	Release Right Temporomandibular Joint, Open Approach
0RNC3ZZ	Release Right Temporomandibular Joint, Percutaneous Approach
0RNC4ZZ	Release Right Temporomandibular Joint, Percutaneous Endoscopic Approach
0RNCXZZ	Release Right Temporomandibular Joint, External Approach
0RND0ZZ	Release Left Temporomandibular Joint, Open Approach
0RND3ZZ	Release Left Temporomandibular Joint, Percutaneous Approach
0RND4ZZ	Release Left Temporomandibular Joint, Percutaneous Endoscopic Approach
0RNDXZZ	Release Left Temporomandibular Joint, External Approach
0RNE0ZZ	Release Right Sternoclavicular Joint, Open Approach
0RNE3ZZ	Release Right Sternoclavicular Joint, Percutaneous Approach
0RNE4ZZ	Release Right Sternoclavicular Joint, Percutaneous Endoscopic Approach
0RNEXZZ	Release Right Sternoclavicular Joint, External Approach
0RNF0ZZ	Release Left Sternoclavicular Joint, Open Approach
0RNF3ZZ	Release Left Sternoclavicular Joint, Percutaneous Approach
0RNF4ZZ	Release Left Sternoclavicular Joint, Percutaneous Endoscopic Approach
0RNFXZZ	Release Left Sternoclavicular Joint, External Approach
0RNG0ZZ	Release Right Acromioclavicular Joint, Open Approach
0RNG3ZZ	Release Right Acromioclavicular Joint, Percutaneous Approach
0RNG4ZZ	Release Right Acromioclavicular Joint, Percutaneous Endoscopic Approach
0RNGXZZ	Release Right Acromioclavicular Joint, External Approach
0RNH0ZZ	Release Left Acromioclavicular Joint, Open Approach
0RNH3ZZ	Release Left Acromioclavicular Joint, Percutaneous Approach
0RNH4ZZ	Release Left Acromioclavicular Joint, Percutaneous Endoscopic Approach
0RNHXZZ	Release Left Acromioclavicular Joint, External Approach
0RNJ0ZZ	Release Right Shoulder Joint, Open Approach
0RNJ3ZZ	Release Right Shoulder Joint, Percutaneous Approach
0RNJ4ZZ	Release Right Shoulder Joint, Percutaneous Endoscopic Approach
	AHA CC: 3Q, 2016, 32-33
0RNJXZZ	Release Right Shoulder Joint, External Approach
0RNK0ZZ	Release Left Shoulder Joint, Open Approach
0RNK3ZZ	Release Left Shoulder Joint, Percutaneous Approach
0RNK4ZZ	Release Left Shoulder Joint, Percutaneous Endoscopic Approach
	AHA CC: 2Q, 2015, 22-23
0RNKXZZ	Release Left Shoulder Joint, External Approach
0RNL0ZZ	Release Right Elbow Joint, Open Approach
0RNL3ZZ	Release Right Elbow Joint, Percutaneous Approach
0RNL4ZZ	Release Right Elbow Joint, Percutaneous Endoscopic Approach
0RNLXZZ	Release Right Elbow Joint, External Approach
0RNM0ZZ	Release Left Elbow Joint, Open Approach
0RNM3ZZ	Release Left Elbow Joint, Percutaneous Approach
0RNM4ZZ	Release Left Elbow Joint, Percutaneous Endoscopic Approach
0RNMXZZ	Release Left Elbow Joint, External Approach
0RNN0ZZ	Release Right Wrist Joint, Open Approach
0RNN3ZZ	Release Right Wrist Joint, Percutaneous Approach
0RNN4ZZ	Release Right Wrist Joint, Percutaneous Endoscopic Approach
0RNNXZZ	Release Right Wrist Joint, External Approach
0RNP0ZZ	Release Left Wrist Joint, Open Approach
0RNP3ZZ	Release Left Wrist Joint, Percutaneous Approach
0RNP4ZZ	Release Left Wrist Joint, Percutaneous Endoscopic Approach
0RNPXZZ	Release Left Wrist Joint, External Approach
0RNQ0ZZ	Release Right Carpal Joint, Open Approach
0RNQ3ZZ	Release Right Carpal Joint, Percutaneous Approach
0RNQ4ZZ	Release Right Carpal Joint, Percutaneous Endoscopic Approach
0RNQXZZ	Release Right Carpal Joint, External Approach
0RNR0ZZ	Release Left Carpal Joint, Open Approach
0RNR3ZZ	Release Left Carpal Joint, Percutaneous Approach
0RNR4ZZ	Release Left Carpal Joint, Percutaneous Endoscopic Approach
0RNRXZZ	Release Left Carpal Joint, External Approach
0RNS0ZZ	Release Right Carpometacarpal Joint, Open Approach
0RNS3ZZ	Release Right Carpometacarpal Joint, Percutaneous Approach
0RNS4ZZ	Release Right Carpometacarpal Joint, Percutaneous Endoscopic Approach
0RNSXZZ	Release Right Carpometacarpal Joint, External Approach
0RNT0ZZ	Release Left Carpometacarpal Joint, Open Approach
0RNT3ZZ	Release Left Carpometacarpal Joint, Percutaneous Approach
0RNT4ZZ	Release Left Carpometacarpal Joint, Percutaneous Endoscopic Approach
0RNTXZZ	Release Left Carpometacarpal Joint, External Approach
0RNU0ZZ	Release Right Metacarpophalangeal Joint, Open Approach
0RNU3ZZ	Release Right Metacarpophalangeal Joint, Percutaneous Approach
0RNU4ZZ	Release Right Metacarpophalangeal Joint, Percutaneous Endoscopic Approach
0RNUXZZ	Release Right Metacarpophalangeal Joint, External Approach
0RNV0ZZ	Release Left Metacarpophalangeal Joint, Open Approach
0RNV3ZZ	Release Left Metacarpophalangeal Joint, Percutaneous Approach
0RNV4ZZ	Release Left Metacarpophalangeal Joint, Percutaneous Endoscopic Approach
0RNVXZZ	Release Left Metacarpophalangeal Joint, External Approach
0RNW0ZZ	Release Right Finger Phalangeal Joint, Open Approach
0RNW3ZZ	Release Right Finger Phalangeal Joint, Percutaneous Approach
0RNW4ZZ	Release Right Finger Phalangeal Joint, Percutaneous Endoscopic Approach
0RNWXZZ	Release Right Finger Phalangeal Joint, External Approach
0RNX0ZZ	Release Left Finger Phalangeal Joint, Open Approach
0RNX3ZZ	Release Left Finger Phalangeal Joint, Percutaneous Approach
0RNX4ZZ	Release Left Finger Phalangeal Joint, Percutaneous Endoscopic Approach
0RNXXZZ	Release Left Finger Phalangeal Joint, External Approach

♀ Female-only   ♂ Male-only   ▲ Limited Coverage   ● Non-OR   HAC HAC-associated procedure   ▲ Non-covered procedures   ✚ Cluster

Review Coding Guideline B6.1c

0RP000Z Removal of Drainage Device from Occipital-cervical Joint, Open Approach

0RP003Z Removal of Infusion Device from Occipital-cervical Joint, Open Approach

0RP004Z Removal of Internal Fixation Device from Occipital-cervical Joint, Open Approach

0RP007Z Removal of Autologous Tissue Substitute from Occipital-cervical Joint, Open Approach

0RP008Z Removal of Spacer from Occipital-cervical Joint, Open Approach

0RP00AZ Removal of Interbody Fusion Device from Occipital-cervical Joint, Open Approach

0RP00JZ Removal of Synthetic Substitute from Occipital-cervical Joint, Open Approach

0RP00KZ Removal of Nonautologous Tissue Substitute from Occipital-cervical Joint, Open Approach

0RP030Z Removal of Drainage Device from Occipital-cervical Joint, Percutaneous Approach

0RP033Z Removal of Infusion Device from Occipital-cervical Joint, Percutaneous Approach

0RP034Z Removal of Internal Fixation Device from Occipital-cervical Joint, Percutaneous Approach

0RP037Z Removal of Autologous Tissue Substitute from Occipital-cervical Joint, Percutaneous Approach

0RP038Z Removal of Spacer from Occipital-cervical Joint, Percutaneous Approach

0RP03AZ Removal of Interbody Fusion Device from Occipital-cervical Joint, Percutaneous Approach

0RP03JZ Removal of Synthetic Substitute from Occipital-cervical Joint, Percutaneous Approach

0RP03KZ Removal of Nonautologous Tissue Substitute from Occipital-cervical Joint, Percutaneous Approach

0RP040Z Removal of Drainage Device from Occipital-cervical Joint, Percutaneous Endoscopic Approach

0RP043Z Removal of Infusion Device from Occipital-cervical Joint, Percutaneous Endoscopic Approach

0RP044Z Removal of Internal Fixation Device from Occipital-cervical Joint, Percutaneous Endoscopic Approach

0RP047Z Removal of Autologous Tissue Substitute from Occipital-cervical Joint, Percutaneous Endoscopic Approach

0RP048Z Removal of Spacer from Occipital-cervical Joint, Percutaneous Endoscopic Approach

0RP04AZ Removal of Interbody Fusion Device from Occipital-cervical Joint, Percutaneous Endoscopic Approach

0RP04JZ Removal of Synthetic Substitute from Occipital-cervical Joint, Percutaneous Endoscopic Approach

0RP04KZ Removal of Nonautologous Tissue Substitute from Occipital-cervical Joint, Percutaneous Endoscopic Approach

0RP0X0Z Removal of Drainage Device from Occipital-cervical Joint, External Approach

0RP0X3Z Removal of Infusion Device from Occipital-cervical Joint, External Approach

0RP0X4Z Removal of Internal Fixation Device from Occipital-cervical Joint, External Approach

0RP100Z Removal of Drainage Device from Cervical Vertebral Joint, Open Approach

0RP103Z Removal of Infusion Device from Cervical Vertebral Joint, Open Approach

0RP104Z Removal of Internal Fixation Device from Cervical Vertebral Joint, Open Approach

0RP107Z Removal of Autologous Tissue Substitute from Cervical Vertebral Joint, Open Approach

0RP108Z Removal of Spacer from Cervical Vertebral Joint, Open Approach

0RP10AZ Removal of Interbody Fusion Device from Cervical Vertebral Joint, Open Approach

0RP10JZ Removal of Synthetic Substitute from Cervical Vertebral Joint, Open Approach

0RP10KZ Removal of Nonautologous Tissue Substitute from Cervical Vertebral Joint, Open Approach

0RP130Z Removal of Drainage Device from Cervical Vertebral Joint, Percutaneous Approach

0RP133Z Removal of Infusion Device from Cervical Vertebral Joint, Percutaneous Approach

0RP134Z Removal of Internal Fixation Device from Cervical Vertebral Joint, Percutaneous Approach

0RP137Z Removal of Autologous Tissue Substitute from Cervical Vertebral Joint, Percutaneous Approach

0RP138Z Removal of Spacer from Cervical Vertebral Joint, Percutaneous Approach

0RP13AZ Removal of Interbody Fusion Device from Cervical Vertebral Joint, Percutaneous Approach

0RP13JZ Removal of Synthetic Substitute from Cervical Vertebral Joint, Percutaneous Approach

0RP13KZ Removal of Nonautologous Tissue Substitute from Cervical Vertebral Joint, Percutaneous Approach

0RP140Z Removal of Drainage Device from Cervical Vertebral Joint, Percutaneous Endoscopic Approach

0RP143Z Removal of Infusion Device from Cervical Vertebral Joint, Percutaneous Endoscopic Approach

0RP144Z Removal of Internal Fixation Device from Cervical Vertebral Joint, Percutaneous Endoscopic Approach

0RP147Z Removal of Autologous Tissue Substitute from Cervical Vertebral Joint, Percutaneous Endoscopic Approach

0RP148Z Removal of Spacer from Cervical Vertebral Joint, Percutaneous Endoscopic Approach

0RP14AZ Removal of Interbody Fusion Device from Cervical Vertebral Joint, Percutaneous Endoscopic Approach

0RP14JZ Removal of Synthetic Substitute from Cervical Vertebral Joint, Percutaneous Endoscopic Approach

0RP14KZ Removal of Nonautologous Tissue Substitute from Cervical Vertebral Joint, Percutaneous Endoscopic Approach

0RP1X0Z Removal of Drainage Device from Cervical Vertebral Joint, External Approach

0RP1X3Z Removal of Infusion Device from Cervical Vertebral Joint, External Approach

0RP1X4Z Removal of Internal Fixation Device from Cervical Vertebral Joint, External Approach

0RP300Z Removal of Drainage Device from Cervical Vertebral Disc, Open Approach

0RP303Z Removal of Infusion Device from Cervical Vertebral Disc, Open Approach

0RP307Z Removal of Autologous Tissue Substitute from Cervical Vertebral Disc, Open Approach

0RP30JZ Removal of Synthetic Substitute from Cervical Vertebral Disc, Open Approach

0RP30KZ Removal of Nonautologous Tissue Substitute from Cervical Vertebral Disc, Open Approach

0RP330Z Removal of Drainage Device from Cervical Vertebral Disc, Percutaneous Approach

0RP333Z Removal of Infusion Device from Cervical Vertebral Disc, Percutaneous Approach

0RP337Z Removal of Autologous Tissue Substitute from Cervical Vertebral Disc, Percutaneous Approach

0RP33JZ Removal of Synthetic Substitute from Cervical Vertebral Disc, Percutaneous Approach

0RP33KZ Removal of Nonautologous Tissue Substitute from Cervical Vertebral Disc, Percutaneous Approach

0RP340Z Removal of Drainage Device from Cervical Vertebral Disc, Percutaneous Endoscopic Approach

0RP343Z Removal of Infusion Device from Cervical Vertebral Disc, Percutaneous Endoscopic Approach

0RP347Z Removal of Autologous Tissue Substitute from Cervical Vertebral Disc, Percutaneous Endoscopic Approach

0RP34JZ Removal of Synthetic Substitute from Cervical Vertebral Disc, Percutaneous Endoscopic Approach

0RP34KZ Removal of Nonautologous Tissue Substitute from Cervical Vertebral Disc, Percutaneous Endoscopic Approach

0RP3X0Z Removal of Drainage Device from Cervical Vertebral Disc, External Approach

0RP3X3Z Removal of Infusion Device from Cervical Vertebral Disc, External Approach

0RP400Z Removal of Drainage Device from Cervicothoracic Vertebral Joint, Open Approach

0RP403Z Removal of Infusion Device from Cervicothoracic Vertebral Joint, Open Approach

0RP404Z Removal of Internal Fixation Device from Cervicothoracic Vertebral Joint, Open Approach

0RP407Z Removal of Autologous Tissue Substitute from Cervicothoracic Vertebral Joint, Open Approach

0RP408Z Removal of Spacer from Cervicothoracic Vertebral Joint, Open Approach

0RP40AZ Removal of Interbody Fusion Device from Cervicothoracic Vertebral Joint, Open Approach

0RP40JZ Removal of Synthetic Substitute from Cervicothoracic Vertebral Joint, Open Approach

0RP40KZ Removal of Nonautologous Tissue Substitute from Cervicothoracic Vertebral Joint, Open Approach

0RP430Z Removal of Drainage Device from Cervicothoracic Vertebral Joint, Percutaneous Approach

0RP433Z Removal of Infusion Device from Cervicothoracic Vertebral Joint, Percutaneous Approach

0RP434Z Removal of Internal Fixation Device from Cervicothoracic Vertebral Joint, Percutaneous Approach

0RP437Z Removal of Autologous Tissue Substitute from Cervicothoracic Vertebral Joint, Percutaneous Approach

0RP438Z Removal of Spacer from Cervicothoracic Vertebral Joint, Percutaneous Approach

0RP43AZ Removal of Interbody Fusion Device from Cervicothoracic Vertebral Joint, Percutaneous Approach

0RP43JZ Removal of Synthetic Substitute from Cervicothoracic Vertebral Joint, Percutaneous Approach

0RP43KZ Removal of Nonautologous Tissue Substitute from Cervicothoracic Vertebral Joint, Percutaneous Approach

0RP440Z Removal of Drainage Device from Cervicothoracic Vertebral Joint, Percutaneous Endoscopic Approach

0RP443Z Removal of Infusion Device from Cervicothoracic Vertebral Joint, Percutaneous Endoscopic Approach

0RP444Z Removal of Internal Fixation Device from Cervicothoracic Vertebral Joint, Percutaneous Endoscopic Approach

0RP447Z Removal of Autologous Tissue Substitute from Cervicothoracic Vertebral Joint, Percutaneous Endoscopic Approach

0RP448Z Removal of Spacer from Cervicothoracic Vertebral Joint, Percutaneous Endoscopic Approach

0RP44AZ Removal of Interbody Fusion Device from Cervicothoracic Vertebral Joint, Percutaneous Endoscopic Approach

0RP44JZ Removal of Synthetic Substitute from Cervicothoracic Vertebral Joint, Percutaneous Endoscopic Approach

0RP44KZ Removal of Nonautologous Tissue Substitute from Cervicothoracic Vertebral Joint, Percutaneous Endoscopic Approach

0RP4X0Z Removal of Drainage Device from Cervicothoracic Vertebral Joint, External Approach

0RP4X3Z Removal of Infusion Device from Cervicothoracic Vertebral Joint, External Approach

0RP4X4Z Removal of Internal Fixation Device from Cervicothoracic Vertebral Joint, External Approach

0RP500Z Removal of Drainage Device from Cervicothoracic Vertebral Disc, Open Approach

0RP503Z Removal of Infusion Device from Cervicothoracic Vertebral Disc, Open Approach

0RP507Z Removal of Autologous Tissue Substitute from Cervicothoracic Vertebral Disc, Open Approach

0RP50JZ Removal of Synthetic Substitute from Cervicothoracic Vertebral Disc, Open Approach

0RP50KZ Removal of Nonautologous Tissue Substitute from Cervicothoracic Vertebral Disc, Open Approach

0RP530Z Removal of Drainage Device from Cervicothoracic Vertebral Disc, Percutaneous Approach

0RP533Z Removal of Infusion Device from Cervicothoracic Vertebral Disc, Percutaneous Approach

0RP537Z Removal of Autologous Tissue Substitute from Cervicothoracic Vertebral Disc, Percutaneous Approach

0RP53JZ Removal of Synthetic Substitute from Cervicothoracic Vertebral Disc, Percutaneous Approach

0RP53KZ Removal of Nonautologous Tissue Substitute from Cervicothoracic Vertebral Disc, Percutaneous Approach

0RP540Z Removal of Drainage Device from Cervicothoracic Vertebral Disc, Percutaneous Endoscopic Approach

0RP543Z Removal of Infusion Device from Cervicothoracic Vertebral Disc, Percutaneous Endoscopic Approach

0RP547Z Removal of Autologous Tissue Substitute from Cervicothoracic Vertebral Disc, Percutaneous Endoscopic Approach

0RP54JZ Removal of Synthetic Substitute from Cervicothoracic Vertebral Disc, Percutaneous Endoscopic Approach

0RP54KZ Removal of Nonautologous Tissue Substitute from Cervicothoracic Vertebral Disc, Percutaneous Endoscopic Approach

0RP5X0Z Removal of Drainage Device from Cervicothoracic Vertebral Disc, External Approach

0RP5X3Z Removal of Infusion Device from Cervicothoracic Vertebral Disc, External Approach

0RP600Z Removal of Drainage Device from Thoracic Vertebral Joint, Open Approach

0RP603Z Removal of Infusion Device from Thoracic Vertebral Joint, Open Approach

0RP604Z Removal of Internal Fixation Device from Thoracic Vertebral Joint, Open Approach

0RP607Z Removal of Autologous Tissue Substitute from Thoracic Vertebral Joint, Open Approach

0RP608Z Removal of Spacer from Thoracic Vertebral Joint, Open Approach

0RP60AZ Removal of Interbody Fusion Device from Thoracic Vertebral Joint, Open Approach

0RP60JZ Removal of Synthetic Substitute from Thoracic Vertebral Joint, Open Approach

0RP60KZ Removal of Nonautologous Tissue Substitute from Thoracic Vertebral Joint, Open Approach

0RP630Z Removal of Drainage Device from Thoracic Vertebral Joint, Percutaneous Approach

0RP633Z Removal of Infusion Device from Thoracic Vertebral Joint, Percutaneous Approach

0RP634Z Removal of Internal Fixation Device from Thoracic Vertebral Joint, Percutaneous Approach

0RP637Z Removal of Autologous Tissue Substitute from Thoracic Vertebral Joint, Percutaneous Approach

0RP638Z Removal of Spacer from Thoracic Vertebral Joint, Percutaneous Approach

0RP63AZ Removal of Interbody Fusion Device from Thoracic Vertebral Joint, Percutaneous Approach

0RP63JZ Removal of Synthetic Substitute from Thoracic Vertebral Joint, Percutaneous Approach

0RP63KZ Removal of Nonautologous Tissue Substitute from Thoracic Vertebral Joint, Percutaneous Approach

0RP640Z Removal of Drainage Device from Thoracic Vertebral Joint, Percutaneous Endoscopic Approach

0RP643Z Removal of Infusion Device from Thoracic Vertebral Joint, Percutaneous Endoscopic Approach

0RP644Z Removal of Internal Fixation Device from Thoracic Vertebral Joint, Percutaneous Endoscopic Approach

0RP647Z Removal of Autologous Tissue Substitute from Thoracic Vertebral Joint, Percutaneous Endoscopic Approach

0RP648Z Removal of Spacer from Thoracic Vertebral Joint, Percutaneous Endoscopic Approach

0RP64AZ Removal of Interbody Fusion Device from Thoracic Vertebral Joint, Percutaneous Endoscopic Approach

0RP64JZ Removal of Synthetic Substitute from Thoracic Vertebral Joint, Percutaneous Endoscopic Approach

0RP64KZ Removal of Nonautologous Tissue Substitute from Thoracic Vertebral Joint, Percutaneous Endoscopic Approach

0RP6X0Z Removal of Drainage Device from Thoracic Vertebral Joint, External Approach

0RP6X3Z Removal of Infusion Device from Thoracic Vertebral Joint, External Approach

0RP6X4Z Removal of Internal Fixation Device from Thoracic Vertebral Joint, External Approach

0RP900Z Removal of Drainage Device from Thoracic Vertebral Disc, Open Approach

0RP903Z Removal of Infusion Device from Thoracic Vertebral Disc, Open Approach

0RP907Z Removal of Autologous Tissue Substitute from Thoracic Vertebral Disc, Open Approach

♀ Female-only   ♂ Male-only   ▲ Limited Coverage   ● Non-OR   HAC HAC-associated procedure   ▲ Non-covered procedures   ✚ Cluster

0RP90JZ Removal of Synthetic Substitute from Thoracic Vertebral Disc, Open Approach

0RP90KZ Removal of Nonautologous Tissue Substitute from Thoracic Vertebral Disc, Open Approach

0RP930Z Removal of Drainage Device from Thoracic Vertebral Disc, Percutaneous Approach

0RP933Z Removal of Infusion Device from Thoracic Vertebral Disc, Percutaneous Approach

0RP937Z Removal of Autologous Tissue Substitute from Thoracic Vertebral Disc, Percutaneous Approach

0RP93JZ Removal of Synthetic Substitute from Thoracic Vertebral Disc, Percutaneous Approach

0RP93KZ Removal of Nonautologous Tissue Substitute from Thoracic Vertebral Disc, Percutaneous Approach

0RP940Z Removal of Drainage Device from Thoracic Vertebral Disc, Percutaneous Endoscopic Approach

0RP943Z Removal of Infusion Device from Thoracic Vertebral Disc, Percutaneous Endoscopic Approach

0RP947Z Removal of Autologous Tissue Substitute from Thoracic Vertebral Disc, Percutaneous Endoscopic Approach

0RP94JZ Removal of Synthetic Substitute from Thoracic Vertebral Disc, Percutaneous Endoscopic Approach

0RP94KZ Removal of Nonautologous Tissue Substitute from Thoracic Vertebral Disc, Percutaneous Endoscopic Approach

0RP9X0Z Removal of Drainage Device from Thoracic Vertebral Disc, External Approach

0RP9X3Z Removal of Infusion Device from Thoracic Vertebral Disc, External Approach

0RPA00Z Removal of Drainage Device from Thoracolumbar Vertebral Joint, Open Approach

0RPA03Z Removal of Infusion Device from Thoracolumbar Vertebral Joint, Open Approach

0RPA04Z Removal of Internal Fixation Device from Thoracolumbar Vertebral Joint, Open Approach

0RPA07Z Removal of Autologous Tissue Substitute from Thoracolumbar Vertebral Joint, Open Approach

0RPA08Z Removal of Spacer from Thoracolumbar Vertebral Joint, Open Approach

0RPA0AZ Removal of Interbody Fusion Device from Thoracolumbar Vertebral Joint, Open Approach

0RPA0JZ Removal of Synthetic Substitute from Thoracolumbar Vertebral Joint, Open Approach

0RPA0KZ Removal of Nonautologous Tissue Substitute from Thoracolumbar Vertebral Joint, Open Approach

0RPA30Z Removal of Drainage Device from Thoracolumbar Vertebral Joint, Percutaneous Approach

0RPA33Z Removal of Infusion Device from Thoracolumbar Vertebral Joint, Percutaneous Approach

0RPA34Z Removal of Internal Fixation Device from Thoracolumbar Vertebral Joint, Percutaneous Approach

0RPA37Z Removal of Autologous Tissue Substitute from Thoracolumbar Vertebral Joint, Percutaneous Approach

0RPA38Z Removal of Spacer from Thoracolumbar Vertebral Joint, Percutaneous Approach

0RPA3AZ Removal of Interbody Fusion Device from Thoracolumbar Vertebral Joint, Percutaneous Approach

0RPA3JZ Removal of Synthetic Substitute from Thoracolumbar Vertebral Joint, Percutaneous Approach

0RPA3KZ Removal of Nonautologous Tissue Substitute from Thoracolumbar Vertebral Joint, Percutaneous Approach

0RPA40Z Removal of Drainage Device from Thoracolumbar Vertebral Joint, Percutaneous Endoscopic Approach

0RPA43Z Removal of Infusion Device from Thoracolumbar Vertebral Joint, Percutaneous Endoscopic Approach

0RPA44Z Removal of Internal Fixation Device from Thoracolumbar Vertebral Joint, Percutaneous Endoscopic Approach

0RPA47Z Removal of Autologous Tissue Substitute from Thoracolumbar Vertebral Joint, Percutaneous Endoscopic Approach

0RPA48Z Removal of Spacer from Thoracolumbar Vertebral Joint, Percutaneous Endoscopic Approach

0RPA4AZ Removal of Interbody Fusion Device from Thoracolumbar Vertebral Joint, Percutaneous Endoscopic Approach

0RPA4JZ Removal of Synthetic Substitute from Thoracolumbar Vertebral Joint, Percutaneous Endoscopic Approach

0RPA4KZ Removal of Nonautologous Tissue Substitute from Thoracolumbar Vertebral Joint, Percutaneous Endoscopic Approach

0RPAX0Z Removal of Drainage Device from Thoracolumbar Vertebral Joint, External Approach

0RPAX3Z Removal of Infusion Device from Thoracolumbar Vertebral Joint, External Approach

0RPAX4Z Removal of Internal Fixation Device from Thoracolumbar Vertebral Joint, External Approach

0RPB00Z Removal of Drainage Device from Thoracolumbar Vertebral Disc, Open Approach

0RPB03Z Removal of Infusion Device from Thoracolumbar Vertebral Disc, Open Approach

0RPB07Z Removal of Autologous Tissue Substitute from Thoracolumbar Vertebral Disc, Open Approach

0RPB0JZ Removal of Synthetic Substitute from Thoracolumbar Vertebral Disc, Open Approach

0RPB0KZ Removal of Nonautologous Tissue Substitute from Thoracolumbar Vertebral Disc, Open Approach

0RPB30Z Removal of Drainage Device from Thoracolumbar Vertebral Disc, Percutaneous Approach

0RPB33Z Removal of Infusion Device from Thoracolumbar Vertebral Disc, Percutaneous Approach

0RPB37Z Removal of Autologous Tissue Substitute from Thoracolumbar Vertebral Disc, Percutaneous Approach

0RPB3JZ Removal of Synthetic Substitute from Thoracolumbar Vertebral Disc, Percutaneous Approach

0RPB3KZ Removal of Nonautologous Tissue Substitute from Thoracolumbar Vertebral Disc, Percutaneous Approach

0RPB40Z Removal of Drainage Device from Thoracolumbar Vertebral Disc, Percutaneous Endoscopic Approach

0RPB43Z Removal of Infusion Device from Thoracolumbar Vertebral Disc, Percutaneous Endoscopic Approach

0RPB47Z Removal of Autologous Tissue Substitute from Thoracolumbar Vertebral Disc, Percutaneous Endoscopic Approach

0RPB4JZ Removal of Synthetic Substitute from Thoracolumbar Vertebral Disc, Percutaneous Endoscopic Approach

0RPB4KZ Removal of Nonautologous Tissue Substitute from Thoracolumbar Vertebral Disc, Percutaneous Endoscopic Approach

0RPBX0Z Removal of Drainage Device from Thoracolumbar Vertebral Disc, External Approach

0RPBX3Z Removal of Infusion Device from Thoracolumbar Vertebral Disc, External Approach

0RPC00Z Removal of Drainage Device from Right Temporomandibular Joint, Open Approach

0RPC03Z Removal of Infusion Device from Right Temporomandibular Joint, Open Approach

0RPC04Z Removal of Internal Fixation Device from Right Temporomandibular Joint, Open Approach

0RPC07Z Removal of Autologous Tissue Substitute from Right Temporomandibular Joint, Open Approach

0RPC08Z Removal of Spacer from Right Temporomandibular Joint, Open Approach

0RPC0JZ Removal of Synthetic Substitute from Right Temporomandibular Joint, Open Approach

0RPC0KZ Removal of Nonautologous Tissue Substitute from Right Temporomandibular Joint, Open Approach

0RPC30Z Removal of Drainage Device from Right Temporomandibular Joint, Percutaneous Approach

0RPC33Z Removal of Infusion Device from Right Temporomandibular Joint, Percutaneous Approach

0RPC34Z Removal of Internal Fixation Device from Right Temporomandibular Joint, Percutaneous Approach

0RPC37Z Removal of Autologous Tissue Substitute from Right Temporomandibular Joint, Percutaneous Approach

0RPC38Z Removal of Spacer from Right Temporomandibular Joint, Percutaneous Approach

0RPC3JZ Removal of Synthetic Substitute from Right Temporomandibular Joint, Percutaneous Approach

0RPC3KZ Removal of Nonautologous Tissue Substitute from Right Temporomandibular Joint, Percutaneous Approach

0RPC40Z Removal of Drainage Device from Right Temporomandibular Joint, Percutaneous Endoscopic Approach

0RPC43Z Removal of Infusion Device from Right Temporomandibular Joint, Percutaneous Endoscopic Approach

0RPC44Z Removal of Internal Fixation Device from Right Temporomandibular Joint, Percutaneous Endoscopic Approach

0RPC47Z Removal of Autologous Tissue Substitute from Right Temporomandibular Joint, Percutaneous Endoscopic Approach

0RPC48Z Removal of Spacer from Right Temporomandibular Joint, Percutaneous Endoscopic Approach

0RPC4JZ Removal of Synthetic Substitute from Right Temporomandibular Joint, Percutaneous Endoscopic Approach

0RPC4KZ Removal of Nonautologous Tissue Substitute from Right Temporomandibular Joint, Percutaneous Endoscopic Approach

0RPCX0Z Removal of Drainage Device from Right Temporomandibular Joint, External Approach

0RPCX3Z Removal of Infusion Device from Right Temporomandibular Joint, External Approach

0RPCX4Z Removal of Internal Fixation Device from Right Temporomandibular Joint, External Approach

0RPD00Z Removal of Drainage Device from Left Temporomandibular Joint, Open Approach

0RPD03Z Removal of Infusion Device from Left Temporomandibular Joint, Open Approach

0RPD04Z Removal of Internal Fixation Device from Left Temporomandibular Joint, Open Approach

0RPD07Z Removal of Autologous Tissue Substitute from Left Temporomandibular Joint, Open Approach

0RPD08Z Removal of Spacer from Left Temporomandibular Joint, Open Approach

0RPD0JZ Removal of Synthetic Substitute from Left Temporomandibular Joint, Open Approach

0RPD0KZ Removal of Nonautologous Tissue Substitute from Left Temporomandibular Joint, Open Approach

0RPD30Z Removal of Drainage Device from Left Temporomandibular Joint, Percutaneous Approach

0RPD33Z Removal of Infusion Device from Left Temporomandibular Joint, Percutaneous Approach

0RPD34Z Removal of Internal Fixation Device from Left Temporomandibular Joint, Percutaneous Approach

0RPD37Z Removal of Autologous Tissue Substitute from Left Temporomandibular Joint, Percutaneous Approach

0RPD38Z Removal of Spacer from Left Temporomandibular Joint, Percutaneous Approach

0RPD3JZ Removal of Synthetic Substitute from Left Temporomandibular Joint, Percutaneous Approach

0RPD3KZ Removal of Nonautologous Tissue Substitute from Left Temporomandibular Joint, Percutaneous Approach

0RPD40Z Removal of Drainage Device from Left Temporomandibular Joint, Percutaneous Endoscopic Approach

0RPD43Z Removal of Infusion Device from Left Temporomandibular Joint, Percutaneous Endoscopic Approach

0RPD44Z Removal of Internal Fixation Device from Left Temporomandibular Joint, Percutaneous Endoscopic Approach

0RPD47Z Removal of Autologous Tissue Substitute from Left Temporomandibular Joint, Percutaneous Endoscopic Approach

0RPD48Z Removal of Spacer from Left Temporomandibular Joint, Percutaneous Endoscopic Approach

0RPD4JZ Removal of Synthetic Substitute from Left Temporomandibular Joint, Percutaneous Endoscopic Approach

0RPD4KZ Removal of Nonautologous Tissue Substitute from Left Temporomandibular Joint, Percutaneous Endoscopic Approach

0RPDX0Z Removal of Drainage Device from Left Temporomandibular Joint, External Approach

0RPDX3Z Removal of Infusion Device from Left Temporomandibular Joint, External Approach

0RPDX4Z Removal of Internal Fixation Device from Left Temporomandibular Joint, External Approach

0RPE00Z Removal of Drainage Device from Right Sternoclavicular Joint, Open Approach

0RPE03Z Removal of Infusion Device from Right Sternoclavicular Joint, Open Approach

0RPE04Z Removal of Internal Fixation Device from Right Sternoclavicular Joint, Open Approach

0RPE07Z Removal of Autologous Tissue Substitute from Right Sternoclavicular Joint, Open Approach

0RPE08Z Removal of Spacer from Right Sternoclavicular Joint, Open Approach

0RPE0JZ Removal of Synthetic Substitute from Right Sternoclavicular Joint, Open Approach

0RPE0KZ Removal of Nonautologous Tissue Substitute from Right Sternoclavicular Joint, Open Approach

0RPE30Z Removal of Drainage Device from Right Sternoclavicular Joint, Percutaneous Approach

0RPE33Z Removal of Infusion Device from Right Sternoclavicular Joint, Percutaneous Approach

0RPE34Z Removal of Internal Fixation Device from Right Sternoclavicular Joint, Percutaneous Approach

0RPE37Z Removal of Autologous Tissue Substitute from Right Sternoclavicular Joint, Percutaneous Approach

0RPE38Z Removal of Spacer from Right Sternoclavicular Joint, Percutaneous Approach

0RPE3JZ Removal of Synthetic Substitute from Right Sternoclavicular Joint, Percutaneous Approach

0RPE3KZ Removal of Nonautologous Tissue Substitute from Right Sternoclavicular Joint, Percutaneous Approach

0RPE40Z Removal of Drainage Device from Right Sternoclavicular Joint, Percutaneous Endoscopic Approach

0RPE43Z Removal of Infusion Device from Right Sternoclavicular Joint, Percutaneous Endoscopic Approach

0RPE44Z Removal of Internal Fixation Device from Right Sternoclavicular Joint, Percutaneous Endoscopic Approach

0RPE47Z Removal of Autologous Tissue Substitute from Right Sternoclavicular Joint, Percutaneous Endoscopic Approach

0RPE48Z Removal of Spacer from Right Sternoclavicular Joint, Percutaneous Endoscopic Approach

0RPE4JZ Removal of Synthetic Substitute from Right Sternoclavicular Joint, Percutaneous Endoscopic Approach

0RPE4KZ Removal of Nonautologous Tissue Substitute from Right Sternoclavicular Joint, Percutaneous Endoscopic Approach

0RPEX0Z Removal of Drainage Device from Right Sternoclavicular Joint, External Approach

0RPEX3Z Removal of Infusion Device from Right Sternoclavicular Joint, External Approach

0RPEX4Z Removal of Internal Fixation Device from Right Sternoclavicular Joint, External Approach

0RPF00Z Removal of Drainage Device from Left Sternoclavicular Joint, Open Approach

0RPF03Z Removal of Infusion Device from Left Sternoclavicular Joint, Open Approach

0RPF04Z Removal of Internal Fixation Device from Left Sternoclavicular Joint, Open Approach

0RPF07Z Removal of Autologous Tissue Substitute from Left Sternoclavicular Joint, Open Approach

0RPF08Z Removal of Spacer from Left Sternoclavicular Joint, Open Approach

0RPF0JZ Removal of Synthetic Substitute from Left Sternoclavicular Joint, Open Approach

0RPF0KZ Removal of Nonautologous Tissue Substitute from Left Sternoclavicular Joint, Open Approach

0RPF30Z Removal of Drainage Device from Left Sternoclavicular Joint, Percutaneous Approach

0RPF33Z Removal of Infusion Device from Left Sternoclavicular Joint, Percutaneous Approach

0RPF34Z Removal of Internal Fixation Device from Left Sternoclavicular Joint, Percutaneous Approach

0RPF37Z Removal of Autologous Tissue Substitute from Left Sternoclavicular Joint, Percutaneous Approach

0RPF38Z Removal of Spacer from Left Sternoclavicular Joint, Percutaneous Approach

0RPF3JZ Removal of Synthetic Substitute from Left Sternoclavicular Joint, Percutaneous Approach

0RPF3KZ Removal of Nonautologous Tissue Substitute from Left Sternoclavicular Joint, Percutaneous Approach

♀ Female-only   ♂ Male-only   ▲ Limited Coverage   ● Non-OR   **HAC** HAC-associated procedure   ▲ Non-covered procedures   ✚ Cluster

0RPF40Z Removal of Drainage Device from Left Sternoclavicular Joint, Percutaneous Endoscopic Approach

0RPF43Z Removal of Infusion Device from Left Sternoclavicular Joint, Percutaneous Endoscopic Approach

0RPF44Z Removal of Internal Fixation Device from Left Sternoclavicular Joint, Percutaneous Endoscopic Approach

0RPF47Z Removal of Autologous Tissue Substitute from Left Sternoclavicular Joint, Percutaneous Endoscopic Approach

0RPF48Z Removal of Spacer from Left Sternoclavicular Joint, Percutaneous Endoscopic Approach

0RPF4JZ Removal of Synthetic Substitute from Left Sternoclavicular Joint, Percutaneous Endoscopic Approach

0RPF4KZ Removal of Nonautologous Tissue Substitute from Left Sternoclavicular Joint, Percutaneous Endoscopic Approach

0RPFX0Z Removal of Drainage Device from Left Sternoclavicular Joint, External Approach

0RPFX3Z Removal of Infusion Device from Left Sternoclavicular Joint, External Approach

0RPFX4Z Removal of Internal Fixation Device from Left Sternoclavicular Joint, External Approach

0RPG00Z Removal of Drainage Device from Right Acromioclavicular Joint, Open Approach

0RPG03Z Removal of Infusion Device from Right Acromioclavicular Joint, Open Approach

0RPG04Z Removal of Internal Fixation Device from Right Acromioclavicular Joint, Open Approach

0RPG07Z Removal of Autologous Tissue Substitute from Right Acromioclavicular Joint, Open Approach

0RPG08Z Removal of Spacer from Right Acromioclavicular Joint, Open Approach

0RPG0JZ Removal of Synthetic Substitute from Right Acromioclavicular Joint, Open Approach

0RPG0KZ Removal of Nonautologous Tissue Substitute from Right Acromioclavicular Joint, Open Approach

0RPG30Z Removal of Drainage Device from Right Acromioclavicular Joint, Percutaneous Approach

0RPG33Z Removal of Infusion Device from Right Acromioclavicular Joint, Percutaneous Approach

0RPG34Z Removal of Internal Fixation Device from Right Acromioclavicular Joint, Percutaneous Approach

0RPG37Z Removal of Autologous Tissue Substitute from Right Acromioclavicular Joint, Percutaneous Approach

0RPG38Z Removal of Spacer from Right Acromioclavicular Joint, Percutaneous Approach

0RPG3JZ Removal of Synthetic Substitute from Right Acromioclavicular Joint, Percutaneous Approach

0RPG3KZ Removal of Nonautologous Tissue Substitute from Right Acromioclavicular Joint, Percutaneous Approach

0RPG40Z Removal of Drainage Device from Right Acromioclavicular Joint, Percutaneous Endoscopic Approach

0RPG43Z Removal of Infusion Device from Right Acromioclavicular Joint, Percutaneous Endoscopic Approach

0RPG44Z Removal of Internal Fixation Device from Right Acromioclavicular Joint, Percutaneous Endoscopic Approach

0RPG47Z Removal of Autologous Tissue Substitute from Right Acromioclavicular Joint, Percutaneous Endoscopic Approach

0RPG48Z Removal of Spacer from Right Acromioclavicular Joint, Percutaneous Endoscopic Approach

0RPG4JZ Removal of Synthetic Substitute from Right Acromioclavicular Joint, Percutaneous Endoscopic Approach

0RPG4KZ Removal of Nonautologous Tissue Substitute from Right Acromioclavicular Joint, Percutaneous Endoscopic Approach

0RPGX0Z Removal of Drainage Device from Right Acromioclavicular Joint, External Approach

0RPGX3Z Removal of Infusion Device from Right Acromioclavicular Joint, External Approach

0RPGX4Z Removal of Internal Fixation Device from Right Acromioclavicular Joint, External Approach

0RPH00Z Removal of Drainage Device from Left Acromioclavicular Joint, Open Approach

0RPH03Z Removal of Infusion Device from Left Acromioclavicular Joint, Open Approach

0RPH04Z Removal of Internal Fixation Device from Left Acromioclavicular Joint, Open Approach

0RPH07Z Removal of Autologous Tissue Substitute from Left Acromioclavicular Joint, Open Approach

0RPH08Z Removal of Spacer from Left Acromioclavicular Joint, Open Approach

0RPH0JZ Removal of Synthetic Substitute from Left Acromioclavicular Joint, Open Approach

0RPH0KZ Removal of Nonautologous Tissue Substitute from Left Acromioclavicular Joint, Open Approach

0RPH30Z Removal of Drainage Device from Left Acromioclavicular Joint, Percutaneous Approach

0RPH33Z Removal of Infusion Device from Left Acromioclavicular Joint, Percutaneous Approach

0RPH34Z Removal of Internal Fixation Device from Left Acromioclavicular Joint, Percutaneous Approach

0RPH37Z Removal of Autologous Tissue Substitute from Left Acromioclavicular Joint, Percutaneous Approach

0RPH38Z Removal of Spacer from Left Acromioclavicular Joint, Percutaneous Approach

0RPH3JZ Removal of Synthetic Substitute from Left Acromioclavicular Joint, Percutaneous Approach

0RPH3KZ Removal of Nonautologous Tissue Substitute from Left Acromioclavicular Joint, Percutaneous Approach

0RPH40Z Removal of Drainage Device from Left Acromioclavicular Joint, Percutaneous Endoscopic Approach

0RPH43Z Removal of Infusion Device from Left Acromioclavicular Joint, Percutaneous Endoscopic Approach

0RPH44Z Removal of Internal Fixation Device from Left Acromioclavicular Joint, Percutaneous Endoscopic Approach

0RPH47Z Removal of Autologous Tissue Substitute from Left Acromioclavicular Joint, Percutaneous Endoscopic Approach

0RPH48Z Removal of Spacer from Left Acromioclavicular Joint, Percutaneous Endoscopic Approach

0RPH4JZ Removal of Synthetic Substitute from Left Acromioclavicular Joint, Percutaneous Endoscopic Approach

0RPH4KZ Removal of Nonautologous Tissue Substitute from Left Acromioclavicular Joint, Percutaneous Endoscopic Approach

0RPHX0Z Removal of Drainage Device from Left Acromioclavicular Joint, External Approach

0RPHX3Z Removal of Infusion Device from Left Acromioclavicular Joint, External Approach

0RPHX4Z Removal of Internal Fixation Device from Left Acromioclavicular Joint, External Approach

0RPJ00Z Removal of Drainage Device from Right Shoulder Joint, Open Approach

0RPJ03Z Removal of Infusion Device from Right Shoulder Joint, Open Approach

0RPJ04Z Removal of Internal Fixation Device from Right Shoulder Joint, Open Approach

0RPJ07Z Removal of Autologous Tissue Substitute from Right Shoulder Joint, Open Approach

0RPJ08Z Removal of Spacer from Right Shoulder Joint, Open Approach

0RPJ0J6 Removal of Synthetic Substitute from Right Shoulder Joint, Humeral Surface, Open Approach

0RPJ0J7 Removal of Synthetic Substitute from Right Shoulder Joint, Glenoid Surface, Open Approach

0RPJ0JZ Removal of Synthetic Substitute from Right Shoulder Joint, Open Approach

0RPJ0KZ Removal of Nonautologous Tissue Substitute from Right Shoulder Joint, Open Approach

0RPJ30Z Removal of Drainage Device from Right Shoulder Joint, Percutaneous Approach

0RPJ33Z Removal of Infusion Device from Right Shoulder Joint, Percutaneous Approach

0RPJ34Z Removal of Internal Fixation Device from Right Shoulder Joint, Percutaneous Approach

0RPJ37Z Removal of Autologous Tissue Substitute from Right Shoulder Joint, Percutaneous Approach

0RPJ38Z Removal of Spacer from Right Shoulder Joint, Percutaneous Approach

0RPJ3J6 Removal of Synthetic Substitute from Right Shoulder Joint, Humeral Surface, Percutaneous Approach

0RPJ3J7 Removal of Synthetic Substitute from Right Shoulder Joint, Glenoid Surface, Percutaneous Approach

0RPJ3JZ Removal of Synthetic Substitute from Right Shoulder Joint, Percutaneous Approach

0RPJ3KZ Removal of Nonautologous Tissue Substitute from Right Shoulder Joint, Percutaneous Approach

0RPJ40Z Removal of Drainage Device from Right Shoulder Joint, Percutaneous Endoscopic Approach

0RPJ43Z Removal of Infusion Device from Right Shoulder Joint, Percutaneous Endoscopic Approach

0RPJ44Z Removal of Internal Fixation Device from Right Shoulder Joint, Percutaneous Endoscopic Approach

0RPJ47Z Removal of Autologous Tissue Substitute from Right Shoulder Joint, Percutaneous Endoscopic Approach

0RPJ48Z Removal of Spacer from Right Shoulder Joint, Percutaneous Endoscopic Approach

0RPJ4J6 Removal of Synthetic Substitute from Right Shoulder Joint, Humeral Surface, Percutaneous Endoscopic Approach

0RPJ4J7 Removal of Synthetic Substitute from Right Shoulder Joint, Glenoid Surface, Percutaneous Endoscopic Approach

0RPJ4JZ Removal of Synthetic Substitute from Right Shoulder Joint, Percutaneous Endoscopic Approach

0RPJ4KZ Removal of Nonautologous Tissue Substitute from Right Shoulder Joint, Percutaneous Endoscopic Approach

0RPJX0Z Removal of Drainage Device from Right Shoulder Joint, External Approach

0RPJX3Z Removal of Infusion Device from Right Shoulder Joint, External Approach

0RPJX4Z Removal of Internal Fixation Device from Right Shoulder Joint, External Approach

0RPK00Z Removal of Drainage Device from Left Shoulder Joint, Open Approach

0RPK03Z Removal of Infusion Device from Left Shoulder Joint, Open Approach

0RPK04Z Removal of Internal Fixation Device from Left Shoulder Joint, Open Approach

0RPK07Z Removal of Autologous Tissue Substitute from Left Shoulder Joint, Open Approach

0RPK08Z Removal of Spacer from Left Shoulder Joint, Open Approach

0RPK0J6 Removal of Synthetic Substitute from Left Shoulder Joint, Humeral Surface, Open Approach

0RPK0J7 Removal of Synthetic Substitute from Left Shoulder Joint, Glenoid Surface, Open Approach

0RPK0JZ Removal of Synthetic Substitute from Left Shoulder Joint, Open Approach

0RPK0KZ Removal of Nonautologous Tissue Substitute from Left Shoulder Joint, Open Approach

0RPK30Z Removal of Drainage Device from Left Shoulder Joint, Percutaneous Approach

0RPK33Z Removal of Infusion Device from Left Shoulder Joint, Percutaneous Approach

0RPK34Z Removal of Internal Fixation Device from Left Shoulder Joint, Percutaneous Approach

0RPK37Z Removal of Autologous Tissue Substitute from Left Shoulder Joint, Percutaneous Approach

0RPK38Z Removal of Spacer from Left Shoulder Joint, Percutaneous Approach

0RPK3J6 Removal of Synthetic Substitute from Left Shoulder Joint, Humeral Surface, Percutaneous Approach

0RPK3J7 Removal of Synthetic Substitute from Left Shoulder Joint, Glenoid Surface, Percutaneous Approach

0RPK3JZ Removal of Synthetic Substitute from Left Shoulder Joint, Percutaneous Approach

0RPK3KZ Removal of Nonautologous Tissue Substitute from Left Shoulder Joint, Percutaneous Approach

0RPK40Z Removal of Drainage Device from Left Shoulder Joint, Percutaneous Endoscopic Approach

0RPK43Z Removal of Infusion Device from Left Shoulder Joint, Percutaneous Endoscopic Approach

0RPK44Z Removal of Internal Fixation Device from Left Shoulder Joint, Percutaneous Endoscopic Approach

0RPK47Z Removal of Autologous Tissue Substitute from Left Shoulder Joint, Percutaneous Endoscopic Approach

0RPK48Z Removal of Spacer from Left Shoulder Joint, Percutaneous Endoscopic Approach

0RPK4J6 Removal of Synthetic Substitute from Left Shoulder Joint, Humeral Surface, Percutaneous Endoscopic Approach

0RPK4J7 Removal of Synthetic Substitute from Left Shoulder Joint, Glenoid Surface, Percutaneous Endoscopic Approach

0RPK4JZ Removal of Synthetic Substitute from Left Shoulder Joint, Percutaneous Endoscopic Approach

0RPK4KZ Removal of Nonautologous Tissue Substitute from Left Shoulder Joint, Percutaneous Endoscopic Approach

0RPKX0Z Removal of Drainage Device from Left Shoulder Joint, External Approach

0RPKX3Z Removal of Infusion Device from Left Shoulder Joint, External Approach

0RPKX4Z Removal of Internal Fixation Device from Left Shoulder Joint, External Approach

0RPL00Z Removal of Drainage Device from Right Elbow Joint, Open Approach

0RPL03Z Removal of Infusion Device from Right Elbow Joint, Open Approach

0RPL04Z Removal of Internal Fixation Device from Right Elbow Joint, Open Approach

0RPL05Z Removal of External Fixation Device from Right Elbow Joint, Open Approach

0RPL07Z Removal of Autologous Tissue Substitute from Right Elbow Joint, Open Approach

0RPL08Z Removal of Spacer from Right Elbow Joint, Open Approach

0RPL0JZ Removal of Synthetic Substitute from Right Elbow Joint, Open Approach

0RPL0KZ Removal of Nonautologous Tissue Substitute from Right Elbow Joint, Open Approach

0RPL30Z Removal of Drainage Device from Right Elbow Joint, Percutaneous Approach

0RPL33Z Removal of Infusion Device from Right Elbow Joint, Percutaneous Approach

0RPL34Z Removal of Internal Fixation Device from Right Elbow Joint, Percutaneous Approach

0RPL35Z Removal of External Fixation Device from Right Elbow Joint, Percutaneous Approach

0RPL37Z Removal of Autologous Tissue Substitute from Right Elbow Joint, Percutaneous Approach

0RPL38Z Removal of Spacer from Right Elbow Joint, Percutaneous Approach

0RPL3JZ Removal of Synthetic Substitute from Right Elbow Joint, Percutaneous Approach

0RPL3KZ Removal of Nonautologous Tissue Substitute from Right Elbow Joint, Percutaneous Approach

0RPL40Z Removal of Drainage Device from Right Elbow Joint, Percutaneous Endoscopic Approach

0RPL43Z Removal of Infusion Device from Right Elbow Joint, Percutaneous Endoscopic Approach

0RPL44Z Removal of Internal Fixation Device from Right Elbow Joint, Percutaneous Endoscopic Approach

0RPL45Z Removal of External Fixation Device from Right Elbow Joint, Percutaneous Endoscopic Approach

0RPL47Z Removal of Autologous Tissue Substitute from Right Elbow Joint, Percutaneous Endoscopic Approach

0RPL48Z Removal of Spacer from Right Elbow Joint, Percutaneous Endoscopic Approach

0RPL4JZ Removal of Synthetic Substitute from Right Elbow Joint, Percutaneous Endoscopic Approach

0RPL4KZ Removal of Nonautologous Tissue Substitute from Right Elbow Joint, Percutaneous Endoscopic Approach

0RPLX0Z Removal of Drainage Device from Right Elbow Joint, External Approach

0RPLX3Z Removal of Infusion Device from Right Elbow Joint, External Approach

0RPLX4Z Removal of Internal Fixation Device from Right Elbow Joint, External Approach

0RPLX5Z Removal of External Fixation Device from Right Elbow Joint, External Approach

0RPM00Z Removal of Drainage Device from Left Elbow Joint, Open Approach

0RPM03Z Removal of Infusion Device from Left Elbow Joint, Open Approach

0RPM04Z Removal of Internal Fixation Device from Left Elbow Joint, Open Approach

0RPM05Z Removal of External Fixation Device from Left Elbow Joint, Open Approach

0RPM07Z Removal of Autologous Tissue Substitute from Left Elbow Joint, Open Approach

0RPM08Z Removal of Spacer from Left Elbow Joint, Open Approach

0RPM0JZ Removal of Synthetic Substitute from Left Elbow Joint, Open Approach

0RPM0KZ Removal of Nonautologous Tissue Substitute from Left Elbow Joint, Open Approach

0RPM30Z Removal of Drainage Device from Left Elbow Joint, Percutaneous Approach

0RPM33Z Removal of Infusion Device from Left Elbow Joint, Percutaneous Approach

0RPM34Z Removal of Internal Fixation Device from Left Elbow Joint, Percutaneous Approach

0RPM35Z Removal of External Fixation Device from Left Elbow Joint, Percutaneous Approach

♀ Female-only   ♂ Male-only   ▲ Limited Coverage   ● Non-OR   HAC HAC-associated procedure   ▲ Non-covered procedures   ✚ Cluster

0RPM37Z   Removal of Autologous Tissue Substitute from Left Elbow Joint, Percutaneous Approach

0RPM38Z   Removal of Spacer from Left Elbow Joint, Percutaneous Approach

0RPM3JZ   Removal of Synthetic Substitute from Left Elbow Joint, Percutaneous Approach

0RPM3KZ   Removal of Nonautologous Tissue Substitute from Left Elbow Joint, Percutaneous Approach

0RPM40Z   Removal of Drainage Device from Left Elbow Joint, Percutaneous Endoscopic Approach

0RPM43Z   Removal of Infusion Device from Left Elbow Joint, Percutaneous Endoscopic Approach

0RPM44Z   Removal of Internal Fixation Device from Left Elbow Joint, Percutaneous Endoscopic Approach

0RPM45Z   Removal of External Fixation Device from Left Elbow Joint, Percutaneous Endoscopic Approach

0RPM47Z   Removal of Autologous Tissue Substitute from Left Elbow Joint, Percutaneous Endoscopic Approach

0RPM48Z   Removal of Spacer from Left Elbow Joint, Percutaneous Endoscopic Approach

0RPM4JZ   Removal of Synthetic Substitute from Left Elbow Joint, Percutaneous Endoscopic Approach

0RPM4KZ   Removal of Nonautologous Tissue Substitute from Left Elbow Joint, Percutaneous Endoscopic Approach

0RPMX0Z   Removal of Drainage Device from Left Elbow Joint, External Approach

0RPMX3Z   Removal of Infusion Device from Left Elbow Joint, External Approach

0RPMX4Z   Removal of Internal Fixation Device from Left Elbow Joint, External Approach

0RPMX5Z   Removal of External Fixation Device from Left Elbow Joint, External Approach

0RPN00Z   Removal of Drainage Device from Right Wrist Joint, Open Approach

0RPN03Z   Removal of Infusion Device from Right Wrist Joint, Open Approach

0RPN04Z   Removal of Internal Fixation Device from Right Wrist Joint, Open Approach

0RPN05Z   Removal of External Fixation Device from Right Wrist Joint, Open Approach

0RPN07Z   Removal of Autologous Tissue Substitute from Right Wrist Joint, Open Approach

0RPN08Z   Removal of Spacer from Right Wrist Joint, Open Approach

0RPN0JZ   Removal of Synthetic Substitute from Right Wrist Joint, Open Approach

0RPN0KZ   Removal of Nonautologous Tissue Substitute from Right Wrist Joint, Open Approach

0RPN30Z   Removal of Drainage Device from Right Wrist Joint, Percutaneous Approach

0RPN33Z   Removal of Infusion Device from Right Wrist Joint, Percutaneous Approach

0RPN34Z   Removal of Internal Fixation Device from Right Wrist Joint, Percutaneous Approach

0RPN35Z   Removal of External Fixation Device from Right Wrist Joint, Percutaneous Approach

0RPN37Z   Removal of Autologous Tissue Substitute from Right Wrist Joint, Percutaneous Approach

0RPN38Z   Removal of Spacer from Right Wrist Joint, Percutaneous Approach

0RPN3JZ   Removal of Synthetic Substitute from Right Wrist Joint, Percutaneous Approach

0RPN3KZ   Removal of Nonautologous Tissue Substitute from Right Wrist Joint, Percutaneous Approach

0RPN40Z   Removal of Drainage Device from Right Wrist Joint, Percutaneous Endoscopic Approach

0RPN43Z   Removal of Infusion Device from Right Wrist Joint, Percutaneous Endoscopic Approach

0RPN44Z   Removal of Internal Fixation Device from Right Wrist Joint, Percutaneous Endoscopic Approach

0RPN45Z   Removal of External Fixation Device from Right Wrist Joint, Percutaneous Endoscopic Approach

0RPN47Z   Removal of Autologous Tissue Substitute from Right Wrist Joint, Percutaneous Endoscopic Approach

0RPN48Z   Removal of Spacer from Right Wrist Joint, Percutaneous Endoscopic Approach

0RPN4JZ   Removal of Synthetic Substitute from Right Wrist Joint, Percutaneous Endoscopic Approach

0RPN4KZ   Removal of Nonautologous Tissue Substitute from Right Wrist Joint, Percutaneous Endoscopic Approach

0RPNX0Z   Removal of Drainage Device from Right Wrist Joint, External Approach

0RPNX3Z   Removal of Infusion Device from Right Wrist Joint, External Approach

0RPNX4Z   Removal of Internal Fixation Device from Right Wrist Joint, External Approach

0RPNX5Z   Removal of External Fixation Device from Right Wrist Joint, External Approach

0RPP00Z   Removal of Drainage Device from Left Wrist Joint, Open Approach

0RPP03Z   Removal of Infusion Device from Left Wrist Joint, Open Approach

0RPP04Z   Removal of Internal Fixation Device from Left Wrist Joint, Open Approach

0RPP05Z   Removal of External Fixation Device from Left Wrist Joint, Open Approach

0RPP07Z   Removal of Autologous Tissue Substitute from Left Wrist Joint, Open Approach

0RPP08Z   Removal of Spacer from Left Wrist Joint, Open Approach

0RPP0JZ   Removal of Synthetic Substitute from Left Wrist Joint, Open Approach

0RPP0KZ   Removal of Nonautologous Tissue Substitute from Left Wrist Joint, Open Approach

0RPP30Z   Removal of Drainage Device from Left Wrist Joint, Percutaneous Approach

0RPP33Z   Removal of Infusion Device from Left Wrist Joint, Percutaneous Approach

0RPP34Z   Removal of Internal Fixation Device from Left Wrist Joint, Percutaneous Approach

0RPP35Z   Removal of External Fixation Device from Left Wrist Joint, Percutaneous Approach

0RPP37Z   Removal of Autologous Tissue Substitute from Left Wrist Joint, Percutaneous Approach

0RPP38Z   Removal of Spacer from Left Wrist Joint, Percutaneous Approach

0RPP3JZ   Removal of Synthetic Substitute from Left Wrist Joint, Percutaneous Approach

0RPP3KZ   Removal of Nonautologous Tissue Substitute from Left Wrist Joint, Percutaneous Approach

0RPP40Z   Removal of Drainage Device from Left Wrist Joint, Percutaneous Endoscopic Approach

0RPP43Z   Removal of Infusion Device from Left Wrist Joint, Percutaneous Endoscopic Approach

0RPP44Z   Removal of Internal Fixation Device from Left Wrist Joint, Percutaneous Endoscopic Approach

0RPP45Z   Removal of External Fixation Device from Left Wrist Joint, Percutaneous Endoscopic Approach

0RPP47Z   Removal of Autologous Tissue Substitute from Left Wrist Joint, Percutaneous Endoscopic Approach

0RPP48Z   Removal of Spacer from Left Wrist Joint, Percutaneous Endoscopic Approach

0RPP4JZ   Removal of Synthetic Substitute from Left Wrist Joint, Percutaneous Endoscopic Approach

0RPP4KZ   Removal of Nonautologous Tissue Substitute from Left Wrist Joint, Percutaneous Endoscopic Approach

0RPPX0Z   Removal of Drainage Device from Left Wrist Joint, External Approach

0RPPX3Z   Removal of Infusion Device from Left Wrist Joint, External Approach

0RPPX4Z   Removal of Internal Fixation Device from Left Wrist Joint, External Approach

0RPPX5Z   Removal of External Fixation Device from Left Wrist Joint, External Approach

0RPQ00Z   Removal of Drainage Device from Right Carpal Joint, Open Approach

0RPQ03Z   Removal of Infusion Device from Right Carpal Joint, Open Approach

0RPQ04Z   Removal of Internal Fixation Device from Right Carpal Joint, Open Approach

0RPQ05Z   Removal of External Fixation Device from Right Carpal Joint, Open Approach

0RPQ07Z   Removal of Autologous Tissue Substitute from Right Carpal Joint, Open Approach

0RPQ08Z   Removal of Spacer from Right Carpal Joint, Open Approach

0RPQ0JZ   Removal of Synthetic Substitute from Right Carpal Joint, Open Approach

0RPQ0KZ   Removal of Nonautologous Tissue Substitute from Right Carpal Joint, Open Approach

0RPQ30Z   Removal of Drainage Device from Right Carpal Joint, Percutaneous Approach

0RPQ33Z   Removal of Infusion Device from Right Carpal Joint, Percutaneous Approach

0RPQ34Z   Removal of Internal Fixation Device from Right Carpal Joint, Percutaneous Approach

0RPQ35Z   Removal of External Fixation Device from Right Carpal Joint, Percutaneous Approach

♀ Female-only   ♂ Male-only   ▲ Limited Coverage   ● Non-OR   ▨ HAC-associated procedure   ▲ Non-covered procedures   ✚ Cluster   1095

Medical and Surgical, Upper Joints Code Listings

0RPQ37Z Removal of Autologous Tissue Substitute from Right Carpal Joint, Percutaneous Approach

0RPQ38Z Removal of Spacer from Right Carpal Joint, Percutaneous Approach

0RPQ3JZ Removal of Synthetic Substitute from Right Carpal Joint, Percutaneous Approach

0RPQ3KZ Removal of Nonautologous Tissue Substitute from Right Carpal Joint, Percutaneous Approach

0RPQ40Z Removal of Drainage Device from Right Carpal Joint, Percutaneous Endoscopic Approach

0RPQ43Z Removal of Infusion Device from Right Carpal Joint, Percutaneous Endoscopic Approach

0RPQ44Z Removal of Internal Fixation Device from Right Carpal Joint, Percutaneous Endoscopic Approach

0RPQ45Z Removal of External Fixation Device from Right Carpal Joint, Percutaneous Endoscopic Approach

0RPQ47Z Removal of Autologous Tissue Substitute from Right Carpal Joint, Percutaneous Endoscopic Approach

0RPQ48Z Removal of Spacer from Right Carpal Joint, Percutaneous Endoscopic Approach

0RPQ4JZ Removal of Synthetic Substitute from Right Carpal Joint, Percutaneous Endoscopic Approach

0RPQ4KZ Removal of Nonautologous Tissue Substitute from Right Carpal Joint, Percutaneous Endoscopic Approach

0RPQX0Z Removal of Drainage Device from Right Carpal Joint, External Approach

0RPQX3Z Removal of Infusion Device from Right Carpal Joint, External Approach

0RPQX4Z Removal of Internal Fixation Device from Right Carpal Joint, External Approach

0RPQX5Z Removal of External Fixation Device from Right Carpal Joint, External Approach

0RPR00Z Removal of Drainage Device from Left Carpal Joint, Open Approach

0RPR03Z Removal of Infusion Device from Left Carpal Joint, Open Approach

0RPR04Z Removal of Internal Fixation Device from Left Carpal Joint, Open Approach

0RPR05Z Removal of External Fixation Device from Left Carpal Joint, Open Approach

0RPR07Z Removal of Autologous Tissue Substitute from Left Carpal Joint, Open Approach

0RPR08Z Removal of Spacer from Left Carpal Joint, Open Approach

0RPR0JZ Removal of Synthetic Substitute from Left Carpal Joint, Open Approach

0RPR0KZ Removal of Nonautologous Tissue Substitute from Left Carpal Joint, Open Approach

0RPR30Z Removal of Drainage Device from Left Carpal Joint, Percutaneous Approach

0RPR33Z Removal of Infusion Device from Left Carpal Joint, Percutaneous Approach

0RPR34Z Removal of Internal Fixation Device from Left Carpal Joint, Percutaneous Approach

0RPR35Z Removal of External Fixation Device from Left Carpal Joint, Percutaneous Approach

0RPR37Z Removal of Autologous Tissue Substitute from Left Carpal Joint, Percutaneous Approach

0RPR38Z Removal of Spacer from Left Carpal Joint, Percutaneous Approach

0RPR3JZ Removal of Synthetic Substitute from Left Carpal Joint, Percutaneous Approach

0RPR3KZ Removal of Nonautologous Tissue Substitute from Left Carpal Joint, Percutaneous Approach

0RPR40Z Removal of Drainage Device from Left Carpal Joint, Percutaneous Endoscopic Approach

0RPR43Z Removal of Infusion Device from Left Carpal Joint, Percutaneous Endoscopic Approach

0RPR44Z Removal of Internal Fixation Device from Left Carpal Joint, Percutaneous Endoscopic Approach

0RPR45Z Removal of External Fixation Device from Left Carpal Joint, Percutaneous Endoscopic Approach

0RPR47Z Removal of Autologous Tissue Substitute from Left Carpal Joint, Percutaneous Endoscopic Approach

0RPR48Z Removal of Spacer from Left Carpal Joint, Percutaneous Endoscopic Approach

0RPR4JZ Removal of Synthetic Substitute from Left Carpal Joint, Percutaneous Endoscopic Approach

0RPR4KZ Removal of Nonautologous Tissue Substitute from Left Carpal Joint, Percutaneous Endoscopic Approach

0RPRX0Z Removal of Drainage Device from Left Carpal Joint, External Approach

0RPRX3Z Removal of Infusion Device from Left Carpal Joint, External Approach

0RPRX4Z Removal of Internal Fixation Device from Left Carpal Joint, External Approach

0RPRX5Z Removal of External Fixation Device from Left Carpal Joint, External Approach

0RPS00Z Removal of Drainage Device from Right Carpometacarpal Joint, Open Approach

0RPS03Z Removal of Infusion Device from Right Carpometacarpal Joint, Open Approach

0RPS04Z Removal of Internal Fixation Device from Right Carpometacarpal Joint, Open Approach

0RPS05Z Removal of External Fixation Device from Right Carpometacarpal Joint, Open Approach

0RPS07Z Removal of Autologous Tissue Substitute from Right Carpometacarpal Joint, Open Approach

0RPS08Z Removal of Spacer from Right Carpometacarpal Joint, Open Approach

0RPS0JZ Removal of Synthetic Substitute from Right Carpometacarpal Joint, Open Approach

0RPS0KZ Removal of Nonautologous Tissue Substitute from Right Carpometacarpal Joint, Open Approach

0RPS30Z Removal of Drainage Device from Right Carpometacarpal Joint, Percutaneous Approach

0RPS33Z Removal of Infusion Device from Right Carpometacarpal Joint, Percutaneous Approach

0RPS34Z Removal of Internal Fixation Device from Right Carpometacarpal Joint, Percutaneous Approach

0RPS35Z Removal of External Fixation Device from Right Carpometacarpal Joint, Percutaneous Approach

0RPS37Z Removal of Autologous Tissue Substitute from Right Carpometacarpal Joint, Percutaneous Approach

0RPS38Z Removal of Spacer from Right Carpometacarpal Joint, Percutaneous Approach

0RPS3JZ Removal of Synthetic Substitute from Right Carpometacarpal Joint, Percutaneous Approach

0RPS3KZ Removal of Nonautologous Tissue Substitute from Right Carpometacarpal Joint, Percutaneous Approach

0RPS40Z Removal of Drainage Device from Right Carpometacarpal Joint, Percutaneous Endoscopic Approach

0RPS43Z Removal of Infusion Device from Right Carpometacarpal Joint, Percutaneous Endoscopic Approach

0RPS44Z Removal of Internal Fixation Device from Right Carpometacarpal Joint, Percutaneous Endoscopic Approach

0RPS45Z Removal of External Fixation Device from Right Carpometacarpal Joint, Percutaneous Endoscopic Approach

0RPS47Z Removal of Autologous Tissue Substitute from Right Carpometacarpal Joint, Percutaneous Endoscopic Approach

0RPS48Z Removal of Spacer from Right Carpometacarpal Joint, Percutaneous Endoscopic Approach

0RPS4JZ Removal of Synthetic Substitute from Right Carpometacarpal Joint, Percutaneous Endoscopic Approach

0RPS4KZ Removal of Nonautologous Tissue Substitute from Right Carpometacarpal Joint, Percutaneous Endoscopic Approach

0RPSX0Z Removal of Drainage Device from Right Carpometacarpal Joint, External Approach

0RPSX3Z Removal of Infusion Device from Right Carpometacarpal Joint, External Approach

0RPSX4Z Removal of Internal Fixation Device from Right Carpometacarpal Joint, External Approach

0RPSX5Z Removal of External Fixation Device from Right Carpometacarpal Joint, External Approach

0RPT00Z Removal of Drainage Device from Left Carpometacarpal Joint, Open Approach

0RPT03Z Removal of Infusion Device from Left Carpometacarpal Joint, Open Approach

0RPT04Z Removal of Internal Fixation Device from Left Carpometacarpal Joint, Open Approach

0RPT05Z Removal of External Fixation Device from Left Carpometacarpal Joint, Open Approach

0RPT07Z Removal of Autologous Tissue Substitute from Left Carpometacarpal Joint, Open Approach

0RPT08Z Removal of Spacer from Left Carpometacarpal Joint, Open Approach

0RPT0JZ Removal of Synthetic Substitute from Left Carpometacarpal Joint, Open Approach

0RPT0KZ Removal of Nonautologous Tissue Substitute from Left Carpometacarpal Joint, Open Approach

0RPT30Z Removal of Drainage Device from Left Carpometacarpal Joint, Percutaneous Approach

0RPT33Z Removal of Infusion Device from Left Carpometacarpal Joint, Percutaneous Approach

0RPT34Z Removal of Internal Fixation Device from Left Carpometacarpal Joint, Percutaneous Approach

0RPT35Z Removal of External Fixation Device from Left Carpometacarpal Joint, Percutaneous Approach

0RPT37Z Removal of Autologous Tissue Substitute from Left Carpometacarpal Joint, Percutaneous Approach

0RPT38Z Removal of Spacer from Left Carpometacarpal Joint, Percutaneous Approach

0RPT3JZ Removal of Synthetic Substitute from Left Carpometacarpal Joint, Percutaneous Approach

0RPT3KZ Removal of Nonautologous Tissue Substitute from Left Carpometacarpal Joint, Percutaneous Approach

0RPT40Z Removal of Drainage Device from Left Carpometacarpal Joint, Percutaneous Endoscopic Approach

0RPT43Z Removal of Infusion Device from Left Carpometacarpal Joint, Percutaneous Endoscopic Approach

0RPT44Z Removal of Internal Fixation Device from Left Carpometacarpal Joint, Percutaneous Endoscopic Approach

0RPT45Z Removal of External Fixation Device from Left Carpometacarpal Joint, Percutaneous Endoscopic Approach

0RPT47Z Removal of Autologous Tissue Substitute from Left Carpometacarpal Joint, Percutaneous Endoscopic Approach

0RPT48Z Removal of Spacer from Left Carpometacarpal Joint, Percutaneous Endoscopic Approach

0RPT4JZ Removal of Synthetic Substitute from Left Carpometacarpal Joint, Percutaneous Endoscopic Approach

0RPT4KZ Removal of Nonautologous Tissue Substitute from Left Carpometacarpal Joint, Percutaneous Endoscopic Approach

0RPTX0Z Removal of Drainage Device from Left Carpometacarpal Joint, External Approach

0RPTX3Z Removal of Infusion Device from Left Carpometacarpal Joint, External Approach

0RPTX4Z Removal of Internal Fixation Device from Left Carpometacarpal Joint, External Approach

0RPTX5Z Removal of External Fixation Device from Left Carpometacarpal Joint, External Approach

0RPU00Z Removal of Drainage Device from Right Metacarpophalangeal Joint, Open Approach

0RPU03Z Removal of Infusion Device from Right Metacarpophalangeal Joint, Open Approach

0RPU04Z Removal of Internal Fixation Device from Right Metacarpophalangeal Joint, Open Approach

0RPU05Z Removal of External Fixation Device from Right Metacarpophalangeal Joint, Open Approach

0RPU07Z Removal of Autologous Tissue Substitute from Right Metacarpophalangeal Joint, Open Approach

0RPU08Z Removal of Spacer from Right Metacarpophalangeal Joint, Open Approach

0RPU0JZ Removal of Synthetic Substitute from Right Metacarpophalangeal Joint, Open Approach

0RPU0KZ Removal of Nonautologous Tissue Substitute from Right Metacarpophalangeal Joint, Open Approach

0RPU30Z Removal of Drainage Device from Right Metacarpophalangeal Joint, Percutaneous Approach

0RPU33Z Removal of Infusion Device from Right Metacarpophalangeal Joint, Percutaneous Approach

0RPU34Z Removal of Internal Fixation Device from Right Metacarpophalangeal Joint, Percutaneous Approach

0RPU35Z Removal of External Fixation Device from Right Metacarpophalangeal Joint, Percutaneous Approach

0RPU37Z Removal of Autologous Tissue Substitute from Right Metacarpophalangeal Joint, Percutaneous Approach

0RPU38Z Removal of Spacer from Right Metacarpophalangeal Joint, Percutaneous Approach

0RPU3JZ Removal of Synthetic Substitute from Right Metacarpophalangeal Joint, Percutaneous Approach

0RPU3KZ Removal of Nonautologous Tissue Substitute from Right Metacarpophalangeal Joint, Percutaneous Approach

0RPU40Z Removal of Drainage Device from Right Metacarpophalangeal Joint, Percutaneous Endoscopic Approach

0RPU43Z Removal of Infusion Device from Right Metacarpophalangeal Joint, Percutaneous Endoscopic Approach

0RPU44Z Removal of Internal Fixation Device from Right Metacarpophalangeal Joint, Percutaneous Endoscopic Approach

0RPU45Z Removal of External Fixation Device from Right Metacarpophalangeal Joint, Percutaneous Endoscopic Approach

0RPU47Z Removal of Autologous Tissue Substitute from Right Metacarpophalangeal Joint, Percutaneous Endoscopic Approach

0RPU48Z Removal of Spacer from Right Metacarpophalangeal Joint, Percutaneous Endoscopic Approach

0RPU4JZ Removal of Synthetic Substitute from Right Metacarpophalangeal Joint, Percutaneous Endoscopic Approach

0RPU4KZ Removal of Nonautologous Tissue Substitute from Right Metacarpophalangeal Joint, Percutaneous Endoscopic Approach

0RPUX0Z Removal of Drainage Device from Right Metacarpophalangeal Joint, External Approach

0RPUX3Z Removal of Infusion Device from Right Metacarpophalangeal Joint, External Approach

0RPUX4Z Removal of Internal Fixation Device from Right Metacarpophalangeal Joint, External Approach

0RPUX5Z Removal of External Fixation Device from Right Metacarpophalangeal Joint, External Approach

0RPV00Z Removal of Drainage Device from Left Metacarpophalangeal Joint, Open Approach

0RPV03Z Removal of Infusion Device from Left Metacarpophalangeal Joint, Open Approach

0RPV04Z Removal of Internal Fixation Device from Left Metacarpophalangeal Joint, Open Approach

0RPV05Z Removal of External Fixation Device from Left Metacarpophalangeal Joint, Open Approach

0RPV07Z Removal of Autologous Tissue Substitute from Left Metacarpophalangeal Joint, Open Approach

0RPV08Z Removal of Spacer from Left Metacarpophalangeal Joint, Open Approach

0RPV0JZ Removal of Synthetic Substitute from Left Metacarpophalangeal Joint, Open Approach

0RPV0KZ Removal of Nonautologous Tissue Substitute from Left Metacarpophalangeal Joint, Open Approach

0RPV30Z Removal of Drainage Device from Left Metacarpophalangeal Joint, Percutaneous Approach

0RPV33Z Removal of Infusion Device from Left Metacarpophalangeal Joint, Percutaneous Approach

0RPV34Z Removal of Internal Fixation Device from Left Metacarpophalangeal Joint, Percutaneous Approach

0RPV35Z Removal of External Fixation Device from Left Metacarpophalangeal Joint, Percutaneous Approach

0RPV37Z Removal of Autologous Tissue Substitute from Left Metacarpophalangeal Joint, Percutaneous Approach

0RPV38Z Removal of Spacer from Left Metacarpophalangeal Joint, Percutaneous Approach

0RPV3JZ Removal of Synthetic Substitute from Left Metacarpophalangeal Joint, Percutaneous Approach

0RPV3KZ Removal of Nonautologous Tissue Substitute from Left Metacarpophalangeal Joint, Percutaneous Approach

0RPV40Z Removal of Drainage Device from Left Metacarpophalangeal Joint, Percutaneous Endoscopic Approach

0RPV43Z Removal of Infusion Device from Left Metacarpophalangeal Joint, Percutaneous Endoscopic Approach

0RPV44Z Removal of Internal Fixation Device from Left Metacarpophalangeal Joint, Percutaneous Endoscopic Approach

0RPV45Z Removal of External Fixation Device from Left Metacarpophalangeal Joint, Percutaneous Endoscopic Approach

0RPV47Z Removal of Autologous Tissue Substitute from Left Metacarpophalangeal Joint, Percutaneous Endoscopic Approach

0RPV48Z Removal of Spacer from Left Metacarpophalangeal Joint, Percutaneous Endoscopic Approach

0RPV4JZ Removal of Synthetic Substitute from Left Metacarpophalangeal Joint, Percutaneous Endoscopic Approach

0RPV4KZ Removal of Nonautologous Tissue Substitute from Left Metacarpophalangeal Joint, Percutaneous Endoscopic Approach

0RPVX0Z Removal of Drainage Device from Left Metacarpophalangeal Joint, External Approach

0RPVX3Z Removal of Infusion Device from Left Metacarpophalangeal Joint, External Approach

0RPVX4Z Removal of Internal Fixation Device from Left Metacarpophalangeal Joint, External Approach

0RPVX5Z Removal of External Fixation Device from Left Metacarpophalangeal Joint, External Approach

0RPW00Z Removal of Drainage Device from Right Finger Phalangeal Joint, Open Approach

0RPW03Z Removal of Infusion Device from Right Finger Phalangeal Joint, Open Approach

0RPW04Z Removal of Internal Fixation Device from Right Finger Phalangeal Joint, Open Approach

0RPW05Z Removal of External Fixation Device from Right Finger Phalangeal Joint, Open Approach

0RPW07Z Removal of Autologous Tissue Substitute from Right Finger Phalangeal Joint, Open Approach

0RPW08Z Removal of Spacer from Right Finger Phalangeal Joint, Open Approach

0RPW0JZ Removal of Synthetic Substitute from Right Finger Phalangeal Joint, Open Approach

0RPW0KZ Removal of Nonautologous Tissue Substitute from Right Finger Phalangeal Joint, Open Approach

0RPW30Z Removal of Drainage Device from Right Finger Phalangeal Joint, Percutaneous Approach

0RPW33Z Removal of Infusion Device from Right Finger Phalangeal Joint, Percutaneous Approach

0RPW34Z Removal of Internal Fixation Device from Right Finger Phalangeal Joint, Percutaneous Approach

0RPW35Z Removal of External Fixation Device from Right Finger Phalangeal Joint, Percutaneous Approach

0RPW37Z Removal of Autologous Tissue Substitute from Right Finger Phalangeal Joint, Percutaneous Approach

0RPW38Z Removal of Spacer from Right Finger Phalangeal Joint, Percutaneous Approach

0RPW3JZ Removal of Synthetic Substitute from Right Finger Phalangeal Joint, Percutaneous Approach

0RPW3KZ Removal of Nonautologous Tissue Substitute from Right Finger Phalangeal Joint, Percutaneous Approach

0RPW40Z Removal of Drainage Device from Right Finger Phalangeal Joint, Percutaneous Endoscopic Approach

0RPW43Z Removal of Infusion Device from Right Finger Phalangeal Joint, Percutaneous Endoscopic Approach

0RPW44Z Removal of Internal Fixation Device from Right Finger Phalangeal Joint, Percutaneous Endoscopic Approach

0RPW45Z Removal of External Fixation Device from Right Finger Phalangeal Joint, Percutaneous Endoscopic Approach

0RPW47Z Removal of Autologous Tissue Substitute from Right Finger Phalangeal Joint, Percutaneous Endoscopic Approach

0RPW48Z Removal of Spacer from Right Finger Phalangeal Joint, Percutaneous Endoscopic Approach

0RPW4JZ Removal of Synthetic Substitute from Right Finger Phalangeal Joint, Percutaneous Endoscopic Approach

0RPW4KZ Removal of Nonautologous Tissue Substitute from Right Finger Phalangeal Joint, Percutaneous Endoscopic Approach

0RPWX0Z Removal of Drainage Device from Right Finger Phalangeal Joint, External Approach

0RPWX3Z Removal of Infusion Device from Right Finger Phalangeal Joint, External Approach

0RPWX4Z Removal of Internal Fixation Device from Right Finger Phalangeal Joint, External Approach

0RPWX5Z Removal of External Fixation Device from Right Finger Phalangeal Joint, External Approach

0RPX00Z Removal of Drainage Device from Left Finger Phalangeal Joint, Open Approach

0RPX03Z Removal of Infusion Device from Left Finger Phalangeal Joint, Open Approach

0RPX04Z Removal of Internal Fixation Device from Left Finger Phalangeal Joint, Open Approach

0RPX05Z Removal of External Fixation Device from Left Finger Phalangeal Joint, Open Approach

0RPX07Z Removal of Autologous Tissue Substitute from Left Finger Phalangeal Joint, Open Approach

0RPX08Z Removal of Spacer from Left Finger Phalangeal Joint, Open Approach

0RPX0JZ Removal of Synthetic Substitute from Left Finger Phalangeal Joint, Open Approach

0RPX0KZ Removal of Nonautologous Tissue Substitute from Left Finger Phalangeal Joint, Open Approach

0RPX30Z Removal of Drainage Device from Left Finger Phalangeal Joint, Percutaneous Approach

0RPX33Z Removal of Infusion Device from Left Finger Phalangeal Joint, Percutaneous Approach

0RPX34Z Removal of Internal Fixation Device from Left Finger Phalangeal Joint, Percutaneous Approach

0RPX35Z Removal of External Fixation Device from Left Finger Phalangeal Joint, Percutaneous Approach

0RPX37Z Removal of Autologous Tissue Substitute from Left Finger Phalangeal Joint, Percutaneous Approach

0RPX38Z Removal of Spacer from Left Finger Phalangeal Joint, Percutaneous Approach

0RPX3JZ Removal of Synthetic Substitute from Left Finger Phalangeal Joint, Percutaneous Approach

0RPX3KZ Removal of Nonautologous Tissue Substitute from Left Finger Phalangeal Joint, Percutaneous Approach

0RPX40Z Removal of Drainage Device from Left Finger Phalangeal Joint, Percutaneous Endoscopic Approach

0RPX43Z Removal of Infusion Device from Left Finger Phalangeal Joint, Percutaneous Endoscopic Approach

0RPX44Z Removal of Internal Fixation Device from Left Finger Phalangeal Joint, Percutaneous Endoscopic Approach

0RPX45Z Removal of External Fixation Device from Left Finger Phalangeal Joint, Percutaneous Endoscopic Approach

0RPX47Z Removal of Autologous Tissue Substitute from Left Finger Phalangeal Joint, Percutaneous Endoscopic Approach

0RPX48Z Removal of Spacer from Left Finger Phalangeal Joint, Percutaneous Endoscopic Approach

0RPX4JZ Removal of Synthetic Substitute from Left Finger Phalangeal Joint, Percutaneous Endoscopic Approach

0RPX4KZ Removal of Nonautologous Tissue Substitute from Left Finger Phalangeal Joint, Percutaneous Endoscopic Approach

0RPXX0Z Removal of Drainage Device from Left Finger Phalangeal Joint, External Approach

0RPXX3Z Removal of Infusion Device from Left Finger Phalangeal Joint, External Approach

0RPXX4Z Removal of Internal Fixation Device from Left Finger Phalangeal Joint, External Approach

0RPXX5Z Removal of External Fixation Device from Left Finger Phalangeal Joint, External Approach

0RQ – Upper Joints, Repair

Review Coding Guideline B3.5

0RQ00ZZ Repair Occipital-cervical Joint, Open Approach

0RQ03ZZ Repair Occipital-cervical Joint, Percutaneous Approach

0RQ04ZZ Repair Occipital-cervical Joint, Percutaneous Endoscopic Approach

♀ Female-only   ♂ Male-only   ▲ Limited Coverage   ● Non-OR   HAC HAC-associated procedure   ▲ Non-covered procedures   ➕ Cluster

0RQ0XZZ Repair Occipital-cervical Joint, External Approach

0RQ10ZZ Repair Cervical Vertebral Joint, Open Approach

0RQ13ZZ Repair Cervical Vertebral Joint, Percutaneous Approach

0RQ14ZZ Repair Cervical Vertebral Joint, Percutaneous Endoscopic Approach

0RQ1XZZ Repair Cervical Vertebral Joint, External Approach

0RQ30ZZ Repair Cervical Vertebral Disc, Open Approach

0RQ33ZZ Repair Cervical Vertebral Disc, Percutaneous Approach

0RQ34ZZ Repair Cervical Vertebral Disc, Percutaneous Endoscopic Approach

0RQ3XZZ Repair Cervical Vertebral Disc, External Approach

0RQ40ZZ Repair Cervicothoracic Vertebral Joint, Open Approach

0RQ43ZZ Repair Cervicothoracic Vertebral Joint, Percutaneous Approach

0RQ44ZZ Repair Cervicothoracic Vertebral Joint, Percutaneous Endoscopic Approach

0RQ4XZZ Repair Cervicothoracic Vertebral Joint, External Approach

0RQ50ZZ Repair Cervicothoracic Vertebral Disc, Open Approach

0RQ53ZZ Repair Cervicothoracic Vertebral Disc, Percutaneous Approach

0RQ54ZZ Repair Cervicothoracic Vertebral Disc, Percutaneous Endoscopic Approach

0RQ5XZZ Repair Cervicothoracic Vertebral Disc, External Approach

0RQ60ZZ Repair Thoracic Vertebral Joint, Open Approach

0RQ63ZZ Repair Thoracic Vertebral Joint, Percutaneous Approach

0RQ64ZZ Repair Thoracic Vertebral Joint, Percutaneous Endoscopic Approach

0RQ6XZZ Repair Thoracic Vertebral Joint, External Approach

0RQ90ZZ Repair Thoracic Vertebral Disc, Open Approach

0RQ93ZZ Repair Thoracic Vertebral Disc, Percutaneous Approach

0RQ94ZZ Repair Thoracic Vertebral Disc, Percutaneous Endoscopic Approach

0RQ9XZZ Repair Thoracic Vertebral Disc, External Approach

0RQA0ZZ Repair Thoracolumbar Vertebral Joint, Open Approach

0RQA3ZZ Repair Thoracolumbar Vertebral Joint, Percutaneous Approach

0RQA4ZZ Repair Thoracolumbar Vertebral Joint, Percutaneous Endoscopic Approach

0RQAXZZ Repair Thoracolumbar Vertebral Joint, External Approach

0RQB0ZZ Repair Thoracolumbar Vertebral Disc, Open Approach

0RQB3ZZ Repair Thoracolumbar Vertebral Disc, Percutaneous Approach

0RQB4ZZ Repair Thoracolumbar Vertebral Disc, Percutaneous Endoscopic Approach

0RQBXZZ Repair Thoracolumbar Vertebral Disc, External Approach

0RQC0ZZ Repair Right Temporomandibular Joint, Open Approach

0RQC3ZZ Repair Right Temporomandibular Joint, Percutaneous Approach

0RQC4ZZ Repair Right Temporomandibular Joint, Percutaneous Endoscopic Approach

0RQCXZZ Repair Right Temporomandibular Joint, External Approach

0RQD0ZZ Repair Left Temporomandibular Joint, Open Approach

0RQD3ZZ Repair Left Temporomandibular Joint, Percutaneous Approach

0RQD4ZZ Repair Left Temporomandibular Joint, Percutaneous Endoscopic Approach

0RQDXZZ Repair Left Temporomandibular Joint, External Approach

0RQE0ZZ Repair Right Sternoclavicular Joint, Open Approach

HAC When reported with secondary diagnosis code K68.11, T81.40XA, T81.41XA, T81.42XA, T81.43XA, T81.44XA, T81.49XA, T84.60XA, T84.610A, T84.611A, T84.612A, T84.613A, T84.614A, T84.615A, T84.619A, T84.63XA, T84.69XA, T84.7XXA

0RQE3ZZ Repair Right Sternoclavicular Joint, Percutaneous Approach

HAC When reported with secondary diagnosis code K68.11, T81.40XA, T81.41XA, T81.42XA, T81.43XA, T81.44XA, T81.49XA, T84.60XA, T84.610A, T84.611A, T84.612A, T84.613A, T84.614A, T84.615A, T84.619A, T84.63XA, T84.69XA, T84.7XXA

0RQE4ZZ Repair Right Sternoclavicular Joint, Percutaneous Endoscopic Approach

HAC When reported with secondary diagnosis code K68.11, T81.40XA, T81.41XA, T81.42XA, T81.43XA, T81.44XA, T81.49XA, T84.60XA, T84.610A, T84.611A, T84.612A, T84.613A, T84.614A, T84.615A, T84.619A, T84.63XA, T84.69XA, T84.7XXA

0RQEXZZ Repair Right Sternoclavicular Joint, External Approach

HAC When reported with secondary diagnosis code K68.11, T81.40XA, T81.41XA, T81.42XA, T81.43XA, T81.44XA, T81.49XA, T84.60XA, T84.610A, T84.611A, T84.612A, T84.613A, T84.614A, T84.615A, T84.619A, T84.63XA, T84.69XA, T84.7XXA

0RQF0ZZ Repair Left Sternoclavicular Joint, Open Approach

HAC When reported with secondary diagnosis code K68.11, T81.40XA, T81.41XA, T81.42XA, T81.43XA, T81.44XA, T81.49XA, T84.60XA, T84.610A, T84.611A, T84.612A, T84.613A, T84.614A, T84.615A, T84.619A, T84.63XA, T84.69XA, T84.7XXA

0RQF3ZZ Repair Left Sternoclavicular Joint, Percutaneous Approach

HAC When reported with secondary diagnosis code K68.11, T81.40XA, T81.41XA, T81.42XA, T81.43XA, T81.44XA, T81.49XA, T84.60XA, T84.610A, T84.611A, T84.612A, T84.613A, T84.614A, T84.615A, T84.619A, T84.63XA, T84.69XA, T84.7XXA

0RQF4ZZ Repair Left Sternoclavicular Joint, Percutaneous Endoscopic Approach

HAC When reported with secondary diagnosis code K68.11, T81.40XA,

T81.41XA, T81.42XA, T81.43XA, T81.44XA, T81.49XA, T84.60XA, T84.610A, T84.611A, T84.612A, T84.613A, T84.614A, T84.615A, T84.619A, T84.63XA, T84.69XA, T84.7XXA

0RQFXZZ Repair Left Sternoclavicular Joint, External Approach

HAC When reported with secondary diagnosis code K68.11, T81.40XA, T81.41XA, T81.42XA, T81.43XA, T81.44XA, T81.49XA, T84.60XA, T84.610A, T84.611A, T84.612A, T84.613A, T84.614A, T84.615A, T84.619A, T84.63XA, T84.69XA, T84.7XXA

0RQG0ZZ Repair Right Acromioclavicular Joint, Open Approach

HAC When reported with secondary diagnosis code K68.11, T81.40XA, T81.41XA, T81.42XA, T81.43XA, T81.44XA, T81.49XA, T84.60XA, T84.610A, T84.611A, T84.612A, T84.613A, T84.614A, T84.615A, T84.619A, T84.63XA, T84.69XA, T84.7XXA

0RQG3ZZ Repair Right Acromioclavicular Joint, Percutaneous Approach

HAC When reported with secondary diagnosis code K68.11, T81.40XA, T81.41XA, T81.42XA, T81.43XA, T81.44XA, T81.49XA, T84.60XA, T84.610A, T84.611A, T84.612A, T84.613A, T84.614A, T84.615A, T84.619A, T84.63XA, T84.69XA, T84.7XXA

0RQG4ZZ Repair Right Acromioclavicular Joint, Percutaneous Endoscopic Approach

HAC When reported with secondary diagnosis code K68.11, T81.40XA, T81.41XA, T81.42XA, T81.43XA, T81.44XA, T81.49XA, T84.60XA, T84.610A, T84.611A, T84.612A, T84.613A, T84.614A, T84.615A, T84.619A, T84.63XA, T84.69XA, T84.7XXA

0RQGXZZ Repair Right Acromioclavicular Joint, External Approach

HAC When reported with secondary diagnosis code K68.11, T81.40XA, T81.41XA, T81.42XA, T81.43XA, T81.44XA, T81.49XA, T84.60XA, T84.610A, T84.611A, T84.612A, T84.613A, T84.614A, T84.615A, T84.619A, T84.63XA, T84.69XA, T84.7XXA

0RQH0ZZ Repair Left Acromioclavicular Joint, Open Approach

HAC When reported with secondary diagnosis code K68.11, T81.40XA, T81.41XA, T81.42XA, T81.43XA, T81.44XA, T81.49XA, T84.60XA, T84.610A, T84.611A, T84.612A, T84.613A, T84.614A, T84.615A, T84.619A, T84.63XA, T84.69XA, T84.7XXA

0RQH3ZZ Repair Left Acromioclavicular Joint, Percutaneous Approach

HAC When reported with secondary diagnosis code K68.11, T81.40XA, T81.41XA, T81.42XA, T81.43XA, T81.44XA, T81.49XA, T84.60XA, T84.610A, T84.611A, T84.612A, T84.613A, T84.614A, T84.615A, T84.619A, T84.63XA, T84.69XA, T84.7XXA

♀ Female-only   ♂ Male-only   ▲ Limited Coverage   ● Non-OR   HAC HAC-associated procedure   ▲ Non-covered procedures   ➕ Cluster

0RQH4ZZ Repair Left Acromioclavicular Joint, Percutaneous Endoscopic Approach

HAC When reported with secondary diagnosis code K68.11, T81.40XA, T81.41XA, T81.42XA, T81.43XA, T81.44XA, T81.49XA, T84.60XA, T84.610A, T84.611A, T84.612A, T84.613A, T84.614A, T84.615A, T84.619A, T84.63XA, T84.69XA, T84.7XXA

0RQHXZZ Repair Left Acromioclavicular Joint, External Approach

HAC When reported with secondary diagnosis code K68.11, T81.40XA, T81.41XA, T81.42XA, T81.43XA, T81.44XA, T81.49XA, T84.60XA, T84.610A, T84.611A, T84.612A, T84.613A, T84.614A, T84.615A, T84.619A, T84.63XA, T84.69XA, T84.7XXA

0RQJ0ZZ Repair Right Shoulder Joint, Open Approach

HAC When reported with secondary diagnosis code K68.11, T81.40XA, T81.41XA, T81.42XA, T81.43XA, T81.44XA, T81.49XA, T84.60XA, T84.610A, T84.611A, T84.612A, T84.613A, T84.614A, T84.615A, T84.619A, T84.63XA, T84.69XA, T84.7XXA

0RQJ3ZZ Repair Right Shoulder Joint, Percutaneous Approach

HAC When reported with secondary diagnosis code K68.11, T81.40XA, T81.41XA, T81.42XA, T81.43XA, T81.44XA, T81.49XA, T84.60XA, T84.610A, T84.611A, T84.612A, T84.613A, T84.614A, T84.615A, T84.619A, T84.63XA, T84.69XA, T84.7XXA

0RQJ4ZZ Repair Right Shoulder Joint, Percutaneous Endoscopic Approach

HAC When reported with secondary diagnosis code K68.11, T81.40XA, T81.41XA, T81.42XA, T81.43XA, T81.44XA, T81.49XA, T84.60XA, T84.610A, T84.611A, T84.612A, T84.613A, T84.614A, T84.615A, T84.619A, T84.63XA, T84.69XA, T84.7XXA

AHA CC: 1Q, 2016, 30-31

0RQJXZZ Repair Right Shoulder Joint, External Approach

HAC When reported with secondary diagnosis code K68.11, T81.40XA, T81.41XA, T81.42XA, T81.43XA, T81.44XA, T81.49XA, T84.60XA, T84.610A, T84.611A, T84.612A, T84.613A, T84.614A, T84.615A, T84.619A, T84.63XA, T84.69XA, T84.7XXA

0RQK0ZZ Repair Left Shoulder Joint, Open Approach

HAC When reported with secondary diagnosis code K68.11, T81.40XA, T81.41XA, T81.42XA, T81.43XA, T81.44XA, T81.49XA, T84.60XA, T84.610A, T84.611A, T84.612A, T84.613A, T84.614A, T84.615A, T84.619A, T84.63XA, T84.69XA, T84.7XXA

0RQK3ZZ Repair Left Shoulder Joint, Percutaneous Approach

HAC When reported with secondary diagnosis code K68.11, T81.40XA, T81.41XA, T81.42XA, T81.43XA, T81.44XA, T81.49XA, T84.60XA, T84.610A, T84.611A, T84.612A, T84.613A, T84.614A, T84.615A, T84.619A, T84.63XA, T84.69XA, T84.7XXA

0RQK4ZZ Repair Left Shoulder Joint, Percutaneous Endoscopic Approach

HAC When reported with secondary diagnosis code K68.11, T81.40XA, T81.41XA, T81.42XA, T81.43XA, T81.44XA, T81.49XA, T84.60XA, T84.610A, T84.611A, T84.612A, T84.613A, T84.614A, T84.615A, T84.619A, T84.63XA, T84.69XA, T84.7XXA

0RQKXZZ Repair Left Shoulder Joint, External Approach

HAC When reported with secondary diagnosis code K68.11, T81.40XA, T81.41XA, T81.42XA, T81.43XA, T81.44XA, T81.49XA, T84.60XA, T84.610A, T84.611A, T84.612A, T84.613A, T84.614A, T84.615A, T84.619A, T84.63XA, T84.69XA, T84.7XXA

0RQL0ZZ Repair Right Elbow Joint, Open Approach

HAC When reported with secondary diagnosis code K68.11, T81.40XA, T81.41XA, T81.42XA, T81.43XA, T81.44XA, T81.49XA, T84.60XA, T84.610A, T84.611A, T84.612A, T84.613A, T84.614A, T84.615A, T84.619A, T84.63XA, T84.69XA, T84.7XXA

0RQL3ZZ Repair Right Elbow Joint, Percutaneous Approach

HAC When reported with secondary diagnosis code K68.11, T81.40XA, T81.41XA, T81.42XA, T81.43XA, T81.44XA, T81.49XA, T84.60XA, T84.610A, T84.611A, T84.612A, T84.613A, T84.614A, T84.615A, T84.619A, T84.63XA, T84.69XA, T84.7XXA

0RQL4ZZ Repair Right Elbow Joint, Percutaneous Endoscopic Approach

HAC When reported with secondary diagnosis code K68.11, T81.40XA, T81.41XA, T81.42XA, T81.43XA, T81.44XA, T81.49XA, T84.60XA, T84.610A, T84.611A, T84.612A, T84.613A, T84.614A, T84.615A, T84.619A, T84.63XA, T84.69XA, T84.7XXA

0RQLXZZ Repair Right Elbow Joint, External Approach

HAC When reported with secondary diagnosis code T84.60XA, T84.610A, T84.611A, T84.612A, T84.613A, T84.614A, T84.615A, T84.619A, T84.63XA, T84.69XA, T84.7XXA

0RQM0ZZ Repair Left Elbow Joint, Open Approach

HAC When reported with secondary diagnosis code T84.60XA, T84.610A, T84.611A, T84.612A, T84.613A, T84.614A, T84.615A, T84.619A, T84.63XA, T84.69XA, T84.7XXA

0RQM3ZZ Repair Left Elbow Joint, Percutaneous Approach

0RQM4ZZ Repair Left Elbow Joint, Percutaneous Endoscopic Approach

HAC When reported with secondary diagnosis code K68.11, T81.40XA, T81.41XA, T81.42XA, T81.43XA, T81.44XA, T81.49XA, T84.60XA, T84.610A, T84.611A, T84.612A, T84.613A, T84.614A, T84.615A, T84.619A, T84.63XA, T84.69XA, T84.7XXA

0RQMXZZ Repair Left Elbow Joint, External Approach

HAC When reported with secondary diagnosis code K68.11, T81.40XA, T81.41XA, T81.42XA, T81.43XA, T81.44XA, T81.49XA, T84.60XA, T84.610A, T84.611A, T84.612A, T84.613A, T84.614A, T84.615A, T84.619A, T84.63XA, T84.69XA, T84.7XXA

0RQN0ZZ Repair Right Wrist Joint, Open Approach

0RQN3ZZ Repair Right Wrist Joint, Percutaneous Approach

0RQN4ZZ Repair Right Wrist Joint, Percutaneous Endoscopic Approach

0RQNXZZ Repair Right Wrist Joint, External Approach

0RQP0ZZ Repair Left Wrist Joint, Open Approach

0RQP3ZZ Repair Left Wrist Joint, Percutaneous Approach

0RQP4ZZ Repair Left Wrist Joint, Percutaneous Endoscopic Approach

0RQPXZZ Repair Left Wrist Joint, External Approach

0RQQ0ZZ Repair Right Carpal Joint, Open Approach

0RQQ3ZZ Repair Right Carpal Joint, Percutaneous Approach

0RQQ4ZZ Repair Right Carpal Joint, Percutaneous Endoscopic Approach

0RQQXZZ Repair Right Carpal Joint, External Approach

0RQR0ZZ Repair Left Carpal Joint, Open Approach

0RQR3ZZ Repair Left Carpal Joint, Percutaneous Approach

0RQR4ZZ Repair Left Carpal Joint, Percutaneous Endoscopic Approach

0RQRXZZ Repair Left Carpal Joint, External Approach

0RQS0ZZ Repair Right Carpometacarpal Joint, Open Approach

0RQS3ZZ Repair Right Carpometacarpal Joint, Percutaneous Approach

0RQS4ZZ Repair Right Carpometacarpal Joint, Percutaneous Endoscopic Approach

0RQSXZZ Repair Right Carpometacarpal Joint, External Approach

0RQT0ZZ Repair Left Carpometacarpal Joint, Open Approach

0RQT3ZZ Repair Left Carpometacarpal Joint, Percutaneous Approach

0RQT4ZZ Repair Left Carpometacarpal Joint, Percutaneous Endoscopic Approach

0RQTXZZ Repair Left Carpometacarpal Joint, External Approach

♀ Female-only   ♂ Male-only   ▲ Limited Coverage   ● Non-OR   HAC HAC-associated procedure   ▲ Non-covered procedures   ✚ Cluster

0RQU0ZZ	Repair Right Metacarpophalangeal Joint, Open Approach
0RQU3ZZ	Repair Right Metacarpophalangeal Joint, Percutaneous Approach
0RQU4ZZ	Repair Right Metacarpophalangeal Joint, Percutaneous Endoscopic Approach
0RQUXZZ	Repair Right Metacarpophalangeal Joint, External Approach
0RQV0ZZ	Repair Left Metacarpophalangeal Joint, Open Approach
0RQV3ZZ	Repair Left Metacarpophalangeal Joint, Percutaneous Approach
0RQV4ZZ	Repair Left Metacarpophalangeal Joint, Percutaneous Endoscopic Approach
0RQVXZZ	Repair Left Metacarpophalangeal Joint, External Approach
0RQW0ZZ	Repair Right Finger Phalangeal Joint, Open Approach
0RQW3ZZ	Repair Right Finger Phalangeal Joint, Percutaneous Approach
0RQW4ZZ	Repair Right Finger Phalangeal Joint, Percutaneous Endoscopic Approach
0RQWXZZ	Repair Right Finger Phalangeal Joint, External Approach
0RQX0ZZ	Repair Left Finger Phalangeal Joint, Open Approach
0RQX3ZZ	Repair Left Finger Phalangeal Joint, Percutaneous Approach
0RQX4ZZ	Repair Left Finger Phalangeal Joint, Percutaneous Endoscopic Approach
0RQXXZZ	Repair Left Finger Phalangeal Joint, External Approach

0RR – Upper Joints, Replacement

Review Coding Guideline B3.18

0RR007Z	Replacement of Occipital-cervical Joint with Autologous Tissue Substitute, Open Approach
0RR00JZ	Replacement of Occipital-cervical Joint with Synthetic Substitute, Open Approach
0RR00KZ	Replacement of Occipital-cervical Joint with Nonautologous Tissue Substitute, Open Approach
0RR107Z	Replacement of Cervical Vertebral Joint with Autologous Tissue Substitute, Open Approach
0RR10JZ	Replacement of Cervical Vertebral Joint with Synthetic Substitute, Open Approach
0RR10KZ	Replacement of Cervical Vertebral Joint with Nonautologous Tissue Substitute, Open Approach
0RR307Z	Replacement of Cervical Vertebral Disc with Autologous Tissue Substitute, Open Approach
0RR30JZ	Replacement of Cervical Vertebral Disc with Synthetic Substitute, Open Approach
0RR30KZ	Replacement of Cervical Vertebral Disc with Nonautologous Tissue Substitute, Open Approach
0RR407Z	Replacement of Cervicothoracic Vertebral Joint with Autologous Tissue Substitute, Open Approach
0RR40JZ	Replacement of Cervicothoracic Vertebral Joint with Synthetic Substitute, Open Approach
0RR40KZ	Replacement of Cervicothoracic Vertebral Joint with Nonautologous Tissue Substitute, Open Approach
0RR507Z	Replacement of Cervicothoracic Vertebral Disc with Autologous Tissue Substitute, Open Approach
0RR50JZ	Replacement of Cervicothoracic Vertebral Disc with Synthetic Substitute, Open Approach
0RR50KZ	Replacement of Cervicothoracic Vertebral Disc with Nonautologous Tissue Substitute, Open Approach
0RR607Z	Replacement of Thoracic Vertebral Joint with Autologous Tissue Substitute, Open Approach
0RR60JZ	Replacement of Thoracic Vertebral Joint with Synthetic Substitute, Open Approach
0RR60KZ	Replacement of Thoracic Vertebral Joint with Nonautologous Tissue Substitute, Open Approach

0RR907Z	Replacement of Thoracic Vertebral Disc with Autologous Tissue Substitute, Open Approach
0RR90JZ	Replacement of Thoracic Vertebral Disc with Synthetic Substitute, Open Approach
0RR90KZ	Replacement of Thoracic Vertebral Disc with Nonautologous Tissue Substitute, Open Approach
0RRA07Z	Replacement of Thoracolumbar Vertebral Joint with Autologous Tissue Substitute, Open Approach
0RRA0JZ	Replacement of Thoracolumbar Vertebral Joint with Synthetic Substitute, Open Approach
0RRA0KZ	Replacement of Thoracolumbar Vertebral Joint with Nonautologous Tissue Substitute, Open Approach
0RRB07Z	Replacement of Thoracolumbar Vertebral Disc with Autologous Tissue Substitute, Open Approach
0RRB0JZ	Replacement of Thoracolumbar Vertebral Disc with Synthetic Substitute, Open Approach
0RRB0KZ	Replacement of Thoracolumbar Vertebral Disc with Nonautologous Tissue Substitute, Open Approach
0RRC07Z	Replacement of Right Temporomandibular Joint with Autologous Tissue Substitute, Open Approach
0RRC0JZ	Replacement of Right Temporomandibular Joint with Synthetic Substitute, Open Approach
0RRC0KZ	Replacement of Right Temporomandibular Joint with Nonautologous Tissue Substitute, Open Approach
0RRD07Z	Replacement of Left Temporomandibular Joint with Autologous Tissue Substitute, Open Approach
0RRD0JZ	Replacement of Left Temporomandibular Joint with Synthetic Substitute, Open Approach
0RRD0KZ	Replacement of Left Temporomandibular Joint with Nonautologous Tissue Substitute, Open Approach
0RRE07Z	Replacement of Right Sternoclavicular Joint with Autologous Tissue Substitute, Open Approach
0RRE0JZ	Replacement of Right Sternoclavicular Joint with Synthetic Substitute, Open Approach

0RRE0KZ	Replacement of Right Sternoclavicular Joint with Nonautologous Tissue Substitute, Open Approach
0RRF07Z	Replacement of Left Sternoclavicular Joint with Autologous Tissue Substitute, Open Approach
0RRF0JZ	Replacement of Left Sternoclavicular Joint with Synthetic Substitute, Open Approach
0RRF0KZ	Replacement of Left Sternoclavicular Joint with Nonautologous Tissue Substitute, Open Approach
0RRG07Z	Replacement of Right Acromioclavicular Joint with Autologous Tissue Substitute, Open Approach
0RRG0JZ	Replacement of Right Acromioclavicular Joint with Synthetic Substitute, Open Approach
0RRG0KZ	Replacement of Right Acromioclavicular Joint with Nonautologous Tissue Substitute, Open Approach
0RRH07Z	Replacement of Left Acromioclavicular Joint with Autologous Tissue Substitute, Open Approach
0RRH0JZ	Replacement of Left Acromioclavicular Joint with Synthetic Substitute, Open Approach
0RRH0KZ	Replacement of Left Acromioclavicular Joint with Nonautologous Tissue Substitute, Open Approach
0RRJ00Z	Replacement of Right Shoulder Joint with Reverse Ball and Socket Synthetic Substitute, Open Approach
	AHA CC: 1Q, 2015, 27
0RRJ07Z	Replacement of Right Shoulder Joint with Autologous Tissue Substitute, Open Approach
0RRJ0J6	Replacement of Right Shoulder Joint with Synthetic Substitute, Humeral Surface, Open Approach
0RRJ0J7	Replacement of Right Shoulder Joint with Synthetic Substitute, Glenoid Surface, Open Approach
0RRJ0JZ	Replacement of Right Shoulder Joint with Synthetic Substitute, Open Approach
0RRJ0KZ	Replacement of Right Shoulder Joint with Nonautologous Tissue Substitute, Open Approach
0RRK00Z	Replacement of Left Shoulder Joint with Reverse Ball and Socket Synthetic Substitute, Open Approach
0RRK07Z	Replacement of Left Shoulder Joint with Autologous Tissue Substitute, Open Approach

0RRK0J6 Replacement of Left Shoulder Joint with Synthetic Substitute, Humeral Surface, Open Approach
AHA CC: 3Q, 2015, 14-15

0RRK0J7 Replacement of Left Shoulder Joint with Synthetic Substitute, Glenoid Surface, Open Approach

0RRK0JZ Replacement of Left Shoulder Joint with Synthetic Substitute, Open Approach

0RRK0KZ Replacement of Left Shoulder Joint with Nonautologous Tissue Substitute, Open Approach

0RRL07Z Replacement of Right Elbow Joint with Autologous Tissue Substitute, Open Approach

0RRL0JZ Replacement of Right Elbow Joint with Synthetic Substitute, Open Approach

0RRL0KZ Replacement of Right Elbow Joint with Nonautologous Tissue Substitute, Open Approach

0RRM07Z Replacement of Left Elbow Joint with Autologous Tissue Substitute, Open Approach

0RRM0JZ Replacement of Left Elbow Joint with Synthetic Substitute, Open Approach

0RRM0KZ Replacement of Left Elbow Joint with Nonautologous Tissue Substitute, Open Approach

0RRN07Z Replacement of Right Wrist Joint with Autologous Tissue Substitute, Open Approach

0RRN0JZ Replacement of Right Wrist Joint with Synthetic Substitute, Open Approach

0RRN0KZ Replacement of Right Wrist Joint with Nonautologous Tissue Substitute, Open Approach

0RRP07Z Replacement of Left Wrist Joint with Autologous Tissue Substitute, Open Approach

0RRP0JZ Replacement of Left Wrist Joint with Synthetic Substitute, Open Approach

0RRP0KZ Replacement of Left Wrist Joint with Nonautologous Tissue Substitute, Open Approach

0RRQ07Z Replacement of Right Carpal Joint with Autologous Tissue Substitute, Open Approach

0RRQ0JZ Replacement of Right Carpal Joint with Synthetic Substitute, Open Approach

0RRQ0KZ Replacement of Right Carpal Joint with Nonautologous Tissue Substitute, Open Approach

0RRR07Z Replacement of Left Carpal Joint with Autologous Tissue Substitute, Open Approach

0RRR0JZ Replacement of Left Carpal Joint with Synthetic Substitute, Open Approach

0RRR0KZ Replacement of Left Carpal Joint with Nonautologous Tissue Substitute, Open Approach

0RRS07Z Replacement of Right Carpometacarpal Joint with Autologous Tissue Substitute, Open Approach

0RRS0JZ Replacement of Right Carpometacarpal Joint with Synthetic Substitute, Open Approach

0RRS0KZ Replacement of Right Carpometacarpal Joint with Nonautologous Tissue Substitute, Open Approach

0RRT07Z Replacement of Left Carpometacarpal Joint with Autologous Tissue Substitute, Open Approach

0RRT0JZ Replacement of Left Carpometacarpal Joint with Synthetic Substitute, Open Approach

0RRT0KZ Replacement of Left Carpometacarpal Joint with Nonautologous Tissue Substitute, Open Approach

0RRU07Z Replacement of Right Metacarpophalangeal Joint with Autologous Tissue Substitute, Open Approach

0RRU0JZ Replacement of Right Metacarpophalangeal Joint with Synthetic Substitute, Open Approach

0RRU0KZ Replacement of Right Metacarpophalangeal Joint with Nonautologous Tissue Substitute, Open Approach

0RRV07Z Replacement of Left Metacarpophalangeal Joint with Autologous Tissue Substitute, Open Approach

0RRV0JZ Replacement of Left Metacarpophalangeal Joint with Synthetic Substitute, Open Approach

0RRV0KZ Replacement of Left Metacarpophalangeal Joint with Nonautologous Tissue Substitute, Open Approach

0RRW07Z Replacement of Right Finger Phalangeal Joint with Autologous Tissue Substitute, Open Approach

0RRW0JZ Replacement of Right Finger Phalangeal Joint with Synthetic Substitute, Open Approach

0RRW0KZ Replacement of Right Finger Phalangeal Joint with Nonautologous Tissue Substitute, Open Approach

0RRX07Z Replacement of Left Finger Phalangeal Joint with Autologous Tissue Substitute, Open Approach

0RRX0JZ Replacement of Left Finger Phalangeal Joint with Synthetic Substitute, Open Approach

0RRX0KZ Replacement of Left Finger Phalangeal Joint with Nonautologous Tissue Substitute, Open Approach

0RS – Upper Joints, Reposition

0RS004Z Reposition Occipital-cervical Joint with Internal Fixation Device, Open Approach

0RS00ZZ Reposition Occipital-cervical Joint, Open Approach

0RS034Z Reposition Occipital-cervical Joint with Internal Fixation Device, Percutaneous Approach

0RS03ZZ Reposition Occipital-cervical Joint, Percutaneous Approach

0RS044Z Reposition Occipital-cervical Joint with Internal Fixation Device, Percutaneous Endoscopic Approach

0RS04ZZ Reposition Occipital-cervical Joint, Percutaneous Endoscopic Approach

0RS0X4Z Reposition Occipital-cervical Joint with Internal Fixation Device, External Approach

0RS0XZZ Reposition Occipital-cervical Joint, External Approach

0RS104Z Reposition Cervical Vertebral Joint with Internal Fixation Device, Open Approach

0RS10ZZ Reposition Cervical Vertebral Joint, Open Approach

0RS134Z Reposition Cervical Vertebral Joint with Internal Fixation Device, Percutaneous Approach

0RS13ZZ Reposition Cervical Vertebral Joint, Percutaneous Approach

0RS144Z Reposition Cervical Vertebral Joint with Internal Fixation Device, Percutaneous Endoscopic Approach

0RS14ZZ Reposition Cervical Vertebral Joint, Percutaneous Endoscopic Approach

0RS1X4Z Reposition Cervical Vertebral Joint with Internal Fixation Device, External Approach

0RS1XZZ Reposition Cervical Vertebral Joint, External Approach

0RS404Z Reposition Cervicothoracic Vertebral Joint with Internal Fixation Device, Open Approach

0RS40ZZ Reposition Cervicothoracic Vertebral Joint, Open Approach

0RS434Z Reposition Cervicothoracic Vertebral Joint with Internal Fixation Device, Percutaneous Approach

0RS43ZZ Reposition Cervicothoracic Vertebral Joint, Percutaneous Approach

0RS444Z Reposition Cervicothoracic Vertebral Joint with Internal Fixation Device, Percutaneous Endoscopic Approach

0RS44ZZ Reposition Cervicothoracic Vertebral Joint, Percutaneous Endoscopic Approach

0RS4X4Z Reposition Cervicothoracic Vertebral Joint with Internal Fixation Device, External Approach

0RS4XZZ Reposition Cervicothoracic Vertebral Joint, External Approach

0RS604Z Reposition Thoracic Vertebral Joint with Internal Fixation Device, Open Approach

0RS60ZZ Reposition Thoracic Vertebral Joint, Open Approach

0RS634Z Reposition Thoracic Vertebral Joint with Internal Fixation Device, Percutaneous Approach

0RS63ZZ Reposition Thoracic Vertebral Joint, Percutaneous Approach

0RS644Z Reposition Thoracic Vertebral Joint with Internal Fixation Device, Percutaneous Endoscopic Approach

0RS64ZZ Reposition Thoracic Vertebral Joint, Percutaneous Endoscopic Approach

0RS6X4Z Reposition Thoracic Vertebral Joint with Internal Fixation Device, External Approach

0RS6XZZ Reposition Thoracic Vertebral Joint, External Approach

0RSA04Z Reposition Thoracolumbar Vertebral Joint with Internal Fixation Device, Open Approach

0RSA0ZZ Reposition Thoracolumbar Vertebral Joint, Open Approach

0RSA34Z	Reposition Thoracolumbar Vertebral Joint with Internal Fixation Device, Percutaneous Approach
0RSA3ZZ	Reposition Thoracolumbar Vertebral Joint, Percutaneous Approach
0RSA44Z	Reposition Thoracolumbar Vertebral Joint with Internal Fixation Device, Percutaneous Endoscopic Approach
0RSA4ZZ	Reposition Thoracolumbar Vertebral Joint, Percutaneous Endoscopic Approach
0RSAX4Z	Reposition Thoracolumbar Vertebral Joint with Internal Fixation Device, External Approach
0RSAXZZ	Reposition Thoracolumbar Vertebral Joint, External Approach
0RSC04Z	Reposition Right Temporomandibular Joint with Internal Fixation Device, Open Approach
0RSC0ZZ	Reposition Right Temporomandibular Joint, Open Approach
0RSC34Z	Reposition Right Temporomandibular Joint with Internal Fixation Device, Percutaneous Approach
0RSC3ZZ	Reposition Right Temporomandibular Joint, Percutaneous Approach
0RSC44Z	Reposition Right Temporomandibular Joint with Internal Fixation Device, Percutaneous Endoscopic Approach
0RSC4ZZ	Reposition Right Temporomandibular Joint, Percutaneous Endoscopic Approach
0RSCX4Z	Reposition Right Temporomandibular Joint with Internal Fixation Device, External Approach
0RSCXZZ	Reposition Right Temporomandibular Joint, External Approach
0RSD04Z	Reposition Left Temporomandibular Joint with Internal Fixation Device, Open Approach
0RSD0ZZ	Reposition Left Temporomandibular Joint, Open Approach
0RSD34Z	Reposition Left Temporomandibular Joint with Internal Fixation Device, Percutaneous Approach
0RSD3ZZ	Reposition Left Temporomandibular Joint, Percutaneous Approach
0RSD44Z	Reposition Left Temporomandibular Joint with Internal Fixation Device, Percutaneous Endoscopic Approach
0RSD4ZZ	Reposition Left Temporomandibular Joint, Percutaneous Endoscopic Approach
0RSDX4Z	Reposition Left Temporomandibular Joint with Internal Fixation Device, External Approach
0RSDXZZ	Reposition Left Temporomandibular Joint, External Approach
0RSE04Z	Reposition Right Sternoclavicular Joint with Internal Fixation Device, Open Approach
0RSE0ZZ	Reposition Right Sternoclavicular Joint, Open Approach
0RSE34Z	Reposition Right Sternoclavicular Joint with Internal Fixation Device, Percutaneous Approach
0RSE3ZZ	Reposition Right Sternoclavicular Joint, Percutaneous Approach
0RSE44Z	Reposition Right Sternoclavicular Joint with Internal Fixation Device, Percutaneous Endoscopic Approach
0RSE4ZZ	Reposition Right Sternoclavicular Joint, Percutaneous Endoscopic Approach

0RSEX4Z	Reposition Right Sternoclavicular Joint with Internal Fixation Device, External Approach
0RSEXZZ	Reposition Right Sternoclavicular Joint, External Approach
0RSF04Z	Reposition Left Sternoclavicular Joint with Internal Fixation Device, Open Approach
0RSF0ZZ	Reposition Left Sternoclavicular Joint, Open Approach
0RSF34Z	Reposition Left Sternoclavicular Joint with Internal Fixation Device, Percutaneous Approach
0RSF3ZZ	Reposition Left Sternoclavicular Joint, Percutaneous Approach
0RSF44Z	Reposition Left Sternoclavicular Joint with Internal Fixation Device, Percutaneous Endoscopic Approach
0RSF4ZZ	Reposition Left Sternoclavicular Joint, Percutaneous Endoscopic Approach
0RSFX4Z	Reposition Left Sternoclavicular Joint with Internal Fixation Device, External Approach
0RSFXZZ	Reposition Left Sternoclavicular Joint, External Approach
0RSG04Z	Reposition Right Acromioclavicular Joint with Internal Fixation Device, Open Approach
0RSG0ZZ	Reposition Right Acromioclavicular Joint, Open Approach
0RSG34Z	Reposition Right Acromioclavicular Joint with Internal Fixation Device, Percutaneous Approach
0RSG3ZZ	Reposition Right Acromioclavicular Joint, Percutaneous Approach
0RSG44Z	Reposition Right Acromioclavicular Joint with Internal Fixation Device, Percutaneous Endoscopic Approach
0RSG4ZZ	Reposition Right Acromioclavicular Joint, Percutaneous Endoscopic Approach
0RSGX4Z	Reposition Right Acromioclavicular Joint with Internal Fixation Device, External Approach
0RSGXZZ	Reposition Right Acromioclavicular Joint, External Approach
0RSH04Z	Reposition Left Acromioclavicular Joint with Internal Fixation Device, Open Approach
	AHA CC: 3Q, 2019, 26-27
0RSH0ZZ	Reposition Left Acromioclavicular Joint, Open Approach
0RSH34Z	Reposition Left Acromioclavicular Joint with Internal Fixation Device, Percutaneous Approach
0RSH3ZZ	Reposition Left Acromioclavicular Joint, Percutaneous Approach
0RSH44Z	Reposition Left Acromioclavicular Joint with Internal Fixation Device, Percutaneous Endoscopic Approach
0RSH4ZZ	Reposition Left Acromioclavicular Joint, Percutaneous Endoscopic Approach
0RSHX4Z	Reposition Left Acromioclavicular Joint with Internal Fixation Device, External Approach
0RSHXZZ	Reposition Left Acromioclavicular Joint, External Approach
0RSJ04Z	Reposition Right Shoulder Joint with Internal Fixation Device, Open Approach
0RSJ0ZZ	Reposition Right Shoulder Joint, Open Approach
0RSJ34Z	Reposition Right Shoulder Joint with Internal Fixation Device, Percutaneous Approach

0RSJ3ZZ	Reposition Right Shoulder Joint, Percutaneous Approach
0RSJ44Z	Reposition Right Shoulder Joint with Internal Fixation Device, Percutaneous Endoscopic Approach
0RSJ4ZZ	Reposition Right Shoulder Joint, Percutaneous Endoscopic Approach
0RSJX4Z	Reposition Right Shoulder Joint with Internal Fixation Device, External Approach
0RSJXZZ	Reposition Right Shoulder Joint, External Approach
0RSK04Z	Reposition Left Shoulder Joint with Internal Fixation Device, Open Approach
0RSK0ZZ	Reposition Left Shoulder Joint, Open Approach
0RSK34Z	Reposition Left Shoulder Joint with Internal Fixation Device, Percutaneous Approach
0RSK3ZZ	Reposition Left Shoulder Joint, Percutaneous Approach
0RSK44Z	Reposition Left Shoulder Joint with Internal Fixation Device, Percutaneous Endoscopic Approach
0RSK4ZZ	Reposition Left Shoulder Joint with Internal Fixation Device, Percutaneous Endoscopic Approach
0RSKX4Z	Reposition Left Shoulder Joint with Internal Fixation Device, External Approach
0RSKXZZ	Reposition Left Shoulder Joint, External Approach
0RSL04Z	Reposition Right Elbow Joint with Internal Fixation Device, Open Approach
0RSL05Z	Reposition Right Elbow Joint with External Fixation Device, Open Approach
0RSL0ZZ	Reposition Right Elbow Joint, Open Approach
0RSL34Z	Reposition Right Elbow Joint with Internal Fixation Device, Percutaneous Approach
0RSL35Z	Reposition Right Elbow Joint with External Fixation Device, Percutaneous Approach
0RSL3ZZ	Reposition Right Elbow Joint, Percutaneous Approach
0RSL44Z	Reposition Right Elbow Joint with Internal Fixation Device, Percutaneous Endoscopic Approach
0RSL45Z	Reposition Right Elbow Joint with External Fixation Device, Percutaneous Endoscopic Approach
0RSL4ZZ	Reposition Right Elbow Joint, Percutaneous Endoscopic Approach
0RSLX4Z	Reposition Right Elbow Joint with Internal Fixation Device, External Approach
0RSLX5Z	Reposition Right Elbow Joint with External Fixation Device, External Approach
0RSLXZZ	Reposition Right Elbow Joint, External Approach
0RSM04Z	Reposition Left Elbow Joint with Internal Fixation Device, Open Approach
0RSM05Z	Reposition Left Elbow Joint with External Fixation Device, Open Approach
0RSM0ZZ	Reposition Left Elbow Joint, Open Approach
0RSM34Z	Reposition Left Elbow Joint with Internal Fixation Device, Percutaneous Approach

0RSM35Z Reposition Left Elbow Joint with External Fixation Device, Percutaneous Approach

0RSM3ZZ Reposition Left Elbow Joint, Percutaneous Approach

0RSM44Z Reposition Left Elbow Joint with Internal Fixation Device, Percutaneous Endoscopic Approach

0RSM45Z Reposition Left Elbow Joint with External Fixation Device, Percutaneous Endoscopic Approach

0RSM4ZZ Reposition Left Elbow Joint, Percutaneous Endoscopic Approach

0RSMX4Z Reposition Left Elbow Joint with Internal Fixation Device, External Approach

0RSMX5Z Reposition Left Elbow Joint with External Fixation Device, External Approach

0RSMXZZ Reposition Left Elbow Joint, External Approach

0RSN04Z Reposition Right Wrist Joint with Internal Fixation Device, Open Approach

0RSN05Z Reposition Right Wrist Joint with External Fixation Device, Open Approach

0RSN0ZZ Reposition Right Wrist Joint, Open Approach

0RSN34Z Reposition Right Wrist Joint with Internal Fixation Device, Percutaneous Approach

0RSN35Z Reposition Right Wrist Joint with External Fixation Device, Percutaneous Approach

0RSN3ZZ Reposition Right Wrist Joint, Percutaneous Approach

0RSN44Z Reposition Right Wrist Joint with Internal Fixation Device, Percutaneous Endoscopic Approach

0RSN45Z Reposition Right Wrist Joint with External Fixation Device, Percutaneous Endoscopic Approach

0RSN4ZZ Reposition Right Wrist Joint, Percutaneous Endoscopic Approach

0RSNX4Z Reposition Right Wrist Joint with Internal Fixation Device, External Approach

0RSNX5Z Reposition Right Wrist Joint with External Fixation Device, External Approach

0RSNXZZ Reposition Right Wrist Joint, External Approach

0RSP04Z Reposition Left Wrist Joint with Internal Fixation Device, Open Approach

0RSP05Z Reposition Left Wrist Joint with External Fixation Device, Open Approach

0RSP0ZZ Reposition Left Wrist Joint, Open Approach

0RSP34Z Reposition Left Wrist Joint with Internal Fixation Device, Percutaneous Approach

0RSP35Z Reposition Left Wrist Joint with External Fixation Device, Percutaneous Approach

0RSP3ZZ Reposition Left Wrist Joint, Percutaneous Approach

0RSP44Z Reposition Left Wrist Joint with Internal Fixation Device, Percutaneous Endoscopic Approach

0RSP45Z Reposition Left Wrist Joint with External Fixation Device, Percutaneous Endoscopic Approach

0RSP4ZZ Reposition Left Wrist Joint, Percutaneous Endoscopic Approach

0RSPX4Z Reposition Left Wrist Joint with Internal Fixation Device, External Approach

0RSPX5Z Reposition Left Wrist Joint with External Fixation Device, External Approach

0RSPXZZ Reposition Left Wrist Joint, External Approach

AHA CC: 4Q, 2014, 32-33

0RSQ04Z Reposition Right Carpal Joint with Internal Fixation Device, Open Approach

0RSQ05Z Reposition Right Carpal Joint with External Fixation Device, Open Approach

0RSQ0ZZ Reposition Right Carpal Joint, Open Approach

0RSQ34Z Reposition Right Carpal Joint with Internal Fixation Device, Percutaneous Approach

0RSQ35Z Reposition Right Carpal Joint with External Fixation Device, Percutaneous Approach

0RSQ3ZZ Reposition Right Carpal Joint, Percutaneous Approach

0RSQ44Z Reposition Right Carpal Joint with Internal Fixation Device, Percutaneous Endoscopic Approach

0RSQ45Z Reposition Right Carpal Joint with External Fixation Device, Percutaneous Endoscopic Approach

0RSQ4ZZ Reposition Right Carpal Joint, Percutaneous Endoscopic Approach

0RSQX4Z Reposition Right Carpal Joint with Internal Fixation Device, External Approach

0RSQX5Z Reposition Right Carpal Joint with External Fixation Device, External Approach

0RSQXZZ Reposition Right Carpal Joint, External Approach

0RSR04Z Reposition Left Carpal Joint with Internal Fixation Device, Open Approach

AHA CC: 3Q, 2014, 33-34

0RSR05Z Reposition Left Carpal Joint with External Fixation Device, Open Approach

0RSR0ZZ Reposition Left Carpal Joint, Open Approach

0RSR34Z Reposition Left Carpal Joint with Internal Fixation Device, Percutaneous Approach

0RSR35Z Reposition Left Carpal Joint with External Fixation Device, Percutaneous Approach

0RSR3ZZ Reposition Left Carpal Joint, Percutaneous Approach

0RSR44Z Reposition Left Carpal Joint with Internal Fixation Device, Percutaneous Endoscopic Approach

0RSR45Z Reposition Left Carpal Joint with External Fixation Device, Percutaneous Endoscopic Approach

0RSR4ZZ Reposition Left Carpal Joint, Percutaneous Endoscopic Approach

0RSRX4Z Reposition Left Carpal Joint with Internal Fixation Device, External Approach

0RSRX5Z Reposition Left Carpal Joint with External Fixation Device, External Approach

0RSRXZZ Reposition Left Carpal Joint, External Approach

0RSS04Z Reposition Right Carpometacarpal Joint with Internal Fixation Device, Open Approach

0RSS05Z Reposition Right Carpometacarpal Joint with External Fixation Device, Open Approach

0RSS0ZZ Reposition Right Carpometacarpal Joint, Open Approach

0RSS34Z Reposition Right Carpometacarpal Joint with Internal Fixation Device, Percutaneous Approach

0RSS35Z Reposition Right Carpometacarpal Joint with External Fixation Device, Percutaneous Approach

0RSS3ZZ Reposition Right Carpometacarpal Joint, Percutaneous Approach

0RSS44Z Reposition Right Carpometacarpal Joint with Internal Fixation Device, Percutaneous Endoscopic Approach

0RSS45Z Reposition Right Carpometacarpal Joint with External Fixation Device, Percutaneous Endoscopic Approach

0RSS4ZZ Reposition Right Carpometacarpal Joint, Percutaneous Endoscopic Approach

0RSSX4Z Reposition Right Carpometacarpal Joint with Internal Fixation Device, External Approach

0RSSX5Z Reposition Right Carpometacarpal Joint with External Fixation Device, External Approach

0RSSXZZ Reposition Right Carpometacarpal Joint, External Approach

0RST04Z Reposition Left Carpometacarpal Joint with Internal Fixation Device, Open Approach

0RST05Z Reposition Left Carpometacarpal Joint with External Fixation Device, Open Approach

0RST0ZZ Reposition Left Carpometacarpal Joint, Open Approach

0RST34Z Reposition Left Carpometacarpal Joint with Internal Fixation Device, Percutaneous Approach

0RST35Z Reposition Left Carpometacarpal Joint with External Fixation Device, Percutaneous Approach

0RST3ZZ Reposition Left Carpometacarpal Joint, Percutaneous Approach

0RST44Z Reposition Left Carpometacarpal Joint with Internal Fixation Device, Percutaneous Endoscopic Approach

0RST45Z Reposition Left Carpometacarpal Joint with External Fixation Device, Percutaneous Endoscopic Approach

0RST4ZZ Reposition Left Carpometacarpal Joint, Percutaneous Endoscopic Approach

0RSTX4Z Reposition Left Carpometacarpal Joint with Internal Fixation Device, External Approach

0RSTX5Z Reposition Left Carpometacarpal Joint with External Fixation Device, External Approach

0RSTXZZ Reposition Left Carpometacarpal Joint, External Approach

0RSU04Z Reposition Right Metacarpophalangeal Joint with Internal Fixation Device, Open Approach

0RSU05Z Reposition Right Metacarpophalangeal Joint with External Fixation Device, Open Approach

0RSU0ZZ Reposition Right Metacarpophalangeal Joint, Open Approach

0RSU34Z Reposition Right Metacarpophalangeal Joint with Internal Fixation Device, Percutaneous Approach

♀ Female-only   ♂ Male-only   ▲ Limited Coverage   ● Non-OR   ■ HAC-associated procedure   ▲ Non-covered procedures   ✚ Cluster

0RSU35Z	Reposition Right Metacarpophalangeal Joint with External Fixation Device, Percutaneous Approach
0RSU3ZZ	Reposition Right Metacarpophalangeal Joint, Percutaneous Approach
0RSU44Z	Reposition Right Metacarpophalangeal Joint with Internal Fixation Device, Percutaneous Endoscopic Approach
0RSU45Z	Reposition Right Metacarpophalangeal Joint with External Fixation Device, Percutaneous Endoscopic Approach
0RSU4ZZ	Reposition Right Metacarpophalangeal Joint, Percutaneous Endoscopic Approach
0RSUX4Z	Reposition Right Metacarpophalangeal Joint with Internal Fixation Device, External Approach
0RSUX5Z	Reposition Right Metacarpophalangeal Joint with External Fixation Device, External Approach
0RSUXZZ	Reposition Right Metacarpophalangeal Joint, External Approach
0RSV04Z	Reposition Left Metacarpophalangeal Joint with Internal Fixation Device, Open Approach
0RSV05Z	Reposition Left Metacarpophalangeal Joint with External Fixation Device, Open Approach
0RSV0ZZ	Reposition Left Metacarpophalangeal Joint, Open Approach
0RSV34Z	Reposition Left Metacarpophalangeal Joint with Internal Fixation Device, Percutaneous Approach
0RSV35Z	Reposition Left Metacarpophalangeal Joint with External Fixation Device, Percutaneous Approach
0RSV3ZZ	Reposition Left Metacarpophalangeal Joint, Percutaneous Approach
0RSV44Z	Reposition Left Metacarpophalangeal Joint with Internal Fixation

0RSV45Z	Reposition Left Metacarpophalangeal Joint with External Fixation Device, Percutaneous Endoscopic Approach
0RSV4ZZ	Reposition Left Metacarpophalangeal Joint, Percutaneous Endoscopic Approach
0RSVX4Z	Reposition Left Metacarpophalangeal Joint with Internal Fixation Device, External Approach
0RSVX5Z	Reposition Left Metacarpophalangeal Joint with External Fixation Device, External Approach
0RSVXZZ	Reposition Left Metacarpophalangeal Joint, External Approach
0RSW04Z	Reposition Right Finger Phalangeal Joint with Internal Fixation Device, Open Approach
0RSW05Z	Reposition Right Finger Phalangeal Joint with External Fixation Device, Open Approach
0RSW0ZZ	Reposition Right Finger Phalangeal Joint, Open Approach
0RSW34Z	Reposition Right Finger Phalangeal Joint with Internal Fixation Device, Percutaneous Approach
0RSW35Z	Reposition Right Finger Phalangeal Joint with External Fixation Device, Percutaneous Approach
0RSW3ZZ	Reposition Right Finger Phalangeal Joint, Percutaneous Approach
0RSW44Z	Reposition Right Finger Phalangeal Joint with Internal Fixation Device, Percutaneous Endoscopic Approach
0RSW45Z	Reposition Right Finger Phalangeal Joint with External Fixation Device, Percutaneous Endoscopic Approach
0RSW4ZZ	Reposition Right Finger Phalangeal Joint, Percutaneous Endoscopic Approach

0RSWX4Z	Reposition Right Finger Phalangeal Joint with Internal Fixation Device, External Approach
0RSWX5Z	Reposition Right Finger Phalangeal Joint with External Fixation Device, External Approach
0RSWXZZ	Reposition Right Finger Phalangeal Joint, External Approach
0RSX04Z	Reposition Left Finger Phalangeal Joint with Internal Fixation Device, Open Approach
0RSX05Z	Reposition Left Finger Phalangeal Joint with External Fixation Device, Open Approach
0RSX0ZZ	Reposition Left Finger Phalangeal Joint, Open Approach
0RSX34Z	Reposition Left Finger Phalangeal Joint with Internal Fixation Device, Percutaneous Approach
0RSX35Z	Reposition Left Finger Phalangeal Joint with External Fixation Device, Percutaneous Approach
0RSX3ZZ	Reposition Left Finger Phalangeal Joint, Percutaneous Approach
0RSX44Z	Reposition Left Finger Phalangeal Joint with Internal Fixation Device, Percutaneous Endoscopic Approach
0RSX45Z	Reposition Left Finger Phalangeal Joint with External Fixation Device, Percutaneous Endoscopic Approach
0RSX4ZZ	Reposition Left Finger Phalangeal Joint, Percutaneous Endoscopic Approach
0RSXX4Z	Reposition Left Finger Phalangeal Joint with Internal Fixation Device, External Approach
0RSXX5Z	Reposition Left Finger Phalangeal Joint with External Fixation Device, External Approach
0RSXXZZ	Reposition Left Finger Phalangeal Joint, External Approach

0RT – Upper Joints, Resection

Review Coding Guideline B3.8

Review Coding Guideline B3.18

0RT30ZZ	Resection of Cervical Vertebral Disc, Open Approach
0RT40ZZ	Resection of Cervicothoracic Vertebral Joint, Open Approach
0RT50ZZ	Resection of Cervicothoracic Vertebral Disc, Open Approach
	AHA CC: 2Q, 2014, 7-8
0RT90ZZ	Resection of Thoracic Vertebral Disc, Open Approach
0RTB0ZZ	Resection of Thoracolumbar Vertebral Disc, Open Approach
0RTC0ZZ	Resection of Right Temporomandibular Joint, Open Approach
0RTD0ZZ	Resection of Left Temporomandibular Joint, Open Approach
0RTE0ZZ	Resection of Right Sternoclavicular Joint, Open Approach

0RTF0ZZ	Resection of Left Sternoclavicular Joint, Open Approach
0RTG0ZZ	Resection of Right Acromioclavicular Joint, Open Approach
0RTH0ZZ	Resection of Left Acromioclavicular Joint, Open Approach
0RTJ0ZZ	Resection of Right Shoulder Joint, Open Approach
0RTK0ZZ	Resection of Left Shoulder Joint, Open Approach
0RTL0ZZ	Resection of Right Elbow Joint, Open Approach
0RTM0ZZ	Resection of Left Elbow Joint, Open Approach
0RTN0ZZ	Resection of Right Wrist Joint, Open Approach
0RTP0ZZ	Resection of Left Wrist Joint, Open Approach

0RTQ0ZZ	Resection of Right Carpal Joint, Open Approach
0RTR0ZZ	Resection of Left Carpal Joint, Open Approach
0RTS0ZZ	Resection of Right Carpometacarpal Joint, Open Approach
0RTT0ZZ	Resection of Left Carpometacarpal Joint, Open Approach
0RTU0ZZ	Resection of Right Metacarpophalangeal Joint, Open Approach
0RTV0ZZ	Resection of Left Metacarpophalangeal Joint, Open Approach
0RTW0ZZ	Resection of Right Finger Phalangeal Joint, Open Approach
0RTX0ZZ	Resection of Left Finger Phalangeal Joint, Open Approach

0RU – Upper Joints, Supplement

| 0RU007Z | Supplement Occipital-cervical Joint with Autologous Tissue Substitute, Open Approach |
| 0RU00JZ | Supplement Occipital-cervical Joint with Synthetic Substitute, Open Approach |

| 0RU00KZ | Supplement Occipital-cervical Joint with Nonautologous Tissue Substitute, Open Approach |
| 0RU037Z | Supplement Occipital-cervical Joint with Autologous Tissue Substitute, Percutaneous Approach |

| 0RU03JZ | Supplement Occipital-cervical Joint with Synthetic Substitute, Percutaneous Approach |
| 0RU03KZ | Supplement Occipital-cervical Joint with Nonautologous Tissue Substitute, Percutaneous Approach |

0RU047Z Supplement Occipital-cervical Joint with Autologous Tissue Substitute, Percutaneous Endoscopic Approach

0RU04JZ Supplement Occipital-cervical Joint with Synthetic Substitute, Percutaneous Endoscopic Approach

0RU04KZ Supplement Occipital-cervical Joint with Nonautologous Tissue Substitute, Percutaneous Endoscopic Approach

0RU107Z Supplement Cervical Vertebral Joint with Autologous Tissue Substitute, Open Approach

0RU10JZ Supplement Cervical Vertebral Joint with Synthetic Substitute, Open Approach

0RU10KZ Supplement Cervical Vertebral Joint with Nonautologous Tissue Substitute, Open Approach

0RU137Z Supplement Cervical Vertebral Joint with Autologous Tissue Substitute, Percutaneous Approach

0RU13JZ Supplement Cervical Vertebral Joint with Synthetic Substitute, Percutaneous Approach

0RU13KZ Supplement Cervical Vertebral Joint with Nonautologous Tissue Substitute, Percutaneous Approach

0RU147Z Supplement Cervical Vertebral Joint with Autologous Tissue Substitute, Percutaneous Endoscopic Approach

0RU14JZ Supplement Cervical Vertebral Joint with Synthetic Substitute, Percutaneous Endoscopic Approach

0RU14KZ Supplement Cervical Vertebral Joint with Nonautologous Tissue Substitute, Percutaneous Endoscopic Approach

0RU307Z Supplement Cervical Vertebral Disc with Autologous Tissue Substitute, Open Approach

0RU30JZ Supplement Cervical Vertebral Disc with Synthetic Substitute, Open Approach

0RU30KZ Supplement Cervical Vertebral Disc with Nonautologous Tissue Substitute, Open Approach

0RU337Z Supplement Cervical Vertebral Disc with Autologous Tissue Substitute, Percutaneous Approach

0RU33JZ Supplement Cervical Vertebral Disc with Synthetic Substitute, Percutaneous Approach

0RU33KZ Supplement Cervical Vertebral Disc with Nonautologous Tissue Substitute, Percutaneous Approach

0RU347Z Supplement Cervical Vertebral Disc with Autologous Tissue Substitute, Percutaneous Endoscopic Approach

0RU34JZ Supplement Cervical Vertebral Disc with Synthetic Substitute, Percutaneous Endoscopic Approach

0RU34KZ Supplement Cervical Vertebral Disc with Nonautologous Tissue Substitute, Percutaneous Endoscopic Approach

0RU407Z Supplement Cervicothoracic Vertebral Joint with Autologous Tissue Substitute, Open Approach

0RU40JZ Supplement Cervicothoracic Vertebral Joint with Synthetic Substitute, Open Approach

0RU40KZ Supplement Cervicothoracic Vertebral Joint with Nonautologous Tissue Substitute, Open Approach

0RU437Z Supplement Cervicothoracic Vertebral Joint with Autologous Tissue Substitute, Percutaneous Approach

0RU43JZ Supplement Cervicothoracic Vertebral Joint with Synthetic Substitute, Percutaneous Approach

0RU43KZ Supplement Cervicothoracic Vertebral Joint with Nonautologous Tissue Substitute, Percutaneous Approach

0RU447Z Supplement Cervicothoracic Vertebral Joint with Autologous Tissue Substitute, Percutaneous Endoscopic Approach

0RU44JZ Supplement Cervicothoracic Vertebral Joint with Synthetic Substitute, Percutaneous Endoscopic Approach

0RU44KZ Supplement Cervicothoracic Vertebral Joint with Nonautologous Tissue Substitute, Percutaneous Endoscopic Approach

0RU507Z Supplement Cervicothoracic Vertebral Disc with Autologous Tissue Substitute, Open Approach

0RU50JZ Supplement Cervicothoracic Vertebral Disc with Synthetic Substitute, Open Approach

0RU50KZ Supplement Cervicothoracic Vertebral Disc with Nonautologous Tissue Substitute, Open Approach

0RU537Z Supplement Cervicothoracic Vertebral Disc with Autologous Tissue Substitute, Percutaneous Approach

0RU53JZ Supplement Cervicothoracic Vertebral Disc with Synthetic Substitute, Percutaneous Approach

0RU53KZ Supplement Cervicothoracic Vertebral Disc with Nonautologous Tissue Substitute, Percutaneous Approach

0RU547Z Supplement Cervicothoracic Vertebral Disc with Autologous Tissue Substitute, Percutaneous Endoscopic Approach

0RU54JZ Supplement Cervicothoracic Vertebral Disc with Synthetic Substitute, Percutaneous Endoscopic Approach

0RU54KZ Supplement Cervicothoracic Vertebral Disc with Nonautologous Tissue Substitute, Percutaneous Endoscopic Approach

0RU607Z Supplement Thoracic Vertebral Joint with Autologous Tissue Substitute, Open Approach

0RU60JZ Supplement Thoracic Vertebral Joint with Synthetic Substitute, Open Approach

0RU60KZ Supplement Thoracic Vertebral Joint with Nonautologous Tissue Substitute, Open Approach

0RU637Z Supplement Thoracic Vertebral Joint with Autologous Tissue Substitute, Percutaneous Approach

0RU63JZ Supplement Thoracic Vertebral Joint with Synthetic Substitute, Percutaneous Approach

0RU63KZ Supplement Thoracic Vertebral Joint with Nonautologous Tissue Substitute, Percutaneous Approach

0RU647Z Supplement Thoracic Vertebral Joint with Autologous Tissue Substitute, Percutaneous Endoscopic Approach

0RU64JZ Supplement Thoracic Vertebral Joint with Synthetic Substitute, Percutaneous Endoscopic Approach

0RU64KZ Supplement Thoracic Vertebral Joint with Nonautologous Tissue Substitute, Percutaneous Endoscopic Approach

0RU907Z Supplement Thoracic Vertebral Disc with Autologous Tissue Substitute, Open Approach

0RU90JZ Supplement Thoracic Vertebral Disc with Synthetic Substitute, Open Approach

0RU90KZ Supplement Thoracic Vertebral Disc with Nonautologous Tissue Substitute, Open Approach

0RU937Z Supplement Thoracic Vertebral Disc with Autologous Tissue Substitute, Percutaneous Approach

0RU93JZ Supplement Thoracic Vertebral Disc with Synthetic Substitute, Percutaneous Approach

0RU93KZ Supplement Thoracic Vertebral Disc with Nonautologous Tissue Substitute, Percutaneous Approach

0RU947Z Supplement Thoracic Vertebral Disc with Autologous Tissue Substitute, Percutaneous Endoscopic Approach

0RU94JZ Supplement Thoracic Vertebral Disc with Synthetic Substitute, Percutaneous Endoscopic Approach

0RU94KZ Supplement Thoracic Vertebral Disc with Nonautologous Tissue Substitute, Percutaneous Endoscopic Approach

0RUA07Z Supplement Thoracolumbar Vertebral Joint with Autologous Tissue Substitute, Open Approach

0RUA0JZ Supplement Thoracolumbar Vertebral Joint with Synthetic Substitute, Open Approach

0RUA0KZ Supplement Thoracolumbar Vertebral Joint with Nonautologous Tissue Substitute, Open Approach

0RUA37Z Supplement Thoracolumbar Vertebral Joint with Autologous Tissue Substitute, Percutaneous Approach

0RUA3JZ Supplement Thoracolumbar Vertebral Joint with Synthetic Substitute, Percutaneous Approach

0RUA3KZ Supplement Thoracolumbar Vertebral Joint with Nonautologous Tissue Substitute, Percutaneous Approach

0RUA47Z Supplement Thoracolumbar Vertebral Joint with Autologous Tissue Substitute, Percutaneous Endoscopic Approach

0RUA4JZ Supplement Thoracolumbar Vertebral Joint with Synthetic Substitute, Percutaneous Endoscopic Approach

0RUA4KZ Supplement Thoracolumbar Vertebral Joint with Nonautologous Tissue Substitute, Percutaneous Endoscopic Approach

0RUB07Z Supplement Thoracolumbar Vertebral Disc with Autologous Tissue Substitute, Open Approach

0RUB0JZ Supplement Thoracolumbar Vertebral Disc with Synthetic Substitute, Open Approach

0RUB0KZ Supplement Thoracolumbar Vertebral Disc with Nonautologous Tissue Substitute, Open Approach

0RUB37Z Supplement Thoracolumbar Vertebral Disc with Autologous Tissue Substitute, Percutaneous Approach

0RUB3JZ Supplement Thoracolumbar Vertebral Disc with Synthetic Substitute, Percutaneous Approach

0RUB3KZ Supplement Thoracolumbar Vertebral Disc with Nonautologous Tissue Substitute, Percutaneous Approach

♀ Female-only　　♂ Male-only　　▲ Limited Coverage　　● Non-OR　　■ HAC-associated procedure　　▲ Non-covered procedures　　✚ Cluster

0RUB47Z Supplement Thoracolumbar Vertebral Disc with Autologous Tissue Substitute, Percutaneous Endoscopic Approach

0RUB4JZ Supplement Thoracolumbar Vertebral Disc with Synthetic Substitute, Percutaneous Endoscopic Approach

0RUB4KZ Supplement Thoracolumbar Vertebral Disc with Nonautologous Tissue Substitute, Percutaneous Endoscopic Approach

0RUC07Z Supplement Right Temporomandibular Joint with Autologous Tissue Substitute, Open Approach

0RUC0JZ Supplement Right Temporomandibular Joint with Synthetic Substitute, Open Approach

0RUC0KZ Supplement Right Temporomandibular Joint with Nonautologous Tissue Substitute, Open Approach

0RUC37Z Supplement Right Temporomandibular Joint with Autologous Tissue Substitute, Percutaneous Approach

0RUC3JZ Supplement Right Temporomandibular Joint with Synthetic Substitute, Percutaneous Approach

0RUC3KZ Supplement Right Temporomandibular Joint with Nonautologous Tissue Substitute, Percutaneous Approach

0RUC47Z Supplement Right Temporomandibular Joint with Autologous Tissue Substitute, Percutaneous Endoscopic Approach

0RUC4JZ Supplement Right Temporomandibular Joint with Synthetic Substitute, Percutaneous Endoscopic Approach

0RUC4KZ Supplement Right Temporomandibular Joint with Nonautologous Tissue Substitute, Percutaneous Endoscopic Approach

0RUD07Z Supplement Left Temporomandibular Joint with Autologous Tissue Substitute, Open Approach

0RUD0JZ Supplement Left Temporomandibular Joint with Synthetic Substitute, Open Approach

0RUD0KZ Supplement Left Temporomandibular Joint with Nonautologous Tissue Substitute, Open Approach

0RUD37Z Supplement Left Temporomandibular Joint with Autologous Tissue Substitute, Percutaneous Approach

0RUD3JZ Supplement Left Temporomandibular Joint with Synthetic Substitute, Percutaneous Approach

0RUD3KZ Supplement Left Temporomandibular Joint with Nonautologous Tissue Substitute, Percutaneous Approach

0RUD47Z Supplement Left Temporomandibular Joint with Autologous Tissue Substitute, Percutaneous Endoscopic Approach

0RUD4JZ Supplement Left Temporomandibular Joint with Synthetic Substitute, Percutaneous Endoscopic Approach

0RUD4KZ Supplement Left Temporomandibular Joint with Nonautologous Tissue Substitute, Percutaneous Endoscopic Approach

0RUE07Z Supplement Right Sternoclavicular Joint with Autologous Tissue Substitute, Open Approach

HAC When reported with secondary diagnosis code K68.11, T81.40XA, T81.41XA, T81.42XA, T81.43XA, T81.44XA, T81.49XA, T84.60XA,

0RUE0JZ Supplement Right Sternoclavicular Joint with Synthetic Substitute, Open Approach

HAC When reported with secondary diagnosis code K68.11, T81.40XA, T81.41XA, T81.42XA, T81.43XA, T81.44XA, T81.49XA, T84.60XA, T84.610A, T84.611A, T84.612A, T84.613A, T84.614A, T84.615A, T84.619A, T84.63XA, T84.69XA, T84.7XXA

0RUE0KZ Supplement Right Sternoclavicular Joint with Nonautologous Tissue Substitute, Open Approach

HAC When reported with secondary diagnosis code K68.11, T81.40XA, T81.41XA, T81.42XA, T81.43XA, T81.44XA, T81.49XA, T84.60XA, T84.610A, T84.611A, T84.612A, T84.613A, T84.614A, T84.615A, T84.619A, T84.63XA, T84.69XA, T84.7XXA

0RUE37Z Supplement Right Sternoclavicular Joint with Autologous Tissue Substitute, Percutaneous Approach

HAC When reported with secondary diagnosis code K68.11, T81.40XA, T81.41XA, T81.42XA, T81.43XA, T81.44XA, T81.49XA, T84.60XA, T84.610A, T84.611A, T84.612A, T84.613A, T84.614A, T84.615A, T84.619A, T84.63XA, T84.69XA, T84.7XXA

0RUE3JZ Supplement Right Sternoclavicular Joint with Synthetic Substitute, Percutaneous Approach

HAC When reported with secondary diagnosis code K68.11, T81.40XA, T81.41XA, T81.42XA, T81.43XA, T81.44XA, T81.49XA, T84.60XA, T84.610A, T84.611A, T84.612A, T84.613A, T84.614A, T84.615A, T84.619A, T84.63XA, T84.69XA, T84.7XXA

0RUE3KZ Supplement Right Sternoclavicular Joint with Nonautologous Tissue Substitute, Percutaneous Approach

HAC When reported with secondary diagnosis code K68.11, T81.40XA, T81.41XA, T81.42XA, T81.43XA, T81.44XA, T81.49XA, T84.60XA, T84.610A, T84.611A, T84.612A, T84.613A, T84.614A, T84.615A, T84.619A, T84.63XA, T84.69XA, T84.7XXA

0RUE47Z Supplement Right Sternoclavicular Joint with Autologous Tissue Substitute, Percutaneous Endoscopic Approach

HAC When reported with secondary diagnosis code K68.11, T81.40XA, T81.41XA, T81.42XA, T81.43XA, T81.44XA, T81.49XA, T84.60XA, T84.610A, T84.611A, T84.612A, T84.613A, T84.614A, T84.615A, T84.619A, T84.63XA, T84.69XA, T84.7XXA

0RUE4JZ Supplement Right Sternoclavicular Joint with Synthetic Substitute, Percutaneous Endoscopic Approach

HAC When reported with secondary diagnosis code K68.11, T81.40XA, T81.41XA, T81.42XA, T81.43XA, T81.44XA, T81.49XA, T84.60XA, T84.610A, T84.611A, T84.612A, T84.613A, T84.614A, T84.615A, T84.619A, T84.63XA, T84.69XA, T84.7XXA

0RUE4KZ Supplement Right Sternoclavicular Joint with Nonautologous Tissue Substitute, Percutaneous Endoscopic Approach

HAC When reported with secondary diagnosis code K68.11, T81.40XA, T81.41XA, T81.42XA, T81.43XA, T81.44XA, T81.49XA, T84.60XA, T84.610A, T84.611A, T84.612A, T84.613A, T84.614A, T84.615A, T84.619A, T84.63XA, T84.69XA, T84.7XXA

0RUF07Z Supplement Left Sternoclavicular Joint with Autologous Tissue Substitute, Open Approach

HAC When reported with secondary diagnosis code K68.11, T81.40XA, T81.41XA, T81.42XA, T81.43XA, T81.44XA, T81.49XA, T84.60XA, T84.610A, T84.611A, T84.612A, T84.613A, T84.614A, T84.615A, T84.619A, T84.63XA, T84.69XA, T84.7XXA

0RUF0JZ Supplement Left Sternoclavicular Joint with Synthetic Substitute, Open Approach

HAC When reported with secondary diagnosis code K68.11, T81.40XA, T81.41XA, T81.42XA, T81.43XA, T81.44XA, T81.49XA, T84.60XA, T84.610A, T84.611A, T84.612A, T84.613A, T84.614A, T84.615A, T84.619A, T84.63XA, T84.69XA, T84.7XXA

0RUF0KZ Supplement Left Sternoclavicular Joint with Nonautologous Tissue Substitute, Open Approach

HAC When reported with secondary diagnosis code K68.11, T81.40XA, T81.41XA, T81.42XA, T81.43XA, T81.44XA, T81.49XA, T84.60XA, T84.610A, T84.611A, T84.612A, T84.613A, T84.614A, T84.615A, T84.619A, T84.63XA, T84.69XA, T84.7XXA

0RUF37Z Supplement Left Sternoclavicular Joint with Autologous Tissue Substitute, Percutaneous Approach

HAC When reported with secondary diagnosis code K68.11, T81.40XA, T81.41XA, T81.42XA, T81.43XA, T81.44XA, T81.49XA, T84.60XA, T84.610A, T84.611A, T84.612A, T84.613A, T84.614A, T84.615A, T84.619A, T84.63XA, T84.69XA, T84.7XXA

0RUF3JZ Supplement Left Sternoclavicular Joint with Synthetic Substitute, Percutaneous Approach

HAC When reported with secondary diagnosis code K68.11, T81.40XA, T81.41XA, T81.42XA, T81.43XA, T81.44XA, T81.49XA, T84.60XA, T84.610A, T84.611A, T84.612A, T84.613A, T84.614A, T84.615A, T84.619A, T84.63XA, T84.69XA, T84.7XXA

0RUF3KZ Supplement Left Sternoclavicular Joint with Nonautologous Tissue Substitute, Percutaneous Approach

---

♀ Female-only   ♂ Male-only   ▲ Limited Coverage   ● Non-OR   HAC HAC-associated procedure   ▲ Non-covered procedures   ✚ Cluster

HAC When reported with secondary diagnosis code K68.11, T81.40XA, T81.41XA, T81.42XA, T81.43XA, T81.44XA, T81.49XA, T84.60XA, T84.610A, T84.611A, T84.612A, T84.613A, T84.614A, T84.615A, T84.619A, T84.63XA, T84.69XA, T84.7XXA

0RUF47Z Supplement Left Sternoclavicular Joint with Autologous Tissue Substitute, Percutaneous Endoscopic Approach

HAC When reported with secondary diagnosis code K68.11, T81.40XA, T81.41XA, T81.42XA, T81.43XA, T81.44XA, T81.49XA, T84.60XA, T84.610A, T84.611A, T84.612A, T84.613A, T84.614A, T84.615A, T84.619A, T84.63XA, T84.69XA, T84.7XXA

0RUF4JZ Supplement Left Sternoclavicular Joint with Synthetic Substitute, Percutaneous Endoscopic Approach

HAC When reported with secondary diagnosis code K68.11, T81.40XA, T81.41XA, T81.42XA, T81.43XA, T81.44XA, T81.49XA, T84.60XA, T84.610A, T84.611A, T84.612A, T84.613A, T84.614A, T84.615A, T84.619A, T84.63XA, T84.69XA, T84.7XXA

0RUF4KZ Supplement Left Sternoclavicular Joint with Nonautologous Tissue Substitute, Percutaneous Endoscopic Approach

HAC When reported with secondary diagnosis code K68.11, T81.40XA, T81.41XA, T81.42XA, T81.43XA, T81.44XA, T81.49XA, T84.60XA, T84.610A, T84.611A, T84.612A, T84.613A, T84.614A, T84.615A, T84.619A, T84.63XA, T84.69XA, T84.7XXA

0RUG07Z Supplement Right Acromioclavicular Joint with Autologous Tissue Substitute, Open Approach

HAC When reported with secondary diagnosis code K68.11, T81.40XA, T81.41XA, T81.42XA, T81.43XA, T81.44XA, T81.49XA, T84.60XA, T84.610A, T84.611A, T84.612A, T84.613A, T84.614A, T84.615A, T84.619A, T84.63XA, T84.69XA, T84.7XXA

0RUG0JZ Supplement Right Acromioclavicular Joint with Synthetic Substitute, Open Approach

HAC When reported with secondary diagnosis code K68.11, T81.40XA, T81.41XA, T81.42XA, T81.43XA, T81.44XA, T81.49XA, T84.60XA, T84.610A, T84.611A, T84.612A, T84.613A, T84.614A, T84.615A, T84.619A, T84.63XA, T84.69XA, T84.7XXA

0RUG0KZ Supplement Right Acromioclavicular Joint with Nonautologous Tissue Substitute, Open Approach

HAC When reported with secondary diagnosis code K68.11, T81.40XA, T81.41XA, T81.42XA, T81.43XA, T81.44XA, T81.49XA, T84.60XA, T84.610A, T84.611A, T84.612A, T84.613A, T84.614A, T84.615A, T84.619A, T84.63XA, T84.69XA, T84.7XXA

0RUG37Z Supplement Right Acromioclavicular Joint with Autologous Tissue Substitute, Percutaneous Approach

HAC When reported with secondary diagnosis code K68.11, T81.40XA, T81.41XA, T81.42XA, T81.43XA, T81.44XA, T81.49XA, T84.60XA, T84.610A, T84.611A, T84.612A, T84.613A, T84.614A, T84.615A, T84.619A, T84.63XA, T84.69XA, T84.7XXA

0RUG3JZ Supplement Right Acromioclavicular Joint with Synthetic Substitute, Percutaneous Approach

HAC When reported with secondary diagnosis code K68.11, T81.40XA, T81.41XA, T81.42XA, T81.43XA, T81.44XA, T81.49XA, T84.60XA, T84.610A, T84.611A, T84.612A, T84.613A, T84.614A, T84.615A, T84.619A, T84.63XA, T84.69XA, T84.7XXA

0RUG3KZ Supplement Right Acromioclavicular Joint with Nonautologous Tissue Substitute, Percutaneous Approach

HAC When reported with secondary diagnosis code K68.11, T81.40XA, T81.41XA, T81.42XA, T81.43XA, T81.44XA, T81.49XA, T84.60XA, T84.610A, T84.611A, T84.612A, T84.613A, T84.614A, T84.615A, T84.619A, T84.63XA, T84.69XA, T84.7XXA

0RUG47Z Supplement Right Acromioclavicular Joint with Autologous Tissue Substitute, Percutaneous Endoscopic Approach

HAC When reported with secondary diagnosis code K68.11, T81.40XA, T81.41XA, T81.42XA, T81.43XA, T81.44XA, T81.49XA, T84.60XA, T84.610A, T84.611A, T84.612A, T84.613A, T84.614A, T84.615A, T84.619A, T84.63XA, T84.69XA, T84.7XXA

0RUG4JZ Supplement Right Acromioclavicular Joint with Synthetic Substitute, Percutaneous Endoscopic Approach

HAC When reported with secondary diagnosis code K68.11, T81.40XA, T81.41XA, T81.42XA, T81.43XA, T81.44XA, T81.49XA, T84.60XA, T84.610A, T84.611A, T84.612A, T84.613A, T84.614A, T84.615A, T84.619A, T84.63XA, T84.69XA, T84.7XXA

0RUG4KZ Supplement Right Acromioclavicular Joint with Nonautologous Tissue Substitute, Percutaneous Endoscopic Approach

HAC When reported with secondary diagnosis code K68.11, T81.40XA, T81.41XA, T81.42XA, T81.43XA, T81.44XA, T81.49XA, T84.60XA, T84.610A, T84.611A, T84.612A, T84.613A, T84.614A, T84.615A, T84.619A, T84.63XA, T84.69XA, T84.7XXA

0RUH07Z Supplement Left Acromioclavicular Joint with Autologous Tissue Substitute, Open Approach

HAC When reported with secondary diagnosis code K68.11, T81.40XA, T81.41XA, T81.42XA, T81.43XA, T81.44XA, T81.49XA, T84.60XA, T84.610A, T84.611A, T84.612A,

T84.613A, T84.614A, T84.615A, T84.619A, T84.63XA, T84.69XA, T84.7XXA

0RUH0JZ Supplement Left Acromioclavicular Joint with Synthetic Substitute, Open Approach

HAC When reported with secondary diagnosis code K68.11, T81.40XA, T81.41XA, T81.42XA, T81.43XA, T81.44XA, T81.49XA, T84.60XA, T84.610A, T84.611A, T84.612A, T84.613A, T84.614A, T84.615A, T84.619A, T84.63XA, T84.69XA, T84.7XXA

0RUH0KZ Supplement Left Acromioclavicular Joint with Nonautologous Tissue Substitute, Open Approach

AHA CC: 3Q, 2019, 26-27

HAC When reported with secondary diagnosis code K68.11, T81.40XA, T81.41XA, T81.42XA, T81.43XA, T81.44XA, T81.49XA, T84.60XA, T84.610A, T84.611A, T84.612A, T84.613A, T84.614A, T84.615A, T84.619A, T84.63XA, T84.69XA, T84.7XXA

0RUH37Z Supplement Left Acromioclavicular Joint with Autologous Tissue Substitute, Percutaneous Approach

HAC When reported with secondary diagnosis code K68.11, T81.40XA, T81.41XA, T81.42XA, T81.43XA, T81.44XA, T81.49XA, T84.60XA, T84.610A, T84.611A, T84.612A, T84.613A, T84.614A, T84.615A, T84.619A, T84.63XA, T84.69XA, T84.7XXA

0RUH3JZ Supplement Left Acromioclavicular Joint with Synthetic Substitute, Percutaneous Approach

HAC When reported with secondary diagnosis code K68.11, T81.40XA, T81.41XA, T81.42XA, T81.43XA, T81.44XA, T81.49XA, T84.60XA, T84.610A, T84.611A, T84.612A, T84.613A, T84.614A, T84.615A, T84.619A, T84.63XA, T84.69XA, T84.7XXA

0RUH3KZ Supplement Left Acromioclavicular Joint with Nonautologous Tissue Substitute, Percutaneous Approach

HAC When reported with secondary diagnosis code K68.11, T81.40XA, T81.41XA, T81.42XA, T81.43XA, T81.44XA, T81.49XA, T84.60XA, T84.610A, T84.611A, T84.612A, T84.613A, T84.614A, T84.615A, T84.619A, T84.63XA, T84.69XA, T84.7XXA

0RUH47Z Supplement Left Acromioclavicular Joint with Autologous Tissue Substitute, Percutaneous Endoscopic Approach

HAC When reported with secondary diagnosis code K68.11, T81.40XA, T81.41XA, T81.42XA, T81.43XA, T81.44XA, T81.49XA, T84.60XA, T84.610A, T84.611A, T84.612A, T84.613A, T84.614A, T84.615A, T84.619A, T84.63XA, T84.69XA, T84.7XXA

0RUH4JZ Supplement Left Acromioclavicular Joint with Synthetic Substitute, Percutaneous Endoscopic Approach

HAC When reported with secondary diagnosis code K68.11, T81.40XA,

♀ Female-only ♂ Male-only ▲ Limited Coverage ● Non-OR HAC HAC-associated procedure ▲ Non-covered procedures ✚ Cluster

T81.41XA, T81.42XA, T81.43XA,
T81.44XA, T81.49XA, T84.60XA,
T84.610A, T84.611A, T84.612A,
T84.613A, T84.614A, T84.615A,
T84.619A, T84.63XA, T84.69XA,
T84.7XXA

0RUH4KZ Supplement Left Acromioclavicular
Joint with Nonautologous Tissue
Substitute, Percutaneous Endoscopic
Approach

HAC When reported with secondary
diagnosis code K68.11, T81.40XA,
T81.41XA, T81.42XA, T81.43XA,
T81.44XA, T81.49XA, T84.60XA,
T84.610A, T84.611A, T84.612A,
T84.613A, T84.614A, T84.615A,
T84.619A, T84.63XA, T84.69XA,
T84.7XXA

0RUJ07Z Supplement Right Shoulder Joint with
Autologous Tissue Substitute, Open
Approach

HAC When reported with secondary
diagnosis code K68.11, T81.40XA,
T81.41XA, T81.42XA, T81.43XA,
T81.44XA, T81.49XA, T84.60XA,
T84.610A, T84.611A, T84.612A,
T84.613A, T84.614A, T84.615A,
T84.619A, T84.63XA, T84.69XA,
T84.7XXA

0RUJ0JZ Supplement Right Shoulder Joint
with Synthetic Substitute, Open
Approach

HAC When reported with secondary
diagnosis code K68.11, T81.40XA,
T81.41XA, T81.42XA, T81.43XA,
T81.44XA, T81.49XA, T84.60XA,
T84.610A, T84.611A, T84.612A,
T84.613A, T84.614A, T84.615A,
T84.619A, T84.63XA, T84.69XA,
T84.7XXA

0RUJ0KZ Supplement Right Shoulder Joint with
Nonautologous Tissue Substitute,
Open Approach

HAC When reported with secondary
diagnosis code K68.11, T81.40XA,
T81.41XA, T81.42XA, T81.43XA,
T81.44XA, T81.49XA, T84.60XA,
T84.610A, T84.611A, T84.612A,
T84.613A, T84.614A, T84.615A,
T84.619A, T84.63XA, T84.69XA,
T84.7XXA

0RUJ37Z Supplement Right Shoulder Joint
with Autologous Tissue Substitute,
Percutaneous Approach

HAC When reported with secondary
diagnosis code K68.11, T81.40XA,
T81.41XA, T81.42XA, T81.43XA,
T81.44XA, T81.49XA, T84.60XA,
T84.610A, T84.611A, T84.612A,
T84.613A, T84.614A, T84.615A,
T84.619A, T84.63XA, T84.69XA,
T84.7XXA

0RUJ3JZ Supplement Right Shoulder Joint with
Synthetic Substitute, Percutaneous
Approach

HAC When reported with secondary
diagnosis code K68.11, T81.40XA,
T81.41XA, T81.42XA, T81.43XA,
T81.44XA, T81.49XA, T84.60XA,
T84.610A, T84.611A, T84.612A,
T84.613A, T84.614A, T84.615A,
T84.619A, T84.63XA, T84.69XA,
T84.7XXA

0RUJ3KZ Supplement Right Shoulder Joint with
Nonautologous Tissue Substitute,
Percutaneous Approach

HAC When reported with secondary
diagnosis code K68.11, T81.40XA,
T81.41XA, T81.42XA, T81.43XA,
T81.44XA, T81.49XA, T84.60XA,
T84.610A, T84.611A, T84.612A,
T84.613A, T84.614A, T84.615A,
T84.619A, T84.63XA, T84.69XA,
T84.7XXA

0RUJ47Z Supplement Right Shoulder Joint
with Autologous Tissue Substitute,
Percutaneous Endoscopic Approach

HAC When reported with secondary
diagnosis code K68.11, T81.40XA,
T81.41XA, T81.42XA, T81.43XA,
T81.44XA, T81.49XA, T84.60XA,
T84.610A, T84.611A, T84.612A,
T84.613A, T84.614A, T84.615A,
T84.619A, T84.63XA, T84.69XA,
T84.7XXA

0RUJ4JZ Supplement Right Shoulder Joint with
Synthetic Substitute, Percutaneous
Endoscopic Approach

HAC When reported with secondary
diagnosis code K68.11, T81.40XA,
T81.41XA, T81.42XA, T81.43XA,
T81.44XA, T81.49XA, T84.60XA,
T84.610A, T84.611A, T84.612A,
T84.613A, T84.614A, T84.615A,
T84.619A, T84.63XA, T84.69XA,
T84.7XXA

0RUJ4KZ Supplement Right Shoulder Joint with
Nonautologous Tissue Substitute,
Percutaneous Endoscopic Approach

HAC When reported with secondary
diagnosis code K68.11, T81.40XA,
T81.41XA, T81.42XA, T81.43XA,
T81.44XA, T81.49XA, T84.60XA,
T84.610A, T84.611A, T84.612A,
T84.613A, T84.614A, T84.615A,
T84.619A, T84.63XA, T84.69XA,
T84.7XXA

0RUK07Z Supplement Left Shoulder Joint with
Autologous Tissue Substitute, Open
Approach

HAC When reported with secondary
diagnosis code K68.11, T81.40XA,
T81.41XA, T81.42XA, T81.43XA,
T81.44XA, T81.49XA, T84.60XA,
T84.610A, T84.611A, T84.612A,
T84.613A, T84.614A, T84.615A,
T84.619A, T84.63XA, T84.69XA,
T84.7XXA

0RUK0JZ Supplement Left Shoulder Joint with
Synthetic Substitute, Open Approach

HAC When reported with secondary
diagnosis code K68.11, T81.40XA,
T81.41XA, T81.42XA, T81.43XA,
T81.44XA, T81.49XA, T84.60XA,
T84.610A, T84.611A, T84.612A,
T84.613A, T84.614A, T84.615A,
T84.619A, T84.63XA, T84.69XA,
T84.7XXA

0RUK0KZ Supplement Left Shoulder Joint with
Nonautologous Tissue Substitute,
Open Approach

HAC When reported with secondary
diagnosis code K68.11, T81.40XA,
T81.41XA, T81.42XA, T81.43XA,
T81.44XA, T81.49XA, T84.60XA,
T84.610A, T84.611A, T84.612A,
T84.613A, T84.614A, T84.615A,
T84.619A, T84.63XA, T84.69XA,
T84.7XXA

0RUK37Z Supplement Left Shoulder Joint
with Autologous Tissue Substitute,
Percutaneous Approach

HAC When reported with secondary
diagnosis code K68.11, T81.40XA,
T81.41XA, T81.42XA, T81.43XA,
T81.44XA, T81.49XA, T84.60XA,
T84.610A, T84.611A, T84.612A,
T84.613A, T84.614A, T84.615A,
T84.619A, T84.63XA, T84.69XA,
T84.7XXA

0RUK3JZ Supplement Left Shoulder Joint with
Synthetic Substitute, Percutaneous
Approach

HAC When reported with secondary
diagnosis code K68.11, T81.40XA,
T81.41XA, T81.42XA, T81.43XA,
T81.44XA, T81.49XA, T84.60XA,
T84.610A, T84.611A, T84.612A,
T84.613A, T84.614A, T84.615A,
T84.619A, T84.63XA, T84.69XA,
T84.7XXA

0RUK3KZ Supplement Left Shoulder Joint with
Nonautologous Tissue Substitute,
Percutaneous Approach

HAC When reported with secondary
diagnosis code K68.11, T81.40XA,
T81.41XA, T81.42XA, T81.43XA,
T81.44XA, T81.49XA, T84.60XA,
T84.610A, T84.611A, T84.612A,
T84.613A, T84.614A, T84.615A,
T84.619A, T84.63XA, T84.69XA,
T84.7XXA

0RUK47Z Supplement Left Shoulder Joint
with Autologous Tissue Substitute,
Percutaneous Endoscopic
Approach

HAC When reported with secondary
diagnosis code K68.11, T81.40XA,
T81.41XA, T81.42XA, T81.43XA,
T81.44XA, T81.49XA, T84.60XA,
T84.610A, T84.611A, T84.612A,
T84.613A, T84.614A, T84.615A,
T84.619A, T84.63XA, T84.69XA,
T84.7XXA

0RUK4JZ Supplement Left Shoulder Joint with
Synthetic Substitute, Percutaneous
Endoscopic Approach

HAC When reported with secondary
diagnosis code K68.11, T81.40XA,
T81.41XA, T81.42XA, T81.43XA,
T81.44XA, T81.49XA, T84.60XA,
T84.610A, T84.611A, T84.612A,
T84.613A, T84.614A, T84.615A,
T84.619A, T84.63XA, T84.69XA,
T84.7XXA

0RUK4KZ Supplement Left Shoulder Joint
with Nonautologous Tissue
Substitute, Percutaneous Endoscopic
Approach

HAC When reported with secondary
diagnosis code K68.11, T81.40XA,
T81.41XA, T81.42XA, T81.43XA,
T81.44XA, T81.49XA, T84.60XA,
T84.610A, T84.611A, T84.612A,
T84.613A, T84.614A, T84.615A,
T84.619A, T84.63XA, T84.69XA,
T84.7XXA

0RUL07Z Supplement Right Elbow Joint with
Autologous Tissue Substitute, Open
Approach

HAC When reported with secondary
diagnosis code K68.11, T81.40XA,
T81.41XA, T81.42XA, T81.43XA,
T81.44XA, T81.49XA, T84.60XA,
T84.610A, T84.611A, T84.612A,
T84.613A, T84.614A, T84.615A,
T84.619A, T84.63XA, T84.69XA,
T84.7XXA

♀ Female-only   ♂ Male-only   ▲ Limited Coverage   ● Non-OR   HAC HAC-associated procedure   ▲ Non-covered procedures   ✚ Cluster   **1109**

Medical and Surgical, Upper Joints Code Listings

0RUL0JZ Supplement Right Elbow Joint with Synthetic Substitute, Open Approach

HAC When reported with secondary diagnosis code K68.11, T81.40XA, T81.41XA, T81.42XA, T81.43XA, T81.44XA, T81.49XA, T84.60XA, T84.610A, T84.611A, T84.612A, T84.613A, T84.614A, T84.615A, T84.619A, T84.63XA, T84.69XA, T84.7XXA

0RUL0KZ Supplement Right Elbow Joint with Nonautologous Tissue Substitute, Open Approach

HAC When reported with secondary diagnosis code K68.11, T81.40XA, T81.41XA, T81.42XA, T81.43XA, T81.44XA, T81.49XA, T84.60XA, T84.610A, T84.611A, T84.612A, T84.613A, T84.614A, T84.615A, T84.619A, T84.63XA, T84.69XA, T84.7XXA

0RUL37Z Supplement Right Elbow Joint with Autologous Tissue Substitute, Percutaneous Approach

HAC When reported with secondary diagnosis code K68.11, T81.40XA, T81.41XA, T81.42XA, T81.43XA, T81.44XA, T81.49XA, T84.60XA, T84.610A, T84.611A, T84.612A, T84.613A, T84.614A, T84.615A, T84.619A, T84.63XA, T84.69XA, T84.7XXA

0RUL3JZ Supplement Right Elbow Joint with Synthetic Substitute, Percutaneous Approach

HAC When reported with secondary diagnosis code K68.11, T81.40XA, T81.41XA, T81.42XA, T81.43XA, T81.44XA, T81.49XA, T84.60XA, T84.610A, T84.611A, T84.612A, T84.613A, T84.614A, T84.615A, T84.619A, T84.63XA, T84.69XA, T84.7XXA

0RUL3KZ Supplement Right Elbow Joint with Nonautologous Tissue Substitute, Percutaneous Approach

HAC When reported with secondary diagnosis code K68.11, T81.40XA, T81.41XA, T81.42XA, T81.43XA, T81.44XA, T81.49XA, T84.60XA, T84.610A, T84.611A, T84.612A, T84.613A, T84.614A, T84.615A, T84.619A, T84.63XA, T84.69XA, T84.7XXA

0RUL47Z Supplement Right Elbow Joint with Autologous Tissue Substitute, Percutaneous Endoscopic Approach

HAC When reported with secondary diagnosis code K68.11, T81.40XA, T81.41XA, T81.42XA, T81.43XA, T81.44XA, T81.49XA, T84.60XA, T84.610A, T84.611A, T84.612A, T84.613A, T84.614A, T84.615A, T84.619A, T84.63XA, T84.69XA, T84.7XXA

0RUL4JZ Supplement Right Elbow Joint with Synthetic Substitute, Percutaneous Endoscopic Approach

HAC When reported with secondary diagnosis code K68.11, T81.40XA, T81.41XA, T81.42XA, T81.43XA, T81.44XA, T81.49XA, T84.60XA, T84.610A, T84.611A, T84.612A, T84.613A, T84.614A, T84.615A, T84.619A, T84.63XA, T84.69XA, T84.7XXA

0RUL4KZ Supplement Right Elbow Joint with Nonautologous Tissue Substitute, Percutaneous Endoscopic Approach

HAC When reported with secondary diagnosis code K68.11, T81.40XA, T81.41XA, T81.42XA, T81.43XA, T81.44XA, T81.49XA, T84.60XA, T84.610A, T84.611A, T84.612A, T84.613A, T84.614A, T84.615A, T84.619A, T84.63XA, T84.69XA, T84.7XXA

0RUM07Z Supplement Left Elbow Joint with Autologous Tissue Substitute, Open Approach

HAC When reported with secondary diagnosis code K68.11, T81.40XA, T81.41XA, T81.42XA, T81.43XA, T81.44XA, T81.49XA, T84.60XA, T84.610A, T84.611A, T84.612A, T84.613A, T84.614A, T84.615A, T84.619A, T84.63XA, T84.69XA, T84.7XXA

0RUM0JZ Supplement Left Elbow Joint with Synthetic Substitute, Open Approach

HAC When reported with secondary diagnosis code K68.11, T81.40XA, T81.41XA, T81.42XA, T81.43XA, T81.44XA, T81.49XA, T84.60XA, T84.610A, T84.611A, T84.612A, T84.613A, T84.614A, T84.615A, T84.619A, T84.63XA, T84.69XA, T84.7XXA

0RUM0KZ Supplement Left Elbow Joint with Nonautologous Tissue Substitute, Open Approach

HAC When reported with secondary diagnosis code K68.11, T81.40XA, T81.41XA, T81.42XA, T81.43XA, T81.44XA, T81.49XA, T84.60XA, T84.610A, T84.611A, T84.612A, T84.613A, T84.614A, T84.615A, T84.619A, T84.63XA, T84.69XA, T84.7XXA

0RUM37Z Supplement Left Elbow Joint with Autologous Tissue Substitute, Percutaneous Approach

HAC When reported with secondary diagnosis code K68.11, T81.40XA, T81.41XA, T81.42XA, T81.43XA, T81.44XA, T81.49XA, T84.60XA, T84.610A, T84.611A, T84.612A, T84.613A, T84.614A, T84.615A, T84.619A, T84.63XA, T84.69XA, T84.7XXA

0RUM3JZ Supplement Left Elbow Joint with Synthetic Substitute, Percutaneous Approach

HAC When reported with secondary diagnosis code K68.11, T81.40XA, T81.41XA, T81.42XA, T81.43XA, T81.44XA, T81.49XA, T84.60XA, T84.610A, T84.611A, T84.612A, T84.613A, T84.614A, T84.615A, T84.619A, T84.63XA, T84.69XA, T84.7XXA

0RUM3KZ Supplement Left Elbow Joint with Nonautologous Tissue Substitute, Percutaneous Approach

HAC When reported with secondary diagnosis code K68.11, T81.40XA, T81.41XA, T81.42XA, T81.43XA, T81.44XA, T81.49XA, T84.60XA, T84.610A, T84.611A, T84.612A, T84.613A, T84.614A, T84.615A, T84.619A, T84.63XA, T84.69XA, T84.7XXA

0RUM47Z Supplement Left Elbow Joint with Autologous Tissue Substitute, Percutaneous Endoscopic Approach

HAC When reported with secondary diagnosis code K68.11, T81.40XA, T81.41XA, T81.42XA, T81.43XA, T81.44XA, T81.49XA, T84.60XA, T84.610A, T84.611A, T84.612A, T84.613A, T84.614A, T84.615A, T84.619A, T84.63XA, T84.69XA, T84.7XXA

0RUM4JZ Supplement Left Elbow Joint with Synthetic Substitute, Percutaneous Endoscopic Approach

HAC When reported with secondary diagnosis code K68.11, T81.40XA, T81.41XA, T81.42XA, T81.43XA, T81.44XA, T81.49XA, T84.60XA, T84.610A, T84.611A, T84.612A, T84.613A, T84.614A, T84.615A, T84.619A, T84.63XA, T84.69XA, T84.7XXA

0RUM4KZ Supplement Left Elbow Joint with Nonautologous Tissue Substitute, Percutaneous Endoscopic Approach

HAC When reported with secondary diagnosis code K68.11, T81.40XA, T81.41XA, T81.42XA, T81.43XA, T81.44XA, T81.49XA, T84.60XA, T84.610A, T84.611A, T84.612A, T84.613A, T84.614A, T84.615A, T84.619A, T84.63XA, T84.69XA, T84.7XXA

0RUN07Z Supplement Right Wrist Joint with Autologous Tissue Substitute, Open Approach

0RUN0JZ Supplement Right Wrist Joint with Synthetic Substitute, Open Approach

0RUN0KZ Supplement Right Wrist Joint with Nonautologous Tissue Substitute, Open Approach

0RUN37Z Supplement Right Wrist Joint with Autologous Tissue Substitute, Percutaneous Approach

0RUN3JZ Supplement Right Wrist Joint with Synthetic Substitute, Percutaneous Approach

0RUN3KZ Supplement Right Wrist Joint with Nonautologous Tissue Substitute, Percutaneous Approach

0RUN47Z Supplement Right Wrist Joint with Autologous Tissue Substitute, Percutaneous Endoscopic Approach

0RUN4JZ Supplement Right Wrist Joint with Synthetic Substitute, Percutaneous Endoscopic Approach

0RUN4KZ Supplement Right Wrist Joint with Nonautologous Tissue Substitute, Percutaneous Endoscopic Approach

0RUP07Z Supplement Left Wrist Joint with Autologous Tissue Substitute, Open Approach

0RUP0JZ Supplement Left Wrist Joint with Synthetic Substitute, Open Approach

0RUP0KZ Supplement Left Wrist Joint with Nonautologous Tissue Substitute, Open Approach

0RUP37Z Supplement Left Wrist Joint with Autologous Tissue Substitute, Percutaneous Approach

0RUP3JZ Supplement Left Wrist Joint with Synthetic Substitute, Percutaneous Approach

0RUP3KZ Supplement Left Wrist Joint with Nonautologous Tissue Substitute, Percutaneous Approach

0RUP47Z Supplement Left Wrist Joint with Autologous Tissue Substitute, Percutaneous Endoscopic Approach

0RUP4JZ Supplement Left Wrist Joint with Synthetic Substitute, Percutaneous Endoscopic Approach

0RUP4KZ Supplement Left Wrist Joint with Nonautologous Tissue Substitute, Percutaneous Endoscopic Approach

0RUQ07Z Supplement Right Carpal Joint with Autologous Tissue Substitute, Open Approach

0RUQ0JZ Supplement Right Carpal Joint with Synthetic Substitute, Open Approach

0RUQ0KZ Supplement Right Carpal Joint with Nonautologous Tissue Substitute, Open Approach

0RUQ37Z Supplement Right Carpal Joint with Autologous Tissue Substitute, Percutaneous Approach

0RUQ3JZ Supplement Right Carpal Joint with Synthetic Substitute, Percutaneous Approach

0RUQ3KZ Supplement Right Carpal Joint with Nonautologous Tissue Substitute, Percutaneous Approach

0RUQ47Z Supplement Right Carpal Joint with Autologous Tissue Substitute, Percutaneous Endoscopic Approach

0RUQ4JZ Supplement Right Carpal Joint with Synthetic Substitute, Percutaneous Endoscopic Approach

0RUQ4KZ Supplement Right Carpal Joint with Nonautologous Tissue Substitute, Percutaneous Endoscopic Approach

0RUR07Z Supplement Left Carpal Joint with Autologous Tissue Substitute, Open Approach

0RUR0JZ Supplement Left Carpal Joint with Synthetic Substitute, Open Approach

0RUR0KZ Supplement Left Carpal Joint with Nonautologous Tissue Substitute, Open Approach

0RUR37Z Supplement Left Carpal Joint with Autologous Tissue Substitute, Percutaneous Approach

0RUR3JZ Supplement Left Carpal Joint with Synthetic Substitute, Percutaneous Approach

0RUR3KZ Supplement Left Carpal Joint with Nonautologous Tissue Substitute, Percutaneous Approach

0RUR47Z Supplement Left Carpal Joint with Autologous Tissue Substitute, Percutaneous Endoscopic Approach

0RUR4JZ Supplement Left Carpal Joint with Synthetic Substitute, Percutaneous Endoscopic Approach

0RUR4KZ Supplement Left Carpal Joint with Nonautologous Tissue Substitute, Percutaneous Endoscopic Approach

0RUS07Z Supplement Right Carpometacarpal Joint with Autologous Tissue Substitute, Open Approach

0RUS0JZ Supplement Right Carpometacarpal Joint with Synthetic Substitute, Open Approach

0RUS0KZ Supplement Right Carpometacarpal Joint with Nonautologous Tissue Substitute, Open Approach

0RUS37Z Supplement Right Carpometacarpal Joint with Autologous Tissue Substitute, Percutaneous Approach

0RUS3JZ Supplement Right Carpometacarpal Joint with Synthetic Substitute, Percutaneous Approach

0RUS3KZ Supplement Right Carpometacarpal Joint with Nonautologous Tissue Substitute, Percutaneous Approach

0RUS47Z Supplement Right Carpometacarpal Joint with Autologous Tissue Substitute, Percutaneous Endoscopic Approach

0RUS4JZ Supplement Right Carpometacarpal Joint with Synthetic Substitute, Percutaneous Endoscopic Approach

0RUS4KZ Supplement Right Carpometacarpal Joint with Nonautologous Tissue Substitute, Percutaneous Endoscopic Approach

0RUT07Z Supplement Left Carpometacarpal Joint with Autologous Tissue Substitute, Open Approach

AHA CC: 3Q, 2015, 26-27

0RUT0JZ Supplement Left Carpometacarpal Joint with Synthetic Substitute, Open Approach

0RUT0KZ Supplement Left Carpometacarpal Joint with Nonautologous Tissue Substitute, Open Approach

0RUT37Z Supplement Left Carpometacarpal Joint with Autologous Tissue Substitute, Percutaneous Approach

0RUT3JZ Supplement Left Carpometacarpal Joint with Synthetic Substitute, Percutaneous Approach

0RUT3KZ Supplement Left Carpometacarpal Joint with Nonautologous Tissue Substitute, Percutaneous Approach

0RUT47Z Supplement Left Carpometacarpal Joint with Autologous Tissue Substitute, Percutaneous Endoscopic Approach

0RUT4JZ Supplement Left Carpometacarpal Joint with Synthetic Substitute, Percutaneous Endoscopic Approach

0RUT4KZ Supplement Left Carpometacarpal Joint with Nonautologous Tissue Substitute, Percutaneous Endoscopic Approach

0RUU07Z Supplement Right Metacarpophalangeal Joint with Autologous Tissue Substitute, Open Approach

0RUU0JZ Supplement Right Metacarpophalangeal Joint with Synthetic Substitute, Open Approach

0RUU0KZ Supplement Right Metacarpophalangeal Joint with Nonautologous Tissue Substitute, Open Approach

0RUU37Z Supplement Right Metacarpophalangeal Joint with Autologous Tissue Substitute, Percutaneous Approach

0RUU3JZ Supplement Right Metacarpophalangeal Joint with Synthetic Substitute, Percutaneous Approach

0RUU3KZ Supplement Right Metacarpophalangeal Joint with Nonautologous Tissue Substitute, Percutaneous Approach

0RUU47Z Supplement Right Metacarpophalangeal Joint with Autologous Tissue Substitute, Percutaneous Endoscopic Approach

0RUU4JZ Supplement Right Metacarpophalangeal Joint with

Synthetic Substitute, Percutaneous Endoscopic Approach

0RUU4KZ Supplement Right Metacarpophalangeal Joint with Nonautologous Tissue Substitute, Percutaneous Endoscopic Approach

0RUV07Z Supplement Left Metacarpophalangeal Joint with Autologous Tissue Substitute, Open Approach

0RUV0JZ Supplement Left Metacarpophalangeal Joint with Synthetic Substitute, Open Approach

0RUV0KZ Supplement Left Metacarpophalangeal Joint with Nonautologous Tissue Substitute, Open Approach

0RUV37Z Supplement Left Metacarpophalangeal Joint with Autologous Tissue Substitute, Percutaneous Approach

0RUV3JZ Supplement Left Metacarpophalangeal Joint with Synthetic Substitute, Percutaneous Approach

0RUV3KZ Supplement Left Metacarpophalangeal Joint with Nonautologous Tissue Substitute, Percutaneous Approach

0RUV47Z Supplement Left Metacarpophalangeal Joint with Autologous Tissue Substitute, Percutaneous Endoscopic Approach

0RUV4JZ Supplement Left Metacarpophalangeal Joint with Synthetic Substitute, Percutaneous Endoscopic Approach

0RUV4KZ Supplement Left Metacarpophalangeal Joint with Nonautologous Tissue Substitute, Percutaneous Endoscopic Approach

0RUW07Z Supplement Right Finger Phalangeal Joint with Autologous Tissue Substitute, Open Approach

0RUW0JZ Supplement Right Finger Phalangeal Joint with Synthetic Substitute, Open Approach

0RUW0KZ Supplement Right Finger Phalangeal Joint with Nonautologous Tissue Substitute, Open Approach

0RUW37Z Supplement Right Finger Phalangeal Joint with Autologous Tissue Substitute, Percutaneous Approach

0RUW3JZ Supplement Right Finger Phalangeal Joint with Synthetic Substitute, Percutaneous Approach

0RUW3KZ Supplement Right Finger Phalangeal Joint with Nonautologous Tissue Substitute, Percutaneous Approach

0RUW47Z Supplement Right Finger Phalangeal Joint with Autologous Tissue Substitute, Percutaneous Endoscopic Approach

0RUW4JZ Supplement Right Finger Phalangeal Joint with Synthetic Substitute, Percutaneous Endoscopic Approach

0RUW4KZ Supplement Right Finger Phalangeal Joint with Nonautologous Tissue Substitute, Percutaneous Endoscopic Approach

0RUX07Z Supplement Left Finger Phalangeal Joint with Autologous Tissue Substitute, Open Approach

0RUX0JZ Supplement Left Finger Phalangeal Joint with Synthetic Substitute, Open Approach

0RUX0KZ Supplement Left Finger Phalangeal Joint with Nonautologous Tissue Substitute, Open Approach

0RUX37Z Supplement Left Finger Phalangeal Joint with Autologous Tissue Substitute, Percutaneous Approach

0RUX3JZ Supplement Left Finger Phalangeal Joint with Synthetic Substitute, Percutaneous Approach

0RUX3KZ Supplement Left Finger Phalangeal Joint with Nonautologous Tissue Substitute, Percutaneous Approach

0RUX47Z Supplement Left Finger Phalangeal Joint with Autologous Tissue Substitute, Percutaneous Endoscopic Approach

0RUX4JZ Supplement Left Finger Phalangeal Joint with Synthetic

Substitute, Percutaneous Endoscopic Approach

0RUX4KZ Supplement Left Finger Phalangeal Joint with Nonautologous Tissue Substitute, Percutaneous Endoscopic Approach

0RW – Upper Joints, Revision

Review Coding Guideline B6.1c

0RW000Z Revision of Drainage Device in Occipital-cervical Joint, Open Approach

0RW003Z Revision of Infusion Device in Occipital-cervical Joint, Open Approach

0RW004Z Revision of Internal Fixation Device in Occipital-cervical Joint, Open Approach

0RW007Z Revision of Autologous Tissue Substitute in Occipital-cervical Joint, Open Approach

0RW008Z Revision of Spacer in Occipital-cervical Joint, Open Approach

0RW00AZ Revision of Interbody Fusion Device in Occipital-cervical Joint, Open Approach

0RW00JZ Revision of Synthetic Substitute in Occipital-cervical Joint, Open Approach

0RW00KZ Revision of Nonautologous Tissue Substitute in Occipital-cervical Joint, Open Approach

0RW030Z Revision of Drainage Device in Occipital-cervical Joint, Percutaneous Approach

0RW033Z Revision of Infusion Device in Occipital-cervical Joint, Percutaneous Approach

0RW034Z Revision of Internal Fixation Device in Occipital-cervical Joint, Percutaneous Approach

0RW037Z Revision of Autologous Tissue Substitute in Occipital-cervical Joint, Percutaneous Approach

0RW038Z Revision of Spacer in Occipital-cervical Joint, Percutaneous Approach

0RW03AZ Revision of Interbody Fusion Device in Occipital-cervical Joint, Percutaneous Approach

0RW03JZ Revision of Synthetic Substitute in Occipital-cervical Joint, Percutaneous Approach

0RW03KZ Revision of Nonautologous Tissue Substitute in Occipital-cervical Joint, Percutaneous Approach

0RW040Z Revision of Drainage Device in Occipital-cervical Joint, Percutaneous Endoscopic Approach

0RW043Z Revision of Infusion Device in Occipital-cervical Joint, Percutaneous Endoscopic Approach

0RW044Z Revision of Internal Fixation Device in Occipital-cervical Joint, Percutaneous Endoscopic Approach

0RW047Z Revision of Autologous Tissue Substitute in Occipital-cervical Joint, Percutaneous Endoscopic Approach

0RW048Z Revision of Spacer in Occipital-cervical Joint, Percutaneous Endoscopic Approach

0RW04AZ Revision of Interbody Fusion Device in Occipital-cervical Joint, Percutaneous Endoscopic Approach

0RW04JZ Revision of Synthetic Substitute in Occipital-cervical Joint, Percutaneous Endoscopic Approach

0RW04KZ Revision of Nonautologous Tissue Substitute in Occipital-cervical Joint, Percutaneous Endoscopic Approach

0RW0X0Z Revision of Drainage Device in Occipital-cervical Joint, External Approach

0RW0X3Z Revision of Infusion Device in Occipital-cervical Joint, External Approach

0RW0X4Z Revision of Internal Fixation Device in Occipital-cervical Joint, External Approach

0RW0X7Z Revision of Autologous Tissue Substitute in Occipital-cervical Joint, External Approach

0RW0X8Z Revision of Spacer in Occipital-cervical Joint, External Approach

0RW0XAZ Revision of Interbody Fusion Device in Occipital-cervical Joint, External Approach

0RW0XJZ Revision of Synthetic Substitute in Occipital-cervical Joint, External Approach

0RW0XKZ Revision of Nonautologous Tissue Substitute in Occipital-cervical Joint, External Approach

0RW100Z Revision of Drainage Device in Cervical Vertebral Joint, Open Approach

0RW103Z Revision of Infusion Device in Cervical Vertebral Joint, Open Approach

0RW104Z Revision of Internal Fixation Device in Cervical Vertebral Joint, Open Approach

0RW107Z Revision of Autologous Tissue Substitute in Cervical Vertebral Joint, Open Approach

0RW108Z Revision of Spacer in Cervical Vertebral Joint, Open Approach

0RW10AZ Revision of Interbody Fusion Device in Cervical Vertebral Joint, Open Approach

0RW10JZ Revision of Synthetic Substitute in Cervical Vertebral Joint, Open Approach

0RW10KZ Revision of Nonautologous Tissue Substitute in Cervical Vertebral Joint, Open Approach

0RW130Z Revision of Drainage Device in Cervical Vertebral Joint, Percutaneous Approach

0RW133Z Revision of Infusion Device in Cervical Vertebral Joint, Percutaneous Approach

0RW134Z Revision of Internal Fixation Device in Cervical Vertebral Joint, Percutaneous Approach

0RW137Z Revision of Autologous Tissue Substitute in Cervical Vertebral Joint, Percutaneous Approach

0RW138Z Revision of Spacer in Cervical Vertebral Joint, Percutaneous Approach

0RW13AZ Revision of Interbody Fusion Device in Cervical Vertebral Joint, Percutaneous Approach

0RW13JZ Revision of Synthetic Substitute in Cervical Vertebral Joint, Percutaneous Approach

0RW13KZ Revision of Nonautologous Tissue Substitute in Cervical Vertebral Joint, Percutaneous Approach

0RW140Z Revision of Drainage Device in Cervical Vertebral Joint, Percutaneous Endoscopic Approach

0RW143Z Revision of Infusion Device in Cervical Vertebral Joint, Percutaneous Endoscopic Approach

0RW144Z Revision of Internal Fixation Device in Cervical Vertebral Joint, Percutaneous Endoscopic Approach

0RW147Z Revision of Autologous Tissue Substitute in Cervical Vertebral Joint, Percutaneous Endoscopic Approach

0RW148Z Revision of Spacer in Cervical Vertebral Joint, Percutaneous Endoscopic Approach

0RW14AZ Revision of Interbody Fusion Device in Cervical Vertebral Joint, Percutaneous Endoscopic Approach

0RW14JZ Revision of Synthetic Substitute in Cervical Vertebral Joint, Percutaneous Endoscopic Approach

0RW14KZ Revision of Nonautologous Tissue Substitute in Cervical Vertebral Joint, Percutaneous Endoscopic Approach

0RW1X0Z Revision of Drainage Device in Cervical Vertebral Joint, External Approach

0RW1X3Z Revision of Infusion Device in Cervical Vertebral Joint, External Approach

0RW1X4Z Revision of Internal Fixation Device in Cervical Vertebral Joint, External Approach

0RW1X7Z Revision of Autologous Tissue Substitute in Cervical Vertebral Joint, External Approach

0RW1X8Z Revision of Spacer in Cervical Vertebral Joint, External Approach

0RW1XAZ Revision of Interbody Fusion Device in Cervical Vertebral Joint, External Approach

0RW1XJZ Revision of Synthetic Substitute in Cervical Vertebral Joint, External Approach

0RW1XKZ Revision of Nonautologous Tissue Substitute in Cervical Vertebral Joint, External Approach

0RW300Z Revision of Drainage Device in Cervical Vertebral Disc, Open Approach

0RW303Z Revision of Infusion Device in Cervical Vertebral Disc, Open Approach

♀ Female-only   ♂ Male-only   ▲ Limited Coverage   ● Non-OR   ᴴᴬᶜ HAC-associated procedure   ▲ Non-covered procedures   ✚ Cluster

0RW307Z   Revision of Autologous Tissue Substitute in Cervical Vertebral Disc, Open Approach

0RW30JZ   Revision of Synthetic Substitute in Cervical Vertebral Disc, Open Approach

0RW30KZ   Revision of Nonautologous Tissue Substitute in Cervical Vertebral Disc, Open Approach

0RW330Z   Revision of Drainage Device in Cervical Vertebral Disc, Percutaneous Approach

0RW333Z   Revision of Infusion Device in Cervical Vertebral Disc, Percutaneous Approach

0RW337Z   Revision of Autologous Tissue Substitute in Cervical Vertebral Disc, Percutaneous Approach

0RW33JZ   Revision of Synthetic Substitute in Cervical Vertebral Disc, Percutaneous Approach

0RW33KZ   Revision of Nonautologous Tissue Substitute in Cervical Vertebral Disc, Percutaneous Approach

0RW340Z   Revision of Drainage Device in Cervical Vertebral Disc, Percutaneous Endoscopic Approach

0RW343Z   Revision of Infusion Device in Cervical Vertebral Disc, Percutaneous Endoscopic Approach

0RW347Z   Revision of Autologous Tissue Substitute in Cervical Vertebral Disc, Percutaneous Endoscopic Approach

0RW34JZ   Revision of Synthetic Substitute in Cervical Vertebral Disc, Percutaneous Endoscopic Approach

0RW34KZ   Revision of Nonautologous Tissue Substitute in Cervical Vertebral Disc, Percutaneous Endoscopic Approach

0RW3X0Z   Revision of Drainage Device in Cervical Vertebral Disc, External Approach

0RW3X3Z   Revision of Infusion Device in Cervical Vertebral Disc, External Approach

0RW3X7Z   Revision of Autologous Tissue Substitute in Cervical Vertebral Disc, External Approach

0RW3XJZ   Revision of Synthetic Substitute in Cervical Vertebral Disc, External Approach

0RW3XKZ   Revision of Nonautologous Tissue Substitute in Cervical Vertebral Disc, External Approach

0RW400Z   Revision of Drainage Device in Cervicothoracic Vertebral Joint, Open Approach

0RW403Z   Revision of Infusion Device in Cervicothoracic Vertebral Joint, Open Approach

0RW404Z   Revision of Internal Fixation Device in Cervicothoracic Vertebral Joint, Open Approach

0RW407Z   Revision of Autologous Tissue Substitute in Cervicothoracic Vertebral Joint, Open Approach

0RW408Z   Revision of Spacer in Cervicothoracic Vertebral Joint, Open Approach

0RW40AZ   Revision of Interbody Fusion Device in Cervicothoracic Vertebral Joint, Open Approach

0RW40JZ   Revision of Synthetic Substitute in Cervicothoracic Vertebral Joint, Open Approach

0RW40KZ   Revision of Nonautologous Tissue Substitute in Cervicothoracic Vertebral Joint, Open Approach

0RW430Z   Revision of Drainage Device in Cervicothoracic Vertebral Joint, Percutaneous Approach

0RW433Z   Revision of Infusion Device in Cervicothoracic Vertebral Joint, Percutaneous Approach

0RW434Z   Revision of Internal Fixation Device in Cervicothoracic Vertebral Joint, Percutaneous Approach

0RW437Z   Revision of Autologous Tissue Substitute in Cervicothoracic Vertebral Joint, Percutaneous Approach

0RW438Z   Revision of Spacer in Cervicothoracic Vertebral Joint, Percutaneous Approach

0RW43AZ   Revision of Interbody Fusion Device in Cervicothoracic Vertebral Joint, Percutaneous Approach

0RW43JZ   Revision of Synthetic Substitute in Cervicothoracic Vertebral Joint, Percutaneous Approach

0RW43KZ   Revision of Nonautologous Tissue Substitute in Cervicothoracic Vertebral Joint, Percutaneous Approach

0RW440Z   Revision of Drainage Device in Cervicothoracic Vertebral Joint, Percutaneous Endoscopic Approach

0RW443Z   Revision of Infusion Device in Cervicothoracic Vertebral Joint, Percutaneous Endoscopic Approach

0RW444Z   Revision of Internal Fixation Device in Cervicothoracic Vertebral Joint, Percutaneous Endoscopic Approach

0RW447Z   Revision of Autologous Tissue Substitute in Cervicothoracic Vertebral Joint, Percutaneous Endoscopic Approach

0RW448Z   Revision of Spacer in Cervicothoracic Vertebral Joint, Percutaneous Endoscopic Approach

0RW44AZ   Revision of Interbody Fusion Device in Cervicothoracic Vertebral Joint, Percutaneous Endoscopic Approach

0RW44JZ   Revision of Synthetic Substitute in Cervicothoracic Vertebral Joint, Percutaneous Endoscopic Approach

0RW44KZ   Revision of Nonautologous Tissue Substitute in Cervicothoracic Vertebral Joint, Percutaneous Endoscopic Approach

0RW4X0Z   Revision of Drainage Device in Cervicothoracic Vertebral Joint, External Approach

0RW4X3Z   Revision of Infusion Device in Cervicothoracic Vertebral Joint, External Approach

0RW4X4Z   Revision of Internal Fixation Device in Cervicothoracic Vertebral Joint, External Approach

0RW4X7Z   Revision of Autologous Tissue Substitute in Cervicothoracic Vertebral Joint, External Approach

0RW4X8Z   Revision of Spacer in Cervicothoracic Vertebral Joint, External Approach

0RW4XAZ   Revision of Interbody Fusion Device in Cervicothoracic Vertebral Joint, External Approach

0RW4XJZ   Revision of Synthetic Substitute in Cervicothoracic Vertebral Joint, External Approach

0RW4XKZ   Revision of Nonautologous Tissue Substitute in Cervicothoracic Vertebral Joint, External Approach

0RW500Z   Revision of Drainage Device in Cervicothoracic Vertebral Disc, Open Approach

0RW503Z   Revision of Infusion Device in Cervicothoracic Vertebral Disc, Open Approach

0RW507Z   Revision of Autologous Tissue Substitute in Cervicothoracic Vertebral Disc, Open Approach

0RW50JZ   Revision of Synthetic Substitute in Cervicothoracic Vertebral Disc, Open Approach

0RW50KZ   Revision of Nonautologous Tissue Substitute in Cervicothoracic Vertebral Disc, Open Approach

0RW530Z   Revision of Drainage Device in Cervicothoracic Vertebral Disc, Percutaneous Approach

0RW533Z   Revision of Infusion Device in Cervicothoracic Vertebral Disc, Percutaneous Approach

0RW537Z   Revision of Autologous Tissue Substitute in Cervicothoracic Vertebral Disc, Percutaneous Approach

0RW53JZ   Revision of Synthetic Substitute in Cervicothoracic Vertebral Disc, Percutaneous Approach

0RW53KZ   Revision of Nonautologous Tissue Substitute in Cervicothoracic Vertebral Disc, Percutaneous Approach

0RW540Z   Revision of Drainage Device in Cervicothoracic Vertebral Disc, Percutaneous Endoscopic Approach

0RW543Z   Revision of Infusion Device in Cervicothoracic Vertebral Disc, Percutaneous Endoscopic Approach

0RW547Z   Revision of Autologous Tissue Substitute in Cervicothoracic Vertebral Disc, Percutaneous Endoscopic Approach

0RW54JZ   Revision of Synthetic Substitute in Cervicothoracic Vertebral Disc, Percutaneous Endoscopic Approach

0RW54KZ   Revision of Nonautologous Tissue Substitute in Cervicothoracic Vertebral Disc, Percutaneous Endoscopic Approach

0RW5X0Z   Revision of Drainage Device in Cervicothoracic Vertebral Disc, External Approach

0RW5X3Z   Revision of Infusion Device in Cervicothoracic Vertebral Disc, External Approach

0RW5X7Z   Revision of Autologous Tissue Substitute in Cervicothoracic Vertebral Disc, External Approach

0RW5XJZ   Revision of Synthetic Substitute in Cervicothoracic Vertebral Disc, External Approach

0RW5XKZ   Revision of Nonautologous Tissue Substitute in Cervicothoracic Vertebral Disc, External Approach

0RW600Z   Revision of Drainage Device in Thoracic Vertebral Joint, Open Approach

0RW603Z   Revision of Infusion Device in Thoracic Vertebral Joint, Open Approach

0RW604Z   Revision of Internal Fixation Device in Thoracic Vertebral Joint, Open Approach

0RW607Z   Revision of Autologous Tissue Substitute in Thoracic Vertebral Joint, Open Approach

0RW608Z   Revision of Spacer in Thoracic Vertebral Joint, Open Approach

---

♀ Female-only   ♂ Male-only   ▲ Limited Coverage   ● Non-OR   ■ HAC-associated procedure   ▲ Non-covered procedures   ✛ Cluster

0RW60AZ	Revision of Interbody Fusion Device in Thoracic Vertebral Joint, Open Approach	**0RW6XJZ**	Revision of Synthetic Substitute in Thoracic Vertebral Joint, External Approach	**0RWA07Z**	Revision of Autologous Tissue Substitute in Thoracolumbar Vertebral Joint, Open Approach
0RW60JZ	Revision of Synthetic Substitute in Thoracic Vertebral Joint, Open Approach	**0RW6XKZ**	Revision of Nonautologous Tissue Substitute in Thoracic Vertebral Joint, External Approach	**0RWA08Z**	Revision of Spacer in Thoracolumbar Vertebral Joint, Open Approach
0RW60KZ	Revision of Nonautologous Tissue Substitute in Thoracic Vertebral Joint, Open Approach	**0RW900Z**	Revision of Drainage Device in Thoracic Vertebral Disc, Open Approach	**0RWA0AZ**	Revision of Interbody Fusion Device in Thoracolumbar Vertebral Joint, Open Approach
0RW630Z	Revision of Drainage Device in Thoracic Vertebral Joint, Percutaneous Approach	**0RW903Z**	Revision of Infusion Device in Thoracic Vertebral Disc, Open Approach	**0RWA0JZ**	Revision of Synthetic Substitute in Thoracolumbar Vertebral Joint, Open Approach
0RW633Z	Revision of Infusion Device in Thoracic Vertebral Joint, Percutaneous Approach	**0RW907Z**	Revision of Autologous Tissue Substitute in Thoracic Vertebral Disc, Open Approach	**0RWA0KZ**	Revision of Nonautologous Tissue Substitute in Thoracolumbar Vertebral Joint, Open Approach
0RW634Z	Revision of Internal Fixation Device in Thoracic Vertebral Joint, Percutaneous Approach	**0RW90JZ**	Revision of Synthetic Substitute in Thoracic Vertebral Disc, Open Approach	**0RWA30Z**	Revision of Drainage Device in Thoracolumbar Vertebral Joint, Percutaneous Approach
0RW637Z	Revision of Autologous Tissue Substitute in Thoracic Vertebral Joint, Percutaneous Approach	**0RW90KZ**	Revision of Nonautologous Tissue Substitute in Thoracic Vertebral Disc, Open Approach	**0RWA33Z**	Revision of Infusion Device in Thoracolumbar Vertebral Joint, Percutaneous Approach
0RW638Z	Revision of Spacer in Thoracic Vertebral Joint, Percutaneous Approach	**0RW930Z**	Revision of Drainage Device in Thoracic Vertebral Disc, Percutaneous Approach	**0RWA34Z**	Revision of Internal Fixation Device in Thoracolumbar Vertebral Joint, Percutaneous Approach
0RW63AZ	Revision of Interbody Fusion Device in Thoracic Vertebral Joint, Percutaneous Approach	**0RW933Z**	Revision of Infusion Device in Thoracic Vertebral Disc, Percutaneous Approach	**0RWA37Z**	Revision of Autologous Tissue Substitute in Thoracolumbar Vertebral Joint, Percutaneous Approach
0RW63JZ	Revision of Synthetic Substitute in Thoracic Vertebral Joint, Percutaneous Approach	**0RW937Z**	Revision of Autologous Tissue Substitute in Thoracic Vertebral Disc, Percutaneous Approach	**0RWA38Z**	Revision of Spacer in Thoracolumbar Vertebral Joint, Percutaneous Approach
0RW63KZ	Revision of Nonautologous Tissue Substitute in Thoracic Vertebral Joint, Percutaneous Approach	**0RW93JZ**	Revision of Synthetic Substitute in Thoracic Vertebral Disc, Percutaneous Approach	**0RWA3AZ**	Revision of Interbody Fusion Device in Thoracolumbar Vertebral Joint, Percutaneous Approach
0RW640Z	Revision of Drainage Device in Thoracic Vertebral Joint, Percutaneous Endoscopic Approach	**0RW93KZ**	Revision of Nonautologous Tissue Substitute in Thoracic Vertebral Disc, Percutaneous Approach	**0RWA3JZ**	Revision of Synthetic Substitute in Thoracolumbar Vertebral Joint, Percutaneous Approach
0RW643Z	Revision of Infusion Device in Thoracic Vertebral Joint, Percutaneous Endoscopic Approach	**0RW940Z**	Revision of Drainage Device in Thoracic Vertebral Disc, Percutaneous Endoscopic Approach	**0RWA3KZ**	Revision of Nonautologous Tissue Substitute in Thoracolumbar Vertebral Joint, Percutaneous Approach
0RW644Z	Revision of Internal Fixation Device in Thoracic Vertebral Joint, Percutaneous Endoscopic Approach	**0RW943Z**	Revision of Infusion Device in Thoracic Vertebral Disc, Percutaneous Endoscopic Approach	**0RWA40Z**	Revision of Drainage Device in Thoracolumbar Vertebral Joint, Percutaneous Endoscopic Approach
0RW647Z	Revision of Autologous Tissue Substitute in Thoracic Vertebral Joint, Percutaneous Endoscopic Approach	**0RW947Z**	Revision of Autologous Tissue Substitute in Thoracic Vertebral Disc, Percutaneous Endoscopic Approach	**0RWA43Z**	Revision of Infusion Device in Thoracolumbar Vertebral Joint, Percutaneous Endoscopic Approach
0RW648Z	Revision of Spacer in Thoracic Vertebral Joint, Percutaneous Endoscopic Approach	**0RW94JZ**	Revision of Synthetic Substitute in Thoracic Vertebral Disc, Percutaneous Endoscopic Approach	**0RWA44Z**	Revision of Internal Fixation Device in Thoracolumbar Vertebral Joint, Percutaneous Endoscopic Approach
0RW64AZ	Revision of Interbody Fusion Device in Thoracic Vertebral Joint, Percutaneous Endoscopic Approach	**0RW94KZ**	Revision of Nonautologous Tissue Substitute in Thoracic Vertebral Disc, Percutaneous Endoscopic Approach	**0RWA47Z**	Revision of Autologous Tissue Substitute in Thoracolumbar Vertebral Joint, Percutaneous Endoscopic Approach
0RW64JZ	Revision of Synthetic Substitute in Thoracic Vertebral Joint, Percutaneous Endoscopic Approach	**0RW9X0Z**	Revision of Drainage Device in Thoracic Vertebral Disc, External Approach	**0RWA48Z**	Revision of Spacer in Thoracolumbar Vertebral Joint, Percutaneous Endoscopic Approach
0RW64KZ	Revision of Nonautologous Tissue Substitute in Thoracic Vertebral Joint, Percutaneous Endoscopic Approach	**0RW9X3Z**	Revision of Infusion Device in Thoracic Vertebral Disc, External Approach	**0RWA4AZ**	Revision of Interbody Fusion Device in Thoracolumbar Vertebral Joint, Percutaneous Endoscopic Approach
0RW6X0Z	Revision of Drainage Device in Thoracic Vertebral Joint, External Approach	**0RW9X7Z**	Revision of Autologous Tissue Substitute in Thoracic Vertebral Disc, External Approach	**0RWA4JZ**	Revision of Synthetic Substitute in Thoracolumbar Vertebral Joint, Percutaneous Endoscopic Approach
0RW6X3Z	Revision of Infusion Device in Thoracic Vertebral Joint, External Approach	**0RW9XJZ**	Revision of Synthetic Substitute in Thoracic Vertebral Disc, External Approach	**0RWA4KZ**	Revision of Nonautologous Tissue Substitute in Thoracolumbar Vertebral Joint, Percutaneous Endoscopic Approach
0RW6X4Z	Revision of Internal Fixation Device in Thoracic Vertebral Joint, External Approach	**0RW9XKZ**	Revision of Nonautologous Tissue Substitute in Thoracic Vertebral Disc, External Approach	**0RWAX0Z**	Revision of Drainage Device in Thoracolumbar Vertebral Joint, External Approach
0RW6X7Z	Revision of Autologous Tissue Substitute in Thoracic Vertebral Joint, External Approach	**0RWA00Z**	Revision of Drainage Device in Thoracolumbar Vertebral Joint, Open Approach	**0RWAX3Z**	Revision of Infusion Device in Thoracolumbar Vertebral Joint, External Approach
0RW6X8Z	Revision of Spacer in Thoracic Vertebral Joint, External Approach	**0RWA03Z**	Revision of Infusion Device in Thoracolumbar Vertebral Joint, Open Approach	**0RWAX4Z**	Revision of Internal Fixation Device in Thoracolumbar Vertebral Joint, External Approach
0RW6XAZ	Revision of Interbody Fusion Device in Thoracic Vertebral Joint, External Approach	**0RWA04Z**	Revision of Internal Fixation Device in Thoracolumbar Vertebral Joint, Open Approach	**0RWAX7Z**	Revision of Autologous Tissue Substitute in Thoracolumbar Vertebral Joint, External Approach

♀ Female-only   ♂ Male-only   ▲ Limited Coverage   ● Non-OR   **HAC** HAC-associated procedure   ▲ Non-covered procedures   ✚ Cluster

0RWAX8Z	Revision of Spacer in Thoracolumbar Vertebral Joint, External Approach
0RWAXAZ	Revision of Interbody Fusion Device in Thoracolumbar Vertebral Joint, External Approach
0RWAXJZ	Revision of Synthetic Substitute in Thoracolumbar Vertebral Joint, External Approach
0RWAXKZ	Revision of Nonautologous Tissue Substitute in Thoracolumbar Vertebral Joint, External Approach
0RWB00Z	Revision of Drainage Device in Thoracolumbar Vertebral Disc, Open Approach
0RWB03Z	Revision of Infusion Device in Thoracolumbar Vertebral Disc, Open Approach
0RWB07Z	Revision of Autologous Tissue Substitute in Thoracolumbar Vertebral Disc, Open Approach
0RWB0JZ	Revision of Synthetic Substitute in Thoracolumbar Vertebral Disc, Open Approach
0RWB0KZ	Revision of Nonautologous Tissue Substitute in Thoracolumbar Vertebral Disc, Open Approach
0RWB30Z	Revision of Drainage Device in Thoracolumbar Vertebral Disc, Percutaneous Approach
0RWB33Z	Revision of Infusion Device in Thoracolumbar Vertebral Disc, Percutaneous Approach
0RWB37Z	Revision of Autologous Tissue Substitute in Thoracolumbar Vertebral Disc, Percutaneous Approach
0RWB3JZ	Revision of Synthetic Substitute in Thoracolumbar Vertebral Disc, Percutaneous Approach
0RWB3KZ	Revision of Nonautologous Tissue Substitute in Thoracolumbar Vertebral Disc, Percutaneous Approach
0RWB40Z	Revision of Drainage Device in Thoracolumbar Vertebral Disc, Percutaneous Endoscopic Approach
0RWB43Z	Revision of Infusion Device in Thoracolumbar Vertebral Disc, Percutaneous Endoscopic Approach
0RWB47Z	Revision of Autologous Tissue Substitute in Thoracolumbar Vertebral Disc, Percutaneous Endoscopic Approach
0RWB4JZ	Revision of Synthetic Substitute in Thoracolumbar Vertebral Disc, Percutaneous Endoscopic Approach
0RWB4KZ	Revision of Nonautologous Tissue Substitute in Thoracolumbar Vertebral Disc, Percutaneous Endoscopic Approach
0RWBX0Z	Revision of Drainage Device in Thoracolumbar Vertebral Disc, External Approach
0RWBX3Z	Revision of Infusion Device in Thoracolumbar Vertebral Disc, External Approach
0RWBX7Z	Revision of Autologous Tissue Substitute in Thoracolumbar Vertebral Disc, External Approach
0RWBXJZ	Revision of Synthetic Substitute in Thoracolumbar Vertebral Disc, External Approach
0RWBXKZ	Revision of Nonautologous Tissue Substitute in Thoracolumbar Vertebral Disc, External Approach
0RWC00Z	Revision of Drainage Device in Right Temporomandibular Joint, Open Approach
0RWC03Z	Revision of Infusion Device in Right Temporomandibular Joint, Open Approach
0RWC04Z	Revision of Internal Fixation Device in Right Temporomandibular Joint, Open Approach
0RWC07Z	Revision of Autologous Tissue Substitute in Right Temporomandibular Joint, Open Approach
0RWC08Z	Revision of Spacer in Right Temporomandibular Joint, Open Approach
0RWC0JZ	Revision of Synthetic Substitute in Right Temporomandibular Joint, Open Approach
0RWC0KZ	Revision of Nonautologous Tissue Substitute in Right Temporomandibular Joint, Open Approach
0RWC30Z	Revision of Drainage Device in Right Temporomandibular Joint, Percutaneous Approach
0RWC33Z	Revision of Infusion Device in Right Temporomandibular Joint, Percutaneous Approach
0RWC34Z	Revision of Internal Fixation Device in Right Temporomandibular Joint, Percutaneous Approach
0RWC37Z	Revision of Autologous Tissue Substitute in Right Temporomandibular Joint, Percutaneous Approach
0RWC38Z	Revision of Spacer in Right Temporomandibular Joint, Percutaneous Approach
0RWC3JZ	Revision of Synthetic Substitute in Right Temporomandibular Joint, Percutaneous Approach
0RWC3KZ	Revision of Nonautologous Tissue Substitute in Right Temporomandibular Joint, Percutaneous Approach
0RWC40Z	Revision of Drainage Device in Right Temporomandibular Joint, Percutaneous Endoscopic Approach
0RWC43Z	Revision of Infusion Device in Right Temporomandibular Joint, Percutaneous Endoscopic Approach
0RWC44Z	Revision of Internal Fixation Device in Right Temporomandibular Joint, Percutaneous Endoscopic Approach
0RWC47Z	Revision of Autologous Tissue Substitute in Right Temporomandibular Joint, Percutaneous Endoscopic Approach
0RWC48Z	Revision of Spacer in Right Temporomandibular Joint, Percutaneous Endoscopic Approach
0RWC4JZ	Revision of Synthetic Substitute in Right Temporomandibular Joint, Percutaneous Endoscopic Approach
0RWC4KZ	Revision of Nonautologous Tissue Substitute in Right Temporomandibular Joint, Percutaneous Endoscopic Approach
0RWCX0Z	Revision of Drainage Device in Right Temporomandibular Joint, External Approach
0RWCX3Z	Revision of Infusion Device in Right Temporomandibular Joint, External Approach
0RWCX4Z	Revision of Internal Fixation Device in Right Temporomandibular Joint, External Approach
0RWCX7Z	Revision of Autologous Tissue Substitute in Right Temporomandibular Joint, External Approach
0RWCX8Z	Revision of Spacer in Right Temporomandibular Joint, External Approach
0RWCXJZ	Revision of Synthetic Substitute in Right Temporomandibular Joint, External Approach
0RWCXKZ	Revision of Nonautologous Tissue Substitute in Right Temporomandibular Joint, External Approach
0RWD00Z	Revision of Drainage Device in Left Temporomandibular Joint, Open Approach
0RWD03Z	Revision of Infusion Device in Left Temporomandibular Joint, Open Approach
0RWD04Z	Revision of Internal Fixation Device in Left Temporomandibular Joint, Open Approach
0RWD07Z	Revision of Autologous Tissue Substitute in Left Temporomandibular Joint, Open Approach
0RWD08Z	Revision of Spacer in Left Temporomandibular Joint, Open Approach
0RWD0JZ	Revision of Synthetic Substitute in Left Temporomandibular Joint, Open Approach
0RWD0KZ	Revision of Nonautologous Tissue Substitute in Left Temporomandibular Joint, Open Approach
0RWD30Z	Revision of Drainage Device in Left Temporomandibular Joint, Percutaneous Approach
0RWD33Z	Revision of Infusion Device in Left Temporomandibular Joint, Percutaneous Approach
0RWD34Z	Revision of Internal Fixation Device in Left Temporomandibular Joint, Percutaneous Approach
0RWD37Z	Revision of Autologous Tissue Substitute in Left Temporomandibular Joint, Percutaneous Approach
0RWD38Z	Revision of Spacer in Left Temporomandibular Joint, Percutaneous Approach
0RWD3JZ	Revision of Synthetic Substitute in Left Temporomandibular Joint, Percutaneous Approach
0RWD3KZ	Revision of Nonautologous Tissue Substitute in Left Temporomandibular Joint, Percutaneous Approach
0RWD40Z	Revision of Drainage Device in Left Temporomandibular Joint, Percutaneous Endoscopic Approach
0RWD43Z	Revision of Infusion Device in Left Temporomandibular Joint, Percutaneous Endoscopic Approach
0RWD44Z	Revision of Internal Fixation Device in Left Temporomandibular Joint, Percutaneous Endoscopic Approach
0RWD47Z	Revision of Autologous Tissue Substitute in Left Temporomandibular Joint, Percutaneous Endoscopic Approach
0RWD48Z	Revision of Spacer in Left Temporomandibular Joint, Percutaneous Endoscopic Approach

0RWD4JZ Revision of Synthetic Substitute in Left Temporomandibular Joint, Percutaneous Endoscopic Approach

0RWD4KZ Revision of Nonautologous Tissue Substitute in Left Temporomandibular Joint, Percutaneous Endoscopic Approach

0RWDX0Z Revision of Drainage Device in Left Temporomandibular Joint, External Approach

0RWDX3Z Revision of Infusion Device in Left Temporomandibular Joint, External Approach

0RWDX4Z Revision of Internal Fixation Device in Left Temporomandibular Joint, External Approach

0RWDX7Z Revision of Autologous Tissue Substitute in Left Temporomandibular Joint, External Approach

0RWDX8Z Revision of Spacer in Left Temporomandibular Joint, External Approach

0RWDXJZ Revision of Synthetic Substitute in Left Temporomandibular Joint, External Approach

0RWDXKZ Revision of Nonautologous Tissue Substitute in Left Temporomandibular Joint, External Approach

0RWE00Z Revision of Drainage Device in Right Sternoclavicular Joint, Open Approach

0RWE03Z Revision of Infusion Device in Right Sternoclavicular Joint, Open Approach

0RWE04Z Revision of Internal Fixation Device in Right Sternoclavicular Joint, Open Approach

0RWE07Z Revision of Autologous Tissue Substitute in Right Sternoclavicular Joint, Open Approach

0RWE08Z Revision of Spacer in Right Sternoclavicular Joint, Open Approach

0RWE0JZ Revision of Synthetic Substitute in Right Sternoclavicular Joint, Open Approach

0RWE0KZ Revision of Nonautologous Tissue Substitute in Right Sternoclavicular Joint, Open Approach

0RWE30Z Revision of Drainage Device in Right Sternoclavicular Joint, Percutaneous Approach

0RWE33Z Revision of Infusion Device in Right Sternoclavicular Joint, Percutaneous Approach

0RWE34Z Revision of Internal Fixation Device in Right Sternoclavicular Joint, Percutaneous Approach

0RWE37Z Revision of Autologous Tissue Substitute in Right Sternoclavicular Joint, Percutaneous Approach

0RWE38Z Revision of Spacer in Right Sternoclavicular Joint, Percutaneous Approach

0RWE3JZ Revision of Synthetic Substitute in Right Sternoclavicular Joint, Percutaneous Approach

0RWE3KZ Revision of Nonautologous Tissue Substitute in Right Sternoclavicular Joint, Percutaneous Approach

0RWE40Z Revision of Drainage Device in Right Sternoclavicular Joint, Percutaneous Endoscopic Approach

0RWE43Z Revision of Infusion Device in Right Sternoclavicular Joint, Percutaneous Endoscopic Approach

0RWE44Z Revision of Internal Fixation Device in Right Sternoclavicular Joint, Percutaneous Endoscopic Approach

0RWE47Z Revision of Autologous Tissue Substitute in Right Sternoclavicular Joint, Percutaneous Endoscopic Approach

0RWE48Z Revision of Spacer in Right Sternoclavicular Joint, Percutaneous Endoscopic Approach

0RWE4JZ Revision of Synthetic Substitute in Right Sternoclavicular Joint, Percutaneous Endoscopic Approach

0RWE4KZ Revision of Nonautologous Tissue Substitute in Right Sternoclavicular Joint, Percutaneous Endoscopic Approach

0RWEX0Z Revision of Drainage Device in Right Sternoclavicular Joint, External Approach

0RWEX3Z Revision of Infusion Device in Right Sternoclavicular Joint, External Approach

0RWEX4Z Revision of Internal Fixation Device in Right Sternoclavicular Joint, External Approach

0RWEX7Z Revision of Autologous Tissue Substitute in Right Sternoclavicular Joint, External Approach

0RWEX8Z Revision of Spacer in Right Sternoclavicular Joint, External Approach

0RWEXJZ Revision of Synthetic Substitute in Right Sternoclavicular Joint, External Approach

0RWEXKZ Revision of Nonautologous Tissue Substitute in Right Sternoclavicular Joint, External Approach

0RWF00Z Revision of Drainage Device in Left Sternoclavicular Joint, Open Approach

0RWF03Z Revision of Infusion Device in Left Sternoclavicular Joint, Open Approach

0RWF04Z Revision of Internal Fixation Device in Left Sternoclavicular Joint, Open Approach

0RWF07Z Revision of Autologous Tissue Substitute in Left Sternoclavicular Joint, Open Approach

0RWF08Z Revision of Spacer in Left Sternoclavicular Joint, Open Approach

0RWF0JZ Revision of Synthetic Substitute in Left Sternoclavicular Joint, Open Approach

0RWF0KZ Revision of Nonautologous Tissue Substitute in Left Sternoclavicular Joint, Open Approach

0RWF30Z Revision of Drainage Device in Left Sternoclavicular Joint, Percutaneous Approach

0RWF33Z Revision of Infusion Device in Left Sternoclavicular Joint, Percutaneous Approach

0RWF34Z Revision of Internal Fixation Device in Left Sternoclavicular Joint, Percutaneous Approach

0RWF37Z Revision of Autologous Tissue Substitute in Left Sternoclavicular Joint, Percutaneous Approach

0RWF38Z Revision of Spacer in Left Sternoclavicular Joint, Percutaneous Approach

0RWF3JZ Revision of Synthetic Substitute in Left Sternoclavicular Joint, Percutaneous Approach

0RWF3KZ Revision of Nonautologous Tissue Substitute in Left Sternoclavicular Joint, Percutaneous Approach

0RWF40Z Revision of Drainage Device in Left Sternoclavicular Joint, Percutaneous Endoscopic Approach

0RWF43Z Revision of Infusion Device in Left Sternoclavicular Joint, Percutaneous Endoscopic Approach

0RWF44Z Revision of Internal Fixation Device in Left Sternoclavicular Joint, Percutaneous Endoscopic Approach

0RWF47Z Revision of Autologous Tissue Substitute in Left Sternoclavicular Joint, Percutaneous Endoscopic Approach

0RWF48Z Revision of Spacer in Left Sternoclavicular Joint, Percutaneous Endoscopic Approach

0RWF4JZ Revision of Synthetic Substitute in Left Sternoclavicular Joint, Percutaneous Endoscopic Approach

0RWF4KZ Revision of Nonautologous Tissue Substitute in Left Sternoclavicular Joint, Percutaneous Endoscopic Approach

0RWFX0Z Revision of Drainage Device in Left Sternoclavicular Joint, External Approach

0RWFX3Z Revision of Infusion Device in Left Sternoclavicular Joint, External Approach

0RWFX4Z Revision of Internal Fixation Device in Left Sternoclavicular Joint, External Approach

0RWFX7Z Revision of Autologous Tissue Substitute in Left Sternoclavicular Joint, External Approach

0RWFX8Z Revision of Spacer in Left Sternoclavicular Joint, External Approach

0RWFXJZ Revision of Synthetic Substitute in Left Sternoclavicular Joint, External Approach

0RWFXKZ Revision of Nonautologous Tissue Substitute in Left Sternoclavicular Joint, External Approach

0RWG00Z Revision of Drainage Device in Right Acromioclavicular Joint, Open Approach

0RWG03Z Revision of Infusion Device in Right Acromioclavicular Joint, Open Approach

0RWG04Z Revision of Internal Fixation Device in Right Acromioclavicular Joint, Open Approach

0RWG07Z Revision of Autologous Tissue Substitute in Right Acromioclavicular Joint, Open Approach

0RWG08Z Revision of Spacer in Right Acromioclavicular Joint, Open Approach

0RWG0JZ Revision of Synthetic Substitute in Right Acromioclavicular Joint, Open Approach

0RWG0KZ Revision of Nonautologous Tissue Substitute in Right Acromioclavicular Joint, Open Approach

0RWG30Z Revision of Drainage Device in Right Acromioclavicular Joint, Percutaneous Approach

0RWG33Z Revision of Infusion Device in Right Acromioclavicular Joint, Percutaneous Approach

0RWG34Z Revision of Internal Fixation Device in Right Acromioclavicular Joint, Percutaneous Approach

♀ Female-only   ♂ Male-only   ▲ Limited Coverage   ● Non-OR   HAC-associated procedure   ▲ Non-covered procedures   ✚ Cluster

0RWG37Z Revision of Autologous Tissue Substitute in Right Acromioclavicular Joint, Percutaneous Approach

0RWG38Z Revision of Spacer in Right Acromioclavicular Joint, Percutaneous Approach

0RWG3JZ Revision of Synthetic Substitute in Right Acromioclavicular Joint, Percutaneous Approach

0RWG3KZ Revision of Nonautologous Tissue Substitute in Right Acromioclavicular Joint, Percutaneous Approach

0RWG40Z Revision of Drainage Device in Right Acromioclavicular Joint, Percutaneous Endoscopic Approach

0RWG43Z Revision of Infusion Device in Right Acromioclavicular Joint, Percutaneous Endoscopic Approach

0RWG44Z Revision of Internal Fixation Device in Right Acromioclavicular Joint, Percutaneous Endoscopic Approach

0RWG47Z Revision of Autologous Tissue Substitute in Right Acromioclavicular Joint, Percutaneous Endoscopic Approach

0RWG48Z Revision of Spacer in Right Acromioclavicular Joint, Percutaneous Endoscopic Approach

0RWG4JZ Revision of Synthetic Substitute in Right Acromioclavicular Joint, Percutaneous Endoscopic Approach

0RWG4KZ Revision of Nonautologous Tissue Substitute in Right Acromioclavicular Joint, Percutaneous Endoscopic Approach

0RWGX0Z Revision of Drainage Device in Right Acromioclavicular Joint, External Approach

0RWGX3Z Revision of Infusion Device in Right Acromioclavicular Joint, External Approach

0RWGX4Z Revision of Internal Fixation Device in Right Acromioclavicular Joint, External Approach

0RWGX7Z Revision of Autologous Tissue Substitute in Right Acromioclavicular Joint, External Approach

0RWGX8Z Revision of Spacer in Right Acromioclavicular Joint, External Approach

0RWGXJZ Revision of Synthetic Substitute in Right Acromioclavicular Joint, External Approach

0RWGXKZ Revision of Nonautologous Tissue Substitute in Right Acromioclavicular Joint, External Approach

0RWH00Z Revision of Drainage Device in Left Acromioclavicular Joint, Open Approach

0RWH03Z Revision of Infusion Device in Left Acromioclavicular Joint, Open Approach

0RWH04Z Revision of Internal Fixation Device in Left Acromioclavicular Joint, Open Approach

0RWH07Z Revision of Autologous Tissue Substitute in Left Acromioclavicular Joint, Open Approach

0RWH08Z Revision of Spacer in Left Acromioclavicular Joint, Open Approach

0RWH0JZ Revision of Synthetic Substitute in Left Acromioclavicular Joint, Open Approach

0RWH0KZ Revision of Nonautologous Tissue Substitute in Left Acromioclavicular Joint, Open Approach

0RWH30Z Revision of Drainage Device in Left Acromioclavicular Joint, Percutaneous Approach

0RWH33Z Revision of Infusion Device in Left Acromioclavicular Joint, Percutaneous Approach

0RWH34Z Revision of Internal Fixation Device in Left Acromioclavicular Joint, Percutaneous Approach

0RWH37Z Revision of Autologous Tissue Substitute in Left Acromioclavicular Joint, Percutaneous Approach

0RWH38Z Revision of Spacer in Left Acromioclavicular Joint, Percutaneous Approach

0RWH3JZ Revision of Synthetic Substitute in Left Acromioclavicular Joint, Percutaneous Approach

0RWH3KZ Revision of Nonautologous Tissue Substitute in Left Acromioclavicular Joint, Percutaneous Approach

0RWH40Z Revision of Drainage Device in Left Acromioclavicular Joint, Percutaneous Endoscopic Approach

0RWH43Z Revision of Infusion Device in Left Acromioclavicular Joint, Percutaneous Endoscopic Approach

0RWH44Z Revision of Internal Fixation Device in Left Acromioclavicular Joint, Percutaneous Endoscopic Approach

0RWH47Z Revision of Autologous Tissue Substitute in Left Acromioclavicular Joint, Percutaneous Endoscopic Approach

0RWH48Z Revision of Spacer in Left Acromioclavicular Joint, Percutaneous Endoscopic Approach

0RWH4JZ Revision of Synthetic Substitute in Left Acromioclavicular Joint, Percutaneous Endoscopic Approach

0RWH4KZ Revision of Nonautologous Tissue Substitute in Left Acromioclavicular Joint, Percutaneous Endoscopic Approach

0RWHX0Z Revision of Drainage Device in Left Acromioclavicular Joint, External Approach

0RWHX3Z Revision of Infusion Device in Left Acromioclavicular Joint, External Approach

0RWHX4Z Revision of Internal Fixation Device in Left Acromioclavicular Joint, External Approach

0RWHX7Z Revision of Autologous Tissue Substitute in Left Acromioclavicular Joint, External Approach

0RWHX8Z Revision of Spacer in Left Acromioclavicular Joint, External Approach

0RWHXJZ Revision of Synthetic Substitute in Left Acromioclavicular Joint, External Approach

0RWHXKZ Revision of Nonautologous Tissue Substitute in Left Acromioclavicular Joint, External Approach

0RWJ00Z Revision of Drainage Device in Right Shoulder Joint, Open Approach

0RWJ03Z Revision of Infusion Device in Right Shoulder Joint, Open Approach

0RWJ04Z Revision of Internal Fixation Device in Right Shoulder Joint, Open Approach

0RWJ07Z Revision of Autologous Tissue Substitute in Right Shoulder Joint, Open Approach

0RWJ08Z Revision of Spacer in Right Shoulder Joint, Open Approach

0RWJ0J6 Revision of Synthetic Substitute in Right Shoulder Joint, Humeral Surface, Open Approach

0RWJ0J7 Revision of Synthetic Substitute in Right Shoulder Joint, Glenoid Surface, Open Approach

0RWJ0JZ Revision of Synthetic Substitute in Right Shoulder Joint, Open Approach

0RWJ0KZ Revision of Nonautologous Tissue Substitute in Right Shoulder Joint, Open Approach

0RWJ30Z Revision of Drainage Device in Right Shoulder Joint, Percutaneous Approach

0RWJ33Z Revision of Infusion Device in Right Shoulder Joint, Percutaneous Approach

0RWJ34Z Revision of Internal Fixation Device in Right Shoulder Joint, Percutaneous Approach

0RWJ37Z Revision of Autologous Tissue Substitute in Right Shoulder Joint, Percutaneous Approach

0RWJ38Z Revision of Spacer in Right Shoulder Joint, Percutaneous Approach

0RWJ3J6 Revision of Synthetic Substitute in Right Shoulder Joint, Humeral Surface, Percutaneous Approach

0RWJ3J7 Revision of Synthetic Substitute in Right Shoulder Joint, Glenoid Surface, Percutaneous Approach

0RWJ3JZ Revision of Synthetic Substitute in Right Shoulder Joint, Percutaneous Approach

0RWJ3KZ Revision of Nonautologous Tissue Substitute in Right Shoulder Joint, Percutaneous Approach

0RWJ40Z Revision of Drainage Device in Right Shoulder Joint, Percutaneous Endoscopic Approach

0RWJ43Z Revision of Infusion Device in Right Shoulder Joint, Percutaneous Endoscopic Approach

0RWJ44Z Revision of Internal Fixation Device in Right Shoulder Joint, Percutaneous Endoscopic Approach

0RWJ47Z Revision of Autologous Tissue Substitute in Right Shoulder Joint, Percutaneous Endoscopic Approach

0RWJ48Z Revision of Spacer in Right Shoulder Joint, Percutaneous Endoscopic Approach

0RWJ4J6 Revision of Synthetic Substitute in Right Shoulder Joint, Humeral Surface, Percutaneous Endoscopic Approach

0RWJ4J7 Revision of Synthetic Substitute in Right Shoulder Joint, Glenoid Surface, Percutaneous Endoscopic Approach

0RWJ4JZ Revision of Synthetic Substitute in Right Shoulder Joint, Percutaneous Endoscopic Approach

0RWJ4KZ Revision of Nonautologous Tissue Substitute in Right Shoulder Joint, Percutaneous Endoscopic Approach

0RWJX0Z Revision of Drainage Device in Right Shoulder Joint, External Approach

0RWJX3Z Revision of Infusion Device in Right Shoulder Joint, External Approach

0RWJX4Z Revision of Internal Fixation Device in Right Shoulder Joint, External Approach

0RWJX7Z Revision of Autologous Tissue Substitute in Right Shoulder Joint, External Approach

0RWJX8Z Revision of Spacer in Right Shoulder Joint, External Approach

0RWJXJ6 Revision of Synthetic Substitute in Right Shoulder Joint, Humeral Surface, External Approach

0RWJXJ7 Revision of Synthetic Substitute in Right Shoulder Joint, Glenoid Surface, External Approach

0RWJXJZ Revision of Synthetic Substitute in Right Shoulder Joint, External Approach

0RWJXKZ Revision of Nonautologous Tissue Substitute in Right Shoulder Joint, External Approach

0RWK00Z Revision of Drainage Device in Left Shoulder Joint, Open Approach

0RWK03Z Revision of Infusion Device in Left Shoulder Joint, Open Approach

0RWK04Z Revision of Internal Fixation Device in Left Shoulder Joint, Open Approach

0RWK07Z Revision of Autologous Tissue Substitute in Left Shoulder Joint, Open Approach

0RWK08Z Revision of Spacer in Left Shoulder Joint, Open Approach

0RWK0J6 Revision of Synthetic Substitute in Left Shoulder Joint, Humeral Surface, Open Approach

0RWK0J7 Revision of Synthetic Substitute in Left Shoulder Joint, Glenoid Surface, Open Approach

0RWK0JZ Revision of Synthetic Substitute in Left Shoulder Joint, Open Approach

0RWK0KZ Revision of Nonautologous Tissue Substitute in Left Shoulder Joint, Open Approach

0RWK30Z Revision of Drainage Device in Left Shoulder Joint, Percutaneous Approach

0RWK33Z Revision of Infusion Device in Left Shoulder Joint, Percutaneous Approach

0RWK34Z Revision of Internal Fixation Device in Left Shoulder Joint, Percutaneous Approach

0RWK37Z Revision of Autologous Tissue Substitute in Left Shoulder Joint, Percutaneous Approach

0RWK38Z Revision of Spacer in Left Shoulder Joint, Percutaneous Approach

0RWK3J6 Revision of Synthetic Substitute in Left Shoulder Joint, Humeral Surface, Percutaneous Approach

0RWK3J7 Revision of Synthetic Substitute in Left Shoulder Joint, Glenoid Surface, Percutaneous Approach

0RWK3JZ Revision of Synthetic Substitute in Left Shoulder Joint, Percutaneous Approach

0RWK3KZ Revision of Nonautologous Tissue Substitute in Left Shoulder Joint, Percutaneous Approach

0RWK40Z Revision of Drainage Device in Left Shoulder Joint, Percutaneous Endoscopic Approach

0RWK43Z Revision of Infusion Device in Left Shoulder Joint, Percutaneous Endoscopic Approach

0RWK44Z Revision of Internal Fixation Device in Left Shoulder Joint, Percutaneous Endoscopic Approach

0RWK47Z Revision of Autologous Tissue Substitute in Left Shoulder Joint, Percutaneous Endoscopic Approach

0RWK48Z Revision of Spacer in Left Shoulder Joint, Percutaneous Endoscopic Approach

0RWK4J6 Revision of Synthetic Substitute in Left Shoulder Joint, Humeral Surface, Percutaneous Endoscopic Approach

0RWK4J7 Revision of Synthetic Substitute in Left Shoulder Joint, Glenoid Surface, Percutaneous Endoscopic Approach

0RWK4JZ Revision of Synthetic Substitute in Left Shoulder Joint, Percutaneous Endoscopic Approach

0RWK4KZ Revision of Nonautologous Tissue Substitute in Left Shoulder Joint, Percutaneous Endoscopic Approach

0RWKX0Z Revision of Drainage Device in Left Shoulder Joint, External Approach

0RWKX3Z Revision of Infusion Device in Left Shoulder Joint, External Approach

0RWKX4Z Revision of Internal Fixation Device in Left Shoulder Joint, External Approach

0RWKX7Z Revision of Autologous Tissue Substitute in Left Shoulder Joint, External Approach

0RWKX8Z Revision of Spacer in Left Shoulder Joint, External Approach

0RWKXJ6 Revision of Synthetic Substitute in Left Shoulder Joint, Humeral Surface, External Approach

0RWKXJ7 Revision of Synthetic Substitute in Left Shoulder Joint, Glenoid Surface, External Approach

0RWKXJZ Revision of Synthetic Substitute in Left Shoulder Joint, External Approach

0RWKXKZ Revision of Nonautologous Tissue Substitute in Left Shoulder Joint, External Approach

0RWL00Z Revision of Drainage Device in Right Elbow Joint, Open Approach

0RWL03Z Revision of Infusion Device in Right Elbow Joint, Open Approach

0RWL04Z Revision of Internal Fixation Device in Right Elbow Joint, Open Approach

0RWL05Z Revision of External Fixation Device in Right Elbow Joint, Open Approach

0RWL07Z Revision of Autologous Tissue Substitute in Right Elbow Joint, Open Approach

0RWL08Z Revision of Spacer in Right Elbow Joint, Open Approach

0RWL0JZ Revision of Synthetic Substitute in Right Elbow Joint, Open Approach

0RWL0KZ Revision of Nonautologous Tissue Substitute in Right Elbow Joint, Open Approach

0RWL30Z Revision of Drainage Device in Right Elbow Joint, Percutaneous Approach

0RWL33Z Revision of Infusion Device in Right Elbow Joint, Percutaneous Approach

0RWL34Z Revision of Internal Fixation Device in Right Elbow Joint, Percutaneous Approach

0RWL35Z Revision of External Fixation Device in Right Elbow Joint, Percutaneous Approach

0RWL37Z Revision of Autologous Tissue Substitute in Right Elbow Joint, Percutaneous Approach

0RWL38Z Revision of Spacer in Right Elbow Joint, Percutaneous Approach

0RWL3JZ Revision of Synthetic Substitute in Right Elbow Joint, Percutaneous Approach

0RWL3KZ Revision of Nonautologous Tissue Substitute in Right Elbow Joint, Percutaneous Approach

0RWL40Z Revision of Drainage Device in Right Elbow Joint, Percutaneous Endoscopic Approach

0RWL43Z Revision of Infusion Device in Right Elbow Joint, Percutaneous Endoscopic Approach

0RWL44Z Revision of Internal Fixation Device in Right Elbow Joint, Percutaneous Endoscopic Approach

0RWL45Z Revision of External Fixation Device in Right Elbow Joint, Percutaneous Endoscopic Approach

0RWL47Z Revision of Autologous Tissue Substitute in Right Elbow Joint, Percutaneous Endoscopic Approach

0RWL48Z Revision of Spacer in Right Elbow Joint, Percutaneous Endoscopic Approach

0RWL4JZ Revision of Synthetic Substitute in Right Elbow Joint, Percutaneous Endoscopic Approach

0RWL4KZ Revision of Nonautologous Tissue Substitute in Right Elbow Joint, Percutaneous Endoscopic Approach

0RWLX0Z Revision of Drainage Device in Right Elbow Joint, External Approach

0RWLX3Z Revision of Infusion Device in Right Elbow Joint, External Approach

0RWLX4Z Revision of Internal Fixation Device in Right Elbow Joint, External Approach

0RWLX5Z Revision of External Fixation Device in Right Elbow Joint, External Approach

0RWLX7Z Revision of Autologous Tissue Substitute in Right Elbow Joint, External Approach

0RWLX8Z Revision of Spacer in Right Elbow Joint, External Approach

0RWLXJZ Revision of Synthetic Substitute in Right Elbow Joint, External Approach

0RWLXKZ Revision of Nonautologous Tissue Substitute in Right Elbow Joint, External Approach

0RWM00Z Revision of Drainage Device in Left Elbow Joint, Open Approach

0RWM03Z Revision of Infusion Device in Left Elbow Joint, Open Approach

0RWM04Z Revision of Internal Fixation Device in Left Elbow Joint, Open Approach

0RWM05Z Revision of External Fixation Device in Left Elbow Joint, Open Approach

0RWM07Z Revision of Autologous Tissue Substitute in Left Elbow Joint, Open Approach

0RWM08Z Revision of Spacer in Left Elbow Joint, Open Approach

0RWM0JZ Revision of Synthetic Substitute in Left Elbow Joint, Open Approach

0RWM0KZ Revision of Nonautologous Tissue Substitute in Left Elbow Joint, Open Approach

0RWM30Z Revision of Drainage Device in Left Elbow Joint, Percutaneous Approach

0RWM33Z Revision of Infusion Device in Left Elbow Joint, Percutaneous Approach

♀ Female-only   ♂ Male-only   ▲ Limited Coverage   ● Non-OR   ʜᴀᴄ HAC-associated procedure   ▲ Non-covered procedures   ✚ Cluster

0RWM34Z Revision of Internal Fixation Device in Left Elbow Joint, Percutaneous Approach

0RWM35Z Revision of External Fixation Device in Left Elbow Joint, Percutaneous Approach

0RWM37Z Revision of Autologous Tissue Substitute in Left Elbow Joint, Percutaneous Approach

0RWM38Z Revision of Spacer in Left Elbow Joint, Percutaneous Approach

0RWM3JZ Revision of Synthetic Substitute in Left Elbow Joint, Percutaneous Approach

0RWM3KZ Revision of Nonautologous Tissue Substitute in Left Elbow Joint, Percutaneous Approach

0RWM40Z Revision of Drainage Device in Left Elbow Joint, Percutaneous Endoscopic Approach

0RWM43Z Revision of Infusion Device in Left Elbow Joint, Percutaneous Endoscopic Approach

0RWM44Z Revision of Internal Fixation Device in Left Elbow Joint, Percutaneous Endoscopic Approach

0RWM45Z Revision of External Fixation Device in Left Elbow Joint, Percutaneous Endoscopic Approach

0RWM47Z Revision of Autologous Tissue Substitute in Left Elbow Joint, Percutaneous Endoscopic Approach

0RWM48Z Revision of Spacer in Left Elbow Joint, Percutaneous Endoscopic Approach

0RWM4JZ Revision of Synthetic Substitute in Left Elbow Joint, Percutaneous Endoscopic Approach

0RWM4KZ Revision of Nonautologous Tissue Substitute in Left Elbow Joint, Percutaneous Endoscopic Approach

0RWMX0Z Revision of Drainage Device in Left Elbow Joint, External Approach

0RWMX3Z Revision of Infusion Device in Left Elbow Joint, External Approach

0RWMX4Z Revision of Internal Fixation Device in Left Elbow Joint, External Approach

0RWMX5Z Revision of External Fixation Device in Left Elbow Joint, External Approach

0RWMX7Z Revision of Autologous Tissue Substitute in Left Elbow Joint, External Approach

0RWMX8Z Revision of Spacer in Left Elbow Joint, External Approach

0RWMXJZ Revision of Synthetic Substitute in Left Elbow Joint, External Approach

0RWMXKZ Revision of Nonautologous Tissue Substitute in Left Elbow Joint, External Approach

0RWN00Z Revision of Drainage Device in Right Wrist Joint, Open Approach

0RWN03Z Revision of Infusion Device in Right Wrist Joint, Open Approach

0RWN04Z Revision of Internal Fixation Device in Right Wrist Joint, Open Approach

0RWN05Z Revision of External Fixation Device in Right Wrist Joint, Open Approach

0RWN07Z Revision of Autologous Tissue Substitute in Right Wrist Joint, Open Approach

0RWN08Z Revision of Spacer in Right Wrist Joint, Open Approach

0RWN0JZ Revision of Synthetic Substitute in Right Wrist Joint, Open Approach

0RWN0KZ Revision of Nonautologous Tissue Substitute in Right Wrist Joint, Open Approach

0RWN30Z Revision of Drainage Device in Right Wrist Joint, Percutaneous Approach

0RWN33Z Revision of Infusion Device in Right Wrist Joint, Percutaneous Approach

0RWN34Z Revision of Internal Fixation Device in Right Wrist Joint, Percutaneous Approach

0RWN35Z Revision of External Fixation Device in Right Wrist Joint, Percutaneous Approach

0RWN37Z Revision of Autologous Tissue Substitute in Right Wrist Joint, Percutaneous Approach

0RWN38Z Revision of Spacer in Right Wrist Joint, Percutaneous Approach

0RWN3JZ Revision of Synthetic Substitute in Right Wrist Joint, Percutaneous Approach

0RWN3KZ Revision of Nonautologous Tissue Substitute in Right Wrist Joint, Percutaneous Approach

0RWN40Z Revision of Drainage Device in Right Wrist Joint, Percutaneous Endoscopic Approach

0RWN43Z Revision of Infusion Device in Right Wrist Joint, Percutaneous Endoscopic Approach

0RWN44Z Revision of Internal Fixation Device in Right Wrist Joint, Percutaneous Endoscopic Approach

0RWN45Z Revision of External Fixation Device in Right Wrist Joint, Percutaneous Endoscopic Approach

0RWN47Z Revision of Autologous Tissue Substitute in Right Wrist Joint, Percutaneous Endoscopic Approach

0RWN48Z Revision of Spacer in Right Wrist Joint, Percutaneous Endoscopic Approach

0RWN4JZ Revision of Synthetic Substitute in Right Wrist Joint, Percutaneous Endoscopic Approach

0RWN4KZ Revision of Nonautologous Tissue Substitute in Right Wrist Joint, Percutaneous Endoscopic Approach

0RWNX0Z Revision of Drainage Device in Right Wrist Joint, External Approach

0RWNX3Z Revision of Infusion Device in Right Wrist Joint, External Approach

0RWNX4Z Revision of Internal Fixation Device in Right Wrist Joint, External Approach

0RWNX5Z Revision of External Fixation Device in Right Wrist Joint, External Approach

0RWNX7Z Revision of Autologous Tissue Substitute in Right Wrist Joint, External Approach

0RWNX8Z Revision of Spacer in Right Wrist Joint, External Approach

0RWNXJZ Revision of Synthetic Substitute in Right Wrist Joint, External Approach

0RWNXKZ Revision of Nonautologous Tissue Substitute in Right Wrist Joint, External Approach

0RWP00Z Revision of Drainage Device in Left Wrist Joint, Open Approach

0RWP03Z Revision of Infusion Device in Left Wrist Joint, Open Approach

0RWP04Z Revision of Internal Fixation Device in Left Wrist Joint, Open Approach

0RWP05Z Revision of External Fixation Device in Left Wrist Joint, Open Approach

0RWP07Z Revision of Autologous Tissue Substitute in Left Wrist Joint, Open Approach

0RWP08Z Revision of Spacer in Left Wrist Joint, Open Approach

0RWP0JZ Revision of Synthetic Substitute in Left Wrist Joint, Open Approach

0RWP0KZ Revision of Nonautologous Tissue Substitute in Left Wrist Joint, Open Approach

0RWP30Z Revision of Drainage Device in Left Wrist Joint, Percutaneous Approach

0RWP33Z Revision of Infusion Device in Left Wrist Joint, Percutaneous Approach

0RWP34Z Revision of Internal Fixation Device in Left Wrist Joint, Percutaneous Approach

0RWP35Z Revision of External Fixation Device in Left Wrist Joint, Percutaneous Approach

0RWP37Z Revision of Autologous Tissue Substitute in Left Wrist Joint, Percutaneous Approach

0RWP38Z Revision of Spacer in Left Wrist Joint, Percutaneous Approach

0RWP3JZ Revision of Synthetic Substitute in Left Wrist Joint, Percutaneous Approach

0RWP3KZ Revision of Nonautologous Tissue Substitute in Left Wrist Joint, Percutaneous Approach

0RWP40Z Revision of Drainage Device in Left Wrist Joint, Percutaneous Endoscopic Approach

0RWP43Z Revision of Infusion Device in Left Wrist Joint, Percutaneous Endoscopic Approach

0RWP44Z Revision of Internal Fixation Device in Left Wrist Joint, Percutaneous Endoscopic Approach

0RWP45Z Revision of External Fixation Device in Left Wrist Joint, Percutaneous Endoscopic Approach

0RWP47Z Revision of Autologous Tissue Substitute in Left Wrist Joint, Percutaneous Endoscopic Approach

0RWP48Z Revision of Spacer in Left Wrist Joint, Percutaneous Endoscopic Approach

0RWP4JZ Revision of Synthetic Substitute in Left Wrist Joint, Percutaneous Endoscopic Approach

0RWP4KZ Revision of Nonautologous Tissue Substitute in Left Wrist Joint, Percutaneous Endoscopic Approach

0RWPX0Z Revision of Drainage Device in Left Wrist Joint, External Approach

0RWPX3Z Revision of Infusion Device in Left Wrist Joint, External Approach

0RWPX4Z Revision of Internal Fixation Device in Left Wrist Joint, External Approach

0RWPX5Z Revision of External Fixation Device in Left Wrist Joint, External Approach

0RWPX7Z Revision of Autologous Tissue Substitute in Left Wrist Joint, External Approach

0RWPX8Z Revision of Spacer in Left Wrist Joint, External Approach

0RWPXJZ Revision of Synthetic Substitute in Left Wrist Joint, External Approach

0RWPXKZ Revision of Nonautologous Tissue Substitute in Left Wrist Joint, External Approach

0RWQ00Z Revision of Drainage Device in Right Carpal Joint, Open Approach

0RWQ03Z Revision of Infusion Device in Right Carpal Joint, Open Approach

0RWQ04Z Revision of Internal Fixation Device in Right Carpal Joint, Open Approach

0RWQ05Z Revision of External Fixation Device in Right Carpal Joint, Open Approach

0RWQ07Z Revision of Autologous Tissue Substitute in Right Carpal Joint, Open Approach

0RWQ08Z Revision of Spacer in Right Carpal Joint, Open Approach

0RWQ0JZ Revision of Synthetic Substitute in Right Carpal Joint, Open Approach

0RWQ0KZ Revision of Nonautologous Tissue Substitute in Right Carpal Joint, Open Approach

0RWQ30Z Revision of Drainage Device in Right Carpal Joint, Percutaneous Approach

0RWQ33Z Revision of Infusion Device in Right Carpal Joint, Percutaneous Approach

0RWQ34Z Revision of Internal Fixation Device in Right Carpal Joint, Percutaneous Approach

0RWQ35Z Revision of External Fixation Device in Right Carpal Joint, Percutaneous Approach

0RWQ37Z Revision of Autologous Tissue Substitute in Right Carpal Joint, Percutaneous Approach

0RWQ38Z Revision of Spacer in Right Carpal Joint, Percutaneous Approach

0RWQ3JZ Revision of Synthetic Substitute in Right Carpal Joint, Percutaneous Approach

0RWQ3KZ Revision of Nonautologous Tissue Substitute in Right Carpal Joint, Percutaneous Approach

0RWQ40Z Revision of Drainage Device in Right Carpal Joint, Percutaneous Endoscopic Approach

0RWQ43Z Revision of Infusion Device in Right Carpal Joint, Percutaneous Endoscopic Approach

0RWQ44Z Revision of Internal Fixation Device in Right Carpal Joint, Percutaneous Endoscopic Approach

0RWQ45Z Revision of External Fixation Device in Right Carpal Joint, Percutaneous Endoscopic Approach

0RWQ47Z Revision of Autologous Tissue Substitute in Right Carpal Joint, Percutaneous Endoscopic Approach

0RWQ48Z Revision of Spacer in Right Carpal Joint, Percutaneous Endoscopic Approach

0RWQ4JZ Revision of Synthetic Substitute in Right Carpal Joint, Percutaneous Endoscopic Approach

0RWQ4KZ Revision of Nonautologous Tissue Substitute in Right Carpal Joint, Percutaneous Endoscopic Approach

0RWQX0Z Revision of Drainage Device in Right Carpal Joint, External Approach

0RWQX3Z Revision of Infusion Device in Right Carpal Joint, External Approach

0RWQX4Z Revision of Internal Fixation Device in Right Carpal Joint, External Approach

0RWQX5Z Revision of External Fixation Device in Right Carpal Joint, External Approach

0RWQX7Z Revision of Autologous Tissue Substitute in Right Carpal Joint, External Approach

0RWQX8Z Revision of Spacer in Right Carpal Joint, External Approach

0RWQXJZ Revision of Synthetic Substitute in Right Carpal Joint, External Approach

0RWQXKZ Revision of Nonautologous Tissue Substitute in Right Carpal Joint, External Approach

0RWR00Z Revision of Drainage Device in Left Carpal Joint, Open Approach

0RWR03Z Revision of Infusion Device in Left Carpal Joint, Open Approach

0RWR04Z Revision of Internal Fixation Device in Left Carpal Joint, Open Approach

0RWR05Z Revision of External Fixation Device in Left Carpal Joint, Open Approach

0RWR07Z Revision of Autologous Tissue Substitute in Left Carpal Joint, Open Approach

0RWR08Z Revision of Spacer in Left Carpal Joint, Open Approach

0RWR0JZ Revision of Synthetic Substitute in Left Carpal Joint, Open Approach

0RWR0KZ Revision of Nonautologous Tissue Substitute in Left Carpal Joint, Open Approach

0RWR30Z Revision of Drainage Device in Left Carpal Joint, Percutaneous Approach

0RWR33Z Revision of Infusion Device in Left Carpal Joint, Percutaneous Approach

0RWR34Z Revision of Internal Fixation Device in Left Carpal Joint, Percutaneous Approach

0RWR35Z Revision of External Fixation Device in Left Carpal Joint, Percutaneous Approach

0RWR37Z Revision of Autologous Tissue Substitute in Left Carpal Joint, Percutaneous Approach

0RWR38Z Revision of Spacer in Left Carpal Joint, Percutaneous Approach

0RWR3JZ Revision of Synthetic Substitute in Left Carpal Joint, Percutaneous Approach

0RWR3KZ Revision of Nonautologous Tissue Substitute in Left Carpal Joint, Percutaneous Approach

0RWR40Z Revision of Drainage Device in Left Carpal Joint, Percutaneous Endoscopic Approach

0RWR43Z Revision of Infusion Device in Left Carpal Joint, Percutaneous Endoscopic Approach

0RWR44Z Revision of Internal Fixation Device in Left Carpal Joint, Percutaneous Endoscopic Approach

0RWR45Z Revision of External Fixation Device in Left Carpal Joint, Percutaneous Endoscopic Approach

0RWR47Z Revision of Autologous Tissue Substitute in Left Carpal Joint, Percutaneous Endoscopic Approach

0RWR48Z Revision of Spacer in Left Carpal Joint, Percutaneous Endoscopic Approach

0RWR4JZ Revision of Synthetic Substitute in Left Carpal Joint, Percutaneous Endoscopic Approach

0RWR4KZ Revision of Nonautologous Tissue Substitute in Left Carpal Joint, Percutaneous Endoscopic Approach

0RWRX0Z Revision of Drainage Device in Left Carpal Joint, External Approach

0RWRX3Z Revision of Infusion Device in Left Carpal Joint, External Approach

0RWRX4Z Revision of Internal Fixation Device in Left Carpal Joint, External Approach

0RWRX5Z Revision of External Fixation Device in Left Carpal Joint, External Approach

0RWRX7Z Revision of Autologous Tissue Substitute in Left Carpal Joint, External Approach

0RWRX8Z Revision of Spacer in Left Carpal Joint, External Approach

0RWRXJZ Revision of Synthetic Substitute in Left Carpal Joint, External Approach

0RWRXKZ Revision of Nonautologous Tissue Substitute in Left Carpal Joint, External Approach

0RWS00Z Revision of Drainage Device in Right Carpometacarpal Joint, Open Approach

0RWS03Z Revision of Infusion Device in Right Carpometacarpal Joint, Open Approach

0RWS04Z Revision of Internal Fixation Device in Right Carpometacarpal Joint, Open Approach

0RWS05Z Revision of External Fixation Device in Right Carpometacarpal Joint, Open Approach

0RWS07Z Revision of Autologous Tissue Substitute in Right Carpometacarpal Joint, Open Approach

0RWS08Z Revision of Spacer in Right Carpometacarpal Joint, Open Approach

0RWS0JZ Revision of Synthetic Substitute in Right Carpometacarpal Joint, Open Approach

0RWS0KZ Revision of Nonautologous Tissue Substitute in Right Carpometacarpal Joint, Open Approach

0RWS30Z Revision of Drainage Device in Right Carpometacarpal Joint, Percutaneous Approach

0RWS33Z Revision of Infusion Device in Right Carpometacarpal Joint, Percutaneous Approach

0RWS34Z Revision of Internal Fixation Device in Right Carpometacarpal Joint, Percutaneous Approach

0RWS35Z Revision of External Fixation Device in Right Carpometacarpal Joint, Percutaneous Approach

0RWS37Z Revision of Autologous Tissue Substitute in Right Carpometacarpal Joint, Percutaneous Approach

0RWS38Z Revision of Spacer in Right Carpometacarpal Joint, Percutaneous Approach

0RWS3JZ Revision of Synthetic Substitute in Right Carpometacarpal Joint, Percutaneous Approach

0RWS3KZ Revision of Nonautologous Tissue Substitute in Right Carpometacarpal Joint, Percutaneous Approach

0RWS40Z Revision of Drainage Device in Right Carpometacarpal Joint, Percutaneous Endoscopic Approach

0RWS43Z	Revision of Infusion Device in Right Carpometacarpal Joint, Percutaneous Endoscopic Approach
0RWS44Z	Revision of Internal Fixation Device in Right Carpometacarpal Joint, Percutaneous Endoscopic Approach
0RWS45Z	Revision of External Fixation Device in Right Carpometacarpal Joint, Percutaneous Endoscopic Approach
0RWS47Z	Revision of Autologous Tissue Substitute in Right Carpometacarpal Joint, Percutaneous Endoscopic Approach
0RWS48Z	Revision of Spacer in Right Carpometacarpal Joint, Percutaneous Endoscopic Approach
0RWS4JZ	Revision of Synthetic Substitute in Right Carpometacarpal Joint, Percutaneous Endoscopic Approach
0RWS4KZ	Revision of Nonautologous Tissue Substitute in Right Carpometacarpal Joint, Percutaneous Endoscopic Approach
0RWSX0Z	Revision of Drainage Device in Right Carpometacarpal Joint, External Approach
0RWSX3Z	Revision of Infusion Device in Right Carpometacarpal Joint, External Approach
0RWSX4Z	Revision of Internal Fixation Device in Right Carpometacarpal Joint, External Approach
0RWSX5Z	Revision of External Fixation Device in Right Carpometacarpal Joint, External Approach
0RWSX7Z	Revision of Autologous Tissue Substitute in Right Carpometacarpal Joint, External Approach
0RWSX8Z	Revision of Spacer in Right Carpometacarpal Joint, External Approach
0RWSXJZ	Revision of Synthetic Substitute in Right Carpometacarpal Joint, External Approach
0RWSXKZ	Revision of Nonautologous Tissue Substitute in Right Carpometacarpal Joint, External Approach
0RWT00Z	Revision of Drainage Device in Left Carpometacarpal Joint, Open Approach
0RWT03Z	Revision of Infusion Device in Left Carpometacarpal Joint, Open Approach
0RWT04Z	Revision of Internal Fixation Device in Left Carpometacarpal Joint, Open Approach
0RWT05Z	Revision of External Fixation Device in Left Carpometacarpal Joint, Open Approach
0RWT07Z	Revision of Autologous Tissue Substitute in Left Carpometacarpal Joint, Open Approach
0RWT08Z	Revision of Spacer in Left Carpometacarpal Joint, Open Approach
0RWT0JZ	Revision of Synthetic Substitute in Left Carpometacarpal Joint, Open Approach
0RWT0KZ	Revision of Nonautologous Tissue Substitute in Left Carpometacarpal Joint, Open Approach
0RWT30Z	Revision of Drainage Device in Left Carpometacarpal Joint, Percutaneous Approach
0RWT33Z	Revision of Infusion Device in Left Carpometacarpal Joint, Percutaneous Approach
0RWT34Z	Revision of Internal Fixation Device in Left Carpometacarpal Joint, Percutaneous Approach
0RWT35Z	Revision of External Fixation Device in Left Carpometacarpal Joint, Percutaneous Approach
0RWT37Z	Revision of Autologous Tissue Substitute in Left Carpometacarpal Joint, Percutaneous Approach
0RWT38Z	Revision of Spacer in Left Carpometacarpal Joint, Percutaneous Approach
0RWT3JZ	Revision of Synthetic Substitute in Left Carpometacarpal Joint, Percutaneous Approach
0RWT3KZ	Revision of Nonautologous Tissue Substitute in Left Carpometacarpal Joint, Percutaneous Approach
0RWT40Z	Revision of Drainage Device in Left Carpometacarpal Joint, Percutaneous Endoscopic Approach
0RWT43Z	Revision of Infusion Device in Left Carpometacarpal Joint, Percutaneous Endoscopic Approach
0RWT44Z	Revision of Internal Fixation Device in Left Carpometacarpal Joint, Percutaneous Endoscopic Approach
0RWT45Z	Revision of External Fixation Device in Left Carpometacarpal Joint, Percutaneous Endoscopic Approach
0RWT47Z	Revision of Autologous Tissue Substitute in Left Carpometacarpal Joint, Percutaneous Endoscopic Approach
0RWT48Z	Revision of Spacer in Left Carpometacarpal Joint, Percutaneous Endoscopic Approach
0RWT4JZ	Revision of Synthetic Substitute in Left Carpometacarpal Joint, Percutaneous Endoscopic Approach
0RWT4KZ	Revision of Nonautologous Tissue Substitute in Left Carpometacarpal Joint, Percutaneous Endoscopic Approach
0RWTX0Z	Revision of Drainage Device in Left Carpometacarpal Joint, External Approach
0RWTX3Z	Revision of Infusion Device in Left Carpometacarpal Joint, External Approach
0RWTX4Z	Revision of Internal Fixation Device in Left Carpometacarpal Joint, External Approach
0RWTX5Z	Revision of External Fixation Device in Left Carpometacarpal Joint, External Approach
0RWTX7Z	Revision of Autologous Tissue Substitute in Left Carpometacarpal Joint, External Approach
0RWTX8Z	Revision of Spacer in Left Carpometacarpal Joint, External Approach
0RWTXJZ	Revision of Synthetic Substitute in Left Carpometacarpal Joint, External Approach
0RWTXKZ	Revision of Nonautologous Tissue Substitute in Left Carpometacarpal Joint, External Approach
0RWU00Z	Revision of Drainage Device in Right Metacarpophalangeal Joint, Open Approach
0RWU03Z	Revision of Infusion Device in Right Metacarpophalangeal Joint, Open Approach
0RWU04Z	Revision of Internal Fixation Device in Right Metacarpophalangeal Joint, Open Approach
0RWU05Z	Revision of External Fixation Device in Right Metacarpophalangeal Joint, Open Approach
0RWU07Z	Revision of Autologous Tissue Substitute in Right Metacarpophalangeal Joint, Open Approach
0RWU08Z	Revision of Spacer in Right Metacarpophalangeal Joint, Open Approach
0RWU0JZ	Revision of Synthetic Substitute in Right Metacarpophalangeal Joint, Open Approach
0RWU0KZ	Revision of Nonautologous Tissue Substitute in Right Metacarpophalangeal Joint, Open Approach
0RWU30Z	Revision of Drainage Device in Right Metacarpophalangeal Joint, Percutaneous Approach
0RWU33Z	Revision of Infusion Device in Right Metacarpophalangeal Joint, Percutaneous Approach
0RWU34Z	Revision of Internal Fixation Device in Right Metacarpophalangeal Joint, Percutaneous Approach
0RWU35Z	Revision of External Fixation Device in Right Metacarpophalangeal Joint, Percutaneous Approach
0RWU37Z	Revision of Autologous Tissue Substitute in Right Metacarpophalangeal Joint, Percutaneous Approach
0RWU38Z	Revision of Spacer in Right Metacarpophalangeal Joint, Percutaneous Approach
0RWU3JZ	Revision of Synthetic Substitute in Right Metacarpophalangeal Joint, Percutaneous Approach
0RWU3KZ	Revision of Nonautologous Tissue Substitute in Right Metacarpophalangeal Joint, Percutaneous Approach
0RWU40Z	Revision of Drainage Device in Right Metacarpophalangeal Joint, Percutaneous Endoscopic Approach
0RWU43Z	Revision of Infusion Device in Right Metacarpophalangeal Joint, Percutaneous Endoscopic Approach
0RWU44Z	Revision of Internal Fixation Device in Right Metacarpophalangeal Joint, Percutaneous Endoscopic Approach
0RWU45Z	Revision of External Fixation Device in Right Metacarpophalangeal Joint, Percutaneous Endoscopic Approach
0RWU47Z	Revision of Autologous Tissue Substitute in Right Metacarpophalangeal Joint, Percutaneous Endoscopic Approach
0RWU48Z	Revision of Spacer in Right Metacarpophalangeal Joint, Percutaneous Endoscopic Approach
0RWU4JZ	Revision of Synthetic Substitute in Right Metacarpophalangeal Joint, Percutaneous Endoscopic Approach

0RWU4KZ   Revision of Nonautologous Tissue Substitute in Right Metacarpophalangeal Joint, Percutaneous Endoscopic Approach

0RWUX0Z   Revision of Drainage Device in Right Metacarpophalangeal Joint, External Approach

0RWUX3Z   Revision of Infusion Device in Right Metacarpophalangeal Joint, External Approach

0RWUX4Z   Revision of Internal Fixation Device in Right Metacarpophalangeal Joint, External Approach

0RWUX5Z   Revision of External Fixation Device in Right Metacarpophalangeal Joint, External Approach

0RWUX7Z   Revision of Autologous Tissue Substitute in Right Metacarpophalangeal Joint, External Approach

0RWUX8Z   Revision of Spacer in Right Metacarpophalangeal Joint, External Approach

0RWUXJZ   Revision of Synthetic Substitute in Right Metacarpophalangeal Joint, External Approach

0RWUXKZ   Revision of Nonautologous Tissue Substitute in Right Metacarpophalangeal Joint, External Approach

0RWV00Z   Revision of Drainage Device in Left Metacarpophalangeal Joint, Open Approach

0RWV03Z   Revision of Infusion Device in Left Metacarpophalangeal Joint, Open Approach

0RWV04Z   Revision of Internal Fixation Device in Left Metacarpophalangeal Joint, Open Approach

0RWV05Z   Revision of External Fixation Device in Left Metacarpophalangeal Joint, Open Approach

0RWV07Z   Revision of Autologous Tissue Substitute in Left Metacarpophalangeal Joint, Open Approach

0RWV08Z   Revision of Spacer in Left Metacarpophalangeal Joint, Open Approach

0RWV0JZ   Revision of Synthetic Substitute in Left Metacarpophalangeal Joint, Open Approach

0RWV0KZ   Revision of Nonautologous Tissue Substitute in Left Metacarpophalangeal Joint, Open Approach

0RWV30Z   Revision of Drainage Device in Left Metacarpophalangeal Joint, Percutaneous Approach

0RWV33Z   Revision of Infusion Device in Left Metacarpophalangeal Joint, Percutaneous Approach

0RWV34Z   Revision of Internal Fixation Device in Left Metacarpophalangeal Joint, Percutaneous Approach

0RWV35Z   Revision of External Fixation Device in Left Metacarpophalangeal Joint, Percutaneous Approach

0RWV37Z   Revision of Autologous Tissue Substitute in Left Metacarpophalangeal Joint, Percutaneous Approach

0RWV38Z   Revision of Spacer in Left Metacarpophalangeal Joint, Percutaneous Approach

0RWV3JZ   Revision of Synthetic Substitute in Left Metacarpophalangeal Joint, Percutaneous Approach

0RWV3KZ   Revision of Nonautologous Tissue Substitute in Left Metacarpophalangeal Joint, Percutaneous Approach

0RWV40Z   Revision of Drainage Device in Left Metacarpophalangeal Joint, Percutaneous Endoscopic Approach

0RWV43Z   Revision of Infusion Device in Left Metacarpophalangeal Joint, Percutaneous Endoscopic Approach

0RWV44Z   Revision of Internal Fixation Device in Left Metacarpophalangeal Joint, Percutaneous Endoscopic Approach

0RWV45Z   Revision of External Fixation Device in Left Metacarpophalangeal Joint, Percutaneous Endoscopic Approach

0RWV47Z   Revision of Autologous Tissue Substitute in Left Metacarpophalangeal Joint, Percutaneous Endoscopic Approach

0RWV48Z   Revision of Spacer in Left Metacarpophalangeal Joint, Percutaneous Endoscopic Approach

0RWV4JZ   Revision of Synthetic Substitute in Left Metacarpophalangeal Joint, Percutaneous Endoscopic Approach

0RWV4KZ   Revision of Nonautologous Tissue Substitute in Left Metacarpophalangeal Joint, Percutaneous Endoscopic Approach

0RWVX0Z   Revision of Drainage Device in Left Metacarpophalangeal Joint, External Approach

0RWVX3Z   Revision of Infusion Device in Left Metacarpophalangeal Joint, External Approach

0RWVX4Z   Revision of Internal Fixation Device in Left Metacarpophalangeal Joint, External Approach

0RWVX5Z   Revision of External Fixation Device in Left Metacarpophalangeal Joint, External Approach

0RWVX7Z   Revision of Autologous Tissue Substitute in Left Metacarpophalangeal Joint, External Approach

0RWVX8Z   Revision of Spacer in Left Metacarpophalangeal Joint, External Approach

0RWVXJZ   Revision of Synthetic Substitute in Left Metacarpophalangeal Joint, External Approach

0RWVXKZ   Revision of Nonautologous Tissue Substitute in Left Metacarpophalangeal Joint, External Approach

0RWW00Z   Revision of Drainage Device in Right Finger Phalangeal Joint, Open Approach

0RWW03Z   Revision of Infusion Device in Right Finger Phalangeal Joint, Open Approach

0RWW04Z   Revision of Internal Fixation Device in Right Finger Phalangeal Joint, Open Approach

0RWW05Z   Revision of External Fixation Device in Right Finger Phalangeal Joint, Open Approach

0RWW07Z   Revision of Autologous Tissue Substitute in Right Finger Phalangeal Joint, Open Approach

0RWW08Z   Revision of Spacer in Right Finger Phalangeal Joint, Open Approach

0RWW0JZ   Revision of Synthetic Substitute in Right Finger Phalangeal Joint, Open Approach

0RWW0KZ   Revision of Nonautologous Tissue Substitute in Right Finger Phalangeal Joint, Open Approach

0RWW30Z   Revision of Drainage Device in Right Finger Phalangeal Joint, Percutaneous Approach

0RWW33Z   Revision of Infusion Device in Right Finger Phalangeal Joint, Percutaneous Approach

0RWW34Z   Revision of Internal Fixation Device in Right Finger Phalangeal Joint, Percutaneous Approach

0RWW35Z   Revision of External Fixation Device in Right Finger Phalangeal Joint, Percutaneous Approach

0RWW37Z   Revision of Autologous Tissue Substitute in Right Finger Phalangeal Joint, Percutaneous Approach

0RWW38Z   Revision of Spacer in Right Finger Phalangeal Joint, Percutaneous Approach

0RWW3JZ   Revision of Synthetic Substitute in Right Finger Phalangeal Joint, Percutaneous Approach

0RWW3KZ   Revision of Nonautologous Tissue Substitute in Right Finger Phalangeal Joint, Percutaneous Approach

0RWW40Z   Revision of Drainage Device in Right Finger Phalangeal Joint, Percutaneous Endoscopic Approach

0RWW43Z   Revision of Infusion Device in Right Finger Phalangeal Joint, Percutaneous Endoscopic Approach

0RWW44Z   Revision of Internal Fixation Device in Right Finger Phalangeal Joint, Percutaneous Endoscopic Approach

0RWW45Z   Revision of External Fixation Device in Right Finger Phalangeal Joint, Percutaneous Endoscopic Approach

0RWW47Z   Revision of Autologous Tissue Substitute in Right Finger Phalangeal Joint, Percutaneous Endoscopic Approach

0RWW48Z   Revision of Spacer in Right Finger Phalangeal Joint, Percutaneous Endoscopic Approach

0RWW4JZ   Revision of Synthetic Substitute in Right Finger Phalangeal Joint, Percutaneous Endoscopic Approach

0RWW4KZ   Revision of Nonautologous Tissue Substitute in Right Finger Phalangeal Joint, Percutaneous Endoscopic Approach

0RWWX0Z   Revision of Drainage Device in Right Finger Phalangeal Joint, External Approach

0RWWX3Z   Revision of Infusion Device in Right Finger Phalangeal Joint, External Approach

0RWWX4Z   Revision of Internal Fixation Device in Right Finger Phalangeal Joint, External Approach

0RWWX5Z   Revision of External Fixation Device in Right Finger Phalangeal Joint, External Approach

♀ Female-only   ♂ Male-only   ▲ Limited Coverage   ● Non-OR   HAC HAC-associated procedure   ▲ Non-covered procedures   ✚ Cluster

0RWWX7Z Revision of Autologous Tissue Substitute in Right Finger Phalangeal Joint, External Approach

0RWWX8Z Revision of Spacer in Right Finger Phalangeal Joint, External Approach

0RWWXJZ Revision of Synthetic Substitute in Right Finger Phalangeal Joint, External Approach

0RWWXKZ Revision of Nonautologous Tissue Substitute in Right Finger Phalangeal Joint, External Approach

0RWX00Z Revision of Drainage Device in Left Finger Phalangeal Joint, Open Approach

0RWX03Z Revision of Infusion Device in Left Finger Phalangeal Joint, Open Approach

0RWX04Z Revision of Internal Fixation Device in Left Finger Phalangeal Joint, Open Approach

0RWX05Z Revision of External Fixation Device in Left Finger Phalangeal Joint, Open Approach

0RWX07Z Revision of Autologous Tissue Substitute in Left Finger Phalangeal Joint, Open Approach

0RWX08Z Revision of Spacer in Left Finger Phalangeal Joint, Open Approach

0RWX0JZ Revision of Synthetic Substitute in Left Finger Phalangeal Joint, Open Approach

0RWX0KZ Revision of Nonautologous Tissue Substitute in Left Finger Phalangeal Joint, Open Approach

0RWX30Z Revision of Drainage Device in Left Finger Phalangeal Joint, Percutaneous Approach

0RWX33Z Revision of Infusion Device in Left Finger Phalangeal Joint, Percutaneous Approach

0RWX34Z Revision of Internal Fixation Device in Left Finger Phalangeal Joint, Percutaneous Approach

0RWX35Z Revision of External Fixation Device in Left Finger Phalangeal Joint, Percutaneous Approach

0RWX37Z Revision of Autologous Tissue Substitute in Left Finger Phalangeal Joint, Percutaneous Approach

0RWX38Z Revision of Spacer in Left Finger Phalangeal Joint, Percutaneous Approach

0RWX3JZ Revision of Synthetic Substitute in Left Finger Phalangeal Joint, Percutaneous Approach

0RWX3KZ Revision of Nonautologous Tissue Substitute in Left Finger Phalangeal Joint, Percutaneous Approach

0RWX40Z Revision of Drainage Device in Left Finger Phalangeal Joint, Percutaneous Endoscopic Approach

0RWX43Z Revision of Infusion Device in Left Finger Phalangeal Joint, Percutaneous Endoscopic Approach

0RWX44Z Revision of Internal Fixation Device in Left Finger Phalangeal Joint, Percutaneous Endoscopic Approach

0RWX45Z Revision of External Fixation Device in Left Finger Phalangeal Joint, Percutaneous Endoscopic Approach

0RWX47Z Revision of Autologous Tissue Substitute in Left Finger Phalangeal Joint, Percutaneous Endoscopic Approach

0RWX48Z Revision of Spacer in Left Finger Phalangeal Joint, Percutaneous Endoscopic Approach

0RWX4JZ Revision of Synthetic Substitute in Left Finger Phalangeal Joint, Percutaneous Endoscopic Approach

0RWX4KZ Revision of Nonautologous Tissue Substitute in Left Finger Phalangeal Joint, Percutaneous Endoscopic Approach

0RWXX0Z Revision of Drainage Device in Left Finger Phalangeal Joint, External Approach

0RWXX3Z Revision of Infusion Device in Left Finger Phalangeal Joint, External Approach

0RWXX4Z Revision of Internal Fixation Device in Left Finger Phalangeal Joint, External Approach

0RWXX5Z Revision of External Fixation Device in Left Finger Phalangeal Joint, External Approach

0RWXX7Z Revision of Autologous Tissue Substitute in Left Finger Phalangeal Joint, External Approach

0RWXX8Z Revision of Spacer in Left Finger Phalangeal Joint, External Approach

0RWXXJZ Revision of Synthetic Substitute in Left Finger Phalangeal Joint, External Approach

0RWXXKZ Revision of Nonautologous Tissue Substitute in Left Finger Phalangeal Joint, External Approach

---

♀ Female-only   ♂ Male-only   ▲ Limited Coverage   ● Non-OR   ▦ HAC-associated procedure   ▲ Non-covered procedures   ✚ Cluster

Intervertebral Joint

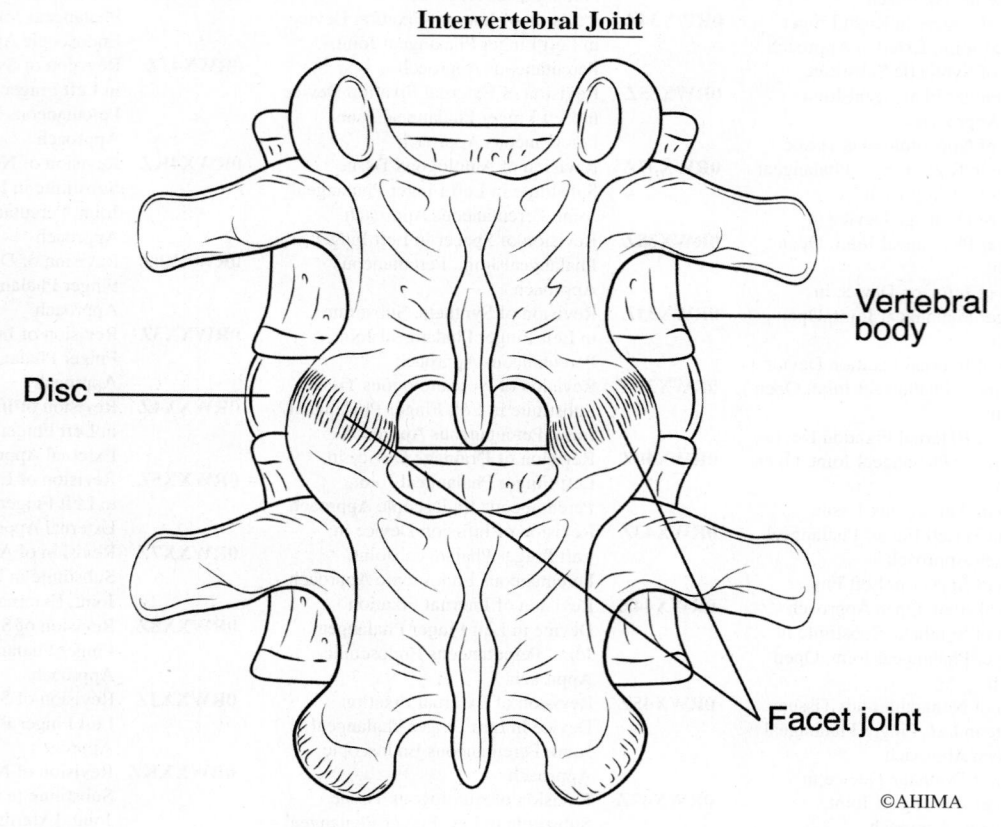

Vertebral body

Disc

Facet joint

©AHIMA

Hip

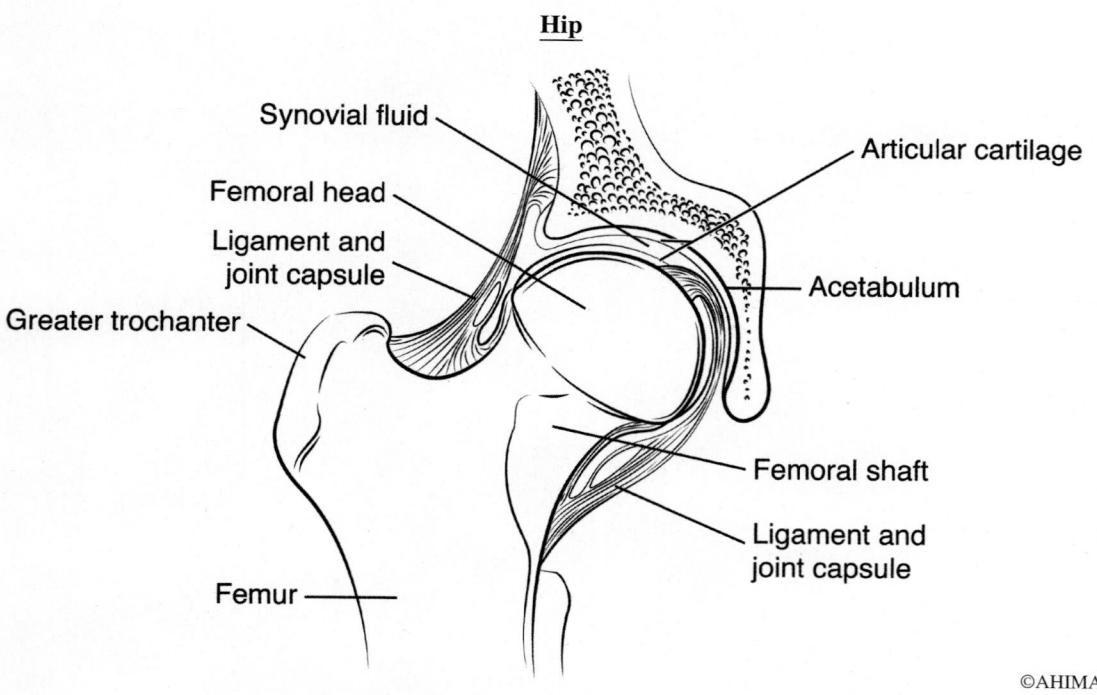

Synovial fluid

Femoral head

Ligament and joint capsule

Greater trochanter

Femur

Articular cartilage

Acetabulum

Femoral shaft

Ligament and joint capsule

©AHIMA

Knee Joint

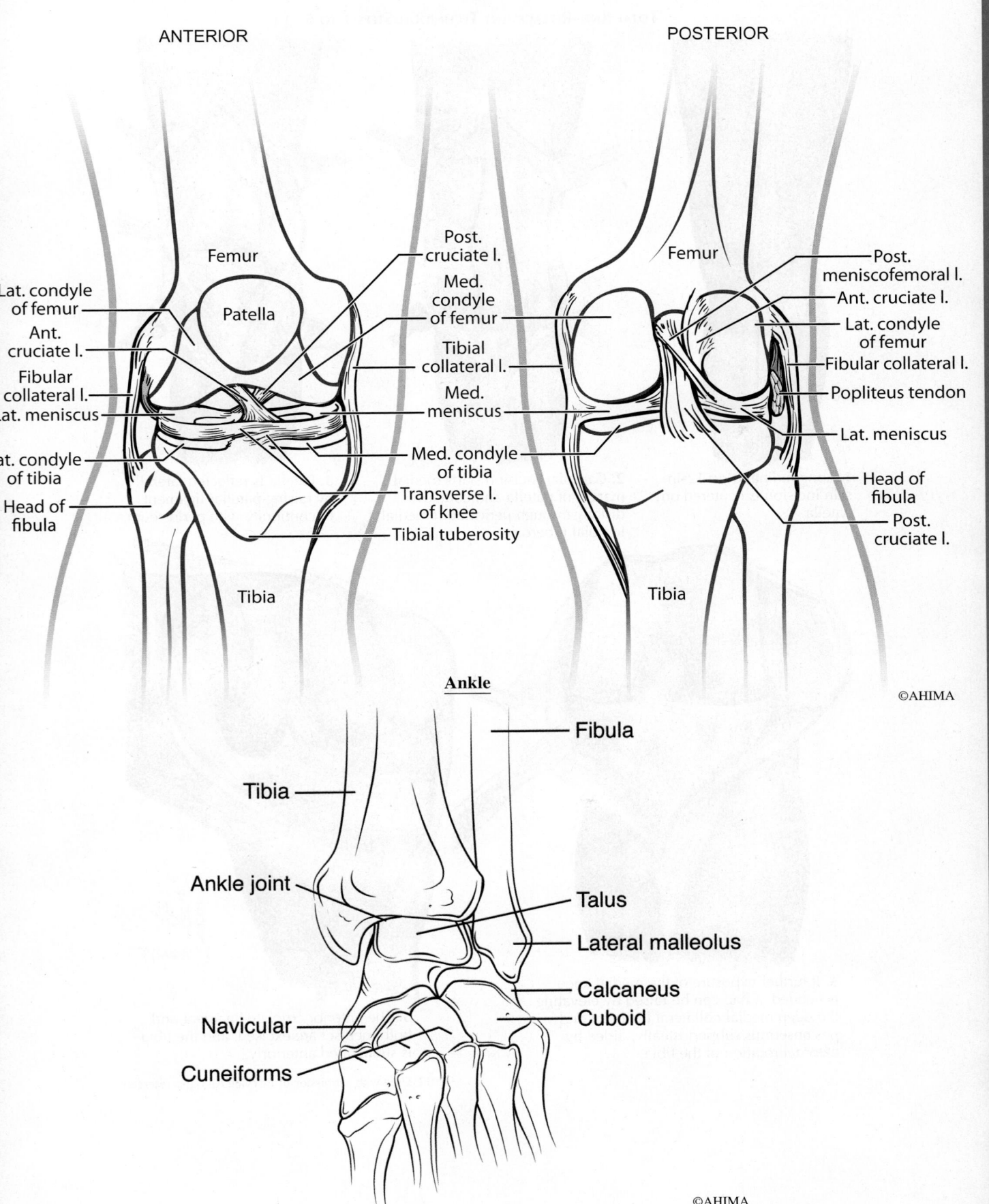

ANTERIOR

POSTERIOR

Femur

Patella

Lat. condyle
of femur

Ant.
cruciate l.

Fibular
collateral l.

Lat. meniscus

Lat. condyle
of tibia

Head of
fibula

Tibia

Post.
cruciate l.

Med.
condyle
of femur

Tibial
collateral l.

Med.
meniscus

Med. condyle
of tibia

Transverse l.
of knee

Tibial tuberosity

Femur

Post.
meniscofemoral l.

Ant. cruciate l.

Lat. condyle
of femur

Fibular collateral l.

Popliteus tendon

Lat. meniscus

Head of
fibula

Post.
cruciate l.

Tibia

©AHIMA

Ankle

Fibula

Tibia

Ankle joint

Navicular

Cuneiforms

Talus

Lateral malleolus

Calcaneus

Cuboid

©AHIMA

TOTAL KNEE REPLACEMENT TECHNIQUE: STEPS 1 TO 5

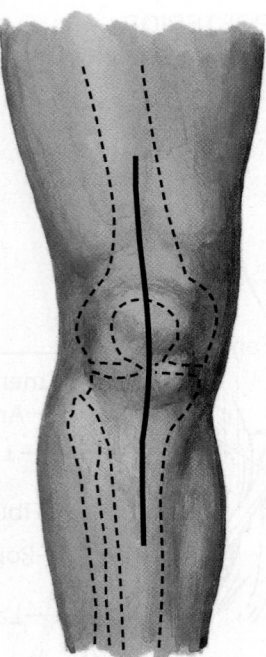

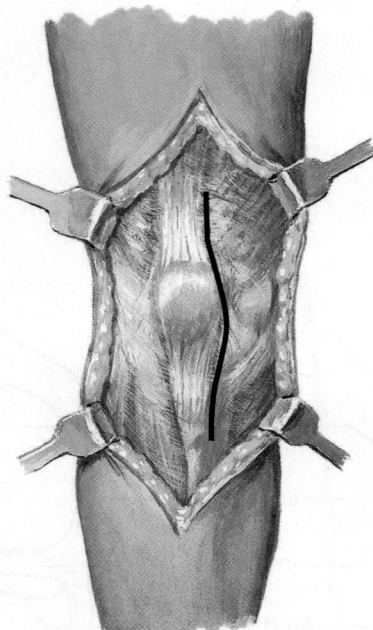

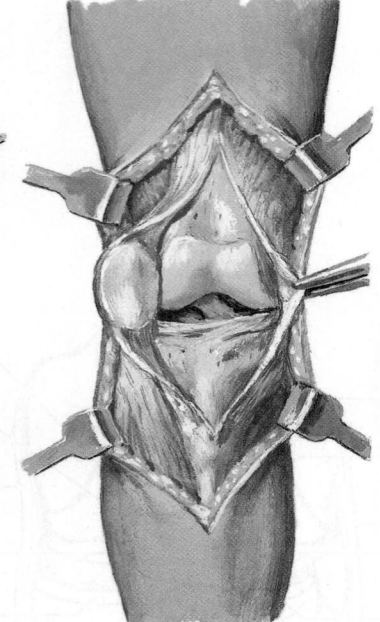

1. Longitudinal 8- to 12-in. skin incision is centered on patella.

2. Capsular incision skirts medial margin of patella and courses distally through periosteum medial to tibial tuberosity.

3. Patella is reflected laterally by raising patellar ligament in continuity with periosteum.

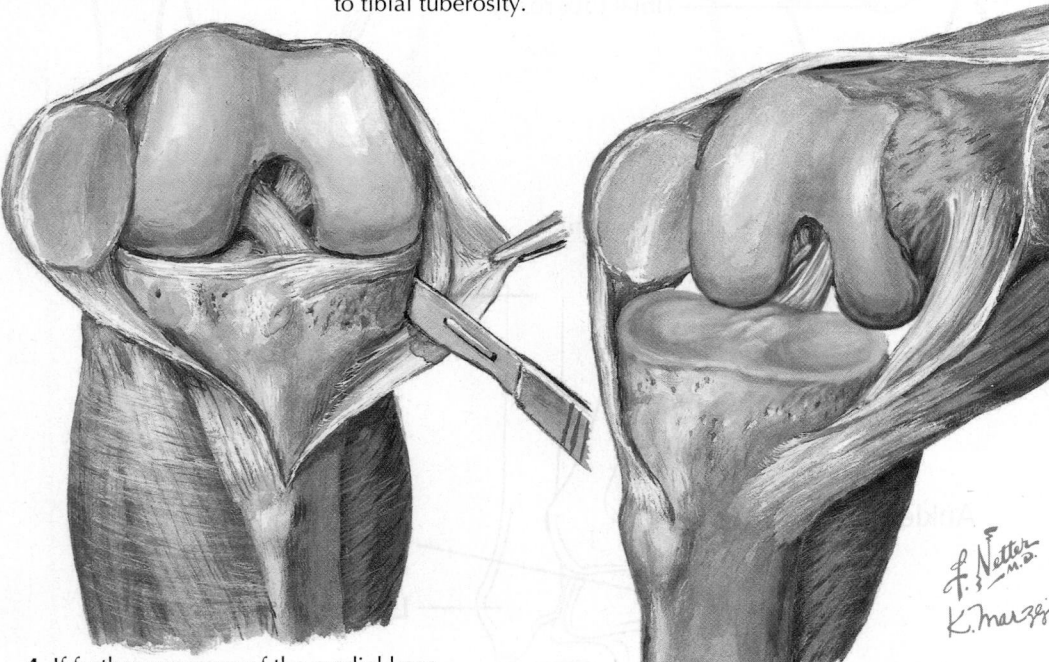

4. If further exposure of the medial knee is needed, a flap can be raised by elevating the deep medial collateral ligament and pes anserinus subperiosteally, aided by external rotation of the tibia.

5. The anterior cruciate ligament and both menisci are excised, and the tibia is subluxated anteriorly.

6. The femoral canal is accessed for placement of guide for distal femoral resections.

7. Femoral size guide is used to determine implant size and rotation.

8. Femoral cutting block is used for anterior, posterior, and chamfer cuts.

9. Tibial cutting block is placed using the aid of an extramedullary alignment rod (pictured, may also use an intramedullary device). The bar can be used to assess slope and alignment of the cut.

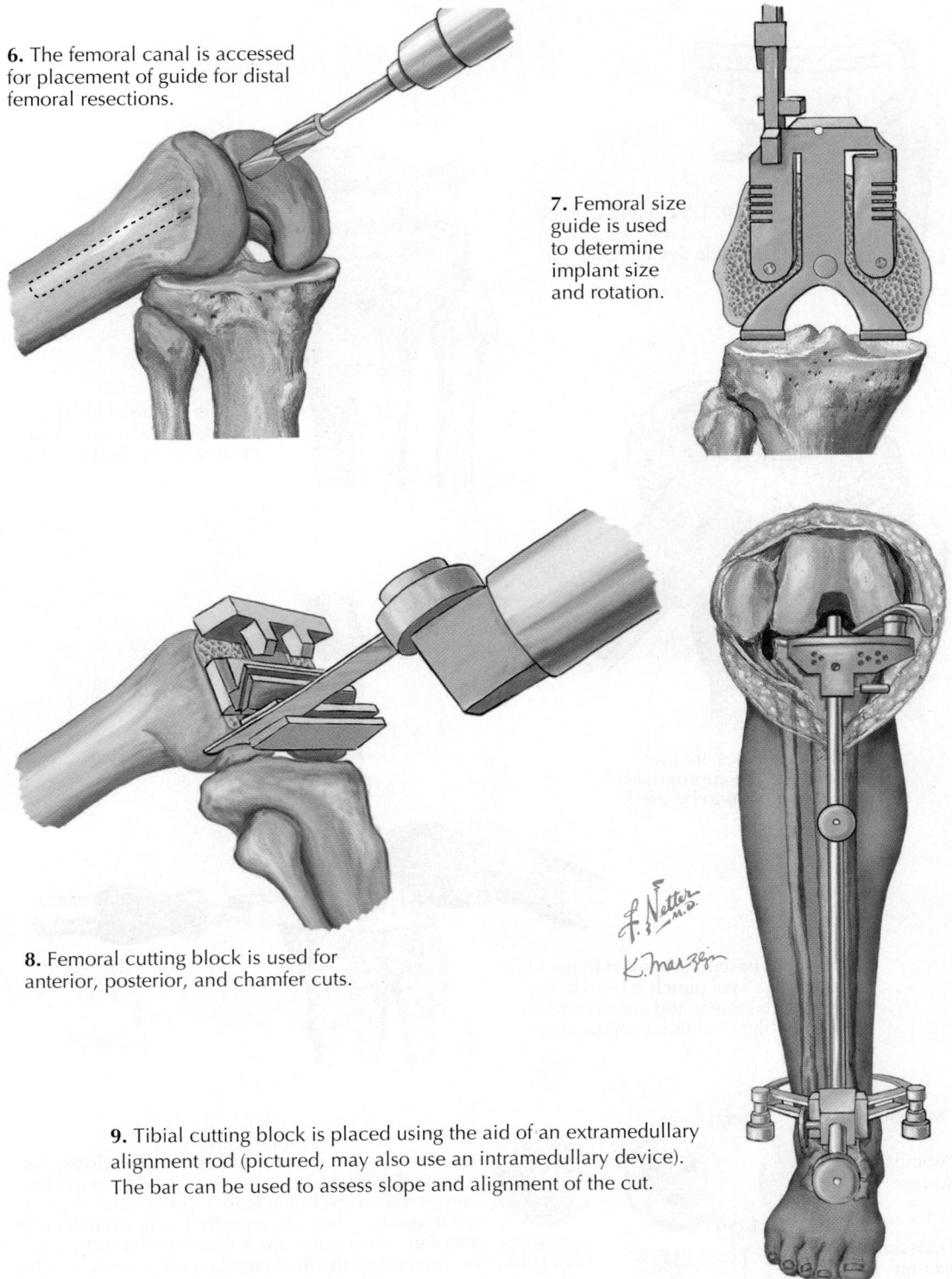

Medical and Surgical, Lower Joints, Total Knee Replacement Technique

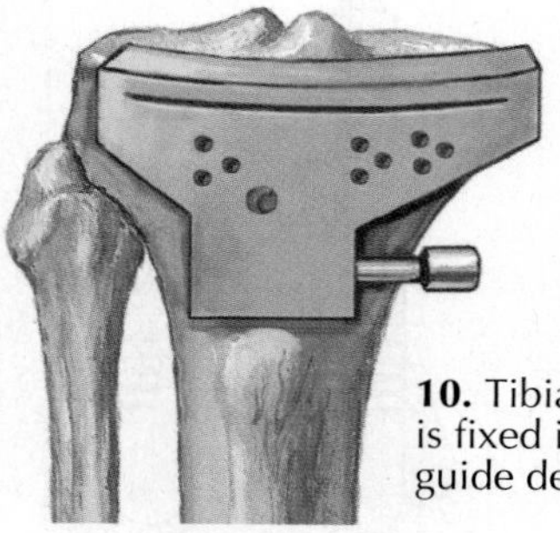

10. Tibial cutting block is fixed into place and guide device removed.

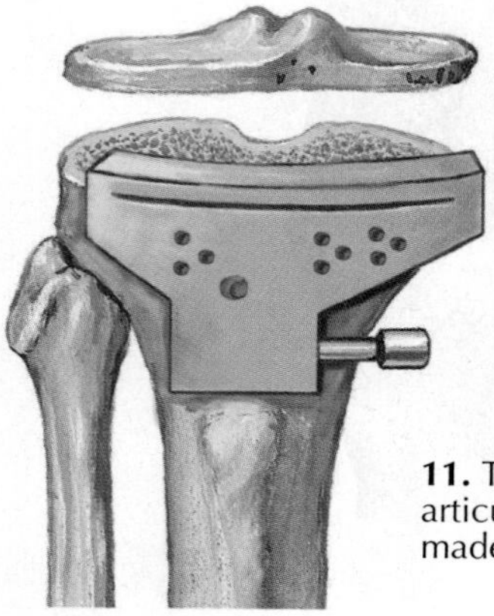

11. The proximal tibial articular surface cut is then made with oscillating saw.

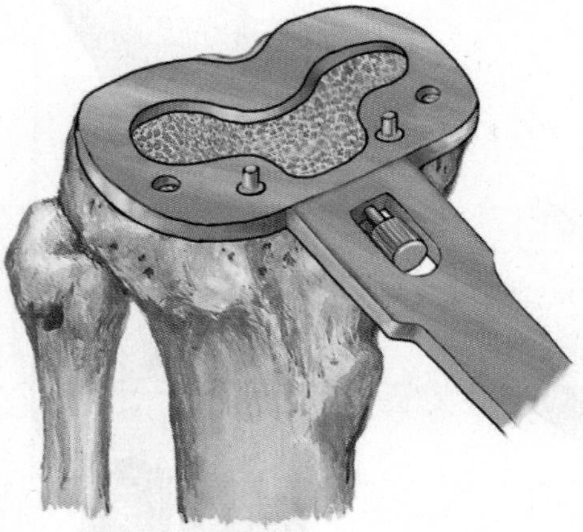

12. Trial baseplates are then used to assess the appropriate size of the implant to be used.

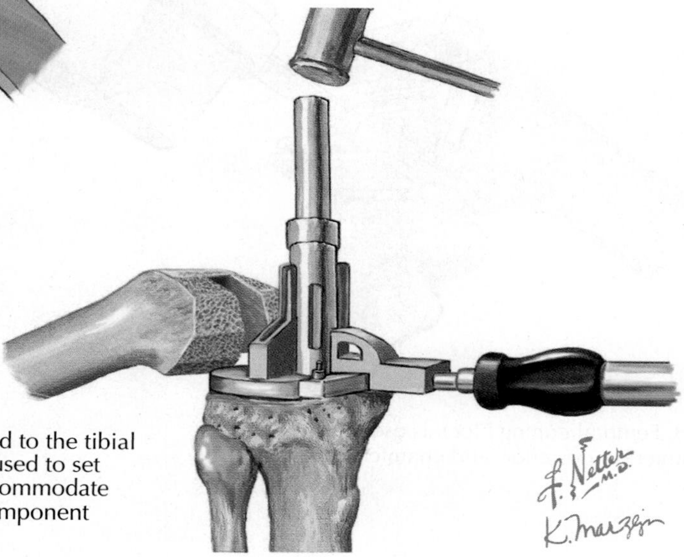

13. The trial baseplate is fixed to the tibial surface and a keel punch is used to set rotational alignment and accommodate the stem of the final tibial component

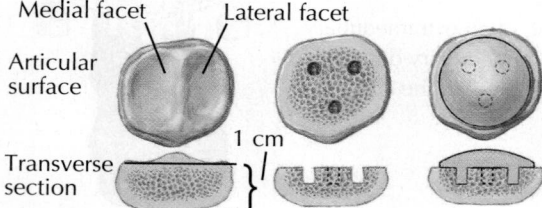

Medial facet   Lateral facet

Articular surface

Transverse section

1 cm

14. Articular surface of patella resected to leave flat surface. Equal amounts to be removed from medial and lateral facets, but at least 1 cm of bone must be left to ensure adequate strength. Using a patella drill template, three holes are drilled into the surface to accommodate the final patellar component, which is cemented in place.

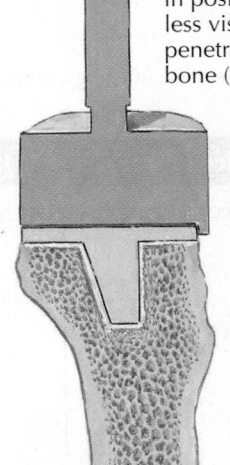

15. Cement is applied to tibial component and cut surfaces of tibia, and component is placed in position. Cement is somewhat less viscous to facilitate penetration into trabecular bone (sagittal section).

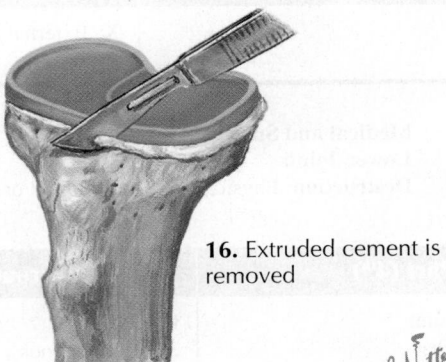

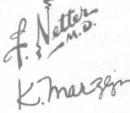

16. Extruded cement is removed

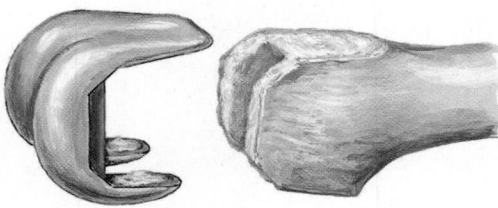

17. Cement is applied to posterior limb of femoral component and spread evenly over beveled ends of femur

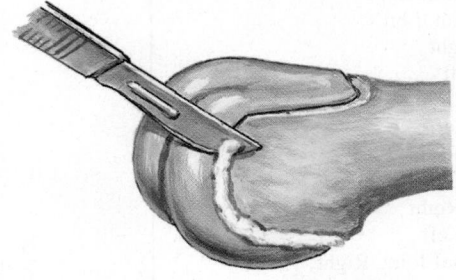

18. Extruded cement is removed

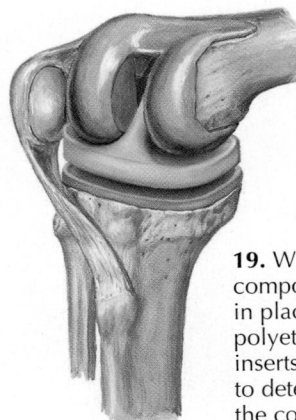

19. With all components in place, trial polyethylene inserts are used to determine the correct size.

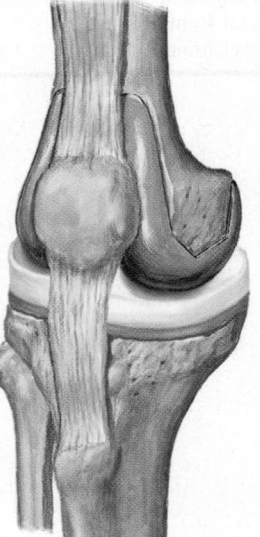

20. Once the final components are in place, the knee is placed through a range of motion and appropriate stress tests. The knee is then irrigated, hemostasis achieved, and the wound is closed.

Lower Joints Tables 0S2–0SW

Section	0	Medical and Surgical
Body System	S	Lower Joints
Operation	2	**Change:** Taking out or off a device from a body part and putting back an identical or similar device in or on the same body part without cutting or puncturing the skin or a mucous membrane

Body Part (4th)	Approach (5th)	Device (6th)	Qualifier (7th)
Y Lower Joint	**X** External	**0** Drainage Device **Y** Other Device	**Z** No Qualifier

Section	0	Medical and Surgical
Body System	S	Lower Joints
Operation	5	**Destruction:** Physical eradication of all or a portion of a body part by the direct use of energy, force, or a destructive agent

Body Part (4th)	Approach (5th)	Device (6th)	Qualifier (7th)
0 Lumbar Vertebral Joint **2** Lumbar Vertebral Disc **3** Lumbosacral Joint **4** Lumbosacral Disc **5** Sacrococcygeal Joint **6** Coccygeal Joint **7** Sacroiliac Joint, Right **8** Sacroiliac Joint, Left **9** Hip Joint, Right **B** Hip Joint, Left **C** Knee Joint, Right **D** Knee Joint, Left **F** Ankle Joint, Right **G** Ankle Joint, Left **H** Tarsal Joint, Right **J** Tarsal Joint, Left **K** Tarsometatarsal Joint, Right **L** Tarsometatarsal Joint, Left **M** Metatarsal-Phalangeal Joint, Right **N** Metatarsal-Phalangeal Joint, Left **P** Toe Phalangeal Joint, Right **Q** Toe Phalangeal Joint, Left	**0** Open **3** Percutaneous **4** Percutaneous Endoscopic	**Z** No Device	**Z** No Qualifier

Section	0	**Medical and Surgical**
Body System	S	**Lower Joints**
Operation	9	**Drainage:** Taking or letting out fluids and/or gases from a body part

Body Part (4ᵗʰ)	Approach (5ᵗʰ)	Device (6ᵗʰ)	Qualifier (7ᵗʰ)
0 Lumbar Vertebral Joint 2 Lumbar Vertebral Disc 3 Lumbosacral Joint 4 Lumbosacral Disc 5 Sacrococcygeal Joint 6 Coccygeal Joint 7 Sacroiliac Joint, Right 8 Sacroiliac Joint, Left 9 Hip Joint, Right B Hip Joint, Left C Knee Joint, Right D Knee Joint, Left F Ankle Joint, Right G Ankle Joint, Left H Tarsal Joint, Right J Tarsal Joint, Left K Tarsometatarsal Joint, Right L Tarsometatarsal Joint, Left M Metatarsal-Phalangeal Joint, Right N Metatarsal-Phalangeal Joint, Left P Toe Phalangeal Joint, Right Q Toe Phalangeal Joint, Left	0 Open 3 Percutaneous 4 Percutaneous Endoscopic	0 Drainage Device	Z No Qualifier
0 Lumbar Vertebral Joint 2 Lumbar Vertebral Disc 3 Lumbosacral Joint 4 Lumbosacral Disc 5 Sacrococcygeal Joint 6 Coccygeal Joint 7 Sacroiliac Joint, Right 8 Sacroiliac Joint, Left 9 Hip Joint, Right B Hip Joint, Left C Knee Joint, Right D Knee Joint, Left F Ankle Joint, Right G Ankle Joint, Left H Tarsal Joint, Right J Tarsal Joint, Left K Tarsometatarsal Joint, Right L Tarsometatarsal Joint, Left M Metatarsal-Phalangeal Joint, Right N Metatarsal-Phalangeal Joint, Left P Toe Phalangeal Joint, Right Q Toe Phalangeal Joint, Left	0 Open 3 Percutaneous 4 Percutaneous Endoscopic	Z No Device	X Diagnostic Z No Qualifier

Section	0	Medical and Surgical
Body System	S	Lower Joints
Operation	B	Excision: Cutting out or off, without replacement, a portion of a body part

Body Part (4th)	Approach (5th)	Device (6th)	Qualifier (7th)
0 Lumbar Vertebral Joint 2 Lumbar Vertebral Disc 3 Lumbosacral Joint 4 Lumbosacral Disc 5 Sacrococcygeal Joint 6 Coccygeal Joint 7 Sacroiliac Joint, Right 8 Sacroiliac Joint, Left 9 Hip Joint, Right B Hip Joint, Left C Knee Joint, Right D Knee Joint, Left F Ankle Joint, Right G Ankle Joint, Left H Tarsal Joint, Right J Tarsal Joint, Left K Tarsometatarsal Joint, Right L Tarsometatarsal Joint, Left M Metatarsal-Phalangeal Joint, Right N Metatarsal-Phalangeal Joint, Left P Toe Phalangeal Joint, Right Q Toe Phalangeal Joint, Left	0 Open 3 Percutaneous 4 Percutaneous Endoscopic	Z No Device	X Diagnostic Z No Qualifier

Section	0	Medical and Surgical
Body System	S	Lower Joints
Operation	C	Extirpation: Taking or cutting out solid matter from a body part

Body Part (4th)	Approach (5th)	Device (6th)	Qualifier (7th)
0 Lumbar Vertebral Joint 2 Lumbar Vertebral Disc 3 Lumbosacral Joint 4 Lumbosacral Disc 5 Sacrococcygeal Joint 6 Coccygeal Joint 7 Sacroiliac Joint, Right 8 Sacroiliac Joint, Left 9 Hip Joint, Right B Hip Joint, Left C Knee Joint, Right D Knee Joint, Left F Ankle Joint, Right G Ankle Joint, Left H Tarsal Joint, Right J Tarsal Joint, Left K Tarsometatarsal Joint, Right L Tarsometatarsal Joint, Left M Metatarsal-Phalangeal Joint, Right N Metatarsal-Phalangeal Joint, Left P Toe Phalangeal Joint, Right Q Toe Phalangeal Joint, Left	0 Open 3 Percutaneous 4 Percutaneous Endoscopic	Z No Device	Z No Qualifier

Section	0	Medical and Surgical
Body System	S	Lower Joints
Operation	G	Fusion: Joining together portions of an articular body part rendering the articular body part immobile

Body Part (4th)	Approach (5th)	Device (6th)	Qualifier (7th)
0 Lumbar Vertebral Joint 1 Lumbar Vertebral Joints, 2 or more 3 Lumbosacral Joint	0 Open 3 Percutaneous 4 Percutaneous Endoscopic	7 Autologous Tissue Substitute J Synthetic Substitute K Nonautologous Tissue Substitute	0 Anterior Approach, Anterior Column 1 Posterior Approach, Posterior Column J Posterior Approach, Anterior Column
0 Lumbar Vertebral Joint 1 Lumbar Vertebral Joints, 2 or more 3 Lumbosacral Joint	0 Open 3 Percutaneous 4 Percutaneous Endoscopic	A Interbody Fusion Device	0 Anterior Approach, Anterior Column J Posterior Approach, Anterior Column
5 Sacrococcygeal Joint 6 Coccygeal Joint 7 Sacroiliac Joint, Right 8 Sacroiliac Joint, Left	0 Open 3 Percutaneous 4 Percutaneous Endoscopic	4 Internal Fixation Device 7 Autologous Tissue Substitute J Synthetic Substitute K Nonautologous Tissue Substitute	Z No Qualifier
9 Hip Joint, Right B Hip Joint, Left C Knee Joint, Right D Knee Joint, Left F Ankle Joint, Right G Ankle Joint, Left H Tarsal Joint, Right J Tarsal Joint, Left K Tarsometatarsal Joint, Right L Tarsometatarsal Joint, Left M Metatarsal-Phalangeal Joint, Right N Metatarsal-Phalangeal Joint, Left P Toe Phalangeal Joint, Right Q Toe Phalangeal Joint, Left	0 Open 3 Percutaneous 4 Percutaneous Endoscopic	3 Internal Fixation Device, Sustained Compression 4 Internal Fixation Device 5 External Fixation Device 7 Autologous Tissue Substitute J Synthetic Substitute K Nonautologous Tissue Substitute	Z No Qualifier

Section	0	Medical and Surgical
Body System	S	Lower Joints
Operation	H	Insertion: Putting in a nonbiological appliance that monitors, assists, performs, or prevents a physiological function but does not physically take the place of a body part

Body Part (4th)	Approach (5th)	Device (6th)	Qualifier (7th)
0 Lumbar Vertebral Joint 3 Lumbosacral Joint	0 Open 3 Percutaneous 4 Percutaneous Endoscopic	3 Infusion Device 4 Internal Fixation Device 8 Spacer B Spinal Stabilization Device, Interspinous Process C Spinal Stabilization Device, Pedicle-Based D Spinal Stabilization Device, Facet Replacement	Z No Qualifier
2 Lumbar Vertebral Disc 4 Lumbosacral Disc	0 Open 3 Percutaneous 4 Percutaneous Endoscopic	3 Infusion Device 8 Spacer	Z No Qualifier
5 Sacrococcygeal Joint 6 Coccygeal Joint 7 Sacroiliac Joint, Right 8 Sacroiliac Joint, Left	0 Open 3 Percutaneous 4 Percutaneous Endoscopic	3 Infusion Device 4 Internal Fixation Device 8 Spacer	Z No Qualifier

Continued →

Section	0	Medical and Surgical
Body System	S	Lower Joints
Operation	H	**Insertion:** Putting in a nonbiological appliance that monitors, assists, performs, or prevents a physiological function but does not physically take the place of a body part

Body Part (4th)	Approach (5th)	Device (6th)	Qualifier (7th)
9 Hip Joint, Right B Hip Joint, Left C Knee Joint, Right D Knee Joint, Left F Ankle Joint, Right G Ankle Joint, Left H Tarsal Joint, Right J Tarsal Joint, Left K Tarsometatarsal Joint, Right L Tarsometatarsal Joint, Left M Metatarsal-Phalangeal Joint, Right N Metatarsal-Phalangeal Joint, Left P Toe Phalangeal Joint, Right Q Toe Phalangeal Joint, Left	0 Open 3 Percutaneous 4 Percutaneous Endoscopic	3 Infusion Device 4 Internal Fixation Device 5 External Fixation Device 8 Spacer	Z No Qualifier

Section	0	Medical and Surgical
Body System	S	Lower Joints
Operation	J	**Inspection:** Visually and/or manually exploring a body part

Body Part (4th)	Approach (5th)	Device (6th)	Qualifier (7th)
0 Lumbar Vertebral Joint 2 Lumbar Vertebral Disc 3 Lumbosacral Joint 4 Lumbosacral Disc 5 Sacrococcygeal Joint 6 Coccygeal Joint 7 Sacroiliac Joint, Right 8 Sacroiliac Joint, Left 9 Hip Joint, Right B Hip Joint, Left C Knee Joint, Right D Knee Joint, Left F Ankle Joint, Right G Ankle Joint, Left H Tarsal Joint, Right J Tarsal Joint, Left K Tarsometatarsal Joint, Right L Tarsometatarsal Joint, Left M Metatarsal-Phalangeal Joint, Right N Metatarsal-Phalangeal Joint, Left P Toe Phalangeal Joint, Right Q Toe Phalangeal Joint, Left	0 Open 3 Percutaneous 4 Percutaneous Endoscopic X External	Z No Device	Z No Qualifier

Section 0 **Medical and Surgical**
Body System S **Lower Joints**
Operation N **Release:** Freeing a body part from an abnormal physical constraint by cutting or by the use of force

Body Part (4ᵗʰ)	Approach (5ᵗʰ)	Device (6ᵗʰ)	Qualifier (7ᵗʰ)
0 Lumbar Vertebral Joint 2 Lumbar Vertebral Disc 3 Lumbosacral Joint 4 Lumbosacral Disc 5 Sacrococcygeal Joint 6 Coccygeal Joint 7 Sacroiliac Joint, Right 8 Sacroiliac Joint, Left 9 Hip Joint, Right B Hip Joint, Left C Knee Joint, Right D Knee Joint, Left F Ankle Joint, Right G Ankle Joint, Left H Tarsal Joint, Right J Tarsal Joint, Left K Tarsometatarsal Joint, Right L Tarsometatarsal Joint, Left M Metatarsal-Phalangeal Joint, Right N Metatarsal-Phalangeal Joint, Left P Toe Phalangeal Joint, Right Q Toe Phalangeal Joint, Left	0 Open 3 Percutaneous 4 Percutaneous Endoscopic X External	Z No Device	Z No Qualifier

Section 0 **Medical and Surgical**
Body System S **Lower Joints**
Operation P **Removal:** Taking out or off a device from a body part

Body Part (4ᵗʰ)	Approach (5ᵗʰ)	Device (6ᵗʰ)	Qualifier (7ᵗʰ)
0 Lumbar Vertebral Joint 3 Lumbosacral Joint	0 Open 3 Percutaneous 4 Percutaneous Endoscopic	0 Drainage Device 3 Infusion Device 4 Internal Fixation Device 7 Autologous Tissue Substitute 8 Spacer A Interbody Fusion Device J Synthetic Substitute K Nonautologous Tissue Substitute	Z No Qualifier
0 Lumbar Vertebral Joint 3 Lumbosacral Joint	X External	0 Drainage Device 3 Infusion Device 4 Internal Fixation Device	Z No Qualifier
2 Lumbar Vertebral Disc 4 Lumbosacral Disc	0 Open 3 Percutaneous 4 Percutaneous Endoscopic	0 Drainage Device 3 Infusion Device 7 Autologous Tissue Substitute J Synthetic Substitute K Nonautologous Tissue Substitute	Z No Qualifier
2 Lumbar Vertebral Disc 4 Lumbosacral Disc	X External	0 Drainage Device 3 Infusion Device	Z No Qualifier
5 Sacrococcygeal Joint 6 Coccygeal Joint 7 Sacroiliac Joint, Right 8 Sacroiliac Joint, Left	0 Open 3 Percutaneous 4 Percutaneous Endoscopic	0 Drainage Device 3 Infusion Device 4 Internal Fixation Device 7 Autologous Tissue Substitute 8 Spacer J Synthetic Substitute K Nonautologous Tissue Substitute	Z No Qualifier
5 Sacrococcygeal Joint 6 Coccygeal Joint 7 Sacroiliac Joint, Right 8 Sacroiliac Joint, Left	X External	0 Drainage Device 3 Infusion Device 4 Internal Fixation Device	Z No Qualifier

Continued →

Section **0** **Medical and Surgical**
Body System **S** **Lower Joints**
Operation **P** **Removal:** Taking out or off a device from a body part

Body Part (4th)	Approach (5th)	Device (6th)	Qualifier (7th)
9 Hip Joint, Right **B** Hip Joint, Left	**0** Open	**0** Drainage Device **3** Infusion Device **4** Internal Fixation Device **5** External Fixation Device **7** Autologous Tissue Substitute **8** Spacer **9** Liner **B** Resurfacing Device **E** Articulating Spacer **J** Synthetic Substitute **K** Nonautologous Tissue Substitute	**Z** No Qualifier
9 Hip Joint, Right **B** Hip Joint, Left	**3** Percutaneous **4** Percutaneous Endoscopic	**0** Drainage Device **3** Infusion Device **4** Internal Fixation Device **5** External Fixation Device **7** Autologous Tissue Substitute **8** Spacer **J** Synthetic Substitute **K** Nonautologous Tissue Substitute	**Z** No Qualifier
9 Hip Joint, Right **B** Hip Joint, Left	**X** External	**0** Drainage Device **3** Infusion Device **4** Internal Fixation Device **5** External Fixation Device	**Z** No Qualifier
A Hip Joint, Acetabular Surface, Right **E** Hip Joint, Acetabular Surface, Left **R** Hip Joint, Femoral Surface, Right **S** Hip Joint, Femoral Surface, Left **T** Knee Joint, Femoral Surface, Right **U** Knee Joint, Femoral Surface, Left **V** Knee Joint, Tibial Surface, Right **W** Knee Joint, Tibial Surface, Left	**0** Open **3** Percutaneous **4** Percutaneous Endoscopic	**J** Synthetic Substitute	**Z** No Qualifier
C Knee Joint, Right **D** Knee Joint, Left	**0** Open	**0** Drainage Device **3** Infusion Device **4** Internal Fixation Device **5** External Fixation Device **7** Autologous Tissue Substitute **8** Spacer **9** Liner **E** Articulating Spacer **K** Nonautologous Tissue Substitute **L** Synthetic Substitute, Unicondylar Medial **M** Synthetic Substitute, Unicondylar Lateral **N** Synthetic Substitute, Unicondylar Patellofemoral	**Z** No Qualifier
C Knee Joint, Right **D** Knee Joint, Left	**0** Open	**J** Synthetic Substitute	**C** Patellar Surface **Z** No Qualifier
C Knee Joint, Right **D** Knee Joint, Left	**3** Percutaneous **4** Percutaneous Endoscopic	**0** Drainage Device **3** Infusion Device **4** Internal Fixation Device **5** External Fixation Device **7** Autologous Tissue Substitute **8** Spacer **K** Nonautologous Tissue Substitute **L** Synthetic Substitute, Unicondylar Medial **M** Synthetic Substitute, Unicondylar Lateral **N** Synthetic Substitute, Unicondylar Patellofemoral	**Z** No Qualifier

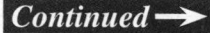

Continued →

Section	0	Medical and Surgical
Body System	S	Lower Joints
Operation	P	Removal: Taking out or off a device from a body part

Body Part (4th)	Approach (5th)	Device (6th)	Qualifier (7th)
C Knee Joint, Right D Knee Joint, Left	3 Percutaneous 4 Percutaneous Endoscopic	J Synthetic Substitute	C Patellar Surface Z No Qualifier
C Knee Joint, Right D Knee Joint, Left	X External	0 Drainage Device 3 Infusion Device 4 Internal Fixation Device 5 External Fixation Device	Z No Qualifier
F Ankle Joint, Right G Ankle Joint, Left H Tarsal Joint, Right J Tarsal Joint, Left K Tarsometatarsal Joint, Right L Tarsometatarsal Joint, Left M Metatarsal-Phalangeal Joint, Right N Metatarsal-Phalangeal Joint, Left P Toe Phalangeal Joint, Right Q Toe Phalangeal Joint, Left	0 Open 3 Percutaneous 4 Percutaneous Endoscopic	0 Drainage Device 3 Infusion Device 4 Internal Fixation Device 5 External Fixation Device 7 Autologous Tissue Substitute 8 Spacer J Synthetic Substitute K Nonautologous Tissue Substitute	Z No Qualifier
F Ankle Joint, Right G Ankle Joint, Left H Tarsal Joint, Right J Tarsal Joint, Left K Tarsometatarsal Joint, Right L Tarsometatarsal Joint, Left M Metatarsal-Phalangeal Joint, Right N Metatarsal-Phalangeal Joint, Left P Toe Phalangeal Joint, Right Q Toe Phalangeal Joint, Left	X External	0 Drainage Device 3 Infusion Device 4 Internal Fixation Device 5 External Fixation Device	Z No Qualifier

Section	0	Medical and Surgical
Body System	S	Lower Joints
Operation	Q	Repair: Restoring, to the extent possible, a body part to its normal anatomic structure and function

Body Part (4th)	Approach (5th)	Device (6th)	Qualifier (7th)
0 Lumbar Vertebral Joint 2 Lumbar Vertebral Disc 3 Lumbosacral Joint 4 Lumbosacral Disc 5 Sacrococcygeal Joint 6 Coccygeal Joint 7 Sacroiliac Joint, Right 8 Sacroiliac Joint, Left 9 Hip Joint, Right B Hip Joint, Left C Knee Joint, Right D Knee Joint, Left F Ankle Joint, Right G Ankle Joint, Left H Tarsal Joint, Right J Tarsal Joint, Left K Tarsometatarsal Joint, Right L Tarsometatarsal Joint, Left M Metatarsal-Phalangeal Joint, Right N Metatarsal-Phalangeal Joint, Left P Toe Phalangeal Joint, Right Q Toe Phalangeal Joint, Left	0 Open 3 Percutaneous 4 Percutaneous Endoscopic X External	Z No Device	Z No Qualifier

Section	0	**Medical and Surgical**
Body System	S	**Lower Joints**
Operation	R	**Replacement:** Putting in or on biological or synthetic material that physically takes the place and/or function of all or a portion of a body part

Body Part (4th)	Approach (5th)	Device (6th)	Qualifier (7th)
0 Lumbar Vertebral Joint 2 Lumbar Vertebral Disc 3 Lumbosacral Joint 4 Lumbosacral Disc 5 Sacrococcygeal Joint 6 Coccygeal Joint 7 Sacroiliac Joint, Right 8 Sacroiliac Joint, Left H Tarsal Joint, Right J Tarsal Joint, Left K Tarsometatarsal Joint, Right L Tarsometatarsal Joint, Left M Metatarsal-Phalangeal Joint, Right N Metatarsal-Phalangeal Joint, Left P Toe Phalangeal Joint, Right Q Toe Phalangeal Joint, Left	0 Open	7 Autologous Tissue Substitute J Synthetic Substitute K Nonautologous Tissue Substitute	Z No Qualifier
9 Hip Joint, Right B Hip Joint, Left	0 Open	1 Synthetic Substitute, Metal 2 Synthetic Substitute, Metal on Polyethylene 3 Synthetic Substitute, Ceramic 4 Synthetic Substitute, Ceramic on Polyethylene 6 Synthetic Substitute, Oxidized Zirconium on Polyethylene J Synthetic Substitute	9 Cemented A Uncemented Z No Qualifier
9 Hip Joint, Right B Hip Joint, Left	0 Open	7 Autologous Tissue Substitute E Articulating Spacer K Nonautologous Tissue Substitute	Z No Qualifier
A Hip Joint, Acetabular Surface, Right E Hip Joint, Acetabular Surface, Left	0 Open	0 Synthetic Substitute, Polyethylene 1 Synthetic Substitute, Metal 3 Synthetic Substitute, Ceramic J Synthetic Substitute	9 Cemented A Uncemented Z No Qualifier
A Hip Joint, Acetabular Surface, Right E Hip Joint, Acetabular Surface, Left	0 Open	7 Autologous Tissue Substitute K Nonautologous Tissue Substitute	Z No Qualifier
C Knee Joint, Right D Knee Joint, Left	0 Open	6 Synthetic Substitute, Oxidized Zirconium on Polyethylene J Synthetic Substitute L Synthetic Substitute, Unicondylar Medial M Synthetic Substitute, Unicondylar Lateral N Synthetic Substitute, Unicondylar Patellofemoral	9 Cemented A Uncemented Z No Qualifier
C Knee Joint, Right D Knee Joint, Left	0 Open	7 Autologous Tissue Substitute E Articulating Spacer K Nonautologous Tissue Substitute	Z No Qualifier
F Ankle Joint, Right G Ankle Joint, Left T Knee Joint, Femoral Surface, Right U Knee Joint, Femoral Surface, Left V Knee Joint, Tibial Surface, Right W Knee Joint, Tibial Surface, Left	0 Open	7 Autologous Tissue Substitute K Nonautologous Tissue Substitute	Z No Qualifier
F Ankle Joint, Right G Ankle Joint, Left T Knee Joint, Femoral Surface, Right U Knee Joint, Femoral Surface, Left V Knee Joint, Tibial Surface, Right W Knee Joint, Tibial Surface, Left	0 Open	J Synthetic Substitute	9 Cemented A Uncemented Z No Qualifier
R Hip Joint, Femoral Surface, Right S Hip Joint, Femoral Surface, Left	0 Open	1 Synthetic Substitute, Metal 3 Synthetic Substitute, Ceramic J Synthetic Substitute	9 Cemented A Uncemented Z No Qualifier
R Hip Joint, Femoral Surface, Right S Hip Joint, Femoral Surface, Left	0 Open	7 Autologous Tissue Substitute K Nonautologous Tissue Substitute	Z No Qualifier

Section　　　**0**　　**Medical and Surgical**
Body System　**S**　　**Lower Joints**
Operation　　**S**　　**Reposition:** Moving to its normal location, or other suitable location, all or a portion of a body part

Body Part (4ᵗʰ)	Approach (5ᵗʰ)	Device (6ᵗʰ)	Qualifier (7ᵗʰ)
0 Lumbar Vertebral Joint **3** Lumbosacral Joint **5** Sacrococcygeal Joint **6** Coccygeal Joint **7** Sacroiliac Joint, Right **8** Sacroiliac Joint, Left	**0** Open **3** Percutaneous **4** Percutaneous Endoscopic **X** External	**4** Internal Fixation Device **Z** No Device	**Z** No Qualifier
9 Hip Joint, Right **B** Hip Joint, Left **C** Knee Joint, Right **D** Knee Joint, Left **F** Ankle Joint, Right **G** Ankle Joint, Left **H** Tarsal Joint, Right **J** Tarsal Joint, Left **K** Tarsometatarsal Joint, Right **L** Tarsometatarsal Joint, Left **M** Metatarsal-Phalangeal Joint, Right **N** Metatarsal-Phalangeal Joint, Left **P** Toe Phalangeal Joint, Right **Q** Toe Phalangeal Joint, Left	**0** Open **3** Percutaneous **4** Percutaneous Endoscopic **X** External	**4** Internal Fixation Device **5** External Fixation Device **Z** No Device	**Z** No Qualifier

Section　　　**0**　　**Medical and Surgical**
Body System　**S**　　**Lower Joints**
Operation　　**T**　　**Resection:** Cutting out or off, without replacement, all of a body part

Body Part (4ᵗʰ)	Approach (5ᵗʰ)	Device (6ᵗʰ)	Qualifier (7ᵗʰ)
2 Lumbar Vertebral Disc **4** Lumbosacral Disc **5** Sacrococcygeal Joint **6** Coccygeal Joint **7** Sacroiliac Joint, Right **8** Sacroiliac Joint, Left **9** Hip Joint, Right **B** Hip Joint, Left **C** Knee Joint, Right **D** Knee Joint, Left **F** Ankle Joint, Right **G** Ankle Joint, Left **H** Tarsal Joint, Right **J** Tarsal Joint, Left **K** Tarsometatarsal Joint, Right **L** Tarsometatarsal Joint, Left **M** Metatarsal-Phalangeal Joint, Right **N** Metatarsal-Phalangeal Joint, Left **P** Toe Phalangeal Joint, Right **Q** Toe Phalangeal Joint, Left	**0** Open	**Z** No Device	**Z** No Qualifier

Section	0	Medical and Surgical
Body System	S	Lower Joints
Operation	U	**Supplement:** Putting in or on biological or synthetic material that physically reinforces and/or augments the function of a portion of a body part

Body Part (4th)	Approach (5th)	Device (6th)	Qualifier (7th)
0 Lumbar Vertebral Joint **2** Lumbar Vertebral Disc **3** Lumbosacral Joint **4** Lumbosacral Disc **5** Sacrococcygeal Joint **6** Coccygeal Joint **7** Sacroiliac Joint, Right **8** Sacroiliac Joint, Left **F** Ankle Joint, Right **G** Ankle Joint, Left **H** Tarsal Joint, Right **J** Tarsal Joint, Left **K** Tarsometatarsal Joint, Right **L** Tarsometatarsal Joint, Left **M** Metatarsal-Phalangeal Joint, Right **N** Metatarsal-Phalangeal Joint, Left **P** Toe Phalangeal Joint, Right **Q** Toe Phalangeal Joint, Left	**0** Open **3** Percutaneous **4** Percutaneous Endoscopic	**7** Autologous Tissue Substitute **J** Synthetic Substitute **K** Nonautologous Tissue Substitute	**Z** No Qualifier
9 Hip Joint, Right **B** Hip Joint, Left	**0** Open	**7** Autologous Tissue Substitute **9** Liner **B** Resurfacing Device **J** Synthetic Substitute **K** Nonautologous Tissue Substitute	**Z** No Qualifier
9 Hip Joint, Right **B** Hip Joint, Left	**3** Percutaneous **4** Percutaneous Endoscopic	**7** Autologous Tissue Substitute **J** Synthetic Substitute **K** Nonautologous Tissue Substitute	**Z** No Qualifier
A Hip Joint, Acetabular Surface, Right **E** Hip Joint, Acetabular Surface, Left **R** Hip Joint, Femoral Surface, Right **S** Hip Joint, Femoral Surface, Left	**0** Open	**9** Liner **B** Resurfacing Device	**Z** No Qualifier
C Knee Joint, Right **D** Knee Joint, Left	**0** Open	**7** Autologous Tissue Substitute **J** Synthetic Substitute **K** Nonautologous Tissue Substitute	**Z** No Qualifier
C Knee Joint, Right **D** Knee Joint, Left	**0** Open	**9** Liner	**C** Patellar Surface **Z** No Qualifier
C Knee Joint, Right **D** Knee Joint, Left	**3** Percutaneous **4** Percutaneous Endoscopic	**7** Autologous Tissue Substitute **J** Synthetic Substitute **K** Nonautologous Tissue Substitute	**Z** No Qualifier
T Knee Joint, Femoral Surface, Right **U** Knee Joint, Femoral Surface, Left **V** Knee Joint, Tibial Surface, Right **W** Knee Joint, Tibial Surface, Left	**0** Open	**9** Liner	**Z** No Qualifier

	Section	0	Medical and Surgical
Body System	S	Lower Joints
Operation	W	Revision: Correcting, to the extent possible, a portion of a malfunctioning device or the position of a displaced device

Body Part (4ᵗʰ)	Approach (5ᵗʰ)	Device (6ᵗʰ)	Qualifier (7ᵗʰ)
0 Lumbar Vertebral Joint 3 Lumbosacral Joint	0 Open 3 Percutaneous 4 Percutaneous Endoscopic X External	0 Drainage Device 3 Infusion Device 4 Internal Fixation Device 7 Autologous Tissue Substitute 8 Spacer A Interbody Fusion Device J Synthetic Substitute K Nonautologous Tissue Substitute	Z No Qualifier
2 Lumbar Vertebral Disc 4 Lumbosacral Disc	0 Open 3 Percutaneous 4 Percutaneous Endoscopic X External	0 Drainage Device 3 Infusion Device 7 Autologous Tissue Substitute J Synthetic Substitute K Nonautologous Tissue Substitute	Z No Qualifier
5 Sacrococcygeal Joint 6 Coccygeal Joint 7 Sacroiliac Joint, Right 8 Sacroiliac Joint, Left	0 Open 3 Percutaneous 4 Percutaneous Endoscopic X External	0 Drainage Device 3 Infusion Device 4 Internal Fixation Device 7 Autologous Tissue Substitute 8 Spacer J Synthetic Substitute K Nonautologous Tissue Substitute	Z No Qualifier
9 Hip Joint, Right B Hip Joint, Left	0 Open	0 Drainage Device 3 Infusion Device 4 Internal Fixation Device 5 External Fixation Device 7 Autologous Tissue Substitute 8 Spacer 9 Liner B Resurfacing Device J Synthetic Substitute K Nonautologous Tissue Substitute	Z No Qualifier
9 Hip Joint, Right B Hip Joint, Left	3 Percutaneous 4 Percutaneous Endoscopic X External	0 Drainage Device 3 Infusion Device 4 Internal Fixation Device 5 External Fixation Device 7 Autologous Tissue Substitute 8 Spacer J Synthetic Substitute K Nonautologous Tissue Substitute	Z No Qualifier
A Hip Joint, Acetabular Surface, Right E Hip Joint, Acetabular Surface, Left R Hip Joint, Femoral Surface, Right S Hip Joint, Femoral Surface, Left T Knee Joint, Femoral Surface, Right U Knee Joint, Femoral Surface, Left V Knee Joint, Tibial Surface, Right W Knee Joint, Tibial Surface, Left	0 Open 3 Percutaneous 4 Percutaneous Endoscopic X External	J Synthetic Substitute	Z No Qualifier
C Knee Joint, Right D Knee Joint, Left	0 Open	0 Drainage Device 3 Infusion Device 4 Internal Fixation Device 5 External Fixation Device 7 Autologous Tissue Substitute 8 Spacer 9 Liner K Nonautologous Tissue Substitute	Z No Qualifier

Continued →

Section	0	Medical and Surgical
Body System	S	Lower Joints
Operation	W	Revision: Correcting, to the extent possible, a portion of a malfunctioning device or the position of a displaced device

Body Part (4th)	Approach (5th)	Device (6th)	Qualifier (7th)
C Knee Joint, Right D Knee Joint, Left	0 Open	J Synthetic Substitute	C Patellar Surface Z No Qualifier
C Knee Joint, Right D Knee Joint, Left	3 Percutaneous 4 Percutaneous Endoscopic X External	0 Drainage Device 3 Infusion Device 4 Internal Fixation Device 5 External Fixation Device 7 Autologous Tissue Substitute 8 Spacer K Nonautologous Tissue Substitute	Z No Qualifier
C Knee Joint, Right E Knee Joint, Left	3 Percutaneous 4 Percutaneous Endoscopic X External	J Synthetic Substitute	C Patellar Surface Z No Qualifier
F Ankle Joint, Right G Ankle Joint, Left H Tarsal Joint, Right J Tarsal Joint, Left K Tarsometatarsal Joint, Right L Tarsometatarsal Joint, Left M Metatarsal-Phalangeal Joint, Right N Metatarsal-Phalangeal Joint, Left P Toe Phalangeal Joint, Right Q Toe Phalangeal Joint, Left	0 Open 3 Percutaneous 4 Percutaneous Endoscopic X External	0 Drainage Device 3 Infusion Device 4 Internal Fixation Device 5 External Fixation Device 7 Autologous Tissue Substitute 8 Spacer J Synthetic Substitute K Nonautologous Tissue Substitute	Z No Qualifier

Lower Joints Code Listing 0S2–0SW

Review Coding Guideline B4.5

0S2 – Lower Joints, Change

Review Coding Guideline B6.1c

0S2YX0Z Change Drainage Device in Lower Joint, External Approach

0S2YXYZ Change Other Device in Lower Joint, External Approach

0S5 – Lower Joints, Destruction

0S500ZZ Destruction of Lumbar Vertebral Joint, Open Approach
0S503ZZ Destruction of Lumbar Vertebral Joint, Percutaneous Approach
0S504ZZ Destruction of Lumbar Vertebral Joint, Percutaneous Endoscopic Approach
0S520ZZ Destruction of Lumbar Vertebral Disc, Open Approach
0S523ZZ Destruction of Lumbar Vertebral Disc, Percutaneous Approach
0S524ZZ Destruction of Lumbar Vertebral Disc, Percutaneous Endoscopic Approach
0S530ZZ Destruction of Lumbosacral Joint, Open Approach
0S533ZZ Destruction of Lumbosacral Joint, Percutaneous Approach
0S534ZZ Destruction of Lumbosacral Joint, Percutaneous Endoscopic Approach
0S540ZZ Destruction of Lumbosacral Disc, Open Approach
0S543ZZ Destruction of Lumbosacral Disc, Percutaneous Approach

0S544ZZ Destruction of Lumbosacral Disc, Percutaneous Endoscopic Approach
0S550ZZ Destruction of Sacrococcygeal Joint, Open Approach
0S553ZZ Destruction of Sacrococcygeal Joint, Percutaneous Approach
0S554ZZ Destruction of Sacrococcygeal Joint, Percutaneous Endoscopic Approach
0S560ZZ Destruction of Coccygeal Joint, Open Approach
0S563ZZ Destruction of Coccygeal Joint, Percutaneous Approach
0S564ZZ Destruction of Coccygeal Joint, Percutaneous Endoscopic Approach
0S570ZZ Destruction of Right Sacroiliac Joint, Open Approach
0S573ZZ Destruction of Right Sacroiliac Joint, Percutaneous Approach
0S574ZZ Destruction of Right Sacroiliac Joint, Percutaneous Endoscopic Approach
0S580ZZ Destruction of Left Sacroiliac Joint, Open Approach

0S583ZZ Destruction of Left Sacroiliac Joint, Percutaneous Approach
0S584ZZ Destruction of Left Sacroiliac Joint, Percutaneous Endoscopic Approach
0S590ZZ Destruction of Right Hip Joint, Open Approach
0S593ZZ Destruction of Right Hip Joint, Percutaneous Approach
0S594ZZ Destruction of Right Hip Joint, Percutaneous Endoscopic Approach
0S5B0ZZ Destruction of Left Hip Joint, Open Approach
0S5B3ZZ Destruction of Left Hip Joint, Percutaneous Approach
0S5B4ZZ Destruction of Left Hip Joint, Percutaneous Endoscopic Approach
0S5C0ZZ Destruction of Right Knee Joint, Open Approach
0S5C3ZZ Destruction of Right Knee Joint, Percutaneous Approach
0S5C4ZZ Destruction of Right Knee Joint, Percutaneous Endoscopic Approach

♀ Female-only   ♂ Male-only   ▲ Limited Coverage   ● Non-OR   HAC HAC-associated procedure   ▲ Non-covered procedures   ✚ Cluster

0S5D0ZZ	Destruction of Left Knee Joint, Open Approach	
0S5D3ZZ	Destruction of Left Knee Joint, Percutaneous Approach	
0S5D4ZZ	Destruction of Left Knee Joint, Percutaneous Endoscopic Approach	
0S5F0ZZ	Destruction of Right Ankle Joint, Open Approach	
0S5F3ZZ	Destruction of Right Ankle Joint, Percutaneous Approach	
0S5F4ZZ	Destruction of Right Ankle Joint, Percutaneous Endoscopic Approach	
0S5G0ZZ	Destruction of Left Ankle Joint, Open Approach	
0S5G3ZZ	Destruction of Left Ankle Joint, Percutaneous Approach	
0S5G4ZZ	Destruction of Left Ankle Joint, Percutaneous Endoscopic Approach	
0S5H0ZZ	Destruction of Right Tarsal Joint, Open Approach	
0S5H3ZZ	Destruction of Right Tarsal Joint, Percutaneous Approach	
0S5H4ZZ	Destruction of Right Tarsal Joint, Percutaneous Endoscopic Approach	
0S5J0ZZ	Destruction of Left Tarsal Joint, Open Approach	
0S5J3ZZ	Destruction of Left Tarsal Joint, Percutaneous Approach	
0S5J4ZZ	Destruction of Left Tarsal Joint, Percutaneous Endoscopic Approach	
0S5K0ZZ	Destruction of Right Tarsometatarsal Joint, Open Approach	
0S5K3ZZ	Destruction of Right Tarsometatarsal Joint, Percutaneous Approach	
0S5K4ZZ	Destruction of Right Tarsometatarsal Joint, Percutaneous Endoscopic Approach	
0S5L0ZZ	Destruction of Left Tarsometatarsal Joint, Open Approach	
0S5L3ZZ	Destruction of Left Tarsometatarsal Joint, Percutaneous Approach	
0S5L4ZZ	Destruction of Left Tarsometatarsal Joint, Percutaneous Endoscopic Approach	
0S5M0ZZ	Destruction of Right Metatarsal-Phalangeal Joint, Open Approach	
0S5M3ZZ	Destruction of Right Metatarsal-Phalangeal Joint, Percutaneous Approach	
0S5M4ZZ	Destruction of Right Metatarsal-Phalangeal Joint, Percutaneous Endoscopic Approach	
0S5N0ZZ	Destruction of Left Metatarsal-Phalangeal Joint, Open Approach	
0S5N3ZZ	Destruction of Left Metatarsal-Phalangeal Joint, Percutaneous Approach	
0S5N4ZZ	Destruction of Left Metatarsal-Phalangeal Joint, Percutaneous Endoscopic Approach	
0S5P0ZZ	Destruction of Right Toe Phalangeal Joint, Open Approach	
0S5P3ZZ	Destruction of Right Toe Phalangeal Joint, Percutaneous Approach	
0S5P4ZZ	Destruction of Right Toe Phalangeal Joint, Percutaneous Endoscopic Approach	
0S5Q0ZZ	Destruction of Left Toe Phalangeal Joint, Open Approach	
0S5Q3ZZ	Destruction of Left Toe Phalangeal Joint, Percutaneous Approach	
0S5Q4ZZ	Destruction of Left Toe Phalangeal Joint, Percutaneous Endoscopic Approach	

0S9 – Lower Joints, Drainage

Review Coding Guidelines B3.4a and B3.4b

Review Coding Guideline B6.2

0S9000Z	Drainage of Lumbar Vertebral Joint with Drainage Device, Open Approach
0S900ZX	Drainage of Lumbar Vertebral Joint, Open Approach, Diagnostic
0S900ZZ	Drainage of Lumbar Vertebral Joint, Open Approach
0S9030Z	Drainage of Lumbar Vertebral Joint with Drainage Device, Percutaneous Approach
0S903ZX	Drainage of Lumbar Vertebral Joint, Percutaneous Approach, Diagnostic
0S903ZZ	Drainage of Lumbar Vertebral Joint, Percutaneous Approach
0S9040Z	Drainage of Lumbar Vertebral Joint with Drainage Device, Percutaneous Endoscopic Approach
0S904ZX	Drainage of Lumbar Vertebral Joint, Percutaneous Endoscopic Approach, Diagnostic
0S904ZZ	Drainage of Lumbar Vertebral Joint, Percutaneous Endoscopic Approach
0S9200Z	Drainage of Lumbar Vertebral Disc with Drainage Device, Open Approach
0S920ZX	Drainage of Lumbar Vertebral Disc, Open Approach, Diagnostic
0S920ZZ	Drainage of Lumbar Vertebral Disc, Open Approach
0S9230Z	Drainage of Lumbar Vertebral Disc with Drainage Device, Percutaneous Approach
0S923ZX	Drainage of Lumbar Vertebral Disc, Percutaneous Approach, Diagnostic
0S923ZZ	Drainage of Lumbar Vertebral Disc, Percutaneous Approach
0S9240Z	Drainage of Lumbar Vertebral Disc with Drainage Device, Percutaneous Endoscopic Approach
0S924ZX	Drainage of Lumbar Vertebral Disc, Percutaneous Endoscopic Approach, Diagnostic
0S924ZZ	Drainage of Lumbar Vertebral Disc, Percutaneous Endoscopic Approach
0S9300Z	Drainage of Lumbosacral Joint with Drainage Device, Open Approach
0S930ZX	Drainage of Lumbosacral Joint, Open Approach, Diagnostic
0S930ZZ	Drainage of Lumbosacral Joint, Open Approach
0S9330Z	Drainage of Lumbosacral Joint with Drainage Device, Percutaneous Approach
0S933ZX	Drainage of Lumbosacral Joint, Percutaneous Approach, Diagnostic
0S933ZZ	Drainage of Lumbosacral Joint, Percutaneous Approach
0S9340Z	Drainage of Lumbosacral Joint with Drainage Device, Percutaneous Endoscopic Approach
0S934ZX	Drainage of Lumbosacral Joint, Percutaneous Endoscopic Approach, Diagnostic
0S934ZZ	Drainage of Lumbosacral Joint, Percutaneous Endoscopic Approach
0S9400Z	Drainage of Lumbosacral Disc with Drainage Device, Open Approach
0S940ZX	Drainage of Lumbosacral Disc, Open Approach, Diagnostic
0S940ZZ	Drainage of Lumbosacral Disc, Open Approach
0S9430Z	Drainage of Lumbosacral Disc with Drainage Device, Percutaneous Approach
0S943ZX	Drainage of Lumbosacral Disc, Percutaneous Approach, Diagnostic
0S943ZZ	Drainage of Lumbosacral Disc, Percutaneous Approach
0S9440Z	Drainage of Lumbosacral Disc with Drainage Device, Percutaneous Endoscopic Approach
0S944ZX	Drainage of Lumbosacral Disc, Percutaneous Endoscopic Approach, Diagnostic
0S944ZZ	Drainage of Lumbosacral Disc, Percutaneous Endoscopic Approach
0S9500Z	Drainage of Sacrococcygeal Joint with Drainage Device, Open Approach
0S950ZX	Drainage of Sacrococcygeal Joint, Open Approach, Diagnostic
0S950ZZ	Drainage of Sacrococcygeal Joint, Open Approach
0S9530Z	Drainage of Sacrococcygeal Joint with Drainage Device, Percutaneous Approach
0S953ZX	Drainage of Sacrococcygeal Joint, Percutaneous Approach, Diagnostic
0S953ZZ	Drainage of Sacrococcygeal Joint, Percutaneous Approach
0S9540Z	Drainage of Sacrococcygeal Joint with Drainage Device, Percutaneous Endoscopic Approach
0S954ZX	Drainage of Sacrococcygeal Joint, Percutaneous Endoscopic Approach, Diagnostic
0S954ZZ	Drainage of Sacrococcygeal Joint, Percutaneous Endoscopic Approach
0S9600Z	Drainage of Coccygeal Joint with Drainage Device, Open Approach
0S960ZX	Drainage of Coccygeal Joint, Open Approach, Diagnostic
0S960ZZ	Drainage of Coccygeal Joint, Open Approach
0S9630Z	Drainage of Coccygeal Joint with Drainage Device, Percutaneous Approach
0S963ZX	Drainage of Coccygeal Joint, Percutaneous Approach, Diagnostic
0S963ZZ	Drainage of Coccygeal Joint, Percutaneous Approach
0S9640Z	Drainage of Coccygeal Joint with Drainage Device, Percutaneous Endoscopic Approach
0S964ZX	Drainage of Coccygeal Joint, Percutaneous Endoscopic Approach, Diagnostic
0S964ZZ	Drainage of Coccygeal Joint, Percutaneous Endoscopic Approach
0S9700Z	Drainage of Right Sacroiliac Joint with Drainage Device, Open Approach
0S970ZX	Drainage of Right Sacroiliac Joint, Open Approach, Diagnostic
0S970ZZ	Drainage of Right Sacroiliac Joint, Open Approach

0S9730Z Drainage of Right Sacroiliac Joint with Drainage Device, Percutaneous Approach

0S973ZX Drainage of Right Sacroiliac Joint, Percutaneous Approach, Diagnostic

0S973ZZ Drainage of Right Sacroiliac Joint, Percutaneous Approach

0S9740Z Drainage of Right Sacroiliac Joint with Drainage Device, Percutaneous Endoscopic Approach

0S974ZX Drainage of Right Sacroiliac Joint, Percutaneous Endoscopic Approach, Diagnostic

0S974ZZ Drainage of Right Sacroiliac Joint, Percutaneous Endoscopic Approach

0S9800Z Drainage of Left Sacroiliac Joint with Drainage Device, Open Approach

0S980ZX Drainage of Left Sacroiliac Joint, Open Approach, Diagnostic

0S980ZZ Drainage of Left Sacroiliac Joint, Open Approach

0S9830Z Drainage of Left Sacroiliac Joint with Drainage Device, Percutaneous Approach

0S983ZX Drainage of Left Sacroiliac Joint, Percutaneous Approach, Diagnostic

0S983ZZ Drainage of Left Sacroiliac Joint, Percutaneous Approach

0S9840Z Drainage of Left Sacroiliac Joint with Drainage Device, Percutaneous Endoscopic Approach

0S984ZX Drainage of Left Sacroiliac Joint, Percutaneous Endoscopic Approach, Diagnostic

0S984ZZ Drainage of Left Sacroiliac Joint, Percutaneous Endoscopic Approach

0S9900Z Drainage of Right Hip Joint with Drainage Device, Open Approach

0S990ZX Drainage of Right Hip Joint, Open Approach, Diagnostic

0S990ZZ Drainage of Right Hip Joint, Open Approach

0S9930Z Drainage of Right Hip Joint with Drainage Device, Percutaneous Approach

0S993ZX Drainage of Right Hip Joint, Percutaneous Approach, Diagnostic

0S993ZZ Drainage of Right Hip Joint, Percutaneous Approach

0S9940Z Drainage of Right Hip Joint with Drainage Device, Percutaneous Endoscopic Approach

0S994ZX Drainage of Right Hip Joint, Percutaneous Endoscopic Approach, Diagnostic

0S994ZZ Drainage of Right Hip Joint, Percutaneous Endoscopic Approach

0S9B00Z Drainage of Left Hip Joint with Drainage Device, Open Approach

0S9B0ZX Drainage of Left Hip Joint, Open Approach, Diagnostic

0S9B0ZZ Drainage of Left Hip Joint, Open Approach

0S9B30Z Drainage of Left Hip Joint with Drainage Device, Percutaneous Approach

0S9B3ZX Drainage of Left Hip Joint, Percutaneous Approach, Diagnostic

0S9B3ZZ Drainage of Left Hip Joint, Percutaneous Approach

0S9B40Z Drainage of Left Hip Joint with Drainage Device, Percutaneous Endoscopic Approach

0S9B4ZX Drainage of Left Hip Joint, Percutaneous Endoscopic Approach, Diagnostic

0S9B4ZZ Drainage of Left Hip Joint, Percutaneous Endoscopic Approach

0S9C00Z Drainage of Right Knee Joint with Drainage Device, Open Approach

0S9C0ZX Drainage of Right Knee Joint, Open Approach, Diagnostic

0S9C0ZZ Drainage of Right Knee Joint, Open Approach

0S9C30Z Drainage of Right Knee Joint with Drainage Device, Percutaneous Approach

0S9C3ZX Drainage of Right Knee Joint, Percutaneous Approach, Diagnostic

0S9C3ZZ Drainage of Right Knee Joint, Percutaneous Approach

0S9C40Z Drainage of Right Knee Joint with Drainage Device, Percutaneous Endoscopic Approach

0S9C4ZX Drainage of Right Knee Joint, Percutaneous Endoscopic Approach, Diagnostic

0S9C4ZZ Drainage of Right Knee Joint, Percutaneous Endoscopic Approach

0S9D00Z Drainage of Left Knee Joint with Drainage Device, Open Approach

0S9D0ZX Drainage of Left Knee Joint, Open Approach, Diagnostic

0S9D0ZZ Drainage of Left Knee Joint, Open Approach

0S9D30Z Drainage of Left Knee Joint with Drainage Device, Percutaneous Approach

0S9D3ZX Drainage of Left Knee Joint, Percutaneous Approach, Diagnostic

0S9D3ZZ Drainage of Left Knee Joint, Percutaneous Approach

0S9D40Z Drainage of Left Knee Joint with Drainage Device, Percutaneous Endoscopic Approach

0S9D4ZX Drainage of Left Knee Joint, Percutaneous Endoscopic Approach, Diagnostic

0S9D4ZZ Drainage of Left Knee Joint, Percutaneous Endoscopic Approach

AHA CC: 2Q, 2018, 17

0S9F00Z Drainage of Right Ankle Joint with Drainage Device, Open Approach

0S9F0ZX Drainage of Right Ankle Joint, Open Approach, Diagnostic

0S9F0ZZ Drainage of Right Ankle Joint, Open Approach

0S9F30Z Drainage of Right Ankle Joint with Drainage Device, Percutaneous Approach

0S9F3ZX Drainage of Right Ankle Joint, Percutaneous Approach, Diagnostic

0S9F3ZZ Drainage of Right Ankle Joint, Percutaneous Approach

0S9F40Z Drainage of Right Ankle Joint with Drainage Device, Percutaneous Endoscopic Approach

0S9F4ZX Drainage of Right Ankle Joint, Percutaneous Endoscopic Approach, Diagnostic

0S9F4ZZ Drainage of Right Ankle Joint, Percutaneous Endoscopic Approach

0S9G00Z Drainage of Left Ankle Joint with Drainage Device, Open Approach

0S9G0ZX Drainage of Left Ankle Joint, Open Approach, Diagnostic

0S9G0ZZ Drainage of Left Ankle Joint, Open Approach

0S9G30Z Drainage of Left Ankle Joint with Drainage Device, Percutaneous Approach

0S9G3ZX Drainage of Left Ankle Joint, Percutaneous Approach, Diagnostic

0S9G3ZZ Drainage of Left Ankle Joint, Percutaneous Approach

0S9G40Z Drainage of Left Ankle Joint with Drainage Device, Percutaneous Endoscopic Approach

0S9G4ZX Drainage of Left Ankle Joint, Percutaneous Endoscopic Approach, Diagnostic

0S9G4ZZ Drainage of Left Ankle Joint, Percutaneous Endoscopic Approach

0S9H00Z Drainage of Right Tarsal Joint with Drainage Device, Open Approach

0S9H0ZX Drainage of Right Tarsal Joint, Open Approach, Diagnostic

0S9H0ZZ Drainage of Right Tarsal Joint, Open Approach

0S9H30Z Drainage of Right Tarsal Joint with Drainage Device, Percutaneous Approach

0S9H3ZX Drainage of Right Tarsal Joint, Percutaneous Approach, Diagnostic

0S9H3ZZ Drainage of Right Tarsal Joint, Percutaneous Approach

0S9H40Z Drainage of Right Tarsal Joint with Drainage Device, Percutaneous Endoscopic Approach

0S9H4ZX Drainage of Right Tarsal Joint, Percutaneous Endoscopic Approach, Diagnostic

0S9H4ZZ Drainage of Right Tarsal Joint, Percutaneous Endoscopic Approach

0S9J00Z Drainage of Left Tarsal Joint with Drainage Device, Open Approach

0S9J0ZX Drainage of Left Tarsal Joint, Open Approach, Diagnostic

0S9J0ZZ Drainage of Left Tarsal Joint, Open Approach

0S9J30Z Drainage of Left Tarsal Joint with Drainage Device, Percutaneous Approach

0S9J3ZX Drainage of Left Tarsal Joint, Percutaneous Approach, Diagnostic

0S9J3ZZ Drainage of Left Tarsal Joint, Percutaneous Approach

0S9J40Z Drainage of Left Tarsal Joint with Drainage Device, Percutaneous Endoscopic Approach

0S9J4ZX Drainage of Left Tarsal Joint, Percutaneous Endoscopic Approach, Diagnostic

0S9J4ZZ Drainage of Left Tarsal Joint, Percutaneous Endoscopic Approach

0S9K00Z Drainage of Right Tarsometatarsal Joint with Drainage Device, Open Approach

0S9K0ZX Drainage of Right Tarsometatarsal Joint, Open Approach, Diagnostic

0S9K0ZZ Drainage of Right Tarsometatarsal Joint, Open Approach

0S9K30Z Drainage of Right Tarsometatarsal Joint with Drainage Device, Percutaneous Approach

0S9K3ZX Drainage of Right Tarsometatarsal Joint, Percutaneous Approach, Diagnostic

0S9K3ZZ Drainage of Right Tarsometatarsal Joint, Percutaneous Approach

0S9K40Z Drainage of Right Tarsometatarsal Joint with Drainage Device, Percutaneous Endoscopic Approach

0S9K4ZX Drainage of Right Tarsometatarsal Joint, Percutaneous Endoscopic Approach, Diagnostic

0S9K4ZZ Drainage of Right Tarsometatarsal Joint, Percutaneous Endoscopic Approach

♀ Female-only   ♂ Male-only   ▲ Limited Coverage   ● Non-OR   🅷🅰🅲 HAC-associated procedure   ▲ Non-covered procedures   ➕ Cluster

0S9L00Z	Drainage of Left Tarsometatarsal Joint with Drainage Device, Open Approach
0S9L0ZZ	Drainage of Left Tarsometatarsal Joint, Open Approach
0S9L30Z	Drainage of Left Tarsometatarsal Joint with Drainage Device, Percutaneous Approach
0S9L3ZX	Drainage of Left Tarsometatarsal Joint, Percutaneous Approach, Diagnostic
0S9L3ZZ	Drainage of Left Tarsometatarsal Joint, Percutaneous Approach
0S9L40Z	Drainage of Left Tarsometatarsal Joint with Drainage Device, Percutaneous Endoscopic Approach
0S9L4ZX	Drainage of Left Tarsometatarsal Joint, Percutaneous Endoscopic Approach, Diagnostic
0S9L4ZZ	Drainage of Left Tarsometatarsal Joint, Percutaneous Endoscopic Approach
0S9M00Z	Drainage of Right Metatarsal-Phalangeal Joint with Drainage Device, Open Approach
0S9M0ZX	Drainage of Right Metatarsal-Phalangeal Joint, Open Approach, Diagnostic
0S9M0ZZ	Drainage of Right Metatarsal-Phalangeal Joint, Open Approach
0S9M30Z	Drainage of Right Metatarsal-Phalangeal Joint with Drainage Device, Percutaneous Approach
0S9M3ZX	Drainage of Right Metatarsal-Phalangeal Joint, Percutaneous Approach, Diagnostic
0S9M3ZZ	Drainage of Right Metatarsal-Phalangeal Joint, Percutaneous Approach
0S9M40Z	Drainage of Right Metatarsal-Phalangeal Joint with Drainage Device, Percutaneous Endoscopic Approach

0S9M4ZX	Drainage of Right Metatarsal-Phalangeal Joint, Percutaneous Endoscopic Approach, Diagnostic
0S9M4ZZ	Drainage of Right Metatarsal-Phalangeal Joint, Percutaneous Endoscopic Approach
0S9N00Z	Drainage of Left Metatarsal-Phalangeal Joint with Drainage Device, Open Approach
0S9N0ZX	Drainage of Left Metatarsal-Phalangeal Joint, Open Approach, Diagnostic
0S9N0ZZ	Drainage of Left Metatarsal-Phalangeal Joint, Open Approach
0S9N30Z	Drainage of Left Metatarsal-Phalangeal Joint with Drainage Device, Percutaneous Approach
0S9N3ZX	Drainage of Left Metatarsal-Phalangeal Joint, Percutaneous Approach, Diagnostic
0S9N3ZZ	Drainage of Left Metatarsal-Phalangeal Joint, Percutaneous Approach
0S9N40Z	Drainage of Left Metatarsal-Phalangeal Joint with Drainage Device, Percutaneous Endoscopic Approach
0S9N4ZX	Drainage of Left Metatarsal-Phalangeal Joint, Percutaneous Endoscopic Approach, Diagnostic
0S9N4ZZ	Drainage of Left Metatarsal-Phalangeal Joint, Percutaneous Endoscopic Approach
0S9P00Z	Drainage of Right Toe Phalangeal Joint with Drainage Device, Open Approach
0S9P0ZX	Drainage of Right Toe Phalangeal Joint, Open Approach, Diagnostic
0S9P0ZZ	Drainage of Right Toe Phalangeal Joint, Open Approach

0S9P30Z	Drainage of Right Toe Phalangeal Joint with Drainage Device, Percutaneous Approach
0S9P3ZX	Drainage of Right Toe Phalangeal Joint, Percutaneous Approach, Diagnostic
0S9P3ZZ	Drainage of Right Toe Phalangeal Joint, Percutaneous Approach
0S9P40Z	Drainage of Right Toe Phalangeal Joint with Drainage Device, Percutaneous Endoscopic Approach
0S9P4ZX	Drainage of Right Toe Phalangeal Joint, Percutaneous Endoscopic Approach, Diagnostic
0S9P4ZZ	Drainage of Right Toe Phalangeal Joint, Percutaneous Endoscopic Approach
0S9Q00Z	Drainage of Left Toe Phalangeal Joint with Drainage Device, Open Approach
0S9Q0ZX	Drainage of Left Toe Phalangeal Joint, Open Approach, Diagnostic
0S9Q0ZZ	Drainage of Left Toe Phalangeal Joint, Open Approach
0S9Q30Z	Drainage of Left Toe Phalangeal Joint with Drainage Device, Percutaneous Approach
0S9Q3ZX	Drainage of Left Toe Phalangeal Joint, Percutaneous Approach, Diagnostic
0S9Q3ZZ	Drainage of Left Toe Phalangeal Joint, Percutaneous Approach
0S9Q40Z	Drainage of Left Toe Phalangeal Joint with Drainage Device, Percutaneous Endoscopic Approach
0S9Q4ZX	Drainage of Left Toe Phalangeal Joint, Percutaneous Endoscopic Approach, Diagnostic
0S9Q4ZZ	Drainage of Left Toe Phalangeal Joint, Percutaneous Endoscopic Approach

0SB – Lower Joints, Excision

Review Coding Guidelines B3.4a and B3.4b

Review Coding Guideline B3.5

Review Coding Guideline B3.8

Review Coding Guideline B3.18

0SB00ZX	Excision of Lumbar Vertebral Joint, Open Approach, Diagnostic
0SB00ZZ	Excision of Lumbar Vertebral Joint, Open Approach
0SB03ZX	Excision of Lumbar Vertebral Joint, Percutaneous Approach, Diagnostic
0SB03ZZ	Excision of Lumbar Vertebral Joint, Percutaneous Approach
0SB04ZX	Excision of Lumbar Vertebral Joint, Percutaneous Endoscopic Approach, Diagnostic
0SB04ZZ	Excision of Lumbar Vertebral Joint, Percutaneous Endoscopic Approach
0SB20ZX	Excision of Lumbar Vertebral Disc, Open Approach, Diagnostic
0SB20ZZ	Excision of Lumbar Vertebral Disc, Open Approach
	AHA CC: 2Q, 2014, 6-7; 2Q, 2016, 16; 4Q, 2017, 76-77
0SB23ZX	Excision of Lumbar Vertebral Disc, Percutaneous Approach, Diagnostic
0SB23ZZ	Excision of Lumbar Vertebral Disc, Percutaneous Approach
0SB24ZX	Excision of Lumbar Vertebral Disc, Percutaneous Endoscopic Approach, Diagnostic

0SB24ZZ	Excision of Lumbar Vertebral Disc, Percutaneous Endoscopic Approach
0SB30ZX	Excision of Lumbosacral Joint, Open Approach, Diagnostic
0SB30ZZ	Excision of Lumbosacral Joint, Open Approach
0SB33ZX	Excision of Lumbosacral Joint, Percutaneous Approach, Diagnostic
0SB33ZZ	Excision of Lumbosacral Joint, Percutaneous Approach
0SB34ZX	Excision of Lumbosacral Joint, Percutaneous Endoscopic Approach, Diagnostic
0SB34ZZ	Excision of Lumbosacral Joint, Percutaneous Endoscopic Approach
0SB40ZX	Excision of Lumbosacral Disc, Open Approach, Diagnostic
0SB40ZZ	Excision of Lumbosacral Disc, Open Approach
	AHA CC: 4Q, 2017, 76-77
0SB43ZX	Excision of Lumbosacral Disc, Percutaneous Approach, Diagnostic
0SB43ZZ	Excision of Lumbosacral Disc, Percutaneous Approach

0SB44ZX	Excision of Lumbosacral Disc, Percutaneous Endoscopic Approach, Diagnostic
0SB44ZZ	Excision of Lumbosacral Disc, Percutaneous Endoscopic Approach
0SB50ZX	Excision of Sacrococcygeal Joint, Open Approach, Diagnostic
0SB50ZZ	Excision of Sacrococcygeal Joint, Open Approach
0SB53ZX	Excision of Sacrococcygeal Joint, Percutaneous Approach, Diagnostic
0SB53ZZ	Excision of Sacrococcygeal Joint, Percutaneous Approach
0SB54ZX	Excision of Sacrococcygeal Joint, Percutaneous Endoscopic Approach, Diagnostic
0SB54ZZ	Excision of Sacrococcygeal Joint, Percutaneous Endoscopic Approach
0SB60ZX	Excision of Coccygeal Joint, Open Approach, Diagnostic
0SB60ZZ	Excision of Coccygeal Joint, Open Approach
0SB63ZX	Excision of Coccygeal Joint, Percutaneous Approach, Diagnostic
0SB63ZZ	Excision of Coccygeal Joint, Percutaneous Approach

♀ Female-only   ♂ Male-only   ▲ Limited Coverage   ● Non-OR   ▦ HAC-associated procedure   ▲ Non-covered procedures   ✚ Cluster   **1145**

Medical and Surgical, Lower Joints Code Listings

0SB64ZX Excision of Coccygeal Joint, Percutaneous Endoscopic Approach, Diagnostic

0SB64ZZ Excision of Coccygeal Joint, Percutaneous Endoscopic Approach

0SB70ZX Excision of Right Sacroiliac Joint, Open Approach, Diagnostic

0SB70ZZ Excision of Right Sacroiliac Joint, Open Approach

0SB73ZX Excision of Right Sacroiliac Joint, Percutaneous Approach, Diagnostic

0SB73ZZ Excision of Right Sacroiliac Joint, Percutaneous Approach

0SB74ZX Excision of Right Sacroiliac Joint, Percutaneous Endoscopic Approach, Diagnostic

0SB74ZZ Excision of Right Sacroiliac Joint, Percutaneous Endoscopic Approach

0SB80ZX Excision of Left Sacroiliac Joint, Open Approach, Diagnostic

0SB80ZZ Excision of Left Sacroiliac Joint, Open Approach

0SB83ZX Excision of Left Sacroiliac Joint, Percutaneous Approach, Diagnostic

0SB83ZZ Excision of Left Sacroiliac Joint, Percutaneous Approach

0SB84ZX Excision of Left Sacroiliac Joint, Percutaneous Endoscopic Approach, Diagnostic

0SB84ZZ Excision of Left Sacroiliac Joint, Percutaneous Endoscopic Approach

0SB90ZX Excision of Right Hip Joint, Open Approach, Diagnostic

0SB90ZZ Excision of Right Hip Joint, Open Approach

0SB93ZX Excision of Right Hip Joint, Percutaneous Approach, Diagnostic

0SB93ZZ Excision of Right Hip Joint, Percutaneous Approach

0SB94ZX Excision of Right Hip Joint, Percutaneous Endoscopic Approach, Diagnostic

0SB94ZZ Excision of Right Hip Joint, Percutaneous Endoscopic Approach

0SBB0ZX Excision of Left Hip Joint, Open Approach, Diagnostic

0SBB0ZZ Excision of Left Hip Joint, Open Approach

0SBB3ZX Excision of Left Hip Joint, Percutaneous Approach, Diagnostic

0SBB3ZZ Excision of Left Hip Joint, Percutaneous Approach

0SBB4ZX Excision of Left Hip Joint, Percutaneous Endoscopic Approach, Diagnostic

0SBB4ZZ Excision of Left Hip Joint, Percutaneous Endoscopic Approach

0SBC0ZX Excision of Right Knee Joint, Open Approach, Diagnostic

0SBC0ZZ Excision of Right Knee Joint, Open Approach

0SBC3ZX Excision of Right Knee Joint, Percutaneous Approach, Diagnostic

0SBC3ZZ Excision of Right Knee Joint, Percutaneous Approach

0SBC4ZX Excision of Right Knee Joint, Percutaneous Endoscopic Approach, Diagnostic

0SBC4ZZ Excision of Right Knee Joint, Percutaneous Endoscopic Approach

0SBD0ZX Excision of Left Knee Joint, Open Approach, Diagnostic

0SBD0ZZ Excision of Left Knee Joint, Open Approach

0SBD3ZX Excision of Left Knee Joint, Percutaneous Approach, Diagnostic

0SBD3ZZ Excision of Left Knee Joint, Percutaneous Approach

0SBD4ZX Excision of Left Knee Joint, Percutaneous Endoscopic Approach, Diagnostic

0SBD4ZZ Excision of Left Knee Joint, Percutaneous Endoscopic Approach

AHA CC: 1Q, 2015, 34

0SBF0ZX Excision of Right Ankle Joint, Open Approach, Diagnostic

0SBF0ZZ Excision of Right Ankle Joint, Open Approach

0SBF3ZX Excision of Right Ankle Joint, Percutaneous Approach, Diagnostic

0SBF3ZZ Excision of Right Ankle Joint, Percutaneous Approach

0SBF4ZX Excision of Right Ankle Joint, Percutaneous Endoscopic Approach, Diagnostic

0SBF4ZZ Excision of Right Ankle Joint, Percutaneous Endoscopic Approach

0SBG0ZX Excision of Left Ankle Joint, Open Approach, Diagnostic

0SBG0ZZ Excision of Left Ankle Joint, Open Approach

0SBG3ZX Excision of Left Ankle Joint, Percutaneous Approach, Diagnostic

0SBG3ZZ Excision of Left Ankle Joint, Percutaneous Approach

0SBG4ZX Excision of Left Ankle Joint, Percutaneous Endoscopic Approach, Diagnostic

0SBG4ZZ Excision of Left Ankle Joint, Percutaneous Endoscopic Approach

0SBH0ZX Excision of Right Tarsal Joint, Open Approach, Diagnostic

0SBH0ZZ Excision of Right Tarsal Joint, Open Approach

0SBH3ZX Excision of Right Tarsal Joint, Percutaneous Approach, Diagnostic

0SBH3ZZ Excision of Right Tarsal Joint, Percutaneous Approach

0SBH4ZX Excision of Right Tarsal Joint, Percutaneous Endoscopic Approach, Diagnostic

0SBH4ZZ Excision of Right Tarsal Joint, Percutaneous Endoscopic Approach

0SBJ0ZX Excision of Left Tarsal Joint, Open Approach, Diagnostic

0SBJ0ZZ Excision of Left Tarsal Joint, Open Approach

0SBJ3ZX Excision of Left Tarsal Joint, Percutaneous Approach, Diagnostic

0SBJ3ZZ Excision of Left Tarsal Joint, Percutaneous Approach

0SBJ4ZX Excision of Left Tarsal Joint, Percutaneous Endoscopic Approach, Diagnostic

0SBJ4ZZ Excision of Left Tarsal Joint, Percutaneous Endoscopic Approach

0SBK0ZX Excision of Right Tarsometatarsal Joint, Open Approach, Diagnostic

0SBK0ZZ Excision of Right Tarsometatarsal Joint, Open Approach

0SBK3ZX Excision of Right Tarsometatarsal Joint, Percutaneous Approach, Diagnostic

0SBK3ZZ Excision of Right Tarsometatarsal Joint, Percutaneous Approach

0SBK4ZX Excision of Right Tarsometatarsal Joint, Percutaneous Endoscopic Approach, Diagnostic

0SBK4ZZ Excision of Right Tarsometatarsal Joint, Percutaneous Endoscopic Approach

0SBL0ZX Excision of Left Tarsometatarsal Joint, Open Approach, Diagnostic

0SBL0ZZ Excision of Left Tarsometatarsal Joint, Open Approach

0SBL3ZX Excision of Left Tarsometatarsal Joint, Percutaneous Approach, Diagnostic

0SBL3ZZ Excision of Left Tarsometatarsal Joint, Percutaneous Approach

0SBL4ZX Excision of Left Tarsometatarsal Joint, Percutaneous Endoscopic Approach, Diagnostic

0SBL4ZZ Excision of Left Tarsometatarsal Joint, Percutaneous Endoscopic Approach

0SBM0ZX Excision of Right Metatarsal-Phalangeal Joint, Open Approach, Diagnostic

0SBM0ZZ Excision of Right Metatarsal-Phalangeal Joint, Open Approach

0SBM3ZX Excision of Right Metatarsal-Phalangeal Joint, Percutaneous Approach, Diagnostic

0SBM3ZZ Excision of Right Metatarsal-Phalangeal Joint, Percutaneous Approach

0SBM4ZX Excision of Right Metatarsal-Phalangeal Joint, Percutaneous Endoscopic Approach, Diagnostic

0SBM4ZZ Excision of Right Metatarsal-Phalangeal Joint, Percutaneous Endoscopic Approach

0SBN0ZX Excision of Left Metatarsal-Phalangeal Joint, Open Approach, Diagnostic

0SBN0ZZ Excision of Left Metatarsal-Phalangeal Joint, Open Approach

0SBN3ZX Excision of Left Metatarsal-Phalangeal Joint, Percutaneous Approach, Diagnostic

0SBN3ZZ Excision of Left Metatarsal-Phalangeal Joint, Percutaneous Approach

0SBN4ZX Excision of Left Metatarsal-Phalangeal Joint, Percutaneous Endoscopic Approach, Diagnostic

0SBN4ZZ Excision of Left Metatarsal-Phalangeal Joint, Percutaneous Endoscopic Approach

0SBP0ZX Excision of Right Toe Phalangeal Joint, Open Approach, Diagnostic

0SBP0ZZ Excision of Right Toe Phalangeal Joint, Open Approach

0SBP3ZX Excision of Right Toe Phalangeal Joint, Percutaneous Approach, Diagnostic

0SBP3ZZ Excision of Right Toe Phalangeal Joint, Percutaneous Approach

0SBP4ZX Excision of Right Toe Phalangeal Joint, Percutaneous Endoscopic Approach, Diagnostic

0SBP4ZZ Excision of Right Toe Phalangeal Joint, Percutaneous Endoscopic Approach

0SBQ0ZX Excision of Left Toe Phalangeal Joint, Open Approach, Diagnostic

0SBQ0ZZ Excision of Left Toe Phalangeal Joint, Open Approach

0SBQ3ZX Excision of Left Toe Phalangeal Joint, Percutaneous Approach, Diagnostic

0SBQ3ZZ Excision of Left Toe Phalangeal Joint, Percutaneous Approach

0SBQ4ZX Excision of Left Toe Phalangeal Joint, Percutaneous Endoscopic Approach, Diagnostic

0SBQ4ZZ Excision of Left Toe Phalangeal Joint, Percutaneous Endoscopic Approach

♀ Female-only ♂ Male-only ▲ Limited Coverage ● Non-OR ▆ HAC-associated procedure ▲ Non-covered procedures ✚ Cluster

0SC – Lower Joints, Extirpation

0SC00ZZ	Extirpation of Matter from Lumbar Vertebral Joint, Open Approach	**0SC84ZZ**	Extirpation of Matter from Left Sacroiliac Joint, Percutaneous Endoscopic Approach	**0SCJ4ZZ**	Extirpation of Matter from Left Tarsal Joint, Percutaneous Endoscopic Approach
0SC03ZZ	Extirpation of Matter from Lumbar Vertebral Joint, Percutaneous Approach	**0SC90ZZ**	Extirpation of Matter from Right Hip Joint, Open Approach	**0SCK0ZZ**	Extirpation of Matter from Right Tarsometatarsal Joint, Open Approach
0SC04ZZ	Extirpation of Matter from Lumbar Vertebral Joint, Percutaneous Endoscopic Approach	**0SC93ZZ**	Extirpation of Matter from Right Hip Joint, Percutaneous Approach	**0SCK3ZZ**	Extirpation of Matter from Right Tarsometatarsal Joint, Percutaneous Approach
0SC20ZZ	Extirpation of Matter from Lumbar Vertebral Disc, Open Approach	**0SC94ZZ**	Extirpation of Matter from Right Hip Joint, Percutaneous Endoscopic Approach	**0SCK4ZZ**	Extirpation of Matter from Right Tarsometatarsal Joint, Percutaneous Endoscopic Approach
0SC23ZZ	Extirpation of Matter from Lumbar Vertebral Disc, Percutaneous Approach	**0SCB0ZZ**	Extirpation of Matter from Left Hip Joint, Open Approach	**0SCL0ZZ**	Extirpation of Matter from Left Tarsometatarsal Joint, Open Approach
0SC24ZZ	Extirpation of Matter from Lumbar Vertebral Disc, Percutaneous Endoscopic Approach	**0SCB3ZZ**	Extirpation of Matter from Left Hip Joint, Percutaneous Approach	**0SCL3ZZ**	Extirpation of Matter from Left Tarsometatarsal Joint, Percutaneous Approach
0SC30ZZ	Extirpation of Matter from Lumbosacral Joint, Open Approach	**0SCB4ZZ**	Extirpation of Matter from Left Hip Joint, Percutaneous Endoscopic Approach	**0SCL4ZZ**	Extirpation of Matter from Left Tarsometatarsal Joint, Percutaneous Endoscopic Approach
0SC33ZZ	Extirpation of Matter from Lumbosacral Joint, Percutaneous Approach	**0SCC0ZZ**	Extirpation of Matter from Right Knee Joint, Open Approach	**0SCM0ZZ**	Extirpation of Matter from Right Metatarsal-Phalangeal Joint, Open Approach
0SC34ZZ	Extirpation of Matter from Lumbosacral Joint, Percutaneous Endoscopic Approach	**0SCC3ZZ**	Extirpation of Matter from Right Knee Joint, Percutaneous Approach	**0SCM3ZZ**	Extirpation of Matter from Right Metatarsal-Phalangeal Joint, Percutaneous Approach
0SC40ZZ	Extirpation of Matter from Lumbosacral Disc, Open Approach	**0SCC4ZZ**	Extirpation of Matter from Right Knee Joint, Percutaneous Endoscopic Approach	**0SCM4ZZ**	Extirpation of Matter from Right Metatarsal-Phalangeal Joint, Percutaneous Endoscopic Approach
0SC43ZZ	Extirpation of Matter from Lumbosacral Disc, Percutaneous Approach	**0SCD0ZZ**	Extirpation of Matter from Left Knee Joint, Open Approach	**0SCN0ZZ**	Extirpation of Matter from Left Metatarsal-Phalangeal Joint, Open Approach
0SC44ZZ	Extirpation of Matter from Lumbosacral Disc, Percutaneous Endoscopic Approach	**0SCD3ZZ**	Extirpation of Matter from Left Knee Joint, Percutaneous Approach	**0SCN3ZZ**	Extirpation of Matter from Left Metatarsal-Phalangeal Joint, Percutaneous Approach
0SC50ZZ	Extirpation of Matter from Sacrococcygeal Joint, Open Approach	**0SCD4ZZ**	Extirpation of Matter from Left Knee Joint, Percutaneous Endoscopic Approach	**0SCN4ZZ**	Extirpation of Matter from Left Metatarsal-Phalangeal Joint, Percutaneous Endoscopic Approach
0SC53ZZ	Extirpation of Matter from Sacrococcygeal Joint, Percutaneous Approach	**0SCF0ZZ**	Extirpation of Matter from Right Ankle Joint, Open Approach	**0SCP0ZZ**	Extirpation of Matter from Right Toe Phalangeal Joint, Open Approach
0SC54ZZ	Extirpation of Matter from Sacrococcygeal Joint, Percutaneous Endoscopic Approach	**0SCF3ZZ**	Extirpation of Matter from Right Ankle Joint, Percutaneous Approach	**0SCP3ZZ**	Extirpation of Matter from Right Toe Phalangeal Joint, Percutaneous Approach
0SC60ZZ	Extirpation of Matter from Coccygeal Joint, Open Approach	**0SCF4ZZ**	Extirpation of Matter from Right Ankle Joint, Percutaneous Endoscopic Approach	**0SCP4ZZ**	Extirpation of Matter from Right Toe Phalangeal Joint, Percutaneous Endoscopic Approach
0SC63ZZ	Extirpation of Matter from Coccygeal Joint, Percutaneous Approach	**0SCG0ZZ**	Extirpation of Matter from Left Ankle Joint, Open Approach	**0SCQ0ZZ**	Extirpation of Matter from Left Toe Phalangeal Joint, Open Approach
0SC64ZZ	Extirpation of Matter from Coccygeal Joint, Percutaneous Endoscopic Approach	**0SCG3ZZ**	Extirpation of Matter from Left Ankle Joint, Percutaneous Approach	**0SCQ3ZZ**	Extirpation of Matter from Left Toe Phalangeal Joint, Percutaneous Approach
0SC70ZZ	Extirpation of Matter from Right Sacroiliac Joint, Open Approach	**0SCG4ZZ**	Extirpation of Matter from Left Ankle Joint, Percutaneous Endoscopic Approach	**0SCQ4ZZ**	Extirpation of Matter from Left Toe Phalangeal Joint, Percutaneous Endoscopic Approach
0SC73ZZ	Extirpation of Matter from Right Sacroiliac Joint, Percutaneous Approach	**0SCH0ZZ**	Extirpation of Matter from Right Tarsal Joint, Open Approach		
0SC74ZZ	Extirpation of Matter from Right Sacroiliac Joint, Percutaneous Endoscopic Approach	**0SCH3ZZ**	Extirpation of Matter from Right Tarsal Joint, Percutaneous Approach		
0SC80ZZ	Extirpation of Matter from Left Sacroiliac Joint, Open Approach	**0SCH4ZZ**	Extirpation of Matter from Right Tarsal Joint, Percutaneous Endoscopic Approach		
0SC83ZZ	Extirpation of Matter from Left Sacroiliac Joint, Percutaneous Approach	**0SCJ0ZZ**	Extirpation of Matter from Left Tarsal Joint, Open Approach		
		0SCJ3ZZ	Extirpation of Matter from Left Tarsal Joint, Percutaneous Approach		

0SG – Lower Joints, Fusion

For Fusion procedures involving the vertebral joints

Review Coding Guidelines B3.10a, B3.10b and B3.10c

0SG0070	Fusion of Lumbar Vertebral Joint with Autologous Tissue Substitute, Anterior Approach, Anterior Column, Open Approach	**0SG0071**	Fusion of Lumbar Vertebral Joint with Autologous Tissue Substitute, Posterior Approach, Posterior Column, Open Approach	**0SG007J**	Fusion of Lumbar Vertebral Joint with Autologous Tissue Substitute, Posterior Approach, Anterior Column, Open Approach
	HAC When reported with secondary diagnosis code K68.11, T81.40XA, T81.41XA, T81.42XA, T81.43XA, T81.44XA or T81.49XA, T84.60XA, T84.610A, T84.611A, T84.612A, T84.613A, T84.614A, T84.615A, T84.619A, T84.63XA, T84.69XA, T84.7XXA		*AHA CC: 1Q, 2013, 21-23; 3Q, 2013, 25-26* **HAC** When reported with secondary diagnosis code K68.11, T81.40XA, T81.41XA, T81.42XA, T81.43XA, T81.44XA or T81.49XA, T84.60XA, T84.610A, T84.611A, T84.612A, T84.613A, T84.614A, T84.615A, T84.619A, T84.63XA, T84.69XA, T84.7XXA		**HAC** When reported with secondary diagnosis code K68.11, T81.40XA, T81.41XA, T81.42XA, T81.43XA, T81.44XA or T81.49XA, T84.60XA, T84.610A, T84.611A, T84.612A, T84.613A, T84.614A, T84.615A, T84.619A, T84.63XA, T84.69XA, T84.7XXA

0SG00A0 Fusion of Lumbar Vertebral Joint with Interbody Fusion Device, Anterior Approach, Anterior Column, Open Approach

HAC When reported with secondary diagnosis code K68.11, T81.40XA, T81.41XA, T81.42XA, T81.43XA, T81.44XA or T81.49XA, T84.60XA, T84.610A, T84.611A, T84.612A, T84.613A, T84.614A, T84.615A, T84.619A, T84.63XA, T84.69XA, T84.7XXA

0SG00AJ Fusion of Lumbar Vertebral Joint with Interbody Fusion Device, Posterior Approach, Anterior Column, Open Approach

AHA CC: 3Q, 2013, 25-26

HAC When reported with secondary diagnosis code K68.11, T81.40XA, T81.41XA, T81.42XA, T81.43XA, T81.44XA or T81.49XA, T84.60XA, T84.610A, T84.611A, T84.612A, T84.613A, T84.614A, T84.615A, T84.619A, T84.63XA, T84.69XA, T84.7XXA

0SG00J0 Fusion of Lumbar Vertebral Joint with Synthetic Substitute, Anterior Approach, Anterior Column, Open Approach

HAC When reported with secondary diagnosis code K68.11, T81.40XA, T81.41XA, T81.42XA, T81.43XA, T81.44XA or T81.49XA, T84.60XA, T84.610A, T84.611A, T84.612A, T84.613A, T84.614A, T84.615A, T84.619A, T84.63XA, T84.69XA, T84.7XXA

0SG00J1 Fusion of Lumbar Vertebral Joint with Synthetic Substitute, Posterior Approach, Posterior Column, Open Approach

HAC When reported with secondary diagnosis code K68.11, T81.40XA, T81.41XA, T81.42XA, T81.43XA, T81.44XA or T81.49XA, T84.60XA, T84.610A, T84.611A, T84.612A, T84.613A, T84.614A, T84.615A, T84.619A, T84.63XA, T84.69XA, T84.7XXA

0SG00JJ Fusion of Lumbar Vertebral Joint with Synthetic Substitute, Posterior Approach, Anterior Column, Open Approach

HAC When reported with secondary diagnosis code K68.11, T81.40XA, T81.41XA, T81.42XA, T81.43XA, T81.44XA or T81.49XA, T84.60XA, T84.610A, T84.611A, T84.612A, T84.613A, T84.614A, T84.615A, T84.619A, T84.63XA, T84.69XA, T84.7XXA

0SG00K0 Fusion of Lumbar Vertebral Joint with Nonautologous Tissue Substitute, Anterior Approach, Anterior Column, Open Approach

HAC When reported with secondary diagnosis code K68.11, T81.40XA, T81.41XA, T81.42XA, T81.43XA, T81.44XA or T81.49XA, T84.60XA, T84.610A, T84.611A, T84.612A, T84.613A, T84.614A, T84.615A, T84.619A, T84.63XA, T84.69XA, T84.7XXA

0SG00K1 Fusion of Lumbar Vertebral Joint with Nonautologous Tissue Substitute, Posterior Approach, Posterior Column, Open Approach

HAC When reported with secondary diagnosis code K68.11, T81.40XA, T81.41XA, T81.42XA, T81.43XA, T81.44XA or T81.49XA, T84.60XA, T84.610A, T84.611A, T84.612A, T84.613A, T84.614A, T84.615A, T84.619A, T84.63XA, T84.69XA, T84.7XXA

0SG00KJ Fusion of Lumbar Vertebral Joint with Nonautologous Tissue Substitute, Posterior Approach, Anterior Column, Open Approach

HAC When reported with secondary diagnosis code K68.11, T81.40XA, T81.41XA, T81.42XA, T81.43XA, T81.44XA or T81.49XA, T84.60XA, T84.610A, T84.611A, T84.612A, T84.613A, T84.614A, T84.615A, T84.619A, T84.63XA, T84.69XA, T84.7XXA

0SG0370 Fusion of Lumbar Vertebral Joint with Autologous Tissue Substitute, Anterior Approach, Anterior Column, Percutaneous Approach

HAC When reported with secondary diagnosis code K68.11, T81.40XA, T81.41XA, T81.42XA, T81.43XA, T81.44XA or T81.49XA, T84.60XA, T84.610A, T84.611A, T84.612A, T84.613A, T84.614A, T84.615A, T84.619A, T84.63XA, T84.69XA, T84.7XXA

0SG0371 Fusion of Lumbar Vertebral Joint with Autologous Tissue Substitute, Posterior Approach, Posterior Column, Percutaneous Approach

HAC When reported with secondary diagnosis code K68.11, T81.40XA, T81.41XA, T81.42XA, T81.43XA, T81.44XA or T81.49XA, T84.60XA, T84.610A, T84.611A, T84.612A, T84.613A, T84.614A, T84.615A, T84.619A, T84.63XA, T84.69XA, T84.7XXA

0SG037J Fusion of Lumbar Vertebral Joint with Autologous Tissue Substitute, Posterior Approach, Anterior Column, Percutaneous Approach

HAC When reported with secondary diagnosis code K68.11, T81.40XA, T81.41XA, T81.42XA, T81.43XA, T81.44XA or T81.49XA, T84.60XA, T84.610A, T84.611A, T84.612A, T84.613A, T84.614A, T84.615A, T84.619A, T84.63XA, T84.69XA, T84.7XXA

0SG03A0 Fusion of Lumbar Vertebral Joint with Interbody Fusion Device, Anterior Approach, Anterior Column, Percutaneous Approach

HAC When reported with secondary diagnosis code K68.11, T81.40XA, T81.41XA, T81.42XA, T81.43XA, T81.44XA or T81.49XA, T84.60XA, T84.610A, T84.611A, T84.612A, T84.613A, T84.614A, T84.615A, T84.619A, T84.63XA, T84.69XA, T84.7XXA

0SG03AJ Fusion of Lumbar Vertebral Joint with Interbody Fusion Device, Posterior Approach, Anterior Column, Percutaneous Approach

HAC When reported with secondary diagnosis code K68.11, T81.40XA, T81.41XA, T81.42XA, T81.43XA, T81.44XA or T81.49XA, T84.60XA, T84.610A, T84.611A, T84.612A, T84.613A, T84.614A, T84.615A, T84.619A, T84.63XA, T84.69XA, T84.7XXA

0SG03J0 Fusion of Lumbar Vertebral Joint with Synthetic Substitute, Anterior Approach, Anterior Column, Percutaneous Approach

HAC When reported with secondary diagnosis code K68.11, T81.40XA, T81.41XA, T81.42XA, T81.43XA, T81.44XA or T81.49XA, T84.60XA, T84.610A, T84.611A, T84.612A, T84.613A, T84.614A, T84.615A, T84.619A, T84.63XA, T84.69XA, T84.7XXA

0SG03J1 Fusion of Lumbar Vertebral Joint with Synthetic Substitute, Posterior Approach, Posterior Column, Percutaneous Approach

HAC When reported with secondary diagnosis code K68.11, T81.40XA, T81.41XA, T81.42XA, T81.43XA, T81.44XA or T81.49XA, T84.60XA, T84.610A, T84.611A, T84.612A, T84.613A, T84.614A, T84.615A, T84.619A, T84.63XA, T84.69XA, T84.7XXA

0SG03JJ Fusion of Lumbar Vertebral Joint with Synthetic Substitute, Posterior Approach, Anterior Column, Percutaneous Approach

HAC When reported with secondary diagnosis code K68.11, T81.40XA, T81.41XA, T81.42XA, T81.43XA, T81.44XA or T81.49XA, T84.60XA, T84.610A, T84.611A, T84.612A, T84.613A, T84.614A, T84.615A, T84.619A, T84.63XA, T84.69XA, T84.7XXA

0SG03K0 Fusion of Lumbar Vertebral Joint with Nonautologous Tissue Substitute, Anterior Approach, Anterior Column, Percutaneous Approach

HAC When reported with secondary diagnosis code K68.11, T81.40XA, T81.41XA, T81.42XA, T81.43XA, T81.44XA or T81.49XA, T84.60XA, T84.610A, T84.611A, T84.612A, T84.613A, T84.614A, T84.615A, T84.619A, T84.63XA, T84.69XA, T84.7XXA

0SG03K1 Fusion of Lumbar Vertebral Joint with Nonautologous Tissue Substitute, Posterior Approach, Posterior Column, Percutaneous Approach

HAC When reported with secondary diagnosis code K68.11, T81.40XA, T81.41XA, T81.42XA, T81.43XA, T81.44XA or T81.49XA, T84.60XA, T84.610A, T84.611A, T84.612A, T84.613A, T84.614A, T84.615A, T84.619A, T84.63XA, T84.69XA, T84.7XXA

0SG03KJ Fusion of Lumbar Vertebral Joint with Nonautologous Tissue Substitute, Posterior Approach, Anterior Column, Percutaneous Approach

HAC When reported with secondary diagnosis code K68.11, T81.40XA, T81.41XA, T81.42XA, T81.43XA, T81.44XA or T81.49XA, T84.60XA, T84.610A, T84.611A, T84.612A, T84.613A, T84.614A, T84.615A, T84.619A, T84.63XA, T84.69XA, T84.7XXA

♀ Female-only   ♂ Male-only   ▲ Limited Coverage   ● Non-OR   HAC HAC-associated procedure   ▲ Non-covered procedures   ✚ Cluster

0SG0470 Fusion of Lumbar Vertebral Joint with Autologous Tissue Substitute, Anterior Approach, Anterior Column, Percutaneous Endoscopic Approach

HAC When reported with secondary diagnosis code K68.11, T81.40XA, T81.41XA, T81.42XA, T81.43XA, T81.44XA or T81.49XA, T84.60XA, T84.610A, T84.611A, T84.612A, T84.613A, T84.614A, T84.615A, T84.619A, T84.63XA, T84.69XA, T84.7XXA

0SG0471 Fusion of Lumbar Vertebral Joint with Autologous Tissue Substitute, Posterior Approach, Posterior Column, Percutaneous Endoscopic Approach

HAC When reported with secondary diagnosis code K68.11, T81.40XA, T81.41XA, T81.42XA, T81.43XA, T81.44XA or T81.49XA, T84.60XA, T84.610A, T84.611A, T84.612A, T84.613A, T84.614A, T84.615A, T84.619A, T84.63XA, T84.69XA, T84.7XXA

0SG047J Fusion of Lumbar Vertebral Joint with Autologous Tissue Substitute, Posterior Approach, Anterior Column, Percutaneous Endoscopic Approach

HAC When reported with secondary diagnosis code K68.11, T81.40XA, T81.41XA, T81.42XA, T81.43XA, T81.44XA or T81.49XA, T84.60XA, T84.610A, T84.611A, T84.612A, T84.613A, T84.614A, T84.615A, T84.619A, T84.63XA, T84.69XA, T84.7XXA

0SG04A0 Fusion of Lumbar Vertebral Joint with Interbody Fusion Device, Anterior Approach, Anterior Column, Percutaneous Endoscopic Approach

HAC When reported with secondary diagnosis code K68.11, T81.40XA, T81.41XA, T81.42XA, T81.43XA, T81.44XA or T81.49XA, T84.60XA, T84.610A, T84.611A, T84.612A, T84.613A, T84.614A, T84.615A, T84.619A, T84.63XA, T84.69XA, T84.7XXA

0SG04AJ Fusion of Lumbar Vertebral Joint with Interbody Fusion Device, Posterior Approach, Anterior Column, Percutaneous Endoscopic Approach

HAC When reported with secondary diagnosis code K68.11, T81.40XA, T81.41XA, T81.42XA, T81.43XA, T81.44XA or T81.49XA, T84.60XA, T84.610A, T84.611A, T84.612A, T84.613A, T84.614A, T84.615A, T84.619A, T84.63XA, T84.69XA, T84.7XXA

0SG04J0 Fusion of Lumbar Vertebral Joint with Synthetic Substitute, Anterior Approach, Anterior Column, Percutaneous Endoscopic Approach

HAC When reported with secondary diagnosis code K68.11, T81.40XA, T81.41XA, T81.42XA, T81.43XA, T81.44XA or T81.49XA, T84.60XA, T84.610A, T84.611A, T84.612A, T84.613A, T84.614A, T84.615A, T84.619A, T84.63XA, T84.69XA, T84.7XXA

0SG04J1 Fusion of Lumbar Vertebral Joint with Synthetic Substitute, Posterior Approach, Posterior Column, Percutaneous Endoscopic Approach

HAC When reported with secondary diagnosis code K68.11, T81.40XA, T81.41XA, T81.42XA, T81.43XA, T81.44XA or T81.49XA, T84.60XA, T84.610A, T84.611A, T84.612A, T84.613A, T84.614A, T84.615A, T84.619A, T84.63XA, T84.69XA, T84.7XXA

0SG04JJ Fusion of Lumbar Vertebral Joint with Synthetic Substitute, Posterior Approach, Anterior Column, Percutaneous Endoscopic Approach

HAC When reported with secondary diagnosis code K68.11, T81.40XA, T81.41XA, T81.42XA, T81.43XA, T81.44XA or T81.49XA, T84.60XA, T84.610A, T84.611A, T84.612A, T84.613A, T84.614A, T84.615A, T84.619A, T84.63XA, T84.69XA, T84.7XXA

0SG04K0 Fusion of Lumbar Vertebral Joint with Nonautologous Tissue Substitute, Anterior Approach, Anterior Column, Percutaneous Endoscopic Approach

HAC When reported with secondary diagnosis code K68.11, T81.40XA, T81.41XA, T81.42XA, T81.43XA, T81.44XA or T81.49XA, T84.60XA, T84.610A, T84.611A, T84.612A, T84.613A, T84.614A, T84.615A, T84.619A, T84.63XA, T84.69XA, T84.7XXA

0SG04K1 Fusion of Lumbar Vertebral Joint with Nonautologous Tissue Substitute, Posterior Approach, Posterior Column, Percutaneous Endoscopic Approach

HAC When reported with secondary diagnosis code K68.11, T81.40XA, T81.41XA, T81.42XA, T81.43XA, T81.44XA or T81.49XA, T84.60XA, T84.610A, T84.611A, T84.612A, T84.613A, T84.614A, T84.615A, T84.619A, T84.63XA, T84.69XA, T84.7XXA

0SG04KJ Fusion of Lumbar Vertebral Joint with Nonautologous Tissue Substitute, Posterior Approach, Anterior Column, Percutaneous Endoscopic Approach

HAC When reported with secondary diagnosis code K68.11, T81.40XA, T81.41XA, T81.42XA, T81.43XA, T81.44XA or T81.49XA, T84.60XA, T84.610A, T84.611A, T84.612A, T84.613A, T84.614A, T84.615A, T84.619A, T84.63XA, T84.69XA, T84.7XXA

0SG1070 Fusion of 2 or more Lumbar Vertebral Joints with Autologous Tissue Substitute, Anterior Approach, Anterior Column, Open Approach

HAC When reported with secondary diagnosis code K68.11, T81.40XA, T81.41XA, T81.42XA, T81.43XA, T81.44XA or T81.49XA, T84.60XA, T84.610A, T84.611A, T84.612A, T84.613A, T84.614A, T84.615A, T84.619A, T84.63XA, T84.69XA, T84.7XXA

0SG1071 Fusion of 2 or more Lumbar Vertebral Joints with Autologous Tissue Substitute, Posterior Approach, Posterior Column, Open Approach

HAC When reported with secondary diagnosis code K68.11, T81.40XA, T81.41XA, T81.42XA, T81.43XA, T81.44XA or T81.49XA, T84.60XA,

T84.610A, T84.611A, T84.612A, T84.613A, T84.614A, T84.615A, T84.619A, T84.63XA, T84.69XA, T84.7XXA

0SG107J Fusion of 2 or more Lumbar Vertebral Joints with Autologous Tissue Substitute, Posterior Approach, Anterior Column, Open Approach

AHA CC: 3Q, 2014, 36

HAC When reported with secondary diagnosis code K68.11, T81.40XA, T81.41XA, T81.42XA, T81.43XA, T81.44XA or T81.49XA, T84.60XA, T84.610A, T84.611A, T84.612A, T84.613A, T84.614A, T84.615A, T84.619A, T84.63XA, T84.69XA, T84.7XXA

0SG10A0 Fusion of 2 or more Lumbar Vertebral Joints with Interbody Fusion Device, Anterior Approach, Anterior Column, Open Approach

HAC When reported with secondary diagnosis code K68.11, T81.40XA, T81.41XA, T81.42XA, T81.43XA, T81.44XA or T81.49XA, T84.60XA, T84.610A, T84.611A, T84.612A, T84.613A, T84.614A, T84.615A, T84.619A, T84.63XA, T84.69XA, T84.7XXA

0SG10AJ Fusion of 2 or more Lumbar Vertebral Joints with Interbody Fusion Device, Posterior Approach, Anterior Column, Open Approach

HAC When reported with secondary diagnosis code K68.11, T81.40XA, T81.41XA, T81.42XA, T81.43XA, T81.44XA or T81.49XA, T84.60XA, T84.610A, T84.611A, T84.612A, T84.613A, T84.614A, T84.615A, T84.619A, T84.63XA, T84.69XA, T84.7XXA

0SG10J0 Fusion of 2 or more Lumbar Vertebral Joints with Synthetic Substitute, Anterior Approach, Anterior Column, Open Approach

HAC When reported with secondary diagnosis code K68.11, T81.40XA, T81.41XA, T81.42XA, T81.43XA, T81.44XA or T81.49XA, T84.60XA, T84.610A, T84.611A, T84.612A, T84.613A, T84.614A, T84.615A, T84.619A, T84.63XA, T84.69XA, T84.7XXA

0SG10J1 Fusion of 2 or more Lumbar Vertebral Joints with Synthetic Substitute, Posterior Approach, Posterior Column, Open Approach

HAC When reported with secondary diagnosis code K68.11, T81.40XA, T81.41XA, T81.42XA, T81.43XA, T81.44XA or T81.49XA, T84.60XA, T84.610A, T84.611A, T84.612A, T84.613A, T84.614A, T84.615A, T84.619A, T84.63XA, T84.69XA, T84.7XXA

0SG10JJ Fusion of 2 or more Lumbar Vertebral Joints with Synthetic Substitute, Posterior Approach, Anterior Column, Open Approach

HAC When reported with secondary diagnosis code K68.11, T81.40XA, T81.41XA, T81.42XA, T81.43XA, T81.44XA or T81.49XA, T84.60XA, T84.610A, T84.611A, T84.612A, T84.613A, T84.614A, T84.615A, T84.619A, T84.63XA, T84.69XA, T84.7XXA

0SG10K0 Fusion of 2 or more Lumbar Vertebral Joints with Nonautologous Tissue Substitute, Anterior Approach, Anterior Column, Open Approach

HAC When reported with secondary diagnosis code K68.11, T81.40XA, T81.41XA, T81.42XA, T81.43XA, T81.44XA or T81.49XA, T84.60XA, T84.610A, T84.611A, T84.612A, T84.613A, T84.614A, T84.615A, T84.619A, T84.63XA, T84.69XA, T84.7XXA

0SG10K1 Fusion of 2 or more Lumbar Vertebral Joints with Nonautologous Tissue Substitute, Posterior Approach, Posterior Column, Open Approach

HAC When reported with secondary diagnosis code K68.11, T81.40XA, T81.41XA, T81.42XA, T81.43XA, T81.44XA or T81.49XA, T84.60XA, T84.610A, T84.611A, T84.612A, T84.613A, T84.614A, T84.615A, T84.619A, T84.63XA, T84.69XA, T84.7XXA

0SG10KJ Fusion of 2 or more Lumbar Vertebral Joints with Nonautologous Tissue Substitute, Posterior Approach, Anterior Column, Open Approach

HAC When reported with secondary diagnosis code K68.11, T81.40XA, T81.41XA, T81.42XA, T81.43XA, T81.44XA or T81.49XA, T84.60XA, T84.610A, T84.611A, T84.612A, T84.613A, T84.614A, T84.615A, T84.619A, T84.63XA, T84.69XA, T84.7XXA

0SG1370 Fusion of 2 or more Lumbar Vertebral Joints with Autologous Tissue Substitute, Anterior Approach, Anterior Column, Percutaneous Approach

HAC When reported with secondary diagnosis code K68.11, T81.40XA, T81.41XA, T81.42XA, T81.43XA, T81.44XA or T81.49XA, T84.60XA, T84.610A, T84.611A, T84.612A, T84.613A, T84.614A, T84.615A, T84.619A, T84.63XA, T84.69XA, T84.7XXA

0SG1371 Fusion of 2 or more Lumbar Vertebral Joints with Autologous Tissue Substitute, Posterior Approach, Posterior Column, Percutaneous Approach

HAC When reported with secondary diagnosis code K68.11, T81.40XA, T81.41XA, T81.42XA, T81.43XA, T81.44XA or T81.49XA, T84.60XA, T84.610A, T84.611A, T84.612A, T84.613A, T84.614A, T84.615A, T84.619A, T84.63XA, T84.69XA, T84.7XXA

0SG137J Fusion of 2 or more Lumbar Vertebral Joints with Autologous Tissue Substitute, Posterior Approach, Anterior Column, Percutaneous Approach

HAC When reported with secondary diagnosis code K68.11, T81.40XA, T81.41XA, T81.42XA, T81.43XA, T81.44XA or T81.49XA, T84.60XA, T84.610A, T84.611A, T84.612A, T84.613A, T84.614A, T84.615A, T84.619A, T84.63XA, T84.69XA, T84.7XXA

0SG13A0 Fusion of 2 or more Lumbar Vertebral Joints with Interbody Fusion Device, Anterior Approach, Anterior Column, Percutaneous Approach

HAC When reported with secondary diagnosis code K68.11, T81.40XA, T81.41XA, T81.42XA, T81.43XA, T81.44XA or T81.49XA, T84.60XA, T84.610A, T84.611A, T84.612A, T84.613A, T84.614A, T84.615A, T84.619A, T84.63XA, T84.69XA, T84.7XXA

0SG13AJ Fusion of 2 or more Lumbar Vertebral Joints with Interbody Fusion Device, Posterior Approach, Anterior Column, Percutaneous Approach

HAC When reported with secondary diagnosis code K68.11, T81.40XA, T81.41XA, T81.42XA, T81.43XA, T81.44XA or T81.49XA, T84.60XA, T84.610A, T84.611A, T84.612A, T84.613A, T84.614A, T84.615A, T84.619A, T84.63XA, T84.69XA, T84.7XXA

0SG13J0 Fusion of 2 or more Lumbar Vertebral Joints with Synthetic Substitute, Anterior Approach, Anterior Column, Percutaneous Approach

HAC When reported with secondary diagnosis code K68.11, T81.40XA, T81.41XA, T81.42XA, T81.43XA, T81.44XA or T81.49XA, T84.60XA, T84.610A, T84.611A, T84.612A, T84.613A, T84.614A, T84.615A, T84.619A, T84.63XA, T84.69XA, T84.7XXA

0SG13J1 Fusion of 2 or more Lumbar Vertebral Joints with Synthetic Substitute, Posterior Approach, Posterior Column, Percutaneous Approach

HAC When reported with secondary diagnosis code K68.11, T81.40XA, T81.41XA, T81.42XA, T81.43XA, T81.44XA or T81.49XA, T84.60XA, T84.610A, T84.611A, T84.612A, T84.613A, T84.614A, T84.615A, T84.619A, T84.63XA, T84.69XA, T84.7XXA

0SG13JJ Fusion of 2 or more Lumbar Vertebral Joints with Synthetic Substitute, Posterior Approach, Anterior Column, Percutaneous Approach

HAC When reported with secondary diagnosis code K68.11, T81.40XA, T81.41XA, T81.42XA, T81.43XA, T81.44XA or T81.49XA, T84.60XA, T84.610A, T84.611A, T84.612A, T84.613A, T84.614A, T84.615A, T84.619A, T84.63XA, T84.69XA, T84.7XXA

0SG13K0 Fusion of 2 or more Lumbar Vertebral Joints with Nonautologous Tissue Substitute, Anterior Approach, Anterior Column, Percutaneous Approach

HAC When reported with secondary diagnosis code K68.11, T81.40XA, T81.41XA, T81.42XA, T81.43XA, T81.44XA or T81.49XA, T84.60XA, T84.610A, T84.611A, T84.612A, T84.613A, T84.614A, T84.615A, T84.619A, T84.63XA, T84.69XA, T84.7XXA

0SG13K1 Fusion of 2 or more Lumbar Vertebral Joints with Nonautologous Tissue Substitute, Posterior Approach, Posterior Column, Percutaneous Approach

HAC When reported with secondary diagnosis code K68.11, T81.40XA, T81.41XA, T81.42XA, T81.43XA, T81.44XA or T81.49XA, T84.60XA, T84.610A, T84.611A, T84.612A, T84.613A, T84.614A, T84.615A, T84.619A, T84.63XA, T84.69XA, T84.7XXA

0SG13KJ Fusion of 2 or more Lumbar Vertebral Joints with Nonautologous Tissue Substitute, Posterior Approach, Anterior Column, Percutaneous Approach

HAC When reported with secondary diagnosis code K68.11, T81.40XA, T81.41XA, T81.42XA, T81.43XA, T81.44XA or T81.49XA, T84.60XA, T84.610A, T84.611A, T84.612A, T84.613A, T84.614A, T84.615A, T84.619A, T84.63XA, T84.69XA, T84.7XXA

0SG1470 Fusion of 2 or more Lumbar Vertebral Joints with Autologous Tissue Substitute, Anterior Approach, Anterior Column, Percutaneous Endoscopic Approach

HAC When reported with secondary diagnosis code K68.11, T81.40XA, T81.41XA, T81.42XA, T81.43XA, T81.44XA or T81.49XA, T84.60XA, T84.610A, T84.611A, T84.612A, T84.613A, T84.614A, T84.615A, T84.619A, T84.63XA, T84.69XA, T84.7XXA

0SG1471 Fusion of 2 or more Lumbar Vertebral Joints with Autologous Tissue Substitute, Posterior Approach, Posterior Column, Percutaneous Endoscopic Approach

HAC When reported with secondary diagnosis code K68.11, T81.40XA, T81.41XA, T81.42XA, T81.43XA, T81.44XA or T81.49XA, T84.60XA, T84.610A, T84.611A, T84.612A, T84.613A, T84.614A, T84.615A, T84.619A, T84.63XA, T84.69XA, T84.7XXA

0SG147J Fusion of 2 or more Lumbar Vertebral Joints with Autologous Tissue Substitute, Posterior Approach, Anterior Column, Percutaneous Endoscopic Approach

HAC When reported with secondary diagnosis code K68.11, T81.40XA, T81.41XA, T81.42XA, T81.43XA, T81.44XA or T81.49XA, T84.60XA, T84.610A, T84.611A, T84.612A, T84.613A, T84.614A, T84.615A, T84.619A, T84.63XA, T84.69XA, T84.7XXA

0SG14A0 Fusion of 2 or more Lumbar Vertebral Joints with Interbody Fusion Device, Anterior Approach, Anterior Column, Percutaneous Endoscopic Approach

HAC When reported with secondary diagnosis code K68.11, T81.40XA, T81.41XA, T81.42XA, T81.43XA, T81.44XA or T81.49XA, T84.60XA, T84.610A, T84.611A, T84.612A, T84.613A, T84.614A, T84.615A, T84.619A, T84.63XA, T84.69XA, T84.7XXA

0SG14AJ Fusion of 2 or more Lumbar Vertebral Joints with Interbody Fusion Device, Posterior Approach, Anterior Column, Percutaneous Endoscopic Approach

♀ Female-only   ♂ Male-only   ▲ Limited Coverage   ● Non-OR   HAC HAC-associated procedure   ▲ Non-covered procedures   ✚ Cluster

[HAC] When reported with secondary diagnosis code K68.11, T81.40XA, T81.41XA, T81.42XA, T81.43XA, T81.44XA or T81.49XA, T84.60XA, T84.610A, T84.611A, T84.612A, T84.613A, T84.614A, T84.615A, T84.619A, T84.63XA, T84.69XA, T84.7XXA

0SG14J0 Fusion of 2 or more Lumbar Vertebral Joints with Synthetic Substitute, Anterior Approach, Anterior Column, Percutaneous Endoscopic Approach

[HAC] When reported with secondary diagnosis code K68.11, T81.40XA, T81.41XA, T81.42XA, T81.43XA, T81.44XA or T81.49XA, T84.60XA, T84.610A, T84.611A, T84.612A, T84.613A, T84.614A, T84.615A, T84.619A, T84.63XA, T84.69XA, T84.7XXA

0SG14J1 Fusion of 2 or more Lumbar Vertebral Joints with Synthetic Substitute, Posterior Approach, Posterior Column, Percutaneous Endoscopic Approach

[HAC] When reported with secondary diagnosis code K68.11, T81.40XA, T81.41XA, T81.42XA, T81.43XA, T81.44XA or T81.49XA, T84.60XA, T84.610A, T84.611A, T84.612A, T84.613A, T84.614A, T84.615A, T84.619A, T84.63XA, T84.69XA, T84.7XXA

0SG14JJ Fusion of 2 or more Lumbar Vertebral Joints with Synthetic Substitute, Posterior Approach, Anterior Column, Percutaneous Endoscopic Approach

[HAC] When reported with secondary diagnosis code K68.11, T81.40XA, T81.41XA, T81.42XA, T81.43XA, T81.44XA or T81.49XA, T84.60XA, T84.610A, T84.611A, T84.612A, T84.613A, T84.614A, T84.615A, T84.619A, T84.63XA, T84.69XA, T84.7XXA

0SG14K0 Fusion of 2 or more Lumbar Vertebral Joints with Nonautologous Tissue Substitute, Anterior Approach, Anterior Column, Percutaneous Endoscopic Approach

[HAC] When reported with secondary diagnosis code K68.11, T81.40XA, T81.41XA, T81.42XA, T81.43XA, T81.44XA or T81.49XA, T84.60XA, T84.610A, T84.611A, T84.612A, T84.613A, T84.614A, T84.615A, T84.619A, T84.63XA, T84.69XA, T84.7XXA

0SG14K1 Fusion of 2 or more Lumbar Vertebral Joints with Nonautologous Tissue Substitute, Posterior Approach, Posterior Column, Percutaneous Endoscopic Approach

[HAC] When reported with secondary diagnosis code K68.11, T81.40XA, T81.41XA, T81.42XA, T81.43XA, T81.44XA or T81.49XA, T84.60XA, T84.610A, T84.611A, T84.612A, T84.613A, T84.614A, T84.615A, T84.619A, T84.63XA, T84.69XA, T84.7XXA

0SG14KJ Fusion of 2 or more Lumbar Vertebral Joints with Nonautologous Tissue Substitute, Posterior Approach, Anterior Column, Percutaneous Endoscopic Approach

[HAC] When reported with secondary diagnosis code K68.11, T81.40XA, T81.41XA, T81.42XA, T81.43XA, T81.44XA or T81.49XA, T84.60XA, T84.610A, T84.611A, T84.612A, T84.613A, T84.614A, T84.615A, T84.619A, T84.63XA, T84.69XA, T84.7XXA

0SG3070 Fusion of Lumbosacral Joint with Autologous Tissue Substitute, Anterior Approach, Anterior Column, Open Approach

[HAC] When reported with secondary diagnosis code K68.11, T81.40XA, T81.41XA, T81.42XA, T81.43XA, T81.44XA or T81.49XA, T84.60XA, T84.610A, T84.611A, T84.612A, T84.613A, T84.614A, T84.615A, T84.619A, T84.63XA, T84.69XA, T84.7XXA

0SG3071 Fusion of Lumbosacral Joint with Autologous Tissue Substitute, Posterior Approach, Posterior Column, Open Approach

[HAC] When reported with secondary diagnosis code K68.11, T81.40XA, T81.41XA, T81.42XA, T81.43XA, T81.44XA or T81.49XA, T84.60XA, T84.610A, T84.611A, T84.612A, T84.613A, T84.614A, T84.615A, T84.619A, T84.63XA, T84.69XA, T84.7XXA

0SG307J Fusion of Lumbosacral Joint with Autologous Tissue Substitute, Posterior Approach, Anterior Column, Open Approach

[HAC] When reported with secondary diagnosis code K68.11, T81.40XA, T81.41XA, T81.42XA, T81.43XA, T81.44XA or T81.49XA, T84.60XA, T84.610A, T84.611A, T84.612A, T84.613A, T84.614A, T84.615A, T84.619A, T84.63XA, T84.69XA, T84.7XXA

0SG30A0 Fusion of Lumbosacral Joint with Interbody Fusion Device, Anterior Approach, Anterior Column, Open Approach

[HAC] When reported with secondary diagnosis code K68.11, T81.40XA, T81.41XA, T81.42XA, T81.43XA, T81.44XA or T81.49XA, T84.60XA, T84.610A, T84.611A, T84.612A, T84.613A, T84.614A, T84.615A, T84.619A, T84.63XA, T84.69XA, T84.7XXA

0SG30AJ Fusion of Lumbosacral Joint with Interbody Fusion Device, Posterior Approach, Anterior Column, Open Approach

[HAC] When reported with secondary diagnosis code K68.11, T81.40XA, T81.41XA, T81.42XA, T81.43XA, T81.44XA or T81.49XA, T84.60XA, T84.610A, T84.611A, T84.612A, T84.613A, T84.614A, T84.615A, T84.619A, T84.63XA, T84.69XA, T84.7XXA

0SG30J0 Fusion of Lumbosacral Joint with Synthetic Substitute, Anterior Approach, Anterior Column, Open Approach

[HAC] When reported with secondary diagnosis code K68.11, T81.40XA, T81.41XA, T81.42XA, T81.43XA, T81.44XA or T81.49XA, T84.60XA,

T84.610A, T84.611A, T84.612A, T84.613A, T84.614A, T84.615A, T84.619A, T84.63XA, T84.69XA, T84.7XXA

0SG30J1 Fusion of Lumbosacral Joint with Synthetic Substitute, Posterior Approach, Posterior Column, Open Approach

[HAC] When reported with secondary diagnosis code K68.11, T81.40XA, T81.41XA, T81.42XA, T81.43XA, T81.44XA or T81.49XA, T84.60XA, T84.610A, T84.611A, T84.612A, T84.613A, T84.614A, T84.615A, T84.619A, T84.63XA, T84.69XA, T84.7XXA

0SG30JJ Fusion of Lumbosacral Joint with Synthetic Substitute, Posterior Approach, Anterior Column, Open Approach

[HAC] When reported with secondary diagnosis code K68.11, T81.40XA, T81.41XA, T81.42XA, T81.43XA, T81.44XA or T81.49XA, T84.60XA, T84.610A, T84.611A, T84.612A, T84.613A, T84.614A, T84.615A, T84.619A, T84.63XA, T84.69XA, T84.7XXA

0SG30K0 Fusion of Lumbosacral Joint with Nonautologous Tissue Substitute, Anterior Approach, Anterior Column, Open Approach

[HAC] When reported with secondary diagnosis code K68.11, T81.40XA, T81.41XA, T81.42XA, T81.43XA, T81.44XA or T81.49XA, T84.60XA, T84.610A, T84.611A, T84.612A, T84.613A, T84.614A, T84.615A, T84.619A, T84.63XA, T84.69XA, T84.7XXA

0SG30K1 Fusion of Lumbosacral Joint with Nonautologous Tissue Substitute, Posterior Approach, Posterior Column, Open Approach

[HAC] When reported with secondary diagnosis code K68.11, T81.40XA, T81.41XA, T81.42XA, T81.43XA, T81.44XA or T81.49XA, T84.60XA, T84.610A, T84.611A, T84.612A, T84.613A, T84.614A, T84.615A, T84.619A, T84.63XA, T84.69XA, T84.7XXA

0SG30KJ Fusion of Lumbosacral Joint with Nonautologous Tissue Substitute, Posterior Approach, Anterior Column, Open Approach

[HAC] When reported with secondary diagnosis code K68.11, T81.40XA, T81.41XA, T81.42XA, T81.43XA, T81.44XA or T81.49XA, T84.60XA, T84.610A, T84.611A, T84.612A, T84.613A, T84.614A, T84.615A, T84.619A, T84.63XA, T84.69XA, T84.7XXA

0SG3370 Fusion of Lumbosacral Joint with Autologous Tissue Substitute, Anterior Approach, Anterior Column, Percutaneous Approach

[HAC] When reported with secondary diagnosis code K68.11, T81.40XA, T81.41XA, T81.42XA, T81.43XA, T81.44XA or T81.49XA, T84.60XA, T84.610A, T84.611A, T84.612A, T84.613A, T84.614A, T84.615A, T84.619A, T84.63XA, T84.69XA, T84.7XXA

♀ Female-only   ♂ Male-only   ▲ Limited Coverage   ● Non-OR   [HAC] HAC-associated procedure   ▲ Non-covered procedures   ✚ Cluster

0SG3371 Fusion of Lumbosacral Joint with Autologous Tissue Substitute, Posterior Approach, Posterior Column, Percutaneous Approach

HAC When reported with secondary diagnosis code K68.11, T81.40XA, T81.41XA, T81.42XA, T81.43XA, T81.44XA or T81.49XA, T84.60XA, T84.610A, T84.611A, T84.612A, T84.613A, T84.614A, T84.615A, T84.619A, T84.63XA, T84.69XA, T84.7XXA

0SG337J Fusion of Lumbosacral Joint with Autologous Tissue Substitute, Posterior Approach, Anterior Column, Percutaneous Approach

HAC When reported with secondary diagnosis code K68.11, T81.40XA, T81.41XA, T81.42XA, T81.43XA, T81.44XA or T81.49XA, T84.60XA, T84.610A, T84.611A, T84.612A, T84.613A, T84.614A, T84.615A, T84.619A, T84.63XA, T84.69XA, T84.7XXA

0SG33A0 Fusion of Lumbosacral Joint with Interbody Fusion Device, Anterior Approach, Anterior Column, Percutaneous Approach

HAC When reported with secondary diagnosis code K68.11, T81.40XA, T81.41XA, T81.42XA, T81.43XA, T81.44XA or T81.49XA, T84.60XA, T84.610A, T84.611A, T84.612A, T84.613A, T84.614A, T84.615A, T84.619A, T84.63XA, T84.69XA, T84.7XXA

0SG33AJ Fusion of Lumbosacral Joint with Interbody Fusion Device, Posterior Approach, Anterior Column, Percutaneous Approach

HAC When reported with secondary diagnosis code K68.11, T81.40XA, T81.41XA, T81.42XA, T81.43XA, T81.44XA or T81.49XA, T84.60XA, T84.610A, T84.611A, T84.612A, T84.613A, T84.614A, T84.615A, T84.619A, T84.63XA, T84.69XA, T84.7XXA

0SG33J0 Fusion of Lumbosacral Joint with Synthetic Substitute, Anterior Approach, Anterior Column, Percutaneous Approach

HAC When reported with secondary diagnosis code K68.11, T81.40XA, T81.41XA, T81.42XA, T81.43XA, T81.44XA or T81.49XA, T84.60XA, T84.610A, T84.611A, T84.612A, T84.613A, T84.614A, T84.615A, T84.619A, T84.63XA, T84.69XA, T84.7XXA

0SG33J1 Fusion of Lumbosacral Joint with Synthetic Substitute, Posterior Approach, Posterior Column, Percutaneous Approach

HAC When reported with secondary diagnosis code K68.11, T81.40XA, T81.41XA, T81.42XA, T81.43XA, T81.44XA or T81.49XA, T84.60XA, T84.610A, T84.611A, T84.612A, T84.613A, T84.614A, T84.615A, T84.619A, T84.63XA, T84.69XA, T84.7XXA

0SG33JJ Fusion of Lumbosacral Joint with Synthetic Substitute, Posterior Approach, Anterior Column, Percutaneous Approach

HAC When reported with secondary diagnosis code K68.11, T81.40XA, T81.41XA, T81.42XA, T81.43XA, T81.44XA or T81.49XA, T84.60XA, T84.610A, T84.611A, T84.612A, T84.613A, T84.614A, T84.615A, T84.619A, T84.63XA, T84.69XA, T84.7XXA

0SG33K0 Fusion of Lumbosacral Joint with Nonautologous Tissue Substitute, Anterior Approach, Anterior Column, Percutaneous Approach

HAC When reported with secondary diagnosis code K68.11, T81.40XA, T81.41XA, T81.42XA, T81.43XA, T81.44XA or T81.49XA, T84.60XA, T84.610A, T84.611A, T84.612A, T84.613A, T84.614A, T84.615A, T84.619A, T84.63XA, T84.69XA, T84.7XXA

0SG33K1 Fusion of Lumbosacral Joint with Nonautologous Tissue Substitute, Posterior Approach, Posterior Column, Percutaneous Approach

HAC When reported with secondary diagnosis code K68.11, T81.40XA, T81.41XA, T81.42XA, T81.43XA, T81.44XA or T81.49XA, T84.60XA, T84.610A, T84.611A, T84.612A, T84.613A, T84.614A, T84.615A, T84.619A, T84.63XA, T84.69XA, T84.7XXA

0SG33KJ Fusion of Lumbosacral Joint with Nonautologous Tissue Substitute, Posterior Approach, Anterior Column, Percutaneous Approach

HAC When reported with secondary diagnosis code K68.11, T81.40XA, T81.41XA, T81.42XA, T81.43XA, T81.44XA or T81.49XA, T84.60XA, T84.610A, T84.611A, T84.612A, T84.613A, T84.614A, T84.615A, T84.619A, T84.63XA, T84.69XA, T84.7XXA

0SG3470 Fusion of Lumbosacral Joint with Autologous Tissue Substitute, Anterior Approach, Anterior Column, Percutaneous Endoscopic Approach

HAC When reported with secondary diagnosis code K68.11, T81.40XA, T81.41XA, T81.42XA, T81.43XA, T81.44XA or T81.49XA, T84.60XA, T84.610A, T84.611A, T84.612A, T84.613A, T84.614A, T84.615A, T84.619A, T84.63XA, T84.69XA, T84.7XXA

0SG3471 Fusion of Lumbosacral Joint with Autologous Tissue Substitute, Posterior Approach, Posterior Column, Percutaneous Endoscopic Approach

HAC When reported with secondary diagnosis code K68.11, T81.40XA, T81.41XA, T81.42XA, T81.43XA, T81.44XA or T81.49XA, T84.60XA, T84.610A, T84.611A, T84.612A, T84.613A, T84.614A, T84.615A, T84.619A, T84.63XA, T84.69XA, T84.7XXA

0SG347J Fusion of Lumbosacral Joint with Autologous Tissue Substitute, Posterior Approach, Anterior Column, Percutaneous Endoscopic Approach

HAC When reported with secondary diagnosis code K68.11, T81.40XA, T81.41XA, T81.42XA, T81.43XA, T81.44XA or T81.49XA, T84.60XA, T84.610A, T84.611A, T84.612A, T84.613A, T84.614A, T84.615A, T84.619A, T84.63XA, T84.69XA, T84.7XXA

0SG34A0 Fusion of Lumbosacral Joint with Interbody Fusion Device, Anterior Approach, Anterior Column, Percutaneous Endoscopic Approach

HAC When reported with secondary diagnosis code K68.11, T81.40XA, T81.41XA, T81.42XA, T81.43XA, T81.44XA or T81.49XA, T84.60XA, T84.610A, T84.611A, T84.612A, T84.613A, T84.614A, T84.615A, T84.619A, T84.63XA, T84.69XA, T84.7XXA

0SG34AJ Fusion of Lumbosacral Joint with Interbody Fusion Device, Posterior Approach, Anterior Column, Percutaneous Endoscopic Approach

HAC When reported with secondary diagnosis code K68.11, T81.40XA, T81.41XA, T81.42XA, T81.43XA, T81.44XA or T81.49XA, T84.60XA, T84.610A, T84.611A, T84.612A, T84.613A, T84.614A, T84.615A, T84.619A, T84.63XA, T84.69XA, T84.7XXA

0SG34J0 Fusion of Lumbosacral Joint with Synthetic Substitute, Anterior Approach, Anterior Column, Percutaneous Endoscopic Approach

HAC When reported with secondary diagnosis code K68.11, T81.40XA, T81.41XA, T81.42XA, T81.43XA, T81.44XA or T81.49XA, T84.60XA, T84.610A, T84.611A, T84.612A, T84.613A, T84.614A, T84.615A, T84.619A, T84.63XA, T84.69XA, T84.7XXA

0SG34J1 Fusion of Lumbosacral Joint with Synthetic Substitute, Posterior Approach, Posterior Column, Percutaneous Endoscopic Approach

HAC When reported with secondary diagnosis code K68.11, T81.40XA, T81.41XA, T81.42XA, T81.43XA, T81.44XA or T81.49XA, T84.60XA, T84.610A, T84.611A, T84.612A, T84.613A, T84.614A, T84.615A, T84.619A, T84.63XA, T84.69XA, T84.7XXA

0SG34JJ Fusion of Lumbosacral Joint with Synthetic Substitute, Posterior Approach, Anterior Column, Percutaneous Endoscopic Approach

HAC When reported with secondary diagnosis code K68.11, T81.40XA, T81.41XA, T81.42XA, T81.43XA, T81.44XA or T81.49XA, T84.60XA, T84.610A, T84.611A, T84.612A, T84.613A, T84.614A, T84.615A, T84.619A, T84.63XA, T84.69XA, T84.7XXA

0SG34K0 Fusion of Lumbosacral Joint with Nonautologous Tissue Substitute, Anterior Approach, Anterior Column, Percutaneous Endoscopic Approach

HAC When reported with secondary diagnosis code K68.11, T81.40XA, T81.41XA, T81.42XA, T81.43XA, T81.44XA or T81.49XA, T84.60XA, T84.610A, T84.611A, T84.612A, T84.613A, T84.614A, T84.615A, T84.619A, T84.63XA, T84.69XA, T84.7XXA

♀ Female-only ♂ Male-only ▲ Limited Coverage ● Non-OR HAC HAC-associated procedure ▲ Non-covered procedures ✚ Cluster

0SG34K1 Fusion of Lumbosacral Joint with Nonautologous Tissue Substitute, Posterior Approach, Posterior Column, Percutaneous Endoscopic Approach

HAC When reported with secondary diagnosis code K68.11, T81.40XA, T81.41XA, T81.42XA, T81.43XA, T81.44XA or T81.49XA, T84.60XA, T84.610A, T84.611A, T84.612A, T84.613A, T84.614A, T84.615A, T84.619A, T84.63XA, T84.69XA, T84.7XXA

0SG34KJ Fusion of Lumbosacral Joint with Nonautologous Tissue Substitute, Posterior Approach, Anterior Column, Percutaneous Endoscopic Approach

HAC When reported with secondary diagnosis code K68.11, T81.40XA, T81.41XA, T81.42XA, T81.43XA, T81.44XA or T81.49XA, T84.60XA, T84.610A, T84.611A, T84.612A, T84.613A, T84.614A, T84.615A, T84.619A, T84.63XA, T84.69XA, T84.7XXA

0SG504Z Fusion of Sacrococcygeal Joint with Internal Fixation Device, Open Approach

0SG507Z Fusion of Sacrococcygeal Joint with Autologous Tissue Substitute, Open Approach

0SG50JZ Fusion of Sacrococcygeal Joint with Synthetic Substitute, Open Approach

0SG50KZ Fusion of Sacrococcygeal Joint with Nonautologous Tissue Substitute, Open Approach

0SG534Z Fusion of Sacrococcygeal Joint with Internal Fixation Device, Percutaneous Approach

0SG537Z Fusion of Sacrococcygeal Joint with Autologous Tissue Substitute, Percutaneous Approach

0SG53JZ Fusion of Sacrococcygeal Joint with Synthetic Substitute, Percutaneous Approach

0SG53KZ Fusion of Sacrococcygeal Joint with Nonautologous Tissue Substitute, Percutaneous Approach

0SG544Z Fusion of Sacrococcygeal Joint with Internal Fixation Device, Percutaneous Endoscopic Approach

0SG547Z Fusion of Sacrococcygeal Joint with Autologous Tissue Substitute, Percutaneous Endoscopic Approach

0SG54JZ Fusion of Sacrococcygeal Joint with Synthetic Substitute, Percutaneous Endoscopic Approach

0SG54KZ Fusion of Sacrococcygeal Joint with Nonautologous Tissue Substitute, Percutaneous Endoscopic Approach

0SG604Z Fusion of Coccygeal Joint with Internal Fixation Device, Open Approach

0SG607Z Fusion of Coccygeal Joint with Autologous Tissue Substitute, Open Approach

0SG60JZ Fusion of Coccygeal Joint with Synthetic Substitute, Open Approach

0SG60KZ Fusion of Coccygeal Joint with Nonautologous Tissue Substitute, Open Approach

0SG634Z Fusion of Coccygeal Joint with Internal Fixation Device, Percutaneous Approach

0SG637Z Fusion of Coccygeal Joint with Autologous Tissue Substitute, Percutaneous Approach

0SG63JZ Fusion of Coccygeal Joint with Synthetic Substitute, Percutaneous Approach

0SG63KZ Fusion of Coccygeal Joint with Nonautologous Tissue Substitute, Percutaneous Approach

0SG644Z Fusion of Coccygeal Joint with Internal Fixation Device, Percutaneous Endoscopic Approach

0SG647Z Fusion of Coccygeal Joint with Autologous Tissue Substitute, Percutaneous Endoscopic Approach

0SG64JZ Fusion of Coccygeal Joint with Synthetic Substitute, Percutaneous Endoscopic Approach

0SG64KZ Fusion of Coccygeal Joint with Nonautologous Tissue Substitute, Percutaneous Endoscopic Approach

0SG704Z Fusion of Right Sacroiliac Joint with Internal Fixation Device, Open Approach

HAC When reported with secondary diagnosis code K68.11, T81.40XA, T81.41XA, T81.42XA, T81.43XA, T81.44XA or T81.49XA, T84.60XA, T84.610A, T84.611A, T84.612A, T84.613A, T84.614A, T84.615A, T84.619A, T84.63XA, T84.69XA, T84.7XXA

0SG707Z Fusion of Right Sacroiliac Joint with Autologous Tissue Substitute, Open Approach

HAC When reported with secondary diagnosis code K68.11, T81.40XA, T81.41XA, T81.42XA, T81.43XA, T81.44XA or T81.49XA, T84.60XA, T84.610A, T84.611A, T84.612A, T84.613A, T84.614A, T84.615A, T84.619A, T84.63XA, T84.69XA, T84.7XXA

0SG70JZ Fusion of Right Sacroiliac Joint with Synthetic Substitute, Open Approach

HAC When reported with secondary diagnosis code K68.11, T81.40XA, T81.41XA, T81.42XA, T81.43XA, T81.44XA or T81.49XA, T84.60XA, T84.610A, T84.611A, T84.612A, T84.613A, T84.614A, T84.615A, T84.619A, T84.63XA, T84.69XA, T84.7XXA

0SG70KZ Fusion of Right Sacroiliac Joint with Nonautologous Tissue Substitute, Open Approach

HAC When reported with secondary diagnosis code K68.11, T81.40XA, T81.41XA, T81.42XA, T81.43XA, T81.44XA or T81.49XA, T84.60XA, T84.610A, T84.611A, T84.612A, T84.613A, T84.614A, T84.615A, T84.619A, T84.63XA, T84.69XA, T84.7XXA

0SG734Z Fusion of Right Sacroiliac Joint with Internal Fixation Device, Percutaneous Approach

HAC When reported with secondary diagnosis code K68.11, T81.40XA, T81.41XA, T81.42XA, T81.43XA, T81.44XA or T81.49XA, T84.60XA, T84.610A, T84.611A, T84.612A, T84.613A, T84.614A, T84.615A, T84.619A, T84.63XA, T84.69XA, T84.7XXA

0SG737Z Fusion of Right Sacroiliac Joint with Autologous Tissue Substitute, Percutaneous Approach

HAC When reported with secondary diagnosis code K68.11, T81.40XA, T81.41XA, T81.42XA, T81.43XA, T81.44XA or T81.49XA, T84.60XA, T84.610A, T84.611A, T84.612A, T84.613A, T84.614A, T84.615A, T84.619A, T84.63XA, T84.69XA, T84.7XXA

0SG73JZ Fusion of Right Sacroiliac Joint with Synthetic Substitute, Percutaneous Approach

HAC When reported with secondary diagnosis code K68.11, T81.40XA, T81.41XA, T81.42XA, T81.43XA, T81.44XA or T81.49XA, T84.60XA, T84.610A, T84.611A, T84.612A, T84.613A, T84.614A, T84.615A, T84.619A, T84.63XA, T84.69XA, T84.7XXA

0SG73KZ Fusion of Right Sacroiliac Joint with Nonautologous Tissue Substitute, Percutaneous Approach

HAC When reported with secondary diagnosis code K68.11, T81.40XA, T81.41XA, T81.42XA, T81.43XA, T81.44XA or T81.49XA, T84.60XA, T84.610A, T84.611A, T84.612A, T84.613A, T84.614A, T84.615A, T84.619A, T84.63XA, T84.69XA, T84.7XXA

0SG744Z Fusion of Right Sacroiliac Joint with Internal Fixation Device, Percutaneous Endoscopic Approach

HAC When reported with secondary diagnosis code K68.11, T81.40XA, T81.41XA, T81.42XA, T81.43XA, T81.44XA or T81.49XA, T84.60XA, T84.610A, T84.611A, T84.612A, T84.613A, T84.614A, T84.615A, T84.619A, T84.63XA, T84.69XA, T84.7XXA

0SG747Z Fusion of Right Sacroiliac Joint with Autologous Tissue Substitute, Percutaneous Endoscopic Approach

HAC When reported with secondary diagnosis code K68.11, T81.40XA, T81.41XA, T81.42XA, T81.43XA, T81.44XA or T81.49XA, T84.60XA, T84.610A, T84.611A, T84.612A, T84.613A, T84.614A, T84.615A, T84.619A, T84.63XA, T84.69XA, T84.7XXA

0SG74JZ Fusion of Right Sacroiliac Joint with Synthetic Substitute, Percutaneous Endoscopic Approach

HAC When reported with secondary diagnosis code K68.11, T81.40XA, T81.41XA, T81.42XA, T81.43XA, T81.44XA or T81.49XA, T84.60XA, T84.610A, T84.611A, T84.612A, T84.613A, T84.614A, T84.615A, T84.619A, T84.63XA, T84.69XA, T84.7XXA

0SG74KZ Fusion of Right Sacroiliac Joint with Nonautologous Tissue Substitute, Percutaneous Endoscopic Approach

HAC When reported with secondary diagnosis code K68.11, T81.40XA, T81.41XA, T81.42XA, T81.43XA, T81.44XA or T81.49XA, T84.60XA, T84.610A, T84.611A, T84.612A, T84.613A, T84.614A, T84.615A, T84.619A, T84.63XA, T84.69XA, T84.7XXA

0SG804Z Fusion of Left Sacroiliac Joint with Internal Fixation Device, Open Approach

HAC When reported with secondary diagnosis code K68.11, T81.40XA, T81.41XA, T81.42XA, T81.43XA, T81.44XA or T81.49XA, T84.60XA, T84.610A, T84.611A, T84.612A, T84.613A, T84.614A, T84.615A, T84.619A, T84.63XA, T84.69XA, T84.7XXA

0SG807Z Fusion of Left Sacroiliac Joint with Autologous Tissue Substitute, Open Approach

HAC When reported with secondary diagnosis code K68.11, T81.40XA, T81.41XA, T81.42XA, T81.43XA, T81.44XA or T81.49XA, T84.60XA, T84.610A, T84.611A, T84.612A, T84.613A, T84.614A, T84.615A, T84.619A, T84.63XA, T84.69XA, T84.7XXA

0SG80JZ Fusion of Left Sacroiliac Joint with Synthetic Substitute, Open Approach

HAC When reported with secondary diagnosis code K68.11, T81.40XA, T81.41XA, T81.42XA, T81.43XA, T81.44XA or T81.49XA, T84.60XA, T84.610A, T84.611A, T84.612A, T84.613A, T84.614A, T84.615A, T84.619A, T84.63XA, T84.69XA, T84.7XXA

0SG80KZ Fusion of Left Sacroiliac Joint with Nonautologous Tissue Substitute, Open Approach

HAC When reported with secondary diagnosis code K68.11, T81.40XA, T81.41XA, T81.42XA, T81.43XA, T81.44XA or T81.49XA, T84.60XA, T84.610A, T84.611A, T84.612A, T84.613A, T84.614A, T84.615A, T84.619A, T84.63XA, T84.69XA, T84.7XXA

0SG834Z Fusion of Left Sacroiliac Joint with Internal Fixation Device, Percutaneous Approach

HAC When reported with secondary diagnosis code K68.11, T81.40XA, T81.41XA, T81.42XA, T81.43XA, T81.44XA or T81.49XA, T84.60XA, T84.610A, T84.611A, T84.612A, T84.613A, T84.614A, T84.615A, T84.619A, T84.63XA, T84.69XA, T84.7XXA

0SG837Z Fusion of Left Sacroiliac Joint with Autologous Tissue Substitute, Percutaneous Approach

HAC When reported with secondary diagnosis code K68.11, T81.40XA, T81.41XA, T81.42XA, T81.43XA, T81.44XA or T81.49XA, T84.60XA, T84.610A, T84.611A, T84.612A, T84.613A, T84.614A, T84.615A, T84.619A, T84.63XA, T84.69XA, T84.7XXA

0SG83JZ Fusion of Left Sacroiliac Joint with Synthetic Substitute, Percutaneous Approach

HAC When reported with secondary diagnosis code K68.11, T81.40XA, T81.41XA, T81.42XA, T81.43XA, T81.44XA or T81.49XA, T84.60XA, T84.610A, T84.611A, T84.612A, T84.613A, T84.614A, T84.615A, T84.619A, T84.63XA, T84.69XA, T84.7XXA

0SG83KZ Fusion of Left Sacroiliac Joint with Nonautologous Tissue Substitute, Percutaneous Approach

HAC When reported with secondary diagnosis code K68.11, T81.40XA, T81.41XA, T81.42XA, T81.43XA, T81.44XA or T81.49XA, T84.60XA, T84.610A, T84.611A, T84.612A, T84.613A, T84.614A, T84.615A, T84.619A, T84.63XA, T84.69XA, T84.7XXA

0SG844Z Fusion of Left Sacroiliac Joint with Internal Fixation Device, Percutaneous Endoscopic Approach

HAC When reported with secondary diagnosis code K68.11, T81.40XA, T81.41XA, T81.42XA, T81.43XA, T81.44XA or T81.49XA, T84.60XA, T84.610A, T84.611A, T84.612A, T84.613A, T84.614A, T84.615A, T84.619A, T84.63XA, T84.69XA, T84.7XXA

0SG847Z Fusion of Left Sacroiliac Joint with Autologous Tissue Substitute, Percutaneous Endoscopic Approach

HAC When reported with secondary diagnosis code K68.11, T81.40XA, T81.41XA, T81.42XA, T81.43XA, T81.44XA or T81.49XA, T84.60XA, T84.610A, T84.611A, T84.612A, T84.613A, T84.614A, T84.615A, T84.619A, T84.63XA, T84.69XA, T84.7XXA

0SG84JZ Fusion of Left Sacroiliac Joint with Synthetic Substitute, Percutaneous Endoscopic Approach

HAC When reported with secondary diagnosis code K68.11, T81.41XA, T81.42XA, T81.43XA, T81.44XA or T81.49XA, T84.60XA, T84.610A, T84.611A, T84.612A, T84.613A, T84.614A, T84.615A, T84.619A, T84.63XA, T84.69XA, T84.7XXA

0SG84KZ Fusion of Left Sacroiliac Joint with Nonautologous Tissue Substitute, Percutaneous Endoscopic Approach

HAC When reported with secondary diagnosis code K68.11, T81.40XA, T81.41XA, T81.42XA, T81.43XA, T81.44XA or T81.49XA, T84.60XA, T84.610A, T84.611A, T84.612A, T84.613A, T84.614A, T84.615A, T84.619A, T84.63XA, T84.69XA, T84.7XXA

0SG903Z Fusion of Right Hip Joint with Sustained Compression Internal Fixation Device, Open Approach

0SG904Z Fusion of Right Hip Joint with Internal Fixation Device, Open Approach

0SG905Z Fusion of Right Hip Joint with External Fixation Device, Open Approach

0SG907Z Fusion of Right Hip Joint with Autologous Tissue Substitute, Open Approach

0SG90JZ Fusion of Right Hip Joint with Synthetic Substitute, Open Approach

0SG90KZ Fusion of Right Hip Joint with Nonautologous Tissue Substitute, Open Approach

0SG933Z Fusion of Right Hip Joint with Sustained Compression Internal Fixation Device, Percutaneous Approach

0SG934Z Fusion of Right Hip Joint with Internal Fixation Device, Percutaneous Approach

0SG935Z Fusion of Right Hip Joint with External Fixation Device, Percutaneous Approach

0SG937Z Fusion of Right Hip Joint with Autologous Tissue Substitute, Percutaneous Approach

0SG93JZ Fusion of Right Hip Joint with Synthetic Substitute, Percutaneous Approach

0SG93KZ Fusion of Right Hip Joint with Nonautologous Tissue Substitute, Percutaneous Approach

0SG943Z Fusion of Right Hip Joint with Sustained Compression Internal Fixation Device, Percutaneous Endoscopic Approach

0SG944Z Fusion of Right Hip Joint with Internal Fixation Device, Percutaneous Endoscopic Approach

0SG945Z Fusion of Right Hip Joint with External Fixation Device, Percutaneous Endoscopic Approach

0SG947Z Fusion of Right Hip Joint with Autologous Tissue Substitute, Percutaneous Endoscopic Approach

0SG94JZ Fusion of Right Hip Joint with Synthetic Substitute, Percutaneous Endoscopic Approach

0SG94KZ Fusion of Right Hip Joint with Nonautologous Tissue Substitute, Percutaneous Endoscopic Approach

0SGB03Z Fusion of Left Hip Joint with Sustained Compression Internal Fixation Device, Open Approach

0SGB04Z Fusion of Left Hip Joint with Internal Fixation Device, Open Approach

0SGB05Z Fusion of Left Hip Joint with External Fixation Device, Open Approach

0SGB07Z Fusion of Left Hip Joint with Autologous Tissue Substitute, Open Approach

0SGB0JZ Fusion of Left Hip Joint with Synthetic Substitute, Open Approach

0SGB0KZ Fusion of Left Hip Joint with Nonautologous Tissue Substitute, Open Approach

0SGB33Z Fusion of Left Hip Joint with Sustained Compression Internal Fixation Device, Percutaneous Approach

0SGB34Z Fusion of Left Hip Joint with Internal Fixation Device, Percutaneous Approach

0SGB35Z Fusion of Left Hip Joint with External Fixation Device, Percutaneous Approach

0SGB37Z Fusion of Left Hip Joint with Autologous Tissue Substitute, Percutaneous Approach

0SGB3JZ Fusion of Left Hip Joint with Synthetic Substitute, Percutaneous Approach

0SGB3KZ Fusion of Left Hip Joint with Nonautologous Tissue Substitute, Percutaneous Approach

0SGB43Z Fusion of Left Hip Joint with Sustained Compression Internal Fixation Device, Percutaneous Endoscopic Approach

0SGB44Z Fusion of Left Hip Joint with Internal Fixation Device, Percutaneous Endoscopic Approach

0SGB45Z Fusion of Left Hip Joint with External Fixation Device, Percutaneous Endoscopic Approach

0SGB47Z Fusion of Left Hip Joint with Autologous Tissue Substitute, Percutaneous Endoscopic Approach

♀ Female-only   ♂ Male-only   ▲ Limited Coverage   ● Non-OR   HAC HAC-associated procedure   ▲ Non-covered procedures   ✛ Cluster

0SGB4JZ Fusion of Left Hip Joint with Synthetic Substitute, Percutaneous Endoscopic Approach

0SGB4KZ Fusion of Left Hip Joint with Nonautologous Tissue Substitute, Percutaneous Endoscopic Approach

0SGC03Z Fusion of Right Knee Joint with Sustained Compression Internal Fixation Device, Open Approach

0SGC04Z Fusion of Right Knee Joint with Internal Fixation Device, Open Approach

0SGC05Z Fusion of Right Knee Joint with External Fixation Device, Open Approach

0SGC07Z Fusion of Right Knee Joint with Autologous Tissue Substitute, Open Approach

0SGC0JZ Fusion of Right Knee Joint with Synthetic Substitute, Open Approach

0SGC0KZ Fusion of Right Knee Joint with Nonautologous Tissue Substitute, Open Approach

0SGC33Z Fusion of Right Knee Joint with Sustained Compression Internal Fixation Device, Percutaneous Approach

0SGC34Z Fusion of Right Knee Joint with Internal Fixation Device, Percutaneous Approach

0SGC35Z Fusion of Right Knee Joint with External Fixation Device, Percutaneous Approach

0SGC37Z Fusion of Right Knee Joint with Autologous Tissue Substitute, Percutaneous Approach

0SGC3JZ Fusion of Right Knee Joint with Synthetic Substitute, Percutaneous Approach

0SGC3KZ Fusion of Right Knee Joint with Nonautologous Tissue Substitute, Percutaneous Approach

0SGC43Z Fusion of Right Knee Joint with Sustained Compression Internal Fixation Device, Percutaneous Endoscopic Approach

0SGC44Z Fusion of Right Knee Joint with Internal Fixation Device, Percutaneous Endoscopic Approach

0SGC45Z Fusion of Right Knee Joint with External Fixation Device, Percutaneous Endoscopic Approach

0SGC47Z Fusion of Right Knee Joint with Autologous Tissue Substitute, Percutaneous Endoscopic Approach

0SGC4JZ Fusion of Right Knee Joint with Synthetic Substitute, Percutaneous Endoscopic Approach

0SGC4KZ Fusion of Right Knee Joint with Nonautologous Tissue Substitute, Percutaneous Endoscopic Approach

0SGD03Z Fusion of Left Knee Joint with Sustained Compression Internal Fixation Device, Open Approach

0SGD04Z Fusion of Left Knee Joint with Internal Fixation Device, Open Approach

0SGD05Z Fusion of Left Knee Joint with External Fixation Device, Open Approach

0SGD07Z Fusion of Left Knee Joint with Autologous Tissue Substitute, Open Approach

0SGD0JZ Fusion of Left Knee Joint with Synthetic Substitute, Open Approach

0SGD0KZ Fusion of Left Knee Joint with Nonautologous Tissue Substitute, Open Approach

0SGD33Z Fusion of Left Knee Joint with Sustained Compression Internal Fixation Device, Percutaneous Approach

0SGD34Z Fusion of Left Knee Joint with Internal Fixation Device, Percutaneous Approach

0SGD35Z Fusion of Left Knee Joint with External Fixation Device, Percutaneous Approach

0SGD37Z Fusion of Left Knee Joint with Autologous Tissue Substitute, Percutaneous Approach

0SGD3JZ Fusion of Left Knee Joint with Synthetic Substitute, Percutaneous Approach

0SGD3KZ Fusion of Left Knee Joint with Nonautologous Tissue Substitute, Percutaneous Approach

0SGD43Z Fusion of Left Knee Joint with Sustained Compression Internal Fixation Device, Percutaneous Endoscopic Approach

0SGD44Z Fusion of Left Knee Joint with Internal Fixation Device, Percutaneous Endoscopic Approach

0SGD45Z Fusion of Left Knee Joint with External Fixation Device, Percutaneous Endoscopic Approach

0SGD47Z Fusion of Left Knee Joint with Autologous Tissue Substitute, Percutaneous Endoscopic Approach

0SGD4JZ Fusion of Left Knee Joint with Synthetic Substitute, Percutaneous Endoscopic Approach

0SGD4KZ Fusion of Left Knee Joint with Nonautologous Tissue Substitute, Percutaneous Endoscopic Approach

0SGF03Z Fusion of Right Ankle Joint with Sustained Compression Internal Fixation Device, Open Approach

0SGF04Z Fusion of Right Ankle Joint with Internal Fixation Device, Open Approach

0SGF05Z Fusion of Right Ankle Joint with External Fixation Device, Open Approach

0SGF07Z Fusion of Right Ankle Joint with Autologous Tissue Substitute, Open Approach

0SGF0JZ Fusion of Right Ankle Joint with Synthetic Substitute, Open Approach

0SGF0KZ Fusion of Right Ankle Joint with Nonautologous Tissue Substitute, Open Approach

0SGF33Z Fusion of Right Ankle Joint with Sustained Compression Internal Fixation Device, Percutaneous Approach

0SGF34Z Fusion of Right Ankle Joint with Internal Fixation Device, Percutaneous Approach

0SGF35Z Fusion of Right Ankle Joint with External Fixation Device, Percutaneous Approach

0SGF37Z Fusion of Right Ankle Joint with Autologous Tissue Substitute, Percutaneous Approach

0SGF3JZ Fusion of Right Ankle Joint with Synthetic Substitute, Percutaneous Approach

0SGF3KZ Fusion of Right Ankle Joint with Nonautologous Tissue Substitute, Percutaneous Approach

0SGF43Z Fusion of Right Ankle Joint with Sustained Compression Internal Fixation Device, Percutaneous Endoscopic Approach

0SGF44Z Fusion of Right Ankle Joint with Internal Fixation Device, Percutaneous Endoscopic Approach

0SGF45Z Fusion of Right Ankle Joint with External Fixation Device, Percutaneous Endoscopic Approach

0SGF47Z Fusion of Right Ankle Joint with Autologous Tissue Substitute, Percutaneous Endoscopic Approach

0SGF4JZ Fusion of Right Ankle Joint with Synthetic Substitute, Percutaneous Endoscopic Approach

0SGF4KZ Fusion of Right Ankle Joint with Nonautologous Tissue Substitute, Percutaneous Endoscopic Approach

0SGG03Z Fusion of Left Ankle Joint with Sustained Compression Internal Fixation Device, Open Approach

0SGG04Z Fusion of Left Ankle Joint with Internal Fixation Device, Open Approach
AHA CC: 2Q, 2013, 39-40

0SGG05Z Fusion of Left Ankle Joint with External Fixation Device, Open Approach

0SGG07Z Fusion of Left Ankle Joint with Autologous Tissue Substitute, Open Approach
AHA CC: 2Q, 2013, 39-40

0SGG0JZ Fusion of Left Ankle Joint with Synthetic Substitute, Open Approach

0SGG0KZ Fusion of Left Ankle Joint with Nonautologous Tissue Substitute, Open Approach

0SGG33Z Fusion of Left Ankle Joint with Sustained Compression Internal Fixation Device, Percutaneous Approach

0SGG34Z Fusion of Left Ankle Joint with Internal Fixation Device, Percutaneous Approach

0SGG35Z Fusion of Left Ankle Joint with External Fixation Device, Percutaneous Approach

0SGG37Z Fusion of Left Ankle Joint with Autologous Tissue Substitute, Percutaneous Approach

0SGG3JZ Fusion of Left Ankle Joint with Synthetic Substitute, Percutaneous Approach

0SGG3KZ Fusion of Left Ankle Joint with Nonautologous Tissue Substitute, Percutaneous Approach

0SGG43Z Fusion of Left Ankle Joint with Sustained Compression Internal Fixation Device, Percutaneous Endoscopic Approach

0SGG44Z Fusion of Left Ankle Joint with Internal Fixation Device, Percutaneous Endoscopic Approach

0SGG45Z Fusion of Left Ankle Joint with External Fixation Device, Percutaneous Endoscopic Approach

0SGG47Z Fusion of Left Ankle Joint with Autologous Tissue Substitute, Percutaneous Endoscopic Approach

0SGG4JZ Fusion of Left Ankle Joint with Synthetic Substitute, Percutaneous Endoscopic Approach

0SGG4KZ Fusion of Left Ankle Joint with Nonautologous Tissue Substitute, Percutaneous Endoscopic Approach

0SGH03Z Fusion of Right Tarsal Joint with Sustained Compression Internal Fixation Device, Open Approach

0SGH04Z Fusion of Right Tarsal Joint with Internal Fixation Device, Open Approach

0SGH05Z Fusion of Right Tarsal Joint with External Fixation Device, Open Approach

0SGH07Z Fusion of Right Tarsal Joint with Autologous Tissue Substitute, Open Approach

0SGH0JZ Fusion of Right Tarsal Joint with Synthetic Substitute, Open Approach

0SGH0KZ Fusion of Right Tarsal Joint with Nonautologous Tissue Substitute, Open Approach

0SGH33Z Fusion of Right Tarsal Joint with Sustained Compression Internal Fixation Device, Percutaneous Approach

0SGH34Z Fusion of Right Tarsal Joint with Internal Fixation Device, Percutaneous Approach

0SGH35Z Fusion of Right Tarsal Joint with External Fixation Device, Percutaneous Approach

0SGH37Z Fusion of Right Tarsal Joint with Autologous Tissue Substitute, Percutaneous Approach

0SGH3JZ Fusion of Right Tarsal Joint with Synthetic Substitute, Percutaneous Approach

0SGH3KZ Fusion of Right Tarsal Joint with Nonautologous Tissue Substitute, Percutaneous Approach

0SGH43Z Fusion of Right Tarsal Joint with Sustained Compression Internal Fixation Device, Percutaneous Endoscopic Approach

0SGH44Z Fusion of Right Tarsal Joint with Internal Fixation Device, Percutaneous Endoscopic Approach

0SGH45Z Fusion of Right Tarsal Joint with External Fixation Device, Percutaneous Endoscopic Approach

0SGH47Z Fusion of Right Tarsal Joint with Autologous Tissue Substitute, Percutaneous Endoscopic Approach

0SGH4JZ Fusion of Right Tarsal Joint with Synthetic Substitute, Percutaneous Endoscopic Approach

0SGH4KZ Fusion of Right Tarsal Joint with Nonautologous Tissue Substitute, Percutaneous Endoscopic Approach

0SGJ03Z Fusion of Left Tarsal Joint with Sustained Compression Internal Fixation Device, Open Approach

0SGJ04Z Fusion of Left Tarsal Joint with Internal Fixation Device, Open Approach

0SGJ05Z Fusion of Left Tarsal Joint with External Fixation Device, Open Approach

0SGJ07Z Fusion of Left Tarsal Joint with Autologous Tissue Substitute, Open Approach

0SGJ0JZ Fusion of Left Tarsal Joint with Synthetic Substitute, Open Approach

0SGJ0KZ Fusion of Left Tarsal Joint with Nonautologous Tissue Substitute, Open Approach

0SGJ33Z Fusion of Left Tarsal Joint with Sustained Compression Internal Fixation Device, Percutaneous Approach

0SGJ34Z Fusion of Left Tarsal Joint with Internal Fixation Device, Percutaneous Approach

0SGJ35Z Fusion of Left Tarsal Joint with External Fixation Device, Percutaneous Approach

0SGJ37Z Fusion of Left Tarsal Joint with Autologous Tissue Substitute, Percutaneous Approach

0SGJ3JZ Fusion of Left Tarsal Joint with Synthetic Substitute, Percutaneous Approach

0SGJ3KZ Fusion of Left Tarsal Joint with Nonautologous Tissue Substitute, Percutaneous Approach

0SGJ43Z Fusion of Left Tarsal Joint with Sustained Compression Internal Fixation Device, Percutaneous Endoscopic Approach

0SGJ44Z Fusion of Left Tarsal Joint with Internal Fixation Device, Percutaneous Endoscopic Approach

0SGJ45Z Fusion of Left Tarsal Joint with External Fixation Device, Percutaneous Endoscopic Approach

0SGJ47Z Fusion of Left Tarsal Joint with Autologous Tissue Substitute, Percutaneous Endoscopic Approach

0SGJ4JZ Fusion of Left Tarsal Joint with Synthetic Substitute, Percutaneous Endoscopic Approach

0SGJ4KZ Fusion of Left Tarsal Joint with Nonautologous Tissue Substitute, Percutaneous Endoscopic Approach

0SGK03Z Fusion of Right Tarsometatarsal Joint with Sustained Compression Internal Fixation Device, Open Approach

0SGK04Z Fusion of Right Tarsometatarsal Joint with Internal Fixation Device, Open Approach

0SGK05Z Fusion of Right Tarsometatarsal Joint with External Fixation Device, Open Approach

0SGK07Z Fusion of Right Tarsometatarsal Joint with Autologous Tissue Substitute, Open Approach

0SGK0JZ Fusion of Right Tarsometatarsal Joint with Synthetic Substitute, Open Approach

0SGK0KZ Fusion of Right Tarsometatarsal Joint with Nonautologous Tissue Substitute, Open Approach

0SGK33Z Fusion of Right Tarsometatarsal Joint with Sustained Compression Internal Fixation Device, Percutaneous Approach

0SGK34Z Fusion of Right Tarsometatarsal Joint with Internal Fixation Device, Percutaneous Approach

0SGK35Z Fusion of Right Tarsometatarsal Joint with External Fixation Device, Percutaneous Approach

0SGK37Z Fusion of Right Tarsometatarsal Joint with Autologous Tissue Substitute, Percutaneous Approach

0SGK3JZ Fusion of Right Tarsometatarsal Joint with Synthetic Substitute, Percutaneous Approach

0SGK3KZ Fusion of Right Tarsometatarsal Joint with Nonautologous Tissue Substitute, Percutaneous Approach

0SGK43Z Fusion of Right Tarsometatarsal Joint with Sustained Compression Internal Fixation Device, Percutaneous Endoscopic Approach

0SGK44Z Fusion of Right Tarsometatarsal Joint with Internal Fixation Device, Percutaneous Endoscopic Approach

0SGK45Z Fusion of Right Tarsometatarsal Joint with External Fixation Device, Percutaneous Endoscopic Approach

0SGK47Z Fusion of Right Tarsometatarsal Joint with Autologous Tissue Substitute, Percutaneous Endoscopic Approach

0SGK4JZ Fusion of Right Tarsometatarsal Joint with Synthetic Substitute, Percutaneous Endoscopic Approach

0SGK4KZ Fusion of Right Tarsometatarsal Joint with Nonautologous Tissue Substitute, Percutaneous Endoscopic Approach

0SGL03Z Fusion of Left Tarsometatarsal Joint with Sustained Compression Internal Fixation Device, Open Approach

0SGL04Z Fusion of Left Tarsometatarsal Joint with Internal Fixation Device, Open Approach

0SGL05Z Fusion of Left Tarsometatarsal Joint with External Fixation Device, Open Approach

0SGL07Z Fusion of Left Tarsometatarsal Joint with Autologous Tissue Substitute, Open Approach

0SGL0JZ Fusion of Left Tarsometatarsal Joint with Synthetic Substitute, Open Approach

0SGL0KZ Fusion of Left Tarsometatarsal Joint with Nonautologous Tissue Substitute, Open Approach

0SGL33Z Fusion of Left Tarsometatarsal Joint with Sustained Compression Internal Fixation Device, Percutaneous Approach

0SGL34Z Fusion of Left Tarsometatarsal Joint with Internal Fixation Device, Percutaneous Approach

0SGL35Z Fusion of Left Tarsometatarsal Joint with External Fixation Device, Percutaneous Approach

0SGL37Z Fusion of Left Tarsometatarsal Joint with Autologous Tissue Substitute, Percutaneous Approach

0SGL3JZ Fusion of Left Tarsometatarsal Joint with Synthetic Substitute, Percutaneous Approach

0SGL3KZ Fusion of Left Tarsometatarsal Joint with Nonautologous Tissue Substitute, Percutaneous Approach

0SGL43Z Fusion of Left Tarsometatarsal Joint with Sustained Compression Internal Fixation Device, Percutaneous Endoscopic Approach

0SGL44Z Fusion of Left Tarsometatarsal Joint with Internal Fixation Device, Percutaneous Endoscopic Approach

0SGL45Z Fusion of Left Tarsometatarsal Joint with External Fixation Device, Percutaneous Endoscopic Approach

0SGL47Z Fusion of Left Tarsometatarsal Joint with Autologous Tissue Substitute, Percutaneous Endoscopic Approach

0SGL4JZ Fusion of Left Tarsometatarsal Joint with Synthetic Substitute, Percutaneous Endoscopic Approach

0SGL4KZ Fusion of Left Tarsometatarsal Joint with Nonautologous Tissue Substitute, Percutaneous Endoscopic Approach

0SGM03Z Fusion of Right Metatarsal-Phalangeal Joint with Sustained Compression Internal Fixation Device, Open Approach

♀ Female-only   ♂ Male-only   ▲ Limited Coverage   ● Non-OR   ▨ HAC-associated procedure   ▲ Non-covered procedures   ✚ Cluster

0SGM04Z Fusion of Right Metatarsal-Phalangeal Joint with Internal Fixation Device, Open Approach

0SGM05Z Fusion of Right Metatarsal-Phalangeal Joint with External Fixation Device, Open Approach

0SGM07Z Fusion of Right Metatarsal-Phalangeal Joint with Autologous Tissue Substitute, Open Approach

0SGM0JZ Fusion of Right Metatarsal-Phalangeal Joint with Synthetic Substitute, Open Approach

0SGM0KZ Fusion of Right Metatarsal-Phalangeal Joint with Nonautologous Tissue Substitute, Open Approach

0SGM33Z Fusion of Right Metatarsal-Phalangeal Joint with Sustained Compression Internal Fixation Device, Percutaneous Approach

0SGM34Z Fusion of Right Metatarsal-Phalangeal Joint with Internal Fixation Device, Percutaneous Approach

0SGM35Z Fusion of Right Metatarsal-Phalangeal Joint with External Fixation Device, Percutaneous Approach

0SGM37Z Fusion of Right Metatarsal-Phalangeal Joint with Autologous Tissue Substitute, Percutaneous Approach

0SGM3JZ Fusion of Right Metatarsal-Phalangeal Joint with Synthetic Substitute, Percutaneous Approach

0SGM3KZ Fusion of Right Metatarsal-Phalangeal Joint with Nonautologous Tissue Substitute, Percutaneous Approach

0SGM43Z Fusion of Right Metatarsal-Phalangeal Joint with Sustained Compression Internal Fixation Device, Percutaneous Endoscopic Approach

0SGM44Z Fusion of Right Metatarsal-Phalangeal Joint with Internal Fixation Device, Percutaneous Endoscopic Approach

0SGM45Z Fusion of Right Metatarsal-Phalangeal Joint with External Fixation Device, Percutaneous Endoscopic Approach

0SGM47Z Fusion of Right Metatarsal-Phalangeal Joint with Autologous Tissue Substitute, Percutaneous Endoscopic Approach

0SGM4JZ Fusion of Right Metatarsal-Phalangeal Joint with Synthetic Substitute, Percutaneous Endoscopic Approach

0SGM4KZ Fusion of Right Metatarsal-Phalangeal Joint with Nonautologous Tissue Substitute, Percutaneous Endoscopic Approach

0SGN03Z Fusion of Left Metatarsal-Phalangeal Joint with Sustained Compression Internal Fixation Device, Open Approach

0SGN04Z Fusion of Left Metatarsal-Phalangeal Joint with Internal Fixation Device, Open Approach

0SGN05Z Fusion of Left Metatarsal-Phalangeal Joint with External Fixation Device, Open Approach

0SGN07Z Fusion of Left Metatarsal-Phalangeal Joint with Autologous Tissue Substitute, Open Approach

0SGN0JZ Fusion of Left Metatarsal-Phalangeal Joint with Synthetic Substitute, Open Approach

0SGN0KZ Fusion of Left Metatarsal-Phalangeal Joint with Nonautologous Tissue Substitute, Open Approach

0SGN33Z Fusion of Left Metatarsal-Phalangeal Joint with Sustained Compression

0SGN34Z Internal Fixation Device, Percutaneous Approach

0SGN34Z Fusion of Left Metatarsal-Phalangeal Joint with Internal Fixation Device, Percutaneous Approach

0SGN35Z Fusion of Left Metatarsal-Phalangeal Joint with External Fixation Device, Percutaneous Approach

0SGN37Z Fusion of Left Metatarsal-Phalangeal Joint with Autologous Tissue Substitute, Percutaneous Approach

0SGN3JZ Fusion of Left Metatarsal-Phalangeal Joint with Synthetic Substitute, Percutaneous Approach

0SGN3KZ Fusion of Left Metatarsal-Phalangeal Joint with Nonautologous Tissue Substitute, Percutaneous Approach

0SGN43Z Fusion of Left Metatarsal-Phalangeal Joint with Sustained Compression Internal Fixation Device, Percutaneous Endoscopic Approach

0SGN44Z Fusion of Left Metatarsal-Phalangeal Joint with Internal Fixation Device, Percutaneous Endoscopic Approach

0SGN45Z Fusion of Left Metatarsal-Phalangeal Joint with External Fixation Device, Percutaneous Endoscopic Approach

0SGN47Z Fusion of Left Metatarsal-Phalangeal Joint with Autologous Tissue Substitute, Percutaneous Endoscopic Approach

0SGN4JZ Fusion of Left Metatarsal-Phalangeal Joint with Synthetic Substitute, Percutaneous Endoscopic Approach

0SGN4KZ Fusion of Left Metatarsal-Phalangeal Joint with Nonautologous Tissue Substitute, Percutaneous Endoscopic Approach

0SGP03Z Fusion of Right Toe Phalangeal Joint with Sustained Compression Internal Fixation Device, Open Approach

0SGP04Z Fusion of Right Toe Phalangeal Joint with Internal Fixation Device, Open Approach

0SGP05Z Fusion of Right Toe Phalangeal Joint with External Fixation Device, Open Approach

0SGP07Z Fusion of Right Toe Phalangeal Joint with Autologous Tissue Substitute, Open Approach

0SGP0JZ Fusion of Right Toe Phalangeal Joint with Synthetic Substitute, Open Approach

0SGP0KZ Fusion of Right Toe Phalangeal Joint with Nonautologous Tissue Substitute, Open Approach

0SGP33Z Fusion of Right Toe Phalangeal Joint with Sustained Compression Internal Fixation Device, Percutaneous Approach

0SGP34Z Fusion of Right Toe Phalangeal Joint with Internal Fixation Device, Percutaneous Approach

0SGP35Z Fusion of Right Toe Phalangeal Joint with External Fixation Device, Percutaneous Approach

0SGP37Z Fusion of Right Toe Phalangeal Joint with Autologous Tissue Substitute, Percutaneous Approach

0SGP3JZ Fusion of Right Toe Phalangeal Joint with Synthetic Substitute, Percutaneous Approach

0SGP3KZ Fusion of Right Toe Phalangeal Joint with Nonautologous Tissue Substitute, Percutaneous Approach

0SGP43Z Fusion of Right Toe Phalangeal Joint with Sustained Compression Internal Fixation Device, Percutaneous Endoscopic Approach

0SGP44Z Fusion of Right Toe Phalangeal Joint with Internal Fixation Device, Percutaneous Endoscopic Approach

0SGP45Z Fusion of Right Toe Phalangeal Joint with External Fixation Device, Percutaneous Endoscopic Approach

0SGP47Z Fusion of Right Toe Phalangeal Joint with Autologous Tissue Substitute, Percutaneous Endoscopic Approach

0SGP4JZ Fusion of Right Toe Phalangeal Joint with Synthetic Substitute, Percutaneous Endoscopic Approach

0SGP4KZ Fusion of Right Toe Phalangeal Joint with Nonautologous Tissue Substitute, Percutaneous Endoscopic Approach

0SGQ03Z Fusion of Left Toe Phalangeal Joint with Sustained Compression Internal Fixation Device, Open Approach

0SGQ04Z Fusion of Left Toe Phalangeal Joint with Internal Fixation Device, Open Approach

0SGQ05Z Fusion of Left Toe Phalangeal Joint with External Fixation Device, Open Approach

0SGQ07Z Fusion of Left Toe Phalangeal Joint with Autologous Tissue Substitute, Open Approach

0SGQ0JZ Fusion of Left Toe Phalangeal Joint with Synthetic Substitute, Open Approach

0SGQ0KZ Fusion of Left Toe Phalangeal Joint with Nonautologous Tissue Substitute, Open Approach

0SGQ33Z Fusion of Left Toe Phalangeal Joint with Sustained Compression Internal Fixation Device, Percutaneous Approach

0SGQ34Z Fusion of Left Toe Phalangeal Joint with Internal Fixation Device, Percutaneous Approach

0SGQ35Z Fusion of Left Toe Phalangeal Joint with External Fixation Device, Percutaneous Approach

0SGQ37Z Fusion of Left Toe Phalangeal Joint with Autologous Tissue Substitute, Percutaneous Approach

0SGQ3JZ Fusion of Left Toe Phalangeal Joint with Synthetic Substitute, Percutaneous Approach

0SGQ3KZ Fusion of Left Toe Phalangeal Joint with Nonautologous Tissue Substitute, Percutaneous Approach

0SGQ43Z Fusion of Left Toe Phalangeal Joint with Sustained Compression Internal Fixation Device, Percutaneous Endoscopic Approach

0SGQ44Z Fusion of Left Toe Phalangeal Joint with Internal Fixation Device, Percutaneous Endoscopic Approach

0SGQ45Z Fusion of Left Toe Phalangeal Joint with External Fixation Device, Percutaneous Endoscopic Approach

0SGQ47Z Fusion of Left Toe Phalangeal Joint with Autologous Tissue Substitute, Percutaneous Endoscopic Approach

0SGQ4JZ Fusion of Left Toe Phalangeal Joint with Synthetic Substitute, Percutaneous Endoscopic Approach

0SGQ4KZ Fusion of Left Toe Phalangeal Joint with Nonautologous Tissue Substitute, Percutaneous Endoscopic Approach

0SH – Lower Joints, Insertion

0SH003Z Insertion of Infusion Device into Lumbar Vertebral Joint, Open Approach

0SH004Z Insertion of Internal Fixation Device into Lumbar Vertebral Joint, Open Approach

0SH008Z Insertion of Spacer into Lumbar Vertebral Joint, Open Approach

0SH00BZ Insertion of Interspinous Process Spinal Stabilization Device into Lumbar Vertebral Joint, Open Approach

0SH00CZ Insertion of Pedicle-Based Spinal Stabilization Device into Lumbar Vertebral Joint, Open Approach

0SH00DZ Insertion of Facet Replacement Spinal Stabilization Device into Lumbar Vertebral Joint, Open Approach

0SH033Z Insertion of Infusion Device into Lumbar Vertebral Joint, Percutaneous Approach

0SH034Z Insertion of Internal Fixation Device into Lumbar Vertebral Joint, Percutaneous Approach

0SH038Z Insertion of Spacer into Lumbar Vertebral Joint, Percutaneous Approach

0SH03BZ Insertion of Interspinous Process Spinal Stabilization Device into Lumbar Vertebral Joint, Percutaneous Approach

0SH03CZ Insertion of Pedicle-Based Spinal Stabilization Device into Lumbar Vertebral Joint, Percutaneous Approach

0SH03DZ Insertion of Facet Replacement Spinal Stabilization Device into Lumbar Vertebral Joint, Percutaneous Approach

0SH043Z Insertion of Infusion Device into Lumbar Vertebral Joint, Percutaneous Endoscopic Approach

0SH044Z Insertion of Internal Fixation Device into Lumbar Vertebral Joint, Percutaneous Endoscopic Approach

0SH048Z Insertion of Spacer into Lumbar Vertebral Joint, Percutaneous Endoscopic Approach

0SH04BZ Insertion of Interspinous Process Spinal Stabilization Device into Lumbar Vertebral Joint, Percutaneous Endoscopic Approach

0SH04CZ Insertion of Pedicle-Based Spinal Stabilization Device into Lumbar Vertebral Joint, Percutaneous Endoscopic Approach

0SH04DZ Insertion of Facet Replacement Spinal Stabilization Device into Lumbar Vertebral Joint, Percutaneous Endoscopic Approach

0SH203Z Insertion of Infusion Device into Lumbar Vertebral Disc, Open Approach

0SH208Z Insertion of Spacer into Lumbar Vertebral Disc, Open Approach

0SH233Z Insertion of Infusion Device into Lumbar Vertebral Disc, Percutaneous Approach

0SH238Z Insertion of Spacer into Lumbar Vertebral Disc, Percutaneous Approach

0SH243Z Insertion of Infusion Device into Lumbar Vertebral Disc, Percutaneous Endoscopic Approach

0SH248Z Insertion of Spacer into Lumbar Vertebral Disc, Percutaneous Endoscopic Approach

0SH303Z Insertion of Infusion Device into Lumbosacral Joint, Open Approach

0SH304Z Insertion of Internal Fixation Device into Lumbosacral Joint, Open Approach

0SH308Z Insertion of Spacer into Lumbosacral Joint, Open Approach

0SH30BZ Insertion of Interspinous Process Spinal Stabilization Device into Lumbosacral Joint, Open Approach

0SH30CZ Insertion of Pedicle-Based Spinal Stabilization Device into Lumbosacral Joint, Open Approach

0SH30DZ Insertion of Facet Replacement Spinal Stabilization Device into Lumbosacral Joint, Open Approach

0SH333Z Insertion of Infusion Device into Lumbosacral Joint, Percutaneous Approach

0SH334Z Insertion of Internal Fixation Device into Lumbosacral Joint, Percutaneous Approach

0SH338Z Insertion of Spacer into Lumbosacral Joint, Percutaneous Approach

0SH33BZ Insertion of Interspinous Process Spinal Stabilization Device into Lumbosacral Joint, Percutaneous Approach

0SH33CZ Insertion of Pedicle-Based Spinal Stabilization Device into Lumbosacral Joint, Percutaneous Approach

0SH33DZ Insertion of Facet Replacement Spinal Stabilization Device into Lumbosacral Joint, Percutaneous Approach

0SH343Z Insertion of Infusion Device into Lumbosacral Joint, Percutaneous Endoscopic Approach

0SH344Z Insertion of Internal Fixation Device into Lumbosacral Joint, Percutaneous Endoscopic Approach

0SH348Z Insertion of Spacer into Lumbosacral Joint, Percutaneous Endoscopic Approach

0SH34BZ Insertion of Interspinous Process Spinal Stabilization Device into Lumbosacral Joint, Percutaneous Endoscopic Approach

0SH34CZ Insertion of Pedicle-Based Spinal Stabilization Device into Lumbosacral Joint, Percutaneous Endoscopic Approach

0SH34DZ Insertion of Facet Replacement Spinal Stabilization Device into Lumbosacral Joint, Percutaneous Endoscopic Approach

0SH403Z Insertion of Infusion Device into Lumbosacral Disc, Open Approach

0SH408Z Insertion of Spacer into Lumbosacral Disc, Open Approach

AHA CC: 1Q, 2021, 18-19

0SH433Z Insertion of Infusion Device into Lumbosacral Disc, Percutaneous Approach

0SH438Z Insertion of Spacer into Lumbosacral Disc, Percutaneous Approach

0SH443Z Insertion of Infusion Device into Lumbosacral Disc, Percutaneous Endoscopic Approach

0SH448Z Insertion of Spacer into Lumbosacral Disc, Percutaneous Endoscopic Approach

0SH503Z Insertion of Infusion Device into Sacrococcygeal Joint, Open Approach

0SH504Z Insertion of Internal Fixation Device into Sacrococcygeal Joint, Open Approach

0SH508Z Insertion of Spacer into Sacrococcygeal Joint, Open Approach

0SH533Z Insertion of Infusion Device into Sacrococcygeal Joint, Percutaneous Approach

0SH534Z Insertion of Internal Fixation Device into Sacrococcygeal Joint, Percutaneous Approach

0SH538Z Insertion of Spacer into Sacrococcygeal Joint, Percutaneous Approach

0SH543Z Insertion of Infusion Device into Sacrococcygeal Joint, Percutaneous Endoscopic Approach

0SH544Z Insertion of Internal Fixation Device into Sacrococcygeal Joint, Percutaneous Endoscopic Approach

0SH548Z Insertion of Spacer into Sacrococcygeal Joint, Percutaneous Endoscopic Approach

0SH603Z Insertion of Infusion Device into Coccygeal Joint, Open Approach

0SH604Z Insertion of Internal Fixation Device into Coccygeal Joint, Open Approach

0SH608Z Insertion of Spacer into Coccygeal Joint, Open Approach

0SH633Z Insertion of Infusion Device into Coccygeal Joint, Percutaneous Approach

0SH634Z Insertion of Internal Fixation Device into Coccygeal Joint, Percutaneous Approach

0SH638Z Insertion of Spacer into Coccygeal Joint, Percutaneous Approach

0SH643Z Insertion of Infusion Device into Coccygeal Joint, Percutaneous Endoscopic Approach

0SH644Z Insertion of Internal Fixation Device into Coccygeal Joint, Percutaneous Endoscopic Approach

0SH648Z Insertion of Spacer into Coccygeal Joint, Percutaneous Endoscopic Approach

0SH703Z Insertion of Infusion Device into Right Sacroiliac Joint, Open Approach

0SH704Z Insertion of Internal Fixation Device into Right Sacroiliac Joint, Open Approach

0SH708Z Insertion of Spacer into Right Sacroiliac Joint, Open Approach

0SH733Z Insertion of Infusion Device into Right Sacroiliac Joint, Percutaneous Approach

0SH734Z Insertion of Internal Fixation Device into Right Sacroiliac Joint, Percutaneous Approach

0SH738Z Insertion of Spacer into Right Sacroiliac Joint, Percutaneous Approach

0SH743Z Insertion of Infusion Device into Right Sacroiliac Joint, Percutaneous Endoscopic Approach

0SH744Z Insertion of Internal Fixation Device into Right Sacroiliac Joint, Percutaneous Endoscopic Approach

0SH748Z Insertion of Spacer into Right Sacroiliac Joint, Percutaneous Endoscopic Approach

♀ Female-only   ♂ Male-only   ▲ Limited Coverage   ● Non-OR   🅷🅰🅲 HAC-associated procedure   ▲ Non-covered procedures   ✚ Cluster

0SH803Z	Insertion of Infusion Device into Left Sacroiliac Joint, Open Approach
0SH804Z	Insertion of Internal Fixation Device into Left Sacroiliac Joint, Open Approach
0SH808Z	Insertion of Spacer into Left Sacroiliac Joint, Open Approach
0SH833Z	Insertion of Infusion Device into Left Sacroiliac Joint, Percutaneous Approach
0SH834Z	Insertion of Internal Fixation Device into Left Sacroiliac Joint, Percutaneous Approach
0SH838Z	Insertion of Spacer into Left Sacroiliac Joint, Percutaneous Approach
0SH843Z	Insertion of Infusion Device into Left Sacroiliac Joint, Percutaneous Endoscopic Approach
0SH844Z	Insertion of Internal Fixation Device into Left Sacroiliac Joint, Percutaneous Endoscopic Approach
0SH848Z	Insertion of Spacer into Left Sacroiliac Joint, Percutaneous Endoscopic Approach
0SH903Z	Insertion of Infusion Device into Right Hip Joint, Open Approach
0SH904Z	Insertion of Internal Fixation Device into Right Hip Joint, Open Approach
0SH905Z	Insertion of External Fixation Device into Right Hip Joint, Open Approach
0SH908Z	Insertion of Spacer into Right Hip Joint, Open Approach
0SH933Z	Insertion of Infusion Device into Right Hip Joint, Percutaneous Approach
0SH934Z	Insertion of Internal Fixation Device into Right Hip Joint, Percutaneous Approach
0SH935Z	Insertion of External Fixation Device into Right Hip Joint, Percutaneous Approach
0SH938Z	Insertion of Spacer into Right Hip Joint, Percutaneous Approach
0SH943Z	Insertion of Infusion Device into Right Hip Joint, Percutaneous Endoscopic Approach
0SH944Z	Insertion of Internal Fixation Device into Right Hip Joint, Percutaneous Endoscopic Approach
0SH945Z	Insertion of External Fixation Device into Right Hip Joint, Percutaneous Endoscopic Approach
0SH948Z	Insertion of Spacer into Right Hip Joint, Percutaneous Endoscopic Approach
0SHB03Z	Insertion of Infusion Device into Left Hip Joint, Open Approach
0SHB04Z	Insertion of Internal Fixation Device into Left Hip Joint, Open Approach
0SHB05Z	Insertion of External Fixation Device into Left Hip Joint, Open Approach
0SHB08Z	Insertion of Spacer into Left Hip Joint, Open Approach
0SHB33Z	Insertion of Infusion Device into Left Hip Joint, Percutaneous Approach
0SHB34Z	Insertion of Internal Fixation Device into Left Hip Joint, Percutaneous Approach
0SHB35Z	Insertion of External Fixation Device into Left Hip Joint, Percutaneous Approach
0SHB38Z	Insertion of Spacer into Left Hip Joint, Percutaneous Approach
0SHB43Z	Insertion of Infusion Device into Left Hip Joint, Percutaneous Endoscopic Approach
0SHB44Z	Insertion of Internal Fixation Device into Left Hip Joint, Percutaneous Endoscopic Approach
0SHB45Z	Insertion of External Fixation Device into Left Hip Joint, Percutaneous Endoscopic Approach
0SHB48Z	Insertion of Spacer into Left Hip Joint, Percutaneous Endoscopic Approach
0SHC03Z	Insertion of Infusion Device into Right Knee Joint, Open Approach
0SHC04Z	Insertion of Internal Fixation Device into Right Knee Joint, Open Approach
0SHC05Z	Insertion of External Fixation Device into Right Knee Joint, Open Approach
0SHC08Z	Insertion of Spacer into Right Knee Joint, Open Approach
0SHC33Z	Insertion of Infusion Device into Right Knee Joint, Percutaneous Approach
0SHC34Z	Insertion of Internal Fixation Device into Right Knee Joint, Percutaneous Approach
0SHC35Z	Insertion of External Fixation Device into Right Knee Joint, Percutaneous Approach
0SHC38Z	Insertion of Spacer into Right Knee Joint, Percutaneous Approach
0SHC43Z	Insertion of Infusion Device into Right Knee Joint, Percutaneous Endoscopic Approach
0SHC44Z	Insertion of Internal Fixation Device into Right Knee Joint, Percutaneous Endoscopic Approach
0SHC45Z	Insertion of External Fixation Device into Right Knee Joint, Percutaneous Endoscopic Approach
0SHC48Z	Insertion of Spacer into Right Knee Joint, Percutaneous Endoscopic Approach
0SHD03Z	Insertion of Infusion Device into Left Knee Joint, Open Approach
0SHD04Z	Insertion of Internal Fixation Device into Left Knee Joint, Open Approach
0SHD05Z	Insertion of External Fixation Device into Left Knee Joint, Open Approach
0SHD08Z	Insertion of Spacer into Left Knee Joint, Open Approach
0SHD33Z	Insertion of Infusion Device into Left Knee Joint, Percutaneous Approach
0SHD34Z	Insertion of Internal Fixation Device into Left Knee Joint, Percutaneous Approach
0SHD35Z	Insertion of External Fixation Device into Left Knee Joint, Percutaneous Approach
0SHD38Z	Insertion of Spacer into Left Knee Joint, Percutaneous Approach
0SHD43Z	Insertion of Infusion Device into Left Knee Joint, Percutaneous Endoscopic Approach
0SHD44Z	Insertion of Internal Fixation Device into Left Knee Joint, Percutaneous Endoscopic Approach
0SHD45Z	Insertion of External Fixation Device into Left Knee Joint, Percutaneous Endoscopic Approach
0SHD48Z	Insertion of Spacer into Left Knee Joint, Percutaneous Endoscopic Approach
0SHF03Z	Insertion of Infusion Device into Right Ankle Joint, Open Approach
0SHF04Z	Insertion of Internal Fixation Device into Right Ankle Joint, Open Approach
0SHF05Z	Insertion of External Fixation Device into Right Ankle Joint, Open Approach
0SHF08Z	Insertion of Spacer into Right Ankle Joint, Open Approach
0SHF33Z	Insertion of Infusion Device into Right Ankle Joint, Percutaneous Approach
0SHF34Z	Insertion of Internal Fixation Device into Right Ankle Joint, Percutaneous Approach
0SHF35Z	Insertion of External Fixation Device into Right Ankle Joint, Percutaneous Approach
0SHF38Z	Insertion of Spacer into Right Ankle Joint, Percutaneous Approach
0SHF43Z	Insertion of Infusion Device into Right Ankle Joint, Percutaneous Endoscopic Approach
0SHF44Z	Insertion of Internal Fixation Device into Right Ankle Joint, Percutaneous Endoscopic Approach
0SHF45Z	Insertion of External Fixation Device into Right Ankle Joint, Percutaneous Endoscopic Approach
0SHF48Z	Insertion of Spacer into Right Ankle Joint, Percutaneous Endoscopic Approach
0SHG03Z	Insertion of Infusion Device into Left Ankle Joint, Open Approach
0SHG04Z	Insertion of Internal Fixation Device into Left Ankle Joint, Open Approach
0SHG05Z	Insertion of External Fixation Device into Left Ankle Joint, Open Approach
0SHG08Z	Insertion of Spacer into Left Ankle Joint, Open Approach
0SHG33Z	Insertion of Infusion Device into Left Ankle Joint, Percutaneous Approach
0SHG34Z	Insertion of Internal Fixation Device into Left Ankle Joint, Percutaneous Approach
0SHG35Z	Insertion of External Fixation Device into Left Ankle Joint, Percutaneous Approach
0SHG38Z	Insertion of Spacer into Left Ankle Joint, Percutaneous Approach
0SHG43Z	Insertion of Infusion Device into Left Ankle Joint, Percutaneous Endoscopic Approach
0SHG44Z	Insertion of Internal Fixation Device into Left Ankle Joint, Percutaneous Endoscopic Approach
0SHG45Z	Insertion of External Fixation Device into Left Ankle Joint, Percutaneous Endoscopic Approach
0SHG48Z	Insertion of Spacer into Left Ankle Joint, Percutaneous Endoscopic Approach
0SHH03Z	Insertion of Infusion Device into Right Tarsal Joint, Open Approach
0SHH04Z	Insertion of Internal Fixation Device into Right Tarsal Joint, Open Approach
0SHH05Z	Insertion of External Fixation Device into Right Tarsal Joint, Open Approach
0SHH08Z	Insertion of Spacer into Right Tarsal Joint, Open Approach
● **0SHH33Z**	Insertion of Infusion Device into Right Tarsal Joint, Percutaneous Approach
0SHH34Z	Insertion of Internal Fixation Device into Right Tarsal Joint, Percutaneous Approach
0SHH35Z	Insertion of External Fixation Device into Right Tarsal Joint, Percutaneous Approach
0SHH38Z	Insertion of Spacer into Right Tarsal Joint, Percutaneous Approach
0SHH43Z	Insertion of Infusion Device into Right Tarsal Joint, Percutaneous Endoscopic Approach

0SHH44Z Insertion of Internal Fixation Device into Right Tarsal Joint, Percutaneous Endoscopic Approach

0SHH45Z Insertion of External Fixation Device into Right Tarsal Joint, Percutaneous Endoscopic Approach

0SHH48Z Insertion of Spacer into Right Tarsal Joint, Percutaneous Endoscopic Approach

0SHJ03Z Insertion of Infusion Device into Left Tarsal Joint, Open Approach

0SHJ04Z Insertion of Internal Fixation Device into Left Tarsal Joint, Open Approach

0SHJ05Z Insertion of External Fixation Device into Left Tarsal Joint, Open Approach

0SHJ08Z Insertion of Spacer into Left Tarsal Joint, Open Approach

0SHJ33Z Insertion of Infusion Device into Left Tarsal Joint, Percutaneous Approach

0SHJ34Z Insertion of Internal Fixation Device into Left Tarsal Joint, Percutaneous Approach

0SHJ35Z Insertion of External Fixation Device into Left Tarsal Joint, Percutaneous Approach

0SHJ38Z Insertion of Spacer into Left Tarsal Joint, Percutaneous Approach

0SHJ43Z Insertion of Infusion Device into Left Tarsal Joint, Percutaneous Endoscopic Approach

0SHJ44Z Insertion of Internal Fixation Device into Left Tarsal Joint, Percutaneous Endoscopic Approach

0SHJ45Z Insertion of External Fixation Device into Left Tarsal Joint, Percutaneous Endoscopic Approach

0SHJ48Z Insertion of Spacer into Left Tarsal Joint, Percutaneous Endoscopic Approach

0SHK03Z Insertion of Infusion Device into Right Tarsometatarsal Joint, Open Approach

0SHK04Z Insertion of Internal Fixation Device into Right Tarsometatarsal Joint, Open Approach

0SHK05Z Insertion of External Fixation Device into Right Tarsometatarsal Joint, Open Approach

0SHK08Z Insertion of Spacer into Right Tarsometatarsal Joint, Open Approach

0SHK33Z Insertion of Infusion Device into Right Tarsometatarsal Joint, Percutaneous Approach

0SHK34Z Insertion of Internal Fixation Device into Right Tarsometatarsal Joint, Percutaneous Approach

0SHK35Z Insertion of External Fixation Device into Right Tarsometatarsal Joint, Percutaneous Approach

0SHK38Z Insertion of Spacer into Right Tarsometatarsal Joint, Percutaneous Approach

0SHK43Z Insertion of Infusion Device into Right Tarsometatarsal Joint, Percutaneous Endoscopic Approach

0SHK44Z Insertion of Internal Fixation Device into Right Tarsometatarsal Joint, Percutaneous Endoscopic Approach

0SHK45Z Insertion of External Fixation Device into Right Tarsometatarsal Joint, Percutaneous Endoscopic Approach

0SHK48Z Insertion of Spacer into Right Tarsometatarsal Joint, Percutaneous Endoscopic Approach

0SHL03Z Insertion of Infusion Device into Left Tarsometatarsal Joint, Open Approach

0SHL04Z Insertion of Internal Fixation Device into Left Tarsometatarsal Joint, Open Approach

0SHL05Z Insertion of External Fixation Device into Left Tarsometatarsal Joint, Open Approach

0SHL08Z Insertion of Spacer into Left Tarsometatarsal Joint, Open Approach

0SHL33Z Insertion of Infusion Device into Left Tarsometatarsal Joint, Percutaneous Approach

0SHL34Z Insertion of Internal Fixation Device into Left Tarsometatarsal Joint, Percutaneous Approach

0SHL35Z Insertion of External Fixation Device into Left Tarsometatarsal Joint, Percutaneous Approach

0SHL38Z Insertion of Spacer into Left Tarsometatarsal Joint, Percutaneous Approach

0SHL43Z Insertion of Infusion Device into Left Tarsometatarsal Joint, Percutaneous Endoscopic Approach

0SHL44Z Insertion of Internal Fixation Device into Left Tarsometatarsal Joint, Percutaneous Endoscopic Approach

0SHL45Z Insertion of External Fixation Device into Left Tarsometatarsal Joint, Percutaneous Endoscopic Approach

0SHL48Z Insertion of Spacer into Left Tarsometatarsal Joint, Percutaneous Endoscopic Approach

0SHM03Z Insertion of Infusion Device into Right Metatarsal-Phalangeal Joint, Open Approach

0SHM04Z Insertion of Internal Fixation Device into Right Metatarsal-Phalangeal Joint, Open Approach

0SHM05Z Insertion of External Fixation Device into Right Metatarsal-Phalangeal Joint, Open Approach

0SHM08Z Insertion of Spacer into Right Metatarsal-Phalangeal Joint, Open Approach

0SHM33Z Insertion of Infusion Device into Right Metatarsal-Phalangeal Joint, Percutaneous Approach

0SHM34Z Insertion of Internal Fixation Device into Right Metatarsal-Phalangeal Joint, Percutaneous Approach

0SHM35Z Insertion of External Fixation Device into Right Metatarsal-Phalangeal Joint, Percutaneous Approach

0SHM38Z Insertion of Spacer into Right Metatarsal-Phalangeal Joint, Percutaneous Approach

0SHM43Z Insertion of Infusion Device into Right Metatarsal-Phalangeal Joint, Percutaneous Endoscopic Approach

0SHM44Z Insertion of Internal Fixation Device into Right Metatarsal-Phalangeal Joint, Percutaneous Endoscopic Approach

0SHM45Z Insertion of External Fixation Device into Right Metatarsal-Phalangeal Joint, Percutaneous Endoscopic Approach

0SHM48Z Insertion of Spacer into Right Metatarsal-Phalangeal Joint, Percutaneous Endoscopic Approach

0SHN03Z Insertion of Infusion Device into Left Metatarsal-Phalangeal Joint, Open Approach

0SHN04Z Insertion of Internal Fixation Device into Left Metatarsal-Phalangeal Joint, Open Approach

0SHN05Z Insertion of External Fixation Device into Left Metatarsal-Phalangeal Joint, Open Approach

0SHN08Z Insertion of Spacer into Left Metatarsal-Phalangeal Joint, Open Approach

0SHN33Z Insertion of Infusion Device into Left Metatarsal-Phalangeal Joint, Percutaneous Approach

0SHN34Z Insertion of Internal Fixation Device into Left Metatarsal-Phalangeal Joint, Percutaneous Approach

0SHN35Z Insertion of External Fixation Device into Left Metatarsal-Phalangeal Joint, Percutaneous Approach

0SHN38Z Insertion of Spacer into Left Metatarsal-Phalangeal Joint, Percutaneous Approach

0SHN43Z Insertion of Infusion Device into Left Metatarsal-Phalangeal Joint, Percutaneous Endoscopic Approach

0SHN44Z Insertion of Internal Fixation Device into Left Metatarsal-Phalangeal Joint, Percutaneous Endoscopic Approach

0SHN45Z Insertion of External Fixation Device into Left Metatarsal-Phalangeal Joint, Percutaneous Endoscopic Approach

0SHN48Z Insertion of Spacer into Left Metatarsal-Phalangeal Joint, Percutaneous Endoscopic Approach

0SHP03Z Insertion of Infusion Device into Right Toe Phalangeal Joint, Open Approach

0SHP04Z Insertion of Internal Fixation Device into Right Toe Phalangeal Joint, Open Approach

0SHP05Z Insertion of External Fixation Device into Right Toe Phalangeal Joint, Open Approach

0SHP08Z Insertion of Spacer into Right Toe Phalangeal Joint, Open Approach

0SHP33Z Insertion of Infusion Device into Right Toe Phalangeal Joint, Percutaneous Approach

0SHP34Z Insertion of Internal Fixation Device into Right Toe Phalangeal Joint, Percutaneous Approach

0SHP35Z Insertion of External Fixation Device into Right Toe Phalangeal Joint, Percutaneous Approach

0SHP38Z Insertion of Spacer into Right Toe Phalangeal Joint, Percutaneous Approach

0SHP43Z Insertion of Infusion Device into Right Toe Phalangeal Joint, Percutaneous Endoscopic Approach

0SHP44Z Insertion of Internal Fixation Device into Right Toe Phalangeal Joint, Percutaneous Endoscopic Approach

0SHP45Z Insertion of External Fixation Device into Right Toe Phalangeal Joint, Percutaneous Endoscopic Approach

0SHP48Z Insertion of Spacer into Right Toe Phalangeal Joint, Percutaneous Endoscopic Approach

0SHQ03Z Insertion of Infusion Device into Left Toe Phalangeal Joint, Open Approach

0SHQ04Z Insertion of Internal Fixation Device into Left Toe Phalangeal Joint, Open Approach

0SHQ05Z Insertion of External Fixation Device into Left Toe Phalangeal Joint, Open Approach

0SHQ08Z Insertion of Spacer into Left Toe Phalangeal Joint, Open Approach

0SHQ33Z Insertion of Infusion Device into Left Toe Phalangeal Joint, Percutaneous Approach

0SHQ34Z Insertion of Internal Fixation Device into Left Toe Phalangeal Joint, Percutaneous Approach

♀ Female-only   ♂ Male-only   ▲ Limited Coverage   ● Non-OR   ▦ HAC-associated procedure   ▲ Non-covered procedures   ✚ Cluster

0SHQ35Z   Insertion of External Fixation Device into Left Toe Phalangeal Joint, Percutaneous Approach
0SHQ38Z   Insertion of Spacer into Left Toe Phalangeal Joint, Percutaneous Approach

0SHQ43Z   Insertion of Infusion Device into Left Toe Phalangeal Joint, Percutaneous Endoscopic Approach
0SHQ44Z   Insertion of Internal Fixation Device into Left Toe Phalangeal Joint, Percutaneous Endoscopic Approach

0SHQ45Z   Insertion of External Fixation Device into Left Toe Phalangeal Joint, Percutaneous Endoscopic Approach
0SHQ48Z   Insertion of Spacer into Left Toe Phalangeal Joint, Percutaneous Endoscopic Approach

0SJ – Lower Joints, Inspection

Review Coding Guideline B3.5

Review Coding Guidelines B3.11a, B3.11b and B3.11c

0SJ00ZZ   Inspection of Lumbar Vertebral Joint, Open Approach
0SJ03ZZ   Inspection of Lumbar Vertebral Joint, Percutaneous Approach
0SJ04ZZ   Inspection of Lumbar Vertebral Joint, Percutaneous Endoscopic Approach
0SJ0XZZ   Inspection of Lumbar Vertebral Joint, External Approach
0SJ20ZZ   Inspection of Lumbar Vertebral Disc, Open Approach
0SJ23ZZ   Inspection of Lumbar Vertebral Disc, Percutaneous Approach
0SJ24ZZ   Inspection of Lumbar Vertebral Disc, Percutaneous Endoscopic Approach
0SJ2XZZ   Inspection of Lumbar Vertebral Disc, External Approach
0SJ30ZZ   Inspection of Lumbosacral Joint, Open Approach
0SJ33ZZ   Inspection of Lumbosacral Joint, Percutaneous Approach
0SJ34ZZ   Inspection of Lumbosacral Joint, Percutaneous Endoscopic Approach
0SJ3XZZ   Inspection of Lumbosacral Joint, External Approach
0SJ40ZZ   Inspection of Lumbosacral Disc, Open Approach
0SJ43ZZ   Inspection of Lumbosacral Disc, Percutaneous Approach
0SJ44ZZ   Inspection of Lumbosacral Disc, Percutaneous Endoscopic Approach
0SJ4XZZ   Inspection of Lumbosacral Disc, External Approach
0SJ50ZZ   Inspection of Sacrococcygeal Joint, Open Approach
0SJ53ZZ   Inspection of Sacrococcygeal Joint, Percutaneous Approach
0SJ54ZZ   Inspection of Sacrococcygeal Joint, Percutaneous Endoscopic Approach
0SJ5XZZ   Inspection of Sacrococcygeal Joint, External Approach
0SJ60ZZ   Inspection of Coccygeal Joint, Open Approach
0SJ63ZZ   Inspection of Coccygeal Joint, Percutaneous Approach
0SJ64ZZ   Inspection of Coccygeal Joint, Percutaneous Endoscopic Approach
0SJ6XZZ   Inspection of Coccygeal Joint, External Approach
0SJ70ZZ   Inspection of Right Sacroiliac Joint, Open Approach
0SJ73ZZ   Inspection of Right Sacroiliac Joint, Percutaneous Approach
0SJ74ZZ   Inspection of Right Sacroiliac Joint, Percutaneous Endoscopic Approach
0SJ7XZZ   Inspection of Right Sacroiliac Joint, External Approach
0SJ80ZZ   Inspection of Left Sacroiliac Joint, Open Approach
0SJ83ZZ   Inspection of Left Sacroiliac Joint, Percutaneous Approach
0SJ84ZZ   Inspection of Left Sacroiliac Joint, Percutaneous Endoscopic Approach

0SJ8XZZ   Inspection of Left Sacroiliac Joint, External Approach
0SJ90ZZ   Inspection of Right Hip Joint, Open Approach
0SJ93ZZ   Inspection of Right Hip Joint, Percutaneous Approach
0SJ94ZZ   Inspection of Right Hip Joint, Percutaneous Endoscopic Approach
0SJ9XZZ   Inspection of Right Hip Joint, External Approach
0SJB0ZZ   Inspection of Left Hip Joint, Open Approach
0SJB3ZZ   Inspection of Left Hip Joint, Percutaneous Approach
0SJB4ZZ   Inspection of Left Hip Joint, Percutaneous Endoscopic Approach
0SJBXZZ   Inspection of Left Hip Joint, External Approach
0SJC0ZZ   Inspection of Right Knee Joint, Open Approach
0SJC3ZZ   Inspection of Right Knee Joint, Percutaneous Approach
0SJC4ZZ   Inspection of Right Knee Joint, Percutaneous Endoscopic Approach
0SJCXZZ   Inspection of Right Knee Joint, External Approach
0SJD0ZZ   Inspection of Left Knee Joint, Open Approach
0SJD3ZZ   Inspection of Left Knee Joint, Percutaneous Approach
0SJD4ZZ   Inspection of Left Knee Joint, Percutaneous Endoscopic Approach
0SJDXZZ   Inspection of Left Knee Joint, External Approach
0SJF0ZZ   Inspection of Right Ankle Joint, Open Approach
0SJF3ZZ   Inspection of Right Ankle Joint, Percutaneous Approach
0SJF4ZZ   Inspection of Right Ankle Joint, Percutaneous Endoscopic Approach
0SJFXZZ   Inspection of Right Ankle Joint, External Approach
0SJG0ZZ   Inspection of Left Ankle Joint, Open Approach
0SJG3ZZ   Inspection of Left Ankle Joint, Percutaneous Approach
   AHA CC: 1Q, 2017, 50
0SJG4ZZ   Inspection of Left Ankle Joint, Percutaneous Endoscopic Approach
0SJGXZZ   Inspection of Left Ankle Joint, External Approach
0SJH0ZZ   Inspection of Right Tarsal Joint, Open Approach
0SJH3ZZ   Inspection of Right Tarsal Joint, Percutaneous Approach
0SJH4ZZ   Inspection of Right Tarsal Joint, Percutaneous Endoscopic Approach
0SJHXZZ   Inspection of Right Tarsal Joint, External Approach
0SJJ0ZZ   Inspection of Left Tarsal Joint, Open Approach
0SJJ3ZZ   Inspection of Left Tarsal Joint, Percutaneous Approach

0SJJ4ZZ   Inspection of Left Tarsal Joint, Percutaneous Endoscopic Approach
0SJJXZZ   Inspection of Left Tarsal Joint, External Approach
0SJK0ZZ   Inspection of Right Tarsometatarsal Joint, Open Approach
0SJK3ZZ   Inspection of Right Tarsometatarsal Joint, Percutaneous Approach
0SJK4ZZ   Inspection of Right Tarsometatarsal Joint, Percutaneous Endoscopic Approach
0SJKXZZ   Inspection of Right Tarsometatarsal Joint, External Approach
0SJL0ZZ   Inspection of Left Tarsometatarsal Joint, Open Approach
0SJL3ZZ   Inspection of Left Tarsometatarsal Joint, Percutaneous Approach
0SJL4ZZ   Inspection of Left Tarsometatarsal Joint, Percutaneous Endoscopic Approach
0SJLXZZ   Inspection of Left Tarsometatarsal Joint, External Approach
0SJM0ZZ   Inspection of Right Metatarsal-Phalangeal Joint, Open Approach
0SJM3ZZ   Inspection of Right Metatarsal-Phalangeal Joint, Percutaneous Approach
0SJM4ZZ   Inspection of Right Metatarsal-Phalangeal Joint, Percutaneous Endoscopic Approach
0SJMXZZ   Inspection of Right Metatarsal-Phalangeal Joint, External Approach
0SJN0ZZ   Inspection of Left Metatarsal-Phalangeal Joint, Open Approach
0SJN3ZZ   Inspection of Left Metatarsal-Phalangeal Joint, Percutaneous Approach
0SJN4ZZ   Inspection of Left Metatarsal-Phalangeal Joint, Percutaneous Endoscopic Approach
0SJNXZZ   Inspection of Left Metatarsal-Phalangeal Joint, External Approach
0SJP0ZZ   Inspection of Right Toe Phalangeal Joint, Open Approach
0SJP3ZZ   Inspection of Right Toe Phalangeal Joint, Percutaneous Approach
0SJP4ZZ   Inspection of Right Toe Phalangeal Joint, Percutaneous Endoscopic Approach
0SJPXZZ   Inspection of Right Toe Phalangeal Joint, External Approach
0SJQ0ZZ   Inspection of Left Toe Phalangeal Joint, Open Approach
0SJQ3ZZ   Inspection of Left Toe Phalangeal Joint, Percutaneous Approach
0SJQ4ZZ   Inspection of Left Toe Phalangeal Joint, Percutaneous Endoscopic Approach
0SJQXZZ   Inspection of Left Toe Phalangeal Joint, External Approach

---

♀ Female-only   ♂ Male-only   ▲ Limited Coverage   ● Non-OR   🅷🅰🅲 HAC-associated procedure   ▲ Non-covered procedures   ✚ Cluster

0SN – Lower Joints, Release

Review Coding Guideline B3.13

0SN00ZZ	Release Lumbar Vertebral Joint, Open Approach
0SN03ZZ	Release Lumbar Vertebral Joint, Percutaneous Approach
0SN04ZZ	Release Lumbar Vertebral Joint, Percutaneous Endoscopic Approach
0SN0XZZ	Release Lumbar Vertebral Joint, External Approach
0SN20ZZ	Release Lumbar Vertebral Disc, Open Approach
0SN23ZZ	Release Lumbar Vertebral Disc, Percutaneous Approach
0SN24ZZ	Release Lumbar Vertebral Disc, Percutaneous Endoscopic Approach
0SN2XZZ	Release Lumbar Vertebral Disc, External Approach
0SN30ZZ	Release Lumbosacral Joint, Open Approach
0SN33ZZ	Release Lumbosacral Joint, Percutaneous Approach
0SN34ZZ	Release Lumbosacral Joint, Percutaneous Endoscopic Approach
0SN3XZZ	Release Lumbosacral Joint, External Approach
0SN40ZZ	Release Lumbosacral Disc, Open Approach
0SN43ZZ	Release Lumbosacral Disc, Percutaneous Approach
0SN44ZZ	Release Lumbosacral Disc, Percutaneous Endoscopic Approach
0SN4XZZ	Release Lumbosacral Disc, External Approach
0SN50ZZ	Release Sacrococcygeal Joint, Open Approach
0SN53ZZ	Release Sacrococcygeal Joint, Percutaneous Approach
0SN54ZZ	Release Sacrococcygeal Joint, Percutaneous Endoscopic Approach
0SN5XZZ	Release Sacrococcygeal Joint, External Approach
0SN60ZZ	Release Coccygeal Joint, Open Approach
0SN63ZZ	Release Coccygeal Joint, Percutaneous Approach
0SN64ZZ	Release Coccygeal Joint, Percutaneous Endoscopic Approach
0SN6XZZ	Release Coccygeal Joint, External Approach
0SN70ZZ	Release Right Sacroiliac Joint, Open Approach
0SN73ZZ	Release Right Sacroiliac Joint, Percutaneous Approach
0SN74ZZ	Release Right Sacroiliac Joint, Percutaneous Endoscopic Approach
0SN7XZZ	Release Right Sacroiliac Joint, External Approach
0SN80ZZ	Release Left Sacroiliac Joint, Open Approach
0SN83ZZ	Release Left Sacroiliac Joint, Percutaneous Approach
0SN84ZZ	Release Left Sacroiliac Joint, Percutaneous Endoscopic Approach
0SN8XZZ	Release Left Sacroiliac Joint, External Approach
0SN90ZZ	Release Right Hip Joint, Open Approach
0SN93ZZ	Release Right Hip Joint, Percutaneous Approach
0SN94ZZ	Release Right Hip Joint, Percutaneous Endoscopic Approach
0SN9XZZ	Release Right Hip Joint, External Approach
0SNB0ZZ	Release Left Hip Joint, Open Approach
0SNB3ZZ	Release Left Hip Joint, Percutaneous Approach
0SNB4ZZ	Release Left Hip Joint, Percutaneous Endoscopic Approach
0SNBXZZ	Release Left Hip Joint, External Approach
0SNC0ZZ	Release Right Knee Joint, Open Approach
0SNC3ZZ	Release Right Knee Joint, Percutaneous Approach
0SNC4ZZ	Release Right Knee Joint, Percutaneous Endoscopic Approach
	AHA CC: 2Q, 2020, 26-27
0SNCXZZ	Release Right Knee Joint, External Approach
0SND0ZZ	Release Left Knee Joint, Open Approach
0SND3ZZ	Release Left Knee Joint, Percutaneous Approach
0SND4ZZ	Release Left Knee Joint, Percutaneous Endoscopic Approach
0SNDXZZ	Release Left Knee Joint, External Approach
0SNF0ZZ	Release Right Ankle Joint, Open Approach
0SNF3ZZ	Release Right Ankle Joint, Percutaneous Approach
0SNF4ZZ	Release Right Ankle Joint, Percutaneous Endoscopic Approach
0SNFXZZ	Release Right Ankle Joint, External Approach
0SNG0ZZ	Release Left Ankle Joint, Open Approach
0SNG3ZZ	Release Left Ankle Joint, Percutaneous Approach
0SNG4ZZ	Release Left Ankle Joint, Percutaneous Endoscopic Approach
0SNGXZZ	Release Left Ankle Joint, External Approach
0SNH0ZZ	Release Right Tarsal Joint, Open Approach
0SNH3ZZ	Release Right Tarsal Joint, Percutaneous Approach
0SNH4ZZ	Release Right Tarsal Joint, Percutaneous Endoscopic Approach
0SNHXZZ	Release Right Tarsal Joint, External Approach
0SNJ0ZZ	Release Left Tarsal Joint, Open Approach
0SNJ3ZZ	Release Left Tarsal Joint, Percutaneous Approach
0SNJ4ZZ	Release Left Tarsal Joint, Percutaneous Endoscopic Approach
0SNJXZZ	Release Left Tarsal Joint, External Approach
0SNK0ZZ	Release Right Tarsometatarsal Joint, Open Approach
0SNK3ZZ	Release Right Tarsometatarsal Joint, Percutaneous Approach
0SNK4ZZ	Release Right Tarsometatarsal Joint, Percutaneous Endoscopic Approach
0SNKXZZ	Release Right Tarsometatarsal Joint, External Approach
0SNL0ZZ	Release Left Tarsometatarsal Joint, Open Approach
0SNL3ZZ	Release Left Tarsometatarsal Joint, Percutaneous Approach
0SNL4ZZ	Release Left Tarsometatarsal Joint, Percutaneous Endoscopic Approach
0SNLXZZ	Release Left Tarsometatarsal Joint, External Approach
0SNM0ZZ	Release Right Metatarsal-Phalangeal Joint, Open Approach
0SNM3ZZ	Release Right Metatarsal-Phalangeal Joint, Percutaneous Approach
0SNM4ZZ	Release Right Metatarsal-Phalangeal Joint, Percutaneous Endoscopic Approach
0SNMXZZ	Release Right Metatarsal-Phalangeal Joint, External Approach
0SNN0ZZ	Release Left Metatarsal-Phalangeal Joint, Open Approach
0SNN3ZZ	Release Left Metatarsal-Phalangeal Joint, Percutaneous Approach
0SNN4ZZ	Release Left Metatarsal-Phalangeal Joint, Percutaneous Endoscopic Approach
0SNNXZZ	Release Left Metatarsal-Phalangeal Joint, External Approach
0SNP0ZZ	Release Right Toe Phalangeal Joint, Open Approach
0SNP3ZZ	Release Right Toe Phalangeal Joint, Percutaneous Approach
0SNP4ZZ	Release Right Toe Phalangeal Joint, Percutaneous Endoscopic Approach
0SNPXZZ	Release Right Toe Phalangeal Joint, External Approach
0SNQ0ZZ	Release Left Toe Phalangeal Joint, Open Approach
0SNQ3ZZ	Release Left Toe Phalangeal Joint, Percutaneous Approach
0SNQ4ZZ	Release Left Toe Phalangeal Joint, Percutaneous Endoscopic Approach
0SNQXZZ	Release Left Toe Phalangeal Joint, External Approach

0SP – Lower Joints, Removal

Review Coding Guideline B6.1c

0SP000Z	Removal of Drainage Device from Lumbar Vertebral Joint, Open Approach
0SP003Z	Removal of Infusion Device from Lumbar Vertebral Joint, Open Approach
0SP004Z	Removal of Internal Fixation Device from Lumbar Vertebral Joint, Open Approach
0SP007Z	Removal of Autologous Tissue Substitute from Lumbar Vertebral Joint, Open Approach
0SP008Z	Removal of Spacer from Lumbar Vertebral Joint, Open Approach
0SP00AZ	Removal of Interbody Fusion Device from Lumbar Vertebral Joint, Open Approach
0SP00JZ	Removal of Synthetic Substitute from Lumbar Vertebral Joint, Open Approach
0SP00KZ	Removal of Nonautologous Tissue Substitute from Lumbar Vertebral Joint, Open Approach
0SP030Z	Removal of Drainage Device from Lumbar Vertebral Joint, Percutaneous Approach

♀ Female-only ♂ Male-only ▲ Limited Coverage ● Non-OR ▨ HAC-associated procedure ▲ Non-covered procedures ✚ Cluster

0SP033Z Removal of Infusion Device from Lumbar Vertebral Joint, Percutaneous Approach

0SP034Z Removal of Internal Fixation Device from Lumbar Vertebral Joint, Percutaneous Approach

0SP037Z Removal of Autologous Tissue Substitute from Lumbar Vertebral Joint, Percutaneous Approach

0SP038Z Removal of Spacer from Lumbar Vertebral Joint, Percutaneous Approach

0SP03AZ Removal of Interbody Fusion Device from Lumbar Vertebral Joint, Percutaneous Approach

0SP03JZ Removal of Synthetic Substitute from Lumbar Vertebral Joint, Percutaneous Approach

0SP03KZ Removal of Nonautologous Tissue Substitute from Lumbar Vertebral Joint, Percutaneous Approach

0SP040Z Removal of Drainage Device from Lumbar Vertebral Joint, Percutaneous Endoscopic Approach

0SP043Z Removal of Infusion Device from Lumbar Vertebral Joint, Percutaneous Endoscopic Approach

0SP044Z Removal of Internal Fixation Device from Lumbar Vertebral Joint, Percutaneous Endoscopic Approach

0SP047Z Removal of Autologous Tissue Substitute from Lumbar Vertebral Joint, Percutaneous Endoscopic Approach

0SP048Z Removal of Spacer from Lumbar Vertebral Joint, Percutaneous Endoscopic Approach

0SP04AZ Removal of Interbody Fusion Device from Lumbar Vertebral Joint, Percutaneous Endoscopic Approach

0SP04JZ Removal of Synthetic Substitute from Lumbar Vertebral Joint, Percutaneous Endoscopic Approach

0SP04KZ Removal of Nonautologous Tissue Substitute from Lumbar Vertebral Joint, Percutaneous Endoscopic Approach

0SP0X0Z Removal of Drainage Device from Lumbar Vertebral Joint, External Approach

0SP0X3Z Removal of Infusion Device from Lumbar Vertebral Joint, External Approach

0SP0X4Z Removal of Internal Fixation Device from Lumbar Vertebral Joint, External Approach

0SP200Z Removal of Drainage Device from Lumbar Vertebral Disc, Open Approach

0SP203Z Removal of Infusion Device from Lumbar Vertebral Disc, Open Approach

0SP207Z Removal of Autologous Tissue Substitute from Lumbar Vertebral Disc, Open Approach

0SP20JZ Removal of Synthetic Substitute from Lumbar Vertebral Disc, Open Approach

0SP20KZ Removal of Nonautologous Tissue Substitute from Lumbar Vertebral Disc, Open Approach

0SP230Z Removal of Drainage Device from Lumbar Vertebral Disc, Percutaneous Approach

0SP233Z Removal of Infusion Device from Lumbar Vertebral Disc, Percutaneous Approach

0SP237Z Removal of Autologous Tissue Substitute from Lumbar Vertebral Disc, Percutaneous Approach

0SP23JZ Removal of Synthetic Substitute from Lumbar Vertebral Disc, Percutaneous Approach

0SP23KZ Removal of Nonautologous Tissue Substitute from Lumbar Vertebral Disc, Percutaneous Approach

0SP240Z Removal of Drainage Device from Lumbar Vertebral Disc, Percutaneous Endoscopic Approach

0SP243Z Removal of Infusion Device from Lumbar Vertebral Disc, Percutaneous Endoscopic Approach

0SP247Z Removal of Autologous Tissue Substitute from Lumbar Vertebral Disc, Percutaneous Endoscopic Approach

0SP24JZ Removal of Synthetic Substitute from Lumbar Vertebral Disc, Percutaneous Endoscopic Approach

0SP24KZ Removal of Nonautologous Tissue Substitute from Lumbar Vertebral Disc, Percutaneous Endoscopic Approach

0SP2X0Z Removal of Drainage Device from Lumbar Vertebral Disc, External Approach

0SP2X3Z Removal of Infusion Device from Lumbar Vertebral Disc, External Approach

0SP300Z Removal of Drainage Device from Lumbosacral Joint, Open Approach

0SP303Z Removal of Infusion Device from Lumbosacral Joint, Open Approach

0SP304Z Removal of Internal Fixation Device from Lumbosacral Joint, Open Approach

0SP307Z Removal of Autologous Tissue Substitute from Lumbosacral Joint, Open Approach

0SP308Z Removal of Spacer from Lumbosacral Joint, Open Approach

0SP30AZ Removal of Interbody Fusion Device from Lumbosacral Joint, Open Approach

0SP30JZ Removal of Synthetic Substitute from Lumbosacral Joint, Open Approach

0SP30KZ Removal of Nonautologous Tissue Substitute from Lumbosacral Joint, Open Approach

0SP330Z Removal of Drainage Device from Lumbosacral Joint, Percutaneous Approach

0SP333Z Removal of Infusion Device from Lumbosacral Joint, Percutaneous Approach

0SP334Z Removal of Internal Fixation Device from Lumbosacral Joint, Percutaneous Approach

0SP337Z Removal of Autologous Tissue Substitute from Lumbosacral Joint, Percutaneous Approach

0SP338Z Removal of Spacer from Lumbosacral Joint, Percutaneous Approach

0SP33AZ Removal of Interbody Fusion Device from Lumbosacral Joint, Percutaneous Approach

0SP33JZ Removal of Synthetic Substitute from Lumbosacral Joint, Percutaneous Approach

0SP33KZ Removal of Nonautologous Tissue Substitute from Lumbosacral Joint, Percutaneous Approach

0SP340Z Removal of Drainage Device from Lumbosacral Joint, Percutaneous Endoscopic Approach

0SP343Z Removal of Infusion Device from Lumbosacral Joint, Percutaneous Endoscopic Approach

0SP344Z Removal of Internal Fixation Device from Lumbosacral Joint, Percutaneous Endoscopic Approach

0SP347Z Removal of Autologous Tissue Substitute from Lumbosacral Joint, Percutaneous Endoscopic Approach

0SP348Z Removal of Spacer from Lumbosacral Joint, Percutaneous Endoscopic Approach

0SP34AZ Removal of Interbody Fusion Device from Lumbosacral Joint, Percutaneous Endoscopic Approach

0SP34JZ Removal of Synthetic Substitute from Lumbosacral Joint, Percutaneous Endoscopic Approach

0SP34KZ Removal of Nonautologous Tissue Substitute from Lumbosacral Joint, Percutaneous Endoscopic Approach

0SP3X0Z Removal of Drainage Device from Lumbosacral Joint, External Approach

0SP3X3Z Removal of Infusion Device from Lumbosacral Joint, External Approach

0SP3X4Z Removal of Internal Fixation Device from Lumbosacral Joint, External Approach

0SP400Z Removal of Drainage Device from Lumbosacral Disc, Open Approach

0SP403Z Removal of Infusion Device from Lumbosacral Disc, Open Approach

0SP407Z Removal of Autologous Tissue Substitute from Lumbosacral Disc, Open Approach

0SP40JZ Removal of Synthetic Substitute from Lumbosacral Disc, Open Approach

0SP40KZ Removal of Nonautologous Tissue Substitute from Lumbosacral Disc, Open Approach

0SP430Z Removal of Drainage Device from Lumbosacral Disc, Percutaneous Approach

0SP433Z Removal of Infusion Device from Lumbosacral Disc, Percutaneous Approach

0SP437Z Removal of Autologous Tissue Substitute from Lumbosacral Disc, Percutaneous Approach

0SP43JZ Removal of Synthetic Substitute from Lumbosacral Disc, Percutaneous Approach

0SP43KZ Removal of Nonautologous Tissue Substitute from Lumbosacral Disc, Percutaneous Approach

0SP440Z Removal of Drainage Device from Lumbosacral Disc, Percutaneous Endoscopic Approach

0SP443Z Removal of Infusion Device from Lumbosacral Disc, Percutaneous Endoscopic Approach

0SP447Z Removal of Autologous Tissue Substitute from Lumbosacral Disc, Percutaneous Endoscopic Approach

0SP44JZ Removal of Synthetic Substitute from Lumbosacral Disc, Percutaneous Endoscopic Approach

0SP44KZ Removal of Nonautologous Tissue Substitute from Lumbosacral Disc, Percutaneous Endoscopic Approach

0SP4X0Z Removal of Drainage Device from Lumbosacral Disc, External Approach

0SP4X3Z Removal of Infusion Device from Lumbosacral Disc, External Approach

0SP500Z Removal of Drainage Device from Sacrococcygeal Joint, Open Approach

0SP503Z Removal of Infusion Device from Sacrococcygeal Joint, Open Approach

0SP504Z Removal of Internal Fixation Device from Sacrococcygeal Joint, Open Approach

0SP507Z Removal of Autologous Tissue Substitute from Sacrococcygeal Joint, Open Approach

0SP508Z Removal of Spacer from Sacrococcygeal Joint, Open Approach

0SP50JZ Removal of Synthetic Substitute from Sacrococcygeal Joint, Open Approach

0SP50KZ Removal of Nonautologous Tissue Substitute from Sacrococcygeal Joint, Open Approach

0SP530Z Removal of Drainage Device from Sacrococcygeal Joint, Percutaneous Approach

0SP533Z Removal of Infusion Device from Sacrococcygeal Joint, Percutaneous Approach

0SP534Z Removal of Internal Fixation Device from Sacrococcygeal Joint, Percutaneous Approach

0SP537Z Removal of Autologous Tissue Substitute from Sacrococcygeal Joint, Percutaneous Approach

0SP538Z Removal of Spacer from Sacrococcygeal Joint, Percutaneous Approach

0SP53JZ Removal of Synthetic Substitute from Sacrococcygeal Joint, Percutaneous Approach

0SP53KZ Removal of Nonautologous Tissue Substitute from Sacrococcygeal Joint, Percutaneous Approach

0SP540Z Removal of Drainage Device from Sacrococcygeal Joint, Percutaneous Endoscopic Approach

0SP543Z Removal of Infusion Device from Sacrococcygeal Joint, Percutaneous Endoscopic Approach

0SP544Z Removal of Internal Fixation Device from Sacrococcygeal Joint, Percutaneous Endoscopic Approach

0SP547Z Removal of Autologous Tissue Substitute from Sacrococcygeal Joint, Percutaneous Endoscopic Approach

0SP548Z Removal of Spacer from Sacrococcygeal Joint, Percutaneous Endoscopic Approach

0SP54JZ Removal of Synthetic Substitute from Sacrococcygeal Joint, Percutaneous Endoscopic Approach

0SP54KZ Removal of Nonautologous Tissue Substitute from Sacrococcygeal Joint, Percutaneous Endoscopic Approach

0SP5X0Z Removal of Drainage Device from Sacrococcygeal Joint, External Approach

0SP5X3Z Removal of Infusion Device from Sacrococcygeal Joint, External Approach

0SP5X4Z Removal of Internal Fixation Device from Sacrococcygeal Joint, External Approach

0SP600Z Removal of Drainage Device from Coccygeal Joint, Open Approach

0SP603Z Removal of Infusion Device from Coccygeal Joint, Open Approach

0SP604Z Removal of Internal Fixation Device from Coccygeal Joint, Open Approach

0SP607Z Removal of Autologous Tissue Substitute from Coccygeal Joint, Open Approach

0SP608Z Removal of Spacer from Coccygeal Joint, Open Approach

0SP60JZ Removal of Synthetic Substitute from Coccygeal Joint, Open Approach

0SP60KZ Removal of Nonautologous Tissue Substitute from Coccygeal Joint, Open Approach

0SP630Z Removal of Drainage Device from Coccygeal Joint, Percutaneous Approach

0SP633Z Removal of Infusion Device from Coccygeal Joint, Percutaneous Approach

0SP634Z Removal of Internal Fixation Device from Coccygeal Joint, Percutaneous Approach

0SP637Z Removal of Autologous Tissue Substitute from Coccygeal Joint, Percutaneous Approach

0SP638Z Removal of Spacer from Coccygeal Joint, Percutaneous Approach

0SP63JZ Removal of Synthetic Substitute from Coccygeal Joint, Percutaneous Approach

0SP63KZ Removal of Nonautologous Tissue Substitute from Coccygeal Joint, Percutaneous Approach

0SP640Z Removal of Drainage Device from Coccygeal Joint, Percutaneous Endoscopic Approach

0SP643Z Removal of Infusion Device from Coccygeal Joint, Percutaneous Endoscopic Approach

0SP644Z Removal of Internal Fixation Device from Coccygeal Joint, Percutaneous Endoscopic Approach

0SP647Z Removal of Autologous Tissue Substitute from Coccygeal Joint, Percutaneous Endoscopic Approach

0SP648Z Removal of Spacer from Coccygeal Joint, Percutaneous Endoscopic Approach

0SP64JZ Removal of Synthetic Substitute from Coccygeal Joint, Percutaneous Endoscopic Approach

0SP64KZ Removal of Nonautologous Tissue Substitute from Coccygeal Joint, Percutaneous Endoscopic Approach

0SP6X0Z Removal of Drainage Device from Coccygeal Joint, External Approach

0SP6X3Z Removal of Infusion Device from Coccygeal Joint, External Approach

0SP6X4Z Removal of Internal Fixation Device from Coccygeal Joint, External Approach

0SP700Z Removal of Drainage Device from Right Sacroiliac Joint, Open Approach

0SP703Z Removal of Infusion Device from Right Sacroiliac Joint, Open Approach

0SP704Z Removal of Internal Fixation Device from Right Sacroiliac Joint, Open Approach

0SP707Z Removal of Autologous Tissue Substitute from Right Sacroiliac Joint, Open Approach

0SP708Z Removal of Spacer from Right Sacroiliac Joint, Open Approach

0SP70JZ Removal of Synthetic Substitute from Right Sacroiliac Joint, Open Approach

0SP70KZ Removal of Nonautologous Tissue Substitute from Right Sacroiliac Joint, Open Approach

0SP730Z Removal of Drainage Device from Right Sacroiliac Joint, Percutaneous Approach

0SP733Z Removal of Infusion Device from Right Sacroiliac Joint, Percutaneous Approach

0SP734Z Removal of Internal Fixation Device from Right Sacroiliac Joint, Percutaneous Approach

0SP737Z Removal of Autologous Tissue Substitute from Right Sacroiliac Joint, Percutaneous Approach

0SP738Z Removal of Spacer from Right Sacroiliac Joint, Percutaneous Approach

0SP73JZ Removal of Synthetic Substitute from Right Sacroiliac Joint, Percutaneous Approach

0SP73KZ Removal of Nonautologous Tissue Substitute from Right Sacroiliac Joint, Percutaneous Approach

0SP740Z Removal of Drainage Device from Right Sacroiliac Joint, Percutaneous Endoscopic Approach

0SP743Z Removal of Infusion Device from Right Sacroiliac Joint, Percutaneous Endoscopic Approach

0SP744Z Removal of Internal Fixation Device from Right Sacroiliac Joint, Percutaneous Endoscopic Approach

0SP747Z Removal of Autologous Tissue Substitute from Right Sacroiliac Joint, Percutaneous Endoscopic Approach

0SP748Z Removal of Spacer from Right Sacroiliac Joint, Percutaneous Endoscopic Approach

0SP74JZ Removal of Synthetic Substitute from Right Sacroiliac Joint, Percutaneous Endoscopic Approach

0SP74KZ Removal of Nonautologous Tissue Substitute from Right Sacroiliac Joint, Percutaneous Endoscopic Approach

0SP7X0Z Removal of Drainage Device from Right Sacroiliac Joint, External Approach

0SP7X3Z Removal of Infusion Device from Right Sacroiliac Joint, External Approach

0SP7X4Z Removal of Internal Fixation Device from Right Sacroiliac Joint, External Approach

0SP800Z Removal of Drainage Device from Left Sacroiliac Joint, Open Approach

0SP803Z Removal of Infusion Device from Left Sacroiliac Joint, Open Approach

0SP804Z Removal of Internal Fixation Device from Left Sacroiliac Joint, Open Approach

0SP807Z Removal of Autologous Tissue Substitute from Left Sacroiliac Joint, Open Approach

0SP808Z Removal of Spacer from Left Sacroiliac Joint, Open Approach

0SP80JZ Removal of Synthetic Substitute from Left Sacroiliac Joint, Open Approach

0SP80KZ Removal of Nonautologous Tissue Substitute from Left Sacroiliac Joint, Open Approach

0SP830Z Removal of Drainage Device from Left Sacroiliac Joint, Percutaneous Approach

0SP833Z Removal of Infusion Device from Left Sacroiliac Joint, Percutaneous Approach

0SP834Z Removal of Internal Fixation Device from Left Sacroiliac Joint, Percutaneous Approach

0SP837Z Removal of Autologous Tissue Substitute from Left Sacroiliac Joint, Percutaneous Approach

0SP838Z Removal of Spacer from Left Sacroiliac Joint, Percutaneous Approach

♀ Female-only   ♂ Male-only   ▲ Limited Coverage   ● Non-OR   HAC HAC-associated procedure   ▲ Non-covered procedures   ✚ Cluster

0SP83JZ Removal of Synthetic Substitute from Left Sacroiliac Joint, Percutaneous Approach

0SP83KZ Removal of Nonautologous Tissue Substitute from Left Sacroiliac Joint, Percutaneous Approach

0SP840Z Removal of Drainage Device from Left Sacroiliac Joint, Percutaneous Endoscopic Approach

0SP843Z Removal of Infusion Device from Left Sacroiliac Joint, Percutaneous Endoscopic Approach

0SP844Z Removal of Internal Fixation Device from Left Sacroiliac Joint, Percutaneous Endoscopic Approach

0SP847Z Removal of Autologous Tissue Substitute from Left Sacroiliac Joint, Percutaneous Endoscopic Approach

0SP848Z Removal of Spacer from Left Sacroiliac Joint, Percutaneous Endoscopic Approach

0SP84JZ Removal of Synthetic Substitute from Left Sacroiliac Joint, Percutaneous Endoscopic Approach

0SP84KZ Removal of Nonautologous Tissue Substitute from Left Sacroiliac Joint, Percutaneous Endoscopic Approach

0SP8X0Z Removal of Drainage Device from Left Sacroiliac Joint, External Approach

0SP8X3Z Removal of Infusion Device from Left Sacroiliac Joint, External Approach

0SP8X4Z Removal of Internal Fixation Device from Left Sacroiliac Joint, External Approach

0SP900Z Removal of Drainage Device from Right Hip Joint, Open Approach

0SP903Z Removal of Infusion Device from Right Hip Joint, Open Approach

0SP904Z Removal of Internal Fixation Device from Right Hip Joint, Open Approach

0SP905Z Removal of External Fixation Device from Right Hip Joint, Open Approach

0SP907Z Removal of Autologous Tissue Substitute from Right Hip Joint, Open Approach

0SP908Z Removal of Spacer from Right Hip Joint, Open Approach

➕ *If replacement, see table 0SR to construct a code for Replacement of the device.*

0SP909Z Removal of Liner from Right Hip Joint, Open Approach

➕ *If replacement, see table 0SR to construct a code for Replacement of the device or see table 0SU to construct a code for Supplement with liner.*
AHA CC: 2Q, 2015, 19-20; 4Q, 2016, 111-112

0SP90BZ Removal of Resurfacing Device from Right Hip Joint, Open Approach

➕ *If replacement, see table 0SR to construct a code for Replacement of the device.*

0SP90EZ Removal of Articulating Spacer from Right Hip Joint, Open Approach

0SP90JZ Removal of Synthetic Substitute from Right Hip Joint, Open Approach

➕ *If replacement see table 0SR to construct a code for Replacement of the device.*
AHA CC: 2Q, 2015, 19-20

0SP90KZ Removal of Nonautologous Tissue Substitute from Right Hip Joint, Open Approach

0SP930Z Removal of Drainage Device from Right Hip Joint, Percutaneous Approach

0SP933Z Removal of Infusion Device from Right Hip Joint, Percutaneous Approach

0SP934Z Removal of Internal Fixation Device from Right Hip Joint, Percutaneous Approach

0SP935Z Removal of External Fixation Device from Right Hip Joint, Percutaneous Approach

0SP937Z Removal of Autologous Tissue Substitute from Right Hip Joint, Percutaneous Approach

0SP938Z Removal of Spacer from Right Hip Joint, Percutaneous Approach

0SP93JZ Removal of Synthetic Substitute from Right Hip Joint, Percutaneous Approach

0SP93KZ Removal of Nonautologous Tissue Substitute from Right Hip Joint, Percutaneous Approach

0SP940Z Removal of Drainage Device from Right Hip Joint, Percutaneous Endoscopic Approach

0SP943Z Removal of Infusion Device from Right Hip Joint, Percutaneous Endoscopic Approach

0SP944Z Removal of Internal Fixation Device from Right Hip Joint, Percutaneous Endoscopic Approach

0SP945Z Removal of External Fixation Device from Right Hip Joint, Percutaneous Endoscopic Approach

0SP947Z Removal of Autologous Tissue Substitute from Right Hip Joint, Percutaneous Endoscopic Approach

● **0SP948Z** Removal of Spacer from Right Hip Joint, Percutaneous Endoscopic Approach

➕ *If replacement, see table 0SR to construct a code for Replacement of the device.*

0SP94JZ Removal of Synthetic Substitute from Right Hip Joint, Percutaneous Endoscopic Approach

➕ *If replacement, see table 0SR to construct a code for Replacement of the device.*

0SP94KZ Removal of Nonautologous Tissue Substitute from Right Hip Joint, Percutaneous Endoscopic Approach

0SP9X0Z Removal of Drainage Device from Right Hip Joint, External Approach

0SP9X3Z Removal of Infusion Device from Right Hip Joint, External Approach

0SP9X4Z Removal of Internal Fixation Device from Right Hip Joint, External Approach

0SP9X5Z Removal of External Fixation Device from Right Hip Joint, External Approach

0SPA0JZ Removal of Synthetic Substitute from Right Hip Joint, Acetabular Surface, Open Approach

➕ *If replacement, see table 0SR to construct a code for Replacement of the device.*

0SPA3JZ Removal of Synthetic Substitute from Right Hip Joint, Acetabular Surface, Percutaneous Approach

0SPA4JZ Removal of Synthetic Substitute from Right Hip Joint, Acetabular Surface, Percutaneous Endoscopic Approach

➕ *If replacement, see table 0SR to construct a code for Replacement of the device.*

0SPB00Z Removal of Drainage Device from Left Hip Joint, Open Approach

0SPB03Z Removal of Infusion Device from Left Hip Joint, Open Approach

0SPB04Z Removal of Internal Fixation Device from Left Hip Joint, Open Approach

0SPB05Z Removal of External Fixation Device from Left Hip Joint, Open Approach

0SPB07Z Removal of Autologous Tissue Substitute from Left Hip Joint, Open Approach

0SPB08Z Removal of Spacer from Left Hip Joint, Open Approach

➕ *If replacement, see table 0SR to construct a code for Replacement of the device.*

0SPB09Z Removal of Liner from Left Hip Joint, Open Approach

➕ *If replacement, see table 0SR to construct a code for Replacement of the device or see table 0SU to construct a code for Supplement with liner.*

0SPB0BZ Removal of Resurfacing Device from Left Hip Joint, Open Approach

➕ *If replacement, see table 0SR to construct a code for Replacement of the device.*

0SPB0EZ Removal of Articulating Spacer from Left Hip Joint, Open Approach

0SPB0JZ Removal of Synthetic Substitute from Left Hip Joint, Open Approach

➕ *If replacement see table 0SR to construct a code for the Replacement of the device.*

0SPB0KZ Removal of Nonautologous Tissue Substitute from Left Hip Joint, Open Approach

0SPB30Z Removal of Drainage Device from Left Hip Joint, Percutaneous Approach

0SPB33Z Removal of Infusion Device from Left Hip Joint, Percutaneous Approach

0SPB34Z Removal of Internal Fixation Device from Left Hip Joint, Percutaneous Approach

0SPB35Z Removal of External Fixation Device from Left Hip Joint, Percutaneous Approach

0SPB37Z Removal of Autologous Tissue Substitute from Left Hip Joint, Percutaneous Approach

0SPB38Z Removal of Spacer from Left Hip Joint, Percutaneous Approach

0SPB3JZ Removal of Synthetic Substitute from Left Hip Joint, Percutaneous Approach

0SPB3KZ Removal of Nonautologous Tissue Substitute from Left Hip Joint, Percutaneous Approach

0SPB40Z Removal of Drainage Device from Left Hip Joint, Percutaneous Endoscopic Approach

0SPB43Z Removal of Infusion Device from Left Hip Joint, Percutaneous Endoscopic Approach

0SPB44Z Removal of Internal Fixation Device from Left Hip Joint, Percutaneous Endoscopic Approach

0SPB45Z Removal of External Fixation Device from Left Hip Joint, Percutaneous Endoscopic Approach

0SPB47Z Removal of Autologous Tissue Substitute from Left Hip Joint, Percutaneous Endoscopic Approach

● **0SPB48Z** Removal of Spacer from Left Hip Joint, Percutaneous Endoscopic Approach

➕ *If replacement, see table 0SR to construct a code for Replacement of the device.*

♀ Female-only   ♂ Male-only   ▲ Limited Coverage   ● Non-OR   🄷🄰🄲 HAC-associated procedure   ▲ Non-covered procedures   ➕ Cluster

0SPB4JZ Removal of Synthetic Substitute from Left Hip Joint, Percutaneous Endoscopic Approach

⊞ *If replacement, see table 0SR to construct a code for Replacement of the device.*

0SPB4KZ Removal of Nonautologous Tissue Substitute from Left Hip Joint, Percutaneous Endoscopic Approach

0SPBX0Z Removal of Drainage Device from Left Hip Joint, External Approach

0SPBX3Z Removal of Infusion Device from Left Hip Joint, External Approach

0SPBX4Z Removal of Internal Fixation Device from Left Hip Joint, External Approach

0SPBX5Z Removal of External Fixation Device from Left Hip Joint, External Approach

0SPC00Z Removal of Drainage Device from Right Knee Joint, Open Approach

0SPC03Z Removal of Infusion Device from Right Knee Joint, Open Approach

0SPC04Z Removal of Internal Fixation Device from Right Knee Joint, Open Approach

0SPC05Z Removal of External Fixation Device from Right Knee Joint, Open Approach

0SPC07Z Removal of Autologous Tissue Substitute from Right Knee Joint, Open Approach

0SPC08Z Removal of Spacer from Right Knee Joint, Open Approach

⊞ *If revision, see table 0SR to construct a code for Replacement of joint.*

0SPC09Z Removal of Liner from Right Knee Joint, Open Approach

⊞ *If replacement, see table 0SU to construct a code for Supplement with liner.*

0SPC0EZ Removal of Articulating Spacer from Right Knee Joint, Open Approach

0SPC0JC Removal of Synthetic Substitute from Right Knee Joint, Patellar Surface, Open Approach

⊞ *If replacement, see table 0SR to construct a code for Replacement of the device.*

0SPC0JZ Removal of Synthetic Substitute from Right Knee Joint, Open Approach

⊞ *If replacement see table 0SR to construct a code for the Replacement of the device.*

AHA CC: 2Q, 2015, 18-19

0SPC0KZ Removal of Nonautologous Tissue Substitute from Right Knee Joint, Open Approach

0SPC0LZ Removal of Medial Unicondylar Synthetic Substitute from Right Knee Joint, Open Approach

0SPC0MZ Removal of Lateral Unicondylar Synthetic Substitute from Right Knee Joint, Open Approach

0SPC0NZ Removal of Patellofemoral Synthetic Substitute from Right Knee Joint, Open Approach

0SPC30Z Removal of Drainage Device from Right Knee Joint, Percutaneous Approach

0SPC33Z Removal of Infusion Device from Right Knee Joint, Percutaneous Approach

0SPC34Z Removal of Internal Fixation Device from Right Knee Joint, Percutaneous Approach

0SPC35Z Removal of External Fixation Device from Right Knee Joint, Percutaneous Approach

0SPC37Z Removal of Autologous Tissue Substitute from Right Knee Joint, Percutaneous Approach

● **0SPC38Z** Removal of Spacer from Right Knee Joint, Percutaneous Approach

⊞ *If revision, see table 0SR to construct a code for Replacement of joint.*

0SPC3JC Removal of Synthetic Substitute from Right Knee Joint, Patellar Surface, Percutaneous Approac

0SPC3JZ Removal of Synthetic Substitute from Right Knee Joint, Percutaneous Approach

0SPC3KZ Removal of Nonautologous Tissue Substitute from Right Knee Joint, Percutaneous Approach

0SPC3LZ Removal of Medial Unicondylar Synthetic Substitute from Right Knee Joint, Percutaneous Approach

0SPC3MZ Removal of Lateral Unicondylar Synthetic Substitute from Right Knee Joint, Percutaneous Approach

0SPC3NZ Removal of Patellofemoral Synthetic Substitute from Right Knee Joint, Percutaneous Approach

0SPC40Z Removal of Drainage Device from Right Knee Joint, Percutaneous Endoscopic Approach

0SPC43Z Removal of Infusion Device from Right Knee Joint, Percutaneous Endoscopic Approach

0SPC44Z Removal of Internal Fixation Device from Right Knee Joint, Percutaneous Endoscopic Approach

0SPC45Z Removal of External Fixation Device from Right Knee Joint, Percutaneous Endoscopic Approach

0SPC47Z Removal of Autologous Tissue Substitute from Right Knee Joint, Percutaneous Endoscopic Approach

● **0SPC48Z** Removal of Spacer from Right Knee Joint, Percutaneous Endoscopic Approach

⊞ *If revision, see table 0SR to construct a code for Replacement of joint.*

0SPC4JC Removal of Synthetic Substitute from Right Knee Joint, Patellar Surface, Percutaneous Endoscopic Approach

⊞ *If replacement, see table 0SR to construct a code for Replacement of the device.*

0SPC4JZ Removal of Synthetic Substitute from Right Knee Joint, Percutaneous Endoscopic Approach

⊞ *If replacement see table 0SR to construct a code for the Replacement of the device.*

0SPC4KZ Removal of Nonautologous Tissue Substitute from Right Knee Joint, Percutaneous Endoscopic Approach

0SPC4LZ Removal of Medial Unicondylar Synthetic Substitute from Right Knee Joint, Percutaneous Endoscopic Approach

0SPC4MZ Removal of Lateral Unicondylar Synthetic Substitute from Right Knee Joint, Percutaneous Endoscopic Approach

0SPC4NZ Removal of Patellofemoral Synthetic Substitute from Right Knee Joint, Percutaneous Endoscopic Approach

0SPCX0Z Removal of Drainage Device from Right Knee Joint, External Approach

0SPCX3Z Removal of Infusion Device from Right Knee Joint, External Approach

0SPCX4Z Removal of Internal Fixation Device from Right Knee Joint, External Approach

0SPCX5Z Removal of External Fixation Device from Right Knee Joint, External Approach

0SPD00Z Removal of Drainage Device from Left Knee Joint, Open Approach

0SPD03Z Removal of Infusion Device from Left Knee Joint, Open Approach

0SPD04Z Removal of Internal Fixation Device from Left Knee Joint, Open Approach

0SPD05Z Removal of External Fixation Device from Left Knee Joint, Open Approach

0SPD07Z Removal of Autologous Tissue Substitute from Left Knee Joint, Open Approach

0SPD08Z Removal of Spacer from Left Knee Joint, Open Approach

⊞ *If revision, see table 0SR to construct a code for Replacement of joint.*

0SPD09Z Removal of Liner from Left Knee Joint, Open Approach

⊞ *If replacement, see table 0SU to construct a code for Supplement with liner.*

0SPD0EZ Removal of Articulating Spacer from Left Knee Joint, Open Approach

0SPD0JC Removal of Synthetic Substitute from Left Knee Joint, Patellar Surface, Open Approach

⊞ *If replacement, see table 0SR to construct a code for Replacement of the device.*

0SPD0JZ Removal of Synthetic Substitute from Left Knee Joint, Open Approach

⊞ *If replacement see table 0SR to construct a code for the Replacement of the device.*

0SPD0KZ Removal of Nonautologous Tissue Substitute from Left Knee Joint, Open Approach

0SPD0LZ Removal of Medial Unicondylar Synthetic Substitute from Left Knee Joint, Open Approach

0SPD0MZ Removal of Lateral Unicondylar Synthetic Substitute from Left Knee Joint, Open Approach

0SPD0NZ Removal of Patellofemoral Synthetic Substitute from Left Knee Joint, Open Approach

● **0SPD30Z** Removal of Drainage Device from Left Knee Joint, Percutaneous Approach

● **0SPD33Z** Removal of Infusion Device from Left Knee Joint, Percutaneous Approach

0SPD34Z Removal of Internal Fixation Device from Left Knee Joint, Percutaneous Approach

0SPD35Z Removal of External Fixation Device from Left Knee Joint, Percutaneous Approach

0SPD37Z Removal of Autologous Tissue Substitute from Left Knee Joint, Percutaneous Approach

● **0SPD38Z** Removal of Spacer from Left Knee Joint, Percutaneous Approach

⊞ *If revision, see table 0SR to construct a code for Replacement of joint.*

0SPD3JC Removal of Synthetic Substitute from Left Knee Joint, Patellar Surface, Percutaneous Approach

0SPD3JZ Removal of Synthetic Substitute from Left Knee Joint, Percutaneous Approach

0SPD3KZ Removal of Nonautologous Tissue Substitute from Left Knee Joint, Percutaneous Approach

0SPD3LZ Removal of Medial Unicondylar Synthetic Substitute from Left Knee Joint, Percutaneous Approach

♀ Female-only   ♂ Male-only   ▲ Limited Coverage   ● Non-OR   ▨ HAC-associated procedure   ▲ Non-covered procedures   ⊞ Cluster

0SPD3MZ Removal of Lateral Unicondylar Synthetic Substitute from Left Knee Joint, Percutaneous Approach

0SPD3NZ Removal of Patellofemoral Synthetic Substitute from Left Knee Joint, Percutaneous Approach

0SPD40Z Removal of Drainage Device from Left Knee Joint, Percutaneous Endoscopic Approach

0SPD43Z Removal of Infusion Device from Left Knee Joint, Percutaneous Endoscopic Approach

0SPD44Z Removal of Internal Fixation Device from Left Knee Joint, Percutaneous Endoscopic Approach

0SPD45Z Removal of External Fixation Device from Left Knee Joint, Percutaneous Endoscopic Approach

0SPD47Z Removal of Autologous Tissue Substitute from Left Knee Joint, Percutaneous Endoscopic Approach

● **0SPD48Z** Removal of Spacer from Left Knee Joint, Percutaneous Endoscopic Approach

➕ *If revision, see table 0SR to construct a code for Replacement of joint.*

0SPD4JC Removal of Synthetic Substitute from Left Knee Joint, Patellar Surface, Percutaneous Endoscopic Approach

➕ *If replacement, see table 0SR to construct a code for Replacement of the device.*

0SPD4JZ Removal of Synthetic Substitute from Left Knee Joint, Percutaneous Endoscopic Approach

➕ *If replacement see table 0SR to construct a code for the Replacement of the device.*

0SPD4KZ Removal of Nonautologous Tissue Substitute from Left Knee Joint, Percutaneous Endoscopic Approach

0SPD4LZ Removal of Medial Unicondylar Synthetic Substitute from Left Knee Joint, Percutaneous Endoscopic Approach

0SPD4MZ Removal of Lateral Unicondylar Synthetic Substitute from Left Knee Joint, Percutaneous Endoscopic Approach

0SPD4NZ Removal of Patellofemoral Synthetic Substitute from Left Knee Joint, Percutaneous Endoscopic Approach

0SPDX0Z Removal of Drainage Device from Left Knee Joint, External Approach

0SPDX3Z Removal of Infusion Device from Left Knee Joint, External Approach

0SPDX4Z Removal of Internal Fixation Device from Left Knee Joint, External Approach

0SPDX5Z Removal of External Fixation Device from Left Knee Joint, External Approach

0SPE0JZ Removal of Synthetic Substitute from Left Hip Joint, Acetabular Surface, Open Approach

➕ *If replacement, see table 0SR to construct a code for Replacement of the device.*

0SPE3JZ Removal of Synthetic Substitute from Left Hip Joint, Acetabular Surface, Percutaneous Approach

0SPE4JZ Removal of Synthetic Substitute from Left Hip Joint, Acetabular Surface, Percutaneous Endoscopic Approach

➕ *If replacement, see table 0SR to construct a code for Replacement of the device.*

0SPF00Z Removal of Drainage Device from Right Ankle Joint, Open Approach

0SPF03Z Removal of Infusion Device from Right Ankle Joint, Open Approach

0SPF04Z Removal of Internal Fixation Device from Right Ankle Joint, Open Approach

0SPF05Z Removal of External Fixation Device from Right Ankle Joint, Open Approach

0SPF07Z Removal of Autologous Tissue Substitute from Right Ankle Joint, Open Approach

0SPF08Z Removal of Spacer from Right Ankle Joint, Open Approach

0SPF0JZ Removal of Synthetic Substitute from Right Ankle Joint, Open Approach

AHA CC: 4Q, 2017, 107-108; 1Q, 2021, 17-18

0SPF0KZ Removal of Nonautologous Tissue Substitute from Right Ankle Joint, Open Approach

0SPF30Z Removal of Drainage Device from Right Ankle Joint, Percutaneous Approach

0SPF33Z Removal of Infusion Device from Right Ankle Joint, Percutaneous Approach

0SPF34Z Removal of Internal Fixation Device from Right Ankle Joint, Percutaneous Approach

0SPF35Z Removal of External Fixation Device from Right Ankle Joint, Percutaneous Approach

0SPF37Z Removal of Autologous Tissue Substitute from Right Ankle Joint, Percutaneous Approach

0SPF38Z Removal of Spacer from Right Ankle Joint, Percutaneous Approach

0SPF3JZ Removal of Synthetic Substitute from Right Ankle Joint, Percutaneous Approach

0SPF3KZ Removal of Nonautologous Tissue Substitute from Right Ankle Joint, Percutaneous Approach

0SPF40Z Removal of Drainage Device from Right Ankle Joint, Percutaneous Endoscopic Approach

0SPF43Z Removal of Infusion Device from Right Ankle Joint, Percutaneous Endoscopic Approach

0SPF44Z Removal of Internal Fixation Device from Right Ankle Joint, Percutaneous Endoscopic Approach

0SPF45Z Removal of External Fixation Device from Right Ankle Joint, Percutaneous Endoscopic Approach

0SPF47Z Removal of Autologous Tissue Substitute from Right Ankle Joint, Percutaneous Endoscopic Approach

0SPF48Z Removal of Spacer from Right Ankle Joint, Percutaneous Endoscopic Approach

0SPF4JZ Removal of Synthetic Substitute from Right Ankle Joint, Percutaneous Endoscopic Approach

0SPF4KZ Removal of Nonautologous Tissue Substitute from Right Ankle Joint, Percutaneous Endoscopic Approach

0SPFX0Z Removal of Drainage Device from Right Ankle Joint, External Approach

0SPFX3Z Removal of Infusion Device from Right Ankle Joint, External Approach

0SPFX4Z Removal of Internal Fixation Device from Right Ankle Joint, External Approach

0SPFX5Z Removal of External Fixation Device from Right Ankle Joint, External Approach

0SPG00Z Removal of Drainage Device from Left Ankle Joint, Open Approach

0SPG03Z Removal of Infusion Device from Left Ankle Joint, Open Approach

0SPG04Z Removal of Internal Fixation Device from Left Ankle Joint, Open Approach

AHA CC: 2Q, 2013, 39-40

0SPG05Z Removal of External Fixation Device from Left Ankle Joint, Open Approach

0SPG07Z Removal of Autologous Tissue Substitute from Left Ankle Joint, Open Approach

0SPG08Z Removal of Spacer from Left Ankle Joint, Open Approach

0SPG0JZ Removal of Synthetic Substitute from Left Ankle Joint, Open Approach

0SPG0KZ Removal of Nonautologous Tissue Substitute from Left Ankle Joint, Open Approach

0SPG30Z Removal of Drainage Device from Left Ankle Joint, Percutaneous Approach

0SPG33Z Removal of Infusion Device from Left Ankle Joint, Percutaneous Approach

0SPG34Z Removal of Internal Fixation Device from Left Ankle Joint, Percutaneous Approach

0SPG35Z Removal of External Fixation Device from Left Ankle Joint, Percutaneous Approach

0SPG37Z Removal of Autologous Tissue Substitute from Left Ankle Joint, Percutaneous Approach

0SPG38Z Removal of Spacer from Left Ankle Joint, Percutaneous Approach

0SPG3JZ Removal of Synthetic Substitute from Left Ankle Joint, Percutaneous Approach

0SPG3KZ Removal of Nonautologous Tissue Substitute from Left Ankle Joint, Percutaneous Approach

0SPG40Z Removal of Drainage Device from Left Ankle Joint, Percutaneous Endoscopic Approach

0SPG43Z Removal of Infusion Device from Left Ankle Joint, Percutaneous Endoscopic Approach

0SPG44Z Removal of Internal Fixation Device from Left Ankle Joint, Percutaneous Endoscopic Approach

0SPG45Z Removal of External Fixation Device from Left Ankle Joint, Percutaneous Endoscopic Approach

0SPG47Z Removal of Autologous Tissue Substitute from Left Ankle Joint, Percutaneous Endoscopic Approach

0SPG48Z Removal of Spacer from Left Ankle Joint, Percutaneous Endoscopic Approach

0SPG4JZ Removal of Synthetic Substitute from Left Ankle Joint, Percutaneous Endoscopic Approach

0SPG4KZ Removal of Nonautologous Tissue Substitute from Left Ankle Joint, Percutaneous Endoscopic Approach

0SPGX0Z Removal of Drainage Device from Left Ankle Joint, External Approach

0SPGX3Z Removal of Infusion Device from Left Ankle Joint, External Approach

0SPGX4Z Removal of Internal Fixation Device from Left Ankle Joint, External Approach

0SPGX5Z Removal of External Fixation Device from Left Ankle Joint, External Approach

0SPH00Z Removal of Drainage Device from Right Tarsal Joint, Open Approach

---

♀ Female-only   ♂ Male-only   ▲ Limited Coverage   ● Non-OR   🄷🄰🄲 HAC-associated procedure   ▲ Non-covered procedures   ➕ Cluster   **1167**

0SPH03Z Removal of Infusion Device from Right Tarsal Joint, Open Approach

0SPH04Z Removal of Internal Fixation Device from Right Tarsal Joint, Open Approach

0SPH05Z Removal of External Fixation Device from Right Tarsal Joint, Open Approach

0SPH07Z Removal of Autologous Tissue Substitute from Right Tarsal Joint, Open Approach

0SPH08Z Removal of Spacer from Right Tarsal Joint, Open Approach

0SPH0JZ Removal of Synthetic Substitute from Right Tarsal Joint, Open Approach

0SPH0KZ Removal of Nonautologous Tissue Substitute from Right Tarsal Joint, Open Approach

0SPH30Z Removal of Drainage Device from Right Tarsal Joint, Percutaneous Approach

0SPH33Z Removal of Infusion Device from Right Tarsal Joint, Percutaneous Approach

0SPH34Z Removal of Internal Fixation Device from Right Tarsal Joint, Percutaneous Approach

0SPH35Z Removal of External Fixation Device from Right Tarsal Joint, Percutaneous Approach

0SPH37Z Removal of Autologous Tissue Substitute from Right Tarsal Joint, Percutaneous Approach

0SPH38Z Removal of Spacer from Right Tarsal Joint, Percutaneous Approach

0SPH3JZ Removal of Synthetic Substitute from Right Tarsal Joint, Percutaneous Approach

0SPH3KZ Removal of Nonautologous Tissue Substitute from Right Tarsal Joint, Percutaneous Approach

0SPH40Z Removal of Drainage Device from Right Tarsal Joint, Percutaneous Endoscopic Approach

0SPH43Z Removal of Infusion Device from Right Tarsal Joint, Percutaneous Endoscopic Approach

0SPH44Z Removal of Internal Fixation Device from Right Tarsal Joint, Percutaneous Endoscopic Approach

0SPH45Z Removal of External Fixation Device from Right Tarsal Joint, Percutaneous Endoscopic Approach

0SPH47Z Removal of Autologous Tissue Substitute from Right Tarsal Joint, Percutaneous Endoscopic Approach

0SPH48Z Removal of Spacer from Right Tarsal Joint, Percutaneous Endoscopic Approach

0SPH4JZ Removal of Synthetic Substitute from Right Tarsal Joint, Percutaneous Endoscopic Approach

0SPH4KZ Removal of Nonautologous Tissue Substitute from Right Tarsal Joint, Percutaneous Endoscopic Approach

0SPHX0Z Removal of Drainage Device from Right Tarsal Joint, External Approach

0SPHX3Z Removal of Infusion Device from Right Tarsal Joint, External Approach

0SPHX4Z Removal of Internal Fixation Device from Right Tarsal Joint, External Approach

0SPHX5Z Removal of External Fixation Device from Right Tarsal Joint, External Approach

0SPJ00Z Removal of Drainage Device from Left Tarsal Joint, Open Approach

0SPJ03Z Removal of Infusion Device from Left Tarsal Joint, Open Approach

0SPJ04Z Removal of Internal Fixation Device from Left Tarsal Joint, Open Approach

0SPJ05Z Removal of External Fixation Device from Left Tarsal Joint, Open Approach

0SPJ07Z Removal of Autologous Tissue Substitute from Left Tarsal Joint, Open Approach

0SPJ08Z Removal of Spacer from Left Tarsal Joint, Open Approach

0SPJ0JZ Removal of Synthetic Substitute from Left Tarsal Joint, Open Approach

0SPJ0KZ Removal of Nonautologous Tissue Substitute from Left Tarsal Joint, Open Approach

0SPJ30Z Removal of Drainage Device from Left Tarsal Joint, Percutaneous Approach

0SPJ33Z Removal of Infusion Device from Left Tarsal Joint, Percutaneous Approach

0SPJ34Z Removal of Internal Fixation Device from Left Tarsal Joint, Percutaneous Approach

0SPJ35Z Removal of External Fixation Device from Left Tarsal Joint, Percutaneous Approach

0SPJ37Z Removal of Autologous Tissue Substitute from Left Tarsal Joint, Percutaneous Approach

0SPJ38Z Removal of Spacer from Left Tarsal Joint, Percutaneous Approach

0SPJ3JZ Removal of Synthetic Substitute from Left Tarsal Joint, Percutaneous Approach

0SPJ3KZ Removal of Nonautologous Tissue Substitute from Left Tarsal Joint, Percutaneous Approach

0SPJ40Z Removal of Drainage Device from Left Tarsal Joint, Percutaneous Endoscopic Approach

0SPJ43Z Removal of Infusion Device from Left Tarsal Joint, Percutaneous Endoscopic Approach

0SPJ44Z Removal of Internal Fixation Device from Left Tarsal Joint, Percutaneous Endoscopic Approach

0SPJ45Z Removal of External Fixation Device from Left Tarsal Joint, Percutaneous Endoscopic Approach

0SPJ47Z Removal of Autologous Tissue Substitute from Left Tarsal Joint, Percutaneous Endoscopic Approach

0SPJ48Z Removal of Spacer from Left Tarsal Joint, Percutaneous Endoscopic Approach

0SPJ4JZ Removal of Synthetic Substitute from Left Tarsal Joint, Percutaneous Endoscopic Approach

0SPJ4KZ Removal of Nonautologous Tissue Substitute from Left Tarsal Joint, Percutaneous Endoscopic Approach

0SPJX0Z Removal of Drainage Device from Left Tarsal Joint, External Approach

0SPJX3Z Removal of Infusion Device from Left Tarsal Joint, External Approach

0SPJX4Z Removal of Internal Fixation Device from Left Tarsal Joint, External Approach

0SPJX5Z Removal of External Fixation Device from Left Tarsal Joint, External Approach

0SPK00Z Removal of Drainage Device from Right Tarsometatarsal Joint, Open Approach

0SPK03Z Removal of Infusion Device from Right Tarsometatarsal Joint, Open Approach

0SPK04Z Removal of Internal Fixation Device from Right Tarsometatarsal Joint, Open Approach

0SPK05Z Removal of External Fixation Device from Right Tarsometatarsal Joint, Open Approach

0SPK07Z Removal of Autologous Tissue Substitute from Right Tarsometatarsal Joint, Open Approach

0SPK08Z Removal of Spacer from Right Tarsometatarsal Joint, Open Approach

0SPK0JZ Removal of Synthetic Substitute from Right Tarsometatarsal Joint, Open Approach

0SPK0KZ Removal of Nonautologous Tissue Substitute from Right Tarsometatarsal Joint, Open Approach

0SPK30Z Removal of Drainage Device from Right Tarsometatarsal Joint, Percutaneous Approach

0SPK33Z Removal of Infusion Device from Right Tarsometatarsal Joint, Percutaneous Approach

0SPK34Z Removal of Internal Fixation Device from Right Tarsometatarsal Joint, Percutaneous Approach

0SPK35Z Removal of External Fixation Device from Right Tarsometatarsal Joint, Percutaneous Approach

0SPK37Z Removal of Autologous Tissue Substitute from Right Tarsometatarsal Joint, Percutaneous Approach

0SPK38Z Removal of Spacer from Right Tarsometatarsal Joint, Percutaneous Approach

0SPK3JZ Removal of Synthetic Substitute from Right Tarsometatarsal Joint, Percutaneous Approach

0SPK3KZ Removal of Nonautologous Tissue Substitute from Right Tarsometatarsal Joint, Percutaneous Approach

0SPK40Z Removal of Drainage Device from Right Tarsometatarsal Joint, Percutaneous Endoscopic Approach

0SPK43Z Removal of Infusion Device from Right Tarsometatarsal Joint, Percutaneous Endoscopic Approach

0SPK44Z Removal of Internal Fixation Device from Right Tarsometatarsal Joint, Percutaneous Endoscopic Approach

0SPK45Z Removal of External Fixation Device from Right Tarsometatarsal Joint, Percutaneous Endoscopic Approach

0SPK47Z Removal of Autologous Tissue Substitute from Right Tarsometatarsal Joint, Percutaneous Endoscopic Approach

0SPK48Z Removal of Spacer from Right Tarsometatarsal Joint, Percutaneous Endoscopic Approach

0SPK4JZ Removal of Synthetic Substitute from Right Tarsometatarsal Joint, Percutaneous Endoscopic Approach

0SPK4KZ Removal of Nonautologous Tissue Substitute from Right Tarsometatarsal Joint, Percutaneous Endoscopic Approach

0SPKX0Z Removal of Drainage Device from Right Tarsometatarsal Joint, External Approach

0SPKX3Z Removal of Infusion Device from Right Tarsometatarsal Joint, External Approach

0SPKX4Z Removal of Internal Fixation Device from Right Tarsometatarsal Joint, External Approach

♀ Female-only   ♂ Male-only   ▲ Limited Coverage   ● Non-OR   HAC HAC-associated procedure   ▲ Non-covered procedures   ✚ Cluster

0SPKX5Z Removal of External Fixation Device from Right Tarsometatarsal Joint, External Approach

0SPL00Z Removal of Drainage Device from Left Tarsometatarsal Joint, Open Approach

0SPL03Z Removal of Infusion Device from Left Tarsometatarsal Joint, Open Approach

0SPL04Z Removal of Internal Fixation Device from Left Tarsometatarsal Joint, Open Approach

0SPL05Z Removal of External Fixation Device from Left Tarsometatarsal Joint, Open Approach

0SPL07Z Removal of Autologous Tissue Substitute from Left Tarsometatarsal Joint, Open Approach

0SPL08Z Removal of Spacer from Left Tarsometatarsal Joint, Open Approach

0SPL0JZ Removal of Synthetic Substitute from Left Tarsometatarsal Joint, Open Approach

0SPL0KZ Removal of Nonautologous Tissue Substitute from Left Tarsometatarsal Joint, Open Approach

0SPL30Z Removal of Drainage Device from Left Tarsometatarsal Joint, Percutaneous Approach

0SPL33Z Removal of Infusion Device from Left Tarsometatarsal Joint, Percutaneous Approach

0SPL34Z Removal of Internal Fixation Device from Left Tarsometatarsal Joint, Percutaneous Approach

0SPL35Z Removal of External Fixation Device from Left Tarsometatarsal Joint, Percutaneous Approach

0SPL37Z Removal of Autologous Tissue Substitute from Left Tarsometatarsal Joint, Percutaneous Approach

0SPL38Z Removal of Spacer from Left Tarsometatarsal Joint, Percutaneous Approach

0SPL3JZ Removal of Synthetic Substitute from Left Tarsometatarsal Joint, Percutaneous Approach

0SPL3KZ Removal of Nonautologous Tissue Substitute from Left Tarsometatarsal Joint, Percutaneous Approach

0SPL40Z Removal of Drainage Device from Left Tarsometatarsal Joint, Percutaneous Endoscopic Approach

0SPL43Z Removal of Infusion Device from Left Tarsometatarsal Joint, Percutaneous Endoscopic Approach

0SPL44Z Removal of Internal Fixation Device from Left Tarsometatarsal Joint, Percutaneous Endoscopic Approach

0SPL45Z Removal of External Fixation Device from Left Tarsometatarsal Joint, Percutaneous Endoscopic Approach

0SPL47Z Removal of Autologous Tissue Substitute from Left Tarsometatarsal Joint, Percutaneous Endoscopic Approach

0SPL48Z Removal of Spacer from Left Tarsometatarsal Joint, Percutaneous Endoscopic Approach

0SPL4JZ Removal of Synthetic Substitute from Left Tarsometatarsal Joint, Percutaneous Endoscopic Approach

0SPL4KZ Removal of Nonautologous Tissue Substitute from Left Tarsometatarsal Joint, Percutaneous Endoscopic Approach

0SPLX0Z Removal of Drainage Device from Left Tarsometatarsal Joint, External Approach

0SPLX3Z Removal of Infusion Device from Left Tarsometatarsal Joint, External Approach

0SPLX4Z Removal of Internal Fixation Device from Left Tarsometatarsal Joint, External Approach

0SPLX5Z Removal of External Fixation Device from Left Tarsometatarsal Joint, External Approach

0SPM00Z Removal of Drainage Device from Right Metatarsal-Phalangeal Joint, Open Approach

0SPM03Z Removal of Infusion Device from Right Metatarsal-Phalangeal Joint, Open Approach

0SPM04Z Removal of Internal Fixation Device from Right Metatarsal-Phalangeal Joint, Open Approach

0SPM05Z Removal of External Fixation Device from Right Metatarsal-Phalangeal Joint, Open Approach

0SPM07Z Removal of Autologous Tissue Substitute from Right Metatarsal-Phalangeal Joint, Open Approach

0SPM08Z Removal of Spacer from Right Metatarsal-Phalangeal Joint, Open Approach

0SPM0JZ Removal of Synthetic Substitute from Right Metatarsal-Phalangeal Joint, Open Approach

0SPM0KZ Removal of Nonautologous Tissue Substitute from Right Metatarsal-Phalangeal Joint, Open Approach

0SPM30Z Removal of Drainage Device from Right Metatarsal-Phalangeal Joint, Percutaneous Approach

0SPM33Z Removal of Infusion Device from Right Metatarsal-Phalangeal Joint, Percutaneous Approach

0SPM34Z Removal of Internal Fixation Device from Right Metatarsal-Phalangeal Joint, Percutaneous Approach

0SPM35Z Removal of External Fixation Device from Right Metatarsal-Phalangeal Joint, Percutaneous Approach

0SPM37Z Removal of Autologous Tissue Substitute from Right Metatarsal-Phalangeal Joint, Percutaneous Approach

0SPM38Z Removal of Spacer from Right Metatarsal-Phalangeal Joint, Percutaneous Approach

0SPM3JZ Removal of Synthetic Substitute from Right Metatarsal-Phalangeal Joint, Percutaneous Approach

0SPM3KZ Removal of Nonautologous Tissue Substitute from Right Metatarsal-Phalangeal Joint, Percutaneous Approach

0SPM40Z Removal of Drainage Device from Right Metatarsal-Phalangeal Joint, Percutaneous Endoscopic Approach

0SPM43Z Removal of Infusion Device from Right Metatarsal-Phalangeal Joint, Percutaneous Endoscopic Approach

0SPM44Z Removal of Internal Fixation Device from Right Metatarsal-Phalangeal Joint, Percutaneous Endoscopic Approach

0SPM45Z Removal of External Fixation Device from Right Metatarsal-Phalangeal Joint, Percutaneous Endoscopic Approach

0SPM47Z Removal of Autologous Tissue Substitute from Right Metatarsal-Phalangeal Joint, Percutaneous Endoscopic Approach

0SPM48Z Removal of Spacer from Right Metatarsal-Phalangeal Joint, Percutaneous Endoscopic Approach

0SPM4JZ Removal of Synthetic Substitute from Right Metatarsal-Phalangeal Joint, Percutaneous Endoscopic Approach

0SPM4KZ Removal of Nonautologous Tissue Substitute from Right Metatarsal-Phalangeal Joint, Percutaneous Endoscopic Approach

0SPMX0Z Removal of Drainage Device from Right Metatarsal-Phalangeal Joint, External Approach

0SPMX3Z Removal of Infusion Device from Right Metatarsal-Phalangeal Joint, External Approach

0SPMX4Z Removal of Internal Fixation Device from Right Metatarsal-Phalangeal Joint, External Approach

0SPMX5Z Removal of External Fixation Device from Right Metatarsal-Phalangeal Joint, External Approach

0SPN00Z Removal of Drainage Device from Left Metatarsal-Phalangeal Joint, Open Approach

0SPN03Z Removal of Infusion Device from Left Metatarsal-Phalangeal Joint, Open Approach

0SPN04Z Removal of Internal Fixation Device from Left Metatarsal-Phalangeal Joint, Open Approach

0SPN05Z Removal of External Fixation Device from Left Metatarsal-Phalangeal Joint, Open Approach

0SPN07Z Removal of Autologous Tissue Substitute from Left Metatarsal-Phalangeal Joint, Open Approach

0SPN08Z Removal of Spacer from Left Metatarsal-Phalangeal Joint, Open Approach

0SPN0JZ Removal of Synthetic Substitute from Left Metatarsal-Phalangeal Joint, Open Approach

0SPN0KZ Removal of Nonautologous Tissue Substitute from Left Metatarsal-Phalangeal Joint, Open Approach

0SPN30Z Removal of Drainage Device from Left Metatarsal-Phalangeal Joint, Percutaneous Approach

0SPN33Z Removal of Infusion Device from Left Metatarsal-Phalangeal Joint, Percutaneous Approach

0SPN34Z Removal of Internal Fixation Device from Left Metatarsal-Phalangeal Joint, Percutaneous Approach

0SPN35Z Removal of External Fixation Device from Left Metatarsal-Phalangeal Joint, Percutaneous Approach

0SPN37Z Removal of Autologous Tissue Substitute from Left Metatarsal-Phalangeal Joint, Percutaneous Approach

0SPN38Z Removal of Spacer from Left Metatarsal-Phalangeal Joint, Percutaneous Approach

0SPN3JZ Removal of Synthetic Substitute from Left Metatarsal-Phalangeal Joint, Percutaneous Approach

0SPN3KZ Removal of Nonautologous Tissue Substitute from Left Metatarsal-Phalangeal Joint, Percutaneous Approach

0SPN40Z Removal of Drainage Device from Left Metatarsal-Phalangeal Joint, Percutaneous Endoscopic Approach

0SPN43Z Removal of Infusion Device from Left Metatarsal-Phalangeal Joint, Percutaneous Endoscopic Approach

0SPN44Z Removal of Internal Fixation Device from Left Metatarsal-Phalangeal Joint, Percutaneous Endoscopic Approach

0SPN45Z Removal of External Fixation Device from Left Metatarsal-Phalangeal Joint, Percutaneous Endoscopic Approach

0SPN47Z Removal of Autologous Tissue Substitute from Left Metatarsal-Phalangeal Joint, Percutaneous Endoscopic Approach

0SPN48Z Removal of Spacer from Left Metatarsal-Phalangeal Joint, Percutaneous Endoscopic Approach

0SPN4JZ Removal of Synthetic Substitute from Left Metatarsal-Phalangeal Joint, Percutaneous Endoscopic Approach

0SPN4KZ Removal of Nonautologous Tissue Substitute from Left Metatarsal-Phalangeal Joint, Percutaneous Endoscopic Approach

0SPNX0Z Removal of Drainage Device from Left Metatarsal-Phalangeal Joint, External Approach

0SPNX3Z Removal of Infusion Device from Left Metatarsal-Phalangeal Joint, External Approach

0SPNX4Z Removal of Internal Fixation Device from Left Metatarsal-Phalangeal Joint, External Approach

0SPNX5Z Removal of External Fixation Device from Left Metatarsal-Phalangeal Joint, External Approach

0SPP00Z Removal of Drainage Device from Right Toe Phalangeal Joint, Open Approach

0SPP03Z Removal of Infusion Device from Right Toe Phalangeal Joint, Open Approach

0SPP04Z Removal of Internal Fixation Device from Right Toe Phalangeal Joint, Open Approach

0SPP05Z Removal of External Fixation Device from Right Toe Phalangeal Joint, Open Approach

0SPP07Z Removal of Autologous Tissue Substitute from Right Toe Phalangeal Joint, Open Approach

0SPP08Z Removal of Spacer from Right Toe Phalangeal Joint, Open Approach

0SPP0JZ Removal of Synthetic Substitute from Right Toe Phalangeal Joint, Open Approach

0SPP0KZ Removal of Nonautologous Tissue Substitute from Right Toe Phalangeal Joint, Open Approach

0SPP30Z Removal of Drainage Device from Right Toe Phalangeal Joint, Percutaneous Approach

0SPP33Z Removal of Infusion Device from Right Toe Phalangeal Joint, Percutaneous Approach

0SPP34Z Removal of Internal Fixation Device from Right Toe Phalangeal Joint, Percutaneous Approach

0SPP35Z Removal of External Fixation Device from Right Toe Phalangeal Joint, Percutaneous Approach

0SPP37Z Removal of Autologous Tissue Substitute from Right Toe Phalangeal Joint, Percutaneous Approach

0SPP38Z Removal of Spacer from Right Toe Phalangeal Joint, Percutaneous Approach

0SPP3JZ Removal of Synthetic Substitute from Right Toe Phalangeal Joint, Percutaneous Approach

0SPP3KZ Removal of Nonautologous Tissue Substitute from Right Toe Phalangeal Joint, Percutaneous Approach

0SPP40Z Removal of Drainage Device from Right Toe Phalangeal Joint, Percutaneous Endoscopic Approach

0SPP43Z Removal of Infusion Device from Right Toe Phalangeal Joint, Percutaneous Endoscopic Approach

0SPP44Z Removal of Internal Fixation Device from Right Toe Phalangeal Joint, Percutaneous Endoscopic Approach

0SPP45Z Removal of External Fixation Device from Right Toe Phalangeal Joint, Percutaneous Endoscopic Approach

0SPP47Z Removal of Autologous Tissue Substitute from Right Toe Phalangeal Joint, Percutaneous Endoscopic Approach

0SPP48Z Removal of Spacer from Right Toe Phalangeal Joint, Percutaneous Endoscopic Approach

0SPP4JZ Removal of Synthetic Substitute from Right Toe Phalangeal Joint, Percutaneous Endoscopic Approach

0SPP4KZ Removal of Nonautologous Tissue Substitute from Right Toe Phalangeal Joint, Percutaneous Endoscopic Approach

0SPPX0Z Removal of Drainage Device from Right Toe Phalangeal Joint, External Approach

0SPPX3Z Removal of Infusion Device from Right Toe Phalangeal Joint, External Approach

0SPPX4Z Removal of Internal Fixation Device from Right Toe Phalangeal Joint, External Approach

0SPPX5Z Removal of External Fixation Device from Right Toe Phalangeal Joint, External Approach

0SPQ00Z Removal of Drainage Device from Left Toe Phalangeal Joint, Open Approach

0SPQ03Z Removal of Infusion Device from Left Toe Phalangeal Joint, Open Approach

0SPQ04Z Removal of Internal Fixation Device from Left Toe Phalangeal Joint, Open Approach

0SPQ05Z Removal of External Fixation Device from Left Toe Phalangeal Joint, Open Approach

0SPQ07Z Removal of Autologous Tissue Substitute from Left Toe Phalangeal Joint, Open Approach

0SPQ08Z Removal of Spacer from Left Toe Phalangeal Joint, Open Approach

0SPQ0JZ Removal of Synthetic Substitute from Left Toe Phalangeal Joint, Open Approach

0SPQ0KZ Removal of Nonautologous Tissue Substitute from Left Toe Phalangeal Joint, Open Approach

0SPQ30Z Removal of Drainage Device from Left Toe Phalangeal Joint, Percutaneous Approach

0SPQ33Z Removal of Infusion Device from Left Toe Phalangeal Joint, Percutaneous Approach

0SPQ34Z Removal of Internal Fixation Device from Left Toe Phalangeal Joint, Percutaneous Approach

0SPQ35Z Removal of External Fixation Device from Left Toe Phalangeal Joint, Percutaneous Approach

0SPQ37Z Removal of Autologous Tissue Substitute from Left Toe Phalangeal Joint, Percutaneous Approach

0SPQ38Z Removal of Spacer from Left Toe Phalangeal Joint, Percutaneous Approach

0SPQ3JZ Removal of Synthetic Substitute from Left Toe Phalangeal Joint, Percutaneous Approach

0SPQ3KZ Removal of Nonautologous Tissue Substitute from Left Toe Phalangeal Joint, Percutaneous Approach

0SPQ40Z Removal of Drainage Device from Left Toe Phalangeal Joint, Percutaneous Endoscopic Approach

0SPQ43Z Removal of Infusion Device from Left Toe Phalangeal Joint, Percutaneous Endoscopic Approach

0SPQ44Z Removal of Internal Fixation Device from Left Toe Phalangeal Joint, Percutaneous Endoscopic Approach

0SPQ45Z Removal of External Fixation Device from Left Toe Phalangeal Joint, Percutaneous Endoscopic Approach

0SPQ47Z Removal of Autologous Tissue Substitute from Left Toe Phalangeal Joint, Percutaneous Endoscopic Approach

0SPQ48Z Removal of Spacer from Left Toe Phalangeal Joint, Percutaneous Endoscopic Approach

0SPQ4JZ Removal of Synthetic Substitute from Left Toe Phalangeal Joint, Percutaneous Endoscopic Approach

0SPQ4KZ Removal of Nonautologous Tissue Substitute from Left Toe Phalangeal Joint, Percutaneous Endoscopic Approach

0SPQX0Z Removal of Drainage Device from Left Toe Phalangeal Joint, External Approach

0SPQX3Z Removal of Infusion Device from Left Toe Phalangeal Joint, External Approach

0SPQX4Z Removal of Internal Fixation Device from Left Toe Phalangeal Joint, External Approach

0SPQX5Z Removal of External Fixation Device from Left Toe Phalangeal Joint, External Approach

0SPR0JZ Removal of Synthetic Substitute from Right Hip Joint, Femoral Surface, Open Approach

➕ *If replacement, see table 0SR to construct a code for Replacement of the device.*

AHA CC: 4Q, 2016, 111-112

0SPR3JZ Removal of Synthetic Substitute from Right Hip Joint, Femoral Surface, Percutaneous Approach

0SPR4JZ Removal of Synthetic Substitute from Right Hip Joint, Femoral Surface, Percutaneous Endoscopic Approach

➕ *If replacement, see table 0SR to construct a code for Replacement of the device.*

♀ Female-only   ♂ Male-only   ▲ Limited Coverage   ● Non-OR   ▣ HAC-associated procedure   ▲ Non-covered procedures   ➕ Cluster

0SPS0JZ Removal of Synthetic Substitute from Left Hip Joint, Femoral Surface, Open Approach

   ⊞ *If replacement, see table 0SR to construct a code for Replacement of the device.*

0SPS3JZ Removal of Synthetic Substitute from Left Hip Joint, Femoral Surface, Percutaneous Approach

0SPS4JZ Removal of Synthetic Substitute from Left Hip Joint, Femoral Surface, Percutaneous Endoscopic Approach

   ⊞ *If replacement, see table 0SR to construct a code for Replacement of the device.*

0SPT0JZ Removal of Synthetic Substitute from Right Knee Joint, Femoral Surface, Open Approach

   ⊞ *If replacement, see table 0SR to construct a code for Replacement of the device.*

0SPT3JZ Removal of Synthetic Substitute from Right Knee Joint, Femoral Surface, Percutaneous Approach

0SPT4JZ Removal of Synthetic Substitute from Right Knee Joint, Femoral Surface, Percutaneous Endoscopic Approach

   ⊞ *If replacement, see table 0SR to construct a code for Replacement of the device.*

0SPU0JZ Removal of Synthetic Substitute from Left Knee Joint, Femoral Surface, Open Approach

   ⊞ *If replacement, see table 0SR to construct a code for Replacement of the device.*

0SPU3JZ Removal of Synthetic Substitute from Left Knee Joint, Femoral Surface, Percutaneous Approach

0SPU4JZ Removal of Synthetic Substitute from Left Knee Joint, Femoral Surface, Percutaneous Endoscopic Approach

   ⊞ *If replacement, see table 0SR to construct a code for Replacement of the device.*

0SPV0JZ Removal of Synthetic Substitute from Right Knee Joint, Tibial Surface, Open Approach

   ⊞ *If replacement, see table 0SR to construct a code for Replacement of the device.*

0SPV3JZ Removal of Synthetic Substitute from Right Knee Joint, Tibial Surface, Percutaneous Approach

0SPV4JZ Removal of Synthetic Substitute from Right Knee Joint, Tibial Surface, Percutaneous Endoscopic Approach

   ⊞ *If replacement, see table 0SR to construct a code for Replacement of the device.*

0SPW0JZ Removal of Synthetic Substitute from Left Knee Joint, Tibial Surface, Open Approach

   ⊞ *If replacement, see table 0SR to construct a code for Replacement of the device.*

   AHA CC: 2Q, 2018, 16-17

0SPW3JZ Removal of Synthetic Substitute from Left Knee Joint, Tibial Surface, Percutaneous Approach

0SPW4JZ Removal of Synthetic Substitute from Left Knee Joint, Tibial Surface, Percutaneous Endoscopic Approach

   ⊞ *If replacement, see table 0SR to construct a code for Replacement of the device.*

0SQ – Lower Joints, Repair

Review Coding Guideline B3.5

0SQ00ZZ Repair Lumbar Vertebral Joint, Open Approach

0SQ03ZZ Repair Lumbar Vertebral Joint, Percutaneous Approach

0SQ04ZZ Repair Lumbar Vertebral Joint, Percutaneous Endoscopic Approach

● **0SQ0XZZ** Repair Lumbar Vertebral Joint, External Approach

0SQ20ZZ Repair Lumbar Vertebral Disc, Open Approach

0SQ23ZZ Repair Lumbar Vertebral Disc, Percutaneous Approach

0SQ24ZZ Repair Lumbar Vertebral Disc, Percutaneous Endoscopic Approach

0SQ2XZZ Repair Lumbar Vertebral Disc, External Approach

0SQ30ZZ Repair Lumbosacral Joint, Open Approach

0SQ33ZZ Repair Lumbosacral Joint, Percutaneous Approach

0SQ34ZZ Repair Lumbosacral Joint, Percutaneous Endoscopic Approach

0SQ3XZZ Repair Lumbosacral Joint, External Approach

0SQ40ZZ Repair Lumbosacral Disc, Open Approach

0SQ43ZZ Repair Lumbosacral Disc, Percutaneous Approach

0SQ44ZZ Repair Lumbosacral Disc, Percutaneous Endoscopic Approach

0SQ4XZZ Repair Lumbosacral Disc, External Approach

0SQ50ZZ Repair Sacrococcygeal Joint, Open Approach

0SQ53ZZ Repair Sacrococcygeal Joint, Percutaneous Approach

0SQ54ZZ Repair Sacrococcygeal Joint, Percutaneous Endoscopic Approach

0SQ5XZZ Repair Sacrococcygeal Joint, External Approach

0SQ60ZZ Repair Coccygeal Joint, Open Approach

0SQ63ZZ Repair Coccygeal Joint, Percutaneous Approach

0SQ64ZZ Repair Coccygeal Joint, Percutaneous Endoscopic Approach

0SQ6XZZ Repair Coccygeal Joint, External Approach

0SQ70ZZ Repair Right Sacroiliac Joint, Open Approach

0SQ73ZZ Repair Right Sacroiliac Joint, Percutaneous Approach

0SQ74ZZ Repair Right Sacroiliac Joint, Percutaneous Endoscopic Approach

0SQ7XZZ Repair Right Sacroiliac Joint, External Approach

0SQ80ZZ Repair Left Sacroiliac Joint, Open Approach

0SQ83ZZ Repair Left Sacroiliac Joint, Percutaneous Approach

0SQ84ZZ Repair Left Sacroiliac Joint, Percutaneous Endoscopic Approach

0SQ8XZZ Repair Left Sacroiliac Joint, External Approach

0SQ90ZZ Repair Right Hip Joint, Open Approach

0SQ93ZZ Repair Right Hip Joint, Percutaneous Approach

0SQ94ZZ Repair Right Hip Joint, Percutaneous Endoscopic Approach

0SQ9XZZ Repair Right Hip Joint, External Approach

0SQB0ZZ Repair Left Hip Joint, Open Approach

0SQB3ZZ Repair Left Hip Joint, Percutaneous Approach

0SQB4ZZ Repair Left Hip Joint, Percutaneous Endoscopic Approach

   AHA CC: 4Q, 2014, 25-26

0SQBXZZ Repair Left Hip Joint, External Approach

0SQC0ZZ Repair Right Knee Joint, Open Approach

0SQC3ZZ Repair Right Knee Joint, Percutaneous Approach

0SQC4ZZ Repair Right Knee Joint, Percutaneous Endoscopic Approach

0SQCXZZ Repair Right Knee Joint, External Approach

0SQD0ZZ Repair Left Knee Joint, Open Approach

0SQD3ZZ Repair Left Knee Joint, Percutaneous Approach

0SQD4ZZ Repair Left Knee Joint, Percutaneous Endoscopic Approach

0SQDXZZ Repair Left Knee Joint, External Approach

0SQF0ZZ Repair Right Ankle Joint, Open Approach

0SQF3ZZ Repair Right Ankle Joint, Percutaneous Approach

0SQF4ZZ Repair Right Ankle Joint, Percutaneous Endoscopic Approach

0SQFXZZ Repair Right Ankle Joint, External Approach

0SQG0ZZ Repair Left Ankle Joint, Open Approach

0SQG3ZZ Repair Left Ankle Joint, Percutaneous Approach

0SQG4ZZ Repair Left Ankle Joint, Percutaneous Endoscopic Approach

0SQGXZZ Repair Left Ankle Joint, External Approach

0SQH0ZZ Repair Right Tarsal Joint, Open Approach

0SQH3ZZ Repair Right Tarsal Joint, Percutaneous Approach

0SQH4ZZ Repair Right Tarsal Joint, Percutaneous Endoscopic Approach

0SQHXZZ Repair Right Tarsal Joint, External Approach

0SQJ0ZZ Repair Left Tarsal Joint, Open Approach

0SQJ3ZZ Repair Left Tarsal Joint, Percutaneous Approach

0SQJ4ZZ Repair Left Tarsal Joint, Percutaneous Endoscopic Approach

0SQJXZZ Repair Left Tarsal Joint, External Approach

0SQK0ZZ Repair Right Tarsometatarsal Joint, Open Approach

0SQK3ZZ Repair Right Tarsometatarsal Joint, Percutaneous Approach

♀ Female-only   ♂ Male-only   ▲ Limited Coverage   ● Non-OR   ▇ HAC-associated procedure   ▲ Non-covered procedures   ⊞ Cluster   **1171**

Medical and Surgical, Lower Joints Code Listings

0SQK4ZZ	Repair Right Tarsometatarsal Joint, Percutaneous Endoscopic Approach	0SQM4ZZ	Repair Right Metatarsal-Phalangeal Joint, Percutaneous Endoscopic Approach	0SQP3ZZ	Repair Right Toe Phalangeal Joint, Percutaneous Approach
0SQKXZZ	Repair Right Tarsometatarsal Joint, External Approach	0SQMXZZ	Repair Right Metatarsal-Phalangeal Joint, External Approach	0SQP4ZZ	Repair Right Toe Phalangeal Joint, Percutaneous Endoscopic Approach
0SQL0ZZ	Repair Left Tarsometatarsal Joint, Open Approach	0SQN0ZZ	Repair Left Metatarsal-Phalangeal Joint, Open Approach	0SQPXZZ	Repair Right Toe Phalangeal Joint, External Approach
0SQL3ZZ	Repair Left Tarsometatarsal Joint, Percutaneous Approach	0SQN3ZZ	Repair Left Metatarsal-Phalangeal Joint, Percutaneous Approach	0SQQ0ZZ	Repair Left Toe Phalangeal Joint, Open Approach
0SQL4ZZ	Repair Left Tarsometatarsal Joint, Percutaneous Endoscopic Approach	0SQN4ZZ	Repair Left Metatarsal-Phalangeal Joint, Percutaneous Endoscopic Approach	0SQQ3ZZ	Repair Left Toe Phalangeal Joint, Percutaneous Approach
0SQLXZZ	Repair Left Tarsometatarsal Joint, External Approach	0SQNXZZ	Repair Left Metatarsal-Phalangeal Joint, External Approach	0SQQ4ZZ	Repair Left Toe Phalangeal Joint, Percutaneous Endoscopic Approach
0SQM0ZZ	Repair Right Metatarsal-Phalangeal Joint, Open Approach	0SQP0ZZ	Repair Right Toe Phalangeal Joint, Open Approach	0SQQXZZ	Repair Left Toe Phalangeal Joint, External Approach
0SQM3ZZ	Repair Right Metatarsal-Phalangeal Joint, Percutaneous Approach				

0SR – Lower Joints, Replacement

Review Coding Guideline B3.18

0SR007Z	Replacement of Lumbar Vertebral Joint with Autologous Tissue Substitute, Open Approach	0SR707Z	Replacement of Right Sacroiliac Joint with Autologous Tissue Substitute, Open Approach	0SR9039	Replacement of Right Hip Joint with Ceramic Synthetic Substitute, Cemented, Open Approach
0SR00JZ	Replacement of Lumbar Vertebral Joint with Synthetic Substitute, Open Approach	0SR70JZ	Replacement of Right Sacroiliac Joint with Synthetic Substitute, Open Approach	HAC	When reported with secondary diagnosis code I26.02, I26.09, I26.92-I26.99, I82.401-I82.4Z9
0SR00KZ	Replacement of Lumbar Vertebral Joint with Nonautologous Tissue Substitute, Open Approach	0SR70KZ	Replacement of Right Sacroiliac Joint with Nonautologous Tissue Substitute, Open Approach	0SR903A	Replacement of Right Hip Joint with Ceramic Synthetic Substitute, Uncemented, Open Approach
0SR207Z	Replacement of Lumbar Vertebral Disc with Autologous Tissue Substitute, Open Approach	0SR807Z	Replacement of Left Sacroiliac Joint with Autologous Tissue Substitute, Open Approach	HAC	When reported with secondary diagnosis code I26.02, I26.09, I26.92-I26.99, I82.401-I82.4Z9
0SR20JZ	Replacement of Lumbar Vertebral Disc with Synthetic Substitute, Open Approach	0SR80JZ	Replacement of Left Sacroiliac Joint with Synthetic Substitute, Open Approach	0SR903Z	Replacement of Right Hip Joint with Ceramic Synthetic Substitute, Open Approach
▲	When the patients age is greater than 60 years old	0SR80KZ	Replacement of Left Sacroiliac Joint with Nonautologous Tissue Substitute, Open Approach	HAC	When reported with secondary diagnosis code I26.02, I26.09, I26.92-I26.99, I82.401-I82.4Z9
0SR20KZ	Replacement of Lumbar Vertebral Disc with Nonautologous Tissue Substitute, Open Approach	0SR9019	Replacement of Right Hip Joint with Metal Synthetic Substitute, Cemented, Open Approach	0SR9049	Replacement of Right Hip Joint with Ceramic on Polyethylene Synthetic Substitute, Cemented, Open Approach
0SR307Z	Replacement of Lumbosacral Joint with Autologous Tissue Substitute, Open Approach	HAC	When reported with secondary diagnosis code I26.02, I26.09, I26.92-I26.99, I82.401-I82.4Z9	HAC	When reported with secondary diagnosis code I26.02, I26.09, I26.92-I26.99, I82.401-I82.4Z9
0SR30JZ	Replacement of Lumbosacral Joint with Synthetic Substitute, Open Approach	0SR901A	Replacement of Right Hip Joint with Metal Synthetic Substitute, Uncemented, Open Approach	0SR904A	Replacement of Right Hip Joint with Ceramic on Polyethylene Synthetic Substitute, Uncemented, Open Approach
0SR30KZ	Replacement of Lumbosacral Joint with Nonautologous Tissue Substitute, Open Approach	HAC	When reported with secondary diagnosis code I26.02, I26.09, I26.92-I26.99, I82.401-I82.4Z9	HAC	When reported with secondary diagnosis code I26.02, I26.09, I26.92-I26.99, I82.401-I82.4Z9
0SR407Z	Replacement of Lumbosacral Disc with Autologous Tissue Substitute, Open Approach	0SR901Z	Replacement of Right Hip Joint with Metal Synthetic Substitute, Open Approach	0SR904Z	Replacement of Right Hip Joint with Ceramic on Polyethylene Synthetic Substitute, Open Approach
0SR40JZ	Replacement of Lumbosacral Disc with Synthetic Substitute, Open Approach	HAC	When reported with secondary diagnosis code I26.02, I26.09, I26.92-I26.99, I82.401-I82.4Z9	HAC	When reported with secondary diagnosis code I26.02, I26.09, I26.92-I26.99, I82.401-I82.4Z9
▲	When the patients age is greater than 60 years old	0SR9029	Replacement of Right Hip Joint with Metal on Polyethylene Synthetic Substitute, Cemented, Open Approach	0SR9069	Replacement of Right Hip Joint with Oxidized Zirconium on Polyethylene Synthetic Substitute, Cemented, Open Approach
0SR40KZ	Replacement of Lumbosacral Disc with Nonautologous Tissue Substitute, Open Approach	HAC	When reported with secondary diagnosis code I26.02, I26.09, I26.92-I26.99, I82.401-I82.4Z9	HAC	When reported with secondary diagnosis code I26.02, I26.09, I26.92-I26.99, I82.401-I82.4Z9
0SR507Z	Replacement of Sacrococcygeal Joint with Autologous Tissue Substitute, Open Approach		AHA CC: 3Q, 2020, 33-34	0SR906A	Replacement of Right Hip Joint with Oxidized Zirconium on Polyethylene Synthetic Substitute, Uncemented, Open Approach
0SR50JZ	Replacement of Sacrococcygeal Joint with Synthetic Substitute, Open Approach	0SR902A	Replacement of Right Hip Joint with Metal on Polyethylene Synthetic Substitute, Uncemented, Open Approach	HAC	When reported with secondary diagnosis code I26.02, I26.09, I26.92-I26.99, I82.401-I82.4Z9
0SR50KZ	Replacement of Sacrococcygeal Joint with Nonautologous Tissue Substitute, Open Approach	HAC	When reported with secondary diagnosis code I26.02, I26.09, I26.92-I26.99, I82.401-I82.4Z9	0SR906Z	Replacement of Right Hip Joint with Oxidized Zirconium on Polyethylene Synthetic Substitute, Open Approach
0SR607Z	Replacement of Coccygeal Joint with Autologous Tissue Substitute, Open Approach	0SR902Z	Replacement of Right Hip Joint with Metal on Polyethylene Synthetic Substitute, Open Approach		
0SR60JZ	Replacement of Coccygeal Joint with Synthetic Substitute, Open Approach	HAC	When reported with secondary diagnosis code I26.02, I26.09, I26.92-I26.99, I82.401-I82.4Z9		
0SR60KZ	Replacement of Coccygeal Joint with Nonautologous Tissue Substitute, Open Approach				

♀ Female-only   ♂ Male-only   ▲ Limited Coverage   ● Non-OR   HAC HAC-associated procedure   ▲ Non-covered procedures   ➕ Cluster

HAC When reported with secondary diagnosis code I26.02, I26.09, I26.92-I26.99, I82.401-I82.4Z9

0SR907Z Replacement of Right Hip Joint with Autologous Tissue Substitute, Open Approach

HAC When reported with secondary diagnosis code I26.02, I26.09, I26.92-I26.99, I82.401-I82.4Z9

0SR90EZ Replacement of Right Hip Joint with Articulating Spacer, Open Approach

HAC When reported with secondary diagnosis code I26.02, I26.09, I26.92-I26.99, I82.401-I82.4Z9

0SR90J9 Replacement of Right Hip Joint with Synthetic Substitute, Cemented, Open Approach

HAC When reported with secondary diagnosis code I26.02, I26.09, I26.92-I26.99, I82.401-I82.4Z9

0SR90JA Replacement of Right Hip Joint with Synthetic Substitute, Uncemented, Open Approach

HAC When reported with secondary diagnosis code I26.02, I26.09, I26.92-I26.99, I82.401-I82.4Z9

0SR90JZ Replacement of Right Hip Joint with Synthetic Substitute, Open Approach

HAC When reported with secondary diagnosis code I26.02, I26.09, I26.92-I26.99, I82.401-I82.4Z9

0SR90KZ Replacement of Right Hip Joint with Nonautologous Tissue Substitute, Open Approach

HAC When reported with secondary diagnosis code I26.02, I26.09, I26.92-I26.99, I82.401-I82.4Z9

0SRA009 Replacement of Right Hip Joint, Acetabular Surface with Polyethylene Synthetic Substitute, Cemented, Open Approach

HAC When reported with secondary diagnosis code I26.02, I26.09, I26.92-I26.99, I82.401-I82.4Z9

0SRA00A Replacement of Right Hip Joint, Acetabular Surface with Polyethylene Synthetic Substitute, Uncemented, Open Approach

HAC When reported with secondary diagnosis code I26.02, I26.09, I26.92-I26.99, I82.401-I82.4Z9

0SRA00Z Replacement of Right Hip Joint, Acetabular Surface with Polyethylene Synthetic Substitute, Open Approach

HAC When reported with secondary diagnosis code I26.02, I26.09, I26.92-I26.99, I82.401-I82.4Z9

0SRA019 Replacement of Right Hip Joint, Acetabular Surface with Metal Synthetic Substitute, Cemented, Open Approach

HAC When reported with secondary diagnosis code I26.02, I26.09, I26.92-I26.99, I82.401-I82.4Z9

0SRA01A Replacement of Right Hip Joint, Acetabular Surface with Metal Synthetic Substitute, Uncemented, Open Approach

HAC When reported with secondary diagnosis code I26.02, I26.09, I26.92-I26.99, I82.401-I82.4Z9

0SRA01Z Replacement of Right Hip Joint, Acetabular Surface with Metal Synthetic Substitute, Open Approach

HAC When reported with secondary diagnosis code I26.02, I26.09, I26.92-I26.99, I82.401-I82.4Z9

0SRA039 Replacement of Right Hip Joint, Acetabular Surface with Ceramic Synthetic Substitute, Cemented, Open Approach

HAC When reported with secondary diagnosis code I26.02, I26.09, I26.92-I26.99, I82.401-I82.4Z9

0SRA03A Replacement of Right Hip Joint, Acetabular Surface with Ceramic Synthetic Substitute, Uncemented, Open Approach

HAC When reported with secondary diagnosis code I26.02, I26.09, I26.92-I26.99, I82.401-I82.4Z9

0SRA03Z Replacement of Right Hip Joint, Acetabular Surface with Ceramic Synthetic Substitute, Open Approach

HAC When reported with secondary diagnosis code I26.02, I26.09, I26.92-I26.99, I82.401-I82.4Z9

0SRA07Z Replacement of Right Hip Joint, Acetabular Surface with Autologous Tissue Substitute, Open Approach

HAC When reported with secondary diagnosis code I26.02, I26.09, I26.92-I26.99, I82.401-I82.4Z9

0SRA0J9 Replacement of Right Hip Joint, Acetabular Surface with Synthetic Substitute, Cemented, Open Approach

HAC When reported with secondary diagnosis code I26.02, I26.09, I26.92-I26.99, I82.401-I82.4Z9

0SRA0JA Replacement of Right Hip Joint, Acetabular Surface with Synthetic Substitute, Uncemented, Open Approach

HAC When reported with secondary diagnosis code I26.02, I26.09, I26.92-I26.99, I82.401-I82.4Z9

0SRA0JZ Replacement of Right Hip Joint, Acetabular Surface with Synthetic Substitute, Open Approach

HAC When reported with secondary diagnosis code I26.02, I26.09, I26.92-I26.99, I82.401-I82.4Z9

0SRA0KZ Replacement of Right Hip Joint, Acetabular Surface with Nonautologous Tissue Substitute, Open Approach

HAC When reported with secondary diagnosis code I26.02, I26.09, I26.92-I26.99, I82.401-I82.4Z9

0SRB019 Replacement of Left Hip Joint with Metal Synthetic Substitute, Cemented, Open Approach

HAC When reported with secondary diagnosis code I26.02, I26.09, I26.92-I26.99, I82.401-I82.4Z9

0SRB01A Replacement of Left Hip Joint with Metal Synthetic Substitute, Uncemented, Open Approach

HAC When reported with secondary diagnosis code I26.02, I26.09, I26.92-I26.99, I82.401-I82.4Z9

0SRB01Z Replacement of Left Hip Joint with Metal Synthetic Substitute, Open Approach

HAC When reported with secondary diagnosis code I26.02, I26.09, I26.92-I26.99, I82.401-I82.4Z9

0SRB029 Replacement of Left Hip Joint with Metal on Polyethylene Synthetic Substitute, Cemented, Open Approach

HAC When reported with secondary diagnosis code I26.02, I26.09, I26.92-I26.99, I82.401-I82.4Z9

0SRB02A Replacement of Left Hip Joint with Metal on Polyethylene Synthetic Substitute, Uncemented, Open Approach

HAC When reported with secondary diagnosis code I26.02, I26.09, I26.92-I26.99, I82.401-I82.4Z9

0SRB02Z Replacement of Left Hip Joint with Metal on Polyethylene Synthetic Substitute, Open Approach

HAC When reported with secondary diagnosis code I26.02, I26.09, I26.92-I26.99, I82.401-I82.4Z9

0SRB039 Replacement of Left Hip Joint with Ceramic Synthetic Substitute, Cemented, Open Approach

HAC When reported with secondary diagnosis code I26.02, I26.09, I26.92-I26.99, I82.401-I82.4Z9

0SRB03A Replacement of Left Hip Joint with Ceramic Synthetic Substitute, Uncemented, Open Approach

HAC When reported with secondary diagnosis code I26.02, I26.09, I26.92-I26.99, I82.401-I82.4Z9

0SRB03Z Replacement of Left Hip Joint with Ceramic Synthetic Substitute, Open Approach

HAC When reported with secondary diagnosis code I26.02, I26.09, I26.92-I26.99, I82.401-I82.4Z9

0SRB049 Replacement of Left Hip Joint with Ceramic on Polyethylene Synthetic Substitute, Cemented, Open Approach

HAC When reported with secondary diagnosis code I26.02, I26.09, I26.92-I26.99, I82.401-I82.4Z9

0SRB04A Replacement of Left Hip Joint with Ceramic on Polyethylene Synthetic Substitute, Uncemented, Open Approach

HAC When reported with secondary diagnosis code I26.02, I26.09, I26.92-I26.99, I82.401-I82.4Z9

0SRB04Z Replacement of Left Hip Joint with Ceramic on Polyethylene Synthetic Substitute, Open Approach

HAC When reported with secondary diagnosis code I26.02, I26.09, I26.92-I26.99, I82.401-I82.4Z9

0SRB069 Replacement of Left Hip Joint with Oxidized Zirconium on Polyethylene Synthetic Substitute, Cemented, Open Approach

HAC When reported with secondary diagnosis code I26.02, I26.09, I26.92-I26.99, I82.401-I82.4Z9

0SRB06A Replacement of Left Hip Joint with Oxidized Zirconium on Polyethylene Synthetic Substitute, Uncemented, Open Approach

HAC When reported with secondary diagnosis code I26.02, I26.09, I26.92-I26.99, I82.401-I82.4Z9

0SRB06Z Replacement of Left Hip Joint with Oxidized Zirconium on Polyethylene Synthetic Substitute, Open Approach

AHA CC: 4Q, 2017, 39

HAC When reported with secondary diagnosis code I26.02, I26.09, I26.92-I26.99, I82.401-I82.4Z9

0SRB07Z Replacement of Left Hip Joint with Autologous Tissue Substitute, Open Approach
- HAC When reported with secondary diagnosis code I26.02, I26.09, I26.92-I26.99, I82.401-I82.4Z9

0SRB0EZ Replacement of Left Hip Joint with Articulating Spacer, Open Approach
- HAC When reported with secondary diagnosis code I26.02, I26.09, I26.92-I26.99, I82.401-I82.4Z9

0SRB0J9 Replacement of Left Hip Joint with Synthetic Substitute, Cemented, Open Approach
- *AHA CC: 3Q, 2015, 18-19*
- HAC When reported with secondary diagnosis code I26.02, I26.09, I26.92-I26.99, I82.401-I82.4Z9

0SRB0JA Replacement of Left Hip Joint with Synthetic Substitute, Uncemented, Open Approach
- HAC When reported with secondary diagnosis code I26.02, I26.09, I26.92-I26.99, I82.401-I82.4Z9

0SRB0JZ Replacement of Left Hip Joint with Synthetic Substitute, Open Approach
- HAC When reported with secondary diagnosis code I26.02, I26.09, I26.92-I26.99, I82.401-I82.4Z9

0SRB0KZ Replacement of Left Hip Joint with Nonautologous Tissue Substitute, Open Approach
- HAC When reported with secondary diagnosis code I26.02, I26.09, I26.92-I26.99, I82.401-I82.4Z9

0SRC069 Replacement of Right Knee Joint with Oxidized Zirconium on Polyethylene Synthetic Substitute, Cemented, Open Approach
- HAC When reported with secondary diagnosis code I26.02, I26.09, I26.92-I26.99, I82.401-I82.4Z9

0SRC06A Replacement of Right Knee Joint with Oxidized Zirconium on Polyethylene Synthetic Substitute, Uncemented, Open Approach
- HAC When reported with secondary diagnosis code I26.02, I26.09, I26.92-I26.99, I82.401-I82.4Z9

0SRC06Z Replacement of Right Knee Joint with Oxidized Zirconium on Polyethylene Synthetic Substitute, Open Approach
- HAC When reported with secondary diagnosis code I26.02, I26.09, I26.92-I26.99, I82.401-I82.4Z9

0SRC07Z Replacement of Right Knee Joint with Autologous Tissue Substitute, Open Approach
- HAC When reported with secondary diagnosis code I26.02, I26.09, I26.92-I26.99, I82.401-I82.4Z9

0SRC0EZ Replacement of Right Knee Joint with Articulating Spacer, Open Approach
- HAC When reported with secondary diagnosis code I26.02, I26.09, I26.92-I26.99, I82.401-I82.4Z9

0SRC0J9 Replacement of Right Knee Joint with Synthetic Substitute, Cemented, Open Approach
- *AHA CC: 2Q, 2015, 18-19*
- HAC When reported with secondary diagnosis code I26.02, I26.09, I26.92-I26.99, I82.401-I82.4Z9

0SRC0JA Replacement of Right Knee Joint with Synthetic Substitute, Uncemented, Open Approach

0SRC0JZ Replacement of Right Knee Joint with Synthetic Substitute, Open Approach
- HAC When reported with secondary diagnosis code I26.02, I26.09, I26.92-I26.99, I82.401-I82.4Z9

0SRC0KZ Replacement of Right Knee Joint with Nonautologous Tissue Substitute, Open Approach
- HAC When reported with secondary diagnosis code I26.02, I26.09, I26.92-I26.99, I82.401-I82.4Z9

0SRC0L9 Replacement of Right Knee Joint with Medial Unicondylar Synthetic Substitute, Cemented, Open Approach
- HAC When reported with secondary diagnosis code I26.02, I26.09, I26.92-I26.99, I82.401-I82.4Z9

0SRC0LA Replacement of Right Knee Joint with Medial Unicondylar Synthetic Substitute, Uncemented, Open Approach
- HAC When reported with secondary diagnosis code I26.02, I26.09, I26.92-I26.99, I82.401-I82.4Z9

0SRC0LZ Replacement of Right Knee Joint with Medial Unicondylar Synthetic Substitute, Open Approach
- HAC When reported with secondary diagnosis code I26.02, I26.09, I26.92-I26.99, I82.401-I82.4Z9

0SRC0M9 Replacement of Right Knee Joint with Lateral Unicondylar Synthetic Substitute, Cemented, Open Approach
- HAC When reported with secondary diagnosis code I26.02, I26.09, I26.92-I26.99, I82.401-I82.4Z9

0SRC0MA Replacement of Right Knee Joint with Lateral Unicondylar Synthetic Substitute, Uncemented, Open Approach
- HAC When reported with secondary diagnosis code I26.02, I26.09, I26.92-I26.99, I82.401-I82.4Z9

0SRC0MZ Replacement of Right Knee Joint with Lateral Unicondylar Synthetic Substitute, Open Approach
- HAC When reported with secondary diagnosis code I26.02, I26.09, I26.92-I26.99, I82.401-I82.4Z9

0SRC0N9 Replacement of Right Knee Joint with Patellofemoral Synthetic Substitute, Cemented, Open Approach
- HAC When reported with secondary diagnosis code I26.02, I26.09, I26.92-I26.99, I82.401-I82.4Z9

0SRC0NA Replacement of Right Knee Joint with Patellofemoral Synthetic Substitute, Uncemented, Open Approach
- HAC When reported with secondary diagnosis code I26.02, I26.09, I26.92-I26.99, I82.401-I82.4Z9

0SRC0NZ Replacement of Right Knee Joint with Patellofemoral Synthetic Substitute, Open Approach
- HAC When reported with secondary diagnosis code I26.02, I26.09, I26.92-I26.99, I82.401-I82.4Z9

0SRD069 Replacement of Left Knee Joint with Oxidized Zirconium on Polyethylene Synthetic Substitute, Cemented, Open Approach
- HAC When reported with secondary diagnosis code I26.02, I26.09, I26.92-I26.99, I82.401-I82.4Z9

0SRD06A Replacement of Left Knee Joint with Oxidized Zirconium on Polyethylene Synthetic Substitute, Uncemented, Open Approach
- HAC When reported with secondary diagnosis code I26.02, I26.09, I26.92-I26.99, I82.401-I82.4Z9

0SRD06Z Replacement of Left Knee Joint with Oxidized Zirconium on Polyethylene Synthetic Substitute, Open Approach
- HAC When reported with secondary diagnosis code I26.02, I26.09, I26.92-I26.99, I82.401-I82.4Z9

0SRD07Z Replacement of Left Knee Joint with Autologous Tissue Substitute, Open Approach
- HAC When reported with secondary diagnosis code I26.02, I26.09, I26.92-I26.99, I82.401-I82.4Z9

0SRD0EZ Replacement of Left Knee Joint with Articulating Spacer, Open Approach
- HAC When reported with secondary diagnosis code I26.02, I26.09, I26.92-I26.99, I82.401-I82.4Z9

0SRD0J9 Replacement of Left Knee Joint with Synthetic Substitute, Cemented, Open Approach
- HAC When reported with secondary diagnosis code I26.02, I26.09, I26.92-I26.99, I82.401-I82.4Z9

0SRD0JA Replacement of Left Knee Joint with Synthetic Substitute, Uncemented, Open Approach
- HAC When reported with secondary diagnosis code I26.02, I26.09, I26.92-I26.99, I82.401-I82.4Z9

0SRD0JZ Replacement of Left Knee Joint with Synthetic Substitute, Open Approach
- *AHA CC: 4Q, 2016, 109-110*
- HAC When reported with secondary diagnosis code I26.02, I26.09, I26.92-I26.99, I82.401-I82.4Z9

0SRD0KZ Replacement of Left Knee Joint with Nonautologous Tissue Substitute, Open Approach
- HAC When reported with secondary diagnosis code I26.02, I26.09, I26.92-I26.99, I82.401-I82.4Z9

0SRD0L9 Replacement of Left Knee Joint with Medial Unicondylar Synthetic Substitute, Cemented, Open Approach
- HAC When reported with secondary diagnosis code I26.02, I26.09, I26.92-I26.99, I82.401-I82.4Z9

0SRD0LA Replacement of Left Knee Joint with Medial Unicondylar Synthetic Substitute, Uncemented, Open Approach
- HAC When reported with secondary diagnosis code I26.02, I26.09, I26.92-I26.99, I82.401-I82.4Z9

0SRD0LZ Replacement of Left Knee Joint with Medial Unicondylar Synthetic Substitute, Open Approach
- *AHA CC: 4Q, 2016, 110*
- HAC When reported with secondary diagnosis code I26.02, I26.09, I26.92-I26.99, I82.401-I82.4Z9

0SRD0M9 Replacement of Left Knee Joint with Lateral Unicondylar Synthetic Substitute, Cemented, Open Approach
- HAC When reported with secondary diagnosis code I26.02, I26.09, I26.92-I26.99, I82.401-I82.4Z9

0SRD0MA Replacement of Left Knee Joint with Lateral Unicondylar Synthetic Substitute, Uncemented, Open Approach
HAC When reported with secondary diagnosis code I26.02, I26.09, I26.92-I26.99, I82.401-I82.4Z9

0SRD0MZ Replacement of Left Knee Joint with Lateral Unicondylar Synthetic Substitute, Open Approach
HAC When reported with secondary diagnosis code I26.02, I26.09, I26.92-I26.99, I82.401-I82.4Z9

0SRD0N9 Replacement of Left Knee Joint with Patellofemoral Synthetic Substitute, Cemented, Open Approach
HAC When reported with secondary diagnosis code I26.02, I26.09, I26.92-I26.99, I82.401-I82.4Z9

0SRD0NA Replacement of Left Knee Joint with Patellofemoral Synthetic Substitute, Uncemented, Open Approach
HAC When reported with secondary diagnosis code I26.02, I26.09, I26.92-I26.99, I82.401-I82.4Z9

0SRD0NZ Replacement of Left Knee Joint with Patellofemoral Synthetic Substitute, Open Approach
HAC When reported with secondary diagnosis code I26.02, I26.09, I26.92-I26.99, I82.401-I82.4Z9

0SRE009 Replacement of Left Hip Joint, Acetabular Surface with Polyethylene Synthetic Substitute, Cemented, Open Approach
HAC When reported with secondary diagnosis code I26.02, I26.09, I26.92-I26.99, I82.401-I82.4Z9

0SRE00A Replacement of Left Hip Joint, Acetabular Surface with Polyethylene Synthetic Substitute, Uncemented, Open Approach
HAC When reported with secondary diagnosis code I26.02, I26.09, I26.92-I26.99, I82.401-I82.4Z9

0SRE00Z Replacement of Left Hip Joint, Acetabular Surface with Polyethylene Synthetic Substitute, Open Approach
HAC When reported with secondary diagnosis code I26.02, I26.09, I26.92-I26.99, I82.401-I82.4Z9

0SRE019 Replacement of Left Hip Joint, Acetabular Surface with Metal Synthetic Substitute, Cemented, Open Approach
HAC When reported with secondary diagnosis code I26.02, I26.09, I26.92-I26.99, I82.401-I82.4Z9

0SRE01A Replacement of Left Hip Joint, Acetabular Surface with Metal Synthetic Substitute, Uncemented, Open Approach
HAC When reported with secondary diagnosis code I26.02, I26.09, I26.92-I26.99, I82.401-I82.4Z9

0SRE01Z Replacement of Left Hip Joint, Acetabular Surface with Metal Synthetic Substitute, Open Approach
HAC When reported with secondary diagnosis code I26.02, I26.09, I26.92-I26.99, I82.401-I82.4Z9

0SRE039 Replacement of Left Hip Joint, Acetabular Surface with Ceramic Synthetic Substitute, Cemented, Open Approach
HAC When reported with secondary diagnosis code I26.02, I26.09, I26.92-I26.99, I82.401-I82.4Z9

0SRE03A Replacement of Left Hip Joint, Acetabular Surface with Ceramic Synthetic Substitute, Uncemented, Open Approach
HAC When reported with secondary diagnosis code I26.02, I26.09, I26.92-I26.99, I82.401-I82.4Z9

0SRE03Z Replacement of Left Hip Joint, Acetabular Surface with Ceramic Synthetic Substitute, Open Approach
HAC When reported with secondary diagnosis code I26.02, I26.09, I26.92-I26.99, I82.401-I82.4Z9

0SRE07Z Replacement of Left Hip Joint, Acetabular Surface with Autologous Tissue Substitute, Open Approach
HAC When reported with secondary diagnosis code I26.02, I26.09, I26.92-I26.99, I82.401-I82.4Z9

0SRE0J9 Replacement of Left Hip Joint, Acetabular Surface with Synthetic Substitute, Cemented, Open Approach
HAC When reported with secondary diagnosis code I26.02, I26.09, I26.92-I26.99, I82.401-I82.4Z9

0SRE0JA Replacement of Left Hip Joint, Acetabular Surface with Synthetic Substitute, Uncemented, Open Approach
HAC When reported with secondary diagnosis code I26.02, I26.09, I26.92-I26.99, I82.401-I82.4Z9

0SRE0JZ Replacement of Left Hip Joint, Acetabular Surface with Synthetic Substitute, Open Approach
HAC When reported with secondary diagnosis code I26.02, I26.09, I26.92-I26.99, I82.401-I82.4Z9

0SRE0KZ Replacement of Left Hip Joint, Acetabular Surface with Nonautologous Tissue Substitute, Open Approach
HAC When reported with secondary diagnosis code I26.02, I26.09, I26.92-I26.99, I82.401-I82.4Z9

0SRF07Z Replacement of Right Ankle Joint with Autologous Tissue Substitute, Open Approach

0SRF0J9 Replacement of Right Ankle Joint with Synthetic Substitute, Cemented, Open Approach

0SRF0JA Replacement of Right Ankle Joint with Synthetic Substitute, Uncemented, Open Approach
AHA CC: 4Q, 2017, 107-108

0SRF0JZ Replacement of Right Ankle Joint with Synthetic Substitute, Open Approach

0SRF0KZ Replacement of Right Ankle Joint with Nonautologous Tissue Substitute, Open Approach

0SRG07Z Replacement of Left Ankle Joint with Autologous Tissue Substitute, Open Approach

0SRG0J9 Replacement of Left Ankle Joint with Synthetic Substitute, Cemented, Open Approach

0SRG0JA Replacement of Left Ankle Joint with Synthetic Substitute, Uncemented, Open Approach

0SRG0JZ Replacement of Left Ankle Joint with Synthetic Substitute, Open Approach

0SRG0KZ Replacement of Left Ankle Joint with Nonautologous Tissue Substitute, Open Approach

0SRH07Z Replacement of Right Tarsal Joint with Autologous Tissue Substitute, Open Approach

0SRH0JZ Replacement of Right Tarsal Joint with Synthetic Substitute, Open Approach

0SRH0KZ Replacement of Right Tarsal Joint with Nonautologous Tissue Substitute, Open Approach

0SRJ07Z Replacement of Left Tarsal Joint with Autologous Tissue Substitute, Open Approach

0SRJ0JZ Replacement of Left Tarsal Joint with Synthetic Substitute, Open Approach

0SRJ0KZ Replacement of Left Tarsal Joint with Nonautologous Tissue Substitute, Open Approach

0SRK07Z Replacement of Right Tarsometatarsal Joint with Autologous Tissue Substitute, Open Approach

0SRK0JZ Replacement of Right Tarsometatarsal Joint with Synthetic Substitute, Open Approach

0SRK0KZ Replacement of Right Tarsometatarsal Joint with Nonautologous Tissue Substitute, Open Approach

0SRL07Z Replacement of Left Tarsometatarsal Joint with Autologous Tissue Substitute, Open Approach

0SRL0JZ Replacement of Left Tarsometatarsal Joint with Synthetic Substitute, Open Approach

0SRL0KZ Replacement of Left Tarsometatarsal Joint with Nonautologous Tissue Substitute, Open Approach

0SRM07Z Replacement of Right Metatarsal-Phalangeal Joint with Autologous Tissue Substitute, Open Approach

0SRM0JZ Replacement of Right Metatarsal-Phalangeal Joint with Synthetic Substitute, Open Approach

0SRM0KZ Replacement of Right Metatarsal-Phalangeal Joint with Nonautologous Tissue Substitute, Open Approach

0SRN07Z Replacement of Left Metatarsal-Phalangeal Joint with Autologous Tissue Substitute, Open Approach

0SRN0JZ Replacement of Left Metatarsal-Phalangeal Joint with Synthetic Substitute, Open Approach

0SRN0KZ Replacement of Left Metatarsal-Phalangeal Joint with Nonautologous Tissue Substitute, Open Approach

0SRP07Z Replacement of Right Toe Phalangeal Joint with Autologous Tissue Substitute, Open Approach

0SRP0JZ Replacement of Right Toe Phalangeal Joint with Synthetic Substitute, Open Approach

0SRP0KZ Replacement of Right Toe Phalangeal Joint with Nonautologous Tissue Substitute, Open Approach

0SRQ07Z Replacement of Left Toe Phalangeal Joint with Autologous Tissue Substitute, Open Approach

0SRQ0JZ Replacement of Left Toe Phalangeal Joint with Synthetic Substitute, Open Approach

0SRQ0KZ Replacement of Left Toe Phalangeal Joint with Nonautologous Tissue Substitute, Open Approach

0SRR019 Replacement of Right Hip Joint, Femoral Surface with Metal Synthetic Substitute, Cemented, Open Approach
HAC When reported with secondary diagnosis code I26.02, I26.09, I26.92-I26.99, I82.401-I82.4Z9

0SRR01A Replacement of Right Hip Joint, Femoral Surface with Metal Synthetic Substitute, Uncemented, Open Approach

 HAC When reported with secondary diagnosis code I26.02, I26.09, I26.92-I26.99, I82.401-I82.4Z9

0SRR01Z Replacement of Right Hip Joint, Femoral Surface with Metal Synthetic Substitute, Open Approach

 HAC When reported with secondary diagnosis code I26.02, I26.09, I26.92-I26.99, I82.401-I82.4Z9

0SRR039 Replacement of Right Hip Joint, Femoral Surface with Ceramic Synthetic Substitute, Cemented, Open Approach

 HAC When reported with secondary diagnosis code I26.02, I26.09, I26.92-I26.99, I82.401-I82.4Z9

0SRR03A Replacement of Right Hip Joint, Femoral Surface with Ceramic Synthetic Substitute, Uncemented, Open Approach

AHA CC: 2Q, 2015, 19-20

 HAC When reported with secondary diagnosis code I26.02, I26.09, I26.92-I26.99, I82.401-I82.4Z9

0SRR03Z Replacement of Right Hip Joint, Femoral Surface with Ceramic Synthetic Substitute, Open Approach

 HAC When reported with secondary diagnosis code I26.02, I26.09, I26.92-I26.99, I82.401-I82.4Z9

0SRR07Z Replacement of Right Hip Joint, Femoral Surface with Autologous Tissue Substitute, Open Approach

 HAC When reported with secondary diagnosis code I26.02, I26.09, I26.92-I26.99, I82.401-I82.4Z9

0SRR0J9 Replacement of Right Hip Joint, Femoral Surface with Synthetic Substitute, Cemented, Open Approach

AHA CC: 4Q, 2016, 111-112

 HAC When reported with secondary diagnosis code I26.02, I26.09, I26.92-I26.99, I82.401-I82.4Z9

0SRR0JA Replacement of Right Hip Joint, Femoral Surface with Synthetic Substitute, Uncemented, Open Approach

 HAC When reported with secondary diagnosis code I26.02, I26.09, I26.92-I26.99, I82.401-I82.4Z9

0SRR0JZ Replacement of Right Hip Joint, Femoral Surface with Synthetic Substitute, Open Approach

 HAC When reported with secondary diagnosis code I26.02, I26.09, I26.92-I26.99, I82.401-I82.4Z9

0SRR0KZ Replacement of Right Hip Joint, Femoral Surface with Nonautologous Tissue Substitute, Open Approach

 HAC When reported with secondary diagnosis code I26.02, I26.09, I26.92-I26.99, I82.401-I82.4Z9

0SRS019 Replacement of Left Hip Joint, Femoral Surface with Metal Synthetic Substitute, Cemented, Open Approach

 HAC When reported with secondary diagnosis code I26.02, I26.09, I26.92-I26.99, I82.401-I82.4Z9

0SRS01A Replacement of Left Hip Joint, Femoral Surface with Metal Synthetic Substitute, Uncemented, Open Approach

 HAC When reported with secondary diagnosis code I26.02, I26.09, I26.92-I26.99, I82.401-I82.4Z9

0SRS01Z Replacement of Left Hip Joint, Femoral Surface with Metal Synthetic Substitute, Open Approach

 HAC When reported with secondary diagnosis code I26.02, I26.09, I26.92-I26.99, I82.401-I82.4Z9

0SRS039 Replacement of Left Hip Joint, Femoral Surface with Ceramic Synthetic Substitute, Cemented, Open Approach

 HAC When reported with secondary diagnosis code I26.02, I26.09, I26.92-I26.99, I82.401-I82.4Z9

0SRS03A Replacement of Left Hip Joint, Femoral Surface with Ceramic Synthetic Substitute, Uncemented, Open Approach

 HAC When reported with secondary diagnosis code I26.02, I26.09, I26.92-I26.99, I82.401-I82.4Z9

0SRS03Z Replacement of Left Hip Joint, Femoral Surface with Ceramic Synthetic Substitute, Open Approach

 HAC When reported with secondary diagnosis code I26.02, I26.09, I26.92-I26.99, I82.401-I82.4Z9

0SRS07Z Replacement of Left Hip Joint, Femoral Surface with Autologous Tissue Substitute, Open Approach

 HAC When reported with secondary diagnosis code I26.02, I26.09, I26.92-I26.99, I82.401-I82.4Z9

0SRS0J9 Replacement of Left Hip Joint, Femoral Surface with Synthetic Substitute, Cemented, Open Approach

 HAC When reported with secondary diagnosis code I26.02, I26.09, I26.92-I26.99, I82.401-I82.4Z9

0SRS0JA Replacement of Left Hip Joint, Femoral Surface with Synthetic Substitute, Uncemented, Open Approach

 HAC When reported with secondary diagnosis code I26.02, I26.09, I26.92-I26.99, I82.401-I82.4Z9

0SRS0JZ Replacement of Left Hip Joint, Femoral Surface with Synthetic Substitute, Open Approach

 HAC When reported with secondary diagnosis code I26.02; I26.09, I26.92-I26.99, I82.401-I82.4Z9

0SRS0KZ Replacement of Left Hip Joint, Femoral Surface with Nonautologous Tissue Substitute, Open Approach

 HAC When reported with secondary diagnosis code I26.02, I26.09, I26.92-I26.99, I82.401-I82.4Z9

0SRT07Z Replacement of Right Knee Joint, Femoral Surface with Autologous Tissue Substitute, Open Approach

 HAC When reported with secondary diagnosis code I26.02, I26.09, I26.92-I26.99, I82.401-I82.4Z9

0SRT0J9 Replacement of Right Knee Joint, Femoral Surface with Synthetic Substitute, Cemented, Open Approach

 HAC When reported with secondary diagnosis code I26.02, I26.09, I26.92-I26.99, I82.401-I82.4Z9

0SRT0JA Replacement of Right Knee Joint, Femoral Surface with Synthetic Substitute, Uncemented, Open Approach

 HAC When reported with secondary diagnosis code I26.02, I26.09, I26.92-I26.99, I82.401-I82.4Z9

0SRT0JZ Replacement of Right Knee Joint, Femoral Surface with Synthetic Substitute, Open Approach

 HAC When reported with secondary diagnosis code I26.02, I26.09, I26.92-I26.99, I82.401-I82.4Z9

0SRT0KZ Replacement of Right Knee Joint, Femoral Surface with Nonautologous Tissue Substitute, Open Approach

 HAC When reported with secondary diagnosis code I26.02, I26.09, I26.92-I26.99, I82.401-I82.4Z9

0SRU07Z Replacement of Left Knee Joint, Femoral Surface with Autologous Tissue Substitute, Open Approach

 HAC When reported with secondary diagnosis code I26.02, I26.09, I26.92-I26.99, I82.401-I82.4Z9

0SRU0J9 Replacement of Left Knee Joint, Femoral Surface with Synthetic Substitute, Cemented, Open Approach

 HAC When reported with secondary diagnosis code I26.02, I26.09, I26.92-I26.99, I82.401-I82.4Z9

0SRU0JA Replacement of Left Knee Joint, Femoral Surface with Synthetic Substitute, Uncemented, Open Approach

 HAC When reported with secondary diagnosis code I26.02, I26.09, I26.92-I26.99, I82.401-I82.4Z9

0SRU0JZ Replacement of Left Knee Joint, Femoral Surface with Synthetic Substitute, Open Approach

 HAC When reported with secondary diagnosis code I26.02, I26.09, I26.92-I26.99, I82.401-I82.4Z9

0SRU0KZ Replacement of Left Knee Joint, Femoral Surface with Nonautologous Tissue Substitute, Open Approach

 HAC When reported with secondary diagnosis code I26.02, I26.09, I26.92-I26.99, I82.401-I82.4Z9

0SRV07Z Replacement of Right Knee Joint, Tibial Surface with Autologous Tissue Substitute, Open Approach

 HAC When reported with secondary diagnosis code I26.02, I26.09, I26.92-I26.99, I82.401-I82.4Z9

0SRV0J9 Replacement of Right Knee Joint, Tibial Surface with Synthetic Substitute, Cemented, Open Approach

 HAC When reported with secondary diagnosis code I26.02, I26.09, I26.92-I26.99, I82.401-I82.4Z9

0SRV0JA Replacement of Right Knee Joint, Tibial Surface with Synthetic Substitute, Uncemented, Open Approach

 HAC When reported with secondary diagnosis code I26.02, I26.09, I26.92-I26.99, I82.401-I82.4Z9

0SRV0JZ Replacement of Right Knee Joint, Tibial Surface with Synthetic Substitute, Open Approach

 HAC When reported with secondary diagnosis code I26.02, I26.09, I26.92-I26.99, I82.401-I82.4Z9

0SRV0KZ Replacement of Right Knee Joint, Tibial Surface with Nonautologous Tissue Substitute, Open Approach

 HAC When reported with secondary diagnosis code I26.02, I26.09, I26.92-I26.99, I82.401-I82.4Z9

♀ Female-only ♂ Male-only ▲ Limited Coverage ● Non-OR HAC HAC-associated procedure ▲ Non-covered procedures ✚ Cluster

0SRW07Z Replacement of Left Knee Joint, Tibial Surface with Autologous Tissue Substitute, Open Approach
- When reported with secondary diagnosis code I26.02, I26.09, I26.92-I26.99, I82.401-I82.4Z9

0SRW0J9 Replacement of Left Knee Joint, Tibial Surface with Synthetic Substitute, Cemented, Open Approach
- When reported with secondary diagnosis code I26.02, I26.09, I26.92-I26.99, I82.401-I82.4Z9

0SRW0JA Replacement of Left Knee Joint, Tibial Surface with Synthetic Substitute, Uncemented, Open Approach
- When reported with secondary diagnosis code I26.02, I26.09, I26.92-I26.99, I82.401-I82.4Z9

0SRW0JZ Replacement of Left Knee Joint, Tibial Surface with Synthetic Substitute, Open Approach
- *AHA CC: 2Q, 2018, 16-17*

0SRW0KZ Replacement of Left Knee Joint, Tibial Surface with Nonautologous Tissue Substitute, Open Approach
- When reported with secondary diagnosis code I26.02, I26.09, I26.92-I26.99, I82.401-I82.4Z9

0SS – Lower Joints, Reposition

0SS004Z Reposition Lumbar Vertebral Joint with Internal Fixation Device, Open Approach

0SS00ZZ Reposition Lumbar Vertebral Joint, Open Approach

0SS034Z Reposition Lumbar Vertebral Joint with Internal Fixation Device, Percutaneous Approach

0SS03ZZ Reposition Lumbar Vertebral Joint, Percutaneous Approach

0SS044Z Reposition Lumbar Vertebral Joint with Internal Fixation Device, Percutaneous Endoscopic Approach

0SS04ZZ Reposition Lumbar Vertebral Joint, Percutaneous Endoscopic Approach

0SS0X4Z Reposition Lumbar Vertebral Joint with Internal Fixation Device, External Approach

0SS0XZZ Reposition Lumbar Vertebral Joint, External Approach

0SS304Z Reposition Lumbosacral Joint with Internal Fixation Device, Open Approach

0SS30ZZ Reposition Lumbosacral Joint, Open Approach

0SS334Z Reposition Lumbosacral Joint with Internal Fixation Device, Percutaneous Approach

0SS33ZZ Reposition Lumbosacral Joint, Percutaneous Approach

0SS344Z Reposition Lumbosacral Joint with Internal Fixation Device, Percutaneous Endoscopic Approach

0SS34ZZ Reposition Lumbosacral Joint, Percutaneous Endoscopic Approach

0SS3X4Z Reposition Lumbosacral Joint with Internal Fixation Device, External Approach

0SS3XZZ Reposition Lumbosacral Joint, External Approach

0SS504Z Reposition Sacrococcygeal Joint with Internal Fixation Device, Open Approach

0SS50ZZ Reposition Sacrococcygeal Joint, Open Approach

0SS534Z Reposition Sacrococcygeal Joint with Internal Fixation Device, Percutaneous Approach

0SS53ZZ Reposition Sacrococcygeal Joint, Percutaneous Approach

0SS544Z Reposition Sacrococcygeal Joint with Internal Fixation Device, Percutaneous Endoscopic Approach

0SS54ZZ Reposition Sacrococcygeal Joint, Percutaneous Endoscopic Approach

0SS5X4Z Reposition Sacrococcygeal Joint with Internal Fixation Device, External Approach

0SS5XZZ Reposition Sacrococcygeal Joint, External Approach

0SS604Z Reposition Coccygeal Joint with Internal Fixation Device, Open Approach

0SS60ZZ Reposition Coccygeal Joint, Open Approach

0SS634Z Reposition Coccygeal Joint with Internal Fixation Device, Percutaneous Approach

0SS63ZZ Reposition Coccygeal Joint, Percutaneous Approach

0SS644Z Reposition Coccygeal Joint with Internal Fixation Device, Percutaneous Endoscopic Approach

0SS64ZZ Reposition Coccygeal Joint, Percutaneous Endoscopic Approach

0SS6X4Z Reposition Coccygeal Joint with Internal Fixation Device, External Approach

0SS6XZZ Reposition Coccygeal Joint, External Approach

0SS704Z Reposition Right Sacroiliac Joint with Internal Fixation Device, Open Approach

0SS70ZZ Reposition Right Sacroiliac Joint, Open Approach

0SS734Z Reposition Right Sacroiliac Joint with Internal Fixation Device, Percutaneous Approach

0SS73ZZ Reposition Right Sacroiliac Joint, Percutaneous Approach

0SS744Z Reposition Right Sacroiliac Joint with Internal Fixation Device, Percutaneous Endoscopic Approach

0SS74ZZ Reposition Right Sacroiliac Joint, Percutaneous Endoscopic Approach

0SS7X4Z Reposition Right Sacroiliac Joint with Internal Fixation Device, External Approach

0SS7XZZ Reposition Right Sacroiliac Joint, External Approach

0SS804Z Reposition Left Sacroiliac Joint with Internal Fixation Device, Open Approach

0SS80ZZ Reposition Left Sacroiliac Joint, Open Approach

0SS834Z Reposition Left Sacroiliac Joint with Internal Fixation Device, Percutaneous Approach

0SS83ZZ Reposition Left Sacroiliac Joint, Percutaneous Approach

0SS844Z Reposition Left Sacroiliac Joint with Internal Fixation Device, Percutaneous Endoscopic Approach

0SS84ZZ Reposition Left Sacroiliac Joint, Percutaneous Endoscopic Approach

0SS8X4Z Reposition Left Sacroiliac Joint with Internal Fixation Device, External Approach

0SS8XZZ Reposition Left Sacroiliac Joint, External Approach

0SS904Z Reposition Right Hip Joint with Internal Fixation Device, Open Approach

0SS905Z Reposition Right Hip Joint with External Fixation Device, Open Approach

0SS90ZZ Reposition Right Hip Joint, Open Approach

0SS934Z Reposition Right Hip Joint with Internal Fixation Device, Percutaneous Approach

0SS935Z Reposition Right Hip Joint with External Fixation Device, Percutaneous Approach

0SS93ZZ Reposition Right Hip Joint, Percutaneous Approach

0SS944Z Reposition Right Hip Joint with Internal Fixation Device, Percutaneous Endoscopic Approach

0SS945Z Reposition Right Hip Joint with External Fixation Device, Percutaneous Endoscopic Approach

0SS94ZZ Reposition Right Hip Joint, Percutaneous Endoscopic Approach

0SS9X4Z Reposition Right Hip Joint with Internal Fixation Device, External Approach

0SS9X5Z Reposition Right Hip Joint with External Fixation Device, External Approach

0SS9XZZ Reposition Right Hip Joint, External Approach

0SSB04Z Reposition Left Hip Joint with Internal Fixation Device, Open Approach

0SSB05Z Reposition Left Hip Joint with External Fixation Device, Open Approach

0SSB0ZZ Reposition Left Hip Joint, Open Approach

0SSB34Z Reposition Left Hip Joint with Internal Fixation Device, Percutaneous Approach

0SSB35Z Reposition Left Hip Joint with External Fixation Device, Percutaneous Approach

0SSB3ZZ Reposition Left Hip Joint, Percutaneous Approach

0SSB44Z Reposition Left Hip Joint with Internal Fixation Device, Percutaneous Endoscopic Approach

0SSB45Z Reposition Left Hip Joint with External Fixation Device, Percutaneous Endoscopic Approach

0SSB4ZZ Reposition Left Hip Joint, Percutaneous Endoscopic Approach

0SSBX4Z Reposition Left Hip Joint with Internal Fixation Device, External Approach

0SSBX5Z Reposition Left Hip Joint with External Fixation Device, External Approach

0SSBXZZ Reposition Left Hip Joint, External Approach

0SSC04Z Reposition Right Knee Joint with Internal Fixation Device, Open Approach

0SSC05Z Reposition Right Knee Joint with External Fixation Device, Open Approach

0SSC0ZZ	Reposition Right Knee Joint, Open Approach
0SSC34Z	Reposition Right Knee Joint with Internal Fixation Device, Percutaneous Approach
0SSC35Z	Reposition Right Knee Joint with External Fixation Device, Percutaneous Approach
0SSC3ZZ	Reposition Right Knee Joint, Percutaneous Approach
0SSC44Z	Reposition Right Knee Joint with Internal Fixation Device, Percutaneous Endoscopic Approach
0SSC45Z	Reposition Right Knee Joint with External Fixation Device, Percutaneous Endoscopic Approach
0SSC4ZZ	Reposition Right Knee Joint, Percutaneous Endoscopic Approach
0SSCX4Z	Reposition Right Knee Joint with Internal Fixation Device, External Approach
0SSCX5Z	Reposition Right Knee Joint with External Fixation Device, External Approach
0SSCXZZ	Reposition Right Knee Joint, External Approach
0SSD04Z	Reposition Left Knee Joint with Internal Fixation Device, Open Approach
0SSD05Z	Reposition Left Knee Joint with External Fixation Device, Open Approach
0SSD0ZZ	Reposition Left Knee Joint, Open Approach
0SSD34Z	Reposition Left Knee Joint with Internal Fixation Device, Percutaneous Approach
0SSD35Z	Reposition Left Knee Joint with External Fixation Device, Percutaneous Approach
0SSD3ZZ	Reposition Left Knee Joint, Percutaneous Approach
0SSD44Z	Reposition Left Knee Joint with Internal Fixation Device, Percutaneous Endoscopic Approach
0SSD45Z	Reposition Left Knee Joint with External Fixation Device, Percutaneous Endoscopic Approach
0SSD4ZZ	Reposition Left Knee Joint, Percutaneous Endoscopic Approach
0SSDX4Z	Reposition Left Knee Joint with Internal Fixation Device, External Approach
0SSDX5Z	Reposition Left Knee Joint with External Fixation Device, External Approach
0SSDXZZ	Reposition Left Knee Joint, External Approach
0SSF04Z	Reposition Right Ankle Joint with Internal Fixation Device, Open Approach
0SSF05Z	Reposition Right Ankle Joint with External Fixation Device, Open Approach
0SSF0ZZ	Reposition Right Ankle Joint, Open Approach
0SSF34Z	Reposition Right Ankle Joint with Internal Fixation Device, Percutaneous Approach
0SSF35Z	Reposition Right Ankle Joint with External Fixation Device, Percutaneous Approach
0SSF3ZZ	Reposition Right Ankle Joint, Percutaneous Approach
0SSF44Z	Reposition Right Ankle Joint with Internal Fixation Device, Percutaneous Endoscopic Approach
0SSF45Z	Reposition Right Ankle Joint with External Fixation Device, Percutaneous Endoscopic Approach
0SSF4ZZ	Reposition Right Ankle Joint, Percutaneous Endoscopic Approach
0SSFX4Z	Reposition Right Ankle Joint with Internal Fixation Device, External Approach
0SSFX5Z	Reposition Right Ankle Joint with External Fixation Device, External Approach
0SSFXZZ	Reposition Right Ankle Joint, External Approach
0SSG04Z	Reposition Left Ankle Joint with Internal Fixation Device, Open Approach
0SSG05Z	Reposition Left Ankle Joint with External Fixation Device, Open Approach
0SSG0ZZ	Reposition Left Ankle Joint, Open Approach
0SSG34Z	Reposition Left Ankle Joint with Internal Fixation Device, Percutaneous Approach
0SSG35Z	Reposition Left Ankle Joint with External Fixation Device, Percutaneous Approach
0SSG3ZZ	Reposition Left Ankle Joint, Percutaneous Approach
0SSG44Z	Reposition Left Ankle Joint with Internal Fixation Device, Percutaneous Endoscopic Approach
0SSG45Z	Reposition Left Ankle Joint with External Fixation Device, Percutaneous Endoscopic Approach
0SSG4ZZ	Reposition Left Ankle Joint, Percutaneous Endoscopic Approach
0SSGX4Z	Reposition Left Ankle Joint with Internal Fixation Device, External Approach
0SSGX5Z	Reposition Left Ankle Joint with External Fixation Device, External Approach
0SSGXZZ	Reposition Left Ankle Joint, External Approach
0SSH04Z	Reposition Right Tarsal Joint with Internal Fixation Device, Open Approach
0SSH05Z	Reposition Right Tarsal Joint with External Fixation Device, Open Approach
0SSH0ZZ	Reposition Right Tarsal Joint, Open Approach
0SSH34Z	Reposition Right Tarsal Joint with Internal Fixation Device, Percutaneous Approach
0SSH35Z	Reposition Right Tarsal Joint with External Fixation Device, Percutaneous Approach
0SSH3ZZ	Reposition Right Tarsal Joint, Percutaneous Approach
0SSH44Z	Reposition Right Tarsal Joint with Internal Fixation Device, Percutaneous Endoscopic Approach
0SSH45Z	Reposition Right Tarsal Joint with External Fixation Device, Percutaneous Endoscopic Approach
0SSH4ZZ	Reposition Right Tarsal Joint, Percutaneous Endoscopic Approach
0SSHX4Z	Reposition Right Tarsal Joint with Internal Fixation Device, External Approach
0SSHX5Z	Reposition Right Tarsal Joint with External Fixation Device, External Approach
0SSHXZZ	Reposition Right Tarsal Joint, External Approach
0SSJ04Z	Reposition Left Tarsal Joint with Internal Fixation Device, Open Approach
0SSJ05Z	Reposition Left Tarsal Joint with External Fixation Device, Open Approach
0SSJ0ZZ	Reposition Left Tarsal Joint, Open Approach
0SSJ34Z	Reposition Left Tarsal Joint with Internal Fixation Device, Percutaneous Approach
0SSJ35Z	Reposition Left Tarsal Joint with External Fixation Device, Percutaneous Approach
0SSJ3ZZ	Reposition Left Tarsal Joint, Percutaneous Approach
0SSJ44Z	Reposition Left Tarsal Joint with Internal Fixation Device, Percutaneous Endoscopic Approach
0SSJ45Z	Reposition Left Tarsal Joint with External Fixation Device, Percutaneous Endoscopic Approach
0SSJ4ZZ	Reposition Left Tarsal Joint, Percutaneous Endoscopic Approach
0SSJX4Z	Reposition Left Tarsal Joint with Internal Fixation Device, External Approach
0SSJX5Z	Reposition Left Tarsal Joint with External Fixation Device, External Approach
0SSJXZZ	Reposition Left Tarsal Joint, External Approach
0SSK04Z	Reposition Right Tarsometatarsal Joint with Internal Fixation Device, Open Approach
0SSK05Z	Reposition Right Tarsometatarsal Joint with External Fixation Device, Open Approach
0SSK0ZZ	Reposition Right Tarsometatarsal Joint, Open Approach
0SSK34Z	Reposition Right Tarsometatarsal Joint with Internal Fixation Device, Percutaneous Approach
0SSK35Z	Reposition Right Tarsometatarsal Joint with External Fixation Device, Percutaneous Approach
0SSK3ZZ	Reposition Right Tarsometatarsal Joint, Percutaneous Approach
0SSK44Z	Reposition Right Tarsometatarsal Joint with Internal Fixation Device, Percutaneous Endoscopic Approach
0SSK45Z	Reposition Right Tarsometatarsal Joint with External Fixation Device, Percutaneous Endoscopic Approach
0SSK4ZZ	Reposition Right Tarsometatarsal Joint, Percutaneous Endoscopic Approach
0SSKX4Z	Reposition Right Tarsometatarsal Joint with Internal Fixation Device, External Approach
0SSKX5Z	Reposition Right Tarsometatarsal Joint with External Fixation Device, External Approach
0SSKXZZ	Reposition Right Tarsometatarsal Joint, External Approach
0SSL04Z	Reposition Left Tarsometatarsal Joint with Internal Fixation Device, Open Approach
0SSL05Z	Reposition Left Tarsometatarsal Joint with External Fixation Device, Open Approach
0SSL0ZZ	Reposition Left Tarsometatarsal Joint, Open Approach
0SSL34Z	Reposition Left Tarsometatarsal Joint with Internal Fixation Device, Percutaneous Approach

♀ Female-only ♂ Male-only ▲ Limited Coverage ● Non-OR ▨ HAC-associated procedure ▲ Non-covered procedures ✛ Cluster

0SSL35Z	Reposition Left Tarsometatarsal Joint with External Fixation Device, Percutaneous Approach
0SSL3ZZ	Reposition Left Tarsometatarsal Joint, Percutaneous Approach
0SSL44Z	Reposition Left Tarsometatarsal Joint with Internal Fixation Device, Percutaneous Endoscopic Approach
0SSL45Z	Reposition Left Tarsometatarsal Joint with External Fixation Device, Percutaneous Endoscopic Approach
0SSL4ZZ	Reposition Left Tarsometatarsal Joint, Percutaneous Endoscopic Approach
0SSLX4Z	Reposition Left Tarsometatarsal Joint with Internal Fixation Device, External Approach
0SSLX5Z	Reposition Left Tarsometatarsal Joint with External Fixation Device, External Approach
0SSLXZZ	Reposition Left Tarsometatarsal Joint, External Approach
0SSM04Z	Reposition Right Metatarsal-Phalangeal Joint with Internal Fixation Device, Open Approach
0SSM05Z	Reposition Right Metatarsal-Phalangeal Joint with External Fixation Device, Open Approach
0SSM0ZZ	Reposition Right Metatarsal-Phalangeal Joint, Open Approach
0SSM34Z	Reposition Right Metatarsal-Phalangeal Joint with Internal Fixation Device, Percutaneous Approach
0SSM35Z	Reposition Right Metatarsal-Phalangeal Joint with External Fixation Device, Percutaneous Approach
0SSM3ZZ	Reposition Right Metatarsal-Phalangeal Joint, Percutaneous Approach
0SSM44Z	Reposition Right Metatarsal-Phalangeal Joint with Internal Fixation Device, Percutaneous Endoscopic Approach
0SSM45Z	Reposition Right Metatarsal-Phalangeal Joint with External Fixation Device, Percutaneous Endoscopic Approach
0SSM4ZZ	Reposition Right Metatarsal-Phalangeal Joint, Percutaneous Endoscopic Approach
0SSMX4Z	Reposition Right Metatarsal-Phalangeal Joint with Internal Fixation Device, External Approach

0SSMX5Z	Reposition Right Metatarsal-Phalangeal Joint with External Fixation Device, External Approach
0SSMXZZ	Reposition Right Metatarsal-Phalangeal Joint, External Approach
0SSN04Z	Reposition Left Metatarsal-Phalangeal Joint with Internal Fixation Device, Open Approach
0SSN05Z	Reposition Left Metatarsal-Phalangeal Joint with External Fixation Device, Open Approach
0SSN0ZZ	Reposition Left Metatarsal-Phalangeal Joint, Open Approach
0SSN34Z	Reposition Left Metatarsal-Phalangeal Joint with Internal Fixation Device, Percutaneous Approach
0SSN35Z	Reposition Left Metatarsal-Phalangeal Joint with External Fixation Device, Percutaneous Approach
0SSN3ZZ	Reposition Left Metatarsal-Phalangeal Joint, Percutaneous Approach
0SSN44Z	Reposition Left Metatarsal-Phalangeal Joint with Internal Fixation Device, Percutaneous Endoscopic Approach
0SSN45Z	Reposition Left Metatarsal-Phalangeal Joint with External Fixation Device, Percutaneous Endoscopic Approach
0SSN4ZZ	Reposition Left Metatarsal-Phalangeal Joint, Percutaneous Endoscopic Approach
0SSNX4Z	Reposition Left Metatarsal-Phalangeal Joint with Internal Fixation Device, External Approach
0SSNX5Z	Reposition Left Metatarsal-Phalangeal Joint with External Fixation Device, External Approach
0SSNXZZ	Reposition Left Metatarsal-Phalangeal Joint, External Approach
0SSP04Z	Reposition Right Toe Phalangeal Joint with Internal Fixation Device, Open Approach
0SSP05Z	Reposition Right Toe Phalangeal Joint with External Fixation Device, Open Approach
0SSP0ZZ	Reposition Right Toe Phalangeal Joint, Open Approach
0SSP34Z	Reposition Right Toe Phalangeal Joint with Internal Fixation Device, Percutaneous Approach
0SSP35Z	Reposition Right Toe Phalangeal Joint with External Fixation Device, Percutaneous Approach

0SSP3ZZ	Reposition Right Toe Phalangeal Joint, Percutaneous Approach
0SSP44Z	Reposition Right Toe Phalangeal Joint with Internal Fixation Device, Percutaneous Endoscopic Approach
0SSP45Z	Reposition Right Toe Phalangeal Joint with External Fixation Device, Percutaneous Endoscopic Approach
0SSP4ZZ	Reposition Right Toe Phalangeal Joint, Percutaneous Endoscopic Approach
0SSPX4Z	Reposition Right Toe Phalangeal Joint with Internal Fixation Device, External Approach
0SSPX5Z	Reposition Right Toe Phalangeal Joint with External Fixation Device, External Approach
0SSPXZZ	Reposition Right Toe Phalangeal Joint, External Approach
0SSQ04Z	Reposition Left Toe Phalangeal Joint with Internal Fixation Device, Open Approach
0SSQ05Z	Reposition Left Toe Phalangeal Joint with External Fixation Device, Open Approach
0SSQ0ZZ	Reposition Left Toe Phalangeal Joint, Open Approach
0SSQ34Z	Reposition Left Toe Phalangeal Joint with Internal Fixation Device, Percutaneous Approach
0SSQ35Z	Reposition Left Toe Phalangeal Joint with External Fixation Device, Percutaneous Approach
0SSQ3ZZ	Reposition Left Toe Phalangeal Joint, Percutaneous Approach
0SSQ44Z	Reposition Left Toe Phalangeal Joint with Internal Fixation Device, Percutaneous Endoscopic Approach
0SSQ45Z	Reposition Left Toe Phalangeal Joint with External Fixation Device, Percutaneous Endoscopic Approach
0SSQ4ZZ	Reposition Left Toe Phalangeal Joint, Percutaneous Endoscopic Approach
0SSQX4Z	Reposition Left Toe Phalangeal Joint with Internal Fixation Device, External Approach
0SSQX5Z	Reposition Left Toe Phalangeal Joint with External Fixation Device, External Approach
0SSQXZZ	Reposition Left Toe Phalangeal Joint, External Approach

0ST – Lower Joints, Resection

Review Coding Guideline B3.8

Review Coding Guideline B3.18

0ST20ZZ	Resection of Lumbar Vertebral Disc, Open Approach
0ST40ZZ	Resection of Lumbosacral Disc, Open Approach
0ST50ZZ	Resection of Sacrococcygeal Joint, Open Approach
0ST60ZZ	Resection of Coccygeal Joint, Open Approach
0ST70ZZ	Resection of Right Sacroiliac Joint, Open Approach
0ST80ZZ	Resection of Left Sacroiliac Joint, Open Approach
0ST90ZZ	Resection of Right Hip Joint, Open Approach

0STB0ZZ	Resection of Left Hip Joint, Open Approach
0STC0ZZ	Resection of Right Knee Joint, Open Approach
0STD0ZZ	Resection of Left Knee Joint, Open Approach
	AHA CC: 4Q, 2014, 30-31
0STF0ZZ	Resection of Right Ankle Joint, Open Approach
0STG0ZZ	Resection of Left Ankle Joint, Open Approach
0STH0ZZ	Resection of Right Tarsal Joint, Open Approach
0STJ0ZZ	Resection of Left Tarsal Joint, Open Approach

0STK0ZZ	Resection of Right Tarsometatarsal Joint, Open Approach
0STL0ZZ	Resection of Left Tarsometatarsal Joint, Open Approach
0STM0ZZ	Resection of Right Metatarsal-Phalangeal Joint, Open Approach
	AHA CC: 1Q, 2016, 20-21
0STN0ZZ	Resection of Left Metatarsal-Phalangeal Joint, Open Approach
0STP0ZZ	Resection of Right Toe Phalangeal Joint, Open Approach
0STQ0ZZ	Resection of Left Toe Phalangeal Joint, Open Approach

0SU – Lower Joints, Supplement

0SU007Z Supplement Lumbar Vertebral Joint with Autologous Tissue Substitute, Open Approach

0SU00JZ Supplement Lumbar Vertebral Joint with Synthetic Substitute, Open Approach

0SU00KZ Supplement Lumbar Vertebral Joint with Nonautologous Tissue Substitute, Open Approach

0SU037Z Supplement Lumbar Vertebral Joint with Autologous Tissue Substitute, Percutaneous Approach

0SU03JZ Supplement Lumbar Vertebral Joint with Synthetic Substitute, Percutaneous Approach

0SU03KZ Supplement Lumbar Vertebral Joint with Nonautologous Tissue Substitute, Percutaneous Approach

0SU047Z Supplement Lumbar Vertebral Joint with Autologous Tissue Substitute, Percutaneous Endoscopic Approach

0SU04JZ Supplement Lumbar Vertebral Joint with Synthetic Substitute, Percutaneous Endoscopic Approach

0SU04KZ Supplement Lumbar Vertebral Joint with Nonautologous Tissue Substitute, Percutaneous Endoscopic Approach

0SU207Z Supplement Lumbar Vertebral Disc with Autologous Tissue Substitute, Open Approach

0SU20JZ Supplement Lumbar Vertebral Disc with Synthetic Substitute, Open Approach

0SU20KZ Supplement Lumbar Vertebral Disc with Nonautologous Tissue Substitute, Open Approach

0SU237Z Supplement Lumbar Vertebral Disc with Autologous Tissue Substitute, Percutaneous Approach

0SU23JZ Supplement Lumbar Vertebral Disc with Synthetic Substitute, Percutaneous Approach

0SU23KZ Supplement Lumbar Vertebral Disc with Nonautologous Tissue Substitute, Percutaneous Approach

0SU247Z Supplement Lumbar Vertebral Disc with Autologous Tissue Substitute, Percutaneous Endoscopic Approach

0SU24JZ Supplement Lumbar Vertebral Disc with Synthetic Substitute, Percutaneous Endoscopic Approach

0SU24KZ Supplement Lumbar Vertebral Disc with Nonautologous Tissue Substitute, Percutaneous Endoscopic Approach

0SU307Z Supplement Lumbosacral Joint with Autologous Tissue Substitute, Open Approach

0SU30JZ Supplement Lumbosacral Joint with Synthetic Substitute, Open Approach

0SU30KZ Supplement Lumbosacral Joint with Nonautologous Tissue Substitute, Open Approach

0SU337Z Supplement Lumbosacral Joint with Autologous Tissue Substitute, Percutaneous Approach

0SU33JZ Supplement Lumbosacral Joint with Synthetic Substitute, Percutaneous Approach

0SU33KZ Supplement Lumbosacral Joint with Nonautologous Tissue Substitute, Percutaneous Approach

0SU347Z Supplement Lumbosacral Joint with Autologous Tissue Substitute, Percutaneous Endoscopic Approach

0SU34JZ Supplement Lumbosacral Joint with Synthetic Substitute, Percutaneous Endoscopic Approach

0SU34KZ Supplement Lumbosacral Joint with Nonautologous Tissue Substitute, Percutaneous Endoscopic Approach

0SU407Z Supplement Lumbosacral Disc with Autologous Tissue Substitute, Open Approach

0SU40JZ Supplement Lumbosacral Disc with Synthetic Substitute, Open Approach

0SU40KZ Supplement Lumbosacral Disc with Nonautologous Tissue Substitute, Open Approach

0SU437Z Supplement Lumbosacral Disc with Autologous Tissue Substitute, Percutaneous Approach

0SU43JZ Supplement Lumbosacral Disc with Synthetic Substitute, Percutaneous Approach

0SU43KZ Supplement Lumbosacral Disc with Nonautologous Tissue Substitute, Percutaneous Approach

0SU447Z Supplement Lumbosacral Disc with Autologous Tissue Substitute, Percutaneous Endoscopic Approach

0SU44JZ Supplement Lumbosacral Disc with Synthetic Substitute, Percutaneous Endoscopic Approach

0SU44KZ Supplement Lumbosacral Disc with Nonautologous Tissue Substitute, Percutaneous Endoscopic Approach

0SU507Z Supplement Sacrococcygeal Joint with Autologous Tissue Substitute, Open Approach

0SU50JZ Supplement Sacrococcygeal Joint with Synthetic Substitute, Open Approach

0SU50KZ Supplement Sacrococcygeal Joint with Nonautologous Tissue Substitute, Open Approach

0SU537Z Supplement Sacrococcygeal Joint with Autologous Tissue Substitute, Percutaneous Approach

0SU53JZ Supplement Sacrococcygeal Joint with Synthetic Substitute, Percutaneous Approach

0SU53KZ Supplement Sacrococcygeal Joint with Nonautologous Tissue Substitute, Percutaneous Approach

0SU547Z Supplement Sacrococcygeal Joint with Autologous Tissue Substitute, Percutaneous Endoscopic Approach

0SU54JZ Supplement Sacrococcygeal Joint with Synthetic Substitute, Percutaneous Endoscopic Approach

0SU54KZ Supplement Sacrococcygeal Joint with Nonautologous Tissue Substitute, Percutaneous Endoscopic Approach

0SU607Z Supplement Coccygeal Joint with Autologous Tissue Substitute, Open Approach

0SU60JZ Supplement Coccygeal Joint with Synthetic Substitute, Open Approach

0SU60KZ Supplement Coccygeal Joint with Nonautologous Tissue Substitute, Open Approach

0SU637Z Supplement Coccygeal Joint with Autologous Tissue Substitute, Percutaneous Approach

0SU63JZ Supplement Coccygeal Joint with Synthetic Substitute, Percutaneous Approach

0SU63KZ Supplement Coccygeal Joint with Nonautologous Tissue Substitute, Percutaneous Approach

0SU647Z Supplement Coccygeal Joint with Autologous Tissue Substitute, Percutaneous Endoscopic Approach

0SU64JZ Supplement Coccygeal Joint with Synthetic Substitute, Percutaneous Endoscopic Approach

0SU64KZ Supplement Coccygeal Joint with Nonautologous Tissue Substitute, Percutaneous Endoscopic Approach

0SU707Z Supplement Right Sacroiliac Joint with Autologous Tissue Substitute, Open Approach

0SU70JZ Supplement Right Sacroiliac Joint with Synthetic Substitute, Open Approach

0SU70KZ Supplement Right Sacroiliac Joint with Nonautologous Tissue Substitute, Open Approach

0SU737Z Supplement Right Sacroiliac Joint with Autologous Tissue Substitute, Percutaneous Approach

0SU73JZ Supplement Right Sacroiliac Joint with Synthetic Substitute, Percutaneous Approach

0SU73KZ Supplement Right Sacroiliac Joint with Nonautologous Tissue Substitute, Percutaneous Approach

0SU747Z Supplement Right Sacroiliac Joint with Autologous Tissue Substitute, Percutaneous Endoscopic Approach

0SU74JZ Supplement Right Sacroiliac Joint with Synthetic Substitute, Percutaneous Endoscopic Approach

0SU74KZ Supplement Right Sacroiliac Joint with Nonautologous Tissue Substitute, Percutaneous Endoscopic Approach

0SU807Z Supplement Left Sacroiliac Joint with Autologous Tissue Substitute, Open Approach

0SU80JZ Supplement Left Sacroiliac Joint with Synthetic Substitute, Open Approach

0SU80KZ Supplement Left Sacroiliac Joint with Nonautologous Tissue Substitute, Open Approach

0SU837Z Supplement Left Sacroiliac Joint with Autologous Tissue Substitute, Percutaneous Approach

0SU83JZ Supplement Left Sacroiliac Joint with Synthetic Substitute, Percutaneous Approach

0SU83KZ Supplement Left Sacroiliac Joint with Nonautologous Tissue Substitute, Percutaneous Approach

0SU847Z Supplement Left Sacroiliac Joint with Autologous Tissue Substitute, Percutaneous Endoscopic Approach

0SU84JZ Supplement Left Sacroiliac Joint with Synthetic Substitute, Percutaneous Endoscopic Approach

0SU84KZ Supplement Left Sacroiliac Joint with Nonautologous Tissue Substitute, Percutaneous Endoscopic Approach

0SU907Z Supplement Right Hip Joint with Autologous Tissue Substitute, Open Approach

♀ Female-only   ♂ Male-only   ▲ Limited Coverage   ● Non-OR   ▒ HAC-associated procedure   ▲ Non-covered procedures   ✚ Cluster

0SU909Z Supplement Right Hip Joint with Liner, Open Approach

0SU90BZ Supplement Right Hip Joint with Resurfacing Device, Open Approach
- HAC When reported with secondary diagnosis code I26.02, I26.09, I26.92-I26.99, I82.401-I82.4Z9

0SU90JZ Supplement Right Hip Joint with Synthetic Substitute, Open Approach

0SU90KZ Supplement Right Hip Joint with Nonautologous Tissue Substitute, Open Approach

0SU937Z Supplement Right Hip Joint with Autologous Tissue Substitute, Percutaneous Approach

0SU93JZ Supplement Right Hip Joint with Synthetic Substitute, Percutaneous Approach

0SU93KZ Supplement Right Hip Joint with Nonautologous Tissue Substitute, Percutaneous Approach

0SU947Z Supplement Right Hip Joint with Autologous Tissue Substitute, Percutaneous Endoscopic Approach

0SU94JZ Supplement Right Hip Joint with Synthetic Substitute, Percutaneous Endoscopic Approach

0SU94KZ Supplement Right Hip Joint with Nonautologous Tissue Substitute, Percutaneous Endoscopic Approach

0SUA09Z Supplement Right Hip Joint, Acetabular Surface with Liner, Open Approach
AHA CC: 2Q, 2015, 19-20; 4Q, 2016, 111-112

0SUA0BZ Supplement Right Hip Joint, Acetabular Surface with Resurfacing Device, Open Approach
- HAC When reported with secondary diagnosis code I26.02, I26.09, I26.92-I26.99, I82.401-I82.4Z9

0SUB07Z Supplement Left Hip Joint with Autologous Tissue Substitute, Open Approach

0SUB09Z Supplement Left Hip Joint with Liner, Open Approach

0SUB0BZ Supplement Left Hip Joint with Resurfacing Device, Open Approach
- HAC When reported with secondary diagnosis code I26.02, I26.09, I26.92-I26.99, I82.401-I82.4Z9

0SUB0JZ Supplement Left Hip Joint with Synthetic Substitute, Open Approach

0SUB0KZ Supplement Left Hip Joint with Nonautologous Tissue Substitute, Open Approach

0SUB37Z Supplement Left Hip Joint with Autologous Tissue Substitute, Percutaneous Approach

0SUB3JZ Supplement Left Hip Joint with Synthetic Substitute, Percutaneous Approach

0SUB3KZ Supplement Left Hip Joint with Nonautologous Tissue Substitute, Percutaneous Approach

0SUB47Z Supplement Left Hip Joint with Autologous Tissue Substitute, Percutaneous Endoscopic Approach

0SUB4JZ Supplement Left Hip Joint with Synthetic Substitute, Percutaneous Endoscopic Approach

0SUB4KZ Supplement Left Hip Joint with Nonautologous Tissue Substitute, Percutaneous Endoscopic Approach

0SUC07Z Supplement Right Knee Joint with Autologous Tissue Substitute, Open Approach

0SUC09C Supplement Right Knee Joint with Liner, Patellar Surface, Open Approach

0SUC09Z Supplement Right Knee Joint with Liner, Open Approach

0SUC0JZ Supplement Right Knee Joint with Synthetic Substitute, Open Approach

0SUC0KZ Supplement Right Knee Joint with Nonautologous Tissue Substitute, Open Approach

0SUC37Z Supplement Right Knee Joint with Autologous Tissue Substitute, Percutaneous Approach

0SUC3JZ Supplement Right Knee Joint with Synthetic Substitute, Percutaneous Approach

0SUC3KZ Supplement Right Knee Joint with Nonautologous Tissue Substitute, Percutaneous Approach

0SUC47Z Supplement Right Knee Joint with Autologous Tissue Substitute, Percutaneous Endoscopic Approach

0SUC4JZ Supplement Right Knee Joint with Synthetic Substitute, Percutaneous Endoscopic Approach

0SUC4KZ Supplement Right Knee Joint with Nonautologous Tissue Substitute, Percutaneous Endoscopic Approach

0SUD07Z Supplement Left Knee Joint with Autologous Tissue Substitute, Open Approach

0SUD09C Supplement Left Knee Joint with Liner, Patellar Surface, Open Approach

0SUD09Z Supplement Left Knee Joint with Liner, Open Approach

0SUD0JZ Supplement Left Knee Joint with Synthetic Substitute, Open Approach

0SUD0KZ Supplement Left Knee Joint with Nonautologous Tissue Substitute, Open Approach

0SUD37Z Supplement Left Knee Joint with Autologous Tissue Substitute, Percutaneous Approach

0SUD3JZ Supplement Left Knee Joint with Synthetic Substitute, Percutaneous Approach

0SUD3KZ Supplement Left Knee Joint with Nonautologous Tissue Substitute, Percutaneous Approach

0SUD47Z Supplement Left Knee Joint with Autologous Tissue Substitute, Percutaneous Endoscopic Approach

0SUD4JZ Supplement Left Knee Joint with Synthetic Substitute, Percutaneous Endoscopic Approach

0SUD4KZ Supplement Left Knee Joint with Nonautologous Tissue Substitute, Percutaneous Endoscopic Approach

0SUE09Z Supplement Left Hip Joint, Acetabular Surface with Liner, Open Approach

0SUE0BZ Supplement Left Hip Joint, Acetabular Surface with Resurfacing Device, Open Approach
- HAC When reported with secondary diagnosis code I26.02, I26.09, I26.92-I26.99, I82.401-I82.4Z9

0SUF07Z Supplement Right Ankle Joint with Autologous Tissue Substitute, Open Approach

0SUF0JZ Supplement Right Ankle Joint with Synthetic Substitute, Open Approach
AHA CC: 1Q, 2021, 17-18

0SUF0KZ Supplement Right Ankle Joint with Nonautologous Tissue Substitute, Open Approach

0SUF37Z Supplement Right Ankle Joint with Autologous Tissue Substitute, Percutaneous Approach

0SUF3JZ Supplement Right Ankle Joint with Synthetic Substitute, Percutaneous Approach

0SUF3KZ Supplement Right Ankle Joint with Nonautologous Tissue Substitute, Percutaneous Approach

0SUF47Z Supplement Right Ankle Joint with Autologous Tissue Substitute, Percutaneous Endoscopic Approach

0SUF4JZ Supplement Right Ankle Joint with Synthetic Substitute, Percutaneous Endoscopic Approach

0SUF4KZ Supplement Right Ankle Joint with Nonautologous Tissue Substitute, Percutaneous Endoscopic Approach

0SUG07Z Supplement Left Ankle Joint with Autologous Tissue Substitute, Open Approach

0SUG0JZ Supplement Left Ankle Joint with Synthetic Substitute, Open Approach

0SUG0KZ Supplement Left Ankle Joint with Nonautologous Tissue Substitute, Open Approach

0SUG37Z Supplement Left Ankle Joint with Autologous Tissue Substitute, Percutaneous Approach

0SUG3JZ Supplement Left Ankle Joint with Synthetic Substitute, Percutaneous Approach

0SUG3KZ Supplement Left Ankle Joint with Nonautologous Tissue Substitute, Percutaneous Approach

0SUG47Z Supplement Left Ankle Joint with Autologous Tissue Substitute, Percutaneous Endoscopic Approach

0SUG4JZ Supplement Left Ankle Joint with Synthetic Substitute, Percutaneous Endoscopic Approach

0SUG4KZ Supplement Left Ankle Joint with Nonautologous Tissue Substitute, Percutaneous Endoscopic Approach

0SUH07Z Supplement Right Tarsal Joint with Autologous Tissue Substitute, Open Approach

0SUH0JZ Supplement Right Tarsal Joint with Synthetic Substitute, Open Approach

0SUH0KZ Supplement Right Tarsal Joint with Nonautologous Tissue Substitute, Open Approach

0SUH37Z Supplement Right Tarsal Joint with Autologous Tissue Substitute, Percutaneous Approach

0SUH3JZ Supplement Right Tarsal Joint with Synthetic Substitute, Percutaneous Approach

0SUH3KZ Supplement Right Tarsal Joint with Nonautologous Tissue Substitute, Percutaneous Approach

0SUH47Z Supplement Right Tarsal Joint with Autologous Tissue Substitute, Percutaneous Endoscopic Approach

0SUH4JZ Supplement Right Tarsal Joint with Synthetic Substitute, Percutaneous Endoscopic Approach

0SUH4KZ Supplement Right Tarsal Joint with Nonautologous Tissue Substitute, Percutaneous Endoscopic Approach

0SUJ07Z Supplement Left Tarsal Joint with Autologous Tissue Substitute, Open Approach

0SUJ0JZ Supplement Left Tarsal Joint with Synthetic Substitute, Open Approach

0SUJ0KZ Supplement Left Tarsal Joint with Nonautologous Tissue Substitute, Open Approach

0SUJ37Z Supplement Left Tarsal Joint with Autologous Tissue Substitute, Percutaneous Approach

0SUJ3JZ Supplement Left Tarsal Joint with Synthetic Substitute, Percutaneous Approach

0SUJ3KZ Supplement Left Tarsal Joint with Nonautologous Tissue Substitute, Percutaneous Approach

0SUJ47Z Supplement Left Tarsal Joint with Autologous Tissue Substitute, Percutaneous Endoscopic Approach

0SUJ4JZ Supplement Left Tarsal Joint with Synthetic Substitute, Percutaneous Endoscopic Approach

0SUJ4KZ Supplement Left Tarsal Joint with Nonautologous Tissue Substitute, Percutaneous Endoscopic Approach

0SUK07Z Supplement Right Tarsometatarsal Joint with Autologous Tissue Substitute, Open Approach

0SUK0JZ Supplement Right Tarsometatarsal Joint with Synthetic Substitute, Open Approach

0SUK0KZ Supplement Right Tarsometatarsal Joint with Nonautologous Tissue Substitute, Open Approach

0SUK37Z Supplement Right Tarsometatarsal Joint with Autologous Tissue Substitute, Percutaneous Approach

0SUK3JZ Supplement Right Tarsometatarsal Joint with Synthetic Substitute, Percutaneous Approach

0SUK3KZ Supplement Right Tarsometatarsal Joint with Nonautologous Tissue Substitute, Percutaneous Approach

0SUK47Z Supplement Right Tarsometatarsal Joint with Autologous Tissue Substitute, Percutaneous Endoscopic Approach

0SUK4JZ Supplement Right Tarsometatarsal Joint with Synthetic Substitute, Percutaneous Endoscopic Approach

0SUK4KZ Supplement Right Tarsometatarsal Joint with Nonautologous Tissue Substitute, Percutaneous Endoscopic Approach

0SUL07Z Supplement Left Tarsometatarsal Joint with Autologous Tissue Substitute, Open Approach

0SUL0JZ Supplement Left Tarsometatarsal Joint with Synthetic Substitute, Open Approach

0SUL0KZ Supplement Left Tarsometatarsal Joint with Nonautologous Tissue Substitute, Open Approach

0SUL37Z Supplement Left Tarsometatarsal Joint with Autologous Tissue Substitute, Percutaneous Approach

0SUL3JZ Supplement Left Tarsometatarsal Joint with Synthetic Substitute, Percutaneous Approach

0SUL3KZ Supplement Left Tarsometatarsal Joint with Nonautologous Tissue Substitute, Percutaneous Approach

0SUL47Z Supplement Left Tarsometatarsal Joint with Autologous Tissue Substitute, Percutaneous Endoscopic Approach

0SUL4JZ Supplement Left Tarsometatarsal Joint with Synthetic Substitute, Percutaneous Endoscopic Approach

0SUL4KZ Supplement Left Tarsometatarsal Joint with Nonautologous Tissue Substitute, Percutaneous Endoscopic Approach

0SUM07Z Supplement Right Metatarsal-Phalangeal Joint with Autologous Tissue Substitute, Open Approach

0SUM0JZ Supplement Right Metatarsal-Phalangeal Joint with Synthetic Substitute, Open Approach

0SUM0KZ Supplement Right Metatarsal-Phalangeal Joint with Nonautologous Tissue Substitute, Open Approach

0SUM37Z Supplement Right Metatarsal-Phalangeal Joint with Autologous Tissue Substitute, Percutaneous Approach

0SUM3JZ Supplement Right Metatarsal-Phalangeal Joint with Synthetic Substitute, Percutaneous Approach

0SUM3KZ Supplement Right Metatarsal-Phalangeal Joint with Nonautologous Tissue Substitute, Percutaneous Approach

0SUM47Z Supplement Right Metatarsal-Phalangeal Joint with Autologous Tissue Substitute, Percutaneous Endoscopic Approach

0SUM4JZ Supplement Right Metatarsal-Phalangeal Joint with Synthetic Substitute, Percutaneous Endoscopic Approach

0SUM4KZ Supplement Right Metatarsal-Phalangeal Joint with Nonautologous Tissue Substitute, Percutaneous Endoscopic Approach

0SUN07Z Supplement Left Metatarsal-Phalangeal Joint with Autologous Tissue Substitute, Open Approach

0SUN0JZ Supplement Left Metatarsal-Phalangeal Joint with Synthetic Substitute, Open Approach

0SUN0KZ Supplement Left Metatarsal-Phalangeal Joint with Nonautologous Tissue Substitute, Open Approach

0SUN37Z Supplement Left Metatarsal-Phalangeal Joint with Autologous Tissue Substitute, Percutaneous Approach

0SUN3JZ Supplement Left Metatarsal-Phalangeal Joint with Synthetic Substitute, Percutaneous Approach

0SUN3KZ Supplement Left Metatarsal-Phalangeal Joint with Nonautologous Tissue Substitute, Percutaneous Approach

0SUN47Z Supplement Left Metatarsal-Phalangeal Joint with Autologous Tissue Substitute, Percutaneous Endoscopic Approach

0SUN4JZ Supplement Left Metatarsal-Phalangeal Joint with Synthetic Substitute, Percutaneous Endoscopic Approach

0SUN4KZ Supplement Left Metatarsal-Phalangeal Joint with Nonautologous Tissue Substitute, Percutaneous Endoscopic Approach

0SUP07Z Supplement Right Toe Phalangeal Joint with Autologous Tissue Substitute, Open Approach

0SUP0JZ Supplement Right Toe Phalangeal Joint with Synthetic Substitute, Open Approach

0SUP0KZ Supplement Right Toe Phalangeal Joint with Nonautologous Tissue Substitute, Open Approach

0SUP37Z Supplement Right Toe Phalangeal Joint with Autologous Tissue Substitute, Percutaneous Approach

0SUP3JZ Supplement Right Toe Phalangeal Joint with Synthetic Substitute, Percutaneous Approach

0SUP3KZ Supplement Right Toe Phalangeal Joint with Nonautologous Tissue Substitute, Percutaneous Approach

0SUP47Z Supplement Right Toe Phalangeal Joint with Autologous Tissue Substitute, Percutaneous Endoscopic Approach

0SUP4JZ Supplement Right Toe Phalangeal Joint with Synthetic Substitute, Percutaneous Endoscopic Approach

0SUP4KZ Supplement Right Toe Phalangeal Joint with Nonautologous Tissue Substitute, Percutaneous Endoscopic Approach

0SUQ07Z Supplement Left Toe Phalangeal Joint with Autologous Tissue Substitute, Open Approach

0SUQ0JZ Supplement Left Toe Phalangeal Joint with Synthetic Substitute, Open Approach

0SUQ0KZ Supplement Left Toe Phalangeal Joint with Nonautologous Tissue Substitute, Open Approach

0SUQ37Z Supplement Left Toe Phalangeal Joint with Autologous Tissue Substitute, Percutaneous Approach

0SUQ3JZ Supplement Left Toe Phalangeal Joint with Synthetic Substitute, Percutaneous Approach

0SUQ3KZ Supplement Left Toe Phalangeal Joint with Nonautologous Tissue Substitute, Percutaneous Approach

0SUQ47Z Supplement Left Toe Phalangeal Joint with Autologous Tissue Substitute, Percutaneous Endoscopic Approach

0SUQ4JZ Supplement Left Toe Phalangeal Joint with Synthetic Substitute, Percutaneous Endoscopic Approach

0SUQ4KZ Supplement Left Toe Phalangeal Joint with Nonautologous Tissue Substitute, Percutaneous Endoscopic Approach

0SUR09Z Supplement Right Hip Joint, Femoral Surface with Liner, Open Approach

0SUR0BZ Supplement Right Hip Joint, Femoral Surface with Resurfacing Device, Open Approach

HAC When reported with secondary diagnosis code I26.02, I26.09, I26.92-I26.99, I82.401-I82.4Z9

0SUS09Z Supplement Left Hip Joint, Femoral Surface with Liner, Open Approach

0SUS0BZ Supplement Left Hip Joint, Femoral Surface with Resurfacing Device, Open Approach

HAC When reported with secondary diagnosis code I26.02, I26.09, I26.92-I26.99, I82.401-I82.4Z9

0SUT09Z Supplement Right Knee Joint, Femoral Surface with Liner, Open Approach

0SUU09Z Supplement Left Knee Joint, Femoral Surface with Liner, Open Approach

0SUV09Z Supplement Right Knee Joint, Tibial Surface with Liner, Open Approach

0SUW09Z Supplement Left Knee Joint, Tibial Surface with Liner, Open Approach

♀ Female-only   ♂ Male-only   ▲ Limited Coverage   ● Non-OR   HAC HAC-associated procedure   ▲ Non-covered procedures   ✚ Cluster

Review Coding Guideline B6.1c

0SW000Z Revision of Drainage Device in Lumbar Vertebral Joint, Open Approach

0SW003Z Revision of Infusion Device in Lumbar Vertebral Joint, Open Approach

0SW004Z Revision of Internal Fixation Device in Lumbar Vertebral Joint, Open Approach

0SW007Z Revision of Autologous Tissue Substitute in Lumbar Vertebral Joint, Open Approach

0SW008Z Revision of Spacer in Lumbar Vertebral Joint, Open Approach

0SW00AZ Revision of Interbody Fusion Device in Lumbar Vertebral Joint, Open Approach

0SW00JZ Revision of Synthetic Substitute in Lumbar Vertebral Joint, Open Approach

0SW00KZ Revision of Nonautologous Tissue Substitute in Lumbar Vertebral Joint, Open Approach

0SW030Z Revision of Drainage Device in Lumbar Vertebral Joint, Percutaneous Approach

0SW033Z Revision of Infusion Device in Lumbar Vertebral Joint, Percutaneous Approach

0SW034Z Revision of Internal Fixation Device in Lumbar Vertebral Joint, Percutaneous Approach

0SW037Z Revision of Autologous Tissue Substitute in Lumbar Vertebral Joint, Percutaneous Approach

0SW038Z Revision of Spacer in Lumbar Vertebral Joint, Percutaneous Approach

0SW03AZ Revision of Interbody Fusion Device in Lumbar Vertebral Joint, Percutaneous Approach

0SW03JZ Revision of Synthetic Substitute in Lumbar Vertebral Joint, Percutaneous Approach

0SW03KZ Revision of Nonautologous Tissue Substitute in Lumbar Vertebral Joint, Percutaneous Approach

0SW040Z Revision of Drainage Device in Lumbar Vertebral Joint, Percutaneous Endoscopic Approach

0SW043Z Revision of Infusion Device in Lumbar Vertebral Joint, Percutaneous Endoscopic Approach

0SW044Z Revision of Internal Fixation Device in Lumbar Vertebral Joint, Percutaneous Endoscopic Approach

0SW047Z Revision of Autologous Tissue Substitute in Lumbar Vertebral Joint, Percutaneous Endoscopic Approach

0SW048Z Revision of Spacer in Lumbar Vertebral Joint, Percutaneous Endoscopic Approach

0SW04AZ Revision of Interbody Fusion Device in Lumbar Vertebral Joint, Percutaneous Endoscopic Approach

0SW04JZ Revision of Synthetic Substitute in Lumbar Vertebral Joint, Percutaneous Endoscopic Approach

0SW04KZ Revision of Nonautologous Tissue Substitute in Lumbar Vertebral Joint, Percutaneous Endoscopic Approach

0SW0X0Z Revision of Drainage Device in Lumbar Vertebral Joint, External Approach

0SW0X3Z Revision of Infusion Device in Lumbar Vertebral Joint, External Approach

0SW0X4Z Revision of Internal Fixation Device in Lumbar Vertebral Joint, External Approach

0SW0X7Z Revision of Autologous Tissue Substitute in Lumbar Vertebral Joint, External Approach

0SW0X8Z Revision of Spacer in Lumbar Vertebral Joint, External Approach

0SW0XAZ Revision of Interbody Fusion Device in Lumbar Vertebral Joint, External Approach

0SW0XJZ Revision of Synthetic Substitute in Lumbar Vertebral Joint, External Approach

0SW0XKZ Revision of Nonautologous Tissue Substitute in Lumbar Vertebral Joint, External Approach

0SW200Z Revision of Drainage Device in Lumbar Vertebral Disc, Open Approach

0SW203Z Revision of Infusion Device in Lumbar Vertebral Disc, Open Approach

0SW207Z Revision of Autologous Tissue Substitute in Lumbar Vertebral Disc, Open Approach

0SW20JZ Revision of Synthetic Substitute in Lumbar Vertebral Disc, Open Approach

0SW20KZ Revision of Nonautologous Tissue Substitute in Lumbar Vertebral Disc, Open Approach

0SW230Z Revision of Drainage Device in Lumbar Vertebral Disc, Percutaneous Approach

0SW233Z Revision of Infusion Device in Lumbar Vertebral Disc, Percutaneous Approach

0SW237Z Revision of Autologous Tissue Substitute in Lumbar Vertebral Disc, Percutaneous Approach

0SW23JZ Revision of Synthetic Substitute in Lumbar Vertebral Disc, Percutaneous Approach

0SW23KZ Revision of Nonautologous Tissue Substitute in Lumbar Vertebral Disc, Percutaneous Approach

0SW240Z Revision of Drainage Device in Lumbar Vertebral Disc, Percutaneous Endoscopic Approach

0SW243Z Revision of Infusion Device in Lumbar Vertebral Disc, Percutaneous Endoscopic Approach

0SW247Z Revision of Autologous Tissue Substitute in Lumbar Vertebral Disc, Percutaneous Endoscopic Approach

0SW24JZ Revision of Synthetic Substitute in Lumbar Vertebral Disc, Percutaneous Endoscopic Approach

0SW24KZ Revision of Nonautologous Tissue Substitute in Lumbar Vertebral Disc, Percutaneous Endoscopic Approach

0SW2X0Z Revision of Drainage Device in Lumbar Vertebral Disc, External Approach

0SW2X3Z Revision of Infusion Device in Lumbar Vertebral Disc, External Approach

0SW2X7Z Revision of Autologous Tissue Substitute in Lumbar Vertebral Disc, External Approach

0SW2XJZ Revision of Synthetic Substitute in Lumbar Vertebral Disc, External Approach

0SW2XKZ Revision of Nonautologous Tissue Substitute in Lumbar Vertebral Disc, External Approach

0SW300Z Revision of Drainage Device in Lumbosacral Joint, Open Approach

0SW303Z Revision of Infusion Device in Lumbosacral Joint, Open Approach

0SW304Z Revision of Internal Fixation Device in Lumbosacral Joint, Open Approach

0SW307Z Revision of Autologous Tissue Substitute in Lumbosacral Joint, Open Approach

0SW308Z Revision of Spacer in Lumbosacral Joint, Open Approach

0SW30AZ Revision of Interbody Fusion Device in Lumbosacral Joint, Open Approach

0SW30JZ Revision of Synthetic Substitute in Lumbosacral Joint, Open Approach

0SW30KZ Revision of Nonautologous Tissue Substitute in Lumbosacral Joint, Open Approach

0SW330Z Revision of Drainage Device in Lumbosacral Joint, Percutaneous Approach

0SW333Z Revision of Infusion Device in Lumbosacral Joint, Percutaneous Approach

0SW334Z Revision of Internal Fixation Device in Lumbosacral Joint, Percutaneous Approach

0SW337Z Revision of Autologous Tissue Substitute in Lumbosacral Joint, Percutaneous Approach

0SW338Z Revision of Spacer in Lumbosacral Joint, Percutaneous Approach

0SW33AZ Revision of Interbody Fusion Device in Lumbosacral Joint, Percutaneous Approach

0SW33JZ Revision of Synthetic Substitute in Lumbosacral Joint, Percutaneous Approach

0SW33KZ Revision of Nonautologous Tissue Substitute in Lumbosacral Joint, Percutaneous Approach

0SW340Z Revision of Drainage Device in Lumbosacral Joint, Percutaneous Endoscopic Approach

0SW343Z Revision of Infusion Device in Lumbosacral Joint, Percutaneous Endoscopic Approach

0SW344Z Revision of Internal Fixation Device in Lumbosacral Joint, Percutaneous Endoscopic Approach

0SW347Z Revision of Autologous Tissue Substitute in Lumbosacral Joint, Percutaneous Endoscopic Approach

0SW348Z Revision of Spacer in Lumbosacral Joint, Percutaneous Endoscopic Approach

0SW34AZ Revision of Interbody Fusion Device in Lumbosacral Joint, Percutaneous Endoscopic Approach

0SW34JZ Revision of Synthetic Substitute in Lumbosacral Joint, Percutaneous Endoscopic Approach

0SW34KZ Revision of Nonautologous Tissue Substitute in Lumbosacral Joint, Percutaneous Endoscopic Approach

0SW3X0Z Revision of Drainage Device in Lumbosacral Joint, External Approach

0SW3X3Z Revision of Infusion Device in Lumbosacral Joint, External Approach

0SW3X4Z Revision of Internal Fixation Device in Lumbosacral Joint, External Approach

0SW3X7Z Revision of Autologous Tissue Substitute in Lumbosacral Joint, External Approach

0SW3X8Z Revision of Spacer in Lumbosacral Joint, External Approach

0SW3XAZ Revision of Interbody Fusion Device in Lumbosacral Joint, External Approach

0SW3XJZ Revision of Synthetic Substitute in Lumbosacral Joint, External Approach

0SW3XKZ Revision of Nonautologous Tissue Substitute in Lumbosacral Joint, External Approach

0SW400Z Revision of Drainage Device in Lumbosacral Disc, Open Approach

0SW403Z Revision of Infusion Device in Lumbosacral Disc, Open Approach

0SW407Z Revision of Autologous Tissue Substitute in Lumbosacral Disc, Open Approach

0SW40JZ Revision of Synthetic Substitute in Lumbosacral Disc, Open Approach

0SW40KZ Revision of Nonautologous Tissue Substitute in Lumbosacral Disc, Open Approach

0SW430Z Revision of Drainage Device in Lumbosacral Disc, Percutaneous Approach

0SW433Z Revision of Infusion Device in Lumbosacral Disc, Percutaneous Approach

0SW437Z Revision of Autologous Tissue Substitute in Lumbosacral Disc, Percutaneous Approach

0SW43JZ Revision of Synthetic Substitute in Lumbosacral Disc, Percutaneous Approach

0SW43KZ Revision of Nonautologous Tissue Substitute in Lumbosacral Disc, Percutaneous Approach

0SW440Z Revision of Drainage Device in Lumbosacral Disc, Percutaneous Endoscopic Approach

0SW443Z Revision of Infusion Device in Lumbosacral Disc, Percutaneous Endoscopic Approach

0SW447Z Revision of Autologous Tissue Substitute in Lumbosacral Disc, Percutaneous Endoscopic Approach

0SW44JZ Revision of Synthetic Substitute in Lumbosacral Disc, Percutaneous Endoscopic Approach

0SW44KZ Revision of Nonautologous Tissue Substitute in Lumbosacral Disc, Percutaneous Endoscopic Approach

0SW4X0Z Revision of Drainage Device in Lumbosacral Disc, External Approach

0SW4X3Z Revision of Infusion Device in Lumbosacral Disc, External Approach

0SW4X7Z Revision of Autologous Tissue Substitute in Lumbosacral Disc, External Approach

0SW4XJZ Revision of Synthetic Substitute in Lumbosacral Disc, External Approach

0SW4XKZ Revision of Nonautologous Tissue Substitute in Lumbosacral Disc, External Approach

0SW500Z Revision of Drainage Device in Sacrococcygeal Joint, Open Approach

0SW503Z Revision of Infusion Device in Sacrococcygeal Joint, Open Approach

0SW504Z Revision of Internal Fixation Device in Sacrococcygeal Joint, Open Approach

0SW507Z Revision of Autologous Tissue Substitute in Sacrococcygeal Joint, Open Approach

0SW508Z Revision of Spacer in Sacrococcygeal Joint, Open Approach

0SW50JZ Revision of Synthetic Substitute in Sacrococcygeal Joint, Open Approach

0SW50KZ Revision of Nonautologous Tissue Substitute in Sacrococcygeal Joint, Open Approach

0SW530Z Revision of Drainage Device in Sacrococcygeal Joint, Percutaneous Approach

0SW533Z Revision of Infusion Device in Sacrococcygeal Joint, Percutaneous Approach

0SW534Z Revision of Internal Fixation Device in Sacrococcygeal Joint, Percutaneous Approach

0SW537Z Revision of Autologous Tissue Substitute in Sacrococcygeal Joint, Percutaneous Approach

0SW538Z Revision of Spacer in Sacrococcygeal Joint, Percutaneous Approach

0SW53JZ Revision of Synthetic Substitute in Sacrococcygeal Joint, Percutaneous Approach

0SW53KZ Revision of Nonautologous Tissue Substitute in Sacrococcygeal Joint, Percutaneous Approach

0SW540Z Revision of Drainage Device in Sacrococcygeal Joint, Percutaneous Endoscopic Approach

0SW543Z Revision of Infusion Device in Sacrococcygeal Joint, Percutaneous Endoscopic Approach

0SW544Z Revision of Internal Fixation Device in Sacrococcygeal Joint, Percutaneous Endoscopic Approach

0SW547Z Revision of Autologous Tissue Substitute in Sacrococcygeal Joint, Percutaneous Endoscopic Approach

0SW548Z Revision of Spacer in Sacrococcygeal Joint, Percutaneous Endoscopic Approach

0SW54JZ Revision of Synthetic Substitute in Sacrococcygeal Joint, Percutaneous Endoscopic Approach

0SW54KZ Revision of Nonautologous Tissue Substitute in Sacrococcygeal Joint, Percutaneous Endoscopic Approach

0SW5X0Z Revision of Drainage Device in Sacrococcygeal Joint, External Approach

0SW5X3Z Revision of Infusion Device in Sacrococcygeal Joint, External Approach

0SW5X4Z Revision of Internal Fixation Device in Sacrococcygeal Joint, External Approach

0SW5X7Z Revision of Autologous Tissue Substitute in Sacrococcygeal Joint, External Approach

0SW5X8Z Revision of Spacer in Sacrococcygeal Joint, External Approach

0SW5XJZ Revision of Synthetic Substitute in Sacrococcygeal Joint, External Approach

0SW5XKZ Revision of Nonautologous Tissue Substitute in Sacrococcygeal Joint, External Approach

0SW600Z Revision of Drainage Device in Coccygeal Joint, Open Approach

0SW603Z Revision of Infusion Device in Coccygeal Joint, Open Approach

0SW604Z Revision of Internal Fixation Device in Coccygeal Joint, Open Approach

0SW607Z Revision of Autologous Tissue Substitute in Coccygeal Joint, Open Approach

0SW608Z Revision of Spacer in Coccygeal Joint, Open Approach

0SW60JZ Revision of Synthetic Substitute in Coccygeal Joint, Open Approach

0SW60KZ Revision of Nonautologous Tissue Substitute in Coccygeal Joint, Open Approach

0SW630Z Revision of Drainage Device in Coccygeal Joint, Percutaneous Approach

0SW633Z Revision of Infusion Device in Coccygeal Joint, Percutaneous Approach

0SW634Z Revision of Internal Fixation Device in Coccygeal Joint, Percutaneous Approach

0SW637Z Revision of Autologous Tissue Substitute in Coccygeal Joint, Percutaneous Approach

0SW638Z Revision of Spacer in Coccygeal Joint, Percutaneous Approach

0SW63JZ Revision of Synthetic Substitute in Coccygeal Joint, Percutaneous Approach

0SW63KZ Revision of Nonautologous Tissue Substitute in Coccygeal Joint, Percutaneous Approach

0SW640Z Revision of Drainage Device in Coccygeal Joint, Percutaneous Endoscopic Approach

0SW643Z Revision of Infusion Device in Coccygeal Joint, Percutaneous Endoscopic Approach

0SW644Z Revision of Internal Fixation Device in Coccygeal Joint, Percutaneous Endoscopic Approach

0SW647Z Revision of Autologous Tissue Substitute in Coccygeal Joint, Percutaneous Endoscopic Approach

0SW648Z Revision of Spacer in Coccygeal Joint, Percutaneous Endoscopic Approach

0SW64JZ Revision of Synthetic Substitute in Coccygeal Joint, Percutaneous Endoscopic Approach

0SW64KZ Revision of Nonautologous Tissue Substitute in Coccygeal Joint, Percutaneous Endoscopic Approach

0SW6X0Z Revision of Drainage Device in Coccygeal Joint, External Approach

0SW6X3Z Revision of Infusion Device in Coccygeal Joint, External Approach

0SW6X4Z Revision of Internal Fixation Device in Coccygeal Joint, External Approach

0SW6X7Z Revision of Autologous Tissue Substitute in Coccygeal Joint, External Approach

0SW6X8Z Revision of Spacer in Coccygeal Joint, External Approach

0SW6XJZ Revision of Synthetic Substitute in Coccygeal Joint, External Approach

0SW6XKZ Revision of Nonautologous Tissue Substitute in Coccygeal Joint, External Approach

♀ Female-only   ♂ Male-only   ▲ Limited Coverage   ● Non-OR   ▨ HAC-associated procedure   ▲ Non-covered procedures   ✛ Cluster

0SW700Z	Revision of Drainage Device in Right Sacroiliac Joint, Open Approach	**0SW800Z**	Revision of Drainage Device in Left Sacroiliac Joint, Open Approach	**0SW900Z**	Revision of Drainage Device in Right Hip Joint, Open Approach
0SW703Z	Revision of Infusion Device in Right Sacroiliac Joint, Open Approach	**0SW803Z**	Revision of Infusion Device in Left Sacroiliac Joint, Open Approach	**0SW903Z**	Revision of Infusion Device in Right Hip Joint, Open Approach
0SW704Z	Revision of Internal Fixation Device in Right Sacroiliac Joint, Open Approach	**0SW804Z**	Revision of Internal Fixation Device in Left Sacroiliac Joint, Open Approach	**0SW904Z**	Revision of Internal Fixation Device in Right Hip Joint, Open Approach
0SW707Z	Revision of Autologous Tissue Substitute in Right Sacroiliac Joint, Open Approach	**0SW807Z**	Revision of Autologous Tissue Substitute in Left Sacroiliac Joint, Open Approach	**0SW905Z**	Revision of External Fixation Device in Right Hip Joint, Open Approach
0SW708Z	Revision of Spacer in Right Sacroiliac Joint, Open Approach	**0SW808Z**	Revision of Spacer in Left Sacroiliac Joint, Open Approach	**0SW907Z**	Revision of Autologous Tissue Substitute in Right Hip Joint, Open Approach
0SW70JZ	Revision of Synthetic Substitute in Right Sacroiliac Joint, Open Approach	**0SW80JZ**	Revision of Synthetic Substitute in Left Sacroiliac Joint, Open Approach	**0SW908Z**	Revision of Spacer in Right Hip Joint, Open Approach
0SW70KZ	Revision of Nonautologous Tissue Substitute in Right Sacroiliac Joint, Open Approach	**0SW80KZ**	Revision of Nonautologous Tissue Substitute in Left Sacroiliac Joint, Open Approach	**0SW909Z**	Revision of Liner in Right Hip Joint, Open Approach
0SW730Z	Revision of Drainage Device in Right Sacroiliac Joint, Percutaneous Approach	**0SW830Z**	Revision of Drainage Device in Left Sacroiliac Joint, Percutaneous Approach	**0SW90BZ**	Revision of Resurfacing Device in Right Hip Joint, Open Approach
0SW733Z	Revision of Infusion Device in Right Sacroiliac Joint, Percutaneous Approach	**0SW833Z**	Revision of Infusion Device in Left Sacroiliac Joint, Percutaneous Approach	**0SW90JZ**	Revision of Synthetic Substitute in Right Hip Joint, Open Approach
0SW734Z	Revision of Internal Fixation Device in Right Sacroiliac Joint, Percutaneous Approach	**0SW834Z**	Revision of Internal Fixation Device in Left Sacroiliac Joint, Percutaneous Approach	**0SW90KZ**	Revision of Nonautologous Tissue Substitute in Right Hip Joint, Open Approach
0SW737Z	Revision of Autologous Tissue Substitute in Right Sacroiliac Joint, Percutaneous Approach	**0SW837Z**	Revision of Autologous Tissue Substitute in Left Sacroiliac Joint, Percutaneous Approach	**0SW930Z**	Revision of Drainage Device in Right Hip Joint, Percutaneous Approach
0SW738Z	Revision of Spacer in Right Sacroiliac Joint, Percutaneous Approach	**0SW838Z**	Revision of Spacer in Left Sacroiliac Joint, Percutaneous Approach	**0SW933Z**	Revision of Infusion Device in Right Hip Joint, Percutaneous Approach
0SW73JZ	Revision of Synthetic Substitute in Right Sacroiliac Joint, Percutaneous Approach	**0SW83JZ**	Revision of Synthetic Substitute in Left Sacroiliac Joint, Percutaneous Approach	**0SW934Z**	Revision of Internal Fixation Device in Right Hip Joint, Percutaneous Approach
0SW73KZ	Revision of Nonautologous Tissue Substitute in Right Sacroiliac Joint, Percutaneous Approach	**0SW83KZ**	Revision of Nonautologous Tissue Substitute in Left Sacroiliac Joint, Percutaneous Approach	**0SW935Z**	Revision of External Fixation Device in Right Hip Joint, Percutaneous Approach
0SW740Z	Revision of Drainage Device in Right Sacroiliac Joint, Percutaneous Endoscopic Approach	**0SW840Z**	Revision of Drainage Device in Left Sacroiliac Joint, Percutaneous Endoscopic Approach	**0SW937Z**	Revision of Autologous Tissue Substitute in Right Hip Joint, Percutaneous Approach
0SW743Z	Revision of Infusion Device in Right Sacroiliac Joint, Percutaneous Endoscopic Approach	**0SW843Z**	Revision of Infusion Device in Left Sacroiliac Joint, Percutaneous Endoscopic Approach	**0SW938Z**	Revision of Spacer in Right Hip Joint, Percutaneous Approach
0SW744Z	Revision of Internal Fixation Device in Right Sacroiliac Joint, Percutaneous Endoscopic Approach	**0SW844Z**	Revision of Internal Fixation Device in Left Sacroiliac Joint, Percutaneous Endoscopic Approach	**0SW93JZ**	Revision of Synthetic Substitute in Right Hip Joint, Percutaneous Approach
0SW747Z	Revision of Autologous Tissue Substitute in Right Sacroiliac Joint, Percutaneous Endoscopic Approach	**0SW847Z**	Revision of Autologous Tissue Substitute in Left Sacroiliac Joint, Percutaneous Endoscopic Approach	**0SW93KZ**	Revision of Nonautologous Tissue Substitute in Right Hip Joint, Percutaneous Approach
0SW748Z	Revision of Spacer in Right Sacroiliac Joint, Percutaneous Endoscopic Approach	**0SW848Z**	Revision of Spacer in Left Sacroiliac Joint, Percutaneous Endoscopic Approach	**0SW940Z**	Revision of Drainage Device in Right Hip Joint, Percutaneous Endoscopic Approach
0SW74JZ	Revision of Synthetic Substitute in Right Sacroiliac Joint, Percutaneous Endoscopic Approach	**0SW84JZ**	Revision of Synthetic Substitute in Left Sacroiliac Joint, Percutaneous Endoscopic Approach	**0SW943Z**	Revision of Infusion Device in Right Hip Joint, Percutaneous Endoscopic Approach
0SW74KZ	Revision of Nonautologous Tissue Substitute in Right Sacroiliac Joint, Percutaneous Endoscopic Approach	**0SW84KZ**	Revision of Nonautologous Tissue Substitute in Left Sacroiliac Joint, Percutaneous Endoscopic Approach	**0SW944Z**	Revision of Internal Fixation Device in Right Hip Joint, Percutaneous Endoscopic Approach
0SW7X0Z	Revision of Drainage Device in Right Sacroiliac Joint, External Approach	**0SW8X0Z**	Revision of Drainage Device in Left Sacroiliac Joint, External Approach	**0SW945Z**	Revision of External Fixation Device in Right Hip Joint, Percutaneous Endoscopic Approach
0SW7X3Z	Revision of Infusion Device in Right Sacroiliac Joint, External Approach	**0SW8X3Z**	Revision of Infusion Device in Left Sacroiliac Joint, External Approach	**0SW947Z**	Revision of Autologous Tissue Substitute in Right Hip Joint, Percutaneous Endoscopic Approach
0SW7X4Z	Revision of Internal Fixation Device in Right Sacroiliac Joint, External Approach	**0SW8X4Z**	Revision of Internal Fixation Device in Left Sacroiliac Joint, External Approach	**0SW948Z**	Revision of Spacer in Right Hip Joint, Percutaneous Endoscopic Approach
0SW7X7Z	Revision of Autologous Tissue Substitute in Right Sacroiliac Joint, External Approach	**0SW8X7Z**	Revision of Autologous Tissue Substitute in Left Sacroiliac Joint, External Approach	**0SW94JZ**	Revision of Synthetic Substitute in Right Hip Joint, Percutaneous Endoscopic Approach
0SW7X8Z	Revision of Spacer in Right Sacroiliac Joint, External Approach	**0SW8X8Z**	Revision of Spacer in Left Sacroiliac Joint, External Approach	**0SW94KZ**	Revision of Nonautologous Tissue Substitute in Right Hip Joint, Percutaneous Endoscopic Approach
0SW7XJZ	Revision of Synthetic Substitute in Right Sacroiliac Joint, External Approach	**0SW8XJZ**	Revision of Synthetic Substitute in Left Sacroiliac Joint, External Approach	**0SW9X0Z**	Revision of Drainage Device in Right Hip Joint, External Approach
0SW7XKZ	Revision of Nonautologous Tissue Substitute in Right Sacroiliac Joint, External Approach	**0SW8XKZ**	Revision of Nonautologous Tissue Substitute in Left Sacroiliac Joint, External Approach	**0SW9X3Z**	Revision of Infusion Device in Right Hip Joint, External Approach
				0SW9X4Z	Revision of Internal Fixation Device in Right Hip Joint, External Approach
				0SW9X5Z	Revision of External Fixation Device in Right Hip Joint, External Approach

♀ Female-only ♂ Male-only ▲ Limited Coverage ● Non-OR ▨ HAC-associated procedure ▲ Non-covered procedures ✚ Cluster

0SW9X7Z Revision of Autologous Tissue Substitute in Right Hip Joint, External Approach

0SW9X8Z Revision of Spacer in Right Hip Joint, External Approach

0SW9XJZ Revision of Synthetic Substitute in Right Hip Joint, External Approach

0SW9XKZ Revision of Nonautologous Tissue Substitute in Right Hip Joint, External Approach

0SWA0JZ Revision of Synthetic Substitute in Right Hip Joint, Acetabular Surface, Open Approach

0SWA3JZ Revision of Synthetic Substitute in Right Hip Joint, Acetabular Surface, Percutaneous Approach

0SWA4JZ Revision of Synthetic Substitute in Right Hip Joint, Acetabular Surface, Percutaneous Endoscopic Approach

0SWAXJZ Revision of Synthetic Substitute in Right Hip Joint, Acetabular Surface, External Approach

0SWB00Z Revision of Drainage Device in Left Hip Joint, Open Approach

0SWB03Z Revision of Infusion Device in Left Hip Joint, Open Approach

0SWB04Z Revision of Internal Fixation Device in Left Hip Joint, Open Approach

0SWB05Z Revision of External Fixation Device in Left Hip Joint, Open Approach

0SWB07Z Revision of Autologous Tissue Substitute in Left Hip Joint, Open Approach

0SWB08Z Revision of Spacer in Left Hip Joint, Open Approach

0SWB09Z Revision of Liner in Left Hip Joint, Open Approach

0SWB0BZ Revision of Resurfacing Device in Left Hip Joint, Open Approach

0SWB0JZ Revision of Synthetic Substitute in Left Hip Joint, Open Approach

0SWB0KZ Revision of Nonautologous Tissue Substitute in Left Hip Joint, Open Approach

0SWB30Z Revision of Drainage Device in Left Hip Joint, Percutaneous Approach

0SWB33Z Revision of Infusion Device in Left Hip Joint, Percutaneous Approach

0SWB34Z Revision of Internal Fixation Device in Left Hip Joint, Percutaneous Approach

0SWB35Z Revision of External Fixation Device in Left Hip Joint, Percutaneous Approach

0SWB37Z Revision of Autologous Tissue Substitute in Left Hip Joint, Percutaneous Approach

0SWB38Z Revision of Spacer in Left Hip Joint, Percutaneous Approach

0SWB3JZ Revision of Synthetic Substitute in Left Hip Joint, Percutaneous Approach

0SWB3KZ Revision of Nonautologous Tissue Substitute in Left Hip Joint, Percutaneous Approach

0SWB40Z Revision of Drainage Device in Left Hip Joint, Percutaneous Endoscopic Approach

0SWB43Z Revision of Infusion Device in Left Hip Joint, Percutaneous Endoscopic Approach

0SWB44Z Revision of Internal Fixation Device in Left Hip Joint, Percutaneous Endoscopic Approach

0SWB45Z Revision of External Fixation Device in Left Hip Joint, Percutaneous Endoscopic Approach

0SWB47Z Revision of Autologous Tissue Substitute in Left Hip Joint, Percutaneous Endoscopic Approach

0SWB48Z Revision of Spacer in Left Hip Joint, Percutaneous Endoscopic Approach

0SWB4JZ Revision of Synthetic Substitute in Left Hip Joint, Percutaneous Endoscopic Approach

0SWB4KZ Revision of Nonautologous Tissue Substitute in Left Hip Joint, Percutaneous Endoscopic Approach

0SWBX0Z Revision of Drainage Device in Left Hip Joint, External Approach

0SWBX3Z Revision of Infusion Device in Left Hip Joint, External Approach

0SWBX4Z Revision of Internal Fixation Device in Left Hip Joint, External Approach

0SWBX5Z Revision of External Fixation Device in Left Hip Joint, External Approach

0SWBX7Z Revision of Autologous Tissue Substitute in Left Hip Joint, External Approach

0SWBX8Z Revision of Spacer in Left Hip Joint, External Approach

0SWBXJZ Revision of Synthetic Substitute in Left Hip Joint, External Approach

0SWBXKZ Revision of Nonautologous Tissue Substitute in Left Hip Joint, External Approach

0SWC00Z Revision of Drainage Device in Right Knee Joint, Open Approach

0SWC03Z Revision of Infusion Device in Right Knee Joint, Open Approach

0SWC04Z Revision of Internal Fixation Device in Right Knee Joint, Open Approach

0SWC05Z Revision of External Fixation Device in Right Knee Joint, Open Approach

0SWC07Z Revision of Autologous Tissue Substitute in Right Knee Joint, Open Approach

0SWC08Z Revision of Spacer in Right Knee Joint, Open Approach

0SWC09Z Revision of Liner in Right Knee Joint, Open Approach

0SWC0JC Revision of Synthetic Substitute in Right Knee Joint, Patellar Surface, Open Approach

0SWC0JZ Revision of Synthetic Substitute in Right Knee Joint, Open Approach

0SWC0KZ Revision of Nonautologous Tissue Substitute in Right Knee Joint, Open Approach

0SWC30Z Revision of Drainage Device in Right Knee Joint, Percutaneous Approach

0SWC33Z Revision of Infusion Device in Right Knee Joint, Percutaneous Approach

0SWC34Z Revision of Internal Fixation Device in Right Knee Joint, Percutaneous Approach

0SWC35Z Revision of External Fixation Device in Right Knee Joint, Percutaneous Approach

0SWC37Z Revision of Autologous Tissue Substitute in Right Knee Joint, Percutaneous Approach

0SWC38Z Revision of Spacer in Right Knee Joint, Percutaneous Approach

0SWC3JC Revision of Synthetic Substitute in Right Knee Joint, Patellar Surface, Percutaneous Approach

0SWC3JZ Revision of Synthetic Substitute in Right Knee Joint, Percutaneous Approach

0SWC3KZ Revision of Nonautologous Tissue Substitute in Right Knee Joint, Percutaneous Approach

0SWC40Z Revision of Drainage Device in Right Knee Joint, Percutaneous Endoscopic Approach

0SWC43Z Revision of Infusion Device in Right Knee Joint, Percutaneous Endoscopic Approach

0SWC44Z Revision of Internal Fixation Device in Right Knee Joint, Percutaneous Endoscopic Approach

0SWC45Z Revision of External Fixation Device in Right Knee Joint, Percutaneous Endoscopic Approach

0SWC47Z Revision of Autologous Tissue Substitute in Right Knee Joint, Percutaneous Endoscopic Approach

0SWC48Z Revision of Spacer in Right Knee Joint, Percutaneous Endoscopic Approach

0SWC4JC Revision of Synthetic Substitute in Right Knee Joint, Patellar Surface, Percutaneous Endoscopic Approach

0SWC4JZ Revision of Synthetic Substitute in Right Knee Joint, Percutaneous Endoscopic Approach

0SWC4KZ Revision of Nonautologous Tissue Substitute in Right Knee Joint, Percutaneous Endoscopic Approach

0SWCX0Z Revision of Drainage Device in Right Knee Joint, External Approach

0SWCX3Z Revision of Infusion Device in Right Knee Joint, External Approach

0SWCX4Z Revision of Internal Fixation Device in Right Knee Joint, External Approach

0SWCX5Z Revision of External Fixation Device in Right Knee Joint, External Approach

0SWCX7Z Revision of Autologous Tissue Substitute in Right Knee Joint, External Approach

0SWCX8Z Revision of Spacer in Right Knee Joint, External Approach

0SWCXJC Revision of Synthetic Substitute in Right Knee Joint, Patellar Surface, External Approach

0SWCXJZ Revision of Synthetic Substitute in Right Knee Joint, External Approach

0SWCXKZ Revision of Nonautologous Tissue Substitute in Right Knee Joint, External Approach

0SWD00Z Revision of Drainage Device in Left Knee Joint, Open Approach

0SWD03Z Revision of Infusion Device in Left Knee Joint, Open Approach

0SWD04Z Revision of Internal Fixation Device in Left Knee Joint, Open Approach

0SWD05Z Revision of External Fixation Device in Left Knee Joint, Open Approach

0SWD07Z Revision of Autologous Tissue Substitute in Left Knee Joint, Open Approach

0SWD08Z Revision of Spacer in Left Knee Joint, Open Approach

0SWD09Z Revision of Liner in Left Knee Joint, Open Approach

0SWD0JC Revision of Synthetic Substitute in Left Knee Joint, Patellar Surface, Open Approach

0SWD0JZ Revision of Synthetic Substitute in Left Knee Joint, Open Approach

♀ Female-only   ♂ Male-only   ▲ Limited Coverage   ● Non-OR   [HAC] HAC-associated procedure   ▲ Non-covered procedures   ✚ Cluster

0SWD0KZ Revision of Nonautologous Tissue Substitute in Left Knee Joint, Open Approach

0SWD30Z Revision of Drainage Device in Left Knee Joint, Percutaneous Approach

0SWD33Z Revision of Infusion Device in Left Knee Joint, Percutaneous Approach

0SWD34Z Revision of Internal Fixation Device in Left Knee Joint, Percutaneous Approach

0SWD35Z Revision of External Fixation Device in Left Knee Joint, Percutaneous Approach

0SWD37Z Revision of Autologous Tissue Substitute in Left Knee Joint, Percutaneous Approach

0SWD38Z Revision of Spacer in Left Knee Joint, Percutaneous Approach

0SWD3JC Revision of Synthetic Substitute in Left Knee Joint, Patellar Surface, Percutaneous Approach

0SWD3JZ Revision of Synthetic Substitute in Left Knee Joint, Percutaneous Approach

0SWD3KZ Revision of Nonautologous Tissue Substitute in Left Knee Joint, Percutaneous Approach

0SWD40Z Revision of Drainage Device in Left Knee Joint, Percutaneous Endoscopic Approach

0SWD43Z Revision of Infusion Device in Left Knee Joint, Percutaneous Endoscopic Approach

0SWD44Z Revision of Internal Fixation Device in Left Knee Joint, Percutaneous Endoscopic Approach

0SWD45Z Revision of External Fixation Device in Left Knee Joint, Percutaneous Endoscopic Approach

0SWD47Z Revision of Autologous Tissue Substitute in Left Knee Joint, Percutaneous Endoscopic Approach

0SWD48Z Revision of Spacer in Left Knee Joint, Percutaneous Endoscopic Approach

0SWD4JC Revision of Synthetic Substitute in Left Knee Joint, Patellar Surface, Percutaneous Endoscopic Approach

0SWD4JZ Revision of Synthetic Substitute in Left Knee Joint, Percutaneous Endoscopic Approach

0SWD4KZ Revision of Nonautologous Tissue Substitute in Left Knee Joint, Percutaneous Endoscopic Approach

0SWDX0Z Revision of Drainage Device in Left Knee Joint, External Approach

0SWDX3Z Revision of Infusion Device in Left Knee Joint, External Approach

0SWDX4Z Revision of Internal Fixation Device in Left Knee Joint, External Approach

0SWDX5Z Revision of External Fixation Device in Left Knee Joint, External Approach

0SWDX7Z Revision of Autologous Tissue Substitute in Left Knee Joint, External Approach

0SWDX8Z Revision of Spacer in Left Knee Joint, External Approach

0SWDXJC Revision of Synthetic Substitute in Left Knee Joint, Patellar Surface, External Approach

0SWDXJZ Revision of Synthetic Substitute in Left Knee Joint, External Approach

0SWDXKZ Revision of Nonautologous Tissue Substitute in Left Knee Joint, External Approach

0SWE0JZ Revision of Synthetic Substitute in Left Hip Joint, Acetabular Surface, Open Approach

0SWE3JZ Revision of Synthetic Substitute in Left Hip Joint, Acetabular Surface, Percutaneous Approach

0SWE4JZ Revision of Synthetic Substitute in Left Hip Joint, Acetabular Surface, Percutaneous Endoscopic Approach

0SWEXJZ Revision of Synthetic Substitute in Left Hip Joint, Acetabular Surface, External Approach

0SWF00Z Revision of Drainage Device in Right Ankle Joint, Open Approach

0SWF03Z Revision of Infusion Device in Right Ankle Joint, Open Approach

0SWF04Z Revision of Internal Fixation Device in Right Ankle Joint, Open Approach

0SWF05Z Revision of External Fixation Device in Right Ankle Joint, Open Approach

0SWF07Z Revision of Autologous Tissue Substitute in Right Ankle Joint, Open Approach

0SWF08Z Revision of Spacer in Right Ankle Joint, Open Approach

0SWF0JZ Revision of Synthetic Substitute in Right Ankle Joint, Open Approach

AHA CC: 4Q, 2017, 107-108

0SWF0KZ Revision of Nonautologous Tissue Substitute in Right Ankle Joint, Open Approach

0SWF30Z Revision of Drainage Device in Right Ankle Joint, Percutaneous Approach

0SWF33Z Revision of Infusion Device in Right Ankle Joint, Percutaneous Approach

0SWF34Z Revision of Internal Fixation Device in Right Ankle Joint, Percutaneous Approach

0SWF35Z Revision of External Fixation Device in Right Ankle Joint, Percutaneous Approach

0SWF37Z Revision of Autologous Tissue Substitute in Right Ankle Joint, Percutaneous Approach

0SWF38Z Revision of Spacer in Right Ankle Joint, Percutaneous Approach

0SWF3JZ Revision of Synthetic Substitute in Right Ankle Joint, Percutaneous Approach

0SWF3KZ Revision of Nonautologous Tissue Substitute in Right Ankle Joint, Percutaneous Approach

0SWF40Z Revision of Drainage Device in Right Ankle Joint, Percutaneous Endoscopic Approach

0SWF43Z Revision of Infusion Device in Right Ankle Joint, Percutaneous Endoscopic Approach

0SWF44Z Revision of Internal Fixation Device in Right Ankle Joint, Percutaneous Endoscopic Approach

0SWF45Z Revision of External Fixation Device in Right Ankle Joint, Percutaneous Endoscopic Approach

0SWF47Z Revision of Autologous Tissue Substitute in Right Ankle Joint, Percutaneous Endoscopic Approach

0SWF48Z Revision of Spacer in Right Ankle Joint, Percutaneous Endoscopic Approach

0SWF4JZ Revision of Synthetic Substitute in Right Ankle Joint, Percutaneous Endoscopic Approach

0SWF4KZ Revision of Nonautologous Tissue Substitute in Right Ankle Joint, Percutaneous Endoscopic Approach

0SWFX0Z Revision of Drainage Device in Right Ankle Joint, External Approach

0SWFX3Z Revision of Infusion Device in Right Ankle Joint, External Approach

0SWFX4Z Revision of Internal Fixation Device in Right Ankle Joint, External Approach

0SWFX5Z Revision of External Fixation Device in Right Ankle Joint, External Approach

0SWFX7Z Revision of Autologous Tissue Substitute in Right Ankle Joint, External Approach

0SWFX8Z Revision of Spacer in Right Ankle Joint, External Approach

0SWFXJZ Revision of Synthetic Substitute in Right Ankle Joint, External Approach

0SWFXKZ Revision of Nonautologous Tissue Substitute in Right Ankle Joint, External Approach

0SWG00Z Revision of Drainage Device in Left Ankle Joint, Open Approach

0SWG03Z Revision of Infusion Device in Left Ankle Joint, Open Approach

0SWG04Z Revision of Internal Fixation Device in Left Ankle Joint, Open Approach

0SWG05Z Revision of External Fixation Device in Left Ankle Joint, Open Approach

0SWG07Z Revision of Autologous Tissue Substitute in Left Ankle Joint, Open Approach

0SWG08Z Revision of Spacer in Left Ankle Joint, Open Approach

0SWG0JZ Revision of Synthetic Substitute in Left Ankle Joint, Open Approach

0SWG0KZ Revision of Nonautologous Tissue Substitute in Left Ankle Joint, Open Approach

0SWG30Z Revision of Drainage Device in Left Ankle Joint, Percutaneous Approach

0SWG33Z Revision of Infusion Device in Left Ankle Joint, Percutaneous Approach

0SWG34Z Revision of Internal Fixation Device in Left Ankle Joint, Percutaneous Approach

0SWG35Z Revision of External Fixation Device in Left Ankle Joint, Percutaneous Approach

0SWG37Z Revision of Autologous Tissue Substitute in Left Ankle Joint, Percutaneous Approach

0SWG38Z Revision of Spacer in Left Ankle Joint, Percutaneous Approach

0SWG3JZ Revision of Synthetic Substitute in Left Ankle Joint, Percutaneous Approach

0SWG3KZ Revision of Nonautologous Tissue Substitute in Left Ankle Joint, Percutaneous Approach

0SWG40Z Revision of Drainage Device in Left Ankle Joint, Percutaneous Endoscopic Approach

0SWG43Z Revision of Infusion Device in Left Ankle Joint, Percutaneous Endoscopic Approach

0SWG44Z Revision of Internal Fixation Device in Left Ankle Joint, Percutaneous Endoscopic Approach

0SWG45Z Revision of External Fixation Device in Left Ankle Joint, Percutaneous Endoscopic Approach

0SWG47Z	Revision of Autologous Tissue Substitute in Left Ankle Joint, Percutaneous Endoscopic Approach
0SWG48Z	Revision of Spacer in Left Ankle Joint, Percutaneous Endoscopic Approach
0SWG4JZ	Revision of Synthetic Substitute in Left Ankle Joint, Percutaneous Endoscopic Approach
0SWG4KZ	Revision of Nonautologous Tissue Substitute in Left Ankle Joint, Percutaneous Endoscopic Approach
0SWGX0Z	Revision of Drainage Device in Left Ankle Joint, External Approach
0SWGX3Z	Revision of Infusion Device in Left Ankle Joint, External Approach
0SWGX4Z	Revision of Internal Fixation Device in Left Ankle Joint, External Approach
0SWGX5Z	Revision of External Fixation Device in Left Ankle Joint, External Approach
0SWGX7Z	Revision of Autologous Tissue Substitute in Left Ankle Joint, External Approach
0SWGX8Z	Revision of Spacer in Left Ankle Joint, External Approach
0SWGXJZ	Revision of Synthetic Substitute in Left Ankle Joint, External Approach
0SWGXKZ	Revision of Nonautologous Tissue Substitute in Left Ankle Joint, External Approach
0SWH00Z	Revision of Drainage Device in Right Tarsal Joint, Open Approach
0SWH03Z	Revision of Infusion Device in Right Tarsal Joint, Open Approach
0SWH04Z	Revision of Internal Fixation Device in Right Tarsal Joint, Open Approach
0SWH05Z	Revision of External Fixation Device in Right Tarsal Joint, Open Approach
0SWH07Z	Revision of Autologous Tissue Substitute in Right Tarsal Joint, Open Approach
0SWH08Z	Revision of Spacer in Right Tarsal Joint, Open Approach
0SWH0JZ	Revision of Synthetic Substitute in Right Tarsal Joint, Open Approach
0SWH0KZ	Revision of Nonautologous Tissue Substitute in Right Tarsal Joint, Open Approach
0SWH30Z	Revision of Drainage Device in Right Tarsal Joint, Percutaneous Approach
0SWH33Z	Revision of Infusion Device in Right Tarsal Joint, Percutaneous Approach
0SWH34Z	Revision of Internal Fixation Device in Right Tarsal Joint, Percutaneous Approach
0SWH35Z	Revision of External Fixation Device in Right Tarsal Joint, Percutaneous Approach
0SWH37Z	Revision of Autologous Tissue Substitute in Right Tarsal Joint, Percutaneous Approach
0SWH38Z	Revision of Spacer in Right Tarsal Joint, Percutaneous Approach
0SWH3JZ	Revision of Synthetic Substitute in Right Tarsal Joint, Percutaneous Approach
0SWH3KZ	Revision of Nonautologous Tissue Substitute in Right Tarsal Joint, Percutaneous Approach
0SWH40Z	Revision of Drainage Device in Right Tarsal Joint, Percutaneous Endoscopic Approach

0SWH43Z	Revision of Infusion Device in Right Tarsal Joint, Percutaneous Endoscopic Approach
0SWH44Z	Revision of Internal Fixation Device in Right Tarsal Joint, Percutaneous Endoscopic Approach
0SWH45Z	Revision of External Fixation Device in Right Tarsal Joint, Percutaneous Endoscopic Approach
0SWH47Z	Revision of Autologous Tissue Substitute in Right Tarsal Joint, Percutaneous Endoscopic Approach
0SWH48Z	Revision of Spacer in Right Tarsal Joint, Percutaneous Endoscopic Approach
0SWH4JZ	Revision of Synthetic Substitute in Right Tarsal Joint, Percutaneous Endoscopic Approach
0SWH4KZ	Revision of Nonautologous Tissue Substitute in Right Tarsal Joint, Percutaneous Endoscopic Approach
0SWHX0Z	Revision of Drainage Device in Right Tarsal Joint, External Approach
0SWHX3Z	Revision of Infusion Device in Right Tarsal Joint, External Approach
0SWHX4Z	Revision of Internal Fixation Device in Right Tarsal Joint, External Approach
0SWHX5Z	Revision of External Fixation Device in Right Tarsal Joint, External Approach
0SWHX7Z	Revision of Autologous Tissue Substitute in Right Tarsal Joint, External Approach
0SWHX8Z	Revision of Spacer in Right Tarsal Joint, External Approach
0SWHXJZ	Revision of Synthetic Substitute in Right Tarsal Joint, External Approach
0SWHXKZ	Revision of Nonautologous Tissue Substitute in Right Tarsal Joint, External Approach
0SWJ00Z	Revision of Drainage Device in Left Tarsal Joint, Open Approach
0SWJ03Z	Revision of Infusion Device in Left Tarsal Joint, Open Approach
0SWJ04Z	Revision of Internal Fixation Device in Left Tarsal Joint, Open Approach
0SWJ05Z	Revision of External Fixation Device in Left Tarsal Joint, Open Approach
0SWJ07Z	Revision of Autologous Tissue Substitute in Left Tarsal Joint, Open Approach
0SWJ08Z	Revision of Spacer in Left Tarsal Joint, Open Approach
0SWJ0JZ	Revision of Synthetic Substitute in Left Tarsal Joint, Open Approach
0SWJ0KZ	Revision of Nonautologous Tissue Substitute in Left Tarsal Joint, Open Approach
0SWJ30Z	Revision of Drainage Device in Left Tarsal Joint, Percutaneous Approach
0SWJ33Z	Revision of Infusion Device in Left Tarsal Joint, Percutaneous Approach
0SWJ34Z	Revision of Internal Fixation Device in Left Tarsal Joint, Percutaneous Approach
0SWJ35Z	Revision of External Fixation Device in Left Tarsal Joint, Percutaneous Approach
0SWJ37Z	Revision of Autologous Tissue Substitute in Left Tarsal Joint, Percutaneous Approach
0SWJ38Z	Revision of Spacer in Left Tarsal Joint, Percutaneous Approach

0SWJ3JZ	Revision of Synthetic Substitute in Left Tarsal Joint, Percutaneous Approach
0SWJ3KZ	Revision of Nonautologous Tissue Substitute in Left Tarsal Joint, Percutaneous Approach
0SWJ40Z	Revision of Drainage Device in Left Tarsal Joint, Percutaneous Endoscopic Approach
0SWJ43Z	Revision of Infusion Device in Left Tarsal Joint, Percutaneous Endoscopic Approach
0SWJ44Z	Revision of Internal Fixation Device in Left Tarsal Joint, Percutaneous Endoscopic Approach
0SWJ45Z	Revision of External Fixation Device in Left Tarsal Joint, Percutaneous Endoscopic Approach
0SWJ47Z	Revision of Autologous Tissue Substitute in Left Tarsal Joint, Percutaneous Endoscopic Approach
0SWJ48Z	Revision of Spacer in Left Tarsal Joint, Percutaneous Endoscopic Approach
0SWJ4JZ	Revision of Synthetic Substitute in Left Tarsal Joint, Percutaneous Endoscopic Approach
0SWJ4KZ	Revision of Nonautologous Tissue Substitute in Left Tarsal Joint, Percutaneous Endoscopic Approach
0SWJX0Z	Revision of Drainage Device in Left Tarsal Joint, External Approach
0SWJX3Z	Revision of Infusion Device in Left Tarsal Joint, External Approach
0SWJX4Z	Revision of Internal Fixation Device in Left Tarsal Joint, External Approach
0SWJX5Z	Revision of External Fixation Device in Left Tarsal Joint, External Approach
0SWJX7Z	Revision of Autologous Tissue Substitute in Left Tarsal Joint, External Approach
0SWJX8Z	Revision of Spacer in Left Tarsal Joint, External Approach
0SWJXJZ	Revision of Synthetic Substitute in Left Tarsal Joint, External Approach
0SWJXKZ	Revision of Nonautologous Tissue Substitute in Left Tarsal Joint, External Approach
0SWK00Z	Revision of Drainage Device in Right Tarsometatarsal Joint, Open Approach
0SWK03Z	Revision of Infusion Device in Right Tarsometatarsal Joint, Open Approach
0SWK04Z	Revision of Internal Fixation Device in Right Tarsometatarsal Joint, Open Approach
0SWK05Z	Revision of External Fixation Device in Right Tarsometatarsal Joint, Open Approach
0SWK07Z	Revision of Autologous Tissue Substitute in Right Tarsometatarsal Joint, Open Approach
0SWK08Z	Revision of Spacer in Right Tarsometatarsal Joint, Open Approach
0SWK0JZ	Revision of Synthetic Substitute in Right Tarsometatarsal Joint, Open Approach
0SWK0KZ	Revision of Nonautologous Tissue Substitute in Right Tarsometatarsal Joint, Open Approach
0SWK30Z	Revision of Drainage Device in Right Tarsometatarsal Joint, Percutaneous Approach

♀ Female-only   ♂ Male-only   ▲ Limited Coverage   ● Non-OR   HAC HAC-associated procedure   ▲ Non-covered procedures   ✛ Cluster

0SWK33Z Revision of Infusion Device in Right Tarsometatarsal Joint, Percutaneous Approach

0SWK34Z Revision of Internal Fixation Device in Right Tarsometatarsal Joint, Percutaneous Approach

0SWK35Z Revision of External Fixation Device in Right Tarsometatarsal Joint, Percutaneous Approach

0SWK37Z Revision of Autologous Tissue Substitute in Right Tarsometatarsal Joint, Percutaneous Approach

0SWK38Z Revision of Spacer in Right Tarsometatarsal Joint, Percutaneous Approach

0SWK3JZ Revision of Synthetic Substitute in Right Tarsometatarsal Joint, Percutaneous Approach

0SWK3KZ Revision of Nonautologous Tissue Substitute in Right Tarsometatarsal Joint, Percutaneous Approach

0SWK40Z Revision of Drainage Device in Right Tarsometatarsal Joint, Percutaneous Endoscopic Approach

0SWK43Z Revision of Infusion Device in Right Tarsometatarsal Joint, Percutaneous Endoscopic Approach

0SWK44Z Revision of Internal Fixation Device in Right Tarsometatarsal Joint, Percutaneous Endoscopic Approach

0SWK45Z Revision of External Fixation Device in Right Tarsometatarsal Joint, Percutaneous Endoscopic Approach

0SWK47Z Revision of Autologous Tissue Substitute in Right Tarsometatarsal Joint, Percutaneous Endoscopic Approach

0SWK48Z Revision of Spacer in Right Tarsometatarsal Joint, Percutaneous Endoscopic Approach

0SWK4JZ Revision of Synthetic Substitute in Right Tarsometatarsal Joint, Percutaneous Endoscopic Approach

0SWK4KZ Revision of Nonautologous Tissue Substitute in Right Tarsometatarsal Joint, Percutaneous Endoscopic Approach

0SWKX0Z Revision of Drainage Device in Right Tarsometatarsal Joint, External Approach

0SWKX3Z Revision of Infusion Device in Right Tarsometatarsal Joint, External Approach

0SWKX4Z Revision of Internal Fixation Device in Right Tarsometatarsal Joint, External Approach

0SWKX5Z Revision of External Fixation Device in Right Tarsometatarsal Joint, External Approach

0SWKX7Z Revision of Autologous Tissue Substitute in Right Tarsometatarsal Joint, External Approach

0SWKX8Z Revision of Spacer in Right Tarsometatarsal Joint, External Approach

0SWKXJZ Revision of Synthetic Substitute in Right Tarsometatarsal Joint, External Approach

0SWKXKZ Revision of Nonautologous Tissue Substitute in Right Tarsometatarsal Joint, External Approach

0SWL00Z Revision of Drainage Device in Left Tarsometatarsal Joint, Open Approach

0SWL03Z Revision of Infusion Device in Left Tarsometatarsal Joint, Open Approach

0SWL04Z Revision of Internal Fixation Device in Left Tarsometatarsal Joint, Open Approach

0SWL05Z Revision of External Fixation Device in Left Tarsometatarsal Joint, Open Approach

0SWL07Z Revision of Autologous Tissue Substitute in Left Tarsometatarsal Joint, Open Approach

0SWL08Z Revision of Spacer in Left Tarsometatarsal Joint, Open Approach

0SWL0JZ Revision of Synthetic Substitute in Left Tarsometatarsal Joint, Open Approach

0SWL0KZ Revision of Nonautologous Tissue Substitute in Left Tarsometatarsal Joint, Open Approach

0SWL30Z Revision of Drainage Device in Left Tarsometatarsal Joint, Percutaneous Approach

0SWL33Z Revision of Infusion Device in Left Tarsometatarsal Joint, Percutaneous Approach

0SWL34Z Revision of Internal Fixation Device in Left Tarsometatarsal Joint, Percutaneous Approach

0SWL35Z Revision of External Fixation Device in Left Tarsometatarsal Joint, Percutaneous Approach

0SWL37Z Revision of Autologous Tissue Substitute in Left Tarsometatarsal Joint, Percutaneous Approach

0SWL38Z Revision of Spacer in Left Tarsometatarsal Joint, Percutaneous Approach

0SWL3JZ Revision of Synthetic Substitute in Left Tarsometatarsal Joint, Percutaneous Approach

0SWL3KZ Revision of Nonautologous Tissue Substitute in Left Tarsometatarsal Joint, Percutaneous Approach

0SWL40Z Revision of Drainage Device in Left Tarsometatarsal Joint, Percutaneous Endoscopic Approach

0SWL43Z Revision of Infusion Device in Left Tarsometatarsal Joint, Percutaneous Endoscopic Approach

0SWL44Z Revision of Internal Fixation Device in Left Tarsometatarsal Joint, Percutaneous Endoscopic Approach

0SWL45Z Revision of External Fixation Device in Left Tarsometatarsal Joint, Percutaneous Endoscopic Approach

0SWL47Z Revision of Autologous Tissue Substitute in Left Tarsometatarsal Joint, Percutaneous Endoscopic Approach

0SWL48Z Revision of Spacer in Left Tarsometatarsal Joint, Percutaneous Endoscopic Approach

0SWL4JZ Revision of Synthetic Substitute in Left Tarsometatarsal Joint, Percutaneous Endoscopic Approach

0SWL4KZ Revision of Nonautologous Tissue Substitute in Left Tarsometatarsal Joint, Percutaneous Endoscopic Approach

0SWLX0Z Revision of Drainage Device in Left Tarsometatarsal Joint, External Approach

0SWLX3Z Revision of Infusion Device in Left Tarsometatarsal Joint, External Approach

0SWLX4Z Revision of Internal Fixation Device in Left Tarsometatarsal Joint, External Approach

0SWLX5Z Revision of External Fixation Device in Left Tarsometatarsal Joint, External Approach

0SWLX7Z Revision of Autologous Tissue Substitute in Left Tarsometatarsal Joint, External Approach

0SWLX8Z Revision of Spacer in Left Tarsometatarsal Joint, External Approach

0SWLXJZ Revision of Synthetic Substitute in Left Tarsometatarsal Joint, External Approach

0SWLXKZ Revision of Nonautologous Tissue Substitute in Left Tarsometatarsal Joint, External Approach

0SWM00Z Revision of Drainage Device in Right Metatarsal-Phalangeal Joint, Open Approach

0SWM03Z Revision of Infusion Device in Right Metatarsal-Phalangeal Joint, Open Approach

0SWM04Z Revision of Internal Fixation Device in Right Metatarsal-Phalangeal Joint, Open Approach

0SWM05Z Revision of External Fixation Device in Right Metatarsal-Phalangeal Joint, Open Approach

0SWM07Z Revision of Autologous Tissue Substitute in Right Metatarsal-Phalangeal Joint, Open Approach

0SWM08Z Revision of Spacer in Right Metatarsal-Phalangeal Joint, Open Approach

0SWM0JZ Revision of Synthetic Substitute in Right Metatarsal-Phalangeal Joint, Open Approach

0SWM0KZ Revision of Nonautologous Tissue Substitute in Right Metatarsal-Phalangeal Joint, Open Approach

0SWM30Z Revision of Drainage Device in Right Metatarsal-Phalangeal Joint, Percutaneous Approach

0SWM33Z Revision of Infusion Device in Right Metatarsal-Phalangeal Joint, Percutaneous Approach

0SWM34Z Revision of Internal Fixation Device in Right Metatarsal-Phalangeal Joint, Percutaneous Approach

0SWM35Z Revision of External Fixation Device in Right Metatarsal-Phalangeal Joint, Percutaneous Approach

0SWM37Z Revision of Autologous Tissue Substitute in Right Metatarsal-Phalangeal Joint, Percutaneous Approach

0SWM38Z Revision of Spacer in Right Metatarsal-Phalangeal Joint, Percutaneous Approach

0SWM3JZ Revision of Synthetic Substitute in Right Metatarsal-Phalangeal Joint, Percutaneous Approach

0SWM3KZ Revision of Nonautologous Tissue Substitute in Right Metatarsal-Phalangeal Joint, Percutaneous Approach

0SWM40Z Revision of Drainage Device in Right Metatarsal-Phalangeal Joint, Percutaneous Endoscopic Approach

0SWM43Z Revision of Infusion Device in Right Metatarsal-Phalangeal Joint, Percutaneous Endoscopic Approach

0SWM44Z Revision of Internal Fixation Device in Right Metatarsal-Phalangeal Joint, Percutaneous Endoscopic Approach

♀ Female-only   ♂ Male-only   ▲ Limited Coverage   ● Non-OR   HAC HAC-associated procedure   ▲ Non-covered procedures   ✚ Cluster   1189

Medical and Surgical, Lower Joints Code Listings

0SWM45Z Revision of External Fixation Device in Right Metatarsal-Phalangeal Joint, Percutaneous Endoscopic Approach

0SWM47Z Revision of Autologous Tissue Substitute in Right Metatarsal-Phalangeal Joint, Percutaneous Endoscopic Approach

0SWM48Z Revision of Spacer in Right Metatarsal-Phalangeal Joint, Percutaneous Endoscopic Approach

0SWM4JZ Revision of Synthetic Substitute in Right Metatarsal-Phalangeal Joint, Percutaneous Endoscopic Approach

0SWM4KZ Revision of Nonautologous Tissue Substitute in Right Metatarsal-Phalangeal Joint, Percutaneous Endoscopic Approach

0SWMX0Z Revision of Drainage Device in Right Metatarsal-Phalangeal Joint, External Approach

0SWMX3Z Revision of Infusion Device in Right Metatarsal-Phalangeal Joint, External Approach

0SWMX4Z Revision of Internal Fixation Device in Right Metatarsal-Phalangeal Joint, External Approach

0SWMX5Z Revision of External Fixation Device in Right Metatarsal-Phalangeal Joint, External Approach

0SWMX7Z Revision of Autologous Tissue Substitute in Right Metatarsal-Phalangeal Joint, External Approach

0SWMX8Z Revision of Spacer in Right Metatarsal-Phalangeal Joint, External Approach

0SWMXJZ Revision of Synthetic Substitute in Right Metatarsal-Phalangeal Joint, External Approach

0SWMXKZ Revision of Nonautologous Tissue Substitute in Right Metatarsal-Phalangeal Joint, External Approach

0SWN00Z Revision of Drainage Device in Left Metatarsal-Phalangeal Joint, Open Approach

0SWN03Z Revision of Infusion Device in Left Metatarsal-Phalangeal Joint, Open Approach

0SWN04Z Revision of Internal Fixation Device in Left Metatarsal-Phalangeal Joint, Open Approach

0SWN05Z Revision of External Fixation Device in Left Metatarsal-Phalangeal Joint, Open Approach

0SWN07Z Revision of Autologous Tissue Substitute in Left Metatarsal-Phalangeal Joint, Open Approach

0SWN08Z Revision of Spacer in Left Metatarsal-Phalangeal Joint, Open Approach

0SWN0JZ Revision of Synthetic Substitute in Left Metatarsal-Phalangeal Joint, Open Approach

0SWN0KZ Revision of Nonautologous Tissue Substitute in Left Metatarsal-Phalangeal Joint, Open Approach

0SWN30Z Revision of Drainage Device in Left Metatarsal-Phalangeal Joint, Percutaneous Approach

0SWN33Z Revision of Infusion Device in Left Metatarsal-Phalangeal Joint, Percutaneous Approach

0SWN34Z Revision of Internal Fixation Device in Left Metatarsal-Phalangeal Joint, Percutaneous Approach

0SWN35Z Revision of External Fixation Device in Left Metatarsal-Phalangeal Joint, Percutaneous Approach

0SWN37Z Revision of Autologous Tissue Substitute in Left Metatarsal-Phalangeal Joint, Percutaneous Approach

0SWN38Z Revision of Spacer in Left Metatarsal-Phalangeal Joint, Percutaneous Approach

0SWN3JZ Revision of Synthetic Substitute in Left Metatarsal-Phalangeal Joint, Percutaneous Approach

0SWN3KZ Revision of Nonautologous Tissue Substitute in Left Metatarsal-Phalangeal Joint, Percutaneous Approach

0SWN40Z Revision of Drainage Device in Left Metatarsal-Phalangeal Joint, Percutaneous Endoscopic Approach

0SWN43Z Revision of Infusion Device in Left Metatarsal-Phalangeal Joint, Percutaneous Endoscopic Approach

0SWN44Z Revision of Internal Fixation Device in Left Metatarsal-Phalangeal Joint, Percutaneous Endoscopic Approach

0SWN45Z Revision of External Fixation Device in Left Metatarsal-Phalangeal Joint, Percutaneous Endoscopic Approach

0SWN47Z Revision of Autologous Tissue Substitute in Left Metatarsal-Phalangeal Joint, Percutaneous Endoscopic Approach

0SWN48Z Revision of Spacer in Left Metatarsal-Phalangeal Joint, Percutaneous Endoscopic Approach

0SWN4JZ Revision of Synthetic Substitute in Left Metatarsal-Phalangeal Joint, Percutaneous Endoscopic Approach

0SWN4KZ Revision of Nonautologous Tissue Substitute in Left Metatarsal-Phalangeal Joint, Percutaneous Endoscopic Approach

0SWNX0Z Revision of Drainage Device in Left Metatarsal-Phalangeal Joint, External Approach

0SWNX3Z Revision of Infusion Device in Left Metatarsal-Phalangeal Joint, External Approach

0SWNX4Z Revision of Internal Fixation Device in Left Metatarsal-Phalangeal Joint, External Approach

0SWNX5Z Revision of External Fixation Device in Left Metatarsal-Phalangeal Joint, External Approach

0SWNX7Z Revision of Autologous Tissue Substitute in Left Metatarsal-Phalangeal Joint, External Approach

0SWNX8Z Revision of Spacer in Left Metatarsal-Phalangeal Joint, External Approach

0SWNXJZ Revision of Synthetic Substitute in Left Metatarsal-Phalangeal Joint, External Approach

0SWNXKZ Revision of Nonautologous Tissue Substitute in Left Metatarsal-Phalangeal Joint, External Approach

0SWP00Z Revision of Drainage Device in Right Toe Phalangeal Joint, Open Approach

0SWP03Z Revision of Infusion Device in Right Toe Phalangeal Joint, Open Approach

0SWP04Z Revision of Internal Fixation Device in Right Toe Phalangeal Joint, Open Approach

0SWP05Z Revision of External Fixation Device in Right Toe Phalangeal Joint, Open Approach

0SWP07Z Revision of Autologous Tissue Substitute in Right Toe Phalangeal Joint, Open Approach

0SWP08Z Revision of Spacer in Right Toe Phalangeal Joint, Open Approach

0SWP0JZ Revision of Synthetic Substitute in Right Toe Phalangeal Joint, Open Approach

0SWP0KZ Revision of Nonautologous Tissue Substitute in Right Toe Phalangeal Joint, Open Approach

0SWP30Z Revision of Drainage Device in Right Toe Phalangeal Joint, Percutaneous Approach

0SWP33Z Revision of Infusion Device in Right Toe Phalangeal Joint, Percutaneous Approach

0SWP34Z Revision of Internal Fixation Device in Right Toe Phalangeal Joint, Percutaneous Approach

0SWP35Z Revision of External Fixation Device in Right Toe Phalangeal Joint, Percutaneous Approach

0SWP37Z Revision of Autologous Tissue Substitute in Right Toe Phalangeal Joint, Percutaneous Approach

0SWP38Z Revision of Spacer in Right Toe Phalangeal Joint, Percutaneous Approach

0SWP3JZ Revision of Synthetic Substitute in Right Toe Phalangeal Joint, Percutaneous Approach

0SWP3KZ Revision of Nonautologous Tissue Substitute in Right Toe Phalangeal Joint, Percutaneous Approach

0SWP40Z Revision of Drainage Device in Right Toe Phalangeal Joint, Percutaneous Endoscopic Approach

0SWP43Z Revision of Infusion Device in Right Toe Phalangeal Joint, Percutaneous Endoscopic Approach

0SWP44Z Revision of Internal Fixation Device in Right Toe Phalangeal Joint, Percutaneous Endoscopic Approach

0SWP45Z Revision of External Fixation Device in Right Toe Phalangeal Joint, Percutaneous Endoscopic Approach

0SWP47Z Revision of Autologous Tissue Substitute in Right Toe Phalangeal Joint, Percutaneous Endoscopic Approach

0SWP48Z Revision of Spacer in Right Toe Phalangeal Joint, Percutaneous Endoscopic Approach

0SWP4JZ Revision of Synthetic Substitute in Right Toe Phalangeal Joint, Percutaneous Endoscopic Approach

0SWP4KZ Revision of Nonautologous Tissue Substitute in Right Toe Phalangeal Joint, Percutaneous Endoscopic Approach

0SWPX0Z Revision of Drainage Device in Right Toe Phalangeal Joint, External Approach

0SWPX3Z Revision of Infusion Device in Right Toe Phalangeal Joint, External Approach

0SWPX4Z Revision of Internal Fixation Device in Right Toe Phalangeal Joint, External Approach

0SWPX5Z Revision of External Fixation Device in Right Toe Phalangeal Joint, External Approach

0SWPX7Z Revision of Autologous Tissue Substitute in Right Toe Phalangeal Joint, External Approach

♀ Female-only   ♂ Male-only   ▲ Limited Coverage   ● Non-OR   HAC HAC-associated procedure   ▲ Non-covered procedures   ✚ Cluster

0SWPX8Z Revision of Spacer in Right Toe Phalangeal Joint, External Approach

0SWPXJZ Revision of Synthetic Substitute in Right Toe Phalangeal Joint, External Approach

0SWPXKZ Revision of Nonautologous Tissue Substitute in Right Toe Phalangeal Joint, External Approach

0SWQ00Z Revision of Drainage Device in Left Toe Phalangeal Joint, Open Approach

0SWQ03Z Revision of Infusion Device in Left Toe Phalangeal Joint, Open Approach

0SWQ04Z Revision of Internal Fixation Device in Left Toe Phalangeal Joint, Open Approach

0SWQ05Z Revision of External Fixation Device in Left Toe Phalangeal Joint, Open Approach

0SWQ07Z Revision of Autologous Tissue Substitute in Left Toe Phalangeal Joint, Open Approach

0SWQ08Z Revision of Spacer in Left Toe Phalangeal Joint, Open Approach

0SWQ0JZ Revision of Synthetic Substitute in Left Toe Phalangeal Joint, Open Approach

0SWQ0KZ Revision of Nonautologous Tissue Substitute in Left Toe Phalangeal Joint, Open Approach

0SWQ30Z Revision of Drainage Device in Left Toe Phalangeal Joint, Percutaneous Approach

0SWQ33Z Revision of Infusion Device in Left Toe Phalangeal Joint, Percutaneous Approach

0SWQ34Z Revision of Internal Fixation Device in Left Toe Phalangeal Joint, Percutaneous Approach

0SWQ35Z Revision of External Fixation Device in Left Toe Phalangeal Joint, Percutaneous Approach

0SWQ37Z Revision of Autologous Tissue Substitute in Left Toe Phalangeal Joint, Percutaneous Approach

0SWQ38Z Revision of Spacer in Left Toe Phalangeal Joint, Percutaneous Approach

0SWQ3JZ Revision of Synthetic Substitute in Left Toe Phalangeal Joint, Percutaneous Approach

0SWQ3KZ Revision of Nonautologous Tissue Substitute in Left Toe Phalangeal Joint, Percutaneous Approach

0SWQ40Z Revision of Drainage Device in Left Toe Phalangeal Joint, Percutaneous Endoscopic Approach

0SWQ43Z Revision of Infusion Device in Left Toe Phalangeal Joint, Percutaneous Endoscopic Approach

0SWQ44Z Revision of Internal Fixation Device in Left Toe Phalangeal Joint, Percutaneous Endoscopic Approach

0SWQ45Z Revision of External Fixation Device in Left Toe Phalangeal Joint, Percutaneous Endoscopic Approach

0SWQ47Z Revision of Autologous Tissue Substitute in Left Toe Phalangeal Joint, Percutaneous Endoscopic Approach

0SWQ48Z Revision of Spacer in Left Toe Phalangeal Joint, Percutaneous Endoscopic Approach

0SWQ4JZ Revision of Synthetic Substitute in Left Toe Phalangeal Joint, Percutaneous Endoscopic Approach

0SWQ4KZ Revision of Nonautologous Tissue Substitute in Left Toe Phalangeal Joint, Percutaneous Endoscopic Approach

0SWQX0Z Revision of Drainage Device in Left Toe Phalangeal Joint, External Approach

0SWQX3Z Revision of Infusion Device in Left Toe Phalangeal Joint, External Approach

0SWQX4Z Revision of Internal Fixation Device in Left Toe Phalangeal Joint, External Approach

0SWQX5Z Revision of External Fixation Device in Left Toe Phalangeal Joint, External Approach

0SWQX7Z Revision of Autologous Tissue Substitute in Left Toe Phalangeal Joint, External Approach

0SWQX8Z Revision of Spacer in Left Toe Phalangeal Joint, External Approach

0SWQXJZ Revision of Synthetic Substitute in Left Toe Phalangeal Joint, External Approach

0SWQXKZ Revision of Nonautologous Tissue Substitute in Left Toe Phalangeal Joint, External Approach

0SWR0JZ Revision of Synthetic Substitute in Right Hip Joint, Femoral Surface, Open Approach

0SWR3JZ Revision of Synthetic Substitute in Right Hip Joint, Femoral Surface, Percutaneous Approach

0SWR4JZ Revision of Synthetic Substitute in Right Hip Joint, Femoral Surface, Percutaneous Endoscopic Approach

0SWRXJZ Revision of Synthetic Substitute in Right Hip Joint, Femoral Surface, External Approach

0SWS0JZ Revision of Synthetic Substitute in Left Hip Joint, Femoral Surface, Open Approach

0SWS3JZ Revision of Synthetic Substitute in Left Hip Joint, Femoral Surface, Percutaneous Approach

0SWS4JZ Revision of Synthetic Substitute in Left Hip Joint, Femoral Surface, Percutaneous Endoscopic Approach

0SWSXJZ Revision of Synthetic Substitute in Left Hip Joint, Femoral Surface, External Approach

0SWT0JZ Revision of Synthetic Substitute in Right Knee Joint, Femoral Surface, Open Approach

0SWT3JZ Revision of Synthetic Substitute in Right Knee Joint, Femoral Surface, Percutaneous Approach

0SWT4JZ Revision of Synthetic Substitute in Right Knee Joint, Femoral Surface, Percutaneous Endoscopic Approach

0SWTXJZ Revision of Synthetic Substitute in Right Knee Joint, Femoral Surface, External Approach

0SWU0JZ Revision of Synthetic Substitute in Left Knee Joint, Femoral Surface, Open Approach

0SWU3JZ Revision of Synthetic Substitute in Left Knee Joint, Femoral Surface, Percutaneous Approach

0SWU4JZ Revision of Synthetic Substitute in Left Knee Joint, Femoral Surface, Percutaneous Endoscopic Approach

0SWUXJZ Revision of Synthetic Substitute in Left Knee Joint, Femoral Surface, External Approach

0SWV0JZ Revision of Synthetic Substitute in Right Knee Joint, Tibial Surface, Open Approach

0SWV3JZ Revision of Synthetic Substitute in Right Knee Joint, Tibial Surface, Percutaneous Approach

0SWV4JZ Revision of Synthetic Substitute in Right Knee Joint, Tibial Surface, Percutaneous Endoscopic Approach

0SWVXJZ Revision of Synthetic Substitute in Right Knee Joint, Tibial Surface, External Approach

0SWW0JZ Revision of Synthetic Substitute in Left Knee Joint, Tibial Surface, Open Approach
AHA CC: 4Q, 2016, 112

0SWW3JZ Revision of Synthetic Substitute in Left Knee Joint, Tibial Surface, Percutaneous Approach

0SWW4JZ Revision of Synthetic Substitute in Left Knee Joint, Tibial Surface, Percutaneous Endoscopic Approach

0SWWXJZ Revision of Synthetic Substitute in Left Knee Joint, Tibial Surface, External Approach

Urinary System

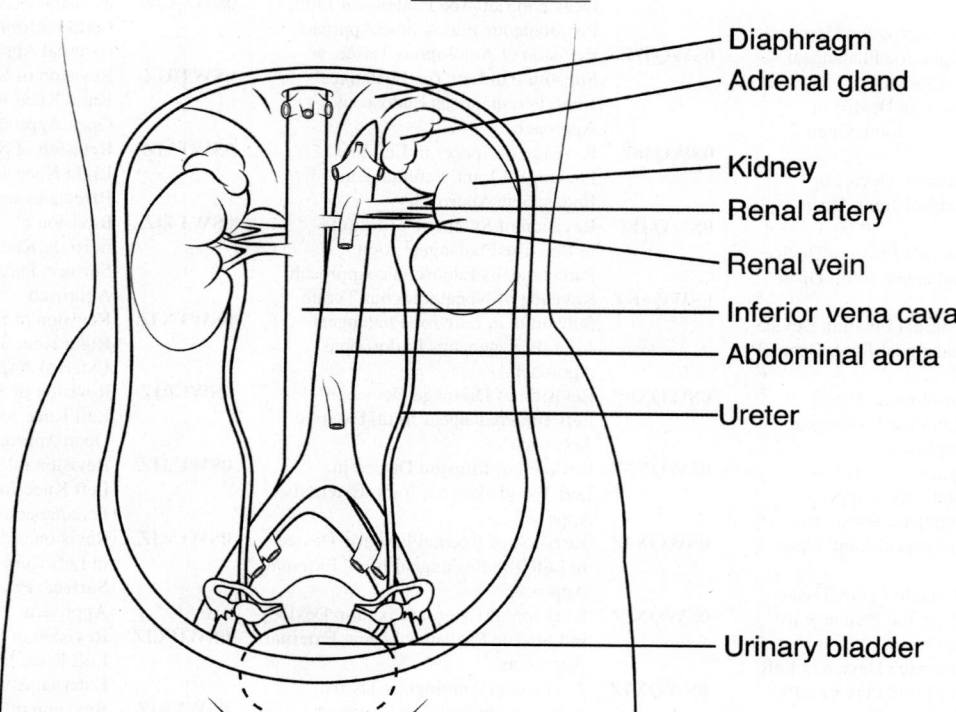

- Diaphragm
- Adrenal gland
- Kidney
- Renal artery
- Renal vein
- Inferior vena cava
- Abdominal aorta
- Ureter
- Urinary bladder
- Urethra

©AHIMA

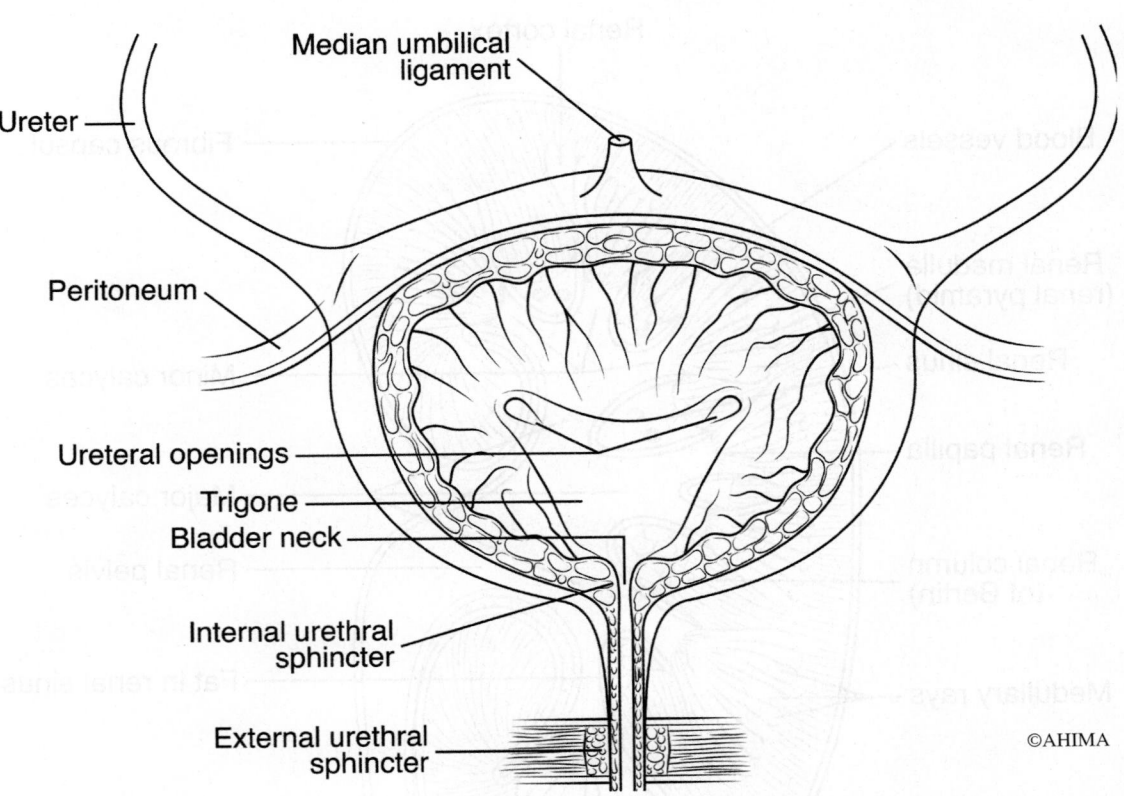

Median umbilical
ligament

Ureter

Peritoneum

Ureteral openings

Trigone

Bladder neck

Internal urethral
sphincter

External urethral
sphincter

©AHIMA

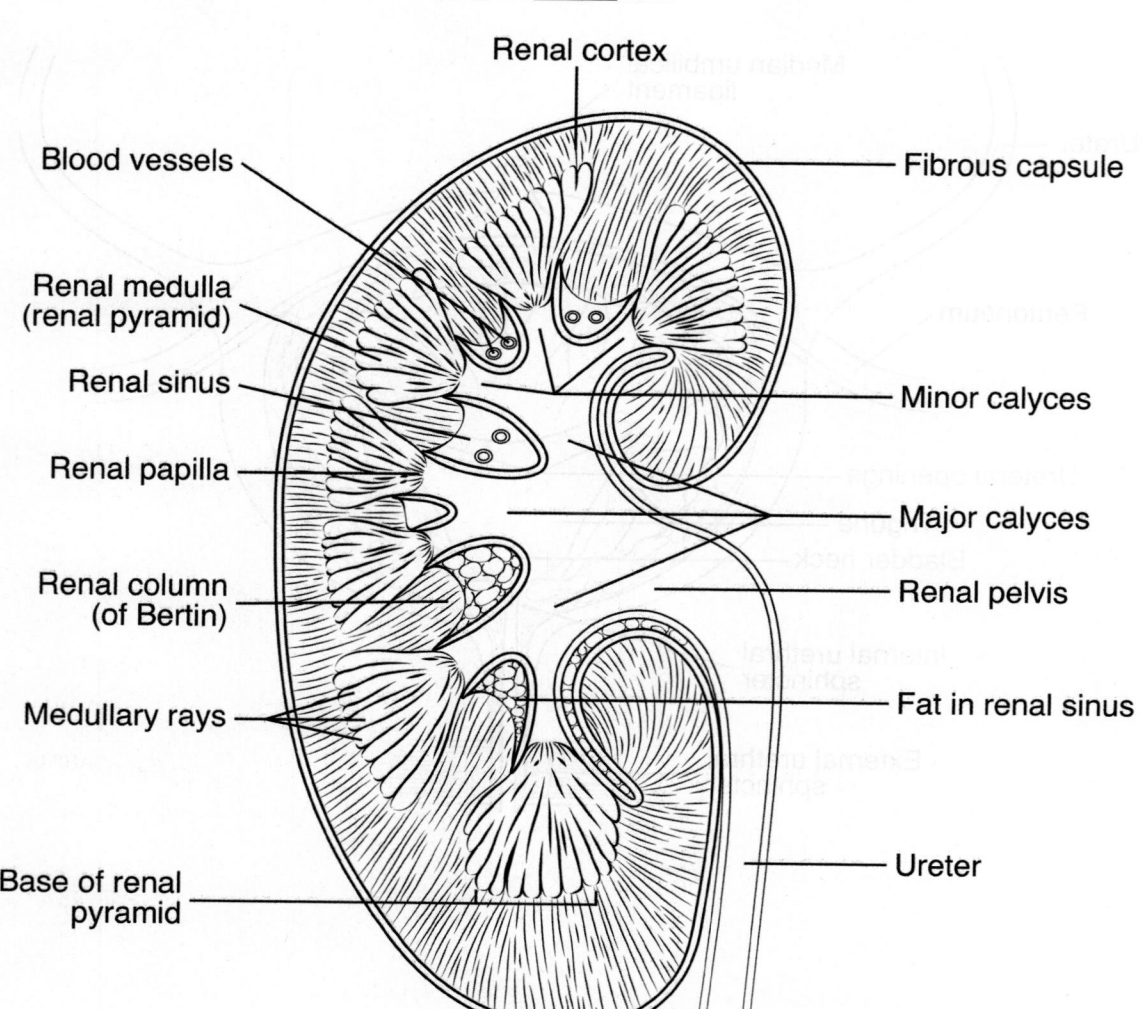

Renal cortex

Blood vessels

Fibrous capsule

Renal medulla
(renal pyramid)

Renal sinus

Minor calyces

Renal papilla

Major calyces

Renal column
(of Bertin)

Renal pelvis

Fat in renal sinus

Medullary rays

Base of renal
pyramid

Ureter

©AHIMA

Renal Revascularization

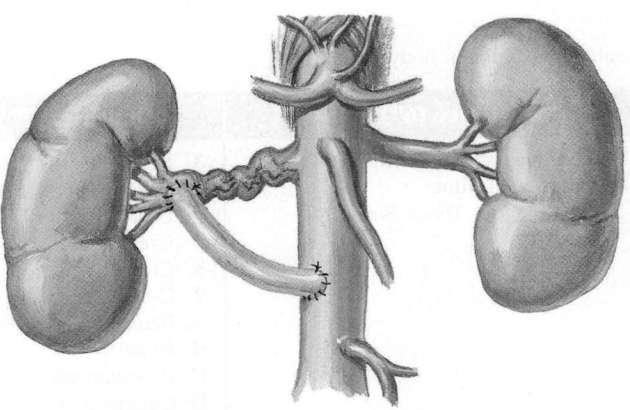

Bypass to distal extremity of renal artery
beyond extensive fibromuscular hyperplasia,
employing segment of saphenous vein

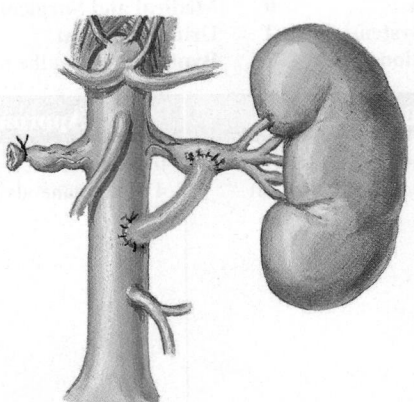

Renal artery bypass plus
contralateral nephrectomy

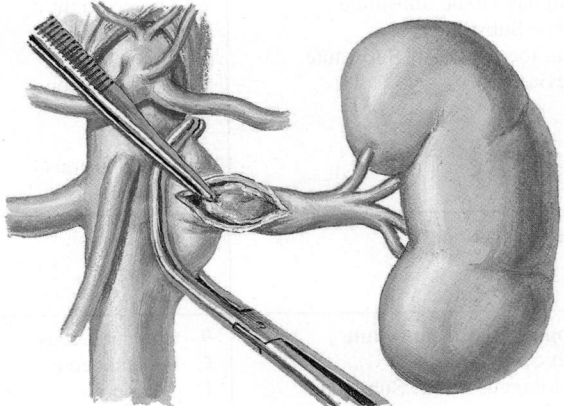

Endarterectomy

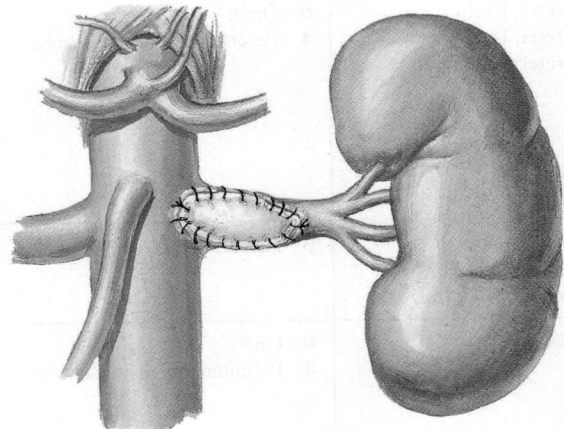

Patch graft with or without
endarterectomy

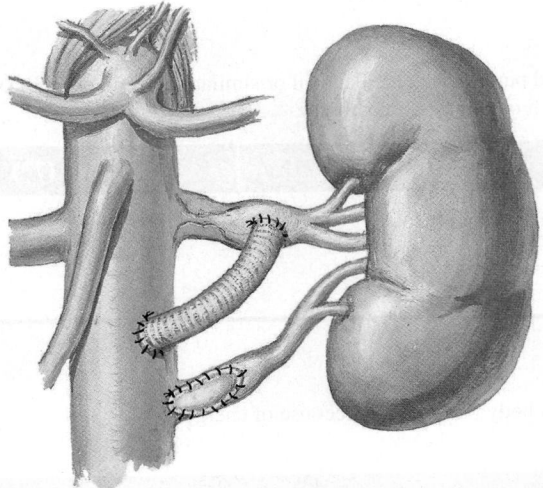

Renal artery bypass plus patch graft
to accessory renal artery

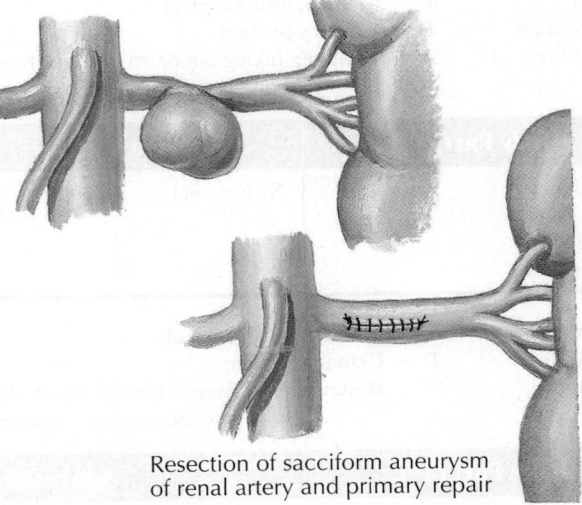

Resection of sacciform aneurysm
of renal artery and primary repair

Medical and Surgical, Urinary System

Urinary System Tables 0T1–0TY

Section	0	Medical and Surgical
Body System	T	Urinary System
Operation	1	**Bypass:** Altering the route of passage of the contents of a tubular body part

Body Part (4th)	Approach (5th)	Device (6th)	Qualifier (7th)
3 Kidney Pelvis, Right 4 Kidney Pelvis, Left	0 Open 4 Percutaneous Endoscopic	7 Autologous Tissue Substitute J Synthetic Substitute K Nonautologous Tissue Substitute Z No Device	3 Kidney Pelvis, Right 4 Kidney Pelvis, Left 6 Ureter, Right 7 Ureter, Left 8 Colon 9 Colocutaneous A Ileum B Bladder C Ileocutaneous D Cutaneous
3 Kidney Pelvis, Right 4 Kidney Pelvis, Left	3 Percutaneous	J Synthetic Substitute	D Cutaneous
6 Ureter, Right 7 Ureter, Left 8 Ureters, Bilateral	0 Open 4 Percutaneous Endoscopic	7 Autologous Tissue Substitute J Synthetic Substitute K Nonautologous Tissue Substitute Z No Device	6 Ureter, Right 7 Ureter, Left 8 Colon 9 Colocutaneous A Ileum B Bladder C Ileocutaneous D Cutaneous
6 Ureter, Right 7 Ureter, Left 8 Ureters, Bilateral	3 Percutaneous	J Synthetic Substitute	D Cutaneous
B Bladder	0 Open 4 Percutaneous Endoscopic	7 Autologous Tissue Substitute J Synthetic Substitute K Nonautologous Tissue Substitute Z No Device	9 Colocutaneous C Ileocutaneous D Cutaneous
B Bladder	3 Percutaneous	J Synthetic Substitute	D Cutaneous

Section	0	Medical and Surgical
Body System	T	Urinary System
Operation	2	**Change:** Taking out or off a device from a body part and putting back an identical or similar device in or on the same body part without cutting or puncturing the skin or a mucous membrane

Body Part (4th)	Approach (5th)	Device (6th)	Qualifier (7th)
5 Kidney 9 Ureter B Bladder D Urethra	X External	0 Drainage Device Y Other Device	Z No Qualifier

Section	0	Medical and Surgical
Body System	T	Urinary System
Operation	5	**Destruction:** Physical eradication of all or a portion of a body part by the direct use of energy, force, or a destructive agent

Body Part (4th)	Approach (5th)	Device (6th)	Qualifier (7th)
0 Kidney, Right 1 Kidney, Left 3 Kidney Pelvis, Right 4 Kidney Pelvis, Left 6 Ureter, Right 7 Ureter, Left B Bladder C Bladder Neck	0 Open 3 Percutaneous 4 Percutaneous Endoscopic 7 Via Natural or Artificial Opening 8 Via Natural or Artificial Opening Endoscopic	Z No Device	Z No Qualifier

Continued →

Section   **0**   **Medical and Surgical**
Body System   **T**   **Urinary System**
Operation   **5**   **Destruction:** Physical eradication of all or a portion of a body part by the direct use of energy, force, or a destructive agent

Body Part (4ᵗʰ)	Approach (5ᵗʰ)	Device (6ᵗʰ)	Qualifier (7ᵗʰ)
D Urethra	0 Open 3 Percutaneous 4 Percutaneous Endoscopic 7 Via Natural or Artificial Opening 8 Via Natural or Artificial Opening Endoscopic X External	Z No Device	Z No Qualifier

Section   **0**   **Medical and Surgical**
Body System   **T**   **Urinary System**
Operation   **7**   **Dilation:** Expanding an orifice or the lumen of a tubular body part

Body Part (4ᵗʰ)	Approach (5ᵗʰ)	Device (6ᵗʰ)	Qualifier (7ᵗʰ)
3 Kidney Pelvis, Right 4 Kidney Pelvis, Left 6 Ureter, Right 7 Ureter, Left 8 Ureters, Bilateral B Bladder C Bladder Neck D Urethra	0 Open 3 Percutaneous 4 Percutaneous Endoscopic 7 Via Natural or Artificial Opening 8 Via Natural or Artificial Opening Endoscopic	D Intraluminal Device Z No Device	Z No Qualifier

Section   **0**   **Medical and Surgical**
Body System   **T**   **Urinary System**
Operation   **8**   **Division:** Cutting into a body part, without draining fluids and/or gases from the body part, in order to separate or transect a body part

Body Part (4ᵗʰ)	Approach (5ᵗʰ)	Device (6ᵗʰ)	Qualifier (7ᵗʰ)
2 Kidneys, Bilateral C Bladder Neck	0 Open 3 Percutaneous 4 Percutaneous Endoscopic	Z No Device	Z No Qualifier

Section   **0**   **Medical and Surgical**
Body System   **T**   **Urinary System**
Operation   **9**   **Drainage:** Taking or letting out fluids and/or gases from a body part

Body Part (4ᵗʰ)	Approach (5ᵗʰ)	Device (6ᵗʰ)	Qualifier (7ᵗʰ)
0 Kidney, Right 1 Kidney, Left 3 Kidney Pelvis, Right 4 Kidney Pelvis, Left 6 Ureter, Right 7 Ureter, Left 8 Ureters, Bilateral B Bladder C Bladder Neck	0 Open 3 Percutaneous 4 Percutaneous Endoscopic 7 Via Natural or Artificial Opening 8 Via Natural or Artificial Opening Endoscopic	0 Drainage Device	Z No Qualifier
0 Kidney, Right 1 Kidney, Left 3 Kidney Pelvis, Right 4 Kidney Pelvis, Left 6 Ureter, Right 7 Ureter, Left 8 Ureters, Bilateral B Bladder C Bladder Neck	0 Open 3 Percutaneous 4 Percutaneous Endoscopic 7 Via Natural or Artificial Opening 8 Via Natural or Artificial Opening Endoscopic	Z No Device	X Diagnostic Z No Qualifier

Continued →

Section 0 **Medical and Surgical**
Body System T **Urinary System**
Operation 9 **Drainage:** Taking or letting out fluids and/or gases from a body part

Body Part (4th)	Approach (5th)	Device (6th)	Qualifier (7th)
D Urethra	**0** Open **3** Percutaneous **4** Percutaneous Endoscopic **7** Via Natural or Artificial Opening **8** Via Natural or Artificial Opening Endoscopic **X** External	**0** Drainage Device	**Z** No Qualifier
D Urethra	**0** Open **3** Percutaneous **4** Percutaneous Endoscopic **7** Via Natural or Artificial Opening **8** Via Natural or Artificial Opening Endoscopic **X** External	**Z** No Device	**X** Diagnostic **Z** No Qualifier

Section 0 **Medical and Surgical**
Body System T **Urinary System**
Operation B **Excision:** Cutting out or off, without replacement, a portion of a body part

Body Part (4th)	Approach (5th)	Device (6th)	Qualifier (7th)
0 Kidney, Right **1** Kidney, Left **3** Kidney Pelvis, Right **4** Kidney Pelvis, Left **6** Ureter, Right **7** Ureter, Left **B** Bladder **C** Bladder Neck	**0** Open **3** Percutaneous **4** Percutaneous Endoscopic **7** Via Natural or Artificial Opening **8** Via Natural or Artificial Opening Endoscopic	**Z** No Device	**X** Diagnostic **Z** No Qualifier
D Urethra	**0** Open **3** Percutaneous **4** Percutaneous Endoscopic **7** Via Natural or Artificial Opening **8** Via Natural or Artificial Opening Endoscopic **X** External	**Z** No Device	**X** Diagnostic **Z** No Qualifier

Section 0 **Medical and Surgical**
Body System T **Urinary System**
Operation C **Extirpation:** Taking or cutting out solid matter from a body part

Body Part (4th)	Approach (5th)	Device (6th)	Qualifier (7th)
0 Kidney, Right **1** Kidney, Left **3** Kidney Pelvis, Right **4** Kidney Pelvis, Left **6** Ureter, Right **7** Ureter, Left **B** Bladder **C** Bladder Neck	**0** Open **3** Percutaneous **4** Percutaneous Endoscopic **7** Via Natural or Artificial Opening **8** Via Natural or Artificial Opening Endoscopic	**Z** No Device	**Z** No Qualifier
D Urethra	**0** Open **3** Percutaneous **4** Percutaneous Endoscopic **7** Via Natural or Artificial Opening **8** Via Natural or Artificial Opening Endoscopic **X** External	**Z** No Device	**Z** No Qualifier

Section	0	Medical and Surgical
Body System	T	Urinary System
Operation	D	**Extraction:** Pulling or stripping out or off all or a portion of a body part by the use of force

Body Part (4ᵗʰ)	Approach (5ᵗʰ)	Device (6ᵗʰ)	Qualifier (7ᵗʰ)
0 Kidney, Right 1 Kidney, Left	0 Open 3 Percutaneous 4 Percutaneous Endoscopic	Z No Device	Z No Qualifier

Section	0	Medical and Surgical
Body System	T	Urinary System
Operation	F	**Fragmentation:** Breaking solid matter in a body part into pieces

Body Part (4ᵗʰ)	Approach (5ᵗʰ)	Device (6ᵗʰ)	Qualifier (7ᵗʰ)
3 Kidney Pelvis, Right 4 Kidney Pelvis, Left 6 Ureter, Right 7 Ureter, Left B Bladder C Bladder Neck D Urethra	0 Open 3 Percutaneous 4 Percutaneous Endoscopic 7 Via Natural or Artificial Opening 8 Via Natural or Artificial Opening Endoscopic X External	Z No Device	Z No Qualifier

Section	0	Medical and Surgical
Body System	T	Urinary System
Operation	H	**Insertion:** Putting in a nonbiological appliance that monitors, assists, performs, or prevents a physiological function but does not physically take the place of a body part

Body Part (4ᵗʰ)	Approach (5ᵗʰ)	Device (6ᵗʰ)	Qualifier (7ᵗʰ)
5 Kidney	0 Open 3 Percutaneous 4 Percutaneous Endoscopic 7 Via Natural or Artificial Opening 8 Via Natural or Artificial Opening Endoscopic	1 Radioactive Element 2 Monitoring Device 3 Infusion Device Y Other Device	Z No Qualifier
9 Ureter	0 Open 3 Percutaneous 4 Percutaneous Endoscopic 7 Via Natural or Artificial Opening 8 Via Natural or Artificial Opening Endoscopic	1 Radioactive Element 2 Monitoring Device 3 Infusion Device M Stimulator Lead Y Other Device	Z No Qualifier
B Bladder	0 Open 3 Percutaneous 4 Percutaneous Endoscopic 7 Via Natural or Artificial Opening 8 Via Natural or Artificial Opening Endoscopic	1 Radioactive Element 2 Monitoring Device 3 Infusion Device L Artificial Sphincter M Stimulator Lead Y Other Device	Z No Qualifier
C Bladder Neck	0 Open 3 Percutaneous 4 Percutaneous Endoscopic 7 Via Natural or Artificial Opening 8 Via Natural or Artificial Opening Endoscopic	L Artificial Sphincter	Z No Qualifier
D Urethra	0 Open 3 Percutaneous 4 Percutaneous Endoscopic 7 Via Natural or Artificial Opening 8 Via Natural or Artificial Opening Endoscopic	1 Radioactive Element 2 Monitoring Device 3 Infusion Device L Artificial Sphincter Y Other Device	Z No Qualifier
D Urethra	X External	2 Monitoring Device 3 Infusion Device L Artificial Sphincter	Z No Qualifier

Section	0	Medical and Surgical
Body System	T	Urinary System
Operation	J	**Inspection:** Visually and/or manually exploring a body part

Body Part (4th)	Approach (5th)	Device (6th)	Qualifier (7th)
5 Kidney 9 Ureter B Bladder D Urethra	0 Open 3 Percutaneous 4 Percutaneous Endoscopic 7 Via Natural or Artificial Opening 8 Via Natural or Artificial Opening Endoscopic X External	Z No Device	Z No Qualifier

Section	0	Medical and Surgical
Body System	T	Urinary System
Operation	L	**Occlusion:** Completely closing an orifice or the lumen of a tubular body part

Body Part (4th)	Approach (5th)	Device (6th)	Qualifier (7th)
3 Kidney Pelvis, Right 4 Kidney Pelvis, Left 6 Ureter, Right 7 Ureter, Left B Bladder C Bladder Neck	0 Open 3 Percutaneous 4 Percutaneous Endoscopic	C Extraluminal Device D Intraluminal Device Z No Device	Z No Qualifier
3 Kidney Pelvis, Right 4 Kidney Pelvis, Left 6 Ureter, Right 7 Ureter, Left B Bladder C Bladder Neck	7 Via Natural or Artificial Opening 8 Via Natural or Artificial Opening Endoscopic	D Intraluminal Device Z No Device	Z No Qualifier
D Urethra	0 Open 3 Percutaneous 4 Percutaneous Endoscopic X External	C Extraluminal Device D Intraluminal Device Z No Device	Z No Qualifier
D Urethra	7 Via Natural or Artificial Opening 8 Via Natural or Artificial Opening Endoscopic	D Intraluminal Device Z No Device	Z No Qualifier

Section	0	Medical and Surgical
Body System	T	Urinary System
Operation	M	**Reattachment:** Putting back in or on all or a portion of a separated body part to its normal location or other suitable location

Body Part (4th)	Approach (5th)	Device (6th)	Qualifier (7th)
0 Kidney, Right 1 Kidney, Left 2 Kidneys, Bilateral 3 Kidney Pelvis, Right 4 Kidney Pelvis, Left 6 Ureter, Right 7 Ureter, Left 8 Ureters, Bilateral B Bladder C Bladder Neck D Urethra	0 Open 4 Percutaneous Endoscopic	Z No Device	Z No Qualifier

Section	0	Medical and Surgical
Body System	T	Urinary System
Operation	N	Release: Freeing a body part from an abnormal physical constraint by cutting or by the use of force

Body Part (4th)	Approach (5th)	Device (6th)	Qualifier (7th)
0 Kidney, Right 1 Kidney, Left 3 Kidney Pelvis, Right 4 Kidney Pelvis, Left 6 Ureter, Right 7 Ureter, Left B Bladder C Bladder Neck	0 Open 3 Percutaneous 4 Percutaneous Endoscopic 7 Via Natural or Artificial Opening 8 Via Natural or Artificial Opening Endoscopic	Z No Device	Z No Qualifier
D Urethra	0 Open 3 Percutaneous 4 Percutaneous Endoscopic 7 Via Natural or Artificial Opening 8 Via Natural or Artificial Opening Endoscopic X External	Z No Device	Z No Qualifier

Section	0	Medical and Surgical
Body System	T	Urinary System
Operation	P	Removal: Taking out or off a device from a body part

Body Part (4th)	Approach (5th)	Device (6th)	Qualifier (7th)
5 Kidney	0 Open 3 Percutaneous 4 Percutaneous Endoscopic 7 Via Natural or Artificial Opening 8 Via Natural or Artificial Opening Endoscopic	0 Drainage Device 2 Monitoring Device 3 Infusion Device 7 Autologous Tissue Substitute C Extraluminal Device D Intraluminal Device J Synthetic Substitute K Nonautologous Tissue Substitute Y Other Device	Z No Qualifier
5 Kidney	X External	0 Drainage Device 2 Monitoring Device 3 Infusion Device D Intraluminal Device	Z No Qualifier
9 Ureter	0 Open 3 Percutaneous 4 Percutaneous Endoscopic 7 Via Natural or Artificial Opening 8 Via Natural or Artificial Opening Endoscopic	0 Drainage Device 2 Monitoring Device 3 Infusion Device 7 Autologous Tissue Substitute C Extraluminal Device D Intraluminal Device J Synthetic Substitute K Nonautologous Tissue Substitute M Stimulator Lead Y Other Device	Z No Qualifier
9 Ureter	X External	0 Drainage Device 2 Monitoring Device 3 Infusion Device D Intraluminal Device M Stimulator Lead	Z No Qualifier

Continued →

Section   **0**   **Medical and Surgical**
Body System   **T**   **Urinary System**
Operation   **P**   **Removal:** Taking out or off a device from a body part

Body Part (4ᵗʰ)	Approach (5ᵗʰ)	Device (6ᵗʰ)	Qualifier (7ᵗʰ)
B Bladder	0 Open 3 Percutaneous 4 Percutaneous Endoscopic 7 Via Natural or Artificial Opening 8 Via Natural or Artificial Opening Endoscopic	0 Drainage Device 2 Monitoring Device 3 Infusion Device 7 Autologous Tissue Substitute C Extraluminal Device D Intraluminal Device J Synthetic Substitute K Nonautologous Tissue Substitute L Artificial Sphincter M Stimulator Lead Y Other Device	Z No Qualifier
B Bladder	X External	0 Drainage Device 2 Monitoring Device 3 Infusion Device D Intraluminal Device L Artificial Sphincter M Stimulator Lead	Z No Qualifier
D Urethra	0 Open 3 Percutaneous 4 Percutaneous Endoscopic 7 Via Natural or Artificial Opening 8 Via Natural or Artificial Opening Endoscopic	0 Drainage Device 2 Monitoring Device 3 Infusion Device 7 Autologous Tissue Substitute C Extraluminal Device D Intraluminal Device J Synthetic Substitute K Nonautologous Tissue Substitute L Artificial Sphincter Y Other Device	Z No Qualifier
D Urethra	X External	0 Drainage Device 2 Monitoring Device 3 Infusion Device D Intraluminal Device L Artificial Sphincter	Z No Qualifier

Section   **0**   **Medical and Surgical**
Body System   **T**   **Urinary System**
Operation   **Q**   **Repair:** Restoring, to the extent possible, a body part to its normal anatomic structure and function

Body Part (4ᵗʰ)	Approach (5ᵗʰ)	Device (6ᵗʰ)	Qualifier (7ᵗʰ)
0 Kidney, Right 1 Kidney, Left 3 Kidney Pelvis, Right 4 Kidney Pelvis, Left 6 Ureter, Right 7 Ureter, Left B Bladder C Bladder Neck	0 Open 3 Percutaneous 4 Percutaneous Endoscopic 7 Via Natural or Artificial Opening 8 Via Natural or Artificial Opening Endoscopic	Z No Device	Z No Qualifier
D Urethra	0 Open 3 Percutaneous 4 Percutaneous Endoscopic 7 Via Natural or Artificial Opening 8 Via Natural or Artificial Opening Endoscopic X External	Z No Device	Z No Qualifier

Section   **0**   **Medical and Surgical**
Body System   **T**   **Urinary System**
Operation   **R**   **Replacement:** Putting in or on biological or synthetic material that physically takes the place and/or function of all or a portion of a body part

Body Part (4th)	Approach (5th)	Device (6th)	Qualifier (7th)
3 Kidney Pelvis, Right 4 Kidney Pelvis, Left 6 Ureter, Right 7 Ureter, Left B Bladder C Bladder Neck	0 Open 4 Percutaneous Endoscopic 7 Via Natural or Artificial Opening 8 Via Natural or Artificial Opening Endoscopic	7 Autologous Tissue Substitute J Synthetic Substitute K Nonautologous Tissue Substitute	Z No Qualifier
D Urethra	0 Open 4 Percutaneous Endoscopic 7 Via Natural or Artificial Opening 8 Via Natural or Artificial Opening Endoscopic X External	7 Autologous Tissue Substitute J Synthetic Substitute K Nonautologous Tissue Substitute	Z No Qualifier

Section   **0**   **Medical and Surgical**
Body System   **T**   **Urinary System**
Operation   **S**   **Reposition:** Moving to its normal location, or other suitable location, all or a portion of a body part

Body Part (4th)	Approach (5th)	Device (6th)	Qualifier (7th)
0 Kidney, Right 1 Kidney, Left 2 Kidneys, Bilateral 3 Kidney Pelvis, Right 4 Kidney Pelvis, Left 6 Ureter, Right 7 Ureter, Left 8 Ureters, Bilateral B Bladder C Bladder Neck D Urethra	0 Open 4 Percutaneous Endoscopic	Z No Device	Z No Qualifier

Section   **0**   **Medical and Surgical**
Body System   **T**   **Urinary System**
Operation   **T**   **Resection:** Cutting out or off, without replacement, all of a body part

Body Part (4th)	Approach (5th)	Device (6th)	Qualifier (7th)
0 Kidney, Right 1 Kidney, Left 2 Kidneys, Bilateral	0 Open 4 Percutaneous Endoscopic	Z No Device	Z No Qualifier
3 Kidney Pelvis, Right 4 Kidney Pelvis, Left 6 Ureter, Right 7 Ureter, Left B Bladder C Bladder Neck D Urethra	0 Open 4 Percutaneous Endoscopic 7 Via Natural or Artificial Opening 8 Via Natural or Artificial Opening Endoscopic	Z No Device	Z No Qualifier

Section   0   Medical and Surgical
Body System   T   Urinary System
Operation   U   **Supplement:** Putting in or on biological or synthetic material that physically reinforces and/or augments the function of a portion of a body part

Body Part (4th)	Approach (5th)	Device (6th)	Qualifier (7th)
3 Kidney Pelvis, Right 4 Kidney Pelvis, Left 6 Ureter, Right 7 Ureter, Left B Bladder C Bladder Neck	0 Open 4 Percutaneous Endoscopic 7 Via Natural or Artificial Opening 8 Via Natural or Artificial Opening Endoscopic	7 Autologous Tissue Substitute J Synthetic Substitute K Nonautologous Tissue Substitute	Z No Qualifier
D Urethra	0 Open 4 Percutaneous Endoscopic 7 Via Natural or Artificial Opening 8 Via Natural or Artificial Opening Endoscopic X External	7 Autologous Tissue Substitute J Synthetic Substitute K Nonautologous Tissue Substitute	Z No Qualifier

Section   0   Medical and Surgical
Body System   T   Urinary System
Operation   V   **Restriction:** Partially closing an orifice or the lumen of a tubular body part

Body Part (4th)	Approach (5th)	Device (6th)	Qualifier (7th)
3 Kidney Pelvis, Right 4 Kidney Pelvis, Left 6 Ureter, Right 7 Ureter, Left B Bladder C Bladder Neck	0 Open 3 Percutaneous 4 Percutaneous Endoscopic	C Extraluminal Device D Intraluminal Device Z No Device	Z No Qualifier
3 Kidney Pelvis, Right 4 Kidney Pelvis, Left 6 Ureter, Right 7 Ureter, Left B Bladder C Bladder Neck	7 Via Natural or Artificial Opening 8 Via Natural or Artificial Opening Endoscopic	D Intraluminal Device Z No Device	Z No Qualifier
D Urethra	0 Open 3 Percutaneous 4 Percutaneous Endoscopic	C Extraluminal Device D Intraluminal Device Z No Device	Z No Qualifier
D Urethra	7 Via Natural or Artificial Opening 8 Via Natural or Artificial Opening Endoscopic	D Intraluminal Device Z No Device	Z No Qualifier
D Urethra	X External	Z No Device	Z No Qualifier

Section   0   Medical and Surgical
Body System   T   Urinary System
Operation   W   **Revision:** Correcting, to the extent possible, a portion of a malfunctioning device or the position of a displaced device

Body Part (4th)	Approach (5th)	Device (6th)	Qualifier (7th)
5 Kidney	0 Open 3 Percutaneous 4 Percutaneous Endoscopic 7 Via Natural or Artificial Opening 8 Via Natural or Artificial Opening Endoscopic	0 Drainage Device 2 Monitoring Device 3 Infusion Device 7 Autologous Tissue Substitute C Extraluminal Device D Intraluminal Device J Synthetic Substitute K Nonautologous Tissue Substitute Y Other Device	Z No Qualifier

Continued →

Section	0	Medical and Surgical
Body System	T	Urinary System
Operation	W	**Revision:** Correcting, to the extent possible, a portion of a malfunctioning device or the position of a displaced device

Body Part (4th)	Approach (5th)	Device (6th)	Qualifier (7th)
5 Kidney	X External	0 Drainage Device 2 Monitoring Device 3 Infusion Device 7 Autologous Tissue Substitute C Extraluminal Device D Intraluminal Device J Synthetic Substitute K Nonautologous Tissue Substitute	Z No Qualifier
9 Ureter	0 Open 3 Percutaneous 4 Percutaneous Endoscopic 7 Via Natural or Artificial Opening 8 Via Natural or Artificial Opening Endoscopic	0 Drainage Device 2 Monitoring Device 3 Infusion Device 7 Autologous Tissue Substitute C Extraluminal Device D Intraluminal Device J Synthetic Substitute K Nonautologous Tissue Substitute M Stimulator Lead Y Other Device	Z No Qualifier
9 Ureter	X External	0 Drainage Device 2 Monitoring Device 3 Infusion Device 7 Autologous Tissue Substitute C Extraluminal Device D Intraluminal Device J Synthetic Substitute K Nonautologous Tissue Substitute M Stimulator Lead	Z No Qualifier
B Bladder	0 Open 3 Percutaneous 4 Percutaneous Endoscopic 7 Via Natural or Artificial Opening 8 Via Natural or Artificial Opening Endoscopic	0 Drainage Device 2 Monitoring Device 3 Infusion Device 7 Autologous Tissue Substitute C Extraluminal Device D Intraluminal Device J Synthetic Substitute K Nonautologous Tissue Substitute L Artificial Sphincter M Stimulator Lead Y Other Device	Z No Qualifier
B Bladder	X External	0 Drainage Device 2 Monitoring Device 3 Infusion Device 7 Autologous Tissue Substitute C Extraluminal Device D Intraluminal Device J Synthetic Substitute K Nonautologous Tissue Substitute L Artificial Sphincter M Stimulator Lead	Z No Qualifier
D Urethra	0 Open 3 Percutaneous 4 Percutaneous Endoscopic 7 Via Natural or Artificial Opening 8 Via Natural or Artificial Opening Endoscopic	0 Drainage Device 2 Monitoring Device 3 Infusion Device 7 Autologous Tissue Substitute C Extraluminal Device D Intraluminal Device J Synthetic Substitute K Nonautologous Tissue Substitute L Artificial Sphincter Y Other Device	Z No Qualifier

Continued →

Section	0	Medical and Surgical
Body System	T	Urinary System
Operation	W	Revision: Correcting, to the extent possible, a portion of a malfunctioning device or the position of a displaced device

Body Part (4th)	Approach (5th)	Device (6th)	Qualifier (7th)
D Urethra	X External	0 Drainage Device 2 Monitoring Device 3 Infusion Device 7 Autologous Tissue Substitute C Extraluminal Device D Intraluminal Device J Synthetic Substitute K Nonautologous Tissue Substitute L Artificial Sphincter	Z No Qualifier

Section	0	Medical and Surgical
Body System	T	Urinary System
Operation	Y	Transplantation: Putting in or on all or a portion of a living body part taken from another individual or animal to physically take the place and/or function of all or a portion of a similar body part

Body Part (4th)	Approach (5th)	Device (6th)	Qualifier (7th)
0 Kidney, Right 1 Kidney, Left	0 Open	Z No Device	0 Allogeneic 1 Syngeneic 2 Zooplastic

Urinary System Code Listing 0T1–0TY

0T1 – Urinary System, Bypass

Review Coding Guideline B3.6a

0T13073 Bypass Right Kidney Pelvis to Right Kidney Pelvis with Autologous Tissue Substitute, Open Approach

0T13074 Bypass Right Kidney Pelvis to Left Kidney Pelvis with Autologous Tissue Substitute, Open Approach

0T13076 Bypass Right Kidney Pelvis to Right Ureter with Autologous Tissue Substitute, Open Approach

0T13077 Bypass Right Kidney Pelvis to Left Ureter with Autologous Tissue Substitute, Open Approach

0T13078 Bypass Right Kidney Pelvis to Colon with Autologous Tissue Substitute, Open Approach

0T13079 Bypass Right Kidney Pelvis to Colocutaneous with Autologous Tissue Substitute, Open Approach

0T1307A Bypass Right Kidney Pelvis to Ileum with Autologous Tissue Substitute, Open Approach

0T1307B Bypass Right Kidney Pelvis to Bladder with Autologous Tissue Substitute, Open Approach

0T1307C Bypass Right Kidney Pelvis to Ileocutaneous with Autologous Tissue Substitute, Open Approach

0T1307D Bypass Right Kidney Pelvis to Cutaneous with Autologous Tissue Substitute, Open Approach

0T130J3 Bypass Right Kidney Pelvis to Right Kidney Pelvis with Synthetic Substitute, Open Approach

0T130J4 Bypass Right Kidney Pelvis to Left Kidney Pelvis with Synthetic Substitute, Open Approach

0T130J6 Bypass Right Kidney Pelvis to Right Ureter with Synthetic Substitute, Open Approach

0T130J7 Bypass Right Kidney Pelvis to Left Ureter with Synthetic Substitute, Open Approach

0T130J8 Bypass Right Kidney Pelvis to Colon with Synthetic Substitute, Open Approach

0T130J9 Bypass Right Kidney Pelvis to Colocutaneous with Synthetic Substitute, Open Approach

0T130JA Bypass Right Kidney Pelvis to Ileum with Synthetic Substitute, Open Approach

0T130JB Bypass Right Kidney Pelvis to Bladder with Synthetic Substitute, Open Approach

0T130JC Bypass Right Kidney Pelvis to Ileocutaneous with Synthetic Substitute, Open Approach

0T130JD Bypass Right Kidney Pelvis to Cutaneous with Synthetic Substitute, Open Approach

0T130K3 Bypass Right Kidney Pelvis to Right Kidney Pelvis with Nonautologous Tissue Substitute, Open Approach

0T130K4 Bypass Right Kidney Pelvis to Left Kidney Pelvis with Nonautologous Tissue Substitute, Open Approach

0T130K6 Bypass Right Kidney Pelvis to Right Ureter with Nonautologous Tissue Substitute, Open Approach

0T130K7 Bypass Right Kidney Pelvis to Left Ureter with Nonautologous Tissue Substitute, Open Approach

0T130K8 Bypass Right Kidney Pelvis to Colon with Nonautologous Tissue Substitute, Open Approach

0T130K9 Bypass Right Kidney Pelvis to Colocutaneous with Nonautologous Tissue Substitute, Open Approach

0T130KA Bypass Right Kidney Pelvis to Ileum with Nonautologous Tissue Substitute, Open Approach

0T130KB Bypass Right Kidney Pelvis to Bladder with Nonautologous Tissue Substitute, Open Approach

0T130KC Bypass Right Kidney Pelvis to Ileocutaneous with Nonautologous Tissue Substitute, Open Approach

0T130KD Bypass Right Kidney Pelvis to Cutaneous with Nonautologous Tissue Substitute, Open Approach

0T130Z3 Bypass Right Kidney Pelvis to Right Kidney Pelvis, Open Approach

0T130Z4 Bypass Right Kidney Pelvis to Left Kidney Pelvis, Open Approach

0T130Z6 Bypass Right Kidney Pelvis to Right Ureter, Open Approach

0T130Z7 Bypass Right Kidney Pelvis to Left Ureter, Open Approach

0T130Z8 Bypass Right Kidney Pelvis to Colon, Open Approach

0T130Z9 Bypass Right Kidney Pelvis to Colocutaneous, Open Approach

0T130ZA Bypass Right Kidney Pelvis to Ileum, Open Approach

0T130ZB Bypass Right Kidney Pelvis to Bladder, Open Approach

0T130ZC Bypass Right Kidney Pelvis to Ileocutaneous, Open Approach

0T130ZD Bypass Right Kidney Pelvis to Cutaneous, Open Approach

0T133JD Bypass Right Kidney Pelvis to Cutaneous with Synthetic Substitute, Percutaneous Approach

0T13473 Bypass Right Kidney Pelvis to Right Kidney Pelvis with Autologous Tissue Substitute, Percutaneous Endoscopic Approach

♀ Female-only   ♂ Male-only   ▲ Limited Coverage   ● Non-OR   HAC HAC-associated procedure   ▲ Non-covered procedures   ✚ Cluster

0T13474	Bypass Right Kidney Pelvis to Left Kidney Pelvis with Autologous Tissue Substitute, Percutaneous Endoscopic Approach
0T13476	Bypass Right Kidney Pelvis to Right Ureter with Autologous Tissue Substitute, Percutaneous Endoscopic Approach
0T13477	Bypass Right Kidney Pelvis to Left Ureter with Autologous Tissue Substitute, Percutaneous Endoscopic Approach
0T13478	Bypass Right Kidney Pelvis to Colon with Autologous Tissue Substitute, Percutaneous Endoscopic Approach
0T13479	Bypass Right Kidney Pelvis to Colocutaneous with Autologous Tissue Substitute, Percutaneous Endoscopic Approach
0T1347A	Bypass Right Kidney Pelvis to Ileum with Autologous Tissue Substitute, Percutaneous Endoscopic Approach
0T1347B	Bypass Right Kidney Pelvis to Bladder with Autologous Tissue Substitute, Percutaneous Endoscopic Approach
0T1347C	Bypass Right Kidney Pelvis to Ileocutaneous with Autologous Tissue Substitute, Percutaneous Endoscopic Approach
0T1347D	Bypass Right Kidney Pelvis to Cutaneous with Autologous Tissue Substitute, Percutaneous Endoscopic Approach
0T134J3	Bypass Right Kidney Pelvis to Right Kidney Pelvis with Synthetic Substitute, Percutaneous Endoscopic Approach
0T134J4	Bypass Right Kidney Pelvis to Left Kidney Pelvis with Synthetic Substitute, Percutaneous Endoscopic Approach
0T134J6	Bypass Right Kidney Pelvis to Right Ureter with Synthetic Substitute, Percutaneous Endoscopic Approach
0T134J7	Bypass Right Kidney Pelvis to Left Ureter with Synthetic Substitute, Percutaneous Endoscopic Approach
0T134J8	Bypass Right Kidney Pelvis to Colon with Synthetic Substitute, Percutaneous Endoscopic Approach
0T134J9	Bypass Right Kidney Pelvis to Colocutaneous with Synthetic Substitute, Percutaneous Endoscopic Approach
0T134JA	Bypass Right Kidney Pelvis to Ileum with Synthetic Substitute, Percutaneous Endoscopic Approach
0T134JB	Bypass Right Kidney Pelvis to Bladder with Synthetic Substitute, Percutaneous Endoscopic Approach
0T134JC	Bypass Right Kidney Pelvis to Ileocutaneous with Synthetic Substitute, Percutaneous Endoscopic Approach
0T134JD	Bypass Right Kidney Pelvis to Cutaneous with Synthetic Substitute, Percutaneous Endoscopic Approach
0T134K3	Bypass Right Kidney Pelvis to Right Kidney Pelvis with Nonautologous Tissue Substitute, Percutaneous Endoscopic Approach
0T134K4	Bypass Right Kidney Pelvis to Left Kidney Pelvis with Nonautologous Tissue Substitute, Percutaneous Endoscopic Approach
0T134K6	Bypass Right Kidney Pelvis to Right Ureter with Nonautologous Tissue Substitute, Percutaneous Endoscopic Approach
0T134K7	Bypass Right Kidney Pelvis to Left Ureter with Nonautologous Tissue Substitute, Percutaneous Endoscopic Approach
0T134K8	Bypass Right Kidney Pelvis to Colon with Nonautologous Tissue Substitute, Percutaneous Endoscopic Approach
0T134K9	Bypass Right Kidney Pelvis to Colocutaneous with Nonautologous Tissue Substitute, Percutaneous Endoscopic Approach
0T134KA	Bypass Right Kidney Pelvis to Ileum with Nonautologous Tissue Substitute, Percutaneous Endoscopic Approach
0T134KB	Bypass Right Kidney Pelvis to Bladder with Nonautologous Tissue Substitute, Percutaneous Endoscopic Approach
0T134KC	Bypass Right Kidney Pelvis to Ileocutaneous with Nonautologous Tissue Substitute, Percutaneous Endoscopic Approach
0T134KD	Bypass Right Kidney Pelvis to Cutaneous with Nonautologous Tissue Substitute, Percutaneous Endoscopic Approach
0T134Z3	Bypass Right Kidney Pelvis to Right Kidney Pelvis, Percutaneous Endoscopic Approach
0T134Z4	Bypass Right Kidney Pelvis to Left Kidney Pelvis, Percutaneous Endoscopic Approach
0T134Z6	Bypass Right Kidney Pelvis to Right Ureter, Percutaneous Endoscopic Approach
0T134Z7	Bypass Right Kidney Pelvis to Left Ureter, Percutaneous Endoscopic Approach
0T134Z8	Bypass Right Kidney Pelvis to Colon, Percutaneous Endoscopic Approach
0T134Z9	Bypass Right Kidney Pelvis to Colocutaneous, Percutaneous Endoscopic Approach
0T134ZA	Bypass Right Kidney Pelvis to Ileum, Percutaneous Endoscopic Approach
0T134ZB	Bypass Right Kidney Pelvis to Bladder, Percutaneous Endoscopic Approach
0T134ZC	Bypass Right Kidney Pelvis to Ileocutaneous, Percutaneous Endoscopic Approach
0T134ZD	Bypass Right Kidney Pelvis to Cutaneous, Percutaneous Endoscopic Approach
0T14073	Bypass Left Kidney Pelvis to Right Kidney Pelvis with Autologous Tissue Substitute, Open Approach
0T14074	Bypass Left Kidney Pelvis to Left Kidney Pelvis with Autologous Tissue Substitute, Open Approach
0T14076	Bypass Left Kidney Pelvis to Right Ureter with Autologous Tissue Substitute, Open Approach
0T14077	Bypass Left Kidney Pelvis to Left Ureter with Autologous Tissue Substitute, Open Approach
0T14078	Bypass Left Kidney Pelvis to Colon with Autologous Tissue Substitute, Open Approach
0T14079	Bypass Left Kidney Pelvis to Colocutaneous with Autologous Tissue Substitute, Open Approach
0T1407A	Bypass Left Kidney Pelvis to Ileum with Autologous Tissue Substitute, Open Approach
0T1407B	Bypass Left Kidney Pelvis to Bladder with Autologous Tissue Substitute, Open Approach
0T1407C	Bypass Left Kidney Pelvis to Ileocutaneous with Autologous Tissue Substitute, Open Approach
0T1407D	Bypass Left Kidney Pelvis to Cutaneous with Autologous Tissue Substitute, Open Approach
0T140J3	Bypass Left Kidney Pelvis to Right Kidney Pelvis with Synthetic Substitute, Open Approach
0T140J4	Bypass Left Kidney Pelvis to Left Kidney Pelvis with Synthetic Substitute, Open Approach
0T140J6	Bypass Left Kidney Pelvis to Right Ureter with Synthetic Substitute, Open Approach
0T140J7	Bypass Left Kidney Pelvis to Left Ureter with Synthetic Substitute, Open Approach
0T140J8	Bypass Left Kidney Pelvis to Colon with Synthetic Substitute, Open Approach
0T140J9	Bypass Left Kidney Pelvis to Colocutaneous with Synthetic Substitute, Open Approach
0T140JA	Bypass Left Kidney Pelvis to Ileum with Synthetic Substitute, Open Approach
0T140JB	Bypass Left Kidney Pelvis to Bladder with Synthetic Substitute, Open Approach
0T140JC	Bypass Left Kidney Pelvis to Ileocutaneous with Synthetic Substitute, Open Approach
0T140JD	Bypass Left Kidney Pelvis to Cutaneous with Synthetic Substitute, Open Approach
0T140K3	Bypass Left Kidney Pelvis to Right Kidney Pelvis with Nonautologous Tissue Substitute, Open Approach
0T140K4	Bypass Left Kidney Pelvis to Left Kidney Pelvis with Nonautologous Tissue Substitute, Open Approach
0T140K6	Bypass Left Kidney Pelvis to Right Ureter with Nonautologous Tissue Substitute, Open Approach
0T140K7	Bypass Left Kidney Pelvis to Left Ureter with Nonautologous Tissue Substitute, Open Approach
0T140K8	Bypass Left Kidney Pelvis to Colon with Nonautologous Tissue Substitute, Open Approach
0T140K9	Bypass Left Kidney Pelvis to Colocutaneous with Nonautologous Tissue Substitute, Open Approach
0T140KA	Bypass Left Kidney Pelvis to Ileum with Nonautologous Tissue Substitute, Open Approach
0T140KB	Bypass Left Kidney Pelvis to Bladder with Nonautologous Tissue Substitute, Open Approach
0T140KC	Bypass Left Kidney Pelvis to Ileocutaneous with Nonautologous Tissue Substitute, Open Approach
0T140KD	Bypass Left Kidney Pelvis to Cutaneous with Nonautologous Tissue Substitute, Open Approach
0T140Z3	Bypass Left Kidney Pelvis to Right Kidney Pelvis, Open Approach
0T140Z4	Bypass Left Kidney Pelvis to Left Kidney Pelvis, Open Approach

0T140Z6 Bypass Left Kidney Pelvis to Right Ureter, Open Approach

0T140Z7 Bypass Left Kidney Pelvis to Left Ureter, Open Approach

0T140Z8 Bypass Left Kidney Pelvis to Colon, Open Approach

0T140Z9 Bypass Left Kidney Pelvis to Colocutaneous, Open Approach

0T140ZA Bypass Left Kidney Pelvis to Ileum, Open Approach

0T140ZB Bypass Left Kidney Pelvis to Bladder, Open Approach

0T140ZC Bypass Left Kidney Pelvis to Ileocutaneous, Open Approach

0T140ZD Bypass Left Kidney Pelvis to Cutaneous, Open Approach

0T143JD Bypass Left Kidney Pelvis to Cutaneous with Synthetic Substitute, Percutaneous Approach

0T14473 Bypass Left Kidney Pelvis to Right Kidney Pelvis with Autologous Tissue Substitute, Percutaneous Endoscopic Approach

0T14474 Bypass Left Kidney Pelvis to Left Kidney Pelvis with Autologous Tissue Substitute, Percutaneous Endoscopic Approach

0T14476 Bypass Left Kidney Pelvis to Right Ureter with Autologous Tissue Substitute, Percutaneous Endoscopic Approach

0T14477 Bypass Left Kidney Pelvis to Left Ureter with Autologous Tissue Substitute, Percutaneous Endoscopic Approach

0T14478 Bypass Left Kidney Pelvis to Colon with Autologous Tissue Substitute, Percutaneous Endoscopic Approach

0T14479 Bypass Left Kidney Pelvis to Colocutaneous with Autologous Tissue Substitute, Percutaneous Endoscopic Approach

0T1447A Bypass Left Kidney Pelvis to Ileum with Autologous Tissue Substitute, Percutaneous Endoscopic Approach

0T1447B Bypass Left Kidney Pelvis to Bladder with Autologous Tissue Substitute, Percutaneous Endoscopic Approach

0T1447C Bypass Left Kidney Pelvis to Ileocutaneous with Autologous Tissue Substitute, Percutaneous Endoscopic Approach

0T1447D Bypass Left Kidney Pelvis to Cutaneous with Autologous Tissue Substitute, Percutaneous Endoscopic Approach

0T144J3 Bypass Left Kidney Pelvis to Right Kidney Pelvis with Synthetic Substitute, Percutaneous Endoscopic Approach

0T144J4 Bypass Left Kidney Pelvis to Left Kidney Pelvis with Synthetic Substitute, Percutaneous Endoscopic Approach

0T144J6 Bypass Left Kidney Pelvis to Right Ureter with Synthetic Substitute, Percutaneous Endoscopic Approach

0T144J7 Bypass Left Kidney Pelvis to Left Ureter with Synthetic Substitute, Percutaneous Endoscopic Approach

0T144J8 Bypass Left Kidney Pelvis to Colon with Synthetic Substitute, Percutaneous Endoscopic Approach

0T144J9 Bypass Left Kidney Pelvis to Colocutaneous with Synthetic Substitute, Percutaneous Endoscopic Approach

0T144JA Bypass Left Kidney Pelvis to Ileum with Synthetic Substitute, Percutaneous Endoscopic Approach

0T144JB Bypass Left Kidney Pelvis to Bladder with Synthetic Substitute, Percutaneous Endoscopic Approach

0T144JC Bypass Left Kidney Pelvis to Ileocutaneous with Synthetic Substitute, Percutaneous Endoscopic Approach

0T144JD Bypass Left Kidney Pelvis to Cutaneous with Synthetic Substitute, Percutaneous Endoscopic Approach

0T144K3 Bypass Left Kidney Pelvis to Right Kidney Pelvis with Nonautologous Tissue Substitute, Percutaneous Endoscopic Approach

0T144K4 Bypass Left Kidney Pelvis to Left Kidney Pelvis with Nonautologous Tissue Substitute, Percutaneous Endoscopic Approach

0T144K6 Bypass Left Kidney Pelvis to Right Ureter with Nonautologous Tissue Substitute, Percutaneous Endoscopic Approach

0T144K7 Bypass Left Kidney Pelvis to Left Ureter with Nonautologous Tissue Substitute, Percutaneous Endoscopic Approach

0T144K8 Bypass Left Kidney Pelvis to Colon with Nonautologous Tissue Substitute, Percutaneous Endoscopic Approach

0T144K9 Bypass Left Kidney Pelvis to Colocutaneous with Nonautologous Tissue Substitute, Percutaneous Endoscopic Approach

0T144KA Bypass Left Kidney Pelvis to Ileum with Nonautologous Tissue Substitute, Percutaneous Endoscopic Approach

0T144KB Bypass Left Kidney Pelvis to Bladder with Nonautologous Tissue Substitute, Percutaneous Endoscopic Approach

0T144KC Bypass Left Kidney Pelvis to Ileocutaneous with Nonautologous Tissue Substitute, Percutaneous Endoscopic Approach

0T144KD Bypass Left Kidney Pelvis to Cutaneous with Nonautologous Tissue Substitute, Percutaneous Endoscopic Approach

0T144Z3 Bypass Left Kidney Pelvis to Right Kidney Pelvis, Percutaneous Endoscopic Approach

0T144Z4 Bypass Left Kidney Pelvis to Left Kidney Pelvis, Percutaneous Endoscopic Approach

0T144Z6 Bypass Left Kidney Pelvis to Right Ureter, Percutaneous Endoscopic Approach

0T144Z7 Bypass Left Kidney Pelvis to Left Ureter, Percutaneous Endoscopic Approach

0T144Z8 Bypass Left Kidney Pelvis to Colon, Percutaneous Endoscopic Approach

0T144Z9 Bypass Left Kidney Pelvis to Colocutaneous, Percutaneous Endoscopic Approach

0T144ZA Bypass Left Kidney Pelvis to Ileum, Percutaneous Endoscopic Approach

0T144ZB Bypass Left Kidney Pelvis to Bladder, Percutaneous Endoscopic Approach

0T144ZC Bypass Left Kidney Pelvis to Ileocutaneous, Percutaneous Endoscopic Approach

0T144ZD Bypass Left Kidney Pelvis to Cutaneous, Percutaneous Endoscopic Approach

0T16076 Bypass Right Ureter to Right Ureter with Autologous Tissue Substitute, Open Approach

0T16077 Bypass Right Ureter to Left Ureter with Autologous Tissue Substitute, Open Approach

0T16078 Bypass Right Ureter to Colon with Autologous Tissue Substitute, Open Approach

0T16079 Bypass Right Ureter to Colocutaneous with Autologous Tissue Substitute, Open Approach

0T1607A Bypass Right Ureter to Ileum with Autologous Tissue Substitute, Open Approach

0T1607B Bypass Right Ureter to Bladder with Autologous Tissue Substitute, Open Approach

0T1607C Bypass Right Ureter to Ileocutaneous with Autologous Tissue Substitute, Open Approach

0T1607D Bypass Right Ureter to Cutaneous with Autologous Tissue Substitute, Open Approach

0T160J6 Bypass Right Ureter to Right Ureter with Synthetic Substitute, Open Approach

0T160J7 Bypass Right Ureter to Left Ureter with Synthetic Substitute, Open Approach

0T160J8 Bypass Right Ureter to Colon with Synthetic Substitute, Open Approach

0T160J9 Bypass Right Ureter to Colocutaneous with Synthetic Substitute, Open Approach

0T160JA Bypass Right Ureter to Ileum with Synthetic Substitute, Open Approach

0T160JB Bypass Right Ureter to Bladder with Synthetic Substitute, Open Approach

0T160JC Bypass Right Ureter to Ileocutaneous with Synthetic Substitute, Open Approach

0T160JD Bypass Right Ureter to Cutaneous with Synthetic Substitute, Open Approach

0T160K6 Bypass Right Ureter to Right Ureter with Nonautologous Tissue Substitute, Open Approach

0T160K7 Bypass Right Ureter to Left Ureter with Nonautologous Tissue Substitute, Open Approach

0T160K8 Bypass Right Ureter to Colon with Nonautologous Tissue Substitute, Open Approach

0T160K9 Bypass Right Ureter to Colocutaneous with Nonautologous Tissue Substitute, Open Approach

0T160KA Bypass Right Ureter to Ileum with Nonautologous Tissue Substitute, Open Approach

0T160KB Bypass Right Ureter to Bladder with Nonautologous Tissue Substitute, Open Approach

0T160KC Bypass Right Ureter to Ileocutaneous with Nonautologous Tissue Substitute, Open Approach

0T160KD Bypass Right Ureter to Cutaneous with Nonautologous Tissue Substitute, Open Approach

0T160Z6 Bypass Right Ureter to Right Ureter, Open Approach

0T160Z7 Bypass Right Ureter to Left Ureter, Open Approach

♀ Female-only   ♂ Male-only   ▲ Limited Coverage   ● Non-OR   ᴴᴬᶜ HAC-associated procedure   ▲ Non-covered procedures   ✚ Cluster

0T160Z8 Bypass Right Ureter to Colon, Open Approach

0T160Z9 Bypass Right Ureter to Colocutaneous, Open Approach

0T160ZA Bypass Right Ureter to Ileum, Open Approach

0T160ZB Bypass Right Ureter to Bladder, Open Approach

0T160ZC Bypass Right Ureter to Ileocutaneous, Open Approach

0T160ZD Bypass Right Ureter to Cutaneous, Open Approach

0T163JD Bypass Right Ureter to Cutaneous with Synthetic Substitute, Percutaneous Approach

0T16476 Bypass Right Ureter to Right Ureter with Autologous Tissue Substitute, Percutaneous Endoscopic Approach

0T16477 Bypass Right Ureter to Left Ureter with Autologous Tissue Substitute, Percutaneous Endoscopic Approach

0T16478 Bypass Right Ureter to Colon with Autologous Tissue Substitute, Percutaneous Endoscopic Approach

0T16479 Bypass Right Ureter to Colocutaneous with Autologous Tissue Substitute, Percutaneous Endoscopic Approach

0T1647A Bypass Right Ureter to Ileum with Autologous Tissue Substitute, Percutaneous Endoscopic Approach

0T1647B Bypass Right Ureter to Bladder with Autologous Tissue Substitute, Percutaneous Endoscopic Approach

0T1647C Bypass Right Ureter to Ileocutaneous with Autologous Tissue Substitute, Percutaneous Endoscopic Approach

0T1647D Bypass Right Ureter to Cutaneous with Autologous Tissue Substitute, Percutaneous Endoscopic Approach

0T164J6 Bypass Right Ureter to Right Ureter with Synthetic Substitute, Percutaneous Endoscopic Approach

0T164J7 Bypass Right Ureter to Left Ureter with Synthetic Substitute, Percutaneous Endoscopic Approach

0T164J8 Bypass Right Ureter to Colon with Synthetic Substitute, Percutaneous Endoscopic Approach

0T164J9 Bypass Right Ureter to Colocutaneous with Synthetic Substitute, Percutaneous Endoscopic Approach

0T164JA Bypass Right Ureter to Ileum with Synthetic Substitute, Percutaneous Endoscopic Approach

0T164JB Bypass Right Ureter to Bladder with Synthetic Substitute, Percutaneous Endoscopic Approach

0T164JC Bypass Right Ureter to Ileocutaneous with Synthetic Substitute, Percutaneous Endoscopic Approach

0T164JD Bypass Right Ureter to Cutaneous with Synthetic Substitute, Percutaneous Endoscopic Approach

0T164K6 Bypass Right Ureter to Right Ureter with Nonautologous Tissue Substitute, Percutaneous Endoscopic Approach

0T164K7 Bypass Right Ureter to Left Ureter with Nonautologous Tissue Substitute, Percutaneous Endoscopic Approach

0T164K8 Bypass Right Ureter to Colon with Nonautologous Tissue Substitute, Percutaneous Endoscopic Approach

0T164K9 Bypass Right Ureter to Colocutaneous with Nonautologous Tissue Substitute, Percutaneous Endoscopic Approach

0T164KA Bypass Right Ureter to Ileum with Nonautologous Tissue Substitute, Percutaneous Endoscopic Approach

0T164KB Bypass Right Ureter to Bladder with Nonautologous Tissue Substitute, Percutaneous Endoscopic Approach

0T164KC Bypass Right Ureter to Ileocutaneous with Nonautologous Tissue Substitute, Percutaneous Endoscopic Approach

0T164KD Bypass Right Ureter to Cutaneous with Nonautologous Tissue Substitute, Percutaneous Endoscopic Approach

0T164Z6 Bypass Right Ureter to Right Ureter, Percutaneous Endoscopic Approach

0T164Z7 Bypass Right Ureter to Left Ureter, Percutaneous Endoscopic Approach

0T164Z8 Bypass Right Ureter to Colon, Percutaneous Endoscopic Approach

0T164Z9 Bypass Right Ureter to Colocutaneous, Percutaneous Endoscopic Approach

0T164ZA Bypass Right Ureter to Ileum, Percutaneous Endoscopic Approach

0T164ZB Bypass Right Ureter to Bladder, Percutaneous Endoscopic Approach

0T164ZC Bypass Right Ureter to Ileocutaneous, Percutaneous Endoscopic Approach

0T164ZD Bypass Right Ureter to Cutaneous, Percutaneous Endoscopic Approach

0T17076 Bypass Left Ureter to Right Ureter with Autologous Tissue Substitute, Open Approach

0T17077 Bypass Left Ureter to Left Ureter with Autologous Tissue Substitute, Open Approach

0T17078 Bypass Left Ureter to Colon with Autologous Tissue Substitute, Open Approach

0T17079 Bypass Left Ureter to Colocutaneous with Autologous Tissue Substitute, Open Approach

0T1707A Bypass Left Ureter to Ileum with Autologous Tissue Substitute, Open Approach

0T1707B Bypass Left Ureter to Bladder with Autologous Tissue Substitute, Open Approach

0T1707C Bypass Left Ureter to Ileocutaneous with Autologous Tissue Substitute, Open Approach

0T1707D Bypass Left Ureter to Cutaneous with Autologous Tissue Substitute, Open Approach

0T170J6 Bypass Left Ureter to Right Ureter with Synthetic Substitute, Open Approach

0T170J7 Bypass Left Ureter to Left Ureter with Synthetic Substitute, Open Approach

0T170J8 Bypass Left Ureter to Colon with Synthetic Substitute, Open Approach

0T170J9 Bypass Left Ureter to Colocutaneous with Synthetic Substitute, Open Approach

0T170JA Bypass Left Ureter to Ileum with Synthetic Substitute, Open Approach

0T170JB Bypass Left Ureter to Bladder with Synthetic Substitute, Open Approach

0T170JC Bypass Left Ureter to Ileocutaneous with Synthetic Substitute, Open Approach

0T170JD Bypass Left Ureter to Cutaneous with Synthetic Substitute, Open Approach

0T170K6 Bypass Left Ureter to Right Ureter with Nonautologous Tissue Substitute, Open Approach

0T170K7 Bypass Left Ureter to Left Ureter with Nonautologous Tissue Substitute, Open Approach

0T170K8 Bypass Left Ureter to Colon with Nonautologous Tissue Substitute, Open Approach

0T170K9 Bypass Left Ureter to Colocutaneous with Nonautologous Tissue Substitute, Open Approach

0T170KA Bypass Left Ureter to Ileum with Nonautologous Tissue Substitute, Open Approach

0T170KB Bypass Left Ureter to Bladder with Nonautologous Tissue Substitute, Open Approach

0T170KC Bypass Left Ureter to Ileocutaneous with Nonautologous Tissue Substitute, Open Approach

0T170KD Bypass Left Ureter to Cutaneous with Nonautologous Tissue Substitute, Open Approach

0T170Z6 Bypass Left Ureter to Right Ureter, Open Approach

0T170Z7 Bypass Left Ureter to Left Ureter, Open Approach

0T170Z8 Bypass Left Ureter to Colon, Open Approach

0T170Z9 Bypass Left Ureter to Colocutaneous, Open Approach

0T170ZA Bypass Left Ureter to Ileum, Open Approach

0T170ZB Bypass Left Ureter to Bladder, Open Approach

AHA CC: 3Q, 2015, 34-35

0T170ZC Bypass Left Ureter to Ileocutaneous, Open Approach

0T170ZD Bypass Left Ureter to Cutaneous, Open Approach

0T173JD Bypass Left Ureter to Cutaneous with Synthetic Substitute, Percutaneous Approach

0T17476 Bypass Left Ureter to Right Ureter with Autologous Tissue Substitute, Percutaneous Endoscopic Approach

0T17477 Bypass Left Ureter to Left Ureter with Autologous Tissue Substitute, Percutaneous Endoscopic Approach

0T17478 Bypass Left Ureter to Colon with Autologous Tissue Substitute, Percutaneous Endoscopic Approach

0T17479 Bypass Left Ureter to Colocutaneous with Autologous Tissue Substitute, Percutaneous Endoscopic Approach

0T1747A Bypass Left Ureter to Ileum with Autologous Tissue Substitute, Percutaneous Endoscopic Approach

0T1747B Bypass Left Ureter to Bladder with Autologous Tissue Substitute, Percutaneous Endoscopic Approach

0T1747C Bypass Left Ureter to Ileocutaneous with Autologous Tissue Substitute, Percutaneous Endoscopic Approach

0T1747D Bypass Left Ureter to Cutaneous with Autologous Tissue Substitute, Percutaneous Endoscopic Approach

0T174J6 Bypass Left Ureter to Right Ureter with Synthetic Substitute, Percutaneous Endoscopic Approach

0T174J7 Bypass Left Ureter to Left Ureter with Synthetic Substitute, Percutaneous Endoscopic Approach

0T174J8 Bypass Left Ureter to Colon with Synthetic Substitute, Percutaneous Endoscopic Approach

0T174J9 Bypass Left Ureter to Colocutaneous with Synthetic Substitute, Percutaneous Endoscopic Approach

0T174JA Bypass Left Ureter to Ileum with Synthetic Substitute, Percutaneous Endoscopic Approach

0T174JB Bypass Left Ureter to Bladder with Synthetic Substitute, Percutaneous Endoscopic Approach

0T174JC Bypass Left Ureter to Ileocutaneous with Synthetic Substitute, Percutaneous Endoscopic Approach

0T174JD Bypass Left Ureter to Cutaneous with Synthetic Substitute, Percutaneous Endoscopic Approach

0T174K6 Bypass Left Ureter to Right Ureter with Nonautologous Tissue Substitute, Percutaneous Endoscopic Approach

0T174K7 Bypass Left Ureter to Left Ureter with Nonautologous Tissue Substitute, Percutaneous Endoscopic Approach

0T174K8 Bypass Left Ureter to Colon with Nonautologous Tissue Substitute, Percutaneous Endoscopic Approach

0T174K9 Bypass Left Ureter to Colocutaneous with Nonautologous Tissue Substitute, Percutaneous Endoscopic Approach

0T174KA Bypass Left Ureter to Ileum with Nonautologous Tissue Substitute, Percutaneous Endoscopic Approach

0T174KB Bypass Left Ureter to Bladder with Nonautologous Tissue Substitute, Percutaneous Endoscopic Approach

0T174KC Bypass Left Ureter to Ileocutaneous with Nonautologous Tissue Substitute, Percutaneous Endoscopic Approach

0T174KD Bypass Left Ureter to Cutaneous with Nonautologous Tissue Substitute, Percutaneous Endoscopic Approach

0T174Z6 Bypass Left Ureter to Right Ureter, Percutaneous Endoscopic Approach

0T174Z7 Bypass Left Ureter to Left Ureter, Percutaneous Endoscopic Approach

0T174Z8 Bypass Left Ureter to Colon, Percutaneous Endoscopic Approach

0T174Z9 Bypass Left Ureter to Colocutaneous, Percutaneous Endoscopic Approach

0T174ZA Bypass Left Ureter to Ileum, Percutaneous Endoscopic Approach

0T174ZB Bypass Left Ureter to Bladder, Percutaneous Endoscopic Approach

0T174ZC Bypass Left Ureter to Ileocutaneous, Percutaneous Endoscopic Approach

0T174ZD Bypass Left Ureter to Cutaneous, Percutaneous Endoscopic Approach

0T18076 Bypass Bilateral Ureters to Right Ureter with Autologous Tissue Substitute, Open Approach

0T18077 Bypass Bilateral Ureters to Left Ureter with Autologous Tissue Substitute, Open Approach

0T18078 Bypass Bilateral Ureters to Colon with Autologous Tissue Substitute, Open Approach

0T18079 Bypass Bilateral Ureters to Colocutaneous with Autologous Tissue Substitute, Open Approach

0T1807A Bypass Bilateral Ureters to Ileum with Autologous Tissue Substitute, Open Approach

0T1807B Bypass Bilateral Ureters to Bladder with Autologous Tissue Substitute, Open Approach

0T1807C Bypass Bilateral Ureters to Ileocutaneous with Autologous Tissue Substitute, Open Approach

0T1807D Bypass Bilateral Ureters to Cutaneous with Autologous Tissue Substitute, Open Approach

0T180J6 Bypass Bilateral Ureters to Right Ureter with Synthetic Substitute, Open Approach

0T180J7 Bypass Bilateral Ureters to Left Ureter with Synthetic Substitute, Open Approach

0T180J8 Bypass Bilateral Ureters to Colon with Synthetic Substitute, Open Approach

0T180J9 Bypass Bilateral Ureters to Colocutaneous with Synthetic Substitute, Open Approach

0T180JA Bypass Bilateral Ureters to Ileum with Synthetic Substitute, Open Approach

0T180JB Bypass Bilateral Ureters to Bladder with Synthetic Substitute, Open Approach

0T180JC Bypass Bilateral Ureters to Ileocutaneous with Synthetic Substitute, Open Approach

0T180JD Bypass Bilateral Ureters to Cutaneous with Synthetic Substitute, Open Approach

0T180K6 Bypass Bilateral Ureters to Right Ureter with Nonautologous Tissue Substitute, Open Approach

0T180K7 Bypass Bilateral Ureters to Left Ureter with Nonautologous Tissue Substitute, Open Approach

0T180K8 Bypass Bilateral Ureters to Colon with Nonautologous Tissue Substitute, Open Approach

0T180K9 Bypass Bilateral Ureters to Colocutaneous with Nonautologous Tissue Substitute, Open Approach

0T180KA Bypass Bilateral Ureters to Ileum with Nonautologous Tissue Substitute, Open Approach

0T180KB Bypass Bilateral Ureters to Bladder with Nonautologous Tissue Substitute, Open Approach

0T180KC Bypass Bilateral Ureters to Ileocutaneous with Nonautologous Tissue Substitute, Open Approach

0T180KD Bypass Bilateral Ureters to Cutaneous with Nonautologous Tissue Substitute, Open Approach

0T180Z6 Bypass Bilateral Ureters to Right Ureter, Open Approach

0T180Z7 Bypass Bilateral Ureters to Left Ureter, Open Approach

0T180Z8 Bypass Bilateral Ureters to Colon, Open Approach

0T180Z9 Bypass Bilateral Ureters to Colocutaneous, Open Approach

0T180ZA Bypass Bilateral Ureters to Ileum, Open Approach

0T180ZB Bypass Bilateral Ureters to Bladder, Open Approach

0T180ZC Bypass Bilateral Ureters to Ileocutaneous, Open Approach

AHA CC: 3Q, 2017, 20-21

0T180ZD Bypass Bilateral Ureters to Cutaneous, Open Approach

0T183JD Bypass Bilateral Ureters to Cutaneous with Synthetic Substitute, Percutaneous Approach

0T18476 Bypass Bilateral Ureters to Right Ureter with Autologous Tissue Substitute, Percutaneous Endoscopic Approach

0T18477 Bypass Bilateral Ureters to Left Ureter with Autologous Tissue Substitute, Percutaneous Endoscopic Approach

0T18478 Bypass Bilateral Ureters to Colon with Autologous Tissue Substitute, Percutaneous Endoscopic Approach

0T18479 Bypass Bilateral Ureters to Colocutaneous with Autologous Tissue Substitute, Percutaneous Endoscopic Approach

0T1847A Bypass Bilateral Ureters to Ileum with Autologous Tissue Substitute, Percutaneous Endoscopic Approach

0T1847B Bypass Bilateral Ureters to Bladder with Autologous Tissue Substitute, Percutaneous Endoscopic Approach

0T1847C Bypass Bilateral Ureters to Ileocutaneous with Autologous Tissue Substitute, Percutaneous Endoscopic Approach

0T1847D Bypass Bilateral Ureters to Cutaneous with Autologous Tissue Substitute, Percutaneous Endoscopic Approach

0T184J6 Bypass Bilateral Ureters to Right Ureter with Synthetic Substitute, Percutaneous Endoscopic Approach

0T184J7 Bypass Bilateral Ureters to Left Ureter with Synthetic Substitute, Percutaneous Endoscopic Approach

0T184J8 Bypass Bilateral Ureters to Colon with Synthetic Substitute, Percutaneous Endoscopic Approach

0T184J9 Bypass Bilateral Ureters to Colocutaneous with Synthetic Substitute, Percutaneous Endoscopic Approach

0T184JA Bypass Bilateral Ureters to Ileum with Synthetic Substitute, Percutaneous Endoscopic Approach

0T184JB Bypass Bilateral Ureters to Bladder with Synthetic Substitute, Percutaneous Endoscopic Approach

0T184JC Bypass Bilateral Ureters to Ileocutaneous with Synthetic Substitute, Percutaneous Endoscopic Approach

0T184JD Bypass Bilateral Ureters to Cutaneous with Synthetic Substitute, Percutaneous Endoscopic Approach

0T184K6 Bypass Bilateral Ureters to Right Ureter with Nonautologous Tissue Substitute, Percutaneous Endoscopic Approach

0T184K7 Bypass Bilateral Ureters to Left Ureter with Nonautologous Tissue Substitute, Percutaneous Endoscopic Approach

0T184K8 Bypass Bilateral Ureters to Colon with Nonautologous Tissue Substitute, Percutaneous Endoscopic Approach

0T184K9 Bypass Bilateral Ureters to Colocutaneous with Nonautologous Tissue Substitute, Percutaneous Endoscopic Approach

0T184KA Bypass Bilateral Ureters to Ileum with Nonautologous Tissue Substitute, Percutaneous Endoscopic Approach

0T184KB Bypass Bilateral Ureters to Bladder with Nonautologous Tissue Substitute, Percutaneous Endoscopic Approach

0T184KC Bypass Bilateral Ureters to Ileocutaneous with Nonautologous Tissue Substitute, Percutaneous Endoscopic Approach

0T184KD Bypass Bilateral Ureters to Cutaneous with Nonautologous Tissue Substitute, Percutaneous Endoscopic Approach

♀ Female-only   ♂ Male-only   ▲ Limited Coverage   ● Non-OR   ▨ HAC-associated procedure   ▲ Non-covered procedures   ✚ Cluster

0T184Z6	Bypass Bilateral Ureters to Right Ureter, Percutaneous Endoscopic Approach
0T184Z7	Bypass Bilateral Ureters to Left Ureter, Percutaneous Endoscopic Approach
0T184Z8	Bypass Bilateral Ureters to Colon, Percutaneous Endoscopic Approach
0T184Z9	Bypass Bilateral Ureters to Colocutaneous, Percutaneous Endoscopic Approach
0T184ZA	Bypass Bilateral Ureters to Ileum, Percutaneous Endoscopic Approach
0T184ZB	Bypass Bilateral Ureters to Bladder, Percutaneous Endoscopic Approach
0T184ZC	Bypass Bilateral Ureters to Ileocutaneous, Percutaneous Endoscopic Approach
0T184ZD	Bypass Bilateral Ureters to Cutaneous, Percutaneous Endoscopic Approach
0T1B079	Bypass Bladder to Colocutaneous with Autologous Tissue Substitute, Open Approach
0T1B07C	Bypass Bladder to Ileocutaneous with Autologous Tissue Substitute, Open Approach
0T1B07D	Bypass Bladder to Cutaneous with Autologous Tissue Substitute, Open Approach
0T1B0J9	Bypass Bladder to Colocutaneous with Synthetic Substitute, Open Approach

0T1B0JC	Bypass Bladder to Ileocutaneous with Synthetic Substitute, Open Approach
0T1B0JD	Bypass Bladder to Cutaneous with Synthetic Substitute, Open Approach
0T1B0K9	Bypass Bladder to Colocutaneous with Nonautologous Tissue Substitute, Open Approach
0T1B0KC	Bypass Bladder to Ileocutaneous with Nonautologous Tissue Substitute, Open Approach
0T1B0KD	Bypass Bladder to Cutaneous with Nonautologous Tissue Substitute, Open Approach
0T1B0Z9	Bypass Bladder to Colocutaneous, Open Approach
	AHA CC: 3Q, 2017, 21-22
0T1B0ZC	Bypass Bladder to Ileocutaneous, Open Approach
0T1B0ZD	Bypass Bladder to Cutaneous, Open Approach
0T1B3JD	Bypass Bladder to Cutaneous with Synthetic Substitute, Percutaneous Approach
0T1B479	Bypass Bladder to Colocutaneous with Autologous Tissue Substitute, Percutaneous Endoscopic Approach
0T1B47C	Bypass Bladder to Ileocutaneous with Autologous Tissue Substitute, Percutaneous Endoscopic Approach

0T1B47D	Bypass Bladder to Cutaneous with Autologous Tissue Substitute, Percutaneous Endoscopic Approach
0T1B4J9	Bypass Bladder to Colocutaneous with Synthetic Substitute, Percutaneous Endoscopic Approach
0T1B4JC	Bypass Bladder to Ileocutaneous with Synthetic Substitute, Percutaneous Endoscopic Approach
0T1B4JD	Bypass Bladder to Cutaneous with Synthetic Substitute, Percutaneous Endoscopic Approach
0T1B4K9	Bypass Bladder to Colocutaneous with Nonautologous Tissue Substitute, Percutaneous Endoscopic Approach
0T1B4KC	Bypass Bladder to Ileocutaneous with Nonautologous Tissue Substitute, Percutaneous Endoscopic Approach
0T1B4KD	Bypass Bladder to Cutaneous with Nonautologous Tissue Substitute, Percutaneous Endoscopic Approach
0T1B4Z9	Bypass Bladder to Colocutaneous, Percutaneous Endoscopic Approach
0T1B4ZC	Bypass Bladder to Ileocutaneous, Percutaneous Endoscopic Approach
0T1B4ZD	Bypass Bladder to Cutaneous, Percutaneous Endoscopic Approach

0T2 – Urinary System, Change

Review Coding Guideline B6.1c

0T25X0Z	Change Drainage Device in Kidney, External Approach
0T25XYZ	Change Other Device in Kidney, External Approach
0T29X0Z	Change Drainage Device in Ureter, External Approach

0T29XYZ	Change Other Device in Ureter, External Approach
0T2BX0Z	Change Drainage Device in Bladder, External Approach
0T2BXYZ	Change Other Device in Bladder, External Approach

| 0T2DX0Z | Change Drainage Device in Urethra, External Approach |
| 0T2DXYZ | Change Other Device in Urethra, External Approach |

0T5 – Urinary System, Destruction

0T500ZZ	Destruction of Right Kidney, Open Approach
0T503ZZ	Destruction of Right Kidney, Percutaneous Approach
0T504ZZ	Destruction of Right Kidney, Percutaneous Endoscopic Approach
0T507ZZ	Destruction of Right Kidney, Via Natural or Artificial Opening
0T508ZZ	Destruction of Right Kidney, Via Natural or Artificial Opening Endoscopic
0T510ZZ	Destruction of Left Kidney, Open Approach
0T513ZZ	Destruction of Left Kidney, Percutaneous Approach
0T514ZZ	Destruction of Left Kidney, Percutaneous Endoscopic Approach
0T517ZZ	Destruction of Left Kidney, Via Natural or Artificial Opening
0T518ZZ	Destruction of Left Kidney, Via Natural or Artificial Opening Endoscopic
0T530ZZ	Destruction of Right Kidney Pelvis, Open Approach
0T533ZZ	Destruction of Right Kidney Pelvis, Percutaneous Approach
0T534ZZ	Destruction of Right Kidney Pelvis, Percutaneous Endoscopic Approach
0T537ZZ	Destruction of Right Kidney Pelvis, Via Natural or Artificial Opening
0T538ZZ	Destruction of Right Kidney Pelvis, Via Natural or Artificial Opening Endoscopic

0T540ZZ	Destruction of Left Kidney Pelvis, Open Approach
0T543ZZ	Destruction of Left Kidney Pelvis, Percutaneous Approach
0T544ZZ	Destruction of Left Kidney Pelvis, Percutaneous Endoscopic Approach
0T547ZZ	Destruction of Left Kidney Pelvis, Via Natural or Artificial Opening
0T548ZZ	Destruction of Left Kidney Pelvis, Via Natural or Artificial Opening Endoscopic
0T560ZZ	Destruction of Right Ureter, Open Approach
0T563ZZ	Destruction of Right Ureter, Percutaneous Approach
0T564ZZ	Destruction of Right Ureter, Percutaneous Endoscopic Approach
0T567ZZ	Destruction of Right Ureter, Via Natural or Artificial Opening
0T568ZZ	Destruction of Right Ureter, Via Natural or Artificial Opening Endoscopic
0T570ZZ	Destruction of Left Ureter, Open Approach
0T573ZZ	Destruction of Left Ureter, Percutaneous Approach
0T574ZZ	Destruction of Left Ureter, Percutaneous Endoscopic Approach
0T577ZZ	Destruction of Left Ureter, Via Natural or Artificial Opening
0T578ZZ	Destruction of Left Ureter, Via Natural or Artificial Opening Endoscopic

0T5B0ZZ	Destruction of Bladder, Open Approach
0T5B3ZZ	Destruction of Bladder, Percutaneous Approach
0T5B4ZZ	Destruction of Bladder, Percutaneous Endoscopic Approach
0T5B7ZZ	Destruction of Bladder, Via Natural or Artificial Opening
0T5B8ZZ	Destruction of Bladder, Via Natural or Artificial Opening Endoscopic
0T5C0ZZ	Destruction of Bladder Neck, Open Approach
0T5C3ZZ	Destruction of Bladder Neck, Percutaneous Approach
0T5C4ZZ	Destruction of Bladder Neck, Percutaneous Endoscopic Approach
0T5C7ZZ	Destruction of Bladder Neck, Via Natural or Artificial Opening
0T5C8ZZ	Destruction of Bladder Neck, Via Natural or Artificial Opening Endoscopic
0T5D0ZZ	Destruction of Urethra, Open Approach
0T5D3ZZ	Destruction of Urethra, Percutaneous Approach
0T5D4ZZ	Destruction of Urethra, Percutaneous Endoscopic Approach
0T5D7ZZ	Destruction of Urethra, Via Natural or Artificial Opening
0T5D8ZZ	Destruction of Urethra, Via Natural or Artificial Opening Endoscopic
0T5DXZZ	Destruction of Urethra, External Approach

0T7 – Urinary System, Dilation

0T730DZ	Dilation of Right Kidney Pelvis with Intraluminal Device, Open Approach
0T730ZZ	Dilation of Right Kidney Pelvis, Open Approach
0T733DZ	Dilation of Right Kidney Pelvis with Intraluminal Device, Percutaneous Approach
0T733ZZ	Dilation of Right Kidney Pelvis, Percutaneous Approach
0T734DZ	Dilation of Right Kidney Pelvis with Intraluminal Device, Percutaneous Endoscopic Approach
0T734ZZ	Dilation of Right Kidney Pelvis, Percutaneous Endoscopic Approach
0T737DZ	Dilation of Right Kidney Pelvis with Intraluminal Device, Via Natural or Artificial Opening
0T737ZZ	Dilation of Right Kidney Pelvis, Via Natural or Artificial Opening
0T738DZ	Dilation of Right Kidney Pelvis with Intraluminal Device, Via Natural or Artificial Opening Endoscopic
0T738ZZ	Dilation of Right Kidney Pelvis, Via Natural or Artificial Opening Endoscopic
0T740DZ	Dilation of Left Kidney Pelvis with Intraluminal Device, Open Approach
0T740ZZ	Dilation of Left Kidney Pelvis, Open Approach
0T743DZ	Dilation of Left Kidney Pelvis with Intraluminal Device, Percutaneous Approach
0T743ZZ	Dilation of Left Kidney Pelvis, Percutaneous Approach
0T744DZ	Dilation of Left Kidney Pelvis with Intraluminal Device, Percutaneous Endoscopic Approach
0T744ZZ	Dilation of Left Kidney Pelvis, Percutaneous Endoscopic Approach
0T747DZ	Dilation of Left Kidney Pelvis with Intraluminal Device, Via Natural or Artificial Opening
0T747ZZ	Dilation of Left Kidney Pelvis, Via Natural or Artificial Opening
0T748DZ	Dilation of Left Kidney Pelvis with Intraluminal Device, Via Natural or Artificial Opening Endoscopic
0T748ZZ	Dilation of Left Kidney Pelvis, Via Natural or Artificial Opening Endoscopic
0T760DZ	Dilation of Right Ureter with Intraluminal Device, Open Approach
0T760ZZ	Dilation of Right Ureter, Open Approach
0T763DZ	Dilation of Right Ureter with Intraluminal Device, Percutaneous Approach
0T763ZZ	Dilation of Right Ureter, Percutaneous Approach
0T764DZ	Dilation of Right Ureter with Intraluminal Device, Percutaneous Endoscopic Approach
0T764ZZ	Dilation of Right Ureter, Percutaneous Endoscopic Approach

0T767DZ	Dilation of Right Ureter with Intraluminal Device, Via Natural or Artificial Opening
0T767ZZ	Dilation of Right Ureter, Via Natural or Artificial Opening
0T768DZ	Dilation of Right Ureter with Intraluminal Device, Via Natural or Artificial Opening Endoscopic
	AHA CC: 2Q, 2016, 27-28; 4Q, 2017, 111
0T768ZZ	Dilation of Right Ureter, Via Natural or Artificial Opening Endoscopic
0T770DZ	Dilation of Left Ureter with Intraluminal Device, Open Approach
0T770ZZ	Dilation of Left Ureter, Open Approach
0T773DZ	Dilation of Left Ureter with Intraluminal Device, Percutaneous Approach
0T773ZZ	Dilation of Left Ureter, Percutaneous Approach
0T774DZ	Dilation of Left Ureter with Intraluminal Device, Percutaneous Endoscopic Approach
0T774ZZ	Dilation of Left Ureter, Percutaneous Endoscopic Approach
0T777DZ	Dilation of Left Ureter with Intraluminal Device, Via Natural or Artificial Opening
0T777ZZ	Dilation of Left Ureter, Via Natural or Artificial Opening
0T778DZ	Dilation of Left Ureter with Intraluminal Device, Via Natural or Artificial Opening Endoscopic
	AHA CC: 2Q, 2015, 8-9
0T778ZZ	Dilation of Left Ureter, Via Natural or Artificial Opening Endoscopic
0T780DZ	Dilation of Bilateral Ureters with Intraluminal Device, Open Approach
0T780ZZ	Dilation of Bilateral Ureters, Open Approach
0T783DZ	Dilation of Bilateral Ureters with Intraluminal Device, Percutaneous Approach
0T783ZZ	Dilation of Bilateral Ureters, Percutaneous Approach
0T784DZ	Dilation of Bilateral Ureters with Intraluminal Device, Percutaneous Endoscopic Approach
0T784ZZ	Dilation of Bilateral Ureters, Percutaneous Endoscopic Approach
0T787DZ	Dilation of Bilateral Ureters with Intraluminal Device, Via Natural or Artificial Opening
0T787ZZ	Dilation of Bilateral Ureters, Via Natural or Artificial Opening
0T788DZ	Dilation of Bilateral Ureters with Intraluminal Device, Via Natural or Artificial Opening Endoscopic
0T788ZZ	Dilation of Bilateral Ureters, Via Natural or Artificial Opening Endoscopic
0T7B0DZ	Dilation of Bladder with Intraluminal Device, Open Approach
0T7B0ZZ	Dilation of Bladder, Open Approach
0T7B3DZ	Dilation of Bladder with Intraluminal Device, Percutaneous Approach

0T7B3ZZ	Dilation of Bladder, Percutaneous Approach
0T7B4DZ	Dilation of Bladder with Intraluminal Device, Percutaneous Endoscopic Approach
0T7B4ZZ	Dilation of Bladder, Percutaneous Endoscopic Approach
0T7B7DZ	Dilation of Bladder with Intraluminal Device, Via Natural or Artificial Opening
0T7B7ZZ	Dilation of Bladder, Via Natural or Artificial Opening
0T7B8DZ	Dilation of Bladder with Intraluminal Device, Via Natural or Artificial Opening Endoscopic
0T7B8ZZ	Dilation of Bladder, Via Natural or Artificial Opening Endoscopic
0T7C0DZ	Dilation of Bladder Neck with Intraluminal Device, Open Approach
0T7C0ZZ	Dilation of Bladder Neck, Open Approach
0T7C3DZ	Dilation of Bladder Neck with Intraluminal Device, Percutaneous Approach
0T7C3ZZ	Dilation of Bladder Neck, Percutaneous Approach
0T7C4DZ	Dilation of Bladder Neck with Intraluminal Device, Percutaneous Endoscopic Approach
0T7C4ZZ	Dilation of Bladder Neck, Percutaneous Endoscopic Approach
0T7C7DZ	Dilation of Bladder Neck with Intraluminal Device, Via Natural or Artificial Opening
0T7C7ZZ	Dilation of Bladder Neck, Via Natural or Artificial Opening
0T7C8DZ	Dilation of Bladder Neck with Intraluminal Device, Via Natural or Artificial Opening Endoscopic
0T7C8ZZ	Dilation of Bladder Neck, Via Natural or Artificial Opening Endoscopic
0T7D0DZ	Dilation of Urethra with Intraluminal Device, Open Approach
0T7D0ZZ	Dilation of Urethra, Open Approach
0T7D3DZ	Dilation of Urethra with Intraluminal Device, Percutaneous Approach
0T7D3ZZ	Dilation of Urethra, Percutaneous Approach
0T7D4DZ	Dilation of Urethra with Intraluminal Device, Percutaneous Endoscopic Approach
0T7D4ZZ	Dilation of Urethra, Percutaneous Endoscopic Approach
0T7D7DZ	Dilation of Urethra with Intraluminal Device, Via Natural or Artificial Opening
0T7D7ZZ	Dilation of Urethra, Via Natural or Artificial Opening
0T7D8DZ	Dilation of Urethra with Intraluminal Device, Via Natural or Artificial Opening Endoscopic
	AHA CC: 4Q, 2013, 123
0T7D8ZZ	Dilation of Urethra, Via Natural or Artificial Opening Endoscopic

0T8 – Urinary System, Division

Review Coding Guideline B3.14

0T820ZZ	Division of Bilateral Kidneys, Open Approach
0T823ZZ	Division of Bilateral Kidneys, Percutaneous Approach
0T824ZZ	Division of Bilateral Kidneys, Percutaneous Endoscopic Approach
0T8C0ZZ	Division of Bladder Neck, Open Approach
0T8C3ZZ	Division of Bladder Neck, Percutaneous Approach
0T8C4ZZ	Division of Bladder Neck, Percutaneous Endoscopic Approach

♀ Female-only   ♂ Male-only   ▲ Limited Coverage   ● Non-OR   ▨ HAC-associated procedure   ▲ Non-covered procedures   ✚ Cluster

0T9 – Urinary System, Drainage

Review Coding Guidelines B3.4a and B3.4b

Review Coding Guideline B6.2

0T9000Z Drainage of Right Kidney with Drainage Device, Open Approach
0T900ZX Drainage of Right Kidney, Open Approach, Diagnostic
0T900ZZ Drainage of Right Kidney, Open Approach
0T9030Z Drainage of Right Kidney with Drainage Device, Percutaneous Approach
0T903ZX Drainage of Right Kidney, Percutaneous Approach, Diagnostic
0T903ZZ Drainage of Right Kidney, Percutaneous Approach
0T9040Z Drainage of Right Kidney with Drainage Device, Percutaneous Endoscopic Approach
0T904ZX Drainage of Right Kidney, Percutaneous Endoscopic Approach, Diagnostic
0T904ZZ Drainage of Right Kidney, Percutaneous Endoscopic Approach
0T9070Z Drainage of Right Kidney with Drainage Device, Via Natural or Artificial Opening
0T907ZX Drainage of Right Kidney, Via Natural or Artificial Opening, Diagnostic
0T907ZZ Drainage of Right Kidney, Via Natural or Artificial Opening
0T9080Z Drainage of Right Kidney with Drainage Device, Via Natural or Artificial Opening Endoscopic
0T908ZX Drainage of Right Kidney, Via Natural or Artificial Opening Endoscopic, Diagnostic
0T908ZZ Drainage of Right Kidney, Via Natural or Artificial Opening Endoscopic
0T9100Z Drainage of Left Kidney with Drainage Device, Open Approach
0T910ZX Drainage of Left Kidney, Open Approach, Diagnostic
0T910ZZ Drainage of Left Kidney, Open Approach
0T9130Z Drainage of Left Kidney with Drainage Device, Percutaneous Approach
0T913ZX Drainage of Left Kidney, Percutaneous Approach, Diagnostic
0T913ZZ Drainage of Left Kidney, Percutaneous Approach
0T9140Z Drainage of Left Kidney with Drainage Device, Percutaneous Endoscopic Approach
0T914ZX Drainage of Left Kidney, Percutaneous Endoscopic Approach, Diagnostic
0T914ZZ Drainage of Left Kidney, Percutaneous Endoscopic Approach
0T9170Z Drainage of Left Kidney with Drainage Device, Via Natural or Artificial Opening
0T917ZX Drainage of Left Kidney, Via Natural or Artificial Opening, Diagnostic
0T917ZZ Drainage of Left Kidney, Via Natural or Artificial Opening
0T9180Z Drainage of Left Kidney with Drainage Device, Via Natural or Artificial Opening Endoscopic
0T918ZX Drainage of Left Kidney, Via Natural or Artificial Opening Endoscopic, Diagnostic
0T918ZZ Drainage of Left Kidney, Via Natural or Artificial Opening Endoscopic

0T9300Z Drainage of Right Kidney Pelvis with Drainage Device, Open Approach
0T930ZX Drainage of Right Kidney Pelvis, Open Approach, Diagnostic
0T930ZZ Drainage of Right Kidney Pelvis, Open Approach
0T9330Z Drainage of Right Kidney Pelvis with Drainage Device, Percutaneous Approach
0T933ZX Drainage of Right Kidney Pelvis, Percutaneous Approach, Diagnostic
0T933ZZ Drainage of Right Kidney Pelvis, Percutaneous Approach
0T9340Z Drainage of Right Kidney Pelvis with Drainage Device, Percutaneous Endoscopic Approach
0T934ZX Drainage of Right Kidney Pelvis, Percutaneous Endoscopic Approach, Diagnostic
0T934ZZ Drainage of Right Kidney Pelvis, Percutaneous Endoscopic Approach
0T9370Z Drainage of Right Kidney Pelvis with Drainage Device, Via Natural or Artificial Opening
0T937ZX Drainage of Right Kidney Pelvis, Via Natural or Artificial Opening, Diagnostic
0T937ZZ Drainage of Right Kidney Pelvis, Via Natural or Artificial Opening
0T9380Z Drainage of Right Kidney Pelvis with Drainage Device, Via Natural or Artificial Opening Endoscopic
0T938ZX Drainage of Right Kidney Pelvis, Via Natural or Artificial Opening Endoscopic, Diagnostic
0T938ZZ Drainage of Right Kidney Pelvis, Via Natural or Artificial Opening Endoscopic
0T9400Z Drainage of Left Kidney Pelvis with Drainage Device, Open Approach
0T940ZX Drainage of Left Kidney Pelvis, Open Approach, Diagnostic
0T940ZZ Drainage of Left Kidney Pelvis, Open Approach
0T9430Z Drainage of Left Kidney Pelvis with Drainage Device, Percutaneous Approach
0T943ZX Drainage of Left Kidney Pelvis, Percutaneous Approach, Diagnostic
0T943ZZ Drainage of Left Kidney Pelvis, Percutaneous Approach
0T9440Z Drainage of Left Kidney Pelvis with Drainage Device, Percutaneous Endoscopic Approach
0T944ZX Drainage of Left Kidney Pelvis, Percutaneous Endoscopic Approach, Diagnostic
0T944ZZ Drainage of Left Kidney Pelvis, Percutaneous Endoscopic Approach
0T9470Z Drainage of Left Kidney Pelvis with Drainage Device, Via Natural or Artificial Opening
0T947ZX Drainage of Left Kidney Pelvis, Via Natural or Artificial Opening, Diagnostic
0T947ZZ Drainage of Left Kidney Pelvis, Via Natural or Artificial Opening
0T9480Z Drainage of Left Kidney Pelvis with Drainage Device, Via Natural or Artificial Opening Endoscopic

0T948ZX Drainage of Left Kidney Pelvis, Via Natural or Artificial Opening Endoscopic, Diagnostic
0T948ZZ Drainage of Left Kidney Pelvis, Via Natural or Artificial Opening Endoscopic
0T9600Z Drainage of Right Ureter with Drainage Device, Open Approach
0T960ZX Drainage of Right Ureter, Open Approach, Diagnostic
0T960ZZ Drainage of Right Ureter, Open Approach
0T9630Z Drainage of Right Ureter with Drainage Device, Percutaneous Approach
0T963ZX Drainage of Right Ureter, Percutaneous Approach, Diagnostic
0T963ZZ Drainage of Right Ureter, Percutaneous Approach
0T9640Z Drainage of Right Ureter with Drainage Device, Percutaneous Endoscopic Approach
0T964ZX Drainage of Right Ureter, Percutaneous Endoscopic Approach, Diagnostic
0T964ZZ Drainage of Right Ureter, Percutaneous Endoscopic Approach
0T9670Z Drainage of Right Ureter with Drainage Device, Via Natural or Artificial Opening
0T967ZX Drainage of Right Ureter, Via Natural or Artificial Opening, Diagnostic
0T967ZZ Drainage of Right Ureter, Via Natural or Artificial Opening
0T9680Z Drainage of Right Ureter with Drainage Device, Via Natural or Artificial Opening Endoscopic

AHA CC: 3Q, 2017, 19-20

0T968ZX Drainage of Right Ureter, Via Natural or Artificial Opening Endoscopic, Diagnostic
0T968ZZ Drainage of Right Ureter, Via Natural or Artificial Opening Endoscopic
0T9700Z Drainage of Left Ureter with Drainage Device, Open Approach
0T970ZX Drainage of Left Ureter, Open Approach, Diagnostic
0T970ZZ Drainage of Left Ureter, Open Approach
0T9730Z Drainage of Left Ureter with Drainage Device, Percutaneous Approach
0T973ZX Drainage of Left Ureter, Percutaneous Approach, Diagnostic
0T973ZZ Drainage of Left Ureter, Percutaneous Approach
0T9740Z Drainage of Left Ureter with Drainage Device, Percutaneous Endoscopic Approach
0T974ZX Drainage of Left Ureter, Percutaneous Endoscopic Approach, Diagnostic
0T974ZZ Drainage of Left Ureter, Percutaneous Endoscopic Approach
0T9770Z Drainage of Left Ureter with Drainage Device, Via Natural or Artificial Opening
0T977ZX Drainage of Left Ureter, Via Natural or Artificial Opening, Diagnostic
0T977ZZ Drainage of Left Ureter, Via Natural or Artificial Opening
0T9780Z Drainage of Left Ureter with Drainage Device, Via Natural or Artificial Opening Endoscopic

0T978ZX	Drainage of Left Ureter, Via Natural or Artificial Opening Endoscopic, Diagnostic
0T978ZZ	Drainage of Left Ureter, Via Natural or Artificial Opening Endoscopic
0T9800Z	Drainage of Bilateral Ureters with Drainage Device, Open Approach
0T980ZX	Drainage of Bilateral Ureters, Open Approach, Diagnostic
0T980ZZ	Drainage of Bilateral Ureters, Open Approach
0T9830Z	Drainage of Bilateral Ureters with Drainage Device, Percutaneous Approach
0T983ZX	Drainage of Bilateral Ureters, Percutaneous Approach, Diagnostic
0T983ZZ	Drainage of Bilateral Ureters, Percutaneous Approach
0T9840Z	Drainage of Bilateral Ureters with Drainage Device, Percutaneous Endoscopic Approach
0T984ZX	Drainage of Bilateral Ureters, Percutaneous Endoscopic Approach, Diagnostic
0T984ZZ	Drainage of Bilateral Ureters, Percutaneous Endoscopic Approach
0T9870Z	Drainage of Bilateral Ureters with Drainage Device, Via Natural or Artificial Opening
0T987ZX	Drainage of Bilateral Ureters, Via Natural or Artificial Opening, Diagnostic
0T987ZZ	Drainage of Bilateral Ureters, Via Natural or Artificial Opening
0T9880Z	Drainage of Bilateral Ureters with Drainage Device, Via Natural or Artificial Opening Endoscopic
0T988ZX	Drainage of Bilateral Ureters, Via Natural or Artificial Opening Endoscopic, Diagnostic
0T988ZZ	Drainage of Bilateral Ureters, Via Natural or Artificial Opening Endoscopic
0T9B00Z	Drainage of Bladder with Drainage Device, Open Approach
0T9B0ZX	Drainage of Bladder, Open Approach, Diagnostic
0T9B0ZZ	Drainage of Bladder, Open Approach
0T9B30Z	Drainage of Bladder with Drainage Device, Percutaneous Approach
0T9B3ZX	Drainage of Bladder, Percutaneous Approach, Diagnostic
0T9B3ZZ	Drainage of Bladder, Percutaneous Approach
0T9B40Z	Drainage of Bladder with Drainage Device, Percutaneous Endoscopic Approach
0T9B4ZX	Drainage of Bladder, Percutaneous Endoscopic Approach, Diagnostic
0T9B4ZZ	Drainage of Bladder, Percutaneous Endoscopic Approach
0T9B70Z	Drainage of Bladder with Drainage Device, Via Natural or Artificial Opening
0T9B7ZX	Drainage of Bladder, Via Natural or Artificial Opening, Diagnostic
0T9B7ZZ	Drainage of Bladder, Via Natural or Artificial Opening
0T9B80Z	Drainage of Bladder with Drainage Device, Via Natural or Artificial Opening Endoscopic
0T9B8ZX	Drainage of Bladder, Via Natural or Artificial Opening Endoscopic, Diagnostic
0T9B8ZZ	Drainage of Bladder, Via Natural or Artificial Opening Endoscopic
0T9C00Z	Drainage of Bladder Neck with Drainage Device, Open Approach
0T9C0ZX	Drainage of Bladder Neck, Open Approach, Diagnostic
0T9C0ZZ	Drainage of Bladder Neck, Open Approach
0T9C30Z	Drainage of Bladder Neck with Drainage Device, Percutaneous Approach
0T9C3ZX	Drainage of Bladder Neck, Percutaneous Approach, Diagnostic
0T9C3ZZ	Drainage of Bladder Neck, Percutaneous Approach
0T9C40Z	Drainage of Bladder Neck with Drainage Device, Percutaneous Endoscopic Approach
0T9C4ZX	Drainage of Bladder Neck, Percutaneous Endoscopic Approach, Diagnostic
0T9C4ZZ	Drainage of Bladder Neck, Percutaneous Endoscopic Approach
0T9C70Z	Drainage of Bladder Neck with Drainage Device, Via Natural or Artificial Opening
0T9C7ZX	Drainage of Bladder Neck, Via Natural or Artificial Opening, Diagnostic
0T9C7ZZ	Drainage of Bladder Neck, Via Natural or Artificial Opening
0T9C80Z	Drainage of Bladder Neck with Drainage Device, Via Natural or Artificial Opening Endoscopic
0T9C8ZX	Drainage of Bladder Neck, Via Natural or Artificial Opening Endoscopic, Diagnostic
0T9C8ZZ	Drainage of Bladder Neck, Via Natural or Artificial Opening Endoscopic
0T9D00Z	Drainage of Urethra with Drainage Device, Open Approach
0T9D0ZX	Drainage of Urethra, Open Approach, Diagnostic
0T9D0ZZ	Drainage of Urethra, Open Approach
0T9D30Z	Drainage of Urethra with Drainage Device, Percutaneous Approach
0T9D3ZX	Drainage of Urethra, Percutaneous Approach, Diagnostic
0T9D3ZZ	Drainage of Urethra, Percutaneous Approach
0T9D40Z	Drainage of Urethra with Drainage Device, Percutaneous Endoscopic Approach
0T9D4ZX	Drainage of Urethra, Percutaneous Endoscopic Approach, Diagnostic
0T9D4ZZ	Drainage of Urethra, Percutaneous Endoscopic Approach
0T9D70Z	Drainage of Urethra with Drainage Device, Via Natural or Artificial Opening
0T9D7ZX	Drainage of Urethra, Via Natural or Artificial Opening, Diagnostic
0T9D7ZZ	Drainage of Urethra, Via Natural or Artificial Opening
0T9D80Z	Drainage of Urethra with Drainage Device, Via Natural or Artificial Opening Endoscopic
0T9D8ZX	Drainage of Urethra, Via Natural or Artificial Opening Endoscopic, Diagnostic
0T9D8ZZ	Drainage of Urethra, Via Natural or Artificial Opening Endoscopic
0T9DX0Z	Drainage of Urethra with Drainage Device, External Approach
0T9DXZX	Drainage of Urethra, External Approach, Diagnostic
0T9DXZZ	Drainage of Urethra, External Approach

0TB – Urinary System, Excision

Review Coding Guidelines B3.4a and B3.4b

Review Coding Guideline B3.8

Review Coding Guideline B3.18

0TB00ZX	Excision of Right Kidney, Open Approach, Diagnostic
0TB00ZZ	Excision of Right Kidney, Open Approach
0TB03ZX	Excision of Right Kidney, Percutaneous Approach, Diagnostic
0TB03ZZ	Excision of Right Kidney, Percutaneous Approach
0TB04ZX	Excision of Right Kidney, Percutaneous Endoscopic Approach, Diagnostic
0TB04ZZ	Excision of Right Kidney, Percutaneous Endoscopic Approach
0TB07ZX	Excision of Right Kidney, Via Natural or Artificial Opening, Diagnostic
0TB07ZZ	Excision of Right Kidney, Via Natural or Artificial Opening
0TB08ZX	Excision of Right Kidney, Via Natural or Artificial Opening Endoscopic, Diagnostic
0TB08ZZ	Excision of Right Kidney, Via Natural or Artificial Opening Endoscopic
0TB10ZX	Excision of Left Kidney, Open Approach, Diagnostic
0TB10ZZ	Excision of Left Kidney, Open Approach
0TB13ZX	Excision of Left Kidney, Percutaneous Approach, Diagnostic
0TB13ZZ	Excision of Left Kidney, Percutaneous Approach
0TB14ZX	Excision of Left Kidney, Percutaneous Endoscopic Approach, Diagnostic
0TB14ZZ	Excision of Left Kidney, Percutaneous Endoscopic Approach
0TB17ZX	Excision of Left Kidney, Via Natural or Artificial Opening, Diagnostic
0TB17ZZ	Excision of Left Kidney, Via Natural or Artificial Opening
0TB18ZX	Excision of Left Kidney, Via Natural or Artificial Opening Endoscopic, Diagnostic
0TB18ZZ	Excision of Left Kidney, Via Natural or Artificial Opening Endoscopic
0TB30ZX	Excision of Right Kidney Pelvis, Open Approach, Diagnostic
0TB30ZZ	Excision of Right Kidney Pelvis, Open Approach
0TB33ZX	Excision of Right Kidney Pelvis, Percutaneous Approach, Diagnostic

0TB33ZZ	Excision of Right Kidney Pelvis, Percutaneous Approach
0TB34ZX	Excision of Right Kidney Pelvis, Percutaneous Endoscopic Approach, Diagnostic
0TB34ZZ	Excision of Right Kidney Pelvis, Percutaneous Endoscopic Approach
0TB37ZX	Excision of Right Kidney Pelvis, Via Natural or Artificial Opening, Diagnostic
0TB37ZZ	Excision of Right Kidney Pelvis, Via Natural or Artificial Opening
0TB38ZX	Excision of Right Kidney Pelvis, Via Natural or Artificial Opening Endoscopic, Diagnostic
0TB38ZZ	Excision of Right Kidney Pelvis, Via Natural or Artificial Opening Endoscopic
0TB40ZX	Excision of Left Kidney Pelvis, Open Approach, Diagnostic
0TB40ZZ	Excision of Left Kidney Pelvis, Open Approach
0TB43ZX	Excision of Left Kidney Pelvis, Percutaneous Approach, Diagnostic
0TB43ZZ	Excision of Left Kidney Pelvis, Percutaneous Approach
0TB44ZX	Excision of Left Kidney Pelvis, Percutaneous Endoscopic Approach, Diagnostic
0TB44ZZ	Excision of Left Kidney Pelvis, Percutaneous Endoscopic Approach
0TB47ZX	Excision of Left Kidney Pelvis, Via Natural or Artificial Opening, Diagnostic
0TB47ZZ	Excision of Left Kidney Pelvis, Via Natural or Artificial Opening
0TB48ZX	Excision of Left Kidney Pelvis, Via Natural or Artificial Opening Endoscopic, Diagnostic
0TB48ZZ	Excision of Left Kidney Pelvis, Via Natural or Artificial Opening Endoscopic
0TB60ZX	Excision of Right Ureter, Open Approach, Diagnostic
0TB60ZZ	Excision of Right Ureter, Open Approach
0TB63ZX	Excision of Right Ureter, Percutaneous Approach, Diagnostic
0TB63ZZ	Excision of Right Ureter, Percutaneous Approach
0TB64ZX	Excision of Right Ureter, Percutaneous Endoscopic Approach, Diagnostic
0TB64ZZ	Excision of Right Ureter, Percutaneous Endoscopic Approach
0TB67ZX	Excision of Right Ureter, Via Natural or Artificial Opening, Diagnostic
0TB67ZZ	Excision of Right Ureter, Via Natural or Artificial Opening
0TB68ZX	Excision of Right Ureter, Via Natural or Artificial Opening Endoscopic, Diagnostic
0TB68ZZ	Excision of Right Ureter, Via Natural or Artificial Opening Endoscopic
0TB70ZX	Excision of Left Ureter, Open Approach, Diagnostic
0TB70ZZ	Excision of Left Ureter, Open Approach
0TB73ZX	Excision of Left Ureter, Percutaneous Approach, Diagnostic
0TB73ZZ	Excision of Left Ureter, Percutaneous Approach
0TB74ZX	Excision of Left Ureter, Percutaneous Endoscopic Approach, Diagnostic
0TB74ZZ	Excision of Left Ureter, Percutaneous Endoscopic Approach
0TB77ZX	Excision of Left Ureter, Via Natural or Artificial Opening, Diagnostic
0TB77ZZ	Excision of Left Ureter, Via Natural or Artificial Opening
0TB78ZX	Excision of Left Ureter, Via Natural or Artificial Opening Endoscopic, Diagnostic
0TB78ZZ	Excision of Left Ureter, Via Natural or Artificial Opening Endoscopic
0TBB0ZX	Excision of Bladder, Open Approach, Diagnostic
0TBB0ZZ	Excision of Bladder, Open Approach
0TBB3ZX	Excision of Bladder, Percutaneous Approach, Diagnostic
0TBB3ZZ	Excision of Bladder, Percutaneous Approach
0TBB4ZX	Excision of Bladder, Percutaneous Endoscopic Approach, Diagnostic
0TBB4ZZ	Excision of Bladder, Percutaneous Endoscopic Approach
0TBB7ZX	Excision of Bladder, Via Natural or Artificial Opening, Diagnostic
0TBB7ZZ	Excision of Bladder, Via Natural or Artificial Opening
0TBB8ZX	Excision of Bladder, Via Natural or Artificial Opening Endoscopic, Diagnostic

AHA CC: 1Q, 2016, 19

0TBB8ZZ	Excision of Bladder, Via Natural or Artificial Opening Endoscopic

AHA CC: 2Q, 2014, 8

0TBC0ZX	Excision of Bladder Neck, Open Approach, Diagnostic
0TBC0ZZ	Excision of Bladder Neck, Open Approach
0TBC3ZX	Excision of Bladder Neck, Percutaneous Approach, Diagnostic
0TBC3ZZ	Excision of Bladder Neck, Percutaneous Approach
0TBC4ZX	Excision of Bladder Neck, Percutaneous Endoscopic Approach, Diagnostic
0TBC4ZZ	Excision of Bladder Neck, Percutaneous Endoscopic Approach
0TBC7ZX	Excision of Bladder Neck, Via Natural or Artificial Opening, Diagnostic
0TBC7ZZ	Excision of Bladder Neck, Via Natural or Artificial Opening
0TBC8ZX	Excision of Bladder Neck, Via Natural or Artificial Opening Endoscopic, Diagnostic
0TBC8ZZ	Excision of Bladder Neck, Via Natural or Artificial Opening Endoscopic
0TBD0ZX	Excision of Urethra, Open Approach, Diagnostic
0TBD0ZZ	Excision of Urethra, Open Approach
0TBD3ZX	Excision of Urethra, Percutaneous Approach, Diagnostic
0TBD3ZZ	Excision of Urethra, Percutaneous Approach
0TBD4ZX	Excision of Urethra, Percutaneous Endoscopic Approach, Diagnostic
0TBD4ZZ	Excision of Urethra, Percutaneous Endoscopic Approach
0TBD7ZX	Excision of Urethra, Via Natural or Artificial Opening, Diagnostic
0TBD7ZZ	Excision of Urethra, Via Natural or Artificial Opening
0TBD8ZX	Excision of Urethra, Via Natural or Artificial Opening Endoscopic, Diagnostic
0TBD8ZZ	Excision of Urethra, Via Natural or Artificial Opening Endoscopic

AHA CC: 3Q, 2015, 34

0TBDXZX	Excision of Urethra, External Approach, Diagnostic
0TBDXZZ	Excision of Urethra, External Approach

0TC – Urinary System, Extirpation

0TC00ZZ	Extirpation of Matter from Right Kidney, Open Approach
0TC03ZZ	Extirpation of Matter from Right Kidney, Percutaneous Approach
0TC04ZZ	Extirpation of Matter from Right Kidney, Percutaneous Endoscopic Approach
0TC07ZZ	Extirpation of Matter from Right Kidney, Via Natural or Artificial Opening
0TC08ZZ	Extirpation of Matter from Right Kidney, Via Natural or Artificial Opening Endoscopic
0TC10ZZ	Extirpation of Matter from Left Kidney, Open Approach
0TC13ZZ	Extirpation of Matter from Left Kidney, Percutaneous Approach
0TC14ZZ	Extirpation of Matter from Left Kidney, Percutaneous Endoscopic Approach
0TC17ZZ	Extirpation of Matter from Left Kidney, Via Natural or Artificial Opening
0TC18ZZ	Extirpation of Matter from Left Kidney, Via Natural or Artificial Opening Endoscopic

AHA CC: 2Q, 2015, 8-9

0TC30ZZ	Extirpation of Matter from Right Kidney Pelvis, Open Approach
0TC33ZZ	Extirpation of Matter from Right Kidney Pelvis, Percutaneous Approach
0TC34ZZ	Extirpation of Matter from Right Kidney Pelvis, Percutaneous Endoscopic Approach
0TC37ZZ	Extirpation of Matter from Right Kidney Pelvis, Via Natural or Artificial Opening
0TC38ZZ	Extirpation of Matter from Right Kidney Pelvis, Via Natural or Artificial Opening Endoscopic
0TC40ZZ	Extirpation of Matter from Left Kidney Pelvis, Open Approach
0TC43ZZ	Extirpation of Matter from Left Kidney Pelvis, Percutaneous Approach
0TC44ZZ	Extirpation of Matter from Left Kidney Pelvis, Percutaneous Endoscopic Approach
0TC47ZZ	Extirpation of Matter from Left Kidney Pelvis, Via Natural or Artificial Opening
0TC48ZZ	Extirpation of Matter from Left Kidney Pelvis, Via Natural or Artificial Opening Endoscopic

AHA CC: 2Q, 2015, 7-8

0TC60ZZ	Extirpation of Matter from Right Ureter, Open Approach
0TC63ZZ	Extirpation of Matter from Right Ureter, Percutaneous Approach
0TC64ZZ	Extirpation of Matter from Right Ureter, Percutaneous Endoscopic Approach

0TC67ZZ Extirpation of Matter from Right Ureter, Via Natural or Artificial Opening

0TC68ZZ Extirpation of Matter from Right Ureter, Via Natural or Artificial Opening Endoscopic
AHA CC: 4Q, 2013, 122-123

0TC70ZZ Extirpation of Matter from Left Ureter, Open Approach

0TC73ZZ Extirpation of Matter from Left Ureter, Percutaneous Approach

0TC74ZZ Extirpation of Matter from Left Ureter, Percutaneous Endoscopic Approach

0TC77ZZ Extirpation of Matter from Left Ureter, Via Natural or Artificial Opening

0TC78ZZ Extirpation of Matter from Left Ureter, Via Natural or Artificial Opening Endoscopic
AHA CC: 2Q, 2015, 8-9

0TCB0ZZ Extirpation of Matter from Bladder, Open Approach

0TCB3ZZ Extirpation of Matter from Bladder, Percutaneous Approach

0TCB4ZZ Extirpation of Matter from Bladder, Percutaneous Endoscopic Approach

0TCB7ZZ Extirpation of Matter from Bladder, Via Natural or Artificial Opening

0TCB8ZZ Extirpation of Matter from Bladder, Via Natural or Artificial Opening Endoscopic
AHA CC: 2Q, 2015, 8-9; 3Q, 2016, 23-24; 3Q, 2019, 4

0TCC0ZZ Extirpation of Matter from Bladder Neck, Open Approach

0TCC3ZZ Extirpation of Matter from Bladder Neck, Percutaneous Approach

0TCC4ZZ Extirpation of Matter from Bladder Neck, Percutaneous Endoscopic Approach

0TCC7ZZ Extirpation of Matter from Bladder Neck, Via Natural or Artificial Opening

0TCC8ZZ Extirpation of Matter from Bladder Neck, Via Natural or Artificial Opening Endoscopic

0TCD0ZZ Extirpation of Matter from Urethra, Open Approach

0TCD3ZZ Extirpation of Matter from Urethra, Percutaneous Approach

0TCD4ZZ Extirpation of Matter from Urethra, Percutaneous Endoscopic Approach

0TCD7ZZ Extirpation of Matter from Urethra, Via Natural or Artificial Opening

0TCD8ZZ Extirpation of Matter from Urethra, Via Natural or Artificial Opening Endoscopic

0TCDXZZ Extirpation of Matter from Urethra, External Approach

0TD – Urinary System, Extraction

0TD00ZZ Extraction of Right Kidney, Open Approach

0TD03ZZ Extraction of Right Kidney, Percutaneous Approach

0TD04ZZ Extraction of Right Kidney, Percutaneous Endoscopic Approach

0TD10ZZ Extraction of Left Kidney, Open Approach

0TD13ZZ Extraction of Left Kidney, Percutaneous Approach

0TD14ZZ Extraction of Left Kidney, Percutaneous Endoscopic Approach

0TF – Urinary System, Fragmentation

0TF30ZZ Fragmentation in Right Kidney Pelvis, Open Approach

0TF33ZZ Fragmentation in Right Kidney Pelvis, Percutaneous Approach

0TF34ZZ Fragmentation in Right Kidney Pelvis, Percutaneous Endoscopic Approach

0TF37ZZ Fragmentation in Right Kidney Pelvis, Via Natural or Artificial Opening

0TF38ZZ Fragmentation in Right Kidney Pelvis, Via Natural or Artificial Opening Endoscopic

● **0TF3XZZ** Fragmentation in Right Kidney Pelvis, External Approach
AHA CC: 4Q, 2013, 122

0TF40ZZ Fragmentation in Left Kidney Pelvis, Open Approach

0TF43ZZ Fragmentation in Left Kidney Pelvis, Percutaneous Approach

0TF44ZZ Fragmentation in Left Kidney Pelvis, Percutaneous Endoscopic Approach

0TF47ZZ Fragmentation in Left Kidney Pelvis, Via Natural or Artificial Opening

0TF48ZZ Fragmentation in Left Kidney Pelvis, Via Natural or Artificial Opening Endoscopic

● **0TF4XZZ** Fragmentation in Left Kidney Pelvis, External Approach

0TF60ZZ Fragmentation in Right Ureter, Open Approach

0TF63ZZ Fragmentation in Right Ureter, Percutaneous Approach

0TF64ZZ Fragmentation in Right Ureter, Percutaneous Endoscopic Approach

0TF67ZZ Fragmentation in Right Ureter, Via Natural or Artificial Opening

0TF68ZZ Fragmentation in Right Ureter, Via Natural or Artificial Opening Endoscopic

● **0TF6XZZ** Fragmentation in Right Ureter, External Approach

0TF70ZZ Fragmentation in Left Ureter, Open Approach

0TF73ZZ Fragmentation in Left Ureter, Percutaneous Approach

0TF74ZZ Fragmentation in Left Ureter, Percutaneous Endoscopic Approach

0TF77ZZ Fragmentation in Left Ureter, Via Natural or Artificial Opening

0TF78ZZ Fragmentation in Left Ureter, Via Natural or Artificial Opening Endoscopic

● **0TF7XZZ** Fragmentation in Left Ureter, External Approach

0TFB0ZZ Fragmentation in Bladder, Open Approach

0TFB3ZZ Fragmentation in Bladder, Percutaneous Approach

0TFB4ZZ Fragmentation in Bladder, Percutaneous Endoscopic Approach

0TFB7ZZ Fragmentation in Bladder, Via Natural or Artificial Opening

0TFB8ZZ Fragmentation in Bladder, Via Natural or Artificial Opening Endoscopic

● **0TFBXZZ** Fragmentation in Bladder, External Approach

0TFC0ZZ Fragmentation in Bladder Neck, Open Approach

0TFC3ZZ Fragmentation in Bladder Neck, Percutaneous Approach

0TFC4ZZ Fragmentation in Bladder Neck, Percutaneous Endoscopic Approach

0TFC7ZZ Fragmentation in Bladder Neck, Via Natural or Artificial Opening

0TFC8ZZ Fragmentation in Bladder Neck, Via Natural or Artificial Opening Endoscopic

● **0TFCXZZ** Fragmentation in Bladder Neck, External Approach

0TFD0ZZ Fragmentation in Urethra, Open Approach

0TFD3ZZ Fragmentation in Urethra, Percutaneous Approach

0TFD4ZZ Fragmentation in Urethra, Percutaneous Endoscopic Approach

0TFD7ZZ Fragmentation in Urethra, Via Natural or Artificial Opening

0TFD8ZZ Fragmentation in Urethra, Via Natural or Artificial Opening Endoscopic

▲ **0TFDXZZ** Fragmentation in Urethra, External Approach

0TH – Urinary System, Insertion

0TH501Z Insertion of Radioactive Element into Kidney, Open Approach

0TH502Z Insertion of Monitoring Device into Kidney, Open Approach

0TH503Z Insertion of Infusion Device into Kidney, Open Approach

0TH50YZ Insertion of Other Device into Kidney, Open Approach

0TH531Z Insertion of Radioactive Element into Kidney, Percutaneous Approach

0TH532Z Insertion of Monitoring Device into Kidney, Percutaneous Approach

0TH533Z Insertion of Infusion Device into Kidney, Percutaneous Approach

0TH53YZ Insertion of Other Device into Kidney, Percutaneous Approach

0TH541Z Insertion of Radioactive Element into Kidney, Percutaneous Endoscopic Approach

0TH542Z Insertion of Monitoring Device into Kidney, Percutaneous Endoscopic Approach

0TH543Z Insertion of Infusion Device into Kidney, Percutaneous Endoscopic Approach

0TH54YZ Insertion of Other Device into Kidney, Percutaneous Endoscopic Approach

0TH571Z Insertion of Radioactive Element into Kidney, Via Natural or Artificial Opening

♀ Female-only ♂ Male-only ▲ Limited Coverage ● Non-OR [HAC] HAC-associated procedure ▲ Non-covered procedures ✛ Cluster

0TH572Z Insertion of Monitoring Device into Kidney, Via Natural or Artificial Opening

0TH573Z Insertion of Infusion Device into Kidney, Via Natural or Artificial Opening

0TH57YZ Insertion of Other Device into Kidney, Via Natural or Artificial Opening

0TH581Z Insertion of Radioactive Element into Kidney, Via Natural or Artificial Opening Endoscopic

0TH582Z Insertion of Monitoring Device into Kidney, Via Natural or Artificial Opening Endoscopic

0TH583Z Insertion of Infusion Device into Kidney, Via Natural or Artificial Opening Endoscopic

0TH58YZ Insertion of Other Device into Kidney, Via Natural or Artificial Opening Endoscopic

0TH901Z Insertion of Radioactive Element into Ureter, Open Approach

0TH902Z Insertion of Monitoring Device into Ureter, Open Approach

0TH903Z Insertion of Infusion Device into Ureter, Open Approach

0TH90MZ Insertion of Stimulator Lead into Ureter, Open Approach

0TH90YZ Insertion of Other Device into Ureter, Open Approach

0TH931Z Insertion of Radioactive Element into Ureter, Percutaneous Approach

0TH932Z Insertion of Monitoring Device into Ureter, Percutaneous Approach

0TH933Z Insertion of Infusion Device into Ureter, Percutaneous Approach

0TH93MZ Insertion of Stimulator Lead into Ureter, Percutaneous Approach

0TH93YZ Insertion of Other Device into Ureter, Percutaneous Approach

0TH941Z Insertion of Radioactive Element into Ureter, Percutaneous Endoscopic Approach

0TH942Z Insertion of Monitoring Device into Ureter, Percutaneous Endoscopic Approach

0TH943Z Insertion of Infusion Device into Ureter, Percutaneous Endoscopic Approach

0TH94MZ Insertion of Stimulator Lead into Ureter, Percutaneous Endoscopic Approach

0TH94YZ Insertion of Other Device into Ureter, Percutaneous Endoscopic Approach

0TH971Z Insertion of Radioactive Element into Ureter, Via Natural or Artificial Opening

0TH972Z Insertion of Monitoring Device into Ureter, Via Natural or Artificial Opening

0TH973Z Insertion of Infusion Device into Ureter, Via Natural or Artificial Opening

0TH97MZ Insertion of Stimulator Lead into Ureter, Via Natural or Artificial Opening

0TH97YZ Insertion of Other Device into Ureter, Via Natural or Artificial Opening

0TH981Z Insertion of Radioactive Element into Ureter, Via Natural or Artificial Opening Endoscopic

0TH982Z Insertion of Monitoring Device into Ureter, Via Natural or Artificial Opening Endoscopic

0TH983Z Insertion of Infusion Device into Ureter, Via Natural or Artificial Opening Endoscopic

0TH98MZ Insertion of Stimulator Lead into Ureter, Via Natural or Artificial Opening Endoscopic

0TH98YZ Insertion of Other Device into Ureter, Via Natural or Artificial Opening Endoscopic

0THB01Z Insertion of Radioactive Element into Bladder, Open Approach

0THB02Z Insertion of Monitoring Device into Bladder, Open Approach

0THB03Z Insertion of Infusion Device into Bladder, Open Approach

0THB0LZ Insertion of Artificial Sphincter into Bladder, Open Approach

▲ **0THB0MZ** Insertion of Stimulator Lead into Bladder, Open Approach

0THB0YZ Insertion of Other Device into Bladder, Open Approach

0THB31Z Insertion of Radioactive Element into Bladder, Percutaneous Approach

0THB32Z Insertion of Monitoring Device into Bladder, Percutaneous Approach

0THB33Z Insertion of Infusion Device into Bladder, Percutaneous Approach

0THB3LZ Insertion of Artificial Sphincter into Bladder, Percutaneous Approach

▲ **0THB3MZ** Insertion of Stimulator Lead into Bladder, Percutaneous Approach

0THB3YZ Insertion of Other Device into Bladder, Percutaneous Approach

0THB41Z Insertion of Radioactive Element into Bladder, Percutaneous Endoscopic Approach

0THB42Z Insertion of Monitoring Device into Bladder, Percutaneous Endoscopic Approach

0THB43Z Insertion of Infusion Device into Bladder, Percutaneous Endoscopic Approach

0THB4LZ Insertion of Artificial Sphincter into Bladder, Percutaneous Endoscopic Approach

▲ **0THB4MZ** Insertion of Stimulator Lead into Bladder, Percutaneous Endoscopic Approach

0THB4YZ Insertion of Other Device into Bladder, Percutaneous Endoscopic Approach

0THB71Z Insertion of Radioactive Element into Bladder, Via Natural or Artificial Opening

0THB72Z Insertion of Monitoring Device into Bladder, Via Natural or Artificial Opening

0THB73Z Insertion of Infusion Device into Bladder, Via Natural or Artificial Opening

0THB7LZ Insertion of Artificial Sphincter into Bladder, Via Natural or Artificial Opening

▲ **0THB7MZ** Insertion of Stimulator Lead into Bladder, Via Natural or Artificial Opening

0THB7YZ Insertion of Other Device into Bladder, Via Natural or Artificial Opening

0THB81Z Insertion of Radioactive Element into Bladder, Via Natural or Artificial Opening Endoscopic

0THB82Z Insertion of Monitoring Device into Bladder, Via Natural or Artificial Opening Endoscopic

0THB83Z Insertion of Infusion Device into Bladder, Via Natural or Artificial Opening Endoscopic

0THB8LZ Insertion of Artificial Sphincter into Bladder, Via Natural or Artificial Opening Endoscopic

▲ **0THB8MZ** Insertion of Stimulator Lead into Bladder, Via Natural or Artificial Opening Endoscopic

0THB8YZ Insertion of Other Device into Bladder, Via Natural or Artificial Opening Endoscopic

0THC0LZ Insertion of Artificial Sphincter into Bladder Neck, Open Approach

0THC3LZ Insertion of Artificial Sphincter into Bladder Neck, Percutaneous Approach

0THC4LZ Insertion of Artificial Sphincter into Bladder Neck, Percutaneous Endoscopic Approach

0THC7LZ Insertion of Artificial Sphincter into Bladder Neck, Via Natural or Artificial Opening

0THC8LZ Insertion of Artificial Sphincter into Bladder Neck, Via Natural or Artificial Opening Endoscopic

0THD01Z Insertion of Radioactive Element into Urethra, Open Approach

0THD02Z Insertion of Monitoring Device into Urethra, Open Approach

0THD03Z Insertion of Infusion Device into Urethra, Open Approach

0THD0LZ Insertion of Artificial Sphincter into Urethra, Open Approach

0THD0YZ Insertion of Other Device into Urethra, Open Approach

0THD31Z Insertion of Radioactive Element into Urethra, Percutaneous Approach

0THD32Z Insertion of Monitoring Device into Urethra, Percutaneous Approach

0THD33Z Insertion of Infusion Device into Urethra, Percutaneous Approach

0THD3LZ Insertion of Artificial Sphincter into Urethra, Percutaneous Approach

0THD3YZ Insertion of Other Device into Urethra, Percutaneous Approach

0THD41Z Insertion of Radioactive Element into Urethra, Percutaneous Endoscopic Approach

0THD42Z Insertion of Monitoring Device into Urethra, Percutaneous Endoscopic Approach

0THD43Z Insertion of Infusion Device into Urethra, Percutaneous Endoscopic Approach

0THD4LZ Insertion of Artificial Sphincter into Urethra, Percutaneous Endoscopic Approach

0THD4YZ Insertion of Other Device into Urethra, Percutaneous Endoscopic Approach

0THD71Z Insertion of Radioactive Element into Urethra, Via Natural or Artificial Opening

0THD72Z Insertion of Monitoring Device into Urethra, Via Natural or Artificial Opening

0THD73Z Insertion of Infusion Device into Urethra, Via Natural or Artificial Opening

0THD7LZ Insertion of Artificial Sphincter into Urethra, Via Natural or Artificial Opening

0THD7YZ Insertion of Other Device into Urethra, Via Natural or Artificial Opening

0THD81Z Insertion of Radioactive Element into Urethra, Via Natural or Artificial Opening Endoscopic

0THD82Z   Insertion of Monitoring Device into Urethra, Via Natural or Artificial Opening Endoscopic
0THD83Z   Insertion of Infusion Device into Urethra, Via Natural or Artificial Opening Endoscopic

0THD8LZ   Insertion of Artificial Sphincter into Urethra, Via Natural or Artificial Opening Endoscopic
0THD8YZ   Insertion of Other Device into Urethra, Via Natural or Artificial Opening Endoscopic

0THDX2Z   Insertion of Monitoring Device into Urethra, External Approach
0THDX3Z   Insertion of Infusion Device into Urethra, External Approach
0THDXLZ   Insertion of Artificial Sphincter into Urethra, External Approach

0TJ – Urinary System, Inspection

Review Coding Guidelines B3.11a, B3.11b and B3.11c

0TJ50ZZ   Inspection of Kidney, Open Approach
0TJ53ZZ   Inspection of Kidney, Percutaneous Approach
0TJ54ZZ   Inspection of Kidney, Percutaneous Endoscopic Approach
0TJ57ZZ   Inspection of Kidney, Via Natural or Artificial Opening
0TJ58ZZ   Inspection of Kidney, Via Natural or Artificial Opening Endoscopic
0TJ5XZZ   Inspection of Kidney, External Approach
0TJ90ZZ   Inspection of Ureter, Open Approach
0TJ93ZZ   Inspection of Ureter, Percutaneous Approach

0TJ94ZZ   Inspection of Ureter, Percutaneous Endoscopic Approach
0TJ97ZZ   Inspection of Ureter, Via Natural or Artificial Opening
0TJ98ZZ   Inspection of Ureter, Via Natural or Artificial Opening Endoscopic
0TJ9XZZ   Inspection of Ureter, External Approach
0TJB0ZZ   Inspection of Bladder, Open Approach
0TJB3ZZ   Inspection of Bladder, Percutaneous Approach
0TJB4ZZ   Inspection of Bladder, Percutaneous Endoscopic Approach
0TJB7ZZ   Inspection of Bladder, Via Natural or Artificial Opening

0TJB8ZZ   Inspection of Bladder, Via Natural or Artificial Opening Endoscopic
0TJBXZZ   Inspection of Bladder, External Approach
0TJD0ZZ   Inspection of Urethra, Open Approach
0TJD3ZZ   Inspection of Urethra, Percutaneous Approach
0TJD4ZZ   Inspection of Urethra, Percutaneous Endoscopic Approach
0TJD7ZZ   Inspection of Urethra, Via Natural or Artificial Opening
0TJD8ZZ   Inspection of Urethra, Via Natural or Artificial Opening Endoscopic
0TJDXZZ   Inspection of Urethra, External Approach

0TL – Urinary System, Occlusion

0TL30CZ   Occlusion of Right Kidney Pelvis with Extraluminal Device, Open Approach
0TL30DZ   Occlusion of Right Kidney Pelvis with Intraluminal Device, Open Approach
0TL30ZZ   Occlusion of Right Kidney Pelvis, Open Approach
0TL33CZ   Occlusion of Right Kidney Pelvis with Extraluminal Device, Percutaneous Approach
0TL33DZ   Occlusion of Right Kidney Pelvis with Intraluminal Device, Percutaneous Approach
0TL33ZZ   Occlusion of Right Kidney Pelvis, Percutaneous Approach
0TL34CZ   Occlusion of Right Kidney Pelvis with Extraluminal Device, Percutaneous Endoscopic Approach
0TL34DZ   Occlusion of Right Kidney Pelvis with Intraluminal Device, Percutaneous Endoscopic Approach
0TL34ZZ   Occlusion of Right Kidney Pelvis, Percutaneous Endoscopic Approach
0TL37DZ   Occlusion of Right Kidney Pelvis with Intraluminal Device, Via Natural or Artificial Opening
0TL37ZZ   Occlusion of Right Kidney Pelvis, Via Natural or Artificial Opening
0TL38DZ   Occlusion of Right Kidney Pelvis with Intraluminal Device, Via Natural or Artificial Opening Endoscopic
0TL38ZZ   Occlusion of Right Kidney Pelvis, Via Natural or Artificial Opening Endoscopic
0TL40CZ   Occlusion of Left Kidney Pelvis with Extraluminal Device, Open Approach
0TL40DZ   Occlusion of Left Kidney Pelvis with Intraluminal Device, Open Approach
0TL40ZZ   Occlusion of Left Kidney Pelvis, Open Approach
0TL43CZ   Occlusion of Left Kidney Pelvis with Extraluminal Device, Percutaneous Approach
0TL43DZ   Occlusion of Left Kidney Pelvis with Intraluminal Device, Percutaneous Approach

0TL43ZZ   Occlusion of Left Kidney Pelvis, Percutaneous Approach
0TL44CZ   Occlusion of Left Kidney Pelvis with Extraluminal Device, Percutaneous Endoscopic Approach
0TL44DZ   Occlusion of Left Kidney Pelvis with Intraluminal Device, Percutaneous Endoscopic Approach
0TL44ZZ   Occlusion of Left Kidney Pelvis, Percutaneous Endoscopic Approach
0TL47DZ   Occlusion of Left Kidney Pelvis with Intraluminal Device, Via Natural or Artificial Opening
0TL47ZZ   Occlusion of Left Kidney Pelvis, Via Natural or Artificial Opening
0TL48DZ   Occlusion of Left Kidney Pelvis with Intraluminal Device, Via Natural or Artificial Opening Endoscopic
0TL48ZZ   Occlusion of Left Kidney Pelvis, Via Natural or Artificial Opening Endoscopic
0TL60CZ   Occlusion of Right Ureter with Extraluminal Device, Open Approach
0TL60DZ   Occlusion of Right Ureter with Intraluminal Device, Open Approach
0TL60ZZ   Occlusion of Right Ureter, Open Approach
0TL63CZ   Occlusion of Right Ureter with Extraluminal Device, Percutaneous Approach
0TL63DZ   Occlusion of Right Ureter with Intraluminal Device, Percutaneous Approach
0TL63ZZ   Occlusion of Right Ureter, Percutaneous Approach
0TL64CZ   Occlusion of Right Ureter with Extraluminal Device, Percutaneous Endoscopic Approach
0TL64DZ   Occlusion of Right Ureter with Intraluminal Device, Percutaneous Endoscopic Approach
0TL64ZZ   Occlusion of Right Ureter, Percutaneous Endoscopic Approach
0TL67DZ   Occlusion of Right Ureter with Intraluminal Device, Via Natural or Artificial Opening

0TL67ZZ   Occlusion of Right Ureter, Via Natural or Artificial Opening
0TL68DZ   Occlusion of Right Ureter with Intraluminal Device, Via Natural or Artificial Opening Endoscopic
0TL68ZZ   Occlusion of Right Ureter, Via Natural or Artificial Opening Endoscopic
0TL70CZ   Occlusion of Left Ureter with Extraluminal Device, Open Approach
0TL70DZ   Occlusion of Left Ureter with Intraluminal Device, Open Approach
0TL70ZZ   Occlusion of Left Ureter, Open Approach
0TL73CZ   Occlusion of Left Ureter with Extraluminal Device, Percutaneous Approach
0TL73DZ   Occlusion of Left Ureter with Intraluminal Device, Percutaneous Approach
0TL73ZZ   Occlusion of Left Ureter, Percutaneous Approach
0TL74CZ   Occlusion of Left Ureter with Extraluminal Device, Percutaneous Endoscopic Approach
0TL74DZ   Occlusion of Left Ureter with Intraluminal Device, Percutaneous Endoscopic Approach
0TL74ZZ   Occlusion of Left Ureter, Percutaneous Endoscopic Approach
0TL77DZ   Occlusion of Left Ureter with Intraluminal Device, Via Natural or Artificial Opening
0TL77ZZ   Occlusion of Left Ureter, Via Natural or Artificial Opening
0TL78DZ   Occlusion of Left Ureter with Intraluminal Device, Via Natural or Artificial Opening Endoscopic
0TL78ZZ   Occlusion of Left Ureter, Via Natural or Artificial Opening Endoscopic
0TLB0CZ   Occlusion of Bladder with Extraluminal Device, Open Approach
0TLB0DZ   Occlusion of Bladder with Intraluminal Device, Open Approach
0TLB0ZZ   Occlusion of Bladder, Open Approach

♀ Female-only   ♂ Male-only   ▲ Limited Coverage   ● Non-OR   HAC HAC-associated procedure   ▲ Non-covered procedures   ✚ Cluster

0TLB3CZ Occlusion of Bladder with Extraluminal Device, Percutaneous Approach
0TLB3DZ Occlusion of Bladder with Intraluminal Device, Percutaneous Approach
0TLB3ZZ Occlusion of Bladder, Percutaneous Approach
0TLB4CZ Occlusion of Bladder with Extraluminal Device, Percutaneous Endoscopic Approach
0TLB4DZ Occlusion of Bladder with Intraluminal Device, Percutaneous Endoscopic Approach
0TLB4ZZ Occlusion of Bladder, Percutaneous Endoscopic Approach
0TLB7DZ Occlusion of Bladder with Intraluminal Device, Via Natural or Artificial Opening
0TLB7ZZ Occlusion of Bladder, Via Natural or Artificial Opening
0TLB8DZ Occlusion of Bladder with Intraluminal Device, Via Natural or Artificial Opening Endoscopic
0TLB8ZZ Occlusion of Bladder, Via Natural or Artificial Opening Endoscopic
0TLC0CZ Occlusion of Bladder Neck with Extraluminal Device, Open Approach
0TLC0DZ Occlusion of Bladder Neck with Intraluminal Device, Open Approach
0TLC0ZZ Occlusion of Bladder Neck, Open Approach

0TLC3CZ Occlusion of Bladder Neck with Extraluminal Device, Percutaneous Approach
0TLC3DZ Occlusion of Bladder Neck with Intraluminal Device, Percutaneous Approach
0TLC3ZZ Occlusion of Bladder Neck, Percutaneous Approach
0TLC4CZ Occlusion of Bladder Neck with Extraluminal Device, Percutaneous Endoscopic Approach
0TLC4DZ Occlusion of Bladder Neck with Intraluminal Device, Percutaneous Endoscopic Approach
0TLC4ZZ Occlusion of Bladder Neck, Percutaneous Endoscopic Approach
0TLC7DZ Occlusion of Bladder Neck with Intraluminal Device, Via Natural or Artificial Opening
0TLC7ZZ Occlusion of Bladder Neck, Via Natural or Artificial Opening
0TLC8DZ Occlusion of Bladder Neck with Intraluminal Device, Via Natural or Artificial Opening Endoscopic
0TLC8ZZ Occlusion of Bladder Neck, Via Natural or Artificial Opening Endoscopic
0TLD0CZ Occlusion of Urethra with Extraluminal Device, Open Approach
0TLD0DZ Occlusion of Urethra with Intraluminal Device, Open Approach
0TLD0ZZ Occlusion of Urethra, Open Approach

0TLD3CZ Occlusion of Urethra with Extraluminal Device, Percutaneous Approach
0TLD3DZ Occlusion of Urethra with Intraluminal Device, Percutaneous Approach
0TLD3ZZ Occlusion of Urethra, Percutaneous Approach
0TLD4CZ Occlusion of Urethra with Extraluminal Device, Percutaneous Endoscopic Approach
0TLD4DZ Occlusion of Urethra with Intraluminal Device, Percutaneous Endoscopic Approach
0TLD4ZZ Occlusion of Urethra, Percutaneous Endoscopic Approach
0TLD7DZ Occlusion of Urethra with Intraluminal Device, Via Natural or Artificial Opening
0TLD7ZZ Occlusion of Urethra, Via Natural or Artificial Opening
0TLD8DZ Occlusion of Urethra with Intraluminal Device, Via Natural or Artificial Opening Endoscopic
0TLD8ZZ Occlusion of Urethra, Via Natural or Artificial Opening Endoscopic
0TLDXCZ Occlusion of Urethra with Extraluminal Device, External Approach
0TLDXDZ Occlusion of Urethra with Intraluminal Device, External Approach
0TLDXZZ Occlusion of Urethra, External Approach

0TM – Urinary System, Reattachment

0TM00ZZ Reattachment of Right Kidney, Open Approach
0TM04ZZ Reattachment of Right Kidney, Percutaneous Endoscopic Approach
0TM10ZZ Reattachment of Left Kidney, Open Approach
0TM14ZZ Reattachment of Left Kidney, Percutaneous Endoscopic Approach
0TM20ZZ Reattachment of Bilateral Kidneys, Open Approach
0TM24ZZ Reattachment of Bilateral Kidneys, Percutaneous Endoscopic Approach
0TM30ZZ Reattachment of Right Kidney Pelvis, Open Approach

0TM34ZZ Reattachment of Right Kidney Pelvis, Percutaneous Endoscopic Approach
0TM40ZZ Reattachment of Left Kidney Pelvis, Open Approach
0TM44ZZ Reattachment of Left Kidney Pelvis, Percutaneous Endoscopic Approach
0TM60ZZ Reattachment of Right Ureter, Open Approach
0TM64ZZ Reattachment of Right Ureter, Percutaneous Endoscopic Approach
0TM70ZZ Reattachment of Left Ureter, Open Approach
0TM74ZZ Reattachment of Left Ureter, Percutaneous Endoscopic Approach

0TM80ZZ Reattachment of Bilateral Ureters, Open Approach
0TM84ZZ Reattachment of Bilateral Ureters, Percutaneous Endoscopic Approach
0TMB0ZZ Reattachment of Bladder, Open Approach
0TMB4ZZ Reattachment of Bladder, Percutaneous Endoscopic Approach
0TMC0ZZ Reattachment of Bladder Neck, Open Approach
0TMC4ZZ Reattachment of Bladder Neck, Percutaneous Endoscopic Approach
0TMD0ZZ Reattachment of Urethra, Open Approach
0TMD4ZZ Reattachment of Urethra, Percutaneous Endoscopic Approach

0TN – Urinary System, Release

Review Coding Guideline B3.13

Review Coding Guideline B3.14

0TN00ZZ Release Right Kidney, Open Approach
0TN03ZZ Release Right Kidney, Percutaneous Approach
0TN04ZZ Release Right Kidney, Percutaneous Endoscopic Approach
0TN07ZZ Release Right Kidney, Via Natural or Artificial Opening
0TN08ZZ Release Right Kidney, Via Natural or Artificial Opening Endoscopic
0TN10ZZ Release Left Kidney, Open Approach
0TN13ZZ Release Left Kidney, Percutaneous Approach
0TN14ZZ Release Left Kidney, Percutaneous Endoscopic Approach
0TN17ZZ Release Left Kidney, Via Natural or Artificial Opening

0TN18ZZ Release Left Kidney, Via Natural or Artificial Opening Endoscopic
0TN30ZZ Release Right Kidney Pelvis, Open Approach
0TN33ZZ Release Right Kidney Pelvis, Percutaneous Approach
0TN34ZZ Release Right Kidney Pelvis, Percutaneous Endoscopic Approach
0TN37ZZ Release Right Kidney Pelvis, Via Natural or Artificial Opening
0TN38ZZ Release Right Kidney Pelvis, Via Natural or Artificial Opening Endoscopic
0TN40ZZ Release Left Kidney Pelvis, Open Approach
0TN43ZZ Release Left Kidney Pelvis, Percutaneous Approach

0TN44ZZ Release Left Kidney Pelvis, Percutaneous Endoscopic Approach
0TN47ZZ Release Left Kidney Pelvis, Via Natural or Artificial Opening
0TN48ZZ Release Left Kidney Pelvis, Via Natural or Artificial Opening Endoscopic
0TN60ZZ Release Right Ureter, Open Approach
0TN63ZZ Release Right Ureter, Percutaneous Approach
0TN64ZZ Release Right Ureter, Percutaneous Endoscopic Approach
0TN67ZZ Release Right Ureter, Via Natural or Artificial Opening
0TN68ZZ Release Right Ureter, Via Natural or Artificial Opening Endoscopic
0TN70ZZ Release Left Ureter, Open Approach

0TN73ZZ	Release Left Ureter, Percutaneous Approach	0TNB7ZZ	Release Bladder, Via Natural or Artificial Opening
0TN74ZZ	Release Left Ureter, Percutaneous Endoscopic Approach	0TNB8ZZ	Release Bladder, Via Natural or Artificial Opening Endoscopic
0TN77ZZ	Release Left Ureter, Via Natural or Artificial Opening	0TNC0ZZ	Release Bladder Neck, Open Approach
0TN78ZZ	Release Left Ureter, Via Natural or Artificial Opening Endoscopic	0TNC3ZZ	Release Bladder Neck, Percutaneous Approach
0TNB0ZZ	Release Bladder, Open Approach	0TNC4ZZ	Release Bladder Neck, Percutaneous Endoscopic Approach
0TNB3ZZ	Release Bladder, Percutaneous Approach	0TNC7ZZ	Release Bladder Neck, Via Natural or Artificial Opening
0TNB4ZZ	Release Bladder, Percutaneous Endoscopic Approach	0TNC8ZZ	Release Bladder Neck, Via Natural or Artificial Opening Endoscopic

0TND0ZZ	Release Urethra, Open Approach
0TND3ZZ	Release Urethra, Percutaneous Approach
0TND4ZZ	Release Urethra, Percutaneous Endoscopic Approach
0TND7ZZ	Release Urethra, Via Natural or Artificial Opening
0TND8ZZ	Release Urethra, Via Natural or Artificial Opening Endoscopic
0TNDXZZ	Release Urethra, External Approach

0TP – Urinary System, Removal

Review Coding Guideline B6.1c

0TP500Z	Removal of Drainage Device from Kidney, Open Approach	0TP54JZ	Removal of Synthetic Substitute from Kidney, Percutaneous Endoscopic Approach	0TP58YZ	Removal of Other Device from Kidney, Via Natural or Artificial Opening Endoscopic
0TP502Z	Removal of Monitoring Device from Kidney, Open Approach	0TP54KZ	Removal of Nonautologous Tissue Substitute from Kidney, Percutaneous Endoscopic Approach	0TP5X0Z	Removal of Drainage Device from Kidney, External Approach
0TP503Z	Removal of Infusion Device from Kidney, Open Approach	0TP54YZ	Removal of Other Device from Kidney, Percutaneous Endoscopic Approach	0TP5X2Z	Removal of Monitoring Device from Kidney, External Approach
0TP507Z	Removal of Autologous Tissue Substitute from Kidney, Open Approach	0TP570Z	Removal of Drainage Device from Kidney, Via Natural or Artificial Opening	0TP5X3Z	Removal of Infusion Device from Kidney, External Approach
0TP50CZ	Removal of Extraluminal Device from Kidney, Open Approach	0TP572Z	Removal of Monitoring Device from Kidney, Via Natural or Artificial Opening	0TP5XDZ	Removal of Intraluminal Device from Kidney, External Approach
0TP50DZ	Removal of Intraluminal Device from Kidney, Open Approach	0TP573Z	Removal of Infusion Device from Kidney, Via Natural or Artificial Opening	0TP900Z	Removal of Drainage Device from Ureter, Open Approach
0TP50JZ	Removal of Synthetic Substitute from Kidney, Open Approach	0TP577Z	Removal of Autologous Tissue Substitute from Kidney, Via Natural or Artificial Opening	0TP902Z	Removal of Monitoring Device from Ureter, Open Approach
0TP50KZ	Removal of Nonautologous Tissue Substitute from Kidney, Open Approach	0TP57CZ	Removal of Extraluminal Device from Kidney, Via Natural or Artificial Opening	0TP903Z	Removal of Infusion Device from Ureter, Open Approach
0TP50YZ	Removal of Other Device from Kidney, Open Approach	0TP57DZ	Removal of Intraluminal Device from Kidney, Via Natural or Artificial Opening	0TP907Z	Removal of Autologous Tissue Substitute from Ureter, Open Approach
0TP530Z	Removal of Drainage Device from Kidney, Percutaneous Approach	0TP57JZ	Removal of Synthetic Substitute from Kidney, Via Natural or Artificial Opening	0TP90CZ	Removal of Extraluminal Device from Ureter, Open Approach
0TP532Z	Removal of Monitoring Device from Kidney, Percutaneous Approach	0TP57KZ	Removal of Nonautologous Tissue Substitute from Kidney, Via Natural or Artificial Opening	0TP90DZ	Removal of Intraluminal Device from Ureter, Open Approach
0TP533Z	Removal of Infusion Device from Kidney, Percutaneous Approach	0TP57YZ	Removal of Other Device from Kidney, Via Natural or Artificial Opening	0TP90JZ	Removal of Synthetic Substitute from Ureter, Open Approach
0TP537Z	Removal of Autologous Tissue Substitute from Kidney, Percutaneous Approach	0TP580Z	Removal of Drainage Device from Kidney, Via Natural or Artificial Opening Endoscopic	0TP90KZ	Removal of Nonautologous Tissue Substitute from Ureter, Open Approach
0TP53CZ	Removal of Extraluminal Device from Kidney, Percutaneous Approach	0TP582Z	Removal of Monitoring Device from Kidney, Via Natural or Artificial Opening Endoscopic	0TP90MZ	Removal of Stimulator Lead from Ureter, Open Approach
0TP53DZ	Removal of Intraluminal Device from Kidney, Percutaneous Approach	0TP583Z	Removal of Infusion Device from Kidney, Via Natural or Artificial Opening Endoscopic	0TP90YZ	Removal of Other Device from Ureter, Open Approach
0TP53JZ	Removal of Synthetic Substitute from Kidney, Percutaneous Approach	0TP587Z	Removal of Autologous Tissue Substitute from Kidney, Via Natural or Artificial Opening Endoscopic	0TP930Z	Removal of Drainage Device from Ureter, Percutaneous Approach
0TP53KZ	Removal of Nonautologous Tissue Substitute from Kidney, Percutaneous Approach	0TP58CZ	Removal of Extraluminal Device from Kidney, Via Natural or Artificial Opening Endoscopic	0TP932Z	Removal of Monitoring Device from Ureter, Percutaneous Approach
0TP53YZ	Removal of Other Device from Kidney, Percutaneous Approach	0TP58DZ	Removal of Intraluminal Device from Kidney, Via Natural or Artificial Opening Endoscopic	0TP933Z	Removal of Infusion Device from Ureter, Percutaneous Approach
0TP540Z	Removal of Drainage Device from Kidney, Percutaneous Endoscopic Approach	0TP58JZ	Removal of Synthetic Substitute from Kidney, Via Natural or Artificial Opening Endoscopic	0TP937Z	Removal of Autologous Tissue Substitute from Ureter, Percutaneous Approach
0TP542Z	Removal of Monitoring Device from Kidney, Percutaneous Endoscopic Approach	0TP58KZ	Removal of Nonautologous Tissue Substitute from Kidney, Via Natural or Artificial Opening Endoscopic	0TP93CZ	Removal of Extraluminal Device from Ureter, Percutaneous Approach
0TP543Z	Removal of Infusion Device from Kidney, Percutaneous Endoscopic Approach			0TP93DZ	Removal of Intraluminal Device from Ureter, Percutaneous Approach
0TP547Z	Removal of Autologous Tissue Substitute from Kidney, Percutaneous Endoscopic Approach			0TP93JZ	Removal of Synthetic Substitute from Ureter, Percutaneous Approach
0TP54CZ	Removal of Extraluminal Device from Kidney, Percutaneous Endoscopic Approach			0TP93KZ	Removal of Nonautologous Tissue Substitute from Ureter, Percutaneous Approach
0TP54DZ	Removal of Intraluminal Device from Kidney, Percutaneous Endoscopic Approach			0TP93MZ	Removal of Stimulator Lead from Ureter, Percutaneous Approach
				0TP93YZ	Removal of Other Device from Ureter, Percutaneous Approach
				0TP940Z	Removal of Drainage Device from Ureter, Percutaneous Endoscopic Approach

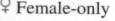

0TP942Z Removal of Monitoring Device from Ureter, Percutaneous Endoscopic Approach

0TP943Z Removal of Infusion Device from Ureter, Percutaneous Endoscopic Approach

0TP947Z Removal of Autologous Tissue Substitute from Ureter, Percutaneous Endoscopic Approach

0TP94CZ Removal of Extraluminal Device from Ureter, Percutaneous Endoscopic Approach

0TP94DZ Removal of Intraluminal Device from Ureter, Percutaneous Endoscopic Approach

0TP94JZ Removal of Synthetic Substitute from Ureter, Percutaneous Endoscopic Approach

0TP94KZ Removal of Nonautologous Tissue Substitute from Ureter, Percutaneous Endoscopic Approach

0TP94MZ Removal of Stimulator Lead from Ureter, Percutaneous Endoscopic Approach

0TP94YZ Removal of Other Device from Ureter, Percutaneous Endoscopic Approach

0TP970Z Removal of Drainage Device from Ureter, Via Natural or Artificial Opening

0TP972Z Removal of Monitoring Device from Ureter, Via Natural or Artificial Opening

0TP973Z Removal of Infusion Device from Ureter, Via Natural or Artificial Opening

0TP977Z Removal of Autologous Tissue Substitute from Ureter, Via Natural or Artificial Opening

0TP97CZ Removal of Extraluminal Device from Ureter, Via Natural or Artificial Opening

0TP97DZ Removal of Intraluminal Device from Ureter, Via Natural or Artificial Opening

0TP97JZ Removal of Synthetic Substitute from Ureter, Via Natural or Artificial Opening

0TP97KZ Removal of Nonautologous Tissue Substitute from Ureter, Via Natural or Artificial Opening

0TP97MZ Removal of Stimulator Lead from Ureter, Via Natural or Artificial Opening

0TP97YZ Removal of Other Device from Ureter, Via Natural or Artificial Opening

0TP980Z Removal of Drainage Device from Ureter, Via Natural or Artificial Opening Endoscopic

0TP982Z Removal of Monitoring Device from Ureter, Via Natural or Artificial Opening Endoscopic

0TP983Z Removal of Infusion Device from Ureter, Via Natural or Artificial Opening Endoscopic

0TP987Z Removal of Autologous Tissue Substitute from Ureter, Via Natural or Artificial Opening Endoscopic

0TP98CZ Removal of Extraluminal Device from Ureter, Via Natural or Artificial Opening Endoscopic

0TP98DZ Removal of Intraluminal Device from Ureter, Via Natural or Artificial Opening Endoscopic

AHA CC: 2Q, 2016, 27-28

0TP98JZ Removal of Synthetic Substitute from Ureter, Via Natural or Artificial Opening Endoscopic

0TP98KZ Removal of Nonautologous Tissue Substitute from Ureter, Via Natural or Artificial Opening Endoscopic

0TP98MZ Removal of Stimulator Lead from Ureter, Via Natural or Artificial Opening Endoscopic

0TP98YZ Removal of Other Device from Ureter, Via Natural or Artificial Opening Endoscopic

0TP9X0Z Removal of Drainage Device from Ureter, External Approach

0TP9X2Z Removal of Monitoring Device from Ureter, External Approach

0TP9X3Z Removal of Infusion Device from Ureter, External Approach

0TP9XDZ Removal of Intraluminal Device from Ureter, External Approach

0TP9XMZ Removal of Stimulator Lead from Ureter, External Approach

0TPB00Z Removal of Drainage Device from Bladder, Open Approach

0TPB02Z Removal of Monitoring Device from Bladder, Open Approach

0TPB03Z Removal of Infusion Device from Bladder, Open Approach

0TPB07Z Removal of Autologous Tissue Substitute from Bladder, Open Approach

0TPB0CZ Removal of Extraluminal Device from Bladder, Open Approach

0TPB0DZ Removal of Intraluminal Device from Bladder, Open Approach

0TPB0JZ Removal of Synthetic Substitute from Bladder, Open Approach

0TPB0KZ Removal of Nonautologous Tissue Substitute from Bladder, Open Approach

0TPB0LZ Removal of Artificial Sphincter from Bladder, Open Approach

▲ **0TPB0MZ** Removal of Stimulator Lead from Bladder, Open Approach

0TPB0YZ Removal of Other Device from Bladder, Open Approach

0TPB30Z Removal of Drainage Device from Bladder, Percutaneous Approach

0TPB32Z Removal of Monitoring Device from Bladder, Percutaneous Approach

0TPB33Z Removal of Infusion Device from Bladder, Percutaneous Approach

0TPB37Z Removal of Autologous Tissue Substitute from Bladder, Percutaneous Approach

0TPB3CZ Removal of Extraluminal Device from Bladder, Percutaneous Approach

0TPB3DZ Removal of Intraluminal Device from Bladder, Percutaneous Approach

0TPB3JZ Removal of Synthetic Substitute from Bladder, Percutaneous Approach

0TPB3KZ Removal of Nonautologous Tissue Substitute from Bladder, Percutaneous Approach

0TPB3LZ Removal of Artificial Sphincter from Bladder, Percutaneous Approach

▲ **0TPB3MZ** Removal of Stimulator Lead from Bladder, Percutaneous Approach

0TPB3YZ Removal of Other Device from Bladder, Percutaneous Approach

0TPB40Z Removal of Drainage Device from Bladder, Percutaneous Endoscopic Approach

0TPB42Z Removal of Monitoring Device from Bladder, Percutaneous Endoscopic Approach

0TPB43Z Removal of Infusion Device from Bladder, Percutaneous Endoscopic Approach

0TPB47Z Removal of Autologous Tissue Substitute from Bladder, Percutaneous Endoscopic Approach

0TPB4CZ Removal of Extraluminal Device from Bladder, Percutaneous Endoscopic Approach

0TPB4DZ Removal of Intraluminal Device from Bladder, Percutaneous Endoscopic Approach

0TPB4JZ Removal of Synthetic Substitute from Bladder, Percutaneous Endoscopic Approach

0TPB4KZ Removal of Nonautologous Tissue Substitute from Bladder, Percutaneous Endoscopic Approach

0TPB4LZ Removal of Artificial Sphincter from Bladder, Percutaneous Endoscopic Approach

▲ **0TPB4MZ** Removal of Stimulator Lead from Bladder, Percutaneous Endoscopic Approach

0TPB4YZ Removal of Other Device from Bladder, Percutaneous Endoscopic Approach

0TPB70Z Removal of Drainage Device from Bladder, Via Natural or Artificial Opening

0TPB72Z Removal of Monitoring Device from Bladder, Via Natural or Artificial Opening

0TPB73Z Removal of Infusion Device from Bladder, Via Natural or Artificial Opening

0TPB77Z Removal of Autologous Tissue Substitute from Bladder, Via Natural or Artificial Opening

0TPB7CZ Removal of Extraluminal Device from Bladder, Via Natural or Artificial Opening

0TPB7DZ Removal of Intraluminal Device from Bladder, Via Natural or Artificial Opening

0TPB7JZ Removal of Synthetic Substitute from Bladder, Via Natural or Artificial Opening

0TPB7KZ Removal of Nonautologous Tissue Substitute from Bladder, Via Natural or Artificial Opening

0TPB7LZ Removal of Artificial Sphincter from Bladder, Via Natural or Artificial Opening

▲ **0TPB7MZ** Removal of Stimulator Lead from Bladder, Via Natural or Artificial Opening

0TPB7YZ Removal of Other Device from Bladder, Via Natural or Artificial Opening

0TPB80Z Removal of Drainage Device from Bladder, Via Natural or Artificial Opening Endoscopic

0TPB82Z Removal of Monitoring Device from Bladder, Via Natural or Artificial Opening Endoscopic

0TPB83Z Removal of Infusion Device from Bladder, Via Natural or Artificial Opening Endoscopic

0TPB87Z Removal of Autologous Tissue Substitute from Bladder, Via Natural or Artificial Opening Endoscopic

0TPB8CZ Removal of Extraluminal Device from Bladder, Via Natural or Artificial Opening Endoscopic

0TPB8DZ Removal of Intraluminal Device from Bladder, Via Natural or Artificial Opening Endoscopic

0TPB8JZ Removal of Synthetic Substitute from Bladder, Via Natural or Artificial Opening Endoscopic

0TPB8KZ	Removal of Nonautologous Tissue Substitute from Bladder, Via Natural or Artificial Opening Endoscopic
0TPB8LZ	Removal of Artificial Sphincter from Bladder, Via Natural or Artificial Opening Endoscopic
▲ 0TPB8MZ	Removal of Stimulator Lead from Bladder, Via Natural or Artificial Opening Endoscopic
0TPB8YZ	Removal of Other Device from Bladder, Via Natural or Artificial Opening Endoscopic
0TPBX0Z	Removal of Drainage Device from Bladder, External Approach
0TPBX2Z	Removal of Monitoring Device from Bladder, External Approach
0TPBX3Z	Removal of Infusion Device from Bladder, External Approach
0TPBXDZ	Removal of Intraluminal Device from Bladder, External Approach
0TPBXLZ	Removal of Artificial Sphincter from Bladder, External Approach
0TPBXMZ	Removal of Stimulator Lead from Bladder, External Approach
0TPD00Z	Removal of Drainage Device from Urethra, Open Approach
0TPD02Z	Removal of Monitoring Device from Urethra, Open Approach
0TPD03Z	Removal of Infusion Device from Urethra, Open Approach
0TPD07Z	Removal of Autologous Tissue Substitute from Urethra, Open Approach
0TPD0CZ	Removal of Extraluminal Device from Urethra, Open Approach
0TPD0DZ	Removal of Intraluminal Device from Urethra, Open Approach
0TPD0JZ	Removal of Synthetic Substitute from Urethra, Open Approach
0TPD0KZ	Removal of Nonautologous Tissue Substitute from Urethra, Open Approach
0TPD0LZ	Removal of Artificial Sphincter from Urethra, Open Approach
0TPD0YZ	Removal of Other Device from Urethra, Open Approach
0TPD30Z	Removal of Drainage Device from Urethra, Percutaneous Approach
0TPD32Z	Removal of Monitoring Device from Urethra, Percutaneous Approach
0TPD33Z	Removal of Infusion Device from Urethra, Percutaneous Approach
0TPD37Z	Removal of Autologous Tissue Substitute from Urethra, Percutaneous Approach
0TPD3CZ	Removal of Extraluminal Device from Urethra, Percutaneous Approach

0TPD3DZ	Removal of Intraluminal Device from Urethra, Percutaneous Approach
0TPD3JZ	Removal of Synthetic Substitute from Urethra, Percutaneous Approach
0TPD3KZ	Removal of Nonautologous Tissue Substitute from Urethra, Percutaneous Approach
0TPD3LZ	Removal of Artificial Sphincter from Urethra, Percutaneous Approach
0TPD3YZ	Removal of Other Device from Urethra, Percutaneous Approach
0TPD40Z	Removal of Drainage Device from Urethra, Percutaneous Endoscopic Approach
0TPD42Z	Removal of Monitoring Device from Urethra, Percutaneous Endoscopic Approach
0TPD43Z	Removal of Infusion Device from Urethra, Percutaneous Endoscopic Approach
0TPD47Z	Removal of Autologous Tissue Substitute from Urethra, Percutaneous Endoscopic Approach
0TPD4CZ	Removal of Extraluminal Device from Urethra, Percutaneous Endoscopic Approach
0TPD4DZ	Removal of Intraluminal Device from Urethra, Percutaneous Endoscopic Approach
0TPD4JZ	Removal of Synthetic Substitute from Urethra, Percutaneous Endoscopic Approach
0TPD4KZ	Removal of Nonautologous Tissue Substitute from Urethra, Percutaneous Endoscopic Approach
0TPD4LZ	Removal of Artificial Sphincter from Urethra, Percutaneous Endoscopic Approach
0TPD4YZ	Removal of Other Device from Urethra, Percutaneous Endoscopic Approach
0TPD70Z	Removal of Drainage Device from Urethra, Via Natural or Artificial Opening
0TPD72Z	Removal of Monitoring Device from Urethra, Via Natural or Artificial Opening
0TPD73Z	Removal of Infusion Device from Urethra, Via Natural or Artificial Opening
0TPD77Z	Removal of Autologous Tissue Substitute from Urethra, Via Natural or Artificial Opening
0TPD7CZ	Removal of Extraluminal Device from Urethra, Via Natural or Artificial Opening

0TPD7DZ	Removal of Intraluminal Device from Urethra, Via Natural or Artificial Opening
0TPD7JZ	Removal of Synthetic Substitute from Urethra, Via Natural or Artificial Opening
0TPD7KZ	Removal of Nonautologous Tissue Substitute from Urethra, Via Natural or Artificial Opening
0TPD7LZ	Removal of Artificial Sphincter from Urethra, Via Natural or Artificial Opening
0TPD7YZ	Removal of Other Device from Urethra, Via Natural or Artificial Opening
0TPD80Z	Removal of Drainage Device from Urethra, Via Natural or Artificial Opening Endoscopic
0TPD82Z	Removal of Monitoring Device from Urethra, Via Natural or Artificial Opening Endoscopic
0TPD83Z	Removal of Infusion Device from Urethra, Via Natural or Artificial Opening Endoscopic
0TPD87Z	Removal of Autologous Tissue Substitute from Urethra, Via Natural or Artificial Opening Endoscopic
0TPD8CZ	Removal of Extraluminal Device from Urethra, Via Natural or Artificial Opening Endoscopic
0TPD8DZ	Removal of Intraluminal Device from Urethra, Via Natural or Artificial Opening Endoscopic
0TPD8JZ	Removal of Synthetic Substitute from Urethra, Via Natural or Artificial Opening Endoscopic
0TPD8KZ	Removal of Nonautologous Tissue Substitute from Urethra, Via Natural or Artificial Opening Endoscopic
0TPD8LZ	Removal of Artificial Sphincter from Urethra, Via Natural or Artificial Opening Endoscopic
0TPD8YZ	Removal of Other Device from Urethra, Via Natural or Artificial Opening Endoscopic
0TPDX0Z	Removal of Drainage Device from Urethra, External Approach
0TPDX2Z	Removal of Monitoring Device from Urethra, External Approach
0TPDX3Z	Removal of Infusion Device from Urethra, External Approach
0TPDXDZ	Removal of Intraluminal Device from Urethra, External Approach
0TPDXLZ	Removal of Artificial Sphincter from Urethra, External Approach

0TQ – Urinary System, Repair

| 0TQ00ZZ | Repair Right Kidney, Open Approach |
| 0TQ03ZZ | Repair Right Kidney, Percutaneous Approach |

AHA CC: 1Q, 2017, 36-37; 2Q, 2018, 27

0TQ04ZZ	Repair Right Kidney, Percutaneous Endoscopic Approach
0TQ07ZZ	Repair Right Kidney, Via Natural or Artificial Opening
0TQ08ZZ	Repair Right Kidney, Via Natural or Artificial Opening Endoscopic
0TQ10ZZ	Repair Left Kidney, Open Approach
0TQ13ZZ	Repair Left Kidney, Percutaneous Approach
0TQ14ZZ	Repair Left Kidney, Percutaneous Endoscopic Approach
0TQ17ZZ	Repair Left Kidney, Via Natural or Artificial Opening

0TQ18ZZ	Repair Left Kidney, Via Natural or Artificial Opening Endoscopic
0TQ30ZZ	Repair Right Kidney Pelvis, Open Approach
0TQ33ZZ	Repair Right Kidney Pelvis, Percutaneous Approach
0TQ34ZZ	Repair Right Kidney Pelvis, Percutaneous Endoscopic Approach
0TQ37ZZ	Repair Right Kidney Pelvis, Via Natural or Artificial Opening
0TQ38ZZ	Repair Right Kidney Pelvis, Via Natural or Artificial Opening Endoscopic
0TQ40ZZ	Repair Left Kidney Pelvis, Open Approach
0TQ43ZZ	Repair Left Kidney Pelvis, Percutaneous Approach

0TQ44ZZ	Repair Left Kidney Pelvis, Percutaneous Endoscopic Approach
0TQ47ZZ	Repair Left Kidney Pelvis, Via Natural or Artificial Opening
0TQ48ZZ	Repair Left Kidney Pelvis, Via Natural or Artificial Opening Endoscopic
0TQ60ZZ	Repair Right Ureter, Open Approach
0TQ63ZZ	Repair Right Ureter, Percutaneous Approach
0TQ64ZZ	Repair Right Ureter, Percutaneous Endoscopic Approach
0TQ67ZZ	Repair Right Ureter, Via Natural or Artificial Opening
0TQ68ZZ	Repair Right Ureter, Via Natural or Artificial Opening Endoscopic
0TQ70ZZ	Repair Left Ureter, Open Approach

♀ Female-only   ♂ Male-only   ▲ Limited Coverage   ● Non-OR   ᴴᴬᶜ HAC-associated procedure   ▲ Non-covered procedures   ✚ Cluster

0TQ73ZZ	Repair Left Ureter, Percutaneous Approach
0TQ74ZZ	Repair Left Ureter, Percutaneous Endoscopic Approach
0TQ77ZZ	Repair Left Ureter, Via Natural or Artificial Opening
0TQ78ZZ	Repair Left Ureter, Via Natural or Artificial Opening Endoscopic
0TQB0ZZ	Repair Bladder, Open Approach
⊞	Urostomy takedown when performed with code 0WQFXZ2, Repair of abdominal wall, stoma, external approach or 0WQFXZZ, Repair of abdominal wall, external approach.
0TQB3ZZ	Repair Bladder, Percutaneous Approach
⊞	Urostomy takedown when performed with code 0WQFXZ2, Repair of

	abdominal wall, stoma, external approach or 0WQFXZZ, Repair of abdominal wall, external approach.
0TQB4ZZ	Repair Bladder, Percutaneous Endoscopic Approach
⊞	Urostomy takedown when performed with code 0WQFXZ2, Repair of abdominal wall, stoma, external approach or 0WQFXZZ, Repair of abdominal wall, external approach.
0TQB7ZZ	Repair Bladder, Via Natural or Artificial Opening
0TQB8ZZ	Repair Bladder, Via Natural or Artificial Opening Endoscopic
0TQC0ZZ	Repair Bladder Neck, Open Approach
0TQC3ZZ	Repair Bladder Neck, Percutaneous Approach

0TQC4ZZ	Repair Bladder Neck, Percutaneous Endoscopic Approach
0TQC7ZZ	Repair Bladder Neck, Via Natural or Artificial Opening
0TQC8ZZ	Repair Bladder Neck, Via Natural or Artificial Opening Endoscopic
0TQD0ZZ	Repair Urethra, Open Approach
	AHA CC: 1Q, 2017, 37-38
0TQD3ZZ	Repair Urethra, Percutaneous Approach
0TQD4ZZ	Repair Urethra, Percutaneous Endoscopic Approach
0TQD7ZZ	Repair Urethra, Via Natural or Artificial Opening
0TQD8ZZ	Repair Urethra, Via Natural or Artificial Opening Endoscopic
0TQDXZZ	Repair Urethra, External Approach

0TR – Urinary System, Replacement

Review Coding Guideline B3.18

0TR307Z	Replacement of Right Kidney Pelvis with Autologous Tissue Substitute, Open Approach
0TR30JZ	Replacement of Right Kidney Pelvis with Synthetic Substitute, Open Approach
0TR30KZ	Replacement of Right Kidney Pelvis with Nonautologous Tissue Substitute, Open Approach
0TR347Z	Replacement of Right Kidney Pelvis with Autologous Tissue Substitute, Percutaneous Endoscopic Approach
0TR34JZ	Replacement of Right Kidney Pelvis with Synthetic Substitute, Percutaneous Endoscopic Approach
0TR34KZ	Replacement of Right Kidney Pelvis with Nonautologous Tissue Substitute, Percutaneous Endoscopic Approach
0TR377Z	Replacement of Right Kidney Pelvis with Autologous Tissue Substitute, Via Natural or Artificial Opening
0TR37JZ	Replacement of Right Kidney Pelvis with Synthetic Substitute, Via Natural or Artificial Opening
0TR37KZ	Replacement of Right Kidney Pelvis with Nonautologous Tissue Substitute, Via Natural or Artificial Opening
0TR387Z	Replacement of Right Kidney Pelvis with Autologous Tissue Substitute, Via Natural or Artificial Opening Endoscopic
0TR38JZ	Replacement of Right Kidney Pelvis with Synthetic Substitute, Via Natural or Artificial Opening Endoscopic
0TR38KZ	Replacement of Right Kidney Pelvis with Nonautologous Tissue Substitute, Via Natural or Artificial Opening Endoscopic
0TR407Z	Replacement of Left Kidney Pelvis with Autologous Tissue Substitute, Open Approach
0TR40JZ	Replacement of Left Kidney Pelvis with Synthetic Substitute, Open Approach
0TR40KZ	Replacement of Left Kidney Pelvis with Nonautologous Tissue Substitute, Open Approach
0TR447Z	Replacement of Left Kidney Pelvis with Autologous Tissue Substitute, Percutaneous Endoscopic Approach
0TR44JZ	Replacement of Left Kidney Pelvis with Synthetic Substitute, Percutaneous Endoscopic Approach

0TR44KZ	Replacement of Left Kidney Pelvis with Nonautologous Tissue Substitute, Percutaneous Endoscopic Approach
0TR477Z	Replacement of Left Kidney Pelvis with Autologous Tissue Substitute, Via Natural or Artificial Opening
0TR47JZ	Replacement of Left Kidney Pelvis with Synthetic Substitute, Via Natural or Artificial Opening
0TR47KZ	Replacement of Left Kidney Pelvis with Nonautologous Tissue Substitute, Via Natural or Artificial Opening
0TR487Z	Replacement of Left Kidney Pelvis with Autologous Tissue Substitute, Via Natural or Artificial Opening Endoscopic
0TR48JZ	Replacement of Left Kidney Pelvis with Synthetic Substitute, Via Natural or Artificial Opening Endoscopic
0TR48KZ	Replacement of Left Kidney Pelvis with Nonautologous Tissue Substitute, Via Natural or Artificial Opening Endoscopic
0TR607Z	Replacement of Right Ureter with Autologous Tissue Substitute, Open Approach
0TR60JZ	Replacement of Right Ureter with Synthetic Substitute, Open Approach
0TR60KZ	Replacement of Right Ureter with Nonautologous Tissue Substitute, Open Approach
0TR647Z	Replacement of Right Ureter with Autologous Tissue Substitute, Percutaneous Endoscopic Approach
0TR64JZ	Replacement of Right Ureter with Synthetic Substitute, Percutaneous Endoscopic Approach
0TR64KZ	Replacement of Right Ureter with Nonautologous Tissue Substitute, Percutaneous Endoscopic Approach
0TR677Z	Replacement of Right Ureter with Autologous Tissue Substitute, Via Natural or Artificial Opening
0TR67JZ	Replacement of Right Ureter with Synthetic Substitute, Via Natural or Artificial Opening
0TR67KZ	Replacement of Right Ureter with Nonautologous Tissue Substitute, Via Natural or Artificial Opening
0TR687Z	Replacement of Right Ureter with Autologous Tissue Substitute, Via Natural or Artificial Opening Endoscopic

0TR68JZ	Replacement of Right Ureter with Synthetic Substitute, Via Natural or Artificial Opening Endoscopic
0TR68KZ	Replacement of Right Ureter with Nonautologous Tissue Substitute, Via Natural or Artificial Opening Endoscopic
0TR707Z	Replacement of Left Ureter with Autologous Tissue Substitute, Open Approach
0TR70JZ	Replacement of Left Ureter with Synthetic Substitute, Open Approach
0TR70KZ	Replacement of Left Ureter with Nonautologous Tissue Substitute, Open Approach
0TR747Z	Replacement of Left Ureter with Autologous Tissue Substitute, Percutaneous Endoscopic Approach
0TR74JZ	Replacement of Left Ureter with Synthetic Substitute, Percutaneous Endoscopic Approach
0TR74KZ	Replacement of Left Ureter with Nonautologous Tissue Substitute, Percutaneous Endoscopic Approach
0TR777Z	Replacement of Left Ureter with Autologous Tissue Substitute, Via Natural or Artificial Opening
0TR77JZ	Replacement of Left Ureter with Synthetic Substitute, Via Natural or Artificial Opening
0TR77KZ	Replacement of Left Ureter with Nonautologous Tissue Substitute, Via Natural or Artificial Opening
0TR787Z	Replacement of Left Ureter with Autologous Tissue Substitute, Via Natural or Artificial Opening Endoscopic
0TR78JZ	Replacement of Left Ureter with Synthetic Substitute, Via Natural or Artificial Opening Endoscopic
0TR78KZ	Replacement of Left Ureter with Nonautologous Tissue Substitute, Via Natural or Artificial Opening Endoscopic
0TRB07Z	Replacement of Bladder with Autologous Tissue Substitute, Open Approach
	AHA CC: 3Q, 2017, 20-21
0TRB0JZ	Replacement of Bladder with Synthetic Substitute, Open Approach
0TRB0KZ	Replacement of Bladder with Nonautologous Tissue Substitute, Open Approach

0TRB47Z	Replacement of Bladder with Autologous Tissue Substitute, Percutaneous Endoscopic Approach	0TRC47Z	Replacement of Bladder Neck with Autologous Tissue Substitute, Percutaneous Endoscopic Approach	0TRD47Z	Replacement of Urethra with Autologous Tissue Substitute, Percutaneous Endoscopic Approach
0TRB4JZ	Replacement of Bladder with Synthetic Substitute, Percutaneous Endoscopic Approach	0TRC4JZ	Replacement of Bladder Neck with Synthetic Substitute, Percutaneous Endoscopic Approach	0TRD4JZ	Replacement of Urethra with Synthetic Substitute, Percutaneous Endoscopic Approach
0TRB4KZ	Replacement of Bladder with Nonautologous Tissue Substitute, Percutaneous Endoscopic Approach	0TRC4KZ	Replacement of Bladder Neck with Nonautologous Tissue Substitute, Percutaneous Endoscopic Approach	0TRD4KZ	Replacement of Urethra with Nonautologous Tissue Substitute, Percutaneous Endoscopic Approach
0TRB77Z	Replacement of Bladder with Autologous Tissue Substitute, Via Natural or Artificial Opening	0TRC77Z	Replacement of Bladder Neck with Autologous Tissue Substitute, Via Natural or Artificial Opening	0TRD77Z	Replacement of Urethra with Autologous Tissue Substitute, Via Natural or Artificial Opening
0TRB7JZ	Replacement of Bladder with Synthetic Substitute, Via Natural or Artificial Opening	0TRC7JZ	Replacement of Bladder Neck with Synthetic Substitute, Via Natural or Artificial Opening	0TRD7JZ	Replacement of Urethra with Synthetic Substitute, Via Natural or Artificial Opening
0TRB7KZ	Replacement of Bladder with Nonautologous Tissue Substitute, Via Natural or Artificial Opening	0TRC7KZ	Replacement of Bladder Neck with Nonautologous Tissue Substitute, Via Natural or Artificial Opening	0TRD7KZ	Replacement of Urethra with Nonautologous Tissue Substitute, Via Natural or Artificial Opening
0TRB87Z	Replacement of Bladder with Autologous Tissue Substitute, Via Natural or Artificial Opening Endoscopic	0TRC87Z	Replacement of Bladder Neck with Autologous Tissue Substitute, Via Natural or Artificial Opening Endoscopic	0TRD87Z	Replacement of Urethra with Autologous Tissue Substitute, Via Natural or Artificial Opening Endoscopic
0TRB8JZ	Replacement of Bladder with Synthetic Substitute, Via Natural or Artificial Opening Endoscopic	0TRC8JZ	Replacement of Bladder Neck with Synthetic Substitute, Via Natural or Artificial Opening Endoscopic	0TRD8JZ	Replacement of Urethra with Synthetic Substitute, Via Natural or Artificial Opening Endoscopic
0TRB8KZ	Replacement of Bladder with Nonautologous Tissue Substitute, Via Natural or Artificial Opening Endoscopic	0TRC8KZ	Replacement of Bladder Neck with Nonautologous Tissue Substitute, Via Natural or Artificial Opening Endoscopic	0TRD8KZ	Replacement of Urethra with Nonautologous Tissue Substitute, Via Natural or Artificial Opening Endoscopic
0TRC07Z	Replacement of Bladder Neck with Autologous Tissue Substitute, Open Approach	0TRD07Z	Replacement of Urethra with Autologous Tissue Substitute, Open Approach	0TRDX7Z	Replacement of Urethra with Autologous Tissue Substitute, External Approach
0TRC0JZ	Replacement of Bladder Neck with Synthetic Substitute, Open Approach	0TRD0JZ	Replacement of Urethra with Synthetic Substitute, Open Approach	0TRDXJZ	Replacement of Urethra with Synthetic Substitute, External Approach
0TRC0KZ	Replacement of Bladder Neck with Nonautologous Tissue Substitute, Open Approach	0TRD0KZ	Replacement of Urethra with Nonautologous Tissue Substitute, Open Approach	0TRDXKZ	Replacement of Urethra with Nonautologous Tissue Substitute, External Approach

0TS – Urinary System, Reposition

0TS00ZZ	Reposition Right Kidney, Open Approach	0TS34ZZ	Reposition Right Kidney Pelvis, Percutaneous Endoscopic Approach	0TS80ZZ	Reposition Bilateral Ureters, Open Approach
0TS04ZZ	Reposition Right Kidney, Percutaneous Endoscopic Approach	0TS40ZZ	Reposition Left Kidney Pelvis, Open Approach	0TS84ZZ	Reposition Bilateral Ureters, Percutaneous Endoscopic Approach
0TS10ZZ	Reposition Left Kidney, Open Approach	0TS44ZZ	Reposition Left Kidney Pelvis, Percutaneous Endoscopic Approach	0TSB0ZZ	Reposition Bladder, Open Approach
0TS14ZZ	Reposition Left Kidney, Percutaneous Endoscopic Approach	0TS60ZZ	Reposition Right Ureter, Open Approach	0TSB4ZZ	Reposition Bladder, Percutaneous Endoscopic Approach
0TS20ZZ	Reposition Bilateral Kidneys, Open Approach		*AHA CC: 1Q, 2019, 29-30*	0TSC0ZZ	Reposition Bladder Neck, Open Approach
0TS24ZZ	Reposition Bilateral Kidneys, Percutaneous Endoscopic Approach	0TS64ZZ	Reposition Right Ureter, Percutaneous Endoscopic Approach	0TSC4ZZ	Reposition Bladder Neck, Percutaneous Endoscopic Approach
0TS30ZZ	Reposition Right Kidney Pelvis, Open Approach	0TS70ZZ	Reposition Left Ureter, Open Approach	0TSD0ZZ	Reposition Urethra, Open Approach
		0TS74ZZ	Reposition Left Ureter, Percutaneous Endoscopic Approach		*AHA CC: 1Q, 2016, 15-16*
				0TSD4ZZ	Reposition Urethra, Percutaneous Endoscopic Approach

0TT – Urinary System, Resection

Review Coding Guideline B3.8

Review Coding Guideline B3.18

0TT00ZZ	Resection of Right Kidney, Open Approach	0TT30ZZ	Resection of Right Kidney Pelvis, Open Approach	0TT47ZZ	Resection of Left Kidney Pelvis, Via Natural or Artificial Opening
0TT04ZZ	Resection of Right Kidney, Percutaneous Endoscopic Approach	0TT34ZZ	Resection of Right Kidney Pelvis, Percutaneous Endoscopic Approach	0TT48ZZ	Resection of Left Kidney Pelvis, Via Natural or Artificial Opening Endoscopic
0TT10ZZ	Resection of Left Kidney, Open Approach	0TT37ZZ	Resection of Right Kidney Pelvis, Via Natural or Artificial Opening	0TT60ZZ	Resection of Right Ureter, Open Approach
	AHA CC: 3Q, 2014, 16	0TT38ZZ	Resection of Right Kidney Pelvis, Via Natural or Artificial Opening Endoscopic	0TT64ZZ	Resection of Right Ureter, Percutaneous Endoscopic Approach
0TT14ZZ	Resection of Left Kidney, Percutaneous Endoscopic Approach	0TT40ZZ	Resection of Left Kidney Pelvis, Open Approach	0TT67ZZ	Resection of Right Ureter, Via Natural or Artificial Opening
0TT20ZZ	Resection of Bilateral Kidneys, Open Approach	0TT44ZZ	Resection of Left Kidney Pelvis, Percutaneous Endoscopic Approach	0TT68ZZ	Resection of Right Ureter, Via Natural or Artificial Opening Endoscopic
0TT24ZZ	Resection of Bilateral Kidneys, Percutaneous Endoscopic Approach				

 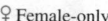

♀ Female-only   ♂ Male-only   ▲ Limited Coverage   ● Non-OR   **HAC** HAC-associated procedure   ▲ Non-covered procedures   ✛ Cluster

0TT70ZZ Resection of Left Ureter, Open Approach

AHA CC: 3Q, 2014, 16

0TT74ZZ Resection of Left Ureter, Percutaneous Endoscopic Approach

0TT77ZZ Resection of Left Ureter, Via Natural or Artificial Opening

0TT78ZZ Resection of Left Ureter, Via Natural or Artificial Opening Endoscopic

0TTB0ZZ Resection of Bladder, Open Approach

➕ Pelvic evisceration when reported with Resection of urethra, bilateral ovaries, bilateral fallopian tubes, uterus, cervix and vagina. *See tables 0TT and 0UT to construct the Resection codes.*

0TTB4ZZ Resection of Bladder, Percutaneous Endoscopic Approach

0TTB7ZZ Resection of Bladder, Via Natural or Artificial Opening

0TTB8ZZ Resection of Bladder, Via Natural or Artificial Opening Endoscopic

0TTC0ZZ Resection of Bladder Neck, Open Approach

0TTC4ZZ Resection of Bladder Neck, Percutaneous Endoscopic Approach

0TTC7ZZ Resection of Bladder Neck, Via Natural or Artificial Opening

0TTC8ZZ Resection of Bladder Neck, Via Natural or Artificial Opening Endoscopic

● **0TTD0ZZ** Resection of Urethra, Open Approach

➕ Pelvic evisceration when reported with Resection of bladder, bilateral ovaries, bilateral fallopian tubes, uterus, cervix and vagina. *See tables 0TT and 0UT to construct the Resection codes.*

0TTD4ZZ Resection of Urethra, Percutaneous Endoscopic Approach

0TTD7ZZ Resection of Urethra, Via Natural or Artificial Opening

0TTD8ZZ Resection of Urethra, Via Natural or Artificial Opening Endoscopic

0TU – Urinary System, Supplement

0TU307Z Supplement Right Kidney Pelvis with Autologous Tissue Substitute, Open Approach

0TU30JZ Supplement Right Kidney Pelvis with Synthetic Substitute, Open Approach

0TU30KZ Supplement Right Kidney Pelvis with Nonautologous Tissue Substitute, Open Approach

0TU347Z Supplement Right Kidney Pelvis with Autologous Tissue Substitute, Percutaneous Endoscopic Approach

0TU34JZ Supplement Right Kidney Pelvis with Synthetic Substitute, Percutaneous Endoscopic Approach

0TU34KZ Supplement Right Kidney Pelvis with Nonautologous Tissue Substitute, Percutaneous Endoscopic Approach

0TU377Z Supplement Right Kidney Pelvis with Autologous Tissue Substitute, Via Natural or Artificial Opening

0TU37JZ Supplement Right Kidney Pelvis with Synthetic Substitute, Via Natural or Artificial Opening

0TU37KZ Supplement Right Kidney Pelvis with Nonautologous Tissue Substitute, Via Natural or Artificial Opening

0TU387Z Supplement Right Kidney Pelvis with Autologous Tissue Substitute, Via Natural or Artificial Opening Endoscopic

0TU38JZ Supplement Right Kidney Pelvis with Synthetic Substitute, Via Natural or Artificial Opening Endoscopic

0TU38KZ Supplement Right Kidney Pelvis with Nonautologous Tissue Substitute, Via Natural or Artificial Opening Endoscopic

0TU407Z Supplement Left Kidney Pelvis with Autologous Tissue Substitute, Open Approach

0TU40JZ Supplement Left Kidney Pelvis with Synthetic Substitute, Open Approach

0TU40KZ Supplement Left Kidney Pelvis with Nonautologous Tissue Substitute, Open Approach

0TU447Z Supplement Left Kidney Pelvis with Autologous Tissue Substitute, Percutaneous Endoscopic Approach

0TU44JZ Supplement Left Kidney Pelvis with Synthetic Substitute, Percutaneous Endoscopic Approach

0TU44KZ Supplement Left Kidney Pelvis with Nonautologous Tissue Substitute, Percutaneous Endoscopic Approach

0TU477Z Supplement Left Kidney Pelvis with Autologous Tissue Substitute, Via Natural or Artificial Opening

0TU47JZ Supplement Left Kidney Pelvis with Synthetic Substitute, Via Natural or Artificial Opening

0TU47KZ Supplement Left Kidney Pelvis with Nonautologous Tissue Substitute, Via Natural or Artificial Opening

0TU487Z Supplement Left Kidney Pelvis with Autologous Tissue Substitute, Via Natural or Artificial Opening Endoscopic

0TU48JZ Supplement Left Kidney Pelvis with Synthetic Substitute, Via Natural or Artificial Opening Endoscopic

0TU48KZ Supplement Left Kidney Pelvis with Nonautologous Tissue Substitute, Via Natural or Artificial Opening Endoscopic

0TU607Z Supplement Right Ureter with Autologous Tissue Substitute, Open Approach

0TU60JZ Supplement Right Ureter with Synthetic Substitute, Open Approach

0TU60KZ Supplement Right Ureter with Nonautologous Tissue Substitute, Open Approach

0TU647Z Supplement Right Ureter with Autologous Tissue Substitute, Percutaneous Endoscopic Approach

0TU64JZ Supplement Right Ureter with Synthetic Substitute, Percutaneous Endoscopic Approach

0TU64KZ Supplement Right Ureter with Nonautologous Tissue Substitute, Percutaneous Endoscopic Approach

0TU677Z Supplement Right Ureter with Autologous Tissue Substitute, Via Natural or Artificial Opening

0TU67JZ Supplement Right Ureter with Synthetic Substitute, Via Natural or Artificial Opening

0TU67KZ Supplement Right Ureter with Nonautologous Tissue Substitute, Via Natural or Artificial Opening

0TU687Z Supplement Right Ureter with Autologous Tissue Substitute, Via Natural or Artificial Opening Endoscopic

0TU68JZ Supplement Right Ureter with Synthetic Substitute, Via Natural or Artificial Opening Endoscopic

0TU68KZ Supplement Right Ureter with Nonautologous Tissue Substitute, Via Natural or Artificial Opening Endoscopic

0TU707Z Supplement Left Ureter with Autologous Tissue Substitute, Open Approach

0TU70JZ Supplement Left Ureter with Synthetic Substitute, Open Approach

0TU70KZ Supplement Left Ureter with Nonautologous Tissue Substitute, Open Approach

0TU747Z Supplement Left Ureter with Autologous Tissue Substitute, Percutaneous Endoscopic Approach

0TU74JZ Supplement Left Ureter with Synthetic Substitute, Percutaneous Endoscopic Approach

0TU74KZ Supplement Left Ureter with Nonautologous Tissue Substitute, Percutaneous Endoscopic Approach

0TU777Z Supplement Left Ureter with Autologous Tissue Substitute, Via Natural or Artificial Opening

0TU77JZ Supplement Left Ureter with Synthetic Substitute, Via Natural or Artificial Opening

0TU77KZ Supplement Left Ureter with Nonautologous Tissue Substitute, Via Natural or Artificial Opening

0TU787Z Supplement Left Ureter with Autologous Tissue Substitute, Via Natural or Artificial Opening Endoscopic

0TU78JZ Supplement Left Ureter with Synthetic Substitute, Via Natural or Artificial Opening Endoscopic

0TU78KZ Supplement Left Ureter with Nonautologous Tissue Substitute, Via Natural or Artificial Opening Endoscopic

0TUB07Z Supplement Bladder with Autologous Tissue Substitute, Open Approach

AHA CC: 3Q, 2017, 21-22

0TUB0JZ Supplement Bladder with Synthetic Substitute, Open Approach

0TUB0KZ Supplement Bladder with Nonautologous Tissue Substitute, Open Approach

0TUB47Z Supplement Bladder with Autologous Tissue Substitute, Percutaneous Endoscopic Approach

0TUB4JZ Supplement Bladder with Synthetic Substitute, Percutaneous Endoscopic Approach

0TUB4KZ Supplement Bladder with Nonautologous Tissue Substitute, Percutaneous Endoscopic Approach

0TUB77Z Supplement Bladder with Autologous Tissue Substitute, Via Natural or Artificial Opening

0TUB7JZ Supplement Bladder with Synthetic Substitute, Via Natural or Artificial Opening

0TUB7KZ Supplement Bladder with Nonautologous Tissue Substitute, Via Natural or Artificial Opening

0TUB87Z Supplement Bladder with Autologous Tissue Substitute, Via Natural or Artificial Opening Endoscopic

0TUB8JZ Supplement Bladder with Synthetic Substitute, Via Natural or Artificial Opening Endoscopic

0TUB8KZ Supplement Bladder with Nonautologous Tissue Substitute, Via Natural or Artificial Opening Endoscopic

0TUC07Z Supplement Bladder Neck with Autologous Tissue Substitute, Open Approach

0TUC0JZ Supplement Bladder Neck with Synthetic Substitute, Open Approach

0TUC0KZ Supplement Bladder Neck with Nonautologous Tissue Substitute, Open Approach

0TUC47Z Supplement Bladder Neck with Autologous Tissue Substitute, Percutaneous Endoscopic Approach

0TUC4JZ Supplement Bladder Neck with Synthetic Substitute, Percutaneous Endoscopic Approach

0TUC4KZ Supplement Bladder Neck with Nonautologous Tissue Substitute, Percutaneous Endoscopic Approach

0TUC77Z Supplement Bladder Neck with Autologous Tissue Substitute, Via Natural or Artificial Opening

0TUC7JZ Supplement Bladder Neck with Synthetic Substitute, Via Natural or Artificial Opening

0TUC7KZ Supplement Bladder Neck with Nonautologous Tissue Substitute, Via Natural or Artificial Opening

0TUC87Z Supplement Bladder Neck with Autologous Tissue Substitute, Via Natural or Artificial Opening Endoscopic

0TUC8JZ Supplement Bladder Neck with Synthetic Substitute, Via Natural or Artificial Opening Endoscopic

0TUC8KZ Supplement Bladder Neck with Nonautologous Tissue Substitute, Via Natural or Artificial Opening Endoscopic

0TUD07Z Supplement Urethra with Autologous Tissue Substitute, Open Approach
AHA CC: 1Q, 2019, 29-30

0TUD0JZ Supplement Urethra with Synthetic Substitute, Open Approach

0TUD0KZ Supplement Urethra with Nonautologous Tissue Substitute, Open Approach

0TUD47Z Supplement Urethra with Autologous Tissue Substitute, Percutaneous Endoscopic Approach

0TUD4JZ Supplement Urethra with Synthetic Substitute, Percutaneous Endoscopic Approach

0TUD4KZ Supplement Urethra with Nonautologous Tissue Substitute, Percutaneous Endoscopic Approach

0TUD77Z Supplement Urethra with Autologous Tissue Substitute, Via Natural or Artificial Opening

0TUD7JZ Supplement Urethra with Synthetic Substitute, Via Natural or Artificial Opening

0TUD7KZ Supplement Urethra with Nonautologous Tissue Substitute, Via Natural or Artificial Opening

0TUD87Z Supplement Urethra with Autologous Tissue Substitute, Via Natural or Artificial Opening Endoscopic

0TUD8JZ Supplement Urethra with Synthetic Substitute, Via Natural or Artificial Opening Endoscopic

0TUD8KZ Supplement Urethra with Nonautologous Tissue Substitute, Via Natural or Artificial Opening Endoscopic

0TUDX7Z Supplement Urethra with Autologous Tissue Substitute, External Approach

0TUDXJZ Supplement Urethra with Synthetic Substitute, External Approach

0TUDXKZ Supplement Urethra with Nonautologous Tissue Substitute, External Approach

0TV – Urinary System, Restriction

0TV30CZ Restriction of Right Kidney Pelvis with Extraluminal Device, Open Approach

0TV30DZ Restriction of Right Kidney Pelvis with Intraluminal Device, Open Approach

0TV30ZZ Restriction of Right Kidney Pelvis, Open Approach

0TV33CZ Restriction of Right Kidney Pelvis with Extraluminal Device, Percutaneous Approach

0TV33DZ Restriction of Right Kidney Pelvis with Intraluminal Device, Percutaneous Approach

0TV33ZZ Restriction of Right Kidney Pelvis, Percutaneous Approach

0TV34CZ Restriction of Right Kidney Pelvis with Extraluminal Device, Percutaneous Endoscopic Approach

0TV34DZ Restriction of Right Kidney Pelvis with Intraluminal Device, Percutaneous Endoscopic Approach

0TV34ZZ Restriction of Right Kidney Pelvis, Percutaneous Endoscopic Approach

0TV37DZ Restriction of Right Kidney Pelvis with Intraluminal Device, Via Natural or Artificial Opening

0TV37ZZ Restriction of Right Kidney Pelvis, Via Natural or Artificial Opening

0TV38DZ Restriction of Right Kidney Pelvis with Intraluminal Device, Via Natural or Artificial Opening Endoscopic

0TV38ZZ Restriction of Right Kidney Pelvis, Via Natural or Artificial Opening Endoscopic

0TV40CZ Restriction of Left Kidney Pelvis with Extraluminal Device, Open Approach

0TV40DZ Restriction of Left Kidney Pelvis with Intraluminal Device, Open Approach

0TV40ZZ Restriction of Left Kidney Pelvis, Open Approach

0TV43CZ Restriction of Left Kidney Pelvis with Extraluminal Device, Percutaneous Approach

0TV43DZ Restriction of Left Kidney Pelvis with Intraluminal Device, Percutaneous Approach

0TV43ZZ Restriction of Left Kidney Pelvis, Percutaneous Approach

0TV44CZ Restriction of Left Kidney Pelvis with Extraluminal Device, Percutaneous Endoscopic Approach

0TV44DZ Restriction of Left Kidney Pelvis with Intraluminal Device, Percutaneous Endoscopic Approach

0TV44ZZ Restriction of Left Kidney Pelvis, Percutaneous Endoscopic Approach

0TV47DZ Restriction of Left Kidney Pelvis with Intraluminal Device, Via Natural or Artificial Opening

0TV47ZZ Restriction of Left Kidney Pelvis, Via Natural or Artificial Opening

0TV48DZ Restriction of Left Kidney Pelvis with Intraluminal Device, Via Natural or Artificial Opening Endoscopic

0TV48ZZ Restriction of Left Kidney Pelvis, Via Natural or Artificial Opening Endoscopic

0TV60CZ Restriction of Right Ureter with Extraluminal Device, Open Approach

0TV60DZ Restriction of Right Ureter with Intraluminal Device, Open Approach

0TV60ZZ Restriction of Right Ureter, Open Approach

0TV63CZ Restriction of Right Ureter with Extraluminal Device, Percutaneous Approach

0TV63DZ Restriction of Right Ureter with Intraluminal Device, Percutaneous Approach

0TV63ZZ Restriction of Right Ureter, Percutaneous Approach

0TV64CZ Restriction of Right Ureter with Extraluminal Device, Percutaneous Endoscopic Approach

0TV64DZ Restriction of Right Ureter with Intraluminal Device, Percutaneous Endoscopic Approach

0TV64ZZ Restriction of Right Ureter, Percutaneous Endoscopic Approach

0TV67DZ Restriction of Right Ureter with Intraluminal Device, Via Natural or Artificial Opening

0TV67ZZ Restriction of Right Ureter, Via Natural or Artificial Opening

0TV68DZ Restriction of Right Ureter with Intraluminal Device, Via Natural or Artificial Opening Endoscopic

0TV68ZZ Restriction of Right Ureter, Via Natural or Artificial Opening Endoscopic
AHA CC: 2Q, 2015, 11-12

0TV70CZ Restriction of Left Ureter with Extraluminal Device, Open Approach

0TV70DZ Restriction of Left Ureter with Intraluminal Device, Open Approach

0TV70ZZ Restriction of Left Ureter, Open Approach

0TV73CZ Restriction of Left Ureter with Extraluminal Device, Percutaneous Approach

0TV73DZ Restriction of Left Ureter with Intraluminal Device, Percutaneous Approach

0TV73ZZ Restriction of Left Ureter, Percutaneous Approach

0TV74CZ Restriction of Left Ureter with Extraluminal Device, Percutaneous Endoscopic Approach

0TV74DZ Restriction of Left Ureter with Intraluminal Device, Percutaneous Endoscopic Approach

♀ Female-only　♂ Male-only　▲ Limited Coverage　● Non-OR　HAC HAC-associated procedure　▲ Non-covered procedures　✚ Cluster

0TV74ZZ	Restriction of Left Ureter, Percutaneous Endoscopic Approach
0TV77DZ	Restriction of Left Ureter with Intraluminal Device, Via Natural or Artificial Opening
0TV77ZZ	Restriction of Left Ureter, Via Natural or Artificial Opening
0TV78DZ	Restriction of Left Ureter with Intraluminal Device, Via Natural or Artificial Opening Endoscopic
0TV78ZZ	Restriction of Left Ureter, Via Natural or Artificial Opening Endoscopic

AHA CC: 2Q, 2015, 11-12

0TVB0CZ	Restriction of Bladder with Extraluminal Device, Open Approach
0TVB0DZ	Restriction of Bladder with Intraluminal Device, Open Approach
0TVB0ZZ	Restriction of Bladder, Open Approach
0TVB3CZ	Restriction of Bladder with Extraluminal Device, Percutaneous Approach
0TVB3DZ	Restriction of Bladder with Intraluminal Device, Percutaneous Approach
0TVB3ZZ	Restriction of Bladder, Percutaneous Approach
0TVB4CZ	Restriction of Bladder with Extraluminal Device, Percutaneous Endoscopic Approach
0TVB4DZ	Restriction of Bladder with Intraluminal Device, Percutaneous Endoscopic Approach
0TVB4ZZ	Restriction of Bladder, Percutaneous Endoscopic Approach
0TVB7DZ	Restriction of Bladder with Intraluminal Device, Via Natural or Artificial Opening

0TVB7ZZ	Restriction of Bladder, Via Natural or Artificial Opening
0TVB8DZ	Restriction of Bladder with Intraluminal Device, Via Natural or Artificial Opening Endoscopic
0TVB8ZZ	Restriction of Bladder, Via Natural or Artificial Opening Endoscopic
0TVC0CZ	Restriction of Bladder Neck with Extraluminal Device, Open Approach
0TVC0DZ	Restriction of Bladder Neck with Intraluminal Device, Open Approach
0TVC0ZZ	Restriction of Bladder Neck, Open Approach
0TVC3CZ	Restriction of Bladder Neck with Extraluminal Device, Percutaneous Approach
0TVC3DZ	Restriction of Bladder Neck with Intraluminal Device, Percutaneous Approach
0TVC3ZZ	Restriction of Bladder Neck, Percutaneous Approach
0TVC4CZ	Restriction of Bladder Neck with Extraluminal Device, Percutaneous Endoscopic Approach
0TVC4DZ	Restriction of Bladder Neck with Intraluminal Device, Percutaneous Endoscopic Approach
0TVC4ZZ	Restriction of Bladder Neck, Percutaneous Endoscopic Approach
0TVC7DZ	Restriction of Bladder Neck with Intraluminal Device, Via Natural or Artificial Opening
0TVC7ZZ	Restriction of Bladder Neck, Via Natural or Artificial Opening
0TVC8DZ	Restriction of Bladder Neck with Intraluminal Device, Via Natural or Artificial Opening Endoscopic

0TVC8ZZ	Restriction of Bladder Neck, Via Natural or Artificial Opening Endoscopic
0TVD0CZ	Restriction of Urethra with Extraluminal Device, Open Approach
0TVD0DZ	Restriction of Urethra with Intraluminal Device, Open Approach
0TVD0ZZ	Restriction of Urethra, Open Approach
0TVD3CZ	Restriction of Urethra with Extraluminal Device, Percutaneous Approach
0TVD3DZ	Restriction of Urethra with Intraluminal Device, Percutaneous Approach
0TVD3ZZ	Restriction of Urethra, Percutaneous Approach
0TVD4CZ	Restriction of Urethra with Extraluminal Device, Percutaneous Endoscopic Approach
0TVD4DZ	Restriction of Urethra with Intraluminal Device, Percutaneous Endoscopic Approach
0TVD4ZZ	Restriction of Urethra, Percutaneous Endoscopic Approach
0TVD7DZ	Restriction of Urethra with Intraluminal Device, Via Natural or Artificial Opening
0TVD7ZZ	Restriction of Urethra, Via Natural or Artificial Opening
0TVD8DZ	Restriction of Urethra with Intraluminal Device, Via Natural or Artificial Opening Endoscopic
0TVD8ZZ	Restriction of Urethra, Via Natural or Artificial Opening Endoscopic
0TVDXZZ	Restriction of Urethra, External Approach

0TW – Urinary System, Revision

Review Coding Guideline B6.1c

0TW500Z	Revision of Drainage Device in Kidney, Open Approach
0TW502Z	Revision of Monitoring Device in Kidney, Open Approach
0TW503Z	Revision of Infusion Device in Kidney, Open Approach
0TW507Z	Revision of Autologous Tissue Substitute in Kidney, Open Approach
0TW50CZ	Revision of Extraluminal Device in Kidney, Open Approach
0TW50DZ	Revision of Intraluminal Device in Kidney, Open Approach
0TW50JZ	Revision of Synthetic Substitute in Kidney, Open Approach
0TW50KZ	Revision of Nonautologous Tissue Substitute in Kidney, Open Approach
0TW50YZ	Revision of Other Device in Kidney, Open Approach
0TW530Z	Revision of Drainage Device in Kidney, Percutaneous Approach
0TW532Z	Revision of Monitoring Device in Kidney, Percutaneous Approach
0TW533Z	Revision of Infusion Device in Kidney, Percutaneous Approach
0TW537Z	Revision of Autologous Tissue Substitute in Kidney, Percutaneous Approach
0TW53CZ	Revision of Extraluminal Device in Kidney, Percutaneous Approach
0TW53DZ	Revision of Intraluminal Device in Kidney, Percutaneous Approach
0TW53JZ	Revision of Synthetic Substitute in Kidney, Percutaneous Approach

0TW53KZ	Revision of Nonautologous Tissue Substitute in Kidney, Percutaneous Approach
0TW53YZ	Revision of Other Device in Kidney, Percutaneous Approach
0TW540Z	Revision of Drainage Device in Kidney, Percutaneous Endoscopic Approach
0TW542Z	Revision of Monitoring Device in Kidney, Percutaneous Endoscopic Approach
0TW543Z	Revision of Infusion Device in Kidney, Percutaneous Endoscopic Approach
0TW547Z	Revision of Autologous Tissue Substitute in Kidney, Percutaneous Endoscopic Approach
0TW54CZ	Revision of Extraluminal Device in Kidney, Percutaneous Endoscopic Approach
0TW54DZ	Revision of Intraluminal Device in Kidney, Percutaneous Endoscopic Approach
0TW54JZ	Revision of Synthetic Substitute in Kidney, Percutaneous Endoscopic Approach
0TW54KZ	Revision of Nonautologous Tissue Substitute in Kidney, Percutaneous Endoscopic Approach
0TW54YZ	Revision of Other Device in Kidney, Percutaneous Endoscopic Approach
0TW570Z	Revision of Drainage Device in Kidney, Via Natural or Artificial Opening

0TW570Z	Revision of Monitoring Device in Kidney, Via Natural or Artificial Opening
0TW573Z	Revision of Infusion Device in Kidney, Via Natural or Artificial Opening
0TW577Z	Revision of Autologous Tissue Substitute in Kidney, Via Natural or Artificial Opening
0TW57CZ	Revision of Extraluminal Device in Kidney, Via Natural or Artificial Opening
0TW57DZ	Revision of Intraluminal Device in Kidney, Via Natural or Artificial Opening
0TW57JZ	Revision of Synthetic Substitute in Kidney, Via Natural or Artificial Opening
0TW57KZ	Revision of Nonautologous Tissue Substitute in Kidney, Via Natural or Artificial Opening
0TW57YZ	Revision of Other Device in Kidney, Via Natural or Artificial Opening
0TW580Z	Revision of Drainage Device in Kidney, Via Natural or Artificial Opening Endoscopic
0TW582Z	Revision of Monitoring Device in Kidney, Via Natural or Artificial Opening Endoscopic
0TW583Z	Revision of Infusion Device in Kidney, Via Natural or Artificial Opening Endoscopic
0TW587Z	Revision of Autologous Tissue Substitute in Kidney, Via Natural or Artificial Opening Endoscopic

♀ Female-only   ♂ Male-only   ▲ Limited Coverage   ● Non-OR   **HAC** HAC-associated procedure   ▲ Non-covered procedures   ✚ Cluster

0TW58CZ	Revision of Extraluminal Device in Kidney, Via Natural or Artificial Opening Endoscopic
0TW58DZ	Revision of Intraluminal Device in Kidney, Via Natural or Artificial Opening Endoscopic
0TW58JZ	Revision of Synthetic Substitute in Kidney, Via Natural or Artificial Opening Endoscopic
0TW58KZ	Revision of Nonautologous Tissue Substitute in Kidney, Via Natural or Artificial Opening Endoscopic
0TW58YZ	Revision of Other Device in Kidney, Via Natural or Artificial Opening Endoscopic
0TW5X0Z	Revision of Drainage Device in Kidney, External Approach
0TW5X2Z	Revision of Monitoring Device in Kidney, External Approach
0TW5X3Z	Revision of Infusion Device in Kidney, External Approach
0TW5X7Z	Revision of Autologous Tissue Substitute in Kidney, External Approach
0TW5XCZ	Revision of Extraluminal Device in Kidney, External Approach
0TW5XDZ	Revision of Intraluminal Device in Kidney, External Approach
0TW5XJZ	Revision of Synthetic Substitute in Kidney, External Approach
0TW5XKZ	Revision of Nonautologous Tissue Substitute in Kidney, External Approach
0TW900Z	Revision of Drainage Device in Ureter, Open Approach
0TW902Z	Revision of Monitoring Device in Ureter, Open Approach
0TW903Z	Revision of Infusion Device in Ureter, Open Approach
0TW907Z	Revision of Autologous Tissue Substitute in Ureter, Open Approach
0TW90CZ	Revision of Extraluminal Device in Ureter, Open Approach
0TW90DZ	Revision of Intraluminal Device in Ureter, Open Approach
0TW90JZ	Revision of Synthetic Substitute in Ureter, Open Approach
0TW90KZ	Revision of Nonautologous Tissue Substitute in Ureter, Open Approach
0TW90MZ	Revision of Stimulator Lead in Ureter, Open Approach
0TW90YZ	Revision of Other Device in Ureter, Open Approach
0TW930Z	Revision of Drainage Device in Ureter, Percutaneous Approach
0TW932Z	Revision of Monitoring Device in Ureter, Percutaneous Approach
0TW933Z	Revision of Infusion Device in Ureter, Percutaneous Approach
0TW937Z	Revision of Autologous Tissue Substitute in Ureter, Percutaneous Approach
0TW93CZ	Revision of Extraluminal Device in Ureter, Percutaneous Approach
0TW93DZ	Revision of Intraluminal Device in Ureter, Percutaneous Approach
0TW93JZ	Revision of Synthetic Substitute in Ureter, Percutaneous Approach
0TW93KZ	Revision of Nonautologous Tissue Substitute in Ureter, Percutaneous Approach
0TW93MZ	Revision of Stimulator Lead in Ureter, Percutaneous Approach
0TW93YZ	Revision of Other Device in Ureter, Percutaneous Approach
0TW940Z	Revision of Drainage Device in Ureter, Percutaneous Endoscopic Approach
0TW942Z	Revision of Monitoring Device in Ureter, Percutaneous Endoscopic Approach
0TW943Z	Revision of Infusion Device in Ureter, Percutaneous Endoscopic Approach
0TW947Z	Revision of Autologous Tissue Substitute in Ureter, Percutaneous Endoscopic Approach
0TW94CZ	Revision of Extraluminal Device in Ureter, Percutaneous Endoscopic Approach
0TW94DZ	Revision of Intraluminal Device in Ureter, Percutaneous Endoscopic Approach
0TW94JZ	Revision of Synthetic Substitute in Ureter, Percutaneous Endoscopic Approach
0TW94KZ	Revision of Nonautologous Tissue Substitute in Ureter, Percutaneous Endoscopic Approach
0TW94MZ	Revision of Stimulator Lead in Ureter, Percutaneous Endoscopic Approach
0TW94YZ	Revision of Other Device in Ureter, Percutaneous Endoscopic Approach
0TW970Z	Revision of Drainage Device in Ureter, Via Natural or Artificial Opening
0TW972Z	Revision of Monitoring Device in Ureter, Via Natural or Artificial Opening
0TW973Z	Revision of Infusion Device in Ureter, Via Natural or Artificial Opening
0TW977Z	Revision of Autologous Tissue Substitute in Ureter, Via Natural or Artificial Opening
0TW97CZ	Revision of Extraluminal Device in Ureter, Via Natural or Artificial Opening
0TW97DZ	Revision of Intraluminal Device in Ureter, Via Natural or Artificial Opening
0TW97JZ	Revision of Synthetic Substitute in Ureter, Via Natural or Artificial Opening
0TW97KZ	Revision of Nonautologous Tissue Substitute in Ureter, Via Natural or Artificial Opening
0TW97MZ	Revision of Stimulator Lead in Ureter, Via Natural or Artificial Opening
0TW97YZ	Revision of Other Device in Ureter, Via Natural or Artificial Opening
0TW980Z	Revision of Drainage Device in Ureter, Via Natural or Artificial Opening Endoscopic
0TW982Z	Revision of Monitoring Device in Ureter, Via Natural or Artificial Opening Endoscopic
0TW983Z	Revision of Infusion Device in Ureter, Via Natural or Artificial Opening Endoscopic
0TW987Z	Revision of Autologous Tissue Substitute in Ureter, Via Natural or Artificial Opening Endoscopic
0TW98CZ	Revision of Extraluminal Device in Ureter, Via Natural or Artificial Opening Endoscopic
0TW98DZ	Revision of Intraluminal Device in Ureter, Via Natural or Artificial Opening Endoscopic
0TW98JZ	Revision of Synthetic Substitute in Ureter, Via Natural or Artificial Opening Endoscopic
0TW98KZ	Revision of Nonautologous Tissue Substitute in Ureter, Via Natural or Artificial Opening Endoscopic
0TW98MZ	Revision of Stimulator Lead in Ureter, Via Natural or Artificial Opening Endoscopic
0TW98YZ	Revision of Other Device in Ureter, Via Natural or Artificial Opening Endoscopic
0TW9X0Z	Revision of Drainage Device in Ureter, External Approach
0TW9X2Z	Revision of Monitoring Device in Ureter, External Approach
0TW9X3Z	Revision of Infusion Device in Ureter, External Approach
0TW9X7Z	Revision of Autologous Tissue Substitute in Ureter, External Approach
0TW9XCZ	Revision of Extraluminal Device in Ureter, External Approach
0TW9XDZ	Revision of Intraluminal Device in Ureter, External Approach
0TW9XJZ	Revision of Synthetic Substitute in Ureter, External Approach
0TW9XKZ	Revision of Nonautologous Tissue Substitute in Ureter, External Approach
0TW9XMZ	Revision of Stimulator Lead in Ureter, External Approach
0TWB00Z	Revision of Drainage Device in Bladder, Open Approach
0TWB02Z	Revision of Monitoring Device in Bladder, Open Approach
0TWB03Z	Revision of Infusion Device in Bladder, Open Approach
0TWB07Z	Revision of Autologous Tissue Substitute in Bladder, Open Approach
0TWB0CZ	Revision of Extraluminal Device in Bladder, Open Approach
0TWB0DZ	Revision of Intraluminal Device in Bladder, Open Approach
0TWB0JZ	Revision of Synthetic Substitute in Bladder, Open Approach
0TWB0KZ	Revision of Nonautologous Tissue Substitute in Bladder, Open Approach
0TWB0LZ	Revision of Artificial Sphincter in Bladder, Open Approach
0TWB0MZ	Revision of Stimulator Lead in Bladder, Open Approach
0TWB0YZ	Revision of Other Device in Bladder, Open Approach
0TWB30Z	Revision of Drainage Device in Bladder, Percutaneous Approach
0TWB32Z	Revision of Monitoring Device in Bladder, Percutaneous Approach
0TWB33Z	Revision of Infusion Device in Bladder, Percutaneous Approach
0TWB37Z	Revision of Autologous Tissue Substitute in Bladder, Percutaneous Approach
0TWB3CZ	Revision of Extraluminal Device in Bladder, Percutaneous Approach
0TWB3DZ	Revision of Intraluminal Device in Bladder, Percutaneous Approach
0TWB3JZ	Revision of Synthetic Substitute in Bladder, Percutaneous Approach
0TWB3KZ	Revision of Nonautologous Tissue Substitute in Bladder, Percutaneous Approach
0TWB3LZ	Revision of Artificial Sphincter in Bladder, Percutaneous Approach
0TWB3MZ	Revision of Stimulator Lead in Bladder, Percutaneous Approach
0TWB3YZ	Revision of Other Device in Bladder, Percutaneous Approach

♀ Female-only   ♂ Male-only   ▲ Limited Coverage   ● Non-OR   ᴴᴬᶜ HAC-associated procedure   ▲ Non-covered procedures   ✚ Cluster

0TWB40Z	Revision of Drainage Device in Bladder, Percutaneous Endoscopic Approach
0TWB42Z	Revision of Monitoring Device in Bladder, Percutaneous Endoscopic Approach
0TWB43Z	Revision of Infusion Device in Bladder, Percutaneous Endoscopic Approach
0TWB47Z	Revision of Autologous Tissue Substitute in Bladder, Percutaneous Endoscopic Approach
0TWB4CZ	Revision of Extraluminal Device in Bladder, Percutaneous Endoscopic Approach
0TWB4DZ	Revision of Intraluminal Device in Bladder, Percutaneous Endoscopic Approach
0TWB4JZ	Revision of Synthetic Substitute in Bladder, Percutaneous Endoscopic Approach
0TWB4KZ	Revision of Nonautologous Tissue Substitute in Bladder, Percutaneous Endoscopic Approach
0TWB4LZ	Revision of Artificial Sphincter in Bladder, Percutaneous Endoscopic Approach
0TWB4MZ	Revision of Stimulator Lead in Bladder, Percutaneous Endoscopic Approach
0TWB4YZ	Revision of Other Device in Bladder, Percutaneous Endoscopic Approach
0TWB70Z	Revision of Drainage Device in Bladder, Via Natural or Artificial Opening
0TWB72Z	Revision of Monitoring Device in Bladder, Via Natural or Artificial Opening
0TWB73Z	Revision of Infusion Device in Bladder, Via Natural or Artificial Opening
0TWB77Z	Revision of Autologous Tissue Substitute in Bladder, Via Natural or Artificial Opening
0TWB7CZ	Revision of Extraluminal Device in Bladder, Via Natural or Artificial Opening
0TWB7DZ	Revision of Intraluminal Device in Bladder, Via Natural or Artificial Opening
0TWB7JZ	Revision of Synthetic Substitute in Bladder, Via Natural or Artificial Opening
0TWB7KZ	Revision of Nonautologous Tissue Substitute in Bladder, Via Natural or Artificial Opening
0TWB7LZ	Revision of Artificial Sphincter in Bladder, Via Natural or Artificial Opening
0TWB7MZ	Revision of Stimulator Lead in Bladder, Via Natural or Artificial Opening
0TWB7YZ	Revision of Other Device in Bladder, Via Natural or Artificial Opening
0TWB80Z	Revision of Drainage Device in Bladder, Via Natural or Artificial Opening Endoscopic
0TWB82Z	Revision of Monitoring Device in Bladder, Via Natural or Artificial Opening Endoscopic
0TWB83Z	Revision of Infusion Device in Bladder, Via Natural or Artificial Opening Endoscopic
0TWB87Z	Revision of Autologous Tissue Substitute in Bladder, Via Natural or Artificial Opening Endoscopic

0TWB8CZ	Revision of Extraluminal Device in Bladder, Via Natural or Artificial Opening Endoscopic
0TWB8DZ	Revision of Intraluminal Device in Bladder, Via Natural or Artificial Opening Endoscopic
0TWB8JZ	Revision of Synthetic Substitute in Bladder, Via Natural or Artificial Opening Endoscopic
0TWB8KZ	Revision of Nonautologous Tissue Substitute in Bladder, Via Natural or Artificial Opening Endoscopic
0TWB8LZ	Revision of Artificial Sphincter in Bladder, Via Natural or Artificial Opening Endoscopic
0TWB8MZ	Revision of Stimulator Lead in Bladder, Via Natural or Artificial Opening Endoscopic
0TWB8YZ	Revision of Other Device in Bladder, Via Natural or Artificial Opening Endoscopic
0TWBX0Z	Revision of Drainage Device in Bladder, External Approach
0TWBX2Z	Revision of Monitoring Device in Bladder, External Approach
0TWBX3Z	Revision of Infusion Device in Bladder, External Approach
0TWBX7Z	Revision of Autologous Tissue Substitute in Bladder, External Approach
0TWBXCZ	Revision of Extraluminal Device in Bladder, External Approach
0TWBXDZ	Revision of Intraluminal Device in Bladder, External Approach
0TWBXJZ	Revision of Synthetic Substitute in Bladder, External Approach
0TWBXKZ	Revision of Nonautologous Tissue Substitute in Bladder, External Approach
0TWBXLZ	Revision of Artificial Sphincter in Bladder, External Approach
0TWBXMZ	Revision of Stimulator Lead in Bladder, External Approach
0TWD00Z	Revision of Drainage Device in Urethra, Open Approach
0TWD02Z	Revision of Monitoring Device in Urethra, Open Approach
0TWD03Z	Revision of Infusion Device in Urethra, Open Approach
0TWD07Z	Revision of Autologous Tissue Substitute in Urethra, Open Approach
0TWD0CZ	Revision of Extraluminal Device in Urethra, Open Approach
0TWD0DZ	Revision of Intraluminal Device in Urethra, Open Approach
0TWD0JZ	Revision of Synthetic Substitute in Urethra, Open Approach
0TWD0KZ	Revision of Nonautologous Tissue Substitute in Urethra, Open Approach
0TWD0LZ	Revision of Artificial Sphincter in Urethra, Open Approach
0TWD0YZ	Revision of Other Device in Urethra, Open Approach
0TWD30Z	Revision of Drainage Device in Urethra, Percutaneous Approach
0TWD32Z	Revision of Monitoring Device in Urethra, Percutaneous Approach
0TWD33Z	Revision of Infusion Device in Urethra, Percutaneous Approach
0TWD37Z	Revision of Autologous Tissue Substitute in Urethra, Percutaneous Approach
0TWD3CZ	Revision of Extraluminal Device in Urethra, Percutaneous Approach

0TWD3DZ	Revision of Intraluminal Device in Urethra, Percutaneous Approach
0TWD3JZ	Revision of Synthetic Substitute in Urethra, Percutaneous Approach
0TWD3KZ	Revision of Nonautologous Tissue Substitute in Urethra, Percutaneous Approach
0TWD3LZ	Revision of Artificial Sphincter in Urethra, Percutaneous Approach
0TWD3YZ	Revision of Other Device in Urethra, Percutaneous Approach
0TWD40Z	Revision of Drainage Device in Urethra, Percutaneous Endoscopic Approach
0TWD42Z	Revision of Monitoring Device in Urethra, Percutaneous Endoscopic Approach
0TWD43Z	Revision of Infusion Device in Urethra, Percutaneous Endoscopic Approach
0TWD47Z	Revision of Autologous Tissue Substitute in Urethra, Percutaneous Endoscopic Approach
0TWD4CZ	Revision of Extraluminal Device in Urethra, Percutaneous Endoscopic Approach
0TWD4DZ	Revision of Intraluminal Device in Urethra, Percutaneous Endoscopic Approach
0TWD4JZ	Revision of Synthetic Substitute in Urethra, Percutaneous Endoscopic Approach
0TWD4KZ	Revision of Nonautologous Tissue Substitute in Urethra, Percutaneous Endoscopic Approach
0TWD4LZ	Revision of Artificial Sphincter in Urethra, Percutaneous Endoscopic Approach
0TWD4YZ	Revision of Other Device in Urethra, Percutaneous Endoscopic Approach
0TWD70Z	Revision of Drainage Device in Urethra, Via Natural or Artificial Opening
0TWD72Z	Revision of Monitoring Device in Urethra, Via Natural or Artificial Opening
0TWD73Z	Revision of Infusion Device in Urethra, Via Natural or Artificial Opening
0TWD77Z	Revision of Autologous Tissue Substitute in Urethra, Via Natural or Artificial Opening
0TWD7CZ	Revision of Extraluminal Device in Urethra, Via Natural or Artificial Opening
0TWD7DZ	Revision of Intraluminal Device in Urethra, Via Natural or Artificial Opening
0TWD7JZ	Revision of Synthetic Substitute in Urethra, Via Natural or Artificial Opening
0TWD7KZ	Revision of Nonautologous Tissue Substitute in Urethra, Via Natural or Artificial Opening
0TWD7LZ	Revision of Artificial Sphincter in Urethra, Via Natural or Artificial Opening
0TWD7YZ	Revision of Other Device in Urethra, Via Natural or Artificial Opening
0TWD80Z	Revision of Drainage Device in Urethra, Via Natural or Artificial Opening Endoscopic
0TWD82Z	Revision of Monitoring Device in Urethra, Via Natural or Artificial Opening Endoscopic

♀ Female-only   ♂ Male-only   ▲ Limited Coverage   ● Non-OR   HAC HAC-associated procedure   ▲ Non-covered procedures   ➕ Cluster   **1229**

Medical and Surgical, Urinary System Code Listings

0TWD83Z	Revision of Infusion Device in Urethra, Via Natural or Artificial Opening Endoscopic
0TWD87Z	Revision of Autologous Tissue Substitute in Urethra, Via Natural or Artificial Opening Endoscopic
0TWD8CZ	Revision of Extraluminal Device in Urethra, Via Natural or Artificial Opening Endoscopic
0TWD8DZ	Revision of Intraluminal Device in Urethra, Via Natural or Artificial Opening Endoscopic
0TWD8JZ	Revision of Synthetic Substitute in Urethra, Via Natural or Artificial Opening Endoscopic

0TWD8KZ	Revision of Nonautologous Tissue Substitute in Urethra, Via Natural or Artificial Opening Endoscopic
0TWD8LZ	Revision of Artificial Sphincter in Urethra, Via Natural or Artificial Opening Endoscopic
0TWD8YZ	Revision of Other Device in Urethra, Via Natural or Artificial Opening Endoscopic
0TWDX0Z	Revision of Drainage Device in Urethra, External Approach
0TWDX2Z	Revision of Monitoring Device in Urethra, External Approach
0TWDX3Z	Revision of Infusion Device in Urethra, External Approach

0TWDX7Z	Revision of Autologous Tissue Substitute in Urethra, External Approach
0TWDXCZ	Revision of Extraluminal Device in Urethra, External Approach
0TWDXDZ	Revision of Intraluminal Device in Urethra, External Approach
0TWDXJZ	Revision of Synthetic Substitute in Urethra, External Approach
0TWDXKZ	Revision of Nonautologous Tissue Substitute in Urethra, External Approach
0TWDXLZ	Revision of Artificial Sphincter in Urethra, External Approach

0TY – Urinary System, Transplantation

Review Coding Guideline B3.16

▲ **0TY00Z0** Transplantation of Right Kidney, Allogeneic, Open Approach
  ➕ Kidney/Pancreas transplant when reported with Transplant of the Pancreas. *See table 0FY to construct the Transplantation code.*

▲ **0TY00Z1** Transplantation of Right Kidney, Syngeneic, Open Approach
  ➕ Kidney/Pancreas transplant when reported with Transplant of the Pancreas. *See table 0FY to construct the Transplantation code.*

▲ **0TY00Z2** Transplantation of Right Kidney, Zooplastic, Open Approach
  ➕ Kidney/Pancreas transplant when reported with Transplant of the Pancreas. *See table 0FY to construct the Transplantation code.*

▲ **0TY10Z0** Transplantation of Left Kidney, Allogeneic, Open Approach
  ➕ Kidney/Pancreas transplant when reported with Transplant of the Pancreas. *See table 0FY to construct the Transplantation code.*

▲ **0TY10Z1** Transplantation of Left Kidney, Syngeneic, Open Approach
  ➕ Kidney/Pancreas transplant when reported with Transplant of the Pancreas. *See table 0FY to construct the Transplantation code.*

▲ **0TY10Z2** Transplantation of Left Kidney, Zooplastic, Open Approach
  ➕ Kidney/Pancreas transplant when reported with Transplant of the Pancreas. *See table 0FY to construct the Transplantation code.*

Female Reproductive System

Female Reproductive System

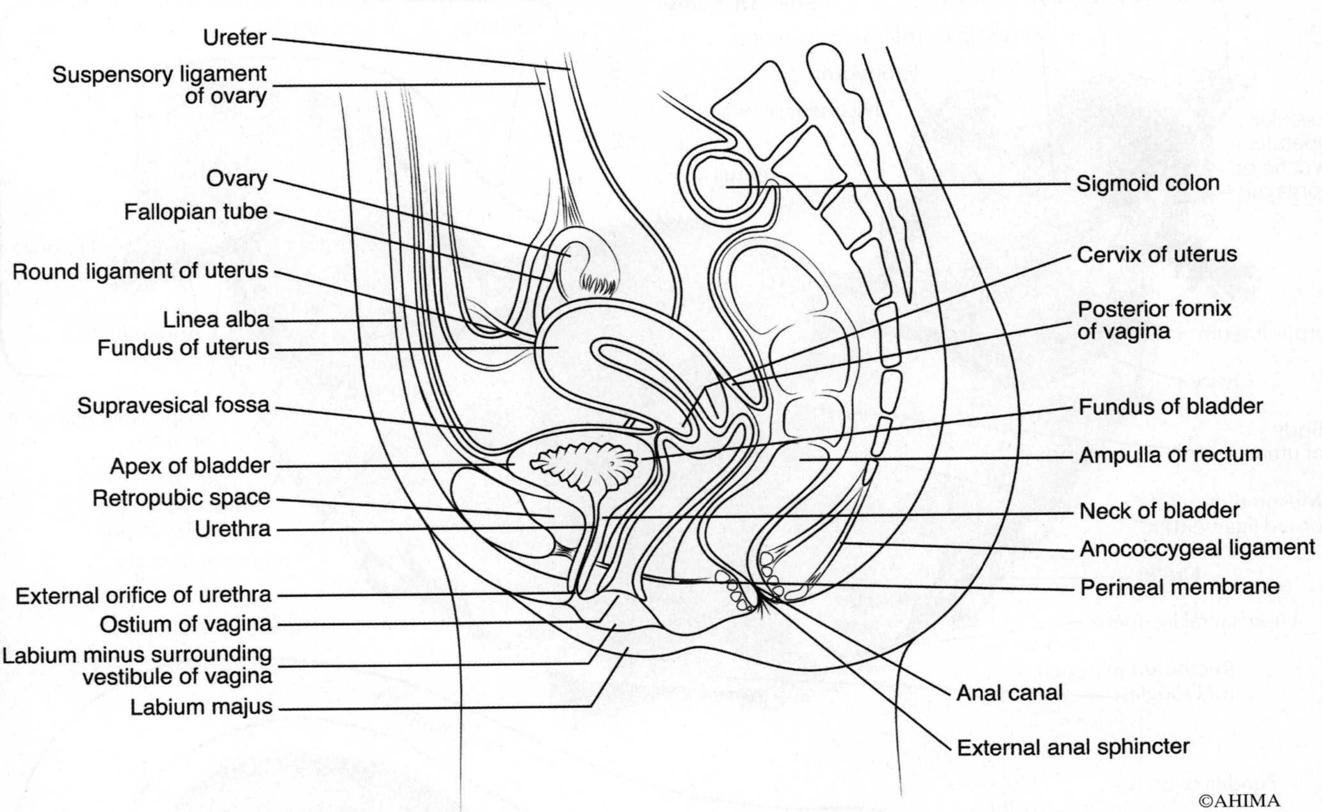

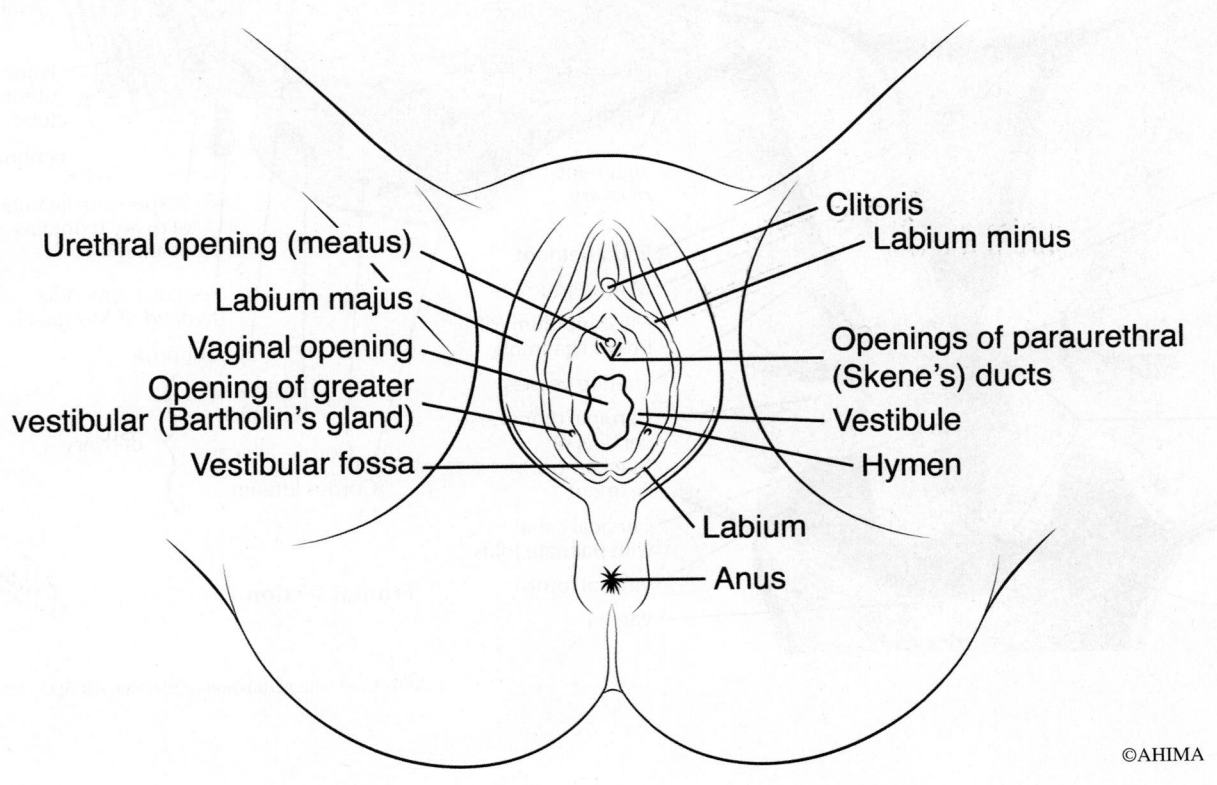

Ureter

Suspensory ligament of ovary

Ovary

Fallopian tube

Round ligament of uterus

Linea alba

Fundus of uterus

Supravesical fossa

Apex of bladder

Retropubic space

Urethra

External orifice of urethra

Ostium of vagina

Labium minus surrounding vestibule of vagina

Labium majus

Sigmoid colon

Cervix of uterus

Posterior fornix of vagina

Fundus of bladder

Ampulla of rectum

Neck of bladder

Anococcygeal ligament

Perineal membrane

Anal canal

External anal sphincter

©AHIMA

Urethral opening (meatus)

Labium majus

Vaginal opening

Opening of greater vestibular (Bartholin's gland)

Vestibular fossa

Clitoris

Labium minus

Openings of paraurethral (Skene's) ducts

Vestibule

Hymen

Labium

Anus

©AHIMA

Uterus, Ovaries and Uterine Tubes

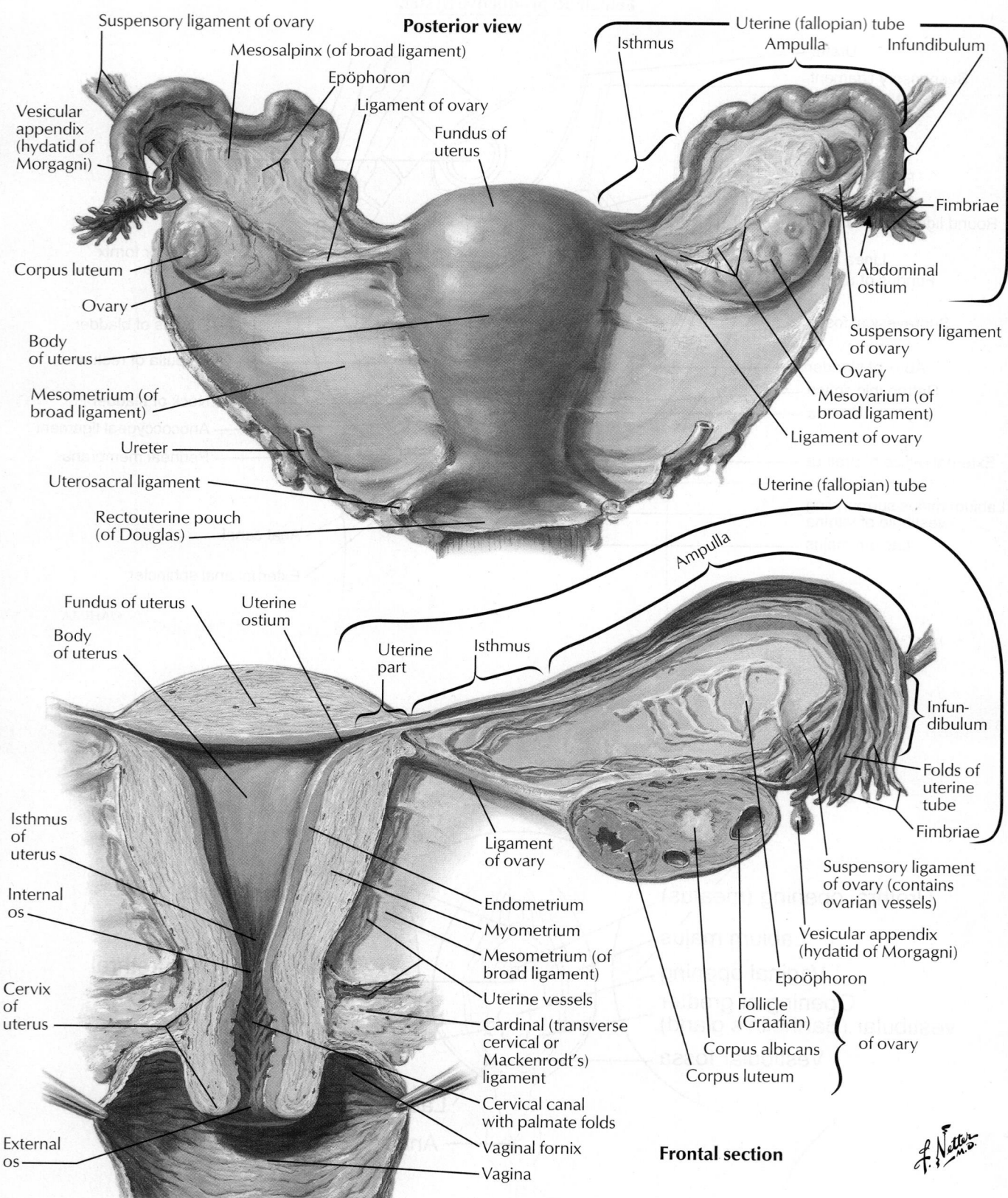

Posterior view

Suspensory ligament of ovary

Mesosalpinx (of broad ligament)

Epöphoron

Vesicular appendix (hydatid of Morgagni)

Ligament of ovary

Fundus of uterus

Corpus luteum

Ovary

Body of uterus

Mesometrium (of broad ligament)

Ureter

Uterosacral ligament

Rectouterine pouch (of Douglas)

Isthmus

Uterine (fallopian) tube

Ampulla

Infundibulum

Fimbriae

Abdominal ostium

Suspensory ligament of ovary

Ovary

Mesovarium (of broad ligament)

Ligament of ovary

Uterine (fallopian) tube

Ampulla

Fundus of uterus

Uterine ostium

Body of uterus

Uterine part

Isthmus

Infundibulum

Isthmus of uterus

Internal os

Cervix of uterus

External os

Ligament of ovary

Endometrium

Myometrium

Mesometrium (of broad ligament)

Uterine vessels

Cardinal (transverse cervical or Mackenrodt's) ligament

Cervical canal with palmate folds

Vaginal fornix

Vagina

Folds of uterine tube

Fimbriae

Suspensory ligament of ovary (contains ovarian vessels)

Vesicular appendix (hydatid of Morgagni)

Epoöphoron

Follicle (Graafian)

Corpus albicans

Corpus luteum

of ovary

Frontal section

f. Netter m.s.

Female Reproductive System Tables 0U1–0UY

Section	0	Medical and Surgical
Body System	U	Female Reproductive System
Operation	1	Bypass: Altering the route of passage of the contents of a tubular body part

Body Part (4th)	Approach (5th)	Device (6th)	Qualifier (7th)
5 Fallopian Tube, Right 6 Fallopian Tube, Left	0 Open 4 Percutaneous Endoscopic	7 Autologous Tissue Substitute J Synthetic Substitute K Nonautologous Tissue Substitute Z No Device	5 Fallopian Tube, Right 6 Fallopian Tube, Left 9 Uterus

Section	0	Medical and Surgical
Body System	U	Female Reproductive System
Operation	2	Change: Taking out or off a device from a body part and putting back an identical or similar device in or on the same body part without cutting or puncturing the skin or a mucous membrane

Body Part (4th)	Approach (5th)	Device (6th)	Qualifier (7th)
3 Ovary 8 Fallopian Tube M Vulva	X External	0 Drainage Device Y Other Device	Z No Qualifier
D Uterus and Cervix	X External	0 Drainage Device H Contraceptive Device Y Other Device	Z No Qualifier
H Vagina and Cul-de-sac	X External	0 Drainage Device G Intraluminal Device, Pessary Y Other Device	Z No Qualifier

Section	0	Medical and Surgical
Body System	U	Female Reproductive System
Operation	5	Destruction: Physical eradication of all or a portion of a body part by the direct use of energy, force, or a destructive agent

Body Part (4th)	Approach (5th)	Device (6th)	Qualifier (7th)
0 Ovary, Right 1 Ovary, Left 2 Ovaries, Bilateral 4 Uterine Supporting Structure	0 Open 3 Percutaneous 4 Percutaneous Endoscopic 8 Via Natural or Artificial Opening Endoscopic	Z No Device	Z No Qualifier
5 Fallopian Tube, Right 6 Fallopian Tube, Left 7 Fallopian Tubes, Bilateral 9 Uterus B Endometrium C Cervix F Cul-de-sac	0 Open 3 Percutaneous 4 Percutaneous Endoscopic 7 Via Natural or Artificial Opening 8 Via Natural or Artificial Opening Endoscopic	Z No Device	Z No Qualifier
G Vagina K Hymen	0 Open 3 Percutaneous 4 Percutaneous Endoscopic 7 Via Natural or Artificial Opening 8 Via Natural or Artificial Opening Endoscopic X External	Z No Device	Z No Qualifier
J Clitoris L Vestibular Gland M Vulva	0 Open X External	Z No Device	Z No Qualifier

Section   0   **Medical and Surgical**
Body System   U   **Female Reproductive System**
Operation   7   **Dilation:** Expanding an orifice or the lumen of a tubular body part

Body Part (4th)	Approach (5th)	Device (6th)	Qualifier (7th)
5 Fallopian Tube, Right 6 Fallopian Tube, Left 7 Fallopian Tubes, Bilateral 9 Uterus C Cervix G Vagina	0 Open 3 Percutaneous 4 Percutaneous Endoscopic 7 Via Natural or Artificial Opening 8 Via Natural or Artificial Opening Endoscopic	D Intraluminal Device Z No Device	Z No Qualifier
K Hymen	0 Open 3 Percutaneous 4 Percutaneous Endoscopic 7 Via Natural or Artificial Opening 8 Via Natural or Artificial Opening Endoscopic X External	D Intraluminal Device Z No Device	Z No Qualifier

Section   0   **Medical and Surgical**
Body System   U   **Female Reproductive System**
Operation   8   **Division:** Cutting into a body part, without draining fluids and/or gases from the body part, in order to separate or transect a body part

Body Part (4th)	Approach (5th)	Device (6th)	Qualifier (7th)
0 Ovary, Right 1 Ovary, Left 2 Ovaries, Bilateral 4 Uterine Supporting Structure	0 Open 3 Percutaneous 4 Percutaneous Endoscopic	Z No Device	Z No Qualifier
K Hymen	7 Via Natural or Artificial Opening 8 Via Natural or Artificial Opening Endoscopic X External	Z No Device	Z No Qualifier

Section   0   **Medical and Surgical**
Body System   U   **Female Reproductive System**
Operation   9   **Drainage:** Taking or letting out fluids and/or gases from a body part

Body Part (4th)	Approach (5th)	Device (6th)	Qualifier (7th)
0 Ovary, Right 1 Ovary, Left 2 Ovaries, Bilateral	0 Open 3 Percutaneous 4 Percutaneous Endoscopic 8 Via Natural or Artificial Opening Endoscopic	0 Drainage Device	Z No Qualifier
0 Ovary, Right 1 Ovary, Left 2 Ovaries, Bilateral	0 Open 3 Percutaneous 4 Percutaneous Endoscopic 8 Via Natural or Artificial Opening Endoscopic	Z No Device	X Diagnostic Z No Qualifier
0 Ovary, Right 1 Ovary, Left 2 Ovaries, Bilateral	X External	Z No Device	Z No Qualifier
4 Uterine Supporting Structure	0 Open 3 Percutaneous 4 Percutaneous Endoscopic 8 Via Natural or Artificial Opening Endoscopic	0 Drainage Device	Z No Qualifier
4 Uterine Supporting Structure	0 Open 3 Percutaneous 4 Percutaneous Endoscopic 8 Via Natural or Artificial Opening Endoscopic	Z No Device	X Diagnostic Z No Qualifier

Continued →

Section	0	Medical and Surgical
Body System	U	Female Reproductive System
Operation	9	Drainage: Taking or letting out fluids and/or gases from a body part

Body Part (4th)	Approach (5th)	Device (6th)	Qualifier (7th)
5 Fallopian Tube, Right 6 Fallopian Tube, Left 7 Fallopian Tubes, Bilateral 9 Uterus C Cervix F Cul-de-sac	0 Open 3 Percutaneous 4 Percutaneous Endoscopic 7 Via Natural or Artificial Opening 8 Via Natural or Artificial Opening Endoscopic	0 Drainage Device	Z No Qualifier
5 Fallopian Tube, Right 6 Fallopian Tube, Left 7 Fallopian Tubes, Bilateral 9 Uterus C Cervix F Cul-de-sac	0 Open 3 Percutaneous 4 Percutaneous Endoscopic 7 Via Natural or Artificial Opening 8 Via Natural or Artificial Opening Endoscopic	Z No Device	X Diagnostic Z No Qualifier
G Vagina K Hymen	0 Open 3 Percutaneous 4 Percutaneous Endoscopic 7 Via Natural or Artificial Opening 8 Via Natural or Artificial Opening Endoscopic X External	0 Drainage Device	Z No Qualifier
G Vagina K Hymen	0 Open 3 Percutaneous 4 Percutaneous Endoscopic 7 Via Natural or Artificial Opening 8 Via Natural or Artificial Opening Endoscopic X External	Z No Device	X Diagnostic Z No Qualifier
J Clitoris L Vestibular Gland M Vulva	0 Open X External	0 Drainage Device	Z No Qualifier
J Clitoris L Vestibular Gland M Vulva	0 Open X External	Z No Device	X Diagnostic Z No Qualifier

Section	0	Medical and Surgical
Body System	U	Female Reproductive System
Operation	B	Excision: Cutting out or off, without replacement, a portion of a body part

Body Part (4th)	Approach (5th)	Device (6th)	Qualifier (7th)
0 Ovary, Right 1 Ovary, Left 2 Ovaries, Bilateral 4 Uterine Supporting Structure 5 Fallopian Tube, Right 6 Fallopian Tube, Left 7 Fallopian Tubes, Bilateral 9 Uterus C Cervix F Cul-de-sac	0 Open 3 Percutaneous 4 Percutaneous Endoscopic 7 Via Natural or Artificial Opening 8 Via Natural or Artificial Opening Endoscopic	Z No Device	X Diagnostic Z No Qualifier

Continued →

Section   **0**   **Medical and Surgical**
Body System   **U**   **Female Reproductive System**
Operation   **B**   **Excision:** Cutting out or off, without replacement, a portion of a body part

Body Part (4ᵗʰ)	Approach (5ᵗʰ)	Device (6ᵗʰ)	Qualifier (7ᵗʰ)
G Vagina **K** Hymen	**0** Open **3** Percutaneous **4** Percutaneous Endoscopic **7** Via Natural or Artificial Opening **8** Via Natural or Artificial Opening Endoscopic **X** External	**Z** No Device	**X** Diagnostic **Z** No Qualifier
J Clitoris **L** Vestibular Gland **M** Vulva	**0** Open **X** External	**Z** No Device	**X** Diagnostic **Z** No Qualifier

Section   **0**   **Medical and Surgical**
Body System   **U**   **Female Reproductive System**
Operation   **C**   **Extirpation:** Taking or cutting out solid matter from a body part

Body Part (4ᵗʰ)	Approach (5ᵗʰ)	Device (6ᵗʰ)	Qualifier (7ᵗʰ)
0 Ovary, Right **1** Ovary, Left **2** Ovaries, Bilateral **4** Uterine Supporting Structure	**0** Open **3** Percutaneous **4** Percutaneous Endoscopic **8** Via Natural or Artificial Opening Endoscopic	**Z** No Device	**Z** No Qualifier
5 Fallopian Tube, Right **6** Fallopian Tube, Left **7** Fallopian Tubes, Bilateral **9** Uterus **B** Endometrium **C** Cervix **F** Cul-de-sac	**0** Open **3** Percutaneous **4** Percutaneous Endoscopic **7** Via Natural or Artificial Opening **8** Via Natural or Artificial Opening Endoscopic	**Z** No Device	**Z** No Qualifier
G Vagina **K** Hymen	**0** Open **3** Percutaneous **4** Percutaneous Endoscopic **7** Via Natural or Artificial Opening **8** Via Natural or Artificial Opening Endoscopic **X** External	**Z** No Device	**Z** No Qualifier
J Clitoris **L** Vestibular Gland **M** Vulva	**0** Open **X** External	**Z** No Device	**Z** No Qualifier

Section   **0**   **Medical and Surgical**
Body System   **U**   **Female Reproductive System**
Operation   **D**   **Extraction:** Pulling or stripping out or off all or a portion of a body part by the use of force

Body Part (4ᵗʰ)	Approach (5ᵗʰ)	Device (6ᵗʰ)	Qualifier (7ᵗʰ)
B Endometrium	**7** Via Natural or Artificial Opening **8** Via Natural or Artificial Opening Endoscopic	**Z** No Device	**X** Diagnostic **Z** No Qualifier
N Ova	**0** Open **3** Percutaneous **4** Percutaneous Endoscopic	**Z** No Device	**Z** No Qualifier

Section 0 **Medical and Surgical**
Body System U **Female Reproductive System**
Operation F **Fragmentation:** Breaking solid matter in a body part into pieces

Body Part (4th)	Approach (5th)	Device (6th)	Qualifier (7th)
5 Fallopian Tube, Right 6 Fallopian Tube, Left 7 Fallopian Tubes, Bilateral 9 Uterus	0 Open 3 Percutaneous 4 Percutaneous Endoscopic 7 Via Natural or Artificial Opening 8 Via Natural or Artificial Opening Endoscopic X External	Z No Device	Z No Qualifier

Section 0 **Medical and Surgical**
Body System U **Female Reproductive System**
Operation H **Insertion:** Putting in a nonbiological appliance that monitors, assists, performs, or prevents a physiological function but does not physically take the place of a body part

Body Part (4th)	Approach (5th)	Device (6th)	Qualifier (7th)
3 Ovary	0 Open 3 Percutaneous 4 Percutaneous Endoscopic	1 Radioactive Element 3 Infusion Device Y Other Device	Z No Qualifier
3 Ovary	7 Via Natural or Artificial Opening 8 Via Natural or Artificial Opening Endoscopic	1 Radioactive Element Y Other Device	Z No Qualifier
8 Fallopian Tube D Uterus and Cervix H Vagina and Cul-de-sac	0 Open 3 Percutaneous 4 Percutaneous Endoscopic 7 Via Natural or Artificial Opening 8 Via Natural or Artificial Opening Endoscopic	3 Infusion Device Y Other Device	Z No Qualifier
9 Uterus	0 Open 7 Via Natural or Artificial Opening 8 Via Natural or Artificial Opening Endoscopic	1 Radioactive Element H Contraceptive Device	Z No Qualifier
C Cervix	0 Open 3 Percutaneous 4 Percutaneous Endoscopic	1 Radioactive Element	Z No Qualifier
C Cervix	7 Via Natural or Artificial Opening 8 Via Natural or Artificial Opening Endoscopic	1 Radioactive Element H Contraceptive Device	Z No Qualifier
F Cul-de-sac	7 Via Natural or Artificial Opening 8 Via Natural or Artificial Opening Endoscopic	G Intraluminal Device, Pessary	Z No Qualifier
G Vagina	0 Open 3 Percutaneous 4 Percutaneous Endoscopic X External	1 Radioactive Element	Z No Qualifier
G Vagina	7 Via Natural or Artificial Opening 8 Via Natural or Artificial Opening Endoscopic	1 Radioactive Element G Intraluminal Device, Pessary	Z No Qualifier

Section 0 **Medical and Surgical**
Body System U **Female Reproductive System**
Operation J **Inspection:** Visually and/or manually exploring a body part

Body Part (4th)	Approach (5th)	Device (6th)	Qualifier (7th)
3 Ovary	0 Open 3 Percutaneous 4 Percutaneous Endoscopic 8 Via Natural or Artificial Opening Endoscopic X External	Z No Device	Z No Qualifier

Continued →

Section	0	Medical and Surgical
Body System	U	Female Reproductive System
Operation	J	**Inspection:** Visually and/or manually exploring a body part

Body Part (4th)	Approach (5th)	Device (6th)	Qualifier (7th)
8 Fallopian Tube D Uterus and Cervix H Vagina and Cul-de-sac	0 Open 3 Percutaneous 4 Percutaneous Endoscopic 7 Via Natural or Artificial Opening 8 Via Natural or Artificial Opening Endoscopic X External	Z No Device	Z No Qualifier
M Vulva	0 Open X External	Z No Device	Z No Qualifier

Section	0	Medical and Surgical
Body System	U	Female Reproductive System
Operation	L	**Occlusion:** Completely closing an orifice or the lumen of a tubular body part

Body Part (4th)	Approach (5th)	Device (6th)	Qualifier (7th)
5 Fallopian Tube, Right 6 Fallopian Tube, Left 7 Fallopian Tubes, Bilateral	0 Open 3 Percutaneous 4 Percutaneous Endoscopic	C Extraluminal Device D Intraluminal Device Z No Device	Z No Qualifier
5 Fallopian Tube, Right 6 Fallopian Tube, Left 7 Fallopian Tubes, Bilateral	7 Via Natural or Artificial Opening 8 Via Natural or Artificial Opening Endoscopic	D Intraluminal Device Z No Device	Z No Qualifier
F Cul-de-sac G Vagina	7 Via Natural or Artificial Opening 8 Via Natural or Artificial Opening Endoscopic	D Intraluminal Device Z No Device	Z No Qualifier

Section	0	Medical and Surgical
Body System	U	Female Reproductive System
Operation	M	**Reattachment:** Putting back in or on all or a portion of a separated body part to its normal location or other suitable location

Body Part (4th)	Approach (5th)	Device (6th)	Qualifier (7th)
0 Ovary, Right 1 Ovary, Left 2 Ovaries, Bilateral 4 Uterine Supporting Structure 5 Fallopian Tube, Right 6 Fallopian Tube, Left 7 Fallopian Tubes, Bilateral 9 Uterus C Cervix F Cul-de-sac G Vagina	0 Open 4 Percutaneous Endoscopic	Z No Device	Z No Qualifier
J Clitoris M Vulva	X External	Z No Device	Z No Qualifier
K Hymen	0 Open 4 Percutaneous Endoscopic X External	Z No Device	Z No Qualifier

Section   **0**   **Medical and Surgical**
Body System   **U**   **Female Reproductive System**
Operation   **N**   **Release:** Freeing a body part from an abnormal physical constraint by cutting or by the use of force

Body Part (4ᵗʰ)	Approach (5ᵗʰ)	Device (6ᵗʰ)	Qualifier (7ᵗʰ)
0 Ovary, Right 1 Ovary, Left 2 Ovaries, Bilateral 4 Uterine Supporting Structure	0 Open 3 Percutaneous 4 Percutaneous Endoscopic 8 Via Natural or Artificial Opening Endoscopic	Z No Device	Z No Qualifier
5 Fallopian Tube, Right 6 Fallopian Tube, Left 7 Fallopian Tubes, Bilateral 9 Uterus C Cervix F Cul-de-sac	0 Open 3 Percutaneous 4 Percutaneous Endoscopic 7 Via Natural or Artificial Opening 8 Via Natural or Artificial Opening Endoscopic	Z No Device	Z No Qualifier
G Vagina K Hymen	0 Open 3 Percutaneous 4 Percutaneous Endoscopic 7 Via Natural or Artificial Opening 8 Via Natural or Artificial Opening Endoscopic X External	Z No Device	Z No Qualifier
J Clitoris L Vestibular Gland M Vulva	0 Open X External	Z No Device	Z No Qualifier

Section   **0**   **Medical and Surgical**
Body System   **U**   **Female Reproductive System**
Operation   **P**   **Removal:** Taking out or off a device from a body part

Body Part (4ᵗʰ)	Approach (5ᵗʰ)	Device (6ᵗʰ)	Qualifier (7ᵗʰ)
3 Ovary	0 Open 3 Percutaneous 4 Percutaneous Endoscopic	0 Drainage Device 3 Infusion Device Y Other Device	Z No Qualifier
3 Ovary	7 Via Natural or Artificial Opening 8 Via Natural or Artificial Opening Endoscopic	Y Other Device	Z No Qualifier
3 Ovary	X External	0 Drainage Device 3 Infusion Device	Z No Qualifier
8 Fallopian Tube	0 Open 3 Percutaneous 4 Percutaneous Endoscopic 7 Via Natural or Artificial Opening 8 Via Natural or Artificial Opening Endoscopic	0 Drainage Device 3 Infusion Device 7 Autologous Tissue Substitute C Extraluminal Device D Intraluminal Device J Synthetic Substitute K Nonautologous Tissue Substitute Y Other Device	Z No Qualifier
8 Fallopian Tube	X External	0 Drainage Device 3 Infusion Device D Intraluminal Device	Z No Qualifier
D Uterus and Cervix	0 Open 3 Percutaneous 4 Percutaneous Endoscopic 7 Via Natural or Artificial Opening 8 Via Natural or Artificial Opening Endoscopic	0 Drainage Device 1 Radioactive Element 3 Infusion Device 7 Autologous Tissue Substitute C Extraluminal Device D Intraluminal Device H Contraceptive Device J Synthetic Substitute K Nonautologous Tissue Substitute Y Other Device	Z No Qualifier

Continued →

Section	0	Medical and Surgical
Body System	U	Female Reproductive System
Operation	P	**Removal:** Taking out or off a device from a body part

Body Part (4ᵗʰ)	Approach (5ᵗʰ)	Device (6ᵗʰ)	Qualifier (7ᵗʰ)
D Uterus and Cervix	X External	0 Drainage Device 3 Infusion Device D Intraluminal Device H Contraceptive Device	Z No Qualifier
H Vagina and Cul-de-sac	0 Open 3 Percutaneous 4 Percutaneous Endoscopic 7 Via Natural or Artificial Opening 8 Via Natural or Artificial Opening Endoscopic	0 Drainage Device 1 Radioactive Element 3 Infusion Device 7 Autologous Tissue Substitute D Intraluminal Device J Synthetic Substitute K Nonautologous Tissue Substitute Y Other Device	Z No Qualifier
H Vagina and Cul-de-sac	X External	0 Drainage Device 1 Radioactive Element 3 Infusion Device D Intraluminal Device	Z No Qualifier
M Vulva	0 Open	0 Drainage Device 7 Autologous Tissue Substitute J Synthetic Substitute K Nonautologous Tissue Substitute	Z No Qualifier
M Vulva	X External	0 Drainage Device	Z No Qualifier

Section	0	Medical and Surgical
Body System	U	Female Reproductive System
Operation	Q	**Repair:** Restoring, to the extent possible, a body part to its normal anatomic structure and function

Body Part (4ᵗʰ)	Approach (5ᵗʰ)	Device (6ᵗʰ)	Qualifier (7ᵗʰ)
0 Ovary, Right 1 Ovary, Left 2 Ovaries, Bilateral 4 Uterine Supporting Structure	0 Open 3 Percutaneous 4 Percutaneous Endoscopic 8 Via Natural or Artificial Opening Endoscopic	Z No Device	Z No Qualifier
5 Fallopian Tube, Right 6 Fallopian Tube, Left 7 Fallopian Tubes, Bilateral 9 Uterus C Cervix F Cul-de-sac	0 Open 3 Percutaneous 4 Percutaneous Endoscopic 7 Via Natural or Artificial Opening 8 Via Natural or Artificial Opening Endoscopic	Z No Device	Z No Qualifier
G Vagina K Hymen	0 Open 3 Percutaneous 4 Percutaneous Endoscopic 7 Via Natural or Artificial Opening 8 Via Natural or Artificial Opening Endoscopic X External	Z No Device	Z No Qualifier
J Clitoris L Vestibular Gland M Vulva	0 Open X External	Z No Device	Z No Qualifier

Section	0	Medical and Surgical
Body System	U	Female Reproductive System
Operation	S	Reposition: Moving to its normal location, or other suitable location, all or a portion of a body part

Body Part (4th)	Approach (5th)	Device (6th)	Qualifier (7th)
0 Ovary, Right 1 Ovary, Left 2 Ovaries, Bilateral 4 Uterine Supporting Structure 5 Fallopian Tube, Right 6 Fallopian Tube, Left 7 Fallopian Tubes, Bilateral C Cervix F Cul-de-sac	0 Open 4 Percutaneous Endoscopic 8 Via Natural or Artificial Opening Endoscopic	Z No Device	Z No Qualifier
9 Uterus G Vagina	0 Open 4 Percutaneous Endoscopic 7 Via Natural or Artificial Opening 8 Via Natural or Artificial Opening Endoscopic X External	Z No Device	Z No Qualifier

Section	0	Medical and Surgical
Body System	U	Female Reproductive System
Operation	T	Resection: Cutting out or off, without replacement, all of a body part

Body Part (4th)	Approach (5th)	Device (6th)	Qualifier (7th)
0 Ovary, Right 1 Ovary, Left 2 Ovaries, Bilateral 5 Fallopian Tube, Right 6 Fallopian Tube, Left 7 Fallopian Tubes, Bilateral	0 Open 4 Percutaneous Endoscopic 7 Via Natural or Artificial Opening 8 Via Natural or Artificial Opening Endoscopic F Via Natural or Artificial Opening With Percutaneous Endoscopic Assistance	Z No Device	Z No Qualifier
4 Uterine Supporting Structure C Cervix F Cul-de-sac G Vagina	0 Open 4 Percutaneous Endoscopic 7 Via Natural or Artificial Opening 8 Via Natural or Artificial Opening Endoscopic	Z No Device	Z No Qualifier
9 Uterus	0 Open 4 Percutaneous Endoscopic 7 Via Natural or Artificial Opening 8 Via Natural or Artificial Opening Endoscopic F Via Natural or Artificial Opening with Percutaneous Endoscopic Assistance	Z No Device	L Supracervical Z No Qualifier
J Clitoris L Vestibular Gland M Vulva	0 Open X External	Z No Device	Z No Qualifier
K Hymen	0 Open 4 Percutaneous Endoscopic 7 Via Natural or Artificial Opening 8 Via Natural or Artificial Opening Endoscopic X External	Z No Device	Z No Qualifier

Section	0	Medical and Surgical
Body System	U	Female Reproductive System
Operation	U	Supplement: Putting in or on biological or synthetic material that physically reinforces and/or augments the function of a portion of a body part

Body Part (4th)	Approach (5th)	Device (6th)	Qualifier (7th)
4 Uterine Supporting Structure	0 Open 4 Percutaneous Endoscopic	7 Autologous Tissue Substitute J Synthetic Substitute K Nonautologous Tissue Substitute	Z No Qualifier
5 Fallopian Tube, Right 6 Fallopian Tube, Left 7 Fallopian Tubes, Bilateral F Cul-de-sac	0 Open 4 Percutaneous Endoscopic 7 Via Natural or Artificial Opening 8 Via Natural or Artificial Opening Endoscopic	7 Autologous Tissue Substitute J Synthetic Substitute K Nonautologous Tissue Substitute	Z No Qualifier
G Vagina K Hymen	0 Open 4 Percutaneous Endoscopic 7 Via Natural or Artificial Opening 8 Via Natural or Artificial Opening Endoscopic X External	7 Autologous Tissue Substitute J Synthetic Substitute K Nonautologous Tissue Substitute	Z No Qualifier
J Clitoris M Vulva	0 Open X External	7 Autologous Tissue Substitute J Synthetic Substitute K Nonautologous Tissue Substitute	Z No Qualifier

Section	0	Medical and Surgical
Body System	U	Female Reproductive System
Operation	V	Restriction: Partially closing an orifice or the lumen of a tubular body part

Body Part (4th)	Approach (5th)	Device (6th)	Qualifier (7th)
C Cervix	0 Open 3 Percutaneous 4 Percutaneous Endoscopic	C Extraluminal Device D Intraluminal Device Z No Device	Z No Qualifier
C Cervix	7 Via Natural or Artificial Opening 8 Via Natural or Artificial Opening Endoscopic	D Intraluminal Device Z No Device	Z No Qualifier

Section	0	Medical and Surgical
Body System	U	Female Reproductive System
Operation	W	Revision: Correcting, to the extent possible, a portion of a malfunctioning device or the position of a displaced device

Body Part (4th)	Approach (5th)	Device (6th)	Qualifier (7th)
3 Ovary	0 Open 3 Percutaneous 4 Percutaneous Endoscopic	0 Drainage Device 3 Infusion Device Y Other Device	Z No Qualifier
3 Ovary	7 Via Natural or Artificial Opening 8 Via Natural or Artificial Opening Endoscopic	Y Other Device	Z No Qualifier
3 Ovary	X External	0 Drainage Device 3 Infusion Device	Z No Qualifier
8 Fallopian Tube	0 Open 3 Percutaneous 4 Percutaneous Endoscopic 7 Via Natural or Artificial Opening 8 Via Natural or Artificial Opening Endoscopic X External	0 Drainage Device 3 Infusion Device 7 Autologous Tissue Substitute C Extraluminal Device D Intraluminal Device J Synthetic Substitute K Nonautologous Tissue Substitute Y Other Device	Z No Qualifier

Continued →

Section	0	Medical and Surgical
Body System	U	Female Reproductive System
Operation	W	Revision: Correcting, to the extent possible, a portion of a malfunctioning device or the position of a displaced device

Body Part (4th)	Approach (5th)	Device (6th)	Qualifier (7th)
8 Fallopian Tube	X External	0 Drainage Device 3 Infusion Device 7 Autologous Tissue Substitute C Extraluminal Device D Intraluminal Device J Synthetic Substitute K Nonautologous Tissue Substitute	Z No Qualifier
D Uterus and Cervix	0 Open 3 Percutaneous 4 Percutaneous Endoscopic 7 Via Natural or Artificial Opening 8 Via Natural or Artificial Opening Endoscopic	0 Drainage Device 1 Radioactive Element 3 Infusion Device 7 Autologous Tissue Substitute C Extraluminal Device D Intraluminal Device H Contraceptive Device J Synthetic Substitute K Nonautologous Tissue Substitute Y Other Device	Z No Qualifier
D Uterus and Cervix	X External	0 Drainage Device 3 Infusion Device 7 Autologous Tissue Substitute C Extraluminal Device D Intraluminal Device H Contraceptive Device J Synthetic Substitute K Nonautologous Tissue Substitute	Z No Qualifier
H Vagina and Cul-de-sac	0 Open 3 Percutaneous 4 Percutaneous Endoscopic 7 Via Natural or Artificial Opening 8 Via Natural or Artificial Opening Endoscopic	0 Drainage Device 1 Radioactive Element 3 Infusion Device 7 Autologous Tissue Substitute D Intraluminal Device J Synthetic Substitute K Nonautologous Tissue Substitute Y Other Device	Z No Qualifier
H Vagina and Cul-de-sac	X External	0 Drainage Device 3 Infusion Device 7 Autologous Tissue Substitute D Intraluminal Device J Synthetic Substitute K Nonautologous Tissue Substitute	Z No Qualifier
M Vulva	0 Open X External	0 Drainage Device 7 Autologous Tissue Substitute J Synthetic Substitute K Nonautologous Tissue Substitute	Z No Qualifier

Section	0	Medical and Surgical
Body System	U	Female Reproductive System
Operation	Y	Transplantation: Putting in or on all or a portion of a living body part taken from another individual or animal to physically take the place and/or function of all or a portion of a similar body part

Body Part (4th)	Approach (5th)	Device (6th)	Qualifier (7th)
0 Ovary, Right 1 Ovary, Left 9 Uterus	0 Open	Z No Device	0 Allogeneic 1 Syngeneic 2 Zooplastic

Female Reproductive System Code Listing 0U1–0UY

0U1 – Female Reproductive System, Bypass

Review Coding Guideline B3.6a

♀ **0U15075** Bypass Right Fallopian Tube to Right Fallopian Tube with Autologous Tissue Substitute, Open Approach

♀ **0U15076** Bypass Right Fallopian Tube to Left Fallopian Tube with Autologous Tissue Substitute, Open Approach

♀ **0U15079** Bypass Right Fallopian Tube to Uterus with Autologous Tissue Substitute, Open Approach

♀ **0U150J5** Bypass Right Fallopian Tube to Right Fallopian Tube with Synthetic Substitute, Open Approach

♀ **0U150J6** Bypass Right Fallopian Tube to Left Fallopian Tube with Synthetic Substitute, Open Approach

♀ **0U150J9** Bypass Right Fallopian Tube to Uterus with Synthetic Substitute, Open Approach

♀ **0U150K5** Bypass Right Fallopian Tube to Right Fallopian Tube with Nonautologous Tissue Substitute, Open Approach

♀ **0U150K6** Bypass Right Fallopian Tube to Left Fallopian Tube with Nonautologous Tissue Substitute, Open Approach

♀ **0U150K9** Bypass Right Fallopian Tube to Uterus with Nonautologous Tissue Substitute, Open Approach

♀ **0U150Z5** Bypass Right Fallopian Tube to Right Fallopian Tube, Open Approach

♀ **0U150Z6** Bypass Right Fallopian Tube to Left Fallopian Tube, Open Approach

♀ **0U150Z9** Bypass Right Fallopian Tube to Uterus, Open Approach

♀ **0U15475** Bypass Right Fallopian Tube to Right Fallopian Tube with Autologous Tissue Substitute, Percutaneous Endoscopic Approach

♀ **0U15476** Bypass Right Fallopian Tube to Left Fallopian Tube with Autologous Tissue Substitute, Percutaneous Endoscopic Approach

♀ **0U15479** Bypass Right Fallopian Tube to Uterus with Autologous Tissue Substitute, Percutaneous Endoscopic Approach

♀ **0U154J5** Bypass Right Fallopian Tube to Right Fallopian Tube with Synthetic Substitute, Percutaneous Endoscopic Approach

♀ **0U154J6** Bypass Right Fallopian Tube to Left Fallopian Tube with Synthetic Substitute, Percutaneous Endoscopic Approach

♀ **0U154J9** Bypass Right Fallopian Tube to Uterus with Synthetic Substitute, Percutaneous Endoscopic Approach

♀ **0U154K5** Bypass Right Fallopian Tube to Right Fallopian Tube with Nonautologous Tissue Substitute, Percutaneous Endoscopic Approach

♀ **0U154K6** Bypass Right Fallopian Tube to Left Fallopian Tube with Nonautologous Tissue Substitute, Percutaneous Endoscopic Approach

♀ **0U154K9** Bypass Right Fallopian Tube to Uterus with Nonautologous Tissue Substitute, Percutaneous Endoscopic Approach

♀ **0U154Z5** Bypass Right Fallopian Tube to Right Fallopian Tube, Percutaneous Endoscopic Approach

♀ **0U154Z6** Bypass Right Fallopian Tube to Left Fallopian Tube, Percutaneous Endoscopic Approach

♀ **0U154Z9** Bypass Right Fallopian Tube to Uterus, Percutaneous Endoscopic Approach

♀ **0U16075** Bypass Left Fallopian Tube to Right Fallopian Tube with Autologous Tissue Substitute, Open Approach

♀ **0U16076** Bypass Left Fallopian Tube to Left Fallopian Tube with Autologous Tissue Substitute, Open Approach

♀ **0U16079** Bypass Left Fallopian Tube to Uterus with Autologous Tissue Substitute, Open Approach

♀ **0U160J5** Bypass Left Fallopian Tube to Right Fallopian Tube with Synthetic Substitute, Open Approach

♀ **0U160J6** Bypass Left Fallopian Tube to Left Fallopian Tube with Synthetic Substitute, Open Approach

♀ **0U160J9** Bypass Left Fallopian Tube to Uterus with Synthetic Substitute, Open Approach

♀ **0U160K5** Bypass Left Fallopian Tube to Right Fallopian Tube with Nonautologous Tissue Substitute, Open Approach

♀ **0U160K6** Bypass Left Fallopian Tube to Left Fallopian Tube with Nonautologous Tissue Substitute, Open Approach

♀ **0U160K9** Bypass Left Fallopian Tube to Uterus with Nonautologous Tissue Substitute, Open Approach

♀ **0U160Z5** Bypass Left Fallopian Tube to Right Fallopian Tube, Open Approach

♀ **0U160Z6** Bypass Left Fallopian Tube to Left Fallopian Tube, Open Approach

♀ **0U160Z9** Bypass Left Fallopian Tube to Uterus, Open Approach

♀ **0U16475** Bypass Left Fallopian Tube to Right Fallopian Tube with Autologous Tissue Substitute, Percutaneous Endoscopic Approach

♀ **0U16476** Bypass Left Fallopian Tube to Left Fallopian Tube with Autologous Tissue Substitute, Percutaneous Endoscopic Approach

♀ **0U16479** Bypass Left Fallopian Tube to Uterus with Autologous Tissue Substitute, Percutaneous Endoscopic Approach

♀ **0U164J5** Bypass Left Fallopian Tube to Right Fallopian Tube with Synthetic Substitute, Percutaneous Endoscopic Approach

♀ **0U164J6** Bypass Left Fallopian Tube to Left Fallopian Tube with Synthetic Substitute, Percutaneous Endoscopic Approach

♀ **0U164J9** Bypass Left Fallopian Tube to Uterus with Synthetic Substitute, Percutaneous Endoscopic Approach

♀ **0U164K5** Bypass Left Fallopian Tube to Right Fallopian Tube with Nonautologous Tissue Substitute, Percutaneous Endoscopic Approach

♀ **0U164K6** Bypass Left Fallopian Tube to Left Fallopian Tube with Nonautologous Tissue Substitute, Percutaneous Endoscopic Approach

♀ **0U164K9** Bypass Left Fallopian Tube to Uterus with Nonautologous Tissue Substitute, Percutaneous Endoscopic Approach

♀ **0U164Z5** Bypass Left Fallopian Tube to Right Fallopian Tube, Percutaneous Endoscopic Approach

♀ **0U164Z6** Bypass Left Fallopian Tube to Left Fallopian Tube, Percutaneous Endoscopic Approach

♀ **0U164Z9** Bypass Left Fallopian Tube to Uterus, Percutaneous Endoscopic Approach

0U2 – Female Reproductive System, Change

Review Coding Guideline B6.1c

♀ **0U23X0Z** Change Drainage Device in Ovary, External Approach

♀ **0U23XYZ** Change Other Device in Ovary, External Approach

♀ **0U28X0Z** Change Drainage Device in Fallopian Tube, External Approach

♀ **0U28XYZ** Change Other Device in Fallopian Tube, External Approach

♀ **0U2DX0Z** Change Drainage Device in Uterus and Cervix, External Approach

♀ **0U2DXHZ** Change Contraceptive Device in Uterus and Cervix, External Approach

♀ **0U2DXYZ** Change Other Device in Uterus and Cervix, External Approach

♀ **0U2HX0Z** Change Drainage Device in Vagina and Cul-de-sac, External Approach

♀ **0U2HXGZ** Change Pessary in Vagina and Cul-de-sac, External Approach

♀ **0U2HXYZ** Change Other Device in Vagina and Cul-de-sac, External Approach

♀ **0U2MX0Z** Change Drainage Device in Vulva, External Approach

♀ **0U2MXYZ** Change Other Device in Vulva, External Approach

0U5 – Female Reproductive System, Destruction

♀ **0U500ZZ** Destruction of Right Ovary, Open Approach

♀ **0U503ZZ** Destruction of Right Ovary, Percutaneous Approach

♀ **0U504ZZ** Destruction of Right Ovary, Percutaneous Endoscopic Approach

♀ **0U508ZZ** Destruction of Right Ovary, Via Natural or Artificial Opening Endoscopic

♀ **0U510ZZ** Destruction of Left Ovary, Open Approach

♀ **0U513ZZ** Destruction of Left Ovary, Percutaneous Approach

♀ Female-only   ♂ Male-only   ▲ Limited Coverage   ● Non-OR   ▨ HAC HAC-associated procedure   ▲ Non-covered procedures   ✚ Cluster

♀ **0U514ZZ** Destruction of Left Ovary, Percutaneous Endoscopic Approach

♀ **0U518ZZ** Destruction of Left Ovary, Via Natural or Artificial Opening Endoscopic

♀ **0U520ZZ** Destruction of Bilateral Ovaries, Open Approach

♀ **0U523ZZ** Destruction of Bilateral Ovaries, Percutaneous Approach

♀ **0U524ZZ** Destruction of Bilateral Ovaries, Percutaneous Endoscopic Approach

♀ **0U528ZZ** Destruction of Bilateral Ovaries, Via Natural or Artificial Opening Endoscopic

♀ **0U540ZZ** Destruction of Uterine Supporting Structure, Open Approach

♀ **0U543ZZ** Destruction of Uterine Supporting Structure, Percutaneous Approach

♀ **0U544ZZ** Destruction of Uterine Supporting Structure, Percutaneous Endoscopic Approach

♀ **0U548ZZ** Destruction of Uterine Supporting Structure, Via Natural or Artificial Opening Endoscopic

♀ **0U550ZZ** Destruction of Right Fallopian Tube, Open Approach

♀ **0U553ZZ** Destruction of Right Fallopian Tube, Percutaneous Approach

♀ **0U554ZZ** Destruction of Right Fallopian Tube, Percutaneous Endoscopic Approach

♀ **0U557ZZ** Destruction of Right Fallopian Tube, Via Natural or Artificial Opening

♀ **0U558ZZ** Destruction of Right Fallopian Tube, Via Natural or Artificial Opening Endoscopic

♀ **0U560ZZ** Destruction of Left Fallopian Tube, Open Approach

♀ **0U563ZZ** Destruction of Left Fallopian Tube, Percutaneous Approach

♀ **0U564ZZ** Destruction of Left Fallopian Tube, Percutaneous Endoscopic Approach

♀ **0U567ZZ** Destruction of Left Fallopian Tube, Via Natural or Artificial Opening

♀ **0U568ZZ** Destruction of Left Fallopian Tube, Via Natural or Artificial Opening Endoscopic

♀ **0U570ZZ** Destruction of Bilateral Fallopian Tubes, Open Approach
  ▲ *When reported with diagnosis code Z30.2*

♀ **0U573ZZ** Destruction of Bilateral Fallopian Tubes, Percutaneous Approach
  ▲ *When reported with diagnosis code Z30.2*

♀ **0U574ZZ** Destruction of Bilateral Fallopian Tubes, Percutaneous Endoscopic Approach
  ▲ *When reported with diagnosis code Z30.2*

♀ **0U577ZZ** Destruction of Bilateral Fallopian Tubes, Via Natural or Artificial Opening
  ▲ *When reported with diagnosis code Z30.2*

♀ **0U578ZZ** Destruction of Bilateral Fallopian Tubes, Via Natural or Artificial Opening Endoscopic
  ▲ *When reported with diagnosis code Z30.2*

♀ **0U590ZZ** Destruction of Uterus, Open Approach

♀ **0U593ZZ** Destruction of Uterus, Percutaneous Approach

♀ **0U594ZZ** Destruction of Uterus, Percutaneous Endoscopic Approach

♀ **0U597ZZ** Destruction of Uterus, Via Natural or Artificial Opening

♀ **0U598ZZ** Destruction of Uterus, Via Natural or Artificial Opening Endoscopic

♀ **0U5B0ZZ** Destruction of Endometrium, Open Approach

♀ **0U5B3ZZ** Destruction of Endometrium, Percutaneous Approach

♀ **0U5B4ZZ** Destruction of Endometrium, Percutaneous Endoscopic Approach

♀ **0U5B7ZZ** Destruction of Endometrium, Via Natural or Artificial Opening

♀ **0U5B8ZZ** Destruction of Endometrium, Via Natural or Artificial Opening Endoscopic

♀ **0U5C0ZZ** Destruction of Cervix, Open Approach

♀ **0U5C3ZZ** Destruction of Cervix, Percutaneous Approach

♀ **0U5C4ZZ** Destruction of Cervix, Percutaneous Endoscopic Approach

♀ **0U5C7ZZ** Destruction of Cervix, Via Natural or Artificial Opening

♀ **0U5C8ZZ** Destruction of Cervix, Via Natural or Artificial Opening Endoscopic

♀ **0U5F0ZZ** Destruction of Cul-de-sac, Open Approach

♀ **0U5F3ZZ** Destruction of Cul-de-sac, Percutaneous Approach

♀ **0U5F4ZZ** Destruction of Cul-de-sac, Percutaneous Endoscopic Approach

♀ **0U5F7ZZ** Destruction of Cul-de-sac, Via Natural or Artificial Opening

♀ **0U5F8ZZ** Destruction of Cul-de-sac, Via Natural or Artificial Opening Endoscopic

♀ **0U5G0ZZ** Destruction of Vagina, Open Approach

♀ **0U5G3ZZ** Destruction of Vagina, Percutaneous Approach

♀ **0U5G4ZZ** Destruction of Vagina, Percutaneous Endoscopic Approach

♀ **0U5G7ZZ** Destruction of Vagina, Via Natural or Artificial Opening

♀ **0U5G8ZZ** Destruction of Vagina, Via Natural or Artificial Opening Endoscopic

♀ **0U5GXZZ** Destruction of Vagina, External Approach

♀ **0U5J0ZZ** Destruction of Clitoris, Open Approach

♀ **0U5JXZZ** Destruction of Clitoris, External Approach

♀ **0U5K0ZZ** Destruction of Hymen, Open Approach

♀ **0U5K3ZZ** Destruction of Hymen, Percutaneous Approach

♀ **0U5K4ZZ** Destruction of Hymen, Percutaneous Endoscopic Approach

♀ **0U5K7ZZ** Destruction of Hymen, Via Natural or Artificial Opening

♀ **0U5K8ZZ** Destruction of Hymen, Via Natural or Artificial Opening Endoscopic
  ▲

♀ **0U5KXZZ** Destruction of Hymen, External Approach

♀ **0U5L0ZZ** Destruction of Vestibular Gland, Open Approach

♀ **0U5LXZZ** Destruction of Vestibular Gland, External Approach

♀ **0U5M0ZZ** Destruction of Vulva, Open Approach

♀ **0U5MXZZ** Destruction of Vulva, External Approach

0U7 – Female Reproductive System, Dilation

♀ **0U750DZ** Dilation of Right Fallopian Tube with Intraluminal Device, Open Approach

♀ **0U750ZZ** Dilation of Right Fallopian Tube, Open Approach

♀ **0U753DZ** Dilation of Right Fallopian Tube with Intraluminal Device, Percutaneous Approach

♀ **0U753ZZ** Dilation of Right Fallopian Tube, Percutaneous Approach

♀ **0U754DZ** Dilation of Right Fallopian Tube with Intraluminal Device, Percutaneous Endoscopic Approach

♀ **0U754ZZ** Dilation of Right Fallopian Tube, Percutaneous Endoscopic Approach

♀ **0U757DZ** Dilation of Right Fallopian Tube with Intraluminal Device, Via Natural or Artificial Opening

♀ **0U757ZZ** Dilation of Right Fallopian Tube, Via Natural or Artificial Opening

♀ **0U758DZ** Dilation of Right Fallopian Tube with Intraluminal Device, Via Natural or Artificial Opening Endoscopic

♀ **0U758ZZ** Dilation of Right Fallopian Tube, Via Natural or Artificial Opening Endoscopic

♀ **0U760DZ** Dilation of Left Fallopian Tube with Intraluminal Device, Open Approach

♀ **0U760ZZ** Dilation of Left Fallopian Tube, Open Approach

♀ **0U763DZ** Dilation of Left Fallopian Tube with Intraluminal Device, Percutaneous Approach

♀ **0U763ZZ** Dilation of Left Fallopian Tube, Percutaneous Approach

♀ **0U764DZ** Dilation of Left Fallopian Tube with Intraluminal Device, Percutaneous Endoscopic Approach

♀ **0U764ZZ** Dilation of Left Fallopian Tube, Percutaneous Endoscopic Approach

♀ **0U767DZ** Dilation of Left Fallopian Tube with Intraluminal Device, Via Natural or Artificial Opening

♀ **0U767ZZ** Dilation of Left Fallopian Tube, Via Natural or Artificial Opening

♀ **0U768DZ** Dilation of Left Fallopian Tube with Intraluminal Device, Via Natural or Artificial Opening Endoscopic

♀ **0U768ZZ** Dilation of Left Fallopian Tube, Via Natural or Artificial Opening Endoscopic

♀ **0U770DZ** Dilation of Bilateral Fallopian Tubes with Intraluminal Device, Open Approach

♀ **0U770ZZ** Dilation of Bilateral Fallopian Tubes, Open Approach

♀ **0U773DZ** Dilation of Bilateral Fallopian Tubes with Intraluminal Device, Percutaneous Approach

♀ **0U773ZZ** Dilation of Bilateral Fallopian Tubes, Percutaneous Approach

♀ **0U774DZ** Dilation of Bilateral Fallopian Tubes with Intraluminal Device, Percutaneous Endoscopic Approach

♀ **0U774ZZ** Dilation of Bilateral Fallopian Tubes, Percutaneous Endoscopic Approach

♀ **0U777DZ** Dilation of Bilateral Fallopian Tubes with Intraluminal Device, Via Natural or Artificial Opening

♀ **0U777ZZ** Dilation of Bilateral Fallopian Tubes, Via Natural or Artificial Opening

♀ **0U778DZ** Dilation of Bilateral Fallopian Tubes with Intraluminal Device, Via Natural or Artificial Opening Endoscopic

♀ **0U778ZZ** Dilation of Bilateral Fallopian Tubes, Via Natural or Artificial Opening Endoscopic

♀ **0U790DZ** Dilation of Uterus with Intraluminal Device, Open Approach

♀ **0U790ZZ** Dilation of Uterus, Open Approach

♀ **0U793DZ** Dilation of Uterus with Intraluminal Device, Percutaneous Approach

♀ **0U793ZZ** Dilation of Uterus, Percutaneous Approach

♀ **0U794DZ** Dilation of Uterus with Intraluminal Device, Percutaneous Endoscopic Approach

♀ **0U794ZZ** Dilation of Uterus, Percutaneous Endoscopic Approach

♀ **0U797DZ** Dilation of Uterus with Intraluminal Device, Via Natural or Artificial Opening

♀ **0U797ZZ** Dilation of Uterus, Via Natural or Artificial Opening

♀ **0U798DZ** Dilation of Uterus with Intraluminal Device, Via Natural or Artificial Opening Endoscopic

♀ **0U798ZZ** Dilation of Uterus, Via Natural or Artificial Opening Endoscopic

♀ **0U7C0DZ** Dilation of Cervix with Intraluminal Device, Open Approach

♀ **0U7C0ZZ** Dilation of Cervix, Open Approach

♀ **0U7C3DZ** Dilation of Cervix with Intraluminal Device, Percutaneous Approach

♀ **0U7C3ZZ** Dilation of Cervix, Percutaneous Approach

♀ **0U7C4DZ** Dilation of Cervix with Intraluminal Device, Percutaneous Endoscopic Approach

♀ **0U7C4ZZ** Dilation of Cervix, Percutaneous Endoscopic Approach

♀ **0U7C7DZ** Dilation of Cervix with Intraluminal Device, Via Natural or Artificial Opening

♀ **0U7C7ZZ** Dilation of Cervix, Via Natural or Artificial Opening
AHA CC: 2Q, 2020, 30

♀ **0U7C8DZ** Dilation of Cervix with Intraluminal Device, Via Natural or Artificial Opening Endoscopic

♀ **0U7C8ZZ** Dilation of Cervix, Via Natural or Artificial Opening Endoscopic

♀ **0U7G0DZ** Dilation of Vagina with Intraluminal Device, Open Approach

♀ **0U7G0ZZ** Dilation of Vagina, Open Approach

♀ **0U7G3DZ** Dilation of Vagina with Intraluminal Device, Percutaneous Approach

♀ **0U7G3ZZ** Dilation of Vagina, Percutaneous Approach

♀ **0U7G4DZ** Dilation of Vagina with Intraluminal Device, Percutaneous Endoscopic Approach

♀ **0U7G4ZZ** Dilation of Vagina, Percutaneous Endoscopic Approach

♀ **0U7G7DZ** Dilation of Vagina with Intraluminal Device, Via Natural or Artificial Opening

♀ **0U7G7ZZ** Dilation of Vagina, Via Natural or Artificial Opening

♀ **0U7G8DZ** Dilation of Vagina with Intraluminal Device, Via Natural or Artificial Opening Endoscopic

♀ **0U7G8ZZ** Dilation of Vagina, Via Natural or Artificial Opening Endoscopic

♀ **0U7K0DZ** Dilation of Hymen with Intraluminal Device, Open Approach

♀ **0U7K0ZZ** Dilation of Hymen, Open Approach

♀ **0U7K3DZ** Dilation of Hymen with Intraluminal Device, Percutaneous Approach

♀ **0U7K3ZZ** Dilation of Hymen, Percutaneous Approach

♀ **0U7K4DZ** Dilation of Hymen with Intraluminal Device, Percutaneous Endoscopic Approach

♀ **0U7K4ZZ** Dilation of Hymen, Percutaneous Endoscopic Approach

♀ **0U7K7DZ** Dilation of Hymen with Intraluminal Device, Via Natural or Artificial Opening

♀ **0U7K7ZZ** Dilation of Hymen, Via Natural or Artificial Opening

♀ **0U7K8DZ** Dilation of Hymen with Intraluminal Device, Via Natural or Artificial Opening Endoscopic

♀ **0U7K8ZZ** Dilation of Hymen, Via Natural or Artificial Opening Endoscopic

♀ **0U7KXDZ** Dilation of Hymen with Intraluminal Device, External Approach

♀ **0U7KXZZ** Dilation of Hymen, External Approach

0U8 – Female Reproductive System, Division

Review Coding Guideline B3.14

♀ **0U800ZZ** Division of Right Ovary, Open Approach

♀ **0U803ZZ** Division of Right Ovary, Percutaneous Approach

♀ **0U804ZZ** Division of Right Ovary, Percutaneous Endoscopic Approach

♀ **0U810ZZ** Division of Left Ovary, Open Approach

♀ **0U813ZZ** Division of Left Ovary, Percutaneous Approach

♀ **0U814ZZ** Division of Left Ovary, Percutaneous Endoscopic Approach

♀ **0U820ZZ** Division of Bilateral Ovaries, Open Approach

♀ **0U823ZZ** Division of Bilateral Ovaries, Percutaneous Approach

♀ **0U824ZZ** Division of Bilateral Ovaries, Percutaneous Endoscopic Approach

♀ **0U840ZZ** Division of Uterine Supporting Structure, Open Approach

♀ **0U843ZZ** Division of Uterine Supporting Structure, Percutaneous Approach

♀ **0U844ZZ** Division of Uterine Supporting Structure, Percutaneous Endoscopic Approach

♀ **0U8K7ZZ** Division of Hymen, Via Natural or Artificial Opening

♀ **0U8K8ZZ** Division of Hymen, Via Natural or Artificial Opening Endoscopic

♀ **0U8KXZZ** Division of Hymen, External Approach

0U9 – Female Reproductive System, Drainage

Review Coding Guidelines B3.4a and B3.4b

Review Coding Guideline B6.2

♀ **0U9000Z** Drainage of Right Ovary with Drainage Device, Open Approach

♀ **0U900ZX** Drainage of Right Ovary, Open Approach, Diagnostic

♀ **0U900ZZ** Drainage of Right Ovary, Open Approach

♀ **0U9030Z** Drainage of Right Ovary with Drainage Device, Percutaneous Approach

♀ **0U903ZX** Drainage of Right Ovary, Percutaneous Approach, Diagnostic

♀ **0U903ZZ** Drainage of Right Ovary, Percutaneous Approach

♀ **0U9040Z** Drainage of Right Ovary with Drainage Device, Percutaneous Endoscopic Approach

♀ **0U904ZX** Drainage of Right Ovary, Percutaneous Endoscopic Approach, Diagnostic

♀ **0U904ZZ** Drainage of Right Ovary, Percutaneous Endoscopic Approach

♀ **0U9080Z** Drainage of Right Ovary with Drainage Device, Via Natural or Artificial Opening Endoscopic

♀ **0U908ZX** Drainage of Right Ovary, Via Natural or Artificial Opening Endoscopic, Diagnostic

♀ **0U908ZZ** Drainage of Right Ovary, Via Natural or Artificial Opening Endoscopic

♀ **0U90XZZ** Drainage of Right Ovary, External Approach

♀ **0U9100Z** Drainage of Left Ovary with Drainage Device, Open Approach

♀ **0U910ZX** Drainage of Left Ovary, Open Approach, Diagnostic

♀ **0U910ZZ** Drainage of Left Ovary, Open Approach

♀ **0U9130Z** Drainage of Left Ovary with Drainage Device, Percutaneous Approach

♀ **0U913ZX** Drainage of Left Ovary, Percutaneous Approach, Diagnostic

♀ **0U913ZZ** Drainage of Left Ovary, Percutaneous Approach

♀ **0U9140Z** Drainage of Left Ovary with Drainage Device, Percutaneous Endoscopic Approach

♀ **0U914ZX** Drainage of Left Ovary, Percutaneous Endoscopic Approach, Diagnostic

♀ **0U914ZZ** Drainage of Left Ovary, Percutaneous Endoscopic Approach

♀ **0U9180Z** Drainage of Left Ovary with Drainage Device, Via Natural or Artificial Opening Endoscopic

♀ **0U918ZX** Drainage of Left Ovary, Via Natural or Artificial Opening Endoscopic, Diagnostic

♀ **0U918ZZ** Drainage of Left Ovary, Via Natural or Artificial Opening Endoscopic

♀ **0U91XZZ** Drainage of Left Ovary, External Approach

♀ **0U9200Z** Drainage of Bilateral Ovaries with Drainage Device, Open Approach

♀ **0U920ZX** Drainage of Bilateral Ovaries, Open Approach, Diagnostic

♀ **0U920ZZ** Drainage of Bilateral Ovaries, Open Approach

♀ **0U9230Z** Drainage of Bilateral Ovaries with Drainage Device, Percutaneous Approach

♀ **0U923ZX** Drainage of Bilateral Ovaries, Percutaneous Approach, Diagnostic

♀ **0U923ZZ** Drainage of Bilateral Ovaries, Percutaneous Approach

♀ **0U9240Z** Drainage of Bilateral Ovaries with Drainage Device, Percutaneous Endoscopic Approach

♀ **0U924ZX** Drainage of Bilateral Ovaries, Percutaneous Endoscopic Approach, Diagnostic

♀ **0U924ZZ** Drainage of Bilateral Ovaries, Percutaneous Endoscopic Approach

♀ **0U9280Z** Drainage of Bilateral Ovaries with Drainage Device, Via Natural or Artificial Opening Endoscopic

♀ **0U928ZX** Drainage of Bilateral Ovaries, Via Natural or Artificial Opening Endoscopic, Diagnostic

♀ **0U928ZZ** Drainage of Bilateral Ovaries, Via Natural or Artificial Opening Endoscopic

♀ **0U92XZZ** Drainage of Bilateral Ovaries, External Approach

♀ **0U9400Z** Drainage of Uterine Supporting Structure with Drainage Device, Open Approach

♀ **0U940ZX** Drainage of Uterine Supporting Structure, Open Approach, Diagnostic

♀ **0U940ZZ** Drainage of Uterine Supporting Structure, Open Approach

♀ **0U9430Z** Drainage of Uterine Supporting Structure with Drainage Device, Percutaneous Approach

♀ **0U943ZX** Drainage of Uterine Supporting Structure, Percutaneous Approach, Diagnostic

♀ **0U943ZZ** Drainage of Uterine Supporting Structure, Percutaneous Approach

♀ **0U9440Z** Drainage of Uterine Supporting Structure with Drainage Device, Percutaneous Endoscopic Approach

♀ **0U944ZX** Drainage of Uterine Supporting Structure, Percutaneous Endoscopic Approach, Diagnostic

♀ **0U944ZZ** Drainage of Uterine Supporting Structure, Percutaneous Endoscopic Approach

♀ **0U9480Z** Drainage of Uterine Supporting Structure with Drainage Device, Via Natural or Artificial Opening Endoscopic

♀ **0U948ZX** Drainage of Uterine Supporting Structure, Via Natural or Artificial Opening Endoscopic, Diagnostic

♀ **0U948ZZ** Drainage of Uterine Supporting Structure, Via Natural or Artificial Opening Endoscopic

♀ **0U9500Z** Drainage of Right Fallopian Tube with Drainage Device, Open Approach

♀ **0U950ZX** Drainage of Right Fallopian Tube, Open Approach, Diagnostic

♀ **0U950ZZ** Drainage of Right Fallopian Tube, Open Approach

♀ **0U9530Z** Drainage of Right Fallopian Tube with Drainage Device, Percutaneous Approach

♀ **0U953ZX** Drainage of Right Fallopian Tube, Percutaneous Approach, Diagnostic

♀ **0U953ZZ** Drainage of Right Fallopian Tube, Percutaneous Approach

♀ **0U9540Z** Drainage of Right Fallopian Tube with Drainage Device, Percutaneous Endoscopic Approach

♀ **0U954ZX** Drainage of Right Fallopian Tube, Percutaneous Endoscopic Approach, Diagnostic

♀ **0U954ZZ** Drainage of Right Fallopian Tube, Percutaneous Endoscopic Approach

♀ **0U9570Z** Drainage of Right Fallopian Tube with Drainage Device, Via Natural or Artificial Opening

♀ **0U957ZX** Drainage of Right Fallopian Tube, Via Natural or Artificial Opening, Diagnostic

♀ **0U957ZZ** Drainage of Right Fallopian Tube, Via Natural or Artificial Opening

♀ **0U9580Z** Drainage of Right Fallopian Tube with Drainage Device, Via Natural or Artificial Opening Endoscopic

♀ **0U958ZX** Drainage of Right Fallopian Tube, Via Natural or Artificial Opening Endoscopic, Diagnostic

♀ **0U958ZZ** Drainage of Right Fallopian Tube, Via Natural or Artificial Opening Endoscopic

♀ **0U9600Z** Drainage of Left Fallopian Tube with Drainage Device, Open Approach

♀ **0U960ZX** Drainage of Left Fallopian Tube, Open Approach, Diagnostic

♀ **0U960ZZ** Drainage of Left Fallopian Tube, Open Approach

♀ **0U9630Z** Drainage of Left Fallopian Tube with Drainage Device, Percutaneous Approach

♀ **0U963ZX** Drainage of Left Fallopian Tube, Percutaneous Approach, Diagnostic

♀ **0U963ZZ** Drainage of Left Fallopian Tube, Percutaneous Approach

♀ **0U9640Z** Drainage of Left Fallopian Tube with Drainage Device, Percutaneous Endoscopic Approach

♀ **0U964ZX** Drainage of Left Fallopian Tube, Percutaneous Endoscopic Approach, Diagnostic

♀ **0U964ZZ** Drainage of Left Fallopian Tube, Percutaneous Endoscopic Approach

♀ **0U9670Z** Drainage of Left Fallopian Tube with Drainage Device, Via Natural or Artificial Opening

♀ **0U967ZX** Drainage of Left Fallopian Tube, Via Natural or Artificial Opening, Diagnostic

♀ **0U967ZZ** Drainage of Left Fallopian Tube, Via Natural or Artificial Opening

♀ **0U9680Z** Drainage of Left Fallopian Tube with Drainage Device, Via Natural or Artificial Opening Endoscopic

♀ **0U968ZX** Drainage of Left Fallopian Tube, Via Natural or Artificial Opening Endoscopic, Diagnostic

♀ **0U968ZZ** Drainage of Left Fallopian Tube, Via Natural or Artificial Opening Endoscopic

♀ **0U9700Z** Drainage of Bilateral Fallopian Tubes with Drainage Device, Open Approach

♀ **0U970ZX** Drainage of Bilateral Fallopian Tubes, Open Approach, Diagnostic

♀ **0U970ZZ** Drainage of Bilateral Fallopian Tubes, Open Approach

♀ **0U9730Z** Drainage of Bilateral Fallopian Tubes with Drainage Device, Percutaneous Approach

♀ **0U973ZX** Drainage of Bilateral Fallopian Tubes, Percutaneous Approach, Diagnostic

♀ **0U973ZZ** Drainage of Bilateral Fallopian Tubes, Percutaneous Approach

♀ **0U9740Z** Drainage of Bilateral Fallopian Tubes with Drainage Device, Percutaneous Endoscopic Approach

♀ **0U974ZX** Drainage of Bilateral Fallopian Tubes, Percutaneous Endoscopic Approach, Diagnostic

♀ **0U974ZZ** Drainage of Bilateral Fallopian Tubes, Percutaneous Endoscopic Approach

♀ **0U9770Z** Drainage of Bilateral Fallopian Tubes with Drainage Device, Via Natural or Artificial Opening

♀ **0U977ZX** Drainage of Bilateral Fallopian Tubes, Via Natural or Artificial Opening, Diagnostic

♀ **0U977ZZ** Drainage of Bilateral Fallopian Tubes, Via Natural or Artificial Opening

♀ **0U9780Z** Drainage of Bilateral Fallopian Tubes with Drainage Device, Via Natural or Artificial Opening Endoscopic

♀ **0U978ZX** Drainage of Bilateral Fallopian Tubes, Via Natural or Artificial Opening Endoscopic, Diagnostic

♀ **0U978ZZ** Drainage of Bilateral Fallopian Tubes, Via Natural or Artificial Opening Endoscopic

♀ **0U9900Z** Drainage of Uterus with Drainage Device, Open Approach

♀ **0U990ZX** Drainage of Uterus, Open Approach, Diagnostic

♀ **0U990ZZ** Drainage of Uterus, Open Approach

♀ **0U9930Z** Drainage of Uterus with Drainage Device, Percutaneous Approach

♀ **0U993ZX** Drainage of Uterus, Percutaneous Approach, Diagnostic

♀ **0U993ZZ** Drainage of Uterus, Percutaneous Approach

♀ **0U9940Z** Drainage of Uterus with Drainage Device, Percutaneous Endoscopic Approach

♀ **0U994ZX** Drainage of Uterus, Percutaneous Endoscopic Approach, Diagnostic

♀ **0U994ZZ** Drainage of Uterus, Percutaneous Endoscopic Approach

♀ **0U9970Z** Drainage of Uterus with Drainage Device, Via Natural or Artificial Opening

♀ **0U997ZX** Drainage of Uterus, Via Natural or Artificial Opening, Diagnostic

♀ **0U997ZZ** Drainage of Uterus, Via Natural or Artificial Opening

♀ **0U9980Z** Drainage of Uterus with Drainage Device, Via Natural or Artificial Opening Endoscopic

♀ **0U998ZX** Drainage of Uterus, Via Natural or Artificial Opening Endoscopic, Diagnostic

♀ **0U998ZZ** Drainage of Uterus, Via Natural or Artificial Opening Endoscopic

♀ **0U9C00Z** Drainage of Cervix with Drainage Device, Open Approach

♀ **0U9C0ZX** Drainage of Cervix, Open Approach, Diagnostic

♀ **0U9C0ZZ** Drainage of Cervix, Open Approach

♀ **0U9C30Z** Drainage of Cervix with Drainage Device, Percutaneous Approach

♀ **0U9C3ZX** Drainage of Cervix, Percutaneous Approach, Diagnostic

♀ **0U9C3ZZ** Drainage of Cervix, Percutaneous Approach

♀ **0U9C40Z** Drainage of Cervix with Drainage Device, Percutaneous Endoscopic Approach

♀ **0U9C4ZX** Drainage of Cervix, Percutaneous Endoscopic Approach, Diagnostic

♀ **0U9C4ZZ** Drainage of Cervix, Percutaneous Endoscopic Approach

♀ **0U9C70Z** Drainage of Cervix with Drainage Device, Via Natural or Artificial Opening

♀ **0U9C7ZX** Drainage of Cervix, Via Natural or Artificial Opening, Diagnostic

♀ **0U9C7ZZ** Drainage of Cervix, Via Natural or Artificial Opening

♀ **0U9C80Z** Drainage of Cervix with Drainage Device, Via Natural or Artificial Opening Endoscopic

♀ **0U9C8ZX** Drainage of Cervix, Via Natural or Artificial Opening Endoscopic, Diagnostic

♀ **0U9C8ZZ** Drainage of Cervix, Via Natural or Artificial Opening Endoscopic

♀ **0U9F00Z** Drainage of Cul-de-sac with Drainage Device, Open Approach

♀ **0U9F0ZX** Drainage of Cul-de-sac, Open Approach, Diagnostic

♀ **0U9F0ZZ** Drainage of Cul-de-sac, Open Approach

♀ **0U9F30Z** Drainage of Cul-de-sac with Drainage Device, Percutaneous Approach

♀ **0U9F3ZX** Drainage of Cul-de-sac, Percutaneous Approach, Diagnostic

♀ **0U9F3ZZ** Drainage of Cul-de-sac, Percutaneous Approach

♀ **0U9F40Z** Drainage of Cul-de-sac with Drainage Device, Percutaneous Endoscopic Approach

♀ **0U9F4ZX** Drainage of Cul-de-sac, Percutaneous Endoscopic Approach, Diagnostic

♀ **0U9F4ZZ** Drainage of Cul-de-sac, Percutaneous Endoscopic Approach

♀ **0U9F70Z** Drainage of Cul-de-sac with Drainage Device, Via Natural or Artificial Opening

♀ **0U9F7ZX** Drainage of Cul-de-sac, Via Natural or Artificial Opening, Diagnostic

♀ **0U9F7ZZ** Drainage of Cul-de-sac, Via Natural or Artificial Opening

♀ **0U9F80Z** Drainage of Cul-de-sac with Drainage Device, Via Natural or Artificial Opening Endoscopic

♀ **0U9F8ZX** Drainage of Cul-de-sac, Via Natural or Artificial Opening Endoscopic, Diagnostic

♀ **0U9F8ZZ** Drainage of Cul-de-sac, Via Natural or Artificial Opening Endoscopic

♀ **0U9G00Z** Drainage of Vagina with Drainage Device, Open Approach

♀ **0U9G0ZX** Drainage of Vagina, Open Approach, Diagnostic

♀ **0U9G0ZZ** Drainage of Vagina, Open Approach

♀ **0U9G30Z** Drainage of Vagina with Drainage Device, Percutaneous Approach

♀ **0U9G3ZX** Drainage of Vagina, Percutaneous Approach, Diagnostic

♀ **0U9G3ZZ** Drainage of Vagina, Percutaneous Approach

♀ **0U9G40Z** Drainage of Vagina with Drainage Device, Percutaneous Endoscopic Approach

♀ **0U9G4ZX** Drainage of Vagina, Percutaneous Endoscopic Approach, Diagnostic

♀ **0U9G4ZZ** Drainage of Vagina, Percutaneous Endoscopic Approach

♀ **0U9G70Z** Drainage of Vagina with Drainage Device, Via Natural or Artificial Opening

♀ **0U9G7ZX** Drainage of Vagina, Via Natural or Artificial Opening, Diagnostic

♀ **0U9G7ZZ** Drainage of Vagina, Via Natural or Artificial Opening

AHA CC: 4Q, 2016, 58-59

♀ **0U9G80Z** Drainage of Vagina with Drainage Device, Via Natural or Artificial Opening Endoscopic

♀ **0U9G8ZX** Drainage of Vagina, Via Natural or Artificial Opening Endoscopic, Diagnostic

♀ **0U9G8ZZ** Drainage of Vagina, Via Natural or Artificial Opening Endoscopic

♀ **0U9GX0Z** Drainage of Vagina with Drainage Device, External Approach

♀ **0U9GXZX** Drainage of Vagina, External Approach, Diagnostic

♀ **0U9GXZZ** Drainage of Vagina, External Approach

♀ **0U9J00Z** Drainage of Clitoris with Drainage Device, Open Approach

♀ **0U9J0ZX** Drainage of Clitoris, Open Approach, Diagnostic

♀ **0U9J0ZZ** Drainage of Clitoris, Open Approach

♀ **0U9JX0Z** Drainage of Clitoris with Drainage Device, External Approach

♀ **0U9JXZX** Drainage of Clitoris, External Approach, Diagnostic

♀ **0U9JXZZ** Drainage of Clitoris, External Approach

♀ **0U9K00Z** Drainage of Hymen with Drainage Device, Open Approach

♀ **0U9K0ZX** Drainage of Hymen, Open Approach, Diagnostic

♀ **0U9K0ZZ** Drainage of Hymen, Open Approach

♀ **0U9K30Z** Drainage of Hymen with Drainage Device, Percutaneous Approach

♀ **0U9K3ZX** Drainage of Hymen, Percutaneous Approach, Diagnostic

♀ **0U9K3ZZ** Drainage of Hymen, Percutaneous Approach

♀ **0U9K40Z** Drainage of Hymen with Drainage Device, Percutaneous Endoscopic Approach

♀ **0U9K4ZX** Drainage of Hymen, Percutaneous Endoscopic Approach, Diagnostic

♀ **0U9K4ZZ** Drainage of Hymen, Percutaneous Endoscopic Approach

♀ **0U9K70Z** Drainage of Hymen with Drainage Device, Via Natural or Artificial Opening

♀ **0U9K7ZX** Drainage of Hymen, Via Natural or Artificial Opening, Diagnostic

♀ **0U9K7ZZ** Drainage of Hymen, Via Natural or Artificial Opening

♀ **0U9K80Z** Drainage of Hymen with Drainage Device, Via Natural or Artificial Opening Endoscopic

♀ **0U9K8ZX** Drainage of Hymen, Via Natural or Artificial Opening Endoscopic, Diagnostic

♀ **0U9K8ZZ** Drainage of Hymen, Via Natural or Artificial Opening Endoscopic

♀ **0U9KX0Z** Drainage of Hymen with Drainage Device, External Approach

♀ **0U9KXZX** Drainage of Hymen, External Approach, Diagnostic

♀ **0U9KXZZ** Drainage of Hymen, External Approach

♀ **0U9L00Z** Drainage of Vestibular Gland with Drainage Device, Open Approach

♀ **0U9L0ZX** Drainage of Vestibular Gland, Open Approach, Diagnostic

♀ **0U9L0ZZ** Drainage of Vestibular Gland, Open Approach

♀ **0U9LX0Z** Drainage of Vestibular Gland with Drainage Device, External Approach

♀ **0U9LXZX** Drainage of Vestibular Gland, External Approach, Diagnostic

♀ **0U9LXZZ** Drainage of Vestibular Gland, External Approach

♀ **0U9M00Z** Drainage of Vulva with Drainage Device, Open Approach

♀ **0U9M0ZX** Drainage of Vulva, Open Approach, Diagnostic

♀ **0U9M0ZZ** Drainage of Vulva, Open Approach

♀ **0U9MX0Z** Drainage of Vulva with Drainage Device, External Approach

♀ **0U9MXZX** Drainage of Vulva, External Approach, Diagnostic

♀ **0U9MXZZ** Drainage of Vulva, External Approach

0UB – Female Reproductive System, Excision

Review Coding Guidelines B3.4a and B3.4b

Review Coding Guideline B3.8

Review Coding Guideline B3.18

♀ **0UB00ZX** Excision of Right Ovary, Open Approach, Diagnostic

♀ **0UB00ZZ** Excision of Right Ovary, Open Approach

♀ **0UB03ZX** Excision of Right Ovary, Percutaneous Approach, Diagnostic

♀ **0UB03ZZ** Excision of Right Ovary, Percutaneous Approach

♀ **0UB04ZX** Excision of Right Ovary, Percutaneous Endoscopic Approach, Diagnostic

♀ **0UB04ZZ** Excision of Right Ovary, Percutaneous Endoscopic Approach

♀ **0UB07ZX** Excision of Right Ovary, Via Natural or Artificial Opening, Diagnostic

♀ **0UB07ZZ** Excision of Right Ovary, Via Natural or Artificial Opening

♀ **0UB08ZX** Excision of Right Ovary, Via Natural or Artificial Opening Endoscopic, Diagnostic

♀ **0UB08ZZ** Excision of Right Ovary, Via Natural or Artificial Opening Endoscopic

♀ **0UB10ZX** Excision of Left Ovary, Open Approach, Diagnostic

♀ **0UB10ZZ** Excision of Left Ovary, Open Approach

♀ **0UB13ZX** Excision of Left Ovary, Percutaneous Approach, Diagnostic

♀ **0UB13ZZ** Excision of Left Ovary, Percutaneous Approach

♀ **0UB14ZX** Excision of Left Ovary, Percutaneous Endoscopic Approach, Diagnostic

♀ **0UB14ZZ** Excision of Left Ovary, Percutaneous Endoscopic Approach

♀ **0UB17ZX** Excision of Left Ovary, Via Natural or Artificial Opening, Diagnostic

♀ **0UB17ZZ** Excision of Left Ovary, Via Natural or Artificial Opening

♀ Female-only   ♂ Male-only   ▲ Limited Coverage   ● Non-OR   🅷🅰🅲 HAC-associated procedure   ▲ Non-covered procedures   ➕ Cluster

♀ **0UB18ZX** Excision of Left Ovary, Via Natural or Artificial Opening Endoscopic, Diagnostic

♀ **0UB18ZZ** Excision of Left Ovary, Via Natural or Artificial Opening Endoscopic

♀ **0UB20ZX** Excision of Bilateral Ovaries, Open Approach, Diagnostic

♀ **0UB20ZZ** Excision of Bilateral Ovaries, Open Approach

♀ **0UB23ZX** Excision of Bilateral Ovaries, Percutaneous Approach, Diagnostic

♀ **0UB23ZZ** Excision of Bilateral Ovaries, Percutaneous Approach

♀ **0UB24ZX** Excision of Bilateral Ovaries, Percutaneous Endoscopic Approach, Diagnostic

♀ **0UB24ZZ** Excision of Bilateral Ovaries, Percutaneous Endoscopic Approach

♀ **0UB27ZX** Excision of Bilateral Ovaries, Via Natural or Artificial Opening, Diagnostic

♀ **0UB27ZZ** Excision of Bilateral Ovaries, Via Natural or Artificial Opening

♀ **0UB28ZX** Excision of Bilateral Ovaries, Via Natural or Artificial Opening Endoscopic, Diagnostic

♀ **0UB28ZZ** Excision of Bilateral Ovaries, Via Natural or Artificial Opening Endoscopic

♀ **0UB40ZX** Excision of Uterine Supporting Structure, Open Approach, Diagnostic

♀ **0UB40ZZ** Excision of Uterine Supporting Structure, Open Approach

♀ **0UB43ZX** Excision of Uterine Supporting Structure, Percutaneous Approach, Diagnostic

♀ **0UB43ZZ** Excision of Uterine Supporting Structure, Percutaneous Approach

♀ **0UB44ZX** Excision of Uterine Supporting Structure, Percutaneous Endoscopic Approach, Diagnostic

♀ **0UB44ZZ** Excision of Uterine Supporting Structure, Percutaneous Endoscopic Approach

♀ **0UB47ZX** Excision of Uterine Supporting Structure, Via Natural or Artificial Opening, Diagnostic

♀ **0UB47ZZ** Excision of Uterine Supporting Structure, Via Natural or Artificial Opening

♀ **0UB48ZX** Excision of Uterine Supporting Structure, Via Natural or Artificial Opening Endoscopic, Diagnostic

♀ **0UB48ZZ** Excision of Uterine Supporting Structure, Via Natural or Artificial Opening Endoscopic

♀ **0UB50ZX** Excision of Right Fallopian Tube, Open Approach, Diagnostic

♀ **0UB50ZZ** Excision of Right Fallopian Tube, Open Approach

♀ **0UB53ZX** Excision of Right Fallopian Tube, Percutaneous Approach, Diagnostic

♀ **0UB53ZZ** Excision of Right Fallopian Tube, Percutaneous Approach

♀ **0UB54ZX** Excision of Right Fallopian Tube, Percutaneous Endoscopic Approach, Diagnostic

♀ **0UB54ZZ** Excision of Right Fallopian Tube, Percutaneous Endoscopic Approach

♀ **0UB57ZX** Excision of Right Fallopian Tube, Via Natural or Artificial Opening, Diagnostic

♀ **0UB57ZZ** Excision of Right Fallopian Tube, Via Natural or Artificial Opening

♀ **0UB58ZX** Excision of Right Fallopian Tube, Via Natural or Artificial Opening Endoscopic, Diagnostic

♀ **0UB58ZZ** Excision of Right Fallopian Tube, Via Natural or Artificial Opening Endoscopic

♀ **0UB60ZX** Excision of Left Fallopian Tube, Open Approach, Diagnostic

♀ **0UB60ZZ** Excision of Left Fallopian Tube, Open Approach

♀ **0UB63ZX** Excision of Left Fallopian Tube, Percutaneous Approach, Diagnostic

♀ **0UB63ZZ** Excision of Left Fallopian Tube, Percutaneous Approach

♀ **0UB64ZX** Excision of Left Fallopian Tube, Percutaneous Endoscopic Approach, Diagnostic

♀ **0UB64ZZ** Excision of Left Fallopian Tube, Percutaneous Endoscopic Approach

AHA CC: 3Q, 2015, 31-32

♀ **0UB67ZX** Excision of Left Fallopian Tube, Via Natural or Artificial Opening, Diagnostic

♀ **0UB67ZZ** Excision of Left Fallopian Tube, Via Natural or Artificial Opening

♀ **0UB68ZX** Excision of Left Fallopian Tube, Via Natural or Artificial Opening Endoscopic, Diagnostic

♀ **0UB68ZZ** Excision of Left Fallopian Tube, Via Natural or Artificial Opening Endoscopic

♀ **0UB70ZX** Excision of Bilateral Fallopian Tubes, Open Approach, Diagnostic

♀ **0UB70ZZ** Excision of Bilateral Fallopian Tubes, Open Approach

AHA CC: 3Q, 2015, 31

♀ **0UB73ZX** Excision of Bilateral Fallopian Tubes, Percutaneous Approach, Diagnostic

♀ **0UB73ZZ** Excision of Bilateral Fallopian Tubes, Percutaneous Approach

♀ **0UB74ZX** Excision of Bilateral Fallopian Tubes, Percutaneous Endoscopic Approach, Diagnostic

♀ **0UB74ZZ** Excision of Bilateral Fallopian Tubes, Percutaneous Endoscopic Approach

♀ **0UB77ZX** Excision of Bilateral Fallopian Tubes, Via Natural or Artificial Opening, Diagnostic

♀ **0UB77ZZ** Excision of Bilateral Fallopian Tubes, Via Natural or Artificial Opening

♀ **0UB78ZX** Excision of Bilateral Fallopian Tubes, Via Natural or Artificial Opening Endoscopic, Diagnostic

♀ **0UB78ZZ** Excision of Bilateral Fallopian Tubes, Via Natural or Artificial Opening Endoscopic

♀ **0UB90ZX** Excision of Uterus, Open Approach, Diagnostic

♀ **0UB90ZZ** Excision of Uterus, Open Approach

AHA CC: 4Q, 2014, 16

♀ **0UB93ZX** Excision of Uterus, Percutaneous Approach, Diagnostic

♀ **0UB93ZZ** Excision of Uterus, Percutaneous Approach

♀ **0UB94ZX** Excision of Uterus, Percutaneous Endoscopic Approach, Diagnostic

♀ **0UB94ZZ** Excision of Uterus, Percutaneous Endoscopic Approach

♀ **0UB97ZX** Excision of Uterus, Via Natural or Artificial Opening, Diagnostic

♀ **0UB97ZZ** Excision of Uterus, Via Natural or Artificial Opening

♀ **0UB98ZX** Excision of Uterus, Via Natural or Artificial Opening Endoscopic, Diagnostic

♀ **0UB98ZZ** Excision of Uterus, Via Natural or Artificial Opening Endoscopic

♀ **0UBC0ZX** Excision of Cervix, Open Approach, Diagnostic

♀ **0UBC0ZZ** Excision of Cervix, Open Approach

♀ **0UBC3ZX** Excision of Cervix, Percutaneous Approach, Diagnostic

♀ **0UBC3ZZ** Excision of Cervix, Percutaneous Approach

♀ **0UBC4ZX** Excision of Cervix, Percutaneous Endoscopic Approach, Diagnostic

♀ **0UBC4ZZ** Excision of Cervix, Percutaneous Endoscopic Approach

♀ **0UBC7ZX** Excision of Cervix, Via Natural or Artificial Opening, Diagnostic

♀ **0UBC7ZZ** Excision of Cervix, Via Natural or Artificial Opening

♀ **0UBC8ZX** Excision of Cervix, Via Natural or Artificial Opening Endoscopic, Diagnostic

♀ **0UBC8ZZ** Excision of Cervix, Via Natural or Artificial Opening Endoscopic

♀ **0UBF0ZX** Excision of Cul-de-sac, Open Approach, Diagnostic

♀ **0UBF0ZZ** Excision of Cul-de-sac, Open Approach

♀ **0UBF3ZX** Excision of Cul-de-sac, Percutaneous Approach, Diagnostic

♀ **0UBF3ZZ** Excision of Cul-de-sac, Percutaneous Approach

♀ **0UBF4ZX** Excision of Cul-de-sac, Percutaneous Endoscopic Approach, Diagnostic

♀ **0UBF4ZZ** Excision of Cul-de-sac, Percutaneous Endoscopic Approach

♀ **0UBF7ZX** Excision of Cul-de-sac, Via Natural or Artificial Opening, Diagnostic

♀ **0UBF7ZZ** Excision of Cul-de-sac, Via Natural or Artificial Opening

♀ **0UBF8ZX** Excision of Cul-de-sac, Via Natural or Artificial Opening Endoscopic, Diagnostic

♀ **0UBF8ZZ** Excision of Cul-de-sac, Via Natural or Artificial Opening Endoscopic

♀ **0UBG0ZX** Excision of Vagina, Open Approach, Diagnostic

♀ **0UBG0ZZ** Excision of Vagina, Open Approach

♀ **0UBG3ZX** Excision of Vagina, Percutaneous Approach, Diagnostic

♀ **0UBG3ZZ** Excision of Vagina, Percutaneous Approach

♀ **0UBG4ZX** Excision of Vagina, Percutaneous Endoscopic Approach, Diagnostic

♀ **0UBG4ZZ** Excision of Vagina, Percutaneous Endoscopic Approach

♀ **0UBG7ZX** Excision of Vagina, Via Natural or Artificial Opening, Diagnostic

♀ **0UBG7ZZ** Excision of Vagina, Via Natural or Artificial Opening

♀ **0UBG8ZX** Excision of Vagina, Via Natural or Artificial Opening Endoscopic, Diagnostic

♀ **0UBG8ZZ** Excision of Vagina, Via Natural or Artificial Opening Endoscopic

♀ **0UBGXZX** Excision of Vagina, External Approach, Diagnostic

♀ **0UBGXZZ** Excision of Vagina, External Approach

♀ **0UBJ0ZX** Excision of Clitoris, Open Approach, Diagnostic

♀ **0UBJ0ZZ** Excision of Clitoris, Open Approach

♀ **0UBJXZX** Excision of Clitoris, External Approach, Diagnostic

♀ **0UBJXZZ** Excision of Clitoris, External Approach

♀ Female-only   ♂ Male-only   ▲ Limited Coverage   ● Non-OR   **HAC** HAC-associated procedure   ▲ Non-covered procedures   ✚ Cluster

♀ **0UBK0ZX** Excision of Hymen, Open Approach, Diagnostic

♀ **0UBK0ZZ** Excision of Hymen, Open Approach

♀ **0UBK3ZX** Excision of Hymen, Percutaneous Approach, Diagnostic

♀ **0UBK3ZZ** Excision of Hymen, Percutaneous Approach

♀ **0UBK4ZX** Excision of Hymen, Percutaneous Endoscopic Approach, Diagnostic

♀ **0UBK4ZZ** Excision of Hymen, Percutaneous Endoscopic Approach

♀ **0UBK7ZX** Excision of Hymen, Via Natural or Artificial Opening, Diagnostic

♀ **0UBK7ZZ** Excision of Hymen, Via Natural or Artificial Opening

♀ **0UBK8ZX** Excision of Hymen, Via Natural or Artificial Opening Endoscopic, Diagnostic

♀ **0UBK8ZZ** Excision of Hymen, Via Natural or Artificial Opening Endoscopic

♀ **0UBKXZX** Excision of Hymen, External Approach, Diagnostic

♀ **0UBKXZZ** Excision of Hymen, External Approach

♀ **0UBL0ZX** Excision of Vestibular Gland, Open Approach, Diagnostic

♀ **0UBL0ZZ** Excision of Vestibular Gland, Open Approach

♀ **0UBLXZX** Excision of Vestibular Gland, External Approach, Diagnostic

♀ **0UBLXZZ** Excision of Vestibular Gland, External Approach

♀ **0UBM0ZX** Excision of Vulva, Open Approach, Diagnostic

♀ **0UBM0ZZ** Excision of Vulva, Open Approach

♀ **0UBMXZX** Excision of Vulva, External Approach, Diagnostic

♀ **0UBMXZZ** Excision of Vulva, External Approach

AHA CC: 3Q, 2014, 12

0UC – Female Reproductive System, Extirpation

♀ **0UC00ZZ** Extirpation of Matter from Right Ovary, Open Approach

♀ **0UC03ZZ** Extirpation of Matter from Right Ovary, Percutaneous Approach

♀ **0UC04ZZ** Extirpation of Matter from Right Ovary, Percutaneous Endoscopic Approach

♀ **0UC08ZZ** Extirpation of Matter from Right Ovary, Via Natural or Artificial Opening Endoscopic

♀ **0UC10ZZ** Extirpation of Matter from Left Ovary, Open Approach

♀ **0UC13ZZ** Extirpation of Matter from Left Ovary, Percutaneous Approach

♀ **0UC14ZZ** Extirpation of Matter from Left Ovary, Percutaneous Endoscopic Approach

♀ **0UC18ZZ** Extirpation of Matter from Left Ovary, Via Natural or Artificial Opening Endoscopic

♀ **0UC20ZZ** Extirpation of Matter from Bilateral Ovaries, Open Approach

♀ **0UC23ZZ** Extirpation of Matter from Bilateral Ovaries, Percutaneous Approach

♀ **0UC24ZZ** Extirpation of Matter from Bilateral Ovaries, Percutaneous Endoscopic Approach

♀ **0UC28ZZ** Extirpation of Matter from Bilateral Ovaries, Via Natural or Artificial Opening Endoscopic

♀ **0UC40ZZ** Extirpation of Matter from Uterine Supporting Structure, Open Approach

♀ **0UC43ZZ** Extirpation of Matter from Uterine Supporting Structure, Percutaneous Approach

♀ **0UC44ZZ** Extirpation of Matter from Uterine Supporting Structure, Percutaneous Endoscopic Approach

♀ **0UC48ZZ** Extirpation of Matter from Uterine Supporting Structure, Via Natural or Artificial Opening Endoscopic

♀ **0UC50ZZ** Extirpation of Matter from Right Fallopian Tube, Open Approach

♀ **0UC53ZZ** Extirpation of Matter from Right Fallopian Tube, Percutaneous Approach

♀ **0UC54ZZ** Extirpation of Matter from Right Fallopian Tube, Percutaneous Endoscopic Approach

♀ **0UC57ZZ** Extirpation of Matter from Right Fallopian Tube, Via Natural or Artificial Opening

♀ **0UC58ZZ** Extirpation of Matter from Right Fallopian Tube, Via Natural or Artificial Opening Endoscopic

♀ **0UC60ZZ** Extirpation of Matter from Left Fallopian Tube, Open Approach

♀ **0UC63ZZ** Extirpation of Matter from Left Fallopian Tube, Percutaneous Approach

♀ **0UC64ZZ** Extirpation of Matter from Left Fallopian Tube, Percutaneous Endoscopic Approach

♀ **0UC67ZZ** Extirpation of Matter from Left Fallopian Tube, Via Natural or Artificial Opening

♀ **0UC68ZZ** Extirpation of Matter from Left Fallopian Tube, Via Natural or Artificial Opening Endoscopic

♀ **0UC70ZZ** Extirpation of Matter from Bilateral Fallopian Tubes, Open Approach

♀ **0UC73ZZ** Extirpation of Matter from Bilateral Fallopian Tubes, Percutaneous Approach

♀ **0UC74ZZ** Extirpation of Matter from Bilateral Fallopian Tubes, Percutaneous Endoscopic Approach

♀ **0UC77ZZ** Extirpation of Matter from Bilateral Fallopian Tubes, Via Natural or Artificial Opening

♀ **0UC78ZZ** Extirpation of Matter from Bilateral Fallopian Tubes, Via Natural or Artificial Opening Endoscopic

♀ **0UC90ZZ** Extirpation of Matter from Uterus, Open Approach

♀ **0UC93ZZ** Extirpation of Matter from Uterus, Percutaneous Approach

♀ **0UC94ZZ** Extirpation of Matter from Uterus, Percutaneous Endoscopic Approach

♀ **0UC97ZZ** Extirpation of Matter from Uterus, Via Natural or Artificial Opening

AHA CC: 2Q, 2013, 38

♀ **0UC98ZZ** Extirpation of Matter from Uterus, Via Natural or Artificial Opening Endoscopic

♀ **0UCB0ZZ** Extirpation of Matter from Endometrium, Open Approach

♀ **0UCB3ZZ** Extirpation of Matter from Endometrium, Percutaneous Approach

♀ **0UCB4ZZ** Extirpation of Matter from Endometrium, Percutaneous Endoscopic Approach

♀ **0UCB7ZZ** Extirpation of Matter from Endometrium, Via Natural or Artificial Opening

♀ **0UCB8ZZ** Extirpation of Matter from Endometrium, Via Natural or Artificial Opening Endoscopic

♀ **0UCC0ZZ** Extirpation of Matter from Cervix, Open Approach

♀ **0UCC3ZZ** Extirpation of Matter from Cervix, Percutaneous Approach

♀ **0UCC4ZZ** Extirpation of Matter from Cervix, Percutaneous Endoscopic Approach

♀ **0UCC7ZZ** Extirpation of Matter from Cervix, Via Natural or Artificial Opening

AHA CC: 3Q, 2015, 30

♀ **0UCC8ZZ** Extirpation of Matter from Cervix, Via Natural or Artificial Opening Endoscopic

AHA CC: 3Q, 2015, 30-31

♀ **0UCF0ZZ** Extirpation of Matter from Cul-de-sac, Open Approach

♀ **0UCF3ZZ** Extirpation of Matter from Cul-de-sac, Percutaneous Approach

♀ **0UCF4ZZ** Extirpation of Matter from Cul-de-sac, Percutaneous Endoscopic Approach

♀ **0UCF7ZZ** Extirpation of Matter from Cul-de-sac, Via Natural or Artificial Opening

♀ **0UCF8ZZ** Extirpation of Matter from Cul-de-sac, Via Natural or Artificial Opening Endoscopic

♀ **0UCG0ZZ** Extirpation of Matter from Vagina, Open Approach

♀ **0UCG3ZZ** Extirpation of Matter from Vagina, Percutaneous Approach

♀ **0UCG4ZZ** Extirpation of Matter from Vagina, Percutaneous Endoscopic Approach

♀ **0UCG7ZZ** Extirpation of Matter from Vagina, Via Natural or Artificial Opening

♀ **0UCG8ZZ** Extirpation of Matter from Vagina, Via Natural or Artificial Opening Endoscopic

♀ **0UCGXZZ** Extirpation of Matter from Vagina, External Approach

♀ **0UCJ0ZZ** Extirpation of Matter from Clitoris, Open Approach

♀ **0UCJXZZ** Extirpation of Matter from Clitoris, External Approach

♀ **0UCK0ZZ** Extirpation of Matter from Hymen, Open Approach

♀ **0UCK3ZZ** Extirpation of Matter from Hymen, Percutaneous Approach

♀ **0UCK4ZZ** Extirpation of Matter from Hymen, Percutaneous Endoscopic Approach

♀ **0UCK7ZZ** Extirpation of Matter from Hymen, Via Natural or Artificial Opening

♀ **0UCK8ZZ** Extirpation of Matter from Hymen, Via Natural or Artificial Opening Endoscopic

♀ **0UCKXZZ** Extirpation of Matter from Hymen, External Approach

♀ **0UCL0ZZ** Extirpation of Matter from Vestibular Gland, Open Approach

♀ **0UCLXZZ** Extirpation of Matter from Vestibular Gland, External Approach

♀ **0UCM0ZZ** Extirpation of Matter from Vulva, Open Approach

♀ **0UCMXZZ** Extirpation of Matter from Vulva, External Approach

♀ Female-only ♂ Male-only ▲ Limited Coverage ● Non-OR HAC HAC-associated procedure ▲ Non-covered procedures ✚ Cluster

0UD – Female Reproductive System, Extraction

Review Coding Guidelines B3.4a and B3.4b

Review Coding Guideline C2

♀ **0UDB7ZX** Extraction of Endometrium, Via Natural or Artificial Opening, Diagnostic

♀ **0UDB7ZZ** Extraction of Endometrium, Via Natural or Artificial Opening

♀ **0UDB8ZX** Extraction of Endometrium, Via Natural or Artificial Opening Endoscopic, Diagnostic

♀ **0UDB8ZZ** Extraction of Endometrium, Via Natural or Artificial Opening Endoscopic

♀ **0UDN0ZZ** Extraction of Ova, Open

♀ **0UDN3ZZ** Extraction of Ova, Percutaneous

♀ **0UDN4ZZ** Extraction of Ova, Percutaneous Endoscopic

0UF – Female Reproductive System, Fragmentation

♀ **0UF50ZZ** Fragmentation in Right Fallopian Tube, Open Approach

♀ **0UF53ZZ** Fragmentation in Right Fallopian Tube, Percutaneous Approach

♀ **0UF54ZZ** Fragmentation in Right Fallopian Tube, Percutaneous Endoscopic Approach

♀ **0UF57ZZ** Fragmentation in Right Fallopian Tube, Via Natural or Artificial vOpening

♀ **0UF58ZZ** Fragmentation in Right Fallopian Tube, Via Natural or Artificial Opening Endoscopic

♀ ▲ **0UF5XZZ** Fragmentation in Right Fallopian Tube, External Approach

♀ **0UF60ZZ** Fragmentation in Left Fallopian Tube, Open Approach

♀ **0UF63ZZ** Fragmentation in Left Fallopian Tube, Percutaneous Approach

♀ **0UF64ZZ** Fragmentation in Left Fallopian Tube, Percutaneous Endoscopic Approach

♀ **0UF67ZZ** Fragmentation in Left Fallopian Tube, Via Natural or Artificial Opening

♀ **0UF68ZZ** Fragmentation in Left Fallopian Tube, Via Natural or Artificial Opening Endoscopic

♀ ▲ **0UF6XZZ** Fragmentation in Left Fallopian Tube, External Approach

♀ **0UF70ZZ** Fragmentation in Bilateral Fallopian Tubes, Open Approach

♀ **0UF73ZZ** Fragmentation in Bilateral Fallopian Tubes, Percutaneous Approach

♀ **0UF74ZZ** Fragmentation in Bilateral Fallopian Tubes, Percutaneous Endoscopic Approach

♀ **0UF77ZZ** Fragmentation in Bilateral Fallopian Tubes, Via Natural or Artificial Opening

♀ **0UF78ZZ** Fragmentation in Bilateral Fallopian Tubes, Via Natural or Artificial Opening Endoscopic

♀ ▲ **0UF7XZZ** Fragmentation in Bilateral Fallopian Tubes, External Approach

♀ **0UF90ZZ** Fragmentation in Uterus, Open Approach

♀ **0UF93ZZ** Fragmentation in Uterus, Percutaneous Approach

♀ **0UF94ZZ** Fragmentation in Uterus, Percutaneous Endoscopic Approach

♀ **0UF97ZZ** Fragmentation in Uterus, Via Natural or Artificial Opening

♀ **0UF98ZZ** Fragmentation in Uterus, Via Natural or Artificial Opening Endoscopic

♀ ▲ **0UF9XZZ** Fragmentation in Uterus, External Approach

0UH – Female Reproductive System, Insertion

♀ **0UH301Z** Insertion of Radioactive Element into Ovary, Open Approach

♀ **0UH303Z** Insertion of Infusion Device into Ovary, Open Approach

♀ **0UH30YZ** Insertion of Other Device into Ovary, Open Approach

♀ **0UH331Z** Insertion of Radioactive Element into Ovary, Percutaneous Approach

♀ **0UH333Z** Insertion of Infusion Device into Ovary, Percutaneous Approach

♀ **0UH33YZ** Insertion of Other Device into Ovary, Percutaneous Approach

♀ **0UH341Z** Insertion of Radioactive Element into Ovary, Percutaneous Endoscopic Approach

♀ **0UH343Z** Insertion of Infusion Device into Ovary, Percutaneous Endoscopic Approach

♀ **0UH34YZ** Insertion of Other Device into Ovary, Percutaneous Endoscopic Approach

♀ **0UH371Z** Insertion of Radioactive Element into Ovary, Via Natural or Artificial Opening

♀ **0UH37YZ** Insertion of Other Device into Ovary, Via Natural or Artificial Opening

♀ **0UH381Z** Insertion of Radioactive Element into Ovary, Via Natural or Artificial Opening Endoscopic

♀ **0UH38YZ** Insertion of Other Device into Ovary, Via Natural or Artificial Opening Endoscopic

♀ **0UH803Z** Insertion of Infusion Device into Fallopian Tube, Open Approach

♀ **0UH80YZ** Insertion of Other Device into Fallopian Tube, Open Approach

♀ **0UH833Z** Insertion of Infusion Device into Fallopian Tube, Percutaneous Approach

♀ **0UH83YZ** Insertion of Other Device into Fallopian Tube, Percutaneous Approach

♀ **0UH843Z** Insertion of Infusion Device into Fallopian Tube, Percutaneous Endoscopic Approach

♀ **0UH84YZ** Insertion of Other Device into Fallopian Tube, Percutaneous Endoscopic Approach

♀ **0UH873Z** Insertion of Infusion Device into Fallopian Tube, Via Natural or Artificial Opening

♀ **0UH87YZ** Insertion of Other Device into Fallopian Tube, Via Natural or Artificial Opening

♀ **0UH883Z** Insertion of Infusion Device into Fallopian Tube, Via Natural or Artificial Opening Endoscopic

♀ **0UH88YZ** Insertion of Other Device into Fallopian Tube, Via Natural or Artificial Opening Endoscopic

♀ **0UH901Z** Insertion of Radioactive Element into Uterus, Open Approach

♀ **0UH90HZ** Insertion of Contraceptive Device into Uterus, Open Approach

♀ **0UH971Z** Insertion of Radioactive Element into Uterus, Via Natural or Artificial Opening

♀ **0UH97HZ** Insertion of Contraceptive Device into Uterus, Via Natural or Artificial Opening

AHA CC: 2Q, 2013, 34

♀ **0UH981Z** Insertion of Radioactive Element into Uterus, Via Natural or Artificial Opening Endoscopic

♀ **0UH98HZ** Insertion of Contraceptive Device into Uterus, Via Natural or Artificial Opening Endoscopic

♀ **0UHC01Z** Insertion of Radioactive Element into Cervix, Open Approach

♀ **0UHC31Z** Insertion of Radioactive Element into Cervix, Percutaneous Approach

♀ **0UHC41Z** Insertion of Radioactive Element into Cervix, Percutaneous Endoscopic Approach

♀ **0UHC71Z** Insertion of Radioactive Element into Cervix, Via Natural or Artificial Opening

♀ **0UHC7HZ** Insertion of Contraceptive Device into Cervix, Via Natural or Artificial Opening

♀ **0UHC81Z** Insertion of Radioactive Element into Cervix, Via Natural or Artificial Opening Endoscopic

♀ **0UHC8HZ** Insertion of Contraceptive Device into Cervix, Via Natural or Artificial Opening Endoscopic

♀ **0UHD03Z** Insertion of Infusion Device into Uterus and Cervix, Open Approach

♀ **0UHD0YZ** Insertion of Other Device into Uterus and Cervix, Open Approach

♀ **0UHD33Z** Insertion of Infusion Device into Uterus and Cervix, Percutaneous Approach

♀ **0UHD3YZ** Insertion of Other Device into Uterus and Cervix, Percutaneous Approach

♀ **0UHD43Z** Insertion of Infusion Device into Uterus and Cervix, Percutaneous Endoscopic Approach

♀ **0UHD4YZ** Insertion of Other Device into Uterus and Cervix, Percutaneous Endoscopic Approach

♀ **0UHD73Z** Insertion of Infusion Device into Uterus and Cervix, Via Natural or Artificial Opening

♀ **0UHD7YZ** Insertion of Other Device into Uterus and Cervix, Via Natural or Artificial Opening

AHA CC: 4Q, 2017, 104; 1Q, 2018, 25

♀ **0UHD83Z** Insertion of Infusion Device into Uterus and Cervix, Via Natural or Artificial Opening Endoscopic

---

♀ Female-only   ♂ Male-only   ▲ Limited Coverage   ● Non-OR   🅷🅰🅲 HAC-associated procedure   ▲ Non-covered procedures   + Cluster

♀ **0UHD8YZ** Insertion of Other Device into Uterus and Cervix, Via Natural or Artificial Opening Endoscopic

♀ **0UHF7GZ** Insertion of Pessary into Cul-de-sac, Via Natural or Artificial Opening

♀ **0UHF8GZ** Insertion of Pessary into Cul-de-sac, Via Natural or Artificial Opening Endoscopic

♀ **0UHG01Z** Insertion of Radioactive Element into Vagina, Open Approach

♀ **0UHG31Z** Insertion of Radioactive Element into Vagina, Percutaneous Approach

♀ **0UHG41Z** Insertion of Radioactive Element into Vagina, Percutaneous Endoscopic Approach

♀ **0UHG71Z** Insertion of Radioactive Element into Vagina, Via Natural or Artificial Opening

♀ **0UHG7GZ** Insertion of Pessary into Vagina, Via Natural or Artificial Opening

♀ **0UHG81Z** Insertion of Radioactive Element into Vagina, Via Natural or Artificial Opening Endoscopic

♀ **0UHG8GZ** Insertion of Pessary into Vagina, Via Natural or Artificial Opening Endoscopic

♀ **0UHGX1Z** Insertion of Radioactive Element into Vagina, External Approach

♀ **0UHH03Z** Insertion of Infusion Device into Vagina and Cul-de-sac, Open Approach

♀ **0UHH0YZ** Insertion of Other Device into Vagina and Cul-de-sac, Open Approach

♀ **0UHH33Z** Insertion of Infusion Device into Vagina and Cul-de-sac, Percutaneous Approach

♀ **0UHH3YZ** Insertion of Other Device into Vagina and Cul-de-sac, Percutaneous Approach

♀ **0UHH43Z** Insertion of Infusion Device into Vagina and Cul-de-sac, Percutaneous Endoscopic Approach

♀ **0UHH4YZ** Insertion of Other Device into Vagina and Cul-de-sac, Percutaneous Endoscopic Approach

♀ **0UHH73Z** Insertion of Infusion Device into Vagina and Cul-de-sac, Via Natural or Artificial Opening

♀ **0UHH7YZ** Insertion of Other Device into Vagina and Cul-de-sac, Via Natural or Artificial Opening

♀ **0UHH83Z** Insertion of Infusion Device into Vagina and Cul-de-sac, Via Natural or Artificial Opening Endoscopic

♀ **0UHH8YZ** Insertion of Other Device into Vagina and Cul-de-sac, Via Natural or Artificial Opening Endoscopic

0UJ – Female Reproductive System, Inspection

Review Coding Guidelines B3.11a, B3.11b and B3.11c

♀ **0UJ30ZZ** Inspection of Ovary, Open Approach

♀ **0UJ33ZZ** Inspection of Ovary, Percutaneous Approach

♀ **0UJ34ZZ** Inspection of Ovary, Percutaneous Endoscopic Approach

♀ **0UJ38ZZ** Inspection of Ovary, Via Natural or Artificial Opening Endoscopic

♀ **0UJ3XZZ** Inspection of Ovary, External Approach

♀ **0UJ80ZZ** Inspection of Fallopian Tube, Open Approach

♀ **0UJ83ZZ** Inspection of Fallopian Tube, Percutaneous Approach

♀ **0UJ84ZZ** Inspection of Fallopian Tube, Percutaneous Endoscopic Approach

♀ **0UJ87ZZ** Inspection of Fallopian Tube, Via Natural or Artificial Opening

♀ **0UJ88ZZ** Inspection of Fallopian Tube, Via Natural or Artificial Opening Endoscopic

♀ **0UJ8XZZ** Inspection of Fallopian Tube, External Approach

♀ **0UJD0ZZ** Inspection of Uterus and Cervix, Open Approach

♀ **0UJD3ZZ** Inspection of Uterus and Cervix, Percutaneous Approach

♀ **0UJD4ZZ** Inspection of Uterus and Cervix, Percutaneous Endoscopic Approach

AHA CC: 1Q, 2015, 33-34

♀ **0UJD7ZZ** Inspection of Uterus and Cervix, Via Natural or Artificial Opening

♀ **0UJD8ZZ** Inspection of Uterus and Cervix, Via Natural or Artificial Opening Endoscopic

♀ **0UJDXZZ** Inspection of Uterus and Cervix, External Approach

♀ **0UJH0ZZ** Inspection of Vagina and Cul-de-sac, Open Approach

♀ **0UJH3ZZ** Inspection of Vagina and Cul-de-sac, Percutaneous Approach

♀ **0UJH4ZZ** Inspection of Vagina and Cul-de-sac, Percutaneous Endoscopic Approach

♀ **0UJH7ZZ** Inspection of Vagina and Cul-de-sac, Via Natural or Artificial Opening

♀ **0UJH8ZZ** Inspection of Vagina and Cul-de-sac, Via Natural or Artificial Opening Endoscopic

♀ **0UJHXZZ** Inspection of Vagina and Cul-de-sac, External Approach

♀ **0UJM0ZZ** Inspection of Vulva, Open Approach

♀ **0UJMXZZ** Inspection of Vulva, External Approach

0UL – Female Reproductive System, Occlusion

♀ **0UL50CZ** Occlusion of Right Fallopian Tube with Extraluminal Device, Open Approach

♀ **0UL50DZ** Occlusion of Right Fallopian Tube with Intraluminal Device, Open Approach

♀ **0UL50ZZ** Occlusion of Right Fallopian Tube, Open Approach

♀ **0UL53CZ** Occlusion of Right Fallopian Tube with Extraluminal Device, Percutaneous Approach

♀ **0UL53DZ** Occlusion of Right Fallopian Tube with Intraluminal Device, Percutaneous Approach

♀ **0UL53ZZ** Occlusion of Right Fallopian Tube, Percutaneous Approach

♀ **0UL54CZ** Occlusion of Right Fallopian Tube with Extraluminal Device, Percutaneous Endoscopic Approach

♀ **0UL54DZ** Occlusion of Right Fallopian Tube with Intraluminal Device, Percutaneous Endoscopic Approach

♀ **0UL54ZZ** Occlusion of Right Fallopian Tube, Percutaneous Endoscopic Approach

♀ **0UL57DZ** Occlusion of Right Fallopian Tube with Intraluminal Device, Via Natural or Artificial Opening

♀ **0UL57ZZ** Occlusion of Right Fallopian Tube, Via Natural or Artificial Opening

♀ **0UL58DZ** Occlusion of Right Fallopian Tube with Intraluminal Device, Via Natural or Artificial Opening Endoscopic

♀ **0UL58ZZ** Occlusion of Right Fallopian Tube, Via Natural or Artificial Opening Endoscopic

♀ **0UL60CZ** Occlusion of Left Fallopian Tube with Extraluminal Device, Open Approach

♀ **0UL60DZ** Occlusion of Left Fallopian Tube with Intraluminal Device, Open Approach

♀ **0UL60ZZ** Occlusion of Left Fallopian Tube, Open Approach

♀ **0UL63CZ** Occlusion of Left Fallopian Tube with Extraluminal Device, Percutaneous Approach

♀ **0UL63DZ** Occlusion of Left Fallopian Tube with Intraluminal Device, Percutaneous Approach

♀ **0UL63ZZ** Occlusion of Left Fallopian Tube, Percutaneous Approach

♀ **0UL64CZ** Occlusion of Left Fallopian Tube with Extraluminal Device, Percutaneous Endoscopic Approach

♀ **0UL64DZ** Occlusion of Left Fallopian Tube with Intraluminal Device, Percutaneous Endoscopic Approach

♀ **0UL64ZZ** Occlusion of Left Fallopian Tube, Percutaneous Endoscopic Approach

♀ **0UL67DZ** Occlusion of Left Fallopian Tube with Intraluminal Device, Via Natural or Artificial Opening

♀ **0UL67ZZ** Occlusion of Left Fallopian Tube, Via Natural or Artificial Opening

♀ **0UL68DZ** Occlusion of Left Fallopian Tube with Intraluminal Device, Via Natural or Artificial Opening Endoscopic

♀ **0UL68ZZ** Occlusion of Left Fallopian Tube, Via Natural or Artificial Opening Endoscopic

♀ **0UL70CZ** Occlusion of Bilateral Fallopian Tubes with Extraluminal Device, Open Approach

▲ *When reported with diagnosis code Z30.2*

♀ **0UL70DZ** Occlusion of Bilateral Fallopian Tubes with Intraluminal Device, Open Approach

▲ *When reported with diagnosis code Z30.2*

♀ **0UL70ZZ** Occlusion of Bilateral Fallopian Tubes, Open Approach

▲ *When reported with diagnosis code Z30.2*

♀ **0UL73CZ** Occlusion of Bilateral Fallopian Tubes with Extraluminal Device, Percutaneous Approach

▲ *When reported with diagnosis code Z30.2*

♀ **0UL73DZ** Occlusion of Bilateral Fallopian Tubes with Intraluminal Device, Percutaneous Approach

▲ *When reported with diagnosis code Z30.2*

♀ **0UL73ZZ** Occlusion of Bilateral Fallopian Tubes, Percutaneous Approach
▲ *When reported with diagnosis code Z30.2*

♀ **0UL74CZ** Occlusion of Bilateral Fallopian Tubes with Extraluminal Device, Percutaneous Endoscopic Approach
▲ *When reported with diagnosis code Z30.2*

♀ **0UL74DZ** Occlusion of Bilateral Fallopian Tubes with Intraluminal Device, Percutaneous Endoscopic Approach
▲ *When reported with diagnosis code Z30.2*

♀ **0UL74ZZ** Occlusion of Bilateral Fallopian Tubes, Percutaneous Endoscopic Approach
▲ *When reported with diagnosis code Z30.2*

♀ **0UL77DZ** Occlusion of Bilateral Fallopian Tubes with Intraluminal Device, Via Natural or Artificial Opening
▲ *When reported with diagnosis code Z30.2*

♀ **0UL77ZZ** Occlusion of Bilateral Fallopian Tubes, Via Natural or Artificial Opening
▲ *When reported with diagnosis code Z30.2*

♀ **0UL78DZ** Occlusion of Bilateral Fallopian Tubes with Intraluminal Device, Via Natural or Artificial Opening Endoscopic
▲ *When reported with diagnosis code Z30.2*

♀ **0UL78ZZ** Occlusion of Bilateral Fallopian Tubes, Via Natural or Artificial Opening Endoscopic
▲ *When reported with diagnosis code Z30.2*

♀ **0ULF7DZ** Occlusion of Cul-de-sac with Intraluminal Device, Via Natural or Artificial Opening

♀ **0ULF7ZZ** Occlusion of Cul-de-sac, Via Natural or Artificial Opening

♀ **0ULF8DZ** Occlusion of Cul-de-sac with Intraluminal Device, Via Natural or Artificial Opening Endoscopic

♀ **0ULF8ZZ** Occlusion of Cul-de-sac, Via Natural or Artificial Opening Endoscopic

♀ **0ULG7DZ** Occlusion of Vagina with Intraluminal Device, Via Natural or Artificial Opening

♀ **0ULG7ZZ** Occlusion of Vagina, Via Natural or Artificial Opening

♀ **0ULG8DZ** Occlusion of Vagina with Intraluminal Device, Via Natural or Artificial Opening Endoscopic

♀ **0ULG8ZZ** Occlusion of Vagina, Via Natural or Artificial Opening Endoscopic

0UM – Female Reproductive System, Reattachment

♀ **0UM00ZZ** Reattachment of Right Ovary, Open Approach

♀ **0UM04ZZ** Reattachment of Right Ovary, Percutaneous Endoscopic Approach

♀ **0UM10ZZ** Reattachment of Left Ovary, Open Approach

♀ **0UM14ZZ** Reattachment of Left Ovary, Percutaneous Endoscopic Approach

♀ **0UM20ZZ** Reattachment of Bilateral Ovaries, Open Approach

♀ **0UM24ZZ** Reattachment of Bilateral Ovaries, Percutaneous Endoscopic Approach

♀ **0UM40ZZ** Reattachment of Uterine Supporting Structure, Open Approach

♀ **0UM44ZZ** Reattachment of Uterine Supporting Structure, Percutaneous Endoscopic Approach

♀ **0UM50ZZ** Reattachment of Right Fallopian Tube, Open Approach

♀ **0UM54ZZ** Reattachment of Right Fallopian Tube, Percutaneous Endoscopic Approach

♀ **0UM60ZZ** Reattachment of Left Fallopian Tube, Open Approach

♀ **0UM64ZZ** Reattachment of Left Fallopian Tube, Percutaneous Endoscopic Approach

♀ **0UM70ZZ** Reattachment of Bilateral Fallopian Tubes, Open Approach

♀ **0UM74ZZ** Reattachment of Bilateral Fallopian Tubes, Percutaneous Endoscopic Approach

♀ **0UM90ZZ** Reattachment of Uterus, Open Approach

♀ **0UM94ZZ** Reattachment of Uterus, Percutaneous Endoscopic Approach

♀ **0UMC0ZZ** Reattachment of Cervix, Open Approach

♀ **0UMC4ZZ** Reattachment of Cervix, Percutaneous Endoscopic Approach

♀ **0UMF0ZZ** Reattachment of Cul-de-sac, Open Approach

♀ **0UMF4ZZ** Reattachment of Cul-de-sac, Percutaneous Endoscopic Approach

♀ **0UMG0ZZ** Reattachment of Vagina, Open Approach

♀ **0UMG4ZZ** Reattachment of Vagina, Percutaneous Endoscopic Approach

♀ **0UMJXZZ** Reattachment of Clitoris, External Approach

♀ **0UMK0ZZ** Reattachment of Hymen, Open Approach

♀ **0UMK4ZZ** Reattachment of Hymen, Percutaneous Endoscopic Approach

♀ **0UMKXZZ** Reattachment of Hymen, External Approach

♀ **0UMMXZZ** Reattachment of Vulva, External Approach

0UN – Female Reproductive System, Release

Review Coding Guideline B3.13

Review Coding Guideline B3.14

♀ **0UN00ZZ** Release Right Ovary, Open Approach

♀ **0UN03ZZ** Release Right Ovary, Percutaneous Approach

♀ **0UN04ZZ** Release Right Ovary, Percutaneous Endoscopic Approach

♀ **0UN08ZZ** Release Right Ovary, Via Natural or Artificial Opening Endoscopic

♀ **0UN10ZZ** Release Left Ovary, Open Approach

♀ **0UN13ZZ** Release Left Ovary, Percutaneous Approach

♀ **0UN14ZZ** Release Left Ovary, Percutaneous Endoscopic Approach

♀ **0UN18ZZ** Release Left Ovary, Via Natural or Artificial Opening Endoscopic

♀ **0UN20ZZ** Release Bilateral Ovaries, Open Approach

♀ **0UN23ZZ** Release Bilateral Ovaries, Percutaneous Approach

♀ **0UN24ZZ** Release Bilateral Ovaries, Percutaneous Endoscopic Approach

♀ **0UN28ZZ** Release Bilateral Ovaries, Via Natural or Artificial Opening Endoscopic

♀ **0UN40ZZ** Release Uterine Supporting Structure, Open Approach

♀ **0UN43ZZ** Release Uterine Supporting Structure, Percutaneous Approach

♀ **0UN44ZZ** Release Uterine Supporting Structure, Percutaneous Endoscopic Approach

♀ **0UN48ZZ** Release Uterine Supporting Structure, Via Natural or Artificial Opening Endoscopic

♀ **0UN50ZZ** Release Right Fallopian Tube, Open Approach

♀ **0UN53ZZ** Release Right Fallopian Tube, Percutaneous Approach

♀ **0UN54ZZ** Release Right Fallopian Tube, Percutaneous Endoscopic Approach

♀ **0UN57ZZ** Release Right Fallopian Tube, Via Natural or Artificial Opening

♀ **0UN58ZZ** Release Right Fallopian Tube, Via Natural or Artificial Opening Endoscopic

♀ **0UN60ZZ** Release Left Fallopian Tube, Open Approach

♀ **0UN63ZZ** Release Left Fallopian Tube, Percutaneous Approach

♀ **0UN64ZZ** Release Left Fallopian Tube, Percutaneous Endoscopic Approach

♀ **0UN67ZZ** Release Left Fallopian Tube, Via Natural or Artificial Opening

♀ **0UN68ZZ** Release Left Fallopian Tube, Via Natural or Artificial Opening Endoscopic

♀ **0UN70ZZ** Release Bilateral Fallopian Tubes, Open Approach

♀ **0UN73ZZ** Release Bilateral Fallopian Tubes, Percutaneous Approach

♀ **0UN74ZZ** Release Bilateral Fallopian Tubes, Percutaneous Endoscopic Approach

♀ **0UN77ZZ** Release Bilateral Fallopian Tubes, Via Natural or Artificial Opening

♀ **0UN78ZZ** Release Bilateral Fallopian Tubes, Via Natural or Artificial Opening Endoscopic

♀ **0UN90ZZ** Release Uterus, Open Approach

♀ **0UN93ZZ** Release Uterus, Percutaneous Approach

♀ **0UN94ZZ** Release Uterus, Percutaneous Endoscopic Approach

♀ **0UN97ZZ** Release Uterus, Via Natural or Artificial Opening

♀ **0UN98ZZ** Release Uterus, Via Natural or Artificial Opening Endoscopic

♀ **0UNC0ZZ** Release Cervix, Open Approach

♀ **0UNC3ZZ** Release Cervix, Percutaneous Approach

♀ 0UNC4ZZ Release Cervix, Percutaneous Endoscopic Approach
♀ 0UNC7ZZ Release Cervix, Via Natural or Artificial Opening
♀ 0UNC8ZZ Release Cervix, Via Natural or Artificial Opening Endoscopic
♀ 0UNF0ZZ Release Cul-de-sac, Open Approach
♀ 0UNF3ZZ Release Cul-de-sac, Percutaneous Approach
♀ 0UNF4ZZ Release Cul-de-sac, Percutaneous Endoscopic Approach
♀ 0UNF7ZZ Release Cul-de-sac, Via Natural or Artificial Opening
♀ 0UNF8ZZ Release Cul-de-sac, Via Natural or Artificial Opening Endoscopic

♀ 0UNG0ZZ Release Vagina, Open Approach
♀ 0UNG3ZZ Release Vagina, Percutaneous Approach
♀ 0UNG4ZZ Release Vagina, Percutaneous Endoscopic Approach
♀ 0UNG7ZZ Release Vagina, Via Natural or Artificial Opening
♀ 0UNG8ZZ Release Vagina, Via Natural or Artificial Opening Endoscopic
♀ 0UNGXZZ Release Vagina, External Approach
♀ 0UNJ0ZZ Release Clitoris, Open Approach
♀ 0UNJXZZ Release Clitoris, External Approach
♀ 0UNK0ZZ Release Hymen, Open Approach
♀ 0UNK3ZZ Release Hymen, Percutaneous Approach

♀ 0UNK4ZZ Release Hymen, Percutaneous Endoscopic Approach
♀ 0UNK7ZZ Release Hymen, Via Natural or Artificial Opening
♀ 0UNK8ZZ Release Hymen, Via Natural or Artificial Opening Endoscopic
♀ 0UNKXZZ Release Hymen, External Approach
♀ 0UNL0ZZ Release Vestibular Gland, Open Approach
♀ 0UNLXZZ Release Vestibular Gland, External Approach
♀ 0UNM0ZZ Release Vulva, Open Approach
♀ 0UNMXZZ Release Vulva, External Approach

0UP – Female Reproductive System, Removal

Review Coding Guideline B6.1c

♀ 0UP300Z Removal of Drainage Device from Ovary, Open Approach
♀ 0UP303Z Removal of Infusion Device from Ovary, Open Approach
♀ 0UP30YZ Removal of Other Device from Ovary, Open Approach
♀ 0UP330Z Removal of Drainage Device from Ovary, Percutaneous Approach
♀ 0UP333Z Removal of Infusion Device from Ovary, Percutaneous Approach
♀ 0UP33YZ Removal of Other Device from Ovary, Percutaneous Approach
♀ 0UP340Z Removal of Drainage Device from Ovary, Percutaneous Endoscopic Approach
♀ 0UP343Z Removal of Infusion Device from Ovary, Percutaneous Endoscopic Approach
♀ 0UP34YZ Removal of Other Device from Ovary, Percutaneous Endoscopic Approach
♀ 0UP37YZ Removal of Other Device from Ovary, Via Natural or Artificial Opening
♀ 0UP38YZ Removal of Other Device from Ovary, Via Natural or Artificial Opening Endoscopic
♀ 0UP3X0Z Removal of Drainage Device from Ovary, External Approach
♀ 0UP3X3Z Removal of Infusion Device from Ovary, External Approach
♀ 0UP800Z Removal of Drainage Device from Fallopian Tube, Open Approach
♀ 0UP803Z Removal of Infusion Device from Fallopian Tube, Open Approach
♀ 0UP807Z Removal of Autologous Tissue Substitute from Fallopian Tube, Open Approach
♀ 0UP80CZ Removal of Extraluminal Device from Fallopian Tube, Open Approach
♀ 0UP80DZ Removal of Intraluminal Device from Fallopian Tube, Open Approach
♀ 0UP80JZ Removal of Synthetic Substitute from Fallopian Tube, Open Approach
♀ 0UP80KZ Removal of Nonautologous Tissue Substitute from Fallopian Tube, Open Approach
♀ 0UP80YZ Removal of Other Device from Fallopian Tube, Open Approach
♀ 0UP830Z Removal of Drainage Device from Fallopian Tube, Percutaneous Approach
♀ 0UP833Z Removal of Infusion Device from Fallopian Tube, Percutaneous Approach
♀ 0UP837Z Removal of Autologous Tissue Substitute from Fallopian Tube, Percutaneous Approach
♀ 0UP83CZ Removal of Extraluminal Device from Fallopian Tube, Percutaneous Approach

♀ 0UP83DZ Removal of Intraluminal Device from Fallopian Tube, Percutaneous Approach
♀ 0UP83JZ Removal of Synthetic Substitute from Fallopian Tube, Percutaneous Approach
♀ 0UP83KZ Removal of Nonautologous Tissue Substitute from Fallopian Tube, Percutaneous Approach
♀ 0UP83YZ Removal of Other Device from Fallopian Tube, Percutaneous Approach
♀ 0UP840Z Removal of Drainage Device from Fallopian Tube, Percutaneous Endoscopic Approach
♀ 0UP843Z Removal of Infusion Device from Fallopian Tube, Percutaneous Endoscopic Approach
♀ 0UP847Z Removal of Autologous Tissue Substitute from Fallopian Tube, Percutaneous Endoscopic Approach
♀ 0UP84CZ Removal of Extraluminal Device from Fallopian Tube, Percutaneous Endoscopic Approach
♀ 0UP84DZ Removal of Intraluminal Device from Fallopian Tube, Percutaneous Endoscopic Approach
♀ 0UP84JZ Removal of Synthetic Substitute from Fallopian Tube, Percutaneous Endoscopic Approach
♀ 0UP84KZ Removal of Nonautologous Tissue Substitute from Fallopian Tube, Percutaneous Endoscopic Approach
♀ 0UP84YZ Removal of Other Device from Fallopian Tube, Percutaneous Endoscopic Approach
♀ 0UP870Z Removal of Drainage Device from Fallopian Tube, Via Natural or Artificial Opening
♀ 0UP873Z Removal of Infusion Device from Fallopian Tube, Via Natural or Artificial Opening
♀ 0UP877Z Removal of Autologous Tissue Substitute from Fallopian Tube, Via Natural or Artificial Opening
♀ 0UP87CZ Removal of Extraluminal Device from Fallopian Tube, Via Natural or Artificial Opening
♀ 0UP87DZ Removal of Intraluminal Device from Fallopian Tube, Via Natural or Artificial Opening
♀ 0UP87JZ Removal of Synthetic Substitute from Fallopian Tube, Via Natural or Artificial Opening
♀ 0UP87KZ Removal of Nonautologous Tissue Substitute from Fallopian Tube, Via Natural or Artificial Opening
♀ 0UP87YZ Removal of Other Device from Fallopian Tube, Via Natural or Artificial Opening

♀ 0UP880Z Removal of Drainage Device from Fallopian Tube, Via Natural or Artificial Opening Endoscopic
♀ 0UP883Z Removal of Infusion Device from Fallopian Tube, Via Natural or Artificial Opening Endoscopic
♀ 0UP887Z Removal of Autologous Tissue Substitute from Fallopian Tube, Via Natural or Artificial Opening Endoscopic
♀ 0UP88CZ Removal of Extraluminal Device from Fallopian Tube, Via Natural or Artificial Opening Endoscopic
♀ 0UP88DZ Removal of Intraluminal Device from Fallopian Tube, Via Natural or Artificial Opening Endoscopic
♀ 0UP88JZ Removal of Synthetic Substitute from Fallopian Tube, Via Natural or Artificial Opening Endoscopic
♀ 0UP88KZ Removal of Nonautologous Tissue Substitute from Fallopian Tube, Via Natural or Artificial Opening Endoscopic
♀ 0UP88YZ Removal of Other Device from Fallopian Tube, Via Natural or Artificial Opening Endoscopic
♀ 0UP8X0Z Removal of Drainage Device from Fallopian Tube, External Approach
♀ 0UP8X3Z Removal of Infusion Device from Fallopian Tube, External Approach
♀ 0UP8XDZ Removal of Intraluminal Device from Fallopian Tube, External Approach
♀ 0UPD00Z Removal of Drainage Device from Uterus and Cervix, Open Approach
♀ 0UPD01Z Removal of Radioactive Element from Uterus and Cervix, Open Approach
♀ 0UPD03Z Removal of Infusion Device from Uterus and Cervix, Open Approach
♀ 0UPD07Z Removal of Autologous Tissue Substitute from Uterus and Cervix, Open Approach
♀ 0UPD0CZ Removal of Extraluminal Device from Uterus and Cervix, Open Approach
♀ 0UPD0DZ Removal of Intraluminal Device from Uterus and Cervix, Open Approach
♀ 0UPD0HZ Removal of Contraceptive Device from Uterus and Cervix, Open Approach
♀ 0UPD0JZ Removal of Synthetic Substitute from Uterus and Cervix, Open Approach
♀ 0UPD0KZ Removal of Nonautologous Tissue Substitute from Uterus and Cervix, Open Approach
♀ 0UPD0YZ Removal of Other Device from Uterus and Cervix, Open Approach
♀ 0UPD30Z Removal of Drainage Device from Uterus and Cervix, Percutaneous Approach

♀ Female-only   ♂ Male-only   ▲ Limited Coverage   ● Non-OR   HAC HAC-associated procedure   ▲ Non-covered procedures   + Cluster

♀ **0UPD31Z** Removal of Radioactive Element from Uterus and Cervix, Percutaneous Approach

♀ **0UPD33Z** Removal of Infusion Device from Uterus and Cervix, Percutaneous Approach

♀ **0UPD37Z** Removal of Autologous Tissue Substitute from Uterus and Cervix, Percutaneous Approach

♀ **0UPD3CZ** Removal of Extraluminal Device from Uterus and Cervix, Percutaneous Approach

♀ **0UPD3DZ** Removal of Intraluminal Device from Uterus and Cervix, Percutaneous Approach

♀ **0UPD3HZ** Removal of Contraceptive Device from Uterus and Cervix, Percutaneous Approach

♀ **0UPD3JZ** Removal of Synthetic Substitute from Uterus and Cervix, Percutaneous Approach

♀ **0UPD3KZ** Removal of Nonautologous Tissue Substitute from Uterus and Cervix, Percutaneous Approach

♀ **0UPD3YZ** Removal of Other Device from Uterus and Cervix, Percutaneous Approach

♀ **0UPD40Z** Removal of Drainage Device from Uterus and Cervix, Percutaneous Endoscopic Approach

♀ **0UPD41Z** Removal of Radioactive Element from Uterus and Cervix, Percutaneous Endoscopic Approach

♀ **0UPD43Z** Removal of Infusion Device from Uterus and Cervix, Percutaneous Endoscopic Approach

♀ **0UPD47Z** Removal of Autologous Tissue Substitute from Uterus and Cervix, Percutaneous Endoscopic Approach

♀ **0UPD4CZ** Removal of Extraluminal Device from Uterus and Cervix, Percutaneous Endoscopic Approach

♀ **0UPD4DZ** Removal of Intraluminal Device from Uterus and Cervix, Percutaneous Endoscopic Approach

♀ **0UPD4HZ** Removal of Contraceptive Device from Uterus and Cervix, Percutaneous Endoscopic Approach

♀ **0UPD4JZ** Removal of Synthetic Substitute from Uterus and Cervix, Percutaneous Endoscopic Approach

♀ **0UPD4KZ** Removal of Nonautologous Tissue Substitute from Uterus and Cervix, Percutaneous Endoscopic Approach

♀ **0UPD4YZ** Removal of Other Device from Uterus and Cervix, Percutaneous Endoscopic Approach

♀ **0UPD70Z** Removal of Drainage Device from Uterus and Cervix, Via Natural or Artificial Opening

♀ **0UPD71Z** Removal of Radioactive Element from Uterus and Cervix, Via Natural or Artificial Opening

♀ **0UPD73Z** Removal of Infusion Device from Uterus and Cervix, Via Natural or Artificial Opening

♀ **0UPD77Z** Removal of Autologous Tissue Substitute from Uterus and Cervix, Via Natural or Artificial Opening

♀ **0UPD7CZ** Removal of Extraluminal Device from Uterus and Cervix, Via Natural or Artificial Opening

♀ **0UPD7DZ** Removal of Intraluminal Device from Uterus and Cervix, Via Natural or Artificial Opening

♀ **0UPD7HZ** Removal of Contraceptive Device from Uterus and Cervix, Via Natural or Artificial Opening

♀ **0UPD7JZ** Removal of Synthetic Substitute from Uterus and Cervix, Via Natural or Artificial Opening

♀ **0UPD7KZ** Removal of Nonautologous Tissue Substitute from Uterus and Cervix, Via Natural or Artificial Opening

♀ **0UPD7YZ** Removal of Other Device from Uterus and Cervix, Via Natural or Artificial Opening

♀ **0UPD80Z** Removal of Drainage Device from Uterus and Cervix, Via Natural or Artificial Opening Endoscopic

♀ **0UPD81Z** Removal of Radioactive Element from Uterus and Cervix, Via Natural or Artificial Opening Endoscopic

♀ **0UPD83Z** Removal of Infusion Device from Uterus and Cervix, Via Natural or Artificial Opening Endoscopic

♀ **0UPD87Z** Removal of Autologous Tissue Substitute from Uterus and Cervix, Via Natural or Artificial Opening Endoscopic

♀ **0UPD8CZ** Removal of Extraluminal Device from Uterus and Cervix, Via Natural or Artificial Opening Endoscopic

♀ **0UPD8DZ** Removal of Intraluminal Device from Uterus and Cervix, Via Natural or Artificial Opening Endoscopic

♀ **0UPD8HZ** Removal of Contraceptive Device from Uterus and Cervix, Via Natural or Artificial Opening Endoscopic

♀ **0UPD8JZ** Removal of Synthetic Substitute from Uterus and Cervix, Via Natural or Artificial Opening Endoscopic

♀ **0UPD8KZ** Removal of Nonautologous Tissue Substitute from Uterus and Cervix, Via Natural or Artificial Opening Endoscopic

♀ **0UPD8YZ** Removal of Other Device from Uterus and Cervix, Via Natural or Artificial Opening Endoscopic

♀ **0UPDX0Z** Removal of Drainage Device from Uterus and Cervix, External Approach

♀ **0UPDX3Z** Removal of Infusion Device from Uterus and Cervix, External Approach

♀ **0UPDXDZ** Removal of Intraluminal Device from Uterus and Cervix, External Approach

♀ **0UPDXHZ** Removal of Contraceptive Device from Uterus and Cervix, External Approach

♀ **0UPH00Z** Removal of Drainage Device from Vagina and Cul-de-sac, Open Approach

♀ **0UPH01Z** Removal of Radioactive Element from Vagina and Cul-de-sac, Open Approach

♀ **0UPH03Z** Removal of Infusion Device from Vagina and Cul-de-sac, Open Approach

♀ **0UPH07Z** Removal of Autologous Tissue Substitute from Vagina and Cul-de-sac, Open Approach

♀ **0UPH0DZ** Removal of Intraluminal Device from Vagina and Cul-de-sac, Open Approach

♀ **0UPH0JZ** Removal of Synthetic Substitute from Vagina and Cul-de-sac, OpenApproach

♀ **0UPH0KZ** Removal of Nonautologous Tissue Substitute from Vagina and Cul-de-sac, Open Approach

♀ **0UPH0YZ** Removal of Other Device from Vagina and Cul-de-sac, Open Approach

♀ **0UPH30Z** Removal of Drainage Device from Vagina and Cul-de-sac, Percutaneous Approach

♀ **0UPH31Z** Removal of Radioactive Element from Vagina and Cul-de-sac, Percutaneous Approach

♀ **0UPH33Z** Removal of Infusion Device from Vagina and Cul-de-sac, Percutaneous Approach

♀ **0UPH37Z** Removal of Autologous Tissue Substitute from Vagina and Cul-de-sac, Percutaneous Approach

♀ **0UPH3DZ** Removal of Intraluminal Device from Vagina and Cul-de-sac, Percutaneous Approach

♀ **0UPH3JZ** Removal of Synthetic Substitute from Vagina and Cul-de-sac, Percutaneous Approach

♀ **0UPH3KZ** Removal of Nonautologous Tissue Substitute from Vagina and Cul-de-sac, Percutaneous Approach

♀ **0UPH3YZ** Removal of Other Device from Vagina and Cul-de-sac, Percutaneous Approach

♀ **0UPH40Z** Removal of Drainage Device from Vagina and Cul-de-sac, Percutaneous Endoscopic Approach

♀ **0UPH41Z** Removal of Radioactive Element from Vagina and Cul-de-sac, Percutaneous Endoscopic Approach

♀ **0UPH43Z** Removal of Infusion Device from Vagina and Cul-de-sac, Percutaneous Endoscopic Approach

♀ **0UPH47Z** Removal of Autologous Tissue Substitute from Vagina and Cul-de-sac, Percutaneous Endoscopic Approach

♀ **0UPH4DZ** Removal of Intraluminal Device from Vagina and Cul-de-sac, Percutaneous Endoscopic Approach

♀ **0UPH4JZ** Removal of Synthetic Substitute from Vagina and Cul-de-sac, Percutaneous Endoscopic Approach

♀ **0UPH4KZ** Removal of Nonautologous Tissue Substitute from Vagina and Cul-de-sac, Percutaneous Endoscopic Approach

♀ **0UPH4YZ** Removal of Other Device from Vagina and Cul-de-sac, Percutaneous Endoscopic Approach

♀ **0UPH70Z** Removal of Drainage Device from Vagina and Cul-de-sac, Via Natural or Artificial Opening

♀ **0UPH71Z** Removal of Radioactive Element from Vagina and Cul-de-sac, Via Natural or Artificial Opening

♀ **0UPH73Z** Removal of Infusion Device from Vagina and Cul-de-sac, Via Natural or Artificial Opening

♀ **0UPH77Z** Removal of Autologous Tissue Substitute from Vagina and Cul-de-sac, Via Natural or Artificial Opening

♀ **0UPH7DZ** Removal of Intraluminal Device from Vagina and Cul-de-sac, Via Natural or Artificial Opening

♀ **0UPH7JZ** Removal of Synthetic Substitute from Vagina and Cul-de-sac, Via Natural or Artificial Opening

♀ **0UPH7KZ** Removal of Nonautologous Tissue Substitute from Vagina and Cul-de-sac, Via Natural or Artificial Opening

♀ **0UPH7YZ** Removal of Other Device from Vagina and Cul-de-sac, Via Natural or Artificial Opening

♀ **0UPH80Z** Removal of Drainage Device from Vagina and Cul-de-sac, Via Natural or Artificial Opening Endoscopic

♀ **0UPH81Z** Removal of Radioactive Element from Vagina and Cul-de-sac, Via Natural or Artificial Opening Endoscopic

♀ **0UPH83Z** Removal of Infusion Device from Vagina and Cul-de-sac, Via Natural or Artificial Opening Endoscopic

♀ **0UPH87Z** Removal of Autologous Tissue Substitute from Vagina and Cul-de-sac, Via Natural or Artificial Opening Endoscopic

♀ **0UPH8DZ** Removal of Intraluminal Device from Vagina and Cul-de-sac, Via Natural or Artificial Opening Endoscopic

♀ **0UPH8JZ** Removal of Synthetic Substitute from Vagina and Cul-de-sac, Via Natural or Artificial Opening Endoscopic

♀ **0UPH8KZ** Removal of Nonautologous Tissue Substitute from Vagina and Cul-de-sac, Via Natural or Artificial Opening Endoscopic

♀ **0UPH8YZ** Removal of Other Device from Vagina and Cul-de-sac, Via Natural or Artificial Opening Endoscopic

♀ **0UPHX0Z** Removal of Drainage Device from Vagina and Cul-de-sac, External Approach

♀ **0UPHX1Z** Removal of Radioactive Element from Vagina and Cul-de-sac, External Approach

♀ **0UPHX3Z** Removal of Infusion Device from Vagina and Cul-de-sac, External Approach

♀ **0UPHXDZ** Removal of Intraluminal Device from Vagina and Cul-de-sac, External Approach

♀ **0UPM00Z** Removal of Drainage Device from Vulva, Open Approach

♀ **0UPM07Z** Removal of Autologous Tissue Substitute from Vulva, Open Approach

♀ **0UPM0JZ** Removal of Synthetic Substitute from Vulva, Open Approach

♀ **0UPM0KZ** Removal of Nonautologous Tissue Substitute from Vulva, Open Approach

♀ **0UPMX0Z** Removal of Drainage Device from Vulva, External Approach

0UQ – Female Reproductive System, Repair

♀ **0UQ00ZZ** Repair Right Ovary, Open Approach

♀ **0UQ03ZZ** Repair Right Ovary, Percutaneous Approach

♀ **0UQ04ZZ** Repair Right Ovary, Percutaneous Endoscopic Approach

♀ **0UQ08ZZ** Repair Right Ovary, Via Natural or Artificial Opening Endoscopic

♀ **0UQ10ZZ** Repair Left Ovary, Open Approach

♀ **0UQ13ZZ** Repair Left Ovary, Percutaneous Approach

♀ **0UQ14ZZ** Repair Left Ovary, Percutaneous Endoscopic Approach

♀ **0UQ18ZZ** Repair Left Ovary, Via Natural or Artificial Opening Endoscopic

♀ **0UQ20ZZ** Repair Bilateral Ovaries, Open Approach

♀ **0UQ23ZZ** Repair Bilateral Ovaries, Percutaneous Approach

♀ **0UQ24ZZ** Repair Bilateral Ovaries, Percutaneous Endoscopic Approach

♀ **0UQ28ZZ** Repair Bilateral Ovaries, Via Natural or Artificial Opening Endoscopic

♀ **0UQ40ZZ** Repair Uterine Supporting Structure, Open Approach

♀ **0UQ43ZZ** Repair Uterine Supporting Structure, Percutaneous Approach

♀ **0UQ44ZZ** Repair Uterine Supporting Structure, Percutaneous Endoscopic Approach

♀ **0UQ48ZZ** Repair Uterine Supporting Structure, Via Natural or Artificial Opening Endoscopic

♀ **0UQ50ZZ** Repair Right Fallopian Tube, Open Approach

♀ **0UQ53ZZ** Repair Right Fallopian Tube, Percutaneous Approach

♀ **0UQ54ZZ** Repair Right Fallopian Tube, Percutaneous Endoscopic Approach

♀ **0UQ57ZZ** Repair Right Fallopian Tube, Via Natural or Artificial Opening

♀ **0UQ58ZZ** Repair Right Fallopian Tube, Via Natural or Artificial Opening Endoscopic

♀ **0UQ60ZZ** Repair Left Fallopian Tube, Open Approach

AHA CC: 4Q, 2020, 60

♀ **0UQ63ZZ** Repair Left Fallopian Tube, Percutaneous Approach

♀ **0UQ64ZZ** Repair Left Fallopian Tube, Percutaneous Endoscopic Approach

♀ **0UQ67ZZ** Repair Left Fallopian Tube, Via Natural or Artificial Opening

♀ **0UQ68ZZ** Repair Left Fallopian Tube, Via Natural or Artificial Opening Endoscopic

♀ **0UQ70ZZ** Repair Bilateral Fallopian Tubes, Open Approach

♀ **0UQ73ZZ** Repair Bilateral Fallopian Tubes, Percutaneous Approach

♀ **0UQ74ZZ** Repair Bilateral Fallopian Tubes, Percutaneous Endoscopic Approach

♀ **0UQ77ZZ** Repair Bilateral Fallopian Tubes, Via Natural or Artificial Opening

♀ **0UQ78ZZ** Repair Bilateral Fallopian Tubes, Via Natural or Artificial Opening Endoscopic

♀ **0UQ90ZZ** Repair Uterus, Open Approach

♀ **0UQ93ZZ** Repair Uterus, Percutaneous Approach

♀ **0UQ94ZZ** Repair Uterus, Percutaneous Endoscopic Approach

♀ **0UQ97ZZ** Repair Uterus, Via Natural or Artificial Opening

♀ **0UQ98ZZ** Repair Uterus, Via Natural or Artificial Opening Endoscopic

♀ **0UQC0ZZ** Repair Cervix, Open Approach

♀ **0UQC3ZZ** Repair Cervix, Percutaneous Approach

♀ **0UQC4ZZ** Repair Cervix, Percutaneous Endoscopic Approach

♀ **0UQC7ZZ** Repair Cervix, Via Natural or Artificial Opening

♀ **0UQC8ZZ** Repair Cervix, Via Natural or Artificial Opening Endoscopic

♀ **0UQF0ZZ** Repair Cul-de-sac, Open Approach

♀ **0UQF3ZZ** Repair Cul-de-sac, Percutaneous Approach

♀ **0UQF4ZZ** Repair Cul-de-sac, Percutaneous Endoscopic Approach

♀ **0UQF7ZZ** Repair Cul-de-sac, Via Natural or Artificial Opening

♀ **0UQF8ZZ** Repair Cul-de-sac, Via Natural or Artificial Opening Endoscopic

♀ **0UQG0ZZ** Repair Vagina, Open Approach

♀ **0UQG3ZZ** Repair Vagina, Percutaneous Approach

♀ **0UQG4ZZ** Repair Vagina, Percutaneous Endoscopic Approach

♀ **0UQG7ZZ** Repair Vagina, Via Natural or Artificial Opening

♀ **0UQG8ZZ** Repair Vagina, Via Natural or Artificial Opening Endoscopic

♀ **0UQGXZZ** Repair Vagina, External Approach

♀ **0UQJ0ZZ** Repair Clitoris, Open Approach

♀ **0UQJXZZ** Repair Clitoris, External Approach

AHA CC: 4Q, 2013, 120-121

♀ **0UQK0ZZ** Repair Hymen, Open Approach

♀ **0UQK3ZZ** Repair Hymen, Percutaneous Approach

♀ **0UQK4ZZ** Repair Hymen, Percutaneous Endoscopic Approach

♀ **0UQK7ZZ** Repair Hymen, Via Natural or Artificial Opening

♀ **0UQK8ZZ** Repair Hymen, Via Natural or Artificial Opening Endoscopic

♀ **0UQKXZZ** Repair Hymen, External Approach

♀ **0UQL0ZZ** Repair Vestibular Gland, Open Approach

♀ **0UQLXZZ** Repair Vestibular Gland, External Approach

♀ **0UQM0ZZ** Repair Vulva, Open Approach

♀ **0UQMXZZ** Repair Vulva, External Approach

AHA CC: 4Q, 2014, 18-19

0US – Female Reproductive System, Reposition

♀ **0US00ZZ** Reposition Right Ovary, Open Approach

♀ **0US04ZZ** Reposition Right Ovary, Percutaneous Endoscopic Approach

♀ **0US08ZZ** Reposition Right Ovary, Via Natural or Artificial Opening Endoscopic

♀ **0US10ZZ** Reposition Left Ovary, Open Approach

♀ **0US14ZZ** Reposition Left Ovary, Percutaneous Endoscopic Approach

♀ **0US18ZZ** Reposition Left Ovary, Via Natural or Artificial Opening Endoscopic

♀ **0US20ZZ** Reposition Bilateral Ovaries, Open Approach

♀ **0US24ZZ** Reposition Bilateral Ovaries, Percutaneous Endoscopic Approach

♀ **0US28ZZ** Reposition Bilateral Ovaries, Via Natural or Artificial Opening Endoscopic

♀ **0US40ZZ** Reposition Uterine Supporting Structure, Open Approach

♀ **0US44ZZ** Reposition Uterine Supporting Structure, Percutaneous Endoscopic Approach

♀ **0US48ZZ** Reposition Uterine Supporting Structure, Via Natural or Artificial Opening Endoscopic

♀ **0US50ZZ** Reposition Right Fallopian Tube, Open Approach

♀ **0US54ZZ** Reposition Right Fallopian Tube, Percutaneous Endoscopic Approach

♀ **0US58ZZ** Reposition Right Fallopian Tube, Via Natural or Artificial Opening Endoscopic

♀ **0US60ZZ** Reposition Left Fallopian Tube, Open Approach

♀ **0US64ZZ** Reposition Left Fallopian Tube, Percutaneous Endoscopic Approach

♀ **0US68ZZ** Reposition Left Fallopian Tube, Via Natural or Artificial Opening Endoscopic

♀ **0US70ZZ** Reposition Bilateral Fallopian Tubes, Open Approach

♀ **0US74ZZ** Reposition Bilateral Fallopian Tubes, Percutaneous Endoscopic Approach

♀ **0US78ZZ** Reposition Bilateral Fallopian Tubes, Via Natural or Artificial Opening Endoscopic

♀ **0US90ZZ** Reposition Uterus, Open Approach

♀ **0US94ZZ** Reposition Uterus, Percutaneous Endoscopic Approach

♀ **0US97ZZ** Reposition Uterus, Via Natural or Artificial Opening

♀ Female-only ♂ Male-only ▲ Limited Coverage ● Non-OR **HAC** HAC-associated procedure ▲ Non-covered procedures ✚ Cluster

♀ **0US98ZZ** Reposition Uterus, Via Natural or Artificial Opening Endoscopic
♀ **0US9XZZ** Reposition Uterus, External Approach
　AHA CC: 1Q, 2016, 9
♀ **0USC0ZZ** Reposition Cervix, Open Approach
♀ **0USC4ZZ** Reposition Cervix, Percutaneous Endoscopic Approach

♀ **0USC8ZZ** Reposition Cervix, Via Natural or Artificial Opening Endoscopic
♀ **0USF0ZZ** Reposition Cul-de-sac, Open Approach
♀ **0USF4ZZ** Reposition Cul-de-sac, Percutaneous Endoscopic Approach
♀ **0USF8ZZ** Reposition Cul-de-sac, Via Natural or Artificial Opening Endoscopic
♀ **0USG0ZZ** Reposition Vagina, Open Approach

♀ **0USG4ZZ** Reposition Vagina, Percutaneous Endoscopic Approach
♀ **0USG7ZZ** Reposition Vagina, Via Natural or Artificial Opening
♀ **0USG8ZZ** Reposition Vagina, Via Natural or Artificial Opening Endoscopic
♀ **0USGXZZ** Reposition Vagina, External Approach

0UT – Female Reproductive System, Resection

Review Coding Guideline B3.8

Review Coding Guideline B3.18

♀ **0UT00ZZ** Resection of Right Ovary, Open Approach
　AHA CC: 1Q, 2013, 24
♀ **0UT04ZZ** Resection of Right Ovary, Percutaneous Endoscopic Approach
♀ **0UT07ZZ** Resection of Right Ovary, Via Natural or Artificial Opening
♀ **0UT08ZZ** Resection of Right Ovary, Via Natural or Artificial Opening Endoscopic
♀ **0UT0FZZ** Resection of Right Ovary, Via Natural or Artificial Opening With Percutaneous Endoscopic Assistance
♀ **0UT10ZZ** Resection of Left Ovary, Open Approach
♀ **0UT14ZZ** Resection of Left Ovary, Percutaneous Endoscopic Approach
♀ **0UT17ZZ** Resection of Left Ovary, Via Natural or Artificial Opening
♀ **0UT18ZZ** Resection of Left Ovary, Via Natural or Artificial Opening Endoscopic
♀ **0UT1FZZ** Resection of Left Ovary, Via Natural or Artificial Opening With Percutaneous Endoscopic Assistance
♀ **0UT20ZZ** Resection of Bilateral Ovaries, Open Approach
　AHA CC: 1Q, 2015, 33-34
　➕ Pelvic evisceration when reported with Resection of bladder, urethra, bilateral fallopian tubes, uterus, cervix and vagina. *See tables 0TT and 0UT to construct the Resection codes.*
♀ **0UT24ZZ** Resection of Bilateral Ovaries, Percutaneous Endoscopic Approach
♀ **0UT27ZZ** Resection of Bilateral Ovaries, Via Natural or Artificial Opening
♀ **0UT28ZZ** Resection of Bilateral Ovaries, Via Natural or Artificial Opening Endoscopic
♀ **0UT2FZZ** Resection of Bilateral Ovaries, Via Natural or Artificial Opening With Percutaneous Endoscopic Assistance
♀ **0UT40ZZ** Resection of Uterine Supporting Structure, Open Approach
　➕ Radical hysterectomy when reported with resection of the uterus and cervix. *See table 0UT to construct the Resection codes.*
♀ **0UT44ZZ** Resection of Uterine Supporting Structure, Percutaneous Endoscopic Approach
　➕ Radical hysterectomy when reported with resection of the uterus and cervix. *See table 0UT to construct the Resection codes.*
♀ **0UT47ZZ** Resection of Uterine Supporting Structure, Via Natural or Artificial Opening
　➕ Radical hysterectomy when reported with resection of the uterus and cervix. *See table 0UT to construct the Resection codes.*

♀ **0UT48ZZ** Resection of Uterine Supporting Structure, Via Natural or Artificial Opening Endoscopic
　➕ Radical hysterectomy when reported with resection of the uterus and cervix. *See table 0UT to construct the Resection codes.*
♀ **0UT50ZZ** Resection of Right Fallopian Tube, Open Approach
♀ **0UT54ZZ** Resection of Right Fallopian Tube, Percutaneous Endoscopic Approach
♀ **0UT57ZZ** Resection of Right Fallopian Tube, Via Natural or Artificial Opening
♀ **0UT58ZZ** Resection of Right Fallopian Tube, Via Natural or Artificial Opening Endoscopic
♀ **0UT5FZZ** Resection of Right Fallopian Tube, Via Natural or Artificial Opening With Percutaneous Endoscopic Assistance
♀ **0UT60ZZ** Resection of Left Fallopian Tube, Open Approach
♀ **0UT64ZZ** Resection of Left Fallopian Tube, Percutaneous Endoscopic Approach
♀ **0UT67ZZ** Resection of Left Fallopian Tube, Via Natural or Artificial Opening
♀ **0UT68ZZ** Resection of Left Fallopian Tube, Via Natural or Artificial Opening Endoscopic
♀ **0UT6FZZ** Resection of Left Fallopian Tube, Via Natural or Artificial Opening With Percutaneous Endoscopic Assistance
♀ **0UT70ZZ** Resection of Bilateral Fallopian Tubes, Open Approach
　AHA CC: 1Q, 2015, 33-34
　➕ Pelvic evisceration when reported with Resection of bladder, urethra, bilateral ovaries, uterus, cervix and vagina. *See tables 0TT and 0UT to construct the Resection codes.*
♀ **0UT74ZZ** Resection of Bilateral Fallopian Tubes, Percutaneous Endoscopic Approach
♀ **0UT77ZZ** Resection of Bilateral Fallopian Tubes, Via Natural or Artificial Opening
♀ **0UT78ZZ** Resection of Bilateral Fallopian Tubes, Via Natural or Artificial Opening Endoscopic
♀ **0UT7FZZ** Resection of Bilateral Fallopian Tubes, Via Natural or Artificial Opening With Percutaneous Endoscopic Assistance
♀ **0UT90ZL** Resection of Uterus, Supracervical, Open Approach
♀ **0UT90ZZ** Resection of Uterus, Open Approach
　AHA CC: 3Q, 2013, 28; 1Q, 2015, 33-34; 4Q, 2017, 68
　➕ Pelvic evisceration when reported with Resection of bladder, urethra, bilateral ovaries, bilateral fallopian tubes, cervix and vagina. *See tables 0TT and 0UT to construct the Resection codes.*

♀ **0UT94ZL** Resection of Uterus, Supracervical, Percutaneous Endoscopic Approach
♀ **0UT94ZZ** Resection of Uterus, Percutaneous Endoscopic Approach
♀ **0UT97ZL** Resection of Uterus, Supracervical, Via Natural or Artificial Opening
　AHA CC: 4Q, 2017, 68
♀ **0UT97ZZ** Resection of Uterus, Via Natural or Artificial Opening
♀ **0UT98ZL** Resection of Uterus, Supracervical, Via Natural or Artificial Opening Endoscopic
♀ **0UT98ZZ** Resection of Uterus, Via Natural or Artificial Opening Endoscopic
♀ **0UT9FZL** Resection of Uterus, Supracervical, Via Natural or Artificial Opening With Percutaneous Endoscopic Assistance
♀ **0UT9FZZ** Resection of Uterus, Via Natural or Artificial Opening With Percutaneous Endoscopic Assistance
♀ **0UTC0ZZ** Resection of Cervix, Open Approach
　AHA CC: 3Q, 2013, 28; 1Q, 2015, 33-34
　➕ Pelvic evisceration when reported with Resection of bladder, urethra, bilateral ovaries, bilateral fallopian tubes, uterus and vagina. *See tables 0TT and 0UT to construct the Resection codes.*
♀ **0UTC4ZZ** Resection of Cervix, Percutaneous Endoscopic Approach
♀ **0UTC7ZZ** Resection of Cervix, Via Natural or Artificial Opening
♀ **0UTC8ZZ** Resection of Cervix, Via Natural or Artificial Opening Endoscopic
♀ **0UTF0ZZ** Resection of Cul-de-sac, Open Approach
♀ **0UTF4ZZ** Resection of Cul-de-sac, Percutaneous Endoscopic Approach
♀ **0UTF7ZZ** Resection of Cul-de-sac, Via Natural or Artificial Opening
♀ **0UTF8ZZ** Resection of Cul-de-sac, Via Natural or Artificial Opening Endoscopic
♀ **0UTG0ZZ** Resection of Vagina, Open Approach
　➕ Pelvic evisceration when reported with Resection of bladder, urethra, bilateral ovaries, bilateral fallopian tubes, uterus and cervix. *See tables 0TT and 0UT to construct the Resection codes.*
♀ **0UTG4ZZ** Resection of Vagina, Percutaneous Endoscopic Approach
♀ **0UTG7ZZ** Resection of Vagina, Via Natural or Artificial Opening
♀ **0UTG8ZZ** Resection of Vagina, Via Natural or Artificial Opening Endoscopic
♀ **0UTJ0ZZ** Resection of Clitoris, Open Approach
♀ **0UTJXZZ** Resection of Clitoris, External Approach
♀ **0UTK0ZZ** Resection of Hymen, Open Approach
♀ **0UTK4ZZ** Resection of Hymen, Percutaneous Endoscopic Approach

♀ 0UTK7ZZ Resection of Hymen, Via Natural or Artificial Opening
♀ 0UTK8ZZ Resection of Hymen, Via Natural or Artificial Opening Endoscopic
♀ 0UTKXZZ Resection of Hymen, External Approach
♀ 0UTL0ZZ Resection of Vestibular Gland, Open Approach
♀ 0UTLXZZ Resection of Vestibular Gland, External Approach
♀ 0UTM0ZZ Resection of Vulva, Open Approach
♀ 0UTMXZZ Resection of Vulva, External Approach

0UU – Female Reproductive System, Supplement

♀ 0UU407Z Supplement Uterine Supporting Structure with Autologous Tissue Substitute, Open Approach
♀ 0UU40JZ Supplement Uterine Supporting Structure with Synthetic Substitute, Open Approach
♀ 0UU40KZ Supplement Uterine Supporting Structure with Nonautologous Tissue Substitute, Open Approach
♀ 0UU447Z Supplement Uterine Supporting Structure with Autologous Tissue Substitute, Percutaneous Endoscopic Approach
♀ 0UU44JZ Supplement Uterine Supporting Structure with Synthetic Substitute, Percutaneous Endoscopic Approach
♀ 0UU44KZ Supplement Uterine Supporting Structure with Nonautologous Tissue Substitute, Percutaneous Endoscopic Approach
♀ 0UU507Z Supplement Right Fallopian Tube with Autologous Tissue Substitute, Open Approach
♀ 0UU50JZ Supplement Right Fallopian Tube with Synthetic Substitute, Open Approach
♀ 0UU50KZ Supplement Right Fallopian Tube with Nonautologous Tissue Substitute, Open Approach
♀ 0UU547Z Supplement Right Fallopian Tube with Autologous Tissue Substitute, Percutaneous Endoscopic Approach
♀ 0UU54JZ Supplement Right Fallopian Tube with Synthetic Substitute, Percutaneous Endoscopic Approach
♀ 0UU54KZ Supplement Right Fallopian Tube with Nonautologous Tissue Substitute, Percutaneous Endoscopic Approach
♀ 0UU577Z Supplement Right Fallopian Tube with Autologous Tissue Substitute, Via Natural or Artificial Opening
♀ 0UU57JZ Supplement Right Fallopian Tube with Synthetic Substitute, Via Natural or Artificial Opening
♀ 0UU57KZ Supplement Right Fallopian Tube with Nonautologous Tissue Substitute, Via Natural or Artificial Opening
♀ 0UU587Z Supplement Right Fallopian Tube with Autologous Tissue Substitute, Via Natural or Artificial Opening Endoscopic
♀ 0UU58JZ Supplement Right Fallopian Tube with Synthetic Substitute, Via Natural or Artificial Opening Endoscopic
♀ 0UU58KZ Supplement Right Fallopian Tube with Nonautologous Tissue Substitute, Via Natural or Artificial Opening Endoscopic
♀ 0UU607Z Supplement Left Fallopian Tube with Autologous Tissue Substitute, Open Approach
♀ 0UU60JZ Supplement Left Fallopian Tube with Synthetic Substitute, Open Approach
♀ 0UU60KZ Supplement Left Fallopian Tube with Nonautologous Tissue Substitute, Open Approach
♀ 0UU647Z Supplement Left Fallopian Tube with Autologous Tissue Substitute, Percutaneous Endoscopic Approach

♀ 0UU64JZ Supplement Left Fallopian Tube with Synthetic Substitute, Percutaneous Endoscopic Approach
♀ 0UU64KZ Supplement Left Fallopian Tube with Nonautologous Tissue Substitute, Percutaneous Endoscopic Approach
♀ 0UU677Z Supplement Left Fallopian Tube with Autologous Tissue Substitute, Via Natural or Artificial Opening
♀ 0UU67JZ Supplement Left Fallopian Tube with Synthetic Substitute, Via Natural or Artificial Opening
♀ 0UU67KZ Supplement Left Fallopian Tube with Nonautologous Tissue Substitute, Via Natural or Artificial Opening
♀ 0UU687Z Supplement Left Fallopian Tube with Autologous Tissue Substitute, Via Natural or Artificial Opening Endoscopic
♀ 0UU68JZ Supplement Left Fallopian Tube with Synthetic Substitute, Via Natural or Artificial Opening Endoscopic
♀ 0UU68KZ Supplement Left Fallopian Tube with Nonautologous Tissue Substitute, Via Natural or Artificial Opening Endoscopic
♀ 0UU707Z Supplement Bilateral Fallopian Tubes with Autologous Tissue Substitute, Open Approach
♀ 0UU70JZ Supplement Bilateral Fallopian Tubes with Synthetic Substitute, Open Approach
♀ 0UU70KZ Supplement Bilateral Fallopian Tubes with Nonautologous Tissue Substitute, Open Approach
♀ 0UU747Z Supplement Bilateral Fallopian Tubes with Autologous Tissue Substitute, Percutaneous Endoscopic Approach
♀ 0UU74JZ Supplement Bilateral Fallopian Tubes with Synthetic Substitute, Percutaneous Endoscopic Approach
♀ 0UU74KZ Supplement Bilateral Fallopian Tubes with Nonautologous Tissue Substitute, Percutaneous Endoscopic Approach
♀ 0UU777Z Supplement Bilateral Fallopian Tubes with Autologous Tissue Substitute, Via Natural or Artificial Opening
♀ 0UU77JZ Supplement Bilateral Fallopian Tubes with Synthetic Substitute, Via Natural or Artificial Opening
♀ 0UU77KZ Supplement Bilateral Fallopian Tubes with Nonautologous Tissue Substitute, Via Natural or Artificial Opening
♀ 0UU787Z Supplement Bilateral Fallopian Tubes with Autologous Tissue Substitute, Via Natural or Artificial Opening Endoscopic
♀ 0UU78JZ Supplement Bilateral Fallopian Tubes with Synthetic Substitute, Via Natural or Artificial Opening Endoscopic
♀ 0UU78KZ Supplement Bilateral Fallopian Tubes with Nonautologous Tissue Substitute, Via Natural or Artificial Opening Endoscopic
♀ 0UUF07Z Supplement Cul-de-sac with Autologous Tissue Substitute, Open Approach

♀ 0UUF0JZ Supplement Cul-de-sac with Synthetic Substitute, Open Approach
♀ 0UUF0KZ Supplement Cul-de-sac with Nonautologous Tissue Substitute, Open Approach
♀ 0UUF47Z Supplement Cul-de-sac with Autologous Tissue Substitute, Percutaneous Endoscopic Approach
♀ 0UUF4JZ Supplement Cul-de-sac with Synthetic Substitute, Percutaneous Endoscopic Approach
♀ 0UUF4KZ Supplement Cul-de-sac with Nonautologous Tissue Substitute, Percutaneous Endoscopic Approach
♀ 0UUF77Z Supplement Cul-de-sac with Autologous Tissue Substitute, Via Natural or Artificial Opening
♀ 0UUF7JZ Supplement Cul-de-sac with Synthetic Substitute, Via Natural or Artificial Opening
♀ 0UUF7KZ Supplement Cul-de-sac with Nonautologous Tissue Substitute, Via Natural or Artificial Opening
♀ 0UUF87Z Supplement Cul-de-sac with Autologous Tissue Substitute, Via Natural or Artificial Opening Endoscopic
♀ 0UUF8JZ Supplement Cul-de-sac with Synthetic Substitute, Via Natural or Artificial Opening Endoscopic
♀ 0UUF8KZ Supplement Cul-de-sac with Nonautologous Tissue Substitute, Via Natural or Artificial Opening Endoscopic
♀ 0UUG07Z Supplement Vagina with Autologous Tissue Substitute, Open Approach
♀ 0UUG0JZ Supplement Vagina with Synthetic Substitute, Open Approach
♀ 0UUG0KZ Supplement Vagina with Nonautologous Tissue Substitute, Open Approach
♀ 0UUG47Z Supplement Vagina with Autologous Tissue Substitute, Percutaneous Endoscopic Approach
♀ 0UUG4JZ Supplement Vagina with Synthetic Substitute, Percutaneous Endoscopic Approach
♀ 0UUG4KZ Supplement Vagina with Nonautologous Tissue Substitute, Percutaneous Endoscopic Approach
♀ 0UUG77Z Supplement Vagina with Autologous Tissue Substitute, Via Natural or Artificial Opening
♀ 0UUG7JZ Supplement Vagina with Synthetic Substitute, Via Natural or Artificial Opening
♀ 0UUG7KZ Supplement Vagina with Nonautologous Tissue Substitute, Via Natural or Artificial Opening
♀ 0UUG87Z Supplement Vagina with Autologous Tissue Substitute, Via Natural or Artificial Opening Endoscopic
♀ 0UUG8JZ Supplement Vagina with Synthetic Substitute, Via Natural or Artificial Opening Endoscopic
♀ 0UUG8KZ Supplement Vagina with Nonautologous Tissue Substitute, Via Natural or Artificial Opening Endoscopic

♀ Female-only   ♂ Male-only   ▲ Limited Coverage   ● Non-OR   HAC HAC-associated procedure   ▲ Non-covered procedures   ✚ Cluster

♀ **0UUGX7Z** Supplement Vagina with Autologous Tissue Substitute, External Approach
♀ **0UUGXJZ** Supplement Vagina with Synthetic Substitute, External Approach
♀ **0UUGXKZ** Supplement Vagina with Nonautologous Tissue Substitute, External Approach
♀ **0UUJ07Z** Supplement Clitoris with Autologous Tissue Substitute, Open Approach
♀ **0UUJ0JZ** Supplement Clitoris with Synthetic Substitute, Open Approach
♀ **0UUJ0KZ** Supplement Clitoris with Nonautologous Tissue Substitute, Open Approach
♀ **0UUJX7Z** Supplement Clitoris with Autologous Tissue Substitute, External Approach
♀ **0UUJXJZ** Supplement Clitoris with Synthetic Substitute, External Approach
♀ **0UUJXKZ** Supplement Clitoris with Nonautologous Tissue Substitute, External Approach
♀ **0UUK07Z** Supplement Hymen with Autologous Tissue Substitute, Open Approach
♀ **0UUK0JZ** Supplement Hymen with Synthetic Substitute, Open Approach

♀ **0UUK0KZ** Supplement Hymen with Nonautologous Tissue Substitute, Open Approach
♀ **0UUK47Z** Supplement Hymen with Autologous Tissue Substitute, Percutaneous Endoscopic Approach
♀ **0UUK4JZ** Supplement Hymen with Synthetic Substitute, Percutaneous Endoscopic Approach
♀ **0UUK4KZ** Supplement Hymen with Nonautologous Tissue Substitute, Percutaneous Endoscopic Approach
♀ **0UUK77Z** Supplement Hymen with Autologous Tissue Substitute, Via Natural or Artificial Opening
♀ **0UUK7JZ** Supplement Hymen with Synthetic Substitute, Via Natural or Artificial Opening
♀ **0UUK7KZ** Supplement Hymen with Nonautologous Tissue Substitute, Via Natural or Artificial Opening
♀ **0UUK87Z** Supplement Hymen with Autologous Tissue Substitute, Via Natural or Artificial Opening Endoscopic
♀ **0UUK8JZ** Supplement Hymen with Synthetic Substitute, Via Natural or Artificial Opening Endoscopic

♀ **0UUK8KZ** Supplement Hymen with Nonautologous Tissue Substitute, Via Natural or Artificial Opening Endoscopic
♀ **0UUKX7Z** Supplement Hymen with Autologous Tissue Substitute, External Approach
♀ **0UUKXJZ** Supplement Hymen with Synthetic Substitute, External Approach
♀ **0UUKXKZ** Supplement Hymen with Nonautologous Tissue Substitute, External Approach
♀ **0UUM07Z** Supplement Vulva with Autologous Tissue Substitute, Open Approach
♀ **0UUM0JZ** Supplement Vulva with Synthetic Substitute, Open Approach
♀ **0UUM0KZ** Supplement Vulva with Nonautologous Tissue Substitute, Open Approach
♀ **0UUMX7Z** Supplement Vulva with Autologous Tissue Substitute, External Approach
♀ **0UUMXJZ** Supplement Vulva with Synthetic Substitute, External Approach
♀ **0UUMXKZ** Supplement Vulva with Nonautologous Tissue Substitute, External Approach

0UV – Female Reproductive System, Restriction

♀ **0UVC0CZ** Restriction of Cervix with Extraluminal Device, Open Approach
♀ **0UVC0DZ** Restriction of Cervix with Intraluminal Device, Open Approach
♀ **0UVC0ZZ** Restriction of Cervix, Open Approach
♀ **0UVC3CZ** Restriction of Cervix with Extraluminal Device, Percutaneous Approach
♀ **0UVC3DZ** Restriction of Cervix with Intraluminal Device, Percutaneous Approach

♀ **0UVC3ZZ** Restriction of Cervix, Percutaneous Approach
♀ **0UVC4CZ** Restriction of Cervix with Extraluminal Device, Percutaneous Endoscopic Approach
♀ **0UVC4DZ** Restriction of Cervix with Intraluminal Device, Percutaneous Endoscopic Approach
♀ **0UVC4ZZ** Restriction of Cervix, Percutaneous Endoscopic Approach

♀ **0UVC7DZ** Restriction of Cervix with Intraluminal Device, Via Natural or Artificial Opening
♀ **0UVC7ZZ** Restriction of Cervix, Via Natural or Artificial Opening
AHA CC: 3Q, 2015, 30
♀ **0UVC8DZ** Restriction of Cervix with Intraluminal Device, Via Natural or Artificial Opening Endoscopic
♀ **0UVC8ZZ** Restriction of Cervix, Via Natural or Artificial Opening Endoscopic

0UW – Female Reproductive System, Revision

Review Coding Guideline B6.1c

♀ **0UW300Z** Revision of Drainage Device in Ovary, Open Approach
♀ **0UW303Z** Revision of Infusion Device in Ovary, Open Approach
♀ **0UW30YZ** Revision of Other Device in Ovary, Open Approach
♀ **0UW330Z** Revision of Drainage Device in Ovary, Percutaneous Approach
♀ **0UW333Z** Revision of Infusion Device in Ovary, Percutaneous Approach
♀ **0UW33YZ** Revision of Other Device in Ovary, Percutaneous Approach
♀ **0UW340Z** Revision of Drainage Device in Ovary, Percutaneous Endoscopic Approach
♀ **0UW343Z** Revision of Infusion Device in Ovary, Percutaneous Endoscopic Approach
♀ **0UW34YZ** Revision of Other Device in Ovary, Percutaneous Endoscopic Approach
♀ **0UW37YZ** Revision of Other Device in Ovary, Via Natural or Artificial Opening
♀ **0UW38YZ** Revision of Other Device in Ovary, Via Natural or Artificial Opening Endoscopic
♀ **0UW3X0Z** Revision of Drainage Device in Ovary, External Approach
♀ **0UW3X3Z** Revision of Infusion Device in Ovary, External Approach
♀ **0UW800Z** Revision of Drainage Device in Fallopian Tube, Open Approach

♀ **0UW803Z** Revision of Infusion Device in Fallopian Tube, Open Approach
♀ **0UW807Z** Revision of Autologous Tissue Substitute in Fallopian Tube, Open Approach
♀ **0UW80CZ** Revision of Extraluminal Device in Fallopian Tube, Open Approach
♀ **0UW80DZ** Revision of Intraluminal Device in Fallopian Tube, Open Approach
♀ **0UW80JZ** Revision of Synthetic Substitute in Fallopian Tube, Open Approach
♀ **0UW80KZ** Revision of Nonautologous Tissue Substitute in Fallopian Tube, Open Approach
♀ **0UW80YZ** Revision of Other Device in Fallopian Tube, Open Approach
♀ **0UW830Z** Revision of Drainage Device in Fallopian Tube, Percutaneous Approach
♀ **0UW833Z** Revision of Infusion Device in Fallopian Tube, Percutaneous Approach
♀ **0UW837Z** Revision of Autologous Tissue Substitute in Fallopian Tube, Percutaneous Approach
♀ **0UW83CZ** Revision of Extraluminal Device in Fallopian Tube, Percutaneous Approach
♀ **0UW83DZ** Revision of Intraluminal Device in Fallopian Tube, Percutaneous Approach

♀ **0UW83JZ** Revision of Synthetic Substitute in Fallopian Tube, Percutaneous Approach
♀ **0UW83KZ** Revision of Nonautologous Tissue Substitute in Fallopian Tube, Percutaneous Approach
♀ **0UW83YZ** Revision of Other Device in Fallopian Tube, Percutaneous Approach
♀ **0UW840Z** Revision of Drainage Device in Fallopian Tube, Percutaneous Endoscopic Approach
♀ **0UW843Z** Revision of Infusion Device in Fallopian Tube, Percutaneous Endoscopic Approach
♀ **0UW847Z** Revision of Autologous Tissue Substitute in Fallopian Tube, Percutaneous Endoscopic Approach
♀ **0UW84CZ** Revision of Extraluminal Device in Fallopian Tube, Percutaneous Endoscopic Approach
♀ **0UW84DZ** Revision of Intraluminal Device in Fallopian Tube, Percutaneous Endoscopic Approach
♀ **0UW84JZ** Revision of Synthetic Substitute in Fallopian Tube, Percutaneous Endoscopic Approach
♀ **0UW84KZ** Revision of Nonautologous Tissue Substitute in Fallopian Tube, Percutaneous Endoscopic Approach

♀ **0UW84YZ** Revision of Other Device in Fallopian Tube, Percutaneous Endoscopic Approach

♀ **0UW870Z** Revision of Drainage Device in Fallopian Tube, Via Natural or Artificial Opening

♀ **0UW873Z** Revision of Infusion Device in Fallopian Tube, Via Natural or Artificial Opening

♀ **0UW877Z** Revision of Autologous Tissue Substitute in Fallopian Tube, Via Natural or Artificial Opening

♀ **0UW87CZ** Revision of Extraluminal Device in Fallopian Tube, Via Natural or Artificial Opening

♀ **0UW87DZ** Revision of Intraluminal Device in Fallopian Tube, Via Natural or Artificial Opening

♀ **0UW87JZ** Revision of Synthetic Substitute in Fallopian Tube, Via Natural or Artificial Opening

♀ **0UW87KZ** Revision of Nonautologous Tissue Substitute in Fallopian Tube, Via Natural or Artificial Opening

♀ **0UW87YZ** Revision of Other Device in Fallopian Tube, Via Natural or Artificial Opening

♀ **0UW880Z** Revision of Drainage Device in Fallopian Tube, Via Natural or Artificial Opening Endoscopic

♀ **0UW883Z** Revision of Infusion Device in Fallopian Tube, Via Natural or Artificial Opening Endoscopic

♀ **0UW887Z** Revision of Autologous Tissue Substitute in Fallopian Tube, Via Natural or Artificial Opening Endoscopic

♀ **0UW88CZ** Revision of Extraluminal Device in Fallopian Tube, Via Natural or Artificial Opening Endoscopic

♀ **0UW88DZ** Revision of Intraluminal Device in Fallopian Tube, Via Natural or Artificial Opening Endoscopic

♀ **0UW88JZ** Revision of Synthetic Substitute in Fallopian Tube, Via Natural or Artificial Opening Endoscopic

♀ **0UW88KZ** Revision of Nonautologous Tissue Substitute in Fallopian Tube, Via Natural or Artificial Opening Endoscopic

♀ **0UW88YZ** Revision of Other Device in Fallopian Tube, Via Natural or Artificial Opening Endoscopic

♀ **0UW8X0Z** Revision of Drainage Device in Fallopian Tube, External Approach

♀ **0UW8X3Z** Revision of Infusion Device in Fallopian Tube, External Approach

♀ **0UW8X7Z** Revision of Autologous Tissue Substitute in Fallopian Tube, External Approach

♀ **0UW8XCZ** Revision of Extraluminal Device in Fallopian Tube, External Approach

♀ **0UW8XDZ** Revision of Intraluminal Device in Fallopian Tube, External Approach

♀ **0UW8XJZ** Revision of Synthetic Substitute in Fallopian Tube, External Approach

♀ **0UW8XKZ** Revision of Nonautologous Tissue Substitute in Fallopian Tube, External Approach

♀ **0UWD00Z** Revision of Drainage Device in Uterus and Cervix, Open Approach

♀ **0UWD01Z** Revision of Radioactive Element in Uterus and Cervix, Open Approach

♀ **0UWD03Z** Revision of Infusion Device in Uterus and Cervix, Open Approach

♀ **0UWD07Z** Revision of Autologous Tissue Substitute in Uterus and Cervix, Open Approach

♀ **0UWD0CZ** Revision of Extraluminal Device in Uterus and Cervix, Open Approach

♀ **0UWD0DZ** Revision of Intraluminal Device in Uterus and Cervix, Open Approach

♀ **0UWD0HZ** Revision of Contraceptive Device in Uterus and Cervix, Open Approach

♀ **0UWD0JZ** Revision of Synthetic Substitute in Uterus and Cervix, Open Approach

♀ **0UWD0KZ** Revision of Nonautologous Tissue Substitute in Uterus and Cervix, Open Approach

♀ **0UWD0YZ** Revision of Other Device in Uterus and Cervix, Open Approach

♀ **0UWD30Z** Revision of Drainage Device in Uterus and Cervix, Percutaneous Approach

♀ **0UWD31Z** Revision of Radioactive Element in Uterus and Cervix, Percutaneous Approach

♀ **0UWD33Z** Revision of Infusion Device in Uterus and Cervix, Percutaneous Approach

♀ **0UWD37Z** Revision of Autologous Tissue Substitute in Uterus and Cervix, Percutaneous Approach

♀ **0UWD3CZ** Revision of Extraluminal Device in Uterus and Cervix, Percutaneous Approach

♀ **0UWD3DZ** Revision of Intraluminal Device in Uterus and Cervix, Percutaneous Approach

♀ **0UWD3HZ** Revision of Contraceptive Device in Uterus and Cervix, Percutaneous Approach

♀ **0UWD3JZ** Revision of Synthetic Substitute in Uterus and Cervix, Percutaneous Approach

♀ **0UWD3KZ** Revision of Nonautologous Tissue Substitute in Uterus and Cervix, Percutaneous Approach

♀ **0UWD3YZ** Revision of Other Device in Uterus and Cervix, Percutaneous Approach

♀ **0UWD40Z** Revision of Drainage Device in Uterus and Cervix, Percutaneous Endoscopic Approach

♀ **0UWD41Z** Revision of Radioactive Element in Uterus and Cervix, Percutaneous Endoscopic Approach

♀ **0UWD43Z** Revision of Infusion Device in Uterus and Cervix, Percutaneous Endoscopic Approach

♀ **0UWD47Z** Revision of Autologous Tissue Substitute in Uterus and Cervix, Percutaneous Endoscopic Approach

♀ **0UWD4CZ** Revision of Extraluminal Device in Uterus and Cervix, Percutaneous Endoscopic Approach

♀ **0UWD4DZ** Revision of Intraluminal Device in Uterus and Cervix, Percutaneous Endoscopic Approach

♀ **0UWD4HZ** Revision of Contraceptive Device in Uterus and Cervix, Percutaneous Endoscopic Approach

♀ **0UWD4JZ** Revision of Synthetic Substitute in Uterus and Cervix, Percutaneous Endoscopic Approach

♀ **0UWD4KZ** Revision of Nonautologous Tissue Substitute in Uterus and Cervix, Percutaneous Endoscopic Approach

♀ **0UWD4YZ** Revision of Other Device in Uterus and Cervix, Percutaneous Endoscopic Approach

♀ **0UWD70Z** Revision of Drainage Device in Uterus and Cervix, Via Natural or Artificial Opening

♀ **0UWD71Z** Revision of Radioactive Element in Uterus and Cervix, Via Natural or Artificial Opening

♀ **0UWD73Z** Revision of Infusion Device in Uterus and Cervix, Via Natural or Artificial Opening

♀ **0UWD77Z** Revision of Autologous Tissue Substitute in Uterus and Cervix, Via Natural or Artificial Opening

♀ **0UWD7CZ** Revision of Extraluminal Device in Uterus and Cervix, Via Natural or Artificial Opening

♀ **0UWD7DZ** Revision of Intraluminal Device in Uterus and Cervix, Via Natural or Artificial Opening

♀ **0UWD7HZ** Revision of Contraceptive Device in Uterus and Cervix, Via Natural or Artificial Opening

♀ **0UWD7JZ** Revision of Synthetic Substitute in Uterus and Cervix, Via Natural or Artificial Opening

♀ **0UWD7KZ** Revision of Nonautologous Tissue Substitute in Uterus and Cervix, Via Natural or Artificial Opening

♀ **0UWD7YZ** Revision of Other Device in Uterus and Cervix, Via Natural or Artificial Opening

♀ **0UWD80Z** Revision of Drainage Device in Uterus and Cervix, Via Natural or Artificial Opening Endoscopic

♀ **0UWD81Z** Revision of Radioactive Element in Uterus and Cervix, Via Natural or Artificial Opening Endoscopic

♀ **0UWD83Z** Revision of Infusion Device in Uterus and Cervix, Via Natural or Artificial Opening Endoscopic

♀ **0UWD87Z** Revision of Autologous Tissue Substitute in Uterus and Cervix, Via Natural or Artificial Opening Endoscopic

♀ **0UWD8CZ** Revision of Extraluminal Device in Uterus and Cervix, Via Natural or Artificial Opening Endoscopic

♀ **0UWD8DZ** Revision of Intraluminal Device in Uterus and Cervix, Via Natural or Artificial Opening Endoscopic

♀ **0UWD8HZ** Revision of Contraceptive Device in Uterus and Cervix, Via Natural or Artificial Opening Endoscopic

♀ **0UWD8JZ** Revision of Synthetic Substitute in Uterus and Cervix, Via Natural or Artificial Opening Endoscopic

♀ **0UWD8KZ** Revision of Nonautologous Tissue Substitute in Uterus and Cervix, Via Natural or Artificial Opening Endoscopic

♀ **0UWD8YZ** Revision of Other Device in Uterus and Cervix, Via Natural or Artificial Opening Endoscopic

♀ **0UWDX0Z** Revision of Drainage Device in Uterus and Cervix, External Approach

♀ **0UWDX3Z** Revision of Infusion Device in Uterus and Cervix, External Approach

♀ **0UWDX7Z** Revision of Autologous Tissue Substitute in Uterus and Cervix, External Approach

♀ **0UWDXCZ** Revision of Extraluminal Device in Uterus and Cervix, External Approach

♀ **0UWDXDZ** Revision of Intraluminal Device in Uterus and Cervix, External Approach

♀ **0UWDXHZ** Revision of Contraceptive Device in Uterus and Cervix, External Approach

 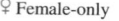
♀ Female-only   ♂ Male-only   ▲ Limited Coverage   ● Non-OR   🅷🅰🅲 HAC-associated procedure   ▲ Non-covered procedures   ✚ Cluster

♀ **0UWDXJZ** Revision of Synthetic Substitute in Uterus and Cervix, External Approach

♀ **0UWDXKZ** Revision of Nonautologous Tissue Substitute in Uterus and Cervix, External Approach

♀ **0UWH00Z** Revision of Drainage Device in Vagina and Cul-de-sac, Open Approach

♀ **0UWH01Z** Revision of Radioactive Element in Vagina and Cul-de-sac, Open Approach

♀ **0UWH03Z** Revision of Infusion Device in Vagina and Cul-de-sac, Open Approach

♀ **0UWH07Z** Revision of Autologous Tissue Substitute in Vagina and Cul-de-sac, Open Approach

♀ **0UWH0DZ** Revision of Intraluminal Device in Vagina and Cul-de-sac, Open Approach

♀ **0UWH0JZ** Revision of Synthetic Substitute in Vagina and Cul-de-sac, Open Approach

♀ **0UWH0KZ** Revision of Nonautologous Tissue Substitute in Vagina and Cul-de-sac, Open Approach

♀ **0UWH0YZ** Revision of Other Device in Vagina and Cul-de-sac, Open Approach

♀ **0UWH30Z** Revision of Drainage Device in Vagina and Cul-de-sac, Percutaneous Approach

♀ **0UWH31Z** Revision of Radioactive Element in Vagina and Cul-de-sac, Percutaneous Approach

♀ **0UWH33Z** Revision of Infusion Device in Vagina and Cul-de-sac, Percutaneous Approach

♀ **0UWH37Z** Revision of Autologous Tissue Substitute in Vagina and Cul-de-sac, Percutaneous Approach

♀ **0UWH3DZ** Revision of Intraluminal Device in Vagina and Cul-de-sac, Percutaneous Approach

♀ **0UWH3JZ** Revision of Synthetic Substitute in Vagina and Cul-de-sac, Percutaneous Approach

♀ **0UWH3KZ** Revision of Nonautologous Tissue Substitute in Vagina and Cul-de-sac, Percutaneous Approach

♀ **0UWH3YZ** Revision of Other Device in Vagina and Cul-de-sac, Percutaneous Approach

♀ **0UWH40Z** Revision of Drainage Device in Vagina and Cul-de-sac, Percutaneous Endoscopic Approach

♀ **0UWH41Z** Revision of Radioactive Element in Vagina and Cul-de-sac, Percutaneous Endoscopic Approach

♀ **0UWH43Z** Revision of Infusion Device in Vagina and Cul-de-sac, Percutaneous Endoscopic Approach

♀ **0UWH47Z** Revision of Autologous Tissue Substitute in Vagina and Cul-de-sac, Percutaneous Endoscopic Approach

♀ **0UWH4DZ** Revision of Intraluminal Device in Vagina and Cul-de-sac, Percutaneous Endoscopic Approach

♀ **0UWH4JZ** Revision of Synthetic Substitute in Vagina and Cul-de-sac, Percutaneous Endoscopic Approach

♀ **0UWH4KZ** Revision of Nonautologous Tissue Substitute in Vagina and Cul-de-sac, Percutaneous Endoscopic Approach

♀ **0UWH4YZ** Revision of Other Device in Vagina and Cul-de-sac, Percutaneous Endoscopic Approach

♀ **0UWH70Z** Revision of Drainage Device in Vagina and Cul-de-sac, Via Natural or Artificial Opening

♀ **0UWH71Z** Revision of Radioactive Element in Vagina and Cul-de-sac, Via Natural or Artificial Opening

♀ **0UWH73Z** Revision of Infusion Device in Vagina and Cul-de-sac, Via Natural or Artificial Opening

♀ **0UWH77Z** Revision of Autologous Tissue Substitute in Vagina and Cul-de-sac, Via Natural or Artificial Opening

♀ **0UWH7DZ** Revision of Intraluminal Device in Vagina and Cul-de-sac, Via Natural or Artificial Opening

♀ **0UWH7JZ** Revision of Synthetic Substitute in Vagina and Cul-de-sac, Via Natural or Artificial Opening

♀ **0UWH7KZ** Revision of Nonautologous Tissue Substitute in Vagina and Cul-de-sac, Via Natural or Artificial Opening

♀ **0UWH7YZ** Revision of Other Device in Vagina and Cul-de-sac, Via Natural or Artificial Opening

♀ **0UWH80Z** Revision of Drainage Device in Vagina and Cul-de-sac, Via Natural or Artificial Opening Endoscopic

♀ **0UWH81Z** Revision of Radioactive Element in Vagina and Cul-de-sac, Via Natural or Artificial Opening Endoscopic

♀ **0UWH83Z** Revision of Infusion Device in Vagina and Cul-de-sac, Via Natural or Artificial Opening Endoscopic

♀ **0UWH87Z** Revision of Autologous Tissue Substitute in Vagina and Cul-de-sac, Via Natural or Artificial Opening Endoscopic

♀ **0UWH8DZ** Revision of Intraluminal Device in Vagina and Cul-de-sac, Via Natural or Artificial Opening Endoscopic

♀ **0UWH8JZ** Revision of Synthetic Substitute in Vagina and Cul-de-sac, Via Natural or Artificial Opening Endoscopic

♀ **0UWH8KZ** Revision of Nonautologous Tissue Substitute in Vagina and Cul-de-sac, Via Natural or Artificial Opening Endoscopic

♀ **0UWH8YZ** Revision of Other Device in Vagina and Cul-de-sac, Via Natural or Artificial Opening Endoscopic

♀ **0UWHX0Z** Revision of Drainage Device in Vagina and Cul-de-sac, External Approach

♀ **0UWHX3Z** Revision of Infusion Device in Vagina and Cul-de-sac, External Approach

♀ **0UWHX7Z** Revision of Autologous Tissue Substitute in Vagina and Cul-de-sac, External Approach

♀ **0UWHXDZ** Revision of Intraluminal Device in Vagina and Cul-de-sac, External Approach

♀ **0UWHXJZ** Revision of Synthetic Substitute in Vagina and Cul-de-sac, External Approach

♀ **0UWHXKZ** Revision of Nonautologous Tissue Substitute in Vagina and Cul-de-sac, External Approach

♀ **0UWM00Z** Revision of Drainage Device in Vulva, Open Approach

♀ **0UWM07Z** Revision of Autologous Tissue Substitute in Vulva, Open Approach

♀ **0UWM0JZ** Revision of Synthetic Substitute in Vulva, Open Approach

♀ **0UWM0KZ** Revision of Nonautologous Tissue Substitute in Vulva, Open Approach

♀ **0UWMX0Z** Revision of Drainage Device in Vulva, External Approach

♀ **0UWMX7Z** Revision of Autologous Tissue Substitute in Vulva, External Approach

♀ **0UWMXJZ** Revision of Synthetic Substitute in Vulva, External Approach

♀ **0UWMXKZ** Revision of Nonautologous Tissue Substitute in Vulva, External Approach

0UY – Female Reproductive System, Transplantation

Review Coding Guideline B3.16

♀ **0UY00Z0** Transplantation of Right Ovary, Allogeneic, Open Approach

♀ **0UY00Z1** Transplantation of Right Ovary, Syngeneic, Open Approach

♀ **0UY00Z2** Transplantation of Right Ovary, Zooplastic, Open Approach

♀ **0UY10Z0** Transplantation of Left Ovary, Allogeneic, Open Approach

♀ **0UY10Z1** Transplantation of Left Ovary, Syngeneic, Open Approach

♀ **0UY10Z2** Transplantation of Left Ovary, Zooplastic, Open Approach

♀ **0UY90Z0** Transplantation of Uterus, Allogeneic, Open Approach

♀ **0UY90Z1** Transplantation of Uterus, Syngeneic, Open Approach

♀ **0UY90Z2** Transplantation of Uterus, Zooplastic, Open Approach

---

♀ Female-only ♂ Male-only ▲ Limited Coverage ● Non-OR ▨ HAC-associated procedure ▲ Non-covered procedures ✚ Cluster

Male Reproductive System

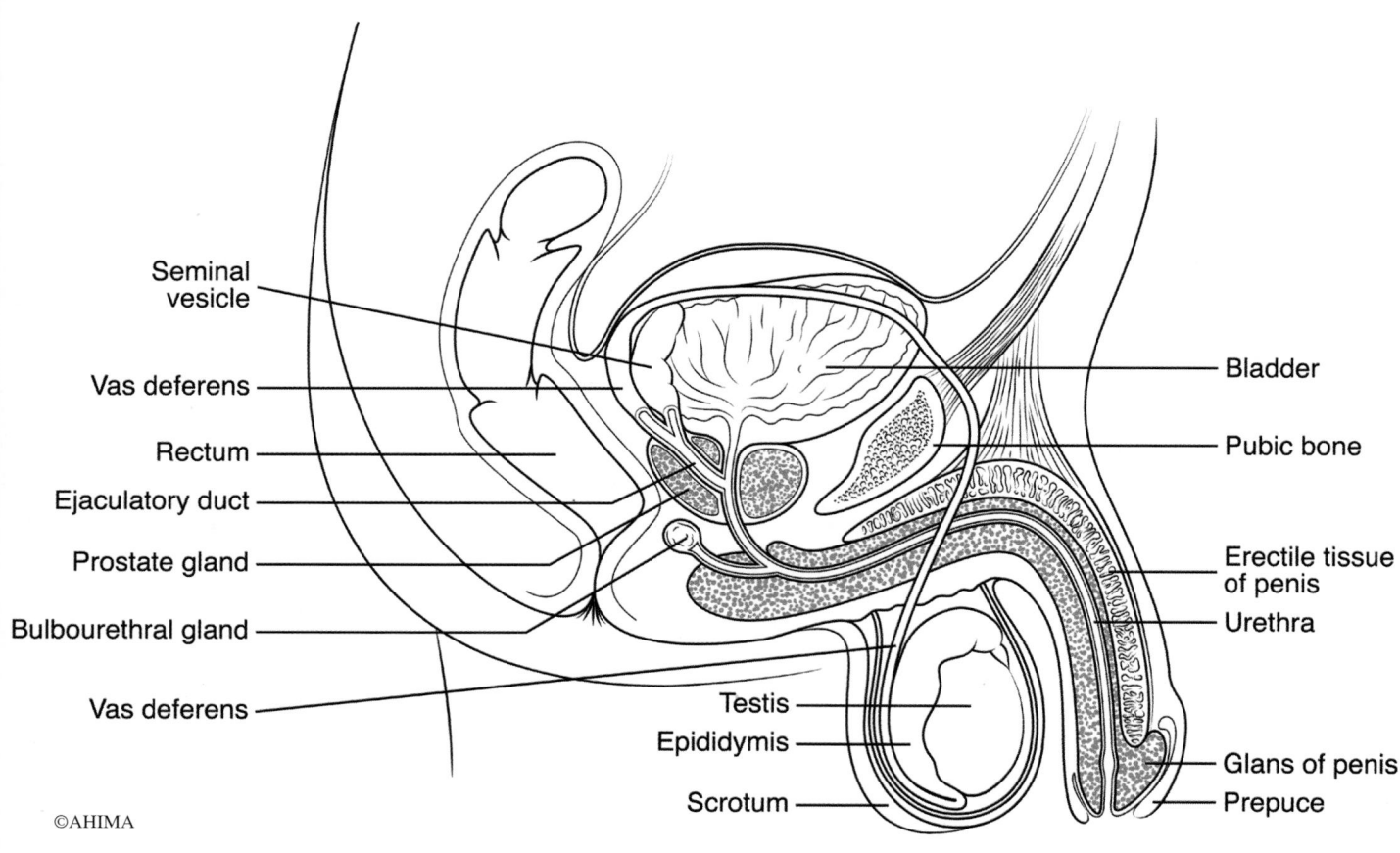

Seminal vesicle

Vas deferens

Rectum

Ejaculatory duct

Prostate gland

Bulbourethral gland

Vas deferens

Testis

Epididymis

Scrotum

©AHIMA

Bladder

Pubic bone

Erectile tissue of penis

Urethra

Glans of penis

Prepuce

Medical and Surgical, Male Reproductive System

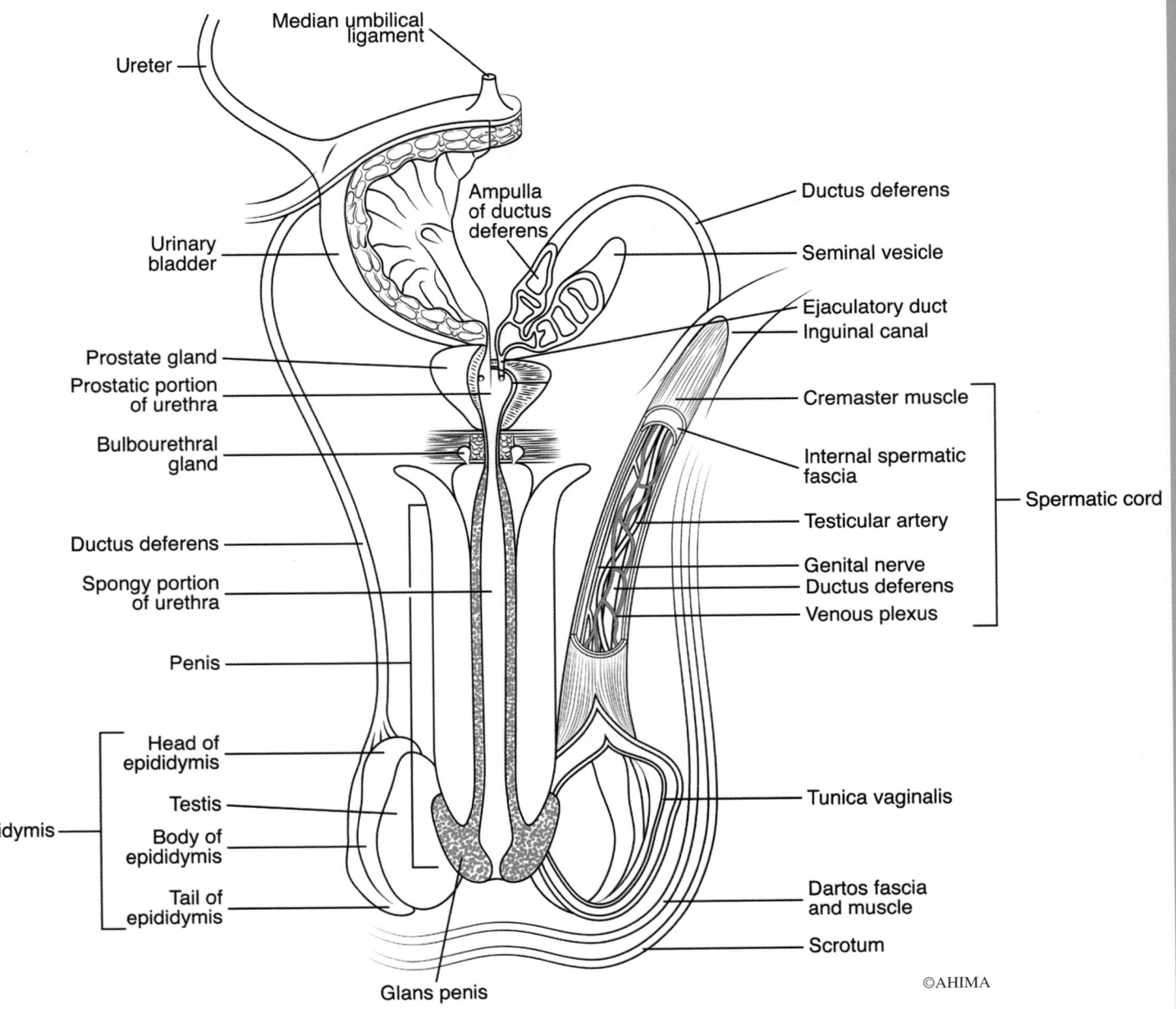

Ureter

Median umbilical ligament

Ampulla of ductus deferens

Ductus deferens

Seminal vesicle

Ejaculatory duct

Inguinal canal

Urinary bladder

Prostate gland

Prostatic portion of urethra

Bulbourethral gland

Ductus deferens

Spongy portion of urethra

Penis

Head of epididymis

Testis

Body of epididymis

Tail of epididymis

Epididymis

Glans penis

Cremaster muscle

Internal spermatic fascia

Testicular artery

Genital nerve

Ductus deferens

Venous plexus

Spermatic cord

Tunica vaginalis

Dartos fascia and muscle

Scrotum

©AHIMA

Section	0	Medical and Surgical
Body System	V	Male Reproductive System
Operation	1	**Bypass:** Altering the route of passage of the contents of a tubular body part

Body Part (4th)	Approach (5th)	Device (6th)	Qualifier (7th)
N Vas Deferens, Right P Vas Deferens, Left Q Vas Deferens, Bilateral	0 Open 4 Percutaneous Endoscopic	7 Autologous Tissue Substitute J Synthetic Substitute K Nonautologous Tissue Substitute Z No Device	J Epididymis, Right K Epididymis, Left N Vas Deferens, Right P Vas Deferens, Left

Section	0	Medical and Surgical
Body System	V	Male Reproductive System
Operation	2	**Change:** Taking out or off a device from a body part and putting back an identical or similar device in or on the same body part without cutting or puncturing the skin or a mucous membrane

Body Part (4th)	Approach (5th)	Device (6th)	Qualifier (7th)
4 Prostate and Seminal Vesicles 8 Scrotum and Tunica Vaginalis D Testis M Epididymis and Spermatic Cord R Vas Deferens S Penis	X External	0 Drainage Device Y Other Device	Z No Qualifier

Section	0	Medical and Surgical
Body System	V	Male Reproductive System
Operation	5	**Destruction:** Physical eradication of all or a portion of a body part by the direct use of energy, force, or a destructive agent

Body Part (4th)	Approach (5th)	Device (6th)	Qualifier (7th)
0 Prostate	0 Open 3 Percutaneous 4 Percutaneous Endoscopic 7 Via Natural or Artificial Opening 8 Via Natural or Artificial Opening Endoscopic	Z No Device	Z No Qualifier
1 Seminal Vesicle, Right 2 Seminal Vesicle, Left 3 Seminal Vesicles, Bilateral 6 Tunica Vaginalis, Right 7 Tunica Vaginalis, Left 9 Testis, Right B Testis, Left C Testes, Bilateral	0 Open 3 Percutaneous 4 Percutaneous Endoscopic	Z No Device	Z No Qualifier
5 Scrotum S Penis T Prepuce	0 Open 3 Percutaneous 4 Percutaneous Endoscopic X External	Z No Device	Z No Qualifier
F Spermatic Cord, Right G Spermatic Cord, Left H Spermatic Cords, Bilateral J Epididymis, Right K Epididymis, Left L Epididymis, Bilateral N Vas Deferens, Right P Vas Deferens, Left Q Vas Deferens, Bilateral	0 Open 3 Percutaneous 4 Percutaneous Endoscopic 8 Via Natural or Artificial Opening Endoscopic	Z No Device	Z No Qualifier

Section	0	Medical and Surgical
Body System	V	Male Reproductive System
Operation	7	**Dilation:** Expanding an orifice or the lumen of a tubular body part

Body Part (4th)	Approach (5th)	Device (6th)	Qualifier (7th)
N Vas Deferens, Right P Vas Deferens, Left Q Vas Deferens, Bilateral	0 Open 3 Percutaneous 4 Percutaneous Endoscopic	D Intraluminal Device Z No Device	Z No Qualifier

Section	0	Medical and Surgical
Body System	V	Male Reproductive System
Operation	9	**Drainage:** Taking or letting out fluids and/or gases from a body part

Body Part (4th)	Approach (5th)	Device (6th)	Qualifier (7th)
0 Prostate	0 Open 3 Percutaneous 4 Percutaneous Endoscopic 7 Via Natural or Artificial Opening 8 Via Natural or Artificial Opening Endoscopic	0 Drainage Device	Z No Qualifier
0 Prostate	0 Open 3 Percutaneous 4 Percutaneous Endoscopic 7 Via Natural or Artificial Opening 8 Via Natural or Artificial Opening Endoscopic	Z No Device	X Diagnostic Z No Qualifier
1 Seminal Vesicle, Right 2 Seminal Vesicle, Left 3 Seminal Vesicles, Bilateral 6 Tunica Vaginalis, Right 7 Tunica Vaginalis, Left 9 Testis, Right B Testis, Left C Testes, Bilateral F Spermatic Cord, Right G Spermatic Cord, Left H Spermatic Cords, Bilateral J Epididymis, Right K Epididymis, Left L Epididymis, Bilateral N Vas Deferens, Right P Vas Deferens, Left Q Vas Deferens, Bilateral	0 Open 3 Percutaneous 4 Percutaneous Endoscopic	0 Drainage Device	Z No Qualifier
1 Seminal Vesicle, Right 2 Seminal Vesicle, Left 3 Seminal Vesicles, Bilateral 6 Tunica Vaginalis, Right 7 Tunica Vaginalis, Left 9 Testis, Right B Testis, Left C Testes, Bilateral F Spermatic Cord, Right G Spermatic Cord, Left H Spermatic Cords, Bilateral J Epididymis, Right K Epididymis, Left L Epididymis, Bilateral N Vas Deferens, Right P Vas Deferens, Left Q Vas Deferens, Bilateral	0 Open 3 Percutaneous 4 Percutaneous Endoscopic	Z No Device	X Diagnostic Z No Qualifier
5 Scrotum S Penis T Prepuce	0 Open 3 Percutaneous 4 Percutaneous Endoscopic X External	0 Drainage Device	Z No Qualifier

Continued →

Section   **0**   **Medical and Surgical**
Body System   **V**   **Male Reproductive System**
Operation   **9**   **Drainage:** Taking or letting out fluids and/or gases from a body part

Body Part (4th)	Approach (5th)	Device (6th)	Qualifier (7th)
5 Scrotum **S** Penis **T** Prepuce	**0** Open **3** Percutaneous **4** Percutaneous Endoscopic **X** External	**Z** No Device	**X** Diagnostic **Z** No Qualifier

Section   **0**   **Medical and Surgical**
Body System   **V**   **Male Reproductive System**
Operation   **B**   **Excision:** Cutting out or off, without replacement, a portion of a body part

Body Part (4th)	Approach (5th)	Device (6th)	Qualifier (7th)
0 Prostate	**0** Open **3** Percutaneous **4** Percutaneous Endoscopic **7** Via Natural or Artificial Opening **8** Via Natural or Artificial Opening Endoscopic	**Z** No Device	**X** Diagnostic **Z** No Qualifier
1 Seminal Vesicle, Right **2** Seminal Vesicle, Left **3** Seminal Vesicles, Bilateral **6** Tunica Vaginalis, Right **7** Tunica Vaginalis, Left **9** Testis, Right **B** Testis, Left **C** Testes, Bilateral	**0** Open **3** Percutaneous **4** Percutaneous Endoscopic	**Z** No Device	**X** Diagnostic **Z** No Qualifier
5 Scrotum **S** Penis **T** Prepuce	**0** Open **3** Percutaneous **4** Percutaneous Endoscopic **X** External	**Z** No Device	**X** Diagnostic **Z** No Qualifier
F Spermatic Cord, Right **G** Spermatic Cord, Left **H** Spermatic Cords, Bilateral **J** Epididymis, Right **K** Epididymis, Left **L** Epididymis, Bilateral **N** Vas Deferens, Right **P** Vas Deferens, Left **Q** Vas Deferens, Bilateral	**0** Open **3** Percutaneous **4** Percutaneous Endoscopic **8** Via Natural or Artificial Opening Endoscopic	**Z** No Device	**X** Diagnostic **Z** No Qualifier

Section   **0**   **Medical and Surgical**
Body System   **V**   **Male Reproductive System**
Operation   **C**   **Extirpation:** Taking or cutting out solid matter from a body part

Body Part (4th)	Approach (5th)	Device (6th)	Qualifier (7th)
0 Prostate	**0** Open **3** Percutaneous **4** Percutaneous Endoscopic **7** Via Natural or Artificial Opening **8** Via Natural or Artificial Opening Endoscopic	**Z** No Device	**Z** No Qualifier

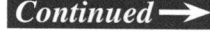
Continued →

Section	0	Medical and Surgical
Body System	V	Male Reproductive System
Operation	C	**Extirpation:** Taking or cutting out solid matter from a body part

Body Part (4th)	Approach (5th)	Device (6th)	Qualifier (7th)
1 Seminal Vesicle, Right 2 Seminal Vesicle, Left 3 Seminal Vesicles, Bilateral 6 Tunica Vaginalis, Right 7 Tunica Vaginalis, Left 9 Testis, Right B Testis, Left C Testes, Bilateral F Spermatic Cord, Right G Spermatic Cord, Left H Spermatic Cords, Bilateral J Epididymis, Right K Epididymis, Left L Epididymis, Bilateral N Vas Deferens, Right P Vas Deferens, Left Q Vas Deferens, Bilateral	0 Open 3 Percutaneous 4 Percutaneous Endoscopic	Z No Device	Z No Qualifier
5 Scrotum S Penis T Prepuce	0 Open 3 Percutaneous 4 Percutaneous Endoscopic X External	Z No Device	Z No Qualifier

Section	0	Medical and Surgical
Body System	V	Male Reproductive System
Operation	H	**Insertion:** Putting in a nonbiological appliance that monitors, assists, performs, or prevents a physiological function but does not physically take the place of a body part

Body Part (4th)	Approach (5th)	Device (6th)	Qualifier (7th)
0 Prostate	0 Open 3 Percutaneous 4 Percutaneous Endoscopic 7 Via Natural or Artificial Opening 8 Via Natural or Artificial Opening Endoscopic	1 Radioactive Element	Z No Qualifier
4 Prostate and Seminal Vesicles 8 Scrotum and Tunica Vaginalis M Epididymis and Spermatic Cord R Vas Deferens	0 Open 3 Percutaneous 4 Percutaneous Endoscopic 7 Via Natural or Artificial Opening 8 Via Natural or Artificial Opening Endoscopic	3 Infusion Device Y Other Device	Z No Qualifier
D Testis	0 Open 3 Percutaneous 4 Percutaneous Endoscopic 7 Via Natural or Artificial Opening 8 Via Natural or Artificial Opening Endoscopic	1 Radioactive Element 3 Infusion Device Y Other Device	Z No Qualifier
S Penis	0 Open 3 Percutaneous 4 Percutaneous Endoscopic	3 Infusion Device Y Other Device	Z No Qualifier
S Penis	7 Via Natural or Artificial Opening 8 Via Natural or Artificial Opening Endoscopic	Y Other Device	Z No Qualifier
S Penis	X External	3 Infusion Device	Z No Qualifier

Section	0	Medical and Surgical
Body System	V	Male Reproductive System
Operation	J	Inspection: Visually and/or manually exploring a body part

Body Part (4th)	Approach (5th)	Device (6th)	Qualifier (7th)
4 Prostate and Seminal Vesicles 8 Scrotum and Tunica Vaginalis D Testis M Epididymis and Spermatic Cord R Vas Deferens S Penis	0 Open 3 Percutaneous 4 Percutaneous Endoscopic X External	Z No Device	Z No Qualifier

Section	0	Medical and Surgical
Body System	V	Male Reproductive System
Operation	L	Occlusion: Completely closing an orifice or the lumen of a tubular body part

Body Part (4th)	Approach (5th)	Device (6th)	Qualifier (7th)
F Spermatic Cord, Right G Spermatic Cord, Left H Spermatic Cords, Bilateral N Vas Deferens, Right P Vas Deferens, Left Q Vas Deferens, Bilateral	0 Open 3 Percutaneous 4 Percutaneous Endoscopic 8 Via Natural or Artificial Opening Endoscopic	C Extraluminal Device D Intraluminal Device Z No Device	Z No Qualifier

Section	0	Medical and Surgical
Body System	V	Male Reproductive System
Operation	M	Reattachment: Putting back in or on all or a portion of a separated body part to its normal location or other suitable location

Body Part (4th)	Approach (5th)	Device (6th)	Qualifier (7th)
5 Scrotum S Penis	X External	Z No Device	Z No Qualifier
6 Tunica Vaginalis, Right 7 Tunica Vaginalis, Left 9 Testis, Right B Testis, Left C Testes, Bilateral F Spermatic Cord, Right G Spermatic Cord, Left H Spermatic Cords, Bilateral	0 Open 4 Percutaneous Endoscopic	Z No Device	Z No Qualifier

Section	0	Medical and Surgical
Body System	V	Male Reproductive System
Operation	N	Release: Freeing a body part from an abnormal physical constraint by cutting or by the use of force

Body Part (4th)	Approach (5th)	Device (6th)	Qualifier (7th)
0 Prostate	0 Open 3 Percutaneous 4 Percutaneous Endoscopic 7 Via Natural or Artificial Opening 8 Via Natural or Artificial Opening Endoscopic	Z No Device	Z No Qualifier
1 Seminal Vesicle, Right 2 Seminal Vesicle, Left 3 Seminal Vesicles, Bilateral 6 Tunica Vaginalis, Right 7 Tunica Vaginalis, Left 9 Testis, Right B Testis, Left C Testes, Bilateral	0 Open 3 Percutaneous 4 Percutaneous Endoscopic	Z No Device	Z No Qualifier

Continued →

Section 0 Medical and Surgical
Body System V Male Reproductive System
Operation N Release: Freeing a body part from an abnormal physical constraint by cutting or by the use of force

Body Part (4th)	Approach (5th)	Device (6th)	Qualifier (7th)
5 Scrotum S Penis T Prepuce	0 Open 3 Percutaneous 4 Percutaneous Endoscopic X External	Z No Device	Z No Qualifier
F Spermatic Cord, Right G Spermatic Cord, Left H Spermatic Cords, Bilateral J Epididymis, Right K Epididymis, Left L Epididymis, Bilateral N Vas Deferens, Right P Vas Deferens, Left Q Vas Deferens, Bilateral	0 Open 3 Percutaneous 4 Percutaneous Endoscopic 8 Via Natural or Artificial Opening Endoscopic	Z No Device	Z No Qualifier

Section 0 Medical and Surgical
Body System V Male Reproductive System
Operation P Removal: Taking out or off a device from a body part

Body Part (4th)	Approach (5th)	Device (6th)	Qualifier (7th)
4 Prostate and Seminal Vesicles	0 Open 3 Percutaneous 4 Percutaneous Endoscopic 7 Via Natural or Artificial Opening 8 Via Natural or Artificial Opening Endoscopic	0 Drainage Device 1 Radioactive Element 3 Infusion Device 7 Autologous Tissue Substitute J Synthetic Substitute K Nonautologous Tissue Substitute Y Other Device	Z No Qualifier
4 Prostate and Seminal Vesicles	X External	0 Drainage Device 1 Radioactive Element 3 Infusion Device	Z No Qualifier
8 Scrotum and Tunica Vaginalis D Testis S Penis	0 Open 3 Percutaneous 4 Percutaneous Endoscopic 7 Via Natural or Artificial Opening 8 Via Natural or Artificial Opening Endoscopic	0 Drainage Device 3 Infusion Device 7 Autologous Tissue Substitute J Synthetic Substitute K Nonautologous Tissue Substitute Y Other Device	Z No Qualifier
8 Scrotum and Tunica Vaginalis D Testis S Penis	X External	0 Drainage Device 3 Infusion Device	Z No Qualifier
M Epididymis and Spermatic Cord	0 Open 3 Percutaneous 4 Percutaneous Endoscopic 7 Via Natural or Artificial Opening 8 Via Natural or Artificial Opening Endoscopic	0 Drainage Device 3 Infusion Device 7 Autologous Tissue Substitute C Extraluminal Device J Synthetic Substitute K Nonautologous Tissue Substitute Y Other Device	Z No Qualifier
M Epididymis and Spermatic Cord	X External	0 Drainage Device 3 Infusion Device	Z No Qualifier
R Vas Deferens	0 Open 3 Percutaneous 4 Percutaneous Endoscopic 7 Via Natural or Artificial Opening 8 Via Natural or Artificial Opening Endoscopic	0 Drainage Device 3 Infusion Device 7 Autologous Tissue Substitute C Extraluminal Device D Intraluminal Device J Synthetic Substitute K Nonautologous Tissue Substitute Y Other Device	Z No Qualifier

Continued ➞

Section	0	Medical and Surgical
Body System	V	Male Reproductive System
Operation	P	**Removal:** Taking out or off a device from a body part

Body Part (4th)	Approach (5th)	Device (6th)	Qualifier (7th)
R Vas Deferens	**X** External	**0** Drainage Device **3** Infusion Device **D** Intraluminal Device	**Z** No Qualifier

Section	0	Medical and Surgical
Body System	V	Male Reproductive System
Operation	Q	**Repair:** Restoring, to the extent possible, a body part to its normal anatomic structure and function

Body Part (4th)	Approach (5th)	Device (6th)	Qualifier (7th)
0 Prostate	**0** Open **3** Percutaneous **4** Percutaneous Endoscopic **7** Via Natural or Artificial Opening **8** Via Natural or Artificial Opening Endoscopic	**Z** No Device	**Z** No Qualifier
1 Seminal Vesicle, Right **2** Seminal Vesicle, Left **3** Seminal Vesicles, Bilateral **6** Tunica Vaginalis, Right **7** Tunica Vaginalis, Left **9** Testis, Right **B** Testis, Left **C** Testes, Bilateral	**0** Open **3** Percutaneous **4** Percutaneous Endoscopic	**Z** No Device	**Z** No Qualifier
5 Scrotum **S** Penis **T** Prepuce	**0** Open **3** Percutaneous **4** Percutaneous Endoscopic **X** External	**Z** No Device	**Z** No Qualifier
F Spermatic Cord, Right **G** Spermatic Cord, Left **H** Spermatic Cords, Bilateral **J** Epididymis, Right **K** Epididymis, Left **L** Epididymis, Bilateral **N** Vas Deferens, Right **P** Vas Deferens, Left **Q** Vas Deferens, Bilateral	**0** Open **3** Percutaneous **4** Percutaneous Endoscopic **8** Via Natural or Artificial Opening Endoscopic	**Z** No Device	**Z** No Qualifier

Section	0	Medical and Surgical
Body System	V	Male Reproductive System
Operation	R	**Replacement:** Putting in or on biological or synthetic material that physically takes the place and/or function of all or a portion of a body part

Body Part (4th)	Approach (5th)	Device (6th)	Qualifier (7th)
9 Testis, Right **B** Testis, Left **C** Testes, Bilateral	**0** Open	**J** Synthetic Substitute	**Z** No Qualifier

Section	0	Medical and Surgical
Body System	V	Male Reproductive System
Operation	S	**Reposition:** Moving to its normal location, or other suitable location, all or a portion of a body part

Body Part (4th)	Approach (5th)	Device (6th)	Qualifier (7th)
9 Testis, Right **B** Testis, Left **C** Testes, Bilateral **F** Spermatic Cord, Right **G** Spermatic Cord, Left **H** Spermatic Cords, Bilateral	**0** Open **3** Percutaneous **4** Percutaneous Endoscopic **8** Via Natural or Artificial Opening Endoscopic	**Z** No Device	**Z** No Qualifier

Section	0	Medical and Surgical
Body System	V	Male Reproductive System
Operation	T	Resection: Cutting out or off, without replacement, all of a body part

Body Part (4th)	Approach (5th)	Device (6th)	Qualifier (7th)
0 Prostate	0 Open 4 Percutaneous Endoscopic 7 Via Natural or Artificial Opening 8 Via Natural or Artificial Opening Endoscopic	Z No Device	Z No Qualifier
1 Seminal Vesicle, Right 2 Seminal Vesicle, Left 3 Seminal Vesicles, Bilateral 6 Tunica Vaginalis, Right 7 Tunica Vaginalis, Left 9 Testis, Right B Testis, Left C Testes, Bilateral F Spermatic Cord, Right G Spermatic Cord, Left H Spermatic Cords, Bilateral J Epididymis, Right K Epididymis, Left L Epididymis, Bilateral N Vas Deferens, Right P Vas Deferens, Left Q Vas Deferens, Bilateral	0 Open 4 Percutaneous Endoscopic	Z No Device	Z No Qualifier
5 Scrotum S Penis T Prepuce	0 Open 4 Percutaneous Endoscopic X External	Z No Device	Z No Qualifier

Section	0	Medical and Surgical
Body System	V	Male Reproductive System
Operation	U	Supplement: Putting in or on biological or synthetic material that physically reinforces and/or augments the function of a portion of a body part

Body Part (4th)	Approach (5th)	Device (6th)	Qualifier (7th)
1 Seminal Vesicle, Right 2 Seminal Vesicle, Left 3 Seminal Vesicles, Bilateral 6 Tunica Vaginalis, Right 7 Tunica Vaginalis, Left F Spermatic Cord, Right G Spermatic Cord, Left H Spermatic Cords, Bilateral J Epididymis, Right K Epididymis, Left L Epididymis, Bilateral N Vas Deferens, Right P Vas Deferens, Left Q Vas Deferens, Bilateral	0 Open 4 Percutaneous Endoscopic 8 Via Natural or Artificial Opening Endoscopic	7 Autologous Tissue Substitute J Synthetic Substitute K Nonautologous Tissue Substitute	Z No Qualifier
5 Scrotum S Penis T Prepuce	0 Open 4 Percutaneous Endoscopic X External	7 Autologous Tissue Substitute J Synthetic Substitute K Nonautologous Tissue Substitute	Z No Qualifier
9 Testis, Right B Testis, Left C Testes, Bilateral	0 Open	7 Autologous Tissue Substitute J Synthetic Substitute K Nonautologous Tissue Substitute	Z No Qualifier

Section	0	Medical and Surgical
Body System	V	Male Reproductive System
Operation	W	**Revision:** Correcting, to the extent possible, a portion of a malfunctioning device or the position of a displaced device

Body Part (4th)	Approach (5th)	Device (6th)	Qualifier (7th)
4 Prostate and Seminal Vesicles 8 Scrotum and Tunica Vaginalis D Testis S Penis	0 Open 3 Percutaneous 4 Percutaneous Endoscopic 7 Via Natural or Artificial Opening 8 Via Natural or Artificial Opening Endoscopic	0 Drainage Device 3 Infusion Device 7 Autologous Tissue Substitute J Synthetic Substitute K Nonautologous Tissue Substitute Y Other Device	Z No Qualifier
4 Prostate and Seminal Vesicles 8 Scrotum and Tunica Vaginalis D Testis S Penis	X External	0 Drainage Device 3 Infusion Device 7 Autologous Tissue Substitute J Synthetic Substitute K Nonautologous Tissue Substitute	Z No Qualifier
M Epididymis and Spermatic Cord	0 Open 3 Percutaneous 4 Percutaneous Endoscopic 7 Via Natural or Artificial Opening 8 Via Natural or Artificial Opening Endoscopic	0 Drainage Device 3 Infusion Device 7 Autologous Tissue Substitute C Extraluminal Device J Synthetic Substitute K Nonautologous Tissue Substitute Y Other Device	Z No Qualifier
M Epididymis and Spermatic Cord	X External	0 Drainage Device 3 Infusion Device 7 Autologous Tissue Substitute C Extraluminal Device J Synthetic Substitute K Nonautologous Tissue Substitute	Z No Qualifier
R Vas Deferens	0 Open 3 Percutaneous 4 Percutaneous Endoscopic 7 Via Natural or Artificial Opening 8 Via Natural or Artificial Opening Endoscopic	0 Drainage Device 3 Infusion Device 7 Autologous Tissue Substitute C Extraluminal Device D Intraluminal Device J Synthetic Substitute K Nonautologous Tissue Substitute Y Other Device	Z No Qualifier
R Vas Deferens	X External	0 Drainage Device 3 Infusion Device 7 Autologous Tissue Substitute C Extraluminal Device C Intraluminal Device J Synthetic Substitute K Nonautologous Tissue Substitute	Z No Qualifier

Section	0	Medical and Surgical
Body System	V	Male Reproductive System
Operation	X	**Transfer:** Moving, without taking out, all or a portion of a body part to another location to take over the function of all or a portion of a body part

Body Part (4th)	Approach (5th)	Device (6th)	Qualifier (7th)
T Prepuce	0 Open X External	Z No Device	D Urethra S Penis

Section	0	Medical and Surgical
Body System	V	Male Reproductive System
Operation	Y	**Transplantation:** Putting in or on all or a portion of a living body part taken from another individual or animal to physically take the place and/or function of all or a portion of a similar body part

Body Part (4th)	Approach (5th)	Device (6th)	Qualifier (7th)
5 Scrotum S Penis	0 Open	Z No Device	0 Allogeneic 1 Syngeneic 2 Zooplastic

Review Coding Guideline B3.6a

♂ **0V1N07J** Bypass Right Vas Deferens to Right Epididymis with Autologous Tissue Substitute, Open Approach

♂ **0V1N07K** Bypass Right Vas Deferens to Left Epididymis with Autologous Tissue Substitute, Open Approach

♂ **0V1N07N** Bypass Right Vas Deferens to Right Vas Deferens with Autologous Tissue Substitute, Open Approach

♂ **0V1N07P** Bypass Right Vas Deferens to Left Vas Deferens with Autologous Tissue Substitute, Open Approach

♂ **0V1N0JJ** Bypass Right Vas Deferens to Right Epididymis with Synthetic Substitute, Open Approach

♂ **0V1N0JK** Bypass Right Vas Deferens to Left Epididymis with Synthetic Substitute, Open Approach

♂ **0V1N0JN** Bypass Right Vas Deferens to Right Vas Deferens with Synthetic Substitute, Open Approach

♂ **0V1N0JP** Bypass Right Vas Deferens to Left Vas Deferens with Synthetic Substitute, Open Approach

♂ **0V1N0KJ** Bypass Right Vas Deferens to Right Epididymis with Nonautologous Tissue Substitute, Open Approach

♂ **0V1N0KK** Bypass Right Vas Deferens to Left Epididymis with Nonautologous Tissue Substitute, Open Approach

♂ **0V1N0KN** Bypass Right Vas Deferens to Right Vas Deferens with Nonautologous Tissue Substitute, Open Approach

♂ **0V1N0KP** Bypass Right Vas Deferens to Left Vas Deferens with Nonautologous Tissue Substitute, Open Approach

♂ **0V1N0ZJ** Bypass Right Vas Deferens to Right Epididymis, Open Approach

♂ **0V1N0ZK** Bypass Right Vas Deferens to Left Epididymis, Open Approach

♂ **0V1N0ZN** Bypass Right Vas Deferens to Right Vas Deferens, Open Approach

♂ **0V1N0ZP** Bypass Right Vas Deferens to Left Vas Deferens, Open Approach

♂ **0V1N47J** Bypass Right Vas Deferens to Right Epididymis with Autologous Tissue Substitute, Percutaneous Endoscopic Approach

♂ **0V1N47K** Bypass Right Vas Deferens to Left Epididymis with Autologous Tissue Substitute, Percutaneous Endoscopic Approach

♂ **0V1N47N** Bypass Right Vas Deferens to Right Vas Deferens with Autologous Tissue Substitute, Percutaneous Endoscopic Approach

♂ **0V1N47P** Bypass Right Vas Deferens to Left Vas Deferens with Autologous Tissue Substitute, Percutaneous Endoscopic Approach

♂ **0V1N4JJ** Bypass Right Vas Deferens to Right Epididymis with Synthetic Substitute, Percutaneous Endoscopic Approach

♂ **0V1N4JK** Bypass Right Vas Deferens to Left Epididymis with Synthetic Substitute, Percutaneous Endoscopic Approach

♂ **0V1N4JN** Bypass Right Vas Deferens to Right Vas Deferens with Synthetic Substitute, Percutaneous Endoscopic Approach

♂ **0V1N4JP** Bypass Right Vas Deferens to Left Vas Deferens with Synthetic Substitute, Percutaneous Endoscopic Approach

♂ **0V1N4KJ** Bypass Right Vas Deferens to Right Epididymis with Nonautologous Tissue Substitute, Percutaneous Endoscopic Approach

♂ **0V1N4KK** Bypass Right Vas Deferens to Left Epididymis with Nonautologous Tissue Substitute, Percutaneous Endoscopic Approach

♂ **0V1N4KN** Bypass Right Vas Deferens to Right Vas Deferens with Nonautologous Tissue Substitute, Percutaneous Endoscopic Approach

♂ **0V1N4KP** Bypass Right Vas Deferens to Left Vas Deferens with Nonautologous Tissue Substitute, Percutaneous Endoscopic Approach

♂ **0V1N4ZJ** Bypass Right Vas Deferens to Right Epididymis, Percutaneous Endoscopic Approach

♂ **0V1N4ZK** Bypass Right Vas Deferens to Left Epididymis, Percutaneous Endoscopic Approach

♂ **0V1N4ZN** Bypass Right Vas Deferens to Right Vas Deferens, Percutaneous Endoscopic Approach

♂ **0V1N4ZP** Bypass Right Vas Deferens to Left Vas Deferens, Percutaneous Endoscopic Approach

♂ **0V1P07J** Bypass Left Vas Deferens to Right Epididymis with Autologous Tissue Substitute, Open Approach

♂ **0V1P07K** Bypass Left Vas Deferens to Left Epididymis with Autologous Tissue Substitute, Open Approach

♂ **0V1P07N** Bypass Left Vas Deferens to Right Vas Deferens with Autologous Tissue Substitute, Open Approach

♂ **0V1P07P** Bypass Left Vas Deferens to Left Vas Deferens with Autologous Tissue Substitute, Open Approach

♂ **0V1P0JJ** Bypass Left Vas Deferens to Right Epididymis with Synthetic Substitute, Open Approach

♂ **0V1P0JK** Bypass Left Vas Deferens to Left Epididymis with Synthetic Substitute, Open Approach

♂ **0V1P0JN** Bypass Left Vas Deferens to Right Vas Deferens with Synthetic Substitute, Open Approach

♂ **0V1P0JP** Bypass Left Vas Deferens to Left Vas Deferens with Synthetic Substitute, Open Approach

♂ **0V1P0KJ** Bypass Left Vas Deferens to Right Epididymis with Nonautologous Tissue Substitute, Open Approach

♂ **0V1P0KK** Bypass Left Vas Deferens to Left Epididymis with Nonautologous Tissue Substitute, Open Approach

♂ **0V1P0KN** Bypass Left Vas Deferens to Right Vas Deferens with Nonautologous Tissue Substitute, Open Approach

♂ **0V1P0KP** Bypass Left Vas Deferens to Left Vas Deferens with Nonautologous Tissue Substitute, Open Approach

♂ **0V1P0ZJ** Bypass Left Vas Deferens to Right Epididymis, Open Approach

♂ **0V1P0ZK** Bypass Left Vas Deferens to Left Epididymis, Open Approach

♂ **0V1P0ZN** Bypass Left Vas Deferens to Right Vas Deferens, Open Approach

♂ **0V1P0ZP** Bypass Left Vas Deferens to Left Vas Deferens, Open Approach

♂ **0V1P47J** Bypass Left Vas Deferens to Right Epididymis with Autologous Tissue Substitute, Percutaneous Endoscopic Approach

♂ **0V1P47K** Bypass Left Vas Deferens to Left Epididymis with Autologous Tissue Substitute, Percutaneous Endoscopic Approach

♂ **0V1P47N** Bypass Left Vas Deferens to Right Vas Deferens with Autologous Tissue Substitute, Percutaneous Endoscopic Approach

♂ **0V1P47P** Bypass Left Vas Deferens to Left Vas Deferens with Autologous Tissue Substitute, Percutaneous Endoscopic Approach

♂ **0V1P4JJ** Bypass Left Vas Deferens to Right Epididymis with Synthetic Substitute, Percutaneous Endoscopic Approach

♂ **0V1P4JK** Bypass Left Vas Deferens to Left Epididymis with Synthetic Substitute, Percutaneous Endoscopic Approach

♂ **0V1P4JN** Bypass Left Vas Deferens to Right Vas Deferens with Synthetic Substitute, Percutaneous Endoscopic Approach

♂ **0V1P4JP** Bypass Left Vas Deferens to Left Vas Deferens with Synthetic Substitute, Percutaneous Endoscopic Approach

♂ **0V1P4KJ** Bypass Left Vas Deferens to Right Epididymis with Nonautologous Tissue Substitute, Percutaneous Endoscopic Approach

♂ **0V1P4KK** Bypass Left Vas Deferens to Left Epididymis with Nonautologous Tissue Substitute, Percutaneous Endoscopic Approach

♂ **0V1P4KN** Bypass Left Vas Deferens to Right Vas Deferens with Nonautologous Tissue Substitute, Percutaneous Endoscopic Approach

♂ **0V1P4KP** Bypass Left Vas Deferens to Left Vas Deferens with Nonautologous Tissue Substitute, Percutaneous Endoscopic Approach

♂ **0V1P4ZJ** Bypass Left Vas Deferens to Right Epididymis, Percutaneous Endoscopic Approach

♂ **0V1P4ZK** Bypass Left Vas Deferens to Left Epididymis, Percutaneous Endoscopic Approach

♂ **0V1P4ZN** Bypass Left Vas Deferens to Right Vas Deferens, Percutaneous Endoscopic Approach

♂ **0V1P4ZP** Bypass Left Vas Deferens to Left Vas Deferens, Percutaneous Endoscopic Approach

♂ **0V1Q07J** Bypass Bilateral Vas Deferens to Right Epididymis with Autologous Tissue Substitute, Open Approach

♂ **0V1Q07K** Bypass Bilateral Vas Deferens to Left Epididymis with Autologous Tissue Substitute, Open Approach

♂ **0V1Q07N** Bypass Bilateral Vas Deferens to Right Vas Deferens with Autologous Tissue Substitute, Open Approach

♂ **0V1Q07P** Bypass Bilateral Vas Deferens to Left Vas Deferens with Autologous Tissue Substitute, Open Approach

♂ **0V1Q0JJ** Bypass Bilateral Vas Deferens to Right Epididymis with Synthetic Substitute, Open Approach

♂ **0V1Q0JK** Bypass Bilateral Vas Deferens to Left Epididymis with Synthetic Substitute, Open Approach

♂ **0V1Q0JN** Bypass Bilateral Vas Deferens to Right Vas Deferens with Synthetic Substitute, Open Approach

♂ **0V1Q0JP** Bypass Bilateral Vas Deferens to Left Vas Deferens with Synthetic Substitute, Open Approach

♂ **0V1Q0KJ** Bypass Bilateral Vas Deferens to Right Epididymis with Nonautologous Tissue Substitute, Open Approach

♂ **0V1Q0KK** Bypass Bilateral Vas Deferens to Left Epididymis with Nonautologous Tissue Substitute, Open Approach

♂ **0V1Q0KN** Bypass Bilateral Vas Deferens to Right Vas Deferens with Nonautologous Tissue Substitute, Open Approach

♂ **0V1Q0KP** Bypass Bilateral Vas Deferens to Left Vas Deferens with Nonautologous Tissue Substitute, Open Approach

♂ **0V1Q0ZJ** Bypass Bilateral Vas Deferens to Right Epididymis, Open Approach

♂ **0V1Q0ZK** Bypass Bilateral Vas Deferens to Left Epididymis, Open Approach

♂ **0V1Q0ZN** Bypass Bilateral Vas Deferens to Right Vas Deferens, Open Approach

♂ **0V1Q0ZP** Bypass Bilateral Vas Deferens to Left Vas Deferens, Open Approach

♂ **0V1Q47J** Bypass Bilateral Vas Deferens to Right Epididymis with Autologous Tissue Substitute, Percutaneous Endoscopic Approach

♂ **0V1Q47K** Bypass Bilateral Vas Deferens to Left Epididymis with Autologous Tissue Substitute, Percutaneous Endoscopic Approach

♂ **0V1Q47N** Bypass Bilateral Vas Deferens to Right Vas Deferens with Autologous Tissue Substitute, Percutaneous Endoscopic Approach

♂ **0V1Q47P** Bypass Bilateral Vas Deferens to Left Vas Deferens with Autologous Tissue Substitute, Percutaneous Endoscopic Approach

♂ **0V1Q4JJ** Bypass Bilateral Vas Deferens to Right Epididymis with Synthetic Substitute, Percutaneous Endoscopic Approach

♂ **0V1Q4JK** Bypass Bilateral Vas Deferens to Left Epididymis with Synthetic Substitute, Percutaneous Endoscopic Approach

♂ **0V1Q4JN** Bypass Bilateral Vas Deferens to Right Vas Deferens with Synthetic Substitute, Percutaneous Endoscopic Approach

♂ **0V1Q4JP** Bypass Bilateral Vas Deferens to Left Vas Deferens with Synthetic Substitute, Percutaneous Endoscopic Approach

♂ **0V1Q4KJ** Bypass Bilateral Vas Deferens to Right Epididymis with Nonautologous Tissue Substitute, Percutaneous Endoscopic Approach

♂ **0V1Q4KK** Bypass Bilateral Vas Deferens to Left Epididymis with Nonautologous Tissue Substitute, Percutaneous Endoscopic Approach

♂ **0V1Q4KN** Bypass Bilateral Vas Deferens to Right Vas Deferens with Nonautologous Tissue Substitute, Percutaneous Endoscopic Approach

♂ **0V1Q4KP** Bypass Bilateral Vas Deferens to Left Vas Deferens with Nonautologous Tissue Substitute, Percutaneous Endoscopic Approach

♂ **0V1Q4ZJ** Bypass Bilateral Vas Deferens to Right Epididymis, Percutaneous Endoscopic Approach

♂ **0V1Q4ZK** Bypass Bilateral Vas Deferens to Left Epididymis, Percutaneous Endoscopic Approach

♂ **0V1Q4ZN** Bypass Bilateral Vas Deferens to Right Vas Deferens, Percutaneous Endoscopic Approach

♂ **0V1Q4ZP** Bypass Bilateral Vas Deferens to Left Vas Deferens, Percutaneous Endoscopic Approach

0V2 – Male Reproductive System, Change

Review Coding Guideline B6.1c

♂ **0V24X0Z** Change Drainage Device in Prostate and Seminal Vesicles, External Approach

♂ **0V24XYZ** Change Other Device in Prostate and Seminal Vesicles, External Approach

♂ **0V28X0Z** Change Drainage Device in Scrotum and Tunica Vaginalis, External Approach

♂ **0V28XYZ** Change Other Device in Scrotum and Tunica Vaginalis, External Approach

♂ **0V2DX0Z** Change Drainage Device in Testis, External Approach

♂ **0V2DXYZ** Change Other Device in Testis, External Approach

♂ **0V2MX0Z** Change Drainage Device in Epididymis and Spermatic Cord, External Approach

♂ **0V2MXYZ** Change Other Device in Epididymis and Spermatic Cord, External Approach

♂ **0V2RX0Z** Change Drainage Device in Vas Deferens, External Approach

♂ **0V2RXYZ** Change Other Device in Vas Deferens, External Approach

♂ **0V2SX0Z** Change Drainage Device in Penis, External Approach

♂ **0V2SXYZ** Change Other Device in Penis, External Approach

0V5 – Male Reproductive System, Destruction

♂ **0V500ZZ** Destruction of Prostate, Open Approach

♂ **0V503ZZ** Destruction of Prostate, Percutaneous Approach

♂ **0V504ZZ** Destruction of Prostate, Percutaneous Endoscopic Approach

♂ **0V507ZZ** Destruction of Prostate, Via Natural or Artificial Opening

♂ **0V508ZZ** Destruction of Prostate, Via Natural or Artificial Opening Endoscopic

♂ **0V510ZZ** Destruction of Right Seminal Vesicle, Open Approach

♂ **0V513ZZ** Destruction of Right Seminal Vesicle, Percutaneous Approach

♂ **0V514ZZ** Destruction of Right Seminal Vesicle, Percutaneous Endoscopic Approach

♂ **0V520ZZ** Destruction of Left Seminal Vesicle, Open Approach

♂ **0V523ZZ** Destruction of Left Seminal Vesicle, Percutaneous Approach

♂ **0V524ZZ** Destruction of Left Seminal Vesicle, Percutaneous Endoscopic Approach

♂ **0V530ZZ** Destruction of Bilateral Seminal Vesicles, Open Approach

♂ **0V533ZZ** Destruction of Bilateral Seminal Vesicles, Percutaneous Approach

♂ **0V534ZZ** Destruction of Bilateral Seminal Vesicles, Percutaneous Endoscopic Approach

♂ **0V550ZZ** Destruction of Scrotum, Open Approach

♂ **0V553ZZ** Destruction of Scrotum, Percutaneous Approach

♂ **0V554ZZ** Destruction of Scrotum, Percutaneous Endoscopic Approach

♂ **0V55XZZ** Destruction of Scrotum, External Approach

♂ **0V560ZZ** Destruction of Right Tunica Vaginalis, Open Approach

♂ **0V563ZZ** Destruction of Right Tunica Vaginalis, Percutaneous Approach

♂ **0V564ZZ** Destruction of Right Tunica Vaginalis, Percutaneous Endoscopic Approach

♂ **0V570ZZ** Destruction of Left Tunica Vaginalis, Open Approach

♂ **0V573ZZ** Destruction of Left Tunica Vaginalis, Percutaneous Approach

♂ **0V574ZZ** Destruction of Left Tunica Vaginalis, Percutaneous Endoscopic Approach

♂ **0V590ZZ** Destruction of Right Testis, Open Approach

♂ **0V593ZZ** Destruction of Right Testis, Percutaneous Approach

♂ **0V594ZZ** Destruction of Right Testis, Percutaneous Endoscopic Approach

♂ **0V5B0ZZ** Destruction of Left Testis, Open Approach

♂ **0V5B3ZZ** Destruction of Left Testis, Percutaneous Approach

♂ **0V5B4ZZ** Destruction of Left Testis, Percutaneous Endoscopic Approach

♂ **0V5C0ZZ** Destruction of Bilateral Testes, Open Approach

♂ **0V5C3ZZ** Destruction of Bilateral Testes, Percutaneous Approach

♂ **0V5C4ZZ** Destruction of Bilateral Testes, Percutaneous Endoscopic Approach

♂ **0V5F0ZZ** Destruction of Right Spermatic Cord, Open Approach

♂ **0V5F3ZZ** Destruction of Right Spermatic Cord, Percutaneous Approach

♂ **0V5F4ZZ** Destruction of Right Spermatic Cord, Percutaneous Endoscopic Approach

♂ **0V5F8ZZ** Destruction of Right Spermatic Cord, Via Natural or Artificial Opening Endoscopic

♂ **0V5G0ZZ** Destruction of Left Spermatic Cord, Open Approach

♂ **0V5G3ZZ** Destruction of Left Spermatic Cord, Percutaneous Approach

 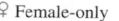

♂ **0V5G4ZZ** Destruction of Left Spermatic Cord, Percutaneous Endoscopic Approach

♂ **0V5G8ZZ** Destruction of Left Spermatic Cord, Via Natural or Artificial Opening Endoscopic

♂ **0V5H0ZZ** Destruction of Bilateral Spermatic Cords, Open Approach

♂ **0V5H3ZZ** Destruction of Bilateral Spermatic Cords, Percutaneous Approach

♂ **0V5H4ZZ** Destruction of Bilateral Spermatic Cords, Percutaneous Endoscopic Approach

♂ **0V5H8ZZ** Destruction of Bilateral Spermatic Cords, Via Natural or Artificial Opening Endoscopic

♂ **0V5J0ZZ** Destruction of Right Epididymis, Open Approach

♂ **0V5J3ZZ** Destruction of Right Epididymis, Percutaneous Approach

♂ **0V5J4ZZ** Destruction of Right Epididymis, Percutaneous Endoscopic Approach

♂ **0V5J8ZZ** Destruction of Right Epididymis, Via Natural or Artificial Opening Endoscopic

♂ **0V5K0ZZ** Destruction of Left Epididymis, Open Approach

♂ **0V5K3ZZ** Destruction of Left Epididymis, Percutaneous Approach

♂ **0V5K4ZZ** Destruction of Left Epididymis, Percutaneous Endoscopic Approach

♂ **0V5K8ZZ** Destruction of Left Epididymis, Via Natural or Artificial Opening Endoscopic

♂ **0V5L0ZZ** Destruction of Bilateral Epididymis, Open Approach

♂ **0V5L3ZZ** Destruction of Bilateral Epididymis, Percutaneous Approach

♂ **0V5L4ZZ** Destruction of Bilateral Epididymis, Percutaneous Endoscopic Approach

♂ **0V5L8ZZ** Destruction of Bilateral Epididymis, Via Natural or Artificial Opening Endoscopic

♂ **0V5N0ZZ** Destruction of Right Vas Deferens, Open Approach
  ▲ *When reported with diagnosis code Z30.2*

♂ **0V5N3ZZ** Destruction of Right Vas Deferens, Percutaneous Approach
  ▲ *When reported with diagnosis code Z30.2*

♂ **0V5N4ZZ** Destruction of Right Vas Deferens, Percutaneous Endoscopic Approach
  ▲ *When reported with diagnosis code Z30.2*

♂ **0V5N8ZZ** Destruction of Right Vas Deferens, Via Natural or Artificial Opening Endoscopic

♂ **0V5P0ZZ** Destruction of Left Vas Deferens, Open Approach
  ▲ *When reported with diagnosis code Z30.2*

♂ **0V5P3ZZ** Destruction of Left Vas Deferens, Percutaneous Approach
  ▲ *When reported with diagnosis code Z30.2*

♂ **0V5P4ZZ** Destruction of Left Vas Deferens, Percutaneous Endoscopic Approach
  ▲ *When reported with diagnosis code Z30.2*

♂ **0V5P8ZZ** Destruction of Left Vas Deferens, Via Natural or Artificial Opening Endoscopic

♂ **0V5Q0ZZ** Destruction of Bilateral Vas Deferens, Open Approach
  ▲ *When reported with diagnosis code Z30.2*

♂ **0V5Q3ZZ** Destruction of Bilateral Vas Deferens, Percutaneous Approach
  ▲ *When reported with diagnosis code Z30.2*

♂ **0V5Q4ZZ** Destruction of Bilateral Vas Deferens, Percutaneous Endoscopic Approach
  ▲ *When reported with diagnosis code Z30.2*

♂ **0V5Q8ZZ** Destruction of Bilateral Vas Deferens, Via Natural or Artificial Opening Endoscopic

♂ **0V5S0ZZ** Destruction of Penis, Open Approach

♂ **0V5S3ZZ** Destruction of Penis, Percutaneous Approach

♂ **0V5S4ZZ** Destruction of Penis, Percutaneous Endoscopic Approach

♂ **0V5SXZZ** Destruction of Penis, External Approach

♂ **0V5T0ZZ** Destruction of Prepuce, Open Approach

♂ **0V5T3ZZ** Destruction of Prepuce, Percutaneous Approach

♂ **0V5T4ZZ** Destruction of Prepuce, Percutaneous Endoscopic Approach

♂ **0V5TXZZ** Destruction of Prepuce, External Approach

0V7 – Male Reproductive System, Dilation

♂ **0V7N0DZ** Dilation of Right Vas Deferens with Intraluminal Device, Open Approach

♂ **0V7N0ZZ** Dilation of Right Vas Deferens, Open Approach

♂ **0V7N3DZ** Dilation of Right Vas Deferens with Intraluminal Device, Percutaneous Approach

♂ **0V7N3ZZ** Dilation of Right Vas Deferens, Percutaneous Approach

♂ **0V7N4DZ** Dilation of Right Vas Deferens with Intraluminal Device, Percutaneous Endoscopic Approach

♂ **0V7N4ZZ** Dilation of Right Vas Deferens, Percutaneous Endoscopic Approach

♂ **0V7P0DZ** Dilation of Left Vas Deferens with Intraluminal Device, Open Approach

♂ **0V7P0ZZ** Dilation of Left Vas Deferens, Open Approach

♂ **0V7P3DZ** Dilation of Left Vas Deferens with Intraluminal Device, Percutaneous Approach

♂ **0V7P3ZZ** Dilation of Left Vas Deferens, Percutaneous Approach

♂ **0V7P4DZ** Dilation of Left Vas Deferens with Intraluminal Device, Percutaneous Endoscopic Approach

♂ **0V7P4ZZ** Dilation of Left Vas Deferens, Percutaneous Endoscopic Approach

♂ **0V7Q0DZ** Dilation of Bilateral Vas Deferens with Intraluminal Device, Open Approach

♂ **0V7Q0ZZ** Dilation of Bilateral Vas Deferens, Open Approach

♂ **0V7Q3DZ** Dilation of Bilateral Vas Deferens with Intraluminal Device, Percutaneous Approach

♂ **0V7Q3ZZ** Dilation of Bilateral Vas Deferens, Percutaneous Approach

♂ **0V7Q4DZ** Dilation of Bilateral Vas Deferens with Intraluminal Device, Percutaneous Endoscopic Approach

♂ **0V7Q4ZZ** Dilation of Bilateral Vas Deferens, Percutaneous Endoscopic Approach

0V9 – Male Reproductive System, Drainage

Review Coding Guidelines B3.4a and B3.4b

Review Coding Guideline B6.2

♂ **0V9000Z** Drainage of Prostate with Drainage Device, Open Approach

♂ **0V900ZX** Drainage of Prostate, Open Approach, Diagnostic

♂ **0V900ZZ** Drainage of Prostate, Open Approach

♂ **0V9030Z** Drainage of Prostate with Drainage Device, Percutaneous Approach

♂ **0V903ZX** Drainage of Prostate, Percutaneous Approach, Diagnostic

♂ **0V903ZZ** Drainage of Prostate, Percutaneous Approach

♂ **0V9040Z** Drainage of Prostate with Drainage Device, Percutaneous Endoscopic Approach

♂ **0V904ZX** Drainage of Prostate, Percutaneous Endoscopic Approach, Diagnostic

♂ **0V904ZZ** Drainage of Prostate, Percutaneous Endoscopic Approach

♂ **0V9070Z** Drainage of Prostate with Drainage Device, Via Natural or Artificial Opening

♂ **0V907ZX** Drainage of Prostate, Via Natural or Artificial Opening, Diagnostic

♂ **0V907ZZ** Drainage of Prostate, Via Natural or Artificial Opening

♂ **0V9080Z** Drainage of Prostate with Drainage Device, Via Natural or Artificial Opening Endoscopic

♂ **0V908ZX** Drainage of Prostate, Via Natural or Artificial Opening Endoscopic, Diagnostic

♂ **0V908ZZ** Drainage of Prostate, Via Natural or Artificial Opening Endoscopic

♂ **0V9100Z** Drainage of Right Seminal Vesicle with Drainage Device, Open Approach

♂ **0V910ZX** Drainage of Right Seminal Vesicle, Open Approach, Diagnostic

♂ **0V910ZZ** Drainage of Right Seminal Vesicle, Open Approach

♂ **0V9130Z** Drainage of Right Seminal Vesicle with Drainage Device, Percutaneous Approach

♂ **0V913ZX** Drainage of Right Seminal Vesicle, Percutaneous Approach, Diagnostic

♂ **0V913ZZ** Drainage of Right Seminal Vesicle, Percutaneous Approach

♂ **0V9140Z** Drainage of Right Seminal Vesicle with Drainage Device, Percutaneous Endoscopic Approach

♂ **0V914ZX** Drainage of Right Seminal Vesicle, Percutaneous Endoscopic Approach, Diagnostic

♂ **0V914ZZ** Drainage of Right Seminal Vesicle, Percutaneous Endoscopic Approach

♂ **0V9200Z** Drainage of Left Seminal Vesicle with Drainage Device, Open Approach

♂ **0V920ZX** Drainage of Left Seminal Vesicle, Open Approach, Diagnostic

♂ **0V920ZZ** Drainage of Left Seminal Vesicle, Open Approach

♂ **0V9230Z** Drainage of Left Seminal Vesicle with Drainage Device, Percutaneous Approach

♂ **0V923ZX** Drainage of Left Seminal Vesicle, Percutaneous Approach, Diagnostic

♂ **0V923ZZ** Drainage of Left Seminal Vesicle, Percutaneous Approach

♂ **0V9240Z** Drainage of Left Seminal Vesicle with Drainage Device, Percutaneous Endoscopic Approach

♂ **0V924ZX** Drainage of Left Seminal Vesicle, Percutaneous Endoscopic Approach, Diagnostic

♂ **0V924ZZ** Drainage of Left Seminal Vesicle, Percutaneous Endoscopic Approach

♂ **0V9300Z** Drainage of Bilateral Seminal Vesicles with Drainage Device, Open Approach

♂ **0V930ZX** Drainage of Bilateral Seminal Vesicles, Open Approach, Diagnostic

♂ **0V930ZZ** Drainage of Bilateral Seminal Vesicles, Open Approach

♂ **0V9330Z** Drainage of Bilateral Seminal Vesicles with Drainage Device, Percutaneous Approach

♂ **0V933ZX** Drainage of Bilateral Seminal Vesicles, Percutaneous Approach, Diagnostic

♂ **0V933ZZ** Drainage of Bilateral Seminal Vesicles, Percutaneous Approach

♂ **0V9340Z** Drainage of Bilateral Seminal Vesicles with Drainage Device, Percutaneous Endoscopic Approach

♂ **0V934ZX** Drainage of Bilateral Seminal Vesicles, Percutaneous Endoscopic Approach, Diagnostic

♂ **0V934ZZ** Drainage of Bilateral Seminal Vesicles, Percutaneous Endoscopic Approach

♂ **0V9500Z** Drainage of Scrotum with Drainage Device, Open Approach

♂ **0V950ZX** Drainage of Scrotum, Open Approach, Diagnostic

♂ **0V950ZZ** Drainage of Scrotum, Open Approach

♂ **0V9530Z** Drainage of Scrotum with Drainage Device, Percutaneous Approach

♂ **0V953ZX** Drainage of Scrotum, Percutaneous Approach, Diagnostic

♂ **0V953ZZ** Drainage of Scrotum, Percutaneous Approach

♂ **0V9540Z** Drainage of Scrotum with Drainage Device, Percutaneous Endoscopic Approach

♂ **0V954ZX** Drainage of Scrotum, Percutaneous Endoscopic Approach, Diagnostic

♂ **0V954ZZ** Drainage of Scrotum, Percutaneous Endoscopic Approach

♂ **0V95X0Z** Drainage of Scrotum with Drainage Device, External Approach

♂ **0V95XZX** Drainage of Scrotum, External Approach, Diagnostic

♂ **0V95XZZ** Drainage of Scrotum, External Approach

♂ **0V9600Z** Drainage of Right Tunica Vaginalis with Drainage Device, Open Approach

♂ **0V960ZX** Drainage of Right Tunica Vaginalis, Open Approach, Diagnostic

♂ **0V960ZZ** Drainage of Right Tunica Vaginalis, Open Approach

♂ **0V9630Z** Drainage of Right Tunica Vaginalis with Drainage Device, Percutaneous Approach

♂ **0V963ZX** Drainage of Right Tunica Vaginalis, Percutaneous Approach, Diagnostic

♂ **0V963ZZ** Drainage of Right Tunica Vaginalis, Percutaneous Approach

♂ **0V9640Z** Drainage of Right Tunica Vaginalis with Drainage Device, Percutaneous Endoscopic Approach

♂ **0V964ZX** Drainage of Right Tunica Vaginalis, Percutaneous Endoscopic Approach, Diagnostic

♂ **0V964ZZ** Drainage of Right Tunica Vaginalis, Percutaneous Endoscopic Approach

♂ **0V9700Z** Drainage of Left Tunica Vaginalis with Drainage Device, Open Approach

♂ **0V970ZX** Drainage of Left Tunica Vaginalis, Open Approach, Diagnostic

♂ **0V970ZZ** Drainage of Left Tunica Vaginalis, Open Approach

♂ **0V9730Z** Drainage of Left Tunica Vaginalis with Drainage Device, Percutaneous Approach

♂ **0V973ZX** Drainage of Left Tunica Vaginalis, Percutaneous Approach, Diagnostic

♂ **0V973ZZ** Drainage of Left Tunica Vaginalis, Percutaneous Approach

♂ **0V9740Z** Drainage of Left Tunica Vaginalis with Drainage Device, Percutaneous Endoscopic Approach

♂ **0V974ZX** Drainage of Left Tunica Vaginalis, Percutaneous Endoscopic Approach, Diagnostic

♂ **0V974ZZ** Drainage of Left Tunica Vaginalis, Percutaneous Endoscopic Approach

♂ **0V9900Z** Drainage of Right Testis with Drainage Device, Open Approach

♂ **0V990ZX** Drainage of Right Testis, Open Approach, Diagnostic

♂ **0V990ZZ** Drainage of Right Testis, Open Approach

♂ **0V9930Z** Drainage of Right Testis with Drainage Device, Percutaneous Approach

♂ **0V993ZX** Drainage of Right Testis, Percutaneous Approach, Diagnostic

♂ **0V993ZZ** Drainage of Right Testis, Percutaneous Approach

♂ **0V9940Z** Drainage of Right Testis with Drainage Device, Percutaneous Endoscopic Approach

♂ **0V994ZX** Drainage of Right Testis, Percutaneous Endoscopic Approach, Diagnostic

♂ **0V994ZZ** Drainage of Right Testis, Percutaneous Endoscopic Approach

♂ **0V9B00Z** Drainage of Left Testis with Drainage Device, Open Approach

♂ **0V9B0ZX** Drainage of Left Testis, Open Approach, Diagnostic

♂ **0V9B0ZZ** Drainage of Left Testis, Open Approach

♂ **0V9B30Z** Drainage of Left Testis with Drainage Device, Percutaneous Approach

♂ **0V9B3ZX** Drainage of Left Testis, Percutaneous Approach, Diagnostic

♂ **0V9B3ZZ** Drainage of Left Testis, Percutaneous Approach

♂ **0V9B40Z** Drainage of Left Testis with Drainage Device, Percutaneous Endoscopic Approach

♂ **0V9B4ZX** Drainage of Left Testis, Percutaneous Endoscopic Approach, Diagnostic

♂ **0V9B4ZZ** Drainage of Left Testis, Percutaneous Endoscopic Approach

♂ **0V9C00Z** Drainage of Bilateral Testes with Drainage Device, Open Approach

♂ **0V9C0ZX** Drainage of Bilateral Testes, Open Approach, Diagnostic

♂ **0V9C0ZZ** Drainage of Bilateral Testes, Open Approach

♂ **0V9C30Z** Drainage of Bilateral Testes with Drainage Device, Percutaneous Approach

♂ **0V9C3ZX** Drainage of Bilateral Testes, Percutaneous Approach, Diagnostic

♂ **0V9C3ZZ** Drainage of Bilateral Testes, Percutaneous Approach

♂ **0V9C40Z** Drainage of Bilateral Testes with Drainage Device, Percutaneous Endoscopic Approach

♂ **0V9C4ZX** Drainage of Bilateral Testes, Percutaneous Endoscopic Approach, Diagnostic

♂ **0V9C4ZZ** Drainage of Bilateral Testes, Percutaneous Endoscopic Approach

♂ **0V9F00Z** Drainage of Right Spermatic Cord with Drainage Device, Open Approach

♂ **0V9F0ZX** Drainage of Right Spermatic Cord, Open Approach, Diagnostic

♂ **0V9F0ZZ** Drainage of Right Spermatic Cord, Open Approach

♂ **0V9F30Z** Drainage of Right Spermatic Cord with Drainage Device, Percutaneous Approach

♂ **0V9F3ZX** Drainage of Right Spermatic Cord, Percutaneous Approach, Diagnostic

♂ **0V9F3ZZ** Drainage of Right Spermatic Cord, Percutaneous Approach

♂ **0V9F40Z** Drainage of Right Spermatic Cord with Drainage Device, Percutaneous Endoscopic Approach

♂ **0V9F4ZX** Drainage of Right Spermatic Cord, Percutaneous Endoscopic Approach, Diagnostic

♂ **0V9F4ZZ** Drainage of Right Spermatic Cord, Percutaneous Endoscopic Approach

♂ **0V9G00Z** Drainage of Left Spermatic Cord with Drainage Device, Open Approach

♂ **0V9G0ZX** Drainage of Left Spermatic Cord, Open Approach, Diagnostic

♂ **0V9G0ZZ** Drainage of Left Spermatic Cord, Open Approach

♂ **0V9G30Z** Drainage of Left Spermatic Cord with Drainage Device, Percutaneous Approach

♂ **0V9G3ZX** Drainage of Left Spermatic Cord, Percutaneous Approach, Diagnostic

♂ **0V9G3ZZ** Drainage of Left Spermatic Cord, Percutaneous Approach

♂ **0V9G40Z** Drainage of Left Spermatic Cord with Drainage Device, Percutaneous Endoscopic Approach

♂ **0V9G4ZX** Drainage of Left Spermatic Cord, Percutaneous Endoscopic Approach, Diagnostic

♂ **0V9G4ZZ** Drainage of Left Spermatic Cord, Percutaneous Endoscopic Approach

♂ **0V9H00Z** Drainage of Bilateral Spermatic Cords with Drainage Device, Open Approach

♂ **0V9H0ZX** Drainage of Bilateral Spermatic Cords, Open Approach, Diagnostic

♂ **0V9H0ZZ** Drainage of Bilateral Spermatic Cords, Open Approach

♂ **0V9H30Z** Drainage of Bilateral Spermatic Cords with Drainage Device, Percutaneous Approach

♂ **0V9H3ZX** Drainage of Bilateral Spermatic Cords, Percutaneous Approach, Diagnostic

♀ Female-only   ♂ Male-only   ▲ Limited Coverage   ● Non-OR   HAC HAC-associated procedure   ▲ Non-covered procedures   ✚ Cluster

♂ 0V9H3ZZ Drainage of Bilateral Spermatic Cords, Percutaneous Approach

♂ 0V9H40Z Drainage of Bilateral Spermatic Cords with Drainage Device, Percutaneous Endoscopic Approach

♂ 0V9H4ZX Drainage of Bilateral Spermatic Cords, Percutaneous Endoscopic Approach, Diagnostic

♂ 0V9H4ZZ Drainage of Bilateral Spermatic Cords, Percutaneous Endoscopic Approach

♂ 0V9J00Z Drainage of Right Epididymis with Drainage Device, Open Approach

♂ 0V9J0ZX Drainage of Right Epididymis, Open Approach, Diagnostic

♂ 0V9J0ZZ Drainage of Right Epididymis, Open Approach

♂ 0V9J30Z Drainage of Right Epididymis with Drainage Device, Percutaneous Approach

♂ 0V9J3ZX Drainage of Right Epididymis, Percutaneous Approach, Diagnostic

♂ 0V9J3ZZ Drainage of Right Epididymis, Percutaneous Approach

♂ 0V9J40Z Drainage of Right Epididymis with Drainage Device, Percutaneous Endoscopic Approach

♂ 0V9J4ZX Drainage of Right Epididymis, Percutaneous Endoscopic Approach, Diagnostic

♂ 0V9J4ZZ Drainage of Right Epididymis, Percutaneous Endoscopic Approach

♂ 0V9K00Z Drainage of Left Epididymis with Drainage Device, Open Approach

♂ 0V9K0ZX Drainage of Left Epididymis, Open Approach, Diagnostic

♂ 0V9K0ZZ Drainage of Left Epididymis, Open Approach

♂ 0V9K30Z Drainage of Left Epididymis with Drainage Device, Percutaneous Approach

♂ 0V9K3ZX Drainage of Left Epididymis, Percutaneous Approach, Diagnostic

♂ 0V9K3ZZ Drainage of Left Epididymis, Percutaneous Approach

♂ 0V9K40Z Drainage of Left Epididymis with Drainage Device, Percutaneous Endoscopic Approach

♂ 0V9K4ZX Drainage of Left Epididymis, Percutaneous Endoscopic Approach, Diagnostic

♂ 0V9K4ZZ Drainage of Left Epididymis, Percutaneous Endoscopic Approach

♂ 0V9L00Z Drainage of Bilateral Epididymis with Drainage Device, Open Approach

♂ 0V9L0ZX Drainage of Bilateral Epididymis, Open Approach, Diagnostic

♂ 0V9L0ZZ Drainage of Bilateral Epididymis, Open Approach

♂ 0V9L30Z Drainage of Bilateral Epididymis with Drainage Device, Percutaneous Approach

♂ 0V9L3ZX Drainage of Bilateral Epididymis, Percutaneous Approach, Diagnostic

♂ 0V9L3ZZ Drainage of Bilateral Epididymis, Percutaneous Approach

♂ 0V9L40Z Drainage of Bilateral Epididymis with Drainage Device, Percutaneous Endoscopic Approach

♂ 0V9L4ZX Drainage of Bilateral Epididymis, Percutaneous Endoscopic Approach, Diagnostic

♂ 0V9L4ZZ Drainage of Bilateral Epididymis, Percutaneous Endoscopic Approach

♂ 0V9N00Z Drainage of Right Vas Deferens with Drainage Device, Open Approach

♂ 0V9N0ZX Drainage of Right Vas Deferens, Open Approach, Diagnostic

♂ 0V9N0ZZ Drainage of Right Vas Deferens, Open Approach

♂ 0V9N30Z Drainage of Right Vas Deferens with Drainage Device, Percutaneous Approach

♂ 0V9N3ZX Drainage of Right Vas Deferens, Percutaneous Approach, Diagnostic

♂ 0V9N3ZZ Drainage of Right Vas Deferens, Percutaneous Approach

♂ 0V9N40Z Drainage of Right Vas Deferens with Drainage Device, Percutaneous Endoscopic Approach

♂ 0V9N4ZX Drainage of Right Vas Deferens, Percutaneous Endoscopic Approach, Diagnostic

♂ 0V9N4ZZ Drainage of Right Vas Deferens, Percutaneous Endoscopic Approach

♂ 0V9P00Z Drainage of Left Vas Deferens with Drainage Device, Open Approach

♂ 0V9P0ZX Drainage of Left Vas Deferens, Open Approach, Diagnostic

♂ 0V9P0ZZ Drainage of Left Vas Deferens, Open Approach

♂ 0V9P30Z Drainage of Left Vas Deferens with Drainage Device, Percutaneous Approach

♂ 0V9P3ZX Drainage of Left Vas Deferens, Percutaneous Approach, Diagnostic

♂ 0V9P3ZZ Drainage of Left Vas Deferens, Percutaneous Approach

♂ 0V9P40Z Drainage of Left Vas Deferens with Drainage Device, Percutaneous Endoscopic Approach

♂ 0V9P4ZX Drainage of Left Vas Deferens, Percutaneous Endoscopic Approach, Diagnostic

♂ 0V9P4ZZ Drainage of Left Vas Deferens, Percutaneous Endoscopic Approach

♂ 0V9Q00Z Drainage of Bilateral Vas Deferens with Drainage Device, Open Approach

♂ 0V9Q0ZX Drainage of Bilateral Vas Deferens, Open Approach, Diagnostic

♂ 0V9Q0ZZ Drainage of Bilateral Vas Deferens, Open Approach

♂ 0V9Q30Z Drainage of Bilateral Vas Deferens with Drainage Device, Percutaneous Approach

♂ 0V9Q3ZX Drainage of Bilateral Vas Deferens, Percutaneous Approach, Diagnostic

♂ 0V9Q3ZZ Drainage of Bilateral Vas Deferens, Percutaneous Approach

♂ 0V9Q40Z Drainage of Bilateral Vas Deferens with Drainage Device, Percutaneous Endoscopic Approach

♂ 0V9Q4ZX Drainage of Bilateral Vas Deferens, Percutaneous Endoscopic Approach, Diagnostic

♂ 0V9Q4ZZ Drainage of Bilateral Vas Deferens, Percutaneous Endoscopic Approach

♂ 0V9S00Z Drainage of Penis with Drainage Device, Open Approach

♂ 0V9S0ZX Drainage of Penis, Open Approach, Diagnostic

♂ 0V9S0ZZ Drainage of Penis, Open Approach

♂ 0V9S30Z Drainage of Penis with Drainage Device, Percutaneous Approach

♂ 0V9S3ZX Drainage of Penis, Percutaneous Approach, Diagnostic

♂ 0V9S3ZZ Drainage of Penis, Percutaneous Approach

♂ 0V9S40Z Drainage of Penis with Drainage Device, Percutaneous Endoscopic Approach

♂ 0V9S4ZX Drainage of Penis, Percutaneous Endoscopic Approach, Diagnostic

♂ 0V9S4ZZ Drainage of Penis, Percutaneous Endoscopic Approach

♂ 0V9SX0Z Drainage of Penis with Drainage Device, External Approach

♂ 0V9SXZX Drainage of Penis, External Approach, Diagnostic

♂ 0V9SXZZ Drainage of Penis, External Approach

♂ 0V9T00Z Drainage of Prepuce with Drainage Device, Open Approach

♂ 0V9T0ZX Drainage of Prepuce, Open Approach, Diagnostic

♂ 0V9T0ZZ Drainage of Prepuce, Open Approach

♂ 0V9T30Z Drainage of Prepuce with Drainage Device, Percutaneous Approach

♂ 0V9T3ZX Drainage of Prepuce, Percutaneous Approach, Diagnostic

♂ 0V9T3ZZ Drainage of Prepuce, Percutaneous Approach

♂ 0V9T40Z Drainage of Prepuce with Drainage Device, Percutaneous Endoscopic Approach

♂ 0V9T4ZX Drainage of Prepuce, Percutaneous Endoscopic Approach, Diagnostic

♂ 0V9T4ZZ Drainage of Prepuce, Percutaneous Endoscopic Approach

♂ 0V9TX0Z Drainage of Prepuce with Drainage Device, External Approach

♂ 0V9TXZX Drainage of Prepuce, External Approach, Diagnostic

♂ 0V9TXZZ Drainage of Prepuce, External Approach

0VB – Male Reproductive System, Excision

Review Coding Guidelines B3.4a and B3.4b

Review Coding Guideline B3.8

Review Coding Guideline B3.18

♂ 0VB00ZX Excision of Prostate, Open Approach, Diagnostic

♂ 0VB00ZZ Excision of Prostate, Open Approach

♂ 0VB03ZX Excision of Prostate, Percutaneous Approach, Diagnostic

♂ 0VB03ZZ Excision of Prostate, Percutaneous Approach

♂ 0VB04ZX Excision of Prostate, Percutaneous Endoscopic Approach, Diagnostic

♂ 0VB04ZZ Excision of Prostate, Percutaneous Endoscopic Approach

♂ 0VB07ZX Excision of Prostate, Via Natural or Artificial Opening, Diagnostic

---

♀ Female-only   ♂ Male-only   ▲ Limited Coverage   ● Non-OR   HAC HAC-associated procedure   ▲ Non-covered procedures   ✚ Cluster

♂ **0VB07ZZ** Excision of Prostate, Via Natural or Artificial Opening

♂ **0VB08ZX** Excision of Prostate, Via Natural or Artificial Opening Endoscopic, Diagnostic

♂ **0VB08ZZ** Excision of Prostate, Via Natural or Artificial Opening Endoscopic

♂ **0VB10ZX** Excision of Right Seminal Vesicle, Open Approach, Diagnostic

♂ **0VB10ZZ** Excision of Right Seminal Vesicle, Open Approach

♂ **0VB13ZX** Excision of Right Seminal Vesicle, Percutaneous Approach, Diagnostic

♂ **0VB13ZZ** Excision of Right Seminal Vesicle, Percutaneous Approach

♂ **0VB14ZX** Excision of Right Seminal Vesicle, Percutaneous Endoscopic Approach, Diagnostic

♂ **0VB14ZZ** Excision of Right Seminal Vesicle, Percutaneous Endoscopic Approach

♂ **0VB20ZX** Excision of Left Seminal Vesicle, Open Approach, Diagnostic

♂ **0VB20ZZ** Excision of Left Seminal Vesicle, Open Approach

♂ **0VB23ZX** Excision of Left Seminal Vesicle, Percutaneous Approach, Diagnostic

♂ **0VB23ZZ** Excision of Left Seminal Vesicle, Percutaneous Approach

♂ **0VB24ZX** Excision of Left Seminal Vesicle, Percutaneous Endoscopic Approach, Diagnostic

♂ **0VB24ZZ** Excision of Left Seminal Vesicle, Percutaneous Endoscopic Approach

♂ **0VB30ZX** Excision of Bilateral Seminal Vesicles, Open Approach, Diagnostic

♂ **0VB30ZZ** Excision of Bilateral Seminal Vesicles, Open Approach

♂ **0VB33ZX** Excision of Bilateral Seminal Vesicles, Percutaneous Approach, Diagnostic

♂ **0VB33ZZ** Excision of Bilateral Seminal Vesicles, Percutaneous Approach

♂ **0VB34ZX** Excision of Bilateral Seminal Vesicles, Percutaneous Endoscopic Approach, Diagnostic

♂ **0VB34ZZ** Excision of Bilateral Seminal Vesicles, Percutaneous Endoscopic Approach

♂ **0VB50ZX** Excision of Scrotum, Open Approach, Diagnostic

♂ **0VB50ZZ** Excision of Scrotum, Open Approach

♂ **0VB53ZX** Excision of Scrotum, Percutaneous Approach, Diagnostic

♂ **0VB53ZZ** Excision of Scrotum, Percutaneous Approach

♂ **0VB54ZX** Excision of Scrotum, Percutaneous Endoscopic Approach, Diagnostic

♂ **0VB54ZZ** Excision of Scrotum, Percutaneous Endoscopic Approach

♂ **0VB5XZX** Excision of Scrotum, External Approach, Diagnostic

♂ **0VB5XZZ** Excision of Scrotum, External Approach

♂ **0VB60ZX** Excision of Right Tunica Vaginalis, Open Approach, Diagnostic

♂ **0VB60ZZ** Excision of Right Tunica Vaginalis, Open Approach

♂ **0VB63ZX** Excision of Right Tunica Vaginalis, Percutaneous Approach, Diagnostic

♂ **0VB63ZZ** Excision of Right Tunica Vaginalis, Percutaneous Approach

♂ **0VB64ZX** Excision of Right Tunica Vaginalis, Percutaneous Endoscopic Approach, Diagnostic

♂ **0VB64ZZ** Excision of Right Tunica Vaginalis, Percutaneous Endoscopic Approach

♂ **0VB70ZX** Excision of Left Tunica Vaginalis, Open Approach, Diagnostic

♂ **0VB70ZZ** Excision of Left Tunica Vaginalis, Open Approach

♂ **0VB73ZX** Excision of Left Tunica Vaginalis, Percutaneous Approach, Diagnostic

♂ **0VB73ZZ** Excision of Left Tunica Vaginalis, Percutaneous Approach

♂ **0VB74ZX** Excision of Left Tunica Vaginalis, Percutaneous Endoscopic Approach, Diagnostic

♂ **0VB74ZZ** Excision of Left Tunica Vaginalis, Percutaneous Endoscopic Approach

♂ **0VB90ZX** Excision of Right Testis, Open Approach, Diagnostic

♂ **0VB90ZZ** Excision of Right Testis, Open Approach

♂ **0VB93ZX** Excision of Right Testis, Percutaneous Approach, Diagnostic

♂ **0VB93ZZ** Excision of Right Testis, Percutaneous Approach

♂ **0VB94ZX** Excision of Right Testis, Percutaneous Endoscopic Approach, Diagnostic

♂ **0VB94ZZ** Excision of Right Testis, Percutaneous Endoscopic Approach

♂ **0VBB0ZX** Excision of Left Testis, Open Approach, Diagnostic

♂ **0VBB0ZZ** Excision of Left Testis, Open Approach

♂ **0VBB3ZX** Excision of Left Testis, Percutaneous Approach, Diagnostic

♂ **0VBB3ZZ** Excision of Left Testis, Percutaneous Approach

♂ **0VBB4ZX** Excision of Left Testis, Percutaneous Endoscopic Approach, Diagnostic

♂ **0VBB4ZZ** Excision of Left Testis, Percutaneous Endoscopic Approach

♂ **0VBC0ZX** Excision of Bilateral Testes, Open Approach, Diagnostic

♂ **0VBC0ZZ** Excision of Bilateral Testes, Open Approach

♂ **0VBC3ZX** Excision of Bilateral Testes, Percutaneous Approach, Diagnostic

♂ **0VBC3ZZ** Excision of Bilateral Testes, Percutaneous Approach

♂ **0VBC4ZX** Excision of Bilateral Testes, Percutaneous Endoscopic Approach, Diagnostic

♂ **0VBC4ZZ** Excision of Bilateral Testes, Percutaneous Endoscopic Approach

♂ **0VBF0ZX** Excision of Right Spermatic Cord, Open Approach, Diagnostic

♂ **0VBF0ZZ** Excision of Right Spermatic Cord, Open Approach

♂ **0VBF3ZX** Excision of Right Spermatic Cord, Percutaneous Approach, Diagnostic

♂ **0VBF3ZZ** Excision of Right Spermatic Cord, Percutaneous Approach

♂ **0VBF4ZX** Excision of Right Spermatic Cord, Percutaneous Endoscopic Approach, Diagnostic

♂ **0VBF4ZZ** Excision of Right Spermatic Cord, Percutaneous Endoscopic Approach

♂ **0VBF8ZX** Excision of Right Spermatic Cord, Via Natural or Artificial Opening Endoscopic, Diagnostic

♂ **0VBF8ZZ** Excision of Right Spermatic Cord, Via Natural or Artificial Opening Endoscopic

♂ **0VBG0ZX** Excision of Left Spermatic Cord, Open Approach, Diagnostic

♂ **0VBG0ZZ** Excision of Left Spermatic Cord, Open Approach

♂ **0VBG3ZX** Excision of Left Spermatic Cord, Percutaneous Approach, Diagnostic

♂ **0VBG3ZZ** Excision of Left Spermatic Cord, Percutaneous Approach

♂ **0VBG4ZX** Excision of Left Spermatic Cord, Percutaneous Endoscopic Approach, Diagnostic

♂ **0VBG4ZZ** Excision of Left Spermatic Cord, Percutaneous Endoscopic Approach

♂ **0VBG8ZX** Excision of Left Spermatic Cord, Via Natural or Artificial Opening Endoscopic, Diagnostic

♂ **0VBG8ZZ** Excision of Left Spermatic Cord, Via Natural or Artificial Opening Endoscopic

♂ **0VBH0ZX** Excision of Bilateral Spermatic Cords, Open Approach, vDiagnostic

♂ **0VBH0ZZ** Excision of Bilateral Spermatic Cords, Open Approach

♂ **0VBH3ZX** Excision of Bilateral Spermatic Cords, Percutaneous Approach, Diagnostic

♂ **0VBH3ZZ** Excision of Bilateral Spermatic Cords, Percutaneous Approach

♂ **0VBH4ZX** Excision of Bilateral Spermatic Cords, Percutaneous Endoscopic Approach, Diagnostic

♂ **0VBH4ZZ** Excision of Bilateral Spermatic Cords, Percutaneous Endoscopic Approach

♂ **0VBH8ZX** Excision of Bilateral Spermatic Cords, Via Natural or Artificial Opening Endoscopic, Diagnostic

♂ **0VBH8ZZ** Excision of Bilateral Spermatic Cords, Via Natural or Artificial Opening Endoscopic

♂ **0VBJ0ZX** Excision of Right Epididymis, Open Approach, Diagnostic

♂ **0VBJ0ZZ** Excision of Right Epididymis, Open Approach

♂ **0VBJ3ZX** Excision of Right Epididymis, Percutaneous Approach, Diagnostic

♂ **0VBJ3ZZ** Excision of Right Epididymis, Percutaneous Approach

♂ **0VBJ4ZX** Excision of Right Epididymis, Percutaneous Endoscopic Approach, Diagnostic

♂ **0VBJ4ZZ** Excision of Right Epididymis, Percutaneous Endoscopic Approach

♂ **0VBJ8ZX** Excision of Right Epididymis, Via Natural or Artificial Opening Endoscopic, Diagnostic

♂ **0VBJ8ZZ** Excision of Right Epididymis, Via Natural or Artificial Opening Endoscopic

♂ **0VBK0ZX** Excision of Left Epididymis, Open Approach, Diagnostic

♂ **0VBK0ZZ** Excision of Left Epididymis, Open Approach

♂ **0VBK3ZX** Excision of Left Epididymis, Percutaneous Approach, Diagnostic

♂ **0VBK3ZZ** Excision of Left Epididymis, Percutaneous Approach

♂ **0VBK4ZX** Excision of Left Epididymis, Percutaneous Endoscopic Approach, Diagnostic

♂ **0VBK4ZZ** Excision of Left Epididymis, Percutaneous Endoscopic Approach

♂ **0VBK8ZX** Excision of Left Epididymis, Via Natural or Artificial Opening Endoscopic, Diagnostic

♂ **0VBK8ZZ** Excision of Left Epididymis, Via Natural or Artificial Opening Endoscopic

♂ **0VBL0ZX** Excision of Bilateral Epididymis, Open Approach, Diagnostic

♂ **0VBL0ZZ** Excision of Bilateral Epididymis, Open Approach

♂ **0VBL3ZX** Excision of Bilateral Epididymis, Percutaneous Approach, Diagnostic

♀ Female-only   ♂ Male-only   ▲ Limited Coverage   ● Non-OR   🄷🄰🄲 HAC-associated procedure   ▲ Non-covered procedures   ✚ Cluster

♂ **0VBL3ZZ** Excision of Bilateral Epididymis, Percutaneous Approach

♂ **0VBL4ZX** Excision of Bilateral Epididymis, Percutaneous Endoscopic Approach, Diagnostic

♂ **0VBL4ZZ** Excision of Bilateral Epididymis, Percutaneous Endoscopic Approach

♂ **0VBL8ZX** Excision of Bilateral Epididymis, Via Natural or Artificial Opening Endoscopic, Diagnostic

♂ **0VBL8ZZ** Excision of Bilateral Epididymis, Via Natural or Artificial Opening Endoscopic

♂ **0VBN0ZX** Excision of Right Vas Deferens, Open Approach, Diagnostic

♂ **0VBN0ZZ** Excision of Right Vas Deferens, Open Approach
  ▲ *When reported with diagnosis code Z30.2*

♂ **0VBN3ZX** Excision of Right Vas Deferens, Percutaneous Approach, Diagnostic

♂ **0VBN3ZZ** Excision of Right Vas Deferens, Percutaneous Approach
  ▲ *When reported with diagnosis code Z30.2*

♂ **0VBN4ZX** Excision of Right Vas Deferens, Percutaneous Endoscopic Approach, Diagnostic

♂ **0VBN4ZZ** Excision of Right Vas Deferens, Percutaneous Endoscopic Approach
  ▲ *When reported with diagnosis code Z30.2*

♂ **0VBN8ZX** Excision of Right Vas Deferens, Via Natural or Artificial Opening Endoscopic, Diagnostic

♂ **0VBN8ZZ** Excision of Right Vas Deferens, Via Natural or Artificial Opening Endoscopic

♂ **0VBP0ZX** Excision of Left Vas Deferens, Open Approach, Diagnostic

♂ **0VBP0ZZ** Excision of Left Vas Deferens, Open Approach

  ▲ *When reported with diagnosis code Z30.2*

♂ **0VBP3ZX** Excision of Left Vas Deferens, Percutaneous Approach, Diagnostic

♂ **0VBP3ZZ** Excision of Left Vas Deferens, Percutaneous Approach
  ▲ *When reported with diagnosis code Z30.2*

♂ **0VBP4ZX** Excision of Left Vas Deferens, Percutaneous Endoscopic Approach, Diagnostic

♂ **0VBP4ZZ** Excision of Left Vas Deferens, Percutaneous Endoscopic Approach
  ▲ *When reported with diagnosis code Z30.2*

♂ **0VBP8ZX** Excision of Left Vas Deferens, Via Natural or Artificial Opening Endoscopic, Diagnostic

♂ **0VBP8ZZ** Excision of Left Vas Deferens, Via Natural or Artificial Opening Endoscopic

♂ **0VBQ0ZX** Excision of Bilateral Vas Deferens, Open Approach, Diagnostic

♂ **0VBQ0ZZ** Excision of Bilateral Vas Deferens, Open Approach
  ▲ *When reported with diagnosis code Z30.2*

♂ **0VBQ3ZX** Excision of Bilateral Vas Deferens, Percutaneous Approach, Diagnostic

♂ **0VBQ3ZZ** Excision of Bilateral Vas Deferens, Percutaneous Approach
  ▲ *When reported with diagnosis code Z30.2*

♂ **0VBQ4ZX** Excision of Bilateral Vas Deferens, Percutaneous Endoscopic Approach, Diagnostic

♂ **0VBQ4ZZ** Excision of Bilateral Vas Deferens, Percutaneous Endoscopic Approach
  ▲ *When reported with diagnosis code Z30.2*

  AHA CC: 4Q, 2014, 33-34; 1Q, 2016, 23

♂ **0VBQ8ZX** Excision of Bilateral Vas Deferens, Via Natural or Artificial Opening Endoscopic, Diagnostic

♂ **0VBQ8ZZ** Excision of Bilateral Vas Deferens, Via Natural or Artificial Opening Endoscopic

♂ **0VBS0ZX** Excision of Penis, Open Approach, Diagnostic

♂ **0VBS0ZZ** Excision of Penis, Open Approach

♂ **0VBS3ZX** Excision of Penis, Percutaneous Approach, Diagnostic

♂ **0VBS3ZZ** Excision of Penis, Percutaneous Approach

♂ **0VBS4ZX** Excision of Penis, Percutaneous Endoscopic Approach, Diagnostic

♂ **0VBS4ZZ** Excision of Penis, Percutaneous Endoscopic Approach

♂ **0VBSXZX** Excision of Penis, External Approach, Diagnostic

♂ **0VBSXZZ** Excision of Penis, External Approach

♂ **0VBT0ZX** Excision of Prepuce, Open Approach, Diagnostic

♂ **0VBT0ZZ** Excision of Prepuce, Open Approach

♂ **0VBT3ZX** Excision of Prepuce, Percutaneous Approach, Diagnostic

♂ **0VBT3ZZ** Excision of Prepuce, Percutaneous Approach

♂ **0VBT4ZX** Excision of Prepuce, Percutaneous Endoscopic Approach, Diagnostic

♂ **0VBT4ZZ** Excision of Prepuce, Percutaneous Endoscopic Approach

♂ **0VBTXZX** Excision of Prepuce, External Approach, Diagnostic

♂ **0VBTXZZ** Excision of Prepuce, External Approach

0VC – Male Reproductive System, Extirpation

♂ **0VC00ZZ** Extirpation of Matter from Prostate, Open Approach

♂ **0VC03ZZ** Extirpation of Matter from Prostate, Percutaneous Approach

♂ **0VC04ZZ** Extirpation of Matter from Prostate, Percutaneous Endoscopic Approach

♂ **0VC07ZZ** Extirpation of Matter from Prostate, Via Natural or Artificial Opening

♂ **0VC08ZZ** Extirpation of Matter from Prostate, Via Natural or Artificial Opening Endoscopic

♂ **0VC10ZZ** Extirpation of Matter from Right Seminal Vesicle, Open Approach

♂ **0VC13ZZ** Extirpation of Matter from Right Seminal Vesicle, Percutaneous Approach

♂ **0VC14ZZ** Extirpation of Matter from Right Seminal Vesicle, Percutaneous Endoscopic Approach

♂ **0VC20ZZ** Extirpation of Matter from Left Seminal Vesicle, Open Approach

♂ **0VC23ZZ** Extirpation of Matter from Left Seminal Vesicle, Percutaneous Approach

♂ **0VC24ZZ** Extirpation of Matter from Left Seminal Vesicle, Percutaneous Endoscopic Approach

♂ **0VC30ZZ** Extirpation of Matter from Bilateral Seminal Vesicles, Open Approach

♂ **0VC33ZZ** Extirpation of Matter from Bilateral Seminal Vesicles, Percutaneous Approach

♂ **0VC34ZZ** Extirpation of Matter from Bilateral Seminal Vesicles, Percutaneous Endoscopic Approach

♂ **0VC50ZZ** Extirpation of Matter from Scrotum, Open Approach

♂ **0VC53ZZ** Extirpation of Matter from Scrotum, Percutaneous Approach

♂ **0VC54ZZ** Extirpation of Matter from Scrotum, Percutaneous Endoscopic Approach

♂ **0VC5XZZ** Extirpation of Matter from Scrotum, External Approach

♂ **0VC60ZZ** Extirpation of Matter from Right Tunica Vaginalis, Open Approach

♂ **0VC63ZZ** Extirpation of Matter from Right Tunica Vaginalis, Percutaneous Approach

♂ **0VC64ZZ** Extirpation of Matter from Right Tunica Vaginalis, Percutaneous Endoscopic Approach

♂ **0VC70ZZ** Extirpation of Matter from Left Tunica Vaginalis, Open Approach

♂ **0VC73ZZ** Extirpation of Matter from Left Tunica Vaginalis, Percutaneous Approach

♂ **0VC74ZZ** Extirpation of Matter from Left Tunica Vaginalis, Percutaneous Endoscopic Approach

♂ **0VC90ZZ** Extirpation of Matter from Right Testis, Open Approach

♂ **0VC93ZZ** Extirpation of Matter from Right Testis, Percutaneous Approach

♂ **0VC94ZZ** Extirpation of Matter from Right Testis, Percutaneous Endoscopic Approach

♂ **0VCB0ZZ** Extirpation of Matter from Left Testis, Open Approach

♂ **0VCB3ZZ** Extirpation of Matter from Left Testis, Percutaneous Approach

♂ **0VCB4ZZ** Extirpation of Matter from Left Testis, Percutaneous Endoscopic Approach

♂ **0VCC0ZZ** Extirpation of Matter from Bilateral Testes, Open Approach

♂ **0VCC3ZZ** Extirpation of Matter from Bilateral Testes, Percutaneous Approach

♂ **0VCC4ZZ** Extirpation of Matter from Bilateral Testes, Percutaneous Endoscopic Approach

♂ **0VCF0ZZ** Extirpation of Matter from Right Spermatic Cord, Open Approach

♂ **0VCF3ZZ** Extirpation of Matter from Right Spermatic Cord, Percutaneous Approach

♂ **0VCF4ZZ** Extirpation of Matter from Right Spermatic Cord, Percutaneous Endoscopic Approach

♂ **0VCG0ZZ** Extirpation of Matter from Left Spermatic Cord, Open Approach

♂ **0VCG3ZZ** Extirpation of Matter from Left Spermatic Cord, Percutaneous Approach

♂ **0VCG4ZZ** Extirpation of Matter from Left Spermatic Cord, Percutaneous Endoscopic Approach

♂ **0VCH0ZZ** Extirpation of Matter from Bilateral Spermatic Cords, Open Approach

♂ **0VCH3ZZ** Extirpation of Matter from Bilateral Spermatic Cords, Percutaneous Approach

♂ **0VCH4ZZ** Extirpation of Matter from Bilateral Spermatic Cords, Percutaneous Endoscopic Approach

♂ **0VCJ0ZZ** Extirpation of Matter from Right Epididymis, Open Approach

♂ **0VCJ3ZZ** Extirpation of Matter from Right Epididymis, Percutaneous Approach

♂ **0VCJ4ZZ** Extirpation of Matter from Right Epididymis, Percutaneous Endoscopic Approach

♂ **0VCK0ZZ** Extirpation of Matter from Left Epididymis, Open Approach

♂ **0VCK3ZZ** Extirpation of Matter from Left Epididymis, Percutaneous Approach

♂ **0VCK4ZZ** Extirpation of Matter from Left Epididymis, Percutaneous Endoscopic Approach

♂ **0VCL0ZZ** Extirpation of Matter from Bilateral Epididymis, Open Approach

♂ **0VCL3ZZ** Extirpation of Matter from Bilateral Epididymis, Percutaneous Approach

♂ **0VCL4ZZ** Extirpation of Matter from Bilateral Epididymis, Percutaneous Endoscopic Approach

♂ **0VCN0ZZ** Extirpation of Matter from Right Vas Deferens, Open Approach

♂ **0VCN3ZZ** Extirpation of Matter from Right Vas Deferens, Percutaneous Approach

♂ **0VCN4ZZ** Extirpation of Matter from Right Vas Deferens, Percutaneous Endoscopic Approach

♂ **0VCP0ZZ** Extirpation of Matter from Left Vas Deferens, Open Approach

♂ **0VCP3ZZ** Extirpation of Matter from Left Vas Deferens, Percutaneous Approach

♂ **0VCP4ZZ** Extirpation of Matter from Left Vas Deferens, Percutaneous Endoscopic Approach

♂ **0VCQ0ZZ** Extirpation of Matter from Bilateral Vas Deferens, Open Approach

♂ **0VCQ3ZZ** Extirpation of Matter from Bilateral Vas Deferens, Percutaneous Approach

♂ **0VCQ4ZZ** Extirpation of Matter from Bilateral Vas Deferens, Percutaneous Endoscopic Approach

♂ **0VCS0ZZ** Extirpation of Matter from Penis, Open Approach

♂ **0VCS3ZZ** Extirpation of Matter from Penis, Percutaneous Approach

♂ **0VCS4ZZ** Extirpation of Matter from Penis, Percutaneous Endoscopic Approach

♂ **0VCSXZZ** Extirpation of Matter from Penis, External Approach

♂ **0VCT0ZZ** Extirpation of Matter from Prepuce, Open Approach

♂ **0VCT3ZZ** Extirpation of Matter from Prepuce, Percutaneous Approach

♂ **0VCT4ZZ** Extirpation of Matter from Prepuce, Percutaneous Endoscopic Approach

♂ **0VCTXZZ** Extirpation of Matter from Prepuce, External Approach

0VH – Male Reproductive System, Insertion

♂ **0VH001Z** Insertion of Radioactive Element into Prostate, Open Approach

♂ **0VH031Z** Insertion of Radioactive Element into Prostate, Percutaneous Approach

♂ **0VH041Z** Insertion of Radioactive Element into Prostate, Percutaneous Endoscopic Approach

♂ **0VH071Z** Insertion of Radioactive Element into Prostate, Via Natural or Artificial Opening

♂ **0VH081Z** Insertion of Radioactive Element into Prostate, Via Natural or Artificial Opening Endoscopic

♂ **0VH403Z** Insertion of Infusion Device into Prostate and Seminal Vesicles, Open Approach

♂ **0VH40YZ** Insertion of Other Device into Prostate and Seminal Vesicles, Open Approach

♂ **0VH433Z** Insertion of Infusion Device into Prostate and Seminal Vesicles, Percutaneous Approach

♂ **0VH43YZ** Insertion of Other Device into Prostate and Seminal Vesicles, Percutaneous Approach

♂ **0VH443Z** Insertion of Infusion Device into Prostate and Seminal Vesicles, Percutaneous Endoscopic Approach

♂ **0VH44YZ** Insertion of Other Device into Prostate and Seminal Vesicles, Percutaneous Endoscopic Approach

♂ **0VH473Z** Insertion of Infusion Device into Prostate and Seminal Vesicles, Via Natural or Artificial Opening

♂ **0VH47YZ** Insertion of Other Device into Prostate and Seminal Vesicles, Via Natural or Artificial Opening

♂ **0VH483Z** Insertion of Infusion Device into Prostate and Seminal Vesicles, Via Natural or Artificial Opening Endoscopic

♂ **0VH48YZ** Insertion of Other Device into Prostate and Seminal Vesicles, Via Natural or Artificial Opening Endoscopic

♂ **0VH803Z** Insertion of Infusion Device into Scrotum and Tunica Vaginalis, Open Approach

♂ **0VH80YZ** Insertion of Other Device into Scrotum and Tunica Vaginalis, Open Approach

♂ **0VH833Z** Insertion of Infusion Device into Scrotum and Tunica Vaginalis, Percutaneous Approach

♂ **0VH83YZ** Insertion of Other Device into Scrotum and Tunica Vaginalis, Percutaneous Approach

♂ **0VH843Z** Insertion of Infusion Device into Scrotum and Tunica Vaginalis, Percutaneous Endoscopic Approach

♂ **0VH84YZ** Insertion of Other Device into Scrotum and Tunica Vaginalis, Percutaneous Endoscopic Approach

♂ **0VH873Z** Insertion of Infusion Device into Scrotum and Tunica Vaginalis, Via Natural or Artificial Opening

♂ **0VH87YZ** Insertion of Other Device into Scrotum and Tunica Vaginalis, Via Natural or Artificial Opening

♂ **0VH883Z** Insertion of Infusion Device into Scrotum and Tunica Vaginalis, Via Natural or Artificial Opening Endoscopic

♂ **0VH88YZ** Insertion of Other Device into Scrotum and Tunica Vaginalis, Via Natural or Artificial Opening Endoscopic

♂ **0VHD01Z** Insertion of Radioactive Element into Testis, Open Approach

♂ **0VHD03Z** Insertion of Infusion Device into Testis, Open Approach

♂ **0VHD0YZ** Insertion of Other Device into Testis, Open Approach

♂ **0VHD31Z** Insertion of Radioactive Element into Testis, Percutaneous Approach

♂ **0VHD33Z** Insertion of Infusion Device into Testis, Percutaneous Approach

♂ **0VHD3YZ** Insertion of Other Device into Testis, Percutaneous Approach

♂ **0VHD41Z** Insertion of Radioactive Element into Testis, Percutaneous Endoscopic Approach

♂ **0VHD43Z** Insertion of Infusion Device into Testis, Percutaneous Endoscopic Approach

♂ **0VHD4YZ** Insertion of Other Device into Testis, Percutaneous Endoscopic Approach

♂ **0VHD71Z** Insertion of Radioactive Element into Testis, Via Natural or Artificial Opening

♂ **0VHD73Z** Insertion of Infusion Device into Testis, Via Natural or Artificial Opening

♂ **0VHD7YZ** Insertion of Other Device into Testis, Via Natural or Artificial Opening

♂ **0VHD81Z** Insertion of Radioactive Element into Testis, Via Natural or Artificial Opening Endoscopic

♂ **0VHD83Z** Insertion of Infusion Device into Testis, Via Natural or Artificial Opening Endoscopic

♂ **0VHD8YZ** Insertion of Other Device into Testis, Via Natural or Artificial Opening Endoscopic

♂ **0VHM03Z** Insertion of Infusion Device into Epididymis and Spermatic Cord, Open Approach

♂ **0VHM0YZ** Insertion of Other Device into Epididymis and Spermatic Cord, Open Approach

♂ **0VHM33Z** Insertion of Infusion Device into Epididymis and Spermatic Cord, Percutaneous Approach

♂ **0VHM3YZ** Insertion of Other Device into Epididymis and Spermatic Cord, Percutaneous Approach

♂ **0VHM43Z** Insertion of Infusion Device into Epididymis and Spermatic Cord, Percutaneous Endoscopic Approach

♂ **0VHM4YZ** Insertion of Other Device into Epididymis and Spermatic Cord, Percutaneous Endoscopic Approach

♂ **0VHM73Z** Insertion of Infusion Device into Epididymis and Spermatic Cord, Via Natural or Artificial Opening

♂ **0VHM7YZ** Insertion of Other Device into Epididymis and Spermatic Cord, Via Natural or Artificial Opening

♂ **0VHM83Z** Insertion of Infusion Device into Epididymis and Spermatic Cord, Via Natural or Artificial Opening Endoscopic

♂ **0VHM8YZ** Insertion of Other Device into Epididymis and Spermatic Cord, Via Natural or Artificial Opening Endoscopic

♂ **0VHR03Z** Insertion of Infusion Device into Vas Deferens, Open Approach

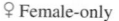

♂ **0VHR0YZ** Insertion of Other Device into Vas Deferens, Open Approach

♂ **0VHR33Z** Insertion of Infusion Device into Vas Deferens, Percutaneous Approach

♂ **0VHR3YZ** Insertion of Other Device into Vas Deferens, Percutaneous Approach

♂ **0VHR43Z** Insertion of Infusion Device into Vas Deferens, Percutaneous Endoscopic Approach

♂ **0VHR4YZ** Insertion of Other Device into Vas Deferens, Percutaneous Endoscopic Approach

♂ **0VHR73Z** Insertion of Infusion Device into Vas Deferens, Via Natural or Artificial Opening

♂ **0VHR7YZ** Insertion of Other Device into Vas Deferens, Via Natural or Artificial Opening

♂ **0VHR83Z** Insertion of Infusion Device into Vas Deferens, Via Natural or Artificial Opening Endoscopic

♂ **0VHR8YZ** Insertion of Other Device into Vas Deferens, Via Natural or Artificial Opening Endoscopic

♂ **0VHS03Z** Insertion of Infusion Device into Penis, Open Approach

♂ **0VHS0YZ** Insertion of Other Device into Penis, Open Approach

♂ **0VHS33Z** Insertion of Infusion Device into Penis, Percutaneous Approach

♂ **0VHS3YZ** Insertion of Other Device into Penis, Percutaneous Approach

♂ **0VHS43Z** Insertion of Infusion Device into Penis, Percutaneous Endoscopic Approach

♂ **0VHS4YZ** Insertion of Other Device into Penis, Percutaneous Endoscopic Approach

♂ **0VHS7YZ** Insertion of Other Device into Penis, Via Natural or Artificial Opening

♂ **0VHS8YZ** Insertion of Other Device into Penis, Via Natural or Artificial Opening Endoscopic

♂ **0VHSX3Z** Insertion of Infusion Device into Penis, External Approach

0VJ – Male Reproductive System, Inspection

Review Coding Guidelines B3.11a, B3.11b and B3.11c

♂ **0VJ40ZZ** Inspection of Prostate and Seminal Vesicles, Open Approach

♂ **0VJ43ZZ** Inspection of Prostate and Seminal Vesicles, Percutaneous Approach

♂ **0VJ44ZZ** Inspection of Prostate and Seminal Vesicles, Percutaneous Endoscopic Approach

♂ **0VJ4XZZ** Inspection of Prostate and Seminal Vesicles, External Approach

♂ **0VJ80ZZ** Inspection of Scrotum and Tunica Vaginalis, Open Approach

♂ **0VJ83ZZ** Inspection of Scrotum and Tunica Vaginalis, Percutaneous Approach

♂ **0VJ84ZZ** Inspection of Scrotum and Tunica Vaginalis, Percutaneous Endoscopic Approach

♂ **0VJ8XZZ** Inspection of Scrotum and Tunica Vaginalis, External Approach

♂ **0VJD0ZZ** Inspection of Testis, Open Approach

♂ **0VJD3ZZ** Inspection of Testis, Percutaneous Approach

♂ **0VJD4ZZ** Inspection of Testis, Percutaneous Endoscopic Approach

♂ **0VJDXZZ** Inspection of Testis, External Approach

♂ **0VJM0ZZ** Inspection of Epididymis and Spermatic Cord, Open Approach

♂ **0VJM3ZZ** Inspection of Epididymis and Spermatic Cord, Percutaneous Approach

♂ **0VJM4ZZ** Inspection of Epididymis and Spermatic Cord, Percutaneous Endoscopic Approach

♂ **0VJMXZZ** Inspection of Epididymis and Spermatic Cord, External Approach

♂ **0VJR0ZZ** Inspection of Vas Deferens, Open Approach

♂ **0VJR3ZZ** Inspection of Vas Deferens, Percutaneous Approach

♂ **0VJR4ZZ** Inspection of Vas Deferens, Percutaneous Endoscopic Approach

♂ **0VJRXZZ** Inspection of Vas Deferens, External Approach

♂ **0VJS0ZZ** Inspection of Penis, Open Approach

♂ **0VJS3ZZ** Inspection of Penis, Percutaneous Approach

♂ **0VJS4ZZ** Inspection of Penis, Percutaneous Endoscopic Approach

♂ **0VJSXZZ** Inspection of Penis, External Approach

0VL – Male Reproductive System, Occlusion

♂ **0VLF0CZ** Occlusion of Right Spermatic Cord with Extraluminal Device, Open Approach
▲ *When reported with diagnosis code Z30.2*

♂ **0VLF0DZ** Occlusion of Right Spermatic Cord with Intraluminal Device, Open Approach
▲ *When reported with diagnosis code Z30.2*

♂ **0VLF0ZZ** Occlusion of Right Spermatic Cord, Open Approach
▲ *When reported with diagnosis code Z30.2*

♂ **0VLF3CZ** Occlusion of Right Spermatic Cord with Extraluminal Device, Percutaneous Approach
▲ *When reported with diagnosis code Z30.2*

♂ **0VLF3DZ** Occlusion of Right Spermatic Cord with Intraluminal Device, Percutaneous Approach
▲ *When reported with diagnosis code Z30.2*

♂ **0VLF3ZZ** Occlusion of Right Spermatic Cord, Percutaneous Approach
▲ *When reported with diagnosis code Z30.2*

♂ **0VLF4CZ** Occlusion of Right Spermatic Cord with Extraluminal Device, Percutaneous Endoscopic Approach
▲ *When reported with diagnosis code Z30.2*

♂ **0VLF4DZ** Occlusion of Right Spermatic Cord with Intraluminal Device, Percutaneous Endoscopic Approach
▲ *When reported with diagnosis code Z30.2*

♂ **0VLF4ZZ** Occlusion of Right Spermatic Cord, Percutaneous Endoscopic Approach
▲ *When reported with diagnosis code Z30.2*

♂ **0VLF8CZ** Occlusion of Right Spermatic Cord with Extraluminal Device, Via Natural or Artificial Opening Endoscopic

♂ **0VLF8DZ** Occlusion of Right Spermatic Cord with Intraluminal Device, Via Natural or Artificial Opening Endoscopic

♂ **0VLF8ZZ** Occlusion of Right Spermatic Cord, Via Natural or Artificial Opening Endoscopic

♂ **0VLG0CZ** Occlusion of Left Spermatic Cord with Extraluminal Device, Open Approach
▲ *When reported with diagnosis code Z30.2*

♂ **0VLG0DZ** Occlusion of Left Spermatic Cord with Intraluminal Device, Open Approach
▲ *When reported with diagnosis code Z30.2*

♂ **0VLG0ZZ** Occlusion of Left Spermatic Cord, Open Approach
▲ *When reported with diagnosis code Z30.2*

♂ **0VLG3CZ** Occlusion of Left Spermatic Cord with Extraluminal Device, Percutaneous Approach
▲ *When reported with diagnosis code Z30.2*

♂ **0VLG3DZ** Occlusion of Left Spermatic Cord with Intraluminal Device, Percutaneous Approach
▲ *When reported with diagnosis code Z30.2*

♂ **0VLG3ZZ** Occlusion of Left Spermatic Cord, Percutaneous Approach
▲ *When reported with diagnosis code Z30.2*

♂ **0VLG4CZ** Occlusion of Left Spermatic Cord with Extraluminal Device, Percutaneous Endoscopic Approach
▲ *When reported with diagnosis code Z30.2*

♂ **0VLG4DZ** Occlusion of Left Spermatic Cord with Intraluminal Device, Percutaneous Endoscopic Approach
▲ *When reported with diagnosis code Z30.2*

♂ **0VLG4ZZ** Occlusion of Left Spermatic Cord, Percutaneous Endoscopic Approach
▲ *When reported with diagnosis code Z30.2*

♂ **0VLG8CZ** Occlusion of Left Spermatic Cord with Extraluminal Device, Via Natural or Artificial Opening Endoscopic

♂ **0VLG8DZ** Occlusion of Left Spermatic Cord with Intraluminal Device, Via Natural or Artificial Opening Endoscopic

♂ **0VLG8ZZ** Occlusion of Left Spermatic Cord, Via Natural or Artificial Opening Endoscopic

♀ Female-only   ♂ Male-only   ▲ Limited Coverage   ● Non-OR   ⬛ HAC-associated procedure   ▲ Non-covered procedures   ➕ Cluster

♂ **0VLH0CZ** Occlusion of Bilateral Spermatic Cords with Extraluminal Device, Open Approach
▲ *When reported with diagnosis code Z30.2*

♂ **0VLH0DZ** Occlusion of Bilateral Spermatic Cords with Intraluminal Device, Open Approach
▲ *When reported with diagnosis code Z30.2*

♂ **0VLH0ZZ** Occlusion of Bilateral Spermatic Cords, Open Approach
▲ *When reported with diagnosis code Z30.2*

♂ **0VLH3CZ** Occlusion of Bilateral Spermatic Cords with Extraluminal Device, Percutaneous Approach
▲ *When reported with diagnosis code Z30.2*

♂ **0VLH3DZ** Occlusion of Bilateral Spermatic Cords with Intraluminal Device, Percutaneous Approach
▲ *When reported with diagnosis code Z30.2*

♂ **0VLH3ZZ** Occlusion of Bilateral Spermatic Cords, Percutaneous Approach
▲ *When reported with diagnosis code Z30.2*

♂ **0VLH4CZ** Occlusion of Bilateral Spermatic Cords with Extraluminal Device, Percutaneous Endoscopic Approach
▲ *When reported with diagnosis code Z30.2*

♂ **0VLH4DZ** Occlusion of Bilateral Spermatic Cords with Intraluminal Device, Percutaneous Endoscopic Approach
▲ *When reported with diagnosis code Z30.2*

♂ **0VLH4ZZ** Occlusion of Bilateral Spermatic Cords, Percutaneous Endoscopic Approach
▲ *When reported with diagnosis code Z30.2*

♂ **0VLH8CZ** Occlusion of Bilateral Spermatic Cords with Extraluminal Device, Via Natural or Artificial Opening Endoscopic

♂ **0VLH8DZ** Occlusion of Bilateral Spermatic Cords with Intraluminal Device, Via Natural or Artificial Opening Endoscopic

♂ **0VLH8ZZ** Occlusion of Bilateral Spermatic Cords, Via Natural or Artificial Opening Endoscopic

♂ **0VLN0CZ** Occlusion of Right Vas Deferens with Extraluminal Device, Open Approach
▲ *When reported with diagnosis code Z30.2*

♂ **0VLN0DZ** Occlusion of Right Vas Deferens with Intraluminal Device, Open Approach

♂ **0VLN0ZZ** Occlusion of Right Vas Deferens, Open Approach

▲ *When reported with diagnosis code Z30.2*

♂ **0VLN3CZ** Occlusion of Right Vas Deferens with Extraluminal Device, Percutaneous Approach
▲ *When reported with diagnosis code Z30.2*

♂ **0VLN3DZ** Occlusion of Right Vas Deferens with Intraluminal Device, Percutaneous Approach

♂ **0VLN3ZZ** Occlusion of Right Vas Deferens, Percutaneous Approach
▲ *When reported with diagnosis code Z30.2*

♂ **0VLN4CZ** Occlusion of Right Vas Deferens with Extraluminal Device, Percutaneous Endoscopic Approach
▲ *When reported with diagnosis code Z30.2*

♂ **0VLN4DZ** Occlusion of Right Vas Deferens with Intraluminal Device, Percutaneous Endoscopic Approach

♂ **0VLN4ZZ** Occlusion of Right Vas Deferens, Percutaneous Endoscopic Approach
▲ *When reported with diagnosis code Z30.2*

♂ **0VLN8CZ** Occlusion of Right Vas Deferens with Extraluminal Device, Via Natural or Artificial Opening Endoscopic

♂ **0VLN8DZ** Occlusion of Right Vas Deferens with Intraluminal Device, Via Natural or Artificial Opening Endoscopic

♂ **0VLN8ZZ** Occlusion of Right Vas Deferens, Via Natural or Artificial Opening Endoscopic

♂ **0VLP0CZ** Occlusion of Left Vas Deferens with Extraluminal Device, Open Approach
▲ *When reported with diagnosis code Z30.2*

♂ **0VLP0DZ** Occlusion of Left Vas Deferens with Intraluminal Device, Open Approach

♂ **0VLP0ZZ** Occlusion of Left Vas Deferens, Open Approach
▲ *When reported with diagnosis code Z30.2*

♂ **0VLP3CZ** Occlusion of Left Vas Deferens with Extraluminal Device, Percutaneous Approach
▲ *When reported with diagnosis code Z30.2*

♂ **0VLP3DZ** Occlusion of Left Vas Deferens with Intraluminal Device, Percutaneous Approach

♂ **0VLP3ZZ** Occlusion of Left Vas Deferens, Percutaneous Approach
▲ *When reported with diagnosis code Z30.2*

♂ **0VLP4CZ** Occlusion of Left Vas Deferens with Extraluminal Device, Percutaneous Endoscopic Approach
▲ *When reported with diagnosis code Z30.2*

♂ **0VLP4DZ** Occlusion of Left Vas Deferens with Intraluminal Device, Percutaneous Endoscopic Approach

♂ **0VLP4ZZ** Occlusion of Left Vas Deferens, Percutaneous Endoscopic Approach
▲ *When reported with diagnosis code Z30.2*

♂ **0VLP8CZ** Occlusion of Left Vas Deferens with Extraluminal Device, Via Natural or Artificial Opening Endoscopic

♂ **0VLP8DZ** Occlusion of Left Vas Deferens with Intraluminal Device, Via Natural or Artificial Opening Endoscopic

♂ **0VLP8ZZ** Occlusion of Left Vas Deferens, Via Natural or Artificial Opening Endoscopic

♂ **0VLQ0CZ** Occlusion of Bilateral Vas Deferens with Extraluminal Device, Open Approach
▲ *When reported with diagnosis code Z30.2*

♂ **0VLQ0DZ** Occlusion of Bilateral Vas Deferens with Intraluminal Device, Open Approach

♂ **0VLQ0ZZ** Occlusion of Bilateral Vas Deferens, Open Approach
▲ *When reported with diagnosis code Z30.2*

♂ **0VLQ3CZ** Occlusion of Bilateral Vas Deferens with Extraluminal Device, Percutaneous Approach
▲ *When reported with diagnosis code Z30.2*

♂ **0VLQ3DZ** Occlusion of Bilateral Vas Deferens with Intraluminal Device, Percutaneous Approach

♂ **0VLQ3ZZ** Occlusion of Bilateral Vas Deferens, Percutaneous Approach
▲ *When reported with diagnosis code Z30.2*

♂ **0VLQ4CZ** Occlusion of Bilateral Vas Deferens with Extraluminal Device, Percutaneous Endoscopic Approach
▲ *When reported with diagnosis code Z30.2*

♂ **0VLQ4DZ** Occlusion of Bilateral Vas Deferens with Intraluminal Device, Percutaneous Endoscopic Approach

♂ **0VLQ4ZZ** Occlusion of Bilateral Vas Deferens, Percutaneous Endoscopic Approach
▲ *When reported with diagnosis code Z30.2*

♂ **0VLQ8CZ** Occlusion of Bilateral Vas Deferens with Extraluminal Device, Via Natural or Artificial Opening Endoscopic

♂ **0VLQ8DZ** Occlusion of Bilateral Vas Deferens with Intraluminal Device, Via Natural or Artificial Opening Endoscopic

♂ **0VLQ8ZZ** Occlusion of Bilateral Vas Deferens, Via Natural or Artificial Opening Endoscopic

0VM – Male Reproductive System, Reattachment

♂ **0VM5XZZ** Reattachment of Scrotum, External Approach

♂ **0VM60ZZ** Reattachment of Right Tunica Vaginalis, Open Approach

♂ **0VM64ZZ** Reattachment of Right Tunica Vaginalis, Percutaneous Endoscopic Approach

♂ **0VM70ZZ** Reattachment of Left Tunica Vaginalis, Open Approach

♂ **0VM74ZZ** Reattachment of Left Tunica Vaginalis, Percutaneous Endoscopic Approach

♂ **0VM90ZZ** Reattachment of Right Testis, Open Approach

♂ **0VM94ZZ** Reattachment of Right Testis, Percutaneous Endoscopic Approach

♂ **0VMB0ZZ** Reattachment of Left Testis, Open Approach

♂ **0VMB4ZZ** Reattachment of Left Testis, Percutaneous Endoscopic Approach

♂ **0VMC0ZZ** Reattachment of Bilateral Testes, Open Approach

♂ **0VMC4ZZ** Reattachment of Bilateral Testes, Percutaneous Endoscopic Approach

♂ **0VMF0ZZ** Reattachment of Right Spermatic Cord, Open Approach

♀ Female-only ♂ Male-only ▲ Limited Coverage ● Non-OR HAC HAC-associated procedure ▲ Non-covered procedures ✚ Cluster

♂ 0VMF4ZZ Reattachment of Right Spermatic Cord, Percutaneous Endoscopic Approach

♂ 0VMG0ZZ Reattachment of Left Spermatic Cord, Open Approach

♂ 0VMG4ZZ Reattachment of Left Spermatic Cord, Percutaneous Endoscopic Approach

♂ 0VMH0ZZ Reattachment of Bilateral Spermatic Cords, Open Approach

♂ 0VMH4ZZ Reattachment of Bilateral Spermatic Cords, Percutaneous Endoscopic Approach

♂ 0VMSXZZ Reattachment of Penis, External Approach

0VN – Male Reproductive System, Release

Review Coding Guideline B3.13

♂ 0VN00ZZ Release Prostate, Open Approach
♂ 0VN03ZZ Release Prostate, Percutaneous Approach
♂ 0VN04ZZ Release Prostate, Percutaneous Endoscopic Approach
♂ 0VN07ZZ Release Prostate, Via Natural or Artificial Opening
♂ 0VN08ZZ Release Prostate, Via Natural or Artificial Opening Endoscopic
♂ 0VN10ZZ Release Right Seminal Vesicle, Open Approach
♂ 0VN13ZZ Release Right Seminal Vesicle, Percutaneous Approach
♂ 0VN14ZZ Release Right Seminal Vesicle, Percutaneous Endoscopic Approach
♂ 0VN20ZZ Release Left Seminal Vesicle, Open Approach
♂ 0VN23ZZ Release Left Seminal Vesicle, Percutaneous Approach
♂ 0VN24ZZ Release Left Seminal Vesicle, Percutaneous Endoscopic Approach
♂ 0VN30ZZ Release Bilateral Seminal Vesicles, Open Approach
♂ 0VN33ZZ Release Bilateral Seminal Vesicles, Percutaneous Approach
♂ 0VN34ZZ Release Bilateral Seminal Vesicles, Percutaneous Endoscopic Approach
♂ 0VN50ZZ Release Scrotum, Open Approach
♂ 0VN53ZZ Release Scrotum, Percutaneous Approach
♂ 0VN54ZZ Release Scrotum, Percutaneous Endoscopic Approach
♂ 0VN5XZZ Release Scrotum, External Approach
♂ 0VN60ZZ Release Right Tunica Vaginalis, Open Approach
♂ 0VN63ZZ Release Right Tunica Vaginalis, Percutaneous Approach
♂ 0VN64ZZ Release Right Tunica Vaginalis, Percutaneous Endoscopic Approach
♂ 0VN70ZZ Release Left Tunica Vaginalis, Open Approach
♂ 0VN73ZZ Release Left Tunica Vaginalis, Percutaneous Approach
♂ 0VN74ZZ Release Left Tunica Vaginalis, Percutaneous Endoscopic Approach
♂ 0VN90ZZ Release Right Testis, Open Approach
♂ 0VN93ZZ Release Right Testis, Percutaneous Approach
♂ 0VN94ZZ Release Right Testis, Percutaneous Endoscopic Approach
♂ 0VNB0ZZ Release Left Testis, Open Approach

♂ 0VNB3ZZ Release Left Testis, Percutaneous Approach
♂ 0VNB4ZZ Release Left Testis, Percutaneous Endoscopic Approach
♂ 0VNC0ZZ Release Bilateral Testes, Open Approach
♂ 0VNC3ZZ Release Bilateral Testes, Percutaneous Approach
♂ 0VNC4ZZ Release Bilateral Testes, Percutaneous Endoscopic Approach
♂ 0VNF0ZZ Release Right Spermatic Cord, Open Approach
♂ 0VNF3ZZ Release Right Spermatic Cord, Percutaneous Approach
♂ 0VNF4ZZ Release Right Spermatic Cord, Percutaneous Endoscopic Approach
♂ 0VNF8ZZ Release Right Spermatic Cord, Via Natural or Artificial Opening Endoscopic
♂ 0VNG0ZZ Release Left Spermatic Cord, Open Approach
♂ 0VNG3ZZ Release Left Spermatic Cord, Percutaneous Approach
♂ 0VNG4ZZ Release Left Spermatic Cord, Percutaneous Endoscopic Approach
♂ 0VNG8ZZ Release Left Spermatic Cord, Via Natural or Artificial Opening Endoscopic
♂ 0VNH0ZZ Release Bilateral Spermatic Cords, Open Approach
♂ 0VNH3ZZ Release Bilateral Spermatic Cords, Percutaneous Approach
♂ 0VNH4ZZ Release Bilateral Spermatic Cords, Percutaneous Endoscopic Approach
♂ 0VNH8ZZ Release Bilateral Spermatic Cords, Via Natural or Artificial Opening Endoscopic
♂ 0VNJ0ZZ Release Right Epididymis, Open Approach
♂ 0VNJ3ZZ Release Right Epididymis, Percutaneous Approach
♂ 0VNJ4ZZ Release Right Epididymis, Percutaneous Endoscopic Approach
♂ 0VNJ8ZZ Release Right Epididymis, Via Natural or Artificial Opening Endoscopic
♂ 0VNK0ZZ Release Left Epididymis, Open Approach
♂ 0VNK3ZZ Release Left Epididymis, Percutaneous Approach
♂ 0VNK4ZZ Release Left Epididymis, Percutaneous Endoscopic Approach

♂ 0VNK8ZZ Release Left Epididymis, Via Natural or Artificial Opening Endoscopic
♂ 0VNL0ZZ Release Bilateral Epididymis, Open Approach
♂ 0VNL3ZZ Release Bilateral Epididymis, Percutaneous Approach
♂ 0VNL4ZZ Release Bilateral Epididymis, Percutaneous Endoscopic Approach
♂ 0VNL8ZZ Release Bilateral Epididymis, Via Natural or Artificial Opening Endoscopic
♂ 0VNN0ZZ Release Right Vas Deferens, Open Approach
♂ 0VNN3ZZ Release Right Vas Deferens, Percutaneous Approach
♂ 0VNN4ZZ Release Right Vas Deferens, Percutaneous Endoscopic Approach
♂ 0VNN8ZZ Release Right Vas Deferens, Via Natural or Artificial Opening Endoscopic
♂ 0VNP0ZZ Release Left Vas Deferens, Open Approach
♂ 0VNP3ZZ Release Left Vas Deferens, Percutaneous Approach
♂ 0VNP4ZZ Release Left Vas Deferens, Percutaneous Endoscopic Approach
♂ 0VNP8ZZ Release Left Vas Deferens, Via Natural or Artificial Opening Endoscopic
♂ 0VNQ0ZZ Release Bilateral Vas Deferens, Open Approach
♂ 0VNQ3ZZ Release Bilateral Vas Deferens, Percutaneous Approach
♂ 0VNQ4ZZ Release Bilateral Vas Deferens, Percutaneous Endoscopic Approach
♂ 0VNQ8ZZ Release Bilateral Vas Deferens, Via Natural or Artificial Opening Endoscopic
♂ 0VNS0ZZ Release Penis, Open Approach
♂ 0VNS3ZZ Release Penis, Percutaneous Approach
♂ 0VNS4ZZ Release Penis, Percutaneous Endoscopic Approach
♂ 0VNSXZZ Release Penis, External Approach
♂ 0VNT0ZZ Release Prepuce, Open Approach
♂ 0VNT3ZZ Release Prepuce, Percutaneous Approach
♂ 0VNT4ZZ Release Prepuce, Percutaneous Endoscopic Approach
♂ 0VNTXZZ Release Prepuce, External Approach

0VP – Male Reproductive System, Removal

Review Coding Guideline B6.1c

♂ 0VP400Z Removal of Drainage Device from Prostate and Seminal Vesicles, Open Approach
♂ 0VP401Z Removal of Radioactive Element from Prostate and Seminal Vesicles, Open Approach
♂ 0VP403Z Removal of Infusion Device from Prostate and Seminal Vesicles, Open Approach

♂ 0VP407Z Removal of Autologous Tissue Substitute from Prostate and Seminal Vesicles, Open Approach
♂ 0VP40JZ Removal of Synthetic Substitute from Prostate and Seminal Vesicles, Open Approach
♂ 0VP40KZ Removal of Nonautologous Tissue Substitute from Prostate and Seminal Vesicles, Open Approach

♂ 0VP40YZ Removal of Other Device from Prostate and Seminal Vesicles, Open Approach
♂ 0VP430Z Removal of Drainage Device from Prostate and Seminal Vesicles, Percutaneous Approach
♂ 0VP431Z Removal of Radioactive Element from Prostate and Seminal Vesicles, Percutaneous Approach

♂ **0VP433Z** Removal of Infusion Device from Prostate and Seminal Vesicles, Percutaneous Approach

♂ **0VP437Z** Removal of Autologous Tissue Substitute from Prostate and Seminal Vesicles, Percutaneous Approach

♂ **0VP43JZ** Removal of Synthetic Substitute from Prostate and Seminal Vesicles, Percutaneous Approach

♂ **0VP43KZ** Removal of Nonautologous Tissue Substitute from Prostate and Seminal Vesicles, Percutaneous Approach

♂ **0VP43YZ** Removal of Other Device from Prostate and Seminal Vesicles, Percutaneous Approach

♂ **0VP440Z** Removal of Drainage Device from Prostate and Seminal Vesicles, Percutaneous Endoscopic Approach

♂ **0VP441Z** Removal of Radioactive Element from Prostate and Seminal Vesicles, Percutaneous Endoscopic Approach

♂ **0VP443Z** Removal of Infusion Device from Prostate and Seminal Vesicles, Percutaneous Endoscopic Approach

♂ **0VP447Z** Removal of Autologous Tissue Substitute from Prostate and Seminal Vesicles, Percutaneous Endoscopic Approach

♂ **0VP44JZ** Removal of Synthetic Substitute from Prostate and Seminal Vesicles, Percutaneous Endoscopic Approach

♂ **0VP44KZ** Removal of Nonautologous Tissue Substitute from Prostate and Seminal Vesicles, Percutaneous Endoscopic Approach

♂ **0VP44YZ** Removal of Other Device from Prostate and Seminal Vesicles, Percutaneous Endoscopic Approach

♂ **0VP470Z** Removal of Drainage Device from Prostate and Seminal Vesicles, Via Natural or Artificial Opening

♂ **0VP471Z** Removal of Radioactive Element from Prostate and Seminal Vesicles, Via Natural or Artificial Opening

♂ **0VP473Z** Removal of Infusion Device from Prostate and Seminal Vesicles, Via Natural or Artificial Opening

♂ **0VP477Z** Removal of Autologous Tissue Substitute from Prostate and Seminal Vesicles, Via Natural or Artificial Opening

♂ **0VP47JZ** Removal of Synthetic Substitute from Prostate and Seminal Vesicles, Via Natural or Artificial Opening

♂ **0VP47KZ** Removal of Nonautologous Tissue Substitute from Prostate and Seminal Vesicles, Via Natural or Artificial Opening

♂ **0VP47YZ** Removal of Other Device from Prostate and Seminal Vesicles, Via Natural or Artificial Opening

♂ **0VP480Z** Removal of Drainage Device from Prostate and Seminal Vesicles, Via Natural or Artificial Opening Endoscopic

♂ **0VP481Z** Removal of Radioactive Element from Prostate and Seminal Vesicles, Via Natural or Artificial Opening Endoscopic

♂ **0VP483Z** Removal of Infusion Device from Prostate and Seminal Vesicles, Via Natural or Artificial Opening Endoscopic

♂ **0VP487Z** Removal of Autologous Tissue Substitute from Prostate and Seminal Vesicles, Via Natural or Artificial Opening Endoscopic

♂ **0VP48JZ** Removal of Synthetic Substitute from Prostate and Seminal Vesicles, Via Natural or Artificial Opening Endoscopic

♂ **0VP48KZ** Removal of Nonautologous Tissue Substitute from Prostate and Seminal Vesicles, Via Natural or Artificial Opening Endoscopic

♂ **0VP48YZ** Removal of Other Device from Prostate and Seminal Vesicles, Via Natural or Artificial Opening Endoscopic

♂ **0VP4X0Z** Removal of Drainage Device from Prostate and Seminal Vesicles, External Approach

♂ **0VP4X1Z** Removal of Radioactive Element from Prostate and Seminal Vesicles, External Approach

♂ **0VP4X3Z** Removal of Infusion Device from Prostate and Seminal Vesicles, External Approach

♂ **0VP800Z** Removal of Drainage Device from Scrotum and Tunica Vaginalis, Open Approach

♂ **0VP803Z** Removal of Infusion Device from Scrotum and Tunica Vaginalis, Open Approach

♂ **0VP807Z** Removal of Autologous Tissue Substitute from Scrotum and Tunica Vaginalis, Open Approach

♂ **0VP80JZ** Removal of Synthetic Substitute from Scrotum and Tunica Vaginalis, Open Approach

♂ **0VP80KZ** Removal of Nonautologous Tissue Substitute from Scrotum and Tunica Vaginalis, Open Approach

♂ **0VP80YZ** Removal of Other Device from Scrotum and Tunica Vaginalis, Open Approach

♂ **0VP830Z** Removal of Drainage Device from Scrotum and Tunica Vaginalis, Percutaneous Approach

♂ **0VP833Z** Removal of Infusion Device from Scrotum and Tunica Vaginalis, Percutaneous Approach

♂ **0VP837Z** Removal of Autologous Tissue Substitute from Scrotum and Tunica Vaginalis, Percutaneous Approach

♂ **0VP83JZ** Removal of Synthetic Substitute from Scrotum and Tunica Vaginalis, Percutaneous Approach

♂ **0VP83KZ** Removal of Nonautologous Tissue Substitute from Scrotum and Tunica Vaginalis, Percutaneous Approach

♂ **0VP83YZ** Removal of Other Device from Scrotum and Tunica Vaginalis, Percutaneous Approach

♂ **0VP840Z** Removal of Drainage Device from Scrotum and Tunica Vaginalis, Percutaneous Endoscopic Approach

♂ **0VP843Z** Removal of Infusion Device from Scrotum and Tunica Vaginalis, Percutaneous Endoscopic Approach

♂ **0VP847Z** Removal of Autologous Tissue Substitute from Scrotum and Tunica Vaginalis, Percutaneous Endoscopic Approach

♂ **0VP84JZ** Removal of Synthetic Substitute from Scrotum and Tunica Vaginalis, Percutaneous Endoscopic Approach

♂ **0VP84KZ** Removal of Nonautologous Tissue Substitute from Scrotum and Tunica Vaginalis, Percutaneous Endoscopic Approach

♂ **0VP84YZ** Removal of Other Device from Scrotum and Tunica Vaginalis, Percutaneous Endoscopic Approach

♂ **0VP870Z** Removal of Drainage Device from Scrotum and Tunica Vaginalis, Via Natural or Artificial Opening

♂ **0VP873Z** Removal of Infusion Device from Scrotum and Tunica Vaginalis, Via Natural or Artificial Opening

♂ **0VP877Z** Removal of Autologous Tissue Substitute from Scrotum and Tunica Vaginalis, Via Natural or Artificial Opening

♂ **0VP87JZ** Removal of Synthetic Substitute from Scrotum and Tunica Vaginalis, Via Natural or Artificial Opening

♂ **0VP87KZ** Removal of Nonautologous Tissue Substitute from Scrotum and Tunica Vaginalis, Via Natural or Artificial Opening

♂ **0VP87YZ** Removal of Other Device from Scrotum and Tunica Vaginalis, Via Natural or Artificial Opening

♂ **0VP880Z** Removal of Drainage Device from Scrotum and Tunica Vaginalis, Via Natural or Artificial Opening Endoscopic

♂ **0VP883Z** Removal of Infusion Device from Scrotum and Tunica Vaginalis, Via Natural or Artificial Opening Endoscopic

♂ **0VP887Z** Removal of Autologous Tissue Substitute from Scrotum and Tunica Vaginalis, Via Natural or Artificial Opening Endoscopic

♂ **0VP88JZ** Removal of Synthetic Substitute from Scrotum and Tunica Vaginalis, Via Natural or Artificial Opening Endoscopic

♂ **0VP88KZ** Removal of Nonautologous Tissue Substitute from Scrotum and Tunica Vaginalis, Via Natural or Artificial Opening Endoscopic

♂ **0VP88YZ** Removal of Other Device from Scrotum and Tunica Vaginalis, Via Natural or Artificial Opening Endoscopic

♂ **0VP8X0Z** Removal of Drainage Device from Scrotum and Tunica Vaginalis, External Approach

♂ **0VP8X3Z** Removal of Infusion Device from Scrotum and Tunica Vaginalis, External Approach

♂ **0VPD00Z** Removal of Drainage Device from Testis, Open Approach

♂ **0VPD03Z** Removal of Infusion Device from Testis, Open Approach

♂ **0VPD07Z** Removal of Autologous Tissue Substitute from Testis, Open Approach

♂ **0VPD0JZ** Removal of Synthetic Substitute from Testis, Open Approach

♂ **0VPD0KZ** Removal of Nonautologous Tissue Substitute from Testis, Open Approach

♂ **0VPD0YZ** Removal of Other Device from Testis, Open Approach

♂ **0VPD30Z** Removal of Drainage Device from Testis, Percutaneous Approach

♂ **0VPD33Z** Removal of Infusion Device from Testis, Percutaneous Approach

♂ **0VPD37Z** Removal of Autologous Tissue Substitute from Testis, Percutaneous Approach

♂ **0VPD3JZ** Removal of Synthetic Substitute from Testis, Percutaneous Approach

♂ **0VPD3KZ** Removal of Nonautologous Tissue Substitute from Testis, Percutaneous Approach

♂ **0VPD3YZ** Removal of Other Device from Testis, Percutaneous Approach

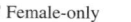 ♀ Female-only   ♂ Male-only   ▲ Limited Coverage   ● Non-OR   ⬛ HAC-associated procedure   ▲ Non-covered procedures   ✚ Cluster

♂ **0VPD40Z** Removal of Drainage Device from Testis, Percutaneous Endoscopic Approach

♂ **0VPD43Z** Removal of Infusion Device from Testis, Percutaneous Endoscopic Approach

♂ **0VPD47Z** Removal of Autologous Tissue Substitute from Testis, Percutaneous Endoscopic Approach

♂ **0VPD4JZ** Removal of Synthetic Substitute from Testis, Percutaneous Endoscopic Approach

♂ **0VPD4KZ** Removal of Nonautologous Tissue Substitute from Testis, Percutaneous Endoscopic Approach

♂ **0VPD4YZ** Removal of Other Device from Testis, Percutaneous Endoscopic Approach

♂ **0VPD70Z** Removal of Drainage Device from Testis, Via Natural or Artificial Opening

♂ **0VPD73Z** Removal of Infusion Device from Testis, Via Natural or Artificial Opening

♂ **0VPD77Z** Removal of Autologous Tissue Substitute from Testis, Via Natural or Artificial Opening

♂ **0VPD7JZ** Removal of Synthetic Substitute from Testis, Via Natural or Artificial Opening

♂ **0VPD7KZ** Removal of Nonautologous Tissue Substitute from Testis, Via Natural or Artificial Opening

♂ **0VPD7YZ** Removal of Other Device from Testis, Via Natural or Artificial Opening

♂ **0VPD80Z** Removal of Drainage Device from Testis, Via Natural or Artificial Opening Endoscopic

♂ **0VPD83Z** Removal of Infusion Device from Testis, Via Natural or Artificial Opening Endoscopic

♂ **0VPD87Z** Removal of Autologous Tissue Substitute from Testis, Via Natural or Artificial Opening Endoscopic

♂ **0VPD8JZ** Removal of Synthetic Substitute from Testis, Via Natural or Artificial Opening Endoscopic

♂ **0VPD8KZ** Removal of Nonautologous Tissue Substitute from Testis, Via Natural or Artificial Opening Endoscopic

♂ **0VPD8YZ** Removal of Other Device from Testis, Via Natural or Artificial Opening Endoscopic

♂ **0VPDX0Z** Removal of Drainage Device from Testis, External Approach

♂ **0VPDX3Z** Removal of Infusion Device from Testis, External Approach

♂ **0VPM00Z** Removal of Drainage Device from Epididymis and Spermatic Cord, Open Approach

♂ **0VPM03Z** Removal of Infusion Device from Epididymis and Spermatic Cord, Open Approach

♂ **0VPM07Z** Removal of Autologous Tissue Substitute from Epididymis and Spermatic Cord, Open Approach

♂ **0VPM0CZ** Removal of Extraluminal Device from Epididymis and Spermatic Cord, Open Approach

♂ **0VPM0JZ** Removal of Synthetic Substitute from Epididymis and Spermatic Cord, Open Approach

♂ **0VPM0KZ** Removal of Nonautologous Tissue Substitute from Epididymis and Spermatic Cord, Open Approach

♂ **0VPM0YZ** Removal of Other Device from Epididymis and Spermatic Cord, Open Approach

♂ **0VPM30Z** Removal of Drainage Device from Epididymis and Spermatic Cord, Percutaneous Approach

♂ **0VPM33Z** Removal of Infusion Device from Epididymis and Spermatic Cord, Percutaneous Approach

♂ **0VPM37Z** Removal of Autologous Tissue Substitute from Epididymis and Spermatic Cord, Percutaneous Approach

♂ **0VPM3CZ** Removal of Extraluminal Device from Epididymis and Spermatic Cord, Percutaneous Approach

♂ **0VPM3JZ** Removal of Synthetic Substitute from Epididymis and Spermatic Cord, Percutaneous Approach

♂ **0VPM3KZ** Removal of Nonautologous Tissue Substitute from Epididymis and Spermatic Cord, Percutaneous Approach

♂ **0VPM3YZ** Removal of Other Device from Epididymis and Spermatic Cord, Percutaneous Approach

♂ **0VPM40Z** Removal of Drainage Device from Epididymis and Spermatic Cord, Percutaneous Endoscopic Approach

♂ **0VPM43Z** Removal of Infusion Device from Epididymis and Spermatic Cord, Percutaneous Endoscopic Approach

♂ **0VPM47Z** Removal of Autologous Tissue Substitute from Epididymis and Spermatic Cord, Percutaneous Endoscopic Approach

♂ **0VPM4CZ** Removal of Extraluminal Device from Epididymis and Spermatic Cord, Percutaneous Endoscopic Approach

♂ **0VPM4JZ** Removal of Synthetic Substitute from Epididymis and Spermatic Cord, Percutaneous Endoscopic Approach

♂ **0VPM4KZ** Removal of Nonautologous Tissue Substitute from Epididymis and Spermatic Cord, Percutaneous Endoscopic Approach

♂ **0VPM4YZ** Removal of Other Device from Epididymis and Spermatic Cord, Percutaneous Endoscopic Approach

♂ **0VPM70Z** Removal of Drainage Device from Epididymis and Spermatic Cord, Via Natural or Artificial Opening

♂ **0VPM73Z** Removal of Infusion Device from Epididymis and Spermatic Cord, Via Natural or Artificial Opening

♂ **0VPM77Z** Removal of Autologous Tissue Substitute from Epididymis and Spermatic Cord, Via Natural or Artificial Opening

♂ **0VPM7CZ** Removal of Extraluminal Device from Epididymis and Spermatic Cord, Via Natural or Artificial Opening

♂ **0VPM7JZ** Removal of Synthetic Substitute from Epididymis and Spermatic Cord, Via Natural or Artificial Opening

♂ **0VPM7KZ** Removal of Nonautologous Tissue Substitute from Epididymis and Spermatic Cord, Via Natural or Artificial Opening

♂ **0VPM7YZ** Removal of Other Device from Epididymis and Spermatic Cord, Via Natural or Artificial Opening

♂ **0VPM80Z** Removal of Drainage Device from Epididymis and Spermatic Cord, Via Natural or Artificial Opening Endoscopic

♂ **0VPM83Z** Removal of Infusion Device from Epididymis and Spermatic Cord, Via Natural or Artificial Opening Endoscopic

♂ **0VPM87Z** Removal of Autologous Tissue Substitute from Epididymis and Spermatic Cord, Via Natural or Artificial Opening Endoscopic

♂ **0VPM8CZ** Removal of Extraluminal Device from Epididymis and Spermatic Cord, Via Natural or Artificial Opening Endoscopic

♂ **0VPM8JZ** Removal of Synthetic Substitute from Epididymis and Spermatic Cord, Via Natural or Artificial Opening Endoscopic

♂ **0VPM8KZ** Removal of Nonautologous Tissue Substitute from Epididymis and Spermatic Cord, Via Natural or Artificial Opening Endoscopic

♂ **0VPM8YZ** Removal of Other Device from Epididymis and Spermatic Cord, Via Natural or Artificial Opening Endoscopic

♂ **0VPMX0Z** Removal of Drainage Device from Epididymis and Spermatic Cord, External Approach

♂ **0VPMX3Z** Removal of Infusion Device from Epididymis and Spermatic Cord, External Approach

♂ **0VPR00Z** Removal of Drainage Device from Vas Deferens, Open Approach

♂ **0VPR03Z** Removal of Infusion Device from Vas Deferens, Open Approach

♂ **0VPR07Z** Removal of Autologous Tissue Substitute from Vas Deferens, Open Approach

♂ **0VPR0CZ** Removal of Extraluminal Device from Vas Deferens, Open Approach

♂ **0VPR0DZ** Removal of Intraluminal Device from Vas Deferens, Open Approach

♂ **0VPR0JZ** Removal of Synthetic Substitute from Vas Deferens, Open Approach

♂ **0VPR0KZ** Removal of Nonautologous Tissue Substitute from Vas Deferens, Open Approach

♂ **0VPR0YZ** Removal of Other Device from Vas Deferens, Open Approach

♂ **0VPR30Z** Removal of Drainage Device from Vas Deferens, Percutaneous Approach

♂ **0VPR33Z** Removal of Infusion Device from Vas Deferens, Percutaneous Approach

♂ **0VPR37Z** Removal of Autologous Tissue Substitute from Vas Deferens, Percutaneous Approach

♂ **0VPR3CZ** Removal of Extraluminal Device from Vas Deferens, Percutaneous Approach

♂ **0VPR3DZ** Removal of Intraluminal Device from Vas Deferens, Percutaneous Approach

♂ **0VPR3JZ** Removal of Synthetic Substitute from Vas Deferens, Percutaneous Approach

♂ **0VPR3KZ** Removal of Nonautologous Tissue Substitute from Vas Deferens, Percutaneous Approach

♂ **0VPR3YZ** Removal of Other Device from Vas Deferens, Percutaneous Approach

♂ **0VPR40Z** Removal of Drainage Device from Vas Deferens, Percutaneous Endoscopic Approach

♂ **0VPR43Z** Removal of Infusion Device from Vas Deferens, Percutaneous Endoscopic Approach

♂ **0VPR47Z** Removal of Autologous Tissue Substitute from Vas Deferens, Percutaneous Endoscopic Approach

♂ **0VPR4CZ** Removal of Extraluminal Device from Vas Deferens, Percutaneous Endoscopic Approach

♂ **0VPR4DZ** Removal of Intraluminal Device from Vas Deferens, Percutaneous Endoscopic Approach

---

♀ Female-only   ♂ Male-only   ▲ Limited Coverage   ● Non-OR   ▥ HAC-associated procedure   ▲ Non-covered procedures   ➕ Cluster

♂ **0VPR4JZ** Removal of Synthetic Substitute from Vas Deferens, Percutaneous Endoscopic Approach

♂ **0VPR4KZ** Removal of Nonautologous Tissue Substitute from Vas Deferens, Percutaneous Endoscopic Approach

♂ **0VPR4YZ** Removal of Other Device from Vas Deferens, Percutaneous Endoscopic Approach

♂ **0VPR70Z** Removal of Drainage Device from Vas Deferens, Via Natural or Artificial Opening

♂ **0VPR73Z** Removal of Infusion Device from Vas Deferens, Via Natural or Artificial Opening

♂ **0VPR77Z** Removal of Autologous Tissue Substitute from Vas Deferens, Via Natural or Artificial Opening

♂ **0VPR7CZ** Removal of Extraluminal Device from Vas Deferens, Via Natural or Artificial Opening

♂ **0VPR7DZ** Removal of Intraluminal Device from Vas Deferens, Via Natural or Artificial Opening

♂ **0VPR7JZ** Removal of Synthetic Substitute from Vas Deferens, Via Natural or Artificial Opening

♂ **0VPR7KZ** Removal of Nonautologous Tissue Substitute from Vas Deferens, Via Natural or Artificial Opening

♂ **0VPR7YZ** Removal of Other Device from Vas Deferens, Via Natural or Artificial Opening

♂ **0VPR80Z** Removal of Drainage Device from Vas Deferens, Via Natural or Artificial Opening Endoscopic

♂ **0VPR83Z** Removal of Infusion Device from Vas Deferens, Via Natural or Artificial Opening Endoscopic

♂ **0VPR87Z** Removal of Autologous Tissue Substitute from Vas Deferens, Via Natural or Artificial Opening Endoscopic

♂ **0VPR8CZ** Removal of Extraluminal Device from Vas Deferens, Via Natural or Artificial Opening Endoscopic

♂ **0VPR8DZ** Removal of Intraluminal Device from Vas Deferens, Via Natural or Artificial Opening Endoscopic

♂ **0VPR8JZ** Removal of Synthetic Substitute from Vas Deferens, Via Natural or Artificial Opening Endoscopic

♂ **0VPR8KZ** Removal of Nonautologous Tissue Substitute from Vas Deferens, Via Natural or Artificial Opening Endoscopic

♂ **0VPR8YZ** Removal of Other Device from Vas Deferens, Via Natural or Artificial Opening Endoscopic

♂ **0VPRX0Z** Removal of Drainage Device from Vas Deferens, External Approach

♂ **0VPRX3Z** Removal of Infusion Device from Vas Deferens, External Approach

♂ **0VPRXDZ** Removal of Intraluminal Device from Vas Deferens, External Approach

♂ **0VPS00Z** Removal of Drainage Device from Penis, Open Approach

♂ **0VPS03Z** Removal of Infusion Device from Penis, Open Approach

♂ **0VPS07Z** Removal of Autologous Tissue Substitute from Penis, Open Approach

♂ **0VPS0JZ** Removal of Synthetic Substitute from Penis, Open Approach

AHA CC: 2Q, 2016, 28-29

♂ **0VPS0KZ** Removal of Nonautologous Tissue Substitute from Penis, Open Approach

♂ **0VPS0YZ** Removal of Other Device from Penis, Open Approach

♂ **0VPS30Z** Removal of Drainage Device from Penis, Percutaneous Approach

♂ **0VPS33Z** Removal of Infusion Device from Penis, Percutaneous Approach

♂ **0VPS37Z** Removal of Autologous Tissue Substitute from Penis, Percutaneous Approach

♂ **0VPS3JZ** Removal of Synthetic Substitute from Penis, Percutaneous Approach

♂ **0VPS3KZ** Removal of Nonautologous Tissue Substitute from Penis, Percutaneous Approach

♂ **0VPS3YZ** Removal of Other Device from Penis, Percutaneous Approach

♂ **0VPS40Z** Removal of Drainage Device from Penis, Percutaneous Endoscopic Approach

♂ **0VPS43Z** Removal of Infusion Device from Penis, Percutaneous Endoscopic Approach

♂ **0VPS47Z** Removal of Autologous Tissue Substitute from Penis, Percutaneous Endoscopic Approach

♂ **0VPS4JZ** Removal of Synthetic Substitute from Penis, Percutaneous Endoscopic Approach

♂ **0VPS4KZ** Removal of Nonautologous Tissue Substitute from Penis, Percutaneous Endoscopic Approach

♂ **0VPS4YZ** Removal of Other Device from Penis, Percutaneous Endoscopic Approach

♂ **0VPS70Z** Removal of Drainage Device from Penis, Via Natural or Artificial Opening

♂ **0VPS73Z** Removal of Infusion Device from Penis, Via Natural or Artificial Opening

♂ **0VPS77Z** Removal of Autologous Tissue Substitute from Penis, Via Natural or Artificial Opening

♂ **0VPS7JZ** Removal of Synthetic Substitute from Penis, Via Natural or Artificial Opening

♂ **0VPS7KZ** Removal of Nonautologous Tissue Substitute from Penis, Via Natural or Artificial Opening

♂ **0VPS7YZ** Removal of Other Device from Penis, Via Natural or Artificial Opening

♂ **0VPS80Z** Removal of Drainage Device from Penis, Via Natural or Artificial Opening Endoscopic

♂ **0VPS83Z** Removal of Infusion Device from Penis, Via Natural or Artificial Opening Endoscopic

♂ **0VPS87Z** Removal of Autologous Tissue Substitute from Penis, Via Natural or Artificial Opening Endoscopic

♂ **0VPS8JZ** Removal of Synthetic Substitute from Penis, Via Natural or Artificial Opening Endoscopic

♂ **0VPS8KZ** Removal of Nonautologous Tissue Substitute from Penis, Via Natural or Artificial Opening Endoscopic

♂ **0VPS8YZ** Removal of Other Device from Penis, Via Natural or Artificial Opening Endoscopic

♂ **0VPSX0Z** Removal of Drainage Device from Penis, External Approach

♂ **0VPSX3Z** Removal of Infusion Device from Penis, External Approach

0VQ – Male Reproductive System, Repair

♂ **0VQ00ZZ** Repair Prostate, Open Approach

♂ **0VQ03ZZ** Repair Prostate, Percutaneous Approach

♂ **0VQ04ZZ** Repair Prostate, Percutaneous Endoscopic Approach

♂ **0VQ07ZZ** Repair Prostate, Via Natural or Artificial Opening

♂ **0VQ08ZZ** Repair Prostate, Via Natural or Artificial Opening Endoscopic

♂ **0VQ10ZZ** Repair Right Seminal Vesicle, Open Approach

♂ **0VQ13ZZ** Repair Right Seminal Vesicle, Percutaneous Approach

♂ **0VQ14ZZ** Repair Right Seminal Vesicle, Percutaneous Endoscopic Approach

♂ **0VQ20ZZ** Repair Left Seminal Vesicle, Open Approach

♂ **0VQ23ZZ** Repair Left Seminal Vesicle, Percutaneous Approach

♂ **0VQ24ZZ** Repair Left Seminal Vesicle, Percutaneous Endoscopic Approach

♂ **0VQ30ZZ** Repair Bilateral Seminal Vesicles, Open Approach

♂ **0VQ33ZZ** Repair Bilateral Seminal Vesicles, Percutaneous Approach

♂ **0VQ34ZZ** Repair Bilateral Seminal Vesicles, Percutaneous Endoscopic Approach

♂ **0VQ50ZZ** Repair Scrotum, Open Approach

♂ **0VQ53ZZ** Repair Scrotum, Percutaneous Approach

♂ **0VQ54ZZ** Repair Scrotum, Percutaneous Endoscopic Approach

♂ **0VQ5XZZ** Repair Scrotum, External Approach

♂ **0VQ60ZZ** Repair Right Tunica Vaginalis, Open Approach

♂ **0VQ63ZZ** Repair Right Tunica Vaginalis, Percutaneous Approach

♂ **0VQ64ZZ** Repair Right Tunica Vaginalis, Percutaneous Endoscopic Approach

♂ **0VQ70ZZ** Repair Left Tunica Vaginalis, Open Approach

♂ **0VQ73ZZ** Repair Left Tunica Vaginalis, Percutaneous Approach

♂ **0VQ74ZZ** Repair Left Tunica Vaginalis, Percutaneous Endoscopic Approach

♂ **0VQ90ZZ** Repair Right Testis, Open Approach

♂ **0VQ93ZZ** Repair Right Testis, Percutaneous Approach

♂ **0VQ94ZZ** Repair Right Testis, Percutaneous Endoscopic Approach

♂ **0VQB0ZZ** Repair Left Testis, Open Approach

♂ **0VQB3ZZ** Repair Left Testis, Percutaneous Approach

♂ **0VQB4ZZ** Repair Left Testis, Percutaneous Endoscopic Approach

♂ **0VQC0ZZ** Repair Bilateral Testes, Open Approach

♂ **0VQC3ZZ** Repair Bilateral Testes, Percutaneous Approach

♂ **0VQC4ZZ** Repair Bilateral Testes, Percutaneous Endoscopic Approach

♂ **0VQF0ZZ** Repair Right Spermatic Cord, Open Approach

♂ **0VQF3ZZ** Repair Right Spermatic Cord, Percutaneous Approach

♂ **0VQF4ZZ** Repair Right Spermatic Cord, Percutaneous Endoscopic Approach

♀ Female-only   ♂ Male-only   ▲ Limited Coverage   ● Non-OR   HAC HAC-associated procedure   ▲ Non-covered procedures   ✚ Cluster

♂ **0VQF8ZZ** Repair Right Spermatic Cord, Via Natural or Artificial Opening Endoscopic

♂ **0VQG0ZZ** Repair Left Spermatic Cord, Open Approach

♂ **0VQG3ZZ** Repair Left Spermatic Cord, Percutaneous Approach

♂ **0VQG4ZZ** Repair Left Spermatic Cord, Percutaneous Endoscopic Approach

♂ **0VQG8ZZ** Repair Left Spermatic Cord, Via Natural or Artificial Opening Endoscopic

♂ **0VQH0ZZ** Repair Bilateral Spermatic Cords, Open Approach

♂ **0VQH3ZZ** Repair Bilateral Spermatic Cords, Percutaneous Approach

♂ **0VQH4ZZ** Repair Bilateral Spermatic Cords, Percutaneous Endoscopic Approach

♂ **0VQH8ZZ** Repair Bilateral Spermatic Cords, Via Natural or Artificial Opening Endoscopic

♂ **0VQJ0ZZ** Repair Right Epididymis, Open Approach

♂ **0VQJ3ZZ** Repair Right Epididymis, Percutaneous Approach

♂ **0VQJ4ZZ** Repair Right Epididymis, Percutaneous Endoscopic Approach

♂ **0VQJ8ZZ** Repair Right Epididymis, Via Natural or Artificial Opening Endoscopic

♂ **0VQK0ZZ** Repair Left Epididymis, Open Approach

♂ **0VQK3ZZ** Repair Left Epididymis, Percutaneous Approach

♂ **0VQK4ZZ** Repair Left Epididymis, Percutaneous Endoscopic Approach

♂ **0VQK8ZZ** Repair Left Epididymis, Via Natural or Artificial Opening Endoscopic

♂ **0VQL0ZZ** Repair Bilateral Epididymis, Open Approach

♂ **0VQL3ZZ** Repair Bilateral Epididymis, Percutaneous Approach

♂ **0VQL4ZZ** Repair Bilateral Epididymis, Percutaneous Endoscopic Approach

♂ **0VQL8ZZ** Repair Bilateral Epididymis, Via Natural or Artificial Opening Endoscopic

♂ **0VQN0ZZ** Repair Right Vas Deferens, Open Approach

♂ **0VQN3ZZ** Repair Right Vas Deferens, Percutaneous Approach

♂ **0VQN4ZZ** Repair Right Vas Deferens, Percutaneous Endoscopic Approach

♂ **0VQN8ZZ** Repair Right Vas Deferens, Via Natural or Artificial Opening Endoscopic

♂ **0VQP0ZZ** Repair Left Vas Deferens, Open Approach

♂ **0VQP3ZZ** Repair Left Vas Deferens, Percutaneous Approach

♂ **0VQP4ZZ** Repair Left Vas Deferens, Percutaneous Endoscopic Approach

♂ **0VQP8ZZ** Repair Left Vas Deferens, Via Natural or Artificial Opening Endoscopic

♂ **0VQQ0ZZ** Repair Bilateral Vas Deferens, Open Approach

♂ **0VQQ3ZZ** Repair Bilateral Vas Deferens, Percutaneous Approach

♂ **0VQQ4ZZ** Repair Bilateral Vas Deferens, Percutaneous Endoscopic Approach

♂ **0VQQ8ZZ** Repair Bilateral Vas Deferens, Via Natural or Artificial Opening Endoscopic

♂ **0VQS0ZZ** Repair Penis, Open Approach

♂ **0VQS3ZZ** Repair Penis, Percutaneous Approach
AHA CC: 3Q, 2018, 12

♂ **0VQS4ZZ** Repair Penis, Percutaneous Endoscopic Approach

♂ **0VQSXZZ** Repair Penis, External Approach

♂ **0VQT0ZZ** Repair Prepuce, Open Approach

♂ **0VQT3ZZ** Repair Prepuce, Percutaneous Approach

♂ **0VQT4ZZ** Repair Prepuce, Percutaneous Endoscopic Approach

♂ **0VQTXZZ** Repair Prepuce, External Approach

0VR – Male Reproductive System, Replacement

Review Coding Guideline B3.18

♂ **0VR90JZ** Replacement of Right Testis with Synthetic Substitute, Open Approach

♂ **0VRB0JZ** Replacement of Left Testis with Synthetic Substitute, Open Approach

♂ **0VRC0JZ** Replacement of Bilateral Testes with Synthetic Substitute, Open Approach

0VS – Male Reproductive System, Reposition

♂ **0VS90ZZ** Reposition Right Testis, Open Approach

♂ **0VS93ZZ** Reposition Right Testis, Percutaneous Approach

♂ **0VS94ZZ** Reposition Right Testis, Percutaneous Endoscopic Approach

♂ **0VS98ZZ** Reposition Right Testis, Via Natural or Artificial Opening Endoscopic

♂ **0VSB0ZZ** Reposition Left Testis, Open Approach

♂ **0VSB3ZZ** Reposition Left Testis, Percutaneous Approach

♂ **0VSB4ZZ** Reposition Left Testis, Percutaneous Endoscopic Approach

♂ **0VSB8ZZ** Reposition Left Testis, Via Natural or Artificial Opening Endoscopic

♂ **0VSC0ZZ** Reposition Bilateral Testes, Open Approach

♂ **0VSC3ZZ** Reposition Bilateral Testes, Percutaneous Approach

♂ **0VSC4ZZ** Reposition Bilateral Testes, Percutaneous Endoscopic Approach

♂ **0VSC8ZZ** Reposition Bilateral Testes, Via Natural or Artificial Opening Endoscopic

♂ **0VSF0ZZ** Reposition Right Spermatic Cord, Open Approach

♂ **0VSF3ZZ** Reposition Right Spermatic Cord, Percutaneous Approach

♂ **0VSF4ZZ** Reposition Right Spermatic Cord, Percutaneous Endoscopic Approach

♂ **0VSF8ZZ** Reposition Right Spermatic Cord, Via Natural or Artificial Opening Endoscopic

♂ **0VSG0ZZ** Reposition Left Spermatic Cord, Open Approach

♂ **0VSG3ZZ** Reposition Left Spermatic Cord, Percutaneous Approach

♂ **0VSG4ZZ** Reposition Left Spermatic Cord, Percutaneous Endoscopic Approach

♂ **0VSG8ZZ** Reposition Left Spermatic Cord, Via Natural or Artificial Opening Endoscopic

♂ **0VSH0ZZ** Reposition Bilateral Spermatic Cords, Open Approach

♂ **0VSH3ZZ** Reposition Bilateral Spermatic Cords, Percutaneous Approach

♂ **0VSH4ZZ** Reposition Bilateral Spermatic Cords, Percutaneous Endoscopic Approach

♂ **0VSH8ZZ** Reposition Bilateral Spermatic Cords, Via Natural or Artificial Opening Endoscopic

0VT – Male Reproductive System, Resection

Review Coding Guideline B3.8

Review Coding Guideline B3.18

♂ **0VT00ZZ** Resection of Prostate, Open Approach
➕ Radical prostatectomy when reported with Resection of bilateral seminal vesicles. *See table 0VT to construct the Resection code.*

♂ **0VT04ZZ** Resection of Prostate, Percutaneous Endoscopic Approach
➕ Radical prostatectomy when reported with Resection of bilateral seminal vesicles. *See table 0VT to construct the Resection code.*
AHA CC: 4Q, 2014, 33-34

♂ **0VT07ZZ** Resection of Prostate, Via Natural or Artificial Opening
➕ Radical prostatectomy when reported with Resection of bilateral seminal vesicles. *See table 0VT to construct the Resection code.*

♂ **0VT08ZZ** Resection of Prostate, Via Natural or Artificial Opening Endoscopic
➕ Radical prostatectomy when reported with Resection of bilateral seminal vesicles. *See table 0VT to construct the Resection code.*

♂ **0VT10ZZ** Resection of Right Seminal Vesicle, Open Approach

♂ **0VT14ZZ** Resection of Right Seminal Vesicle, Percutaneous Endoscopic Approach

♂ **0VT20ZZ** Resection of Left Seminal Vesicle, Open Approach

♂ **0VT24ZZ** Resection of Left Seminal Vesicle, Percutaneous Endoscopic Approach

♂ **0VT30ZZ** Resection of Bilateral Seminal Vesicles, Open Approach

♂ **0VT34ZZ** Resection of Bilateral Seminal Vesicles, Percutaneous Endoscopic Approach
AHA CC: 4Q, 2014, 33-34

♂ **0VT50ZZ** Resection of Scrotum, Open Approach

♂ **0VT54ZZ** Resection of Scrotum, Percutaneous Endoscopic Approach

♂ **0VT5XZZ** Resection of Scrotum, External Approach

♂ **0VT60ZZ** Resection of Right Tunica Vaginalis, Open Approach

♂ **0VT64ZZ** Resection of Right Tunica Vaginalis, Percutaneous Endoscopic Approach

♂ **0VT70ZZ** Resection of Left Tunica Vaginalis, Open Approach

♂ **0VT74ZZ** Resection of Left Tunica Vaginalis, Percutaneous Endoscopic Approach

♂ **0VT90ZZ** Resection of Right Testis, Open Approach

♂ **0VT94ZZ** Resection of Right Testis, Percutaneous Endoscopic Approach

♂ **0VTB0ZZ** Resection of Left Testis, Open Approach

♂ **0VTB4ZZ** Resection of Left Testis, Percutaneous Endoscopic Approach

♂ **0VTC0ZZ** Resection of Bilateral Testes, Open Approach

♂ **0VTC4ZZ** Resection of Bilateral Testes, Percutaneous Endoscopic Approach

♂ **0VTF0ZZ** Resection of Right Spermatic Cord, Open Approach

♂ **0VTF4ZZ** Resection of Right Spermatic Cord, Percutaneous Endoscopic Approach

♂ **0VTG0ZZ** Resection of Left Spermatic Cord, Open Approach

♂ **0VTG4ZZ** Resection of Left Spermatic Cord, Percutaneous Endoscopic Approach

♂ **0VTH0ZZ** Resection of Bilateral Spermatic Cords, Open Approach

♂ **0VTH4ZZ** Resection of Bilateral Spermatic Cords, Percutaneous Endoscopic Approach

♂ **0VTJ0ZZ** Resection of Right Epididymis, Open Approach

♂ **0VTJ4ZZ** Resection of Right Epididymis, Percutaneous Endoscopic Approach

♂ **0VTK0ZZ** Resection of Left Epididymis, Open Approach

♂ **0VTK4ZZ** Resection of Left Epididymis, Percutaneous Endoscopic Approach

♂ **0VTL0ZZ** Resection of Bilateral Epididymis, Open Approach

♂ **0VTL4ZZ** Resection of Bilateral Epididymis, Percutaneous Endoscopic Approach

♂ **0VTN0ZZ** Resection of Right Vas Deferens, Open Approach
▲ *When reported with diagnosis code Z30.2*

♂ **0VTN4ZZ** Resection of Right Vas Deferens, Percutaneous Endoscopic Approach
▲ *When reported with diagnosis code Z30.2*

♂ **0VTP0ZZ** Resection of Left Vas Deferens, Open Approach
▲ *When reported with diagnosis code Z30.2*

♂ **0VTP4ZZ** Resection of Left Vas Deferens, Percutaneous Endoscopic Approach
▲ *When reported with diagnosis code Z30.2*

♂ **0VTQ0ZZ** Resection of Bilateral Vas Deferens, Open Approach
▲ *When reported with diagnosis code Z30.2*

♂ **0VTQ4ZZ** Resection of Bilateral Vas Deferens, Percutaneous Endoscopic Approach
▲ *When reported with diagnosis code Z30.2*

♂ **0VTS0ZZ** Resection of Penis, Open Approach

♂ **0VTS4ZZ** Resection of Penis, Percutaneous Endoscopic Approach

♂ **0VTSXZZ** Resection of Penis, External Approach

♂ **0VTT0ZZ** Resection of Prepuce, Open Approach

♂ **0VTT4ZZ** Resection of Prepuce, Percutaneous Endoscopic Approach

♂ **0VTTXZZ** Resection of Prepuce, External Approach

0VU – Male Reproductive System, Supplement

♂ **0VU107Z** Supplement Right Seminal Vesicle with Autologous Tissue Substitute, Open Approach

♂ **0VU10JZ** Supplement Right Seminal Vesicle with Synthetic Substitute, Open Approach

♂ **0VU10KZ** Supplement Right Seminal Vesicle with Nonautologous Tissue Substitute, Open Approach

♂ **0VU147Z** Supplement Right Seminal Vesicle with Autologous Tissue Substitute, Percutaneous Endoscopic Approach

♂ **0VU14JZ** Supplement Right Seminal Vesicle with Synthetic Substitute, Percutaneous Endoscopic Approach

♂ **0VU14KZ** Supplement Right Seminal Vesicle with Nonautologous Tissue Substitute, Percutaneous Endoscopic Approach

♂ **0VU187Z** Supplement Right Seminal Vesicle with Autologous Tissue Substitute, Via Natural or Artificial Opening Endoscopic

♂ **0VU18JZ** Supplement Right Seminal Vesicle with Synthetic Substitute, Via Natural or Artificial Opening Endoscopic

♂ **0VU18KZ** Supplement Right Seminal Vesicle with Nonautologous Tissue Substitute, Via Natural or Artificial Opening Endoscopic

♂ **0VU207Z** Supplement Left Seminal Vesicle with Autologous Tissue Substitute, Open Approach

♂ **0VU20JZ** Supplement Left Seminal Vesicle with Synthetic Substitute, Open Approach

♂ **0VU20KZ** Supplement Left Seminal Vesicle with Nonautologous Tissue Substitute, Open Approach

♂ **0VU247Z** Supplement Left Seminal Vesicle with Autologous Tissue Substitute, Percutaneous Endoscopic Approach

♂ **0VU24JZ** Supplement Left Seminal Vesicle with Synthetic Substitute, Percutaneous Endoscopic Approach

♂ **0VU24KZ** Supplement Left Seminal Vesicle with Nonautologous Tissue Substitute, Percutaneous Endoscopic Approach

♂ **0VU287Z** Supplement Left Seminal Vesicle with Autologous Tissue Substitute, Via Natural or Artificial Opening Endoscopic

♂ **0VU28JZ** Supplement Left Seminal Vesicle with Synthetic Substitute, Via Natural or Artificial Opening Endoscopic

♂ **0VU28KZ** Supplement Left Seminal Vesicle with Nonautologous Tissue Substitute, Via Natural or Artificial Opening Endoscopic

♂ **0VU307Z** Supplement Bilateral Seminal Vesicles with Autologous Tissue Substitute, Open Approach

♂ **0VU30JZ** Supplement Bilateral Seminal Vesicles with Synthetic Substitute, Open Approach

♂ **0VU30KZ** Supplement Bilateral Seminal Vesicles with Nonautologous Tissue Substitute, Open Approach

♂ **0VU347Z** Supplement Bilateral Seminal Vesicles with Autologous Tissue Substitute, Percutaneous Endoscopic Approach

♂ **0VU34JZ** Supplement Bilateral Seminal Vesicles with Synthetic Substitute, Percutaneous Endoscopic Approach

♂ **0VU34KZ** Supplement Bilateral Seminal Vesicles with Nonautologous Tissue Substitute, Percutaneous Endoscopic Approach

♂ **0VU387Z** Supplement Bilateral Seminal Vesicles with Autologous Tissue Substitute, Via Natural or Artificial Opening Endoscopic

♂ **0VU38JZ** Supplement Bilateral Seminal Vesicles with Synthetic Substitute, Via Natural or Artificial Opening Endoscopic

♂ **0VU38KZ** Supplement Bilateral Seminal Vesicles with Nonautologous Tissue Substitute, Via Natural or Artificial Opening Endoscopic

♂ **0VU507Z** Supplement Scrotum with Autologous Tissue Substitute, Open Approach

♂ **0VU50JZ** Supplement Scrotum with Synthetic Substitute, Open Approach

♂ **0VU50KZ** Supplement Scrotum with Nonautologous Tissue Substitute, Open Approach

♂ **0VU547Z** Supplement Scrotum with Autologous Tissue Substitute, Percutaneous Endoscopic Approach

♂ **0VU54JZ** Supplement Scrotum with Synthetic Substitute, Percutaneous Endoscopic Approach

♂ **0VU54KZ** Supplement Scrotum with Nonautologous Tissue Substitute, Percutaneous Endoscopic Approach

♂ **0VU5X7Z** Supplement Scrotum with Autologous Tissue Substitute, External Approach

♂ **0VU5XJZ** Supplement Scrotum with Synthetic Substitute, External Approach

♂ **0VU5XKZ** Supplement Scrotum with Nonautologous Tissue Substitute, External Approach

♂ **0VU607Z** Supplement Right Tunica Vaginalis with Autologous Tissue Substitute, Open Approach

♂ **0VU60JZ** Supplement Right Tunica Vaginalis with Synthetic Substitute, Open Approach

♂ **0VU60KZ** Supplement Right Tunica Vaginalis with Nonautologous Tissue Substitute, Open Approach

♂ **0VU647Z** Supplement Right Tunica Vaginalis with Autologous Tissue Substitute, Percutaneous Endoscopic Approach

♂ **0VU64JZ** Supplement Right Tunica Vaginalis with Synthetic Substitute, Percutaneous Endoscopic Approach

♂ **0VU64KZ** Supplement Right Tunica Vaginalis with Nonautologous Tissue Substitute, Percutaneous Endoscopic Approach

♂ **0VU687Z** Supplement Right Tunica Vaginalis with Autologous Tissue Substitute, Via Natural or Artificial Opening Endoscopic

♀ Female-only   ♂ Male-only   ▲ Limited Coverage   ● Non-OR   🅷🅰🅲 HAC-associated procedure   ▲ Non-covered procedures   ✚ Cluster

♂ **0VU68JZ** Supplement Right Tunica Vaginalis with Synthetic Substitute, Via Natural or Artificial Opening Endoscopic

♂ **0VU68KZ** Supplement Right Tunica Vaginalis with Nonautologous Tissue Substitute, Via Natural or Artificial Opening Endoscopic

♂ **0VU707Z** Supplement Left Tunica Vaginalis with Autologous Tissue Substitute, Open Approach

♂ **0VU70JZ** Supplement Left Tunica Vaginalis with Synthetic Substitute, Open Approach

♂ **0VU70KZ** Supplement Left Tunica Vaginalis with Nonautologous Tissue Substitute, Open Approach

♂ **0VU747Z** Supplement Left Tunica Vaginalis with Autologous Tissue Substitute, Percutaneous Endoscopic Approach

♂ **0VU74JZ** Supplement Left Tunica Vaginalis with Synthetic Substitute, Percutaneous Endoscopic Approach

♂ **0VU74KZ** Supplement Left Tunica Vaginalis with Nonautologous Tissue Substitute, Percutaneous Endoscopic Approach

♂ **0VU787Z** Supplement Left Tunica Vaginalis with Autologous Tissue Substitute, Via Natural or Artificial Opening Endoscopic

♂ **0VU78JZ** Supplement Left Tunica Vaginalis with Synthetic Substitute, Via Natural or Artificial Opening Endoscopic

♂ **0VU78KZ** Supplement Left Tunica Vaginalis with Nonautologous Tissue Substitute, Via Natural or Artificial Opening Endoscopic

♂ **0VU907Z** Supplement Right Testis with Autologous Tissue Substitute, Open Approach

♂ **0VU90JZ** Supplement Right Testis with Synthetic Substitute, Open Approach

♂ **0VU90KZ** Supplement Right Testis with Nonautologous Tissue Substitute, Open Approach

♂ **0VUB07Z** Supplement Left Testis with Autologous Tissue Substitute, Open Approach

♂ **0VUB0JZ** Supplement Left Testis with Synthetic Substitute, Open Approach

♂ **0VUB0KZ** Supplement Left Testis with Nonautologous Tissue Substitute, Open Approach

♂ **0VUC07Z** Supplement Bilateral Testes with Autologous Tissue Substitute, Open Approach

♂ **0VUC0JZ** Supplement Bilateral Testes with Synthetic Substitute, Open Approach

♂ **0VUC0KZ** Supplement Bilateral Testes with Nonautologous Tissue Substitute, Open Approach

♂ **0VUF07Z** Supplement Right Spermatic Cord with Autologous Tissue Substitute, Open Approach

♂ **0VUF0JZ** Supplement Right Spermatic Cord with Synthetic Substitute, Open Approach

♂ **0VUF0KZ** Supplement Right Spermatic Cord with Nonautologous Tissue Substitute, Open Approach

♂ **0VUF47Z** Supplement Right Spermatic Cord with Autologous Tissue Substitute, Percutaneous Endoscopic Approach

♂ **0VUF4JZ** Supplement Right Spermatic Cord with Synthetic Substitute, Percutaneous Endoscopic Approach

♂ **0VUF4KZ** Supplement Right Spermatic Cord with Nonautologous Tissue Substitute, Percutaneous Endoscopic Approach

♂ **0VUF87Z** Supplement Right Spermatic Cord with Autologous Tissue Substitute, Via Natural or Artificial Opening Endoscopic

♂ **0VUF8JZ** Supplement Right Spermatic Cord with Synthetic Substitute, Via Natural or Artificial Opening Endoscopic

♂ **0VUF8KZ** Supplement Right Spermatic Cord with Nonautologous Tissue Substitute, Via Natural or Artificial Opening Endoscopic

♂ **0VUG07Z** Supplement Left Spermatic Cord with Autologous Tissue Substitute, Open Approach

♂ **0VUG0JZ** Supplement Left Spermatic Cord with Synthetic Substitute, Open Approach

♂ **0VUG0KZ** Supplement Left Spermatic Cord with Nonautologous Tissue Substitute, Open Approach

♂ **0VUG47Z** Supplement Left Spermatic Cord with Autologous Tissue Substitute, Percutaneous Endoscopic Approach

♂ **0VUG4JZ** Supplement Left Spermatic Cord with Synthetic Substitute, Percutaneous Endoscopic Approach

♂ **0VUG4KZ** Supplement Left Spermatic Cord with Nonautologous Tissue Substitute, Percutaneous Endoscopic Approach

♂ **0VUG87Z** Supplement Left Spermatic Cord with Autologous Tissue Substitute, Via Natural or Artificial Opening Endoscopic

♂ **0VUG8JZ** Supplement Left Spermatic Cord with Synthetic Substitute, Via Natural or Artificial Opening Endoscopic

♂ **0VUG8KZ** Supplement Left Spermatic Cord with Nonautologous Tissue Substitute, Via Natural or Artificial Opening Endoscopic

♂ **0VUH07Z** Supplement Bilateral Spermatic Cords with Autologous Tissue Substitute, Open Approach

♂ **0VUH0JZ** Supplement Bilateral Spermatic Cords with Synthetic Substitute, Open Approach

♂ **0VUH0KZ** Supplement Bilateral Spermatic Cords with Nonautologous Tissue Substitute, Open Approach

♂ **0VUH47Z** Supplement Bilateral Spermatic Cords with Autologous Tissue Substitute, Percutaneous Endoscopic Approach

♂ **0VUH4JZ** Supplement Bilateral Spermatic Cords with Synthetic Substitute, Percutaneous Endoscopic Approach

♂ **0VUH4KZ** Supplement Bilateral Spermatic Cords with Nonautologous Tissue Substitute, Percutaneous Endoscopic Approach

♂ **0VUH87Z** Supplement Bilateral Spermatic Cords with Autologous Tissue Substitute, Via Natural or Artificial Opening Endoscopic

♂ **0VUH8JZ** Supplement Bilateral Spermatic Cords with Synthetic Substitute, Via Natural or Artificial Opening Endoscopic

♂ **0VUH8KZ** Supplement Bilateral Spermatic Cords with Nonautologous Tissue Substitute, Via Natural or Artificial Opening Endoscopic

♂ **0VUJ07Z** Supplement Right Epididymis with Autologous Tissue Substitute, Open Approach

♂ **0VUJ0JZ** Supplement Right Epididymis with Synthetic Substitute, Open Approach

♂ **0VUJ0KZ** Supplement Right Epididymis with Nonautologous Tissue Substitute, Open Approach

♂ **0VUJ47Z** Supplement Right Epididymis with Autologous Tissue Substitute, Percutaneous Endoscopic Approach

♂ **0VUJ4JZ** Supplement Right Epididymis with Synthetic Substitute, Percutaneous Endoscopic Approach

♂ **0VUJ4KZ** Supplement Right Epididymis with Nonautologous Tissue Substitute, Percutaneous Endoscopic Approach

♂ **0VUJ87Z** Supplement Right Epididymis with Autologous Tissue Substitute, Via Natural or Artificial Opening Endoscopic

♂ **0VUJ8JZ** Supplement Right Epididymis with Synthetic Substitute, Via Natural or Artificial Opening Endoscopic

♂ **0VUJ8KZ** Supplement Right Epididymis with Nonautologous Tissue Substitute, Via Natural or Artificial Opening Endoscopic

♂ **0VUK07Z** Supplement Left Epididymis with Autologous Tissue Substitute, Open Approach

♂ **0VUK0JZ** Supplement Left Epididymis with Synthetic Substitute, Open Approach

♂ **0VUK0KZ** Supplement Left Epididymis with Nonautologous Tissue Substitute, Open Approach

♂ **0VUK47Z** Supplement Left Epididymis with Autologous Tissue Substitute, Percutaneous Endoscopic Approach

♂ **0VUK4JZ** Supplement Left Epididymis with Synthetic Substitute, Percutaneous Endoscopic Approach

♂ **0VUK4KZ** Supplement Left Epididymis with Nonautologous Tissue Substitute, Percutaneous Endoscopic Approach

♂ **0VUK87Z** Supplement Left Epididymis with Autologous Tissue Substitute, Via Natural or Artificial Opening Endoscopic

♂ **0VUK8JZ** Supplement Left Epididymis with Synthetic Substitute, Via Natural or Artificial Opening Endoscopic

♂ **0VUK8KZ** Supplement Left Epididymis with Nonautologous Tissue Substitute, Via Natural or Artificial Opening Endoscopic

♂ **0VUL07Z** Supplement Bilateral Epididymis with Autologous Tissue Substitute, Open Approach

♂ **0VUL0JZ** Supplement Bilateral Epididymis with Synthetic Substitute, Open Approach

♂ **0VUL0KZ** Supplement Bilateral Epididymis with Nonautologous Tissue Substitute, Open Approach

♂ **0VUL47Z** Supplement Bilateral Epididymis with Autologous Tissue Substitute, Percutaneous Endoscopic Approach

♂ **0VUL4JZ** Supplement Bilateral Epididymis with Synthetic Substitute, Percutaneous Endoscopic Approach

♂ **0VUL4KZ** Supplement Bilateral Epididymis with Nonautologous Tissue Substitute, Percutaneous Endoscopic Approach

♂ **0VUL87Z** Supplement Bilateral Epididymis with Autologous Tissue Substitute, Via Natural or Artificial Opening Endoscopic

♂ **0VUL8JZ** Supplement Bilateral Epididymis with Synthetic Substitute, Via Natural or Artificial Opening Endoscopic

♂ **0VUL8KZ** Supplement Bilateral Epididymis with Nonautologous Tissue Substitute, Via Natural or Artificial Opening Endoscopic

---

♀ Female-only   ♂ Male-only   ▲ Limited Coverage   ● Non-OR   HAC HAC-associated procedure   ▲ Non-covered procedures   ＋ Cluster

♂ **0VUN07Z** Supplement Right Vas Deferens with Autologous Tissue Substitute, Open Approach

♂ **0VUN0JZ** Supplement Right Vas Deferens with Synthetic Substitute, Open Approach

♂ **0VUN0KZ** Supplement Right Vas Deferens with Nonautologous Tissue Substitute, Open Approach

♂ **0VUN47Z** Supplement Right Vas Deferens with Autologous Tissue Substitute, Percutaneous Endoscopic Approach

♂ **0VUN4JZ** Supplement Right Vas Deferens with Synthetic Substitute, Percutaneous Endoscopic Approach

♂ **0VUN4KZ** Supplement Right Vas Deferens with Nonautologous Tissue Substitute, Percutaneous Endoscopic Approach

♂ **0VUN87Z** Supplement Right Vas Deferens with Autologous Tissue Substitute, Via Natural or Artificial Opening Endoscopic

♂ **0VUN8JZ** Supplement Right Vas Deferens with Synthetic Substitute, Via Natural or Artificial Opening Endoscopic

♂ **0VUN8KZ** Supplement Right Vas Deferens with Nonautologous Tissue Substitute, Via Natural or Artificial Opening Endoscopic

♂ **0VUP07Z** Supplement Left Vas Deferens with Autologous Tissue Substitute, Open Approach

♂ **0VUP0JZ** Supplement Left Vas Deferens with Synthetic Substitute, Open Approach

♂ **0VUP0KZ** Supplement Left Vas Deferens with Nonautologous Tissue Substitute, Open Approach

♂ **0VUP47Z** Supplement Left Vas Deferens with Autologous Tissue Substitute, Percutaneous Endoscopic Approach

♂ **0VUP4JZ** Supplement Left Vas Deferens with Synthetic Substitute, Percutaneous Endoscopic Approach

♂ **0VUP4KZ** Supplement Left Vas Deferens with Nonautologous Tissue Substitute, Percutaneous Endoscopic Approach

♂ **0VUP87Z** Supplement Left Vas Deferens with Autologous Tissue Substitute, Via Natural or Artificial Opening Endoscopic

♂ **0VUP8JZ** Supplement Left Vas Deferens with Synthetic Substitute, Via Natural or Artificial Opening Endoscopic

♂ **0VUP8KZ** Supplement Left Vas Deferens with Nonautologous Tissue Substitute, Via Natural or Artificial Opening Endoscopic

♂ **0VUQ07Z** Supplement Bilateral Vas Deferens with Autologous Tissue Substitute, Open Approach

♂ **0VUQ0JZ** Supplement Bilateral Vas Deferens with Synthetic Substitute, Open Approach

♂ **0VUQ0KZ** Supplement Bilateral Vas Deferens with Nonautologous Tissue Substitute, Open Approach

♂ **0VUQ47Z** Supplement Bilateral Vas Deferens with Autologous Tissue Substitute, Percutaneous Endoscopic Approach

♂ **0VUQ4JZ** Supplement Bilateral Vas Deferens with Synthetic Substitute, Percutaneous Endoscopic Approach

♂ **0VUQ4KZ** Supplement Bilateral Vas Deferens with Nonautologous Tissue Substitute, Percutaneous Endoscopic Approach

♂ **0VUQ87Z** Supplement Bilateral Vas Deferens with Autologous Tissue Substitute, Via Natural or Artificial Opening Endoscopic

♂ **0VUQ8JZ** Supplement Bilateral Vas Deferens with Synthetic Substitute, Via Natural or Artificial Opening Endoscopic

♂ **0VUQ8KZ** Supplement Bilateral Vas Deferens with Nonautologous Tissue Substitute, Via Natural or Artificial Opening Endoscopic

♂ **0VUS07Z** Supplement Penis with Autologous Tissue Substitute, Open Approach
AHA CC: 1Q, 2020, 31-32

♂ **0VUS0JZ** Supplement Penis with Synthetic Substitute, Open Approach
AHA CC: 3Q, 2015, 25; 2Q, 2016, 28-29

♂ **0VUS0KZ** Supplement Penis with Nonautologous Tissue Substitute, Open Approach

♂ **0VUS47Z** Supplement Penis with Autologous Tissue Substitute, Percutaneous Endoscopic Approach

♂ **0VUS4JZ** Supplement Penis with Synthetic Substitute, Percutaneous Endoscopic Approach

♂ **0VUS4KZ** Supplement Penis with Nonautologous Tissue Substitute, Percutaneous Endoscopic Approach

♂ **0VUSX7Z** Supplement Penis with Autologous Tissue Substitute, External Approach

♂ **0VUSXJZ** Supplement Penis with Synthetic Substitute, External Approach

♂ **0VUSXKZ** Supplement Penis with Nonautologous Tissue Substitute, External Approach

♂ **0VUT07Z** Supplement Prepuce with Autologous Tissue Substitute, Open Approach

♂ **0VUT0JZ** Supplement Prepuce with Synthetic Substitute, Open Approach

♂ **0VUT0KZ** Supplement Prepuce with Nonautologous Tissue Substitute, Open Approach

♂ **0VUT47Z** Supplement Prepuce with Autologous Tissue Substitute, Percutaneous Endoscopic Approach

♂ **0VUT4JZ** Supplement Prepuce with Synthetic Substitute, Percutaneous Endoscopic Approach

♂ **0VUT4KZ** Supplement Prepuce with Nonautologous Tissue Substitute, Percutaneous Endoscopic Approach

♂ **0VUTX7Z** Supplement Prepuce with Autologous Tissue Substitute, External Approach

♂ **0VUTXJZ** Supplement Prepuce with Synthetic Substitute, External Approach

♂ **0VUTXKZ** Supplement Prepuce with Nonautologous Tissue Substitute, External Approach

0VW – Male Reproductive System, Revision

Review Coding Guideline B6.1c

♂ **0VW400Z** Revision of Drainage Device in Prostate and Seminal Vesicles, Open Approach

♂ **0VW403Z** Revision of Infusion Device in Prostate and Seminal Vesicles, Open Approach

♂ **0VW407Z** Revision of Autologous Tissue Substitute in Prostate and Seminal Vesicles, Open Approach

♂ **0VW40JZ** Revision of Synthetic Substitute in Prostate and Seminal Vesicles, Open Approach

♂ **0VW40KZ** Revision of Nonautologous Tissue Substitute in Prostate and Seminal Vesicles, Open Approach

♂ **0VW40YZ** Revision of Other Device in Prostate and Seminal Vesicles, Open Approach

♂ **0VW430Z** Revision of Drainage Device in Prostate and Seminal Vesicles, Percutaneous Approach

♂ **0VW433Z** Revision of Infusion Device in Prostate and Seminal Vesicles, Percutaneous Approach

♂ **0VW437Z** Revision of Autologous Tissue Substitute in Prostate and Seminal Vesicles, Percutaneous Approach

♂ **0VW43JZ** Revision of Synthetic Substitute in Prostate and Seminal Vesicles, Percutaneous Approach

♂ **0VW43KZ** Revision of Nonautologous Tissue Substitute in Prostate and Seminal Vesicles, Percutaneous Approach

♂ **0VW43YZ** Revision of Other Device in Prostate and Seminal Vesicles, Percutaneous Approach

♂ **0VW440Z** Revision of Drainage Device in Prostate and Seminal Vesicles, Percutaneous Endoscopic Approach

♂ **0VW443Z** Revision of Infusion Device in Prostate and Seminal Vesicles, Percutaneous Endoscopic Approach

♂ **0VW447Z** Revision of Autologous Tissue Substitute in Prostate and Seminal Vesicles, Percutaneous Endoscopic Approach

♂ **0VW44JZ** Revision of Synthetic Substitute in Prostate and Seminal Vesicles, Percutaneous Endoscopic Approach

♂ **0VW44KZ** Revision of Nonautologous Tissue Substitute in Prostate and Seminal Vesicles, Percutaneous Endoscopic Approach

♂ **0VW44YZ** Revision of Other Device in Prostate and Seminal Vesicles, Percutaneous Endoscopic Approach

♂ **0VW470Z** Revision of Drainage Device in Prostate and Seminal Vesicles, Via Natural or Artificial Opening

♂ **0VW473Z** Revision of Infusion Device in Prostate and Seminal Vesicles, Via Natural or Artificial Opening

♂ **0VW477Z** Revision of Autologous Tissue Substitute in Prostate and Seminal Vesicles, Via Natural or Artificial Opening

♂ **0VW47JZ** Revision of Synthetic Substitute in Prostate and Seminal Vesicles, Via Natural or Artificial Opening

♂ **0VW47KZ** Revision of Nonautologous Tissue Substitute in Prostate and Seminal Vesicles, Via Natural or Artificial Opening

♀ Female-only   ♂ Male-only   ▲ Limited Coverage   ● Non-OR   HAC HAC-associated procedure   ▲ Non-covered procedures   ✚ Cluster

♂ **0VW47YZ** Revision of Other Device in Prostate and Seminal Vesicles, Via Natural or Artificial Opening

♂ **0VW480Z** Revision of Drainage Device in Prostate and Seminal Vesicles, Via Natural or Artificial Opening Endoscopic

♂ **0VW483Z** Revision of Infusion Device in Prostate and Seminal Vesicles, Via Natural or Artificial Opening Endoscopic

♂ **0VW487Z** Revision of Autologous Tissue Substitute in Prostate and Seminal Vesicles, Via Natural or Artificial Opening Endoscopic

♂ **0VW48JZ** Revision of Synthetic Substitute in Prostate and Seminal Vesicles, Via Natural or Artificial Opening Endoscopic

♂ **0VW48KZ** Revision of Nonautologous Tissue Substitute in Prostate and Seminal Vesicles, Via Natural or Artificial Opening Endoscopic

♂ **0VW48YZ** Revision of Other Device in Prostate and Seminal Vesicles, Via Natural or Artificial Opening Endoscopic

♂ **0VW4X0Z** Revision of Drainage Device in Prostate and Seminal Vesicles, External Approach

♂ **0VW4X3Z** Revision of Infusion Device in Prostate and Seminal Vesicles, External Approach

♂ **0VW4X7Z** Revision of Autologous Tissue Substitute in Prostate and Seminal Vesicles, External Approach

♂ **0VW4XJZ** Revision of Synthetic Substitute in Prostate and Seminal Vesicles, External Approach

♂ **0VW4XKZ** Revision of Nonautologous Tissue Substitute in Prostate and Seminal Vesicles, External Approach

♂ **0VW800Z** Revision of Drainage Device in Scrotum and Tunica Vaginalis, Open Approach

♂ **0VW803Z** Revision of Infusion Device in Scrotum and Tunica Vaginalis, Open Approach

♂ **0VW807Z** Revision of Autologous Tissue Substitute in Scrotum and Tunica Vaginalis, Open Approach

♂ **0VW80JZ** Revision of Synthetic Substitute in Scrotum and Tunica Vaginalis, Open Approach

♂ **0VW80KZ** Revision of Nonautologous Tissue Substitute in Scrotum and Tunica Vaginalis, Open Approach

♂ **0VW80YZ** Revision of Other Device in Scrotum and Tunica Vaginalis, Open Approach

♂ **0VW830Z** Revision of Drainage Device in Scrotum and Tunica Vaginalis, Percutaneous Approach

♂ **0VW833Z** Revision of Infusion Device in Scrotum and Tunica Vaginalis, Percutaneous Approach

♂ **0VW837Z** Revision of Autologous Tissue Substitute in Scrotum and Tunica Vaginalis, Percutaneous Approach

♂ **0VW83JZ** Revision of Synthetic Substitute in Scrotum and Tunica Vaginalis, Percutaneous Approach

♂ **0VW83KZ** Revision of Nonautologous Tissue Substitute in Scrotum and Tunica Vaginalis, Percutaneous Approach

♂ **0VW83YZ** Revision of Other Device in Scrotum and Tunica Vaginalis, Percutaneous Approach

♂ **0VW840Z** Revision of Drainage Device in Scrotum and Tunica Vaginalis, Percutaneous Endoscopic Approach

♂ **0VW843Z** Revision of Infusion Device in Scrotum and Tunica Vaginalis, Percutaneous Endoscopic Approach

♂ **0VW847Z** Revision of Autologous Tissue Substitute in Scrotum and Tunica Vaginalis, Percutaneous Endoscopic Approach

♂ **0VW84JZ** Revision of Synthetic Substitute in Scrotum and Tunica Vaginalis, Percutaneous Endoscopic Approach

♂ **0VW84KZ** Revision of Nonautologous Tissue Substitute in Scrotum and Tunica Vaginalis, Percutaneous Endoscopic Approach

♂ **0VW84YZ** Revision of Other Device in Scrotum and Tunica Vaginalis, Percutaneous Endoscopic Approach

♂ **0VW870Z** Revision of Drainage Device in Scrotum and Tunica Vaginalis, Via Natural or Artificial Opening

♂ **0VW873Z** Revision of Infusion Device in Scrotum and Tunica Vaginalis, Via Natural or Artificial Opening

♂ **0VW877Z** Revision of Autologous Tissue Substitute in Scrotum and Tunica Vaginalis, Via Natural or Artificial Opening

♂ **0VW87JZ** Revision of Synthetic Substitute in Scrotum and Tunica Vaginalis, Via Natural or Artificial Opening

♂ **0VW87KZ** Revision of Nonautologous Tissue Substitute in Scrotum and Tunica Vaginalis, Via Natural or Artificial Opening

♂ **0VW87YZ** Revision of Other Device in Scrotum and Tunica Vaginalis, Via Natural or Artificial Opening

♂ **0VW880Z** Revision of Drainage Device in Scrotum and Tunica Vaginalis, Via Natural or Artificial Opening Endoscopic

♂ **0VW883Z** Revision of Infusion Device in Scrotum and Tunica Vaginalis, Via Natural or Artificial Opening Endoscopic

♂ **0VW887Z** Revision of Autologous Tissue Substitute in Scrotum and Tunica Vaginalis, Via Natural or Artificial Opening Endoscopic

♂ **0VW88JZ** Revision of Synthetic Substitute in Scrotum and Tunica Vaginalis, Via Natural or Artificial Opening Endoscopic

♂ **0VW88KZ** Revision of Nonautologous Tissue Substitute in Scrotum and Tunica Vaginalis, Via Natural or Artificial Opening Endoscopic

♂ **0VW88YZ** Revision of Other Device in Scrotum and Tunica Vaginalis, Via Natural or Artificial Opening Endoscopic

♂ **0VW8X0Z** Revision of Drainage Device in Scrotum and Tunica Vaginalis, External Approach

♂ **0VW8X3Z** Revision of Infusion Device in Scrotum and Tunica Vaginalis, External Approach

♂ **0VW8X7Z** Revision of Autologous Tissue Substitute in Scrotum and Tunica Vaginalis, External Approach

♂ **0VW8XJZ** Revision of Synthetic Substitute in Scrotum and Tunica Vaginalis, External Approach

♂ **0VW8XKZ** Revision of Nonautologous Tissue Substitute in Scrotum and Tunica Vaginalis, External Approach

♂ **0VWD00Z** Revision of Drainage Device in Testis, Open Approach

♂ **0VWD03Z** Revision of Infusion Device in Testis, Open Approach

♂ **0VWD07Z** Revision of Autologous Tissue Substitute in Testis, Open Approach

♂ **0VWD0JZ** Revision of Synthetic Substitute in Testis, Open Approach

♂ **0VWD0KZ** Revision of Nonautologous Tissue Substitute in Testis, Open Approach

♂ **0VWD0YZ** Revision of Other Device in Testis, Open Approach

♂ **0VWD30Z** Revision of Drainage Device in Testis, Percutaneous Approach

♂ **0VWD33Z** Revision of Infusion Device in Testis, Percutaneous Approach

♂ **0VWD37Z** Revision of Autologous Tissue Substitute in Testis, Percutaneous Approach

♂ **0VWD3JZ** Revision of Synthetic Substitute in Testis, Percutaneous Approach

♂ **0VWD3KZ** Revision of Nonautologous Tissue Substitute in Testis, Percutaneous Approach

♂ **0VWD3YZ** Revision of Other Device in Testis, Percutaneous Approach

♂ **0VWD40Z** Revision of Drainage Device in Testis, Percutaneous Endoscopic Approach

♂ **0VWD43Z** Revision of Infusion Device in Testis, Percutaneous Endoscopic Approach

♂ **0VWD47Z** Revision of Autologous Tissue Substitute in Testis, Percutaneous Endoscopic Approach

♂ **0VWD4JZ** Revision of Synthetic Substitute in Testis, Percutaneous Endoscopic Approach

♂ **0VWD4KZ** Revision of Nonautologous Tissue Substitute in Testis, Percutaneous Endoscopic Approach

♂ **0VWD4YZ** Revision of Other Device in Testis, Percutaneous Endoscopic Approach

♂ **0VWD70Z** Revision of Drainage Device in Testis, Via Natural or Artificial Opening

♂ **0VWD73Z** Revision of Infusion Device in Testis, Via Natural or Artificial Opening

♂ **0VWD77Z** Revision of Autologous Tissue Substitute in Testis, Via Natural or Artificial Opening

♂ **0VWD7JZ** Revision of Synthetic Substitute in Testis, Via Natural or Artificial Opening

♂ **0VWD7KZ** Revision of Nonautologous Tissue Substitute in Testis, Via Natural or Artificial Opening

♂ **0VWD7YZ** Revision of Other Device in Testis, Via Natural or Artificial Opening

♂ **0VWD80Z** Revision of Drainage Device in Testis, Via Natural or Artificial Opening Endoscopic

♂ **0VWD83Z** Revision of Infusion Device in Testis, Via Natural or Artificial Opening Endoscopic

♂ **0VWD87Z** Revision of Autologous Tissue Substitute in Testis, Via Natural or Artificial Opening Endoscopic

♂ **0VWD8JZ** Revision of Synthetic Substitute in Testis, Via Natural or Artificial Opening Endoscopic

♂ **0VWD8KZ** Revision of Nonautologous Tissue Substitute in Testis, Via Natural or Artificial Opening Endoscopic

---

♀ Female-only   ♂ Male-only   ▲ Limited Coverage   ● Non-OR   **HAC** HAC-associated procedure   ▲ Non-covered procedures   ➕ Cluster

♂ **0VWD8YZ** Revision of Other Device in Testis, Via Natural or Artificial Opening Endoscopic

♂ **0VWDX0Z** Revision of Drainage Device in Testis, External Approach

♂ **0VWDX3Z** Revision of Infusion Device in Testis, External Approach

♂ **0VWDX7Z** Revision of Autologous Tissue Substitute in Testis, External Approach

♂ **0VWDXJZ** Revision of Synthetic Substitute in Testis, External Approach

♂ **0VWDXKZ** Revision of Nonautologous Tissue Substitute in Testis, External Approach

♂ **0VWM00Z** Revision of Drainage Device in Epididymis and Spermatic Cord, Open Approach

♂ **0VWM03Z** Revision of Infusion Device in Epididymis and Spermatic Cord, Open Approach

♂ **0VWM07Z** Revision of Autologous Tissue Substitute in Epididymis and Spermatic Cord, Open Approach

♂ **0VWM0CZ** Revision of Extraluminal Device in Epididymis and Spermatic Cord, Open Approach

♂ **0VWM0JZ** Revision of Synthetic Substitute in Epididymis and Spermatic Cord, Open Approach

♂ **0VWM0KZ** Revision of Nonautologous Tissue Substitute in Epididymis and Spermatic Cord, Open Approach

♂ **0VWM0YZ** Revision of Other Device in Epididymis and Spermatic Cord, Open Approach

♂ **0VWM30Z** Revision of Drainage Device in Epididymis and Spermatic Cord, Percutaneous Approach

♂ **0VWM33Z** Revision of Infusion Device in Epididymis and Spermatic Cord, Percutaneous Approach

♂ **0VWM37Z** Revision of Autologous Tissue Substitute in Epididymis and Spermatic Cord, Percutaneous Approach

♂ **0VWM3CZ** Revision of Extraluminal Device in Epididymis and Spermatic Cord, Percutaneous Approach

♂ **0VWM3JZ** Revision of Synthetic Substitute in Epididymis and Spermatic Cord, Percutaneous Approach

♂ **0VWM3KZ** Revision of Nonautologous Tissue Substitute in Epididymis and Spermatic Cord, Percutaneous Approach

♂ **0VWM3YZ** Revision of Other Device in Epididymis and Spermatic Cord, Percutaneous Approach

♂ **0VWM40Z** Revision of Drainage Device in Epididymis and Spermatic Cord, Percutaneous Endoscopic Approach

♂ **0VWM43Z** Revision of Infusion Device in Epididymis and Spermatic Cord, Percutaneous Endoscopic Approach

♂ **0VWM47Z** Revision of Autologous Tissue Substitute in Epididymis and Spermatic Cord, Percutaneous Endoscopic Approach

♂ **0VWM4CZ** Revision of Extraluminal Device in Epididymis and Spermatic Cord, Percutaneous Endoscopic Approach

♂ **0VWM4JZ** Revision of Synthetic Substitute in Epididymis and Spermatic Cord, Percutaneous Endoscopic Approach

♂ **0VWM4KZ** Revision of Nonautologous Tissue Substitute in Epididymis and

Spermatic Cord, Percutaneous Endoscopic Approach

♂ **0VWM4YZ** Revision of Other Device in Epididymis and Spermatic Cord, Percutaneous Endoscopic Approach

♂ **0VWM70Z** Revision of Drainage Device in Epididymis and Spermatic Cord, Via Natural or Artificial Opening

♂ **0VWM73Z** Revision of Infusion Device in Epididymis and Spermatic Cord, Via Natural or Artificial Opening

♂ **0VWM77Z** Revision of Autologous Tissue Substitute in Epididymis and Spermatic Cord, Via Natural or Artificial Opening

♂ **0VWM7CZ** Revision of Extraluminal Device in Epididymis and Spermatic Cord, Via Natural or Artificial Opening

♂ **0VWM7JZ** Revision of Synthetic Substitute in Epididymis and Spermatic Cord, Via Natural or Artificial Opening

♂ **0VWM7KZ** Revision of Nonautologous Tissue Substitute in Epididymis and Spermatic Cord, Via Natural or Artificial Opening

♂ **0VWM7YZ** Revision of Other Device in Epididymis and Spermatic Cord, Via Natural or Artificial Opening

♂ **0VWM80Z** Revision of Drainage Device in Epididymis and Spermatic Cord, Via Natural or Artificial Opening Endoscopic

♂ **0VWM83Z** Revision of Infusion Device in Epididymis and Spermatic Cord, Via Natural or Artificial Opening Endoscopic

♂ **0VWM87Z** Revision of Autologous Tissue Substitute in Epididymis and Spermatic Cord, Via Natural or Artificial Opening Endoscopic

♂ **0VWM8CZ** Revision of Extraluminal Device in Epididymis and Spermatic Cord, Via Natural or Artificial Opening Endoscopic

♂ **0VWM8JZ** Revision of Synthetic Substitute in Epididymis and Spermatic Cord, Via Natural or Artificial Opening Endoscopic

♂ **0VWM8KZ** Revision of Nonautologous Tissue Substitute in Epididymis and Spermatic Cord, Via Natural or Artificial Opening Endoscopic

♂ **0VWM8YZ** Revision of Other Device in Epididymis and Spermatic Cord, Via Natural or Artificial Opening Endoscopic

♂ **0VWMX0Z** Revision of Drainage Device in Epididymis and Spermatic Cord, External Approach

♂ **0VWMX3Z** Revision of Infusion Device in Epididymis and Spermatic Cord, External Approach

♂ **0VWMX7Z** Revision of Autologous Tissue Substitute in Epididymis and Spermatic Cord, External Approach

♂ **0VWMXCZ** Revision of Extraluminal Device in Epididymis and Spermatic Cord, External Approach

♂ **0VWMXJZ** Revision of Synthetic Substitute in Epididymis and Spermatic Cord, External Approach

♂ **0VWMXKZ** Revision of Nonautologous Tissue Substitute in Epididymis and Spermatic Cord, External Approach

♂ **0VWR00Z** Revision of Drainage Device in Vas Deferens, Open Approach

♂ **0VWR03Z** Revision of Infusion Device in Vas Deferens, Open Approach

♂ **0VWR07Z** Revision of Autologous Tissue Substitute in Vas Deferens, Open Approach

♂ **0VWR0CZ** Revision of Extraluminal Device in Vas Deferens, Open Approach

♂ **0VWR0DZ** Revision of Intraluminal Device in Vas Deferens, Open Approach

♂ **0VWR0JZ** Revision of Synthetic Substitute in Vas Deferens, Open Approach

♂ **0VWR0KZ** Revision of Nonautologous Tissue Substitute in Vas Deferens, Open Approach

♂ **0VWR0YZ** Revision of Other Device in Vas Deferens, Open Approach

♂ **0VWR30Z** Revision of Drainage Device in Vas Deferens, Percutaneous Approach

♂ **0VWR33Z** Revision of Infusion Device in Vas Deferens, Percutaneous Approach

♂ **0VWR37Z** Revision of Autologous Tissue Substitute in Vas Deferens, Percutaneous Approach

♂ **0VWR3CZ** Revision of Extraluminal Device in Vas Deferens, Percutaneous Approach

♂ **0VWR3DZ** Revision of Intraluminal Device in Vas Deferens, Percutaneous Approach

♂ **0VWR3JZ** Revision of Synthetic Substitute in Vas Deferens, Percutaneous Approach

♂ **0VWR3KZ** Revision of Nonautologous Tissue Substitute in Vas Deferens, Percutaneous Approach

♂ **0VWR3YZ** Revision of Other Device in Vas Deferens, Percutaneous Approach

♂ **0VWR40Z** Revision of Drainage Device in Vas Deferens, Percutaneous Endoscopic Approach

♂ **0VWR43Z** Revision of Infusion Device in Vas Deferens, Percutaneous Endoscopic Approach

♂ **0VWR47Z** Revision of Autologous Tissue Substitute in Vas Deferens, Percutaneous Endoscopic Approach

♂ **0VWR4CZ** Revision of Extraluminal Device in Vas Deferens, Percutaneous Endoscopic Approach

♂ **0VWR4DZ** Revision of Intraluminal Device in Vas Deferens, Percutaneous Endoscopic Approach

♂ **0VWR4JZ** Revision of Synthetic Substitute in Vas Deferens, Percutaneous Endoscopic Approach

♂ **0VWR4KZ** Revision of Nonautologous Tissue Substitute in Vas Deferens, Percutaneous Endoscopic Approach

♂ **0VWR4YZ** Revision of Other Device in Vas Deferens, Percutaneous Endoscopic Approach

♂ **0VWR70Z** Revision of Drainage Device in Vas Deferens, Via Natural or Artificial Opening

♂ **0VWR73Z** Revision of Infusion Device in Vas Deferens, Via Natural or Artificial Opening

♂ **0VWR77Z** Revision of Autologous Tissue Substitute in Vas Deferens, Via Natural or Artificial Opening

♂ **0VWR7CZ** Revision of Extraluminal Device in Vas Deferens, Via Natural or Artificial Opening

♂ **0VWR7DZ** Revision of Intraluminal Device in Vas Deferens, Via Natural or Artificial Opening

♀ Female-only   ♂ Male-only   ▲ Limited Coverage   ● Non-OR   🅷🅰🅲 HAC-associated procedure   ▲ Non-covered procedures   ➕ Cluster

♂ 0VWR7JZ Revision of Synthetic Substitute in Vas Deferens, Via Natural or Artificial Opening

♂ 0VWR7KZ Revision of Nonautologous Tissue Substitute in Vas Deferens, Via Natural or Artificial Opening

♂ 0VWR7YZ Revision of Other Device in Vas Deferens, Via Natural or Artificial Opening

♂ 0VWR80Z Revision of Drainage Device in Vas Deferens, Via Natural or Artificial Opening Endoscopic

♂ 0VWR83Z Revision of Infusion Device in Vas Deferens, Via Natural or Artificial Opening Endoscopic

♂ 0VWR87Z Revision of Autologous Tissue Substitute in Vas Deferens, Via Natural or Artificial Opening Endoscopic

♂ 0VWR8CZ Revision of Extraluminal Device in Vas Deferens, Via Natural or Artificial Opening Endoscopic

♂ 0VWR8DZ Revision of Intraluminal Device in Vas Deferens, Via Natural or Artificial Opening Endoscopic

♂ 0VWR8JZ Revision of Synthetic Substitute in Vas Deferens, Via Natural or Artificial Opening Endoscopic

♂ 0VWR8KZ Revision of Nonautologous Tissue Substitute in Vas Deferens, Via Natural or Artificial Opening Endoscopic

♂ 0VWR8YZ Revision of Other Device in Vas Deferens, Via Natural or Artificial Opening Endoscopic

♂ 0VWRX0Z Revision of Drainage Device in Vas Deferens, External Approach

♂ 0VWRX3Z Revision of Infusion Device in Vas Deferens, External Approach

♂ 0VWRX7Z Revision of Autologous Tissue Substitute in Vas Deferens, External Approach

♂ 0VWRXCZ Revision of Extraluminal Device in Vas Deferens, External Approach

♂ 0VWRXDZ Revision of Intraluminal Device in Vas Deferens, External Approach

♂ 0VWRXJZ Revision of Synthetic Substitute in Vas Deferens, External Approach

♂ 0VWRXKZ Revision of Nonautologous Tissue Substitute in Vas Deferens, External Approach

♂ 0VWS00Z Revision of Drainage Device in Penis, Open Approach

♂ 0VWS03Z Revision of Infusion Device in Penis, Open Approach

♂ 0VWS07Z Revision of Autologous Tissue Substitute in Penis, Open Approach

♂ 0VWS0JZ Revision of Synthetic Substitute in Penis, Open Approach

♂ 0VWS0KZ Revision of Nonautologous Tissue Substitute in Penis, Open Approach

♂ 0VWS0YZ Revision of Other Device in Penis, Open Approach

♂ 0VWS30Z Revision of Drainage Device in Penis, Percutaneous Approach

♂ 0VWS33Z Revision of Infusion Device in Penis, Percutaneous Approach

♂ 0VWS37Z Revision of Autologous Tissue Substitute in Penis, Percutaneous Approach

♂ 0VWS3JZ Revision of Synthetic Substitute in Penis, Percutaneous Approach

♂ 0VWS3KZ Revision of Nonautologous Tissue Substitute in Penis, Percutaneous Approach

♂ 0VWS3YZ Revision of Other Device in Penis, Percutaneous Approach

♂ 0VWS40Z Revision of Drainage Device in Penis, Percutaneous Endoscopic Approach

♂ 0VWS43Z Revision of Infusion Device in Penis, Percutaneous Endoscopic Approach

♂ 0VWS47Z Revision of Autologous Tissue Substitute in Penis, Percutaneous Endoscopic Approach

♂ 0VWS4JZ Revision of Synthetic Substitute in Penis, Percutaneous Endoscopic Approach

♂ 0VWS4KZ Revision of Nonautologous Tissue Substitute in Penis, Percutaneous Endoscopic Approach

♂ 0VWS4YZ Revision of Other Device in Penis, Percutaneous Endoscopic Approach

♂ 0VWS70Z Revision of Drainage Device in Penis, Via Natural or Artificial Opening

♂ 0VWS73Z Revision of Infusion Device in Penis, Via Natural or Artificial Opening

♂ 0VWS77Z Revision of Autologous Tissue Substitute in Penis, Via Natural or Artificial Opening

♂ 0VWS7JZ Revision of Synthetic Substitute in Penis, Via Natural or Artificial Opening

♂ 0VWS7KZ Revision of Nonautologous Tissue Substitute in Penis, Via Natural or Artificial Opening

♂ 0VWS7YZ Revision of Other Device in Penis, Via Natural or Artificial Opening

♂ 0VWS80Z Revision of Drainage Device in Penis, Via Natural or Artificial Opening Endoscopic

♂ 0VWS83Z Revision of Infusion Device in Penis, Via Natural or Artificial Opening Endoscopic

♂ 0VWS87Z Revision of Autologous Tissue Substitute in Penis, Via Natural or Artificial Opening Endoscopic

♂ 0VWS8JZ Revision of Synthetic Substitute in Penis, Via Natural or Artificial Opening Endoscopic

♂ 0VWS8KZ Revision of Nonautologous Tissue Substitute in Penis, Via Natural or Artificial Opening Endoscopic

♂ 0VWS8YZ Revision of Other Device in Penis, Via Natural or Artificial Opening Endoscopic

♂ 0VWSX0Z Revision of Drainage Device in Penis, External Approach

♂ 0VWSX3Z Revision of Infusion Device in Penis, External Approach

♂ 0VWSX7Z Revision of Autologous Tissue Substitute in Penis, External Approach

♂ 0VWSXJZ Revision of Synthetic Substitute in Penis, External Approach

♂ 0VWSXKZ Revision of Nonautologous Tissue Substitute in Penis, External Approach

0VX – Male Reproductive System, Transfer

0VXT0ZD Transfer Prepuce to Urethra, Open Approach

0VXT0ZS Transfer Prepuce to Penis, Open Approach

0VXTXZD Transfer Prepuce to Urethra, External Approach

0VXTXZS Transfer Prepuce to Penis, External Approach

0VY – Male Reproductive System, Transplantation

Review Coding Guideline B3.16

0VY50Z0 Transplantation of Scrotum, Allogeneic, Open Approach
AHA CC: 4Q, 2020, 58-59

0VY50Z1 Transplantation of Scrotum, Syngeneic, Open Approach

0VY50Z2 Transplantation of Scrotum, Zooplastic, Open Approach

0VYS0Z0 Transplantation of Penis, Allogeneic, Open Approach
AHA CC: 4Q, 2020, 58-59

0VYS0Z1 Transplantation of Penis, Syngeneic, Open Approach

0VYS0Z2 Transplantation of Penis, Zooplastic, Open Approach

Body Cavities

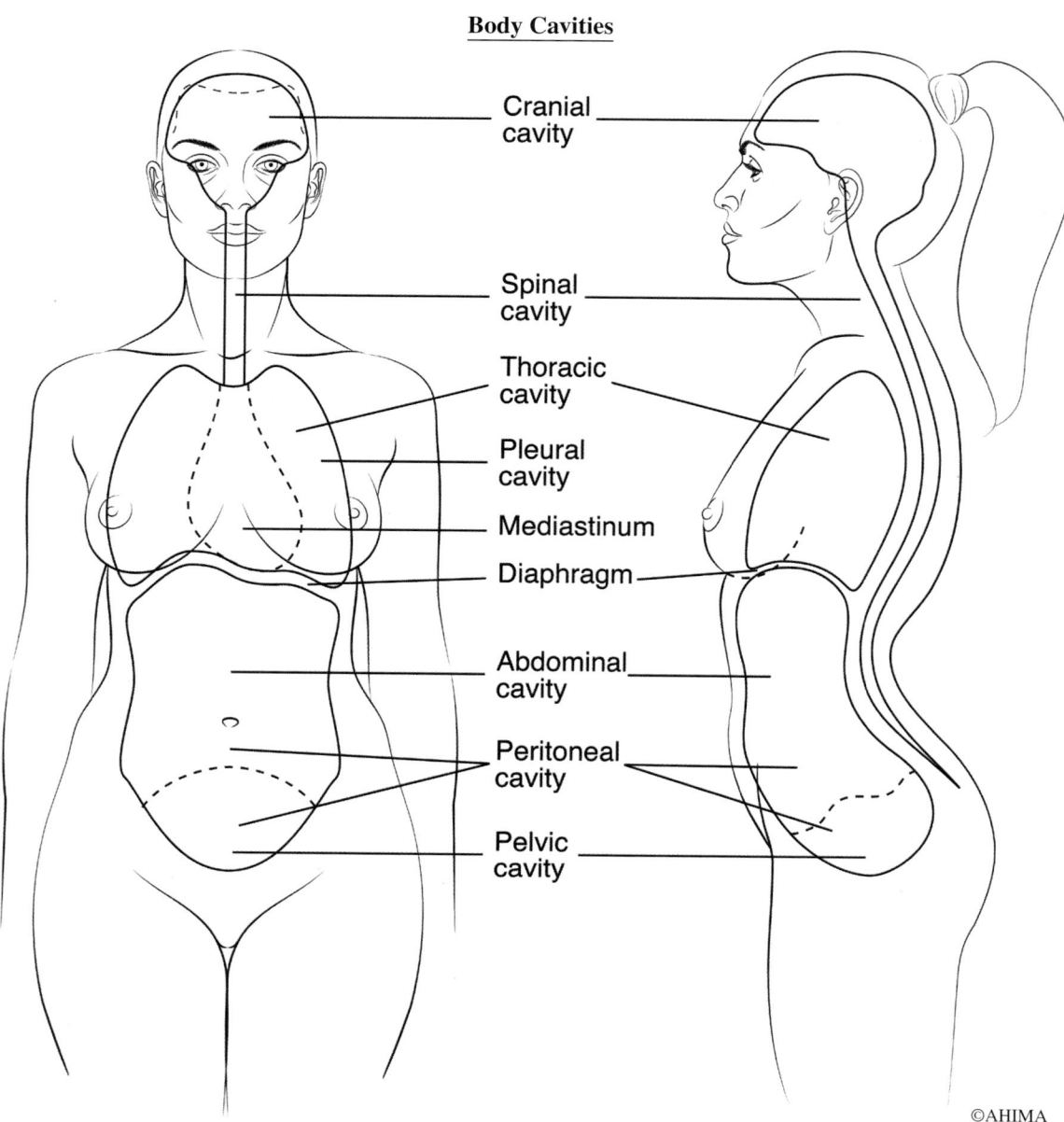

Cranial cavity

Spinal cavity

Thoracic cavity

Pleural cavity

Mediastinum

Diaphragm

Abdominal cavity

Peritoneal cavity

Pelvic cavity

©AHIMA

Body Areas

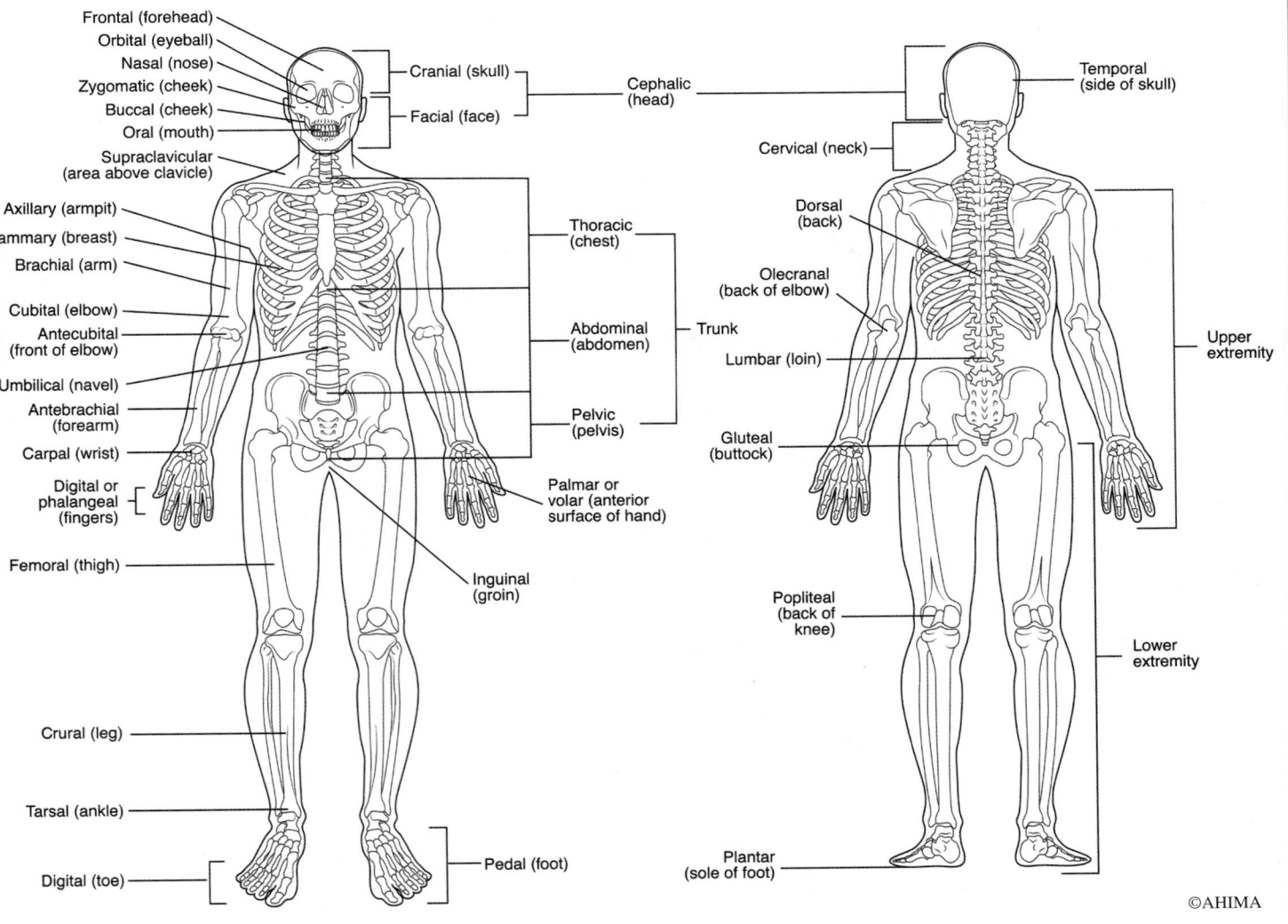

Frontal (forehead)
Orbital (eyeball)
Nasal (nose)
Zygomatic (cheek)
Buccal (cheek)
Oral (mouth)
Supraclavicular
(area above clavicle)
Axillary (armpit)
Mammary (breast)
Brachial (arm)
Cubital (elbow)
Antecubital
(front of elbow)
Umbilical (navel)
Antebrachial
(forearm)
Carpal (wrist)
Digital or
phalangeal
(fingers)
Femoral (thigh)
Crural (leg)
Tarsal (ankle)
Digital (toe)

Cranial (skull)
Facial (face)
Cephalic
(head)

Thoracic
(chest)
Abdominal
(abdomen)   Trunk
Pelvic
(pelvis)
Palmar or
volar (anterior
surface of hand)
Inguinal
(groin)
Pedal (foot)

Temporal
(side of skull)
Cervical (neck)
Dorsal
(back)
Olecranal
(back of elbow)
Lumbar (loin)
Gluteal
(buttock)
Upper
extremity
Popliteal
(back of
knee)
Lower
extremity
Plantar
(sole of foot)

©AHIMA

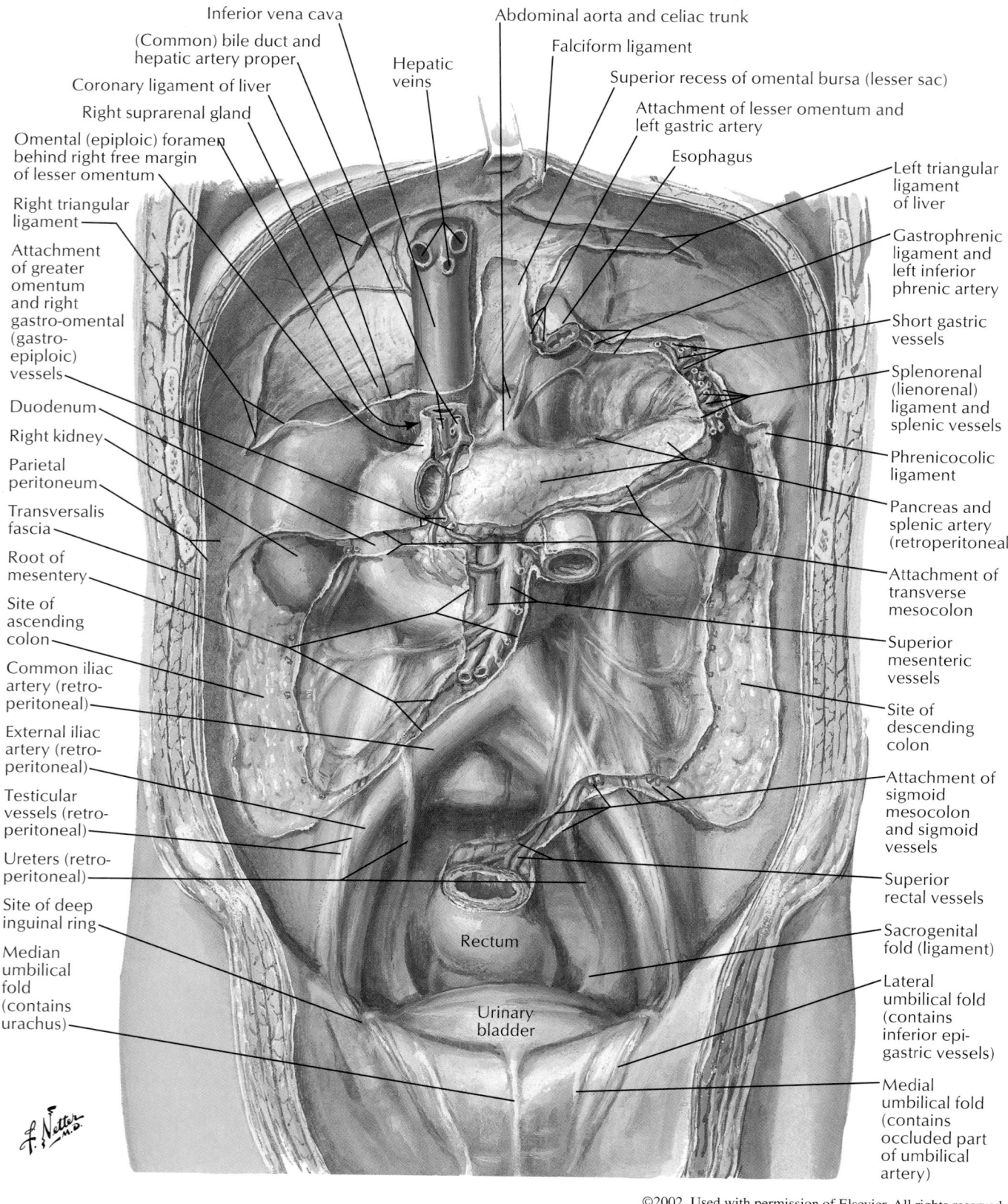

Inferior vena cava

(Common) bile duct and hepatic artery proper

Coronary ligament of liver

Right suprarenal gland

Omental (epiploic) foramen behind right free margin of lesser omentum

Right triangular ligament

Attachment of greater omentum and right gastro-omental (gastro-epiploic) vessels

Duodenum

Right kidney

Parietal peritoneum

Transversalis fascia

Root of mesentery

Site of ascending colon

Common iliac artery (retro-peritoneal)

External iliac artery (retro-peritoneal)

Testicular vessels (retro-peritoneal)

Ureters (retro-peritoneal)

Site of deep inguinal ring

Median umbilical fold (contains urachus)

Hepatic veins

Abdominal aorta and celiac trunk

Falciform ligament

Superior recess of omental bursa (lesser sac)

Attachment of lesser omentum and left gastric artery

Esophagus

Left triangular ligament of liver

Gastrophrenic ligament and left inferior phrenic artery

Short gastric vessels

Splenorenal (lienorenal) ligament and splenic vessels

Phrenicocolic ligament

Pancreas and splenic artery (retroperitoneal)

Attachment of transverse mesocolon

Superior mesenteric vessels

Site of descending colon

Attachment of sigmoid mesocolon and sigmoid vessels

Superior rectal vessels

Sacrogenital fold (ligament)

Lateral umbilical fold (contains inferior epigastric vessels)

Medial umbilical fold (contains occluded part of umbilical artery)

Rectum

Urinary bladder

Medical and Surgical, Anatomical Regions, General

Hernia I - Indirect and Direct Inguinal Hernias

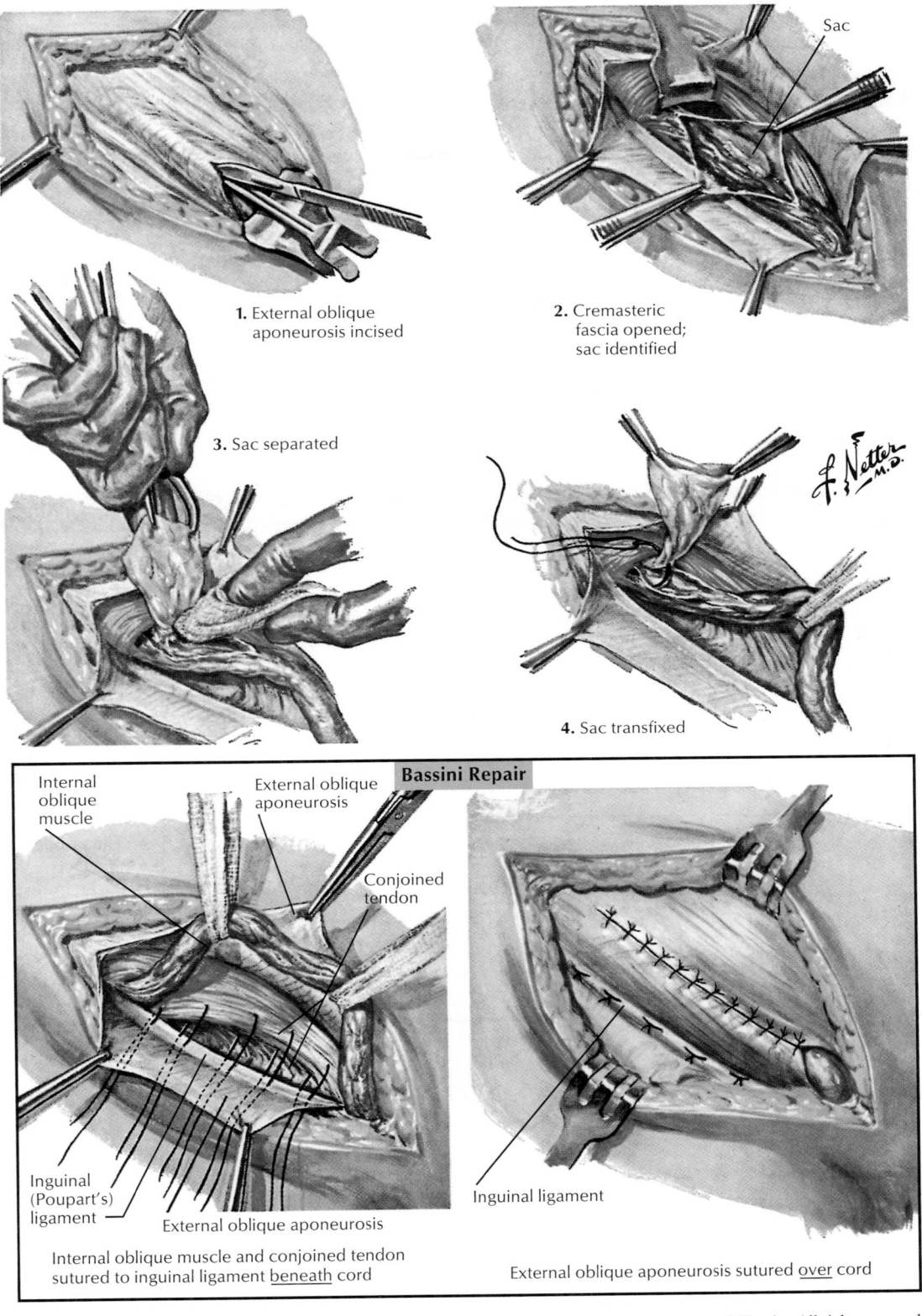

1. External oblique aponeurosis incised

Sac

2. Cremasteric fascia opened; sac identified

3. Sac separated

4. Sac transfixed

Bassini Repair

Internal oblique muscle

External oblique aponeurosis

Conjoined tendon

Inguinal (Poupart's) ligament

External oblique aponeurosis

Internal oblique muscle and conjoined tendon sutured to inguinal ligament <u>beneath</u> cord

Inguinal ligament

External oblique aponeurosis sutured <u>over</u> cord

Medical and Surgical, Anatomical Regions, General

1297

Section	0	Medical and Surgical
Body System	W	Anatomical Regions, General
Operation	0	**Alteration:** Modifying the anatomic structure of a body part without affecting the function of the body part

Body Part (4th)	Approach (5th)	Device (6th)	Qualifier (7th)
0 Head **2** Face **4** Upper Jaw **5** Lower Jaw **6** Neck **8** Chest Wall **F** Abdominal Wall **K** Upper Back **L** Lower Back **M** Perineum, Male **N** Perineum, Female	**0** Open **3** Percutaneous **4** Percutaneous Endoscopic	**7** Autologous Tissue Substitute **J** Synthetic Substitute **K** Nonautologous Tissue Substitute **Z** No Device	**Z** No Qualifier

Section	0	Medical and Surgical
Body System	W	Anatomical Regions, General
Operation	1	**Bypass:** Altering the route of passage of the contents of a tubular body part

Body Part (4th)	Approach (5th)	Device (6th)	Qualifier (7th)
1 Cranial Cavity	**0** Open	**J** Synthetic Substitute	**9** Pleural Cavity, Right **B** Pleural Cavity, Left **G** Peritoneal Cavity **J** Pelvic Cavity
9 Pleural Cavity, Right **B** Pleural Cavity, Left **J** Pelvic Cavity	**0** Open **3** Percutaneous **4** Percutaneous Endoscopic	**J** Synthetic Substitute	**4** Cutaneous **9** Pleural Cavity, Right **B** Pleural Cavity, Left **G** Peritoneal Cavity **J** Pelvic Cavity **W** Upper Vein **Y** Lower Vein
G Peritoneal Cavity	**0** Open **3** Percutaneous **4** Percutaneous Endoscopic	**J** Synthetic Substitute	**4** Cutaneous **6** Bladder **9** Pleural Cavity, Right **B** Pleural Cavity, Left **G** Peritoneal Cavity **J** Pelvic Cavity **W** Upper Vein **Y** Lower Vein

Section	0	Medical and Surgical
Body System	W	Anatomical Regions, General
Operation	2	Change: Taking out or off a device from a body part and putting back an identical or similar device in or on the same body part without cutting or puncturing the skin or a mucous membrane

Body Part (4th)	Approach (5th)	Device (6th)	Qualifier (7th)
0 Head 1 Cranial Cavity 2 Face 4 Upper Jaw 5 Lower Jaw 6 Neck 8 Chest Wall 9 Pleural Cavity, Right B Pleural Cavity, Left C Mediastinum D Pericardial Cavity F Abdominal Wall G Peritoneal Cavity H Retroperitoneum J Pelvic Cavity K Upper Back L Lower Back M Perineum, Male N Perineum, Female	X External	0 Drainage Device Y Other Device	Z No Qualifier

Section	0	Medical and Surgical
Body System	W	Anatomical Regions, General
Operation	3	Control: Stopping, or attempting to stop, postprocedural or other acute bleeding

Body Part (4th)	Approach (5th)	Device (6th)	Qualifier (7th)
0 Head 1 Cranial Cavity 2 Face 4 Upper Jaw 5 Lower Jaw 6 Neck 8 Chest Wall 9 Pleural Cavity, Right B Pleural Cavity, Left C Mediastinum D Pericardial Cavity F Abdominal Wall G Peritoneal Cavity H Retroperitoneum J Pelvic Cavity K Upper Back L Lower Back M Perineum, Male N Perineum, Female	0 Open 3 Percutaneous 4 Percutaneous Endoscopic	Z No Device	Z No Qualifier
3 Oral Cavity and Throat	0 Open 3 Percutaneous 4 Percutaneous Endoscopic 7 Via Natural or Artificial Opening 8 Via Natural or Artificial Opening Endoscopic X External	Z No Device	Z No Qualifier
P Gastrointestinal Tract Q Respiratory Tract R Genitourinary Tract	0 Open 3 Percutaneous 4 Percutaneous Endoscopic 7 Via Natural or Artificial Opening 8 Via Natural or Artificial Opening Endoscopic	Z No Device	Z No Qualifier

Section   0   **Medical and Surgical**
Body System   W   **Anatomical Regions, General**
Operation   4   **Creation:** Putting in or on biological or synthetic material to form a new body part that to the extent possible replicates the anatomic structure or function of an absent body part

Body Part (4ᵗʰ)	Approach (5ᵗʰ)	Device (6ᵗʰ)	Qualifier (7ᵗʰ)
M Perineum, Male	0 Open	7 Autologous Tissue Substitute J Synthetic Substitute K Nonautologous Tissue Substitute	0 Vagina
N Perineum, Female	0 Open	7 Autologous Tissue Substitute J Synthetic Substitute K Nonautologous Tissue Substitute	1 Penis

Section   0   **Medical and Surgical**
Body System   W   **Anatomical Regions, General**
Operation   8   **Division:** Cutting into a body part, without draining fluids and/or gases from the body part, in order to separate or transect a body part

Body Part (4ᵗʰ)	Approach (5ᵗʰ)	Device (6ᵗʰ)	Qualifier (7ᵗʰ)
N Perineum, Female	X External	Z No Device	Z No Qualifier

Section   0   **Medical and Surgical**
Body System   W   **Anatomical Regions, General**
Operation   9   **Drainage:** Taking or letting out fluids and/or gases from a body part

Body Part (4ᵗʰ)	Approach (5ᵗʰ)	Device (6ᵗʰ)	Qualifier (7ᵗʰ)
0 Head 1 Cranial Cavity 2 Face 3 Oral Cavity and Throat 4 Upper Jaw 5 Lower Jaw 6 Neck 8 Chest Wall 9 Pleural Cavity, Right B Pleural Cavity, Left C Mediastinum D Pericardial Cavity F Abdominal Wall G Peritoneal Cavity H Retroperitoneum K Upper Back L Lower Back M Perineum, Male N Perineum, Female	0 Open 3 Percutaneous 4 Percutaneous Endoscopic	0 Drainage Device	Z No Qualifier

Continued →

Body Part (4th)	Approach (5th)	Device (6th)	Qualifier (7th)
0 Head 1 Cranial Cavity 2 Face 3 Oral Cavity and Throat 4 Upper Jaw 5 Lower Jaw 6 Neck 8 Chest Wall 9 Pleural Cavity, Right B Pleural Cavity, Left C Mediastinum D Pericardial Cavity F Abdominal Wall G Peritoneal Cavity H Retroperitoneum K Upper Back L Lower Back M Perineum, Male N Perineum, Female	0 Open 3 Percutaneous 4 Percutaneous Endoscopic	Z No Device	X Diagnostic Z No Qualifier
J Pelvic Cavity	0 Open 3 Percutaneous 4 Percutaneous Endoscopic 7 Via Natural or Artificial Opening 8 Via Natural or Artificial Opening Endoscopic	0 Drainage Device	Z No Qualifier
J Pelvic Cavity	0 Open 3 Percutaneous 4 Percutaneous Endoscopic 7 Via Natural or Artificial Opening 8 Via Natural or Artificial Opening Endoscopic	Z No Device	X Diagnostic Z No Qualifier

Section	0	Medical and Surgical
Body System	W	Anatomical Regions, General
Operation	B	**Excision:** Cutting out or off, without replacement, a portion of a body part

Body Part (4th)	Approach (5th)	Device (6th)	Qualifier (7th)
0 Head 2 Face 3 Oral Cavity and Throat 4 Upper Jaw 5 Lower Jaw 8 Chest Wall K Upper Back L Lower Back M Perineum, Male N Perineum, Female	0 Open 3 Percutaneous 4 Percutaneous Endoscopic X External	Z No Device	X Diagnostic Z No Qualifier
6 Neck F Abdominal Wall	0 Open 3 Percutaneous 4 Percutaneous Endoscopic	Z No Device	X Diagnostic Z No Qualifier
6 Neck F Abdominal Wall	X External	Z No Device	2 Stoma X Diagnostic Z No Qualifier
C Mediastinum H Retroperitoneum	0 Open 3 Percutaneous 4 Percutaneous Endoscopic	Z No Device	X Diagnostic Z No Qualifier

Section	0	Medical and Surgical
Body System	W	Anatomical Regions, General
Operation	C	**Extirpation:** Taking or cutting out solid matter from a body part

Body Part (4th)	Approach (5th)	Device (6th)	Qualifier (7th)
1 Cranial Cavity 3 Oral Cavity and Throat 9 Pleural Cavity, Right B Pleural Cavity, Left C Mediastinum D Pericardial Cavity G Peritoneal Cavity H Retroperitoneum J Pelvic Cavity	0 Open 3 Percutaneous 4 Percutaneous Endoscopic X External	Z No Device	Z No Qualifier
4 Upper Jaw 5 Lower Jaw	0 Open 3 Percutaneous 4 Percutaneous Endoscopic	Z No Device	Z No Qualifier
P Gastrointestinal Tract Q Respiratory Tract R Genitourinary Tract	0 Open 3 Percutaneous 4 Percutaneous Endoscopic 7 Via Natural or Artificial Opening 8 Via Natural or Artificial Opening Endoscopic X External	Z No Device	Z No Qualifier

Section	0	Medical and Surgical
Body System	W	Anatomical Regions, General
Operation	F	Fragmentation: Breaking solid matter in a body part into pieces

Body Part (4th)	Approach (5th)	Device (6th)	Qualifier (7th)
1 Cranial Cavity 3 Oral Cavity and Throat 9 Pleural Cavity, Right B Pleural Cavity, Left C Mediastinum D Pericardial Cavity G Peritoneal Cavity J Pelvic Cavity	0 Open 3 Percutaneous 4 Percutaneous Endoscopic X External	Z No Device	Z No Qualifier
P Gastrointestinal Tract Q Respiratory Tract R Genitourinary Tract	0 Open 3 Percutaneous 4 Percutaneous Endoscopic 7 Via Natural or Artificial Opening 8 Via Natural or Artificial Opening Endoscopic X External	Z No Device	Z No Qualifier

Section	0	Medical and Surgical
Body System	W	Anatomical Regions, General
Operation	H	Insertion: Putting in a nonbiological appliance that monitors, assists, performs, or prevents a physiological function but does not physically take the place of a body part

Body Part (4th)	Approach (5th)	Device (6th)	Qualifier (7th)
0 Head 1 Cranial Cavity 2 Face 3 Oral Cavity and Throat 4 Upper Jaw 5 Lower Jaw 6 Neck 8 Chest Wall 9 Pleural Cavity, Right B Pleural Cavity, Left C Mediastinum D Pericardial Cavity F Abdominal Wall G Peritoneal Cavity H Retroperitoneum J Pelvic Cavity K Upper Back L Lower Back M Perineum, Male N Perineum, Female	0 Open 3 Percutaneous 4 Percutaneous Endoscopic	1 Radioactive Element 3 Infusion Device Y Other Device	Z No Qualifier
P Gastrointestinal Tract Q Respiratory Tract R Genitourinary Tract	0 Open 3 Percutaneous 4 Percutaneous Endoscopic 7 Via Natural or Artificial Opening 8 Via Natural or Artificial Opening Endoscopic	1 Radioactive Element 3 Infusion Device Y Other Device	Z No Qualifier

Section	0	Medical and Surgical
Body System	W	Anatomical Regions, General
Operation	J	Inspection: Visually and/or manually exploring a body part

Body Part (4th)	Approach (5th)	Device (6th)	Qualifier (7th)
0 Head 2 Face 3 Oral Cavity and Throat 4 Upper Jaw 5 Lower Jaw 6 Neck 8 Chest Wall F Abdominal Wall K Upper Back L Lower Back M Perineum, Male N Perineum, Female	0 Open 3 Percutaneous 4 Percutaneous Endoscopic X External	Z No Device	Z No Qualifier
1 Cranial Cavity 9 Pleural Cavity, Right B Pleural Cavity, Left C Mediastinum D Pericardial Cavity G Peritoneal Cavity H Retroperitoneum J Pelvic Cavity	0 Open 3 Percutaneous 4 Percutaneous Endoscopic	Z No Device	Z No Qualifier
P Gastrointestinal Tract Q Respiratory Tract R Genitourinary Tract	0 Open 3 Percutaneous 4 Percutaneous Endoscopic 7 Via Natural or Artificial Opening 8 Via Natural or Artificial Opening Endoscopic	Z No Device	Z No Qualifier

Section	0	Medical and Surgical
Body System	W	Anatomical Regions, General
Operation	M	Reattachment: Putting back in or on all or a portion of a separated body part to its normal location or other suitable location

Body Part (4th)	Approach (5th)	Device (6th)	Qualifier (7th)
2 Face 4 Upper Jaw 5 Lower Jaw 6 Neck 8 Chest Wall F Abdominal Wall K Upper Back L Lower Back M Perineum, Male N Perineum, Female	0 Open	Z No Device	Z No Qualifier

Section	0	Medical and Surgical
Body System	W	Anatomical Regions, General
Operation	P	**Removal:** Taking out or off a device from a body part

Body Part (4th)	Approach (5th)	Device (6th)	Qualifier (7th)
0 Head **2** Face **4** Upper Jaw **5** Lower Jaw **6** Neck **8** Chest Wall **C** Mediastinum **F** Abdominal Wall **K** Upper Back **L** Lower Back **M** Perineum, Male **N** Perineum, Female	**0** Open **3** Percutaneous **4** Percutaneous Endoscopic **X** External	**0** Drainage Device **1** Radioactive Element **3** Infusion Device **7** Autologous Tissue Substitute **J** Synthetic Substitute **K** Nonautologous Tissue Substitute **Y** Other Device	**Z** No Qualifier
1 Cranial Cavity **9** Pleural Cavity, Right **B** Pleural Cavity, Left **G** Peritoneal Cavity **J** Pelvic Cavity	**0** Open **3** Percutaneous **4** Percutaneous Endoscopic	**0** Drainage Device **1** Radioactive Element **3** Infusion Device **J** Synthetic Substitute **Y** Other Device	**Z** No Qualifier
1 Cranial Cavity **9** Pleural Cavity, Right **B** Pleural Cavity, Left **G** Peritoneal Cavity **J** Pelvic Cavity	**X** External	**0** Drainage Device **1** Radioactive Element **3** Infusion Device	**Z** No Qualifier
D Pericardial Cavity **H** Retroperitoneum	**0** Open **3** Percutaneous **4** Percutaneous Endoscopic	**0** Drainage Device **1** Radioactive Element **3** Infusion Device **Y** Other Device	**Z** No Qualifier
D Pericardial Cavity **H** Retroperitoneum	**X** External	**0** Drainage Device **1** Radioactive Element **3** Infusion Device	**Z** No Qualifier
P Gastrointestinal Tract **Q** Respiratory Tract **R** Genitourinary Tract	**0** Open **3** Percutaneous **4** Percutaneous Endoscopic **7** Via Natural or Artificial Opening **8** Via Natural or Artificial Opening Endoscopic **X** External	**1** Radioactive Element **3** Infusion Device **Y** Other Device	**Z** No Qualifier

Section   0   **Medical and Surgical**
Body System   W   **Anatomical Regions, General**
Operation   Q   **Repair:** Restoring, to the extent possible, a body part to its normal anatomic structure and function

Body Part (4th)	Approach (5th)	Device (6th)	Qualifier (7th)
0 Head 2 Face 3 Oral Cavity and Throat 4 Upper Jaw 5 Lower Jaw 8 Chest Wall K Upper Back L Lower Back M Perineum, Male N Perineum, Female	0 Open 3 Percutaneous 4 Percutaneous Endoscopic X External	Z No Device	Z No Qualifier
6 Neck F Abdominal Wall	0 Open 3 Percutaneous 4 Percutaneous Endoscopic	Z No Device	Z No Qualifier
6 Neck F Abdominal Wall	X External	Z No Device	2 Stoma Z No Qualifier
C Mediastinum	0 Open 3 Percutaneous 4 Percutaneous Endoscopic	Z No Device	Z No Qualifier

Section   0   **Medical and Surgical**
Body System   W   **Anatomical Regions, General**
Operation   U   **Supplement:** Putting in or on biological or synthetic material that physically reinforces and/or augments the function of a portion of a body part

Body Part (4th)	Approach (5th)	Device (6th)	Qualifier (7th)
0 Head 2 Face 4 Upper Jaw 5 Lower Jaw 6 Neck 8 Chest Wall C Mediastinum F Abdominal Wall K Upper Back L Lower Back M Perineum, Male N Perineum, Female	0 Open 4 Percutaneous Endoscopic	7 Autologous Tissue Substitute J Synthetic Substitute K Nonautologous Tissue Substitute	Z No Qualifier

Section   0   **Medical and Surgical**
Body System   W   **Anatomical Regions, General**
Operation   W   **Revision:** Correcting, to the extent possible, a portion of a malfunctioning device or the position of a displaced device

Body Part (4th)	Approach (5th)	Device (6th)	Qualifier (7th)
0 Head 2 Face 4 Upper Jaw 5 Lower Jaw 6 Neck 8 Chest Wall C Mediastinum F Abdominal Wall K Upper Back L Lower Back M Perineum, Male N Perineum, Female	0 Open 3 Percutaneous 4 Percutaneous Endoscopic X External	0 Drainage Device 1 Radioactive Element 3 Infusion Device 7 Autologous Tissue Substitute J Synthetic Substitute K Nonautologous Tissue Substitute Y Other Device	Z No Qualifier

Continued →

Section   **0**   **Medical and Surgical**
Body System   **W**   **Anatomical Regions, General**
Operation   **W**   **Revision:** Correcting, to the extent possible, a portion of a malfunctioning device or the position of a displaced device

Body Part (4ᵗʰ)	Approach (5ᵗʰ)	Device (6ᵗʰ)	Qualifier (7ᵗʰ)
1 Cranial Cavity 9 Pleural Cavity, Right B Pleural Cavity, Left G Peritoneal Cavity J Pelvic Cavity	0 Open 3 Percutaneous 4 Percutaneous Endoscopic X External	0 Drainage Device 1 Radioactive Element 3 Infusion Device J Synthetic Substitute Y Other Device	Z No Qualifier
D Pericardial Cavity H Retroperitoneum	0 Open 3 Percutaneous 4 Percutaneous Endoscopic X External	0 Drainage Device 1 Radioactive Element 3 Infusion Device Y Other Device	Z No Qualifier
P Gastrointestinal Tract Q Respiratory Tract R Genitourinary Tract	0 Open 3 Percutaneous 4 Percutaneous Endoscopic 7 Via Natural or Artificial Opening 8 Via Natural or Artificial Opening Endoscopic X External	1 Radioactive Element 3 Infusion Device Y Other Device	Z No Qualifier

Section   **0**   **Medical and Surgical**
Body System   **W**   **Anatomical Regions, General**
Operation   **Y**   **Transplantation:** Putting in or on all or a portion of a living body part taken from another individual or animal to physically take the place and/or function of all or a portion of a similar body part

Body Part (4ᵗʰ)	Approach (5ᵗʰ)	Device (6ᵗʰ)	Qualifier (7th)
2 Face	0 Open	Z No Device	0 Allogeneic 1 Syngeneic

Anatomical Regions, General Code Listing 0W0–0WW

0W0 – Anatomical Regions, General, Alteration

0W0007Z   Alteration of Head with Autologous Tissue Substitute, Open Approach
0W000JZ   Alteration of Head with Synthetic Substitute, Open Approach
0W000KZ   Alteration of Head with Nonautologous Tissue Substitute, Open Approach
0W000ZZ   Alteration of Head, Open Approach
0W0037Z   Alteration of Head with Autologous Tissue Substitute, Percutaneous Approach
0W003JZ   Alteration of Head with Synthetic Substitute, Percutaneous Approach
0W003KZ   Alteration of Head with Nonautologous Tissue Substitute, Percutaneous Approach
0W003ZZ   Alteration of Head, Percutaneous Approach
0W0047Z   Alteration of Head with Autologous Tissue Substitute, Percutaneous Endoscopic Approach
0W004JZ   Alteration of Head with Synthetic Substitute, Percutaneous Endoscopic Approach
0W004KZ   Alteration of Head with Nonautologous Tissue Substitute, Percutaneous Endoscopic Approach
0W004ZZ   Alteration of Head, Percutaneous Endoscopic Approach
0W0207Z   Alteration of Face with Autologous Tissue Substitute, Open Approach

0W020JZ   Alteration of Face with Synthetic Substitute, Open Approach
0W020KZ   Alteration of Face with Nonautologous Tissue Substitute, Open Approach
0W020ZZ   Alteration of Face, Open Approach
AHA CC: 1Q, 2015, 31
0W0237Z   Alteration of Face with Autologous Tissue Substitute, Percutaneous Approach
0W023JZ   Alteration of Face with Synthetic Substitute, Percutaneous Approach
0W023KZ   Alteration of Face with Nonautologous Tissue Substitute, Percutaneous Approach
0W023ZZ   Alteration of Face, Percutaneous Approach
0W0247Z   Alteration of Face with Autologous Tissue Substitute, Percutaneous Endoscopic Approach
0W024JZ   Alteration of Face with Synthetic Substitute, Percutaneous Endoscopic Approach
0W024KZ   Alteration of Face with Nonautologous Tissue Substitute, Percutaneous Endoscopic Approach
0W024ZZ   Alteration of Face, Percutaneous Endoscopic Approach
0W0407Z   Alteration of Upper Jaw with Autologous Tissue Substitute, Open Approach
0W040JZ   Alteration of Upper Jaw with Synthetic Substitute, Open Approach

0W040KZ   Alteration of Upper Jaw with Nonautologous Tissue Substitute, Open Approach
0W040ZZ   Alteration of Upper Jaw, Open Approach
0W0437Z   Alteration of Upper Jaw with Autologous Tissue Substitute, Percutaneous Approach
0W043JZ   Alteration of Upper Jaw with Synthetic Substitute, Percutaneous Approach
0W043KZ   Alteration of Upper Jaw with Nonautologous Tissue Substitute, Percutaneous Approach
0W043ZZ   Alteration of Upper Jaw, Percutaneous Approach
0W0447Z   Alteration of Upper Jaw with Autologous Tissue Substitute, Percutaneous Endoscopic Approach
0W044JZ   Alteration of Upper Jaw with Synthetic Substitute, Percutaneous Endoscopic Approach
0W044KZ   Alteration of Upper Jaw with Nonautologous Tissue Substitute, Percutaneous Endoscopic Approach
0W044ZZ   Alteration of Upper Jaw, Percutaneous Endoscopic Approach
0W0507Z   Alteration of Lower Jaw with Autologous Tissue Substitute, Open Approach
0W050JZ   Alteration of Lower Jaw with Synthetic Substitute, Open Approach

0W050KZ Alteration of Lower Jaw with Nonautologous Tissue Substitute, Open Approach

0W050ZZ Alteration of Lower Jaw, Open Approach

0W0537Z Alteration of Lower Jaw with Autologous Tissue Substitute, Percutaneous Approach

0W053JZ Alteration of Lower Jaw with Synthetic Substitute, Percutaneous Approach

0W053KZ Alteration of Lower Jaw with Nonautologous Tissue Substitute, Percutaneous Approach

0W053ZZ Alteration of Lower Jaw, Percutaneous Approach

0W0547Z Alteration of Lower Jaw with Autologous Tissue Substitute, Percutaneous Endoscopic Approach

0W054JZ Alteration of Lower Jaw with Synthetic Substitute, Percutaneous Endoscopic Approach

0W054KZ Alteration of Lower Jaw with Nonautologous Tissue Substitute, Percutaneous Endoscopic Approach

0W054ZZ Alteration of Lower Jaw, Percutaneous Endoscopic Approach

0W0607Z Alteration of Neck with Autologous Tissue Substitute, Open Approach

0W060JZ Alteration of Neck with Synthetic Substitute, Open Approach

0W060KZ Alteration of Neck with Nonautologous Tissue Substitute, Open Approach

0W060ZZ Alteration of Neck, Open Approach

0W0637Z Alteration of Neck with Autologous Tissue Substitute, Percutaneous Approach

0W063JZ Alteration of Neck with Synthetic Substitute, Percutaneous Approach

0W063KZ Alteration of Neck with Nonautologous Tissue Substitute, Percutaneous Approach

0W063ZZ Alteration of Neck, Percutaneous Approach

0W0647Z Alteration of Neck with Autologous Tissue Substitute, Percutaneous Endoscopic Approach

0W064JZ Alteration of Neck with Synthetic Substitute, Percutaneous Endoscopic Approach

0W064KZ Alteration of Neck with Nonautologous Tissue Substitute, Percutaneous Endoscopic Approach

0W064ZZ Alteration of Neck, Percutaneous Endoscopic Approach

0W0807Z Alteration of Chest Wall with Autologous Tissue Substitute, Open Approach

0W080JZ Alteration of Chest Wall with Synthetic Substitute, Open Approach

0W080KZ Alteration of Chest Wall with Nonautologous Tissue Substitute, Open Approach

0W080ZZ Alteration of Chest Wall, Open Approach

0W0837Z Alteration of Chest Wall with Autologous Tissue Substitute, Percutaneous Approach

0W083JZ Alteration of Chest Wall with Synthetic Substitute, Percutaneous Approach

0W083KZ Alteration of Chest Wall with Nonautologous Tissue Substitute, Percutaneous Approach

0W083ZZ Alteration of Chest Wall, Percutaneous Approach

0W0847Z Alteration of Chest Wall with Autologous Tissue Substitute, Percutaneous Endoscopic Approach

0W084JZ Alteration of Chest Wall with Synthetic Substitute, Percutaneous Endoscopic Approach

0W084KZ Alteration of Chest Wall with Nonautologous Tissue Substitute, Percutaneous Endoscopic Approach

0W084ZZ Alteration of Chest Wall, Percutaneous Endoscopic Approach

0W0F07Z Alteration of Abdominal Wall with Autologous Tissue Substitute, Open Approach

0W0F0JZ Alteration of Abdominal Wall with Synthetic Substitute, Open Approach

0W0F0KZ Alteration of Abdominal Wall with Nonautologous Tissue Substitute, Open Approach

0W0F0ZZ Alteration of Abdominal Wall, Open Approach

0W0F37Z Alteration of Abdominal Wall with Autologous Tissue Substitute, Percutaneous Approach

0W0F3JZ Alteration of Abdominal Wall with Synthetic Substitute, Percutaneous Approach

0W0F3KZ Alteration of Abdominal Wall with Nonautologous Tissue Substitute, Percutaneous Approach

0W0F3ZZ Alteration of Abdominal Wall, Percutaneous Approach

0W0F47Z Alteration of Abdominal Wall with Autologous Tissue Substitute, Percutaneous Endoscopic Approach

0W0F4JZ Alteration of Abdominal Wall with Synthetic Substitute, Percutaneous Endoscopic Approach

0W0F4KZ Alteration of Abdominal Wall with Nonautologous Tissue Substitute, Percutaneous Endoscopic Approach

0W0F4ZZ Alteration of Abdominal Wall, Percutaneous Endoscopic Approach

0W0K07Z Alteration of Upper Back with Autologous Tissue Substitute, Open Approach

0W0K0JZ Alteration of Upper Back with Synthetic Substitute, Open Approach

0W0K0KZ Alteration of Upper Back with Nonautologous Tissue Substitute, Open Approach

0W0K0ZZ Alteration of Upper Back, Open Approach

0W0K37Z Alteration of Upper Back with Autologous Tissue Substitute, Percutaneous Approach

0W0K3JZ Alteration of Upper Back with Synthetic Substitute, Percutaneous Approach

0W0K3KZ Alteration of Upper Back with Nonautologous Tissue Substitute, Percutaneous Approach

0W0K3ZZ Alteration of Upper Back, Percutaneous Approach

0W0K47Z Alteration of Upper Back with Autologous Tissue Substitute, Percutaneous Endoscopic Approach

0W0K4JZ Alteration of Upper Back with Synthetic Substitute, Percutaneous Endoscopic Approach

0W0K4KZ Alteration of Upper Back with Nonautologous Tissue Substitute, Percutaneous Endoscopic Approach

0W0K4ZZ Alteration of Upper Back, Percutaneous Endoscopic Approach

0W0L07Z Alteration of Lower Back with Autologous Tissue Substitute, Open Approach

0W0L0JZ Alteration of Lower Back with Synthetic Substitute, Open Approach

0W0L0KZ Alteration of Lower Back with Nonautologous Tissue Substitute, Open Approach

0W0L0ZZ Alteration of Lower Back, Open Approach

0W0L37Z Alteration of Lower Back with Autologous Tissue Substitute, Percutaneous Approach

0W0L3JZ Alteration of Lower Back with Synthetic Substitute, Percutaneous Approach

0W0L3KZ Alteration of Lower Back with Nonautologous Tissue Substitute, Percutaneous Approach

0W0L3ZZ Alteration of Lower Back, Percutaneous Approach

0W0L47Z Alteration of Lower Back with Autologous Tissue Substitute, Percutaneous Endoscopic Approach

0W0L4JZ Alteration of Lower Back with Synthetic Substitute, Percutaneous Endoscopic Approach

0W0L4KZ Alteration of Lower Back with Nonautologous Tissue Substitute, Percutaneous Endoscopic Approach

0W0L4ZZ Alteration of Lower Back, Percutaneous Endoscopic Approach

♂ **0W0M07Z** Alteration of Male Perineum with Autologous Tissue Substitute, Open Approach

♂ **0W0M0JZ** Alteration of Male Perineum with Synthetic Substitute, Open Approach

♂ **0W0M0KZ** Alteration of Male Perineum with Nonautologous Tissue Substitute, Open Approach

♂ **0W0M0ZZ** Alteration of Male Perineum, Open Approach

♂ **0W0M37Z** Alteration of Male Perineum with Autologous Tissue Substitute, Percutaneous Approach

♂ **0W0M3JZ** Alteration of Male Perineum with Synthetic Substitute, Percutaneous Approach

♂ **0W0M3KZ** Alteration of Male Perineum with Nonautologous Tissue Substitute, Percutaneous Approach

♂ **0W0M3ZZ** Alteration of Male Perineum, Percutaneous Approach

♂ **0W0M47Z** Alteration of Male Perineum with Autologous Tissue Substitute, Percutaneous Endoscopic Approach

♂ **0W0M4JZ** Alteration of Male Perineum with Synthetic Substitute, Percutaneous Endoscopic Approach

♂ **0W0M4KZ** Alteration of Male Perineum with Nonautologous Tissue Substitute, Percutaneous Endoscopic Approach

♂ **0W0M4ZZ** Alteration of Male Perineum, Percutaneous Endoscopic Approach

♀ **0W0N07Z** Alteration of Female Perineum with Autologous Tissue Substitute, Open Approach

♀ **0W0N0JZ** Alteration of Female Perineum with Synthetic Substitute, Open Approach

♀ **0W0N0KZ** Alteration of Female Perineum with Nonautologous Tissue Substitute, Open Approach

♀ **0W0N0ZZ** Alteration of Female Perineum, Open Approach

♀ **0W0N37Z** Alteration of Female Perineum with Autologous Tissue Substitute, Percutaneous Approach

♀ Female-only   ♂ Male-only   ▲ Limited Coverage   ● Non-OR   ᴴᴬᶜ HAC-associated procedure   ▲ Non-covered procedures   ➕ Cluster

♀ **0W0N3JZ** Alteration of Female Perineum with Synthetic Substitute, Percutaneous Approach

♀ **0W0N3KZ** Alteration of Female Perineum with Nonautologous Tissue Substitute, Percutaneous Approach

♀ **0W0N3ZZ** Alteration of Female Perineum, Percutaneous Approach

♀ **0W0N47Z** Alteration of Female Perineum with Autologous Tissue Substitute, Percutaneous Endoscopic Approach

♀ **0W0N4JZ** Alteration of Female Perineum with Synthetic Substitute, Percutaneous Endoscopic Approach

♀ **0W0N4KZ** Alteration of Female Perineum with Nonautologous Tissue Substitute, Percutaneous Endoscopic Approach

♀ **0W0N4ZZ** Alteration of Female Perineum, Percutaneous Endoscopic Approach

0W1 – Anatomical Regions, General, Bypass

Review Coding Guideline B3.6a

0W110J9 Bypass Cranial Cavity to Right Pleural Cavity with Synthetic Substitute, Open Approach

0W110JB Bypass Cranial Cavity to Left Pleural Cavity with Synthetic Substitute, Open Approach

0W110JG Bypass Cranial Cavity to Peritoneal Cavity with Synthetic Substitute, Open Approach

0W110JJ Bypass Cranial Cavity to Pelvic Cavity with Synthetic Substitute, Open Approach

0W190J4 Bypass Right Pleural Cavity to Cutaneous with Synthetic Substitute, Open Approach

0W190J9 Bypass Right Pleural Cavity to Right Pleural Cavity with Synthetic Substitute, Open Approach

0W190JB Bypass Right Pleural Cavity to Left Pleural Cavity with Synthetic Substitute, Open Approach

0W190JG Bypass Right Pleural Cavity to Peritoneal Cavity with Synthetic Substitute, Open Approach

0W190JJ Bypass Right Pleural Cavity to Pelvic Cavity with Synthetic Substitute, Open Approach

0W190JW Bypass Right Pleural Cavity to Upper Vein with Synthetic Substitute, Open Approach

0W190JY Bypass Right Pleural Cavity to Lower Vein with Synthetic Substitute, Open Approach

0W193J4 Bypass Right Pleural Cavity to Cutaneous with Synthetic Substitute, Percutaneous Approach

0W193J9 Bypass Right Pleural Cavity to Right Pleural Cavity with Synthetic Substitute, Percutaneous Approach

0W193JB Bypass Right Pleural Cavity to Left Pleural Cavity with Synthetic Substitute, Percutaneous Approach

0W193JG Bypass Right Pleural Cavity to Peritoneal Cavity with Synthetic Substitute, Percutaneous Approach

0W193JJ Bypass Right Pleural Cavity to Pelvic Cavity with Synthetic Substitute, Percutaneous Approach

0W193JW Bypass Right Pleural Cavity to Upper Vein with Synthetic Substitute, Percutaneous Approach

0W193JY Bypass Right Pleural Cavity to Lower Vein with Synthetic Substitute, Percutaneous Approach

0W194J4 Bypass Right Pleural Cavity to Cutaneous with Synthetic Substitute, Percutaneous Endoscopic Approach

0W194J9 Bypass Right Pleural Cavity to Right Pleural Cavity with Synthetic Substitute, Percutaneous Endoscopic Approach

0W194JB Bypass Right Pleural Cavity to Left Pleural Cavity with Synthetic Substitute, Percutaneous Endoscopic Approach

0W194JG Bypass Right Pleural Cavity to Peritoneal Cavity with Synthetic Substitute, Percutaneous Endoscopic Approach

0W194JJ Bypass Right Pleural Cavity to Pelvic Cavity with Synthetic Substitute, Percutaneous Endoscopic Approach

0W194JW Bypass Right Pleural Cavity to Upper Vein with Synthetic Substitute, Percutaneous Endoscopic Approach

0W194JY Bypass Right Pleural Cavity to Lower Vein with Synthetic Substitute, Percutaneous Endoscopic Approach

0W1B0J4 Bypass Left Pleural Cavity to Cutaneous with Synthetic Substitute, Open Approach

0W1B0J9 Bypass Left Pleural Cavity to Right Pleural Cavity with Synthetic Substitute, Open Approach

0W1B0JB Bypass Left Pleural Cavity to Left Pleural Cavity with Synthetic Substitute, Open Approach

0W1B0JG Bypass Left Pleural Cavity to Peritoneal Cavity with Synthetic Substitute, Open Approach

0W1B0JJ Bypass Left Pleural Cavity to Pelvic Cavity with Synthetic Substitute, Open Approach

0W1B0JW Bypass Left Pleural Cavity to Upper Vein with Synthetic Substitute, Open Approach

0W1B0JY Bypass Left Pleural Cavity to Lower Vein with Synthetic Substitute, Open Approach

0W1B3J4 Bypass Left Pleural Cavity to Cutaneous with Synthetic Substitute, Percutaneous Approach

0W1B3J9 Bypass Left Pleural Cavity to Right Pleural Cavity with Synthetic Substitute, Percutaneous Approach

0W1B3JB Bypass Left Pleural Cavity to Left Pleural Cavity with Synthetic Substitute, Percutaneous Approach

0W1B3JG Bypass Left Pleural Cavity to Peritoneal Cavity with Synthetic Substitute, Percutaneous Approach

0W1B3JJ Bypass Left Pleural Cavity to Pelvic Cavity with Synthetic Substitute, Percutaneous Approach

0W1B3JW Bypass Left Pleural Cavity to Upper Vein with Synthetic Substitute, Percutaneous Approach

0W1B3JY Bypass Left Pleural Cavity to Lower Vein with Synthetic Substitute, Percutaneous Approach

0W1B4J4 Bypass Left Pleural Cavity to Cutaneous with Synthetic Substitute, Percutaneous Endoscopic Approach

0W1B4J9 Bypass Left Pleural Cavity to Right Pleural Cavity with Synthetic Substitute, Percutaneous Endoscopic Approach

0W1B4JB Bypass Left Pleural Cavity to Left Pleural Cavity with Synthetic Substitute, Percutaneous Endoscopic Approach

0W1B4JG Bypass Left Pleural Cavity to Peritoneal Cavity with Synthetic Substitute, Percutaneous Endoscopic Approach

0W1B4JJ Bypass Left Pleural Cavity to Pelvic Cavity with Synthetic Substitute, Percutaneous Endoscopic Approach

0W1B4JW Bypass Left Pleural Cavity to Upper Vein with Synthetic Substitute, Percutaneous Endoscopic Approach

0W1B4JY Bypass Left Pleural Cavity to Lower Vein with Synthetic Substitute, Percutaneous Endoscopic Approach

0W1G0J4 Bypass Peritoneal Cavity to Cutaneous with Synthetic Substitute, Open Approach

0W1G0J6 Bypass Peritoneal Cavity to Bladder with Synthetic Substitute, Open Approach

0W1G0J9 Bypass Peritoneal Cavity to Right Pleural Cavity with Synthetic Substitute, Open Approach

0W1G0JB Bypass Peritoneal Cavity to Left Pleural Cavity with Synthetic Substitute, Open Approach

0W1G0JG Bypass Peritoneal Cavity to Peritoneal Cavity with Synthetic Substitute, Open Approach

0W1G0JJ Bypass Peritoneal Cavity to Pelvic Cavity with Synthetic Substitute, Open Approach

0W1G0JW Bypass Peritoneal Cavity to Upper Vein with Synthetic Substitute, Open Approach

0W1G0JY Bypass Peritoneal Cavity to Lower Vein with Synthetic Substitute, Open Approach

0W1G3J4 Bypass Peritoneal Cavity to Cutaneous with Synthetic Substitute, Percutaneous Approach
AHA CC: 4Q, 2013, 126-127

0W1G3J6 Bypass Peritoneal Cavity to Bladder with Synthetic Substitute, Percutaneous Approach
AHA CC: 4Q, 2020, 55

0W1G3J9 Bypass Peritoneal Cavity to Right Pleural Cavity with Synthetic Substitute, Percutaneous Approach

0W1G3JB Bypass Peritoneal Cavity to Left Pleural Cavity with Synthetic Substitute, Percutaneous Approach

0W1G3JG Bypass Peritoneal Cavity to Peritoneal Cavity with Synthetic Substitute, Percutaneous Approach

0W1G3JJ Bypass Peritoneal Cavity to Pelvic Cavity with Synthetic Substitute, Percutaneous Approach

---

♀ Female-only   ♂ Male-only   ▲ Limited Coverage   ● Non-OR   ▦ HAC-associated procedure   ▲ Non-covered procedures   ➕ Cluster

0W1G3JW Bypass Peritoneal Cavity to Upper Vein with Synthetic Substitute, Percutaneous Approach *AHA CC: 4Q, 2018, 42-43*	**0W1J0J4** Bypass Pelvic Cavity to Cutaneous with Synthetic Substitute, Open Approach	**0W1J3JJ** Bypass Pelvic Cavity to Pelvic Cavity with Synthetic Substitute, Percutaneous Approach
0W1G3JY Bypass Peritoneal Cavity to Lower Vein with Synthetic Substitute, Percutaneous Approach	**0W1J0J9** Bypass Pelvic Cavity to Right Pleural Cavity with Synthetic Substitute, Open Approach	**0W1J3JW** Bypass Pelvic Cavity to Upper Vein with Synthetic Substitute, Percutaneous Approach
0W1G4J4 Bypass Peritoneal Cavity to Cutaneous with Synthetic Substitute, Percutaneous Endoscopic Approach	**0W1J0JB** Bypass Pelvic Cavity to Left Pleural Cavity with Synthetic Substitute, Open Approach	**0W1J3JY** Bypass Pelvic Cavity to Lower Vein with Synthetic Substitute, Percutaneous Approach
0W1G4J6 Bypass Peritoneal Cavity to Bladder with Synthetic Substitute, Percutaneous Endoscopic Approach	**0W1J0JG** Bypass Pelvic Cavity to Peritoneal Cavity with Synthetic Substitute, Open Approach	**0W1J4J4** Bypass Pelvic Cavity to Cutaneous with Synthetic Substitute, Percutaneous Endoscopic Approach
0W1G4J9 Bypass Peritoneal Cavity to Right Pleural Cavity with Synthetic Substitute, Percutaneous Endoscopic Approach	**0W1J0JJ** Bypass Pelvic Cavity to Pelvic Cavity with Synthetic Substitute, Open Approach	**0W1J4J9** Bypass Pelvic Cavity to Right Pleural Cavity with Synthetic Substitute, Percutaneous Endoscopic Approach
0W1G4JB Bypass Peritoneal Cavity to Left Pleural Cavity with Synthetic Substitute, Percutaneous Endoscopic Approach	**0W1J0JW** Bypass Pelvic Cavity to Upper Vein with Synthetic Substitute, Open Approach	**0W1J4JB** Bypass Pelvic Cavity to Left Pleural Cavity with Synthetic Substitute, Percutaneous Endoscopic Approach
0W1G4JG Bypass Peritoneal Cavity to Peritoneal Cavity with Synthetic Substitute, Percutaneous Endoscopic Approach	**0W1J0JY** Bypass Pelvic Cavity to Lower Vein with Synthetic Substitute, Open Approach	**0W1J4JG** Bypass Pelvic Cavity to Peritoneal Cavity with Synthetic Substitute, Percutaneous Endoscopic Approach
0W1G4JJ Bypass Peritoneal Cavity to Pelvic Cavity with Synthetic Substitute, Percutaneous Endoscopic Approach	**0W1J3J4** Bypass Pelvic Cavity to Cutaneous with Synthetic Substitute, Percutaneous Approach	**0W1J4JJ** Bypass Pelvic Cavity to Pelvic Cavity with Synthetic Substitute, Percutaneous Endoscopic Approach
0W1G4JW Bypass Peritoneal Cavity to Upper Vein with Synthetic Substitute, Percutaneous Endoscopic Approach	**0W1J3J9** Bypass Pelvic Cavity to Right Pleural Cavity with Synthetic Substitute, Percutaneous Approach	**0W1J4JW** Bypass Pelvic Cavity to Upper Vein with Synthetic Substitute, Percutaneous Endoscopic Approach
0W1G4JY Bypass Peritoneal Cavity to Lower Vein with Synthetic Substitute, Percutaneous Endoscopic Approach	**0W1J3JB** Bypass Pelvic Cavity to Left Pleural Cavity with Synthetic Substitute, Percutaneous Approach	**0W1J4JY** Bypass Pelvic Cavity to Lower Vein with Synthetic Substitute, Percutaneous Endoscopic Approach
	0W1J3JG Bypass Pelvic Cavity to Peritoneal Cavity with Synthetic Substitute, Percutaneous Approach	

0W2 – Anatomical Regions, General, Change

Review Coding Guideline B6.1c

0W20X0Z Change Drainage Device in Head, External Approach	**0W28XYZ** Change Other Device in Chest Wall, External Approach	**0W2HX0Z** Change Drainage Device in Retroperitoneum, External Approach
0W20XYZ Change Other Device in Head, External Approach	**0W29X0Z** Change Drainage Device in Right Pleural Cavity, External Approach	**0W2HXYZ** Change Other Device in Retroperitoneum, External Approach
0W21X0Z Change Drainage Device in Cranial Cavity, External Approach	**0W29XYZ** Change Other Device in Right Pleural Cavity, External Approach	**0W2JX0Z** Change Drainage Device in Pelvic Cavity, External Approach
0W21XYZ Change Other Device in Cranial Cavity, External Approach	**0W2BX0Z** Change Drainage Device in Left Pleural Cavity, External Approach	**0W2JXYZ** Change Other Device in Pelvic Cavity, External Approach
0W22X0Z Change Drainage Device in Face, External Approach	**0W2BXYZ** Change Other Device in Left Pleural Cavity, External Approach	**0W2KX0Z** Change Drainage Device in Upper Back, External Approach
0W22XYZ Change Other Device in Face, External Approach	**0W2CX0Z** Change Drainage Device in Mediastinum, External Approach	**0W2KXYZ** Change Other Device in Upper Back, External Approach
0W24X0Z Change Drainage Device in Upper Jaw, External Approach	**0W2CXYZ** Change Other Device in Mediastinum, External Approach	**0W2LX0Z** Change Drainage Device in Lower Back, External Approach
0W24XYZ Change Other Device in Upper Jaw, External Approach	**0W2DX0Z** Change Drainage Device in Pericardial Cavity, External Approach	**0W2LXYZ** Change Other Device in Lower Back, External Approach
0W25X0Z Change Drainage Device in Lower Jaw, External Approach	**0W2DXYZ** Change Other Device in Pericardial Cavity, External Approach	♂ **0W2MX0Z** Change Drainage Device in Male Perineum, External Approach
0W25XYZ Change Other Device in Lower Jaw, External Approach	♂ **0W2FX0Z** Change Drainage Device in Abdominal Wall, External Approach	♂ **0W2MXYZ** Change Other Device in Male Perineum, External Approach
0W26X0Z Change Drainage Device in Neck, External Approach	♂ **0W2FXYZ** Change Other Device in Abdominal Wall, External Approach	♀ **0W2NX0Z** Change Drainage Device in Female Perineum, External Approach
0W26XYZ Change Other Device in Neck, External Approach	**0W2GX0Z** Change Drainage Device in Peritoneal Cavity, External Approach	♀ **0W2NXYZ** Change Other Device in Female Perineum, External Approach
0W28X0Z Change Drainage Device in Chest Wall, External Approach	**0W2GXYZ** Change Other Device in Peritoneal Cavity, External Approach	

0W3 – Anatomical Regions, General, Control

Review Coding Guideline B3.7

0W300ZZ Control Bleeding in Head, Open Approach	**0W310ZZ** Control Bleeding in Cranial Cavity, Open Approach *AHA CC: 3Q, 2019, 4-5*	**0W320ZZ** Control Bleeding in Face, Open Approach
0W303ZZ Control Bleeding in Head, Percutaneous Approach	**0W313ZZ** Control Bleeding in Cranial Cavity, Percutaneous Approach	**0W323ZZ** Control Bleeding in Face, Percutaneous Approach
0W304ZZ Control Bleeding in Head, Percutaneous Endoscopic Approach	**0W314ZZ** Control Bleeding in Cranial Cavity, Percutaneous Endoscopic Approach	**0W324ZZ** Control Bleeding in Face, Percutaneous Endoscopic Approach

♀ Female-only   ♂ Male-only   ▲ Limited Coverage   ● Non-OR   **HAC** HAC-associated procedure   ▲ Non-covered procedures   ✛ Cluster

0W330ZZ	Control Bleeding in Oral Cavity and Throat, Open Approach
0W333ZZ	Control Bleeding in Oral Cavity and Throat, Percutaneous Approach
0W334ZZ	Control Bleeding in Oral Cavity and Throat, Percutaneous Endoscopic Approach
0W337ZZ	Control Bleeding in Oral Cavity and Throat, Via Natural or Artificial Opening
0W338ZZ	Control Bleeding in Oral Cavity and Throat, Via Natural or Artificial Opening Endoscopic
0W33XZZ	Control Bleeding in Oral Cavity and Throat, External Approach
0W340ZZ	Control Bleeding in Upper Jaw, Open Approach
0W343ZZ	Control Bleeding in Upper Jaw, Percutaneous Approach
0W344ZZ	Control Bleeding in Upper Jaw, Percutaneous Endoscopic Approach
0W350ZZ	Control Bleeding in Lower Jaw, Open Approach
0W353ZZ	Control Bleeding in Lower Jaw, Percutaneous Approach
0W354ZZ	Control Bleeding in Lower Jaw, Percutaneous Endoscopic Approach
0W360ZZ	Control Bleeding in Neck, Open Approach
0W363ZZ	Control Bleeding in Neck, Percutaneous Approach
0W364ZZ	Control Bleeding in Neck, Percutaneous Endoscopic Approach
0W380ZZ	Control Bleeding in Chest Wall, Open Approach
0W383ZZ	Control Bleeding in Chest Wall, Percutaneous Approach
0W384ZZ	Control Bleeding in Chest Wall, Percutaneous Endoscopic Approach
0W390ZZ	Control Bleeding in Right Pleural Cavity, Open Approach
0W393ZZ	Control Bleeding in Right Pleural Cavity, Percutaneous Approach
0W394ZZ	Control Bleeding in Right Pleural Cavity, Percutaneous Endoscopic Approach
0W3B0ZZ	Control Bleeding in Left Pleural Cavity, Open Approach
0W3B3ZZ	Control Bleeding in Left Pleural Cavity, Percutaneous Approach
0W3B4ZZ	Control Bleeding in Left Pleural Cavity, Percutaneous Endoscopic Approach

0W3C0ZZ	Control Bleeding in Mediastinum, Open Approach
0W3C3ZZ	Control Bleeding in Mediastinum, Percutaneous Approach
0W3C4ZZ	Control Bleeding in Mediastinum, Percutaneous Endoscopic Approach
0W3D0ZZ	Control Bleeding in Pericardial Cavity, Open Approach
0W3D3ZZ	Control Bleeding in Pericardial Cavity, Percutaneous Approach
0W3D4ZZ	Control Bleeding in Pericardial Cavity, Percutaneous Endoscopic Approach
0W3F0ZZ	Control Bleeding in Abdominal Wall, Open Approach

AHA CC: 4Q, 2016, 100-101

0W3F3ZZ	Control Bleeding in Abdominal Wall, Percutaneous Approach
0W3F4ZZ	Control Bleeding in Abdominal Wall, Percutaneous Endoscopic Approach
0W3G0ZZ	Control Bleeding in Peritoneal Cavity, Open Approach
0W3G3ZZ	Control Bleeding in Peritoneal Cavity, Percutaneous Approach
0W3G4ZZ	Control Bleeding in Peritoneal Cavity, Percutaneous Endoscopic Approach
0W3H0ZZ	Control Bleeding in Retroperitoneum, Open Approach
0W3H3ZZ	Control Bleeding in Retroperitoneum, Percutaneous Approach
0W3H4ZZ	Control Bleeding in Retroperitoneum, Percutaneous Endoscopic Approach
0W3J0ZZ	Control Bleeding in Pelvic Cavity, Open Approach
0W3J3ZZ	Control Bleeding in Pelvic Cavity, Percutaneous Approach
0W3J4ZZ	Control Bleeding in Pelvic Cavity, Percutaneous Endoscopic Approach
0W3K0ZZ	Control Bleeding in Upper Back, Open Approach
0W3K3ZZ	Control Bleeding in Upper Back, Percutaneous Approach
0W3K4ZZ	Control Bleeding in Upper Back, Percutaneous Endoscopic Approach
0W3L0ZZ	Control Bleeding in Lower Back, Open Approach
0W3L3ZZ	Control Bleeding in Lower Back, Percutaneous Approach
0W3L4ZZ	Control Bleeding in Lower Back, Percutaneous Endoscopic Approach
♂ 0W3M0ZZ	Control Bleeding in Male Perineum, Open Approach

♂ 0W3M3ZZ	Control Bleeding in Male Perineum, Percutaneous Approach
♂ 0W3M4ZZ	Control Bleeding in Male Perineum, Percutaneous Endoscopic Approach
♀ 0W3N0ZZ	Control Bleeding in Female Perineum, Open Approach
♀ 0W3N3ZZ	Control Bleeding in Female Perineum, Percutaneous Approach
♀ 0W3N4ZZ	Control Bleeding in Female Perineum, Percutaneous Endoscopic Approach
0W3P0ZZ	Control Bleeding in Gastrointestinal Tract, Open Approach
0W3P3ZZ	Control Bleeding in Gastrointestinal Tract, Percutaneous Approach
0W3P4ZZ	Control Bleeding in Gastrointestinal Tract, Percutaneous Endoscopic Approach
0W3P7ZZ	Control Bleeding in Gastrointestinal Tract, Via Natural or Artificial Opening
0W3P8ZZ	Control Bleeding in Gastrointestinal Tract, Via Natural or Artificial Opening Endoscopic

AHA CC: 4Q, 2016, 99-100; 4Q, 2017, 105; 1Q, 2018, 19

0W3Q0ZZ	Control Bleeding in Respiratory Tract, Open Approach
0W3Q3ZZ	Control Bleeding in Respiratory Tract, Percutaneous Approach
0W3Q4ZZ	Control Bleeding in Respiratory Tract, Percutaneous Endoscopic Approach
0W3Q7ZZ	Control Bleeding in Respiratory Tract, Via Natural or Artificial Opening

AHA CC: 4Q, 2017, 106

| 0W3Q8ZZ | Control Bleeding in Respiratory Tract, Via Natural or Artificial Opening Endoscopic |

AHA CC: 1Q, 2018, 19-20

0W3R0ZZ	Control Bleeding in Genitourinary Tract, Open Approach
0W3R3ZZ	Control Bleeding in Genitourinary Tract, Percutaneous Approach
0W3R4ZZ	Control Bleeding in Genitourinary Tract, Percutaneous Endoscopic Approach
0W3R7ZZ	Control Bleeding in Genitourinary Tract, Via Natural or Artificial Opening

AHA CC: 4Q, 2014, 44

| 0W3R8ZZ | Control Bleeding in Genitourinary Tract, Via Natural or Artificial Opening Endoscopic |

0W4 – Anatomical Regions, General, Creation

♂ 0W4M070	Creation of Vagina in Male Perineum with Autologous Tissue Substitute, Open Approach
♂ 0W4M0J0	Creation of Vagina in Male Perineum with Synthetic Substitute, Open Approach
♂ 0W4M0K0	Creation of Vagina in Male Perineum with Nonautologous Tissue Substitute, Open Approach
♀ 0W4N071	Creation of Penis in Female Perineum with Autologous Tissue Substitute, Open Approach
♀ 0W4N0J1	Creation of Penis in Female Perineum with Synthetic Substitute, Open Approach
♀ 0W4N0K1	Creation of Penis in Female Perineum with Nonautologous Tissue Substitute, Open Approach

0W8 – Anatomical Regions, General, Division

| ♀ 0W8NXZZ | Division of Female Perineum, External Approach |

0W9 – Anatomical Regions, General, Drainage

Review Coding Guidelines B3.4a and B3.4b

Review Coding Guideline B6.2

0W9000Z	Drainage of Head with Drainage Device, Open Approach
0W900ZX	Drainage of Head, Open Approach, Diagnostic
0W900ZZ	Drainage of Head, Open Approach

0W9030Z	Drainage of Head with Drainage Device, Percutaneous Approach
0W903ZX	Drainage of Head, Percutaneous Approach, Diagnostic
0W903ZZ	Drainage of Head, Percutaneous Approach
0W9040Z	Drainage of Head with Drainage Device, Percutaneous Endoscopic Approach
0W904ZX	Drainage of Head, Percutaneous Endoscopic Approach, Diagnostic
0W904ZZ	Drainage of Head, Percutaneous Endoscopic Approach
0W9100Z	Drainage of Cranial Cavity with Drainage Device, Open Approach
0W910ZX	Drainage of Cranial Cavity, Open Approach, Diagnostic
0W910ZZ	Drainage of Cranial Cavity, Open Approach
0W9130Z	Drainage of Cranial Cavity with Drainage Device, Percutaneous Approach
0W913ZX	Drainage of Cranial Cavity, Percutaneous Approach, Diagnostic
0W913ZZ	Drainage of Cranial Cavity, Percutaneous Approach
0W9140Z	Drainage of Cranial Cavity with Drainage Device, Percutaneous Endoscopic Approach
0W914ZX	Drainage of Cranial Cavity, Percutaneous Endoscopic Approach, Diagnostic
0W914ZZ	Drainage of Cranial Cavity, Percutaneous Endoscopic Approach
0W9200Z	Drainage of Face with Drainage Device, Open Approach
0W920ZX	Drainage of Face, Open Approach, Diagnostic
0W920ZZ	Drainage of Face, Open Approach
0W9230Z	Drainage of Face with Drainage Device, Percutaneous Approach
0W923ZX	Drainage of Face, Percutaneous Approach, Diagnostic
0W923ZZ	Drainage of Face, Percutaneous Approach
0W9240Z	Drainage of Face with Drainage Device, Percutaneous Endoscopic Approach
0W924ZX	Drainage of Face, Percutaneous Endoscopic Approach, Diagnostic
0W924ZZ	Drainage of Face, Percutaneous Endoscopic Approach
0W9300Z	Drainage of Oral Cavity and Throat with Drainage Device, Open Approach
0W930ZX	Drainage of Oral Cavity and Throat, Open Approach, Diagnostic
0W930ZZ	Drainage of Oral Cavity and Throat, Open Approach
	AHA CC: 2Q, 2017, 16-17
0W9330Z	Drainage of Oral Cavity and Throat with Drainage Device, Percutaneous Approach
0W933ZX	Drainage of Oral Cavity and Throat, Percutaneous Approach, Diagnostic
0W933ZZ	Drainage of Oral Cavity and Throat, Percutaneous Approach
0W9340Z	Drainage of Oral Cavity and Throat with Drainage Device, Percutaneous Endoscopic Approach
0W934ZX	Drainage of Oral Cavity and Throat, Percutaneous Endoscopic Approach, Diagnostic
0W934ZZ	Drainage of Oral Cavity and Throat, Percutaneous Endoscopic Approach
0W9400Z	Drainage of Upper Jaw with Drainage Device, Open Approach
0W940ZX	Drainage of Upper Jaw, Open Approach, Diagnostic
0W940ZZ	Drainage of Upper Jaw, Open Approach
0W9430Z	Drainage of Upper Jaw with Drainage Device, Percutaneous Approach
0W943ZX	Drainage of Upper Jaw, Percutaneous Approach, Diagnostic
0W943ZZ	Drainage of Upper Jaw, Percutaneous Approach
0W9440Z	Drainage of Upper Jaw with Drainage Device, Percutaneous Endoscopic Approach
0W944ZX	Drainage of Upper Jaw, Percutaneous Endoscopic Approach, Diagnostic
0W944ZZ	Drainage of Upper Jaw, Percutaneous Endoscopic Approach
0W9500Z	Drainage of Lower Jaw with Drainage Device, Open Approach
0W950ZX	Drainage of Lower Jaw, Open Approach, Diagnostic
0W950ZZ	Drainage of Lower Jaw, Open Approach
0W9530Z	Drainage of Lower Jaw with Drainage Device, Percutaneous Approach
0W953ZX	Drainage of Lower Jaw, Percutaneous Approach, Diagnostic
0W953ZZ	Drainage of Lower Jaw, Percutaneous Approach
0W9540Z	Drainage of Lower Jaw with Drainage Device, Percutaneous Endoscopic Approach
0W954ZX	Drainage of Lower Jaw, Percutaneous Endoscopic Approach, Diagnostic
0W954ZZ	Drainage of Lower Jaw, Percutaneous Endoscopic Approach
0W9600Z	Drainage of Neck with Drainage Device, Open Approach
0W960ZX	Drainage of Neck, Open Approach, Diagnostic
0W960ZZ	Drainage of Neck, Open Approach
0W9630Z	Drainage of Neck with Drainage Device, Percutaneous Approach
0W963ZX	Drainage of Neck, Percutaneous Approach, Diagnostic
0W963ZZ	Drainage of Neck, Percutaneous Approach
0W9640Z	Drainage of Neck with Drainage Device, Percutaneous Endoscopic Approach
0W964ZX	Drainage of Neck, Percutaneous Endoscopic Approach, Diagnostic
0W964ZZ	Drainage of Neck, Percutaneous Endoscopic Approach
0W9800Z	Drainage of Chest Wall with Drainage Device, Open Approach
0W980ZX	Drainage of Chest Wall, Open Approach, Diagnostic
0W980ZZ	Drainage of Chest Wall, Open Approach
0W9830Z	Drainage of Chest Wall with Drainage Device, Percutaneous Approach
0W983ZX	Drainage of Chest Wall, Percutaneous Approach, Diagnostic
0W983ZZ	Drainage of Chest Wall, Percutaneous Approach
0W9840Z	Drainage of Chest Wall with Drainage Device, Percutaneous Endoscopic Approach
0W984ZX	Drainage of Chest Wall, Percutaneous Endoscopic Approach, Diagnostic
0W984ZZ	Drainage of Chest Wall, Percutaneous Endoscopic Approach
0W9900Z	Drainage of Right Pleural Cavity with Drainage Device, Open Approach
0W990ZX	Drainage of Right Pleural Cavity, Open Approach, Diagnostic
0W990ZZ	Drainage of Right Pleural Cavity, Open Approach
0W9930Z	Drainage of Right Pleural Cavity with Drainage Device, Percutaneous Approach
0W993ZX	Drainage of Right Pleural Cavity, Percutaneous Approach, Diagnostic
0W993ZZ	Drainage of Right Pleural Cavity, Percutaneous Approach
0W9940Z	Drainage of Right Pleural Cavity with Drainage Device, Percutaneous Endoscopic Approach
0W994ZX	Drainage of Right Pleural Cavity, Percutaneous Endoscopic Approach, Diagnostic
0W994ZZ	Drainage of Right Pleural Cavity, Percutaneous Endoscopic Approach
0W9B00Z	Drainage of Left Pleural Cavity with Drainage Device, Open Approach
0W9B0ZX	Drainage of Left Pleural Cavity, Open Approach, Diagnostic
0W9B0ZZ	Drainage of Left Pleural Cavity, Open Approach
0W9B30Z	Drainage of Left Pleural Cavity with Drainage Device, Percutaneous Approach
0W9B3ZX	Drainage of Left Pleural Cavity, Percutaneous Approach, Diagnostic
0W9B3ZZ	Drainage of Left Pleural Cavity, Percutaneous Approach
0W9B40Z	Drainage of Left Pleural Cavity with Drainage Device, Percutaneous Endoscopic Approach
0W9B4ZX	Drainage of Left Pleural Cavity, Percutaneous Endoscopic Approach, Diagnostic
0W9B4ZZ	Drainage of Left Pleural Cavity, Percutaneous Endoscopic Approach
0W9C00Z	Drainage of Mediastinum with Drainage Device, Open Approach
0W9C0ZX	Drainage of Mediastinum, Open Approach, Diagnostic
0W9C0ZZ	Drainage of Mediastinum, Open Approach
0W9C30Z	Drainage of Mediastinum with Drainage Device, Percutaneous Approach
0W9C3ZX	Drainage of Mediastinum, Percutaneous Approach, Diagnostic
0W9C3ZZ	Drainage of Mediastinum, Percutaneous Approach
0W9C40Z	Drainage of Mediastinum with Drainage Device, Percutaneous Endoscopic Approach
0W9C4ZX	Drainage of Mediastinum, Percutaneous Endoscopic Approach, Diagnostic
0W9C4ZZ	Drainage of Mediastinum, Percutaneous Endoscopic Approach
0W9D00Z	Drainage of Pericardial Cavity with Drainage Device, Open Approach
0W9D0ZX	Drainage of Pericardial Cavity, Open Approach, Diagnostic
0W9D0ZZ	Drainage of Pericardial Cavity, Open Approach
0W9D30Z	Drainage of Pericardial Cavity with Drainage Device, Percutaneous Approach
0W9D3ZX	Drainage of Pericardial Cavity, Percutaneous Approach, Diagnostic
0W9D3ZZ	Drainage of Pericardial Cavity, Percutaneous Approach

♀ Female-only   ♂ Male-only   ▲ Limited Coverage   ● Non-OR   🅷🅰🅲 HAC-associated procedure   ▲ Non-covered procedures   ➕ Cluster

0W9D40Z   Drainage of Pericardial Cavity with Drainage Device, Percutaneous Endoscopic Approach

0W9D4ZX   Drainage of Pericardial Cavity, Percutaneous Endoscopic Approach, Diagnostic

0W9D4ZZ   Drainage of Pericardial Cavity, Percutaneous Endoscopic Approach

0W9F00Z   Drainage of Abdominal Wall with Drainage Device, Open Approach

0W9F0ZX   Drainage of Abdominal Wall, Open Approach, Diagnostic

0W9F0ZZ   Drainage of Abdominal Wall, Open Approach

0W9F30Z   Drainage of Abdominal Wall with Drainage Device, Percutaneous Approach

0W9F3ZX   Drainage of Abdominal Wall, Percutaneous Approach, Diagnostic

0W9F3ZZ   Drainage of Abdominal Wall, Percutaneous Approach

0W9F40Z   Drainage of Abdominal Wall with Drainage Device, Percutaneous Endoscopic Approach

0W9F4ZX   Drainage of Abdominal Wall, Percutaneous Endoscopic Approach, Diagnostic

0W9F4ZZ   Drainage of Abdominal Wall, Percutaneous Endoscopic Approach

0W9G00Z   Drainage of Peritoneal Cavity with Drainage Device, Open Approach

0W9G0ZX   Drainage of Peritoneal Cavity, Open Approach, Diagnostic

0W9G0ZZ   Drainage of Peritoneal Cavity, Open Approach

0W9G30Z   Drainage of Peritoneal Cavity with Drainage Device, Percutaneous Approach

0W9G3ZX   Drainage of Peritoneal Cavity, Percutaneous Approach, Diagnostic

0W9G3ZZ   Drainage of Peritoneal Cavity, Percutaneous Approach

AHA CC: 3Q, 2017, 12-13

0W9G40Z   Drainage of Peritoneal Cavity with Drainage Device, Percutaneous Endoscopic Approach

0W9G4ZX   Drainage of Peritoneal Cavity, Percutaneous Endoscopic Approach, Diagnostic

0W9G4ZZ   Drainage of Peritoneal Cavity, Percutaneous Endoscopic Approach

0W9H00Z   Drainage of Retroperitoneum with Drainage Device, Open Approach

0W9H0ZX   Drainage of Retroperitoneum, Open Approach, Diagnostic

0W9H0ZZ   Drainage of Retroperitoneum, Open Approach

0W9H30Z   Drainage of Retroperitoneum with Drainage Device, Percutaneous Approach

0W9H3ZX   Drainage of Retroperitoneum, Percutaneous Approach, Diagnostic

0W9H3ZZ   Drainage of Retroperitoneum, Percutaneous Approach

0W9H40Z   Drainage of Retroperitoneum with Drainage Device, Percutaneous Endoscopic Approach

0W9H4ZX   Drainage of Retroperitoneum, Percutaneous Endoscopic Approach, Diagnostic

0W9H4ZZ   Drainage of Retroperitoneum, Percutaneous Endoscopic Approach

0W9J00Z   Drainage of Pelvic Cavity with Drainage Device, Open Approach

0W9J0ZX   Drainage of Pelvic Cavity, Open Approach, Diagnostic

0W9J0ZZ   Drainage of Pelvic Cavity, Open Approach

0W9J30Z   Drainage of Pelvic Cavity with Drainage Device, Percutaneous Approach

0W9J3ZX   Drainage of Pelvic Cavity, Percutaneous Approach, Diagnostic

0W9J3ZZ   Drainage of Pelvic Cavity, Percutaneous Approach

0W9J40Z   Drainage of Pelvic Cavity with Drainage Device, Percutaneous Endoscopic Approach

0W9J4ZX   Drainage of Pelvic Cavity, Percutaneous Endoscopic Approach, Diagnostic

0W9J4ZZ   Drainage of Pelvic Cavity, Percutaneous Endoscopic Approach

0W9J70Z   Drainage of Pelvic Cavity with Drainage Device, Via Natural or Artificial Opening

0W9J7ZX   Drainage of Pelvic Cavity, Via Natural or Artificial Opening, Diagnostic

0W9J7ZZ   Drainage of Pelvic Cavity, Via Natural or Artificial Opening

0W9J80Z   Drainage of Pelvic Cavity with Drainage Device, Via Natural or Artificial Opening Endoscopic

0W9J8ZX   Drainage of Pelvic Cavity, Via Natural or Artificial Opening Endoscopic, Diagnostic

0W9J8ZZ   Drainage of Pelvic Cavity, Via Natural or Artificial Opening Endoscopic

0W9K00Z   Drainage of Upper Back with Drainage Device, Open Approach

0W9K0ZX   Drainage of Upper Back, Open Approach, Diagnostic

0W9K0ZZ   Drainage of Upper Back, Open Approach

0W9K30Z   Drainage of Upper Back with Drainage Device, Percutaneous Approach

0W9K3ZX   Drainage of Upper Back, Percutaneous Approach, Diagnostic

0W9K3ZZ   Drainage of Upper Back, Percutaneous Approach

0W9K40Z   Drainage of Upper Back with Drainage Device, Percutaneous Endoscopic Approach

0W9K4ZX   Drainage of Upper Back, Percutaneous Endoscopic Approach, Diagnostic

0W9K4ZZ   Drainage of Upper Back, Percutaneous Endoscopic Approach

0W9L00Z   Drainage of Lower Back with Drainage Device, Open Approach

0W9L0ZX   Drainage of Lower Back, Open Approach, Diagnostic

0W9L0ZZ   Drainage of Lower Back, Open Approach

0W9L30Z   Drainage of Lower Back with Drainage Device, Percutaneous Approach

0W9L3ZX   Drainage of Lower Back, Percutaneous Approach, Diagnostic

0W9L3ZZ   Drainage of Lower Back, Percutaneous Approach

0W9L40Z   Drainage of Lower Back with Drainage Device, Percutaneous Endoscopic Approach

0W9L4ZX   Drainage of Lower Back, Percutaneous Endoscopic Approach, Diagnostic

0W9L4ZZ   Drainage of Lower Back, Percutaneous Endoscopic Approach

♂ 0W9M00Z   Drainage of Male Perineum with Drainage Device, Open Approach

♂ 0W9M0ZX   Drainage of Male Perineum, Open Approach, Diagnostic

♂ 0W9M0ZZ   Drainage of Male Perineum, Open Approach

♂ 0W9M30Z   Drainage of Male Perineum with Drainage Device, Percutaneous Approach

♂ 0W9M3ZX   Drainage of Male Perineum, Percutaneous Approach, Diagnostic

♂ 0W9M3ZZ   Drainage of Male Perineum, Percutaneous Approach

♂ 0W9M40Z   Drainage of Male Perineum with Drainage Device, Percutaneous Endoscopic Approach

♂ 0W9M4ZX   Drainage of Male Perineum, Percutaneous Endoscopic Approach, Diagnostic

♂ 0W9M4ZZ   Drainage of Male Perineum, Percutaneous Endoscopic Approach

♀ 0W9N00Z   Drainage of Female Perineum with Drainage Device, Open Approach

♀ 0W9N0ZX   Drainage of Female Perineum, Open Approach, Diagnostic

♀ 0W9N0ZZ   Drainage of Female Perineum, Open Approach

♀ 0W9N30Z   Drainage of Female Perineum with Drainage Device, Percutaneous Approach

♀ 0W9N3ZX   Drainage of Female Perineum, Percutaneous Approach, Diagnostic

♀ 0W9N3ZZ   Drainage of Female Perineum, Percutaneous Approach

♀ 0W9N40Z   Drainage of Female Perineum with Drainage Device, Percutaneous Endoscopic Approach

♀ 0W9N4ZX   Drainage of Female Perineum, Percutaneous Endoscopic Approach, Diagnostic

♀ 0W9N4ZZ   Drainage of Female Perineum, Percutaneous Endoscopic Approach

0WB – Anatomical Regions, General, Excision

Review Coding Guidelines B3.4a and B3.4b

Review Coding Guideline B3.18

0WB00ZX   Excision of Head, Open Approach, Diagnostic

0WB00ZZ   Excision of Head, Open Approach

0WB03ZX   Excision of Head, Percutaneous Approach, Diagnostic

0WB03ZZ   Excision of Head, Percutaneous Approach

0WB04ZX   Excision of Head, Percutaneous Endoscopic Approach, Diagnostic

0WB04ZZ   Excision of Head, Percutaneous Endoscopic Approach

♀ Female-only   ♂ Male-only   ▲ Limited Coverage   ● Non-OR   HAC HAC-associated procedure   ▲ Non-covered procedures   ✚ Cluster

0WB0XZX	Excision of Head, External Approach, Diagnostic
0WB0XZZ	Excision of Head, External Approach
0WB20ZX	Excision of Face, Open Approach, Diagnostic
0WB20ZZ	Excision of Face, Open Approach
0WB23ZX	Excision of Face, Percutaneous Approach, Diagnostic
0WB23ZZ	Excision of Face, Percutaneous Approach
0WB24ZX	Excision of Face, Percutaneous Endoscopic Approach, Diagnostic
0WB24ZZ	Excision of Face, Percutaneous Endoscopic Approach
0WB2XZX	Excision of Face, External Approach, Diagnostic
0WB2XZZ	Excision of Face, External Approach
0WB30ZX	Excision of Oral Cavity and Throat, Open Approach, Diagnostic
0WB30ZZ	Excision of Oral Cavity and Throat, Open Approach
0WB33ZX	Excision of Oral Cavity and Throat, Percutaneous Approach, Diagnostic
0WB33ZZ	Excision of Oral Cavity and Throat, Percutaneous Approach
0WB34ZX	Excision of Oral Cavity and Throat, Percutaneous Endoscopic Approach, Diagnostic
0WB34ZZ	Excision of Oral Cavity and Throat, Percutaneous Endoscopic Approach
0WB3XZX	Excision of Oral Cavity and Throat, External Approach, Diagnostic
0WB3XZZ	Excision of Oral Cavity and Throat, External Approach
0WB40ZX	Excision of Upper Jaw, Open Approach, Diagnostic
0WB40ZZ	Excision of Upper Jaw, Open Approach
0WB43ZX	Excision of Upper Jaw, Percutaneous Approach, Diagnostic
0WB43ZZ	Excision of Upper Jaw, Percutaneous Approach
0WB44ZX	Excision of Upper Jaw, Percutaneous Endoscopic Approach, Diagnostic
0WB44ZZ	Excision of Upper Jaw, Percutaneous Endoscopic Approach
0WB4XZX	Excision of Upper Jaw, External Approach, Diagnostic
0WB4XZZ	Excision of Upper Jaw, External Approach
0WB50ZX	Excision of Lower Jaw, Open Approach, Diagnostic
0WB50ZZ	Excision of Lower Jaw, Open Approach
0WB53ZX	Excision of Lower Jaw, Percutaneous Approach, Diagnostic
0WB53ZZ	Excision of Lower Jaw, Percutaneous Approach
0WB54ZX	Excision of Lower Jaw, Percutaneous Endoscopic Approach, Diagnostic
0WB54ZZ	Excision of Lower Jaw, Percutaneous Endoscopic Approach
0WB5XZX	Excision of Lower Jaw, External Approach, Diagnostic
0WB5XZZ	Excision of Lower Jaw, External Approach
0WB60ZX	Excision of Neck, Open Approach, Diagnostic
0WB60ZZ	Excision of Neck, Open Approach
0WB63ZX	Excision of Neck, Percutaneous Approach, Diagnostic
0WB63ZZ	Excision of Neck, Percutaneous Approach
0WB64ZX	Excision of Neck, Percutaneous Endoscopic Approach, Diagnostic
0WB64ZZ	Excision of Neck, Percutaneous Endoscopic Approach
0WB6XZ2	Excision of Neck, Stoma, External Approach
0WB6XZX	Excision of Neck, External Approach, Diagnostic
0WB6XZZ	Excision of Neck, External Approach
0WB80ZX	Excision of Chest Wall, Open Approach, Diagnostic
0WB80ZZ	Excision of Chest Wall, Open Approach
0WB83ZX	Excision of Chest Wall, Percutaneous Approach, Diagnostic
0WB83ZZ	Excision of Chest Wall, Percutaneous Approach
0WB84ZX	Excision of Chest Wall, Percutaneous Endoscopic Approach, Diagnostic
0WB84ZZ	Excision of Chest Wall, Percutaneous Endoscopic Approach
0WB8XZX	Excision of Chest Wall, External Approach, Diagnostic
0WB8XZZ	Excision of Chest Wall, External Approach
0WBC0ZX	Excision of Mediastinum, Open Approach, Diagnostic
0WBC0ZZ	Excision of Mediastinum, Open Approach
0WBC3ZX	Excision of Mediastinum, Percutaneous Approach, Diagnostic
0WBC3ZZ	Excision of Mediastinum, Percutaneous Approach
0WBC4ZX	Excision of Mediastinum, Percutaneous Endoscopic Approach, Diagnostic
0WBC4ZZ	Excision of Mediastinum, Percutaneous Endoscopic Approach
0WBF0ZX	Excision of Abdominal Wall, Open Approach, Diagnostic
0WBF0ZZ	Excision of Abdominal Wall, Open Approach
0WBF3ZX	Excision of Abdominal Wall, Percutaneous Approach, Diagnostic
0WBF3ZZ	Excision of Abdominal Wall, Percutaneous Approach
0WBF4ZX	Excision of Abdominal Wall, Percutaneous Endoscopic Approach, Diagnostic
0WBF4ZZ	Excision of Abdominal Wall, Percutaneous Endoscopic Approach

AHA CC: 1Q, 2016, 21-22

0WBFXZ2	Excision of Abdominal Wall, Stoma, External Approach
0WBFXZX	Excision of Abdominal Wall, External Approach, Diagnostic
0WBFXZZ	Excision of Abdominal Wall, External Approach
0WBH0ZX	Excision of Retroperitoneum, Open Approach, Diagnostic
0WBH0ZZ	Excision of Retroperitoneum, Open Approach

AHA CC: 1Q, 2019, 27

0WBH3ZX	Excision of Retroperitoneum, Percutaneous Approach, Diagnostic
0WBH3ZZ	Excision of Retroperitoneum, Percutaneous Approach
0WBH4ZX	Excision of Retroperitoneum, Percutaneous Endoscopic Approach, Diagnostic
0WBH4ZZ	Excision of Retroperitoneum, Percutaneous Endoscopic Approach
0WBK0ZX	Excision of Upper Back, Open Approach, Diagnostic
0WBK0ZZ	Excision of Upper Back, Open Approach
0WBK3ZX	Excision of Upper Back, Percutaneous Approach, Diagnostic
0WBK3ZZ	Excision of Upper Back, Percutaneous Approach
0WBK4ZX	Excision of Upper Back, Percutaneous Endoscopic Approach, Diagnostic
0WBK4ZZ	Excision of Upper Back, Percutaneous Endoscopic Approach
0WBKXZX	Excision of Upper Back, External Approach, Diagnostic
0WBKXZZ	Excision of Upper Back, External Approach
0WBL0ZX	Excision of Lower Back, Open Approach, Diagnostic
0WBL0ZZ	Excision of Lower Back, Open Approach
0WBL3ZX	Excision of Lower Back, Percutaneous Approach, Diagnostic
0WBL3ZZ	Excision of Lower Back, Percutaneous Approach
0WBL4ZX	Excision of Lower Back, Percutaneous Endoscopic Approach, Diagnostic
0WBL4ZZ	Excision of Lower Back, Percutaneous Endoscopic Approach
0WBLXZX	Excision of Lower Back, External Approach, Diagnostic
0WBLXZZ	Excision of Lower Back, External Approach
♂ 0WBM0ZX	Excision of Male Perineum, Open Approach, Diagnostic
♂ 0WBM0ZZ	Excision of Male Perineum, Open Approach
♂ 0WBM3ZX	Excision of Male Perineum, Percutaneous Approach, Diagnostic
♂ 0WBM3ZZ	Excision of Male Perineum, Percutaneous Approach
♂ 0WBM4ZX	Excision of Male Perineum, Percutaneous Endoscopic Approach, Diagnostic
♂ 0WBM4ZZ	Excision of Male Perineum, Percutaneous Endoscopic Approach
♂ 0WBMXZX	Excision of Male Perineum, External Approach, Diagnostic
♂ 0WBMXZZ	Excision of Male Perineum, External Approach
♀ 0WBN0ZX	Excision of Female Perineum, Open Approach, Diagnostic
♀ 0WBN0ZZ	Excision of Female Perineum, Open Approach
♀ 0WBN3ZX	Excision of Female Perineum, Percutaneous Approach, Diagnostic
♀ 0WBN3ZZ	Excision of Female Perineum, Percutaneous Approach
♀ 0WBN4ZX	Excision of Female Perineum, Percutaneous Endoscopic Approach, Diagnostic
♀ 0WBN4ZZ	Excision of Female Perineum, Percutaneous Endoscopic Approach
♀ 0WBNXZX	Excision of Female Perineum, External Approach, Diagnostic
♀ 0WBNXZZ	Excision of Female Perineum, External Approach

AHA CC: 4Q, 2013, 119-120

♀ Female-only   ♂ Male-only   ▲ Limited Coverage   ● Non-OR   HAC HAC-associated procedure   ▲ Non-covered procedures   ✚ Cluster

0WC – Anatomical Regions, General, Extirpation

0WC10ZZ	Extirpation of Matter from Cranial Cavity, Open Approach
0WC13ZZ	Extirpation of Matter from Cranial Cavity, Percutaneous Approach
0WC14ZZ	Extirpation of Matter from Cranial Cavity, Percutaneous Endoscopic Approach
0WC1XZZ	Extirpation of Matter from Cranial Cavity, External Approach
0WC30ZZ	Extirpation of Matter from Oral Cavity and Throat, Open Approach
	AHA CC: 2Q, 2017, 16
0WC33ZZ	Extirpation of Matter from Oral Cavity and Throat, Percutaneous Approach
0WC34ZZ	Extirpation of Matter from Oral Cavity and Throat, Percutaneous Endoscopic Approach
0WC3XZZ	Extirpation of Matter from Oral Cavity and Throat, External Approach
0WC40ZZ	Extirpation of Matter from Upper Jaw, Open Approach
0WC43ZZ	Extirpation of Matter from Upper Jaw, Percutaneous Approach
0WC44ZZ	Extirpation of Matter from Upper Jaw, Percutaneous Endoscopic Approach
0WC50ZZ	Extirpation of Matter from Lower Jaw, Open Approach
0WC53ZZ	Extirpation of Matter from Lower Jaw, Percutaneous Approach
0WC54ZZ	Extirpation of Matter from Lower Jaw, Percutaneous Endoscopic Approach
0WC90ZZ	Extirpation of Matter from Right Pleural Cavity, Open Approach
0WC93ZZ	Extirpation of Matter from Right Pleural Cavity, Percutaneous Approach
0WC94ZZ	Extirpation of Matter from Right Pleural Cavity, Percutaneous Endoscopic Approach
0WC9XZZ	Extirpation of Matter from Right Pleural Cavity, External Approach
0WCB0ZZ	Extirpation of Matter from Left Pleural Cavity, Open Approach
0WCB3ZZ	Extirpation of Matter from Left Pleural Cavity, Percutaneous Approach
0WCB4ZZ	Extirpation of Matter from Left Pleural Cavity, Percutaneous Endoscopic Approach
0WCBXZZ	Extirpation of Matter from Left Pleural Cavity, External Approach
0WCC0ZZ	Extirpation of Matter from Mediastinum, Open Approach
0WCC3ZZ	Extirpation of Matter from Mediastinum, Percutaneous Approach
0WCC4ZZ	Extirpation of Matter from Mediastinum, Percutaneous Endoscopic Approach
0WCCXZZ	Extirpation of Matter from Mediastinum, External Approach
0WCD0ZZ	Extirpation of Matter from Pericardial Cavity, Open Approach
0WCD3ZZ	Extirpation of Matter from Pericardial Cavity, Percutaneous Approach
0WCD4ZZ	Extirpation of Matter from Pericardial Cavity, Percutaneous Endoscopic Approach
0WCDXZZ	Extirpation of Matter from Pericardial Cavity, External Approach
0WCG0ZZ	Extirpation of Matter from Peritoneal Cavity, Open Approach
0WCG3ZZ	Extirpation of Matter from Peritoneal Cavity, Percutaneous Approach
0WCG4ZZ	Extirpation of Matter from Peritoneal Cavity, Percutaneous Endoscopic Approach
0WCGXZZ	Extirpation of Matter from Peritoneal Cavity, External Approach
0WCH0ZZ	Extirpation of Matter from Retroperitoneum, Open Approach
0WCH3ZZ	Extirpation of Matter from Retroperitoneum, Percutaneous Approach
0WCH4ZZ	Extirpation of Matter from Retroperitoneum, Percutaneous Endoscopic Approach
0WCHXZZ	Extirpation of Matter from Retroperitoneum, External Approach
0WCJ0ZZ	Extirpation of Matter from Pelvic Cavity, Open Approach
0WCJ3ZZ	Extirpation of Matter from Pelvic Cavity, Percutaneous Approach
0WCJ4ZZ	Extirpation of Matter from Pelvic Cavity, Percutaneous Endoscopic Approach
0WCJXZZ	Extirpation of Matter from Pelvic Cavity, External Approach
0WCP0ZZ	Extirpation of Matter from Gastrointestinal Tract, Open Approach
0WCP3ZZ	Extirpation of Matter from Gastrointestinal Tract, Percutaneous Approach
0WCP4ZZ	Extirpation of Matter from Gastrointestinal Tract, Percutaneous Endoscopic Approach
0WCP7ZZ	Extirpation of Matter from Gastrointestinal Tract, Via Natural or Artificial Opening
0WCP8ZZ	Extirpation of Matter from Gastrointestinal Tract, Via Natural or Artificial Opening Endoscopic
0WCPXZZ	Extirpation of Matter from Gastrointestinal Tract, External Approach
0WCQ0ZZ	Extirpation of Matter from Respiratory Tract, Open Approach
0WCQ3ZZ	Extirpation of Matter from Respiratory Tract, Percutaneous Approach
0WCQ4ZZ	Extirpation of Matter from Respiratory Tract, Percutaneous Endoscopic Approach
0WCQ7ZZ	Extirpation of Matter from Respiratory Tract, Via Natural or Artificial Opening
0WCQ8ZZ	Extirpation of Matter from Respiratory Tract, Via Natural or Artificial Opening Endoscopic
0WCQXZZ	Extirpation of Matter from Respiratory Tract, External Approach
0WCR0ZZ	Extirpation of Matter from Genitourinary Tract, Open Approach
0WCR3ZZ	Extirpation of Matter from Genitourinary Tract, Percutaneous Approach
0WCR4ZZ	Extirpation of Matter from Genitourinary Tract, Percutaneous Endoscopic Approach
0WCR7ZZ	Extirpation of Matter from Genitourinary Tract, Via Natural or Artificial Opening
0WCR8ZZ	Extirpation of Matter from Genitourinary Tract, Via Natural or Artificial Opening Endoscopic
0WCRXZZ	Extirpation of Matter from Genitourinary Tract, External Approach

0WF – Anatomical Regions, General, Fragmentation

0WF10ZZ	Fragmentation in Cranial Cavity, Open Approach
0WF13ZZ	Fragmentation in Cranial Cavity, Percutaneous Approach
0WF14ZZ	Fragmentation in Cranial Cavity, Percutaneous Endoscopic Approach
▲ 0WF1XZZ	Fragmentation in Cranial Cavity, External Approach
0WF30ZZ	Fragmentation in Oral Cavity and Throat, Open Approach
0WF33ZZ	Fragmentation in Oral Cavity and Throat, Percutaneous Approach
0WF34ZZ	Fragmentation in Oral Cavity and Throat, Percutaneous Endoscopic Approach
▲ 0WF3XZZ	Fragmentation in Oral Cavity and Throat, External Approach
0WF90ZZ	Fragmentation in Right Pleural Cavity, Open Approach
0WF93ZZ	Fragmentation in Right Pleural Cavity, Percutaneous Approach
0WF94ZZ	Fragmentation in Right Pleural Cavity, Percutaneous Endoscopic Approach
▲ 0WF9XZZ	Fragmentation in Right Pleural Cavity, External Approach
0WFB0ZZ	Fragmentation in Left Pleural Cavity, Open Approach
0WFB3ZZ	Fragmentation in Left Pleural Cavity, Percutaneous Approach
0WFB4ZZ	Fragmentation in Left Pleural Cavity, Percutaneous Endoscopic Approach
▲ 0WFBXZZ	Fragmentation in Left Pleural Cavity, External Approach
0WFC0ZZ	Fragmentation in Mediastinum, Open Approach
0WFC3ZZ	Fragmentation in Mediastinum, Percutaneous Approach
0WFC4ZZ	Fragmentation in Mediastinum, Percutaneous Endoscopic Approach
▲ 0WFCXZZ	Fragmentation in Mediastinum, External Approach
0WFD0ZZ	Fragmentation in Pericardial Cavity, Open Approach
0WFD3ZZ	Fragmentation in Pericardial Cavity, Percutaneous Approach
0WFD4ZZ	Fragmentation in Pericardial Cavity, Percutaneous Endoscopic Approach
0WFDXZZ	Fragmentation in Pericardial Cavity, External Approach
0WFG0ZZ	Fragmentation in Peritoneal Cavity, Open Approach
0WFG3ZZ	Fragmentation in Peritoneal Cavity, Percutaneous Approach
0WFG4ZZ	Fragmentation in Peritoneal Cavity, Percutaneous Endoscopic Approach

---

♀ Female-only   ♂ Male-only   ▲ Limited Coverage   ● Non-OR   HAC HAC-associated procedure   ▲ Non-covered procedures   ✚ Cluster

▲ 0WFGXZZ Fragmentation in Peritoneal Cavity, External Approach
0WFJ0ZZ Fragmentation in Pelvic Cavity, Open Approach
0WFJ3ZZ Fragmentation in Pelvic Cavity, Percutaneous Approach
0WFJ4ZZ Fragmentation in Pelvic Cavity, Percutaneous Endoscopic Approach
▲ 0WFJXZZ Fragmentation in Pelvic Cavity, External Approach
0WFP0ZZ Fragmentation in Gastrointestinal Tract, Open Approach
0WFP3ZZ Fragmentation in Gastrointestinal Tract, Percutaneous Approach
0WFP4ZZ Fragmentation in Gastrointestinal Tract, Percutaneous Endoscopic Approach

0WFP7ZZ Fragmentation in Gastrointestinal Tract, Via Natural or Artificial Opening
0WFP8ZZ Fragmentation in Gastrointestinal Tract, Via Natural or Artificial Opening Endoscopic
▲ 0WFPXZZ Fragmentation in Gastrointestinal Tract, External Approach
0WFQ0ZZ Fragmentation in Respiratory Tract, Open Approach
0WFQ3ZZ Fragmentation in Respiratory Tract, Percutaneous Approach
0WFQ4ZZ Fragmentation in Respiratory Tract, Percutaneous Endoscopic Approach
0WFQ7ZZ Fragmentation in Respiratory Tract, Via Natural or Artificial Opening

0WFQ8ZZ Fragmentation in Respiratory Tract, Via Natural or Artificial Opening Endoscopic
▲ 0WFQXZZ Fragmentation in Respiratory Tract, External Approach
0WFR0ZZ Fragmentation in Genitourinary Tract, Open Approach
0WFR3ZZ Fragmentation in Genitourinary Tract, Percutaneous Approach
0WFR4ZZ Fragmentation in Genitourinary Tract, Percutaneous Endoscopic Approach
0WFR7ZZ Fragmentation in Genitourinary Tract, Via Natural or Artificial Opening
0WFR8ZZ Fragmentation in Genitourinary Tract, Via Natural or Artificial Opening Endoscopic
● 0WFRXZZ Fragmentation in Genitourinary Tract, External Approach

0WH – Anatomical Regions, General, Insertion

0WH001Z Insertion of Radioactive Element into Head, Open Approach
● 0WH003Z Insertion of Infusion Device into Head, Open Approach
● 0WH00YZ Insertion of Other Device into Head, Open Approach
0WH031Z Insertion of Radioactive Element into Head, Percutaneous Approach
● 0WH033Z Insertion of Infusion Device into Head, Percutaneous Approach
● 0WH03YZ Insertion of Other Device into Head, Percutaneous Approach
0WH041Z Insertion of Radioactive Element into Head, Percutaneous Endoscopic Approach
● 0WH043Z Insertion of Infusion Device into Head, Percutaneous Endoscopic Approach
● 0WH04YZ Insertion of Other Device into Head, Percutaneous Endoscopic Approach
0WH101Z Insertion of Radioactive Element into Cranial Cavity, Open Approach
0WH103Z Insertion of Infusion Device into Cranial Cavity, Open Approach
0WH10YZ Insertion of Other Device into Cranial Cavity, Open Approach
0WH131Z Insertion of Radioactive Element into Cranial Cavity, Percutaneous Approach
0WH133Z Insertion of Infusion Device into Cranial Cavity, Percutaneous Approach
0WH13YZ Insertion of Other Device into Cranial Cavity, Percutaneous Approach
0WH141Z Insertion of Radioactive Element into Cranial Cavity, Percutaneous Endoscopic Approach
0WH143Z Insertion of Infusion Device into Cranial Cavity, Percutaneous Endoscopic Approach
0WH14YZ Insertion of Other Device into Cranial Cavity, Percutaneous Endoscopic Approach
0WH201Z Insertion of Radioactive Element into Face, Open Approach
● 0WH203Z Insertion of Infusion Device into Face, Open Approach
● 0WH20YZ Insertion of Other Device into Face, Open Approach
0WH231Z Insertion of Radioactive Element into Face, Percutaneous Approach
● 0WH233Z Insertion of Infusion Device into Face, Percutaneous Approach
● 0WH23YZ Insertion of Other Device into Face, Percutaneous Approach

0WH241Z Insertion of Radioactive Element into Face, Percutaneous Endoscopic Approach
● 0WH243Z Insertion of Infusion Device into Face, Percutaneous Endoscopic Approach
● 0WH24YZ Insertion of Other Device into Face, Percutaneous Endoscopic Approach
0WH301Z Insertion of Radioactive Element into Oral Cavity and Throat, Open Approach
0WH303Z Insertion of Infusion Device into Oral Cavity and Throat, Open Approach
0WH30YZ Insertion of Other Device into Oral Cavity and Throat, Open Approach
0WH331Z Insertion of Radioactive Element into Oral Cavity and Throat, Percutaneous Approach
0WH333Z Insertion of Infusion Device into Oral Cavity and Throat, Percutaneous Approach
0WH33YZ Insertion of Other Device into Oral Cavity and Throat, Percutaneous Approach
0WH341Z Insertion of Radioactive Element into Oral Cavity and Throat, Percutaneous Endoscopic Approach
0WH343Z Insertion of Infusion Device into Oral Cavity and Throat, Percutaneous Endoscopic Approach
0WH34YZ Insertion of Other Device into Oral Cavity and Throat, Percutaneous Endoscopic Approach
0WH401Z Insertion of Radioactive Element into Upper Jaw, Open Approach
● 0WH403Z Insertion of Infusion Device into Upper Jaw, Open Approach
● 0WH40YZ Insertion of Other Device into Upper Jaw, Open Approach
0WH431Z Insertion of Radioactive Element into Upper Jaw, Percutaneous Approach
● 0WH433Z Insertion of Infusion Device into Upper Jaw, Percutaneous Approach
● 0WH43YZ Insertion of Other Device into Upper Jaw, Percutaneous Approach
0WH441Z Insertion of Radioactive Element into Upper Jaw, Percutaneous Endoscopic Approach
● 0WH443Z Insertion of Infusion Device into Upper Jaw, Percutaneous Endoscopic Approach
● 0WH44YZ Insertion of Other Device into Upper Jaw, Percutaneous Endoscopic Approach

0WH501Z Insertion of Radioactive Element into Lower Jaw, Open Approach
● 0WH503Z Insertion of Infusion Device into Lower Jaw, Open Approach
● 0WH50YZ Insertion of Other Device into Lower Jaw, Open Approach
0WH531Z Insertion of Radioactive Element into Lower Jaw, Percutaneous Approach
● 0WH533Z Insertion of Infusion Device into Lower Jaw, Percutaneous Approach
● 0WH53YZ Insertion of Other Device into Lower Jaw, Percutaneous Approach
0WH541Z Insertion of Radioactive Element into Lower Jaw, Percutaneous Endoscopic Approach
0WH543Z Insertion of Infusion Device into Lower Jaw, Percutaneous Endoscopic Approach
0WH54YZ Insertion of Other Device into Lower Jaw, Percutaneous Endoscopic Approach
0WH601Z Insertion of Radioactive Element into Neck, Open Approach
● 0WH603Z Insertion of Infusion Device into Neck, Open Approach
● 0WH60YZ Insertion of Other Device into Neck, Open Approach
0WH631Z Insertion of Radioactive Element into Neck, Percutaneous Approach
● 0WH633Z Insertion of Infusion Device into Neck, Percutaneous Approach
● 0WH63YZ Insertion of Other Device into Neck, Percutaneous Approach
0WH641Z Insertion of Radioactive Element into Neck, Percutaneous Endoscopic Approach
● 0WH643Z Insertion of Infusion Device into Neck, Percutaneous Endoscopic Approach
● 0WH64YZ Insertion of Other Device into Neck, Percutaneous Endoscopic Approach
0WH801Z Insertion of Radioactive Element into Chest Wall, Open Approach
0WH803Z Insertion of Infusion Device into Chest Wall, Open Approach
0WH80YZ Insertion of Other Device into Chest Wall, Open Approach
0WH831Z Insertion of Radioactive Element into Chest Wall, Percutaneous Approach
0WH833Z Insertion of Infusion Device into Chest Wall, Percutaneous Approach
0WH83YZ Insertion of Other Device into Chest Wall, Percutaneous Approach

♀ Female-only   ♂ Male-only   ▲ Limited Coverage   ● Non-OR   HAC HAC-associated procedure   ▲ Non-covered procedures   ✚ Cluster

0WH841Z   Insertion of Radioactive Element into Chest Wall, Percutaneous Endoscopic Approach

0WH843Z   Insertion of Infusion Device into Chest Wall, Percutaneous Endoscopic Approach

0WH84YZ   Insertion of Other Device into Chest Wall, Percutaneous Endoscopic Approach

0WH901Z   Insertion of Radioactive Element into Right Pleural Cavity, Open Approach

0WH903Z   Insertion of Infusion Device into Right Pleural Cavity, Open Approach

0WH90YZ   Insertion of Other Device into Right Pleural Cavity, Open Approach

0WH931Z   Insertion of Radioactive Element into Right Pleural Cavity, Percutaneous Approach

0WH933Z   Insertion of Infusion Device into Right Pleural Cavity, Percutaneous Approach

0WH93YZ   Insertion of Other Device into Right Pleural Cavity, Percutaneous Approach

0WH941Z   Insertion of Radioactive Element into Right Pleural Cavity, Percutaneous Endoscopic Approach

0WH943Z   Insertion of Infusion Device into Right Pleural Cavity, Percutaneous Endoscopic Approach

0WH94YZ   Insertion of Other Device into Right Pleural Cavity, Percutaneous Endoscopic Approach

0WHB01Z   Insertion of Radioactive Element into Left Pleural Cavity, Open Approach

0WHB03Z   Insertion of Infusion Device into Left Pleural Cavity, Open Approach

0WHB0YZ   Insertion of Other Device into Left Pleural Cavity, Open Approach

0WHB31Z   Insertion of Radioactive Element into Left Pleural Cavity, Percutaneous Approach

0WHB33Z   Insertion of Infusion Device into Left Pleural Cavity, Percutaneous Approach

0WHB3YZ   Insertion of Other Device into Left Pleural Cavity, Percutaneous Approach

0WHB41Z   Insertion of Radioactive Element into Left Pleural Cavity, Percutaneous Endoscopic Approach

0WHB43Z   Insertion of Infusion Device into Left Pleural Cavity, Percutaneous Endoscopic Approach

0WHB4YZ   Insertion of Other Device into Left Pleural Cavity, Percutaneous Endoscopic Approach

0WHC01Z   Insertion of Radioactive Element into Mediastinum, Open Approach

0WHC03Z   Insertion of Infusion Device into Mediastinum, Open Approach

0WHC0YZ   Insertion of Other Device into Mediastinum, Open Approach

0WHC31Z   Insertion of Radioactive Element into Mediastinum, Percutaneous Approach

0WHC33Z   Insertion of Infusion Device into Mediastinum, Percutaneous Approach

0WHC3YZ   Insertion of Other Device into Mediastinum, Percutaneous Approach

0WHC41Z   Insertion of Radioactive Element into Mediastinum, Percutaneous Endoscopic Approach

0WHC43Z   Insertion of Infusion Device into Mediastinum, Percutaneous Endoscopic Approach

0WHC4YZ   Insertion of Other Device into Mediastinum, Percutaneous Endoscopic Approach

0WHD01Z   Insertion of Radioactive Element into Pericardial Cavity, Open Approach

0WHD03Z   Insertion of Infusion Device into Pericardial Cavity, Open Approach

0WHD0YZ   Insertion of Other Device into Pericardial Cavity, Open Approach

0WHD31Z   Insertion of Radioactive Element into Pericardial Cavity, Percutaneous Approach

0WHD33Z   Insertion of Infusion Device into Pericardial Cavity, Percutaneous Approach

0WHD3YZ   Insertion of Other Device into Pericardial Cavity, Percutaneous Approach

0WHD41Z   Insertion of Radioactive Element into Pericardial Cavity, Percutaneous Endoscopic Approach

0WHD43Z   Insertion of Infusion Device into Pericardial Cavity, Percutaneous Endoscopic Approach

0WHD4YZ   Insertion of Other Device into Pericardial Cavity, Percutaneous Endoscopic Approach

0WHF01Z   Insertion of Radioactive Element into Abdominal Wall, Open Approach

0WHF03Z   Insertion of Infusion Device into Abdominal Wall, Open Approach

0WHF0YZ   Insertion of Other Device into Abdominal Wall, Open Approach

0WHF31Z   Insertion of Radioactive Element into Abdominal Wall, Percutaneous Approach

0WHF33Z   Insertion of Infusion Device into Abdominal Wall, Percutaneous Approach

0WHF3YZ   Insertion of Other Device into Abdominal Wall, Percutaneous Approach

0WHF41Z   Insertion of Radioactive Element into Abdominal Wall, Percutaneous Endoscopic Approach

0WHF43Z   Insertion of Infusion Device into Abdominal Wall, Percutaneous Endoscopic Approach

0WHF4YZ   Insertion of Other Device into Abdominal Wall, Percutaneous Endoscopic Approach

0WHG01Z   Insertion of Radioactive Element into Peritoneal Cavity, Open Approach

0WHG03Z   Insertion of Infusion Device into Peritoneal Cavity, Open Approach
AHA CC: 2Q, 2021, 14

0WHG0YZ   Insertion of Other Device into Peritoneal Cavity, Open Approach

0WHG31Z   Insertion of Radioactive Element into Peritoneal Cavity, Percutaneous Approach

0WHG33Z   Insertion of Infusion Device into Peritoneal Cavity, Percutaneous Approach
AHA CC: 2Q, 2015, 36; 2Q, 2016, 14

0WHG3YZ   Insertion of Other Device into Peritoneal Cavity, Percutaneous Approach

0WHG41Z   Insertion of Radioactive Element into Peritoneal Cavity, Percutaneous Endoscopic Approach

0WHG43Z   Insertion of Infusion Device into Peritoneal Cavity, Percutaneous Endoscopic Approach

0WHG4YZ   Insertion of Other Device into Peritoneal Cavity, Percutaneous Endoscopic Approach

0WHH01Z   Insertion of Radioactive Element into Retroperitoneum, Open Approach

0WHH03Z   Insertion of Infusion Device into Retroperitoneum, Open Approach

0WHH0YZ   Insertion of Other Device into Retroperitoneum, Open Approach

0WHH31Z   Insertion of Radioactive Element into Retroperitoneum, Percutaneous Approach

0WHH33Z   Insertion of Infusion Device into Retroperitoneum, Percutaneous Approach

0WHH3YZ   Insertion of Other Device into Retroperitoneum, Percutaneous Approach

0WHH41Z   Insertion of Radioactive Element into Retroperitoneum, Percutaneous Endoscopic Approach

0WHH43Z   Insertion of Infusion Device into Retroperitoneum, Percutaneous Endoscopic Approach

0WHH4YZ   Insertion of Other Device into Retroperitoneum, Percutaneous Endoscopic Approach

0WHJ01Z   Insertion of Radioactive Element into Pelvic Cavity, Open Approach
AHA CC: 4Q, 2019, 43-44

0WHJ03Z   Insertion of Infusion Device into Pelvic Cavity, Open Approach

0WHJ0YZ   Insertion of Other Device into Pelvic Cavity, Open Approach

0WHJ31Z   Insertion of Radioactive Element into Pelvic Cavity, Percutaneous Approach

0WHJ33Z   Insertion of Infusion Device into Pelvic Cavity, Percutaneous Approach

0WHJ3YZ   Insertion of Other Device into Pelvic Cavity, Percutaneous Approach

0WHJ41Z   Insertion of Radioactive Element into Pelvic Cavity, Percutaneous Endoscopic Approach

0WHJ43Z   Insertion of Infusion Device into Pelvic Cavity, Percutaneous Endoscopic Approach

0WHJ4YZ   Insertion of Other Device into Pelvic Cavity, Percutaneous Endoscopic Approach

0WHK01Z   Insertion of Radioactive Element into Upper Back, Open Approach

● 0WHK03Z   Insertion of Infusion Device into Upper Back, Open Approach

● 0WHK0YZ   Insertion of Other Device into Upper Back, Open Approach

0WHK31Z   Insertion of Radioactive Element into Upper Back, Percutaneous Approach

● 0WHK33Z   Insertion of Infusion Device into Upper Back, Percutaneous Approach

● 0WHK3YZ   Insertion of Other Device into Upper Back, Percutaneous Approach

0WHK41Z   Insertion of Radioactive Element into Upper Back, Percutaneous Endoscopic Approach

● 0WHK43Z   Insertion of Infusion Device into Upper Back, Percutaneous Endoscopic Approach

● 0WHK4YZ   Insertion of Other Device into Upper Back, Percutaneous Endoscopic Approach

0WHL01Z   Insertion of Radioactive Element into Lower Back, Open Approach

● **0WHL03Z** Insertion of Infusion Device into Lower Back, Open Approach

● **0WHL0YZ** Insertion of Other Device into Lower Back, Open Approach

0WHL31Z Insertion of Radioactive Element into Lower Back, Percutaneous Approach

● **0WHL33Z** Insertion of Infusion Device into Lower Back, Percutaneous Approach

● **0WHL3YZ** Insertion of Other Device into Lower Back, Percutaneous Approach

0WHL41Z Insertion of Radioactive Element into Lower Back, Percutaneous Endoscopic Approach

● **0WHL43Z** Insertion of Infusion Device into Lower Back, Percutaneous Endoscopic Approach

● **0WHL4YZ** Insertion of Other Device into Lower Back, Percutaneous Endoscopic Approach

♂ **0WHM01Z** Insertion of Radioactive Element into Male Perineum, Open Approach
This is a male-only service, however, it is not included in the male-only edit logic for MCE V36

♂● **0WHM03Z** Insertion of Infusion Device into Male Perineum, Open Approach
This is a male-only service, however, it is not included in the male-only edit logic for MCE V36

♂ **0WHM0YZ** Insertion of Other Device into Male Perineum, Open Approach
This is a male-only service, however, it is not included in the male-only edit logic for MCE V36

♂ **0WHM31Z** Insertion of Radioactive Element into Male Perineum, Percutaneous Approach
This is a male-only service, however, it is not included in the male-only edit logic for MCE V36

♂● **0WHM33Z** Insertion of Infusion Device into Male Perineum, Percutaneous Approach
This is a male-only service, however, it is not included in the male-only edit logic for MCE V36

♂● **0WHM3YZ** Insertion of Other Device into Male Perineum, Percutaneous Approach
This is a male-only service, however, it is not included in the male-only edit logic for MCE V36

♂ **0WHM41Z** Insertion of Radioactive Element into Male Perineum, Percutaneous Endoscopic Approach
This is a male-only service, however, it is not included in the male-only edit logic for MCE V36

♂ **0WHM43Z** Insertion of Infusion Device into Male Perineum, Percutaneous Endoscopic Approach
This is a male-only service, however, it is not included in the male-only edit logic for MCE V36

♂● **0WHM4YZ** Insertion of Other Device into Male Perineum, Percutaneous Endoscopic Approach
This is a male-only service, however, it is not included in the male-only edit logic for MCE V36

♀ **0WHN01Z** Insertion of Radioactive Element into Female Perineum, Open Approach
This is a female-only service, however, it is not included in the female-only edit logic for MCE V36

♀ **0WHN03Z** Insertion of Infusion Device into Female Perineum, Open Approach

♀ **0WHN0YZ** Insertion of Other Device into Female Perineum, Open Approach

♀ **0WHN31Z** Insertion of Radioactive Element into Female Perineum, Percutaneous Approach
This is a female-only service, however, it is not included in the female-only edit logic for MCE V36

♀ **0WHN33Z** Insertion of Infusion Device into Female Perineum, Percutaneous Approach

♀ **0WHN3YZ** Insertion of Other Device into Female Perineum, Percutaneous Approach

♀ **0WHN41Z** Insertion of Radioactive Element into Female Perineum, Percutaneous Endoscopic Approach
This is a female-only service, however, it is not included in the female-only edit logic for MCE V36

♀ **0WHN43Z** Insertion of Infusion Device into Female Perineum, Percutaneous Endoscopic Approach

♀ **0WHN4YZ** Insertion of Other Device into Female Perineum, Percutaneous Endoscopic Approach

0WHP01Z Insertion of Radioactive Element into Gastrointestinal Tract, Open Approach

0WHP03Z Insertion of Infusion Device into Gastrointestinal Tract, Open Approach

0WHP0YZ Insertion of Other Device into Gastrointestinal Tract, Open Approach

0WHP31Z Insertion of Radioactive Element into Gastrointestinal Tract, Percutaneous Approach

0WHP33Z Insertion of Infusion Device into Gastrointestinal Tract, Percutaneous Approach

0WHP3YZ Insertion of Other Device into Gastrointestinal Tract, Percutaneous Approach

0WHP41Z Insertion of Radioactive Element into Gastrointestinal Tract, Percutaneous Endoscopic Approach

0WHP43Z Insertion of Infusion Device into Gastrointestinal Tract, Percutaneous Endoscopic Approach

0WHP4YZ Insertion of Other Device into Gastrointestinal Tract, Percutaneous Endoscopic Approach

0WHP71Z Insertion of Radioactive Element into Gastrointestinal Tract, Via Natural or Artificial Opening

0WHP73Z Insertion of Infusion Device into Gastrointestinal Tract, Via Natural or Artificial Opening

0WHP7YZ Insertion of Other Device into Gastrointestinal Tract, Via Natural or Artificial Opening

0WHP81Z Insertion of Radioactive Element into Gastrointestinal Tract, Via Natural or Artificial Opening Endoscopic

0WHP83Z Insertion of Infusion Device into Gastrointestinal Tract, Via Natural or Artificial Opening Endoscopic

0WHP8YZ Insertion of Other Device into Gastrointestinal Tract, Via Natural or Artificial Opening Endoscopic

0WHQ01Z Insertion of Radioactive Element into Respiratory Tract, Open Approach

0WHQ03Z Insertion of Infusion Device into Respiratory Tract, Open Approach

0WHQ0YZ Insertion of Other Device into Respiratory Tract, Open Approach

0WHQ31Z Insertion of Radioactive Element into Respiratory Tract, Percutaneous Approach

0WHQ33Z Insertion of Infusion Device into Respiratory Tract, Percutaneous Approach

0WHQ3YZ Insertion of Other Device into Respiratory Tract, Percutaneous Approach

0WHQ41Z Insertion of Radioactive Element into Respiratory Tract, Percutaneous Endoscopic Approach

0WHQ43Z Insertion of Infusion Device into Respiratory Tract, Percutaneous Endoscopic Approach

0WHQ4YZ Insertion of Other Device into Respiratory Tract, Percutaneous Endoscopic Approach

0WHQ71Z Insertion of Radioactive Element into Respiratory Tract, Via Natural or Artificial Opening

0WHQ73Z Insertion of Infusion Device into Respiratory Tract, Via Natural or Artificial Opening

0WHQ7YZ Insertion of Other Device into Respiratory Tract, Via Natural or Artificial Opening

0WHQ81Z Insertion of Radioactive Element into Respiratory Tract, Via Natural or Artificial Opening Endoscopic

0WHQ83Z Insertion of Infusion Device into Respiratory Tract, Via Natural or Artificial Opening Endoscopic

0WHQ8YZ Insertion of Other Device into Respiratory Tract, Via Natural or Artificial Opening Endoscopic

0WHR01Z Insertion of Radioactive Element into Genitourinary Tract, Open Approach

0WHR03Z Insertion of Infusion Device into Genitourinary Tract, Open Approach

0WHR0YZ Insertion of Other Device into Genitourinary Tract, Open Approach

0WHR31Z Insertion of Radioactive Element into Genitourinary Tract, Percutaneous Approach

0WHR33Z Insertion of Infusion Device into Genitourinary Tract, Percutaneous Approach

0WHR3YZ Insertion of Other Device into Genitourinary Tract, Percutaneous Approach

0WHR41Z Insertion of Radioactive Element into Genitourinary Tract, Percutaneous Endoscopic Approach

0WHR43Z Insertion of Infusion Device into Genitourinary Tract, Percutaneous Endoscopic Approach

0WHR4YZ Insertion of Other Device into Genitourinary Tract, Percutaneous Endoscopic Approach

0WHR71Z Insertion of Radioactive Element into Genitourinary Tract, Via Natural or Artificial Opening

0WHR73Z Insertion of Infusion Device into Genitourinary Tract, Via Natural or Artificial Opening

0WHR7YZ Insertion of Other Device into Genitourinary Tract, Via Natural or Artificial Opening

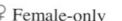 ♀ Female-only   ♂ Male-only   ▲ Limited Coverage   ● Non-OR   ᴴᴬᶜ HAC-associated procedure   ▲ Non-covered procedures   ✚ Cluster

| 0WHR81Z | Insertion of Radioactive Element into Genitourinary Tract, Via Natural or Artificial Opening Endoscopic | 0WHR83Z | Insertion of Infusion Device into Genitourinary Tract, Via Natural or Artificial Opening Endoscopic | 0WHR8YZ | Insertion of Other Device into Genitourinary Tract, Via Natural or Artificial Opening Endoscopic |

0WJ – Anatomical Regions, General, Inspection

Review Coding Guidelines B3.11a, B3.11b and B3.11c

● 0WJ00ZZ — Inspection of Head, Open Approach
0WJ03ZZ — Inspection of Head, Percutaneous Approach
0WJ04ZZ — Inspection of Head, Percutaneous Endoscopic Approach
0WJ0XZZ — Inspection of Head, External Approach
0WJ10ZZ — Inspection of Cranial Cavity, Open Approach
0WJ13ZZ — Inspection of Cranial Cavity, Percutaneous Approach
0WJ14ZZ — Inspection of Cranial Cavity, Percutaneous Endoscopic Approach
● 0WJ20ZZ — Inspection of Face, Open Approach
0WJ23ZZ — Inspection of Face, Percutaneous Approach
0WJ24ZZ — Inspection of Face, Percutaneous Endoscopic Approach
0WJ2XZZ — Inspection of Face, External Approach
0WJ30ZZ — Inspection of Oral Cavity and Throat, Open Approach
0WJ33ZZ — Inspection of Oral Cavity and Throat, Percutaneous Approach
0WJ34ZZ — Inspection of Oral Cavity and Throat, Percutaneous Endoscopic Approach
0WJ3XZZ — Inspection of Oral Cavity and Throat, External Approach
● 0WJ40ZZ — Inspection of Upper Jaw, Open Approach
0WJ43ZZ — Inspection of Upper Jaw, Percutaneous Approach
0WJ44ZZ — Inspection of Upper Jaw, Percutaneous Endoscopic Approach
0WJ4XZZ — Inspection of Upper Jaw, External Approach
● 0WJ50ZZ — Inspection of Lower Jaw, Open Approach
0WJ53ZZ — Inspection of Lower Jaw, Percutaneous Approach
0WJ54ZZ — Inspection of Lower Jaw, Percutaneous Endoscopic Approach
0WJ5XZZ — Inspection of Lower Jaw, External Approach
0WJ60ZZ — Inspection of Neck, Open Approach
0WJ63ZZ — Inspection of Neck, Percutaneous Approach
0WJ64ZZ — Inspection of Neck, Percutaneous Endoscopic Approach
0WJ6XZZ — Inspection of Neck, External Approach
0WJ80ZZ — Inspection of Chest Wall, Open Approach
0WJ83ZZ — Inspection of Chest Wall, Percutaneous Approach
0WJ84ZZ — Inspection of Chest Wall, Percutaneous Endoscopic Approach
0WJ8XZZ — Inspection of Chest Wall, External Approach
0WJ90ZZ — Inspection of Right Pleural Cavity, Open Approach

0WJ93ZZ — Inspection of Right Pleural Cavity, Percutaneous Approach
0WJ94ZZ — Inspection of Right Pleural Cavity, Percutaneous Endoscopic Approach
0WJB0ZZ — Inspection of Left Pleural Cavity, Open Approach
0WJB3ZZ — Inspection of Left Pleural Cavity, Percutaneous Approach
0WJB4ZZ — Inspection of Left Pleural Cavity, Percutaneous Endoscopic Approach
0WJC0ZZ — Inspection of Mediastinum, Open Approach
AHA CC: 3Q, 2018, 29
0WJC3ZZ — Inspection of Mediastinum, Percutaneous Approach
0WJC4ZZ — Inspection of Mediastinum, Percutaneous Endoscopic Approach
0WJD0ZZ — Inspection of Pericardial Cavity, Open Approach
0WJD3ZZ — Inspection of Pericardial Cavity, Percutaneous Approach
0WJD4ZZ — Inspection of Pericardial Cavity, Percutaneous Endoscopic Approach
0WJF0ZZ — Inspection of Abdominal Wall, Open Approach
0WJF3ZZ — Inspection of Abdominal Wall, Percutaneous Approach
0WJF4ZZ — Inspection of Abdominal Wall, Percutaneous Endoscopic Approach
0WJFXZZ — Inspection of Abdominal Wall, External Approach
0WJG0ZZ — Inspection of Peritoneal Cavity, Open Approach
0WJG3ZZ — Inspection of Peritoneal Cavity, Percutaneous Approach
0WJG4ZZ — Inspection of Peritoneal Cavity, Percutaneous Endoscopic Approach
AHA CC: 2Q, 2013, 36-37; 1Q, 2019, 4-5, 25; 2Q, 2021, 19-20
0WJH0ZZ — Inspection of Retroperitoneum, Open Approach
0WJH3ZZ — Inspection of Retroperitoneum, Percutaneous Approach
0WJH4ZZ — Inspection of Retroperitoneum, Percutaneous Endoscopic Approach
0WJJ0ZZ — Inspection of Pelvic Cavity, Open Approach
0WJJ3ZZ — Inspection of Pelvic Cavity, Percutaneous Approach
0WJJ4ZZ — Inspection of Pelvic Cavity, Percutaneous Endoscopic Approach
AHA CC: 4Q, 2016, 58-59
● 0WJK0ZZ — Inspection of Upper Back, Open Approach
0WJK3ZZ — Inspection of Upper Back, Percutaneous Approach
0WJK4ZZ — Inspection of Upper Back, Percutaneous Endoscopic Approach
0WJKXZZ — Inspection of Upper Back, External Approach

● 0WJL0ZZ — Inspection of Lower Back, Open Approach
0WJL3ZZ — Inspection of Lower Back, Percutaneous Approach
0WJL4ZZ — Inspection of Lower Back, Percutaneous Endoscopic Approach
0WJLXZZ — Inspection of Lower Back, External Approach
♂ ● 0WJM0ZZ — Inspection of Male Perineum, Open Approach
♂ 0WJM3ZZ — Inspection of Male Perineum, Percutaneous Approach
♂ ● 0WJM4ZZ — Inspection of Male Perineum, Percutaneous Endoscopic Approach
♂ 0WJMXZZ — Inspection of Male Perineum, External Approach
♀ 0WJN0ZZ — Inspection of Female Perineum, Open Approach
♀ 0WJN3ZZ — Inspection of Female Perineum, Percutaneous Approach
♀ 0WJN4ZZ — Inspection of Female Perineum, Percutaneous Endoscopic Approach
♀ 0WJNXZZ — Inspection of Female Perineum, External Approach
0WJP0ZZ — Inspection of Gastrointestinal Tract, Open Approach
0WJP3ZZ — Inspection of Gastrointestinal Tract, Percutaneous Approach
0WJP4ZZ — Inspection of Gastrointestinal Tract, Percutaneous Endoscopic Approach
0WJP7ZZ — Inspection of Gastrointestinal Tract, Via Natural or Artificial Opening Approach
0WJP8ZZ — Inspection of Gastrointestinal Tract, Via Natural or Artificial Opening Endoscopic Approach
0WJQ0ZZ — Inspection of Respiratory Tract, Open Approach
0WJQ3ZZ — Inspection of Respiratory Tract, Percutaneous Approach
0WJQ4ZZ — Inspection of Respiratory Tract, Percutaneous Endoscopic Approach
0WJQ7ZZ — Inspection of Respiratory Tract, Via Natural or Artificial Opening Approach
0WJQ8ZZ — Inspection of Respiratory Tract, Via Natural or Artificial Opening Endoscopic Approach
0WJR0ZZ — Inspection of Genitourinary Tract, Open Approach
0WJR3ZZ — Inspection of Genitourinary Tract, Percutaneous Approach
0WJR4ZZ — Inspection of Genitourinary Tract, Percutaneous Endoscopic Approach
0WJR7ZZ — Inspection of Genitourinary Tract, Via Natural or Artificial Opening Approach
0WJR8ZZ — Inspection of Genitourinary Tract, Via Natural or Artificial Opening Endoscopic Approach

0WM – Anatomical Regions, General, Reattachment

0WM20ZZ — Reattachment of Face, Open Approach
0WM40ZZ — Reattachment of Upper Jaw, Open Approach

0WM50ZZ — Reattachment of Lower Jaw, Open Approach
0WM60ZZ — Reattachment of Neck, Open Approach

0WM80ZZ — Reattachment of Chest Wall, Open Approach
0WMF0ZZ — Reattachment of Abdominal Wall, Open Approach

0WMK0ZZ   Reattachment of Upper Back, Open Approach

0WML0ZZ   Reattachment of Lower Back, Open Approach

♂ 0WMM0ZZ   Reattachment of Male Perineum, Open Approach

♀ 0WMN0ZZ   Reattachment of Female Perineum, Open Approach

0WP – Anatomical Regions, General, Removal

Review Coding Guideline B6.1c

0WP000Z   Removal of Drainage Device from Head, Open Approach

0WP001Z   Removal of Radioactive Element from Head, Open Approach

0WP003Z   Removal of Infusion Device from Head, Open Approach

0WP007Z   Removal of Autologous Tissue Substitute from Head, Open Approach

0WP00JZ   Removal of Synthetic Substitute from Head, Open Approach

0WP00KZ   Removal of Nonautologous Tissue Substitute from Head, Open Approach

0WP00YZ   Removal of Other Device from Head, Open Approach

0WP030Z   Removal of Drainage Device from Head, Percutaneous Approach

0WP031Z   Removal of Radioactive Element from Head, Percutaneous Approach

0WP033Z   Removal of Infusion Device from Head, Percutaneous Approach

0WP037Z   Removal of Autologous Tissue Substitute from Head, Percutaneous Approach

0WP03JZ   Removal of Synthetic Substitute from Head, Percutaneous Approach

0WP03KZ   Removal of Nonautologous Tissue Substitute from Head, Percutaneous Approach

0WP03YZ   Removal of Other Device from Head, Percutaneous Approach

0WP040Z   Removal of Drainage Device from Head, Percutaneous Endoscopic Approach

0WP041Z   Removal of Radioactive Element from Head, Percutaneous Endoscopic Approach

0WP043Z   Removal of Infusion Device from Head, Percutaneous Endoscopic Approach

0WP047Z   Removal of Autologous Tissue Substitute from Head, Percutaneous Endoscopic Approach

0WP04JZ   Removal of Synthetic Substitute from Head, Percutaneous Endoscopic Approach

0WP04KZ   Removal of Nonautologous Tissue Substitute from Head, Percutaneous Endoscopic Approach

0WP04YZ   Removal of Other Device from Head, Percutaneous Endoscopic Approach

0WP0X0Z   Removal of Drainage Device from Head, External Approach

0WP0X1Z   Removal of Radioactive Element from Head, External Approach

0WP0X3Z   Removal of Infusion Device from Head, External Approach

0WP0X7Z   Removal of Autologous Tissue Substitute from Head, External Approach

0WP0XJZ   Removal of Synthetic Substitute from Head, External Approach

0WP0XKZ   Removal of Nonautologous Tissue Substitute from Head, External Approach

0WP0XYZ   Removal of Other Device from Head, External Approach

0WP100Z   Removal of Drainage Device from Cranial Cavity, Open Approach

0WP101Z   Removal of Radioactive Element from Cranial Cavity, Open Approach

0WP103Z   Removal of Infusion Device from Cranial Cavity, Open Approach

0WP10JZ   Removal of Synthetic Substitute from Cranial Cavity, Open Approach

0WP10YZ   Removal of Other Device from Cranial Cavity, Open Approach

0WP130Z   Removal of Drainage Device from Cranial Cavity, Percutaneous Approach

0WP131Z   Removal of Radioactive Element from Cranial Cavity, Percutaneous Approach

0WP133Z   Removal of Infusion Device from Cranial Cavity, Percutaneous Approach

0WP13JZ   Removal of Synthetic Substitute from Cranial Cavity, Percutaneous Approach

0WP13YZ   Removal of Other Device from Cranial Cavity, Percutaneous Approach

0WP140Z   Removal of Drainage Device from Cranial Cavity, Percutaneous Endoscopic Approach

0WP141Z   Removal of Radioactive Element from Cranial Cavity, Percutaneous Endoscopic Approach

0WP143Z   Removal of Infusion Device from Cranial Cavity, Percutaneous Endoscopic Approach

0WP14JZ   Removal of Synthetic Substitute from Cranial Cavity, Percutaneous Endoscopic Approach

0WP14YZ   Removal of Other Device from Cranial Cavity, Percutaneous Endoscopic Approach

0WP1X0Z   Removal of Drainage Device from Cranial Cavity, External Approach

0WP1X1Z   Removal of Radioactive Element from Cranial Cavity, External Approach

0WP1X3Z   Removal of Infusion Device from Cranial Cavity, External Approach

0WP200Z   Removal of Drainage Device from Face, Open Approach

0WP201Z   Removal of Radioactive Element from Face, Open Approach

0WP203Z   Removal of Infusion Device from Face, Open Approach

0WP207Z   Removal of Autologous Tissue Substitute from Face, Open Approach

0WP20JZ   Removal of Synthetic Substitute from Face, Open Approach

0WP20KZ   Removal of Nonautologous Tissue Substitute from Face, Open Approach

0WP20YZ   Removal of Other Device from Face, Open Approach

0WP230Z   Removal of Drainage Device from Face, Percutaneous Approach

0WP231Z   Removal of Radioactive Element from Face, Percutaneous Approach

0WP233Z   Removal of Infusion Device from Face, Percutaneous Approach

0WP237Z   Removal of Autologous Tissue Substitute from Face, Percutaneous Approach

0WP23JZ   Removal of Synthetic Substitute from Face, Percutaneous Approach

0WP23KZ   Removal of Nonautologous Tissue Substitute from Face, Percutaneous Approach

0WP23YZ   Removal of Other Device from Face, Percutaneous Approach

0WP240Z   Removal of Drainage Device from Face, Percutaneous Endoscopic Approach

0WP241Z   Removal of Radioactive Element from Face, Percutaneous Endoscopic Approach

0WP243Z   Removal of Infusion Device from Face, Percutaneous Endoscopic Approach

0WP247Z   Removal of Autologous Tissue Substitute from Face, Percutaneous Endoscopic Approach

0WP24JZ   Removal of Synthetic Substitute from Face, Percutaneous Endoscopic Approach

0WP24KZ   Removal of Nonautologous Tissue Substitute from Face, Percutaneous Endoscopic Approach

0WP24YZ   Removal of Other Device from Face, Percutaneous Endoscopic Approach

0WP2X0Z   Removal of Drainage Device from Face, External Approach

0WP2X1Z   Removal of Radioactive Element from Face, External Approach

0WP2X3Z   Removal of Infusion Device from Face, External Approach

0WP2X7Z   Removal of Autologous Tissue Substitute from Face, External Approach

0WP2XJZ   Removal of Synthetic Substitute from Face, External Approach

0WP2XKZ   Removal of Nonautologous Tissue Substitute from Face, External Approach

0WP2XYZ   Removal of Other Device from Face, External Approach

0WP400Z   Removal of Drainage Device from Upper Jaw, Open Approach

0WP401Z   Removal of Radioactive Element from Upper Jaw, Open Approach

0WP403Z   Removal of Infusion Device from Upper Jaw, Open Approach

0WP407Z   Removal of Autologous Tissue Substitute from Upper Jaw, Open Approach

0WP40JZ   Removal of Synthetic Substitute from Upper Jaw, Open Approach

0WP40KZ   Removal of Nonautologous Tissue Substitute from Upper Jaw, Open Approach

0WP40YZ   Removal of Other Device from Upper Jaw, Open Approach

0WP430Z Removal of Drainage Device from Upper Jaw, Percutaneous Approach

0WP431Z Removal of Radioactive Element from Upper Jaw, Percutaneous Approach

0WP433Z Removal of Infusion Device from Upper Jaw, Percutaneous Approach

0WP437Z Removal of Autologous Tissue Substitute from Upper Jaw, Percutaneous Approach

0WP43JZ Removal of Synthetic Substitute from Upper Jaw, Percutaneous Approach

0WP43KZ Removal of Nonautologous Tissue Substitute from Upper Jaw, Percutaneous Approach

0WP43YZ Removal of Other Device from Upper Jaw, Percutaneous Approach

0WP440Z Removal of Drainage Device from Upper Jaw, Percutaneous Endoscopic Approach

0WP441Z Removal of Radioactive Element from Upper Jaw, Percutaneous Endoscopic Approach

0WP443Z Removal of Infusion Device from Upper Jaw, Percutaneous Endoscopic Approach

0WP447Z Removal of Autologous Tissue Substitute from Upper Jaw, Percutaneous Endoscopic Approach

0WP44JZ Removal of Synthetic Substitute from Upper Jaw, Percutaneous Endoscopic Approach

0WP44KZ Removal of Nonautologous Tissue Substitute from Upper Jaw, Percutaneous Endoscopic Approach

0WP44YZ Removal of Other Device from Upper Jaw, Percutaneous Endoscopic Approach

0WP4X0Z Removal of Drainage Device from Upper Jaw, External Approach

0WP4X1Z Removal of Radioactive Element from Upper Jaw, External Approach

0WP4X3Z Removal of Infusion Device from Upper Jaw, External Approach

0WP4X7Z Removal of Autologous Tissue Substitute from Upper Jaw, External Approach

0WP4XJZ Removal of Synthetic Substitute from Upper Jaw, External Approach

0WP4XKZ Removal of Nonautologous Tissue Substitute from Upper Jaw, External Approach

0WP4XYZ Removal of Other Device from Upper Jaw, External Approach

0WP500Z Removal of Drainage Device from Lower Jaw, Open Approach

0WP501Z Removal of Radioactive Element from Lower Jaw, Open Approach

0WP503Z Removal of Infusion Device from Lower Jaw, Open Approach

0WP507Z Removal of Autologous Tissue Substitute from Lower Jaw, Open Approach

0WP50JZ Removal of Synthetic Substitute from Lower Jaw, Open Approach

0WP50KZ Removal of Nonautologous Tissue Substitute from Lower Jaw, Open Approach

0WP50YZ Removal of Other Device from Lower Jaw, Open Approach

0WP530Z Removal of Drainage Device from Lower Jaw, Percutaneous Approach

0WP531Z Removal of Radioactive Element from Lower Jaw, Percutaneous Approach

0WP533Z Removal of Infusion Device from Lower Jaw, Percutaneous Approach

0WP537Z Removal of Autologous Tissue Substitute from Lower Jaw, Percutaneous Approach

0WP53JZ Removal of Synthetic Substitute from Lower Jaw, Percutaneous Approach

0WP53KZ Removal of Nonautologous Tissue Substitute from Lower Jaw, Percutaneous Approach

0WP53YZ Removal of Other Device from Lower Jaw, Percutaneous Approach

0WP540Z Removal of Drainage Device from Lower Jaw, Percutaneous Endoscopic Approach

0WP541Z Removal of Radioactive Element from Lower Jaw, Percutaneous Endoscopic Approach

0WP543Z Removal of Infusion Device from Lower Jaw, Percutaneous Endoscopic Approach

0WP547Z Removal of Autologous Tissue Substitute from Lower Jaw, Percutaneous Endoscopic Approach

0WP54JZ Removal of Synthetic Substitute from Lower Jaw, Percutaneous Endoscopic Approach

0WP54KZ Removal of Nonautologous Tissue Substitute from Lower Jaw, Percutaneous Endoscopic Approach

0WP54YZ Removal of Other Device from Lower Jaw, Percutaneous Endoscopic Approach

0WP5X0Z Removal of Drainage Device from Lower Jaw, External Approach

0WP5X1Z Removal of Radioactive Element from Lower Jaw, External Approach

0WP5X3Z Removal of Infusion Device from Lower Jaw, External Approach

0WP5X7Z Removal of Autologous Tissue Substitute from Lower Jaw, External Approach

0WP5XJZ Removal of Synthetic Substitute from Lower Jaw, External Approach

0WP5XKZ Removal of Nonautologous Tissue Substitute from Lower Jaw, External Approach

0WP5XYZ Removal of Other Device from Lower Jaw, External Approach

0WP600Z Removal of Drainage Device from Neck, Open Approach

0WP601Z Removal of Radioactive Element from Neck, Open Approach

0WP603Z Removal of Infusion Device from Neck, Open Approach

0WP607Z Removal of Autologous Tissue Substitute from Neck, Open Approach

0WP60JZ Removal of Synthetic Substitute from Neck, Open Approach

0WP60KZ Removal of Nonautologous Tissue Substitute from Neck, Open Approach

0WP60YZ Removal of Other Device from Neck, Open Approach

0WP630Z Removal of Drainage Device from Neck, Percutaneous Approach

0WP631Z Removal of Radioactive Element from Neck, Percutaneous Approach

0WP633Z Removal of Infusion Device from Neck, Percutaneous Approach

0WP637Z Removal of Autologous Tissue Substitute from Neck, Percutaneous Approach

0WP63JZ Removal of Synthetic Substitute from Neck, Percutaneous Approach

0WP63KZ Removal of Nonautologous Tissue Substitute from Neck, Percutaneous Approach

0WP63YZ Removal of Other Device from Neck, Percutaneous Approach

0WP640Z Removal of Drainage Device from Neck, Percutaneous Endoscopic Approach

0WP641Z Removal of Radioactive Element from Neck, Percutaneous Endoscopic Approach

0WP643Z Removal of Infusion Device from Neck, Percutaneous Endoscopic Approach

0WP647Z Removal of Autologous Tissue Substitute from Neck, Percutaneous Endoscopic Approach

0WP64JZ Removal of Synthetic Substitute from Neck, Percutaneous Endoscopic Approach

0WP64KZ Removal of Nonautologous Tissue Substitute from Neck, Percutaneous Endoscopic Approach

0WP64YZ Removal of Other Device from Neck, Percutaneous Endoscopic Approach

0WP6X0Z Removal of Drainage Device from Neck, External Approach

0WP6X1Z Removal of Radioactive Element from Neck, External Approach

0WP6X3Z Removal of Infusion Device from Neck, External Approach

0WP6X7Z Removal of Autologous Tissue Substitute from Neck, External Approach

0WP6XJZ Removal of Synthetic Substitute from Neck, External Approach

0WP6XKZ Removal of Nonautologous Tissue Substitute from Neck, External Approach

0WP6XYZ Removal of Other Device from Neck, External Approach

0WP800Z Removal of Drainage Device from Chest Wall, Open Approach

0WP801Z Removal of Radioactive Element from Chest Wall, Open Approach

0WP803Z Removal of Infusion Device from Chest Wall, Open Approach

0WP807Z Removal of Autologous Tissue Substitute from Chest Wall, Open Approach

0WP80JZ Removal of Synthetic Substitute from Chest Wall, Open Approach

0WP80KZ Removal of Nonautologous Tissue Substitute from Chest Wall, Open Approach

0WP80YZ Removal of Other Device from Chest Wall, Open Approach

0WP830Z Removal of Drainage Device from Chest Wall, Percutaneous Approach

0WP831Z Removal of Radioactive Element from Chest Wall, Percutaneous Approach

0WP833Z Removal of Infusion Device from Chest Wall, Percutaneous Approach

0WP837Z Removal of Autologous Tissue Substitute from Chest Wall, Percutaneous Approach

0WP83JZ Removal of Synthetic Substitute from Chest Wall, Percutaneous Approach

0WP83KZ Removal of Nonautologous Tissue Substitute from Chest Wall, Percutaneous Approach

0WP83YZ Removal of Other Device from Chest Wall, Percutaneous Approach

0WP840Z Removal of Drainage Device from Chest Wall, Percutaneous Endoscopic Approach

0WP841Z	Removal of Radioactive Element from Chest Wall, Percutaneous Endoscopic Approach
0WP843Z	Removal of Infusion Device from Chest Wall, Percutaneous Endoscopic Approach
0WP847Z	Removal of Autologous Tissue Substitute from Chest Wall, Percutaneous Endoscopic Approach
0WP84JZ	Removal of Synthetic Substitute from Chest Wall, Percutaneous Endoscopic Approach
0WP84KZ	Removal of Nonautologous Tissue Substitute from Chest Wall, Percutaneous Endoscopic Approach
0WP84YZ	Removal of Other Device from Chest Wall, Percutaneous Endoscopic Approach
0WP8X0Z	Removal of Drainage Device from Chest Wall, External Approach
0WP8X1Z	Removal of Radioactive Element from Chest Wall, External Approach
0WP8X3Z	Removal of Infusion Device from Chest Wall, External Approach
0WP8X7Z	Removal of Autologous Tissue Substitute from Chest Wall, External Approach
0WP8XJZ	Removal of Synthetic Substitute from Chest Wall, External Approach
0WP8XKZ	Removal of Nonautologous Tissue Substitute from Chest Wall, External Approach
0WP8XYZ	Removal of Other Device from Chest Wall, External Approach
0WP900Z	Removal of Drainage Device from Right Pleural Cavity, Open Approach
0WP901Z	Removal of Radioactive Element from Right Pleural Cavity, Open Approach
0WP903Z	Removal of Infusion Device from Right Pleural Cavity, Open Approach
0WP90JZ	Removal of Synthetic Substitute from Right Pleural Cavity, Open Approach
0WP90YZ	Removal of Other Device from Right Pleural Cavity, Open Approach
0WP930Z	Removal of Drainage Device from Right Pleural Cavity, Percutaneous Approach
0WP931Z	Removal of Radioactive Element from Right Pleural Cavity, Percutaneous Approach
0WP933Z	Removal of Infusion Device from Right Pleural Cavity, Percutaneous Approach
0WP93JZ	Removal of Synthetic Substitute from Right Pleural Cavity, Percutaneous Approach
0WP93YZ	Removal of Other Device from Right Pleural Cavity, Percutaneous Approach
0WP940Z	Removal of Drainage Device from Right Pleural Cavity, Percutaneous Endoscopic Approach
0WP941Z	Removal of Radioactive Element from Right Pleural Cavity, Percutaneous Endoscopic Approach
0WP943Z	Removal of Infusion Device from Right Pleural Cavity, Percutaneous Endoscopic Approach
0WP94JZ	Removal of Synthetic Substitute from Right Pleural Cavity, Percutaneous Endoscopic Approach
0WP94YZ	Removal of Other Device from Right Pleural Cavity, Percutaneous Endoscopic Approach
0WP9X0Z	Removal of Drainage Device from Right Pleural Cavity, External Approach
0WP9X1Z	Removal of Radioactive Element from Right Pleural Cavity, External Approach
0WP9X3Z	Removal of Infusion Device from Right Pleural Cavity, External Approach
0WPB00Z	Removal of Drainage Device from Left Pleural Cavity, Open Approach
0WPB01Z	Removal of Radioactive Element from Left Pleural Cavity, Open Approach
0WPB03Z	Removal of Infusion Device from Left Pleural Cavity, Open Approach
0WPB0JZ	Removal of Synthetic Substitute from Left Pleural Cavity, Open Approach
0WPB0YZ	Removal of Other Device from Left Pleural Cavity, Open Approach
0WPB30Z	Removal of Drainage Device from Left Pleural Cavity, Percutaneous Approach
0WPB31Z	Removal of Radioactive Element from Left Pleural Cavity, Percutaneous Approach
0WPB33Z	Removal of Infusion Device from Left Pleural Cavity, Percutaneous Approach
0WPB3JZ	Removal of Synthetic Substitute from Left Pleural Cavity, Percutaneous Approach
0WPB3YZ	Removal of Other Device from Left Pleural Cavity, Percutaneous Approach
0WPB40Z	Removal of Drainage Device from Left Pleural Cavity, Percutaneous Endoscopic Approach
0WPB41Z	Removal of Radioactive Element from Left Pleural Cavity, Percutaneous Endoscopic Approach
0WPB43Z	Removal of Infusion Device from Left Pleural Cavity, Percutaneous Endoscopic Approach
0WPB4JZ	Removal of Synthetic Substitute from Left Pleural Cavity, Percutaneous Endoscopic Approach
0WPB4YZ	Removal of Other Device from Left Pleural Cavity, Percutaneous Endoscopic Approach
0WPBX0Z	Removal of Drainage Device from Left Pleural Cavity, External Approach
0WPBX1Z	Removal of Radioactive Element from Left Pleural Cavity, External Approach
0WPBX3Z	Removal of Infusion Device from Left Pleural Cavity, External Approach
0WPC00Z	Removal of Drainage Device from Mediastinum, Open Approach
0WPC01Z	Removal of Radioactive Element from Mediastinum, Open Approach
0WPC03Z	Removal of Infusion Device from Mediastinum, Open Approach
0WPC07Z	Removal of Autologous Tissue Substitute from Mediastinum, Open Approach
0WPC0JZ	Removal of Synthetic Substitute from Mediastinum, Open Approach
0WPC0KZ	Removal of Nonautologous Tissue Substitute from Mediastinum, Open Approach
0WPC0YZ	Removal of Other Device from Mediastinum, Open Approach
0WPC30Z	Removal of Drainage Device from Mediastinum, Percutaneous Approach
0WPC31Z	Removal of Radioactive Element from Mediastinum, Percutaneous Approach
0WPC33Z	Removal of Infusion Device from Mediastinum, Percutaneous Approach
0WPC37Z	Removal of Autologous Tissue Substitute from Mediastinum, Percutaneous Approach
0WPC3JZ	Removal of Synthetic Substitute from Mediastinum, Percutaneous Approach
0WPC3KZ	Removal of Nonautologous Tissue Substitute from Mediastinum, Percutaneous Approach
0WPC3YZ	Removal of Other Device from Mediastinum, Percutaneous Approach
0WPC40Z	Removal of Drainage Device from Mediastinum, Percutaneous Endoscopic Approach
0WPC41Z	Removal of Radioactive Element from Mediastinum, Percutaneous Endoscopic Approach
0WPC43Z	Removal of Infusion Device from Mediastinum, Percutaneous Endoscopic Approach
0WPC47Z	Removal of Autologous Tissue Substitute from Mediastinum, Percutaneous Endoscopic Approach
0WPC4JZ	Removal of Synthetic Substitute from Mediastinum, Percutaneous Endoscopic Approach
0WPC4KZ	Removal of Nonautologous Tissue Substitute from Mediastinum, Percutaneous Endoscopic Approach
0WPC4YZ	Removal of Other Device from Mediastinum, Percutaneous Endoscopic Approach
0WPCX0Z	Removal of Drainage Device from Mediastinum, External Approach
0WPCX1Z	Removal of Radioactive Element from Mediastinum, External Approach
0WPCX3Z	Removal of Infusion Device from Mediastinum, External Approach
0WPCX7Z	Removal of Autologous Tissue Substitute from Mediastinum, External Approach
0WPCXJZ	Removal of Synthetic Substitute from Mediastinum, External Approach
0WPCXKZ	Removal of Nonautologous Tissue Substitute from Mediastinum, External Approach
0WPCXYZ	Removal of Other Device from Mediastinum, External Approach
0WPD00Z	Removal of Drainage Device from Pericardial Cavity, Open Approach
0WPD01Z	Removal of Radioactive Element from Pericardial Cavity, Open Approach
0WPD03Z	Removal of Infusion Device from Pericardial Cavity, Open Approach
0WPD0YZ	Removal of Other Device from Pericardial Cavity, Open Approach
0WPD30Z	Removal of Drainage Device from Pericardial Cavity, Percutaneous Approach
0WPD31Z	Removal of Radioactive Element from Pericardial Cavity, Percutaneous Approach
0WPD33Z	Removal of Infusion Device from Pericardial Cavity, Percutaneous Approach
0WPD3YZ	Removal of Other Device from Pericardial Cavity, Percutaneous Approach
0WPD40Z	Removal of Drainage Device from Pericardial Cavity, Percutaneous Endoscopic Approach

♀ Female-only   ♂ Male-only   ▲ Limited Coverage   ● Non-OR   ▦ HAC-associated procedure   ▲ Non-covered procedures   ✚ Cluster

0WPD41Z Removal of Radioactive Element from Pericardial Cavity, Percutaneous Endoscopic Approach

0WPD43Z Removal of Infusion Device from Pericardial Cavity, Percutaneous Endoscopic Approach

0WPD4YZ Removal of Other Device from Pericardial Cavity, Percutaneous Endoscopic Approach

0WPDX0Z Removal of Drainage Device from Pericardial Cavity, External Approach

0WPDX1Z Removal of Radioactive Element from Pericardial Cavity, External Approach

0WPDX3Z Removal of Infusion Device from Pericardial Cavity, External Approach

0WPF00Z Removal of Drainage Device from Abdominal Wall, Open Approach

0WPF01Z Removal of Radioactive Element from Abdominal Wall, Open Approach

0WPF03Z Removal of Infusion Device from Abdominal Wall, Open Approach

0WPF07Z Removal of Autologous Tissue Substitute from Abdominal Wall, Open Approach

0WPF0JZ Removal of Synthetic Substitute from Abdominal Wall, Open Approach

0WPF0KZ Removal of Nonautologous Tissue Substitute from Abdominal Wall, Open Approach

0WPF0YZ Removal of Other Device from Abdominal Wall, Open Approach

0WPF30Z Removal of Drainage Device from Abdominal Wall, Percutaneous Approach

0WPF31Z Removal of Radioactive Element from Abdominal Wall, Percutaneous Approach

0WPF33Z Removal of Infusion Device from Abdominal Wall, Percutaneous Approach

0WPF37Z Removal of Autologous Tissue Substitute from Abdominal Wall, Percutaneous Approach

0WPF3JZ Removal of Synthetic Substitute from Abdominal Wall, Percutaneous Approach

0WPF3KZ Removal of Nonautologous Tissue Substitute from Abdominal Wall, Percutaneous Approach

0WPF3YZ Removal of Other Device from Abdominal Wall, Percutaneous Approach

0WPF40Z Removal of Drainage Device from Abdominal Wall, Percutaneous Endoscopic Approach

0WPF41Z Removal of Radioactive Element from Abdominal Wall, Percutaneous Endoscopic Approach

0WPF43Z Removal of Infusion Device from Abdominal Wall, Percutaneous Endoscopic Approach

0WPF47Z Removal of Autologous Tissue Substitute from Abdominal Wall, Percutaneous Endoscopic Approach

0WPF4JZ Removal of Synthetic Substitute from Abdominal Wall, Percutaneous Endoscopic Approach

0WPF4KZ Removal of Nonautologous Tissue Substitute from Abdominal Wall, Percutaneous Endoscopic Approach

0WPF4YZ Removal of Other Device from Abdominal Wall, Percutaneous Endoscopic Approach

0WPFX0Z Removal of Drainage Device from Abdominal Wall, External Approach

0WPFX1Z Removal of Radioactive Element from Abdominal Wall, External Approach

0WPFX3Z Removal of Infusion Device from Abdominal Wall, External Approach

0WPFX7Z Removal of Autologous Tissue Substitute from Abdominal Wall, External Approach

0WPFXJZ Removal of Synthetic Substitute from Abdominal Wall, External Approach

0WPFXKZ Removal of Nonautologous Tissue Substitute from Abdominal Wall, External Approach

0WPFXYZ Removal of Other Device from Abdominal Wall, External Approach

0WPG00Z Removal of Drainage Device from Peritoneal Cavity, Open Approach

0WPG01Z Removal of Radioactive Element from Peritoneal Cavity, Open Approach

0WPG03Z Removal of Infusion Device from Peritoneal Cavity, Open Approach

0WPG0JZ Removal of Synthetic Substitute from Peritoneal Cavity, Open Approach

0WPG0YZ Removal of Other Device from Peritoneal Cavity, Open Approach

0WPG30Z Removal of Drainage Device from Peritoneal Cavity, Percutaneous Approach

0WPG31Z Removal of Radioactive Element from Peritoneal Cavity, Percutaneous Approach

0WPG33Z Removal of Infusion Device from Peritoneal Cavity, Percutaneous Approach

0WPG3JZ Removal of Synthetic Substitute from Peritoneal Cavity, Percutaneous Approach

0WPG3YZ Removal of Other Device from Peritoneal Cavity, Percutaneous Approach

0WPG40Z Removal of Drainage Device from Peritoneal Cavity, Percutaneous Endoscopic Approach

0WPG41Z Removal of Radioactive Element from Peritoneal Cavity, Percutaneous Endoscopic Approach

0WPG43Z Removal of Infusion Device from Peritoneal Cavity, Percutaneous Endoscopic Approach

0WPG4JZ Removal of Synthetic Substitute from Peritoneal Cavity, Percutaneous Endoscopic Approach

0WPG4YZ Removal of Other Device from Peritoneal Cavity, Percutaneous Endoscopic Approach

0WPGX0Z Removal of Drainage Device from Peritoneal Cavity, External Approach

0WPGX1Z Removal of Radioactive Element from Peritoneal Cavity, External Approach

0WPGX3Z Removal of Infusion Device from Peritoneal Cavity, External Approach

0WPH00Z Removal of Drainage Device from Retroperitoneum, Open Approach

0WPH01Z Removal of Radioactive Element from Retroperitoneum, Open Approach

0WPH03Z Removal of Infusion Device from Retroperitoneum, Open Approach

0WPH0YZ Removal of Other Device from Retroperitoneum, Open Approach

0WPH30Z Removal of Drainage Device from Retroperitoneum, Percutaneous Approach

0WPH31Z Removal of Radioactive Element from Retroperitoneum, Percutaneous Approach

0WPH33Z Removal of Infusion Device from Retroperitoneum, Percutaneous Approach

0WPH3YZ Removal of Other Device from Retroperitoneum, Percutaneous Approach

0WPH40Z Removal of Drainage Device from Retroperitoneum, Percutaneous Endoscopic Approach

0WPH41Z Removal of Radioactive Element from Retroperitoneum, Percutaneous Endoscopic Approach

0WPH43Z Removal of Infusion Device from Retroperitoneum, Percutaneous Endoscopic Approach

0WPH4YZ Removal of Other Device from Retroperitoneum, Percutaneous Endoscopic Approach

0WPHX0Z Removal of Drainage Device from Retroperitoneum, External Approach

0WPHX1Z Removal of Radioactive Element from Retroperitoneum, External Approach

0WPHX3Z Removal of Infusion Device from Retroperitoneum, External Approach

0WPJ00Z Removal of Drainage Device from Pelvic Cavity, Open Approach

0WPJ01Z Removal of Radioactive Element from Pelvic Cavity, Open Approach

0WPJ03Z Removal of Infusion Device from Pelvic Cavity, Open Approach

0WPJ0JZ Removal of Synthetic Substitute from Pelvic Cavity, Open Approach

0WPJ0YZ Removal of Other Device from Pelvic Cavity, Open Approach

0WPJ30Z Removal of Drainage Device from Pelvic Cavity, Percutaneous Approach

0WPJ31Z Removal of Radioactive Element from Pelvic Cavity, Percutaneous Approach

0WPJ33Z Removal of Infusion Device from Pelvic Cavity, Percutaneous Approach

0WPJ3JZ Removal of Synthetic Substitute from Pelvic Cavity, Percutaneous Approach

0WPJ3YZ Removal of Other Device from Pelvic Cavity, Percutaneous Approach

0WPJ40Z Removal of Drainage Device from Pelvic Cavity, Percutaneous Endoscopic Approach

0WPJ41Z Removal of Radioactive Element from Pelvic Cavity, Percutaneous Endoscopic Approach

0WPJ43Z Removal of Infusion Device from Pelvic Cavity, Percutaneous Endoscopic Approach

0WPJ4JZ Removal of Synthetic Substitute from Pelvic Cavity, Percutaneous Endoscopic Approach

0WPJ4YZ Removal of Other Device from Pelvic Cavity, Percutaneous Endoscopic Approach

0WPJX0Z Removal of Drainage Device from Pelvic Cavity, External Approach

0WPJX1Z Removal of Radioactive Element from Pelvic Cavity, External Approach

0WPJX3Z Removal of Infusion Device from Pelvic Cavity, External Approach

0WPK00Z Removal of Drainage Device from Upper Back, Open Approach

0WPK01Z Removal of Radioactive Element from Upper Back, Open Approach

0WPK03Z Removal of Infusion Device from Upper Back, Open Approach

0WPK07Z Removal of Autologous Tissue Substitute from Upper Back, Open Approach

0WPK0JZ Removal of Synthetic Substitute from Upper Back, Open Approach

0WPK0KZ Removal of Nonautologous Tissue Substitute from Upper Back, Open Approach

0WPK0YZ Removal of Other Device from Upper Back, Open Approach

0WPK30Z Removal of Drainage Device from Upper Back, Percutaneous Approach

0WPK31Z Removal of Radioactive Element from Upper Back, Percutaneous Approach

0WPK33Z Removal of Infusion Device from Upper Back, Percutaneous Approach

0WPK37Z Removal of Autologous Tissue Substitute from Upper Back, Percutaneous Approach

0WPK3JZ Removal of Synthetic Substitute from Upper Back, Percutaneous Approach

0WPK3KZ Removal of Nonautologous Tissue Substitute from Upper Back, Percutaneous Approach

0WPK3YZ Removal of Other Device from Upper Back, Percutaneous Approach

0WPK40Z Removal of Drainage Device from Upper Back, Percutaneous Endoscopic Approach

0WPK41Z Removal of Radioactive Element from Upper Back, Percutaneous Endoscopic Approach

0WPK43Z Removal of Infusion Device from Upper Back, Percutaneous Endoscopic Approach

0WPK47Z Removal of Autologous Tissue Substitute from Upper Back, Percutaneous Endoscopic Approach

0WPK4JZ Removal of Synthetic Substitute from Upper Back, Percutaneous Endoscopic Approach

0WPK4KZ Removal of Nonautologous Tissue Substitute from Upper Back, Percutaneous Endoscopic Approach

0WPK4YZ Removal of Other Device from Upper Back, Percutaneous Endoscopic Approach

0WPKX0Z Removal of Drainage Device from Upper Back, External Approach

0WPKX1Z Removal of Radioactive Element from Upper Back, External Approach

0WPKX3Z Removal of Infusion Device from Upper Back, External Approach

0WPKX7Z Removal of Autologous Tissue Substitute from Upper Back, External Approach

0WPKXJZ Removal of Synthetic Substitute from Upper Back, External Approach

0WPKXKZ Removal of Nonautologous Tissue Substitute from Upper Back, External Approach

0WPKXYZ Removal of Other Device from Upper Back, External Approach

0WPL00Z Removal of Drainage Device from Lower Back, Open Approach

0WPL01Z Removal of Radioactive Element from Lower Back, Open Approach

0WPL03Z Removal of Infusion Device from Lower Back, Open Approach

0WPL07Z Removal of Autologous Tissue Substitute from Lower Back, Open Approach

0WPL0JZ Removal of Synthetic Substitute from Lower Back, Open Approach

0WPL0KZ Removal of Nonautologous Tissue Substitute from Lower Back, Open Approach

0WPL0YZ Removal of Other Device from Lower Back, Open Approach

0WPL30Z Removal of Drainage Device from Lower Back, Percutaneous Approach

0WPL31Z Removal of Radioactive Element from Lower Back, Percutaneous Approach

0WPL33Z Removal of Infusion Device from Lower Back, Percutaneous Approach

0WPL37Z Removal of Autologous Tissue Substitute from Lower Back, Percutaneous Approach

0WPL3JZ Removal of Synthetic Substitute from Lower Back, Percutaneous Approach

0WPL3KZ Removal of Nonautologous Tissue Substitute from Lower Back, Percutaneous Approach

0WPL3YZ Removal of Other Device from Lower Back, Percutaneous Approach

0WPL40Z Removal of Drainage Device from Lower Back, Percutaneous Endoscopic Approach

0WPL41Z Removal of Radioactive Element from Lower Back, Percutaneous Endoscopic Approach

0WPL43Z Removal of Infusion Device from Lower Back, Percutaneous Endoscopic Approach

0WPL47Z Removal of Autologous Tissue Substitute from Lower Back, Percutaneous Endoscopic Approach

0WPL4JZ Removal of Synthetic Substitute from Lower Back, Percutaneous Endoscopic Approach

0WPL4KZ Removal of Nonautologous Tissue Substitute from Lower Back, Percutaneous Endoscopic Approach

0WPL4YZ Removal of Other Device from Lower Back, Percutaneous Endoscopic Approach

0WPLX0Z Removal of Drainage Device from Lower Back, External Approach

0WPLX1Z Removal of Radioactive Element from Lower Back, External Approach

0WPLX3Z Removal of Infusion Device from Lower Back, External Approach

0WPLX7Z Removal of Autologous Tissue Substitute from Lower Back, External Approach

0WPLXJZ Removal of Synthetic Substitute from Lower Back, External Approach

0WPLXKZ Removal of Nonautologous Tissue Substitute from Lower Back, External Approach

0WPLXYZ Removal of Other Device from Lower Back, External Approach

♂ **0WPM00Z** Removal of Drainage Device from Male Perineum, Open Approach

♂ **0WPM01Z** Removal of Radioactive Element from Male Perineum, Open Approach

♂ **0WPM03Z** Removal of Infusion Device from Male Perineum, Open Approach

♂ **0WPM07Z** Removal of Autologous Tissue Substitute from Male Perineum, Open Approach

♂ **0WPM0JZ** Removal of Synthetic Substitute from Male Perineum, Open Approach

♂ **0WPM0KZ** Removal of Nonautologous Tissue Substitute from Male Perineum, Open Approach

♂ **0WPM0YZ** Removal of Other Device from Male Perineum, Open Approach

♂ **0WPM30Z** Removal of Drainage Device from Male Perineum, Percutaneous Approach

♂ **0WPM31Z** Removal of Radioactive Element from Male Perineum, Percutaneous Approach

♂ **0WPM33Z** Removal of Infusion Device from Male Perineum, Percutaneous Approach

♂ **0WPM37Z** Removal of Autologous Tissue Substitute from Male Perineum, Percutaneous Approach

♂ **0WPM3JZ** Removal of Synthetic Substitute from Male Perineum, Percutaneous Approach

♂ **0WPM3KZ** Removal of Nonautologous Tissue Substitute from Male Perineum, Percutaneous Approach

♂ **0WPM3YZ** Removal of Other Device from Male Perineum, Percutaneous Approach

♂ **0WPM40Z** Removal of Drainage Device from Male Perineum, Percutaneous Endoscopic Approach

♂ **0WPM41Z** Removal of Radioactive Element from Male Perineum, Percutaneous Endoscopic Approach

♂ **0WPM43Z** Removal of Infusion Device from Male Perineum, Percutaneous Endoscopic Approach

♂ **0WPM47Z** Removal of Autologous Tissue Substitute from Male Perineum, Percutaneous Endoscopic Approach

♂ **0WPM4JZ** Removal of Synthetic Substitute from Male Perineum, Percutaneous Endoscopic Approach

♂ **0WPM4KZ** Removal of Nonautologous Tissue Substitute from Male Perineum, Percutaneous Endoscopic Approach

♂ **0WPM4YZ** Removal of Other Device from Male Perineum, Percutaneous Endoscopic Approach

♂ **0WPMX0Z** Removal of Drainage Device from Male Perineum, External Approach

♂ **0WPMX1Z** Removal of Radioactive Element from Male Perineum, External Approach

♂ **0WPMX3Z** Removal of Infusion Device from Male Perineum, External Approach

♂ **0WPMX7Z** Removal of Autologous Tissue Substitute from Male Perineum, External Approach

♂ **0WPMXJZ** Removal of Synthetic Substitute from Male Perineum, External Approach

♂ **0WPMXKZ** Removal of Nonautologous Tissue Substitute from Male Perineum, External Approach

♂ **0WPMXYZ** Removal of Other Device from Male Perineum, External Approach

♀ **0WPN00Z** Removal of Drainage Device from Female Perineum, Open Approach

♀ **0WPN01Z** Removal of Radioactive Element from Female Perineum, Open Approach

♀ **0WPN03Z** Removal of Infusion Device from Female Perineum, Open Approach

♀ **0WPN07Z** Removal of Autologous Tissue Substitute from Female Perineum, Open Approach

♀ **0WPN0JZ** Removal of Synthetic Substitute from Female Perineum, Open Approach

♀ **0WPN0KZ** Removal of Nonautologous Tissue Substitute from Female Perineum, Open Approach

♀ **0WPN0YZ** Removal of Other Device from Female Perineum, Open Approach

♀ **0WPN30Z** Removal of Drainage Device from Female Perineum, Percutaneous Approach

♀ **0WPN31Z** Removal of Radioactive Element from Female Perineum, Percutaneous Approach

♀ **0WPN33Z** Removal of Infusion Device from Female Perineum, Percutaneous Approach

♀ Female-only   ♂ Male-only   ▲ Limited Coverage   ● Non-OR   HAC HAC-associated procedure   ▲ Non-covered procedures   ✚ Cluster

♀ **0WPN37Z** Removal of Autologous Tissue Substitute from Female Perineum, Percutaneous Approach

♀ **0WPN3JZ** Removal of Synthetic Substitute from Female Perineum, Percutaneous Approach

♀ **0WPN3KZ** Removal of Nonautologous Tissue Substitute from Female Perineum, Percutaneous Approach

♀ **0WPN3YZ** Removal of Other Device from Female Perineum, Percutaneous Approach

♀ **0WPN40Z** Removal of Drainage Device from Female Perineum, Percutaneous Endoscopic Approach

♀ **0WPN41Z** Removal of Radioactive Element from Female Perineum, Percutaneous Endoscopic Approach

♀ **0WPN43Z** Removal of Infusion Device from Female Perineum, Percutaneous Endoscopic Approach

♀ **0WPN47Z** Removal of Autologous Tissue Substitute from Female Perineum, Percutaneous Endoscopic Approach

♀ **0WPN4JZ** Removal of Synthetic Substitute from Female Perineum, Percutaneous Endoscopic Approach

♀ **0WPN4KZ** Removal of Nonautologous Tissue Substitute from Female Perineum, Percutaneous Endoscopic Approach

♀ **0WPN4YZ** Removal of Other Device from Female Perineum, Percutaneous Endoscopic Approach

♀ **0WPNX0Z** Removal of Drainage Device from Female Perineum, External Approach

♀ **0WPNX1Z** Removal of Radioactive Element from Female Perineum, External Approach

♀ **0WPNX3Z** Removal of Infusion Device from Female Perineum, External Approach

♀ **0WPNX7Z** Removal of Autologous Tissue Substitute from Female Perineum, External Approach

♀ **0WPNXJZ** Removal of Synthetic Substitute from Female Perineum, External Approach

♀ **0WPNXKZ** Removal of Nonautologous Tissue Substitute from Female Perineum, External Approach

♀ **0WPNXYZ** Removal of Other Device from Female Perineum, External Approach

0WPP01Z Removal of Radioactive Element from Gastrointestinal Tract, Open Approach

0WPP03Z Removal of Infusion Device from Gastrointestinal Tract, Open Approach

0WPP0YZ Removal of Other Device from Gastrointestinal Tract, Open Approach

0WPP31Z Removal of Radioactive Element from Gastrointestinal Tract, Percutaneous Approach

0WPP33Z Removal of Infusion Device from Gastrointestinal Tract, Percutaneous Approach

0WPP3YZ Removal of Other Device from Gastrointestinal Tract, Percutaneous Approach

0WPP41Z Removal of Radioactive Element from Gastrointestinal Tract, Percutaneous Endoscopic Approach

0WPP43Z Removal of Infusion Device from Gastrointestinal Tract, Percutaneous Endoscopic Approach

0WPP4YZ Removal of Other Device from Gastrointestinal Tract, Percutaneous Endoscopic Approach

0WPP71Z Removal of Radioactive Element from Gastrointestinal Tract, Via Natural or Artificial Opening

0WPP73Z Removal of Infusion Device from Gastrointestinal Tract, Via Natural or Artificial Opening

0WPP7YZ Removal of Other Device from Gastrointestinal Tract, Via Natural or Artificial Opening

0WPP81Z Removal of Radioactive Element from Gastrointestinal Tract, Via Natural or Artificial Opening Endoscopic

0WPP83Z Removal of Infusion Device from Gastrointestinal Tract, Via Natural or Artificial Opening Endoscopic

0WPP8YZ Removal of Other Device from Gastrointestinal Tract, Via Natural or Artificial Opening Endoscopic

0WPPX1Z Removal of Radioactive Element from Gastrointestinal Tract, External Approach

0WPPX3Z Removal of Infusion Device from Gastrointestinal Tract, External Approach

0WPPXYZ Removal of Other Device from Gastrointestinal Tract, External Approach

0WPQ01Z Removal of Radioactive Element from Respiratory Tract, Open Approach

0WPQ03Z Removal of Infusion Device from Respiratory Tract, Open Approach

0WPQ0YZ Removal of Other Device from Respiratory Tract, Open Approach

0WPQ31Z Removal of Radioactive Element from Respiratory Tract, Percutaneous Approach

0WPQ33Z Removal of Infusion Device from Respiratory Tract, Percutaneous Approach

0WPQ3YZ Removal of Other Device from Respiratory Tract, Percutaneous Approach

0WPQ41Z Removal of Radioactive Element from Respiratory Tract, Percutaneous Endoscopic Approach

0WPQ43Z Removal of Infusion Device from Respiratory Tract, Percutaneous Endoscopic Approach

0WPQ4YZ Removal of Other Device from Respiratory Tract, Percutaneous Endoscopic Approach

0WPQ71Z Removal of Radioactive Element from Respiratory Tract, Via Natural or Artificial Opening

● **0WPQ73Z** Removal of Infusion Device from Respiratory Tract, Via Natural or Artificial Opening

0WPQ7YZ Removal of Other Device from Respiratory Tract, Via Natural or Artificial Opening

0WPQ81Z Removal of Radioactive Element from Respiratory Tract, Via Natural or Artificial Opening Endoscopic

0WPQ83Z Removal of Infusion Device from Respiratory Tract, Via Natural or Artificial Opening Endoscopic

0WPQ8YZ Removal of Other Device from Respiratory Tract, Via Natural or Artificial Opening Endoscopic

0WPQX1Z Removal of Radioactive Element from Respiratory Tract, External Approach

0WPQX3Z Removal of Infusion Device from Respiratory Tract, External Approach

0WPQXYZ Removal of Other Device from Respiratory Tract, External Approach

0WPR01Z Removal of Radioactive Element from Genitourinary Tract, Open Approach

0WPR03Z Removal of Infusion Device from Genitourinary Tract, Open Approach

0WPR0YZ Removal of Other Device from Genitourinary Tract, Open Approach

0WPR31Z Removal of Radioactive Element from Genitourinary Tract, Percutaneous Approach

0WPR33Z Removal of Infusion Device from Genitourinary Tract, Percutaneous Approach

0WPR3YZ Removal of Other Device from Genitourinary Tract, Percutaneous Approach

0WPR41Z Removal of Radioactive Element from Genitourinary Tract, Percutaneous Endoscopic Approach

0WPR43Z Removal of Infusion Device from Genitourinary Tract, Percutaneous Endoscopic Approach

0WPR4YZ Removal of Other Device from Genitourinary Tract, Percutaneous Endoscopic Approach

0WPR71Z Removal of Radioactive Element from Genitourinary Tract, Via Natural or Artificial Opening

0WPR73Z Removal of Infusion Device from Genitourinary Tract, Via Natural or Artificial Opening

0WPR7YZ Removal of Other Device from Genitourinary Tract, Via Natural or Artificial Opening

0WPR81Z Removal of Radioactive Element from Genitourinary Tract, Via Natural or Artificial Opening Endoscopic

0WPR83Z Removal of Infusion Device from Genitourinary Tract, Via Natural or Artificial Opening Endoscopic

0WPR8YZ Removal of Other Device from Genitourinary Tract, Via Natural or Artificial Opening Endoscopic

0WPRX1Z Removal of Radioactive Element from Genitourinary Tract, External Approach

0WPRX3Z Removal of Infusion Device from Genitourinary Tract, External Approach

0WPRXYZ Removal of Other Device from Genitourinary Tract, External Approach

0WQ – Anatomical Regions, General, Repair

0WQ00ZZ Repair Head, Open Approach

0WQ03ZZ Repair Head, Percutaneous Approach

0WQ04ZZ Repair Head, Percutaneous Endoscopic Approach

0WQ0XZZ Repair Head, External Approach

0WQ20ZZ Repair Face, Open Approach

0WQ23ZZ Repair Face, Percutaneous Approach

0WQ24ZZ Repair Face, Percutaneous Endoscopic Approach

0WQ2XZZ Repair Face, External Approach

0WQ30ZZ Repair Oral Cavity and Throat, Open Approach

0WQ33ZZ Repair Oral Cavity and Throat, Percutaneous Approach

0WQ34ZZ	Repair Oral Cavity and Throat, Percutaneous Endoscopic Approach	0WQ84ZZ	Repair Chest Wall, Percutaneous Endoscopic Approach	0WQKXZZ	Repair Upper Back, External Approach
0WQ3XZZ	Repair Oral Cavity and Throat, External Approach	0WQ8XZZ	Repair Chest Wall, External Approach	0WQL0ZZ	Repair Lower Back, Open Approach
0WQ40ZZ	Repair Upper Jaw, Open Approach	0WQC0ZZ	Repair Mediastinum, Open Approach	0WQL3ZZ	Repair Lower Back, Percutaneous Approach
0WQ43ZZ	Repair Upper Jaw, Percutaneous Approach	0WQC3ZZ	Repair Mediastinum, Percutaneous Approach	0WQL4ZZ	Repair Lower Back, Percutaneous Endoscopic Approach
0WQ44ZZ	Repair Upper Jaw, Percutaneous Endoscopic Approach	0WQC4ZZ	Repair Mediastinum, Percutaneous Endoscopic Approach	0WQLXZZ	Repair Lower Back, External Approach
0WQ4XZZ	Repair Upper Jaw, External Approach	0WQF0ZZ	Repair Abdominal Wall, Open Approach	♂ 0WQM0ZZ	Repair Male Perineum, Open Approach
0WQ50ZZ	Repair Lower Jaw, Open Approach		*AHA CC: 4Q, 2014, 38-39; 3Q, 2014, 28-29; 3Q, 2016, 6; 3Q, 2017, 8-9*	♂ 0WQM3ZZ	Repair Male Perineum, Percutaneous Approach
0WQ53ZZ	Repair Lower Jaw, Percutaneous Approach	0WQF3ZZ	Repair Abdominal Wall, Percutaneous Approach	♂ 0WQM4ZZ	Repair Male Perineum, Percutaneous Endoscopic Approach
0WQ54ZZ	Repair Lower Jaw, Percutaneous Endoscopic Approach	0WQF4ZZ	Repair Abdominal Wall, Percutaneous Endoscopic Approach	♂ 0WQMXZZ	Repair Male Perineum, External Approach
0WQ5XZZ	Repair Lower Jaw, External Approach	0WQFXZ2	Repair Abdominal Wall, Stoma, External Approach	♀ 0WQN0ZZ	Repair Female Perineum, Open Approach
0WQ60ZZ	Repair Neck, Open Approach	0WQFXZZ	Repair Abdominal Wall, External Approach	♀ 0WQN3ZZ	Repair Female Perineum, Percutaneous Approach
0WQ63ZZ	Repair Neck, Percutaneous Approach	0WQK0ZZ	Repair Upper Back, Open Approach	♀ 0WQN4ZZ	Repair Female Perineum, Percutaneous Endoscopic Approach
0WQ64ZZ	Repair Neck, Percutaneous Endoscopic Approach	0WQK3ZZ	Repair Upper Back, Percutaneous Approach	♀ 0WQNXZZ	Repair Female Perineum, External Approach
0WQ6XZ2	Repair Neck, Stoma, External Approach	0WQK4ZZ	Repair Upper Back, Percutaneous Endoscopic Approach		
0WQ6XZZ	Repair Neck, External Approach				
0WQ80ZZ	Repair Chest Wall, Open Approach				
0WQ83ZZ	Repair Chest Wall, Percutaneous Approach				

0WU – Anatomical Regions, General, Supplement

0WU007Z	Supplement Head with Autologous Tissue Substitute, Open Approach	0WU44KZ	Supplement Upper Jaw with Nonautologous Tissue Substitute, Percutaneous Endoscopic Approach	0WU847Z	Supplement Chest Wall with Autologous Tissue Substitute, Percutaneous Endoscopic Approach
0WU00JZ	Supplement Head with Synthetic Substitute, Open Approach	0WU507Z	Supplement Lower Jaw with Autologous Tissue Substitute, Open Approach	0WU84JZ	Supplement Chest Wall with Synthetic Substitute, Percutaneous Endoscopic Approach
0WU00KZ	Supplement Head with Nonautologous Tissue Substitute, Open Approach	0WU50JZ	Supplement Lower Jaw with Synthetic Substitute, Open Approach	0WU84KZ	Supplement Chest Wall with Nonautologous Tissue Substitute, Percutaneous Endoscopic Approach
0WU047Z	Supplement Head with Autologous Tissue Substitute, Percutaneous Endoscopic Approach	0WU50KZ	Supplement Lower Jaw with Nonautologous Tissue Substitute, Open Approach	0WUC07Z	Supplement Mediastinum with Autologous Tissue Substitute, Open Approach
0WU04JZ	Supplement Head with Synthetic Substitute, Percutaneous Endoscopic Approach	0WU547Z	Supplement Lower Jaw with Autologous Tissue Substitute, Percutaneous Endoscopic Approach	0WUC0JZ	Supplement Mediastinum with Synthetic Substitute, Open Approach
0WU04KZ	Supplement Head with Nonautologous Tissue Substitute, Percutaneous Endoscopic Approach	0WU54JZ	Supplement Lower Jaw with Synthetic Substitute, Percutaneous Endoscopic Approach	0WUC0KZ	Supplement Mediastinum with Nonautologous Tissue Substitute, Open Approach
0WU207Z	Supplement Face with Autologous Tissue Substitute, Open Approach	0WU54KZ	Supplement Lower Jaw with Nonautologous Tissue Substitute, Percutaneous Endoscopic Approach	0WUC47Z	Supplement Mediastinum with Autologous Tissue Substitute, Percutaneous Endoscopic Approach
0WU20JZ	Supplement Face with Synthetic Substitute, Open Approach	0WU607Z	Supplement Neck with Autologous Tissue Substitute, Open Approach	0WUC4JZ	Supplement Mediastinum with Synthetic Substitute, Percutaneous Endoscopic Approach
0WU20KZ	Supplement Face with Nonautologous Tissue Substitute, Open Approach	0WU60JZ	Supplement Neck with Synthetic Substitute, Open Approach	0WUC4KZ	Supplement Mediastinum with Nonautologous Tissue Substitute, Percutaneous Endoscopic Approach
0WU247Z	Supplement Face with Autologous Tissue Substitute, Percutaneous Endoscopic Approach	0WU60KZ	Supplement Neck with Nonautologous Tissue Substitute, Open Approach	0WUF07Z	Supplement Abdominal Wall with Autologous Tissue Substitute, Open Approach
0WU24JZ	Supplement Face with Synthetic Substitute, Percutaneous Endoscopic Approach	0WU647Z	Supplement Neck with Autologous Tissue Substitute, Percutaneous Endoscopic Approach		*AHA CC: 3Q, 2016, 40-41*
0WU24KZ	Supplement Face with Nonautologous Tissue Substitute, Percutaneous Endoscopic Approach	0WU64JZ	Supplement Neck with Synthetic Substitute, Percutaneous Endoscopic Approach	0WUF0JZ	Supplement Abdominal Wall with Synthetic Substitute, Open Approach
0WU407Z	Supplement Upper Jaw with Autologous Tissue Substitute, Open Approach	0WU64KZ	Supplement Neck with Nonautologous Tissue Substitute, Percutaneous Endoscopic Approach		*AHA CC: 4Q, 2014, 39-40; 3Q, 2017, 8*
0WU40JZ	Supplement Upper Jaw with Synthetic Substitute, Open Approach			0WUF0KZ	Supplement Abdominal Wall with Nonautologous Tissue Substitute, Open Approach
0WU40KZ	Supplement Upper Jaw with Nonautologous Tissue Substitute, Open Approach	0WU807Z	Supplement Chest Wall with Autologous Tissue Substitute, Open Approach	0WUF47Z	Supplement Abdominal Wall with Autologous Tissue Substitute, Percutaneous Endoscopic Approach
0WU447Z	Supplement Upper Jaw with Autologous Tissue Substitute, Percutaneous Endoscopic Approach	0WU80JZ	Supplement Chest Wall with Synthetic Substitute, Open Approach	0WUF4JZ	Supplement Abdominal Wall with Synthetic Substitute, Percutaneous Endoscopic Approach
0WU44JZ	Supplement Upper Jaw with Synthetic Substitute, Percutaneous Endoscopic Approach		*AHA CC: 4Q, 2012, 101-102*	0WUF4KZ	Supplement Abdominal Wall with Nonautologous Tissue Substitute, Percutaneous Endoscopic Approach
		0WU80KZ	Supplement Chest Wall with Nonautologous Tissue Substitute, Open Approach		

♀ Female-only   ♂ Male-only   ▲ Limited Coverage   ● Non-OR   HAC HAC-associated procedure   ▲ Non-covered procedures   ✛ Cluster

0WUK07Z Supplement Upper Back with Autologous Tissue Substitute, Open Approach
0WUK0JZ Supplement Upper Back with Synthetic Substitute, Open Approach
0WUK0KZ Supplement Upper Back with Nonautologous Tissue Substitute, Open Approach
0WUK47Z Supplement Upper Back with Autologous Tissue Substitute, Percutaneous Endoscopic Approach
0WUK4JZ Supplement Upper Back with Synthetic Substitute, Percutaneous Endoscopic Approach
0WUK4KZ Supplement Upper Back with Nonautologous Tissue Substitute, Percutaneous Endoscopic Approach
0WUL07Z Supplement Lower Back with Autologous Tissue Substitute, Open Approach
0WUL0JZ Supplement Lower Back with Synthetic Substitute, Open Approach

0WUL0KZ Supplement Lower Back with Nonautologous Tissue Substitute, Open Approach
0WUL47Z Supplement Lower Back with Autologous Tissue Substitute, Percutaneous Endoscopic Approach
0WUL4JZ Supplement Lower Back with Synthetic Substitute, Percutaneous Endoscopic Approach
0WUL4KZ Supplement Lower Back with Nonautologous Tissue Substitute, Percutaneous Endoscopic Approach
♂ 0WUM07Z Supplement Male Perineum with Autologous Tissue Substitute, Open Approach
♂ 0WUM0JZ Supplement Male Perineum with Synthetic Substitute, Open Approach
♂ 0WUM0KZ Supplement Male Perineum with Nonautologous Tissue Substitute, Open Approach
♂ 0WUM47Z Supplement Male Perineum with Autologous Tissue Substitute, Percutaneous Endoscopic Approach

♂ 0WUM4JZ Supplement Male Perineum with Synthetic Substitute, Percutaneous Endoscopic Approach
♂ 0WUM4KZ Supplement Male Perineum with Nonautologous Tissue Substitute, Percutaneous Endoscopic Approach
♀ 0WUN07Z Supplement Female Perineum with Autologous Tissue Substitute, Open Approach
♀ 0WUN0JZ Supplement Female Perineum with Synthetic Substitute, Open Approach
♀ 0WUN0KZ Supplement Female Perineum with Nonautologous Tissue Substitute, Open Approach
♀ 0WUN47Z Supplement Female Perineum with Autologous Tissue Substitute, Percutaneous Endoscopic Approach
♀ 0WUN4JZ Supplement Female Perineum with Synthetic Substitute, Percutaneous Endoscopic Approach
♀ 0WUN4KZ Supplement Female Perineum with Nonautologous Tissue Substitute, Percutaneous Endoscopic Approach

0WW – Anatomical Regions, General, Revision

Review Coding Guideline B6.1c

● 0WW000Z Revision of Drainage Device in Head, Open Approach
● 0WW001Z Revision of Radioactive Element in Head, Open Approach
● 0WW003Z Revision of Infusion Device in Head, Open Approach
● 0WW007Z Revision of Autologous Tissue Substitute in Head, Open Approach
● 0WW00JZ Revision of Synthetic Substitute in Head, Open Approach
● 0WW00KZ Revision of Nonautologous Tissue Substitute in Head, Open Approach
● 0WW00YZ Revision of Other Device in Head, Open Approach
● 0WW030Z Revision of Drainage Device in Head, Percutaneous Approach
● 0WW031Z Revision of Radioactive Element in Head, Percutaneous Approach
● 0WW033Z Revision of Infusion Device in Head, Percutaneous Approach
● 0WW037Z Revision of Autologous Tissue Substitute in Head, Percutaneous Approach
● 0WW03JZ Revision of Synthetic Substitute in Head, Percutaneous Approach
● 0WW03KZ Revision of Nonautologous Tissue Substitute in Head, Percutaneous Approach
● 0WW03YZ Revision of Other Device in Head, Percutaneous Approach
● 0WW040Z Revision of Drainage Device in Head, Percutaneous Endoscopic Approach
● 0WW041Z Revision of Radioactive Element in Head, Percutaneous Endoscopic Approach
● 0WW043Z Revision of Infusion Device in Head, Percutaneous Endoscopic Approach
● 0WW047Z Revision of Autologous Tissue Substitute in Head, Percutaneous Endoscopic Approach
● 0WW04JZ Revision of Synthetic Substitute in Head, Percutaneous Endoscopic Approach
● 0WW04KZ Revision of Nonautologous Tissue Substitute in Head, Percutaneous Endoscopic Approach

● 0WW04YZ Revision of Other Device in Head, Percutaneous Endoscopic Approach
0WW0X0Z Revision of Drainage Device in Head, External Approach
0WW0X1Z Revision of Radioactive Element in Head, External Approach
0WW0X3Z Revision of Infusion Device in Head, External Approach
0WW0X7Z Revision of Autologous Tissue Substitute in Head, External Approach
0WW0XJZ Revision of Synthetic Substitute in Head, External Approach
0WW0XKZ Revision of Nonautologous Tissue Substitute in Head, External Approach
0WW0XYZ Revision of Other Device in Head, External Approach
0WW100Z Revision of Drainage Device in Cranial Cavity, Open Approach
0WW101Z Revision of Radioactive Element in Cranial Cavity, Open Approach
0WW103Z Revision of Infusion Device in Cranial Cavity, Open Approach
0WW10JZ Revision of Synthetic Substitute in Cranial Cavity, Open Approach
0WW10YZ Revision of Other Device in Cranial Cavity, Open Approach
0WW130Z Revision of Drainage Device in Cranial Cavity, Percutaneous Approach
0WW131Z Revision of Radioactive Element in Cranial Cavity, Percutaneous Approach
0WW133Z Revision of Infusion Device in Cranial Cavity, Percutaneous Approach
0WW13JZ Revision of Synthetic Substitute in Cranial Cavity, Percutaneous Approach
0WW13YZ Revision of Other Device in Cranial Cavity, Percutaneous Approach
0WW140Z Revision of Drainage Device in Cranial Cavity, Percutaneous Endoscopic Approach
0WW141Z Revision of Radioactive Element in Cranial Cavity, Percutaneous Endoscopic Approach

0WW143Z Revision of Infusion Device in Cranial Cavity, Percutaneous Endoscopic Approach
0WW14JZ Revision of Synthetic Substitute in Cranial Cavity, Percutaneous Endoscopic Approach
0WW14YZ Revision of Other Device in Cranial Cavity, Percutaneous Endoscopic Approach
0WW1X0Z Revision of Drainage Device in Cranial Cavity, External Approach
0WW1X1Z Revision of Radioactive Element in Cranial Cavity, External Approach
0WW1X3Z Revision of Infusion Device in Cranial Cavity, External Approach
0WW1XJZ Revision of Synthetic Substitute in Cranial Cavity, External Approach
0WW1XYZ Revision of Other Device in Cranial Cavity, External Approach
● 0WW200Z Revision of Drainage Device in Face, Open Approach
● 0WW201Z Revision of Radioactive Element in Face, Open Approach
● 0WW203Z Revision of Infusion Device in Face, Open Approach
● 0WW207Z Revision of Autologous Tissue Substitute in Face, Open Approach
● 0WW20JZ Revision of Synthetic Substitute in Face, Open Approach
● 0WW20KZ Revision of Nonautologous Tissue Substitute in Face, Open Approach
● 0WW20YZ Revision of Other Device in Face, Open Approach
● 0WW230Z Revision of Drainage Device in Face, Percutaneous Approach
● 0WW231Z Revision of Radioactive Element in Face, Percutaneous Approach
● 0WW233Z Revision of Infusion Device in Face, Percutaneous Approach
● 0WW237Z Revision of Autologous Tissue Substitute in Face, Percutaneous Approach
● 0WW23JZ Revision of Synthetic Substitute in Face, Percutaneous Approach
● 0WW23KZ Revision of Nonautologous Tissue Substitute in Face, Percutaneous Approach

● **0WW23YZ** Revision of Other Device in Face, Percutaneous Approach

● **0WW240Z** Revision of Drainage Device in Face, Percutaneous Endoscopic Approach

● **0WW241Z** Revision of Radioactive Element in Face, Percutaneous Endoscopic Approach

● **0WW243Z** Revision of Infusion Device in Face, Percutaneous Endoscopic Approach

● **0WW247Z** Revision of Autologous Tissue Substitute in Face, Percutaneous Endoscopic Approach

● **0WW24JZ** Revision of Synthetic Substitute in Face, Percutaneous Endoscopic Approach

● **0WW24KZ** Revision of Nonautologous Tissue Substitute in Face, Percutaneous Endoscopic Approach

● **0WW24YZ** Revision of Other Device in Face, Percutaneous Endoscopic Approach

0WW2X0Z Revision of Drainage Device in Face, External Approach

0WW2X1Z Revision of Radioactive Element in Face, External Approach

0WW2X3Z Revision of Infusion Device in Face, External Approach

0WW2X7Z Revision of Autologous Tissue Substitute in Face, External Approach

0WW2XJZ Revision of Synthetic Substitute in Face, External Approach

0WW2XKZ Revision of Nonautologous Tissue Substitute in Face, External Approach

0WW2XYZ Revision of Other Device in Face, External Approach

● **0WW400Z** Revision of Drainage Device in Upper Jaw, Open Approach

● **0WW401Z** Revision of Radioactive Element in Upper Jaw, Open Approach

● **0WW403Z** Revision of Infusion Device in Upper Jaw, Open Approach

● **0WW407Z** Revision of Autologous Tissue Substitute in Upper Jaw, Open Approach

● **0WW40JZ** Revision of Synthetic Substitute in Upper Jaw, Open Approach

● **0WW40KZ** Revision of Nonautologous Tissue Substitute in Upper Jaw, Open Approach

● **0WW40YZ** Revision of Other Device in Upper Jaw, Open Approach

● **0WW430Z** Revision of Drainage Device in Upper Jaw, Percutaneous Approach

● **0WW431Z** Revision of Radioactive Element in Upper Jaw, Percutaneous Approach

● **0WW433Z** Revision of Infusion Device in Upper Jaw, Percutaneous Approach

● **0WW437Z** Revision of Autologous Tissue Substitute in Upper Jaw, Percutaneous Approach

● **0WW43JZ** Revision of Synthetic Substitute in Upper Jaw, Percutaneous Approach

● **0WW43KZ** Revision of Nonautologous Tissue Substitute in Upper Jaw, Percutaneous Approach

● **0WW43YZ** Revision of Other Device in Upper Jaw, Percutaneous Approach

● **0WW440Z** Revision of Drainage Device in Upper Jaw, Percutaneous Endoscopic Approach

● **0WW441Z** Revision of Radioactive Element in Upper Jaw, Percutaneous Endoscopic Approach

● **0WW443Z** Revision of Infusion Device in Upper Jaw, Percutaneous Endoscopic Approach

● **0WW447Z** Revision of Autologous Tissue Substitute in Upper Jaw, Percutaneous Endoscopic Approach

● **0WW44JZ** Revision of Synthetic Substitute in Upper Jaw, Percutaneous Endoscopic Approach

● **0WW44KZ** Revision of Nonautologous Tissue Substitute in Upper Jaw, Percutaneous Endoscopic Approach

● **0WW44YZ** Revision of Other Device in Upper Jaw, Percutaneous Endoscopic Approach

0WW4X0Z Revision of Drainage Device in Upper Jaw, External Approach

0WW4X1Z Revision of Radioactive Element in Upper Jaw, External Approach

0WW4X3Z Revision of Infusion Device in Upper Jaw, External Approach

0WW4X7Z Revision of Autologous Tissue Substitute in Upper Jaw, External Approach

0WW4XJZ Revision of Synthetic Substitute in Upper Jaw, External Approach

0WW4XKZ Revision of Nonautologous Tissue Substitute in Upper Jaw, External Approach

0WW4XYZ Revision of Other Device in Upper Jaw, External Approach

● **0WW500Z** Revision of Drainage Device in Lower Jaw, Open Approach

● **0WW501Z** Revision of Radioactive Element in Lower Jaw, Open Approach

● **0WW503Z** Revision of Infusion Device in Lower Jaw, Open Approach

● **0WW507Z** Revision of Autologous Tissue Substitute in Lower Jaw, Open Approach

● **0WW50JZ** Revision of Synthetic Substitute in Lower Jaw, Open Approach

● **0WW50KZ** Revision of Nonautologous Tissue Substitute in Lower Jaw, Open Approach

● **0WW50YZ** Revision of Other Device in Lower Jaw, Open Approach

● **0WW530Z** Revision of Drainage Device in Lower Jaw, Percutaneous Approach

● **0WW531Z** Revision of Radioactive Element in Lower Jaw, Percutaneous Approach

● **0WW533Z** Revision of Infusion Device in Lower Jaw, Percutaneous Approach

● **0WW537Z** Revision of Autologous Tissue Substitute in Lower Jaw, Percutaneous Approach

● **0WW53JZ** Revision of Synthetic Substitute in Lower Jaw, Percutaneous Approach

● **0WW53KZ** Revision of Nonautologous Tissue Substitute in Lower Jaw, Percutaneous Approach

● **0WW53YZ** Revision of Other Device in Lower Jaw, Percutaneous Approach

● **0WW540Z** Revision of Drainage Device in Lower Jaw, Percutaneous Endoscopic Approach

● **0WW541Z** Revision of Radioactive Element in Lower Jaw, Percutaneous Endoscopic Approach

● **0WW543Z** Revision of Infusion Device in Lower Jaw, Percutaneous Endoscopic Approach

● **0WW547Z** Revision of Autologous Tissue Substitute in Lower Jaw, Percutaneous Endoscopic Approach

● **0WW54JZ** Revision of Synthetic Substitute in Lower Jaw, Percutaneous Endoscopic Approach

● **0WW54KZ** Revision of Nonautologous Tissue Substitute in Lower Jaw, Percutaneous Endoscopic Approach

● **0WW54YZ** Revision of Other Device in Lower Jaw, Percutaneous Endoscopic Approach

0WW5X0Z Revision of Drainage Device in Lower Jaw, External Approach

0WW5X1Z Revision of Radioactive Element in Lower Jaw, External Approach

0WW5X3Z Revision of Infusion Device in Lower Jaw, External Approach

0WW5X7Z Revision of Autologous Tissue Substitute in Lower Jaw, External Approach

0WW5XJZ Revision of Synthetic Substitute in Lower Jaw, External Approach

0WW5XKZ Revision of Nonautologous Tissue Substitute in Lower Jaw, External Approach

0WW5XYZ Revision of Other Device in Lower Jaw, External Approach

● **0WW600Z** Revision of Drainage Device in Neck, Open Approach

● **0WW601Z** Revision of Radioactive Element in Neck, Open Approach

● **0WW603Z** Revision of Infusion Device in Neck, Open Approach

● **0WW607Z** Revision of Autologous Tissue Substitute in Neck, Open Approach

● **0WW60JZ** Revision of Synthetic Substitute in Neck, Open Approach

● **0WW60KZ** Revision of Nonautologous Tissue Substitute in Neck, Open Approach

● **0WW60YZ** Revision of Other Device in Neck, Open Approach

● **0WW630Z** Revision of Drainage Device in Neck, Percutaneous Approach

● **0WW631Z** Revision of Radioactive Element in Neck, Percutaneous Approach

● **0WW633Z** Revision of Infusion Device in Neck, Percutaneous Approach

● **0WW637Z** Revision of Autologous Tissue Substitute in Neck, Percutaneous Approach

● **0WW63JZ** Revision of Synthetic Substitute in Neck, Percutaneous Approach

● **0WW63KZ** Revision of Nonautologous Tissue Substitute in Neck, Percutaneous Approach

● **0WW63YZ** Revision of Other Device in Neck, Percutaneous Approach

● **0WW640Z** Revision of Drainage Device in Neck, Percutaneous Endoscopic Approach

● **0WW641Z** Revision of Radioactive Element in Neck, Percutaneous Endoscopic Approach

● **0WW643Z** Revision of Infusion Device in Neck, Percutaneous Endoscopic Approach

● **0WW647Z** Revision of Autologous Tissue Substitute in Neck, Percutaneous Endoscopic Approach

● **0WW64JZ** Revision of Synthetic Substitute in Neck, Percutaneous Endoscopic Approach

● **0WW64KZ** Revision of Nonautologous Tissue Substitute in Neck, Percutaneous Endoscopic Approach

● **0WW64YZ** Revision of Other Device in Neck, Percutaneous Endoscopic Approach

0WW6X0Z Revision of Drainage Device in Neck, External Approach

0WW6X1Z Revision of Radioactive Element in Neck, External Approach

0WW6X3Z Revision of Infusion Device in Neck, External Approach

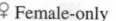 ♀ Female-only   ♂ Male-only   ▲ Limited Coverage   ● Non-OR   **HAC** HAC-associated procedure   ▲ Non-covered procedures   ✚ Cluster

0WW6X7Z Revision of Autologous Tissue Substitute in Neck, External Approach

0WW6XJZ Revision of Synthetic Substitute in Neck, External Approach

0WW6XKZ Revision of Nonautologous Tissue Substitute in Neck, External Approach

0WW6XYZ Revision of Other Device in Neck, External Approach

0WW800Z Revision of Drainage Device in Chest Wall, Open Approach

0WW801Z Revision of Radioactive Element in Chest Wall, Open Approach

0WW803Z Revision of Infusion Device in Chest Wall, Open Approach

0WW807Z Revision of Autologous Tissue Substitute in Chest Wall, Open Approach

0WW80JZ Revision of Synthetic Substitute in Chest Wall, Open Approach

0WW80KZ Revision of Nonautologous Tissue Substitute in Chest Wall, Open Approach

0WW80YZ Revision of Other Device in Chest Wall, Open Approach

0WW830Z Revision of Drainage Device in Chest Wall, Percutaneous Approach

0WW831Z Revision of Radioactive Element in Chest Wall, Percutaneous Approach

0WW833Z Revision of Infusion Device in Chest Wall, Percutaneous Approach

0WW837Z Revision of Autologous Tissue Substitute in Chest Wall, Percutaneous Approach

0WW83JZ Revision of Synthetic Substitute in Chest Wall, Percutaneous Approach

0WW83KZ Revision of Nonautologous Tissue Substitute in Chest Wall, Percutaneous Approach

0WW83YZ Revision of Other Device in Chest Wall, Percutaneous Approach

0WW840Z Revision of Drainage Device in Chest Wall, Percutaneous Endoscopic Approach

0WW841Z Revision of Radioactive Element in Chest Wall, Percutaneous Endoscopic Approach

0WW843Z Revision of Infusion Device in Chest Wall, Percutaneous Endoscopic Approach

0WW847Z Revision of Autologous Tissue Substitute in Chest Wall, Percutaneous Endoscopic Approach

0WW84JZ Revision of Synthetic Substitute in Chest Wall, Percutaneous Endoscopic Approach

0WW84KZ Revision of Nonautologous Tissue Substitute in Chest Wall, Percutaneous Endoscopic Approach

0WW84YZ Revision of Other Device in Chest Wall, Percutaneous Endoscopic Approach

0WW8X0Z Revision of Drainage Device in Chest Wall, External Approach

0WW8X1Z Revision of Radioactive Element in Chest Wall, External Approach

0WW8X3Z Revision of Infusion Device in Chest Wall, External Approach

0WW8X7Z Revision of Autologous Tissue Substitute in Chest Wall, External Approach

0WW8XJZ Revision of Synthetic Substitute in Chest Wall, External Approach

0WW8XKZ Revision of Nonautologous Tissue Substitute in Chest Wall, External Approach

0WW8XYZ Revision of Other Device in Chest Wall, External Approach

0WW900Z Revision of Drainage Device in Right Pleural Cavity, Open Approach

0WW901Z Revision of Radioactive Element in Right Pleural Cavity, Open Approach

0WW903Z Revision of Infusion Device in Right Pleural Cavity, Open Approach

0WW90JZ Revision of Synthetic Substitute in Right Pleural Cavity, Open Approach

0WW90YZ Revision of Other Device in Right Pleural Cavity, Open Approach

0WW930Z Revision of Drainage Device in Right Pleural Cavity, Percutaneous Approach

0WW931Z Revision of Radioactive Element in Right Pleural Cavity, Percutaneous Approach

0WW933Z Revision of Infusion Device in Right Pleural Cavity, Percutaneous Approach

0WW93JZ Revision of Synthetic Substitute in Right Pleural Cavity, Percutaneous Approach

0WW93YZ Revision of Other Device in Right Pleural Cavity, Percutaneous Approach

0WW940Z Revision of Drainage Device in Right Pleural Cavity, Percutaneous Endoscopic Approach

0WW941Z Revision of Radioactive Element in Right Pleural Cavity, Percutaneous Endoscopic Approach

0WW943Z Revision of Infusion Device in Right Pleural Cavity, Percutaneous Endoscopic Approach

0WW94JZ Revision of Synthetic Substitute in Right Pleural Cavity, Percutaneous Endoscopic Approach

0WW94YZ Revision of Other Device in Right Pleural Cavity, Percutaneous Endoscopic Approach

0WW9X0Z Revision of Drainage Device in Right Pleural Cavity, External Approach

0WW9X1Z Revision of Radioactive Element in Right Pleural Cavity, External Approach

0WW9X3Z Revision of Infusion Device in Right Pleural Cavity, External Approach

0WW9XJZ Revision of Synthetic Substitute in Right Pleural Cavity, External Approach

0WW9XYZ Revision of Other Device in Right Pleural Cavity, External Approach

0WWB00Z Revision of Drainage Device in Left Pleural Cavity, Open Approach

0WWB01Z Revision of Radioactive Element in Left Pleural Cavity, Open Approach

0WWB03Z Revision of Infusion Device in Left Pleural Cavity, Open Approach

0WWB0JZ Revision of Synthetic Substitute in Left Pleural Cavity, Open Approach

0WWB0YZ Revision of Other Device in Left Pleural Cavity, Open Approach

0WWB30Z Revision of Drainage Device in Left Pleural Cavity, Percutaneous Approach

0WWB31Z Revision of Radioactive Element in Left Pleural Cavity, Percutaneous Approach

0WWB33Z Revision of Infusion Device in Left Pleural Cavity, Percutaneous Approach

0WWB3JZ Revision of Synthetic Substitute in Left Pleural Cavity, Percutaneous Approach

0WWB3YZ Revision of Other Device in Left Pleural Cavity, Percutaneous Approach

0WWB40Z Revision of Drainage Device in Left Pleural Cavity, Percutaneous Endoscopic Approach

0WWB41Z Revision of Radioactive Element in Left Pleural Cavity, Percutaneous Endoscopic Approach

0WWB43Z Revision of Infusion Device in Left Pleural Cavity, Percutaneous Endoscopic Approach

0WWB4JZ Revision of Synthetic Substitute in Left Pleural Cavity, Percutaneous Endoscopic Approach

0WWB4YZ Revision of Other Device in Left Pleural Cavity, Percutaneous Endoscopic Approach

0WWBX0Z Revision of Drainage Device in Left Pleural Cavity, External Approach

0WWBX1Z Revision of Radioactive Element in Left Pleural Cavity, External Approach

0WWBX3Z Revision of Infusion Device in Left Pleural Cavity, External Approach

0WWBXJZ Revision of Synthetic Substitute in Left Pleural Cavity, External Approach

0WWBXYZ Revision of Other Device in Left Pleural Cavity, External Approach

0WWC00Z Revision of Drainage Device in Mediastinum, Open Approach

0WWC01Z Revision of Radioactive Element in Mediastinum, Open Approach

0WWC03Z Revision of Infusion Device in Mediastinum, Open Approach

0WWC07Z Revision of Autologous Tissue Substitute in Mediastinum, Open Approach

0WWC0JZ Revision of Synthetic Substitute in Mediastinum, Open Approach

0WWC0KZ Revision of Nonautologous Tissue Substitute in Mediastinum, Open Approach

0WWC0YZ Revision of Other Device in Mediastinum, Open Approach

0WWC30Z Revision of Drainage Device in Mediastinum, Percutaneous Approach

0WWC31Z Revision of Radioactive Element in Mediastinum, Percutaneous Approach

0WWC33Z Revision of Infusion Device in Mediastinum, Percutaneous Approach

0WWC37Z Revision of Autologous Tissue Substitute in Mediastinum, Percutaneous Approach

0WWC3JZ Revision of Synthetic Substitute in Mediastinum, Percutaneous Approach

0WWC3KZ Revision of Nonautologous Tissue Substitute in Mediastinum, Percutaneous Approach

0WWC3YZ Revision of Other Device in Mediastinum, Percutaneous Approach

0WWC40Z Revision of Drainage Device in Mediastinum, Percutaneous Endoscopic Approach

0WWC41Z Revision of Radioactive Element in Mediastinum, Percutaneous Endoscopic Approach

0WWC43Z Revision of Infusion Device in Mediastinum, Percutaneous Endoscopic Approach

0WWC47Z Revision of Autologous Tissue Substitute in Mediastinum, Percutaneous Endoscopic Approach

0WWC4JZ Revision of Synthetic Substitute in Mediastinum, Percutaneous Endoscopic Approach

0WWC4KZ Revision of Nonautologous Tissue Substitute in Mediastinum, Percutaneous Endoscopic Approach

0WWC4YZ Revision of Other Device in Mediastinum, Percutaneous Endoscopic Approach

0WWCX0Z Revision of Drainage Device in Mediastinum, External Approach

0WWCX1Z Revision of Radioactive Element in Mediastinum, External Approach

0WWCX3Z Revision of Infusion Device in Mediastinum, External Approach

0WWCX7Z Revision of Autologous Tissue Substitute in Mediastinum, External Approach

0WWCXJZ Revision of Synthetic Substitute in Mediastinum, External Approach

0WWCXKZ Revision of Nonautologous Tissue Substitute in Mediastinum, External Approach

0WWCXYZ Revision of Other Device in Mediastinum, External Approach

0WWD00Z Revision of Drainage Device in Pericardial Cavity, Open Approach

0WWD01Z Revision of Radioactive Element in Pericardial Cavity, Open Approach

0WWD03Z Revision of Infusion Device in Pericardial Cavity, Open Approach

0WWD0YZ Revision of Other Device in Pericardial Cavity, Open Approach

0WWD30Z Revision of Drainage Device in Pericardial Cavity, Percutaneous Approach

0WWD31Z Revision of Radioactive Element in Pericardial Cavity, Percutaneous Approach

0WWD33Z Revision of Infusion Device in Pericardial Cavity, Percutaneous Approach

0WWD3YZ Revision of Other Device in Pericardial Cavity, Percutaneous Approach

0WWD40Z Revision of Drainage Device in Pericardial Cavity, Percutaneous Endoscopic Approach

0WWD41Z Revision of Radioactive Element in Pericardial Cavity, Percutaneous Endoscopic Approach

0WWD43Z Revision of Infusion Device in Pericardial Cavity, Percutaneous Endoscopic Approach

0WWD4YZ Revision of Other Device in Pericardial Cavity, Percutaneous Endoscopic Approach

0WWDX0Z Revision of Drainage Device in Pericardial Cavity, External Approach

0WWDX1Z Revision of Radioactive Element in Pericardial Cavity, External Approach

0WWDX3Z Revision of Infusion Device in Pericardial Cavity, External Approach

0WWDXYZ Revision of Other Device in Pericardial Cavity, External Approach

0WWF00Z Revision of Drainage Device in Abdominal Wall, Open Approach

0WWF01Z Revision of Radioactive Element in Abdominal Wall, Open Approach

0WWF03Z Revision of Infusion Device in Abdominal Wall, Open Approach

0WWF07Z Revision of Autologous Tissue Substitute in Abdominal Wall, Open Approach

0WWF0JZ Revision of Synthetic Substitute in Abdominal Wall, Open Approach

0WWF0KZ Revision of Nonautologous Tissue Substitute in Abdominal Wall, Open Approach

0WWF0YZ Revision of Other Device in Abdominal Wall, Open Approach

0WWF30Z Revision of Drainage Device in Abdominal Wall, Percutaneous Approach

0WWF31Z Revision of Radioactive Element in Abdominal Wall, Percutaneous Approach

0WWF33Z Revision of Infusion Device in Abdominal Wall, Percutaneous Approach

0WWF37Z Revision of Autologous Tissue Substitute in Abdominal Wall, Percutaneous Approach

0WWF3JZ Revision of Synthetic Substitute in Abdominal Wall, Percutaneous Approach

0WWF3KZ Revision of Nonautologous Tissue Substitute in Abdominal Wall, Percutaneous Approach

0WWF3YZ Revision of Other Device in Abdominal Wall, Percutaneous Approach

0WWF40Z Revision of Drainage Device in Abdominal Wall, Percutaneous Endoscopic Approach

0WWF41Z Revision of Radioactive Element in Abdominal Wall, Percutaneous Endoscopic Approach

0WWF43Z Revision of Infusion Device in Abdominal Wall, Percutaneous Endoscopic Approach

0WWF47Z Revision of Autologous Tissue Substitute in Abdominal Wall, Percutaneous Endoscopic Approach

0WWF4JZ Revision of Synthetic Substitute in Abdominal Wall, Percutaneous Endoscopic Approach

0WWF4KZ Revision of Nonautologous Tissue Substitute in Abdominal Wall, Percutaneous Endoscopic Approach

0WWF4YZ Revision of Other Device in Abdominal Wall, Percutaneous Endoscopic Approach

0WWFX0Z Revision of Drainage Device in Abdominal Wall, External Approach

0WWFX1Z Revision of Radioactive Element in Abdominal Wall, External Approach

0WWFX3Z Revision of Infusion Device in Abdominal Wall, External Approach

0WWFX7Z Revision of Autologous Tissue Substitute in Abdominal Wall, External Approach

0WWFXJZ Revision of Synthetic Substitute in Abdominal Wall, External Approach

0WWFXKZ Revision of Nonautologous Tissue Substitute in Abdominal Wall, External Approach

0WWFXYZ Revision of Other Device in Abdominal Wall, External Approach

0WWG00Z Revision of Drainage Device in Peritoneal Cavity, Open Approach

0WWG01Z Revision of Radioactive Element in Peritoneal Cavity, Open Approach

0WWG03Z Revision of Infusion Device in Peritoneal Cavity, Open Approach

0WWG0JZ Revision of Synthetic Substitute in Peritoneal Cavity, Open Approach

0WWG0YZ Revision of Other Device in Peritoneal Cavity, Open Approach

0WWG30Z Revision of Drainage Device in Peritoneal Cavity, Percutaneous Approach

0WWG31Z Revision of Radioactive Element in Peritoneal Cavity, Percutaneous Approach

0WWG33Z Revision of Infusion Device in Peritoneal Cavity, Percutaneous Approach

0WWG3JZ Revision of Synthetic Substitute in Peritoneal Cavity, Percutaneous Approach

0WWG3YZ Revision of Other Device in Peritoneal Cavity, Percutaneous Approach

0WWG40Z Revision of Drainage Device in Peritoneal Cavity, Percutaneous Endoscopic Approach

0WWG41Z Revision of Radioactive Element in Peritoneal Cavity, Percutaneous Endoscopic Approach

0WWG43Z Revision of Infusion Device in Peritoneal Cavity, Percutaneous Endoscopic Approach

0WWG4JZ Revision of Synthetic Substitute in Peritoneal Cavity, Percutaneous Endoscopic Approach

AHA CC: 2Q, 2015, 9-10

0WWG4YZ Revision of Other Device in Peritoneal Cavity, Percutaneous Endoscopic Approach

0WWGX0Z Revision of Drainage Device in Peritoneal Cavity, External Approach

0WWGX1Z Revision of Radioactive Element in Peritoneal Cavity, External Approach

0WWGX3Z Revision of Infusion Device in Peritoneal Cavity, External Approach

0WWGXJZ Revision of Synthetic Substitute in Peritoneal Cavity, External Approach

0WWGXYZ Revision of Other Device in Peritoneal Cavity, External Approach

0WWH00Z Revision of Drainage Device in Retroperitoneum, Open Approach

0WWH01Z Revision of Radioactive Element in Retroperitoneum, Open Approach

0WWH03Z Revision of Infusion Device in Retroperitoneum, Open Approach

0WWH0YZ Revision of Other Device in Retroperitoneum, Open Approach

0WWH30Z Revision of Drainage Device in Retroperitoneum, Percutaneous Approach

0WWH31Z Revision of Radioactive Element in Retroperitoneum, Percutaneous Approach

0WWH33Z Revision of Infusion Device in Retroperitoneum, Percutaneous Approach

0WWH3YZ Revision of Other Device in Retroperitoneum, Percutaneous Approach

0WWH40Z Revision of Drainage Device in Retroperitoneum, Percutaneous Endoscopic Approach

0WWH41Z Revision of Radioactive Element in Retroperitoneum, Percutaneous Endoscopic Approach

♀ Female-only   ♂ Male-only   ▲ Limited Coverage   ● Non-OR   HAC HAC-associated procedure   ▲ Non-covered procedures   ✚ Cluster

0WWH43Z	Revision of Infusion Device in Retroperitoneum, Percutaneous Endoscopic Approach
0WWH4YZ	Revision of Other Device in Retroperitoneum, Percutaneous Endoscopic Approach
0WWHX0Z	Revision of Drainage Device in Retroperitoneum, External Approach
0WWHX1Z	Revision of Radioactive Element in Retroperitoneum, External Approach
0WWHX3Z	Revision of Infusion Device in Retroperitoneum, External Approach
0WWHXYZ	Revision of Other Device in Retroperitoneum, External Approach
0WWJ00Z	Revision of Drainage Device in Pelvic Cavity, Open Approach
0WWJ01Z	Revision of Radioactive Element in Pelvic Cavity, Open Approach
0WWJ03Z	Revision of Infusion Device in Pelvic Cavity, Open Approach
0WWJ0JZ	Revision of Synthetic Substitute in Pelvic Cavity, Open Approach
0WWJ0YZ	Revision of Other Device in Pelvic Cavity, Open Approach
0WWJ30Z	Revision of Drainage Device in Pelvic Cavity, Percutaneous Approach
0WWJ31Z	Revision of Radioactive Element in Pelvic Cavity, Percutaneous Approach
0WWJ33Z	Revision of Infusion Device in Pelvic Cavity, Percutaneous Approach
0WWJ3JZ	Revision of Synthetic Substitute in Pelvic Cavity, Percutaneous Approach
0WWJ3YZ	Revision of Other Device in Pelvic Cavity, Percutaneous Approach
0WWJ40Z	Revision of Drainage Device in Pelvic Cavity, Percutaneous Endoscopic Approach
0WWJ41Z	Revision of Radioactive Element in Pelvic Cavity, Percutaneous Endoscopic Approach
0WWJ43Z	Revision of Infusion Device in Pelvic Cavity, Percutaneous Endoscopic Approach
0WWJ4JZ	Revision of Synthetic Substitute in Pelvic Cavity, Percutaneous Endoscopic Approach
0WWJ4YZ	Revision of Other Device in Pelvic Cavity, Percutaneous Endoscopic Approach
0WWJX0Z	Revision of Drainage Device in Pelvic Cavity, External Approach
0WWJX1Z	Revision of Radioactive Element in Pelvic Cavity, External Approach
0WWJX3Z	Revision of Infusion Device in Pelvic Cavity, External Approach
0WWJXJZ	Revision of Synthetic Substitute in Pelvic Cavity, External Approach
0WWJXYZ	Revision of Other Device in Pelvic Cavity, External Approach
● 0WWK00Z	Revision of Drainage Device in Upper Back, Open Approach
● 0WWK01Z	Revision of Radioactive Element in Upper Back, Open Approach
● 0WWK03Z	Revision of Infusion Device in Upper Back, Open Approach
● 0WWK07Z	Revision of Autologous Tissue Substitute in Upper Back, Open Approach
● 0WWK0JZ	Revision of Synthetic Substitute in Upper Back, Open Approach
● 0WWK0KZ	Revision of Nonautologous Tissue Substitute in Upper Back, Open Approach
● 0WWK0YZ	Revision of Other Device in Upper Back, Open Approach
● 0WWK30Z	Revision of Drainage Device in Upper Back, Percutaneous Approach
● 0WWK31Z	Revision of Radioactive Element in Upper Back, Percutaneous Approach
● 0WWK33Z	Revision of Infusion Device in Upper Back, Percutaneous Approach
● 0WWK37Z	Revision of Autologous Tissue Substitute in Upper Back, Percutaneous Approach
● 0WWK3JZ	Revision of Synthetic Substitute in Upper Back, Percutaneous Approach
● 0WWK3KZ	Revision of Nonautologous Tissue Substitute in Upper Back, Percutaneous Approach
● 0WWK3YZ	Revision of Other Device in Upper Back, Percutaneous Approach
● 0WWK40Z	Revision of Drainage Device in Upper Back, Percutaneous Endoscopic Approach
● 0WWK41Z	Revision of Radioactive Element in Upper Back, Percutaneous Endoscopic Approach
● 0WWK43Z	Revision of Infusion Device in Upper Back, Percutaneous Endoscopic Approach
● 0WWK47Z	Revision of Autologous Tissue Substitute in Upper Back, Percutaneous Endoscopic Approach
● 0WWK4JZ	Revision of Synthetic Substitute in Upper Back, Percutaneous Endoscopic Approach
● 0WWK4KZ	Revision of Nonautologous Tissue Substitute in Upper Back, Percutaneous Endoscopic Approach
● 0WWK4YZ	Revision of Other Device in Upper Back, Percutaneous Endoscopic Approach
0WWKX0Z	Revision of Drainage Device in Upper Back, External Approach
0WWKX1Z	Revision of Radioactive Element in Upper Back, External Approach
0WWKX3Z	Revision of Infusion Device in Upper Back, External Approach
0WWKX7Z	Revision of Autologous Tissue Substitute in Upper Back, External Approach
0WWKXJZ	Revision of Synthetic Substitute in Upper Back, External Approach
0WWKXKZ	Revision of Nonautologous Tissue Substitute in Upper Back, External Approach
0WWKXYZ	Revision of Other Device in Upper Back, External Approach
● 0WWL00Z	Revision of Drainage Device in Lower Back, Open Approach
● 0WWL01Z	Revision of Radioactive Element in Lower Back, Open Approach
● 0WWL03Z	Revision of Infusion Device in Lower Back, Open Approach
● 0WWL07Z	Revision of Autologous Tissue Substitute in Lower Back, Open Approach
● 0WWL0JZ	Revision of Synthetic Substitute in Lower Back, Open Approach
● 0WWL0KZ	Revision of Nonautologous Tissue Substitute in Lower Back, Open Approach
● 0WWL0YZ	Revision of Other Device in Lower Back, Open Approach
● 0WWL30Z	Revision of Drainage Device in Lower Back, Percutaneous Approach
● 0WWL31Z	Revision of Radioactive Element in Lower Back, Percutaneous Approach
● 0WWL33Z	Revision of Infusion Device in Lower Back, Percutaneous Approach
● 0WWL37Z	Revision of Autologous Tissue Substitute in Lower Back, Percutaneous Approach
● 0WWL3JZ	Revision of Synthetic Substitute in Lower Back, Percutaneous Approach
● 0WWL3KZ	Revision of Nonautologous Tissue Substitute in Lower Back, Percutaneous Approach
● 0WWL3YZ	Revision of Other Device in Lower Back, Percutaneous Approach
● 0WWL40Z	Revision of Drainage Device in Lower Back, Percutaneous Endoscopic Approach
● 0WWL41Z	Revision of Radioactive Element in Lower Back, Percutaneous Endoscopic Approach
● 0WWL43Z	Revision of Infusion Device in Lower Back, Percutaneous Endoscopic Approach
● 0WWL47Z	Revision of Autologous Tissue Substitute in Lower Back, Percutaneous Endoscopic Approach
● 0WWL4JZ	Revision of Synthetic Substitute in Lower Back, Percutaneous Endoscopic Approach
● 0WWL4KZ	Revision of Nonautologous Tissue Substitute in Lower Back, Percutaneous Endoscopic Approach
● 0WWL4YZ	Revision of Other Device in Lower Back, Percutaneous Endoscopic Approach
0WWLX0Z	Revision of Drainage Device in Lower Back, External Approach
0WWLX1Z	Revision of Radioactive Element in Lower Back, External Approach
0WWLX3Z	Revision of Infusion Device in Lower Back, External Approach
0WWLX7Z	Revision of Autologous Tissue Substitute in Lower Back, External Approach
0WWLXJZ	Revision of Synthetic Substitute in Lower Back, External Approach
0WWLXKZ	Revision of Nonautologous Tissue Substitute in Lower Back, External Approach
0WWLXYZ	Revision of Other Device in Lower Back, External Approach
♂ 0WWM00Z	Revision of Drainage Device in Male Perineum, Open Approach
♂ 0WWM01Z	Revision of Radioactive Element in Male Perineum, Open Approach
♂ 0WWM03Z	Revision of Infusion Device in Male Perineum, Open Approach
♂ 0WWM07Z	Revision of Autologous Tissue Substitute in Male Perineum, Open Approach
♂ 0WWM0JZ	Revision of Synthetic Substitute in Male Perineum, Open Approach
♂ 0WWM0KZ	Revision of Nonautologous Tissue Substitute in Male Perineum, Open Approach
♂ 0WWM0YZ	Revision of Other Device in Male Perineum, Open Approach
♂ 0WWM30Z	Revision of Drainage Device in Male Perineum, Percutaneous Approach
♂ 0WWM31Z	Revision of Radioactive Element in Male Perineum, Percutaneous Approach

♂ **0WWM33Z** Revision of Infusion Device in Male Perineum, Percutaneous Approach

♂ **0WWM37Z** Revision of Autologous Tissue Substitute in Male Perineum, Percutaneous Approach

♂ **0WWM3JZ** Revision of Synthetic Substitute in Male Perineum, Percutaneous Approach

♂ **0WWM3KZ** Revision of Nonautologous Tissue Substitute in Male Perineum, Percutaneous Approach

♂ **0WWM3YZ** Revision of Other Device in Male Perineum, Percutaneous Approach

♂ **0WWM40Z** Revision of Drainage Device in Male Perineum, Percutaneous Endoscopic Approach

♂ **0WWM41Z** Revision of Radioactive Element in Male Perineum, Percutaneous Endoscopic Approach

♂ **0WWM43Z** Revision of Infusion Device in Male Perineum, Percutaneous Endoscopic Approach

♂ **0WWM47Z** Revision of Autologous Tissue Substitute in Male Perineum, Percutaneous Endoscopic Approach

♂ **0WWM4JZ** Revision of Synthetic Substitute in Male Perineum, Percutaneous Endoscopic Approach

♂ **0WWM4KZ** Revision of Nonautologous Tissue Substitute in Male Perineum, Percutaneous Endoscopic Approach

♂ **0WWM4YZ** Revision of Other Device in Male Perineum, Percutaneous Endoscopic Approach

♂ **0WWMX0Z** Revision of Drainage Device in Male Perineum, External Approach

♂ **0WWMX1Z** Revision of Radioactive Element in Male Perineum, External Approach

♂ **0WWMX3Z** Revision of Infusion Device in Male Perineum, External Approach

♂ **0WWMX7Z** Revision of Autologous Tissue Substitute in Male Perineum, External Approach

♂ **0WWMXJZ** Revision of Synthetic Substitute in Male Perineum, External Approach

♂ **0WWMXKZ** Revision of Nonautologous Tissue Substitute in Male Perineum, External Approach

♂ **0WWMXYZ** Revision of Other Device in Male Perineum, External Approach

♀ **0WWN00Z** Revision of Drainage Device in Female Perineum, Open Approach

♀ **0WWN01Z** Revision of Radioactive Element in Female Perineum, Open Approach

♀ **0WWN03Z** Revision of Infusion Device in Female Perineum, Open Approach

♀ **0WWN07Z** Revision of Autologous Tissue Substitute in Female Perineum, Open Approach

♀ **0WWN0JZ** Revision of Synthetic Substitute in Female Perineum, Open Approach

♀ **0WWN0KZ** Revision of Nonautologous Tissue Substitute in Female Perineum, Open Approach

♀ **0WWN0YZ** Revision of Other Device in Female Perineum, Open Approach

♀ **0WWN30Z** Revision of Drainage Device in Female Perineum, Percutaneous Approach

♀ **0WWN31Z** Revision of Radioactive Element in Female Perineum, Percutaneous Approach

♀ **0WWN33Z** Revision of Infusion Device in Female Perineum, Percutaneous Approach

♀ **0WWN37Z** Revision of Autologous Tissue Substitute in Female Perineum, Percutaneous Approach

♀ **0WWN3JZ** Revision of Synthetic Substitute in Female Perineum, Percutaneous Approach

♀ **0WWN3KZ** Revision of Nonautologous Tissue Substitute in Female Perineum, Percutaneous Approach

♀ **0WWN3YZ** Revision of Other Device in Female Perineum, Percutaneous Approach

♀ **0WWN40Z** Revision of Drainage Device in Female Perineum, Percutaneous Endoscopic Approach

♀ **0WWN41Z** Revision of Radioactive Element in Female Perineum, Percutaneous Endoscopic Approach

♀ **0WWN43Z** Revision of Infusion Device in Female Perineum, Percutaneous Endoscopic Approach

♀ **0WWN47Z** Revision of Autologous Tissue Substitute in Female Perineum, Percutaneous Endoscopic Approach

♀ **0WWN4JZ** Revision of Synthetic Substitute in Female Perineum, Percutaneous Endoscopic Approach

♀ **0WWN4KZ** Revision of Nonautologous Tissue Substitute in Female Perineum, Percutaneous Endoscopic Approach

♀ **0WWN4YZ** Revision of Other Device in Female Perineum, Percutaneous Endoscopic Approach

♀ **0WWNX0Z** Revision of Drainage Device in Female Perineum, External Approach

♀ **0WWNX1Z** Revision of Radioactive Element in Female Perineum, External Approach

♀ **0WWNX3Z** Revision of Infusion Device in Female Perineum, External Approach

♀ **0WWNX7Z** Revision of Autologous Tissue Substitute in Female Perineum, External Approach

♀ **0WWNXJZ** Revision of Synthetic Substitute in Female Perineum, External Approach

♀ **0WWNXKZ** Revision of Nonautologous Tissue Substitute in Female Perineum, External Approach

♀ **0WWNXYZ** Revision of Other Device in Female Perineum, External Approach

0WWP01Z Revision of Radioactive Element in Gastrointestinal Tract, Open Approach

0WWP03Z Revision of Infusion Device in Gastrointestinal Tract, Open Approach

0WWP0YZ Revision of Other Device in Gastrointestinal Tract, Open Approach

0WWP31Z Revision of Radioactive Element in Gastrointestinal Tract, Percutaneous Approach

0WWP33Z Revision of Infusion Device in Gastrointestinal Tract, Percutaneous Approach

0WWP3YZ Revision of Other Device in Gastrointestinal Tract, Percutaneous Approach

0WWP41Z Revision of Radioactive Element in Gastrointestinal Tract, Percutaneous Endoscopic Approach

0WWP43Z Revision of Infusion Device in Gastrointestinal Tract, Percutaneous Endoscopic Approach

0WWP4YZ Revision of Other Device in Gastrointestinal Tract, Percutaneous Endoscopic Approach

0WWP71Z Revision of Radioactive Element in Gastrointestinal Tract, Via Natural or Artificial Opening

0WWP73Z Revision of Infusion Device in Gastrointestinal Tract, Via Natural or Artificial Opening

0WWP7YZ Revision of Other Device in Gastrointestinal Tract, Via Natural or Artificial Opening

0WWP81Z Revision of Radioactive Element in Gastrointestinal Tract, Via Natural or Artificial Opening Endoscopic

0WWP83Z Revision of Infusion Device in Gastrointestinal Tract, Via Natural or Artificial Opening Endoscopic

0WWP8YZ Revision of Other Device in Gastrointestinal Tract, Via Natural or Artificial Opening Endoscopic

0WWPX1Z Revision of Radioactive Element in Gastrointestinal Tract, External Approach

0WWPX3Z Revision of Infusion Device in Gastrointestinal Tract, External Approach

0WWPXYZ Revision of Other Device in Gastrointestinal Tract, External Approach

0WWQ01Z Revision of Radioactive Element in Respiratory Tract, Open Approach

0WWQ03Z Revision of Infusion Device in Respiratory Tract, Open Approach

0WWQ0YZ Revision of Other Device in Respiratory Tract, Open Approach

0WWQ31Z Revision of Radioactive Element in Respiratory Tract, Percutaneous Approach

0WWQ33Z Revision of Infusion Device in Respiratory Tract, Percutaneous Approach

0WWQ3YZ Revision of Other Device in Respiratory Tract, Percutaneous Approach

0WWQ41Z Revision of Radioactive Element in Respiratory Tract, Percutaneous Endoscopic Approach

0WWQ43Z Revision of Infusion Device in Respiratory Tract, Percutaneous Endoscopic Approach

0WWQ4YZ Revision of Other Device in Respiratory Tract, Percutaneous Endoscopic Approach

0WWQ71Z Revision of Radioactive Element in Respiratory Tract, Via Natural or Artificial Opening

0WWQ73Z Revision of Infusion Device in Respiratory Tract, Via Natural or Artificial Opening

0WWQ7YZ Revision of Other Device in Respiratory Tract, Via Natural or Artificial Opening

0WWQ81Z Revision of Radioactive Element in Respiratory Tract, Via Natural or Artificial Opening Endoscopic

0WWQ83Z Revision of Infusion Device in Respiratory Tract, Via Natural or Artificial Opening Endoscopic

0WWQ8YZ Revision of Other Device in Respiratory Tract, Via Natural or Artificial Opening Endoscopic

0WWQX1Z Revision of Radioactive Element in Respiratory Tract, External Approach

0WWQX3Z Revision of Infusion Device in Respiratory Tract, External Approach

♀ Female-only   ♂ Male-only   ▲ Limited Coverage   ● Non-OR   ▦ HAC-associated procedure   ▲ Non-covered procedures   ✚ Cluster

0WWQXYZ	Revision of Other Device in Respiratory Tract, External Approach	0WWR41Z	Revision of Radioactive Element in Genitourinary Tract, Percutaneous Endoscopic Approach	0WWR81Z	Revision of Radioactive Element in Genitourinary Tract, Via Natural or Artificial Opening Endoscopic
0WWR01Z	Revision of Radioactive Element in Genitourinary Tract, Open Approach	0WWR43Z	Revision of Infusion Device in Genitourinary Tract, Percutaneous Endoscopic Approach	0WWR83Z	Revision of Infusion Device in Genitourinary Tract, Via Natural or Artificial Opening Endoscopic
0WWR03Z	Revision of Infusion Device in Genitourinary Tract, Open Approach	0WWR4YZ	Revision of Other Device in Genitourinary Tract, Percutaneous Endoscopic Approach	0WWR8YZ	Revision of Other Device in Genitourinary Tract, Via Natural or Artificial Opening Endoscopic
0WWR0YZ	Revision of Other Device in Genitourinary Tract, Open Approach	0WWR71Z	Revision of Radioactive Element in Genitourinary Tract, Via Natural or Artificial Opening	0WWRX1Z	Revision of Radioactive Element in Genitourinary Tract, External Approach
0WWR31Z	Revision of Radioactive Element in Genitourinary Tract, Percutaneous Approach	0WWR73Z	Revision of Infusion Device in Genitourinary Tract, Via Natural or Artificial Opening	0WWRX3Z	Revision of Infusion Device in Genitourinary Tract, External Approach
0WWR33Z	Revision of Infusion Device in Genitourinary Tract, Percutaneous Approach	0WWR7YZ	Revision of Other Device in Genitourinary Tract, Via Natural or Artificial Opening	0WWRXYZ	Revision of Other Device in Genitourinary Tract, External Approach
0WWR3YZ	Revision of Other Device in Genitourinary Tract, Percutaneous Approach				

0WY – Anatomical Regions, General, Transplantation

| 0WY20Z0 | Transplantation of Face, Allogeneic, Open Approach | 0WY20Z1 | Transplantation of Face, Syngeneic, Open Approach |

♀ Female-only   ♂ Male-only   ▲ Limited Coverage   ● Non-OR   HAC HAC-associated procedure   ▲ Non-covered procedures   ✚ Cluster   1333

0WWQXYZ–0WY20Z1

Medical and Surgical, Anatomical Regions, General Code Listings

Anatomical Regions, Upper Extremities

Anatomical Regions, Upper Extremities Tables 0X0–0XY

Section	0	Medical and Surgical
Body System	X	Anatomical Regions, Upper Extremities
Operation	0	Alteration: Modifying the anatomic structure of a body part without affecting the function of the body part

Body Part (4th)	Approach (5th)	Device (6th)	Qualifier (7th)
2 Shoulder Region, Right 3 Shoulder Region, Left 4 Axilla, Right 5 Axilla, Left 6 Upper Extremity, Right 7 Upper Extremity, Left 8 Upper Arm, Right 9 Upper Arm, Left B Elbow Region, Right C Elbow Region, Left D Lower Arm, Right F Lower Arm, Left G Wrist Region, Right H Wrist Region, Left	0 Open 3 Percutaneous 4 Percutaneous Endoscopic	7 Autologous Tissue Substitute J Synthetic Substitute K Nonautologous Tissue Substitute Z No Device	Z No Qualifier

Section	0	Medical and Surgical
Body System	X	Anatomical Regions, Upper Extremities
Operation	2	Change: Taking out or off a device from a body part and putting back an identical or similar device in or on the same body part without cutting or puncturing the skin or a mucous membrane

Body Part (4th)	Approach (5th)	Device (6th)	Qualifier (7th)
6 Upper Extremity, Right 7 Upper Extremity, Left	X External	0 Drainage Device Y Other Device	Z No Qualifier

Section	0	Medical and Surgical
Body System	X	Anatomical Regions, Upper Extremities
Operation	3	Control: Stopping, or attempting to stop, postprocedural or other acute bleeding

Body Part (4th)	Approach (5th)	Device (6th)	Qualifier (7th)
2 Shoulder Region, Right 3 Shoulder Region, Left 4 Axilla, Right 5 Axilla, Left 6 Upper Extremity, Right 7 Upper Extremity, Left 8 Upper Arm, Right 9 Upper Arm, Left B Elbow Region, Right C Elbow Region, Left D Lower Arm, Right F Lower Arm, Left G Wrist Region, Right H Wrist Region, Left J Hand, Right K Hand, Left	0 Open 3 Percutaneous 4 Percutaneous Endoscopic	Z No Device	Z No Qualifier

Section	0	Medical and Surgical
Body System	X	Anatomical Regions, Upper Extremities
Operation	6	Detachment: Cutting off all or a portion of the upper or lower extremities

Body Part (4th)	Approach (5th)	Device (6th)	Qualifier (7th)
0 Forequarter, Right 1 Forequarter, Left 2 Shoulder Region, Right 3 Shoulder Region, Left B Elbow Region, Right C Elbow Region, Left	0 Open	Z No Device	Z No Qualifier
8 Upper Arm, Right 9 Upper Arm, Left D Lower Arm, Right F Lower Arm, Left	0 Open	Z No Device	1 High 2 Mid 3 Low
J Hand, Right K Hand, Left	0 Open	Z No Device	0 Complete 4 Complete 1st Ray 5 Complete 2nd Ray 6 Complete 3rd Ray 7 Complete 4th Ray 8 Complete 5th Ray 9 Partial 1st Ray B Partial 2nd Ray C Partial 3rd Ray D Partial 4th Ray F Partial 5th Ray
L Thumb, Right M Thumb, Left N Index Finger, Right P Index Finger, Left Q Middle Finger, Right R Middle Finger, Left S Ring Finger, Right T Ring Finger, Left V Little Finger, Right W Little Finger, Left	0 Open	Z No Device	0 Complete 1 High 2 Mid 3 Low

Section	0	Medical and Surgical
Body System	X	Anatomical Regions, Upper Extremities
Operation	9	Drainage: Taking or letting out fluids and/or gases from a body part

Body Part (4th)	Approach (5th)	Device (6th)	Qualifier (7th)
2 Shoulder Region, Right 3 Shoulder Region, Left 4 Axilla, Right 5 Axilla, Left 6 Upper Extremity, Right 7 Upper Extremity, Left 8 Upper Arm, Right 9 Upper Arm, Left B Elbow Region, Right C Elbow Region, Left D Lower Arm, Right F Lower Arm, Left G Wrist Region, Right H Wrist Region, Left J Hand, Right K Hand, Left	0 Open 3 Percutaneous 4 Percutaneous Endoscopic	0 Drainage Device	Z No Qualifier

Continued →

Section   0   **Medical and Surgical**
Body System   X   **Anatomical Regions, Upper Extremities**
Operation   9   **Drainage:** Taking or letting out fluids and/or gases from a body part

Body Part (4ᵗʰ)	Approach (5ᵗʰ)	Device (6ᵗʰ)	Qualifier (7ᵗʰ)
2 Shoulder Region, Right 3 Shoulder Region, Left 4 Axilla, Right 5 Axilla, Left 6 Upper Extremity, Right 7 Upper Extremity, Left 8 Upper Arm, Right 9 Upper Arm, Left B Elbow Region, Right C Elbow Region, Left D Lower Arm, Right F Lower Arm, Left G Wrist Region, Right H Wrist Region, Left J Hand, Right K Hand, Left	0 Open 3 Percutaneous 4 Percutaneous Endoscopic	Z No Device	X Diagnostic Z No Qualifier

Section   0   **Medical and Surgical**
Body System   X   **Anatomical Regions, Upper Extremities**
Operation   B   **Excision:** Cutting out or off, without replacement, a portion of a body part

Body Part (4ᵗʰ)	Approach (5ᵗʰ)	Device (6ᵗʰ)	Qualifier (7ᵗʰ)
2 Shoulder Region, Right 3 Shoulder Region, Left 4 Axilla, Right 5 Axilla, Left 6 Upper Extremity, Right 7 Upper Extremity, Left 8 Upper Arm, Right 9 Upper Arm, Left B Elbow Region, Right C Elbow Region, Left D Lower Arm, Right F Lower Arm, Left G Wrist Region, Right H Wrist Region, Left J Hand, Right K Hand, Left	0 Open 3 Percutaneous 4 Percutaneous Endoscopic	Z No Device	X Diagnostic Z No Qualifier

Section   0   **Medical and Surgical**
Body System   X   **Anatomical Regions, Upper Extremities**
Operation   H   **Insertion:** Putting in a nonbiological appliance that monitors, assists, performs, or prevents a physiological function but does not physically take the place of a body part

Body Part (4ᵗʰ)	Approach (5ᵗʰ)	Device (6ᵗʰ)	Qualifier (7ᵗʰ)
2 Shoulder Region, Right 3 Shoulder Region, Left 4 Axilla, Right 5 Axilla, Left 6 Upper Extremity, Right 7 Upper Extremity, Left 8 Upper Arm, Right 9 Upper Arm, Left B Elbow Region, Right C Elbow Region, Left D Lower Arm, Right F Lower Arm, Left G Wrist Region, Right H Wrist Region, Left J Hand, Right K Hand, Left	0 Open 3 Percutaneous 4 Percutaneous Endoscopic	1 Radioactive Element 3 Infusion Device Y Other Device	Z No Qualifier

Section   0   **Medical and Surgical**
Body System   X   **Anatomical Regions, Upper Extremities**
Operation   J   **Inspection:** Visually and/or manually exploring a body part

Body Part (4th)	Approach (5th)	Device (6th)	Qualifier (7th)
2 Shoulder Region, Right 3 Shoulder Region, Left 4 Axilla, Right 5 Axilla, Left 6 Upper Extremity, Right 7 Upper Extremity, Left 8 Upper Arm, Right 9 Upper Arm, Left B Elbow Region, Right C Elbow Region, Left D Lower Arm, Right F Lower Arm, Left G Wrist Region, Right H Wrist Region, Left J Hand, Right K Hand, Left	0 Open 3 Percutaneous 4 Percutaneous Endoscopic X External	Z No Device	Z No Qualifier

Section   0   **Medical and Surgical**
Body System   X   **Anatomical Regions, Upper Extremities**
Operation   M   **Reattachment:** Putting back in or on all or a portion of a separated body part to its normal location or other suitable location

Body Part (4th)	Approach (5th)	Device (6th)	Qualifier (7th)
0 Forequarter, Right 1 Forequarter, Left 2 Shoulder Region, Right 3 Shoulder Region, Left 4 Axilla, Right 5 Axilla, Left 6 Upper Extremity, Right 7 Upper Extremity, Left 8 Upper Arm, Right 9 Upper Arm, Left B Elbow Region, Right C Elbow Region, Left D Lower Arm, Right F Lower Arm, Left G Wrist Region, Right H Wrist Region, Left J Hand, Right K Hand, Left L Thumb, Right M Thumb, Left N Index Finger, Right P Index Finger, Left Q Middle Finger, Right R Middle Finger, Left S Ring Finger, Right T Ring Finger, Left V Little Finger, Right W Little Finger, Left	0 Open	Z No Device	Z No Qualifier

Section	0	Medical and Surgical
Body System	X	Anatomical Regions, Upper Extremities
Operation	P	Removal: Taking out or off a device from a body part

Body Part (4th)	Approach (5th)	Device (6th)	Qualifier (7th)
6 Upper Extremity, Right 7 Upper Extremity, Left	0 Open 3 Percutaneous 4 Percutaneous Endoscopic X External	0 Drainage Device 1 Radioactive Element 3 Infusion Device 7 Autologous Tissue Substitute J Synthetic Substitute K Nonautologous Tissue Substitute Y Other Device	Z No Qualifier

Section	0	Medical and Surgical
Body System	X	Anatomical Regions, Upper Extremities
Operation	Q	Repair: Restoring, to the extent possible, a body part to its normal anatomic structure and function

Body Part (4th)	Approach (5th)	Device (6th)	Qualifier (7th)
2 Shoulder Region, Right 3 Shoulder Region, Left 4 Axilla, Right 5 Axilla, Left 6 Upper Extremity, Right 7 Upper Extremity, Left 8 Upper Arm, Right 9 Upper Arm, Left B Elbow Region, Right C Elbow Region, Left D Lower Arm, Right F Lower Arm, Left G Wrist Region, Right H Wrist Region, Left J Hand, Right K Hand, Left L Thumb, Right M Thumb, Left N Index Finger, Right P Index Finger, Left Q Middle Finger, Right R Middle Finger, Left S Ring Finger, Right T Ring Finger, Left V Little Finger, Right W Little Finger, Left	0 Open 3 Percutaneous 4 Percutaneous Endoscopic X External	Z No Device	Z No Qualifier

Section	0	Medical and Surgical
Body System	X	Anatomical Regions, Upper Extremities
Operation	R	Replacement: Putting in or on biological or synthetic material that physically takes the place and/or function of all or a portion of a body part

Body Part (4th)	Approach (5th)	Device (6th)	Qualifier (7th)
L Thumb, Right M Thumb, Left	0 Open 4 Percutaneous Endoscopic	7 Autologous Tissue Substitute	N Toe, Right P Toe, Left

Section	0	Medical and Surgical
Body System	X	Anatomical Regions, Upper Extremities
Operation	U	**Supplement:** Putting in or on biological or synthetic material that physically reinforces and/or augments the function of a portion of a body part

Body Part (4th)	Approach (5th)	Device (6th)	Qualifier (7th)
2 Shoulder Region, Right 3 Shoulder Region, Left 4 Axilla, Right 5 Axilla, Left 6 Upper Extremity, Right 7 Upper Extremity, Left 8 Upper Arm, Right 9 Upper Arm, Left B Elbow Region, Right C Elbow Region, Left D Lower Arm, Right F Lower Arm, Left G Wrist Region, Right H Wrist Region, Left J Hand, Right K Hand, Left L Thumb, Right M Thumb, Left N Index Finger, Right P Index Finger, Left Q Middle Finger, Right R Middle Finger, Left S Ring Finger, Right T Ring Finger, Left V Little Finger, Right W Little Finger, Left	0 Open 4 Percutaneous Endoscopic	7 Autologous Tissue Substitute J Synthetic Substitute K Nonautologous Tissue Substitute	Z No Qualifier

Section	0	Medical and Surgical
Body System	X	Anatomical Regions, Upper Extremities
Operation	W	**Revision:** Correcting, to the extent possible, a portion of a malfunctioning device or the position of a displaced device

Body Part (4th)	Approach (5th)	Device (6th)	Qualifier (7th)
6 Upper Extremity, Right 7 Upper Extremity, Left	0 Open 3 Percutaneous 4 Percutaneous Endoscopic X External	0 Drainage Device 3 Infusion Device 7 Autologous Tissue Substitute J Synthetic Substitute K Nonautologous Tissue Substitute Y Other Device	Z No Qualifier

Section	0	Medical and Surgical
Body System	X	Anatomical Regions, Upper Extremities
Operation	X	**Transfer:** Moving, without taking out, all or a portion of a body part to another location to take over the function of all or a portion of a body part

Body Part (4th)	Approach (5th)	Device (6th)	Qualifier (7th)
N Index Finger, Right	0 Open	Z No Device	L Thumb, Right
P Index Finger, Left	0 Open	Z No Device	M Thumb, Left

Section	0	Medical and Surgical
Body System	X	Anatomical Regions, Upper Extremities
Operation	Y	**Transplantation:** Putting in or on all or a portion of a living body part taken from another individual or animal to physically take the place and/or function of all or a portion of a similar body part

Body Part (4th)	Approach (5th)	Device (6th)	Qualifier (7th)
J Hand, Right K Hand, Left	0 Open	Z No Device	0 Allogeneic 1 Syngeneic

Anatomical Regions, Upper Extremities Code Listing 0X0–0XX

0X0 – Anatomical Regions, Upper Extremities, Alteration

0X0207Z Alteration of Right Shoulder Region with Autologous Tissue Substitute, Open Approach

0X020JZ Alteration of Right Shoulder Region with Synthetic Substitute, Open Approach

0X020KZ Alteration of Right Shoulder Region with Nonautologous Tissue Substitute, Open Approach

0X020ZZ Alteration of Right Shoulder Region, Open Approach

0X0237Z Alteration of Right Shoulder Region with Autologous Tissue Substitute, Percutaneous Approach

0X023JZ Alteration of Right Shoulder Region with Synthetic Substitute, Percutaneous Approach

0X023KZ Alteration of Right Shoulder Region with Nonautologous Tissue Substitute, Percutaneous Approach

0X023ZZ Alteration of Right Shoulder Region, Percutaneous Approach

0X0247Z Alteration of Right Shoulder Region with Autologous Tissue Substitute, Percutaneous Endoscopic Approach

0X024JZ Alteration of Right Shoulder Region with Synthetic Substitute, Percutaneous Endoscopic Approach

0X024KZ Alteration of Right Shoulder Region with Nonautologous Tissue Substitute, Percutaneous Endoscopic Approach

0X024ZZ Alteration of Right Shoulder Region, Percutaneous Endoscopic Approach

0X0307Z Alteration of Left Shoulder Region with Autologous Tissue Substitute, Open Approach

0X030JZ Alteration of Left Shoulder Region with Synthetic Substitute, Open Approach

0X030KZ Alteration of Left Shoulder Region with Nonautologous Tissue Substitute, Open Approach

0X030ZZ Alteration of Left Shoulder Region, Open Approach

0X0337Z Alteration of Left Shoulder Region with Autologous Tissue Substitute, Percutaneous Approach

0X033JZ Alteration of Left Shoulder Region with Synthetic Substitute, Percutaneous Approach

0X033KZ Alteration of Left Shoulder Region with Nonautologous Tissue Substitute, Percutaneous Approach

0X033ZZ Alteration of Left Shoulder Region, Percutaneous Approach

0X0347Z Alteration of Left Shoulder Region with Autologous Tissue Substitute, Percutaneous Endoscopic Approach

0X034JZ Alteration of Left Shoulder Region with Synthetic Substitute, Percutaneous Endoscopic Approach

0X034KZ Alteration of Left Shoulder Region with Nonautologous Tissue Substitute, Percutaneous Endoscopic Approach

0X034ZZ Alteration of Left Shoulder Region, Percutaneous Endoscopic Approach

0X0407Z Alteration of Right Axilla with Autologous Tissue Substitute, Open Approach

0X040JZ Alteration of Right Axilla with Synthetic Substitute, Open Approach

0X040KZ Alteration of Right Axilla with Nonautologous Tissue Substitute, Open Approach

0X040ZZ Alteration of Right Axilla, Open Approach

0X0437Z Alteration of Right Axilla with Autologous Tissue Substitute, Percutaneous Approach

0X043JZ Alteration of Right Axilla with Synthetic Substitute, Percutaneous Approach

0X043KZ Alteration of Right Axilla with Nonautologous Tissue Substitute, Percutaneous Approach

0X043ZZ Alteration of Right Axilla, Percutaneous Approach

0X0447Z Alteration of Right Axilla with Autologous Tissue Substitute, Percutaneous Endoscopic Approach

0X044JZ Alteration of Right Axilla with Synthetic Substitute, Percutaneous Endoscopic Approach

0X044KZ Alteration of Right Axilla with Nonautologous Tissue Substitute, Percutaneous Endoscopic Approach

0X044ZZ Alteration of Right Axilla, Percutaneous Endoscopic Approach

0X0507Z Alteration of Left Axilla with Autologous Tissue Substitute, Open Approach

0X050JZ Alteration of Left Axilla with Synthetic Substitute, Open Approach

0X050KZ Alteration of Left Axilla with Nonautologous Tissue Substitute, Open Approach

0X050ZZ Alteration of Left Axilla, Open Approach

0X0537Z Alteration of Left Axilla with Autologous Tissue Substitute, Percutaneous Approach

0X053JZ Alteration of Left Axilla with Synthetic Substitute, Percutaneous Approach

0X053KZ Alteration of Left Axilla with Nonautologous Tissue Substitute, Percutaneous Approach

0X053ZZ Alteration of Left Axilla, Percutaneous Approach

0X0547Z Alteration of Left Axilla with Autologous Tissue Substitute, Percutaneous Endoscopic Approach

0X054JZ Alteration of Left Axilla with Synthetic Substitute, Percutaneous Endoscopic Approach

0X054KZ Alteration of Left Axilla with Nonautologous Tissue Substitute, Percutaneous Endoscopic Approach

0X054ZZ Alteration of Left Axilla, Percutaneous Endoscopic Approach

0X0607Z Alteration of Right Upper Extremity with Autologous Tissue Substitute, Open Approach

0X060JZ Alteration of Right Upper Extremity with Synthetic Substitute, Open Approach

0X060KZ Alteration of Right Upper Extremity with Nonautologous Tissue Substitute, Open Approach

0X060ZZ Alteration of Right Upper Extremity, Open Approach

0X0637Z Alteration of Right Upper Extremity with Autologous Tissue Substitute, Percutaneous Approach

0X063JZ Alteration of Right Upper Extremity with Synthetic Substitute, Percutaneous Approach

0X063KZ Alteration of Right Upper Extremity with Nonautologous Tissue Substitute, Percutaneous Approach

0X063ZZ Alteration of Right Upper Extremity, Percutaneous Approach

0X0647Z Alteration of Right Upper Extremity with Autologous Tissue Substitute, Percutaneous Endoscopic Approach

0X064JZ Alteration of Right Upper Extremity with Synthetic Substitute, Percutaneous Endoscopic Approach

0X064KZ Alteration of Right Upper Extremity with Nonautologous Tissue Substitute, Percutaneous Endoscopic Approach

0X064ZZ Alteration of Right Upper Extremity, Percutaneous Endoscopic Approach

0X0707Z Alteration of Left Upper Extremity with Autologous Tissue Substitute, Open Approach

0X070JZ Alteration of Left Upper Extremity with Synthetic Substitute, Open Approach

0X070KZ Alteration of Left Upper Extremity with Nonautologous Tissue Substitute, Open Approach

0X070ZZ Alteration of Left Upper Extremity, Open Approach

0X0737Z Alteration of Left Upper Extremity with Autologous Tissue Substitute, Percutaneous Approach

0X073JZ Alteration of Left Upper Extremity with Synthetic Substitute, Percutaneous Approach

0X073KZ Alteration of Left Upper Extremity with Nonautologous Tissue Substitute, Percutaneous Approach

0X073ZZ Alteration of Left Upper Extremity, Percutaneous Approach

0X0747Z Alteration of Left Upper Extremity with Autologous Tissue Substitute, Percutaneous Endoscopic Approach

0X074JZ Alteration of Left Upper Extremity with Synthetic Substitute, Percutaneous Endoscopic Approach

0X074KZ Alteration of Left Upper Extremity with Nonautologous Tissue Substitute, Percutaneous Endoscopic Approach

0X074ZZ Alteration of Left Upper Extremity, Percutaneous Endoscopic Approach

0X0807Z Alteration of Right Upper Arm with Autologous Tissue Substitute, Open Approach

0X080JZ Alteration of Right Upper Arm with Synthetic Substitute, Open Approach

0X080KZ Alteration of Right Upper Arm with Nonautologous Tissue Substitute, Open Approach

0X080ZZ Alteration of Right Upper Arm, Open Approach

0X0837Z Alteration of Right Upper Arm with Autologous Tissue Substitute, Percutaneous Approach

0X083JZ Alteration of Right Upper Arm with Synthetic Substitute, Percutaneous Approach

0X083KZ Alteration of Right Upper Arm with Nonautologous Tissue Substitute, Percutaneous Approach

0X083ZZ Alteration of Right Upper Arm, Percutaneous Approach

♀ Female-only   ♂ Male-only   ▲ Limited Coverage   ● Non-OR   HAC HAC-associated procedure   ▲ Non-covered procedures   ✚ Cluster

0X0847Z Alteration of Right Upper Arm with Autologous Tissue Substitute, Percutaneous Endoscopic Approach

0X084JZ Alteration of Right Upper Arm with Synthetic Substitute, Percutaneous Endoscopic Approach

0X084KZ Alteration of Right Upper Arm with Nonautologous Tissue Substitute, Percutaneous Endoscopic Approach

0X084ZZ Alteration of Right Upper Arm, Percutaneous Endoscopic Approach

0X0907Z Alteration of Left Upper Arm with Autologous Tissue Substitute, Open Approach

0X090JZ Alteration of Left Upper Arm with Synthetic Substitute, Open Approach

0X090KZ Alteration of Left Upper Arm with Nonautologous Tissue Substitute, Open Approach

0X090ZZ Alteration of Left Upper Arm, Open Approach

0X0937Z Alteration of Left Upper Arm with Autologous Tissue Substitute, Percutaneous Approach

0X093JZ Alteration of Left Upper Arm with Synthetic Substitute, Percutaneous Approach

0X093KZ Alteration of Left Upper Arm with Nonautologous Tissue Substitute, Percutaneous Approach

0X093ZZ Alteration of Left Upper Arm, Percutaneous Approach

0X0947Z Alteration of Left Upper Arm with Autologous Tissue Substitute, Percutaneous Endoscopic Approach

0X094JZ Alteration of Left Upper Arm with Synthetic Substitute, Percutaneous Endoscopic Approach

0X094KZ Alteration of Left Upper Arm with Nonautologous Tissue Substitute, Percutaneous Endoscopic Approach

0X094ZZ Alteration of Left Upper Arm, Percutaneous Endoscopic Approach

0X0B07Z Alteration of Right Elbow Region with Autologous Tissue Substitute, Open Approach

0X0B0JZ Alteration of Right Elbow Region with Synthetic Substitute, Open Approach

0X0B0KZ Alteration of Right Elbow Region with Nonautologous Tissue Substitute, Open Approach

0X0B0ZZ Alteration of Right Elbow Region, Open Approach

0X0B37Z Alteration of Right Elbow Region with Autologous Tissue Substitute, Percutaneous Approach

0X0B3JZ Alteration of Right Elbow Region with Synthetic Substitute, Percutaneous Approach

0X0B3KZ Alteration of Right Elbow Region with Nonautologous Tissue Substitute, Percutaneous Approach

0X0B3ZZ Alteration of Right Elbow Region, Percutaneous Approach

0X0B47Z Alteration of Right Elbow Region with Autologous Tissue Substitute, Percutaneous Endoscopic Approach

0X0B4JZ Alteration of Right Elbow Region with Synthetic Substitute, Percutaneous Endoscopic Approach

0X0B4KZ Alteration of Right Elbow Region with Nonautologous Tissue Substitute, Percutaneous Endoscopic Approach

0X0B4ZZ Alteration of Right Elbow Region, Percutaneous Endoscopic Approach

0X0C07Z Alteration of Left Elbow Region with Autologous Tissue Substitute, Open Approach

0X0C0JZ Alteration of Left Elbow Region with Synthetic Substitute, Open Approach

0X0C0KZ Alteration of Left Elbow Region with Nonautologous Tissue Substitute, Open Approach

0X0C0ZZ Alteration of Left Elbow Region, Open Approach

0X0C37Z Alteration of Left Elbow Region with Autologous Tissue Substitute, Percutaneous Approach

0X0C3JZ Alteration of Left Elbow Region with Synthetic Substitute, Percutaneous Approach

0X0C3KZ Alteration of Left Elbow Region with Nonautologous Tissue Substitute, Percutaneous Approach

0X0C3ZZ Alteration of Left Elbow Region, Percutaneous Approach

0X0C47Z Alteration of Left Elbow Region with Autologous Tissue Substitute, Percutaneous Endoscopic Approach

0X0C4JZ Alteration of Left Elbow Region with Synthetic Substitute, Percutaneous Endoscopic Approach

0X0C4KZ Alteration of Left Elbow Region with Nonautologous Tissue Substitute, Percutaneous Endoscopic Approach

0X0C4ZZ Alteration of Left Elbow Region, Percutaneous Endoscopic Approach

0X0D07Z Alteration of Right Lower Arm with Autologous Tissue Substitute, Open Approach

0X0D0JZ Alteration of Right Lower Arm with Synthetic Substitute, Open Approach

0X0D0KZ Alteration of Right Lower Arm with Nonautologous Tissue Substitute, Open Approach

0X0D0ZZ Alteration of Right Lower Arm, Open Approach

0X0D37Z Alteration of Right Lower Arm with Autologous Tissue Substitute, Percutaneous Approach

0X0D3JZ Alteration of Right Lower Arm with Synthetic Substitute, Percutaneous Approach

0X0D3KZ Alteration of Right Lower Arm with Nonautologous Tissue Substitute, Percutaneous Approach

0X0D3ZZ Alteration of Right Lower Arm, Percutaneous Approach

0X0D47Z Alteration of Right Lower Arm with Autologous Tissue Substitute, Percutaneous Endoscopic Approach

0X0D4JZ Alteration of Right Lower Arm with Synthetic Substitute, Percutaneous Endoscopic Approach

0X0D4KZ Alteration of Right Lower Arm with Nonautologous Tissue Substitute, Percutaneous Endoscopic Approach

0X0D4ZZ Alteration of Right Lower Arm, Percutaneous Endoscopic Approach

0X0F07Z Alteration of Left Lower Arm with Autologous Tissue Substitute, Open Approach

0X0F0JZ Alteration of Left Lower Arm with Synthetic Substitute, Open Approach

0X0F0KZ Alteration of Left Lower Arm with Nonautologous Tissue Substitute, Open Approach

0X0F0ZZ Alteration of Left Lower Arm, Open Approach

0X0F37Z Alteration of Left Lower Arm with Autologous Tissue Substitute, Percutaneous Approach

0X0F3JZ Alteration of Left Lower Arm with Synthetic Substitute, Percutaneous Approach

0X0F3KZ Alteration of Left Lower Arm with Nonautologous Tissue Substitute, Percutaneous Approach

0X0F3ZZ Alteration of Left Lower Arm, Percutaneous Approach

0X0F47Z Alteration of Left Lower Arm with Autologous Tissue Substitute, Percutaneous Endoscopic Approach

0X0F4JZ Alteration of Left Lower Arm with Synthetic Substitute, Percutaneous Endoscopic Approach

0X0F4KZ Alteration of Left Lower Arm with Nonautologous Tissue Substitute, Percutaneous Endoscopic Approach

0X0F4ZZ Alteration of Left Lower Arm, Percutaneous Endoscopic Approach

0X0G07Z Alteration of Right Wrist Region with Autologous Tissue Substitute, Open Approach

0X0G0JZ Alteration of Right Wrist Region with Synthetic Substitute, Open Approach

0X0G0KZ Alteration of Right Wrist Region with Nonautologous Tissue Substitute, Open Approach

0X0G0ZZ Alteration of Right Wrist Region, Open Approach

0X0G37Z Alteration of Right Wrist Region with Autologous Tissue Substitute, Percutaneous Approach

0X0G3JZ Alteration of Right Wrist Region with Synthetic Substitute, Percutaneous Approach

0X0G3KZ Alteration of Right Wrist Region with Nonautologous Tissue Substitute, Percutaneous Approach

0X0G3ZZ Alteration of Right Wrist Region, Percutaneous Approach

0X0G47Z Alteration of Right Wrist Region with Autologous Tissue Substitute, Percutaneous Endoscopic Approach

0X0G4JZ Alteration of Right Wrist Region with Synthetic Substitute, Percutaneous Endoscopic Approach

0X0G4KZ Alteration of Right Wrist Region with Nonautologous Tissue Substitute, Percutaneous Endoscopic Approach

0X0G4ZZ Alteration of Right Wrist Region, Percutaneous Endoscopic Approach

0X0H07Z Alteration of Left Wrist Region with Autologous Tissue Substitute, Open Approach

0X0H0JZ Alteration of Left Wrist Region with Synthetic Substitute, Open Approach

0X0H0KZ Alteration of Left Wrist Region with Nonautologous Tissue Substitute, Open Approach

0X0H0ZZ Alteration of Left Wrist Region, Open Approach

0X0H37Z Alteration of Left Wrist Region with Autologous Tissue Substitute, Percutaneous Approach

0X0H3JZ Alteration of Left Wrist Region with Synthetic Substitute, Percutaneous Approach

| 0X0H3KZ | Alteration of Left Wrist Region with Nonautologous Tissue Substitute, Percutaneous Approach | 0X0H47Z | Alteration of Left Wrist Region with Autologous Tissue Substitute, Percutaneous Endoscopic Approach | 0X0H4KZ | Alteration of Left Wrist Region with Nonautologous Tissue Substitute, Percutaneous Endoscopic Approach |
| 0X0H3ZZ | Alteration of Left Wrist Region, Percutaneous Approach | 0X0H4JZ | Alteration of Left Wrist Region with Synthetic Substitute, Percutaneous Endoscopic Approach | 0X0H4ZZ | Alteration of Left Wrist Region, Percutaneous Endoscopic Approach |

0X2 – Anatomical Regions, Upper Extremities, Change

Review Coding Guideline B6.1c

| 0X26X0Z | Change Drainage Device in Right Upper Extremity, External Approach | 0X27X0Z | Change Drainage Device in Left Upper Extremity, External Approach | 0X27XYZ | Change Other Device in Left Upper Extremity, External Approach |
| 0X26XYZ | Change Other Device in Right Upper Extremity, External Approach | | | | |

0X3 – Anatomical Regions, Upper Extremities, Control

Review Coding Guideline B3.7

0X320ZZ	Control Bleeding in Right Shoulder Region, Open Approach	0X373ZZ	Control Bleeding in Left Upper Extremity, Percutaneous Approach	0X3F0ZZ	Control Bleeding in Left Lower Arm, Open Approach
0X323ZZ	Control Bleeding in Right Shoulder Region, Percutaneous Approach	0X374ZZ	Control Bleeding in Left Upper Extremity, Percutaneous Endoscopic Approach	0X3F3ZZ	Control Bleeding in Left Lower Arm, Percutaneous Approach
0X324ZZ	Control Bleeding in Right Shoulder Region, Percutaneous Endoscopic Approach	0X380ZZ	Control Bleeding in Right Upper Arm, Open Approach	0X3F4ZZ	Control Bleeding in Left Lower Arm, Percutaneous Endoscopic Approach
0X330ZZ	Control Bleeding in Left Shoulder Region, Open Approach	0X383ZZ	Control Bleeding in Right Upper Arm, Percutaneous Approach	0X3G0ZZ	Control Bleeding in Right Wrist Region, Open Approach
0X333ZZ	Control Bleeding in Left Shoulder Region, Percutaneous Approach	0X384ZZ	Control Bleeding in Right Upper Arm, Percutaneous Endoscopic Approach	0X3G3ZZ	Control Bleeding in Right Wrist Region, Percutaneous Approach
0X334ZZ	Control Bleeding in Left Shoulder Region, Percutaneous Endoscopic Approach	0X390ZZ	Control Bleeding in Left Upper Arm, Open Approach	0X3G4ZZ	Control Bleeding in Right Wrist Region, Percutaneous Endoscopic Approach
0X340ZZ	Control Bleeding in Right Axilla, Open Approach	0X393ZZ	Control Bleeding in Left Upper Arm, Percutaneous Approach	0X3H0ZZ	Control Bleeding in Left Wrist Region, Open Approach
0X343ZZ	Control Bleeding in Right Axilla, Percutaneous Approach	0X394ZZ	Control Bleeding in Left Upper Arm, Percutaneous Endoscopic Approach	0X3H3ZZ	Control Bleeding in Left Wrist Region, Percutaneous Approach
0X344ZZ	Control Bleeding in Right Axilla, Percutaneous Endoscopic Approach	0X3B0ZZ	Control Bleeding in Right Elbow Region, Open Approach	0X3H4ZZ	Control Bleeding in Left Wrist Region, Percutaneous Endoscopic Approach
0X350ZZ	Control Bleeding in Left Axilla, Open Approach	0X3B3ZZ	Control Bleeding in Right Elbow Region, Percutaneous Approach	0X3J0ZZ	Control Bleeding in Right Hand, Open Approach
0X353ZZ	Control Bleeding in Left Axilla, Percutaneous Approach	0X3B4ZZ	Control Bleeding in Right Elbow Region, Percutaneous Endoscopic Approach	0X3J3ZZ	Control Bleeding in Right Hand, Percutaneous Approach
0X354ZZ	Control Bleeding in Left Axilla, Percutaneous Endoscopic Approach	0X3C0ZZ	Control Bleeding in Left Elbow Region, Open Approach	0X3J4ZZ	Control Bleeding in Right Hand, Percutaneous Endoscopic Approach
0X360ZZ	Control Bleeding in Right Upper Extremity, Open Approach	0X3C3ZZ	Control Bleeding in Left Elbow Region, Percutaneous Approach	0X3K0ZZ	Control Bleeding in Left Hand, Open Approach
0X363ZZ	Control Bleeding in Right Upper Extremity, Percutaneous Approach	0X3C4ZZ	Control Bleeding in Left Elbow Region, Percutaneous Endoscopic Approach	0X3K3ZZ	Control Bleeding in Left Hand, Percutaneous Approach
0X364ZZ	Control Bleeding in Right Upper Extremity, Percutaneous Endoscopic Approach	0X3D0ZZ	Control Bleeding in Right Lower Arm, Open Approach	0X3K4ZZ	Control Bleeding in Left Hand, Percutaneous Endoscopic Approach
0X370ZZ	Control Bleeding in Left Upper Extremity, Open Approach	0X3D3ZZ	Control Bleeding in Right Lower Arm, Percutaneous Approach		
	AHA CC: 1Q, 2015, 35	0X3D4ZZ	Control Bleeding in Right Lower Arm, Percutaneous Endoscopic Approach		

0X6 – Anatomical Regions, Upper Extremities, Detachment

0X600ZZ	Detachment at Right Forequarter, Open Approach	0X690Z2	Detachment at Left Upper Arm, Mid, Open Approach	0X6F0Z2	Detachment at Left Lower Arm, Mid, Open Approach
0X610ZZ	Detachment at Left Forequarter, Open Approach	0X690Z3	Detachment at Left Upper Arm, Low, Open Approach	0X6F0Z3	Detachment at Left Lower Arm, Low, Open Approach
0X620ZZ	Detachment at Right Shoulder Region, Open Approach	0X6B0ZZ	Detachment at Right Elbow Region, Open Approach	0X6J0Z0	Detachment at Right Hand, Complete, Open Approach
0X630ZZ	Detachment at Left Shoulder Region, Open Approach	0X6C0ZZ	Detachment at Left Elbow Region, Open Approach	0X6J0Z4	Detachment at Right Hand, Complete 1st Ray, Open Approach
0X680Z1	Detachment at Right Upper Arm, High, Open Approach	0X6D0Z1	Detachment at Right Lower Arm, High, Open Approach	0X6J0Z5	Detachment at Right Hand, Complete 2nd Ray, Open Approach
0X680Z2	Detachment at Right Upper Arm, Mid, Open Approach	0X6D0Z2	Detachment at Right Lower Arm, Mid, Open Approach	0X6J0Z6	Detachment at Right Hand, Complete 3rd Ray, Open Approach
0X680Z3	Detachment at Right Upper Arm, Low, Open Approach	0X6D0Z3	Detachment at Right Lower Arm, Low, Open Approach	0X6J0Z7	Detachment at Right Hand, Complete 4th Ray, Open Approach
0X690Z1	Detachment at Left Upper Arm, High, Open Approach	0X6F0Z1	Detachment at Left Lower Arm, High, Open Approach	0X6J0Z8	Detachment at Right Hand, Complete 5th Ray, Open Approach

♀ Female-only　　♂ Male-only　　▲ Limited Coverage　　● Non-OR　　⬛ HAC-associated procedure　　▲ Non-covered procedures　　✚ Cluster

0X6J0Z9	Detachment at Right Hand, Partial 1st Ray, Open Approach
0X6J0ZB	Detachment at Right Hand, Partial 2nd Ray, Open Approach
0X6J0ZC	Detachment at Right Hand, Partial 3rd Ray, Open Approach
0X6J0ZD	Detachment at Right Hand, Partial 4th Ray, Open Approach
0X6J0ZF	Detachment at Right Hand, Partial 5th Ray, Open Approach
0X6K0Z0	Detachment at Left Hand, Complete, Open Approach
0X6K0Z4	Detachment at Left Hand, Complete 1st Ray, Open Approach
0X6K0Z5	Detachment at Left Hand, Complete 2nd Ray, Open Approach
0X6K0Z6	Detachment at Left Hand, Complete 3rd Ray, Open Approach
0X6K0Z7	Detachment at Left Hand, Complete 4th Ray, Open Approach
0X6K0Z8	Detachment at Left Hand, Complete 5th Ray, Open Approach
0X6K0Z9	Detachment at Left Hand, Partial 1st Ray, Open Approach
0X6K0ZB	Detachment at Left Hand, Partial 2nd Ray, Open Approach
0X6K0ZC	Detachment at Left Hand, Partial 3rd Ray, Open Approach
0X6K0ZD	Detachment at Left Hand, Partial 4th Ray, Open Approach
0X6K0ZF	Detachment at Left Hand, Partial 5th Ray, Open Approach
0X6L0Z0	Detachment at Right Thumb, Complete, Open Approach
0X6L0Z1	Detachment at Right Thumb, High, Open Approach
0X6L0Z2	Detachment at Right Thumb, Mid, Open Approach

0X6L0Z3	Detachment at Right Thumb, Low, Open Approach
0X6M0Z0	Detachment at Left Thumb, Complete, Open Approach
0X6M0Z1	Detachment at Left Thumb, High, Open Approach
0X6M0Z2	Detachment at Left Thumb, Mid, Open Approach
0X6M0Z3	Detachment at Left Thumb, Low, Open Approach
	AHA CC: 3Q, 2016, 33-34; 1Q, 2017, 52
0X6N0Z0	Detachment at Right Index Finger, Complete, Open Approach
0X6N0Z1	Detachment at Right Index Finger, High, Open Approach
0X6N0Z2	Detachment at Right Index Finger, Mid, Open Approach
0X6N0Z3	Detachment at Right Index Finger, Low, Open Approach
0X6P0Z0	Detachment at Left Index Finger, Complete, Open Approach
0X6P0Z1	Detachment at Left Index Finger, High, Open Approach
0X6P0Z2	Detachment at Left Index Finger, Mid, Open Approach
0X6P0Z3	Detachment at Left Index Finger, Low, Open Approach
0X6Q0Z0	Detachment at Right Middle Finger, Complete, Open Approach
0X6Q0Z1	Detachment at Right Middle Finger, High, Open Approach
0X6Q0Z2	Detachment at Right Middle Finger, Mid, Open Approach
0X6Q0Z3	Detachment at Right Middle Finger, Low, Open Approach
0X6R0Z0	Detachment at Left Middle Finger, Complete, Open Approach
0X6R0Z1	Detachment at Left Middle Finger, High, Open Approach

0X6R0Z2	Detachment at Left Middle Finger, Mid, Open Approach
0X6R0Z3	Detachment at Left Middle Finger, Low, Open Approach
0X6S0Z0	Detachment at Right Ring Finger, Complete, Open Approach
0X6S0Z1	Detachment at Right Ring Finger, High, Open Approach
0X6S0Z2	Detachment at Right Ring Finger, Mid, Open Approach
0X6S0Z3	Detachment at Right Ring Finger, Low, Open Approach
0X6T0Z0	Detachment at Left Ring Finger, Complete, Open Approach
0X6T0Z1	Detachment at Left Ring Finger, High, Open Approach
0X6T0Z2	Detachment at Left Ring Finger, Mid, Open Approach
0X6T0Z3	Detachment at Left Ring Finger, Low, Open Approach
	AHA CC: 3Q, 2016, 33-34; 1Q, 2017, 52
0X6V0Z0	Detachment at Right Little Finger, Complete, Open Approach
	AHA CC: 2Q, 2017, 18-19
0X6V0Z1	Detachment at Right Little Finger, High, Open Approach
0X6V0Z2	Detachment at Right Little Finger, Mid, Open Approach
0X6V0Z3	Detachment at Right Little Finger, Low, Open Approach
0X6W0Z0	Detachment at Left Little Finger, Complete, Open Approach
0X6W0Z1	Detachment at Left Little Finger, High, Open Approach
0X6W0Z2	Detachment at Left Little Finger, Mid, Open Approach
0X6W0Z3	Detachment at Left Little Finger, Low, Open Approach
	AHA CC: 3Q, 2016, 33-34; 1Q, 2017, 52

0X9 – Anatomical Regions, Upper Extremities, Drainage

Review Coding Guidelines B3.4a and B3.4b

Review Coding Guideline B6.2

0X9200Z	Drainage of Right Shoulder Region with Drainage Device, Open Approach
0X920ZX	Drainage of Right Shoulder Region, Open Approach, Diagnostic
0X920ZZ	Drainage of Right Shoulder Region, Open Approach
0X9230Z	Drainage of Right Shoulder Region with Drainage Device, Percutaneous Approach
0X923ZX	Drainage of Right Shoulder Region, Percutaneous Approach, Diagnostic
0X923ZZ	Drainage of Right Shoulder Region, Percutaneous Approach
0X9240Z	Drainage of Right Shoulder Region with Drainage Device, Percutaneous Endoscopic Approach
0X924ZX	Drainage of Right Shoulder Region, Percutaneous Endoscopic Approach, Diagnostic
0X924ZZ	Drainage of Right Shoulder Region, Percutaneous Endoscopic Approach
0X9300Z	Drainage of Left Shoulder Region with Drainage Device, Open Approach
0X930ZX	Drainage of Left Shoulder Region, Open Approach, Diagnostic
0X930ZZ	Drainage of Left Shoulder Region, Open Approach
0X9330Z	Drainage of Left Shoulder Region with Drainage Device, Percutaneous Approach

0X933ZX	Drainage of Left Shoulder Region, Percutaneous Approach, Diagnostic
0X933ZZ	Drainage of Left Shoulder Region, Percutaneous Approach
0X9340Z	Drainage of Left Shoulder Region with Drainage Device, Percutaneous Endoscopic Approach
0X934ZX	Drainage of Left Shoulder Region, Percutaneous Endoscopic Approach, Diagnostic
0X934ZZ	Drainage of Left Shoulder Region, Percutaneous Endoscopic Approach
0X9400Z	Drainage of Right Axilla with Drainage Device, Open Approach
0X940ZX	Drainage of Right Axilla, Open Approach, Diagnostic
0X940ZZ	Drainage of Right Axilla, Open Approach
0X9430Z	Drainage of Right Axilla with Drainage Device, Percutaneous Approach
0X943ZX	Drainage of Right Axilla, Percutaneous Approach, Diagnostic
0X943ZZ	Drainage of Right Axilla, Percutaneous Approach
0X9440Z	Drainage of Right Axilla with Drainage Device, Percutaneous Endoscopic Approach
0X944ZX	Drainage of Right Axilla, Percutaneous Endoscopic Approach, Diagnostic

0X944ZZ	Drainage of Right Axilla, Percutaneous Endoscopic Approach
0X9500Z	Drainage of Left Axilla with Drainage Device, Open Approach
0X950ZX	Drainage of Left Axilla, Open Approach, Diagnostic
0X950ZZ	Drainage of Left Axilla, Open Approach
0X9530Z	Drainage of Left Axilla with Drainage Device, Percutaneous Approach
0X953ZX	Drainage of Left Axilla, Percutaneous Approach, Diagnostic
0X953ZZ	Drainage of Left Axilla, Percutaneous Approach
0X9540Z	Drainage of Left Axilla with Drainage Device, Percutaneous Endoscopic Approach
0X954ZX	Drainage of Left Axilla, Percutaneous Endoscopic Approach, Diagnostic
0X954ZZ	Drainage of Left Axilla, Percutaneous Endoscopic Approach
0X9600Z	Drainage of Right Upper Extremity with Drainage Device, Open Approach
0X960ZX	Drainage of Right Upper Extremity, Open Approach, Diagnostic
0X960ZZ	Drainage of Right Upper Extremity, Open Approach
0X9630Z	Drainage of Right Upper Extremity with Drainage Device, Percutaneous Approach

---

♀ Female-only   ♂ Male-only   ▲ Limited Coverage   ● Non-OR   ⬛ HAC-associated procedure   ▲ Non-covered procedures   ✚ Cluster

0X963ZX Drainage of Right Upper Extremity, Percutaneous Approach, Diagnostic

0X963ZZ Drainage of Right Upper Extremity, Percutaneous Approach

0X9640Z Drainage of Right Upper Extremity with Drainage Device, Percutaneous Endoscopic Approach

0X964ZX Drainage of Right Upper Extremity, Percutaneous Endoscopic Approach, Diagnostic

0X964ZZ Drainage of Right Upper Extremity, Percutaneous Endoscopic Approach

0X9700Z Drainage of Left Upper Extremity with Drainage Device, Open Approach

0X970ZX Drainage of Left Upper Extremity, Open Approach, Diagnostic

0X970ZZ Drainage of Left Upper Extremity, Open Approach

0X9730Z Drainage of Left Upper Extremity with Drainage Device, Percutaneous Approach

0X973ZX Drainage of Left Upper Extremity, Percutaneous Approach, Diagnostic

0X973ZZ Drainage of Left Upper Extremity, Percutaneous Approach

0X9740Z Drainage of Left Upper Extremity with Drainage Device, Percutaneous Endoscopic Approach

0X974ZX Drainage of Left Upper Extremity, Percutaneous Endoscopic Approach, Diagnostic

0X974ZZ Drainage of Left Upper Extremity, Percutaneous Endoscopic Approach

0X9800Z Drainage of Right Upper Arm with Drainage Device, Open Approach

0X980ZX Drainage of Right Upper Arm, Open Approach, Diagnostic

0X980ZZ Drainage of Right Upper Arm, Open Approach

0X9830Z Drainage of Right Upper Arm with Drainage Device, Percutaneous Approach

0X983ZX Drainage of Right Upper Arm, Percutaneous Approach, Diagnostic

0X983ZZ Drainage of Right Upper Arm, Percutaneous Approach

0X9840Z Drainage of Right Upper Arm with Drainage Device, Percutaneous Endoscopic Approach

0X984ZX Drainage of Right Upper Arm, Percutaneous Endoscopic Approach, Diagnostic

0X984ZZ Drainage of Right Upper Arm, Percutaneous Endoscopic Approach

0X9900Z Drainage of Left Upper Arm with Drainage Device, Open Approach

0X990ZX Drainage of Left Upper Arm, Open Approach, Diagnostic

0X990ZZ Drainage of Left Upper Arm, Open Approach

0X9930Z Drainage of Left Upper Arm with Drainage Device, Percutaneous Approach

0X993ZX Drainage of Left Upper Arm, Percutaneous Approach, Diagnostic

0X993ZZ Drainage of Left Upper Arm, Percutaneous Approach

0X9940Z Drainage of Left Upper Arm with Drainage Device, Percutaneous Endoscopic Approach

0X994ZX Drainage of Left Upper Arm, Percutaneous Endoscopic Approach, Diagnostic

0X994ZZ Drainage of Left Upper Arm, Percutaneous Endoscopic Approach

0X9B00Z Drainage of Right Elbow Region with Drainage Device, Open Approach

0X9B0ZX Drainage of Right Elbow Region, Open Approach, Diagnostic

0X9B0ZZ Drainage of Right Elbow Region, Open Approach

0X9B30Z Drainage of Right Elbow Region with Drainage Device, Percutaneous Approach

0X9B3ZX Drainage of Right Elbow Region, Percutaneous Approach, Diagnostic

0X9B3ZZ Drainage of Right Elbow Region, Percutaneous Approach

0X9B40Z Drainage of Right Elbow Region with Drainage Device, Percutaneous Endoscopic Approach

0X9B4ZX Drainage of Right Elbow Region, Percutaneous Endoscopic Approach, Diagnostic

0X9B4ZZ Drainage of Right Elbow Region, Percutaneous Endoscopic Approach

0X9C00Z Drainage of Left Elbow Region with Drainage Device, Open Approach

0X9C0ZX Drainage of Left Elbow Region, Open Approach, Diagnostic

0X9C0ZZ Drainage of Left Elbow Region, Open Approach

0X9C30Z Drainage of Left Elbow Region with Drainage Device, Percutaneous Approach

0X9C3ZX Drainage of Left Elbow Region, Percutaneous Approach, Diagnostic

0X9C3ZZ Drainage of Left Elbow Region, Percutaneous Approach

0X9C40Z Drainage of Left Elbow Region with Drainage Device, Percutaneous Endoscopic Approach

0X9C4ZX Drainage of Left Elbow Region, Percutaneous Endoscopic Approach, Diagnostic

0X9C4ZZ Drainage of Left Elbow Region, Percutaneous Endoscopic Approach

0X9D00Z Drainage of Right Lower Arm with Drainage Device, Open Approach

0X9D0ZX Drainage of Right Lower Arm, Open Approach, Diagnostic

0X9D0ZZ Drainage of Right Lower Arm, Open Approach

0X9D30Z Drainage of Right Lower Arm with Drainage Device, Percutaneous Approach

0X9D3ZX Drainage of Right Lower Arm, Percutaneous Approach, Diagnostic

0X9D3ZZ Drainage of Right Lower Arm, Percutaneous Approach

0X9D40Z Drainage of Right Lower Arm with Drainage Device, Percutaneous Endoscopic Approach

0X9D4ZX Drainage of Right Lower Arm, Percutaneous Endoscopic Approach, Diagnostic

0X9D4ZZ Drainage of Right Lower Arm, Percutaneous Endoscopic Approach

0X9F00Z Drainage of Left Lower Arm with Drainage Device, Open Approach

0X9F0ZX Drainage of Left Lower Arm, Open Approach, Diagnostic

0X9F0ZZ Drainage of Left Lower Arm, Open Approach

0X9F30Z Drainage of Left Lower Arm with Drainage Device, Percutaneous Approach

0X9F3ZX Drainage of Left Lower Arm, Percutaneous Approach, Diagnostic

0X9F3ZZ Drainage of Left Lower Arm, Percutaneous Approach

0X9F40Z Drainage of Left Lower Arm with Drainage Device, Percutaneous Endoscopic Approach

0X9F4ZX Drainage of Left Lower Arm, Percutaneous Endoscopic Approach, Diagnostic

0X9F4ZZ Drainage of Left Lower Arm, Percutaneous Endoscopic Approach

0X9G00Z Drainage of Right Wrist Region with Drainage Device, Open Approach

0X9G0ZX Drainage of Right Wrist Region, Open Approach, Diagnostic

0X9G0ZZ Drainage of Right Wrist Region, Open Approach

0X9G30Z Drainage of Right Wrist Region with Drainage Device, Percutaneous Approach

0X9G3ZX Drainage of Right Wrist Region, Percutaneous Approach, Diagnostic

0X9G3ZZ Drainage of Right Wrist Region, Percutaneous Approach

0X9G40Z Drainage of Right Wrist Region with Drainage Device, Percutaneous Endoscopic Approach

0X9G4ZX Drainage of Right Wrist Region, Percutaneous Endoscopic Approach, Diagnostic

0X9G4ZZ Drainage of Right Wrist Region, Percutaneous Endoscopic Approach

0X9H00Z Drainage of Left Wrist Region with Drainage Device, Open Approach

0X9H0ZX Drainage of Left Wrist Region, Open Approach, Diagnostic

0X9H0ZZ Drainage of Left Wrist Region, Open Approach

0X9H30Z Drainage of Left Wrist Region with Drainage Device, Percutaneous Approach

0X9H3ZX Drainage of Left Wrist Region, Percutaneous Approach, Diagnostic

0X9H3ZZ Drainage of Left Wrist Region, Percutaneous Approach

0X9H40Z Drainage of Left Wrist Region with Drainage Device, Percutaneous Endoscopic Approach

0X9H4ZX Drainage of Left Wrist Region, Percutaneous Endoscopic Approach, Diagnostic

0X9H4ZZ Drainage of Left Wrist Region, Percutaneous Endoscopic Approach

0X9J00Z Drainage of Right Hand with Drainage Device, Open Approach

0X9J0ZX Drainage of Right Hand, Open Approach, Diagnostic

0X9J0ZZ Drainage of Right Hand, Open Approach

0X9J30Z Drainage of Right Hand with Drainage Device, Percutaneous Approach

0X9J3ZX Drainage of Right Hand, Percutaneous Approach, Diagnostic

0X9J3ZZ Drainage of Right Hand, Percutaneous Approach

0X9J40Z Drainage of Right Hand with Drainage Device, Percutaneous Endoscopic Approach

0X9J4ZX Drainage of Right Hand, Percutaneous Endoscopic Approach, Diagnostic

0X9J4ZZ Drainage of Right Hand, Percutaneous Endoscopic Approach

0X9K00Z Drainage of Left Hand with Drainage Device, Open Approach

0X9K0ZX Drainage of Left Hand, Open Approach, Diagnostic

0X9K0ZZ Drainage of Left Hand, Open Approach

0X9K30Z Drainage of Left Hand with Drainage Device, Percutaneous Approach

♀ Female-only   ♂ Male-only   ▲ Limited Coverage   ● Non-OR   ▦ HAC-associated procedure   ▲ Non-covered procedures   ✚ Cluster

0X9K3ZX Drainage of Left Hand, Percutaneous Approach, Diagnostic
0X9K3ZZ Drainage of Left Hand, Percutaneous Approach

0X9K40Z Drainage of Left Hand with Drainage Device, Percutaneous Endoscopic Approach

0X9K4ZX Drainage of Left Hand, Percutaneous Endoscopic Approach, Diagnostic
0X9K4ZZ Drainage of Left Hand, Percutaneous Endoscopic Approach

0XB – Anatomical Regions, Upper Extremities, Excision

Review Coding Guidelines B3.4a and B3.4b

Review Coding Guideline B3.18

0XB20ZX Excision of Right Shoulder Region, Open Approach, Diagnostic
0XB20ZZ Excision of Right Shoulder Region, Open Approach
0XB23ZX Excision of Right Shoulder Region, Percutaneous Approach, Diagnostic
0XB23ZZ Excision of Right Shoulder Region, Percutaneous Approach
0XB24ZX Excision of Right Shoulder Region, Percutaneous Endoscopic Approach, Diagnostic
0XB24ZZ Excision of Right Shoulder Region, Percutaneous Endoscopic Approach
0XB30ZX Excision of Left Shoulder Region, Open Approach, Diagnostic
0XB30ZZ Excision of Left Shoulder Region, Open Approach
0XB33ZX Excision of Left Shoulder Region, Percutaneous Approach, Diagnostic
0XB33ZZ Excision of Left Shoulder Region, Percutaneous Approach
0XB34ZX Excision of Left Shoulder Region, Percutaneous Endoscopic Approach, Diagnostic
0XB34ZZ Excision of Left Shoulder Region, Percutaneous Endoscopic Approach
0XB40ZX Excision of Right Axilla, Open Approach, Diagnostic
0XB40ZZ Excision of Right Axilla, Open Approach
0XB43ZX Excision of Right Axilla, Percutaneous Approach, Diagnostic
0XB43ZZ Excision of Right Axilla, Percutaneous Approach
0XB44ZX Excision of Right Axilla, Percutaneous Endoscopic Approach, Diagnostic
0XB44ZZ Excision of Right Axilla, Percutaneous Endoscopic Approach
0XB50ZX Excision of Left Axilla, Open Approach, Diagnostic
0XB50ZZ Excision of Left Axilla, Open Approach
0XB53ZX Excision of Left Axilla, Percutaneous Approach, Diagnostic
0XB53ZZ Excision of Left Axilla, Percutaneous Approach
0XB54ZX Excision of Left Axilla, Percutaneous Endoscopic Approach, Diagnostic
0XB54ZZ Excision of Left Axilla, Percutaneous Endoscopic Approach
0XB60ZX Excision of Right Upper Extremity, Open Approach, Diagnostic
XB60ZZ Excision of Right Upper Extremity, Open Approach
XB63ZX Excision of Right Upper Extremity, Percutaneous Approach, Diagnostic
 363ZZ Excision of Right Upper Extremity, Percutaneous Approach
 64ZX Excision of Right Upper Extremity, Percutaneous Endoscopic Approach, Diagnostic
 ZZ Excision of Right Upper Extremity, Percutaneous Endoscopic Approach
 X Excision of Left Upper Extremity, Open Approach, Diagnostic

0XB70ZZ Excision of Left Upper Extremity, Open Approach
0XB73ZX Excision of Left Upper Extremity, Percutaneous Approach, Diagnostic
0XB73ZZ Excision of Left Upper Extremity, Percutaneous Approach
0XB74ZX Excision of Left Upper Extremity, Percutaneous Endoscopic Approach, Diagnostic
0XB74ZZ Excision of Left Upper Extremity, Percutaneous Endoscopic Approach
0XB80ZX Excision of Right Upper Arm, Open Approach, Diagnostic
0XB80ZZ Excision of Right Upper Arm, Open Approach
0XB83ZX Excision of Right Upper Arm, Percutaneous Approach, Diagnostic
0XB83ZZ Excision of Right Upper Arm, Percutaneous Approach
0XB84ZX Excision of Right Upper Arm, Percutaneous Endoscopic Approach, Diagnostic
0XB84ZZ Excision of Right Upper Arm, Percutaneous Endoscopic Approach
0XB90ZX Excision of Left Upper Arm, Open Approach, Diagnostic
0XB90ZZ Excision of Left Upper Arm, Open Approach
0XB93ZX Excision of Left Upper Arm, Percutaneous Approach, Diagnostic
0XB93ZZ Excision of Left Upper Arm, Percutaneous Approach
0XB94ZX Excision of Left Upper Arm, Percutaneous Endoscopic Approach, Diagnostic
0XB94ZZ Excision of Left Upper Arm, Percutaneous Endoscopic Approach
0XBB0ZX Excision of Right Elbow Region, Open Approach, Diagnostic
0XBB0ZZ Excision of Right Elbow Region, Open Approach
0XBB3ZX Excision of Right Elbow Region, Percutaneous Approach, Diagnostic
0XBB3ZZ Excision of Right Elbow Region, Percutaneous Approach
0XBB4ZX Excision of Right Elbow Region, Percutaneous Endoscopic Approach, Diagnostic
0XBB4ZZ Excision of Right Elbow Region, Percutaneous Endoscopic Approach
0XBC0ZX Excision of Left Elbow Region, Open Approach, Diagnostic
0XBC0ZZ Excision of Left Elbow Region, Open Approach
0XBC3ZX Excision of Left Elbow Region, Percutaneous Approach, Diagnostic
0XBC3ZZ Excision of Left Elbow Region, Percutaneous Approach
0XBC4ZX Excision of Left Elbow Region, Percutaneous Endoscopic Approach, Diagnostic
0XBC4ZZ Excision of Left Elbow Region, Percutaneous Endoscopic Approach

0XBD0ZX Excision of Right Lower Arm, Open Approach, Diagnostic
0XBD0ZZ Excision of Right Lower Arm, Open Approach
0XBD3ZX Excision of Right Lower Arm, Percutaneous Approach, Diagnostic
0XBD3ZZ Excision of Right Lower Arm, Percutaneous Approach
0XBD4ZX Excision of Right Lower Arm, Percutaneous Endoscopic Approach, Diagnostic
0XBD4ZZ Excision of Right Lower Arm, Percutaneous Endoscopic Approach
0XBF0ZX Excision of Left Lower Arm, Open Approach, Diagnostic
0XBF0ZZ Excision of Left Lower Arm, Open Approach
0XBF3ZX Excision of Left Lower Arm, Percutaneous Approach, Diagnostic
0XBF3ZZ Excision of Left Lower Arm, Percutaneous Approach
0XBF4ZX Excision of Left Lower Arm, Percutaneous Endoscopic Approach, Diagnostic
0XBF4ZZ Excision of Left Lower Arm, Percutaneous Endoscopic Approach
0XBG0ZX Excision of Right Wrist Region, Open Approach, Diagnostic
0XBG0ZZ Excision of Right Wrist Region, Open Approach
0XBG3ZX Excision of Right Wrist Region, Percutaneous Approach, Diagnostic
0XBG3ZZ Excision of Right Wrist Region, Percutaneous Approach
0XBG4ZX Excision of Right Wrist Region, Percutaneous Endoscopic Approach, Diagnostic
0XBG4ZZ Excision of Right Wrist Region, Percutaneous Endoscopic Approach
0XBH0ZX Excision of Left Wrist Region, Open Approach, Diagnostic
0XBH0ZZ Excision of Left Wrist Region, Open Approach
0XBH3ZX Excision of Left Wrist Region, Percutaneous Approach, Diagnostic
0XBH3ZZ Excision of Left Wrist Region, Percutaneous Approach
0XBH4ZX Excision of Left Wrist Region, Percutaneous Endoscopic Approach, Diagnostic
0XBH4ZZ Excision of Left Wrist Region, Percutaneous Endoscopic Approach
0XBJ0ZX Excision of Right Hand, Open Approach, Diagnostic
0XBJ0ZZ Excision of Right Hand, Open Approach
0XBJ3ZX Excision of Right Hand, Percutaneous Approach, Diagnostic
0XBJ3ZZ Excision of Right Hand, Percutaneous Approach
0XBJ4ZX Excision of Right Hand, Percutaneous Endoscopic Approach, Diagnostic
0XBJ4ZZ Excision of Right Hand, Percutaneous Endoscopic Approach

0XBK0ZX	Excision of Left Hand, Open Approach, Diagnostic	0XBK3ZX	Excision of Left Hand, Percutaneous Approach, Diagnostic	0XBK4ZX	Excision of Left Hand, Percutaneous Endoscopic Approach, Diagnostic
0XBK0ZZ	Excision of Left Hand, Open Approach	0XBK3ZZ	Excision of Left Hand, Percutaneous Approach	0XBK4ZZ	Excision of Left Hand, Percutaneous Endoscopic Approach

0XH – Anatomical Regions, Upper Extremities, Insertion

0XH201Z	Insertion of Radioactive Element into Right Shoulder Region, Open Approach	● 0XH44YZ	Insertion of Other Device into Right Axilla, Percutaneous Endoscopic Approach	● 0XH743Z	Insertion of Infusion Device into Left Upper Extremity, Percutaneous Endoscopic Approach
● 0XH203Z	Insertion of Infusion Device into Right Shoulder Region, Open Approach	0XH501Z	Insertion of Radioactive Element into Left Axilla, Open Approach	● 0XH74YZ	Insertion of Other Device into Left Upper Extremity, Percutaneous Endoscopic Approach
● 0XH20YZ	Insertion of Other Device into Right Shoulder Region, Open Approach	● 0XH503Z	Insertion of Infusion Device into Left Axilla, Open Approach	0XH801Z	Insertion of Radioactive Element into Right Upper Arm, Open Approach
0XH231Z	Insertion of Radioactive Element into Right Shoulder Region, Percutaneous Approach	● 0XH50YZ	Insertion of Other Device into Left Axilla, Open Approach	● 0XH803Z	Insertion of Infusion Device into Right Upper Arm, Open Approach
● 0XH233Z	Insertion of Infusion Device into Right Shoulder Region, Percutaneous Approach	0XH531Z	Insertion of Radioactive Element into Left Axilla, Percutaneous Approach	● 0XH80YZ	Insertion of Other Device into Right Upper Arm, Open Approach
● 0XH23YZ	Insertion of Other Device into Right Shoulder Region, Percutaneous Approach	● 0XH533Z	Insertion of Infusion Device into Left Axilla, Percutaneous Approach	0XH831Z	Insertion of Radioactive Element into Right Upper Arm, Percutaneous Approach
0XH241Z	Insertion of Radioactive Element into Right Shoulder Region, Percutaneous Endoscopic Approach	● 0XH53YZ	Insertion of Other Device into Left Axilla, Percutaneous Approach	● 0XH833Z	Insertion of Infusion Device into Right Upper Arm, Percutaneous Approach
● 0XH243Z	Insertion of Infusion Device into Right Shoulder Region, Percutaneous Endoscopic Approach	0XH541Z	Insertion of Radioactive Element into Left Axilla, Percutaneous Endoscopic Approach	● 0XH83YZ	Insertion of Other Device into Right Upper Arm, Percutaneous Approach
● 0XH24YZ	Insertion of Other Device into Right Shoulder Region, Percutaneous Endoscopic Approach	● 0XH543Z	Insertion of Infusion Device into Left Axilla, Percutaneous Endoscopic Approach	0XH841Z	Insertion of Radioactive Element into Right Upper Arm, Percutaneous Endoscopic Approach
0XH301Z	Insertion of Radioactive Element into Left Shoulder Region, Open Approach	● 0XH54YZ	Insertion of Other Device into Left Axilla, Percutaneous Endoscopic Approach	● 0XH843Z	Insertion of Infusion Device into Right Upper Arm, Percutaneous Endoscopic Approach
● 0XH303Z	Insertion of Infusion Device into Left Shoulder Region, Open Approach	0XH601Z	Insertion of Radioactive Element into Right Upper Extremity, Open Approach	● 0XH84YZ	Insertion of Other Device into Right Upper Arm, Percutaneous Endoscopic Approach
● 0XH30YZ	Insertion of Other Device into Left Shoulder Region, Open Approach	● 0XH603Z	Insertion of Infusion Device into Right Upper Extremity, Open Approach	0XH901Z	Insertion of Radioactive Element into Left Upper Arm, Open Approach
0XH331Z	Insertion of Radioactive Element into Left Shoulder Region, Percutaneous Approach	● 0XH60YZ	Insertion of Other Device into Right Upper Extremity, Open Approach	● 0XH903Z	Insertion of Infusion Device into Left Upper Arm, Open Approach
● 0XH333Z	Insertion of Infusion Device into Left Shoulder Region, Percutaneous Approach	0XH631Z	Insertion of Radioactive Element into Right Upper Extremity, Percutaneous Approach	● 0XH90YZ	Insertion of Other Device into Left Upper Arm, Open Approach
● 0XH33YZ	Insertion of Other Device into Left Shoulder Region, Percutaneous Approach	● 0XH633Z	Insertion of Infusion Device into Right Upper Extremity, Percutaneous Approach	*AHA CC: 2Q, 2017, 20-21*	
0XH341Z	Insertion of Radioactive Element into Left Shoulder Region, Percutaneous Endoscopic Approach	● 0XH63YZ	Insertion of Other Device into Right Upper Extremity, Percutaneous Approach	0XH931Z	Insertion of Radioactive Element into Left Upper Arm, Percutaneous Approach
● 0XH343Z	Insertion of Infusion Device into Left Shoulder Region, Percutaneous Endoscopic Approach	0XH641Z	Insertion of Radioactive Element into Right Upper Extremity, Percutaneous Endoscopic Approach	● 0XH933Z	Insertion of Infusion Device into Left Upper Arm, Percutaneous Approach
● 0XH34YZ	Insertion of Other Device into Left Shoulder Region, Percutaneous Endoscopic Approach	● 0XH643Z	Insertion of Infusion Device into Right Upper Extremity, Percutaneous Endoscopic Approach	● 0XH93YZ	Insertion of Other Device into Left Upper Arm, Percutaneous Approach
0XH401Z	Insertion of Radioactive Element into Right Axilla, Open Approach	● 0XH64YZ	Insertion of Other Device into Right Upper Extremity, Percutaneous Endoscopic Approach	0XH941Z	Insertion of Radioactive Element into Left Upper Arm, Percutaneous Endoscopic Approach
● 0XH403Z	Insertion of Infusion Device into Right Axilla, Open Approach	0XH701Z	Insertion of Radioactive Element into Left Upper Extremity, Open Approach	● 0XH943Z	Insertion of Infusion Device into Left Upper Arm, Percutaneous Endoscopic Approach
● 0XH40YZ	Insertion of Other Device into Right Axilla, Open Approach	● 0XH703Z	Insertion of Infusion Device into Left Upper Extremity, Open Approach	● 0XH94YZ	Insertion of Other Device into Left Upper Arm, Percutaneous Endoscopic Approach
0XH431Z	Insertion of Radioactive Element into Right Axilla, Percutaneous Approach	● 0XH70YZ	Insertion of Other Device into Left Upper Extremity, Open Approach	0XHB01Z	Insertion of Radioactive Element into Right Elbow Region, Open Approach
● 0XH433Z	Insertion of Infusion Device into Right Axilla, Percutaneous Approach	0XH731Z	Insertion of Radioactive Element into Left Upper Extremity, Percutaneous Approach	● 0XHB03Z	Insertion of Infusion Device into Right Elbow Region, Open Approach
● 0XH43YZ	Insertion of Other Device into Right Axilla, Percutaneous Approach	● 0XH733Z	Insertion of Infusion Device into Left Upper Extremity, Percutaneous Approach	● 0XHB0YZ	Insertion of Other Device into Right Elbow Region, Open Approach
0XH441Z	Insertion of Radioactive Element into Right Axilla, Percutaneous Endoscopic Approach	● 0XH73YZ	Insertion of Other Device into Left Upper Extremity, Percutaneous Approach	0XHB31Z	Insertion of Radioactive Element into Right Elbow Region, Percutaneous Approach
● 0XH443Z	Insertion of Infusion Device into Right Axilla, Percutaneous Endoscopic Approach	0XH741Z	Insertion of Radioactive Element into Left Upper Extremity, Percutaneous Endoscopic Approach	● 0XHB33Z	Insertion of Infusion Device into Right Elbow Region, Percutaneous Approach
				● 0XHB3YZ	Insertion of Other Device into Right Elbow Region, Percutaneous Approach

♀ Female-only   ♂ Male-only   ▲ Limited Coverage   ● Non-OR   🅷🅰🅲 HAC-associated procedure   ▲ Non-covered procedures   ➕ Clus'

0XHB41Z Insertion of Radioactive Element into Right Elbow Region, Percutaneous Endoscopic Approach

● 0XHB43Z Insertion of Infusion Device into Right Elbow Region, Percutaneous Endoscopic Approach

● 0XHB4YZ Insertion of Other Device into Right Elbow Region, Percutaneous Endoscopic Approach

0XHC01Z Insertion of Radioactive Element into Left Elbow Region, Open Approach

● 0XHC03Z Insertion of Infusion Device into Left Elbow Region, Open Approach

● 0XHC0YZ Insertion of Other Device into Left Elbow Region, Open Approach

0XHC31Z Insertion of Radioactive Element into Left Elbow Region, Percutaneous Approach

● 0XHC33Z Insertion of Infusion Device into Left Elbow Region, Percutaneous Approach

● 0XHC3YZ Insertion of Other Device into Left Elbow Region, Percutaneous Approach

0XHC41Z Insertion of Radioactive Element into Left Elbow Region, Percutaneous Endoscopic Approach

● 0XHC43Z Insertion of Infusion Device into Left Elbow Region, Percutaneous Endoscopic Approach

● 0XHC4YZ Insertion of Other Device into Left Elbow Region, Percutaneous Endoscopic Approach

0XHD01Z Insertion of Radioactive Element into Right Lower Arm, Open Approach

● 0XHD03Z Insertion of Infusion Device into Right Lower Arm, Open Approach

● 0XHD0YZ Insertion of Other Device into Right Lower Arm, Open Approach

0XHD31Z Insertion of Radioactive Element into Right Lower Arm, Percutaneous Approach

● 0XHD33Z Insertion of Infusion Device into Right Lower Arm, Percutaneous Approach

● 0XHD3YZ Insertion of Other Device into Right Lower Arm, Percutaneous Approach

0XHD41Z Insertion of Radioactive Element into Right Lower Arm, Percutaneous Endoscopic Approach

● 0XHD43Z Insertion of Infusion Device into Right Lower Arm, Percutaneous Endoscopic Approach

● 0XHD4YZ Insertion of Other Device into Right Lower Arm, Percutaneous Endoscopic Approach

0XHF01Z Insertion of Radioactive Element into Left Lower Arm, Open Approach

● 0XHF03Z Insertion of Infusion Device into Left Lower Arm, Open Approach

● 0XHF0YZ Insertion of Other Device into Left Lower Arm, Open Approach

0XHF31Z Insertion of Radioactive Element into Left Lower Arm, Percutaneous Approach

● 0XHF33Z Insertion of Infusion Device into Left Lower Arm, Percutaneous Approach

● 0XHF3YZ Insertion of Other Device into Left Lower Arm, Percutaneous Approach

0XHF41Z Insertion of Radioactive Element into Left Lower Arm, Percutaneous Endoscopic Approach

● 0XHF43Z Insertion of Infusion Device into Left Lower Arm, Percutaneous Endoscopic Approach

● 0XHF4YZ Insertion of Other Device into Left Lower Arm, Percutaneous Endoscopic Approach

0XHG01Z Insertion of Radioactive Element into Right Wrist Region, Open Approach

● 0XHG03Z Insertion of Infusion Device into Right Wrist Region, Open Approach

● 0XHG0YZ Insertion of Other Device into Right Wrist Region, Open Approach

0XHG31Z Insertion of Radioactive Element into Right Wrist Region, Percutaneous Approach

● 0XHG33Z Insertion of Infusion Device into Right Wrist Region, Percutaneous Approach

● 0XHG3YZ Insertion of Other Device into Right Wrist Region, Percutaneous Approach

0XHG41Z Insertion of Radioactive Element into Right Wrist Region, Percutaneous Endoscopic Approach

● 0XHG43Z Insertion of Infusion Device into Right Wrist Region, Percutaneous Endoscopic Approach

● 0XHG4YZ Insertion of Other Device into Right Wrist Region, Percutaneous Endoscopic Approach

0XHH01Z Insertion of Radioactive Element into Left Wrist Region, Open Approach

● 0XHH03Z Insertion of Infusion Device into Left Wrist Region, Open Approach

● 0XHH0YZ Insertion of Other Device into Left Wrist Region, Open Approach

0XHH31Z Insertion of Radioactive Element into Left Wrist Region, Percutaneous Approach

● 0XHH33Z Insertion of Infusion Device into Left Wrist Region, Percutaneous Approach

● 0XHH3YZ Insertion of Other Device into Left Wrist Region, Percutaneous Approach

0XHH41Z Insertion of Radioactive Element into Left Wrist Region, Percutaneous Endoscopic Approach

● 0XHH43Z Insertion of Infusion Device into Left Wrist Region, Percutaneous Endoscopic Approach

● 0XHH4YZ Insertion of Other Device into Left Wrist Region, Percutaneous Endoscopic Approach

0XHJ01Z Insertion of Radioactive Element into Right Hand, Open Approach

● 0XHJ03Z Insertion of Infusion Device into Right Hand, Open Approach

● 0XHJ0YZ Insertion of Other Device into Right Hand, Open Approach

0XHJ31Z Insertion of Radioactive Element into Right Hand, Percutaneous Approach

● 0XHJ33Z Insertion of Infusion Device into Right Hand, Percutaneous Approach

● 0XHJ3YZ Insertion of Other Device into Right Hand, Percutaneous Approach

0XHJ41Z Insertion of Radioactive Element into Right Hand, Percutaneous Endoscopic Approach

● 0XHJ43Z Insertion of Infusion Device into Right Hand, Percutaneous Endoscopic Approach

● 0XHJ4YZ Insertion of Other Device into Right Hand, Percutaneous Endoscopic Approach

0XHK01Z Insertion of Radioactive Element into Left Hand, Open Approach

● 0XHK03Z Insertion of Infusion Device into Left Hand, Open Approach

● 0XHK0YZ Insertion of Other Device into Left Hand, Open Approach

0XHK31Z Insertion of Radioactive Element into Left Hand, Percutaneous Approach

● 0XHK33Z Insertion of Infusion Device into Left Hand, Percutaneous Approach

● 0XHK3YZ Insertion of Other Device into Left Hand, Percutaneous Approach

0XHK41Z Insertion of Radioactive Element into Left Hand, Percutaneous Endoscopic Approach

● 0XHK43Z Insertion of Infusion Device into Left Hand, Percutaneous Endoscopic Approach

● 0XHK4YZ Insertion of Other Device into Left Hand, Percutaneous Endoscopic Approach

0XJ – Anatomical Regions, Upper Extremities, Inspection

Review Coding Guidelines B3.11a, B3.11b and B3.11c

● 0XJ20ZZ Inspection of Right Shoulder Region, Open Approach

0XJ23ZZ Inspection of Right Shoulder Region, Percutaneous Approach

0XJ24ZZ Inspection of Right Shoulder Region, Percutaneous Endoscopic Approach

0XJ2XZZ Inspection of Right Shoulder Region, External Approach

● 0XJ30ZZ Inspection of Left Shoulder Region, Open Approach

0XJ33ZZ Inspection of Left Shoulder Region, Percutaneous Approach

0XJ34ZZ Inspection of Left Shoulder Region, Percutaneous Endoscopic Approach

0XJ3XZZ Inspection of Left Shoulder Region, External Approach

● 0XJ40ZZ Inspection of Right Axilla, Open Approach

0XJ43ZZ Inspection of Right Axilla, Percutaneous Approach

0XJ44ZZ Inspection of Right Axilla, Percutaneous Endoscopic Approach

0XJ4XZZ Inspection of Right Axilla, External Approach

● 0XJ50ZZ Inspection of Left Axilla, Open Approach

0XJ53ZZ Inspection of Left Axilla, Percutaneous Approach

0XJ54ZZ Inspection of Left Axilla, Percutaneous Endoscopic Approach

0XJ5XZZ Inspection of Left Axilla, External Approach

● 0XJ60ZZ Inspection of Right Upper Extremity, Open Approach

0XJ63ZZ Inspection of Right Upper Extremity, Percutaneous Approach

0XJ64ZZ Inspection of Right Upper Extremity, Percutaneous Endoscopic Approach

0XJ6XZZ Inspection of Right Upper Extremity, External Approach

---

♀ Female-only   ♂ Male-only   ▲ Limited Coverage   ● Non-OR   ▨ HAC-associated procedure   ▲ Non-covered procedures   ✚ Cluster

● 0XJ70ZZ Inspection of Left Upper Extremity, Open Approach
0XJ73ZZ Inspection of Left Upper Extremity, Percutaneous Approach
0XJ74ZZ Inspection of Left Upper Extremity, Percutaneous Endoscopic Approach
0XJ7XZZ Inspection of Left Upper Extremity, External Approach
● 0XJ80ZZ Inspection of Right Upper Arm, Open Approach
0XJ83ZZ Inspection of Right Upper Arm, Percutaneous Approach
0XJ84ZZ Inspection of Right Upper Arm, Percutaneous Endoscopic Approach
0XJ8XZZ Inspection of Right Upper Arm, External Approach
● 0XJ90ZZ Inspection of Left Upper Arm, Open Approach
0XJ93ZZ Inspection of Left Upper Arm, Percutaneous Approach
0XJ94ZZ Inspection of Left Upper Arm, Percutaneous Endoscopic Approach
0XJ9XZZ Inspection of Left Upper Arm, External Approach
● 0XJB0ZZ Inspection of Right Elbow Region, Open Approach
0XJB3ZZ Inspection of Right Elbow Region, Percutaneous Approach
0XJB4ZZ Inspection of Right Elbow Region, Percutaneous Endoscopic Approach

0XJBXZZ Inspection of Right Elbow Region, External Approach
● 0XJC0ZZ Inspection of Left Elbow Region, Open Approach
0XJC3ZZ Inspection of Left Elbow Region, Percutaneous Approach
0XJC4ZZ Inspection of Left Elbow Region, Percutaneous Endoscopic Approach
0XJCXZZ Inspection of Left Elbow Region, External Approach
● 0XJD0ZZ Inspection of Right Lower Arm, Open Approach
0XJD3ZZ Inspection of Right Lower Arm, Percutaneous Approach
0XJD4ZZ Inspection of Right Lower Arm, Percutaneous Endoscopic Approach
0XJDXZZ Inspection of Right Lower Arm, External Approach
● 0XJF0ZZ Inspection of Left Lower Arm, Open Approach
0XJF3ZZ Inspection of Left Lower Arm, Percutaneous Approach
0XJF4ZZ Inspection of Left Lower Arm, Percutaneous Endoscopic Approach
0XJFXZZ Inspection of Left Lower Arm, External Approach
● 0XJG0ZZ Inspection of Right Wrist Region, Open Approach
0XJG3ZZ Inspection of Right Wrist Region, Percutaneous Approach

0XJG4ZZ Inspection of Right Wrist Region, Percutaneous Endoscopic Approach
0XJGXZZ Inspection of Right Wrist Region, External Approach
● 0XJH0ZZ Inspection of Left Wrist Region, Open Approach
0XJH3ZZ Inspection of Left Wrist Region, Percutaneous Approach
0XJH4ZZ Inspection of Left Wrist Region, Percutaneous Endoscopic Approach
0XJHXZZ Inspection of Left Wrist Region, External Approach
● 0XJJ0ZZ Inspection of Right Hand, Open Approach
● 0XJJ3ZZ Inspection of Right Hand, Percutaneous Approach
0XJJ4ZZ Inspection of Right Hand, Percutaneous Endoscopic Approach
0XJJXZZ Inspection of Right Hand, External Approach
● 0XJK0ZZ Inspection of Left Hand, Open Approach
● 0XJK3ZZ Inspection of Left Hand, Percutaneous Approach
0XJK4ZZ Inspection of Left Hand, Percutaneous Endoscopic Approach
0XJKXZZ Inspection of Left Hand, External Approach

0XM – Anatomical Regions, Upper Extremities, Reattachment

0XM00ZZ Reattachment of Right Forequarter, Open Approach
0XM10ZZ Reattachment of Left Forequarter, Open Approach
0XM20ZZ Reattachment of Right Shoulder Region, Open Approach
0XM30ZZ Reattachment of Left Shoulder Region, Open Approach
0XM40ZZ Reattachment of Right Axilla, Open Approach
0XM50ZZ Reattachment of Left Axilla, Open Approach
0XM60ZZ Reattachment of Right Upper Extremity, Open Approach
0XM70ZZ Reattachment of Left Upper Extremity, Open Approach
0XM80ZZ Reattachment of Right Upper Arm, Open Approach
0XM90ZZ Reattachment of Left Upper Arm, Open Approach

0XMB0ZZ Reattachment of Right Elbow Region, Open Approach
0XMC0ZZ Reattachment of Left Elbow Region, Open Approach
0XMD0ZZ Reattachment of Right Lower Arm, Open Approach
0XMF0ZZ Reattachment of Left Lower Arm, Open Approach
0XMG0ZZ Reattachment of Right Wrist Region, Open Approach
0XMH0ZZ Reattachment of Left Wrist Region, Open Approach
0XMJ0ZZ Reattachment of Right Hand, Open Approach
0XMK0ZZ Reattachment of Left Hand, Open Approach
0XML0ZZ Reattachment of Right Thumb, Open Approach
0XMM0ZZ Reattachment of Left Thumb, Open Approach

0XMN0ZZ Reattachment of Right Index Finger, Open Approach
0XMP0ZZ Reattachment of Left Index Finger, Open Approach
0XMQ0ZZ Reattachment of Right Middle Finger, Open Approach
0XMR0ZZ Reattachment of Left Middle Finger, Open Approach
0XMS0ZZ Reattachment of Right Ring Finger, Open Approach
0XMT0ZZ Reattachment of Left Ring Finger, Open Approach
0XMV0ZZ Reattachment of Right Little Finger, Open Approach
0XMW0ZZ Reattachment of Left Little Finger, Open Approach

0XP – Anatomical Regions, Upper Extremities, Removal

Review Coding Guideline B6.1c

0XP600Z Removal of Drainage Device from Right Upper Extremity, Open Approach
0XP601Z Removal of Radioactive Element from Right Upper Extremity, Open Approach
0XP603Z Removal of Infusion Device from Right Upper Extremity, Open Approach
0XP607Z Removal of Autologous Tissue Substitute from Right Upper Extremity, Open Approach
0XP60JZ Removal of Synthetic Substitute from Right Upper Extremity, Open Approach
0XP60KZ Removal of Nonautologous Tissue Substitute from Right Upper Extremity, Open Approach
0XP60YZ Removal of Other Device from Right Upper Extremity, Open Approach

0XP630Z Removal of Drainage Device from Right Upper Extremity, Percutaneous Approach
0XP631Z Removal of Radioactive Element from Right Upper Extremity, Percutaneous Approach
0XP633Z Removal of Infusion Device from Right Upper Extremity, Percutaneous Approach
0XP637Z Removal of Autologous Tissue Substitute from Right Upper Extremity, Percutaneous Approach
0XP63JZ Removal of Synthetic Substitute from Right Upper Extremity, Percutaneous Approach
0XP63KZ Removal of Nonautologous Tissue Substitute from Right Upper Extremity, Percutaneous Approach

0XP63YZ Removal of Other Device from Right Upper Extremity, Percutaneous Approach
0XP640Z Removal of Drainage Device from Right Upper Extremity, Percutaneous Endoscopic Approach
0XP641Z Removal of Radioactive Element from Right Upper Extremity, Percutaneous Endoscopic Approach
0XP643Z Removal of Infusion Device from Right Upper Extremity, Percutaneous Endoscopic Approach
0XP647Z Removal of Autologous Tissue Substitute from Right Upper Extremity, Percutaneous Endoscopic Approach
0XP64JZ Removal of Synthetic Substitute from Right Upper Extremity, Percutaneous Endoscopic Approach

♀ Female-only   ♂ Male-only   ▲ Limited Coverage   ● Non-OR   HAC HAC-associated procedure   ▲ Non-covered procedures   ✛ Cluster

0XP64KZ Removal of Nonautologous Tissue Substitute from Right Upper Extremity, Percutaneous Endoscopic Approach

0XP64YZ Removal of Other Device from Right Upper Extremity, Percutaneous Endoscopic Approach

0XP6X0Z Removal of Drainage Device from Right Upper Extremity, External Approach

0XP6X1Z Removal of Radioactive Element from Right Upper Extremity, External Approach

0XP6X3Z Removal of Infusion Device from Right Upper Extremity, External Approach

0XP6X7Z Removal of Autologous Tissue Substitute from Right Upper Extremity, External Approach

0XP6XJZ Removal of Synthetic Substitute from Right Upper Extremity, External Approach

0XP6XKZ Removal of Nonautologous Tissue Substitute from Right Upper Extremity, External Approach

0XP6XYZ Removal of Other Device from Right Upper Extremity, External Approach

0XP700Z Removal of Drainage Device from Left Upper Extremity, Open Approach

0XP701Z Removal of Radioactive Element from Left Upper Extremity, Open Approach

0XP703Z Removal of Infusion Device from Left Upper Extremity, Open Approach

0XP707Z Removal of Autologous Tissue Substitute from Left Upper Extremity, Open Approach

0XP70JZ Removal of Synthetic Substitute from Left Upper Extremity, Open Approach

0XP70KZ Removal of Nonautologous Tissue Substitute from Left Upper Extremity, Open Approach

0XP70YZ Removal of Other Device from Left Upper Extremity, Open Approach
AHA CC: 2Q, 2017, 20-21

0XP730Z Removal of Drainage Device from Left Upper Extremity, Percutaneous Approach

0XP731Z Removal of Radioactive Element from Left Upper Extremity, Percutaneous Approach

0XP733Z Removal of Infusion Device from Left Upper Extremity, Percutaneous Approach

0XP737Z Removal of Autologous Tissue Substitute from Left Upper Extremity, Percutaneous Approach

0XP73JZ Removal of Synthetic Substitute from Left Upper Extremity, Percutaneous Approach

0XP73KZ Removal of Nonautologous Tissue Substitute from Left Upper Extremity, Percutaneous Approach

0XP73YZ Removal of Other Device from Left Upper Extremity, Percutaneous Approach

0XP740Z Removal of Drainage Device from Left Upper Extremity, Percutaneous Endoscopic Approach

0XP741Z Removal of Radioactive Element from Left Upper Extremity, Percutaneous Endoscopic Approach

0XP743Z Removal of Infusion Device from Left Upper Extremity, Percutaneous Endoscopic Approach

0XP747Z Removal of Autologous Tissue Substitute from Left Upper Extremity, Percutaneous Endoscopic Approach

0XP74JZ Removal of Synthetic Substitute from Left Upper Extremity, Percutaneous Endoscopic Approach

0XP74KZ Removal of Nonautologous Tissue Substitute from Left Upper Extremity, Percutaneous Endoscopic Approach

0XP74YZ Removal of Other Device from Left Upper Extremity, Percutaneous Endoscopic Approach

0XP7X0Z Removal of Drainage Device from Left Upper Extremity, External Approach

0XP7X1Z Removal of Radioactive Element from Left Upper Extremity, External Approach

0XP7X3Z Removal of Infusion Device from Left Upper Extremity, External Approach

0XP7X7Z Removal of Autologous Tissue Substitute from Left Upper Extremity, External Approach

0XP7XJZ Removal of Synthetic Substitute from Left Upper Extremity, External Approach

0XP7XKZ Removal of Nonautologous Tissue Substitute from Left Upper Extremity, External Approach

0XP7XYZ Removal of Other Device from Left Upper Extremity, External Approach

0XQ – Anatomical Regions, Upper Extremities, Repair

0XQ20ZZ Repair Right Shoulder Region, Open Approach

0XQ23ZZ Repair Right Shoulder Region, Percutaneous Approach

0XQ24ZZ Repair Right Shoulder Region, Percutaneous Endoscopic Approach

0XQ2XZZ Repair Right Shoulder Region, External Approach

0XQ30ZZ Repair Left Shoulder Region, Open Approach

0XQ33ZZ Repair Left Shoulder Region, Percutaneous Approach

0XQ34ZZ Repair Left Shoulder Region, Percutaneous Endoscopic Approach

0XQ3XZZ Repair Left Shoulder Region, External Approach

0XQ40ZZ Repair Right Axilla, Open Approach

0XQ43ZZ Repair Right Axilla, Percutaneous Approach

0XQ44ZZ Repair Right Axilla, Percutaneous Endoscopic Approach

0XQ4XZZ Repair Right Axilla, External Approach

0XQ50ZZ Repair Left Axilla, Open Approach

0XQ53ZZ Repair Left Axilla, Percutaneous Approach

0XQ54ZZ Repair Left Axilla, Percutaneous Endoscopic Approach

0XQ5XZZ Repair Left Axilla, External Approach

0XQ60ZZ Repair Right Upper Extremity, Open Approach

0XQ63ZZ Repair Right Upper Extremity, Percutaneous Approach

0XQ64ZZ Repair Right Upper Extremity, Percutaneous Endoscopic Approach

0XQ6XZZ Repair Right Upper Extremity, External Approach

0XQ70ZZ Repair Left Upper Extremity, Open Approach

0XQ73ZZ Repair Left Upper Extremity, Percutaneous Approach

0XQ74ZZ Repair Left Upper Extremity, Percutaneous Endoscopic Approach

0XQ7XZZ Repair Left Upper Extremity, External Approach

0XQ80ZZ Repair Right Upper Arm, Open Approach

0XQ83ZZ Repair Right Upper Arm, Percutaneous Approach

0XQ84ZZ Repair Right Upper Arm, Percutaneous Endoscopic Approach

0XQ8XZZ Repair Right Upper Arm, External Approach

0XQ90ZZ Repair Left Upper Arm, Open Approach

0XQ93ZZ Repair Left Upper Arm, Percutaneous Approach

0XQ94ZZ Repair Left Upper Arm, Percutaneous Endoscopic Approach

0XQ9XZZ Repair Left Upper Arm, External Approach

0XQB0ZZ Repair Right Elbow Region, Open Approach

0XQB3ZZ Repair Right Elbow Region, Percutaneous Approach

0XQB4ZZ Repair Right Elbow Region, Percutaneous Endoscopic Approach

0XQBXZZ Repair Right Elbow Region, External Approach

0XQC0ZZ Repair Left Elbow Region, Open Approach

0XQC3ZZ Repair Left Elbow Region, Percutaneous Approach

0XQC4ZZ Repair Left Elbow Region, Percutaneous Endoscopic Approach

0XQCXZZ Repair Left Elbow Region, External Approach

0XQD0ZZ Repair Right Lower Arm, Open Approach

0XQD3ZZ Repair Right Lower Arm, Percutaneous Approach

0XQD4ZZ Repair Right Lower Arm, Percutaneous Endoscopic Approach

0XQDXZZ Repair Right Lower Arm, External Approach

0XQF0ZZ Repair Left Lower Arm, Open Approach

0XQF3ZZ Repair Left Lower Arm, Percutaneous Approach

0XQF4ZZ Repair Left Lower Arm, Percutaneous Endoscopic Approach

0XQFXZZ Repair Left Lower Arm, External Approach

0XQG0ZZ Repair Right Wrist Region, Open Approach

0XQG3ZZ Repair Right Wrist Region, Percutaneous Approach

0XQG4ZZ Repair Right Wrist Region, Percutaneous Endoscopic Approach

0XQGXZZ Repair Right Wrist Region, External Approach

0XQH0ZZ Repair Left Wrist Region, Open Approach

0XQH3ZZ Repair Left Wrist Region, Percutaneous Approach

0XQH4ZZ Repair Left Wrist Region, Percutaneous Endoscopic Approach

0XQHXZZ Repair Left Wrist Region, External Approach

0XQJ0ZZ Repair Right Hand, Open Approach

0XQJ3ZZ Repair Right Hand, Percutaneous Approach

0XQJ4ZZ	Repair Right Hand, Percutaneous Endoscopic Approach
0XQJXZZ	Repair Right Hand, External Approach
0XQK0ZZ	Repair Left Hand, Open Approach
0XQK3ZZ	Repair Left Hand, Percutaneous Approach
0XQK4ZZ	Repair Left Hand, Percutaneous Endoscopic Approach
0XQKXZZ	Repair Left Hand, External Approach
0XQL0ZZ	Repair Right Thumb, Open Approach
0XQL3ZZ	Repair Right Thumb, Percutaneous Approach
0XQL4ZZ	Repair Right Thumb, Percutaneous Endoscopic Approach
0XQLXZZ	Repair Right Thumb, External Approach
0XQM0ZZ	Repair Left Thumb, Open Approach
0XQM3ZZ	Repair Left Thumb, Percutaneous Approach
0XQM4ZZ	Repair Left Thumb, Percutaneous Endoscopic Approach
0XQMXZZ	Repair Left Thumb, External Approach
0XQN0ZZ	Repair Right Index Finger, Open Approach
0XQN3ZZ	Repair Right Index Finger, Percutaneous Approach
0XQN4ZZ	Repair Right Index Finger, Percutaneous Endoscopic Approach
0XQNXZZ	Repair Right Index Finger, External Approach
0XQP0ZZ	Repair Left Index Finger, Open Approach
0XQP3ZZ	Repair Left Index Finger, Percutaneous Approach
0XQP4ZZ	Repair Left Index Finger, Percutaneous Endoscopic Approach
0XQPXZZ	Repair Left Index Finger, External Approach
0XQQ0ZZ	Repair Right Middle Finger, Open Approach
0XQQ3ZZ	Repair Right Middle Finger, Percutaneous Approach
0XQQ4ZZ	Repair Right Middle Finger, Percutaneous Endoscopic Approach
0XQQXZZ	Repair Right Middle Finger, External Approach
0XQR0ZZ	Repair Left Middle Finger, Open Approach
0XQR3ZZ	Repair Left Middle Finger, Percutaneous Approach
0XQR4ZZ	Repair Left Middle Finger, Percutaneous Endoscopic Approach
0XQRXZZ	Repair Left Middle Finger, External Approach
0XQS0ZZ	Repair Right Ring Finger, Open Approach
0XQS3ZZ	Repair Right Ring Finger, Percutaneous Approach
0XQS4ZZ	Repair Right Ring Finger, Percutaneous Endoscopic Approach
0XQSXZZ	Repair Right Ring Finger, External Approach
0XQT0ZZ	Repair Left Ring Finger, Open Approach
0XQT3ZZ	Repair Left Ring Finger, Percutaneous Approach
0XQT4ZZ	Repair Left Ring Finger, Percutaneous Endoscopic Approach
0XQTXZZ	Repair Left Ring Finger, External Approach
0XQV0ZZ	Repair Right Little Finger, Open Approach
0XQV3ZZ	Repair Right Little Finger, Percutaneous Approach
0XQV4ZZ	Repair Right Little Finger, Percutaneous Endoscopic Approach
0XQVXZZ	Repair Right Little Finger, External Approach
0XQW0ZZ	Repair Left Little Finger, Open Approach
0XQW3ZZ	Repair Left Little Finger, Percutaneous Approach
0XQW4ZZ	Repair Left Little Finger, Percutaneous Endoscopic Approach
0XQWXZZ	Repair Left Little Finger, External Approach

0XR – Anatomical Regions, Upper Extremities, Replacement

0XRL07N	Replacement of Right Thumb with Right Toe, Autologous Tissue Substitute, Open Approach
0XRL07P	Replacement of Right Thumb with Left Toe, Autologous Tissue Substitute, Open Approach
0XRL47N	Replacement of Right Thumb with Right Toe, Autologous Tissue Substitute, Percutaneous Endoscopic Approach
0XRL47P	Replacement of Right Thumb with Left Toe, Autologous Tissue Substitute, Percutaneous Endoscopic Approach
0XRM07N	Replacement of Left Thumb with Right Toe, Autologous Tissue Substitute, Open Approach
0XRM07P	Replacement of Left Thumb with Left Toe, Autologous Tissue Substitute, Open Approach
0XRM47N	Replacement of Left Thumb with Right Toe, Autologous Tissue Substitute, Percutaneous Endoscopic Approach
0XRM47P	Replacement of Left Thumb with Left Toe, Autologous Tissue Substitute, Percutaneous Endoscopic Approach

0XU – Anatomical Regions, Upper Extremities, Supplement

0XU207Z	Supplement Right Shoulder Region with Autologous Tissue Substitute, Open Approach
0XU20JZ	Supplement Right Shoulder Region with Synthetic Substitute, Open Approach
0XU20KZ	Supplement Right Shoulder Region with Nonautologous Tissue Substitute, Open Approach
0XU247Z	Supplement Right Shoulder Region with Autologous Tissue Substitute, Percutaneous Endoscopic Approach
0XU24JZ	Supplement Right Shoulder Region with Synthetic Substitute, Percutaneous Endoscopic Approach
0XU24KZ	Supplement Right Shoulder Region with Nonautologous Tissue Substitute, Percutaneous Endoscopic Approach
0XU307Z	Supplement Left Shoulder Region with Autologous Tissue Substitute, Open Approach
0XU30JZ	Supplement Left Shoulder Region with Synthetic Substitute, Open Approach
0XU30KZ	Supplement Left Shoulder Region with Nonautologous Tissue Substitute, Open Approach
0XU347Z	Supplement Left Shoulder Region with Autologous Tissue Substitute, Percutaneous Endoscopic Approach
0XU34JZ	Supplement Left Shoulder Region with Synthetic Substitute, Percutaneous Endoscopic Approach
0XU34KZ	Supplement Left Shoulder Region with Nonautologous Tissue Substitute, Percutaneous Endoscopic Approach
0XU407Z	Supplement Right Axilla with Autologous Tissue Substitute, Open Approach
0XU40JZ	Supplement Right Axilla with Synthetic Substitute, Open Approach
0XU40KZ	Supplement Right Axilla with Nonautologous Tissue Substitute, Open Approach
0XU447Z	Supplement Right Axilla with Autologous Tissue Substitute, Percutaneous Endoscopic Approach
0XU44JZ	Supplement Right Axilla with Synthetic Substitute, Percutaneous Endoscopic Approach
0XU44KZ	Supplement Right Axilla with Nonautologous Tissue Substitute, Percutaneous Endoscopic Approach
0XU507Z	Supplement Left Axilla with Autologous Tissue Substitute, Open Approach
0XU50JZ	Supplement Left Axilla with Synthetic Substitute, Open Approach
0XU50KZ	Supplement Left Axilla with Nonautologous Tissue Substitute, Open Approach
0XU547Z	Supplement Left Axilla with Autologous Tissue Substitute, Percutaneous Endoscopic Approach
0XU54JZ	Supplement Left Axilla with Synthetic Substitute, Percutaneous Endoscopic Approach
0XU54KZ	Supplement Left Axilla with Nonautologous Tissue Substitute, Percutaneous Endoscopic Approach
0XU607Z	Supplement Right Upper Extremity with Autologous Tissue Substitute, Open Approach
0XU60JZ	Supplement Right Upper Extremity with Synthetic Substitute, Open Approach
0XU60KZ	Supplement Right Upper Extremity with Nonautologous Tissue Substitute, Open Approach
0XU647Z	Supplement Right Upper Extremity with Autologous Tissue Substitute, Percutaneous Endoscopic Approach
0XU64JZ	Supplement Right Upper Extremity with Synthetic Substitute, Percutaneous Endoscopic Approach
0XU64KZ	Supplement Right Upper Extremity with Nonautologous Tissue Substitute, Percutaneous Endoscopic Approach

♀ Female-only ♂ Male-only ▲ Limited Coverage ● Non-OR HAC HAC-associated procedure ▲ Non-covered procedures ✚ Cluster

0XU707Z — Supplement Left Upper Extremity with Autologous Tissue Substitute, Open Approach

0XU70JZ — Supplement Left Upper Extremity with Synthetic Substitute, Open Approach

0XU70KZ — Supplement Left Upper Extremity with Nonautologous Tissue Substitute, Open Approach

0XU747Z — Supplement Left Upper Extremity with Autologous Tissue Substitute, Percutaneous Endoscopic Approach

0XU74JZ — Supplement Left Upper Extremity with Synthetic Substitute, Percutaneous Endoscopic Approach

0XU74KZ — Supplement Left Upper Extremity with Nonautologous Tissue Substitute, Percutaneous Endoscopic Approach

0XU807Z — Supplement Right Upper Arm with Autologous Tissue Substitute, Open Approach

0XU80JZ — Supplement Right Upper Arm with Synthetic Substitute, Open Approach

0XU80KZ — Supplement Right Upper Arm with Nonautologous Tissue Substitute, Open Approach

0XU847Z — Supplement Right Upper Arm with Autologous Tissue Substitute, Percutaneous Endoscopic Approach

0XU84JZ — Supplement Right Upper Arm with Synthetic Substitute, Percutaneous Endoscopic Approach

0XU84KZ — Supplement Right Upper Arm with Nonautologous Tissue Substitute, Percutaneous Endoscopic Approach

0XU907Z — Supplement Left Upper Arm with Autologous Tissue Substitute, Open Approach

0XU90JZ — Supplement Left Upper Arm with Synthetic Substitute, Open Approach

0XU90KZ — Supplement Left Upper Arm with Nonautologous Tissue Substitute, Open Approach

0XU947Z — Supplement Left Upper Arm with Autologous Tissue Substitute, Percutaneous Endoscopic Approach

0XU94JZ — Supplement Left Upper Arm with Synthetic Substitute, Percutaneous Endoscopic Approach

0XU94KZ — Supplement Left Upper Arm with Nonautologous Tissue Substitute, Percutaneous Endoscopic Approach

0XUB07Z — Supplement Right Elbow Region with Autologous Tissue Substitute, Open Approach

0XUB0JZ — Supplement Right Elbow Region with Synthetic Substitute, Open Approach

0XUB0KZ — Supplement Right Elbow Region with Nonautologous Tissue Substitute, Open Approach

0XUB47Z — Supplement Right Elbow Region with Autologous Tissue Substitute, Percutaneous Endoscopic Approach

0XUB4JZ — Supplement Right Elbow Region with Synthetic Substitute, Percutaneous Endoscopic Approach

0XUB4KZ — Supplement Right Elbow Region with Nonautologous Tissue Substitute, Percutaneous Endoscopic Approach

0XUC07Z — Supplement Left Elbow Region with Autologous Tissue Substitute, Open Approach

0XUC0JZ — Supplement Left Elbow Region with Synthetic Substitute, Open Approach

0XUC0KZ — Supplement Left Elbow Region with Nonautologous Tissue Substitute, Open Approach

0XUC47Z — Supplement Left Elbow Region with Autologous Tissue Substitute, Percutaneous Endoscopic Approach

0XUC4JZ — Supplement Left Elbow Region with Synthetic Substitute, Percutaneous Endoscopic Approach

0XUC4KZ — Supplement Left Elbow Region with Nonautologous Tissue Substitute, Percutaneous Endoscopic Approach

0XUD07Z — Supplement Right Lower Arm with Autologous Tissue Substitute, Open Approach

0XUD0JZ — Supplement Right Lower Arm with Synthetic Substitute, Open Approach

0XUD0KZ — Supplement Right Lower Arm with Nonautologous Tissue Substitute, Open Approach

0XUD47Z — Supplement Right Lower Arm with Autologous Tissue Substitute, Percutaneous Endoscopic Approach

0XUD4JZ — Supplement Right Lower Arm with Synthetic Substitute, Percutaneous Endoscopic Approach

0XUD4KZ — Supplement Right Lower Arm with Nonautologous Tissue Substitute, Percutaneous Endoscopic Approach

0XUF07Z — Supplement Left Lower Arm with Autologous Tissue Substitute, Open Approach

0XUF0JZ — Supplement Left Lower Arm with Synthetic Substitute, Open Approach

0XUF0KZ — Supplement Left Lower Arm with Nonautologous Tissue Substitute, Open Approach

0XUF47Z — Supplement Left Lower Arm with Autologous Tissue Substitute, Percutaneous Endoscopic Approach

0XUF4JZ — Supplement Left Lower Arm with Synthetic Substitute, Percutaneous Endoscopic Approach

0XUF4KZ — Supplement Left Lower Arm with Nonautologous Tissue Substitute, Percutaneous Endoscopic Approach

0XUG07Z — Supplement Right Wrist Region with Autologous Tissue Substitute, Open Approach

0XUG0JZ — Supplement Right Wrist Region with Synthetic Substitute, Open Approach

0XUG0KZ — Supplement Right Wrist Region with Nonautologous Tissue Substitute, Open Approach

0XUG47Z — Supplement Right Wrist Region with Autologous Tissue Substitute, Percutaneous Endoscopic Approach

0XUG4JZ — Supplement Right Wrist Region with Synthetic Substitute, Percutaneous Endoscopic Approach

0XUG4KZ — Supplement Right Wrist Region with Nonautologous Tissue Substitute, Percutaneous Endoscopic Approach

0XUH07Z — Supplement Left Wrist Region with Autologous Tissue Substitute, Open Approach

0XUH0JZ — Supplement Left Wrist Region with Synthetic Substitute, Open Approach

0XUH0KZ — Supplement Left Wrist Region with Nonautologous Tissue Substitute, Open Approach

0XUH47Z — Supplement Left Wrist Region with Autologous Tissue Substitute, Percutaneous Endoscopic Approach

0XUH4JZ — Supplement Left Wrist Region with Synthetic Substitute, Percutaneous Endoscopic Approach

0XUH4KZ — Supplement Left Wrist Region with Nonautologous Tissue Substitute, Percutaneous Endoscopic Approach

0XUJ07Z — Supplement Right Hand with Autologous Tissue Substitute, Open Approach

0XUJ0JZ — Supplement Right Hand with Synthetic Substitute, Open Approach

0XUJ0KZ — Supplement Right Hand with Nonautologous Tissue Substitute, Open Approach

0XUJ47Z — Supplement Right Hand with Autologous Tissue Substitute, Percutaneous Endoscopic Approach

0XUJ4JZ — Supplement Right Hand with Synthetic Substitute, Percutaneous Endoscopic Approach

0XUJ4KZ — Supplement Right Hand with Nonautologous Tissue Substitute, Percutaneous Endoscopic Approach

0XUK07Z — Supplement Left Hand with Autologous Tissue Substitute, Open Approach

0XUK0JZ — Supplement Left Hand with Synthetic Substitute, Open Approach

0XUK0KZ — Supplement Left Hand with Nonautologous Tissue Substitute, Open Approach

0XUK47Z — Supplement Left Hand with Autologous Tissue Substitute, Percutaneous Endoscopic Approach

0XUK4JZ — Supplement Left Hand with Synthetic Substitute, Percutaneous Endoscopic Approach

0XUK4KZ — Supplement Left Hand with Nonautologous Tissue Substitute, Percutaneous Endoscopic Approach

0XUL07Z — Supplement Right Thumb with Autologous Tissue Substitute, Open Approach

0XUL0JZ — Supplement Right Thumb with Synthetic Substitute, Open Approach

0XUL0KZ — Supplement Right Thumb with Nonautologous Tissue Substitute, Open Approach

0XUL47Z — Supplement Right Thumb with Autologous Tissue Substitute, Percutaneous Endoscopic Approach

0XUL4JZ — Supplement Right Thumb with Synthetic Substitute, Percutaneous Endoscopic Approach

0XUL4KZ — Supplement Right Thumb with Nonautologous Tissue Substitute, Percutaneous Endoscopic Approach

0XUM07Z — Supplement Left Thumb with Autologous Tissue Substitute, Open Approach

0XUM0JZ — Supplement Left Thumb with Synthetic Substitute, Open Approach

0XUM0KZ — Supplement Left Thumb with Nonautologous Tissue Substitute, Open Approach

0XUM47Z — Supplement Left Thumb with Autologous Tissue Substitute, Percutaneous Endoscopic Approach

0XUM4JZ — Supplement Left Thumb with Synthetic Substitute, Percutaneous Endoscopic Approach

0XUM4KZ Supplement Left Thumb with Nonautologous Tissue Substitute, Percutaneous Endoscopic Approach

0XUN07Z Supplement Right Index Finger with Autologous Tissue Substitute, Open Approach

0XUN0JZ Supplement Right Index Finger with Synthetic Substitute, Open Approach

0XUN0KZ Supplement Right Index Finger with Nonautologous Tissue Substitute, Open Approach

0XUN47Z Supplement Right Index Finger with Autologous Tissue Substitute, Percutaneous Endoscopic Approach

0XUN4JZ Supplement Right Index Finger with Synthetic Substitute, Percutaneous Endoscopic Approach

0XUN4KZ Supplement Right Index Finger with Nonautologous Tissue Substitute, Percutaneous Endoscopic Approach

0XUP07Z Supplement Left Index Finger with Autologous Tissue Substitute, Open Approach

0XUP0JZ Supplement Left Index Finger with Synthetic Substitute, Open Approach

0XUP0KZ Supplement Left Index Finger with Nonautologous Tissue Substitute, Open Approach

0XUP47Z Supplement Left Index Finger with Autologous Tissue Substitute, Percutaneous Endoscopic Approach

0XUP4JZ Supplement Left Index Finger with Synthetic Substitute, Percutaneous Endoscopic Approach

0XUP4KZ Supplement Left Index Finger with Nonautologous Tissue Substitute, Percutaneous Endoscopic Approach

0XUQ07Z Supplement Right Middle Finger with Autologous Tissue Substitute, Open Approach

0XUQ0JZ Supplement Right Middle Finger with Synthetic Substitute, Open Approach

0XUQ0KZ Supplement Right Middle Finger with Nonautologous Tissue Substitute, Open Approach

0XUQ47Z Supplement Right Middle Finger with Autologous Tissue Substitute, Percutaneous Endoscopic Approach

0XUQ4JZ Supplement Right Middle Finger with Synthetic Substitute, Percutaneous Endoscopic Approach

0XUQ4KZ Supplement Right Middle Finger with Nonautologous Tissue Substitute, Percutaneous Endoscopic Approach

0XUR07Z Supplement Left Middle Finger with Autologous Tissue Substitute, Open Approach

0XUR0JZ Supplement Left Middle Finger with Synthetic Substitute, Open Approach

0XUR0KZ Supplement Left Middle Finger with Nonautologous Tissue Substitute, Open Approach

0XUR47Z Supplement Left Middle Finger with Autologous Tissue Substitute, Percutaneous Endoscopic Approach

0XUR4JZ Supplement Left Middle Finger with Synthetic Substitute, Percutaneous Endoscopic Approach

0XUR4KZ Supplement Left Middle Finger with Nonautologous Tissue Substitute, Percutaneous Endoscopic Approach

0XUS07Z Supplement Right Ring Finger with Autologous Tissue Substitute, Open Approach

0XUS0JZ Supplement Right Ring Finger with Synthetic Substitute, Open Approach

0XUS0KZ Supplement Right Ring Finger with Nonautologous Tissue Substitute, Open Approach

0XUS47Z Supplement Right Ring Finger with Autologous Tissue Substitute, Percutaneous Endoscopic Approach

0XUS4JZ Supplement Right Ring Finger with Synthetic Substitute, Percutaneous Endoscopic Approach

0XUS4KZ Supplement Right Ring Finger with Nonautologous Tissue Substitute, Percutaneous Endoscopic Approach

0XUT07Z Supplement Left Ring Finger with Autologous Tissue Substitute, Open Approach

0XUT0JZ Supplement Left Ring Finger with Synthetic Substitute, Open Approach

0XUT0KZ Supplement Left Ring Finger with Nonautologous Tissue Substitute, Open Approach

0XUT47Z Supplement Left Ring Finger with Autologous Tissue Substitute, Percutaneous Endoscopic Approach

0XUT4JZ Supplement Left Ring Finger with Synthetic Substitute, Percutaneous Endoscopic Approach

0XUT4KZ Supplement Left Ring Finger with Nonautologous Tissue Substitute, Percutaneous Endoscopic Approach

0XUV07Z Supplement Right Little Finger with Autologous Tissue Substitute, Open Approach

0XUV0JZ Supplement Right Little Finger with Synthetic Substitute, Open Approach

0XUV0KZ Supplement Right Little Finger with Nonautologous Tissue Substitute, Open Approach

0XUV47Z Supplement Right Little Finger with Autologous Tissue Substitute, Percutaneous Endoscopic Approach

0XUV4JZ Supplement Right Little Finger with Synthetic Substitute, Percutaneous Endoscopic Approach

0XUV4KZ Supplement Right Little Finger with Nonautologous Tissue Substitute, Percutaneous Endoscopic Approach

0XUW07Z Supplement Left Little Finger with Autologous Tissue Substitute, Open Approach

0XUW0JZ Supplement Left Little Finger with Synthetic Substitute, Open Approach

0XUW0KZ Supplement Left Little Finger with Nonautologous Tissue Substitute, Open Approach

0XUW47Z Supplement Left Little Finger with Autologous Tissue Substitute, Percutaneous Endoscopic Approach

0XUW4JZ Supplement Left Little Finger with Synthetic Substitute, Percutaneous Endoscopic Approach

0XUW4KZ Supplement Left Little Finger with Nonautologous Tissue Substitute, Percutaneous Endoscopic Approach

0XW – Anatomical Regions, Upper Extremities, Revision

Review Coding Guideline B6.1c

● **0XW600Z** Revision of Drainage Device in Right Upper Extremity, Open Approach

● **0XW603Z** Revision of Infusion Device in Right Upper Extremity, Open Approach

● **0XW607Z** Revision of Autologous Tissue Substitute in Right Upper Extremity, Open Approach

● **0XW60JZ** Revision of Synthetic Substitute in Right Upper Extremity, Open Approach

● **0XW60KZ** Revision of Nonautologous Tissue Substitute in Right Upper Extremity, Open Approach

● **0XW60YZ** Revision of Other Device in Right Upper Extremity, Open Approach

● **0XW630Z** Revision of Drainage Device in Right Upper Extremity, Percutaneous Approach

● **0XW633Z** Revision of Infusion Device in Right Upper Extremity, Percutaneous Approach

● **0XW637Z** Revision of Autologous Tissue Substitute in Right Upper Extremity, Percutaneous Approach

● **0XW63JZ** Revision of Synthetic Substitute in Right Upper Extremity, Percutaneous Approach

● **0XW63KZ** Revision of Nonautologous Tissue Substitute in Right Upper Extremity, Percutaneous Approach

● **0XW63YZ** Revision of Other Device in Right Upper Extremity, Percutaneous Approach

● **0XW640Z** Revision of Drainage Device in Right Upper Extremity, Percutaneous Endoscopic Approach

● **0XW643Z** Revision of Infusion Device in Right Upper Extremity, Percutaneous Endoscopic Approach

● **0XW647Z** Revision of Autologous Tissue Substitute in Right Upper Extremity, Percutaneous Endoscopic Approach

● **0XW64JZ** Revision of Synthetic Substitute in Right Upper Extremity, Percutaneous Endoscopic Approach

● **0XW64KZ** Revision of Nonautologous Tissue Substitute in Right Upper Extremity, Percutaneous Endoscopic Approach

0XW64YZ Revision of Other Device in Right Upper Extremity, Percutaneous Endoscopic Approach

0XW6X0Z Revision of Drainage Device in Right Upper Extremity, External Approach

0XW6X3Z Revision of Infusion Device in Right Upper Extremity, External Approach

0XW6X7Z Revision of Autologous Tissue Substitute in Right Upper Extremity, External Approach

0XW6XJZ Revision of Synthetic Substitute in Right Upper Extremity, External Approach

0XW6XKZ Revision of Nonautologous Tissue Substitute in Right Upper Extremity, External Approach

0XW6XYZ Revision of Other Device in Right Upper Extremity, External Approach

● **0XW700Z** Revision of Drainage Device in Left Upper Extremity, Open Approach

● **0XW703Z** Revision of Infusion Device in Left Upper Extremity, Open Approach

♀ Female-only   ♂ Male-only   ▲ Limited Coverage   ● Non-OR   HAC HAC-associated procedure   ▲ Non-covered procedures   ✚ Cluster

● **0XW707Z**	Revision of Autologous Tissue Substitute in Left Upper Extremity, Open Approach	● **0XW73KZ**	Revision of Nonautologous Tissue Substitute in Left Upper Extremity, Percutaneous Approach	● **0XW74YZ**	Revision of Other Device in Left Upper Extremity, Percutaneous Endoscopic Approach
● **0XW70JZ**	Revision of Synthetic Substitute in Left Upper Extremity, Open Approach	● **0XW73YZ**	Revision of Other Device in Left Upper Extremity, Percutaneous Approach	**0XW7X0Z**	Revision of Drainage Device in Left Upper Extremity, External Approach
● **0XW70KZ**	Revision of Nonautologous Tissue Substitute in Left Upper Extremity, Open Approach	● **0XW740Z**	Revision of Drainage Device in Left Upper Extremity, Percutaneous Endoscopic Approach	**0XW7X3Z**	Revision of Infusion Device in Left Upper Extremity, External Approach
● **0XW70YZ**	Revision of Other Device in Left Upper Extremity, Open Approach	● **0XW743Z**	Revision of Infusion Device in Left Upper Extremity, Percutaneous Endoscopic Approach	**0XW7X7Z**	Revision of Autologous Tissue Substitute in Left Upper Extremity, External Approach
● **0XW730Z**	Revision of Drainage Device in Left Upper Extremity, Percutaneous Approach	● **0XW747Z**	Revision of Autologous Tissue Substitute in Left Upper Extremity, Percutaneous Endoscopic Approach	**0XW7XJZ**	Revision of Synthetic Substitute in Left Upper Extremity, External Approach
● **0XW733Z**	Revision of Infusion Device in Left Upper Extremity, Percutaneous Approach	● **0XW74JZ**	Revision of Synthetic Substitute in Left Upper Extremity, Percutaneous Endoscopic Approach	**0XW7XKZ**	Revision of Nonautologous Tissue Substitute in Left Upper Extremity, External Approach
● **0XW737Z**	Revision of Autologous Tissue Substitute in Left Upper Extremity, Percutaneous Approach	● **0XW74KZ**	Revision of Nonautologous Tissue Substitute in Left Upper Extremity, Percutaneous Endoscopic Approach	**0XW7XYZ**	Revision of Other Device in Left Upper Extremity, External Approach
● **0XW73JZ**	Revision of Synthetic Substitute in Left Upper Extremity, Percutaneous Approach				

0XX – Anatomical Regions, Upper Extremities, Transfer

0XXN0ZL	Transfer Right Index Finger to Right Thumb, Open Approach	**0XXP0ZM**	Transfer Left Index Finger to Left Thumb, Open Approach

0XY – Anatomical Regions, Upper Extremities, Transplant

0XYJ0Z0	Transplantation of Right Hand, Allogeneic, Open Approach	**0XYK0Z0**	Transplantation of Left Hand, Allogeneic, Open Approach
0XYJ0Z1	Transplantation of Right Hand, Syngeneic, Open Approach	**0XYK0Z1**	Transplantation of Left Hand, Syngeneic, Open Approach

Anatomical Regions, Lower Extremities 0Y0–0YW

Section	0	**Medical and Surgical**
Body System	Y	**Anatomical Regions, Lower Extremities**
Operation	0	**Alteration:** Modifying the anatomic structure of a body part without affecting the function of the body part

Body Part (4th)	Approach (5th)	Device (6th)	Qualifier (7th)
0 Buttock, Right **1** Buttock, Left **9** Lower Extremity, Right **B** Lower Extremity, Left **C** Upper Leg, Right **D** Upper Leg, Left **F** Knee Region, Right **G** Knee Region, Left **H** Lower Leg, Right **J** Lower Leg, Left **K** Ankle Region, Right **L** Ankle Region, Left	**0** Open **3** Percutaneous **4** Percutaneous Endoscopic	**7** Autologous Tissue Substitute **J** Synthetic Substitute **K** Nonautologous Tissue Substitute **Z** No Device	**Z** No Qualifier

Section	0	**Medical and Surgical**
Body System	Y	**Anatomical Regions, Lower Extremities**
Operation	2	**Change:** Taking out or off a device from a body part and putting back an identical or similar device in or on the same body part without cutting or puncturing the skin or a mucous membrane

Body Part (4th)	Approach (5th)	Device (6th)	Qualifier (7th)
9 Lower Extremity, Right **B** Lower Extremity, Left	**X** External	**0** Drainage Device **Y** Other Device	**Z** No Qualifier

Section	0	**Medical and Surgical**
Body System	Y	**Anatomical Regions, Lower Extremities**
Operation	3	**Control:** Stopping, or attempting to stop, postprocedural or other acute bleeding

Body Part (4th)	Approach (5th)	Device (6th)	Qualifier (7th)
0 Buttock, Right **1** Buttock, Left **5** Inguinal Region, Right **6** Inguinal Region, Left **7** Femoral Region, Right **8** Femoral Region, Left **9** Lower Extremity, Right **B** Lower Extremity, Left **C** Upper Leg, Right **D** Upper Leg, Left **F** Knee Region, Right **G** Knee Region, Left **H** Lower Leg, Right **J** Lower Leg, Left **K** Ankle Region, Right **L** Ankle Region, Left **M** Foot, Right **N** Foot, Left	**0** Open **3** Percutaneous **4** Percutaneous Endoscopic	**Z** No Device	**Z** No Qualifier

Section	0	Medical and Surgical
Body System	Y	Anatomical Regions, Lower Extremities
Operation	6	Detachment: Cutting off all or a portion of the upper or lower extremities

Body Part (4th)	Approach (5th)	Device (6th)	Qualifier (7th)
2 Hindquarter, Right 3 Hindquarter, Left 4 Hindquarter, Bilateral 7 Femoral Region, Right 8 Femoral Region, Left F Knee Region, Right G Knee Region, Left	0 Open	Z No Device	Z No Qualifier
C Upper Leg, Right D Upper Leg, Left H Lower Leg, Right J Lower Leg, Left	0 Open	Z No Device	1 High 2 Mid 3 Low
M Foot, Right N Foot, Left	0 Open	Z No Device	0 Complete 4 Complete 1st Ray 5 Complete 2nd Ray 6 Complete 3rd Ray 7 Complete 4th Ray 8 Complete 5th Ray 9 Partial 1st Ray B Partial 2nd Ray C Partial 3rd Ray D Partial 4th Ray F Partial 5th Ray
P 1st Toe, Right Q 1st Toe, Left R 2nd Toe, Right S 2nd Toe, Left T 3rd Toe, Right U 3rd Toe, Left V 4th Toe, Right W 4th Toe, Left X 5th Toe, Right Y 5th Toe, Left	0 Open	Z No Device	0 Complete 1 High 2 Mid 3 Low

Section	0	Medical and Surgical
Body System	Y	Anatomical Regions, Lower Extremities
Operation	9	Drainage: Taking or letting out fluids and/or gases from a body part

Body Part (4th)	Approach (5th)	Device (6th)	Qualifier (7th)
0 Buttock, Right 1 Buttock, Left 5 Inguinal Region, Right 6 Inguinal Region, Left 7 Femoral Region, Right 8 Femoral Region, Left 9 Lower Extremity, Right B Lower Extremity, Left C Upper Leg, Right D Upper Leg, Left F Knee Region, Right G Knee Region, Left H Lower Leg, Right J Lower Leg, Left K Ankle Region, Right L Ankle Region, Left M Foot, Right N Foot, Left	0 Open 3 Percutaneous 4 Percutaneous Endoscopic	0 Drainage Device	Z No Qualifier

Continued →

Section	0	Medical and Surgical
Body System	Y	Anatomical Regions, Lower Extremities
Operation	9	**Drainage:** Taking or letting out fluids and/or gases from a body part

Body Part (4ᵗʰ)	Approach (5ᵗʰ)	Device (6ᵗʰ)	Qualifier (7ᵗʰ)
0 Buttock, Right	0 Open	Z No Device	X Diagnostic
1 Buttock, Left	3 Percutaneous		Z No Qualifier
5 Inguinal Region, Right	4 Percutaneous Endoscopic		
6 Inguinal Region, Left			
7 Femoral Region, Right			
8 Femoral Region, Left			
9 Lower Extremity, Right			
B Lower Extremity, Left			
C Upper Leg, Right			
D Upper Leg, Left			
F Knee Region, Right			
G Knee Region, Left			
H Lower Leg, Right			
J Lower Leg, Left			
K Ankle Region, Right			
L Ankle Region, Left			
M Foot, Right			
N Foot, Left			

Section	0	Medical and Surgical
Body System	Y	Anatomical Regions, Lower Extremities
Operation	B	**Excision:** Cutting out or off, without replacement, a portion of a body part

Body Part (4ᵗʰ)	Approach (5ᵗʰ)	Device (6ᵗʰ)	Qualifier (7ᵗʰ)
0 Buttock, Right	0 Open	Z No Device	X Diagnostic
1 Buttock, Left	3 Percutaneous		Z No Qualifier
5 Inguinal Region, Right	4 Percutaneous Endoscopic		
6 Inguinal Region, Left			
7 Femoral Region, Right			
8 Femoral Region, Left			
9 Lower Extremity, Right			
B Lower Extremity, Left			
C Upper Leg, Right			
D Upper Leg, Left			
F Knee Region, Right			
G Knee Region, Left			
H Lower Leg, Right			
J Lower Leg, Left			
K Ankle Region, Right			
L Ankle Region, Left			
M Foot, Right			
N Foot, Left			

Section 0 Medical and Surgical
Body System Y Anatomical Regions, Lower Extremities
Operation H Insertion: Putting in a nonbiological appliance that monitors, assists, performs, or prevents a physiological function but does not physically take the place of a body part

Body Part (4th)	Approach (5th)	Device (6th)	Qualifier (7th)
0 Buttock, Right 1 Buttock, Left 5 Inguinal Region, Right 6 Inguinal Region, Left 7 Femoral Region, Right 8 Femoral Region, Left 9 Lower Extremity, Right B Lower Extremity, Left C Upper Leg, Right D Upper Leg, Left F Knee Region, Right G Knee Region, Left H Lower Leg, Right J Lower Leg, Left K Ankle Region, Right L Ankle Region, Left M Foot, Right N Foot, Left	0 Open 3 Percutaneous 4 Percutaneous Endoscopic	1 Radioactive Element 3 Infusion Device Y Other Device	Z No Qualifier

Section 0 Medical and Surgical
Body System Y Anatomical Regions, Lower Extremities
Operation J Inspection: Visually and/or manually exploring a body part

Body Part (4th)	Approach (5th)	Device (6th)	Qualifier (7th)
0 Buttock, Right 1 Buttock, Left 5 Inguinal Region, Right 6 Inguinal Region, Left 7 Femoral Region, Right 8 Femoral Region, Left 9 Lower Extremity, Right A Inguinal Region, Bilateral B Lower Extremity, Left C Upper Leg, Right D Upper Leg, Left E Femoral Region, Bilateral F Knee Region, Right G Knee Region, Left H Lower Leg, Right J Lower Leg, Left K Ankle Region, Right L Ankle Region, Left M Foot, Right N Foot, Left	0 Open 3 Percutaneous 4 Percutaneous Endoscopic X External	Z No Device	Z No Qualifier

Section	0	Medical and Surgical
Body System	Y	Anatomical Regions, Lower Extremities
Operation	M	**Reattachment:** Putting back in or on all or a portion of a separated body part to its normal location or other suitable location

Body Part (4th)	Approach (5th)	Device (6th)	Qualifier (7th)
0 Buttock, Right	0 Open	Z No Device	Z No Qualifier
1 Buttock, Left			
2 Hindquarter, Right			
3 Hindquarter, Left			
4 Hindquarter, Bilateral			
5 Inguinal Region, Right			
6 Inguinal Region, Left			
7 Femoral Region, Right			
8 Femoral Region, Left			
9 Lower Extremity, Right			
B Lower Extremity, Left			
C Upper Leg, Right			
D Upper Leg, Left			
F Knee Region, Right			
G Knee Region, Left			
H Lower Leg, Right			
J Lower Leg, Left			
K Ankle Region, Right			
L Ankle Region, Left			
M Foot, Right			
N Foot, Left			
P 1st Toe, Right			
Q 1st Toe, Left			
R 2nd Toe, Right			
S 2nd Toe, Left			
T 3rd Toe, Right			
U 3rd Toe, Left			
V 4th Toe, Right			
W 4th Toe, Left			
X 5th Toe, Right			
Y 5th Toe, Left			

Section	0	Medical and Surgical
Body System	Y	Anatomical Regions, Lower Extremities
Operation	P	**Removal:** Taking out or off a device from a body part

Body Part (4th)	Approach (5th)	Device (6th)	Qualifier (7th)
9 Lower Extremity, Right	0 Open	0 Drainage Device	Z No Qualifier
B Lower Extremity, Left	3 Percutaneous	1 Radioactive Element	
	4 Percutaneous Endoscopic	3 Infusion Device	
	X External	7 Autologous Tissue Substitute	
		J Synthetic Substitute	
		K Nonautologous Tissue Substitute	
		Y Other Device	

Section	0	Medical and Surgical
Body System	Y	Anatomical Regions, Lower Extremities
Operation	Q	Repair: Restoring, to the extent possible, a body part to its normal anatomic structure and function

Body Part (4th)	Approach (5th)	Device (6th)	Qualifier (7th)
0 Buttock, Right 1 Buttock, Left 5 Inguinal Region, Right 6 Inguinal Region, Left 7 Femoral Region, Right 8 Femoral Region, Left 9 Lower Extremity, Right A Inguinal Region, Bilateral B Lower Extremity, Left C Upper Leg, Right D Upper Leg, Left E Femoral Region, Bilateral F Knee Region, Right G Knee Region, Left H Lower Leg, Right J Lower Leg, Left K Ankle Region, Right L Ankle Region, Left M Foot, Right N Foot, Left P 1st Toe, Right Q 1st Toe, Left R 2nd Toe, Right S 2nd Toe, Left T 3rd Toe, Right U 3rd Toe, Left V 4th Toe, Right W 4th Toe, Left X 5th Toe, Right Y 5th Toe, Left	0 Open 3 Percutaneous 4 Percutaneous Endoscopic X External	Z No Device	Z No Qualifier

Section	0	Medical and Surgical
Body System	Y	Anatomical Regions, Lower Extremities
Operation	U	Supplement: Putting in or on biological or synthetic material that physically reinforces and/or augments the function of a portion of a body part

Body Part (4th)	Approach (5th)	Device (6th)	Qualifier (7th)
0 Buttock, Right 1 Buttock, Left 5 Inguinal Region, Right 6 Inguinal Region, Left 7 Femoral Region, Right 8 Femoral Region, Left 9 Lower Extremity, Right A Inguinal Region, Bilateral B Lower Extremity, Left C Upper Leg, Right D Upper Leg, Left E Femoral Region, Bilateral F Knee Region, Right G Knee Region, Left H Lower Leg, Right J Lower Leg, Left K Ankle Region, Right L Ankle Region, Left M Foot, Right N Foot, Left P 1st Toe, Right Q 1st Toe, Left R 2nd Toe, Right S 2nd Toe, Left T 3rd Toe, Right U 3rd Toe, Left V 4th Toe, Right W 4th Toe, Left X 5th Toe, Right Y 5th Toe, Left	0 Open 4 Percutaneous Endoscopic	7 Autologous Tissue Substitute J Synthetic Substitute K Nonautologous Tissue Substitute	Z No Qualifier

Section	0	Medical and Surgical
Body System	Y	Anatomical Regions, Lower Extremities
Operation	W	Revision: Correcting, to the extent possible, a portion of a malfunctioning device or the position of a displaced device

Body Part (4th)	Approach (5th)	Device (6th)	Qualifier (7th)
9 Lower Extremity, Right B Lower Extremity, Left	0 Open 3 Percutaneous 4 Percutaneous Endoscopic X External	0 Drainage Device 3 Infusion Device 7 Autologous Tissue Substitute J Synthetic Substitute K Nonautologous Tissue Substitute Y Other Device	Z No Qualifier

Anatomical Regions, Lower Extremities Code Listing 0Y0–0YW

0Y0 – Anatomical Regions, Lower Extremities, Alteration

0Y0007Z Alteration of Right Buttock with Autologous Tissue Substitute, Open Approach

0Y000JZ Alteration of Right Buttock with Synthetic Substitute, Open Approach

0Y000KZ Alteration of Right Buttock with Nonautologous Tissue Substitute, Open Approach

0Y000ZZ Alteration of Right Buttock, Open Approach

0Y0037Z Alteration of Right Buttock with Autologous Tissue Substitute, Percutaneous Approach

0Y003JZ Alteration of Right Buttock with Synthetic Substitute, Percutaneous Approach

0Y003KZ Alteration of Right Buttock with Nonautologous Tissue Substitute, Percutaneous Approach

0Y003ZZ Alteration of Right Buttock, Percutaneous Approach

0Y0047Z Alteration of Right Buttock with Autologous Tissue Substitute, Percutaneous Endoscopic Approach

0Y004JZ Alteration of Right Buttock with Synthetic Substitute, Percutaneous Endoscopic Approach

0Y004KZ Alteration of Right Buttock with Nonautologous Tissue Substitute, Percutaneous Endoscopic Approach

0Y004ZZ Alteration of Right Buttock, Percutaneous Endoscopic Approach

0Y0107Z Alteration of Left Buttock with Autologous Tissue Substitute, Open Approach

0Y010JZ Alteration of Left Buttock with Synthetic Substitute, Open Approach

0Y010KZ Alteration of Left Buttock with Nonautologous Tissue Substitute, Open Approach

♀ Female-only   ♂ Male-only   ▲ Limited Coverage   ● Non-OR   ▧ HAC-associated procedure   ▲ Non-covered procedures   ✚ Cluster

0Y010ZZ Alteration of Left Buttock, Open Approach

0Y0137Z Alteration of Left Buttock with Autologous Tissue Substitute, Percutaneous Approach

0Y013JZ Alteration of Left Buttock with Synthetic Substitute, Percutaneous Approach

0Y013KZ Alteration of Left Buttock with Nonautologous Tissue Substitute, Percutaneous Approach

0Y013ZZ Alteration of Left Buttock, Percutaneous Approach

0Y0147Z Alteration of Left Buttock with Autologous Tissue Substitute, Percutaneous Endoscopic Approach

0Y014JZ Alteration of Left Buttock with Synthetic Substitute, Percutaneous Endoscopic Approach

0Y014KZ Alteration of Left Buttock with Nonautologous Tissue Substitute, Percutaneous Endoscopic Approach

0Y014ZZ Alteration of Left Buttock, Percutaneous Endoscopic Approach

0Y0907Z Alteration of Right Lower Extremity with Autologous Tissue Substitute, Open Approach

0Y090JZ Alteration of Right Lower Extremity with Synthetic Substitute, Open Approach

0Y090KZ Alteration of Right Lower Extremity with Nonautologous Tissue Substitute, Open Approach

0Y090ZZ Alteration of Right Lower Extremity, Open Approach

0Y0937Z Alteration of Right Lower Extremity with Autologous Tissue Substitute, Percutaneous Approach

0Y093JZ Alteration of Right Lower Extremity with Synthetic Substitute, Percutaneous Approach

0Y093KZ Alteration of Right Lower Extremity with Nonautologous Tissue Substitute, Percutaneous Approach

0Y093ZZ Alteration of Right Lower Extremity, Percutaneous Approach

0Y0947Z Alteration of Right Lower Extremity with Autologous Tissue Substitute, Percutaneous Endoscopic Approach

0Y094JZ Alteration of Right Lower Extremity with Synthetic Substitute, Percutaneous Endoscopic Approach

0Y094KZ Alteration of Right Lower Extremity with Nonautologous Tissue Substitute, Percutaneous Endoscopic Approach

0Y094ZZ Alteration of Right Lower Extremity, Percutaneous Endoscopic Approach

0Y0B07Z Alteration of Left Lower Extremity with Autologous Tissue Substitute, Open Approach

0Y0B0JZ Alteration of Left Lower Extremity with Synthetic Substitute, Open Approach

0Y0B0KZ Alteration of Left Lower Extremity with Nonautologous Tissue Substitute, Open Approach

0Y0B0ZZ Alteration of Left Lower Extremity, Open Approach

0Y0B37Z Alteration of Left Lower Extremity with Autologous Tissue Substitute, Percutaneous Approach

0Y0B3JZ Alteration of Left Lower Extremity with Synthetic Substitute, Percutaneous Approach

0Y0B3KZ Alteration of Left Lower Extremity with Nonautologous Tissue Substitute, Percutaneous Approach

0Y0B3ZZ Alteration of Left Lower Extremity, Percutaneous Approach

0Y0B47Z Alteration of Left Lower Extremity with Autologous Tissue Substitute, Percutaneous Endoscopic Approach

0Y0B4JZ Alteration of Left Lower Extremity with Synthetic Substitute, Percutaneous Endoscopic Approach

0Y0B4KZ Alteration of Left Lower Extremity with Nonautologous Tissue Substitute, Percutaneous Endoscopic Approach

0Y0B4ZZ Alteration of Left Lower Extremity, Percutaneous Endoscopic Approach

0Y0C07Z Alteration of Right Upper Leg with Autologous Tissue Substitute, Open Approach

0Y0C0JZ Alteration of Right Upper Leg with Synthetic Substitute, Open Approach

0Y0C0KZ Alteration of Right Upper Leg with Nonautologous Tissue Substitute, Open Approach

0Y0C0ZZ Alteration of Right Upper Leg, Open Approach

0Y0C37Z Alteration of Right Upper Leg with Autologous Tissue Substitute, Percutaneous Approach

0Y0C3JZ Alteration of Right Upper Leg with Synthetic Substitute, Percutaneous Approach

0Y0C3KZ Alteration of Right Upper Leg with Nonautologous Tissue Substitute, Percutaneous Approach

0Y0C3ZZ Alteration of Right Upper Leg, Percutaneous Approach

0Y0C47Z Alteration of Right Upper Leg with Autologous Tissue Substitute, Percutaneous Endoscopic Approach

0Y0C4JZ Alteration of Right Upper Leg with Synthetic Substitute, Percutaneous Endoscopic Approach

0Y0C4KZ Alteration of Right Upper Leg with Nonautologous Tissue Substitute, Percutaneous Endoscopic Approach

0Y0C4ZZ Alteration of Right Upper Leg, Percutaneous Endoscopic Approach

0Y0D07Z Alteration of Left Upper Leg with Autologous Tissue Substitute, Open Approach

0Y0D0JZ Alteration of Left Upper Leg with Synthetic Substitute, Open Approach

0Y0D0KZ Alteration of Left Upper Leg with Nonautologous Tissue Substitute, Open Approach

0Y0D0ZZ Alteration of Left Upper Leg, Open Approach

0Y0D37Z Alteration of Left Upper Leg with Autologous Tissue Substitute, Percutaneous Approach

0Y0D3JZ Alteration of Left Upper Leg with Synthetic Substitute, Percutaneous Approach

0Y0D3KZ Alteration of Left Upper Leg with Nonautologous Tissue Substitute, Percutaneous Approach

0Y0D3ZZ Alteration of Left Upper Leg, Percutaneous Approach

0Y0D47Z Alteration of Left Upper Leg with Autologous Tissue Substitute, Percutaneous Endoscopic Approach

0Y0D4JZ Alteration of Left Upper Leg with Synthetic Substitute, Percutaneous Endoscopic Approach

0Y0D4KZ Alteration of Left Upper Leg with Nonautologous Tissue Substitute, Percutaneous Endoscopic Approach

0Y0D4ZZ Alteration of Left Upper Leg, Percutaneous Endoscopic Approach

0Y0F07Z Alteration of Right Knee Region with Autologous Tissue Substitute, Open Approach

0Y0F0JZ Alteration of Right Knee Region with Synthetic Substitute, Open Approach

0Y0F0KZ Alteration of Right Knee Region with Nonautologous Tissue Substitute, Open Approach

0Y0F0ZZ Alteration of Right Knee Region, Open Approach

0Y0F37Z Alteration of Right Knee Region with Autologous Tissue Substitute, Percutaneous Approach

0Y0F3JZ Alteration of Right Knee Region with Synthetic Substitute, Percutaneous Approach

0Y0F3KZ Alteration of Right Knee Region with Nonautologous Tissue Substitute, Percutaneous Approach

0Y0F3ZZ Alteration of Right Knee Region, Percutaneous Approach

0Y0F47Z Alteration of Right Knee Region with Autologous Tissue Substitute, Percutaneous Endoscopic Approach

0Y0F4JZ Alteration of Right Knee Region with Synthetic Substitute, Percutaneous Endoscopic Approach

0Y0F4KZ Alteration of Right Knee Region with Nonautologous Tissue Substitute, Percutaneous Endoscopic Approach

0Y0F4ZZ Alteration of Right Knee Region, Percutaneous Endoscopic Approach

0Y0G07Z Alteration of Left Knee Region with Autologous Tissue Substitute, Open Approach

0Y0G0JZ Alteration of Left Knee Region with Synthetic Substitute, Open Approach

0Y0G0KZ Alteration of Left Knee Region with Nonautologous Tissue Substitute, Open Approach

0Y0G0ZZ Alteration of Left Knee Region, Open Approach

0Y0G37Z Alteration of Left Knee Region with Autologous Tissue Substitute, Percutaneous Approach

0Y0G3JZ Alteration of Left Knee Region with Synthetic Substitute, Percutaneous Approach

0Y0G3KZ Alteration of Left Knee Region with Nonautologous Tissue Substitute, Percutaneous Approach

0Y0G3ZZ Alteration of Left Knee Region, Percutaneous Approach

0Y0G47Z Alteration of Left Knee Region with Autologous Tissue Substitute, Percutaneous Endoscopic Approach

0Y0G4JZ Alteration of Left Knee Region with Synthetic Substitute, Percutaneous Endoscopic Approach

0Y0G4KZ Alteration of Left Knee Region with Nonautologous Tissue Substitute, Percutaneous Endoscopic Approach

0Y0G4ZZ Alteration of Left Knee Region, Percutaneous Endoscopic Approach

0Y0H07Z Alteration of Right Lower Leg with Autologous Tissue Substitute, Open Approach

0Y0H0JZ Alteration of Right Lower Leg with Synthetic Substitute, Open Approach

0Y0H0KZ	Alteration of Right Lower Leg with Nonautologous Tissue Substitute, Open Approach	**0Y0J3JZ**	Alteration of Left Lower Leg with Synthetic Substitute, Percutaneous Approach	**0Y0K4JZ**	Alteration of Right Ankle Region with Synthetic Substitute, Percutaneous Endoscopic Approach
0Y0H0ZZ	Alteration of Right Lower Leg, Open Approach	**0Y0J3KZ**	Alteration of Left Lower Leg with Nonautologous Tissue Substitute, Percutaneous Approach	**0Y0K4KZ**	Alteration of Right Ankle Region with Nonautologous Tissue Substitute, Percutaneous Endoscopic Approach
0Y0H37Z	Alteration of Right Lower Leg with Autologous Tissue Substitute, Percutaneous Approach	**0Y0J3ZZ**	Alteration of Left Lower Leg, Percutaneous Approach	**0Y0K4ZZ**	Alteration of Right Ankle Region, Percutaneous Endoscopic Approach
0Y0H3JZ	Alteration of Right Lower Leg with Synthetic Substitute, Percutaneous Approach	**0Y0J47Z**	Alteration of Left Lower Leg with Autologous Tissue Substitute, Percutaneous Endoscopic Approach	**0Y0L07Z**	Alteration of Left Ankle Region with Autologous Tissue Substitute, Open Approach
0Y0H3KZ	Alteration of Right Lower Leg with Nonautologous Tissue Substitute, Percutaneous Approach	**0Y0J4JZ**	Alteration of Left Lower Leg with Synthetic Substitute, Percutaneous Endoscopic Approach	**0Y0L0JZ**	Alteration of Left Ankle Region with Synthetic Substitute, Open Approach
0Y0H3ZZ	Alteration of Right Lower Leg, Percutaneous Approach	**0Y0J4KZ**	Alteration of Left Lower Leg with Nonautologous Tissue Substitute, Percutaneous Endoscopic Approach	**0Y0L0KZ**	Alteration of Left Ankle Region with Nonautologous Tissue Substitute, Open Approach
0Y0H47Z	Alteration of Right Lower Leg with Autologous Tissue Substitute, Percutaneous Endoscopic Approach	**0Y0J4ZZ**	Alteration of Left Lower Leg, Percutaneous Endoscopic Approach	**0Y0L0ZZ**	Alteration of Left Ankle Region, Open Approach
0Y0H4JZ	Alteration of Right Lower Leg with Synthetic Substitute, Percutaneous Endoscopic Approach	**0Y0K07Z**	Alteration of Right Ankle Region with Autologous Tissue Substitute, Open Approach	**0Y0L37Z**	Alteration of Left Ankle Region with Autologous Tissue Substitute, Percutaneous Approach
0Y0H4KZ	Alteration of Right Lower Leg with Nonautologous Tissue Substitute, Percutaneous Endoscopic Approach	**0Y0K0JZ**	Alteration of Right Ankle Region with Synthetic Substitute, Open Approach	**0Y0L3JZ**	Alteration of Left Ankle Region with Synthetic Substitute, Percutaneous Approach
0Y0H4ZZ	Alteration of Right Lower Leg, Percutaneous Endoscopic Approach	**0Y0K0KZ**	Alteration of Right Ankle Region with Nonautologous Tissue Substitute, Open Approach	**0Y0L3KZ**	Alteration of Left Ankle Region with Nonautologous Tissue Substitute, Percutaneous Approach
0Y0J07Z	Alteration of Left Lower Leg with Autologous Tissue Substitute, Open Approach	**0Y0K0ZZ**	Alteration of Right Ankle Region, Open Approach	**0Y0L3ZZ**	Alteration of Left Ankle Region, Percutaneous Approach
0Y0J0JZ	Alteration of Left Lower Leg with Synthetic Substitute, Open Approach	**0Y0K37Z**	Alteration of Right Ankle Region with Autologous Tissue Substitute, Percutaneous Approach	**0Y0L47Z**	Alteration of Left Ankle Region with Autologous Tissue Substitute, Percutaneous Endoscopic Approach
0Y0J0KZ	Alteration of Left Lower Leg with Nonautologous Tissue Substitute, Open Approach	**0Y0K3JZ**	Alteration of Right Ankle Region with Synthetic Substitute, Percutaneous Approach	**0Y0L4JZ**	Alteration of Left Ankle Region with Synthetic Substitute, Percutaneous Endoscopic Approach
0Y0J0ZZ	Alteration of Left Lower Leg, Open Approach	**0Y0K3KZ**	Alteration of Right Ankle Region with Nonautologous Tissue Substitute, Percutaneous Approach	**0Y0L4KZ**	Alteration of Left Ankle Region with Nonautologous Tissue Substitute, Percutaneous Endoscopic Approach
0Y0J37Z	Alteration of Left Lower Leg with Autologous Tissue Substitute, Percutaneous Approach	**0Y0K3ZZ**	Alteration of Right Ankle Region, Percutaneous Approach	**0Y0L4ZZ**	Alteration of Left Ankle Region, Percutaneous Endoscopic Approach
		0Y0K47Z	Alteration of Right Ankle Region with Autologous Tissue Substitute, Percutaneous Endoscopic Approach		

0Y2 – Anatomical Regions, Lower Extremities, Change

Review Coding Guideline B6.1c

0Y29X0Z	Change Drainage Device in Right Lower Extremity, External Approach	**0Y2BX0Z**	Change Drainage Device in Left Lower Extremity, External Approach
0Y29XYZ	Change Other Device in Right Lower Extremity, External Approach	**0Y2BXYZ**	Change Other Device in Left Lower Extremity, External Approach

0Y3 – Anatomical Regions, Lower Extremities, Control

Review Coding Guideline B3.7

0Y300ZZ	Control Bleeding in Right Buttock, Open Approach	**0Y360ZZ**	Control Bleeding in Left Inguinal Region, Open Approach	**0Y384ZZ**	Control Bleeding in Left Femoral Region, Percutaneous Endoscopic Approach
0Y303ZZ	Control Bleeding in Right Buttock, Percutaneous Approach	**0Y363ZZ**	Control Bleeding in Left Inguinal Region, Percutaneous Approach	**0Y390ZZ**	Control Bleeding in Right Lower Extremity, Open Approach
0Y304ZZ	Control Bleeding in Right Buttock, Percutaneous Endoscopic Approach	**0Y364ZZ**	Control Bleeding in Left Inguinal Region, Percutaneous Endoscopic Approach	**0Y393ZZ**	Control Bleeding in Right Lower Extremity, Percutaneous Approach
0Y310ZZ	Control Bleeding in Left Buttock, Open Approach	**0Y370ZZ**	Control Bleeding in Right Femoral Region, Open Approach	**0Y394ZZ**	Control Bleeding in Right Lower Extremity, Percutaneous Endoscopic Approach
0Y313ZZ	Control Bleeding in Left Buttock, Percutaneous Approach	**0Y373ZZ**	Control Bleeding in Right Femoral Region, Percutaneous Approach	**0Y3B0ZZ**	Control Bleeding in Left Lower Extremity, Open Approach
0Y314ZZ	Control Bleeding in Left Buttock, Percutaneous Endoscopic Approach	**0Y374ZZ**	Control Bleeding in Right Femoral Region, Percutaneous Endoscopic Approach	**0Y3B3ZZ**	Control Bleeding in Left Lower Extremity, Percutaneous Approach
0Y350ZZ	Control Bleeding in Right Inguinal Region, Open Approach	**0Y380ZZ**	Control Bleeding in Left Femoral Region, Open Approach	**0Y3B4ZZ**	Control Bleeding in Left Lower Extremity, Percutaneous Endoscopic Approach
0Y353ZZ	Control Bleeding in Right Inguinal Region, Percutaneous Approach	**0Y383ZZ**	Control Bleeding in Left Femoral Region, Percutaneous Approach	**0Y3C0ZZ**	Control Bleeding in Right Upper Leg, Open Approach
0Y354ZZ	Control Bleeding in Right Inguinal Region, Percutaneous Endoscopic Approach				

♀ Female-only   ♂ Male-only   ▲ Limited Coverage   ● Non-OR   ▨ HAC-associated procedure   ▲ Non-covered procedures   ✚ Cluster

0Y3C3ZZ Control Bleeding in Right Upper Leg, Percutaneous Approach

0Y3C4ZZ Control Bleeding in Right Upper Leg, Percutaneous Endoscopic Approach

0Y3D0ZZ Control Bleeding in Left Upper Leg, Open Approach

0Y3D3ZZ Control Bleeding in Left Upper Leg, Percutaneous Approach

0Y3D4ZZ Control Bleeding in Left Upper Leg, Percutaneous Endoscopic Approach

0Y3F0ZZ Control Bleeding in Right Knee Region, Open Approach

0Y3F3ZZ Control Bleeding in Right Knee Region, Percutaneous Approach

0Y3F4ZZ Control Bleeding in Right Knee Region, Percutaneous Endoscopic Approach

0Y3G0ZZ Control Bleeding in Left Knee Region, Open Approach

0Y3G3ZZ Control Bleeding in Left Knee Region, Percutaneous Approach

0Y3G4ZZ Control Bleeding in Left Knee Region, Percutaneous Endoscopic Approach

0Y3H0ZZ Control Bleeding in Right Lower Leg, Open Approach

0Y3H3ZZ Control Bleeding in Right Lower Leg, Percutaneous Approach

0Y3H4ZZ Control Bleeding in Right Lower Leg, Percutaneous Endoscopic Approach

0Y3J0ZZ Control Bleeding in Left Lower Leg, Open Approach

0Y3J3ZZ Control Bleeding in Left Lower Leg, Percutaneous Approach

0Y3J4ZZ Control Bleeding in Left Lower Leg, Percutaneous Endoscopic Approach

0Y3K0ZZ Control Bleeding in Right Ankle Region, Open Approach

0Y3K3ZZ Control Bleeding in Right Ankle Region, Percutaneous Approach

0Y3K4ZZ Control Bleeding in Right Ankle Region, Percutaneous Endoscopic Approach

0Y3L0ZZ Control Bleeding in Left Ankle Region, Open Approach

0Y3L3ZZ Control Bleeding in Left Ankle Region, Percutaneous Approach

0Y3L4ZZ Control Bleeding in Left Ankle Region, Percutaneous Endoscopic Approach

0Y3M0ZZ Control Bleeding in Right Foot, Open Approach

0Y3M3ZZ Control Bleeding in Right Foot, Percutaneous Approach

0Y3M4ZZ Control Bleeding in Right Foot, Percutaneous Endoscopic Approach

0Y3N0ZZ Control Bleeding in Left Foot, Open Approach

0Y3N3ZZ Control Bleeding in Left Foot, Percutaneous Approach

0Y3N4ZZ Control Bleeding in Left Foot, Percutaneous Endoscopic Approach

0Y6 – Anatomical Regions, Lower Extremities, Detachment

0Y620ZZ Detachment at Right Hindquarter, Open Approach

0Y630ZZ Detachment at Left Hindquarter, Open Approach

0Y640ZZ Detachment at Bilateral Hindquarter, Open Approach

0Y670ZZ Detachment at Right Femoral Region, Open Approach

0Y680ZZ Detachment at Left Femoral Region, Open Approach

0Y6C0Z1 Detachment at Right Upper Leg, High, Open Approach

0Y6C0Z2 Detachment at Right Upper Leg, Mid, Open Approach

0Y6C0Z3 Detachment at Right Upper Leg, Low, Open Approach

0Y6D0Z1 Detachment at Left Upper Leg, High, Open Approach

0Y6D0Z2 Detachment at Left Upper Leg, Mid, Open Approach

0Y6D0Z3 Detachment at Left Upper Leg, Low, Open Approach

0Y6F0ZZ Detachment at Right Knee Region, Open Approach

0Y6G0ZZ Detachment at Left Knee Region, Open Approach

0Y6H0Z1 Detachment at Right Lower Leg, High, Open Approach

0Y6H0Z2 Detachment at Right Lower Leg, Mid, Open Approach

0Y6H0Z3 Detachment at Right Lower Leg, Low, Open Approach

0Y6J0Z1 Detachment at Left Lower Leg, High, Open Approach

0Y6J0Z2 Detachment at Left Lower Leg, Mid, Open Approach

0Y6J0Z3 Detachment at Left Lower Leg, Low, Open Approach

0Y6M0Z0 Detachment at Right Foot, Complete, Open Approach

0Y6M0Z4 Detachment at Right Foot, Complete 1st Ray, Open Approach

0Y6M0Z5 Detachment at Right Foot, Complete 2nd Ray, Open Approach

0Y6M0Z6 Detachment at Right Foot, Complete 3rd Ray, Open Approach

0Y6M0Z7 Detachment at Right Foot, Complete 4th Ray, Open Approach

0Y6M0Z8 Detachment at Right Foot, Complete 5th Ray, Open Approach

0Y6M0Z9 Detachment at Right Foot, Partial 1st Ray, Open Approach

0Y6M0ZB Detachment at Right Foot, Partial 2nd Ray, Open Approach

0Y6M0ZC Detachment at Right Foot, Partial 3rd Ray, Open Approach

0Y6M0ZD Detachment at Right Foot, Partial 4th Ray, Open Approach

0Y6M0ZF Detachment at Right Foot, Partial 5th Ray, Open Approach

0Y6N0Z0 Detachment at Left Foot, Complete, Open Approach

AHA CC: 1Q, 2015, 28; 1Q, 2017, 22-23

0Y6N0Z4 Detachment at Left Foot, Complete 1st Ray, Open Approach

0Y6N0Z5 Detachment at Left Foot, Complete 2nd Ray, Open Approach

0Y6N0Z6 Detachment at Left Foot, Complete 3rd Ray, Open Approach

0Y6N0Z7 Detachment at Left Foot, Complete 4th Ray, Open Approach

0Y6N0Z8 Detachment at Left Foot, Complete 5th Ray, Open Approach

0Y6N0Z9 Detachment at Left Foot, Partial 1st Ray, Open Approach

0Y6N0ZB Detachment at Left Foot, Partial 2nd Ray, Open Approach

0Y6N0ZC Detachment at Left Foot, Partial 3rd Ray, Open Approach

0Y6N0ZD Detachment at Left Foot, Partial 4th Ray, Open Approach

0Y6N0ZF Detachment at Left Foot, Partial 5th Ray, Open Approach

0Y6P0Z0 Detachment at Right 1st Toe, Complete, Open Approach

0Y6P0Z1 Detachment at Right 1st Toe, High, Open Approach

0Y6P0Z2 Detachment at Right 1st Toe, Mid, Open Approach

0Y6P0Z3 Detachment at Right 1st Toe, Low, Open Approach

AHA CC: 2Q, 2015, 28-29

0Y6Q0Z0 Detachment at Left 1st Toe, Complete, Open Approach

0Y6Q0Z1 Detachment at Left 1st Toe, High, Open Approach

0Y6Q0Z2 Detachment at Left 1st Toe, Mid, Open Approach

0Y6Q0Z3 Detachment at Left 1st Toe, Low, Open Approach

AHA CC: 2Q, 2015, 28-29

0Y6R0Z0 Detachment at Right 2nd Toe, Complete, Open Approach

0Y6R0Z1 Detachment at Right 2nd Toe, High, Open Approach

0Y6R0Z2 Detachment at Right 2nd Toe, Mid, Open Approach

0Y6R0Z3 Detachment at Right 2nd Toe, Low, Open Approach

0Y6S0Z0 Detachment at Left 2nd Toe, Complete, Open Approach

0Y6S0Z1 Detachment at Left 2nd Toe, High, Open Approach

0Y6S0Z2 Detachment at Left 2nd Toe, Mid, Open Approach

0Y6S0Z3 Detachment at Left 2nd Toe, Low, Open Approach

0Y6T0Z0 Detachment at Right 3rd Toe, Complete, Open Approach

0Y6T0Z1 Detachment at Right 3rd Toe, High, Open Approach

0Y6T0Z2 Detachment at Right 3rd Toe, Mid, Open Approach

0Y6T0Z3 Detachment at Right 3rd Toe, Low, Open Approach

0Y6U0Z0 Detachment at Left 3rd Toe, Complete, Open Approach

0Y6U0Z1 Detachment at Left 3rd Toe, High, Open Approach

0Y6U0Z2 Detachment at Left 3rd Toe, Mid, Open Approach

0Y6U0Z3 Detachment at Left 3rd Toe, Low, Open Approach

0Y6V0Z0 Detachment at Right 4th Toe, Complete, Open Approach

0Y6V0Z1 Detachment at Right 4th Toe, High, Open Approach

0Y6V0Z2 Detachment at Right 4th Toe, Mid, Open Approach

0Y6V0Z3 Detachment at Right 4th Toe, Low, Open Approach

0Y6W0Z0 Detachment at Left 4th Toe, Complete, Open Approach

0Y6W0Z1 Detachment at Left 4th Toe, High, Open Approach

0Y6W0Z2 Detachment at Left 4th Toe, Mid, Open Approach

0Y6W0Z3 Detachment at Left 4th Toe, Low, Open Approach	**0Y6X0Z2** Detachment at Right 5th Toe, Mid, Open Approach	**0Y6Y0Z1** Detachment at Left 5th Toe, High, Open Approach
0Y6X0Z0 Detachment at Right 5th Toe, Complete, Open Approach	**0Y6X0Z3** Detachment at Right 5th Toe, Low, Open Approach	**0Y6Y0Z2** Detachment at Left 5th Toe, Mid, Open Approach
0Y6X0Z1 Detachment at Right 5th Toe, High, Open Approach	**0Y6Y0Z0** Detachment at Left 5th Toe, Complete, Open Approach	**0Y6Y0Z3** Detachment at Left 5th Toe, Low, Open Approach

0Y9 – Anatomical Regions, Lower Extremities, Drainage

Review Coding Guidelines B3.4a and B3.4b

Review Coding Guideline B6.2

0Y9000Z Drainage of Right Buttock with Drainage Device, Open Approach	**0Y9600Z** Drainage of Left Inguinal Region with Drainage Device, Open Approach	**0Y984ZZ** Drainage of Left Femoral Region, Percutaneous Endoscopic Approach
0Y900ZX Drainage of Right Buttock, Open Approach, Diagnostic	**0Y960ZX** Drainage of Left Inguinal Region, Open Approach, Diagnostic	**0Y9900Z** Drainage of Right Lower Extremity with Drainage Device, Open Approach
0Y900ZZ Drainage of Right Buttock, Open Approach	**0Y960ZZ** Drainage of Left Inguinal Region, Open Approach	**0Y990ZX** Drainage of Right Lower Extremity, Open Approach, Diagnostic
0Y9030Z Drainage of Right Buttock with Drainage Device, Percutaneous Approach	**0Y9630Z** Drainage of Left Inguinal Region with Drainage Device, Percutaneous Approach	**0Y990ZZ** Drainage of Right Lower Extremity, Open Approach
0Y903ZX Drainage of Right Buttock, Percutaneous Approach, Diagnostic	**0Y963ZX** Drainage of Left Inguinal Region, Percutaneous Approach, Diagnostic	**0Y9930Z** Drainage of Right Lower Extremity with Drainage Device, Percutaneous Approach
0Y903ZZ Drainage of Right Buttock, Percutaneous Approach	**0Y963ZZ** Drainage of Left Inguinal Region, Percutaneous Approach	**0Y993ZX** Drainage of Right Lower Extremity, Percutaneous Approach, Diagnostic
0Y9040Z Drainage of Right Buttock with Drainage Device, Percutaneous Endoscopic Approach	**0Y9640Z** Drainage of Left Inguinal Region with Drainage Device, Percutaneous Endoscopic Approach	**0Y993ZZ** Drainage of Right Lower Extremity, Percutaneous Approach
0Y904ZX Drainage of Right Buttock, Percutaneous Endoscopic Approach, Diagnostic	**0Y964ZX** Drainage of Left Inguinal Region, Percutaneous Endoscopic Approach, Diagnostic	**0Y9940Z** Drainage of Right Lower Extremity with Drainage Device, Percutaneous Endoscopic Approach
0Y904ZZ Drainage of Right Buttock, Percutaneous Endoscopic Approach	**0Y964ZZ** Drainage of Left Inguinal Region, Percutaneous Endoscopic Approach	**0Y994ZX** Drainage of Right Lower Extremity, Percutaneous Endoscopic Approach, Diagnostic
0Y9100Z Drainage of Left Buttock with Drainage Device, Open Approach	**0Y9700Z** Drainage of Right Femoral Region with Drainage Device, Open Approach	**0Y994ZZ** Drainage of Right Lower Extremity, Percutaneous Endoscopic Approach
0Y910ZX Drainage of Left Buttock, Open Approach, Diagnostic	**0Y970ZX** Drainage of Right Femoral Region, Open Approach, Diagnostic	**0Y9B00Z** Drainage of Left Lower Extremity with Drainage Device, Open Approach
0Y910ZZ Drainage of Left Buttock, Open Approach	**0Y970ZZ** Drainage of Right Femoral Region, Open Approach	**0Y9B0ZX** Drainage of Left Lower Extremity, Open Approach, Diagnostic
0Y9130Z Drainage of Left Buttock with Drainage Device, Percutaneous Approach	**0Y9730Z** Drainage of Right Femoral Region with Drainage Device, Percutaneous Approach	**0Y9B0ZZ** Drainage of Left Lower Extremity, Open Approach
0Y913ZX Drainage of Left Buttock, Percutaneous Approach, Diagnostic	**0Y973ZX** Drainage of Right Femoral Region, Percutaneous Approach, Diagnostic	**0Y9B30Z** Drainage of Left Lower Extremity with Drainage Device, Percutaneous Approach
0Y913ZZ Drainage of Left Buttock, Percutaneous Approach	**0Y973ZZ** Drainage of Right Femoral Region, Percutaneous Approach	**0Y9B3ZX** Drainage of Left Lower Extremity, Percutaneous Approach, Diagnostic
0Y9140Z Drainage of Left Buttock with Drainage Device, Percutaneous Endoscopic Approach	**0Y9740Z** Drainage of Right Femoral Region with Drainage Device, Percutaneous Endoscopic Approach	**0Y9B3ZZ** Drainage of Left Lower Extremity, Percutaneous Approach
0Y914ZX Drainage of Left Buttock, Percutaneous Endoscopic Approach, Diagnostic	**0Y974ZX** Drainage of Right Femoral Region, Percutaneous Endoscopic Approach, Diagnostic	**0Y9B40Z** Drainage of Left Lower Extremity with Drainage Device, Percutaneous Endoscopic Approach
0Y914ZZ Drainage of Left Buttock, Percutaneous Endoscopic Approach	**0Y974ZZ** Drainage of Right Femoral Region, Percutaneous Endoscopic Approach	**0Y9B4ZX** Drainage of Left Lower Extremity, Percutaneous Endoscopic Approach, Diagnostic
0Y9500Z Drainage of Right Inguinal Region with Drainage Device, Open Approach	**0Y9800Z** Drainage of Left Femoral Region with Drainage Device, Open Approach	**0Y9B4ZZ** Drainage of Left Lower Extremity, Percutaneous Endoscopic Approach
0Y950ZX Drainage of Right Inguinal Region, Open Approach, Diagnostic	**0Y980ZX** Drainage of Left Femoral Region, Open Approach, Diagnostic	**0Y9C00Z** Drainage of Right Upper Leg with Drainage Device, Open Approach
0Y950ZZ Drainage of Right Inguinal Region, Open Approach	**0Y980ZZ** Drainage of Left Femoral Region, Open Approach	**0Y9C0ZX** Drainage of Right Upper Leg, Open Approach, Diagnostic
AHA CC: 1Q, 2015, 23	*AHA CC: 1Q, 2015, 22*	**0Y9C0ZZ** Drainage of Right Upper Leg, Open Approach
0Y9530Z Drainage of Right Inguinal Region with Drainage Device, Percutaneous Approach	**0Y9830Z** Drainage of Left Femoral Region with Drainage Device, Percutaneous Approach	**0Y9C30Z** Drainage of Right Upper Leg with Drainage Device, Percutaneous Approach
0Y953ZX Drainage of Right Inguinal Region, Percutaneous Approach, Diagnostic	**0Y983ZX** Drainage of Left Femoral Region, Percutaneous Approach, Diagnostic	**0Y9C3ZX** Drainage of Right Upper Leg, Percutaneous Approach, Diagnostic
0Y953ZZ Drainage of Right Inguinal Region, Percutaneous Approach	**0Y983ZZ** Drainage of Left Femoral Region, Percutaneous Approach	**0Y9C3ZZ** Drainage of Right Upper Leg, Percutaneous Approach
0Y9540Z Drainage of Right Inguinal Region with Drainage Device, Percutaneous Endoscopic Approach	**0Y9840Z** Drainage of Left Femoral Region with Drainage Device, Percutaneous Endoscopic Approach	**0Y9C40Z** Drainage of Right Upper Leg with Drainage Device, Percutaneous Endoscopic Approach
0Y954ZX Drainage of Right Inguinal Region, Percutaneous Endoscopic Approach, Diagnostic	**0Y984ZX** Drainage of Left Femoral Region, Percutaneous Endoscopic Approach, Diagnostic	**0Y9C4ZX** Drainage of Right Upper Leg, Percutaneous Endoscopic Approach, Diagnostic
0Y954ZZ Drainage of Right Inguinal Region, Percutaneous Endoscopic Approach		

♀ Female-only   ♂ Male-only   ▲ Limited Coverage   ● Non-OR   **HAC** HAC-associated procedure   ▲ Non-covered procedures   ✚ Cluster

0Y9C4ZZ Drainage of Right Upper Leg, Percutaneous Endoscopic Approach

0Y9D00Z Drainage of Left Upper Leg with Drainage Device, Open Approach

0Y9D0ZX Drainage of Left Upper Leg, Open Approach, Diagnostic

0Y9D0ZZ Drainage of Left Upper Leg, Open Approach

0Y9D30Z Drainage of Left Upper Leg with Drainage Device, Percutaneous Approach

0Y9D3ZX Drainage of Left Upper Leg, Percutaneous Approach, Diagnostic

0Y9D3ZZ Drainage of Left Upper Leg, Percutaneous Approach

0Y9D40Z Drainage of Left Upper Leg with Drainage Device, Percutaneous Endoscopic Approach

0Y9D4ZX Drainage of Left Upper Leg, Percutaneous Endoscopic Approach, Diagnostic

0Y9D4ZZ Drainage of Left Upper Leg, Percutaneous Endoscopic Approach

0Y9F00Z Drainage of Right Knee Region with Drainage Device, Open Approach

0Y9F0ZX Drainage of Right Knee Region, Open Approach, Diagnostic

0Y9F0ZZ Drainage of Right Knee Region, Open Approach

0Y9F30Z Drainage of Right Knee Region with Drainage Device, Percutaneous Approach

0Y9F3ZX Drainage of Right Knee Region, Percutaneous Approach, Diagnostic

0Y9F3ZZ Drainage of Right Knee Region, Percutaneous Approach

0Y9F40Z Drainage of Right Knee Region with Drainage Device, Percutaneous Endoscopic Approach

0Y9F4ZX Drainage of Right Knee Region, Percutaneous Endoscopic Approach, Diagnostic

0Y9F4ZZ Drainage of Right Knee Region, Percutaneous Endoscopic Approach

0Y9G00Z Drainage of Left Knee Region with Drainage Device, Open Approach

0Y9G0ZX Drainage of Left Knee Region, Open Approach, Diagnostic

0Y9G0ZZ Drainage of Left Knee Region, Open Approach

0Y9G30Z Drainage of Left Knee Region with Drainage Device, Percutaneous Approach

0Y9G3ZX Drainage of Left Knee Region, Percutaneous Approach, Diagnostic

0Y9G3ZZ Drainage of Left Knee Region, Percutaneous Approach

0Y9G40Z Drainage of Left Knee Region with Drainage Device, Percutaneous Endoscopic Approach

0Y9G4ZX Drainage of Left Knee Region, Percutaneous Endoscopic Approach, Diagnostic

0Y9G4ZZ Drainage of Left Knee Region, Percutaneous Endoscopic Approach

0Y9H00Z Drainage of Right Lower Leg with Drainage Device, Open Approach

0Y9H0ZX Drainage of Right Lower Leg, Open Approach, Diagnostic

0Y9H0ZZ Drainage of Right Lower Leg, Open Approach

0Y9H30Z Drainage of Right Lower Leg with Drainage Device, Percutaneous Approach

0Y9H3ZX Drainage of Right Lower Leg, Percutaneous Approach, Diagnostic

0Y9H3ZZ Drainage of Right Lower Leg, Percutaneous Approach

0Y9H40Z Drainage of Right Lower Leg with Drainage Device, Percutaneous Endoscopic Approach

0Y9H4ZX Drainage of Right Lower Leg, Percutaneous Endoscopic Approach, Diagnostic

0Y9H4ZZ Drainage of Right Lower Leg, Percutaneous Endoscopic Approach

0Y9J00Z Drainage of Left Lower Leg with Drainage Device, Open Approach

0Y9J0ZX Drainage of Left Lower Leg, Open Approach, Diagnostic

0Y9J0ZZ Drainage of Left Lower Leg, Open Approach

0Y9J30Z Drainage of Left Lower Leg with Drainage Device, Percutaneous Approach

0Y9J3ZX Drainage of Left Lower Leg, Percutaneous Approach, Diagnostic

0Y9J3ZZ Drainage of Left Lower Leg, Percutaneous Approach

0Y9J40Z Drainage of Left Lower Leg with Drainage Device, Percutaneous Endoscopic Approach

0Y9J4ZX Drainage of Left Lower Leg, Percutaneous Endoscopic Approach, Diagnostic

0Y9J4ZZ Drainage of Left Lower Leg, Percutaneous Endoscopic Approach

0Y9K00Z Drainage of Right Ankle Region with Drainage Device, Open Approach

0Y9K0ZX Drainage of Right Ankle Region, Open Approach, Diagnostic

0Y9K0ZZ Drainage of Right Ankle Region, Open Approach

0Y9K30Z Drainage of Right Ankle Region with Drainage Device, Percutaneous Approach

0Y9K3ZX Drainage of Right Ankle Region, Percutaneous Approach, Diagnostic

0Y9K3ZZ Drainage of Right Ankle Region, Percutaneous Approach

0Y9K40Z Drainage of Right Ankle Region with Drainage Device, Percutaneous Endoscopic Approach

0Y9K4ZX Drainage of Right Ankle Region, Percutaneous Endoscopic Approach, Diagnostic

0Y9K4ZZ Drainage of Right Ankle Region, Percutaneous Endoscopic Approach

0Y9L00Z Drainage of Left Ankle Region with Drainage Device, Open Approach

0Y9L0ZX Drainage of Left Ankle Region, Open Approach, Diagnostic

0Y9L0ZZ Drainage of Left Ankle Region, Open Approach

0Y9L30Z Drainage of Left Ankle Region with Drainage Device, Percutaneous Approach

0Y9L3ZX Drainage of Left Ankle Region, Percutaneous Approach, Diagnostic

0Y9L3ZZ Drainage of Left Ankle Region, Percutaneous Approach

0Y9L40Z Drainage of Left Ankle Region with Drainage Device, Percutaneous Endoscopic Approach

0Y9L4ZX Drainage of Left Ankle Region, Percutaneous Endoscopic Approach, Diagnostic

0Y9L4ZZ Drainage of Left Ankle Region, Percutaneous Endoscopic Approach

0Y9M00Z Drainage of Right Foot with Drainage Device, Open Approach

0Y9M0ZX Drainage of Right Foot, Open Approach, Diagnostic

0Y9M0ZZ Drainage of Right Foot, Open Approach

0Y9M30Z Drainage of Right Foot with Drainage Device, Percutaneous Approach

0Y9M3ZX Drainage of Right Foot, Percutaneous Approach, Diagnostic

0Y9M3ZZ Drainage of Right Foot, Percutaneous Approach

0Y9M40Z Drainage of Right Foot with Drainage Device, Percutaneous Endoscopic Approach

0Y9M4ZX Drainage of Right Foot, Percutaneous Endoscopic Approach, Diagnostic

0Y9M4ZZ Drainage of Right Foot, Percutaneous Endoscopic Approach

0Y9N00Z Drainage of Left Foot with Drainage Device, Open Approach

0Y9N0ZX Drainage of Left Foot, Open Approach, Diagnostic

0Y9N0ZZ Drainage of Left Foot, Open Approach

0Y9N30Z Drainage of Left Foot with Drainage Device, Percutaneous Approach

0Y9N3ZX Drainage of Left Foot, Percutaneous Approach, Diagnostic

0Y9N3ZZ Drainage of Left Foot, Percutaneous Approach

0Y9N40Z Drainage of Left Foot with Drainage Device, Percutaneous Endoscopic Approach

0Y9N4ZX Drainage of Left Foot, Percutaneous Endoscopic Approach, Diagnostic

0Y9N4ZZ Drainage of Left Foot, Percutaneous Endoscopic Approach

0YB – Anatomical Regions, Lower Extremities, Excision

Review Coding Guidelines B3.4a and B3.4b

Review Coding Guideline B3.18

0YB00ZX Excision of Right Buttock, Open Approach, Diagnostic

0YB00ZZ Excision of Right Buttock, Open Approach

0YB03ZX Excision of Right Buttock, Percutaneous Approach, Diagnostic

0YB03ZZ Excision of Right Buttock, Percutaneous Approach

0YB04ZX Excision of Right Buttock, Percutaneous Endoscopic Approach, Diagnostic

0YB04ZZ Excision of Right Buttock, Percutaneous Endoscopic Approach

0YB10ZX Excision of Left Buttock, Open Approach, Diagnostic

0YB10ZZ Excision of Left Buttock, Open Approach

0YB13ZX Excision of Left Buttock, Percutaneous Approach, Diagnostic

0YB13ZZ Excision of Left Buttock, Percutaneous Approach

0YB14ZX Excision of Left Buttock, Percutaneous Endoscopic Approach, Diagnostic

0YB14ZZ Excision of Left Buttock, Percutaneous Endoscopic Approach

0YB50ZX Excision of Right Inguinal Region, Open Approach, Diagnostic
0YB50ZZ Excision of Right Inguinal Region, Open Approach
0YB53ZX Excision of Right Inguinal Region, Percutaneous Approach, Diagnostic
0YB53ZZ Excision of Right Inguinal Region, Percutaneous Approach
0YB54ZX Excision of Right Inguinal Region, Percutaneous Endoscopic Approach, Diagnostic
0YB54ZZ Excision of Right Inguinal Region, Percutaneous Endoscopic Approach
0YB60ZX Excision of Left Inguinal Region, Open Approach, Diagnostic
0YB60ZZ Excision of Left Inguinal Region, Open Approach
0YB63ZX Excision of Left Inguinal Region, Percutaneous Approach, Diagnostic
0YB63ZZ Excision of Left Inguinal Region, Percutaneous Approach
0YB64ZX Excision of Left Inguinal Region, Percutaneous Endoscopic Approach, Diagnostic
0YB64ZZ Excision of Left Inguinal Region, Percutaneous Endoscopic Approach
0YB70ZX Excision of Right Femoral Region, Open Approach, Diagnostic
0YB70ZZ Excision of Right Femoral Region, Open Approach
0YB73ZX Excision of Right Femoral Region, Percutaneous Approach, Diagnostic
0YB73ZZ Excision of Right Femoral Region, Percutaneous Approach
0YB74ZX Excision of Right Femoral Region, Percutaneous Endoscopic Approach, Diagnostic
0YB74ZZ Excision of Right Femoral Region, Percutaneous Endoscopic Approach
0YB80ZX Excision of Left Femoral Region, Open Approach, Diagnostic
0YB80ZZ Excision of Left Femoral Region, Open Approach
0YB83ZX Excision of Left Femoral Region, Percutaneous Approach, Diagnostic
0YB83ZZ Excision of Left Femoral Region, Percutaneous Approach
0YB84ZX Excision of Left Femoral Region, Percutaneous Endoscopic Approach, Diagnostic
0YB84ZZ Excision of Left Femoral Region, Percutaneous Endoscopic Approach
0YB90ZX Excision of Right Lower Extremity, Open Approach, Diagnostic
0YB90ZZ Excision of Right Lower Extremity, Open Approach
0YB93ZX Excision of Right Lower Extremity, Percutaneous Approach, Diagnostic
0YB93ZZ Excision of Right Lower Extremity, Percutaneous Approach
0YB94ZX Excision of Right Lower Extremity, Percutaneous Endoscopic Approach, Diagnostic
0YB94ZZ Excision of Right Lower Extremity, Percutaneous Endoscopic Approach
0YBB0ZX Excision of Left Lower Extremity, Open Approach, Diagnostic
0YBB0ZZ Excision of Left Lower Extremity, Open Approach

0YBB3ZX Excision of Left Lower Extremity, Percutaneous Approach, Diagnostic
0YBB3ZZ Excision of Left Lower Extremity, Percutaneous Approach
0YBB4ZX Excision of Left Lower Extremity, Percutaneous Endoscopic Approach, Diagnostic
0YBB4ZZ Excision of Left Lower Extremity, Percutaneous Endoscopic Approach
0YBC0ZX Excision of Right Upper Leg, Open Approach, Diagnostic
0YBC0ZZ Excision of Right Upper Leg, Open Approach
0YBC3ZX Excision of Right Upper Leg, Percutaneous Approach, Diagnostic
0YBC3ZZ Excision of Right Upper Leg, Percutaneous Approach
0YBC4ZX Excision of Right Upper Leg, Percutaneous Endoscopic Approach, Diagnostic
0YBC4ZZ Excision of Right Upper Leg, Percutaneous Endoscopic Approach
0YBD0ZX Excision of Left Upper Leg, Open Approach, Diagnostic
0YBD0ZZ Excision of Left Upper Leg, Open Approach
0YBD3ZX Excision of Left Upper Leg, Percutaneous Approach, Diagnostic
0YBD3ZZ Excision of Left Upper Leg, Percutaneous Approach
0YBD4ZX Excision of Left Upper Leg, Percutaneous Endoscopic Approach, Diagnostic
0YBD4ZZ Excision of Left Upper Leg, Percutaneous Endoscopic Approach
0YBF0ZX Excision of Right Knee Region, Open Approach, Diagnostic
0YBF0ZZ Excision of Right Knee Region, Open Approach
0YBF3ZX Excision of Right Knee Region, Percutaneous Approach, Diagnostic
0YBF3ZZ Excision of Right Knee Region, Percutaneous Approach
0YBF4ZX Excision of Right Knee Region, Percutaneous Endoscopic Approach, Diagnostic
0YBF4ZZ Excision of Right Knee Region, Percutaneous Endoscopic Approach
0YBG0ZX Excision of Left Knee Region, Open Approach, Diagnostic
0YBG0ZZ Excision of Left Knee Region, Open Approach
0YBG3ZX Excision of Left Knee Region, Percutaneous Approach, Diagnostic
0YBG3ZZ Excision of Left Knee Region, Percutaneous Approach
0YBG4ZX Excision of Left Knee Region, Percutaneous Endoscopic Approach, Diagnostic
0YBG4ZZ Excision of Left Knee Region, Percutaneous Endoscopic Approach
0YBH0ZX Excision of Right Lower Leg, Open Approach, Diagnostic
0YBH0ZZ Excision of Right Lower Leg, Open Approach
0YBH3ZX Excision of Right Lower Leg, Percutaneous Approach, Diagnostic

0YBH3ZZ Excision of Right Lower Leg, Percutaneous Approach
0YBH4ZX Excision of Right Lower Leg, Percutaneous Endoscopic Approach, Diagnostic
0YBH4ZZ Excision of Right Lower Leg, Percutaneous Endoscopic Approach
0YBJ0ZX Excision of Left Lower Leg, Open Approach, Diagnostic
0YBJ0ZZ Excision of Left Lower Leg, Open Approach
0YBJ3ZX Excision of Left Lower Leg, Percutaneous Approach, Diagnostic
0YBJ3ZZ Excision of Left Lower Leg, Percutaneous Approach
0YBJ4ZX Excision of Left Lower Leg, Percutaneous Endoscopic Approach, Diagnostic
0YBJ4ZZ Excision of Left Lower Leg, Percutaneous Endoscopic Approach
0YBK0ZX Excision of Right Ankle Region, Open Approach, Diagnostic
0YBK0ZZ Excision of Right Ankle Region, Open Approach
0YBK3ZX Excision of Right Ankle Region, Percutaneous Approach, Diagnostic
0YBK3ZZ Excision of Right Ankle Region, Percutaneous Approach
0YBK4ZX Excision of Right Ankle Region, Percutaneous Endoscopic Approach, Diagnostic
0YBK4ZZ Excision of Right Ankle Region, Percutaneous Endoscopic Approach
0YBL0ZX Excision of Left Ankle Region, Open Approach, Diagnostic
0YBL0ZZ Excision of Left Ankle Region, Open Approach
0YBL3ZX Excision of Left Ankle Region, Percutaneous Approach, Diagnostic
0YBL3ZZ Excision of Left Ankle Region, Percutaneous Approach
0YBL4ZX Excision of Left Ankle Region, Percutaneous Endoscopic Approach, Diagnostic
0YBL4ZZ Excision of Left Ankle Region, Percutaneous Endoscopic Approach
0YBM0ZX Excision of Right Foot, Open Approach, Diagnostic
0YBM0ZZ Excision of Right Foot, Open Approach
0YBM3ZX Excision of Right Foot, Percutaneous Approach, Diagnostic
0YBM3ZZ Excision of Right Foot, Percutaneous Approach
0YBM4ZX Excision of Right Foot, Percutaneous Endoscopic Approach, Diagnostic
0YBM4ZZ Excision of Right Foot, Percutaneous Endoscopic Approach
0YBN0ZX Excision of Left Foot, Open Approach, Diagnostic
0YBN0ZZ Excision of Left Foot, Open Approach
0YBN3ZX Excision of Left Foot, Percutaneous Approach, Diagnostic
0YBN3ZZ Excision of Left Foot, Percutaneous Approach
0YBN4ZX Excision of Left Foot, Percutaneous Endoscopic Approach, Diagnostic
0YBN4ZZ Excision of Left Foot, Percutaneous Endoscopic Approach

0YH – Anatomical Regions, Lower Extremities, Insertion

0YH001Z Insertion of Radioactive Element into Right Buttock, Open Approach
● **0YH003Z** Insertion of Infusion Device into Right Buttock, Open Approach

● **0YH00YZ** Insertion of Other Device into Right Buttock, Open Approach
0YH031Z Insertion of Radioactive Element into Right Buttock, Percutaneous Approach

● **0YH033Z** Insertion of Infusion Device into Right Buttock, Percutaneous Approach
● **0YH03YZ** Insertion of Other Device into Right Buttock, Percutaneous Approach

♀ Female-only   ♂ Male-only   ▲ Limited Coverage   ● Non-OR   ⬛ HAC-associated procedure   ▲ Non-covered procedures   ✚ Cluster

0YH041Z Insertion of Radioactive Element into Right Buttock, Percutaneous Endoscopic Approach

● **0YH043Z** Insertion of Infusion Device into Right Buttock, Percutaneous Endoscopic Approach

● **0YH04YZ** Insertion of Other Device into Right Buttock, Percutaneous Endoscopic Approach

0YH101Z Insertion of Radioactive Element into Left Buttock, Open Approach

● **0YH103Z** Insertion of Infusion Device into Left Buttock, Open Approach

● **0YH10YZ** Insertion of Other Device into Left Buttock, Open Approach

0YH131Z Insertion of Radioactive Element into Left Buttock, Percutaneous Approach

● **0YH133Z** Insertion of Infusion Device into Left Buttock, Percutaneous Approach

● **0YH13YZ** Insertion of Other Device into Left Buttock, Percutaneous Approach

0YH141Z Insertion of Radioactive Element into Left Buttock, Percutaneous Endoscopic Approach

● **0YH143Z** Insertion of Infusion Device into Left Buttock, Percutaneous Endoscopic Approach

● **0YH14YZ** Insertion of Other Device into Left Buttock, Percutaneous Endoscopic Approach

0YH501Z Insertion of Radioactive Element into Right Inguinal Region, Open Approach

● **0YH503Z** Insertion of Infusion Device into Right Inguinal Region, Open Approach

● **0YH50YZ** Insertion of Other Device into Right Inguinal Region, Open Approach

0YH531Z Insertion of Radioactive Element into Right Inguinal Region, Percutaneous Approach

● **0YH533Z** Insertion of Infusion Device into Right Inguinal Region, Percutaneous Approach

● **0YH53YZ** Insertion of Other Device into Right Inguinal Region, Percutaneous Approach

0YH541Z Insertion of Radioactive Element into Right Inguinal Region, Percutaneous Endoscopic Approach

● **0YH543Z** Insertion of Infusion Device into Right Inguinal Region, Percutaneous Endoscopic Approach

● **0YH54YZ** Insertion of Other Device into Right Inguinal Region, Percutaneous Endoscopic Approach

0YH601Z Insertion of Radioactive Element into Left Inguinal Region, Open Approach

● **0YH603Z** Insertion of Infusion Device into Left Inguinal Region, Open Approach

● **0YH60YZ** Insertion of Other Device into Left Inguinal Region, Open Approach

0YH631Z Insertion of Radioactive Element into Left Inguinal Region, Percutaneous Approach

● **0YH633Z** Insertion of Infusion Device into Left Inguinal Region, Percutaneous Approach

● **0YH63YZ** Insertion of Other Device into Left Inguinal Region, Percutaneous Approach

0YH641Z Insertion of Radioactive Element into Left Inguinal Region, Percutaneous Endoscopic Approach

● **0YH643Z** Insertion of Infusion Device into Left Inguinal Region, Percutaneous Endoscopic Approach

● **0YH64YZ** Insertion of Other Device into Left Inguinal Region, Percutaneous Endoscopic Approach

0YH701Z Insertion of Radioactive Element into Right Femoral Region, Open Approach

● **0YH703Z** Insertion of Infusion Device into Right Femoral Region, Open Approach

● **0YH70YZ** Insertion of Other Device into Right Femoral Region, Open Approach

0YH731Z Insertion of Radioactive Element into Right Femoral Region, Percutaneous Approach

● **0YH733Z** Insertion of Infusion Device into Right Femoral Region, Percutaneous Approach

● **0YH73YZ** Insertion of Other Device into Right Femoral Region, Percutaneous Approach

0YH741Z Insertion of Radioactive Element into Right Femoral Region, Percutaneous Endoscopic Approach

● **0YH743Z** Insertion of Infusion Device into Right Femoral Region, Percutaneous Endoscopic Approach

● **0YH74YZ** Insertion of Other Device into Right Femoral Region, Percutaneous Endoscopic Approach

0YH801Z Insertion of Radioactive Element into Left Femoral Region, Open Approach

● **0YH803Z** Insertion of Infusion Device into Left Femoral Region, Open Approach

● **0YH80YZ** Insertion of Other Device into Left Femoral Region, Open Approach

0YH831Z Insertion of Radioactive Element into Left Femoral Region, Percutaneous Approach

● **0YH833Z** Insertion of Infusion Device into Left Femoral Region, Percutaneous Approach

● **0YH83YZ** Insertion of Other Device into Left Femoral Region, Percutaneous Approach

0YH841Z Insertion of Radioactive Element into Left Femoral Region, Percutaneous Endoscopic Approach

● **0YH843Z** Insertion of Infusion Device into Left Femoral Region, Percutaneous Endoscopic Approach

● **0YH84YZ** Insertion of Other Device into Left Femoral Region, Percutaneous Endoscopic Approach

0YH901Z Insertion of Radioactive Element into Right Lower Extremity, Open Approach

● **0YH903Z** Insertion of Infusion Device into Right Lower Extremity, Open Approach

● **0YH90YZ** Insertion of Other Device into Right Lower Extremity, Open Approach

0YH931Z Insertion of Radioactive Element into Right Lower Extremity, Percutaneous Approach

● **0YH933Z** Insertion of Infusion Device into Right Lower Extremity, Percutaneous Approach

● **0YH93YZ** Insertion of Other Device into Right Lower Extremity, Percutaneous Approach

0YH941Z Insertion of Radioactive Element into Right Lower Extremity, Percutaneous Endoscopic Approach

● **0YH943Z** Insertion of Infusion Device into Right Lower Extremity, Percutaneous Endoscopic Approach

● **0YH94YZ** Insertion of Other Device into Right Lower Extremity, Percutaneous Endoscopic Approach

0YHB01Z Insertion of Radioactive Element into Left Lower Extremity, Open Approach

● **0YHB03Z** Insertion of Infusion Device into Left Lower Extremity, Open Approach

● **0YHB0YZ** Insertion of Other Device into Left Lower Extremity, Open Approach

0YHB31Z Insertion of Radioactive Element into Left Lower Extremity, Percutaneous Approach

● **0YHB33Z** Insertion of Infusion Device into Left Lower Extremity, Percutaneous Approach

● **0YHB3YZ** Insertion of Other Device into Left Lower Extremity, Percutaneous Approach

0YHB41Z Insertion of Radioactive Element into Left Lower Extremity, Percutaneous Endoscopic Approach

● **0YHB43Z** Insertion of Infusion Device into Left Lower Extremity, Percutaneous Endoscopic Approach

● **0YHB4YZ** Insertion of Other Device into Left Lower Extremity, Percutaneous Endoscopic Approach

0YHC01Z Insertion of Radioactive Element into Right Upper Leg, Open Approach

● **0YHC03Z** Insertion of Infusion Device into Right Upper Leg, Open Approach

● **0YHC0YZ** Insertion of Other Device into Right Upper Leg, Open Approach

0YHC31Z Insertion of Radioactive Element into Right Upper Leg, Percutaneous Approach

● **0YHC33Z** Insertion of Infusion Device into Right Upper Leg, Percutaneous Approach

● **0YHC3YZ** Insertion of Other Device into Right Upper Leg, Percutaneous Approach

0YHC41Z Insertion of Radioactive Element into Right Upper Leg, Percutaneous Endoscopic Approach

● **0YHC43Z** Insertion of Infusion Device into Right Upper Leg, Percutaneous Endoscopic Approach

● **0YHC4YZ** Insertion of Other Device into Right Upper Leg, Percutaneous Endoscopic Approach

0YHD01Z Insertion of Radioactive Element into Left Upper Leg, Open Approach

● **0YHD03Z** Insertion of Infusion Device into Left Upper Leg, Open Approach

● **0YHD0YZ** Insertion of Other Device into Left Upper Leg, Open Approach

0YHD31Z Insertion of Radioactive Element into Left Upper Leg, Percutaneous Approach

● **0YHD33Z** Insertion of Infusion Device into Left Upper Leg, Percutaneous Approach

● **0YHD3YZ** Insertion of Other Device into Left Upper Leg, Percutaneous Approach

0YHD41Z Insertion of Radioactive Element into Left Upper Leg, Percutaneous Endoscopic Approach

● **0YHD43Z** Insertion of Infusion Device into Left Upper Leg, Percutaneous Endoscopic Approach

● **0YHD4YZ** Insertion of Other Device into Left Upper Leg, Percutaneous Endoscopic Approach

0YHF01Z Insertion of Radioactive Element into Right Knee Region, Open Approach

● **0YHF03Z** Insertion of Infusion Device into Right Knee Region, Open Approach

● **0YHF0YZ** Insertion of Other Device into Right Knee Region, Open Approach

0YHF31Z Insertion of Radioactive Element into Right Knee Region, Percutaneous Approach

● **0YHF33Z** Insertion of Infusion Device into Right Knee Region, Percutaneous Approach

● 0YHF3YZ Insertion of Other Device into Right Knee Region, Percutaneous Approach

0YHF41Z Insertion of Radioactive Element into Right Knee Region, Percutaneous Endoscopic Approach

● 0YHF43Z Insertion of Infusion Device into Right Knee Region, Percutaneous Endoscopic Approach

● 0YHF4YZ Insertion of Other Device into Right Knee Region, Percutaneous Endoscopic Approach

0YHG01Z Insertion of Radioactive Element into Left Knee Region, Open Approach

● 0YHG03Z Insertion of Infusion Device into Left Knee Region, Open Approach

● 0YHG0YZ Insertion of Other Device into Left Knee Region, Open Approach

0YHG31Z Insertion of Radioactive Element into Left Knee Region, Percutaneous Approach

● 0YHG33Z Insertion of Infusion Device into Left Knee Region, Percutaneous Approach

● 0YHG3YZ Insertion of Other Device into Left Knee Region, Percutaneous Approach

0YHG41Z Insertion of Radioactive Element into Left Knee Region, Percutaneous Endoscopic Approach

● 0YHG43Z Insertion of Infusion Device into Left Knee Region, Percutaneous Endoscopic Approach

● 0YHG4YZ Insertion of Other Device into Left Knee Region, Percutaneous Endoscopic Approach

0YHH01Z Insertion of Radioactive Element into Right Lower Leg, Open Approach

● 0YHH03Z Insertion of Infusion Device into Right Lower Leg, Open Approach

● 0YHH0YZ Insertion of Other Device into Right Lower Leg, Open Approach

0YHH31Z Insertion of Radioactive Element into Right Lower Leg, Percutaneous Approach

● 0YHH33Z Insertion of Infusion Device into Right Lower Leg, Percutaneous Approach

● 0YHH3YZ Insertion of Other Device into Right Lower Leg, Percutaneous Approach

0YHH41Z Insertion of Radioactive Element into Right Lower Leg, Percutaneous Endoscopic Approach

● 0YHH43Z Insertion of Infusion Device into Right Lower Leg, Percutaneous Endoscopic Approach

● 0YHH4YZ Insertion of Other Device into Right Lower Leg, Percutaneous Endoscopic Approach

0YHJ01Z Insertion of Radioactive Element into Left Lower Leg, Open Approach

● 0YHJ03Z Insertion of Infusion Device into Left Lower Leg, Open Approach

● 0YHJ0YZ Insertion of Other Device into Left Lower Leg, Open Approach

0YHJ31Z Insertion of Radioactive Element into Left Lower Leg, Percutaneous Approach

● 0YHJ33Z Insertion of Infusion Device into Left Lower Leg, Percutaneous Approach

● 0YHJ3YZ Insertion of Other Device into Left Lower Leg, Percutaneous Approach

0YHJ41Z Insertion of Radioactive Element into Left Lower Leg, Percutaneous Endoscopic Approach

● 0YHJ43Z Insertion of Infusion Device into Left Lower Leg, Percutaneous Endoscopic Approach

● 0YHJ4YZ Insertion of Other Device into Left Lower Leg, Percutaneous Endoscopic Approach

0YHK01Z Insertion of Radioactive Element into Right Ankle Region, Open Approach

● 0YHK03Z Insertion of Infusion Device into Right Ankle Region, Open Approach

● 0YHK0YZ Insertion of Other Device into Right Ankle Region, Open Approach

0YHK31Z Insertion of Radioactive Element into Right Ankle Region, Percutaneous Approach

● 0YHK33Z Insertion of Infusion Device into Right Ankle Region, Percutaneous Approach

● 0YHK3YZ Insertion of Other Device into Right Ankle Region, Percutaneous Approach

0YHK41Z Insertion of Radioactive Element into Right Ankle Region, Percutaneous Endoscopic Approach

● 0YHK43Z Insertion of Infusion Device into Right Ankle Region, Percutaneous Endoscopic Approach

● 0YHK4YZ Insertion of Other Device into Right Ankle Region, Percutaneous Endoscopic Approach

0YHL01Z Insertion of Radioactive Element into Left Ankle Region, Open Approach

● 0YHL03Z Insertion of Infusion Device into Left Ankle Region, Open Approach

● 0YHL0YZ Insertion of Other Device into Left Ankle Region, Open Approach

0YHL31Z Insertion of Radioactive Element into Left Ankle Region, Percutaneous Approach

● 0YHL33Z Insertion of Infusion Device into Left Ankle Region, Percutaneous Approach

● 0YHL3YZ Insertion of Other Device into Left Ankle Region, Percutaneous Approach

0YHL41Z Insertion of Radioactive Element into Left Ankle Region, Percutaneous Endoscopic Approach

● 0YHL43Z Insertion of Infusion Device into Left Ankle Region, Percutaneous Endoscopic Approach

● 0YHL4YZ Insertion of Other Device into Left Ankle Region, Percutaneous Endoscopic Approach

0YHM01Z Insertion of Radioactive Element into Right Foot, Open Approach

● 0YHM03Z Insertion of Infusion Device into Right Foot, Open Approach

● 0YHM0YZ Insertion of Other Device into Right Foot, Open Approach

0YHM31Z Insertion of Radioactive Element into Right Foot, Percutaneous Approach

● 0YHM33Z Insertion of Infusion Device into Right Foot, Percutaneous Approach

● 0YHM3YZ Insertion of Other Device into Right Foot, Percutaneous Approach

0YHM41Z Insertion of Radioactive Element into Right Foot, Percutaneous Endoscopic Approach

● 0YHM43Z Insertion of Infusion Device into Right Foot, Percutaneous Endoscopic Approach

● 0YHM4YZ Insertion of Other Device into Right Foot, Percutaneous Endoscopic Approach

0YHN01Z Insertion of Radioactive Element into Left Foot, Open Approach

● 0YHN03Z Insertion of Infusion Device into Left Foot, Open Approach

● 0YHN0YZ Insertion of Other Device into Left Foot, Open Approach

0YHN31Z Insertion of Radioactive Element into Left Foot, Percutaneous Approach

● 0YHN33Z Insertion of Infusion Device into Left Foot, Percutaneous Approach

● 0YHN3YZ Insertion of Other Device into Left Foot, Percutaneous Approach

0YHN41Z Insertion of Radioactive Element into Left Foot, Percutaneous Endoscopic Approach

● 0YHN43Z Insertion of Infusion Device into Left Foot, Percutaneous Endoscopic Approach

● 0YHN4YZ Insertion of Other Device into Left Foot, Percutaneous Endoscopic Approach

0YJ – Anatomical Regions, Lower Extremities, Inspection

Review Coding Guidelines B3.11a, B3.11b and B3.11c

● 0YJ00ZZ Inspection of Right Buttock, Open Approach

0YJ03ZZ Inspection of Right Buttock, Percutaneous Approach

0YJ04ZZ Inspection of Right Buttock, Percutaneous Endoscopic Approach

0YJ0XZZ Inspection of Right Buttock, External Approach

● 0YJ10ZZ Inspection of Left Buttock, Open Approach

0YJ13ZZ Inspection of Left Buttock, Percutaneous Approach

0YJ14ZZ Inspection of Left Buttock, Percutaneous Endoscopic Approach

0YJ1XZZ Inspection of Left Buttock, External Approach

0YJ50ZZ Inspection of Right Inguinal Region, Open Approach

0YJ53ZZ Inspection of Right Inguinal Region, Percutaneous Approach

0YJ54ZZ Inspection of Right Inguinal Region, Percutaneous Endoscopic Approach

0YJ5XZZ Inspection of Right Inguinal Region, External Approach

0YJ60ZZ Inspection of Left Inguinal Region, Open Approach

0YJ63ZZ Inspection of Left Inguinal Region, Percutaneous Approach

0YJ64ZZ Inspection of Left Inguinal Region, Percutaneous Endoscopic Approach

0YJ6XZZ Inspection of Left Inguinal Region, External Approach

0YJ70ZZ Inspection of Right Femoral Region, Open Approach

0YJ73ZZ Inspection of Right Femoral Region, Percutaneous Approach

0YJ74ZZ Inspection of Right Femoral Region, Percutaneous Endoscopic Approach

0YJ7XZZ Inspection of Right Femoral Region, External Approach

● 0YJ80ZZ Inspection of Left Femoral Region, Open Approach

♀ Female-only   ♂ Male-only   ▲ Limited Coverage   ● Non-OR   [HAC] HAC-associated procedure   ▲ Non-covered procedures   ✚ Cluster

0YJ83ZZ	Inspection of Left Femoral Region, Percutaneous Approach
0YJ84ZZ	Inspection of Left Femoral Region, Percutaneous Endoscopic Approach
0YJ8XZZ	Inspection of Left Femoral Region, External Approach
● 0YJ90ZZ	Inspection of Right Lower Extremity, Open Approach
0YJ93ZZ	Inspection of Right Lower Extremity, Percutaneous Approach
0YJ94ZZ	Inspection of Right Lower Extremity, Percutaneous Endoscopic Approach
0YJ9XZZ	Inspection of Right Lower Extremity, External Approach
0YJA0ZZ	Inspection of Bilateral Inguinal Region, Open Approach
0YJA3ZZ	Inspection of Bilateral Inguinal Region, Percutaneous Approach
0YJA4ZZ	Inspection of Bilateral Inguinal Region, Percutaneous Endoscopic Approach
0YJAXZZ	Inspection of Bilateral Inguinal Region, External Approach
● 0YJB0ZZ	Inspection of Left Lower Extremity, Open Approach
0YJB3ZZ	Inspection of Left Lower Extremity, Percutaneous Approach
0YJB4ZZ	Inspection of Left Lower Extremity, Percutaneous Endoscopic Approach
0YJBXZZ	Inspection of Left Lower Extremity, External Approach
● 0YJC0ZZ	Inspection of Right Upper Leg, Open Approach
0YJC3ZZ	Inspection of Right Upper Leg, Percutaneous Approach
0YJC4ZZ	Inspection of Right Upper Leg, Percutaneous Endoscopic Approach
0YJCXZZ	Inspection of Right Upper Leg, External Approach
● 0YJD0ZZ	Inspection of Left Upper Leg, Open Approach
0YJD3ZZ	Inspection of Left Upper Leg, Percutaneous Approach
0YJD4ZZ	Inspection of Left Upper Leg, Percutaneous Endoscopic Approach
0YJDXZZ	Inspection of Left Upper Leg, External Approach
● 0YJE0ZZ	Inspection of Bilateral Femoral Region, Open Approach
0YJE3ZZ	Inspection of Bilateral Femoral Region, Percutaneous Approach
0YJE4ZZ	Inspection of Bilateral Femoral Region, Percutaneous Endoscopic Approach
0YJEXZZ	Inspection of Bilateral Femoral Region, External Approach
● 0YJF0ZZ	Inspection of Right Knee Region, Open Approach
0YJF3ZZ	Inspection of Right Knee Region, Percutaneous Approach
0YJF4ZZ	Inspection of Right Knee Region, Percutaneous Endoscopic Approach
0YJFXZZ	Inspection of Right Knee Region, External Approach
● 0YJG0ZZ	Inspection of Left Knee Region, Open Approach
0YJG3ZZ	Inspection of Left Knee Region, Percutaneous Approach
0YJG4ZZ	Inspection of Left Knee Region, Percutaneous Endoscopic Approach
0YJGXZZ	Inspection of Left Knee Region, External Approach
● 0YJH0ZZ	Inspection of Right Lower Leg, Open Approach
0YJH3ZZ	Inspection of Right Lower Leg, Percutaneous Approach
0YJH4ZZ	Inspection of Right Lower Leg, Percutaneous Endoscopic Approach
0YJHXZZ	Inspection of Right Lower Leg, External Approach
● 0YJJ0ZZ	Inspection of Left Lower Leg, Open Approach
0YJJ3ZZ	Inspection of Left Lower Leg, Percutaneous Approach
0YJJ4ZZ	Inspection of Left Lower Leg, Percutaneous Endoscopic Approach
0YJJXZZ	Inspection of Left Lower Leg, External Approach
● 0YJK0ZZ	Inspection of Right Ankle Region, Open Approach
0YJK3ZZ	Inspection of Right Ankle Region, Percutaneous Approach
0YJK4ZZ	Inspection of Right Ankle Region, Percutaneous Endoscopic Approach
0YJKXZZ	Inspection of Right Ankle Region, External Approach
● 0YJL0ZZ	Inspection of Left Ankle Region, Open Approach
0YJL3ZZ	Inspection of Left Ankle Region, Percutaneous Approach
0YJL4ZZ	Inspection of Left Ankle Region, Percutaneous Endoscopic Approach
0YJLXZZ	Inspection of Left Ankle Region, External Approach
● 0YJM0ZZ	Inspection of Right Foot, Open Approach
0YJM3ZZ	Inspection of Right Foot, Percutaneous Approach
0YJM4ZZ	Inspection of Right Foot, Percutaneous Endoscopic Approach
0YJMXZZ	Inspection of Right Foot, External Approach
● 0YJN0ZZ	Inspection of Left Foot, Open Approach
0YJN3ZZ	Inspection of Left Foot, Percutaneous Approach
0YJN4ZZ	Inspection of Left Foot, Percutaneous Endoscopic Approach
0YJNXZZ	Inspection of Left Foot, External Approach

0YM – Anatomical Regions, Lower Extremities, Reattachment

0YM00ZZ	Reattachment of Right Buttock, Open Approach
0YM10ZZ	Reattachment of Left Buttock, Open Approach
0YM20ZZ	Reattachment of Right Hindquarter, Open Approach
0YM30ZZ	Reattachment of Left Hindquarter, Open Approach
0YM40ZZ	Reattachment of Bilateral Hindquarter, Open Approach
0YM50ZZ	Reattachment of Right Inguinal Region, Open Approach
0YM60ZZ	Reattachment of Left Inguinal Region, Open Approach
0YM70ZZ	Reattachment of Right Femoral Region, Open Approach
0YM80ZZ	Reattachment of Left Femoral Region, Open Approach
0YM90ZZ	Reattachment of Right Lower Extremity, Open Approach
0YMB0ZZ	Reattachment of Left Lower Extremity, Open Approach
0YMC0ZZ	Reattachment of Right Upper Leg, Open Approach
0YMD0ZZ	Reattachment of Left Upper Leg, Open Approach
0YMF0ZZ	Reattachment of Right Knee Region, Open Approach
0YMG0ZZ	Reattachment of Left Knee Region, Open Approach
0YMH0ZZ	Reattachment of Right Lower Leg, Open Approach
0YMJ0ZZ	Reattachment of Left Lower Leg, Open Approach
0YMK0ZZ	Reattachment of Right Ankle Region, Open Approach
0YML0ZZ	Reattachment of Left Ankle Region, Open Approach
0YMM0ZZ	Reattachment of Right Foot, Open Approach
0YMN0ZZ	Reattachment of Left Foot, Open Approach
0YMP0ZZ	Reattachment of Right 1st Toe, Open Approach
0YMQ0ZZ	Reattachment of Left 1st Toe, Open Approach
0YMR0ZZ	Reattachment of Right 2nd Toe, Open Approach
0YMS0ZZ	Reattachment of Left 2nd Toe, Open Approach
0YMT0ZZ	Reattachment of Right 3rd Toe, Open Approach
0YMU0ZZ	Reattachment of Left 3rd Toe, Open Approach
0YMV0ZZ	Reattachment of Right 4th Toe, Open Approach
0YMW0ZZ	Reattachment of Left 4th Toe, Open Approach
0YMX0ZZ	Reattachment of Right 5th Toe, Open Approach
0YMY0ZZ	Reattachment of Left 5th Toe, Open Approach

0YP – Anatomical Regions, Lower Extremities, Removal

Review Coding Guideline B6.1c

0YP900Z	Removal of Drainage Device from Right Lower Extremity, Open Approach
0YP901Z	Removal of Radioactive Element from Right Lower Extremity, Open Approach
0YP903Z	Removal of Infusion Device from Right Lower Extremity, Open Approach
0YP907Z	Removal of Autologous Tissue Substitute from Right Lower Extremity, Open Approach
0YP90JZ	Removal of Synthetic Substitute from Right Lower Extremity, Open Approach
0YP90KZ	Removal of Nonautologous Tissue Substitute from Right Lower Extremity, Open Approach

♀ Female-only   ♂ Male-only   ▲ Limited Coverage   ● Non-OR   HAC HAC-associated procedure   ▲ Non-covered procedures   ✚ Cluster

0YP90YZ Removal of Other Device from Right Lower Extremity, Open Approach
0YP930Z Removal of Drainage Device from Right Lower Extremity, Percutaneous Approach
0YP931Z Removal of Radioactive Element from Right Lower Extremity, Percutaneous Approach
0YP933Z Removal of Infusion Device from Right Lower Extremity, Percutaneous Approach
0YP937Z Removal of Autologous Tissue Substitute from Right Lower Extremity, Percutaneous Approach
0YP93JZ Removal of Synthetic Substitute from Right Lower Extremity, Percutaneous Approach
0YP93KZ Removal of Nonautologous Tissue Substitute from Right Lower Extremity, Percutaneous Approach
0YP93YZ Removal of Other Device from Right Lower Extremity, Percutaneous Approach
0YP940Z Removal of Drainage Device from Right Lower Extremity, Percutaneous Endoscopic Approach
0YP941Z Removal of Radioactive Element from Right Lower Extremity, Percutaneous Endoscopic Approach
0YP943Z Removal of Infusion Device from Right Lower Extremity, Percutaneous Endoscopic Approach
0YP947Z Removal of Autologous Tissue Substitute from Right Lower Extremity, Percutaneous Endoscopic Approach
0YP94JZ Removal of Synthetic Substitute from Right Lower Extremity, Percutaneous Endoscopic Approach
0YP94KZ Removal of Nonautologous Tissue Substitute from Right Lower Extremity, Percutaneous Endoscopic Approach
0YP94YZ Removal of Other Device from Right Lower Extremity, Percutaneous Endoscopic Approach
0YP9X0Z Removal of Drainage Device from Right Lower Extremity, External Approach

0YP9X1Z Removal of Radioactive Element from Right Lower Extremity, External Approach
0YP9X3Z Removal of Infusion Device from Right Lower Extremity, External Approach
0YP9X7Z Removal of Autologous Tissue Substitute from Right Lower Extremity, External Approach
0YP9XJZ Removal of Synthetic Substitute from Right Lower Extremity, External Approach
0YP9XKZ Removal of Nonautologous Tissue Substitute from Right Lower Extremity, External Approach
0YP9XYZ Removal of Other Device from Right Lower Extremity, External Approach
0YPB00Z Removal of Drainage Device from Left Lower Extremity, Open Approach
0YPB01Z Removal of Radioactive Element from Left Lower Extremity, Open Approach
0YPB03Z Removal of Infusion Device from Left Lower Extremity, Open Approach
0YPB07Z Removal of Autologous Tissue Substitute from Left Lower Extremity, Open Approach
0YPB0JZ Removal of Synthetic Substitute from Left Lower Extremity, Open Approach
0YPB0KZ Removal of Nonautologous Tissue Substitute from Left Lower Extremity, Open Approach
0YPB0YZ Removal of Other Device from Left Lower Extremity, Open Approach
0YPB30Z Removal of Drainage Device from Left Lower Extremity, Percutaneous Approach
0YPB31Z Removal of Radioactive Element from Left Lower Extremity, Percutaneous Approach
0YPB33Z Removal of Infusion Device from Left Lower Extremity, Percutaneous Approach
0YPB37Z Removal of Autologous Tissue Substitute from Left Lower Extremity, Percutaneous Approach
0YPB3JZ Removal of Synthetic Substitute from Left Lower Extremity, Percutaneous Approach

0YPB3KZ Removal of Nonautologous Tissue Substitute from Left Lower Extremity, Percutaneous Approach
0YPB3YZ Removal of Other Device from Left Lower Extremity, Percutaneous Approach
0YPB40Z Removal of Drainage Device from Left Lower Extremity, Percutaneous Endoscopic Approach
0YPB41Z Removal of Radioactive Element from Left Lower Extremity, Percutaneous Endoscopic Approach
0YPB43Z Removal of Infusion Device from Left Lower Extremity, Percutaneous Endoscopic Approach
0YPB47Z Removal of Autologous Tissue Substitute from Left Lower Extremity, Percutaneous Endoscopic Approach
0YPB4JZ Removal of Synthetic Substitute from Left Lower Extremity, Percutaneous Endoscopic Approach
0YPB4KZ Removal of Nonautologous Tissue Substitute from Left Lower Extremity, Percutaneous Endoscopic Approach
0YPB4YZ Removal of Other Device from Left Lower Extremity, Percutaneous Endoscopic Approach
0YPBX0Z Removal of Drainage Device from Left Lower Extremity, External Approach
0YPBX1Z Removal of Radioactive Element from Left Lower Extremity, External Approach
0YPBX3Z Removal of Infusion Device from Left Lower Extremity, External Approach
0YPBX7Z Removal of Autologous Tissue Substitute from Left Lower Extremity, External Approach
0YPBXJZ Removal of Synthetic Substitute from Left Lower Extremity, External Approach
0YPBXKZ Removal of Nonautologous Tissue Substitute from Left Lower Extremity, External Approach
0YPBXYZ Removal of Other Device from Left Lower Extremity, External Approach

0YQ – Anatomical Regions, Lower Extremities, Repair

0YQ00ZZ Repair Right Buttock, Open Approach
0YQ03ZZ Repair Right Buttock, Percutaneous Approach
0YQ04ZZ Repair Right Buttock, Percutaneous Endoscopic Approach
0YQ0XZZ Repair Right Buttock, External Approach
0YQ10ZZ Repair Left Buttock, Open Approach
0YQ13ZZ Repair Left Buttock, Percutaneous Approach
0YQ14ZZ Repair Left Buttock, Percutaneous Endoscopic Approach
0YQ1XZZ Repair Left Buttock, External Approach
0YQ50ZZ Repair Right Inguinal Region, Open Approach
0YQ53ZZ Repair Right Inguinal Region, Percutaneous Approach
0YQ54ZZ Repair Right Inguinal Region, Percutaneous Endoscopic Approach
0YQ5XZZ Repair Right Inguinal Region, External Approach
0YQ60ZZ Repair Left Inguinal Region, Open Approach

0YQ63ZZ Repair Left Inguinal Region, Percutaneous Approach
0YQ64ZZ Repair Left Inguinal Region, Percutaneous Endoscopic Approach
0YQ6XZZ Repair Left Inguinal Region, External Approach
0YQ70ZZ Repair Right Femoral Region, Open Approach
0YQ73ZZ Repair Right Femoral Region, Percutaneous Approach
0YQ74ZZ Repair Right Femoral Region, Percutaneous Endoscopic Approach
0YQ7XZZ Repair Right Femoral Region, External Approach
0YQ80ZZ Repair Left Femoral Region, Open Approach
0YQ83ZZ Repair Left Femoral Region, Percutaneous Approach
0YQ84ZZ Repair Left Femoral Region, Percutaneous Endoscopic Approach
0YQ8XZZ Repair Left Femoral Region, External Approach
0YQ90ZZ Repair Right Lower Extremity, Open Approach

0YQ93ZZ Repair Right Lower Extremity, Percutaneous Approach
0YQ94ZZ Repair Right Lower Extremity, Percutaneous Endoscopic Approach
0YQ9XZZ Repair Right Lower Extremity, External Approach
0YQA0ZZ Repair Bilateral Inguinal Region, Open Approach
0YQA3ZZ Repair Bilateral Inguinal Region, Percutaneous Approach
0YQA4ZZ Repair Bilateral Inguinal Region, Percutaneous Endoscopic Approach
0YQAXZZ Repair Bilateral Inguinal Region, External Approach
0YQB0ZZ Repair Left Lower Extremity, Open Approach
0YQB3ZZ Repair Left Lower Extremity, Percutaneous Approach
0YQB4ZZ Repair Left Lower Extremity, Percutaneous Endoscopic Approach
0YQBXZZ Repair Left Lower Extremity, External Approach
0YQC0ZZ Repair Right Upper Leg, Open Approach

♀ Female-only   ♂ Male-only   ▲ Limited Coverage   ● Non-OR   ᴴᴬᶜ HAC-associated procedure   ▲ Non-covered procedures   ➕ Cluster

0YQC3ZZ	Repair Right Upper Leg, Percutaneous Approach	0YQJ4ZZ	Repair Left Lower Leg, Percutaneous Endoscopic Approach	0YQRXZZ	Repair Right 2nd Toe, External Approach
0YQC4ZZ	Repair Right Upper Leg, Percutaneous Endoscopic Approach	0YQJXZZ	Repair Left Lower Leg, External Approach	0YQS0ZZ	Repair Left 2nd Toe, Open Approach
0YQCXZZ	Repair Right Upper Leg, External Approach	0YQK0ZZ	Repair Right Ankle Region, Open Approach	0YQS3ZZ	Repair Left 2nd Toe, Percutaneous Approach
0YQD0ZZ	Repair Left Upper Leg, Open Approach	0YQK3ZZ	Repair Right Ankle Region, Percutaneous Approach	0YQS4ZZ	Repair Left 2nd Toe, Percutaneous Endoscopic Approach
0YQD3ZZ	Repair Left Upper Leg, Percutaneous Approach	0YQK4ZZ	Repair Right Ankle Region, Percutaneous Endoscopic Approach	0YQSXZZ	Repair Left 2nd Toe, External Approach
0YQD4ZZ	Repair Left Upper Leg, Percutaneous Endoscopic Approach	0YQKXZZ	Repair Right Ankle Region, External Approach	0YQT0ZZ	Repair Right 3rd Toe, Open Approach
0YQDXZZ	Repair Left Upper Leg, External Approach	0YQL0ZZ	Repair Left Ankle Region, Open Approach	0YQT3ZZ	Repair Right 3rd Toe, Percutaneous Approach
0YQE0ZZ	Repair Bilateral Femoral Region, Open Approach	0YQL3ZZ	Repair Left Ankle Region, Percutaneous Approach	0YQT4ZZ	Repair Right 3rd Toe, Percutaneous Endoscopic Approach
0YQE3ZZ	Repair Bilateral Femoral Region, Percutaneous Approach	0YQL4ZZ	Repair Left Ankle Region, Percutaneous Endoscopic Approach	0YQTXZZ	Repair Right 3rd Toe, External Approach
0YQE4ZZ	Repair Bilateral Femoral Region, Percutaneous Endoscopic Approach	0YQLXZZ	Repair Left Ankle Region, External Approach	0YQU0ZZ	Repair Left 3rd Toe, Open Approach
0YQEXZZ	Repair Bilateral Femoral Region, External Approach	0YQM0ZZ	Repair Right Foot, Open Approach	0YQU3ZZ	Repair Left 3rd Toe, Percutaneous Approach
0YQF0ZZ	Repair Right Knee Region, Open Approach	0YQM3ZZ	Repair Right Foot, Percutaneous Approach	0YQU4ZZ	Repair Left 3rd Toe, Percutaneous Endoscopic Approach
0YQF3ZZ	Repair Right Knee Region, Percutaneous Approach	0YQM4ZZ	Repair Right Foot, Percutaneous Endoscopic Approach	0YQUXZZ	Repair Left 3rd Toe, External Approach
0YQF4ZZ	Repair Right Knee Region, Percutaneous Endoscopic Approach	0YQMXZZ	Repair Right Foot, External Approach	0YQV0ZZ	Repair Right 4th Toe, Open Approach
0YQFXZZ	Repair Right Knee Region, External Approach	0YQN0ZZ	Repair Left Foot, Open Approach	0YQV3ZZ	Repair Right 4th Toe, Percutaneous Approach
0YQG0ZZ	Repair Left Knee Region, Open Approach	0YQN3ZZ	Repair Left Foot, Percutaneous Approach	0YQV4ZZ	Repair Right 4th Toe, Percutaneous Endoscopic Approach
0YQG3ZZ	Repair Left Knee Region, Percutaneous Approach	0YQN4ZZ	Repair Left Foot, Percutaneous Endoscopic Approach	0YQVXZZ	Repair Right 4th Toe, External Approach
0YQG4ZZ	Repair Left Knee Region, Percutaneous Endoscopic Approach	0YQNXZZ	Repair Left Foot, External Approach	0YQW0ZZ	Repair Left 4th Toe, Open Approach
0YQGXZZ	Repair Left Knee Region, External Approach	0YQP0ZZ	Repair Right 1st Toe, Open Approach	0YQW3ZZ	Repair Left 4th Toe, Percutaneous Approach
0YQH0ZZ	Repair Right Lower Leg, Open Approach	0YQP3ZZ	Repair Right 1st Toe, Percutaneous Approach	0YQW4ZZ	Repair Left 4th Toe, Percutaneous Endoscopic Approach
0YQH3ZZ	Repair Right Lower Leg, Percutaneous Approach	0YQP4ZZ	Repair Right 1st Toe, Percutaneous Endoscopic Approach	0YQWXZZ	Repair Left 4th Toe, External Approach
0YQH4ZZ	Repair Right Lower Leg, Percutaneous Endoscopic Approach	0YQPXZZ	Repair Right 1st Toe, External Approach	0YQX0ZZ	Repair Right 5th Toe, Open Approach
0YQHXZZ	Repair Right Lower Leg, External Approach	0YQQ0ZZ	Repair Left 1st Toe, Open Approach	0YQX3ZZ	Repair Right 5th Toe, Percutaneous Approach
0YQJ0ZZ	Repair Left Lower Leg, Open Approach	0YQQ3ZZ	Repair Left 1st Toe, Percutaneous Approach	0YQX4ZZ	Repair Right 5th Toe, Percutaneous Endoscopic Approach
0YQJ3ZZ	Repair Left Lower Leg, Percutaneous Approach	0YQQ4ZZ	Repair Left 1st Toe, Percutaneous Endoscopic Approach	0YQXXZZ	Repair Right 5th Toe, External Approach
		0YQQXZZ	Repair Left 1st Toe, External Approach	0YQY0ZZ	Repair Left 5th Toe, Open Approach
		0YQR0ZZ	Repair Right 2nd Toe, Open Approach	0YQY3ZZ	Repair Left 5th Toe, Percutaneous Approach
		0YQR3ZZ	Repair Right 2nd Toe, Percutaneous Approach	0YQY4ZZ	Repair Left 5th Toe, Percutaneous Endoscopic Approach
		0YQR4ZZ	Repair Right 2nd Toe, Percutaneous Endoscopic Approach	0YQYXZZ	Repair Left 5th Toe, External Approach

0YU – Anatomical Regions, Lower Extremities, Supplement

0YU007Z	Supplement Right Buttock with Autologous Tissue Substitute, Open Approach	0YU10JZ	Supplement Left Buttock with Synthetic Substitute, Open Approach	0YU50KZ	Supplement Right Inguinal Region with Nonautologous Tissue Substitute, Open Approach
0YU00JZ	Supplement Right Buttock with Synthetic Substitute, Open Approach	0YU10KZ	Supplement Left Buttock with Nonautologous Tissue Substitute, Open Approach	0YU547Z	Supplement Right Inguinal Region with Autologous Tissue Substitute, Percutaneous Endoscopic Approach
0YU00KZ	Supplement Right Buttock with Nonautologous Tissue Substitute, Open Approach	0YU147Z	Supplement Left Buttock with Autologous Tissue Substitute, Percutaneous Endoscopic Approach	0YU54JZ	Supplement Right Inguinal Region with Synthetic Substitute, Percutaneous Endoscopic Approach
0YU047Z	Supplement Right Buttock with Autologous Tissue Substitute, Percutaneous Endoscopic Approach	0YU14JZ	Supplement Left Buttock with Synthetic Substitute, Percutaneous Endoscopic Approach	0YU54KZ	Supplement Right Inguinal Region with Nonautologous Tissue Substitute, Percutaneous Endoscopic Approach
0YU04JZ	Supplement Right Buttock with Synthetic Substitute, Percutaneous Endoscopic Approach	0YU14KZ	Supplement Left Buttock with Nonautologous Tissue Substitute, Percutaneous Endoscopic Approach	0YU607Z	Supplement Left Inguinal Region with Autologous Tissue Substitute, Open Approach
0YU04KZ	Supplement Right Buttock with Nonautologous Tissue Substitute, Percutaneous Endoscopic Approach	0YU507Z	Supplement Right Inguinal Region with Autologous Tissue Substitute, Open Approach	0YU60JZ	Supplement Left Inguinal Region with Synthetic Substitute, Open Approach
0YU107Z	Supplement Left Buttock with Autologous Tissue Substitute, Open Approach	0YU50JZ	Supplement Right Inguinal Region with Synthetic Substitute, Open Approach	0YU60KZ	Supplement Left Inguinal Region with Nonautologous Tissue Substitute, Open Approach

0YU647Z Supplement Left Inguinal Region with Autologous Tissue Substitute, Percutaneous Endoscopic Approach

0YU64JZ Supplement Left Inguinal Region with Synthetic Substitute, Percutaneous Endoscopic Approach

0YU64KZ Supplement Left Inguinal Region with Nonautologous Tissue Substitute, Percutaneous Endoscopic Approach

0YU707Z Supplement Right Femoral Region with Autologous Tissue Substitute, Open Approach

0YU70JZ Supplement Right Femoral Region with Synthetic Substitute, Open Approach

0YU70KZ Supplement Right Femoral Region with Nonautologous Tissue Substitute, Open Approach

0YU747Z Supplement Right Femoral Region with Autologous Tissue Substitute, Percutaneous Endoscopic Approach

0YU74JZ Supplement Right Femoral Region with Synthetic Substitute, Percutaneous Endoscopic Approach

0YU74KZ Supplement Right Femoral Region with Nonautologous Tissue Substitute, Percutaneous Endoscopic Approach

0YU807Z Supplement Left Femoral Region with Autologous Tissue Substitute, Open Approach

0YU80JZ Supplement Left Femoral Region with Synthetic Substitute, Open Approach

0YU80KZ Supplement Left Femoral Region with Nonautologous Tissue Substitute, Open Approach

0YU847Z Supplement Left Femoral Region with Autologous Tissue Substitute, Percutaneous Endoscopic Approach

0YU84JZ Supplement Left Femoral Region with Synthetic Substitute, Percutaneous Endoscopic Approach

0YU84KZ Supplement Left Femoral Region with Nonautologous Tissue Substitute, Percutaneous Endoscopic Approach

0YU907Z Supplement Right Lower Extremity with Autologous Tissue Substitute, Open Approach

0YU90JZ Supplement Right Lower Extremity with Synthetic Substitute, Open Approach

0YU90KZ Supplement Right Lower Extremity with Nonautologous Tissue Substitute, Open Approach

0YU947Z Supplement Right Lower Extremity with Autologous Tissue Substitute, Percutaneous Endoscopic Approach

0YU94JZ Supplement Right Lower Extremity with Synthetic Substitute, Percutaneous Endoscopic Approach

0YU94KZ Supplement Right Lower Extremity with Nonautologous Tissue Substitute, Percutaneous Endoscopic Approach

0YUA07Z Supplement Bilateral Inguinal Region with Autologous Tissue Substitute, Open Approach

0YUA0JZ Supplement Bilateral Inguinal Region with Synthetic Substitute, Open Approach

0YUA0KZ Supplement Bilateral Inguinal Region with Nonautologous Tissue Substitute, Open Approach

0YUA47Z Supplement Bilateral Inguinal Region with Autologous Tissue Substitute, Percutaneous Endoscopic Approach

0YUA4JZ Supplement Bilateral Inguinal Region with Synthetic Substitute, Percutaneous Endoscopic Approach

0YUA4KZ Supplement Bilateral Inguinal Region with Nonautologous Tissue Substitute, Percutaneous Endoscopic Approach

0YUB07Z Supplement Left Lower Extremity with Autologous Tissue Substitute, Open Approach

0YUB0JZ Supplement Left Lower Extremity with Synthetic Substitute, Open Approach

0YUB0KZ Supplement Left Lower Extremity with Nonautologous Tissue Substitute, Open Approach

0YUB47Z Supplement Left Lower Extremity with Autologous Tissue Substitute, Percutaneous Endoscopic Approach

0YUB4JZ Supplement Left Lower Extremity with Synthetic Substitute, Percutaneous Endoscopic Approach

0YUB4KZ Supplement Left Lower Extremity with Nonautologous Tissue Substitute, Percutaneous Endoscopic Approach

0YUC07Z Supplement Right Upper Leg with Autologous Tissue Substitute, Open Approach

0YUC0JZ Supplement Right Upper Leg with Synthetic Substitute, Open Approach

0YUC0KZ Supplement Right Upper Leg with Nonautologous Tissue Substitute, Open Approach

0YUC47Z Supplement Right Upper Leg with Autologous Tissue Substitute, Percutaneous Endoscopic Approach

0YUC4JZ Supplement Right Upper Leg with Synthetic Substitute, Percutaneous Endoscopic Approach

0YUC4KZ Supplement Right Upper Leg with Nonautologous Tissue Substitute, Percutaneous Endoscopic Approach

0YUD07Z Supplement Left Upper Leg with Autologous Tissue Substitute, Open Approach

0YUD0JZ Supplement Left Upper Leg with Synthetic Substitute, Open Approach

0YUD0KZ Supplement Left Upper Leg with Nonautologous Tissue Substitute, Open Approach

0YUD47Z Supplement Left Upper Leg with Autologous Tissue Substitute, Percutaneous Endoscopic Approach

0YUD4JZ Supplement Left Upper Leg with Synthetic Substitute, Percutaneous Endoscopic Approach

0YUD4KZ Supplement Left Upper Leg with Nonautologous Tissue Substitute, Percutaneous Endoscopic Approach

0YUE07Z Supplement Bilateral Femoral Region with Autologous Tissue Substitute, Open Approach

0YUE0JZ Supplement Bilateral Femoral Region with Synthetic Substitute, Open Approach

0YUE0KZ Supplement Bilateral Femoral Region with Nonautologous Tissue Substitute, Open Approach

0YUE47Z Supplement Bilateral Femoral Region with Autologous Tissue Substitute, Percutaneous Endoscopic Approach

0YUE4JZ Supplement Bilateral Femoral Region with Synthetic Substitute, Percutaneous Endoscopic Approach

0YUE4KZ Supplement Bilateral Femoral Region with Nonautologous Tissue Substitute, Percutaneous Endoscopic Approach

0YUF07Z Supplement Right Knee Region with Autologous Tissue Substitute, Open Approach

0YUF0JZ Supplement Right Knee Region with Synthetic Substitute, Open Approach

0YUF0KZ Supplement Right Knee Region with Nonautologous Tissue Substitute, Open Approach

0YUF47Z Supplement Right Knee Region with Autologous Tissue Substitute, Percutaneous Endoscopic Approach

0YUF4JZ Supplement Right Knee Region with Synthetic Substitute, Percutaneous Endoscopic Approach

0YUF4KZ Supplement Right Knee Region with Nonautologous Tissue Substitute, Percutaneous Endoscopic Approach

0YUG07Z Supplement Left Knee Region with Autologous Tissue Substitute, Open Approach

0YUG0JZ Supplement Left Knee Region with Synthetic Substitute, Open Approach

0YUG0KZ Supplement Left Knee Region with Nonautologous Tissue Substitute, Open Approach

0YUG47Z Supplement Left Knee Region with Autologous Tissue Substitute, Percutaneous Endoscopic Approach

0YUG4JZ Supplement Left Knee Region with Synthetic Substitute, Percutaneous Endoscopic Approach

0YUG4KZ Supplement Left Knee Region with Nonautologous Tissue Substitute, Percutaneous Endoscopic Approach

0YUH07Z Supplement Right Lower Leg with Autologous Tissue Substitute, Open Approach

0YUH0JZ Supplement Right Lower Leg with Synthetic Substitute, Open Approach

0YUH0KZ Supplement Right Lower Leg with Nonautologous Tissue Substitute, Open Approach

0YUH47Z Supplement Right Lower Leg with Autologous Tissue Substitute, Percutaneous Endoscopic Approach

0YUH4JZ Supplement Right Lower Leg with Synthetic Substitute, Percutaneous Endoscopic Approach

0YUH4KZ Supplement Right Lower Leg with Nonautologous Tissue Substitute, Percutaneous Endoscopic Approach

0YUJ07Z Supplement Left Lower Leg with Autologous Tissue Substitute, Open Approach

0YUJ0JZ Supplement Left Lower Leg with Synthetic Substitute, Open Approach

0YUJ0KZ Supplement Left Lower Leg with Nonautologous Tissue Substitute, Open Approach

0YUJ47Z Supplement Left Lower Leg with Autologous Tissue Substitute, Percutaneous Endoscopic Approach

0YUJ4JZ Supplement Left Lower Leg with Synthetic Substitute, Percutaneous Endoscopic Approach

0YUJ4KZ Supplement Left Lower Leg with Nonautologous Tissue Substitute, Percutaneous Endoscopic Approach

0YUK07Z Supplement Right Ankle Region with Autologous Tissue Substitute, Open Approach

0YUK0JZ Supplement Right Ankle Region with Synthetic Substitute, Open Approach

0YUK0KZ Supplement Right Ankle Region with Nonautologous Tissue Substitute, Open Approach

0YUK47Z Supplement Right Ankle Region with Autologous Tissue Substitute, Percutaneous Endoscopic Approach

♀ Female-only   ♂ Male-only   ▲ Limited Coverage   ● Non-OR   HAC HAC-associated procedure   ▲ Non-covered procedures   ✚ Cluster

0YUK4JZ Supplement Right Ankle Region with Synthetic Substitute, Percutaneous Endoscopic Approach

0YUK4KZ Supplement Right Ankle Region with Nonautologous Tissue Substitute, Percutaneous Endoscopic Approach

0YUL07Z Supplement Left Ankle Region with Autologous Tissue Substitute, Open Approach

0YUL0JZ Supplement Left Ankle Region with Synthetic Substitute, Open Approach

0YUL0KZ Supplement Left Ankle Region with Nonautologous Tissue Substitute, Open Approach

0YUL47Z Supplement Left Ankle Region with Autologous Tissue Substitute, Percutaneous Endoscopic Approach

0YUL4JZ Supplement Left Ankle Region with Synthetic Substitute, Percutaneous Endoscopic Approach

0YUL4KZ Supplement Left Ankle Region with Nonautologous Tissue Substitute, Percutaneous Endoscopic Approach

0YUM07Z Supplement Right Foot with Autologous Tissue Substitute, Open Approach

0YUM0JZ Supplement Right Foot with Synthetic Substitute, Open Approach

0YUM0KZ Supplement Right Foot with Nonautologous Tissue Substitute, Open Approach

0YUM47Z Supplement Right Foot with Autologous Tissue Substitute, Percutaneous Endoscopic Approach

0YUM4JZ Supplement Right Foot with Synthetic Substitute, Percutaneous Endoscopic Approach

0YUM4KZ Supplement Right Foot with Nonautologous Tissue Substitute, Percutaneous Endoscopic Approach

0YUN07Z Supplement Left Foot with Autologous Tissue Substitute, Open Approach

0YUN0JZ Supplement Left Foot with Synthetic Substitute, Open Approach

0YUN0KZ Supplement Left Foot with Nonautologous Tissue Substitute, Open Approach

0YUN47Z Supplement Left Foot with Autologous Tissue Substitute, Percutaneous Endoscopic Approach

0YUN4JZ Supplement Left Foot with Synthetic Substitute, Percutaneous Endoscopic Approach

0YUN4KZ Supplement Left Foot with Nonautologous Tissue Substitute, Percutaneous Endoscopic Approach

0YUP07Z Supplement Right 1st Toe with Autologous Tissue Substitute, Open Approach

0YUP0JZ Supplement Right 1st Toe with Synthetic Substitute, Open Approach

0YUP0KZ Supplement Right 1st Toe with Nonautologous Tissue Substitute, Open Approach

0YUP47Z Supplement Right 1st Toe with Autologous Tissue Substitute, Percutaneous Endoscopic Approach

0YUP4JZ Supplement Right 1st Toe with Synthetic Substitute, Percutaneous Endoscopic Approach

0YUP4KZ Supplement Right 1st Toe with Nonautologous Tissue Substitute, Percutaneous Endoscopic Approach

0YUQ07Z Supplement Left 1st Toe with Autologous Tissue Substitute, Open Approach

0YUQ0JZ Supplement Left 1st Toe with Synthetic Substitute, Open Approach

0YUQ0KZ Supplement Left 1st Toe with Nonautologous Tissue Substitute, Open Approach

0YUQ47Z Supplement Left 1st Toe with Autologous Tissue Substitute, Percutaneous Endoscopic Approach

0YUQ4JZ Supplement Left 1st Toe with Synthetic Substitute, Percutaneous Endoscopic Approach

0YUQ4KZ Supplement Left 1st Toe with Nonautologous Tissue Substitute, Percutaneous Endoscopic Approach

0YUR07Z Supplement Right 2nd Toe with Autologous Tissue Substitute, Open Approach

0YUR0JZ Supplement Right 2nd Toe with Synthetic Substitute, Open Approach

0YUR0KZ Supplement Right 2nd Toe with Nonautologous Tissue Substitute, Open Approach

0YUR47Z Supplement Right 2nd Toe with Autologous Tissue Substitute, Percutaneous Endoscopic Approach

0YUR4JZ Supplement Right 2nd Toe with Synthetic Substitute, Percutaneous Endoscopic Approach

0YUR4KZ Supplement Right 2nd Toe with Nonautologous Tissue Substitute, Percutaneous Endoscopic Approach

0YUS07Z Supplement Left 2nd Toe with Autologous Tissue Substitute, Open Approach

0YUS0JZ Supplement Left 2nd Toe with Synthetic Substitute, Open Approach

0YUS0KZ Supplement Left 2nd Toe with Nonautologous Tissue Substitute, Open Approach

0YUS47Z Supplement Left 2nd Toe with Autologous Tissue Substitute, Percutaneous Endoscopic Approach

0YUS4JZ Supplement Left 2nd Toe with Synthetic Substitute, Percutaneous Endoscopic Approach

0YUS4KZ Supplement Left 2nd Toe with Nonautologous Tissue Substitute, Percutaneous Endoscopic Approach

0YUT07Z Supplement Right 3rd Toe with Autologous Tissue Substitute, Open Approach

0YUT0JZ Supplement Right 3rd Toe with Synthetic Substitute, Open Approach

0YUT0KZ Supplement Right 3rd Toe with Nonautologous Tissue Substitute, Open Approach

0YUT47Z Supplement Right 3rd Toe with Autologous Tissue Substitute, Percutaneous Endoscopic Approach

0YUT4JZ Supplement Right 3rd Toe with Synthetic Substitute, Percutaneous Endoscopic Approach

0YUT4KZ Supplement Right 3rd Toe with Nonautologous Tissue Substitute, Percutaneous Endoscopic Approach

0YUU07Z Supplement Left 3rd Toe with Autologous Tissue Substitute, Open Approach

0YUU0JZ Supplement Left 3rd Toe with Synthetic Substitute, Open Approach

0YUU0KZ Supplement Left 3rd Toe with Nonautologous Tissue Substitute, Open Approach

0YUU47Z Supplement Left 3rd Toe with Autologous Tissue Substitute, Percutaneous Endoscopic Approach

0YUU4JZ Supplement Left 3rd Toe with Synthetic Substitute, Percutaneous Endoscopic Approach

0YUU4KZ Supplement Left 3rd Toe with Nonautologous Tissue Substitute, Percutaneous Endoscopic Approach

0YUV07Z Supplement Right 4th Toe with Autologous Tissue Substitute, Open Approach

0YUV0JZ Supplement Right 4th Toe with Synthetic Substitute, Open Approach

0YUV0KZ Supplement Right 4th Toe with Nonautologous Tissue Substitute, Open Approach

0YUV47Z Supplement Right 4th Toe with Autologous Tissue Substitute, Percutaneous Endoscopic Approach

0YUV4JZ Supplement Right 4th Toe with Synthetic Substitute, Percutaneous Endoscopic Approach

0YUV4KZ Supplement Right 4th Toe with Nonautologous Tissue Substitute, Percutaneous Endoscopic Approach

0YUW07Z Supplement Left 4th Toe with Autologous Tissue Substitute, Open Approach

0YUW0JZ Supplement Left 4th Toe with Synthetic Substitute, Open Approach

0YUW0KZ Supplement Left 4th Toe with Nonautologous Tissue Substitute, Open Approach

0YUW47Z Supplement Left 4th Toe with Autologous Tissue Substitute, Percutaneous Endoscopic Approach

0YUW4JZ Supplement Left 4th Toe with Synthetic Substitute, Percutaneous Endoscopic Approach

0YUW4KZ Supplement Left 4th Toe with Nonautologous Tissue Substitute, Percutaneous Endoscopic Approach

0YUX07Z Supplement Right 5th Toe with Autologous Tissue Substitute, Open Approach

0YUX0JZ Supplement Right 5th Toe with Synthetic Substitute, Open Approach

0YUX0KZ Supplement Right 5th Toe with Nonautologous Tissue Substitute, Open Approach

0YUX47Z Supplement Right 5th Toe with Autologous Tissue Substitute, Percutaneous Endoscopic Approach

0YUX4JZ Supplement Right 5th Toe with Synthetic Substitute, Percutaneous Endoscopic Approach

0YUX4KZ Supplement Right 5th Toe with Nonautologous Tissue Substitute, Percutaneous Endoscopic Approach

0YUY07Z Supplement Left 5th Toe with Autologous Tissue Substitute, Open Approach

0YUY0JZ Supplement Left 5th Toe with Synthetic Substitute, Open Approach

0YUY0KZ Supplement Left 5th Toe with Nonautologous Tissue Substitute, Open Approach

0YUY47Z Supplement Left 5th Toe with Autologous Tissue Substitute, Percutaneous Endoscopic Approach

0YUY4JZ Supplement Left 5th Toe with Synthetic Substitute, Percutaneous Endoscopic Approach

0YUY4KZ Supplement Left 5th Toe with Nonautologous Tissue Substitute, Percutaneous Endoscopic Approach

♀ Female-only   ♂ Male-only   ▲ Limited Coverage   ● Non-OR   HAC HAC-associated procedure   ▲ Non-covered procedures   ✚ Cluster

Review Coding Guideline B6.1c

● **0YW900Z** Revision of Drainage Device in Right Lower Extremity, Open Approach

● **0YW903Z** Revision of Infusion Device in Right Lower Extremity, Open Approach

● **0YW907Z** Revision of Autologous Tissue Substitute in Right Lower Extremity, Open Approach

● **0YW90JZ** Revision of Synthetic Substitute in Right Lower Extremity, Open Approach

● **0YW90KZ** Revision of Nonautologous Tissue Substitute in Right Lower Extremity, Open Approach

● **0YW90YZ** Revision of Other Device in Right Lower Extremity, Open Approach

● **0YW930Z** Revision of Drainage Device in Right Lower Extremity, Percutaneous Approach

● **0YW933Z** Revision of Infusion Device in Right Lower Extremity, Percutaneous Approach

● **0YW937Z** Revision of Autologous Tissue Substitute in Right Lower Extremity, Percutaneous Approach

● **0YW93JZ** Revision of Synthetic Substitute in Right Lower Extremity, Percutaneous Approach

● **0YW93KZ** Revision of Nonautologous Tissue Substitute in Right Lower Extremity, Percutaneous Approach

● **0YW93YZ** Revision of Other Device in Right Lower Extremity, Percutaneous Approach

● **0YW940Z** Revision of Drainage Device in Right Lower Extremity, Percutaneous Endoscopic Approach

● **0YW943Z** Revision of Infusion Device in Right Lower Extremity, Percutaneous Endoscopic Approach

● **0YW947Z** Revision of Autologous Tissue Substitute in Right Lower Extremity, Percutaneous Endoscopic Approach

● **0YW94JZ** Revision of Synthetic Substitute in Right Lower Extremity, Percutaneous Endoscopic Approach

● **0YW94KZ** Revision of Nonautologous Tissue Substitute in Right Lower Extremity, Percutaneous Endoscopic Approach

● **0YW94YZ** Revision of Other Device in Right Lower Extremity, Percutaneous Endoscopic Approach

0YW9X0Z Revision of Drainage Device in Right Lower Extremity, External Approach

0YW9X3Z Revision of Infusion Device in Right Lower Extremity, External Approach

0YW9X7Z Revision of Autologous Tissue Substitute in Right Lower Extremity, External Approach

0YW9XJZ Revision of Synthetic Substitute in Right Lower Extremity, External Approach

0YW9XKZ Revision of Nonautologous Tissue Substitute in Right Lower Extremity, External Approach

0YW9XYZ Revision of Other Device in Right Lower Extremity, External Approach

● **0YWB00Z** Revision of Drainage Device in Left Lower Extremity, Open Approach

● **0YWB03Z** Revision of Infusion Device in Left Lower Extremity, Open Approach

● **0YWB07Z** Revision of Autologous Tissue Substitute in Left Lower Extremity, Open Approach

● **0YWB0JZ** Revision of Synthetic Substitute in Left Lower Extremity, Open Approach

● **0YWB0KZ** Revision of Nonautologous Tissue Substitute in Left Lower Extremity, Open Approach

● **0YWB0YZ** Revision of Other Device in Left Lower Extremity, Open Approach

● **0YWB30Z** Revision of Drainage Device in Left Lower Extremity, Percutaneous Approach

● **0YWB33Z** Revision of Infusion Device in Left Lower Extremity, Percutaneous Approach

● **0YWB37Z** Revision of Autologous Tissue Substitute in Left Lower Extremity, Percutaneous Approach

● **0YWB3JZ** Revision of Synthetic Substitute in Left Lower Extremity, Percutaneous Approach

● **0YWB3KZ** Revision of Nonautologous Tissue Substitute in Left Lower Extremity, Percutaneous Approach

● **0YWB3YZ** Revision of Other Device in Left Lower Extremity, Percutaneous Approach

● **0YWB40Z** Revision of Drainage Device in Left Lower Extremity, Percutaneous Endoscopic Approach

● **0YWB43Z** Revision of Infusion Device in Left Lower Extremity, Percutaneous Endoscopic Approach

● **0YWB47Z** Revision of Autologous Tissue Substitute in Left Lower Extremity, Percutaneous Endoscopic Approach

● **0YWB4JZ** Revision of Synthetic Substitute in Left Lower Extremity, Percutaneous Endoscopic Approach

● **0YWB4KZ** Revision of Nonautologous Tissue Substitute in Left Lower Extremity, Percutaneous Endoscopic Approach

● **0YWB4YZ** Revision of Other Device in Left Lower Extremity, Percutaneous Endoscopic Approach

0YWBX0Z Revision of Drainage Device in Left Lower Extremity, External Approach

0YWBX3Z Revision of Infusion Device in Left Lower Extremity, External Approach

0YWBX7Z Revision of Autologous Tissue Substitute in Left Lower Extremity, External Approach

0YWBXJZ Revision of Synthetic Substitute in Left Lower Extremity, External Approach

0YWBXKZ Revision of Nonautologous Tissue Substitute in Left Lower Extremity, External Approach

0YWBXYZ Revision of Other Device in Left Lower Extremity, External Approach

♀ Female-only   ♂ Male-only   ▲ Limited Coverage   ● Non-OR   ▆ HAC-associated procedure   ▲ Non-covered procedures   ✛ Cluster

Within each section of ICD-10-PCS the characters have different meanings. The seven character meanings for the Obstetrics section are illustrated here through the procedure example of *Manually-assisted delivery*.

Section	Body System	Root Operation	Body Part	Approach	Device	Qualifier
Obstetrics	Pregnancy	Delivery	Products of Conception	External	None	None
1	0	E	0	X	Z	Z

Section (Character 1)

All Obstetric procedure codes have a first character value of 1.

Body System (Character 2)

The alphanumeric character for the body system is placed in the second position. The body system applicable to the Obstetrics section is Pregnancy and has a character value of 0.

Root Operations (Character 3)

The alphanumeric character value for root operations is placed in the third position. Listed below are the root operations applicable to the Obstetrics section with their associated meaning.

Character Value	Root Operation	Root Operation Definition
2	Change	Taking out or off a device from a body part and putting back an identical or similar device in or on the same body part without cutting or puncturing the skin or a mucous membrane
9	Drainage	Taking or letting out fluids and/or gases from a body part
A	Abortion	Artificially terminating a pregnancy
D	Extraction	Pulling or stripping out or off all or a portion of a body part by the use of force
E	Delivery	Assisting the passage of the products of conception from the genital canal
H	Insertion	Putting in a nonbiological appliance that monitors, assists, performs, or prevents a physiological function but does not physically take the place of a body part
J	Inspection	Visually and/or manually exploring a body part
P	Removal	Taking out or off a device from a body part, region or orifice
Q	Repair	Restoring, to the extent possible, a body part to its normal anatomic structure and function
S	Reposition	Moving to its normal location, or other suitable location, all or a portion of a body part
T	Resection	Cutting out or off, without replacement, all of a body part
Y	Transplantation	Putting in or on all or a portion of a living body part taken from another individual or animal to physically take the place and/or function of all or a portion of a similar body part

Body Part (Character 4)

For each body system the applicable body part character values will be available for procedure code construction. An example of a body part is Products of Conception.

Approach (Character 5)

The approach is the technique used to reach the procedure site. The following are the approach character values for the Obstetrics section with the associated definitions.

Character Value	Approach	Approach Definition
0	Open	Cutting through the skin or mucous membrane and any other body layers necessary to expose the site of the procedure

Continued →

Character Value	Approach	Approach Definition
3	Percutaneous	Entry, by puncture or minor incision, of instrumentation through the skin or mucous membrane and any other body layers necessary to reach the site of the procedure
4	Percutaneous Endoscopic	Entry, by puncture or minor incision, of instrumentation through the skin or mucous membrane and any other body layers necessary to reach and visualize the site of the procedure
7	Via Natural or Artificial Opening	Entry of instrumentation through a natural or artificial external opening to reach the site of the procedure
8	Via Natural or Artificial Opening Endoscopic	Entry of instrumentation through a natural or artificial external opening to reach and visualize the site of the procedure
X	External	Procedures performed directly on the skin or mucous membrane and procedures performed indirectly by the application of external force through the skin or mucous membrane

Device (Character 6)

Depending on the procedure performed there may or may not be a device used. There are two types of devices included in the Obstetrics section: monitoring electrode and other device. When a device is not utilized during the procedure, the placeholder Z is the character value that should be reported.

Qualifier (Character 7)

The qualifier represents an additional attribute for the procedure when applicable. For example, drainage procedures in this section include several qualifiers including fetal cerebrospinal fluid that is reported with the character value of A. If there is no qualifier for a procedure, the placeholder Z is the character valve that should be reported.

Obstetric Section Guidelines (section 1)

C. Obstetrics Section

Products of Conception
C1. Procedures performed on the products of conception are coded to the Obstetrics section. Procedures performed on the pregnant female other than the products of conception are coded to the appropriate root operation in the Medical and Surgical section.

Example: Amniocentesis is coded to the products of conception body part in the Obstetrics section. Repair of obstetric urethral laceration is coded to the urethra body part in the Medical and Surgical section.

Procedures following delivery or abortion
C2. Procedures performed following a delivery or abortion for curettage of the endometrium or evacuation of retained products of conception are all coded in the Obstetrics section, to the root operation Extraction and the body part Products of Conception, Retained. Diagnostic or therapeutic dilation and curettage performed during times other than the postpartum or post-abortion period are all coded in the Medical and Surgical section, to the root operation Extraction and the body part Endometrium.

Obstetrics Section Tables and Code Listings

Obstetrics Tables 102–10Y

Section	1	Obstetrics
Body System	0	Pregnancy
Operation	2	**Change:** Taking out or off a device from a body part and putting back an identical or similar device in or on the same body part without cutting or puncturing the skin or a mucous membrane

Body Part (4th)	Approach (5th)	Device (6th)	Qualifier (7th)
0 Products of Conception	7 Via Natural or Artificial Opening	3 Monitoring Electrode Y Other Device	Z No Qualifier

Section	1	Obstetrics
Body System	0	Pregnancy
Operation	9	**Drainage:** Taking or letting out fluids and/or gases from a body part

Body Part (4th)	Approach (5th)	Device (6th)	Qualifier (7th)
0 Products of Conception	0 Open 3 Percutaneous 4 Percutaneous Endoscopic 7 Via Natural or Artificial Opening 8 Via Natural or Artificial Opening Endoscopic	Z No Device	9 Fetal Blood A Fetal Cerebrospinal Fluid B Fetal Fluid, Other C Amniotic Fluid, Therapeutic D Fluid, Other U Amniotic Fluid, Diagnostic

Section	1	Obstetrics
Body System	0	Pregnancy
Operation	A	**Abortion:** Artificially terminating a pregnancy

Body Part (4th)	Approach (5th)	Device (6th)	Qualifier (7th)
0 Products of Conception	0 Open 3 Percutaneous 4 Percutaneous Endoscopic 8 Via Natural or Artificial Opening Endoscopic	Z No Device	Z No Qualifier
0 Products of Conception	7 Via Natural or Artificial Opening	Z No Device	6 Vacuum W Laminaria X Abortifacient Z No Qualifier

Section	1	Obstetrics
Body System	0	Pregnancy
Operation	D	**Extraction:** Pulling or stripping out or off all or a portion of a body part by the use of force

Body Part (4th)	Approach (5th)	Device (6th)	Qualifier (7th)
0 Products of Conception	0 Open	Z No Device	0 High 1 Low 2 Extraperitoneal
0 Products of Conception	7 Via Natural or Artificial Opening	Z No Device	3 Low Forceps 4 Mid Forceps 5 High Forceps 6 Vacuum 7 Internal Version 8 Other
1 Products of Conception, Retained	7 Via Natural or Artificial Opening 8 Via Natural or Artificial Opening Endoscopic	Z No Device	9 Manual Z No Qualifier
2 Products of Conception, Ectopic	0 Open 4 Percutaneous Endoscopic 7 Via Natural or Artificial Opening 8 Via Natural or Artificial Opening Endoscopic	Z No Device	Z No Qualifier

Section	1	Obstetrics
Body System	0	Pregnancy
Operation	E	**Delivery:** Assisting the passage of the products of conception from the genital canal

Body Part (4th)	Approach (5th)	Device (6th)	Qualifier (7th)
0 Products of Conception	X External	Z No Device	Z No Qualifier

Section	1	Obstetrics
Body System	0	Pregnancy
Operation	H	**Insertion:** Putting in a nonbiological appliance that monitors, assists, performs, or prevents a physiological function but does not physically take the place of a body part

Body Part (4th)	Approach (5th)	Device (6th)	Qualifier (7th)
0 Products of Conception	0 Open 7 Via Natural or Artificial Opening	3 Monitoring Electrode Y Other Device	Z No Qualifier

Section	1	Obstetrics
Body System	0	Pregnancy
Operation	J	**Inspection:** Visually and/or manually exploring a body part

Body Part (4th)	Approach (5th)	Device (6th)	Qualifier (7th)
0 Products of Conception 1 Products of Conception, Retained 2 Products of Conception, Ectopic	0 Open 3 Percutaneous 4 Percutaneous Endoscopic 7 Via Natural or Artificial Opening 8 Via Natural or Artificial Opening Endoscopic X External	Z No Device	Z No Qualifier

Section	1	Obstetrics
Body System	0	Pregnancy
Operation	P	**Removal:** Taking out or off a device from a body part, region or orifice

Body Part (4th)	Approach (5th)	Device (6th)	Qualifier (7th)
0 Products of Conception	0 Open 7 Via Natural or Artificial Opening	3 Monitoring Electrode Y Other Device	Z No Qualifier

Section	1	Obstetrics
Body System	0	Pregnancy
Operation	Q	**Repair:** Restoring, to the extent possible, a body part to its normal anatomic structure and function

Body Part (4th)	Approach (5th)	Device (6th)	Qualifier (7th)
0 Products of Conception	0 Open 3 Percutaneous 4 Percutaneous Endoscopic 7 Via Natural or Artificial Opening 8 Via Natural or Artificial Opening Endoscopic	Y Other Device Z No Device	E Nervous System F Cardiovascular System G Lymphatics and Hemic H Eye J Ear, Nose and Sinus K Respiratory System L Mouth and Throat M Gastrointestinal System N Hepatobiliary and Pancreas P Endocrine System Q Skin R Musculoskeletal System S Urinary System T Female Reproductive System V Male Reproductive System Y Other Body System

Section	1	Obstetrics
Body System	0	Pregnancy
Operation	S	**Reposition:** Moving to its normal location, or other suitable location, all or a portion of a body part

Body Part (4ᵗʰ)	Approach (5ᵗʰ)	Device (6ᵗʰ)	Qualifier (7ᵗʰ)
0 Products of Conception	7 Via Natural or Artificial Opening X External	Z No Device	Z No Qualifier
2 Products of Conception, Ectopic	0 Open 3 Percutaneous 4 Percutaneous Endoscopic 7 Via Natural or Artificial Opening 8 Via Natural or Artificial Opening Endoscopic	Z No Device	Z No Qualifier

Section	1	Obstetrics
Body System	0	Pregnancy
Operation	T	**Resection:** Cutting out or off, without replacement, all of a body part

Body Part (4ᵗʰ)	Approach (5ᵗʰ)	Device (6ᵗʰ)	Qualifier (7ᵗʰ)
2 Products of Conception, Ectopic	0 Open 3 Percutaneous 4 Percutaneous Endoscopic 7 Via Natural or Artificial Opening 8 Via Natural or Artificial Opening Endoscopic	Z No Device	Z No Qualifier

Section	1	Obstetrics
Body System	0	Pregnancy
Operation	Y	**Transplantation:** Putting in or on all or a portion of a living body part taken from another individual or animal to physically take the place and/or function of all or a portion of a similar body part

Body Part (4ᵗʰ)	Approach (5ᵗʰ)	Device (6ᵗʰ)	Qualifier (7ᵗʰ)
0 Products of Conception	3 Percutaneous 4 Percutaneous Endoscopic 7 Via Natural or Artificial Opening	Z No Device	E Nervous System F Cardiovascular System G Lymphatics and Hemic H Eye J Ear, Nose and Sinus K Respiratory System L Mouth and Throat M Gastrointestinal System N Hepatobiliary and Pancreas P Endocrine System Q Skin R Musculoskeletal System S Urinary System T Female Reproductive System V Male Reproductive System Y Other Body System

Obstetrics Code Listing 102–10Y

102 – Obstetrics, Pregnancy, Change
Review Coding Guideline C1

♀ **102073Z** Change Monitoring Electrode in Products of Conception, Via Natural or Artificial Opening

♀ **10207YZ** Change Other Device in Products of Conception, Via Natural or Artificial Opening

109 – Obstetrics, Pregnancy, Drainage

♀ **10900Z9** Drainage of Fetal Blood from Products of Conception, Open Approach
♀ **10900ZA** Drainage of Fetal Cerebrospinal Fluid from Products of Conception, Open Approach
♀ **10900ZB** Drainage of Other Fetal Fluid from Products of Conception, Open Approach
♀ **10900ZC** Drainage of Amniotic Fluid, Therapeutic from Products of Conception, Open Approach
♀ **10900ZD** Drainage of Other Fluid from Products of Conception, Open Approach
♀ **10900ZU** Drainage of Amniotic Fluid, Diagnostic from Products of Conception, Open Approach
♀ **10903Z9** Drainage of Fetal Blood from Products of Conception, Percutaneous Approach
♀ **10903ZA** Drainage of Fetal Cerebrospinal Fluid from Products of Conception, Percutaneous Approach
♀ **10903ZB** Drainage of Other Fetal Fluid from Products of Conception, Percutaneous Approach
♀ **10903ZC** Drainage of Amniotic Fluid, Therapeutic from Products of Conception, Percutaneous Approach
♀ **10903ZD** Drainage of Other Fluid from Products of Conception, Percutaneous Approach
♀ **10903ZU** Drainage of Amniotic Fluid, Diagnostic from Products of Conception, Percutaneous Approach

♀ **10904Z9** Drainage of Fetal Blood from Products of Conception, Percutaneous Endoscopic Approach
♀ **10904ZA** Drainage of Fetal Cerebrospinal Fluid from Products of Conception, Percutaneous Endoscopic Approach
♀ **10904ZB** Drainage of Other Fetal Fluid from Products of Conception, Percutaneous Endoscopic Approach
♀ **10904ZC** Drainage of Amniotic Fluid, Therapeutic from Products of Conception, Percutaneous Endoscopic Approach
AHA CC: 3Q, 2014, 12-13
♀ **10904ZD** Drainage of Other Fluid from Products of Conception, Percutaneous Endoscopic Approach
♀ **10904ZU** Drainage of Amniotic Fluid, Diagnostic from Products of Conception, Percutaneous Endoscopic Approach
♀ **10907Z9** Drainage of Fetal Blood from Products of Conception, Via Natural or Artificial Opening
♀ **10907ZA** Drainage of Fetal Cerebrospinal Fluid from Products of Conception, Via Natural or Artificial Opening
♀ **10907ZB** Drainage of Other Fetal Fluid from Products of Conception, Via Natural or Artificial Opening

♀ **10907ZC** Drainage of Amniotic Fluid, Therapeutic from Products of Conception, Via Natural or Artificial Opening
AHA CC: 2Q, 2014, 9-10
♀ **10907ZD** Drainage of Other Fluid from Products of Conception, Via Natural or Artificial Opening
♀ **10907ZU** Drainage of Amniotic Fluid, Diagnostic from Products of Conception, Via Natural or Artificial Opening
♀ **10908Z9** Drainage of Fetal Blood from Products of Conception, Via Natural or Artificial Opening Endoscopic
♀ **10908ZA** Drainage of Fetal Cerebrospinal Fluid from Products of Conception, Via Natural or Artificial Opening Endoscopic
♀ **10908ZB** Drainage of Other Fetal Fluid from Products of Conception, Via Natural or Artificial Opening Endoscopic
♀ **10908ZC** Drainage of Amniotic Fluid, Therapeutic from Products of Conception, Via Natural or Artificial Opening Endoscopic
♀ **10908ZD** Drainage of Other Fluid from Products of Conception, Via Natural or Artificial Opening Endoscopic
♀ **10908ZU** Drainage of Amniotic Fluid, Diagnostic from Products of Conception, Via Natural or Artificial Opening Endoscopic

10A – Obstetrics, Pregnancy, Abortion

♀ **10A00ZZ** Abortion of Products of Conception, Open Approach
♀ **10A03ZZ** Abortion of Products of Conception, Percutaneous Approach
♀ **10A04ZZ** Abortion of Products of Conception, Percutaneous Endoscopic Approach
♀ **10A07Z6** Abortion of Products of Conception, Vacuum, Via Natural or Artificial Opening
♀ **10A07ZW** Abortion of Products of Conception, Laminaria, Via Natural or Artificial Opening
♀ **10A07ZX** Abortion of Products of Conception, Abortifacient, Via Natural or Artificial Opening
♀ **10A07ZZ** Abortion of Products of Conception, Via Natural or Artificial Opening
♀ **10A08ZZ** Abortion of Products of Conception, Via Natural or Artificial Opening Endoscopic

10D – Obstetrics, Pregnancy, Extraction
Review Coding Guideline C2

♀ **10D00Z0** Extraction of Products of Conception, High, Open Approach
AHA CC: 2Q, 2018, 17-18; 4Q, 2018, 51
♀ **10D00Z1** Extraction of Products of Conception, Low, Open Approach
AHA CC: 4Q, 2018, 50-51
♀ **10D00Z2** Extraction of Products of Conception, Extraperitoneal, Open Approach
● ♀ **10D07Z3** Extraction of Products of Conception, Low Forceps, Via Natural or Artificial Opening
AHA CC: 1Q, 2016, 9-10
● ♀ **10D07Z5** Extraction of Products of Conception, High Forceps, Via Natural or Artificial Opening

♀● **10D07Z6** Extraction of Products of Conception, Vacuum, Via Natural or Artificial Opening
AHA CC: 4Q, 2014, 43
♀● **10D07Z7** Extraction of Products of Conception, Internal Version, Via Natural or Artificial Opening
♀● **10D07Z8** Extraction of Products of Conception, Other, Via Natural or Artificial Opening
♀ **10D17Z9** Manual Extraction of Products of Conception, Retained, Via Natural or Artificial Opening
♀ **10D17ZZ** Extraction of Products of Conception, Retained, Via Natural or Artificial Opening
♀ **10D18Z9** Manual Extraction of Products of Conception, Retained, Via Natural or Artificial Opening Endoscopic

♀ **10D18ZZ** Extraction of Products of Conception, Retained, Via Natural or Artificial Opening Endoscopic
♀ **10D20ZZ** Extraction of Products of Conception, Ectopic, Open Approach
AHA CC: 1Q, 2021, 52
♀ **10D24ZZ** Extraction of Products of Conception, Ectopic, Percutaneous Endoscopic Approach
♀ **10D27ZZ** Extraction of Products of Conception, Ectopic, Via Natural or Artificial Opening
AHA CC: 4Q, 2020, 60; 1Q, 2021, 52
♀ **10D28ZZ** Extraction of Products of Conception, Ectopic, Via Natural or Artificial Opening Endoscopic

♀ Female-only　　♂ Male-only　　▲ Limited Coverage　　● Non-OR　　 HAC-associated procedure　　▲ Non-covered procedures　　✛ Cluster

♀ **10E0XZZ** Delivery of Products of Conception,
● External Approach
   AHA CC: 2Q, 2014, 9-10; 4Q, 2014, 17-18; 2Q,
   2016, 34-35; 3Q, 2017, 5

10H – Obstetrics, Pregnancy, Insertion

♀ **10H003Z** Insertion of Monitoring Electrode
into Products of Conception, Open
Approach

♀ **10H00YZ** Insertion of Other Device into Products
of Conception, Open Approach

♀ **10H073Z** Insertion of Monitoring Electrode into
Products of Conception, Via Natural or
Artificial Opening

♀ **10H07YZ** Insertion of Other Device into Products
of Conception, Via Natural or Artificial
Opening
   AHA CC: 2Q, 2013, 36

10J – Obstetrics, Pregnancy, Inspection

♀ **10J00ZZ** Inspection of Products of Conception,
Open Approach

♀ **10J03ZZ** Inspection of Products of Conception,
Percutaneous Approach

♀ **10J04ZZ** Inspection of Products of Conception,
Percutaneous Endoscopic Approach

♀ **10J07ZZ** Inspection of Products of Conception,
Via Natural or Artificial Opening

♀ **10J08ZZ** Inspection of Products of Conception,
Via Natural or Artificial Opening
Endoscopic

♀ **10J0XZZ** Inspection of Products of Conception,
External Approach

♀ **10J10ZZ** Inspection of Products of Conception,
Retained, Open Approach

♀ **10J13ZZ** Inspection of Products of Conception,
Retained, Percutaneous Approach

♀ **10J14ZZ** Inspection of Products of Conception,
Retained, Percutaneous Endoscopic
Approach

♀ **10J17ZZ** Inspection of Products of Conception,
Retained, Via Natural or Artificial
Opening

♀ **10J18ZZ** Inspection of Products of Conception,
Retained, Via Natural or Artificial
Opening Endoscopic

♀ **10J1XZZ** Inspection of Products of Conception,
Retained, External Approach

♀ **10J20ZZ** Inspection of Products of Conception,
Ectopic, Open Approach

♀ **10J23ZZ** Inspection of Products of
Conception, Ectopic, Percutaneous
Approach

♀ **10J24ZZ** Inspection of Products of Conception,
Ectopic, Percutaneous Endoscopic
Approach

♀ **10J27ZZ** Inspection of Products of Conception,
Ectopic, Via Natural or Artificial
Opening

♀ **10J28ZZ** Inspection of Products of
Conception, Ectopic, Via Natural
or Artificial Opening Endoscopic

♀ **10J2XZZ** Inspection of Products of Conception,
Ectopic, External Approach

10P – Obstetrics, Pregnancy, Removal

♀ **10P003Z** Removal of Monitoring Electrode
from Products of Conception, Open
Approach

♀ **10P00YZ** Removal of Other Device from
Products of Conception, Open
Approach

♀ **10P073Z** Removal of Monitoring Electrode from
Products of Conception, Via Natural or
Artificial Opening

♀ **10P07YZ** Removal of Other Device from
Products of Conception, Via Natural or
Artificial Opening

10Q – Obstetrics, Pregnancy, Repair

♀ **10Q00YE** Repair Nervous System in Products of
Conception with Other Device, Open
Approach

♀ **10Q00YF** Repair Cardiovascular System in
Products of Conception with Other
Device, Open Approach

♀ **10Q00YG** Repair Lymphatics and Hemic in
Products of Conception with Other
Device, Open Approach

♀ **10Q00YH** Repair Eye in Products of
Conception with Other Device, Open
Approach

♀ **10Q00YJ** Repair Ear, Nose and Sinus in Products
of Conception with Other Device, Open
Approach

♀ **10Q00YK** Repair Respiratory System in Products
of Conception with Other Device, Open
Approach

♀ **10Q00YL** Repair Mouth and Throat in Products
of Conception with Other Device, Open
Approach

♀ **10Q00YM** Repair Gastrointestinal System in
Products of Conception with Other
Device, Open Approach

♀ **10Q00YN** Repair Hepatobiliary and Pancreas in
Products of Conception with Other
Device, Open Approach

♀ **10Q00YP** Repair Endocrine System in Products
of Conception with Other Device, Open
Approach

♀ **10Q00YQ** Repair Skin in Products of
Conception with Other Device, Open
Approach

♀ **10Q00YR** Repair Musculoskeletal System in
Products of Conception with Other
Device, Open Approach

♀ **10Q00YS** Repair Urinary System in Products of
Conception with Other Device, Open
Approach

♀ **10Q00YT** Repair Female Reproductive System
in Products of Conception with Other
Device, Open Approach

♀ **10Q00YV** Repair Male Reproductive System in
Products of Conception with Other
Device, Open Approach

♀ **10Q00YY** Repair Other Body System in Products
of Conception with Other Device, Open
Approach

♀ **10Q00ZE** Repair Nervous System in Products of
Conception, Open Approach

♀ **10Q00ZF** Repair Cardiovascular System in
Products of Conception, Open
Approach

♀ **10Q00ZG** Repair Lymphatics and Hemic in
Products of Conception, Open
Approach

♀ **10Q00ZH** Repair Eye in Products of Conception,
Open Approach

♀ **10Q00ZJ** Repair Ear, Nose and Sinus in Products
of Conception, Open Approach

♀ **10Q00ZK** Repair Respiratory System in Products
of Conception, Open Approach
   AHA CC: 2Q, 2021, 21-22

♀ **10Q00ZL** Repair Mouth and Throat in Products of
Conception, Open Approach

♀ **10Q00ZM** Repair Gastrointestinal System
in Products of Conception, Open
Approach

♀ **10Q00ZN** Repair Hepatobiliary and Pancreas
in Products of Conception, Open
Approach

♀ **10Q00ZP** Repair Endocrine System in Products of
Conception, Open Approach

♀ **10Q00ZQ** Repair Skin in Products of Conception,
Open Approach

♀ **10Q00ZR** Repair Musculoskeletal System
in Products of Conception, Open
Approach

♀ **10Q00ZS** Repair Urinary System in Products of
Conception, Open Approach

♀ **10Q00ZT** Repair Female Reproductive System in
Products of Conception, Open Approach

♀ **10Q00ZV** Repair Male Reproductive System
in Products of Conception, Open
Approach

♀ **10Q00ZY** Repair Other Body System in Products
of Conception, Open Approach

♀ **10Q03YE** Repair Nervous System in Products
of Conception with Other Device,
Percutaneous Approach

♀ **10Q03YF** Repair Cardiovascular System in Products of Conception with Other Device, Percutaneous Approach

♀ **10Q03YG** Repair Lymphatics and Hemic in Products of Conception with Other Device, Percutaneous Approach

♀ **10Q03YH** Repair Eye in Products of Conception with Other Device, Percutaneous Approach

♀ **10Q03YJ** Repair Ear, Nose and Sinus in Products of Conception with Other Device, Percutaneous Approach

♀ **10Q03YK** Repair Respiratory System in Products of Conception with Other Device, Percutaneous Approach

♀ **10Q03YL** Repair Mouth and Throat in Products of Conception with Other Device, Percutaneous Approach

♀ **10Q03YM** Repair Gastrointestinal System in Products of Conception with Other Device, Percutaneous Approach

♀ **10Q03YN** Repair Hepatobiliary and Pancreas in Products of Conception with Other Device, Percutaneous Approach

♀ **10Q03YP** Repair Endocrine System in Products of Conception with Other Device, Percutaneous Approach

♀ **10Q03YQ** Repair Skin in Products of Conception with Other Device, Percutaneous Approach

♀ **10Q03YR** Repair Musculoskeletal System in Products of Conception with Other Device, Percutaneous Approach

♀ **10Q03YS** Repair Urinary System in Products of Conception with Other Device, Percutaneous Approach

♀ **10Q03YT** Repair Female Reproductive System in Products of Conception with Other Device, Percutaneous Approach

♀ **10Q03YV** Repair Male Reproductive System in Products of Conception with Other Device, Percutaneous Approach

♀ **10Q03YY** Repair Other Body System in Products of Conception with Other Device, Percutaneous Approach

♀ **10Q03ZE** Repair Nervous System in Products of Conception, Percutaneous Approach

♀ **10Q03ZF** Repair Cardiovascular System in Products of Conception, Percutaneous Approach

♀ **10Q03ZG** Repair Lymphatics and Hemic in Products of Conception, Percutaneous Approach

♀ **10Q03ZH** Repair Eye in Products of Conception, Percutaneous Approach

♀ **10Q03ZJ** Repair Ear, Nose and Sinus in Products of Conception, Percutaneous Approach

♀ **10Q03ZK** Repair Respiratory System in Products of Conception, Percutaneous Approach

♀ **10Q03ZL** Repair Mouth and Throat in Products of Conception, Percutaneous Approach

♀ **10Q03ZM** Repair Gastrointestinal System in Products of Conception, Percutaneous Approach

♀ **10Q03ZN** Repair Hepatobiliary and Pancreas in Products of Conception, Percutaneous Approach

♀ **10Q03ZP** Repair Endocrine System in Products of Conception, Percutaneous Approach

♀ **10Q03ZQ** Repair Skin in Products of Conception, Percutaneous Approach

♀ **10Q03ZR** Repair Musculoskeletal System in Products of Conception, Percutaneous Approach

♀ **10Q03ZS** Repair Urinary System in Products of Conception, Percutaneous Approach

♀ **10Q03ZT** Repair Female Reproductive System in Products of Conception, Percutaneous Approach

♀ **10Q03ZV** Repair Male Reproductive System in Products of Conception, Percutaneous Approach

♀ **10Q03ZY** Repair Other Body System in Products of Conception, Percutaneous Approach

♀ **10Q04YE** Repair Nervous System in Products of Conception with Other Device, Percutaneous Endoscopic Approach

♀ **10Q04YF** Repair Cardiovascular System in Products of Conception with Other Device, Percutaneous Endoscopic Approach

♀ **10Q04YG** Repair Lymphatics and Hemic in Products of Conception with Other Device, Percutaneous Endoscopic Approach

♀ **10Q04YH** Repair Eye in Products of Conception with Other Device, Percutaneous Endoscopic Approach

♀ **10Q04YJ** Repair Ear, Nose and Sinus in Products of Conception with Other Device, Percutaneous Endoscopic Approach

♀ **10Q04YK** Repair Respiratory System in Products of Conception with Other Device, Percutaneous Endoscopic Approach

♀ **10Q04YL** Repair Mouth and Throat in Products of Conception with Other Device, Percutaneous Endoscopic Approach

♀ **10Q04YM** Repair Gastrointestinal System in Products of Conception with Other Device, Percutaneous Endoscopic Approach

♀ **10Q04YN** Repair Hepatobiliary and Pancreas in Products of Conception with Other Device, Percutaneous Endoscopic Approach

♀ **10Q04YP** Repair Endocrine System in Products of Conception with Other Device, Percutaneous Endoscopic Approach

♀ **10Q04YQ** Repair Skin in Products of Conception with Other Device, Percutaneous Endoscopic Approach

♀ **10Q04YR** Repair Musculoskeletal System in Products of Conception with Other Device, Percutaneous Endoscopic Approach

♀ **10Q04YS** Repair Urinary System in Products of Conception with Other Device, Percutaneous Endoscopic Approach

♀ **10Q04YT** Repair Female Reproductive System in Products of Conception with Other Device, Percutaneous Endoscopic Approach

♀ **10Q04YV** Repair Male Reproductive System in Products of Conception with Other Device, Percutaneous Endoscopic Approach

♀ **10Q04YY** Repair Other Body System in Products of Conception with Other Device, Percutaneous Endoscopic Approach

♀ **10Q04ZE** Repair Nervous System in Products of Conception, Percutaneous Endoscopic Approach

♀ **10Q04ZF** Repair Cardiovascular System in Products of Conception, Percutaneous Endoscopic Approach

♀ **10Q04ZG** Repair Lymphatics and Hemic in Products of Conception, Percutaneous Endoscopic Approach

♀ **10Q04ZH** Repair Eye in Products of Conception, Percutaneous Endoscopic Approach

♀ **10Q04ZJ** Repair Ear, Nose and Sinus in Products of Conception, Percutaneous Endoscopic Approach

♀ **10Q04ZK** Repair Respiratory System in Products of Conception, Percutaneous Endoscopic Approach

♀ **10Q04ZL** Repair Mouth and Throat in Products of Conception, Percutaneous Endoscopic Approach

♀ **10Q04ZM** Repair Gastrointestinal System in Products of Conception, Percutaneous Endoscopic Approach

♀ **10Q04ZN** Repair Hepatobiliary and Pancreas in Products of Conception, Percutaneous Endoscopic Approach

♀ **10Q04ZP** Repair Endocrine System in Products of Conception, Percutaneous Endoscopic Approach

♀ **10Q04ZQ** Repair Skin in Products of Conception, Percutaneous Endoscopic Approach

♀ **10Q04ZR** Repair Musculoskeletal System in Products of Conception, Percutaneous Endoscopic Approach

♀ **10Q04ZS** Repair Urinary System in Products of Conception, Percutaneous Endoscopic Approach

♀ **10Q04ZT** Repair Female Reproductive System in Products of Conception, Percutaneous Endoscopic Approach

♀ **10Q04ZV** Repair Male Reproductive System in Products of Conception, Percutaneous Endoscopic Approach

♀ **10Q04ZY** Repair Other Body System in Products of Conception, Percutaneous Endoscopic Approach

AHA CC: 3Q, 2014, 12-13

♀ **10Q07YE** Repair Nervous System in Products of Conception with Other Device, Via Natural or Artificial Opening

♀ **10Q07YF** Repair Cardiovascular System in Products of Conception with Other Device, Via Natural or Artificial Opening

♀ **10Q07YG** Repair Lymphatics and Hemic in Products of Conception with Other Device, Via Natural or Artificial Opening

♀ **10Q07YH** Repair Eye in Products of Conception with Other Device, Via Natural or Artificial Opening

♀ **10Q07YJ** Repair Ear, Nose and Sinus in Products of Conception with Other Device, Via Natural or Artificial Opening

♀ **10Q07YK** Repair Respiratory System in Products of Conception with Other Device, Via Natural or Artificial Opening

♀ **10Q07YL** Repair Mouth and Throat in Products of Conception with Other Device, Via Natural or Artificial Opening

♀ **10Q07YM** Repair Gastrointestinal System in Products of Conception with Other Device, Via Natural or Artificial Opening

♀ **10Q07YN** Repair Hepatobiliary and Pancreas in Products of Conception with Other Device, Via Natural or Artificial Opening

♀ **10Q07YP** Repair Endocrine System in Products of Conception with Other Device, Via Natural or Artificial Opening

♀ **10Q07YQ** Repair Skin in Products of Conception with Other Device, Via Natural or Artificial Opening

♀ Female-only   ♂ Male-only   ▲ Limited Coverage   ● Non-OR   ▣ HAC-associated procedure   ▲ Non-covered procedures   ✚ Cluster

♀ **10Q07YR** Repair Musculoskeletal System in Products of Conception with Other Device, Via Natural or Artificial Opening

♀ **10Q07YS** Repair Urinary System in Products of Conception with Other Device, Via Natural or Artificial Opening

♀ **10Q07YT** Repair Female Reproductive System in Products of Conception with Other Device, Via Natural or Artificial Opening

♀ **10Q07YV** Repair Male Reproductive System in Products of Conception with Other Device, Via Natural or Artificial Opening

♀ **10Q07YY** Repair Other Body System in Products of Conception with Other Device, Via Natural or Artificial Opening

♀ **10Q07ZE** Repair Nervous System in Products of Conception, Via Natural or Artificial Opening

♀ **10Q07ZF** Repair Cardiovascular System in Products of Conception, Via Natural or Artificial Opening

♀ **10Q07ZG** Repair Lymphatics and Hemic in Products of Conception, Via Natural or Artificial Opening

♀ **10Q07ZH** Repair Eye in Products of Conception, Via Natural or Artificial Opening

♀ **10Q07ZJ** Repair Ear, Nose and Sinus in Products of Conception, Via Natural or Artificial Opening

♀ **10Q07ZK** Repair Respiratory System in Products of Conception, Via Natural or Artificial Opening

♀ **10Q07ZL** Repair Mouth and Throat in Products of Conception, Via Natural or Artificial Opening

♀ **10Q07ZM** Repair Gastrointestinal System in Products of Conception, Via Natural or Artificial Opening

♀ **10Q07ZN** Repair Hepatobiliary and Pancreas in Products of Conception, Via Natural or Artificial Opening

♀ **10Q07ZP** Repair Endocrine System in Products of Conception, Via Natural or Artificial Opening

♀ **10Q07ZQ** Repair Skin in Products of Conception, Via Natural or Artificial Opening

♀ **10Q07ZR** Repair Musculoskeletal System in Products of Conception, Via Natural or Artificial Opening

♀ **10Q07ZS** Repair Urinary System in Products of Conception, Via Natural or Artificial Opening

♀ **10Q07ZT** Repair Female Reproductive System in Products of Conception, Via Natural or Artificial Opening

♀ **10Q07ZV** Repair Male Reproductive System in Products of Conception, Via Natural or Artificial Opening

♀ **10Q07ZY** Repair Other Body System in Products of Conception, Via Natural or Artificial Opening

♀ **10Q08YE** Repair Nervous System in Products of Conception with Other Device, Via Natural or Artificial Opening Endoscopic

♀ **10Q08YF** Repair Cardiovascular System in Products of Conception with Other Device, Via Natural or Artificial Opening Endoscopic

♀ **10Q08YG** Repair Lymphatics and Hemic in Products of Conception with Other Device, Via Natural or Artificial Opening Endoscopic

♀ **10Q08YH** Repair Eye in Products of Conception with Other Device, Via Natural or Artificial Opening Endoscopic

♀ **10Q08YJ** Repair Ear, Nose and Sinus in Products of Conception with Other Device, Via Natural or Artificial Opening Endoscopic

♀ **10Q08YK** Repair Respiratory System in Products of Conception with Other Device, Via Natural or Artificial Opening Endoscopic

♀ **10Q08YL** Repair Mouth and Throat in Products of Conception with Other Device, Via Natural or Artificial Opening Endoscopic

♀ **10Q08YM** Repair Gastrointestinal System in Products of Conception with Other Device, Via Natural or Artificial Opening Endoscopic

♀ **10Q08YN** Repair Hepatobiliary and Pancreas in Products of Conception with Other Device, Via Natural or Artificial Opening Endoscopic

♀ **10Q08YP** Repair Endocrine System in Products of Conception with Other Device, Via Natural or Artificial Opening Endoscopic

♀ **10Q08YQ** Repair Skin in Products of Conception with Other Device, Via Natural or Artificial Opening Endoscopic

♀ **10Q08YR** Repair Musculoskeletal System in Products of Conception with Other Device, Via Natural or Artificial Opening Endoscopic

♀ **10Q08YS** Repair Urinary System in Products of Conception with Other Device, Via Natural or Artificial Opening Endoscopic

♀ **10Q08YT** Repair Female Reproductive System in Products of Conception with Other Device, Via Natural or Artificial Opening Endoscopic

♀ **10Q08YV** Repair Male Reproductive System in Products of Conception with Other Device, Via Natural or Artificial Opening Endoscopic

♀ **10Q08YY** Repair Other Body System in Products of Conception with Other Device, Via Natural or Artificial Opening Endoscopic

♀ **10Q08ZE** Repair Nervous System in Products of Conception, Via Natural or Artificial Opening Endoscopic

♀ **10Q08ZF** Repair Cardiovascular System in Products of Conception, Via Natural or Artificial Opening Endoscopic

♀ **10Q08ZG** Repair Lymphatics and Hemic in Products of Conception, Via Natural or Artificial Opening Endoscopic

♀ **10Q08ZH** Repair Eye in Products of Conception, Via Natural or Artificial Opening Endoscopic

♀ **10Q08ZJ** Repair Ear, Nose and Sinus in Products of Conception, Via Natural or Artificial Opening Endoscopic

♀ **10Q08ZK** Repair Respiratory System in Products of Conception, Via Natural or Artificial Opening Endoscopic

♀ **10Q08ZL** Repair Mouth and Throat in Products of Conception, Via Natural or Artificial Opening Endoscopic

♀ **10Q08ZM** Repair Gastrointestinal System in Products of Conception, Via Natural or Artificial Opening Endoscopic

♀ **10Q08ZN** Repair Hepatobiliary and Pancreas in Products of Conception, Via Natural or Artificial Opening Endoscopic

♀ **10Q08ZP** Repair Endocrine System in Products of Conception, Via Natural or Artificial Opening Endoscopic

♀ **10Q08ZQ** Repair Skin in Products of Conception, Via Natural or Artificial Opening Endoscopic

♀ **10Q08ZR** Repair Musculoskeletal System in Products of Conception, Via Natural or Artificial Opening Endoscopic

♀ **10Q08ZS** Repair Urinary System in Products of Conception, Via Natural or Artificial Opening Endoscopic

♀ **10Q08ZT** Repair Female Reproductive System in Products of Conception, Via Natural or Artificial Opening Endoscopic

♀ **10Q08ZV** Repair Male Reproductive System in Products of Conception, Via Natural or Artificial Opening Endoscopic

♀ **10Q08ZY** Repair Other Body System in Products of Conception, Via Natural or Artificial Opening Endoscopic

10S – Obstetrics, Pregnancy, Reposition

♀ **10S07ZZ** Reposition Products of Conception, Via Natural or Artificial Opening

♀ **10S0XZZ** Reposition Products of Conception, External Approach

♀ **10S20ZZ** Reposition Products of Conception, Ectopic, Open Approach

♀ **10S23ZZ** Reposition Products of Conception, Ectopic, Percutaneous Approach

♀ **10S24ZZ** Reposition Products of Conception, Ectopic, Percutaneous Endoscopic Approach

♀ **10S27ZZ** Reposition Products of Conception, Ectopic, Via Natural or Artificial Opening

♀ **10S28ZZ** Reposition Products of Conception, Ectopic, Via Natural or Artificial Opening Endoscopic

10T – Obstetrics, Pregnancy, Resection

♀ **10T20ZZ** Resection of Products of Conception, Ectopic, Open Approach

♀ **10T23ZZ** Resection of Products of Conception, Ectopic, Percutaneous Approach

♀ **10T24ZZ** Resection of Products of Conception, Ectopic, Percutaneous Endoscopic Approach
AHA CC: 3Q, 2015, 32; 3Q, 2020, 47

♀ **10T27ZZ** Resection of Products of Conception, Ectopic, Via Natural or Artificial Opening

♀ **10T28ZZ** Resection of Products of Conception, Ectopic, Via Natural or Artificial Opening Endoscopic

♀ **10Y03ZE** Transplantation of Nervous System into Products of Conception, Percutaneous Approach

♀ **10Y03ZF** Transplantation of Cardiovascular System into Products of Conception, Percutaneous Approach

♀ **10Y03ZG** Transplantation of Lymphatics and Hemic into Products of Conception, Percutaneous Approach

♀ **10Y03ZH** Transplantation of Eye into Products of Conception, Percutaneous Approach

♀ **10Y03ZJ** Transplantation of Ear, Nose and Sinus into Products of Conception, Percutaneous Approach

♀ **10Y03ZK** Transplantation of Respiratory System into Products of Conception, Percutaneous Approach

♀ **10Y03ZL** Transplantation of Mouth and Throat into Products of Conception, Percutaneous Approach

♀ **10Y03ZM** Transplantation of Gastrointestinal System into Products of Conception, Percutaneous Approach

♀ **10Y03ZN** Transplantation of Hepatobiliary and Pancreas into Products of Conception, Percutaneous Approach

♀ **10Y03ZP** Transplantation of Endocrine System into Products of Conception, Percutaneous Approach

♀ **10Y03ZQ** Transplantation of Skin into Products of Conception, Percutaneous Approach

♀ **10Y03ZR** Transplantation of Musculoskeletal System into Products of Conception, Percutaneous Approach

♀ **10Y03ZS** Transplantation of Urinary System into Products of Conception, Percutaneous Approach

♀ **10Y03ZT** Transplantation of Female Reproductive System into Products of Conception, Percutaneous Approach

♀ **10Y03ZV** Transplantation of Male Reproductive System into Products of Conception, Percutaneous Approach

♀ **10Y03ZY** Transplantation of Other Body System into Products of Conception, Percutaneous Approach

♀ **10Y04ZE** Transplantation of Nervous System into Products of Conception, Percutaneous Endoscopic Approach

♀ **10Y04ZF** Transplantation of Cardiovascular System into Products of Conception, Percutaneous Endoscopic Approach

♀ **10Y04ZG** Transplantation of Lymphatics and Hemic into Products of Conception, Percutaneous Endoscopic Approach

♀ **10Y04ZH** Transplantation of Eye into Products of Conception, Percutaneous Endoscopic Approach

♀ **10Y04ZJ** Transplantation of Ear, Nose and Sinus into Products of Conception, Percutaneous Endoscopic Approach

♀ **10Y04ZK** Transplantation of Respiratory System into Products of Conception, Percutaneous Endoscopic Approach

♀ **10Y04ZL** Transplantation of Mouth and Throat into Products of Conception, Percutaneous Endoscopic Approach

♀ **10Y04ZM** Transplantation of Gastrointestinal System into Products of Conception, Percutaneous Endoscopic Approach

♀ **10Y04ZN** Transplantation of Hepatobiliary and Pancreas into Products of Conception, Percutaneous Endoscopic Approach

♀ **10Y04ZP** Transplantation of Endocrine System into Products of Conception, Percutaneous Endoscopic Approach

♀ **10Y04ZQ** Transplantation of Skin into Products of Conception, Percutaneous Endoscopic Approach

♀ **10Y04ZR** Transplantation of Musculoskeletal System into Products of Conception, Percutaneous Endoscopic Approach

♀ **10Y04ZS** Transplantation of Urinary System into Products of Conception, Percutaneous Endoscopic Approach

♀ **10Y04ZT** Transplantation of Female Reproductive System into Products of Conception, Percutaneous Endoscopic Approach

♀ **10Y04ZV** Transplantation of Male Reproductive System into Products of Conception, Percutaneous Endoscopic Approach

♀ **10Y04ZY** Transplantation of Other Body System into Products of Conception, Percutaneous Endoscopic Approach

♀ **10Y07ZE** Transplantation of Nervous System into Products of Conception, Via Natural or Artificial Opening

♀ **10Y07ZF** Transplantation of Cardiovascular System into Products of Conception, Via Natural or Artificial Opening

♀ **10Y07ZG** Transplantation of Lymphatics and Hemic into Products of Conception, Via Natural or Artificial Opening

♀ **10Y07ZH** Transplantation of Eye into Products of Conception, Via Natural or Artificial Opening

♀ **10Y07ZJ** Transplantation of Ear, Nose and Sinus into Products of Conception, Via Natural or Artificial Opening

♀ **10Y07ZK** Transplantation of Respiratory System into Products of Conception, Via Natural or Artificial Opening

♀ **10Y07ZL** Transplantation of Mouth and Throat into Products of Conception, Via Natural or Artificial Opening

♀ **10Y07ZM** Transplantation of Gastrointestinal System into Products of Conception, Via Natural or Artificial Opening

♀ **10Y07ZN** Transplantation of Hepatobiliary and Pancreas into Products of Conception, Via Natural or Artificial Opening

♀ **10Y07ZP** Transplantation of Endocrine System into Products of Conception, Via Natural or Artificial Opening

♀ **10Y07ZQ** Transplantation of Skin into Products of Conception, Via Natural or Artificial Opening

♀ **10Y07ZR** Transplantation of Musculoskeletal System into Products of Conception, Via Natural or Artificial Opening

♀ **10Y07ZS** Transplantation of Urinary System into Products of Conception, Via Natural or Artificial Opening

♀ **10Y07ZT** Transplantation of Female Reproductive System into Products of Conception, Via Natural or Artificial Opening

♀ **10Y07ZV** Transplantation of Male Reproductive System into Products of Conception, Via Natural or Artificial Opening

♀ **10Y07ZY** Transplantation of Other Body System into Products of Conception, Via Natural or Artificial Opening

Within each section of ICD-10-PCS the characters have different meanings. The seven character meanings for the Placement section are illustrated below through the procedure example of *Placement of pressure dressing on abdominal wall.*

Section	Body System	Root Operation	Body Region	Approach	Device	Qualifier
Placement	Anatomical Regions	Compression	Abdominal Wall	External	Pressure Dressing	None
2	W	1	3	X	6	Z

Section (Character 1)

All Placement procedure codes have a first character value of 2.

Body System (Character 2)

The alphanumeric character for the body system is placed in the second position. There are two character values applicable for the Placement section. The character value of W is reported for anatomical regions. The character value Y is reported for anatomical orifices.

Root Operations (Character 3)

The alphanumeric character value for root operations is placed in the third position. The following are the root operations applicable to the Placement section with their associated meaning.

Character Value	Root Operation	Root Operation Definition
0	Change	Taking out or off a device from a body part and putting back an identical or similar device in or on the same body part without cutting or puncturing the skin or a mucous membrane
1	Compression	Putting pressure on a body region
2	Dressing	Putting material on a body region for protection
3	Immobilization	Limiting or preventing motion of a body region
4	Packing	Putting material in a body region or orifice
5	Removal	Taking out or off a device from a body part
6	Traction	Exerting a pulling force on a body region in a distal direction

Body Region (Character 4)

For each body system the applicable body part character values will be available for procedure code construction. An example of a body region is Chest Wall.

Approach (Character 5)

The only approach technique utilized for the Placement section is External approach and is reported with the character value of X.

Character Value	Approach	Approach Definition
X	External	Procedures performed directly on the skin or mucous membrane and procedures performed indirectly by the application of external force through the skin or mucous membrane

Device (Character 6)

Depending on the procedure performed there may or may not be a device used. There are several types of devices included in the Placement section. Here is a sample list of the devices included in this section:

- Cast
- Packing material
- Pressure dressing
- Traction apparatus

When a device is not utilized during the procedure, the placeholder Z is the character value that should be reported.

Qualifier (Character 7)

The qualifier represents an additional attribute for the procedure when applicable. Currently, there are no qualifiers in the Placement section; therefore, the placeholder character value of Z should be reported.

Section Notes

Before reporting Change and Removal procedures in this section users should *Review coding guideline B6.1c.*

AHA Coding Clinic

2W60X0Z Traction of Head using Traction Apparatus - AHA CC: 2Q, 2013, 39

2W62X0Z Traction of Neck using Traction Apparatus - AHA CC: 2Q, 2015, 35

2Y41X5Z Packing of Nasal Region using Packing Material - AHA CC: 4Q, 2017, 106; 4Q, 2018, 38

Placement Section Tables

Placement Tables 2W0–2Y5

Section	2	Placement
Body System	W	Anatomical Regions
Operation	0	**Change:** Taking out or off a device from a body part and putting back an identical or similar device in or on the same body part without cutting or puncturing the skin or a mucous membrane

Body Region (4th)	Approach (5th)	Device (6th)	Qualifier (7th)
0 Head 2 Neck 3 Abdominal Wall 4 Chest Wall 5 Back 6 Inguinal Region, Right 7 Inguinal Region, Left 8 Upper Extremity, Right 9 Upper Extremity, Left A Upper Arm, Right B Upper Arm, Left C Lower Arm, Right D Lower Arm, Left E Hand, Right F Hand, Left G Thumb, Right H Thumb, Left J Finger, Right K Finger, Left L Lower Extremity, Right M Lower Extremity, Left N Upper Leg, Right P Upper Leg, Left Q Lower Leg, Right R Lower Leg, Left S Foot, Right T Foot, Left U Toe, Right V Toe, Left	X External	0 Traction Apparatus 1 Splint 2 Cast 3 Brace 4 Bandage 5 Packing Material 6 Pressure Dressing 7 Intermittent Pressure Device Y Other Device	Z No Qualifier
1 Face	X External	0 Traction Apparatus 1 Splint 2 Cast 3 Brace 4 Bandage 5 Packing Material 6 Pressure Dressing 7 Intermittent Pressure Device 9 Wire Y Other Device	Z No Qualifier

Section 2 Placement
Body System W Anatomical Regions
Operation 1 Compression: Putting pressure on a body region

Body Region (4ᵗʰ)	Approach (5ᵗʰ)	Device (6ᵗʰ)	Qualifier (7ᵗʰ)
0 Head	X External	6 Pressure Dressing	Z No Qualifier
1 Face		7 Intermittent Pressure Device	
2 Neck			
3 Abdominal Wall			
4 Chest Wall			
5 Back			
6 Inguinal Region, Right			
7 Inguinal Region, Left			
8 Upper Extremity, Right			
9 Upper Extremity, Left			
A Upper Arm, Right			
B Upper Arm, Left			
C Lower Arm, Right			
D Lower Arm, Left			
E Hand, Right			
F Hand, Left			
G Thumb, Right			
H Thumb, Left			
J Finger, Right			
K Finger, Left			
L Lower Extremity, Right			
M Lower Extremity, Left			
N Upper Leg, Right			
P Upper Leg, Left			
Q Lower Leg, Right			
R Lower Leg, Left			
S Foot, Right			
T Foot, Left			
U Toe, Right			
V Toe, Left			

	Section	2	Placement
Body System	W	Anatomical Regions
Operation	2	**Dressing:** Putting material on a body region for protection

Body Region (4th)	Approach (5th)	Device (6th)	Qualifier (7th)
0 Head	X External	4 Bandage	Z No Qualifier
1 Face			
2 Neck			
3 Abdominal Wall			
4 Chest Wall			
5 Back			
6 Inguinal Region, Right			
7 Inguinal Region, Left			
8 Upper Extremity, Right			
9 Upper Extremity, Left			
A Upper Arm, Right			
B Upper Arm, Left			
C Lower Arm, Right			
D Lower Arm, Left			
E Hand, Right			
F Hand, Left			
G Thumb, Right			
H Thumb, Left			
J Finger, Right			
K Finger, Left			
L Lower Extremity, Right			
M Lower Extremity, Left			
N Upper Leg, Right			
P Upper Leg, Left			
Q Lower Leg, Right			
R Lower Leg, Left			
S Foot, Right			
T Foot, Left			
U Toe, Right			
V Toe, Left			

Section   **2**   **Placement**
Body System   **W**   **Anatomical Regions**
Operation   **3**   **Immobilization:** Limiting or preventing motion of a body region

Body Region (4th)	Approach (5th)	Device (6th)	Qualifier (7th)
0 Head	**X** External	**1** Splint	**Z** No Qualifier
2 Neck		**2** Cast	
3 Abdominal Wall		**3** Brace	
4 Chest Wall		**Y** Other Device	
5 Back			
6 Inguinal Region, Right			
7 Inguinal Region, Left			
8 Upper Extremity, Right			
9 Upper Extremity, Left			
A Upper Arm, Right			
B Upper Arm, Left			
C Lower Arm, Right			
D Lower Arm, Left			
E Hand, Right			
F Hand, Left			
G Thumb, Right			
H Thumb, Left			
J Finger, Right			
K Finger, Left			
L Lower Extremity, Right			
M Lower Extremity, Left			
N Upper Leg, Right			
P Upper Leg, Left			
Q Lower Leg, Right			
R Lower Leg, Left			
S Foot, Right			
T Foot, Left			
U Toe, Right			
V Toe, Left			
1 Face	**X** External	**1** Splint	**Z** No Qualifier
		2 Cast	
		3 Brace	
		9 Wire	
		Y Other Device	

Section	2	Placement
Body System	W	Anatomical Regions
Operation	4	Packing: Putting material in a body region or orifice

Body Region (4th)	Approach (5th)	Device (6th)	Qualifier (7th)
0 Head	X External	5 Packing Material	Z No Qualifier
1 Face			
2 Neck			
3 Abdominal Wall			
4 Chest Wall			
5 Back			
6 Inguinal Region, Right			
7 Inguinal Region, Left			
8 Upper Extremity, Right			
9 Upper Extremity, Left			
A Upper Arm, Right			
B Upper Arm, Left			
C Lower Arm, Right			
D Lower Arm, Left			
E Hand, Right			
F Hand, Left			
G Thumb, Right			
H Thumb, Left			
J Finger, Right			
K Finger, Left			
L Lower Extremity, Right			
M Lower Extremity, Left			
N Upper Leg, Right			
P Upper Leg, Left			
Q Lower Leg, Right			
R Lower Leg, Left			
S Foot, Right			
T Foot, Left			
U Toe, Right			
V Toe, Left			

Section	2	Placement
Body System	W	Anatomical Regions
Operation	5	**Removal:** Taking out or off a device from a body part

Body Region (4th)	Approach (5th)	Device (6th)	Qualifier (7th)
0 Head **2** Neck **3** Abdominal Wall **4** Chest Wall **5** Back **6** Inguinal Region, Right **7** Inguinal Region, Left **8** Upper Extremity, Right **9** Upper Extremity, Left **A** Upper Arm, Right **B** Upper Arm, Left **C** Lower Arm, Right **D** Lower Arm, Left **E** Hand, Right **F** Hand, Left **G** Thumb, Right **H** Thumb, Left **J** Finger, Right **K** Finger, Left **L** Lower Extremity, Right **M** Lower Extremity, Left **N** Upper Leg, Right **P** Upper Leg, Left **Q** Lower Leg, Right **R** Lower Leg, Left **S** Foot, Right **T** Foot, Left **U** Toe, Right **V** Toe, Left	**X** External	**0** Traction Apparatus **1** Splint **2** Cast **3** Brace **4** Bandage **5** Packing Material **6** Pressure Dressing **7** Intermittent Pressure Device **Y** Other Device	**Z** No Qualifier
1 Face	**X** External	**0** Traction Apparatus **1** Splint **2** Cast **3** Brace **4** Bandage **5** Packing Material **6** Pressure Dressing **7** Intermittent Pressure Device **9** Wire **Y** Other Device	**Z** No Qualifier

Section	2	Placement
Body System	W	Anatomical Regions
Operation	6	**Traction:** Exerting a pulling force on a body region in a distal direction

Body Region (4th)	Approach (5th)	Device (6th)	Qualifier (7th)
0 Head **1** Face **2** Neck **3** Abdominal Wall **4** Chest Wall **5** Back **6** Inguinal Region, Right **7** Inguinal Region, Left **8** Upper Extremity, Right **9** Upper Extremity, Left **A** Upper Arm, Right **B** Upper Arm, Left **C** Lower Arm, Right **D** Lower Arm, Left **E** Hand, Right **F** Hand, Left **G** Thumb, Right **H** Thumb, Left **J** Finger, Right **K** Finger, Left **L** Lower Extremity, Right **M** Lower Extremity, Left **N** Upper Leg, Right **P** Upper Leg, Left **Q** Lower Leg, Right **R** Lower Leg, Left **S** Foot, Right **T** Foot, Left **U** Toe, Right **V** Toe, Left	**X** External	**0** Traction Apparatus **Z** No Device	**Z** No Qualifier

Section	2	Placement
Body System	Y	Anatomical Orifices
Operation	0	**Change:** Taking out or off a device from a body part and putting back an identical or similar device in or on the same body part without cutting or puncturing the skin or a mucous membrane

Body Region (4th)	Approach (5th)	Device (6th)	Qualifier (7th)
0 Mouth and Pharynx **1** Nasal **2** Ear **3** Anorectal **4** Female Genital Tract **5** Urethra	**X** External	**5** Packing Material	**Z** No Qualifier

Section	2	Placement
Body System	Y	Anatomical Orifices
Operation	4	**Packing:** Putting material in a body region or orifice

Body Region (4th)	Approach (5th)	Device (6th)	Qualifier (7th)
0 Mouth and Pharynx **1** Nasal **2** Ear **3** Anorectal **4** Female Genital Tract **5** Urethra	**X** External	**5** Packing Material	**Z** No Qualifier

Section	2	Placement
Body System	Y	Anatomical Orifices
Operation	5	Removal: Taking out or off a device from a body part

Body Region (4ᵗʰ)	Approach (5ᵗʰ)	Device (6ᵗʰ)	Qualifier (7ᵗʰ)
0 Mouth and Pharynx **1** Nasal **2** Ear **3** Anorectal **4** Female Genital Tract **5** Urethra	**X** External	**5** Packing Material	**Z** No Qualifier

Within each section of ICD-10-PCS, the characters have different meanings. The seven character meanings for the Administration section are illustrated here through the procedure example of *Nerve block injection to median nerve*.

Section	Body System	Root Operation	Body System/ Region	Approach	Substance	Qualifier
Administration	Physiological System and Anatomical Region	Introduction	Peripheral Nerves and Plexi	Percutaneous	Regional Anesthetic	None
3	E	0	T	3	C	Z

Section (Character 1)

All Administration procedure codes have a first character value of 3.

Body System (Character 2)

The alphanumeric character for the body system is placed in the second position. There are three character values applicable for the Administration section.

Character Value	Character Value Description
0	Circulatory
C	Indwelling Device
E	Physiological System and Anatomical Region

Root Operations (Character 3)

The alphanumeric character value for root operations is placed in the third position. Listed here are the root operations applicable to the Administration section with their associated meaning.

Character Value	Root Operation	Root Operation Definition
0	Introduction	Putting in or on a therapeutic, diagnostic, nutritional, physiological, or prophylactic substance except blood or blood products
1	Irrigation	Putting in or on a cleansing substance
2	Transfusion	Putting in blood or blood products

Body System/Region (Character 4)

For each body system the applicable body part character values will be available for procedure code construction. An example of a body region is upper GI.

Approach (Character 5)

The approach is the technique used to reach the procedure site. Listed here are the approach character values for the Administration with the associated definitions.

Character Value	Approach	Approach Definition
0	Open	Cutting through the skin or mucous membrane and any other body layers necessary to expose the site of the procedure
3	Percutaneous	Entry, by puncture or minor incision, of instrumentation through the skin or mucous membrane and any other body layers necessary to reach the site of the procedure
4	Percutaneous Endoscopic	Entry, by puncture or minor incision, of instrumentation through the skin or mucous membrane and any other body layers necessary to reach and visualize the site of the procedure
7	Via Natural or Artificial Opening	Entry of instrumentation through a natural or artificial external opening to reach the site of the procedure
8	Via Natural or Artificial Opening Endoscopic	Entry of instrumentation through a natural or artificial external opening to reach and visualize the site of the procedure
X	External	Procedures performed directly on the skin or mucous membrane and procedures performed indirectly by the application of external force through the skin or mucous membrane

Substance (Character 6)

In the Administration section a substance is always utilized. The substance is reported in the sixth character position by the type of substance utilized. The following is a sample list of the substances included in this section:

- Anti-inflammatory
- Antineoplastic
- Bone marrow
- Platelet inhibitor
- Whole blood

Qualifier (Character 7)

The qualifier represents an additional attribute for the procedure when applicable. There are several qualifiers included in the Administration section. For example, transfusion procedures in this section include qualifiers including Autologous and Nonautologous that are reported with the character values of 0 and 1, respectively. If there is no qualifier for a procedure, the placeholder Z is the character value that should be reported.

If a coder is unsure of which option to select for the substance qualifier utilized during the procedure, Appendix F can be used to guide the selection. It is important to note that not all substance qualifier categories are provided by CMS in Appendix F. However, for example, the coding scenario indicates that Clolar was introduced percutaneously via the peripheral vein. The coder references Table 3E0 (Introduction in Physiological Systems and Anatomical Regions) under the peripheral vein, percutaneous approach, antineoplastic. Clolar is not a substance qualifier choice. However, the coder can then locate the substance qualifier categories in Appendix F. The category Clofarabine includes Clolar. Therefore, the coder should select P - Clofarabine for the 7th character.

IPPS New Services and Technology Add-On Payment

SPRAVATO (Esketamine)   Maximum reimbursement $1,041.79

3E097GC Introduction of Other Therapeutic Substance into Nose, Via Natural or Artificial Opening

Important Definitions for the Administration Section

Administration Root Operation	Qualifier	Definition
Transfusion (302)	0 - Autologous	Derived or transferred from the same individual's body*
	1 - Nonautologous	Derived or transferred from another individual's body

*Taken from The Free Dictionary by Farlex at www.thefreedictionary.com

Section Notes

Before reporting Transfusion procedures for embryonic stem cells (6th character A), bone marrow (6th character G), cord blood stem cells (6th character X) or hematopoietic stem cells (6th character Y) users should *Review coding guideline B3.16.*

Before reporting Administration codes for all Biliary and Pancreatic Tract (4th character value of J) procedures with a 6th character value of U (Pancreatic Islet Cells), users should *Review coding guideline B3.16.*

Before reporting Irrigation procedures in this section, users should *Review coding guideline B6.1c.*

Medicare Non-Covered Administration Codes

Non-Covered with pdx or sdx C91.00, C92.00, C92.10, C92.11, C92.40, C92.50, C92.60, C92.A0, C93.00, C94.00 or C95.00

30230AZ	30233AZ	30240AZ	30243AZ			
30230G0	30233G0	30240G0	30243G0			
30230Y0	30233Y0	30240Y0	30243Y0			

AHA Coding Clinic

3E013GC Introduction of Other Therapeutic Substance into Subcutaneous Tissue, Percutaneous Approach - AHA CC: 2Q, 2014, 10

3E0234Z Introduction of Serum, Toxoid and Vaccine into Muscle, Percutaneous Approach - AHA CC: 4Q, 2014, 16

3E03317 Introduction of Other Thrombolytic into Peripheral Vein, Percutaneous Approach - AHA CC: 4Q, 2013, 124; 4Q, 2020, 49-50

3E033VJ Introduction of Other Hormone into Peripheral Vein, Percutaneous Approach - AHA CC: 4Q, 2014, 17-18

3E04317 Introduction of Other Thrombolytic into Central Vein, Percutaneous Approach - AHA CC: 4Q, 2020, 49-50

3E05305 Introduction of Other Antineoplastic into Peripheral Artery, Percutaneous Approach - AHA CC: 1Q, 2015, 38

3E05317 Introduction of Other Thrombolytic into Peripheral Artery, Percutaneous Approach - AHA CC: 4Q, 2020, 49-50

3E06305 Introduction of Other Antineoplastic into Central Artery, Percutaneous Approach - AHA CC: 3Q, 2014 26-27

3E06317 Introduction of Other Thrombolytic into Central Artery, Percutaneous Approach - AHA CC: 4Q, 2014, 19-20; 4Q, 2020, 49-50

3E073GC Introduction of Other Therapeutic Substance into Coronary Artery, Percutaneous Approach - AHA CC: 3Q, 2018. 7-8

3E0G76Z Introduction of Nutritional Substance into Upper GI, Via Natural or Artificial Opening - AHA CC: 2Q, 2015, 29

3E0G8GC Introduction of Other Therapeutic Substance into Upper GI, via Natural or Artificial Opening Endoscopic - AHA CC: 3Q, 2015, 24-25

3E0G8TZ Introduction of Destructive Agent into Upper GI, Via Natural or Artificial Opening Endoscopic - AHA CC: 1Q, 2013, 27

Administration Section Tables

Administration Tables 302–3E1

Section	3	Administration
Body System	0	Circulatory
Operation	2	**Transfusion:** Putting in blood or blood products

Body System / Region (4th)	Approach (5th)	Substance (6th)	Qualifier (7th)
3 Peripheral Vein 4 Central Vein	3 Percutaneous	A Stem Cells, Embryonic	Z No Qualifier
3 Peripheral Vein 4 Central Vein	3 Percutaneous	C Hematopoietic Stem/Progenitor Cells, Genetically Modified	0 Autologous
3 Peripheral Vein 4 Central Vein	3 Percutaneous	D Pathogen Reduced Cryoprecipitated Fibrinogen Complex	1 Nonautologous
3 Peripheral Vein 4 Central Vein	3 Percutaneous	G Bone Marrow X Stem Cells, Cord Blood Y Stem Cells, Hematopoietic	0 Autologous 2 Allogeneic, Related 3 Allogeneic, Unrelated 4 Allogeneic, Unspecified
3 Peripheral Vein 4 Central Vein	3 Percutaneous	H Whole Blood J Serum Albumin K Frozen Plasma L Fresh Plasma M Plasma Cryoprecipitate N Red Blood Cells P Frozen Red Cells Q White Cells R Platelets S Globulin T Fibrinogen V Antihemophilic Factors W Factor IX	0 Autologous 1 Nonautologous
3 Peripheral Vein 4 Central Vein	3 Percutaneous	U Stem Cells, T-cell Depleted Hematopoietic	2 Allogeneic, Related 3 Allogeneic, Unrelated 4 Allogeneic, Unspecified
7 Products of Conception, Circulatory	3 Percutaneous 7 Via Natural or Artificial Opening	H Whole Blood J Serum Albumin K Frozen Plasma L Fresh Plasma M Plasma Cryoprecipitate N Red Blood Cells P Frozen Red Cells Q White Cells R Platelets S Globulin T Fibrinogen V Antihemophilic Factors W Factor IX	1 Nonautologous
8 Vein	3 Percutaneous	B 4-Factor Prothrombin Complex Concentrate	1 Nonautologous

Section 3 **Administration**
Body System C **Indwelling Device**
Operation 1 **Irrigation:** Putting in or on a cleansing substance

Body System / Region (4th)	Approach (5th)	Substance (6th)	Qualifier (7th)
Z None	**X** External	**8** Irrigating Substance	**Z** No Qualifier

Section 3 **Administration**
Body System E **Physiological Systems and Anatomical Regions**
Operation 0 **Introduction:** Putting in or on a therapeutic, diagnostic, nutritional, physiological, or prophylactic substance except blood or blood products

Body System / Region (4th)	Approach (5th)	Substance (6th)	Qualifier (7th)
0 Skin and Mucous Membranes	**X** External	**0** Antineoplastic	**5** Other Antineoplastic **M** Monoclonal Antibody
0 Skin and Mucous Membranes	**X** External	**2** Anti-infective	**8** Oxazolidinones **9** Other Anti-infective
0 Skin and Mucous Membranes	**X** External	**3** Anti-inflammatory **B** Anesthetic Agent **K** Other Diagnostic Substance **M** Pigment **N** Analgesics, Hypnotics, Sedatives **T** Destructive Agent	**Z** No Qualifier
0 Skin and Mucous Membranes	**X** External	**G** Other Therapeutic Substance	**C** Other Substance
1 Subcutaneous Tissue	**0** Open	**2** Anti-infective	**A** Anti-Infective Envelope
1 Subcutaneous Tissue	**3** Percutaneous	**0** Antineoplastic	**5** Other Antineoplastic **M** Monoclonal Antibody
1 Subcutaneous Tissue	**3** Percutaneous	**2** Anti-infective	**8** Oxazolidinones **9** Other Anti-infective **A** Anti-Infective Envelope
1 Subcutaneous Tissue	**3** Percutaneous	**3** Anti-inflammatory **6** Nutritional Substance **7** Electrolytic and Water Balance Substance **B** Anesthetic Agent **H** Radioactive Substance **K** Other Diagnostic Substance **N** Analgesics, Hypnotics, Sedatives **T** Destructive Agent	**Z** No Qualifier
1 Subcutaneous Tissue	**3** Percutaneous	**4** Serum, Toxoid and Vaccine	**0** Influenza Vaccine **Z** No Qualifier
1 Subcutaneous Tissue	**3** Percutaneous	**G** Other Therapeutic Substance	**C** Other Substance
1 Subcutaneous Tissue	**3** Percutaneous	**V** Hormone	**G** Insulin **J** Other Hormone
2 Muscle	**3** Percutaneous	**0** Antineoplastic	**5** Other Antineoplastic **M** Monoclonal Antibody
2 Muscle	**3** Percutaneous	**2** Anti-infective	**8** Oxazolidinones **9** Other Anti-infective

Continued →

3E0

Section   3   **Administration**
Body System   E   **Physiological Systems and Anatomical Regions**
Operation   0   **Introduction:** Putting in or on a therapeutic, diagnostic, nutritional, physiological, or prophylactic substance except blood or blood products

3E0 Continued

Body System / Region (4th)	Approach (5th)	Substance (6th)	Qualifier (7th)
2 Muscle	3 Percutaneous	3 Anti-inflammatory 6 Nutritional Substance 7 Electrolytic and Water Balance Substance B Anesthetic Agent H Radioactive Substance K Other Diagnostic Substance N Analgesics, Hypnotics, Sedatives T Destructive Agent	Z No Qualifier
2 Muscle	3 Percutaneous	4 Serum, Toxoid and Vaccine	0 Influenza Vaccine Z No Qualifier
2 Muscle	3 Percutaneous	G Other Therapeutic Substance	C Other Substance
3 Peripheral Vein	0 Open	0 Antineoplastic	2 High-dose Interleukin-2 3 Low-dose Interleukin-2 5 Other Antineoplastic M Monoclonal Antibody P Clofarabine
3 Peripheral Vein	0 Open	1 Thrombolytic	6 Recombinant Human-activated Protein C 7 Other Thrombolytic
3 Peripheral Vein	0 Open	2 Anti-infective	8 Oxazolidinones 9 Other Anti-infective
3 Peripheral Vein	0 Open	3 Anti-inflammatory 4 Serum, Toxoid and Vaccine 6 Nutritional Substance 7 Electrolytic and Water Balance Substance F Intracirculatory Anesthetic H Radioactive Substance K Other Diagnostic Substance N Analgesics, Hypnotics, Sedatives P Platelet Inhibitor R Antiarrhythmic T Destructive Agent X Vasopressor	Z No Qualifier
3 Peripheral Vein	0 Open	G Other Therapeutic Substance	C Other Substance N Blood Brain Barrier Disruption
3 Peripheral Vein	0 Open	U Pancreatic Islet Cells	0 Autologous 1 Nonautologous
3 Peripheral Vein	0 Open	V Hormone	G Insulin H Human B-type Natriuretic Peptide J Other Hormone
3 Peripheral Vein	0 Open	W Immunotherapeutic	K Immunostimulator L Immunosuppressive
3 Peripheral Vein	3 Percutaneous	0 Antineoplastic	2 High-dose Interleukin-2 3 Low-dose Interleukin-2 5 Other Antineoplastic M Monoclonal Antibody P Clofarabine
3 Peripheral Vein	3 Percutaneous	1 Thrombolytic	6 Recombinant Human-activated Protein C 7 Other Thrombolytic

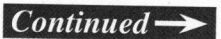

Continued →

Section	3	Administration
Body System	E	Physiological Systems and Anatomical Regions
Operation	0	Introduction: Putting in or on a therapeutic, diagnostic, nutritional, physiological, or prophylactic substance except blood or blood products

Body System / Region (4th)	Approach (5th)	Substance (6th)	Qualifier (7th)
3 Peripheral Vein	3 Percutaneous	2 Anti-infective	8 Oxazolidinones 9 Other Anti-infective
3 Peripheral Vein	3 Percutaneous	3 Anti-inflammatory 4 Serum, Toxoid and Vaccine 6 Nutritional Substance 7 Electrolytic and Water Balance Substance F Intracirculatory Anesthetic H Radioactive Substance K Other Diagnostic Substance N Analgesics, Hypnotics, Sedatives P Platelet Inhibitor R Antiarrhythmic T Destructive Agent X Vasopressor	Z No Qualifier
3 Peripheral Vein	3 Percutaneous	G Other Therapeutic Substance	C Other Substance N Blood Brain Barrier Disruption Q Glucarpidase
3 Peripheral Vein	3 Percutaneous	U Pancreatic Islet Cells	0 Autologous 1 Nonautologous
3 Peripheral Vein	3 Percutaneous	V Hormone	G Insulin H Human B-type Natriuretic Peptide J Other Hormone
3 Peripheral Vein	3 Percutaneous	W Immunotherapeutic	K Immunostimulator L Immunosuppressive
4 Central Vein	0 Open	0 Antineoplastic	2 High-dose Interleukin-2 3 Low-dose Interleukin-2 5 Other Antineoplastic M Monoclonal Antibody P Clofarabine
4 Central Vein	0 Open	1 Thrombolytic	6 Recombinant Human-activated Protein C 7 Other Thrombolytic
4 Central Vein	0 Open	2 Anti-infective	8 Oxazolidinones 9 Other Anti-infective
4 Central Vein	0 Open	3 Anti-inflammatory 4 Serum, Toxoid and Vaccine 6 Nutritional Substance 7 Electrolytic and Water Balance Substance F Intracirculatory Anesthetic H Radioactive Substance K Other Diagnostic Substance N Analgesics, Hypnotics, Sedatives P Platelet Inhibitor R Antiarrhythmic T Destructive Agent X Vasopressor	Z No Qualifier
4 Central Vein	0 Open	G Other Therapeutic Substance	C Other Substance N Blood Brain Barrier Disruption

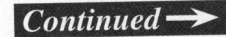
Continued →

Section	3	**Administration**
Body System	E	**Physiological Systems and Anatomical Regions**
Operation	0	**Introduction:** Putting in or on a therapeutic, diagnostic, nutritional, physiological, or prophylactic substance except blood or blood products

Body System / Region (4th)	Approach (5th)	Substance (6th)	Qualifier (7th)
4 Central Vein	0 Open	V Hormone	G Insulin H Human B-type Natriuretic Peptide J Other Hormone
4 Central Vein	0 Open	W Immunotherapeutic	K Immunostimulator L Immunosuppressive
4 Central Vein	3 Percutaneous	0 Antineoplastic	2 High-dose Interleukin-2 3 Low-dose Interleukin-2 5 Other Antineoplastic M Monoclonal Antibody P Clofarabine
4 Central Vein	3 Percutaneous	1 Thrombolytic	6 Recombinant Human-activated Protein C 7 Other Thrombolytic
4 Central Vein	3 Percutaneous	2 Anti-infective	8 Oxazolidinones 9 Other Anti-infective
4 Central Vein	3 Percutaneous	3 Anti-inflammatory 4 Serum, Toxoid and Vaccine 6 Nutritional Substance 7 Electrolytic and Water Balance Substance F Intracirculatory Anesthetic H Radioactive Substance K Other Diagnostic Substance N Analgesics, Hypnotics, Sedatives P Platelet Inhibitor R Antiarrhythmic T Destructive Agent X Vasopressor	Z No Qualifier
4 Central Vein	3 Percutaneous	G Other Therapeutic Substance	C Other Substance N Blood Brain Barrier Disruption Q Glucarpidase
4 Central Vein	3 Percutaneous	V Hormone	G Insulin H Human B-type Natriuretic Peptide J Other Hormone
4 Central Vein	3 Percutaneous	W Immunotherapeutic	K Immunostimulator L Immunosuppressive
5 Peripheral Artery 6 Central Artery	0 Open 3 Percutaneous	0 Antineoplastic	2 High-dose Interleukin-2 3 Low-dose Interleukin-2 5 Other Antineoplastic M Monoclonal Antibody P Clofarabine
5 Peripheral Artery 6 Central Artery	0 Open 3 Percutaneous	1 Thrombolytic	6 Recombinant Human-activated Protein C 7 Other Thrombolytic

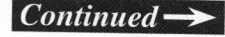

Continued →

Section	3	Administration
Body System	E	Physiological Systems and Anatomical Regions
Operation	0	Introduction: Putting in or on a therapeutic, diagnostic, nutritional, physiological, or prophylactic substance except blood or blood products

Body System / Region (4th)	Approach (5th)	Substance (6th)	Qualifier (7th)
5 Peripheral Artery 6 Central Artery	0 Open 3 Percutaneous	2 Anti-infective	8 Oxazolidinones 9 Other Anti-infective
5 Peripheral Artery 6 Central Artery	0 Open 3 Percutaneous	3 Anti-inflammatory 4 Serum, Toxoid and Vaccine 6 Nutritional Substance 7 Electrolytic and Water Balance Substance F Intracirculatory Anesthetic H Radioactive Substance K Other Diagnostic Substance N Analgesics, Hypnotics, Sedatives P Platelet Inhibitor R Antiarrhythmic T Destructive Agent X Vasopressor	Z No Qualifier
5 Peripheral Artery 6 Central Artery	0 Open 3 Percutaneous	G Other Therapeutic Substance	C Other Substance N Blood Brain Barrier Disruption
5 Peripheral Artery 6 Central Artery	0 Open 3 Percutaneous	V Hormone	G Insulin H Human B-type Natriuretic Peptide J Other Hormone
5 Peripheral Artery 6 Central Artery	0 Open 3 Percutaneous	W Immunotherapeutic	K Immunostimulator L Immunosuppressive
7 Coronary Artery 8 Heart	0 Open 3 Percutaneous	1 Thrombolytic	6 Recombinant Human-activated Protein C 7 Other Thrombolytic
7 Coronary Artery 8 Heart	0 Open 3 Percutaneous	G Other Therapeutic Substance	C Other Substance
7 Coronary Artery 8 Heart	0 Open 3 Percutaneous	K Other Diagnostic Substance P Platelet Inhibitor	Z No Qualifier
7 Coronary Artery 8 Heart	4 Percutaneous Endoscopic	G Other Therapeutic Substance	C Other Substance
9 Nose	3 Percutaneous 7 Via Natural or Artificial Opening X External	0 Antineoplastic	5 Other Antineoplastic M Monoclonal Antibody
9 Nose	3 Percutaneous 7 Via Natural or Artificial Opening X External	2 Anti-infective	8 Oxazolidinones 9 Other Anti-infective
9 Nose	3 Percutaneous 7 Via Natural or Artificial Opening X External	3 Anti-inflammatory 4 Serum, Toxoid and Vaccine B Anesthetic Agent H Radioactive Substance K Other Diagnostic Substance N Analgesics, Hypnotics, Sedatives T Destructive Agent	Z No Qualifier

Continued →

Section	3	Administration
Body System	E	Physiological Systems and Anatomical Regions
Operation	0	Introduction: Putting in or on a therapeutic, diagnostic, nutritional, physiological, or prophylactic substance except blood or blood products

Body System / Region (4ᵗʰ)	Approach (5ᵗʰ)	Substance (6ᵗʰ)	Qualifier (7ᵗʰ)
9 Nose	3 Percutaneous 7 Via Natural or Artificial Opening X External	G Other Therapeutic Substance	C Other Substance
A Bone Marrow	3 Percutaneous	0 Antineoplastic	5 Other Antineoplastic M Monoclonal Antibody
A Bone Marrow	3 Percutaneous	G Other Therapeutic Substance	C Other Substance
B Ear	3 Percutaneous 7 Via Natural or Artificial Opening X External	0 Antineoplastic	4 Liquid Brachytherapy Radioisotope 5 Other Antineoplastic M Monoclonal Antibody
B Ear	3 Percutaneous 7 Via Natural or Artificial Opening X External	2 Anti-infective	8 Oxazolidinones 9 Other Anti-infective
B Ear	3 Percutaneous 7 Via Natural or Artificial Opening X External	3 Anti-inflammatory B Anesthetic Agent H Radioactive Substance K Other Diagnostic Substance N Analgesics, Hypnotics, Sedatives T Destructive Agent	Z No Qualifier
B Ear	3 Percutaneous 7 Via Natural or Artificial Opening X External	G Other Therapeutic Substance	C Other Substance
C Eye	3 Percutaneous 7 Via Natural or Artificial Opening X External	0 Antineoplastic	4 Liquid Brachytherapy Radioisotope 5 Other Antineoplastic M Monoclonal Antibody
C Eye	3 Percutaneous 7 Via Natural or Artificial Opening X External	2 Anti-infective	8 Oxazolidinones 9 Other Anti-infective
C Eye	3 Percutaneous 7 Via Natural or Artificial Opening X External	3 Anti-inflammatory B Anesthetic Agent H Radioactive Substance K Other Diagnostic Substance M Pigment N Analgesics, Hypnotics, Sedatives T Destructive Agent	Z No Qualifier
C Eye	3 Percutaneous 7 Via Natural or Artificial Opening X External	G Other Therapeutic Substance	C Other Substance
C Eye	3 Percutaneous 7 Via Natural or Artificial Opening X External	S Gas	F Other Gas

Continued →

Section	3	Administration
Body System	E	Physiological Systems and Anatomical Regions
Operation	0	Introduction: Putting in or on a therapeutic, diagnostic, nutritional, physiological, or prophylactic substance except blood or blood products

Body System / Region (4th)	Approach (5th)	Substance (6th)	Qualifier (7th)
D Mouth and Pharynx	**3** Percutaneous **7** Via Natural or Artificial Opening **X** External	**0** Antineoplastic	**4** Liquid Brachytherapy Radioisotope **5** Other Antineoplastic **M** Monoclonal Antibody
D Mouth and Pharynx	**3** Percutaneous **7** Via Natural or Artificial Opening **X** External	**2** Anti-infective	**8** Oxazolidinones **9** Other Anti-infective
D Mouth and Pharynx	**3** Percutaneous **7** Via Natural or Artificial Opening **X** External	**3** Anti-inflammatory **4** Serum, Toxoid and Vaccine **6** Nutritional Substance **7** Electrolytic and Water Balance Substance **B** Anesthetic Agent **H** Radioactive Substance **K** Other Diagnostic Substance **N** Analgesics, Hypnotics, Sedatives **R** Antiarrhythmic **T** Destructive Agent	**Z** No Qualifier
D Mouth and Pharynx	**3** Percutaneous **7** Via Natural or Artificial Opening **X** External	**G** Other Therapeutic Substance	**C** Other Substance
E Products of Conception **G** Upper GI **H** Lower GI **K** Genitourinary Tract **N** Male Reproductive	**3** Percutaneous **7** Via Natural or Artificial Opening **8** Via Natural or Artificial Opening Endoscopic	**0** Antineoplastic	**4** Liquid Brachytherapy Radioisotope **5** Other Antineoplastic **M** Monoclonal Antibody
E Products of Conception **G** Upper GI **H** Lower GI **K** Genitourinary Tract **N** Male Reproductive	**3** Percutaneous **7** Via Natural or Artificial Opening **8** Via Natural or Artificial Opening Endoscopic	**2** Anti-infective	**8** Oxazolidinones **9** Other Anti-infective
E Products of Conception **G** Upper GI **H** Lower GI **K** Genitourinary Tract **N** Male Reproductive	**3** Percutaneous **7** Via Natural or Artificial Opening **8** Via Natural or Artificial Opening Endoscopic	**3** Anti-inflammatory **6** Nutritional Substance **7** Electrolytic and Water Balance Substance **B** Anesthetic Agent **H** Radioactive Substance **K** Other Diagnostic Substance **N** Analgesics, Hypnotics, Sedatives **T** Destructive Agent	**Z** No Qualifier
E Products of Conception **G** Upper GI **H** Lower GI **K** Genitourinary Tract **N** Male Reproductive	**3** Percutaneous **7** Via Natural or Artificial Opening **8** Via Natural or Artificial Opening Endoscopic	**G** Other Therapeutic Substance	**C** Other Substance
E Products of Conception **G** Upper GI **H** Lower GI **K** Genitourinary Tract **N** Male Reproductive	**3** Percutaneous **7** Via Natural or Artificial Opening **8** Via Natural or Artificial Opening Endoscopic	**S** Gas	**F** Other Gas

Continued →

3E0

Section	3	Administration
Body System	E	Physiological Systems and Anatomical Regions
Operation	0	Introduction: Putting in or on a therapeutic, diagnostic, nutritional, physiological, or prophylactic substance except blood or blood products

3E0 Continued

Body System / Region (4th)	Approach (5th)	Substance (6th)	Qualifier (7th)
E Products of Conception **G** Upper GI **H** Lower GI **K** Genitourinary Tract **N** Male Reproductive	**4** Percutaneous Endoscopic	**G** Other Therapeutic Substance	**C** Other Substance
F Respiratory Tract	**3** Percutaneous **7** Via Natural or Artificial Opening **8** Via Natural or Artificial Opening Endoscopic	**0** Antineoplastic	**4** Liquid Brachytherapy Radioisotope **5** Other Antineoplastic **M** Monoclonal Antibody
F Respiratory Tract	**3** Percutaneous **7** Via Natural or Artificial Opening **8** Via Natural or Artificial Opening Endoscopic	**2** Anti-infective	**8** Oxazolidinones **9** Other Anti-infective
F Respiratory Tract	**3** Percutaneous **7** Via Natural or Artificial Opening **8** Via Natural or Artificial Opening Endoscopic	**3** Anti-inflammatory **6** Nutritional Substance **7** Electrolytic and Water Balance Substance **B** Anesthetic Agent **H** Radioactive Substance **K** Other Diagnostic Substance **N** Analgesics, Hypnotics, Sedatives **T** Destructive Agent	**Z** No Qualifier
F Respiratory Tract	**3** Percutaneous **7** Via Natural or Artificial Opening **8** Via Natural or Artificial Opening Endoscopic	**G** Other Therapeutic Substance	**C** Other Substance
F Respiratory Tract	**3** Percutaneous **7** Via Natural or Artificial Opening **8** Via Natural or Artificial Opening Endoscopic	**S** Gas	**D** Nitric Oxide **F** Other Gas
F Respiratory Tract	**4** Percutaneous Endoscopic	**G** Other Therapeutic Substance	**C** Other Substance
J Biliary and Pancreatic Tract	**3** Percutaneous **7** Via Natural or Artificial Opening **8** Via Natural or Artificial Opening Endoscopic	**0** Antineoplastic	**4** Liquid Brachytherapy Radioisotope **5** Other Antineoplastic **M** Monoclonal Antibody
J Biliary and Pancreatic Tract	**3** Percutaneous **7** Via Natural or Artificial Opening **8** Via Natural or Artificial Opening Endoscopic	**2** Anti-infective	**8** Oxazolidinones **9** Other Anti-infective

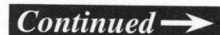

Continued →

Section 3 Administration
Body System E Physiological Systems and Anatomical Regions
Operation 0 Introduction: Putting in or on a therapeutic, diagnostic, nutritional, physiological, or prophylactic substance except blood or blood products

Body System / Region (4th)	Approach (5th)	Substance (6th)	Qualifier (7th)
J Biliary and Pancreatic Tract	3 Percutaneous 7 Via Natural or Artificial Opening 8 Via Natural or Artificial Opening Endoscopic	3 Anti-inflammatory 6 Nutritional Substance 7 Electrolytic and Water Balance Substance B Anesthetic Agent H Radioactive Substance K Other Diagnostic Substance N Analgesics, Hypnotics, Sedatives T Destructive Agent	Z No Qualifier
J Biliary and Pancreatic Tract	3 Percutaneous 7 Via Natural or Artificial Opening 8 Via Natural or Artificial Opening Endoscopic	G Other Therapeutic Substance	C Other Substance
J Biliary and Pancreatic Tract	3 Percutaneous 7 Via Natural or Artificial Opening 8 Via Natural or Artificial Opening Endoscopic	S Gas	F Other Gas
J Biliary and Pancreatic Tract	3 Percutaneous 7 Via Natural or Artificial Opening 8 Via Natural or Artificial Opening Endoscopic	U Pancreatic Islet Cells	0 Autologous 1 Nonautologous
J Biliary and Pancreatic Tract	4 Percutaneous Endoscopic	G Other Therapeutic Substance	C Other Substance
L Pleural Cavity	0 Open	5 Adhesion Barrier	Z No Qualifier
L Pleural Cavity	3 Percutaneous	0 Antineoplastic	4 Liquid Brachytherapy Radioisotope 5 Other Antineoplastic M Monoclonal Antibody
L Pleural Cavity	3 Percutaneous	2 Anti-infective	8 Oxazolidinones 9 Other Anti-infective
L Pleural Cavity	3 Percutaneous	3 Anti-inflammatory 5 Adhesion Barrier 6 Nutritional Substance 7 Electrolytic and Water Balance Substance B Anesthetic Agent H Radioactive Substance K Other Diagnostic Substance N Analgesics, Hypnotics, Sedatives T Destructive Agent	Z No Qualifier
L Pleural Cavity	3 Percutaneous	G Other Therapeutic Substance	C Other Substance
L Pleural Cavity	3 Percutaneous	S Gas	F Other Gas
L Pleural Cavity	4 Percutaneous Endoscopic	5 Adhesion Barrier	Z No Qualifier

Continued →

3E0

Section	3	Administration
Body System	E	**Physiological Systems and Anatomical Regions**
Operation	0	**Introduction:** Putting in or on a therapeutic, diagnostic, nutritional, physiological, or prophylactic substance except blood or blood products

3E0 Continued

Body System / Region (4ᵗʰ)	Approach (5ᵗʰ)	Substance (6ᵗʰ)	Qualifier (7ᵗʰ)
L Pleural Cavity	**4** Percutaneous Endoscopic	**G** Other Therapeutic Substance	**C** Other Substance
L Pleural Cavity	**7** Via Natural or Artificial Opening	**0** Antineoplastic	**4** Liquid Brachytherapy Radioisotope **5** Other Antineoplastic **M** Monoclonal Antibody
L Pleural Cavity	**7** Via Natural or Artificial Opening	**S** Gas	**F** Other Gas
M Peritoneal Cavity	**0** Open	**5** Adhesion Barrier	**Z** No Qualifier
M Peritoneal Cavity	**3** Percutaneous	**0** Antineoplastic	**4** Liquid Brachytherapy Radioisotope **5** Other Antineoplastic **M** Monoclonal Antibody **Y** Hyperthermic
M Peritoneal Cavity	**3** Percutaneous	**2** Anti-infective	**8** Oxazolidinones **9** Other Anti-infective
M Peritoneal Cavity	**3** Percutaneous	**3** Anti-inflammatory **5** Adhesion Barrier **6** Nutritional Substance **7** Electrolytic and Water Balance Substance **B** Anesthetic Agent **H** Radioactive Substance **K** Other Diagnostic Substance **N** Analgesics, Hypnotics, Sedatives **T** Destructive Agent	**Z** No Qualifier
M Peritoneal Cavity	**3** Percutaneous	**G** Other Therapeutic Substance	**C** Other Substance
M Peritoneal Cavity	**3** Percutaneous	**S** Gas	**F** Other Gas
M Peritoneal Cavity	**4** Percutaneous Endoscopic	**5** Adhesion Barrier	**Z** No Qualifier
M Peritoneal Cavity	**4** Percutaneous Endoscopic	**G** Other Therapeutic Substance	**C** Other Substance
M Peritoneal Cavity	**7** Via Natural or Artificial Opening	**0** Antineoplastic	**4** Liquid Brachytherapy Radioisotope **5** Other Antineoplastic **M** Monoclonal Antibody
M Peritoneal Cavity	**7** Via Natural or Artificial Opening	**S** Gas	**F** Other Gas
P Female Reproductive	**0** Open	**5** Adhesion Barrier	**Z** No Qualifier
P Female Reproductive	**3** Percutaneous	**0** Antineoplastic	**4** Liquid Brachytherapy Radioisotope **5** Other Antineoplastic **M** Monoclonal Antibody
P Female Reproductive	**3** Percutaneous	**2** Anti-infective	**8** Oxazolidinones **9** Other Anti-infective

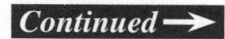
Continued →

Section 3 Administration
Body System E Physiological Systems and Anatomical Regions
Operation 0 Introduction: Putting in or on a therapeutic, diagnostic, nutritional, physiological, or prophylactic substance except blood or blood products

3E0 Continued

3E0

Body System / Region (4th)	Approach (5th)	Substance (6th)	Qualifier (7th)
P Female Reproductive	3 Percutaneous	3 Anti-inflammatory 5 Adhesion Barrier 6 Nutritional Substance 7 Electrolytic and Water Balance Substance B Anesthetic Agent H Radioactive Substance K Other Diagnostic Substance L Sperm N Analgesics, Hypnotics, Sedatives T Destructive Agent V Hormone	Z No Qualifier
P Female Reproductive	3 Percutaneous	G Other Therapeutic Substance	C Other Substance
P Female Reproductive	3 Percutaneous	Q Fertilized Ovum	0 Autologous 1 Nonautologous
P Female Reproductive	3 Percutaneous	S Gas	F Other Gas
P Female Reproductive	4 Percutaneous Endoscopic	5 Adhesion Barrier	Z No Qualifier
P Female Reproductive	4 Percutaneous Endoscopic	G Other Therapeutic Substance	C Other Substance
P Female Reproductive	7 Via Natural or Artificial Opening	0 Antineoplastic	4 Liquid Brachytherapy Radioisotope 5 Other Antineoplastic M Monoclonal Antibody
P Female Reproductive	7 Via Natural or Artificial Opening	2 Anti-infective	8 Oxazolidinones 9 Other Anti-infective
P Female Reproductive	7 Via Natural or Artificial Opening	5 Adhesion Barrier 6 Nutritional Substance 7 Electrolytic and Water Balance Substance B Anesthetic Agent H Radioactive Substance K Other Diagnostic Substance L Sperm N Analgestics, Hypnotics, Sedatives T Destructive Agent V Hormone	Z No Qualifier
P Female Reproductive	7 Via Natural or Artificial Opening	G Other Therapeutic Substance	C Other Substance
P Female Reproductive	7 Via Natural or Artificial Opening	Q Fertilized Ovum	0 Autologous 1 Nonautologous
P Female Reproductive	7 Via Natural or Artificial Opening	S Gas	F Other Gas
P Female Reproductive	8 Via Natural or Artificial Opening Endoscopic	0 Antineoplastic	4 Liquid Brachytherapy Radioisotope 5 Other Antineoplastic M Monoclonal Antibody
P Female Reproductive	8 Via Natural or Artificial Opening Endoscopic	2 Anti-infective	8 Oxazolidinones 9 Other Anti-infective

Continued →

3E0

Section 3 Administration
Body System E Physiological Systems and Anatomical Regions
Operation 0 Introduction: Putting in or on a therapeutic, diagnostic, nutritional, physiological,
or prophylactic substance except blood or blood products

3E0 Continued

Body System / Region (4th)	Approach (5th)	Substance (6th)	Qualifier (7th)
P Female Reproductive	8 Via Natural or Artificial Opening Endoscopic	3 Anti-inflammatory 6 Nutritional Substance 7 Electrolytic and Water Balance Substance B Anesthetic Agent H Radioactive Substance K Other Diagnostic Substance N Analgesics, Hypnotics, Sedatives T Destructive Agent	Z No Qualifier
P Female Reproductive	8 Via Natural or Artificial Opening Endoscopic	G Other Therapeutic Substance	C Other Substance
P Female Reproductive	8 Via Natural or Artificial Opening Endoscopic	S Gas	F Other Gas
Q Cranial Cavity and Brain	0 Open 3 Percutaneous	0 Antineoplastic	4 Liquid Brachytherapy Radioisotope 5 Other Antineoplastic M Monoclonal Antibody
Q Cranial Cavity and Brain	0 Open 3 Percutaneous	2 Anti-infective	8 Oxazolidinones 9 Other Anti-infective
Q Cranial Cavity and Brain	0 Open 3 Percutaneous	3 Anti-inflammatory 6 Nutritional Substitute 7 Electrolytic and Water Balance Substitute A Stem Cells, Embryonic B Anesthetic Agent H Radioactive Substance K Other Diagnostic Substance N Analgesics, Hypnotics, Sedatives T Destructive Agent	Z No Qualifier
Q Cranial Cavity and Brain	0 Open 3 Percutaneous	E Stem Cells, Somatic	0 Autologous 1 Nonautologous
Q Cranial Cavity and Brain	0 Open 3 Percutaneous	G Other Therapeutic Substance	C Other Substance
Q Cranial Cavity and Brain	0 Open 3 Percutaneous	S Gas	F Other Gas
Q Cranial Cavity and Brain	7 Via Natural or Artificial Opening	0 Antineoplastic	4 Liquid Brachytherapy Radioisotope 5 Other Antineoplastic M Monoclonal Antibody
Q Cranial Cavity and Brain	7 Via Natural or Artificial Opening	S Gas	F Other Gas
R Spinal Canal	0 Open	A Stem Cells, Embryonic	Z No Qualifier
R Spinal Canal	0 Open	E Stem Cells, Somatic	0 Autologous 1 Nonautologous
R Spinal Canal	3 Percutaneous	0 Antineoplastic	2 High-dose Interleukin-2 3 Low-dose Interleukin-2 4 Liquid Brachytherapy Radioisotope 5 Other Antineoplastic M Monoclonal Antibody

Continued →

Administration Section Tables

Body System / Region (4ᵗʰ)	Approach (5ᵗʰ)	Substance (6ᵗʰ)	Qualifier (7ᵗʰ)
R Spinal Canal	**3** Percutaneous	**2** Anti-infective	**8** Oxazolidinones **9** Other Anti-infective
R Spinal Canal	**3** Percutaneous	**3** Anti-inflammatory **6** Nutritional Substance **7** Electrolytic and Water Balance Substance **A** Stem Cells, Embryonic **B** Anesthetic Agent **H** Radioactive Substance **K** Other Diagnostic Substance **N** Analgesics, Hypnotics, Sedatives **T** Destructive Agent	**Z** No Qualifier
R Spinal Canal	**3** Percutaneous	**E** Stem Cells, Somatic	**0** Autologous **1** Nonautologous
R Spinal Canal	**3** Percutaneous	**G** Other Therapeutic Substance	**C** Other Substance
R Spinal Canal	**3** Percutaneous	**S** Gas	**F** Other Gas
R Spinal Canal	**7** Via Natural or Artificial Opening	**S** Gas	**F** Other Gas
S Epidural Space	**3** Percutaneous	**0** Antineoplastic	**2** High-dose Interleukin-2 **3** Low-dose Interleukin-2 **4** Liquid Brachytherapy Radioisotope **5** Other Antineoplastic **M** Monoclonal Antibody
S Epidural Space	**3** Percutaneous	**2** Anti-infective	**8** Oxazolidinones **9** Other Anti-infective
S Epidural Space	**3** Percutaneous	**3** Anti-inflammatory **6** Nutritional Substance **7** Electrolytic and Water Balance Substance **B** Anesthetic Agent **H** Radioactive Substance **K** Other Diagnostic Substance **N** Analgesics, Hypnotics, Sedatives **T** Destructive Agent	**Z** No Qualifier
S Epidural Space	**3** Percutaneous	**G** Other Therapeutic Substance	**C** Other Substance
S Epidural Space	**3** Percutaneous	**S** Gas	**F** Other Gas
S Epidural Space	**7** Via Natural or Artificial Opening	**S** Gas	**F** Other Gas
T Peripheral Nerves and Plexi **X** Cranial Nerves	**3** Percutaneous	**3** Anti-inflammatory **B** Anesthetic Agent **T** Destructive Agent	**Z** No Qualifier
T Peripheral Nerves and Plexi **X** Cranial Nerves	**3** Percutaneous	**G** Other Therapeutic Substance	**C** Other Substance
U Joints	**0** Open	**2** Anti-infective	**8** Oxazolidinones **9** Other Anti-infective
U Joints	**0** Open	**G** Other Therapeutic Substance	**B** Recombinant Bone Morphogenetic Protein

Continued →

3E0

Section 3 Administration
Body System E Physiological Systems and Anatomical Regions
Operation 0 Introduction: Putting in or on a therapeutic, diagnostic, nutritional, physiological,
or prophylactic substance except blood or blood products

3E0 Continued

Body System / Region (4th)	Approach (5th)	Substance (6th)	Qualifier (7th)
U Joints	3 Percutaneous	0 Antineoplastic	4 Liquid Brachytherapy Radioisotope 5 Other Antineoplastic M Monoclonal Antibody
U Joints	3 Percutaneous	2 Anti-infective	8 Oxazolidinones 9 Other Anti-infective
U Joints	3 Percutaneous	3 Anti-inflammatory 6 Nutritional Substance 7 Electrolytic and Water Balance Substance B Anesthetic Agent H Radioactive Substance K Other Diagnostic Substance N Analgesics, Hypnotics, Sedatives T Destructive Agent	Z No Qualifier
U Joints	3 Percutaneous	G Other Therapeutic Substance	B Recombinant Bone Morphogenetic Protein C Other Substance
U Joints	3 Percutaneous	S Gas	F Other Gas
U Joints	4 Percutaneous Endoscopic	G Other Therapeutic Substance	C Other Substance
V Bones	0 Open	G Other Therapeutic Substance	B Recombinant Bone Morphogenetic Protein
V Bones	3 Percutaneous	0 Antineoplastic	5 Other Antineoplastic M Monoclonal Antibody
V Bones	3 Percutaneous	2 Anti-infective	8 Oxazolidinones 9 Other Anti-infective
V Bones	3 Percutaneous	3 Anti-inflammatory 6 Nutritional Substance 7 Electrolytic and Water Balance Substance B Anesthetic Agent H Radioactive Substance K Other Diagnostic Substance N Analgesics, Hypnotics, Sedatives T Destructive Agent	Z No Qualifier
V Bones	3 Percutaneous	G Other Therapeutic Substance	B Recombinant Bone Morphogenetic Protein C Other Substance
W Lymphatics	3 Percutaneous	0 Antineoplastic	5 Other Antineoplastic M Monoclonal Antibody
W Lymphatics	3 Percutaneous	2 Anti-infective	8 Oxazolidinones 9 Other Anti-infective

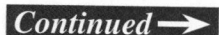

Continued →

Section   3   Administration
Body System   E   Physiological Systems and Anatomical Regions
Operation   0   Introduction: Putting in or on a therapeutic, diagnostic, nutritional, physiological,
                      or prophylactic substance except blood or blood products

Body System / Region (4ᵗʰ)	Approach (5ᵗʰ)	Substance (6ᵗʰ)	Qualifier (7ᵗʰ)
W Lymphatics	**3** Percutaneous	**3** Anti-inflammatory **6** Nutritional Substance **7** Electrolytic and Water Balance Substance **B** Anesthetic Agent **H** Radioactive Substance **K** Other Diagnostic Substance **N** Analgesics, Hypnotics, Sedatives **T** Destructive Agent	**Z** No Qualifier
W Lymphatics	**3** Percutaneous	**G** Other Therapeutic Substance	**C** Other Substance
Y Pericardial Cavity	**3** Percutaneous	**0** Antineoplastic	**4** Liquid Brachytherapy Radioisotope **5** Other Antineoplastic **M** Monoclonal Antibody
Y Pericardial Cavity	**3** Percutaneous	**2** Anti-infective	**8** Oxazolidinones **9** Other Anti-infective
Y Pericardial Cavity	**3** Percutaneous	**3** Anti-inflammatory **6** Nutritional Substance **7** Electrolytic and Water Balance Substance **B** Anesthetic Agent **H** Radioactive Substance **K** Other Diagnostic Substance **N** Analgesics, Hypnotics, Sedatives **T** Destructive Agent	**Z** No Qualifier
Y Pericardial Cavity	**3** Percutaneous	**G** Other Therapeutic Substance	**C** Other Substance
Y Pericardial Cavity	**3** Percutaneous	**S** Gas	**F** Other Gas
Y Pericardial Cavity	**4** Percutaneous Endoscopic	**G** Other Therapeutic Substance	**C** Other Substance
Y Pericardial Cavity	**7** Via Natural or Artificial Opening	**0** Antineoplastic	**4** Liquid Brachytherapy Radioisotope **5** Other Antineoplastic **M** Monoclonal Antibody
Y Pericardial Cavity	**7** Via Natural or Artificial Opening	**S** Gas	**F** Other Gas

Section	3	Administration
Body System	E	**Physiological Systems and Anatomical Regions**
Operation	1	**Irrigation:** Putting in or on a cleansing substance

Body System / Region (4th)	Approach (5th)	Substance (6th)	Qualifier (7th)
0 Skin and Mucous Membranes **C** Eye	**3** Percutaneous **X** External	**8** Irrigating Substance	**X** Diagnostic **Z** No Qualifier
9 Nose **B** Ear **F** Respiratory Tract **G** Upper GI **H** Lower GI **J** Biliary and Pancreatic Tract **K** Genitourinary Tract **N** Male Reproductive **P** Female Reproductive	**3** Percutaneous **7** Via Natural or Artificial Opening **8** Via Natural or Artificial Opening Endoscopic	**8** Irrigating Substance	**X** Diagnostic **Z** No Qualifier
L Pleural Cavity **Q** Cranial Cavity and Brain **R** Spinal Canal **S** Epidural Space **Y** Pericardial Cavity	**3** Percutaneous	**8** Irrigating Substance	**X** Diagnostic **Z** No Qualifier
M Peritoneal Cavity	**3** Percutaneous	**8** Irrigating Substance	**X** Diagnostic **Z** No Qualifier
M Peritoneal Cavity	**3** Percutaneous	**9** Dialysate	**Z** No Qualifier
M Peritoneal Cavity	**4** Percutaneous Endoscopic	**8** Irrigating Substance	**X** Diagnostic **Z** No Qualifier
U Joints	**3** Percutaneous **4** Percutaneous Endoscopic	**8** Irrigating Substance	**X** Diagnostic **Z** No Qualifier

Within each section of ICD-10-PCS the characters have different meanings. The seven character meanings for the Measurement and Monitoring section are illustrated here through the procedure example of *External electrocardiogram (EKG), single reading*.

Section	Body System	Root Operation	Body System	Approach	Function / Device	Qualifier
Measurement and Monitoring	Physiological Systems	Measurement	Cardiac	External	Electrical Activity	None
4	A	0	2	X	4	Z

Section (Character 1)

All Measurement and Monitoring procedure codes have a first character value of 4.

Body System (Character 2)

The alphanumeric character for the body system is placed in the second position. There are two character values applicable for the Measurement and Monitoring section. The character value of A is reported for physiological systems. The character value B is reported for physiological devices.

Root Operations (Character 3)

The alphanumeric character value for root operations is placed in the third position. Listed here are the root operations applicable to the Measurement and Monitoring section with their associated meaning.

Character Value	Root Operation	Root Operation Definition
0	Measurement	Determining the level of a physiological or physical function at a point in time
1	Monitoring	Determining the level of a physiological or physical function repetitively over a period of time

Body System/Region (Character 4)

For each body system the applicable body part character values will be available for procedure code construction. An example of a body region for this section is Respiratory.

Approach (Character 5)

The approach is the technique used to reach the procedure site. The following are the approach character values for the Measurement and Monitoring section with the associated definitions.

Character Value	Approach	Approach Definition
0	Open	Cutting through the skin or mucous membrane and any other body layers necessary to expose the site of the procedure
3	Percutaneous	Entry, by puncture or minor incision, of instrumentation through the skin or mucous membrane and any other body layers necessary to reach the site of the procedure
4	Percutaneous Endoscopic	Entry, by puncture or minor incision, of instrumentation through the skin or mucous membrane and any other body layers necessary to reach and visualize the site of the procedure
7	Via Natural or Artificial Opening	Entry of instrumentation through a natural or artificial external opening to reach the site of the procedure
8	Via Natural or Artificial Opening Endoscopic	Entry of instrumentation through a natural or artificial external opening to reach and visualize the site of the procedure
X	External	Procedures performed directly on the skin or mucous membrane and procedures performed indirectly by the application of external force through the skin or mucous membrane

Function/Device (Character 6)

In the Measurement and Monitoring section a function or device is always utilized. The function or device is reported in the sixth character position by the type of function monitored or measured or by the device utilized. The following is a sample list of the functions and devices included in this section:

- Conductivity
- Flow
- Metabolism
- Pressure
- Sound

Qualifier (Character 7)

The qualifier represents an additional attribute for the procedure when applicable. There are several qualifiers included in the Measurement and Monitoring section. For example, measurement procedures in this section include several qualifiers including stress that is reported with the character value of 4. If there is no qualifier for a procedure, the placeholder Z is the character valve that should be reported.

AHA Coding Clinic

4A023N6 Measurement of Cardiac Sampling and Pressure, Right Heart, Percutaneous Approach - AHA CC: 3Q, 2019, 32

4A023N8 Measurement of Cardiac Sampling and Pressure, Bilateral, Percutaneous Approach - AHA CC: 1Q, 2018, 12-13

4A02X4Z Measurement of Cardiac Electrical Activity, External Approach - AHA CC: 3Q, 2015, 29

4A033BC Measurement of Arterial Pressure, Coronary, Percutaneous Approach - AHA CC: 3Q, 2016, 37

4A0F3BE Measurement of Musculoskeletal Pressure, Compartment, Percutaneous Approach - AHA CC: 4Q, 2020, 63-64

4A103BD Monitoring of Intracranial Pressure, Percutaneous Approach - AHA CC: 2Q, 2016, 29

4A1134G Monitoring of Peripheral Nervous Electrical Activity, Intraoperative, Percutaneous Approach - AHA CC: 4Q, 2014, 28-29

4A11X4G Monitoring of Peripheral Nervous Electrical Activity, Intraoperative, External Approach - AHA CC: 1Q, 2015, 26; 2Q, 2015, 14

4A1239Z Monitoring of Cardiac Output, Percutaneous Approach - AHA CC: 3Q, 2015, 35

4A133B1 Monitoring of Arterial Pressure, Peripheral, Percutaneous Approach, for Continuous Monitoring of Pressure - AHA CC: 2Q, 2016, 33

4A133B3 Monitoring of Arterial Pressure, Pulmonary, Percutaneous Approach - AHA CC: 3Q, 2015, 35

4A133J1 Monitoring of Arterial Pulse, Peripheral, Percutaneous Approach, for Continuous Monitoring of Pulse - AHA CC: 2Q, 2016, 33

Measurement and Monitoring Section Tables

Measurement and Monitoring Tables 4A0–4B0

Section	4	Measurement and Monitoring
Body System	A	Physiological Systems
Operation	0	Measurement: Determining the level of a physiological or physical function at a point in time

Body System (4ᵗʰ)	Approach (5ᵗʰ)	Function / Device (6ᵗʰ)	Qualifier (7ᵗʰ)
0 Central Nervous	0 Open	2 Conductivity 4 Electrical Activity B Pressure	Z No Qualifier
0 Central Nervous	3 Percutaneous 7 Via Natural or Artificial Opening 8 Via Natural or Artificial Opening Endoscopic	4 Electrical Activity	Z No Qualifier
0 Central Nervous	3 Percutaneous 7 Via Natural or Artificial Opening 8 Via Natural or Artificial Opening Endoscopic	B Pressure K Temperature R Saturation	D Intracranial
0 Central Nervous	X External	2 Conductivity 4 Electrical Activity	Z No Qualifier
1 Peripheral Nervous	0 Open 3 Percutaneous 7 Via Natural or Artificial Opening 8 Via Natural or Artificial Opening Endoscopic X External	2 Conductivity	9 Sensory B Motor

Continued →

Section	4	Measurement and Monitoring
Body System	A	Physiological Systems
Operation	0	Measurement: Determining the level of a physiological or physical function at a point in time

Body System (4th)	Approach (5th)	Function / Device (6th)	Qualifier (7th)
1 Peripheral Nervous	0 Open 3 Percutaneous 7 Via Natural or Artificial Opening 8 Via Natural or Artificial Opening Endoscopic X External	4 Electrical Activity	Z No Qualifier
2 Cardiac	0 Open 3 Percutaneous 7 Via Natural or Artificial Opening 8 Via Natural or Artificial Opening Endoscopic	4 Electrical Activity 9 Output C Rate F Rhythm H Sound P Action Currents	Z No Qualifier
2 Cardiac	0 Open 3 Percutaneous 7 Via Natural or Artificial Opening 8 Via Natural or Artificial Opening Endoscopic	N Sampling and Pressure	6 Right Heart 7 Left Heart 8 Bilateral
2 Cardiac	X External	4 Electrical Activity	A Guidance Z No Qualifier
2 Cardiac	X External	9 Output C Rate F Rhythm H Sound P Action Currents	Z No Qualifier
2 Cardiac	X External	M Total Activity	4 Stress
3 Arterial	0 Open 3 Percutaneous	5 Flow J Pulse	1 Peripheral 3 Pulmonary C Coronary
3 Arterial	0 Open 3 Percutaneous	B Pressure	1 Peripheral 3 Pulmonary C Coronary F Other Thoracic
3 Arterial	0 Open 3 Percutaneous	H Sound R Saturation	1 Peripheral
3 Arterial	X External	5 Flow	1 Peripheral D Intracranial
3 Arterial	X External	B Pressure H Sound J Pulse R Saturation	1 Peripheral
4 Venous	0 Open 3 Percutaneous	5 Flow B Pressure J Pulse	0 Central 1 Peripheral 2 Portal 3 Pulmonary
4 Venous	0 Open 3 Percutaneous	R Saturation	1 Peripheral
4 Venous	4 Percutaneous Endoscopic	B Pressure	2 Portal
4 Venous	X External	5 Flow B Pressure J Pulse R Saturation	1 Peripheral
5 Circulatory	X External	L Volume	Z No Qualifier

Continued →

Section 4 **Measurement and Monitoring**
Body System A **Physiological Systems**
Operation 0 **Measurement:** Determining the level of a physiological or physical function at a point in time

Body System (4th)	Approach (5th)	Function / Device (6th)	Qualifier (7th)
6 Lymphatic	0 Open 3 Percutaneous 7 Via Natural or Artificial Opening 8 Via Natural or Artificial Opening Endoscopic	5 Flow B Pressure	Z No Qualifier
7 Visual	X External	0 Acuity 7 Mobility B Pressure	Z No Qualifier
8 Olfactory	X External	0 Acuity	Z No Qualifier
9 Respiratory	7 Via Natural or Artificial Opening 8 Via Natural or Artificial Opening Endoscopic X External	1 Capacity 5 Flow C Rate D Resistance L Volume M Total Activity	Z No Qualifier
B Gastrointestinal	7 Via Natural or Artificial Opening 8 Via Natural or Artificial Opening Endoscopic	8 Motility B Pressure G Secretion	Z No Qualifier
C Biliary	3 Percutaneous 4 Percutaneous Endoscopic 7 Via Natural or Artificial Opening 8 Via Natural or Artificial Opening Endoscopic	5 Flow B Pressure	Z No Qualifier
D Urinary	7 Via Natural or Artificial Opening 8 Via Natural or Artificial Opening Endoscopic	3 Contractility 5 Flow B Pressure D Resistance L Volume	Z No Qualifier
F Musculoskeletal	3 Percutaneous	3 Contractility	Z No Qualifier
F Musculoskeletal	3 Percutaneous	B Pressure	E Compartment
F Musculoskeletal	X External	3 Contractility	Z No Qualifier
H Products of Conception, Cardiac	7 Via Natural or Artificial Opening 8 Via Natural or Artificial Opening Endoscopic X External	4 Electrical Activity C Rate F Rhythm H Sound	Z No Qualifier
J Products of Conception, Nervous	7 Via Natural or Artificial Opening 8 Via Natural or Artificial Opening Endoscopic X External	2 Conductivity 4 Electrical Activity B Pressure	Z No Qualifier
Z None	7 Via Natural or Artificial Opening	6 Metabolism K Temperature	Z No Qualifier
Z None	X External	6 Metabolism K Temperature Q Sleep	Z No Qualifier

Section 4 **Measurement and Monitoring**
Body System A **Physiological Systems**
Operation 1 **Monitoring:** Determining the level of a physiological or physical function repetitively over a period of time

Body System (4th)	Approach (5th)	Function / Device (6th)	Qualifier (7th)
0 Central Nervous	0 Open	2 Conductivity B Pressure	Z No Qualifier

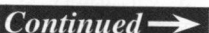

Continued →

Section	4	Measurement and Monitoring
Body System	A	Physiological Systems
Operation	1	Monitoring: Determining the level of a physiological or physical function repetitively over a period of time

Body System (4th)	Approach (5th)	Function / Device (6th)	Qualifier (7th)
0 Central Nervous	0 Open	4 Electrical Activity	G Intraoperative Z No Qualifier
0 Central Nervous	3 Percutaneous 7 Via Natural or Artificial Opening 8 Via Natural or Artificial Opening Endoscopic	4 Electrical Activity	G Intraoperative Z No Qualifier
0 Central Nervous	3 Percutaneous 7 Via Natural or Artificial Opening 8 Via Natural or Artificial Opening Endoscopic	B Pressure K Temperature R Saturation	D Intracranial
0 Central Nervous	X External	2 Conductivity	Z No Qualifier
0 Central Nervous	X External	4 Electrical Activity	G Intraoperative Z No Qualifier
1 Peripheral Nervous	0 Open 3 Percutaneous 7 Via Natural or Artificial Opening 8 Via Natural or Artificial Opening Endoscopic X External	2 Conductivity	9 Sensory B Motor
1 Peripheral Nervous	0 Open 3 Percutaneous 7 Via Natural or Artificial Opening 8 Via Natural or Artificial Opening Endoscopic X External	4 Electrical Activity	G Intraoperative Z No Qualifier
2 Cardiac	0 Open 3 Percutaneous 7 Via Natural or Artificial Opening 8 Via Natural or Artificial Opening Endoscopic	4 Electrical Activity 9 Output C Rate F Rhythm H Sound	Z No Qualifier
2 Cardiac	X External	4 Electrical Activity	5 Ambulatory Z No Qualifier
2 Cardiac	X External	9 Output C Rate F Rhythm H Sound	Z No Qualifier
2 Cardiac	X External	M Total Activity	4 Stress
2 Cardiac	X External	S Vascular Perfusion	H Indocyanine Green Dye
3 Arterial	0 Open 3 Percutaneous	5 Flow B Pressure J Pulse	1 Peripheral 3 Pulmonary C Coronary
3 Arterial	0 Open 3 Percutaneous	H Sound R Saturation	1 Peripheral
3 Arterial	X External	5 Flow B Pressure H Sound J Pulse R Saturation	1 Peripheral

Continued →

4A1

Section	4	**Measurement and Monitoring**	*4A1 Continued*
Body System	A	**Physiological Systems**	
Operation	1	**Monitoring:** Determining the level of a physiological or physical function repetitively over a period of time	

Body System (4th)	Approach (5th)	Function / Device (6th)	Qualifier (7th)
4 Venous	**0** Open **3** Percutaneous	**5** Flow **B** Pressure **J** Pulse	**0** Central **1** Peripheral **2** Portal **3** Pulmonary
4 Venous	**0** Open **3** Percutaneous	**R** Saturation	**0** Central **2** Portal **3** Pulmonary
4 Venous	**X** External	**5** Flow **B** Pressure **J** Pulse	**1** Peripheral
6 Lymphatic	**0** Open **3** Percutaneous **7** Via Natural or Artificial Opening **8** Via Natural or Artificial Opening Endoscopic	**5** Flow	**H** Indocyanine Green Dye **Z** No Qualifier
6 Lymphatic	**0** Open **3** Percutaneous **7** Via Natural or Artificial Opening **8** Via Natural or Artificial Opening Endoscopic	**B** Pressure	**Z** No Qualifier
9 Respiratory	**7** Via Natural or Artificial Opening **X** External	**1** Capacity **5** Flow **C** Rate **D** Resistance **L** Volume	**Z** No Qualifier
B Gastrointestinal	**7** Via Natural or Artificial Opening **8** Via Natural or Artificial Opening Endoscopic	**8** Motility **B** Pressure **G** Secretion	**Z** No Qualifier
B Gastrointestinal	**X** External	**S** Vascular Perfusion	**H** Indocyanine Green Dye
D Urinary	**7** Via Natural or Artificial Opening **8** Via Natural or Artificial Opening Endoscopic	**3** Contractility **5** Flow **B** Pressure **D** Resistance **L** Volume	**Z** No Qualifier
G Skin and Breast	**X** External	**S** Vascular Perfusion	**H** Indocyanine Green Dye
H Products of Conception, Cardiac	**7** Via Natural or Artificial Opening **8** Via Natural or Artificial Opening Endoscopic **X** External	**4** Electrical Activity **C** Rate **F** Rhythm **H** Sound	**Z** No Qualifier
J Products of Conception, Nervous	**7** Via Natural or Artificial Opening **8** Via Natural or Artificial Opening Endoscopic **X** External	**2** Conductivity **4** Electrical Activity **B** Pressure	**Z** No Qualifier
Z None	**7** Via Natural or Artificial Opening	**K** Temperature	**Z** No Qualifier
Z None	**X** External	**K** Temperature **Q** Sleep	**Z** No Qualifier

Section	4	Measurement and Monitoring
Body System	B	Physiological Devices
Operation	0	Measurement: Determining the level of a physiological or physical function at a point in time

Body System (4ᵗʰ)	Approach (5ᵗʰ)	Function / Device (6ᵗʰ)	Qualifier (7ᵗʰ)
0 Central Nervous	**X** External	**V** Stimulator	**Z** No Qualifier
0 Central Nervous	**X** External	**W** Cerebrospinal Fluid Shunt	**0** Wireless Sensor
1 Peripheral Nervous **F** Musculoskeletal	**X** External	**V** Stimulator	**Z** No Qualifier
2 Cardiac	**X** External	**S** Pacemaker **T** Defibrillator	**Z** No Qualifier
9 Respiratory	**X** External	**S** Pacemaker	**Z** No Qualifier

Within each section of ICD-10-PCS the characters have different meanings. The seven character meanings for the Extracorporeal or Systemic Assistance and Performance section are illustrated here through the procedure example of *Hyperbaric oxygenation of wound*.

Section	Body System	Root Operation	Body System	Duration	Function	Qualifier
Extracorporeal or Systemic Assistance and Performance	Physiological Systems	Assistance	Circulatory	Intermittent	Oxygenation	Hyperbaric
5	A	0	5	1	2	1

Section (Character 1)

All Extracorporeal or Systemic Assistance and Performance procedure codes have a first character value of 5.

Body System (Character 2)

The alphanumeric character for the body system is placed in the second position. There is one character value applicable for the Extracorporeal or Systemic Assistance and Performance section. The character value of A is reported for physiological systems.

Root Operations (Character 3)

The alphanumeric character value for root operations is placed in the third position. Listed here are the root operations applicable to the Extracorporeal or Systemic Assistance and Performance section with their associated meaning.

Character Value	Root Operation	Root Operation Definition
0	Assistance	Taking over a portion of a physiological function by extracorporeal means
1	Performance	Completely taking over a physiological function by extracorporeal means
2	Restoration	Returning, or attempting to return, a physiological function to its original state by extracorporeal means

Body System (Character 4)

For each body system, the applicable body part character values will be available for procedure code construction. An example of a body region for this section is respiratory.

Duration (Character 5)

The duration represents the length of time or frequency for which the assistance or performance is utilized. Some examples of duration are Intermittent, Continuous, or Less than 24 consecutive hours.

Function (Character 6)

In the Extracorporeal or Systemic Assistance and Performance section a function is always reported. The function is reported in the sixth character position. The following is a sample list of the functions utilized in this section:

- Output
- Oxygenation
- Pacing
- Ventilation

Qualifier (Character 7)

The qualifier represents an additional attribute for the procedure when applicable. There are several qualifiers included in the Extracorporeal or Systemic Assistance and Performance section. For example, assistance procedures in this section include several qualifiers including Balloon Pump, which is reported with the character value of 0. If there is no qualifier for a procedure, the placeholder Z is the character valve that should be reported.

AHA Coding Clinic

5A02210 Assistance with Cardiac Output using Balloon Pump, Continuous - AHA CC: 3Q, 2013, 18-19; 2Q, 2018, 4-5; 2Q, 2021, 12

5A0221D Assistance with Cardiac Output using Impeller Pump, Continuous - AHA CC: 3Q, 2014, 19; 4Q, 2016, 138-139; 1Q, 2017, 11-12; 4Q, 2017, 43-45

5A09357 Assistance with Respiratory Ventilation, <24 Hrs, CPAP - AHA CC: 4Q, 2014, 9-10; 1Q, 2020, 10-11

5A09457 Assistance with Respiratory Ventilation, 24-96 Hrs, CPAP - AHA CC: 4Q, 2014, 9-10

5A09557 Assistance with Respiratory Ventilation, >96 Hrs, CPAP - AHA CC: 4Q, 2014, 9-10

5A1221Z Performance of Cardiac Output, Continuous - AHA CC: 3Q, 2013, 18-19; 1Q, 2014, 10-11; 3Q, 2014, 16-17, 20-21; 4Q, 2015, 22-25; 1Q, 2016, 27-28; 1Q, 2017, 19-20; 3Q, 2017, 7-8

5A1223Z Performance of Cardiac Pacing, Continuous - AHA CC: 3Q, 2013, 18-19

ECMO, Extracorporeal Oxygenation, Membrane - AHA CC: 3Q, 2019, 19-23; 4Q, 2019, 39-41

5A1522F Extracorporeal Oxygenation, Membrane, Central - AHA CC: 2Q, 2019, 36

5A1522G Extracorporeal Oxygenation, Membrane, Peripheral Veno-arterial - AHA CC: 4Q, 2018, 53-54

5A1522H Extracorporeal Oxygenation, Membrane, Peripheral Veno-venous - AHA CC: 4Q, 2018, 53-54

5A15A2G Extracorporeal Oxygenation, Membrane, Peripheral Veno-arterial, Intraoperative - AHA CC: 4Q, 2019, 39-40

5A1935Z Respiratory Ventilation, Less than 24 Consecutive Hours - AHA CC: 4Q, 2014, 3-15; 1Q, 2018, 13-14

5A1945Z Respiratory Ventilation, 24-96 Consecutive Hours - AHA CC: 4Q, 2014, 3-15

5A1955Z Respiratory Ventilation, Greater than 96 Consecutive Hours - AHA CC: 4Q, 2014, 3-15

5A1C00Z Performance of Biliary Filtration, Single - AHA CC: 1Q, 2016, 28-29

5A1D60Z Performance of Urinary Filtration, Multiple - AHA CC: 1Q, 2016, 29

5A1D70Z Performance of Urinary Filtration, Intermittent, Less than 6 Hours Per Day - AHA CC: 4Q, 2017, 72-73

5A1D80Z Performance of Urinary Filtration, Prolonged Intermittent, 6-18 hours Per Day - AHA CC: 4Q, 2017, 72

5A1D90Z Performance of Urinary Filtration, Continuous, Greater than 18 hours Per Day - AHA CC: 4Q, 2017, 72-73

Extracorporeal or Systemic Assistance and Performance Section Tables

Extracorporeal or Systemic Assistance and Performance Tables 5A0–5A2

Section	5	Extracorporeal or Systemic Assistance and Performance
Body System	A	Physiological Systems
Operation	0	**Assistance:** Taking over a portion of a physiological function by extracorporeal means

Body System (4th)	Duration (5th)	Function (6th)	Qualifier (7th)
2 Cardiac	1 Intermittent 2 Continuous	1 Output	0 Balloon Pump 5 Pulsatile Compression 6 Other Pump D Impeller Pump
5 Circulatory	1 Intermittent 2 Continuous	2 Oxygenation	1 Hyperbaric C Supersaturated
9 Respiratory	2 Continuous	0 Filtration	Z No Qualifier
9 Respiratory	3 Less than 24 Consecutive Hours 4 24-96 Consecutive Hours 5 Greater than 96 Consecutive Hours	5 Ventilation	7 Continuous Positive Airway Pressure 8 Intermittent Positive Airway Pressure 9 Continuous Negative Airway Pressure A High Nasal Flow/Velocity B Intermittent Negative Airway Pressure Z No Qualifier

Section 5 **Extracorporeal or Systemic Assistance and Performance**
Body System A **Physiological Systems**
Operation 1 **Performance:** Completely taking over a physiological function by extracorporeal means

Body System (4th)	Duration (5th)	Function (6th)	Qualifier (7th)
2 Cardiac	**0** Single	**1** Output	**2** Manual
2 Cardiac	**1** Intermittent	**3** Pacing	**Z** No Qualifier
2 Cardiac	**2** Continuous	**1** Output	**J** Automated **Z** No Qualifier
2 Cardiac	**2** Continuous	**3** Pacing	**Z** No Qualifier
5 Circulatory	**2** Continuous **A** Intraoperative	**2** Oxygenation	**F** Membrane, Central **G** Membrane, Peripheral Veno-arterial **H** Membrane, Peripheral Veno-venous
9 Respiratory	**0** Single	**5** Ventilation	**4** Nonmechanical
9 Respiratory	**3** Less than 24 Consecutive Hours **4** 24-96 Consecutive Hours **5** Greater than 96 Consecutive Hours	**5** Ventilation	**Z** No Qualifier
C Biliary	**0** Single **6** Multiple	**0** Filtration	**Z** No Qualifier
D Urinary	**7** Intermittent, Less than 6 Hours Per Day **8** Prolonged Intermittent, 6-18 Hours Per Day **9** Continuous, Greater than 18 Hours Per Day	**0** Filtration	**Z** No Qualifier

Section 5 **Extracorporeal or Systemic Assistance and Performance**
Body System A **Physiological Systems**
Operation 2 **Restoration:** Returning, or attempting to return, a physiological function to its original state by extracorporeal means.

Body System (4th)	Duration (5th)	Function (6th)	Qualifier (7th)
2 Cardiac	**0** Single	**4** Rhythm	**Z** No Qualifier

Within each section of ICD-10-PCS the characters have different meanings. The seven character meanings for the Extracorporeal or Systemic Therapies section are illustrated here through the procedure example of *Ultraviolet light phototherapy, series treatment.*

Section	Body System	Root Operation	Body System	Duration	Qualifier	Qualifier
Extracorporeal or Systemic Therapies	Physiological Systems	UV Light Therapy	Skin	Multiple	None	None
6	A	8	0	1	Z	Z

Section (Character 1)

All Extracorporeal or Systemic Therapies procedure codes have a first character value of 6.

Body System (Character 2)

The alphanumeric character for the body system is placed in the second position. There is one character value applicable for the Extracorporeal or Systemic Therapies section. The character value of A is reported for physiological systems.

Root Operations (Character 3)

The alphanumeric character value for root operations is placed in the third position. Listed below are the root operations applicable to the Extracorporeal or Systemic Therapies section with their associated meaning.

Character Value	Root Operation	Root Operation Definition
0	Atmospheric Control	Extracorporeal control of atmospheric pressure and composition
1	Decompression	Extracorporeal elimination of undissolved gas from body fluids
2	Electromagnetic Therapy	Extracorporeal treatment by electromagnetic rays
3	Hyperthermia	Extracorporeal raising of body temperature
4	Hypothermia	Extracorporeal lowering of body temperature
5	Pheresis	Extracorporeal separation of blood products
6	Phototherapy	Extracorporeal treatment by light rays
7	Ultrasound Therapy	Extracorporeal treatment by ultrasound
8	Ultraviolet Light Therapy	Extracorporeal treatment by ultraviolet light
9	Shock Wave Therapy	Extracorporeal treatment by shock waves
B	Perfusion	Extracorporeal treatment by diffusion of therapeutic fluid

Body System (Character 4)

For each body system the applicable body part character values will be available for procedure code construction. An example of a body region for this section is Skin.

Duration (Character 5)

The duration represents the number of therapy sessions performed. Single is reported with character value 0; Multiple is reported with character value 1.

Qualifier (Character 6)

Character 6 is the first of two qualifier characters for the Extracorporeal or Systemic Therapies section. The qualifier represents an additional attribute for the procedure when applicable. There are currently no qualifier values for the sixth character position, so the character value of Z is always reported.

Qualifier (Character 7)

Character 7 is the second of two qualifier characters for the Extracorporeal or Systemic Therapies section. The qualifier represents an additional attribute for the procedure when applicable. There are some qualifiers included in the Extracorporeal or Systemic Therapies section. For example, pheresis procedures in this section include several qualifiers including Plasma that is reported with the character value of 3. If there is no qualifier for a procedure, the placeholder Z is the character valve that should be reported.

AHA Coding Clinic

6A4Z0ZZ Hypothermia, Single - AHA CC: 2Q, 2019, 17-18
6A750Z7 Ultrasound Therapy of Other Vessels, Single - AHA CC: 4Q, 2014, 19-20

Extracorporeal or Systemic Therapies Section Tables

Extracorporeal or Systemic Therapies Tables 6A0–6AB

Section	6	**Extracorporeal or Systemic Therapies**
Body System	A	**Physiological Systems**
Operation	0	**Atmospheric Control:** Extracorporeal control of atmospheric pressure and composition

Body System (4th)	Duration (5th)	Qualifier (6th)	Qualifier (7th)
Z None	**0** Single **1** Multiple	**Z** No Qualifier	**Z** No Qualifier

Section	6	**Extracorporeal or Systemic Therapies**
Body System	A	**Physiological Systems**
Operation	1	**Decompression:** Extracorporeal elimination of undissolved gas from body fluids

Body System (4th)	Duration (5th)	Qualifier (6th)	Qualifier (7th)
5 Circulatory	**0** Single **1** Multiple	**Z** No Qualifier	**Z** No Qualifier

Section	6	**Extracorporeal or Systemic Therapies**
Body System	A	**Physiological Systems**
Operation	2	**Electromagnetic Therapy:** Extracorporeal treatment by electromagnetic rays

Body System (4th)	Duration (5th)	Qualifier (6th)	Qualifier (7th)
1 Urinary **2** Central Nervous	**0** Single **1** Multiple	**Z** No Qualifier	**Z** No Qualifier

Section	6	**Extracorporeal or Systemic Therapies**
Body System	A	**Physiological Systems**
Operation	3	**Hyperthermia:** Extracorporeal raising of body temperature

Body System (4th)	Duration (5th)	Qualifier (6th)	Qualifier (7th)
Z None	**0** Single **1** Multiple	**Z** No Qualifier	**Z** No Qualifier

Section	6	**Extracorporeal or Systemic Therapies**
Body System	A	**Physiological Systems**
Operation	4	**Hypothermia:** Extracorporeal lowering of body temperature

Body System (4th)	Duration (5th)	Qualifier (6th)	Qualifier (7th)
Z None	**0** Single **1** Multiple	**Z** No Qualifier	**Z** No Qualifier

Section	6	**Extracorporeal or Systemic Therapies**
Body System	A	**Physiological Systems**
Operation	5	**Pheresis:** Extracorporeal separation of blood products

Body System (4th)	Duration (5th)	Qualifier (6th)	Qualifier (7th)
5 Circulatory	**0** Single **1** Multiple	**Z** No Qualifier	**0** Erythrocytes **1** Leukocytes **2** Platelets **3** Plasma **T** Stem Cells, Cord Blood **V** Stem Cells, Hematopoietic

Section   6   **Extracorporeal or Systemic Therapies**
Body System   A   **Physiological Systems**
Operation   6   **Phototherapy:** Extracorporeal treatment by light rays

Body System (4th)	Duration (5th)	Qualifier (6th)	Qualifier (7th)
0 Skin **5** Circulatory	**0** Single **1** Multiple	**Z** No Qualifier	**Z** No Qualifier

Section   6   **Extracorporeal or Systemic Therapies**
Body System   A   **Physiological Systems**
Operation   7   **Ultrasound Therapy:** Extracorporeal treatment by ultrasound

Body System (4th)	Duration (5th)	Qualifier (6th)	Qualifier (7th)
5 Circulatory	**0** Single **1** Multiple	**Z** No Qualifier	**4** Head and Neck Vessels **5** Heart **6** Peripheral Vessels **7** Other Vessels **Z** No Qualifier

Section   6   **Extracorporeal or Systemic Therapies**
Body System   A   **Physiological Systems**
Operation   8   **Ultraviolet Light Therapy:** Extracorporeal treatment by ultraviolet light

Body System (4th)	Duration (5th)	Qualifier (6th)	Qualifier (7th)
0 Skin	**0** Single **1** Multiple	**Z** No Qualifier	**Z** No Qualifier

Section   6   **Extracorporeal or Systemic Therapies**
Body System   A   **Physiological Systems**
Operation   9   **Shock Wave Therapy:** Extracorporeal treatment by shock waves

Body System (4th)	Duration (5th)	Qualifier (6th)	Qualifier (7th)
3 Musculoskeletal	**0** Single **1** Multiple	**Z** No Qualifier	**Z** No Qualifier

Section   6   **Extracorporeal or Systemic Therapies**
Body System   A   **Physiological Systems**
Operation   B   **Perfusion:** Extracorporeal treatment by diffusion of therapeutic fluid

Body System (4th)	Duration (5th)	Qualifier (6th)	Qualifier (7th)
5 Circulatory **B** Respiratory System **F** Hepatobiliary System and Pancreas **T** Urinary System	**0** Single	**B** Donor Organ	**Z** No Qualifier

Within each section of ICD-10-PCS, the characters have different meanings. The seven character meanings for the Osteopathic section are illustrated below through the procedure example of Indirect osteopathic treatment of sacrum.

Section	Body System	Root Operation	Body Region	Approach	Method	Qualifier
Osteopathic	Anatomical Regions	Treatment	Sacrum	External	Indirect	None
7	W	0	4	X	4	Z

Section (Character 1)

All Osteopathic procedure codes have a first character value of 7.

Body System (Character 2)

The alphanumeric character for the body system is placed in the second position. There is one character value applicable for the Osteopathic section. The character value of W is reported for anatomical regions.

Root Operations (Character 3)

The alphanumeric character value for root operations is placed in the third position. Listed here is the root operation applicable to the Osteopathic section with its associated meaning.

Character Value	Root Operation	Root Operation Definition
0	Treatment	Manual treatment to eliminate or alleviate somatic dysfunction and related disorders

Body Region (Character 4)

For each body region the applicable body part character values will be available for procedure code construction. An example of a body region for this section is Head.

Approach (Character 5)

The approach is the technique used to reach the procedure site. The following are the approach character values for the Osteopathic section with the associated definitions.

Character Value	Approach	Approach Definition
X	External	Procedures performed directly on the skin or mucous membrane and procedures performed indirectly by the application of external force through the skin or mucous membrane

Method (Character 6)

The method identifies the treatment method used to complete the osteopathic procedure. The available methods are:

- Articulatory-Raising
- Fascial Release
- General Mobilization
- High Velocity-Low Amplitude
- Indirect
- Low Velocity-High Amplitude
- Lymphatic Pump
- Muscle Energy-Isometric
- Muscle Energy-Isotonic
- Other

Qualifier (Character 7)

The qualifier represents an additional attribute for the procedure when applicable. Currently, there are no qualifiers in the Osteopathic section; therefore, the placeholder character value of Z should be reported.

Osteopathic Section Table

Osteopathic Table 7W0

Section 7 **Osteopathic**
Body System W **Anatomical Regions**
Operation 0 **Treatment:** Manual treatment to eliminate or alleviate somatic dysfunction and related disorders

Body Region (4th)	Approach (5th)	Method (6th)	Qualifier (7th)
0 Head	X External	0 Articulatory-Raising	Z None
1 Cervical		1 Fascial Release	
2 Thoracic		2 General Mobilization	
3 Lumbar		3 High Velocity-Low Amplitude	
4 Sacrum		4 Indirect	
5 Pelvis		5 Low Velocity-High Amplitude	
6 Lower Extremities		6 Lymphatic Pump	
7 Upper Extremities		7 Muscle Energy-Isometric	
8 Rib Cage		8 Muscle Energy-Isotonic	
9 Abdomen		9 Other Method	

Within each section of ICD-10-PCS the characters have different meanings. The seven character meanings for the Other Procedures section are illustrated here through the procedure example of Yoga therapy.

Section	Body System	Root Operation	Body Region	Approach	Method	Qualifier
Other Procedures	Physiological Systems and Anatomical Regions	Other Procedures	None	External	Other Method	Yoga Therapy
8	E	0	Z	X	Y	4

Section (Character 1)

All Other Procedures codes have a first character value of 8.

Body System (Character 2)

The alphanumeric character for the body system is placed in the second position. There are two character values applicable for the Other Procedures section. The character value of C is reported for indwelling device. The character value of E is reported for physiological system and anatomical regions.

Root Operations (Character 3)

The alphanumeric character value for root operations is placed in the third position. Listed here is the root operation applicable to the Other Procedures section with its associated meaning.

Character Value	Root Operation	Root Operation Definition
0	Other Procedures	Methodologies which attempt to remediate or cure a disorder or disease

Body Region (Character 4)

For each body region the applicable body part character values will be available for procedure code construction. An example of a body region for this section is Lower Extremity.

Approach (Character 5)

The approach is the technique used to reach the procedure site. The following are the approach character values for the Other Procedures section with the associated definitions.

Character Value	Approach	Approach Definition
0	Open	Cutting through the skin or mucous membrane and any other body layers necessary to expose the site of the procedure
3	Percutaneous	Entry, by puncture or minor incision, of instrumentation through the skin or mucous membrane and any other body layers necessary to reach the site of the procedure
4	Percutaneous Endoscopic	Entry, by puncture or minor incision, of instrumentation through the skin or mucous membrane and any other body layers necessary to reach and visualize the site of the procedure
7	Via Natural or Artificial Opening	Entry of instrumentation through a natural or artificial external opening to reach the site of the procedure
8	Via Natural or Artificial Opening Endoscopic	Entry of instrumentation through a natural or artificial external opening to reach and visualize the site of the procedure
X	External	Procedures performed directly on the skin or mucous membrane and procedures performed indirectly by the application of external force through the skin or mucous membrane

Method (Character 6)

The method identifies the treatment method used to complete the other procedure. The available methods are:

- Acupuncture
- Collection
- Computer Assisted Procedure
- Near Infrared Spectroscopy
- Robotic Assisted procedure
- Therapeutic Massage
- Other

Qualifier (Character 7)

The qualifier represents an additional attribute for the procedure when applicable. In the preceding example of Yoga therapy, the qualifier of 4 was used to report that the other procedure was Yoga therapy. If there is no qualifier for a procedure, the placeholder Z is the character valve that should be reported.

AHA Coding Clinic

8E09XBZ Computer Assisted Procedure of Head and Neck Region - AHA CC: 2Q, 2021, 19-20

8E0W4CZ Robotic Assisted Procedure of Trunk Region, Percutaneous Endoscopic Approach - AHA CC: 4Q, 2014, 33-34; 1Q, 2015, 33-34; 1Q, 2019, 30-31; 4Q, 2020, 53-54

Other Procedures Section Tables

Other Procedures Tables 8C0–8E0

Section	8	Other Procedures
Body System	C	Indwelling Device
Operation	0	Other Procedures: Methodologies which attempt to remediate or cure a disorder or disease

Body Region (4ᵗʰ)	Approach (5ᵗʰ)	Method (6ᵗʰ)	Qualifier (7ᵗʰ)
1 Nervous System	X External	6 Collection	J Cerebrospinal Fluid L Other Fluid
2 Circulatory System	X External	6 Collection	K Blood L Other Fluid

Section	8	Other Procedures
Body System	E	Physiological Systems and Anatomical Regions
Operation	0	Other Procedures: Methodologies which attempt to remediate or cure a disorder or disease

Body Region (4ᵗʰ)	Approach (5ᵗʰ)	Method (6ᵗʰ)	Qualifier (7ᵗʰ)
1 Nervous System U Female Reproductive System	X External	Y Other Method	7 Examination
2 Circulatory System	3 Percutaneous X External	D Near Infrared Spectroscopy	Z No Qualifier
9 Head and Neck Region	0 Open	C Robotic Assisted Procedure	Z No Qualifier
9 Head and Neck Region	0 Open	E Fluorescence Guided Procedure	M Aminolevulinic Acid Z No Qualifier
9 Head and Neck Region	3 Percutaneous 4 Percutaneous Endoscopic 7 Via Natural or Artificial Opening 8 Via Natural or Artificial Opening Endoscopic	C Robotic Assisted Procedure E Fluorescence Guided Procedure	Z No Qualifier

Continued →

8E0

Section 8 Other Procedures 8E0 Continued
Body System E Physiological Systems and Anatomical Regions
Operation 0 Other Procedures: Methodologies which attempt to remediate or cure a disorder or disease

Body Region (4th)	Approach (5th)	Method (6th)	Qualifier (7th)
9 Head and Neck Region	X External	B Computer Assisted Procedure	F With Fluoroscopy G With Computerized Tomography H With Magnetic Resonance Imaging Z No Qualifier
9 Head and Neck Region	X External	C Robotic Assisted Procedure	Z No Qualifier
9 Head and Neck Region	X External	Y Other Method	8 Suture Removal
H Integumentary System and Breast	3 Percutaneous	0 Acupuncture	0 Anesthesia Z No Qualifier
H Integumentary System and Breast	X External	6 Collection	2 Breast Milk
H Integumentary System and Breast	X External	Y Other Method	9 Piercing
K Musculoskeletal System	X External	1 Therapeutic Massage	Z No Qualifier
K Musculoskeletal System	X External	Y Other Method	7 Examination
V Male Reproductive System	X External	1 Therapeutic Massage	C Prostate D Rectum
V Male Reproductive System	X External	6 Collection	3 Sperm
W Trunk Region	0 Open 3 Percutaneous 4 Percutaneous Endoscopic 7 Via Natural or Artificial Opening 8 Via Natural or Artificial Opening Endoscopic	C Robotic Assisted Procedure E Fluorescence Guided Procedure	Z No Qualifier
W Trunk Region	X External	B Computer Assisted Procedure	F With Fluoroscopy G With Computerized Tomography H With Magnetic Resonance Imaging Z No Qualifier
W Trunk Region	X External	C Robotic Assisted Procedure	Z No Qualifier
W Trunk Region	X External	Y Other Method	8 Suture Removal
X Upper Extremity Y Lower Extremity	0 Open 3 Percutaneous 4 Percutaneous Endoscopic	C Robotic Assisted Procedure E Fluorescence Guided Procedure	Z No Qualifier
X Upper Extremity Y Lower Extremity	X External	B Computer Assisted Procedure	F With Fluoroscopy G With Computerized Tomography H With Magnetic Resonance Imaging Z No Qualifier
X Upper Extremity Y Lower Extremity	X External	C Robotic Assisted Procedure	Z No Qualifier
X Upper Extremity Y Lower Extremity	X External	Y Other Method	8 Suture Removal
Z None	X External	Y Other Method	1 In Vitro Fertilization 4 Yoga Therapy 5 Meditation 6 Isolation

Within each section of ICD-10-PCS the characters have different meanings. The seven character meanings for the Chiropractic section are illustrated here through the procedure example of Chiropractic treatment of cervical spine, short lever specific contact.

Section	Body System	Root Operation	Body Region	Approach	Method	Qualifier
Chiropractic	Anatomical Regions	Manipulation	Cervical	External	Short Lever Specific Contact	None
9	W	B	1	X	H	Z

Section (Character 1)

All Chiropractic procedure codes have a first character value of 9.

Body System (Character 2)

The alphanumeric character for the body system is placed in the second position. There is one character value applicable for the Chiropractic section. The character value of W is reported for anatomical regions.

Root Operations (Character 3)

The alphanumeric character value for root operations is placed in the third position. The following is the root operation applicable to the Chiropractic section with its associated meaning.

Character Value	Root Operation	Root Operation Definition
B	Manipulation	Manual procedure that involves a directed thrust to move a joint past the physiological range of motion, without exceeding the anatomical limit

Body Region (Character 4)

For each body region the applicable body part character values will be available for procedure code construction. An example of a body region for this section is Rib Cage.

Approach (Character 5)

The approach is the technique used to reach the procedure site. The following are the approach character values for the Chiropractic section with the associated definitions.

Character Value	Approach	Approach Definition
X	External	Procedures performed directly on the skin or mucous membrane and procedures performed indirectly by the application of external force through the skin or mucous membrane

Method (Character 6)

The method identifies the treatment method used to complete the chiropractic procedure. The available methods are:

- Non-Manual
- Indirect Visceral
- Extra-Articular
- Direct-Visual
- Long Lever Specific Contact
- Short Lever Specific Contact
- Long and Short Lever Specific Contact
- Mechanically Assisted
- Other

Qualifier (Character 7)

The qualifier represents an additional attribute for the procedure when applicable. Currently, there are no qualifiers in the Chiropractic section; therefore, the placeholder character value of Z should be reported.

Chiropractic Section Table

Chiropractic Table 9WB

Section   **9**   **Chiropractic**
Body System   **W**   **Anatomical Regions**
Operation   **B**   **Manipulation:** Manual procedure that involves a directed thrust to move a joint past the physiological range of motion, without exceeding the anatomical limit

Body Region (4th)	Approach (5th)	Method (6th)	Qualifier (7th)
0 Head 1 Cervical 2 Thoracic 3 Lumbar 4 Sacrum 5 Pelvis 6 Lower Extremities 7 Upper Extremities 8 Rib Cage 9 Abdomen	X External	B Non-Manual C Indirect Visceral D Extra-Articular F Direct Visceral G Long Lever Specific Contact H Short Lever Specific Contact J Long and Short Lever Specific Contact K Mechanically Assisted L Other Method	Z None

Within each section of ICD-10-PCS the characters have different meanings. The seven character meanings for the Imaging section are illustrated here through the procedure example of X-ray right clavicle, limited study.

Section	Body System	Root Type	Body Part	Contrast	Qualifier	Qualifier
Imaging	Non-Axial Upper Bones	Plain Radiography	Clavicle, right	None	None	None
B	P	0	4	Z	Z	Z

Section (Character 1)

All Imaging procedure codes have a first character value of B.

Body System (Character 2)

The alphanumeric character for the body system is placed in the second position. The following are the body systems applicable to the Imaging section.

Character Value	Character Value Description
0	Central Nervous System
2	Heart
3	Upper Arteries
4	Lower Arteries
5	Veins
7	Lymphatic System
8	Eye
9	Ear, Nose, Mouth and Throat
B	Respiratory System
D	Gastrointestinal System
F	Hepatobiliary System and Pancreas
G	Endocrine System
H	Skin, Subcutaneous Tissue and Breast
L	Connective Tissue
N	Skull and Facial Bones
P	Non-Axial Upper Bones
Q	Non-Axial Lower Bones
R	Axial Skeleton, Except Skull and Facial Bones
T	Urinary System
U	Female Reproductive System
V	Male Reproductive System
W	Anatomical Regions
Y	Fetus and Obstetrical

Root Types (Character 3)

The alphanumeric character value for root types is placed in the third position. Listed here are the root types applicable to the Imaging section with their associated meaning.

Character Value	Root Type	Root Type Definition
0	Plain Radiography	Planar display of an image developed from the capture of external ionizing radiation on photographic or photoconductive plate
1	Fluoroscopy	Single plane or bi-plane real time display of an image developed from the capture of external ionizing radiation on a fluorescent screen. The image may also be stored by either digital or analog means

Continued →

Character Value	Root Type	Root Type Definition
2	Computerized Tomography (CT Scan)	Computer reformatted digital display of multiplanar images developed from the capture of multiple exposures of external ionizing radiation
3	Magnetic Resonance Imaging (MRI)	Computer reformatted digital display of multiplanar images developed from the capture of radiofrequency signals emitted by nuclei in a body site excited within a magnetic field
4	Ultrasonography	Real time display of images of anatomy or flow information developed from the capture of reflected and attenuated high frequency sound waves
5	Other Imaging	Other specified modality for visualizing a body part

Body Part (Character 4)

For each body part the applicable body part character values will be available for procedure code construction. An example of a body part for this section is Spinal Cord.

Contrast (Character 5)

When contrast is utilized during an imaging procedure, the corresponding contrast character value should be reported in the fifth character position. The following are the contrast character values for the Imaging section:

- High Osmolar
- Low Osmolar
- Other Contrast

If contrast is not utilized, the placeholder character value of Z should be reported.

Qualifier (Character 6)

This qualifier character specifies when an image taken without contrast is followed by one with contrast. The character value of 0 is reported for Unenhanced and Enhanced.

Qualifier (Character 7)

The qualifier represents an additional attribute for the procedure when applicable. For example, ultrasonography procedures in this section include the qualifier Densitometry that is reported with the character value of 1 for some body parts. If there is no qualifier for a procedure, the placeholder Z is the character valve that should be reported.

AHA Coding Clinic

B2151ZZ Fluoroscopy of Left Heart using Low Osmolar Contrast - AHA CC: 1Q, 2018, 12-13

B518ZZA Fluoroscopy of Superior Vena Cava, Guidance, for Fluoroscopic Guidance used to Place the Renal Dialysis Catheter - AHA CC: 4Q, 2015, 30

BF50200 Other Imaging of Bile Ducts using Fluorescing Agent, Indocyanine Green Dye, Intraoperative - AHA CC: 4Q, 2020, 67-68

Imaging Section Tables

Imaging Tables B00–BY4

Section	B	Imaging
Body System	0	Central Nervous System
Type	0	**Plain Radiography:** Planar display of an image developed from the capture of external ionizing radiation on photographic or photoconductive plate

Body Part (4ᵗʰ)	Contrast (5ᵗʰ)	Qualifier (6ᵗʰ)	Qualifier (7ᵗʰ)
B Spinal Cord	**0** High Osmolar **1** Low Osmolar **Y** Other Contrast **Z** None	**Z** None	**Z** None

Section	B	Imaging
Body System	0	Central Nervous System
Type	1	**Fluoroscopy:** Single plane or bi-plane real time display of an image developed from the capture of external ionizing radiation on a fluorescent screen. The image may also be stored by either digital or analog means

Body Part (4ᵗʰ)	Contrast (5ᵗʰ)	Qualifier (6ᵗʰ)	Qualifier (7ᵗʰ)
B Spinal Cord	**0** High Osmolar **1** Low Osmolar **Y** Other Contrast **Z** None	**Z** None	**Z** None

Section   **B**   **Imaging**
Body System   **0**   **Central Nervous System**
Type   **2**   **Computerized Tomography (CT Scan):** Computer reformatted digital display of multiplanar images developed from the capture of multiple exposures of external ionizing radiation

Body Part (4th)	Contrast (5th)	Qualifier (6th)	Qualifier (7th)
0 Brain **7** Cisterna **8** Cerebral Ventricle(s) **9** Sella Turcica/Pituitary Gland **B** Spinal Cord	**0** High Osmolar **1** Low Osmolar **Y** Other Contrast	**0** Unenhanced and Enhanced **Z** None	**Z** None
0 Brain **7** Cisterna **8** Cerebral Ventricle(s) **9** Sella Turcica/Pituitary Gland **B** Spinal Cord	**Z** None	**Z** None	**Z** None

Section   **B**   **Imaging**
Body System   **0**   **Central Nervous System**
Type   **3**   **Magnetic Resonance Imaging (MRI):** Computer reformatted digital display of multiplanar images developed from the capture of radiofrequency signals emitted by nuclei in a body site excited within a magnetic field

Body Part (4th)	Contrast (5th)	Qualifier (6th)	Qualifier (7th)
0 Brain **9** Sella Turcica/Pituitary Gland **B** Spinal Cord **C** Acoustic Nerves	**Y** Other Contrast	**0** Unenhanced and Enhanced **Z** None	**Z** None
0 Brain **9** Sella Turcica/Pituitary Gland **B** Spinal Cord **C** Acoustic Nerves	**Z** None	**Z** None	**Z** None

Section   **B**   **Imaging**
Body System   **0**   **Central Nervous System**
Type   **4**   **Ultrasonography:** Real time display of images of anatomy or flow information developed from the capture of reflected and attenuated high frequency sound waves

Body Part (4th)	Contrast (5th)	Qualifier (6th)	Qualifier (7th)
0 Brain **B** Spinal Cord	**Z** None	**Z** None	**Z** None

Section   **B**   **Imaging**
Body System   **2**   **Heart**
Type   **0**   **Plain Radiography:** Planar display of an image developed from the capture of external ionizing radiation on photographic or photoconductive plate

Body Part (4th)	Contrast (5th)	Qualifier (6th)	Qualifier (7th)
0 Coronary Artery, Single **1** Coronary Arteries, Multiple **2** Coronary Artery Bypass Graft, Single **3** Coronary Artery Bypass Grafts, Multiple **4** Heart, Right **5** Heart, Left **6** Heart, Right and Left **7** Internal Mammary Bypass Graft, Right **8** Internal Mammary Bypass Graft, Left **F** Bypass Graft, Other	**0** High Osmolar **1** Low Osmolar **Y** Other Contrast	**Z** None	**Z** None

Section	B	Imaging
Body System	2	Heart
Type	1	**Fluoroscopy:** Single plane or bi-plane real time display of an image developed from the capture of external ionizing radiation on a fluorescent screen. The image may also be stored by either digital or analog means

Body Part (4th)	Contrast (5th)	Qualifier (6th)	Qualifier (7th)
0 Coronary Artery, Single 1 Coronary Arteries, Multiple 2 Coronary Artery Bypass Graft, Single 3 Coronary Artery Bypass Grafts, Multiple	0 High Osmolar 1 Low Osmolar Y Other Contrast	1 Laser	0 Intraoperative
0 Coronary Artery, Single 1 Coronary Arteries, Multiple 2 Coronary Artery Bypass Graft, Single 3 Coronary Artery Bypass Grafts, Multiple	0 High Osmolar 1 Low Osmolar Y Other Contrast	Z None	Z None
4 Heart, Right 5 Heart, Left 6 Heart, Right and Left 7 Internal Mammary Bypass Graft, Right 8 Internal Mammary Bypass Graft, Left F Bypass Graft, Other	0 High Osmolar 1 Low Osmolar Y Other Contrast	Z None	Z None

Section	B	Imaging
Body System	2	Heart
Type	2	**Computerized Tomography (CT Scan):** Computer reformatted digital display of multiplanar images developed from the capture of multiple exposures of external ionizing radiation

Body Part (4th)	Contrast (5th)	Qualifier (6th)	Qualifier (7th)
1 Coronary Arteries, Multiple 3 Coronary Artery Bypass Grafts, Multiple 6 Heart, Right and Left	0 High Osmolar 1 Low Osmolar Y Other Contrast	0 Unenhanced and Enhanced Z None	Z None
1 Coronary Arteries, Multiple 3 Coronary Artery Bypass Grafts, Multiple 6 Heart, Right and Left	Z None	2 Intravascular Optical Coherence Z None	Z None

Section	B	Imaging
Body System	2	Heart
Type	3	**Magnetic Resonance Imaging (MRI):** Computer reformatted digital display of multiplanar images developed from the capture of radiofrequency signals emitted by nuclei in a body site excited within a magnetic field

Body Part (4th)	Contrast (5th)	Qualifier (6th)	Qualifier (7th)
1 Coronary Arteries, Multiple 3 Coronary Artery Bypass Grafts, Multiple 6 Heart, Right and Left	Y Other Contrast	0 Unenhanced and Enhanced Z None	Z None
1 Coronary Arteries, Multiple 3 Coronary Artery Bypass Grafts, Multiple 6 Heart, Right and Left	Z None	Z None	Z None

Section	B	Imaging
Body System	2	Heart
Type	4	Ultrasonography: Real time display of images of anatomy or flow information developed from the capture of reflected and attenuated high frequency sound waves

Body Part (4ᵗʰ)	Contrast (5ᵗʰ)	Qualifier (6ᵗʰ)	Qualifier (7ᵗʰ)
0 Coronary Artery, Single 1 Coronary Arteries, Multiple 4 Heart, Right 5 Heart, Left 6 Heart, Right and Left B Heart with Aorta C Pericardium D Pediatric Heart	Y Other Contrast	Z None	Z None
0 Coronary Artery, Single 1 Coronary Arteries, Multiple 4 Heart, Right 5 Heart, Left 6 Heart, Right and Left B Heart with Aorta C Pericardium D Pediatric Heart	Z None	Z None	3 Intravascular 4 Transesophageal Z None

Section	B	Imaging
Body System	3	Upper Arteries
Type	0	Plain Radiography: Planar display of an image developed from the capture of external ionizing radiation on photographic or photoconductive plate

Body Part (4ᵗʰ)	Contrast (5ᵗʰ)	Qualifier (6ᵗʰ)	Qualifier (7ᵗʰ)
0 Thoracic Aorta 1 Brachiocephalic-Subclavian Artery, Right 2 Subclavian Artery, Left 3 Common Carotid Artery, Right 4 Common Carotid Artery, Left 5 Common Carotid Arteries, Bilateral 6 Internal Carotid Artery, Right 7 Internal Carotid Artery, Left 8 Internal Carotid Arteries, Bilateral 9 External Carotid Artery, Right B External Carotid Artery, Left C External Carotid Arteries, Bilateral D Vertebral Artery, Right F Vertebral Artery, Left G Vertebral Arteries, Bilateral H Upper Extremity Arteries, Right J Upper Extremity Arteries, Left K Upper Extremity Arteries, Bilateral L Intercostal and Bronchial Arteries M Spinal Arteries N Upper Arteries, Other P Thoraco-Abdominal Aorta Q Cervico-Cerebral Arch R Intracranial Arteries S Pulmonary Artery, Right T Pulmonary Artery, Left	0 High Osmolar 1 Low Osmolar Y Other Contrast Z None	Z None	Z None

Section   **B**   **Imaging**
Body System   **3**   **Upper Arteries**
Type   **1**   **Fluoroscopy:** Single plane or bi-plane real time display of an image developed from the capture of external ionizing radiation on a fluorescent screen. The image may also be stored by either digital or analog means

Body Part (4ᵗʰ)	Contrast (5ᵗʰ)	Qualifier (6ᵗʰ)	Qualifier (7ᵗʰ)
0 Thoracic Aorta	0 High Osmolar	1 Laser	0 Intraoperative
1 Brachiocephalic-Subclavian Artery, Right	1 Low Osmolar		
2 Subclavian Artery, Left	Y Other Contrast		
3 Common Carotid Artery, Right			
4 Common Carotid Artery, Left			
5 Common Carotid Arteries, Bilateral			
6 Internal Carotid Artery, Right			
7 Internal Carotid Artery, Left			
8 Internal Carotid Arteries, Bilateral			
9 External Carotid Artery, Right			
B External Carotid Artery, Left			
C External Carotid Arteries, Bilateral			
D Vertebral Artery, Right			
F Vertebral Artery, Left			
G Vertebral Arteries, Bilateral			
H Upper Extremity Arteries, Right			
J Upper Extremity Arteries, Left			
K Upper Extremity Arteries, Bilateral			
L Intercostal and Bronchial Arteries			
M Spinal Arteries			
N Upper Arteries, Other			
P Thoraco-Abdominal Aorta			
Q Cervico-Cerebral Arch			
R Intracranial Arteries			
S Pulmonary Artery, Right			
T Pulmonary Artery, Left			
U Pulmonary Trunk			
0 Thoracic Aorta	0 High Osmolar	Z None	Z None
1 Brachiocephalic-Subclavian Artery, Right	1 Low Osmolar		
2 Subclavian Artery, Left	Y Other Contrast		
3 Common Carotid Artery, Right			
4 Common Carotid Artery, Left			
5 Common Carotid Arteries, Bilateral			
6 Internal Carotid Artery, Right			
7 Internal Carotid Artery, Left			
8 Internal Carotid Arteries, Bilateral			
9 External Carotid Artery, Right			
B External Carotid Artery, Left			
C External Carotid Arteries, Bilateral			
D Vertebral Artery, Right			
F Vertebral Artery, Left			
G Vertebral Arteries, Bilateral			
H Upper Extremity Arteries, Right			
J Upper Extremity Arteries, Left			
K Upper Extremity Arteries, Bilateral			
L Intercostal and Bronchial Arteries			
M Spinal Arteries			
N Upper Arteries, Other			
P Thoraco-Abdominal Aorta			
Q Cervico-Cerebral Arch			
R Intracranial Arteries			
S Pulmonary Artery, Right			
T Pulmonary Artery, Left			
U Pulmonary Trunk			

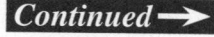 Continued →

Section   **B**   **Imaging**
Body System   **3**   **Upper Arteries**
Type   **1**   **Fluoroscopy:** Single plane or bi-plane real time display of an image developed from the capture of external ionizing radiation on a fluorescent screen. The image may also be stored by either digital or analog means

Body Part (4th)	Contrast (5th)	Qualifier (6th)	Qualifier (7th)
0 Thoracic Aorta 1 Brachiocephalic-Subclavian Artery, Right 2 Subclavian Artery, Left 3 Common Carotid Artery, Right 4 Common Carotid Artery, Left 5 Common Carotid Arteries, Bilateral 6 Internal Carotid Artery, Right 7 Internal Carotid Artery, Left 8 Internal Carotid Arteries, Bilateral 9 External Carotid Artery, Right B External Carotid Artery, Left C External Carotid Arteries, Bilateral D Vertebral Artery, Right F Vertebral Artery, Left G Vertebral Arteries, Bilateral H Upper Extremity Arteries, Right J Upper Extremity Arteries, Left K Upper Extremity Arteries, Bilateral L Intercostal and Bronchial Arteries M Spinal Arteries N Upper Arteries, Other P Thoraco-Abdominal Aorta Q Cervico-Cerebral Arch R Intracranial Arteries S Pulmonary Artery, Right T Pulmonary Artery, Left U Pulmonary Trunk	Z None	Z None	Z None

Section   **B**   **Imaging**
Body System   **3**   **Upper Arteries**
Type   **2**   **Computerized Tomography (CT Scan):** Computer reformatted digital display of multiplanar images developed from the capture of multiple exposures of external ionizing radiation

Body Part (4th)	Contrast (5th)	Qualifier (6th)	Qualifier (7th)
0 Thoracic Aorta 5 Common Carotid Arteries, Bilateral 8 Internal Carotid Arteries, Bilateral G Vertebral Arteries, Bilateral R Intracranial Arteries S Pulmonary Artery, Right T Pulmonary Artery, Left	0 High Osmolar 1 Low Osmolar Y Other Contrast	Z None	Z None
0 Thoracic Aorta 5 Common Carotid Arteries, Bilateral 8 Internal Carotid Arteries, Bilateral G Vertebral Arteries, Bilateral R Intracranial Arteries S Pulmonary Artery, Right T Pulmonary Artery, Left	Z None	2 Intravascular Optical Coherence Z None	Z None

Section	B	Imaging
Body System	3	Upper Arteries
Type	3	**Magnetic Resonance Imaging (MRI):** Computer reformatted digital display of multiplanar images developed from the capture of radiofrequency signals emitted by nuclei in a body site excited within a magnetic field

Body Part (4ᵗʰ)	Contrast (5ᵗʰ)	Qualifier (6ᵗʰ)	Qualifier (7ᵗʰ)
0 Thoracic Aorta 5 Common Carotid Arteries, Bilateral 8 Internal Carotid Arteries, Bilateral G Vertebral Arteries, Bilateral H Upper Extremity Arteries, Right J Upper Extremity Arteries, Left K Upper Extremity Arteries, Bilateral M Spinal Arteries Q Cervico-Cerebral Arch R Intracranial Arteries	Y Other Contrast	0 Unenhanced and Enhanced Z None	Z None
0 Thoracic Aorta 5 Common Carotid Arteries, Bilateral 8 Internal Carotid Arteries, Bilateral G Vertebral Arteries, Bilateral H Upper Extremity Arteries, Right J Upper Extremity Arteries, Left K Upper Extremity Arteries, Bilateral M Spinal Arteries Q Cervico-Cerebral Arch R Intracranial Arteries	Z None	Z None	Z None

Section	B	Imaging
Body System	3	Upper Arteries
Type	4	**Ultrasonography:** Real time display of images of anatomy or flow information developed from the capture of reflected and attenuated high frequency sound waves

Body Part (4ᵗʰ)	Contrast (5ᵗʰ)	Qualifier (6ᵗʰ)	Qualifier (7ᵗʰ)
0 Thoracic Aorta 1 Brachiocephalic-Subclavian Artery, Right 2 Subclavian Artery, Left 3 Common Carotid Artery, Right 4 Common Carotid Artery, Left 5 Common Carotid Arteries, Bilateral 6 Internal Carotid Artery, Right 7 Internal Carotid Artery, Left 8 Internal Carotid Arteries, Bilateral H Upper Extremity Arteries, Right J Upper Extremity Arteries, Left K Upper Extremity Arteries, Bilateral R Intracranial Arteries S Pulmonary Artery, Right T Pulmonary Artery, Left V Ophthalmic Arteries	Z None	Z None	3 Intravascular Z None

Section **B** **Imaging**
Body System **4** **Lower Arteries**
Type **0** **Plain Radiography:** Planar display of an image developed from the capture of external ionizing radiation on photographic or photoconductive plate

Body Part (4th)	Contrast (5th)	Qualifier (6th)	Qualifier (7th)
0 Abdominal Aorta	0 High Osmolar	Z None	Z None
2 Hepatic Artery	1 Low Osmolar		
3 Splenic Arteries	Y Other Contrast		
4 Superior Mesenteric Artery			
5 Inferior Mesenteric Artery			
6 Renal Artery, Right			
7 Renal Artery, Left			
8 Renal Arteries, Bilateral			
9 Lumbar Arteries			
B Intra-Abdominal Arteries, Other			
C Pelvic Arteries			
D Aorta and Bilateral Lower Extremity Arteries			
F Lower Extremity Arteries, Right			
G Lower Extremity Arteries, Left			
J Lower Arteries, Other			
M Renal Artery Transplant			

Section **B** **Imaging**
Body System **4** **Lower Arteries**
Type **1** **Fluoroscopy:** Single plane or bi-plane real time display of an image developed from the capture of external ionizing radiation on a fluorescent screen. The image may also be stored by either digital or analog means

Body Part (4th)	Contrast (5th)	Qualifier (6th)	Qualifier (7th)
0 Abdominal Aorta	0 High Osmolar	1 Laser	0 Intraoperative
2 Hepatic Artery	1 Low Osmolar		
3 Splenic Arteries	Y Other Contrast		
4 Superior Mesenteric Artery			
5 Inferior Mesenteric Artery			
6 Renal Artery, Right			
7 Renal Artery, Left			
8 Renal Arteries, Bilateral			
9 Lumbar Arteries			
B Intra-Abdominal Arteries, Other			
C Pelvic Arteries			
D Aorta and Bilateral Lower Extremity Arteries			
F Lower Extremity Arteries, Right			
G Lower Extremity Arteries, Left			
J Lower Arteries, Other			
0 Abdominal Aorta	0 High Osmolar	Z None	Z None
2 Hepatic Artery	1 Low Osmolar		
3 Splenic Arteries	Y Other Contrast		
4 Superior Mesenteric Artery			
5 Inferior Mesenteric Artery			
6 Renal Artery, Right			
7 Renal Artery, Left			
8 Renal Arteries, Bilateral			
9 Lumbar Arteries			
B Intra-Abdominal Arteries, Other			
C Pelvic Arteries			
D Aorta and Bilateral Lower Extremity Arteries			
F Lower Extremity Arteries, Right			
G Lower Extremity Arteries, Left			
J Lower Arteries, Other			

Continued →

Section **B** Imaging
Body System **4** Lower Arteries
Type **1** **Fluoroscopy:** Single plane or bi-plane real time display of an image developed from the capture of external ionizing radiation on a fluorescent screen. The image may also be stored by either digital or analog means

Body Part (4ᵗʰ)	Contrast (5ᵗʰ)	Qualifier (6ᵗʰ)	Qualifier (7ᵗʰ)
0 Abdominal Aorta **2** Hepatic Artery **3** Splenic Arteries **4** Superior Mesenteric Artery **5** Inferior Mesenteric Artery **6** Renal Artery, Right **7** Renal Artery, Left **8** Renal Arteries, Bilateral **9** Lumbar Arteries **B** Intra-Abdominal Arteries, Other **C** Pelvic Arteries **D** Aorta and Bilateral Lower Extremity Arteries **F** Lower Extremity Arteries, Right **G** Lower Extremity Arteries, Left **J** Lower Arteries, Other	**Z** None	**Z** None	**Z** None

Section **B** Imaging
Body System **4** Lower Arteries
Type **2** **Computerized Tomography (CT Scan):** Computer reformatted digital display of multiplanar images developed from the capture of multiple exposures of external ionizing radiation

Body Part (4ᵗʰ)	Contrast (5ᵗʰ)	Qualifier (6ᵗʰ)	Qualifier (7ᵗʰ)
0 Abdominal Aorta **1** Celiac Artery **4** Superior Mesenteric Artery **8** Renal Arteries, Bilateral **C** Pelvic Arteries **F** Lower Extremity Arteries, Right **G** Lower Extremity Arteries, Left **H** Lower Extremity Arteries, Bilateral **M** Renal Artery Transplant	**0** High Osmolar **1** Low Osmolar **Y** Other Contrast	**Z** None	**Z** None
0 Abdominal Aorta **1** Celiac Artery **4** Superior Mesenteric Artery **8** Renal Arteries, Bilateral **C** Pelvic Arteries **F** Lower Extremity Arteries, Right **G** Lower Extremity Arteries, Left **H** Lower Extremity Arteries, Bilateral **M** Renal Artery Transplant	**Z** None	**2** Intravascular Optical Coherence **Z** None	**Z** None

Section **B** Imaging
Body System **4** Lower Arteries
Type **3** **Magnetic Resonance Imaging (MRI):** Computer reformatted digital display of multiplanar images developed from the capture of radiofrequency signals emitted by nuclei in a body site excited within a magnetic field

Body Part (4ᵗʰ)	Contrast (5ᵗʰ)	Qualifier (6ᵗʰ)	Qualifier (7ᵗʰ)
0 Abdominal Aorta **1** Celiac Artery **4** Superior Mesenteric Artery **8** Renal Arteries, Bilateral **C** Pelvic Arteries **F** Lower Extremity Arteries, Right **G** Lower Extremity Arteries, Left **H** Lower Extremity Arteries, Bilateral	**Y** Other Contrast	**0** Unenhanced and Enhanced **Z** None	**Z** None

Continued →

Section	B	Imaging
Body System	4	Lower Arteries
Type	3	**Magnetic Resonance Imaging (MRI):** Computer reformatted digital display of multiplanar images developed from the capture of radiofrequency signals emitted by nuclei in a body site excited within a magnetic field

Body Part (4th)	Contrast (5th)	Qualifier (6th)	Qualifier (7th)
0 Abdominal Aorta 1 Celiac Artery 4 Superior Mesenteric Artery 8 Renal Arteries, Bilateral C Pelvic Arteries F Lower Extremity Arteries, Right G Lower Extremity Arteries, Left H Lower Extremity Arteries, Bilateral	Z None	Z None	Z None

Section	B	Imaging
Body System	4	Lower Arteries
Type	4	**Ultrasonography:** Real time display of images of anatomy or flow information developed from the capture of reflected and attenuated high frequency sound waves

Body Part (4th)	Contrast (5th)	Qualifier (6th)	Qualifier (7th)
0 Abdominal Aorta 4 Superior Mesenteric Artery 5 Inferior Mesenteric Artery 6 Renal Artery, Right 7 Renal Artery, Left 8 Renal Arteries, Bilateral B Intra-Abdominal Arteries, Other F Lower Extremity Arteries, Right G Lower Extremity Arteries, Left H Lower Extremity Arteries, Bilateral K Celiac and Mesenteric Arteries L Femoral Artery N Penile Arteries	Z None	Z None	3 Intravascular Z None

Section	B	Imaging
Body System	5	Veins
Type	0	**Plain Radiography:** Planar display of an image developed from the capture of external ionizing radiation on photographic or photoconductive plate

Body Part (4th)	Contrast (5th)	Qualifier (6th)	Qualifier (7th)
0 Epidural Veins	0 High Osmolar	Z None	Z None
1 Cerebral and Cerebellar Veins	1 Low Osmolar		
2 Intracranial Sinuses	Y Other Contrast		
3 Jugular Veins, Right			
4 Jugular Veins, Left			
5 Jugular Veins, Bilateral			
6 Subclavian Vein, Right			
7 Subclavian Vein, Left			
8 Superior Vena Cava			
9 Inferior Vena Cava			
B Lower Extremity Veins, Right			
C Lower Extremity Veins, Left			
D Lower Extremity Veins, Bilateral			
F Pelvic (Iliac) Veins, Right			
G Pelvic (Iliac) Veins, Left			
H Pelvic (Iliac) Veins, Bilateral			
J Renal Vein, Right			
K Renal Vein, Left			
L Renal Veins, Bilateral			
M Upper Extremity Veins, Right			
N Upper Extremity Veins, Left			
P Upper Extremity Veins, Bilateral			
Q Pulmonary Vein, Right			
R Pulmonary Vein, Left			
S Pulmonary Veins, Bilateral			
T Portal and Splanchnic Veins			
V Veins, Other			
W Dialysis Shunt/Fistula			

Section	B	Imaging
Body System	5	Veins
Type	1	**Fluoroscopy:** Single plane or bi-plane real time display of an image developed from the capture of external ionizing radiation on a fluorescent screen. The image may also be stored by either digital or analog means

Body Part (4th)	Contrast (5th)	Qualifier (6th)	Qualifier (7th)
0 Epidural Veins	0 High Osmolar	Z None	A Guidance
1 Cerebral and Cerebellar Veins	1 Low Osmolar		Z None
2 Intracranial Sinuses	Y Other Contrast		
3 Jugular Veins, Right	Z None		
4 Jugular Veins, Left			
5 Jugular Veins, Bilateral			
6 Subclavian Vein, Right			
7 Subclavian Vein, Left			
8 Superior Vena Cava			
9 Inferior Vena Cava			
B Lower Extremity Veins, Right			
C Lower Extremity Veins, Left			
D Lower Extremity Veins, Bilateral			
F Pelvic (Iliac) Veins, Right			
G Pelvic (Iliac) Veins, Left			
H Pelvic (Iliac) Veins, Bilateral			
J Renal Vein, Right			
K Renal Vein, Left			
L Renal Veins, Bilateral			
M Upper Extremity Veins, Right			
N Upper Extremity Veins, Left			
P Upper Extremity Veins, Bilateral			
Q Pulmonary Vein, Right			
R Pulmonary Vein, Left			
S Pulmonary Veins, Bilateral			
T Portal and Splanchnic Veins			
V Veins, Other			
W Dialysis Shunt/Fistula			

Section   **B**   Imaging
Body System   **5**   Veins
Type   **2**   **Computerized Tomography (CT Scan):** Computer reformatted digital display of multiplanar images developed from the capture of multiple exposures of external ionizing radiation

Body Part (4th)	Contrast (5th)	Qualifier (6th)	Qualifier (7th)
2 Intracranial Sinuses 8 Superior Vena Cava 9 Inferior Vena Cava F Pelvic (Iliac) Veins, Right G Pelvic (Iliac) Veins, Left H Pelvic (Iliac) Veins, Bilateral J Renal Vein, Right K Renal Vein, Left L Renal Veins, Bilateral Q Pulmonary Vein, Right R Pulmonary Vein, Left S Pulmonary Veins, Bilateral T Portal and Splanchnic Veins	0 High Osmolar 1 Low Osmolar Y Other Contrast	0 Unenhanced and Enhanced Z None	Z None
2 Intracranial Sinuses 8 Superior Vena Cava 9 Inferior Vena Cava F Pelvic (Iliac) Veins, Right G Pelvic (Iliac) Veins, Left H Pelvic (Iliac) Veins, Bilateral J Renal Vein, Right	Z None	2 Intravascular Optical Coherence Z None	Z None
K Renal Vein, Left L Renal Veins, Bilateral Q Pulmonary Vein, Right R Pulmonary Vein, Left S Pulmonary Veins, Bilateral T Portal and Splanchnic Veins			

Section   **B**   Imaging
Body System   **5**   Veins
Type   **3**   **Magnetic Resonance Imaging (MRI):** Computer reformatted digital display of multiplanar images developed from the capture of radiofrequency signals emitted by nuclei in a body site excited within a magnetic field

Body Part (4th)	Contrast (5th)	Qualifier (6th)	Qualifier (7th)
1 Cerebral and Cerebellar Veins 2 Intracranial Sinuses 5 Jugular Veins, Bilateral 8 Superior Vena Cava 9 Inferior Vena Cava B Lower Extremity Veins, Right C Lower Extremity Veins, Left D Lower Extremity Veins, Bilateral H Pelvic (Iliac) Veins, Bilateral L Renal Veins, Bilateral M Upper Extremity Veins, Right N Upper Extremity Veins, Left P Upper Extremity Veins, Bilateral S Pulmonary Veins, Bilateral T Portal and Splanchnic Veins V Veins, Other	Y Other Contrast	0 Unenhanced and Enhanced Z None	Z None

Continued →

Section	B	Imaging
Body System	5	Veins
Type	3	**Magnetic Resonance Imaging (MRI):** Computer reformatted digital display of multiplanar images developed from the capture of radiofrequency signals emitted by nuclei in a body site excited within a magnetic field

Body Part (4th)	Contrast (5th)	Qualifier (6th)	Qualifier (7th)
1 Cerebral and Cerebellar Veins	Z None	Z None	Z None
2 Intracranial Sinuses			
5 Jugular Veins, Bilateral			
8 Superior Vena Cava			
9 Inferior Vena Cava			
B Lower Extremity Veins, Right			
C Lower Extremity Veins, Left			
D Lower Extremity Veins, Bilateral			
H Pelvic (Iliac) Veins, Bilateral			
L Renal Veins, Bilateral			
M Upper Extremity Veins, Right			
N Upper Extremity Veins, Left			
P Upper Extremity Veins, Bilateral			
S Pulmonary Veins, Bilateral			
T Portal and Splanchnic Veins			
V Veins, Other			

Section	B	Imaging
Body System	5	Veins
Type	4	**Ultrasonography:** Real time display of images of anatomy or flow information developed from the capture of reflected and attenuated high frequency sound waves

Body Part (4th)	Contrast (5th)	Qualifier (6th)	Qualifier (7th)
3 Jugular Veins, Right	Z None	Z None	3 Intravascular
4 Jugular Veins, Left			A Guidance
6 Subclavian Vein, Right			Z None
7 Subclavian Vein, Left			
8 Superior Vena Cava			
9 Inferior Vena Cava			
B Lower Extremity Veins, Right			
C Lower Extremity Veins, Left			
D Lower Extremity Veins, Bilateral			
J Renal Vein, Right			
K Renal Vein, Left			
L Renal Veins, Bilateral			
M Upper Extremity Veins, Right			
N Upper Extremity Veins, Left			
P Upper Extremity Veins, Bilateral			
T Portal and Splanchnic Veins			

Section	B	Imaging
Body System	7	Lymphatic System
Type	0	**Plain Radiography:** Planar display of an image developed from the capture of external ionizing radiation on photographic or photoconductive plate

Body Part (4th)	Contrast (5th)	Qualifier (6th)	Qualifier (7th)
0 Abdominal/Retroperitoneal Lymphatics, Unilateral	0 High Osmolar	Z None	Z None
1 Abdominal/Retroperitoneal Lymphatics, Bilateral	1 Low Osmolar		
4 Lymphatics, Head and Neck	Y Other Contrast		
5 Upper Extremity Lymphatics, Right			
6 Upper Extremity Lymphatics, Left			
7 Upper Extremity Lymphatics, Bilateral			
8 Lower Extremity Lymphatics, Right			
9 Lower Extremity Lymphatics, Left			
B Lower Extremity Lymphatics, Bilateral			
C Lymphatics, Pelvic			

Section   B   **Imaging**
Body System   8   **Eye**
Type   0   **Plain Radiography:** Planar display of an image developed from the capture of external ionizing radiation on photographic or photoconductive plate

Body Part (4th)	Contrast (5th)	Qualifier (6th)	Qualifier (7th)
0 Lacrimal Duct, Right 1 Lacrimal Duct, Left 2 Lacrimal Ducts, Bilateral	0 High Osmolar 1 Low Osmolar Y Other Contrast	Z None	Z None
3 Optic Foramina, Right 4 Optic Foramina, Left 5 Eye, Right 6 Eye, Left 7 Eyes, Bilateral	Z None	Z None	Z None

Section   B   **Imaging**
Body System   8   **Eye**
Type   2   **Computerized Tomography (CT Scan):** Computer reformatted digital display of multiplanar images developed from the capture of multiple exposures of external ionizing radiation

Body Part (4th)	Contrast (5th)	Qualifier (6th)	Qualifier (7th)
5 Eye, Right 6 Eye, Left 7 Eyes, Bilateral	0 High Osmolar 1 Low Osmolar Y Other Contrast	0 Unenhanced and Enhanced Z None	Z None
5 Eye, Right 6 Eye, Left 7 Eyes, Bilateral	Z None	Z None	Z None

Section   B   **Imaging**
Body System   8   **Eye**
Type   3   **Magnetic Resonance Imaging (MRI):** Computer reformatted digital display of multiplanar images developed from the capture of radiofrequency signals emitted by nuclei in a body site excited within a magnetic field

Body Part (4th)	Contrast (5th)	Qualifier (6th)	Qualifier (7th)
5 Eye, Right 6 Eye, Left 7 Eyes, Bilateral	Y Other Contrast	0 Unenhanced and Enhanced Z None	Z None
5 Eye, Right 6 Eye, Left 7 Eyes, Bilateral	Z None	Z None	Z None

Section   B   **Imaging**
Body System   8   **Eye**
Type   4   **Ultrasonography:** Real time display of images of anatomy or flow information developed from the capture of reflected and attenuated high frequency sound waves

Body Part (4th)	Contrast (5th)	Qualifier (6th)	Qualifier (7th)
5 Eye, Right 6 Eye, Left 7 Eyes, Bilateral	Z None	Z None	Z None

Section **B** Imaging
Body System **9** Ear, Nose, Mouth and Throat
Type **0** **Plain Radiography:** Planar display of an image developed from the capture of external ionizing radiation on photographic or photoconductive plate

Body Part (4th)	Contrast (5th)	Qualifier (6th)	Qualifier (7th)
2 Paranasal Sinuses **F** Nasopharynx/Oropharynx **H** Mastoids	**Z** None	**Z** None	**Z** None
4 Parotid Gland, Right **5** Parotid Gland, Left **6** Parotid Glands, Bilateral **7** Submandibular Gland, Right **8** Submandibular Gland, Left **9** Submandibular Glands, Bilateral **B** Salivary Gland, Right **C** Salivary Gland, Left **D** Salivary Glands, Bilateral	**0** High Osmolar **1** Low Osmolar **Y** Other Contrast	**Z** None	**Z** None

Section **B** Imaging
Body System **9** Ear, Nose, Mouth and Throat
Type **1** **Fluoroscopy:** Single plane or bi-plane real time display of an image developed from the capture of external ionizing radiation on a fluorescent screen. The image may also be stored by either digital or analog means

Body Part (4th)	Contrast (5th)	Qualifier (6th)	Qualifier (7th)
G Pharynx and Epiglottis **J** Larynx	**Y** Other Contrast **Z** None	**Z** None	**Z** None

Section **B** Imaging
Body System **9** Ear, Nose, Mouth and Throat
Type **2** **Computerized Tomography (CT Scan):** Computer reformatted digital display of multiplanar images developed from the capture of multiple exposures of external ionizing radiation

Body Part (4th)	Contrast (5th)	Qualifier (6th)	Qualifier (7th)
0 Ear **2** Paranasal Sinuses **6** Parotid Glands, Bilateral **9** Submandibular Glands, Bilateral **D** Salivary Glands, Bilateral **F** Nasopharynx/Oropharynx **J** Larynx	**0** High Osmolar **1** Low Osmolar **Y** Other Contrast	**0** Unenhanced and Enhanced **Z** None	**Z** None
0 Ear **2** Paranasal Sinuses **6** Parotid Glands, Bilateral **9** Submandibular Glands, Bilateral **D** Salivary Glands, Bilateral **F** Nasopharynx/Oropharynx **J** Larynx	**Z** None	**Z** None	**Z** None

Section **B** Imaging
Body System **9** Ear, Nose, Mouth and Throat
Type **3** **Magnetic Resonance Imaging (MRI):** Computer reformatted digital display of multiplanar images developed from the capture of radiofrequency signals emitted by nuclei in a body site excited within a magnetic field

Body Part (4th)	Contrast (5th)	Qualifier (6th)	Qualifier (7th)
0 Ear **2** Paranasal Sinuses **6** Parotid Glands, Bilateral **9** Submandibular Glands, Bilateral **D** Salivary Glands, Bilateral **F** Nasopharynx/Oropharynx **J** Larynx	**Y** Other Contrast	**0** Unenhanced and Enhanced **Z** None	**Z** None

Continued →

Section   **B**   **Imaging**
Body System   **9**   **Ear, Nose, Mouth and Throat**
Type   **3**   **Magnetic Resonance Imaging (MRI):** Computer reformatted digital display of multiplanar images developed from the capture of radiofrequency signals emitted by nuclei in a body site excited within a magnetic field

Body Part (4th)	Contrast (5th)	Qualifier (6th)	Qualifier (7th)
0 Ear **2** Paranasal Sinuses **6** Parotid Glands, Bilateral **9** Submandibular Glands, Bilateral **D** Salivary Glands, Bilateral **F** Nasopharynx/Oropharynx **J** Larynx	**Z** None	**Z** None	**Z** None

Section   **B**   **Imaging**
Body System   **B**   **Respiratory System**
Type   **0**   **Plain Radiography:** Planar display of an image developed from the capture of external ionizing radiation on photographic or photoconductive plate

Body Part (4th)	Contrast (5th)	Qualifier (6th)	Qualifier (7th)
7 Tracheobronchial Tree, Right **8** Tracheobronchial Tree, Left **9** Tracheobronchial Trees, Bilateral	**Y** Other Contrast	**Z** None	**Z** None
D Upper Airways	**Z** None	**Z** None	**Z** None

Section   **B**   **Imaging**
Body System   **B**   **Respiratory System**
Type   **1**   **Fluoroscopy:** Single plane or bi-plane real time display of an image developed from the capture of external ionizing radiation on a fluorescent screen. The image may also be stored by either digital or analog means

Body Part (4th)	Contrast (5th)	Qualifier (6th)	Qualifier (7th)
2 Lung, Right **3** Lung, Left **4** Lungs, Bilateral **6** Diaphragm **C** Mediastinum **D** Upper Airways	**Z** None	**Z** None	**Z** None
7 Tracheobronchial Tree, Right **8** Tracheobronchial Tree, Left **9** Tracheobronchial Trees, Bilateral	**Y** Other Contrast	**Z** None	**Z** None

Section   **B**   **Imaging**
Body System   **B**   **Respiratory System**
Type   **2**   **Computerized Tomography (CT Scan):** Computer reformatted digital display of multiplanar images developed from the capture of multiple exposures of external ionizing radiation

Body Part (4th)	Contrast (5th)	Qualifier (6th)	Qualifier (7th)
4 Lungs, Bilateral **7** Tracheobronchial Tree, Right **8** Tracheobronchial Tree, Left **9** Tracheobronchial Trees, Bilateral **F** Trachea/Airways	**0** High Osmolar **1** Low Osmolar **Y** Other Contrast	**0** Unenhanced and Enhanced **Z** None	**Z** None
4 Lungs, Bilateral **7** Tracheobronchial Tree, Right **8** Tracheobronchial Tree, Left **9** Tracheobronchial Trees, Bilateral **F** Trachea/Airways	**Z** None	**Z** None	**Z** None

Section   **B**   **Imaging**
Body System   **B**   **Respiratory System**
Type   **3**   **Magnetic Resonance Imaging (MRI):** Computer reformatted digital display of multiplanar images developed from the capture of radiofrequency signals emitted by nuclei in a body site excited within a magnetic field

Body Part (4th)	Contrast (5th)	Qualifier (6th)	Qualifier (7th)
G Lung Apices	Y Other Contrast	0 Unenhanced and Enhanced Z None	Z None
G Lung Apices	Z None	Z None	Z None

Section   **B**   **Imaging**
Body System   **B**   **Respiratory System**
Type   **4**   **Ultrasonography:** Real time display of images of anatomy or flow information developed from the capture of reflected and attenuated high frequency sound waves

Body Part (4th)	Contrast (5th)	Qualifier (6th)	Qualifier (7th)
B Pleura C Mediastinum	Z None	Z None	Z None

Section   **B**   **Imaging**
Body System   **D**   **Gastrointestinal System**
Type   **1**   **Fluoroscopy:** Single plane or bi-plane real time display of an image developed from the capture of external ionizing radiation on a fluorescent screen. The image may also be stored by either digital or analog means

Body Part (4th)	Contrast (5th)	Qualifier (6th)	Qualifier (7th)
1 Esophagus 2 Stomach 3 Small Bowel 4 Colon 5 Upper GI 6 Upper GI and Small Bowel 9 Duodenum B Mouth/Oropharynx	Y Other Contrast Z None	Z None	Z None

Section   **B**   **Imaging**
Body System   **D**   **Gastrointestinal System**
Type   **2**   **Computerized Tomography (CT Scan):** Computer reformatted digital display of multiplanar images developed from the capture of multiple exposures of external ionizing radiation

Body Part (4th)	Contrast (5th)	Qualifier (6th)	Qualifier (7th)
4 Colon	0 High Osmolar 1 Low Osmolar Y Other Contrast	0 Unenhanced and Enhanced Z None	Z None
4 Colon	Z None	Z None	Z None

Section   **B**   **Imaging**
Body System   **D**   **Gastrointestinal System**
Type   **4**   **Ultrasonography:** Real time display of images of anatomy or flow information developed from the capture of reflected and attenuated high frequency sound waves

Body Part (4th)	Contrast (5th)	Qualifier (6th)	Qualifier (7th)
1 Esophagus 2 Stomach 7 Gastrointestinal Tract 8 Appendix 9 Duodenum C Rectum	Z None	Z None	Z None

Section	B	Imaging
Body System	F	Hepatobiliary System and Pancreas
Type	0	**Plain Radiography:** Planar display of an image developed from the capture of external ionizing radiation on photographic or photoconductive plate

Body Part (4th)	Contrast (5th)	Qualifier (6th)	Qualifier (7th)
0 Bile Ducts **3** Gallbladder and Bile Ducts **C** Hepatobiliary System, All	**0** High Osmolar **1** Low Osmolar **Y** Other Contrast	**Z** None	**Z** None

Section	B	Imaging
Body System	F	Hepatobiliary System and Pancreas
Type	1	**Fluoroscopy:** Single plane or bi-plane real time display of an image developed from the capture of external ionizing radiation on a fluorescent screen. The image may also be stored by either digital or analog means

Body Part (4th)	Contrast (5th)	Qualifier (6th)	Qualifier (7th)
0 Bile Ducts **1** Biliary and Pancreatic Ducts **2** Gallbladder **3** Gallbladder and Bile Ducts **4** Gallbladder, Bile Ducts and Pancreatic Ducts **8** Pancreatic Ducts	**0** High Osmolar **1** Low Osmolar **Y** Other Contrast	**Z** None	**Z** None
5 Liver	**0** High Osmolar **1** Low Osmolar **Y** Other Contrast	**Z** None	**Z** None
5 Liver	**Z** None	**Z** None	**A** Guidance

Section	B	Imaging
Body System	F	Hepatobiliary System and Pancreas
Type	2	**Computerized Tomography (CT Scan):** Computer reformatted digital display of multiplanar images developed from the capture of multiple exposures of external ionizing radiation

Body Part (4th)	Contrast (5th)	Qualifier (6th)	Qualifier (7th)
5 Liver **6** Liver and Spleen **7** Pancreas **C** Hepatobiliary System, All	**0** High Osmolar **1** Low Osmolar **Y** Other Contrast	**0** Unenhanced and Enhanced **Z** None	**Z** None
5 Liver **6** Liver and Spleen **7** Pancreas **C** Hepatobiliary System, All	**Z** None	**Z** None	**Z** None

Section	B	Imaging
Body System	F	Hepatobiliary System and Pancreas
Type	3	**Magnetic Resonance Imaging (MRI):** Computer reformatted digital display of multiplanar images developed from the capture of radiofrequency signals emitted by nuclei in a body site excited within a magnetic field

Body Part (4th)	Contrast (5th)	Qualifier (6th)	Qualifier (7th)
5 Liver **6** Liver and Spleen **7** Pancreas	**Y** Other Contrast	**0** Unenhanced and Enhanced **Z** None	**Z** None
5 Liver **6** Liver and Spleen **7** Pancreas	**Z** None	**Z** None	**Z** None

1451

Section **B** **Imaging**
Body System **F** **Hepatobiliary System and Pancreas**
Type **4** **Ultrasonography:** Real time display of images of anatomy or flow information developed from the capture of reflected and attenuated high frequency sound waves

Body Part (4th)	Contrast (5th)	Qualifier (6th)	Qualifier (7th)
0 Bile Ducts **2** Gallbladder **3** Gallbladder and Bile Ducts **5** Liver **6** Liver and Spleen **7** Pancreas **C** Hepatobiliary System, All	**Z** None	**Z** None	**Z** None

Section **B** **Imaging**
Body System **F** **Hepatobiliary System and Pancreas**
Operation **5** **Other Imaging:** Other specified modality for visualizing a body part

Body Part (4th)	Approach (5th)	Device (6th)	Qualifier (7th)
0 Bile Ducts **2** Gallbladder **3** Gallbladder and Bile Ducts **5** Liver **6** Liver and Spleen **7** Pancreas **C** Hepatobiliary System, All	**2** Fluorescing Agent	**0** Indocyanine Green Dye **Z** None	**0** Intraoperative **Z** None

Section **B** **Imaging**
Body System **G** **Endocrine System**
Type **2** **Computerized Tomography (CT Scan):** Computer reformatted digital display of multiplanar images developed from the capture of multiple exposures of external ionizing radiation

Body Part (4th)	Contrast (5th)	Qualifier (6th)	Qualifier (7th)
2 Adrenal Glands, Bilateral **3** Parathyroid Glands **4** Thyroid Gland	**0** High Osmolar **1** Low Osmolar **Y** Other Contrast	**0** Unenhanced and Enhanced **Z** None	**Z** None
2 Adrenal Glands, Bilateral **3** Parathyroid Glands **4** Thyroid Gland	**Z** None	**Z** None	**Z** None

Section **B** **Imaging**
Body System **G** **Endocrine System**
Type **3** **Magnetic Resonance Imaging (MRI):** Computer reformatted digital display of multiplanar images developed from the capture of radiofrequency signals emitted by nuclei in a body site excited within a magnetic field

Body Part (4th)	Contrast (5th)	Qualifier (6th)	Qualifier (7th)
2 Adrenal Glands, Bilateral **3** Parathyroid Glands **4** Thyroid Gland	**Y** Other Contrast	**0** Unenhanced and Enhanced **Z** None	**Z** None
2 Adrenal Glands, Bilateral **3** Parathyroid Glands **4** Thyroid Gland	**Z** None	**Z** None	**Z** None

Section	B	Imaging
Body System	G	Endocrine System
Type	4	Ultrasonography: Real time display of images of anatomy or flow information developed from the capture of reflected and attenuated high frequency sound waves

Body Part (4th)	Contrast (5th)	Qualifier (6th)	Qualifier (7th)
0 Adrenal Gland, Right 1 Adrenal Gland, Left 2 Adrenal Glands, Bilateral 3 Parathyroid Glands 4 Thyroid Gland	Z None	Z None	Z None

Section	B	Imaging
Body System	H	Skin, Subcutaneous Tissue and Breast
Type	0	Plain Radiography: Planar display of an image developed from the capture of external ionizing radiation on photographic or photoconductive plate

Body Part (4th)	Contrast (5th)	Qualifier (6th)	Qualifier (7th)
0 Breast, Right 1 Breast, Left 2 Breasts, Bilateral	Z None	Z None	Z None
3 Single Mammary Duct, Right 4 Single Mammary Duct, Left 5 Multiple Mammary Ducts, Right 6 Multiple Mammary Ducts, Left	0 High Osmolar 1 Low Osmolar Y Other Contrast Z None	Z None	Z None

Section	B	Imaging
Body System	H	Skin, Subcutaneous Tissue and Breast
Type	3	Magnetic Resonance Imaging (MRI): Computer reformatted digital display of multiplanar images developed from the capture of radiofrequency signals emitted by nuclei in a body site excited within a magnetic field

Body Part (4th)	Contrast (5th)	Qualifier (6th)	Qualifier (7th)
0 Breast, Right 1 Breast, Left 2 Breasts, Bilateral D Subcutaneous Tissue, Head/Neck F Subcutaneous Tissue, Upper Extremity G Subcutaneous Tissue, Thorax H Subcutaneous Tissue, Abdomen and Pelvis J Subcutaneous Tissue, Lower Extremity	Y Other Contrast	0 Unenhanced and Enhanced Z None	Z None
0 Breast, Right 1 Breast, Left 2 Breasts, Bilateral D Subcutaneous Tissue, Head/Neck F Subcutaneous Tissue, Upper Extremity G Subcutaneous Tissue, Thorax H Subcutaneous Tissue, Abdomen and Pelvis J Subcutaneous Tissue, Lower Extremity	Z None	Z None	Z None

Section	B	Imaging
Body System	H	Skin, Subcutaneous Tissue and Breast
Type	4	Ultrasonography: Real time display of images of anatomy or flow information developed from the capture of reflected and attenuated high frequency sound waves

Body Part (4th)	Contrast (5th)	Qualifier (6th)	Qualifier (7th)
0 Breast, Right 1 Breast, Left 2 Breasts, Bilateral 7 Extremity, Upper 8 Extremity, Lower 9 Abdominal Wall B Chest Wall C Head and Neck	Z None	Z None	Z None

Section	B	Imaging
Body System	L	Connective Tissue
Type	3	**Magnetic Resonance Imaging (MRI):** Computer reformatted digital display of multiplanar images developed from the capture of radiofrequency signals emitted by nuclei in a body site excited within a magnetic field

Body Part (4th)	Contrast (5th)	Qualifier (6th)	Qualifier (7th)
0 Connective Tissue, Upper Extremity **1** Connective Tissue, Lower Extremity **2** Tendons, Upper Extremity **3** Tendons, Lower Extremity	**Y** Other Contrast	**0** Unenhanced and Enhanced **Z** None	**Z** None
0 Connective Tissue, Upper Extremity **1** Connective Tissue, Lower Extremity **2** Tendons, Upper Extremity **3** Tendons, Lower Extremity	**Z** None	**Z** None	**Z** None

Section	B	Imaging
Body System	L	Connective Tissue
Type	4	**Ultrasonography:** Real time display of images of anatomy or flow information developed from the capture of reflected and attenuated high frequency sound waves

Body Part (4th)	Contrast (5th)	Qualifier (6th)	Qualifier (7th)
0 Connective Tissue, Upper Extremity **1** Connective Tissue, Lower Extremity **2** Tendons, Upper Extremity **3** Tendons, Lower Extremity	**Z** None	**Z** None	**Z** None

Section	B	Imaging
Body System	N	Skull and Facial Bones
Type	0	**Plain Radiography:** Planar display of an image developed from the capture of external ionizing radiation on photographic or photoconductive plate

Body Part (4th)	Contrast (5th)	Qualifier (6th)	Qualifier (7th)
0 Skull **1** Orbit, Right **2** Orbit, Left **3** Orbits, Bilateral **4** Nasal Bones **5** Facial Bones **6** Mandible **B** Zygomatic Arch, Right **C** Zygomatic Arch, Left **D** Zygomatic Arches, Bilateral **G** Tooth, Single **H** Teeth, Multiple **J** Teeth, All	**Z** None	**Z** None	**Z** None
7 Temporomandibular Joint, Right **8** Temporomandibular Joint, Left **9** Temporomandibular Joints, Bilateral	**0** High Osmolar **1** Low Osmolar **Y** Other Contrast **Z** None	**Z** None	**Z** None

Section	B	Imaging
Body System	N	Skull and Facial Bones
Type	1	**Fluoroscopy:** Single plane or bi-plane real time display of an image developed from the capture of external ionizing radiation on a fluorescent screen. The image may also be stored by either digital or analog means

Body Part (4th)	Contrast (5th)	Qualifier (6th)	Qualifier (7th)
7 Temporomandibular Joint, Right **8** Temporomandibular Joint, Left **9** Temporomandibular Joints, Bilateral	**0** High Osmolar **1** Low Osmolar **Y** Other Contrast **Z** None	**Z** None	**Z** None

Section	B	Imaging
Body System	N	Skull and Facial Bones
Type	2	Computerized Tomography (CT Scan): Computer reformatted digital display of multiplanar images developed from the capture of multiple exposures of external ionizing radiation

Body Part (4th)	Contrast (5th)	Qualifier (6th)	Qualifier (7th)
0 Skull 3 Orbits, Bilateral 5 Facial Bones 6 Mandible 9 Temporomandibular Joints, Bilateral F Temporal Bones	0 High Osmolar 1 Low Osmolar Y Other Contrast Z None	Z None	Z None

Section	B	Imaging
Body System	N	Skull and Facial Bones
Type	3	Magnetic Resonance Imaging (MRI): Computer reformatted digital display of multiplanar images developed from the capture of radiofrequency signals emitted by nuclei in a body site excited within a magnetic field

Body Part (4th)	Contrast (5th)	Qualifier (6th)	Qualifier (7th)
9 Temporomandibular Joints, Bilateral	Y Other Contrast Z None	Z None	Z None

Section	B	Imaging
Body System	P	Non-Axial Upper Bones
Type	0	Plain Radiography: Planar display of an image developed from the capture of external ionizing radiation on photographic or photoconductive plate

Body Part (4th)	Contrast (5th)	Qualifier (6th)	Qualifier (7th)
0 Sternoclavicular Joint, Right 1 Sternoclavicular Joint, Left 2 Sternoclavicular Joints, Bilateral 3 Acromioclavicular Joints, Bilateral 4 Clavicle, Right 5 Clavicle, Left 6 Scapula, Right 7 Scapula, Left A Humerus, Right B Humerus, Left E Upper Arm, Right F Upper Arm, Left J Forearm, Right K Forearm, Left N Hand, Right P Hand, Left R Finger(s), Right S Finger(s), Left X Ribs, Right Y Ribs, Left	Z None	Z None	Z None
8 Shoulder, Right 9 Shoulder, Left C Hand/Finger Joint, Right D Hand/Finger Joint, Left G Elbow, Right H Elbow, Left L Wrist, Right M Wrist, Left	0 High Osmolar 1 Low Osmolar Y Other Contrast Z None	Z None	Z None

Section   **B**   **Imaging**
Body System   **P**   **Non-Axial Upper Bones**
Type   **1**   **Fluoroscopy:** Single plane or bi-plane real time display of an image developed from the capture of external ionizing radiation on a fluorescent screen. The image may also be stored by either digital or analog means

Body Part (4th)	Contrast (5th)	Qualifier (6th)	Qualifier (7th)
0 Sternoclavicular Joint, Right **1** Sternoclavicular Joint, Left **2** Sternoclavicular Joints, Bilateral **3** Acromioclavicular Joints, Bilateral **4** Clavicle, Right **5** Clavicle, Left **6** Scapula, Right **7** Scapula, Left **A** Humerus, Right **B** Humerus, Left **E** Upper Arm, Right **F** Upper Arm, Left **J** Forearm, Right **K** Forearm, Left **N** Hand, Right **P** Hand, Left **R** Finger(s), Right **S** Finger(s), Left **X** Ribs, Right **Y** Ribs, Left	**Z** None	**Z** None	**Z** None
8 Shoulder, Right **9** Shoulder, Left **L** Wrist, Right **M** Wrist, Left	**0** High Osmolar **1** Low Osmolar **Y** Other Contrast **Z** None	**Z** None	**Z** None
C Hand/Finger Joint, Right **D** Hand/Finger Joint, Left **G** Elbow, Right **H** Elbow, Left	**0** High Osmolar **1** Low Osmolar **Y** Other Contrast	**Z** None	**Z** None

Section   **B**   **Imaging**
Body System   **P**   **Non-Axial Upper Bones**
Type   **2**   **Computerized Tomography (CT Scan):** Computer reformatted digital display of multiplanar images developed from the capture of multiple exposures of external ionizing radiation

Body Part (4th)	Contrast (5th)	Qualifier (6th)	Qualifier (7th)
0 Sternoclavicular Joint, Right **1** Sternoclavicular Joint, Left **W** Thorax	**0** High Osmolar **1** Low Osmolar **Y** Other Contrast	**Z** None	**Z** None

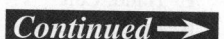
Continued →

Section	B	Imaging
Body System	P	Non-Axial Upper Bones
Type	2	**Computerized Tomography (CT Scan):** Computer reformatted digital display of multiplanar images developed from the capture of multiple exposures of external ionizing radiation

Body Part (4th)	Contrast (5th)	Qualifier (6th)	Qualifier (7th)
2 Sternoclavicular Joints, Bilateral 3 Acromioclavicular Joints, Bilateral 4 Clavicle, Right 5 Clavicle, Left 6 Scapula, Right 7 Scapula, Left 8 Shoulder, Right 9 Shoulder, Left A Humerus, Right B Humerus, Left E Upper Arm, Right F Upper Arm, Left G Elbow, Right H Elbow, Left J Forearm, Right K Forearm, Left L Wrist, Right M Wrist, Left N Hand, Right P Hand, Left Q Hands and Wrists, Bilateral R Finger(s), Right S Finger(s), Left T Upper Extremity, Right U Upper Extremity, Left V Upper Extremities, Bilateral X Ribs, Right Y Ribs, Left	0 High Osmolar 1 Low Osmolar Y Other Contrast Z None	Z None	Z None
C Hand/Finger Joint, Right D Hand/Finger Joint, Left	Z None	Z None	Z None

Section	B	Imaging
Body System	P	Non-Axial Upper Bones
Type	3	**Magnetic Resonance Imaging (MRI):** Computer reformatted digital display of multiplanar images developed from the capture of radiofrequency signals emitted by nuclei in a body site excited within a magnetic field

Body Part (4th)	Contrast (5th)	Qualifier (6th)	Qualifier (7th)
8 Shoulder, Right 9 Shoulder, Left C Hand/Finger Joint, Right D Hand/Finger Joint, Left E Upper Arm, Right F Upper Arm, Left G Elbow, Right H Elbow, Left J Forearm, Right K Forearm, Left L Wrist, Right M Wrist, Left	Y Other Contrast	0 Unenhanced and Enhanced Z None	Z None

Continued →

Section	B	Imaging
Body System	P	Non-Axial Upper Bones
Type	3	Magnetic Resonance Imaging (MRI): Computer reformatted digital display of multiplanar images developed from the capture of radiofrequency signals emitted by nuclei in a body site excited within a magnetic field

Body Part (4th)	Contrast (5th)	Qualifier (6th)	Qualifier (7th)
8 Shoulder, Right 9 Shoulder, Left C Hand/Finger Joint, Right D Hand/Finger Joint, Left E Upper Arm, Right F Upper Arm, Left G Elbow, Right H Elbow, Left J Forearm, Right K Forearm, Left L Wrist, Right M Wrist, Left	Z None	Z None	Z None

Section	B	Imaging
Body System	P	Non-Axial Upper Bones
Type	4	Ultrasonography: Real time display of images of anatomy or flow information developed from the capture of reflected and attenuated high frequency sound waves

Body Part (4th)	Contrast (5th)	Qualifier (6th)	Qualifier (7th)
8 Shoulder, Right 9 Shoulder, Left G Elbow, Right H Elbow, Left L Wrist, Right M Wrist, Left N Hand, Right P Hand, Left	Z None	Z None	1 Densitometry Z None

Section	B	Imaging
Body System	Q	Non-Axial Lower Bones
Type	0	Plain Radiography: Planar display of an image developed from the capture of external ionizing radiation on photographic or photoconductive plate

Body Part (4th)	Contrast (5th)	Qualifier (6th)	Qualifier (7th)
0 Hip, Right 1 Hip, Left	0 High Osmolar 1 Low Osmolar Y Other Contrast	Z None	Z None
0 Hip, Right 1 Hip, Left	Z None	Z None	1 Densitometry Z None
3 Femur, Right 4 Femur, Left	Z None	Z None	1 Densitometry Z None
7 Knee, Right 8 Knee, Left G Ankle, Right H Ankle, Left	0 High Osmolar 1 Low Osmolar Y Other Contrast Z None	Z None	Z None
D Lower Leg, Right F Lower Leg, Left J Calcaneus, Right K Calcaneus, Left L Foot, Right M Foot, Left P Toe(s), Right Q Toe(s), Left V Patella, Right W Patella, Left	Z None	Z None	Z None

Continued →

1458

Section	B	Imaging
Body System	Q	Non-Axial Lower Bones
Type	0	Plain Radiography: Planar display of an image developed from the capture of external ionizing radiation on photographic or photoconductive plate

Body Part (4th)	Contrast (5th)	Qualifier (6th)	Qualifier (7th)
X Foot/Toe Joint, Right Y Foot/Toe Joint, Left	0 High Osmolar 1 Low Osmolar Y Other Contrast	Z None	Z None

Section	B	Imaging
Body System	Q	Non-Axial Lower Bones
Type	1	Fluoroscopy: Single plane or bi-plane real time display of an image developed from the capture of external ionizing radiation on a fluorescent screen. The image may also be stored by either digital or analog means

Body Part (4th)	Contrast (5th)	Qualifier (6th)	Qualifier (7th)
0 Hip, Right 1 Hip, Left 7 Knee, Right 8 Knee, Left G Ankle, Right H Ankle, Left X Foot/Toe Joint, Right Y Foot/Toe Joint, Left	0 High Osmolar 1 Low Osmolar Y Other Contrast Z None	Z None	Z None
3 Femur, Right 4 Femur, Left D Lower Leg, Right F Lower Leg, Left J Calcaneus, Right K Calcaneus, Left L Foot, Right M Foot, Left P Toe(s), Right Q Toe(s), Left V Patella, Right W Patella, Left	Z None	Z None	Z None

Section	B	Imaging
Body System	Q	Non-Axial Lower Bones
Type	2	Computerized Tomography (CT Scan): Computer reformatted digital display of multiplanar images developed from the capture of multiple exposures of external ionizing radiation

Body Part (4th)	Contrast (5th)	Qualifier (6th)	Qualifier (7th)
0 Hip, Right 1 Hip, Left 3 Femur, Right 4 Femur, Left 7 Knee, Right 8 Knee, Left D Lower Leg, Right F Lower Leg, Left G Ankle, Right H Ankle, Left J Calcaneus, Right K Calcaneus, Left L Foot, Right M Foot, Left P Toe(s), Right Q Toe(s), Left R Lower Extremity, Right S Lower Extremity, Left V Patella, Right W Patella, Left X Foot/Toe Joint, Right Y Foot/Toe Joint, Left	0 High Osmolar 1 Low Osmolar Y Other Contrast Z None	Z None	Z None

Continued →

Section	B	Imaging
Body System	Q	**Non-Axial Lower Bones**
Type	2	**Computerized Tomography (CT Scan):** Computer reformatted digital display of multiplanar images developed from the capture of multiple exposures of external ionizing radiation

Body Part (4th)	Contrast (5th)	Qualifier (6th)	Qualifier (7th)
B Tibia/Fibula, Right **C** Tibia/Fibula, Left	**0** High Osmolar **1** Low Osmolar **Y** Other Contrast	**Z** None	**Z** None

Section	B	Imaging
Body System	Q	**Non-Axial Lower Bones**
Type	3	**Magnetic Resonance Imaging (MRI):** Computer reformatted digital display of multiplanar images developed from the capture of radiofrequency signals emitted by nuclei in a body site excited within a magnetic field

Body Part (4th)	Contrast (5th)	Qualifier (6th)	Qualifier (7th)
0 Hip, Right **1** Hip, Left **3** Femur, Right **4** Femur, Left **7** Knee, Right **8** Knee, Left **D** Lower Leg, Right **F** Lower Leg, Left **G** Ankle, Right **H** Ankle, Left **J** Calcaneus, Right **K** Calcaneus, Left **L** Foot, Right **M** Foot, Left **P** Toe(s), Right **Q** Toe(s), Left **V** Patella, Right **W** Patella, Left	**Y** Other Contrast	**0** Unenhanced and Enhanced **Z** None	**Z** None
0 Hip, Right **1** Hip, Left **3** Femur, Right **4** Femur, Left **7** Knee, Right **8** Knee, Left **D** Lower Leg, Right **F** Lower Leg, Left **G** Ankle, Right **H** Ankle, Left **J** Calcaneus, Right **K** Calcaneus, Left **L** Foot, Right **M** Foot, Left **P** Toe(s), Right **Q** Toe(s), Left **V** Patella, Right **W** Patella, Left	**Z** None	**Z** None	**Z** None

Section	B	Imaging
Body System	Q	**Non-Axial Lower Bones**
Type	4	**Ultrasonography:** Real time display of images of anatomy or flow information developed from the capture of reflected and attenuated high frequency sound waves

Body Part (4th)	Contrast (5th)	Qualifier (6th)	Qualifier (7th)
0 Hip, Right 1 Hip, Left 2 Hips, Bilateral 7 Knee, Right 8 Knee, Left 9 Knees, Bilateral	Z None	Z None	Z None

Section	B	Imaging
Body System	R	**Axial Skeleton, Except Skull and Facial Bones**
Type	0	**Plain Radiography:** Planar display of an image developed from the capture of external ionizing radiation on photographic or photoconductive plate

Body Part (4th)	Contrast (5th)	Qualifier (6th)	Qualifier (7th)
0 Cervical Spine 7 Thoracic Spine 9 Lumbar Spine G Whole Spine	Z None	Z None	1 Densitometry Z None
1 Cervical Disc(s) 2 Thoracic Disc(s) 3 Lumbar Disc(s) 4 Cervical Facet Joint(s) 5 Thoracic Facet Joint(s) 6 Lumbar Facet Joint(s) D Sacroiliac Joints	0 High Osmolar 1 Low Osmolar Y Other Contrast Z None	Z None	Z None
8 Thoracolumbar Joint B Lumbosacral Joint C Pelvis F Sacrum and Coccyx H Sternum	Z None	Z None	Z None

Section	B	Imaging
Body System	R	**Axial Skeleton, Except Skull and Facial Bones**
Type	1	**Fluoroscopy:** Single plane or bi-plane real time display of an image developed from the capture of external ionizing radiation on a fluorescent screen. The image may also be stored by either digital or analog means

Body Part (4th)	Contrast (5th)	Qualifier (6th)	Qualifier (7th)
0 Cervical Spine 1 Cervical Disc(s) 2 Thoracic Disc(s) 3 Lumbar Disc(s) 4 Cervical Facet Joint(s) 5 Thoracic Facet Joint(s) 6 Lumbar Facet Joint(s) 7 Thoracic Spine 8 Thoracolumbar Joint 9 Lumbar Spine B Lumbosacral Joint C Pelvis D Sacroiliac Joints F Sacrum and Coccyx G Whole Spine H Sternum	0 High Osmolar 1 Low Osmolar Y Other Contrast Z None	Z None	Z None

Section	B	Imaging
Body System	R	Axial Skeleton, Except Skull and Facial Bones
Type	2	**Computerized Tomography (CT Scan):** Computer reformatted digital display of multiplanar images developed from the capture of multiple exposures of external ionizing radiation

Body Part (4th)	Contrast (5th)	Qualifier (6th)	Qualifier (7th)
0 Cervical Spine 7 Thoracic Spine 9 Lumbar Spine C Pelvis D Sacroiliac Joints F Sacrum and Coccyx	0 High Osmolar 1 Low Osmolar Y Other Contrast Z None	Z None	Z None

Section	B	Imaging
Body System	R	Axial Skeleton, Except Skull and Facial Bones
Type	3	**Magnetic Resonance Imaging (MRI):** Computer reformatted digital display of multiplanar images developed from the capture of radiofrequency signals emitted by nuclei in a body site excited within a magnetic field

Body Part (4th)	Contrast (5th)	Qualifier (6th)	Qualifier (7th)
0 Cervical Spine 1 Cervical Disc(s) 2 Thoracic Disc(s) 3 Lumbar Disc(s) 7 Thoracic Spine 9 Lumbar Spine C Pelvis F Sacrum and Coccyx	Y Other Contrast	0 Unenhanced and Enhanced Z None	Z None
0 Cervical Spine 1 Cervical Disc(s) 2 Thoracic Disc(s) 3 Lumbar Disc(s) 7 Thoracic Spine 9 Lumbar Spine C Pelvis F Sacrum and Coccyx	Z None	Z None	Z None

Section	B	Imaging
Body System	R	Axial Skeleton, Except Skull and Facial Bones
Type	4	**Ultrasonography:** Real time display of images of anatomy or flow information developed from the capture of reflected and attenuated high frequency sound waves

Body Part (4th)	Contrast (5th)	Qualifier (6th)	Qualifier (7th)
0 Cervical Spine 7 Thoracic Spine 9 Lumbar Spine F Sacrum and Coccyx	Z None	Z None	Z None

Section	B	Imaging
Body System	T	Urinary System
Type	0	**Plain Radiography:** Planar display of an image developed from the capture of external ionizing radiation on photographic or photoconductive plate

Body Part (4th)	Contrast (5th)	Qualifier (6th)	Qualifier (7th)
0 Bladder 1 Kidney, Right 2 Kidney, Left 3 Kidneys, Bilateral 4 Kidneys, Ureters and Bladder 5 Urethra 6 Ureter, Right 7 Ureter, Left 8 Ureters, Bilateral B Bladder and Urethra C Ileal Diversion Loop	0 High Osmolar 1 Low Osmolar Y Other Contrast Z None	Z None	Z None

Section   **B**   **Imaging**
Body System   **T**   **Urinary System**
Type   **1**   **Fluoroscopy:** Single plane or bi-plane real time display of an image developed from the capture of external ionizing radiation on a fluorescent screen. The image may also be stored by either digital or analog means

Body Part (4th)	Contrast (5th)	Qualifier (6th)	Qualifier (7th)
0 Bladder 1 Kidney, Right 2 Kidney, Left 3 Kidneys, Bilateral 4 Kidneys, Ureters and Bladder 5 Urethra 6 Ureter, Right 7 Ureter, Left B Bladder and Urethra C Ileal Diversion Loop D Kidney, Ureter and Bladder, Right F Kidney, Ureter and Bladder, Left G Ileal Loop, Ureters and Kidneys	0 High Osmolar 1 Low Osmolar Y Other Contrast Z None	Z None	Z None

Section   **B**   **Imaging**
Body System   **T**   **Urinary System**
Type   **2**   **Computerized Tomography (CT Scan):** Computer reformatted digital display of multiplanar images developed from the capture of multiple exposures of external ionizing radiation

Body Part (4th)	Contrast (5th)	Qualifier (6th)	Qualifier (7th)
0 Bladder 1 Kidney, Right 2 Kidney, Left 3 Kidneys, Bilateral 9 Kidney Transplant	0 High Osmolar 1 Low Osmolar Y Other Contrast	0 Unenhanced and Enhanced Z None	Z None
0 Bladder 1 Kidney, Right 2 Kidney, Left 3 Kidneys, Bilateral 9 Kidney Transplant	Z None	Z None	Z None

Section   **B**   **Imaging**
Body System   **T**   **Urinary System**
Type   **3**   **Magnetic Resonance Imaging (MRI):** Computer reformatted digital display of multiplanar images developed from the capture of radiofrequency signals emitted by nuclei in a body site excited within a magnetic field

Body Part (4th)	Contrast (5th)	Qualifier (6th)	Qualifier (7th)
0 Bladder 1 Kidney, Right 2 Kidney, Left 3 Kidneys, Bilateral 9 Kidney Transplant	Y Other Contrast	0 Unenhanced and Enhanced Z None	Z None
0 Bladder 1 Kidney, Right 2 Kidney, Left 3 Kidneys, Bilateral 9 Kidney Transplant	Z None	Z None	Z None

Section	B	Imaging
Body System	T	Urinary System
Type	4	Ultrasonography: Real time display of images of anatomy or flow information developed from the capture of reflected and attenuated high frequency sound waves

Body Part (4th)	Contrast (5th)	Qualifier (6th)	Qualifier (7th)
0 Bladder 1 Kidney, Right 2 Kidney, Left 3 Kidneys, Bilateral 5 Urethra 6 Ureter, Right 7 Ureter, Left 8 Ureters, Bilateral 9 Kidney Transplant J Kidneys and Bladder	Z None	Z None	Z None

Section	B	Imaging
Body System	U	Female Reproductive System
Type	0	Plain Radiography: Planar display of an image developed from the capture of external ionizing radiation on photographic or photoconductive plate

Body Part (4th)	Contrast (5th)	Qualifier (6th)	Qualifier (7th)
0 Fallopian Tube, Right 1 Fallopian Tube, Left 2 Fallopian Tubes, Bilateral 6 Uterus 8 Uterus and Fallopian Tubes 9 Vagina	0 High Osmolar 1 Low Osmolar Y Other Contrast	Z None	Z None

Section	B	Imaging
Body System	U	Female Reproductive System
Type	1	Fluoroscopy: Single plane or bi-plane real time display of an image developed from the capture of external ionizing radiation on a fluorescent screen. The image may also be stored by either digital or analog means

Body Part (4th)	Contrast (5th)	Qualifier (6th)	Qualifier (7th)
0 Fallopian Tube, Right 1 Fallopian Tube, Left 2 Fallopian Tubes, Bilateral 6 Uterus 8 Uterus and Fallopian Tubes 9 Vagina	0 High Osmolar 1 Low Osmolar Y Other Contrast Z None	Z None	Z None

Section	B	Imaging
Body System	U	Female Reproductive System
Type	3	Magnetic Resonance Imaging (MRI): Computer reformatted digital display of multiplanar images developed from the capture of radiofrequency signals emitted by nuclei in a body site excited within a magnetic field

Body Part (4th)	Contrast (5th)	Qualifier (6th)	Qualifier (7th)
3 Ovary, Right 4 Ovary, Left 5 Ovaries, Bilateral 6 Uterus 9 Vagina B Pregnant Uterus C Uterus and Ovaries	Y Other Contrast	0 Unenhanced and Enhanced Z None	Z None
3 Ovary, Right 4 Ovary, Left 5 Ovaries, Bilateral 6 Uterus 9 Vagina B Pregnant Uterus C Uterus and Ovaries	Z None	Z None	Z None

1464

Section	B	Imaging
Body System	U	Female Reproductive System
Type	4	**Ultrasonography:** Real time display of images of anatomy or flow information developed from the capture of reflected and attenuated high frequency sound waves

Body Part (4th)	Contrast (5th)	Qualifier (6th)	Qualifier (7th)
0 Fallopian Tube, Right 1 Fallopian Tube, Left 2 Fallopian Tubes, Bilateral 3 Ovary, Right 4 Ovary, Left 5 Ovaries, Bilateral 6 Uterus C Uterus and Ovaries	Y Other Contrast Z None	Z None	Z None

Section	B	Imaging
Body System	V	Male Reproductive System
Type	0	**Plain Radiography:** Planar display of an image developed from the capture of external ionizing radiation on photographic or photoconductive plate

Body Part (4th)	Contrast (5th)	Qualifier (6th)	Qualifier (7th)
0 Corpora Cavernosa 1 Epididymis, Right 2 Epididymis, Left 3 Prostate 5 Testicle, Right 6 Testicle, Left 8 Vasa Vasorum	0 High Osmolar 1 Low Osmolar Y Other Contrast	Z None	Z None

Section	B	Imaging
Body System	V	Male Reproductive System
Type	1	**Fluoroscopy:** Single plane or bi-plane real time display of an image developed from the capture of external ionizing radiation on a fluorescent screen. The image may also be stored by either digital or analog means

Body Part (4th)	Contrast (5th)	Qualifier (6th)	Qualifier (7th)
0 Corpora Cavernosa 8 Vasa Vasorum	0 High Osmolar 1 Low Osmolar Y Other Contrast Z None	Z None	Z None

Section	B	Imaging
Body System	V	Male Reproductive System
Type	2	**Computerized Tomography (CT Scan):** Computer reformatted digital display of multiplanar images developed from the capture of multiple exposures of external ionizing radiation

Body Part (4th)	Contrast (5th)	Qualifier (6th)	Qualifier (7th)
3 Prostate	0 High Osmolar 1 Low Osmolar Y Other Contrast	0 Unenhanced and Enhanced Z None	Z None
3 Prostate	Z None	Z None	Z None

Section	B	Imaging
Body System	V	Male Reproductive System
Type	3	Magnetic Resonance Imaging (MRI): Computer reformatted digital display of multiplanar images developed from the capture of radiofrequency signals emitted by nuclei in a body site excited within a magnetic field

Body Part (4th)	Contrast (5th)	Qualifier (6th)	Qualifier (7th)
0 Corpora Cavernosa 3 Prostate 4 Scrotum 5 Testicle, Right 6 Testicle, Left 7 Testicles, Bilateral	Y Other Contrast	0 Unenhanced and Enhanced Z None	Z None
0 Corpora Cavernosa 3 Prostate 4 Scrotum 5 Testicle, Right 6 Testicle, Left 7 Testicles, Bilateral	Z None	Z None	Z None

Section	B	Imaging
Body System	V	Male Reproductive System
Type	4	Ultrasonography: Real time display of images of anatomy or flow information developed from the capture of reflected and attenuated high frequency sound waves

Body Part (4th)	Contrast (5th)	Qualifier (6th)	Qualifier (7th)
4 Scrotum 9 Prostate and Seminal Vesicles B Penis	Z None	Z None	Z None

Section	B	Imaging
Body System	W	Anatomical Regions
Type	0	Plain Radiography: Planar display of an image developed from the capture of external ionizing radiation on photographic or photoconductive plate

Body Part (4th)	Contrast (5th)	Qualifier (6th)	Qualifier (7th)
0 Abdomen 1 Abdomen and Pelvis 3 Chest B Long Bones, All C Lower Extremity J Upper Extremity K Whole Body L Whole Skeleton M Whole Body, Infant	Z None	Z None	Z None

Section	B	Imaging
Body System	W	Anatomical Regions
Type	1	Fluoroscopy: Single plane or bi-plane real time display of an image developed from the capture of external ionizing radiation on a fluorescent screen. The image may also be stored by either digital or analog means

Body Part (4th)	Contrast (5th)	Qualifier (6th)	Qualifier (7th)
1 Abdomen and Pelvis 9 Head and Neck C Lower Extremity J Upper Extremity	0 High Osmolar 1 Low Osmolar Y Other Contrast Z None	Z None	Z None

Section **B** **Imaging**
Body System **W** **Anatomical Regions**
Type **2** **Computerized Tomography (CT Scan):** Computer reformatted digital display of multiplanar images developed from the capture of multiple exposures of external ionizing radiation

Body Part (4th)	Contrast (5th)	Qualifier (6th)	Qualifier (7th)
0 Abdomen **1** Abdomen and Pelvis **4** Chest and Abdomen **5** Chest, Abdomen and Pelvis **8** Head **9** Head and Neck **F** Neck **G** Pelvic Region	**0** High Osmolar **1** Low Osmolar **Y** Other Contrast	**0** Unenhanced and Enhanced **Z** None	**Z** None
0 Abdomen **1** Abdomen and Pelvis **4** Chest and Abdomen **5** Chest, Abdomen and Pelvis **8** Head **9** Head and Neck **F** Neck **G** Pelvic Region	**Z** None	**Z** None	**Z** None

Section **B** **Imaging**
Body System **W** **Anatomical Regions**
Type **3** **Magnetic Resonance Imaging (MRI):** Computer reformatted digital display of multiplanar images developed from the capture of radiofrequency signals emitted by nuclei in a body site excited within a magnetic field

Body Part (4th)	Contrast (5th)	Qualifier (6th)	Qualifier (7th)
0 Abdomen **8** Head **F** Neck **G** Pelvic Region **H** Retroperitoneum **P** Brachial Plexus	**Y** Other Contrast	**0** Unenhanced and Enhanced **Z** None	**Z** None
0 Abdomen **8** Head **F** Neck **G** Pelvic Region **H** Retroperitoneum **P** Brachial Plexus	**Z** None	**Z** None	**Z** None
3 Chest	**Y** Other Contrast	**0** Unenhanced and Enhanced **Z** None	**Z** None

Section **B** **Imaging**
Body System **W** **Anatomical Regions**
Type **4** **Ultrasonography:** Real time display of images of anatomy or flow information developed from the capture of reflected and attenuated high frequency sound waves

Body Part (4th)	Contrast (5th)	Qualifier (6th)	Qualifier (7th)
0 Abdomen **1** Abdomen and Pelvis **F** Neck **G** Pelvic Region	**Z** None	**Z** None	**Z** None

Section	B	Imaging
Body System	W	Anatomical Regions
Operation	5	Other Imaging: Other specified modality for visualizing a body part

Body Part (4th)	Approach (5th)	Device (6th)	Qualifier (7th)
2 Trunk 9 Head and Neck C Lower Extremity J Upper Extremity	Z None	1 Bacterial Autofluorescence	Z None

Section	B	Imaging
Body System	Y	Fetus and Obstetrical
Type	3	Magnetic Resonance Imaging (MRI): Computer reformatted digital display of multiplanar images developed from the capture of radiofrequency signals emitted by nuclei in a body site excited within a magnetic field

Body Part (4th)	Contrast (5th)	Qualifier (6th)	Qualifier (7th)
0 Fetal Head 1 Fetal Heart 2 Fetal Thorax 3 Fetal Abdomen 4 Fetal Spine 5 Fetal Extremities 6 Whole Fetus	Y Other Contrast	0 Unenhanced and Enhanced Z None	Z None
0 Fetal Head 1 Fetal Heart 2 Fetal Thorax 3 Fetal Abdomen 4 Fetal Spine 5 Fetal Extremities 6 Whole Fetus	Z None	Z None	Z None

Section	B	Imaging
Body System	Y	Fetus and Obstetrical
Type	4	Ultrasonography: Real time display of images of anatomy or flow information developed from the capture of reflected and attenuated high frequency sound waves

Body Part (4th)	Contrast (5th)	Qualifier (6th)	Qualifier (7th)
7 Fetal Umbilical Cord 8 Placenta 9 First Trimester, Single Fetus B First Trimester, Multiple Gestation C Second Trimester, Single Fetus D Second Trimester, Multiple Gestation F Third Trimester, Single Fetus G Third Trimester, Multiple Gestation	Z None	Z None	Z None

Within each section of ICD-10-PCS the characters have different meanings. The seven character meanings for the Nuclear Medicine section are illustrated here through the procedure example of *Technetium tomo scan of liver*.

Section	Body System	Root Type	Body Part	Radionuclide	Qualifier	Qualifier
Nuclear Medicine	Hepatobiliary and Pancreas	Tomographic (Tomo)	Liver	Technetium 99m	None	None
C	F	2	5	1	Z	Z

Section (Character 1)

All Nuclear Medicine procedure codes have a first character value of C.

Body System (Character 2)

The alphanumeric character for the body system is placed in the second position. The following are the body systems applicable to the Nuclear Medicine section.

Character Value	Character Value Description
0	Central Nervous System
2	Heart
5	Veins
7	Lymphatic System
8	Eye
9	Ear, Nose, Mouth and Throat
B	Respiratory System
D	Gastrointestinal System
F	Hepatobiliary System and Pancreas
G	Endocrine System
H	Skin, Subcutaneous Tissue and Breast
P	Musculoskeletal
T	Urinary System
V	Male Reproductive System
W	Anatomical Regions

Root Types (Character 3)

The alphanumeric character value for root types is placed in the third position. The following are the root types applicable to the Nuclear Medicine section with their associated meaning.

Character Value	Root Type	Root Type Definition
1	Planar Nuclear Medicine Imaging	Introduction of radioactive materials into the body for single plane display of images developed from the capture of radioactive emissions
2	Tomographic (Tomo) Nuclear Medicine Imaging	Introduction of radioactive materials into the body for three dimensional display of images developed from the capture of radioactive emissions
3	Positron Emission Tomographic (PET) Imaging	Introduction of radioactive materials into the body for three dimensional display of images developed from the simultaneous capture, 180 degrees apart, of radioactive emissions
4	Nonimaging Nuclear Medicine Uptake	Introduction of radioactive materials into the body for measurements of organ function, from the detection of radioactive emissions
5	Nonimaging Nuclear Medicine Probe	Introduction of radioactive materials into the body for the study of distribution and fate of certain substances by the detection of radioactive emissions; or, alternatively, measurement of absorption of radioactive emissions from an external source

Continued →

Character Value	Root Type	Root Type Definition	
6	Nonimaging Nuclear Medicine Assay	Introduction of radioactive materials into the body for the study of body fluids and blood elements, by the detection of radioactive emissions	
7	Systemic Nuclear Medicine Therapy	Introduction of unsealed radioactive materials into the body for treatment	

Body Part (Character 4)

For each body part the applicable body part character values will be available for procedure code construction. An example of a body part is Cerebrospinal Fluid.

Radionuclide (Character 5)

When radionuclide is utilized during a nuclear medicine procedure, the corresponding radionuclide character value should be reported in the fifth character position. The following are examples of the radionuclide character values available for the Nuclear Medicine section.

- Krypton (Kr-81m)
- Technetium 99m (Tc-99m)
- Xenon 127 (Xe-127)
- Xenon 133 (Xe-133)
- Other Radionuclide

If radionuclide is not utilized, the placeholder character value of Z should be reported.

Qualifier (Character 6)

The qualifier represents an additional attribute for the procedure when applicable. Currently, there are no qualifiers in the Nuclear Medicine section; therefore, the placeholder character value of Z should be reported.

Qualifier (Character 7)

The qualifier represents an additional attribute for the procedure when applicable. Currently, there are no qualifiers in the Nuclear Medicine section; therefore, the placeholder character value of Z should be reported.

Nuclear Medicine Section Tables

Nuclear Medicine Tables C01–CW7

Section	C	Nuclear Medicine
Body System	0	Central Nervous System
Type	1	**Planar Nuclear Medicine Imaging:** Introduction of radioactive materials into the body for single plane display of images developed from the capture of radioactive emissions

Body Part (4ᵗʰ)	Radionuclide (5ᵗʰ)	Qualifier (6ᵗʰ)	Qualifier (7ᵗʰ)
0 Brain	1 Technetium 99m (Tc-99m) Y Other Radionuclide	Z None	Z None
5 Cerebrospinal Fluid	D Indium 111 (In-111) Y Other Radionuclide	Z None	Z None
Y Central Nervous System	Y Other Radionuclide	Z None	Z None

Section   **C**   **Nuclear Medicine**
Body System   **0**   **Central Nervous System**
Type   **2**   **Tomographic (Tomo) Nuclear Medicine Imaging:** Introduction of radioactive materials into the body for three dimensional display of images developed from the capture of radioactive emissions

Body Part (4th)	Radionuclide (5th)	Qualifier (6th)	Qualifier (7th)
0 Brain	1 Technetium 99m (Tc-99m) F Iodine 123 (I-123) S Thallium 201 (Tl-201) Y Other Radionuclide	Z None	Z None
5 Cerebrospinal Fluid	D Indium 111 (In-111) Y Other Radionuclide	Z None	Z None
Y Central Nervous System	Y Other Radionuclide	Z None	Z None

Section   **C**   **Nuclear Medicine**
Body System   **0**   **Central Nervous System**
Type   **3**   **Positron Emission Tomographic (PET) Imaging:** Introduction of radioactive materials into the body for three dimensional display of images developed from the simultaneous capture, 180 degrees apart, of radioactive emissions

Body Part (4th)	Radionuclide (5th)	Qualifier (6th)	Qualifier (7th)
0 Brain	B Carbon 11 (C-11) K Fluorine 18 (F-18) M Oxygen 15 (O-15) Y Other Radionuclide	Z None	Z None
Y Central Nervous System	Y Other Radionuclide	Z None	Z None

Section   **C**   **Nuclear Medicine**
Body System   **0**   **Central Nervous System**
Type   **5**   **Nonimaging Nuclear Medicine Probe:** Introduction of radioactive materials into the body for the study of distribution and fate of certain substances by the detection of radioactive emissions; or, alternatively, measurement of absorption of radioactive emissions from an external source

Body Part (4th)	Radionuclide (5th)	Qualifier (6th)	Qualifier (7th)
0 Brain	V Xenon 133 (Xe-133) Y Other Radionuclide	Z None	Z None
Y Central Nervous System	Y Other Radionuclide	Z None	Z None

Section   **C**   **Nuclear Medicine**
Body System   **2**   **Heart**
Type   **1**   **Planar Nuclear Medicine Imaging:** Introduction of radioactive materials into the body for single plane display of images developed from the capture of radioactive emissions

Body Part (4th)	Radionuclide (5th)	Qualifier (6th)	Qualifier (7th)
6 Heart, Right and Left	1 Technetium 99m (Tc-99m) Y Other Radionuclide	Z None	Z None
G Myocardium	1 Technetium 99m (Tc-99m) D Indium 111 (In-111) S Thallium 201 (Tl-201) Y Other Radionuclide Z None	Z None	Z None
Y Heart	Y Other Radionuclide	Z None	Z None

Section	C	Nuclear Medicine
Body System	2	Heart
Type	2	**Tomographic (Tomo) Nuclear Medicine Imaging:** Introduction of radioactive materials into the body for three dimensional display of images developed from the capture of radioactive emissions

Body Part (4th)	Radionuclide (5th)	Qualifier (6th)	Qualifier (7th)
6 Heart, Right and Left	1 Technetium 99m (Tc-99m) Y Other Radionuclide	Z None	Z None
G Myocardium	1 Technetium 99m (Tc-99m) D Indium 111 (In-111) K Fluorine 18 (F-18) S Thallium 201 (Tl-201) Y Other Radionuclide Z None	Z None	Z None
Y Heart	Y Other Radionuclide	Z None	Z None

Section	C	Nuclear Medicine
Body System	2	Heart
Type	3	**Positron Emission Tomographic (PET) Imaging:** Introduction of radioactive materials into the body for three dimensional display of images developed from the simultaneous capture, 180 degrees apart, of radioactive emissions

Body Part (4th)	Radionuclide (5th)	Qualifier (6th)	Qualifier (7th)
G Myocardium	K Fluorine 18 (F-18) M Oxygen 15 (O-15) Q Rubidium 82 (Rb-82) R Nitrogen 13 (N-13) Y Other Radionuclide	Z None	Z None
Y Heart	Y Other Radionuclide	Z None	Z None

Section	C	Nuclear Medicine
Body System	2	Heart
Type	5	**Nonimaging Nuclear Medicine Probe:** Introduction of radioactive materials into the body for the study of distribution and fate of certain substances by the detection of radioactive emissions; or, alternatively, measurement of absorption of radioactive emissions from an external source

Body Part (4th)	Radionuclide (5th)	Qualifier (6th)	Qualifier (7th)
6 Heart, Right and Left	1 Technetium 99m (Tc-99m) Y Other Radionuclide	Z None	Z None
Y Heart	Y Other Radionuclide	Z None	Z None

Section	C	Nuclear Medicine
Body System	5	Veins
Type	1	**Planar Nuclear Medicine Imaging:** Introduction of radioactive materials into the body for single plane display of images developed from the capture of radioactive emissions

Body Part (4th)	Radionuclide (5th)	Qualifier (6th)	Qualifier (7th)
B Lower Extremity Veins, Right C Lower Extremity Veins, Left D Lower Extremity Veins, Bilateral N Upper Extremity Veins, Right P Upper Extremity Veins, Left Q Upper Extremity Veins, Bilateral R Central Veins	1 Technetium 99m (Tc-99m) Y Other Radionuclide	Z None	Z None
Y Veins	Y Other Radionuclide	Z None	Z None

Section   **C**   **Nuclear Medicine**
Body System   **7**   **Lymphatic and Hematologic System**
Type   **1**   **Planar Nuclear Medicine Imaging:** Introduction of radioactive materials into the body for single plane display of images developed from the capture of radioactive emissions

Body Part (4th)	Radionuclide (5th)	Qualifier (6th)	Qualifier (7th)
0 Bone Marrow	**1** Technetium 99m (Tc-99m) **D** Indium 111 (In-111) **Y** Other Radionuclide	**Z** None	**Z** None
2 Spleen **5** Lymphatics, Head and Neck **D** Lymphatics, Pelvic **J** Lymphatics, Head **K** Lymphatics, Neck **L** Lymphatics, Upper Chest **M** Lymphatics, Trunk **N** Lymphatics, Upper Extremity **P** Lymphatics, Lower Extremity	**1** Technetium 99m (Tc-99m) **Y** Other Radionuclide	**Z** None	**Z** None
3 Blood	**D** Indium 111 (In-111) **Y** Other Radionuclide	**Z** None	**Z** None
Y Lymphatic and Hematologic System	**Y** Other Radionuclide	**Z** None	**Z** None

Section   **C**   **Nuclear Medicine**
Body System   **7**   **Lymphatic and Hematologic System**
Type   **2**   **Tomographic (Tomo) Nuclear Medicine Imaging:** Introduction of radioactive materials into the body for three dimensional display of images developed from the capture of radioactive emissions

Body Part (4th)	Radionuclide (5th)	Qualifier (6th)	Qualifier (7th)
2 Spleen	**1** Technetium 99m (Tc-99m) **Y** Other Radionuclide	**Z** None	**Z** None
Y Lymphatic and Hematologic System	**Y** Other Radionuclide	**Z** None	**Z** None

Section   **C**   **Nuclear Medicine**
Body System   **7**   **Lymphatic and Hematologic System**
Type   **5**   **Nonimaging Nuclear Medicine Probe:** Introduction of radioactive materials into the body for the study of distribution and fate of certain substances by the detection of radioactive emissions; or, alternatively, measurement of absorption of radioactive emissions from an external source

Body Part (4th)	Radionuclide (5th)	Qualifier (6th)	Qualifier (7th)
5 Lymphatics, Head and Neck **D** Lymphatics, Pelvic **J** Lymphatics, Head **K** Lymphatics, Neck **L** Lymphatics, Upper Chest **M** Lymphatics, Trunk **N** Lymphatics, Upper Extremity **P** Lymphatics, Lower Extremity	**1** Technetium 99m (Tc-99m) **Y** Other Radionuclide	**Z** None	**Z** None
Y Lymphatic and Hematologic System	**Y** Other Radionuclide	**Z** None	**Z** None

Section	C	Nuclear Medicine
Body System	7	Lymphatic and Hematologic System
Type	6	Nonimaging Nuclear Medicine Assay: Introduction of radioactive materials into the body for the study of body fluids and blood elements, by the detection of radioactive emissions

Body Part (4th)	Radionuclide (5th)	Qualifier (6th)	Qualifier (7th)
3 Blood	1 Technetium 99m (Tc-99m) 7 Cobalt 58 (Co-58) C Cobalt 57 (Co-57) D Indium 111 (In-111) H Iodine 125 (I-125) W Chromium (Cr-51) Y Other Radionuclide	Z None	Z None
Y Lymphatic and Hematologic System	Y Other Radionuclide	Z None	Z None

Section	C	Nuclear Medicine
Body System	8	Eye
Type	1	Planar Nuclear Medicine Imaging: Introduction of radioactive materials into the body for single plane display of images developed from the capture of radioactive emissions

Body Part (4th)	Radionuclide (5th)	Qualifier (6th)	Qualifier (7th)
9 Lacrimal Ducts, Bilateral	1 Technetium 99m (Tc-99m) Y Other Radionuclide	Z None	Z None
Y Eye	Y Other Radionuclide	Z None	Z None

Section	C	Nuclear Medicine
Body System	9	Ear, Nose, Mouth and Throat
Type	1	Planar Nuclear Medicine Imaging: Introduction of radioactive materials into the body for single plane display of images developed from the capture of radioactive emissions

Body Part (4th)	Radionuclide (5th)	Qualifier (6th)	Qualifier (7th)
B Salivary Glands, Bilateral	1 Technetium 99m (Tc-99m) Y Other Radionuclide	Z None	Z None
Y Ear, Nose, Mouth and Throat	Y Other Radionuclide	Z None	Z None

Section	C	Nuclear Medicine
Body System	B	Respiratory System
Type	1	Planar Nuclear Medicine Imaging: Introduction of radioactive materials into the body for single plane display of images developed from the capture of radioactive emissions

Body Part (4th)	Radionuclide (5th)	Qualifier (6th)	Qualifier (7th)
2 Lungs and Bronchi	1 Technetium 99m (Tc-99m) 9 Krypton (Kr-81m) T Xenon 127 (Xe-127) V Xenon 133 (Xe-133) Y Other Radionuclide	Z None	Z None
Y Respiratory System	Y Other Radionuclide	Z None	Z None

Section	C	Nuclear Medicine
Body System	B	Respiratory System
Type	2	Tomographic (Tomo) Nuclear Medicine Imaging: Introduction of radioactive materials into the body for three dimensional display of images developed from the capture of radioactive emissions

Body Part (4th)	Radionuclide (5th)	Qualifier (6th)	Qualifier (7th)
2 Lungs and Bronchi	1 Technetium 99m (Tc-99m) 9 Krypton (Kr-81m) Y Other Radionuclide	Z None	Z None
Y Respiratory System	Y Other Radionuclide	Z None	Z None

Section	C	Nuclear Medicine
Body System	B	Respiratory System
Type	3	Positron Emission Tomographic (PET) Imaging: Introduction of radioactive materials into the body for three dimensional display of images developed from the simultaneous capture, 180 degrees apart, of radioactive emissions

Body Part (4th)	Radionuclide (5th)	Qualifier (6th)	Qualifier (7th)
2 Lungs and Bronchi	K Fluorine 18 (F-18) Y Other Radionuclide	Z None	Z None
Y Respiratory System	Y Other Radionuclide	Z None	Z None

Section	C	Nuclear Medicine
Body System	D	Gastrointestinal System
Type	1	Planar Nuclear Medicine Imaging: Introduction of radioactive materials into the body for single plane display of images developed from the capture of radioactive emissions

Body Part (4th)	Radionuclide (5th)	Qualifier (6th)	Qualifier (7th)
5 Upper Gastrointestinal Tract 7 Gastrointestinal Tract	1 Technetium 99m (Tc-99m) D Indium 111 (In-111) Y Other Radionuclide	Z None	Z None
Y Digestive System	Y Other Radionuclide	Z None	Z None

Section	C	Nuclear Medicine
Body System	D	Gastrointestinal System
Type	2	Tomographic (Tomo) Nuclear Medicine Imaging: Introduction of radioactive materials into the body for three dimensional display of images developed from the capture of radioactive emissions

Body Part (4th)	Radionuclide (5th)	Qualifier (6th)	Qualifier (7th)
7 Gastrointestinal Tract	1 Technetium 99m (Tc-99m) D Indium 111 (In-111) Y Other Radionuclide	Z None	Z None
Y Digestive System	Y Other Radionuclide	Z None	Z None

Section	C	Nuclear Medicine
Body System	F	Hepatobiliary System and Pancreas
Type	1	Planar Nuclear Medicine Imaging: Introduction of radioactive materials into the body for single plane display of images developed from the capture of radioactive emissions

Body Part (4th)	Radionuclide (5th)	Qualifier (6th)	Qualifier (7th)
4 Gallbladder 5 Liver 6 Liver and Spleen C Hepatobiliary System, All	1 Technetium 99m (Tc-99m) Y Other Radionuclide	Z None	Z None
Y Hepatobiliary System and Pancreas	Y Other Radionuclide	Z None	Z None

Section	C	Nuclear Medicine
Body System	F	Hepatobiliary System and Pancreas
Type	2	Tomographic (Tomo) Nuclear Medicine Imaging: Introduction of radioactive materials into the body for three dimensional display of images developed from the capture of radioactive emissions

Body Part (4th)	Radionuclide (5th)	Qualifier (6th)	Qualifier (7th)
4 Gallbladder 5 Liver 6 Liver and Spleen	1 Technetium 99m (Tc-99m) Y Other Radionuclide	Z None	Z None
Y Hepatobiliary System and Pancreas	Y Other Radionuclide	Z None	Z None

Section	C	Nuclear Medicine
Body System	G	Endocrine System
Type	1	Planar Nuclear Medicine Imaging: Introduction of radioactive materials into the body for single plane display of images developed from the capture of radioactive emissions

Body Part (4th)	Radionuclide (5th)	Qualifier (6th)	Qualifier (7th)
1 Parathyroid Glands	1 Technetium 99m (Tc-99m) S Thallium 201 (Tl-201) Y Other Radionuclide	Z None	Z None
2 Thyroid Gland	1 Technetium 99m (Tc-99m) F Iodine 123 (I-123) G Iodine 131 (I-131) Y Other Radionuclide	Z None	Z None
4 Adrenal Glands, Bilateral	G Iodine 131 (I-131) Y Other Radionuclide	Z None	Z None
Y Endocrine System	Y Other Radionuclide	Z None	Z None

Section	C	Nuclear Medicine
Body System	G	Endocrine System
Type	2	Tomographic (Tomo) Nuclear Medicine Imaging: Introduction of radioactive materials into the body for three dimensional display of images developed from the capture of radioactive emissions

Body Part (4th)	Radionuclide (5th)	Qualifier (6th)	Qualifier (7th)
1 Parathyroid Glands	1 Technetium 99m (Tc-99m) S Thallium 201 (Tl-201) Y Other Radionuclide	Z None	Z None
Y Endocrine System	Y Other Radionuclide	Z None	Z None

Section	C	Nuclear Medicine
Body System	G	Endocrine System
Type	4	Nonimaging Nuclear Medicine Uptake: Introduction of radioactive materials into the body for measurements of organ function, from the detection of radioactive emissions

Body Part (4th)	Radionuclide (5th)	Qualifier (6th)	Qualifier (7th)
2 Thyroid Gland	1 Technetium 99m (Tc-99m) F Iodine 123 (I-123) G Iodine 131 (I-131) Y Other Radionuclide	Z None	Z None
Y Endocrine System	Y Other Radionuclide	Z None	Z None

Section	C	Nuclear Medicine
Body System	H	Skin, Subcutaneous Tissue and Breast
Type	1	**Planar Nuclear Medicine Imaging:** Introduction of radioactive materials into the body for single plane display of images developed from the capture of radioactive emissions

Body Part (4th)	Radionuclide (5th)	Qualifier (6th)	Qualifier (7th)
0 Breast, Right **1** Breast, Left **2** Breasts, Bilateral	**1** Technetium 99m (Tc-99m) **S** Thallium 201 (Tl-201) **Y** Other Radionuclide	**Z** None	**Z** None
Y Skin, Subcutaneous Tissue and Breast	**Y** Other Radionuclide	**Z** None	**Z** None

Section	C	Nuclear Medicine
Body System	H	Skin, Subcutaneous Tissue and Breast
Type	2	**Tomographic (Tomo) Nuclear Medicine Imaging:** Introduction of radioactive materials into the body for three dimensional display of images developed from the capture of radioactive emissions

Body Part (4th)	Radionuclide (5th)	Qualifier (6th)	Qualifier (7th)
0 Breast, Right **1** Breast, Left **2** Breasts, Bilateral	**1** Technetium 99m (Tc-99m) **S** Thallium 201 (Tl-201) **Y** Other Radionuclide	**Z** None	**Z** None
Y Skin, Subcutaneous Tissue and Breast	**Y** Other Radionuclide	**Z** None	**Z** None

Section	C	Nuclear Medicine
Body System	P	Musculoskeletal System
Type	1	**Planar Nuclear Medicine Imaging:** Introduction of radioactive materials into the body for single plane display of images developed from the capture of radioactive emissions

Body Part (4th)	Radionuclide (5th)	Qualifier (6th)	Qualifier (7th)
1 Skull **4** Thorax **5** Spine **6** Pelvis **7** Spine and Pelvis **8** Upper Extremity, Right **9** Upper Extremity, Left **B** Upper Extremities, Bilateral **C** Lower Extremity, Right **D** Lower Extremity, Left **F** Lower Extremities, Bilateral **Z** Musculoskeletal System, All	**1** Technetium 99m (Tc-99m) **Y** Other Radionuclide	**Z** None	**Z** None
Y Musculoskeletal System, Other	**Y** Other Radionuclide	**Z** None	**Z** None

Section	C	Nuclear Medicine
Body System	P	Musculoskeletal System
Type	2	**Tomographic (Tomo) Nuclear Medicine Imaging:** Introduction of radioactive materials into the body for three dimensional display of images developed from the capture of radioactive emissions

Body Part (4th)	Radionuclide (5th)	Qualifier (6th)	Qualifier (7th)
1 Skull 2 Cervical Spine 3 Skull and Cervical Spine 4 Thorax 6 Pelvis 7 Spine and Pelvis 8 Upper Extremity, Right 9 Upper Extremity, Left B Upper Extremities, Bilateral C Lower Extremity, Right D Lower Extremity, Left F Lower Extremities, Bilateral G Thoracic Spine H Lumbar Spine J Thoracolumbar Spine	1 Technetium 99m (Tc-99m) Y Other Radionuclide	Z None	Z None
Y Musculoskeletal System, Other	Y Other Radionuclide	Z None	Z None

Section	C	Nuclear Medicine
Body System	P	Musculoskeletal System
Type	5	**Nonimaging Nuclear Medicine Probe:** Introduction of radioactive materials into the body for the study of distribution and fate of certain substances by the detection of radioactive emissions; or, alternatively, measurement of absorption of radioactive emissions from an external source

Body Part (4th)	Radionuclide (5th)	Qualifier (6th)	Qualifier (7th)
5 Spine N Upper Extremities P Lower Extremities	Z None	Z None	Z None
Y Musculoskeletal System, Other	Y Other Radionuclide	Z None	Z None

Section	C	Nuclear Medicine
Body System	T	Urinary System
Type	1	**Planar Nuclear Medicine Imaging:** Introduction of radioactive materials into the body for single plane display of images developed from the capture of radioactive emissions

Body Part (4th)	Radionuclide (5th)	Qualifier (6th)	Qualifier (7th)
3 Kidneys, Ureters and Bladder	1 Technetium 99m (Tc-99m) F Iodine 123 (I-123) G Iodine 131 (I-131) Y Other Radionuclide	Z None	Z None
H Bladder and Ureters	1 Technetium 99m (Tc-99m) Y Other Radionuclide	Z None	Z None
Y Urinary System	Y Other Radionuclide	Z None	Z None

Section	C	Nuclear Medicine
Body System	T	Urinary System
Type	2	**Tomographic (Tomo) Nuclear Medicine Imaging:** Introduction of radioactive materials into the body for three dimensional display of images developed from the capture of radioactive emissions

Body Part (4th)	Radionuclide (5th)	Qualifier (6th)	Qualifier (7th)
3 Kidneys, Ureters and Bladder	1 Technetium 99m (Tc-99m) Y Other Radionuclide	Z None	Z None
Y Urinary System	Y Other Radionuclide	Z None	Z None

Section	C	Nuclear Medicine
Body System	T	Urinary System
Type	6	**Nonimaging Nuclear Medicine Assay:** Introduction of radioactive materials into the body for the study of body fluids and blood elements, by the detection of radioactive emissions

Body Part (4th)	Radionuclide (5th)	Qualifier (6th)	Qualifier (7th)
3 Kidneys, Ureters and Bladder	1 Technetium 99m (Tc-99m) F Iodine 123 (I-123) G Iodine 131 (I-131) H Iodine 125 (I-125) Y Other Radionuclide	Z None	Z None
Y Urinary System	Y Other Radionuclide	Z None	Z None

Section	C	Nuclear Medicine
Body System	V	Male Reproductive System
Type	1	**Planar Nuclear Medicine Imaging:** Introduction of radioactive materials into the body for single plane display of images developed from the capture of radioactive emissions

Body Part (4th)	Radionuclide (5th)	Qualifier (6th)	Qualifier (7th)
9 Testicles, Bilateral	1 Technetium 99m (Tc-99m) Y Other Radionuclide	Z None	Z None
Y Male Reproductive System	Y Other Radionuclide	Z None	Z None

Section	C	Nuclear Medicine
Body System	W	Anatomical Regions
Type	1	**Planar Nuclear Medicine Imaging:** Introduction of radioactive materials into the body for single plane display of images developed from the capture of radioactive emissions

Body Part (4th)	Radionuclide (5th)	Qualifier (6th)	Qualifier (7th)
0 Abdomen 1 Abdomen and Pelvis 4 Chest and Abdomen 6 Chest and Neck B Head and Neck D Lower Extremity J Pelvic Region M Upper Extremity N Whole Body	1 Technetium 99m (Tc-99m) D Indium 111 (In-111) F Iodine 123 (I-123) G Iodine 131 (I-131) L Gallium 67 (Ga-67) S Thallium 201 (Tl-201) Y Other Radionuclide	Z None	Z None
3 Chest	1 Technetium 99m (Tc-99m) D Indium 111 (In-111) F Iodine 123 (I-123) G Iodine 131 (I-131) K Fluorine 18 (F-18) L Gallium 67 (Ga-67) S Thallium 201 (Tl-201) Y Other Radionuclide	Z None	Z None
Y Anatomical Regions, Multiple	Y Other Radionuclide	Z None	Z None
Z Anatomical Region, Other	Z None	Z None	Z None

Section	C	Nuclear Medicine
Body System	W	Anatomical Regions
Type	2	Tomographic (Tomo) Nuclear Medicine Imaging: Introduction of radioactive materials into the body for three dimensional display of images developed from the capture of radioactive emissions

Body Part (4th)	Radionuclide (5th)	Qualifier (6th)	Qualifier (7th)
0 Abdomen 1 Abdomen and Pelvis 3 Chest 4 Chest and Abdomen 6 Chest and Neck B Head and Neck D Lower Extremity J Pelvic Region M Upper Extremity	1 Technetium 99m (Tc-99m) D Indium 111 (In-111) F Iodine 123 (I-123) G Iodine 131 (I-131) K Fluorine 18 (F-18) L Gallium 67 (Ga-67) S Thallium 201 (Tl-201) Y Other Radionuclide	Z None	Z None
Y Anatomical Regions, Multiple	Y Other Radionuclide	Z None	Z None

Section	C	Nuclear Medicine
Body System	W	Anatomical Regions
Type	3	Positron Emission Tomographic (PET) Imaging: Introduction of radioactive materials into the body for three dimensional display of images developed from the simultaneous capture, 180 degrees apart, of radioactive emissions

Body Part (4th)	Radionuclide (5th)	Qualifier (6th)	Qualifier (7th)
N Whole Body	Y Other Radionuclide	Z None	Z None

Section	C	Nuclear Medicine
Body System	W	Anatomical Regions
Type	5	Nonimaging Nuclear Medicine Probe: Introduction of radioactive materials into the body for the study of distribution and fate of certain substances by the detection of radioactive emissions; or, alternatively, measurement of absorption of radioactive emissions from an external source

Body Part (4th)	Radionuclide (5th)	Qualifier (6th)	Qualifier (7th)
0 Abdomen 1 Abdomen and Pelvis 3 Chest 4 Chest and Abdomen 6 Chest and Neck B Head and Neck D Lower Extremity J Pelvic Region M Upper Extremity	1 Technetium 99m (Tc-99m) D Indium 111 (In-111) Y Other Radionuclide	Z None	Z None

Section	C	Nuclear Medicine
Body System	W	Anatomical Regions
Type	7	Systemic Nuclear Medicine Therapy: Introduction of unsealed radioactive materials into the body for treatment

Body Part (4th)	Radionuclide (5th)	Qualifier (6th)	Qualifier (7th)
0 Abdomen 3 Chest	N Phosphorus 32 (P-32) Y Other Radionuclide	Z None	Z None
G Thyroid	G Iodine 131 (I-131) Y Other Radionuclide	Z None	Z None
N Whole Body	8 Samarium 153 (Sm-153) G Iodine 131 (I-131) N Phosphorus 32 (P-32) P Strontium 89 (Sr-89) Y Other Radionuclide	Z None	Z None
Y Anatomical Regions, Multiple	Y Other Radionuclide	Z None	Z None

Within each section of ICD-10-PCS the characters have different meanings. The seven character meanings for the Radiation Therapy section are illustrated here through the procedure example of *HDR brachytherapy of prostate using Palladium 103*.

Section	Body System	Modality	Treatment Site	Modality Qualifier	Isotope	Qualifier
Radiation Therapy	Male Reproductive System	Brachytherapy	Prostate	High Dose Rate (HDR)	Palladium 103	None
D	V	1	0	9	B	Z

Section (Character 1)

All Radiation Therapy procedure codes have a first character value of D.

Body System (Character 2)

The alphanumeric character for the body system is placed in the second position. The following are the body systems applicable to the Radiation Therapy section.

Character Value	Character Value Description
0	Central and Peripheral Nervous System
7	Lymphatic and Hematologic System
8	Eye
9	Ear, Nose, Mouth and Throat
B	Respiratory System
D	Gastrointestinal System
F	Hepatobiliary System and Pancreas
G	Endocrine System
H	Skin
M	Breast
P	Musculoskeletal
T	Urinary System
U	Female Reproductive System
V	Male Reproductive System
W	Anatomical Regions

Modality (Character 3)

The alphanumeric character value for root types is placed in the third position. The following are the root types applicable to the Radiation Therapy section with their associated meaning.

Character Value	Modality	Modality Definition
0	Beam Radiation	The external use of high-energy radiation such as x-rays, photons, electrons, or protons
1	Brachytherapy	The use of radioactive sources placed directly into a tumor bearing area to generate local regions of high intensity radiation
2	Stereotactic Radiosurgery	The use of external radiation sources either from a linear accelerator or a special Cobalt-60 irradiator to deliver many beams of radiation directly to an internal structure in a single fraction
Y	Other Radiation	Other types of radiation therapy such as hyperthermia, contact radiation and plaque radiation. *See Modality qualifier, character 5, for specified types of other radiation.*

Source: CSI Navigator for Radiation Oncology, 2010

Treatment Site (Character 4)

For each treatment site the applicable body part character values will be available for procedure code construction. An example of a treatment site for this section is Brain Stem.

Modality Qualifier (Character 5)

The modality qualifier further specifies the treatment modality. The following are examples of the modality qualifier values available for the Radiation Therapy section:

- Photons >10 MeV
- Neutrons

- Electrons
- High Dose Rate
- Hyperthermia

Isotope (Character 6)

When an isotope is utilized during a radiation oncology procedure, the corresponding isotope character value should be reported in the sixth character position. The following are examples of the isotope character values available for the Radiation Therapy section:

- Iridium 192 (Ir-192)
- Iodine 125 (I-125)
- Californium 252 (Cf-252)

Qualifier (Character 7)

The qualifier represents an additional attribute for the procedure when applicable. For example, beam radiation procedures in this section include the qualifier Intraoperative that is reported with the character value of 0 for some body parts. If there is no qualifier for a procedure, the placeholder Z is the character value that should be reported.

Radiation Therapy Section Guidelines (section D)

Radiation Therapy Section Guidelines (section D)

D. Radiation Therapy Section

Brachytherapy

D1.a Brachytherapy is coded to the modality Brachytherapy in the Radiation Therapy section. When a radioactive brachytherapy source is left in the body at the end of the procedure, it is coded separately to the root operation Insertion with the device value Radioactive Element.

Example: Brachytherapy with implantation of a low dose rate brachytherapy source left in the body at the end of the procedure is coded to the applicable treatment site in section D, Radiation Therapy, with the modality Brachytherapy, the modality qualifier value, Low Dose Rate, and the applicable isotope value and qualifier value. The implantation of the brachytherapy source is coded separately to the device value Radioactive Element in the appropriate Insertion table of the Medical and Surgical section. The Radiation Therapy section code identifies the specific modality and isotope of the brachytherapy, and the root operation Insertion code identifies the implantation of the brachytherapy source that remain in the body at the end of the procedure.

Exception: Implantation of Cesium-131 brachytherapy seeds embedded in a collagen matrix to the treatment site after resection of brain tumor is coded to the root operation Insertion with the device value Radioactive Element, Cesium-131 Collagen Implant. The procedure is coded to the root operation Insertion only, because the device value identifies both the implantation of the radioactive element and a specific brachytherapy isotope that is not included in the Radiation Therapy section tables.

D1.b A separate procedure to place a temporary applicator for delivering the brachytherapy is coded to the root operation Insertion and the device value Other Device.

Examples: Intrauterine brachytherapy applicator placed as a separate procedure from the brachytherapy procedure is coded to Insertion of Other Device, and the brachytherapy is coded separately using the modality Brachytherapy in the Radiation Therapy section. Intrauterine brachytherapy applicator placed concomitantly with delivery of the brachytherapy dose is coded with a single code using the modality Brachytherapy in the Radiation Therapy section.

AHA Coding Clinic

DU11B7Z Low Dose Rate (LDR) Brachytherapy of Cervix using Cesium 137 (Cs-137) - AHA CC: 4Q, 2017, 104

DW16BB1 Low Dose Rate (LDR) Brachytherapy of Pelvic Region using Palladium 103 (Pd-103), Unidirectional Source - AHA CC: 4Q, 2019, 43-44

DWY38ZZ Hyperthermia of Abdomen - AHA CC: 4Q, 2019, 37

Radiation Therapy Section Tables

Radiation Therapy Tables D00–DWY

Section	D	Radiation Therapy
Body System	0	Central and Peripheral Nervous System
Modality	0	Beam Radiation

Treatment Site (4th)	Modality Qualifier (5th)	Isotope (6th)	Qualifier (7th)
0 Brain 1 Brain Stem 6 Spinal Cord 7 Peripheral Nerve	0 Photons <1 MeV 1 Photons 1 - 10 MeV 2 Photons >10 MeV 4 Heavy Particles (Protons,Ions) 5 Neutrons 6 Neutron Capture	Z None	Z None

Continued →

Section	D	Radiation Therapy
Body System	0	Central and Peripheral Nervous System
Modality	0	Beam Radiation

Treatment Site (4th)	Modality Qualifier (5th)	Isotope (6th)	Qualifier (7th)
0 Brain 1 Brain Stem 6 Spinal Cord 7 Peripheral Nerve	3 Electrons	Z None	0 Intraoperative Z None

Section	D	Radiation Therapy
Body System	0	Central and Peripheral Nervous System
Modality	1	Brachytherapy

Treatment Site (4th)	Modality Qualifier (5th)	Isotope (6th)	Qualifier (7th)
0 Brain 1 Brain Stem 6 Spinal Cord 7 Peripheral Nerve	9 High Dose Rate (HDR)	7 Cesium 137 (Cs-137) 8 Iridium 192 (Ir-192) 9 Iodine 125 (I-125) B Palladium 103 (Pd-103) C Californium 252 (Cf-252) Y Other Isotope	Z None
0 Brain 1 Brain Stem 6 Spinal Cord 7 Peripheral Nerve	B Low Dose Rate (LDR)	6 Cesium 131 (Cs-131) 7 Cesium 137 (Cs-137) 8 Iridium 192 (Ir-192) 9 Iodine 125 (I-125) C Californium 252 (Cf-252) Y Other Isotope	Z None
0 Brain 1 Brain Stem 6 Spinal Cord 7 Peripheral Nerve	B Low Dose Rate (LDR)	B Palladium 103 (Pd-103)	1 Unidirectional Source Z None

Section	D	Radiation Therapy
Body System	0	Central and Peripheral Nervous System
Modality	2	Stereotactic Radiosurgery

Treatment Site (4th)	Modality Qualifier (5th)	Isotope (6th)	Qualifier (7th)
0 Brain 1 Brain Stem 6 Spinal Cord 7 Peripheral Nerve	D Stereotactic Other Photon Radiosurgery H Stereotactic Particulate Radiosurgery J Stereotactic Gamma Beam Radiosurgery	Z None	Z None

Section	D	Radiation Therapy
Body System	0	Central and Peripheral Nervous System
Modality	Y	Other Radiation

Treatment Site (4th)	Modality Qualifier (5th)	Isotope (6th)	Qualifier (7th)
0 Brain 1 Brain Stem 6 Spinal Cord 7 Peripheral Nerve	7 Contact Radiation 8 Hyperthermia C Intraoperative Radiation Therapy (IORT) F Plaque Radiation K Laser Interstitial Thermal Therapy	Z None	Z None

Section	D	Radiation Therapy
Body System	7	Lymphatic and Hematologic System
Modality	0	Beam Radiation

Treatment Site (4th)	Modality Qualifier (5th)	Isotope (6th)	Qualifier (7th)
0 Bone Marrow 1 Thymus 2 Spleen 3 Lymphatics, Neck 4 Lymphatics, Axillary 5 Lymphatics, Thorax 6 Lymphatics, Abdomen 7 Lymphatics, Pelvis 8 Lymphatics, Inguinal	0 Photons <1 MeV 1 Photons 1 - 10 MeV 2 Photons >10 MeV 4 Heavy Particles (Protons,Ions) 5 Neutrons 6 Neutron Capture	Z None	Z None
0 Bone Marrow 1 Thymus 2 Spleen 3 Lymphatics, Neck 4 Lymphatics, Axillary 5 Lymphatics, Thorax 6 Lymphatics, Abdomen 7 Lymphatics, Pelvis 8 Lymphatics, Inguinal	3 Electrons	Z None	0 Intraoperative Z None

Section	D	Radiation Therapy
Body System	7	Lymphatic and Hematologic System
Modality	1	Brachytherapy

Treatment Site (4th)	Modality Qualifier (5th)	Isotope (6th)	Qualifier (7th)
0 Bone Marrow 1 Thymus 2 Spleen 3 Lymphatics, Neck 4 Lymphatics, Axillary 5 Lymphatics, Thorax 6 Lymphatics, Abdomen 7 Lymphatics, Pelvis 8 Lymphatics, Inguinal	9 High Dose Rate (HDR)	7 Cesium 137 (Cs-137) 8 Iridium 192 (Ir-192) 9 Iodine 125 (I-125) B Palladium 103 (Pd-103) C Californium 252 (Cf-252) Y Other Isotope	Z None
0 Bone Marrow 1 Thymus 2 Spleen 3 Lymphatics, Neck 4 Lymphatics, Axillary 5 Lymphatics, Thorax 6 Lymphatics, Abdomen 7 Lymphatics, Pelvis 8 Lymphatics, Inguinal	B Low Dose Rate (LDR)	6 Cesium 131 (Cs-131) 7 Cesium 137 (Cs-137) 8 Iridium 192 (Ir-192) 9 Iodine 125 (I-125) C Californium 252 (Cf-252) Y Other Isotope	Z None
0 Bone Marrow 1 Thymus 2 Spleen 3 Lymphatics, Neck 4 Lymphatics, Axillary 5 Lymphatics, Thorax 6 Lymphatics, Abdomen 7 Lymphatics, Pelvis 8 Lymphatics, Inguinal	B Low Dose Rate (LDR)	B Palladium 103 (Pd-103)	1 Unidirectional Source Z None

Section   **D**   **Radiation Therapy**
Body System   **7**   **Lymphatic and Hematologic System**
Modality   **2**   **Stereotactic Radiosurgery**

Treatment Site (4ᵗʰ)	Modality Qualifier (5ᵗʰ)	Isotope (6ᵗʰ)	Qualifier (7ᵗʰ)
0 Bone Marrow 1 Thymus 2 Spleen 3 Lymphatics, Neck 4 Lymphatics, Axillary 5 Lymphatics, Thorax 6 Lymphatics, Abdomen 7 Lymphatics, Pelvis 8 Lymphatics, Inguinal	D Stereotactic Other Photon Radiosurgery H Stereotactic Particulate Radiosurgery J Stereotactic Gamma Beam Radiosurgery	Z None	Z None

Section   **D**   **Radiation Therapy**
Body System   **7**   **Lymphatic and Hematologic System**
Modality   **Y**   **Other Radiation**

Treatment Site (4ᵗʰ)	Modality Qualifier (5ᵗʰ)	Isotope (6ᵗʰ)	Qualifier (7ᵗʰ)
0 Bone Marrow 1 Thymus 2 Spleen 3 Lymphatics, Neck 4 Lymphatics, Axillary 5 Lymphatics, Thorax 6 Lymphatics, Abdomen 7 Lymphatics, Pelvis 8 Lymphatics, Inguinal	8 Hyperthermia F Plaque Radiation	Z None	Z None

Section   **D**   **Radiation Therapy**
Body System   **8**   **Eye**
Modality   **0**   **Beam Radiation**

Treatment Site (4ᵗʰ)	Modality Qualifier (5ᵗʰ)	Isotope (6ᵗʰ)	Qualifier (7ᵗʰ)
0 Eye	0 Photons <1 MeV 1 Photons 1 - 10 MeV 2 Photons >10 MeV 4 Heavy Particles (Protons,Ions) 5 Neutrons 6 Neutron Capture	Z None	Z None
0 Eye	3 Electrons	Z None	0 Intraoperative Z None

Section   **D**   **Radiation Therapy**
Body System   **8**   **Eye**
Modality   **1**   **Brachytherapy**

Treatment Site (4ᵗʰ)	Modality Qualifier (5ᵗʰ)	Isotope (6ᵗʰ)	Qualifier (7ᵗʰ)
0 Eye	9 High Dose Rate (HDR)	7 Cesium 137 (Cs-137) 8 Iridium 192 (Ir-192) 9 Iodine 125 (I-125) B Palladium 103 (Pd-103) C Californium 252 (Cf-252) Y Other Isotope	Z None
0 Eye	B Low Dose Rate (LDR)	6 Cesium 131 (Cs-131) 7 Cesium 137 (Cs-137) 8 Iridium 192 (Ir-192) 9 Iodine 125 (I-125) C Californium 252 (Cf-252) Y Other Isotope	Z None
0 Eye	B Low Dose Rate (LDR)	B Palladium 103 (Pd-103)	1 Unidirectional Source Z None

Section	D	Radiation Therapy
Body System	8	Eye
Modality	2	Stereotactic Radiosurgery

Treatment Site (4th)	Modality Qualifier (5th)	Isotope (6th)	Qualifier (7th)
0 Eye	D Stereotactic Other Photon Radiosurgery H Stereotactic Particulate Radiosurgery J Stereotactic Gamma Beam Radiosurgery	Z None	Z None

Section	D	Radiation Therapy
Body System	8	Eye
Modality	Y	Other Radiation

Treatment Site (4th)	Modality Qualifier (5th)	Isotope (6th)	Qualifier (7th)
0 Eye	7 Contact Radiation 8 Hyperthermia F Plaque Radiation	Z None	Z None

Section	D	Radiation Therapy
Body System	9	Ear, Nose, Mouth and Throat
Modality	0	Beam Radiation

Treatment Site (4th)	Modality Qualifier (5th)	Isotope (6th)	Qualifier (7th)
0 Ear 1 Nose 3 Hypopharynx 4 Mouth 5 Tongue 6 Salivary Glands 7 Sinuses 8 Hard Palate 9 Soft Palate B Larynx D Nasopharynx F Oropharynx	0 Photons <1 MeV 1 Photons 1 - 10 MeV 2 Photons >10 MeV 4 Heavy Particles (Protons,Ions) 5 Neutrons 6 Neutron Capture	Z None	Z None
0 Ear 1 Nose 3 Hypopharynx 4 Mouth 5 Tongue 6 Salivary Glands 7 Sinuses 8 Hard Palate 9 Soft Palate B Larynx D Nasopharynx F Oropharynx	3 Electrons	Z None	0 Intraoperative Z None

Section   **D**   **Radiation Therapy**
Body System   **9**   **Ear, Nose, Mouth and Throat**
Modality   **1**   **Brachytherapy**

Treatment Site (4th)	Modality Qualifier (5th)	Isotope (6th)	Qualifier (7th)
0 Ear 1 Nose 3 Hypopharynx 4 Mouth 5 Tongue 6 Salivary Glands 7 Sinuses 8 Hard Palate 9 Soft Palate B Larynx D Nasopharynx F Oropharynx	9 High Dose Rate (HDR)	7 Cesium 137 (Cs-137) 8 Iridium 192 (Ir-192) 9 Iodine 125 (I-125) B Palladium 103 (Pd-103) C Californium 252 (Cf-252) Y Other Isotope	Z None
0 Ear 1 Nose 3 Hypopharynx 4 Mouth 5 Tongue 6 Salivary Glands 7 Sinuses 8 Hard Palate 9 Soft Palate B Larynx D Nasopharynx F Oropharynx	B Low Dose Rate (LDR)	6 Cesium 131 (Cs-131) 7 Cesium 137 (Cs-137) 8 Iridium 192 (Ir-192) 9 Iodine 125 (I-125) C Californium 252 (Cf-252) Y Other Isotope	Z None
0 Ear 1 Nose 3 Hypopharynx 4 Mouth 5 Tongue 6 Salivary Glands 7 Sinuses 8 Hard Palate 9 Soft Palate B Larynx D Nasopharynx F Oropharynx	B Low Dose Rate (LDR)	B Palladium 103 (Pd-103)	1 Unidirectional Source Z None

Section   **D**   **Radiation Therapy**
Body System   **9**   **Ear, Nose, Mouth and Throat**
Modality   **2**   **Stereotactic Radiosurgery**

Treatment Site (4th)	Modality Qualifier (5th)	Isotope (6th)	Qualifier (7th)
0 Ear 1 Nose 4 Mouth 5 Tongue 6 Salivary Glands 7 Sinuses 8 Hard Palate 9 Soft Palate B Larynx C Pharynx D Nasopharynx	D Stereotactic Other Photon Radiosurgery H Stereotactic Particulate Radiosurgery J Stereotactic Gamma Beam Radiosurgery	Z None	Z None

Section	D	Radiation Therapy
Body System	9	Ear, Nose, Mouth and Throat
Modality	Y	Other Radiation

Treatment Site (4th)	Modality Qualifier (5th)	Isotope (6th)	Qualifier (7th)
0 Ear 1 Nose 5 Tongue 6 Salivary Glands 7 Sinuses 8 Hard Palate 9 Soft Palate	7 Contact Radiation 8 Hyperthermia F Plaque Radiation	Z None	Z None
3 Hypopharynx F Oropharynx	7 Contact Radiation 8 Hyperthermia	Z None	Z None
4 Mouth B Larynx D Nasopharynx	7 Contact Radiation 8 Hyperthermia C Intraoperative Radiation Therapy (IORT) F Plaque Radiation	Z None	Z None
C Pharynx	C Intraoperative Radiation Therapy (IORT) F Plaque Radiation	Z None	Z None

Section	D	Radiation Therapy
Body System	B	Respiratory System
Modality	0	Beam Radiation

Treatment Site (4th)	Modality Qualifier (5th)	Isotope (6th)	Qualifier (7th)
0 Trachea 1 Bronchus 2 Lung 5 Pleura 6 Mediastinum 7 Chest Wall 8 Diaphragm	0 Photons <1 MeV 1 Photons 1 - 10 MeV 2 Photons >10 MeV 4 Heavy Particles (Protons,Ions) 5 Neutrons 6 Neutron Capture	Z None	Z None
0 Trachea 1 Bronchus 2 Lung 5 Pleura 6 Mediastinum 7 Chest Wall 8 Diaphragm	3 Electrons	Z None	0 Intraoperative Z None

Section	D	Radiation Therapy
Body System	B	Respiratory System
Modality	1	Brachytherapy

Treatment Site (4th)	Modality Qualifier (5th)	Isotope (6th)	Qualifier (7th)
0 Trachea 1 Bronchus 2 Lung 5 Pleura 6 Mediastinum 7 Chest Wall 8 Diaphragm	9 High Dose Rate (HDR)	7 Cesium 137 (Cs-137) 8 Iridium 192 (Ir-192) 9 Iodine 125 (I-125) B Palladium 103 (Pd-103) C Californium 252 (Cf-252) Y Other Isotope	Z None

Continued ⟶

Section   D   Radiation Therapy
Body System   B   Respiratory System
Modality   1   Brachytherapy

Treatment Site (4th)	Modality Qualifier (5th)	Isotope (6th)	Qualifier (7th)
0 Trachea 1 Bronchus 2 Lung 5 Pleura 6 Mediastinum 7 Chest Wall 8 Diaphragm	B Low Dose Rate (LDR)	6 Cesium 131 (Cs-131) 7 Cesium 137 (Cs-137) 8 Iridium 192 (Ir-192) 9 Iodine 125 (I-125) C Californium 252 (Cf-252) Y Other Isotope	Z None
0 Trachea 1 Bronchus 2 Lung 5 Pleura 6 Mediastinum 7 Chest Wall 8 Diaphragm	B Low Dose Rate (LDR)	B Palladium 103 (Pd-103)	1 Unidirectional Source Z None

Section   D   Radiation Therapy
Body System   B   Respiratory System
Modality   2   Stereotactic Radiosurgery

Treatment Site (4th)	Modality Qualifier (5th)	Isotope (6th)	Qualifier (7th)
0 Trachea 1 Bronchus 2 Lung 5 Pleura 6 Mediastinum 7 Chest Wall 8 Diaphragm	D Stereotactic Other Photon Radiosurgery H Stereotactic Particulate Radiosurgery J Stereotactic Gamma Beam Radiosurgery	Z None	Z None

Section   D   Radiation Therapy
Body System   B   Respiratory System
Modality   Y   Other Radiation

Treatment Site (4th)	Modality Qualifier (5th)	Isotope (6th)	Qualifier (7th)
0 Trachea 1 Bronchus 2 Lung 5 Pleura 6 Mediastinum 7 Chest Wall 8 Diaphragm	7 Contact Radiation 8 Hyperthermia F Plaque Radiation K Laser Interstitial Thermal Therapy	Z None	Z None

Section   D   **Radiation Therapy**
Body System   D   **Gastrointestinal System**
Modality   0   **Beam Radiation**

Treatment Site (4th)	Modality Qualifier (5th)	Isotope (6th)	Qualifier (7th)
0 Esophagus 1 Stomach 2 Duodenum 3 Jejunum 4 Ileum 5 Colon 7 Rectum	0 Photons <1 MeV 1 Photons 1 - 10 MeV 2 Photons >10 MeV 4 Heavy Particles (Protons,Ions) 5 Neutrons 6 Neutron Capture	Z None	Z None
0 Esophagus 1 Stomach 2 Duodenum 3 Jejunum 4 Ileum 5 Colon 7 Rectum	3 Electrons	Z None	0 Intraoperative Z None

Section   D   **Radiation Therapy**
Body System   D   **Gastrointestinal System**
Modality   1   **Brachytherapy**

Treatment Site (4th)	Modality Qualifier (5th)	Isotope (6th)	Qualifier (7th)
0 Esophagus 1 Stomach 2 Duodenum 3 Jejunum 4 Ileum 5 Colon 7 Rectum	9 High Dose Rate (HDR)	7 Cesium 137 (Cs-137) 8 Iridium 192 (Ir-192) 9 Iodine 125 (I-125) B Palladium 103 (Pd-103) C Californium 252 (Cf-252) Y Other Isotope	Z None
0 Esophagus 1 Stomach 2 Duodenum 3 Jejunum 4 Ileum 5 Colon 7 Rectum	B Low Dose Rate (LDR)	6 Cesium 131 (Cs-131) 7 Cesium 137 (Cs-137) 8 Iridium 192 (Ir-192) 9 Iodine 125 (I-125) C Californium 252 (Cf-252) Y Other Isotope	Z None
0 Esophagus 1 Stomach 2 Duodenum 3 Jejunum 4 Ileum 5 Colon 7 Rectum	B Low Dose Rate (LDR)	B Palladium 103 (Pd-103)	1 Unidirectional Source Z None

Section   D   **Radiation Therapy**
Body System   D   **Gastrointestinal System**
Modality   2   **Stereotactic Radiosurgery**

Treatment Site (4th)	Modality Qualifier (5th)	Isotope (6th)	Qualifier (7th)
0 Esophagus 1 Stomach 2 Duodenum 3 Jejunum 4 Ileum 5 Colon 7 Rectum	D Stereotactic Other Photon Radiosurgery H Stereotactic Particulate Radiosurgery J Stereotactic Gamma Beam Radiosurgery	Z None	Z None

Section	D	Radiation Therapy
Body System	D	Gastrointestinal System
Modality	Y	Other Radiation

Treatment Site (4th)	Modality Qualifier (5th)	Isotope (6th)	Qualifier (7th)
0 Esophagus	7 Contact Radiation 8 Hyperthermia F Plaque Radiation K Laser Interstitial Thermal Therapy	Z None	Z None
1 Stomach 2 Duodenum 3 Jejunum 4 Ileum 5 Colon 7 Rectum	7 Contact Radiation 8 Hyperthermia C Intraoperative Radiation Therapy (IORT) F Plaque Radiation K Laser Interstitial Thermal Therapy	Z None	Z None
8 Anus	C Intraoperative Radiation Therapy (IORT) F Plaque Radiation K Laser Interstitial Thermal Therapy	Z None	Z None

Section	D	Radiation Therapy
Body System	F	Hepatobiliary System and Pancreas
Modality	0	Beam Radiation

Treatment Site (4th)	Modality Qualifier (5th)	Isotope (6th)	Qualifier (7th)
0 Liver 1 Gallbladder 2 Bile Ducts 3 Pancreas	0 Photons <1 MeV 1 Photons 1 - 10 MeV 2 Photons >10 MeV 4 Heavy Particles (Protons,Ions) 5 Neutrons 6 Neutron Capture	Z None	Z None
0 Liver 1 Gallbladder 2 Bile Ducts 3 Pancreas	3 Electrons	Z None	0 Intraoperative Z None

Section	D	Radiation Therapy
Body System	F	Hepatobiliary System and Pancreas
Modality	1	Brachytherapy

Treatment Site (4th)	Modality Qualifier (5th)	Isotope (6th)	Qualifier (7th)
0 Liver 1 Gallbladder 2 Bile Ducts 3 Pancreas	9 High Dose Rate (HDR)	7 Cesium 137 (Cs-137) 8 Iridium 192 (Ir-192) 9 Iodine 125 (I-125) B Palladium 103 (Pd-103) C Californium 252 (Cf-252) Y Other Isotope	Z None
0 Liver 1 Gallbladder 2 Bile Ducts 3 Pancreas	B Low Dose Rate (LDR)	6 Cesium 131 (Cs-131) 7 Cesium 137 (Cs-137) 8 Iridium 192 (Ir-192) 9 Iodine 125 (I-125) C Californium 252 (Cf-252) Y Other Isotope	Z None
0 Liver 1 Gallbladder 2 Bile Ducts 3 Pancreas	B Low Dose Rate (LDR)	B Palladium 103 (Pd-103)	1 Unidirectional Source Z None

Section	D	Radiation Therapy
Body System	F	Hepatobiliary System and Pancreas
Modality	2	Stereotactic Radiosurgery

Treatment Site (4th)	Modality Qualifier (5th)	Isotope (6th)	Qualifier (7th)
0 Liver 1 Gallbladder 2 Bile Ducts 3 Pancreas	D Stereotactic Other Photon Radiosurgery H Stereotactic Particulate Radiosurgery J Stereotactic Gamma Beam Radiosurgery	Z None	Z None

Section	D	Radiation Therapy
Body System	F	Hepatobiliary System and Pancreas
Modality	Y	Other Radiation

Treatment Site (4th)	Modality Qualifier (5th)	Isotope (6th)	Qualifier (7th)
0 Liver 1 Gallbladder 2 Bile Ducts 3 Pancreas	7 Contact Radiation 8 Hyperthermia C Intraoperative Radiation Therapy (IORT) F Plaque Radiation K Laser Interstitial Thermal Therapy	Z None	Z None

Section	D	Radiation Therapy
Body System	G	Endocrine System
Modality	0	Beam Radiation

Treatment Site (4th)	Modality Qualifier (5th)	Isotope (6th)	Qualifier (7th)
0 Pituitary Gland 1 Pineal Body 2 Adrenal Glands 4 Parathyroid Glands 5 Thyroid	0 Photons <1 MeV 1 Photons 1 - 10 MeV 2 Photons >10 MeV 5 Neutrons 6 Neutron Capture	Z None	Z None
0 Pituitary Gland 1 Pineal Body 2 Adrenal Glands 4 Parathyroid Glands 5 Thyroid	3 Electrons	Z None	0 Intraoperative Z None

Section	D	Radiation Therapy
Body System	G	Endocrine System
Modality	1	Brachytherapy

Treatment Site (4th)	Modality Qualifier (5th)	Isotope (6th)	Qualifier (7th)
0 Pituitary Gland 1 Pineal Body 2 Adrenal Glands 4 Parathyroid Glands 5 Thyroid	9 High Dose Rate (HDR)	7 Cesium 137 (Cs-137) 8 Iridium 192 (Ir-192) 9 Iodine 125 (I-125) B Palladium 103 (Pd-103) C Californium 252 (Cf-252) Y Other Isotope	Z None
0 Pituitary Gland 1 Pineal Body 2 Adrenal Glands 4 Parathyroid Glands 5 Thyroid	B Low Dose Rate (LDR)	6 Cesium 131 (Cs-131) 7 Cesium 137 (Cs-137) 8 Iridium 192 (Ir-192) 9 Iodine 125 (I-125) C Californium 252 (Cf-252) Y Other Isotope	Z None
0 Pituitary Gland 1 Pineal Body 2 Adrenal Glands 4 Parathyroid Glands 5 Thyroid	B Low Dose Rate (LDR)	B Palladium 103 (Pd-103)	1 Unidirectional Source Z None

Section	D	Radiation Therapy
Body System	G	Endocrine System
Modality	2	Stereotactic Radiosurgery

Treatment Site (4th)	Modality Qualifier (5th)	Isotope (6th)	Qualifier (7th)
0 Pituitary Gland 1 Pineal Body 2 Adrenal Glands 4 Parathyroid Glands 5 Thyroid	D Stereotactic Other Photon Radiosurgery H Stereotactic Particulate Radiosurgery J Stereotactic Gamma Beam Radiosurgery	Z None	Z None

Section	D	Radiation Therapy
Body System	G	Endocrine System
Modality	Y	Other Radiation

Treatment Site (4th)	Modality Qualifier (5th)	Isotope (6th)	Qualifier (7th)
0 Pituitary Gland 1 Pineal Body 2 Adrenal Glands 4 Parathyroid Glands 5 Thyroid	7 Contact Radiation 8 Hyperthermia F Plaque Radiation K Laser Interstitial Thermal Therapy	Z None	Z None

Section	D	Radiation Therapy
Body System	H	Skin
Modality	0	Beam Radiation

Treatment Site (4th)	Modality Qualifier (5th)	Isotope (6th)	Qualifier (7th)
2 Skin, Face 3 Skin, Neck 4 Skin, Arm 6 Skin, Chest 7 Skin, Back 8 Skin, Abdomen 9 Skin, Buttock B Skin, Leg	0 Photons <1 MeV 1 Photons 1 - 10 MeV 2 Photons >10 MeV 4 Heavy Particles (Protons,Ions) 5 Neutrons 6 Neutron Capture	Z None	Z None
2 Skin, Face 3 Skin, Neck 4 Skin, Arm 6 Skin, Chest 7 Skin, Back 8 Skin, Abdomen 9 Skin, Buttock B Skin, Leg	3 Electrons	Z None	0 Intraoperative Z None

Section	D	Radiation Therapy
Body System	H	Skin
Modality	Y	Other Radiation

Treatment Site (4th)	Modality Qualifier (5th)	Isotope (6th)	Qualifier (7th)
2 Skin, Face 3 Skin, Neck 4 Skin, Arm 6 Skin, Chest 7 Skin, Back 8 Skin, Abdomen 9 Skin, Buttock B Skin, Leg	7 Contact Radiation 8 Hyperthermia F Plaque Radiation	Z None	Z None
5 Skin, Hand C Skin, Foot	F Plaque Radiation	Z None	Z None

Section	D	Radiation Therapy
Body System	M	Breast
Modality	0	Beam Radiation

Treatment Site (4th)	Modality Qualifier (5th)	Isotope (6th)	Qualifier (7th)
0 Breast, Left 1 Breast, Right	0 Photons <1 MeV 1 Photons 1 - 10 MeV 2 Photons >10 MeV 4 Heavy Particles (Protons,Ions) 5 Neutrons 6 Neutron Capture	Z None	Z None
0 Breast, Left 1 Breast, Right	3 Electrons	Z None	0 Intraoperative Z None

Section	D	Radiation Therapy
Body System	M	Breast
Modality	1	Brachytherapy

Treatment Site (4th)	Modality Qualifier (5th)	Isotope (6th)	Qualifier (7th)
0 Breast, Left 1 Breast, Right	9 High Dose Rate (HDR)	7 Cesium 137 (Cs-137) 8 Iridium 192 (Ir-192) 9 Iodine 125 (I-125) B Palladium 103 (Pd-103) C Californium 252 (Cf-252) Y Other Isotope	Z None
0 Breast, Left 1 Breast, Right	B Low Dose Rate (LDR)	6 Cesium 131 (Cs-131) 7 Cesium 137 (Cs-137) 8 Iridium 192 (Ir-192) 9 Iodine 125 (I-125) C Californium 252 (Cf-252) Y Other Isotope	Z None
0 Breast, Left 1 Breast, Right	B Low Dose Rate (LDR)	B Palladium 103 (Pd-103)	1 Unidirectional Source Z None

Section	D	Radiation Therapy
Body System	M	Breast
Modality	2	Stereotactic Radiosurgery

Treatment Site (4th)	Modality Qualifier (5th)	Isotope (6th)	Qualifier (7th)
0 Breast, Left 1 Breast, Right	D Stereotactic Other Photon Radiosurgery H Stereotactic Particulate Radiosurgery J Stereotactic Gamma Beam Radiosurgery	Z None	Z None

Section	D	Radiation Therapy
Body System	M	Breast
Modality	Y	Other Radiation

Treatment Site (4th)	Modality Qualifier (5th)	Isotope (6th)	Qualifier (7th)
0 Breast, Left 1 Breast, Right	7 Contact Radiation 8 Hyperthermia F Plaque Radiation K Laser Interstitial Thermal Therapy	Z None	Z None

Section   **D**   **Radiation Therapy**
Body System   **P**   **Musculoskeletal System**
Modality   **0**   **Beam Radiation**

Treatment Site (4th)	Modality Qualifier (5th)	Isotope (6th)	Qualifier (7th)
0 Skull 2 Maxilla 3 Mandible 4 Sternum 5 Rib(s) 6 Humerus 7 Radius/Ulna 8 Pelvic Bones 9 Femur B Tibia/Fibula C Other Bone	0 Photons <1 MeV 1 Photons 1 - 10 MeV 2 Photons >10 MeV 4 Heavy Particles (Protons,Ions) 5 Neutrons 6 Neutron Capture	Z None	Z None
0 Skull 2 Maxilla 3 Mandible 4 Sternum 5 Rib(s) 6 Humerus 7 Radius/Ulna 8 Pelvic Bones 9 Femur B Tibia/Fibula C Other Bone	3 Electrons	Z None	0 Intraoperative Z None

Section   **D**   **Radiation Therapy**
Body System   **P**   **Musculoskeletal System**
Modality   **Y**   **Other Radiation**

Treatment Site (4th)	Modality Qualifier (5th)	Isotope (6th)	Qualifier (7th)
0 Skull 2 Maxilla 3 Mandible 4 Sternum 5 Rib(s) 6 Humerus 7 Radius/Ulna 8 Pelvic Bones 9 Femur B Tibia/Fibula C Other Bone	7 Contact Radiation 8 Hyperthermia F Plaque Radiation	Z None	Z None

Section   **D**   **Radiation Therapy**
Body System   **T**   **Urinary System**
Modality   **0**   **Beam Radiation**

Treatment Site (4th)	Modality Qualifier (5th)	Isotope (6th)	Qualifier (7th)
0 Kidney 1 Ureter 2 Bladder 3 Urethra	0 Photons <1 MeV 1 Photons 1 - 10 MeV 2 Photons >10 MeV 4 Heavy Particles (Protons,Ions) 5 Neutrons 6 Neutron Capture	Z None	Z None
0 Kidney 1 Ureter 2 Bladder 3 Urethra	3 Electrons	Z None	0 Intraoperative Z None

Section D Radiation Therapy
Body System T Urinary System
Modality 1 Brachytherapy

Treatment Site (4ᵗʰ)	Modality Qualifier (5ᵗʰ)	Isotope (6ᵗʰ)	Qualifier (7ᵗʰ)
0 Kidney 1 Ureter 2 Bladder 3 Urethra	9 High Dose Rate (HDR)	7 Cesium 137 (Cs-137) 8 Iridium 192 (Ir-192) 9 Iodine 125 (I-125) B Palladium 103 (Pd-103) C Californium 252 (Cf-252) Y Other Isotope	Z None
0 Kidney 1 Ureter 2 Bladder 3 Urethra	B Low Dose Rate (LDR)	6 Cesium 131 (Cs-131) 7 Cesium 137 (Cs-137) 8 Iridium 192 (Ir-192) 9 Iodine 125 (I-125) C Californium 252 (Cf-252) Y Other Isotope	Z None
0 Kidney 1 Ureter 2 Bladder 3 Urethra	B Low Dose Rate (LDR)	B Palladium 103 (Pd-103)	1 Unidirectional Source Z None

Section D Radiation Therapy
Body System T Urinary System
Modality 2 Stereotactic Radiosurgery

Treatment Site (4ᵗʰ)	Modality Qualifier (5ᵗʰ)	Isotope (6ᵗʰ)	Qualifier (7ᵗʰ)
0 Kidney 1 Ureter 2 Bladder 3 Urethra	D Stereotactic Other Photon Radiosurgery H Stereotactic Particulate Radiosurgery J Stereotactic Gamma Beam Radiosurgery	Z None	Z None

Section D Radiation Therapy
Body System T Urinary System
Modality Y Other Radiation

Treatment Site (4ᵗʰ)	Modality Qualifier (5ᵗʰ)	Isotope (6ᵗʰ)	Qualifier (7ᵗʰ)
0 Kidney 1 Ureter 2 Bladder 3 Urethra	7 Contact Radiation 8 Hyperthermia C Intraoperative Radiation Therapy (IORT) F Plaque Radiation	Z None	Z None

Section D Radiation Therapy
Body System U Female Reproductive System
Modality 0 Beam Radiation

Treatment Site (4ᵗʰ)	Modality Qualifier (5ᵗʰ)	Isotope (6ᵗʰ)	Qualifier (7ᵗʰ)
0 Ovary 1 Cervix 2 Uterus	0 Photons <1 MeV 1 Photons 1 - 10 MeV 2 Photons >10 MeV 4 Heavy Particles (Protons,Ions) 5 Neutrons 6 Neutron Capture	Z None	Z None

Continued →

Section	D	Radiation Therapy
Body System	U	Female Reproductive System
Modality	0	Beam Radiation

Treatment Site (4th)	Modality Qualifier (5th)	Isotope (6th)	Qualifier (7th)
0 Ovary 1 Cervix 2 Uterus	3 Electrons	Z None	0 Intraoperative Z None

Section	D	Radiation Therapy
Body System	U	Female Reproductive System
Modality	1	Brachytherapy

Treatment Site (4th)	Modality Qualifier (5th)	Isotope (6th)	Qualifier (7th)
0 Ovary 1 Cervix 2 Uterus	9 High Dose Rate (HDR)	7 Cesium 137 (Cs-137) 8 Iridium 192 (Ir-192) 9 Iodine 125 (I-125) B Palladium 103 (Pd-103) C Californium 252 (Cf-252) Y Other Isotope	Z None
0 Ovary 1 Cervix 2 Uterus	B Low Dose Rate (LDR)	6 Cesium 131 (Cs-131) 7 Cesium 137 (Cs-137) 8 Iridium 192 (Ir-192) 9 Iodine 125 (I-125) C Californium 252 (Cf-252) Y Other Isotope	Z None
0 Ovary 1 Cervix 2 Uterus	B Low Dose Rate (LDR)	B Palladium 103 (Pd-103)	1 Unidirectional Source Z None

Section	D	Radiation Therapy
Body System	U	Female Reproductive System
Modality	2	Stereotactic Radiosurgery

Treatment Site (4th)	Modality Qualifier (5th)	Isotope (6th)	Qualifier (7th)
0 Ovary 1 Cervix 2 Uterus	D Stereotactic Other Photon Radiosurgery H Stereotactic Particulate Radiosurgery J Stereotactic Gamma Beam Radiosurgery	Z None	Z None

Section	D	Radiation Therapy
Body System	U	Female Reproductive System
Modality	Y	Other Radiation

Treatment Site (4th)	Modality Qualifier (5th)	Isotope (6th)	Qualifier (7th)
0 Ovary 1 Cervix 2 Uterus	7 Contact Radiation 8 Hyperthermia C Intraoperative Radiation Therapy (IORT) F Plaque Radiation	Z None	Z None

Section   D   **Radiation Therapy**
Body System   V   **Male Reproductive System**
Modality   0   **Beam Radiation**

Treatment Site (4th)	Modality Qualifier (5th)	Isotope (6th)	Qualifier (7th)
0 Prostate 1 Testis	0 Photons <1 MeV 1 Photons 1 - 10 MeV 2 Photons >10 MeV 4 Heavy Particles (Protons,Ions) 5 Neutrons 6 Neutron Capture	Z None	Z None
0 Prostate 1 Testis	3 Electrons	Z None	0 Intraoperative Z None

Section   D   **Radiation Therapy**
Body System   V   **Male Reproductive System**
Modality   1   **Brachytherapy**

Treatment Site (4th)	Modality Qualifier (5th)	Isotope (6th)	Qualifier (7th)
0 Prostate 1 Testis	9 High Dose Rate (HDR)	7 Cesium 137 (Cs-137) 8 Iridium 192 (Ir-192) 9 Iodine 125 (I-125) B Palladium 103 (Pd-103) C Californium 252 (Cf-252) Y Other Isotope	Z None
0 Prostate 1 Testis	B Low Dose Rate (LDR)	6 Cesium 131 (Cs-131) 7 Cesium 137 (Cs-137) 8 Iridium 192 (Ir-192) 9 Iodine 125 (I-125) C Californium 252 (Cf-252) Y Other Isotope	Z None
0 Prostate 1 Testis	B Low Dose Rate (LDR)	B Palladium 103 (Pd-103)	1 Unidirectional Source Z None

Section   D   **Radiation Therapy**
Body System   V   **Male Reproductive System**
Modality   2   **Stereotactic Radiosurgery**

Treatment Site (4th)	Modality Qualifier (5th)	Isotope (6th)	Qualifier (7th)
0 Prostate 1 Testis	D Stereotactic Other Photon Radiosurgery H Stereotactic Particulate Radiosurgery J Stereotactic Gamma Beam Radiosurgery	Z None	Z None

Section   D   **Radiation Therapy**
Body System   V   **Male Reproductive System**
Modality   Y   **Other Radiation**

Treatment Site (4th)	Modality Qualifier (5th)	Isotope (6th)	Qualifier (7th)
0 Prostate	7 Contact Radiation 8 Hyperthermia C Intraoperative Radiation Therapy (IORT) F Plaque Radiation K Laser Interstitial Thermal Therapy	Z None	Z None
1 Testis	7 Contact Radiation 8 Hyperthermia F Plaque Radiation	Z None	Z None

Section   **D**   **Radiation Therapy**
Body System   **W**   **Anatomical Regions**
Modality   **0**   **Beam Radiation**

Treatment Site (4th)	Modality Qualifier (5th)	Isotope (6th)	Qualifier (7th)
1 Head and Neck 2 Chest 3 Abdomen 4 Hemibody 5 Whole Body 6 Pelvic Region	0 Photons <1 MeV 1 Photons 1 - 10 MeV 2 Photons >10 MeV 4 Heavy Particles (Protons,Ions) 5 Neutrons 6 Neutron Capture	Z None	Z None
1 Head and Neck 2 Chest 3 Abdomen 4 Hemibody 5 Whole Body 6 Pelvic Region	3 Electrons	Z None	0 Intraoperative Z None

Section   **D**   **Radiation Therapy**
Body System   **W**   **Anatomical Regions**
Modality   **1**   **Brachytherapy**

Treatment Site (4th)	Modality Qualifier (5th)	Isotope (6th)	Qualifier (7th)
0 Cranial Cavity K Upper Back L Lower Back P Gastrointestinal Track Q Respiratory Track R Genitourinary Track X Upper Extremity Y Lower Extremity	B Low Dose Rate (LDR)	B Palladium 103 (Pd-103)	1 Unidirectional Source Z None
1 Head and Neck 2 Chest 3 Abdomen 6 Pelvic Region	9 High Dose Rate (HDR)	7 Cesium 137 (Cs-137) 8 Iridium 192 (Ir-192) 9 Iodine 125 (I-125) B Palladium 103 (Pd-103) C Californium 252 (Cf-252) Y Other Isotope	Z None
1 Head and Neck 2 Chest 3 Abdomen 6 Pelvic Region	B Low Dose Rate (LDR)	6 Cesium 131 (Cs-131) 7 Cesium 137 (Cs-137) 8 Iridium 192 (Ir-192) 9 Iodine 125 (I-125) C Californium 252 (Cf-252) Y Other Isotope	Z None
1 Head and Neck 2 Chest 3 Abdomen 6 Pelvic Region	B Low Dose Rate (LDR)	B Palladium 103 (Pd-103)	1 Unidirectional Source Z None

Section   **D**   **Radiation Therapy**
Body System   **W**   **Anatomical Regions**
Modality   **2**   **Stereotactic Radiosurgery**

Treatment Site (4th)	Modality Qualifier (5th)	Isotope (6th)	Qualifier (7th)
1 Head and Neck 2 Chest 3 Abdomen 6 Pelvic Region	D Stereotactic Other Photon Radiosurgery H Stereotactic Particulate Radiosurgery J Stereotactic Gamma Beam Radiosurgery	Z None	Z None

Section **D** Radiation Therapy
Body System **W** Anatomical Regions
Modality **Y** Other Radiation

Treatment Site (4ᵗʰ)	Modality Qualifier (5ᵗʰ)	Isotope (6ᵗʰ)	Qualifier (7ᵗʰ)
1 Head and Neck **2** Chest **3** Abdomen **4** Hemibody **6** Pelvic Region	**7** Contact Radiation **8** Hyperthermia **F** Plaque Radiation	**Z** None	**Z** None
5 Whole Body	**7** Contact Radiation **8** Hyperthermia **F** Plaque Radiation	**Z** None	**Z** None
5 Whole Body	**G** Isotope Administration	**D** Iodine 131 (I-131) **F** Phosphorus 32 (P-32) **G** Strontium 89 (Sr-89) **H** Strontium 90 (Sr-90) **Y** Other Isotope	**Z** None

Within each section of ICD-10-PCS the characters have different meanings. The seven character meanings for the Physical Rehabilitation and Diagnostic Audiology section are illustrated below through the procedure example of *Individual fitting of moveable brace, right knee*.

Section	Section Qualifier	Root Type	Body System/ Region	Type Qualifier	Equipment	Qualifier
Physical Rehabilitation and Diagnostic Audiology	Rehabilitation	Device Fitting	None	Dynamic Orthosis	Orthosis	None
F	0	D	Z	6	E	Z

Section (Character 1)

All Physical Rehabilitation and Diagnostic Audiology procedure codes have a first character value of F.

Section Qualifier (Character 2)

The alphanumeric character in the second character position identifies if the procedure is a physical rehabilitation procedure or a diagnostic audiology procedure. Physical rehabilitation is reported with character value 0, and diagnostic audiology is reported with character value 1.

Root Type (Character 3)

The alphanumeric character value for root types is placed in the third position. The following are the root types applicable to the Physical Rehabilitation and Diagnostic Audiology section with their associated meaning.

Character Value	Root Type	Root Type Definition
0	Speech Assessment	Measurement of speech and related functions
1	Motor and/or Nerve Function Assessment	Measurement of motor, nerve, and related functions
2	Activities of Daily Living Assessment	Measurement of functional level for activities of daily living
3	Hearing Assessment	Measurement of hearing and related functions
4	Hearing Aid Assessment	Measurement of the appropriateness and/or effectiveness of a hearing device
5	Vestibular Assessment	Measurement of the vestibular system and related functions
6	Speech Treatment	Application of techniques to improve, augment, or compensate for speech and related functional impairment
7	Motor Treatment	Exercise or activities to increase or facilitate motor function
8	Activities of Daily Living Treatment	Exercise or activities to facilitate functional competence for activities of daily living
9	Hearing Treatment	Application of techniques to improve, augment, or compensate for hearing and related functional impairment
B	Cochlear Implant Treatment	Application of techniques to improve the communication abilities of individuals with cochlear implant
C	Vestibular Treatment	Application of techniques to improve, augment, or compensate for vestibular and related functional impairment
D	Device Fitting	Fitting of a device designed to facilitate or support achievement of a higher level of function
F	Caregiver Training	Training in activities to support patient's optimal level of function

Body System/Region (Character 4)

For each body system/region the applicable body part character values will be available for procedure code construction. An example of a body region for this section is Musculoskeletal System—Lower Back/Lower Extremity.

Type Qualifier (Character 5)

Type qualifier further specifies the root type procedure. For example, the type qualifier of Gait Training/Functional Ambulation is used with Motor Treatment (character value 7) when applicable.

Equipment (Character 6)

If equipment is utilized during the procedure character six is used to report the type. Some examples of equipment are

- Aerobic Endurance and Conditioning
- Electrotherapeutic
- Mechanical
- Orthosis
- Prosthesis

If equipment is not utilized, the placeholder character value of Z should be reported.

Qualifier (Character 7)

The qualifier represents an additional attribute for the procedure when applicable. Currently, there are no qualifiers in the Physical Rehabilitation and Diagnostic Audiology section; therefore, the placeholder character value of Z should be reported.

Physical Rehabilitation and Diagnostic Audiology Section Tables

Physical Rehabilitation and Diagnostic Audiology Tables F00–F15

Section	F	Physical Rehabilitation and Diagnostic Audiology
Section Qualifier	0	Rehabilitation
Type	0	Speech Assessment: Measurement of speech and related functions

Body System / Region (4th)	Type Qualifier (5th)	Equipment (6th)	Qualifier (7th)
3 Neurological System - Whole Body	G Communicative/Cognitive Integration Skills	K Audiovisual M Augmentative / Alternative Communication P Computer Y Other Equipment Z None	Z None
Z None	0 Filtered Speech 3 Staggered Spondaic Word Q Performance Intensity Phonetically Balanced Speech Discrimination R Brief Tone Stimuli S Distorted Speech T Dichotic Stimuli V Temporal Ordering of Stimuli W Masking Patterns	1 Audiometer 2 Sound Field / Booth K Audiovisual Z None	Z None
Z None	1 Speech Threshold 2 Speech/Word Recognition	1 Audiometer 2 Sound Field / Booth 9 Cochlear Implant K Audiovisual Z None	Z None
Z None	4 Sensorineural Acuity Level	1 Audiometer 2 Sound Field / Booth Z None	Z None
Z None	5 Synthetic Sentence Identification	1 Audiometer 2 Sound Field / Booth 9 Cochlear Implant K Audiovisual	Z None
Z None	6 Speech and/or Language Screening 7 Nonspoken Language 8 Receptive/Expressive Language C Aphasia G Communicative/Cognitive Integration Skills L Augmentative/Alternative Communication System	K Audiovisual M Augmentative / Alternative Communication P Computer Y Other Equipment Z None	Z None

Continued →

Section	F	Physical Rehabilitation and Diagnostic Audiology
Section Qualifier	0	Rehabilitation
Type	0	Speech Assessment: Measurement of speech and related functions

Body System / Region (4th)	Type Qualifier (5th)	Equipment (6th)	Qualifier (7th)
Z None	**9** Articulation/Phonology	**K** Audiovisual **P** Computer **Q** Speech Analysis **Y** Other Equipment **Z** None	**Z** None
Z None	**B** Motor Speech	**K** Audiovisual **N** Biosensory Feedback **P** Computer **Q** Speech Analysis **T** Aerodynamic Function **Y** Other Equipment **Z** None	**Z** None
Z None	**D** Fluency	**K** Audiovisual **N** Biosensory Feedback **P** Computer **Q** Speech Analysis **S** Voice Analysis **T** Aerodynamic Function **Y** Other Equipment **Z** None	**Z** None
Z None	**F** Voice	**K** Audiovisual **N** Biosensory Feedback **P** Computer **S** Voice Analysis **T** Aerodynamic Function **Y** Other Equipment **Z** None	**Z** None
Z None	**H** Bedside Swallowing and Oral Function **P** Oral Peripheral Mechanism	**Y** Other Equipment **Z** None	**Z** None
Z None	**J** Instrumental Swallowing and Oral Function	**T** Aerodynamic Function **W** Swallowing **Y** Other Equipment	**Z** None
Z None	**K** Orofacial Myofunctional	**K** Audiovisual **P** Computer **Y** Other Equipment **Z** None	**Z** None
Z None	**M** Voice Prosthetic	**K** Audiovisual **P** Computer **S** Voice Analysis **V** Speech Prosthesis **Y** Other Equipment **Z** None	**Z** None
Z None	**N** Non-invasive Instrumental Status	**N** Biosensory Feedback **P** Computer **Q** Speech Analysis **S** Voice Analysis **T** Aerodynamic Function **Y** Other Equipment	**Z** None
Z None	**X** Other Specified Central Auditory Processing	**Z** None	**Z** None

Section   F   **Physical Rehabilitation and Diagnostic Audiology**
Section Qualifier   0   **Rehabilitation**
Type   1   **Motor and/or Nerve Function Assessment:** Measurement of motor, nerve, and related functions

Body System / Region (4ᵗʰ)	Type Qualifier (5ᵗʰ)	Equipment (6ᵗʰ)	Qualifier (7ᵗʰ)
0 Neurological System - Head and Neck 1 Neurological System - Upper Back / Upper Extremity 2 Neurological System - Lower Back / Lower Extremity 3 Neurological System - Whole Body	0 Muscle Performance	E Orthosis F Assistive, Adaptive, Supportive or Protective U Prosthesis Y Other Equipment Z None	Z None
0 Neurological System - Head and Neck 1 Neurological System - Upper Back / Upper Extremity 2 Neurological System - Lower Back / Lower Extremity 3 Neurological System - Whole Body	1 Integumentary Integrity 3 Coordination/Dexterity 4 Motor Function G Reflex Integrity	Z None	Z None
0 Neurological System - Head and Neck 1 Neurological System - Upper Back / Upper Extremity 2 Neurological System - Lower Back / Lower Extremity 3 Neurological System - Whole Body	5 Range of Motion and Joint Integrity 6 Sensory Awareness/ Processing/Integrity	Y Other Equipment Z None	Z None
D Integumentary System - Head and Neck F Integumentary System - Upper Back / Upper Extremity G Integumentary System - Lower Back / Lower Extremity H Integumentary System - Whole Body J Musculoskeletal System - Head and Neck K Musculoskeletal System - Upper Back / Upper Extremity L Musculoskeletal System - Lower Back / Lower Extremity M Musculoskeletal System - Whole Body	0 Muscle Performance	E Orthosis F Assistive, Adaptive, Supportive or Protective U Prosthesis Y Other Equipment Z None	Z None
D Integumentary System - Head and Neck F Integumentary System - Upper Back / Upper Extremity G Integumentary System - Lower Back / Lower Extremity H Integumentary System - Whole Body J Musculoskeletal System - Head and Neck K Musculoskeletal System - Upper Back / Upper Extremity L Musculoskeletal System - Lower Back / Lower Extremity M Musculoskeletal System - Whole Body	1 Integumentary Integrity	Z None	Z None
D Integumentary System - Head and Neck F Integumentary System - Upper Back / Upper Extremity G Integumentary System - Lower Back / Lower Extremity H Integumentary System - Whole Body J Musculoskeletal System - Head and Neck K Musculoskeletal System - Upper Back / Upper Extremity L Musculoskeletal System - Lower Back / Lower Extremity M Musculoskeletal System - Whole Body	5 Range of Motion and Joint Integrity 6 Sensory Awareness/ Processing/Integrity	Y Other Equipment Z None	Z None

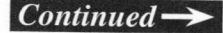

Continued →

Section   F   Physical Rehabilitation and Diagnostic Audiology
Section Qualifier 0   Rehabilitation
Type   1   **Motor and/or Nerve Function Assessment:** Measurement of motor, nerve, and related functions

Body System / Region (4th)	Type Qualifier (5th)	Equipment (6th)	Qualifier (7th)
N Genitourinary System	0 Muscle Performance	E Orthosis F Assistive, Adaptive, Supportive or Protective U Prosthesis Y Other Equipment Z None	Z None
Z None	2 Visual Motor Integration	K Audiovisual M Augmentative / Alternative Communication N Biosensory Feedback P Computer Q Speech Analysis S Voice Analysis Y Other Equipment Z None	Z None
Z None	7 Facial Nerve Function	7 Electrophysiologic	Z None
Z None	9 Somatosensory Evoked Potentials	J Somatosensory	Z None
Z None	B Bed Mobility C Transfer F Wheelchair Mobility	E Orthosis F Assistive, Adaptive, Supportive or Protective U Prosthesis Z None	Z None
Z None	D Gait and/or Balance	E Orthosis F Assistive, Adaptive, Supportive or Protective U Prosthesis Y Other Equipment Z None	Z None

Section   F   Physical Rehabilitation and Diagnostic Audiology
Section Qualifier 0   Rehabilitation
Type   2   **Activities of Daily Living Assessment:** Measurement of functional level for activities of daily living

Body System / Region (4th)	Type Qualifier (5th)	Equipment (6th)	Qualifier (7th)
0 Neurological System - Head and Neck	9 Cranial Nerve Integrity D Neuromotor Development	Y Other Equipment Z None	Z None
1 Neurological System - Upper Back / Upper Extremity 2 Neurological System - Lower Back / Lower Extremity 3 Neurological System - Whole Body	D Neuromotor Development	Y Other Equipment Z None	Z None
4 Circulatory System - Head and Neck 5 Circulatory System - Upper Back / Upper Extremity 6 Circulatory System - Lower Back / Lower Extremity 8 Respiratory System - Head and Neck 9 Respiratory System - Upper Back / Upper Extremity B Respiratory System - Lower Back / Lower Extremity	G Ventilation, Respiration and Circulation	C Mechanical G Aerobic Endurance and Conditioning Y Other Equipment Z None	Z None

Continued →

Section   F   Physical Rehabilitation and Diagnostic Audiology
Section Qualifier 0   Rehabilitation
Type   2   Activities of Daily Living Assessment: Measurement of functional level for activities of daily living

Body System / Region (4th)	Type Qualifier (5th)	Equipment (6th)	Qualifier (7th)
7 Circulatory System - Whole Body C Respiratory System - Whole Body	7 Aerobic Capacity and Endurance	E Orthosis G Aerobic Endurance and Conditioning U Prosthesis Y Other Equipment Z None	Z None
7 Circulatory System - Whole Body C Respiratory System - Whole Body	G Ventilation, Respiration and Circulation	C Mechanical G Aerobic Endurance and Conditioning Y Other Equipment Z None	Z None
Z None	0 Bathing/Showering 1 Dressing 3 Grooming/Personal Hygiene 4 Home Management	E Orthosis F Assistive, Adaptive, Supportive or Protective U Prosthesis Z None	Z None
Z None	2 Feeding/Eating 8 Anthropometric Characteristics F Pain	Y Other Equipment Z None	Z None
Z None	5 Perceptual Processing	K Audiovisual M Augmentative / Alternative Communication N Biosensory Feedback P Computer Q Speech Analysis S Voice Analysis Y Other Equipment Z None	Z None
Z None	6 Psychosocial Skills	Z None	Z None
Z None	B Environmental, Home and Work Barriers C Ergonomics and Body Mechanics	E Orthosis F Assistive, Adaptive, Supportive or Protective U Prosthesis Y Other Equipment Z None	Z None
Z None	H Vocational Activities and Functional Community or Work Reintegration Skills	E Orthosis F Assistive, Adaptive, Supportive or Protective G Aerobic Endurance and Conditioning U Prosthesis Y Other Equipment Z None	Z None

Section   F   Physical Rehabilitation and Diagnostic Audiology
Section Qualifier 0   Rehabilitation
Type   6   Speech Treatment: Application of techniques to improve, augment, or compensate for speech and related functional impairment

Body System / Region (4th)	Type Qualifier (5th)	Equipment (6th)	Qualifier (7th)
3 Neurological System - Whole Body	6 Communicative/Cognitive Integration Skills	K Audiovisual M Augmentative / Alternative Communication P Computer Y Other Equipment Z None	Z None

Continued →

Section | F | **Physical Rehabilitation and Diagnostic Audiology**
Section Qualifier | 0 | **Rehabilitation**
Type | 6 | **Speech Treatment:** Application of techniques to improve, augment, or compensate for speech and related functional impairment

Body System / Region (4th)	Type Qualifier (5th)	Equipment (6th)	Qualifier (7th)
Z None	0 Nonspoken Language 3 Aphasia 6 Communicative/Cognitive Integration Skills	K Audiovisual M Augmentative / Alternative Communication P Computer Y Other Equipment Z None	Z None
Z None	1 Speech-Language Pathology and Related Disorders Counseling 2 Speech-Language Pathology and Related Disorders Prevention	K Audiovisual Z None	Z None
Z None	4 Articulation/Phonology	K Audiovisual P Computer Q Speech Analysis T Aerodynamic Function Y Other Equipment Z None	Z None
Z None	5 Aural Rehabilitation	K Audiovisual L Assistive Listening M Augmentative / Alternative Communication N Biosensory Feedback P Computer Q Speech Analysis S Voice Analysis Y Other Equipment Z None	Z None
Z None	7 Fluency	4 Electroacoustic Immitance / Acoustic Reflex K Audiovisual N Biosensory Feedback Q Speech Analysis S Voice Analysis T Aerodynamic Function Y Other Equipment Z None	Z None
Z None	8 Motor Speech	K Audiovisual N Biosensory Feedback P Computer Q Speech Analysis S Voice Analysis T Aerodynamic Function Y Other Equipment Z None	Z None
Z None	9 Orofacial Myofunctional	K Audiovisual P Computer Y Other Equipment Z None	Z None
Z None	B Receptive/Expressive Language	K Audiovisual L Assistive Listening M Augmentative / Alternative Communication P Computer Y Other Equipment Z None	Z None

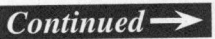

Section	F	Physical Rehabilitation and Diagnostic Audiology
Section Qualifier	0	Rehabilitation
Type	6	**Speech Treatment:** Application of techniques to improve, augment, or compensate for speech and related functional impairment

Body System / Region (4th)	Type Qualifier (5th)	Equipment (6th)	Qualifier (7th)
Z None	**C** Voice	**K** Audiovisual **N** Biosensory Feedback **P** Computer **S** Voice Analysis **T** Aerodynamic Function **V** Speech Prosthesis **Y** Other Equipment **Z** None	**Z** None
Z None	**D** Swallowing Dysfunction	**M** Augmentative / Alternative Communication **T** Aerodynamic Function **V** Speech Prosthesis **Y** Other Equipment **Z** None	**Z** None

Section	F	Physical Rehabilitation and Diagnostic Audiology
Section Qualifier	0	Rehabilitation
Type	7	**Motor Treatment:** Exercise or activities to increase or facilitate motor function

Body System / Region (4th)	Type Qualifier (5th)	Equipment (6th)	Qualifier (7th)
0 Neurological System - Head and Neck **1** Neurological System - Upper Back / Upper Extremity **2** Neurological System - Lower Back / Lower Extremity **3** Neurological System - Whole Body **D** Integumentary System - Head and Neck **F** Integumentary System - Upper Back / Upper Extremity **G** Integumentary System - Lower Back / Lower Extremity **H** Integumentary System - Whole Body **J** Musculoskeletal System - Head and Neck **K** Musculoskeletal System - Upper Back / Upper Extremity **L** Musculoskeletal System - Lower Back / Lower Extremity **M** Musculoskeletal System - Whole Body	**0** Range of Motion and Joint Mobility **1** Muscle Performance **2** Coordination/ Dexterity **3** Motor Function	**E** Orthosis **F** Assistive, Adaptive, Supportive or Protective **U** Prosthesis **Y** Other Equipment **Z** None	**Z** None
0 Neurological System - Head and Neck **1** Neurological System - Upper Back / Upper Extremity **2** Neurological System - Lower Back / Lower Extremity **3** Neurological System - Whole Body **D** Integumentary System - Head and Neck **F** Integumentary System - Upper Back / Upper Extremity **G** Integumentary System - Lower Back / Lower Extremity **H** Integumentary System - Whole Body **J** Musculoskeletal System - Head and Neck **K** Musculoskeletal System - Upper Back / Upper Extremity **L** Musculoskeletal System - Lower Back / Lower Extremity **M** Musculoskeletal System - Whole Body	**6** Therapeutic Exercise	**B** Physical Agents **C** Mechanical **D** Electrotherapeutic **E** Orthosis **F** Assistive, Adaptive, Supportive or Protective **G** Aerobic Endurance and Conditioning **H** Mechanical or Electromechanical **U** Prosthesis **Y** Other Equipment **Z** None	**Z** None

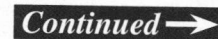

Continued →

Section	F	Physical Rehabilitation and Diagnostic Audiology
Section Qualifier	0	Rehabilitation
Type	7	**Motor Treatment:** Exercise or activities to increase or facilitate motor function

Body System / Region (4th)	Type Qualifier (5th)	Equipment (6th)	Qualifier (7th)
0 Neurological System - Head and Neck 1 Neurological System - Upper Back / Upper Extremity 2 Neurological System - Lower Back / Lower Extremity 3 Neurological System - Whole Body D Integumentary System - Head and Neck F Integumentary System - Upper Back / Upper Extremity G Integumentary System - Lower Back / Lower Extremity H Integumentary System - Whole Body J Musculoskeletal System - Head and Neck K Musculoskeletal System - Upper Back / Upper Extremity L Musculoskeletal System - Lower Back / Lower Extremity M Musculoskeletal System - Whole Body	7 Manual Therapy Techniques	Z None	Z None
4 Circulatory System - Head and Neck 5 Circulatory System - Upper Back / Upper Extremity 6 Circulatory System - Lower Back / Lower Extremity 7 Circulatory System - Whole Body 8 Respiratory System - Head and Neck 9 Respiratory System - Upper Back / Upper Extremity B Respiratory System - Lower Back / Lower Extremity C Respiratory System - Whole Body	6 Therapeutic Exercise	B Physical Agents C Mechanical D Electrotherapeutic E Orthosis F Assistive, Adaptive, Supportive or Protective G Aerobic Endurance and Conditioning H Mechanical or Electromechanical U Prosthesis Y Other Equipment Z None	Z None
N Genitourinary System	1 Muscle Performance	E Orthosis F Assistive, Adaptive, Supportive or Protective U Prosthesis Y Other Equipment Z None	Z None
N Genitourinary System	6 Therapeutic Exercise	B Physical Agents C Mechanical D Electrotherapeutic E Orthosis F Assistive, Adaptive, Supportive or Protective G Aerobic Endurance and Conditioning H Mechanical or Electromechanical U Prosthesis Y Other Equipment Z None	Z None
Z None	4 Wheelchair Mobility	D Electrotherapeutic E Orthosis F Assistive, Adaptive, Supportive or Protective U Prosthesis Y Other Equipment Z None	Z None
Z None	5 Bed Mobility	C Mechanical E Orthosis F Assistive, Adaptive, Supportive or Protective U Prosthesis Y Other Equipment Z None	Z None

Continued →

Section F Physical Rehabilitation and Diagnostic Audiology
Section Qualifier 0 Rehabilitation
Type 7 Motor Treatment: Exercise or activities to increase or facilitate motor function

Body System / Region (4th)	Type Qualifier (5th)	Equipment (6th)	Qualifier (7th)
Z None	8 Transfer Training	C Mechanical D Electrotherapeutic E Orthosis F Assistive, Adaptive, Supportive or Protective U Prosthesis Y Other Equipment Z None	Z None
Z None	9 Gait Training/ Functional Ambulation	C Mechanical D Electrotherapeutic E Orthosis F Assistive, Adaptive, Supportive or Protective G Aerobic Endurance and Conditioning U Prosthesis Y Other Equipment Z None	Z None

Section F Physical Rehabilitation and Diagnostic Audiology
Section Qualifier 0 Rehabilitation
Type 8 Activities of Daily Living Treatment: Exercise or activities to facilitate functional competence for activities of daily living

Body System / Region (4th)	Type Qualifier (5th)	Equipment (6th)	Qualifier (7th)
D Integumentary System - Head and Neck F Integumentary System - Upper Back / Upper Extremity G Integumentary System - Lower Back / Lower Extremity H Integumentary System - Whole Body J Musculoskeletal System - Head and Neck K Musculoskeletal System - Upper Back / Upper Extremity L Musculoskeletal System - Lower Back / Lower Extremity M Musculoskeletal System - Whole Body	5 Wound Management	B Physical Agents C Mechanical D Electrotherapeutic E Orthosis F Assistive, Adaptive, Supportive or Protective U Prosthesis Y Other Equipment Z None	Z None
Z None	0 Bathing/Showering Techniques 1 Dressing Techniques 2 Grooming/Personal Hygiene	E Orthosis F Assistive, Adaptive, Supportive or Protective U Prosthesis Y Other Equipment Z None	Z None
Z None	3 Feeding/Eating	C Mechanical D Electrotherapeutic E Orthosis F Assistive, Adaptive, Supportive or Protective U Prosthesis Y Other Equipment Z None	Z None
Z None	4 Home Management	D Electrotherapeutic E Orthosis F Assistive, Adaptive, Supportive or Protective U Prosthesis Y Other Equipment Z None	Z None

Continued →

Section	F	Physical Rehabilitation and Diagnostic Audiology
Section Qualifier	0	Rehabilitation
Type	8	Activities of Daily Living Treatment: Exercise or activities to facilitate functional competence for activities of daily living

F08 Continued
F08–F0C
Physical Rehabilitation and Diagnostic Audiology Section Tables

Body System / Region (4th)	Type Qualifier (5th)	Equipment (6th)	Qualifier (7th)
Z None	6 Psychosocial Skills	Z None	Z None
Z None	7 Vocational Activities and Functional Community or Work Reintegration Skills	B Physical Agents C Mechanical D Electrotherapeutic E Orthosis F Assistive, Adaptive, Supportive or Protective G Aerobic Endurance and Conditioning U Prosthesis Y Other Equipment Z None	Z None

Section	F	Physical Rehabilitation and Diagnostic Audiology
Section Qualifier	0	Rehabilitation
Type	9	Hearing Treatment: Application of techniques to improve, augment, or compensate for hearing and related functional impairment

Body System / Region (4th)	Type Qualifier (5th)	Equipment (6th)	Qualifier (7th)
Z None	0 Hearing and Related Disorders Counseling 1 Hearing and Related Disorders Prevention	K Audiovisual Z None	Z None
Z None	2 Auditory Processing	K Audiovisual L Assistive Listening P Computer Y Other Equipment Z None	Z None
Z None	3 Cerumen Management	X Cerumen Management Z None	Z None

Section	F	Physical Rehabilitation and Diagnostic Audiology
Section Qualifier	0	Rehabilitation
Type	B	Cochlear Implant Treatment: Application of techniques to improve the communication abilities of individuals with cochlear implant

Body System / Region (4th)	Type Qualifier (5th)	Equipment (6th)	Qualifier (7th)
Z None	0 Cochlear Implant Rehabilitation	1 Audiometer 2 Sound Field / Booth 9 Cochlear Implant K Audiovisual P Computer Y Other Equipment	Z None

Section	F	Physical Rehabilitation and Diagnostic Audiology
Section Qualifier	0	Rehabilitation
Type	C	Vestibular Treatment: Application of techniques to improve, augment, or compensate for vestibular and related functional impairment

Body System / Region (4th)	Type Qualifier (5th)	Equipment (6th)	Qualifier (7th)
3 Neurological System - Whole Body H Integumentary System - Whole Body M Musculoskeletal System - Whole Body	3 Postural Control	E Orthosis F Assistive, Adaptive, Supportive or Protective U Prosthesis Y Other Equipment Z None	Z None

Continued →

Section	F	Physical Rehabilitation and Diagnostic Audiology
Section Qualifier	0	Rehabilitation
Type	C	**Vestibular Treatment:** Application of techniques to improve, augment, or compensate for vestibular and related functional impairment

Body System / Region (4th)	Type Qualifier (5th)	Equipment (6th)	Qualifier (7th)
Z None	**0** Vestibular	**8** Vestibular / Balance **Z** None	**Z** None
Z None	**1** Perceptual Processing **2** Visual Motor Integration	**K** Audiovisual **L** Assistive Listening **N** Biosensory Feedback **P** Computer **Q** Speech Analysis **S** Voice Analysis **T** Aerodynamic Function **Y** Other Equipment **Z** None	**Z** None

Section	F	Physical Rehabilitation and Diagnostic Audiology
Section Qualifier	0	Rehabilitation
Type	D	**Device Fitting:** Fitting of a device designed to facilitate or support achievement of a higher level of function

Body System / Region (4th)	Type Qualifier (5th)	Equipment (6th)	Qualifier (7th)
Z None	**0** Tinnitus Masker	**5** Hearing Aid Selection / Fitting / Test **Z** None	**Z** None
Z None	**1** Monaural Hearing Aid **2** Binaural Hearing Aid **5** Assistive Listening Device	**1** Audiometer **2** Sound Field / Booth **5** Hearing Aid Selection / Fitting / Test **K** Audiovisual **L** Assistive Listening **Z** None	**Z** None
Z None	**3** Augmentative/Alternative Communication System	**M** Augmentative / Alternative Communication	**Z** None
Z None	**4** Voice Prosthetic	**S** Voice Analysis **V** Speech Prosthesis	**Z** None
Z None	**6** Dynamic Orthosis **7** Static Orthosis **8** Prosthesis **9** Assistive, Adaptive, Supportive or Protective Devices	**E** Orthosis **F** Assistive, Adaptive, Supportive or Protective **U** Prosthesis **Z** None	**Z** None

Section F Physical Rehabilitation and Diagnostic Audiology

Section	F	Physical Rehabilitation and Diagnostic Audiology
Section Qualifier	0	Rehabilitation
Type	F	Caregiver Training: Training in activities to support patient's optimal level of function

Body System / Region (4th)	Type Qualifier (5th)	Equipment (6th)	Qualifier (7th)
Z None	**0** Bathing/Showering Technique **1** Dressing **2** Feeding and Eating **3** Grooming/Personal Hygiene **4** Bed Mobility **5** Transfer **6** Wheelchair Mobility **7** Therapeutic Exercise **8** Airway Clearance Techniques **9** Wound Management **B** Vocational Activities and Functional Community or Work Reintegration Skills **C** Gait Training/Functional Ambulation **D** Application, Proper Use and Care of Devices **F** Application, Proper Use and Care of Orthoses **G** Application, Proper Use and Care of Prosthesis **H** Home Management	**E** Orthosis **F** Assistive, Adaptive, Supportive or Protective **U** Prosthesis **Z** None	**Z** None
Z None	**J** Communication Skills	**K** Audiovisual **L** Assistive Listening **M** Augmentative / Alternative Communication **P** Computer **Z** None	**Z** None

Section	F	Physical Rehabilitation and Diagnostic Audiology
Section Qualifier	1	Diagnostic Audiology
Type	3	Hearing Assessment: Measurement of hearing and related functions

Body System / Region (4th)	Type Qualifier (5th)	Equipment (6th)	Qualifier (7th)
Z None	**0** Hearing Screening	**0** Occupational Hearing **1** Audiometer **2** Sound Field / Booth **3** Tympanometer **8** Vestibular / Balance **9** Cochlear Implant **Z** None	**Z** None
Z None	**1** Pure Tone Audiometry, Air **2** Pure Tone Audiometry, Air and Bone	**0** Occupational Hearing **1** Audiometer **2** Sound Field / Booth **Z** None	**Z** None
Z None	**3** Bekesy Audiometry **6** Visual Reinforcement Audiometry **9** Short Increment Sensitivity Index **B** Stenger **C** Pure Tone Stenger	**1** Audiometer **2** Sound Field / Booth **Z** None	**Z** None
Z None	**4** Conditioned Play Audiometry **5** Select Picture Audiometry	**1** Audiometer **2** Sound Field / Booth **K** Audiovisual **Z** None	**Z** None
Z None	**7** Alternate Binaural or Monaural Loudness Balance	**1** Audiometer **K** Audiovisual **Z** None	**Z** None

Continued →

Section   **F**   **Physical Rehabilitation and Diagnostic Audiology**
Section Qualifier   **1**   **Diagnostic Audiology**
Type   **3**   **Hearing Assessment:** Measurement of hearing and related functions

Body System / Region (4th)	Type Qualifier (5th)	Equipment (6th)	Qualifier (7th)
Z None	**8** Tone Decay **D** Tympanometry **F** Eustachian Tube Function **G** Acoustic Reflex Patterns **H** Acoustic Reflex Threshold **J** Acoustic Reflex Decay	**3** Tympanometer **4** Electroacoustic Immitance / Acoustic Reflex **Z** None	**Z** None
Z None	**K** Electrocochleography **L** Auditory Evoked Potentials	**7** Electrophysiologic **Z** None	**Z** None
Z None	**M** Evoked Otoacoustic Emissions, Screening **N** Evoked Otoacoustic Emissions, Diagnostic	**6** Otoacoustic Emission (OAE) **Z** None	**Z** None
Z None	**P** Aural Rehabilitation Status	**1** Audiometer **2** Sound Field / Booth **4** Electroacoustic Immitance / Acoustic Reflex **9** Cochlear Implant **K** Audiovisual **L** Assistive Listening **P** Computer **Z** None	**Z** None
Z None	**Q** Auditory Processing	**K** Audiovisual **P** Computer **Y** Other Equipment **Z** None	**Z** None

Section   **F**   **Physical Rehabilitation and Diagnostic Audiology**
Section Qualifier   **1**   **Diagnostic Audiology**
Type   **4**   **Hearing Aid Assessment:** Measurement of the appropriateness and/or effectiveness of a hearing device

Body System / Region (4th)	Type Qualifier (5th)	Equipment (6th)	Qualifier (7th)
Z None	**0** Cochlear Implant	**1** Audiometer **2** Sound Field / Booth **3** Tympanometer **4** Electroacoustic Immitance / Acoustic Reflex **5** Hearing Aid Selection / Fitting / Test **7** Electrophysiologic **9** Cochlear Implant **K** Audiovisual **L** Assistive Listening **P** Computer **Y** Other Equipment **Z** None	**Z** None
Z None	**1** Ear Canal Probe Microphone **6** Binaural Electroacoustic Hearing Aid Check **8** Monaural Electroacoustic Hearing Aid Check	**5** Hearing Aid Selection / Fitting / Test **Z** None	**Z** None

Continued →

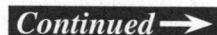

Section	F	Physical Rehabilitation and Diagnostic Audiology
Section Qualifier	1	Diagnostic Audiology
Type	4	Hearing Aid Assessment: Measurement of the appropriateness and/or effectiveness of a hearing device

Body System / Region (4th)	Type Qualifier (5th)	Equipment (6th)	Qualifier (7th)
Z None	2 Monaural Hearing Aid 3 Binaural Hearing Aid	1 Audiometer 2 Sound Field / Booth 3 Tympanometer 4 Electroacoustic Immitance / Acoustic Reflex 5 Hearing Aid Selection / Fitting / Test K Audiovisual L Assistive Listening P Computer Z None	Z None
Z None	4 Assistive Listening System/Device Selection	1 Audiometer 2 Sound Field / Booth 3 Tympanometer 4 Electroacoustic Immitance / Acoustic Reflex K Audiovisual L Assistive Listening Z None	Z None
Z None	5 Sensory Aids	1 Audiometer 2 Sound Field / Booth 3 Tympanometer 4 Electroacoustic Immitance / Acoustic Reflex 5 Hearing Aid Selection / Fitting / Test K Audiovisual L Assistive Listening Z None	Z None
Z None	7 Ear Protector Attentuation	0 Occupational Hearing Z None	Z None

Section	F	Physical Rehabilitation and Diagnostic Audiology
Section Qualifier	1	Diagnostic Audiology
Type	5	Vestibular Assessment: Measurement of the vestibular system and related functions

Body System / Region (4th)	Type Qualifier (5th)	Equipment (6th)	Qualifier (7th)
Z None	0 Bithermal, Binaural Caloric Irrigation 1 Bithermal, Monaural Caloric Irrigation 2 Unithermal Binaural Screen 3 Oscillating Tracking 4 Sinusoidal Vertical Axis Rotational 5 Dix-Hallpike Dynamic 6 Computerized Dynamic Posturography	8 Vestibular / Balance Z None	Z None
Z None	7 Tinnitus Masker	5 Hearing Aid Selection / Fitting / Test Z None	Z None

Within each section of ICD-10-PCS the characters have different meanings. The seven character meanings for the Mental Health section are illustrated here through the procedure example of *Crisis intervention*.

Section	Body System	Root Type	Qualifier	Qualifier	Qualifier	Qualifier
Mental Health	None	Crisis Intervention	None	None	None	None
G	Z	2	Z	Z	Z	Z

Section (Character 1)

All Mental Health procedure codes have a first character value of G.

Body System (Character 2)

The body system is not specified for mental health; therefore, the placeholder character value of Z is reported in the second character position.

Root Type (Character 3)

The alphanumeric character value for root types is placed in the third position. Listed below are the root types applicable to the Mental Health section with their associated meaning.

Character Value	Root Type	Root Type Definition
1	Psychological Tests	The administration and interpretation of standardized psychological tests and measurement instruments for the assessment of psychological function
2	Crisis Intervention	Treatment of a traumatized, acutely disturbed or distressed individual for the purpose of short-term stabilization
3	Medication Management	Monitoring and adjusting the use of medications for the treatment of a mental health disorder
5	Individual Psychotherapy	Treatment of an individual with a mental health disorder by behavioral, cognitive, psychoanalytic, psychodynamic or psychophysiological means to improve functioning or well-being
6	Counseling	The application of psychological methods to treat an individual with normal developmental issues and psychological problems in order to increase function, improve well-being, alleviate distress, maladjustment or resolve crises
7	Family Psychotherapy	Treatment that includes one or more family members of an individual with a mental health disorder by behavioral, cognitive, psychoanalytic, psychodynamic or psychophysiological means to improve functioning or well-being
B	Electroconvulsive Therapy	The application of controlled electrical voltages to treat a mental health disorder
C	Biofeedback	Provision of information from the monitoring and regulating of physiological processes in conjunction with cognitive-behavioral techniques to improve patient functioning or well-being
F	Hypnosis	Induction of a state of heightened suggestibility by auditory, visual and tactile techniques to elicit an emotional or behavioral response
G	Narcosynthesis	Administration of intravenous barbiturates in order to release suppressed or repressed thoughts
H	Group Psychotherapy	Treatment of two or more individuals with a mental health disorder by behavioral, cognitive, psychoanalytic, psychodynamic or psychophysiological means to improve functioning or well-being
J	Light Therapy	Application of specialized light treatments to improve functioning or well-being

Qualifier (Character 4)

This qualifier further specifies the root type procedure. For example, the qualifier of Development further specifies the type of Psychological Tests.

Qualifier (Character 5)

The qualifier represents an additional attribute for the procedure when applicable. Currently, there are no qualifiers in the Mental Health section; therefore, the placeholder character value of Z should be reported.

Qualifier (Character 6)

The qualifier represents an additional attribute for the procedure when applicable. Currently, there are no qualifiers in the Mental Health section; therefore, the placeholder character value of Z should be reported.

Qualifier (Character 7)

The qualifier represents an additional attribute for the procedure when applicable. Currently, there are no qualifiers in the Mental Health section; therefore, the placeholder character value of Z should be reported.

Mental Health Tables

Mental Health Tables GZ1–GZJ

Section	G	Mental Health
Body System	Z	None
Type	1	**Psychological Tests:** The administration and interpretation of standardized psychological tests and measurement instruments for the assessment of psychological function

Qualifier (4th)	Qualifier (5th)	Qualifier (6th)	Qualifier (7th)
0 Developmental 1 Personality and Behavioral 2 Intellectual and Psychoeducational 3 Neuropsychological 4 Neurobehavioral and Cognitive Status	Z None	Z None	Z None

Section	G	Mental Health
Body System	Z	None
Type	2	**Crisis Intervention:** Treatment of a traumatized, acutely disturbed or distressed individual for the purpose of short-term stabilization

Qualifier (4th)	Qualifier (5th)	Qualifier (6th)	Qualifier (7th)
Z None	Z None	Z None	Z None

Section	G	Mental Health
Body System	Z	None
Type	3	**Medication Management:** Monitoring and adjusting the use of medications for the treatment of a mental health disorder

Qualifier (4th)	Qualifier (5th)	Qualifier (6th)	Qualifier (7th)
Z None	Z None	Z None	Z None

Section	G	Mental Health
Body System	Z	None
Type	5	**Individual Psychotherapy:** Treatment of an individual with a mental health disorder by behavioral, cognitive, psychoanalytic, psychodynamic or psychophysiological means to improve functioning or well-being

Qualifier (4th)	Qualifier (5th)	Qualifier (6th)	Qualifier (7th)
0 Interactive 1 Behavioral 2 Cognitive 3 Interpersonal 4 Psychoanalysis 5 Psychodynamic 6 Supportive 8 Cognitive-Behavioral 9 Psychophysiological	Z None	Z None	Z None

Section	G	Mental Health
Body System	Z	None
Type	6	**Counseling:** The application of psychological methods to treat an individual with normal developmental issues and psychological problems in order to increase function, improve well-being, alleviate distress, maladjustment or resolve crises

Qualifier (4ᵗʰ)	Qualifier (5ᵗʰ)	Qualifier (6ᵗʰ)	Qualifier (7ᵗʰ)
0 Educational 1 Vocational 3 Other Counseling	Z None	Z None	Z None

Section	G	Mental Health
Body System	Z	None
Type	7	**Family Psychotherapy:** Treatment that includes one or more family members of an individual with a mental health disorder by behavioral, cognitive, psychoanalytic, psychodynamic or psychophysiological means to improve functioning or well-being

Qualifier (4ᵗʰ)	Qualifier (5ᵗʰ)	Qualifier (6ᵗʰ)	Qualifier (7ᵗʰ)
2 Other Family Psychotherapy	Z None	Z None	Z None

Section	G	Mental Health
Body System	Z	None
Type	B	**Electroconvulsive Therapy:** The application of controlled electrical voltages to treat a mental health disorder

Qualifier (4ᵗʰ)	Qualifier (5ᵗʰ)	Qualifier (6ᵗʰ)	Qualifier (7ᵗʰ)
0 Unilateral-Single Seizure 1 Unilateral-Multiple Seizure 2 Bilateral-Single Seizure 3 Bilateral-Multiple Seizure 4 Other Electroconvulsive Therapy	Z None	Z None	Z None

Section	G	Mental Health
Body System	Z	None
Type	C	**Biofeedback:** Provision of information from the monitoring and regulating of physiological processes in conjunction with cognitive-behavioral techniques to improve patient functioning or well-being

Qualifier (4ᵗʰ)	Qualifier (5ᵗʰ)	Qualifier (6ᵗʰ)	Qualifier (7ᵗʰ)
9 Other Biofeedback	Z None	Z None	Z None

Section	G	Mental Health
Body System	Z	None
Type	F	**Hypnosis:** Induction of a state of heightened suggestibility by auditory, visual and tactile techniques to elicit an emotional or behavioral response

Qualifier (4ᵗʰ)	Qualifier (5ᵗʰ)	Qualifier (6ᵗʰ)	Qualifier (7ᵗʰ)
Z None	Z None	Z None	Z None

Section	G	Mental Health
Body System	Z	None
Type	G	**Narcosynthesis:** Administration of intravenous barbiturates in order to release suppressed or repressed thoughts

Qualifier (4ᵗʰ)	Qualifier (5ᵗʰ)	Qualifier (6ᵗʰ)	Qualifier (7ᵗʰ)
Z None	Z None	Z None	Z None

Section	G	Mental Health
Body System	Z	None
Type	H	**Group Psychotherapy:** Treatment of two or more individuals with a mental health disorder by behavioral, cognitive, psychoanalytic, psychodynamic or psychophysiological means to improve functioning or well-being

Qualifier (4th)	Qualifier (5th)	Qualifier (6th)	Qualifier (7th)
Z None	**Z** None	**Z** None	**Z** None

Section	G	Mental Health
Body System	Z	None
Type	J	**Light Therapy:** Application of specialized light treatments to improve functioning or well-being

Qualifier (4th)	Qualifier (5th)	Qualifier (6th)	Qualifier (7th)
Z None	**Z** None	**Z** None	**Z** None

Within each section of ICD-10-PCS the characters have different meanings. The seven character meanings for the Substance Abuse Treatment section are illustrated below through the procedure example of *Substance abuse family counseling*.

Section	Body System	Root Type	Qualifier	Qualifier	Qualifier	Qualifier
Substance Abuse Treatment	None	Family Counseling	Other Family Counseling	None	None	None
H	Z	6	3	Z	Z	Z

Section (Character 1)

All Substance Abuse Treatment procedure codes have a first character value of H.

Body System (Character 2)

The body system is not specified for substance abuse treatment; therefore, the placeholder character value of Z is reported in the second character position.

Root Type (Character 3)

The alphanumeric character value for root types is placed in the third position. The following are the root types applicable to the Substance Abuse Treatment section with their associated meaning.

Character Value	Root Type	Root Type Definition
2	Detoxification Services	Detoxification from alcohol and/or drugs
3	Individual Counseling	The application of psychological methods to treat an individual with addictive behavior
4	Group Counseling	The application of psychological methods to treat two or more individuals with addictive behavior
5	Individual Psychotherapy	Treatment of an individual with addictive behavior by behavioral, cognitive, psychoanalytic, psychodynamic or psychophysiological means
6	Family Counseling	The application of psychological methods that includes one or more family members to treat an individual with addictive behavior
8	Medication Management	Monitoring and adjusting the use of replacement medications for the treatment of addiction
9	Pharmacotherapy	The use of replacement medications for the treatment of addiction

Qualifier (Character 4)

This qualifier further specifies the root type procedure. For example, the qualifier of Cognitive further specifies the type of Individual counseling.

Qualifier (Character 5)

The qualifier represents an additional attribute for the procedure when applicable. Currently, there are no qualifiers in the Substance Abuse Treatment section; therefore, the placeholder character value of Z should be reported.

Qualifier (Character 6)

The qualifier represents an additional attribute for the procedure when applicable. Currently, there are no qualifiers in the Substance Abuse Treatment section; therefore, the placeholder character value of Z should be reported.

Qualifier (Character 7)

The qualifier represents an additional attribute for the procedure when applicable. Currently, there are no qualifiers in the Substance Abuse Treatment section; therefore, the placeholder character value of Z should be reported.

AHA Coding Clinic

HZ2ZZZZ Detoxification Services for Substance Abuse Treatment - AHA CC: 1Q, 2020, 21-22
HZ98ZZZ Pharmacotherapy for Substance Abuse Treatment, Psychiatric Medication - AHA CC: 1Q, 2020, 21-22

Substance Abuse Treatment Section Tables

Substance Abuse Treatment Tables HZ2–HZ9

Section	H	Substance Abuse Treatment
Body System	Z	None
Type	2	**Detoxification Services:** Detoxification from alcohol and/or drugs

Qualifier (4ᵗʰ)	Qualifier (5ᵗʰ)	Qualifier (6ᵗʰ)	Qualifier (7ᵗʰ)
Z None	**Z** None	**Z** None	**Z** None

Section	H	Substance Abuse Treatment
Body System	Z	None
Type	3	**Individual Counseling:** The application of psychological methods to treat an individual with addictive behavior

Qualifier (4ᵗʰ)	Qualifier (5ᵗʰ)	Qualifier (6ᵗʰ)	Qualifier (7ᵗʰ)
0 Cognitive **1** Behavioral **2** Cognitive-Behavioral **3** 12-Step **4** Interpersonal **5** Vocational **6** Psychoeducation **7** Motivational Enhancement **8** Confrontational **9** Continuing Care **B** Spiritual **C** Pre/Post-Test Infectious Disease	**Z** None	**Z** None	**Z** None

Section	H	Substance Abuse Treatment
Body System	Z	None
Type	4	**Group Counseling:** The application of psychological methods to treat two or more individuals with addictive behavior

Qualifier (4ᵗʰ)	Qualifier (5ᵗʰ)	Qualifier (6ᵗʰ)	Qualifier (7ᵗʰ)
0 Cognitive **1** Behavioral **2** Cognitive-Behavioral **3** 12-Step **4** Interpersonal **5** Vocational **6** Psychoeducation **7** Motivational Enhancement **8** Confrontational **9** Continuing Care **B** Spiritual **C** Pre/Post-Test Infectious Disease	**Z** None	**Z** None	**Z** None

Section	H	Substance Abuse Treatment
Body System	Z	None
Type	5	**Individual Psychotherapy:** Treatment of an individual with addictive behavior by behavioral, cognitive, psychoanalytic, psychodynamic or psychophysiological means

Qualifier (4th)	Qualifier (5th)	Qualifier (6th)	Qualifier (7th)
0 Cognitive	Z None	Z None	Z None
1 Behavioral			
2 Cognitive-Behavioral			
3 12-Step			
4 Interpersonal			
5 Interactive			
6 Psychoeducation			
7 Motivational Enhancement			
8 Confrontational			
9 Supportive			
B Psychoanalysis			
C Psychodynamic			
D Psychophysiological			

Section	H	Substance Abuse Treatment
Body System	Z	None
Type	6	**Family Counseling:** The application of psychological methods that includes one or more family members to treat an individual with addictive behavior

Qualifier (4th)	Qualifier (5th)	Qualifier (6th)	Qualifier (7th)
3 Other Family Counseling	Z None	Z None	Z None

Section	H	Substance Abuse Treatment
Body System	Z	None
Type	8	**Medication Management:** Monitoring and adjusting the use of replacement medications for the treatment of addiction

Qualifier (4th)	Qualifier (5th)	Qualifier (6th)	Qualifier (7th)
0 Nicotine Replacement	Z None	Z None	Z None
1 Methadone Maintenance			
2 Levo-alpha-acetyl-methadol (LAAM)			
3 Antabuse			
4 Naltrexone			
5 Naloxone			
6 Clonidine			
7 Bupropion			
8 Psychiatric Medication			
9 Other Replacement Medication			

Section	H	Substance Abuse Treatment
Body System	Z	None
Type	9	**Pharmacotherapy:** The use of replacement medications for the treatment of addiction

Qualifier (4th)	Qualifier (5th)	Qualifier (6th)	Qualifier (7th)
0 Nicotine Replacement	Z None	Z None	Z None
1 Methadone Maintenance			
2 Levo-alpha-acetyl-methadol (LAAM)			
3 Antabuse			
4 Naltrexone			
5 Naloxone			
6 Clonidine			
7 Bupropion			
8 Psychiatric Medication			
9 Other Replacement Medication			

Within each section of ICD-10-PCS the characters have different meanings. The seven character meanings for the New Technology section are illustrated below through the procedure example of *Introduction of ceftazidime-avibactam anti-infective into peripheral vein, percutaneous approach.*

Section	Body System	Root Operation	Body Part	Approach	Device / Substance / Technology	Qualifier
New Technology	Anatomical Regions	Introduction	Peripheral Vein	Percutaneous	Ceftazidime-Avibactam Anti-infective	New Technology Group 1
X	W	0	3	3	2	1

Section (Character 1)
All New Technology procedure codes have a first character value of X.

Body System (Character 2)
For each body system the applicable body part character values will be available for procedure code construction.

Root Operations (Character 3)
The alphanumeric character value for root operations is placed in the third position. Listed below are the root operations applicable to the New Technology section with their associated meaning.

Character Value	Root Operation	Root Operation Definition
A	Assistance	Taking over a portion of a physiological function by extracorporeal means
C	Extirpation	Taking or cutting out solid matter from a body part
E	Measurement	Determining a level of a physiological or physical function at a point in time
G	Fusion	Joining together portions of an articular body part rendering the articular body part immobile
H	Insertion	Putting in a nonbiological appliance that monitors, assists, performs, or prevents a physiological function bust does not physically take the place of a body part.
J	Inspection	Visually and/or manually exploring a body part
K	Bypass	Altering the route of passage of the contents of a tubular body part
P	Irrigation	Putting in or on a cleansing substance
R	Replacement	Putting in or on biological or synthetic material that physically takes the place and/or function of all or a portion of a body part
S	Reposition	Moving to its normal location, or other suitable location, all or a portion of a body part
U	Supplement	Putting in or on biological or synthetic material that physically reinforces and/or augments the function of a portion of a body part
V	Restriction	Partially closing an orifice or the lumen of a tubular body part
0	Introduction	Putting in or on a therapeutic, diagnostic, nutritional, physiological, or prophylactic substance except blood or blood products
1	Transfusion In Anatomical Regions	Putting in blood or blood products
2	Monitoring In Joints & Urinary System	Determining the level of a physiological or physical function repetitively
2	Transfusion In Anatomical Regions	Putting in blood or blood products
5	Destruction	Physical eradication of all or a portion of a body part by the direct use of energy, force or a destructive agent
7	Dilation	Expanding an orifice or the lumen of a tubular body part

Body Part (Character 4)

For each body system the applicable body part character values will be available for procedure code construction.

Approach (Character 5)

The approach is the technique used to reach the procedure site. Listed below are the approach character values for the New Technology section with the associated definitions.

Character Value	Approach	Approach Definition
0	Open	Cutting through the skin or mucous membrane and any other body layers necessary to expose the site of the procedure
3	Percutaneous	Entry, by puncture or minor incision, of instrumentation through the skin or mucous membrane and any other body layers necessary to reach the site of the procedure
4	Percutaneous Endoscopic	Entry, by puncture or minor incision, of instrumentation through the skin or mucous membrane and any other body layers necessary to reach and visualize the site of the procedure
7	Via Natural or Artificial Opening	Entry of instrumentation through a natural or artificial external opening to reach the site of the procedure
8	Via Natural or Artificial Opening Endoscopic	Entry of instrumentation through a natural or artificial external opening to reach and visualize the site of the procedure
X	External	Procedures performed directly on the skin or mucous membrane and procedures performed indirectly by the application of external force through the skin or mucous membrane

Device/Substance/Technology (Character 6)

The New Technology section created a place within ICD-10-PCS to include procedure codes for new services that utilize a specific new device, substance, or technology. Procedures in this section may be part of the Inpatient Prospective Payment System (IPPS) new technology add-on payment mechanism. Depending on the procedure performed there is either a device, substance, or new technology utilized.

Qualifier (Character 7)

The qualifier represents the category year in which the new device, substance, or technology was added to the coding system. In federal fiscal year 2016 (October 1, 2015) the first group of device, substance, and technology was added and therefore are labeled as New Technology Group 1.

AHA Coding Clinic

X2A5312 Cerebral Embolic Filtration, Dual Filter in Innominate Artery and Left Common Carotid Artery, Percutaneous Approach, New Technology Group 2 - AHA CC: 1Q, 2021, 16-17

X2C0361 Extirpation of Matter from Coronary Artery, One Site Using Orbital Atherectomy Technology, Percutaneous Approach, New Technology Group 1 - AHA CC: 4Q, 2015, 13-14

XNS0032 Reposition of Lumbar Vertebra using Magnetically Controlled Growth Rod(s), Open Approach, New Technology Group 2 - AHA CC: 4Q, 2017, 75

XRGB0F3 Fusion of Lumbar Vertebral Joint using Radiolucent Porous Interbody Fusion Device, Open Approach, New Technology Group 3 - AHA CC: 4Q, 2017, 76-77

XRGD0F3 Fusion of Lumbosacral Joint using Radiolucent Porous Interbody Fusion Device, Open Approach, New Technology Group 3 - AHA CC: 4Q, 2017, 76-77

XV508A4 Destruction of Prostate using Robotic Waterjet Ablation, Via Natural or Artificial Opening Endoscopic, New Technology Group 4 - AHA CC: 4Q, 2018, 55

XW013F5 Introduction of Other New Technology Therapeutic Substance into Subcutaneous Tissue, Percutaneous Approach, New Technology Group 5 - AHA CC: 3Q, 2020, 19-20; 1Q, 2021, 49-51

XW033E5 Introduction of Remdesivir Anti-infective into Peripheral Vein, Percutaneous Approach, New Technology Group 5 - AHA CC: 3Q, 2020, 18-19

XW033F5 Introduction of Other New Technology Therapeutic Substance into Peripheral Vein, Percutaneous Approach, New Technology Group 5 - AHA CC: 3Q, 2020, 19-20; 1Q, 2021, 49-51

XW033G5 Introduction of Sarilumab into Peripheral Vein, Percutaneous Approach, New Technology Group 5 - AHA CC: 3Q, 2020, 18-19

XW033H5 Introduction of Tocilizumab into Peripheral Vein, Percutaneous Approach, New Technology Group 5 - AHA CC: 3Q, 2020, 18-19

XW04331 Introduction of Idarucizumab, Dabigatran Reversal Agent into Central Vein, Percutaneous Approach, New Technology Group 1 - AHA CC: 4Q, 2015, 13

XW04351 Introduction of Blinatumomab Antineoplastic into Central Vein, Percutaneous Approach, New Technology Group 1 - AHA CC: 4Q, 2015, 14-15

XW043E5 Introduction of Remdesivir Anti-infective into Central Vein, Percutaneous Approach, New Technology Group 5 - AHA CC: 3Q, 2020, 18-19

XW043F5 Introduction of Other New Technology Therapeutic Substance into Central Vein, Percutaneous Approach, New Technology Group 5 - AHA CC: 3Q, 2020, 19-20; 1Q, 2021, 49-51

XW043G5 Introduction of Sarilumab into Central Vein, Percutaneous Approach, New Technology Group 5 - AHA CC: 3Q, 2020, 18-19

XW043H5 Introduction of Tocilizumab into Central Vein, Percutaneous Approach, New Technology Group 5 - AHA CC: 3Q, 2020, 18-19

XW0DXF5 Introduction of Other New Technology Therapeutic Substance into Mouth and Pharynx, External Approach, New Technology Group 5 - AHA CC: 3Q, 2020, 19-20; 1Q, 2021, 49-51

XW0Q316 Introduction of Eladocagene exuparvovec into Cranial Cavity and Brain, Percutaneous Approach, New Technology Group 6 - AHA CC: 4Q, 2020, 73

XW13325 Transfusion of Convalescent Plasma (Nonautologous) into Peripheral Vein, Percutaneous Approach, New Technology Group 5 - AHA CC: 3Q, 2020, 19

XW14325 Transfusion of Convalescent Plasma (Nonautologous) into Central Vein, Percutaneous Approach, New Technology Group 5 - AHA CC: 3Q, 2020, 19

Hospital Acquired Conditions Related Procedures

The following codes are HAC procedures when reported with secondary diagnosis code K68.11, T81.4XXA, T84.60XA, T84.610A, T84.611A, T84.612A, T84.613A, T84.614A, T84.615A, T84.619A, T84.63XA, T84.69XA, T84.7XXA

XRG0092 Fusion of Occipital-cervical Joint using Nanotextured Surface Interbody Fusion Device, Open Approach, New Technology Group 2

XRG1092 Fusion of Cervical Vertebral Joint using Nanotextured Surface Interbody Fusion Device, Open Approach, New Technology Group 2

XRG2092 Fusion of 2 or more Cervical Vertebral Joints using Nanotextured Surface Interbody Fusion Device, Open Approach, New Technology Group 2

XRG4092 Fusion of Cervicothoracic Vertebral Joint using Nanotextured Surface Interbody Fusion Device, Open Approach, New Technology Group 2

XRG6092 Fusion of Thoracic Vertebral Joint using Nanotextured Surface Interbody Fusion Device, Open Approach, New Technology Group 2

XRG7092 Fusion of 2 to 7 Thoracic Vertebral Joints using Nanotextured Surface Interbody Fusion Device, Open Approach, New Technology Group 2

XRG8092 Fusion of 8 or more Thoracic Vertebral Joints using Nanotextured Surface Interbody Fusion Device, Open Approach, New Technology Group 2

XRGA092 Fusion of Thoracolumbar Vertebral Joint using Nanotextured Surface Interbody Fusion Device, Open Approach, New Technology Group 2

XRGB092 Fusion of Lumbar Vertebral Joint using Nanotextured Surface Interbody Fusion Device, Open Approach, New Technology Group 2

XRGC092 Fusion of 2 or more Lumbar Vertebral Joints using Nanotextured Surface Interbody Fusion Device, Open Approach, New Technology Group 2

XRGD092 Fusion of Lumbosacral Joint using Nanotextured Surface Interbody Fusion Device, Open Approach, New Technology Group 2

New Technology Section Guidelines (Section X)

E. New Technology Section

General Guidelines

E1.a Section X codes fully represent the specific procedure described in the code title, and do not require any additional codes from other sections of ICD-10-PCS. When section X contains a code title which describes a specific new technology procedure, and it is the only procedure performed, only the X code is reported for the procedure. There is no need to report an additional code in another section of ICD-10-PCS.

Example: XW043A6 Introduction of Cefiderocol Anti-infective into Central Vein, Percutaneous Approach, New Technology Group 6 can be coded to indicate that Cefiderocol Anti-infective was administered via a central vein. A separate code from table 3E0 in the Administration section of ICD-10-PCS is not coded in addition to this code.

E1.b When multiple procedures are performed, New Technology section X codes are coded following the multiple procedures guideline.

Examples: Dual filter cerebral embolic filtration used during transcatheter aortic valve replacement (TAVR), X2A5312 Cerebral Embolic Filtration, Dual Filter in Innominate Artery and Left Common Carotid Artery, Percutaneous Approach, New Technology Group 2, is coded for the cerebral embolic filtration, along with an ICD-10-PCS code for the TAVR procedure. An extracorporeal flow reversal circuit for embolic neuroprotection placed during a transcarotid arterial revascularization procedure, a code from table X2A, Assistance of the Cardiovascular System is coded for the use of the extracoporeal flow reversal circuit, along with an ICD-10-PCS code for the transcarotid arterial revascularization procedure.

New Technology Section Tables

New Technology Tables X27–XY0

Section	X	New Technology
Body System	2	Cardiovascular
Operation	7	**Dilation:** Expanding an orifice or the lumen of a tubular body part

Body Part (4th)	Approach (5th)	Device/Substance/Technology (6th)	Qualifier (7th)
H Femoral Artery, Right J Femoral Artery, Left K Popliteal Artery, Proximal Right L Popliteal Artery, Proximal Left M Popliteal Artery, Distal Right N Popliteal Artery, Distal Left P Anterior Tibial Artery, Right Q Anterior Tibial Artery, Left R Posterior Tibial Artery, Right S Posterior Tibial Artery, Left T Peroneal Tibial Artery, Right U Peroneal Tibial Artery, Left	3 Percutaneous	8 Intraluminal Device, Sustained Release Drug-eluting 9 Intraluminal Device, Sustained Release Drug-eluting, Two B Intraluminal Device, Sustained Release Drug-eluting, Three C Intraluminal Device, Sustained Release Drug-eluting, Four or More	5 New Technology Group 5

Section	X	New Technology
Body System	2	Cardiovascular System
Operation	A	**Assistance:** Taking over a portion of a physiological function by extracorporeal means

Body Part (4th)	Approach (5th)	Device/Substance/Technology (6th)	Qualifier (7th)
5 Innominate Artery and Left Common Carotid Artery	3 Percutaneous	1 Cerebral Embolic Filtration, Dual Filter	2 New Technology Group 2
6 Aortic Arch	3 Percutaneous	2 Cerebral Embolic Filtration, Single Deflection Filter	5 New Technology Group 5
H Common Carotid Artery, Right J Common Carotid Artery, Left	3 Percutaneous	3 Cerebral Embolic Filtration, Extracorporeal Flow Reversal Circuit	6 New Technology Group 6

Section	X	New Technology
Body System	2	Cardiovascular System
Operation	C	**Extirpation:** Taking or cutting out solid matter from a body part

Body Part (4th)	Approach (5th)	Device/Substance/Technology (6th)	Qualifier (7th)
P Abdominal Aorta Q Upper Extremity Vein, Right R Upper Extremity Vein, Left S Lower Extremity Artery, Right T Lower Extremity Artery, Left U Lower Extremity Vein, Right V Lower Extremity Vein, Left Y Great Vessel	3 Percutaneous	T Computer-aided Mechanical Aspiration	7 New Technology Group 7

Section   **X**   **New Technology**
Body System   **2**   **Cardiovascular System**
Operation   **J**   **Inspection:** Visually and/or manually exploring a body part

Body Part (4th)	Approach (5th)	Device/Substance/Technology (6th)	Qualifier (7th)
A Heart	**X** External	**4** Transthoracic Echocardiography Computer-aided Guidance	**7** New Technology Group 7

Section   **X**   **New Technology**
Body System   **2**   **Cardiovascular System**
Operation   **K**   **Bypass:** Altering the route of passage of the contents of a tubular body part

Body Part (4th)	Approach (5th)	Device/Substance/Technology (6th)	Qualifier (7th)
B Radial Artery, Right **C** Radial Artery, Left	**3** Percutaneous	**1** Thermal Resistance Energy	**7** New Technology Group 7

Section   **X**   **New Technology**
Body System   **2**   **Cardiovascular System**
Operation   **R**   **Replacement:** Putting in or on biological or synthetic material that physically takes the place and/or function of all or a portion of a body part

Body Part (4th)	Approach (5th)	Device/Substance/Technology (6th)	Qualifier (7th)
F Aortic Valve	**0** Open **3** Percutaneous **4** Percutaneous Endoscopic	**3** Zooplastic Tissue, Rapid Deployment Technique	**2** New Technology Group 2
X Thoracic Aorta, Arch	**0** Open	**N** Branched Synthetic Substitute with Intraluminal Device	**7** New Technology Group 7

Section   **X**   **New Technology**
Body System   **2**   **Cardiovascular System**
Operation   **V**   **Restriction:** Partially closing an orifice or the lumen of a tubular body part

Body Part (4th)	Approach (5th)	Device/Substance/Technology (6th)	Qualifier (7th)
7 Coronary Sinus	**3** Percutaneous	**Q** Reduction Device	**7** New Technology Group 7
W Thoracic Aorta, Descending	**0** Open	**N** Branched Synthetic Substitute with Intraluminal Device	**7** New Technology Group 7

Section   **X**   **New Technology**
Body System   **D**   **Gastrointestinal System**
Operation   **2**   **Monitoring:** Determining the level of a physiological or physical function repetitively over a period of time

Body Part (4th)	Approach (5th)	Device/Substance/Technology (6th)	Qualifier (7th)
G Upper GI **H** Lower GI	**4** Percutaneous Endoscopic **8** Via Natural or Artificial Opening Endoscopic	**V** Oxygen Saturation	**7** New Technology Group 7

Section	X	New Technology
Body System	D	Gastrointestinal System
Operation	P	**Irrigation:** Putting in or on a cleansing substance

Body Part (4th)	Approach (5th)	Device/Substance/Technology (6th)	Qualifier (7th)
H Lower GI	**8** Via Natural or Artificial Opening Endoscopic	**K** Intraoperative Single-use Oversleeve	**7** New Technology Group 7

Section	X	New Technology
Body System	F	**Hepatobiliary System and Pancreas**
Operation	J	**Inspection:** Visually and/or manually exploring a body part

Body Part (4th)	Approach (5th)	Device/Substance/Technology (6th)	Qualifier (7th)
B Hepatobiliary Duct **D** Pancreatic Duct	**8** Via Natural or Artificial Opening Endoscopic	**A** Single-use Duodenoscope	**7** New Technology Group 7

Section	X	New Technology
Body System	H	**Skin, Subcutaneous Tissue, Fascia and Breast**
Operation	R	**Replacement:** Putting in or on biological or synthetic material that physically takes the place and/or function of all or a portion of a body part

Body Part (4th)	Approach (5th)	Device/Substance/Technology (6th)	Qualifier (7th)
P Skin	**X** External	**F** Bioengineered Allogeneic Construct	**7** New Technology Group 7
P Skin	**X** External	**L** Skin Substitute, Porcine Liver Derived	**2** New Technology Group 2

Section	X	New Technology
Body System	K	**Muscles, Tendons, Bursae and Ligaments**
Operation	0	**Introduction:** Putting in or on a therapeutic, diagnostic, nutritional, physiological, or prophylactic substance except blood or blood products

Body Part (4th)	Approach (5th)	Device/Substance/Technology (6th)	Qualifier (7th)
2 Muscle	**3** Percutaneous	**0** Concentrated Bone Marrow Aspirate	**3** New Technology Group 3

Section	X	New Technology
Body System	N	**Bones**
Operation	S	**Reposition:** Moving to its normal location, or other suitable location, all or a portion of a body part

Body Part (4th)	Approach (5th)	Device/Substance/Technology (6th)	Qualifier (7th)
0 Lumbar Vertebra	**0** Open	**3** Magnetically Controlled Growth Rod(s)	**2** New Technology Group 2
0 Lumbar Vertebra	**0** Open	**C** Posterior (Dynamic) Distraction Device	**7** New Technology Group 7
0 Lumbar Vertebra	**3** Percutaneous	**3** Magnetically Controlled Growth Rod(s)	**2** New Technology Group 2
0 Lumbar Vertebra	**3** Percutaneous	**C** Posterior (Dynamic) Distraction Device	**7** New Technology Group
3 Cervical Vertebra	**0** Open **3** Percutaneous	**3** Magnetically Controlled Growth Rod(s)	**2** New Technology Group 2
4 Thoracic Vertebra	**0** Open	**3** Magnetically Controlled Growth Rod(s)	**2** New Technology Group 2
4 Thoracic Vertebra	**0** Open	**C** Posterior (Dynamic) Distraction Device	**7** New Technology Group 7
4 Thoracic Vertebra	**3** Percutaneous	**3** Magnetically Controlled Growth Rod(s)	**2** New Technology Group 2
4 Thoracic Vertebra	**3** Percutaneous	**C** Posterior (Dynamic) Distraction Device	**7** New Technology Group 7

Section	X	New Technology
Body System	N	Bones
Operation	U	Supplement: Putting in or on biological or synthetic material that physically reinforces and/or augments the function of a portion of a body part

Body Part (4th)	Approach (5th)	Device (6th)	Qualifier (7th)
0 Lumbar Vertebra 4 Thoracic Vertebra	3 Percutaneous	5 Synthetic Substitute, Mechanically Expandable (Paired)	6 New Technology Group 6

Section	X	New Technology
Body System	R	Joints
Operation	G	Fusion: Joining together portions of an articular body part rendering the articular body part immobile

Body Part (4th)	Approach (5th)	Device/Substance/Technology (6th)	Qualifier (7th)
0 Occipital-cervical Joint	0 Open	9 Interbody Fusion Device, Nanotextured Surface	2 New Technology Group 2
0 Occipital-cervical Joint	0 Open	F Interbody Fusion Device, Radiolucent Porous	3 New Technology Group 3
1 Cervical Vertebral Joint	0 Open	9 Interbody Fusion Device, Nanotextured Surface	2 New Technology Group 2
1 Cervical Vertebral Joint	0 Open	F Interbody Fusion Device, Radiolucent Porous	3 New Technology Group 3
2 Cervical Vertebral Joints, 2 or More	0 Open	9 Interbody Fusion Device, Nanotextured Surface	2 New Technology Group 2
2 Cervical Vertebral Joints, 2 or More	0 Open	F Interbody Fusion Device, Radiolucent Porous	3 New Technology Group 3
4 Cervicothoracic Vertebral Joint	0 Open	9 Interbody Fusion Device, Nanotextured Surface	2 New Technology Group 2
4 Cervicothoracic Vertebral Joint	0 Open	F Interbody Fusion Device, Radiolucent Porous	3 New Technology Group 3
6 Thoracic Vertebral Joint	0 Open	9 Interbody Fusion Device, Nanotextured Surface	2 New Technology Group 2
6 Thoracic Vertebral Joint	0 Open	F Interbody Fusion Device, Radiolucent Porous	3 New Technology Group 3
7 Thoracic Vertebral Joints, 2 to 7	0 Open	9 Interbody Fusion Device, Nanotextured Surface	2 New Technology Group 2
7 Thoracic Vertebral Joints. 2 to 7	0 Open	F Interbody Fusion Device, Radiolucent Porous	3 New Technology Group 3
8 Thoracic Vertebral Joints, 8 or More	0 Open	9 Interbody Fusion Device, Nanotextured Surface	2 New Technology Group 2
8 Thoracic Vertebral Joints, 8 or More	0 Open	F Interbody Fusion Device, Radiolucent Porous	3 New Technology Group 3
A Thoracolumbar Vertebral Joint	0 Open	9 Interbody Fusion Device, Nanotextured Surface	2 New Technology Group 2
A Thoracolumbar Vertebral Joint	0 Open	F Interbody Fusion Device, Radiolucent Porous	3 New Technology Group 3
A Thoracolumbar Vertebral Joint	0 Open 3 Percutaneous 4 Percutaneous Endoscopic	R Interbody Fusion Device, Customizable	7 New Technology Group 7

Continued →

Section	X	New Technology
Body System	R	Joints
Operation	G	**Fusion:** Joining together portions of an articular body part rendering the articular body part immobile

Body Part (4th)	Approach (5th)	Device/Substance/Technology (6th)	Qualifier (7th)
B Lumbar Vertebral Joint	**0** Open	**9** Interbody Fusion Device, Nanotextured Surface	**2** New Technology Group 2
B Lumbar Vertebral Joint	**0** Open	**F** Interbody Fusion Device, Radiolucent Porous	**3** New Technology Group 3
B Lumbar Vertebral Joint	**0** Open **3** Percutaneous **4** Percutaneous Endoscopic	**R** Interbody Fusion Device, Customizable	**7** New Technology Group 7
C Lumbar Vertebral Joints, 2 or More	**0** Open	**9** Interbody Fusion Device, Nanotextured Surface	**2** New Technology Group 2
C Lumbar Vertebral Joints, 2 or More	**0** Open	**F** Interbody Fusion Device, Radiolucent Porous	**3** New Technology Group 3
C Lumbar Vertebral Joints, 2 or More	**0** Open **3** Percutaneous **4** Percutaneous Endoscopic	**R** Interbody Fusion Device, Customizable	**7** New Technology Group 7
D Lumbosacral Vertebral Joint	**0** Open	**9** Interbody Fusion Device, Nanotextured Surface	**2** New Technology Group 2
D Lumbosacral Vertebral Joint	**0** Open	**F** Interbody Fusion Device, Radiolucent Porous	**3** New Technology Group 3
D Lumbarosacral Joint	**0** Open **3** Percutaneous **4** Percutaneous Endoscopic	**R** Interbody Fusion Device, Customizable	**7** New Technology Group 7

Section	X	New Technology
Body System	T	Urinary System
Operation	2	**Monitoring:** Determining the level of a physiological or physical function repetitively over a period of time

Body Part (4th)	Approach (5th)	Device/Substance/Technology (6th)	Qualifier (7th)
5 Kidney	**X** External	**E** Fluorescent Pyrazine	**5** New Technology Group 5

Section	X	New Technology
Body System	V	Male Reproductive System
Operation	5	**Destruction:** Physical eradication of all or a portion of a body part by the direct use of energy, force, or a destructive agent

Body Part (4th)	Approach (5th)	Device/Substance/Technology (6th)	Qualifier (7th)
0 Prostate	**8** Via Natural or Artificial Opening Endoscopic	**A** Robotic Waterjet Ablation	**4** New Technology Group 4

Section	X	New Technology
Body System	W	Anatomical Regions
Operation	0	**Introduction:** Putting in or on a therapeutic, diagnostic, nutritional, physiological, or prophylactic substance except blood or blood products

Body Part (4th)	Approach (5th)	Device/Substance/Technology (6th)	Qualifier (7th)
0 Skin	**X** External	**2** Bromelain-enriched Proteolytic Enzyme	**7** New Technology Group 7
1 Subcutaneous Tissue	**3** Percutaneous	**9** Satrailzumab-mwge	**7** New Technology Group 7
1 Subcutaneous Tissue	**3** Percutaneous	**F** Other New Technology Therapeutic Substance	**5** New Technology Group 5
1 Subcutaneous Tissue	**3** Percutaneous	**H** Other New Technology Monoclonal Antibody **K** Leronlimab Monoclonal Antibody **S** COVID-19 Vaccine Dose 1 **T** COVID-19 Vaccine Dose 2 **U** COVID-19 Vaccine	**6** New Technology Group 6
1 Subcutaneous Tissue	**3** Percutaneous	**W** Caplacizumab	**5** New Technology Group 5
1 Subcutaneous Tissue	**X** External	**2** Bromelain-enriched Proteolytic Enzyme	**7** New Technology Group 7
2 Muscle	**3** Percutaneous	**S** COVID-19 Vaccine Dose 1 **T** COVID-19 Vaccine Dose 2 **U** COVID-19 Vaccine	**6** New Technology Group 6
3 Peripheral Vein	**3** Percutaneous	**0** Brexanolone **2** Nerinitide **3** Durvalumab Antineoplastic	**6** New Technology Group 6
3 Peripheral Vein	**3** Percutaneous	**5** Narsoplimab Monoclonal Antibody	**7** New Technology Group 7
3 Peripheral Vein	**3** Percutaneous	**6** Lefamulin Anti-infective	**6** New Technology Group 6
3 Peripheral Vein	**3** Percutaneous	**6** Terlipressin	**7** New Technology Group 7
3 Peripheral Vein	**3** Percutaneous	**7** Coagulation Factor Xa, Inactivated	**2** New Technology Group 2
3 Peripheral Vein	**3** Percutaneous	**7** Trilaciclib **8** Lurbinectedin	**7** New Technology Group 7
3 Peripheral Vein	**3** Percutaneous	**9** Defibrotide Sodium Anticoagulant	**2** New Technology Group 2
3 Peripheral Vein	**3** Percutaneous	**9** Ceftolozane/Tazobactam Anti-infective	**6** New Technology Group 6
3 Peripheral Vein	**3** Percutaneous	**A** Bezlotoxumab Monoclonal Antibody	**3** New Technology Group 3
3 Peripheral Vein	**3** Percutaneous	**A** Cefiderocol Anti-infective	**6** New Technology Group 6
3 Peripheral Vein	**3** Percutaneous	**A** Ciltacabtagene Autoleucel	**7** New Technology Group 7
3 Peripheral Vein	**3** Percutaneous	**B** Cytarabine and Daunorubicin Liposome Antineoplastic	**3** New Technology Group 3
3 Peripheral Vein	**3** Percutaneous	**B** Omadacycline Anti-infective	**6** New Technology Group 6
3 Peripheral Vein	**3** Percutaneous	**B** Amivantamab Monoclonal Antibody	**7** New Technology Group 7
3 Peripheral Vein	**3** Percutaneous	**C** Eculizumab	**6** New Technology Group 6
3 Peripheral Vein	**3** Percutaneous	**C** Engineered Chimeric Antigen Receptor T-cell Immunotherapy, Autologous	**7** New Technology Group 7
3 Peripheral Vein	**3** Peripheral Vein	**D** Atezolizumab Antineoplastic	**6** New Technology Group 6
3 Peripheral Vein	**3** Percutaneous	**E** Remdesivir Anti-infective	**5** New Technology Group 5

Continued →

Section   X   **New Technology**
Body System   W   **Anatomical Regions**
Operation   0   **Introduction:** Putting in or on a therapeutic, diagnostic, nutritional, physiological, or prophylactic substance except blood or blood products

Body Part (4th)	Approach (5th)	Device/Substance/Technology (6th)	Qualifier (7th)
3 Peripheral Vein	3 Percutaneous	E Etesevimab Monoclonal Antibody	6 New Technology Group 6
3 Peripheral Vein	3 Percutaneous	F Other New Technology Therapeutic Substance	3 New Technology Group 3
3 Peripheral Vein	3 Percutaneous	F Other New Technology Therapeutic Substance	5 New Technology Group 5
3 Peripheral Vein	3 Percutaneous	F Bamlanivimab Monoclonal Antibody	6 New Technology Group 6
3 Peripheral Vein	3 Percutaneous	G Plazomicin Anti-infective	4 New Technology Group 4
3 Peripheral Vein	3 Percutaneous	G Sarilumab	5 New Technology Group 5
3 Peripheral Vein	3 Percutaneous	G REGN-COV2 Monoclonal Antibody	6 New Technology Group 6
3 Peripheral Vein	3 Percutaneous	G Engineered Chimeric Antigen Receptor T-cell Immunotherapy, Allogeneic	7 New Technology Group 7
3 Peripheral Vein	3 Percutaneous	H Synthetic Human Angiotensin II	4 New Technology Group 4
3 Peripheral Vein	3 Percutaneous	H Tocilizumab	5 New Technology Group 5
3 Peripheral Vein	3 Percutaneous	H Other New Technology Monoclonal Antibody	6 New Technology Group 6
3 Peripheral Vein	3 Percutaneous	H Axicabtagene Ciloleucel Immunotherapy J Tisagenlecleucel Immunotherapy	7 New Technology Group 7
3 Peripheral Vein	3 Percutaneous	K Fosfomycin Anti-Infective	5 New Technology Group 5
3 Peripheral Vein	3 Percutaneous	K Idecabtagene Vicleucel Immunotherapy	7 New Technology Group 7
3 Peripheral Vein	3 Percutaneous	L CD24Fc Immunomodulator	6 New Technology Group 6
3 Peripheral Vein	3 Percutaneous	L Lifileucel Immunotherapy M Brexucabtagene Autoleucel Immunotherapy	7 New Technology Group 7
3 Peripheral Vein	3 Percutaneous	N Meropenem-vaborbactam Anti-infective	5 New Technology Group 5
3 Peripheral Vein	3 Percutaneous	N Lisocabtagene Maraleucel Immunotherapy	7 New Technology Group 7
3 Peripheral Vein	3 Percutaneous	Q Tagraxofusp-erzs Antineoplastic S Iobenguane I-131 Antineoplastic U Imipenem-cilastatin-relebactam Anti-infective W Caplacizumab	5 New Technology Group 5
4 Central Vein	3 Percutaneous	0 Brexanolone 2 Nerinitide 3 Durvalumab Antineoplastic	6 New Technology Group 6
4 Central Vein	3 Percutaneous	5 Narsoplimab Monoclonal Antibody	7 New Technology Group 7
4 Central Vein	3 Percutaneous	6 Lefamulin Anti-infective	6 New Technology Group 6
4 Central Vein	3 Percutaneous	6 Terlipressin	7 New Technology Group 7
4 Central Vein	3 Percutaneous	7 Coagulation Factor Xa, Inactivated	2 New Technology Group 2
4 Central Vein	3 Percutaneous	7 Trilaciclib 8 Lurbinectedin	7 New Technology Group 7
4 Central Vein	3 Percutaneous	9 Defibrotide Sodium Anticoagulant	2 New Technology Group 2
4 Central Vein	3 Percutaneous	9 Ceftolozane/Tazobactam Anti-infective	6 New Technology Group 6

Continued →

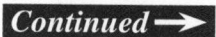

XW0

New Technology Section Tables

Section X New Technology
Body System W Anatomical Regions
Operation 0 Introduction: Putting in or on a therapeutic, diagnostic, nutritional, physiological, or prophylactic substance except blood or blood products

XW0 Continued

XW0

New Technology Section Tables

Body Part (4th)	Approach (5th)	Device/Substance/Technology (6th)	Qualifier (7th)
4 Central Vein	**3** Percutaneous	**A** Bezlotoxumab Monoclonal Antibody	**3** New Technology Group 3
4 Central Vein	**3** Percutaneous	**A** Cefiderocol Anti-infective	**6** New Technology Group 6
4 Central Vein	**3** Percutaneous	**A** Ciltacabtagene Autoleucel	**7** New Technology Group 7
4 Central Vein	**3** Percutaneous	**B** Cytarabine and Daunorubicin Liposome Antineoplastic	**3** New Technology Group 3
4 Central Vein	**3** Percutaneous	**B** Omadacycline Anti-infective	**6** New Technology Group 6
4 Central Vein	**3** Percutaneous	**B** Amivantamab Monoclonal Antibody	**7** New Technology Group 7
4 Central Vein	**3** Percutaneous	**C** Eculizumab	**6** New Technology Group 6
4 Central Vein	**3** Percutaneous	**C** Engineered Chimeric Antigen Receptor T-cell Immunotherapy, Autologous	**7** New Technology Group 7
4 Central Vein	**3** Percutaneous	**D** Atezolizumab Antineoplastic	**6** New Technology Group 6
4 Central Vein	**3** Percutaneous	**E** Remdesivir Anti-infective	**5** New Technology Group 5
4 Central Vein	**3** Percutaneous	**E** Etesevimab Monoclonal Antibody	**6** New Technology Group 6
4 Central Vein	**3** Percutaneous	**F** Other New Technology Therapeutic Substance	**3** New Technology Group 3
4 Central Vein	**3** Percutaneous	**F** Other New Technology Therapeutic Substance	**5** New Technology Group 5
4 Central Vein	**3** Percutaneous	**F** Bamlanivimab Monoclonal Antibody	**6** New Technology Group 6
4 Central Vein	**3** Percutaneous	**G** Plazomicin Anti-infective	**4** New Technology Group 4
4 Central Vein	**3** Percutaneous	**G** Sarilumab	**5** New Technology Group 5
4 Central Vein	**3** Percutaneous	**G** REGN-COV2 Monoclonal Antibody	**6** New Technology Group 6
4 Central Vein	**3** Percutaneous	**G** Engineered Chimeric Antigen Receptor T-cell Immunotherapy, Allogeneic	**7** New Technology Group 7
4 Central Vein	**3** Percutaneous	**H** Synthetic Human Angiotensin II	**4** New Technology Group 4
4 Central Vein	**3** Percutaneous	**H** Tocilizumab	**5** New Technology Group 5
4 Central Vein	**3** Percutaneous	**H** Other New Technology Monoclonal Antibody	**6** New Technology Group 6
4 Central Vein	**3** Percutaneous	**H** Axicabtagene Ciloleucel Immunotherapy **J** Tisagenlecleucel Immunotherapy	**7** New Technology Group 7
4 Central Vein	**3** Percutaneous	**K** Fosfomycin Anti-Infective	**5** New Technology Group 5
4 Central Vein	**3** Percutaneous	**K** Idecabtagene Vicleucel Immunotherapy	**7** New Technology Group 7
4 Central Vein	**3** Percutaneous	**L** CD24Fc Immunomodulator	**6** New Technology Group 6
4 Central Vein	**3** Percutaneous	**L** Lifileucel Immunotherapy **M** Brexucabtagene Autoleucel Immunotherapy	**7** New Technology Group 7
4 Central Vein	**3** Percutaneous	**N** Meropenem-vaborbactam Anti-infective	**5** New Technology Group 5
4 Central Vein	**3** Percutaneous	**N** Lisocabtagene Maraleucel Immunotherapy	**7** New Technology Group 7

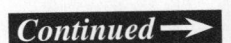

Continued →

Section	X	New Technology
Body System	W	Anatomical Regions
Operation	0	Introduction: Putting in or on a therapeutic, diagnostic, nutritional, physiological, or prophylactic substance except blood or blood products

Body Part (4th)	Approach (5th)	Device/Substance/Technology (6th)	Qualifier (7th)
4 Central Vein	3 Percutaneous	Q Tagraxofusp-erzs Antineoplastic S Iobenguane I-131 Antineoplastic U Imipenem-cilastatin-relebactam Anti-infective W Caplacizumab	5 New Technology Group 5
9 Nose	7 Via Natural or Artificial Opening	M Esketamine Hydrochloride	5 New Technology Group 5
D Mouth and Pharynx	X External	6 Lefamulin Anti-infective	6 New Technology Group 6
D Mouth and Pharynx	X External	8 Uridine Triacetate	2 New Technology Group 2
D Mouth and Pharynx	X External	F Other New Technology Therapeutic Substance J Apalutamide Antienoplastic L Erdafitinib Antineoplastic	5 New Technology Group 5
D Mouth and Pharynx	X External	M Baricitinib	6 New Technology Group 6
D Mouth and Pharynx	X External	R Venetoclax Antineoplastic T Ruxolitinib V Gilteritnib Antineoplastic	5 New Technology Group 5
G Upper GI H Lower GI	7 Via Natural or Artificial Opening	M Baricitinib	6 New Technology Group 6
G Upper GI H Lower GI	8 Via Natural or Artificial Opening Endoscopic	8 Mineral-based Topical Hemostatic Agent	6 New Technology Group 6
Q Cranial Cavity and Brain	3 Percutaneous	1 Eladocagene exuparvovec	6 New Technology Group 6
V Bones	0 Open	P Antibiotic-eluting Bone Void Filler	7 New Technology Group 7

Section	X	New Technology
Body System	W	Anatomical Regions
Operation	1	Transfusion: Putting in blood or blood products

Body Part (4th)	Approach (5th)	Device (6th)	Qualifier (7th)
3 Peripheral Vein	3 Percutaneous	2 Plasma, Convalescent (Nonautologous)	5 New Technology Group 5
3 Peripheral Vein	3 Percutaneous	D High-Dose Intravenous Immune Globulin E Hyperimmune Globulin	7 New Technology Group 7
4 Central Vein	3 Percutaneous	2 Plasma, Convalescent (Nonautologous)	5 New Technology Group 5
4 Central Vein	3 Percutaneous	D High-Dose Intravenous Immune Globulin E Hyperimmune Globulin	7 New Technology Group 7

Section	X	New Technology
Body System	W	Anatomical Regions
Operation	H	Insertion: Putting in a nonbiological appliance that monitors, assists, performs, or prevents a physiological function but does not physically take the place of a body part

Body Part (4th)	Approach (5th)	Device (6th)	Qualifier (7th)
D Mouth and Pharynx	7 Via Natural or Artificial Opening	Q Neurostimulator Lead	7 New Technology Group 7

Section	X	New Technology
Body System	X	Physiological Systems
Operation	E	Measurement: Determining the level of a physiological or physical function at a point in time

Body Part (4th)	Approach (5th)	Device/Substance/Technology (6th)	Qualifier (7th)
0 Central Nervous	X External	0 Intracranial Vascular Activity, Computer-aided Assessment	7 New Technology Group 7
3 Arterial	X External	2 Pulmonary Artery Flow, Computer-aided Triage and Notification	7 New Technology Group 7
5 Circulatory	X External	M Infection, Whole Blood Nucleic Acid-base Microbial Detection	5 New Technology Group 5
5 Circulatory	X External	N Infection, Positive Blood Culture Fluorescence Hybridization for Organism Identification, Concentration and Susceptibility	6 New Technology Group 6
5 Circulatory	X External	R Infection, Mechanical Initial Specimen Diversion Technique Using Active Negative Pressure T Intracranial Arterial Flow, Whole Blood mRNA V Infection, Serum/Plasma Nanoparticle Fluorescence SARS-CoV-2 Antibody Detection	7 New Technology Group 7
9 Nose	7 Via Natural or Artificial Opening	U Infection, Nasopharyngeal Fluid SARS-CoV-2 Polymerase Chain Reaction	7 New Technology Group 7
B Respiratory	X External	Q Infection, Lower Respiratory Fluid Nucleic Acid-base Microbial Detection	6 New Technology Group 6

Section	X	New Technology
Body System	Y	Extracorporeal
Operation	0	Introduction: Putting in or on a therapeutic, diagnostic, nutritional, physiological, or prophylactic substance except blood or blood products

Body Part (4th)	Approach (5th)	Device/Substance/Technology (6th)	Qualifier (7th)
V Vein Graft	X External	8 Endothelial Damage Inhibitor	3 New Technology Group 3
Y Extracorporeal	X External	3 Nafamostat Anticoagulant	7 New Technology Group 7

Appendix A: Root Operations Definitions

Section 0 - Medical and Surgical — Character 3 - Root Operation

Alteration (0)	**Definition:** Modifying the anatomic structure of a body part without affecting the function of the body part **Explanation:** Principal purpose is to improve appearance **Includes/Examples:** Face lift, breast augmentation
Bypass (1)	**Definition:** Altering the route of passage of the contents of a tubular body part **Explanation:** Rerouting contents of a body part to a downstream area of the normal route, to a similar route and body part, or to an abnormal route and dissimilar body part. Includes one or more anastomoses, with or without the use of a device **Includes/Examples:** Coronary artery bypass, colostomy formation
Change (2)	**Definition:** Taking out or off a device from a body part and putting back an identical or similar device in or on the same body part without cutting or puncturing the skin or a mucous membrane **Explanation:** All CHANGE procedures are coded using the approach EXTERNAL **Includes/Examples:** Urinary catheter change, gastrostomy tube change
Control (3)	**Definition:** Stopping, or attempting to stop, postprocedural or other acute bleeding **Includes/Examples:** Control of post-prostatectomy hemorrhage, control of intracranial subdural hemorrhage, control of bleeding duodenal ulcer, control of retroperitoneal hemorrhage
Creation (4)	**Definition:** Putting in or on biological or synthetic material to form a new body part that to the extent possible replicates the anatomic structure or function of an absent body part **Explanation:** Used for gender reassignment surgery and corrective procedures in individuals with congenital anomalies **Includes/Examples:** Creation of vagina in a male, creation of right and left atrioventricular valve from common atrioventricular valve
Destruction (5)	**Definition:** Physical eradication of all or a portion of a body part by the direct use of energy, force, or a destructive agent **Explanation:** None of the body part is physically taken out **Includes/Examples:** Fulguration of rectal polyp, cautery of skin lesion
Detachment (6)	**Definition:** Cutting off all or a portion of the upper or lower extremities **Explanation:** The body part value is the site of the detachment, with a qualifier if applicable to further specify the level where the extremity was detached **Includes/Examples:** Below knee amputation, disarticulation of shoulder
Dilation (7)	**Definition:** Expanding an orifice or the lumen of a tubular body part **Explanation:** The orifice can be a natural orifice or an artificially created orifice. Accomplished by stretching a tubular body part using intraluminal pressure or by cutting part of the orifice or wall of the tubular body part **Includes/Examples:** Percutaneous transluminal angioplasty, internal urethrotomy
Division (8)	**Definition:** Cutting into a body part, without draining fluids and/or gases from the body part, in order to separate or transect a body part **Explanation:** All or a portion of the body part is separated into two or more portions **Includes/Examples:** Spinal cordotomy, osteotomy
Drainage (9)	**Definition:** Taking or letting out fluids and/or gases from a body part **Explanation:** The qualifier DIAGNOSTIC is used to identify drainage procedures that are biopsies **Includes/Examples:** Thoracentesis, incision and drainage
Excision (B)	**Definition:** Cutting out or off, without replacement, a portion of a body part **Explanation:** The qualifier DIAGNOSTIC is used to identify excision procedures that are biopsies **Includes/Examples:** Partial nephrectomy, liver biopsy
Extirpation (C)	**Definition:** Taking or cutting out solid matter from a body part **Explanation:** The solid matter may be an abnormal byproduct of a biological function or a foreign body; it may be imbedded in a body part or in the lumen of a tubular body part. The solid matter may or may not have been previously broken into pieces **Includes/Examples:** Thrombectomy, choledocholithotomy
Extraction (D)	**Definition:** Pulling or stripping out or off all or a portion of a body part by the use of force **Explanation:** The qualifier DIAGNOSTIC is used to identify extraction procedures that are biopsies **Includes/Examples:** Dilation and curettage, vein stripping
Fragmentation (F)	**Definition:** Breaking solid matter in a body part into pieces **Explanation:** Physical force (e.g., manual, ultrasonic) applied directly or indirectly is used to break the solid matter into pieces. The solid matter may be an abnormal byproduct of a biological function or a foreign body. The pieces of solid matter are not taken out **Includes/Examples:** Extracorporeal shockwave lithotripsy, transurethral lithotripsy
Fusion (G)	**Definition:** Joining together portions of an articular body part rendering the articular body part immobile **Explanation:** The body part is joined together by fixation device, bone graft, or other means **Includes/Examples:** Spinal fusion, ankle arthrodesis
Insertion (H)	**Definition:** Putting in a nonbiological appliance that monitors, assists, performs, or prevents a physiological function but does not physically take the place of a body part **Includes/Examples:** Insertion of radioactive implant, insertion of central venous catheter

Continued →

Inspection (J)	**Definition:** Visually and/or manually exploring a body part **Explanation:** Visual exploration may be performed with or without optical instrumentation. Manual exploration may be performed directly or through intervening body layers **Includes/Examples:** Diagnostic arthroscopy, exploratory laparotomy
Map (K)	**Definition:** Locating the route of passage of electrical impulses and/or locating functional areas in a body part **Explanation:** Applicable only to the cardiac conduction mechanism and the central nervous system **Includes/Examples:** Cardiac mapping, cortical mapping
Occlusion (L)	**Definition:** Completely closing an orifice or the lumen of a tubular body part **Explanation:** The orifice can be a natural orifice or an artificially created orifice **Includes/Examples:** Fallopian tube ligation, ligation of inferior vena cava
Reattachment (M)	**Definition:** Putting back in or on all or a portion of a separated body part to its normal location or other suitable location **Explanation:** Vascular circulation and nervous pathways may or may not be reestablished **Includes/Examples:** Reattachment of hand, reattachment of avulsed kidney
Release (N)	**Definition:** Freeing a body part from an abnormal physical constraint by cutting or by the use of force **Explanation:** Some of the restraining tissue may be taken out but none of the body part is taken out **Includes/Examples:** Adhesiolysis, carpal tunnel release
Removal (P)	**Definition:** Taking out or off a device from a body part **Explanation:** If a device is taken out and a similar device put in without cutting or puncturing the skin or mucous membrane, the procedure is coded to the root operation CHANGE. Otherwise, the procedure for taking out a device is coded to the root operation REMOVAL **Includes/Examples:** Drainage tube removal, cardiac pacemaker removal
Repair (Q)	**Definition:** Restoring, to the extent possible, a body part to its normal anatomic structure and function **Explanation:** Used only when the method to accomplish the repair is not one of the other root operations **Includes/Examples:** Colostomy takedown, suture of laceration
Replacement (R)	**Definition:** Putting in or on biological or synthetic material that physically takes the place and/or function of all or a portion of a body part **Explanation:** The body part may have been taken out or replaced, or may be taken out, physically eradicated, or rendered nonfunctional during the Replacement procedure. A Removal procedure is coded for taking out the device used in a previous replacement procedure **Includes/Examples:** Total hip replacement, bone graft, free skin graft
Reposition (S)	**Definition:** Moving to its normal location, or other suitable location, all or a portion of a body part **Explanation:** The body part is moved to a new location from an abnormal location, or from a normal location where it is not functioning correctly. The body part may or may not be cut out or off to be moved to the new location **Includes/Examples:** Reposition of undescended testicle, fracture reduction
Resection (T)	**Definition:** Cutting out or off, without replacement, all of a body part **Includes/Examples:** Total nephrectomy, total lobectomy of lung
Restriction (V)	**Definition:** Partially closing an orifice or the lumen of a tubular body part **Explanation:** The orifice can be a natural orifice or an artificially created orifice **Includes/Examples:** Esophagogastric fundoplication, cervical cerclage
Revision (W)	**Definition:** Correcting, to the extent possible, a portion of a malfunctioning device or the position of a displaced device **Explanation:** Revision can include correcting a malfunctioning or displaced device by taking out or putting in components of the device such as a screw or pin **Includes/Examples:** Adjustment of position of pacemaker lead, recementing of hip prosthesis
Supplement (U)	**Definition:** Putting in or on biological or synthetic material that physically reinforces and/or augments the function of a portion of a body part **Explanation:** The biological material is non-living, or is living and from the same individual. The body part may have been previously replaced, and the Supplement procedure is performed to physically reinforce and/or augment the function of the replaced body part **Includes/Examples:** Herniorrhaphy using mesh, mitral valve ring annuloplasty, put a new acetabular liner in a previous hip replacement
Transfer (X)	**Definition:** Moving, without taking out, all or a portion of a body part to another location to take over the function of all or a portion of a body part **Explanation:** The body part transferred remains connected to its vascular and nervous supply **Includes/Examples:** Tendon transfer, skin pedicle flap transfer
Transplantation (Y)	**Definition:** Putting in or on all or a portion of a living body part taken from another individual or animal to physically take the place and/or function of all or a portion of a similar body part **Explanation:** The native body part may or may not be taken out, and the transplanted body part may take over all or a portion of its function **Includes/Examples:** Kidney transplant, heart transplant

Section 1 - Obstetrics — Character 3 - Root Operations Unique to Obstetrics

Abortion (A)	**Definition:** Artificially terminating a pregnancy **Explanation:** Subdivided according to whether an additional device such as a laminaria or abortifacient is used, or whether the abortion was performed by mechanical means **Includes/Example:** Transvaginal abortion using vacuum aspiration technique

Continued →

Section 1 - Obstetrics — Character 3 - Root Operations Unique to Obstetrics

Delivery (E)	**Definition:** Assisting the passage of the products of conception from the genital canal **Explanation:** Applies only to manually-assisted, vaginal delivery **Includes/Example:** Manually-assisted delivery

Section 2 - Placement — Character 3 - Root Operation

Change (0)	**Definition:** Taking out or off a device from a body part and putting back an identical or similar device in or on the same body part without cutting or puncturing the skin or a mucous membrane **Includes/Example:** Change of vaginal packing
Compression (1)	**Definition:** Putting pressure on a body region **Includes/Example:** Placement of pressure dressing on abdominal wall
Dressing (2)	**Definition:** Putting material on a body region for protection **Includes/Example:** Application of sterile dressing to head wound
Immobilization (3)	**Definition:** Limiting or preventing motion of a body region **Includes/Example:** Placement of splint on left finger
Packing (4)	**Definition:** Putting material in a body region or orifice **Includes/Example:** Placement of nasal packing
Removal (5)	**Definition:** Taking out or off a device from a body part **Includes/Example:** Removal of cast from right lower leg
Traction (6)	**Definition:** Exerting a pulling force on a body region in a distal direction **Includes/Example:** Lumbar traction using motorized split-traction table

Section 3 - Administration — Character 3 - Root Operation

Introduction (0)	**Definition:** Putting in or on a therapeutic, diagnostic, nutritional, physiological, or prophylactic substance except blood or blood products **Includes/Example:** Nerve block injection to median nerve
Irrigation (1)	**Definition:** Putting in or on a cleansing substance **Includes/Example:** Flushing of eye
Transfusion (2)	**Definition:** Putting in blood or blood products **Includes/Example:** Transfusion of cell saver red cells into central venous line

Section 4 - Measurement and Monitoring — Character 3 - Root Operation

Measurement (0)	**Definition:** Determining the level of a physiological or physical function at a point in time **Includes/Example:** External electrocardiogram (EKG), single reading
Monitoring (1)	**Definition:** Determining the level of a physiological or physical function repetitively over a period of time **Includes/Example:** Urinary pressure monitoring

Section 5 - Extracorporeal Assistance and Performance — Character 3 - Root Operation

Assistance (0)	**Definition:** Taking over a portion of a physiological function by extracorporeal means **Includes/Example:** Hyperbaric oxygenation of wound
Performance (1)	**Definition:** Completely taking over a physiological function by extracorporeal means **Includes/Example:** Cardiopulmonary bypass in conjunction with CABG
Restoration (2)	**Definition:** Returning, or attempting to return, a physiological function to its original state by extracorporeal means. **Includes/Example:** Attempted cardiac defibrillation, unsuccessful

Section 6 - Extracorporeal Therapies — Character 3 - Root Operation

Atmospheric Control (0)	**Definition:** Extracorporeal control of atmospheric pressure and composition **Includes/Example:** Atmospheric control, single treatment
Decompression (1)	**Definition:** Extracorporeal elimination of undissolved gas from body fluids **Includes/Example:** Hyperbaric decompression treatment, single
Electromagnetic Therapy (2)	**Definition:** Extracorporeal treatment by electromagnetic rays **Includes/Example:** Electromagnetic therapy, central nervous, multiple treatments
Hyperthermia (3)	**Definition:** Extracorporeal raising of body temperature **Includes/Example:** Hyperthermia, single treatment
Hypothermia (4)	**Definition:** Extracorporeal lowering of body temperature **Includes/Example:** Whole body hypothermia treatment for temperature imbalances, series treatment
Perfusion (B)	**Definition:** Extracorporeal treatment by diffusion of therapeutic fluid

Continued →

Section 6 - Extracorporeal Therapies — Character 3 - Root Operation

Pheresis (5)	**Definition:** Extracorporeal separation of blood products **Includes/Example:** Therapeutic leukopheresis, single treatment
Phototherapy (6)	**Definition:** Extracorporeal treatment by light rays **Includes/Example:** Phototherapy of circulatory system, series treatment
Shock Wave Therapy (7)	**Definition:** Extracorporeal treatment by shock waves **Includes/Example:** Shock wave therapy, musculoskeletal, single treatment
Ultrasound Therapy (8)	**Definition:** Extracorporeal treatment by ultrasound **Includes/Example:** Ultrasound therapy of the heart, single treatment
Ultraviolet Light Therapy (9)	**Definition:** Extracorporeal treatment by ultraviolet light **Includes/Example:** Ultraviolet light phototherapy, series treatment

Section 7 - Osteopathic — Character 3 - Root Operation

Treatment (0)	**Definition:** Manual treatment to eliminate or alleviate somatic dysfunction and related disorders **Includes/Example:** Fascial release of abdomen, osteopathic treatment

Section 8 - Other Procedures — Character 3 - Root Operation

Other Procedures (0)	**Definition:** Methodologies which attempt to remediate or cure a disorder or disease **Includes/Example:** Acupuncture

Section 9 - Chiropractic — Character 3 - Root Operation

Manipulation (B)	**Definition:** Manual procedure that involves a directed thrust to move a joint past the physiological range of motion, without exceeding the anatomical limit **Includes/Example:** Chiropractic treatment of cervical spine, short lever specific contact

Section X - New Technology — Character 3 - Root Operation

Assistance (A)	**Definition:** Taking over a portion of a physiological function by extracorporeal means
Bypass (K)	**Definition:** Altering the route of passage of the contents of a tubular body part
Destruction (5)	**Definition:** Physical eradication of all or a portion of a body part by the direct use of energy, force, or a destructive agent **Explanation:** None of the body part is physically taken out **Includes/Examples:** Fulguration of rectal polyp, cautery of skin lesion
Dilation (7)	**Definition:** Expanding an orifice or the lumen of a tubular body part **Explanation:** The orifice can be a natural orifice or an artificially created orifice. Accomplished by stretching a tubular body part using intraluminal pressure or by cutting part of the orifice or wall of the tubular body part
Extirpation (C)	**Definition:** Taking or cutting out solid matter from a body part **Explanation:** The solid matter may be an abnormal by product of a biological function or a foreign body; it may be imbedded in a body part or in the lumen of a tubular body part. The solid matter may or may not have been previously broken into pieces **Includes/Example:** Thrombectomy, choledocholithotomy
Fusion (G)	**Definition:** Joining together portions of an articular body part rendering the articular body part immobile **Explanation:** The body part is joined together by fixation device, bone graft, or other means **Includes/Examples:** Spinal fusion, ankle arthrodesis
Insertion (H)	**Definition:** Putting in a nonbiological appliance that monitors, assists, performs, or prevents a physiological function bust does not physically take the place of a body part.
Inspection (J)	**Definition:** Visually and/or manually exploring a body part
Introduction (0)	**Definition:** Putting in or on a therapeutic, diagnostic, nutritional, physiological, or prophylactic substance except blood or blood products
Irrigation (P)	**Definition:** Putting in or on a cleansing substance
Measurement (E)	**Definition:** Determining the level of a physiological or physical function at a point in time
Monitoring (2)	**Definition:** Determining the level of a physiological or physical function repetitively over a period of time
Replacement (R)	**Definition:** Putting in or on biological or synthetic material that physically takes the place and/or function of all or a portion of a body part **Explanation:** The body part may have been taken out or replaced, or may be taken out, physically eradicated, or rendered nonfunctional during the Replacement procedure. A Removal procedure is coded for taking out the device used in a previous replacement procedure. **Includes/Examples:** Total hip replacement, bone graft, free skin graft
Reposition (S)	**Definition:** Moving to its normal location, or other suitable location, all or a portion of a body part **Explanation:** The body part is moved to a new location from an abnormal location, or from a normal location where it is not functioning correctly. The body part may or may not be cut out or off to be moved to the new location. **Includes/Examples:** Reposition of undescended testicle, fracture reduction
Restriction (V)	**Definition:** Partially closing an orifice or the lumen of a tubular body part
Supplement (U)	**Definition:** Putting in or on biological or synthetic material that physically reinforces and/or augments the function of a portion of a body part
Transfusion (1&2)	**Definition:** Putting in blood or blood products

Section B - Imaging — Character 3 - Root Type

Computerized Tomography (CT Scan) (2)	**Definition:** Computer reformatted digital display of multiplanar images developed from the capture of multiple exposures of external ionizing radiation
Fluoroscopy (1)	**Definition:** Single plane or bi-plane real time display of an image developed from the capture of external ionizing radiation on a fluorescent screen. The image may also be stored by either digital or analog means
Magnetic Resonance Imaging (MRI) (3)	**Definition:** Computer reformatted digital display of multiplanar images developed from the capture of radiofrequency signals emitted by nuclei in a body site excited within a magnetic field
Other Imaging (5)	**Definition:** Other specified modality for visualizing a body part
Plain Radiography (0)	**Definition:** Planar display of an image developed from the capture of external ionizing radiation on photographic or photoconductive plate
Ultrasonography (4)	**Definition:** Real time display of images of anatomy or flow information developed from the capture of reflected and attenuated high frequency sound waves

Section C - Nuclear Medicine — Character 3 - Root Type

Nonimaging Nuclear Medicine Assay (6)	**Definition:** Introduction of radioactive materials into the body for the study of body fluids and blood elements, by the detection of radioactive emissions
Nonimaging Nuclear Medicine Probe (5)	**Definition:** Introduction of radioactive materials into the body for the study of distribution and fate of certain substances by the detection of radioactive emissions; or, alternatively, measurement of absorption of radioactive emissions from an external source
Nonimaging Nuclear Medicine Uptake (4)	**Definition:** Introduction of radioactive materials into the body for measurements of organ function, from the detection of radioactive emissions
Planar Nuclear Medicine Imaging (1)	**Definition:** Introduction of radioactive materials into the body for single plane display of images developed from the capture of radioactive emissions
Positron Emission Tomographic (PET) Imaging (3)	**Definition:** Introduction of radioactive materials into the body for three dimensional display of images developed from the simultaneous capture, 180 degrees apart, of radioactive emissions
Systemic Nuclear Medicine Therapy (7)	**Definition:** Introduction of unsealed radioactive materials into the body for treatment
Tomographic (Tomo) Nuclear Medicine Imaging (2)	**Definition:** Introduction of radioactive materials into the body for three dimensional display of images developed from the capture of radioactive emissions

Section F - Physical Rehabilitation and Diagnostic Audiology — Character 3 - Root Type

Activities of Daily Living Assessment	**Definition:** Measurement of functional level for activities of daily living
Activities of Daily Living Treatment	**Definition:** Exercise or activities to facilitate functional competence for activities of daily living
Caregiver Training	**Definition:** Training in activities to support patient's optimal level of function
Cochlear Implant Treatment	**Definition:** Application of techniques to improve the communication abilities of individuals with cochlear implant
Device Fitting	**Definition:** Fitting of a device designed to facilitate or support achievement of a higher level of function
Hearing Aid Assessment	**Definition:** Measurement of the appropriateness and/or effectiveness of a hearing device
Hearing Assessment	**Definition:** Measurement of hearing and related functions
Hearing Treatment	**Definition:** Application of techniques to improve, augment, or compensate for hearing and related functional impairment
Motor and/or Nerve Function Assessment	**Definition:** Measurement of motor, nerve, and related functions
Motor Treatment	**Definition:** Exercise or activities to increase or facilitate motor function
Speech Assessment	**Definition:** Measurement of speech and related functions
Speech Treatment	**Definition:** Application of techniques to improve, augment, or compensate for speech and related functional impairment
Vestibular Assessment	**Definition:** Measurement of the vestibular system and related functions
Vestibular Treatment	**Definition:** Application of techniques to improve, augment, or compensate for vestibular and related functional impairment

Acoustic Reflex Decay	**Definition:** Measures reduction in size/strength of acoustic reflex over time **Includes/Examples:** Includes site of lesion test
Acoustic Reflex Patterns	**Definition:** Defines site of lesion based upon presence/absence of acoustic reflexes with ipsilateral vs. contralateral stimulation
Acoustic Reflex Threshold	**Definition:** Determines minimal intensity that acoustic reflex occurs with ipsilateral and/or contralateral stimulation
Aerobic Capacity and Endurance	**Definition:** Measures autonomic responses to positional changes; perceived exertion, dyspnea or angina during activity; performance during exercise protocols; standard vital signs; and blood gas analysis or oxygen consumption
Alternate Binaural or Monaural Loudness Balance	**Definition:** Determines auditory stimulus parameter that yields the same objective sensation **Includes/Examples:** Sound intensities that yield same loudness perception
Anthropometric Characteristics	**Definition:** Measures edema, body fat composition, height, weight, length and girth
Aphasia (Assessment)	**Definition:** Measures expressive and receptive speech and language function including reading and writing
Aphasia (Treatment)	**Definition:** Applying techniques to improve, augment, or compensate for receptive/expressive language impairments
Articulation/Phonology (Assessment)	**Definition:** Measures speech production
Articulation/Phonology (Treatment)	**Definition:** Applying techniques to correct, improve, or compensate for speech productive impairment
Assistive Listening Device	**Definition:** Assists in use of effective and appropriate assistive listening device/system
Assistive Listening System/Device Selection	**Definition:** Measures the effectiveness and appropriateness of assistive listening systems/devices
Assistive, Adaptive, Supportive or Protective Devices	**Explanation:** Devices to facilitate or support achievement of a higher level of function in wheelchair mobility; bed mobility; transfer or ambulation ability; bath and showering ability; dressing; grooming; personal hygiene; play or leisure
Auditory Evoked Potentials	**Definition:** Measures electric responses produced by the VIIIth cranial nerve and brainstem following auditory stimulation
Auditory Processing (Assessment)	**Definition:** Evaluates ability to receive and process auditory information and comprehension of spoken language
Auditory Processing (Treatment)	**Definition:** Applying techniques to improve the receiving and processing of auditory information and comprehension of spoken language
Augmentative/Alternative Communication System (Assessment)	**Definition:** Determines the appropriateness of aids, techniques, symbols, and/or strategies to augment or replace speech and enhance communication **Includes/Examples:** Includes the use of telephones, writing equipment, emergency equipment, and TDD
Augmentative/Alternative Communication System (Treatment)	**Includes/Examples:** Includes augmentative communication devices and aids
Aural Rehabilitation	**Definition:** Applying techniques to improve the communication abilities associated with hearing loss
Aural Rehabilitation Status	**Definition:** Measures impact of a hearing loss including evaluation of receptive and expressive communication skills
Bathing/Showering	**Includes/Examples:** Includes obtaining and using supplies; soaping, rinsing, and drying body parts; maintaining bathing position; and transferring to and from bathing positions
Bathing/Showering Techniques	**Definition:** Activities to facilitate obtaining and using supplies, soaping, rinsing and drying body parts, maintaining bathing position, and transferring to and from bathing positions
Bed Mobility (Assessment)	**Definition:** Transitional movement within bed
Bed Mobility (Treatment)	**Definition:** Exercise or activities to facilitate transitional movements within bed
Bedside Swallowing and Oral Function	**Includes/Examples:** Bedside swallowing includes assessment of sucking, masticating, coughing, and swallowing. Oral function includes assessment of musculature for controlled movements, structures and functions to determine coordination and phonation
Bekesy Audiometry	**Definition:** Uses an instrument that provides a choice of discrete or continuously varying pure tones; choice of pulsed or continuous signal
Binaural Electroacoustic Hearing Aid Check	**Definition:** Determines mechanical and electroacoustic function of bilateral hearing aids using hearing aid test box
Binaural Hearing Aid (Assessment)	**Definition:** Measures the candidacy, effectiveness, and appropriateness of a hearing aids **Explanation:** Measures bilateral fit

Continued →

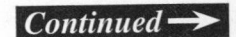

Binaural Hearing Aid (Treatment)	**Explanation:** Assists in achieving maximum understanding and performance
Bithermal, Binaural Caloric Irrigation	**Definition:** Measures the rhythmic eye movements stimulated by changing the temperature of the vestibular system
Bithermal, Monaural Caloric Irrigation	**Definition:** Measures the rhythmic eye movements stimulated by changing the temperature of the vestibular system in one ear
Brief Tone Stimuli	**Definition:** Measures specific central auditory process
Cerumen Management	**Definition:** Includes examination of external auditory canal and tympanic membrane and removal of cerumen from external ear canal
Cochlear Implant	**Definition:** Measures candidacy for cochlear implant
Cochlear Implant Rehabilitation	**Definition:** Applying techniques to improve the communication abilities of individuals with cochlear implant; includes programming the device, providing patients/families with information
Communicative/Cognitive Integration Skills (Assessment)	**Definition:** Measures ability to use higher cortical functions **Includes/Examples:** Includes orientation, recognition, attention span, initiation and termination of activity, memory, sequencing, categorizing, concept formation, spatial operations, judgment, problem solving, generalization and pragmatic communication
Communicative/Cognitive Integration Skills (Treatment)	**Definition:** Activities to facilitate the use of higher cortical functions **Includes/Examples:** Includes level of arousal, orientation, recognition, attention span, initiation and termination of activity, memory sequencing, judgment and problem solving, learning and generalization, and pragmatic communication
Computerized Dynamic Posturography	**Definition:** Measures the status of the peripheral and central vestibular system and the sensory/motor component of balance; evaluates the efficacy of vestibular rehabilitation
Conditioned Play Audiometry	**Definition:** Behavioral measures using nonspeech and speech stimuli to obtain frequency-specific and ear-specific information on auditory status from the patient **Explanation:** Obtains speech reception threshold by having patient point to pictures of spondaic words
Coordination/Dexterity (Assessment)	**Definition:** Measures large and small muscle groups for controlled goal-directed movements **Explanation:** Dexterity includes object manipulation
Coordination/Dexterity (Treatment)	**Definition:** Exercise or activities to facilitate gross coordination and fine coordination
Cranial Nerve Integrity	**Definition:** Measures cranial nerve sensory and motor functions, including tastes, smell and facial expression
Dichotic Stimuli	**Definition:** Measures specific central auditory process
Distorted Speech	**Definition:** Measures specific central auditory process
Dix-Hallpike Dynamic	**Definition:** Measures nystagmus following Dix-Hallpike maneuver
Dressing	**Includes/Examples:** Includes selecting clothing and accessories, obtaining clothing from storage, dressing, fastening and adjusting clothing and shoes, and applying and removing personal devices, prosthesis or orthosis
Dressing Techniques	**Definition:** Activities to facilitate selecting clothing and accessories, dressing and undressing, adjusting clothing and shoes, applying and removing devices, prostheses or orthoses
Dynamic Orthosis	**Includes/Examples:** Includes customized and prefabricated splints, inhibitory casts, spinal and other braces, and protective devices; allows motion through transfer of movement from other body parts or by use of outside forces
Ear Canal Probe Microphone	**Definition:** Real ear measures
Ear Protector Attentuation	**Definition:** Measures ear protector fit and effectiveness
Electrocochleography	**Definition:** Measures the VIIIth cranial nerve action potential
Environmental, Home and Work Barriers	**Definition:** Measures current and potential barriers to optimal function, including safety hazards, access problems and home or office design
Ergonomics and Body Mechanics	**Definition:** Ergonomic measurement of job tasks, work hardening or work conditioning needs; functional capacity; and body mechanics
Eustachian Tube Function	**Definition:** Measures eustachian tube function and patency of eustachian tube
Evoked Otoacoustic Emissions, Diagnostic	**Definition:** Measures auditory evoked potentials in a diagnostic format
Evoked Otoacoustic Emissions, Screening	**Definition:** Measures auditory evoked potentials in a screening format
Facial Nerve Function	**Definition:** Measures electrical activity of the VIIth cranial nerve (facial nerve)
Feeding/Eating (Assessment)	**Includes/Examples:** Includes setting up food, selecting and using utensils and tableware, bringing food or drink to mouth, cleaning face, hands, and clothing, and management of alternative methods of nourishment

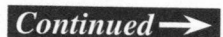

Continued →

Appendix B

Feeding/Eating (Treatment)	**Definition:** Exercise or activities to facilitate setting up food, selecting and using utensils and tableware, bringing food or drink to mouth, cleaning face, hands, and clothing, and management of alternative methods of nourishment
Filtered Speech	**Definition:** Uses high or low pass filtered speech stimuli to assess central auditory processing disorders, site of lesion testing
Fluency (Assessment)	**Definition:** Measures speech fluency or stuttering
Fluency (Treatment)	**Definition:** Applying techniques to improve and augment fluent speech
Gait and/or Balance	**Definition:** Measures biomechanical, arthrokinematic and other spatial and temporal characteristics of gait and balance
Gait Training/Functional Ambulation	**Definition:** Exercise or activities to facilitate ambulation on a variety of surfaces and in a variety of environments
Grooming/Personal Hygiene (Assessment)	**Includes/Examples:** Includes ability to obtain and use supplies in a sequential fashion, general grooming, oral hygiene, toilet hygiene, personal care devices, including care for artificial airways
Grooming/Personal Hygiene (Treatment)	**Definition:** Activities to facilitate obtaining and using supplies in a sequential fashion: general grooming, oral hygiene, toilet hygiene, cleaning body, and personal care devices, including artificial airways
Hearing and Related Disorders Counseling	**Definition:** Provides patients/families/caregivers with information, support, referrals to facilitate recovery from a communication disorder **Includes/Examples:** Includes strategies for psychosocial adjustment to hearing loss for clients and families/caregivers
Hearing and Related Disorders Prevention	**Definition:** Provides patients/families/caregivers with information and support to prevent communication disorders
Hearing Screening	**Definition:** Pass/refer measures designed to identify need for further audiologic assessment
Home Management (Assessment)	**Definition:** Obtaining and maintaining personal and household possessions and environment **Includes/Examples:** Includes clothing care, cleaning, meal preparation and cleanup, shopping, money management, household maintenance, safety procedures, and childcare/parenting
Home Management (Treatment)	**Definition:** Activities to facilitate obtaining and maintaining personal household possessions and environment **Includes/Examples:** Includes clothing care, cleaning, meal preparation and clean-up, shopping, money management, household maintenance, safety procedures, childcare/parenting
Instrumental Swallowing and Oral Function	**Definition:** Measures swallowing function using instrumental diagnostic procedures **Explanation:** Methods include videofluoroscopy, ultrasound, manometry, endoscopy
Integumentary Integrity	**Includes/Examples:** Includes burns, skin conditions, ecchymosis, bleeding, blisters, scar tissue, wounds and other traumas, tissue mobility, turgor and texture
Manual Therapy Techniques	**Definition:** Techniques in which the therapist uses his/her hands to administer skilled movements **Includes/Examples:** Includes connective tissue massage, joint mobilization and manipulation, manual lymph drainage, manual traction, soft tissue mobilization and manipulation
Masking Patterns	**Definition:** Measures central auditory processing status
Monaural Electroacoustic Hearing Aid Check	**Definition:** Determines mechanical and electroacoustic function of one hearing aid using hearing aid test box
Monaural Hearing Aid (Assessment)	**Definition:** Measures the candidacy, effectiveness, and appropriateness of a hearing aid **Explanation:** Measures unilateral fit
Monaural Hearing Aid (Treatment)	**Explanation:** Assists in achieving maximum understanding and performance
Motor Function (Assessment)	**Definition:** Measures the body's functional and versatile movement patterns **Includes/Examples:** Includes motor assessment scales, analysis of head, trunk and limb movement, and assessment of motor learning
Motor Function (Treatment)	**Definition:** Exercise or activities to facilitate crossing midline, laterality, bilateral integration, praxis, neuromuscular relaxation, inhibition, facilitation, motor function and motor learning
Motor Speech (Assessment)	**Definition:** Measures neurological motor aspects of speech production
Motor Speech (Treatment)	**Definition:** Applying techniques to improve and augment the impaired neurological motor aspects of speech production
Muscle Performance (Assessment)	**Definition:** Measures muscle strength, power and endurance using manual testing, dynamometry or computer-assisted electromechanical muscle test; functional muscle strength, power and endurance; muscle pain, tone, or soreness; or pelvic-floor musculature **Explanation:** Muscle endurance refers to the ability to contract a muscle repeatedly over time

Continued →

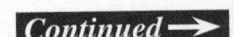

Muscle Performance (Treatment)	**Definition:** Exercise or activities to increase the capacity of a muscle to do work in terms of strength, power, and/or endurance **Explanation:** Muscle strength is the force exerted to overcome resistance in one maximal effort. Muscle power is work produced per unit of time, or the product of strength and speed. Muscle endurance is the ability to contract a muscle repeatedly over time
Neuromotor Development	**Definition:** Measures motor development, righting and equilibrium reactions, and reflex and equilibrium reactions
Non-invasive Instrumental Status	**Definition:** Instrumental measures of oral, nasal, vocal, and velopharyngeal functions as they pertain to speech production
Nonspoken Language (Assessment)	**Definition:** Measures nonspoken language (print, sign, symbols) for communication
Nonspoken Language (Treatment)	**Definition:** Applying techniques that improve, augment, or compensate spoken communication
Oral Peripheral Mechanism	**Definition:** Structural measures of face, jaw, lips, tongue, teeth, hard and soft palate, pharynx as related to speech production
Orofacial Myofunctional (Assessment)	**Definition:** Measures orofacial myofunctional patterns for speech and related functions
Orofacial Myofunctional (Treatment)	**Definition:** Applying techniques to improve, alter, or augment impaired orofacial myofunctional patterns and related speech production errors
Oscillating Tracking	**Definition:** Measures ability to visually track
Pain	**Definition:** Measures muscle soreness, pain and soreness with joint movement, and pain perception **Includes/Examples:** Includes questionnaires, graphs, symptom magnification scales or visual analog scales
Perceptual Processing (Assessment)	**Definition:** Measures stereognosis, kinesthesia, body schema, right-left discrimination, form constancy, position in space, visual closure, figure-ground, depth perception, spatial relations and topographical orientation
Perceptual Processing (Treatment)	**Definition:** Exercise and activities to facilitate perceptual processing **Explanation:** Includes stereognosis, kinesthesia, body schema, right-left discrimination, form constancy, position in space, visual closure, figure-ground, depth perception, spatial relations, and topographical orientation **Includes/Examples:** Includes stereognosis, kinesthesia, body schema, right-left discrimination, form constancy, position in space, visual closure, figure-ground, depth perception, spatial relations, and topographical orientation
Performance Intensity Phonetically Balanced Speech Discrimination	**Definition:** Measures word recognition over varying intensity levels
Postural Control	**Definition:** Exercise or activities to increase postural alignment and control
Prosthesis	**Definition:** Artificial substitutes for missing body parts that augment performance or function **Includes/Examples:** Limb prosthesis, ocular prosthesis
Psychosocial Skills (Assessment)	**Definition:** The ability to interact in society and to process emotions **Includes/Examples:** Includes psychological (values, interests, self-concept); social (role performance, social conduct, interpersonal skills, self expression); self-management (coping skills, time management, self-control)
Psychosocial Skills (Treatment)	**Definition:** The ability to interact in society and to process emotions **Includes/Examples:** Includes psychological (values, interests, self-concept); social (role performance, social conduct, interpersonal skills, self expression); self-management (coping skills, time management, self-control)
Pure Tone Audiometry, Air	**Definition:** Air-conduction pure tone threshold measures with appropriate masking
Pure Tone Audiometry, Air and Bone	**Definition:** Air-conduction and bone-conduction pure tone threshold measures with appropriate masking
Pure Tone Stenger	**Definition:** Measures unilateral nonorganic hearing loss based on simultaneous presentation of pure tones of differing volume
Range of Motion and Joint Integrity	**Definition:** Measures quantity, quality, grade, and classification of joint movement and/or mobility **Explanation:** Range of Motion is the space, distance or angle through which movement occurs at a joint or series of joints. Joint integrity is the conformance of joints to expected anatomic, biomechanical and kinematic norms
Range of Motion and Joint Mobility	**Definition:** Exercise or activities to increase muscle length and joint mobility
Receptive/Expressive Language (Assessment)	**Definition:** Measures receptive and expressive language
Receptive/Expressive Language (Treatment)	**Definition:** Applying techniques to improve and augment receptive/expressive language

Continued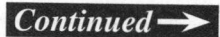

Section F - Physical Rehabilitation and Diagnostic Audiology — Character 5 - Type Qualifier

Reflex Integrity	**Definition:** Measures the presence, absence, or exaggeration of developmentally appropriate, pathologic or normal reflexes
Select Picture Audiometry	**Definition:** Establishes hearing threshold levels for speech using pictures
Sensorineural Acuity Level	**Definition:** Measures sensorineural acuity masking presented via bone conduction
Sensory Aids	**Definition:** Determines the appropriateness of a sensory prosthetic device, other than a hearing aid or assistive listening system/device
Sensory Awareness/Processing/Integrity	**Includes/Examples:** Includes light touch, pressure, temperature, pain, sharp/dull, proprioception, vestibular, visual, auditory, gustatory, and olfactory
Short Increment Sensitivity Index	**Definition:** Measures the ear's ability to detect small intensity changes; site of lesion test requiring a behavioral response
Sinusoidal Vertical Axis Rotational	**Definition:** Measures nystagmus following rotation
Somatosensory Evoked Potentials	**Definition:** Measures neural activity from sites throughout the body
Speech and/or Language Screening	**Definition:** Identifies need for further speech and/or language evaluation
Speech Threshold	**Definition:** Measures minimal intensity needed to repeat spondaic words
Speech-Language Pathology and Related Disorders Counseling	**Definition:** Provides patients/families with information, support, referrals to facilitate recovery from a communication disorder
Speech-Language Pathology and Related Disorders Prevention	**Definition:** Applying techniques to avoid or minimize onset and/or development of a communication disorder
Speech/Word Recognition	**Definition:** Measures ability to repeat/identify single syllable words; scores given as a percentage; includes word recognition/speech discrimination
Staggered Spondaic Word	**Definition:** Measures central auditory processing site of lesion based upon dichotic presentation of spondaic words
Static Orthosis	**Includes/Examples:** Includes customized and prefabricated splints, inhibitory casts, spinal and other braces, and protective devices; has no moving parts, maintains joint(s) in desired position
Stenger	**Definition:** Measures unilateral nonorganic hearing loss based on simultaneous presentation of signals of differing volume
Swallowing Dysfunction	**Definition:** Activities to improve swallowing function in coordination with respiratory function **Includes/Examples:** Includes function and coordination of sucking, mastication, coughing, swallowing
Synthetic Sentence Identification	**Definition:** Measures central auditory dysfunction using identification of third order approximations of sentences and competing messages
Temporal Ordering of Stimuli	**Definition:** Measures specific central auditory process
Therapeutic Exercise	**Definition:** Exercise or activities to facilitate sensory awareness, sensory processing, sensory integration, balance training, conditioning, reconditioning **Includes/Examples:** Includes developmental activities, breathing exercises, aerobic endurance activities, aquatic exercises, stretching and ventilatory muscle training
Tinnitus Masker (Assessment)	**Definition:** Determines candidacy for tinnitus masker
Tinnitus Masker (Treatment)	**Explanation:** Used to verify physical fit, acoustic appropriateness, and benefit; assists in achieving maximum benefit
Tone Decay	**Definition:** Measures decrease in hearing sensitivity to a tone; site of lesion test requiring a behavioral response
Transfer	**Definition:** Transitional movement from one surface to another
Transfer Training	**Definition:** Exercise or activities to facilitate movement from one surface to another
Tympanometry	**Definition:** Measures the integrity of the middle ear; measures ease at which sound flows through the tympanic membrane while air pressure against the membrane is varied
Unithermal Binaural Screen	**Definition:** Measures the rhythmic eye movements stimulated by changing the temperature of the vestibular system in both ears using warm water, screening format
Ventilation, Respiration and Circulation	**Definition:** Measures ventilatory muscle strength, power and endurance, pulmonary function and ventilatory mechanics **Includes/Examples:** Includes ability to clear airway, activities that aggravate or relieve edema, pain, dyspnea or other symptoms, chest wall mobility, cardiopulmonary response to performance of ADL and IAD, cough and sputum, standard vital signs
Vestibular	**Definition:** Applying techniques to compensate for balance disorders; includes habituation, exercise therapy, and balance retraining

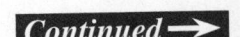

Appendix B

Section F - Physical Rehabilitation and Diagnostic Audiology — Character 5 - Type Qualifier

Visual Motor Integration (Assessment)	**Definition:** Coordinating the interaction of information from the eyes with body movement during activity
Visual Motor Integration (Treatment)	**Definition:** Exercise or activities to facilitate coordinating the interaction of information from eyes with body movement during activity
Visual Reinforcement Audiometry	**Definition:** Behavioral measures using nonspeech and speech stimuli to obtain frequency/ear-specific information on auditory status **Includes/Examples:** Includes a conditioned response of looking toward a visual reinforcer (e.g., lights, animated toy) every time auditory stimuli are heard
Vocational Activities and Functional Community or Work Reintegration Skills (Assessment)	**Definition:** Measures environmental, home, work (job/school/play) barriers that keep patients from functioning optimally in their environment **Includes/Examples:** Includes assessment of vocational skill and interests, environment of work (job/school/play), injury potential and injury prevention or reduction, ergonomic stressors, transportation skills, and ability to access and use community resources
Vocational Activities and Functional Community or Work Reintegration Skills (Treatment)	**Definition:** Activities to facilitate vocational exploration, body mechanics training, job acquisition, and environmental or work (job/school/play) task adaptation **Includes/Examples:** Includes injury prevention and reduction, ergonomic stressor reduction, job coaching and simulation, work hardening and conditioning, driving training, transportation skills, and use of community resources
Voice (Assessment)	**Definition:** Measures vocal structure, function and production
Voice (Treatment)	**Definition:** Applying techniques to improve voice and vocal function
Voice Prosthetic (Assessment)	**Definition:** Determines the appropriateness of voice prosthetic/adaptive device to enhance or facilitate communication
Voice Prosthetic (Treatment)	**Includes/Examples:** Includes electrolarynx, and other assistive, adaptive, supportive devices
Wheelchair Mobility (Assessment)	**Definition:** Measures fit and functional abilities within wheelchair in a variety of environments
Wheelchair Mobility (Treatment)	**Definition:** Management, maintenance and controlled operation of a wheelchair, scooter or other device, in and on a variety of surfaces and environments
Wound Management	**Includes/Examples:** Includes non-selective and selective debridement (enzymes, autolysis, sharp debridement), dressings (wound coverings, hydrogel, vacuum-assisted closure), topical agents, etc.

Section G - Mental Health — Character 3 - Root Type

Biofeedback	**Definition:** Provision of information from the monitoring and regulating of physiological processes in conjunction with cognitive-behavioral techniques to improve patient functioning or well-being **Includes/Examples:** Includes EEG, blood pressure, skin temperature or peripheral blood flow, ECG, electrooculogram, EMG, respirometry or capnometry, GSR/EDR, perineometry to monitor/regulate bowel/bladder activity, electrogastrogram to monitor/regulate gastric motility
Counseling	**Definition:** The application of psychological methods to treat an individual with normal developmental issues and psychological problems in order to increase function, improve well-being, alleviate distress, maladjustment or resolve crises
Crisis Intervention	**Definition:** Treatment of a traumatized, acutely disturbed or distressed individual for the purpose of short-term stabilization **Includes/Examples:** Includes defusing, debriefing, counseling, psychotherapy and/or coordination of care with other providers or agencies
Electroconvulsive Therapy	**Definition:** The application of controlled electrical voltages to treat a mental health disorder **Includes/Examples:** Includes appropriate sedation and other preparation of the individual
Family Psychotherapy	**Definition:** Treatment that includes one or more family members of an individual with a mental health disorder by behavioral, cognitive, psychoanalytic, psychodynamic or psychophysiological means to improve functioning or well-being **Explanation:** Remediation of emotional or behavioral problems presented by one or more family members in cases where psychotherapy with more than one family member is indicated
Group Psychotherapy	**Definition:** Treatment of two or more individuals with a mental health disorder by behavioral, cognitive, psychoanalytic, psychodynamic or psychophysiological means to improve functioning or well-being
Hypnosis	**Definition:** Induction of a state of heightened suggestibility by auditory, visual and tactile techniques to elicit an emotional or behavioral response
Individual Psychotherapy	**Definition:** Treatment of an individual with a mental health disorder by behavioral, cognitive, psychoanalytic, psychodynamic or psychophysiological means to improve functioning or well-being
Light Therapy	**Definition:** Application of specialized light treatments to improve functioning or well-being

Continued →

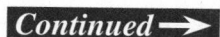

Section G - Mental Health — Character 3 - Root Type

Medication Management	**Definition:** Monitoring and adjusting the use of medications for the treatment of a mental health disorder
Narcosynthesis	**Definition:** Administration of intravenous barbiturates in order to release suppressed or repressed thoughts
Psychological Tests	**Definition:** The administration and interpretation of standardized psychological tests and measurement instruments for the assessment of psychological function

Section G - Mental Health — Character 4 - Type Qualifier

Behavioral	**Definition:** Primarily to modify behavior **Includes/Examples:** Includes modeling and role playing, positive reinforcement of target behaviors, response cost, and training of self-management skills
Cognitive	**Definition:** Primarily to correct cognitive distortions and errors
Cognitive-Behavioral	**Definition:** Combining cognitive and behavioral treatment strategies to improve functioning **Explanation:** Maladaptive responses are examined to determine how cognitions relate to behavior patterns in response to an event. Uses learning principles and information-processing models
Developmental	**Definition:** Age-normed developmental status of cognitive, social and adaptive behavior skills
Intellectual and Psychoeducational	**Definition:** Intellectual abilities, academic achievement and learning capabilities (including behaviors and emotional factors affecting learning)
Interactive	**Definition:** Uses primarily physical aids and other forms of non-oral interaction with a patient who is physically, psychologically or developmentally unable to use ordinary language for communication **Includes/Examples:** Includes the use of toys in symbolic play
Interpersonal	**Definition:** Helps an individual make changes in interpersonal behaviors to reduce psychological dysfunction **Includes/Examples:** Includes exploratory techniques, encouragement of affective expression, clarification of patient statements, analysis of communication patterns, use of therapy relationship and behavior change techniques
Neurobehavioral and Cognitive Status	**Definition:** Includes neurobehavioral status exam, interview(s), and observation for the clinical assessment of thinking, reasoning and judgment, acquired knowledge, attention, memory, visual spatial abilities, language functions, and planning
Neuropsychological	**Definition:** Thinking, reasoning and judgment, acquired knowledge, attention, memory, visual spatial abilities, language functions, planning
Personality and Behavioral	**Definition:** Mood, emotion, behavior, social functioning, psychopathological conditions, personality traits and characteristics
Psychoanalysis	**Definition:** Methods of obtaining a detailed account of past and present mental and emotional experiences to determine the source and eliminate or diminish the undesirable effects of unconscious conflicts **Explanation:** Accomplished by making the individual aware of their existence, origin, and inappropriate expression in emotions and behavior
Psychodynamic	**Definition:** Exploration of past and present emotional experiences to understand motives and drives using insight-oriented techniques to reduce the undesirable effects of internal conflicts on emotions and behavior **Explanation:** Techniques include empathetic listening, clarifying self-defeating behavior patterns, and exploring adaptive alternatives
Psychophysiological	**Definition:** Monitoring and alteration of physiological processes to help the individual associate physiological reactions combined with cognitive and behavioral strategies to gain improved control of these processes to help the individual cope more effectively
Supportive	**Definition:** Formation of therapeutic relationship primarily for providing emotional support to prevent further deterioration in functioning during periods of particular stress **Explanation:** Often used in conjunction with other therapeutic approaches
Vocational	**Definition:** Exploration of vocational interests, aptitudes and required adaptive behavior skills to develop and carry out a plan for achieving a successful vocational placement **Includes/Examples:** Includes enhancing work related adjustment and/or pursuing viable options in training education or preparation

Section H - Substance Abuse Treatment — Character 3 - Root Type

Detoxification Services	**Definition:** Detoxification from alcohol and/or drugs **Explanation:** Not a treatment modality, but helps the patient stabilize physically and psychologically until the body becomes free of drugs and the effects of alcohol
Family Counseling	**Definition:** The application of psychological methods that includes one or more family members to treat an individual with addictive behavior **Explanation:** Provides support and education for family members of addicted individuals. Family member participation is seen as a critical area of substance abuse treatment

Continued →

Section H - Substance Abuse Treatment — Character 3 - Root Type

Group Counseling	**Definition:** The application of psychological methods to treat two or more individuals with addictive behavior **Explanation:** Provides structured group counseling sessions and healing power through the connection with others
Individual Counseling	**Definition:** The application of psychological methods to treat an individual with addictive behavior **Explanation:** Comprised of several different techniques, which apply various strategies to address drug addiction
Individual Psychotherapy	**Definition:** Treatment of an individual with addictive behavior by behavioral, cognitive, psychoanalytic, psychodynamic or psychophysiological means
Medication Management	**Definition:** Monitoring and adjusting the use of replacement medications for the treatment of addiction
Pharmacotherapy	**Definition:** The use of replacement medications for the treatment of addiction

Appendix C: Approach Definitions

Section 0 - Medical and Surgical — Character 5 - Approach

External (X)	**Definition:** Procedures performed directly on the skin or mucous membrane and procedures performed indirectly by the application of external force through the skin or mucous membrane
Open (0)	**Definition:** Cutting through the skin or mucous membrane and any other body layers necessary to expose the site of the procedure
Percutaneous (3)	**Definition:** Entry, by puncture or minor incision, of instrumentation through the skin or mucous membrane and any other body layers necessary to reach the site of the procedure
Percutaneous Endoscopic (4)	**Definition:** Entry, by puncture or minor incision, of instrumentation through the skin or mucous membrane and any other body layers necessary to reach and visualize the site of the procedure
Via Natural or Artificial Opening (7)	**Definition:** Entry of instrumentation through a natural or artificial external opening to reach the site of the procedure
Via Natural or Artificial Opening Endoscopic (8)	**Definition:** Entry of instrumentation through a natural or artificial external opening to reach and visualize the site of the procedure
Via Natural or Artificial Opening With Percutaneous Endoscopic Assistance (F)	**Definition:** Entry of instrumentation through a natural or artificial external opening and entry, by puncture or minor incision, of instrumentation through the skin or mucous membrane and any other body layers necessary to aid in the performance of the procedure

Section 1 - Obstetrics — Character 5 - Approach

External (X)	**Definition:** Procedures performed directly on the skin or mucous membrane and procedures performed indirectly by the application of external force through the skin or mucous membrane
Open (0)	**Definition:** Cutting through the skin or mucous membrane and any other body layers necessary to expose the site of the procedure
Percutaneous (3)	**Definition:** Entry, by puncture or minor incision, of instrumentation through the skin or mucous membrane and any other body layers necessary to reach the site of the procedure
Percutaneous Endoscopic (4)	**Definition:** Entry, by puncture or minor incision, of instrumentation through the skin or mucous membrane and any other body layers necessary to reach and visualize the site of the procedure
Via Natural or Artificial Opening (7)	**Definition:** Entry of instrumentation through a natural or artificial external opening to reach the site of the procedure
Via Natural or Artificial Opening Endoscopic (8)	**Definition:** Entry of instrumentation through a natural or artificial external opening to reach and visualize the site of the procedure

Section 2 - Placement — Character 5 - Approach

External (X)	**Definition:** Procedures performed directly on the skin or mucous membrane and procedures performed indirectly by the application of external force through the skin or mucous membrane

Section 3 - Administration — Character 5 - Approach

External (X)	**Definition:** Procedures performed directly on the skin or mucous membrane and procedures performed indirectly by the application of external force through the skin or mucous membrane
Open (0)	**Definition:** Cutting through the skin or mucous membrane and any other body layers necessary to expose the site of the procedure

Continued →

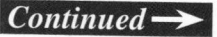

Section 3 - Administration — Character 5 - Approach

Percutaneous (3)	**Definition:** Entry, by puncture or minor incision, of instrumentation through the skin or mucous membrane and any other body layers necessary to reach the site of the procedure
Percutaneous Endoscopic (4)	**Definition:** Entry, by puncture or minor incision, of instrumentation through the skin or mucous membrane and any other body layers necessary to reach and visualize the site of the procedure
Via Natural or Artificial Opening (7)	**Definition:** Entry of instrumentation through a natural or artificial external opening to reach the site of the procedure
Via Natural or Artificial Opening Endoscopic (8)	**Definition:** Entry of instrumentation through a natural or artificial external opening to reach and visualize the site of the procedure

Section 4 - Measurement and Monitoring — Character 5 - Approach

External (X)	**Definition:** Procedures performed directly on the skin or mucous membrane and procedures performed indirectly by the application of external force through the skin or mucous membrane
Open (0)	**Definition:** Cutting through the skin or mucous membrane and any other body layers necessary to expose the site of the procedure
Percutaneous (3)	**Definition:** Entry, by puncture or minor incision, of instrumentation through the skin or mucous membrane and any other body layers necessary to reach the site of the procedure
Percutaneous Endoscopic (4)	**Definition:** Entry, by puncture or minor incision, of instrumentation through the skin or mucous membrane and any other body layers necessary to reach and visualize the site of the procedure
Via Natural or Artificial Opening (7)	**Definition:** Entry of instrumentation through a natural or artificial external opening to reach the site of the procedure
Via Natural or Artificial Opening Endoscopic (8)	**Definition:** Entry of instrumentation through a natural or artificial external opening to reach and visualize the site of the procedure

Section 7 - Osteopathic — Character 5 - Approach

External (X)	**Definition:** Procedures performed directly on the skin or mucous membrane and procedures performed indirectly by the application of external force through the skin or mucous membrane

Section 8 - Other Procedures — Character 5 - Approach

External (X)	**Definition:** Procedures performed directly on the skin or mucous membrane and procedures performed indirectly by the application of external force through the skin or mucous membrane
Open (0)	**Definition:** Cutting through the skin or mucous membrane and any other body layers necessary to expose the site of the procedure
Percutaneous (3)	**Definition:** Entry, by puncture or minor incision, of instrumentation through the skin or mucous membrane and any other body layers necessary to reach the site of the procedure
Percutaneous Endoscopic (4)	**Definition:** Entry, by puncture or minor incision, of instrumentation through the skin or mucous membrane and any other body layers necessary to reach and visualize the site of the procedure
Via Natural or Artificial Opening (7)	**Definition:** Entry of instrumentation through a natural or artificial external opening to reach the site of the procedure
Via Natural or Artificial Opening Endoscopic (8)	**Definition:** Entry of instrumentation through a natural or artificial external opening to reach and visualize the site of the procedure

Section 9 - Chiropractic — Character 5 - Approach

External (X)	**Definition:** Procedures performed directly on the skin or mucous membrane and procedures performed indirectly by the application of external force through the skin or mucous membrane

Section X - New Technology — Character 5 - Approach

External (X)	**Definition:** Procedures performed directly on the skin or mucous membrane and procedures performed indirectly by the application of external force through the skin or mucous membrane
Open (0)	**Definition:** Cutting through the skin or mucous membrane and any other body layers necessary to expose the site of the procedure
Percutaneous (3)	**Definition:** Entry, by puncture or minor incision, of instrumentation through the skin or mucous membrane and any other body layers necessary to reach the site of the procedure
Percutaneous Endoscopic (4)	**Definition:** Entry, by puncture or minor incision, of instrumentation through the skin or mucous membrane and any other body layers necessary to reach and visualize the site of the procedure
Via Natural or Artificial Opening (7)	**Definition:** Entry of instrumentation through a natural or artificial external opening to reach the site of the procedure
Via Natural or Artificial Opening Endoscopic (8)	**Definition:** Entry of instrumentation through a natural or artificial external opening to reach and visualize the site of the procedure

Appendix D: Medical and Surgical Body Parts

Appendices D–F are structured to assist coders with confirming character selections within the Tables. For example, if the coder is considering the body part of Abdomen Muscle, appendix D can be referenced to identify all of the muscles that are included in the body part Abdomen Muscle (see row 2 in the table below). After reviewing the information, the coder can determine if the body part under consideration is correct or if another body part should be reviewed. The same process can be followed for devices which are included in appendix E and substances which are included in appendix F.

Section 0 - Medical and Surgical — Character 4 - Body Part

Body Part	Includes
1st Toe, Left **1st** Toe, Right	**Includes:** Hallux
Abdomen Muscle, Left **Abdomen** Muscle, Right	**Includes:** External oblique muscle Internal oblique muscle Pyramidalis muscle Rectus abdominis muscle Transversus abdominis muscle
Abdominal Aorta	**Includes:** Inferior phrenic artery Lumbar artery Median sacral artery Middle suprarenal artery Ovarian artery Testicular artery
Abdominal Sympathetic Nerve	**Includes:** Abdominal aortic plexus Auerbach's (myenteric) plexus Celiac (solar) plexus Celiac ganglion Gastric plexus Hepatic plexus Inferior hypogastric plexus Inferior mesenteric ganglion Inferior mesenteric plexus Meissner's (submucous) plexus Myenteric (Auerbach's) plexus Pancreatic plexus Pelvic splanchnic nerve Renal nerve Renal plexus Solar (celiac) plexus Splenic plexus Submucous (Meissner's) plexus Superior hypogastric plexus Superior mesenteric ganglion Superior mesenteric plexus Suprarenal plexus
Abducens Nerve	**Includes:** Sixth cranial nerve
Accessory Nerve	**Includes:** Eleventh cranial nerve
Acoustic Nerve	**Includes:** Cochlear nerve Eighth cranial nerve Scarpa's (vestibular) ganglion Spiral ganglion Vestibular (Scarpa's) ganglion Vestibular nerve Vestibulocochlear nerve
Adenoids	**Includes:** Pharyngeal tonsil

Section 0 - Medical and Surgical — Character 4 - Body Part

Body Part	Includes
Adrenal Gland **Adrenal** Gland, Left **Adrenal** Gland, Right **Adrenal** Glands, Bilateral	**Includes:** Suprarenal gland
Ampulla of Vater	**Includes:** Duodenal ampulla Hepatopancreatic ampulla
Anal Sphincter	**Includes:** External anal sphincter Internal anal sphincter
Ankle Bursa and Ligament, Left **Ankle** Bursa and Ligament, Right	**Includes:** Calcaneofibular ligament Deltoid ligament Ligament of the lateral malleolus Talofibular ligament
Ankle Joint, Left **Ankle** Joint, Right	**Includes:** Inferior tibiofibular joint Talocrural joint
Anterior Chamber, Left **Anterior** Chamber, Right	**Includes:** Aqueous humour
Anterior Tibial Artery, Left **Anterior** Tibial Artery, Right	**Includes:** Anterior lateral malleolar artery Anterior medial malleolar artery Anterior tibial recurrent artery Dorsalis pedis artery Posterior tibial recurrent artery
Anus	**Includes:** Anal orifice
Aortic Valve	**Includes:** Aortic annulus
Appendix	**Includes:** Vermiform appendix
Atrial Septum	**Includes:** Interatrial septum
Atrium, Left	**Includes:** Atrium pulmonale Left auricular appendix
Atrium, Right	**Includes:** Atrium dextrum cordis Right auricular appendix Sinus venosus
Auditory Ossicle, Left **Auditory** Ossicle, Right	**Includes:** Incus Malleus Stapes

Continued →

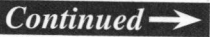

Axillary Artery, Left **Axillary** Artery, Right	**Includes:** Anterior circumflex humeral artery Lateral thoracic artery Posterior circumflex humeral artery Subscapular artery Superior thoracic artery Thoracoacromial artery
Azygos Vein	**Includes:** Right ascending lumbar vein Right subcostal vein
Basal Ganglia	**Includes:** Basal nuclei Claustrum Corpus striatum Globus pallidus Substantia nigra Subthalamic nucleus
Basilic Vein, Left **Basilic** Vein, Right	**Includes:** Median antebrachial vein Median cubital vein
Bladder	**Includes:** Trigone of bladder
Brachial Artery, Left **Brachial** Artery, Right	**Includes:** Inferior ulnar collateral artery Profunda brachii Superior ulnar collateral artery
Brachial Plexus	**Includes:** Axillary nerve Dorsal scapular nerve First intercostal nerve Long thoracic nerve Musculocutaneous nerve Subclavius nerve Suprascapular nerve
Brachial Vein, Left **Brachial** Vein, Right	**Includes:** Radial vein Ulnar vein
Brain	**Includes:** Cerebrum Corpus callosum Encephalon
Breast, Bilateral **Breast,** Left **Breast,** Right	**Includes:** Mammary duct Mammary gland
Buccal Mucosa	**Includes:** Buccal gland Molar gland Palatine gland
Carotid Bodies, Bilateral **Carotid** Body, Left **Carotid** Body, Right	**Includes:** Carotid glomus
Carpal Joint, Left **Carpal** Joint, Right	**Includes:** Intercarpal joint Midcarpal joint

Carpal, Left **Carpal,** Right	**Includes:** Capitate bone Hamate bone Lunate bone Pisiform bone Scaphoid bone Trapezium bone Trapezoid bone Triquetral bone
Celiac Artery	**Includes:** Celiac trunk
Cephalic Vein, Left **Cephalic** Vein, Right	**Includes:** Accessory cephalic vein
Cerebellum	**Includes:** Culmen
Cerebral Hemisphere	**Includes:** Frontal lobe Occipital lobe Parietal lobe Temporal lobe
Cerebral Meninges	**Includes:** Arachnoid mater, intracranial Leptomeninges, intracranial Pia mater, intracranial
Cerebral Ventricle	**Includes:** Aqueduct of Sylvius Cerebral aqueduct (Sylvius) Choroid plexus Ependyma Foramen of Monro (intraventricular) Fourth ventricle Interventricular foramen (Monro) Left lateral ventricle Right lateral ventricle Third ventricle
Cervical Nerve	**Includes:** Greater occipital nerve Spinal nerve, cervical Suboccipital nerve Third occipital nerve
Cervical Plexus	**Includes:** Ansa cervicalis Cutaneous (transverse) cervical nerve Great auricular nerve Lesser occipital nerve Supraclavicular nerve Transverse (cutaneous) cervical nerve
Cervical Spinal Cord	**Includes:** Dorsal root ganglion
Cervical Vertebra	**Includes:** Dens Odontoid process Spinous process Transverse foramen Transverse process Vertebral arch Vertebral body Vertebral foramen Vertebral lamina Vertebral pedicle

Continued →

Cervical Vertebral Joint	**Includes:** Atlantoaxial joint Cervical facet joint
Cervical Vertebral Joints, 2 or more	**Includes:** Cervical facet joint
Cervicothoracic Vertebral Joint	**Includes:** Cervicothoracic facet joint
Cisterna Chyli	**Includes:** Intestinal lymphatic trunk Lumbar lymphatic trunk
Coccygeal Glomus	**Includes:** Coccygeal body
Colic Vein	**Includes:** Ileocolic vein Left colic vein Middle colic vein Right colic vein
Conduction Mechanism	**Includes:** Atrioventricular node Bundle of His Bundle of Kent Sinoatrial node
Conjunctiva, Left **Conjunctiva,** Right	**Includes:** Plica semilunaris
Dura Mater	**Includes:** Diaphragma sellae Dura mater, intracranial Falx cerebri Tentorium cerebelli
Elbow Bursa and Ligament, Left **Elbow** Bursa and Ligament, Right	**Includes:** Annular ligament Olecranon bursa Radial collateral ligament Ulnar collateral ligament
Elbow Joint, Left **Elbow** Joint, Right	**Includes:** Distal humerus, involving joint Humeroradial joint Humeroulnar joint Proximal radioulnar joint
Epidural Space, Intracranial	**Includes:** Extradural space, intracranial
Epiglottis	**Includes:** Glossoepiglottic fold
Esophagogastric Junction	**Includes:** Cardia Cardioesophageal junction Gastroesophageal (GE) junction
Esophagus, Lower	**Includes:** Abdominal esophagus
Esophagus, Middle	**Includes:** Thoracic esophagus
Esophagus, Upper	**Includes:** Cervical esophagus
Ethmoid Bone, Left **Ethmoid** Bone, Right	**Includes:** Cribriform plate
Ethmoid Sinus, Left **Ethmoid** Sinus, Right	**Includes:** Ethmoidal air cell

Eustachian Tube, Left **Eustachian** Tube, Right	**Includes:** Auditory tube Pharyngotympanic tube
External Auditory Canal, Left **External** Auditory Canal, Right	**Includes:** External auditory meatus
External Carotid Artery, Left **External** Carotid Artery, Right	**Includes:** Ascending pharyngeal artery Internal maxillary artery Lingual artery Maxillary artery Occipital artery Posterior auricular artery Superior thyroid artery
External Ear, Bilateral **External** Ear, Left **External** Ear, Right	**Includes:** Antihelix Antitragus Auricle Earlobe Helix Pinna Tragus
External Iliac Artery, Left **External** Iliac Artery, Right	**Includes:** Deep circumflex iliac artery Inferior epigastric artery
External Jugular Vein, Left **External** Jugular Vein, Right	**Includes:** Posterior auricular vein
Extraocular Muscle, Left **Extraocular** Muscle, Right	**Includes:** Inferior oblique muscle Inferior rectus muscle Lateral rectus muscle Medial rectus muscle Superior oblique muscle Superior rectus muscle
Eye, Left **Eye,** Right	**Includes:** Ciliary body Posterior chamber
Face Artery	**Includes:** Angular artery Ascending palatine artery External maxillary artery Facial artery Inferior labial artery Submental artery Superior labial artery
Face Vein, Left **Face** Vein, Right	**Includes:** Angular vein Anterior facial vein Common facial vein Deep facial vein Frontal vein Posterior facial (retromandibular) vein Supraorbital vein
Facial Muscle	**Includes:** Buccinator muscle Corrugator supercilii muscle Depressor anguli oris muscle Depressor labii inferioris muscle

Continued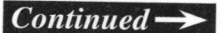

	Depressor septi nasi muscle Depressor supercilii muscle Levator anguli oris muscle Levator labii superioris alaeque nasi Levator labii superioris alaeque nasi Levator labii superioris alaeque nasi Levator labii superioris muscle Mentalis muscle Nasalis muscle Occipitofrontalis muscle Orbicularis oris muscle Procerus muscle Risorius muscle Zygomaticus muscle
Facial Nerve	**Includes:** Chorda tympani Geniculate ganglion Greater superficial petrosal nerve Nerve to the stapedius Parotid plexus Posterior auricular nerve Seventh cranial nerve Submandibular ganglion
Fallopian Tube, Left **Fallopian** Tube, Right	**Includes:** Oviduct Salpinx Uterine tube
Femoral Artery, Left **Femoral** Artery, Right	**Includes:** Circumflex iliac artery Deep femoral artery Descending genicular artery External pudendal artery Superficial epigastric artery
Femoral Nerve	**Includes:** Anterior crural nerve Saphenous nerve
Femoral Shaft, Left **Femoral** Shaft, Right	**Includes:** Body of femur
Femoral Vein, Left **Femoral** Vein, Right	**Includes:** Deep femoral (profunda femoris) vein Popliteal vein Profunda femoris (deep femoral) vein
Fibula, Left **Fibula,** Right	**Includes:** Body of fibula Head of fibula Lateral malleolus
Finger Nail	**Includes:** Nail bed Nail plate
Finger Phalangeal Joint, Left **Finger** Phalangeal Joint, Right	**Includes:** Interphalangeal (IP) joint
Foot Artery, Left **Foot** Artery, Right	**Includes:** Arcuate artery Dorsal metatarsal artery Lateral plantar artery Lateral tarsal artery Medial plantar artery

Foot Bursa and Ligament, Left **Foot** Bursa and Ligament, Right	**Includes:** Calcaneocuboid ligament Cuneonavicular ligament Intercuneiform ligament Interphalangeal ligament Metatarsal ligament Metatarsophalangeal ligament Subtalar ligament Talocalcaneal ligament Talocalcaneonavicular ligament Tarsometatarsal ligament
Foot Muscle, Left **Foot** Muscle, Right	**Includes:** Abductor hallucis muscle Adductor hallucis muscle Extensor digitorum brevis muscle Extensor hallucis brevis muscle Flexor digitorum brevis muscle Flexor hallucis brevis muscle Quadratus plantae muscle
Foot Vein, Left **Foot** Vein, Right	**Includes:** Common digital vein Dorsal metatarsal vein Dorsal venous arch Plantar digital vein Plantar metatarsal vein Plantar venous arch
Frontal Bone	**Includes:** Zygomatic process of frontal bone
Gastric Artery	**Includes:** Left gastric artery Right gastric artery
Glenoid Cavity, Left **Glenoid** Cavity, Right	**Includes:** Glenoid fossa (of scapula)
Glomus Jugulare	**Includes:** Jugular body
Glossopharyngeal Nerve	**Includes:** Carotid sinus nerve Ninth cranial nerve Tympanic nerve
Hand Artery, Left **Hand** Artery, Right	**Includes:** Deep palmar arch Princeps pollicis artery Radialis indicis Superficial palmar arch
Hand Bursa and Ligament, Left **Hand** Bursa and Ligament, Right	**Includes:** Carpometacarpal ligament Intercarpal ligament Interphalangeal ligament Lunotriquetral ligament Metacarpal ligament Metacarpophalangeal ligament Pisohamate ligament Pisometacarpal ligament Scaphotrapezium ligament
Hand Muscle, Left **Hand** Muscle, Right	**Includes:** Hypothenar muscle Palmar interosseous muscle Thenar muscle

Continued →

Hand Vein, Left **Hand** Vein, Right	**Includes:** Dorsal metacarpal vein Palmar (volar) digital vein Palmar (volar) metacarpal vein Superficial palmar venous arch Volar (palmar) digital vein Volar (palmar) metacarpal vein
Head and Neck Bursa and Ligament	**Includes:** Alar ligament of axis Cervical interspinous ligament Cervical intertransverse ligament Cervical ligamentum flavum Interspinous ligament, cervical Intertransverse ligament, cervical Lateral temporomandibular ligament Ligamentum flavum, cervical Sphenomandibular ligament Stylomandibular ligament Transverse ligament of atlas
Head and Neck Sympathetic Nerve	**Includes:** Cavernous plexus Cervical ganglion Ciliary ganglion Internal carotid plexus Otic ganglion Pterygopalatine (sphenopalatine) ganglion Sphenopalatine (pterygopalatine) ganglion Stellate ganglion Submandibular ganglion Submaxillary ganglion
Head Muscle	**Includes:** Auricularis muscle Masseter muscle Pterygoid muscle Splenius capitis muscle Temporalis muscle Temporoparietalis muscle
Heart, Left	**Includes:** Left coronary sulcus Obtuse margin
Heart, Right	**Includes:** Right coronary sulcus
Hemiazygos Vein	**Includes:** Left ascending lumbar vein Left subcostal vein
Hepatic Artery	**Includes:** Common hepatic artery Gastroduodenal artery Hepatic artery proper
Hip Bursa and Ligament, Left **Hip** Bursa and Ligament, Right	**Includes:** Iliofemoral ligament Ischiofemoral ligament Pubofemoral ligament Transverse acetabular ligament Trochanteric bursa
Hip Joint, Left **Hip** Joint, Right	**Includes:** Acetabulofemoral joint

Hip Muscle, Left **Hip** Muscle, Right	**Includes:** Gemellus muscle Gluteus maximus muscle Gluteus medius muscle Gluteus minimus muscle Iliacus muscle Obturator muscle Piriformis muscle Psoas muscle Quadratus femoris muscle Tensor fasciae latae muscle
Humeral Head, Left **Humeral** Head, Right	**Includes:** Greater tuberosity Lesser tuberosity Neck of humerus (anatomical) (surgical)
Humeral Shaft, Left **Humeral** Shaft, Right	**Includes:** Distal humerus Humerus, distal Lateral epicondyle of humerus Medial epicondyle of humerus
Hypogastric Vein, Left **Hypogastric** Vein, Right	**Includes:** Gluteal vein Internal iliac vein Internal pudendal vein Lateral sacral vein Middle hemorrhoidal vein Obturator vein Uterine vein Vaginal vein Vesical vein
Hypoglossal Nerve	**Includes:** Twelfth cranial nerve
Hypothalamus	**Includes:** Mammillary body
Inferior Mesenteric Artery	**Includes:** Sigmoid artery Superior rectal artery
Inferior Mesenteric Vein	**Includes:** Sigmoid vein Superior rectal vein
Inferior Vena Cava	**Includes:** Postcava Right inferior phrenic vein Right ovarian vein Right second lumbar vein Right suprarenal vein Right testicular vein
Inguinal Region, Bilateral **Inguinal** Region, Left **Inguinal** Region, Right	**Includes:** Inguinal canal Inguinal triangle
Inner Ear, Left **Inner** Ear, Right	**Includes:** Bony labyrinth Bony vestibule Cochlea Round window Semicircular canal

Continued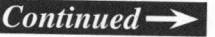

Innominate Artery	Includes: Brachiocephalic artery Brachiocephalic trunk
Innominate Vein, Left Innominate Vein, Right	Includes: Brachiocephalic vein Inferior thyroid vein
Internal Carotid Artery, Left Internal Carotid Artery, Right	Includes: Caroticotympanic artery Carotid sinus
Internal Iliac Artery, Left Internal Iliac Artery, Right	Includes: Deferential artery Hypogastric artery Iliolumbar artery Inferior gluteal artery Inferior vesical artery Internal pudendal artery Lateral sacral artery Middle rectal artery Obturator artery Superior gluteal artery Umbilical artery Uterine artery Vaginal artery
Internal Mammary Artery, Left Internal Mammary Artery, Right	Includes: Anterior intercostal artery Internal thoracic artery Musculophrenic artery Pericardiophrenic artery Superior epigastric artery
Intracranial Artery	Includes: Anterior cerebral artery Anterior choroidal artery Anterior communicating artery Basilar artery Circle of Willis Internal carotid artery, intracranial portion Middle cerebral artery Ophthalmic artery Posterior cerebral artery Posterior communicating artery Posterior inferior cerebellar artery (PICA)
Intracranial Vein	Includes: Anterior cerebral vein Basal (internal) cerebral vein Dural venous sinus Great cerebral vein Inferior cerebellar vein Inferior cerebral vein Internal (basal) cerebral vein Middle cerebral vein Ophthalmic vein Superior cerebellar vein Superior cerebral vein
Jejunum	Includes: Duodenojejunal flexure

Kidney	Includes: Renal calyx Renal capsule Renal cortex Renal segment
Kidney Pelvis, Left Kidney Pelvis, Right	Includes: Ureteropelvic junction (UPJ)
Kidney, Left Kidney, Right Kidneys, Bilateral	Includes: Renal calyx Renal capsule Renal cortex Renal segment
Knee Bursa and Ligament, Left Knee Bursa and Ligament, Right	Includes: Anterior cruciate ligament (ACL) Lateral collateral ligament (LCL) Ligament of head of fibula Medial collateral ligament (MCL) Patellar ligament Popliteal ligament Posterior cruciate ligament (PCL) Prepatellar bursa
Knee Joint, Femoral Surface, Left Knee Joint, Femoral Surface, Right	Includes: Femoropatellar joint Patellofemoral joint
Knee Joint, Left Knee Joint, Right	Includes: Femoropatellar joint Femorotibial joint Lateral meniscus Medial meniscus Patellofemoral joint Tibiofemoral joint
Knee Joint, Tibial Surface, Left Knee Joint, Tibial Surface, Right	Includes: Femorotibial joint Tibiofemoral joint
Knee Tendon, Left Knee Tendon, Right	Includes: Patellar tendon
Lacrimal Duct, Left Lacrimal Duct, Right	Includes: Lacrimal canaliculus Lacrimal punctum Lacrimal sac Nasolacrimal duct
Larynx	Includes: Aryepiglottic fold Arytenoid cartilage Corniculate cartilage Cuneiform cartilage False vocal cord Glottis Rima glottidis Thyroid cartilage Ventricular fold
Lens, Left Lens, Right	Includes: Zonule of Zinn
Liver	Includes: Quadrate lobe

Continued →

Lower Arm and Wrist Muscle, Left **Lower** Arm and Wrist Muscle, Right	**Includes:** Anatomical snuffbox Brachioradialis muscle Extensor carpi radialis muscle Extensor carpi ulnaris muscle Flexor carpi radialis muscle Flexor carpi ulnaris muscle Flexor pollicis longus muscle Palmaris longus muscle Pronator quadratus muscle Pronator teres muscle
Lower Artery	Umbilical artery
Lower Eyelid, Left **Lower** Eyelid, Right	**Includes:** Inferior tarsal plate Medial canthus
Lower Femur, Left **Lower** Femur, Right	**Includes:** Lateral condyle of femur Lateral epicondyle of femur Medial condyle of femur Medial epicondyle of femur
Lower Leg Muscle, Left **Lower** Leg Muscle, Right	**Includes:** Extensor digitorum longus muscle Extensor hallucis longus muscle Fibularis brevis muscle Fibularis longus muscle Flexor digitorum longus muscle Flexor hallucis longus muscle Gastrocnemius muscle Peroneus brevis muscle Peroneus longus muscle Popliteus muscle Soleus muscle Tibialis anterior muscle Tibialis posterior muscle
Lower Leg Tendon, Left **Lower** Leg Tendon, Right	**Includes:** Achilles tendon
Lower Lip	**Includes:** Frenulum labii inferioris Labial gland Vermilion border
Lower Spine Bursa and Ligament	Iliolumbar ligament Interspinous ligament, lumbar Intertransverse ligament, lumbar Ligamentum flavum, lumbar Sacrococcygeal ligament Sacroiliac ligament Sacrospinous ligament Sacrotuberous ligament Supraspinous ligament
Lumbar Nerve	**Includes:** Lumbosacral trunk Spinal nerve, lumbar Superior clunic (cluneal) nerve
Lumbar Plexus	**Includes:** Accessory obturator nerve Genitofemoral nerve Iliohypogastric nerve Ilioinguinal nerve Lateral femoral cutaneous nerve Obturator nerve Superior gluteal nerve

Section 0 - Medical and Surgical —
Character 4 - Body Part

Lumbar Spinal Cord	**Includes:** Cauda equina Conus medullaris Dorsal root ganglion
Lumbar Sympathetic Nerve	**Includes:** Lumbar ganglion Lumbar splanchnic nerve
Lumbar Vertebra	**Includes:** Spinous process Transverse process Vertebral arch Vertebral body Vertebral foramen Vertebral lamina Vertebral pedicle
Lumbar Vertebral Joint	**Includes:** Lumbar facet joint
Lumbosacral Joint	**Includes:** Lumbosacral facet joint
Lymphatic, Aortic	**Includes:** Celiac lymph node Gastric lymph node Hepatic lymph node Lumbar lymph node Pancreaticosplenic lymph node Paraaortic lymph node Retroperitoneal lymph node
Lymphatic, Head	**Includes:** Buccinator lymph node Infraauricular lymph node Infraparotid lymph node Parotid lymph node Preauricular lymph node Submandibular lymph node Submaxillary lymph node Submental lymph node Subparotid lymph node Suprahyoid lymph node
Lymphatic, Left Axillary	**Includes:** Anterior (pectoral) lymph node Apical (subclavicular) lymph node Brachial (lateral) lymph node Central axillary lymph node Lateral (brachial) lymph node Pectoral (anterior) lymph node Posterior (subscapular) lymph node Subclavicular (apical) lymph node Subscapular (posterior) lymph node
Lymphatic, Left Lower Extremity	**Includes:** Femoral lymph node Popliteal lymph node
Lymphatic, Left Neck	**Includes:** Cervical lymph node Jugular lymph node Mastoid (postauricular) lymph node Occipital lymph node Postauricular (mastoid) lymph node Retropharyngeal lymph node Supraclavicular (Virchow's) lymph node Virchow's (supraclavicular) lymph node

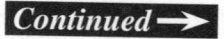
Continued →

Lymphatic, Left Upper Extremity	**Includes:** Cubital lymph node Deltopectoral (infraclavicular) lymph node Epitrochlear lymph node Infraclavicular (deltopectoral) lymph node Supratrochlear lymph node	**Main** Bronchus, Right	**Includes:** Bronchus Intermedius Intermediate bronchus
Lymphatic, Mesenteric	**Includes:** Inferior mesenteric lymph node Pararectal lymph node Superior mesenteric lymph node	**Mandible,** Left **Mandible,** Right	**Includes:** Alveolar process of mandible Condyloid process Mandibular notch Mental foramen
Lymphatic, Pelvis	**Includes:** Common iliac (subaortic) lymph node Gluteal lymph node Iliac lymph node Inferior epigastric lymph node Obturator lymph node Sacral lymph node Subaortic (common iliac) lymph node Suprainguinal lymph node	**Mastoid** Sinus, Left **Mastoid** Sinus, Right	**Includes:** Mastoid air cells
		Maxilla	**Includes:** Alveolar process of maxilla
		Maxillary Sinus, Left **Maxillary** Sinus, Right	**Includes:** Antrum of Highmore
Lymphatic, Right Axillary	**Includes:** Anterior (pectoral) lymph node Apical (subclavicular) lymph node Brachial (lateral) lymph node Central axillary lymph node Lateral (brachial) lymph node Pectoral (anterior) lymph node Posterior (subscapular) lymph node Subclavicular (apical) lymph node Subscapular (posterior) lymph node	**Median** Nerve	**Includes:** Anterior interosseous nerve Palmar cutaneous nerve
		Mediastinum	Mediastinal cavity Mediastinal space
		Medulla Oblongata	**Includes:** Myelencephalon
		Mesentery	**Includes:** Mesoappendix Mesocolon
Lymphatic, Right Lower Extremity	**Includes:** Femoral lymph node Popliteal lymph node	**Metatarsal,** Left **Metatarsal,** Right	**Includes:** Fibular sesamoid Tibial sesamoid
Lymphatic, Right Neck	**Includes:** Cervical lymph node Jugular lymph node Mastoid (postauricular) lymph node Occipital lymph node Postauricular (mastoid) lymph node Retropharyngeal lymph node Right jugular trunk Right lymphatic duct Right subclavian trunk Supraclavicular (Virchow's) lymph node Virchow's (supraclavicular) lymph node	**Metatarsal-Phalangeal** Joint, Left **Metatarsal-Phalangeal** Joint, Right	**Includes:** Metatarsophalangeal (MTP) joint
		Middle Ear, Left **Middle** Ear, Right	**Includes:** Oval window Tympanic cavity
		Minor Salivary Gland	**Includes:** Anterior lingual gland
		Mitral Valve	**Includes:** Bicuspid valve Left atrioventricular valve Mitral annulus
		Nasal Bone	**Includes:** Vomer of nasal septum
Lymphatic, Right Upper Extremity	**Includes:** Cubital lymph node Deltopectoral (infraclavicular) lymph node Epitrochlear lymph node Infraclavicular (deltopectoral) lymph node Supratrochlear lymph node	**Nasal** Mucosa and Soft Tissue	Columella External naris Greater alar cartilage Internal naris Lateral nasal cartilage Lesser alar cartilage Nasal cavity Nostril
		Nasal Septum	**Includes:** Quadrangular cartilage Septal cartilage Vomer bone
Lymphatic, Thorax	**Includes:** Intercostal lymph node Mediastinal lymph node Parasternal lymph node Paratracheal lymph node Tracheobronchial lymph node	**Nasal** Turbinate	**Includes:** Inferior turbinate Middle turbinate Nasal concha Superior turbinate

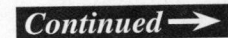

Continued →

Appendix D

Nasopharynx	**Includes:** Choana Fossa of Rosenmuller Pharyngeal recess Rhinopharynx
Neck	Parapharyngeal space Retropharyngeal space
Neck Muscle, Left **Neck** Muscle, Right	**Includes:** Anterior vertebral muscle Arytenoid muscle Cricothyroid muscle Infrahyoid muscle Levator scapulae muscle Platysma muscle Scalene muscle Splenius cervicis muscle Sternocleidomastoid muscle Suprahyoid muscle Thyroarytenoid muscle
Nipple, Left **Nipple,** Right	**Includes:** Areola
Occipital Bone	**Includes:** Foramen magnum
Oculomotor Nerve	**Includes:** Third cranial nerve
Olfactory Nerve	**Includes:** First cranial nerve Olfactory bulb
Omentum	Gastrocolic ligament Gastrocolic omentum Gastrohepatic omentum Gastrophrenic ligament Gastrosplenic ligament Greater Omentum Hepatogastric liagment Lesser Omentum
Optic Nerve	**Includes:** Optic chiasma Second cranial nerve
Orbit, Left **Orbit,** Right	**Includes:** Bony orbit Orbital portion of ethmoid bone Orbital portion of frontal bone Orbital portion of lacrimal bone Orbital portion of maxilla Orbital portion of palatine bone Orbital portion of sphenoid bone Orbital portion of zygomatic bone
Pancreatic Duct	**Includes:** Duct of Wirsung
Pancreatic Duct, Accessory	**Includes:** Duct of Santorini
Parotid Duct, Left **Parotid** Duct, Right	**Includes:** Stensen's duct
Pelvic Bone, Left **Pelvic** Bone, Right	**Includes:** Iliac crest Ilium Ischium Pubis

Pelvic Cavity	**Includes:** Retropubic space
Penis	**Includes:** Corpus cavernosum Corpus spongiosum
Perineum Muscle	**Includes:** Bulbospongiosus muscle Cremaster muscle Deep transverse perineal muscle Ischiocavernosus muscle Levator ani muscle Superficial transverse perineal muscle
Peritoneum	**Includes:** Epiploic foramen
Peroneal Artery, Left **Peroneal** Artery, Right	**Includes:** Fibular artery
Peroneal Nerve	**Includes:** Common fibular nerve Common peroneal nerve External popliteal nerve Lateral sural cutaneous nerve
Pharynx	**Includes:** Base of Tongue Hypopharynx Laryngopharynx Lignual tonsil Oropharynx Piriform recess (sinus) Tongue, base of
Phrenic Nerve	**Includes:** Accessory phrenic nerve
Pituitary Gland	**Includes:** Adenohypophysis Hypophysis Neurohypophysis
Pons	**Includes:** Apneustic center Basis pontis Locus ceruleus Pneumotaxic center Pontine tegmentum Superior olivary nucleus
Popliteal Artery, Left **Popliteal** Artery, Right	**Includes:** Inferior genicular artery Middle genicular artery Superior genicular artery Sural artery Tibioperoneal trunk
Portal Vein	**Includes:** Hepatic portal vein
Prepuce	**Includes:** Foreskin Glans penis
Pudendal Nerve	**Includes:** Posterior labial nerve Posterior scrotal nerve
Pulmonary Artery, Left	**Includes:** Arterial canal (duct) Botallo's duct Pulmoaortic canal

Continued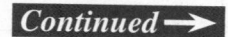

Pulmonary Valve	**Includes:** Pulmonary annulus Pulmonic valve
Pulmonary Vein, Left	**Includes:** Left inferior pulmonary vein Left superior pulmonary vein
Pulmonary Vein, Right	**Includes:** Right inferior pulmonary vein Right superior pulmonary vein
Radial Artery, Left **Radial** Artery, Right	**Includes:** Radial recurrent artery
Radial Nerve	**Includes:** Dorsal digital nerve Musculospiral nerve Palmar cutaneous nerve Posterior interosseous nerve
Radius, Left **Radius,** Right	**Includes:** Ulnar notch
Rectum	**Includes:** Anorectal junction
Renal Artery, Left **Renal** Artery, Right	**Includes:** Inferior suprarenal artery Renal segmental artery
Renal Vein, Left	**Includes:** Left inferior phrenic vein Left ovarian vein Left second lumbar vein Left suprarenal vein Left testicular vein
Retina, Left **Retina,** Right	**Includes:** Fovea Macula Optic disc
Retroperitoneum	**Includes:** Retroperitoneal cavity Retroperitoneal space
Rib(s) Bursa and Ligament	Costotransverse ligament
Sacral Nerve	**Includes:** Spinal nerve, sacral
Sacral Plexus	**Includes:** Inferior gluteal nerve Posterior femoral cutaneous nerve Pudendal nerve
Sacral Sympathetic Nerve	**Includes:** Ganglion impar (ganglion of Walther) Pelvic splanchnic nerve Sacral ganglion Sacral splanchnic nerve
Sacrococcygeal Joint	**Includes:** Sacrococcygeal symphysis
Saphenous Vein, Left **Saphenous** Vein, Right	External pudendal vein Great(er) saphenous vein Lesser saphenous vein Small saphenous vein Superficial circumflex iliac vein Superficial epigastric vein
Scapula, Left **Scapula,** Right	**Includes:** Acromion (process) Coracoid process

Sciatic Nerve	**Includes:** Ischiatic nerve
Shoulder Bursa and Ligament, Left **Shoulder** Bursa and Ligament, Right	**Includes:** Acromioclavicular ligament Coracoacromial ligament Coracoclavicular ligament Coracohumeral ligament Costoclavicular ligament Glenohumeral ligament Interclavicular ligament Sternoclavicular ligament Subacromial bursa Transverse humeral ligament Transverse scapular ligament
Shoulder Joint, Left **Shoulder** Joint, Right	**Includes:** Glenohumeral joint Glenoid ligament (labrum)
Shoulder Muscle, Left **Shoulder** Muscle, Right	**Includes:** Deltoid muscle Infraspinatus muscle Subscapularis muscle Supraspinatus muscle Teres major muscle Teres minor muscle
Sigmoid Colon	**Includes:** Rectosigmoid junction Sigmoid flexure
Skin	**Includes:** Dermis Epidermis Sebaceous gland Sweat gland
Skin, Chest	Breast procedures, skin only
Sphenoid Bone	**Includes:** Greater wing Lesser wing Optic foramen Pterygoid process Sella turcica
Spinal Canal	**Includes:** Epidural space, spinal Extradural space, spinal Subarachnoid space, spinal Subdural space, spinal Vertebral canal
Spinal Cord	**Includes:** Dorsal root ganglion
Spinal Meninges	**Includes:** Arachnoid mater, spinal Denticulate (dentate) ligament Dura mater, spinal Filum terminale Leptomeninges, spinal Pia mater, spinal
Spleen	**Includes:** Accessory spleen
Splenic Artery	**Includes:** Left gastroepiploic artery Pancreatic artery Short gastric artery

Continued →

Splenic Vein	**Includes:** Left gastroepiploic vein Pancreatic vein
Sternum	**Includes:** Manubrium Suprasternal notch Xiphoid process
Sternum Bursa and Ligament	Costoxiphoid ligament Sternocostal ligament
Stomach, Pylorus	**Includes:** Pyloric antrum Pyloric canal Pyloric sphincter
Subclavian Artery, Left **Subclavian** Artery, Right	**Includes:** Costocervical trunk Dorsal scapular artery Internal thoracic artery
Subcutaneous Tissue and Fascia, Chest	**Includes:** Pectoral fascia
Subcutaneous Tissue and Fascia, Face	**Includes:** Masseteric fascia Orbital fascia Submandibular space
Subcutaneous Tissue and Fascia, Left Foot	**Includes:** Plantar fascia (aponeurosis)
Subcutaneous Tissue and Fascia, Left Hand	**Includes:** Palmar fascia (aponeurosis)
Subcutaneous Tissue and Fascia, Left Lower Arm	**Includes:** Antebrachial fascia Bicipital aponeurosis
Subcutaneous Tissue and Fascia, Left Neck	Deep cervical fascia Pretracheal fascia Prevertebral fascia
Subcutaneous Tissue and Fascia, Left Upper Arm	**Includes:** Axillary fascia Deltoid fascia Infraspinatus fascia Subscapular aponeurosis Supraspinatus fascia
Subcutaneous Tissue and Fascia, Left Upper Leg	**Includes:** Crural fascia Fascia lata Iliac fascia Iliotibial tract (band)
Subcutaneous Tissue and Fascia, Right Foot	**Includes:** Plantar fascia (aponeurosis)
Subcutaneous Tissue and Fascia, Right Hand	**Includes:** Palmar fascia (aponeurosis)
Subcutaneous Tissue and Fascia, Right Lower Arm	**Includes:** Antebrachial fascia Bicipital aponeurosis
Subcutaneous Tissue and Fascia, Right Neck	Deep cervical fascia Pretracheal fascia Prevertebral fascia

Subcutaneous Tissue and Fascia, Right Upper Arm	**Includes:** Axillary fascia Deltoid fascia Infraspinatus fascia Subscapular aponeurosis Supraspinatus fascia
Subcutaneous Tissue and Fascia, Right Upper Leg	**Includes:** Crural fascia Fascia lata Iliac fascia Iliotibial tract (band)
Subcutaneous Tissue and Fascia, Scalp	**Includes:** Galea aponeurotica
Subcutaneous Tissue and Fascia, Trunk	**Includes:** External oblique aponeurosis Transversalis fascia
Submaxillary Gland, Left **Submaxillary** Gland, Right	**Includes:** Submandibular gland
Superior Mesenteric Artery	**Includes:** Ileal artery Ileocolic artery Inferior pancreaticoduodenal artery Jejunal artery
Superior Mesenteric Vein	**Includes:** Right gastroepiploic vein
Superior Vena Cava	**Includes:** Precava
Tarsal Joint, Left **Tarsal** Joint, Right	**Includes:** Calcaneocuboid joint Cuboideonavicular joint Cuneonavicular joint Intercuneiform joint Subtalar (talocalcaneal) joint Talocalcaneal (subtalar) joint Talocalcaneonavicular joint
Tarsal, Left **Tarsal,** Right	**Includes:** Calcaneus Cuboid bone Intermediate cuneiform bone Lateral cuneiform bone Medial cuneiform bone Navicular bone Talus bone
Temporal Artery, Left **Temporal** Artery, Right	**Includes:** Middle temporal artery Superficial temporal artery Transverse facial artery
Temporal Bone, Left **Temporal** Bone, Right	**Includes:** Mastoid process Petrous part of temporal bone Tympanic part of temoporal bone Zygomatic process of temporal bone

Continued →

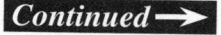

Thalamus	**Includes:** Epithalamus Geniculate nucleus Metathalamus Pulvinar
Thoracic Aorta Ascending/Arch	**Includes:** Aortic arch Ascending aorta
Thoracic Duct	**Includes:** Left jugular trunk Left subclavian trunk
Thoracic Nerve	**Includes:** Intercostal nerve Intercostobrachial nerve Spinal nerve, thoracic Subcostal nerve
Thoracic Spinal Cord	**Includes:** Dorsal root ganglion
Thoracic Sympathetic Nerve	**Includes:** Cardiac plexus Esophageal plexus Greater splanchnic nerve Inferior cardiac nerve Least splanchnic nerve Lesser splanchnic nerve Middle cardiac nerve Pulmonary plexus Superior cardiac nerve Thoracic aortic plexus Thoracic ganglion
Thoracic Vertebra	**Includes:** Spinous process Transverse process Vertebral arch Vertebral body Vertebral foramen Vertebral lamina Vertebral pedicle
Thoracic Vertebral Joint	**Includes:** Costotransverse joint Costovertebral joint Thoracic facet joint
Thoracolumbar Vertebral Joint	**Includes:** Thoracolumbar facet joint
Thorax Muscle, Left **Thorax** Muscle, Right	**Includes:** Intercostal muscle Levatores costarum muscle Pectoralis major muscle Pectoralis minor muscle Serratus anterior muscle Subclavius muscle Subcostal muscle Transverse thoracis muscle
Thymus	**Includes:** Thymus gland

Thyroid Artery, Left **Thyroid** Artery, Right	**Includes:** Cricothyroid artery Hyoid artery Sternocleidomastoid artery Superior laryngeal artery Superior thyroid artery Thyrocervical trunk
Tibia, Left **Tibia**, Right	**Includes:** Lateral condyle of tibia Medial condyle of tibia Medial malleolus
Tibial Nerve	**Includes:** Lateral plantar nerve Medial plantar nerve Medial popliteal nerve Medial sural cutaneous nerve
Toe Nail	**Includes:** Nail bed Nail plate
Toe Phalangeal Joint, Left **Toe** Phalangeal Joint, Right	**Includes:** Interphalangeal (IP) joint
Tongue	**Includes:** Frenulum linguae
Tongue, Palate, Pharynx Muscle	**Includes:** Chondroglossus muscle Genioglossus muscle Hyoglossus muscle Inferior longitudinal muscle Levator veli palatini muscle Palatoglossal muscle Palatopharyngeal muscle Pharyngeal constrictor muscle Salpingopharyngeus muscle Styloglossus muscle Stylopharyngeus muscle Superior longitudinal muscle Tensor veli palatini muscle
Tonsils	**Includes:** Palatine tonsil
Trachea	**Includes:** Cricoid cartilage
Transverse Colon	**Includes:** Hepatic flexure Splenic flexure
Tricuspid Valve	**Includes:** Right atrioventricular valve Tricuspid annulus
Trigeminal Nerve	**Includes:** Fifth cranial nerve Gasserian ganglion Mandibular nerve Maxillary nerve Ophthalmic nerve Trifacial nerve
Trochlear Nerve	**Includes:** Fourth cranial nerve

Continued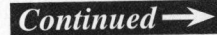

Appendix D

Section 0 - Medical and Surgical — Character 4 - Body Part

Trunk Muscle, Left **Trunk** Muscle, Right	**Includes:** Coccygeus muscle Erector spinae muscle Interspinalis muscle Intertransversarius muscle Latissimus dorsi muscle Quadratus lumborum muscle Rhomboid major muscle Rhomboid minor muscle Serratus posterior muscle Transversospinalis muscle Trapezius muscle
Tympanic Membrane, Left **Tympanic** Membrane, Right	**Includes:** Pars flaccida
Ulna, Left **Ulna,** Right	**Includes:** Olecranon process Radial notch
Ulnar Artery, Left **Ulnar** Artery, Right	**Includes:** Anterior ulnar recurrent artery Common interosseous artery Posterior ulnar recurrent artery
Ulnar Nerve	**Includes:** Cubital nerve
Upper Arm Muscle, Left **Upper** Arm Muscle, Right	**Includes:** Biceps brachii muscle Brachialis muscle Coracobrachialis muscle Triceps brachii muscle
Upper Artery	**Includes:** Aortic intercostal artery Bronchial artery Esophageal artery Subcostal artery
Upper Eyelid, Left **Upper** Eyelid, Right	**Includes:** Lateral canthus Levator palpebrae superioris muscle Orbicularis oculi muscle Superior tarsal plate
Upper Femur, Left **Upper** Femur, Right	**Includes:** Femoral head Greater trochanter Lesser trochanter Neck of femur
Upper Leg Muscle, Left **Upper** Leg Muscle, Right	**Includes:** Adductor brevis muscle Adductor longus muscle Adductor magnus muscle Biceps femoris muscle Gracilis muscle Pectineus muscle Quadriceps (femoris) Rectus femoris muscle Sartorius muscle Semimembranosus muscle Semitendinosus muscle Vastus intermedius muscle Vastus lateralis muscle Vastus medialis muscle

Section 0 - Medical and Surgical — Character 4 - Body Part

Upper Lip	**Includes:** Frenulum labii superioris Labial gland Vermilion border
Upper Spine Bursa and Ligament	Interspinous ligament, thoracic Intertransverse ligament, thoracic Ligamentum flavum, thoracic Supraspinous ligament
Ureter **Ureter,** Left **Ureter,** Right **Ureters,** Bilateral	**Includes:** Ureteral orifice Ureterovesical orifice
Urethra	**Includes:** Bulbourethral (Cowper's) gland Cowper's (bulbourethral) gland External urethral sphincter Internal urethral sphincter Membranous urethra Penile urethra Prostatic urethra
Uterine Supporting Structure	**Includes:** Broad ligament Infundibulopelvic ligament Ovarian ligament Round ligament of uterus
Uterus	**Includes:** Fundus uteri Myometrium Perimetrium Uterine cornu
Uvula	**Includes:** Palatine uvula
Vagus Nerve	**Includes:** Anterior vagal trunk Pharyngeal plexus Pneumogastric nerve Posterior vagal trunk Pulmonary plexus Recurrent laryngeal nerve Superior laryngeal nerve Tenth cranial nerve
Vas Deferens **Vas** Deferens, Bilateral **Vas** Deferens, Left **Vas** Deferens, Right	**Includes:** Ductus deferens Ejaculatory duct
Ventricle, Right	**Includes:** Conus arteriosus
Ventricular Septum	**Includes:** Interventricular septum
Vertebral Artery, Left **Vertebral** Artery, Right	**Includes:** Anterior spinal artery Posterior spinal artery
Vertebral Vein, Left **Vertebral** Vein, Right	**Includes:** Deep cervical vein Suboccipital venous plexus

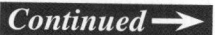

Continued →

Section 0 - Medical and Surgical —
Character 4 - Body Part

Vestibular Gland	**Includes:** Bartholin's (greater vestibular) gland Greater vestibular (Bartholin's) gland Paraurethral (Skene's) gland Skene's (paraurethral) gland
Vitreous, Left **Vitreous,** Right	**Includes:** Vitreous body
Vocal Cord, Left **Vocal** Cord, Right	**Includes:** Vocal fold
Vulva	**Includes:** Labia majora Labia minora
Wrist Bursa and Ligament, Left **Wrist** Bursa and Ligament, Right	**Includes:** Palmar ulnocarpal ligament Radial collateral carpal ligament Radiocarpal ligament Radioulnar ligament Scapholunate ligament Ulnar collateral carpal ligament
Wrist Joint, Left **Wrist** Joint, Right	**Includes:** Distal radioulnar joint Radiocarpal joint

Appendix E: Medical and Surgical Device Table (Device Key) and Device Aggregation Table

Section 0 - Medical and Surgical — Character 6 - Device

Articulating Spacer in Lower Joints	**Includes:** Articulating Spacer (Antibiotic) Spacer, Articulating (Antibiotic)
Artificial Sphincter in Gastrointestinal System	**Includes:** Artificial anal sphincter (AAS) Artificial bowel sphincter (neosphincter)
Artificial Sphincter in Urinary System	**Includes:** AMS 800® Urinary Control System Artificial urinary sphincter (AUS)
Autologous Arterial Tissue in Heart and Great Vessels	**Includes:** Autologous artery graft
Autologous Arterial Tissue in Lower Arteries	**Includes:** Autologous artery graft
Autologous Arterial Tissue in Lower Veins	**Includes:** Autologous artery graft
Autologous Arterial Tissue in Upper Arteries	**Includes:** Autologous artery graft
Autologous Arterial Tissue in Upper Veins	**Includes:** Autologous artery graft
Autologous Tissue Substitute	**Includes:** Autograft Cultured epidermal cell autograft Epicel® cultured epidermal autograft
Autologous Venous Tissue in Heart and Great Vessels	**Includes:** Autologous vein graft
Autologous Venous Tissue in Lower Arteries	**Includes:** Autologous vein graft
Autologous Venous Tissue in Lower Veins	**Includes:** Autologous vein graft
Autologous Venous Tissue in Upper Arteries	**Includes:** Autologous vein graft
Autologous Venous Tissue in Upper Veins	**Includes:** Autologous vein graft
Biologic with Synthetic Substitute, Autoregulated Electrohydraulic for Replacement in Heart and Great Vessels	**Includes:** Carmat total artificial heart (TAH)
Bone Growth Stimulator in Head and Facial Bones	**Includes:** Electrical bone growth stimulator (EBGS) Ultrasonic osteogenic stimulator Ultrasound bone healing system
Bone Growth Stimulator in Lower Bones	**Includes:** Electrical bone growth stimulator (EBGS) Ultrasonic osteogenic stimulator Ultrasound bone healing system

Section 0 - Medical and Surgical — Character 6 - Device

Bone Growth Stimulator in Upper Bones	**Includes:** Electrical bone growth stimulator (EBGS) Ultrasonic osteogenic stimulator Ultrasound bone healing system
Cardiac Lead in Heart and Great Vessels	**Includes:** Cardiac contractility modulation lead
Cardiac Lead, Defibrillator for Insertion in Heart and Great Vessels	**Includes:** ACUITY™ Steerable Lead Attain Ability® lead Attain StarFix® (OTW) lead Cardiac resynchronization therapy (CRT) lead Corox (OTW) Bipolar Lead Durata® Defibrillation Lead ENDOTAK RELIANCE® (G) Defibrillation Lead
Cardiac Lead, Pacemaker for Insertion in Heart and Great Vessels	**Includes:** ACUITY™ Steerable Lead Attain Ability® lead Attain StarFix® (OTW) lead Cardiac resynchronization therapy (CRT) lead Corox (OTW) Bipolar Lead
Cardiac Resynchronization Defibrillator Pulse Generator for Insertion in Subcutaneous Tissue and Fascia	**Includes:** COGNIS® CRT-D Concerto II CRT-D Consulta CRT-D CONTAK RENEWAL® 3 RF (HE) CRT-D LIVIAN™ CRT-D Maximo II DR CRT-D Ovatio™ CRT-D Protecta XT CRT-D Viva (XT)(S)
Cardiac Resynchronization Pacemaker Pulse Generator for Insertion in Subcutaneous Tissue and Fascia	**Includes:** Consulta CRT-P Stratos LV Synchra CRT-P
Contraceptive Device in Female Reproductive System	**Includes:** Intrauterine device (IUD)
Contraceptive Device in Subcutaneous Tissue and Fascia	**Includes:** Subdermal progesterone implant
Contractility Modulation Device for Insertion in Subcutaneous Tissue and Fascia	**Includes:** Optimizer™ III implantable pulse generator

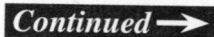
Continued →

Defibrillator Generator for Insertion in Subcutaneous Tissue and Fascia	**Includes:** Evera (XT)(S)(DR/VR) Implantable cardioverter-defibrillator (ICD) Maximo II DR (VR) Protecta XT DR (XT VR) Secura (DR) (VR) Virtuoso (II) (DR) (VR)
Diaphragmatic Pacemaker Lead in Respiratory System	**Includes:** Phrenic nerve stimulator lead
Drainage Device	**Includes:** Cystostomy tube Foley catheter Percutaneous nephrostomy catheter Thoracostomy tube
External Fixation Device in Head and Facial Bones	**Includes:** External fixator
External Fixation Device in Lower Bones	**Includes:** External fixator
External Fixation Device in Lower Joints	**Includes:** External fixator
External Fixation Device in Upper Bones	**Includes:** External fixator
External Fixation Device in Upper Joints	**Includes:** External fixator
External Fixation Device, Hybrid for Insertion in Upper Bones	**Includes:** Delta frame external fixator Sheffield hybrid external fixator
External Fixation Device, Hybrid for Insertion in Lower Bones	**Includes:** Delta frame external fixator Sheffield hybrid external fixator
External Fixation Device, Hybrid for Reposition in Upper Bones	**Includes:** Delta frame external fixator Sheffield hybrid external fixator
External Fixation Device, Hybrid for Reposition in Lower Bones	**Includes:** Delta frame external fixator Sheffield hybrid external fixator
External Fixation Device, Limb Lengthening for Insertion in Upper Bones	**Includes:** Ilizarov-Vecklich device
External Fixation Device, Limb Lengthening for Insertion in Lower Bones	**Includes:** Ilizarov-Vecklich device
External Fixation Device, Monoplanar for Insertion in Upper Bones	**Includes:** Uniplanar external fixator
External Fixation Device, Monoplanar for Insertion in Lower Bones	**Includes:** Uniplanar external fixator
External Fixation Device, Monoplanar for Reposition in Upper Bones	**Includes:** Uniplanar external fixator
External Fixation Device, Monoplanar for Reposition in Lower Bones	**Includes:** Uniplanar external fixator

External Fixation Device, Ring for Insertion in Upper Bones	**Includes:** Ilizarov external fixator Sheffield ring external fixator
External Fixation Device, Ring for Insertion in Lower Bones	**Includes:** Ilizarov external fixator Sheffield ring external fixator
External Fixation Device, Ring for Reposition in Upper Bones	**Includes:** Ilizarov external fixator Sheffield ring external fixator
External Fixation Device, Ring for Reposition in Lower Bones	**Includes:** Ilizarov external fixator Sheffield ring external fixator
Extraluminal Device	**Includes:** AtriClip LAA Exclusion System LAP-BAND® adjustable gastric banding system REALIZE® Adjustable Gastric Band
Feeding Device in Gastrointestinal System	**Includes:** Percutaneous endoscopic gastrojejunostomy (PEG/J) tube Percutaneous endoscopic gastrostomy (PEG) tube
Hearing Device in Ear, Nose, Sinus	**Includes:** Esteem® implantable hearing system
Hearing Device in Head and Facial Bones	**Includes:** Bone anchored hearing device
Hearing Device, Bone Conduction for Insertion in Ear, Nose, Sinus	**Includes:** Bone anchored hearing device
Hearing Device, Multiple Channel Cochlear Prosthesis for Insertion in Ear, Nose, Sinus	**Includes:** Cochlear implant (CI), multiple channel (electrode)
Hearing Device, Single Channel Cochlear Prosthesis for Insertion in Ear, Nose, Sinus	**Includes:** Cochlear implant (CI), single channel (electrode)
Implantable Heart Assist System in Heart and Great Vessels	**Includes:** Berlin Heart Ventricular Assist Device DeBakey Left Ventricular Assist Device DuraHeart Left Ventricular Assist System HeartMate II® Left Ventricular Assist Device (LVAD) HeartMate 3® LVAS HeartMate XVE® Left Ventricular Assist Device (LVAD) MicroMed HeartAssist Novacor Left Ventricular Assist Device Thoratec IVAD (Implantable Ventricular Assist Device)
Infusion Device	**Includes:** Ascenda Intrathecal Catheter InDura, intrathecal catheter (1P) (spinal) Non-tunneled central venous catheter Peripherally inserted central catheter (PICC) Tunneled spinal (intrathecal) catheter

Continued →

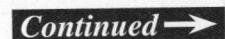

Infusion Device, Pump in Subcutaneous Tissue and Fascia	**Includes:** Implantable drug infusion pump (anti-spasmodic)(chemotherapy)(pain) Injection reservoir, pump Pump reservoir Subcutaneous injection reservoir, pump SynchroMed pump
Interbody Fusion Device in Lower Joints	**Includes:** Axial Lumbar Interbody Fusion System AxiaLIF® System CoRoent® XL Direct Lateral Interbody Fusion (DLIF) device EXtreme Lateral Interbody Fusion (XLIF) device Interbody fusion (spine) cage XLIF® System
Interbody Fusion Device in Upper Joints	**Includes:** BAK/C® Interbody Cervical Fusion System Interbody fusion (spine) cage
Internal Fixation Device in Head and Facial Bones	**Includes:** Bone screw (interlocking)(lag)(pedicle)(recessed) Kirschner wire (K-wire) Neutralization plate
Internal Fixation Device in Lower Bones	**Includes:** Bone screw (interlocking)(lag)(pedicle)(recessed) Clamp and rod internal fixation system (CRIF) Kirschner wire (K-wire) Neutralization plate
Internal Fixation Device in Lower Joints	**Includes:** Fusion screw (compression)(lag)(locking) Joint fixation plate Kirschner wire (K-wire)
Internal Fixation Device in Upper Bones	**Includes:** Bone screw (interlocking)(lag)(pedicle)(recessed) Clamp and rod internal fixation system (CRIF) Kirschner wire (K-wire) Neutralization plate
Internal Fixation Device in Upper Joints	**Includes:** Fusion screw (compression)(lag)(locking) Joint fixation plate Kirschner wire (K-wire)
Internal Fixation Device, Intramedullary in Lower Bones	**Includes:** Intramedullary (IM) rod (nail) Intramedullary skeletal kinetic distractor (ISKD) Kuntscher nail
Internal Fixation Device, Intramedullary in Upper Bones	**Includes:** Intramedullary (IM) rod (nail) Intramedullary skeletal kinetic distractor (ISKD) Kuntscher nail

Internal Fixation Device, Intramedullary Limb Lengthening for Insertion in Lower Bones	PRECICE intramedullary limb lengthening system
Internal Fixation Device, Intramedullary Limb Lengthening for Insertion in Upper Bones	PRECICE intramedullary limb lengthening system
Internal Fixation Device, Rigid Plate for Insertion in Upper Bones	**Includes:** Titanium Sternal Fixation System (TSFS)
Internal Fixation Device, Rigid Plate for Reposition in Upper Bones	**Includes:** Titanium Sternal Fixation System (TSFS)
Internal Fixation Device, Sustained Compression for Fusion in Lower Joints	**Includes:** DynaNail® DynaNail Mini®
Internal Fixation Device, Sustained Compression for Fusion in Upper Joints	**Includes:** DynaNail® DynaNail Mini®
Intraluminal Device	**Includes:** Absolute Pro Vascular (OTW) Self-Expanding Stent System Acculink (RX) Carotid Stent System AFX® Endovascular AAA System AneuRx® AAA Advantage® Assurant (Cobalt) stent Carotid WALLSTENT® Monorail® Endoprosthesis CoAxia NeuroFlo catheter Colonic Z-Stent® Complete (SE) stent Cook Zenith AAA Endovascular Graft Driver stent (RX) (OTW) E-Luminexx™ (Biliary)(Vascular) Stent Embolization coil(s) Endologix AFX® Endovascular AAA System Endurant® II AAA stent graft system Endurant® Endovascular Stent Graft EXCLUDER® AAA Endoprosthesis Express® (LD) Premounted Stent System Express® Biliary SD Monorail® Premounted Stent System Express® SD Renal Monorail® Premounted Stent System FLAIR® Endovascular Stent Graft Formula™ Balloon-Expandable Renal Stent System GORE EXCLUDER® AAA Endoprosthesis GORE TAG® Thoracic Endoprosthesis Herculink (RX) Elite Renal Stent System LifeStent® (Flexstar)(XL) Vascular Stent System Medtronic Endurant® II AAA stent graft system

Continued →
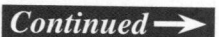

	Micro-Driver stent (RX) (OTW) MULTI-LINK (VISION)(MINI-VISION)(ULTRA) Coronary Stent System Omnilink Elite Vascular Balloon Expandable Stent System Protégé® RX Carotid Stent System Stent, intraluminal (cardiovascular) (gastrointestinal)(hepatobiliary) (urinary) Talent® Converter Talent® Occluder Talent® Stent Graft (abdominal) (thoracic) Therapeutic occlusion coil(s) Ultraflex™ Precision Colonic Stent System Valiant Thoracic Stent Graft WALLSTENT® Endoprosthesis Xact Carotid Stent System Zenith AAA Endovascular Graft Zenith Flex® AAA Endovascular Graft Zenith® Renu™ AAA Ancillary Graft Zenith TX2® TAA Endovascular Graft
Intraluminal Device, Airway in Ear, Nose, Sinus	**Includes:** Nasopharyngeal airway (NPA)
Intraluminal Device, Airway in Gastrointestinal System	**Includes:** Esophageal obturator airway (EOA)
Intraluminal Device, Airway in Mouth and Throat	**Includes:** Guedel airway Oropharyngeal airway (OPA)
Intraluminal Device, Bioactive in Upper Arteries	**Includes:** Bioactive embolization coil(s) Micrus CERECYTE microcoil
Intraluminal Device, Branched or Fenestrated, One or Two Arteries for Restriction in Lower Arteries	**Includes:** Cook Zenith® Fenestrated AAA Endovascular Graft EXCLUDER® AAA Endoprosthesis EXCLUDER® IBE Endoprosthesis GORE EXCLUDER® AAA Endoprosthesis GORE EXCLUDER® IBE Endoprosthesis Zenith® Fenestrated AAA Endovascular Graft
Intraluminal Device, Branched or Fenestrated, Three or More Arteries for Restriction in Lower Arteries	**Includes:** Cook Zenith® Fenestrated AAA Endovascular Graft EXCLUDER® AAA Endoprosthesis GORE EXCLUDER® AAA Endoprosthesis Zenith® Fenestrated AAA Endovascular Graft
Intraluminal Device, Drug-eluting in Heart and Great Vessels	**Includes:** CYPHER® Stent Endeavor® (III)(IV) (Sprint) Zotarolimus-eluting Coronary Stent System Everolimus-eluting coronary stent Paclitaxel-eluting coronary stent Sirolimus-eluting coronary stent TAXUS® Liberté® Paclitaxel-eluting Coronary Stent System XIENCE Everolimus Eluting Coronary Stent System Zotarolimus-eluting coronary stent
Intraluminal Device, Drug-eluting in Lower Arteries	**Includes:** Paclitaxel-eluting peripheral stent Zilver® PTX® (paclitaxel) Drug-Eluting Peripheral Stent
Intraluminal Device, Drug-eluting in Upper Arteries	**Includes:** Paclitaxel-eluting peripheral stent Zilver® PTX® (paclitaxel) Drug-Eluting Peripheral Stent
Intraluminal Device, Endobronchial Valve in Respiratory System	**Includes:** Spiration IBV™ Valve System
Intraluminal Device, Flow Diverter for Restriction in Upper Arteries	**Includes:** Flow Diverter embolization device Pipeline™ (Flex) embolization device Surpass Streamline™ Flow Diverter
Intraluminal Device, Pessary in Female Reproductive System	**Includes:** Pessary ring Vaginal pessary
Intraluminal Device, Endotracheal Airway in Respiratory System	**Includes:** Endotracheal tube (cuffed)(double-lumen)
Liner in Lower Joints	**Includes:** Acetabular cup Hip (joint) liner Joint liner (insert) Knee (implant) insert Tibial insert
Monitoring Device	**Includes:** Blood glucose monitoring system Cardiac event recorder Continuous Glucose Monitoring (CGM) device Implantable glucose monitoring device Loop recorder, implantable Reveal (LINQ)(DX)(XT)
Monitoring Device, Hemodynamic for Insertion in Subcutaneous Tissue and Fascia	**Includes:** Implantable hemodynamic monitor (IHM) Implantable hemodynamic monitoring system (IHMS)
Monitoring Device, Pressure Sensor for Insertion in Heart and Great Vessels	**Includes:** CardioMEMS® pressure sensor EndoSure® sensor

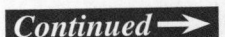

Continued →

Neurostimulator Lead in Central Nervous System and Cranial Nerves	**Includes:** Cortical strip neurostimulator lead DBS lead Deep brain neurostimulator lead RNS System lead Spinal cord neurostimulator lead
Neurostimulator Lead in Peripheral Nervous System	**Includes:** InterStim® Therapy lead
Neurostimulator Generator in Head and Facial Bones	**Includes:** RNS system neurostimulator generator
Nonautologous Tissue Substitute	**Includes:** Acellular Hydrated Dermis Bone bank bone graft Cook Biodesign® Fistula Plug(s) Cook Biodesign® Hernia Graft(s) Cook Biodesign® Layered Graft(s) Cook Zenapro™ Layered Grafts(s) Tissue bank graft
Other Device	**Includes:** Alfapump® system
Pacemaker, Dual Chamber for Insertion in Subcutaneous Tissue and Fascia	**Includes:** Advisa (MRI) EnRhythm Kappa Revo MRI™ SureScan® pacemaker Two lead pacemaker Versa
Pacemaker, Single Chamber for Insertion in Subcutaneous Tissue and Fascia	**Includes:** Single lead pacemaker (atrium) (ventricle)
Pacemaker, Single Chamber Rate Responsive for Insertion in Subcutaneous Tissue and Fascia	**Includes:** Single lead rate responsive pacemaker (atrium)(ventricle)
Radioactive Element	**Includes:** Brachytherapy seeds CivaSheet®
Radioactive Element, Cesium-131 Collagen Implant for Insertion in Central Nervous System and Cranial Nerves	Cesium-131 Collagen Implant GammaTile™
Resurfacing Device in Lower Joints	**Includes:** CONSERVE® PLUS Total Resurfacing Hip System Cormet Hip Resurfacing System
Short-term External Heart Assist System in Heart and Great Vessels	Biventricular external heart assist system BVS 5000 Ventricular Assist Device Centrimag® Blood Pump Impella® heart pump TandemHeart® System Thoratec Paracorporeal Ventricular Assist Device
Spacer in Lower Joints	**Includes:** Joint spacer (antibiotic) Spacer, Static (Antibiotic) Static Spacer (Antibiotic)
Spacer in Upper Joints	**Includes:** Joint spacer (antibiotic)

Spinal Stabilization Device, Facet Replacement for Insertion in Upper Joints	**Includes:** Facet replacement spinal stabilization device
Spinal Stabilization Device, Facet Replacement for Insertion in Lower Joints	**Includes:** Facet replacement spinal stabilization device
Spinal Stabilization Device, Interspinous Process for Insertion in Upper Joints	**Includes:** Interspinous process spinal stabilization device X-STOP® Spacer
Spinal Stabilization Device, Interspinous Process for Insertion in Lower Joints	**Includes:** Interspinous process spinal stabilization device X-STOP® Spacer
Spinal Stabilization Device, Pedicle-Based for Insertion in Upper Joints	**Includes:** Dynesys® Dynamic Stabilization System Pedicle-based dynamic stabilization device
Spinal Stabilization Device, Pedicle-Based for Insertion in Lower Joints	**Includes:** Dynesys® Dynamic Stabilization System Pedicle-based dynamic stabilization device
Stimulator Generator in Subcutaneous Tissue and Fascia	**Includes:** Baroreflex Activation Therapy® (BAT®) Diaphragmatic pacemaker generator Mark IV Breathing Pacemaker System Phrenic nerve stimulator generator Rheos® System device
Stimulator Generator, Multiple Array for Insertion in Subcutaneous Tissue and Fascia	**Includes:** Activa PC neurostimulator Enterra gastric neurostimulator Neurostimulator generator, multiple channel PERCEPT™ PC neurostimulator PrimeAdvanced neurostimulator (SureScan)(MRI Safe)
Stimulator Generator, Multiple Array Rechargeable for Insertion in Subcutaneous Tissue and Fascia	**Includes:** Activa RC neurostimulator Neurostimulator generator, multiple channel rechargeable RestoreAdvanced neurostimulator (SureScan)(MRI Safe) RestoreSensor neurostimulator (SureScan)(MRI Safe) RestoreUltra neurostimulator (SureScan)(MRI Safe)
Stimulator Generator, Single Array for Insertion in Subcutaneous Tissue and Fascia	**Includes:** Activa SC neurostimulator InterStim™ II Therapy neurostimulator Itrel (3)(4) neurostimulator Neurostimulator generator, single channel
Stimulator Generator, Single Array Rechargeable for Insertion in Subcutaneous Tissue and Fascia	**Includes:** InterStim™ Micro Therapy neurostimulator Neurostimulator generator, single channel rechargeable
Stimulator Lead in Gastrointestinal System	**Includes:** Gastric electrical stimulation (GES) lead Gastric pacemaker lead

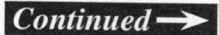

Continued →

Stimulator Lead in Muscles	**Includes:** Electrical muscle stimulation (EMS) lead Electronic muscle stimulator lead Neuromuscular electrical stimulation (NEMS) lead
Stimulator Lead in Upper Arteries	**Includes:** Baroreflex Activation Therapy® (BAT®) Carotid (artery) sinus (baroreceptor) lead Rheos® System lead
Stimulator Lead in Urinary System	**Includes:** Sacral nerve modulation (SNM) lead Sacral neuromodulation lead Urinary incontinence stimulator lead
Subcutaneous Defibrillator Lead in Subcutaneous Tissue and Fascia	S-ICD™ lead
Synthetic Substitute	**Includes:** AbioCor® Total Replacement Heart AMPLATZER® Muscular VSD Occluder Annuloplasty ring Bard® Composix® (E/X)(LP) mesh Bard® Composix® Kugel® patch Bard® Dulex™ mesh Bard® Ventralex™ hernia patch Barricaid® Annular Closure Device (ACD) BRYAN® Cervical Disc System Corvia IASD® Ex-PRESS™ mini glaucoma shunt Flexible Composite Mesh GORE® DUALMESH® Holter valve ventricular shunt IASD® (InterAtrial Shunt Device), Corvia InterAtrial Shunt Device IASD®, Corvia MitraClip valve repair system Nitinol framed polymer mesh Open Pivot Aortic Valve Graft (AVG) Open Pivot (mechanical) valve Partially absorbable mesh PHYSIOMESH™ Flexible Composite Mesh Polymethylmethacrylate (PMMA) Polypropylene mesh PRESTIGE® Cervical Disc PROCEED™ Ventral Patch Prodisc-C Prodisc-L PROLENE Polypropylene Hernia System (PHS) Rebound HRD® (Hernia Repair Device) SynCardia Total Artificial Heart Total artificial (replacement) heart ULTRAPRO Hernia System (UHS) ULTRAPRO Partially Absorbable Lightweight Mesh ULTRAPRO Plug V-WAVE Interatrial Shunt System Ventrio™ Hernia Patch Zimmer® NexGen® LPS Mobile Bearing Knee Zimmer® NexGen® LPS-Flex Mobile Knee
Synthetic Substitute, Ceramic for Replacement in Lower Joints	**Includes:** Ceramic on ceramic bearing surface Novation® Ceramic AHS® (Articulation Hip System)

Synthetic Substitute, Intraocular Telescope for Replacement in Eye	**Includes:** Implantable Miniature Telescope™ (IMT)
Synthetic Substitute, Metal for Replacement in Lower Joints	**Includes:** Cobalt/chromium head and socket Metal on metal bearing surface
Synthetic Substitute, Metal on Polyethylene for Replacement in Lower Joints	**Includes:** Cobalt/chromium head and polyethylene socket
Synthetic Substitute, Oxidized Zirconium on Polyethylene for Replacement in Lower Joints	OXINIUM
Synthetic Substitute, Pneumatic for Replacement in Heart and Great Vessels	**Includes:** SynCardia (temporary) total artificial heart (TAH)
Synthetic Substitute, Polyethylene for Replacement in Lower Joints	**Includes:** Polyethylene socket
Synthetic Substitute, Reverse Ball and Socket for Replacement in Upper Joints	**Includes:** Delta III Reverse shoulder prosthesis Reverse® Shoulder Prosthesis
Tissue Expander in Skin and Breast	**Includes:** Tissue expander (inflatable)(injectable)
Tissue Expander in Subcutaneous Tissue and Fascia	**Includes:** Tissue expander (inflatable)(injectable)
Tracheostomy Device in Respiratory System	**Includes:** Tracheostomy tube
Vascular Access Device, Totally Implantable in Subcutaneous Tissue and Fascia	**Includes:** Implanted (venous)(access) port Injection reservoir, port Subcutaneous injection reservoir, port
Vascular Access Device, Tunneled in Subcutaneous Tissue and Fascia	Tunneled central venous catheter Vectra® Vascular Access Graft
Zooplastic Tissue in Heart and Great Vessels	**Includes:** 3f (Aortic) Bioprosthesis valve Bovine pericardial valve Bovine pericardium graft Contegra Pulmonary Valved Conduit CoreValve transcatheter aortic valve Epic™ Stented Tissue Valve (aortic) Freestyle (Stentless) Aortic Root Bioprosthesis Hancock Bioprosthesis (aortic) (mitral) valve Hancock Bioprosthetic Valved Conduit Melody® transcatheter pulmonary valve Mitroflow® Aortic Pericardial Heart Valve Mosaic Bioprosthesis (aortic) (mitral) valve Porcine (bioprosthetic) valve SAPIEN transcatheter aortic valve SJM Biocor® Stented Valve System Stented tissue valve Trifecta™ Valve (aortic) Xenograft

Device Aggregation Table

Specific Device	for Operation	in Body System	General Device	
Autologous Arterial Tissue	All applicable	Heart and Great Vessels Lower Arteries Lower Veins Upper Arteries Upper Veins	7	Autologous Tissue Substitute
Autologous Venous Tissue	All applicable	Heart and Great Vessels Lower Arteries Lower Veins Upper Arteries Upper Veins	7	Autologous Tissue Substitute
Cardiac Lead, Defibrillator	Insertion	Heart and Great Vessels	M	Cardiac Lead
Cardiac Lead, Pacemaker	Insertion	Heart and Great Vessels	M	Cardiac Lead
Cardiac Resynchronization Defibrillator Pulse Generator	Insertion	Subcutaneous Tissue and Fascia	P	Cardiac Rhythm Related Device
Cardiac Resynchronization Pacemaker Pulse Generator	Insertion	Subcutaneous Tissue and Fascia	P	Cardiac Rhythm Related Device
Contractility Modulation Device	Insertion	Subcutaneous Tissue and Fascia	P	Cardiac Rhythm Related Device
Defibrillator Generator	Insertion	Subcutaneous Tissue and Fascia	P	Cardiac Rhythm Related Device
Epiretinal Visual Prosthesis	All applicable	Eye	J	Synthetic Substitute
External Fixation Device, Hybrid	Insertion	Lower Bones Upper Bones	5	External Fixation Device
External Fixation Device, Hybrid	Reposition	Lower Bones Upper Bones	5	External Fixation Device
External Fixation Device, Limb Lengthening	Insertion	Lower Bones Upper Bones	5	External Fixation Device
External Fixation Device, Monoplanar	Insertion	Lower Bones Upper Bones	5	External Fixation Device
External Fixation Device, Monoplanar	Reposition	Lower Bones Upper Bones	5	External Fixation Device
External Fixation Device, Ring	Insertion	Lower Bones Upper Bones	5	External Fixation Device
External Fixation Device, Ring	Reposition	Lower Bones Upper Bones	5	External Fixation Device
Hearing Device, Bone Conduction	Insertion	Ear, Nose, Sinus	S	Hearing Device
Hearing Device, Multiple Channel Cochlear Prosthesis	Insertion	Ear, Nose, Sinus	S	Hearing Device
Hearing Device, Single Channel Cochlear Prosthesis	Insertion	Ear, Nose, Sinus	S	Hearing Device
Internal Fixation Device, Intramedullary	All applicable	Lower Bones Upper Bones	4	Internal Fixation Device
Internal Fixation Device, Intramedullary Limb Lengthening	Insertion	Lower Bones Upper Bones	6	Internal Fixation Device Intramedullary
Internal Fixation Device, Rigid Plate	Insertion	Upper Bones	4	Internal Fixation Device

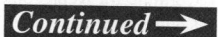
Continued →

Specific Device	for Operation	in Body System	General Device	
Internal Fixation Device, Rigid Plate	Reposition	Upper Bones	**4**	Internal Fixation Device
Intraluminal Device, Airway	All applicable	Ear, Nose, Sinus Gastrointestinal System Mouth and Throat	**D**	Intraluminal Device
Intraluminal Device, Bioactive	All applicable	Upper Arteries	**D**	Intraluminal Device
Intraluminal Device, Branched or Fenestrated, One or Two Arteries	Restriction	Heart and Great Vessels Lower Arteries	**D**	Intraluminal Device
Intraluminal Device, Branched or Fenestrated, Three or More Arteries	Restriction	Heart and Great Vessels Lower Arteries	**D**	Intraluminal Device
Intraluminal Device, Drug-eluting	All applicable	Heart and Great Vessels Lower Arteries Upper Arteries	**D**	Intraluminal Device
Intraluminal Device, Drug-eluting, Four or More	All applicable	Heart and Great Vessels Lower Arteries Upper Arteries	**D**	Intraluminal Device
Intraluminal Device, Drug-eluting, Three	All applicable	Heart and Great Vessels Lower Arteries Upper Arteries	**D**	Intraluminal Device
Intraluminal Device, Drug-eluting, Two	All applicable	Heart and Great Vessels Lower Arteries Upper Arteries	**D**	Intraluminal Device
Intraluminal Device, Endobronchial Valve	All applicable	Respiratory System	**D**	Intraluminal Device
Intraluminal Device, Endotracheal Airway	All applicable	Respiratory System	**D**	Intraluminal Device
Intraluminal Device, Flow Diverter	Restriction	Upper Arteries	**D**	Intraluminal Device
Intraluminal Device, Four or More	All applicable	Heart and Great Vessels Lower Arteries Upper Arteries	**D**	Intraluminal Device
Intraluminal Device, Pessary	All applicable	Female Reproductive System	**D**	Intraluminal Device
Intraluminal Device, Radioactive	All applicable	Heart and Great Vessels	**D**	Intraluminal Device
Intraluminal Device, Three	All applicable	Heart and Great Vessels Lower Arteries Upper Arteries	**D**	Intraluminal Device
Intraluminal Device, Two	All applicable	Heart and Great Vessels Lower Arteries Upper Arteries	**D**	Intraluminal Device
Monitoring Device, Hemodynamic	Insertion	Subcutaneous Tissue and Fascia	**2**	Monitoring Device
Monitoring Device, Pressure Sensor	Insertion	Heart and Great Vessels	**2**	Monitoring Device
Pacemaker, Dual Chamber	Insertion	Subcutaneous Tissue and Fascia	**P**	Cardiac Rhythm Related Device
Pacemaker, Single Chamber	Insertion	Subcutaneous Tissue and Fascia	**P**	Cardiac Rhythm Related Device
Pacemaker, Single Chamber Rate Responsive	Insertion	Subcutaneous Tissue and Fascia	**P**	Cardiac Rhythm Related Device

Continued ➞

Specific Device	for Operation	in Body System	General Device
Spinal Stabilization Device, Facet Replacement	Insertion	Lower Joints Upper Joints	**4** Internal Fixation Device
Spinal Stabilization Device, Interspinous Process	Insertion	Lower Joints Upper Joints	**4** Internal Fixation Device
Spinal Stabilization Device, Pedicle-Based	Insertion	Lower Joints Upper Joints	**4** Internal Fixation Device
Spinal Stabilization Device, Vertebral Body Tether	Reposition	Lower Bones Upper Bones	**4** Internal Fixation Device
Stimulator Generator, Multiple Array	Insertion	Subcutaneous Tissue and Fascia	**M** Stimulator Generator
Stimulator Generator, Multiple Array Rechargeable	Insertion	Subcutaneous Tissue and Fascia	**M** Stimulator Generator
Stimulator Generator, Single Array	Insertion	Subcutaneous Tissue and Fascia	**M** Stimulator Generator
Stimulator Generator, Single Array Rechargeable	Insertion	Subcutaneous Tissue and Fascia	**M** Stimulator Generator
Synthetic Substitute, Ceramic	Replacement	Lower Joints	**J** Synthetic Substitute
Synthetic Substitute, Ceramic on Polyethylene	Replacement	Lower Joints	**J** Synthetic Substitute
Synthetic Substitute, Intraocular Telescope	Replacement	Eye	**J** Synthetic Substitute
Synthetic Substitute, Metal	Replacement	Lower Joints	**J** Synthetic Substitute
Synthetic Substitute, Metal on Polyethylene	Replacement	Lower Joints	**J** Synthetic Substitute
Synthetic Substitute, Oxidized Zirconium on Polyethylene	Replacement	Lower Joints	**J** Synthetic Substitute
Synthetic Substitute, Polyethylene	Replacement	Lower Joints	**J** Synthetic Substitute
Synthetic Substitute, Reverse Ball and Socket	Replacement	Upper Joints	**J** Synthetic Substitute

Section 3 – Administration Character 6 – Substance

4-Factor Prothrombin Complex Concentrate	**Includes:** Kcentra
Adhesion Barrier	**Includes:** Seprafilm
Anti-Infective Envelope	**Includes:** AIGISRx Antibacterial Envelope Antibacterial Envelope (TYRX) (AIGISRx) Antimicrobial envelope TYRX Antibacterial Envelope
Clofarabine	**Includes:** Clolar
Globulin	**Includes:** Gammaglobulin Hyperimmune globulin Immunoglobulin Polyclonal hyperimmune globulin
Glucarpidase	**Includes:** Voraxaze
Hematopoietic Stem/ Progenitor Cells, Genetically Modified	**Includes:** OTL-101 OTL-103
Human B-type Natriuretic Peptide	**Includes:** Nesiritide
Other Anti-infective	**Includes:** AVYCAZ® (ceftazidime-avibactam) Ceftazidime-avibactam CRESEMBA® (isavuconazonium sulfate) Isavuconazole (isavuconazonium sulfate)
Other Antineoplastic	**Includes:** Blinatumomab BLINCYTO® (blinatumomab)
Other Therapeutic Substance	**Includes:** Idarucizumab, Pradaxa® (dabigatran) reversal agent Praxbind® (idarucizumab), Pradaxa® (dabigatran) reversal agent
Other Thrombolytic	**Includes:** Tissue Plasinogen Activator (tPA) (r-tPA)
Oxazolidinones	**Includes:** Zyvox
Pathogen Reduced Cryoprecipitated Fibrinogen Complex	**Includes:** INTERCEPT Blood System for Plasma Pathogen Reduced Cryoprecipitated Fibrinogen Complex INTERCEPT Fibrinogen Complex
Recombinant Bone Morphogenetic Protein	**Includes:** Bone morphogenetic protein 2 (BMP 2) rhBMP-2

Section X - New Technology - Character 6 - Device/Substance/Technology

Antibiotic-eluting Bone Void Filler	CERAMENT® G
Apalutamide Antineoplastic	ERLEADA™
Atezolizumab Antineoplastic	TECENTRIQ®
Axicabtagene Ciloleucel Immunotherapy	Axicabtagene Ciloleucel Yescarta®
Bezlotoxumab Monoclonal Antibody	ZINPLAVA™
Bioengineered Allogeneic Construct	StrataGraft®
Branched Synthetic Substitute with Intraluminal Device in New Technology	Thoraflex™ Hybrid device
Brexanolone	ZULRESSO™
Brexucabtagene Autoleucel Immunotherapy	Brexucabtagene Autoleucel Tecartus™
Bromelain-enriched Proteolytic Enzyme	NexoBrid™
Cefiderocol Anti-infective	FETROJA®
Ceftolozane/Tazobactam Anti-infective	ZERBAXA®
Ciltacabtagene Autoleucel	cilta-cel
Coagulation Factor Xa, Inactivated	Andexanet Alfa, Factor Xa Inhibitor Reversal Agent Andexxa Coagulation Factor Xa, (Recombinant) Inactivated Factor Xa Inhibitor Reversal Agent, Andexanet Alfa
Concentrated Bone Marrow Aspirate	CBMA (Concentrated Bone Marrow Aspirate)
Cytarabine and Daunorubicin Liposome Antineoplastic	VYXEOS™
Defibrotide Sodium Anticoagulant	Defitelio
Durvalumab Antineoplastic	IMFINZI®
Eculizumab	Soliris®
Endothelial Damage Inhibitor	DuraGraft® Endothelial Damage Inhibitor
Esketamine Hydrochloride	SPRAVATO™
Fosfomycin Anti-infective	CONTEPO™ Fosfomycin injection

Continued →

High-Dose Intravenous Immune Globulin	GAMUNEX-C, for COVID-19 treatment hdIVIG (high -dose intravenous immunoglobulin), for COVID-19 treatment High-dose intravenous immunoglobulin (hdIVIG), for COVID-19 treatment Octagam 10%, for COVID-19 treatment
Hyperimmune Globulin	Anti-SARS-CoV-2 hyperimmune globulin HIG (hyperimmune intravenous immunoglobulin), for COVID-19 treatment hIVIG (hyperimmune intravenous immunoglobulin), for COVID-19 treatment Hyperimmune intravenous immunoglobulin (hIVIG), for COVID-19 treatment IGIV-C, for COVID-19 treatment
Idecabtagene Vicleucel Immunotherapy	ABECMA® Ide-cel Idecabtagene Vicleucel
Gilteritinib Antineoplastic	XOSPATA®
Imipenem-cilastatin-relebactam Anti-infective	IMI/REL
Interbody Fusion Device, Customizable in New Technology	aprevo™
Interbody Fusion Device, Nanotextured Surface in New Technology	nanoLOCK™ interbody fusion device
Interbody Fusion Device, Radiolucent Porous in New Technology	COALESCE® radiolucent interbody fusion device COHERE® radiolucent interbody fusion device
Intraluminal Device, Sustained Release Drug-eluting in New Technology	Eluvia™ Drug-Eluting Vascular Stent System SAVAL below-the-knee (BTK) drug-eluting stent system
Intraluminal Device, Sustained Release Drug-eluting, Four or more in New Technology	Eluvia™ Drug-Eluting Vascular Stent System SAVAL below-the-knee (BTK) drug-eluting stent system
Intraluminal Device, Sustained Release Drug-eluting, Three in New Technology	Eluvia™ Drug-Eluting Vascular Stent System SAVAL below-the-knee (BTK) drug-eluting stent system
Intraluminal Device, Sustained Release Drug-eluting, Two in New Technology	Eluvia™ Drug-Eluting Vascular Stent System SAVAL below-the-knee (BTK) drug-eluting stent system
Iobenguane I-131 Antineoplastic	AZEDRA® Iobenguane I-131, High Specific Activity (HSA)
Lefamulin Anti-Infective	XENLETA™
Lifileucel Immunotherapy	Lifileucel
Lisocabtagene Maraleucel Immunotherapy	Lisocabtagene Maraleucel

Lurbinectedin	ZEPZELCA™
Magnetically Controlled Growth Rod(s) in New Technology	MAGEC® Spinal Bracing and Distraction System Spinal growth rods, magnetically controlled
Meropenem-vaborbactam Anti-infective	Vabomere™
Mineral-based Topical Hemostatic Agent	Hemospray® Endoscopic Hemostat
Nafamostat Anticoagulant	LTX Regional Anticoagulant Niyad™
Nerinitide	NA-1 (Nerinitide)
Omadacycline Anti-infective	NUZYRA™
Other New Technology Therapeutic Substance	STELARA® Ustekinumab
Posterior (Dynamic) Distraction Device in New Technology	ApiFix® Minimally Invasive Deformity Correction (MID-C) System
Reduction Device in New Technology	Neovasc Reducer™ Reducer™ System
REGN-COV2 Monoclonal Antibody	Casirivimab (REGN10933) and Imdevimab (REGN10987) Imdevimab (REGN10987) and Casirivimab (REGN10933)
Remdesivir Anti-infective	GS-5734 Veklury
Ruxolitinib	Jakafi®
Sarilumab	KEVZARA®
Satralizumab-mwge	ENSPRYNG™
Skin Substitute, Porcine Liver Derived in New Technology	MIRODERM™ Biologic Wound Matrix
Synthetic Human Angiotensin II	Angiotensin II GIAPREZA™ Human angiotensin II, synthetic
Synthetic Substitute, Mechanically Expandable (Paired) in New Technology	SpineJack® system
Tagraxofusp-erzs Antineoplastic	ELZONRIS™
Terlipressin	TERLIVAZ®
Tisagenlecleucel Immunotherapy	KYMRIAH® Tisagenlecleucel
Tocilizumab	ACTEMRA®
Trilaciclib	COSELA™
Uridine Triacetate	Vistogard®
Venetoclax Antineoplastic	Venclexta®
Zooplastic Tissue, Rapid Deployment Technique in New Technology	EDWARDS INTUITY Elite valve system INTUITY elite valve system, EDWARDS Perceval sutureless valve Sutureless valve, Perceval

Appendix G is provided online in a format suitable for spreadsheet and/or database use. Go to http://ahimapress.org/casto8468/, click the "Online Resources" link, and enter case sensitive password AHIMAQpc1hV2022 to download files.

Appendix H: IPPS New Services and Technology Add-On Payment FY2022

Appendix H is provided online in a format suitable for spreadsheet and/or database use. Go to http://ahimapress.org/casto8468/, click the "Online Resources" link, and enter case sensitive password AHIMAQpc1hV2022 to download files.